P9-DDU-721

MEDICAL-SURGICAL NURSING

A PSYCHOPHYSIOLOGIC APPROACH

Second Edition

JOAN LUCKMANN, R.N., B.S., M.A.

Formerly, Instructor of Nursing, University of Washington, Highline College, Seattle, Oakland City College, and Providence Hospital College of Nursing, Oakland, California

KAREN CREASON SORENSEN, R.N., B.S., M.N.

Formerly, Lecturer in Nursing, University of Washington; Formerly, Instructor of Nursing, Highline College; Formerly, Nurse Clinical Specialist, University Hospital and Firland Sanatorium, Seattle, Washington

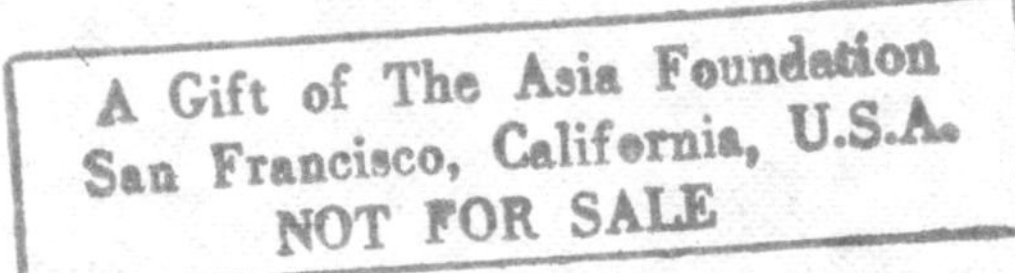

W. B. SAUNDERS COMPANY

Philadelphia London Toronto Mexico City Rio de Janeiro Sydney Tokyo

W. B. Saunders Company: West Washington Square
Philadelphia, PA. 19105

1 St. Anne's Road
Eastbourne, East Sussex BN21 3UN, England

1 Goldthorne Avenue
Toronto, Ontario M8Z 5T9, Canada

Apartado 26370 – Cedro 512
Mexico 4, D.F., Mexico

Rua Coronel Cabrita, 8
Sao Cristovao Caixa Postal 21176
Rio de Janeiro, Brazil

9 Waltham Street
Artarmon, N.S.W. 2064, Australia

Ichibancho, Central Bldg., 22-1 Ichibancho
Chiyoda-Ku, Tokyo 102, Japan

Library of Congress Cataloging in Publication Data

Luckmann, Joan.
Medical-surgical nursing.

Includes bibliographies and index.
1. Nursing. 2. Surgical nursing.
I. Sorensen, Karen Creason, joint author.
II. Title. [DNLM: 1. Medicine–Nursing texts.
2. Nursing care. 3. Surgery–Nursing texts.
WY150 L941m]
RT41.L87 1980 616′.002′4613 77–16973
ISBN 0-7216-5806-7

The reader is advised to review product information, e.g., package inserts for drugs, prior to the administration of any drug or the use of other products. It is assumed that a physician supervises delegated medical care.

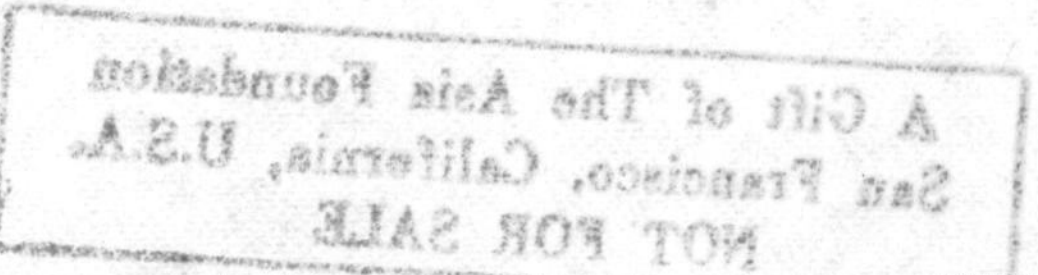

Medical–Surgical Nursing — A Psychophysiologic Approach ISBN 0-7216-5806-7

Print No.: 18 17 16 15 14 13 12 11 10

CONTRIBUTORS, REVISERS AND REVIEWERS

Susan L. Zimmerman Ashburn, R.N., B.S.N., M.S.N.
Formerly Cardiovascular Clinical Specialist, Jewish Hospital of St. Louis, St. Louis

Judith Atwood, R.N., M.N.
Clinical Nurse Specialist—Supervisor, Department of Nursing, Harborview Medical Center, Seattle

Jane Elder Bogle, B.A., M.P.A.
Family Planning and Sexuality Consultant, Seattle

Heather Boyd-Monk, S.R.N., R.N.
Educational Coordinator, Wills Eye Hospital, Philadelphia

Helen Schnell Braun, R.N.
Nurse Coordinator, Burns Plastic Urology Service, Harborview Medical Center, Seattle

Kerry Elizabeth Cavanaugh, R.N., B.S.
Nurse Coordinator, University of Washington Hospital, Seattle

Jonathan Chinn, M.D.
Assistant Clinical Professor, Department of Otolaryngology, School of Medicine, University of Washington, Seattle

Shirley Conwell, R.N.
Nurse Coordinator, Recovery Room, University of Washington Hospital, Seattle

Marie Jeanette Johnson Cowan, Ph.D.
Assistant Professor, Department of Physiological Nursing and Department of Pathology, University of Washington, Seattle

Rosemary J. Craig, B.S., R.N., C.R.T.T., R.R.T.
Clinical Associate, Department of Physiologic Nursing, School of Nursing, University of Washington, Seattle; Technical Director, Respiratory Therapy Department, Swedish Hospital Medical Center, Seattle

Carl B. Dodrill, Ph.D.
Neuropsychologist, Research Assistant Professor, Department of Neurological Surgery, University of Washington, Seattle

Marjorie L. Domenowske
Medical Illustrator

Jean Ellen Espenshade, R.N., M.N.
Formerly Lecturer, School of Nursing, University of Wisconsin – Madison, Full-time graduate student, Department of Psychology, University of Wisconsin – Madison

Patti Sullivan Fenton, R.N.
Staff Nurse, Harborview Burn Center, Harborview Medical Center, Seattle

Henrietta Pauline Gaines, R.N., B.A.
Liaison Nurse, Rancho Los Amigos Hospital, Downey, California

V. Joyce Gauthier, B.Sc.
Candidate in M.D.-Ph.D. Program, University of Washington, Seattle

Bruce G. Gilliland, M.D.
Professor of Medicine, University of Washington; Medical Director, Providence Hospital; Director, Clinical Immunology Laboratory, Seattle

Shirly Jean Harlow, R.N., B.S., B.A., M.A.
Assistant Professor, School of Health Sciences, Seattle Pacific University, Seattle

Dolores Hilden, R.N., M.S.N.
Assistant Professor, University of Pennsylvania, Philadelphia

T. Hongladarom, M.D.
Attending Physiatrist, Mason Clinic, Virginia Mason Hospital, Seattle

Barbara Sue Innes, R.N., B.S., M.S.
Associate Professor, Seattle Pacific University, Seattle

Dolly M. Ito, R.N., B.S., M.A., D.N.Sc.
Professor of Nursing, Seattle University, Seattle

Carolyn Mueller Jarvis, R.N., M.S.N.
Formerly Assistant Professor, School of Nursing, University of Missouri, Columbia

Colleen F. Johnson, R.N.
Clinical Associate, Department of Orthopaedics, University of Washington, Seattle; Consultant, Division of Sports Medicine, University of Washington, Seattle

David G. Johnson, M.D.
Associate Professor and Head of the Section of Endocrinology, University of Arizona Health Sciences Center, Tucson

Judy Johnson, R.N., M.A.
Psychiatric Nurse Consultant, Harborview Medical Center, Seattle

Beatrice Kastenbaum, R.N., B.S.N., M.S.N.
Formerly Instructor, Boston College School of Nursing, Boston

Ruth McCorkle, R.N., Ph.D.
Assistant Professor, School of Nursing, University of Washington, Seattle

Margaret M. McMahon, R.N., B.S.N., CCRN, E.M.T.
Master's Candidate, Department of Physiological Nursing and Department of Psychosocial Nursing, University of Washington, Seattle

Margaret Helen Parkinson, R.N., R.M.N., Dip. N., B.Soc.Sc., M.N.
Formerly Nurse Instructor, School of Nursing, Auckland Technical Institute, Auckland, New Zealand

Phyllis Coindreau Patterson, R.N., M.S.
Clinical Nursing Specialist—Hematology, Nursing Services, University of Michigan Medical Center, Ann Arbor

Walter C. Petersen, M.D.
Clinical Instructor, Department of Ophthalmology, School of Medicine, University of Washington, Seattle

Karen E. Peterson, M.S., M.T. (ASCP)
Research Technologist—Oncology, Arnold Medical Pavilion, Seattle

Rosemary Jeanne Pittman, M.S., C.R.N., F.N.P.
Associate Professor, School of Nursing, University of Washington, Seattle

Wanda Roberts, R.N., M.N.
Assistant Professor, Department of Physiological Nursing, University of Washington, Seattle

Mark Robinson, R.N.
Utilization Review Nurse, Los Angeles County Hospital, Los Angeles

Murali Sivarajan, M.D.
Assistant Professor, Department of Anesthesiology, School of Medicine, University of Washington, Seattle

Kathleen Smith-DiJulio, R.N., M.N.
Assistant Professor, University of Washington, Seattle

Pat R. Starkovich, R.N.
Enterostomal Therapist, Group Health Cooperative of Puget Sound, Seattle; Clinical Faculty, Seattle Pacific University, Seattle

Allan S. Troupin, M.D.
Associate Professor of Neurology, University of Pennsylvania School of Medicine, Philadelphia

Alma Miller Ware, R.N., B.A., M.N.
Consultant, Veterans Administration Hospital, American Lake, Tacoma, Washington; Consultant, private practice, Seattle

Gwen Williams, R.N., M.N.
Formerly Supervisor, Operating Room Recovery Room, University of Washington Hospital, Seattle; Director, Operating Room and Postanesthesia Recovery, Stanford University Medical Center, Palo Alto, California

PREFACE

Dear Reader,

One outstanding hallmark of a profession is the willingness of its members to help one another learn and, thereby, improve the services that the profession performs. A textbook is our means of communicating nursing knowledge both to the student of nursing and to the practicing professional nurse. We are pleased indeed to present this volume to you!

With the publication of this second edition of *Medical-Surgical Nursing: A Psychophysiologic Approach* we achieve the final step of a long-range plan to jointly publish books containing specialized medical-surgical nursing content and fundamental nursing content. This text can be used in conjunction with or independently from our other book, *Basic Nursing: A Psychophysiologic Approach.*

Over the years we have noted large overlaps in some content areas between introductory nursing and medical-surgical nursing texts. Overlaps, with unnecessary repetition, consume reader time and book space—crucial factors in a dynamic profession with a rapidly expanding knowledge base. We have carefully divided content between this edition of our *Medical-Surgical Nursing* text and *Basic Nursing* to avoid unnecessary duplication and yet provide important content bridges, for example, in areas such as nursing process, assessment, fluid and electrolyte balance and imbalances, stress, pain, and emergency life support activities.

The body of knowledge required to practice nursing with expertise is rapidly growing as the nursing profession continues to evolve. The fact that nursing knowledge has increased is reflected in the size of our texts.

Every effort has been made to make your journey through this book an interesting learning experience. Our learning aids, popular with readers in the past, have been strengthened and stylistic clarity has been an important goal. Objectives, overviews, study guides, boxed and arrowed material, tables, and numerous illustrations all combine to make content easy to understand and remember. Comprehensive indexing and frequent cross-referencing between chapters facilitate the effective use of this book. Extensive bibliographies encourage the locating of original sources for additional reading on topics of selected interest. When appropriate, overviews of anatomy and physiology are placed at the beginnings of units along with summaries of typical disorders that may affect the structures being considered. To make learning a dynamic process, learning activities are interspersed throughout the units. For example, periodically the reader is asked to pause to perform various activities or reflect in a directed manner on points emphasized. An accompanying *Teacher's Manual* is a new addition for use by instructors.

Patient care is based upon the holistic intertwining of information from a variety of disciplines, from the physical and social sciences as well as the arts. The professions of nursing and medicine are especially closely interrelated—yet different in important ways. (See Chapter 1). In practicing medical-surgical nursing, nurses are increasingly performing delegated medical tasks, commonly activities formerly carried out by physicians. Some of these activities are highly challenging. Equally challenging is the responsibility of identifying and finding solutions for *nursing* problems in persons experiencing disorders of a medical or surgical nature. It is fortunate for patients that nurses are gaining broader theoretical and clinical expertise, since patients in acute care settings spend more time with nurses than with any other health professionals. Our approach to care includes the belief that patients are most appropriately cared for within their own social network of others significant to them.

As nursing activities become more sophisticated, so must nursing resources. We attempt to keep pace with current nursing practice by providing comprehensive textbooks with a psychophysiologic approach. This text has been thoroughly revised and expanded with the help of experienced professionals. Important new additions (discussed later) have also been made.

This text is designed for use by students in any professional nursing program and as a reference for all nurses. We combine a systems approach with a conceptual model, believing that both frameworks have a place in providing clarity and meaning to the presentation of nursing knowledge.

Because it is essential to keep foremost in mind that we are nurses and the goals of our profession, we open this edition with a unit focusing on *The Unique Contributions of Nursing to Patient Care.* This unit examines the caring art of nursing and summarizes the nursing process. We then proceed to explore a holistic approach to illness, stress and illness, mind-body interaction in illness, and responses to disturbances in homeostasis. These areas all comprise the first section: *Unifying Concepts Basic to Advanced Nursing Practice.*

Section Two: Psychosocial and Physical Assessment is new. It is imperative that nursing actions be based on sound assessments. While assessment is emphasized throughout the book, overviews of psychosocial and physical assessment are presented in this section.

The final section of this book, the majority of text, examines *Specific Problems in Medical-Surgical Nursing Practice.* This section begins with units focusing on such general areas of practice as nursing people experiencing surgery and nursing people experiencing neoplastic disorders. Early in section three is a unit that examines the complex problem of pain. The clinical care of persons experiencing specific disorders of the various body systems and structures is discussed in section three. The book concludes with two new units: *Nursing People Experiencing Dependency on Alcohol and Other Drugs* and *Nursing People Experiencing Medical-Surgical Emergencies.* The latter unit provides a comprehensive review of emergency care. To facilitate its use, an outline is located in this unit's introduction.

Throughout this book we have attempted to explain logically the reasons for observations and clinical actions. Advanced nursing activities are discussed in detail. Health maintenance activities, preventive care and clinical care (including rehabilitation and follow-up care, of course) of patients and their significant others is heavily emphasized. Basic guiding principles of care are applicable in whatever setting a patient is located. While this text presents suggested approaches to care, in actual practice effective care must be individualized depending upon factors such as the patient's circumstances and preferences, physician philosophy, agency guidelines, and current practices. Since opinions vary and changes occur concerning "appropriate" practice, we advise the reader to closely follow current professional literature and to participate in other professional activities. Prior to administering drugs and using other products, drug and other product information sheets and brochures should be read carefully. Also, familiarize yourself with laboratory values considered "normal" in the health care system within which you function.

ACKNOWLEDGMENTS

We acknowledge and thank the numerous people who have helped with the preparation of this book. Countless persons have contributed in indirect, yet vital ways through their contributions to the pool of literature from which we draw in the process of our research. Other professionals have contributed more directly by authoring, reviewing or participating in the revision of specific content areas. We have tried to mention each of these people by name or reference in appropriate places throughout the book.

Marjorie Domenowske has carefully prepared most of our original illustrations. We deeply appreciate her thoughtful, even approach to this work. Once again we also acknowledge with very special thanks Margaret Parkinson and Ilze Rader for their competent and professional "supportive services." Margaret has worked closely with the authors, making important contributions as consultant, author and proofreader. At the W. B. Saunders Company, Ilze has given our work the special, meticulous editing unique to her. Both Margaret and Ilze have given exhaustively of their time and interest and have formed essential bridges between our various offices. Our new editor, Katherine Pitcoff has been a delightful and creative "facilitator," contributing to the publication of this book in varied and interesting ways. Margaret McMahon has been a valued coworker and author. Special thanks also to Kerry Cavanaugh and Mary Chelgren for their help. Finally, our thanks to the Production Department at the W. B. Saunders Company and Production Manager Laura Tarves for the smooth, speedy production of this volume.

Joan Luckmann

JOAN LUCKMANN

Karen Creason Sorensen

KAREN CREASON SORENSEN

CONTENTS

SECTION ONE

UNIFYING CONCEPTS BASIC TO ADVANCED NURSING PRACTICE

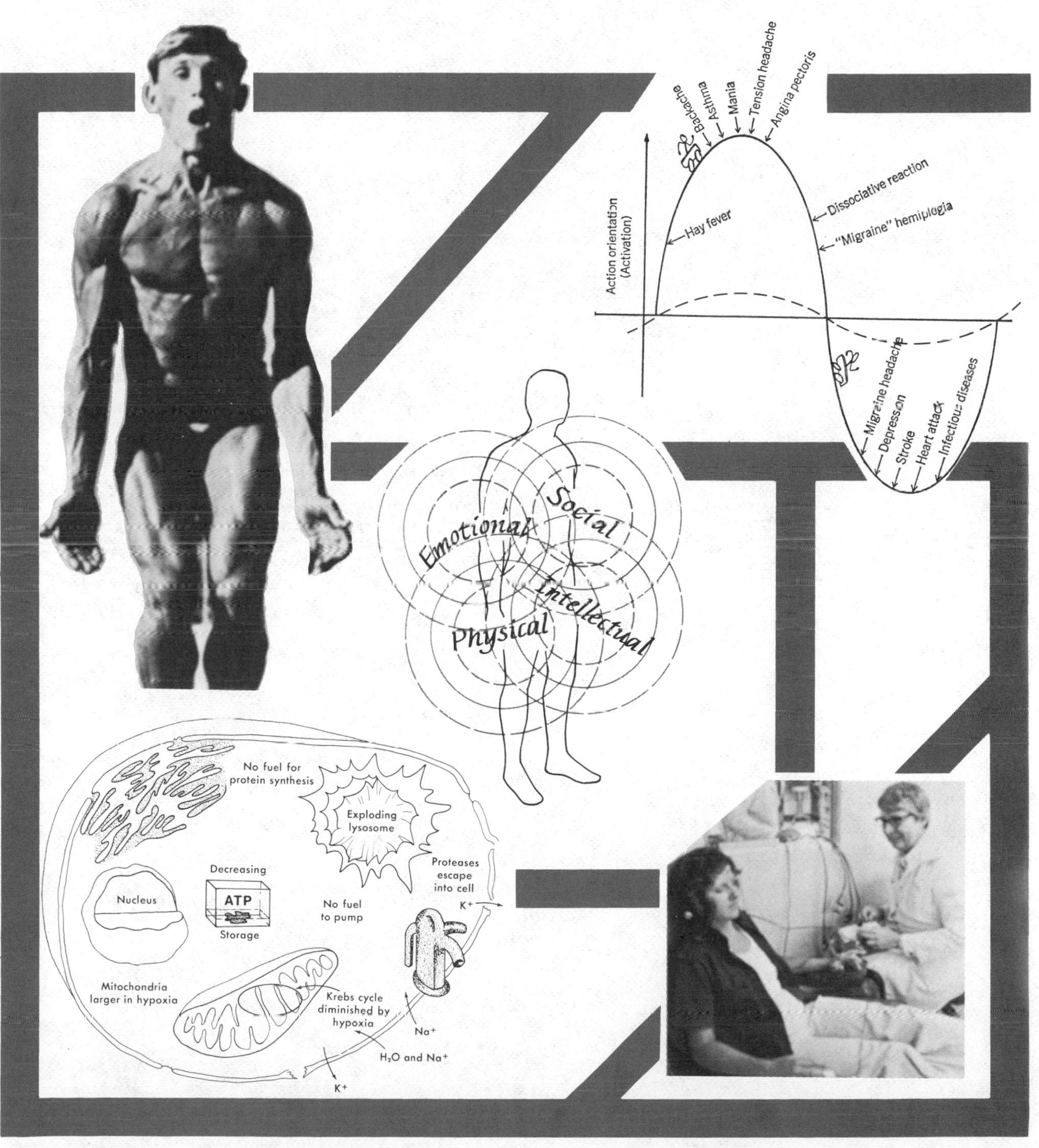

UNIT I

THE UNIQUE CONTRIBUTIONS OF NURSING TO PATIENT CARE

by Margaret Helen Parkinson, R.N., R.M.N., Dip.N., B. Soc. Sc., M.N.

In watching disease, both in private houses and in public hospitals, the thing which strikes the experienced observer most forcibly is this, that the symptoms or the sufferings generally considered to be inevitable and incident to the disease are very often not symptoms of the disease at all, but of something quite different – of the want of fresh air, or of light, or of warmth, or of quiet, or of cleanliness, or of punctuality and care in the administration of diet, of each or all of these.

FLORENCE NIGHTINGALE[59]

INTRODUCTION AND STUDY GUIDE

This is a book about medical-surgical nursing. Yet, nursing is only associated with, not defined by, medicine and surgery. Medicine and surgery have to do with the diagnosis and treatment of disease or pathologic conditions in human beings. *Nursing, on the other hand, has primarily to do with the care, comfort, and support of people whose patterns of daily life are in some way threatened.* A disease process that requires medical or surgical therapeutic intervention is *one* of the stresses that can interfere with normal human functioning. This means that people experiencing disease and medical-surgical therapeutic regimens often require nursing care. For these reasons, medical-surgical practices and nursing practices often (although not always) occur side by side and in an interrelated fashion.

This unit is placed at the beginning of the book to encourage you to consider some of the concepts central to the practice of nursing before you become immersed in the detailed and perhaps more concrete issues related to the nursing care and delegated medical care of the "medical-surgical" patient. In working with the material of Unit I (Chapters 1 and 2) you will, over time, achieve the following objectives. You will be able to:

- ► Appreciate the unique caring role of the nurse as the central core of nursing practice
- ► Identify differences and similarities between the practice of nursing and the practice of medicine
- ► Express an understanding of the holistic nature of human beings
- ► Compare several theoretical frameworks of basic human needs
- ► Understand concepts basic to the nursing process as a problem-solving activity

- Apply the nursing process in clinical situations

The following suggestions for learning activities may be useful as you work toward attainment of the above objectives.

1. Write down in your own words your understanding of the following terms:

health care system	accountability
unique professional functions	dependent nursing functions
general professional functions	interdependent nursing functions
delegated professional functions	independent nursing functions
primary nursing focus	nursing process
care	problem solving
cure	nursing assessment
basic human needs	nursing problem
physical needs	nursing diagnosis
social needs	data gathering
intellectual needs	nursing history
emotional needs	setting nursing priorities
Maslow's hierarchy of basic human needs	nursing objectives
	nursing management
patient independence	nursing care plans
nursing mastery	nursing intervention
responsibility	evaluation of nursing care

2. Spend some time thinking through your own ideas about the following questions:

What do I believe about the nature of human beings?
Are human beings basically "good" or basically "bad"? Or are they neither "good" nor "bad"?
What causes human behavior?
What is health?
What is illness?
How does nursing differ from medicine?
How is nursing similar to medicine?
What effect could my responses to each of the above questions have upon my behavior toward individual patients?

Such questions are never answered conclusively. They require repeated consideration throughout professional life.

3. Write out your own definition of the unique function of nursing. Discuss your definition with colleagues and teachers.

4. Read a number of philosophies of nursing. Go to the original source for each one you read. The bibliography at the end of Unit I (p. 21) gives many such references.

5. Take one framework of basic human needs and, over a two-day period, keep notes about how you achieved satisfaction of each need or group of needs included in the framework. Did you require help from other people to satisfy any needs? Were some needs unsatisfied? If so, what obstructed your need satisfaction? This exercise will give you some subjective experience of need and problem identification.

6. Practice setting long-term and short-term objectives for your own daily living. Evaluate your performance after set periods of time. This will help you assess how specific your objectives were and how well you used behavioral terms. Remember, objective setting takes practice. The more practice you can get, the more skillful you will become.

7. Most important of all, *always* use the nursing process and prepare a nursing care plan when taking care of anyone during your clinical experience in medical-surgical nursing. Continually seek the critique of your colleagues, teachers, and patients.

CHAPTER 1

NURSING: THE CARING ART

Love and caring can't be quantified or measured. They probably would not yield to demands for precision in questionnaires or scales. Can anyone, though, deny their existence and the impact on each of our lives? We have all been touched by the serenity, even joy, of patients and their families who experienced nursing and health care delivered in warm, caring ways.[63]

You have entered a profession of "artists." The "art" you are learning, and will become more and more skilled in practicing, is the *art of caring.* Just as painters work with paint, brushes and pallette and potters create beauty from clay and glazes, so a nurse's art involves the feelings, needs, and experiences of people under stress. When you decided to become a nurse you gained the opportunity to support and assist people experiencing life crises. You will be there when babies are born and when old people die; you will comfort and reassure as you immunize a child; you will teach, you will examine, you will aid. You will always be needed whenever human beings are ill or injured, and you will stay beside them during the experience whether they recover or whether they die. The effectiveness of your service will depend upon the extent to which you learn and become skilled in the caring art of nursing.

In this chapter we consider the components of the caring art of nursing and some of the ways this art contributes to the total health care patients receive. The human love and care of an excellent nurse can bring some sense of peace and meaning to extremely stressful experiences for patients and their significant others.

You, as a nurse, are a part of the *health care system,* that is, the organization of services intended to assist people with problems of health and illness. The health care system is composed of interrelated subsystems each representing specific health-related professions. Each profession or subsystem has both specific and general functions. The "specific functions" are those services that are *unique* to a particular professional group. The "general functions" are those services that are *shared* by all health professional groups and are aimed at the overall goals of health promotion and health maintenance.

To help clarify these points let us look at some of the specific, unique functions of certain professionals. A physician is responsible for diagnosing and planning treatment regimens for pathological conditions. A radiographer is specifically prepared to take clear and appropriate x-ray films. A pharmacist is the person most skilled at preparing and giving advice on medication prescriptions. A chaplain offers religious services and spiritual support. These health professionals may have other specific and unique functions as well. They also have functions that they share with each other.

Functions common to all health professionals include the following:

- *maintenance of the patient and significant others as central in all services*
- *preservation of the dignity and sense of personal control of the patient and significant others*
- *communication with other health professionals to ensure co-ordination of services for the patient's advantage*

Nurses, in addition to shared and unique functions, also have *delegated* functions. This is particularly true for nurses who work in hospitals. Delegated functions are those services that are part of one group's unique function and are performed by another professional group. Nurses carry out many delegated medical care tasks which relate to the physician's unique functions. Examples of such delegated medical functions are the administration of medicines and the removal of surgical sutures. Nurses may also, at times, perform tasks delegated by other health professionals. Such delegation occurs because nurses belong to the professional group that typically spends the most time in closest contact with the patient, e.g., in hospitals nurses maintain a 24 hour patient coverage and attend to the patient's personal needs. It is appropriate for nurses to undertake tasks delegated from other professionals provided that while doing so they do not neglect their own unique functions.

THE UNIQUE FUNCTIONS OF NURSING

Many nurses have attempted to define the unique functions of nursing by identifying areas of nursing practice over which the nurse has authority; areas of nursing practice in which the nurse is the expert, and areas of nursing practice for which the nurse should be legally responsible. Henderson has written a definition that bears consideration.

> *The unique function of the nurse is to assist the individual sick or well, in the performance of those activities contributing to health or its recovery (or to a peaceful death) that he would do unaided if he had the necessary strength, will or knowledge. And to do this in such a way as to help him gain independence as rapidly as possible. This aspect of her work, this part of her function, she initiates and controls; of this she is master.*
>
> *Virginia Henderson*[33]

Let us paraphrase Henderson's definition so that we can look more closely at each component of it:

The unique function of the nurse is to

- assist the individual, sick or well
- meet basic human needs
- and gain independence.

In doing so, the nurse demonstrates

- mastery of nursing.

Assist the Individual

The nurse who is expertly carrying out the unique nursing functions does not rigidly perform routines without reference to the personality, concerns, and desires of the individual patient. *The excellent nurse works "with" the patient (rather than "for" or "on" the patient) in a partnership that encourages and supports the patient's individuality and sense of control.*

Sick or Well

A nurse is not exclusively concerned with the sick person. In fact, it is not simple to differentiate between health and illness. Nor is the excellent nurse exclusively concerned with the restoration of health. *True nursing emerges from a "care" domain rather than a "cure" domain.* In providing nursing care, a nurse assists people to satisfy basic human needs whether they are sick or well, whether they are going to die, fully recover, or retain residual, long-term disabilities. The nurse's concern is to identify with a person that person's unmet needs; discover the problems that are blocking need satisfaction and plan ways of ordering present circumstances so that the individual's basic human needs can be met satisfactorily.

This does not mean, of course, that a nurse is not at all concerned with cure. The *primary* nursing focus is toward *care.* This does not exclude a *secondary* role concerned with future *cure.* Figure 1–1 illustrates the relationship and interdependence of the care and cure roles of nurses and doctors. In fact, a nurse has a very important contribution to make in the cure domain. As Bowers-Ferres says:

> *Nursing's role with the cure component is not to help the physician, but to help the patient make use of the physician's help in whatever way that patient can most successfully do so.*[15]

Meeting Basic Human Needs

The phrase *basic human needs* expresses what Henderson calls "those activities contributing to health or its recovery (or to a peaceful death) that [a person] would do unaided if he had the necessary strength, will or knowledge."[33] Basic human needs are those requirements common

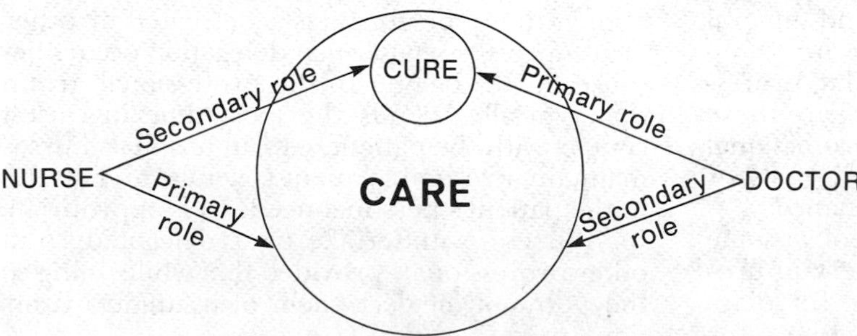

Figure 1–1. Care-cure model, showing the coordination of care and cure functions and the associated responsibilities of the nurse and the doctor. Cure roles are encompassed within the broader base of care roles. Caring is the fundamental, minute-by-minute attention to an individual's basic human needs that will provide an environment for a cure to take place, if a cure is possible or desirable.

to all human beings regardless of culture, race, sex or age. Basic human needs are conditions that must be either supplied or relieved. While methods of fulfilling may vary from person to person, and even from circumstance to circumstance in the same individual, the fact that all human beings have certain common needs remains true.

Every human being is a composite of physical, social, emotional, and intellectual needs.

- Physical needs involve all the physiologic processes of a human being, e.g., breathing, eliminating body wastes, cardiac and circulatory processes, movement.
- Social needs relate to the interactions and interconnections a human being has with other people, e.g., communication processes, the sense of belonging to and being loved by others.
- Emotional needs are concerned with the feelings that a person experiences throughout life, e.g., fear, anxiety, joy, happiness, loneliness.
- Intellectual needs focus on thoughts and rationality, e.g., learning, reasoning, problem solving.

You can think of these components as interconnecting circles, ever changing and in constant dynamic interaction. In health, the components are maintained in a state of balance, equilibrium or homeostasis. *A person who has adequate physiologic functioning, who has a satisfying and productive social network, who is aware of and able to express thoughts and feelings, and who is able to exercise intellectual skills is a person who is functioning in a healthy way.*

A human being is not a static phenomenon; life brings about constant and continuous changes. Each component of a human being is more a process than a fact. Each component involves function both within itself and in relation to the other three components. These interaction patterns occur both in health and in illness. For example, consider Bob, a healthy individual and a university nursing student. Bob has been working hard at his studies all day. During his 4–6 PM class however, he finds it difficult to concentrate on what the lecturer is saying (*intellectual* component); he finds his thoughts stray to the date he has planned for the evening and he realizes he is nervous about it (*emotional* component); he wonders if he is dressed appropriately and if his behavior will be acceptable to his friend (*social* component); and he becomes aware that he is moving restlessly in his chair and that he is hungry (*physical* component). For the moment, Bob's intellectual component is receding as his physical, social, emotional aspects expand. Even our commonplace experiences — difficulty concentrating — are easier to understand when we consider all four aspects.

Likewise, in illness the components interact and influence each other. Pause and remember the last time you experienced a cold. You were made aware of your physical aspect by your runny nose, sneezing, and maybe a cough and sore throat. Additionally, it is likely that you found it difficult to be sociable and you may have tended to be irritable and short tempered. You may also recall that your problem-solving skills were diminished and that it was hard to concentrate on work. Clearly your respiratory infection was more than a physiologic problem!

THEORIES OF BASIC HUMAN NEEDS

The caring art of nursing involves the identification of the needs that a patient is having difficulty meeting and the development of sensitive and skillful ways in which to assist the patient in satisfying those needs. If an old man is

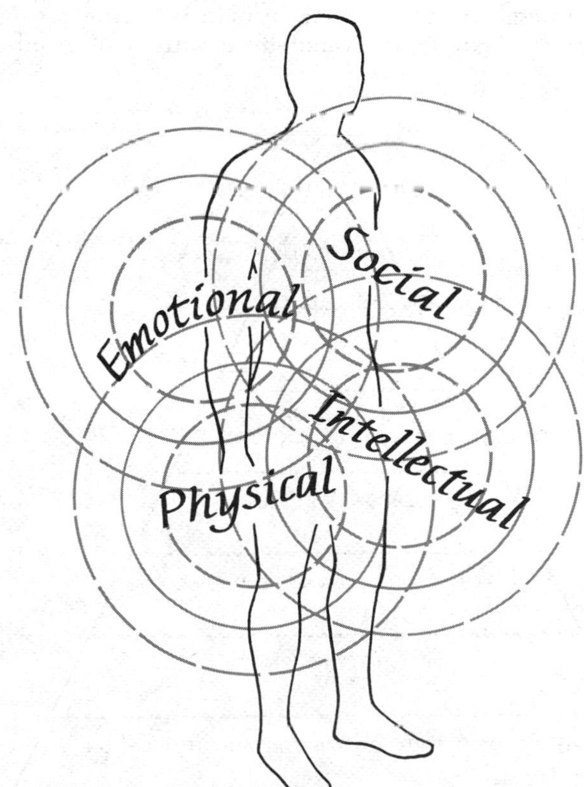

Figure 1–2. Human beings from a holistic viewpoint. The ever-expanding and receding circles represent the dynamic interaction of the physical, social, emotional, and intellectual needs that constitute humanness.

too weak to feed himself, a nurse assists him; if a small boy cannot walk to look out the window, a nurse provides another way for him to move; if a woman feels useless and unloved, a nurse finds ways to lift her self-esteem.

To be effective in identifying patients' needs, the nurse must understand what the basic human needs are. Various theorists have put forward models to explain what the basic human needs are and to organize them in ways that encompass the whole human being. Studying these models can provide you with a framework within which to identify needs and can help you in planning nursing care.

Maslow. A well known model with which you may be familiar is the hierarchy of basic human needs developed by Abraham Maslow.[54] Maslow described a hierarchy, or pyramid, of needs with primary or physiologic needs at the base and secondary or nonphysiologic needs at the higher levels (Fig. 1–3). Maslow states that the basic human needs are organized into a *hierarchy of relative prepotency*. Expressed simply, this means that new needs emerge when those lower on the hierarchy have been relatively well gratified. In other words, human behavior is to a large extent motivated by a system of needs.

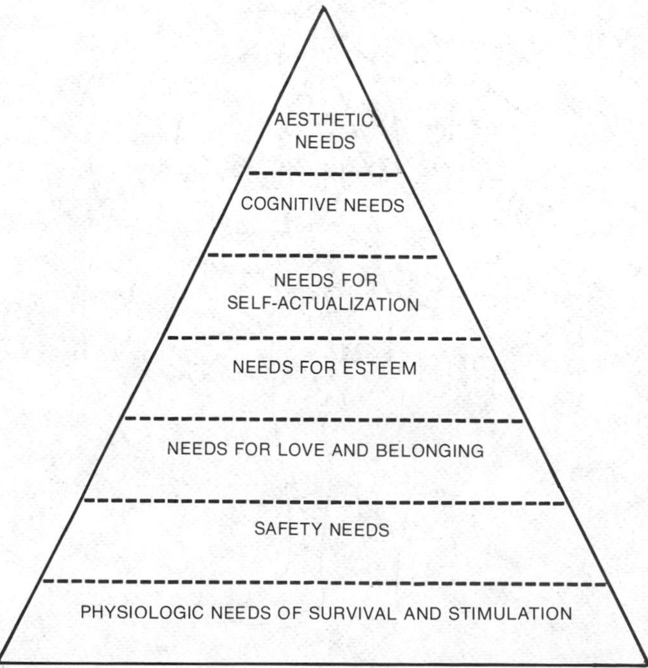

Figure 1–3. Diagrammatic representation of Maslow's hierarchy of basic human needs.

While all needs are present at all times, a person will attempt to satisfy those needs lower on the hierarchy to at least a minimal degree before focusing on those higher up.

The needs described in Maslow's model are, in ascending order:

(a) Survival needs, e.g., food, air, water, temperature, elimination, rest, pain avoidance.

(b) Stimulation needs, e.g., sex, activity, exploration, manipulation, novelty.

(c) Safety and security needs, e.g., safety, security, protection.

(d) Love needs, e.g., love, belonging, closeness, intimacy.

(e) Esteem needs, e.g., value and respect from others, value and respect of self (self-esteem)

(f) Self-actualization needs, e.g., the process of making maximum use of one's abilities.

(g) Cognitive needs, e.g., seeking knowledge, discovering things, working with ideas, knowing and understanding.

(h) Aesthetic needs, e.g., the desire for beauty.

Henderson. Another model of basic human needs has been compiled by Virginia Henderson.[33] She suggests that there are 14 needs of patients with which the nurse should be concerned. Figure 1–4 lists these needs and identifies the various pathologic and nonpathologic conditions that can affect the basic needs. Notice that Henderson refers to the 14 "needs" as the *components of basic nursing*. Study Figure 1–4 and try to think of examples in your own life and in your clinical experiences where each of the conditions that are always present and each of the pathological states listed have affected the achievement of basic human needs. For example, how might age affect one's need to breathe normally; how might anxiety affect one's ability to sleep and rest; what influence might exposure to cold have upon one's ability to move; and how would immobilization affect one's need to keep the body clean?

Kraegel. Kraegel[42] and her associates developed a model of patient needs which they used in studying a system for providing patient care. This model identifies 22 needs within three broad classifications: *physical, sociopsychological,* and *environment.* Physical and sociopsychological needs are grouped as *patient health needs.*

Comparison of Models. As you study these models, you will notice some similarities in them. Compare the three models carefully and identify their similarities and differences. Maslow, Henderson, and Kraegel are describing the same things. Each of their models are attempts to describe the elements of existence that are common to and necessary for all human beings. Figure 1–6 compares the various models and can help you clarify your concepts of basic human needs.

Patient Independence

Henderson's definition states not only what nursing *is* but also gives some indication of *how* nursing should be practiced.

> *The goal of nursing practice is always to encourage and facilitate patient independence.*

The balance between what the nurse does and what the patient does is always changing. While it is the nurse's responsibility to do for people what they cannot do independently, the excellent nurse never continues to attend to all or part of a basic human need once a person can manage this alone. In fact, the nurse tries to modify the environment in such a way that patients can take increasing responsibility for themselves as quickly as possible. It is for this reason that rigid routine has very little place in excellent nursing practice.

Figure 1–4. Needs of all patients usually met by the nurse and how modified by conditions always present and sometimes present. Compiled by Virginia Henderson. (*From* Henderson, V.: *Basic Principles of Nursing Care.* Geneva: International Council of Nurses, 1960 (revised printing 1969) pp. 12–13.

Components of basic nursing	*Conditions always present that affect basic needs*	*Pathological states (as contrasted with specific diseases) that modify basic needs*
Assisting the patient with these functions or providing conditions that will enable him to: 1. Breathe normally 2. Eat and drink adequately 3. Eliminate by all avenues of elimination 4. Move and maintain desirable posture (walking, sitting, lying and changing from one to the other) 5. Sleep and rest 6. Select suitable clothing, dress and undress 7. Maintain body temperature within normal range by adjusting clothing and modifying the environment 8. Keep the body clean and well groomed and protect the integument 9. Avoid dangers in the environment and avoid injuring others 10. Communicate with others in expressing emotions, needs, fears 11. Worship according to his faith 12. Work at something that provides a sense of accomplishment 13. Play, or participate in various forms of recreation 14. Learn, discover, or satisfy the curiosity that leads to "normal" development and health	1. Age: new born, child, youth, adult, middle aged, aged, and dying 2. Temperament, emotional state, or passing mood: a) 'normal' or b) euphoric and hyperactive c) anxious, fearful, agitated or hysterical or d) depressed and hypoactive 3. Social or cultural status: A member of a family unit with friends and status, or a person relatively alone and/or or maladjusted, destitute 4. Physical and intellectual capacity: a) normal weight b) underweight c) overweight d) normal mentality e) sub-normal mentality f) gifted mentality g) normal sense of hearing, sight, equilibrium and touch h) loss of special sense i) normal motor power j) loss of motor power	1. Marked disturbances of fluid and electrolyte balance including starvation states, pernicious vomiting, and diarrhoea 2. Acute oxygen want 3. Shock (including 'collapse' and haemorrhage) 4. Disturbances of consciousness—fainting coma, delirium 5. Exposure to cold and heat causing markedly abnormal body temperatures 6. Acute febrile states (all causes) 7. A local injury, wound and/or infection 8. A communicable condition 9. Pre-operative state 10. Post-operative state 11. Immobilisation from disease or prescribed as treatment 12. Persistent or intractable pain

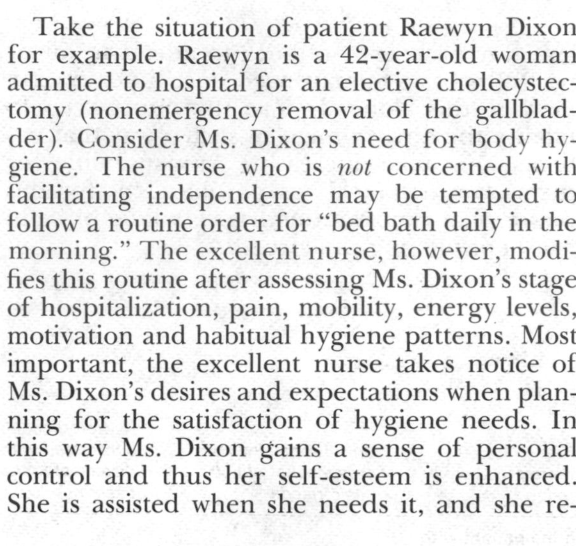

Take the situation of patient Raewyn Dixon for example. Raewyn is a 42-year-old woman admitted to hospital for an elective cholecystectomy (nonemergency removal of the gallbladder). Consider Ms. Dixon's need for body hygiene. The nurse who is *not* concerned with facilitating independence may be tempted to follow a routine order for "bed bath daily in the morning." The excellent nurse, however, modifies this routine after assessing Ms. Dixon's stage of hospitalization, pain, mobility, energy levels, motivation and habitual hygiene patterns. Most important, the excellent nurse takes notice of Ms. Dixon's desires and expectations when planning for the satisfaction of hygiene needs. In this way Ms. Dixon gains a sense of personal control and thus her self-esteem is enhanced. She is assisted when she needs it, and she regains independence as soon as she is ready for it. Such is the essence of fine nursing practice!

Nursing Mastery

> *Nurses must always be* responsible *and* accountable *for what they do in clinical practice.*

Being responsible and accountable means that nursing practice must be based on sound scientific and humanitarian principles. Nurses must be knowledgeable and skilled in the services they provide and must be willing to have their services evaluated. Such are the hallmarks of true professionals.

Responsibility and accountability are vital for dependent, interdependent and independent nursing functions. Dependent and interdependent nursing functions are delegated functions that either entirely or partially arise from the authority of another professional group (often medical practitioners). These functions are usually cure or treatment related. Independent nursing func-

1. Air
2. Rest
3. Sleep
4. Food
5. Fluids
6. Elimination
7. Maintenance of Body Heat
8. Maintenance of Integument
   a. Physical Hygiene
   b. Bodily Safety
9. Quiet
10. Mobility
11. Freedom from Pain and Discomfort
12. Sensory Stimulation

→ PHYSIOLOGICAL

13. Autonomy (Choice, Control)
14. Challenge and Achievement
15. Security
16. Cognitive Clarity (Knowledge upon Which to Act)
    a. Orientation
    b. Health Education
    c. Communication
17. Humanism (Recognition, Acceptance, Respect, Approval)
    a. Status
    b. Success
    c. Self-Esteem
    d. Dignity
    e. Identity
    f. Kindly Concern by Others
    g. Privacy
       i. Physical
       ii. Information

→ SOCIO-PSYCHOLOGICAL

PHYSIOLOGICAL + SOCIO-PSYCHOLOGICAL → PATIENT HEALTH NEEDS

18. Reliability
19. Simplicity
20. Flexibility
21. Cost
    a. Economic
    b. Societal
22. Safety to Human Agents

→ ENVIRONMENTAL NEEDS

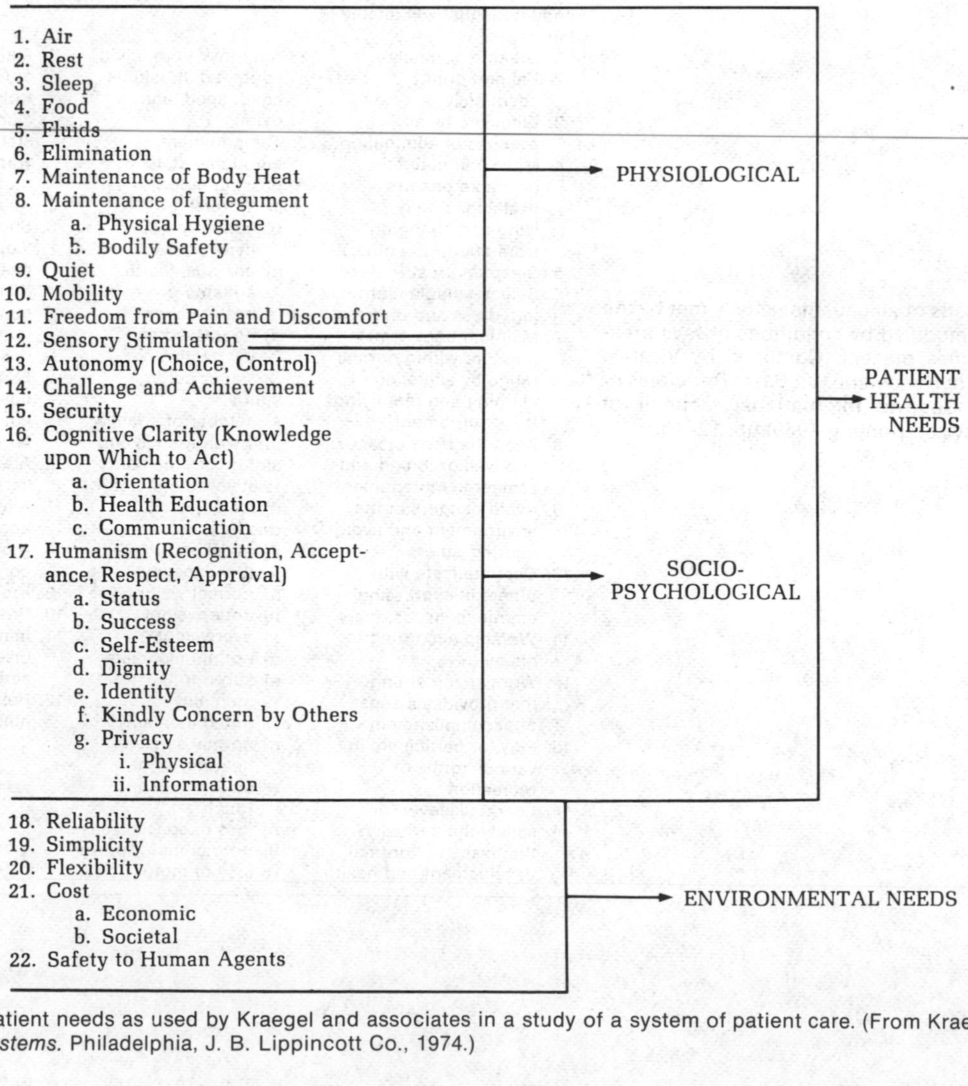

Figure 1–5. Patient needs as used by Kraegel and associates in a study of a system of patient care. (From Kraegel, J. M., et al.: *Patient Care Systems.* Philadelphia, J. B. Lippincott Co., 1974.)

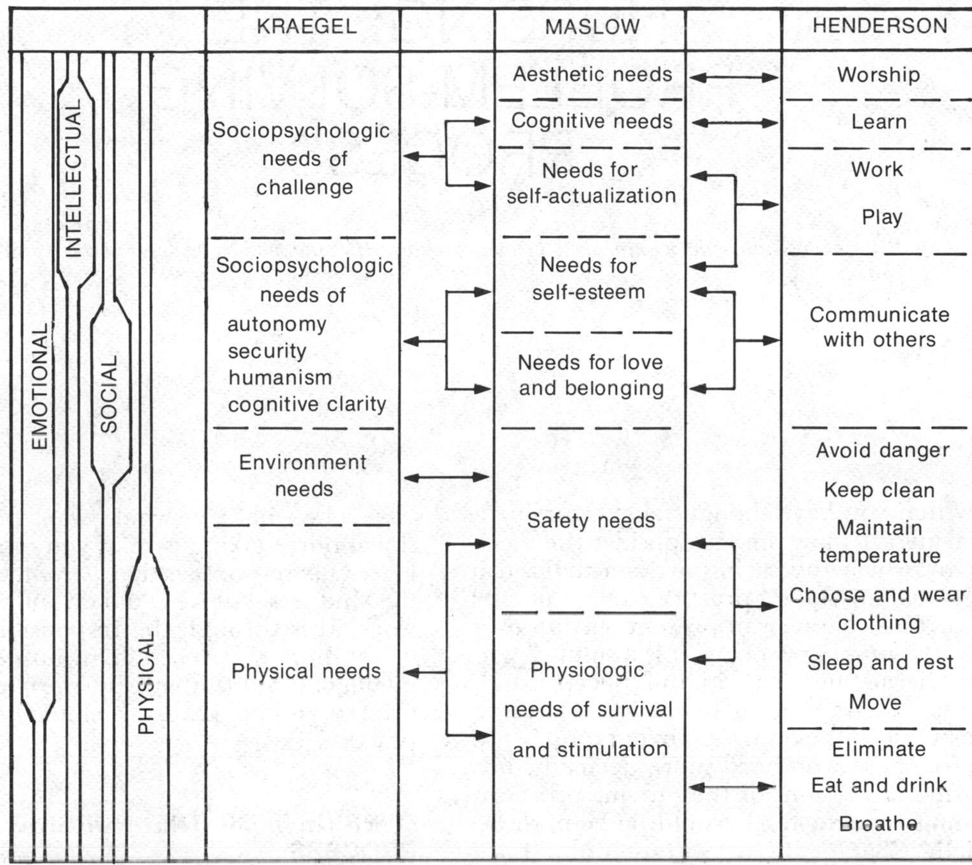

Figure 1–6. The interactions and intersections between Kraegel's, Maslow's, and Henderson's models of basic human needs. On the left is a schematic representation of how the four general components (emotional, intellectual, social, and physical) relate to the various models.

tions are *care* related. Nurses are experts (masters) in caring activities. Excellent nurses initiate and control caring activities (this is "responsibility") and encourage evaluation and feedback about the effectiveness of their caring activities (this is "accountability").

NURSING IS BOTH AN ART AND A SCIENCE

Nursing is a professional service that has a sound knowledge base gleaned from both physical and social sciences. Knowledge alone, however, is not enough. Nursing is expressed through the deliberate and intelligent *application* of knowledge.

> *Nursing is the* art *of applying scientific principles in an intelligent humanitarian way to the care of people experiencing potentially maladaptive stress.*

Such a process requires not only the knowledge a nurse has but also *self-involvement* in a personal relationship with people wanting help.

CONCLUSION

In this chapter various issues have been presented concerning the unique, caring contribution of nursing to patient care. Excellent nurses consider and reconsider such issues throughout their professional careers because they realize that what they *believe* about the nature of nursing, i.e., their own philosophy of nursing, really does determine their day-by-day practice. A number of references pertaining to the philosophy of nursing are provided in the bibliography for Unit I (p. 21). We strongly encourage you to read this material and to keep up to date, through current periodicals and professional discussions, with the ongoing development of a theoretical framework for nursing.

CHAPTER 2

NURSING: THE PROBLEM-SOLVING PROCESS

Prior to the change the man needs to ponder carefully. After the change, he needs to check his results.

I-CHING

Now that you have thought about nursing as "the caring art," it is time to consider the mechanism by which the caring art is actualized in professional nursing practice — the nursing process. This chapter can present only an overview of the nursing process. It is a summary for readers already familiar with the concepts, and a mere introduction for anyone who has not studied this topic. An extensive bibliography is provided for those who need more detailed study. Reviewing discussions of the nursing process in beginning nursing texts would be helpful. See especially Chapter 17 in Sorensen and Luckmann, *Basic Nursing: A Psychophysiologic Approach.*

The nursing process is central to all nursing practice, and we believe that the study of medical-surgical nursing should not begin without a consideration of it. The nursing process is the vehicle for the professional application of nursing knowledge. This chapter gives you a framework for the practical organization of the knowledge you will gain in studying medical-surgical nursing.

Certain myths or fallacies tend to persist about nursing. One such myth is that "nurses are born and not made." You may have heard this expressed in various ways, e.g., "She was such a good nurse, but she just could not pass the examinations," or "It is not the academically clever students who make the best nurses." Such statements imply that nurses do not need to be educated; that good nursing is kindness based on intuition rather than thought; that nursing is mere common sense and can be done by anybody; that nursing actions are simply the "doing of the obvious." Pause for a few moments and consider how a nurse who has kindly intentions but lacks knowledge and relies heavily on intuition would behave in practice. Would such behavior be what you would want from a professional nurse taking care of you or someone you love? Our response is that we would like some of the kindness, but we could do without *any* guesswork! It is through the responsible application of the nursing process by a humanitarian and intelligent nurse that appropriate kindness is offered and guesswork is eliminated in nursing practice.

OVERVIEW OF THE NURSING PROCESS

The nursing process is a system of interrelated and interdependent problem-solving steps directed toward meeting the needs of patients and their significant others. It is most appropriately carried out cooperatively by the nurse, with the patient and the patient's significant others. The nurse offers expertise in the process as well as a professional knowledge of basic human need attainment, while the patient and significant others supply the information about the individual situation — which only they can do.

In nursing literature, the steps of the nursing process are described in a variety of ways. Whatever terms are used, the concepts are the same. Do not let differing terminology confuse you when you read about the nursing process. Instead, remind yourself that the nursing process is really a simple, practical tool, and look for the fundamental concepts that underlie all descriptions.

We find it convenient to consider the nursing process in terms of *nursing assessment,* which determines *nursing management.* (Fig. 2–1) Nursing assessment is the term used to describe all the factors that go into making a *nursing diagnosis,* i.e., *gathering data* so that a patient's *unmet needs can be identified* and the *nursing problems* determined; so that *priorities can be established* and *long- and short-term objectives set.* With these assessment activities carefully done, excellent nursing management can be instituted through *the implementation of planned intervention* and careful *evaluation* of the entire process. Each of these steps is discussed in this chapter.

Look again at Figure 2–1. Note that the patient-nurse partnership is at the center of the diagram, emphasizing that the nurse and the patient work *together* through all stages of the process. Note that while the patient and the nurse are the "principal characters," they each have "supporting artists"! The patient's significant others may include friends, family, and colleagues. The nurse, too, has significant others to rely on — other members of the nursing, medical, and paramedical teams. Significant others are very important, and their influence on the patient-nurse partnership should be acknowledged and utilized.

Notice, too, that Figure 2–1 depicts circular movement. This emphasizes that the nursing process is ongoing and continuous. Evaluation leads into further assessment, which may produce new data that suggest more interventions, which lead to fresh evaluation. Spend some time examining Figure 2–1 and discuss it with your colleagues and teachers until you believe that you understand each concept. Think through each step in terms of your nursing experiences. You may, in fact, wish to add to the diagram to make it show more clearly what the nursing process means to you.

NURSING ASSESSMENT

Nursing assessment is the systematic collection and ordering of information that allows a nurse to make a *nursing diagnosis.* A nursing diagnosis is made when a nurse accurately identifies a patient's unmet needs and the associated nursing problems. Let us look now at what is meant by "nursing problems."

Nursing Problems

The nursing process is a system for problem solving. The problems that nurses work with are the obstacles people meet in satisfying their basic human needs. As described in Chapter 1, a fundamental part of being human is to be continually recognizing basic human needs and seeking to satisfy them. Recognizing a need does not necessarily mean it can be satisfied. Obstacles may arise that must be overcome before a need can be met. A person's ability to overcome such obstacles is called *adaptability.* In optimum health, a person can overcome (or adapt to) such obstacles and achieve need satisfaction without professional help.

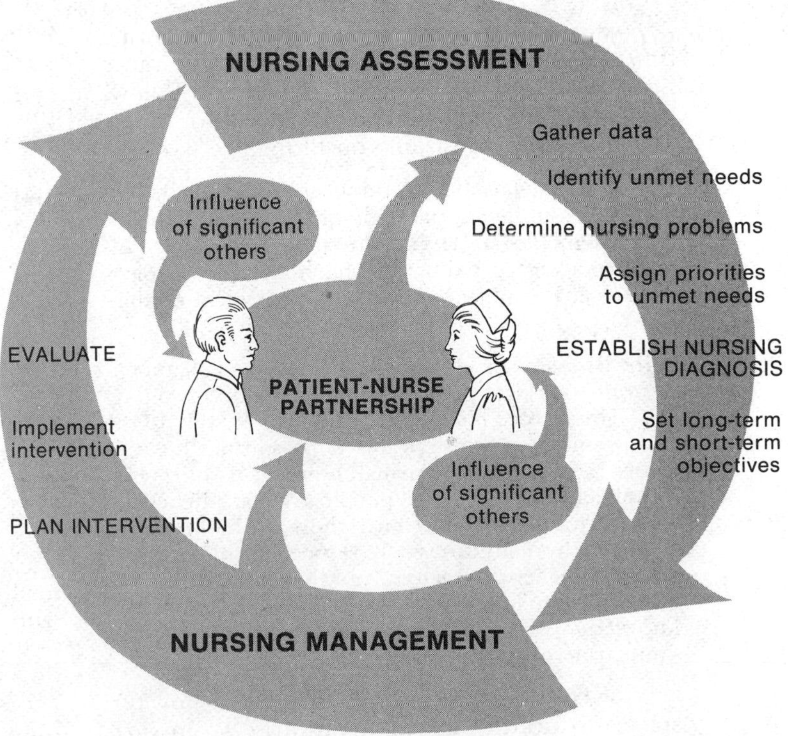

Figure 2–1. The nursing process. The patient-nurse partnership is central to the entire process.

Nursing problem *is a term describing an obstacle that prevents a patient from experiencing satisfaction of a basic human need. Nursing action is directed toward the solution of nursing problems.*

The sources of obstacles to need satisfaction are various:

- *Physiologic,* e.g., illness, fatigue, pain, immobility
- *Emotional,* e.g., anxiety, excitement, fear
- *Intellectual,* e.g., lack of information, knowledge and/or understanding
- *Social,* e.g., strained interpersonal relationships, fear of another person's power, intimidation by a professional person, shyness in the company of strangers, reduced social network
- *Environmental,* e.g., temperature, unfamiliar surroundings (such as a hospital), time, air pollution
- *Personality,* e.g., habits, beliefs, values, and life experiences of the individual
- *Cultural,* e.g., values, beliefs, practices, and habits particular to a group of people

Obstacles to need satisfaction may come from one source or from several sources at the same time, or the sources of obstruction to the same need may vary over time. Consider the following examples focusing on the need to "move and maintain a desirable position."[33]

Mr. White has had a cerebral vascular accident (stroke) resulting in paralysis of the left side of his body (hemeplegia). His need to move and change his position is obstructed by a problem from a physiologic source, i.e., illness and resultant physical disability.

Joe Brown is an 11-year-old boy who had an appendectomy (surgical removal of the appendix) two days ago. To increase his activity, he is told to walk to the bathroom whenever he wants to pass urine. Joe continues to use a bedside urinal, however. It hurts him to walk, and he has heard people say that stitches can "burst." Joe actually isn't sure where the bathroom is, and he is too shy to ask. Joe's need to move is obstructed by several factors: physiologic (pain), emotional (fear), intellectual (lack of information and knowledge), social (shyness), and environmental (unfamiliar accommodation).

Now consider an example that shows how obstacles to need satisfaction can arise from various sources over time. Take the need to "eat and drink adequately."[33]

Mrs. Smith, an elderly woman, is admitted to the hospital unconscious in a diabetic coma (a severe condition resulting from impaired carbohydrate metabolism). At this time her unconsciousness prevents eating and drinking (physiologic source).

Mrs. Smith regains consciousness after emergency care is given, and later an appropriate diet is prescribed for her.The diet includes meat, however, and Mrs. Smith does not tell anyone that she does not eat meat. She leaves on her plate any meat that she is served. The satisfaction of her need to eat and drink adequately now is obstructed by personality (dietary preference and habit), social factors (possibly shy of professionals), and environmental factors (choices of food and control of eating are limited in an institutional environment).

Later Mrs. Smith is discharged from the hospital, with instructions to keep to the diet prescribed. Although she received some teaching about her diet, she does not fully understand how to prepare the food at home. Now, her eating and drinking need is unmet because of an intellectual obstacle (lack of knowledge and understanding).

It is a nursing responsibility to direct care toward the unmet needs of the individual patient. The obstacles to satisfying Mrs. Smith's needs for eating and drinking were easy to discern when she was unconscious. As the sources of obstruction changed, they became less obvious. It is part of nursing assessment to insure that unmet needs and the accompanying nursing problems are identified.

Importance of Nursing Assessment

It is sometimes difficult to convince nurses that careful nursing assessment is necessary. Practicing nurses can be tempted to believe that they do not have time for careful assessment, and they may rely on institutional routines and generalized, nonpersonal nursing care plans. This is most often a result of lack of knowledge and skill in the assessment process, coupled with little personal incentive to acquire the knowledge and skills. In addition, the nursing process is sometimes presented in an unnecessarily complicated way that can deter people from making use of it. Nursing actions can be performed without assessment, but when this is done the nurse cannot know whether the actions are appropriate and helpful to the particular individual.

Consider the following example from another health profession: Suppose you went to a dentist who said to you in words or actions, "I do not really know how to do a dental assessment and I do not really think such a thing is altogether necessary. I *do know* how to drill and fill teeth, however, so I'll do some of that and hope I may help you a little." Would you feel confident with such a dentist?

What would you think of a lawyer who stated that there was no time to find out what you had come for, but there was time to file a divorce suit so that was what you would get? Would this lawyer be a help to you? Of course not, yet there is little difference between such a lawyer and a nurse who rushes through the routine of bathing several patients without first finding out what (if any) help each person requires in satisfying their needs for hygiene.

Data Gathering

Adequate data (or information) must be collected if an accurate nursing diagnosis is to be made.

> *The excellent nurse is an observant person and constantly seeks information about patients.*

The nurse has three sources of information: *primary, secondary, and tertiary.*

Primary Source. The *primary source* is, of course, the patient. The patient provides both verbal and nonverbal information. Thus, an excellent nurse learns to listen to verbal messages and to observe nonverbal behavior. Interpretations of nonverbal behavior must be verified verbally with the patient before they can be considered really accurate information. Likewise when a nurse observes a discrepancy between the verbal response and the nonverbal behavior of a patient, the discrepancy should be discussed with the patient. For example, consider Mr. Robinson, who is admitted to a surgical unit in a hospital, with severe abdominal pain. He may say, "I am so relieved to be in the hospital where something can be done to help me." Nonverbally, however, Mr. Robinson may communicate signs of anxiety, e.g., he may be restless, be unable to remember information, avoid eye contact with the nurse, and have difficulty expressing himself. The skillful nurse may say "I can understand your relief at getting some help. You also appear rather restless and uneasy. Are you feeling anxious about anything?" The patient may express his feelings more directly then. Mr. Robinson may say, "Well, my stomach hurts and I'm nervous about being in the hospital for the first time in my life." By talking with the patient, information that may appear to be inconsistent can be clarified and further information can be obtained.

Primary information can be obtained during any interaction between the patient and the nurse. In addition, structured interviewing is advisable, especially when a patient first enters

the hospital or some other health care system.* Included in such an interview is the *nursing history*.

A nursing history is one way of gathering information about a patient. A good nursing history, taken by a skillful and sensitive nurse within the context of a careful interview, seeks information about:

- A patient's understanding of current health problems
- Physical, mental, social and emotional reactions to the current health problems the patient is experiencing (if in fact a health problem does exist)
- A patient's usual living environment including home, work, and significant others
- A patient's patterns of daily living and the ways basic human needs are normally met
- A patient's perception of current obstacles to the satisfaction of basic human needs
- Any particular worries or stresses the patient is experiencing
- A patient's previous experiences with illness and/or the health care system
- The kinds of physical, social, emotional, intellectual and financial resources available to the patient
- Adaptive and maladaptive responses a patient habitually uses in coping with stress
- Any particular likes and dislikes a patient has concerning any basic human needs

Various nursing history formats have been developed. Some are simple guidelines of topics to be covered in an interview. Others are somewhat more detailed "questionnaire" type forms. It is a useful exercise to develop your own nursing history format, trying to include ways of gaining all the kinds of information mentioned above. After you complete your history format, you may find that seeking the criticism of your colleagues and teachers can be valuable, as well as testing it in a clinical area. The comments and suggestions of some patients may well be the most valuable critique you could get.

The act of conducting a patient interview and taking a nursing history holds the potential for

*The reader is strongly encouraged to consult detailed material on the art of interviewing and on the skills involved in the helping relationship. See, for example, Sorensen and Luckmann, *Basic Nursing: A Psychophysiologic Approach,* Chapters 3 and 17.

establishing rapport with the patient and developing trust within the nurse-patient relationship. If rapport and trust are achieved, patients will experience less anxiety and more of their energies will be available for other purposes. Subsequent nursing care planning may well be easier, as the nurse and the patient will be more comfortable in working together.

Secondary Sources. Information from *secondary sources* includes: (a) data recorded on a patient's chart, (b) information from a patient's significant others, and (c) information from other health personnel who have had contact with the patient. The observations of other people can be very useful in understanding a patient's needs. People who become clients of a health care system are often stressed and have limited energy. It is important not to tax their energy levels unnecessarily by seeking information that has already been gathered by someone else. Secondary sources of information are very important from this point of view. Sometimes, because of a patient's physical, emotional or intellectual state, the primary information available is limited. Secondary sources are essential at such times.

Always remember, however, that all information from secondary sources is subject to the invalidity of the interpretation of others. Excellent nurses verify secondary information with the patient whenever possible and use such information carefully to be sure that they do not make unvalidated assumptions about the patients they care for.

Tertiary Sources. Information from *tertiary sources* is not specific to an individual patient. This is the general information available in textbooks and professional literature. Always remember, however, that no individual is a "textbook patient" and no individual is "typical." Tertiary information provides guidelines only, and excellent nurses modify such knowledge according to the individuality of every patient.

(For further discussion on assessment, see Chapters 14 and 15. Other information about specific assessments is found throughout this book.)

Nursing Diagnosis

With adequate data gathering, a nurse is in a position to make a *nursing diagnosis,* i.e., the identification of a patient's unmet needs and the determination of associated nursing problems. A nursing diagnosis is made by considering the following question: *"Based on the information I have available to me, what are the needs this patient has that require some help from me to be satisified?"* A good nursing history will provide information about a patient's habitual patterns of need satisfaction. The next step is to consider whether there are any present circumstances that are making it difficult for a patient to utilize habitual patterns and/or whether any of the patient's habitual patterns are in fact obstructing need satisfaction rather than facilitating it.

One way of making a nursing diagnosis that may be useful to a beginning nurse or a nursing student is to use one (or several) of the theoretical frameworks of basic human needs that are available (see Chapter 1, p. 7) together with a list of possible sources of nursing problems (p. 14) and systematically apply each item to the particular patient for whom care is being planned. This is a way of reducing the possibility of oversights occurring.

A nurse might, for example, be planning the care of Ms. Marilyn Boyle, a 68-year-old woman admitted to the hospital for assessment and stabilization of her medication regimen, prescribed for a neurological condition. A nurse might refer to Figure 1–6 (p. 11) and consider each need or class of needs individually in relation to Ms. Boyle. Does Ms. Boyle have difficulty with any physical needs — breathing, eating, drinking, eliminating, moving, resting, dressing, keeping warm (or cool), keeping clean, avoiding physical danger? Does Ms. Boyle have any difficulty with social needs — communicating with others, maintaining desired privacy, feeling welcome and accepted, contacting significant others? Does Ms. Boyle have any difficulty meeting any emotional needs — trusting others, being free from anxiety, maintaining a sense of autonomy and control, feeling a comfortable level of self-esteem? Does Ms. Boyle have any difficulty satisfying any intellectual needs — seeking and receiving information, giving input into decisions which concern her.

A list of Ms. Boyle's unmet needs might result from such an analysis. The nurse can then take each need that is identified as being obstructed and consider the source(s) of the obstructions (see p. 14). For example, Ms. Boyle may be unable to meet her elimination needs without help because she experiences some incontinence of feces and because she finds it difficult to walk the distance from her room to the patient's bathroom. One of Ms. Boyle's unmet needs is elimination, and the nursing problems are her incontinence of feces and her difficulty in walking. On the basis of this nursing diagnosis, nursing intervention would be planned.

When a patient's unmet or partially met needs are identified, along with the specific source of need obstruction (i.e., nursing problem), a nursing diagnosis has been made. Only then is it valid to consider intervention.

Setting Priorities

Sometimes a nurse will be in the ideal situation where the time, energy, and resources are available to give attention to all the nursing problems identified for each patient. This is wonderful when it happens — and in reality it does not happen often. Perhaps the most difficult decisions that nurses have to make repeatedly are decisions about what to do for a patient and what not to do when it is impossible to do everything. Maslow's hierarchy of needs is helpful in determining priorities (see p. 8). There is a danger with this tool, however, in assuming that physiologic needs should always be given a higher priority than other needs on the hierarchy. While life-threatening crises take precedence over everything else, "routinized physical care" is not always of primary importance. In all cases, the individual circumstances and desires of each patient must be considered.

In your daily nursing practice, what criteria might you use to decide on what to do and what to leave until later? Take some time to develop a list of criteria that seem justified to you. What are some of the possible good and bad outcomes of the application of your criteria? Try to think of situations where any of your criteria may be dangerous. Share and discuss issues of priority setting with a group of colleagues. It would be interesting and helpful to ask practicing professional nurses how they go about making decisions about priority. Analyze what you hear from colleagues, professional nurses and nurse-teachers and what you read in nursing literature. Consider the consequences of each guideline for priority setting suggested to you. Evaluate each suggestion in the light of your knowledge and understanding of the unique function of nursing.

The following criteria are suggested by Bower to assist with priority setting in nursing practice.[16] She suggests an appropriate hierarchy of importance to be:

1. Threats to the life, dignity and integrity of the individual, significant others or community.
2. Threats that may destructively change the individual, significant others or community.
3. Problems that may affect the normal developmental growth of the individual, significant others and community.

Bower suggests additional criteria that may be helpful in setting priorities in situations where nurses are faced with more than one client or more than one group of clients.[16]

1. Safety
   A. Severity of health problems
   B. Potential for recovery
   C. Attainment of high-level wellness
2. Efficiency — time needed by client, nurse or health team
3. Cost — expense in money and energy to client, nurse, agency, society
4. Receptivity to care

Critically examine both of the above sets of criteria. Are there any needs or groups of people that may be ignored by the application of such criteria?

It is a fact of life that priorities must be set. This does not mean, however, that some needs or some people are unimportant and can be ignored. Periodic evaluation of clinical practice is necessary to make sure that the same areas are not being given low priority consistently.

Nursing Objectives*

> *A* nursing objective *is a short statement that describes in detailed behavioral terms the expected outcomes toward which specific nursing intervention is planned.*

A well written nursing objective achieves two aims. First, it enables everyone concerned with the care of a patient to know what a planned nursing intervention is to achieve. Second, it provides indicators that will enable everyone involved to know whether or not the nursing intervention has been successful.

The following are some guidelines that may help you prepare useful and practical objectives:

- *Nursing objectives are specific to a particular patient at a particular time.* Generalized objectives for all patients experiencing the same medical condition are not appropriate. They do not take into account the many factors that make one person's experience different from that of another person.
- *Nursing objectives are written in clear, simple and concise language.* Objectives are used in clinical situations where time matters. They must be able to be read and understood in seconds.
- *Nursing objectives are expressed in terms of the patient's behavior.* Objectives are patient centered. They

*In nursing literature, the terms "goals" and "objectives" are often used interchangeably. Although some descriptions of the nursing process differentiate between them, both terms refer to the anticipated *end product* of planned nursing action. In practice, objectives are usually expressed in more specific terms than are goals. Therefore, it is probably more useful to express the anticipated end products or expected result of planned nursing actions as *objectives* rather than as goals.

state how the patient will behave if the nursing intervention is successful.

- *Nursing objectives are expressed in as specific terms as possible.* The more specific an objective is about patient behavior, the more evident success or failure of the nursing intervention will be.
- *Nursing objectives include details of "who," "how," and "when."* For example, "Ms. Brown (patient) will take five consecutive deep breaths each hour from 7 AM till 9 PM on her first postoperative day."
- *Nursing objectives are known to the patient and (if the patient wishes) to the patient's significant others.* Whenever possible, the patient should participate in the writing of nursing objectives. If the patient agrees with the objectives and sees them as attainable, the consequent nursing intervention is more likely to be successful.
- *Nursing objectives are never written in isolation from each other, nor are they written in isolation from the rest of the nursing process.* Nursing objectives are a part of the total nursing process in which all parts are interrelated.
- The poorly written objective is a waste of time and energy — and most damaging — it promotes the belief that the entire nursing process is merely an academic exercise, not relevant to daily nursing practice.

> Nursing objectives *are statements of successful outcomes toward which nursing intervention is planned. Objectives are expressed in terms of patient behavior. They are based on very careful nursing assessment, and they describe the* evidence that will indicate *when a nursing problem(s) has been overcome and a patient's basic human need(s) satisfied.*

Long-Term and Short-Term Objectives. It is often useful to write both *short- and long-term objectives.* Long-term objectives express a final outcome. Short-term objectives express achievements that build toward the long-term objective. Study the following series of objectives that might be set for a man who needs daily urine tests and also wishes to be independent. The long-term objective would be set early in the patient-nurse partnership. The short-term objectives would be set over time in such a way that their cumulative effect would lead to the achievement of the long-term overall objective.

Long-term objective. Mr Jones will test his own urine daily, record the results, and make sound judgments about his need for medical consultation.

Short-term objective. Mr Jones will:

1.1 Discuss with the nurse the need for daily urine tests.
1.2 Take instruction from the nurse about the procedure for testing urine.
1.3 Watch the nurse test his urine and record the results.
1.4 Test his own urine in the nurse's company and record the results.
1.5 Discuss with the nurse the significance of the possible results of the urine test.
1.6 Discuss with the nurse the appropriate actions he would take in response to the various possible results of the urine tests.

We have presented a rather brief discussion of nursing objectives to reinforce your previous learning and the experiences you have had with objective setting while planning nursing care. There is a great deal written about goals and objectives in the nursing literature as well as the literature of other fields, e.g., education. It takes some time and practice to become skilled in the use of objectives. It is worth the effort!

It is important, however, to remember that *nursing objectives must work for you and the patients you take care of.* Do not get so immersed in the details of "correct" objective setting that you lose sight of their practical purpose. A useful objective is simply a statement of what you intend to achieve by the nursing care you plan to offer. That is all. To turn nursing objectives into something more complicated than that is a waste of time and energy!

Summary

To summarize, nursing assessment occurs within a patient-nurse relationship and involves the systematic collection of information from primary, secondary, and tertiary sources. It is from a solid data base that a patient's unmet needs and the associated nursing problems are identified (i.e., a nursing diagnosis made). Long- and short-term objectives are set, based on the nursing diagnosis, to guide the planning of nursing intervention and to establish criteria for evaluation.

NURSING MANAGEMENT

In this chapter we have used the term *nursing management* for those parts of the nursing process that refer to the implementation of nursing care. Obviously however, nursing assessment and nursing management are interrelated. While assessment is being made through a nursing history, for example, nursing management is also happening as the nurse facilitates development of trust within the patient-nurse relationship. It is for convenience and clarity that we describe nursing assessment and nursing management separately.

Planning Nursing Intervention

With a nursing diagnosis made and nursing objectives set, it is now time to choose appropriate nursing interventions. Much of the remainder of this book will describe the many interventions that have been found to be useful for people experiencing various stresses of a health-illness nature. In practice, the skill comes in making sound nursing judgments as to just what *nursing interventions* are appropriate for "this patient" at "this time" and in "these circumstances." Careful application of the steps involved in nursing assessment will help you to make valid decisions.

Nursing Care Plans

Nursing care plans are one way of making concrete the decisions made through the nursing process. *A nursing care plan is a written document that states in specific terms the nursing interventions planned for a particular patient.*

There is no one "correct" format for nursing care plans. It is probably appropriate that forms are developed suitable to the situation in which they are to be used. There are certain principles, however, that apply to any nursing care plan, whatever the format:

- *Nursing care plans focus on nursing problems and have a nursing approach.* While care delegated from other health professionals may well be included, a nursing approach and emphasis will ensure that the *patient* remains central — not the disease or technique.
- *Nursing care plans are written in clear, specific, and "actionable" terms.* If a plan cannot be used, it has no place in clinical practice. Vague statements such as "reassure the patient" communicate nothing. Behavioral descriptions such as "explain the x-ray procedure to the patient and give him time to ask questions — return after one hour and offer to repeat the explanation or discuss any further questions" tell a nurse exactly what to do.
- *Nursing care plans are short and concise.* If it takes all day to read or to write a nursing care plan, there will be no time to implement the plan! It is nursing actions that really count!
- *Nursing care plans show the patient needs and nursing problems that are receiving attention as well as the long- and short-term objectives that the interventions are designed to accomplish.* This prevents the plan from becoming merely a list of tasks. It provides the rationale for planned intervention and the basis for evaluation and therefore facilitates modification and change in the plan.
- *Nursing care plans are written in a "non permanent" fashion.* Pencil may be the most appropriate medium. Nursing care is a very fluid, delicate phenomenon. A nursing care plan must be able to be changed quickly and easily.

Figure 2–2 shows part of a nursing care plan that incorporates all of the above principles. The plan is designed for Mr. Moore, a 40-year-old man who is hospitalized following a myocardial infarction (heart attack). Mr. Moore is married, has five children, and is a taxi proprietor who has recently been experiencing considerable worry about his business. The plan shown is based on a thorough nursing assessment — details of which would probably appear on this record.

Figure 2–2 is an incomplete plan. It is included to illustrate the factors included in a nursing care plan. Other needs and nursing problems would of course be included as appropriate.

> Nursing interventions *are planned nursing actions, usually recorded in a nursing care plan, that are intended to reduce nursing problems so that a patient's basic human needs may be satisified and nursing objectives achieved.*

Evaluation

As you read and think about the nursing process, it should become clear that an evaluation procedure is an inherent part of the process. The excellent nurse is continually assessing whether a nursing intervention is successful in helping a patient. This is done both informally, in the thought processes of the nurse, and in periodic formal reviews and revisions of nursing care plans. When evaluating nursing action, it is helpful to ask yourself the following questions:

- Did I implement nursing actions for this patient as planned? *If not,* what were the reasons for the changes I made? Were the changes based on information available only after the plan was made?
- Did my nursing actions solve the nursing problems this patient has? Were the patient's basic human needs met? Were the short term objectives met?
- If the answer to any of these questions is no, what is the reason? Were the nursing interventions inappropriate to the problems, needs or objectives? Were the nursing interventions expressed in vague terms and therefore "unactionable"?
- Do I have further information now that I did not have when I planned this intervention? What changes in circumstance have occurred for this

Name: Mr. Charles Moore
Name patient prefers to be called: Chas

Long-term objective: Chas will return home, recovered from the acute stages of his myocardial infarction having the knowledge and understanding of health practices that help reduce the likelihood of future infarctions.

Short-term objectives:
Chas will state that he understands the reasons for the medical regimen he is on.
Chas will contribute to the planning of his nursing care by providing information about his likes and dislikes.
Chas will be able to rest.
Chas will be able to express his anxieties in words.

NEEDS	NURSING PROBLEMS	NURSING INTERVENTION
Rest	Strange bed & environment Anxiety about heart about work about family about his horse Habitual difficulty in resting or sleeping during the day time Pain	Describe the physical environment carefully. Allow time for questions. Repeat the explanation (without impatience) over the first day until Chas expresses easiness about his environment. Discuss the bed with Chas. Find out if there are any factors that would make it more like the comfort of his bed at home, e.g., number of pillows, which side the bedside stand should be on, the height of the bed. Explain all procedures and treatments–before, during, and after. Facilitate questioning and expression of concerns. Talk with his wife about his concern over his work, family, and horse. Encourage her to discuss them with him and make arrangements together. Encourage visits from others who can help in relieving anxieties.

Figure 2–2. Part of one kind of nursing care plan.

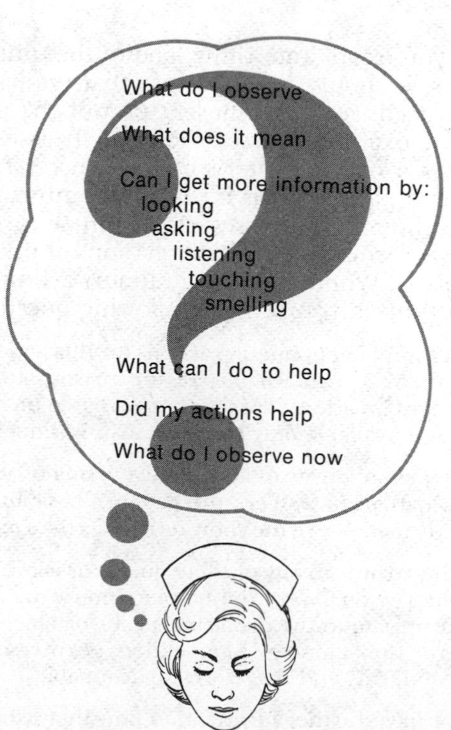

Figure 2–3. The nursing process is a way of thinking.

patient? (Note that the assessment stage of the nursing process is occurring again.)

- What is the next step toward the long-term objective? Do I need to change or alter the objectives?
- What are the needs this patient requires help to satisfy now?

The answers to these questions will help in modifying the nursing care plan so that the nursing care the patient receives will be more likely to be helpful.

THE NURSING PROCESS AS A WAY OF THINKING

So far we have described the nursing process in terms of planning the entire care a patient requires. The nursing process is also useful moment by moment, as a problem-solving way of thinking. With practice, nurses can bring a problem-solving frame of mind to every situation. Such an approach, utilized well, reduces a number of dangers.

- Nursing process avoids the danger of making nursing decisions based on intuition and guesswork.
- Nursing process avoids the danger of taking nursing actions out of routine or habit.

- Nursing process avoids the danger of nursing actions based on generalizations about patients — their disease, age, or any other category.

> *The* nursing process, *well utilized, promotes individualized, sensitive, rational, relevant, and effective nursing care.*

CONCLUSION

The remainder of this book will provide you with an enormous knowledge base from which to plan nursing interventions. As you study the chapters ahead, you will acquire a lot of medical facts and nursing facts. You will gain understanding of disease processes, diagnostic procedures, therapeutic regimens. Such material is fascinating and, without question, essential knowledge for the professional nurse. Always remember, however, that it is *how* you apply such knowledge, within the delicate human interactions of the patient-nurse relationship, that really matters.

It is sometimes tempting for nurses to become so interested in the medical and technical aspects of their education and practice that they forget the reason that nursing exists — the person in need.

As you enter the field of medical-surgical nursing, you may do well to remember the caution Bates gives to Nurse Practitioners.

> By expanding into medicine, you will need — more than ever before — to increase your consciousness of what nursing is all about. The values of nursing must not get lost in the dominant medical culture. If they do, you justly risk the epithet of junior doctor. Our patients do not need junior doctors. They need the knowledge and skills of both medicine and nursing. By combining these, you have the opportunity to practice not only in the highest traditions of medicine, but also in the highest traditions of nursing.[8]

BIBLIOGRAPHY (Unit I)

1. Archer, C. O., and D. Swearingen: Application of Benjamin Franklin's decision-making model to the clinical setting. *Nursing Forum,* XVI:319, Nos. 3 and 4, 1977.
2. Aspinall, M. J.: Nursing diagnosis — The weak link. *Nursing Outlook,* 24:433, July 1976.
3. Baer, E. D., M. N. McGowan, and D. O. McGivern: How to take a health history. *The American Journal of Nursing,* 77:1190, July 1977.
4. Bailey, J. T., and K. E. Claus: *Decision Making in Nursing: Tools for Change.* St. Louis: C. V. Mosby Co., 1975.
5. Bakdash, D. P.: Becoming an assertive nurse. *The American Journal of Nursing,* 78:1710, Oct. 1978.
6. Barba, M., et al.: The evaluation of patient care through use of ANA's Standards of Nursing Practice. *Supervisor Nurse,* 9:42, Jan. 1978.
7. Bartos, L. T., and M. R. Knight: Documentation of nursing process. *Supervisor Nurse,* 9:41, July 1978.
8. Bates, B.: Twelve paradoxes. A message for nurse practitioners. *Nursing Outlook,* 22:686, Nov. 1974.
9. Becknell, E., and D. M. Smith: *System of Nursing Practice — A Clinical Nursing Assessment Tool.* Philadelphia: F. A. Davis Co., 1975.
10. Bennett, L. R.: This I believe . . . that nurses may become extinct. *Nursing Outlook,* 18:28, Jan. 1970.
11. Berggren, H. J., and A. D. Zagornik: Teaching nursing process to beginning students. *Nursing Outlook,* 16:32, July 1968.
12. Billings, C. V.: Documentation — The supervisors dream. *Supervisor Nurse,* 9:16, Oct. 1978.
13. Bloch, D.: Some crucial terms in nursing: What do they really mean? *Nursing Outlook,* 22:689, Nov. 1974.
14. Blount, M., S. S. Green, A. Harmony, A. B. Kinney, and C. W. Sanborn: Documenting with the problem-oriented record system. *The American Journal of Nursing,* 78:1539, Sept. 1978.
15. Bowar-Ferres, S.: Loeb Center and its philosophy of nursing. *The American Journal of Nursing,* 75:810, May 1975.
16. Bower, F. L.: *The Process of Planning Nursing Care,* St. Louis: C. V. Mosby Co., 1972.
17. Browning, M. H.: *The Nursing Process in Practice.* New York: American Journal of Nursing Co., 1974.
18. Byrnc, M. L., and L. F. Thompson: *Key Concepts for the Study and Practice of Nursing.* St. Louis: C. V. Mosby Co., 1972.
19. Cady, J. W., D. J. Froehman, and R. B. Norby: *Taking the Pain Out of Care Planning.* Chicago: Medicus/Nursing Care Systems, 1975.
20. Coffman, C. A.: Nursing care plans for the "Older" graduate. *Supervisor Nurse,* 9:66, July 1978.
21. Daubenmire, M. J., and I. M. King: Nursing process models: A system approach. *Nursing Outlook,* 21:512, Aug. 1973.
22. Dayani, E.: Focus on health. Concepts of wellness. *Nurse Practitioner,* 4:31, Jan./Feb. 1979.
23. Donaldson, S. K., and D. M. Crowley: The discipline of nursing. *Nursing Outlook,* 26:113, Feb. 1978.
24. Donovan, H. M.: Toward a definition of nursing. *Supervisor Nurse,* 1:12, Oct. 1970.
25. Durand, M., and R. Prince: Nursing diagnosis: Process and decision. *Nursing Forum,* V:50, No. 4, 1966.
26. Eggland, E. T.: How to take a meaningful nursing history. *Nursing '77,* 7:21, July 1977.
27. Francis, G. M.: This thing called problem solving. *In* Marriner, A.: *The Nursing Process: A Scientific Approach to Nursing Care.* St. Louis: C. V. Mosby Co., 1975.
28. Gebbie, K., and M. A. Lavin: Clasifying nursing diagnoses. *The American Journal of Nursing,* 74:250, Feb. 1974.
29. Gooding, M.: If you think care plans are a nuisance, read this. *RN,* 41:95, Oct. 1978.
30. Gordon, M.: Nursing diagnosis and the diagnostic process. *The American Journal of Nursing,* 76:1298, Aug. 1976.
31. Grubbs, J.: An interpretation of the Johnson behavioral system model for nursing practice. *In* Riehl, J. P., and Sister C. Roy (Eds.): *Conceptual Models for Nursing Practice.* New York: Appleton-Century-Crofts, 1974.
32. Henderson, V.: *Basic Principles of Nursing Care.* Geneva: International Council of Nurses, 1960 (Revised printing, 1969).
33. Henderson, V.: The nature of nursing. *The American Journal of Nursing,* 64:62, Aug. 1964.
34. Henderson, V.: *The Nature of Nursing: A Definition and Its*

Implications for Practice, Research and Education. New York: MacMillan Company, 1966.
35. Hoyman, H. S.: Models of human nature and their impact on health education. *Nursing Digest,* Vol. III, Sept.-Oct. 1975, p. 36.
36. Hushower, G., D. Gamberg, and N. Smith: The nursing process in discharge planning. *Supervisor Nurse,* 9:55, Sept. 1978.
37. Jackson, C., V. Edmundson, and D. R. Green: Promoting written care plans. *Supervisor Nurse,* 9:43, Aug. 1978.
38. Johnson, D. E.: Development of theory: A requisite for nursing as a primary health profession. *Nursing Research,* 23:372, Sept.-Oct. 1974.
39. Johnson, M. M., and H. W. Martin: A sociological analysis of the nurse role. *The American Journal of Nursing,* 58:373, Mar. 1958.
40. Jones, P. S.: An adaptation model for nursing practice. *The American Journal of Nursing,* 78:1900, Nov. 1978.
41. King, I.: *Toward a Theory for Nursing.* New York: John Wiley and Sons, 1971.
42. Kraegel, J. M., et al.: *Patient Care Systems.* Philadelphia: J. B. Lippincott Co., 1974.
43. Kreuter, F. R. What is good nursing care? *Nursing Outlook,* 5:302, May 1957.
44. Langford, T.: Establishing a nursing contract. *Nursing Outlook,* 26:386, June 1978.
45. Laros, J.: Deriving outcome criteria from a conceptual model. *Nursing Outlook,* 25:333, May 1977.
46. Lewis, L.: This I believe . . . about nursing process — Key to care. 16:26, May 1968.
47. Little, D. E., and D. L. Carnevali: *Nursing Care Planning,* 2nd ed. Philadelphia: J. B. Lippincott Co., 1976.
48. Little, D. E.; and D. L. Carnevali: The nursing care planning system. *Nursing Outlook,* 19:164, Mar. 1971.
49. Lowe, G. M.: Let's have more humane nursing care. *Nursing '74,* 4:10, Jan. 1974.
50. Mager, R. F.: *Goal Analysis.* Belmont, Cal., Fearon Publishers, 1972.
51. Mager, R. F.: *Preparing Instructional Objectives.* Palo Alto, Cal.: Fearon Publishers, 1962.
52. Malloy, J. L.: Taking exception to problem-oriented nursing care. *The American Journal of Nursing,* 76:582, Apr. 1976.
53. Marriner, A.: *The Nursing Process: A Scientific Approach to Nursing Care.* St. Louis: C. V. Mosby Co., 1975.
54. Maslow, A. H.: *Motivation and Personality.* New York: Harper and Row, 1954.
55. Mayers, M.: *A Systematic Approach to the Nursing Care Plan.* New York: Appleton-Century-Crofts, 1972.
56. McCain, R. F.: Nursing by assessment — Not intuition. *In* Marriner, A.: *The Nursing Process: A Scientific Approach to Nursing Care.* St. Louis: C. V. Mosby Co., 1975.
57. McCloskey, J. C.: The nursing care plan: past, present and uncertain future — A review of the literature. *Nursing Forum,* XIV:364, No. 4, 1975.
58. Neuman, B.: Betty Neuman health-care system model: A total person approach to patient problems. *In* Riehl, J. P., and Sister C. Roy (Eds.): *Conceptual Models for Nursing Practice.* New York: Appleton-Century-Crofts, 1974.
59. Nightingale, F.: *Notes on Nursing.* Harrison and Sons, 1859. Reprint edition. London: Gerald Duckworth and Company Limited, 1970.
60. Niles, A. G., and A. E. Paulen: A humanistic approach to nursing care. *Supervisor Nurse,* 4:42, July 1973.
61. Norris, C. M. Delusions that trap nurses. . . . *Canadian Nurse,* 69:37, June 1973.
62. Orem, D. E.: *Nursing: Concepts of Practice.* New York: McGraw-Hill Book Co., 1971.
63. Partridge, K. B.: Nursing values in a changing society. *Nursing Outlook,* 26:356, June 1978.
64. Patrick, G.: Forgotten patients on the medical ward. *Canadian Nurse,* 68:27, Mar. 1972.
65. Porter, A., P. Moschel, B. Liederman, and M. Pope: Patient needs on admission. *The American Journal of Nursing,* 77:112, Jan. 1977.
66. Pumphrey, J. B.: Recognizing your patient's spiritual needs. *Nursing '77,* 7:64, Dec. 1977.
67. Reinkemeyer, Sister A. M.: The myths by which we live. *International Nursing Review,* 16:39, 1969.
68. Riehl, J. P., and Sister C. Roy (Eds.): *Conceptual Models for Nursing Practice.* New York: Appleton-Century-Crofts, 1974.
69. Rogers, M. E.: *Introduction to the Theoretical Basis of Nursing.* Philadelphia: F. A. Davis Co., 1970.
70. Roy, Sister C.: *Introduction to Nursing: An Adaptation Model.* Englewood Cliffs, N. J.: Prentice-Hall, Inc., 1976.
71. Roy, Sister C.: The impact of nursing diagnosis. *Nursing Digest,* 4:67, Summer 1976.
72. Rubel, Sister M.: Coming to grips with the nursing process. *Supervisor Nurse,* 7:30, Feb. 1976.
73. Ryden, M. B.: Energy: A crucial consideration in the nursing process. *Nursing Forum,* XVI:71, No. 1, 1977.
74. Schaefer, J.: The interrelatedness of decision making and the nursing process. *American Journal of Nursing,* 74:1852, Oct. 1974.
75. Scottish National Nursing and Midwifery Consultative Committee. A new concept of nursing. 1. The process of nursing. *Nursing Times,* April 8, 1976, pp. 49–52.
76. Scottish National and Midwifery Consultative Committee. A new concept of nursing. 2. Research. *Nursing Times,* April 15, 1976, pp. 53–56.
77. Smith, D. M.: Writing objectives as a nursing practice skill. *The American Journal of Nursing,* 71:319, Feb., 1971.
78. Snyder, P. J.: Goal setting. *Supervisor Nurse,* 9:61, Sept. 1978.
79. Sorensen, K. C., and J. Luckmann: *Basic Nursing: A Psychophysiologic Approach.* Philadelphia: W. B. Saunders Co., 1979.
80. Tapia, J. A.: The nursing process in family health. *The American Journal of Nursing,* 20:267, Apr. 1972.
81. Wiley, L. (Ed.): The nursing care plan. A communication system that really works. *Nursing '78,* 8:28, Aug. 1978.
82. Wolff, H., and R. Erickson: The assessment man. *Nursing Outlook,* 25:103, Feb. 1977.
83. Yura, H., and M. B. Walsh: *The Nursing Process,* 2nd ed. New York: Appleton-Century-Crofts, 1973.
84. Zimmerman, D. S., and C. Gohrke: The goal directed nursing approach. *The American Journal of Nursing,* 70:306, Feb. 1970.

UNIT II

A HOLISTIC APPROACH TO ILLNESS

It is more important to know what sort of person has a disease than to know what sort of disease a person has.

HIPPOCRATES

Unit I focused on the unique contribution of nursing to patient care. In that unit the functions of nursing were distinguished from medical functions, and it was emphasized that nursing is the "caring" art, best practiced in a problem-solving way. Unit I introduced you to holistic concepts of human beings. You were encouraged to think through systems of basic human needs that are common to every person. It was emphasized that attention to basic human needs is the central focus of excellent nursing care. One experience that can obstruct human need gratification is illness. Unit II, therefore, focuses on a holistic approach to illness.

This unit consists of two chapters. Chapter 3 is titled "Mind-Body (Psyche-Soma) Interaction." An understanding of illness and the ill person is based upon the knowledge that the mind does *not* exist separately from the body, or vice versa. We repeatedly emphasize this point because we believe that in order to understand and care for an ill person, it is imperative for the nurse to realize the following:

> *Every ill person is experiencing* both *physiologic and psychologic imbalances. Physiologic imbalances create an emotional disequilibrium, and emotional imbalances cause physiologic disturbances. Physiologic and psychologic needs must be considered together if nursing care is to be successful.*

Chapter 4 is titled "Modern Unified Theories of Disease." The question of what factors cause disease has given rise to many theories over the centuries, some of which are, in part, acceptable today. Traditionally, each theory has traced the origin of disease to one single cause — an approach that has fragmented the individual, separating mind from body. For example, Descartes, a seventeenth century philosopher, believed that disease resulted from the breakdown of the "body machine." In old medical writings, an imbalance of the "body humors" was blamed for illness. During the Middle Ages and later, theologians expounded that sickness was caused by God's curse or devil possession. Later, Pasteur developed the "germ theory," which holds that microorganisms were the culprits that triggered the development of disease. In contrast, modern unified theories of disease attempt to explain illness in broad holistic terms. These theories view disease as resulting from a collage of physical, psychologic, social, and cultural factors. The modern hypotheses described in Chapter 4 are multidimensional in scope; they encompass the total range of stressors to which human beings are vulnerable.

We wish to emphasize in this introduction that while we use such terms as "mental," "psyche," "emotional," "psychologic," "soma," "somatic," and "physiologic," it is not actually possible to dichotomize (separate) a person into such entities. These terms have filtered down from the time in history when it was incorrectly believed that a separation did exist between mind and body and, consequently, between mental and physical illness. We continue to find evidence of this ancient idea of mind-body separation expressed daily in materials we read and in statements we hear, such as, "I like medical-surgical nursing because I don't like to work with patients who have mental problems." A statement such as this indicates a belief that it is possible to classify patients as *either* physically sick *or* emotionally sick. As we have indicated, this is simply not true. Illness is not an "either-or" matter that involves either physical or mental problems; ultimately, illness involves a combination of both physical and mental factors, interacting to produce symptoms and perhaps pathologic changes.

CHAPTER 3

MIND-BODY (PSYCHE-SOMA) INTERACTION

Our present day Psyche-Soma Complex affects not only our scientific thinking and our research but also our diagnostic systems, our etiological thinking and our therapy. But, even more than that, it influences our cultural and social functioning.[101]

INTRODUCTION AND STUDY GUIDE

Anyone practicing in the health care professions needs to ask certain difficult questions that have been pondered for centuries: "What is mind?" "What is body?" "Are they separate or related?" "Do mind and body affect one another? If so, in what ways?" "Does one control the other?" "How does the mind-body issue influence my professional practice?" "How does it influence illness?"

The questions become increasingly complex and have been answered in a variety of ways. Your answers powerfully influence your view of illness. Ultimately, your answers lead to your personal acceptance or rejection of theories of psychosomatic medicine. The term *psychosomatic* expresses the "mind-body" relationship in medical language: "psycho" refers to the "psychologic" and "somatic" refers to the "physical."

Psychosomatic disorders are those with bodily (physical) symptoms that are *psychogenic* (emotional or psychologic) in origin. There may or may not be demonstrable structural or physiologic changes in the body. The psychogenic theory of disease differs from the *physicogenic* theory. In the latter, the bodily symptoms are viewed as purely organic (physical) in origin. These matters are discussed more completely in the following pages and in Chapters 4 through 8.

Despite the fact that the mind-body relationship has a direct bearing on illness, and thus on nursing and other health care fields, the issue has been slow to affect daily clinical practice. Personal views of the problem are rarely stated. An understanding of mind-body interaction is important in viewing disturbed homeostasis and resultant illness as they effect the total individual. Thus, far from being an "academic issue," the mind-body question has practical significance for nurses. Many health concerns have psychosomatic components.

> *Indeed, in society at large, the view each of us holds about mind-body interaction affects the way we look at our own illnesses and the illnesses of others.*

Study Guide

After studying this chapter you can expect to be able to:

1. Understand the historical origins of our tendency to view "mind" and "body" as separate entities.
2. Differentiate among some of the major mind-body theories.
3. Describe some of the "proofs" used to validate the mind-body interaction theory.
4. Appreciate the implications that individual and professional beliefs about the "mind-body problem" have for nursing practice.

The following *terms* may be new to you as you read this chapter.

psychosomatic	dichotomize
psychogenic	Cartesian dualism
physicogenic	interactionism
soma	independence theory
somatic	

When you have completed this chapter you should be familiar with the following concepts:

- mind-body interaction and its relevance to nursing
- evidences of mind-body interaction
- theories of mind-body interaction
- voodooism
- hypnosis
- meditation
- flight-or-fight response

The following exercises may be useful to do while you are considering this chapter.

1. *Before* reading this chapter write two or three paragraphs about your own ideas about the relationship of the mind to the body. You might want to address such questions as
   What is the mind?
   How does the mind influence the body?
   Which is more important — the mind or the body?

Try to write what you *really* think and not what you think you *should* think. After you have written your paragraphs, compare your ideas with those expressed in this chapter.

2. Recall a time when you were ill. Make a list of the physical symptoms you experienced. Does the list adequately describe your experience? What additional factors would you want to add?

3. Think back to times when you took a day off work or school or cancelled a planned engagement. Make a list of the reasons for such cancellations that make you feel guilty and those that you consider to be OK. These lists may give you some ideas of what you really think of mind-body issues.

4. You might want to take advantage of the knowledge we do have about the interaction of the mind and the body and try meditation. You can do this by either taking instruction or by teaching yourself through books and personal experimentation. It is worth the try!

When you reach the appropriate places in the chapter, pause to carefully think about how you tend to act and feel when anxious. Can you sort out your "mental" feelings from your "physical" ones? You may also find it interesting to talk with your significant others and classmates about how anxiety causes them to feel and react. This may be a group discussion topic.

If you are interested in doing additional reading on the mind-body question, refer to the bibliography for this chapter. It is located at the end of Chapter 8.

HISTORICAL BACKGROUND

At different times in history, the mind and body have been viewed as either interrelated or divided (dichotomous). The belief that the mind and body are both involved in illness, is no new discovery — Hippocrates clearly asserted it in the late fifth century B.C. However, the belief that mind and body both are factors in illness was lost for a period in Western history. How this belief was lost deserves study because it has a direct relation to our attitudes today.

It appears that in primitive society no division was made between physical and mental disease. Ancient healers sometimes used instruments to make holes surgically in their clients' heads. These "trephine holes" found in some ancient skulls indicate attempts to treat disease by making physical entry into the brain (Fig. 3–1). It is speculated that trephine holes were made to enable evil spirits (believed to cause disease) to leave the body.

A holistic approach to disease in human beings, recognizing the importance of the interrelationship of mind and body, was present throughout the Babylonian-Assyrian, Greek, and Roman civilizations, and during the Middle Ages. The nature of the mind-body interrelationship was, however, in keeping with the cultural and religious beliefs of those times. For example, during the Middle Ages in the West, the psyche was viewed as a mystical and irrational force.

Later, during the Renaissance, the "mind" and "body" were separated, so to say. The "mind" was claimed as the proper concern of religion and philosophy, and the "body" became the property of medicine. The mind-body model of Cartesian dualism exemplifies the thinking that became prevalent at this time.

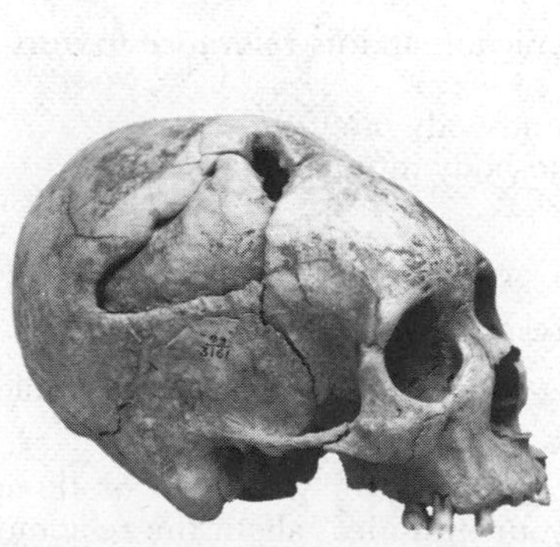
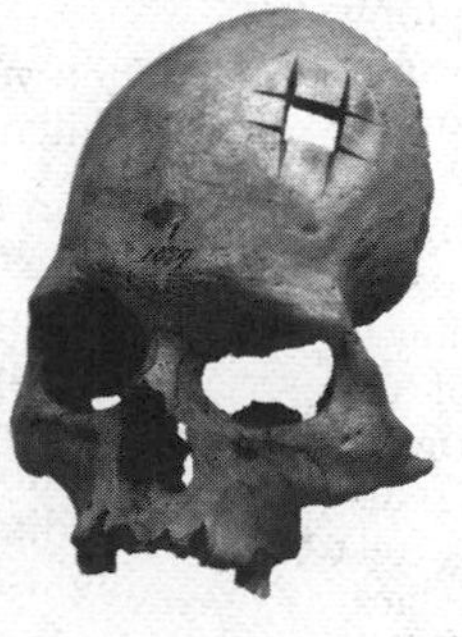
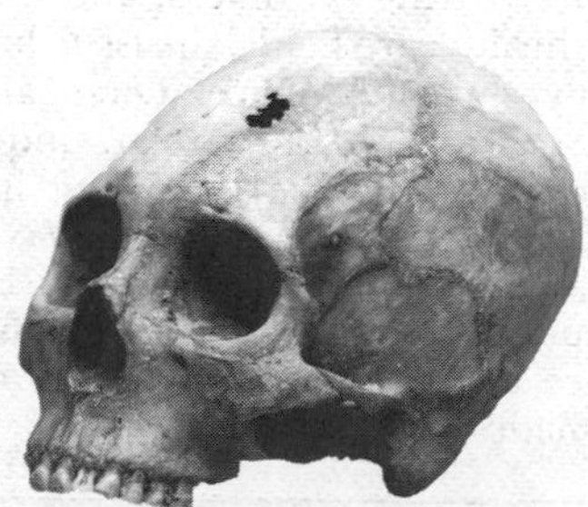

Figure 3–1. Skull with trephine holes. Such holes were made surgically in ancient times in an attempt to treat disease by making an opening over the brain. The purpose of the holes was to enable evil spirits, believed to cause disease, to leave the body. Ancient skulls show that patients sometimes survived even though very large trephine holes were made. In fact, some skulls show multiple large holes which had healed. (Courtesy American Museum of Natural History.)

René Descartes conceived of this dichotomous model in the 17th century, as an attempt to solve the mind-body problem. In essence it stated that a clean cut dualism or separation existed between soul (mind) and body (soma). The soul was thought of as conscious and the body as inanimate. For Descartes, mind and body were two distinct, unrelated entities. Each was subject to different laws of operation and principles of causality. The belief that mind and body are interrelated was rejected. It is the influence of this kind of thinking that we are still trying to overcome in nursing and other health care fields today.

Descartes' model made a tremendous impact on Western thought at that time concerning the nature of humanness. However, a great deal has transpired in scientific thought since the 17th century. When Freud postulated the unconscious element of human mental life, the model of Cartesian dualism was destroyed. Descartes had not conceived of the unconscious, and therefore, it was not considered in his model.

Regardless of how Freudian psychology is viewed today, it must be recognized that Freud's work led to a reversal of the Cartesian trend by increasing our awareness of the importance of emotions in producing mental and physical imbalances. The task of "reuniting" the divided person in Western thought has been difficult and is by no means completed.

> *Mind and body are interrelated, not separate entities.*

MAJOR MIND-BODY THEORIES

Over the centuries a wide variety of theories have attempted to answer the mind-body question. Today, new theories continue to try to resolve the riddle. Unfortunately considerable confusion still exists, and much of the current research deals with the problem in a very inconsistent manner.

Two major groups of theories that should be discussed briefly are the theories of *interactionism* and of *independence* of mind and body. *Interactionist* theories maintain that the mind and body do somehow interact. There have been a variety of ideas about just where and how this interaction takes place. Hippocrates was the first interactionist. Although he derived the psychic from the somatic he nevertheless recognized, with his typical astuteness, that emotions in turn have physical effects. Theories of *independence* maintain that mind and body exist completely separately and do not interact. Today, most people tend to believe that, in ways which are not yet understood, mind and body interact. Theories of independence are rarely openly supported by anyone.

ATTITUDES TOWARD ILLNESS

While most people appear to believe *in theory* that mind and body interact, it often seems that *in practice* or in daily living they believe that mind and body are separate entities. Theories of mind-body independence continue to permeate many persons' attitudes toward illness, as in this quotation:

> Typically, the doctor and his patient oscillate between two mind-body theories — namely, interactionism and independence. If the ordinary physician is specifically asked to state his position, he will usually give an interactionist answer, such as "The body influences the mind and the mind influences the body." He may also include references to "psychosomatic versus somatopsychic." In less guarded moments he is likely to reveal a belief in mind-body independence, with a remark like "There is nothing physically wrong with you, it's all mental." Probably no one who has had experience with the contemporary medical scene could fail to recognize both of these as statements he has heard many times.[45]

While this quotation refers specifically to physicians and patients, it is unfortunately just as applicable to nurse and patient.

Perhaps in your attitudes toward your own illnesses as well as those of others you find yourself sometimes thinking, "This is all just really 'mental.' It's just silly not to 'shape up' and feel better." Or perhaps you've thought the opposite, "This is a 'real' illness, nothing mental about it." Listen carefully to the way you hear people talking about their symptoms. Often one hears such descriptions begin, "I'm not sure if I'm just imagining this or not but I feel . . . ."

Often the implication is that if symptoms (illnesses) are "physical" in origin they are more "acceptable" than if there is a mental component in their origin. Many people thus often try to identify and focus on what they view as the "physical" symptoms they experience and to discount or negate any "mental or emotional" factors. We have all heard (or made) statements such as, "It's not just that I have an exam this morning. I really don't feel well. My stomach *is* cramping. My head *does* ache."

NURSING IMPLICATIONS

An ambivalent viewpoint about the mind-body issue presents definite problems in nursing and related fields. Conscientious nurses think seriously about their individual beliefs about this issue. They also periodically examine their behaviors to see if their actions are consistent with their intellectual beliefs. It is not uncommon in human behavior to say we believe in certain things, but to act in ways that are not in accordance with our stated beliefs. This can be a serious matter when one's behaviors are part of one's professional practice.

It is desirable for nurses to believe in interactionist mind-body theories and for nursing actions to reflect such a belief. In this way, the "total person" is considered and cared for.

> *When thinking about the psychologic factors in a person's illness, do not exclude consideration of physical factors . . . and vice versa.*

If a nurse considers psychologic elements as *the* basic cause of illness, then the physical elements may be neglected in patient care or they may assume secondary importance. The opposite is also true. If illness is viewed only in "physical" ways, then psychologic factors may be overlooked. Such omissions may be crucial to the welfare of patients.

The mind-body problem is often a conceptual barrier that poses problems in nursing and allied health care practices. To overcome such obstacles, unifying concepts are needed rather than concepts that break a human being into parts (e.g., physical and mental) and then name and focus on the divisions. We need cohesive models that enable us to view mind and body as one indivisible monistic event, i.e., to view a human being as a reality — one unitary whole — within the environment. The holistic view of the nature of humanness, as presented in Chapter 1, and its application through the nursing process, as discussed in Chapter 2, are effective working models of such theories within nursing.

We do a disservice to clients if we view them on an exclusively physical or exclusively mental basis. Surely we would not want ourselves to be viewed in this manner.

"PROOFS" OF MIND-BODY INTERACTION

Our personal experience tells us that our mind and body *are* unitary in nature — that we do experience them together. We experience our "self" as a combination of physical and mental phenomena. Sometimes we may be more aware of our body (e.g., with gastric distress) and at other times our mind (e.g., when recalling the day's events), but we cannot experience one without the other. For example, we cannot normally experience our body sensations (e.g., pain) without consciousness, and we cannot experience consciousness without our body's anatomic and physiologic brain functions.

Evidence of the *interaction* of mind and body can be provided by recalling manifestations of anxiety. If you are not convinced that mind and body interact, assess how you feel "physically" the next time you are "mentally" anxious. You will find it most difficult (indeed impossible) to separate your feelings into "physical" and "mental." It is likely that as well as "worrying" or having difficulty focusing your thoughts you may also experience interrelated symptoms such as restlessness, muscular tension, shortness of breath, and perhaps varied gastrointestinal disturbances. Some persons will experience a headache. Possibly you will also feel the need to pass urine frequently.

Pause for a moment and try to identify as accurately as possible what *your* mind and body reactions are when you are anxious — how do you feel, think, and act? By gaining insight into one's own experiences when anxious, it is possible to more readily understand the psychosomatic and somatopsychic illnesses that are discussed in Chapter 7 and the concepts of stress and illness presented in Unit III. Also, you will be able to examine more critically the theories of disease summarized in the following chapter.

Let us now briefly consider some additional manifestations of mind-body interaction:

1. *Apathy* (a spiritless state characterized by lack of interest, concern, feeling or emotion) of prisoners of war[130] has been known to lead to death even though there was no evidence of physical illness and food was available (Fig. 3–2).

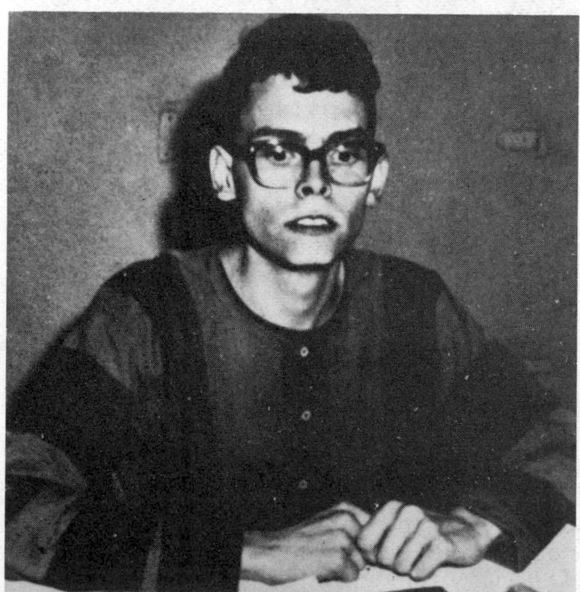

Figure 3–2. Prisoners of war frequently experience prolonged stresses that affect their psychological and physical health. (Courtesy Captain D. Rigby, U.S. Air Force.)

This occurred in prisoners with no evidence of psychotic reaction. Wild, healthy animals have also been known to die tragically when confined (e.g., in zoos), apparently from apathy.

2. The *tickle*[90] is an interesting example of mind-body interaction. Have you noticed that you cannot tickle yourself? The response depends on more than mere touch. Certain mental interactions are necessary to make a "touch" a "tickle." As Darwin observed, someone other than the tickled must do the tickling.

3. *Voodoo* may provide additional evidence of the monistic (united) nature of mind and body. While the actual practice assumes many forms, in essence voodoo, or "hexing," represents a "magical" suggestion that can produce illness and even death. Voodoo could be said to demonstrate mind-body interaction when an individual is aware of being hexed by another person and subsequently develops physical problems. It has been suggested that the voodoo deaths of folklore were psychologically provoked through the development of psychosomatic disease.[82] Belief in such magical suggestion is not limited to the past. For example, "rootwork"[136] appears to be a North American derivative of voodoo that is still in practice. Many questions about voodoo remain unanswered. The central question is, of course, whether the individual becomes ill from the curse or whether the illness might have resulted anyway, from other causes?

4. *Hypnosis* also demonstrates some fascinating connections between mind and body. For example, one study demonstrates that it was apparently possible to produce ecchymotic (bruise-like) lesions in specific locations on the subject's body through the use of hypnotic suggestion.[1]

5. The *couvade syndrome* (from the French verb *couver,* meaning to hatch or to brood) is a relatively recently recognized phenomenon in which a psychophysiologic reaction to pregnancy occurs in a *male* who experiences symptoms very similar to those occurring in his pregnant woman life partner. He may suffer from nausea, vomiting, cramps or appetite change early in the pregnancy or close to the time of the expected birth.[146]

6. Studies of meditation (a highly relaxed condition, not the same as sleep) show that this practice can decrease heart and breathing rates as well as reduce the rate of metabolism. Figure 3–3 shows a yogi (a person highly skilled in the

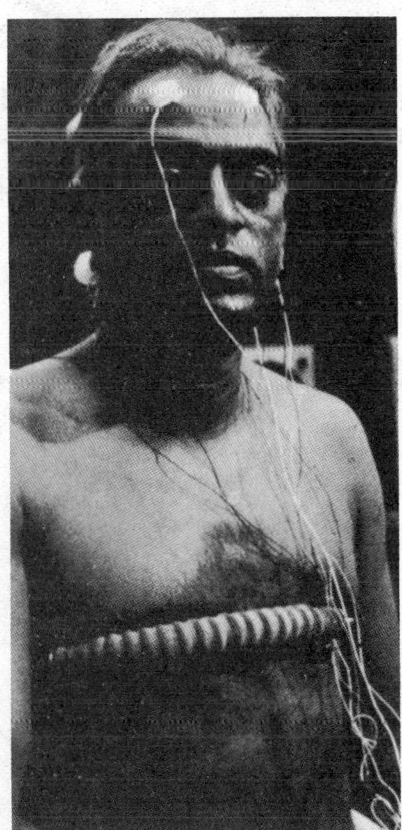

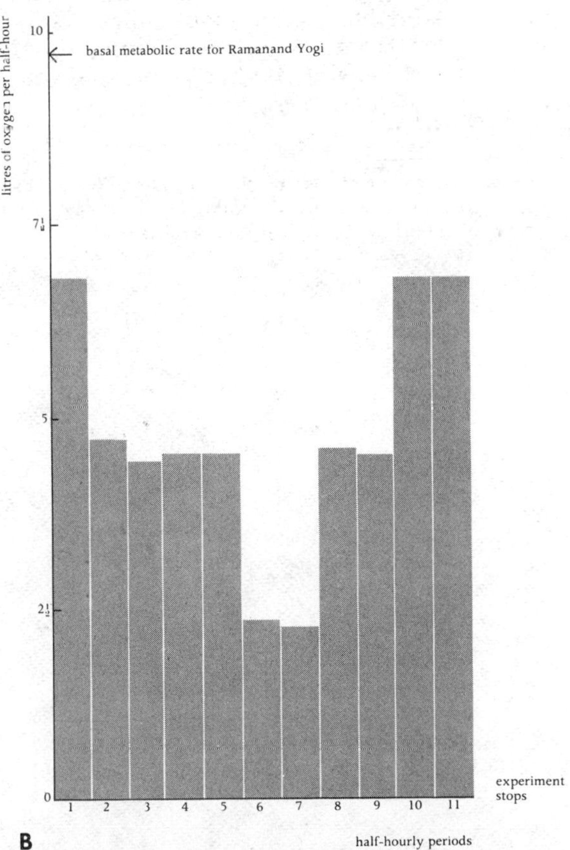

Figure 3–3. Research has shown that yoga techniques can reduce the body's oxygen requirements. **A.** Ramanand Yogi, "wired up" in preparation for a test of his ability to reduce his body's demand for oxygen. **B.** Graphed results of Ramanand Yogi's oxygen consumption during meditation. (From Calder, N.: *The Mind of Man.* New York: Viking Press, Inc. 1970. Photo by Phillip Daly, BBC program producer.)

practice of yoga) being tested to determine his ability to lower his body oxygen requirements during a meditative trance. Research has shown that other forms of meditation and relaxation, such as transcendental meditation (TM), the practices of Zen Buddhism, and autogenic training, also produce measurable physiologic changes, including decreased heart and respiration rates, lowered oxygen consumption, and reduced blood lactate levels.* The fact that a person can use conscious techniques to induce such physiologic changes is clear support for the theories of mind-body interaction. These physiologic changes are of such benefit to all body systems that the techniques for eliciting them have become of considerable interest to the health professions. Chapter 6 deals in detail with relaxation exercises and the changes they can bring about.

7. One of the most important evidences of the mind-body interaction is the *fight-or-flight response,* which occurs when a person is faced with certain situations that demand behavioral adjustments. "Fight or flight" is a primitive response, apparently originally serving just that purpose — enabling a person either to fight with or flee from an enemy. During this response the following bodily changes involuntarily occur: increased heart and breathing rates, increased rate of metabolism (blood flow to the muscles increases markedly), and increased blood pressure. In human beings today, the fight-or-flight response is often repeatedly and inappropriately elicited in situations where the person can neither fight nor run away. The physiologic changes involved in the fight-or-flight response, if frequently elicited or maintained for prolonged periods, can take a serious toll on health.[8] The consequences and control of the fight-or-flight response are an important topic and are discussed from various aspects in later chapters.

*Blood lactate, produced by skeletal muscle metabolism, appears to be associated with anxiety, i.e., increased lactate levels may experimentally elicit anxiety attacks.

Conclusion

Mind-body (psyche-soma) interactions are really the foundation of the next chapters, which deal with theories of disease, the relationship of stress and illness, the responses to stress, the theories of psychosomatic and somatopsychic illness, and the treatment of psychosomatic disorders.

The examples of mind-body interaction discussed in this chapter demonstrate that the so-called borders between our conscious, unconscious, and physical selves are not rigid. Indeed, there well may be no "borders" at all, but rather complicated interrelationships. While mind-body interactions occur that are not clearly understood at this time, it is nevertheless clear that mind and body exist together and are not separate entities.

BIBLIOGRAPHY

The bibliography for this chapter is at the end of Chapter 8, p. 92.

CHAPTER 4

MODERN UNIFIED THEORIES OF DISEASE

. . . disease is not the simple result of simple causes, but rather the complex result of an infinite range of human ecological factors.[39]

INTRODUCTION AND STUDY GUIDE

Disease is a predictable aspect of human life; it touches all of us in one form or another. Thus, disease and health concern us both personally and professionally. Diseases, injuries, and homeostatic imbalances — those painful adaptive failures that cause us so much misery — are present everywhere. Moreover, their number is staggering, their definitions variable, their causations multiple and complex, their symptoms numerous and sometimes apparently unrelated, their treatments subject to constant change and revision, and their prevention often questionable or unknown. It is no wonder that mankind has so desperately sought a theory of disease that is broad and comprehensive and which serves to unify the many divergent theories of causation that have been postulated over the years.

Indeed, a unified theory of disease has been the dream of scientists since the beginning of medical history. A perfectly unified disease theory, however, appears impossible because of the tremendous variety of diseases and the endless number of factors in their causation. Nevertheless, certain physicians and other scientists have attempted to establish modern theories of disease causation that are broad enough to encompass a large percentage of the diseases as well as a majority of the causative factors. Scientists such as Bernard, Cannon, Selye, Harold Wolff, Stewart Wolf, Holmes, Rahe, Dudley, Friedman, and Rosenman, in particular, are responsible for the development of unified concepts of disease with which you should be familiar.

As a student of nursing, you may wonder why it is necessary to have a detailed theoretic knowledge of disease causation. Such knowledge is necessary because theory is not something that remains restricted to a book or laboratory; theories are eventually applied to patients. *You* are the vital link between a hypothesis formed in the mind of a scientist and the actual practical benefits which that hypothesis provides for sick individuals. In other words, you are the person who will help to put the theory into practice. Thus, you can never know too much about disease or why it occurs. Your whole professional life will revolve around questions of causation and treatment. By understanding what scientists presently believe to be true about disease you can better contribute to total patient care.

Study Guide

Upon completing this chapter you should be able to generally discuss the following theories of disease:

1. Bernard's theory of the disturbed internal milieu
2. Cannon's theory of homeostatic imbalance
3. Selye's theory of stress
4. Harold Wolff's theory of inappropriate and harmful organ responses to stressful situations
5. Stewart Wolf's theory of "disease as a way of life"
6. Theory of the brain's role in regulating, causing and preventing disease (theories of Wolff and Wolf)
7. Holmes, Rahe and associates' theory of life change and resultant illness
8. Dudley's theory of cycling (or coastering) behavior and resultant illness
9. Friedman and Roseman's theory of behavior patterns as a factor in the causation of coronary artery disease
10. The systems theory of disease

Important terms and key concepts with which you should become familiar in this chapter are:

internal milieu
homeostasis
"fight-or-flight" reaction to stress
adaptive hormones
general adaptation syndrome (GAS)
local adaptation syndrome (LAS)
stress
nonspecific response
stressors

diseases of adaptation
life change units
social readjustment rating scale (SRRS)
life change profile
"Coltar coaster"
A and B type behavior patterns system
feedback
feedback linkage
downward and upward disruption

Let us now briefly summarize the important hypothesis of disease causation that modern scientists have formulated.

THE THEORIES OF BERNARD AND CANNON[25, 37]

Claude Bernard, nineteenth century French physiologist, laid the foundation for the modern concept of disease causation with his experiments and hypotheses. His contributions to medicine and nursing are multiple. First, Bernard had a unique view of the human being, whom he described as "a piece of constancy moving in a world of variables." He saw the human organism not as a being set apart from its environment, but rather as an integral part of the environment.

Second, it was Bernard who originally described the *internal milieu*, or the internal environment of the body. He hypothesized correctly that if an organism is to live, it must have the capacity to maintain its internal milieu in a relative state of constancy. As a result of his experiments, Bernard was able to describe some of the mechanisms that regulate the balance of our internal body fluids.

Third, Bernard saw illness in a new and enlightening way. He argued that sickness was the result of (1) imbalances in the internal environment of the body and (2) breaks in the vital communication that must exist between the internal milieu and the external environment.

As a fourth contribution, Bernard described disease not only as a disturbance of the body's internal environmental balance, but also as an *adaptive attempt* to restore balance. He taught that these adaptive attempts at balance were appropriate in kind, but were incorrect in magnitude. For example, an individual with pneumonia suffers from a lack of oxygen. In response to this deficit, the bone marrow produces more red blood cells, these being the oxygen-carrying cells of the body. These excess erythrocytes, however, thicken the blood, making it more difficult for the heart to pump blood through the lungs. Congestive heart failure may then result from the body's response, which, while appropriate to the situation, is excessive for the good of the total organism.

Today we carry Bernard's theory of adaptive responses a step further. We now believe that the body's adaptive reactions not only may be excessive but may also be inappropriate to the situation. We will elaborate more on this modern concept when we discuss the theories of Hans Selye and Harold Wolff.

The first physician to expand radically upon Bernard's hypotheses was Walter Cannon, who taught physiology at Harvard in the early part of this century. Cannon was especially interested in the body's *coordinated self-regulating physiologic process*, which, as he stated, "maintain most of the steady states in the organism." It was Cannon who in 1939 coined the term "homeostasis" from the Greek words *homoios,* meaning "like," and *stasis* meaning "standing."

Basically, Cannon conceived of homeostasis as a type of *dynamic* equilibrium as opposed to a static condition. His use of the term "homeostasis" applied mainly to the self-regulation of such internal physiologic processes as body temperature, blood pressure, water balance, blood sugar concentration, and blood oxygen and carbon dioxide levels. In particular, Cannon explored the "fight-or-flight" reactions of the body to emergency situations, and the nervous and adrenal mechanisms involved in these reactions. On the whole, this American physiologist was more concerned with the body's ability to satisfactorily regulate itself, than with breakdowns in physiologic processes, i.e., Cannon was more interested in health than in disease. Thus, it was not until Hans Selye formulated his famous theory of stress that Bernard's contributions were fully applied to the problem of disease causation.

SELYE'S GENERAL THEORY OF STRESS[119, 120, 121, 123]

Hans Selye is regarded by many as the "father" of modern stress theory. Selye, in the late 1930's and 1940's, did many of the first extensive studies on stress responses. In 1950, Selye published a famous book entitled *Stress* — a massive treatise that influenced stress research throughout the world. From his hypotheses concerning stress, Selye developed the modern unified theory of disease that we discuss here.

Before presenting Selye's theory, let us pause and consider a few crucial definitions, beginning with the term *stress*. In 1974, Selye defined stress as follows:

Stress. In biology the *nonspecific response* of the *body to any demand made upon it*. For general orientation, it suffices to keep in mind that *by stress* the *physician means the common results of exposure to any stimulus*. For example, the bodily changes produced whether a person is exposed to *nervous tension, physical injury, infection, cold, heat, x-rays, or anything else are what we call stress.*[121]

Nonspecific response is defined by Selye as "... one which affects all or most parts of a system without selectivity." Thus, when Selye writes of the "nonspecific response of the body" to stimuli, he means that the *entire* body or the majority of its systems must try to adjust to any specific agent that places demands upon it. The *agents* placing demands upon the body which can precipitate stress are termed *"stressors."* Stressors may be of a beneficial or a harmful nature depending upon the individual, the total situation, and the intensity of the stressor. Examples of stressors include nervous tension, physical injury, physical exertion (as in jogging), cold, heat, infection, and x-rays. According to Selye, the multiple and constant stressors to which one is exposed throughout life result in the "wear and tear" on the body that produces the physical and physiologic signs of *aging*. As aging continues in response to stress, the individual finally becomes "worn down" and ceases to respond to the continuous challenges. Thus the person dies.

Selye's interest in formulating a general theory of stress and disease causation began when, as a medical student, he noted that most diseases are characterized by only a *few* specific signs, and that almost all maladies share *many signs and symptoms in common*; for example, weight loss, fatigue, malaise, aches and pains, gastrointestinal upsets. In other words, he observed that almost all patients, regardless of diagnosis, share the same pathologic changes. Selye subsequently called this phenomenon the "syndrome of just being sick." Later, after years of experimentation, he renamed it the *stress syndrome* or *general adaptation syndrome* (GAS). Furthermore, he suggested that certain hormones, called *adaptive hormones*, are released during stress, and that these hormones help to create the common symptoms seen in all patients. From his observations, Selye concluded that stress plays a role in every disease process regardless of causation.

According to Selye, the GAS appears whenever an organism is subjected to long-continued stress. Some of the manifestations of the GAS may include: the stimulation of the adrenal glands, with a release of hormones; the development of gastrointestinal ulcers; and the shrinkage of lymphatic tissues. The stressors that may bring about the GAS are nonspecific in nature and may be trauma, infection, burns, severe colds, emotional upsets, or other common events.

In addition to the body's general systemic response to stress, Selye proposed that the body can also adapt to local stressors. He has called this process of local response, which takes place within a single organ or specific section of the body, the *local adaptation syndrome* (LAS). An example of LAS is inflammation.

Selye suggested that both the GAS and the LAS develop in three distinct stages: (1) an alarm reaction, (2) the stage of resistance, and (3) the stage of exhaustion. These three phases are elaborated in Figure 4–1.

Balancing and Conditioning Factors

What coordinates and regulates the GAS and LAS? Selye writes that many organs and systems contribute to the regulation of these stress syndromes; most important are the brain, the central and autonomic nervous systems, and the pituitary and adrenal glands. The adrenal and pituitary glands are particularly crucial to adaptation, for they release hormones that specifically combat stress and that inhibit or stimulate the body's defense mechanisms are necessary. Selye calls the hormones produced by the adrenal and pituitary glands *adaptive hormones*. The group of adaptive hormones that *inhibit* excessively defensive activities on the part of the body have been termed *anti-inflammatory corticoids* or *glucocorticoids*. The release of glucocorticoids into the blood stream is stimulated by the pituitary hormone ACTH. An example of a glucocorticoid is cortisone, one of the hormones secreted by the adrenal cortex. The other group of adaptive

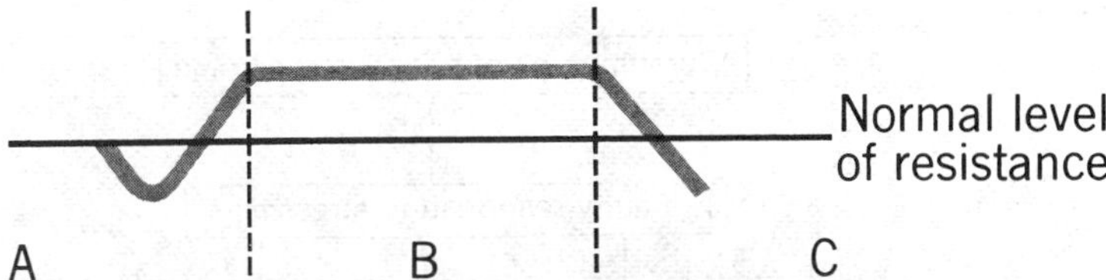

Figure 4–1. The three phases of the general adaptation syndrome (GAS). **A.** *Alarm reaction.* The body shows the changes characteristic of the first exposure to a stressor. At the same time, its resistance is diminished and, if the stressor is sufficiently strong (severe burns, extremes of temperature), death may result. **B.** *Stage of resistance.* Resistance ensues if continued exposure to the stressor is compatible with adaptation. The bodily signs characteristic of the alarm reaction have virtually disappeared, and resistance rises above normal. **C.** *Stage of exhaustion.* Following long-continued exposure to the same stressor, to which the body had become adjusted, eventually adaptation energy is exhausted. The signs of the alarm reaction reappear, but now they are irreversible, and the individual dies. (From Selye, H.: *Stress Without Distress.* New York: New American Library, 1974.)

hormones *stimulate* the body's defenses. These secretions are known as *pro-inflammatory corticoids,* or *mineralocorticoids*. An example of a mineralocorticoid is aldosterone, also secreted by the adrenal cortex.

The body's ability to resist stress and adapt to noxious forces depends upon a proper balance of these essential chemical substances. In turn, the effect of these adaptive hormones upon the body's resistance to stress depends upon certain *conditioning factors*, i.e., circumstances that influence the course of the GAS without being a part of it. The most important conditioning factors are diet, climate, heredity, past experience, and past exposure to stressors. Such conditioning factors are responsible for the varying individual ways in which different persons react to the same degree of stress.

Diseases of Adaptation

What specifically is the relationship of the GAS to disease? First, as we have said, Selye theorizes that the GAS is an integral part of all pathologic processes, no matter what their cause; i.e., adaptation to stress on the part of the body plays a role in *every* disease. Second, Selye states that *faulty adaptation*, in itself, can cause disease. Selye has named these "derailments" of the adaptive syndrome the *diseases of adaptation*. These maladies are not due to any specific pathogen, but instead they are the direct result of a faulty response to a stressor. Usually, adaptation to stressors involves a balanced blend of defense and submission on the part of the body. When the body overdefends itself and there is a surplus of pro-inflammatory hormones, such diseases as arthritis, allergy, and asthma develop. When the body does not defend itself sufficiently, as a result of the release or injection of too much anti-inflammatory hormone, then the individual may succumb to overwhelming infection. Further, sometimes adaptation can be faulty or inappropriate and result in such conditions as stomach ulcers, a disorder we discuss below in connection with the theories of Harold Wolff.

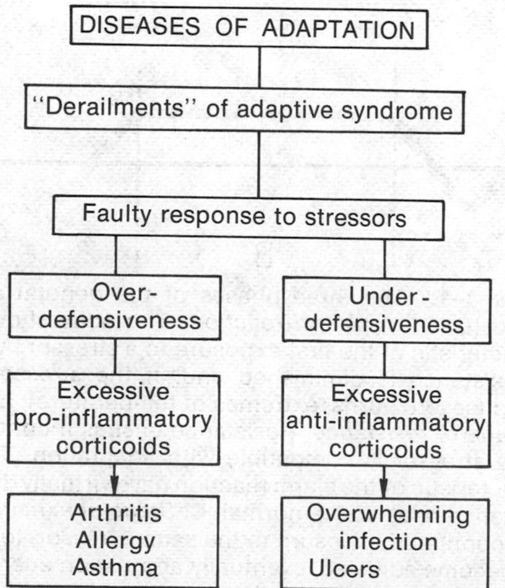

Figure 4–2. Selye's scheme of the major diseases of adaptation and the pathophysiologic factors that precipitate them.

HAROLD WOLFF'S THEORY OF STRESS, DISEASE, AND ORGAN MALADAPTATION[160, 161, 162]

Both Selye and Harold Wolff, a New York psychiatrist, have been interested in how people respond to stress, and how these responses, in themselves, can subsequently lead to a breakdown in homeostasis. Selye, however, was mainly concerned with *physiologic* processes and the responses of the body to such *acute* stressors as hemorrhage, burns, trauma, and shock. Wolff, on the other hand, was more interested in the responses of individuals, both *physiologically and psychologically*, to such *chronic* stressors as a frustrating job situation or an unhappy home life. Wolff believed that a person's "total life situation," with its sorrows, joys, successes, and frustrations, could profoundly affect the person's susceptibility to disease. Wolff's research in this area helped to lay the foundation for some modern theories of psychosomatic medicine.

Like Selye, Wolff based much of his thinking on the concepts developed by Claude Bernard. As you will recall, Bernard believed that disease was often the result of adaptive attempts on the part of the body to restore homeostasis — attempts that were appropriate in kind but incorrect in magnitude. Wolff's research in this area helped to lay the research methods, that adaptive responses are not only incorrect in magnitude but are also frequently blundering and *inappropriate* to the situation. He theorized that inappropriate attempts at adaptation occur in humans for several reasons. First, a human being has a *highly developed nervous system and cerebral cortex.* Consequently human beings can symbolize, recall the past, and project themselves into the future. Therefore, *threats* of possible danger and *symbols* of danger are just as important in human disease causation as are noxious microbial, chemical, and mechanical forces. Second, humans are essentially *tribal creatures.* That is, they depend upon other people for many of their satisfactions in life. Stresses may be created by the need to work and to associate successfully with other people, many of whom differ radically from the individual concerned. Often a person responds inappropriately to other individuals because of an unrealistic and distorted perception of certain human relationships; this distortion results, again, from the human ability to symbolize and to consider both past and future.

Distorted perception of a situation involving human relations can eventually lead to illness. For example, consider the following situation.

A husband and wife come home from a long day at their respective jobs. Both are exhausted and still preoccupied with the day's business. Upon arriving home, they are greeted by their teenage son, who is anxious to discuss some problems which developed during his school day. The father, at this point, feels an overwhelming desire to just sit down and relax for a while with a newspaper and a drink. The mother, equally tired, wants to unwind for a few minutes in a hot bath. Unfortunately, their son, who has been waiting for hours to talk with his family, perceives his parents' fatigue as a sign of disinterest in him. He thinks, "Oh well, they don't care *about me* and my problems. They're just interested in their jobs and themselves." By dinner time, which is late, the son feels neglected and withdrawn. His resultant attitude at the dinner table is interpreted by his parents as pouty and hostile toward *them*, and they, in response, become angry with their son. Moreover, the parents — hurt and irritated — may even attempt to blame each other for their son's antagonistic behavior. This communication breakdown results in a headache for the son, gastric distress and diarrhea for the father, and insomnia that night for the mother. If this scenario is re-enacted night after night, the stress feelings engendered may eventually lead to serious physical or mental illness in one or all members of this family.

To summarize, in this family's case essentially four things have happened: *First*, there was a distorted evaluation by three people of each other's behavior; *second*, this distortion resulted in blocked communication and guarded hostility; *third*, these negative reactions, in turn, led to further inappropriate responses on the part of all parties. *Finally*, out of the frustration, disappointment, and anger came physiologic symptoms which further added to their unhappiness.

Wolff's research indicates that certain individuals consistently respond to such frustrating situations through a *particular* body organ or system, perhaps the stomach, back, colon, or nasal membrane. The organ involved varies from person to person and seems to follow a pattern specific for the individual. Mucous membranes (whether of the nose, stomach, rectum, bladder, or vagina) seem to be particularly susceptible to stress, probably because these tissues comprise one of the body's main lines of defense against stressful invaders from without the body. Mucous membranes can exhibit a variety of stress reactions: for instance, engorgement, edema, hemorrhage, ischemia, increased friability, faulty absorption, ulceration, inflammation, and altered reactions to chemical substances. Such pathologic changes occur frequently in response to traumatic personal situations. If these changes are habitual and are combined with other noxious, chemical, or physical stressors, such responses can eventually lead to irreversible tissue damage.

Selye points out that every organ responds in its *own particular way* to stress. For example, the liver may develop an abscess in response to stress, but it will never develop an ulcer no matter how great a stressor it is exposed to. Wolff carried the point further and proved that organs not only respond to stress in their own particular way, but they, like people, may also respond *inappropriately* to stressful situations; that is, organ functions such as digestion and elimination, which ordinarily are beneficial, may be activated inappropriately in response to a stimulus or need that these functions *are not equipped to satisfy or control*. Such troublesome patterns of organ response cannot help an individual achieve goals or control the environment; instead, if prolonged, they may lead to serious illness. For example, when something irritates the colon (e.g., castor oil), diarrhea tends to develop and the noxious substance is expelled. Such a response is appropriate and expected. It is inappropriate, however, to develop diarrhea as a result of unsatisfactory interpersonal relationships (e.g., forced association with a hated person). No matter how severe the diarrhea, it is not possible to get rid of the hated person in this way.

Let us now summarize the essentials of Wolff's theory:

(1) The development of illness is related to the total life pattern of an individual.

(2) We, as individuals with highly developed nervous systems, are capable of symbolizing and reacting to these symbols. Consequently we may react inappropriately to situations, especially those involving interpersonal relationships.

(3) Organs themselves can react *inappropriately* in a stressful situation, activating functions that cannot vanquish the stressor.

(4) Such inappropriate organ response, if prolonged, can result in disability, disease, and death.

STEWART WOLF'S CONCEPT OF DISEASE AS A WAY OF LIFE[157, 158, 159]

Stewart Wolf, like his former colleague Harold Wolff, views disease causation from many aspects — physiologic, psychologic, and cultural. He has contributed important research on the role of the brain and nervous system in the regulation of the body's processes and in causation of disease. Some of Stewart Wolf's important findings can be summarized as follows:

1. The brain is important both in maintaining our *internal* milieu and in aiding us to adapt to our *external* surroundings.

2. We use our brain to *interpret* the external environment, including the many sights, odors, and noises surrounding us. Depending upon our past mental associations, these sights, odors, and noises (including spoken words) can produce symptoms of disease. For example, a person who fears pregnancy can become nauseated at the mere mention of pregnancy. Eating something with a disgusting taste of smelling a noxious odor can also create nausea. This phenomenon is related to the activity of the brain and nervous system and the *meaning* that it gives certain experiences.

According to Wolf, a person's ability to respond to symbols actually determines whether that person will remain healthy or become diseased. Because people's responses to stresses of a symbolic nature involve their goals, aspirations and values, these responses actually constitute their "way of life." Thus, if a person's responses are essentially and consistently negative and maladaptive in nature, *disease becomes a way of life* for that individual.

3. While neural processes can *cause* disease manifestations to appear, the power of the brain also can *relieve* the symptoms of disease and mitigate injury. For example, consider the *placebo effect* — a well known phenomenon in medicine. This occurs when, in certain cases, patients in severe pain are given injections of sterile water or normal saline ("the placebo"), which they believe to be morphine sulfate or some other narcotic. The placebo may produce definite pain relief. Moreover, placebo administration, whether pill, injection, or procedure, has at times been followed by "substantial and measurable changes in bodily mechanisms."[157] According to Wolf, a placebo works not because of any pharmacologic properties but because of the way in which the *brain interprets the therapeutic effort*, and the significance and meaning to the patient of the *total situation* surrounding that effort, e.g., the hospital environment and the attitudes of doctors and nurses.

Studies with *hypnosis* provide yet another example of the brain's ability to mitigate tissue damage. In an impressive experiment by Chapman and associates, subjects were exposed to thermal stimuli in precise quantities which were sufficient to produce burns. These stimuli were applied to both of their forearms. In the control group, no hypnotic suggestion was given and the right and left forearms of each subject developed virtually identical burns as a result of the stimulus. In the experimental group, however, the subjects were first placed under hypnosis and, while hypnotized, were told that the left arm would be impervious to the stimulus, but the right arm would be particularly vulnerable. Then the thermal stimulus was applied. In 30 out of 40 trials, the left arm of the subject showed only a small burned area while the right arm incurred a substantial area of tissue damage. In these cases, mental suggestion and neural integrative action actually determined, in part, the response of the body tissues to an external stressor.[156]

4. In addition to the fact that the brain can create and mitigate the development of disease, the brain itself can be damaged by faulty interaction between an individual and the environment. This faulty interaction, in turn, leads to further maladaptation. Brain damage as a result of environmental stress has been particularly noted in prisoners of war. Such damage has been irreversible in some instances.

For example, a group of 100 Norwegian war veterans of World War II, who had been interned in concentration camps for three years, were examined 12 years after liberation. These men (all of whom had experienced humiliation, deprivation, isolation, beatings, floggings, and threats of execution) were found to suffer from a "more or less gross loss of brain substance."[160] In reviewing the life histories of these abused men following their release from prison and from the service, it was found that the men could not readjust to civilian life and that they complained of fatigue, irritability, mood swings, sleeplessness, memory loss, lack of initiative, and headache. Thus, for these men, the highly traumatic situation of internment had led to brain damage that resulted in a poor adjustment to civilian life.

5. If the cerebral hemispheres are destroyed, removed, or damaged, the signs and symptoms of systemic disease are greatly changed. For example, a cat without its cerebral cortex, but with brain stem and hypothalamus intact, will not respond with fever to the injection of pyogenic substances. Thus, the brain affects not only the development of disease but the manifestations of disease.

In sum, Wolf sees the brain as an integral part of the total organism or individual. In turn, he envisions the total individual as an integral part of the total environment. This environment includes all of the sights, sounds, and symbols, both pleasing and noxious, that surround each person, and which each individual interprets and makes meaningful through the use of the brain. Disease, then, cannot be separated from the total person, including the person's way of life and interpretation of what life means. For this reason, Wolf believes that such terms as "psychogenic" disease, "functional" disease, and "organic" disease are inaccurate and misleading. All disease affects the function of some organ or system, and no disease can be completely divorced from the influence of the nervous system, the higher mental centers, and the meaning that these bodily components give to the stimuli and stresses that are a part of life.

THEORIES OF LIFE CHANGE AND SUBSEQUENT ONSET OF ILLNESS (HOLMES, RAHE, AND ASSOCIATES)

As we all know from personal experience, *change* is a form of stress to which we must adapt psychologically and physically. Life changes vary greatly in their universality and in their intensity. Some changes affect all human beings — regardless of race, culture, geographic location or station in life, e.g., biologic changes such as the processes of maturation and aging, development of a self-image, the experience of pain. Other changes affect certain individuals and fail to touch others, e.g., the death of a parent during one's childhood, severe accident or disability, birth of a child.[93] Finally, certain changes are more difficult to adapt to than are other changes. For instance, in most cultures the death of a spouse appears to be more stressful than any other type of life change.

Adaptation to change, of whatever nature, requires expenditure of energy over and above that required for the maintenance of a "steady state" of life. Therefore, if an individual is called upon to cope with many significant changes within a *short period of time,* it is likely that the person will be overextended and expend too much adaptive energy and, consequently, become ill.

Philosophers and scientists have for many centuries theorized that life change and illness are linked in some way. However, only recently has this link been systematically studied and irrevocably confirmed. In this section we will briefly consider the definitive studies of Thomas Holmes and others (Rahe, Arthur, Heisel, S.T. Holmes, Paykel, Wyler, and Masuda) concerning the critical relationship between life change and illness. We will also discuss the implications of these studies for patient assessment and care.

Historical Background[67, 110, 111]

As we implied above, the belief that disease and life change are strongly linked is very old. Indeed, the astute clinician or nurse often noted that patients with recently developed physical ailments had undergone a clustering of psychosocial changes in their lives prior to the onset of symptoms, e.g., changes in the patient's personal, mental, family, career, economic, recreational, religious and/or social spheres. However, these observations were undocumented until approximately 25 years ago when Thomas Holmes began to systematically study the relationship between change and illness.

At the University of Washington in Seattle, Holmes and associates developed a questionnaire entitled *Schedule of Recent Experience* (SRE) which they initially administered to patients in a nearby tuberculosis sanitarium. This paper and pencil self-administered questionnaire had the subjects list life changes by the year of occurrence. The researchers discovered that the patients at the sanitarium had experienced a definite clustering of psychosocial changes in their lives prior to the onset of their disease.

Next, Holmes and associates attempted to qualify life experiences in terms of their *impact* on an individual, i.e., graduation from college is not as radical a change as is the death of a spouse or the birth of a baby. To rate life changes in terms of their significance, Holmes and Rahe listed 43 different life changes ranging in magnitude from minor violations of the law to death of a spouse. The researchers first arbitrarily assigned a numerical weight of 50 to "marriage" and then asked their subjects to assign numerical values (ranging from 1 to 100) to the other items on the list. Holmes and Rahe obtained the opinions of thousands of American and Japanese subjects from all walks of life. To their astonishment, the investigators discovered that despite differences in lifestyles, education and economic status, people tended to agree on the numerical values that should be assigned to various life changes. From this information, Holmes and Rahe developed their Social Readjustment Rating Scale (SRRS) (Table 4–1). Note that the SRRS ranks each life event according to *life change units* (LCU). For example, death of a spouse (ranked highest in stress) is worth 100 LCU's while a vacation (ranked number 41) is worth only 12 LCU's.

Holmes and Rahe began to use their new tool (the SRRS) to explore the relationship between the *amount* of change in a person's life and *subsequent illness.* To do this, Holmes and Rahe obtained *life change scores* from thousands of people by asking each subject to write down the number of times each life event had occurred over the past two years. The researchers then added up the units and obtained a score. For example, if a person had undergone the death of a spouse (100 units), remarriage (50 units), 3 minor violations of the law (33 units), 2 changes in residence (40 units), and a change in financial status (38 units), that person's score would be 361 units of change. Next, Holmes and Rahe compared these scores with the subjects' medical histories and found that the *higher the life change score the more likelihood that the individual would develop an illness in the near future.*

To help in predicting the possibility of illness, life change scores (based on the most recent two years) have been rated as follows:

1–150	No significant life change
150–199	Mild life change (33% chance of illness)
200–299	Moderate life change (50% chance of illness)
300 +	Major life change (80% chance of illness)[105]

Thus the individual in our example above, with a life change score of 361 units, has an 80 per cent chance of developing a serious illness within the following year.

The positive correlation between change and disease, as well as the accuracy of the SRRS for predicting onset of illness, was confirmed in a study designed by Rahe and Arthur in 1965. The purpose of this study was to predict illness patterns in a group of 2500 navy men on a 6-month ocean cruise. Using the SRE questionnaire and obtaining live change scores with the use of the SRRS, researchers found that the men who had scored in the top 10 per cent of life change units suffered from one-and-a-half to two times as much illness as those in the lower 10 per cent of scores. In addition, the higher the scores, the more serious the illness.[110]

Since these classic studies, other investigators have researched further aspects of the change–illness relationship.

Additional Studies

Researchers have studied the effects of both a single significant life event and multiple life events on susceptibility to illness. Some interesting research findings concerning the relationship between *one or two life events* and illness onset are as follows:

- Widows and widowers are far more susceptible to illness during the year after the death of their spouses than are control subjects; they also suffer from greatly increased mortality rates during the first 6 months following bereavement.[167, 100, 111]
- Persons with poor marital adjustment frequently suffer illness shortly after the development of problems with their spouses.[124]
- Job loss and unemployment may be associated with a subsequent rise in blood pressure.[76]
- Persons who have experienced accelerated job and residential mobility are significantly more susceptible to coronary heart disease than are persons with more stable jobs and residences.[139]

TABLE 4–1. SOCIAL READJUSTMENT RATING SCALE

Rank	Life Event	Life Change Units	Rank	Life Event	Life Change Units
1	Death of spouse	100	23	Son or daughter leaving home	29
2	Divorce	73	24	Trouble with in-laws	29
3	Marital separation	65	25	Outstanding personal achievement	28
4	Jail term	63	26	Wife begins or stops work	26
5	Death of close family member	63	27	Begin or end school	26
6	Personal injury or illness	53	28	Change in living conditions	25
7	Marriage	50	29	Revision of personal habits	24
8	Fired at work	47	30	Trouble with boss	23
9	Marital reconciliation	45	31	Change in work hours or conditions	20
10	Retirement	45	32	Change in residence	20
11	Change in health of family member	44	33	Change in school	20
12	Pregnancy	40	34	Change in recreation	19
13	Sex difficulties	39	35	Change in church activities	19
14	Gain of new family member	39	36	Change in social activities	18
15	Business readjustment	39	37	Mortgage or loan less than $10,000	17
16	Change in financial state	38	38	Change in sleeping habits	16
17	Death of close friend	37	39	Change in number of family get-togethers	15
18	Change to different line of work	36	40	Change in eating habits	15
19	Change in number of arguments with spouse	35	41	Vacation	13
20	Mortgage over $10,000	31	42	Christmas	12
21	Foreclosure of mortgage or loan	30	43	Minor violations of the law	11
22	Change in responsibilities at work	29			

(Adapted from Holmes, T. H., and R. H. Rahe: The social readjustment rating scale. *Journal of Psychosomatic Medicine, 14*:121, 1970.)

Turning to studies of *multiple life events* and subsequent illness, we find that researchers have studied different patient populations as well as different types of life change. Below we consider three studies relevant to patient care.

Illness in Children and Life Events. The hypothesis underlying this study conducted by Heisel et al. (1973) was that "children in any patient population experience more significant 'life events' preceding an illness than is to be expected in a healthy population."[63] The investigations, developed a life change scale similar to that of Holmes and Rahe, but geared to the lives of children at different age levels (Table 4–2). The researchers used the birth of a sibling as a standard (rather than marriage, as did Holmes), giving sibling birth a value of 50. Next, the number of life changes occurring in a healthy population of 3500 children was compared with a variety of patient populations. They found that the data confirmed their hypothesis, i.e., "Major life changes had been experienced by twice as many children with disease as would have been expected in a control population of healthy children."[63] One other interesting finding emerged from this study. Children with psychiatric disorders had *not* experienced any more "traumatic external events" than had children with medical-surgical problems. The authors thus reasoned that the child who copes with change must adjust both physically and psychologically. Consequently, when adjustment fails the child may develop *either* a mental or a physical illness.

Attempted Suicide and Life Events.[103, 104] Paykel and associates (1975) investigated the relationship between life events and suicide attempts. The researchers administered a list of significant life events to three groups: (1) persons who had attempted suicide, (2) depressed patients, and (3) a control group drawn from the general population. Participants were asked to indicate events in their lives over the preceding 6 months. The findings were as follows:

> Suicide attempters reported four times as many events as were reported by subjects from the general population and 1½ times as many as were reported by depressed patients prior to depressive onset. A substantial peaking of events occurred in the month before the attempt.[104]

This peaking of number of life events in the lives of suicide attempters is clearly indicated in Figure 4–4. These results support the belief that people who attempt suicide may do so in reaction to an overwhelming number of life changes within a relatively brief period of time. Consequently Hiesel et al. emphasized that the "identification and control" of rapidly changing life events is central to the care of persons who have attempted suicide or who are possibly planning an attempt.

Seriousness of Illness and Magnitude of Life Change.[165, 39, 108] In 1968, Wyler, Masuda, and Holmes published an important new scale en-

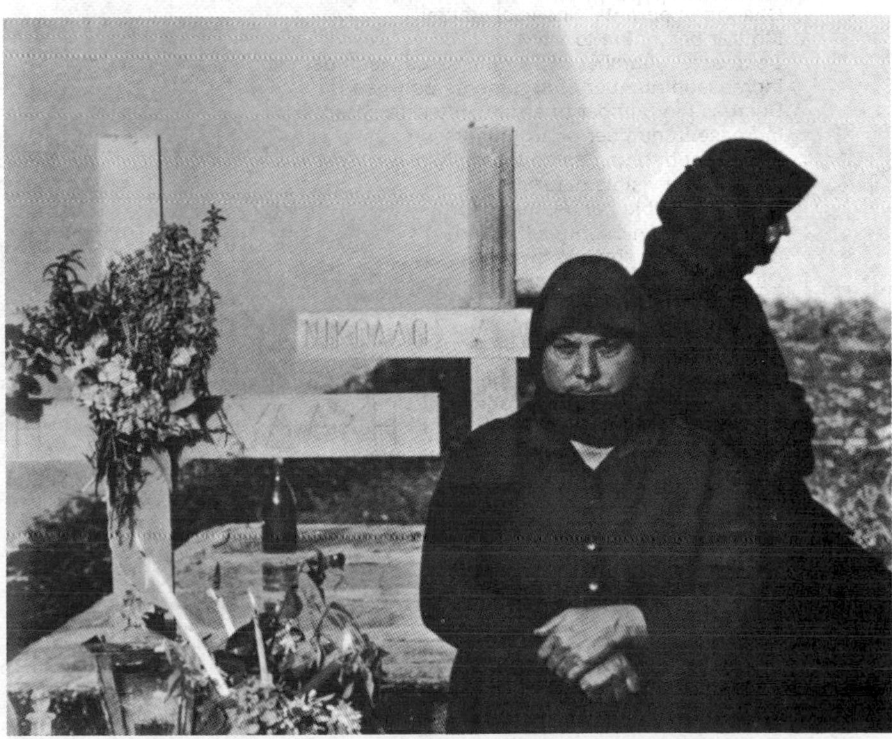

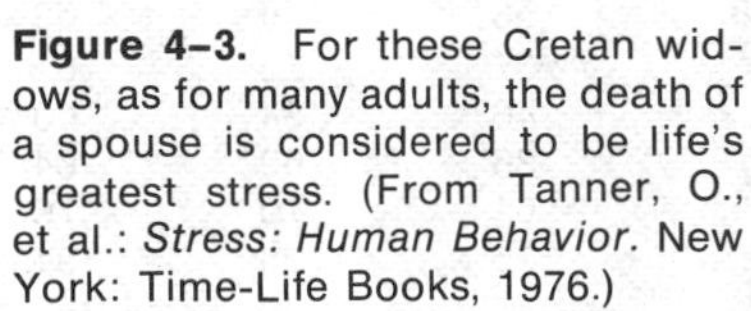

Figure 4–3. For these Cretan widows, as for many adults, the death of a spouse is considered to be life's greatest stress. (From Tanner, O., et al.: *Stress: Human Behavior.* New York: Time-Life Books, 1976.)

titled the Seriousness of Illness Rating Scale (SIRS). To develop this scale, the authors asked participants to rank a list of 126 illnesses according to what they believed to be the relative "seriousness" of each disease (a sampling of these illnesses is shown in Table 4–3). The researchers gave peptic ulcer a rating of 500 SIU (Seriousness of Illness Units). The study participants were to rate each of the 126 illnesses against peptic ulcer. In making their decisions, participants were asked to consider such factors as the degree of discomfort, amount of disability involved, duration of the illness, the prognosis, and whether or not the illness was life threatening. As shown in Table 4–3, participants ranked dandruff as the least serious illness and leukemia as the most serious.

Next, the researchers studied the relationship between the amount of life change experienced by 232 randomly-selected subjects and the seriousness of illnesses they had developed. They discovered that the *greater the amount of life change experienced by the subject, the more serious was the illness developed.* In addition, persons who had a large number of life change units were more likely to develop chronic illness, whereas subjects with lower life change units tended to develop more acute illnesses which were relatively minor in nature. Dudley and Welke present the

TABLE 4–2. LIFE EVENT SCORES (IN LIFE CHANGE) BY AGE GROUP

Life events	Preschool	Elementary	Junior high	Senior high
Beginning nursery school, first grade, seventh grade, or high school	42	46	45	42
Change to a different school	33	46	52	56
Birth or adoption of a brother or sister	50	50	50	50
Brother or sister leaving home	39	36	33	37
Hospitalization of brother or sister	37	41	44	41
Death of brother or sister	59	68	71	68
Change of father's occupation requiring increased absence from home	36	45	42	38
Loss of job by a parent	23	38	48	46
Marital separation of parents	74	78	77	69
Divorce of parents	78	84	84	77
Hospitalization of parent (serious illness)	51	55	54	55
Death of a parent	89	91	94	87
Death of a grandparent	30	38	35	36
Marriage of parent to stepparent	62	65	63	63
Jail sentence of parent for 30 days or less	34	44	50	53
Jail sentence of parent for 1 year or more	67	67	76	75
Addition of third adult to family (e.g., grandparent)	39	41	34	34
Change in parents' financial status	21	29	40	45
Mother beginning to work	47	44	36	26
Decrease in number of arguments between parents	21	25	29	27
Increase in number of arguments between parents	44	51	48	46
Decrease in number of arguments with parents	22	27	29	26
Increase in number of arguments with parents	39	47	46	47
Discovery of being an adopted child	33	52	70	64
Acquiring a visible deformity	52	69	83	81
Having a visible congenital deformity	39	60	70	62
Hospitalization of yourself (child)	59	62	59	58
Change in acceptance by peers	38	51	68	67
Outstanding personal achievement	23	39	45	46
Death of a close friend (child's friend)	38	53	65	63
Failure of a year in school		57	62	56
Suspension from school		46	54	50
Pregnancy in unwed teen-age sister		36	60	64
Becoming involved with drugs or alcohol		61	70	76
Becoming a full-fledged member of a church/synagogue		25	28	31
Not making an extracurricular activity you wanted to be involved in (i.e., athletic team, band)			49	55
Breaking up with a boyfriend or girlfriend			47	53
Beginning to date			55	51
Fathering an unwed pregnancy			76	77
Unwed pregnancy			95	92
Being accepted to a college of your choice				43
Getting married				101

(From Heisel, J. S., et al.: The significance of life events as contributing factors in the diseases of children. *The Journal of Pediatrics, 83*:119, July 1973, p. 120.)

most dramatic findings from this study in Table 4–4. Note the significant difference in the mean average life change units in persons developing headache as compared with life change units in persons later developing cancer.

Basic Concepts Concerning Life Changes and Illness

1. The *rate, magnitude* and *variability* of life changes affect one's state of health.

2. The greater the *number of life changes* within a one- to two-year period, the more likely a person will become ill in the near future; thus disease tends to follow a *clustering* of life changes.

3. The greater the *number* of life changes and the more *severe* the life changes, the greater the risk that a severe illness will develop.

4. Life changes do *not* have to be unfortunate or undesirable to precipitate illness. People must adapt to happy events (e.g., marriage, job promotion, or birth of a baby), just as they do to sad events (e.g., death of a loved one or job loss).

5. Life changes do not have to be great in magnitude to result in illness. Small changes in daily routine (traffic tieups, minor arguments, staying up late, welcome but unexpected visitors) may result in minor health changes (stomach upsets, skin rashes, minor accidents, sneezing and coughing). Organs that are particularly susceptible to symptoms are the skin, ears, eyes, nose, throat, gastrointestinal tract, and musculoskeletal system. These organs are in continuous contact with the external environment and thus are more vulnerable than internal organs.[66]

6. Multiple life changes in a person's psychosocial spheres may result in the development of not only *psychosomatic disorders* (i.e., ulcers, bronchial asthma) but also "classical" *medical entities* such as coronary heart disease, infectious illnesses, "accidents," or hernias.[111]

7. Multiple life changes within a brief period of time may be linked not only to illness onset but also to *untimely death*. For example, we reported earlier that the mortality rate among the widowed is very high during the first 6 months following bereavement. With the research of Holmes et al., a question has emerged: Is it grief that kills the widowed or is the numerous major life changes which the surviving spouse must suddenly make following the death of a husband or wife? Increasingly, researchers believe that rapid changes in residence, finances, occupation, personal habits (eating, sleeping, sexual, social), and family constellation coupled with grief may be the precipitating factors in the premature deaths of the widowed.

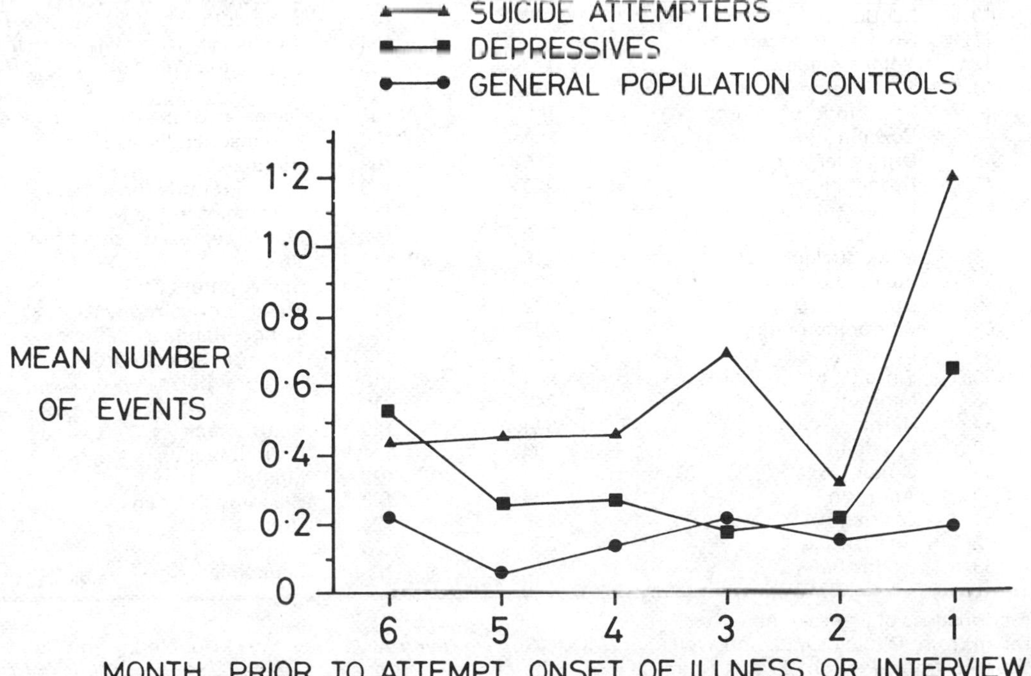

Figure 4–4. Mean number of events reported over each one-month period. (From Paykel, E. S.: Life stress, depression and suicide. *Journal of Human Stress*, 2:2, Sept. 1976, p. 10.)

TABLE 4-3. SERIOUSNESS OF ILLNESS RATING SCALE (SIRS)

Rank	Disease	SIU*	Rank	Disease	SIU*
1.	Dandruff	21	64.	Irregular heartbeats	302
2.	Warts	32	65.	Overweight	309
3.	Coldsore, canker sore	43	66.	Anemia	312
4.	Corns	46	67.	Anxiety reaction	315
5.	Hiccups	48	68.	Gout	322
6.	Bad breath	49	69.	Snake bite	324
7.	Sty	59	70.	Appendicitis	337
8.	Common cold	62	71.	Pneumonia	338
9.	Farsightedness	72	72.	Depression	344
10.	Nosebleed	73	73.	Frigidity	347
11.	Sore throat	74	74.	Burns	348
12.	Nearsightedness	75	75.	Kidney infection	374
13.	Sunburn	80	76.	Inability for sexual intercourse	382
14.	Constipation	81	77.	Hyperthyroidism	393
15.	Astigmatism	83	78.	Asthma	413
16.	Laryngitis	84	79.	Glaucoma	426
17.	Ringworm	85	80.	Sexual deviation	446
18.	Headache	88	81.	Gallstones	454
19.	Scabies	89	82.	Arthritis	468
20.	Boils	96	83.	Starvation	473
21.	Heartburn	98	84.	Syphilis	474
22.	Acne	103	85.	Accidental poisoning	480
23.	Abscessed tooth	108	86.	Slipped disk	487
24.	Color blindness	109	87.	Hepatitis	488
25.	Tonsillitis	117	88.	Kidney stones	499
26.	Diarrhea	118	89.	Peptic ulcer	500
27.	Carbuncle	122	90.	Pancreatitis	514
28.	Chicken pox	134	91.	High blood pressure	520
29.	Menopause	140	92.	Smallpox	530
30.	Mumps	148	93.	Deafness	533
31.	Dizziness	149	94.	Collapsed lung	536
32.	Sinus infection	150	95.	Shark bite	545
33.	Bedsores	153	96.	Epilepsy	582
34.	Increased menstrual flow	154	97.	Chest pain	609
35.	Fainting	155	98.	Nervous breakdown	610
36.	Measles	159	99.	Diabetes	621
37.	Painful menstruation	163	100.	Blood clot in vessels	631
38.	Infection of the middle ear	164	101.	Hardening of the arteries	635
39.	Varicose veins	173	102.	Emphysema	636
40.	Psoriasis	174	103.	Tuberculosis	645
41.	No menstrual period	175	104.	Alcoholism	688
42.	Hemorrhoids	177	105.	Drug addiction	722
43.	Hay fever	185	106.	Coma	725
44.	Low blood pressure	189	107.	Cirrhosis of the liver	733
45.	Eczema	204	108.	Parkinson's disease	734
46.	Drug allergy	206	109.	Blindness	737
47.	Bronchitis	210	110.	Mental retardation	745
48.	Hyperventilation	211	111.	Blood clot in the lung	753
49.	Shingles	212	112.	Manic depressive psychosis	766
50.	Mononucleosis	216	113.	Stroke	774
51.	Infected eye	220	114.	Schizophrenia	785
52.	Bursitis	222	115.	Muscular dystrophy	785
53.	Whooping cough	230	116.	Congenital heart defects	794
54.	Lumbago	231	117.	Tumor in spinal cord	800
55.	Fibroids of the uterus	234	118.	Cerebral palsy	805
56.	Migraine	242	119.	Heart failure	824
57.	Hernia	244	120.	Heart attack	855
58.	Frostbite	263	121.	Brain infection	872
59.	Goiter	283	122.	Multiple sclerosis	875
60.	Abortion	284	123.	Bleeding in brain	913
61.	Ovarian cyst	288	124.	Uremia	963
62.	Heat stroke	293	125.	Cancer	1020
63.	Gonorrhea	296	126.	Leukemia	1080

*Seriousness of illness units.
Taken from: Dudley, D. L., and Welke, E. *How to Survive Being Alive*. New York: Doubleday and Co., 1977, pp. 52–5. Adapted from: Petrich, J., and Holmes, T. H. "Life change and onset of illness", *Medical Clinics of North America, 61*:954, October, 1977. pp. 831–3.

Uses and Limitations of Life Change Profiles

Life-change scales and questionnaires are proving to be useful clinical tools in two ways. First, the SRRS and similar scales are being used to *predict* the changes of a person developing illness. You recall that predictions are based on an individual's life change score and that the higher the person's score, the greater the risk of ensuing illness. However, despite the general accuracy of these scales as prognostic aids, they do have their limitations.

For example, while researchers can predict statistically that a certain *percentage* of people with a high life change score will become ill, they cannot yet predict *which individuals* will fall ill. In other words, why some persons become sick with a life change score of only 150 and others remain healthy with a score of over 300 units remains unknown.[105]

Another limitation of these scales as a predictive aid is that they measure only *one dimension* of a person's life stress; namely, recent changes in the psychosocial sphere. Rahe points out that each of us faces not only immediate stresses to which we must adjust, but long-term *chronic* problems (e.g., chronic financial stresses) and *anticipated* changes and stresses (e.g., a possible divorce, job change). When considering disease causation, chronic stresses and anticipated future stress must be evaluated along with recent stressful changes. Unfortunately, there is no way yet to measure the effects of all three factors on a person's health status.[110]

Despite these limitations, life-change scales are being used for a second purpose: to *counsel patients* in a effort to *prevent disease.** For instance, a new widow can be counseled to keep life changes at a minimum for at least a year following the death of her spouse. The family of a teenager who threatens suicide can be helped to stabilize their child's life, thereby preventing a suicide attempt. The newly divorced can be advised to wait before moving, going on a radical diet, changing jobs, seeking new friends, or making other changes.

Finally, Petrich and Holmes offer this general prescription to patients to help them reduce illness brought on by life change:[108]

> 1. *Become familiar with the life events and the amounts of change they require.*
> 2. *With practice you can recognize when a life event happens.*
> 3. *Think about the meaning of the event for you and try to identify some of the feelings you experience.*
> 4. *Think about the different ways in which you might best adjust to the event.*
> 5. *Take your time in arriving at decisions.*
> 6. *If possible, anticipate life changes and plan for them well in advance.*
> 7. *Pace yourself. It can be done even if you are in a hurry.*
> 8. *Look at the accomplishment of a task as a part of daily living and avoid looking at such an achievement as a "stopping point" or "a time for letting down."*
> 9. *Remember, the more change you have, the more likely you are to get sick.*

*Methods for reducing illnesses brought on by too many life changes are described in Chapter 6.

TABLE 4–4. SUMMARY OF SIGNIFICANT DATA FROM SERIOUSNESS OF ILLNESS AND MAGNITUDE OF LIFE CHANGE RESEARCH BY WYLER, MASUDA AND HOLMES

Illness	*Seriousness of illness units in parentheses*	*Mean average life change units in the 2 years preceding the illness*
Headache	(88)	209
Acne	(103)	311
Psoriasis	(174)	317
Eczema	(204)	231
Bronchitis	(210)	322
Hernia	(244)	457
Anemia	(312)	325
Anxiety reaction	(315)	482
Gallstones	(454)	563
Peptic ulcer	(500)	603
High blood pressure	(520)	405
Chest pain	(609)	638
Diabetes	(621)	599
Alcoholism	(688)	688
Manic-depressive psychosis	(766)	753
Schizophrenia	(785)	609
Heart failure	(824)	772
Cancer	(1020)	777

(Modified from Dudley, D. L., and E. Welke: *How to Survive Being Alive.* New York: Doubleday and Co., 1977, p. 56.)

The skilled nurse can substantially reduce the threat of illness or even death in clients by teaching them about the importance of regulating life change.

CYCLING BEHAVIOR (ACTIVITY VERSUS WITHDRAWAL) AS A FACTOR IN DISEASE CAUSATION[39, 99]

In their book, *How To Survive Being Alive*, Dudley and Welke emphasize that illness may result when a person's lifestyle swings back and forth between periods of heavy activity and periods of nonaction or withdrawal. To depict these swings or cycles, they have constructed a graph model they call the *Coltar Coaster* (Fig. 4–5). The coaster is named after John Coltar, a famous "mountain man" and a member of the Lewis and Clark expedition to the Pacific Coast. Coltar led a life marked by periods of great activity — escaping from hostile Indians, active exploration of new territory — followed by periods of letdown and withdrawal. Coltar finally died from an infectious disease following his semiretirement from mountain life to farm life. Dudley and Welke believe that what really overcame Coltar was *stress* engendered by his coastering behavior.

They emphasize that it is the wide swings from activity to inactivity and not the specific activities or attitudes themselves that finally cause illness. Their term for activity is "action orientation," which can include "vigorous exercise, anger, anxiety, euphoria, or excitement." The withdrawal or "non-action orientation" portion of the coaster may be "sleep, depression, apathy, or a conditioned inhibition of activity." Note in Figure 4–5 that certain diseases are linked with different parts of the coaster (e.g., increased activation with tension headache; withdrawal with migraine headache).

There are many examples of the negative effects of coastering. For instance, the highly active, job-oriented person who abruptly retires may become ill or even die prematurely. The person with a sedentary job who overexerts on the weekend is known for developing all sorts of ailments. As a student, you may have experienced the phenomenon of coastering just before, during, and following final examinations. When preparing for and taking exams, you may have felt "keyed up" and anxious. You may have studied more hours than normal or stayed up all

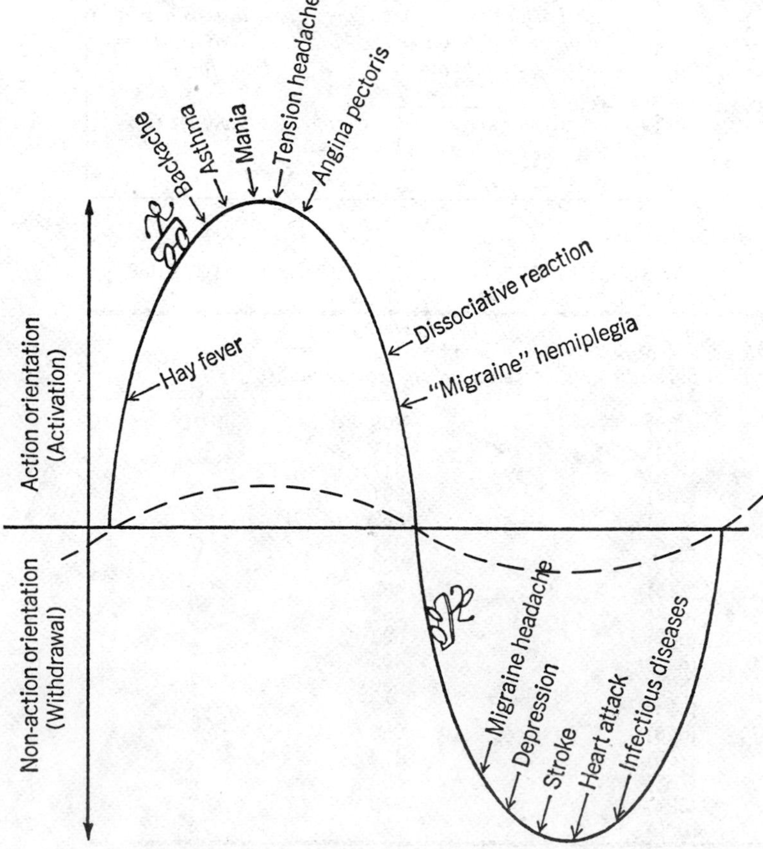

Figure 4–5. Coltar Coaster. Some of the diseases that fit into the coastering phenomenon. Most diseases vary in intensity with wide changes in activity and/or begin during the extreme high or low periods. The dotted line indicates how Dudley and Welke recommend that a person minimize illness – by modulating activities and "flattening out" the Coltar Coaster. (Modified from Dudley, D. L., and E. Welke: *How to Survive Being Alive.* New York: Doubleday & Co., 1977, p. 77.)

night cramming; you may have had a term project due the same week. Very possibly you suffered from tension headache. Following the exam week, while you may have felt relieved, you may also have had a sense of "letdown" and depression. Possibly you even developed a migraine headache or a cold. If you became ill during or following exam week, you were probably experiencing the effects of severe coastering.

Dudley and Welke recommend keeping the coaster "as flat as possible," as shown by the dotted line in Figure 4–5. The person nearing retirement can reduce job activities gradually, while planning ahead for new "action-oriented" retirement activities. For the student, the way to manage exam week may be to spread out the work load, by beginning projects and studying earlier in the semester. If you are depressed after exams are over, don't sit around your room trying to "recover." As Dudley and Welke say,

> . . . the last thing in the world you need if you are depressed is more non-action orientation. Instead, get moving. Run around the block, chop wood, go to a baseball game, make love, but don't sit and fret . . . If you can achieve the point of view that the goal of life is to be adequate to the tasks ahead, your Coltar Coaster will just about manage itself.[39]

FRIEDMAN'S AND ROSENMAN'S THEORY OF BEHAVIOR PATTERNS AND SUSCEPTIBILITY TO CORONARY ARTERY DISEASE[34, 46, 52, 53, 96, 135, 137, 139]

Heart disease is currently the foremost cause of death in the United States. Indeed, over 100 million Americans possibly suffer from some degree of coronary artery disease.* In 1975 an estimated 675,000 Americans died from heart attacks; 175,000 of these persons were under 65 years of age.[53] Because heart disease is the number one health problem for Americans, we are including here Friedman and Rosenman's theory on the causation of coronary artery disease — a theory that links behavior, stress, and life-threatening illness.†

Since the 1950's, Friedman and Rosenman have extensively studied the relationship between certain patterns of behavior and susceptibility of subjects to coronary artery disease. Before the 1950's, most physicians assumed that heart disease probably resulted from faulty diet (e.g., over consumption of foods high in fat and cholesterol), lack of proper rest and exercise, excessive smoking, and a family history of heart disease. With the work of Friedman and Rosenman, a new theory of heart disease developed: the hypothesis that *heart disease can evolve as a consequence of a certain type of behavior pattern.*

In their widely read book, *Type A Behavior and Heart Disease*, Friedman and Rosenman discuss their theory that there are two basic types of behavior patterns: Type A and Type B. The type A personality characterizes individuals who are constantly mobilizing inner resources to combat real or imagined stresses. They are aggressive, often hostile, hard-driving deadline-ridden people with a chronic sense of time urgency. The type A personality feels vaguely guilty when relaxing, characteristically moves, walks, and eats rapidly, and frequently strives to do or think about two or more things at once (polyphasic thinking).

Type A behavior is at present typically displayed by *men* in American society. Job position does not appear to be a factor: type A behavior is common to urbanites of all occupations — bank presidents, janitors, middle-class business executives, shoe salespersons.

The type B personality is just the opposite. The type B subject tends to take life with all of its stresses in stride. Although this type of person is often intelligent and ambitious, the type B personality is not "driven" by ambition and does not allow activity to become self-destructive. The person is able to relax without guilt and work without a sense of time urgency. Whatever the person's occupation or responsibilities, the basic attitude toward life is calm, optimistic, and self-confident.

A person who displays type A behavior patterns, is, according to Friedman and Rosenman, in grave danger of developing coronary artery disease and a subsequent life-threatening heart attack. They base this conclusion upon years of patient observation, including a study of 3500 healthy men who were followed from 1960 to 1970. These men were interviewed, given physical examinations, and classified by behavior pattern as either type A or type B. Then their health was carefully monitored for the following 10 years. In 1974, Friedman and Rosenman published their findings, which showed that the man who had exhibited a type A behavior pattern in 1960 (and who was over 35 and under 60 years old) "was almost three times more likely than a type B man to get coronary heart disease in the subsequent decade." On the other hand, individuals who had displayed type B behavior patterns in 1960 did not develop heart problems even though their diet was high in fat and cho-

*Coronary artery disease as Friedman and Rosenman use the term is "a symptomless disorder characterized and identified by the thickening and deterioration of the blood-supply conduits to the heart."[46]

†Stress-induced heart attacks and the physiologic effects of the Type A behavior pattern upon the cardiovascular system are discussed in Chapter 36.

lesterol, they smoked cigarettes, they were overweight, and coronary artery disease was present in their parents. Thus, the researchers concluded that type B personality types appear to be almost immune to the onset of coronary artery disease.[46, 140]

The work of Friedman, Rosenman, and other researchers has prompted informed patients and their physicians and nurses to look at the effect of behavior patterns on susceptibility to heart disease. Also, from their work has come incentive for the coronary-prone type A personality to change behavior patterns to type B, thereby possibly averting heart damage. Friedman and Rosenman suggest various "drills" for combatting "hurry sickness," hostility, and the sense that quantity is always more important than quality. They believe that the practice of such drills will not only prevent heart disease, but also will make life more interesting and meaningful. Today, psychologists and physicians are trying to help people convert from type A to type B behavior through such practices as relaxation exercises and behavior modification techniques.*

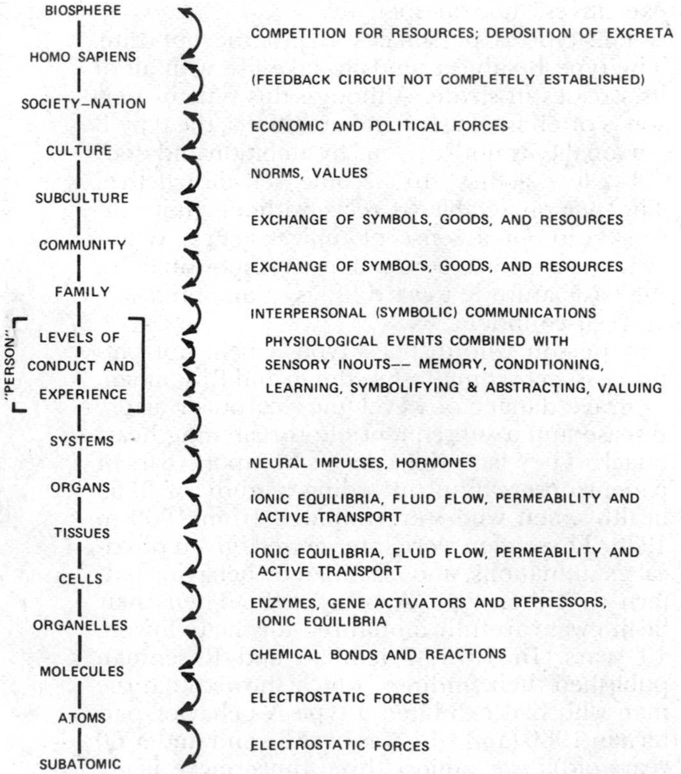

BIOSPHERE — COMPETITION FOR RESOURCES; DEPOSITION OF EXCRETA
HOMO SAPIENS — (FEEDBACK CIRCUIT NOT COMPLETELY ESTABLISHED)
SOCIETY–NATION — ECONOMIC AND POLITICAL FORCES
CULTURE — NORMS, VALUES
SUBCULTURE — EXCHANGE OF SYMBOLS, GOODS, AND RESOURCES
COMMUNITY — EXCHANGE OF SYMBOLS, GOODS, AND RESOURCES
FAMILY — INTERPERSONAL (SYMBOLIC) COMMUNICATIONS
"PERSON": LEVELS OF CONDUCT AND EXPERIENCE — PHYSIOLOGICAL EVENTS COMBINED WITH SENSORY INOUTS-- MEMORY, CONDITIONING, LEARNING, SYMBOLIFYING & ABSTRACTING, VALUING
SYSTEMS — NEURAL IMPULSES, HORMONES
ORGANS — IONIC EQUILIBRIA, FLUID FLOW, PERMEABILITY AND ACTIVE TRANSPORT
TISSUES — IONIC EQUILIBRIA, FLUID FLOW, PERMEABILITY AND ACTIVE TRANSPORT
CELLS — ENZYMES, GENE ACTIVATORS AND REPRESSORS, IONIC EQUILIBRIA
ORGANELLES — CHEMICAL BONDS AND REACTIONS
MOLECULES — ELECTROSTATIC FORCES
ATOMS — ELECTROSTATIC FORCES
SUBATOMIC PARTICLES — (?)
QUARKS (?)

Figure 4–6. Nature of feedback signals at various interlevel feedback loops in the "Man" hierarchy. (From Brody, H.: Systems view of man. *Perspectives in Biology and Medicine,* Autumn 1973, p. 77.)

The area of behavior and disease causation is clearly a fertile one for research. Many questions need exploration. For example, to what degree can heart damage be reversed by a change in behavior patterns? What are the implications of Friedman's and Rosenman's research for our educational system — which tends to promote and reward type A behavior? In what ways are the behavior patterns related to the causation of conditions other than coronary artery disease; for example, gastric ulcers and hypertension? With the pioneering work of Friedman and Rosenman as a foundation, the answers to these vital questions hopefully lie in the near future.

THE SYSTEMS THEORY OF DISEASE

The systems theory of disease is derived historically from: (a) Bernard's principle of the disturbed internal milieu, (b) Cannon's concept of upset homeostasis, (c) general systems theory, and (d) modern concepts of cybernetics and feedback. The ideas of Bernard and Cannon are briefly considered on p. 32. Before proceeding, let us quickly review the concepts of systems theory, cybernetics and feedback — all terms with which you are possibly familiar.

Basically, *systems theory* is a unifying approach to the study of life which can be applied to any structure in the universe from a planet to a subatomic particle.

> *In essence, a* system *(which can be natural or manmade) is "a relatively stable whole" composed of various components which are integrated and coordinated in their activities by a* communications network."[2]

The activities of a system are always directed toward particular ends — states or *goals*. For a system to attain a goal, it must interact continuously and adaptively with its environment; also its various components must interact correctly.

Highly complex systems (e.g., our solar system) are characterized by subcomponents (e.g., the various planets). Each subcomponent, in turn, is a natural system in its own right, as well as part of a greater system. Also each subcomponent can itself be broken down into smaller and simpler systems, thus forming a *hierarchy of systems* ranging from the complex to the simple.[17]

*Techniques for coping with stress and converting type A behavior to type B behavior are considered in Chapters 6 and 36.

Using the systems approach, an individual human being is defined as a *natural system within a hierarchy of natural systems* that range from the biosphere to subatomic particles (Fig. 4–6). Note in the left portion of Figure 4–6 that the "Man" hierarchy encompasses and integrates biologic, social and cultural aspects of human life. Note also in Figure 4–6 that the part of the hierarchy labeled "Person" corresponds to each individual woman, man, or child with all of each person's memories, goals, needs, and aspirations. For, like all other systems, humans are basically *goal oriented*. That is, all of our activities are directed toward the achievement of certain biologic, cultural or social end-states, e.g., the satisfaction of basic needs for oxygen, safety, love, or acceptance by the group.

Let us next consider the terms cybernetics and feedback. *Cybernetics* — a word coined by Norbert Weiner — is defined as the science of the processes of communication and control in the animal and in the machine. *Feedback* basically involves reinserting (or feeding back) into an organism or a machine that results of its past performance in order to control its present and future performance. In other words, feedback is the mechanism that enables a self-regulating system to sense the degree to which it is deviating from the set norm and to make the adjustments necessary to correct the detected deviation.

In essence, then, the systems theory of disease springs from the concept that a human being is a hierarchy of natural systems, which is integrated, coordinated, and self regulated by means of signals transmitted through feedback loops (see Figure 4–6). The systems theory thus explains disease in terms of various perturbations and disruptions that develop within the vast natural systems of which people are a part, and which cause disturbances in signals and breaks within feedback linkage.[17]

Note in Figure 4–6 that the function of each individual "person" depends upon the nature and stability of the feedback linkage which connects "the person" to other levels of the hierarchy. Consequently, when feedback signals break down anywhere within this hierarchy, disruption spreads "down" through the hierarchy, and to a more limited extent, "up" through the hierarchy. For instance, a "person" may be adversely affected by a perturbation higher in the hierarchy; in the case of the unemployed aerospace engineer described in Figure 4–7, the perturbation was at the national level. As a result of *downward* disruption, the "person" may experience economic and emotional stress at the family level followed by a breakdown of homeostatic self-regulation of body systems; then organs, then tissues, then cells, and so on. In other words, i.e., the individual becomes ill. As a result of *upward* disruption, the sick person's conduct and ability to communicate with others may deteriorate. Significant others may suffer even more financially and psychologically; the person may be too ill to work at gainful employment. Financial assistance may be needed from government; in extreme cases, the person may even threaten the safety of the community. Generally speaking, disruption infrequently spreads upward into the natural level.

Fortunately, disease-producing disruption can be halted or at least limited in its destructiveness if (a) the initial perturbation is not too great, (b) the means of adaptation to disturbance and change are adequate, and (c) the hierarchical levels immediately above and below the point of disruption can quickly remove or inactivate the disruptive force before it spreads havoc into other parts of the overall system. However, when disease-producing disruption *cannot* be halted in its rapid spread downward through the hierarchy, the "ultimate disruption of the person by death" results. Thus, in summary, this theory explains disease and death as a breakdown of feedback linkage, resulting in an upset in homeostasis within the human hierarchy.

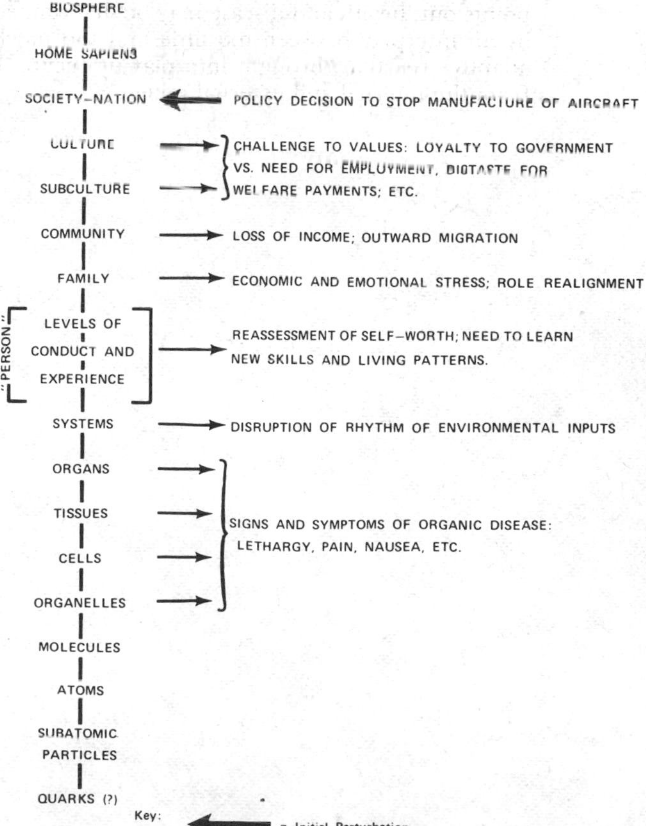

Figure 4–7. Disease example. Stress-related psychosomatic illness in an unemployed aerospace engineer: Example of spread of disruption downward through the hierarchy. (From Brody, H.: Systems view of man. *Perspectives in Biology and Medicine*, Autumn 1973, p. 80.)

Conclusion

The systems theory of disease and the concept of feedback plays an important role in all of the modern theories of disease which we have discussed. As you quickly review each theory, identify how feedback is a part of the theory.

- *Selye* writes of the body's attempts to restore homeostatic balance by means of adaptive hormones. He explores the problems engendered by too little hormone, too much hormone, or an inappropriate release of hormones in response to stressors. He describes the stages and consequences of the General Adaptation Syndrome (GAS).
- *Harold Wolff* hypothesized that individuals attempt to adapt to or to correct situations that are experienced by them as deviant or abnormal. In their attempt to adapt, organ functions are often used inappropriately and to the detriment of the individuals.
- *Stewart Wolf* concentrates on the action of the brain and the nervous system in upsetting the body's balance and in mitigating imbalances. As Wolf points out, health and disease may be determined by an interplay between too little and too much adaptive reaction "brought into play by feedback from the internal and external milieu."
- *Thomas Holmes* and his associates emphasize that serious illnesses may result when an individual must adapt to many life changes within a short period of time, i.e., one to two years. Recent studies concerning the correlation between illness and life change, have shown that the onset of minor ailments, serious diseases, depression, and suicidal attempts have followed a clustering of both positive and negative life changes.
- *Dudley* writes that illness may result from a lifestyle which is characterized by swings between periods of heavy activity and withdrawal. Such a lifestyle is characterized by cycling behavior. Dudley depicts this type of behavior as a type of "roller coaster," which he terms the Coltar Coaster. This theory emphasizes that "coastering" behavior must be modulated and controlled if an individual is t remain healthy.
- *Friedman and Rosenman* point out that a person' behavior patterns can affect the heart. They hav shown that there are two major types of behavi patterns: Type A (hostile, hurried, deadlin ridden behavior patterns) and type B (calm, r laxed, nonaggressive behavior patterns). Th studies show that type A personalities are at le three times more prone to coronary artery dise (and the danger of a heart attack) than are typ personalities. They believe that type A perso ities can learn to adapt to stress and thus pre further heart damage.

BIBLIOGRAPHY

The bibliography for this chapter is at the end of Unit III, p. 73.

UNIT III

STRESS AND ILLNESS

INTRODUCTION AND STUDY GUIDE

In Chapter 4, we presented several modern theories of disease causation. While all of the theories discussed differ in their special emphasis (e.g., life change is emphasized by Holmes, fluctuations in activity by Dudley, the stress response by Selye, personality type by Friedman and Rosenman), the various hypotheses seem to agree upon one point:

> *Most disease is related in some way to* stress.

In this unit we pursue the link between stress and disease in more detail. Chapter 5 describes the various factors or *stressors* that can result in illness, e.g., physical factors, psychologic factors, cultural changes, job-related stresses. Chapter 6 explains the various ways in which human beings *respond* to stress-producing factors. In Chapter 6, we present physiologic and behavioral responses to physical and psychologic stressors. We also point out that responses to stressors may be either maladaptive or adaptive, and we present some methods recommended by experts in stress control for achieving the latter. Finally, after describing holistic concepts of illness, the unit closes with a brief discussion of why disease must be prevented and treated with a *multidimensional* approach to healing — an approach vital for the modern nurse to understand and pursue.

Upon completion of Chapters 5 and 6, you should be able to discuss the following:

1. Disease as a failure of adaptation to stress
2. Stressors and five general ways in which they affect people
3. Ten major factors involved in the causation of disease
4. The body's response to physical injury
5. The anatomic and chemical divisions of the autonomic nervous system (ANS); the role of each division in mediating stress responses
6. The effect of psychologic stimuli on the autonomic nervous system
7. The specific effects of autonomic nervous system function and emotion upon the endocrine system, the circulatory system, the digestive system, the bladder, and the muscles
8. Pleasurable emotion and physiologic changes
9. Six behavioral responses to stress
10. The differences between children and adults in their responses to stress
11. Maladaptive responses to stress
12. Methods for controlling the stressors in one's life and one's reactions to them
13. Nursing and a holistic approach to disease — its cure and prevention
14. Nursing and medicine as social sciences

CHAPTER 5

STRESS AND DISEASE: MAJOR CAUSATIVE FACTORS

Among the day-to-day problems, triumphs, and events we all experience, there is an infinite range of stressors. From bitter coffee at dawn to unresolved problems at dusk, from great personal achievements to life's tragedies, all of us must cope with a constant mix of stressful events . . . .[39]

As indicated in the previous chapter, many factors are involved in disease causation. The nurse needs a precise knowledge of these factors to fulfill the role of mitigating and preventing illness. To more fully appreciate the complexity of disease causation and the difficulty of controlling it, it is necessary to look at human beings and their environment from many different aspects — the physical, the chemical, the biologic, the psychocultural, and the ecologic.

GENERAL CONSIDERATIONS

Before considering specific factors in disease causation, let us first briefly discuss *stressors.* We shall define stressors as agents or factors that challenge the adaptive capacities of an individual, placing a strain upon the person that may result in stress and disease. Below we consider five general statements about stressors that are of special importance in the study of health and disease.

1. Stressors affect different people in different ways.

These differences in reaction depend upon the following factors:

a. *The stressor itself,* how suddenly it appears, how long it lasts, how forceful it is and whether it occurs alone or in combination with other stressors. A person may be able to cope successfully with one serious stressor but may fail to adapt to several milder stressors that occur simultaneously or in rapid sequence (see Holmes et al. studies, Chapter 4). Furthermore, a very stressful situation that is short-lived may be better tolerated than a less stressful situation that tends to be chronic. This is because chronic stress demands continuous adaptive efforts. Eventually, because of constant wear and tear of a chronic nature, the individual actually changes, physically and psychologically, and becomes more vulnerable to other stressors. If the stress has been both chronic and severe, the individual may be permanently and adversely altered.

b. The reaction to a stressor depends also upon the *limitations and potentialities of the individual* for dealing with stress. These two factors, in turn, depend upon the person's genetic constitution, personality type, state of physical and mental health, past history of adapting to stressful situations, the social system under which the person lives, and the group and family support available. For example, a person with diabetes mellitus, a hereditary disease of metabolism, is far less able to resist infection than one who does not have diabetes. An individual with a large and supportive network of family and friends is better able to withstand the death of a spouse than is the person who is a newcomer to a city or country. Thus, the effect of a stressor is always *relative* and never absolute; it is relative to the individual undergoing stress and, in particular, to his or her adaptive capabilities.

c. Certain stresses have more *meaning* and *importance* in the lives of some individuals than in the lives of others. This variation depends upon the person's family background and environment, and upon the values developed as a result. For instance, the child from a family in which education is highly valued may find poor school grades very distressing. On the other hand, the youngster from a family in which academic learning is not important may find low grades somewhat disappointing but not devastating.

2. Whenever people encounter stress, from whatever source, they attempt to adapt to it.

If adaptation is successful, the individual's balance will not be disturbed or will be restored. Indeed, many people gain confidence in themselves, achieve goals, and develop new potentials as a result of a stressful encounter . . . to which they have successfully adapted. Others are not successful in their adaptation to stressors. If adaptation is consistently faulty, these people will become ill.

3. Any one stressor is, in itself, a source of new stresses.

As we pointed out earlier, people often find themselves caught in a chain of events stemming from one original upset. For example, a woman with a communicable disease is undergoing stress because she is ill. She is usually placed in an isolation unit, which constitutes another stressor. Consequently, she may become upset with the staff and they, in turn, with her. As a result, a third stressor is created. These stresses, put together, may slow down her recovery. She is hospitalized longer, her finances are affected adversely, her job is threatened, her family is upset, and so one stressor leads to another. Unfortunately the patient must adapt herself to many diverse stresses during a time she lacks the resources to do so.

4. No one stressor or etiologic factor can, by itself, cause a disease.

When a person is ill, one factor involved in the illness may be of greater importance than any other factor. This factor may be highly specific to the causation of the disease; indeed, it may be absolutely necessary for the development of the disease. However, *no one factor is both necessary and sufficient* for the development of a particular malady.[40]

For example, consider the nurse who develops staphylococcal boils as a result of working with a patient with a staphylococcus wound infection. For this nurse to become infected, exposure to staphylococci must occur. The staphylococcus, then, is a *necessary* agent in this case of contamination. However, the exposure to the staphylococcus, alone, is *not* an adequate reason for the development of an infection. Nurses are exposed daily to this organism, yet they do not become infected! One or more other factors must be present for infection to occur, e.g., lowered resistance to disease, fatigue, emotional stress, inadequate handwashing or poor dressing technique that allows contact with contaminated equipment. In sum, it takes *both* exposure to the staphylococcus *and* some of these other factors to provide necessary and sufficient cause for the development of a staphylococcic infection.

In chronic diseases, such as cancer and heart disease, it is even more difficult to find the contributing causes necessary for their development. Exactly which etiologic factors must be present, and in what particular combination, for any one chronic disease to evolve remains a mystery.

5. Stress, of whatever nature, if too prolonged and too severe, can eventually overwhelm any person, no matter how well developed the person's adaptive capabilities are.

Research on the effect of combat duty and concentration camp experiences on the individual soldier has more than proved the eventual overwhelming effect of constant stress. Harold Wolff, for example, writes concerning the effects of battle:

> . . . it may be inferred that everyone has his breaking point, that there are stresses that no man can withstand. Conflict in excess of an individual's current integrative capacity may be a precipitating factor in such a "break." Conversely, whatever reduces integrative capacity may increase the possibility of an individual being overwhelmed by frustrations and conflicts, hitherto managed successfully. Loss of sleep, exhaustion, pain, very loud noises, starvation, malnutrition, infection, sepsis and intoxication, by decreasing integrative capacity, make conflict relatively excessive. Likewise, acts that terrorize, humiliate, destroy self-esteem and create a conviction of being isolated, abandoned or unwanted may reduce integrative effectiveness.[160]

We can summarize by making these general statements concerning stressful factors and their effects.

- People react in different ways to stressors, depending upon the stressor itself, the limitations and potentialities of the individual, and the special meaning that the stressor has for that individual.

- Persons always attempt to adapt to stress.
- These attempts at adaptation inevitably lead to new stresses.
- No single stress, by itself, is both necessary and sufficient to cause disease.
- There are stresses that are either so severe or so prolonged that they can eventually overwhelm the adaptive capabilities of the best-adjusted individual.

Let us now turn to a discussion of specific stress-producing factors.

TYPES OF STRESSFUL FACTORS THAT CAUSE DISEASE

There are numerous stressors that can elicit an alarm reaction and subsequent adaptive activities by the organism, e.g., trauma due to surgery or accidents, burns, fasting, extreme rage or fear, and reduced oxygen tension. We can divide stressful stimuli into the following groups to facilitate consideration of their relationship to disease: (1) genetic factors, (2) physical and chemical factors, (3) microorganisms, (4) psychologic factors, (5) cultural factors, (6) "future shock," (7) migrations, (8) ecologic factors, (9) occupational factors and (10) stressful factors resulting specifically from life in a technologic society.

Genetic Factors

Genes — the biological units of heredity — influence the biochemical structure of the entire body. They also "set the stage" for the growth and development of each of the body's cells and systems. Genes consequently have a powerful effect on our appearance and longevity, as well as our vulnerability to stresses and susceptibility to disease.

The relationship between genetic inheritance and disease is an area of current scientific investigation. We know that defective or abnormal biochemical systems can be transmitted through the genes. Such defective systems or "inborn errors of metabolism" give rise to structural and developmental defects in the individual who inherits them. Sometimes these defects appear in the newborn child and adversely affect the individual's entire life. Other inherited defects become evident only under certain conditions. For example, sickle cell anemia is a hereditary disease seen predominantly in blacks. Clinical manifestations of the disease tend to appear when the individual is exposed to a lowered oxygen tension. Thus, many blacks who were soldiers and airmen in World War II did not realize that they had sickle cell anemia until they flew at high altitudes in nonpressurized planes; only then did dramatic symptoms of this hereditary malady appear. In other types of hereditary disease, symptoms may not appear or become troublesome unless precipitated by such factors as diet, climate, or emotional stress.

Whereas genetic factors influence our state of health and susceptibility to disease, environmental factors may influence the *extent* to which our heredity controls us. For example, individuals may lengthen or shorten their life span by their mode of living. The person who is inclined to obesity, and consequently to other maladies such as hypertension, can choose to diet and exercise or the person can choose to overeat and underdo. Maladaptive and detrimental traits of character can be overcome by learning new behavior patterns.

In other words, we are all born with a certain inherited potential for self-realization or self-destruction. What we do with this potential depends upon ourselves and upon the environment in which we live. Therefore, even diseases that are inherited need not inevitably maim, disable, or kill. As a result of modern medicine and better education of the lay public, many of these inborn maladies are being identified and controlled.

Physical and Chemical Factors

Factors that can injure us because of their physical or chemical properties fall into the following groups:

a. Dangerous substances or forces that impinge upon our bodies from the *external environment.* Examples include: poisons, heat, cold, radiation, electricity, high or low atmospheric pressure, industrial poisons, and drugs. The extent to which these substances can injure us depends, in turn, upon three additional factors. First, the *individual's tolerance and ability to adapt* to certain stressors. For example, tall, thin persons are less able to adapt to an extremely cold climate than are persons with a short, heavy body build. Second, *social and psychologic factors* may be significant. For example, a person's work may require contact with dangerous chemicals or machinery. The impulsive or accident-prone individual may be far more susceptible to mechanical injuries than the cautious person. Third, the *virulence of the factor itself* is of critical importance. For instance, some highly concentrated chemicals kill a person on contact. Likewise, a severe enough electric shock can quickly prove fatal.

b. Substances or forces within our bodies (i.e., *within the internal environment*) can injure by being excessive or in contact with organs that are particularly sensitive to them. Excessive insulin production that results in insulin shock, excessive cholesterol storage in the arteries that leads to arteriosclerosis, and the action of refluxed gastric juices on the esophagus, that results in ulcerations, are all examples of how our own internal secretions and products can injure us.

c. Physical or chemical substances *required* by the body may be *insufficient in amount or unavailable.* Lack of such vital substances can result in physiologic deprivation and injury. Examples of deprivation are many; the individual who has oxygen hunger, the person who does not receive proper vitamins and nutrients, the child who is severely dehydrated, and the patient with an electrolyte loss through vomiting or diarrhea are all suffering from the consequences of deprivation.

Microorganisms and Parasites

The extent to which microorganisms and parasites are capable of producing disease in another living organism depends upon their source, their ability to enter the body of the host and establish themselves in a tissue, organ, cell, or body fluid, their potency and virulence, and their number (especially in the case of parasites).

Microorganisms vary in their ability to infect a host; some can infect almost anyone exposed to them for the first time. For example, measles and smallpox viruses, prior to the development of vaccines, caused epidemics affecting thousands of people. Other microorganisms affect only a few persons out of many exposed; still others harmlessly occupy the tissues of the host, becoming destructive only when the individual's resistance is lowered. Such factors as fatigue, poor diet, psychologic stress or the presence of another disease condition, such as diabetes mellitus or leukemia, can lower a person's defenses, causing extreme susceptibility to infection. To sum up, the characteristics of the microorganism or parasite, the adaptive ability of the host, and those environmental stresses currently affecting the host influence the causation of infectious or parasitic disease.

Psychologic Factors

Engel states that "psychological stress refers to all processes, whether originating in the external environment or within the person, which impose a demand or requirement upon the organism, the resolution or handling of which necessitates work or activity of the mental apparatus before any other system is involved or activated."[40] Psychologic factors, then, differ markedly from the various physical and chemical agents we have mentioned in their effect on the individual. The latter affect a biochemical or physiologic system *first;* after the physiologic reaction, these stressors may *then* be perceived by the mind as stressful. Conversely, psychologic factors *first* affect the brain and central nervous system; physiologic changes, often pathologic, may then follow as a *secondary* reaction to the psychologic trauma.

Age and Sex. The causes and effects of psychologic stresses vary with *age.* Thus all

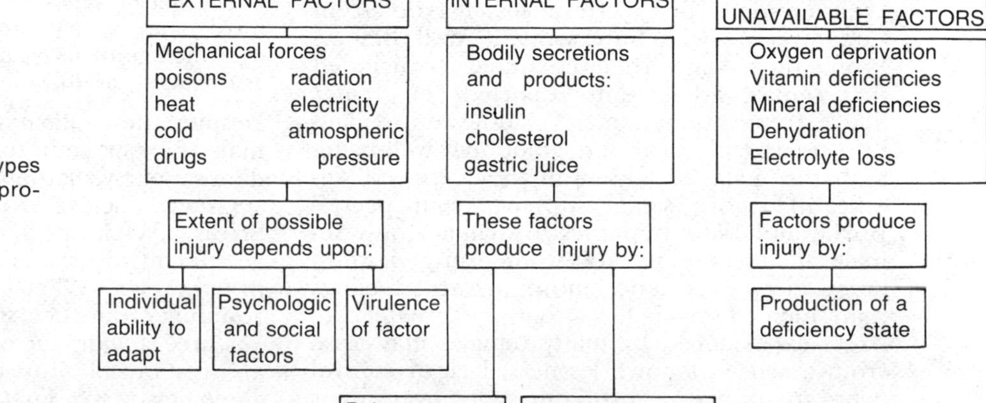

Figure 5–1. The three major types of physical stressors that can produce disease in people.

persons are affected by maturational crises, which are described as "normal processes of growth and development."[3] The active life of adolescents makes them particularly vulnerable to infection and to accidents; the competitive, exhausting existence of middle-class adults makes them susceptible to such problems as stress ulcers, hypertension, heart disease, and alcoholism. The elderly person, perhaps lonely, with diminished hopes, often lapses into an inactive existence accompanied by various degenerative disorders. In sum, the coming of puberty with its physiologic changes, the adult years of responsibility, the advent of the climacteric and menopause, the years of retirement and aging, and the slow decline thereafter — all present unique psychologic stresses to which the individual must adapt.

In addition to age, the origins and consequences of psychologic stress vary with *sex*. Both men and women experience societal pressure to conform to certain traditional roles. This pressure, in turn, can apparently result in mental and physical illness.

In recent years, the feminist movement has encouraged many studies and books concerning the stressors affecting women. Marecek and Kravetz in their review of the literature on women and mental health found that "the social conditions arising from traditional cultural conceptions of women have had a detrimental effect on women's psychological health and personal growth."[87] According to these authors, the traditional view of women holds that the activities and accomplishments of women are less valuable than those of men. This negative view of women has resulted in a poor female self-image, psychologic conflicts, and poorer mental health.

The poorer mental health of young females was further described in a study by Burke and Weir entitled "Sex Differences in Adolescent Life Stress, Social Support and Well Being." From their data the researchers concluded that female adolescents reported (1) greater life stress than male adolescents and (2) "poorer physical and emotional well-being than the males . . . although they received significantly more social support from peers." Burke and Weir hypothesize that not only female adolescents but also women in general in our society experience more stressful feelings than men. They believe that the greater life stress experienced by many females may arise from a sense of powerlessness, lack of control over their lives, and confusion over their role.[20]

In contrast to these studies, some authors present another side of the picture of life stress and sex — the male side. Goldberg reminds us with numerous statistics concerning male disease and death rates that men pay a heavy price for their supposed privileges and greater choice and power. As Goldberg emphasizes, the traditional males roles of breadwinner, family protector, soldier, etc., place men under tremendous stress.[54] And yet, men who wish to maintain their strong "masculine image" cannot openly discuss the stresses of their lives without diminishing that image in their own eyes and in the eyes of others. As a result of this dilemma, men develop more physical and mental ailments than do women, who are freer to discuss problems and who receive more support from family and friends.

Some revealing statistics that support the theory that males of all ages are highly vulnerable to stress and disease are as follows:

There are approximately 150 per cent more boys than girls in state and county hospital units for children.[54]

Among children under 15 years old, boys are diagnosed as schizophrenics 42 per cent more frequently.[54]

Twice as many men die from cardiovascular disease and cirrhosis of the liver as women. Men die 40 per cent more often from hypertension than do women and 64 per cent more often from pneumonia and influenza. Four to five times as many males are likely to die from bronchitis, emphysema, and asthma as females. After the age of 24 years, the male death rate due to all causes is approximately twice as high as that of the female.[144, 146]

The male population of tuberculosis hospitals is 150 per cent higher than the female population, and the male population of chronic disease hospitals is 50 per cent higher.[19]

In men between 15 and 25 years of age, the cause of death in three out of four cases is an accident, suicide, or homicide.[85]

Divorced men suffer from a death rate which is 3.16 times the rate for divorced women.[54]

Men are six times more likely than women to be arrested for possession of narcotics and 13 times more likely for drunkeness.[42]

The suicide rate of males under 24 years is over three times as high as that of females, and men over the age of 65 years commit suicide five times as frequently as do women.[145]

Despite these alarming health statistics, men make 25 per cent fewer visits to doctors and dentists per year than do women.[145]

Other Factors Resulting in Psychologic Stress. What specific factors lead to the development of psychologic stress at any age and in either sex? What is the possibility of disease resulting from such stresses?

Three major factors, as Engel points out, are responsible for the development of psychologic stress.[40] First of all, we are psychologically traumatized if we *lose* or fear losing something that we value or love and which is especially important to us and to our self-concept. Persons, ideals, hopes, valued possessions, a prized job, the body image, social role, home, and country all represent objects of worth for different individuals. The loss of any one of these may result in a variety of psychologic experiences, ranging from depression, grief, and mourning to feelings of anger and frustration.

Second, *injury and pain, or threats of the same,* almost always give rise to psychologic stress. One reason for this is that pain and injury are closely linked with loss and fear of loss.

Strain and Grossman have listed the following seven types of psychologic stress to which the critically ill patient is vulnerable.[132, 133]

1. The basic threat to narcissistic integrity
2. Fear of strangers
3. Separation anxiety
4. Fear of the loss of love and approval
5. Fear of the loss of control of developmentally achieved functions (e.g., bowel and bladder control, regulation and appropriate modulation of feeling states)
6. Fear of loss of, or injury to, body parts (castration anxiety)
7. Reactivation of feelings of guilt and shame, and the accompanying fears of retaliation for past transgressions

How well the patient copes with these stresses depends upon the exact nature of the stress, the person's characteristic way of coping with stress and prior experience with stress, illness, doctors, hospitals, etc. In general, persons respond to injury and stress by attempting to protect themselves and by making the most appropriate adaptations possible. According to Strain and Grossman, successful adaptation to the stresses of critical illness depends upon the following:[132, 133]

1. The patient's ability to regress adequately in the service of recovery
2. His ability to maintain adequate defenses against the stresses evoked by critical illness
3. Access to his feelings and fantasies, and the ability to communicate his needs
4. A basic trust in his medical caretakers
5. The services of an empathetic and flexible critical care team

Frustration of drives is the third factor that gives rise to psychologic stress. Drives are frustrated for a number of reasons. During childhood, we learn that certain drives must be controlled, for example, the sexual drive. The need to control drives, however, often conflicts with the need to express them; if no appropriate outlet can be found for this expression, frustration and possibly illness result.

The fact that *the human being is essentially a tribal animal* also results in the frustration of drives. People want and need the approval of their peers. Consequently a person is often willing to suppress certain drives to please other individuals. On the other hand, people want to express themselves freely and to be themselves; they want to fulfill their own desires, often at the expense of the group. These two divergent needs set up conflict that results in a sense of frustration.

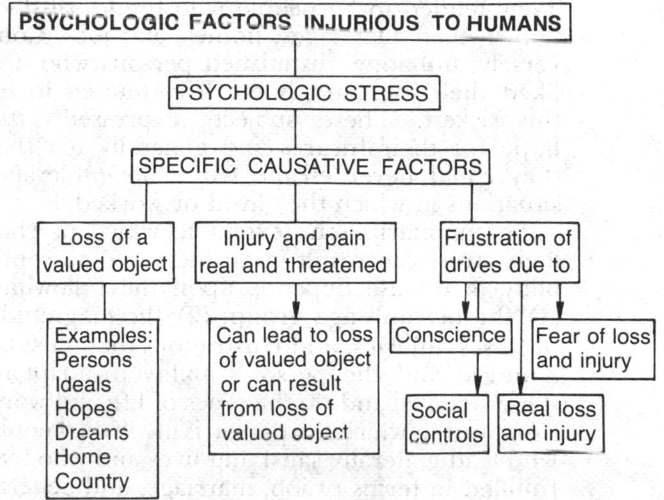

Figure 5–2. The three major types of psychologic stressors that can produce disease in people.

Drives, moreover, can be thwarted because we feel *loss or injury* if we attempt to fulfill them. For example, an unmarried woman may hesitate to satisfy her sexual desires because she fears an unwanted pregnancy, a venereal infection, or the loss of her good reputation. Finally, an *injury* can, in itself, cause drives to be thwarted. For instance, the veteran who is paraplegic as a result of a war injury may be impotent and unable to satisfy his sexual drive.

The conflict engendered by frustrated drives demands some resolution. As Engel points out, stress arises because the individual, feels compelled to satisfy these inner needs and yet can find no satisfactory or safe outlet for these drives. As a result, the drive goes unfulfilled, the conflict is unresolved, psychologic stress builds up, physiologic processes break down, and, finally, physical and mental diseases develop.

Although loss of a loved object, fear of injury, and drive frustration can all lead to psychologic stress, the *total life situation* of a person also has a most profound effect upon that individual's mental and physical well-being. In his classic study of various groups of workers, Hinkle[65] found that the healthiest individuals were also the happiest in their personal lives.

They tended to be people who found satisfaction in their marriages, homes, and jobs. Conversely, unhappy, dissatisfied persons who disliked their jobs and home lives tended to be the sickest. These subjects expressed little hope for their futures and generally felt that they could never escape from the intolerable situations in which they lived or worked.

To summarize, the extent to which psychologic stress can result in an increased susceptibility to disease depends upon the following: (1) the person's age group; (2) the magnitude of losses, injuries, and frustrations that must be endured and the person's ability to adapt to these stresses; and (3) the types of life and work situations in which the person is involved. People who lead generally satisfying lives and who feel fulfilled in terms of job, marriage, and general aspirations suffer from fewer illnesses than people who feel consistently frustrated in their present existence and are without hope for the future.

Cultural Factors

In large part, our particular way of viewing life and the world surrounding us originates in our cultural heritage. Cultural attitudes, beliefs, and traditions are deeply ingrained in each of us and can affect all aspects of our personality and life, including our attitudes toward health and disease.

Cultures vary widely in their traditions. It is not surprising, then, that cultural attitudes toward disease and injury vary throughout the world, and that a disease or injury that is considered serious in one culture may be looked on as trivial in another.

Conflicting cultural values are prevalent in the United States and in Europe; in certain instances, these conflicts lead to illness. For example, in the United States the individual is encouraged from earliest childhood to be competitive, to earn good grades, to reach goals, and to achieve high pay and an elevated status. The very human need to be dependent on other people is discouraged. Thus, a conflict is created between the American cultural values of assertiveness and independence, and the need to be loved and cared for. According to Parsons, one way in which an American can honorably resolve this conflict without losing face is to become legitimately ill.[101] Thus, in our culture, the "sick role" has become an accepted defense against conflict. The person who is sick and who "*tries* to get well" can have dependency needs met without seriously jeopardizing her or his place in American society.

Rapidly changing cultural values also can create a major source of anxiety. Old and traditional cultures appear to produce less stress and disease than newer, more radical societies. Values in traditional societies change little, and there are sanctioned ways for resolving anxieties and conflict. On the other hand, in societies where the "old ways" of life are breaking down and the "new ways" have not yet been fully established, stress and disease tend to become more prevalent. Indeed, disease can become "a way of life" in a society, like our own, which is rapidly changing, where nothing is defined and nothing is sacred, where everyone is potentially mobile, and where there is open choice and constant conflict.

Culture shock, an upsetting psychologic phenomenon, can have a temporary but devastating effect upon the individual who moves into a new cultural environment. The disorientation and confusion that are characteristic of "culture shock" arise whenever a person leaves a familiar country, region, lifestyle, or occupation and enters an environment where dress, customs, beliefs, etc., are radically different. In this age of jet travel and high residential and occupational mobility, the problem of "culture shock" is common.

Future Shock

While "culture shock" results from entry into a new and radically different culture, "future shock" results from the "premature arrival of the future" within *one's own culture.* Alvin Toffler's development of the term "future shock" has gained wide acceptance. In essence, Toffler says:

> We may define future shock as the distress, both physical and psychological, that arises from an overload of the human organism's physical adaptive systems and its decision-making processes. Put more simply, future shock is the human response to overstimulation.[143]

Toffler points out that *overstimulation* can result from the environment, from information overload, and from what he terms "decision stress." *Environmental overstimulation* plagues the city dweller almost constantly. Speeding traffic, blaring music, the roar of aircraft, the din from crowds of people all assault our senses. Moreover, the multiplicity of choices within a modern urban environment can be overwhelming; consider the numbers of restaurants, shops, movie houses, clubs, classes, sporting events, etc., that demand our attention each day. While such an array of choices makes life interesting, it also makes life exhausting.

Information overload is related to the mass

media. Newspapers, books, magazines, television, and radio constantly present information — true or false — for assimilation. Scientific research, along with the demand that professors "publish or perish," brings more articles to read and more new facts and hypotheses to ponder. Technology — copying machines, word processors — and the "knowledge explosion" may get more information to us faster, but this does not mean we can comprehend or assimilate any faster.

Decision stress arises directly from the number of choices each of us faces daily. Innumerable decisions are required during both one's public life (the work or school day) and one's personal life (recreation and relaxation).

For example, consider an evening in the life of Richard M. — a hard working business executive. Richard comes home from work, where he has made many decisions concerning his product and his employees. Tired, he decides not to cook tonight but instead to go out for dinner. First, he must choose a restaurant from among the numerous good ones nearby. Once there, Richard must decide what to eat and drink; thus, he must ponder a long and elaborate menu and a wine list. The meal finished, he must consider whether to tip the waiter and how much. He must also decide what to do the rest of the evening. Go to a movie? Which one? Maybe bowling? To a local bar? To a friend's house? Home to watch television? Richard finally decides to go home, but even there he must decide which program to watch. Finally, at the end of this evening of trying to relax, Richard falls asleep during his selected program. The next day he will get up to face another round of decision making.

As Toffler emphasizes, overstimulation and the rapid-paced lifestyle it promotes can result in both mental and physical illness. Human beings can cope with limited amounts of novelty, change, new information, and "decision stress," but if these amounts are exceeded, coping mechanisms break down. *Mentally,* the overstimulated person may become anxious, hostile or even violent; on the other hand, the person may emotionally withdraw from life and fall into a state of deep depression or apathy. *Physically,* the overstimulated individual can develop all types of ailments. You will recall from Chapter 4 the findings of Holmes et al.: *rapid change within a short period of time is definitely linked with both physical and mental illness.* Thus Toffler warns: future shock is the disease of change and "it may well be the most important disease of tomorrow."

Migrations

Migration as an important stressor and consequent cause of disease is becoming a vital area of research. An editorial in the *Medical Journal of Australia* makes some interesting generalizations about migration and health:

. . . migration in one form or another is such a universal activity of modern man that the health implications have a very wide bearing. People do not migrate only across oceans and national borders — they migrate between rural and urban areas, between small towns and large cities, from suburb to suburb, and from one social or economic class to another. They also migrate, in a sense, through the seven ages of man.[94]

Migrations, according to Michlin, result in several stressful life changes:[93]

- Migrations cause people to lose touch with their "roots" and with familiar and trusted life support systems, i.e., family, friends, schoolmates, working associates.
- Within the new land or social circle, the migrant must strive to form new ties and associations.
- The migrant may have to adjust to a different set of norms and values in his new location — an adjustment that can lead to psychologic conflicts.
- Methods and opportunities for satisfying needs and achieving personal goals may differ between the individual's place of origin and his new abode.

Such losses, changes and stresses, particularly if they occur with any frequency, can lead to a breakdown in health.

One study of "social" coronary risk factors has demonstrated that migration, considered in the broad sense discussed above, plays an important role in the causation of heart disease. Some of the relevant factors named in the study are: (1) recent migration to an urban center, (2) high residential mobility, (3) high occupational mobility, (4) great discontinuity between childhood and adult environment and situation, (5) status incongruity (individuals high on one social status dimension and low on another), (6) residence in an area undergoing rapid increase in its degree of urbanization, (7) recent first entrance to an industrial occupation.[93]

Migration, like other stressors, causes neuroendocrine changes that result in physiologic and psychologic imbalances in the individual which, in turn, can lead to a greater susceptibility to illness. Thus, migration undoubtedly plays an underlying role in many of the ills that distress people today.

Ecologic Factors

Ecology can be defined as the branch of biology dealing with the mutual relations between organisms and their environment. *Human ecology,* a science that particularly interests us in nursing, is the scientific study of the interrelationships between human beings and their environment.

In essence, human ecology implies a certain mutuality and balance between individual human beings and people and nature. When humans are in a state of ecologic balance, they are healthy; conversely, when they are out of balance with the environment and with other humans and are no longer able to make successful adaptations, they are ill.

Ecologic balance is most easily maintained in environments that are stable and fairly settled, so that stresses and the need for change are at a minimum. However, when people must exist under environmental conditions that are upset, unsettled, or highly complex, ecologic balance tends to break down and morbidity and mortality rates rise.

War, for example, tends to upset the ecologic balance of both human beings and nature. War and disease are closely linked; over the centuries epidemics and plagues have followed battles, killing large numbers of the remaining populace. Even today, warfare and disease are inseparable. The large numbers of displaced persons, often poorly clothed and crowded together; the incapacitation of public health facilities with resultant pollution and general lack of sanitation; the problems of food production and food supply; the cultural and psychologic deprivation; and the lack of medical care can all seriously upset the ecologic balance of a wartorn country. Such imbalances increase the vulnerability of a population to serious epidemics.

Second, large-scale migrations and explorations also upset the ecologic balance. Whenever two different peoples come together, each group is exposed to new diseases for which they have developed no immunity. Many isolated primitive populations have had remarkably high levels of health until explorers exposed them to diseases from the outside world, against which the primitive people had no defense.

Third, people's attempts to control the environment through technologic innovation have also disturbed the ecologic balance. The problem of technology as a stressful factor in modern society is considered below.

Occupational Factors

While most jobs produce stress, some occupations are apparently more stressful than others. In a study of job-related stress, Russet compiled data on 14,000 people in 14 categories of jobs. He rated the various occupations according to their "possible stressfulness" and the likelihood of their producing illnesses. His research showed some interesting relationships: For example, general practitioners were found to work under more stress than dermatologists and pathologists, and the general practitioners suffered three to four times more heart attacks than did the specialists. Trial lawyers experienced three times as many heart attacks as did patent attorneys and real estate lawyers, whose work, apparently, is less stressful. Security traders between 40 and 69 years old developed twice as many heart attacks as did security analysts within the same age group; again, security traders are apparently in a more stressful occupation.[48]

The stressful nature of critical care nursing was discussed by Benoliel in a symposium on stress. She pointed out that in intensive care and coronary care units, nurses are exposed to heavy work loads, great responsibility for others, repeated exposure to death and dying, constant contact with pain and distress, crowded work spaces, and communications problems with staff, patients, and families. Nurses working under these conditions experience considerably more stress and pressure than do nurses working in less demanding units. For these reasons, Benoliel advises critical care nurses to develop specific ways of coping with their stress-producing work.[12]

On the other hand, while the deadlines and heavy responsibility in some occupations produce stress, boring, repetitive work is also stressful. According to Frankenhaeuser, workers in mechanized industrial settings (e.g., on assembly lines) experience machine-paced repetitive work and greatly lessened opportunities for social intercourse; these dehumanizing conditions can eventually lead to illness.[44, 45]

Thus high levels of stress are associated both with jobs that are too varied and demanding and jobs that are boring. However, in the last analysis, most researchers agree that it is the individual's *response* to the pressures and problems of the job rather than the job itself that produces ulcers, heart disease, and other stress-related disorders.

Stressful Factors Within Technologic Societies

Within technologic societies such as ours, one finds almost all the stressful factors we have already discussed. Over and above these factors, however, there are other agents that particularly affect technologic societies and that are mainly responsible for the prevalence of chronic degenerative diseases within Western culture. Many of these underlying factors have been created, unwittingly, by human beings as they attempt to control disease, the environment, life and civilization.

More specifically, the major stressful factors within technologic societies are (1) products of our industrial technology, (2) products of our medical technology, and (3) the result of social conditions. Additional agents result from an interplay between social and technologic factors. Let us briefly discuss each of these areas.

Products of Industrial Technology. Some of the industrial technologic factors that contribute to the development of disease are: (1) pollution of air and water with gases, wastes, and poisons — for example, the dangerous byproducts of factories, automobile exhausts, and cigarette smoking; (2) overuse of lethal insecticides and weedkillers, contaminating our water and food; and (3) use of dangerous radioactive materials by science and industry.

Products of Medical Technology. Medical technology, while alleviating many disease factors, has at the same time created perplexing problems by (1) developing numerous dangerous and powerful drugs and other forms of therapy and (2) lengthening the human life span. The number of drugs and medicinal preparations available today is staggering. Ninety per cent of the drugs prescribed by the modern doctor did not exist 20 years ago. Many of these medications, while seemingly safe, have not been subjected to the long test of time. Consequently they may have some unexpected and frightening consequences. For example, young women who have been exposed to diethylstilbestrol (DES) prenatally are highly prone to the development of gynecologic abnormalities and diseases, including carcinoma.[58]

Even those drugs that have been in use for a long time often have dangerous side effects. Allergies to penicillin can be fatal. Chloromycetin, a broad-spectrum antibiotic, has frequently produced aplastic anemia — a potentially deadly disease in which the bone marrow ceases to produce blood cells. Moreover, certain antibiotics and sulfa drugs can destroy the natural flora of the intestinal tract or the vagina, thereby upsetting the ecologic balance of the body. Even aspirin, if taken in too large doses or too frequently, can be poisonous. High doses of phenacetin (a drug frequently combined with aspirin) may cause damage to kidney tissue. Tranquilizers, sleeping pills, weight reduction pills, contraceptive pills, along with thousands of other prescribed drugs, have their dangers. It is no wonder that, according to public health officials, over a million Americans every year are incapacitated for at least one day — sometimes requiring medical aid — because of the side effects and untoward effects of drugs.[38]

Although drugs are the commonest offenders in terms of untoward effects, other medical therapies are not exempt from being potentially dangerous. Let us look at a few examples. Patients can develop serum hepatitis from a blood transfusion; intravenous fluids can overload the circulation, resulting in a filling of the lungs with fluid; irradiation can precipitate leukemia; prescribed bed rest can result in such complications as kidney stones, blood clots, and decubitus ulcers. Disease caused by physicians in an effort to treat the patient is called *iatrogenic disease*.

Modern medicine, moreover, has created certain problems by *extending the average person's life span* in Western society to around 70 years. A long life has always been the dream of people everywhere but the increased longevity in technologic societies is unfortunately associated with a high incidence of chronic and degenerative diseases. Millions of Americans suffer from the chronic disorders of heart disease, cerebrovascular lesions, arthritis, and diabetes — all conditions that tend to appear in their most dangerous form *after* the age of 50. Doctors speculate that these degenerative conditions seem to be related, in some way, to longevity as well as to the person's way of life.

Social Conditions. The urban way of life and the social conditions under which we live constitute the third agent responsible for disease-producing stresses in technologic societies. People in technologic societies tend to live in cities, where they are subjected to certain social stresses. Crowding, vehicular traffic, conflicting life styles, crushing loneliness, racial upheavals, as well as the breakdown of traditional values, eventually take their toll in disease of body and mind. The alienated workman, the disillusioned teacher, the angry slum dweller, the lonely old person aware of obsolescence, the neurotic, the alcoholic, and the drug addict are common to our technologic society. These alienated products of urban life may be our friends and our patients; indeed, they may even be ourselves. As Eric and Mary Josephson express it in *Man Alone:*

> The alienated man is every man, and no man, drifting in a world that has little meaning for him and over which he exercises no power; a stranger to himself and to others . . .[73]

Although our whole society is affected by social stresses, certain groups *within* the society seem to be affected more than others. People of the lower socioeconomic and working classes, as well as certain minority groups, suffer from a higher incidence of disease than do members of the middle and upper classes. In the United States, infections, chronic disease, mental disease, dental caries, cancer, and tuberculosis all occur more commonly among the poor. The higher incidences of these conditions among the economically disadvantaged seem to be related to social isolation, malnutrition, ignorance, poor housing, and a generally low standard of living. Then too, single, widowed and divorced persons also suffer from increased morbidity and mortality rates. As Lynch emphasizes:

> It is a striking fact that U.S. mortality rates for all causes of death, not just heart disease, are consistently higher for divorced, single, and widowed individuals of both sexes and all races. Some of the increased death rates in unmarried individuals are astounding, rising as high as ten times the rates for married individuals of comparable ages.[85]

Many of the agents that underlie chronic disease are the result of an *interplay* among several different factors within our society. One example of such interplay is *obesity* — an important predisposing condition in hypertension and heart disease. The problem of obesity is related to overeating and lack of exercise, both of which are the result of technologic developments and/or emotional and social maladjustment. Technologically, modern farming and marketing methods have made potentially fattening foods easily available; also, the use of the automobile and various labor-saving devices has reduced physical exertion to a minimum for the average American. From a social viewpoint, our society is one in which many people are lonely, nervous, and under emotional stress. Often such people tend to chronically overeat and become obese. Thus, food, made readily available by modern technology, becomes a dangerous solace for those who live sedentary lives under stressful social conditions.

To summarize, while the urban way of life has reduced some health problems, it has obviously produced new problems that are equally serious. On the one hand, we live in a society in which technology gives us a long life, sanitation, pure food and drugs, and comparative freedom from infectious disease. On the other hand, this same society burdens us with pollution, iatrogenic disease, the pain of chronic maladies, and the evils of human alienation, mental illness, and prolonged old age.

BIBLIOGRAPHY

The bibliography for this chapter is located at the end of Unit III, p. 73.

CHAPTER 6

RESPONSES TO STRESS-PRODUCING FACTORS

Trapped in jobs we want to escape, or locked into contracts that seem to bind, or graced by life patterns that breed euphoria, too many of us subsequently overreact, underreact, or react inappropriately, thus providing the stage setting in which illness occurs.[39]

As we have seen, many stressful agents can precipitate disease. However, it is our *individual reaction* to these stressors that ultimately determines the *extent* to which a potentially dangerous stressor can cause a breakdown of tissues, organs, or mental apparatus. Consider now the area of human response from the following standpoints:

- The body's response to physical injury
- The body's response to psychologic stimuli
- Behavioral responses to stress
- Responses productive of disease
- Methods for developing adaptive responses to stress

THE BODY'S RESPONSE TO PHYSICAL INJURY

Providing a degree of protection against bodily injury is one of the major functions of our skin, bones, gastrointestinal tract, blood, liver, and nervous system. For example, the *skin* is the first line of defense against invasion by microorganisms; moreover, its pigmentation protects humans from the adverse effects of certain types of radiation. The *bones* protect the vital organs; the *gastrointestinal tract* neutralizes certain poisons by means of mucous secretions; the *blood* contains antibacterial and antiviral substances; the *liver* detoxifies poisons and dangerous drugs; and, finally, the *nervous system* provides protective reflexes and instincts as well as with the reasoning and intelligence necessary to fight or to flee from stressful and dangerous situations.

Should the protective functions of these structures fail, and the individual subsequently develop a disease or injury, the body continues to respond in a protective manner, this time against the effects of injury and disease.

The body exhibits only a few types of reactions to physical injury. Selye has pointed out that the major reactions elicited by injury are *inflammation, sclerosis, increased capillary permeability, hormonal responses,* and certain *fluid* and *electrolyte shifts.* In cases of infection, *antibodies* are usually built up as a defense against the troublesome organisms. When there has been a long-continued exposure to infectious disease, an *immune* reaction may develop as yet another type of bodily defense. An immune response involves the development of protective proteins in response to an invasion of the body by foreign and dangerous protein substances. In addition, the *nervous system and brain* continue to defend us against the effects of injury by promoting helpful adaptations and through the use of intelligence, knowledge, and will.

Inflammation is the most typical response by the body to tissue injury from whatever cause. Inflammation is defined as an immediate aggressive response by the body to the injury of or potential destruction of its cells and tissues. The classic signs of inflammation are redness, heat, pain, and swelling. Because inflammation tends to remain localized, it is the outstanding example of the body's ability to respond to stress on a *limited basis,* or, according to Selye's stress theory, by means of the local adaptation syndrome (LAS). When stresses become overwhelming, the body *responds as a whole,* with the release of pituitary and adrenal hormones, an increase in blood sugar, and changes in blood pressure and temperature. In terms of Selye's theory, these responses are manifestations of the alarm reaction or first stage of the GAS, in which the entire body mobilizes for action.

In sum, body tissues and organs have only a limited number of defensive responses against a destructive stressor or against the effects of injury and disease. Responses may develop either at a local site undergoing stress, or they may involve the entire organism in an "all-out" encounter against the stressful invader. (See Fig. 6–1.)

THE BODY'S RESPONSE TO PSYCHOLOGIC STIMULI*

The body is remarkably sensitive to even slight psychologic stimuli, responding in observable ways to almost every perceptible variation in the environment. Because the *autonomic nervous system* (ANS) mediates these responses, one must understand (a) the effects of psychologic stimuli upon ANS functions, i.e., those functions that are controlled by the sympathetic and parasympathetic nervous systems and (b) the effects of the ANS upon other body systems. We review briefly here the anatomy and physiology of the ANS to help you understand the vital role it plays in the stress responses.†

Role of the Autonomic Nervous System

The autonomic nervous system is one of the major systems that helps the brain maintain unity of body function. It is the autonomic nervous system that controls the *visceral functions* of the body. The ANS is activated mainly in the hypothalamus, spinal cord, and brain stem. The peripheral motor portions of the autonomic nervous system are made up of preganglionic and postganglionic neurons.

Basically, the ANS is an *involuntary* system. It innervates (a) the smooth muscle found in the digestive tract, air passages of the lung, urinary bladder, uterus, blood vessels, and the eye; (b) cardiac muscle; and (c) the secreting glands, sweat glands, and digestive glands. Thus the ANS helps to regulate arterial blood pressure, heart rate, dilation and constriction of the bronchial tubes, gastrointestinal secretion and motility, urinary output, sweating, body temperature, and the size of the pupil of the eye. The overall function of the autonomic nervous system appears to be maintaining homeostasis of the internal environment.

Anatomically, the ANS is divided into two parts: the sympathetic and parasympathetic nervous systems. *Chemically,* the ANS is also divided into two sections: the cholinergic and adrenergic systems.

Anatomic Divisions of the ANS

1. *The sympathetic nervous system* (SNS). The SNS originates from all the thoracic and the first three lumbar segments of the spinal cord. The SNS is a two neuron system. The nerve fiber that leaves the spinal cord stops in a sympathetic ganglion; it is called the the preganglionic fiber. The second fiber starts from the ganglion, extends to the termination at smooth muscle, and is called the postganglionic fiber.

When nerve impulses reach the end of the postganglionic nerve fiber, they bring about the release of the chemical substance called *norepinephrine.* The release of norepinephrine triggers either a contraction or relaxation of smooth muscle — depending upon whether it is an excitory or inhibitory nerve ending. In the case of sweat glands and some blood vessels, *acetylcholine* (ACH) is released instead of norepinephrine.

*We appreciate the valuable information contributed by Alma Ware, R.N., M.N., concerning the autonomic nervous system.

†The anatomy and physiology of the ANS is also discussed in Unit X; the anatomy is illustrated on p. 492.

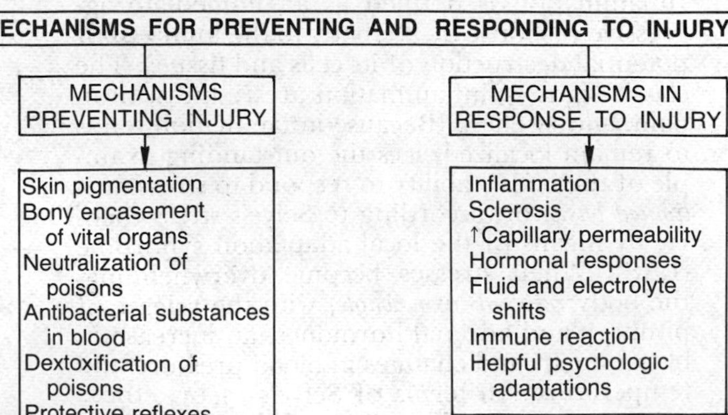

Figure 6–1. Major body mechanisms that prevent injury and defend a person against injury once it occurs.

Also, when nerve impulses pass along the preganglionic sympathetic fibers leading to the *adrenal medulla,* both norepinephrine and epinephrine are released as hormones. When these two hormones reach the sympathetic nerve terminations via the blood stream, they augment the local sympathetic action.

The major action of the SNS is the constriction of blood vessels. In addition, increased SNS activity causes the heart to speed up and the force of the ventricle contractions to increase. This leads to increased blood pressure; the eye pupils dilate; sweating occurs; and the contractions of the arrectores pilorum muscles cause the "hair to stand on end" and goose pimples to form. Blood glucose and free fatty acid levels increase, and movements of the digestive tract are reduced. Furthermore, the air passages dilate (thereby allowing for a fuller intake of oxygen), since the bronchi and bronchioles are composed of smooth muscle, which is relaxed by sympathetic nervous system action.

> *The SNS is particularly active when the body is responding to perceived states of* disequilibrium. *Thus the SNS is associated with the "fight-or-flight" "aggression-versus-avoidance" reactions.*

2. *The parasympathetic nervous system* (PNS). Like the SNS, the PNS is also a two neuron system. The outflow nerve fibers originate in the cranial nerves and in the sacral region of the spinal cord. The cranial nerves that contain parasympathetic fibers innervate the visceral structures in the face, neck, head, thorax, upper abdomen, heart, lungs, and almost all abdominal organs. The sacral outflow supplies the pelvic viscera, colon, rectum, and bladder.

When the PNS nerve impulse reaches its termination, the chemical substance *acetylcholine* is released. The released acetylcholine may bring about either contraction or relaxation of the muscle. Unlike SNS activity, which is augmented by the adrenal medulla, there is no endocrine gland that augments the activity of the PNS by hormone release.

In direct opposition to SNS action, the PNS is associated with "repose" and the more "vegetative" or maintenance functions of the body. It acts primarily on glands, smooth muscles, and in the gut. It slows the heart, lowers blood pressure, constricts the pupils and air passages, speeds up digestion of food, and plays an important part in defecation and micturition. It stimulates the production of saliva, gastric juice, and pancreatic juice; increases the motility of the digestive tract; and, at the same time, relaxes the digestive tract sphincters. It appears to be a more discrete system than the sympathetic; that is, its activity, at any given time, may be restricted to certain organs of the body.

Chemical Divisions of the ANS. The ANS is divided chemically into the cholinergic and adrenergic divisions, based on which specific chemical substance — either acetylcholine or epinephrine — is released at the ganglionic synapses and effector end organs upon transmission of ANS impulses.

1. *Adrenergic division.* Autonomic fibers that release epinephrine are called adrenergic fibers; these fibers are also sympathetic fibers. Adrenergic fibers generally *excite* activity, except in the gastrointestinal tract, where they inhibit activity.

2. *Cholinergic division.* Autonomic fibers that release acetylcholine are called cholinergic fibers; cholinergic fibers are also parasympathetic fibers. These fibers basically *inhibit* activity, except in the gastrointestinal tract where they increase activity.

Specific Effects of Emotion and ANS Activity upon Body Systems

The Endocrine System. During the stress response (the fight-or-flight reaction), two of the major hormones released are epinephrine and norepinephrine. These two hormones (also called adrenaline and noradrenalin, respectively) are referred to collectively as catecholamines. The levels of catecholamine secretion reflect the state of the human organism and the influence of the environment upon that organism. The level of urinary excretion of catecholamines indicates the degree to which the person is psychologically aroused, i.e., the intensity of the person's feelings.[43] Peripheral release of catecholamines allows the individual to cope both mentally and physically with stressful environments. However, chronic elevations of catecholamines may result in permanent pathologic changes within the body tissues. For example, persons with type A personalities (whose fight-or-flight response is continually being aroused) tend to secrete more epinephrine and norepinephrine than do type B personalities. Recall from Chapter 4 that type A individuals suffer more heart disease than do non–type A persons.

Many studies have been published that clearly indicate that catecholamine excretion varies according to an individual's *activity level, stimulation level, mood,* and *personality.*

- Concerning *activity,* when a person is inactive and resting, epinephrine secretion is low. With ordinary daily activities, secretion levels rise to twice the resting level. In active and moderately stressful situations, secretion rates may be three to five times resting levels.

- In a study of *stimulation levels* and stress, persons who were *either* understimulated or overstimulated were found to suffer more stress and were shown to release greater amounts of catecholamines than those persons who were moderately stimulated.[43]
- The effect of a person's *mood* upon catecholamine secretion was studied by Wyatt and associates. Wyatt found that persons with periods of anxiety and depression lasting 6 months or longer had significantly higher total plasma catecholamine levels than the levels in control subjects. It was also found that epinephrine output definitely increases when a person is angry or fearful.[77]
- Some studies indicate that certain *personality* types — psychopaths and criminally deviant persons — are also deviant in autonomic responses to stress. Apparently, unlike more normal personality types, psychopaths do not react to threat with a higher than normal catecholamine secretion until danger is imminent. This finding correlates with the belief that psychopathic personalities lack the ability to plan and to fantasize future happenings and their reactions to them.[83, 161]

Other hormones whose secretion increases as a result of stress include adrenocorticotropin (ACTH), the glucocorticoids, aldosterone, and antidiuretic hormone (ADH).*

ACTH is a pituitary hormone that regulates the activity of the adrenal cortex and, consequently, the secretion of *cortisol* — the most important of the glucocorticoids.

The *glucocorticoids,* in turn, influence the secretion of ACTH and the metabolism of glucose, protein, and fat. During the stress response, cortisol (a) increases the rate of amino acid metabolism, (b) converts proteins and fats into glucose that provides the body with needed energy, and (c) enhances the effects of the catecholamines upon the heart.

Aldosterone, a mineralocorticoid secreted by the adrenal cortex, promotes sodium retention, which in turn, increases extracellular fluid volume. A major stimulus for the release of aldosterone is hemorrhage.

Antidiuretic hormone (ADH), which is secreted by the pituitary gland, conserves body water. Its release is stimulated by the following factors: reduced circulatory blood volume, pain, morphine sulfate injections, barbiturates, emotional stress, anesthetics, surgical trauma, and trauma due to accidents.

The Circulatory System. Slight changes in the environment are capable of affecting the heart rate, arteriole size, muscle tone of veins, and circulating blood volume. For example, hearing a door creak open can produce noticeable changes in arterial pressure, and driving even in moderate traffic can cause alarming elevations of blood pressure. Thus, fairly minor and routine stimuli can result in noticeable physiologic responses.

Although emotions do not have to be intense to produce an autonomic nervous system response, the type of emotional response is related to the type of circulatory change evoked. For example, when we feel angry, hostile, and anxious, the arterioles in the skin and kidneys and throughout the body constrict. This constriction of vessels, in turn, makes the heart beat faster, alters heart rhythm, and causes the arterial blood pressure to rise. On the other hand, when we feel fearful, depressed, or in despair, the opposite reactions occur: heart rate slows and blood pressure falls. If life seems truly bleak or shocking, we may attempt to escape it entirely by fainting.

Observable *local* changes also result from disturbances in the circulation due to emotional stimuli. Who has not observed the flush of anger, the pallor of fear, or the blush of embarrassment? All these color changes of the skin are under autonomic nervous system control, and thus are accompanied by alterations in blood pressure.

The Digestive System. The digestive system, like the circulatory system, responds differently to different sets of emotional stimuli. For example, when one feels angry and hostile, the gastric mucosa reddens and the secretions and movements of the stomach increase in volume and magnitude. Moreover, the colon flushes and may become continuously spastic. Conversely, such feelings as sorrow, disappointment, and fear cause the mucosa of stomach and colon to pale and the movements of these organs to slow or cease. Anorexia, nausea, and vomiting may result. Even the salivary glands are affected by emotion. We all know that the mouth becomes very dry when we are afraid and that it literally "waters" when we are anticipating something pleasant, for example, a good meal. Thus, the body does not lie; through its response to psychologic stimuli it gives us a good indication of how we truly feel about a situation.

Other Systems. The *bladder* also responds in predictable ways to opposing sets of emotions. For example, the person who feels resentful, frustrated, or upset tends to have an increase in bladder contraction and a resultant sense of urgency. Conversely, a sense of dejection or depression causes the bladder wall to

*ACTH and glucocorticoids are discussed in Chapter 74; aldosterone and ADH are considered in Chapter 12.

relax and urine is retained. Fear can cause incontinence of urine in both children and adults.

The *pupil of the eye* is affected by emotion. It tends to become smaller when we are sleepy or uninterested in our environment and, conversely, to enlarge when we are stimulated, afraid, or in a state of rage; hence, the descriptive expression "wide-eyed with fear." The *bronchial muscle*, the *sweat glands*, and the *temperature-regulating mechanisms* are also subject to changes due to psychologic stress. We all know that breathing alters with excitement, sweating can result from fear or passion, and we can feel cold or hot depending upon the immediate events in our lives.

The body's *musculature* also responds to psychologic stress. In Figure 6–2, observe the tautness of this Olympic swimmer's muscles [illegible] he waits to enter into w[illegible] may be the most significant competitive event [illegible] his life.[140] Now compare the swimmer with [illegible] Figure 6–3. This woman, wit[illegible] stunned [illegible]vastation of [illegible] [illegible]quake, shows a [illegible] decrease in muscle tone. Her mouth, jaw, face, shoulders and entire body sag as she gazes upon a situation with which she is momentarily unable to cope. According to Engel and Schmale, the victim in this particular picture has entered a protective, primary biologic state that they term "conservation-withdrawal." Conservation-withdrawal is characterized by relative immobility, quiescence, and unresponsiveness to the environment; its most common manifestation is a "sustained decrease in muscle tone, especially of anti-gravity muscles." The conservation-withdrawal response is a protective mechanism to help sustain us in situations that threaten our psychological survival.[41]

Variations and Inconsistencies in Responses

It is important to note that these autonomic responses to stimuli are typical responses; in other words, people generally react in these particular ways to certain stressors. However, two different people can react to similar psychologic stresses in directly opposite ways. For example, one person caught in a stressful situation might prepare physiologically for a fight; another person of different temperament and upbringing might faint when under comparable emotional pressure. Indeed, the *same* person may respond to similar predicaments in different ways at different times, depending upon the person's perception of the stressor and defensive resources at the moment. In sum, the decision as to whether we should "stand and fight" or "faint and flee" depends upon our personality, our background, our

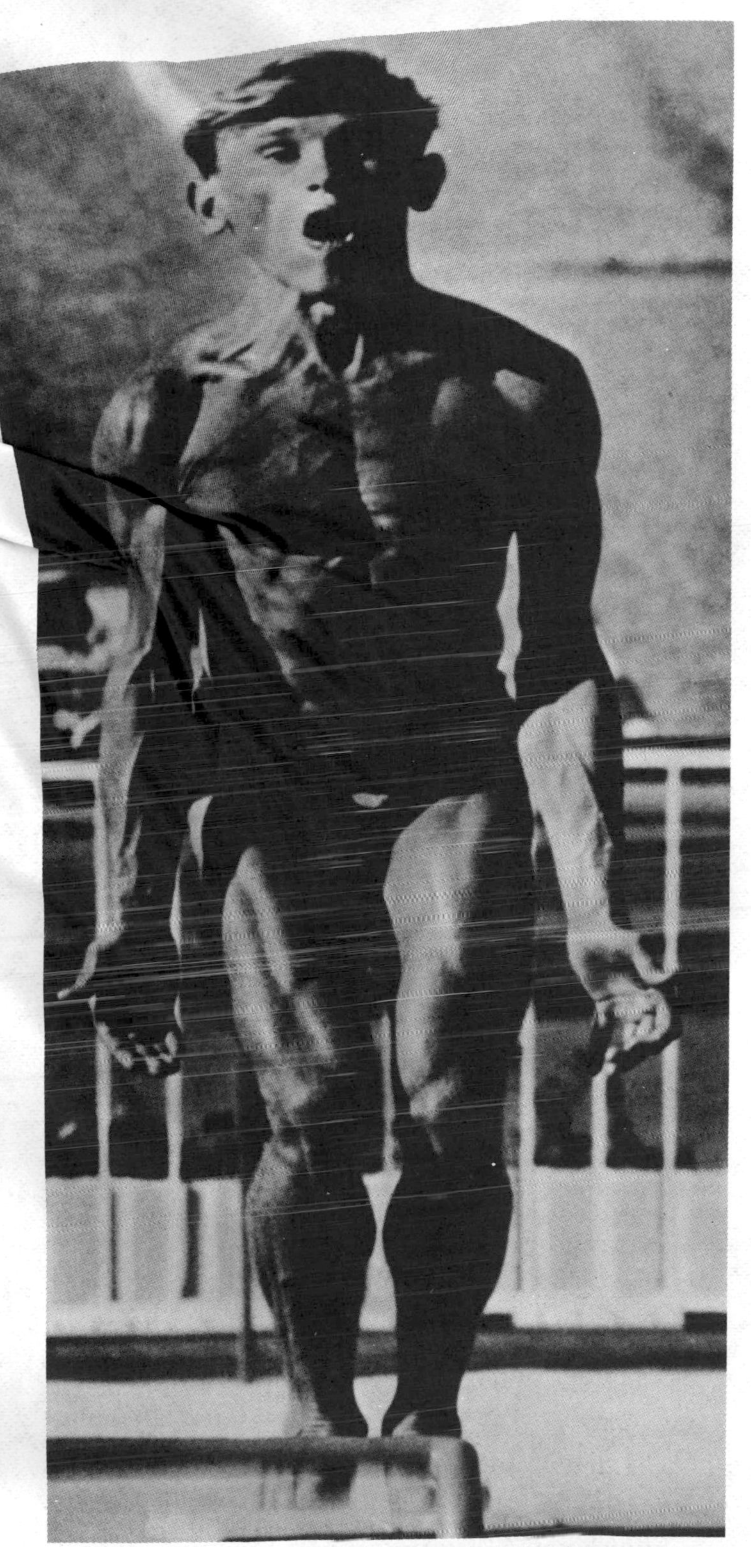

Figure 6–2. An example of muscle tensing and bulging in response to the stress of competitive sports. (From Tanner, O.: *Stress: Time-Life Library of Human Behavior.* New York: Time-Life Books, 1976, p. 16.)

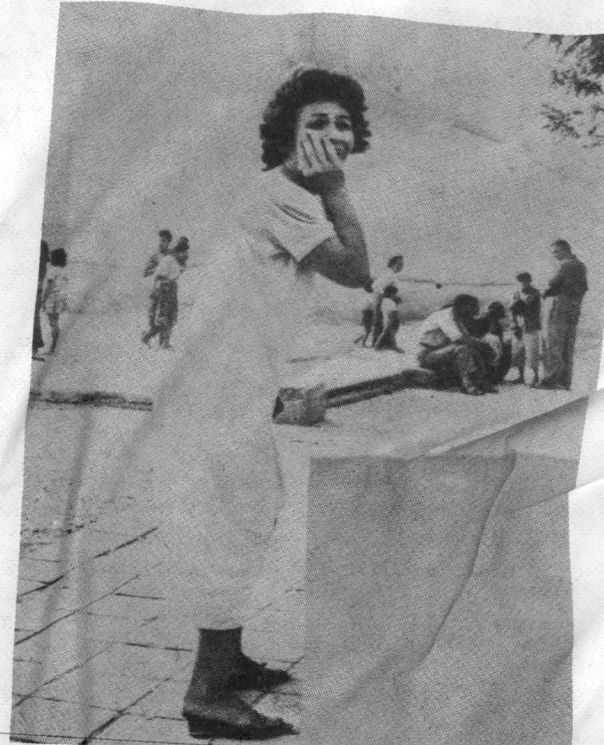

Figure 6–3. An example of muscle sagging in response to stress generated by viewing earthquake devastation. Note the slack jaw, rounded shoulders, and hand supporting head. (From Engel, G. L., and Schmale, A. H.: Conservation-withdrawal. A primary process for organismic homeostasis. *CIBA Foundation Symposium*, 8:57, 1972, p. 68.)

level of vitality at the moment, the circumstances immediately surrounding us, and the way in which our brain perceives and interprets the situation.

Just as the uncomfortable emotions of grief, depression, anger, hostility, and fear all produce body responses, *pleasurable emotions* such as joy, love, and happiness can also lead to physical changes. For example, some people weep "tears of joy" or "scream with joy" when they feel a sense of extreme relief or happy emotion; individuals passionately in love experience changes in heart rate and rhythm, breathing, and muscle tone; a person who feels satisfied after a meal with pleasant companions tends to relax and even to sleep.

Unpleasant bodily responses may also rise on joyful occasions. These undesirable somatic changes appear to be related to one of two factors: First, joy may be mingled with a sense of fear or anxiety; for example, a man may *believe* that he feels happy in a certain situation when in reality he feels *both* happy and anxious—the anxiety leading to many upsetting symptoms. For example, as you recall from Chapter 4, a young man on his wedding day may express feelings of happiness and joy. However, he may also be experiencing various doubts, fears for the future, anxieties concerning parenthood, and so forth. It is these essentially unpleasant emotions, then, rather than the sense of joy or happiness, that give rise to the unpleasant bodily sensations.

Second, unpleasant bodily changes in response to joy may also occur in individuals who are physically too weak or ill to adapt to any intense emotion, [illegible]en great happiness. Upon occasion su[illegible] people have literally died in a trans[illegible] joy. For example, pris[illegible] of N[illegible] many who were [illegible] weakened by [illegible] known to di[illegible] liberated. As one writer observed during just such a liberation:

> All these prisoners lit up with ineffable joy and hope when they saw the white Red Cross busses turn into the concrete square and grasped that they were to leave in them. For many, it was too much altogether, they hadn't the strength to grapple with so fantastic, so marvelous a prospect—they collapsed and died—literally—of joy.[131]

In summary, then, our bodies respond to emotional stimuli with certain definite physiologic changes which may be perceived by the individual as either pleasant or unpleasant. The sympathetic division of the ANS, in particular, plays a vital role in the body's response to stressors through the regulation of heart action, blood pressure, pulse, sensory changes, digestive tract function, bladder function, temperature regulation, and musculature. The degree of functional change in these tissues and organs depends upon the *type* of stressor impinging upon the person and also upon its magnitude and force.

BEHAVIORAL RESPONSES TO STRESS

An individual responds to stressors not only with physiologic changes but also with behavioral changes. Bryne and Thompson describe the following major behavioral changes that occur in response to stress:[21]

1. *Increased use of one specific form of behavior.* For example, when people feel pressured, they may "raid the icebox," drink or smoke excessively, sleep longer hours than normal, or extend their work day. Ask yourself what activity *you* perform excessively when you feel pressured.

2. *Change in the number of activities performed.* Some individuals become hyperactive when they feel stressed, whereas others attempt to cope by conserving their energies and decreasing their activities.

3. *Disorganized behavior which may deteriorate to the point of regression.* Most of us react to severe crises (e.g., an accident, illness, death of a loved one) by becoming somewhat disorganized in our activities, misassigning priorities, and neglecting details. Seriously ill or disturbed persons sometimes regress to childish behavior such as whining or temper tantrums.

4. *A lower frustration tolerance and increased irritability.* You probably know from your own experience that it takes very little to irritate someone who is feeling excessively pressured by life's problems. A person who is normally tolerant of others may, when sufficiently stressed, "blow up" in response to the slightest provocation.

5. *Noticeable physiologic changes that are correlated to behavioral changes.* For example, people suffering a stress reaction may breathe harder, their muscles may twitch or sag depending on the situation, the pupils of their eyes usually dilate, and their skin may redden or pale.

6. *Distortion of reality and decreased ability to problem solve.* Stressful situations sometimes cause people to lose their "grip on reality," i.e., these individuals temporarily lose their ability to accurately assess their situation and employ rational problem-solving methods. Persons undergoing severe crises may develop delusions and/or hallucinations; in other cases, they may become depressed to the point of suicide.

CHILDREN'S RESPONSES TO STRESS

Like adults, children must cope with stressful situations every day. The *physiologic* responses of children are basically the same as are those of adults, e.g., increased heart rate, increased rate and depth of respirations, pallor, cold and clammy skin, enlarged pupil size. However, children's *behavioral* responses to stress differ significantly from those of their elders. Furthermore, youngsters respond to stress differently at different ages and maturational stages. The major fears of children and their responses to stress by age group include:[11]

- Older infant and toddler: *Major fear*—separation from mother. *Verbal responses*—protests ("No"), cries, screams. *Nonverbal responses*—clings to mother; tries to escape; seeks mother with eyes if separated; turns away; avoids eye contact; rejects anyone except mother or father; kicks, flails, bites.
- Preschooler: *Major fear*—mutilation or body harm. *Verbal responses*—protests, cries, screams; uses words to express pain, anger, or fear; tries to postpone treatment in order to escape it ("Wait a minute"); groans, whines, whimpers. *Nonverbal responses*—preoccupied with injury and with actions of personnel; reaches for help, support; seeks body contact (usually with parent); tries to escape; holds rigidly still; turns away; kicks, flails, bites; frowns, clenches teeth; shuts eyes or keeps wide open.
- School-age child: *Major fear*—loss of self-control. *Verbal responses*—protests; uses words or sentences to express pain, anger or fear; tries to postpone treatment (to be in control and to appear brave); cries, screams, groans, whimpers. *Nonverbal responses*—may sit or lie quietly (to have control and appear brave); passively seeks help, body contact (usually will not ask for help but gladly accepts when offered); tries to escape; holds rigidly still; turns or pulls away; kicks, bangs hands or feet against stretcher table.

To cope with stress successfully, children who are frightened, sick, or injured need supportive care from nurses just as adults do. Children are entitled to a positive approach from the nurse, simple explanations of procedures, honest answers to their questions, and the chance to verbalize or vocalize their feelings without being reprimanded or punished.

MALADAPTIVE RESPONSES PRODUCTIVE OF DISEASE

Although many of our attempts to adapt to life's stresses prove satisfactory, some efforts tend to "backfire," causing injury and disease; still other attempts at adaptation fail because they are either inadequate or too chaotic to cope successfully with a stressful situation. Such maladaptive responses lie at the base of many illnesses.

Four major responses to stress that can be extremely damaging to an individual's health are the following: (1) the distorted anticipatory response, (2) the excessive response, (3) the deficient response, and (4) the inappropriate response.

The Distorted Anticipatory Response

Human reactions in anticipation of certain events can be helpful and protective if they are appropriate. For example, as we pointed out earlier, saliva and gastric juices tend to flow in anticipation of a meal, or epinephrine is released and the pupil of the eye enlarges in anticipation of danger. These are appropriate adaptive responses. However, the anticipatory response can be overused, misused, and badly distorted. For instance, when a person thinks intensely about something unpleasant that *might* happen, the body reacts physiologically *as if* that unpleasant thing were actually taking place.

According to Stewart Wolf, faulty reactions "in anticipation" give rise to a group of diseases that he calls the "as if" disorders.[155] One example of an "as if" disorder is the gastric ulcer. Evidently individuals with gastric ulcers consistently behave physiologically "as if" they were going to kill and eat individuals with whom they are in conflict; i.e., their stomachs prepare for a meal whenever they are faced with a hated opponent. Wolf hypothesizes that such a reaction was appropriate under prehistoric conditions, since a primitive man probably *did* want to kill and eat a dangerous opponent. Today, of course, cannibalism is inappropriate, and such behavior on the part of the stomach will not enable an individual to successfully handle a traumatic interpersonal relationship. The inappropriate digestive secretions will instead, over a period of time, lead to the development of gastric ulcers that will further aggravate the individual's life adjustment.

The Excessive Response

Excessive responses are those "apparent attempts at adaptation which either destroy by sheer excess or that, in correcting one defect, involve the organism in other complications caused directly by this same homeostatic effort."[112] Examples of such reactions abound in medical literature. Anaphylactic shock resulting from an overdose of a drug to which one is sensitive; fibrosis and the overgrowth of scar tissue; and the collagen disease, arthritis, are all disorders resulting from excessive attempts by the body to adapt to stress. In the area of mental disorder, excessive response is evident in persons with manic behavior and in individuals who are obsessive, overly compulsive, hyperactive, or hypersensitive to small stimuli. The person with a type A behavior pattern (discussed in Chapter 4) is an individual who responds excessively to stressful situations and who consequently develops heart disease.

The Deficient Response

Feebleness, inadequacy, and failure characterize the deficient response to stressors. In essence, the deficient reaction is representative of a person's weakness of mind and body and vulnerability to the endless stresses of life.

There are numerous examples of inadequate responses in human pathology. For instance, secondary infections represent a failure of tissue response; congenital malformation represents a failure of prenatal development. Nutritional deficiency, starvation, paralysis, atrophy, ischemia, necrosis, hypofunction, endocrine failure, impotence, and senility are all common examples of the body's inadequacy and failure to adapt because of deficient responses. The deficient response is characteristic of even the most vigorous people; everyone has an Achilles' heel—an area of special vulnerability. For instance, such problems as poor eyesight, poor digestion, and inadequate coordination are common.

The Inappropriate Response

In terms of human physiology and psychology, this type of response can be defined as "an ill-timed, inopportune, misguided, inappropriate, blundering reaction of whatever kind."[112] This is the type of reaction that tends to worsen an already stressful situation. One example of an inappropriate response is the body's tendency, when in heart failure, to absorb large amounts of salt and water—a response which only aggravates matters by overloading an already weakened heart with fluid. Another example of an inappropriate response is hysteria, or conversion reaction, in which an individual develops physical symptoms (e.g., blindness, deafness, or partial paralysis) in reaction to psychologic trauma or conflict which is difficult to solve. Again, this response because it is inappropriate, worsens the situation by further incapacitating the stressed individual.

Summary of Responses to Stress

Let us now generally summarize the topic of human response to stress-producing factors. First of all, the body's organs and structures not only serve to protect us against injury, but they also serve to protect us once injury develops. The body responds to *physical injury* by means of inflammation, increased capillary permeability, sclerosis, fluid and electrolyte shifts, the production of antibodies, and the development of the immune reaction against infection. Body reactions to stressors—physical, chemical, or bacterial—may be local or generalized.

Second, the body also responds physiologically to *psychologic stimuli.* Changes in endocrine function; heart action, rate, and rhythm; changes in digestive and urinary tract function; and changes in muscle tone and body temperature all represent physical responses to both negative and positive emotional states. Many of these responses are mediated by the autonomic nervous system.

Third, an individual responds not only physiologically to stress but also with changes in behavior. Finally, *maladaptive attempts* to adapt to stress can lead to serious consequences for the health of the individual. Responses that are distorted, excessive, deficient, or inappropriate are all maladaptations that can result in injury, disease, and death.

As Wolf sums it up:

> Disease, then, may reflect too much or too little of certain adaptive functions, resulting in essentially inappropriate physiologic behavior.
>
> Virtually, every disease becomes a disease, then, on the basis of quantitative considerations.[157]

DEVELOPING ADAPTIVE RESPONSES TO STRESS

Because stressful factors are a part of our lives, it is essential to develop adaptive responses to stress — thereby minimizing illness and generating health. How to adapt to stress is a growing area of research. Numerous academic and popular publications today promote various methods of stress control. Some of the current techniques include (a) relaxation techniques, (b) biofeedback training, (c) stress reduction programs, and (d) development of a rational philosophy of life. Below we briefly touch upon some of these techniques — some of which may help you in controlling the stress of your own life.*

Relaxation Techniques

There are many relaxation techniques available that result in "a set of integrated physiologic changes" (e.g., lowered vital signs).[13] These changes apparently act to (a) reduce the damaging psychophysiologic effects of stress and (b) promote a sense of physical and mental well being.

Some of the methods most commonly taught include Benson's relaxation response, transcendental meditation (TM), autogenic training, progressive relaxation, hypnotic suggestion, and yoga. These techniques appear to have the following characteristics in common:

1. They result in an *altered state of consciousness.*
2. They produce a *decrease in sympathetic nervous system activity,* which consequently counterbalances the fight-flight emergency reaction to real or imagined threats or stressors. Specific physiologic changes resulting from relaxation techniques include decreased oxygen consumption, blood pressure, pulse, respirations, arterial blood lactate as well as a slightly increased blood flow to the resting forearm muscle. In addition, the relaxation response involves an increase in intensity of slow alpha waves and some theta wave activity.
3. They each require *four basic elements* for the relaxation response to take place.[14]
   A. A calm quiet environment with minimal distractions.
   B. A mental device, e.g., a mantra sound or single syllable word which is repeated over and over; mental imagery.
   C. A passive attitude, i.e., the individual does not try to force relaxation but simply allows relaxation "to happen." Distracting thoughts and sounds are gently "pushed aside."
   D. A comfortable position that helps to reduce the need for muscular effort. Ideally, the individual's head and arms should be supported, clothing loose and nonrestrictive, and shoes off.

*Specific methods for modifying type A behavior patterns are described in Chapter 36.

The various techniques differ in the degree to which they concentrate upon either somatic (bodily) aspects of relaxation or upon cognitive (mental) aspects. They also vary in the precise steps for achieving a relaxed state. Some of the specific techniques and their characteristics are:

Benson's Relaxation Response. This is a very simple procedure, which does not rely upon religious or cultic beliefs and does not require a change in lifestyle. It was developed by Harold Benson. His method for achieving the relaxation response involves six basic steps:

> *1. Sit quietly in a comfortable position.*
>
> *2. Close your eyes.*
>
> *3. Deeply relax all your muscles, beginning at your feet and progressing up to your face. Keep them deeply relaxed.*
>
> *4. Breathe through your nose. Become aware of your breathing. As you breathe out, say the word "one" silently to yourself. For example, breathe in . . . out, "one;" in . . . out, "one;" etc.*
>
> *5. Continue for 20 minutes. You may open your eyes to check the time, but do not use an alarm. When you finish, sit quietly for several minutes at first with eyes closed and later with eyes open.*
>
> *6. Do not worry about whether you are successful in achieving a deep level of relaxation. Maintain a passive attitude and permit relaxation to occur at its own pace. When distracting thoughts occur, ignore them and continue repeating "one." With practice, the response should come with little effort. Practice the technique once or twice daily, and not within 2 hours after any meal, since the digestive processes seem to interfere with the elicitation of anticipated changes.*[15]

Transcendental Meditation. Originally developed by the Maharishi Mahesh Yogi, an Indian scholar and teacher, TM is not learned from a book or written instructions. Instead, the new "meditator" is instructed individually and is given a specific mantra, or sound, to repeat throughout meditation periods. Persons who use TM regularly, meditate with their mantra for 20 minutes twice a day.

Autogenic Training. Originated by the neuropsychiatrist J. H. Schultz in the early 1900's, the basis of autogenic training is *passive attention* to the body. The subject begins by sitting quietly in a comfortable chair and then proceeds through the following six exercises:[32]

1. Inducing sensations of heaviness of limbs. To do this, the person thinks "My right arm is heavy; my left arm is heavy."
2. Inducing sensations of warmth in the limbs. "My right arm is warm."
3. Cardiac regulation. "Heartbeat calm and regular."
4. Respiratory regulations. "It breathes me."
5. Induction of sense of upper abdominal warmth. "My solar plexus is warm."
6. Induction of sense of coolness in the forehead. "My forehead is cool."

Apparently, students of autogenic regulation require between 4 and 10 months to develop the sense of passive concentration needed to receive optimum benefits from the exercises.

Progressive Relaxation. Originated by Jacobson, this is possibly the most widely used relaxation technique today. According to Jacobson, "anxiety and muscular relaxation produce opposite physiologic states, and therefore cannot exist together."[13, 70] Jacobson's method teaches the subject to concentrate upon various gross muscle groups in the body—first tensing and then relaxing each group.

Steps in Progressive Muscle Relaxation

1. Take your time; plan to spend about 20 to 30 minutes relaxing each time you do the exercise.
2. Find a comfortable place to relax. Make sure that no unwanted distractions are likely to occur. During the day, darkening the room may help. At night, be prepared to go to sleep right away.
3. During the tension part of the cycle, tense the muscle vigorously and hold the muscle tense for a slow count of 5 to 7 seconds (1001, 1002, 1003, 1004, 1005, 1006, 1007). Notice what the tension feels like.
4. During the relaxation part of the cycle, relax the muscle quickly and completely. Let your mind relax and appreciate how relaxed the muscle is feeling.
5. Tense and relax each muscle group twice. After you have completed the entire sequence, go back and tense and relax specific muscles where you still feel tension.
6. Try to keep all other muscles relaxed as you relax specific muscle groups.
7. Follow the order for tensing and relaxing the muscle groups:
    - Dominant hand and forearm
    - Dominant biceps
    - Nondominant hand and forearm
    - Nondominant biceps
    - Forehead
    - Eyes
    - Mouth and jaws
    - Neck and throat (shoulders forward; shoulders back; shrug shoulders)
    - Upper back (both ways)
    - Chest
    - Stomach
    - Buttocks
    - Thighs
    - Calves (feet pointed down; feet pointed up)
    - Feet (pointed out; pointed up)
8. Don't forget to use your favorite self-suggestions.

Hypnosis. Hypnotic suggestion to induce relaxation depends upon the use of *vivid imagery.* For example, once the subject is comfortable, the hypnotherapist may say: "Imagine descending in an elevator. As you pass each floor on the way down, you feel a little more relaxed." Or "imagine that you are at the seashore on vacation. The sun is warm and there is a pleasant breeze. You feel warm and drowsy." A hypnotic state may be induced either by a hypnotist or by the subject alone (auto-hypnosis). Individuals vary in their ability to be hypnotized. Susceptibility to hypnotic suggestion apparently depends upon the subject's ability to concentrate, imaginative powers, motivation to be hypnotized, faith in the therapist, and age. Persons under the age of six and elderly senile individuals make poor subjects.

Yoga. Yoga techniques have been employed within the Hindu culture for thousands of years. Yoga involves the practice of both physical exercises (hatha yoga) and meditation (raja yoga). Physical exercises concentrate on various postures, breathing techniques, and development of an erect and flexible spine. Mental exercises utilize mantras and imagery. The correct performance of yoga results in deep relaxation without drowsiness or sleep.

All of these techniques are clinically useful, especially in conditions caused by increased sympathetic nervous system activity. Disorders that respond particularly well to relaxation techniques are hypertension, certain arrhythmias, migraine headache, anxiety neuroses, and drug abuse.

Biofeedback Training

Biofeedback training enables selected subjects to become aware of and control one or surrounded by a thin nuclear membrane. The major functions of the nucleus are: (1) the regulation of enzymes produced by the cytoplasm, (2) cellular reproduction or mitosis, and (3) the control of an organism's hereditary characteristics through the transmission of genetic information. These functions are the responsibility of the nucleolus and the chromosomes — structures within the nucleus.

Nucleolus. The word "nucleolus" comes from the Latin word for *little kernel.* This spherical body is evidently composed of rows of bead-like particles or granules, loosely bound together and not encircled by a membrane. One function of the nucleolus is in the production of ribosomes (see section on endoplasmic reticulum). It is also known that the nucleolus contains *nucleic acid*—a vital substance composed of nitrogen bases, sugars, and phosphoric acid. Nucleic acid within the nucleolus exists in the form of *ribonucleic* acid, or RNA, while within the chromosomes it exists in the form of *deoxyribonucleic* acid, or DNA. RNA acts as a messenger by carrying vital information concerning enzyme construction from the DNA of the nucleus to the cytoplasm, where enzymes are produced.

Chromosomes. Within the nucleus of the human cell there are 46 chromosomes, which are grouped into 23 pairs, one member of the pair originating from the father and the other from the mother. The chromosomes themselves are composed of 50,000 to 100,000 genes. The genes carry hereditary information concerning both the species and the individual characteristics of an organism and transmit this information from generation to generation.

The genes are composed of DNA, which exists in a linear chain; two strands of DNA are intertwined in a "double helix." Many genes exist on a single DNA molecule. In order for these long molecules to fit into a small package such as the nucleus, they must coil many times over—much like a super-twisted telephone receiver cord. These coils are stabilized by proteins, which may also play roles in regulating the expression of these genes. Thus, these supercoiled DNA-protein structures appear in the nucleus as coarse, intensely staining granular materials that are referred to by microscopists as *chromatin.* Since each cell carries all the genes the organism possesses, and yet each cell needs to use only a small proportion of those genes, regulation of genetic material is necessary. The genes that the cell *does* use define the functions it performs and the structures it assumes. Regulation of genetic material, then, is the basis for differentiation of cells into various cell types; i.e. blood cells, kidney cells, liver cells and other types.

When a cell divides by *mitosis,* the chromosomes first make doubles of themselves. Mitosis is the process by which the cells of the body multiply. It is a continuous process that involves four complex phases: the prophase, the metaphase, the anaphase, and the telophase. The replicas migrate to opposite sides of the cell and when the cell splits and divides, each daughter cell is identical in every way to the parent cell. DNA, then, acts as the one single key to the once mysterious door of heredity.

DNA transcribes its message by producing an RNA molecule capable of translating the message into the form of a functional protein that can carry out the desired task. Thus the message is in the safekeeping of DNA throughout the life of the cell. One can see that damage to this permanent copy would be a serious loss to the cell.

In such a complex operation as the transmission of heredity, it is not surprising that mistakes are made in the process of duplicating cells. Genes can be lost or they can change in ways that are usually unfavorable to the welfare of the organism. Such a change is called a *mutation.* Lost genes and abnormal genes can lead to inborn errors of metabolism and resultant diseases, as well as to organisms that are physically abnormal in appearance. Examples of diseases caused by an inborn error of metabolism are phenylketonuria (PKU) and sickle cell anemia. An example of a harmless abnormality produced by a genetic mishap is albinism — a nonpathologic condition characterized by an abnormal absence of pigment from the skin, hair, and eyes.

The Cytoplasm. The cytoplasm, a fine, granular substance, is separated from the environment external to it by the cell membrane. Within the cytoplasm is the nucleus of the cell as well as specialized structures called *organelles.* The most important organelle is the mitochondrion. Other organelles are the endoplasmic reticulum, the Golgi apparatus, the lysosomes, microtubules, and microfilaments, and the centrioles.

Mitochondrion. The mitochondrion is often referred to as the "power-house" of the cell, or as a tiny cell-within-a-cell. The mitochondria are extremely complex chemical structures that are to the cell what an engine is to an automobile; they provide the cell with the energy it needs to perform its many activities (Fig. 9–4).

The number of mitochondria per cell varies from a few hundred to a few thousand, depending upon

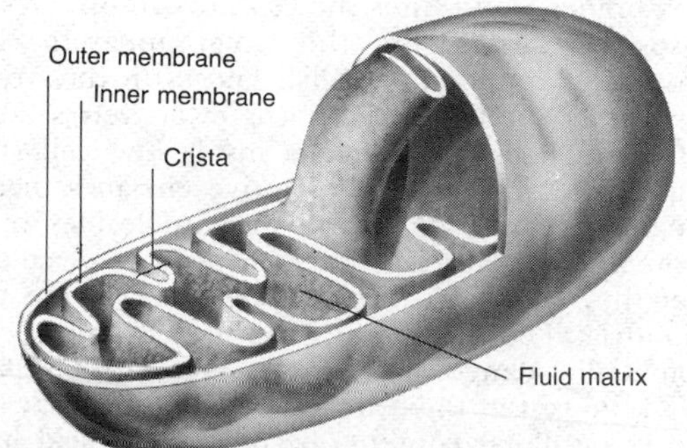

Figure 9–4. Structure of mitochondrion is basically that of a fluid filled vessel with an involuted wall. The wall consists of a double membrane, with infoldings of the inner one forming cristae. (Clark, M. E.: *Contemporary Biology,* 2nd ed. Philadelphia: W. B. Saunders Co., 1979, p. 114.)

the energy requirements of the particular cell. Notably, the erythrocyte is the only cell that does not contain mitochondria. Mitochondria, while highly organized and compartmentalized, are not static structures but are instead very dynamic. They replicate independently of the rest of the cell, and it has been postulated that they were at one time totally independent organisms much like bacteria.

The major function of the mitochondria is the oxidation of foodstuffs and the changing of energy released by oxidation into adenosine triphosphate (ATP), a substance which supplies most of the energy needed by the cell in its daily work and which is necessary for protein synthesis.

Endoplasmic Reticulum. The endoplasmic reticulum (ER) is composed of a fine network of tiny hollow tunnels that branch like miniature arteries throughout the inside of the cell. The ER, along with its other functions, evidently operates somewhat like a pipeline transporting materials throughout the cell as needed.

Studding some of the ER tunnels (*rough ER*) are the *ribosomes* — tiny spherical granular particles with a diameter of slightly less than one-millionth of an inch. The ribosomes, some of which float free in the cytoplasm, are the "factory hands" of the cell; they synthesize proteins. The proteins manufactured by the ribosomes are next transported into the ER tunnels and then on to the Golgi complex, the next station in the protein manufacturing assembly line.

Another type of ER, *smooth ER,* has no ribosomes. It binds enzymes to its surface and is involved with drug metabolism or degradation.

Golgi Apparatus. The Golgi apparatus is a group of miniature sacs filled with protein, which "package" proteins into vesicles. Many of these vesicles contain substances to be released at the cell surface as needed. It is known that the Golgi apparatus is involved in the bonding of carbohydrates to proteins; however, there is still much to be learned about the total role of this structure.

Lysosomes. The lysosome, a vesicle surrounded by membranes, constitutes the cell's organ of digestion. Lysosomes arise from the Golgi apparatus by a process of budding. Unlike most of the vesicles formed by the Golgi apparatus in actively secreting cells, the lysosomes remain inside the cell. Lysosomes contain powerful digestive enzymes that are capable of breaking down large molecules of fat, protein, and nucleic acid into small molecules so that they can be oxidized for energy by the mitochondria. The membranes of the lysosome keep its potentially dangerous digestive enzymes separate from the rest of the cell. Sometimes, however, when the intracellular contents become more acid in nature (e.g., as the result of a severe injury), the lysosome membranes rupture. The outpouring enzymes then destroy the cell as well as the bacteria — if any — that have created the lethal cellular disturbance.

While they obviously can be dangerous to the cell, lysosomes more often act as physiologic defense mechanisms. Authorities now believe that the polymorphonuclear white cells have the power to digest engulfed bacteria because they contain lysosomes within their cytoplasm. Lysosomes also perform the function of removing injured cells or cell parts from damaged tissues so that new cells can replace the old ones in the process of repair.

Microtubules and Microfilaments. The microtubules and microfilaments are filamentous structures within the cytoplasm that are involved in support and cell locomotion. They are often referred to as the cytoskeleton and the contractile forces of the cell. They have also been implicated in communication between the cell membrane and nucleus. Research in this field is only beginning to sort out the functions assigned to these structures.

Centriole. The centriole is a tiny body that plays a role in cell division and reproduction.

In review, the cell is composed of many highly complex, minute structures that work together in a coordinated manner.

Special Cell Units

Cells, while tiny compact worlds within themselves, do not exist in isolation; instead, cells bond together, according to their special functions, and form definite units or structures called *tissues.* In turn, tissues unite to form individual *organs.* The four major specialized types of cells of the body that we find united into larger tissue units are as follows:

- *Epithelial cells* are arranged in sheets. They cover the outside of the body and form the absorptive covering that lines the inside of the body's cavities and tubular structures.
- *Nerve cells* form the highly specialized, irritable, and conductive nerve tissue. Injured or destroyed nerve cells cannot be replaced.
- *Muscle cells,* by contracting and relaxing, do the physical work of the body.
- *Connective tissue cells* bind together and support other cells and tissues; they include blood cells and skeletal cells. *Blood cells* carry oxygen to the tissues, and carry carbon dioxide and wastes from the tissues. Also, they defend the body against microorganisms. *Structural cells* build the bony scaffolding and form the critical intercellular proteins that bind together the cells of the body. Collagen is the most important of these connective tissue proteins.

The fact that groups of cells are *specialized* in function presents critical problems for the total organism when any one group of cells breaks down. For example, the entire body depends upon the ability of the heart muscle to contract and to propel the body's circulation. Should the cells of the heart muscle be damaged or destroyed, the total organism and all relax and urine is retained. Fear can cause incontinence of urine in both children and adults.

The *pupil of the eye* is affected by emotion. It tends to become smaller when we are sleepy or uninterested in our environment and, conversely, to enlarge when we are stimulated, afraid, or in a state of rage; hence, the descriptive expression "wide-eyed with fear." The *bronchial muscle,* the *sweat glands,* and the *temperature-regulating mechanisms* are also subject to changes due to psychologic stress. We all know that breathing alters with excitement, sweating can result from fear or passion, and we can feel cold or hot depending upon the immediate events in our lives.

The body's *musculature* also responds to psychologic stress. In Figure 6–2, observe the tautness of this Olympic swimmer's muscles as he waits to enter into what may be the most significant competitive event of his life.[140] Now compare the swimmer with the stunned woman in Figure 6–3. This woman, witnessing for the first time the total devastation of her neighborhood from an earthquake, shows a remarkable decrease in muscle tone. Her mouth, jaw, face, shoulders and entire body sag as she gazes upon a situation with which she is momentarily unable to cope. According to Engel and Schmale, the victim in this particular picture has entered a protective, primary biologic state that they term "conservation-withdrawal." Conservation-withdrawal is characterized by relative immobility, quiescence, and unresponsiveness to the environment; its most common manifestation is a "sustained decrease in muscle tone, especially of anti-gravity muscles." The conservation-withdrawal response is a protective mechanism to help sustain us in situations that threaten our psychological survival.[41]

Variations and Inconsistencies in Responses

It is important to note that these autonomic responses to stimuli are typical responses; in other words, people generally react in these particular ways to certain stressors. However, two different people can react to similar psychologic stresses in directly opposite ways. For example, one person caught in a stressful situation might prepare physiologically for a fight; another person of different temperament and upbringing might faint when under comparable emotional pressure. Indeed, the *same* person may respond to similar predicaments in different ways at different times, depending upon the person's perception of the stressor and defensive resources at the moment. In sum, the decision as to whether we should "stand and fight" or "faint and flee" depends upon our personality, our background, our

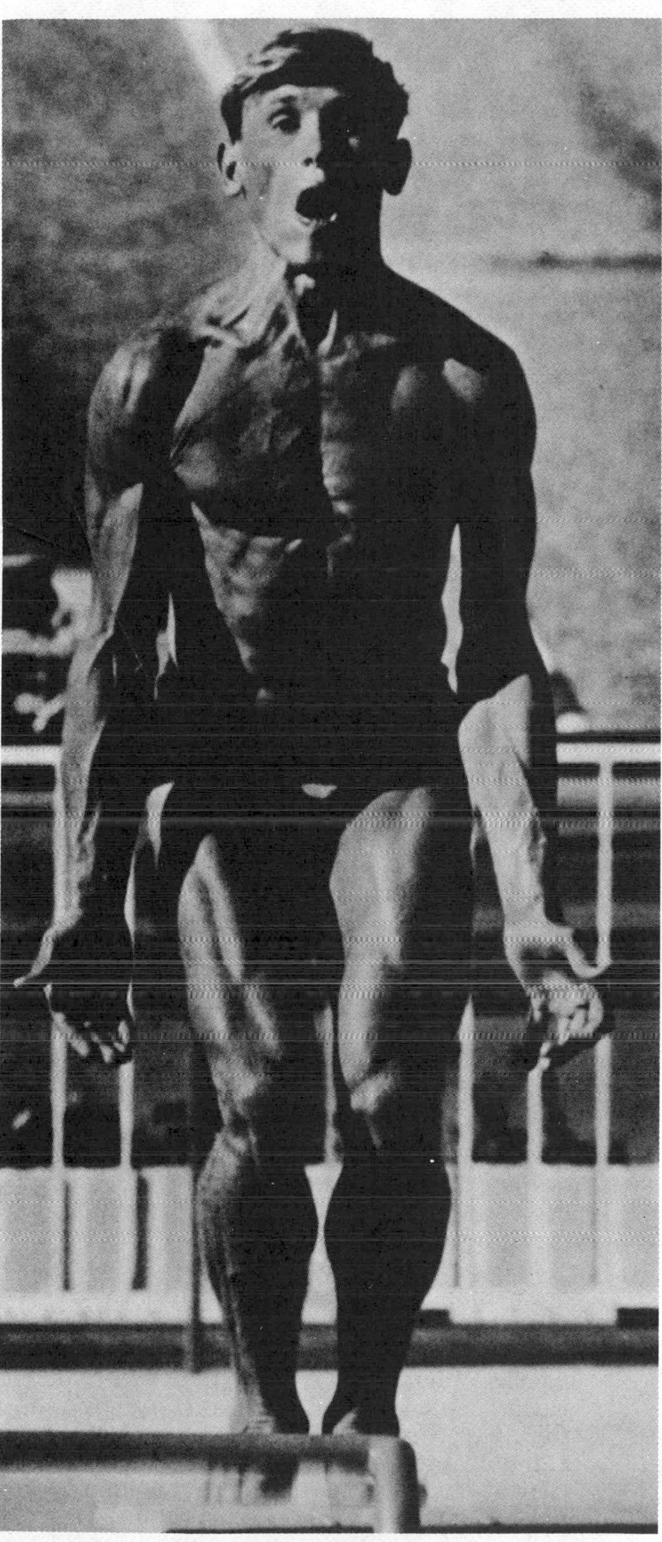

Figure 6–2. An example of muscle tensing and bulging in response to the stress of competitive sports. (From Tanner, O.: *Stress: Time-Life Library of Human Behavior.* New York: Time-Life Books, 1976, p. 16.)

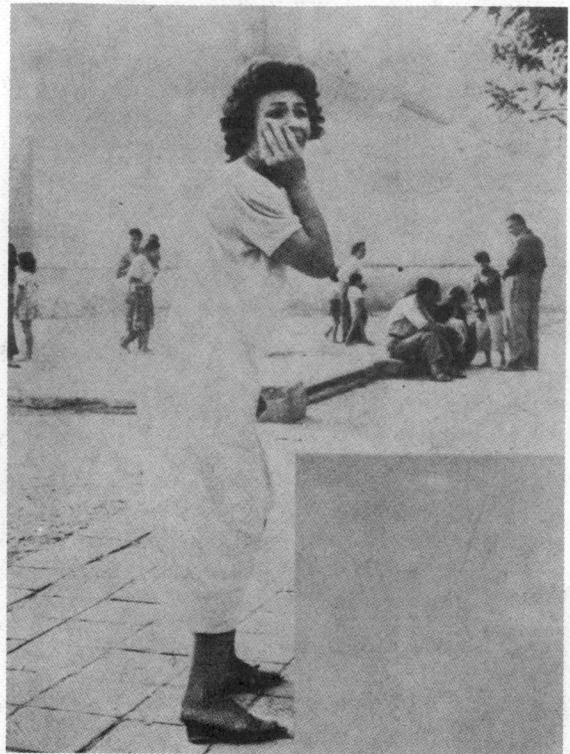

Figure 6–3. An example of muscle sagging in response to stress generated by viewing earthquake devastation. Note the slack jaw, rounded shoulders, and hand supporting head. (From Engel, G. L., and Schmale, A. H.: Conservation-withdrawal. A primary process for organismic homeostasis. *CIBA Foundation Symposium,* 8:57, 1972, p. 68.)

level of vitality at the moment, the circumstances immediately surrounding us, and the way in which our brain perceives and interprets the situation.

Just as the uncomfortable emotions of grief, depression, anger, hostility, and fear all produce body responses, *pleasurable emotions* such as joy, love, and happiness can also lead to physical changes. For example, some people weep "tears of joy" or "scream with joy" when they feel a sense of extreme relief or happy emotion; individuals passionately in love experience changes in heart rate and rhythm, breathing, and muscle tone; a person who feels satisfied after a meal with pleasant companions tends to relax and even to sleep.

Unpleasant bodily responses may also rise on joyful occasions. These undesirable somatic changes appear to be related to one of two factors: First, joy may be mingled with a sense of fear or anxiety; for example, a man may *believe* that he feels happy in a certain situation when in reality he feels *both* happy and anxious — the anxiety leading to many upsetting symptoms. For example, as you recall from Chapter 4, a young man on his wedding day may express feelings of happiness and joy. However, he may also be experiencing various doubts, fears for the future, anxieties concerning parenthood, and so forth. It is these essentially unpleasant emotions, then, rather than the sense of joy or happiness, that give rise to the unpleasant bodily sensations.

Second, unpleasant bodily changes in response to joy may also occur in individuals who are physically too weak or ill to adapt to any intense emotion, even great happiness. Upon occasion such people have literally died in a transport of joy. For example, prisoners of Nazi Germany who were beaten, starved, and weakened by their stressful life were known to die during the excitement of being liberated. As one writer observed during just such a liberation:

> All these prisoners lit up with ineffable joy and hope when they saw the white Red Cross busses turn into the concrete square and grasped that they were to leave in them. For many, it was too much altogether, they hadn't the strength to grapple with so fantastic, so marvelous a prospect — they collapsed and died — literally — of joy.[131]

In summary, then, our bodies respond to emotional stimuli with certain definite physiologic changes which may be perceived by the individual as either pleasant or unpleasant. The sympathetic division of the ANS, in particular, plays a vital role in the body's response to stressors through the regulation of heart action, blood pressure, pulse, sensory changes, digestive tract function, bladder function, temperature regulation, and musculature. The degree of functional change in these tissues and organs depends upon the *type* of stressor impinging upon the person and also upon its magnitude and force.

BEHAVIORAL RESPONSES TO STRESS

An individual responds to stressors not only with physiologic changes but also with behavioral changes. Bryne and Thompson describe the following major behavioral changes that occur in response to stress:[21]

1. *Increased use of one specific form of behavior.* For example, when people feel pressured, they may "raid the icebox," drink or smoke excessively, sleep longer hours than normal, or extend their work day. Ask yourself what activity *you* perform excessively when you feel pressured.

2. *Change in the number of activities performed.* Some individuals become hyperactive when they feel stressed, whereas others attempt to cope by conserving their energies and decreasing their activities.

3. *Disorganized behavior which may deteriorate to the point of regression.* Most of us react to severe crises (e.g., an accident, illness, death of a loved one) by becoming somewhat disorganized in our activities, misassigning priorities, and neglecting details. Seriously ill or disturbed persons sometimes regress to childish behavior such as whining or temper tantrums.

4. *A lower frustration tolerance and increased irritability.* You probably know from your own experience that it takes very little to irritate someone who is feeling excessively pressured by life's problems. A person who is normally tolerant of others may, when sufficiently stressed, "blow up" in response to the slightest provocation.

5. *Noticeable physiologic changes that are correlated to behavioral changes.* For example, people suffering a stress reaction may breathe harder, their muscles may twitch or sag depending on the situation, the pupils of their eyes usually dilate, and their skin may redden or pale.

6. *Distortion of reality and decreased ability to problem solve.* Stressful situations sometimes cause people to lose their "grip on reality," i.e., these individuals temporarily lose their ability to accurately assess their situation and employ rational problem-solving methods. Persons undergoing severe crises may develop delusions and/or hallucinations; in other cases, they may become depressed to the point of suicide.

CHILDREN'S RESPONSES TO STRESS

Like adults, children must cope with stressful situations every day. The *physiologic* responses of children are basically the same as are those of adults, e.g., increased heart rate, increased rate and depth of respirations, pallor, cold and clammy skin, enlarged pupil size. However, children's *behavioral* responses to stress differ significantly from those of their elders. Furthermore, youngsters respond to stress differently at different ages and maturational stages. The major fears of children and their responses to stress by age group include:[11]

- Older infant and toddler: *Major fear*—separation from mother. *Verbal responses*—protests ("No"), cries, screams. *Nonverbal responses*—clings to mother; tries to escape; seeks mother with eyes if separated; turns away; avoids eye contact; rejects anyone except mother or father; kicks, flails, bites.
- Preschooler: *Major fear*—mutilation or body harm. *Verbal responses*—protests, cries, screams; uses words to express pain, anger, or fear; tries to postpone treatment in order to escape it ("Wait a minute"); groans, whines, whimpers. *Nonverbal responses*—preoccupied with injury and with actions of personnel; reaches for help, support; seeks body contact (usually with parent); tries to escape; holds rigidly still; turns away; kicks, flails, bites; frowns, clenches teeth; shuts eyes or keeps wide open.
- School-age child: *Major fear*—loss of self-control. *Verbal responses*—protests; uses words or sentences to express pain, anger or fear; tries to postpone treatment (to be in control and to appear brave); cries, screams, groans, whimpers. *Nonverbal responses*—may sit or lie quietly (to have control and appear brave); passively seeks help, body contact (usually will not ask for help but gladly accepts when offered); tries to escape; holds rigidly still; turns or pulls away; kicks, bangs hands or feet against stretcher table.

To cope with stress successfully, children who are frightened, sick, or injured need supportive care from nurses just as adults do. Children are entitled to a positive approach from the nurse, simple explanations of procedures, honest answers to their questions, and the chance to verbalize or vocalize their feelings without being reprimanded or punished.

MALADAPTIVE RESPONSES PRODUCTIVE OF DISEASE

Although many of our attempts to adapt to life's stresses prove satisfactory, some efforts tend to "backfire," causing injury and disease; still other attempts at adaptation fail because they are either inadequate or too chaotic to cope successfully with a stressful situation. Such maladaptive responses lie at the base of many illnesses.

Four major responses to stress that can be extremely damaging to an individual's health are the following: (1) the distorted anticipatory response, (2) the excessive response, (3) the deficient response, and (4) the inappropriate response.

The Distorted Anticipatory Response

Human reactions in anticipation of certain events can be helpful and protective if they are appropriate. For example, as we pointed out earlier, saliva and gastric juices tend to flow in anticipation of a meal, or epinephrine is released and the pupil of the eye enlarges in anticipation of danger. These are appropriate adaptive responses. However, the anticipatory response can be overused, misused, and badly distorted. For instance, when a person thinks intensely about something unpleasant that *might* happen, the body reacts physiologically *as if* that unpleasant thing were actually taking place.

According to Stewart Wolf, faulty reactions "in anticipation" give rise to a group of diseases that he calls the "as if" disorders.[155] One example of an "as if" disorder is the gastric ulcer. Evidently individuals with gastric ulcers consistently behave physiologically "as if" they were going to kill and eat individuals with whom they are in conflict; i.e., their stomachs prepare for a meal whenever they are faced with a hated opponent. Wolf hypothesizes that such a reaction was appropriate under prehistoric conditions, since a primitive man probably *did* want to kill and eat a dangerous opponent. Today, of course, cannibalism is inappropriate, and such behavior on the part of the stomach will not enable an individual to successfully handle a traumatic interpersonal relationship. The inappropriate digestive secretions will instead, over a period of time, lead to the development of gastric ulcers that will further aggravate the individual's life adjustment.

The Excessive Response

Excessive responses are those "apparent attempts at adaptation which either destroy by sheer excess or that, in correcting one defect, involve the organism in other complications caused directly by this same homeostatic effort."[112] Examples of such reactions abound in medical literature. Anaphylactic shock resulting from an overdose of a drug to which one is sensitive; fibrosis and the overgrowth of scar tissue; and the collagen disease, arthritis, are all disorders resulting from excessive attempts by the body to adapt to stress. In the area of mental disorder, excessive response is evident in persons with manic behavior and in individuals who are obsessive, overly compulsive, hyperactive, or hypersensitive to small stimuli. The person with a type A behavior pattern (discussed in Chapter 4) is an individual who responds excessively to stressful situations and who consequently develops heart disease.

The Deficient Response

Feebleness, inadequacy, and failure characterize the deficient response to stressors. In essence, the deficient reaction is representative of a person's weakness of mind and body and vulnerability to the endless stresses of life.

There are numerous examples of inadequate responses in human pathology. For instance, secondary infections represent a failure of tissue response; congenital malformation represents a failure of prenatal development. Nutritional deficiency, starvation, paralysis, atrophy, ischemia, necrosis, hypofunction, endocrine failure, impotence, and senility are all common examples of the body's inadequacy and failure to adapt because of deficient responses. The deficient response is characteristic of even the most vigorous people; everyone has an Achilles' heel — an area of special vulnerability. For instance, such problems as poor eyesight, poor digestion, and inadequate coordination are common.

The Inappropriate Response

In terms of human physiology and psychology, this type of response can be defined as "an ill-timed, inopportune, misguided, inappropriate, blundering reaction of whatever kind."[112] This is the type of reaction that tends to worsen an already stressful situation. One example of an inappropriate response is the body's tendency, when in heart failure, to absorb large amounts of salt and water — a response which only aggravates matters by overloading an already weakened heart with fluid. Another example of an inappropriate response is hysteria, or conversion reaction, in which an individual develops physical symptoms (e.g., blindness, deafness, or partial paralysis) in reaction to psychologic trauma or conflict which is difficult to solve. Again, this response because it is inappropriate, worsens the situation by further incapacitating the stressed individual.

Summary of Responses to Stress

Let us now generally summarize the topic of human response to stress-producing factors. First of all, the body's organs and structures not only serve to protect us against injury, but they also serve to protect us once injury develops. The body responds to *physical injury* by means of inflammation, increased capillary permeability, sclerosis, fluid and electrolyte shifts, the production of antibodies, and the development of the immune reaction against infection. Body reactions to stressors — physical, chemical, or bacterial — may be local or generalized.

Second, the body also responds physiologically to *psychologic stimuli.* Changes in endocrine function; heart action, rate, and rhythm; changes in digestive and urinary tract function; and changes in muscle tone and body temperature all represent physical responses to both negative and positive emotional states. Many of these responses are mediated by the autonomic nervous system.

Third, an individual responds not only physiologically to stress but also with changes in behavior. Finally, *maladaptive attempts* to adapt to stress can lead to serious consequences for the health of the individual. Responses that are distorted, excessive, deficient, or inappropriate are all maladaptations that can result in injury, disease, and death.

more of their "involuntary" functions, e.g., heart rate, blood pressure, brain waves, muscle relaxation or tension, and skin temperature. Biofeedback training differs from relaxation techniques in two ways: (1) a monitoring device (e.g., an electrocardiogram) is needed to measure the involuntary function and to "feed back" this information to the subject and (2) the subject is helped to monitor and control one physiologic process at a time (whereas relaxation techniques affect various visceral functions at the same time). Because of the need for special equipment, biofeedback training is not as practical as is training in relaxation techniques.

Development of a Stress Reduction Program

When attempting to cope with stressful life problems, many people resort to such short-term coping measures as overeating, drinking excessive alcohol, taking drugs, or sleeping too much. These methods may relieve tension for a short time; however, in the long run, such measures are ineffective and are even dangerous to the health of the individual.

On the other hand, stress reduction programs are based upon the development of a clear and specific *problem-solving approach* for stressful situations. The use of such a program provides the individual with constructive realistic ways for coping with problems. Although various programs differ in details, all problem solving involves these essential steps:

1. Identify the problem
2. Assess the cause of the problem
3. Become aware of personal behavior patterns that contribute to the problem
4. Develop a plan of action
5. Put plan into action
6. Evaluate the plan and modify it as necessary

Development of a Rational Philosophy of Life

The ancient Greeks advocated moderation in all things. The I Ching, the Taoist Book of Days, points out that a calm and rational approach to the stress and change of life is needed. It states:

> *Change is a necessary process of nature. To master it, one must not act prematurely or ruthlessly. Neither can one be excessively conservative or unduly hesitant.*
> *. . . Ponder well and accomplish things.*

Our modern scientists are also recommending moderation and rationality in dealing with stress and change. In essence, the goal is *plan and pace one's life and activities* in order to achieve maximum psychosocial and psychophysiologic well being. To help individuals pace their lives in a healthful way, Dudley and Welke have developed a "Checklist for Survival" (Fig. 6–4). Use this checklist to help you with your own life stress; also you may wish to present the list to those stressed patients who would benefit from it.

THE MULTIDIMENSIONAL APPROACH TO HEALING

We have emphasized throughout this unit the multidimensional aspects of disease. We have pointed out that disease is not only the product of those noxious forces that impinge upon a person from the external world, but that disease also results from the personal responses to various external stressors. We have attempted to discuss disease and the individual's reaction to it from the standpoint of multiple disciplines, namely, physiology, biology, medical science, anthropology, psychology, and human ecology.

If disease is the result of multiple factors, both in humans and in the environment, it follows that the healing and the treatment of disease by nurses and physicians must also take place on multidimensional levels. Healing in one dimension, whether physical, psychologic or social, is limited healing; it results in what Paul Tillich calls "unhealthy health."[142] This phenomenon of "unhealthy health" occurs if and when "healing under one dimension is successful but does not take into consideration the other dimensions in which health is lacking or even imperiled by the particular healing."

For example, consider the care of the patient with hypertension (high blood pressure). To permanently lower an individual's blood pressure to a normal reading (for age), a multidimensional approach to healing is essential. Thus ideally, nursing and medical care of the hypertensive person should involve the following:

- *Weight control* — a lean body weight recommended
- *Diet control,* with sodium and (if needed) caloric restrictions
- *Moderate exercise* — brisk walking, jogging, swimming
- Sufficient mental and physical *rest*

- *Drug therapy* with diuretics and antihypertensive agents
- *Relaxation exercises* — mantra meditation, autohypnosis, autogenic training
- *Biofeedback training* to lower blood pressure, if equipment and facilities are available
- *Patient education* concerning hypertension and its control
- *Professional counseling* if a patient is having difficulty adjusting to or changing a stressful life situation

Nursing, then, must be comprehensive in its scope and in its goals. The educated nurse must be able to understand basic human needs, and the multiple forces that impinge upon people, as well as the many adaptive and maladaptive techniques that we use in meeting stress.

☐ Be aware that your emotional and physical health are one and the same.

☐ Avoid excessive life change, for too much life change produces stress and disease.

☐ Avoid great swings in activity levels; instead maintain a steady level of productive activity at work and play. Pace yourself.

☐ If you are uncomfortable, examine and consider changing your attitudes about life and your present circumstances. If you are ill, examine and consider your attitude about your illness.

☐ Remember that illness and discomfort are relative events, not absolute events. You are probably better off than you previously thought you were.

☐ Study those around you who appear to cope well with the problems of life, and mimic their coping behaviors if you can do so comfortably.

☐ Learn to understand what people are communicating to you non-verbally as well as verbally. Insight into the feelings of others can help minimize tensions in interpersonal transactions.

☐ Realize you are your own best physiological laboratory. Pay attention to how you react to events and circumstances. When you feel uncomfortable, try to alter your reaction and/or the situation.

☐ Never forget that your frame of mind can enormously influence your health, well being, and survival. The idea that a positive attitude is healthy is more than just a cliché–it can save your life.

Figure 6–4. Checklist for survival. (From Dudley, D. L., and E. Welke: *How to Survive Being Alive.* New York: Doubleday and Co. Inc., 1977, p. 162.)

Moreover, the modern nurse and doctor must recognize that curing disease and injury is not enough. Today we need to think in terms of a person's *total life situation* and the personal *meaning* that that situation holds. We must consider the individual's adjustment to the environment and to society, as well as the effect of that adjustment or maladjustment on disease causation, cure, and eradication. This is why modern nursing and medicine are not only biologic sciences; they are also *social sciences.* The aims and goals of nursing today center around not just physiologic needs or psychocultural needs, but the *total* person — the total patient.

BIBLIOGRAPHY (Chapters 4, 5, and 6)

1. Aagaard, G.: Hypertension, a response to stress. Presentation given at the *Symposium On Stress* in Seattle, Mar. 1976. Presentation sponsored by the Pugent Sound Chapter of the American Association of Critical-Care Nurses.
2. Aakster, C. W.: Psycho-social stress and health disturbances. *Social Science in Medicine*, 8:77, Feb. 1974.
3. Aguilera, D., et al.: *Crises Intervention: Theory* and *Methodology*. St. Louis: C. V. Mosby Co., 1970.
4. American Cancer Society data cited in *Associated Press Almanac 1973,* p. 292.
5. Astor, M. H.: An introduction to biofeedback. *American Journal of Orthopsychiatry*, 47:615, Oct. 1977.
6. Bailey, D.: The effects of stress. *NLN Publication*, 16–1674.1, 1977.
7. Barber, T. X. (Ed.): *Advances in Altered States of Consciousness and Human Potentialities* Vol. 1. New York: Psychological Dimensions, 1977.
8. Barber, T. X.: *Hypnosis: A Scientific Approach*. New York: Psychological Dimensions, 1977.
9. Beiman, I., et al.: During training and post-training effects of live and taped extended progressive relaxation, self-relaxation, and electromyogram biofeedback. *Journal of Consulting and Clinical Psychiatry*, 46:314, Apr. 1978.
10. Bell, J. M.: Stressful life events and coping methods in mental illness and wellness behaviors. *Nursing Research*, Mar.-Apr. 1977.
11. Bellack, J. P.: Helping a child cope with the stress of injury. *American Journal of Nursing*, 74:1491, Aug. 1974.
12. Benoliel, J. Q.: "Staff responses to stress." A presentation given at the *Symposium on Stress* in Seattle, Washington, Mar. 31 and Apr. 1, 1976. Presentation sponsored by the Puget Sound Chapter of the American Association of Critical-Care Nurses.
13. Benson, H.: *The Relaxation Response*. New York: William Marrow, 1975.
14. Benson, H.: Your innate asset for combating stress. *Nursing Digest*, May-June 1975, p. 38.
15. Benson, H., et al.: The relaxation response: a bridge between psychiatry and medicine. *Medical Clinics of North America*, 61:929, July 1977.
16. Benson, H., et al.: Historical and clinical considerations of the relaxation response. *American Scientist*, 65:441, July-Aug. 1977.
17. Brody, H.: The systems view of man: Implications for medicine, science, and ethics. *Prospectives in Biology and Medicine*, 17:71, Autumn 1973.
18. Brown, B. B.: *Stress and the Art of Biofeedback*. New York: Harper & Row 1977.
19. Bureau of the Census, U.S. Census of Population, 1960, Vol II, Part PC (2)-8A, cited in U.S. Public Health Service information and unpublished data, *Statistical Abstracts of the United States* 1972, Washington, D.C.: Government Printing Office, 1972, p. 43.
20. Burke, R. J., and T. Weir: Sex differences in adolescent life stress, social support, and well-being. *Journal of Psychology*, 98 (Second Half):277, Mar. 1978.
21. Byrne, M. L. and L. F. Thompson: *Key Concepts for the Study and Practice of Nursing*. St. Louis: C. V. Mosby Co., 1972.
22. Cadoret, R. J., et al.: Depressive disease: Life events and onset of illness. *Archives of General Psychiatry*, 26:133, Feb. 1972.
23. Caldwell, E.: The psychologic impact of trauma, *Nursing Clinics of North American*, 13:2, June 1978.
24. Calhoun, L. G., et al.: *Dealing with Crises: A Guide to Life Problems*. New Jersey: Prentice-Hall, Inc., 1976.
25. Cannon, W. F.: *The Wisdom of the Body*. New York: W. W. Norton & Co., Inc., 1939.
26. Cannon, W.: Quoted by Ingelfinger, F., in The wisdom of the body, reconsidered. *Human Nature*, 1:28, 1978.
27. Carson, R.: *Silent Spring*. Boston: Houghton Mifflin Co., 1962.
28. Cline, D. W., and J. J. Chosy: A prospective study of life changes and subsequent health changes, *Archives of General Psychiatry*, 27:51, Jul. 1972.
29. Coates, T., and C. Thoresen: *How to Sleep Better*. Englewood Cliffs, N.J.: Prentice-Hall, Inc. 1977.
30. Cohen, D. H., and P. A. Obrist: Interactions between behavior and the cardiovascular system. *Circulation Research*, 37:693, 1975.
31. Craven, R. F., and B. H. Sharp: The effects of illness on family functions. *Nursing Forum*, 11:187, 1972.
32. Davidson, R. J., and G. E. Schwartz: Matching relaxation therapies of types of anxiety: A patterning approach. *In* White, J., and J. Fadiman (Eds.): *Relax: How You Can Feel Better, Reduce Stress and Overcome Tension*. The Confucian Press, 1976.
33. Davis, M.: Disease and its treatment: Values in medicine and psychiatry. *Comprehensive Psychiatry*, 18:231, May-June 1977.
34. Dembroski, T. M., et al.: Physiologic reactions to social challenge in persons evidencing the Type A coronary-prone behavior pattern. *Journal of Human Stress*, 3:2, 1977.
35. Donaldson, S.: Physiological responses to stress. Presentation given at the *Symposium On Stress* in Seattle, Mar. 1976. Presentation sponsored by the Puget Sound Chapter of the American Association of Critical-Care Nurses.
36. Dubos, R.: Health and creative adaptation. *Human Nature*, 1:74, 1978.
37. Dubos, R.: *Man Adapting*. New Haven: Yale University Press, 1965.
38. Dubos, R., and M. Pines: *Health and Disease*. Life Science Library, New York: Time-Life, Inc., 1965.
39. Dudley, D. L., and E. Welke: *How to Survive Being Alive*. New York: Doubleday and Co., Inc., 1977.
40. Engel, G. L.: A unified concept of health and disease. *Perspectives in Biology and Medicine*, 3:459, Spring 1960.
41. Engel, G. L., and A. H. Schmale: Conservation-withdrawal: A primary regulatory process for organismic homeostasis. *CIBA Foundation Symposium*. 8:57, 1972.

42. Federal Bureau of Investigation, *Uniform Crime Reports for the United States*, 1970, cited in *Statistical Abstracts of the United States*, 1972, Washington, D.C.: Government Printing Office, 1972, p. 150.
43. Frankenhaeuser, M.: Experimental approaches to the study of catecholamines and emotion. *In* Levi, L. (Ed.): *Emotions: Their Parameters and Measurement*. New York: Raven Press, 1975.
44. Frankenhaeuser, M.: Job demands, health and wellbeing. *Journal of Psychosomatic Research*, 21:313, 1977.
45. Frankenhaeuser, M.: Underload and overload in working life: outline of a multidisciplinary approach. *Journal of Human Stress*, 2:3, Sept. 1976.
46. Friedman, M., and R. H. Rosenman: *Type A Behavior and Your Heart*. Greenwich: Fawcett Publications, Inc., 1974.
47. Galdston, I. (Ed.): *Beyond the Germ Theory; the Roles of Deprivation and Stress in Health and Disease*. New York: Health Education Council, 1954.
48. Galton, L.: *How Long Will I Live?* New York: MacMillan Publishing Co., 1976.
49. Gelhorm, E., and W. F. Kiely: Mystical states of consciousness: neurophysiological and clinical aspects. *Journal of Nervous and Mental Disease*, 154:399, 1972.
50. Gilmore, J.: Physiology of stress. *In* Eliot, R., and M. Kisco: *Stress and the Heart*. New York: Futura Publishing Co., 1974.
51. Glasgow, R. E., and G. M. Rosen: Behavioral bibliotherapy: a review of self-help behavior therapy manuals. *Psychological Bulletin*, 85:1, Jan. 1978.
52. Glass, D. C.: *Behavior Patterns, Stress and Coronary Disease*. New York: John Wiley & Sons, Halsted Press Division, 1977.
53. Glass, D. C.: Stress, competition and heart attacks. *Psychology Today*, 10:54, Dec. 1976.
54. Goldberg, H.: *The Hazards of Being Male: Surviving the Myth of Masculine Privilege*. New York: Nash Publishing, 1976.
55. Gomes-Schwartz, B., et al.: Individual psychotherapy and behavior therapy. *Annual Review of Psychology*, 29:435, 1978.
56. Green, E.: Biofeedback for mind-body-self regulation: Healing and creativity, *In Biofeedback and Self-Control: 1972*. Chicago: Aldine Publishing Co., 1973, p. 152.
57. Green, E. E., A. M. Green, and E. D. Walters: Biofeedback training for anxiety tension reduction. *In* White, J., and J. Fadiman (Eds.): *Relax: How You Can Feel Better, Reduce Stress and Overcome Tension*. The Confucian Press, 1976.
58. Green, T. H.: *Gynecology: Essentials of Clinical Practice*. 3rd ed. Boston: Little, Brown and Co., 1977.
59. Groen, J. J.: The measurement of emotion and arousal in the clinical physiological laboratory and in medical practice. In Levi, L. (Ed.): *Emotions: Their Parameters and Measurement*. New York: Raven Press, 1975.
60. Gruchow, H. W.: Socialization and the human physiologic response to crowding. *American Journal of Public Health*, 67:45, May 1977.
61. Hackett, T. P.: Patient responses to stress. Presentation given at the *Symposium on Stress* in Seattle, Mar. 1976. Presentation sponsored by the Puget Sound Chapter of the American Association of Critical Care Nurses.
62. Hazzard, W.: Metabolic responses to stress. Presentation given at the *Symposium on Stress* in Seattle, Mar. 1976. Presentation sponsored by the Puget Sound Chapter of the American Association of Critical Care Nurses.
63. Heisel, J. S., et al.: The significance of life events as contributing factors in the diseases of children. *The Journal of Pediatrics*, 83:119, July 1973.
64. Hinkle, L. E., Jr.: The concept of stress in the biological and social sciences. *Science, Medicine, and Man*, 1:31, Apr. 1973.
65. Hinkle, L. E.: Normal stress in normal experience. In Galdston, I. (Ed.): *Beyond The Germ Theory*. New York Health Education Council, 1954.
66. Holmes, T. S., and T. H. Holmes: Short-term intrusions into the life style routine. *Journal of Psychosomatic Research*, 14:121, 1970.
67. Holmes, T. H., and R. H. Rahe: The social readjustment rating scale. *Journal of Psychosomatic Research*, 11:213, 1967.
68. Horowitz, M. J.: *Stress Response Syndromes*. New York: Jason Aronson, Inc., 1976.
69. Jacobson, A. M.: Biofeedback: a new treatment for psychosomatic and functional disorders? *Comprehensive Psychiatry*, 19:275, May-June 1978.
70. Jacobson, E.: *Progressive Relaxation*. University of Chicago Press, 1938.
71. Jonas, G.: *Visceral Learning: Toward a Science of Self Control*. New York: Cornerstone Library, 1974.
72. Jones, P. S.: An adaptation model for nursing practice. *American Journal of Nursing*, 78:1900, Nov. 1978.
73. Josephson, E., and M. Josephson: *Man Alone: Alienation in Modern Society*. New York: Dell Publishing Co., 1962.
74. Kagan, A.: Epidemiology, disease, and emotion. *In* Levi, L. (Ed.): *Emotions: Their Parameters and Measurement*. New York: Raven Press, 1975.
75. Kahana, R. J.: Personality and response to physical illness. *Advances in Psychosomatic Medicine*, 8:42, 1972.
76. Kasl, S. V., and S. Cob: Blood pressure changes in men undergoing job loss: a preliminary report. *Psychosomatic Medicine*, 32:19, 1970.
77. Kopin, I. J., et al.: Plasma levels of norepinephrine. *Annals of Internal Medicine*, 88:671, May 1978.
78. Kroger, W. S.: *Clinical and Experimental Hypnosis*. 2nd ed. Philadelphia: J. B. Lippincott Co., 1977.
79. Kroger, W. S., and Fezler, W. D.: *Hypnosis and Behavior Modification: Imagery Conditioning*. Philadelphia: J. B. Lippincott Co., 1976.
80. Lader, M., and P. Tyrer: Vegetative system and emotion. *In* Levi, L. (Ed.) *Emotions: Their Parameters and Measurement*. New York: Raven Press, 1975.
81. Lande, N.: *Mindstyles/Lifestyles*. Los Angeles: Price, Stern, and Sloan Publishers, Inc., 1976.
82. Levine, S.: Stress and behavior. *Scientific American*, 224:26, Jan. 1971.
83. Lidberg, L. A., et al.: Urinary catecholamines, stress, and psychopathy: a study of arrested men awaiting trial. *Psychosomatic Medicine*, 40:116, Mar. 1978.
84. Luce, G. G.: *Body Time: Physiological Rhythms and Social Stress*. New York: Bantam Books, Inc., 1973.
85. Lynch, J. J.: *The Broken Heart: The Medical Consequences of Loneliness*. New York: Basic Books, Inc., 1977.
86. Magid, A.: Stress reduction. *Journal of Practical Nursing*. 28:32, Mar. 1978.
87. Maracek, J., and D. Kravetz: Women and mental health: a review of feminist change efforts. *Psychiatry*, 40:323, Nov. 1977.
88. Mason, J. W.: A historical view of stress field. *Journal of Human Stress*, 1:22, June, 1975.
89. Mason, J. W.: Emotion as reflected in patterns of endocrine integration. *In* Levi, L. (Ed.): *Emotions: Their Parameters and Measurement*. New York: Raven Press, 1975.

90. Meecham, W. C., and H. G. Smith: Decibels and nervous breakdowns. *Human Behavior* (School of Engineering & Applied Science, UCLA.) Nov. 1977, p. 50.
91. Melton, C. E., et al.: Stress in air traffic personnel: low-density towers and flight service stations. *Aviation, Space, and Environmental Medicine*, 49:724, May 1978.
92. Michaels, R. R., et al.: Evaluation of transcendental meditation as a method of reducing stress. *Science*, 192:1242, June 1976.
93. Micklin, M., and C. Leon: Life change and psychiatric disturbance in a South American city: The effects of geographic and social mobility. *Journal of Health and Social Behavior*, 19:92, Mar. 1978.
94. Migration, stress and disease. *The Medical Journal of Australia*, 1:765, June 1975.
95. Miller, N.: Learning of glandular and visceral responses. *In Biofeedback and Self-Control: 1972*. Chicago: Aldine Publishing Company, 1973, p. 90.
96. Miller, R. N.: Stress and its effects. NLN Publication, 1674:21, 1977.
97. Monat, A. and R. Lazarus: *Stress and Coping: An Anthology*. New York: Columbia University Press, 1977.
98. Monjan, A. A., and M. I. Collector: Stress-induced modulation of the immune response. *Science*, 196:307, Apr. 1977.
99. Most illness is stress-related, physician says. *Health Science Review*. W. G. Magnuson Health Science Center, University of Washington, Seattle. Summer, 1978.
100. Parkes, C. M., et al.: Broken heart: a statistical study of increased mortality among widowers. *British Medical Journal*, I:740, 1969.
101. Parsons, T.: *The Social System*. Glencoe, Ill.: The Free Press, 1951.
102. Patel, C.: 12 month follow-up of yoga and biofeedback in the management of hypertension. *Lancet*, II:62, 1975.
103. Paskel, E. S.: Life stress, depression and attempted suicide. *Journal of Human Stress*, 2:3, Sept. 1976.
104. Paykel, E. S., B. A. Prusoff, and Myers, J. K.: Suicide attempts and recent life events. *Archives of General Psychiatry*, 32:327, Mar. 1975.
105. Pesznecker, B.: Life change: a challenge for nurse practitioners. *Nurse Practitioner*, 1:21, Sept.-Oct. 1975.
106. Peters, R. K.: Daily relaxation response breaks in a working population: I. Effects on self-reported measures of health, performance, and well-being. *American Journal of Public Health*, 67:946, Oct. 1977.
107. Peters, R. K., et al.: Daily relaxation response breaks in a working population: II. Effects on blood pressure. *American Journal of Public Health*, 67:954, Oct. 1977.
108. Petrich, J., and T. H. Holmes: Life change and onset of illness. *Medical Clinics of North America*, 61:825, July 1977.
109. Price, V.: Helping men manage stress: reducing Type A behavior. *The Counseling Psychologist*, 1978.
110. Rahe, R. H.: Subjects' recent life changes and their near-future illness reports. *Annals of Clinical Research*, 4:250, 1972.
111. Rahe, R. H.: Subjects' recent life changes and their near-future illness susceptibility. *Advances in Psychosomatic Medicine*, 8:19, 1972.
112. Richards, D.: Homeostasis: its dislocations and perturbations. *Perspectives in Biology and Medicine*, 3:238, Winter 1960.
113. Rosenman, R. H., and M. Friedman: Modifying Type A behavior pattern. *Journal of Psychosomatic Research*, 21:323, 1977.
114. Roskies, E., et al.: Changing the coronary-prone (Type A) behavior pattern in a non-clinical population. *Journal of Behavioral Medicine*, 1978, in press.
115. Russek, H. I.: Behavior patterns, stress and coronary heart disease. *American Family Physician*, 9:122, Apr. 1974.
116. Scherr, A. M.: Transcendental meditation as a means of handling stress. *N.L.N. Publication*, 1674:57, 1977.
117. Schless, A. P., et al.: Life events and illness: a three year prospective study. *British Journal of Psychiatry*, 131:26. Jul. 1977.
118. Schweitzer, L., and Wen-Huey Su: Population density and the rate of mental illness. *American Journal of Public Health*, 67:1165, 1977.
119. Selye, H.: *The Physiology and Pathology of Exposure to Stress; A Treatise Based on the Concepts of the General Adaptation Syndrome and the Diseases of Adaptation*. Montreal, Acta, 1950.
120. Selye, H.: *Stress in Health and Disease*, Reading, Mass.: Butterworths, 1976.
121. Selye, H.: *Stress Without Distress*. Philadelphia: J. B. Lippincott Co., 1974.
122. Selye, H.: *The Stress of My Life*. New York: Harcourt Brace Jovanovich, 1978. Autobiography.
123. Selye, H.: *The Stress of Life*. New York: McGraw-Hill Book Co., Inc., 1956.
124. Sheldon, A. and Hopper, D.: An inquiry into health and ill health adjustment in early marriage. *Journal of Psychosomatic Research*, 13:95, 1969.
125. Shubin, S.: Rx for stress — your stress. Nursing '79, 9:53, Jan. 1979.
126. Shumate, M.: Transcendental meditation: its application to the stress of life. *NLN Publication*, 1674:63, 1977.
127. Snyder, S. H.: *The Troubled Mind: A Guide to Release From Distress*, New York: McGraw-Hill Book Co., 1976.
128. Statistical Abstracts 1974. United States Department of Commerce, Bureau of the Census, 1974.
129. Stephenson, C. A.: Stress in critically ill patients. *American Journal of Nursing*, 77:1806, Nov. 1977.
130. Sterman, L. T.: Clinical biofeedback. *American Journal of Nursing*, 75:2006, Nov. 1975.
131. Stevenson, I.: Physical symptoms during pleasurable emotional states. *Psychosomatic Medicine*, 12:98, Mar.-Apr. 1950.
132. Strain, J. J.: Psychological reactions to acute medical illness and critical care. *Critical Care Medicine*, 6:39, Jan.-Feb. 1978.
133. Strain, J. J. and Grossman, S.: *Psychological Care of the Medically Ill: A Primer in Liaison Psychiatry*. New York: Appleton-Century-Crofts, 1975.
134. Stress — making it work for you. *NLN Publication*, 1674:III, 1977.
135. Suinn, R. M.: How to break the vicious cycle of stress. *Psychology Today*, 10:59, Dec. 1976.
136. Suinn, R. M.: Pattern A behaviors and heart disease: intervention approaches. *In* Ferguson & Taylor (Eds.): *Advances in Behavioral Medicine*, in press.
137. Suinn, R. M.: Type A behavior pattern. *In* R. B. Williams and Gentry, W. D. (Eds.): *Behavioral Approaches to Medical Treatment*. Cambridge, Mass: Ballinger, 1977.
138. Suinn, R. M. and Bloom, L. J.: Anxiety management training for Type A persons. *Journal of Behavioral Medicine*, 1978, in press.
138a. Sutterly, D. C., and G. S. Donnelly (Eds.): Stress management. *Topics in Clinical Nursing*, 1:1–104. Apr. 1979.

139. Syme, S. L., *et al.*: Some social and cultural factors associated with the occurence of coronary heart disease. *Journal of Chronic Disease*, 17:277, 1968.
140. Tanner, O.: *Stress*. Time-Life Library of Human Behavior. New York: Time-Life Books, 1976.
141. Taylor, F. K.: The medical model of the disease concept. *British Journal of Psychiatry*, 128:588. June 1976.
142. Tillich, P.: The meaning of health. Belgum, D. (ed.): *Religion and Medicine: Essays on Meanings, Values and Health*. Ames, Iowa: Iowa State University Press, 1967.
143. Toffler, A.: *Future Shock*. New York, Random House, Inc., 1970.
144. U.S. National Center for Health Statistics, unpublished data cited in *Statistical Abstracts of the United States*. 1973, p. 63.
145. U.S. Public Health Service information and published data in *Statistical Abstracts of the United States, 1972* Washington, D.C.: Government Printing Office, 1972, p. 74.
146. U.S. Public Health Service Information cited in *Associated Press Alamanac*, 1973, p. 290.
147. Wallace, J. M.: Living with stress. *Nursing Times*, 74:457, Mar. 1978.
148. Wegman, D. H.: The environmentalist's challenge. *American Journal of Public Health*, 68:540, June 1978.
149. Westermeyer, J., et al.: A review of the relationship between dysphoria, pleasure, and human bonding. *Journal of Clinical Psychiatry*, 39:415, May 1978.
150. Wiener, N.: *Cybernetics*. 2nd edition. Cambridge: Massachusetts Institiue of Technology Press, 1961.
151. Wiener, N.: *The Human Use of Human Beings: Cybernetics Society*. Garden City, New York: Doubleday Co., 1956.
152. Williams, C. C., et al.: Pregnancy and life change. *Journal of Psychosomatic Research*, 19:123, 1975.
153. Williams, R. B.: What are the psychophysiologic differences between the Types (A and B) that may lead to CHD? *In* Dembroski, T. *et al.*, *Forum on Coronary-Prone Behavior*, monograph to be published by NHLBI, DHEW, Washington, D.C. 1978.
154. Winer, L. R.: Biofeedback: a guide to the clinical literature. *American Journal of Orthopsychiatry*, 47:626, Oct. 1977.
155. Wolf, S.: Disease as a way of life. *Perspectives in Biology and Medicine*, 4:288, Spring 1961.
156. Wolf, S.: A new view of disease. *Journal of American Medical Association*, 84:129, Apr. 13, 1963.
157. Wolf, S.: Regulatory mechanisms and tissue pathology. In Levi, L. (ed.) *Emotions: Their Parameters and Measurement.* New York: Raven Press, 1975.
158. Wolff, H. G.: A concept of disease in man. *Psychosomatic Medicine*, 24:25, Jan.-Feb., 1962.
159. Wolff, H. G.: Life situations, emotions, and bodily disease. *Symposium on Stress*, Mar. 1, 1953, p. 132.
160. Wolff, H. G.: *Stress and Disease*. 2nd ed. Springfield, Illinois: Charles C Thomas, 1968.
161. Woodman, D. D., J. W. Hinton, and M. T. O'Neill: Cortisol secretion and stress in maximum security hospital patients. *Journal of Psychosomatic Research*, 22:133, 1978.
162. *World Health Organization (WHO) Demographic Year Book, 1975*. Department of Economic and Social Affairs, United Nations Statistical Office, 1975.
163. Wyler, A. R., M. Masuda, and T. H. Holmes: The seriousness of illness rating scale: reproducibility. *Journal of Psychosomatic Research*, 14:59, 1970.
164. Yeracaris, L. L. B. and Kim, J. H.: Socioeconomic differentials in selected causes of death. *American Journal of Public Health*, 68:342, Apr. 1978.
165. Young, M., et al.: The mortality of widowers. *Lancet*, Aug. 31, 1963, p. 454.

UNIT IV

MIND-BODY INTERACTION IN ILLNESS

INTRODUCTION AND STUDY GUIDE

The two chapters in this unit consider the powerful effects of mind-body interaction that occur during illness. The general classifications of *somatopsychic* and *psychosomatic* disorders are discussed in Chapter 7. Chapter 8 focuses on the treatment of psychosomatic disorders. Bibliography for this unit is presented at the end of Chapter 8.

Perhaps you wonder why emphasis on mind-body interactions is given in a medical-surgical nursing textbook. Many people, including some nurses (unfortunately), believe that medical-surgical nursing is a practice concerned exclusively with caring for the "physically" ill. If you are a sensitive, aware student of nursing, you will frequently note the far-reaching effects of mind-body interactions in all persons within your care. It has been estimated that out of *all* patients seen in medical practice for "medical" disorders, one third have psychosomatic disorders and another third have somatic (physical) disorders that are complicated by some psychosocial problems. Clearly, then, the nurse who practices "medical-surgical" nursing is not caring for patients who have *purely* physical problems. Perhaps there is no such thing as a "purely physical problem"! (Can *you* identify such a problem?)

Before reading this unit, you may want to review Chapter 3, "Mind-Body (Psyche-Soma) Interaction."

This unit is written with several objectives in mind. After studying carefully the material in this unit you can expect to be able to:

- ▶ Appreciate that physical and psychosocial factors are involved in all disease processes
- ▶ Differentiate between somatopsychic and psychosomatic illness and between functional and psychophysiologic illness
- ▶ Understand the central position of anxiety and stress in theories of psychosomatic etiology
- ▶ Identify therapeutic regimens currently used for the prevention and treatment of psychosomatic illness
- ▶ Offer appropriate, nonjudgmental nursing care to people experiencing functional and psychophysiologic illnesses
- ▶ Remain sensitive, gentle and sympathetic when caring for such people, recognizing that etiology and symptomatology are complex and only scantily understood.

The following suggestions for learning activities may be useful as you work toward the attainment of the above objectives.

1. Write down, in your own words, your understanding of the following terms:

- somatopsychic illness
- psychosomatic illness
- functional illness
- psychophysiologic illness
- theory of multiple causality
- syndrome shift
- psychotherapy
- relaxation therapy
- psychoanalytic psychotherapy
- group psychotherapy
- family therapy
- behavior therapy
- biofeedback
- autogenic therapy
- pharmacotherapy

2. Have group discussions with your colleagues about the concepts mentioned above. Share your understandings with each other.

3. Seek group discussions with your teachers and some practicing professional nurses. They would be able to add knowledge gained from clinical experience to your discussions.

4. Identify the psychotherapy and relaxation therapy services that are available in your community. Are any of the "therapists" nurses?

5. Attempt to consciously identify environmental, physical, and psychosocial factors (and their interaction) in the illness experience of every individual you care for in clinical practice. Because excellent nursing *always* involves assessment of this kind, you will want it to become an integral part of your practice. (Units VI and VII discuss psychosocial and physical assessments.)

CHAPTER 7

PSYCHOSOMATIC AND SOMATOPSYCHIC ILLNESS

It is generally recognized that emotional factors do contribute to physical disease, and that physical symptoms do have emotional consequences. However, the exact mechanisms of the interaction of mind and body are not clearly understood. Indeed, discussions of these mechanisms are often heated and controversial. Both "psychosomatic illnesses" and "somatopsychic illnesses" involve mental and physical disturbances. They are similar in this respect, but they do differ significantly in other ways, as you will see in the following discussion. (Unit II has focused in detail on stress and disease. Chapter 4 presented a careful overview of theories of disease.)

BASIC CONCEPTS OF SOMATOPSYCHIC AND PSYCHOSOMATIC ILLNESS

> Broadly speaking, somatopsychic *disorders are physical disorders that influence mental activity, and* psychosomatic *disorders are extreme or prolonged emotional states that influence body functioning.*

Disorders that you will find in your clinical practice will seldom be as distinct as the above statement may suggest. Cause-effect relationships in illness are often complex and obscure. At our present state of knowledge, the "mind" and the "body" seem so interrelated that the problem is rather like the proverbial "chicken and egg" . . . it is difficult to know which came first.

Figure 7–1 illustrates the tight interconnections that apparently operate when human beings are viewed in a "bio-psycho-social field."[107] For example, the diagram shows energy and information exchanges occurring freely between the physical environment, the body's cellular structure, the mind, and the social environment. The brain appears to be the mediating structure between the body and the mind. Study this diagram carefully and discuss it with your colleagues and teachers. It could help you to understand more clearly how physical factors and psychosocial factors may interact in human function and dysfunction.

Somatopsychic Illness

In *somatopsychic illnesses* the *physical* problems or physical maladaptations *precede* and contribute to the emotional, behavioral problems or maladaptations. Organic disease is primary (that is, "first") and it causes or is associated with personality deviations and their related emotional and psychologic disturbances. Somatopsychic disorders thus include systemic disorders in which central nervous system symptoms, particularly behavioral change, are prominent. In such disorders the emotional complaints have a systemic, organic basis. Examples of such somatopsychic illnesses (in which a person's behavior may be markedly influenced by a physical condition) are: inborn errors of metabolism, intrinsic or extrinsic intoxications, nutritional deficiencies, and disorders of the endocrine glands.

Consider another example of somatopsychic illness that illustrates, in a slightly different manner, the ways a physical disorder might affect a person mentally. Suppose Mr. Robinson is told by his physician that he has cancer. When he realizes that this diagnosis is true, he becomes very despondent and withdrawn from his friends and family. The realization of his seriously ill physical state produces depression. There is an obvious relationship between Mr. Robinson's organic disease (the cancer) and his emotional disturbance (the depression). Notice, also, that in this example of somatopsychic illness the *organic* disease *precedes* the emotional disturbance. The opposite situation is present in psychosomatic disorders.

Psychosomatic Illness

In *psychosomatic illness* the *emotional* problems or maladaptations are believed to *precede* physical disorders in such a manner that the physical maladaptive process is said to be "*psychogenic*" in origin. By psychogenic we mean that the

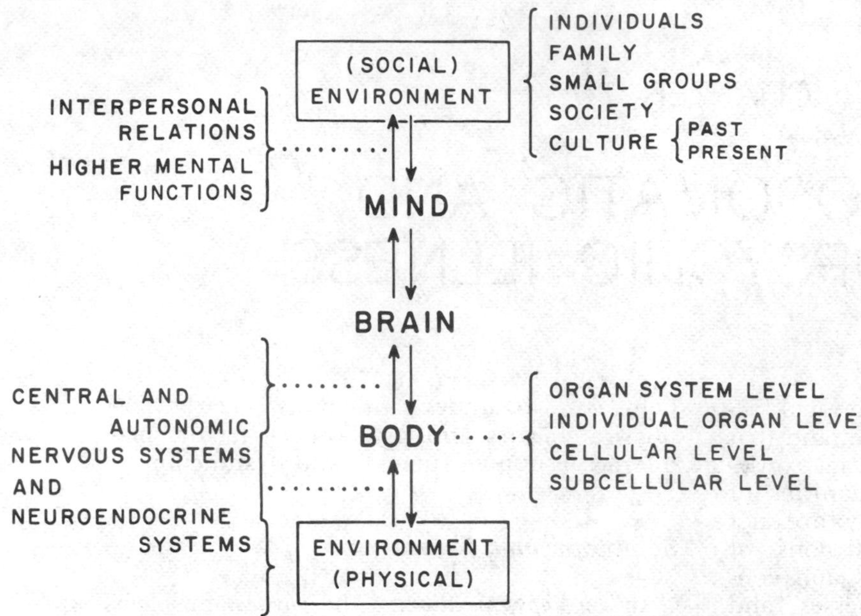

Figure 7–1. The bio-psycho-social field. (*From* Reiser, M.F.: Organic disorders and psychosomatic medicine, *In* Arieti, S. (ed.): *American Handbook of Psychiatry,* 2nd ed. New York: Basic Books, Inc. 1975, Vol. 4, Chap. 21, p. 493.)

illness results from prolonged emotional or psychologic stress.

There is some evidence to indicate that particular "personality types" may be associated with certain psychosomatic disorders. Table 7–1 illustrates this point. As with all classification systems there is danger in applying this information too literally to patients. It is interesting, however, and may help us to understand a bit more about why some persons may develop one particular disorder and other people develop another.

A broad view of psychosomatic etiology states that emotional factors have a role in producing or aggravating many physical disorders. The exact mechanism of psychosomatic interaction is unknown at present. To use a familiar simile, psychosomatic illnesses are comparable to an iceberg: the symptoms and disorders that are observable are similar to the visible part of the iceberg; the multiple unobservable factors of stress represent the much larger mass of ice below the surface of the sea (Fig. 7–2).

> To summarize: Somatopsychic illnesses *are caused by nonpsychogenic factors and result in physical diseases that precede and contribute to psychologic problems.* Psychosomatic illnesses *are psychogenic in origin and, thus, psychologic maladaptions precede and aggravate physical disorders.*

TABLE 7–1. HYPOTHESIZED PERSONALITY PATTERNS IN SELECTED PSYCHOSOMATIC DISORDERS

Disorder	Personality
Asthma	Suppresses cry for maternal help. Fears abandonment or rejection. Overdependent, demanding, hostile toward loved ones.
Colitis	Obsessive, hypersensitive, depressive. Turns hostility inward. Feels conflict over desire to please and resentment.
Hypertension	On guard against feelings of continual threat. Suppressed rage. Underlying insecurity and dependency lead to chronic hostility or anxiety. High achievement needs.
Migraine	Perfectionistic, rigid, intelligent, with achievement needs so high they cannot be met. Unaware of hostile feelings.
Neurodermatitis	Feels conflict involving hostility to and dependency on authority figures. Feels helpless and unfairly treated. Guilt over felt inadequacies. Low self-esteem.
Stomach ulcer	Overemphasizes independence but has strong underlying dependency needs. Chronic hostility, anxiety, insecurity. Represses vengeful feelings.

(From Martin, B.: *Abnormal Psychology. Clinical Scientific Perspectives,* New York: Holt, Rinehart and Winston, 1977, p. 318.)

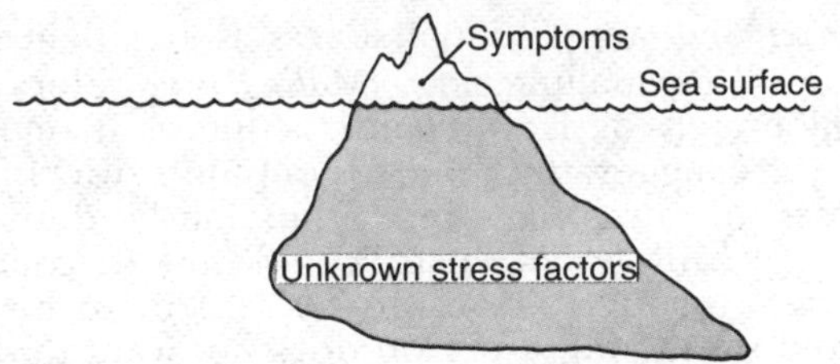

Figure 7–2. The iceberg simile of psychosomatic illness. Observable symptoms represent only a small part of the total disorder.

Psychosomatic illnesses may be divided into two groups, both psychogenic in origin: (1) *functional illnesses* and (2) *psychophysiologic illnesses.* The presence or absence of bodily structural changes (that is, tissue changes or organic damage) constitutes a major difference between functional and psychophysiologic disease. Whereas functional problems result in no demonstrable organic pathologic changes, psychophysiologic disorders do produce demonstrable pathologic changes. Figure 7–3 illustrates schematically the etiology of somatopsychic, psychosomatic, functional, and psychophysiologic illnesses.

FUNCTIONAL ILLNESS

Illnesses are termed *functional* when organic pathologic changes cannot be demonstrated as a basis for a person's symptoms. It has been estimated that one third of the patients who consult physicians are ill but have no definite bodily disease to account for their illness. Nurses thus meet many patients with functional disorders. Such patients are reacting to stress in the sense that they experience physical symptoms (pains, flutterings, and so forth), but structural tissue change has not taken place.

> Functional disorders *are psychogenic disorders which involve no demonstrable structural changes in the body tissue, but which produce problems in the* function *of the area involved.*

Authorities emphasize that the diagnosis of functional illness must be established not simply by the exclusion of organic disease, but by its own characteristics as well. When there is no demonstrable physical basis for a patient's symptoms, serious attempts should be made to understand the symptoms in terms of their *meanings* for the patient and their behavioral significance. This *may* involve careful, thorough psychiatric investigation, since functional

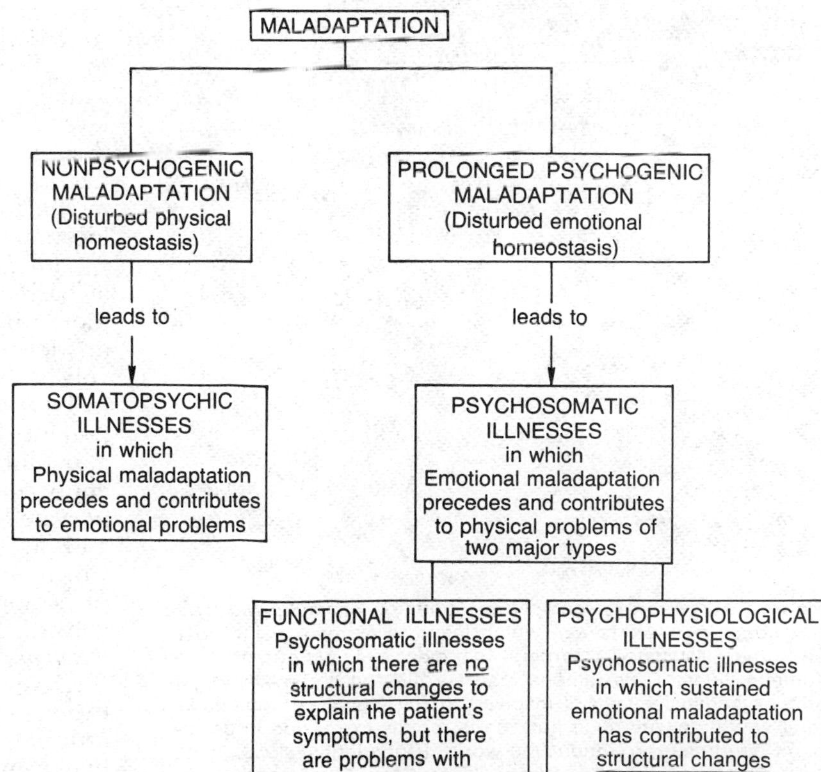

Figure 7–3. The etiology of somatopsychic, psychosomatic, functional, and psychophysiologic illness.

problems may have a symbolic meaning to the patient.

Disorders that are *sometimes* of functional origin include: irritable bowel syndrome, hyperventilation, constipation, enteritis, headaches, anorexia nervosa, disorders of menstruation, sexual disorders (e.g., impotence, orgasmic dysfunction), and psychogenic pain.

Be sure you understand that not everyone who experiences one of the above disorders has a functional psychosomatic illness. It is also very important to realize that true functional illnesses are *not* "put on." A person experiencing a functional illness is not deliberately ill or malingering. (*Malingering* refers to deliberately or fraudulently acting as if one is ill or exaggerating one's symptoms for purposes of attaining some consciously desired goal. Examples of such "goals" are to collect money through an insurance settlement or to avoid something a person does not want to do, such as working or taking an exam.)

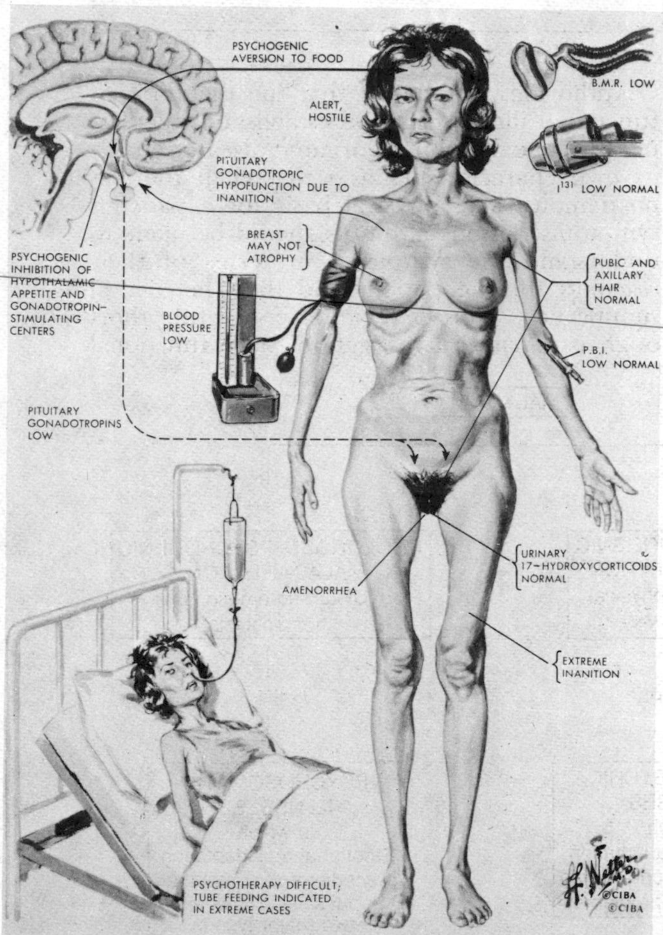

N61 62 VOLUME 4—ENDOCRINE SYSTEM PITUITARY GLAND ANOREXIA NERVOSADR. EZRIN

Figure 7–4. Anorexia nervosa (a condition characterized by a *psychogenic failure to eat,* which leads to extreme weight loss and other associated disorders) is a clear example of a psychosomatic illness. This famous diagram illustrates some physical and psychosocial factors involved in this complex, sometimes fatal condition. Anorexia nervosa is rapidly increasing in developed countries throughout the world. (Copyright © 1959, 1972, CIBA Pharmaceutical Co., Div. of CIBA–Geigy Corp. Reproduced with permission from Clinical Symposia. Illustrated by Frank H. Netter, M.D.)

The psychologic factors involved in functional illness are largely unconscious. The causes of such an illness are complex, and the symptoms manifested are very real and distressing to the patient. Functional disorders require the serious attention and concern of health professionals. Unfortunately, instances occur of patients being ignored, ridiculed, or berated because they have been assigned the diagnostic label of "functional illness." This is, of course, unpleasant for the patient and may also be dangerous, e.g., the patient may retreat from seeking help. Diagnosis of a functional disorder must *never* be made lightly, and once it is made, the patient's problems *must* be given serious attention.

PSYCHOPHYSIOLOGIC ILLNESS

As previously stated, in *psychophysiologic* disorders pathologic changes actually do occur in the structure of tissue composing the organ affected. *The symptoms experienced by the patient are believed by many to be the result of prolonged repression of emotion, which disturbs normal physiologic balance.* Eventually this prolonged malfunctioning produces actual structural changes in visceral organs. The patient's defense against anxiety is said to be on a physiologic level, with affect (mood) being expressed through the body viscera. Thus, psychologic factors are believed to play an important part in the formation or aggravation of the pathologic anatomic-physiologic changes that occur.

Chronic anxiety is the most common emotional basis of psychophysiologic disorders. Other more specific affective reactions, such as rage or depression, are much less commonly involved. The *autonomic nervous system* is believed to be involved in producing the organic component of psychophysiologic reactions. The gastrointestinal, respiratory, cardiovascular, endocrine, and genitourinary systems are innervated by the autonomic nervous system and are thus frequently locations of illness which may commonly be classified as psychophysiologic. The skin also may often be involved. Thus a few of the disorders that are *sometimes* of psychophysiologic origin are: ulcerative colitis, duodenal ulcer, obesity, some headaches, many skin disorders, bronchial asthma, some endocrine disorders, essential hypertension, coronary heart disease, and accident proneness. Recent research has also indicated that emotional factors may be significant

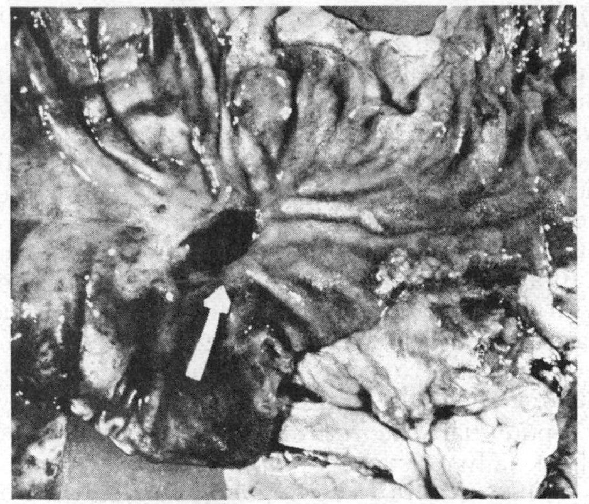

Figure 7–5. Psychophysiological disorders can produce actual tissue damage. In this photograph of an autopsy specimen, the arrow points to an ulcer in the duodenum (that portion of the small intestine that joins to the stomach), which has perforated into the pancreas, seen to the right and below. (From Martin, B.: *Abnormal Psychology. Clinical and Scientific Perspectives.* New York: Holt, Rinehart, and Winston, 1977, p. 309.)

in the etiology of pulmonary tuberculosis and cancer of various types.

Classification Problems. In discussing functional, psychophysiologic, and somatopsychic illnesses we have attempted to list some "typical" illnesses. It should be recognized, however, that wide varieties of opinion exist concerning the placement of illnesses in these various categories. Classifying psychosomatic disorders is indeed difficult and clear diagnostic guidelines are often absent. Some researchers believe that almost every illness can be thought of as psychophysiologic; others place only a few selected diseases in this classification. Shulkin summarizes the problem of classification in his statement.

> Frankly speaking, classification in psychophysiological conditions is a modern day Tower of Babel. There is a joyous disregard for the usual orderliness of science; physicians commonly use lay terms in referring to these disease syndromes. . . Efforts toward classification of psychophysiologic disorders have been very unrewarding.[123]

It is argued by some that it is theoretically possible for psychophysiologic disease to occur in *any* body organ system because "the mind" depends upon nervous system activity, and the nervous system has complex interrelationships with all the organ systems of the body. However, as we have just indicated, the classic position is that the autonomic nervous system mediates the organic component of psychophysiologic reactions, and the somatic nervous symptoms that occur are the end products of psychologic stresses and conflicts. The psychophysiologic symptom is not generally believed to have symbolic significance for the patient. Of course, a tremendous variation is noted between individuals in terms of differences in the degree, nature, and duration of the expression of emotion through disturbances in various body organs.

Theories of Psychophysiologic Etiology. Systems of classification of disease often derive from theories of etiology. Let us now focus our discussion specifically on *psychophysiologic* disorders and consider some etiologic theories.*

In the early days of "psychosomatics" each specialized profession (i.e., psychology, psychoanalysis, neurology) had its own school of thought about the problem and there was little communication between the disciplines — each group held fiercely to its own point of view, believing its theory could not be improved by knowledge from other fields. At this time, a state of cordial relations appears to be developing between the various disciplines studying psychophysiologic conditions. Knowledge from epidemiology, biochemistry, physiology, psychiatry, psychology, neurology, pathology, and other related fields, is being "pooled" with greater frequency. Out of this interdisciplinary approach, eclectic theories are increasingly beginning to emerge, i.e., theories made up of elements drawn from a variety of sources.

Today much of the volatile theorizing and many of the sweeping generalizations which characterized psychosomatic discussions in their infancy are being replaced by a more careful, scientifically delineated, experimental approach. However, much remains unclear, and a great deal of work remains to be done. At present the theories of psychophysiologic illness are still comparable to winds blowing in all directions at once, and while such winds continue to blow, it is impossible to identify what the true causes of psychophysiologic problems may be. Because of the wide variety of etiologic theories of psychophysiologic illness, it is difficult to group them in all-inclusive, meaningful manner. However, certain points are rather commonly agreed upon.

Certainly a great boost toward interdisciplinary understanding came with the introduction of the concept of multiple causes of disease, and it is generally accepted today that the basic model of psychophysiologic disease is the *theory of multi-causality.* The concept was discussed in Chapter 4. In terms of psychophysio-

*We omit a theoretical discussion of the etiology of functional disorders, since these are primarily discussed in psychiatric terminology, which is too involved to present in a medical-surgical textbook.

logic disorders, the theory means that psychic factors *interact* with somatic factors (i.e., nutritional status, constitution, organ pathology) to produce the disease. Although psychic factors have a significant influence on the etiology of psychophysiologic illnesses, they are not considered the *only* causative factors. Psychophysiologic illnesses are thus commonly believed to result from the interaction of *many* determinants — organs, psychologic, and environmental. Let us examine some of these determinants more carefully.

> *In all theories of psychophysiologic etiology,* anxiety or stress *is an initial factor. (See Unit III).*

Patients with psychophysiologic illnesses are considered to be *organically vulnerable* to the physiologic concomitants of emotional arousal in a way that other people are not. In other words, psychic factors in themselves are not the only causative determinant of such disorders, since many people who experience anxiety do not develop somatic illness. A specific interaction of psychic factors with somatic factors, such as nutritional status, constitution, and organ vulnerability, is necessary to produce the disease state.

Although this basic theoretic model is generally accepted, debate exists concerning the interpretation of the model clinically as well as theoretically. For example, there are several theories about the issue of "symptom choice"; that is, why a person develops certain symptoms or pathology rather than developing other symptoms (see also Chapter 4). Why is it that a particular organ is affected by emotional stress more than other organs in a given individual? In other words, why does one person react to stress with stomach trouble while another becomes hypertensive?

There are three general approaches to answering the question of symptom choice in psychophysiologic illnesses: (1) that *specific* psychologic stresses produce *specific* symptoms; (2) that stress *in general* (rather than specific stresses) produces symptoms; and (3) that a wide range of stimuli may evoke a pattern of emotional arousal that consists of specific, consistent physiologic responses which are *characteristic of that individual* (i.e., the symptoms depend upon the individual's typical response pattern rather than the nature of the stimulus).

It can be seen that numerous psychophysiologic theories exist, and the reader is cautioned to remember that, at present, many questions about illnesses of this nature remain unanswered. Nurses' individual attitudes toward psychophysiologic conditions are reflected to the thousands of patients with these conditions as they receive nursing care. Therefore, generalizations, misinterpretations, or reliance on outdated theories by nurses can create unhappiness for many. Speculative theories carry with them both dangers and promises! The careful nurse holds on to the inherent promise, critically reappraising it from time to time. Such a nurse also simultaneously remains alert to potential theoretical dangers which can affect daily practice.

Nurses need, of course, to keep informed of changes in theories that pertain to their area of practice. We cannot wait for clarity to emerge in the field of psychosomatic medicine before we begin to care for those persons who suffer from psychosomatic illnesses. These patients are with us each day; we cannot ignore the psychosomatic problems experienced by many patients. These individuals deserve sensitive, knowledgeable care.

Nurses must constantly explore the uncharted territory of mind-body interaction, keeping company with physicians, scientists, and philosophers. We all look forward to the time when order and definitive answers will emerge from the present admixture of psychosomatic theories, and suffering can be more effectively reduced or prevented. In the interval, we share the hope and professional concern of Michael Polanyi, philosopher of science, that it might be possible "to establish a better foundation than we now possess for holding the beliefs by which we live and must live, though unable adequately to justify them today."[98]

Psychophysiologic Symptoms: Maladaptive or Adaptive? Are the psychophysiologic symptoms that a patient develops maladaptive or adaptive? Do they tend to destroy the individual or do they instead help with adaptation to life? These questions will be discussed from both points of view.

Let us first consider briefly how psychophysiologic symptoms might be *adaptive*. It has been stated that while psychophysiologic symptoms have pathologic aspects (i.e., they produce structural changes in body organs and tissues which are caused by or cause disease), they may serve a positive and constructive function in the patient's adjustment to the conflicts and anxieties of life.[112] For example, by permitting a protective integration of the patient's personality, the symptoms may offer protection from a total mental breakdown. The physical symptom thus represents a more easily tolerated pain than the pain of anxiety. Psychophysiologic symptoms might in this sense be considered as a means of adjustment and could be helpful to the patient. In his discussion of social class and illness, Jurgen Ruesch[113] states that for the lower middle class the only possible solution for unsolved psychologic conflicts lies in physical symptoms. Thus it could be postulated that physical symptoms are actually serving a protective or restitutive function for this highly repressed group of people.

Other authorities, writing on the adaptive function of psychophysiologic symptoms, maintain that the homeostasis of the total organism (person) may be achieved at the expense of the integrity of one part of the organism.[48] Thus, one part saves the whole. This viewpoint is illustrated by the fact that a patient with psychophysiologic symptoms may become emotionally disturbed, possibly even psychotic, when the somatic aspects of the illness are resolved.

If symptoms can be viewed as adaptive, the nurse can consider the patient as a whole person whose behavior and symptom formation are not just random events but are actually a meaningful search for identity and stability in a difficult world.

On the other hand, psychophysiologic illnesses can also be considered from a *maladaptive* perspective. Thus, while it is possible to think of psychophysiologic symptoms as defensive physical adaptations to maintain psychologic homeostasis, it is debatable whether or not such symptoms can actually be considered "helpful."[134] Some psychophysiologic problems are so severe that they interfere with the afflicted person's ability to survive. Clearly it is doubtful whether somatic symptoms of this magnitude are "protecting" or "helping" the patient.

Some investigators maintain that psychophysiologic symptoms do *not* diminish anxiety or tension and thus do *not* serve as psychologic defense mechanisms. Instead, they maintain that the symptoms appear when the psychologic defenses *fail* to reduce anxiety. The symptoms, thus, actually represent the physiologic concomitants of anxiety.

Finally, still other experts believe that it may be a matter of (1) the severity of a symptom (its degree of usage by the patient) or (2) how the symptom fits into the patient's total life situation that determines whether psychophysiologic symptoms are adaptive or maladaptive for a given individual.

Incidence of Psychosomatic Conditions. As previously cautioned, it is erroneous to assume that everyone who develops an illness that might be classified as psychosomatic actually has a psychosomatic disorder. Headaches, for example, can result from a brain tumor as well as from mental stress. Likewise, back pain may arise from a herniated disk in the spine as well as from anxiety. Evidence of disturbed psychologic adaptation must *precede* the ailment for an accurate psychosomatic diagnosis to be made; bodily symptoms alone do not constitute a psychosomatic diagnosis.

Although it is difficult to obtain accurate statistics on psychosomatic problems, illnesses of this nature clearly appear to be great in number and are responsible for much suffering and death. It has been estimated that close to *one million* persons die annually from disorders that are primarily emotional in origin! Naturally, much greater numbers of living persons are assumed to be afflicted with such disorders. Let us repeat our earlier statement:

> *It has been estimated that one third of all patients seen in medical practice today have psychosomatic disorders and that another third have somatic problems complicated by psychiatric problems.*[116]

An understanding of psychosomatic conditions is obviously of great importance. These illnesses must be prevented when possible and recognized and treated when they do occur.

BIBLIOGRAPHY

Bibliography for this chapter is located at the end of Chapter 8, p. 92.

CHAPTER 8

TREATMENT OF PSYCHOSOMATIC DISORDERS

Inclusion of an illness in the psychosomatic group implies that, in a high percentage of cases, emotional conflict in one form or another has contributed to the causation of the disorder. Because psychosomatic illnesses involve both psychologic and physiologic factors, their ideal treatment includes attention to both physical and psychologic maladaptations.

A professional attempt to identify and understand the stress that the patient is subject to is an integral part of successful therapy. Unless the ill individual can adapt successfully to life stresses, psychosomatic conditions may recur or the illness may shift from one symptom to another. Successful treatment of psychosomatic conditions is extremely complex because, at present (1) there is no single conclusive answer to the question of etiology; (2) it is not agreed which illnesses should be considered psychosomatic; and, furthermore, (3) it is not known what specifically constitutes treatment of psychosomatic disorders.

Table 8–1 defines some common forms of illnesses that are often viewed as psychosomatic disorders. Recall that psychosomatic conditions may be divided into two groups (1) *functional* illnesses, and (2) *psychophysiologic* illnesses.

FUNCTIONAL DISORDERS AND THEIR TREATMENT

You will recall that *with functional disorders the problem is primarily one of psychologic imbalance expressed in physical symptoms. Also, no physical structural change is present to account for the original symptoms.* Remember, people experiencing functional disorders are ill even though they have no organic pathology. They are definitely in a state of maladaptation, believed to be precipitated by stress, which creates an imbalance in psychologic homeostasis. Because of their discomfort, persons with functional disorders seek medical help. They are unaware that their illness does not have an organic basis. Persons with functional disorders are often met by nurses in clinics and doctors' offices, as well as in hospitals where the patient may be undergoing a diagnostic work-up.

It is recommended that once a physician is satisfied that a patient has no organic disease to account for the presenting symptoms (i.e., after a thorough diagnostic work-up), the examinations should be stopped. Then the fact that no organic disease has been found should be *sensitively discussed with* the patient, i.e., the patient is not merely "told" that this is the situation. Further help for the patient is then discussed, e.g., psychotherapy and/or relaxation therapy, as appropriate. It is not enough to merely rule out physical disease and send the patient home. Appropriate referral or plans must be made for specific therapy. This may best be done at the time the patient is told that no organic basis for symptoms has been found. Thus, the patient may leave the discussion with some sense of hope about future treatment instead of leaving feeling like "just a hypochondriac" who must be resigned to "putting up with the symptoms."

In the course of psychiatric aid, the patient is helped to understand how the mind influences the body in terms of simple illustrations, e.g., blushing. Gradually the therapist encourages discussion of the patient's life problems. This is best accomplished indirectly rather than asking outright, "Are you worried about anything?" The therapist needs to come to know each patient as a human being. The therapist assesses the patient's ability to adjust to the stresses in life, the amount of anxiety the patient habitually experiences and the nature and seriousness of ongoing conflicts. A genuine understanding of these factors involves far more than merely making a cursory examination of the patient's life and discovering "a problem." Discovering a problem does not mean that the present illness can be explained in terms of that problem. The psychiatric treatment of patients with functional illnesses is complex and specialized. Untrained persons should not attempt to "treat" such a patient, although it can be very reassuring if others indicate that they know the patient is

TABLE 8–1. SOME COMMON FORMS OF PSYCHOSOMATIC DISORDERS*

I. SKIN

Eczema. An inflammatory skin disease most common on hands and face. Lesions vary greatly in different patients: There may be dry patches, red patches, blisters, oozing, edema (swelling), scales, crusts, or pustules from secondary infection.

Urticaria (hives). A skin eruption (often in response to allergenic substances such as shellfish, penicillin, or insect bite) characterized by large, smooth, circular wheals either redder or paler than surrounding skin. Itching may be severe.

Neurodermatitis (Lichen simplex). A chronic, itching, lichen-like outbreak of the skin most typically on the nape of the neck, inner thighs, pubic region, or backs of hands. The skin lesion is commonly dark brown or purple in color with deep creases caused by constant rubbing and irritation.

II. MUSCULOSKELETAL

Backache

Muscle cramps

Tension headache. Headache caused by chronic tension in muscles of the neck and scalp.

III. RESPIRATORY

Hiccoughs

Sighing

Hyperventilation. Overbreathing; excessive rapid and deep breathing.

Bronchial asthma. Attacks of difficult breathing associated with cough, feeling of tightness in chest, and wheezing on expiration of breath. Chest may be held almost fully extended in effort to breathe. Low fever may be present.

IV. CARDIOVASCULAR

Paroxysmal tachycardia. The heart speeds up (*tachycardia* is Greek for "fast heart") to over 100 beats per minute in erratic fits.

Hypertension. High blood pressure, either erratic or chronic. May be no symptoms until damage is severe. May lead to heart and kidney failure, retinal damage, or a stroke.

Vasospasm. Sudden, involuntary contraction of the blood vessels, narrowing the passage for blood flow

Raynaud's phenomenon or disease. Spasmodic obstruction of peripheral arteries. Fingers (sometimes toes) become white or lead-blue, cold, and numb, and sometimes ache. Later blood flow is excessive; fingers become blotchy, turn red, and throb or tingle. In severe cases, gangrene may result.

Migraine. Periodic vascular headache, usually one-sided and accompanied by nausea.

Angina pectoris. Spasmodic choking or suffocating pain in the chest with feeling of impending death caused usually by insufficient oxygenation of the heart wall precipitated by effort or excitement.

Heart attack (myocardial infarction). Blood clot (thrombus) blocks vessel supplying the heart, leading to inadequate blood supply and death of muscle tissue. Pain or tightness in center of chest may radiate to arms, throat, or jaw. Patient may be white and perspiring, blood pressure may fall, and pulse may be rapid and shallow.

V. GASTROINTESTINAL

Gastritis. Inflammation of the stomach. Symptoms include gastric discomfort or pain, nausea, loss of appetite, belching, and distention of the stomach with gas.

Peptic or duodenal ulcer. An open sore on the wall of the esophagus, stomach, or duodenum caused in part by excessive production of pepsin and hydrochloric acid. Symptoms include nausea, discomfort or sharp pain an hour or two after eating, and, in severe cases, bleeding, which may be noted in vomitus or the passing of tarry-black stools.

Colitis. Inflammation of the colon leading in *ulcerative* colitis to ulcers and bleeding with symptoms such as lower abdominal pain, diarrhea, constipation, anemia, and sometimes fever. In *mucous* colitis, mucus is passed in the stools. Symptoms include indigestion, poor appetite, and less often, gas formation and resulting distension.

Hyperacidity. Excessive production of hydrochloric acid in the stomach.

Heartburn. A burning sensation in the esophagus and stomach, often with sour belching.

Nervous eructation. Nervous belching after air swallowing.

Spastic colon. The descending colon contracts tightly, causing vague attacks of abdominal pain and diarrhea.

Chronic constipation or diarrhea

VI. GENITOURINARY

Menstrual Disorders

Amenorrhea. Absence or abnormal stoppage of menstrual flow.

Menorrhagia. Excessive flow during menstruation.

Polymenorrhea. Abnormally frequent menstrual periods.

Dysmenorrhea. Painful menstruation.

Disturbances of Sexuality

Impotence. Sexual inadequacy in the male typified by either failure of penile erection, failure to maintain an erection, failure to ejaculate semen, or premature ejaculation.

Orgasmic dysfunction. Failure of sexual response in the female, ranging from sexual indifference to inability to achieve orgasm.

Vaginismus. Spasm of the vagina making sexual intercourse difficult, painful, or impossible, depending on its extent. *Dyspareunia* (from the Greek for "badly mated") is the general term for difficult or painful intercourse in women.

Urinary Disorders

Dysurea. Painful or difficult urination. *Psychic* dysurea is inability or difficulty in passing urine in the presence of other persons.

Polyurea. Passing of excessive amounts of urine.

Enuresis. Involuntary urination, especially during sleep; bedwetting.

VII. ENDOCRINE

Diabetes mellitus. A metabolic disorder in which pancreatic production of insulin is insufficient so that carbohydrate metabolism is impaired. Symptoms include thirst, frequent urination, loss of weight, fatigue and weakness, sugar in the urine, skin infections, and itching.

Hyperthyroidism. A condition caused by overproduction of thyroid hormone. Symptoms include nervousness, weight loss, protrusion of the eyes, thyroid enlargement, dislike of hot weather, and, in women, irregulatory of menstruation.

Myxedema (hypothyroidism). A condition caused by insufficient thyroid output and characterized by a peculiarly swollen face, flushed cheeks, dry skin, loss of hair (especially the outer eyebrows), anemia, low blood pressure, dislike of the cold, dizziness, hoarseness, constipation, and slowing of thought processes.

Note: Not all disorders included in this list are caused primarily by psychological factors. (From Martin, B.: *Abnormal Psychology; Clinical and Scientific Perspectives*. New York: Holt, Rinehart and Winston, 1977.)

uncomfortable. The illness may, in some way, be psychologically protective for the individual, and the patient's adaptive mechanisms must be treated with respect, knowledge, and sensitivity.

PSYCHOPHYSIOLOGIC DISORDERS AND THEIR TREATMENT

Etiology and Progression

Let us quickly review what we might consider to be the "typical" development and progression of psychophysiologic disorders. As discussed earlier, it is well known that bodily changes, such as an increased heart rate, are concomitant with anxiety. When the body's stress mechanisms function at a heightened level for a *prolonged* period of time, the eventual result may be overreaction and organ damage or malfunction. Prolonged psychophysiologic reactions can produce chronic disease and death, although, in many instances, remission or recovery is possible. Schematically we can portray the possible progressions of psychophysiologic disease as shown in Figure 8–1.

An understanding of etiology is basic to successful treatment. In attempting to understand the causation of a psychophysiologic illness, it is helpful to speculate about the following three questions:[50] (1) Why did this patient become ill in the particular manner in which the illness is presenting? (2) What kind of person is this individual that this behavior should occur in this way? (3) Why did the illness occur when it did? These questions lead us to speculate about: (a) the *physiologic* mechanism of a patient's illness, or what has happened physically; (b) the *individual,* in terms of what kind of person this particular patient is and what physical and psychologic predispositions this person tends to have; and (c) this patient's *physical and psychosocial environment* from the perspective of what the person has met with generally, e.g., food, social, and psychologic problems, irritants. When these three fields can be related to one another, we may say that the illness is explained. (The reader may find it helpful to refer back to Fig. 7–1 in the previous chapter, p. 80. Also, refer to Chapter 4, "Modern Unified Theories of Disease").

Establishing Diagnosis

In establishing a psychophysiologic *diagnosis,* a complete physical examination should be carried out. A careful physical examination, in itself, can often be therapeutically valuable to a patient, especially when accompanied by appropriate reassurance and concern. An examination typically includes radiology, electrocardiography, and laboratory work. In addition, a clinical history and a personal history of personality development should be taken. From these findings, the physician searches for evidence to support a psychophysiologic diagnosis.

Treatment Guidelines

What is the proper *treatment* of a psychophysiologic disorder? Clearly, when a patient with a

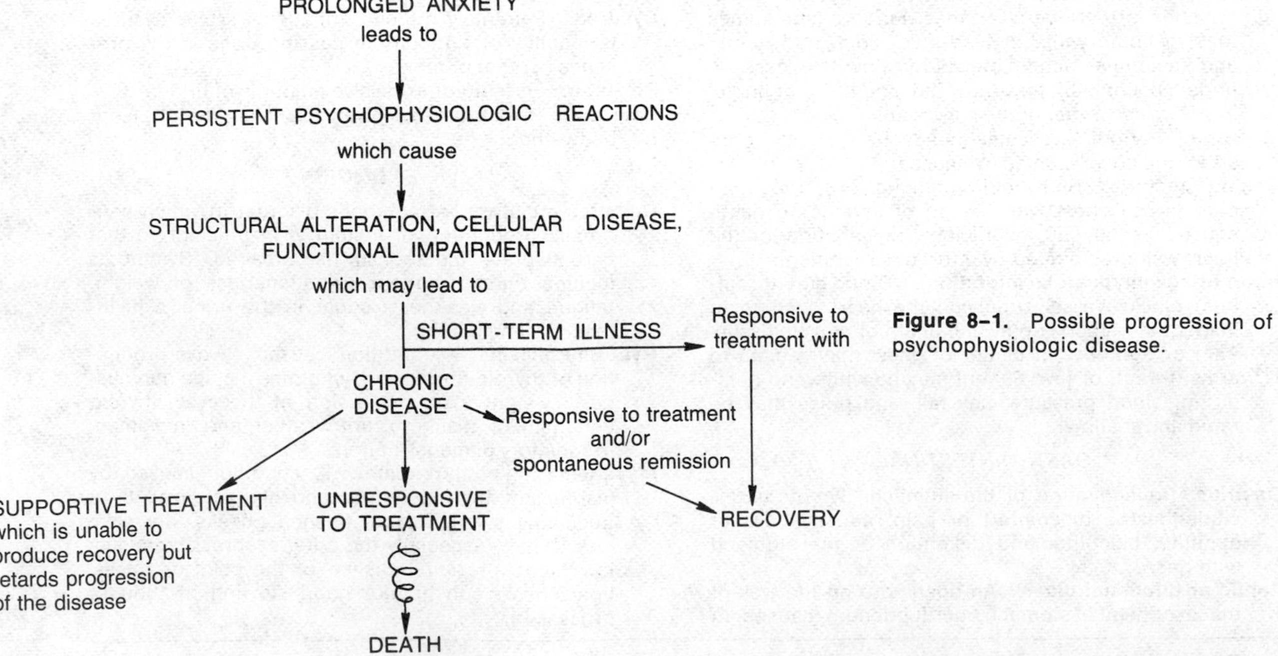

Figure 8–1. Possible progression of psychophysiologic disease.

*psycho*physiologic condition has organic pathologic changes, it is not sufficient to assess and care for the physical problem only. Purely physically oriented treatment could only produce a temporary removal of symptoms, since the individual's emotional capacity to cope with the same or new adverse situations may be unaltered or possibly even worsened. Ideally therefore, in addition to physical care, the patient needs to receive coordinated psychologic help that can focus on emotional difficulties and behavioral patterns. Other therapies, e.g., relaxation therapies, may also be helpful.

If patients with psychophysiologic disturbances are not provided with *both* physical and psychologic care, they may remain vulnerable to emotional conflict even though their physical problem appears to be corrected. Such vulnerability may mean recurrent attacks of the original psychophysiologic illness, or "*syndrome shift*" may occur, with the consecutive replacement of one syndrome by another and the production of a progression of various psychophysiologic illnesses, each differing from its precursor. *It should be recognized, however, that many patients recover from psychophysiologic disorders without either recurrence or syndrome shift.*

We do not discuss the *medical treatment* in this section of the text; rather, the various specific treatments are discussed later in the book in relation to specific medical and surgical conditions. Let us look briefly, however, at the approach of psychotherapy.

Vagueness shrouds many statements in the literature about the *psychiatric treatment* of psychophysiologic disorders. Little is published on the *specific* psychiatric treatment of these illnesses, and thus the field of therapy is permeated with generalizations. This lack of direction, in part, reflects a lack of specific etiologic knowledge. In spite of the problems, some guidelines for the psychotherapy of psychophysiologic disorders do exist.

For example, it is generally accepted by psychiatric experts that psychiatric therapy must be carefully managed so that it does not produce an emotional state that could aggravate the patient's psychophysiologic condition. The broad goal of psychiatric care is to reduce the patient's anxiety. To achieve this goal, much of the care during acute illness consists of support, reinforcement of defenses, reassurance, and gratification of dependency needs when appropriate. Tranquilizers may also be prescribed. Unfortunately, psychotherapy has not proved to be as helpful in treating psychophysiologic disorders as it was originally hoped it would be.

SOME TREATMENT MODALITIES FOR PSYCHOSOMATIC DISORDERS

To this point we have discussed the general principles of treatment for functional and psychophysiologic illnesses. Here we identify and discuss some of the various treatment modalities that may be used for any psychosomatic (i.e., functional and/or psychophysiologic) disorder.

As the evidence of the significance of mind-body interaction in disease processes becomes more abundant, increases are occurring in the kinds of therapies available to prevent stress-related illnesses and/or to offer relief to the psychophysiologically ill person. The various therapeutic methods available arise from several sources, e.g., medicine, psychiatry, psychology, pharmacotherapy. However, there are two main focuses: psychotherapy and relaxation techniques. Those therapeutic methods that take a *psychotherapeutic approach* aim at treating an underlying psychoneurosis. Through some form of psychotherapy it is hoped that change can be facilitated not only in the affected person's habitual lifestyle but also possibly in the individual's personality. In this way, the individual who has effectively participated in psychotherapy may be able to develop defense and coping mechanisms (to deal with anxiety) that do not require the development of physical disorders. In other words, the person is helped to gain behavioral insight and to learn more healthy ways of adjusting to life stresses.

As has been pointed out, anxiety almost always underlies the development of psychosomatic disorders. Anxious people are usually tense. *Relaxation therapies* may therefore be of considerable help. The following are brief descriptions of some psychotherapies and relaxation therapies that may be used either singly or in combination to prevent or treat psychosomatic disorders. (The bibliography at the end of this chapter provides detailed sources.)

Psychoanalytic Psychotherapy. Psychoanalytic psychotherapy is typically conducted in a long-term, one-to-one situation where the patient interacts with a therapist (usually a psychiatrist) who has been trained in the psychoanalytic doctrine. Although therapists may differ somewhat in their approach, the basic aim of this kind of therapy is to bring into the patient's consciousness those unconscious factors that are maintaining illness.

Group Psychotherapy. As the name implies, "group" psychotherapy occurs when a number of persons work together with one (or sometimes more than one) therapist(s). Through group discussions and other group activities, the participants can express themselves and receive help in clarifying and understanding their life conflicts. In a group situation the involved persons are able to meet with others who are experiencing similar problems and share problem-related concerns. In this way the feelings of isolation and guilt that often accompany psychosomatic disorders may be minimized or relieved. Individual group members can plan new ways of dealing with their problems, practice new behaviors in a safe environment, and receive feedback and constructive criticism from others. Most importantly, successful group therapy (a) gives each person the experience of being accepted and valued as an individual and (b) provides an environment in which truthful communication is not only possible but is actually encouraged and supported.

Family Therapy. Family therapy may be viewed as a "kind of group therapy" except that the group includes not only the person identified as "the patient" but also the people who are significant in the personal life of the patient. These significant others usually, although not always, include the patient's family. Family therapy is based upon the beliefs (and upon certain evidences) that: (a) habitual family interaction patterns may support psychophysiologic processes in individuals, and (b) families may (usually unintentionally) use the illness of one member as an "adapting mechanism" for the whole group. Typically, family therapy involves the entire family and two therapists. Work is done by the group (a) to identify the ways family members may be triggering psychosomatic responses in the patient, (b) to identify the dysfunctional use family members may make of the patient's illness, and (c) to develop more healthy ways of interaction.

Behavior Therapy. Behavior therapy is a therapeutic approach based upon learning theory. In treating a person experiencing psychosomatic disease, a behavior therapist tries to understand what the patient *thinks, feels* and *does* in particular life situations. The therapist does not concentrate on the patient's deep personality traits that may be contributing to the condition. Treatment is based on the principle that if certain behaviors can be learned, then they can be "unlearned" (or alternative behaviors can be learned to replace maladaptive behaviors). Careful assessment is always done to identify the patient's maladaptive behaviors. A variety of techniques can be used to help individuals learn more healthy behavioral patterns.

Biofeedback. As discussed in Chapter 6, biofeedback is a way of enabling individuals to exercise some control over their own physiologic processes. Electronic sensors with amplification systems are used to give the patient information (i.e., "feedback") about autonomic functioning, e.g., muscle tension, brain wave activity, skin temperature, blood pressure, heart rate. Although the mechanism involved is not completely clear, it has been found that with experience in receiving such information, a person can actually learn to bring about changes in those biologic processes that have been previously thought of as entirely "involuntary." Thus, particular body functions may be modified. Biofeedback training is relatively new and seems to be helpful for some people suffering from disorders such as hypertension, premature ventricular contractions, headaches and epilepsy.[12, 43, 103a] Figure 8–2 shows a biofeedback session.

Autogenic Therapies. Autogenic therapy is a therapeutic approach based on the belief that human beings have "inbuilt," natural, self-healing mechanisms. The purpose of such therapy is to place the individual in a position where "homeostatic self-regulatory brain mechanisms"[79] can be facilitated. A number of therapeutic approaches can be generally classified as autogenic approaches in so far as they all emphasize the self-healing ability of individuals. Most also promote relaxation and therefore reduce tension. Examples include: *autogenic training, Benson's relaxation response,*[8] *transcendental meditation,*[43] *yoga, autohypnosis* and *systematic relaxation.*

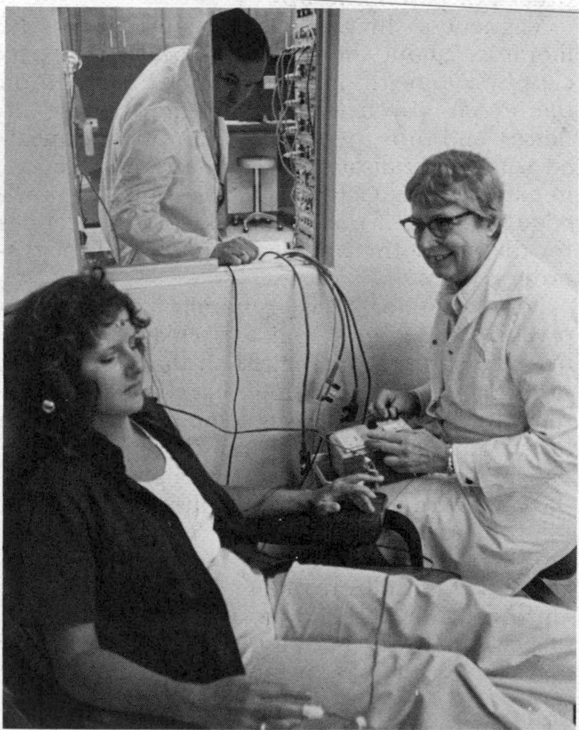

Figure 8–2. Biofeedback session. While the patient listens to relaxation tapes, the nurse therapist determines baseline data for skin temperature, heart rate, and muscle tension. (From Putt, A.M.: A biofeedback service by nurses. *American Journal of Nursing,* 79:88, 1979, p. 88.)

Pharmacotherapy. Medication may be selectively used in the treatment of psychosomatic problems and does bring relief for some people. Prescribing in this situation may place heavy demands upon the physician for many reasons, including: (a) the etiology of psychosomatic disease is unclear and complicated; (b) the use of psychotropic medication requires specialized knowledge that the non-psychiatric physician may not have, and (c) each individual patient is unique in symptom presentation and symptom combination. In addition, today many people have come to expect and even demand pharmacologic treatment whenever they consult a doctor. For these reasons a physician needs to be well informed about both the patient being treated and the drug being prescribed before making the necessary difficult decisions concerning medication prescriptions. This is essential for effective treatment.

Environmental Prescriptions. Environmental prescriptions are guides for therapeutically manipulating the patient's environment. There are times when, for example, the doctor may recommend a change in the patient's basic family environment or job situation. Obviously, such manipulations could alter the patient's life markedly, so they must be made only after an extensive assessment. For such changes to be really effective, the patient must have considerable control in such major life decisions.

Other Therapeutic Approaches. *Self-help groups, hypnosis,* and *Morita therapy* are a few of the other therapeutic approaches that may be helpful for some people experiencing psychosomatic disorders.

NURSING IMPLICATIONS

Nurses meet people with functional and psychophysiologic disorders in a variety of settings, e.g., offices, clinics, on home visits, in hospitals, possibly over the back yard fence. Patients with these disorders pose complex diagnostic and management problems for physicians. They also require skillful nursing care that involves attention to both physical and mental needs. *Physical care* varies with the area of involvement and the severity of the condition; it is discussed in detail throughout the remainder of this text in relation to specific disorders. The *general emotional nursing care* that patients with psychosomatic disorders require is not complicated *and* it does require thought.

Patients with psychosomatic conditions generally require a "giving" *attitude* on the part of those persons supplying care: an attitude of caring, support, understanding, warmth, and comfort.

The major goal of emotional care for a person with a psychosomatic disorder is to reduce anxiety.

This may involve allowing the patient to be dependent, and supporting the patient's mental defense patterns. Allowing people to be dependent does *not* mean keeping them dependent, fostering dependency, or allowing dependency to bring about physical problems or complications. Therapeutic dependency does not place a patient's physical condition in jeopardy, e.g., allowing a patient to develop pneumonia from not coughing and not moving about in bed.

Patients with psychosomatic problems are often extremely sensitive to attitudes that others have toward them. Feelings of rejection may readily intensify these patient's basic anxieties. It is of vital importance for nurses to understand that patients suffering from psychosomatic disorders are *not* "pretending" to be ill. They are *not* malingering . . . they *are* ill, perhaps suffering. A nurse's responsibility is to acknowledge a patient's discomfort and to offer comfort, support, and understanding. These patients are often not conscious of the emotional problems or stresses that may be perpetuating their illnesses. Even when the emotional problem is believed to have been identified, the relationship between the emotional situation and the pathophysiology involved may not be clearly understood — as testified by the variety of etiologic theories that currently exist.

Usually persons suffering from psychosomatic disorders genuinely desire relief from their illness and from the life problems involved in their illness. They want to adapt to life without illness. Unfortunately *some* patients with illnesses of this nature have unmet needs (for love, dependency, attention, and so forth) that cause them to *unconsciously* remain physically ill so that these needs may be partially met. In essence, they are unable to adapt their needs to "wellness" and may be unable to successfully "give up" their symptoms.

A nurse is in a position to carry out *environmental manipulation* for the psychosomatic patient within the hospital. Since a major goal of care during the acute phase of psychosomatic illness is to reduce anxiety, the nurse will want to provide a restful environment. The nurse is also in a key position to make professional *observations* concerning the patient's physical condition and his behavior. Attempts should be made to understand the patient's personality so that circumstances that may provoke anxiety can be anticipated. When anxiety-provoking situations cannot be prevented, the nurse can give appropriate emotional support. The nurse can also observe how a patient expresses anxiety and reacts to it. Patients need to be helped to express anxiety verbally whenever possible.

Nurses may effectively incorporate *relaxation techniques* into their practices in a variety of situations, e.g., to achieve pain reduction, to promote rest and sleep, in health maintenance teaching. Providing clear *patient-family teaching* of such techniques is an integral part of providing professional total care.

Of course, a nurse needs to be familiar with any *psychopharmacologic agents* that a patient receives. Patients with psychosomatic disorders may be anxious and also have an underlying depression. Drug prescriptions must therefore be carefully made and closely supervised. We are becoming increasingly aware of the need for careful supervision of the administration of psychopharmacologic agents, because of their potent nature, complex interactions, and possible serious side effects. The nurse's observations of a patient's responses to such medications are extremely important as attempts are made to determine which agents and which dosages are most helpful to the patient in relieving distressing symptoms.

Finally, let us remind you again, that the careful assessment, planning, and evaluation that is the *nursing process* is essential in the care of patients with psychosomatic illnesses. In circumstances as complex as these disorders, the systematic approach of the nursing process will reduce the possibility of overlooking or ignoring significant factors.

CONCLUSION

It is hoped that Units II, III and IV have helped you to realize that concepts of mind-body interaction are in a state of tumult. However, such tumult should not be viewed with disdain, for some theories, although admittedly fragmentary at present, hold great promise for a future understanding of human beings.

The area of mind-body interaction in the production of disease is of great importance to nursing. Increasingly it is recognized that we cannot think of the ill person as being only physically ill; concomitant mental reactions must also be considered. Concepts of psychophysiologic and psychosomatic disease are gaining an established place in health care fields. These concepts are far more complicated that they were once believed to be. Psychosomatic medicine is a field quite new to the sciences. As such it currently suffers from problems of definitions, classifications, and interpretations. Even the experts are confused. However, such confusion is part of any new scientific approach. We should be reminded that in the science of chemistry it took over a century of research before a clear definition of an element was formulated!

Realizing that some of our discussion has been very theoretical in nature, we caution you to avoid making narrow interpretations of "psychosomatic" problems in nursing practice. It is more helpful to remember that:

> *Patients can best be served if those caring for them assume that illnesses and problems arise from a* multicausal *basis. View illness as a process of* homeostatic disturbances *composed of delicate* psychophysiologic imbalances, *and keep an inquiring mind about the etiology of such imbalances.*

BIBLIOGRAPHY (Chapters 3, 7, and 8)

1. Agle, D., O. Ratnoff, and M. Wasman: Studies in autoerythrocyte sensitization. *Psychosomatic Medicine*, 29:491, Sept.-Oct. 1967.
2. Alexander, F.: *Psychosomatic Medicine: Its Principles and Applications.* New York: W. W. Norton Company, Inc., 1950.
3. Alexander, F., T. M. French, and G. H. Pollock (Eds.): *Psychosomatic Specificity.* Chicago: University of Chicago Press, 1968.
4. Altman, N.: Helping the hypochondriac. *American Family Physician,* 17:107, June 1978.
5. Arce, L.: Somatopsychic disease. *Psychosomatics,* 8:191, May–June 1972.
6. Barrins, P. C.: What nurses need to know about hypnosis. *RN,* 38:37, Jan. 1975.
7. Benson, D. F., and D. Blumer (Ed.): *Psychiatric Aspects of Neurologic Disease.* New York: Grune & Stratton, 1975.
8. Benson, H.: *The Relaxation Response.* New York: Avon Books, 1976.
9. Birk, L. (Ed.): *Behavioral Medicine: The Clinical Uses of Biofeedback.* New York: Grune & Stratton, 1973.
10. Blanchard, E. B., and L. D. Young: Clinical applications of biofeedback training. *Archives General Psychiatry,* 30:573, May 1974.
11. Bloomfield, H. H.: Transcendental meditation as an aid to medical practice. *Nursing Digest,* 4:18, Winter 1976.
12. Breeden, S. A., and C. Kondo: Using biofeedback to reduce tension. *American Journal of Nursing,* 75:2010, Nov. 1975.
13. Brena, S.: *Yoga and Medicine.* Baltimore: Penguin Books, Inc., 1972.
14. Bronner-Huszar, J.: The psychological aspects of cancer in man. *Psychosomatics,* 12:133, Mar.–Apr. 1971.
15. Brophy, J. J.: Psychiatric disorders. *In* Krupp, M. A., and M. J. Chatton: *Current Medical Diagnosis & Treatment 1977.* Los Altos, Cal.: Lange Medical Publications, 1977 (Chapter 17).
16. Buchan, D. J.: Mind-body relationships in gastrointestinal disease. *The Canadian Nurse,* 67:35, Mar. 1971.
17. Budzynski, T. H.: Biofeedback procedures in the clinic. *Seminars in Psychiatry,* 5:537, Nov. 1973.
18. Calder, N.: *The Mind of Man.* New York: The Viking Press, 1970.
19. Carella, M. J.: Psychoanalysis and the mind-body problem. *Psychoanalytic Review,* 61:53, Spring 1974.

20. Cloudsley, T., and J. Leonard: *Animal Conflict and Adaptation.* Chester Springs, Penn.: Dufour Editions, 1965.
21. DeLuca, J. C.: The ulcerative colitis personality. *Nursing Clinics of North America, 5*:23, March 1970.
22. Destounis, N.: Aggression: culture and psychosomatic medicine. *Psychotherapy and Psychosomatics,* 24:123, 1974.
23. Dimond, S. J.: *Introducing Neuropsychology: The Study of Mind and Brain.* Springfield, Ill.: Charles C Thomas, 1978.
24. Dimsdale, J. E., et al.: Emotional correlates of type A behavior pattern. *Psychosomatic Medicine,* 40:580, Nov. 1978.
25. Dohrenwend, B. S., and B. P. Dohrenwend (Eds.): *Stressful Life Events: Their Nature and Effects.* New York: Wiley, 1974.
26. Dorfman, W.: *Closing the Gap Between Medicine and Psychiatry.* Springfield, Ill.: Charles C Thomas, 1966.
27. Doyle, D. K.: A case study in hypnotherapy. *American Journal of Nursing,* 77:806, May 1977.
28. Dudley, D. L., and E. Welke: *How to Survive Being Alive.* Garden City, New York: Doubleday, 1977.
29. Dudley, D. L., and E. Welke: You are how you cope. *Working Woman,* 2:60, Sept. 1977.
30. Dunbar, F.: *Mind and Body: Psychosomatic Medicine.* New York. Random House, 1947.
31. Editorial: A retrospective look at psychosomatic medicine. *Canadian Psychiatric Association Journal,* 17:1, Feb. 1972.
32. Engel, G.: Emotional stress and sudden death. *Psychology Today,* 11:114, Nov. 1977.
33. Field, W. E., Jr.: Treating psychosomatic disorders with behavior therapy: nursing implications. *Nursing Digest,* 3:17, Nov.–Dec. 1975.
34. Fischer, H. K., et al.: Psychosomatic medicine. *Progress in Neurology and Psychiatry,* 25:409, 1970.
35. Fordyce, W. E.: *Behavioral methods for chronic pain and illness.* St. Louis: C. V. Mosby Co., 1976.
36. Frank, J. D.: The faith that heals. *Johns Hopkins Medical Journal,* 137:127, Mar. 1975.
37. Frazer, A., and A. Winokur: *Biological Bases of Psychiatric Disorders.* New York: SP Books Division of Spectrum Publications, 1977.
38. Freedman, A. M., H. I. Kaplan, and B. J. Sadock (Eds.): *Comprehensive Textbook of Psychiatry,* 2nd Ed. 2 Vols. Baltimore: Williams & Wilkins Co., 1975.
39. Freedman, A. M., H. I. Kaplan and B. J. Sadock: *Modern Synopsis of Comprehensive Textbook of Psychiatry II,* 2nd Ed. Baltimore: Williams & Wilkins Co., 1976.
40. Garfinkel, P. E., et al.: Body awareness in anorexia nervosa: disturbances in "body image" and "satiety." *Psychosomatic Medicine,* 40:487, Oct. 1978.
41. Globus, G. G., G. Maxwell, and I. Savodnik, (Eds.): *Consciousness and the Brain: A Scientific and Philosophical Inquiry.* New York: Plenum Press, 1976.
42. Gold, D. D., Jr.: Psychological factors associated with obesity. *American Family Physician,* 13:87, June 1976.
43. Gorman, M. L.: Conscious repatterning of human behavior. *American Journal of Nursing,* 75:1752, Oct. 1975.
44. Gottschalk, L. A.: Psychosomatic medicine today: An overview. *Psychosomatics,* 19:89, Feb. 1978.
45. Graham, D. T.: Health, disease, and the mind-body problem: Linguistic parallelism. *Psychosomatic Medicine,* 29:52, Jan.–Feb. 1967.
46. Graham, D. T.: Psychophysiology and medicine. *Psychophysiology,* 8:121, Mar. 1971.
47. Grenell, R. G., and S. Gabay: *Biological Foundations of Psychiatry.* New York: Raven Press, 1976.
48. Grinker, R. R., and F. P. Robbins: *Psychosomatic Casebook.* New York: Blakiston Division, McGraw-Hill Book Co., Inc. 1954.
49. Groen, J. J.: The challenge of the future: The prevention of psychosomatic disorders. *Psychotherapy and Psychosomatics,* 23:283, 1974.
50. Halliday, J. L.: Concept of a psychosomatic affectation. *Lancet,* 2:692, 1943.
51. Hayter, J.: Patients who have Alzheimer's disease. *American Journal of Nursing,* 74:1460, Aug. 1974.
52. Heim, E., A. Moser, and R. Adler: Defense mechanisms and coping behavior in terminal illness: An overview. *Psychotherapy and Psychosomatics,* 30:1, No. 1, 1978.
53. Herz, F.: The psychiatric clinical specialist in the general hospital: A view. *Supervisor Nurse,* 2:75–81, May 1971.
54. Hurst, M. W., C. D. Jenkins, and R. M. Rose: The assessment of life change stress: A comparative and methodological inquiry. *Psychosomatic Medicine,* 40:127, Mar. 1978.
55. In sickness and in health. *Emergency Medicine,* 9:61, May 1977.
56. Jacobs, L. I.: Emotionally caused neurasthenia. *Consultant,* 17:57, Oct. 1977.
57. Jacobson, E.: *Self-Operations Control: A Manual of Tension Control.* Chicago: National Foundation for Progressive Relaxation, 1964.
58. Jones, A. C.: Life change and psychological distress as predictors of pregnancy outcome. *Psychosomatic Medicine,* 40:401, Aug. 1978.
59. Karlin, M., and L. M. Andrews: *Biofeedback: Turning on the Powers of Your Mind.* Philadelphia: J. B. Lippincott Co., 1972.
60. Kessel, N., and A. Munro: Epidemiological studies in psychosomatic medicine. *Journal of Psychosomatic Research,* 8:67, July 1964.
61. Kimball, C. P.: Conceptual developments in psychosomatic medicine: 1939–1969. *Annals of Internal Medicine,* 73:307, Aug. 1970.
62. Knapp, P. H.: The psychosomatic field. *Psychosomatic Medicine,* 32:425, July–Aug. 1970.
63. Kot, P. A.: The physiology of TM. *American Family Physician,* 14:155, Nov. 1976.
64. Krieger, D.: Therapeutic touch: The imprimatur of nursing. *American Journal of Nursing,* 75:784, May 1975.
65. Kroger, W. S.: *Clinical and Experimental Hypnosis.* Philadelphia: J. B. Lippincott Co., 1963.
66. Lachman, S. J.: *Psychosomatic Disorders.* New York: John Wiley & Sons, 1972.
67. Leigh, H.: Self-Control, biofeedback and change in 'psychosomatic' approach. *Psychotherapy and Psychosomatics,* 30:130, No. 2, 1978.
68. Leshner, A. I.: *An Introduction to Behavioral Endocrinology.* New York: Oxford University Press, 1978.
69. Levine, M. E.: Holistic nursing. *Nursing Clinics of North America,* 6:253, June 1971.
70. Lewis, H. R., and M. E. Lewis: *Psychosomatics: How Your Emotions Can Damage Your Health.* New York: Pinnacle Books, 1975.
71. Lipowski, Z. J.: Introduction. *In* Lipowski, Z. J. (Ed.): *Psychosocial Aspects of Physical Illness. Advances in Psychosomatic Medicine.* Vol. 8. New York: S. Karger, 1972.
72. Lipowski, Z. J.: New perspectives in psychosomatic

medicine. *Canadian Psychiatric Association Journal,* 15:515, Dec. 1970.
73. Lipowski, Z. J.: Psychiatry of somatic diseases: Epidemiology, pathogenesis, classification. *Comprehensive Psychiatry,* 16:105, Mar./Apr. 1975.
74. Lipowski, Z. J. (Ed.): *Psychosocial Aspects of Physical Illness. Advances in Psychosomatic Medicine,* Vol. 8. New York: S. Karger, 1972.
75. Lipowski, Z. J.: Psychosomatic medicine in the seventies: An overview. *American Journal Psychiatry,* 134:233, Mar. 1977.
76. Lipowski, Z. J., and R. Z. Kiriakos: Borderlands between neurology and psychiatry: Observations in a neurological hospital. *Psychiatry in Medicine,* 3:131, Apr. 1972.
77. Lipsitt, D. R.: Some problems in the teaching of psychosomatic medicine. *International Journal Psychiatry in Medicine,* 6:317, Vol. 1/2, 1975.
78. Lucia, S. P.: The psyche of man and his illness. *Medical Times,* 99:140, Aug. 1971.
79. Luthe, W., and J. H. Schultz: *Autogenic Therapy. Medical Applications.* New York: Grune & Stratton, 1970.
80. Lysebeth, A. V.: *Yoga Self-Taught.* New York: Barnes and Noble, 1973.
81. Martin, B.: *Abnormal Psychology: Clinical and Scientific Perspectives.* New York: Holt, Rinehart and Winston, 1977.
82. Mathis, J. L.: A sophisticated version of voodoo death: Report of a case. *Psychosomatic Medicine,* 26:104, Mar.–Apr. 1964.
83. Matthews, K. A., and F. E. Saal: Relationship of the type A coronary-prone behavior pattern to achievement, power and affiliation motives. *Psychosomatic Medicine,* 40:631, Dec. 1978.
84. Maultsby, M. C., Jr., and P. Winkler: Directed rational self-counseling (A new approach to mass mental health). *ANA Clinical Sessions 1972.* New York: Appleton-Century-Crofts, 1973.
85. McKenzie, J. L., and N. J. Chrisman: Healing herbs, gods, and magic: Folk health beliefs among Filipino-Americans. *Nursing Outlook,* 77:326, May 1977.
86. Melton, J. H.: A boy with anorexia nervosa. *American Journal of Nursing,* 74:1649, Sept. 1974.
87. Menninger, W.: Biofeedback training can help to cure migraines. *The Seattle Times,* Sunday, November 6, 1977 (Copyright 1977, Universal Press Syndicate).
88. Meyers, S. T.: You *Have* to Find Time to Nurse the Mind, Too. *RN,* 41:63, Jan. 1978.
89. Miller, N., et al. (Eds.): *Biofeedback and Self-Control 1973.* (An Aldine Annual on the regulation of bodily processes and consciousness.) Chicago: Aldine Publishing Co., 1974.
90. Mintz, T.: Tickle — The itch that moves: A psychophysiological hypothesis. *Psychosomatic Medicine,* 29:606, Nov.–Dec. 1967.
91. Minuchin, S., B. L. Rosman, and L. Baker: *Psychosomatic Families: Anorexia Nervosa in Context.* Cambridge, Mass.: Harvard University Press, 1978.
92. Morehouse, L. E., and L. Gross: How you can have the most ENERGY. *Working Woman,* 2:26, Sept. 1977.
93. Mowchenko, G.: Care of patients with GI diseases that have a psychological component. *Canadian Nurse,* 38:40, Mar. 1971.
94. Norton, W. A.: Mind, body and language. *Canadian Psychiatric Association Journal,* 12:93, Apr. 1967.
95. Nourse, A. E., and Editors of the Time-Life Books. *The Body.* (Life Science Library). New York: Time-Life Books, 1964 (Revised 1968).
96. Parker, B., et al.: Finding medical reasons for psychiatric behavior. *Geriatrics,* 31:87, June 1976.
97. Pelletier, K. R.: *Mind as Healer, Mind as Slayer: A Holistic Approach to Preventing Stress Disorders.* New York: Delacourt Press: Seymore Lawrence, 1977.
98. Polanyi, M.: The mind-body relation. *In* Rogers, C., and W. Clauson (Eds.): *Man and the Science of Man.* Columbus, Ohio: Charles E. Merrill Publishing Co., 1968.
99. Polonia, P.: Mind-mind problems from an empirical point of view. *British Journal of Psychiatry,* 118:7, Jan. 1971.
100. Porter, R., and J. Knight (Eds.): *Physiology, Emotion, and Psychosomatic Illness.* CIBA Foundation Symposium 8. New York: Associated Scientific Publishers, 1972.
101. Pos, R.: The psyche-soma complex: An exercise in symbolic logic. *Canadian Psychiatric Association Journal,* 12:125, Apr. 1967.
102. Price, K. P.: A biofeedback service by nurses. *American Journal of Nursing,* 79:88, Jan. 1979.
103. Profile: Vivian Meehan brings hope to victims of anorexia. *American Journal of Nursing,* 79:340, Feb. 1979.
103a. Putt, A. M.: A biofeedback service by nurses. *American Journal of Nursing,* 79:88, Jan. 1979.
104. Raskin, M., et al.: Chronic anxiety treated by feedback-induced muscle relaxation. *Archives General Psychiatry,* 28:263, Feb. 1973.
105. Reading, A.: Illness and disease. *Medical Clinics of North America,* 61:703, July 1977.
106. Reece, R. M.: Anorexia Nervosa. *American Family Physician,* 13:121, Apr. 1976.
107. Reiser, M. F.: Changing theoretical concepts in psychosomatic medicine. *In* Arieti, S. (Ed. in Chief): *American Handbook of Psychiatry,* 2nd Ed. (Vol. 4, *Organic Disorders and Psychosomatic Medicine.*) New York: Basic Books, Inc., 1975, Chapter 21.
108. Rittelmeyer, L. F.: Caring for the hypochondriac. *American Family Physician,* 14:98, Sept. 1976.
109. Roseman, T. B.: Schizophrenics get sick too. *RN,* 40:39, Dec. 1977.
110. Rosin, A. J.: The influence of emotional reaction on the course of fatal illness. *Geriatrics,* 31:87, July 1976.
111. Rowlett, D. B., and D. L. Dudley: COPD: Psychosocial and psychophysiological issues. *Psychosomatics,* 19:273, May 1978.
112. Rubin, J.: Positive functions of psychosomatic symptoms. *Medical Times,* 93:769, July 1965.
113. Ruesch, J.: Social technique, social status, and social change in illness. *In* Kluckholn, C., and H. Murray (Eds.): *Personality in Nature, Society and Culture.* New York: Alfred A. Knopf, 1959.
114. Russell, R.: Use mind control to ease your patient's ills. *RN,* 39:32, May 1976.
115. Ryan, B. J.: Biofeedback training: The voluntary control of mind over body and mind. *Nursing Forum.* 14:48, No. 1, 1975.
116. Schecter, N.: Management of emotional illnesses in general practice. *Psychosomatics,* 6:132, May–June 1965.
117. Schmidt, M. P. W., and B. A. B. Duncan: Modifying eating behavior in anorexia nervosa. *American Journal of Nursing,* 74:1646, Sept. 1974.
118. Schneider, D. E.: *Revolution in the Body-Mind.* Easthampton, N.Y.: Alexa Press, 1977.
119. Schuster, M. M.: Gastrointestinal tract dysfunctions respond to biofeedback. *Geriatrics,* 32:32, June 1977.
120. Schwab, J. J.: Enlarging our view of psychosomatic medicine. *Psychosomatics,* 12:16, Jan.–Feb. 1971.

121. Schwab, J. J., and R. B. Schwab: Social psychiatry and psychosomatics. *Psychosomatics,* 16:151, Oct.–Nov.–Dec. 1975.
122. Sheehan, D. V., and T. P. Hackett: Psychosomatic disorders. *In* Nicholi, A. M., Jr. (Ed.): *The Harvard Guide to Modern Psychiatry.* Cambridge, Mass.: The Belknap Press of Harvard University Press, 1978.
123. Shulkin, M. W.: Classification of psychophysiologic conditions. *In* Nodine, J. H., and J. H. Moyer (Eds.): *Psychosomatic Medicine.* Philadelphia: Lea & Febiger, 1962.
124. Smart, A.: Conscious control of physical and mental states. *Menninger Perspective,* 1:22 Apr.–May, 1970.
125. Snow, L. F.: Folk medical beliefs and their implications for the care of patients. *Annals of Internal Medicine,* 81:82, July 1974.
126. Spiro, H. M.: The tools of our trade — Some comments on disease and disorder. *New England Journal of Medicine,* 292:575, 1975.
127. Steger, H. G.: Understanding the psychologic factors in rehabilitation. *Geriatrics,* 31:68, May 1976.
128. Sterman, L. T.: Clinical biofeedback. *American Journal of Nursing,* 75:2006, Nov. 1975.
129. Stewart, B. M.: Biochemical aspects of schizophrenia. *American Journal of Nursing,* 75:2176, Dec. 1975.
130. Strassman, H. D., M. B. Thalder, and E. H. Schein: A prisoner of war syndrome: Apathy as a reaction to severe stress. *American Journal of Psychiatry,* 112:998 1956.
131. Stubbert, J., et al.: Physical fitness: A key to emotional health. *RN,* 38:30, Aug. 1975.
132. Taylor, F. K.: The medical model of the disease concept. *British Journal of Psychiatry,* 128:588, June 1976.
133. Taylor, G. J.: The mind-body dichotomy. *Psychosomatics,* 19:264, May 1978.
134. Teitelbaum, H. A.: *Psychosomatic Neurology.* New York: Grune & Stratton, Inc., 1964.
135. The inside story of a patient's ills. *Emergency Medicine,* 10:229, Nov. 1978.
136. Tinling, D. C.: Voodoo, root work, and medicine. *Psychosomatic Medicine,* 29:483, Sept.–Oct. 1967.
137. Vaillant, G. E.: Natural history of male psychological health, IV: What kinds of men do not get psychosomatic illness. *Psychosomatic Medicine.* 40:420, Aug. 1978.
138. Vanderpool, J. P., et al.: Empathy: Towards a psychophysiological definition. *Diseases of the Nervous System,* 31:464, July 1970.
139. Von Bertalanffy, L.: The mind-body problem: A new view. *Psychosomatic Medicine,* 26:29, Jan.–Feb. 1964.
140. Wallace, R. K., and H. Benson: The physiology of meditation. *In* Ornstein, R. E. (Ed.): *The Nature of Human Consciousness: A Book of Readings.* San Francisco: W. H. Freeman and Company, 1973.
141. Warner, R.: The relationship between language and disease concepts. *International Journal of Psychiatry in Medicine,* 7:57, No. 1., 1976–1977.
142. Webster, T. G.: Learning processes in physician education: Integrating psyche and soma. *Psychiatry in Medicine,* 2:67, Jan. 1971.
143. Weiner, H. M.: *Psychobiology and Human Disease.* New York: Elsevier, 1977.
144. Weiner, H.: Toward a mind-body therapy. *Psychoanalytic Review,* 61:45, Spring 1974.
145. Werth, G. R.: The hives dilemma. *American Family Physician,* 17:139, May 1978.
146. Wilson, L. G.: The couvade syndrome. *American Family Physician,* 15:157, May 1977.
147. Wilson, R. L.: An introduction to yoga. *American Journal of Nursing,* 76:261, Feb. 1976.
148. Wilson, R. R., and the Editors of Time-Life Books. *The Mind.* (Life Science Library). New York: Time-Life Books, 1969.
149. Wise, T. N.: Pain: The most common psychosomatic problem. *Medical Clinics of North America,* 61:771, July 1977.
150. Wittkower, E. D.: Some selected psychosomatic problems of current interest. *Psychosomatics,* 12:21, Jan.–Feb. 1971.
151. Wittkower, E. D., and H. Warnes (Eds.): *Psychosomatic Medicine: Its Clinical Applications.* Hagerstown, Maryland: Harper & Row, 1977.
152. Wittkower, E. D., and H. Warnes: Transcultural psychosomatics. *Psychotherapy and Psychosomatics,* 23:1 1974.
153. White, J., and J. Fadiman (Eds.): *Relax: How You Can Feel Better, Reduce Stress and Overcome Tension.* The Confucian Press, Inc., 1976.
154. Worden, J. W., and H. J. Sobel: Ego strength and psychosocial adaptation to cancer. *Psychosomatic Medicine,* 40:585, Dec. 1978.

UNIT V

THE BODY'S RESPONSE TO DISTURBANCES IN HOMEOSTASIS

A wide variety of physiologic imbalances can occur that can disturb bodily homeostasis. Some of these imbalances are listed below:

1. Cellular disturbances
2. Inflammation
3. Drug intoxication*
4. Fluid and electrolyte imbalances
5. Hydrogen ion imbalance
6. Anoxia and asphyxia*
7. Tissue repair and regeneration (the body's response to injury and infection)
8. Physiologic shock
9. Infection*
10. Immunity and hypersensitivity
11. Auto-immunity
12. Nutritional imbalance*
13. Genetic defects*
14. Disturbances in blood flow*
15. Hemorrhage*
16. Extremes in temperature,* and burns*
17. Ionizing radiation*

The starred items are discussed in other units of the text. This unit will focus on the following major areas of discussion, all of which are basic to nursing care.

- ▶ The cell and cellular disturbances
- ▶ Responses to injury (inflammation and repair)
- ▶ The immune system (immunity, hypersensitivity, and auto-immune disorders)
- ▶ Fluid and electrolyte and hydrogen ion imbalances
- ▶ Shock

CHAPTER 9*

THE NORMAL CELL AND CELLULAR DISTURBANCES

Whatever its form, however it behaves, the cell is the basic unit of a living matter. In the cell, nature has enclosed in a microscopic package all the parts and processes necessary to the survival of life in an ever-changing world.

John Pfeiffer, *The Cell*[11]

INTRODUCTION AND STUDY GUIDE

Cells are the basic units or building blocks of all living organisms. Within the adult human body there are approximately 60,000 billion cells — each of them energetically multiplying, reacting to stimuli, producing enzymes, and carrying out many precise and highly specialized functions. Dynamic, frantically active, and yet orderly in its workings, the healthy cell exists as a miniature chemistry laboratory, powerhouse, factory, and duplicating machine — perfectly reproducing itself over and over again. Of course, when aging, illness, and injury strike the cell, as they inevitably will, pathologic changes develop which alter both cellular structure and function. As a consequence, the cell's ability to work and produce is curtailed, to the detriment of the total organism.

In this chapter, we review briefly the structure and function of the normal healthy cell as well as some of the major pathologic problems that affect, damage, and destroy cells. To aid you in your study of the cell, we refer you to the following guide:

1. Upon completion of this chapter, you should be aware of the definitions of the following key terms:

cytoplasm	mitochondria
cell membrane	ribosomes
"receptor theory"	endoplasmic reticulum
nucleus	smooth ER
nucleoli	rough ER
chromosomes	lysosome
chromatin	phagocytosis
nucleic acid	pinocytosis
DNA	degeneration
RNA	infiltration
chromatin	necrosis
organelles	cell death

2. You should be able to discuss generally the following subjects:

a. Major components and composition of cells
b. General functions of cells
c. Major specialized cell groups
d. Causes of cellular damage
e. Major types of degenerations
f. Major types of disturbances in cell growth
g. Major types of cellular necrosis

THE LIVING CELL: A STRUCTURAL AND PHYSIOLOGIC UNIT

Cellular Composition

Cells are composed of protoplasm, a heavy, thick colloidal material that actively exhibits the basic properties of all living matter, namely, growth, movement, reproduction, secretion, irritability, ingestion, and assimilation.

A highly complex substance, protoplasm is composed of many different chemical materials. The most important are the following:

Water. 70 to 85 per cent of protoplasm is water, which acts both as a universal solvent for cellular chemicals and as a fluid medium in which chemical reactions can take place.

Protein. 10 to 25 per cent of protoplasm is composed of protein, which, in turn, is made up of atoms of hydrogen, oxygen, nitrogen, carbon and sulfur. *Structural proteins* make up the surrounding membranes of the cell as well

*Joyce Gauthier, B.Sc. in Bacteriology, critically reviewed and assisted with the revision of this chapter.

as the membranes of many of the tiny structures that exist within the cell. *Enzymes* (which are a type of protein) are also found within the cell. These extremely important protein substances have the power to catalyze chemical reactions, thereby accelerating the speed of vital cellular activities.

Electrolytes. You will recall from chemistry that an electrolyte is a substance or compound composed of atoms which, when placed in solution, break up into separate, charged particles called ions. The most important intracellular electrolytes are potassium, magnesium, phosphate, sulfate, and bicarbonate. The role of these cellular electrolytes will be discussed in detail in Chapter 12.

Lipids. These fatty or fat-like substances, which are generally insoluble in water, make up approximately 2 to 3 per cent of protoplasm. One of the clinically most important cellular lipids is cholesterol.

Carbohydrates. Only about 1 per cent of the protoplasm is composed of carbohydrate. *Glycogen* is a form of carbohydrate frequently stored within liver and skeletal muscle cells. It is readily available for utilization in the production of energy. Also, carbohydrates may be attached to certain proteins that are incorporated into the cell membrane.

The Major Components of the Cell: Their Structure and Function

The cell is composed of three major parts: (1) the cell membrane, (2) the nucleus, and (3) the cytoplasm (Fig. 9–1). The cytoplasm, in turn, holds within its jelly-like substance several tiny, vitally important structures called organelles ("little organs"). Because each of these cellular structures performs specialized functions vital to the metabolism of both the individual cell and the total organism, we shall briefly consider them individually.

The Cell Membrane. This porous, thin, elastic membrane is composed mainly of protein and lipid substances. Only 100 angstrom units (one angstrom unit equals 1 ten-millionth of a millimeter) thick, the cell membrane firmly encircles and encloses the cytoplasm. The cell membrane acts (a) to control the passage of substances into and out of the cell and (b) in information processing.

The cellular membrane is a highly selective structure which allows only certain substances to enter and leave the internal environment of the cell. The cell itself works to maintain this controlled inward and outward flow of substances both actively and passively. Actively, it expends its energy to transport electrolytes and other materials across the membrane in either direction; passively, it allows certain substances to seep through the membranes in accordance with the laws of filtration, diffusion, and osmosis.* Potassium tends to be held within the cell, while most sodium ions and plasma are actively excluded from the cell. Water and food pass freely through the cell's semipermeable membrane, while waste products flow, unhindered, outward into the external environment.

The cell membrane, although structurally flimsy, acts as a highly selective and effective casing for the cellular contents; thus, it is a

*Fluid movement is discussed in Chapter 12.

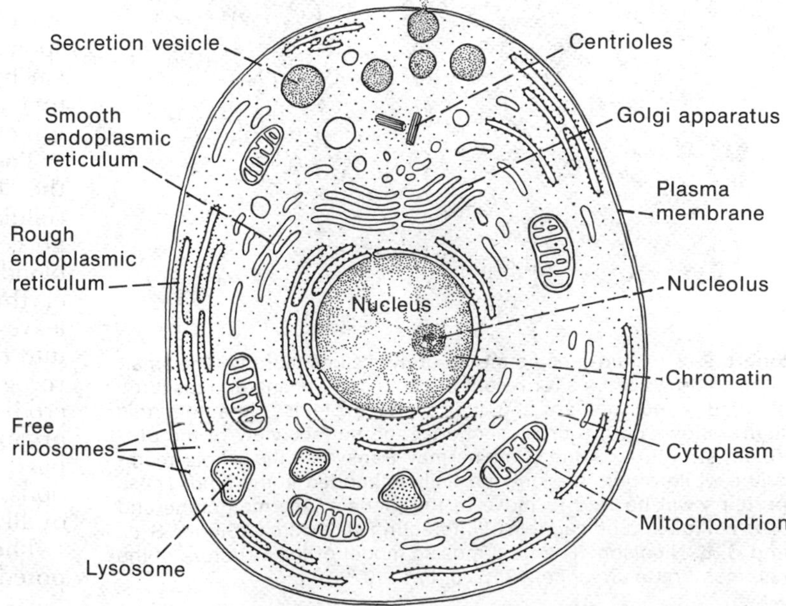

Figure 9–1. Diagram of a generalized animal cell. Although this is a round cell, animal cells may have many shapes. Note the secretion vesicle at the top of the cell, expelling its contents to the external environment.

major line of protection against intrusion into the cell by disruptive forces.

It is fortunate indeed, that the vital cell membrane can regenerate itself should it tear or rupture. Exactly how the cell membrane is repaired remains unknown. However, authorities do recognize that cellular membrane repair will not occur, following rupture, if there are an abnormally low number of calcium ions within the body fluid; calcium evidently helps to promote the health of the cell membrane, as well as the safety of the cytoplasm and the tiny nucleus that it envelops.

The cell membrane's role in the procedure by which information is received, processed, and responded to within the individual cell remains somewhat of a mystery. Scientists do know that the cell membrane is not a rigid structure. Rather, it can be described as a "fluid mosaic" embedded in a sea of lipid (Fig. 9–2). This fluid nature allows for a dynamic and ever-changing pattern on the cell membrane. The proteins at the cell surface are able to move much as dancers meeting and parting on a ballroom floor. Interactions between proteins on the cell surface are critical in stimulating cells to perform their functions.

To understand the interactons of cells with drugs, chemicals, and other cells, you must first understand the concept of *receptor theory.* This theory proposes the presence of cell membrane structures — termed *receptors* —capable of interacting with stimuli. In order to be affected by a specific stimulus (e.g., epinephrine), the cell must possess on its surface a receptor for that stimulus (Fig. 9–3).

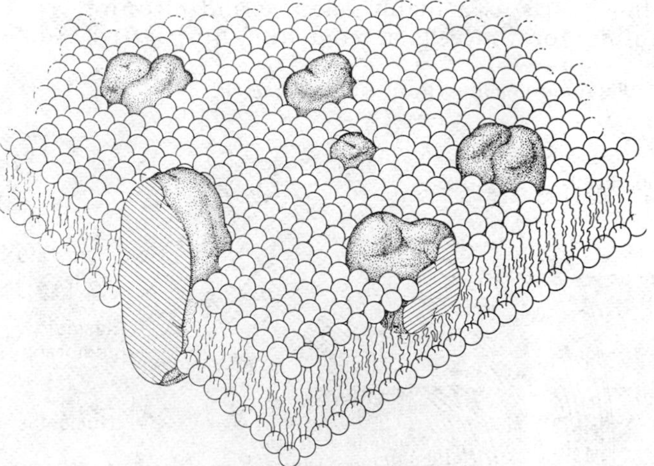

Figure 9–2. Fluid-mosaic model of the cell membrane. The small circles and wavy lines represent the lipid component, and the large stippled structures are the membrane proteins. Note that this figure shows both a cross-sectional and surface view of the proposed structure. Some proteins may transverse the whole membrane while others are only partially imbedded in the lipid. These proteins will be free to move in the plane of the membrane and thus collide and be capable of interacting at this time. (Singer, S. J., and G. L. Nicolson: The fluid mosaic model of the structure of the cell membrane. *Science,* 175:720, Feb. 1972.)

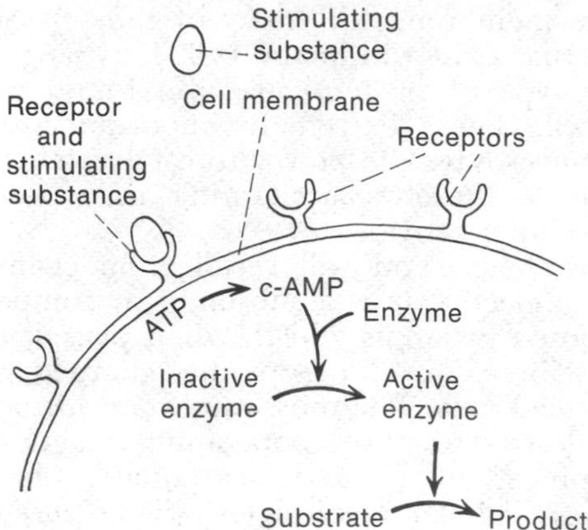

Figure 9–3. *Receptor theory.* One example of how the cell membrane functions in information processing. Note that in this illustration (representative of *some* hormones; e.g., epinephrine, insulin) the stimulating substance never enters the cell. In the case of steroid hormones (e.g., estrogen, progesterone, testosterone), the hormone is believed to enter the cell and react with receptors in the cytoplasm and/or nucleus.

Since the cell membrane represents the interface of the cell with its environment, you can appreciate that information coming into the cell must cross the cell membrane, although the stimulator substance may itself never enter the cell. Information is most commonly relayed from the cell membrane through an internal communication system composed of *chemical pathways.* One of the most common of these "communication chemicals" is cyclic adenosine monophosphate (c-AMP). Typically, c-AMP is produced in response to changes at the membrane surface (such as the binding of a hormone to its receptor), at which time it acts to stimulate or inhibit metabolic pathways in the cell.

The Nucleus. The nucleus has been called the "brain" of the cell because it is so vital to cellular life. Indeed, it was once believed that no cell, with the exception of the mature red blood cell, could live without its nucleus. (An erythrocyte loses its nucleus just before it leaves the bone marrow for its maiden voyage into the general circulation.) However, we now recognize, through experiments involving microdissection of cells, that certain unicellular organisms can live even though their nuclei have been removed. Other than a few exceptions, the nucleus is essential to the existence of all cells.

The nucleus is a spherical structure composed of a substance called nucleoplasm and

the cells that compose it will suffer because of the failure of the heart as a pump, and the resulting disruption in the circulation of oxygenated blood.

Major Characteristics and Activities of Cells

Although cells have their own unique special functions and attributes, they also share many characteristics. All cells reproduce, react to stimuli, and move either by ameboid motion or by means of cilia. The most important activities of cells are:

- Synthesis of protein molecules.
- Production of energy for cellular work.
- Maintenance of a homeostatic environment within the cell.
- Ingestion and assimilation by the cell of materials from the outside environment by means of active and passive transport, pinocytosis, and phagocytosis.*
- Reproduction within unicellular organisms (by means of simple division) and in higher organisms (by means of mitotic division). All cells of the human body divide and reproduce, with the exception of the cells of the brain, spinal cord, glomerulus of the kidney, and striated and cardiac muscles. These cells, which cannot be replaced, are called *permanent cells.* As you will see later, the process of mitosis contains implications for the problem of cancer.
- Differentiation of cells to produce a multicellular organism. Basically a given cell contains all the genetic material an organism has. Through unknown mechanisms, a given cell will express some of the abilities contained in its genetic material and inhibit others. Thus cells in a multicellular organism express different structures and functions despite the fact that they all evolved from a single fertilized ovum. For example, a liver cell functions and looks different from a white blood cell or a bone cell. In cancer, cells begin to dedifferentiate, or lose their special structural and functional identity.

In essence, the body cells—like the body itself—must eat, drink, digest and assimilate substances, protect themselves by reacting to stimuli, reproduce, build products, and expend energy. Also, like the total organism, cells age, become sick and injured, lose their ability to function and to generate energy, die, and finally decay.

**Pinocytosis,* is the engulfment and ingestion of *liquid* droplets by the cell, whereas *phagocytosis* is the engulfment and ingestion of such large particles of matter as bacteria and other cells. Pinocytosis is derived from the Greek word that means *to drink,* while phagocytosis is taken from the Greek word meaning *to eat.*

AGING AND INJURY OF THE CELL

The Aging Cell

Like the human beings they compose, cells age, wither, and die. In a young healthy person, cells are constantly and rapidly multiplying and dividing, and they function efficiently. With aging, however, a person's cells tend to multiply more sluggishly and to perform their tasks with less perfection. Thus, as time passes and people grow old, they usually suffer from a deficiency of cells, and they must also rely upon cells that function less effectively.

What happens to our cells as they age? Many different untoward changes occur; for example, with aging, cells shrink in size, protein synthesis slows, the Golgi complexes begin to break apart, and the mitochondria may fragment into pieces. Ultimately the aged cell dies and disappears—its nucleus disintegrating and its cytoplasm liquefying.

Different types of cells have different life spans. For example, those epithelial cells lining the intestinal tract live only about a day and a half; red blood cells can live for 120 days. At the opposite extreme are nerve cells, which have a potential life expectancy of 100 years.

The Injured Cell

To ascertain whether a cell is healthy or sick, alive or dead, is often a difficult task for the pathologist. Dead cells do not immediately show distinct necrotic changes. Often, injured cells do not demonstrate any external evidence of disease or injury until the injury is far advanced. In other cases, the enzymes that the cell produces are poisoned, while the cell itself appears to be functioning satisfactorily. In addition, when injuries to the cell have been slight, cellular functions and structure remain essentially unchanged. Thus, despite the building of elaborate apparatuses for cellular study, the actual signs of sickness, and even of cellular death, may at times remain obscure.

THE CAUSES OF CELL INJURY

The extent to which any stress can injure or kill cells depends on the following three factors: (1) the *intensity* of the stress upon the cell, (2) the *length of time* during which the cell has been under stress, and (3) the *type* of cell under stress. Some cells are more vulnerable to injury or are more susceptible to certain stresses than other cells.

The major stresses that can injure cells seriously are: ischemia due to infarction or cessation of the blood flow, physical agents, chemical agents, microbial agents, and genetic disorders. These five categories were considered in Chapter 5 under the general causes of disease.

Ischemia. Ischemia injures and kills cells by depriving them of the oxygen they need in order to perform their metabolic functions. Ischemia is usually caused by blood clots of sufficient size to occlude a vessel, thereby depriving the cells and tissues served by that blood vessel of oxygen. Ischemia can also result from peripheral vascular disorders in which the arteries become so narrowed and tortuous that they no longer allow oxygenated blood to reach the tissues.

Physical Agents. Physical agents such as heat, cold, trauma, radiation, and electrical shock can also damage cells.

Heat and Cold. Extreme heat damages cells by literally "cooking them," thereby coagulating the protein within their cytoplasm. Even mild heat can result in permanent cellular damage if it is applied over a prolonged period of time to persons with peripheral vascular disorders. Irreversible damage occurs in these cases because heat increases the metabolic needs of cells and tissues — a dangerous situation when the circulation of oxygen to the cells is deficient and when waste products from increased metabolism cannot be carried away.

Cold injures cells by constricting the blood vessels, thereby decreasing the circulation of blood and oxygen to tissue cells. Freezing temperatures, which result in frostbite, permanently injure involved vessels. Also, cold temperatures can cause blood to form by slowing the circulation. The blood clots can occlude arteries, resulting in ischemia of those cells deprived of oxygen. Cellular death and necrosis will be the final consequence.

Trauma. Trauma injures cells by ripping their membranes and by displacing the organelles of the cell.

Radiation. Radiation can cause mutations, damage enzymes systems, and interrupt the process of cell division. The fact that radiation can stop mitosis makes radiation therapy important in the treatment of cancer — a disease involving pathologic cell growth. While all cells can die as a result of radiation, certain cells are more susceptible than others. Germ cells, bone marrow cells, and lymphocytes are highly sensitive to radiation, while the cells of the cartilage, muscle, brain, kidney, liver, thyroid, pancreas, pituitary gland, adrenal gland, and parathyroid gland are relatively insensitive. Persons who are likely candidates for cellular damage from radiation are those who work with radioactive materials, nuclear fission reactors, or are receiving therapeutic radiation treatment.

Electrical Shock. If severe, electrical shock can cause inflammatory reactions in nerve cells and nerve fibers, which will later be followed by degenerative changes. Damage to the brain may be permanent or temporary. The cells of other vital organs of the body are, of course, also damaged by a jolt of electricity. When voltages are high, the heart muscle may quiver or fibrillate rather than contract, and a usually fatal condition called *ventricular fibrillation* may result. Voltages too low to cause ventricular fibrillation can impair the action of the muscles of the respiratory system and the jolted individual may die of anoxia.

Chemicals. Chemical agents harm cells by destroying or injuring their delicate structures and by disrupting their metabolism. The capacity of any chemical to produce cell injury depends upon the strength and toxicity of the chemical, and upon the susceptibility of the cell to the chemical. Thus salt water, which is normally considered harmless, can, in high concentrations, cause cells to shrivel and die. A small amount of cyanide kills cells because of its extreme toxicity. Carbon tetrachloride is notorious for its affinity to liver cells, while mercury is particularly dangerous to kidney cells. Certain drugs such as LSD and thalidomide are believed to cause genetic changes or to influence embryonic development. The major portals of entry for chemicals toxic to cells are the lungs, the skin and mucous membranes, and the gastrointestinal tract.

Microorganisms. Microorganisms such as bacteria injure cells mainly by means of the *toxins* they produce, either endotoxins or exotoxins. An endotoxin is a toxic substance produced within a microorganism and is released when the cell in which it was produced is destroyed. An exotoxin is excreted by a microorganism into a surrounding medium. Other organisms, like certain of the viruses, produce no toxins, but live as obligatory parasites on the energy of living cells. Viruses are like cells in that they are replicating; however, they lack the ability to do so without the facilities of the cells. Thus, viruses penetrate cells, take over their enzyme systems, and then proceed to drain the doomed cell of its vitality and energy.

Genetic Disturbances. If a cell carries a genetic abnormality either newly acquired or passed on from ancestors, it may manifest in the cell as a disturbance of normal function. Thus disorders which are of genetic cause will not be apparent in the cell until the mutated gene is needed and is seen to be either nonfunctional or only partially functional.

MAJOR TYPES OF CELL DISORDERS

There are several types of cell disorders. The major forms are degenerations and infiltrations and disorders of cell growth, including cancerous growth, atrophy, and hypertrophy.

Degenerations and Infiltrations. Pathologists can generally identify injured cells by means of observable changes within their cytoplasm and nucleus. Some of the commonest pathologic changes are the result of either degeneration or infiltration. Sometimes both conditions occur together, as is the case in fatty change and glycogen degeneration. These two major cellular disturbances generally result from nonfatal injuries, and their unhealthy effects upon the cell can usually be erased in time. Nevertheless, the tell-tale signs of degeneration or infiltration within the cells give the pathologist a basic clue that all is not well within the total organism. Such adverse cellular changes, according to Boyd,[2] truly represent the "fingerprints of disease."

The term *degeneration* implies that the cellular structures are in a state of deterioration or impairment. On the other hand, *infiltration* means that a substance that is *external* to the cell filters into the cell and damages its ability to function. For example, when large amounts of fat globules are deposited within the cell as the result of a metabolic systemic illness, the process is called "fatty infiltration."

While infiltration and degeneration can be distinguished in terms of the process involved, they both represent disorders of the cell's basic biochemistry, resulting from such variable stresses as genetic disorders, metabolic disease, anoxia, and so forth.

The major types of degenerations and infiltrations are: cloudy swelling, fatty change, and glycogen infiltration and degeneration. The major pathologic changes, the causes, and the prognosis for each of the above processes are included in Table 9–1.

Disturbances of Cell Growth. Some major disturbances of cellular growth involve the problems of atrophy, hypertrophy, and cancer.* We shall briefly define these terms as they specifically apply to cellular and tissue pathology.

Atrophy is defined as the wasting of a tissue or organ and a *decrease* in its size *following* both maturity and a normal development. This wasting condition is due to either a decrease in the *number* of cells composing the tissue or a decrease in the actual *size* of the cells themselves. Atrophy may follow disuse of an organ, disorders of a tissue due to disease, circulatory deficiencies, compression of a tissue or part, and nerve damage. Atrophy, although found in connection with many disorders, can also be a *normal* physiologic process that occurs as the individual ages. Thus, the thymus gland atrophies when the child matures, and the ovaries

*The cancer cell is discussed in detail in Unit IX.

TABLE 9–1. DEGENERATIONS AND INFILTRATIONS: A SUMMARY OF IMPORTANT CONSIDERATIONS

Name of Degeneration or Infiltration	Conditions in Which Found	Pathologic Changes Within The Cell	Prognosis
Cloudy swelling	Infectious disease, fever, poisoning, anoxia, malnutrition, kidney, liver, heart, and glandular disorders	1. Protein substances become cloudy 2. Cells tend to swell owing to an increase in intracellular water 3. Protein metabolism is disturbed	Changes are rarely permanent
Fatty change	Starvation, malnutrition, cirrhosis of the liver, infectious hepatitis, poisoning with arsenic, bismuth, gold, or silver, liver intoxication due to chloroform or carbon tetrachloride	1. Excess fat accumulates within the cytoplasm following either disruption of enzyme systems within the cell, leading to faulty fat metabolism by the mitochondria, or infiltration of fat into the cell as a result of starvation or metabolic disease 2. Organs mainly affected by fatty change are the liver, kidney, and myocardium of the heart	This condition is usually reversible; however, it does indicate serious cell injury that may terminate in cellular death
Glycogen infiltration and degeneration	Diabetes mellitus	1. Abnormal accumulation of glycogen within the cells, especially of the kidney and heart 2. Usually there is no disruption of cellular function	Prognosis is good, as most changes are reversible

atrophy as the mature woman passes into the menopause.

Hypertrophy is an increase in the size of an organ or tissue. This increased bulk is *not* the result of additional cells; instead it is the result of an *increase in size* of the cells which already make up the organ. Hypertrophy may represent the response of an organ to a greater load of work. For example, when the heart is subjected to great strain, the left ventricle of the heart enlarges, or hypertrophies, in order to handle the additional stress. A second example of hypertrophy is the increase in size of the biceps muscle in individuals engaged in hard physical labor.

Hypertrophy may occur in any tissue or organ; however, it most commonly affects the heart, kidney, endocrine glands, skeletal muscles, and the smooth muscles of the intestinal tract.

Cancer is a disease in which cellular growth is disturbed and chaotic, and in which normal cellular function becomes modified and physiologically maladaptive. Of cancer cells, Boyd states, "Cancer cells are the anarchists of the body, for they know no law, pay no regard for the commonwealth, serve no useful function, and cause disharmony and death in their surroundings."[2] Cancer cells, moreover, are capable of migrating to different parts of the body, thereby causing the spread, or metastasis, of malignant tumors or neoplasms, which further disrupt and destroy the body's life-sustaining functions. The causes of cancer as well as the measures that will cure and prevent this disorder are still mysteries that are being slowly and relentlessly unraveled by determined scientists.

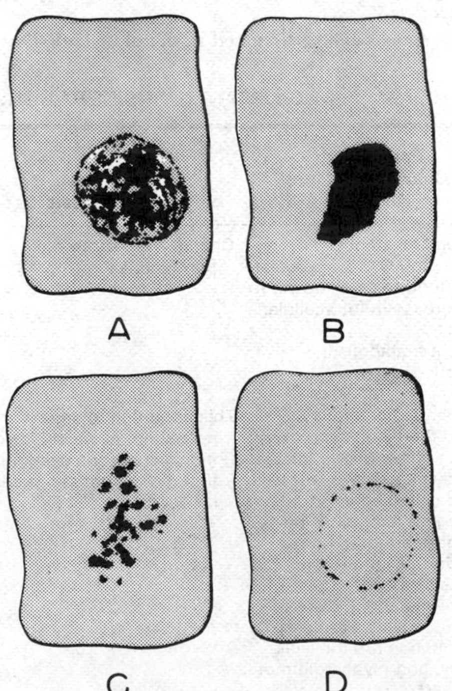

Figure 9–5. The morphological changes that most clearly indicate cell death involve the nucleus. *A.* Normal nucleus. *B.* Pyknotic nucleus. *C.* Karyorrhectic nucleus. *D.* A nucleus that has undergone karyolysis. (Redrawn from Price, S., and L. C. Wilson: *Pathophysiology: Clinical Concepts of Disease Processes.* New York: McGraw-Hill Book Co., Inc., 1978.)

CELL DEATH AND CELLULAR NECROSIS

It is important *not* to use the terms "cell death" and "cell necrosis" interchangeably. *Cell death* occurs when the vital functions of the cell cease; *cell necrosis* follows cell death and includes morphologic changes that eventually result in the lysis and dissolving of the cell. Thus, cells evidently die long before signs of their death become apparent under the pathologist's microscope. Because of this fact, it is as difficult to accurately distinguish between an injured cell and a dead one as it is to differentiate between a normal cell and an injured cell. Thus, it may be difficult for a pathologist to determine the extent of damage caused by a disease process; sometimes only the signs of cellular necrosis can confirm the pathologist's suspicion of cellular death.

Cell Death. Cells die as a result of chemical poisons, bacterial toxins, anoxia due to thrombosis and infarctions, and powerful physical agents such as irradiation. As cells die, their vital functions may cease gradually, one by one, making it impossible for the pathologist to state the exact moment of cellular death.

Following the death of the cell, the process of cell necrosis begins, the nucleus breaks up, and the cytoplasm becomes liquefied. Finally, the dead cell loses its identity as a separate entity and the process of autolysis is complete. The seven major stages of cell injury and death are diagrammed in Figure 9–5.

Cell Necrosis. The process of cell necrosis *follows* the death of the cell. Enzymes within the cell as well as those exterior to it cause the necrotic breakdown. The morphologic changes involved in cell necrosis depend upon which type of necrosis the cell has undergone. The four major *types* of cellular necrosis are: coagulation necrosis, liquefaction necrosis, caseous necrosis, and gangrenous necrosis.

Coagulation Necrosis. The generally results from *anoxia* of the cell, which, in turn, may be caused by a loss of blood supply to the cell. An outstanding characteristic of coagulation necrosis is that a shadowy outline of the cell remains distinct for days or weeks following the death of the cell and the escape of its vital inner contents. This cell, then, can be compared to a rag doll which has lost all its stuffings.

Liquefaction Necrosis. A rapid and *total* destruction of the entire cell, including the cell's membrane, this type of necrosis most commonly affects the cells of the brain and cells that have been invaded by pus-forming bacteria.

Caseous Necrosis. Generally associated with cellular destruction resulting from tuberculosis, the dead cell develops a characteristic appearance of soft cheese. This form of necrosis is very distinctive and can be readily identified in the laboratory.

Gangrenous Necrosis. This necrosis results from ischemia of the cell, coupled with an infection by bacteria which can live only in ischemic tissue.

BIBLIOGRAPHY (Chapter 9)

1. Bloom, W., and D. W. Fawcett: *A Textbook of Histology,* 9th ed. Philadelphia: W. B. Saunders Co., 1968.
2. Boyd, W.: *An Introduction to the Study of Disease.* Philadelphia: Lea & Febiger, 1962.
3. Capaldi, R. A.: A dynamic model of cell membranes. *Scientific American,* 230:26, Mar. 1974.
4. Fox, C. F.: The structure of cell membranes. *Scientific American,* 226:30, Feb. 1972.
5. Kappas, A., and A. P. Alvares: How the liver metabolizes foreign substances. *Scientific American,* 232:22, Jun. 1975.
6. Guyton, A. C.: *Basic Human Physiology; Normal Function and Mechanisms of Disease,* 2nd ed. Philadelphia: W. B. Saunders Co., 1977.
7. Mazia, D.: The cell cycle. *Scientific American,* 230:54, Jan. 1974.
8. O'Malley, B. W., and W. T. Schrader: The receptors of steroid hormones. *Scientific American,* 234:32, Feb. 1976.
9. Pastan, I.: Cyclic AMP. *Scientific American,* 227:97, Aug. 1972.
10. Pepine, C. J., et al.: Guideline to evaluation and management of shock. *Hospital Medicine,* 15:95, Mar. 1979.
11. Pfeiffer, J.: *The Cell.* Life Science Library. New York, Time, Inc., 1964.
12. Reisfeld, R. A., and B. D. Kahan: Markers of biologic individuality. *Scientific American,* 226:28, June 1972.
13. Robbins, S. L.: *Pathological Basis of Disease.* Philadelphia: W. B. Saunders Co., 1974.
14. Robbins, S. L., and M. Angell: *Basic Pathology,* 2nd ed. Philadelphia, W. B. Saunders Co., 1976.
15. Satir, B.: The final steps in secretion. *Scientific American,* 223:28, Oct. 1975.
16. Singer, S. J., and G. L. Nicolson: The fluid mosaic model of the structure of the cell membranes. *Science,* 175(4023):720, Feb. 18, 1972.
17. Sodeman, W. A., and W. A. Sodeman: *Pathologic Physiology,* 5th ed. Philadelphia: W. B. Saunders Co., 1974.
18. Staehelin, L. A., and B. E. Hull: Junctions between living cells. *Scientific American,* 238:140, May 1978.
19. Stent, G. S.: Cellular communication. *Scientific American,* 227:42, Sept. 1972.
20. Wessells, N. K.: How living cells change shape. *Scientific American,* 225:76, Oct. 1971.

CHAPTER 10*

RESPONSES TO INJURY

INTRODUCTION AND STUDY GUIDE

Stress and the individual's response to stress with healthy or faulty adaptation are the pivotal points of any discussion of health and disease. These factors determine whether a given disturbance will result in an individual living or dying.

To some extent, we have already considered these areas in earlier units. First of all, in both Units II and III we discussed many of the multiple stressful factors that continuously impinge upon humans. You will remember that the most important physiologic stressors challenging the adaptive resources of a person are: (1) physical stressors such as heat, cold, radiation, and trauma, (2) chemical irritants such as strong acids, alkalis, and poisons, as well as certain substances which people manufacture within their own bodies, and (3) bacterial agents and microorganisms.

Second, we pointed out that if a person is to survive, response to these stressors must be made with all the protective and adaptive mechanisms at the person's disposal. The major defensive systems, providing a high degree of protection against physical injury, are the intact skin, the mucous membranes, the bones, the blood, the gastrointestinal tract, the reticuloendothelial system, the endocrine system and the nervous system.

Third, we emphasized that despite the hundreds of stressors that can assault us, and despite the complexity of our protective systems, the human animal actually has a very limited repertoire of *physiologic reactions* specifically designed to counter physical stress. You will recall that those major reactions are inflammation, sclerosis, increased capillary permeability, hormonal responses, the immune response (the production of antibodies in reaction to antigens), and fluid and electrolyte shifts. Finally, we stated that *inflammation* is the most typical example of the body's ability to respond to tissue injury or bacterial invasion.

In this section of Unit V we explore the various means by which the body defends itself against attack and injury. The following areas are discussed:

1. The body's defensive cells:
   Cells of the reticuloendothelial system
   Leukocytes
2. The body's major defensive organs:
   Lymph nodes
   Spleen
   Bone marrow
   Liver
3. The body's major physiologic responses to injury:
   Inflammation
   Repair

In discussing these areas we review the work of the reticulum cell, the white blood cell, and the macrophage; the purpose of capillary permeability; and the role of humoral and hormonal defenses in resisting infection. In the later chapters of this unit, we shall look at the immune reaction and at those fluid and electrolyte shifts that occur as a reaction to stress.

Upon completion of this chapter, you should be aware of the meaning of the following key terms:

reticuloendothelial system
reticulum cell
tissue histiocyte
polymorphonuclear leukocyte
lymphocytes
B-cells
T-cells
monocytes
macrophages
phagocytosis
chemotaxis
chemical mediator
histamine
leukocytosis
leukopenia
leukocytosis-promoting factor
agranulocytosis
opsonins
antitoxins
inflammatory lymph
fibroblast
abscess
cellulitis
ulcer
fistula
boil
carbuncle
resolution
repair
parenchymal tissue
connective tissue
permanent cells
granulation tissue
scar tissue
primary union
secondary union
keloid
Hemovac

You should also be able to discuss generally the following topics:

1. The role of the reticuloendothelial system and leukocytes in protecting the body against invasion by dangerous aliens
2. Distinguishing differences between the mor-

*Margaret M. McMahon, R.N., B.S.N., CCRN, critically reviewed and assisted with the revision of this chapter.

phology and physiologic functions of the various leukocytes

3. The roles of the liver, spleen, lymph nodes, and bone marrow in body defense
4. The causes of inflammation
5. The major components of the inflammatory response
6. The overall characteristics of the inflammatory response to injury — the different defenses at work
7. The different types or classes of inflammatory response
8. Major factors affecting the outcome of inflammation
9. Types of tissue repair
10. The rate of wound healing in different types of tissues
11. Factors that distinguish primary union from secondary union
12. The formation of scar tissue
13. Abnormalities that can result from a secondary union and from the formation of excessive scar tissue
14. Treatment of the contaminated wound and other wound complications
15. Factors that govern the success of the repair process
16. The goals of medical and nursing care
17. The psychophysiologic responses to injury
18. The patient/family teaching relative to wound care

THE DEFENSIVE CELLS OF THE BODY

The Cells of the Reticuloendothelial System

While the typical inflammatory response can be likened to a fast-moving, hard-fought battle, the role of the reticuloendothelial system against injury is comparable to that of a vigilant national guard in a country that is currently peaceful, yet under constant threat of annihilation. Like silent sentries, the cells of the reticuloendothelial system are located strategically throughout the body, awaiting possible action should disruption or invasion by foreign material occur. Some cells are stationary, seizing and killing potential invaders before they can enter the circulatory system, which is the body's mainstream. Other cells, such as the tissue histiocyte, are usually stationary, but can change quickly as the need arises, becoming powerful, motile, bacteria-ingesting macrophages. The cells of the reticuloendothelial system are capable not only of capturing and annihilating intruders, but they can also form immune bodies that serve to safeguard the body against future generations of the invaders.

Where is this remarkable protective system located? Of what is it composed? How does it operate?

The reticuloendothelial system is not localized to any one part of the body but is widely dispersed throughout many body organs. Its cells line blood vessels and lymph channels; they are found in the spleen, liver, lymph nodes, and bone marrow.

The major cells of the reticuloendothelial system are the *reticulum cells.* These cells perform two vital functions: first, they are the precursors of the body's erythrocytes and granulocytes; and second, they perform the essential task of phagocytosis. In addition, reticulum cells that are located within the bone marrow operate as efficient "fine filters," removing from the blood such tiny particles as protein toxin.

Reticulum cells are remarkable for their ability to differentiate into many different types of cells and are truly the chameleons of the body. For instance, reticulum cells can change themselves into the following varied forms: hemocytoblasts, which later become red blood cells; myeloblasts, which eventually evolve into leukocytes; lymphocytes, which are a form of leukocyte; plasma cells, which play an important role in immune body formation; and tissue histiocytes.

The *tissue histiocyte* is so useful in the body's defense that it deserves special mention. This versatile cell is found scattered widely throughout the body's tissues, its function being to ingest debris and foreign bodies. Being both fixed and motile, tissue histiocytes are capable of swelling up, leaving their stationary posts, and traveling to the site of inflammatory action, where they then phagocytize invaders. When tissue histiocytes behave in this manner, they are called *macrophages.* Tissue histiocytes can also change into fibroblasts, cells that are capable of laying down collagen or connective tissue fibers. Fibroblasts are formed when inflamed tissue needs to be walled off from healthy tissue by means of a collagen barrier, and when tissue damage needs to be repaired.

In sum, the cells of the reticuloendothelial system are both stationary and wandering. They are highly efficient in their efforts to corner and devour invaders and all manner of foreign materials. Moreover, they are efficient in the production of antibodies.

The Leukocytes

THE CLASSIFICATION AND FUNCTION OF WHITE BLOOD CELLS

The leukocytes, or white blood cells (WBC's), compose another motile unit of the body's defense system. One of the outstanding characteristics of leukocytes is their ability to go *immediately* to the scene of injury and to deal with harmful invaders in an on-the-spot death struggle.

These remarkable protective cells are divided into the following two major groups: (1) the *polymorphonuclear leukocytes,* which include neutrophils, eosinophils, and basophils; and (2) the *mononuclear leukocytes,* which include lymphocytes and monocytes. The relative numbers of the different white blood cells (average differential count for adults) are shown in Table 10–1.

Polymorphonuclear Leukocytes ("Polys"). The poly group is composed of three subgroups of cells: the neutrophil, the eosinophil, and the basophil. While each group has its own distinctive qualities, they also share several characteristics.

First of all, as the name implies, *poly*morphonuclear leukocytes have a *many-shaped* or formed (morpho) (poly) *nucleus.* A second important characteristic of the poly group is their *granular* appearance when viewed under a microscope. Third, all polys are formed in the *bone marrow* and consequently they are sometimes referred to as *myelogenous cells* [*myelo* = bone marrow]. Finally, polys (neutrophils in particular) function to give the body *rapid* protection against any outside invaders. Thus, the polys are the "shock troops" of the body, because they arrive early at the scene of battle and bear the major brunt of the physiologic warfare. In a serious infection, polys may live only 1 or 2 hours before dying in the fray. Normally this group of leukocytes remains alive about 14 hours; at times, however, polys have been known to live for several days before disintegrating.

TABLE 10–1. THE AVERAGE DIFFERENTIAL WHITE COUNT FOR ADULTS

Cell	Number of Cells per Every 100 White Cells
Neutrophils	62.0
Eosinophils	2.3
Basophils	0.4 to 1.0
Lymphocytes	30.0
Monocytes	5.3

While all polys have similar origins and functions, each group has its own specialized tasks in the mechanism of defense.

THE NEUTROPHIL. These polys are the most important and the most numerous of the white cells, composing 50 to 70 per cent of all circulating leukocytes. Neutrophils are small, motile, highly phagocytic cells, for which reason they are sometimes called microphages.

Neutrophils play a vital role in the body's local inflammatory reaction because they are both the first and most numerous type of cell at any area of disease or tissue injury. Also, neutrophils play an important role as "scavengers," by cleaning up the debris that accumulates as a result of the inflammatory "battle." Even in death, neutrophils serve a useful purpose. By releasing a proteolytic enzyme, the dead and disintegrating neutrophil digests not only surrounding bacteria and dead cells but also *itself,* thus cleansing "the inflammatory battlefield" of even its own remains.

While inflammation is the major condition causing a neutrophilia (an increase in neutrophils), *any factor* that leads to the destruction of cells and tissue can give rise to an increase in the neutrophil count. Consequently, cancer, extreme fatigue, acute hemorrhage, a myocardial infarction with resultant necrosis of the heart muscle, poisons, surgery, and injections of foreign protein into the body all result in a degree of neutrophilia. In the case of a myocardial infarction, neutrophilia constitutes an important diagnostic sign.

Neutrophils, over and above their task in abating local tissue injury, may also play a part in the overall *systemic* reaction to the tissue destruction. Some authorities postulate that neutrophils possibly release a substance that produces *fever* — an important general symptom of inflammation and infection.

EOSINOPHILS. The eosinophil differs markedly from its sister cell, the neutrophil. We have contrasted the characteristics and functions of the two cells in Table 10–2.

Eosinophils are apparently a very important cell group in *parasitic* and *allergic* conditions, in which they may increase to form over 50 per cent of the total differential count. Their role in these conditions is quite obscure. Eosinophils apparently enter the circulation whenever foreign proteins are injected into the blood; they are also found in substantial numbers at the sites of antigen-antibody reactions. Moreover, some authors postulate that eosinophils evidently have the capacity to detoxify those harmful protein substances released by parasites. This theory helps to explain the increase of eosinophils in parasitic reactions.

Eosinophils appear to be under the control of the *adrenocortical hormones.* Selye and other scientists have found that eosinophils tend to disappear from the circulation whenever there is an excessive release of the cortical hormones as a result of stress, or when patients are receiving cortisone injections.

BASOPHILS. When stained and viewed under a microscope, basophils can be distinguished by the appearance of blue-black granules in their cytoplasm. This group of polys represents the smallest proportion of the white blood cells, making up no more than 1 per cent of the total differential. This means that out of 1000 leukocytes, approximately 4 are basophils.

What are the functions of this white blood cell minority group? First, basophils, like eosinophils, increase in number during the healing phase of inflammation. Second, basophils evidently play an important role in proper blood circulation by releasing *heparin,* a powerful anticoagulant. It is theorized that the basophil's ability to liberate heparin causes a decrease in cell clumping and other aspects of blood coagulation that occur during the inflammatory process. Also, basophils apparently help to maintain proper circulation by eliminating from the blood those excess fat particles that accumulate following the ingestion of a high-fat meal.

Mononuclear Leukocytes. In contrast to the polys, mononuclear leukocytes do not have granules in their cytoplasm — a fact that has earned them the name of *nongranular* or agranular leukocytes. Also, mononuclear leukocytes are not produced in the bone marrow as polys are, but instead stem from *lymphatic tissue* such as that found in the lymph nodes and spleen.

This second major group of leukocytes is composed of the subgroups lymphocytes and monocytes.

LYMPHOCYTES. A much smaller blood cell than a poly, the lymphocyte is formed mainly in the lymph nodes and, to some extent, in the small lymphoid follicles of the tonsils, intestines, and bone marrow. In the event of an infectious or toxic condition, these lymphogenous tissues tend to hypertrophy greatly. Who has not, at some point in life, experienced swollen, painful nodes in the armpits, groin, or neck as a result of some infection or toxic condition?

Lymphocytes are fairly numerous, forming 25 to 33 per cent of the differential. When no infection exists within the body, there are approximately 2100 lymphocytes per cubic millimeter. However, with certain infections — for example, whooping cough — the lymphocyte count can go as high as 100,000 per cu. mm., although such a high count is generally quite rare!

Like the eosinophils, lymphocytes are under the control of the *adrenocortical hormones.* This statement holds important implications for the nurse working with patients on *steroid therapy.* A patient who is receiving steroid therapy will experience a decrease in the number of lymphocytes being produced as well as a shrinking of lymphoidal tissues. This combination leaves the patient receiving adrenocortical hormones dangerously susceptible to infection.

The lymphocyte is important to the body's well-being. One outstanding function is the *release of immunoglobulins* — a vital task that we shall discuss under the immune reaction. Lymphocytes that are involved in immunoglobulin synthesis are called *bursal-equivalent lymphocytes* or *B-cells.* B-cells are the producers of *humoral* immunity and are primarily involved in the destruction of bacterial pathogens.

A second important function of lymphocytes is the production of *cellular immunity.* Lymphocytes that provide cellular immunity are called *thymus-dependent lymphocytes* or *T cells* (see Chapter 11). T-cells are capable of directly killing foreign invaders. Like B-cells, T-cells carry a "memory" of past contact with specific antigens. These cells also play a vital role in the control of cancer cell growth (see Unit IX), in transplant rejection, and in delayed hypersensitivity reactions. In addition, T-cells release chemical substances called *lymphokines* which are powerful mediators of the immune response.

The life span of these highly useful white

TABLE 10-2. CHARACTERISTICS OF NEUTROPHILS AND EOSINOPHILS

Neutrophils	Eosinophils
1. When stained and viewed under the microscope, granules in them appear as *gray.*	1. When stained and viewed under the microscope, granules in them appear *bright, pinkish red*
2. Make up 50 to 70% of leukocytes	2. Make up 1 to 2 per cent of leukocytes
3. Motile, fast-moving	3. Motile, but sluggish
4. The *first* cells to arrive at the site of inflammation	4. One of the *last* cells to arrive at the inflammatory site — often coming after healing has started
5. Excellent, effective phagocytes	5. Very weak phagocytes

cells is usually only a few hours. However, radioactive studies have shown that when tissue needs are minimal, lymphocytes can live 100 to 200 days.

MONOCYTES. These cells form 4 to 6 per cent of the white blood cell differential count. Their numbers rise mainly in such conditions as tuberculosis and malaria. Like the lymphocyte, monocytes are formed in lymphoid tissue. Their potential life span and ultimate fate remain a mystery.

Monocytes are closely related to the phagocytic macrophages of the reticuloendothelial system. Along with the reticuloendothelial cells, the monocyte forms the *second line of defense* against bacterial invasion by following close "on the heels" of the polys — the first line of defense. Thus, the monocytes arrive at the scene of battle after the initial encounter.

Once at the inflammatory site, the monocytes can act as powerful macrophages, ingesting much larger particles than can the neutrophil, as well as at least five times as many particles in one ingestion. Tougher and less vulnerable than the neutrophils, or microphages, the monocyte is able to survive the polys and live on into the late stages of the acute inflammation as well as into the chronic stages. Thus, like lymphocytes, increased numbers of monocytes are typically observed in *chronic inflammatory conditions.*

Monocytes also play an important part in the "clean up" procedures that follow any inflammatory battle. Active hungry scavengers, monocytes are capable of ingesting dead bacteria, wornout polys, and large amounts of protein debris, thereby clearing and preparing the field for the process of repair and healing.

WHITE BLOOD CELL COUNT (TOTAL WBC)

The normal range for the total WBC in adults is 6000 to 9000 per cu.mm. In infections the total WBC in adults can increase to 30,000 per cu.mm. When such a radical increase in the circulating white cells occurs, the condition is called *leukocytosis.* Pneumonia, myocardial infarctions, malignant disease, and infections can all lead to high leukocyte counts. Conversely, the total WBC can become abnormally low. A marked decrease in the leukocyte count is called *leukopenia.* For obscure reasons, a leukopenia sometimes develops in typhoid fever and occasionally in tuberculosis. Leukopenia may also result from a decreased production of white blood cells owing to extreme debilitation or severe deficits of vitamins, folic acid, and amino acids — those materials that are used extensively by the body in the formation of leukocytes. Finally, since the bone marrow produces a major portion of the body's leukocytes, any damage to the bone marrow can result in the suppression of white blood cell formation and in an extremely dangerous, often fatal, form of leukopenia called agranulocytosis. (See Unit XIV.)

Plasma Cells

The small, round, irregularly shaped plasma cells are probably derived from either lymphocytes or reticulum cells. They exist predominantly in the connective tissue of the walls of the intestinal tract, as well as in the lymph nodes, spleen, and bone marrow. Large numbers of plasma cells are found when inflammatory reactions become chronic. As with the lymphocyte and monocyte, plasma cells are increased in syphilitic conditions.

The actual role and function of plasma cells is somewhat obscure. However, it is generally believed that they are a primary source of antibody production.

In summary, the major defensive cells of the body are the cells of the reticuloendothelial system, the leukocytes, and the plasma cells. Major facts about each cell type are summarized in Table 10–3.

BODY ORGANS INVOLVED IN DEFENSE: THE STRUCTURES OF THE RETICULOENDOTHELIAL SYSTEM

The major organs involved directly in body defense and in the production of protective cells are the *lymph nodes,* the *spleen,* the *liver,* and the *bone marrow.* These structures serve as efficient factories for the production and maturation of reticulum cells and leukocytes; moreover, they work as blood purifiers, filtering out the soot, foreign bodies, microorganisms and defective or malignant cells that threaten to harm or destroy the body. These organs, then, are vitally responsible for the *prevention* of *infection* and *disease.* Because of their important services, the body is often spared the pain and trauma of an inflammatory reaction, as well as the threat of annihilation by the many dangerous forces that continuously assault it.

The Lymph Nodes

All foreign matter and all microbial, bacterial, and viral invaders must pass through the lymphatic system on their way to the general circulation. Strategically located along the

TABLE 10–3. THE BODY'S DEFENSIVE CELLS: A SUMMARY

Cell Type	Number in Health and Disease	Place of Origin	Distinguishing Characteristics	Function
A. Reticulum cell	Large numbers line blood vessels and lymph nodes; also found in spleen, liver, lymph nodes, and bone marrow	Reticuloendothelial system	1. Both stationary and motile 2. Capable of differentiating into different cells as the need arises, e.g., into a tissue histiocyte and then into a fibroblast 3. Can become macrophages	1. Phagocytosis 2. Helpful in process of repair 3. Body's second line of defense against invasion
B. Leukocyte	1. In health, 6000-9000/cu. mm. 2. Increase up to 30,000/cu.mm.in infection			Motile unit of the body's defensive system
1. Polymorphonuclear leukocytes		Formed in bone marrow (myelogenous cells)	1. Many-shaped nucleus 2. Granular appearance under microscope	Give body rapid protection against outside invaders
a. Neutrophils (microphages)	1. In health, 50 to 70% of all circulating white cells 2. High counts in *acute* inflammation and whenever there is tissue damage (myocardial infarction)		1. Small 2. Motile 3. Highly phagocytic 4. Gray granules under a microscope	1. First cell type to arrive at inflammatory site (first line of defense) 2. Phagocytosis 3. Act as scavengers, cleaning inflammatory site 4. Possibly cause fever
b. Eosinophils	1. In health, 1 to 2% of circulating white cells 2. High counts in parasitic infestations and allergic conditions and during healing phase of inflammation		1. Granules stain red under microscope 2. Motile but sluggish 3. Phagocytic 4. Under control of adrenocortical hormones	1. Weak phagocytes 2. Can possibly detoxify foreign protein substances
c. Basophils	1. In health, 1% of circulating cells 2. Increase during healing phase of inflammation		Blue-black granules under a microscope	Release of heparin, which possibly causes a decrease in cell clumping during the inflammatory process
2. Mononuclear leukocytes		Produced in lymphatic tissue such as the lymph nodes and spleen	Nongranular appearance under the microscope	Important defensive cells in chronic inflammation
a. Lymphocytes	1. In health, 25 to 33% of all circulating white cells 2. Increase to great numbers in certain infections 3. Increase late in inflammatory process and in *chronic* inflammation	Formed mainly in lymph nodes and lymphoid follicles	1. Much smaller cell than the poly 2. Under the control of the adrenocortical hormones 3. Classified as B cells or T cells	1. Production of gammaglobulins 2. Phagocytosis 3. Cell-mediated reactions 4. Release of lymphokines
b. Monocytes	1. In health, 4 to 6% of total circulating white cells 2. Numbers increase in tuberculosis and malaria and in chronic inflammatory conditions	Formed in lymphoid tissue	1. Large "tough" cells 2. Capacity to ingest large numbers of bacteria at one time	1. Along with reticulum cell, forms second line of defense against bacterial invasion 2. Phagocytosis 3. Act as scavengers, cleaning inflammatory site
c. Plasma cells	1. Normally found in large numbers in the walls of the intestinal tract, lymph nodes, spleen, and bone marrow 2. Increase in chronic inflammation	Probably derived from either lymphocytes or reticulum cells	1. Small 2. Round 3. Irregularly shaped	1. Role obscure 2. Possibly active in antibody formation

course of the lymphatics are clusters of small structures called lymph nodes, or lymph glands. Some of these oval structures are as small as the head of a pin; others are as large as a lima bean. Rarely solitary, most lymph nodes are found in discrete groups. The major groups of lymph nodes and their locations are as follows:

1. *Submental* and *submaxillary nodes,* in the mouth.
2. *Superficial cervical glands,* in the neck.
3. *Superficial cubital nodes,* which can be found just above the bend of the elbow.
4. *Axillary nodes,* which are located under the arm and in the upper chest regions; 20 to 30 large nodes make up this important group.
5. *Inguinal nodes,* within the groin.

Small lymphoid follicles are also found in the tonsils, intestinal tract, and bone marrow. The anatomic locations of the most important lymph nodes are illustrated in Figure 10–1.

Lymph nodes serve three important functions: First, they contain "passageways" or sinus channels for the transport of the important watery substance called *lymph.* Second, these same passageways also function as vital defensive systems. Lined heavily with reticulum cells, the lymph sinuses are able to filter out and devour dangerous foreign materials. Finally, the lymph node serves as "parent and nursery" for the birth and growth of lymphocytes and monocytes. Thus, if you were to examine tissue from a lymph node, you would find it densely packed with lymphocytes.

Under normal conditions the lymph nodes serve as efficient filters. However, the body is sometimes invaded by hordes of virulent microorganisms. When this happens, the nodes may be so overworked and overtaxed that they themselves succumb to infection. An infection of a lymph node is called *lymphadenitis* while *lymphangitis* is an inflammation of a lymphatic channel. Both are characterized by the signs and symptoms of inflammation that we discuss shortly.

The Spleen*

This highly vascular, bean-shaped, glandlike organ lies beneath the diaphragm, and behind and to the left of the stomach. While the spleen serves many functions, its unique anatomic structure makes it highly valuable as a defensive organ. Basically the spleen is composed of a fibrous tissue capsule that surrounds a network or framework of fibers. In the interstices of these fibers is found a material called the *red pulp,* a substance composed of red blood cells, white blood cells, and macrophages. This red pulp helps to purify the blood and rid it of dangerous substances.

Blood comes into the splenic pulp for cleansing via the splenic artery. From the pulp the nearly purified blood passes into the spleen's venules, which are also loaded with phagocytic cells. The venules eventually unite into the splenic vein, which then carries the blood to the liver. Within the liver, as you will see, the blood undergoes further purifying processes before being released into the general circulation.

The Liver

A highly adaptive and versatile organ, the liver is involved in literally hundreds of the body's functions. The one major function of the liver that concerns us here is defense against noxious invaders. Like the lymph nodes and spleen, the liver is lined with many sinus channels that are filled with reticulum cells or fixed macrophages. Such cells, when they occur in the liver, are called *Kupffer cells.* Like all macrophages, Kupffer cells seize and devour potentially harmful intruders.

Along with the spleen, the liver ranks as an important blood filter and purifier. A large organ, the liver serves as a mighty sieve, cleansing the blood from the *portal circulatory system* before it enters the general circulation. Physiologically the portal system transports blood from the spleen, stomach, pancreas, and intestines — a large and important territory. This means, then, that most adventurous bacteria that have invaded the body by passing from the gastrointestinal mucosa into the portal blood, or have escaped the hazards of the splenic pulp, will still not reach the general circulation. Instead, they will meet swift death in a Kupffer cell.

In reviewing these few facts about the liver as a protective organ, one can readily see the effect of liver disease upon the body's defense against microorganisms. Indeed, these points explain why individuals with cirrhosis of the liver — a condition involving destruction and scarring of the liver tissue — are so vulnerable to overwhelming infection.

The Bone Marrow

The lymphatic tissues and the myeloid tissues (or red bone marrow) are the *hemopoietic* (also called hematopoietic) tissues of the body;

*The spleen and its functions will be discussed in greater detail in Chapter 46.

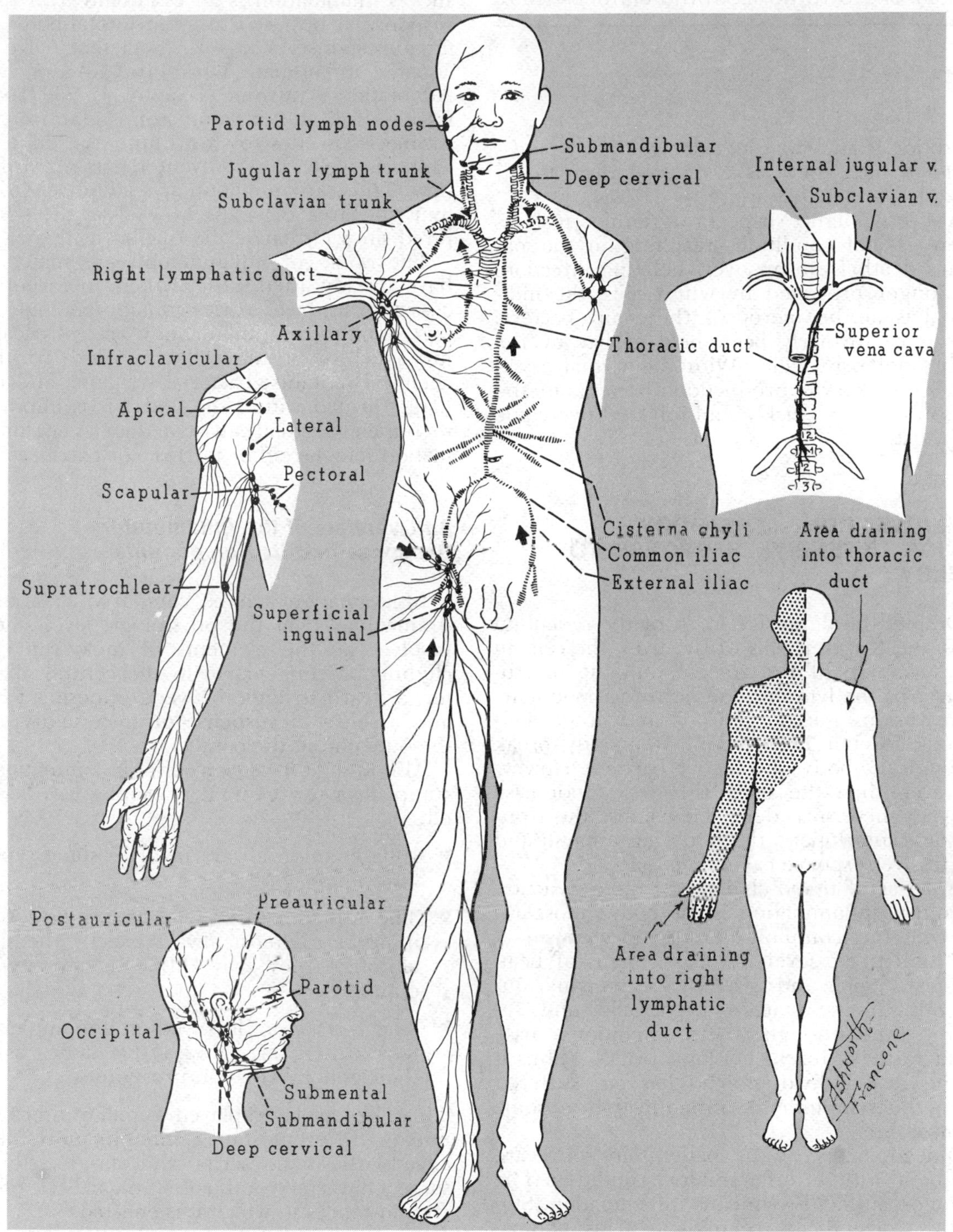

Figure 10–1. The lymphatic system and drainage. (From Jacob, S. W., C. A. Francone, and W. J. Lossow: *Structure and Function in Man*, 4th ed. Philadelphia: W. B. Saunders Co., 1978, p. 410.)

i.e., they produce blood cells. In the adult human the red bone marrow is located only in certain bones, namely, the ribs, sternum, and the ends of the long bones such as the femur. This scattered myeloid tissue produces vast numbers of reticulum cells, remarkable cells discussed earlier on page 109.

It is unfortunately true that this vital bone marrow can, under certain conditions, cease to function. Such a depression of bone marrow activity sometimes affects individuals receiving x-ray therapy, nitrogen mustard, or chloromycetin. When the bone marrow does not produce its usual number of blood cells, the condition is known as *agranulocytosis* or *granulocytopenia;* i.e., there is a marked decrease in granulocyte production.

As you might suspect, agranulocytosis is often a fatal condition, resulting in the patient's death from an overwhelming infection. No longer protected by white cells, the individual is at the mercy of the many bacteria that have formerly been held at bay by the body's defensive cells. With the virtual cessation of leukocyte production, bacteria in the person's tissues quickly multiply and overcome their victim.

INFLAMMATION — THE BODY'S MAJOR DEFENSIVE RESPONSE TO INJURY

Despite the defensive work of the reticulum cells, the Kupffer cells of the liver, the cells in the red pulp of the spleen, and the macrophages of the lymph nodes and the bone marrow, various microorganisms and other dangerous foreign invaders *do* frequently break through the body's protective barriers. However, even then the body tissues are not easy prey to these intruders. To combat the troublesome interlopers, the body has a harsh and aggressive response called *inflammation.*

A series of tissue changes in direct reaction to injury, inflammation is the body's most important and common defense mechanism at the local tissue level. Its classic signs of heat, redness, pain, and swelling accompany numerous disease states — both mild and severe — even though these conditions arise from vastly different etiologic origins. Thus it is the rare individual who has not suffered from the symptoms of inflammation at some point in life.

Indeed, many of the patients in your care will be ill with an inflammatory condition. The common suffix "itis" means inflammation. Stomatitis, appendicitis, cellulitis, gastritis, nephritis, vaginitis, and colitis are all inflammatory conditions.

Since the subject of inflammation is so relevant to the everyday clinical situation, it is necessary to explore it more fully.

Definition, Effect, and Causation

Inflammation can be defined as an immediate, aggressive response by the body to the injury or potential destruction of its cells and tissues. Inflammation is an essentially *local* tissue response as opposed to a more total-body, systemic response. You will recall that Selye has equated inflammation with the LAS or Local Adaptation Syndrome (Chapter 4). The specific *effect* of the inflammatory adaptive syndrome is to destroy or dilute the injurious agent as well as to prevent the spread of injury. Thus, inflammation acts adaptively to delimit the area of stress by walling off the injured site with barricades of fibrous tissue.

The *causes* of inflammation are many. We have already listed most of them in earlier discussions. In brief review, major etiologic factors resulting in inflammation are: physical injury such as trauma, burns, and frostbite; chemical irritants; bacterial irritants; and exudates formed within the body. It is important to remember that causative factors in inflammation may be either intrinsic or extrinsic.

An Overview of the Inflammatory Response and its Components

Inflammation can be compared to a melodrama played at the physiologic level since it involves all the elements of melodrama, including potential harm to the central character, a death struggle between opposing forces, and a sense of suspense or uncertainty as to the outcome of the conflict.

Although the subject of inflammation is complex, a few general principles can be stated:

- ▶ Inflammation always involves some type of *tissue injury.*
- ▶ The inflammatory *events* that follow tissue injury are almost always exactly the same, although they may differ in severity and outcome.
- ▶ The *components* involved in the inflammatory drama are always the same, as are their general roles and responses.

Thus, like a play replayed a million times on a million different stages, inflammation follows exactly the same script and has exactly the same characters and roles, regardless of the circumstances in which it is enacted.

The major *components* involved in inflammation are: (1) the blood vessels, (2) the blood itself, (3) the inflammatory exudate, (4) the defensive cells, including microphages and macrophages, (5) antibodies, and (6) the surrounding connective tissue. The major *responses* that characterize inflammation and that involve the above components include: (1) the vascular response, (2) the formation of the inflammatory exudate, (3) the defensive cell response, (4) the fibrin response, (5) the humoral response, and (6) the hormonal response.

THE VASCULAR RESPONSE

When a person's tissues are injured, blood vessels respond in the following manner:

1. The blood vessels *momentarily constrict* and then quickly *dilate.* These changes in the diameter of the blood vessels are believed to be due to the release of vasoactive substances at the site of injury. The first blood vessels to dilate are the arterioles, followed by the venules and, finally, the capillaries.

2. As a result of the vasodilatation of the blood vessels, more blood is quickly brought to the injured part. The *hyperemia* produced, in turn, results in the redness and heat so characteristic of inflamed tissues.

3. Not only do the blood vessels dilate during an inflammatory reaction, but the capillaries become highly *permeable* as well. The increased capillary permeability, in turn, leads to the passage of water, colloids, ions, and the body's defensive cells into the area of injury.* This fluid is usually called the *inflammatory exudate.*

What exactly causes this increased capillary permeability is still a matter for researchers to ponder. Thus far, scientists believe that when cells are damaged they manufacture and discharge certain substances that compel the capillaries to dilate. These substances are called *chemical mediators.* An important chemical mediator is histamine, a substance that evidently *initiates* the vascular response. However, since it is unable to sustain the increase in capillary permeability for any prolonged length of time, histamine is called a short-acting chemical mediator.

Physiologists are now searching for chemical mediators that play a role in delayed and sustained vascular reactions such as those that follow injury from ultraviolet rays and radiation. Bradykinin is believed to act in this way.

4. The blood flow, which has been rapid during the initial phase of inflammation, slows and may even stagnate. This *stasis of the blood* is the result of the packing of red cells in the capillaries; blood clots because of the heavy concentration of red blood cells and the pressure of the inflammatory exudate. Additionally, the blood stasis also causes decreased oxygenation of the area. Anaerobic metabolism may occur with the build up of acid end products; blood clots more rapidly in acidotic environments.

THE FORMATION OF THE INFLAMMATORY EXUDATE

The inflammatory exudate, as we just stated, is generally composed of water, colloids, ions, and defensive cells. This lymph-like substance collects readily at any site of tissue injury. In mild injuries the inflammatory exudate is mainly composed of serum; in more acute inflammations, however, the exudate contains fibrin and even red blood cells, which gives the exudate a hemorrhagic appearance.

Three factors are responsible for the formation of the exudate: one is the hyperemia that occurs after injury; a second is the increased capillary permeability; and a final cause is the increased filtration pressure created by hyperemia as the increased blood volume presses against the vessel wall. This increased pressure forces some of the blood and some of the cells out into the tissue spaces.

The inflammatory exudate has certain functions once it reaches the area of injury: (1) to dilute the toxins released by bacteria; (2) to bring to the site certain nutrients necessary for tissue repair, and (3) to carry the protective cells that will phagocytize and destroy bacteria.

While the inflammatory exudate is very useful to the body, it can and often does create serious problems for the injured person. First of all, the additional fluid in the area of injury causes swelling, and the swelling causes pain and sometimes immobility. This *swelling or edema,* which is often severe, can constitute a serious problem for the person whose injured arm or leg is in a cast that does not provide room to accommodate the swollen tissues. For these individuals the swelling and compression may result in a closing off of arterial flow to the damaged part as well as a restriction of venous return. Such symptoms as coldness, blueness, and swelling of the extremity may occur, along with sensations of pain, tingling, and numbness. Elevation of the swollen part usually helps to increase venous return and to relieve the edema. At times a hole may have to be cut out of the cast, or the cast may have to be split (bivalved) and then taped together to allow for the swelling.

A second group of patients for whom inflammatory edema constitutes a dangerous problem are those with *head injuries.* When the tissues of the brain swell, the hard bony cranium cannot enlarge to make room for its increased contents. As a result, the patient develops an *increased intracranial pressure,* a neurologic complex of signs discussed in Unit X.

THE DEFENSIVE CELL RESPONSE

The inflammatory exudate that leaks into inflamed tissues as a result of increased capillary permeability is loaded with white blood

*The terms "ion" and "colloid" are defined and discussed in Chapter 12.

cells and with macrophages of the reticuloendothelial system. This response by the body-protecting cells is highly complex and still somewhat of a mystery. The major components of the response are: (1) pavementing of leukocytes, (2) the migration of protective cells, (3) phagocytosis by the protective cells, and (4) leukocytosis — systemic reaction.

Pavementing of Leukocytes. As stated under the *vascular response,* the blood flow tends to be rapid during the first part of the inflammatory response; then the circulation slows and even stagnates. With the slowing of the blood flow, the leukocytes (mainly neutrophils) leave the center of the blood stream in order to line the walls of the capillaries. When neutrophils stick to the vessel walls in this manner, the result is called *margination* or *pavementing* of leukocytes.

The Migration of Protective Cells. From this position, lining the vessel walls, the white cells begin their process of *migration* to the site of injury. Squeezing through the vessel walls by a process known as diapedesis, and slithering through the tissue spaces by means of ameboid motion, the vast army of phagocytic cells begins its journey to the site of invasion.

Even when a person is in a state of health, white blood cells are always migrating to the tissues in small numbers. Injury simply *speeds* this process of migration and greatly increases the number of defensive cells that are "on the move." A very important defense mechanism in injury, this migration of defensive cells serves three purposes: (1) to destroy injurious agents, (2) to neutralize the toxins produced by these agents, and (3) to remove the inflammatory debris of dead cells and dead bacteria. Migration begins within a few minutes after injury.

As we pointed out earlier, all the different types of defensive cells *do not* migrate to the site of injury at the same time. Instead, migration is quite *selective,* with some cells (like the neutrophils and macrophages of the reticuloendothelial system) coming early, while other cells (like the monocyte, lymphocyte, and plasma cell) arrive later.

What is the force that attracts these cells, drawing them like a magnet to the site of injury? One theory, questioned by some authorities, is that of *chemotaxis.* This hypothesis simply states that when certain chemicals are released by the tissues, defensive cells are either drawn *toward* the source of the chemical (positive chemotaxis) or they are propelled *away* from the source of the chemical (negative chemotaxis). The chemicals that evidently are responsible for chemotaxis in the inflammatory reaction are bacterial toxins, as well as the *polysaccharides* that are released by the injured tissues.

Phagocytosis. One of the most important tasks of the body's defensive cells is phagocytosis; the engulfing and ingestion of harmful foreign substances. The material ingested may be bacteria, parasites, dead cells, or foreign matter such as soot. The phagocyte digests its prey by means of the proteolytic enzymes that it produces. White cells also release bactericidal agents, such as lysozyme, which kill the bacteria before the bacteria can kill the white cell.

It is its own gluttony, however, rather than the foreign objects, that finally destroys the phagocyte. As the defensive cell ingests bacteria and other foreign particles, breakdown products accumulate within its cytoplasm. These breakdown products are harmful to the phagocyte and, by accumulating, they eventually bring its life to an end.

Leukocytosis – The Systemic Reaction. As we stated earlier, most infectious and inflammatory conditions are characterized by a marked increase in circulating white blood cells, called leukocytosis. The count may climb from between 6000 and 10,000 per cu. mm. up to 30,000 per cu. mm.

One explanation for this intensification of leukocyte production and release is that the inflammatory exudate contains a substance which is a *leukocytosis-promoting factor* (LPF). It is possible that this globulin factor promotes a hyperplasia of bone marrow tissue which, in turn, increases white blood cell production and release.

A second theory explaining leukocytosis is that the disintegrated white blood cells at the site of inflammation release a substance that promotes leukocytosis. Some physiologists believe that this substance is actually a form of the LPF.

In any event, leukocytosis is a cardinal sign, always present when inflammation occurs, and usually subsiding with the disappearance of the inflammatory reaction.

THE FIBRIN BARRIER

Like the migration of leukocytes and macrophages, the formation of a fibrin barrier or net is a vital physiologic defense mechanism against the further spread of infection and inflammation. Exactly how this fibrin barrier works is still a mystery. Does it form a wall surrounding the inflamed area and encircling the bacteria, thereby trapping these undesirable aliens and making them available to the action of the phagocytes? Does it form a heavy net that catches dangerous intruders as a net catches fish? Or is it a bewildering maze in which the bacteria, on their way to new tissue territories, become endlessly lost and thus more vulnerable than ever to the hungry macrophages? No one knows for certain which answer is correct. We do know, however, that without the fibrin barrier, a simple local infection can easily spread to become a dangerous, even fatal, systemic malady.

How is this valuable fibrinous material formed? First of all, you will recall that both tissue histiocytes and lymphocytes are capable of transforming themselves into fibroblasts, thereby helping to form the fibrin mesh. Second, in the process of inflammation, fibrinogen escapes from the blood. Fibrinogen, an important blood component involved in the clotting mechanism, is then converted to fibrin.

The fibrin barrier, like all physiologic defenses, creates certain problems for the body, the most significant of which is the formation of *adhesions.* When such fibrous bonds or adhesions form between adjacent loops of bowel, they are an important cause of intestinal obstruction. Adhesions can also cause respiratory problems when they form between the pleura covering the lungs and the lining of the chest wall.

THE HUMORAL DEFENSE

While defensive cells phagocytize bacteria, and the fibrin mesh checks the spread of bacteria, the *humoral defense* fights and *neutralizes bacterial toxins.* This defense mechanism depends upon the antitoxins and antibodies that are contained within the inflammatory serum. These powerful substances are involved in the important antibody-antigen reaction, to be discussed in more detail in Chapter 11.

THE HORMONAL RESPONSE

You will recall from Unit II that Selye designated inflammation as the prime example of the Local Adaptation Syndrome or LAS. The LAS, like the GAS, depends on the action of the brain and central nervous system and upon the hormones of the adrenal and pituitary glands. According to Selye, some hormones, such as cortisone, are *anti-inflammatory,* suppressing the formation of eosinophils and lymphocytes and causing the shrinkage of lymphoid tissue. As a consequence, these hormones *limit* the spread of the inflammatory reaction. Other hormones, such as *aldosterone,* are *pro-inflammatory* corticoids that stimulate the body's defensive activities and thereby promote and support the inflammatory reaction.[27]

In sum, there are many factors at the body's disposal for defensive purposes. Each factor has its own particular role to play, yet each factor must work in coordination with several other factors if the defense is to be successful.

SIGNS AND SYMPTOMS OF INFLAMMATION

The major local and systemic manifestations of inflammation and their causation are listed on the following page.

WAYS OF CLASSIFYING INFLAMMATORY REACTIONS

While all inflammatory reactions share to some degree the same general and local manifestations, inflammatory reactions also *differ* from one another in a number of important ways. We find that there are four major ways of classifying inflammatory reactions, each type of reaction being distinguished by certain characteristics. Major criteria used in classifying inflammatory reactions are as follows: causation; duration (acute or chronic); type of exudate produced (serous, fibrinous, catarrhal, purulent, and hemorrhagic); and location and type of tissue involved (abscesses, cellulitis, and ulcers).

Causation

As stated earlier, inflammation can be caused by any agent that is capable of injuring or killing tissues and cells.

Duration

Inflammatory reactions are classified as *acute* or *chronic,* mainly in terms of the length of time they have been in existence. However, chronic and acute inflammatory reactions also have many other distinctive and differentiating characteristics. In Table 10–4 we outline some of the most distinctive features of each.

One important type of chronic inflammation is *granulomatous chronic inflammation.* This inflammatory reaction develops in the following conditions: tuberculosis, syphilis, leprosy, brucellosis, and fungus infections. Characterized by a tumor-like proliferation of cells at the site of injury, granulomatous inflammations may eventually be replaced by large amounts of scar tissue.

It is important to remember that these classifications of inflammation, while useful, are nevertheless arbitrary. Acute inflammation can subside and become chronic, while chronic inflammations may develop as a low-grade reac-

Pathophysiologic Basis	Signs and Symptoms
Local Reaction	
Blood vessels dilate and blood is brought rapidly to injured area; hyperemia results	Heat (calor) and redness (rubor) around the area of injury
Exudation of inflammatory lymph produces local edema around injured area	Swelling (tumor)
Nerve endings in the area of inflammation are painfully stimulated by both the pressure of the inflammatory lymph and the chemicals that are released by the damaged cells	Pain (dolor)
Pain and discomfort resulting from nerve ending involvement cause the patient to hold the injured part as immobile as possible; muscle spasms around the area of injury help to splint motion	Loss of function and the involuntary cessation of movement
Systemic Reactions	
Neutrophils may release enzymes that are fever-producing; in infections, bacteria release toxins that are absorbed into the circulation and then act upon the hypothalamus to produce fever	Fever accompanied by increased pulse and respiration rates; adults may experience chills; children may suffer from convulsions
Increased numbers of WBC are released from the bone marrow and lymph nodes into the blood; this is possibly the result of the leukocytosis-promoting factors (LPF)	Leukocytosis
A chilly sensation commonly precedes fever; it also is accompanied by a lowered skin temperature, which is caused, in turn, by marked vasoconstriction; the chill and shivering cause an increase in body metabolism and heat production; it is speculated that there may be a shivering center in the hypothalamus	Chills and "gooseflesh"
A thermoreceptive center in the hypothalamus is probably responsible for diaphoresis; this symptom usually accompanies fever and usually heralds the beginning of a fall in body temperature	Sweating
The exact cause for a decrease in appetite in inflammatory and infectious conditions is not known; environmental problems such as nauseating odors and sights and psychologic problems such as worry and depression probably contribute to the development of this problem	Anorexia
Fever, anorexia, and nausea predispose to a loss of weight	Weight loss
The exact cause for the achy, exhausted feeling accompanying inflammation and infection is not known	General malaise, "aches and pains," "feeling terrible"
Muscle groups are sometimes directly invaded by organisms; also, the inactivity of muscles that generally accompanies inflammation may lead to atrophy of the muscle and further weakening	Generalized weakness and an inability to sustain normal activity
High fever, sweating, and dehydration contribute to a sense of lethargy and depression; however, other factors of emotional origin are undoubtedly at work	Depression and a loss of enthusiasm
Some authorities believe that the general systemic symptoms that occur in inflammation are the result of the general adaptation syndrome (GAS); Selye states that persons suffering from such symptoms are involved in the "syndrome of just being sick"[25]	"The syndrome of just being sick"

tion to toxicity and never become an acute response.

Exudate

The major types of exudate produced in inflammatory reactions — serous, fibrinous, catarrhal, purulent, and hemorrhagic — are compared and contrasted in Table 10-5.

The type of exudate produced in an inflammatory reaction often serves as an excellent guide to diagnosis. The physician may request that the laboratory take a smear of the exudate from an inflamed area, especially if the

TABLE 10-4. DISTINGUISHING CHARACTERISTICS OF ACUTE AND CHRONIC INFLAMMATORY REACTIONS

Distinguishing Characteristics	Acute Inflammatory Reactions	Chronic Inflammatory Reactions
Duration	Generally last from a few days to a few weeks; if inflammation lasts more than a few weeks, it is termed chronic	Generally persist over many weeks and may last for several months
Important anatomic changes	Vascular congestion; exudation of inflammatory lymph and defensive cells	Proliferative cell multiplication; proliferation mainly fibroblastic, which leads to scarring
Dominant cell at the site of injury	Polymorphonuclear leukocytes, with neutrophils arriving first	Mononuclear cells, especially lymphocytes and plasma cells
Symptoms	Redness, heat, pain, swelling, and all the general systemic signs	Symptoms may not be severe; because of proliferation of fibroblasts, scarring, deformities, and adhesions may develop, with *permanent* tissue damage

presence of bacteria is suspected. The smear of material obtained is then used for a bacterial culture. From the culture it is possible to identify the type of organism present, as well as the antibiotics to which it is sensitive and susceptible.

Location and Position

Inflammatory reactions are also classified according to their *location* within the body and according to the particular *organ* they affect. Thus, the term "myocarditis" signifies inflammation of the heart muscle; "appendicitis," an inflammation of the appendix; "nephritis," an inflammation of the kidney nephron; and so forth.

A final way to group inflammatory conditions is according to the *position* that an inflamed area occupies within the particular tissue involved. Three distinct types of inflammatory reactions are based upon this

TABLE 10-5. A SUMMARY OF THE VARIOUS TYPES OF INFLAMMATORY EXUDATES

Type	Characteristics	Derivation	Typical Conditions in Which Exudate Appears
Serous	A watery, low protein fluid that is generally produced in large amounts	From blood serum and from the cells lining the peritoneal, pleural, and pericardial cavities and joint spaces	Skin blisters Pericarditis Pulmonary tuberculosis with effusion
Fibrinous	Exudate filled with large amounts of fibrinogen, which results in the precipitation of fibrin	If capillaries are damaged, the increase in their permeability leads to the escape of the large fibrinogen molecule into the inflammatory exudate	Occurs in severe acute inflammations Pneumococcal pneumonia
Catarrhal	Mucinous secretion	Released from tissues that are mucus-producing (nasopharynx, lungs, intestinal tract, uterus)	Common cold Smog may cause watering of eyes and nose
Purulent or suppurative	Characterized by the presence of *pus,* which is a thick fluid composed of partly liquefied necrotic tissue debris plus large numbers of dead and living bacteria and polys	Pus is mainly produced by such pus-producing (pyogenic) bacteria as staphylococci, pneumococci, meningococci, gonococci and certain streptococci; certain chemicals such as silver nitrate may also cause suppurative inflammations	Acute appendicitis Gonorrhea Abscesses Boils and carbuncles
Hemorrhagic	Red blood cells escape into the exudate; patients suffer from tiny hemorrhages into their skin and tissues (petechiae); the skin may be covered with small red areas; in severe cases, the patient's coloring may be very dusky	Results from damage to capillaries and blood vessels due to severe infection	Fulminating infection Subacute bacterial endocarditis The "black smallpox"

classification and need clarification: abscesses, cellulitis, and ulcers.

Abscesses. An abscess is defined as a "localized collection of pus caused by suppuration in a tissue, organ, or confined space." Abscesses are usually formed as the result of tissue invasion by pyogenic bacteria. As you will recall, the pus produced is a mixture of bacteria and polys. Abscesses are also characterized by parenchymal and stromal cell destruction which, in turn, leads to scar tissue and to the production of permanent deformities.

Boils and carbuncles are common examples of the inflammatory abscess. A *boil* is an abscess of the root of a hair follicle; it results from bacterial infection. Staphylococci are the pyogenic organisms most frequently involved in the etiology of a boil. A *carbuncle* is a group of boils adjacent to one another. Because this type of abscess extends into the subcutaneous tissue, carbuncles are much more serious than boils. Suppuration is deeper and more extensive, healing is slower, and scarring may be quite extensive.

Abscesses may terminate in a variety of ways. First, some abscesses may extend from the involved organ or tissue to the surface of the body, where the accumulated pus is released. Abscesses frequently extend to the surface by means of either a sinus or a fistula. A *sinus* is a tract that drains pus to the outside from an abscess that is fairly deep within the tissues. A *fistula* is an abnormal tract that may form between two hollow organs or between a hollow organ and the skin. Examples of fistulas are the channels that form between the rectum and vagina or between the interior of the bowel and the skin surface. Second, abscesses may burst *within* the body, releasing pus into a body cavity and thereby creating serious complications for the patient. For example, an appendix may rupture from an inflammatory process; as a result, the contents of the inflamed appendix flow into the peritoneal cavity, causing peritonitis. Third, small abscesses may be terminated by the process called *resolution,* in which the pus and debris of inflammation are simply digested by the macrophages rather than draining out or bursting forth from the area of tissue damage. Finally, as stated earlier, abscesses tend almost always to result in some permanent damage to the involved cell and in the formation of scar tissue.

Since abscesses are common in clinical practice and can be very dangerous, a few words of caution are in order. In working with patients with abscesses, remember these points:

1. Never squeeze a pimple or boil forcefully, as this may cause the infection to extend.

2. Instruct persons with boils around the nose and within the nostrils to seek medical aid, as neglect can produce such serious complications as sinus thrombosis, meningitis, and septicemia.

3. The use of careful technique in the changing and discarding of dressings from patients with abscesses will prevent the transmission of infection to yourself or to other patients. Be sure to wear gloves or to use forceps when removing contaminated dressings.

Cellulitis. Any inflammatory process that is poorly defined and diffuse and has a marked tendency to spread through solid tissues is called cellulitis. This type of inflammation usually involves the skin and subcutaneous tissues, although it may also extend to deeper tissues, as occurs in pelvic cellulitis. Any pathogen that can invade the body's tissue can cause cellulitis, although the *hemolytic streptococcus* is the most common and virulent cause.

Ulcers. An ulcer is a superficial defect of the surface of an organ or tissue that is caused by the sloughing of necrotic tissues destroyed by the inflammatory process. Ulcers are commonly found in the mucosa of the stomach, mouth, and intestines. For example, the gastric or stomach ulcer is frequently encountered. Persons with poor circulation as a result of peripheral vascular disease may develop multiple stasis ulcers on their legs. A third common site for ulcer formation is the cervix of the uterus. Each of these types of ulcer formation will be considered in appropriate sections of the text.

THE OUTCOME OF THE INFLAMMATORY PROCESS

The Results of Inflammation

An inflammatory process can eventually terminate in several ways — some adaptive and some maladaptive.

- ▶ Mild inflammatory reactions are often *resolved* and heal quickly with no complications.
- ▶ Inflammation may be *inadequate* as a response to stressors. The inflammatory defenses may be unable to contain infectious agents to a limited area. Intruders may escape, enter the general circulation, and cause a serious *bacteremia.* If the bacteria increase in number in the blood stream, a fatal *septicemia* may ensue.

- Development of inflammation may result in *over-reaction* by the body to a stressor. For example, arthritis and polyarteritis nodosa may be linked to overly virulent and extensive inflammatory reaction.
- Inflammation can result in *pathologic changes* that cause serious and lasting problems for the persons, e.g., peritonitis, fistulas, ulcers, boils, adhesions, and permanent scars.

Factors that Affect the Outcome of the Inflammatory Process

The eventual outcome of inflammation rests upon (1) the nature of the stressor and (2) the patient's ability to respond adaptively to that stressor. You will recall from Unit III that if the stressor is very powerful or if the patient's resistance is poor, the patient may be overcome and the stressor may emerge the victor over a weakened or dead host. Conversely, if the stressor is weak or the patient has strong resistance, the stressor will be weakened or eliminated, and the patient will continue to live and hopefully will regain strength.

THE NATURE OF THE STRESSOR

Several factors may tip the scales in favor of victory for the stressor.

Number or Amount. The number of invading organisms or the amount of stressor (e.g., the dose of radiation that a person receives). Generally the *greater* the amount of the stressor, the more likelihood of serious or possibly fatal illness in the patient.

Virulence. The virulence or *strength* of the invader. Even a brief exposure to strong radiation can give rise to serious burns. Infection by a few powerful (highly virulent) pyogenic organisms, such as the streptococci, can be more threatening than a similar invasion by a greater number of less virulent organisms.

The Spreading Factor. The ability of certain organisms to *spread* through tissue and to *dissolve fibrin barriers* enables those organisms to undermine the adequacy of the inflammatory process. The streptococcus and the staphylococcus, in particular, have this ability. Both these microorganisms are able to produce an enzyme called *hyaluronidase,* sometimes called the "spreading factor." Hyaluronidase, along with other factors, helps to increase the permeability of tissues and the consequent spread of organisms from diseased tissue to healthy tissue.

Resistance to Phagocytosis. The ability of certain organisms to resist phagocytosis increases their ability to live and to multiply. For example, it is believed that some bacteria are enclosed in a polysaccharide capsule that protects them from polys and macrophages.

THE NATURE OF THE PATIENT AND THE ABILITY TO RESPOND TO STRESS*

The presence of certain factors within a given patient modifies that patient's response to microorganisms and to other stressors. Consider these case histories of two infected patients with inflammatory responses — one who lived and one who died. See if you can select those influences that made the crucial difference between recovery and death.

The Case of the Businessman's Son

One winter, Carl Young, the 19-year-old son of a well-to-do businessman, developed a case of the Asian flu, complicated by a severely inflamed throat. Carl, who had rarely been ill in his life, felt sick enough to go to bed. Carl's mother called their family physician, who told her to bring Carl into his office that afternoon. After examining Carl and taking a smear for a throat culture, the physician ordered cough medicines, antihistamines, a mild pain medication, and an antibiotic. Carl went home to bed. His mother cooked him meat broths and gave him juices to drink. Within a few days Carl was feeling much better, and by the end of a week he felt well enough to return to his college classes.

The Case of the Retired Gardener

Philip Oldster, 68, lived in one room of a boarding house. He was barely existing on his meager savings, money that he had carefully put away during his many years as a gardener. During his prime, Mr. Oldster had been a good gardener and had made a reasonable living. However, when he grew older the bachelor had to give up his livelihood because of the development of severe diabetes and a gradual worsening of his arthritic condition. As a result of such problems, this once active man had to radically change his lifestyle, being forced to live on his savings and sometimes on welfare. Unable to afford the apartment he had lived in, Mr. Oldster moved to the least expensive room he could find. He found he could not afford fresh fruits, meats, and vegetables. Exhausted, crippled, and with only a hot plate for cooking, he was unable to prepare good meals. Increasingly he ate only bread, cereal, eggs, and macaroni or spaghetti. Besides, as he used to admit to himself, if he did cook, who would he eat with anyway?

As you might suspect, Mr. Oldster had few social contacts with the exception of his landlady, whom he saw briefly almost daily. One week, the landlady missed seeing Mr. Oldster for several days and decid-

*Physical and psychological responses to stress and to injury are discussed in Chapter 6.

ed to check on her tenant. She found him ill and feverish, almost delirious, and he was taken by ambulance to the county hospital. The young intern at the hospital decided that Mr. Oldster probably had Asian flu and had developed pneumonia. Despite the efforts of doctors and nurses, antibiotics, and IV's, Mr. Oldster died within 24 hours of admission to the hospital. Mr. Oldster's landlady was the only person who had to be notified of his death

As you review these histories, you can see several reasons why one patient overcame infection while the other succumbed:

Age. The younger the patient the more likely is successful adaptation to stressors that create inflammation.

Nutrition. Patients who have received adequate protein and vitamin C tend to be less predisposed to tissue damage and are better candidiates for healing and repair.

Economic Standing. Persons with adequate incomes tend to survive illness far better than the poor. Patients like Carl Young can afford *immediate* medical care from experienced physicians. On the other hand, patients like Mr. Oldster often will not seek care because of its expense or because they have no transportation to a doctor. Only when critically ill are they taken to a public hospital, where they are sometimes treated by inexperienced interns.

Social Setting. Persons who live in comfortable surroundings and who have a family that cares about them survive illness better than those who live alone in an unpleasant environment, as did Mr. Oldster.

The Tissue Affected. Some tissues are more vulnerable to infectious disease than are other tissues. As you will recall, Mr. Oldster's *lungs* were affected by his infection. Lung tissue is loose tissue filled with large spaces that allow infectious processes to spread rapidly despite inflammatory defenses. Infections also disseminate rapidly in peritoneal, pericardial, pleural, and joint spaces.

The Presence of Other Diseases. Individuals having chronic diseases, such as arthritis, tend to succumb more easily to infections since their resistance is lowered from years of illness.

The Presence of Diabetes. The diabetic is less able to resist infection, because diabetics tend to have a poor vascular response to even slight invasions of microorganisms. Also, the diabetic's elevated blood sugar creates a good medium for the growth and multiplication of bacteria.

Other important factors affecting a host's responses to infections (which were not mentioned in our case histories) are:

The Presence of Arteriosclerosis. Persons with vascular diseases have great difficulty in resisting infections, especially of the lower extremities. Often patients with sclerosed blood vessels, and a resultant inadequate blood supply, develop severe leg ulcers that do not heal.

Immunity. Individuals are more highly resistive to certain infections if they have either a natural or an acquired immunity to the organism causing the infection. Immunity will be discussed in the next chapter of this unit.

Ionizing Radiation (X-radiation). Exposure to ionizing radiation causes a lowered resistance to infection and impaired inflammatory defenses. This is because x-radiation causes the death of many of the body's cells, including the valuable lymphocyte. Moreover, x-radiation suppresses antibody formation. These facts were pitifully demonstrated at Hiroshima and Nagasaki, where many survivors of the blast from the atomic bomb died from overwhelming infection a few days later, because of their exposure to excessive radiation.

Cortical Hormones. Patients who either are receiving cortisone medicinally or are producing too much cortisone in their body have an increased susceptibility to infection. The exact reasons for this increased susceptibility are considered in the discussion of the endocrine system in Unit XIX.

All the factors we have listed are important not only to the patient's ability to *resist* disease, but also to the body's ability to repair damaged tissue. Obviously both resistance and repair must take place for recovery to occur. Let us now consider the processes of repair and healing.

REPAIR AND HEALING

Repair is defined as the "replacement of dead or damaged cells by new healthy cells derived either from the parenchymal or connective tissue stromal elements of the injured tissue."[5] You will recall from physiology that the *parenchymal tissues* are the important, predominant, and functional tissues of an organ or gland, while the "connective tissue stromal elements" make up the framework that supports and contains the parenchymal tissues.

The steps involved in wound healing are complex and involve many biochemical reactions. We shall attempt to summarize those steps as simply as possible. The initial injury, e.g., incision made by a scalpel, puncture wound, etc., evokes an inflammatory response in the injured tissue. Included in the inflammatory response are an exudate, which contains fibrinogen, and an increase in the number of neutrophilic granulocytes. The neutrophilic granulocytes release vasoactive substances that increase capillary permeability. Macrophages also enter the area to remove dead cells and debris. The fibrinogen in the inflammatory exudate stimulates the formation of a fibrin strand, and ultimately, a *fibrin network.* Fibroblasts, in the presence of the fibrin strand, manufacture and secrete a *ground substance,* which is made up of protein polysaccharides and various glycoproteins. Eventually, there is collagen synthesis, the substance of wound tensile strength. Collagen synthesis usually starts about 4 days after the injury and continues for 6 months or longer. The fact that collagen synthesis continues for so long a period is extremely important for the nurse to understand in order to provide good patient/family teaching. Quite often a wound, especially a traumatic wound, appears much worse when the sutures are removed than it did when first sustained. Patients need to understand that wounds change over time, by contracting and relaxing, and that there should be no consideration of plastic surgery for most wounds until 6 months have passed.

The time required for wound healing varies. In addition to the patient factors discussed above, there are also different rates of healing in different parts of the body. Sutures placed in the face, for example, are normally removed after 3 days, while sutures placed in the hands or feet usually remain for 10 to 14 days. This is because the face has a better vascular supply than the extremities and heals faster. This information may need to be included in patient/family teaching so that the sutures are not removed too soon (often by the patient) or too late. Premature removal of sutures can result in poor wound healing; late removal of sutures can lead to wound infection and/or scarring due to granulation around the suture hole. Usually, additional support is given to wounds that require early suture removal by the application of paper adhesive strips.

Because of the many components involved, repair produces different results in different cases, depending upon the type of tissue involved, the extent of tissue injury, and the general condition of the patient. For some patients, repair may lead to almost perfect healing of a wound, with minimal or no scarring; such excellent repair results from the healing of tissues that contain parenchymal elements. In other cases, in which healing is by connective tissue elements, the patient may be left with deforming, disabling, and permanent scars.

To better grasp the process of repair, it is helpful to explore the following six areas: types of repair, types of tissues and their regenerative capacity, types of repair by connective tissue — primary, secondary, and tertiary intention — complications of the repair process, factors that affect the repair process, and the treatment of wounds and injuries.

Types of Repair

Injured tissues may be repaired either by the process of *regeneration* or by the formation of *scar tissue.* Regeneration occurs when injured cells and tissues are replaced by new cells and tissues that are identical or quite similar in nature and function to the damaged cells. Regeneration can follow both minor and serious tissue injuries. The ability of injured tissues to regenerate depends mainly upon two factors: the ability of the cells of the injured tissues to multiply, and the ability of the newly formed cells to coalesce into units that can function physiologically. For proper function, newly formed units must be equipped with a normal blood, lymph, and nerve supply.

A second type of repair is by means of scar tissue formation. Collagenous scars may form in the healing of tendons, fascia, connective tissue, and collagenous structures. Also, nonfunctioning fibrous scars may patch tissues that cannot be regenerated; for example, damaged heart muscle, brain, and some nerve tissue cannot regenerate and, therefore, these vital structures can heal only by scar tissue formation.

Types of Tissue and Their Regenerative Capacity

Tissues that Heal by Regeneration of Identical Tissue. Upon injury, the following tissues are able to heal with perfect regeneration of the injured parts:

Epithelial Tissues. Squamous surfaces of the skin, interior of the mouth, vagina, and cervix; the lining of the salivary glands, pancreas, and biliary tract; the vascular epithelium, the cellular layer of the cornea, the tubular epithelium of the kidney; the epithelium of the digestive and respiratory tracts. For the perfect reconstruction of epithelial tissue, the underlying structures that provide support for the epithelium must be intact.

Splenic and Lymphoidal Tissues. Periodic injury of these tissues results in scarring.

Hemopoietic Tissues. The bone marrow tissues.

Parenchymal Tissues of the Glands. The parenchymal elements of the liver, salivary glands, sebaceous glands, pancreas, and endocrine glands are all highly capable of regeneration. However, repair of the parenchymal tissues of glands cannot take place if the underlying framework of the gland is in poor condition or if the gland has been *completely destroyed.* For example, if the sweat glands or the sebaceous glands of a patient have been completely destroyed by a severe burn, they will never regenerate.

Tissues Replaced and Successfully "Mimicked" by Collagenous Scar Tissue. Tendons, fascia, connective tissue, and collagenous tissues heal by means of fibroblastic activity. The result of such healing is a tissue that closely resembles the original structure.

Tissues Replaced by Nonfunctioning Scar Tissue. Unfortunately some of the most vital tissues of the body, if injured, cannot be replaced by either identical or similar cells and tissues. The tissues of the brain; the neurons of the central nervous system; the renal glomeruli; and striated, cardiac, and smooth tissue must last throughout a person's lifetime. All of these are highly specialized tissues with functions of a precise nature that cannot be simulated by other tissues. Moreover, these structures are composed of cells (sometimes called permanent cells) that are unable to undergo mitotic division except in utero. Consequently when these cells are severely injured or destroyed, the tissues that the cells have built are replaced by fibrous scars that do not contribute to the physiologic functioning of the organism.

For example, when an individual suffers a myocardial infarction, a part of the heart muscle dies. As the necrotic area heals, a nonfunctioning fibrous scar replaces the specialized heart muscle tissue. As a result, the individual who recovers from a myocardial infarction has a heart that is damaged in its efficiency as a circulatory pump. If this same patient should have several more small infarctions, the heart may become so scarred with fibrous tissue that its function is seriously impaired. Consequently, the patient who has suffered from multiple infarctions may die in congestive heart failure.

Types of Repair by Connective Tissue: Primary, Secondary and Tertiary Intention

In most injuries both parenchymal and stromal cells are damaged or destroyed. Consequently healing *normally* involves not only the regeneration of parenchymal cells, but also the proliferation of fibroblasts and the resultant building of connective tissue. A repair by connective tissue also occurs whenever an injury has been very large or extensive; the fibrous scar tissue covers the large central area of the defect, and parenchymal regeneration occurs around the edges of the injured site. Finally, as you will recall, fibrous scar tissue is used in the repair of highly specialized tissue composed of permanent cells (e.g., the heart muscle).

Connective tissue repair can be beneficial to the patient in several ways: (1) it fills in defects after extensive injury; (2) it repairs areas damaged by thrombosis and infarction; (3) it gives added strength to blood vessels damaged by aneurysms;* and (4) it helps to form barricades between damaged, inflamed, and infected tissues and healthy tissues.

On the other hand, connective tissue repair can be as damaging as it is helpful. Crippling scars, obstructed blood vessels and nerve pathways, and permanent disfigurement are some of the complications of healing by fibrous tissue growth.

There are two major types of repair by connective tissue: The first is called *primary healing or union.* Primary union, such as the repair of a clean surgical incision by connective tissue elements, is often referred to as healing by *primary* or *first intention.* The second type of connective tissue repair is called *secondary union.* When this refers to the repair of contaminated surgical wounds, a secondary union is called healing by *secondary intention.* Tertiary intention involves *delayed primary closure* (DPC) of a wound which is initially felt to be too contaminated to close. DPC is usually accomplished surgically 4 or 5 days after the injury is first sustained. The three types of union are illustrated in Figure 10–2.

As a brief comparison of the major characteristics of repair by first intention and by second intention, we quote from Cameron:[5]

> In essence, union by second intention differs from union by first intention in the following respects:
> 1. Loss of a greater amount of tissue.
> 2. Production of necrotic debris and inflammatory exudate requiring removal.
> 3. Formation of larger amounts of granulation tissue to fill the defect.
> 4. Slower replacement of the destroyed elements.
> 5. Production of larger amounts of scar.

Complications of the Repair Process

Like all body responses to injury, the process of repair can sometimes end in new injury and in further disease for the patient. Repair as a response to infection and inflammation can be frustrated by the appearance of a new stressor, for example, a fresh invasion by bacteria or dangerous foreign substances. Repair can be inadequate, leading to poor healing of a wound with the formation of unstable and weak scars. Repair can also be excessive, resulting in large amounts of ugly nonfunctional scar tissue that eventually strangles blood vessels and nerve pathways in its fibrous grip. Because such complications can lead to serious, often irreversible problems for patients, let us briefly explore some of the most important types of pathologic healing.

*An aneurysm is an outpouching of the wall of a blood vessel due to weakness of the vessel wall.

Contaminated Surgical Wounds. Sometimes a clean wound that has been closed and properly sutured becomes infected. An infection of this type is often the result of cross-contamination from other patients or of poor handwashing or dressing technique on the part of the attending doctors or nurses. Such a wound will fill with pus and will need to be cleansed of foreign debris and necrotic tissue before healing by second intention is possible. Sometimes the surgeon will elect to close the wound and resuture it. Following this procedure, which is called *secondary closure,* the wound will then heal by *third intention.*

Unstable Scars. When an injury is quite large, the edges of the open wound may not be able to meet and mend properly. As a result, the new young vascular tissue that has been "granulating in" to fill the defect remains exposed. Eventually its blood supply diminishes, and the granulation tissue stops growing and slowly changes into an avascular unstable scar. Covered by a thin and delicate sheet of epithelial cells, this poorly nourished scar tissue is vulnerable to both ulceration and further injury. If, over several decades, ulceration occurs again and again, the patient with an unstable scar may eventually develop a squamous carcinoma called *Marjolin's ulcer* at the site of ulceration. To prevent the formation of an unstable scar and its complications, the surgeon may employ a split skin graft or a pedicle graft to close the open wound and to cover the unprotected granulation tissue.

Excessive Granulation Tissue. When granulation tissue is unusually abundant and also swollen and edematous, it is called "proud flesh." Such an abnormal growth of granulation tissue can upset the process of repair by hindering the growth of epithelium over the wound.

Keloids. These huge, ugly, tumor-like overgrowths of scar tissue occur mainly among people with highly pigmented skins, particularly blacks. Certain areas of the body are more prone to the development of keloids, with the neck, chest and the deltoid areas most commonly involved. Keloids can be excised; however, they have an infamous capacity for recurring following surgical removal. A rather large keloid is pictured in Figure 10–3.

Hypertrophied Scars. Because they are red, large, raised, and hard, hypertrophied scars have an unpleasant appearance (Fig. 10–4). Moreover, they produce an uncomfortable itching. Hypertrophied scars sometimes develop following inaccurate wound closure. The ugly appearance of these scars can be minimized to some extent by surgical revision.

Contractures. Contracture of scar tissue leading to disability and severe deformity occurs mainly when severe injuries are located on the face or over a joint and are healing by secondary union. Early surgical closure of open injuries by skin grafts can help to prevent contractures. However, in some cases the skin grafts themselves develop contractures unless splints and physical therapy are ordered by the physician. An example of a severe contracture resulting from burns, and the results of surgical efforts to release the contracture are pictured in Figure 10–5.

Interference with Organ Function. Scar tissue, when excessive, can definitely interfere with an organ's physiologic functioning. Function can be impaired or destroyed when the scar

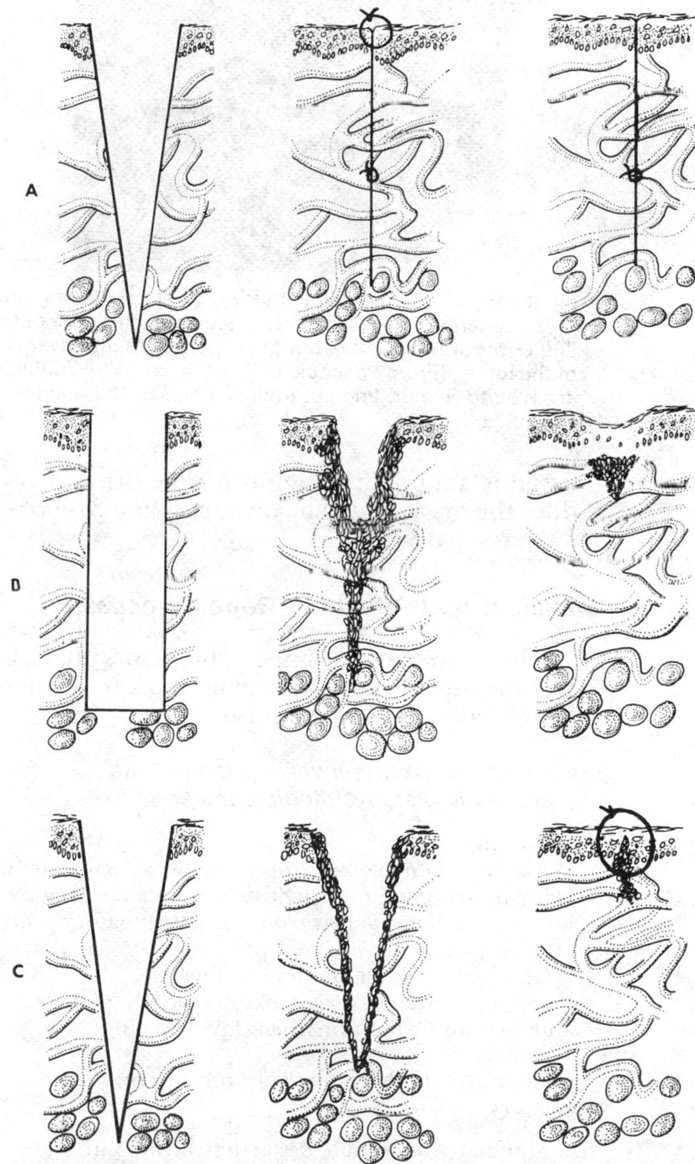

Figure 10–2. **A,** Primary, **B,** secondary, and, **C,** tertiary intention wound healing. (From Sproul, C. W., and P.J. Mullanney: *Emergency Care: Assessment and Intervention.* St. Louis: C. V. Mosby Co., 1974, p. 33.)

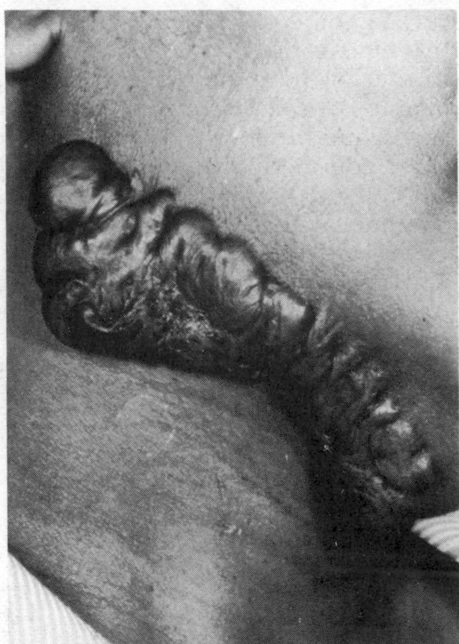

Figure 10–3. Typical keloid following a simple laceration of the anterior neck. Scar tissue does not follow the outline of the wound and is out of proportion to the severity of the injury. (From Peacock, E. E., Jr., and W. Van Winkle, Jr.: *Wound Repair,* 2nd ed. Philadelphia: W. B. Saunders Co., 1976, p. 233.)

tissue is abundant enough to close off and reduce the organ's vital blood supply and to choke its nerve pathways.

Factors that Affect the Repair Process

There are several important factors that affect the outcome of the healing process — some beneficially and some injuriously.

Favorable factors involving the patient and patient's physiologic condition:

Youth.

An adequate blood supply to the affected area, bringing oxygen and nutritive elements and removing the waste and debris from the inflammatory process.

Good general health and stamina.

Adequate nutritional intake, especially of protein and vitamin C, both of which favor healing.

Favorable factors involving the site of injury:

Minimal or moderate tissue destruction rather than extensive destruction.

An intact underlying framework upon which new tissues can be reconstructed.

The presence of tissues that are capable of regeneration.

The absence of infection with its accompanying exudate of pus and necrotic debris.

Immobilization and rest of the injured part.

Adverse factors involving the patient and patient's physiologic condition:

Old age.

Easy fatigability and poor physical condition.

An inadequate blood supply to the affected area due to severe peripheral vascular disease, varicose veins, excessive scarring from earlier injuries, edema around the injured area and/or venous stasis.

The presence of diabetes mellitus, a condition that favors the development of severe infections.

An excess of adrenocortical steroids within the body due to disease of either the pituitary gland or adrenal gland or due to chemotherapy with steroids. Excess steroids in the blood seem to depress the inflammatory reparative process.

Protein and ascorbic acid deficiencies.

Adverse factors involving the site of injury:

Total destruction of a complete physiologic unit (for example, a kidney nephron or a sweat gland). Once destroyed, individual physiologic and anatomic units cannot be regenerated.

Destruction of the underlying framework upon which new tissues can be reconstructed. Such destruction leads, unfortunately, to extensive growth of scar tissue.

The absence of tissues that can be regenerated.

The presence of infection, with its accompanying pus and tissue debris.

Excessive motion of injured parts and tissues.

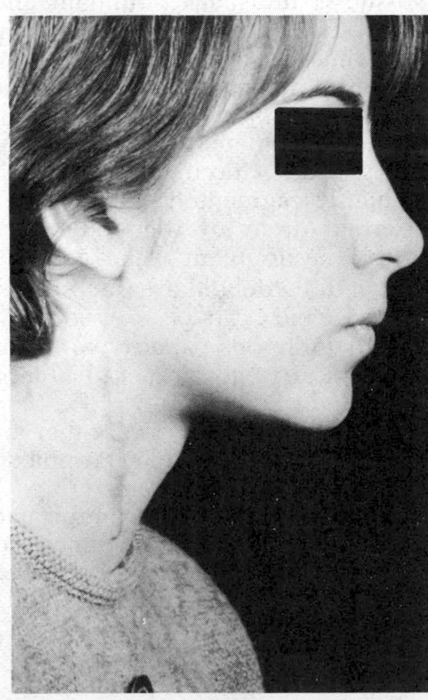

Figure 10–4. Hypertrophic scar which is not producing any functional disability and which follows the outline of the wound accurately. (From Peacock, E. E., Jr., and W. Van Winkle, Jr.: *Wound Repair,* 2nd ed. Philadelphia: W. B. Saunders Co., 1976, p. 232.)

The use of large numbers of sutures in repairing an injury. Sutures, when used to close a wound, tend to act as foreign bodies.

Paralysis of the limb in which the injured tissue is located.

Hematomas, seromas, and severe trauma around the site of the wound.

*Treatment of Wounds and Injuries**

By employing knowledgeable clinical care, doctors and nurses can greatly aid the work of nature in the inflammatory-reparative process. Ten major principles that we can employ in the care of patients with wounds in order to aid reparative process are:

1. Immobilize and rest the injured tissues. Rest ensures better utilization of oxygen and nutrients by the body's injured tissues,

*See Chapter 80 for treatment of wounds and burns.

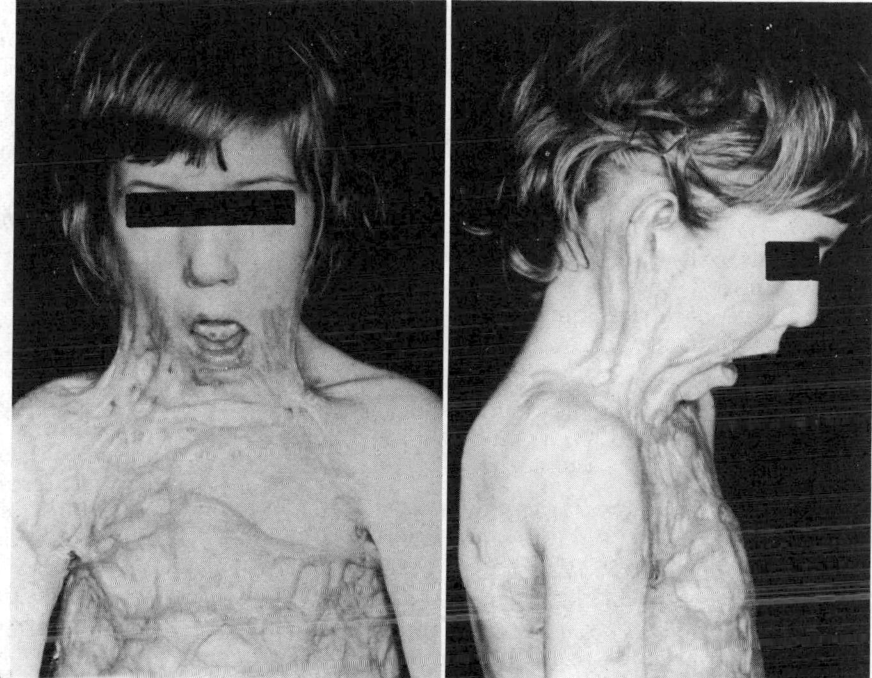

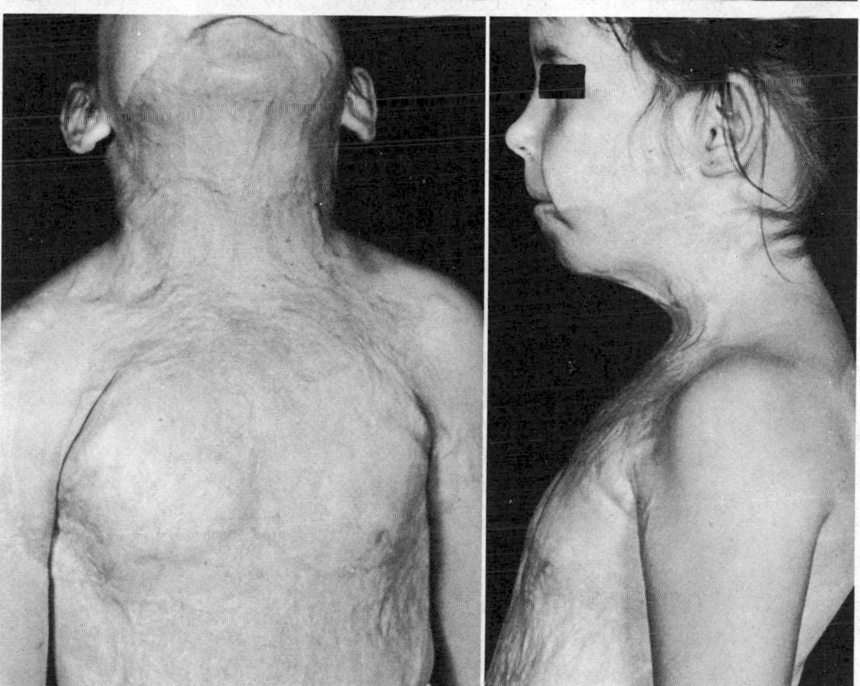

Figure 10–5. **A** and **B**. Full thickness of the anterior chest, which was allowed to heal by wound contraction, resulting in an anterior deformity of the neck and distortion of the facial features. **C** and **D**. Relief of deformity by excision of products of wound healing and resurfacing of the defect with large split-thickness grafts. (From Peacock, E. E., Jr., and W. Van Winkle, Jr.: *Wound Repair,* 2nd ed. Philadelphia: W. B. Saunders Co., 1976, p. 245.)

whereas activity increases the metabolic needs of tissues. Also, activity creates additional waste products at the site of injury and irritates already inflamed tissues. Moreover, activity tends to foster the harmful migration of microorganisms from injured tissues into healthy ones by breaking down the fibrin barriers — major defenses against the spread of infection. To immobilize and rest injured tissues, we place broken legs in casts and injured arms in slings, we shade and bandage damaged eyes, and we place the patient with a damaged heart muscle on total bed rest.

2. Convert the contaminated wound into a clean wound before surgical closure. As we said earlier, injured tissues that are filled with pus and necrotic debris cannot heal properly. Such wounds must be cleaned of foreign materials. Also, stagnant clotted blood must be removed because blood clots can become filled with bacteria. Some methods used for cleansing wounds are:

- Irrigation of the wound with sterile solutions of saline to wash out tissue debris and to reduce the number of bacteria.
- Surgical *debridement* of the wound, that is, excising by scalpel dead tissue and tissues in which foreign materials are embedded.
- Incision and drainage in order to remove from the wound *abnormal collections* of exudate, which act adversely to retard healing, to promote bacterial growth, and to cause pressure on organs nearby the injured area. Penrose drains of soft rubber are frequently used to drain out abnormal fluid collections. When a great deal of fluid is present within the injured area, the drain may be attached to low suction. A special device called a *Hemovac* may be used to provide (a) constant suction, (b) continuous drainage of a wound, or (c) wound irrigation with or without an antibiotic added to the irrigating solution. The Hemovac is commonly used following surgery — especially orthopedic surgery. The Hemovac is also sometimes employed following prostatectomy, radical vulvectomy, mastectomy and plastic and reconstructive surgery. A typical suction device is pictured in Figure 10–6. The Hemovac is described in more detail in Unit VIII.
- *Hemostasis.* The surgeon always endeavors a) to control bleeding into the wounded area and b) to remove old, clotted, and possibly contaminated blood from the site of injury. The nurse has the responsibility to watch for signs of bleeding on a patient's dressing or cast, and to report the appearance of blood drainage or frank blood to the physician.
- *Hyperbarically administered oxygen* may be prescribed for patients with anaerobic infections, e.g., gas gangrene, or patients who have poor healing, e.g., stasis ulcers. The procedure for administration of oxygen under conditions of increased pressure within a hyperbaric chamber is described in detail in Chapter 13.

3. Protect the wound from further injury and infection. The meticulous use of sterile technique in dressing and in irrigating wounds is of the greatest importance in preventing infection. A second factor in preventing wound contamination is isolation of patients with clean wounds from those with contaminated wounds. Finally, to prevent further injury, physicians and nurses usually strive to manipulate injured tissues as little as possible. Unnecessary manipulations and procedures can destroy new granulation tissue and break down fibrin barriers, thereby promoting the spread of bacteria.

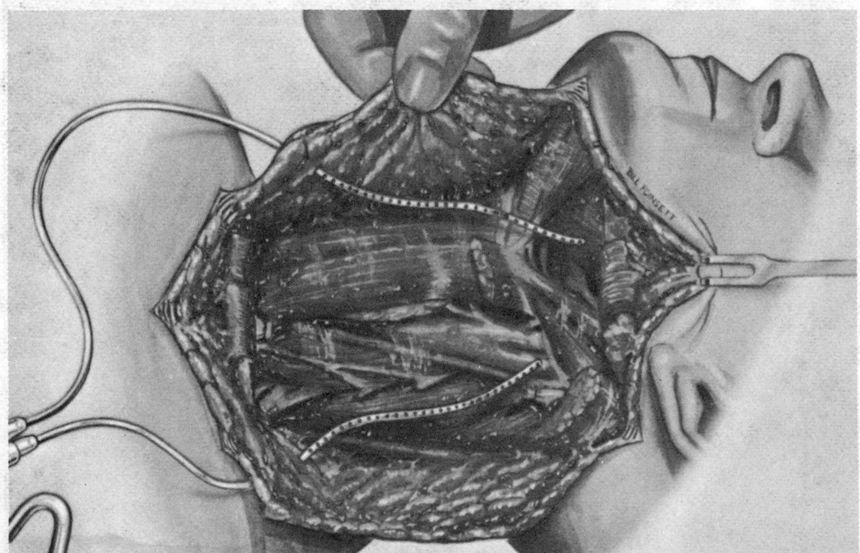

Figure 10–6. The use of the Synder Hemovac. This device provides constant suction to aid in infection control. Note that the tubes lying within the wound have multiple openings for purposes of collecting wound drainage and/or irrigating the wound with an irrigating solution. A simple spring device within the Hemovac unit establishes gentle wound suction, and wound drainage collects within the plastic Hemovac unit. Additional accessories are used for wound irrigation. (From *Synder Hemovac Brochure.* Zimmer USA: Warsaw, Ind. 46580.)

4. Administer antibiotics. To prevent and control infection, physicians often order penicillin or sulfonamides or one of the broad-spectrum antibiotics.

5. Administer steroids. In a few carefully selected cases, steroids may be given to reduce the virulence of the inflammatory reaction to injury, and to limit the spread of inflammation from injured tissues to healthy tissues. For example, cortisone may be given to reduce the severity of a serious eye inflammation.

6. Preserve the blood supply to the injured tissues. It is important to check bandages, casts, and splints for excessive tightness around an injured limb. If poorly applied, or in the presence of excessive tissue swelling, a splint can act as a tourniquet, completely shutting off the blood supply to the involved extremity. Also, tight surgical dressings that encircle an extremity can reduce circulation.

The application of warmth to an injured area *increases* the circulation to damaged tissues. Heat causes the blood vessels and capillaries to dilate; as a result, increased numbers of leukocytes and other natural defense factors are brought to the site of injury.

7. Elevate the injured part. Elevation of injured extremities helps to increase the venous return of blood to the heart; it also contributes to maintenance of proper wound drainage.

8. Promote adequate nutrition. An adequate intake of protein calories and vitamin C tends to speed and to facilitate the reparative process.

9. Relieve pain. Patients who have suffered injury or who have recently undergone surgery will naturally suffer some pain. Pain must be relieved in injured and postoperative patients, since discomfort can cause the additional problems of restlessness, insomnia, and anxiety — all factors that can act adversely on the healing process. For the various methods of pain relief, see Unit XI.

10. Give psychological support. Patients whose bodies are undergoing the process of repair are often emotionally upset. A patient with a broken limb may have to lie in a cast for weeks, losing time from work or school and family. An individual who has developed a severe inflammation of the eye may face the possibility of permanently impaired vision. The person who has suffered severe injuries in an accident will probably fear scarring, deformity, and life-long disability. These are just a few of the worries that patients may have; it is not surprising that many injured persons suffer also from fear, depression, and despair, and look to their doctors and nurses for support.

How do you alleviate their anxiety? A few helpful actions that you can employ are: (1) listen to your patient's concerns and do not minimize the worries expressed. (2) Answer a patient's questions concerning the injury as honestly as possible. Consult with the physician as to what has been told the patient concerning the prognosis, so that your comments do not conflict with the doctor's. (3) Convey the patient's questions to the doctor so that a discussion of these concerns with the patient is possible at the first opportunity. Patients may be afraid to talk with doctors, feeling doctors are too busy to be interested in their questions. It is the nurse's responsibility to strengthen communication patterns between the patient and doctor. (4) Watch your patient carefully for signs of severe depression. A patient who is scarred and crippled for life may think of suicide as an alternative to facing the difficulties of readjustment and the problems of rehabilitation. Such a patient should be brought quickly to the attention of the attending physician. Tranquilizers, antidepressants, and psychotherapy may be ordered for these troubled individuals. (5) Recognize that a patient who is convalescing from serious injuries or surgery may be very hostile or angry at times. Furthermore, the anger may be directed against you — an innocent bystander! Try to accept such a patient's hostility as gracefully as possible; recognize that these outbursts are probably temporary, and that they will pass as the person slowly regains control and a sense of hope for the future.

BIBLIOGRAPHY (Chapter 10)

1. Agris, J.: Traumatic tattooing. *Journal of Trauma,* 16:798, Oct. 1976.
2. Auld, M. E., et al.: Wound healing. *Nursing '72,* 2:36, Oct. 1972.
3. Ballinger, W. F., II, et al.: *The Management of Trauma.* Philadelphia: W. B. Saunders Co., 1975.
4. Boggs, D. R., and A. Winkelstein: *White Cell Manual,* 3rd ed. Philadelphia: F. A. Davis Co., 1975.
5. Cameron, R.: Inflammation and repair. *In* Robbins, S. L.: *Pathology.* Philadelphia: W. B. Saunders Co., 1967.
6. Castle, M.: Wound care: clear-cut ways to speed healing. *Nursing '75,* 40–44, Aug. 1975.
7. Ciancutti, A. R.: *Emergency Care Handbook. How To Deal With People in Emergencies.* Westport, Conn.: Technomic Publishing Co., Inc., 1977.
8. Cosabb, W., and J. W. Smith: *Plastic Surgery.* Boston, Little, Brown and Co., 1973.
9. Faddis, D., et al.: Tissue toxicity of antiseptic solutions. *Journal of Trauma, 17*:895, Dec. 1977.
10. Galvin, J. R., and D. De Simone: Infection rate of simple suturing. *Journal of the American College of Emergency Physicians,* 5:332, May 1976.
11. Ganong, W. F.: *Review of Medical Physiology,* 8th ed. Los Altos: Lange Medical Publications, 1977.
12. Gemberling, R. M., et al.: Dressing comparison in the healing of donor sites. *Journal of Trauma,* 16:812, Oct. 1976.
13. Guyton, A. C.: *Textbook of Medical Physiology,* 5th ed. Philadelphia: W. B. Saunders Co., 1976.
14. Harker, L. A.: *Hemostasis Manual,* 2nd Ed. Philadelphia: F. A. Davis Co., 1974.

15. Katz, R.: The painful ecstasy of healing. *Psychology Today,* Dec. 1976, p. 81–86.
16. Kerner, M., et al.: Gas gangrene complicating limb trauma. *Journal of Trauma,* 16:106, Feb. 1976.
17. Lang, A. G., and H. A. Peterson: Osteomyelitis following puncture wounds of the foot in children. *Journal of Trauma,* 16:993, Dec. 1976.
18. Levine, N. S., et al.: The quantitative swab culture and smear: a quick simple method for determining the number of viable aerobic bacteria on open wounds. *Journal of Trauma,* 16:89, Feb. 1976.
19. Noe, J. M., and S. Kalish: *Wound Care.* Greenwich, Conn.: Cheesebrough-Ponds, Inc., 1975.
20. Pathology of injury. *Lancet,* 2:911, Oct. 28, 1972.
21. Peacock, E. E., Jr., and W. Van Winkle, Jr.: *Wound Repair,* 2nd Ed. Philadelphia: W. B. Saunders Co., 1976.
22. Pesanti, E. L.: When phagocytic dysfunction increases susceptibility to infectious diseases. *Geriatrics,* 32:110, Mar. 1977.
23. Roberts, D.: Wound healing: A scientific review. *Applied Therapeutics,* 12:10, Apr. 1970.
24. Ryan, G. B.: Inflammation and localization of infection. *Surgical Clinics of North America,* 56(4):831, Aug. 1976.
25. Schwartz, C.: Developing foundations for healing grief. *Journal of Emergency Nursing,* 3:29, Jan.–Feb. 1977.
26. Selye, H.: *The Stress of Life.* New York: McGraw-Hill Book Co., Inc. 1956.
27. Sproul, C. W., and P. J. Mullanney: *Emergency Care: Assessment and Intervention.* St. Louis: C. V. Mosby Co., 1974.
28. Stevenson, T. R., et al.: Damage to tissue defenses by vasoconstrictors. *Journal of the American College of Emergency Physicians,* 4:532, Nov.–Dec., 1975.
29. Stevenson, T. R., et al.: Cleansing the traumatic wound by high pressure syringe irrigation. *Journal of the American College of Emergency Physicians,* 5:17, Jan., 1976.
30. Wischman, J., and M. M. McMahon: *The Patient With Surface Trauma.* (unpublished paper).

CHAPTER 11*

THE MECHANISM OF IMMUNITY — NORMAL AND PATHOLOGIC RESPONSES

The immune response is an exquisitely specific yet highly versatile two-edged sword. Although it is vital for survival in the often hostile microbiologic environment, an immune reaction may cause fatal disease, as in the case of an overwhelming hypersensitivity reaction to the sting of a bee.[86]

INTRODUCTION AND STUDY GUIDE

Since the earliest times, both humans and animals have been plagued by unseen enemies — parasites, bacteria, viruses — that have sought to enter and ravage the inner world of their bodies. Against these minute and dangerous living organisms, animals and humans have had to develop some means of defense if they were to live and reproduce their own kind. Thus, over eons of time, there has evolved the homeostatic mechanism called *immunity* — a mysterious and complex process that protects human beings and animals against attacks by such tiny alien invaders as bacteria and viruses.

The subject of immunity raises many questions, some of which are only partially answerable at this time. Questions concerning immunity that are of particular concern in nursing are as follows:

1. What exactly is immunity and how and why did it evolve in the individual and in the species?
2. What are the major components of the immune response?
3. What theories are available to explain the development of immunity and the production of antibodies?
4. What are the major types of immunity?
5. How can immunity be actively and passively acquired by a person? How, specifically, is immunity acquired by vaccination?
6. What happens to the body when the immune response becomes pathologic?
7. In what ways can the immune response be suppressed when it is either pathologic or disruptive to the success of such therapeutic measures as organ and tissue transplantation?

In order to answer these questions, the material in this chapter will focus upon the following areas:

- ▶ The immune response and its components
- ▶ Types of immunity (natural and acquired: active, passive, humoral, cellular)
- ▶ The immune response and its components
- ▶ Pathologic conditions associated with the immune response
- ▶ Immunologic aspects of transplant rejection

Study Guide

Because the subject of immunity is difficult, challenging, and filled with many technical terms and confusing theories, we urge you to make use of the following study guide:

1. Upon completion of this chapter, you should be able to define generally the terms listed below.

acquired immunity	atopic allergies
active immunity	atopy
agammaglobulinemia	autologous antigens
agglutination	autograft
allergen	autoimmune diseases
"allergic salute"	blocking antibodies
allergy	bursal-equivalent cells (B-cells)
allograft	cellular immunity
allograft reaction	clone
anaphylaxis	collagen diseases
antibody	complement
antigen	desensitization
antilymphocyte serum (ALS)	eosinophilia
Arthus reaction	exogenous antigen

*Karen Peterson, B.S., M.T. (ASCP), critically reviewed and assisted with the revision of this chapter. The content and accuracy of this revision was checked by Bruce G. Gilliland, M.D., Professor of Medicine with the University of Washington, Medical Director of Providence Hospital, and Director of Clinical Immunology Laboratory, Seattle, Washington.

gamma globulin
hapten
hay fever
histamine
histocompatibility antigens (HL-A)
homologous antigen
humoral immunity
hypersensitivity
hypogammaglobulinemia
hyposensitization
immune response
immunity
immunogen
immunogenicity
immunoglobulins
immunologic tolerance
immunologically competent cells (ICC)
immunodeficiency disorders
immunopathy
immunosuppressive techniques
immunotherapy
isotransplant
lymphocytes
lymphokines
lysis
mast cells
neutralization
opsonization
passive immunity
precipitation
primary humoral response
properdin
reagins
secondary humoral response
self-tolerance
self-antigen
"self-markers"
serum sickness
specificity
species immunity
thymus-dependent system cells (T-cells)
toxoids
tuberculin reaction
urticaria
vaccine
xenograft
vaccination

2. You should also be able to discuss, in general terms, the following concepts and theories:
   a. "Self" tolerance or immunologic tolerance
   b. The role of the humoral immune response
   c. The role of the cellular immune response
   d. Mediators of the immune response
   e. Mast cell degranulation
   f. The four mechanisms of immunologic injury
   g. The "instructive theory"
   h. The "clonal selective" theory
   i. The difference between an immune response and an allergic response
   j. Etiologic theories of autoimmunity
   k. The physiologic basis for transplant rejection
   l. Types of transplants
   m. Suppression and prevention of graft rejection

3. Describe tests used for diagnosis of diseases associated with the immune system:
   a. Differential white count
   b. Absolute leukocyte count
   c. Sheep erythrocyte rosette test
   d. Radioimmunoassay
   e. Radioallergosorbent test (RAST)
   f. Skin tests for Types I, II, and III hypersensitivity reactions
   g. Skin tests for Type IV delayed-hypersensitivity reactions
   h. Prausnitz-Küstner (P-K) reaction induction
   i. DNCB skin test
   j. Patch test

4. Describe the etiology, symptoms, and clinical care for the following immunopathies:
   a. Hypogammaglobulinemia
   b. Multiple myeloma
   c. Anaphylaxis
   d. Serum sickness
   e. Hay fever
   f. Urticaria
   g. Bronchial asthma
   h. Systemic lupus erythematosus (SLE)
   i. Contact dermatitis

5. State the uses and side effects of the following medications:
   a. Antihistamines (in particular, diphenhydramine hydrochloride)
   b. Sympathomimetics (epinephrine)
   c. Xanthines (Aminophylline)
   d. Corticosteroids
   e. Cromolyn sodium
   f. Levarterenol bitartrate (Levophed)
   g. Metaraminol bitartrate (Aramine)
   h. Cytotoxic drugs (azathioprine)
   i. Antilymphocyte serum

6. After carefully studying this chapter and relating it to your own clinical observations, you can expect to be able to:
   a. Discuss knowledgeably with patients the need to maintain current immunizations, as well as which immunizations are required.
   b. Observe important guidelines for protecting against dangerous infections patients with hypogammaglobulinemia.
   c. Assess the patient with an allergy in terms of the following: past history of allergic problems, family history of allergic problems, the physical environment in which the patient lives, food intake, types of drugs ingested, and what circumstances seem to precipitate allergic reactions (e.g., emotional stress, fatigue).
   d. Perform a physical assessment of the patient, observing in particular the skin, eyes, nose, mouth, pharynx, ears, and neck in particular for signs of hypersensitivity reactions.
   e. Assist in the administration of skin tests for allergies.
   f. Instruct the patient in methods for avoiding specific allergens; e.g., removal of certain rugs or blankets from the home, daily damp dusting if dust acts as an allergen.
   g. Participate in a hyposensitization program, observing safety precautions at all times.
   h. Know the signs of an anaphylactic reaction and be prepared to secure help immediately if such a reaction should occur.
   i. Know and observe safety precautions, should Levophed or Aramine be required for the treatment of anaphylactic shock.
   j. Use preventive measures against the possibility of an anaphylactic reaction, e.g., obtain a history of the patient's drug allergies before administering certain medications, note drug allergies on the patient's chart and Kardex.
   k. Be prepared to observe for and report signs of transplant rejection.
   l. Be aware of the dangerous side effects of corticosteroids — immunosuppressive agents that are used in the treatment of some hypersensitivity reactions and autoimmune diseases and are also employed to help prevent transplant rejection.

IMMUNITY AS A NORMAL ADAPTIVE RESPONSE

Definition

Since ancient times, observant individuals have noted that people recovering from certain infectious diseases become resistant to reinfection by that same disease. From these observations have come the fundamental concepts underlying the complex and ever-evolving field of immunobiology.

Immunity is comprehensively defined by Mackay and Burnet as follows:

> In the broadest terms, immunity is the essential function by which vertebrate organisms maintain their functional integrity insofar as this is threatened by the entry or appearance of foreign chemical substances in the body.[64]

More specifically, immunity implies: (1) specific protection against foreign invaders of the body and subsequent resistance to reinfection by that foreign substance; (2) a heightened responsiveness to antigenic substances, which may be chemicals, foreign proteins, viruses, or bacteria; (3) a response that involves the production of antibodies (*humoral* immunity) and the activation of cytotoxic cellular components (*cellular* immunity), and (4) the capacity to distinguish foreign agents from body constituents — a capacity known as *self-tolerance.*

Immunity, then, is a homeostatic characteristic of vertebrate animals that ensures their survival; a complex group of biologic processes that protects the body against foreign invaders; and a process that builds up resistance in an organism, sometimes thereby preventing that organism from being infected *twice* by the same foreign protein matter. The general effects of immunity are to: (1) neutralize and destroy alien organisms, (2) build up resistance to further attacks by alien proteins, (3) accept or reject cells and tissues from other living beings, as occurs in organ transplants and blood transfusions, and (4) prevent the development and spread of cells that have become malignant.

The Immune Response

Whenever the body recognizes the presence of an invading organism or a protein material that it cannot identify as a part of itself, the body normally protects itself by developing an *immune response.* Normally, the immune system responds to an invasion of foreign and dangerous substances (antigens or immunogens) by producing immune response components, i.e., antibodies and sensitized lymphocytes. However, in an immune system damaged by *pathologic* changes, an immune response may occur in response to certain of the body's *own* proteins, resulting in the production of autoantibodies. Those pathologic conditions in which the body directs the immune response against itself are called *autoimmune* diseases and will be discussed in more detail later.

Antigens and Immunogens

Our immune system recognizes most proteins, bacteria, viruses, and parasites that are not part of the normal body environment as "foreign" and will initiate an immune response. Those substances capable of eliciting an immune response are called *antigens* or *immunogens.* An *antigen* is a substance that, due to its chemical configuration, is capable of reacting with an antibody. An *immunogen* is any substance that induces a detectable immune response (humoral, cellular, or both) when introduced into a host.

Specifically, antigens are chemical substances that are nearly always protein in nature and that are viewed by the body as an attacking force. Thus, we find that the structures of antigenic microorganisms such as bacteria and viruses are protein, as are almost all the toxins that they manufacture and release. Microorganisms and their toxins are termed "antigenic" because they stimulate the immune response.

To be an antigen, a substance must have a high molecular weight — 8000 or more. However, there is an important exception to this rule. There are substances of low molecular weight, called *haptens,* against which the body can develop immunity under certain conditions. Haptens include drugs, chemical constituents in dust, breakdown products of animal dander, some industrial chemicals, and other such substances. To stimulate an immune response, a hapten must first combine with an antigenic substance. *Together,* the hapten and antigen stimulate the body to produce antibodies and sensitized lymphocytes against themselves — which results in their destruction. As a result, if the individual is exposed for a *second* time to *either* the antigen or hapten, an immune response will be elicited. Thus, at this point, the hapten is capable of acting as an antigen.[45]

Self-Tolerance

In order for the immune system to do its job efficiently, there must be a way to distinguish foreign agents from body constituents. The exact mechanism involved has eluded investigators for years and is still unclear. However, a refined hypothesis has emerged and warrants a brief description.

Several decades ago Burnet postulated that the problem of distinguishing between self and non-self could be explained by the "self-marker hypothesis."[16] That is, the body's own proteins have a particular molecular configuration that is marked "self." The cells of the immune system somehow learn to recognize this configuration as such, and produce antibodies only when the "self-marker" is not there. It is important to remember that the cells involved in the inflammatory response rid the body of its own dead cells (as well as foreign protein and bacteria), so it is essential that this process *not* elicit an immune response.[87]

In recent years, investigators have identified immunoglobulins (antibodies) present on the surface of lymphocytes.[66, 9] Although the mechanism is uncertain, one theory states that lymphocytes with immunoglobulins capable of reacting with self-components are eliminated early in life, leaving only those cells with immunoglobulins that recognize non-self determinants and react with substances that are *non-self*[90] (Fig. 11–1).

> *In sum, immunity depends upon the body's ability to recognize differences in the chemical structure of substances. As it comes to recognize what is "self" as compared to what is "non-self," the body develops* self-tolerance *or* immunologic tolerance.

The concept of self as distinguished from non-self contains important implications for the diagnosis and care of patients. For many years, *autoimmune disease* has been thought to be associated with a breakdown of the immune system's ability to recognize self, thus leading to the production of autoantibodies. While this is still considered to be true, some investigators suspect a cross-reacting mechanism in a few cases. That is, antibodies may be produced to an immunogen with a structure very similar to that of a red blood cell. The immune response directed toward that immunogen will react with the red cell structure as well, giving the appearance of development of autoimmunity to "self" red blood cells.

Recently the field of *tumor immunology* gained a new burst of interest when researchers observed that tumor cells had antigens on their surfaces and were thus recognized as non-self by the host immune system. Many tumor-associated antigens have been discovered, and this theory proposes that: (a) malignant cells are constantly arising in all individuals and (b) the immune system cells are continuously patrolling the host to seek out and destroy these malignant cells before they become clinically significant tumors.[28, 90] (See Unit IX.)

Another aspect of the concept of self and non-self arises in transplant surgery; it is the *successful recognition* by the body of foreign tissues as being different from self that results in transplant rejection. Thus, foreign tissues that are sutured to the body's tissues hold for a time only; they then are soon rejected by the body's immune system because they are non-self. It is indeed ironic that a homeostatic mechanism such as the immune reaction can ultimately work against medical efforts to treat our maladies and handicaps.

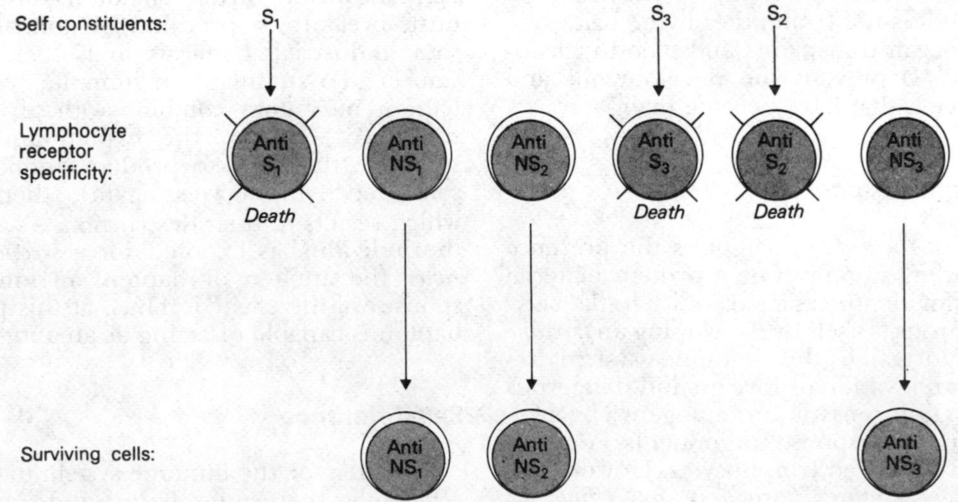

Figure 11–1. Induction of tolerance to self-constituents (S_1–S_3) by selective elimination of lymphocytes with self-reacting surface receptors. These cells are either killed or inactivated. Surviving cells are able to react only with non-self (NS) foreign antigens of specificity NS_1, NS_2, NS_3, etc. (From Roitt, I.: *Essential Immunology*, 3rd ed. Oxford: Blackwell Scientific Publications, 1977, p. 110.)

Traditionally, immunity has been classified as either natural or acquired. Acquired immunity is currently classified as humoral or cellular and as active or passive.

Natural (Innate) Immunity

The terms "natural" or "innate" immunity are commonly used to describe those aspects of our immune system which are the least clearly defined, e.g., the way in which different species or races respond to the same antigen and inheritance of "natural resistance" to illness. Perhaps it is most accurate to define natural immunity as *those immune responses that exist without apparent prior contact with an immunogen* (i.e., any substance that is capable of triggering an immune response).

There are many examples of natural immunity. For instance, one person may have a high natural resistance throughout life to colds and flu, whereas another person becomes ill with colds every winter. Natural immunity may also characterize a race or species. Indeed, the best example of natural immunity is *species immunity.* Because of species immunity, one species of animal will be highly resistant to an invading organism, whereas another species may be extremely vulnerable to that *same* organism. To illustrate, consider these examples: many bacteria have little effect on the human body, i.e., the human organism is highly resistant to them. Thus, humans are totally resistant to distemper, a disease that kills 25 to 75 per cent of all dogs that contract it. On the other hand, human beings are susceptible to certain diseases that other animals resist. For example, while humans have been plagued by gonorrhea and typhoid fever for centuries, these diseases are not found among other species. Also, while innumerable human beings have died from tuberculosis, the rat is highly resistant to this infection.

Substances that play important roles in natural immunity are the following: (1) immunoglobulins, which act to destroy bacteria; (2) lysozyme, which acts to dissolve bacteria; (3) basic polypeptides, which inactivate certain types of gram-positive bacteria; (4) white blood cells and reticuloendothelial cells, which phagocytose bacteria and other foreign agents; (5) gastric acid secretions and digestive enzymes, which destroy invading organisms; and (6) properdin, a serum protein of high molecular weight, which acts directly with gram-negative bacteria and kills them. In addition, the intact skin of uninjured humans acts as the first line of defense against bacterial invasion. However, remember that a person's natural resistance to infectious diseases and the ability to produce immune bodies can be greatly enhanced or reduced by such factors as diet, environment, body metabolism, state of mental health, and the virulence of the invading microorganism.[45]

Acquired or Adaptive Immunity

Acquired or adaptive immunity enables the body to protect itself against foreign organisms and protein substances for which it does not have natural immunity. The body does this by: (a) the production and release of *antibodies* that act to destroy the foreign antigen (*humoral immunity*) and (b) the production of *sensitized lymphocytes*, which attack and destroy the invading antigens (*cell-mediated immunity*). Thus, in acquired immunity, the individual is not born with an inherited resistance to a particular organism; instead she or he *develops* immunity against an organism. This is done by either: (a) *actively* producing his or her own antibodies and sensitized lymphocytes (*active immunity*) or (b) by *passively* receiving immune response components that have been manufactured within the bodies of other people or animals (*passive immunity*). Natural and acquired immunity are compared to each other in Figure 11–2.

Acquired Active and Passive Immunity. Acquired immunity may develop *naturally* with an individual's body or develop *artificially* as a result of vaccination (inoculation) or by injection of immune serum. When immunity develops artificially, it may be acquired either *passively* or *actively*.

1. Acquired Active Immunity. When active acquired immunity develops *naturally*, it results from a disease process within the body. This form of immunity is produced during the *initial* attack by the causative bacteria or viruses and is probably one reason that the sick individual recovers.

To acquire immunity naturally, the patient depends, then, upon an innate ability to develop immune bodies against particular viruses or bacteria. Thus, when the individual's body is invaded by a specific organism for the first time, serious effects may develop (which we recognize as "illness"). However, antibodies and sensitized lymphocytes are built up against the initial invasion of this organism. A "memory" of the antigens produced by the invading organism is passed on to successive generations of body cells. As a result, when the body is attacked a second time by the same antigen, effects will be very slight or possibly none will take place at all. Thus, the individual has *acquired* an immunity to an organism against which there is no natural immunity. This type of immunity, once developed, persists for years or even for life. For example, both smallpox and measles confer lifelong immunity upon their victims. However, as every cold sufferer knows, colds and many types of flu confer no immunity at all.

In some unfortunate cases, individuals can develop an acquired immunity against a particular organism, even though they still harbor the organism within their bodies. This organism, then, while harmless to its carrier, can be transmitted to other individuals and can infect them. The classic example of this situation is the *typhoid carrier*. In the case of a typhoid carrier, antibodies against typhoid are present in the blood, although typhoid bacilli continue to live in the gallbladder and intestinal tract. Thus, these individuals, while protected by their own antibodies, remain highly infective to other susceptible individuals.

Active acquired immunity is conferred *artificially* by means of vaccination or inoculation. In the late 1700's, physicians unknowingly discovered the important principle of inducing immunity by inoculating humans with a dose of *low virulence* pathogen, which established a lifelong immunity to the *fully virulent* infectious agent. An English physician, Edward Jenner, injected cowpox into human volunteers, who then became immune to smallpox.

Immunity acquired by vaccination is established by the production of (a) sufficient levels of antibody and (b) a primed population of sensitized lymphocytes (T-cells) that can rapidly proliferate upon *second* exposure to the immunogen. The initial reaction is slow; it takes about 7 days for antibodies to appear in the blood. Peak antibody concentrations occur 10 to 14 days following immunization and then begin to drop. A booster injection, following the primary response, will cause a more rapid secondary response with longer immunity. It is important that the first exposure to the immunogen not be harmful; thus, the pathogens used for immunization are usually altered by methods that reduce their virulence but retain their immunogenicity. Preparations include the following:[3, 39]

1. *Killed organisms.* Typhoid, cholera, and the injected poliomyelitis (Salk) vaccines are examples of bacteria and viruses that are *killed* prior to immuniza-

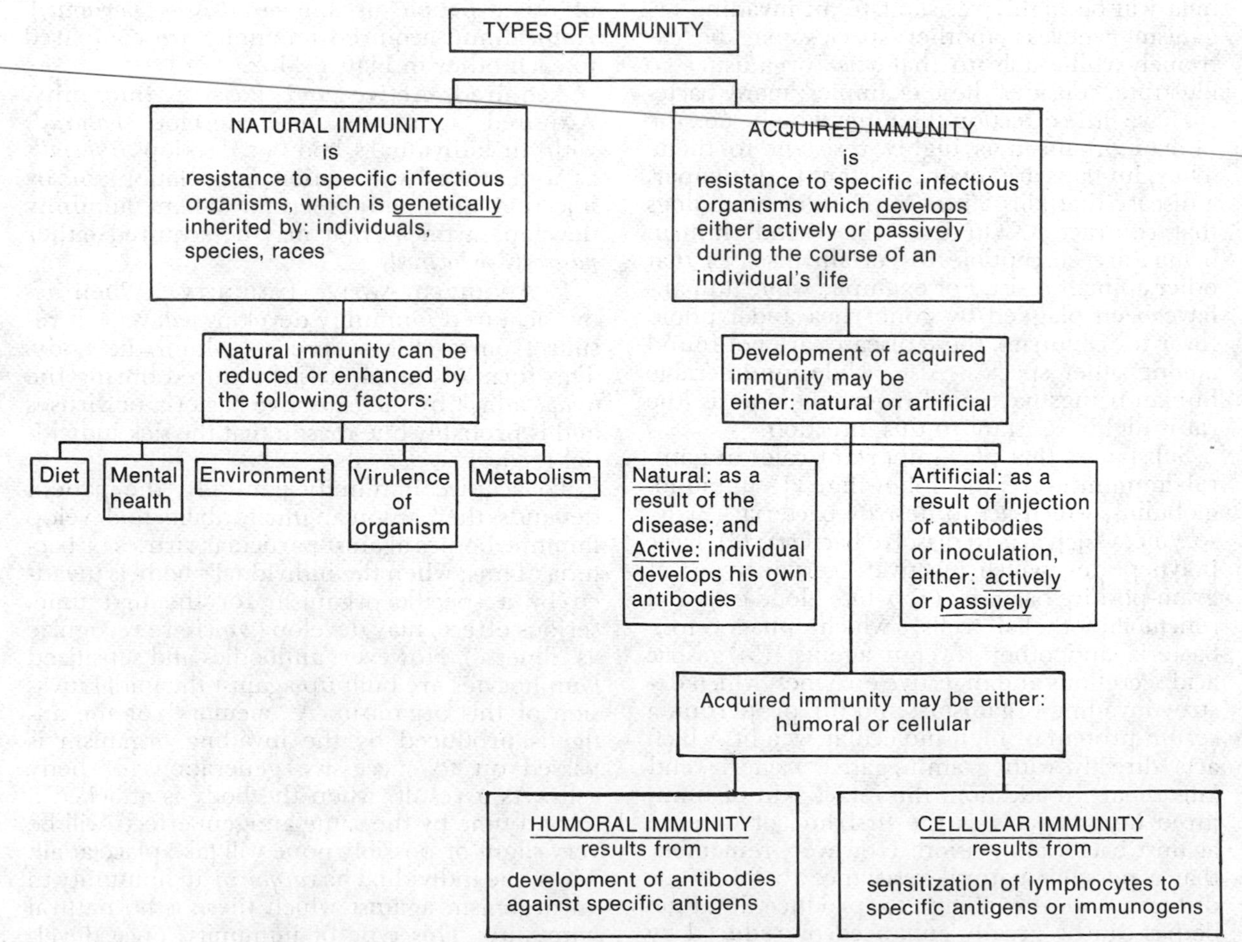

Figure 11–2. A comparison between natural and acquired immunity.

TABLE 11–1. VACCINES GIVEN ROUTINELY AND IN SPECIAL RISK SITUATIONS

Vaccines Given Routinely	Vaccines Given in Special Risk Situations*
Trivalent Oral Polio Vaccine (TOPV)	Cholera
Measles-Mumps-Rubella combination vaccine (MMR)	Influenza
Diphtheria-Pertussis-Tetanus combination vaccine (DPT)	Meningococcal
Adult Diphtheria-Tetanus (Td) booster	*Hemophilus influenzae* type B
	Plague
	Pneumococcus
	Rabies
	Rocky Mountain Spotted Fever
	Smallpox
	Typhus
	Yellow Fever

*Special risk situations and persons include: foreign travel to areas where the infective agent is endemic or where sanitation is poor; prior to possible epidemics (e.g., flu epidemics); within the armed forces (e.g., meningococcal vaccine); very young, aged, or chronically ill persons and persons who may be exposed to an organism in their work (e.g., preexposure rabies immunization may be given to veterinarians or zoo employees).

tion. The immunity conferred by killed organisms is generally inferior to that resulting from infection with living organisms. This may partly be the result of the relatively rapid growth rate of living organisms in the body.

2. *Live, attenuated organisms.* Oral poliomyelitis (Sabin), measles, rubella, and *Mycobacterium tuberculosis* are examples of attenuated vaccines. Attenuation is accomplished by repeated passage of the strains in embryonated eggs, tissue culture, or animals until the organism is rendered nonvirulent. Genetic recombination is a technique being used recently to generate attenuated strains of influenza virus.[79, 98] This method utilizes the parenteral administration of a recombinant virus with the appropriate antigenic properties, but which lacks some virulent characteristics. The partial immunity provided still permits natural infection but prevents the development of disease.

3. *Toxoids.* Bacterial exotoxins such as diphtheria and tetanus bacilli can be detoxified by formaldehyde treatment without destroying their immunogenicity. The immune response to the toxoid generates antibodies that can neutralize the virulent toxins and encourage phagocytosis.

Table 11–1 lists vaccines routinely administered and those recommended in special circumstances. Table 11–2 presents an immunization schedule for infants and children, and Table 11–3 states guidelines for use of common immunizing materials.

Immunization programs have nearly eliminated diseases such as diphtheria, smallpox, and poliomyelitis from communities, but people should still be aware of potential risks involved in being immunized.[39] Generally, the risks of complications should be weighed against the chances of acquiring the disease. For example, encephalitis is a rare but serious occurrence following rabies or smallpox vaccinations. Also, before administering immunizations, it is important to screen patients for immunodeficiency disorders. A child with an impaired cell-mediated response who receives a tuberculin injection may become overwhelmed by infection and die. Also genetic recombination as a means of attenuation of viruses poses many ethical questions, with risks of inaccurate viral nucleic acid incorporation into the host's genes.

Currently, experimental programs in active immunotherapy for the treatment of cancer are being developed. Patients are given vaccines prepared from their own tumors, the tumors of donors, or from live attenuated tumor cells.[28] Active immunotherapy is considered in Chapter 23.

2. Acquired Passive Immunity. In contrast to active immunity, passive immunity is a type of acquired immunity in which the individual receives or is given antibodies that have been manufactured in the bodies of other individuals or animals. Thus, the body cells of the individual who passively accepts immunity will not undergo the changes that take place in the production of active immunity. For example, an unborn child may receive antibodies from the mother through the placental circulation. Or individuals may receive injections of serum containing antibodies that have been actively developed in the bodies of other people or in animals. Like active immunotherapy, passive immunotherapy is being used on an experimental basis for the treatment of cancer patients. Patients are given antitumor antibodies or sensitized lymphocytes from a donor, who is usually a person who is

TABLE 11–2. IMMUNIZATION SCHEDULE

Age	Vaccines
2 months	Diphtheria-Pertussis-Tetanus (DPT) and Trivalent Oral Polio Vaccine (TOPV)
4 months	DPT and TOPV
6 months	DPT and TOPV (TOPV optional)
12 months	Tuberculin Skin Test
15 months	Measles-Mumps-Rubella (MMR)
18 months	DPT and TOPV
4–6 years	Tuberculin skin test at some time or followed by DPT and TOPV booster doses
14–16 years	Adult Diphtheria-Tetanus (Td) booster

From Bader, M.: Infection control: Immunization. *Topics in Clinical Nursing,* 1:7, July 1979.

TABLE 11–3. GUIDELINES FOR USE OF COMMON IMMUNIZING MATERIALS

Diphtheria toxoid
Do not give full doses of adult formulation to anyone >6 years of age. Instead, use pediatric formulation containing one fourth to one fifteenth as much toxoid

Measles vaccine, live, attenuated
Do not administer vaccine to individuals who are immunodeficient (owing to congenital defect, immunosuppressive therapy, lymphatic malignant disease, or other disorder limiting immune responsiveness). Caution is urged in administration of vaccine to individuals who have received killed measles virus vaccine in the past. Serious reactions (local or, occasionally, systemic) may ensue. A method that I have used is to administer 0.1 ml of live measles virus vaccine intradermally to such individuals. Antibody responses have regularly occurred, with very low reaction rates. Whether administration of vaccine in this manner will provide lifelong protection is not known. (Killed measles virus vaccine was used extensively in Canada from 1963 until just a few years ago and was used in the United States from 1963 to 1965. It was usually administered in three doses at monthly intervals or in two monthly doses followed in one month by administration of live vaccine)

Mumps vaccine
The general precautions in the use of live vaccines should be observed

Pertussis vaccine
The World Health Organization's suggestion that a family history of convulsions is a contraindication to pertussis immunization is not accepted in the United States. However, any individual with a personal history of convulsive disorder or with progressive neurologic disease should not receive the vaccine. If any of the following reactions to pertussis vaccine has occurred previously, do not give more of the vaccine: (1) marked febrile response (105 F or greater), especially if associated with excessive lethargy, irritability, or screaming, (2) any central nervous system symptom or sign (altered consciousness and convulsions are most frequent), (3) screaming fits (occurring occasionally in infants and marked by screaming continuing for hours after immunization), which may reflect cerebral irritability, (4) thrombocytopenia, and (5) shock. If a lesser reaction has occurred (fever, local pain, induration, irritability, fretfulness, excessive lethargy short of stupor or coma), the amount of pertussis vaccine may be reduced by half and the vaccine given separately from full doses of diphtheria and tetanus toxoids

Poliovirus vaccine, trivalent
Do not give vaccine to individuals known to have immunodeficiency (antibody, cell-mediated, or combined). Except in epidemics, avoidance of administration of vaccine to pregnant women is advisable

Rubella vaccine, live
Apart from general contraindications, live rubella virus vaccine should not be administered to females who are pregnant or are likely to become pregnant soon.[1] Before administering vaccine to a female of childbearing age, the physician should (1) determine rubella antibody titer when feasible and practical (ideally, only susceptible [seronegative] females beyond puberty should receive the vaccine), (2) insist on pregnancy test if history is doubtful, (3) obtain assurance that effective contraception will be practiced for at least two and preferably for three months after immunization, and (4) carefully explain the high rate of arthralgia as a side effect (as high as 40% in some series)

Tetanus toxoid
Individuals who have received many doses of tetanus toxoid may have severe local Arthus reactions to this material. Follow guidelines to routine use in wound management.[2] Avoid excessive use

From Fulginiti, V. A.: Immunization practice: Some important guidelines. *Postgraduate Medicine,* 60:62, Oct. 1976, p. 66.

[1]*Report of the Committee on Infectious Diseases.* American Academy of Pediatrics. Evanston, Ill., 1974.

[2]Modlin, J. F., Brandling-Bennett, A. D., Witte, J. J., et al.: A review of five years' experience with rubella vaccine in the United States. *Pediatrics, 55*:20–29, 1975.

cured of cancer or in remission. (See Chapter 23.)

The major advantage of passive immunity is that it is *immediate* in its reaction, rescuing the patient almost at once from the adverse effects of an invading antigen. Even though the patient's body has not had time to form antibodies, the patient is protected from the attacking antigen. The major disadvantage of passive immunity is that it is *temporary,* usually lasting for only a few weeks or months. How long passive immunity will last depends upon the source of the antibody, and also upon how well the antibody-producing mechanism of the individual works. Antibodies transmitted from a mother to her child in utero seem to last the longest of any type of passive immunity. Antibodies acquired in this fashion may circulate in the newborn child's blood for as long as 6 months. The fact that a newborn child receives antibodies from the mother is advantageous, because newborn children are unable to efficiently synthesize antibodies. Passive immunity that has been received from another adult tends to last from a few weeks to a few months. Immunoglobulins are destroyed most rapidly when passive immunity has been transferred from an animal source to an adult; this type of immunity lasts from 10 days to 2 weeks.

In addition to the temporary nature of passive immunity, a second disadvantage is that an injection of immune serum can cause the patient to develop an allergic reaction called *serum sickness.* The symptoms of serum sickness and its treatment will be discussed later in this chapter. Active and passive immunity are compared to each other in Figure 11–3.

Acquired Humoral and Cellular Immunity. In the past, those who studied immunology were sharply divided into schools of thought: one school was the humoral school of immunity, and the other was the cellular school. Advocates of the humoral school believed that immunity resulted from antibodies present in the body's *serum* rather than in the body's cells. Advocates of the cellular school stressed the notion that immunity relied solely upon *cells,* such as the small lymphocyte, for its transmission. Today these two schools of thought have merged. Modern immunologists now believe that *both* cells and factors in the serum must be present and normal if the immune process is to function successfully. Thus, both humoral and cellular immunity are important components in the body's complex system of defense. Indeed, humoral and cellular immunity are such vital components of the immune response that in the next section we consider them in detail: their origins, development, and specific functions.

THE IMMUNE RESPONSE AND ITS COMPONENTS

The Development of Humoral and Cellular Immunity.[28, 45, 72, 80, 87, 115] The capacity to respond to immunologic stimuli (i.e., antigens) rests principally in cells of the lymphatic tissue. During embryonic life, a *stem cell* develops in the fetal liver and other organs. This stem cell resides in the bone marrow in postnatal life. These stem cells may differentiate into cells of the red cell series, granulocyte series, or lymphocyte series. The bone marrow sheds cells into the circulation, from which they migrate to the lymphatic tissue (i.e., spleen, lymph nodes, thymus, appendix, tonsils).

The *thymus* serves as the site for proliferation and maturation of *T-lymphocytes* (thymus-dependent cells), which make up 60 to 70 per cent of circulating lymphocytes. When receptors on the T-lymphocytes are exposed to antigen, they are transformed into *sensitized* lymphocytes, which perform specific functions and release chemical factors to provide *cellular immunity*. Examples of cellular immunity include transplant rejection, tuberculin injection reactions, and contact allergy reactions. Moreover, T-cells are primarily involved with the development of immunity to tumor cells, viruses, and mycobacterial pathogens.

The bursa of Fabricius in birds is the site for maturation of *B-lymphocytes* (bursal-equivalent or thymus-independent cells), but no equivalent organ is known to exist in humans. Rather, development of B-cells seems to be associated with various organ systems: particularly the gut and bronchial-associated lymphoid tissues (e.g., tonsils, Peyer's patches, appendix, peritoneal cavi-

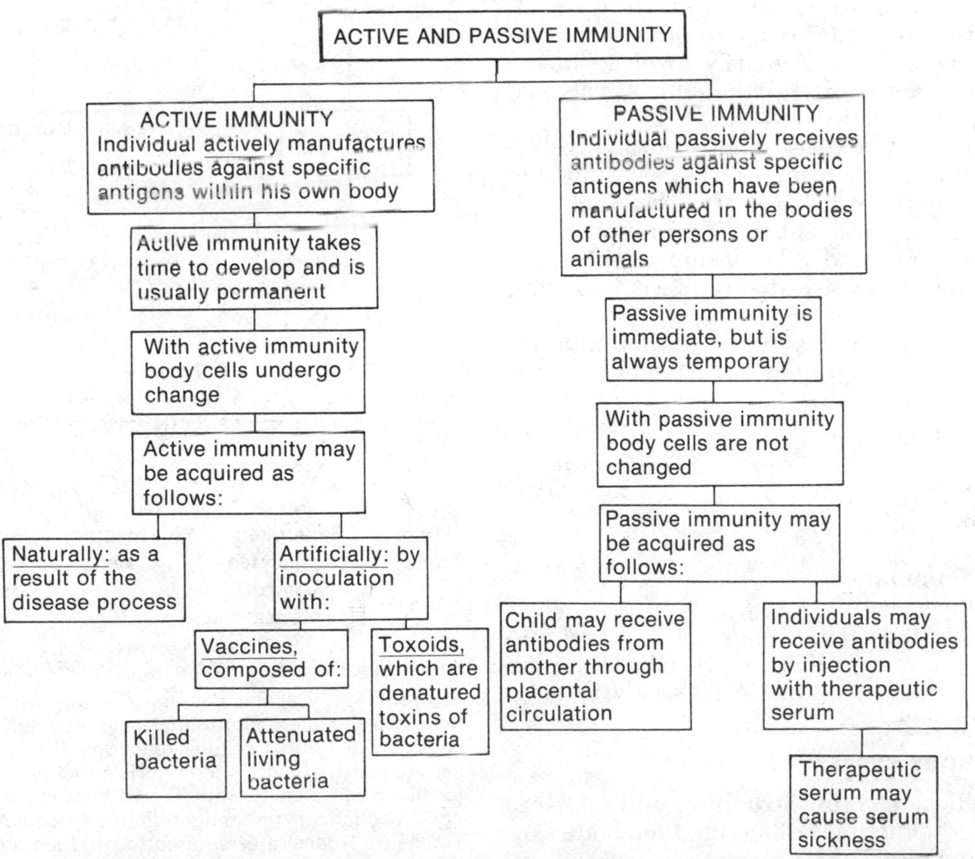

Figure 11–3. A comparison of active and passive immunity.

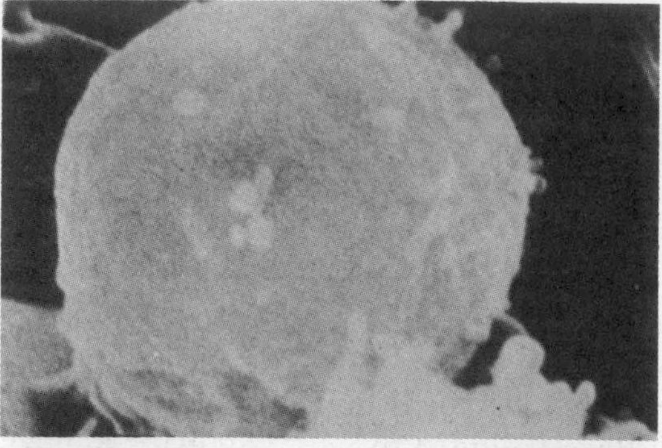

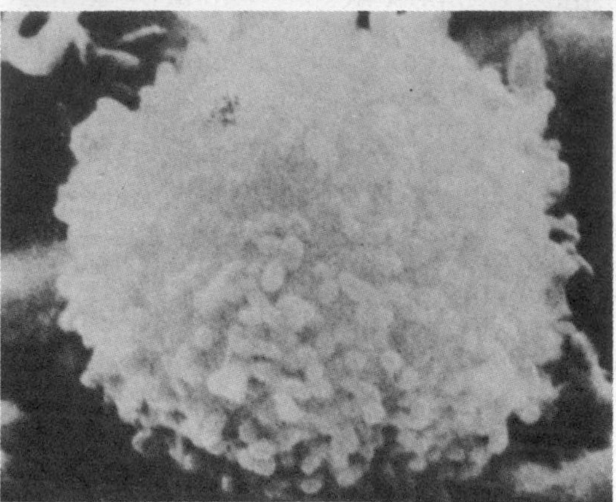

Figure 11–4. T-cell and B-cell. (From Nysather, J. O., et al.: The immune system: Its development and functions. *American Journal of Nursing,* 76:1615, Oct. 1976.)

ty). In response to contact with antigen, B-lymphocytes form *antibodies* and provide *humoral immunity*. B-cells are primarily involved in the destruction of bacterial pathogens. T-cells and B-cells are depicted in Figure 11–4.

In sum, immunologic responsiveness involves two effector mechanisms: humoral antibodies derived from the B-lymphocyte system and cell-mediated mechanisms of the T-lymphocyte system. The origin and relationship of these two immune responses are diagrammed in Figure 11–5.

The following discussion of the immune response and its components is divided into three main parts:

- ▶ Humoral immunity
- ▶ Cellular immunity
- ▶ Mediators of the immune response

Humoral Immunity

Recall that the establishment of humoral immunity is the responsibility of B-cells. Humoral immunity is based upon the antibody system, described below.

THE ANTIBODY SYSTEM

Antibodies: Origin, Structure, and Classes. Antibodies, sometimes called immune bodies or immunoglobulins, are protective substances composed of protein that can be detected in the serum. Antibodies are formed by plasma cells that arise when antigen-specific groups, or clones, of B-cells come in contact with an antigen.

Antibody molecules are *immunoglobulins,* which constitute a part of the body's serum proteins known as gamma globulins. Antibodies are made by the body in response to invading antigens. It is the interaction of antibodies with antigen that renders the invaders helpless. There are five classes of immunoglobulins, which are classified according to their different antibody properties: namely, IgG, IgM, IgA, IgD, and IgE. These are summarized in Table 11–4.

Note in Table 11–4 that *IgG* is the major immunoglobulin and constitutes 80 per cent of the immunoglobulins in the serum. Also IgG is the principal antibody of the *secondary* humoral immune response (discussed below) and the only immunoglobulin that can cross the placental barrier to confer passive immunity to the newborn infant. The structure of a typical immunoglobulin molecule is depicted in Figure 11–6.

IgM is the mainstay of the *primary* immune response. It also forms the antibodies to ABO blood group antigens. *IgA* is present in the serum

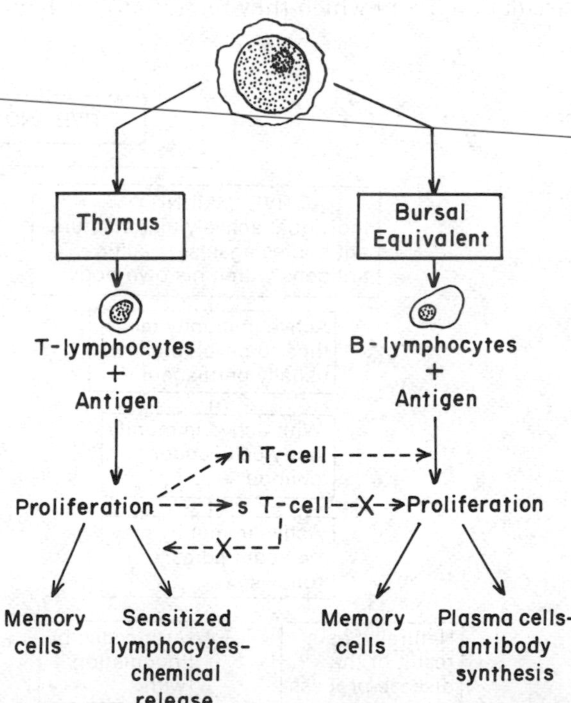

Figure 11–5. Cellular immune response: development, response and interaction with B-cells. Thymus-dependent cells (T-cells) effect cellular reactions. Bursal-equivalent cells (B-cells) are involved in the production of antibodies for humoral defense. Both T- and B-cells have a "memory" mechanism for antigen-antibody contacts. Helper T-cells (h T-cells) are required to produce antibodies to a few antigens. Suppressor T-cells (s T-cells) act to inhibit antibody production and also cellular production.

TABLE 11–4. PROPERTIES OF MAJOR HUMAN IMMUNOGLOBULIN CLASSES

Class	% Total Immunoglobulin	Major Characteristics	Complement* Fixation	Cross Placenta	Fix to Mast Cells†
IgG	80%	Most abundant Ig of extracellular fluid and intravascular fluid. Produced late in immune responses.	++	+	−
IgM	6%	Produced early in immune responses. Mainly intravascular.	++++	−	−
IgA	13%	Most abundant Ig in body secretions.	−	−	−
IgD	1%	Present on lymphocyte surface.	−	−	−
IgE	0.002%	Responsible for symptoms of atopic allergies.	−	−	+

*Complement fixation discussed on p. 146.
†Mast cells discussed on p. 146.

in small amounts but is the predominant immunoglobulin in body secretions (tears, saliva, colostrum, intestinal and bronchial secretions). Its presence offers protection to the mucous membrane surfaces of the GI and respiratory tracts. The breast-fed infant receives IgA, which serves to control pathogenic bacteria in the intestinal tract. *IgD* occurs in minute amounts, and its exact function is not known. However, it has been found on the surface of some lymphocytes.[91] *IgE,* or *reaginic antibody,* is normally present in trace amounts in serum, detectable only by very sensitive methods. With an affinity for *mast cells* (connective tissue cells), it lives primarily in the tissues and is important in allergic, atopic, and anaphylactic reactions to be discussed later.

Immunogenicity (i.e., ability to evoke an immune response) is *not* an inherent property of the immunoglobulin molecule, but depends on the antigen, the mode of entry into the host, and the host itself. More specifically, this includes the size and complexity of the antigen, the ability of the host's immune response to distinguish self from non-self, and the genetic characteristics of the host.

Antibody Function and Specificity. The major *function* of antibodies is to defend the body from foreign antigenic substances. By destroying invading microorganisms, antibodies also protect the body against the effects of these noxious toxins released by antigens.

The most striking feature of antibodies is their great *selectivity in antigen-antibody reactions;* the ability to combine most strongly with certain structures, less strongly with even closely related structures, and poorly with more distantly related structures. This selectivity of reaction is called *specificity,* because the antibodies can *distinguish* between antigenic structures. Note in Figure 11–6 that the antigen binds at two different sites on the variable portions of the chains forming the antibody. The variable portions of each specific antibody molecule are composed of an amino acid sequence that is *specific* to a particular antigen and which thus enables the antibody to attach to that specific antigen. Guyton explains the process this way:

> Each antibody that is specific for a particular antigen has a different organization of amino acid residues in the variable portions of both the light and heavy chains. These have a specific steric shape for each antigen specificity so that when an antigen comes in contact with it, the prosthetic radicals of the antigen fit as a mirror image with those of the antibody, thus allowing a rapid and tight chemical bond between the antibody and the antigen.[45]

This specificity of antibody for antigen or im-

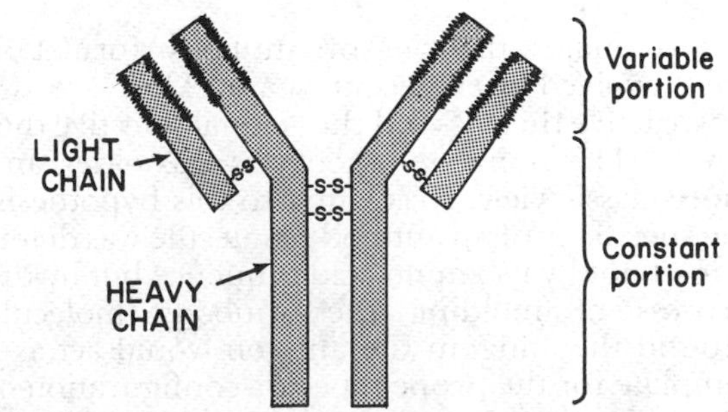

Figure 11–6. Structure of the typical immunoglobulin molecule, showing it to be composed of two heavy polypeptide chains and two light polypeptide chains. The antigen binds at two different sites on the variable portions of the chains. The constant portion of the antibody is responsible for the antibody's gross physical and chemical characteristics, its mobility, and so forth. (From Guyton, A. C.: *Textbook of Medical Physiology,* 5th ed. Philadelphia: W. B. Saunders Co., 1976, p. 82.)

munogen is accomplished by means of the reactions described below.

Antigen-Antibody Reactions. Some of the most important types of antigen-antibody reactions are:

- *Agglutination:* Antibodies disarm bacteria and then render them harmless by causing them to clump together.
- *Precipitation:* Antibodies react with soluble antigens, resulting in a visible lattice formation, i.e., antigens and antibodies cluster together in a viable mass.
- *Opsonization:* Antibodies coat bacteria and increase their susceptibility to phagocytosis (ingestion by certain white blood cells).
- *Lysis:* Antibodies cause invading bacteria to dissolve or liquefy. After interaction of bacteria or red blood cells with antibody, these cells or bacteria may be destroyed through the action of *complement,* another group of serum proteins. Complement exerts its effects primarily on cell membranes after being bound to the cell by antibody. A functional "hole" is punched in the membrane, causing loss of osmotic integrity and eventual cell death. (See p. 146 for further discussion.)
- *Neutralization:* Antibodies combine with the toxins released by some infectious agents, neutralizing their effects. Reticuloendothelial cells then phagocytize the complex and remove it from the blood or tissues.

Current Theories of Antibody Formation. How antibodies are actually formed within the body is a question to which no definitive answer as yet exists. It is clear that immunologically competent cells (i.e., B-cells and sensitized T-cells) underlie immune reactions, whether they are humoral or cellular in nature.*

Two major theories of antibody formation have evolved over recent years. They are the "instructive theory" and the "clonal selective theory."[16] The *instructive* theory is the older and more classic view. According to this hypothesis, the specificity of an antibody molecule was determined not by its amino acid sequence but by the process of molding the antibody molecule around the antigen; the antigen would act as a template for the proper specific configuration of the antibody. However, this theory lost favor when it became apparent that the antibody specificity was a function of amino acid sequence dictated by DNA.

At present, the *clonal selection* theory is widely accepted. It holds that an immunologically responsive cell (i.e., a T-cell or B-cell) can respond to only *one* antigen or a closely related group of antigens and that this property is inherent in the cell *before* the antigen is encountered. Accordingly, each individual is endowed with a very large pool of lymphocytes, each of which is capable of responding to a different antigen. When the antigen enters the body, it is picked up by a macrophage and either directly or indirectly presented to the lymphocyte that has the best "fit" for that antigen by virtue of a surface receptor. The antigen binds to this antibody-like receptor, and the cell is stimulated to proliferate and form a clone of cells. Thus, selected B-cells quickly differentiate into plasma cells and secrete antibody specific for the immunogen that served as the original stimulant.

The initial step in antibody formation is the *phagocytosis of antigen by macrophages.* These cells do not form antibody, but they present antigen in some form (perhaps sticking to their surface) to B-cells. Stimulated B-cells differentiate into plasma cells, and immunoglobulin synthesis commences. Some stimulated B-cells become *memory cells,* which are long-lived lymphocytes that circulate and can rapidly differentiate into specific plasma cells upon *re-exposure* to the same immunogen. (See discussion below.)

PRIMARY AND SECONDARY HUMORAL IMMUNE RESPONSES

When an animal or person contacts or is injected with an antigen for the *first* time, there is a rise in detectable antibody in the serum within several days, depending on the route of injection and the dose and nature of the antigen. The antibody concentration peaks within 1 to 10 weeks, then drops, and may fall below detectable levels. When an animal contacts or is *re-injected* with the same antigen weeks, months, or even years after the primary antibody levels have subsided, there is a *more rapid* antibody response to a *higher level* and for a *longer interval* than in the primary response. This is presumably based on persistence of a substantial number of antigen-sensitive *memory cells* from initial contact with the antigen. The memory for secondary antibody responses resides in B-cells and for certain antigens in both B- and T-cells. The mechanism for memory production in B-cells remains obscure. Possibly the clone of B-cells that produces a specific antibody greatly expands upon first exposure to an antigen; consequently, the antibody is produced more quickly and in greater amounts upon second exposure to the antigen and thus lifelong memory against that antigen is produced (Fig. 11–7).

*Immunologically competent cells are defined as specialized cellular elements that, owing to their particular morphology and physiology, are concerned with immune functions. The formation of antibodies against specific antigens is but one of their many roles. While ICC are not always actively engaged in a direct response to an antigen, they are fully competent to do so should the need arise.

During the evolution of the antibody response to a new antigen, IgM-producing cells and *IgM* antibodies are preferentially represented early in the response. It is only later that *IgG* synthesis increases markedly and IgM antibody levels decrease. There is still controversy on whether this switch from IgM to IgG synthesis occurs in individual antibody-producing cells, in members of a single clone of antigen-stimulated sensitized cells, or in separate populations of B-cells committed to either IgM or IgG production.[38, 41, 90]

Cellular Immunity

Although antibodies arise in response to immunogens, they often play only a minor role in the defense of the organism against invading cells. The central position in such defenses is occupied by *cell-mediated immune responses.* T-cells, as you recall, are small lymphocytes shed from the thymus that circulate until they recognize a foreign substance. The T-cells then undergo transformation to a blast state and are capable of division and production of cellular components. T-cells do not secrete appreciable amounts of antibody. Instead, the sensitized cells fight immunogens by evolving into the following: "killer" T-cells, "memory" T-cells, "helper" T-cells, and "suppressor" T-cells.

- ▶ *Killer T-cells* vanquish immunogens by releasing antigen-specific cytotoxic agents.
- ▶ *Memory T-cells* are formed in the same manner in which "memory" cells develop in the humoral system. Upon exposure to a specific antigen and activation of T-cells, a large number of T-cells belonging to that clone of cells remains in the lymphoid tissue. In this way the number of that type of T-cell is enhanced. When the body is again invaded by the same antigen, T-cells sensitized to that antigen are released in far greater numbers and much more rapidly than in the first encounter with the antigen.[45]
- ▶ *Helper T-cells* "instruct" certain B-cells to respond to antigens. Apparently, some immunogenic antigens are not capable of switching on B-cells. However, in the presence of helper T-cells, these antigens can elicit an antibody response. (See Figure 11–5.)
- ▶ *Suppressor T-cells* act as inhibitors of antibody response and cell-mediated responses. The mechanism by which suppressor T-cells operate is unclear.

In addition to differentiating into these cell forms, sensitized lymphocytes also produce and release chemical substances *(lymphokines)* that help promote nonspecific destruction of immunogens. Lymphokines are mediators of the immune response and are considered below.

Sensitized lymphocytes may continue to survive in the tissues for as long as 10 years, whereas hormonal antibodies may circulate for only a few months and rarely a few years. Thus cellular immunity is more persistent than is humoral immunity.[38, 41, 87, 90]

Mediators of the Immune Response

The following substances act as mediators in the immune response. They are components of *both* humoral and cellular immunity, and they participate in the actual mechanism of cell or tissue destruction in response to foreign invasion. These mediators include: complement, mediators of allergic reactions, lymphokines, and cells of the reticuloendothelial system.

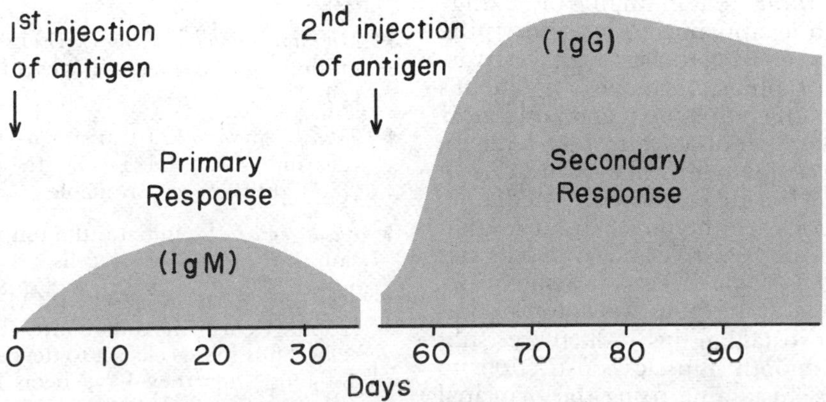

Figure 11–7. Primary and secondary antibody response. The second exposure of an antigen to the host causes a more rapid, stronger, and longer acting response than the first exposure, owing to the presence of "memory cells." IgM is most often produced in the primary response, whereas IgG is more likely to be produced predominantly in the secondary response.

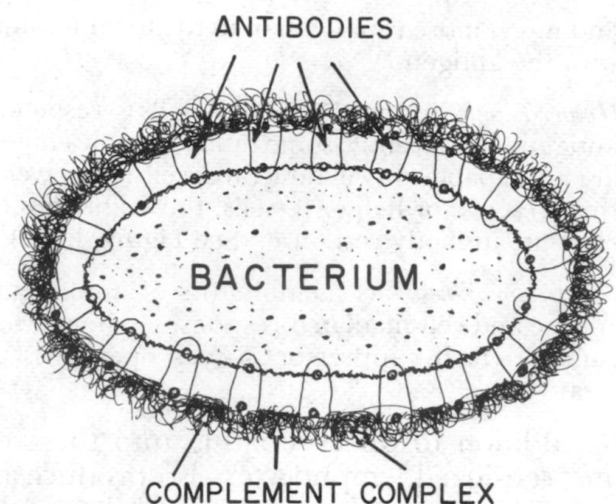

Figure 11–8. Activation of the complement complex. (From Guyton, A. C.: *Textbook of Medical Physiology,* 5th ed. Philadelphia: W. B. Saunders Co., 1976, p. 83.)

Complement. Complement refers to a group of serum proteins of which there are currently 15 known components. These proteins are present in serum in an inactive state until activated or "fixed" by an antibody molecule in an antigen-antibody complex (Fig. 11–8). Complement can also be activated by some lipopolysaccharide structures (e.g., bacterial cell walls). Once complement fixation or activation takes place, the antigen, antibody, and complement become bound together, and the antigen is destroyed. Indeed, complement is thought to be responsible for the actual destruction of antigen, with subsequent formation of potent biologic products that contribute to inflammation. Specific actions of complement are: destruction of cell membranes, promotion of phagocytosis, fixation of antigen-antibody substances, attraction of white cells to the reaction site, and increased capillary permeability.

The role of complement in uniting or "fixing" an antibody with its appropriate antibody is the basis for *complement-fixation* tests; e.g., the Wassermann test for syphilis. A sample of a patient's blood is mixed with complement and antigen. If the serum contains antibodies to that antigen, fixation of the complement will take place.

Mediators of Allergic Reactions. Mediators of allergic reactions are chemical substances that are present in the body or released from cells and that have pharmacologic effects on tissues. Specifically, they include histamine, serotonin, bradykinin, and prostaglandins. All these substances cause smooth muscle constriction to varying degrees, histamine being the principal effector in allergic responses. Bradykinin and prostaglandins are slower to respond and are involved in secondary reactions. *Bradykinin,* although not involved in the immediate allergic reaction, causes slow smooth muscle contraction and stimulates pain fibers. *Prostaglandins* are naturally occurring substances that may participate in asthmatic conditions, but also act against the kinins to alter the pain threshold.[40, 58] *Serotonin* is a vasoconstrictor found in the blood, nervous system, and other tissues. It acts as a smooth muscle stimulator and a neurotransmitter. All of these substances increase capillary permeability and capillary dilatation, with histamine causing edema and erythematosis (redness of the skin caused by capillary dilatation in the lower layers of skin) during anaphylactic reactions.

The granules of *mast cells* and *basophils* serve as the major storage sites for histamine and serotonin, the primary mediators of the allergic reaction. The mechanism by which the mast cell forms and releases the mediators is important for understanding the pharmacologic treatment of allergic reactions. When an antibody-antigen reaction takes place, the mast cell receives a signal to alter its metabolic status and "degranulate," thus releasing histamine and serotonin. The cell's metabolism and, consequently, *degranulation* is controlled by 3′,5′-adenosine monophosphate (cAMP). A *fall* in cAMP enhances chemical release, whereas a *rise* in cAMP reduces it. An enzyme called phosphodiesterase normally acts to inhibit cAMP. Treatment of hypersensitivity reactions, then, can be controlled by hormones or drugs that affect not only the chemicals and enzymes released but also those that affect the levels of cAMP in the mast cell.[18, 58] These effects are summarized in Figure 11–9 and will be discussed in more detail later in the chapter.

Lymphokines. Lymphokines are soluble mediators released by sensitized lymphocytes (T-cells) that are capable of recruiting host inflammatory cells, activating them and keeping them at the reaction site. Lymphokines include the following factors:[38, 80]

- *Chemotactic factor* causes macrophages and sensitized T-cells to migrate to the area of the antigen.
- *Migratory inhibition factor* (MIF) inhibits further migration of the macrophages and sensitized T-cells.
- *Transfer factor* (TF) transforms nonsensitized T-cells into sensitized T-cells, thereby augmenting "the fighting force" available.
- *Blastogenic factor* initiates the mitosis or rapid division of the sensitized T-cells.
- *Macrophage activation factor* (MAF) transforms macrophages near the antigen into highly phagocytic cells. Thus these cells act to devour the remains of antigens after they have been killed by the T-cells.

The Reticuloendothelial System. The reticuloendothelial system refers to the phagocytic system of macrophages and polymorphonuclear cells in the spleen, liver, and lymphoid tissues. (See Chapter 10.)

The principal cellular components are the macrophages and polymorphonuclear cells, which help mediate cellular immunity. In an immune response, the macrophage is often the first cell to respond to the foreign material. It may phagocytize or somehow present the antigen to a circulating lymphocyte, which then may respond, be it via a humoral or cellular mechanism. Some microorganisms, such as tubercle and leprosy bacilli, are capable of reproducing even after phagocytosis. The cellular mediated immune system is then needed to kill the intracellular organism.

PATHOLOGIC CONDITIONS ASSOCIATED WITH THE IMMUNE RESPONSE

Normally the immune response is a homeostatic measure that protects the body from invasion by foreign, antigenic substances. However, the immune response can become pathologic when immune responses are either deficient, excessive, inappropriate, or abnormal.

In light of the immunologic components and systems thus far discussed, we can now examine some of the immunologic diseases that result when the immune system is deficient or malfunctions. While we cannot, in this chapter, begin to cover the wide spectrum of possible immune disorders, we do present diseases of the immune system that are representative of those you are likely to encounter. Specifically, we discuss the following:

1. Immunodeficiency disorders
2. The gammopathies
3. Disorders associated with hypersensitivity reactions
4. Autoimmune disorders

1. Immunodeficiency Disorders

These disorders can be *inherited* or *acquired* and may involve the *humoral* components (B-cells, plasma cells, immunoglobulins), the *cellular* components (T-cells), or both. Also, these diseases may be *primary* or they may be *secondary* to

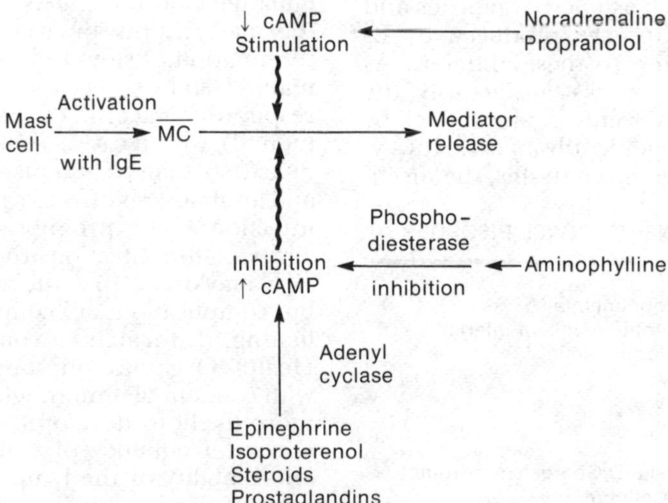

Figure 11-9. Factors concerned with the degranulation of mast cells. Mast cell mediator release is enhanced by a decrease in cAMP, and inhibited by an increase in cAMP. Phosphodiesterase is an enzyme that normally inhibits cAMP. Aminophylline is a drug used to inhibit this enzyme, thereby allowing a rise in cAMP. Epinephrine, on the other hand, is a drug that indirectly acts to stabilize the adenyl cyclase–cAMP system, allowing an increase in cAMP.

malnutrition, infection, cancer, renal diseases, Hodgkin's disease, and the administration of immunosuppressive drugs (e.g., cortisone). Furthermore, *stress* can suppress the immune response by promoting the release of plasma cortisol, which acts to destroy lymphocytes; *cigarette smoking* and *alcohol* also destroy lymphocytes — thereby weakening the immune response.[28]

Age also plays a role in the development of immunologic deficiencies. At birth the infant is partially protected by a supply of IgG from the maternal circulation; adult levels of IgG and IgM are not reached until about 12 months of age and the immunoglobulin system is not fully developed until about age 16 months.[26] Furthermore, with advancing age, humoral immunity markedly declines. Exactly why this decline takes place in aging persons is unknown and is an area of important current research.

Although primary immunodeficiency states are relatively rare, they may have a devastating effect upon the patient and can end in a fatal infection. Secondary states are more common but less often directly result in death.

Major categories of immunodeficiency disorders are outlined in Table 11–5. For this text we have selected to discuss hypogammaglobulinemia (deficiency of immunoglobins) as a representative immunodeficiency disorder.

HYPO- OR AGAMMAGLOBULINEMIA

As we have seen, immunoglobulins, as antibodies, defend the body against the invasion of foreign antigens such as microorganisms and toxins; immunoglobulins are produced by B-lymphocytes in response to these antigens. As long as this mechanism works satisfactorily, the body remains relatively secure against attack by dangerous foreign antigenic substances. However, as with all protective mechanisms, the mechanism of immunoglobulin synthesis can fail or be so inadequate that it is unable to meet the defensive needs of the body. When immunosynthesis fails, the spectrum of resulting disorders ranges from complete absence of all classes of immunoglobulins (agammaglobulinemia) to a selective deficiency of a single immunoglobulin class. Generally those patients with hypogammaglobulinemia become symptomatic earlier and have more severe disease than those with selected immunoglobulin deficiencies.[65]

TABLE 11–5. IMMUNE RESPONSE DISORDERS

Humoral
X-linked hypogammaglobulinemia
Transient hypogammaglobulinemia of infancy
Acquired hypogammaglobulinemia
Selective IgA deficiency
Selective IgM deficiency
Selective IgG deficiency
Cellular
Congenital thymic aplasia (DiGeorge's syndrome)
Combined Humoral and Cellular
Wiskott-Aldrich syndrome
Ataxia-telangiectasia
Severe combined immunodeficiency disease
Nezelof's syndrome
Graft vs. host disease

Agammaglobulinemia, the complete failure of immunoglobulin synthesis, is a congenital defect and may be due to defective development of the stem cells. Without the ability to respond to infections, an infant has a short life unless raised in strict protective isolation without direct physical contact with other people.[29]

Hypogammaglobulinemia is a decrease in the levels of circulating immunoglobulins and may result from (a) decreased synthesis of one or more immunoglobulins, (b) increased catabolism (rare), or (c) increased loss of immunoglobulins through gastrointestinal disease or increased glomerular permeability in the kidneys.

There are two major types of hypogammaglobulinemia — congenital and acquired. Individuals with the *congenital* form usually suffer from an atrophy of lymphoid tissue, and they may die during childhood from trivial infections. This condition usually appears after the third month of life when the antibodies (IgG) that the mother has passed to her child through the placental circulation have been used up, and the child has lost this valuable form of passive acquired immunity for self-protection. At this time it becomes apparent that the child's humoral immune response is ineffective at producing antibodies to protect itself from microorganisms.

Persons with congenital hypogammaglobulinemia have no B-cells. As we saw in Figure 11–5, the malfunction apparently occurs in the differentiation of stem cell to B-cell. The disease is manifested by severe recurrent upper and lower respiratory tract infections, and arthritis is common. In most cases, cellular immunity is still intact, so that treatment with gamma globulin and antibodies is effective in controlling bacterial infections. The prognosis depends on the severity of the infections the child develops. Survival may occur up to the second or third decade, but complications are common and usually debilitating. Information collected by the World Health Organization suggests that individuals with congenital immunoglobulin deficiencies are more likely to develop cancer, owing to an increased frequency of cancer cell development and inability of the lymphoid system to rid the body of these cells.[59] Fortunately, congenital hypogammaglobulinemia is rare.

Individuals with *acquired* hypogammaglobulinemia usually do not become symptomatic until 15 to 35 years of age. Increased susceptibility to bacterial infections is common because these people lack the antibodies to fight microorganisms. Diarrhea and malabsorption occur, presumably secondary to bacterial overgrowth of normal flora. There is also a high incidence of autoimmune disease in these people. However, because such people are still capable of cellular immunity, they may experience delayed hypersensitivity reactions and they reject transplants.

The cause of acquired hypogammaglobulinemia is unknown. However, these patients usually have normal numbers of peripheral B-cells, indicating a malfunction of differentiation from B-cell to plasma cell. (See Figure 11–5.) This suggests possible etiologies of (1) B-cell malignancy, resulting in impaired immunoglobulin synthesis, (2) loss of immunoglobulins through the gastrointestinal tract or the urinary tract, or (3) increased catabolism of the immunoglobulins.

Diagnosis of all types of hypogammaglobulinemia can be established from serum levels of immunoglobulins, and function of B-cells and T-cells if indicated. Measurement of serum immunoglobulin levels will not identify the mechanism involved in the etiology of the disease, but it will distinguish between severe hypogammaglobulinemia and selected immunoglobulin deficiencies.

Selected deficiencies have been noted with IgA, IgM, and IgG. X-linked and non–X linked IgG and IgA deficiencies present similar clinical symptoms to the above with severe pyogenic infections, cyclic neutropenia, thrombocytopenia, and hemolytic anemia. (See Unit XIV, which discusses blood disorders.) IgA deficiency is the most common and is the result of genetic defects, or it can be produced by congenital rubella virus, cytomegalovirus, or *Toxoplasma gondii* infections.

> *Treatment of hypogammaglobulinemia patients is aimed at controlling and preventing bacterial infections.*

Continuous use of *antibiotics* may be necessary. Broad-spectrum antibiotics such as ampicillin in low to moderate doses may be effective in controlling recurrent infections. Regular intramuscular injections of *human gamma globulin* help to increase resistance to infections and, in conjunction with antibiotics, provide an effective means of treatment. However, selected immunoglobulin deficiencies should *not* be treated with gamma globulin. The production of other immunoglobulins is normal, thus the gamma globulin fraction containing the deficient immunoglobulin may be recognized by the body as *foreign* and increase the risks of anaphylactoid reactions.

When nursing patients with hypogammaglobulinemia, it is your responsibility to guard them against dangerous infections. Some guidelines in caring for these individuals are shown in Table 11–6.*

2. The Gammopathies

The gammopathies, also called gammaglobulinopathies, involve "abnormal proliferation of the lymphoid cells producing immunoglobulins."[72] Examples of gammopathies include multiple myeloma, macroglobulinemia, and Hodgkin's disease. We will briefly consider multiple myeloma here; also, multiple myeloma and Hodgkin's disease are discussed in detail in Unit XIV.

MULTIPLE MYELOMA (PLASMA CELL MYELOMA)

As the derivative of the name implies, plasma cell myeloma (*myelos,* marrow, and *oma,* tumor) is

*Caring for persons requiring protective isolation is discussed in detail in Sorensen and Luckmann, *Basic Nursing: A Psychophysiologic Approach,* Chapter 45.

TABLE 11–6. CARING FOR PATIENTS WITH HYPOGAMMAGLOBULINEMIA

1. Isolate patients with hypogammaglobulinemia from all patients with infectious diseases or with contaminated wounds.
2. Do not take care of patients with this diagnosis if you are suffering from a cold, flu, or even a minor infection.
3. Screen visitors for colds or infections.
4. Explain the rationale for and instruct the patient and visitors in isolation and protective procedures.
5. To avoid cross-contamination, give nursing care to these patients *first,* before giving care to your other patients.
6. Observe good handwashing technique!
7. Protect the integrity of the skin and mucous membranes (e.g., promote good hydration and circulation).
8. Use sterile technique in catheterizations, IV changes, and in dressing changes.
9. Use disposable equipment whenever possible.
10. Encourage good nutrition and adequate rest.
11. Observe for and report promptly any temperature elevation or any sign of infection or illness, so that antibiotic therapy may be instituted immediately.
12. Isolation, both physical and social, can be a real problem for the immunosuppressed. It is imperative that psychosocial nursing activities be included in the patient's daily plan of care.

a tumor or neoplasm of the bone marrow. The bone marrow is a tissue that is composed of vast numbers of plasma cells. This disease is marked by excessive production of one type of immunoglobulin by a *malignant plasma cell* – usually *IgG* or *IgA*. In addition, synthesis of normal immunoglobulins is decreased. Furthermore, this condition results in the spread of the neoplasm from the zone of origin to other bones — thus the term "multiple myeloma." It should be noted that a diffuse increase in production of all immunoglobulins (polyclonal gammopathy) is commonly seen in cirrhosis, connective tissue diseases, and infections; it should not be confused with the monoclonal production in multiple myeloma.

Multiple myeloma is characterized by the presence in the serum or urine of a *monoclonal immunoglobulin,* also called a "paraprotein," "M protein," or a "myeloma protein." This protein is derived from one clone of plasma cell. (Malignancies developing in more than one clone of plasma cell are very rare.) Measurement of individual immunoglobulin levels may reveal a marked increase in the class being produced by the abnormal plasma cell.

Clinically, the patient presents with the following:

- *Recurrent infections* due to the uselessness of the monoclonal immunoglobulin.
- *Anemia* because the normal cells residing in the bone marrow are crowded out by abnormal cells.
- *Bone lesions* and severe *bone pain* due to metastasized malignant plasma cells.
- *Pathologic fractures* due to bone destruction.

Supportive management is essential. Bone pain may be controlled with *analgesics.* It is important to maintain adequate *fluid intake* and to encourage *ambulation* whenever possible to avoid further bone loss and hypercalcemia. *Antibiotics* control bacterial infections, particularly pneumonia and some gram-negative organisms. Local *radiation therapy* is useful for relief of pain and reduction of tumor mass for localized bony lesions. *Cytotoxic chemotherapy,* along with general management, will achieve good therapeutic responses in about 70 per cent of patients with multiple myeloma and will produce increases in length and quality of life. *Melphalan,* with or without prednisone, is the drug of choice for the initial treatment of multiple myeloma. *Cyclophosphamide* is also a widely used alkylating agent for the treatment of multiple myeloma, but has the additional side-effects of sterility and baldness. It is generally used in patients who have become refractory to melphalan. Seventy per cent of patients with multiple myeloma respond to therapy. Those who respond have a mean overall survival rate of more than 30 months. The prognosis is worse, of course, for those patients with more severe disease.

3. Diseases Associated with Hypersensitivity Reactions

Whereas the immune response is a protective adaptive response designed to guard the body against the invasion of dangerous, toxic substances, the allergic response is an *oversensitive* and often harmful response on the part of the body against foreign substances that may actually be *harmless,* e.g., plant pollens. In other words, in the immune response the body's protective cells *appropriately* recognize dangerous intruders, fight them, and often destroy them. Conversely, in an allergic response, the body's protective cells *"overestimate"* the danger from a harmless intruder, start a battle and, in the end, produce needless damage to the body's tissues. As Hans Selye points out: "Whether to fight or not to fight depends upon circumstances. . . . Yet all biologic groups from the microscopic to the geographic are singularly short-sighted when it comes to this alternative."[96] The body, then, like a person or a nation, can make a mistake in sizing up its foes. In the case of a nation, a small and foolish incident can lead to a deadly war. Similarly, in the case of the body, a pollen can lead to severe dyspnea and a tiny bee sting can end in death.

Definitions. The word "allergy" (from *allos,* other, and *ergon,* energy) signifies that the activity of an individual or the energy of the body has in some way been altered.[12]

To the general public, an allergy is an idiosyncrasy that usually develops in response to a pollen, food, dust, plant, or animal hair. Such allergies are widespread in our population. Indeed, they account for many of the constant complaints that we hear around us, such as "Keep the cat away from me. I can't stand cat hair — it makes me sneeze," "Don't give me any strawberries! I break out all over," or "My mother-in-law had a dose of penicillin and nearly died."

Although the term "allergy" is widely used by the public, the word *hypersensitivity* is more appropriate to designate those allergic conditions in which a definite immunologic mechanism has been active. The term "atopy" is used to distinguish those people who seem to have familial tendencies for allergies. The term has no clinical relevance to disease processes, but refers to a person's *predisposition* to disease.

Types of Allergens. An *allergen* can be defined as any substance with the capacity to induce hypersensitivity. Although allergens are highly variable in their chemical makeup, most are protein in nature. However, there are a few nonprotein allergens. For example, some nonprotein drugs and some plant oils have the capacity to cause allergic contact dermatitis.

Major types of allergens can be categorized as inhalants, ingestants, contactants, injectants, and infectants.

Inhalants include plant pollens and dusts. They may create such problems as seasonal hay fever, seasonal asthma, and allergic rhinitis. Tissues that are particularly vulnerable to inhalants are the conjunctival mucosa, nasal mucosa, and bronchial mucosa.

Ingestants include foods and drugs. Allergies to ingestants may manifest themselves as allergic rhinitis, asthma, diarrhea, colitis, abdominal pain, dermatitis, urticaria, and migraine headaches. The major organs and tissues affected by ingestants are, therefore, the nasal mucosa, the bronchial mucosa, the gastrointestinal mucosa, the skin, and the brain.

Contactants include soaps and plants and mainly affect the skin, resulting in such problems as contact dermatitis.

Injectants include such preparations as foreign sera and drugs; these substances can affect any tissue in the body, causing drug allergy and serum sickness.

Infectants or *bacteria* can also infect any tissue in the body and can lead to bacterial allergy.

A final and mysterious group of allergens are called *self-allergens* or *autologous antigens.* These allergens develop *within* the body rather than entering the body as foreign substances from the outside environment. Autologous allergens apparently play an important role in causing *autoimmune disease* (discussed on p. 164).

Antibodies Characteristic of Hypersensitivity Reactions. Immunoglobulin E (IgE) antibodies, sometimes called *reagins* or *sensitizing antibodies,* are particularly characteristic of hypersensitivity reactions. Reagins function only when they are attached to mast cells or basophils. When an allergen reacts with a specific type of IgE reagin antibody, an allergen-reagin reaction develops, followed by an immediate or *anaphylactic* response that damages body cells. In addition to IgE antibody, IgM and IgG antibodies play a role in other types of hypersensitivity reactions. These antibodies and their damaging reactions with allergens are discussed in more detail later in this chapter.

Mechanisms of Immunologic Injury.[87, 41] Hypersensitivity reactions may be classified in many different ways. Below we present three basic classifications:

1. Classification according to a *time sequence.* According to this classification (which was popular in the past), the response to allergens is classified as *immediate* or *delayed.* While this classification is sometimes valid, of more significance are the next following two classifications.

2. Classification according to the *source of the antigen.* Thus the antigen may be *exogenous* (originating outside of the organism, or in the environment), *homologous* (being introduced from an animal of the same species but of a different genotype), and *autologous* (originating within the organism itself). Examples of these three types of antigens are presented in Table 11–7.

3. Classification according to the *basic immunologic* mechanism underlying the immune injury. This classification is highly valuable because it clarifies exactly how a faulty immune response can result in tissue injury and death. These mechanisms can basically be divided into *antibody-mediated* responses and *cell-mediated* responses. Gell and Coombs[41] have expanded this idea into the four categories presented in Figure 11–10 and in the discussion below. Note that Types I, II, and III are *antibody-mediated* and Type IV is *cell-mediated.*

Type I – Anaphylactic

The hallmark of the anaphylactic response is the reaction of an antigen with a reaginic antibody (IgE antibody), which, as you recall, has an affinity for mast cells. An anaphylactic reaction will take place *only* in the individual who has been *sensitized* — i.e., antibody formation has been stimulated by exposure to low doses of antigen such as insect venoms, drugs, vaccines, or foods.[14, 44] Often the sensitizing agent or actual time of exposure is unknown. Upon *second* exposure to the immunogen, the cell-bound antibody recognizes it and reacts *immediately.* Mast cell degranulation occurs with the release of histamine and serotonin, causing rapid smooth muscle constriction, increased vascular permeability, and vasodilatation. If the allergen is inhaled (pollen, for example), the smooth muscle of the bronchi is the primary target. Peripheral vasodilatation may lead to pooling of blood and a decrease in the output of the heart. Subsequent events of extreme importance include *shock,* which may be life-threatening.

The types of reactions seen via this mechanism include anaphylactic shock, most often due to drug reactions, and the more common atopic allergies such as hay fever, asthma, and urticaria (hives).

Type II – Cytotoxic or Cytolytic

These reactions are considered to be cytolytic (causing cell lysis) or cytotoxic (direct destruction without

TABLE 11–7. IMMUNE DISORDERS CLASSIFIED BY SOURCE OF ANTIGEN

Exogenous
Atopic diseases (e.g., poison ivy contact dermatitis; reactions to plant pollens, sera, and drugs)

Homologous
Reactions to isoantigens (e.g., transfusion reactions, erythroblastosis fetalis, transplantation rejection)

Autologous
Autoimmune diseases (e.g., systemic lupus erythematosus, rheumatoid arthritis, Sjögren's syndrome)

From Robbins, S. L., and M. Angell (Eds.): *Basic Pathology,* 2nd ed. Philadelphia: W. B. Saunders Co., 1976, p. 172.

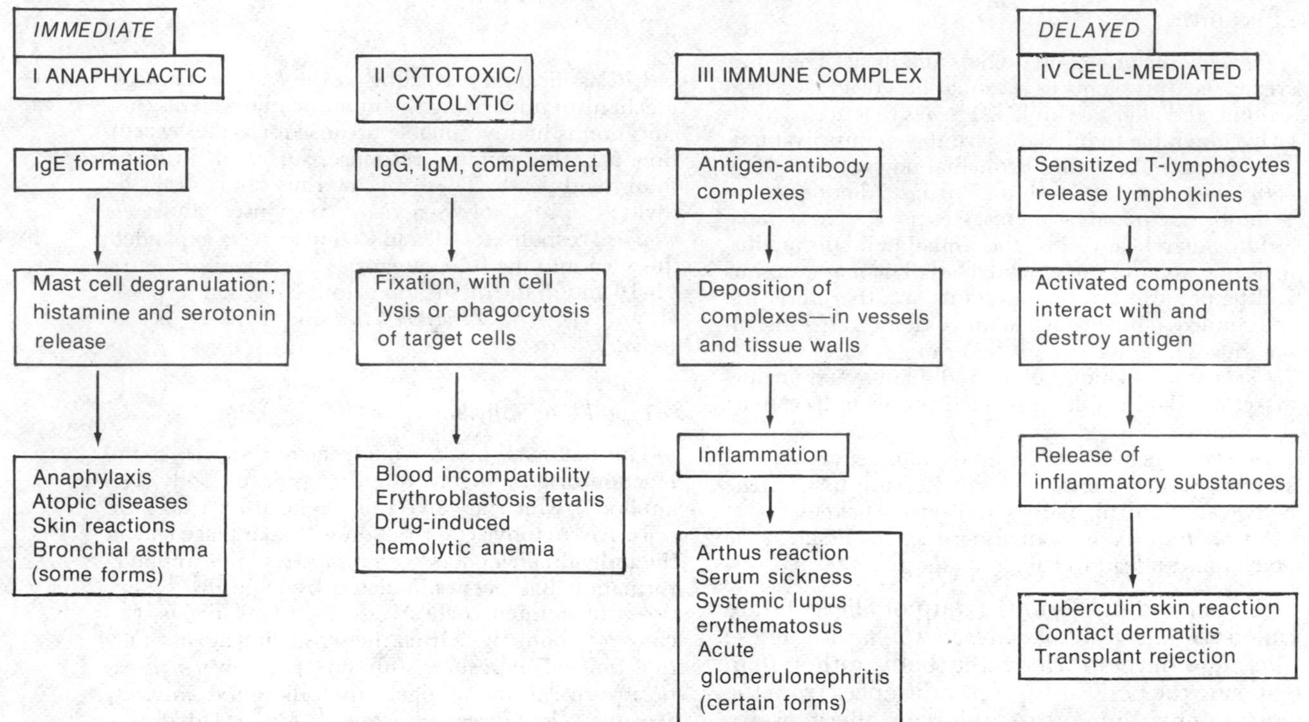

Figure 11–10. Hypersensitivity reactions: types, mediators, mechanisms, responses, and examples of diseases. (Based on Table 6–3 in Robbins, S. L., and M. Angell (Eds.): *Basic Pathology.* Philadelphia: W. B. Saunders Co., 1976, p. 173.)

lysis). Antibody molecules (IgG, IgM) combine with antigens that are part of a cell membrane, e.g., blood type antigens, drugs. Complement may be bound to the cell by the antibody reaction and lead to lysis of the cell. If complement is not bound, phagocytosis of the target cells may still occur because of the antibody on the cell membrane. Red blood cells are common target cells in this type of hypersensitivity reaction, as in the transfusion of grossly incompatible blood, which results in intravascular hemolysis. Other examples include erythroblastosis fetalis and drug-induced hemolytic anemias. (See Unit XIV.)

Type III – Immune Complex Disorders

Reactions of this type are secondary to the formation of antigen-antibody complexes and their subsequent deposition and reaction within the tissues. The following sequence of events leads to the reaction: (a) a soluble immunogen meets with a circulating specific antibody; (b) the immunogen and antibody form a complex; and (c) the complex is deposited in the tissue or vessel walls. Fixation of complement and the activity of macrophages and polymorphonuclear leukocytes leads to inflammation. Eventually the complexes are phagocytized.

Disorders characteristic of this mechanism include the *Arthus reaction,* a cutaneous form of the immune complex in which inflammation of vessels walls (vasculitis) and formation of blood clots (thrombi) lead to focal areas of inflammation until the immune complexes are phagocytized.

Serum sickness, a systemic form of this mechanism, is a self-limiting condition most often caused by sensitivity to prophylactic injections of immune sera. One to two weeks following exposure to the antigen, symptoms of fever, enlarged lymph glands, hives, and painful joints occur. Additionally, patients may also develop myocarditis, glomerulonephritis, arthritis, and neuritis (rarely). Again, phagocytosis is the mechanism that eventually controls the condition (see p. 162).

More serious immune complex diseases such as systemic lupus erythematosus, rheumatoid arthritis, and Hashimoto's thyroiditis are discussed later.

Type IV – Cell-mediated

Cell-mediated immune reactions occur as the result of sensitized lymphocyte interactions with specific antigen. This mechanism does *not* require the presence of humoral antibody or complement. Instead, the sensitized lymphocytes release their mediators of inflammation (lymphokines), which are largely responsible for macrophage infiltration and destruction of the antigen. This process takes 24 to 48 hours, and thus another name for it is a *delayed* reaction.

The cell-mediated reaction is best typified by the *tuberculin skin reaction,* where the typical wheal and flare of inflammation is observed in a couple of days, following the injection of tubercle bacilli. The tuberculin test is used to detect the presence of tuberculosis infection in humans, and it is based upon a positive reaction to an injection of tuberculin. Tuberculin is a sterile preparation of a bacterial protein obtained from a culture medium. Tuberculin is either injected intradermally, as in the Mantoux test; rubbed onto the skin, as in the von Pirquet test; or applied to the skin on a piece of gauze as in the Vollmer patch test. If the individual being tested does not have tuberculosis, there will be no reaction to these tests. However, if the patient is or has been infected by the tubercle bacillus, a local inflammatory reaction will occur on the skin within 48 to 96 hours. The fact that an individual with tuberculosis reacts in a positive manner to the tuberculin test indicates that his or her cells have become sensitized to the tubercle bacillus.

Other types of delayed reaction allergies are (1) *contact sensitivities,* which result from contact with such allergens as poison ivy; (2) *drug sensitivities* due to the administration of sulfonamides, penicillin, and other antibiotics, and (3) *infection allergies* due to contact with certain bacteria, viruses, spirochetes, and parasites.[23, 45] Transplant rejection is also a cell-mediated mechanism. In all these conditions, humoral antibodies within the plasma are relatively unimportant and have little effect; the hypersensitive reaction takes place on the surface of, or within, cells that have previously been sensitized by contact with an allergen.

General Etiologic Factors. The precise factors causing hypersensitivity reactions are not known; however, *heredity, congenital factors,* and *contact* between an individual and an allergen are known to play important roles in the development of allergic reactions.

First of all, heredity has been linked with the etiology of allergy because some allergics definitely appear to run in families. Also, allergies appear to affect one tenth of the population more frequently and more severely than other individuals within the population. Moreover, heredity evidently not only determines that a particular individual will be allergic, but also determines the type of allergy the person will experience, as well as the precise allergens to which he or she will be susceptible. The exact manner in which heredity influences the development of allergic manifestations in a patient is still not clearly understood.

Congenital factors can influence an individual's susceptibility to allergens, because allergens can be passed to the fetus via the placental circulation. Such an allergic sensitivity is *not* the result of hereditary transmission but is *acquired,* the fetus being actively sensitized during prenatal life. For example, if a mother, during pregnancy, eats large amounts of a high protein food, the child may become overly sensitized to that particular protein while it is within its mother's uterus. After birth, when the child comes into contact with that protein food, he or she may manifest certain clinical signs of allergy.

A final important etiologic factor in hypersensitivity is *contact* between the patient and a particular offending allergen. Although heredity plays a role in predisposing an individual to the development of a particular allergy, heredity alone *cannot* cause a person to become allergic. Contact with an allergen is *essential* to the development of any allergy. On the other hand, in certain allergies such as atopic dermatitis, seasonal hay fever, and allergic asthma, contact with the allergen is not sufficient in itself to produce the allergy, because heredity is a major factor. For example, although thousands of people are exposed to certain seasonal pollens every year, only a limited number of persons, with a certain hereditary predisposition toward allergic reactions, develop seasonal hay fever.

There are certain *precipitating or modifying* factors that also influence the development of allergies. The most important of these are psychic stress, infection, endocrine disturbances and, in some instances, pregnancy. Such factors can upset the homeostatic balance between an individual with a hereditary predisposition toward the development of allergy and the allergenic surroundings. For example, some women when pregnant experience severe bronchial asthma attacks for the first time in their lives. Following pregnancy, the same women may have no further attacks. Similarly, certain individuals, when under great nervous stress, will break out in hives. Even the suggestion of an allergic condition can sometimes precipitate the development of an allergic attack. For example, a typist of our acquaintance developed a serious attack of hives while typing a paper on the subject! Thus, the mental state of an individual and the person's physiologic status *both* profoundly influence whether an individual with a hereditary predisposition toward allergy will actually develop the allergy.

Specific Etiologic Factors. The manifestations of any hypersensitive state will depend upon a number of specific factors in addition to the general factors just discussed. The most important are:

1. *The nature of the allergen.* What *type* of allergen is involved? Is it a pollen, dust, food, drug, or microorganism?
2. *The concentration of the allergen.* For example, did the patient receive a large dose of a drug (i.e., penicillin) or only a small dose? Did an individual with a food allergy eat a large portion of a food or only a bite of it? (Incidentally, chocolate and strawberries are common allergic foods.) Naturally the concentration or amount of the allergen taken in or ingested will make a great difference in the severity of the symptoms.
3. *The type of antibody involved in the reaction.* Is the antibody involved reagin (IgE antibody) or is it IgM or IgG? As you recall, each type of antibody is important in a particular type of hypersensitivity state.
4. *The type of organ or tissue that is affected by the allergen.* Almost any tissue in the body can be affected. Particularly vulnerable are the brain, skin, gastrointes-

tinal tract, and the mucosa of the conjunctiva, the nose, and the bronchials. The organ affected will greatly influence the type of symptoms produced. Thus, an allergy affecting the gastrointestinal tract will produce diarrhea, nausea, and vomiting; a skin allergy may erupt into eczema and urticaria; and when the brain is affected, the patient may suffer a migraine headache.

5. *The toxic substances released as a result of the allergen-antibody reaction.* The major substances released through an allergic reaction are histamine, or histamine-like materials, bradykinin, serotonin, prostaglandins, and lysosomal enzymes.

DIAGNOSIS OF ALLERGIC CONDITIONS

To discover whether a person has an allergy and, if so, exactly what allergen is creating the problem, it is necessary for the doctor, nurse, and patient all to act as detectives. Together they will need to explore the patient's past history, present health status, home environment, social habits, and working conditions. To diagnose the presence of an allergy as well as the causative allergen involved, the following three avenues of investigation must be carefully pursued: (1) a complete history, including a medical history, family history, and a social history; (2) a complete physical examination, including certain laboratory procedures; and (3) allergy tests.

The Complete History. The complete history will include a past medical history, a family history, and a social history. We have listed some pertinent questions that should be answered concerning the patient's past and present life and state of health.

I. *Past History of Allergic Problems*
1. Has the patient experienced an allergic reaction to such typical allergens as pollens, plants, certain foods, cat or dog hair, cleansing fluids, soaps, or face powders?
2. Has the patient noted any seasonal bouts of sneezing, wheezing, tearing, asthmatic attacks, or sensitivity to particular foods? Are the attacks seasonal, semiyearly, or yearly?
3. Has the patient been particularly prone to colds and flus over the years?
4. If the patient is presently experiencing allergic symptoms, has he or she experienced these same symptoms in the past?
5. Where was the patient living and what was the patient's occupation when the symptoms of allergy were first experienced?
6. What has been the course of the allergy since the first attack?

If the patient is a woman, you will want to ask her the following:

7. Did the patient develop her allergy during pregnancy? Do the symptoms of allergy appear during *every* pregnancy? Do the symptoms of allergy disappear following the child's birth?
8. Does the patient notice a change in her symptoms when she is menstruating?
9. Did the allergy first develop during the patient's menopause?

II. *Family History of Allergic Problems*
1. Does the patient have any relatives who have similar symptoms as a result of contact with particular allergens?
2. Have any relatives of the patient had to be treated for allergic conditions?
3. Specifically, what types of allergic conditions have family members suffered?

III. *Social and Environmental History*
1. In what type of physical environment does the patient live? In the country where he or she would contact various animal danders, or in a factory area where various soots and pollutants might be in the air? In a heavily forested area where the air, during certain seasons, is heavy with pollens, or in a very windy location where dusts and pollens are constantly circulating in the air? Is the home located on a tree-lined street or are there trees surrounding the house — trees that might carry a pollen to which the patient is allergic?
2. Does the patient have a pet cat, dog, or horse, and are there many animals in the neighborhood?
3. What types of fabrics are used in the patient's home? Does the patient have cotton or wool blankets on the bed? Of what material are the curtains made? What types of rugs are on the floors?
4. What type of heating does the patient have at home? Is air conditioning used, or are the windows left open in the summer?
5. What types of foods does the patient enjoy? Does the patient eat a great deal of chocolate, eggs, shellfish, strawberries, or wheat products — all foods that can act on certain patients as allergens? If the patient does ingest these types of foods, has there been any reaction after eating them?
6. What types of drugs does the patient take? If he or she takes any particular drug continually, has the person ever had a reaction to that drug? Has he or she ever experienced an allergic reaction to *any* drug?
7. Does the patient notice the appearance of allergic symptoms when overly tired or when under emotional tension or strain?

The answers to these questions can provide valuable clues as to whether a patient is experiencing an allergy and what the allergen involved might be. In no other condition is it of greater importance to take a thorough history and to investigate as many aspects of the patient's immediate and past environment as possible.

The Physical Examination. Following history taking, the patient will next be given a complete physical examination, with special attention being paid to the site of symptoms. For example, if the patient has hay fever, the doctor will want

TABLE 11–8. DATA SUGGESTIVE OF ALLERGIES IN CHILDREN

Objective Data

Skin	*Nose (Continued)*
dryness, scaliness	rhinitis
irritations, inflammations	sniffling, paroxysmal sneezing, snorting
pallor	swollen nasal passages
rashes (note symmetry, location)	transverse nasal crease
scratches	*Mouth and Pharynx*
urticaria	allergic gaping
Eyes	continual throat clearing
allergic shiners (discolorations under eyes)	geographic tongue
conjunctivitis	gingival hyperplasia
inflammation	mouth wrinkling with facial grimaces
lacrimation	orofacial dental deformities
long, silky eyelashes	redness of throat
rubbing or excessive blinking	swollen lips or tongue
styes	*Ears*
Nose	decreased hearing
allergic salute	drainage
nasal polyps	immobile or scarred tympanic membrane
nasal voice	absence of cone of light
nose twitching	*Neck*
pale, boggy mucous membranes	palpable lymph nodes

Subjective Data

History of	*History of* (Continued)
failure to gain weight	unusual reactions to drugs, insect bites or stings, inhalants (odors and fumes)
tiring readily upon moderate exertion	recurrent respiratory problems
wheezing or shortness of breath upon moderate exertion	recurrent otitis media
food intolerances	specific problems, such as itching, rashes, hives, recurrent nosebleeds, headaches
colic, cramping, vomiting, diarrhea (in absence of general illness)	seasonal exacerbations of any symptoms
alterations in taste, smell, hearing	behavior or learning problems

From Bridgewater, S. C., R. R. Voignier, and C. S. Smith: Allergies in children: Recognition. *American Journal of Nursing,* 78:613, Apr. 1978, p. 616.

to examine the mucous membranes of the nose very carefully. If the patient has hives, naturally the doctor will want to examine the skin. When a patient experiences dyspnea and asthma, the doctor may wish to order an electrocardiogram to rule out the possibility that the attacks of dyspnea are due to a heart condition. Finally, the doctor may also want to check the patient's sinuses, tonsils, and teeth to learn if these organs are acting as foci for infection.

Because children so frequently suffer from allergies, we have included an assessment guide containing objective and subjective data suggestive of allergy in youngsters (Table 11–8). The "allergic salute" noted in Table 11–8 is shown in Figure 11–11.

Laboratory Tests. *Laboratory work* is an important part of the physical examination of the allergic patient. Be prepared for the doctor to order a urinalysis, blood serology, and a complete blood count. In addition, a differential white count will probably be ordered to detect *eosinophilia* (an increase in eosinophils), a condition that occurs in allergic reactions. In some cases the patient's nasal secretions and sputum may be examined for the presence of eosinophils.

The differential white count also includes an *absolute lymphocyte count,* which can be used to estimate the number of circulating lymphocytes. A count of below 1200 lymphocytes per cu. mm. is considered subnormal. Also, by means of the *sheep erythrocyte rosette test,* numbers of circulating T-cells can be quantified. T-lymphocytes bind immediately to unaltered sheep erythrocytes to form rosettes composed of at least three sheep erythrocytes attached to the surface of the lymphocyte. Normally 60 to 80 per cent of peripheral blood lymphocytes form rosettes. If the test indicates that fewer than 60 per cent of lymphocytes are T-cells, then cellular immunity is deficient.[85]

The laboratory also measures *serum level of IgE* (reagin, sensitizing antibody, or immunoglobulin E).[13, 72, 101] Measures of IgE are important because, as you recall, IgE underlies acute allergic reactions; also, the serum level of IgE is elevated in many allergic conditions. Normally, the IgE serum level is very low — ranging from 0 to 150 international units (one international unit equals 2.4 nanograms). When IgE is elevated, it is still present in miniscule amounts.

Currently, IgE levels can be measured in two ways: (1) by *radioimmunoassay,* which is an immunoassay test using a radioactive-labeled substance to react with the substance being tested and (2) by the *radioallergosorbent* test (RAST). RAST measures the level of IgE antibodies that

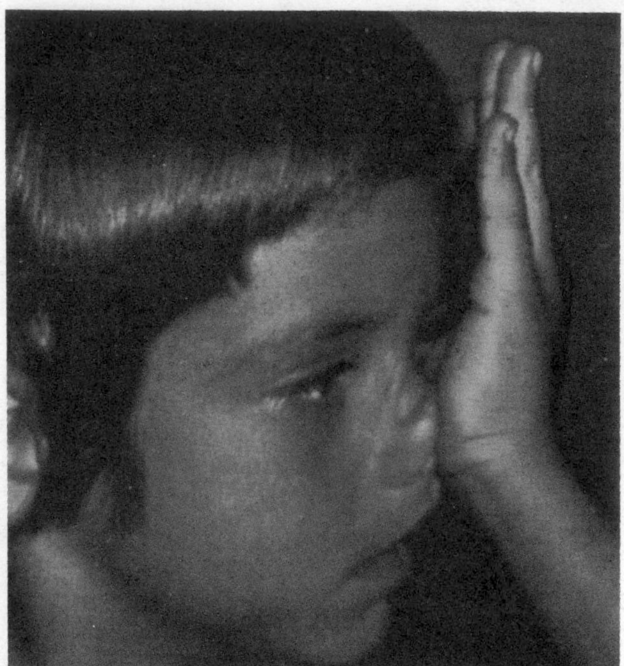

Figure 11–11. "Allergic salute" in a nine-year-old boy with chronic nasal allergy and bronchial asthma from infancy. The patient uses the "heel" of the palm to relieve the itching and free the boggy nasal turbinates from the septum, thus allowing easy ingress of air. (From Marks, M. B.: Recognizing the allergic person. *American Family Physician.* 16:72, July 1977.)

are directed against a *specific* antigen; e.g., pollens, animal dander, food, venoms, insect stings from the Hymenoptera group. To date, not all antigens can be tested for by RAST.

The two major advantages of RAST are its accuracy and safety. It is safer than skin testing (discussed below) — a diagnostic method which sometimes involves the administration of a potentially dangerous substance (e.g., penicillin) to an allergic individual. Also, patients do not have to discontinue their prescribed anti-allergy drugs with RAST as they do with skin testing. The major disadvantage of RAST is its expense.

Tests for Allergies. Major types of allergy tests are: skin tests, food diaries, and elimination diets.

Skin Tests. If the patient's history and physical examination point to the possibility of an allergic condition, the doctor will probably order skin tests to *confirm* that possibility. Skin tests are generally done in a series: for example, the first allergen to be used in testing might be made up from pollens, the second allergen from weeds, the third from dusts, the fourth from horse dander, and so forth.

1. Skin Tests for Types I, II, and III Hypersensitivity Reactions (Antibody-Mediated). With the exception of Type IV hypersensitivity reactions (cell-mediated), sensitization is systemic, meaning that the allergic individual reacts whenever contact with the allergen occurs. Injection of minute quantities of allergens into the skin produces a wheal in 10 to 15 minutes in persons with IgE antibodies. However, a positive skin test does not prove that the patient's symptoms are related to the allergen provoking the skin response.

Skin tests include scratch tests or intradermal (intracutaneous) injections. These tests are performed to confirm a suspicion that a specific allergy exists. Allergen extracts are prepared for skin testing by diluting the allergen in question in a prescribed amount of solution or diluent. The degree of reactivity to the allergen extract will be proportional to the amount of IgE the patient has on mast cells. Intradermal tests are more sensitive than scratch tests, but are also more likely to cause an anaphylactoid reaction.

The scratch and intracutaneous tests depend upon the use of a control site and a test site. A small amount of allergen is placed on or into the test site, while only the diluent is used on the control site. After a predetermined time period, both sites are compared and the test is read as either positive or negative.

To administer a *scratch* test, the doctor or nurse first makes a small superficial test scratch approximately an eighth of an inch long on the patient's forearm or on the inner aspect of the arm, and a *control scratch* on the other arm. Next, the allergen is applied to the test scratch in either liquid, paste, or powdered form. When the allergen is in powdered form, a diluent is first placed on the test site and then the powdered allergen. Diluent only is placed on the control scratch. In approximately 10 to 30 minutes, the test scratch and the control scratch are compared. If the patient has had a reaction to the allergen, both a wheal and a zone of redness will appear around the test site. If the patient has had no reaction to the allergen being tested, both the control and the test sites will appear the same.

With the *intracutaneous test,* the allergen is diluted and then injected into and not through the epidermis. The equipment you will need to gather for an intracutaneous (or intradermal) test is as follows.

- ▶ Sterile liquid allergen
- ▶ A tuberculin syringe
- ▶ A small needle, 26 gauge, ¼ inch long

The intracutaneous test is similar to the scratch test in that a test site and a control site are used. To administer the test, the allergen is injected into the epidermis of the test site and only diluent is injected into the epidermis of the control site. After about 10 minutes, both the control site and the test site are checked for a reaction. As with the scratch test, a positive reaction generally involves the appearance of a wheal and an area of redness that surrounds the test site. When it is not possible to perform skin tests (as in the case of very young children), the *Prausnitz-Küstner* (P-K) reaction may be induced. This test involves passive transfer of the serum of the allergic person into the skin of a healthy (nonallergic) volunteer. The skin of the healthy person becomes sensitized to the donor's antigen, and if the volunteer is exposed to the antigen 24 hours later, a wheal and flare response results. The risk of hepatitis and the availability of lab tests to measure histamine and IgE minimize the use of this test.

2. *Skin Tests for Type IV Delayed Hypersensitivity (Cell-Mediated) Reactions.*[85] It is now possible—by using the delayed hypersensitivity skin tests—to measure the capability of T-lymphocytes to "remember" an antigen that they have previously encountered. Table 11–9 presents the procedure, types of antigens used for testing, and results of Type IV skin tests. A *positive* reaction to the delayed hypersensitivity skin test, utilizing multiple antigens for testing, implies that the cell-mediated immune system is operating satisfactorily. However, if a person has a positive reaction to only *one* antigen, that person may be suffering decreased cellular immunity; i.e., diminished hypersensitivity. Diminished hypersensitivity is characteristic of persons with Hodgkin's disease, immune deficiency disease, leukemia, or acute infection (viral, bacterial, or fungal). Also, diminished hypersensitivity reactions occur in persons who are taking immunosuppressive drugs, undergoing radiation therapy, or who have recently received a viral vaccination.

In addition to testing for secondary (delayed) hypersensitivity reactions, it is also possible to skin test for *primary* immune response; i.e., the ability of the cell-mediated immune system to respond to unfamiliar antigens. The chemical dinitrochlorobenzene (DNCB) is used in this test. First, DNCB is put directly onto the skin of the upper arm in a small plastic ring. The solution is allowed to dry and then covered with gauze for 48 hours. Two weeks later DNCB is applied to the volar surface of the forearm as a challenge dose. 48 hours later a positive reading (redness and induration present) indicates that cellular immunity is intact. The use of the DNCB skin test as a diagnostic test for cancer is discussed in Chapter 22.

Food Diaries and Elimination Diets. Patients who appear to be suffering from a food allergy may be asked to keep a food diary in order to ascertain the particular food or foods to

TABLE 11–9. DELAYED-HYPERSENSITIVITY SKIN TESTING

There are several ways to evaluate cell mediated immunity. Delayed-hypersensitivity skin testing is the best available procedure for routine use, since it is convenient, sensitive, and reproducible.

Procedure

Inject 0.1 ml of each antigen intradermally. The volar surface of the forearm is the preferred site; if necessary, the upper arm or thigh may be used.

First-strength tests

The following antigens are used:

- Purified protein derivative (PPD). Intermediate strength is used, except for patients with active tuberculosis, who get first strength.
- Mumps as supplied in skin-test antigen, or as a 1:8 dilution of inactivated mumps vaccine in normal saline. Mumps antigen should not be used for patients who are allergic to eggs. Since the antigen is incubated in eggs, immediate hypersensitivity reactions may occur in sensitized patients.
- *Tricophyton* in a 1:100 dilution (a 1:10 dilution of the antigen as supplied in normal saline).
- Streptokinase/streptodornase (SK/SD), 10 units SK/2.5 units SD diluted as follows: add 10 ml of normal saline to vial, then prepare a 1:20 dilution in normal saline. Do not shake. Enzymes are highly labile, and bubbling induces denaturation. Do not store the dilution for more than 2 weeks.
- *Candida* in a 1:100 dilution (a 1:10 dilution of antigen as supplied in normal saline).

Second-strength tests

It is preferable to use the arm not used for the first-strength tests, when applying these antigens:

- SK/SD, 20 units SK/5 units SD diluted as follows: add 10 ml of normal saline to vial as supplied, then prepare a 1:10 dilution in normal saline. Do not store longer than 2 weeks.
- *Candida* 1:50 dilution (a 1:5 dilution of antigen as supplied in normal saline).
- If a patient has a reaction to either *Candida* or SK/SD when tested with the first-strength reagents, second-strength injections are not given. An extreme Arthus reaction could result.

Reading

Results of delayed-hypersensitivity skin tests are read at 24 and 48 hours. Two diameters of the area of induration are recorded in millimeters. Erythema is not measured.

A positive response requires induration of at least 5 mm. in diameter present at 48 hours. If the reaction disappears after the first 24 hours, it is considered an Arthus reaction and not an indication of delayed hypersensitivity.

From Rabin, B. S., and T. L. Whiteside: Evaluating cellular immunity. *Consultant,* 19:72, June 1979. p. 77.

which they are allergic. In this method of testing, the patient first keeps a daily written record for a week or more of all foods eaten. Then the physician will ask the patient to not eat one specific food or type of food for a designated period. For example, the patient may be asked not to eat wheat products for a period of 1 week. If the patient continues to have allergic symptoms, all milk products may be removed from the diet for a similar period. If the symptoms still persist, foods containing chocolate may be omitted, and so on, until at last the specific allergen causing the problem is found. Sometimes elimination programs similar to this are used to eliminate cosmetics and clothing believed to act as allergens. Such a program can be tiring and sometimes disappointing to the patient. Therefore, it may be up to you as a nurse to encourage the patient to continue in the search for the allergen that is creating symptoms. Often you will be the person designated to explain to the patient the process of an elimination diet, and perhaps even to set up a specific program for the individual.

In sum, the process of searching for a causative allergen in an allergic condition is an exhaustive, meticulous, and precise procedure. The time involved in diagnosing the allergen responsible for an allergy may run into weeks or even months. Once the allergen itself has been found, then the long process of treatment must begin.

GENERAL PRINCIPLES OF TREATMENT IN ALLERGIC CONDITIONS

Although the treatment of individual allergies will be presented in appropriate sections of this chapter and throughout the text, we outline here some general principles of treatment used in many allergic conditions. Basically, treatment is directed toward avoiding the allergen once it is defined, modifying the state of hypersensitivity, and lessening the symptoms. Specific therapeutic measures include (a) avoidance of specific allergens, (b) drug therapy, and (c) immunotherapy.

Avoidance of Specific Allergens. Despite the fact that a specific allergen may cause a patient to suffer a multitude of miserable symptoms, the avoidance of that allergen may, nevertheless, cause considerable upheaval in the patient's life. Although avoiding the allergen may relieve symptoms, such avoidance may also mean that patients may have to change their place of residence, change their job, or give up certain personal enjoyments (for example, pets). Some of the most common means by which persons avoid specific allergens are as follows:

- The individual may move from his or her neighborhood or, in extreme cases, may even move from one part of the country to another part (i.e., from a wet area of the country like Seattle where pollens abound, to a hot dry section of the country such as Arizona).
- The person may be forced to change occupation. For example, if the patient sells fabrics and is allergic to certain types of materials or to the lint from the material, it may be necessary to change to another type of sales work.
- A change in eating habits is a common solution to allergic conditions. Such well-liked foods as shellfish, chocolate, and cakes and cookies made from wheat products may have to be totally eliminated from the diet.
- People may be forced to give up pets, such as a favorite cat or dog. Persons allergic to animal dander, despite their love for animals, may never be able to have a pet in their homes.
- The use of another soap or cleansing agent is oftentimes a simple solution to an attack of dermatitis-type allergy. Sometimes it is necessary to experiment to find a soap that does not create symptoms.
- Individuals with allergies to certain drugs will naturally have to avoid these drugs. If, on the other hand, it is essential that the drug be taken, it will be necessary to desensitize the person to that medication.
- Certain changes may have to be made within the allergic person's home environment. Damp dusting may have to be done daily, pillows filled with feathers may have to be changed to those made of sponge rubber; cotton blankets may have to be used instead of wool; favorite drapes and rugs may have to be removed.
- The avoidance of colds, flu, and infections is very important in the prevention of allergy. Thus, persons troubled with allergies must take special care to avoid infectious individuals, as well as to dress warmly in cold, damp weather.
- Since emotional upsets and extreme fatigue are important precipitating factors in allergy, patients must try to avoid the occurrence of such problems as much as possible. Adequate rest and a calm outlook on life's problems are helpful in decreasing the number and severity of attacks. When an individual is extremely disturbed mentally, the physician may decide on referral to a psychotherapist for treatment.

Drug Therapy. Patients generally require some drug therapy when suffering from allergic attacks. Drugs that provide systematic relief from allergic attacks include antihistamines, epinephrine, ACTH, cortisone, bronchodilators, sedatives, and tranquilizers.

Antihistamines play a vital role in the treatment of all allergies, but especially in the treatment of anaphylactic shock, serum sickness, hay fever, and urticaria. Antihistaminic drugs commonly employed in the treatment of allergy are:

Chlorpheniramine (Chlor-Trimeton, Teldrin)
Tripelennamine (Pyribenzamine)
Promethazine (Phenergan)
Diphenhydramine hydrochloride (Benadryl)
Doxylamine (Decapryn)
Methapyrilene (Semikon, Histadyl, Thenylene)
Thonzylamine (Anahist, Neohetramine)
Triprolidine (Actifed)

A number of side effects can be caused by the use of antihistamines; the major side effect is sedation or drowsiness. Other side effects are weakness, dizziness, gastrointestinal upsets, a dry mouth, and blurred vision. When large doses are given, excitement and insomnia may sometimes develop.

Immunotherapy (Hyposensitization). When it is not possible to control hypersensitivity by separating the patient from the offending allergen, immunotherapy may be tried. "Immunotherapy is the injection of small quantities of allergens in increasing strengths . . . and at regular intervals . . . until tolerance is achieved."[13] By tolerance we mean *hyposensitization* (lessening of sensitivity) to the allergen — *not* desensitization. Desensitization or total elimination of sensitivity to an allergen is impossible. The dose of allergen that finally produces hyposensitization is administered in the future as the *maintenance dose.* To achieve a maintenance dose can take from a few months to a year.

Why exactly does hyposensitization work? The administration of allergen increases the production of IgG antibodies. IgG antibodies have a greater capacity for combining with allergens than do other immunoglobulins. Thus these IgG antibodies act as "blocking antibodies"; i.e., they compete with IgE antibodies for the allergen. By binding with allergen, the IgG antibodies leave fewer reactive sites on the allergen for IgE antibodies. IgE antibodies are less active, and cellular sensitivity to the antigen (and consequently allergic symptoms) is reduced. By keeping the patient on a schedule of immunotherapy (giving increasing doses at regular intervals), high levels of IgG are obtained. The *maintenance* dose of allergen maintains these high levels of IgG and keeps levels of IgE low.[13, 101]

An immunotherapy program involves the following: (a) extracts of the allergen to which the patient is allergic are prepared from commercial extracts; (b) a starting strength of the allergen is determined; and (c) the allergen is then injected biweekly or weekly — usually subcutaneously. Once a maintenance dose is reached, injections are usually given every 2 to 8 weeks. A hypothetical schedule of immunotherapy for a patient with inhalant allergies is presented in Table 11–10.

Immunotherapy may be given year round (perennial) or on a preseasonal or occasional basis. The therapeutic program usually continues for 3 to 5 years, and in some cases (e.g., insect sting allergies and severe allergies) for a lifetime.

Basic rules and practices to remember when assisting with the administration of immunotherapy:

1. Store vials of allergen *upright* in the *refrigerator.* Vials stored on their sides may leak, and the extract may become contaminated if it contacts the rubber and metal portions of the vial. Refrigeration of the extract prolongs its shelf life.

TABLE 11–10. HYPOTHETICAL SCHEDULE OF IMMUNOTHERAPY FOR A PATIENT WITH INHALANT ALLERGIES

Starting strength (1:100,000), once weekly
.05 ml.
.10 ml.
.15 ml.
.20 ml.
.25 ml.
.30 ml.
.35 ml.
.40 ml.
.45 ml.
.50 ml
Second strength (1:10,000), once weekly
.05 ml.
.10 ml.
.15 ml.
.20 ml.
.25 ml.
.30 ml.
.35 ml.
.40 ml.
.45 ml.
.50 ml.
Third strength (1:1,000), once weekly
.05 ml.
.10 ml.
.15 ml.
.20 ml.
.25 ml.
.30 ml.
.35 ml.
.40 ml.
.45 ml.
.50 ml.
Fourth strength (1:100), once weekly
.05 ml.
.10 ml.
.15 ml.
.20 ml.
.25 ml.
.30 ml.
.35 ml.
.35 ml. (becomes maintenance dose)

From Bridgewater, S. C., et al.: Allergies in children: Recognition. *American Journal of Nursing,* 78:613, Apr. 1978, p. 618.

2. Make certain that *emergency equipment* is on hand in case the patient should develop an anaphylactic reaction to the extract. Emergency procedures for treating anaphylactic shock are described in Unit XXVI.

3. Before administering a dose of allergen, check the *patient's identity*, check the *vial* for the name of the allergen and its strength, and check the *amount* and *date* of the last injection.

4. Ask the patient if he or she suffered a *reaction* to the last injection. Redness and swelling that exceed the size of a nickel (in a child) or a fifty-cent piece (in an adult) indicates that the dosage was too large. Withhold the current dose if the patient had a reaction of the above magnitude to the preceding dose. Note on the patient's record that the dose was withheld and why. Notify the allergist.

5. Check whether the patient has missed two or more consecutive appointments. If so, consult with the allergist before administering the allergen. The allergen may need to be rediluted or the dosage reduced.

6. Preferably give the injection in the upper outer arm. *Always use an extremity* so that a tourniquet can be applied to slow absorption of the allergen in case an anaphylactic reaction should occur. Rotate sites each appointment.[13]

7. For accurate measurement use a *tuberculin syringe*. Needles used for immunotherapy include a 26 gauge, ¼-inch needle; a 26 gauge, ⅜-inch needle; or a 25 gauge, ⅝-inch needle.

8. Before administering the allergen always remember to check that the *needle is in the subcutaneous tissues and not in a blood vessel*. Administration of an allergen directly into the blood stream could cause a deadly anaphylactic reaction.

9. Carefully observe the patient for at least 20 minutes following the injection for itching of the head, palms or soles, urticaria, a feeling of impending doom, laryngeal edema, and shock. Take appropriate action immediately should these symptoms of a systemic reaction develop.

DISEASES ASSOCIATED WITH HYPERSENSITIVITY REACTIONS

We have mentioned these diseases in our previous discussion. With an understanding of underlying mechanisms, diagnosis, and general treatment of hypersensitivity, it is now possible to examine such disorders and their specific management in more detail.* Of particular interest are anaphylaxis, serum sickness, hay fever, urticaria (hives), bronchial asthma, systemic lupus erythematosus, and contact dermatitis.

Anaphylaxis. Anaphylaxis is one of the most dramatic and feared of the allergic reactions. It can occur in any species of animal — humans, dogs, and guinea pigs, to name but a few. Fortunately it is relatively rare in humans.

Anaphylaxis is a systemic form of *immediate hypersensitivity* (Type I) usually precipitated by *injection of a drug* or by an *insect sting* to a *sensitized* individual. The reaction occurs rapidly and may result in death through respiratory obstruction or vascular collapse. A list of important agents causing anaphylaxis is shown in Table 11–11.

TABLE 11–11. AGENTS ASSOCIATED WITH ANAPHYLAXIS

Drugs
Penicillins
Cephalosporins
Streptomycin
Tetracyclines
Sulfonamides
Dextran
Insulin
Chemotherapy agents
ACTH
Opiates (direct histamine release)
Foods
Eggs
Nuts (Brazil nut, black walnut, pecan, hazel nut, hickory nut, pistachio, chestnut, English walnut, almond)
Legumes (peanut, chickpea, pinto bean, soybean, kidney bean)
Fish
Shellfish
Seeds (sesame, cottonseed, flax seed, poppy seed, sunflower seed, caraway)
Insect Venoms
Hymenoptera (bees, hornets, wasps, yellow jackets, fire ants)
Horse Serum
Tetanus antitoxin
Diphtheria antitoxin
Antilymphocyte globulin
Rabies antitoxin
Snake venom antitoxin
Allergenic Extracts
Skin testing agents
Allergic immunotherapy (hyposensitization)
Blood Products
Whole blood
Plasma
Platelets
Gamma globulin
Cryoprecipitate
Other clotting factor preparations
Other blood constituents

From Lockey, R. F., and R. W. Fox: Allergic emergencies. *Hospital Medicine,* 15:67, June 1979, by permission.

As you recall, the reaction is mediated by IgE antibodies on mast cells, which release histamine and serotonin. The *cardiovascular* response to these chemicals includes hypotension and shock due to vasodilatation and increased vascular permeability; the *respiratory* tract response involves the nasal passages, larynx, and bronchi where edema and bronchospasm lead to obstruction of airways. Edema and constriction of smooth muscle in the *gastrointestinal* tract and *skin* are less life-threatening symptoms, yet may persist for weeks following an acute anaphylaxis reaction.

TREATMENT. The *treatment* of anaphylactic shock depends on the organ systems involved, but speed is essential in all cases. Anaphylaxis is

*Anaphylactic shock is discussed further in Unit XXVI, bronchial asthma in Unit XVI, and systemic lupus erythematosus and contact dermatitis in Chapter 79.

an emergency. There is no time to waste — the patient may die in minutes! The major therapies employed in anaphylactic shock are outlined below:

1. *Drug therapy to counteract histamine*
   a. *Epinephrine, a sympathomimetic drug, has an immediate counteraction against histamine.*
   b. *Antihistamines block histamine action peripherally*
   c. *Corticosteroids aid in recovery from initial shock*
   d. *Aminophylline, a xanthine, is used to treat bronchospasm*
2. *Oxygen therapy to counteract asphyxia*
3. *Maintenance of an airway*
4. *Correct hypotension and shock*
   a. *Levarterenol bitartrate*
   b. *Metaraminol bitartrate*
   c. *Monitor blood pressure*

Drug Therapy. The major drugs used to treat anaphylactic reactions include sympathomimetics, antihistamines, corticosteroids, and aminophylline. The action of these drugs will be described briefly.

► *Sympathomimetics.* These drugs include epinephrine, isoproterenol, and ephedrine sulfate. Their actions on the body are directly opposite to that of histamine and can halt anaphylactic symptoms in emergency situations. The most important sympathomimetic drug used in the treatment of anaphylaxis is *epinephrine*. Side effects of the sympathomimetics include nervousness, muscle twitching, insomnia, palpitations, tachycardia, sweating, and anxiety. Hypertension is an important secondary effect of epinephrine, and the blood pressure of the patient should be monitored closely.

► *Antihistamines.* These drugs act as competitive inhibitors of histamine, and they help to reverse some of the life-threatening symptoms associated with anaphylaxis. However, the primary usefulness of antihistamines lies in the management of the urticaria and angioedema (appearance of large edematous wheals on skin and mucous membranes) precipitated by serum sickness.[103a] Antihistamines most commonly used are Benadryl (diphenhydramine hydrochloride) IV and Chlor-Trimeton (chlorpheniramine maleate).

► *Corticosteroids.* Steroids have an anti-inflammatory action and in high doses suppress the immune response. Corticosteroids are rarely used in the immediate treatment of anaphylaxis because their action onset is slow. However, steroids can be prescribed for individuals with severe respiratory distress or hypotension that remains unresponsive to other forms of treatment.[103a] These potent drugs are dangerous because they affect all aspects of the body's immune system as well as the hypersensitive responses, leaving the patient susceptible to many threatening situations. Side effects include Cushingoid features, due to sodium retention and edema, and osteoporesis (softening of the bone). Steroids commonly used are hydrocortisone sodium succinate (Solu-Cortef) and prednisolone hemisuccinate (Metacortelone).

► *Xanthines.* These drugs act as bronchodilators; they inhibit phosphodiesterase, allowing a high level of cAMP, which results in the relaxation of smooth muscle tissue. (See Fig. 11–9.) *Aminophylline* is used to dilate the bronchi of patients in anaphylaxis if wheezing is present without hypotension. The drug is most effective when used with sympathomimetics.

Oxygen Therapy. Since patients with anaphylaxis suffer from bronchial constriction and asphyxia, their need for oxygen is great. The use of a nasal catheter or of positive pressure oxygen therapy is effective if necessary. Monitoring blood gases is essential in the course of the treatment.

Maintenance of an Open Airway. The attending nurse or physician should be prepared to give mouth-to-mouth resuscitation should the patient become cyanotic.

Correction of Shock. Restoration of circulating fluid volume is accomplished with physiologic saline, plasma, or whole blood if the patient is in profound shock. Vasopressors such as levarterenol bitartrate (Levophed) and metaraminol bitartrate (Aramine) given IV may be used. Monitor the blood pressure.

Both Levophed and Aramine are extremely dangerous drugs. Both are capable of causing sloughing of the tissues around the needle site as well as a severe elevation in blood pressure. In caring for patients on these vasopressor drugs, remember the following:*

1. *Check the injection site every few minutes for signs of infiltration of the medication. Remember that infiltration of Levophed or Aramine can cause tissue sloughing and gangrene!*
2. *Continually monitor the blood pressure and pulse of patients on these drugs. Adjust the rate of flow to maintain a constant blood pressure at the level ordered by the doctor.*
3. *Never leave a patient on Aramine or Levophed unattended. During your absence from the bedside, the IV drip may begin to accelerate or the needle may slip out of the vein, causing this necrotizing solution to infiltrate into the patient's tissues.*

PREVENTION. Obviously it is far better to *prevent* the development of anaphylactic shock than

*Levophed and Aramine are discussed in Chapter 13, "Shock," and in the care of the patient with myocardial infarction, Chapter 36.

to be forced to treat it. There are several precautionary measures that physicians and nurses can take to prevent anaphylactic shock. First of all, physicians should use *caution* in the prescription of potentially dangerous drugs, especially if the patient under their care has a history of such allergies as hay fever or bronchial asthma. Second, it is the doctor's and nurse's responsibility to ask the patient whether she or he has suffered from allergic attacks in the past whenever *any* drug is to be administered parenterally, or penicillin is to be given *either* orally or parenterally. Some important questions that you might specifically ask your patient *prior* to the administration of these drug preparations are:

1. *Have you ever been troubled by hay fever, asthma, dermatitis, or any other type of allergy?*
2. *Have you ever had an injection of the drug that I am now going to administer?*
3. *Have you ever experienced an allergic reaction to the particular drug I am preparing to give you?*

Carefully evaluate the patient's answers to these questions, and be prepared to take the following actions:

▶ 1. If the patient does have a definite history of allergy, check with the physician *before* you give the drug to make sure that the doctor is aware of this fact.

▶ 2. If the patient has had a prior allergic reaction to the particular drug that you are now going to give, *do not give the drug* either orally or parenterally! Report your findings immediately to the physician.

Prior to diagnostic procedure using radiopaque contrast media, inquire if the patient is sensitive to iodine-containing substances or has ever had a reaction to contrast media.[8] Before administering a vaccine grown in egg embryo (rubella, mumps, influenza, yellow fever, and rabies, ask if the patient has a history of egg hypersensitivity.[8]

▶ 3. If the patient has a history of allergy to *any* drug, mark this information *clearly* on the patient's chart, on the Kardex, and at the patient's bedside. Remember that a sick individual may not always be able to inform nurses and other personnel of her or his vulnerable allergic state.

There is a third major preventive measure against anaphylactic shock. When you are preparing to give any drug parenterally or to administer penicillin either orally or parenterally, be certain that *emergency drugs are readily available.* (See Unit XXVI.)

As a fourth precaution, patients should be instructed to obtain and wear a medical information *bracelet* or medallion that states the drugs or allergens to which they are allergic. Patients can also carry medical identification cards.

As a final preventive measure, if a patient is definitely allergic to a drug that he or she *must* receive, physicians will then attempt to *hyposensitize* the patient against the allergic effects of the drug (see p. 159).

Special Precautions for Persons Sensitive to Hymenoptera Stings. Since anaphylactic shock may develop from *bee* or other *insect stings* as well as from drugs, let us briefly consider some precautionary measures that persons susceptible to such stings should be taught to observe. Hypersensitive persons must avoid: (1) wearing perfume and bright colors, as these attract insects; (2) excessive exposure of their skin, especially around the neck; (3) sitting or lying down on the grass in areas where there are many bushes, hedges, flowers, and trees; and (4) going barefoot. Moreover, persons susceptible to insect stings should carry emergency insect bite kits and know how to use them.[8] One authority recommends that hypersensitive persons learn to administer epinephrine to themselves. At least, epinephrine should be carried by the individual along with a card stating that he or she is allergic to insect stings and should have *immediate* care if stung. Finally, victims of insect stings should be skin tested and then desensitized against the particular species of insect to which they are allergic.

Serum Sickness. In contrast to anaphylactic shock, *serum sickness* is a generally nonfatal, self-limiting ailment that occurs within 1 to 3 weeks following exposure to an antigenic drug substance. On the other hand, serum sickness is similar to anaphylactic shock in that it can occur after the administration of *any* drug and after the administration of any foreign (usually equine) serum. Currently serum sickness is most commonly induced by penicillin. The use of human serum (especially human antitetanus serum) has reduced the incidence of this disorder.[8]

Since serum sickness does not develop immediately, you may wonder why it is classified, along with anaphylactic shock, as an "immediate" hypersensitivity. Serum sickness is classified as an immediate rather than as a delayed reaction because it is attributable to the presence of *humoral antibodies* and not to the presence of cellular antibodies.

Let us briefly consider the *pathogenesis* of serum sickness. The usual course of events that ultimately lead to serum sickness is as follows: (1) A patient is injected with a particular serum or is given a particular drug against which he or she has no immune bodies. (Note how serum sickness differs from anaphylaxis in that the individual has *not* been previously sensitized to the drug or serum.) (2) Within 10 days, antibodies have formed against the foreign antigen, which still continues to be present in the blood. (3) An extensive, overall allergic reaction takes place.

The *treatment* of serum sickness depends upon the severity of the reaction. The drugs generally used in mild reactions are antihistamines and aspirin. In more severe types of serum sickness reactions, not only antihistamines are given, but epinephrine and cortisone as well. Very severe forms of serum sickness should be treated in the same manner as anaphylactic shock.

Serum sickness can be prevented by the same precautions that prevent anaphylactic shock. In review, to prevent either of these reactions, remember the following rules:

1. *Know your patient's past history of allergy.*
2. *Know specifically what drugs your patient has been allergic to in the past.*
3. *Immediately report any unusual findings concerning the patient's allergic history to the doctor.*
4. *If the patient has a history of allergy, mark this information clearly on the chart, the Kardex, and at the bedside.*

Allergic Rhinitis (Hay Fever). Hay fever is a seasonal allergy that is caused by contact with such allergens as tree pollens, grasses, or plants, e.g., ragweed. Hay fever is an example of a localized Type I anaphylactic (atopic) reaction that involves IgE antibodies. The major problem in hay fever is edema and congestion of the mucous membranes of the nose as a result of the release of histamine. Major signs and symptoms of hay fever are: inflammation of the conjunctivae and tearing, bouts of violent sneezing, and discharge of watery substance from the nose. Hay fever can be treated by first skin testing the patient to see to what particular substances he or she is allergic, and then slowly hyposensitizing him or her against the particular allergen. The drugs of choice in the treatment of hay fever are *antihistamines,* which help to counteract the effects of histamines upon the blood vessels and thereby help to prevent the symptoms of hay fever. Sympathomimetic drugs such as ephedrine and phenylpropanolamine may also be ordered, either alone or in combination with antihistamines. In severe uncontrolled hay fever, the patient may require corticosteroids to ease symptoms.

Urticaria. Urticaria comes from the Latin *urtica,* nettle. This atopic allergy, which is sometimes called "the hives," is the result of contact between a person with a hereditary predisposition and such allergens as plants, foods, pollens, certain drugs, and insect venom. The most common immunologic mechanism underlying urticaria is a Type I hypersensitivity reaction mediated by IgE. Externally urticaria is distinguished by the appearance of large welts or wheals, and internally by small areas of edema that appear throughout the internal organs. The signs of urticaria are probably due to the dilatation of arterioles and to the leakage of fluid out of the capillaries into the tissue spaces. Treatment involves avoidance of the allergen, and drug therapy with antihistaminic drugs. For certain patients the doctor may order epinephrine or ephedrine subcutaneously. Cortisone is sometimes used in more severe cases of hives. Starch baths twice daily and the application of calamine lotion also help relieve *itching* — the classic symptom of urticaria.

Bronchial Asthma. Bronchial asthma, also known as allergic asthma, is a Type I hypersensitivity reaction. This common condition affects individuals who have a hereditary predisposition to the development of allergy. In this type of asthma, the bronchial walls are hypersensitive to foreign substances such as egg whites, plant pollens, vegetable dust, and pet hairs. In addition, there can be sensitivity to certain bacteria that normally dwell within the respiratory tract. Thus, the individual may be hypersensitive to both intrinsic and extrinsic agents. Upon exposure to these antigenic agents, individuals prone to bronchial asthma suffer from constriction of bronchial passages and edema of the mucous membranes of the bronchi. Bronchial constriction and edema are the basis of such symptoms as dyspnea (especially upon exertion), severe wheezing, and a sense of suffocation.

In the treatment of bronchial asthma, antihistamines are of little value. For mild and moderate attacks, *epinephrine* is the drug of choice. The effective drugs for asthma include:

- *Epinephrine* injection (1:1000) 0.2 to 0.5 ml. subcutaneously, repeated every 1 to 2 hours in moderate attacks. Epinephrine may also be used in spray form.
- *Aminophylline.* Another important drug in the treatment of bronchial asthma, aminophylline is especially effective when used in conjunction with epinephrine. Aminophylline is liable to cause gastric irritation or central nervous stimulation manifested as tachycardia, insomnia, or possibly seizures. There are other preparations on the market that may be better tolerated in terms of less gastrointestinal distress and longer duration of activity. These include Slo-Phyllin, Elixophyllin, and Aerolate.[20] These drugs must be given around-the-clock for full benefit.
- *Cromolyn sodium.* This is a powder administered in 20 mg. doses by inhalation. It is not a bronchodilator, but inhibits the release of histamine from mast cells by stabilizing the mast cell, preventing degranulation. It is used as long-term prophylactic therapy in bronchial asthma and is more effective in younger asthmatic patients than in adults. It has no effect in acute attacks of asthma.

Other drugs that are used in the treatment of bronchial asthma are ephedrine, ACTH, and beclomethasone (a steroid inhalant). As in other atopic allergies, it is important for the patient to avoid, as much as possible, the specific allergen that is causing the problem.

Systemic Lupus Erythematosus (SLE). SLE is a chronic inflammatory disease of unknown origin that affects many organ systems. It is characterized by autoantibodies to nuclear constituents — particularly DNA. These constituents form complexes with the antibody and localize within blood vessels and tissues. Deposition of complexes (Type III mechanism) is manifested by fever, an erythematous rash on the face and hands, and involvement of joints, central nervous system, skin, red blood cells, and platelets with these complexes. Renal failure is a frequent and serious feature of SLE. Because SLE is characterized by *both* the formation and deposition of antigen-antibody complexes and the formation of autoantibodies, it is classified as both an autoimmune disorder and a Type III sensitivity reaction (immune complex disorder).

At the onset of SLE, there is no characteristic pattern of clinical features nor is there any consistency in the course of the illness. SLE has a high incidence in women, and it usually appears in the second decade of life. The most common cutaneous feature of SLE is an *erythematous rash* on the cheeks, crossing the bridge of the nose. This is termed the "butterfly rash." These rashes are not confined to just the face but occur in any well-vascularized tissue and they seem to be especially acute upon exposure to sunlight. *Polyarthralgia* or arthritis occurs in 90 per cent of patients and frequently is the initial symptom of SLE. Any joint can be affected. In most cases, joint symptoms are transient and respond rapidly to treatment.

Lupus nephritis is a very frequent and a most serious feature of SLE. Renal involvement usually appears early in the course of the illness, in the form of microscopic hematuria, proteinuria, and red cell casts. Renal lesions may be identified with kidney biopsy material.

Diagnosis of SLE is made on the basis of the above clinical symptoms, but diagnosis is difficult to verify without appropriate lab tests. The presence of serum antibodies against DNA and DNA proteins is strong evidence for SLE. Their presence must be tested for before treatment with steroids.

Treatment of SLE is generally individual, depending on the patient's symptoms.[111] If arthritis is the main symptom, *salicylates* in high doses are usually the treatment of choice. Administration of *steroids* in severe SLE can suppress disease activity by suppressing inflammation. SLE can range from a mild discomfort to a fatal disease. *Renal failure* and *infections* have been the leading cause of death. However, the 5-year survival rate has markedly improved over the last decade, and is now approaching 80 to 90 per cent.

Contact Dermatitis. Contact dermatitis is perhaps the only example of a pathologic process that is wholly the result of a *delayed skin reaction* (Type IV hypersensitivity reaction). It is the most common immunologic disease encountered by dermatologists. The potential allergens involved include drugs, dyes, preservatives, and metals. Contact dermatitis is an *eczematous* reaction, characterized by erythema, edema, and vesiculation, and, perhaps later on, by scaling. The lesions involve perivascular macrophage infiltration. Eczematous reactions are not exclusive to allergic contact dermatitis. Thus, proper diagnosis of this disease requires a *patch test* for confirmation. The suspected antigen is placed in low concentration on the patient's skin and covered with a dressing; the dressing is removed after 48 hours. An eczematous reaction at the site of the patch test constitutes a positive response.

Avoidance of the suspected or known allergens is the best method of treatment. Symptomatic therapy consists of the application of wet dressings, employing Burow's solution plus a 1% hypercortisone cream or lotion. Very severe cases may require the use of steroids.[20]

4. Autoimmune Diseases

In the past immunologists believed that the body reacted with an immune response only against proteins of foreign origin. Physiologists took it for granted that the body would always recognize its *own* proteins and would never make the frightening error of responding to its own materials by the formation of antibodies. The repellency of the very notion that the body might react against its own "self" is expressed clearly in Paul Ehrlich's descriptive term "horror autotoxicus."

Today we realize that it is possible for certain of our own body proteins to be regarded as not-self by the body, and consequently to be reacted against by the body's immunologic system. When such an unfortunate failure to distinguish self from non-self occurs and autoantibodies are formed, the pathologic condition is called an *autoimmune disorder*. The mechanisms underlying autoimmune disease are the same as those of normal immune responses, involving both humoral and cellular components. Normally, antibody and complement together destroy cells, and lymphocytes exert cytotoxic effects both directly and from a distance — thus protecting the individual against foreign invaders. However, in autoimmune diseases, there is a marked *abnormal or excessive activity* on the part of these components. It is still unclear whether this is the fault of the T-cells and B-cells themselves or of faulty regulation of the immune system. Autoimmunity plays a role in a wide range of clinical situations, including aging, response to infections, organ-specific immune diseases (e.g., thyroiditis), and generalized systemic immune disorders (SLE and rheumatoid arthritis).[42]

Theories of Autoimmune Disease. In viewing the evolutionary background of human beings, it is generally true that those factors that are maladaptive have been eliminated, while factors which have adaptive value have been retained. If this is the case, why do autoimmune reactions still exist when they are so maladaptive in nature?

This is not an easy question to answer. As Robbins and Angell point out:

> It is obvious that autoimmunity implies loss of self tolerance. . . . With our imperfect understanding of the nature of self tolerance it is no surprise that a multiplicity of theories have been invoked to explain its loss and the consequent emergence of autoimmune reactions.[87]

Some of the more widely accepted theories of autoimmune disease that have been proposed are the following:

- *Release of sequestered self antigens* may trigger a reaction. Some antigens are sequestered within organs, and consequently, the immune system never has a chance to establish immunologic tolerance to them. Tissue damage of certain organs may release these antigens into the circulation, provoking production of autoantibodies.
- *A pathologic condition or exogenous agent* (e.g., drug, virus, bacteria, radiant energy) may alter the body's tissues so that they are no longer recognized by the body's protective antibodies as "self." For instance, the inflammation that accompanies chronic infection may alter the configuration of a tissue's molecules.
- *The structure of some infectious agents* may be so similar to those of certain tissue components that the normal antibody response to the infectious agent is unable to recognize the self tissues as forbidden reaction territory.
- *Virus infections* may cause certain autoimmune disorders. Recent investigations have shown that viruses damage T-cells, rendering the helper and suppressor T-cell populations incapable of controlling antibody synthesis.[81]
- *A clone of cells may emerge* that is reactive against the self, owing to a *mutation* of an *immunocompetent cell* (i.e., a T-cell or a B cell). Investigators have noted that "frequency of autoantibodies in the general population rises progressively with age, and this is possibly related to an increasing predisposition to mutational events in the later years of life."
- *The combining of a hapten with a body protein* may be one basis of autoimmune disease. You recall that a hapten is a normally nonantigenic substance that has the capacity to combine with a body protein. Evidently, once a hapten combines with a body protein, the body protein can be modified in such a way that it will act as a foreign antigen. Important haptens that may possibly elicit autoimmune reactions are drugs, industrial chemicals, constituents in dust, and breakdown products from horse dander. Remember that the items listed are not in themselves antigenic to the body. It is only when a particular drug or chemical, for example, an antibiotic, combines with a body protein, and only slightly modifies it, that the drug or chemical can cause the body to react immunologically.
- *The genetic instructions for antibody production* might be altered so that the specificity of the resultant immunoglobulin is directed toward self components. Some individuals seem to have a genetic predisposition toward autoimmune disease. For example, there is a higher incidence of these diseases in women; some strains of animals are more vulnerable to autoimmune disorders than other strains; healthy close relatives of persons with autoimmune diseases have a high incidence of circulating autoantibodies.
- A change in the body's metabolism, a disease, or an injury may so *alter an immunocompetent cell* that its specificity for an antigen is directed against self.

It must be evident from the above that the field of autoimmune disease abounds with theories but has few confirmed, established facts. Furthermore, not only is the cause of autoimmune disease uncertain, but even which diseases are truly autoimmune in origin is controversial. Nevertheless, some known autoimmune diseases are listed in Table 11–12, along with the antigen against which the body has produced autoantibodies. The etiology of these diseases is as yet unknown, despite the discovery of some of the antigens.

Sometimes you will find that the terms "diffuse collagen disease" and "connective tissue disease" are used in referring to the following conditions: systemic lupus erythematosus, polyarteritis nodosa, rheumatic fever, rheumatoid arthritis, and scleroderma. These disorders are called collagen diseases because they are generally characterized by changes in collagenous connective tissue — a type of tissue that is widely scattered throughout the body. The term "collagen disease," therefore, refers to the *site of involvement,* while the term "autoimmune disease" refers to the *cause* of the condition.

General Treatment of Autoimmune Conditions. We shall be discussing the treatment of patients with specific autoimmune diseases as appropriate throughout this textbook. While

TABLE 11–12. AUTOIMMUNE DISEASES, ANTIGEN, AND DISEASE PROCESS

Disease	Antigen	Disease process
Autoimmune hemolytic anemia	Red cell	RBC destruction
Idiopathic thrombocytopenia purpura	Platelet	Platelet destruction
Male infertility (some cases)	Sperm	Agglutination of spermatoza
Hashimoto's disease	Thyroid surface antigen	Cytotoxic effect on thyroid cells in culture
Goodpasture's syndrome	Lung and glomeruli basement membrane	Complement-mediated damage
SLE	DNA and others?	Immune complex-mediated damage
Rheumatoid arthritis	IgG	Arthritis

treatment does vary for each condition, we can make a few general statements concerning the care of persons afflicted by any type of autoimmune disease. The treatment of autoimmune conditions is always potentially dangerous. Unfortunately, most of the effective methods of suppressing the formation of autoantibodies also suppresses the immune system in general. Thus in attempting to eliminate the body's antigenic reaction against itself, we cannot help but upset those homeostatic mechanisms of immunity that serve to protect against foreign invaders.

The most commonly used general measures in autoimmune disease are: (1) the administration of corticosteroids and (2) the administration of salicylates. The *corticosteroids* are highly beneficial in the treatment of autoimmune diseases because they produce anti-inflammatory effects, promote lymphocytolysis, suppress antibody production, and weaken or inhibit the effects of antigen-antibody interaction. On the other hand, corticosteroids are dangerous in that they lower the patient's resistance to new infections. Moreover, since the corticosteroids suppress inflammatory reactions, the patient taking corticosteroids, who is also concomitantly suffering from an infection, may be without those symptoms (redness, heat, fever, pain, swelling) that would call attention to the infection.

The *salicylates* have been used for years by physicians in their attempts to relieve the symptoms of rheumatic fever and rheumatoid arthritis. While aspirin is helpful in the relief of symptoms, it is not curative.

In sum, there is as yet no cure for autoimmune disease nor is there any way to prevent it from developing. As immunologists focus more sharply upon the possible causes of autoimmune diseases, there may emerge in the next 10 to 15 years some breakthroughs in the care of persons with these as yet mysterious diseases.

Rheumatoid Arthritis: An Autoimmune Disease. Our representative autoimmune disease is rheumatoid arthritis, which is considered in detail in Unit XX. Briefly, rheumatoid arthritis is a chronic inflammatory disease that occurs when individuals make autoantibodies to their own IgG immunoglobulins. The resulting complexes cause pathologic changes in joints, eventually crippling the individual. The etiology of this disease is unknown, although researchers speculate that chronic bacterial or viral infections may alter the IgG molecules so that they are no longer recognized as self. The disease affects 1 to 3 per cent of Americans yearly, with a female-to-male ratio of 3:1. The usual age of onset is between 20 and 40 years, with symptoms of joint pain, malaise, and fatigue. *Salicylates* are the treatment of choice to reduce inflammation. This disease can be devastating psychologically to the patient and treatment must be holistic — involving medical treatment, physical therapy, comfort measures, and psychologic counseling.[9, 30, 31, 119]

IMMUNOLOGIC ASPECTS OF TRANSPLANT REJECTION

The successful transplantation of organs and tissues as a means of preserving life, correcting deformities, and repairing organic damage has been an age-old dream of physicians. In recent years, as a result of scientific advances in both surgery and physiology, that dream seems to be coming true. As a result of new discoveries in the field of immunology, complex types of transplant surgery have become more common, and these techniques are today a subject of intense interest and concern for professional personnel and laymen alike. Indeed, transplants have been highly newsworthy since December 1967, when the first heart transplant was performed in South Africa.

The major problem in transplanting organs and tissues from one body to another has not been the technical difficulties of surgery; rather the difficulty is that the body, because of the homeostatic mechanism of immunity, tends to immediately reject anything that is not self. Thus, when an attempt is made to transplant an organ, such as the kidney or heart, from one person to another, the transplantation surgery is successful for only a brief time. Then, with deadly efficiency, rejection ultimately begins, and the transplanted tissue shrivels and dies.

Let us now focus our attention briefly on the actual *mechanism* of transplant rejection; which *types* of transplants are most likely to be quickly rejected; *therapeutic measures* that can be taken to suppress the transplant rejection reaction; and the future of transplant surgery.

The Vocabulary of Transplantation Surgery

As you read about transplantation surgery, you will discover a number of terms that may be new to you. The most important terms that you need to know are:

- *Autograft* (autogenous transplant). This term is derived from "auto," which means *self*. An autograft is tissue that is transplanted from one part of a person's body to another part of his or her body —for example, a skin graft with a pedicle flap. This type of transplant, made of the patient's own tissues, is usually successful.
- *Allograft* (homotransplant or homograft) is a transplant that is made between *nonidentical* members of the same species; for example, a heart transplant between two nonrelated people. These transplants are usually unsuccessful unless potent immunosuppressive measures are taken. However, there are pronounced differences in the extent and type of allograft rejection that follows transplantation. As you will see, corneal transplants as well as bone and blood vessel grafts are much less adversely affected than are heart and kidney transplants.

- *Isotransplant* (isograft) is a tissue exchange between *identical* twins. Isotransplants have a greater history of success than do allografts.
- *Xenografts* (heterografts) are tissues that are transplanted between species; for example, from a dog to a cat, or from a rat to a mouse. Xenografts are rapidly rejected because vascular anastomoses are almost never established.

The vocabulary of transplantation surgery involves not only types of grafts but also the possible outcome of the surgery. A few words that you may read or hear include:

- *"Take"* is a successful transplantation in which the wound heals and the transplant functions effectively.
- *Allograft reaction* is the customary type of transplant rejection, in which the allograft transplant is initially accepted and then rejected by the body and ultimately destroyed.
- *White graft reaction* is a rapid form of transplant rejection that occurs between species. For example, a skin graft that is transplanted between species is always white and bloodless in appearance. It soon dies, shrivels, and is then discarded, as a scale.

Mechanism of Allograft Rejection

Although a cause for considerable consternation among surgeons and physicians, allograft rejection is actually a normal homeostatic function of the body. Because an allograft is clearly not-self, allograft rejection is expected in a healthy organism. As stated earlier, the body's adverse reactions to transplants are evidently mediated by the lymphoid system and are a form of *cellular immunity* rather than humoral immunity.

Allografts of skin seem to be more susceptible to rejection than are grafts of most other tissues or organs. The early healing processes in primary skin allografts are similar to those of autografts. Except in rare cases, there is no immediate response. Allografts soon become infiltrated with lymphocytes, macrophages, and plasma cells. Within a week, the rejection apparently has begun.

During the inflammatory process, venules within the graft are the first blood vessels to be damaged, followed by the capillaries, and, finally, the small and then the large arteries. Because of injury and damage to the blood vessels, *ischemia* (a local anemia caused by the obstruction of circulation) develops, and cell damage and necrosis soon ensue. Thus, the graft is destroyed. This whole dramatic rejection process takes approximately 10 days. Should the host receive a *second* transplant from the *same* donor, his or her "sensitized" lymphocytes will quickly produce antibodies against the tissues of the donor, and the second transplant will be rejected even more rapidly than the first — within 4 to 5 days as opposed to 10 days. This accelerated rejection response to the second transplant from the same donor is known as a *second set reaction.*

As stated earlier, the extent of the allograft rejection process as well as the damage produced depends upon the *type* of tissue that is being transplanted between two unrelated members of the same species. For instance, *corneal transplants* are highly successful and are rarely rejected. There are two reasons that corneal transplants take so well. First of all, the cornea is poorly vascularized. Because of a lack of vascular connection between host and donor, the recognition or afferent arc of the rejection process is nullified, since without *recognition* of foreignness there can be no reaction. Second, the cornea contains few cells, and therefore little antigen can be released by the transplanted tissues. Thus, corneal transplants tend to survive the body's usually relentless immunologic mechanism.

In contrast to a corneal transplant, a kidney transplant between an unrelated donor and host typifies the allograft rejection process with all its swift deadliness. For the first few days following the kidney transplant, the kidney is able to put out urine and it tends to function satisfactorily. However, when the rejection process begins, urine output diminishes dramatically, and the renal tissue becomes tender, swollen, and dusky in appearance. Within approximately 10 days the transplanted kidney will cease to be viable unless potent immunosuppressive techniques are employed.

With bone, fascia, and blood vessel grafts, the tissues do not survive the rejection process, *but* the transplant is nevertheless successful. In these types of grafts, the dead cells of the transplanted tissue simply serve as a "scaffolding" over which the patient's own tissues will eventually grow by means of a process called "creeping substitution."

While rejection rarely occurs in corneal transplants, and generally does not affect the success of bone, fascia, and blood vessel grafts, allograft rejection is the major problem surgeons face when performing any other type of transplant procedure.

Overcoming Transplant Rejection Postoperatively

To date there is no one method that is completely successful in overcoming the allograft rejection process. However, surgeons and immunologists are conducting extensive research to discover a method that will make the problem of organ and transplant rejection a concern of the past. Some of the major techniques that surgeons employ for suppressing and preventing rejection are briefly discussed below.

Immunosuppressive Techniques. These do not prevent transplant rejection from occurring; they simply suppress rejection once the process has started. All the following immunosuppressive agents are used to decrease the amount of lymphoid tissue in the body and to lower the number of circulating lymphocytes.

Corticosteroids suppress the destructive inflammatory reaction that occurs at the site of the transplant. Unfortunately the corticosteroids affect *all cells* rather than just lymphoid cells; moreover, they are capable of suppressing all immune responses and not just the rejection response, making the patient more susceptible to infections. Thus, when corticosteroids are used for immunosuppressive purposes, physicians and nurses must use *flawless* sterile techniques during the surgical procedure and after it; also, they must carefully observe the patient for signs of such postoperative infectious complications as pneumonia.

Cytotoxic drugs also serve to reduce the potency of the immune response by destroying or suppressing lymphoid tissue. Perhaps the most commonly used drug is this field in azathioprine (Imuran). Besides immunosuppression, this drug also inhibits inflammation. Methotrexate, a folic acid antagonist, is also used to inhibit the synthesis of nucleic acids.

Antilymphocyte serum (ALS) is an important immunosuppressive agent, especially when used in conjunction with prednisone and azathioprine. ALS is prepared in horses by immunizing them with human T-cells. *Antilymphocyte globulin* (ALG) refers to any ALS that is prepared against various types of lymphocytes; that is, lymph node lymphocytes, thymocytes, and thoracic duct cells. If given to an animal that has been sensitized by graft rejection, ALS can erase the memory of the primary contact with the antigen by depleting the animal of its sensitized lymphocytes (T-cells). The exact mechanism is unclear, but ALS appears to neutralize the T-cells or their soluble factors. The major advantage of ALS over other immunosuppressive agents is that it affects *only those lymphocytes that are involved in graft rejection*, while lymphocytes that protect the body against bacterial invasion are spared.[37]

Prevention of Transplant Rejection Preoperatively

Tissue typing techniques are currently used with success prior to transplant surgery, as a preventive measure against allograft rejection. The purpose of tissue typing is to match graft donors and graft recipients as closely as possible in order to reduce the severity of the rejection response. Thus, tissue typing is much like blood typing; in both instances an attempt is made to match donor and recipient and thereby minimize adverse reactions. The antigens that cause graft rejection are called *histocompatibility antigens (HL-A)* and are present on every living cell in our bodies.[10] Although any cell may theoretically be used for HL-typing, the most readily available are white blood cells and platelets of the blood. Currently, all HL-A typing is done with lymphocytes. While its usefulness is unquestioned, better definition of histocompatibility antigens is necessary, and the search for further antigen loci on chromosomes continues.

Second, the administration of *blood transfusions* to *prospective* organ transplant recipients apparently has a positive effect upon graft survival. Salvatierra and his research team reported that in their experience "kidney recipients who received more than five blood transfusions before transplantation had a 62 per cent survival rate at 12 months in contrast to a 51 per cent graft survival for those receiving five or fewer transfusions" and a 31 per cent survival rate in those recipients receiving no transfusions prior to transplant. Graft protection by blood transfusion administration is being reported worldwide. However, there are risks in the indiscriminate use of blood transfusions, and further investigations are underway.[55]

Ethical Considerations and Transplants

Once the transplant procedure becomes relatively easy and safe technically, there are still many ethical problems that must be considered in its use. Is the replacement of old and damaged organs in an elderly person a humane procedure? What are the ethical considerations in the use of donors? If vital organs are removed from a dying donor, how can the moment of death be precisely determined, so that removal of the organ will not cause the donor's death, and yet the removed tissues will be viable enough to become functional within the recipient's body? How will the widespread use of transplants ultimately affect the human species in terms of adaptation and evolution? These questions are among the major ethical dilemmas that physicians and nurses must face and solve.

BIBLIOGRAPHY (Chapter 11)

1. Allergies, Junior Style. *Emergency Medicine,* 11:106, Apr. 1979.
2. Allison, A. C., et al.: Self-tolerance and autoimmunity. *British Medical Bulletin,* 32:124, May 1976.
3. Armstrong, D.: Whom to vaccinate — and when. *Consultant,* 16:21, Oct. 1976.
4. Asperheim, M. K., and L. A. Eisenhauer: *The Pharmacologic Basis of Patient Care,* 3rd ed. Philadelphia: W. B. Saunders Co., 1977.
5. Asthma, Parts 1 and 2. *In* "Handbook for the Asthmatic." The Allergy Foundation of America, 801 Second Ave., New York, N.Y. 10017.

5a. Bader, M.: Infection control: Immunization. *Topics in Clinical Nursing.* 1:7, July 1979.

6. Barbee, R. A., et al.: Immediate skin test reactivity in a general population sample. *Annals of Internal Medicine,* 84:129, Feb. 1976.
7. Benacerraf, B., et al.: The histocompatibility-linked immune response genes. *Advances in Cancer Research,* 21:121, 1975.

8. Blue, J. A.: Anaphylaxis and serum sickness. *In* Conn, H. F. (Ed.): *Current Therapy*. Philadelphia: W. B. Saunders Co., 1979.
9. Bluestone, R.: Core curriculum symposium #13: Rheumatoid variants. *Postgraduate Medicine,* 61:123, Jan. 1977.
10. Bodmer, W. F.: The HL-A system and its association with immune response and disease. *In* Dumonde, D. C. (Ed.): *Infection and Immunity in the Rheumatic Diseases.* Oxford: Blackwell Scientific, 1976.
11. Bouchard-Kurtz, R., and N. F. Owens: *Nursing Care of the Cancer Patient,* 3rd ed. St. Louis: C. V. Mosby Co., 1976.
12. Boyd, W.: *An Introduction to the Study of Disease.* Philadelphia: Lea and Febiger, 1952.
13. Bridgewater, S. C., et al.: Allergies in children: Recognition. *American Journal of Nursing,* 78:613, Apr. 1978.
14. Brody, J.: Insect bites and stings. *Nursing Care,* June 1977.
15. Burnet, Sir F. M.: How antibodies are made. *Scientific American,* Nov. 1954.
16. Burnet, Sir F. M.: The evolution of receptors and recognition in the immune system. *In* Cuatrecasas, P., and M. F. Greaves (Eds.): *Receptors and Recognition,* Series A. London: Chapman and Hall, 1976.
17. Calne, R. Y.: Mechanisms in the acceptance of organ grafts. *British Medical Bulletin,* 32:107, May 1976.
18. Chaudry, I. H., and A. E. Baue: Depletion or replenishment of cellular cyclic adenosine monophosphate in hemorrhagic shock. *Surgery, Gynecology and Obstetrics,* 145:877, Dec. 1977.
19. Conn, H. F., et al. (Eds.): *Family Practice,* 2nd ed. Philadelphia: W. B. Saunders Co., 1978.
20. Conn, H. F. (Ed.): *Current Therapy.* Philadelphia: W. B. Saunders Co., 1979.
21. Cooper, M. D., et al.: T- and B- cell interactions in auto-immune syndromes. *Annals of the New York Academy of Science,* 256:105, June 1975.
22. Craven, R. F.: Anaphylactic shock. *American Journal of Nursing,* 72:718, Apr. 1972.
23. Crowle, A. J.: *Delayed Hypersensitivity in Health and Disease.* Springfield, Ill.: Charles C Thomas, 1962.
24. Cunningham, B. A.: The structure and function of histocompatibility antigens. *Scientific American,* 237:96, 1977.
25. Dave, V. K.: Contact dermatitis. *Nursing Times,* 67:504, Apr. 1971.
26. DeAngelis, C.: *Basic Pediatrics for the Primary Health Care Provider.* Boston: Little, Brown, and Co., 1975.
27. Dharan, M.: Immunoglobulin abnormalities. *American Journal of Nursing,* 76:1626, Oct. 1976.
28. Dodd, M. J.: Theoretical bases of immunotherapy. *American Journal of Nursing,* 79:310, Feb. 1979.
29. Donley, D. L.: Nursing the patient who is immunosuppressed. *American Journal of Nursing,* 76:1619, Oct. 1976.
30. Driscoll, P. W.: Rheumatoid arthritis: Understanding it more fully. *Nursing '75,* 5:26, Dec. 1975.
31. Driscoll, P. W.: Rheumatoid arthritis: Managing it more successfully. *Nursing '75,* 5:29, Dec. 1975.
32. Edelman, I. S.: Mechanism of action of steroid hormones. *J. Steroid Biochemistry,* 6:147, Mar.–Apr. 1975.
33. Faulk, W. P., et al.: Some effects of malnutrition on immune response in man. *American Journal of Clinical Nutrition,* 27:638, June 1974.
34. Feldman, J.: Graft rejection. *Archives of Internal Medicine,* 123:713, June 1969.
35. Fisher, A. A.: Allergic reactions to topical medication. *Consultant,* 19:146, June 1979.
36. Flavell, S. G.: Asthma. *Nursing Mirror,* 134:19, May 1972.
37. Francis, B. J.: Current concepts in immunization. *American Journal of Nursing,* 73:646, Apr. 1973.
38. Fudenberg, H. H., et al. (Eds.): *Basic and Clinical Immunology.* Los Altos, Calif.: Lange Medical Publishers, 1976.
39. Fulginiti, V. A.: Controversies in current immunization policy and practices: One physician's viewpoint. *Current Problems in Pediatrics,* 6:3, Apr. 1976.
40. Fulgraff, G.: Prostaglandins and inflammation. *Advances in Clinical Pharmacology,* 6:39, 1974.
41. Gell, P. G. H., et al. (Eds.): *Clinical Aspects of Immunology,* 3rd ed. Oxford: Blackwell Scientific Publications, 1975.
42. Glasser, R.: How the body works against itself — autoimmune diseases. *Nursing '77,* 7:38, Sept. 1977. (From Glasser, R.: *The Body is the Hero.* Random House, Inc., 1976.)
43. Gravis, G.: Allergies: A guide to practical diagnostic observations. *Journal of the New York State Nurses Teachers Association,* 3:27, Winter 1972.
44. Greaves, M. W.: The immunopharmacology of the immediate allergic response in the skin. *Clinical Experiments in Dermatology,* 1:83, Mar. 1976.
45. Guyton, A. C.: *Textbook of Medical Physiology,* 5th ed. Philadelphia: W. B. Saunders Co., 1976.
46. Hamburger, J.: Recent advances in the understanding of rejection. *Journal of Advances in Nephrology,* 5:101, 1975.
47. Harvard, C. W. H.: Function of the thymus. *Nursing Mirror,* 134:29, June 1972.
48. Harvey, A. M., et al.: *The Principles and Practice of Medicine,* 19th ed. New York: Appleton-Century-Crofts, 1976.
49. Hermans, P. E., et al.: Idiopathic late-onset immunoglobulin deficiency: Clinical observations in fifty patients. *American Journal of Medicine,* 61:221, Aug. 1976.
50. Hill, J. S.: Urticaria and angioedema: Common clinical problems. *Postgraduate Medicine,* 65:83, Apr. 1979.
51. Hong, R.: The physiology of immunity. *Minnesota Medicine,* 52:1377, Sept. 1969.
52. Houck, J. C.: Inflammation: A quarter century of progress. *Journal of Investigative Dermatology,* 67:124, July 1976.
53. Hutchinson, R.: What to do and what to worry about when treating stings and bites. *Nursing '77,* 7:69, June 1977.
54. Jerne, N. K.: The immune system. *Scientific American,* 229:52, 1973.
55. Jonasson, O.: What's new in surgery: Transplantation. *Emergency Medicine,* 11:143, June 1979.
56. Juhlin, L.: There's more to aspirin sensitivity than aspirin. *Consultant,* 16:212, Oct. 1976.
57. Juliani, L.: Kidney transplant: Your role in aftercare. *Nursing '77,* 7:46, Oct. 1977.
58. Kahn, R. H., and W. E. Lands (Eds.): *Prostaglandins and Cyclic AMP.* New York: Academic Press, 1973.
59. Kersey, J. H., et al.: Primary immunodeficiency diseases and cancer: The immunodeficiency-cancer registry. *International Journal of Cancer,* 12:333, Sept. 1973.
60. Kobrzycki, P.: Renal transplant complications. *American Journal of Nursing,* 77:641, Apr. 1977.
61. Kramer, R. (chairman): Radiation therapy and immunotherapy. *Cancer,* 37:2108, Apr. 1976.
62. Krupp, M. A., and M. J. Chatton: *Current Medical Diagnosis and Treament.* Los Altos, Calif.: Lange Medical Publications, 1978.
63. Lockey, R. F., and R. W. Fox: Allergic emergencies. *Hospital Medicine.* 15:67, June 1979.

64. Mackay, I., and F. M. Burnet: *Autoimmune Diseases: Pathogenesis, Chemistry and Therapy.* Springfield, Ill.: Charles C Thomas, 1963.
65. Mandell, G. L.: When to suspect immune defects. *Consultant,* 19:83, Apr. 1979.
66. Marchalonis, J. J.: Lymphocyte surface immunoglobulins. *Science,* 190:20, Oct. 1975.
67. Marks, M. B.: Recognizing the allergic person. *American Family Practitioner,* 17:72, July 1977.
68. Mass, R. E.: Brief review: diagnosing and managing plasma cell (multiple) myeloma. *Geriatrics,* 33:53, July 1978.
69. McCalla, J.: Immunotherapy: Concepts and nursing implications. *Nursing Clinics of North America,* 11:59, Mar. 1976.
70. McGovern, J. P.: 25 questions patients most often ask . . . about allergic asthma. *Consultant,* 19:112, June 1979.
71. Meyers, F. H., et al.: *Review of Medical Pharmacology,* 5th ed. Los Altos, Calif.: Lange Medical Publications, 1976.
72. Miller, B. F., and C. B. Keane: *Encyclopedia and Dictionary of Medicine, Nursing and Allied Health,* 2nd ed. Philadelphia: W. B. Saunders Co., 1978.
73. Monaco, A. P., et al.: Survey of the current status of the clinical uses of ALS. *Surgery, Gynecology and Obstetrics,* 142:417, Mar. 1976.
74. Mullarkey, M. F.: Allergic and nonallergic rhinitis: Diagnosis and management. *Postgraduate Medicine,* 65:97, Apr. 1979.
75. Newton, D., et al.: You can minimize the hazards of corticosteroids. *Nursing '77,* 7:26, Jun. 1977.
76. Nizami, R. M., et al.: Hyposensitization therapy in allergic disease. *Annals of Allergy,* 53:296, Nov. 1975.
77. Nonsteroidal anti-inflammatory agents: Review and update. *Geriatrics,* 34:112, June 1979.
78. Notkins, A. L., et al.: How the immune response to a virus can cause disease. *Scientific American,* 228:22, Feb. 1973.
79. Notkins, A. L. (Ed.): *Viral Immunology and Immunopathology.* New York: Academic Press, 1975.
80. Nysather, J., et al.: The immune system: Its development and functions. *American Journal of Nursing,* 76:1614, Oct. 1976.
81. Phillips, P. E.: The virus hypothesis in SLE. *Annals of Internal Medicine,* 83:709, Nov. 1975.
82. Pitorak, E. F.: Rheumatoid arthritis: Living with it more comfortably. *Nursing '75,* 5:33, Dec. 1975.
83. Price, S. A., and L. M. Wilson: *Pathophysiology: Clinical Concepts of Disease Processes.* New York: McGraw-Hill Book Co., Inc., 1978.
84. Queng, J. T., and J. P. McGovern: Acute anaphylaxis. *Hospital Medicine,* 12:31, Sept. 1976.
85. Rabin, B. S., and T. L. Whiteside: Evaluating cellular immunity. *Consultant,* 19:72, June 1979.
86. Robbins, S. L., and R. C. Cotran: *Pathologic Basis of Disease,* 2nd ed. Philadelphia: W. B. Saunders Co., 1979.
87. Robbins, S. L., and M. Angell (Eds.): *Basic Pathology,* 2nd ed. Philadelphia: W. B. Saunders Co., 1976.
88. Roberts, A. C.: Modern materials, their contribution and use in the human body. *Nursing Mirror,* Dec. 29, 1967, p.1.
89. Rodman, M. S.: Drugs for allergic disorders: anaphylaxis, asthma. Part 1. *R.N.,* 34:63, June 1971.
90. Roitt, I.: *Essential Immunology,* 3rd ed. Oxford: Blackwell Scientific Publications, 1977.
91. Rowe, D. S., et al.: Immunoglobulin D as a lymphocyte receptor. *Journal of Experimental Medicine,* 138:965, 1973.
92. Rubens, R. D.: Short review: Prospectus for cancer immunochemotherapy. *Cancer Treatment Review,* 1:305, Dec. 1974.
93. Sbarra, A. J., et al.: Bactericidal activities of phagocytes in health and disease. *American Journal of Clinical Nutrition,* 27:629, June 1974.
94. Schechter, D. C.: Transplantation glossary. *New York State Journal of Medicine,* 72:3013, Dec. 1972.
95. Scoggin, C. H., et al.: Status asthmaticus. J.A.M.A., 238:1158, Sept. 1977.
96. Selye, H.: *The Stress of Life.* New York, McGraw-Hill Book Co., Inc., 1956.
97. Settipane, G. A.: Adverse reactions to drugs: hypersensitivity. *In* Conn, H. F. (Ed.): *Current Therapy.* Philadelphia: W. B. Saunders Co., 1978.
98. Shvartsman, Y. S.: Secretory anti-influenza immunity. *Advances in Immunology,* 22:291, 1976.
99. Silverstein, M.: Cancer immunotherapy. *American Journal of Nursing,* 73:1178, July 1973.
100. Simmons, R. S., et al.: Immunosuppressive assay of antilymphoblast globulin in man: Effect of dose, histocompatibility, and serologic response to house gamma globulin. *Surgery,* 68:62, July 1970.
101. Slavin, R. G.: Immunotherapy: A safe and effective way to treat allergies. *Consultant,* 19:117, Mar. 1979.
102. Stevens, J. J.: Allergic rhinitis due to inhalant factors. *In* Conn, H. F. (Ed.): *Current Therapy.* Philadelphia: W. B. Saunders Co., 1978.
103. Taylor, H. E.: The clinical application of antilymphocyte globulin. *Medical Clinics of North America,* 56:419, Mar. 1972.
103a. Tennenbaum, J. L.: Anaphylaxis and serum sickness. *In* Conn, H. F. (Ed.): *1978 Current Therapy.* Philadelphia: W. B. Saunders Co., 1978.
104. The immune system. *American Journal of Nursing,* 76:1613, Oct. 1976.
105. Thorn, G. W., et al. (Eds.): *Harrison's Principles of Internal Medicine,* 8th ed. New York: McGraw-Hill Book Co., Inc., 1977.
106. Urman, J. D., and N. F. Rothfield: Corticosteroid treatment in SLE. J.A.M.A., 238:2272, Nov. 1977.
107. VanThiel, D. H., et al.: A syndrome of immunoglobulin A deficiency, diabetes mellitus, malabsorption, and a common HLA haplotype. *Annals of Internal Medicine,* 86:10, Jan. 1977.
108. Walt, A. J.: The treatment of shock. *Advances in Surgery,* 9:1, 1975.
109. Webb, D. R.: Beclomethasone in steroid-dependent asthma. *J.A.M.A.,* 238:1508, Oct. 1977.
110. Webb, D. R.: Drug allergy in clinical practice. *Postgraduate Medicine,* 65:62, Apr. 1979.
111. White, J. F.: Teaching patients to manage SLE. *Nursing '78,* 8:26, Sept. 1978.
112. Wilkinson, R.: Gamma globulins in health and disease. *Nursing Times,* 64:725, May 1968.
113. Williams, G. M.: What's new in surgery: Transplantation. *Surgery, Gynecology and Obstetrics,* 136:212, Feb. 1973.
114. Wilson, R. E.: Transplantation. *Surgery, Gynecology and Obstetrics,* 142:219, Feb. 1976.
115. Winkelstein, A.: An overview of immune deficiency disorders. *Consultant,* 18:118, Oct. 1978.
116. Winkelstein, A. et al.: Immunosuppressive therapy. *American Journal of Medical Science,* 265:92, May 1973.
117. Wolf, A. F.: Hypersensitivity states. *Hospital Medicine,* 12:56, Nov. 1976.
118. Wolf, Z. R.: What patients awaiting kidney transplant want to know. *American Journal of Nursing,* 76:92, Jan. 1976.
119. Wright, V.: Communicataing with the rheumatic patient. *Nursing Times,* 73:1308, Aug. 1977.
120. Zimmerman, S., et al.: Bone marrow transplantation. *American Journal of Nursing,* 77:1311, Aug. 1977.
121. Zukoski, C. F.: Transplantation. *Surgery, Gynecology and Obstetrics.* 134:280, Feb. 1972.

CHAPTER 12*

FLUID AND ELECTROLYTE IMBALANCES

INTRODUCTION AND STUDY GUIDE

Fluid and electrolyte imbalances exist as dangerous and ever-potential threats to any person sick enough to be hospitalized with any illness; moreover, imbalances affect unhospitalized persons who eat inadequate or faulty diets or who take certain medications, e.g., diuretics and cortisone preparations. Thus an understanding of fluid and electrolyte imbalances is absolutely essential for every qualified practitioner of nursing. But first, before you being reading about imbalances, it is important to review what you already know about *normal* fluid and electrolyte balance.† To help you in this review, we have provided a glossary of important terms and concepts at the end of the study guide. Also, throughout this chapter, we outline basic facts concerning normal fluid balance, the various electrolytes — their distribution and functions, the concept of osmolality, and the homeostatic mechanisms controlling fluid and electrolyte metabolism.

The goal of this chapter, then, is to apply the general concepts of fluid and electrolyte balance both to persons suffering from specific imbalances and to groups of patients who are particularly *prone* to imbalances, e.g., patients who are burned, vomiting, or undergoing surgical treatment. Guidance is given in the process of assessing patients with suspected imbalances as well as in caring for them once an imbalance is diagnosed. Throughout the chapter, prevention of imbalances will be discussed, for preventive care is always one of a nurse's most essential tasks.

The necessity for preventive care is clearly emphasized by the following study:

In a survey of 6,199 consecutive medical patients, 27 deaths were found attributable to drug therapy, representing 3.6 per cent of all deaths in the hospital. Five deaths were related to hyperkalemia (potassium excess) secondary to potassium supplementation, four to fluid overload, and two to dehydration and electrolyte depletion. Thus, 11 of 27 drug deaths were attributable to fluid and electrolyte imbalance which might have been avoided.[55]

The major topics included in this chapter are:

- ▶ General concepts of fluid and electrolyte imbalance
- ▶ Specific fluid and electrolyte imbalances
- ▶ General principles of diagnosis, management, and treatment of various imbalances
- ▶ The care of patients particularly susceptible to imbalances

Study Guide

1. As you study this chapter, familiarize yourself with the following terms:

acidosis
alkalosis
anasarca
ascites
buffer
carbon dioxide narcosis
central venous pressure
chloride shift
Chvostek's sign
circulatory overload
dehydration
delirium tremens
edema
  dependent
  pitting
  refractory
extracellular fluid (ECF)
hypercalcemic crisis
hyperkalemia
hypernatremia
hyperosmolar
hypervolemia
hypodermoclysis
hypokalemia
hyponatremia
hypo-osmolar
hypoproteinemia
hypovolemia
interstitial fluid
intracellular fluid (ICF)
negative nitrogen balance
osmolar
paralytic ileus
parenteral hyperalimentation
pCO_2
pH
pO_2
primary and compensatory H^+ imbalances
saline
steady state regulator
tetany
Trousseau's phenomenon
volume deficit
volume excess
water intoxication

*Dolly Ito, R.N. D.N.Sc., and Wanda Roberts, R.N., B.S.N., M.N., critically reviewed and assisted with the revision of this chapter.

†We assume that the reader has taken at least one course involving fluid and electrolyte balance. We suggest reviewing class notes as well as a basic nursing text. Chapter 24 in *Basic Nursing: A Psychophysiologic Approach* by Sorensen and Luckmann may be particularly helpful because some of the discussions in this chapter elaborate on that material.

2. Endeavor to become acquainted with the following medications and solutions:

colloidal solutions
noncolloidal solutions
amino acid preparations
fat emulsions
alcohol preparations
electrolyte solutions
diuretics (mercurial and thiazide)
potassium chloride
potassium triplex
potassium citrate
IV calcium salts
calcium gluconate
adrenocortical medications
0.9 per cent ammonium chloride

3. Upon completion of this chapter, you should be able to apply this knowledge to patients in your care. Thus, in the clinical situation:

a. Identify those patients assigned to you who are likely candidates for developing an imbalance.

b. *Prevent* imbalances from developing in your patients.

c. Look for the early signs of imbalance and report them accurately.

d. Assess patients' needs in terms of fluids and diet.

e. Participate knowledgeably in the treatment of fluid and electrolyte imbalances, being fully aware of the medical problems that medical treatment can create.

REVIEW OF TERMS RELATED TO FLUID AND ELECTROLYTE BALANCE

I. TERMS RELATED TO BODY WATER AND BODY FLUID

Body water. The aqueous medium of the body minus electrolytes; the major constituent of the body. Total body water (TBW) is the percentage of an individual's weight that is composed of water.

Body fluid. Body water in which electrolytes are dissolved (e.g., Na^+, K^+, Cl^-). Body fluid is divided into intracellular fluid and extracellular fluid.

Intracellular fluid (ICF). Body fluid that is located *within the cells.* 70% of total body water is normally within the *intracellular fluid compartment.* The *ICF* provides the cell with the internal aqueous medium necessary for its chemical functions.

Extracellular fluid (ECF). Body fluid that is located *outside the cells,* within the *extracellular fluid compartment.* 30% of total body water is located within the ECF. The *ECF* serves as the body's transportation system, carrying water, electrolytes, nutrients, and oxygen to the cells and removing the waste products of cellular metabolism. ECF is composed of interstitial fluid and plasma.

Interstitial fluid. Extracellular fluid that lies outside both the vascular space and the cells; it provides the cells with the external medium necessary for cellular metabolism. Interstitial fluid makes up 24% of ECF.

Plasma. Extracellular fluid that contains colloids or plasma proteins and is the liquid part of the blood; along with red blood cells, it maintains vascular volume. Plasma makes up 6% of ECF.

II. TERMS RELATED TO ELECTROLYTES AND PLASMA PROTEINS

Electrolyte. A substance or compound composed of atoms, which, when placed in a solvent such as water, break up into separately charged particles called *ions.*

Ion. An atom or group of atoms having a charge of positive (cation) or negative (anion) electricity by virtue of having gained or lost an electron; ions form one of the elements of an electrolyte.

Cation. *Positively* charged ion; within the body fluid, important cations are sodium (Na^+), potassium (K^+), calcium (Ca^{++}), and magnesium (Mg^{++}).

II. TERMS RELATED TO ELECTROLYTES AND PLASMA PROTEINS (Continued)

Anion. *Negatively* charged ion; within the body fluids, important anions are chloride (Cl^-), bicarbonate (HCO_3^-), phosphate ($HPO_4^=$), and sulfate ($SO_4^=$).

Nonelectrolyte. A substance that does not ionize, dissociate in solution, or carry an electric charge. Glucose is an example of a nonelectrolyte.

Proteinate. Protein that is located within the protoplasm of the cells. Proteinate is an anion.

Colloids. Macromolecules of protein that are located within the *plasma* and that principally function to hold water within the blood vessels.

III. TERMS RELATED TO FLUID AND ELECTROLYTE MEASUREMENT

Liter (L.), milliliter (ml.), or cubic centimeter (cc.). Measures of *volume;* a cc. is equivalent to a ml., 1000 ml. are equivalent to a L.

Gram (Gm.) and milligram (mg.). Units of *weight;* 1000 mg. equal one Gm.

Milliequivalent (mEq.). The measure of the *chemical activity or chemical combining power of an ion.* The milliequivalent is a measure of the power of a cation to combine with an anion, thus forming a molecule. The electrolyte content within a water compartment can be most accurately expressed in terms of milliequivalents per liter (mEq./L.).

IV. TERMS RELATED TO FLUID AND ELECTROLYTE MOVEMENT

Osmolality. The total number of dissolved particles (solute) per liter of solvent. Osmolality controls *water movement and distribution* between and within body fluid compartments.

Hyperosmolality. Decrease in water *relative* to solute concentration or increase in solutes *relative* to water.

Hypo-osmolality. Increase in water *relative* to solute concentration or decrease in solute *relative* to water.

IV. TERMS RELATED TO FLUID AND ELECTROLYTE MOVEMENT (Continued)

Active transport. Work or energy required to *transport ions* across a cellular membrane against concentration or chemical or electrical gradients. One special type of active transport, dealing with sodium and potassium (and operating to keep these ions in their respective compartments) is the *sodium pump*.

Blood hydrostatic pressure (BHP). Pressure of the blood cells and plasma within the capillaries. BHP helps *maintain blood volume* and *prevent edema;* it is dependent upon (a) the level of the arterial blood pressure, (b) the rate of blood flow through the capillaries, and (c) the venous pressure.

Colloid osmotic pressure (also called "oncotic pressure," OP). Pressure exerted by the plasma proteins, which acts to (a) *hold water* within the vessels, and (b) *suck back* water that escapes from the vessels. Normally, colloid osmotic pressure within the capillary is around 22 mm. Hg.

Filtration pressure (FP). Pressure of the blood in the blood vessels minus the colloid osmotic pressure.

V. TERMS RELATED TO HORMONES THAT ACT TO MAINTAIN FLUID AND ELECTROLYTE BALANCE

Antidiuretic hormone (ADH) or vasopressin. A hormone that is released from the posterior lobes of the pituitary gland and acts to *control water reabsorption* by maintaining osmotic pressure within normal limits. ADH acts to prevent the body (under certain circumstances) from losing fluid. Circumstances leading to release of ADH include: reduced circulating blood volume; presence of pain; following administration of morphine sulfate, barbiturates, and anesthetic agents; and during periods of emotional and physiologic stress.

Aldosterone. A hormone released from the zona gomerulosa of the adrenal cortex, which acts to *maintain sodium ion concentration* which, in turn, regulates ECF volume. Circumstances stimulating release of aldosterone include: sodium depletion, pitting edema, dehydration, hemorrhage, stress, large doses of ACTH, and constriction of the carotid and renal arteries.

V. TERMS RELATED TO HORMONES THAT ACT TO MAINTAIN FLUID AND ELECTROLYTE BALANCE (Continued)

Thyroid hormone. A hormone that is secreted by the thyroid gland and is important for normal diuresis and calcium regulation and for release of the hormones tetraiodothyronine (T_4) and triiodothyronine (T_3). These two hormones increase cardiac output sufficiently for adequate perfusion of the nephron as well as increasing the volume of glomerular filtrate, hence urinary output. The hormone thyrocalcitonin helps maintain calcium balance.

Parathormone. A hormone that is secreted by the parathyroid gland and controls calcium and phosphate metabolism; that is, it regulates calcium and phosphate ion concentration by increasing or decreasing the ionization of calcium from bones to maintain normal serum calcium levels. An inverse relationship between serum calcium and phosphate is maintained to foster normal excitability of nerves and muscles.

VI. TERMS RELATED TO HYDROGEN ION BALANCE

Acid. A hydrogen ion (proton) donor; i.e., an acid loses hydrogen ions to a base, thereby neutralizing or lessening the strength of the base.

Base. A hydrogen ion (proton) acceptor; i.e., a base accepts hydrogen ions from an acid, thereby causing the acid to become weaker.

pH. Chemical shorthand for the *negative logarithm* of the hydrogen ion concentration. Neutral pH is a H^+ concentration of 0.0000001 Gm./L., which is 10^{-7} Gm./L. or a pH of 7. The pH scale extends from 0 to 14, with 7 being neutral. pH describes the acidity and alkalinity of a solution.

Buffers. "Buffers are chemicals that act as sponges which can give off or take on hydrogen ions as needed to maintain arterial blood pH at 7.35 to 7.45."[74] Within the body, the major buffer system is the *base bicarbonate* (HCO_3)–*carbonic acid* (H_2CO_3) *system.* This system acts to regulate H^+ concentration of body fluids by maintaining a *ratio* of 20 parts (normally 20 mEq.) base bicarbonate to 1 part (normally 1 mEq.) carbonic acid.

GENERAL CONCEPTS OF FLUID AND ELECTROLYTE IMBALANCE

The Major Types of Imbalances

Fluid and electrolyte imbalances can be categorized into three types of conditions, according to cause: (1) a *deficit* or an *excess* of any one of the substances of which the body is composed, (2) a nutritional deficiency, and (3) an abnormal shift of fluid from one compartment to another.

▶ Disorders that can be caused by a *deficit or excess of essential body substances* are:
Water-sodium imbalances
Hydrogen ion imbalances
Potassium imbalances
Calcium imbalances
Magnesium imbalances

▶ Disorders caused by *nutritional deficiencies* are:
Protein deficiency
Caloric deficiency

▶ The two important *fluid shifts* are:
Plasma shifts to the interstitial space
Interstitial fluid shifts into the plasma

A given patient may have one imbalance or a combination of imbalances. For example, water and sodium deficit, potassium deficit and acidosis (hydrogen ion excess) may all occur together in a patient suffering from severe diarrhea.

Patients Most Likely to Develop Imbalances

Almost *every* patient, regardless of diagnosis, who is sick enough to be in the hospital is susceptible to water and electrolyte imbalances. This is because illness, by its very nature, upsets the body's delicate homeostatic mechanisms, thereby making imbalances inevitable. Certain patients, because of their particular illnesses, are especially vulnerable to fluid and electrolyte upsets. Persons suffering from the following conditions or undergoing the following therapies need special vigilance on the part of the nurse:

Conditions Contributing to Imbalances	Therapies Contributing to Imbalances
Ulcerative colitis	Surgery
Kidney disease	Diuretic therapy
Burns	Low sodium diets
Congestive heart failure	Hormonal therapy
Cirrhosis of the liver	Intravenous therapy
Severe diabetes	
Hormonal disorders	
Pulmonary disease	

These and all other patients whose conditions are serious or critical warrant a careful intake and output record, as well as continuous observation for symptoms of imbalance.

Major Factors Causing Imbalances

Deviations of fluid and electrolyte balance from normal are caused by alterations in the *volume of water* in one or all of the body's fluid compartments, and alterations in the *concentrations of electrolytes* within the fluid media (osmolality). The major causes for such deviations are listed below:

A. Fluids and electrolytes may be *deficient*.
   1. Intake may be below the minimum requirements of the body.
   2. Excretion or loss of fluid and electrolytes may be increased.
   3. Important substances or chemicals may undergo destruction within the body.

B. Fluids and electrolytes may be in *excess* of the body's needs.
   1. Intake may be greater in amount than a healthy body can excrete.
   2. Excretion may be impossible because of kidney or liver disease.
   3. Excessive amounts of electrolytes may *accumulate* in the body of the patient suffering from an extensive death of tissue, e.g., from burns or other severe injury.

C. Water and electrolytes may undergo *fixation* within the body. For example, in *ascites*, fluid collects within the abdomen; in *edema*, fluid accumulates within the interstitial spaces. In both these conditions, fluids are lost from the body's circulatory system. As a result, the patient with ascites or edema, or both conditions, actually suffers from a fluid volume deficit even though appearing to be "water-logged."

D. The body may *increase its use* of fluids and electrolytes in the presence of high fever and infection.

E. Upsets in *homeostatic balance* or the breakdown of homeostatic-regulating mechanisms such as the kidney nephron may result in severe imbalance.

Physiologic Changes Due to Imbalances

> *Fluid and electrolyte imbalances, once they develop, tend to affect* every *system of the body.*

Calcium imbalances affects the bones, kidneys, and gastrointestinal tract; potassium imbalance affects the heart, musculoskeletal system, and nervous system; sodium imbalance affects blood volume and blood pressure as well as the nervous system. A water imbalance affects the entire body, including the eyeballs, the body tissues, and the brain. In sum, while the various imbalances do have specific causes, the *physiologic effects* of the imbalances tend to be somewhat nonspecific and to involve the total organism.

WATER-SODIUM BALANCE AND IMBALANCE

Because body fluids contain *both* water and sodium, and because variations in the water component affect the sodium component and vice versa, water and sodium balances and imbalances must be considered *together* and in *relationship* to each other.* Before describing disturbed relationships between water and sodium, normal water and sodium balance should be understood. Important facts concerning body water are reviewed in Table 12–1.

Sodium (Na^+) Metabolism

Sodium is the major *cation* in the *extracellular* fluid. Because sodium has the ability to *attract* water, it is the primary factor that determines the *volume* of the extracellular space. Therefore, sodium disorders are considered extracellular volume disorders.

Table 12–2 summarizes basic facts concerning Na^+ balance.

The following *general* statements can be made about sodium imbalance from the essential facts listed. First, deficiencies or excesses of body sodium result in the following problems:

*Sodium, potassium, calcium, hydrogen, and so forth, exist in the body in ionized form. Consequently, when we discuss sodium in this chapter, we are referring to the sodium ion (Na^+).

1. Plasma volume changes:
Na^+ deficit → plasma volume deficit (hypovolemia)
Na^+ excess → plasma volume excess (hypervolemia)
2. Blood pressure changes:
Na^+ deficit → hypotension
Na^+ excess → hypertension
3. Hormonal changes:
Na^+ deficit → increased aldosterone secretion
Na^+ excess → decreased aldosterone secretion
4. Disturbances in muscle contractility
5. Changes in neuromuscular irritability
6. H^+ disturbances*

*Pathologic changes 4, 5, and 6 occur in varying degrees in both Na^+ deficit and Na^+ excess.

TABLE 12–1. BODY WATER (H_2O)—A SUMMARY OF BASIC FACTS

I. The body of the "normal" human being consists of from 77% to 47% water, varying with age, sex, and individual characteristics. The rest of the body is composed of solids.
  A. Body water as a percentage of body weight declines with age.
    1. A baby's body is 77% water.
    2. An elderly adult's body is around 47% water.
  B. Variations in percentage of body water in adults are due primarily to the amount of fat in a person's body, since fat is essentially water-free.
  C. Body water as a percentage of body weight differs significantly between men and women, because the "average" woman's body has more fat than the "average" man's body. The average woman's body contains 50% to 54% water; the average man's, 60% to 70%. For example, a normal male adult of 70 kg. (154 lbs.) contains 45 liters of water.

II. *Distribution* of water between two fluid compartments.
  A. 70% of total body water is located in the intracellular fluid (ICF) compartment.
  B. 30% of total body water is located within the extracellular fluid (ECF) compartment.
    1. 24% of water in ECF compartment occupies the tissue spaces as interstitial fluid.
    2. 6% of water in ECF compartment occupies the vascular space, as plasma.

III. *Functions* of water
  A. Provides an aqueous medium for cellular metabolism.
  B. Transports materials to and from cells.
  C. Acts as a solvent in which are dissolved the many solutes available for cell function.
  D. Regulates body temperature.
  E. Maintains the physical and chemical constancy of the intracellular and extracellular fluids.
  F. Maintains the vascular (plasma) volume.
  G. Aids in the digestion of food through hydrolysis, which is the breakdown of molecules through the addition of water.
  H. Provides a medium for the excretion of waste from the body.

IV. Water balance and imbalance
  A. Water *balance* depends upon a balance between water intake and water output, i.e., gains in body water must equal losses in body water. Normally an individual has a water intake of 2600 ml. per day and a water output of 2600 ml. per day.
    1. Average daily amount and sources of water *intake* are:
      (a) 1200 ml./day as water or liquids ingested in beverages.
      (b) 1100 ml./day "hidden" water ingested in foods.
      (c) 300 ml./day as water of oxidation, i.e., water produced during metabolic processes.
    2. Average daily amounts and sources of water *output* are:
      (a) 1500 ml./day water eliminated from kidneys as urine.
      (b) 1000 ml./day water eliminated from skin and lungs as insensible or evaporated water loss.
      (c) 100 ml./day eliminated from gastrointestinal tract in the feces.
  B. Water *imbalance* exists when water intake and output are unequal, and gains in body water exceed losses or losses exceed gains.

V. Water *requirements* for life
  A. Normally, a person needs 2600 ml. of fluid per day to meet the body's water requirements.
  B. The absolute minimum amount of water required per day (in a person who is healthy, relatively inactive, and living in a temperate climate) is 1500 ml. per day.
  C. Adults can live up to 10 days and children 5 days without water, provided that weather conditions are moderate.

VI. The *homeostatic regulation* of water
  A. *Antidiuretic hormone* (ADH), under certain conditions, prevents the body from losing water, by regulating water reabsorption or excretion. ADH release is stimulated by increased osmolality.
  B. The *GI tract* absorbs fluids from dietary intake, as well as approximately 7–9 L. of glandular and gastrointestinal tract secretions per day; it thus replenishes fluids lost from the body through the skin, respiratory tract, and kidney.
  C. The *kidneys* maintain the volume and concentration of urine—thus controlling water output.
  D. The *brain* has two mechanisms for regulating body water volume.
    1. The *volumetric monitoring system* in the midbrain works as follows:
      (a) It receives information concerning body water volume from receptors in the walls of the great veins, arteries, and atria.
      (b) It relays this information to the control systems that govern ADH release, thirst and release of aldosterone.
    2. The *thirst center* in the hypothalamus may be turned on or off by changes in body fluid osmolality.

Second, hormonal imbalances, impaired Na^+ intake, or excessive losses of Na^+ in urine, sweat, feces, or gastric, pancreatic, or intestinal tract secretions all predispose the individual to sodium imbalance (either a deficiency or an excess) which, in turn, leads to extracellular volume imbalances.

Osmolality

Osmolality is the number of dissolved particles per unit of water. Electrolytes contribute the largest number of particles to osmolality; sodium and chloride are most abundant in the extracellular fluid, and potassium and phosphate are most abundant within the cells.

Water moves relatively freely from one fluid compartment to another in order to insure equal osmolality (iso-osmolality) between compartments. When the amount of water decreases in relation to the number of particles, or solutes, within either compartment, the osmolality of *both* compartments *increases*, i.e., the compartments become concentrated. When the amount of water increases relative to solutes, the osmolality *decreases* and the compartments become diluted. Because it is *water movement* that determines solute concentration, disorders of water balance are considered osmolar disorders.

TYPES OF WATER-SODIUM IMBALANCES

Water-sodium imbalances can be broken into the following subgroups:

1. Osmolar imbalances
   a. *Hyperosmolar* imbalance, in which there is a decrease in water relative to solutes or an increase in solutes relative to water. This disturbance leads to the *shrinking* of cells.
   b. *Hypo-osmolar* imbalance, in which there is an increase in water relative to solutes or a decrease in solutes relative to water. This disturbance causes *swollen* cells.
2. Volume imbalances (sodium, saline, isotonic imbalances)
   a. *Hypervolemia*, in which sodium, chloride, and water are gained *together*. This disturbance causes an expansion of the extracellular space.
   b. *Hypovolemia*, in which sodium, chloride, and water (saline) are lost *together*. This disorder leads to a decrease in the size of the extracellular space.

These major imbalances and their subgroups are diagrammatically represented in Figure 12–1.

Osmolar Imbalances

Osmolar imbalances involve disturbances in osmolality, and consequently water distribution, throughout the body's fluid compartments. We stated earlier that osmolality is the total number of dissolved particles per unit of water. Osmolality affects body water distribution because water always moves from areas of *lesser* solute concen-

TABLE 12–2. BODY SODIUM (Na^+)–A SUMMARY OF BASIC FACTS

I. The body of a "normal" male of 70 kg. (154 lb.) contains 2700 to 3000 mEq. of Na^+.
II. Sodium is found in all fluid compartments.
   A. ECF contains 140 mEq./L. of Na^+. Na^+ is the dominant ion of the ECF compartment.
   B. ICF contains 10 mEq./L. of Na^+.
   C. Gastric mucus, bile, intestinal juices, and pancreatic juice all contain substantial amounts of Na^+.
III. Na^+ performs the following vital functions:
   A. Regulates fluid *volume* within the fluid compartments.
      1. Thereby regulates the *size* of the fluid compartments.
      2. Principally regulates the size of the *ECF compartment* where Na^+ is the dominant ion.
   B. Maintains plasma volume and regulates the size of the vascular space.
   C. Controls body water distribution by maintaining an *osmotic* equilibrium between the ECF and the ICF.
   D. Increases cell membrane permeability.
   E. Acts as a buffer base (discussed under H^+ balance).
   F. Aids in the conduction of nerve impulses.
   G. Helps to control muscle contractility, especially heart muscle.
   H. Assists in the maintenance of neuromuscular irritability.
IV. Na^+ requirements for life:
   A. Normally, a person needs 4.5 Gm. of Na^+ per day.
   B. These needs are usually met by a normal diet and by adding salt to food.
   C. Na^+ excretion in sweat, urine, and feces approximates intake.
V. The homeostatic regulation of sodium:
   A. Aldosterone, a mineralocorticoid, controls the excretion and retention of sodium. Aldosterone is probably controlled, in turn, by a midbrain volume receptor.
   B. The GI tract controls Na^+ excretion in the presence of Na^+ depletion.
   C. The corticosteroids promote Na^+ reabsorption by the kidney tubules.

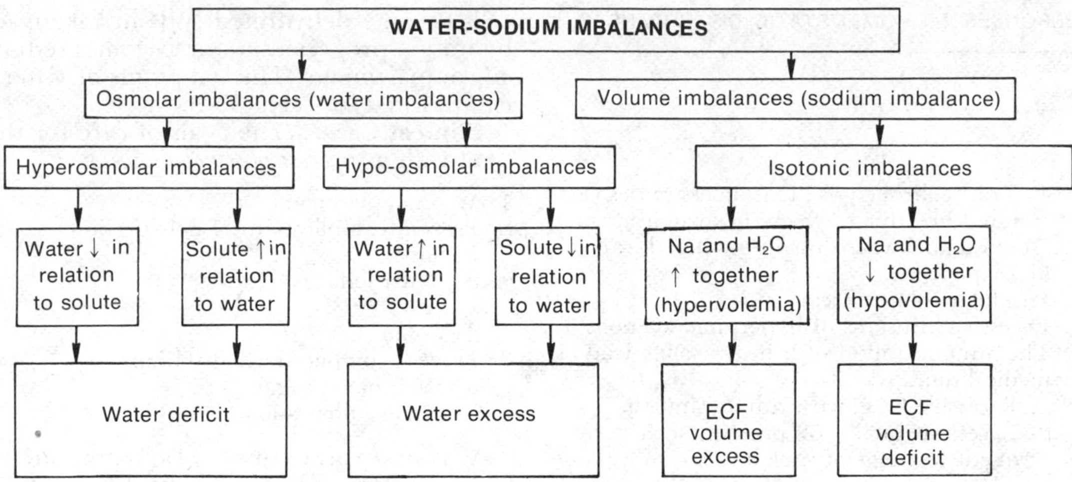

Figure 12–1. Summary of water-sodium imbalances.

tration (low osmolality) to areas of *greater* solute concentration (high osmolality). A change in the osmolality of one fluid compartment will *always* alter the osmolality of the other compartment, until both are equal. A loss or gain of water relative to solute or a loss or gain of solute relative to water will cause osmolar imbalances.

To measure osmolality, and therefore diagnose osmolar imbalances, the concentration of solutes per unit of water must be calculated. Sodium is the easiest solute to measure, because it is abundant and readily accessible in the vascular space (serum). An *elevated serum sodium* value (hypernatremia) indicates a state of hyperosmolality. A *lowered serum sodium* (hyponatremia) indicates hypo-osmolality.

It should be emphasized that the serum sodium value *does not* indicate the amount of sodium (salt) in the extracellular fluid. It only indicates the amount of water in which the sodium is dissolved. To illustrate this point, consider two glasses of water, one full and one half full (Fig. 12–2). To each add one teaspoon of salt. If you were to taste the solution in each glass, the one on the right would taste saltier,yet you know it contains the same amount of salt as the glass on the left. The solution in the glass on the right is just more concentrated; that is, there is less water for the same amount of salt.

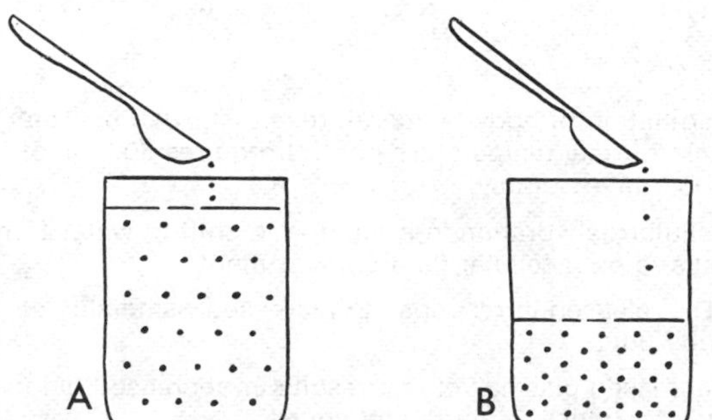

Figure 12–2. The effect of a changing water volume on osmolality. Although the actual salt content in both glasses is the same, glass *B* has a higher osmolality because it contains less water.

The outstanding symptoms in osmolar disturbances are manifestations of *cerebral dysfunction*, e.g., confusion, agitation, depression, and coma. These symptoms develop in response to the *shrinking* of cells during hyperosmolar disturbances and the *swelling* of cells in the presence of hypo-osmolar disturbances. Treatment in osmolar imbalances generally involves *giving water* to correct hyperosmolar disturbances and *restricting water* during hypo-osmolar disturbances.

HYPEROSMOLAR IMBALANCES

Etiology. Hyperosmolar imbalances result from either a water deficit or an extracellular solute overload. In water deficit the concentration of solutes is normal, but they are dissolved in too little water. In solute excess, there are too many particles per unit of water. Both water deficit and solute excess cause hyperosmolality, shrinking of cells, and dehydration. Major causes of H_2O deficit and solute excess are outlined below:

Etiologic factors in hyperosmolality due to either water deficit or solute excess

I. Water deficit
   A. Decreased water intake due to:
      1. Difficulty in swallowing.
      2. Impaired thirst (cerebral injury).
      3. Coma or semicoma.
      4. Unavailability of water.
      5. Extreme debility.
   B. Increased water output due to:
      1. Watery diarrhea.
      2. Diabetes insipidus.*
      3. Diabetic acidosis.*

*Both diabetes insipidus and diabetic acidosis (a complication of diabetes mellitus) will be considered in detail in Unit XIX.

4. Tracheobronchitis (This illness causes very rapid breathing, which, in turn, leads to a substantial water loss in the breath vapor.)
5. Diaphoresis.

II. Extracellular solute excess
   A. Excessive infusions of hypertonic solutions
   B. The administration of a heavy solute load as medical therapy
      1. Excessive IV glucose administration.
      2. Excessive intake of protein, such as frequent feedings of milk and cream without adequate water replacement, or high-protein tube feedings. (These heavy solute loads cause an obligatory loss of water by the kidney and thus dehydration.)
      3. Excessive IV sodium bicarbonate administration.

Bases of Symptoms. The symptoms of hyperosmolar imbalances are primarily symptoms of *dehydration,* since water is *decreased* relative to solutes. In dehydration resulting from decreased water intake, excessive water output, or a heavy solute load, the ECF becomes *hypertonic* (the ECF has a greater osmolality than the ICF). As a result of hypertonicity, water leaves the cells and passes into the extracellular fluid. The cells become dehydrated and shrunken. As dehydration progresses, water becomes reduced in *all* compartments. The symptoms of water deficit are listed in Table 12–3.

Clinical Care. The goals of care for the patient with a *hyperosmolar imbalance* are:

1. Water replacement
2. Prevent complications of dehydration:
   a. Shock
   b. Renal failure
   c. Fever
   d. Coma
3. Prevent complications of therapy:
   a. High blood sugar
   b. Water intoxication

WATER REPLACEMENT. Dehydration due to water deficit or solute overload is treated with water. If dehydration is mild, oral fluids may suffice; if dehydration is severe, intravenous infusions of 5 per cent glucose in water are usually recommended. If hyperosmolality is due to excessive infusions of hypertonic solutions, intravenous therapy with saline solutions is discontinued.

The amount of fluid given to each patient depends upon (1) the degree of dehydration, (2) whether the patient is also losing water through vomiting or diarrhea, (3) the patient's size and weight, and (4) the presence of fever. (A high fever requires more water because fluid is lost through diaphoresis and increased respirations.

TABLE 12–3. SIGNS AND SYMPTOMS OF WATER DEFICIT

Signs and Symptoms	Bases
Thirst in mentally alert patients	Cells shrink, stimulating "thirst" osmoreceptors in the hypothalamus
Poor skin turgor (especially over forehead and upper chest); skin that is pinched over these sites remains in the pinched position for several seconds (severe deficit)	Loss of normal elasticity of skin
Dryness of skin and mucous membranes; tongue dry and furrowed	Cells of the skin and mucous membranes "dry out"
Eyeballs soft and sunken (severe cases)	Water tension in eyeballs decreases
Mild cases result in 2% loss of total body weight; *moderate to severe* cases result in 6% loss of total body weight; *very severe* cases result in 7% to 14% loss of total body weight	Water losses are not being replenished through proper intake
Elevated temperature	Regulation of body temperature is disturbed by water lack (normal temperature control requires 800 ml. of H_2O intake per day)
Apprehension and restlessness; coma in severe cases	Cellular dehydration in brain due to shift of water from cells to extracellular fluid compartment
Concentrated urine and a high specific gravity above 1.030	ADH released in response to increased osmolality of body fluids
Renal shutdown in severe dehydration	Decreased plasma volume results in decreased blood flow to kidney; oliguria and anuria
Laboratory findings: Elevated hemoglobin	Red blood cells shrink as water decreases, concentrating hemoglobin
Elevated serum Na^+ above 150 mEq (hypernatremia)	Osmolality of plasma increases

A high fever may increase insensible fluid losses by 500 to 1500 ml. per day.)

The nurse's role in treating patients with a hyperosmolar imbalance includes:

- ▶ Check weight upon admission and daily.
- ▶ Keep an accurate record of I and O. Measure and record oral, nasogastric, and IV intake. Measure and record output of urine, liquid stools, wound drainage, emesis, bleeding, and suction. Estimate losses from incontinence. Report oliguria or anuria.
- ▶ Check vital signs upon admission and every 2 to 4 hours.
- ▶ Carefully check IV infusions for proper flow rate. Guard against infiltration and infection.
- ▶ Administer adequate fluids (by route ordered) to patients who are comatose or paralyzed, or who are taking tube feedings. Offer oral fluids when appropriate.
- ▶ Monitor the serum sodium and hemoglobin values.
- ▶ Insure that patients with high solute intake receive adequate water.
- ▶ Preserve the integrity of the skin and mucous membranes. Patients who are dehydrated often have decreased body secretions. Nursing measures should include: application of lotion to the patient's skin at least three times a day, less frequent bathing, frequent position change, and keeping mouth, nose and lips clean and moist.

When fluid replacement is adequate, and if other disease conditions are not present, urinary output, body temperature, blood pressure, serum Na^+, and weight all return to normal.

PREVENT THE COMPLICATIONS OF DEHYDRATION. To prevent severe shock, renal failure, and fever from developing in dehydrated patients, the nurse needs to take the following actions:

Shock. Check the vital signs at least every 2 hours (pulse, blood pressure, respiration). Report a drop of blood pressure below normal for the patient, and any rise in pulse or respiratory rate.

Renal failure. Check the urinary output at least every 2 hours if the patient is severely dehydrated. The patient will probably need an indwelling catheter.

> *Report a urinary output of* less than *30 ml. per hour or 500 ml. in a 24-hour period.*

Fever. Report any elevation of temperature over 38.2°C. (101°F.) In the severely dehydrated patient, check the temperature at least every 2 hours.

Coma. Administer ordered fluids promptly and on schedule. Report any decreases in level of conciousness.

PREVENT THE COMPLICATIONS OF THERAPY. Watch for indications of a *high blood sugar* when giving IV glucose in water: thirst, fatigue, large urinary output, and sugar in the urine. Prolonged intravenous feeding with sugar solutions may overtax the islet tissue of the pancreas. This, in turn, may lead to a lowered production of insulin.

Watch also for signs of water intoxication when a patient is receiving IV therapy. The symptoms of water intoxication are discussed below.

HYPO-OSMOLAR IMBALANCES

Etiology. Hypo-osmolar imbalances result from either water excess or solute deficit. In water excess the number of solutes is normal, but they are diluted in *too much water*. In solute deficit, the amount of water in the body may be normal, but there are *too few* particles per unit of water. Both H_2O excess and solute deficit are characterized by *swollen cells*. Major causes of H_2O excess and solute deficit are outlined below:

Etiologic factors in hypo-osmolality due to either water excess or solute deficit

I. Water excess (water intoxication) may be due to:
   A. Excessive intake.
      1. Schizophrenics may drink excessively while hallucinating.
      2. Alcoholics may develop water intoxication on a drinking bout.
   B. Inability to excrete water excesses due to:
      1. Kidney disease
      2. Brain injury or disease.
   C. Iatrogenic problems.
      1. Forcing hypotonic fluids (IV or oral) on patients with increased ADH secretion.
         a. Following surgery or trauma.
         b. Following injections of morphine sulfate.
         c. Following anesthesia.
      2. Excessive infusions of 5 per cent dextrose in water.
      3. Excessive tap water enemas.
         a. Tap water is hypotonic and is absorbed by the bowel.
         b. As a result, the extracellular fluid is diluted and osmolality is lowered.

II. Solute deficit may be due to:
   A. Poor salt (NaCl) intake.
   B. Iatrogenic problems.
      1. Diuretics.
      2. Low salt diet.
      3. Replacement of H_2O and Na^+ losses with *water only*:
         a. Allowing patients to drink large amounts of plain water when perspiring and losing Na^+.

b. Irrigating nasal gastric tubes with *plain water* (this causes Na^+ to be literally washed out and suctioned from the stomach).
c. Giving ice chips made of *plain water* to a patient who is vomiting; again, Na^+ is washed out of the stomach with no replacement.

Bases of Symptoms. In hypo-osmolar imbalances, the cells swell with water, and neuromuscular symptoms predominate. Common symptoms of hypo-osmolar imbalance are listed in Table 12–4, along with their causative factors.

Clinical Care. To treat hypo-osmolar disturbances, it is necessary to *restrict water intake* by mouth and intravenously. In rare instances, when cerebral edema is severe and when renal failure is not a problem, hypertonic solutions may be given IV.

To *prevent* the needless development of water excess, remember these rules:

- Do not give excessive tap water enemas.
- Do not overload patients, especially renal, neurologic, or postoperative patients, with intravenous fluids.
- Do not force fluids on patients with increased ADH secretion. Keep careful track of intake and output to prevent excessive intake.
- Obtain daily weight.
- Do not replace losses of both sodium and water with plain water alone! Replacements should be made with isotonic IV solutions and/or oral liquids containing both electrolytes *and* water, e.g., isotonic ice chips, bouillon, fruit juices.
- Do not irrigate a nasogastric tube with plain water. Instead use *normal saline* for irrigations.

Isotonic Disturbances

In isotonic or volume imbalances (sodium imbalances), Na^+ and H_2O increase or decrease *together* in roughly the same proportions as found in the extracellular fluid, rather than *disproportionately* as in osmolar imbalances. Consequently, when Na^+ is retained, H_2O is also retained, and the extracellular volume increases. Conversely, when Na^+ is lost, proportionate amounts of H_2O are also lost, and the extracellular volume becomes depleted.

Consider again a full glass of water with a teaspoon of salt dissolved in it (Fig. 12–3). If we emptied one-half of the salt solution out of the glass, the total volume would be depleted by one-half, but, the concentration of the salt in the remaining solution would have the same concentration as the part of the solution discarded. This is what occurs in isotonic extracellular volume depletion. The volume of the extracellular space decreases, but the concentration of the solutes (osmolality) remains the same. Therefore, the serum sodium value would be normal.

Volume (isotonic) imbalances, then, are characterized by fluctuations of the ECF volume. When ECF volume *increases*, circulatory overload and edema result. When ECF volume *decreases*, circulatory collapse can result. Since osmolality throughout the body fluid compartments remains unchanged, the cells neither shrink nor swell; consequently, there are *no* cerebral symptoms in isotonic imbalances as there are in osmolar imbalances.

Changes in extracellular fluid volume are detected by means of the physical examination, history, hematocrit, serum protein levels, and urine chloride. Clinical care involves the administration of isotonic fluid in volume depletion and the restriction of fluid in volume excess.

EXTRACELLULAR VOLUME DEPLETION

Etiology. Extracellular volume depletion results from losses of both Na^+ *and* water. The majority of ECF losses are from the gastrointestinal tract and skin. Conditions which can result in large and unusual losses of Na^+ and H_2O include hemorrhage, diarrhea, vomiting, kidney disease, excessive sweating, burns, draining fistulas and abscesses, fever, decreased production of aldosterone, and internal sequestration

TABLE 12–4. SIGNS AND SYMPTOMS OF WATER EXCESS

Signs and Symptoms	Bases
Absence of thirst (in contrast to the thirst present during hyperosmolar imbalances)	Cells swell, inhibiting "thirst" osmoreceptors in the hypothalamus
Polyuria if kidneys are healthy, oliguria if kidneys are diseased; oliguria further contributes to H_2O excess	Release of ADH inhibited
Twitching; hyperirritability; mental disturbances; disorientation; convulsions; coma	Cells swell with fluid, which gives rise to cerebral edema
Laboratory findings: Serum Na^+ level depressed below 120 mEq./L. (hyponatremia); decreased hemoglobin	Plasma osmolality decreases; hemoglobin is diluted in the red blood cell

of fluids—peritonitis, and edema fluid under burns.

It is important to realize that *individuals vary markedly in the rapidity with which volume depletion occurs*. Generally it is recognized that losses from *frequent* diarrhea and vomiting can deplete the *extracellular* fluid within a *few hours*, leading to fatal shock. Gradual losses of intestinal secretions may not deplete the body's store of extracellular fluid for *several days*. Initially, in isotonic volume depletion, there is no shift of fluid from the cellular space, since body osmolality remains the same. However, if extracellular water and electrolytes continue to be lost, eventually water will be drawn from the cells. Thus, prolonged isotonic volume depletion results in depletion of cellular fluid as well.[58]

Bases of Symptoms. The symptoms of extracellular volume deficit are mainly *symptoms of hypovolemia*. Common symptoms and their causation are listed in Table 12–5.

Clinical Care. Extracellular volume depletion is usually treated by *intravenous infusions of isotonic solutions*.

> *Close observation of patients receiving isotonic IV solutions is imperative. If the infusion is given too rapidly, patients with reduced cardiac or renal function can develop circulatory overload leading to congestive heart failure with resultant pulmonary edema. If treatment is delayed, patients with severe extracellular volume depletion can suffer shock or renal failure.*

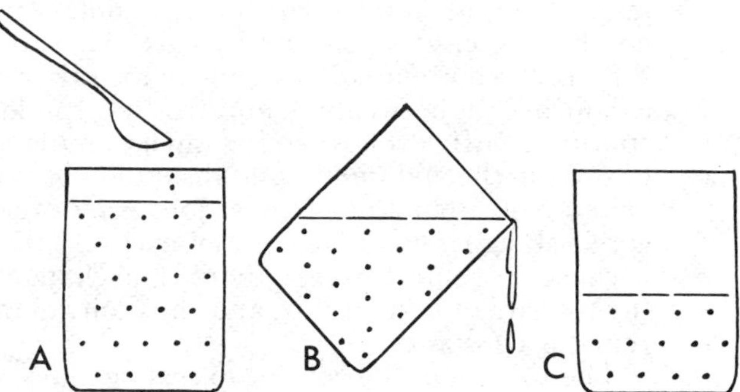

Figure 12–3. Representation of isotonic extracellular volume depletion. Although the volume of the solution decreases as some is poured out, the osmolality of the solution remains the same.

EXTRACELLULAR VOLUME EXCESS

This condition is sometimes called *circulatory overload* or *hypervolemia*. Both water and Na^+ are significantly *increased* in roughly the same proportions. Extracellular volume excess can occur in the following groups of patients:

- ▶ Patients who have received IV *saline* in excessive amounts, too rapidly, or at night when they are sleeping and renal function is normally reduced
- ▶ Patients with *cardiac failure, chronic kidney failure, liver disease*, or *cerebral damage*.
- ▶ Patients who receive *cortisone injections*. (Sodium and water retention is a frequent side effect of cortisone injections.)

The main signs and symptoms of extracellular fluid excess are: weight gain; pitting edema

TABLE 12–5. SIGNS AND SYMPTOMS OF EXTRACELLULAR VOLUME DEPLETION

Signs and Symptoms	Bases
Weakness; nausea; vomiting; weight loss; anorexia	H_2O and Na^+ are deficient in the extracellular fluid compartment, resulting in hypovolemia
Decrease in fullness of the neck veins when patient lies flat*	Venous pressure is decreased owing to loss of plasma volume
A postural systolic blood pressure fall greater than 15 mm. and a diastolic fall greater than 10 mm. Hg†	Plasma volume is inadequate
Oliguria and anuria (in severe cases)	Decreased plasma volume, resulting in decreased blood flow to kidney
Shock	Circulatory collapse as a result of severe plasma volume depletion
No thirst usually	Osmolality of the cells is not disturbed
Laboratory findings: Elevated hemotocrit and protein concentration	Plasma volume is reduced
Urine chloride excretion below 50 mEq./L.	Chloride is being retained with sodium by the kidneys
Normal serum Na^+ concentration	Na^+ and H_2O are lost proportionately

*How to correctly "read" neck vein fullness is discussed in the unit on the heart.

†Postural changes in blood pressure can be detected by taking the patient's blood pressure first in the supine (flat) position, and then in the seated or standing position.

(expansion of interstitial spaces); pulmonary edema (a condition caused by excessive serous fluid in the alveolar spaces and characterized by dyspnea, cough, sweating, and frothy or pinkish sputum); puffy eyelids; ascites (an accumulation of fluid in the abdomen); and distention of neck veins. Note that the patient does *not* develop cerebral signs, as during water excess. This is because, in volume excess, there is no change in the tonicity of body fluids, and thus cell volume remains constant.

The treatment for volume excess includes the administration of *diuretics* and the *restriction of sodium*. Procedures useful in the correction of this condition include weighing the patient daily, strict monitoring of IV infusions, recording and evaluating intake and output, and postural blood pressure measurements.

To *prevent* a volume excess from developing, remember these rules:

> *1. Do not, on your own impulse, increase the rate of drip of an IV infusion simply because the IV is behind schedule. Instead, consult the patient's doctor concerning the possibility of a new IV schedule.*
>
> *2. Attempt to plan your patient's IV schedule with the doctor so that the majority of the fluid is given during the day. Do not overload the "resting kidney" by running IV infusions too rapidly during the night.*

HYDROGEN ION (H^+) BALANCE

Hydrogen ion (H^+) balance is vital to human life and health. Some essential factors concerning the hydrogen ion — its normal concentration within the body fluids, functions, production, measurement, excretion via the kidneys and lungs, and homeostatic regulation — are outlined in Table 12–6.

Because the homeostatic mechanisms regulating H^+ concentration are extremely complex, we shall explore these in detail.

Homeostatic Regulation of Hydrogen

DILUTION OF H^+ EXCESS

H^+ can become heavily concentrated in a single tissue or area of the body. For example, if you exercise your arm excessively, H^+ builds up in the arm muscles. When such a build-up occurs, the excess H^+ are quickly whisked away by the rapidly moving circulation so that they can be distributed more evenly throughout the body fluids. Dilution is a rapid-acting mechanism sometimes termed the *first line of defense* against a shift in pH.

BUFFERS AND BUFFER SYSTEMS

A buffer system of body fluids is composed of a weak acid that coexists with its salt. Buffer systems circulate throughout the body's fluid systems: within the plasma, within the cells, and throughout the extracellular fluid. Three major buffer systems operate to control these vital fluids: (1) the carbonic acid-bicarbonate system, (2) the protein buffer system, and (3) the phosphate buffer system.

The efficiency of all the buffer systems working together is truly remarkable. Out of every one million hydrogen ions added to the body fluids, all but five are successfully and rapidly buffered. However, buffer systems have their limitations in handling the body's acids and bases. Hydrogen ions that the buffers fail to control become the responsibility of the lungs and kidneys.

In its broadest sense, a buffer is a type of "shield" within the body fluids that acts to protect the body against fluctuations of H^+ concentration. Buffers chemically inactivate excess H^+ and OH^-, thereby maintaining the pH of the body within the normal range.*

This sponge-like action of the buffer removes the additional acid or alkaline ions from the circulation. As a result, these ions are unable to affect, to any great degree, the pH of the solution.

For example, note the equation below. If a strong acid† like HCl is added to a buffered solution, the result is a weaker acid and a salt.

$$\underset{\text{(strong acid)}}{\underset{\text{Hydrochloric acid}}{HCl}} + \underset{\text{(strong buffer base)}}{\underset{\text{Sodium bicarbonate}}{NaHCO_3}} \longrightarrow \underset{\text{(weak acid)}}{\underset{\text{Carbonic acid}}{H_2CO_3}} + \underset{\text{(salt)}}{\underset{\text{Sodium chloride}}{NaCl}}$$

The additional hydrogen ions released by the strongly ionized hydrochloric acid are used in forming weak carbonic acid. Because carbonic acid ionizes only slightly in solution, the H^+ donated by the HCl remain "tied up" within the newly formed H_2CO_3 and the pH change of the solution remains within the normal range.

The same general rule applies if a *strong* base, such as sodium hydroxide, is added to a buffered solution; the result is the production of a weaker base and water:

$$\underset{\text{(strong base)}}{\underset{\text{Sodium hydroxide}}{NaOH}} + \underset{\text{(acidic buffer)}}{\underset{\text{Carbonic acid}}{H_2CO_3}} \rightarrow \underset{\text{(weak base)}}{\underset{\text{Sodium bicarbonate}}{NaHCO_3}} + \underset{\text{Water}}{H_2O}$$

*Hydroxyl ions (OH^-) are *released* when a base dissociates in water.

†Strong acids and bases ionize readily in an aqueous solution, whereas weak acids and bases do not.

TABLE 12-6. HYDROGEN ION (H^+) BALANCE–A SUMMARY OF BASIC FACTS

I. H^+ is normally present in body fluids in a concentration of 0.00004 mEq. per liter.
  A. H^+ exists in far lower concentrations within the body fluids than do other ions, e.g., Cl^- and K^+.
  B. The normal body compensates for fluctuations of H^+ better than it does for fluctuations of other ions.

II. H^+ is found in both the intracellular and extracellular fluids.

III. H^+ plays a vital role in the regulation of the following biochemical and metabolic activities for proper cellular function:
  A. Is necessary for the efficient function of enzyme systems.
  B. Is essential for the binding of oxygen by hemoglobin.

IV. H^+ concentration determines the relative *acidity* or *alkalinity* of a solution.
  A. The greater the number of H^+ present, the more *acid* the solution.
  B. The smaller the number of H^+ present, the more *alkaline* the solution.

V. The acidity and alkalinity of a solution (i.e., H^+ concentration within a solution) is measured in terms of pH.
  A. pH is chemical shorthand for the *negative* logarithm of the hydrogen ion (H^+) concentration.
  B. Neutral pH is a H^+ concentration of 0.0000001 Gram per liter or 10^{-7} Gram per liter or a pH of 7.
  C. The total pH scale extends from 0 to 14, with 7 being neutral.
  D. The *higher* the pH the *lower* the H^+ concentration of a solution and vice versa.
    1. A solution with a pH less than 7 is *acid.*
    2. A solution with a pH greater than 7 is *alkaline.*

VI. The pH's of some of the body fluids are as follows:
  A. The *blood* pH is between 7.36 and 7.44.
    1. When the pH of the blood drops *below* 7.36, the individual has *acidosis.*
    2. When the pH of the blood rises *above* 7.44, the individual has *alkalosis.*
    3. The range of blood pH compatible with life is from 6.8 to 7.8.
  B. pH for important transcellular fluids:
    1. Urine pH is approximately 6.0.
    2. Central spinal fluid pH is from 7.36 to 7.44.
    3. Pure gastric juice pH is from 1.0 to 2.0.
    4. Intestinal juice pH is from 6.5 to 7.6.
    5. Bile from gallbladder pH is from 5.0 to 6.0.
    6. Liver bile pH is 7.4.
    7. Pancreatic juice pH is from 7.6 to 8.2.

VII. The body obtains H^+ in the following ways:
  A. The largest number of H^+ arise from the body's many complex metabolic processes.
    1. The metabolic process that produces *volatile* H^+ is the complete metabolism of fat and carbohydrate to CO_2 and H_2O, which yields nearly 14,000 mEq. of carbonic acid daily.
    2. Some of the metabolic processes that yield *nonvolatile* H^+ are:
      a. The incomplete breakdown of carbohydrates and fats to form lactic acid, pyruvic acid, acetoacetic acid, and citric acid.
      b. The oxidation of nucleoproteins and phosphoproteins.
      c. The oxidation of sulfur-containing amino acids to yield sulfuric acid residues.
  B. Excess H^+ can be produced as a consequence of *disease.*
    1. Excess H^+ may be released in cases of trauma and burns as a result of tissue damage and protein breakdown.
    2. H^+ retention and excess occur in respiratory and renal diseases.
  C. Additional loads of H^+ may be ingested by means of *medications* that contain ammonium or mineral salts.
  D. A small amount of H^+ is ingested in the normal diet.

VIII. H^+ circulates throughout the body fluids in the following two forms:
  A. *Volatile* H^+ of carbonic acid.
    1. Volatile H^+ are found mainly in the form of CO_2 and water.
    2. Volatile H^+ must be constantly excreted in gaseous form from the lungs.
  B. *Nonvolatile* H^+ (or metabolic H^+).
    1. Nonvolatile H^+ are produced as the result of various metabolic processes within the body.
      a. Some H^+ are produced in the form of organic acids, e.g., uric acid.
      b. Other H^+ are found in the form of sulfuric and phosphoric acids.
    2. Normally a person ingesting a balanced diet will produce 50 to 100 mEq. of nonvolatile H^+ daily.
    3. Nonvolatile H^+ are eliminated by the kidney.

IX. H^+ are excreted from the body as follows:
  A. The *lungs* primarily eliminate the volatile H^+ of carbonic acid as CO_2 and H_2O.
  B. The *kidneys* excrete nonvolatile H^+ in the following three forms:
    1. A very small amount of *free* H^+ is excreted in the urine. These ions determine the urine pH, which ranges from 4.0 to 8.0.
    2. Sixty per cent of nonvolatile H^+ is excreted as ammonium ions [NH_4^+].
    3. Forty per cent of nonvolatile H^+ is excreted in the form of weak acids.

X. H^+ concentration within the body fluids is homeostatically regulated by means of the following mechanisms:
  A. Dilution of H^+ excess by the extracellular fluid.
  B. Buffering by the following buffer systems:
    1. The H_2CO_3-$NaHCO_3$ buffer system.
    2. Protein buffer system.
    3. Phosphate buffer system.
  C. Respiratory control of volatile H^+.
  D. Renal control of nonvolatile H^+.

In this instance, the additional hydroxyl ions are used in forming a large amount of weak sodium bicarbonate. Again, as a result of buffering, the pH of the solution remains stable despite the addition of a strong base.

Within the body fluids, H_2CO_3 and $NaHCO_3$ operate *together* as a *buffer system*, protecting the body from overwhelming amounts of acid or alkali. The weak acid is H_2CO_3, which ionizes slightly to H^+ and HCO_3^-. The salt of the acid is $NaHCO_3$, which ionizes freely to Na^+ and HCO_3^-.

The H_2CO_3–$NaHCO_3$ Buffer System. The H_2CO_3–$NaHCO_3$ buffer system is the most important system of the ECF, but is the least important buffer operating inside the cell. This system buffers up to 90 per cent of the H^+ of the extracellular fluid. It is closely regulated by the lungs and kidneys, the lungs excreting H_2CO_3 and the kidneys excreting $NaHCO_3$.

The most important thing to remember about the H_2CO_3–$NaHCO_3$ system is that it is *not* the *absolute* amounts of each component of the system that regulates H^+ concentration; rather, it is the *ratio* of H_2CO_3 to $NaHCO_3$ that controls H^+ equilibrium. For example, the normal ECF concentration of H_2CO_3 is 1.37 mEq./L., while the concentration of $NaHCO_3$ is approximately 27 mEq./L. The concentrations of these two chemical components represent a 1:20 ratio—20 parts of $NaHCO_3$ to every 1 part of H_2CO_3. Remember:

> *The 1:20 ratio of H_2CO_3 to $NaHCO_3$ is crucial to H^+ balance. When the ratio is disturbed, balance is upset.*

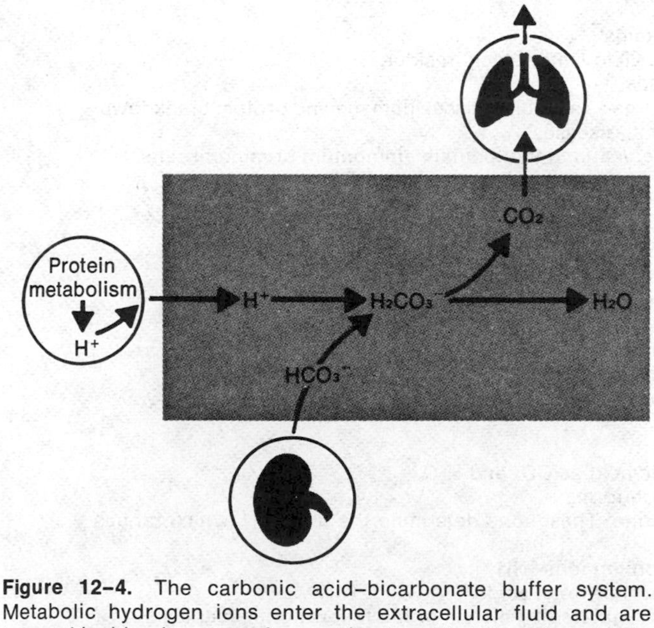

This means, then, that the pH of the body fluids will remain within normal limits even if absolute amounts of each chemical vary. The ratio could conceivably be 2:40 or 0.05/0.10 and still be considered normal. Of course, there are several factors that can disturb the H_2CO_3–$NaHCO_3$ ratio. These upsetting factors will be considered in detail under H^+ imbalances.

Phosphate Buffer System. The phosphate buffer system is almost identical in its actions to the bicarbonate system. The major components of the system are NaH_2PO_4 and Na_2HPO_4. The phosphate buffer is abundant within the cell; thus, it plays a more important role within the cell than within the ECF.

Protein Buffer System. The protein buffer is a very powerful buffer, being active intracellularly as well as extracellularly. Within the cell, it is the hemoglobin of the erythrocyte (a protein substance) that provides nearly three fourths of the chemical buffering power of the body's fluids. Proteins are powerful buffers because they are highly versatile, performing either as acid or base, as the occasion demands.

Figure 12–4. The carbonic acid–bicarbonate buffer system. Metabolic hydrogen ions enter the extracellular fluid and are trapped by bicarbonate to form carbonic acid. Although carbonic acid is a strong acid, it has only a fleeting existence before being converted to carbon dioxide and water. The lungs, by controlling pCO_2, indirectly control carbonic acid levels. The kidneys maintain bicarbonate levels. They reclaim filtered bicarbonate and, in addition, produce new bicarbonate to replace that consumed in buffering. (From Bricker, N. (Ed.): *The Sea Within Us.* New York: Science and Medicine Publishing Co., Inc., for Searle and Co., 1975, p. 38.)

RESPIRATORY CONTROL OF H^+ BALANCE.

The following areas need to be studied in order to understand the role the lungs play:

1. Blood gases
2. CO_2 transport to and elimination from the lungs
3. Chemical feedback control of CO_2 elimination
4. Limitations of the lungs as H^+ regulators

The Blood Gases. The two basic requirements for cellular metabolism are: (a) continuous delivery of oxygen (O_2) from the atmosphere to the tissues and (b) delivery of carbon dioxide (CO_2) from the tissues to the atmosphere. Carbon dioxide is constantly produced in large amounts as a byproduct of the body's metabolic activities. The entire physiologic process of CO_2 transport normally takes only a few minutes, from the production of CO_2 at the cellular level to the time of final release of CO_2 from the lungs.

The respiratory center controls the H_2CO_3 part of the H_2CO_3–$NaHCO_3$ buffer system. This control is exercised by means of a feedback mechanism operating between the respiratory center in the medulla and the lungs. When the bicarbonate side of the 1:20 ratio increases or the acid side decreases, the pH of the plasma rises above 7.44, the base side of the H_2CO_3–$NaHCO_3$ ratio decreases, and the pCO_2 (partial pressure of carbon dioxide) is *lowered*. As a result, the person affected breathes *more slowly* than usual (hypoventilation) and CO_2 is held back and not released from the lungs. CO_2 then combines with H_2O, and more H_2CO_3 is formed, which then *increases* the H^+ concentration of body fluids. These events which occur following CO_2 build-up and excretion are summarized in Figure 12–5.

The lungs are vital regulators of H^+ balance because they have an enormous surface area from which CO_2 can be readily diffused; they can bring about *rapid* changes in H^+ concentration when necessary.

Blood Gas Measurements. The amounts of blood gases in the body are usually measured in terms of their partial pressures. The *partial pressure of a gas* is defined as "the pressure which any one gas exerts, whether it is alone or mixed with other gases." The pressure that any one gas exerts will determine that gas's chemical and physiologic activities.

The partial pressure of *carbon dioxide* (pCO_2) is usually referred to as carbon dioxide pressure or carbon dioxide tension. Likewise, the partial pressure of *oxygen* (pO_2) is called oxygen tension. In the normal resting adult (breathing quietly) the pCO_2 of the alveolar air and venous blood is 40 mm. Hg, while the pCO_2 of the *arterial* blood is 35 to 38 mm. Hg. The pO_2 of *arterial blood* is 75–100 mm. Hg (depending on age), while that of *venous blood* is between 35 and 40 mm. Hg. When the pCO_2 becomes elevated owing either to CO_2 retention or to an overly great CO_2 production, the condition is called *hypercapnia*. When the pCO_2 becomes abnormally low due to excessive "blowing off" of CO_2, the condition is called *hypocapnia*. Finally, a decrease of pO_2 is called *hypoxia*.

The Transport of CO_2 and Its Elimination from the Lungs. Because CO_2 is a potentially deadly acidic substance, it *must* be eliminated via the lungs. But how does CO_2 reach the lungs for elimination and what happens to CO_2 while en route? The major steps in the formation and transport of CO_2 to the lungs are: (1) CO_2 is formed by various intracellular and metabolic processes; (2) CO_2 is then released into the interstitial fluids from which it passes into the plasma, with some CO_2 passing into the erythrocytes; and (3) from the plasma, CO_2 goes to the lungs where it is released into the air. However, CO_2, during the transport period, goes through a number of important processes, which occur within the plasma and red blood cells.

Three things can happen to CO_2 when it enters the *plasma* from the interstitial fluid:[17]

I. A part of CO_2 remains *dissolved* in the blood where it can be measured in terms of the pCO_2.
   A. Dissolved CO_2 reacts with water to form H_2CO_3 (carbonic acid):

$$CO_2 + H_2O \leftrightarrow H_2CO_3$$

   B. H_2CO_3 ionizes into H^+ and bicarbonate (HCO_3^-) in the presence of carbonic anhydrase

$$H_2CO_3 \leftrightarrow H^+ + HCO_3^-$$

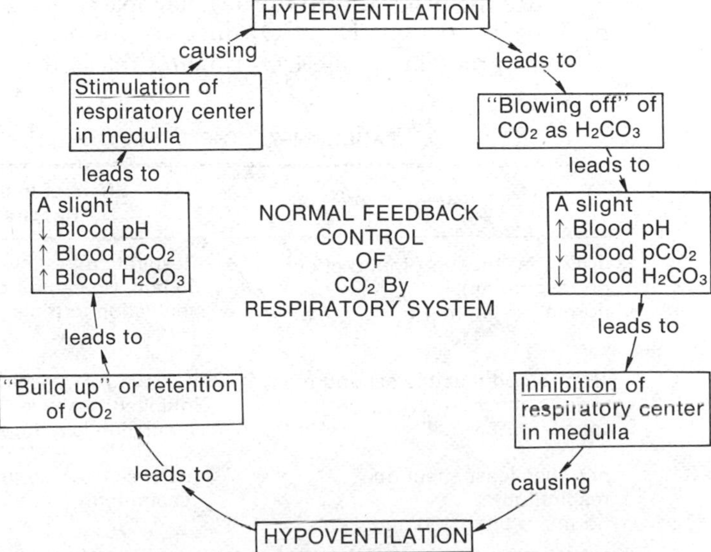

Figure 12–5. Feedback control of H^+ concentration and the elimination of CO_2.

C. The hydrogen ions, which are added to the circulation, are buffered by plasma buffers.
D. As a result, little change in H^+ concentration occurs.

II. A part of CO_2 joins with the proteins of the blood to form *carbamino compounds*.
III. A large proportion of CO_2 passes into the erythrocytes.

Within the erythrocytes, CO_2 again undergoes three distinct processes:

I. Some CO_2 simply remains *dissolved* within the red blood cells.
II. A substantial amount of CO_2 combines with hemoglobin to form *carbamino compounds*.
III. The largest part of the CO_2 combines with water to form H_2CO_3.
   A. H_2CO_3 then ionizes to yield H^+ and HCO_3^-.
   B. The hydrogen ions are buffered by hemoglobin, while the majority of bicarbonate ions pass into plasma in exchange for Cl^-. This exchange of ions is called the *chloride shift* and serves three purposes:
      1. The exchange of negatively charged ions preserves the electrical neutrality of the cells and plasma.
      2. The passage of HCO_3^- into the plasma helps to maintain the 1:20 ratio of H_2CO_3 to $NaHCO_3$.
      3. The transfer of HCO_3^- into the plasma allows large amounts of CO_2 to be carried to the lungs in the form of bicarbonate ions. Thus, the pH of the blood is only slightly disturbed by the additional CO_2.

Following these complex processes, CO_2, mainly in the form of HCO_3^- and carbamino compounds, finally reaches the lungs via the venous blood at a partial pressure of 46 mm. Hg. Since the pCO_2 within the alveolar spaces of the lung is 40 mm. Hg, CO_2 diffuses down a pressure gradient. While CO_2 is being released into the alveolar spaces for expiration, a "reverse chloride shift" takes place within the body fluids. In this process, all the reactions involved in CO_2 transport reverse themselves:

1. Cl^- returns into the plasma in exchange for HCO_3^-.
2. H_2CO_3 diffuses back into the cells where it ionizes into CO_2 and water.
3. The CO_2 thus formed quickly diffuses into the plasma.
4. From the plasma, the CO_2 passes into the alveolar air where it joins the CO_2 from the venous blood.
5. The CO_2 thus accumulated from these two sources is finally excreted from the alveoli into the atmosphere.

Feedback Mechanisms in the Regulation of CO_2 Excretion. The H^+ concentration of the blood and the amount of CO_2 build-up within the body fluids both have a direct effect upon respiration through the respiratory center, thereby maintaining the pH within the normal range. The three major factors that affect the respiratory center in the medulla are the pH of the blood, the pCO_2 and the pO_2. As shown in Table 12–7, increases or decreases of these factors result in significant alterations in pulmonary ventilation.

The influence of plasma pH and CO_2 on pulmonary ventilation through the respiratory center is well integrated. Consider the body's response to a build-up of CO_2, possibly resulting from exercise. When CO_2 within the body fluid increases, the pH of the blood drops below 7.36, the acid side of the H_2CO_3–$NaHCO_3$ ratio increases, and the pCO_2 increases. As a result, the individual responds by breathing more rapidly than usual (hyperventilates) and the extra CO_2 is thereby excreted from the lungs. Because the air expired is moist, CO_2 is actually eliminated as H_2CO_3, thus lowering the concentration of H^+ within the body fluids.

Note that the negative feedback control system governing H_2CO_3 concentration and the elimination of CO_2 is of the *servomechanism* type. The levels of CO_2 and H_2CO_3 are continuously

TABLE 12–7. THE EFFECT OF pH, pCO_2 AND pO_2 UPON RESPIRATION

Factor	Effect of Increase on Respiration	Effect of Decrease on Respiration
pCO_2 (has most profound effect on respiration): normal = 40 mm. Hg	Respiration is stimulated; pCO_2 of 50 mm. Hg causes pulmonary ventilation to triple	Respiration is inhibited; pCO_2 of 30 mm. Hg causes pulmonary ventilation to decrease to one fourth of normal
pH of blood (has the second most serious effect on respiration): normal = 7.35–7.45	If above 7.41, respiration is inhibited; if above 7.50, pulmonary ventilation is reduced by one half	If below 7.41, respiration is stimulated; if below 7.20, pulmonary ventilation quadruples
pO_2 (has least effect on respiration): normal = 98 to 100 mm. Hg	Increase has very little effect on respiration	Respiration is stimulated and CO_2 is blown off

shifting, thereby requiring constant monitoring. If this system is disturbed for even very brief periods of time, H^+ balance is seriously upset.

The Limitations of the Lungs as Steady State Regulators. The lungs have definite limitations in maintaining pH within the normal range. The lungs can excrete, retain, or inactivate only the H^+ of H_2CO_3. Handling the HCO_3^- that results becomes a function of the kidneys. The lungs can help to compensate only *temporarily* for changes in H^+ concentration. If the problem in H^+ balance is secondary to other than pulmonary ventilation, ionic concentration is maintained by renal function. The respiratory tract can only *partially* correct deviations in pH from normal. For example, if the pH of the blood should fall from the normal of 7.36 to 7.0, the lungs will be able to restore the pH to around 7.2 or 7.3 within a minute or so. However, they cannot restore the pH of the blood to 7.36.

Renal Control of H^+ Concentration

The *kidneys* regulate the $NaHCO_3$ part of the $H_2CO_3^-$ buffer system. The kidney eliminates *nonvolatile* H^+, whereas the lung eliminates *volatile* H^+. Also, unlike the lungs, the kidneys work slowly, taking up to half a day to correct an imbalance. However, the renal system is powerful and efficient, neutralizing *almost completely* any excess acid or base that is disturbing the delicate balance of the body fluids. To compensate for H^+ imbalances, the kidney alters the *rate* of excretion of various electrolytes such as H^+, Na^+, and K^+, thereby correcting the concentrations of H^+ and other electrolytes within the body fluids.

Five major processes are involved in the kidney's regulation of H^+ homeostasis:

1. H^+ secretion by the proximal and distal tubules.
2. Exchange of H^+ and Na^+ in the tubular urine.
3. Excretion of H^+ as an ammonium compound.
4. Suppression of H^+ and Na^+ exchange.
5. Increased production of NH_3.

Secretion of H^+. When CO_2 joins with water, hydrogen ions are released along with bicarbonate ions.

$$CO_2 + H_2O \xleftrightarrow{\text{carbonic anhydrase}} H^+ + HCO_3^-$$

The hydrogen ions thus formed are secreted by the epithelial cells of the proximal tubules, distal tubules, and collecting ducts of the kidneys into the urine for excretion.

The exact mechanism that controls H^+ secretion is unknown. However, scientists agree that H^+ secretion is regulated mainly by the *concentration of CO_2 in the ECF*. Thus, the greater the concentration of CO_2 in the ECF, the faster hydrogen ions are secreted; conversely, the lower the concentration of CO_2 in the ECF, the fewer the hydrogen ions secreted.

Hydrogen Ion–Sodium Ion Exchange. As H^+ are secreted from the tubular cells into the tubular urine, they are *exchanged* for sodium ions and then excreted. The *sodium ions* within the tubular urine are usually in partnership with an anion — either HCO_3^- or HPO_4^{--}. When H^+ ions are secreted into the urine, the Na^+ ions are exchanged (to maintain electrical neutrality) from the urine filtrate and from their partner anions by the kidney cells and returned to the plasma. Within the plasma, the reabsorbed sodium ions are reunited with HCO_3^- to again form the compound $NaHCO_3$. Thus, as a result of the H^+–Na^+ exchange, $NaHCO_3$ is regenerated and the H_2CO_3–$NaHCO_3$ ratio is held steady.

And what happens to the secreted hydrogen ions? Their fate ultimately depends upon which anion Na^+ is linked with while in the tubular urine. For example, if the anion is HCO_3^-, as is frequently the case, the following reaction will take place:

HCO_3^- Bicarbonate ion – released from its partnership with Na^+	+	H^+ Secreted hydrogen ions	→	CO_2 Carbon dioxide which diffuses into cell	+	H_2O Water excreted as urine

The *rate* of H^+–Na^+ exchange and HCO_3^- reabsorption is influenced by several factors. Chloride deficiency (hypochloremia), an increased pCO_2, and an increased aldosterone secretion (which causes Na^+ retention) all *stimulate* the exchange process. Conversely, a decrease in the pCO_2 and a decrease in aldosterone secretion both *inhibit* H^+–Na^+ exchange.

A final influence on the exchange mechanism is the *pH of the urine*. If the pH of the urine reaches between 4.0 and 4.5, H^+ secretion stops. This, in turn, halts the H^+–Na^+ exchange. At this critical point, the body must rely upon the *ammonia mechanism* for continued H^+ secretion.

Ammonia Mechanism. Upon the breakdown of certain amino acids, ammonia (NH_3) is formed within the distal tubular cells of the kidney. When the NH_3 formed diffuses from the cells into the urine, it reacts with some of the free H^+ present in the urine to form ammonium molecules (NH_4^+). The NH_4^+ molecules then join with anions such as chloride or sulfate ions, and together they (NH_4^++ anion) are excreted in the urine. The overall effect of this mechan-

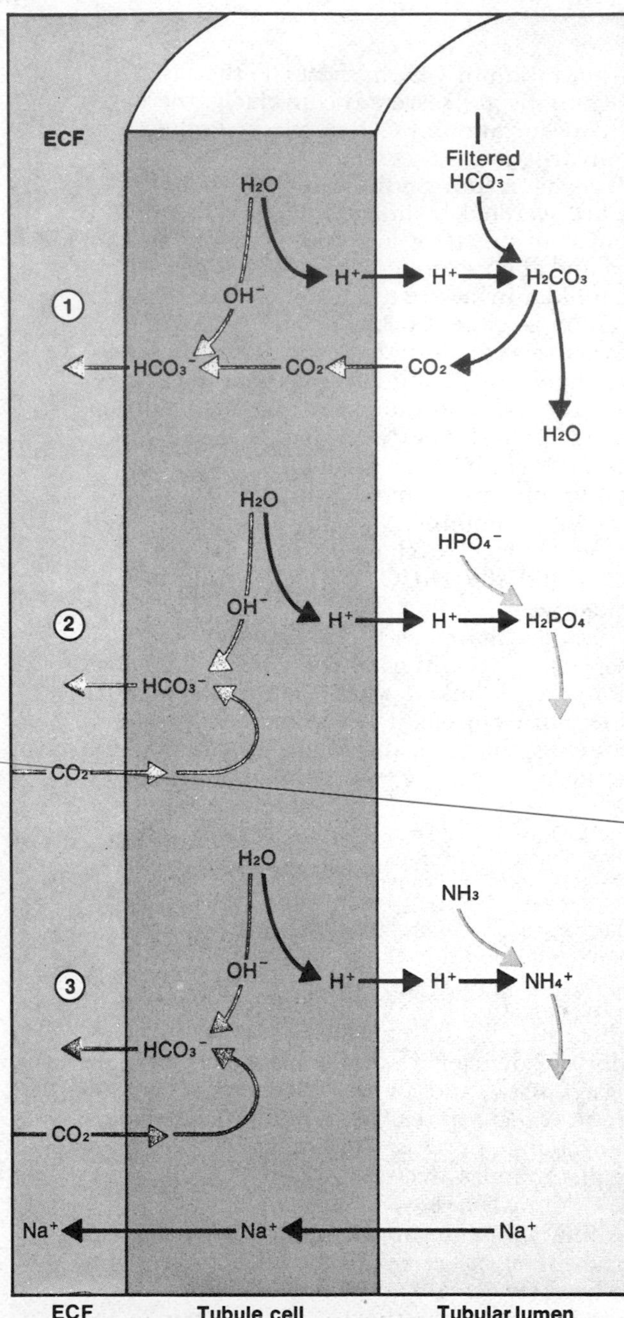

Figure 12–6. Renal handling of bicarbonate–reclamation and regeneration. In the tubular cell, H_2O is split into H^+ ions and OH^- ions. The H^+ is transported into the lumen, where it is trapped by luminal buffers. The OH^- is then free to combine with CO_2 (under the catalytic influence of carbonic anhydrase) to form HCO_3^-, which enters peritubular capillaries. In reaction 1 (at top of diagram), OH^- combines with CO_2 derived from filtered bicarbonate. The bicarbonate formed in this way represents reclaimed bicarbonate. There is also evidence that some filtered bicarbonate is reabsorbed directly as such. In reactions 2 and 3, the OH^- combines with CO_2 from extracellular fluid. The bicarbonate formed in this way represents newly generated bicarbonate. (From Bricker, N. (Ed.): *The Sea Within Us.* New York: Science and Medicine Publishing Co., Inc., for Searle and Co., 1975, p. 40.)

ism is to *increase* the bicarbonate side of the H_2CO_3–$NaHCO_3$ ratio by eliminating excess H^+.

Also, as stated earlier, the ammonia mechanism controls H^+ secretion when the urine pH rises too high. In this case, the mechanism operates by binding the free H^+ in the urine, thus *lowering* the urinary pH. As a result, the renal tubular cells are soon able to operate again in their job of secreting H^+ into the urine for H^+–Na^+ exchange.

Summary of Renal Control Mechanisms

In sum, the kidney (like the lungs) has several ways of coping efficiently with the acid-alkali load, being able to remove substantial amounts of acids or alkali daily. As long as the kidneys and lungs remain healthy, and the acid-alkali loads are not too great, pulmonary and renal systems serve as a powerful line of defense against H^+ imbalance.

HYDROGEN ION (H^+) IMBALANCES

The maintenance of H^+ balance depends upon the healthy function of the kidneys, lungs, and brain as well as normal buffering agents, which include normal serum proteins and hemoglobin concentrations. These remarkable systems can normally adjust swiftly and efficiently to fluctuations of H^+ concentration. However, when subjected to unusually heavy loads of acid or alkali, or in the presence of renal, respiratory, or brain disease, malnutrition, or severe unreplaced blood loss. The body's ability to cope with H^+ regulation fails and imbalances result. The imbalances created are of two major types: *acidosis* or *alkalosis*.

Definitions

> Acidosis *is a condition in which the H^+ concentration is elevated above normal, or the alkali reserve of the body is reduced below normal.*
>
> Alkalosis *is a condition in which the H^+ concentration of the body fluid is decreased below normal or the body base is increased above normal.*

If the basic failure rests with the *pulmonary* system, the condition is called *respiratory acidosis* or *alkalosis*. In respiratory acidosis, H^+ is increased because insufficient CO_2 is being expelled ($H_2O + CO_2 \longleftrightarrow H^+ + HCO_3^-$). In respiratory alkalosis, the converse is true; CO_2 and H_2O are being exhaled too rapidly.

When the basic failure is *renal* in nature, the imbalance is called *metabolic acidosis* or *alkalosis*. In *metabolic acidosis* excessive nonvolatile or metabolic H^+ are being retained or produced within the body fluids, or HCO_3^- is being lost in abnormally large amounts from the kidneys. Conversely, in *metabolic alkalosis* there is either an abnormal loss of nonvolatile H^+ from the body or an abnormal gain in HCO_3^- by the ECF. These various conditions are represented graphically in Figure 12–7.

There are several different names for the four major imbalances that you may find in use on patients' charts. The most representative are listed in Table 12–8.

Besides being classified on a physiologic basis, imbalances may also be grouped as *primary* imbalances, *secondary* or *compensatory* imbalances, and *mixed* imbalances. A primary imbalance is one arising *directly* from an acid or base overload or from disease of the lungs or kidneys. A secondary imbalance occurs in response to compensatory mechanisms attempting to maintain pH within the normal range. Imbalances can also be *mixed*, i.e., a patient can conceivably have two primary imbalances, one metabolic and one respiratory. In *mixed* conditions, neither imbalance is compensating for the other; instead, both imbalances are the result of two distinct disease processes or their complications. For example, a patient could have a primary respiratory acidosis resulting from lung disease *and* a primary metabolic alkalosis as the result of a gastric disorder causing excessive vomiting of HCl or as a result of ingesting systemic alkaline substances such as $NaHCO_3$ or baking soda.

The Effect of H^+ Imbalance

The following points will facilitate learning the signs and symptoms of the different imbalances.

1. *All the major signs and symptoms are the result of disturbances of the central nervous system* (CNS).
2. *In* acidosis *(either respiratory or metabolic) the major problem is depression of the CNS: decrease in mental capacity, delirium, coma may result. Death is not uncommon.*
3. *In* alkalosis *the major problem is* overexcitability *of the CNS. Extreme nervousness, overexcitability, tetany, and convulsions may develop. Death is rare; however, it may follow tetany of the respiratory muscles.*

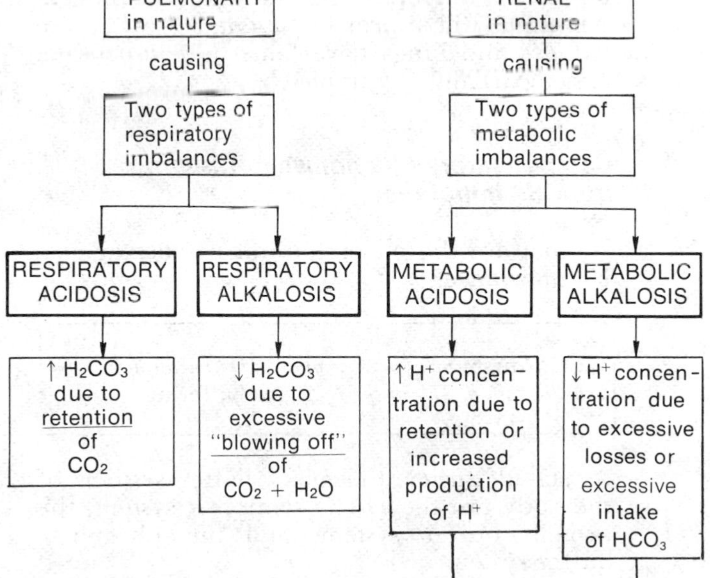

Figure 12–7. Classification of the four major H^+ imbalances.

TABLE 12–8. TERMS COMMONLY APPLIED TO THE FOUR MAJOR IMBALANCES

Imbalance	Names in Common Usage
Metabolic acidosis	Nonrespiratory acidosis Primary base bicarbonate deficiency
Metabolic alkalosis	Nonrespiratory alkalosis Primary base bicarbonate excess
Respiratory acidosis	Primary CO_2 excess Carbon dioxide retention Hypercapnea Hypoventilation
Respiratory alkalosis	Primary CO_2 deficiency Hyperventilation

The number of symptoms seen in an imbalance and their severity depend largely upon the *length of time* the patient has suffered the imbalance, the *magnitude* of the H^+ or HCO_3^- deviation, and the efficiency of the kidneys and lungs in compensating for the imbalance. For example, a patient may die as a result of a rapidly developing, severe imbalance that overwhelms the body's compensatory mechanisms. Conversely, a patient suffering from a mild imbalance over a long period of time may experience few or no symptoms because of the development of compensatory mechanisms. Indeed, symptoms will appear in patients *only* when the kidneys and lungs have failed to compensate, either partially or completely.

Compensatory Mechanisms Resulting from H^+ Imbalance

What are the major lines of defense against H^+ imbalance?

> *The* first *line of defense against H^+ imbalances is the dilution of H^+ in the ECF and* buffering.

As stated earlier, the major buffer systems of the body are the H_2CO_3–$NaHCO_3$ system, the protein buffer system, and the phosphate buffer system.

> *The* second *line of defense against H^+ imbalances is the* respiratory system.

If the patient has a lowered pH or elevated pCO_2, the lungs compensate for the acidosis by increasing respirations. Conversely, if the blood pH is elevated or pCO_2 is lowered, the lungs compensate for the presence of alkalosis by decreasing the rate of respiration.

> *The* third *line of defense against H^+ imbalances is the* renal system.

The five major ways in which the kidneys regulate H^+ concentration are listed on page 187. Diseased kidneys are ineffective in excreting nonvolatile acids. To compensate for the kidney's failure, the *lungs* attempt to lower the body's total acid content by increasing the rate of CO_2 excretion. By eliminating some of the body's volatile acid, the lungs, in the absence of proper renal function, help to raise the pH of the blood toward normal. If the lungs become diseased, the kidneys compensate for increased acid retention by excreting nonvolatile acids more rapidly, thereby lowering the body's total acid content.

The Diagnosis of H^+ Imbalance

Disturbances of H^+ balance are difficult to diagnose for at least three reasons. First of all, H^+ imbalances rarely appear spontaneously; they are almost always the result of *primary underlying conditions* such as diabetes mellitus or emphysema, which must be diagnosed before the H^+ imbalance can be treated effectively. Second, the symptoms of the primary imbalance are often *masked* by the symptoms of a *compensatory imbalance*. For example, a patient who is hyperventilating may have a respiratory alkalosis resulting from hysteria. Hyperventilation, in this case, is a *symptom* of respiratory alkalosis. On the other hand, a rapidly breathing patient might have a metabolic acidosis. Hyperventilation in this latter case represents a *compensatory* reaction to the build-up of H_2CO_3 within the body. A third difficulty in diagnosis is that definite signs and symptoms of imbalance may be minimal or absent for long periods, during which compensatory mechanisms are functioning adequately.

Because of these problems in diagnosis, doctors must rely heavily upon the following laboratory tests when working with patients suffering from H^+ disorders:

- *Blood pH*. Determines whether a H^+ imbalance exists. Although the test confirms the presence of either an acidosis or alkalosis, it *does not* tell whether the imbalance is respiratory or metaboliic. The *normal* blood pH reading is between 7.36

and 7.44. An *elevated* pH indicates alkalosis; a *lowered* pH indicates acidosis.

- *pCO_2 determination*. Measures the amount of *carbon dioxide dissolved in the plasma*. Normally carbon dioxide pressure is 35 to 50 mm. Hg. The pCO_2 is *elevated* when the acid part of the H_2CO_3–$NaHCO_3$ ratio is increased and *acidosis* is present. The pCO_2 is *lowered* when the acid part of the H_2CO_3–$NaHCO_3$ ratio is decreased and *alkalosis* is present.
- *CO_2 combining power*. Essentially measures the amount of serum bicarbonate alone. The *normal* value is between 52 to 58 vol. of CO_2 per ml. serum (22–30 mEq./L) *An elevated* CO_2 combining power indicates *alkalosis*, whereas a depressed CO_2 combining power indicates *acidosis*. The test is easy to obtain and perform but can yield inaccurate data.
- *Plasma total CO_2 content*. This test measures the sum of bicarbonate, carbonic acid, and dissolved CO_2. The collection of the specimen necessitates little or no contact with outside air, thus rendering results more accurate. *Normal* plasma CO_2 content is between 20 and 30 mEq. per L. An *elevation* of plasma CO_2 content indicates alkalosis; a *depression* of plasma CO_2 content indicates acidosis.

The changes in pH, pCO_2, and CO_2 content resulting from H^+ imbalances are shown in Table 12–9.

Basic Clinical Care in H^+ Imbalances

However complex the various imbalances are, five basic rules of care apply to all of them:

1. Treat, and if possible remove, the primary disease or disorder that is creating the imbalance.
2. Through supportive medical and nursing care, aid the renal and respiratory systems in their struggle to compensate for imbalance.
3. Observe and record rate and depth of respiration.
4. Observe abnormal behavior.
5. Medicate with drugs that will neutralize excess acid or base, as the condition warrants.

TABLE 12–9. BLOOD PARAMETERS OF ACID-BASE IMBALANCES DURING MIDDLE PHASE OF COMPENSATION

	Blood Parameters		
Imbalance	*pH*	*pCO_2*	*CO_2 Content*
Metabolic acidosis	↓	↓	↓
Metabolic alkalosis	↑	↑	↑
Respiratory acidosis	↓	↑	↑
Respiratory alkalosis	↑	↓	↓

Note: *The arrows of pCO_2 and CO_2 point in same direction as the pH arrows in metabolic acid-base imbalances, but in the opposite direction from the pH arrows in respiratory imbalances.*

From Sharer, J. E.: Reviewing acid-base balance. *American Journal of Nursing,* 75:982, June 1975. Adapted from *Fluid and Electrolytes,* Abbott Laboratories, North Chicago, Ill., 1970, p. 24.

In acidosis, acids are most commonly neutralized by such drugs as *sodium bicarbonate, sodium lactate*, and *sodium gluconate*. The neutralization of excess base may be achieved by administering *ammonium chloride*, either orally or intravenously.

Now let us consider the specific imbalances.

Metabolic Acidosis

Etiology. The basic causes of metabolic acidosis are: (1) an abnormal loss of $NaHCO_3$, which decreases both the base side of the H_2CO_3–$NaHCO_3$ ratio and the pH of the body fluids; and (2) a heavy production of nonvolatile acids, which overloads the kidneys and exceeds renal capacity for the secretion of excess acid. Major causative factors resulting in these defects are:

Overproduction of Metabolically Produced Acids. In conditions such as diabetes mellitus, hyperthyroidism, starvation, severe infections with fever, and prolonged fasting or vomiting, proteins and fats are burned for energy instead of carbohydrates. The result is an accumulation of ketone bodies, which create an acidosis.

Some studies state that *anesthesia* can also cause acidosis in certain individuals. Because anesthesia is a stress that increases the body's metabolism markedly, additional proteins and fats are burned, causing the production of increased acid.

Excessive Ingestion of Metabolic Acids. Patients on ketogenic and high-fat, low-carbohydrate diets can develop acidosis. Also, the oral ingestion of such organic acids as salicylic acid or boric acid will result in the formation of excess H^+. Finally, excessive ingestion of such medications as ammonium chloride, ferrous sulfate, and paraldehyde (a drug commonly used in treating acute alcoholism) all promote the development of H^+ overload.

Inadequate Renal Function. In renal disease the kidney loses its ability to compensate adequately for acid overloads. Thus, H^+ are not excreted at a normal rate, nor is $NaHCO_3$ sufficiently conserved.

Abnormal Losses of Alkali. Severe diarrhea and the loss of pancreatic, biliary, and lower bowel secretions result in acidosis. In these cases, HCO_3^- is being lost in large amounts from the body. *Prolonged vomiting* of *deep* gastrointestinal contents also causes acidosis owing to loss of base. In contrast, acute vomiting of *stomach contents* results in *alkalosis* owing to the loss of HCl.

SEVERE TISSUE ANOXIA. Anaerobic metabolism, resulting in excessive production of lactic acid, occurs in patients, e.g., who suffer from pulmonary disorders, hepatic diseases, or serious anemia. The circulation of large amounts of lactic acid in the blood can result in a critical metabolic acidosis termed *lactic acidosis.* The onset of lactic acidosis is usually sudden, and the prognosis is almost always poor, since this condition is highly resistive to treatment.

Compensatory Mechanisms. The body fights metabolic acidosis in the following ways:

RESPIRATORY DEFENSE

Kussmaul respirations (air hunger)

1. Breathing increases in rate and depth.
2. Excess H_2CO_3 is "blown off."
3. *Result:* H^+ concentration of ECF is lowered.

RENAL DEFENSE

1. Na^+–H^+ exchange is increased, which results in the excretion of H^+ in the urine with K^+ reabsorbed to maintain electroneutrality.
2. Rate of the ammonia mechanism is increased.
3. *Result*
   a. An acid urine is produced.
   b. Large numbers of H^+ are excreted as NH_4.
   c. There is a greater return of HCO_3^- to the ECF where it joins with Na^+ to form $NaHCO_3$.
   d. The base side of the H_2CO_3–$NaHCO_3$ ratio is increased.

If the acidosis is compensated, H^+ levels in the ECF will decrease and the plasma bicarbonate level will rise.

Bases of Symptoms. The symptoms seen in metabolic acidosis are the result of both the primary imbalance and the compensatory reaction of the body. In Table 12–10 major symptoms are listed along with the causes.

Clinical Care. The major goals of clinical care for patients with metabolic acidosis are:

1. The restoration of proper blood volume and osmolality
2. The correction of HCO_3^- deficit
3. Prevention of electrolyte imbalances

THE RESTORATION OF PROPER BLOOD VOLUME AND OSMOLALITY. Patients with acidosis are often seriously dehydrated, from vomiting, diarrhea, and other problems. Consequently, precise records of fluctuations of the patient's weight as well as a record of intake and output are essential. An indwelling catheter will be ordered, and in severe cases, hourly urine measurements may be necessary to observe for fluid depletion. Also, an isotonic solution such as sodium chloride or Ringer's lactate is usually administered intravenously to compensate for fluid losses.

THE CORRECTION OF THE HCO_3^- DEFICIT. $NaHCO_3$, or molar Na lactate, is often added to the IV solution to help restore H_2CO_3–$NaHCO_3$ ratio. In patients with severe acidosis, large—potentially dangerous—doses of $NaHCO_3$ may be administered.

PREVENTION OF ELECTROLYTE IMBALANCES. Patients with metabolic acidosis can develop hyperkalemia. A common reason is reabsorption of K^+ in place of H^+ excreted, to maintain electro-neutrality. Another cause is severe tissue damage, which can be secondary to anaerobic metabolism. Because a serious K^+ excess can result in cardiac arrest, every effort must be made to reduce K^+ in the plasma.

The general treatment listed above can expose the patient to new dangers. One common complication of therapy in metabolic acidosis is *re-*

TABLE 12–10. SIGNS AND SYMPTOMS OF METABOLIC ACIDOSIS

Signs and Symptoms	Bases
Apathy; disorientation; delirium; weakness; stupor; coma	Central nervous system depression resulting from elevated H^+ concentration secondary to increased H^+ production and accumulation or loss of HCO_3^-
Kussmaul respirations	Compensatory reaction by the lung
Laboratory findings:	
Blood pH below 7.36, plasma HCO_3^- below 25 mEq./L.	Accumulation of H^+ or loss of base from the plasma
Acid urine with pH below 4.5.	Compensatory reaction by the kidney; H^+ secretion and Na^+–H^+ exchange increased
Severe arrhythmias; cardiac arrest	K^+ reabsorbed in exchange for H^+ to maintain electroneutrality across tubular epithelium; intracellular K^+ shifts into the plasma in acidosis and with severe tissue damage

bound respiratory alkalosis. This imbalance commonly occurs following $NaHCO_3$ replacement. A second complication of therapy is *tetany* due to hypocalcemia. This imbalance occurs upon correction of the metabolic acidosis for the following reasons.

When body fluids are acid (or when the patient is acidotic), calcium exists in its ionized form, which is the more effective form for maintaining proper transmission of impulses for neuromuscular activity. If the patient is suffering from a Ca^{++} deficit, symptoms will *not* appear, because the body's Ca^{++} is being utilized. Once the acidosis is corrected and the patient's body fluids return to normal limits of pH, fewer Ca^{++} will then exist in the ionized form, and *neuromuscular irritability* and *tetany* may develop. The treatment of choice is the intravenous administration of calcium gluconate. (See p. 204 for precautions in the administration of this drug.)

Nursing Implications. When caring for patients with metabolic acidosis, watch for the following symptoms: (1) altered respiratory excursion (rate and depth of respiration), (2) CNS depression (delirium and coma), and (3) neuromuscular signs of K^+ excess (weakness, flaccid paralysis, and cardiac arrest). Following therapy, observe for hypoventilation. Take safety precautions when working with patients in metabolic acidosis. Do not leave a delirious patient unattended. Always make certain that the side rails are up if you must leave the bedside. Remember that disorientation and weakness may cause the acidotic patient to fall from the bed, causing serious injury and further physical complications.

Metabolic Alkalosis

Etiology. The basic problems characterizing metabolic alkalosis are (1) an abnormal rise in the base bicarbonate of the plasma that increases the alkali side of the H_2CO_3–$NaHCO_3$ ratio; and/or (2) a decrease in the H^+ concentration of the plasma, with a resultant rise in blood pH.

EXCESSIVE LOSS OF H^+ FROM THE BODY. Patients who are particularly susceptible to H^+ depletion are: (1) those who are vomiting stomach contents (not intestinal contents as in metabolic acidosis) and (2) those on gastric suction who are losing electrolytes and who are *not* receiving adequate electrolyte replacement. In both of these situations patients are *losing large amounts of HCl,* which leads to the following problems:

- The loss of excessive H^+ from the body in emesis or drainage.
- The loss of Cl^-, which leaves Na^+ unattached and free to unite with HCO_3^- to form $NaHCO_3$.
- The conservation of the anion HCO_3^-, which serves to replace the lost anion Cl^-, and thus preserve the electrical neutrality of the body.

As a result of these chemical changes, H^+ is lost and excesses of $NaHCO_3$ are produced; consequently, the 1:20 ratio of buffer acid to buffer base is upset in favor of buffer base. To make matters worse, if the body has been subjected to severe trauma or stress, Na^+ is retained in unusually large amounts because of an increased secretion of aldosterone. The increased Na^+ in the body fluids combines readily with HCO_3^- to form a heavy alkaline load.

EXCESSIVE INGESTION OF ALKALI. Patients with peptic ulcers or "acid stomach" often take ordinary baking soda or milk of magnesia, thinking that self-medication with alkaline substances will relieve their symptoms.* Actually baking soda, indiscriminately used, often causes an "acid rebound" as a result of the release of CO_2. This reaction causes increased acidity. The patient is uncomfortable and consequently ingests more baking soda, and a vicious circle begins that finally ends in metabolic alkalosis. Ulcer patients who are *both* vomiting and ingesting alkali medications are particularly vulnerable to this imbalance, as they are losing H^+ in the emesis at the same time that they are ingesting HCO_3^-.

Compensatory Mechanisms. Major ways in which the body tries to compensate for metabolic alkalosis are as follows:

THE BUFFER DEFENSE. As HCO_3^- increases in the ECF, it reacts with acid buffer salts. This results in a decrease in bicarbonate and an increase in the carbonic acid partner of the H_2CO_3–$NaHCO_3$ ratio.

RESPIRATORY DEFENSE. Hypoventilation is the major defense; this conserves CO_2, which increases the pCO_2; therefore, H^+ concentration of the ECF increases. Two complications can result from hypoventilation: (1) secondary respiratory acidosis owing to retention of CO_2; and (2) decreased O_2 intake, resulting in hypoxia and possible anaerobic metabolism leading to lactic acidemia.

RENAL DEFENSE. H^+ is conserved and large amounts of K^+ and Na^+ are excreted with the excess of HCO_3^-. This can produce a dangerous K^+ deficit. Ammonia production slows, and H^+ is conserved. This results in an alkaline urine rather than the normal slightly acid urine.

Note how the compensatory mechanisms used by the body to fight metabolic alkalosis are almost exactly the opposite of those used to ward off metabolic acidosis. In acidosis the person hyper-

*For a more complete discussion of the relationship of the milk-alkali syndrome and metabolic alkalosis to peptic ulcer, see the discussion of gastrointestinal tract disorders, Unit XVII.

ventilates and excretes an acid urine. In alkalosis the person hypoventilates and excretes an alkaline urine. In both, any malfunctioning of buffers, lungs, or kidneys results in an imbalance that is uncompensated and dangerous.

Bases of Symptoms. The signs and symptoms of metabolic alkalosis appear in the lungs, neuromuscular system, kidneys, and heart. As in metabolic acidosis, symptoms are the result of both the primary imbalance and compensatory mechanisms. Major symptoms and their causative factors are listed in Table 12–11.

Clinical Care. To correct the metabolic alkalosis and alleviate the symptoms, the following therapeutic steps are necessary.

TREATING THE PRIMARY CONDITION. The major causative factors in alkalosis are loss of acid, overingestion of alkali, and loss of electrolytes, especially Cl^- and K^+.

First, patients who are losing acid because of vomiting or gastric suction will need appropriate replacement fluids. Second, to prevent electrolyte losses, irrigate the patient's gastric tube with isotonic solution rather than with plain water, and always give the patient isotonic fluid to drink when fluids are ordered. Third, ulcer and other patients must be instructed *not to medicate themselves* by taking large amounts of baking soda at home.

Warn ulcer patients who are taking *prescribed* alkaline substances at home to stop the medication and call their physician should they develop a distaste for milk, dryness of mouth, anorexia, weakness, and lethargy. These are signs of the milk-alkali syndrome.

CORRECTION OF ALKALOSIS. Alkalosis is usually treated by giving Ringer's solution, which contains 10 mEq./L. of chloride. This solution not only corrects the alkalosis, but alleviates the chloride deficit as well. In severe cases the doctor may order 0.9 per cent ammonium chloride (NH_4Cl) intravenously. This drug causes the release of HCl, thus restoring both the normal H^+ concentration of the ECF and normal Cl^- levels. Ammonium chloride 0.9 per cent is an *extremely dangerous* medication. When administering this drug intravenously, remember these points:

> 1. *Give 0.9 per cent ammonium chloride (NH_4Cl) at a rate of 1 liter in 4 hours or 2–3 ml/minute. A faster rate of administration may result in* hemolysis of the red blood cells.
> 2. *Do not give NH_4Cl to patients with hepatic or renal diseases.*
> 3. *Excessive administration of NH_4Cl may cause metabolic acidosis.*
> 4. *Observe for signs and symptoms of hyperkalemia.*

The use of 0.9 per cent NH_4Cl intravenously is a somewhat controversial subject. Some physicians think that the drug is worthwhile despite its dangers, while others believe that its toxic effects negate its value as a corrective drug in alkalosis.

CORRECTION OF H_2O, Na^+, Cl^-, AND K^+ DEFICITS. Sodium, H_2O, and Cl^- deficits are usually corrected by administering normal saline. To correct K^+ deficits, KCl is given IV; cathartics may be withheld and thiazide-type diuretics discontinued.

The correction of K^+ deficits is particularly important in the treatment of alkalosis. K^+ deficits that have developed prior to or during the course of metabolic alkalosis must be replaced before H^+ balance can be restored, for the following reasons:

1. When body fluids become too alkaline, the kidneys fight to preserve H^+ by *substituting* K^+ for H^+ in the H^+–Na^+ exchange. Thus, large amounts of K^+ are excreted in the urine. The result is *extracellular K^+ loss.*
2. If these extracellular losses of K^+ are not corrected, K^+ is then pulled from the cells to replace the extracellular losses. This results in *intracellular K^+ loss.*
3. In response to decreasing amounts of intracellu-

TABLE 12–11. SIGNS AND SYMPTOMS OF METABOLIC ALKALOSIS

Signs and Symptoms	Bases
Belligerence; irritability; disorientation; lethargy; tetany; convulsions	Altered H_2CO_3–$NaHCO_3$ ratio secondary to accumulation of bicarbonate and loss of H^+
Shallow, slow respirations; decreased thoracic movements; cyanosis; periods of apnea	Compensatory mechanism by the lungs
Irregular pulse; muscle twitch; paralytic ileus, cardiac arrest	Abnormal losses of K^+ from the ECF in exchange for H^+
Laboratory findings: Plasma pH 7.45; plasma bicarbonate above 29 mEq./L.	Increase in HCO_3^- side of H_2CO_3–$NaHCO_3$ ratio due to loss of H^+ from H_2CO_3 side of equation
Urine pH above 7.0 (alkaline)	Compensatory reaction by the kidney

lar K^+, the Na^+ and H^+ enter the cell in order to balance the losses and thus preserve the electric neutrality of the body fluids. The result can be an *intracellular acidosis* and an *extracellular alkalosis.*

The metabolic alkalosis that has contributed to the development of a K^+ deficit in the first place is now complicated further by the problems listed below:

- When a K^+ deficit occurs, the kidneys (for unknown reasons) are unable to excrete HCO_3^-.
- When K^+ losses are severe, the kidney strives to preserve K^+ at the expense of H^+, which it excretes. The loss of H^+ then, coupled with the retention of HCO_3^-, worsens the alkalosis that is already present. To correct the alkalosis, K^+ *deficits* must be immediately replaced. Moreover, to sustain the body's K^+ at a normal level, the alkalosis must be corrected.

The patient's response to therapy can be followed on the basis of a daily electrolyte analysis, weight, and intake and output. Serum K^+ levels must be monitored carefully, for once alkalosis has been corrected, hyperkalemia may result. Generally it takes 12 to 24 hours to correct the NaCl and water deficits, around 42 hours to correct the K^+ deficit, and between 48 and 72 hours to fully reverse the alkalosis.

The findings in metabolic acid-base disturbance are summarized in Table 12–12.

Respiratory Acidosis

Etiology. As the name suggests, respiratory acidosis is an imbalance in which abnormalities of pulmonary ventilation cause an increase in the H^+ concentration of the body fluids. The problem in metabolic acidosis is an excessive loss of sodium bicarbonate coupled with overproduction and retention of nonvolatile acids. In *respiratory* acidosis, *excessive retention of* CO_2 results in: (1) combining of increasingly formed or produced CO_2 with H_2O to form H_2CO_3; (2) a decrease in H_2CO_3–$NaHCO_3$ ratio; (3) increase in H^+ concentration, whereas pCO_2 may be elevated or within normal limits; (4) lowered serum pH; and (5) CO_2 content/combining power may be within limits or lowered.

Several factors can create this situation. First, respiratory acidosis can be voluntarily caused by *breath holding*. This is rare, because the person will become unconscious, thereby losing voluntary control over breathing. Excessive retention of CO_2 is more commonly the result of respiratory diseases that (a) halt or hinder the gaseous exchanges normally occurring between the blood and alveolar air or (b) that cause obstruction, preventing exhalation of CO_2 into the atmosphere. Major physiologic disorders resulting in the reduction of CO_2 and O_2 exchange in the alveoli are:

- Changes in the respiratory center in the medulla
- A decrease in the surface area of the lung, which, in turn, reduces the diffusion of gases.
- Obstruction of the passageways of the respiratory tract

There are many diseases and injuries that can produce the changes just listed. The major conditions are: emphysema, bronchiectasis, pneumothorax, hemothorax, bronchial asthma, drug intoxication (resulting in respiratory depression), bronchial pneumonia, poliomyelitis, pulmonary fibrosis, acute alcoholism, burns of the respiratory tract, congestive heart failure, and major surgery. The development of respiratory acidosis during surgery is discussed in Unit VIII.

Compensatory Mechanisms. The major ways in which the body attempts to compensate for respiratory acidosis are as listed for acidosis in general and are:

DEFENSE BY THE BUFFER SYSTEM. The body increases the *rate of the chloride shift* and a larger than normal number of chloride ions pass into the red blood cells from the plasma in exchange for HCO_3^-, which passes into the blood. The result is that excess H_2CO_3 is neutralized, and the increased proportion of H_2CO_3 to $NaHCO_3$ is corrected and the normal 1:20 ratio is restored.

TABLE 12–12. SUMMARY OF METABOLIC ACID-BASE DISTURBANCES

	Normal	Uncompensated Acidosis	Partially Compensated Acidosis	Uncompensated Alkalosis	Partially Compensated Alkalosis
HCO_3^-	24.0 mEq./L.	15.0	17.2	38.0	34.5
H_2CO_3	1.2 mEq./L.	1.2	0.9	1.2	1.33
Ratio	20:1	12.5:1	19:1	31.6:1	25.9:1
pCO_2	40.0 mm. Hg	40.0	30.0	40.0	45.0
pH	7.4	7.2	7.38	7.6	7.5

From Burke, S.: *The Composition and Function of Body Fluids*, 2nd ed. St. Louis: C. V. Mosby Co., 1976, p. 80.

RESPIRATORY DEFENSE. Hyperventilation, the main defense occurring in response to the increased pCO_2 and lowered pH of the plasma, may not be effective in the presence of pulmonary pathology. If operative, the result is that large amounts of CO_2 and H_2O (H_2CO_3) are "blown off," pCO_2 drops toward normal, and the pH rises.

RENAL DEFENSE. The kidneys labor to lower the concentration of H^+ in the body fluids by: (1) increasing the rate of H^+–Na^+ exchange (this results in H^+ excretion and reabsorption of Na^+, which joins with HCO_3^- to form $NaHCO_3$) and (2) increased formation of ammonia, which results in an increased H^+ excretion. The total result of renal defense is that excess H^+ ions are excreted in an acid urine, and the base portion of the H_2CO_3–$NaHCO_3$ ratio is increased. Compensation by the kidney is complete; however, it takes about half a day for a plasma pH to return to normal.

The individual with pulmonary disease must rely heavily upon the renal compensatory mechanisms for the control of respiratory acidosis. However, in severe cases, the kidney with its slow but steady regulation of blood pH may not be able to act quickly enough to compensate for the acidosis. Thus, the pH may drop to dangerously low levels before compensation finally takes place.

Bases of Symptoms. The major symptoms of respiratory acidosis are cardiopulmonary. Often the only sign of imbalance is *dyspnea upon exertion.* However, other serious symptoms may occur. These are listed in Table 12–13 along with their causative bases.

A patient with chronic lung disease (e.g., emphysema) may develop a severe complication called *CO_2 narcosis.* This condition is the result of the following chain of pathologic events:

1. The diseased lung cannot excrete CO_2 in large amounts
2. CO_2 accumulates within the blood
3. The pCO_2 rises and the pH falls
4. The respiratory center in the medulla is overwhelmed by the rising CO_2 concentration of the body fluids
5. The respiratory center loses its sensitivity to the elevated CO_2 concentrations and fails to respond (the medulla responds to slight changes in blood pH or CO_2; CO_2 concentrations of over 9 per cent cause depression of the respiratory center)
6. The patient, instead of breathing rapidly in order to "blow off" CO_2, now hypoventilates, although rapid, shallow breathing only moves air back and forth in the dead air spaces
7. CO_2 builds up in the body fluids and chronically remains elevated
8. The constant elevation of CO_2 levels in the body fluids leads to the condition of CO_2 narcosis

Symptoms of CO_2 narcosis are the result of huge accumulations of CO_2 within the blood. They involve the respiratory center, the heart, and the neuromuscular system. The major symptoms are:

CNS: drowsiness, irritability, depression, hallucinations, coma, paralysis, convulsions, facial tremors.
Respiratory system: poor ventilation, shallow respirations
Heart: tachycardia, arrhythmias

> Remember:
> *CO_2 narcosis can be precipitated by giving excessive oxygen therapy to patients with poor ventilation (e.g., postoperative patients and patients with emphysema).*

These people, because their respiratory centers are no longer responding adequately to plasma CO_2 concentrations, depend upon *hypoxia* or *anoxia* as their major respiratory stimulus. Therefore, when too high a concentration of O_2 is given to such patients, they lose their *one* reason for breathing, namely, the *need to correct O_2 lack.* As a result, the patient may cease to breathe altogether and will die! Thus, there is need to use caution and judgment when administering O_2 to dyspneic patients.

Clinical Care. In respiratory acidosis the

TABLE 12–13. SIGNS AND SYMPTOMS OF RESPIRATORY ACIDOSIS

Signs and Symptoms	Bases
Respiratory: Severe dyspnea; wheezing; hyperventilation at rest	Inadequate pulmonary ventilation and hindrance of the normal O_2–CO_2 exchange between the blood and alveolar air
CNS: Disorientation; coma may follow	CNS depression; hypoxemia
Cardiac: Tachycardia; arrhythmias	Inadequate pulmonary ventilation and hindrance of the normal O_2–CO_2 exchange between the blood and alveolar air
Laboratory findings: Plasma pH below 7.36; plasma bicarbonate 29 mEq./L.; urine pH 4.5	Results of buffer and renal compensation

major problem is *poor ventilation* and the consequent accumulation of CO_2, resulting in elevated levels of CO_2 within the serum. Therefore, the major goal of therapy is to *improve ventilation* by correcting the respiratory disease. Other goals of therapy are to *neutralize the excessive acid,* and *correct H_2O, K^+,* and *Cl^- imbalances* if they exist.

IMPROVEMENT OF RESPIRATORY FUNCTION.* Some of the typical treatments often ordered to improve respiratory efficiency are antibiotics to curb respiratory infections; postural drainage; bronchodilators and detergents; inhalation therapy with nebulization; breathing exercises that increase the efficiency of respiration; mechanical ventilators; and oxygen, administered with extreme caution.

CORRECTION OF THE ACIDOSIS. Important drugs and solutions used in treating respiratory acidosis are:

- Ringer's lactate solution IV is given in severe cases of respiratory acidosis.
- Sodium bicarbonate orally or intravenously.
- One sixth molar solution of sodium lactate, 20 mg./kg. of body weight, IV until the urine has an alkaline reaction.

These drugs and solutions need to be administered with caution. As you will recall, the intravenous administration of sodium bicarbonate to patients with acidosis may result in *tetany* once the acidosis is corrected and the body fluids become more alkaline. Thus, as in metabolic acidosis, *calcium gluconate* should be on hand in the event of this complication. Some doctors may order a prophylactic dose of 10 ml. of 10 per cent calcium gluconate to be given intravenously *before* sodium bicarbonate administration, thereby alleviating the possibility of tetany.

Occasionally, in addition to the above drugs and solutions, patients may be placed on *gastric suction* to remove excess HCl, thereby raising the pH of the body fluids.

THE CORRECTION OF WATER AND ELECTROLYTE IMBALANCES. To correct dehydration, the doctor may order the intravenous administration of hypotonic solutions containing carbohydrates and electrolytes. If K^+ levels are elevated, appropriate measures will be taken to correct the hyperkalemia.

As with all the imbalances discussed, treatment unfortunately can create new complications. In respiratory acidosis, three iatrogenic conditions may occur as a result of therapy: (1) *tetany,* which results from the administration of $NaHCO_3$ and the consequent correction of the lowered pH of the blood; (2) *CO_2 narcosis*, which results from the administration of large quantities of O_2 to patients with longstanding chronic CO_2 retention; and (3) *rebound respiratory alkalosis,* which results from too rapid compensation of respiratory acidosis, overzealous use of mechanical respirators, and the excessively rapid administration of $NaHCO_3$.

*Methods of treating respiratory problems are discussed in detail in Unit XVI.

Respiratory Alkalosis

Etiology. The major problem that characterizes respiratory alkalosis is the *excessive loss of CO_2*, which results in (1) a decrease in the H^+ concentration of the body fluid, (2) a decrease in the pCO_2, (3) an increase in the ratio of $NaHCO_3$ to H_2CO_3, and (4) a rise in the blood pH.

These disturbances are almost always the result of (1) hyperventilation and (2) overstimulation of the respiratory center in the brain. The following are the most common causes of *hyperventilation,* with consequent respiratory alkalosis:

- Hysteria and anxiety reactions
- The aftermath of severe exercise
- Hypoxia at high altitudes, which leads to increased respirations and an increased loss of CO_2
- Poorly adjusted rate on automatic ventilators which cause patients to hyperventilate

Overstimulation of the respiratory center in the brain can result from:

- Fever
- CNS diseases (e.g., meningitis and encephalitis)
- Intracranial surgery
- Aspirin poisoning

Both respiratory alkalosis and acidosis are imbalances that can be caused voluntarily. For example, acidosis can be caused by purposely holding one's breath, and alkalosis can be caused by voluntary hyperventilation. However, while respiratory acidosis is caused by definite physiologic disorders that interfere with pulmonary ventilation, respiratory alkalosis is more often the result of psychologic and environmental factors and diseases that are not necessarily respiratory in nature.

Compensatory Mechanisms. The body strives to correct respiratory alkalosis with the same three mechanisms, namely:

DEFENSE BY THE BUFFER SYSTEM. The body increases plasma content of organic acids, and the acids react with excess bicarbonate ions. The result is that excessive base is neutralized, and there is restoration of the normal 1:20 ratio of H_2CO_3 to $NaHCO_3$.

RESPIRATORY DEFENSE. Respirations decrease or even cease until CO_2 levels rise to a high enough level to again stimulate respiration. The result is that the decrease in plasma H_2CO_3 is compensated and a H^+ excess results. The excess H^+ is then excreted by the kidneys as necessary.

RENAL COMPENSATION. The kidney halts the reabsorption of HCO_3^- and hastens its excretion; it also diminishes the production of NH_3. The result is that H^+ is retained in the body until the normal 1:20 ratio of H_2CO_3–$NaHCO_3$ is restored.

Thus, the body compensates for respiratory alkalosis by using available buffers in the serum by decreasing respiration and producing an alkaline urine.

Bases of Symptoms. The most outstanding characteristic of respiratory alkalosis is *increased neuromuscular irritability*. Therefore, patients develop hyperreflexia, a positive Chvostek's sign, and muscular twitch. Generalized convulsions sometimes occur. Characteristic laboratory findings are alkaline urine with pH above 7.0 and plasma pH above 7.44. Sometimes K^+ depletion may occur if the attack of respiratory alkalosis is prolonged over several days. Hypokalemia, in this case, can be controlled by administering 1 mEq. of K^+/kg. of body weight per day.

Clinical Care. In treating respiratory alkalosis, eliminate the cause of the hyperventilation and help the patient breathe more slowly and deeply. Psychotherapy may be required for the hysterical or highly anxious patient. Hysterical patients can rebreathe their own CO_2 from a paper bag, thus increasing the H^+ concentration of their blood. Patients suffering from neurologic disorders or from aspirin poisoning require treatment of the primary condition. Ventilators should be checked hourly and adjusted as needed for optimal ventilation.

The findings in respiratory acid-base disturbance are summarized in Table 12–14.

POTASSIUM BALANCE

Essential facts concerning potassium [K^+] balance are summarized in Table 12–15.

In reviewing the outline in Table 12–15, it is apparent that *anything that reduces the integrity of the cell will produce a K^+* imbalance. For example, trauma, burns, and starvation are all factors that impair cellular metabolism, thereby creating potassium disorders. When potassium imbalances do occur, symptoms involving *cardiac, cellular* and *neuromuscular function* develop. *Kidney function* is also disturbed, since the kidney is the major organ of potassium excretion.

POTASSIUM IMBALANCES

Potassium Deficit (Hypokalemia)

This is a common imbalance and one that is potentially deadly in its pathologic effects.

Etiology. The major causes of potassium deficit are summarized in Table 12–16.

Bases of Symptoms. A potassium deficit of the ECF (hypokalemia) basically affects *cellular metabolism,* which in turn, affects the functions of the neuromuscular system, cardiovascular system, gastrointestinal tract, respiratory tract, and kidney. H^+ balance is also affected. These disturbances are listed in Table 12–17 along with the specific symptoms they produce.

The diagnosis of a potassium deficit is usually made on the basis of these signs and symptoms and the patient's history. Also, the serum K^+ value will usually reflect the degree of intracellular K^+ deficit as long as acid-base status is normal. In alkalosis, K^+ shifts from the serum into the cell, resulting in hypokalemia, even though intracellular K^+ content actually increases. Potassium replacement therapy must take this fact into account. Regardless of the cause, hypokalemia is significant because of its potentially lethal effects; it must be diagnosed and treated swiftly.

Prevention of K^+ Deficit. One of the principle goals of nursing care is prevention of K^+ deficit in susceptible patients. Some specific ways

TABLE 12–14. SUMMARY OF RESPIRATORY ACID-BASE IMBALANCE

	Normal	Uncompensated Acidosis	Partially Compensated Acidosis	Uncompensated Alkalosis	Partially Compensated Alkalosis
HCO_3^-	24.0 mEq./L.	24.0	38.1	24.0	20.0
H_2CO_3	1.2 mEq./L.	2.7	2.5	0.6	0.8
Ratio	20:1	8.8:1	15.2:1	40:1	25:1
pCO_2	40.0 mm. Hg	90.0	80.0	20.0	25.0
pH	7.4	7.2	7.3	7.55	7.52

From Burke, S.: *The Composition and Function of Body Fluids*, 2nd ed. St. Louis: C. V. Mosby Co., 1976, p. 76.

TABLE 12–15. BODY POTASSIUM (K^+)—A SUMMARY OF BASIC FACTS

I. The body of a normal 70 kg. (154 lb.) male contains approximately 3500 mEq. of K^+.
II. K^+ is found in all fluid compartments.
  A. It is the dominant ion of cellular fluid (which contains approximately 98% of the body's K^+).
  B. The extracellular fluid contains only about 2% of the body's K^+.
  C. The normal serum K^+ concentration ranges from 3.5 to 5.5 mEq./L.
III. K^+ performs the following valuable functions:
  A. Regulates the intracellular osmolality.
  B. Promotes cellular growth.
  C. Helps to promote the conduction of nerve impulses.
  D. Helps to promote proper skeletal muscle function.
  E. Helps to promote proper heart muscle activity.
  F. Assists in maintenance of acid-base balance by cellular exchange with H^+.
IV. K^+ ingestion and excretion.
  A. Normally a person requires 40 mEq. of K^+ per day.
  B. Eighty to 90% of ingested K^+ is excreted in the urine while 10 to 20% is excreted in the stools.
  C. Under the influence of aldosterone, K^+ is lost while Na^+ is retained.
V. The conservation of cellular K^+.
  A. The amount of K^+ in the cell depends upon the following factors:
    1. The integrity or general health of the cell.
    2. The sodium pump, which maintains a high K^+ cellular content by actively excluding Na^+.
    3. The ability of the kidney to conserve K^+ to some degree when the cells become depleted.
  B. K^+ moves *into* the cells when glucose is being metabolized by the body and during alkalosis.
  C. K^+ moves *out* of the cells under these conditions:
    1. During strenuous exercise.
    2. When cellular metabolism is impaired.
    3. When the cell dies.
    4. During acidosis.
  D. When K^+ *is lost* from the cell, the following happens:
    1. Other ions shift into the cell in order to maintain cellular tonicity, e.g., Na^+ and H^+ ions shift into the cell from the ECF to replace lost K^+.
    2. The cell, due to the H^+, then becomes more acid while the ECF becomes more alkaline.

TABLE 12–16. CAUSES OF POTASSIUM DEFICIT

I. Inadequate intake of K^+ due to:
  A. Poor dietary habits.
  B. Nausea.
  C. Poor appetite.
  D. Acute alcoholism.
  E. Extreme dieting.
  F. Parenteral fluids that are low in K^+ and high in Na^+. The kidneys and cells are unable to conserve K^+ when the body is deprived of a K^+ intake at the same time that it is receiving a large Na^+ load. The body tends to conserve Na^+ at the expense of K^+.
II. Increased utilization of K^+ during the healing phase of burns.
III. Excessive loss of K^+ due to:
  A. Therapies.
    1. Diuretics (e.g., thiazides, mercurials, Lasix) inhibit reabsorption of K^+.
    2. Adrenal steroid therapy, causing Na^+ retention and increased K^+ excretion.
    3. Excessive infusions of IV solutions (especially saline) without adequate K^+ replacement.
    4. Excessive enemas and laxatives leading to inadequate absorption time for K^+.
    5. Gastric and intestinal suction.
    6. Operations in which large amounts of K^+ are lost in the drainage from the surgical site, e.g., colostomies, ileostomies, large or small bowel resections.
  B. Conditions of the gastrointestinal tract.
    1. Vomiting, because K^+ is lost with the regurgitated mucus and gastric secretions.
    2. Ulcerative colitis and diarrhea.
    3. Fistulas of the small or large intestine.
  C. Metabolic disorders.
    1. The stress syndrome:
      a. Occurs in response to fear, severe psychologic upsets, burns, extensive surgery, and tissue cell damage.
      b. Affects adrenal and pituitary gland secretions.
      c. Mobilizes K^+ from tissue cells and excretes it in large amounts.
    2. Conditions causing an increased corticosteroid production, e.g., Cushing's syndrome.
    3. Diabetic ketoacidosis.
  D. Alkalosis due to K^+ shift into cell in exchange for H^+.
  E. Renal disorders.
    1. K^+ losing nephropathies.
    2. Diuretic phase of acute renal failure.

of preventing the development of hypokalemia include:

- Know the following facts about your patient in order to anticipate losses and the need for replacement: What medications are being taken? Diuretics? Cortisone? Has vomiting been present? If so, what is the amount and color of the vomitus? Is diarrhea present? How many stools per day? What kind of foods are being selected? Are they adequate in K^+ content? What is the amount of urinary output? What is the acid-base status? Do the patient's IV fluids contain K^+?
- Carefully observe patients undergoing emotional or physical stress, as well as postoperative patients, for signs and symptoms of K^+ deficit. Monitor the pulse and electrocardiogram.
- Chart and report to the physician any findings that may suggest a K^+ deficiency.
- Always irrigate nasogastric tubes and intestinal drainage tubes with normal saline to prevent a washout of K^+.

Clinical Care. In cases where K^+ loss cannot be prevented, therapy directed at correcting the K^+ deficit is the goal. Potassium can be replaced by diet or medications.

ORAL REPLACEMENT OF POTASSIUM. It is generally agreed that it is less dangerous to use the oral route in replacing K^+ than the more rapid-acting intravenous route. The most natural way to correct a K^+ deficit is through a high-potassium diet. Some dietary sources of K^+ are listed in Table 12–18.

A second important method of K^+ replacement is with *oral medications.* Some of the most common medications are the following:

1. Potassium chloride (KCl) 5–10 Gm. per day. Since potassium and chloride deficiencies often coexist, KCl is the drug of choice in many cases of hypokalemia. Potassium is very irritating to the gastric mucosa and can cause nausea, vomiting, or diarrhea. More seriously, it has been reported that patients ingesting KCl can develop stenosis and ulcers of the small intestine. To reduce gastric irritation, remind patients to drink a full glass of water when taking oral potassium preparations.

2. Potassium triplex, 5 ml. (15 mEq. K^+) orally, 3 times daily. Potassium triplex, a liquid medication, contains equal amounts of potassium acetate, potassium bicarbonate, and potassium citrate. Because this drug is also irritating to the gastric mucosa and has an unpleasant taste, it is best administered in juice and after meals.

3. Potassium citrate, 1 or 2 Gm. orally, daily in divided doses.

4. Potassium gluconate (Kaon), 30 ml. (40 mEq.) orally, daily.

In dispensing oral medications containing potassium, implement the following rules to ensure safety:

> *1. Dispense oral medications containing K^+ with caution, since potassium excess can result from excessive dosages. Frequent monitoring of serum K^+ and the patient's clinical status are important.*
>
> *2. Watch carefully for oliguria in patients receiving K^+ supplements (K^+ may be retained if renal output is poor).*
>
> *3. Carefully observe for signs and symptoms of hyperkalemia.*

INTRAVENOUS ADMINISTRATION. K^+ is administered by means of commercially prepared electrolyte IV solutions containing K^+, or by ampules of liquid potassium that are added to IV fluids such as 5 or 10 per cent glucose in water. Since potassium is potentially highly toxic, the nurse needs to observe carefully the following general rules pertaining to its administration:

- Do *not* give K^+ in concentrated form directly into the vein: *Cardiac arrest can result!* K^+ must be diluted in solution when given by IV drip.
- Carefully watch the *rate* of drip of solutions containing potassium. Usually no more than 20 mEq.

TABLE 12–17. SIGNS AND SYMPTOMS OF POTASSIUM DEFICIT

Signs and Symptoms	Bases
Weakness; speech changes; flaccid paralysis; shallow respirations; decreased intestinal motility; abdominal distention; anorexia; vomiting; flatulence; paralytic ileus	Decreased muscular function
Arrhythmias; rapid, weak, irregular pulse; hypotension; low, flat T wave and U wave on electrocardiogram; cardiac arrest	Weakness of cardiovascular smooth muscle and prolongation of myocardial repolarization
Lethargy; apathy; irritability; mental confusion; tetany; paresthesia	Decreased neuromuscular irritability
Polyuria; nocturia	Inability of kidney to concentrate urine; tubular degeneration
Laboratory findings: Serum K^+ less than 3.5 mEq./L.	Loss of K^+

TABLE 12–18. POTASSIUM CONTENT OF SELECTED FOODS

	Mg.	mEq.
Beverages (8 oz.)		
Apple juice, canned	250	6.4
Apricot juice	372	9.5
Coffee, instant, 2 Gm.	238	6.1
Grape juice, canned, sweetened	387	5.5
Grapefruit juice, canned	405	10.4
Milk, whole	356	9.1
Milk, nonfat	278	7.1
Orange juice, fresh	496	12.7
Pineapple juice, canned	379	9.7
Prune juice, canned	563	14.4
Tea	66	1.7
Tomato juice	544	14.0
Foods		
Apricots, raw, 2 or 3 medium	277	7.1
Banana, fresh, 1 medium	628	16.1
Bouillon, 1 meat-extract cube	108	2.8
Bouillon, 1 vegetable-extract cube	138	3.3
Cantaloupe, ½, 5-in. diameter	230	5.9
Cauliflower, raw, 1¼ cups (10 oz.)	500	12.8
Dates, dried, 3 or 4	226	5.8
Figs, dried, 7 small	780	20.0
Fruit cocktail, canned, sweetened	410	10.5
Molasses, 1 tablespoonful	269	6.9
Peaches, raw, dried, ½ cup (4 oz.)	1,100	28.2
Pear, raw, 1 (2½ by 2 in.)	180	4.6
Prunes, raw, 5 large	300	7.7
Raisins, raw, 2 tablespoonfuls	144	3.7
Strawberries, raw, 8 oz.	265	6.8
Watermelon, ½ slice (¾ by 10 in.)	380	9.7
Wheat germ, 100 Gm.	737	18.9

Adapted from MacLeod, S. M.: The rational use of potassium supplements. *Nursing Digest.* Summer, 1976, p. 88.

of potassium per hour should be given to an adult patient. *A faster rate of infusion can lead to cardiac arrest* due to the effect of K^+ on cardiac muscle cells.

- ▶ Severe pain can develop along the vein used for the K^+ infusion. This usually occurs with high concentrations of K^+ and may be controlled by slowing the drip rate or by diluting the K^+ in a larger volume of fluid.
- ▶ Do not give IV potassium solutions *unless renal flow is adequate,* since K^+ is primarily excreted by the kidneys.
- ▶ Potassium toxicity with impending cardiac arrest is clearly heralded by T and QRS wave changes on EKG. Patients receiving large IV doses of K^+ should be placed on a cardiac monitor.

It usually requires several days to correct a potassium deficit, especially in the presence of large intracellular losses.

Other Precautions. Care must be exercised when administering certain drugs, such as digitalis preparations (cardiac glycosides), to patients with hypokalemia. When K^+ is low, the possibility of digitalis toxicity is greatly enhanced, even though the patient may be receiving nontoxic doses of the drug.

Patients with cardiac disease who are also receiving diuretics in addition to digitalis are particularly vulnerable to hypokalemia and digitalis toxicity. Manifestations of the toxic effects of digitalis are nausea, vomiting, anorexia, and arrhythmias preceding heart block.

Potassium Excess (Hyperkalemia)

Etiology. The major causes of potassium excess are:

Retention of K^+ Within the Body. Patients who are particularly affected are those in renal failure, postoperative patients with a poor renal output, and those with adrenocortical insufficiency.

Excessive Release of K^+ from the Cells. Patients suffering from serious burns, crushing injuries, infection, or acidosis may face the problem of potassium excess, especially when renal function is reduced.

Intravenous Infusions Containing K^+. Rapid administration of IV fluids containing K^+ can lead to hyperkalemia even with normal renal function.

Bases of Symptoms. The major systems affected by K^+ excess are the cardiac, renal, and neuromuscular, as shown in Table 12–19.

Clinical Care. The goals of nursing care are: (a) to prevent hyperkalemia in patients at risk and (b) to support medical therapy aimed at lowering the serum K^+ in patients with hyperkalemia. The treatment of potassium excess depends upon the severity of the imbalance.

A seriously elevated serum potassium constitutes a medical emergency. Cardiac arrest may be imminent.

To promote reduction of serum K^+ levels, the factors that cause potassium excess should be eliminated.

Promotion of K^+ Excretion or Redistribution. Serum K^+ is reduced by promoting a greater urinary output, which may include encouraging adequate fluid intake. In the event of renal shutdown, the artificial kidney may be used for *hemodialysis.* In some cases, *peritoneal dialysis* is instituted (see Unit XIII) to eliminate excess K^+.

Another way to remove excess K^+ from the body is through the use of *ion exchange resins,* such as Kayexalate, which act to remove K^+ in the

TABLE 12–19. SIGNS AND SYMPTOMS OF POTASSIUM EXCESS

Signs and Symptoms	Bases
Bradycardia proceeding to cardiac standstill; ventricular fibrillation; EKG changes of tall, tented T waves; widening QRS; ST segment depression	Depression of cardiac conduction
Intestinal colic; diarrhea; and muscle twitching proceeding to weakness; flaccid muscle paralysis	Increased neuromuscular irritability in slight to moderate hyperkalemia; reduced neuromuscular irritability in severe hyperkalemia
Oliguria; anuria	Renal impairment
Laboratory findings: Serum K^+ greater than 5.5 mEq./L.	Retention of K^+

gastrointestinal tract. They are administered by enema or by mouth and retained for a period of time. Resins, which are not absorbed in the gastrointestinal tract, exchange Na^+ and H^+ for K^+; K^+ is then excreted in the feces.

A reduction in serum K^+ can also be achieved by a *redistribution of K^+ from the serum to the cells.* One method used is the infusion of *glucose and insulin.* Glucose and insulin increase glycogen storage, pulling K^+ along with glycogen into the cell. Also, administration of *sodium bicarbonate* results in an elevation of blood pH, or a state of alkalosis, which promotes K^+ movement into the cells in exchange for H^+. The additional amount of Na^+ also tends to encourage K^+ excretion.

Minimization of Excessive Release of Potassium. K^+ is minimized by controlling the breakdown of tissue. Tissue breakdown is prevented by *controlling infection* and ensuring intake of *adequate calories and carbohydrates.* Such actions serve to spare protein and, consequently, to eliminate the wasting of tissue.

Elimination of Excessive K^+ Intake. Excessive K^+ is eliminated by stopping *all* sources of potassium — oral and parenteral.

Hyperkalemia can best be prevented by limiting K^+ intake in patients susceptible to its development. Close observation of patients for *early* signs and symptoms of K^+ excess may prevent the life-threatening effects produced by severely high K^+ levels.

The fate of the patient with potassium excess depends ultimately upon the speed of diagnosis and the promptness with which the corrective measures are carried out.

CALCIUM BALANCE

Table 12–20 summarizes some important facts about calcium.

TABLE 12–20. BODY CALCIUM (Ca^{++})—A SUMMARY OF BASIC FACTS

I. Normal serum Ca^{++} is approximately 4–5 mEq./L. or 9–11 mg. per cent.
II. Distribution of Ca^{++}.
   A. Nearly 99% in the bones.
   B. Fraction of Ca^{++} in the blood plasma.
III. Ca^{++} performs the following functions:
   A. Promotes normal neuromuscular irritability.
   B. Strengthens capillary membranes.
   C. Promotes normal muscle contractility.
   D. Promotes transmission of nerve impulses.
   E. Essential for blood clotting.
   F. Essential for building of bones and teeth.
IV. Ca^{++} requirements.
   A. Adult requires 0.8 Gm. Ca^{++} daily.
   B. Children and infants require 0.7 to 1.4 Gm. daily.
   C. Pregnant and lactating women require 1.3 to 1.5 Gm. per day.
V. Ca^{++} intake, absorption, and excretion.
   A. Food intake.
      1. Three fourths of Ca^{++} requirement is supplied by milk and milk products.
      2. One fourth of Ca^{++} is supplied by vegetables and fruit.
   B. Absorption of Ca^{++}.
      1. Depends in part upon the presence of vitamin D.
      2. Controlled by the parathyroid glands.
   C. Ca^{++} is excreted in the urine and feces.
VI. Inverse relationship exists between calcium and phosphorus, for obscure reasons.
   A. When calcium is elevated, blood level of phosphorus is low.
   B. When blood level of calcium is low, phosphorus level is elevated.
VII. The regulation of serum Ca^{++}.
   A. Controlled by parathormone [PTH], a parathyroid hormone.
   B. Release of PTH depends upon the level of serum calcium. (The effect of fluctuation in the serum Ca^{++} upon PTH is diagrammed in Figure 12–8.

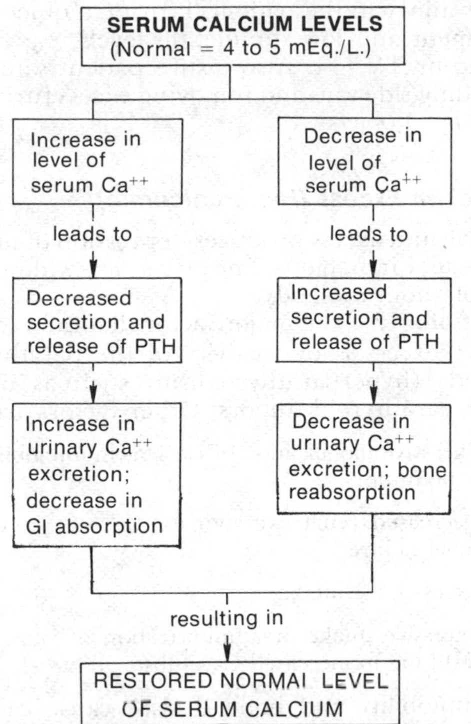

Figure 12–8. The effect of the serum calcium level upon the excretion of parathormone (PTH).

The maintenance of a normal serum calcium depends upon proper intake of calcium and vitamin D, the level of blood phosphorus, and the proper functioning of the parathyroid glands and kidneys (Fig. 12–8). In specific imbalances — either excesses or deficiencies — we can expect symptoms involving the *neuromuscular system,* the *heart,* and the *bones* — all systems in which the Ca^{++} ion is vitally involved. The *kidneys* are also affected, particularly in excesses, because it is the kidney that excretes calcium.

CALCIUM IMBALANCES

Calcium Deficit (Hypocalcemia)

Etiology. A calcium deficit can occur in one or more of the following instances:

- An excessive loss of Ca^{++} from the body. This problem often arises in acute pancreatitis, diarrhea, hypoparathyroidism, and renal disorders.
- Following a *thyroidectomy* in which one or more of the parathyroid glands are accidentally removed.
- During *pregnancy* and *lactation* when Ca^{++} requirements are higher and dietary intake is insufficient.
- When there is an inadequate intake of vitamin D.
- Following the *correction of acidosis* or during alkalosis.

Calcium deficiencies can lead to rickets, osteomalacia, or osteoporosis.

Bases of Symptoms. Hypocalcemia produces an increase in neuromuscular irritability, resulting in a condition called *tetany.* Tetany is characterized by the symptoms listed in Table 12–21.

Both Trousseau's sign and Chvostek's sign are important diagnostic tests for tetany. To test for *Trousseau's sign,* a blood pressure cuff is inflated on the patient's arm (creating enough pressure to stop venous circulation) for 1 to 5 minutes. If contractions of the fingers and hands (carpal spasms) develop, tetany is present. To test for *Chvostek's sign,* tap the patient's face just below the temple where the facial nerve emerges. If there is a momentary contraction of the lip, nose, or side of the face, Chvostek's sign is positive. A positive finding indicates *hyperirritability of the facial nerve* — an important sign of tetany.

Clinical Care. Calcium deficiency is corrected by oral, intramuscular, or intravenous administration of calcium salts. When hypocalcemia is mild and is *not* accompanied by tetany, the following drugs can be given orally.

1. Calcium lactate

TABLE 12–21. SIGNS AND SYMPTOMS OF CALCIUM DEFICIT

Signs and Symptoms	Bases
Painful tonic muscle spasms; facial spasms ("tetany facies"); grimacing; fatigue; laryngospasm; Trousseau's sign; positive Chvostek's sign; convulsions	Increased neuromuscular irritability producing hyperreaction of motor and sensory nerves to stimuli
Tingling and numbness of fingers and circumoral region	Increased irritability of vascular smooth muscle and nerves
Definitive ECG tracing; palpitations; arrhythmias	Decreased cardiac contractility
Laboratory findings: Serum Ca^{++} decreased below 4.5 mEq./L.; serum phosphorus elevated; Sulkowitch urine test shows no precipitation. (For the Sulkowitch test, a 24-hr urine sample is collected and tested for Ca^{++} ions.)	Loss of Ca^{++} from serum, decreased Ca^{++} excretion

2. Calcium chloride. Calcium chloride can be given intravenously as well as orally; however, it should not be given intramuscularly, as it is irritating to tissues.

3. Calcium gluconate. This drug may also be given IV and IM. Give medication containing calcium one half hour before meals and/or at bedtime for best absorption. Often the doctor will order large doses of vitamin D to be given in conjunction with the calcium since vitamin D is necessary for GI absorption of Ca^{++}.

In patients in whom tetany is anticipated or actually present, prompt treatment with IV medication is necessary. One drug commonly used is 10 per cent calcium gluconate solution, IV. Calcium gluconate should be administered slowly. In patients with severe hypocalcemia, 80 ml. of 10 per cent calcium gluconate may have to be added to each liter of 5 per cent glucose in water until the signs of tetany disappear.

The following are guidelines for working with intravenous infusions containing calcium:

> 1. *Guard against the infiltration of IV solutions containing calcium. Tissue hypoxia and sloughing can result.*
> 2. *Do not add calcium to solutions containing carbonate or phosphate.* Dangerous precipitates *will form.*
> 3. *Question giving IV calcium therapy to patients receiving digitalis. Calcium ions have an action similar to that of digitalis and* digitalis toxicity *can result.*
> 4. *Watch for signs of hypercalcemia. Intravenous calcium therapy can result in* cardiac arrest.

Since tetany and convulsions can result from hypocalcemia, precautions must be taken to prevent injury to the patient. Provide a quiet environment and low stimulation levels, e.g., keep radio or TV low. Also insure patient safety by padding side rails and removing excess furniture and hard objects.

Calcium Excess (Hypercalcemia)

Calcium excess produces depression of neuromuscular irritability. The effects are widespread throughout the body.

Etiology. The major factor that can create a Ca^{++} excess is overactivity of the parathyroid glands (hyperparathyroidism) such as occurs with parathyroid tumors. Other factors are:

- Excessive mobilization of Ca^{++} as in immobility or bone tumors.
- Decreased renal excretion of Ca^{++} as occurs in renal failure.
- Excess Ca^{++} intake.
- Excessive intake or administration of vitamin D, resulting in increased Ca^{++} absorption.

Immobility and bone disease cause calcium movement from the bones to the serum, thus raising the serum Ca^{++} level (Fig. 12–9). Also, patients receiving thiazide diuretics may develop a mild hypercalcemia, owing to a decrease in urinary calcium excretion. Patients who have ulcers and drink large amounts of milk daily, as well as taking various alkaline medications, frequently develop hypercalcemia as a part of the milk-alkali syndrome.

Bases of Symptoms. When there is calcium excess in the body, blood calcium levels become abnormally high while serum phosphorus levels become low. These abnormal blood levels, in turn, give rise to many diversified symptoms. Note, in Table 12–22, that the pathologic

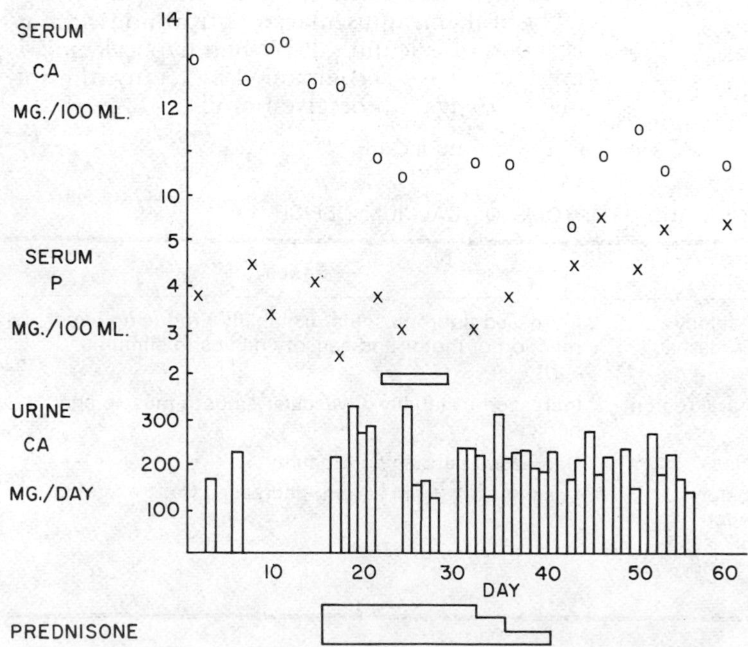

Figure 12–9. Immobilization hypercalcemia. Response of serum calcium concentration to corticosteroid treatment. (From Harrison, H. E., and H. C. Harrison: *Disorders of Calcium and Phosphate Metabolism in Childhood and Adolescence.* Philadelphia: W. B. Saunders Co., 1979.)

changes produced by calcium excess are chiefly related to the *gastrointestinal* tract, the *kidneys,* the *neuromuscular* system, and the *skeletal* tissues.

Because of these many and varied symptoms, it is often difficult to detect Ca^{++} excess and to differentiate it from other disorders. The only reliable way to diagnose Ca^{++} excess is by means of laboratory studies of Ca^{++} and phosphate. Since such studies are not always ordered, patients may be ill for months and even years with an undiagnosed calcium excess. Moreover, a few patients may develop the critical problem of hypercalcemic crisis before treatment is instituted. *Hypercalcemic crisis* is heralded by: severe nausea and vomiting, dehydration, mental confusion, coma, and renal failure. This condition constitutes a *medical emergency* and demands immediate care.

Clinical Care. Treatment of hypercalcemia is aimed at preventing or eliminating the causes. Mobility is encouraged, as much as is permissible, to prevent calcium leaving the bones. Limiting Ca^{++} and vitamin D intake in susceptible patients will also help prevent Ca^{++} excess. Certain measures promote Ca^{++} excretion from the kidneys, such as isotonic saline infusions, disodium phosphate or sodium sulfate, and diuretics. Steroids inhibit the absorption of Ca^{++}. However, these medications can result in hypocalcemia and tetany as well as minor disturbances of K^+, Mg^{++}, and Na^+. Monitor manifestations of these disorders closely. Also remember that the muscle weakness associated with hypercalcemia predisposes the patient to injury; provide for the patient's safety by assisting in ambulation, putting up side rails, keeping the bed lowered, and taking other precautions as necessary.

MAGNESIUM (Mg^{++}) BALANCE

Only recently has the importance of a proper intake of Mg^{++} in the daily diet and the clinical problems of Mg^{++} deficit been explored. Even though Mg^{++} is the second most abundant intracellular cation, its role is still poorly understood, especially in relation to the mechanisms and effects of depletion. Some important facts are available concerning normal Mg^{++} metabolism; they are summarized in Table 12–23.

Because Mg^{++} is essential for neuromuscular integration, disturbances in Mg^{++} balance produce disturbances in *neuromuscular function. Deficits* of Mg^{++} produce increased neuromuscular irritability, convulsions, and extreme behavioral changes (e.g., wild combative actions), similar to hypocalcemia. Mg^{++} *excess* can produce paralysis, hypotension, and sedation of the neuromuscular system, similar to a severe K^+ excess.

MAGNESIUM IMBALANCES

Magnesium Deficiency

Etiology. Depletion is the most common Mg^{++} disorder encountered. A low intake of Mg^{++} over a long period without adequate Mg^{++} replacement, coupled with prolonged and abnormal losses of magnesium from the gastrointestinal tract or kidney is a major cause of Mg^{++} deficit. These problems are commonly seen in *surgical* patients.

Other groups of patients particularly prone to Mg^{++} deficiency are persons with the following: chronic and severe malnutrition, chronic alcoholism, chronic nephritis, prolonged severe diarrhea, prolonged IV therapy without Mg^{++} replacement, intestinal malabsorption, hypoparathyroidism, prolonged diuretic therapy, or patients who are in the diuretic phase of acute renal failure.

Since Mg^{++} is abundant in many of the foods that we normally eat, Mg^{++} deficiency is rarely the result of inadequate diet. When Mg^{++} deficit

TABLE 12–22. SIGNS AND SYMPTOMS OF CALCIUM EXCESS

Signs and Symptoms	Bases
Bone pain; osteoporosis; osteomalacia (softening of bone); pathologic fractures	Decalcification of bones (calcium moves from the bones into the blood)
Flank pain; kidney infection; kidney stones; polyuria; renal failure, which may result in death	Hypercalciuria due to increased Ca^{++} deposits in the renal pelvis and parenchyma; kidney loses its ability to concentrate urine
Diarrhea; constipation; atony of intestinal tract; peptic ulcer (in 8 per cent of patients); anorexia; nausea; vomiting	Gastrointestinal disorders due to an increase of Ca^{++} ions in sympathetic ganglia; this impedes transmission of afferent stimuli
Lethargy; exhaustion; mental confusion; loss of interest in surroundings; irritability, coma	Behavioral changes due to neurologic hypofunction
Laboratory findings: Plasma calcium levels above 5.8 mEq./L.; definitive ECG tracing; serum phosphorus decreased; Sulkowitch urine test shows increased Ca^{++} precipitation	Increased Ca^{++} in serum; increased Ca^{++} excretion; increased cardiac contractility

TABLE 12–23. BODY MAGNESIUM (Mg^{++})—A SUMMARY OF BASIC FACTS

I. A "normal adult male body" contains approximately 25 Gm. of Mg^{++}.
II. Distribution of Mg^{++}:
  A. 70% of Mg^{++} is combined with Ca^{++} and P^{+} in the bones.
  B. 30% of Mg^{++} is in the soft tissues and body fluids.
  C. Predominantly an intracellular ion, with a concentration of 28 mEq./L.
  D. Extracellular concentration of Mg^{++} approximately 1.5–2.5 mEq./L.
III. Mg^{++} performs the following functions:
  A. Essential for integrity of neuromuscular system.
  B. Activates many enzyme reactions especially important in carbohydrate metabolism.
  C. Promotes regulation of blood phosphorus level.
IV. Mg^{++} ingestion, absorption, and excretion:
  A. Ingestion:
    1. Adults normally require 200 to 300 mg. of Mg^{++} per day.
    2. Mg^{++} is abundant in food; it is a vital constituent of chlorophyll.
    3. Nuts, soybeans, cocoa, seafood, whole grains, dried beans, and peas are excellent sources of Mg^{++}.
  B. Absorption:
    1. 45% of ingested Mg^{++} is absorbed while the remainder is excreted in the feces.
    2. Factors inhibiting Mg^{++} *absorption* are the presence of excess fat, phosphates, Ca^{++}, and alkalosis.
    3. Increased absorption of Mg^{++} by the intestinal tract is stimulated by parathyroid hormone (PTH).
  C. Excretion:
    1. 55% of Mg^{++} is excreted in the feces.
    2. Renal excretion of Mg^{++} is low, because kidney conserves Mg^{++} efficiently.

does occur due to nutritional problems, it tends to develop over a prolonged period of time; the dietary inadequacies are extreme; and the effects of the deficit tend to be cumulative.

Bases of Symptoms. Mg^{++} deficiency is characterized by *increased muscular and nervous system irritability*. Table 12–24 lists the major pathologic effects of Mg^{++} deficit and the corresponding symptoms.

Magnesium deficit may be hard to diagnose on the basis of symptoms alone, because the tetany produced by Mg^{++} deficit is almost indistinguishable from that produced by Ca^{++} deficit. In addition Mg^{++} and Ca^{++} deficits frequently coexist. The patient's history may provide some clues to the possibility of a Mg^{++} deficit, but the serum Mg^{++} level is the best means of diagnosis.

Clinical Care. The goals of care in Mg^{++} deficit are:

1. To replace the Mg^{++} deficiency.
2. To replace continuing Mg^{++} losses.
3. To quickly control symptoms.
4. To prevent further losses.

When rapid effect is desired, the parenteral route, especially IV, is the treatment of choice. Oral replacement can be given prophylactically to patients who are at risk of developing Mg^{++} deficit.

Magnesium sulfate is the most commonly used drug for the parenteral treatment of Mg^{++} depletion. When given intramuscularly, therapeutic action starts in 1 hour. This injection is painful and should be given deep in the gluteal muscle, followed by massage to enhance absorption. Intravenous administration of Mg^{++} produces therapeutic effects immediately.

Certain precautions should be observed when administering magnesium sulfate, especially by the intravenous route:

> Remember:
> 1. *Question giving IV magnesium to any patient with poor renal function. Magnesium excess may result.*
> 2. *Assess patient at least hourly and stop the IV infusion at once if the following signs of Mg^{++} toxicity develop:*
>   a. *The patient states "I feel hot all over," or "I'm very thirsty."*
>   b. *Flushing or sweating.*
>   c. *Anxiety followed by drowsiness, lethargy, and decreased motor function (can progress to coma).*
>   d. *A fall in blood pressure.*
>   e. *Weak or absent deep tendon reflexes (e.g., ankle jerk).*
> 3. *Have injectable calcium gluconate available. Calcium antagonizes the action of magnesium and will reverse the above symptoms.*

TABLE 12–24. SIGNS AND SYMPTOMS OF MAGNESIUM DEFICIENCY

Signs and Symptoms	Bases
Tetany; hyperactive reflexes; positive Chvostek's sign; facial twitching; jerking; convulsions	Neuromuscular irritability is increased
Hallucinations; delusions; extreme confusion; aggressive behavior; irritability	Central nervous system is greatly stimulated
Tachycardia; hypotension	Decreased cardiac muscle function
Laboratory findings: Serum Mg^{++} less than 1 mEq./L.	Loss of Mg^{++} from serum

The prevention of Mg^{++} deficiency is a major goal of patient care today. Preventive care should include frequent assessment of vulnerable patients for signs and symptoms of Mg^{++} deficit and the provision of Mg^{++}, either by diet or by medication.

Magnesium Excess

This imbalance may be caused by the following conditions:

- Renal insufficiency, causing Mg^{++} retention
- Overdoses of Mg^{++} during replacement therapy
- Severe dehydration, resulting in oliguria and retention of Mg^{++}
- Repeated enemas with magnesium sulfate (epsom salt), a potent saline cathartic
- Use of antacids containing Mg^{++} by patients with renal failure (e.g., Gelusil, magnesium oxide, and hydrated magnesium aluminate)

The main physiologic alteration in Mg^{++} excess, as in K^+ excess, is *a pronounced reduction in neuromuscular irritability.* Major signs and symptoms are:

- A warm sensation throughout the body.
- Decreased deep tendon reflexes leading to flaccid paralysis.
- Hypotension.
- Drowsiness and lethargy leading to coma.
- Depressed respirations.
- Cardiac arrhythmias progressing to arrest.
- Serum Mg^{++} greater than 3 mEq./L.

Clinical Care. The goals of care for patients with a Mg^{++} excess are: (1) to treat underlying causative conditions or circumstances that are creating a Mg^{++} excess and (2) to offset the toxicity and life-threatening symptoms of Mg^{++} excess.

TREATMENT OF UNDERLYING CONDITIONS. Patients suffering from renal failure are treated with peritoneal dialysis or hemodialysis, whereas dehydrated patients are given fluids. These measures increase urinary output and, consequently, Mg^{++} excretion. Moreover, any medications or compounds containing Mg^{++} (enemas, antacids, IV solutions) are withheld from patients with suspected or confirmed Mg^{++} imbalances or with renal failure.

TREATMENT OF Mg^{++} TOXICITY. Patients with symptoms of Mg^{++} excess are given 10 per cent calcium gluconate immediately. This medication antagonizes the action of Mg^{++}, reversing the symptoms of toxicity.

FLUID SHIFTS

Fluid shifts are basically position changes of the extracellular fluid and electrolytes. There are two main types of fluid shifts: (1) plasma to interstitial fluid shift and (2) interstitial space to plasma fluid shift.

Little is known today about the dynamics of fluid shifts or their purpose in the body's reaction to trauma and disease. As Metheny and Snively stated, "These mysterious tides of disease represent a curious response to unseen, unfathomed forces set in motion by certain illnesses and injuries."[58] Despite their elusive nature, the shifts create very real and dramatic changes within the traumatized human body.

In Table 12–25, the two major fluid shifts are compared and contrasted with each other in terms of characteristics, cause, symptoms, and clinical care.

Nursing Implications

Fluid shifts are potentially dangerous mechanisms: a plasma to interstitial fluid shift can result in *shock*; an interstitial fluid to plasma shift can lead to *pulmonary edema* — both critical, life-threatening complications.

In caring for patients particularly subject to the development of fluid shifts, you need to consider the following points in mapping out a plan of care. First, be aware of *which type* of fluid shift your patient may develop as well as its major signs and symptoms.

Second, be aware of specific ways to protect patients from developing further complications as a result of fluid shifts. With patients suffering from a *plasma to interstitial fluid shift,* the *major goals of preventive care are:* (1) to prevent irreversible shock; (2) to prevent tissue breakdown and decubitus ulcer formation; and (3) to prevent iatrogenic complications of therapy.

> Remember:
> 1. *A patient who has just recently suffered a serious burn, trauma, or obstruction will develop a* plasma to interstitial fluid shift. *The main signs will be those of* circulatory collapse.
> 2. *A patient who has suffered a burn or crushing injury 3 to 5 days earlier will develop an* interstitial fluid to plasma shift. *The main signs will be those of* circulatory overload.

Prevent Irreversible Shock and Renal Failure.* The shock that typifies a plasma to interstitial fluid shift is due to the sudden fluid loss

*For a further discussion of shock, see Chapter 13; renal failure is considered in Chapter 43.

from the vascular system. Such a fluid loss from the blood stream into the tissues can be just as serious and deadly as a hemorrhagic loss of fluid from the body. Vital signs, urinary output, and the patient's sensorium are all profoundly affected. Consequently, in your plan of care for patients with this condition, you should:

- ▶ Check blood pressure at least every 1 to 2 hours for hypotension. (Be sure that you have a baseline blood pressure with which to compare subsequent blood pressures.)
- ▶ Check pulse at least every 1 to 2 hours for tachycardia or for a pulse over 100 beats per minute. Check the *quality* of pulse. A thready, weak pulse may be a sign of shock.
- ▶ Check the patient's state of consciousness. Confusion and decreasing alertness to the environment may indicate shock.
- ▶ Check urinary output hourly; oliguria or anuria are important signs of circulatory collapse.
- ▶ Check the patient's skin color and temperature. A cold moist skin and an ashen pallor may be indicative of shock.
- ▶ Check for dyspnea, restlessness, or cyanosis of the lips or oral mucosa, which may indicate inadequate tissue oxygenation.

Be certain to chart your findings carefully. Re-

TABLE 12–25. FLUID SHIFTS—A COMPARISON OF CHARACTERISTICS, CAUSATIVE FACTORS, SYMPTOMS, AND CLINICAL CARE

Plasma to Interstitial Fluid Shift	**Interstitial Fluid to Plasma Shift**
I. Characteristics A. Following severe trauma or injury, fluid, electrolytes, proteins, and bicarbonate shift from the injured areas into noninjured areas B. Fluid also shifts from the plasma into the peritoneum and into the pleura II. Causative factors A. Massive crushing injuries B. Burns (shift occurs on the first or second day following injury) C. Following perforation of a peptic ulcer D. Intestinal obstruction E. Lymphatic obstruction F. Venous thrombosis G. Obstruction of major vessel III. Bases of symptoms A. Mechanism causing shift is obscure, but it is possibly of neurogenic origin B. The shift results in: 1. Loss of fluid from the vascular space, which leads to shock 2. Edema of noninjured areas 3. Dehydration of the injured cells IV. Common symptoms A. Signs of *shock:* 1. Pallor 2. Hypotension 3. Tachycardia 4. Weak to absent pulse 5. Cold extremities 6. Oliguria 7. Decreased level of consciousness 8. *No* weight loss, as fluid is not lost from the body B. Laboratory findings due to the loss of fluid from the plasma: 1. Hematocrit elevation 2. Red blood cell count elevated 3. Elevated BUN V. Clinical care A. The specific factors causing the shift are treated (e.g., burns, injury, obstruction) B. Fluids, electrolytes and proteins lost from the plasma are *judiciously* replaced. Pulmonary edema and circulatory overload can result when the interstitial fluid to plasma shift occurs on the third to fifth post-trauma day.	I. Characteristics: Fluid and electrolytes shift from the interstitial spaces into the vascular system. II. Causative factors A. Remobilization of edema fluid following burn or severe injury (occurs on third to fifth day) B. Compensation following internal or external hemorrhage C. Excessive infusions of hypertonic solutions: 1. Albumin 2. Plasma 3. Dextran III. Bases of symptoms A. Mechanism causing shift following burns and injury is obscure B. Excessive infusions of hypertonic solutions increase the osmolality of the plasma, consequently drawing fluid from the interstitial spaces and cells IV. Common symptoms A. Following loss of whole blood, signs are similar to shock: 1. Weakness 2. Pallor 3. Tachycardia 4. Hypotension B. Following shift of fluid resulting from administration of hypertonic solution or from burns, the vascular system is overloaded and these signs result: 1. Bounding pulse 2. Pulmonary edema 3. Hypertension 4. Cardiac enlargement 5. Engorgement of peripheral veins C. Laboratory findings due to shift of fluid into plasma: 1. Hematocrit decreased 2. BUN decreased V. Clinical care A. Generally excess fluid is excreted naturally, if the patient has normal heart and kidney function B. In the presence of heart or renal disease, other measures, such as diuretics, dialysis or rotating tourniquets may be necessary to reduce the hypervolemia C. Following hemorrhage, a blood transfusion may be ordered

port to the physician significant changes or observations immediately. Careful, frequent observations are essential during the critical periods of shock, to prevent irreversible damage.

Prevent Tissue Breakdown. Remember that in a plasma to interstitial fluid shift, the injured area becomes *dehydrated* while the noninjured area becomes *edematous.* Because edematous tissue receives less oxygen, it is prone to breakdown and to decubitus ulcer formation. Noninjured areas of the body in a plasma to interstitial fluid shift must be carefully observed for *beginning* signs of breakdown such as redness and tenderness, especially on the skin overlying the sacrum, hips, and other bony prominences. Turn and move the patient every hour on a *specific schedule.* Position properly with pillows.

Prevent Iatrogenic Complications of Therapy. Patients suffering from a plasma to interstitial fluid shift are usually treated with IV fluids. Remember that volume overload may result when the inevitable interstitial to plasma fluid shift occurs on the third to fifth day post trauma. The IV infusion rate may have to be decreased. Observe for signs of pulmonary edema.

Second, to prevent interstitial fluid to plasma shift, never overload *any* patient with hypertonic saline solution.

NUTRITIONAL DEFICIENCIES*

No discussion of fluid and electrolyte imbalance would be complete without considering caloric and protein deficits. These important nutritional deficiencies have spelled misery for human beings over the centuries and continue to plague people even in this modern age. Persons in underdeveloped countries still face starvation; vast numbers of people in the United States do not eat correctly owing to poverty or ignorance concerning proper diet. It is often unrecognized that patients in hospitals require additional proteins, vitamins, and calories for recovery.

Despite many gaps in our knowledge, we are becoming increasingly aware of the role of nutrition and diet in the promotion of health and in the causation of disease. Today, we recognize that the health of an individual may, to a large extent, depend upon what is eaten, how much is eaten, and how well the food is digested, absorbed, and utilized.

While all aspects of nutrition are pertinent to the study of health and disease, the following problems in nutrition are particularly relevant to the area of fluid and electrolyte balance.

Caloric Metabolism

When we eat, our bodies convert the ingested foodstuffs into energy. Energy is measured in terms of *heat equivalents* or calories. The outline in Table 12–26 summarizes a few essential facts about calories.

Caloric Deficit

Major causes of caloric deficit serious enough to create symptoms are:

- *Decrease in caloric intake.* Decreased intake is found in persons suffering from starvation, or those undergoing strenuous therapeutic reducing diets. A lowered caloric intake also results from nausea, vomiting, anorexia nervosa and other gastrointestinal disorders.
- *Abnormally increased utilization of calories.* This problem arises in persons with a higher than normal metabolic rate, e.g., in hyperthyroidism, cancer, and infection. For every degree of fever as measured on the centigrade scale, the basal metabolic rate rises 7 per cent. Thus, patients with fever require a greater caloric intake. Hypertension, anemia, burns, and dyspnea can also cause an increase in the BMR and in caloric needs.
- *Faulty absorption and utilization of food.* Even if food intake is normal, the person who cannot properly absorb or metabolize food actually suffers from a form of starvation. For example, an individual with diabetes mellitus cannot properly metabolize carbohydrates. Consequently, the person burns protein and fat in place of carbohydrates to meet energy needs.

The major physiologic result of any caloric deficit is a *protein* deficit. In the absence of adequate calories, body tissues are burned to supply needed energy for metabolic processes.

The most important *symptoms* of a caloric deficit are, mental depression, shortness of breath (SOB), loss of muscle tone and mass, increased acetone in the urine, weakness, fatigue, weight loss, and malaise.

The prevention of caloric deficits, and consequently of protein deficits, is of importance in the treatment of all patients, but especially those who are burned, have had surgery, or are bedridden. Individuals who are unconscious or NPO must have nutritional replacements carefully calculated in terms of calories.

Protein Metabolism

The word protein is derived from the Greek word *proteios* meaning "primary" or "holding first place." Indeed, protein does hold first place in the human body because it is the essential substance of living cells and tissues. Major facts

*Owing to problems of space, no attempt has been made to present nutritional disorders in detail in this textbook.

concerning protein that are pertinent to patient care are summarized in Table 12–27.

Within this outline of normal protein metabolism, certain points demand reemphasis because they contain vital implications for patient care.

First, essential proteins cannot be made within the body. This means that a person must eat a certain amount of essential protein substance or a deficiency develops. If an individual is *ill,* appetite decreases, nausea and vomiting may occur, and, as a result, sufficient protein for the body's needs may not be ingested. Without adequate diet or parenteral replacement, a state of *hypoproteinemia* and *negative nitrogen balance* develops, further jeopardizing health. Protein replacements and protein-sparing nutrients should be considered when working with the anorexic or nauseated patient. (Protein-sparing nutrients are foods high in carbohydrates or fat content. These foods are used by the body for energy in place of protein; thus, the term, "protein sparing.")

Second, protein is absolutely necessary for the *building of tissues.* Following injury, surgery, or a severe burn, the body desperately needs protein to rebuild those tissues that have been traumatized. Unfortunately patients may be unconscious, unable to eat, or anorexic at the time they are in need of additional protein. The prevention of hypoproteinemia is, thus, a matter of vital clinical concern during these critical periods.

Protein Deficit

The main causes of a protein deficit are as follows:

1. Inadequate intake of protein.
2. Severe loss of protein, e.g., hemorrhage, burns, draining ulcers, ascites.
3. Increased utilization of protein for the rebuilding of tissues, e.g., following burns or trauma.
4. Increased catabolism, e.g., fever, elevated BMR, infection, malignancy.

The major physiologic result of protein deficit is a breakdown of the body tissue protein for use to meet the body's needs. Some outstanding symptoms are: weight loss, fatigue, anemia, decreased hemoglobin, anorexia, loss of muscle mass and tone, and decreased plasma albumin level below 3 Gm./100 ml. (hypoproteinemia). In addition, surgical patients with protein deficiencies also suffer from *retarded healing* of incisions and may develop a condition called *nutritional edema,* a complication resulting from a lowered colloid osmotic pressure owing to inadequate serum proteins. Lowered colloid osmotic pressure results in a loss of fluid from the

TABLE 12–26. THE CALORIE—A BRIEF SUMMARY OF BASIC FACTS

I. The calorie (Latin *calor,* heat) is a measure of heat.
   A. The calorie measures the energy value that a definite proportion of food will yield upon oxidation within the body or upon being burned within a laboratory.
   B. The large calorie or kilocalorie is the unit of measurement used in dietetic laboratories and studies. The kilocalorie is equal to the amount of heat needed to raise 1 kg. of water 1°C.
II. Calories are drawn from the following three major groups of nutrients.
   A. Proteins
      1. One gram of protein is equivalent to 4 calories.
      2. Proteins supply approximately 15% of the average daily caloric intake.
   B. Fats
      1. One gram of fat is equivalent to 9 calories.
      2. Fats supply 40% of the average daily caloric intake.
   C. Carbohydrates
      1. One gram of carbohydrate is equivalent to 4 calories.
      2. Carbohydrates supply approximately 45% of the average dietary intake.
III. The caloric needs of the healthy individual vary with the following factors:
   A. Basal metabolic rate (BMR)
      1. Defined as the amount of energy that a physically, mentally, and emotionally relaxed person must expend in order to maintain the basic physical processes of life.
      2. The BMR, and therefore caloric need, is higher in men than in women; it is increased during periods of growth, during pregnancy and lactation, and during emotional upsets.
      3. The BMR is lower in elderly persons, and in conditions of starvation and malnutrition.
   B. Surface area of the body
      1. Surface area is a measurement that takes both height and weight into account. It can be computed from specially designed tables.
      2. A large person has a greater surface area, greater metabolic rate, and greater need for calories than a smaller individual.
   C. Activity
      1. Sedentary activity requires fewer calories than physical activity.
      2. Mental activity, however difficult and demanding, requires very few calories.

TABLE 12–27. PROTEIN – A BRIEF SUMMARY OF PERTINENT FACTS

I. Protein is an *organic* substance composed of carbon, hydrogen, oxygen, and nitrogen.
II. When proteins are digested, they break down into *amino acids,* the basic structural units of proteins.
III. Amino acids are classified as either *essential* or *nonessential.*
  A. Essential amino acids:
    1. Are absolutely necessary for body growth and cellular life.
    2. Must be *obtained in food,* as they are not produced in the body.
  B. Nonessential amino acids:
    1. Are not absolutely necessary for body health and growth.
    2. Can be manufactured within the body.
IV. Proteins are classified as either *complete* or *incomplete,* according to the type of amino acids they contain.
  A. Proteins that contain all the essential amino acids are *complete proteins,* e.g., those found in meats and dairy foods.*
  B. Proteins missing one or more of the essential amino acids are *incomplete proteins,* e.g., those in grains and vegetables. Diets containing only incomplete proteins are adequate if carefully balanced to include *complementary proteins* which do provide all the essential amino acids.
V. The *functions* of protein:
  A. The most basic and vital constituent of living cells.
  B. Comprises bulk of muscle, visceral, and epithelial tissue.
  C. Important constituent of plasma, hemoglobin, blood cells, and antibodies.
  D. Essential for body growth.
  E. Essential for maintenance and repair of tissue.
VI. Dietary requirement of protein: One gram of protein daily per kg. of body weight is recommended in the United States.†
VII. Phases of protein metabolism:
  A. Anabolism:
    1. Following absorption, amino acids are incorporated into the body tissue protein (tissue protein synthesis).
    2. In this process, complex substances are built up from simpler substances and *energy is used.*
  B. Catabolism: Complete protein substances are broken down into simpler substances, oxidized, and excreted; energy is released.
VIII. The concept of *nitrogen balance:*
  A. Nitrogen is present in protein substances and in nonprotein substances such as urea, uric acid, ammonia, and creatinine.
  B. Nitrogen from all the above sources (both protein nitrogen and nonprotein nitrogen) comprises the *total nitrogen balance.*
  C. Negative nitrogen balance exists when the *output* of nitrogen exceeds *intake.*
  D. Positive nitrogen balance exists when *intake* of nitrogen-containing substances exceeds the *output.*

*The Food and Agriculture Organization, a division of WHO, has ranked eggs and milk as the most complete protein foods; i.e., eggs and milk contain the largest amount of those amino acids that are absolutely necessary for health.

†Protein, 0.85 Gm. daily per kg. of body weight, is recommended by the World Health Organization (WHO). People in underdeveloped countries, however, are surviving on far less protein than this.

vascular system into the interstitial tissues, which then become edematous.

How can protein deficits be *prevented,* especially in patients who are burned, critically ill, or undergoing surgery? The following orders may assist in returning the patient to a positive nitrogen balance:

- ▶ A regular diet that is appetizing to the patient and that is high in carbohydrates is a vital protein sparer. A high-carbohydrate diet rather than one high in protein is ordered because diets high in protein also have a high satiety value; consequently, patients may fail to eat a large enough portion of their food.
- ▶ *Protein hydrolysates,* either parenterally or by tube feeding, can provide essential amino acids with less digestive work.

You, as the nurse, can help to prevent protein deficiencies by carefully evaluating patients' daily dietary intake and needs:

- ▶ Make patient rounds during mealtimes and note the following: The patient's food likes and dislikes with respect to temperature, consistency, texture, and proportions. Whether the meal is balanced, with adequate carbohydrates, protein, fats, and vitamins. Whether dentures fit properly and are provided. Whether motor or sensory deficits, pain, nausea, or emotional stress prevent the patient from eating.
- ▶ Check the timing of your patients' meals. Meals that coincide with uncomfortable procedures may cause a loss of appetite. Some persons prefer six small meals a day rather than the traditional three large meals.
- ▶ Ask the dietitian to consult with you and the patient to determine ways in which dietary intake can be improved within the patient's environmental, financial, or social limitations and considering personal preferences.
- ▶ Make certain that before discharge both patient and persons in the patient's household understand the diet and the need for adequate protein.

Adequate protein should cause weight to stabilize, muscle tone and mass to improve, and wounds to heal without painful time-consuming, expensive complications.

GENERAL PRINCIPLES OF ASSESSMENT, MANAGEMENT, AND TREATMENT OF FLUID AND ELECTROLYTE AND H^+ IMBALANCES

In this section we shall draw upon our knowledge of specific imbalances to consider some general principles for observing, assessing, and treating *any* patient believed to have imbalances, as well as preventing imbalances. Our discussion will explore the following basic steps that nurses and physicians observe in caring for patients with imbalances.

Step 1: Assess patients for fluid and electrolyte balance, and H^+ balance.

Step 2: Arrive at a medical and nursing diagnosis.

Step 3: Develop a plan to care for patients with imbalances and to prevent imbalances.

Step 4: Support medical therapy.

These topics will be discussed in terms of *both* medical and nursing actions, for physicians and nurses today must function as a coordinated team to ensure successful diagnosis and treatment.

Assessing the Patient

In assessing a patient for possible imbalances, many different avenues of inquiry must be explored. Learning about the patient's usual living patterns and past complaints, present signs and symptoms, and actual physical status (through diagnostic and laboratory studies) is important. Such information is then used by the physician to diagnose the patient's particular imbalance, and by the nurse to diagnose the needs of the patient resulting from that imbalance.

In evaluating a patient for possible imbalances, the following should be considered, e.g.:

1. Have there been abnormalities in the volume of ECF? increase? decrease?
2. Have there been abnormalities in the electrolyte composition of the ECF? Are the serum concentrations of Na^+, K^+, Ca^{++}, Mg^{++}, and $NaHCO_3$ normal, excessive, or deficient?
3. Have there been abnormalities in the position of the ECF? fluid shifts?
4. Does the patient show evidence of nutritional deficiency?
5. Are there changes in CBC, MCV (mean corpuscular volume), MCH (mean corpuscular hemoglobin), or MCHC (mean corpuscular hemoglobin concentration)?*
6. Are there changes in pH, pCO_2?
7. Does the patient show signs or symptoms of abnormal neuromuscular, cardiac, gastrointestinal, or respiratory function?

*See Unit XIV.

To answer these questions, a detailed history, a thorough physical examination, and careful evaluation of the patient's fluid balance record and laboratory studies are necessary. The nurse should make sure that laboratory tests are carried out; that these tests are explained to the patient and significant others; that fluids, foods and medications are withheld as necessary; and that unusual laboratory findings are reported to the physician.

THE PATIENT'S HISTORY

The patient is asked for facts about past health:

- ▶ Has the patient recently gained or lost weight?
- ▶ Has the patient been taking any drugs, e.g., cathartics, thiazide diuretics, cortisone, or electrolyte supplements?
- ▶ Has the patient been on any restricted or unusual diets, e.g., a low calorie or low sodium diet?
- ▶ Is there any disease condition present that might upset the body's balance, e.g., endocrine or metabolic disease?
- ▶ Has the patient received any therapeutic fluids intravenously or by tube feeding?
- ▶ Does the patient seem to have a satisfactory intake and output balance record?
- ▶ Does the patient suffer from incontinence, excessive diaphoresis, vomiting, or wound drainage?
- ▶ Has the patient undergone excessive, unaccustomed activity?

When talking with the patient, note sensorium, affect, and level of energy. Does the patient seem confused, belligerent, lethargic, or unusually fatigued? These signs can be important diagnostic observations related to imbalance.

PHYSICAL EXAMINATION

Following the history, the patient is usually examined for clinical signs and symptoms of imbalance. Symptoms may be minimal or prominent. Symptoms of different imbalances are often similar. To offset such confusion, any patient examination, whether a formal physical examination or a daily nursing evaluation, must be systematic and thorough.

Evaluation for deviations from normal include the following factors:

blood pressure (supine and upright)
pulse
respirations

temperature
odor of the skin
moistness or dryness of the skin
skin turgor
appetite for food
thirst (presence or absence)
weight
behavioral changes
changes in urinary
volume and concentration
sensation (e.g., tingling or numbness)
condition of the mucous membranes
breath odor
heart action
neuromuscular function (include deep tendon reflexes)
gastrointestinal function
circulatory changes
neck vein distention
edema
skeletal changes

These factors, as mentioned earlier, vary distinctively with the different imbalances.

FLUID BALANCE RECORD

The fluid balance record is a record maintained for a given patient showing fluid intake (oral, parenteral, and by feeding tube) and fluid output (urine, stool, gastric suction, wound drainage, vomiting, and perspiration). When accurate, the fluid balance record is a valuable aid in diagnosing and anticipating imbalances and in calculating fluid replacement needs. Unfortunately fluid intake and output are not always precisely measured, nor are the findings always accurately recorded.

One study has shown that a significant proportion of the patient's daily fluid intake is with oral medications. Indeed, daily fluid intake with medicines was found to range from approximately 219 to 472 ml. This study further demonstrated that, in some patients, water intake with medicines actually *exceeded* by 30 per cent the daily intake order for the patient. Failure to measure and record water given to patients on medicine rounds can result in a serious fluid overload.[44]

Other errors in recording intake and output include the following:

(1) Bottles of intravenous solutions may actually contain 1100 ml. of fluid rather than the usual 1000 ml. (an additional 100 ml. of fluid).

(2) Bottles of blood or intravenous solution may contain 600 ml. of solution rather than 500 ml.

(3) Small sips of water or mouth rinsing, when repeated throughout the day, can actually total 1000 ml. per 24 hours.

One can see that it is possible for a patient's intake record to be in error by as much as 2000 ml.! Such a lack of accuracy can result in serious consequences for patients with certain conditions, e.g., kidney disease, burns, severe diarrhea.

Other common sources of error, in evaluating and recording intake and output, involve the following:[58]

Poor communication among staff members about which patients are on intake and output recordings.

Failure to communicate with patients and visitors recording intake and output.

Guessing at intake and output measurements rather than actually measuring fluids.

Failure to record fluid taken in as ice chips (a 200-ml. glass of ice chips equals approximately 100 ml. of water).

Failure to record intake of solid foods (recall that solid foods also contain water).

Failure to indicate loss of water by perspiration (i.e., whether patient is perspiring excessively, moderately, or mildly).

Failure to estimate fluid loss from incontinence of stool or urine, or from wound exudate.

Failure to measure fluid used as irrigating solutions (e.g., for bladder or wounds).

Failure to accurately weigh a patient at the same time every day on the same scale and in clothing of the same approximate weight (remember: daily weights are one of the best indicators of fluid gain or loss).

Although a recording of intake and output is not ordered for every patient, *every* patient does require evaluation of the state of fluid balance. In caring for patients not on intake and output measurement, oversights can be avoided by asking yourself the following questions, e.g.,

- Is the patient drinking at least 1500 ml. of fluid per day?
- Is urine voided at least once every 8-hour shift? How much?
- Is the skin dry and loose?
- Is a fever present?
- Is the patient perspiring excessively?
- Is the patient's urine concentrated?
- Is there excessive drainage anywhere?

If the answers to these questions produce doubts about the patient's state of hydration, the situation should be discussed with the doctor, and accurate measurement of intake and output started.

DIAGNOSTIC TESTS

Although a general estimate of the patient's problem can be made from the history and physical examination, laboratory tests are regularly used to confirm or establish a diagnosis or to distinguish one imbalance from another. Standard laboratory tests include:

- *Complete blood count* (CBC). This includes estimates of hemoglobin and hematocrit. Hemoglobin values can be increased with dehydration and decreased with overhydration (normals at sea level: women = 13.0–15.5 Gm./100 ml. blood; men = 14.5–16.5 Gm./100 ml. blood). Hematocrit values can be increased with extracellular volume depletion and decreased with volume excess. (Normals at sea level: women=37%–47%; men=40%–54%.)
- *Urinalysis.* This includes a description of the odor of the urine, amount of sedimentation, pH, specific gravity, and tests for protein and glucose.
- *Electrolyte concentration.* Analysis of electrolyte concentrations generally includes the serum concentrations of Na^+, K^+, Ca^{++}, Mg^{++}, H^+ (pH), and protein. In Table 12–28 dangerously high and low levels of these electrolytes in plasma are recorded.
- *Arterial blood gases.* These include a measurement of pH, pCO_2, and pO_2.
- CO_2 *content* or combining power.
- *Blood urea nitrogen (BUN).* Normal range varies from 8 to 28 mg. per 100 ml. blood; BUN fluctuates with level of hydration; it tends to be elevated during water and Na^+ depletion and when kidney function is poor.
- *Plasma proteins.* The normal amount of plasma protein in blood is approximately 6 Gm. per cent. When the amount of plasma protein is below normal, fluids are retained in the interstitial space because of the plasma's decreased colloidal osmotic pressure.
- *Arterial blood gases.* The normal range of pH for arterial blood in 7.36–7.44. Any deviation from this range indicates an acid-base disorder. The pCO_2 value determines the contribution of the respiratory system to the imbalance. The plasma CO_2 content or combining power will show the contribution of the renal (or metabolic) system to the imbalance.
- *Electrocardiogram (ECG).* This is especially important in diagnosing K^+, Mg^{++}, and Ca^{++} imbalances; when these imbalances are severe, an ECG can give warning of impending cardiac arrest. The nurse should make use of laboratory test results in periodically evaluating a patient's progress and in planning daily care. They are a vital part of ongoing assessment.

MAKING THE DIAGNOSIS

A diagnosis results from synthesizing all available data, considering the patient as a whole. That is, the patient should be considered greater than the summation of collected data.

The following examples illustrate how appropriate information concerning patients is gathered and fit together to diagnose and treat fluid and electrolyte imbalances.

Clinical Case No. 1. Mr. M., an elderly man, is admitted during a severe flu epidemic. He tells you that for 2 days he has been too nauseated to eat or drink, has had severe vomiting and diarrhea, and has been sweating a great deal. His admission record indicates a 10-pound weight loss in the past week. He has a temperature of 38.8°C. (102°F.), a supine blood pressure of 130/92 and sitting measurement of 115/80, and his mouth is very dry. He seems tired and lethargic. Laboratory studies report an elevated hemoglobin and hematocrit, BUN, and serum Na^+. Also, the specific gravity of his urine is high, indicating a concentrated urine.

Analysis of the data indicates extracellular volume deficit and a water deficit. With this knowledge, you can surmise that daily weights, intake and output recordings, and IV replacement fluids will all be a part of the care of this patient.

Clinical Case No. 2. Ms. R. has been admitted on numerous occasions highly intoxicated. When she is admitted today, Ms. R. is semistuporous; however, as

TABLE 12–28. DANGEROUS HIGH AND LOW LEVELS OF SOLUTES IN PLASMA*

	Too High		Too Low	
	Mild to Moderate Symptoms	*Severe Symptoms*	*Mild to Moderate Symptoms*	*Severe Symptoms*
Sodium (mEq./L.)	155–170	>170	120–130	<120
Potassium (mEq./L.)	7–9	>9	2.2–3.0	<2.2
Calcium (mEq./L.)	6–7	>7	3–4	<3
Magnesium (mEq./L.)	>5	>10(?)	1 and below(?)	<1(?)
Hydrogen ion, as pH	7.5–7.6	>7.6	7.0–7.5	<7.0
Glucose (Mg. %)	1000 or above(?)	–	40–60	<40
Protein (Gm. %)	–	–	3.4–5	<3

*From Keitel, H. G.: *Consultant* 3:42–47, February, 1963.

the day progresses, she becomes increasingly belligerent and confused and appears to have various visual and auditory hallucinations. In addition, her face is twitching and she plucks almost incessantly at the bedclothes. The patient's serum Mg^{++} levels are at 1.25 mEq./L., a common finding in cases of delirium tremens.

From this data, Ms. R. is diagnosed as a chronic alcoholic in delirium tremens with a Mg^{++} deficiency. You can surmise that intravenous replacements of Mg^{++} will be ordered, and you can thus review the relevant nursing care before starting the medication.

We have greatly oversimplified the case of Ms. R. Actually, as a severe alcoholic she is probably suffering not only from a Mg^{++} deficiency, but also from water, protein, and vitamin deficits.

Having considered how to assess a patient in terms of imbalance, we shall now proceed to discuss the goal of all diagnoses, laboratory work, and systematic assessment, namely, clinical care.

Composing a Plan of Care

The Emergency Patient. Severely dehydrated or saline depleted persons, burned patients, hemorrhaging patients, and accident victims will die in a state of fluid and electrolyte imbalance if they do not receive adequate and prompt treatment. Some important lifesaving measures are as follows:

- ▶ Treat *shock* immediately. Keep a constant check on the vital signs, on the patient's state of consciousness, and on neuromuscular function.
- ▶ Prepare for the doctor to order an electrolyte analysis followed by IV replacement therapy for any serious electrolyte deficits.
- ▶ For a patient with severe extracellular fluid deficit and oliguria, while awaiting orders (a) start an intravenous fluid infusion with normal saline, or (b) place a heparin lock on the needle placed in the vein. The important thing is to enter the vein *before the patient becomes too hypotensive.*
- ▶ Insert indwelling catheter to monitor urinary output measurements hourly.

Patients with severe life-threatening imbalances will need constant *planned* nursing observations and care until the vital signs stabilize and urinary output is adequate, i.e., at least 30 ml. per hour.

Observations vary with underlying causes, and plans should remain flexible.

The Seriously Ill Patient with an Imbalance. Any seriously ill person is a potential candidate for fluid and electrolyte imbalances. Consequently, in your plan of care for any seriously ill person, whether suffering from acute or chronic illness, be certain to include the following tasks, summarized from preceding material:

- ▶ Evaluate daily the patient's food intake compared with nutritional needs. For example, a postoperative patient needs protein to rebuild tissues and to encourage wound healing. Does this patient order and eat foods high in protein? A patient with diarrhea loses large amounts of K^+. Does the patient eat foods high in K^+, e.g., bananas and orange juice? What is the patient's serum K^+? Any symptoms of hypokalemia?
- ▶ Daily *evaluate* the patient's intake and output record. Is intake adequate in relationship to output and vice versa? An accurate record of intake and output is not useful unless it is reviewed to identify and correct significant discrepancies or deviations from normal.
- ▶ Evaluate the patient's need for fluids, electrolytes, and foods, considering the presence of fever, severe dyspnea, nausea, vomiting, anorexia, and draining wounds. Do not forget that severe emotional stress can also seriously affect the fluid and electrolyte balance.
- ▶ Daily examine the patient in relationship to the multiple factors listed under the physical examination. Remember that new fluid and electrolyte imbalances may develop at any time during the course of an illness. You, as the nurse, often are in a position to make the *first* observations of an early imbalance and to take the first steps in preventing an imbalance.
- ▶ Observe for response to stress, e.g., does the patient have increased ADH and aldosterone secretion? Does the patient have increased K^+ loss?

A Guide to Fluid Replacement

Major goals of fluid replacement are:

1. Correct preexisting deficits of water and electrolytes, and restore, as quickly as possible, the *vascular fluid volume,* thus preventing shock and dehydration.
2. Meet the patient's maintenance (or life-sustaining) needs for fluids, electrolytes, and calories.
3. Replace *dynamic* or *concurrent losses* of fluid and electrolytes from suctioning, vomiting, diarrhea, and so forth.

In ordering fluids, the following should be considered: (1) the individual patient's clinical record, (2) the *route* of fluid administration, (3) the *type* of solution to be given, and (4) the *rate* of administration.

Some general guides for providing fluid replacements based on the *patient's clinical status* are:

- ▶ The patient's appearance, complaints, daily weight, and vital signs

- Daily intake and output requirements
- The laboratory reports

The major *routes* for fluid replacement are oral, rectal, and parenteral.

ORAL ROUTE

Replacement of fluids and electrolytes by mouth is generally considered to be the safest method. Oral replacement should be used when the patient is not vomiting, does not have dysphagia, is conscious, has normal bowel tones, and when the situation is *not* an emergency. During emergencies, fluids are generally administered parenterally for rapid absorption.

Patients receiving oral fluid replacements should be given *prescribed* amounts of water, milk, fresh fruit juice, and beef extracts. These fluids supply needed calories, proteins, sodium, and potassium, as well as serving to replace any fluid volume deficit.

Because oral fluid replacement is considered "safe," doctors' orders and nurses' records concerning oral fluid replacement are not always as precise as they should be. As a result, the patient may not receive the proper type or necessary amount of fluid.

> In caring for patients receiving oral liquids:
> 1. *Question vague orders concerning fluid replacement (e.g., "fluids ad lib" and "force fluids").*
> 2. *Know the* exact *amount and type of fluid a patient should receive for replacement purposes.*
> 3. *Know desired patient outcomes as result of prescriptions.*

For patients unable to drink fluids, the doctor may order tube feedings as an oral fluid replacement procedure. (See Chapter 59 for discussion of tube feeding.)

RECTAL FLUID REPLACEMENT

Proctoclysis, or rectal fluid replacement, is not a very reliable method for replacing an electrolyte deficit so it is infrequently used today. Since only water, sodium, and chloride are absorbed by the large intestine, proctoclysis cannot be relied upon to meet a patient's caloric needs and, consequently, is not used for maintenance purposes.

PARENTERAL ADMINISTRATION

The parenteral route is the most controlled and expedient method of fluid administration, because the solutions go directly into the extracellular compartment. It is also the most dangerous method of fluid administration, giving rise to potential complications which are often rapid and may rival in severity the imbalance being treated. Nevertheless, parenteral fluid replacements frequently are absolutely necessary; therefore, you must be fully acquainted with the subject in order to handle the procedure safely and effectively.

Because parenteral solutions are fast acting and potentially dangerous, specific questions need to be answered concerning their use, e.g.:

1. Under what circumstances are parenteral fluids administered?
2. What major principles serve as guides in parenteral fluid administration?
3. What routes can be used for parenteral fluid replacement? What are the advantages and disadvantages of each method?
4. What are the major types of solutions that can be ordered?
5. Upon what bases are parenteral fluid requirements determined? What are desired outcomes?
6. What data should the fluid order contain? What are the nurse's responsibilities in carrying out a fluid order?

In the discussion below, we shall briefly explore the answers to these questions.

Why Parenteral Fluids Are Ordered. Parenteral fluid replacements are generally ordered under the following circumstances:

- The patient is NPO, has swallowing difficulties, or is physically incapable of taking oral liquids, or when the patient's gastrointestinal tract is not functioning, e.g., paralytic ileus with hypokalemia, shift of blood away from gastrointestinal circulation with hypovolemia.
- The patient requires *rapid* fluid and electrolyte replacements.
- The patient requires a medication that will be destroyed by the gastric juices if it is administered orally.
- The patient requires a medication that, if given orally, cannot be absorbed by the GI tract.

Guiding Principles in Parenteral Fluid Administration. Some important considerations when giving parenteral fluids are as follows:

- *Adequacy of renal function* is the single most important factor to consider in parenteral fluid administration.

> Remember, during parenteral fluid administration:
> *If a patient suffers from any form of renal disease, careful observations of flow rate, meticulous recording of intake and output, and prevention of circulatory overload and pulmonary edema are vitally important!*

- Whenever possible, fluids and electrolytes should be given by the *oral route* in preference to the parenteral route.
- Daily measurement of *weight* is a helpful guide in evaluating a patient's hydration. Sudden weight shifts are highly significant. Any sudden variation in a patient's weight in excess of 5 per cent is usually the result of body fluid loss or retention. The degree of weight change serves as a guide for the amount of fluid that needs to be replaced or removed.
- When a seriously ill patient is receiving parenteral fluids, the insertion of an indwelling catheter and measurements of the *hourly urine volume* provide a useful indication of hydration.
- When a patient must receive IV parenteral fluids for a period of days or even weeks, do all you can to keep the patient comfortable, prevent infiltration of fluid into the tissues, prevent infection at the site of administration, and preserve the patient's veins. Also be aware of potential mechanisms for contamination of IV infusion systems (see Fig. 12–10). These topics are considered below.
- Postoperative patients, patients with a history of cardiac insufficiency, and patients with head injuries or craniotomies should be kept slightly dehydrated.

Major Routes for Parenteral Fluid Therapy and Their Dangers. The two major routes used for administering parenteral fluids are the subcutaneous route (hypodermoclysis) and the intravenous route.

SUBCUTANEOUS ROUTE: HYPODERMOCLYSIS. Like proctoclysis, hypodermoclysis is infrequently used. Subcutaneous fluids, when employed, are mainly given to obese patients, young children, and aged patients with badly sclerosed veins. In such patients, hypodermoclysis is advantageous because it is easier to start and maintain than an intravenous infusion.

Commonly used sites for subcutaneous infusions are the lateral and anterior aspects of the thigh, the abdomen, the lateral chest, the buttocks, and beneath the breasts.

Few fluids are suitable for hypodermoclysis administration, since they must closely resemble the plasma in tonicity and electrolyte content. In Table 12–29 we identify some solutions as either suitable or unsuitable for subcutaneous infusion.

When given subcutaneously, hypertonic solutions that do not contain electrolytes dilute intravascular volume and draw electrolytes intracellularly, thus leading to water intoxication. Hypertonic solutions tend to pull water from the plasma into the subcutaneous spaces because of their high osmotic pressure; this also results in plasma volume reduction causing hypotension. Alcohol, amino acids, and fat emulsions are irritating to tissues, while gastric replacement solutions differ considerably from the normal pH of the body. *Always question* the subcutaneous administration of any of these solutions.

In adults receiving hypodermoclysis, solutions are infused at a rate dependent on fluid needs and the absorptive ability of tissues. When absorption is somewhat slow, the enzyme *hyaluronidase* (Wydase) may be given to facilitate dispersion and absorption of the solution. Wydase is usually injected either into the tissues surrounding the clysis site or into the clysis tubing. When using Wydase watch for signs of *allergic reaction* at the injection site as well as a volume *overload* due to rapid absorption of the clysis fluid.

While a hypodermoclysis is relatively easy to

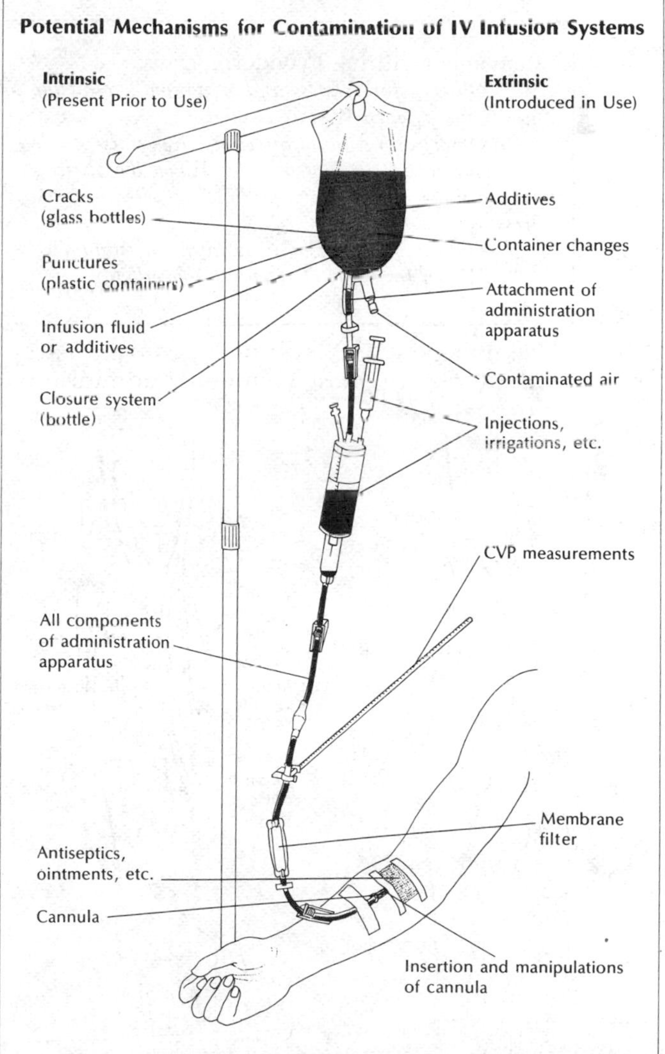

Figure 12–10. Potential mechanisms for contamination of IV infusion systems. (From Maki, D. G.: Preventing infection in intravenous therapy. *Hospital Practice*, 11:97, Apr. 1976.)

TABLE 12–29. A COMPARISON OF SAFE AND CONTRAINDICATED SOLUTIONS IN HYPODERMOCLYSIS

Safe Solutions	Contraindicated Solutions
1. Isotonic saline 0.9%	1. Electrolyte-free solutions
2. Half-isotonic saline (0.45%) with 21% dextrose	2. Hypertonic solutions
3. Ringer's solution	3. Alcohol
4. Lactated Ringer's solution	4. Amino acids
5. Darrow's solution	5. Fat emulsions
	6. Gastric replacement solution

start and does supply needed fluids, it can lead to dangerous complications. Infections with abscess formation, tissue sloughing, and extreme discomfort from stimulation of nerve endings (depending on placement of needle and amount of interstitial pressure) can occur at the infusion site.

> Remember, during hypodermoclysis:
> *1. Observe for redness and irritation around the injection site when Wydase is used.*
> *2. Observe for signs of infection. Always use sterile technique when starting a clysis. When the clysis is discontinued, cover the injection site with a sterile dressing.*
> *3. Observe for swelling around the injection site.*
> *4. Watch for signs of circulatory overload.*

PERIPHERAL INTRAVENOUS ROUTE. Parenteral fluids are most commonly administered intravenously. This is often a lifesaving procedure in hemorrhage or shock because the fluids enter the vascular system directly, thereby immediately increasing the plasma volume. Also, IV fluids can be given to patients over long periods of time if necessary. Fluids given by this route can be calculated daily to supply needed calories, carbohydrates, proteins, vitamins, electrolytes, and water.

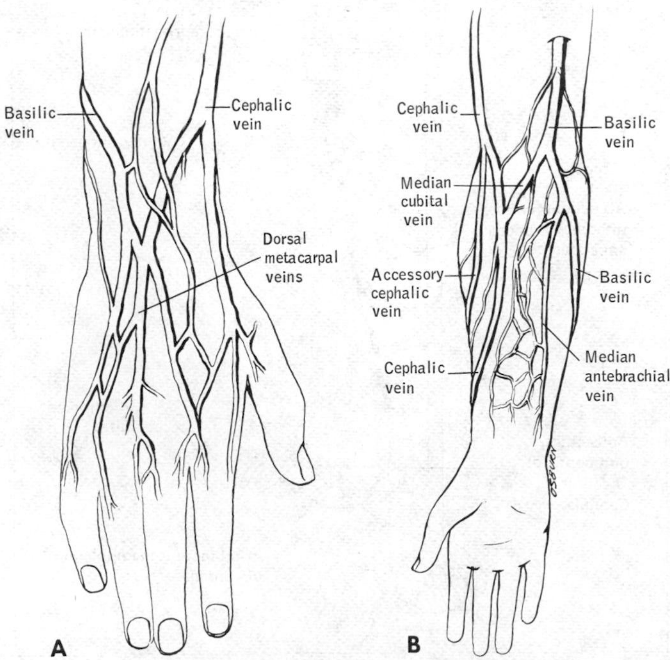

Figure 12–11. A, Superficial veins of the dorsal aspect of the hand. **B,** Superficial veins of the forearm. (From Sutton, A. L.: *Bedside Nursing Techniques in Medicine and Surgery.* Philadelphia: W. B. Saunders Co., 1969, p. 85.)

Choice of site for IV infusions depends upon (a) the length of time and type of IV therapy that will be required and (b) the availability of suitable veins. The accessory cephalii, median antebrachial on the flat surface of the forearm, and the veins on the dorsum of the hands can be used, particularly for prolonged therapy (Fig. 12–11). Both the *antecubital and leg veins should be avoided;* the leg veins because of the risk of thrombophlebitis, and the antecubital vein because of the need for prolonged immobilization at the elbow to insure proper flow rate.

While IV therapy may indeed be lifesaving, it clearly involves multiple dangers. Major complications of IV therapy are:

- *Infiltration* of IV solutions into the tissue spaces, possibly resulting in a hematoma. Infiltration of certain medications (Levophed, Aramine, calcium gluconate, and antineoplastic drugs) can cause dangerous tissue sloughs.
- *Thrombophlebitis* owing to trauma of the vein.
- A *pyogenic reaction due to contaminated fluids or equipment.*
- *Speed shock,* a severe systemic reaction to too rapid administration of IV fluids containing drugs.
- *Air embolism,* which results from entry of air into arterial or central venous line.
- *Circulatory overload.*

Symptoms of these complications as well as nursing actions are summarized in Table 12–30. Figure 12–12 shows effects of possible complications.

CENTRAL INTRAVENOUS ROUTE. Certain IV solutions, because of their hypertonicity, cannot be administered safely through a peripheral vein. In this case a *central* vein, usually the subclavian or superior vena cava, is used. The high blood flow and large diameter of these vessels is sufficient to dilute hypertonic fluids and prevent the pain, irritation, and phlebitis encountered with peripheral infusions. *Total parenteral nutrition* (TPN), or intravenous hyperalimentation, is a recently developed form of nutritional therapy that requires infusion of hypertonic glucose and protein solutions into a central vein.*

TPN was developed to promote anabolism and a positive nitrogen balance in patients who are unable to assimilate sufficient calories, proteins, and other nutrients by conventional means. For

*TPN is discussed in detail in Chapter 59.

example, patients with intestinal malabsorption syndromes, bowel resections, or ulcerative colitis are unable to absorb adequate nutrients from the gastrointestinal tract. Comatose patients cannot physically respond to the need for food. Patients who are undergoing severe stress, such as after trauma, infection or cancer, require tremendous amounts of nutrients to meet the accelerated metabolic needs of the tissues. In general, TPN is indicated in patients with evidence of muscle wasting, decubitus ulcers, nonhealing wounds, persistent weight loss, decreased serum albumin and total proteins, and decreased white blood cell function.

Intravenous hyperalimentation fluids contain hypertonic glucose (10 to 30 per cent), protein (hydrolysates or crystalline amino acids), and vitamins. Electrolytes, such as sodium, chloride, potassium, magnesium, calcium, and phosphate, are also added, based on each patient's individual requirements. Since the glucose is in a highly concentrated form, the administration of exogenous insulin usually accompanies the infusion in order to facilitate transport of glucose and protein into the cells. Additional insulin may be necessary, depending on the urinary glucose levels, which are routinely measured every 4 to 6 hours.

The major complications of TPN therapy include infection, hyperglycemia, hypoglycemia, and infiltration of the infusion catheter.

Bone Marrow Transfusions.[60, 85] Bone marrow transfusions are currently being used in emergency situations when the patient needs

TABLE 12–30. THE COMPLICATIONS OF IV THERAPY–SYMPTOMS AND RELEVANT NURSING ACTIONS

Complication	Symptoms	Nursing Actions
I. *Infiltration of IV solution*	A. Infusion rate slows or stops completely B. Swelling, hardness, and pain around the needle site C. A feeling of coldness around the injection site D. When the bottle is lowered below the level of the needle, blood fails to return into the tubing (not a reliable sign in presence of hypotension) E. Signs of tissue necrosis (with irritating solutions or vasoconstricting drugs)	1. Immediately stop the infusion 2. Apply warm towels to the swollen area 3. If necessary, restart the infusion at another site
II. *Thrombophlebitis*	A. Pain along the vein B. Area of redness and swelling around the affected vein	1. Stop infusion 2. If necessary, restart the infusion at another site 3. Apply warm moist compresses 4. Do *not* massage or rub the affected limb
III. *Pyogenic reaction*	A. Symptoms generally appear 30 min. after the infusion is started B. Temperature elevation and chills C. Headache D. Nausea and vomiting E. Circulatory collapse, if severe	1. Immediately stop infusion 2. Check vital signs 3. Notify doctor 4. Save IV solution so that it can be examined for pathogens 5. Do *not* give any solution that is cloudy
IV. *Speed shock*	A. Pounding headache B. Hypertension with possible loss of consciousness C. Rapid pulse D. Apprehension E. Chills F. Dyspnea Symptoms are variable and will depend upon the drug being used.	1. Stop or slow infusion, depending upon the severity of the symptoms 2. Check vital signs, neurologic and pulmonary functions 3. Notify physician
V. *Air embolism*	The main problem is sudden vascular collapse due to occlusion of vessel by embolism; as a result, tissues which are normally supplied with blood by the involved vessel will not receive adequate oxygen. Signs are: cyanosis, low blood pressure, tachycardia, rise in venous pressure, unconsciousness	1. Check vital signs 2. Administer oxygen 3. To prevent this complication: a. Make certain air does not enter arterial or central venous catheters. Secure all IV connections with adhesive tape. b. Have the patient perform a Valsalva maneuver or place the patient's head below heart level while you are changing tubing on central venous lines.
VI. *Circulatory overload*	This problem was discussed on p. 181.	

fluid *immediately,* and it is not possible (due to collapsed veins or limited time) to cannulize a vein. In a report by Valdez, a long, sharp, 14-gauge needle was inserted into the bone marrow of the tibial malleolus (ankle) at an angle of 20 degrees. Apparently, the patient reported little pain during the procedure. During a 30-day period, the patient's bone marrow was infused with approximately 42 liters of fluid. During this time, not a single infection developed nor were there any signs of embolism.

Nevertheless, when the bone marrow route is used for infusions, it is essential to observe for signs of infection and tissue slough around the site of injection as well as for embolism. Meticulous aseptic technique is mandatory both when inserting the needle into the bone marrow and while caring for the injection site. To keep the infusion open, the needle must be flushed daily with normal saline.

Major Types of Parenteral Solutions.* Many different types of parenteral fluids are available today. Each of the important groups of parenteral fluids is briefly considered in Table 12–31. The table does not, of course, list all the IV solutions available.

Out of the great number of available solutions, how does the doctor know which solution to

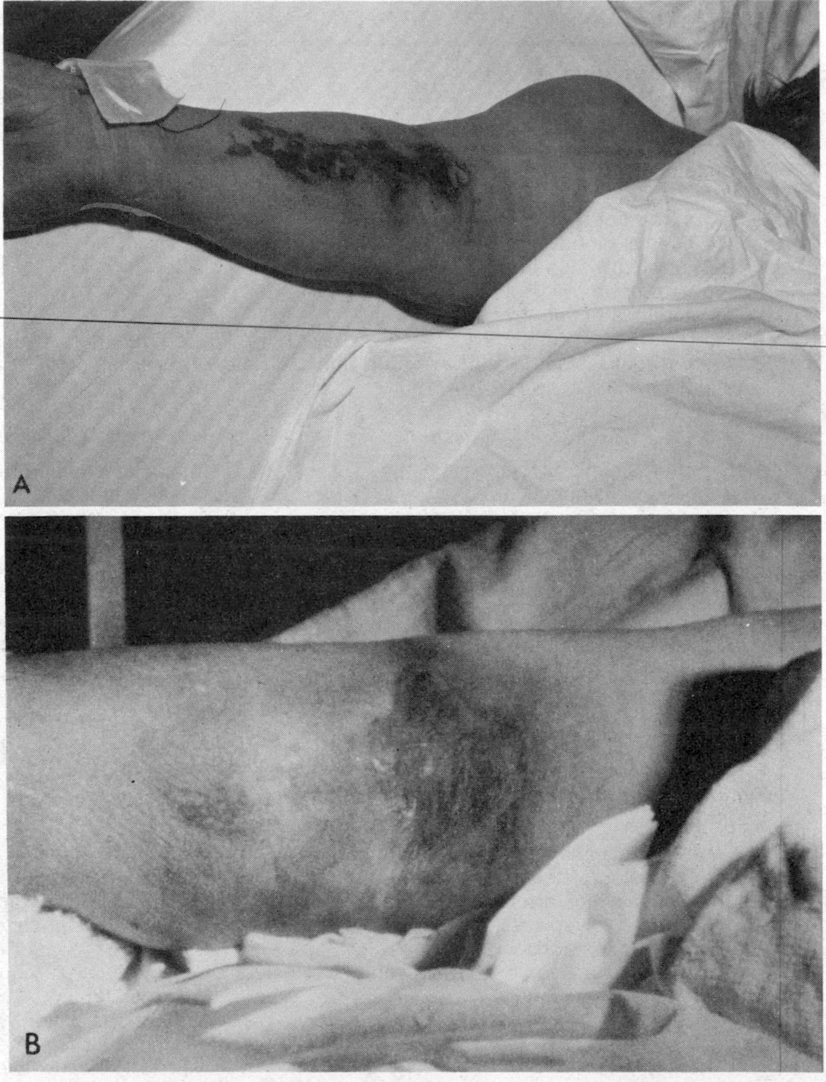

Figure 12–12. A, Necrosis of tissues resulting from infiltration of concentrated solution of potassium chloride. **B,** Necrosis from infiltration of hypertonic solution. (From Plumer, A. L.: *Principles and Practice of Intravenous Therapy,* 2nd ed. Boston: Little, Brown, and Co., 1975, p. 87.)

choose for the patient? How are the patient's replacement needs evaluated? What observations must be made as part of the assessment of fluid needs?

Evaluating the Patient's Parenteral Fluid and Electrolyte Needs. As stated earlier, a patient's fluid requirements fall roughly into three broad groups: (1) fluids to meet basal requirements or maintenance needs, (2) fluids to keep pace with dynamic or continuing losses, and (3) fluids to replace any old or *prior* losses. In Table 12–32 we present some of the major areas generally considered in assessing a patient's fluid needs and in developing a plan of care. Once the patient's fluid and electrolyte needs are assessed, a fluid order is written. To help you understand the assessment process better, we now consider some of the common conditions that make patients especially susceptible to fluid and electrolyte imbalances.

PATIENTS ESPECIALLY SUSCEPTIBLE TO FLUID AND ELECTROLYTE IMBALANCES

Fluid and electrolyte imbalances affect everyone at certain points in their existence. Some individuals, because of particular ailments, are more vulnerable to imbalances than other persons are. Ill persons who especially require careful evaluation and observation are: (1) patients with diarrhea, (2) patients who are vomiting, (3) patients with edema, (4) postoperative patients, (5) patients with burns, and (6) patients with pulmonary, cardiac, or renal problems.

When caring for patients with these special problems, carefully review the sections of this chapter that describe the imbalances to which these individuals are susceptible; particularly note preventive and nursing care measures for each imbalance.

The Patient with Diarrhea

Diarrhea is a commonly encountered clinical problem, occurring both in the hospital and at home. Some common causes of diarrhea are intestinal infections, toxic poisoning, drugs, fecal impactions, carcinoma, ulcerative colitis, pancreatic insufficiency, and certain neurologic diseases such as tabes dorsalis and diabetic neuropathy.

Diarrhea causes four major fluid and electrolyte imbalances:

- Dehydration
- Na^+ deficit (extracellular volume deficit)
- K^+ deficit
- Acidosis (This problem develops in response to decreased kidney function and Na^+ and HCO_3^- loss.)

Diarrhea causes decreases in both plasma volume and electrolytes. The major homeostatic mechanisms that occur in response to diarrhea are the fluid shift mechanism, the aldosterone mechanism, and the ADH mechanism (Fig. 12–13).

The Patient with Losses from Vomiting or Suction

The patient who is vomiting and the patient receiving gastric suction may suffer from large losses of fluid and electrolytes. For example, in 24 hours a patient may lose up to 2500 ml. of gastric fluid plus an additional loss of 1500 ml. of saliva. Water, H^+, Na^+, K^+, Cl^-, and small amounts of Mg^{++} are all present in gastric juice; consequently, deficits of these ions cause the different types of imbalances that result from vomiting.

Vomiting and gastric suction cause:

- Water deficit
- NaCl deficit
- K^+ deficit
- Metabolic alkalosis (H^+ and Cl^- are lost in vomiting. HCO_3^-, a base, is retained to compensate for the Cl^- loss.)
- Mg^{++} deficit
- Ketosis of starvation

These imbalances can be prevented or at least minimized with nursing care.

The Patient with Edema

Edema, an abnormal fluid retention within the body, has five major causes:

1. Damage to the capillary wall due to release of histamine and other substances, which results from burns, trauma, and allergic reactions.

*For a more thorough discussion of parenteral fluids, it is helpful to consult the pamphlets on water and electrolyte balance published by the major drug houses. Both Abbott and Baxter Laboratories have published informative brochures on the different solutions they manufacture.

TABLE 12–31. MAJOR TYPES OF PARENTERAL SOLUTIONS

- I. Carbohydrate solutions
  - A. Purposes and advantages
    1. Provide needed calories and nutrition
    2. Provide water replacement for the body's need for oxidation
    3. Increase the glycogen content of the liver
    4. Act as a protein sparer
    5. Prevent starvation ketosis
  - B. Limitations
    1. Dextrose solutions do not replace electrolyte losses
    2. Dextrose solutions alone are of no value in correcting fluid deficit.
  - C. Major types of solutions available
    1. 2.5%, 5%, 10% and 15% dextrose in water
    2. 5 and 10% dextrose in saline
    3. 50% glucose
       - a. This solution is sometimes given to individuals who need calories but are unable to cope with large amounts of fluid, e.g., patients with severe cardiac or kidney problems.
       - b. Such a concentrated solution should be given *very slowly.*
  - D. Untoward effects
    1. Concentrated carbohydrate solutions (over 5% dextrose in water or saline) may irritate the veins and cause thrombophlebitis.
    2. Rapid administration of hypertonic glucose solution can cause osmotic diuresis with subsequent loss of water and electrolytes. Glucosuria will be evident.
    3. A high blood sugar may result.
- II. Electrolyte solutions containing sodium
  - A. Purposes
    1. Treatment of sodium deficit
    2. Satisfy daily salt requirements
    3. Treatment of shock
    4. Treatment of H^+ imbalances
  - B. Limitations: Will not correct multiple electrolyte imbalances
  - C. Major types of solutions available
    1. Physiologic solution of sodium chloride (normal saline 0.9%).
    2. Hypotonic saline (0.45 or 0.2% saline).
    3. Hypertonic saline in strengths of 3% and 5%.
    4. One-sixth molar sodium lactate (to treat acidosis)
  - D. Complications
    1. Circulatory overload
    2. Sodium overload
    3. Potassium deficit
- III. Special purpose electrolyte solutions
  - A. Examples of solutions available
    1. Potassium solutions
    2. Ringer's solution
       - a. A normal saline solution to which K^+ and Ca^{++} have been added in place of some of the Na^+
       - b. Used in extracellular volume depletion and electrolyte deficits due to vomiting, diarrhea, and gastric suction
    3. Lactated Ringer's solution
       - a. Similar to plasma
       - b. Supplies lactate ions
    4. Multiple electrolyte solutions, for example, Butler's and Darrow's solutions
    5. Gastric replacement solution: replaces losses due to vomiting or gastric suction
- IV. Protein hydrolysates (also called amino acid solutions)
  - A. Purposes
    1. Supply proteins for tissue repair
    2. Correct negative nitrogen balance states
  - B. Contraindications
    1. Should not be given to patients with severe renal disease or hepatic disease (other forms of amino acid are given to these patients)
    2. Give with caution to patients with *liver* disease or with history of *allergy.*
  - C. Types of solutions available
    1. Amigen
    2. Aminosol
    3. Stuart amino acids
  - D. Untoward effects
    1. Fever
    2. Nausea and vomiting
    3. Headache
    4. Thrombophlebitis or infection at the infusion site
    5. Hypo- or hyperglycemia
    6. Hypokalemia
    7. Hypophosphatemia
  - E. Special precautions for greater safety in administration

TABLE 12–31. MAJOR TYPES OF PARENTERAL SOLUTIONS (*Continued*)

> **Remember, in administering protein hydrolysates:**
> 1. **Do not** *keep a solution in the refrigerator once it has been opened. Use at once or discard!*
> 2. **Do not** *use solutions that are cloudy or contain precipitate matter.*
> 3. **Do not** *add other mixtures or medications to amino acid solutions.*
> 4. *Give* **slowly.** *The usual dose of amino acid is 100 to 200 Gm. per 24 hours.*
> 5. *Provide air filter when hanging in room (solution provides good culture media).*
> 6. *Give only in central vein.*

V. Fat emulsions
- A. Purposes and advantages
  1. Provide excellent source of calories
  2. Can be used for severe nutritional disorders coupled with a poor oral intake
  3. Is isotonic so it can be infused into a peripheral vein
- B. Types of solutions available:
  1. Lipomul: Contains cottonseed oil; provides 800 calories in 500 ml
  2. Intralipid: Contains soybean oil
- C. Possible contraindications
  1. Fat emulsions *should always be used with caution.*
  2. Observe patients with liver diseases, coagulation problems, or acidosis meticulously for side effects.
- D. Adverse side effects (especially to Lipomul)
  1. Early reaction
     - a. Apparently due to introduction of colloids into the blood stream
     - b. Characterized by a shock-like syndrome, severe back pain, cyanosis, urticara
  2. Later reaction
     - a. Occurs around the third week following the infusion
     - b. Characterized by anemia, blood clotting, and hemorrhage
- E. Special precautions to observe

> **Remember, in administering fat emulsions:**
> 1. *Give* **slowly** *according to the following schedule:*
>   *First 5 minutes — 10 gtts./min.*
>   *Next 25 minutes — 40 gtts./min.*
>   *Then — 60 gtts./min.*
> 2. *Use sets developed for Lipomul infusion.*
> 3. **Do not** *mix Lipomul with other medicines or liquids.*

VI. Solutions containing alcohol
- A. Indications and advantages
  1. Gives the patient needed calories while sparing the patient's body fats, proteins, and carbohydrates
  2. Has a sedative effect
  3. Gives an increased sense of well-being
  4. May act as an analgesic
- B. Examples of solutions available:
  1. 5% alcohol, 5% dextrose in water
  2. 5% alcohol, 5% dextrose in saline
  3. 10% alcohol, 10% glucose in water
  4. Trinidex, 5% alcohol, 5% dextrose with vitamins in water
- C. Contraindications: Patients with epilepsy, liver, or kidney or neurologic diseases or in shock should not receive alcohol solutions.
- D. Dosage and rate
  1. 200 to 300 ml. of a 5% solution per hour provides sedation without intoxication.
  2. On the average, patients are given 1 to 2 liters of alcohol solutions in 24 hours.
- E. Side effects
  1. Cerebral depression
  2. Loss of alertness
  3. Restlessness and coma (in an overdose)
- F. Special precautions
  1. Watch carefully for signs of infiltration; tissue slough can result.
  2. Observe for signs of phlebitis around the injection site.

VII. Colloidal solutions*
- A. Indications
  1. Expansion of a depleted plasma volume
  2. Support of the plasma osmotic pressure
  3. Prevention of shock and circulatory collapse
- B. Examples of solutions available
  1. Plasma
  2. Human serum albumin
  3. Plasma expanders (dextran and gelatin)

*The giving of blood and plasma will be discussed more fully in the unit on blood, Unit XIV.

2. Interference with the venous return owing to tight garters, thrombophlebitis, lack of exercise, or obesity.

3. Decrease in plasma proteins and plasma oncotic pressure. This problem is found in malnutrition (lack of protein), kidney disease (loss of protein), cirrhosis of the liver (lack of protein), profuse serous drainage (loss of protein), and hemorrhage (loss of protein).

4. Rise in plasma hydrostatic pressure, which causes fluid to be squeezed into the tissues. This problem is due to circulatory overload and occurs in the following conditions: heart failure (due to salt and water retention), kidney failure (due to salt and water retention), and excessive infusions of hypertonic solutions.

5. Obstruction of the lymphatic system, which may follow a radical mastectomy.

Symptoms that commonly accompany edema are weight gain, high blood pressure, and dyspnea.

The principal types of edema that can be identified in clinical practice are: pitting, dependent, and refractory. The major factors that distinguish one form of edema from another are listed below:

Pitting Edema. To test for pitting edema, press the edematous area of the patient, usually the ankles or sacrum, with your finger. If the indentation from your finger remains in the patient's flesh for a period of time, pitting edema is present.

Dependent Edema. This type of edema is related to gravity and to the patient's position. Fluid accumulates in dependent parts of the body. In observing for dependent edema:

1. Check the sacral area and buttocks of patients on *bed rest.* Because the patient is in a supine position, the tissues of the buttocks and sacrum are the dependent areas.

2. Check the ankles and buttocks of patients who

TABLE 12–32. ASSESSING THE PATIENT'S PARENTERAL FLUID NEEDS

I. Basal requirements. To assess a patient's basal requirements, evaluate the patient's needs for water, electrolytes, carbohydrates, and vitamins.

A. Water requirements: Patients require approximately 1500 to 2500 ml. of water per day if they are not sweating excessively, high fever is not present, and renal function is normal. In writing individualized parenteral fluid orders, the following are considered:
   1. The basal metabolic rate, taking into account:
      a. The patient's age, sex, activity, thyroid function, and diagnosis.
      b. Conditions that increase the patient's metabolic rate (i.e., fever, hot weather) or decrease metabolic rate (i.e., cardiac failure, renal shock).
   2. Water losses from the following sources:
      a. Urine
      b. Perspiration (sensible and insensible)
      c. Feces
      d. Respiratory tract
      e. Abnormal drainage (transudate and exudate)
   3. The intake and output record in terms of balance and the adequacy of both intake and output
   4. Daily weight:
      a. An important aid in calculating those water losses that cannot be readily measured (i.e., from sweating or incontinence).
      b. The *ideal* weight should be used in calculating water requirements for patients who are obese or edematous.
   5. Body surface area: Calculated from tables based on height and weight measurements.
   6. Solute loads: Postoperative patients and patients with metabolic disorders need more water intake to excrete wastes, toxins, and excess sugar.
   7. Central venous pressure (CVP):
      a. The pressure of blood within the right atrium is the central venous pressure. It can be measured in the peripheral veins of the arms or in the neck
      b. The CVP procedure provides a most accurate guide in body fluid replacement because it is a good index of the body's circulating blood volume*
      c. A rise in CVP (from baseline) indicates overloading of the circulatory system
      d. A fall in CVP (from baseline) indicates inadequate circulatory volume
      e. CVP is normally performed on oliguric patients receiving parenteral fluids, to prevent fluid overload

B. Basic electrolyte requirements
   1. General, daily electrolyte requirements (variations occur under stress):

Na^+	60 to 1000 mEq./day
K^+	40 to 75 mEq./day
Cl^-	80 to 110 mEq./day
NaCl	3.5 to 6.0 Gm./day (average 4.5 Gm.)

   2. To evaluate needs, physicians use the clinical history, the physical examination, and laboratory findings
   3. Following surgery, use caution in prescribing NaCl solutions, especially if patients are old, debilitated, or have renal or cardiac dysfunction.
   4. Precautions always used when prescribing K^+ solutions or additives

*The procedure for CVP is discussed in the unit on the circulatory system, Unit XII.

have been *sitting* or standing for extended periods of time.

Refractory Edema. Edema that persists despite diuretic therapy and salt-restricted diets is said to be "refractory." Patients with this type of edema will also tend to have persistent weight gain and hypertension.

Location of Edema. While edema may be described as pitting, dependent, or refractory, it can also be classified in relation to *where* it develops within the body. Some words used to describe edema in terms of location include:

1. Anasarca — severe *generalized* edema.
2. Ascites — an excessive accumulation of fluid within the peritoneal cavity.
3. Pulmonary edema — excess fluid within the lung tissue.
4. Interstitial edema — excessive fluid in the interstitial spaces. This condition is common in heart failure.
5. Hydrothorax — effusions of fluid into the pleural cavity resulting in lung collapse.
6. Hydropericardium — effusions of fluid into the pericardial cavity.
7. Pleural effusion — edema fluid in the pleural space.

Edema can be controlled medically by diuretic therapy, the prescription of low-salt diets, and occasionally by the parenteral administration of salt-poor proteins. Water may also be moderately restricted.

There are several points to remember in giving nursing care to patients with edema.

1. Carefully regulate the IV fluids that you administer to patients with edema, especially those having pulmonary edema.

TABLE 12-32. ASSESSING THE PATIENT'S PARENTERAL FLUID NEEDS (Continued)

- C. Basic carbohydrate requirements
  - 1. A 70-kg. patient requires approximately 1800 calories per day for nourishment, to prevent starvation ketosis, and to spare protein.
  - 2. The physician usually orders the carbohydrates to be given in the form of 5 or 10% glucose in water or saline.
  - 3. Glucose solution *alone* cannot supply a patient's total caloric needs over a sustained period of time.
    - a. One liter of 5% glucose in water supplies only 50 Gm. of glucose or 200 calories.
    - b. Generally, patients receive 2500 ml. of glucose in water or saline per day. This amounts to only 500 *calories per day*—not sufficient to meet the 1800 calories required by a patient over a 24 hr. period.
    - c. For long-term patients, physicians may order in addition to glucose solution, the following calorie-supplying preparations: protein hydrolysates, emulsified fat preparations, solutions containing alcohol, or tube feedings.
    - d. For those patients requiring parenteral nutrition for only a few days, physicians are concerned mainly with *fluid* replacement rather than caloric requirements.
- D. Basic vitamin requirements
  - 1. Vitamin supplements are usually ordered for patients:
    - a. Who are NPO and receiving parenteral therapy for more than 3 days
    - b. Who are severely malnourished, e.g., alcoholics
    - c. With acute illnesses or infections
    - d. Who are recovering from surgery
    - e. Who are burned
  - 2. Vitamin C and the vitamin B complex are commonly administered parenterally.

II. Replacing dynamic losses (losses over and above basal losses of fluids and electrolytes)
- A. Main causes
  - 1. Vomiting
  - 2. Diarrhea
  - 3. Gastric or intestinal suction
  - 4. Wound drainage
  - 5. Fluid shifts between compartments as seen in patients with burns and trauma
- B. Special purpose electrolyte solutions often ordered for replacing continuing gastrointestinal tract losses.

III. Replacing prior losses
- A. Prior deficits represent those deficiencies or imbalances of fluids and electrolytes that the patient had *prior* to current treatment.
- B. Major types of prior deficits
  - 1. Water depletion
  - 2. Electrolyte deficits or imbalances
  - 3. Red blood cell mass deficit
  - 4. Deficiency of plasma proteins.
- C. Solution used in treatment
  - 1. Glucose and water solutions
  - 2. General or special purpose electrolyte solutions
  - 3. Whole blood to replace red cell mass
  - 4. Salt-poor human albumin to replace plasma proteins

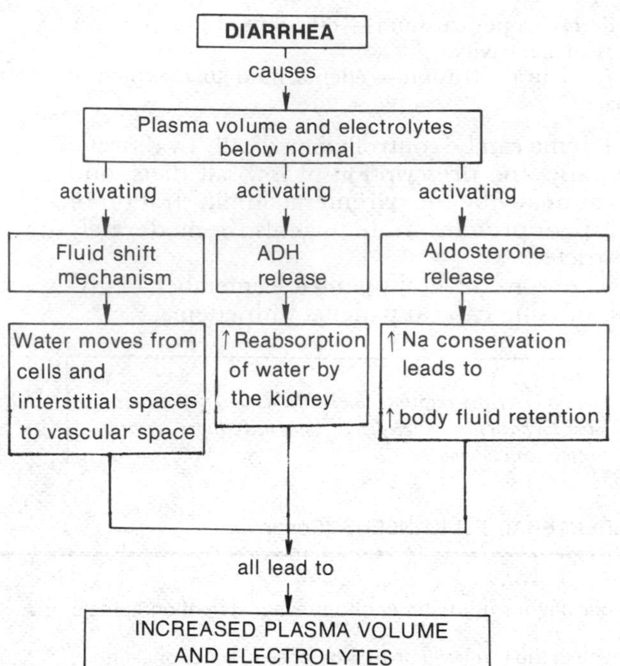

Figure 12–13. Homeostatic mechanisms that help to counteract the fluid and electrolyte imbalances created by diarrhea.

2. Observe carefully and frequently for decubitus ulcer formation, since edematous tissue is fragile and prone to breakdown. Patients with edema require frequent position changes. If possible, procure an alternating pressure mattress or other means of alternating pressure such as water beds, or eggshell mattresses.

3. Edematous patients are usually malnourished. Unless contraindicated, encourage these patients to eat substantial amounts of protein.

4. Observe edematous patients for thirst and hypovolemia. You will recall that edema fluid is trapped in the tissues and thus may not be available to the cells or circulation.

5. Take care when giving subcutaneous or IM injections.

6. Prevent shearing effect when moving patients.

As with any condition, patients being treated for edema are subject to iatrogenic complications. The most important iatrogenic problems are: (1) low salt syndrome resulting from the low-sodium diet causing increased aldosterone release, thereby maintaining the edematous state and (2) hypokalemia, or K^+ deficit, resulting from the administration of diuretics.

The Surgical Patient

During the preoperative period, the major imbalances facing surgical patients are water and salt deficits due to losses of ECF. These losses are usually the result of vomiting, diarrhea, gastrointestinal tract drainage, and intestinal obstructions (in which fluid is trapped in the obstructed loops of bowel). Also, the enemas received by most patients cause further isotonic deficits. Because of such problems, patients often are treated with vigorous IV therapy *before* surgery can be performed.

During the first 24 to 48 hours of the postoperative period, you can expect certain characteristic shifts in the patient's fluids and electrolytes. These adjustments seem to be related to the stress reaction of the GAS as described by Selye. During the early *postoperative period* the following adjustments occur:

- ADH is released.
- Urine volume is *decreased* regardless of intake, and water is retained.
- Aldosterone secretion is increased (especially following major surgery).
- Na^+ is retained (and thus water).
- K^+ excretion is increased.

Patients who vomit or who are on gastric suction following surgery may develop the imbalances discussed on p. 221, whereas those with intestinal drainage or suction will probably present a clinical picture similar to that described for diarrhea on p. 221. Postoperative patients who are NPO, nauseated, or anorexic also face the crucial problems of caloric, protein, and vitamin deficiencies unless these nutrients are replaced.

In sum, the most typical complications following major surgery are:

1. Water excess (due to ↑ ADH)
2. Extracellular volume excess (due to ↑ NaCl by aldosterone)
3. Abdominal distention } (due to K^+ deficit)
4. Paralytic ileus }
5. Shallow respirations
6. Hemorrhage and shock (due to bleeding)
7. Acute renal insufficiency (due to hypovolemia)
8. Signs of tetany (due to ↓ Ca^{++})
9. Arrhythmias (due to ↓ K^+ and ↓ Ca^{++})
10. Respiratory acidosis (generally due to hypoventilation during surgery and to pain and splinting following surgery)

The Burn Patient

Individuals suffering from serious burns are prime candidates for multiple severe imbalances.

Important imbalances that may develop as a result of burns are:

- Water deficit
- Sodium deficit

- ▶ K^+ excess during first 48 hours (due to cellular trauma)
- ▶ K^+ deficit after first 48 hours (due to shifts of K^+ from ECF into cells and increased renal losses)
- ▶ Metabolic acidosis
- ▶ Plasma to interstitial fluid shift (during first 48 hours)
- ▶ Interstitial fluid to plasma shift (following first 48 hours)
- ▶ Ca^{++} deficit
- ▶ Negative nitrogen balance

Immediate recognition and care of the above imbalances and fluid and electrolyte shifting mechanisms are essential to save the life of the severely burned individual.

BIBLIOGRAPHY (Chapter 12)

1. Albanese, A. A.: Calcium nutrition in the elderly. *Postgraduate Medicine,* 63:167, Mar. 1978.
2. Antacid acceptability: Is it the taste that counts? *Nurse's Drug Alert,* 1:82, June 1977.
3. Antacids after all. *Emergency Medicine,* 9:12, Dec. 1977.
4. Asperheim, M. K., and L. A. Eisenhauer: *The Pharmacologic Basis of Patient Care,* 3rd ed. Philadelphia: W. B. Saunders Co., 1977.
5. Aspinall, M. J.: A simplified guide to managing patients with hyponatremia. *Nursing 78,* 8:32, Dec. 1978.
6. Ayres, S. M., et al.: Pulmonary physiology at the bedside: Oxygen and carbon dioxide abnormalities. *Cardiovascular Nursing,* 9:1, Jan. Feb. 1973.
7. Bailey, R.: Diuretics in the elderly. *British Medical Journal,* 1:1618, June 1978.
8. Bay, W. H., and T. F. Ferris: Hypernatremia and hyponatremia: Disorders of tonicity. *Geriatrics,* 31:53, Aug. 1976.
9. Beaumont, F.: The new infusion pumps. *Nursing 77,* 7:31, July 1977.
10. Berkow and Talbott (Eds.): *The Merck Manual, 13th ed.* Rahway, N.J.: Merck and Co., Inc., 1977.
11. Beyers, M., and S. Dudas: *The Clinical Practice of Medical-Surgical Nursing.* Boston: Little, Brown & Co., 1977.
12. Borgen, L.: Total parenteral nutrition in adults. *American Journal of Nursing,* 78:224, Feb. 1978.
13. Bransome, E. D., Jr.: Polyuria and water intoxication: Disorders of antidiuretic hormone. *Consultant,* 18:29, Oct. 1977.
14. Brin, M., and J. C. Bauernfeind: Vitamin needs of the elderly. *Postgraduate Medicine,* 63:155, Mar. 1978.
15. Brundage, J.: *Nursing Management of Renal Problems.* St. Louis: C. V. Mosby Co., 1976.
16. Burke, M.: Electrolyte studies: Potassium, chloride, and acid-base. *Postgraduate Medicine,* 64:205, Nov. 1978.
17. Burke, M. D.: Blood gas measurements. *Postgraduate Medicine,* 64:163, Dec. 1978.
18. Burke, S. R.: *The Composition and Function of Body Fluids.* St. Louis: C. V. Mosby Co., 1976.
19. Butts, P.: Magnesium sulfate in the treatment of toxemia. *The American Journal of Nursing,* 77:1294, Aug. 1977.
20. Byrne, J.: Tests that measure protein metabolism. *Nursing 77,* 7:13, Oct. 1977.
21. Cameron, S., et al.: *Nephrology for Nurses.* Flushing, N.Y.: Medical Examination Publishing Co., Inc., 1976.
22. Cohen, S.: Metabolic acid-base disorders. Part 1: Chemistry and physiology. Programmed instruction. *American Journal of Nursing,* 77:(PI insert) Oct. 1977.
23. Cohen, S.: Metabolic acid-base disorders. Part 2: Physiological abnormalities and nursing actions. Programmed instruction. *American Journal of Nursing.* 78:(PI p. 1) Jan. 1978.
24. Cohen, S.: Metabolic acid-base disorders. Part 3: Clinical and laboratory findings. *American Journal of Nursing.* 78:(PI p. 1) Mar. 1978.
25. Contiguglia, S. R., et al.: Fluid and Electrolyte Therapy. *In* Friedman, H. H., and S. Papper (Eds.): *Problem-Oriented Medical Diagnosis.* Boston: Little, Brown, and Co., 1975.
26. Davenport, H. W.: *Physiology of the Digestive Tract,* 4th ed. Chicago: Year Book Medical Publishers, Inc., 1977.
27. Del Bueno, D. J.: A quick review on using blood-gas determinations. *RN,* 41:68, Mar. 1978.
28. Del Bueno, G. J.: Electrolyte imbalance: How to recognize and respond to it. Part 1. *RN,* 38:52, Feb. 1975.
29. Diuretics: Adverse reactions and precautions. *Nurse's Drug Alert,* 2:134, Nov. 1978.
30. Dudrick, S. J.: A patient on I.V. therapy need not starve! *Consultant,* 18:142, Feb. 1978.
31. Dudrick, S. J., and J. E. Rhodes: Total intravenous feeding. *Scientific American,* 226:73, May 1972.
32. Elbaum, N.: Detecting and correcting magnesium imbalance. *Nursing 77,* 7:34, Aug. 1977.
33. Feldtman, Maj. R. W., and Maj. R. J. Andrassy: Meeting exceptional nutritional needs: Total parenteral nutrition. *Postgraduate Medicine,* 64:64, Aug. 1978.
34. Fenton, M.: What to do about thirst. *American Journal of Nursing,* 69:1014, May 1969.
35. Fisch, C.: Relation of electrolyte disturbances to cardiac arrhythmias. *Circulation,* 47:488, Feb. 1973.
36. Gill, J. R.: Edema. *Annual Review of Medicine,* 21:273, 1970.
37. Goldberg, M.: Water control and the dysnatremias. *In* Bricker, N. S. (Ed.): *The Sea Within Us.* New York: Searle and Co., Science and Medicine Publishing Co., 1975.
38. Grant, M. M., and W. M. Kubo: Assessing a patient's hydration status. *American Journal of Nursing,* 75:1306, Aug. 1975.
39. Gump, F. E., and J. M. Kinney: Caloric and fluid losses through the burn wound. *Surgical Clinics of North America,* 50:1235, Dec. 1970.
40. Guyton, A. C.: *Textbook of Medical Physiology,* 5th ed. Philadelphia: W. B. Saunders Co., 1976.
41. Hamilton, H. (Ed.): *Monitoring Fluid and Electrolytes Precisely.* Nursing 78 Books. Horsham, Pa.: Intermed Communications, Inc., 1978.
42. Haughney, E. J., and F. M. Sica: Diuretics: How safe can you make them? *Nursing 77,* 7:34, Feb. 1977.
43. Herbert, V.: The megavitamin therapy fad. *Consultant,* 18:70, May, 1977.
44. Holmes, J. H.: Fluid intake with medication. *Archives of Internal Medicine,* 116:813, Nov. 1965.
45. Howells, E. M.: Managing fluids and electrolytes in surgical patients. *Geriatrics,* 32:100, May 1977.
46. Kemp, G., and D. Kemp: Diuretics. *American Journal of Nursing,* 78:1007, June 1978.
47. Khokhar, N.: Inappropriate secretion of antidiuretic hormone. *Postgraduate Medicine,* 62:73, Oct. 1977.
48. Kolb, F. O.: Advances in the treatment of calcium disorders. *Consultant,* 18:131, Sept. 1978.
49. Kosman, M. E.: Management of potassium problems during long-term diuretic therapy. *JAMA,* 230(5):743, 1974.

50. Krueger, J. A., and J. C. Ray: *Endocrine Problems in Nursing.* St. Louis: C. V. Mosby Co., 1976.
51. Lancour, J.: ADH and aldosterone: How to recognize their effects. *Nursing 78,* 8:36, Sept. 1978.
52. Leaf, A., and R. S. Cotran: *Renal Pathophysiology.* New York: Oxford University Press, 1976.
53. Lee, C. A., V. R. Stroot, and C. A. Schaper: What to do when acid-base problems hang in the balance. *Nursing 75,* 5:32, Aug. 1975.
54. Livingston, C.: Assisting with intravenous therapy. *Nursing Process II Syllabus,* Seattle: University of Washington School of Nursing, Summer 1975.
55. Macleod, S. M.: The rational use of potassium supplements. *Nursing Digest,* Summer 1976, p. 88.
56. Manzi, C. C.: Edema: How to tell if it's a danger signal. *Nursing 77,* 7:66, Apr. 1977.
57. Mazzara, J. T., and Ayes, S. M.: Fluid and electrolyte and acid-base disturbances in the coronary care unit. *NCNA,* 7(3):549, 1972.
58. Metheny, N. M., and W. D. Snively: *Nurses Handbook of Fluid Balance.* Philadelphia: J. B. Lippincott Co., 1974.
59. Metheny, N. M., and W. D. Snively: Perioperative fluids and electrolytes. *American Journal of Nursing,* 78:840, May 1978.
60. Michaels, R. M. (Ed.): Bone marrow as an emergency route for fluids. *Nurses Drug Alert,* I:156, Nov. 1977.
61. Molyneux-Luick, M., and J. Knecht: Hypovolemic shock. *Nursing 77,* 7:33, Nov. 1977.
62. Money savers: An inexpensive source of potassium replacement. *Nurse's Drug Alert,* 2:22, Mar. 1978.
63. Munro, H. N., and V. R. Young: Protein metabolism in the elderly: Observations relating to dietary needs. *Postgraduate Medicine,* 63:143, Mar. 1978.
64. Narins, G.: A practical approach to managing hyponatremia. *Consultant,* 19:25, Feb. 1979.
65. Nettles, S.: It's more than just a bottle. *Supervisor Nurse,* 10:38, July 1977.
66. Nugent, C. A.: Answers to questions on the differential diagnosis of hypercalcemia. *Hospital Medicine,* 14:106, Feb. 1978.
67. Oakes, A., and H. Morrow: Understanding blood gases. *Nursing 73,* 3:15, Sept. 1973.
68. Origin and action of aldosterone. *Hospital Medicine,* 12:6, June 1976.
69. Pitts, F.: *Physiology of the Kidney and Body Fluids,* 3rd ed. Chicago: Year Book Medical Publishers, Inc., 1974.
70. Plummer, A. L.: *Principles and Practice of Intravenous Therapy.* Boston: Little, Brown and Co., 1975.
71. Randall, H. T.: Fluid, electrolyte, and acid-base balance. *Surgical Clinics of North America,* 56:1019, Oct. 1976.
72. Reed, G. M.: Confused about potassium? Here's a clear and concise guide. *Nursing 74,* 4:20, Mar. 1974.
73. Reed, G. M., and V. F. Sheppard: *Regulation of Fluid and Electrolyte Balance: A Programmed Instruction in Physiology for Nurses,* 2nd ed. Philadelphia: W. B. Saunders Co., 1977.
74. Sharer, J. E.: Reviewing acid-base balance. *American Journal of Nursing,* 75:980, June 1975.
75. Sieger, P.: The physiologic approach to acid-base balance. *MCNA,* 57:863, July 1973.
76. Slonim, N. B.: Blood-gas and pH abnormalities. *In* Friedman, H. H., and S. Papper (Eds.): *Problem-Oriented Medical Diagnosis.* Boston: Little, Brown and Co., 1975.
77. Sopko, J., and R. Freeman: Salt substitutes as a source of potassium. *JAMA,* 238:608, Aug. 1977.
78. Spencer, R. T.: *Patient Care in Endocrine Problems.* Philadelphia: W. B. Saunders Co., 1973.
79. Sklar, D., and M. Liang: Antacids: Cost, taste and buffering. *New England Journal of Medicine,* 296:1007, Apr. 1977.
80. Stolar, V. (Consultant): *Human Acid-Base Chemistry: A Programmed Instruction.* New York: The American Journal of Nursing Company, 1973.
81. Stroot, V., C. Lee, and C. A. Schaper: *Fluids and Electrolytes: A Practical Approach.* Philadelphia: F. A. Davis Co., 1977.
82. Tepperman, J.: *Metabolic and Endocrine Physiology,* 3rd ed. Chicago: The Year Book Medical Publishers Inc., 1973.
83. Troubles with I.V.'s? *Nursing 78,* 8:78, Oct. 1978.
84. Twombly, M.: The shift into third space. *Nursing 78,* 8:38, June 1978.
85. Valdes, M.: Intraosseous fluid administration in emergencies. *Lancet,* 1:1235, June 1977.
86. Waldron, M. W.: Oxygen transport. *American Journal of Nursing,* 79:272, Feb. 1979.
87. Welling, P. G.: How food and fluid affect drug absorption. *Postgraduate Medicine,* 62:73, July 1977.
88. Williams, F. H.: Potassium overdose. A potential hazard of non-rigid parenteral fluid containers. *British Medical Journal,* 1:714, Mar. 1973.
89. Williams, S. R.: *Nutrition and Diet Therapy,* 3rd ed. St. Louis: C. V. Mosby Co., 1977.
90. Wilson, R. F.: Tips on managing fluid and electrolyte problems. *Consultant,* 17:31, Nov. 1977.

CHAPTER 13*

PHYSIOLOGIC SHOCK

Active research interest in shock dates back to the early years of this century. Awareness of the clinical problem existed much before this. The history of this long effort to determine the true nature of the syndrome provides eloquent testimony to its inherent complexity. For at this moment, the critical shock mechanism still remains an elusive entity.[65]

INTRODUCTION AND STUDY GUIDE

"Is the patient going into shock? Is the patient already in shock?" Nurses often ask themselves these critical questions as they give patient care.

> *In its most basic sense, shock is a* generalized *state of inadequate circulation, resulting in poor tissue perfusion with blood. However, poor blood flow alone is not always the cause. Faulty or inadequate cell metabolism is typically a central problem with shock.*

Patients in shock, or threatening to go into shock, are seriously ill; the nurse must act rapidly and precisely to protect them from the complications and possible fatal outcome of a shocked condition.

Tens of thousands of deaths and an unknown number of permanent injuries occur annually from shock, in the United States alone. Because shock occurs frequently and because shock is a serious, often fatal disorder, it is extremely important that nurses be able to recognize and treat promptly the signs and symptoms of *early* circulatory failure, before severe shock ensues.

Let us emphasize that most of the research conducted on shock mechanisms and treatment is based upon hemorrhagic or traumatic shock. This chapter thus focuses on these forms of shock. Much less information is available regarding shock associated with myocardial infarction than other categories of shock, largely because of the absence of any satisfactory laboratory models. Therefore, myocardial shock is often excluded from general discussions of shock, and is only briefly discussed in this chapter. (Unit XII focuses intensively on disturbances of cardiovascular function and blood flow.)

Because of the basically lethal nature of shock, research on shock is usually performed with laboratory animals rather than human subjects. (Researchers seem less reluctant to use animals for potentially dangerous procedures than they are to use humans.) This poses problems in determining which aspects of the experimental data are valid for application to the treatment of shock in human beings. Nevertheless, it is believed that the basic hemodynamic disturbances caused by prolonged shock, whatever the cause, are similar in the dog (used experimentally), in humans, or in any other of the mammalian species. Apparently, the differences among various members of the species lie in the susceptibility of differing tissues to the basic hemodynamic disturbances shared by them all.

We shall discuss four different types of shock: (1) *hematogenic,* (2) *cardiogenic,* (3) *neurogenic,* and (4) *vasogenic.* Because each type of shock varies in form, it is technically more accurate to refer to specific types of shock, or "patterns of shock,"[18] instead of making general references to "shock." Nonetheless, shock is often discussed in a broad sense in medical literature and in clinical situations. In these instances, *"shock" in general terms refers to a state of generalized inadequate circulation that causes decreased perfusion of the body tissues with blood and produces a wide range of systemic effects.*

Shock may arise from many different etiologies since it can be an untoward effect of numerous disease conditions. Moreover, shock usually is a complex phenomenon to treat because its initiating factors are often multiple, e.g., physical injury plus blood loss plus infection. In addition, each patient's general physical status and medical background are unique, and the physiologic responses of different individuals to similar noxious events are never the same.

In studying the clinical syndrome commonly called "shock," you, as a nurse, will be concerned with four major factors: (1) patient's responses to the particular insults leading to shock (e.g., traumatic hemorrhage), (2) their responses to the shock episode itself, (3) the nature of those responses that determine whether recovery will be possible, and (4) the recognition and management of shock.

*This chapter has been critically reviewed and revised by Margaret M. McMahon, R.N., B.S.N., CCRN.

Objectives

1. After carefully studying this chapter and relating it to your own clinical observations you can expect to be able to:

a. Recall the anatomy and physiology of the circulatory system.

b. Discuss the basic pathological processes involved in shock.

c. Identify the similarities and differences between the various types of shock.

d. Describe the generally recognized stages of shock and the possible consequences of each for the patient.

e. Explain, in detail, the physiologic effects of shock.

f. List the signs and symptoms of shock.

g. Recognize *quickly* signs and symptoms of shock in patients.

h. Write down the major principles upon which treatment for a patient in shock are based.

i. Discuss the various invasive and noninvasive techniques currently used in the assessment of people in shock.

j. Identify the drugs commonly used in the treatment of shock and discuss the administration and function of each.

k. Understand the purposes of various mechanical devices used in the treatment and physiologic support of a person in shock.

l. Assist a professional nurse in developing and implementing an appropriate nursing care plan for a person in shock.

m. Understand the needs of and offer emotional support to the patient and the significant others of a patient in shock.

Suggested Learning Activities

- Make a list of all the terms new to you and write, in your own words, a brief description of each term. You may find it useful to make out a small file card for each term, and in this way, develop a quick, personal reference system.
- Gather information about the drugs used in the treatment of shock. You may find it helpful to make out a file card for each drug and include information such as the generic and trade names, usual dose range, beneficial actions, possible side effects, and any special administrative precautions (review basic pharmacology as necessary).
- Familiarize yourself with the location of the emergency supplies on the unit in which you are having clinical experience. Identify the equipment and drugs that could be used for a person in shock and describe the purpose of each.
- Find out if the facility in which you are having clinical experience has any of the mechanical treatment devices described in this chapter (e.g., antishock trousers, extracorporeal membrane oxygenator). If so, arrange to see those devices and have someone who is familiar with their operation explain them to you.
- Under the direction of your nurse-instructor locate patients who are being assessed by some of the invasive techniques described in this chapter (e.g., central venous pressure; monitoring of arterial pressures). Gather information about the nursing care these persons are receiving. (Do not concentrate exclusively on the "machine," but seek information concerning the total care of the person.) Discuss and critically evaluate the information you gather with your instructor and a group of other students. Would *you* plan to care in any other way? On what basis would you do things differently.
- After you have completed working with the material of this chapter evaluate your learning in light of the objectives for this chapter. Can you in fact, do all the things that the objectives state you can expect to be able to do? What objectives have you not completely met? Such an evaluation will give you an indication of the areas in which you need to do some more work.

CIRCULATION: A BRIEF REVIEW

Several major components or divisions make up the circulatory system: namely, the heart, the large blood vessels, and the microcirculation.* Each of these subdivisions is, in a sense, designed for and concerned with separate and distinct intrinsic activities. Therefore, each encompasses a separate area of homeostasis. However, *the circulation is a closed system,† and all parts of the circulation are interdependent, so that an alteration in one part will have an effect on the other parts.*

The operational activities of the heart and large blood vessels are regulated by the vasomotor center of the brain, the autonomic nervous pathways, and the monitoring devices (baroreceptors and chemoreceptors)‡ in the walls of the heart, and the large vessels. Regulation of the microcirculation, however, is a different matter.

Once the blood flow passes "the arteriolar floodgates"[65] and enters the tissues proper by way of the microcirculation, it is regulated by a completely new set of devices that are primarily of a chemical nature. The microcirculation is governed locally by those substances that are "liberated into the local tissue environment by the metabolic activities of its literally millions of cells."[65] Such local regulation gives the body a sensitive, discriminating mechanism by means of

*Terms used interchangeably with "microcirculation" are "peripheral circulation," "capillary circulation," and "terminal vascular bed."

†Blood does not actually come into direct contact with the cells, other than those lining the blood vessels, except in the sinusoids of the liver and in the spleen.[142]

‡*Baroreceptors* are sensory nerve terminals that are stimulated by changes in pressure. *Chemoreceptors* are receptors or sense organs that are excited by chemical substances.

which the blood flow can be adjusted according to the needs of the tissues from one moment to another.

For adequate circulation of blood, the following three factors must function effectively together:

- *Vascular tone,* or resistance of the blood vessels
- *Blood volume,* or the total amount of blood in the body
- *Cardiac pump,* or the pumping action of the heart

When the body is in a state of health, the volume of the blood, the size of the vascular bed (as determined by vasoconstriction and vasodilation), and the cardiac muscle pump action are all operating in balance with one another. This balanced situation is referred to as a state of "dynamic equilibrium"; that is, all parts of the body are receiving the amount of blood that they need to sustain circulatory health.

As long as two of the basic components are able to maintain satisfactory compensatory action, adequate circulation of the blood can be maintained even though the third component may not be functioning normally. Thus, if one function fails, other parts of the system will put compensatory mechanisms into effect, e.g., vascular tone may increase (thereby causing vasoconstriction and reduced vascular capacity), cardiac pump action may increase, or blood volume may increase. However, when compensatory mechanisms fail or when more than one of the three components malfunction, circulatory failure results, throwing the individual into a state of shock.

DEFINITIONS AND BASIC PATHOLOGY OF SHOCK

Although shock has been recognized for over 100 years, a clear definition and dissection of this complex and devastating state has emerged only slowly.[142]

Much confusion exists concerning the definition and classification of shock. The word "shock" is commonly used to refer to a *group* of signs and symptoms that could be caused by a *variety* of disorders, such as hemorrhage, infarction, or coronary thrombosis. One general definition of shock is presented here:

> *Shock is an abnormal physiologic state in which there is a disproportion between the circulating blood volume and the size of the vascular bed, resulting in circulatory failure and anoxia.*[18]

In most cases of shock the decreased perfusion of the microcirculation is caused by *a fall in the cardiac output.* A variety of factors may be responsible: (1) the myocardium itself may fail, as in coronary thrombosis; (2) the heart chambers may not fill adequately, as in cardiac tamponade; or (3) there may be a decrease in the amount of blood returned to the heart by way of the great veins. *Decreased venous return to the heart* may be due to: (a) an increase in the volume capacity of the veins themselves (that is, vasodilation), as in septic shock which is secondary to severe infection or (b) an actual deficit of available blood, as in shock due to hemorrhage or wounds.

Various situations obviously can occur within the body that disrupt adequate vascular tone, adequate blood volume, and/or cardiac pump action. The events of these vicious circles are diagrammed in Figure 13–1. Failure of both the respiratory and circulatory systems contributes to progressive circulatory failure. Circulatory failure produces ischemia of the tissues. This may result in death if the ischemia is so severe or prolonged that the cells are unable to continue with the metabolic activities necessary to sustain life.

Table 13–1 summarizes the body's major typical reactions to shock. The remainder of this chapter provides more detailed discussions of the basic pathology of shock.

CLASSIFICATIONS OF SHOCK

Although shock can be classified in several different ways, one concise classification is that proposed by Blalock in 1934 and modified by Bordicks:[18]

1. *Hematogenic shock* (decreased blood volume)
   A. Hemorrhagic shock (loss of whole blood)
   B. Burn shock (loss of plasma fluids and electrolytes)
   C. Diabetic shock, acidosis (loss of fluids and electrolytes from all three body compartments)
2. *Cardiogenic shock* (failure of the heart to pump adequately)
   A. Left myocardial infarction
3. *Neurogenic shock* and *vasogenic shock* (an increased size in the vascular bed)
   A. Neurogenic shock
      (1) Spinal anesthesia shock
      (2) Insulin shock
   B. Vasogenic shock
      (1) Anaphylactic shock
      (2) Toxic shock

Note that this classification is based on three major physiologic mechanisms that support adequate circulation: blood volume, cardiac pump action, and vascular tone.

Hematogenic Shock. In hematogenic shock the primary cause is a marked *decreased volume of blood,* so that the metabolic needs of the body cannot be met. Any condition that can cause a marked reduction in the blood volume can cause hematogenic shock. Some prime examples are:

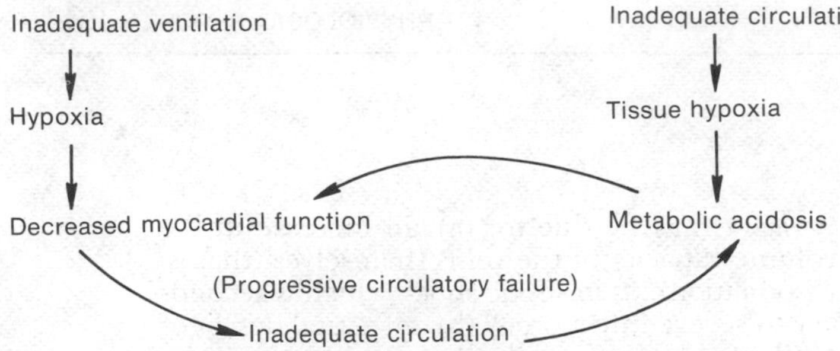

Figure 13–1. Progressive circulatory failure in shock. (From Vandermeer, B. L.: *Journal of the American Association of Anesthetists.* Apr. 1965.)

A. *Hemorrhagic shock,* which is a loss of whole blood. Hemorrhagic shock (also called "hypovolemic shock") develops when a person experiences a reduction in intravascular volume relative to that person's vascular capacity. Hemorrhagic shock can be triggered by a blood volume deficit of 15 to 25 per cent, while loss of 45 per cent or more of a person's blood volume is frequently fatal.[171] Shock will develop fully in a previously healthy person who loses about one-third of normal blood volume. The loss of smaller amounts of blood may result in shock in persons less able to compensate rapidly. Shock following trauma is typically due to hypovolemia.

B. *Burn shock,* also referred to as "electrolyte shock" or "plasma loss shock," is primarily caused by the rapid shift of plasma fluid from the vascular compartment, across heat-damaged capillaries, and into the interstitial compartments and/or the burned area's surface. Also, with burn shock there is a loss of plasma, fluid, and electrolytes from all three body compartments — plasma from the vascular and interstitial compartments (ECF), and potassium from the intracellular compartment.

Regardless of the cause of large losses of plasma, the result is always decreased blood volume and a greatly increased viscosity of the blood, which also adds to the slowness of blood flow.

Burn or electrolyte shock can also be produced in other conditions, e.g., *fistulas* and *diarrhea.* Other disorders in which the loss of plasma may be profuse are severe venous obstruction, nephrotic syndrome, intestinal obstruction, starvation (nutritional hypovolemia), and severe trauma.

C. *Diabetic shock* (acidosis, coma) consists of metabolic acidosis and severe dehydration of all three body compartments — intracellular, interstitial, and vascular. Without insulin replacement, death may result. Once the insulin-glucose-water-electrolyte balance is restored, those metabolic deficiencies that result from insulin insufficiency (dehydration and reduced cellular utilization of glucose for energy) will be corrected.

TABLE 13–1. THE BODY'S REACTION TO SHOCK

1. *Hyperventilation,* caused by the patient's stress, leads to respiratory alkalosis, which is the earliest acid-base change of shock.
2. *Vasoconstriction* occurs in the arteries and veins; the purpose is to shunt the available blood to the heart and brain.
3. *Tachycardia and an increased force of contraction* are the heart's response to shock.
4. *Fluid shifts* occur in an attempt to maintain an effective circulating blood volume.
5. *Cellular changes* contribute to the vascular complications of shock.
6. *Impaired metabolism* occurs when tissue perfusion is inadequate.
7. *Organ function* is impaired in shock.
8. *Disseminated intravascular coagulation* tends to occur with all types of shock, particularly septic shock, if it persists for long periods.

Adapted from Wilson, R. F.: Diagnosis and treatment of shock. *Consultant,* 18:109, Dec. 1978, p. 113.

Cardiogenic Shock. Also called "cardiac shock," this type of shock results from *failure of the cardiac muscle pump.* When the heart muscle can no longer perform adequately (i.e., heart failure), it no longer pumps sufficient blood to all parts of the body. As with all forms of shock, the ultimate result is deficiencies in cellular supplies and waste removal.

Left myocardial failure may cause cardiogenic shock. For example, if a left coronary artery is occluded, an adequate supply of blood cannot reach areas of the left myocardium (*left myocardial infarction*). As a result of tissue hypoxia and lack of nutrients, the left heart muscle becomes increasingly weak and unable to contract forcefully. Blood dams up in the left atrium and left ventricle of the heart and in the pulmonary venous circuit. Pulmonary congestion, pulmonary hypoxia, and marked dyspnea occur.

Other possible causes of cardiogenic shock are rupture of a papillary muscle, rupture of the intraventricular septum, rupture of the free wall of the left ventricle, cardiac tamponade, pulmonary embolus, and cardiac surgery.

Patients in cardiogenic shock generally have a low cardiac output (less than 2.5 l./min./sq. m.). However, this is not always true. For example, 5 to 15 per cent of patients with shock due to a heart attack may have little or no cardiac output reduction.[171]

Neurogenic Shock and Vasogenic Shock. These types of shock result from inadequate vascular tone. Both these forms of shock are caused by an *increase in the size of the vascular bed due to massive vasodilatation.* In both patterns of shock the blood volume remains "normal"; therefore, a disproportion occurs because the normal amount of blood cannot adequately fill the increased size of the capillary area.

Following this extensive vasodilatation there are decreased blood pressure, decreased return of venous blood to the heart, and decreased cardiac output. The end result of these developments is, as in other forms of shock, tissue anoxia and, ultimately, cell destruction.

Although vasodilatation occurs in both neurogenic and vasogenic shock, the mechanisms that cause the vasodilation differ: Neurogenic shock results from a diminished vasomotor tone, hence, a diminished vasoconstrictor tone that produces vasodilatation throughout the body.

Vasogenic shock results from loss of vasomotor activity caused by toxic substances acting directly on the blood vessels, producing vasodilatation.

Neurogenic shock is caused by dilation of the blood vessels secondary to nervous factors. Among the possible causes are brain damage, deep general anesthesia, spinal anesthesia, fainting, and spinal cord injury. Neurogenic shock is characterized by hypotension, warm extremities, and a relatively slow pulse.

Vasogenic shock is caused by dilation of the blood vessels brought about by humoral (vasoactive) substances. Two examples of vasogenic shock are *anaphylactic shock* and *toxic shock* (also known as bacterial shock, septic shock, bacteremic shock, endotoxic shock, or exotoxic shock). Toxic shock can be hyperdynamic (warm, dry skin and normal or increased cardiac output) or hypodynamic (cool, clammy skin, and low cardiac output). The person with a low cardiac output generally has an absolute or relative hypovolemia.[171]

Insulin shock can be classsified as either cardiogenic or neurogenic shock. You will recall that diabetic shock is caused by hyperglycemia, which results from too little insulin (hypoinsulinism) in the body. In insulin shock we find hypoglycemia resulting from too much insulin (hyperinsulinism) in the body. Both the heart and central nervous system are adversely affected by hyperinsulinism. The metabolism of glucose provides essentially all the energy for the central nervous system. Among other problems caused by hyperinsulinism, the vasomotor nerves lose their ability to maintain the tonus of the blood vessels, and vasodilatation with hypotension results.

Summary

We have reviewed some broad basic patterns of shock (hematogenic, cardiogenic, neurogenic, and vasogenic), each of which has a different primary etiology. The pathogenesis of these various types of shock is summarized in Figure 13–2. Of course, some cases of shock are due to combinations of problems and do not fit into a single category. It is becoming increasingly clear that the *initial clinical course and the initial treatment of the various primary events causing shock* (e.g., hemorrhage, infection, coronary thrombosis, immune reaction) *are quite different from one another.** However:

> *Although the circumstances that may initiate shock are many, the underlying common dysfunction is always an inadequacy of tissue perfusion.*

*The specific forms of shock will be discussed in appropriate sections throughout the book in relation to the basic etiology, e.g., burns, myocardial infarction, anaphylaxis, diabetes. The treatment of each type will be included here.

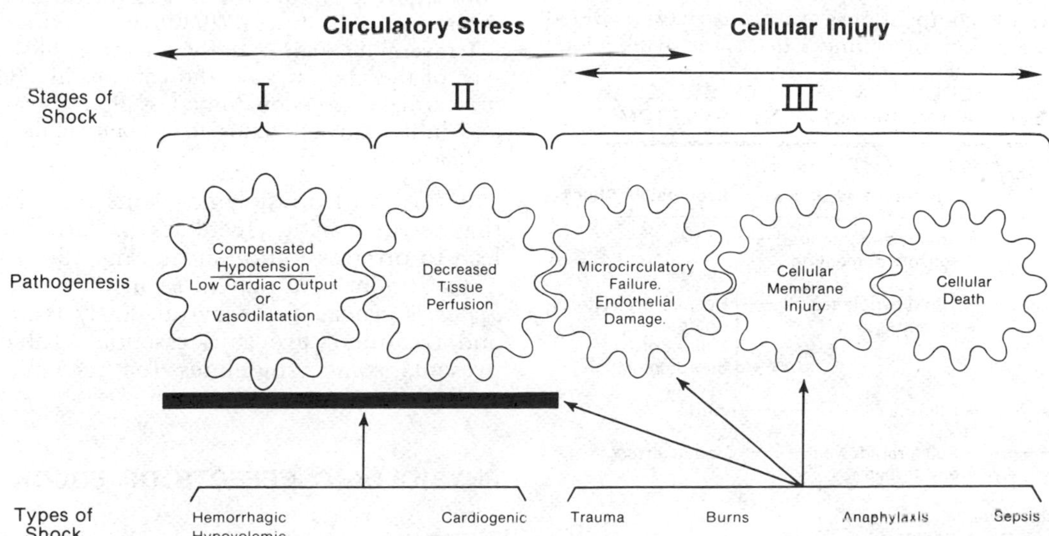

Figure 13–2. Pathophysiology of shock. (From Abboud, F. M.: Shock. In Beeson, P. B., W. McDermott, and J. B. Wyngaarden (Eds.): *Cecil Textbook of Medicine,* 15th ed., Philadelphia: W. B. Saunders Co., 1979.)

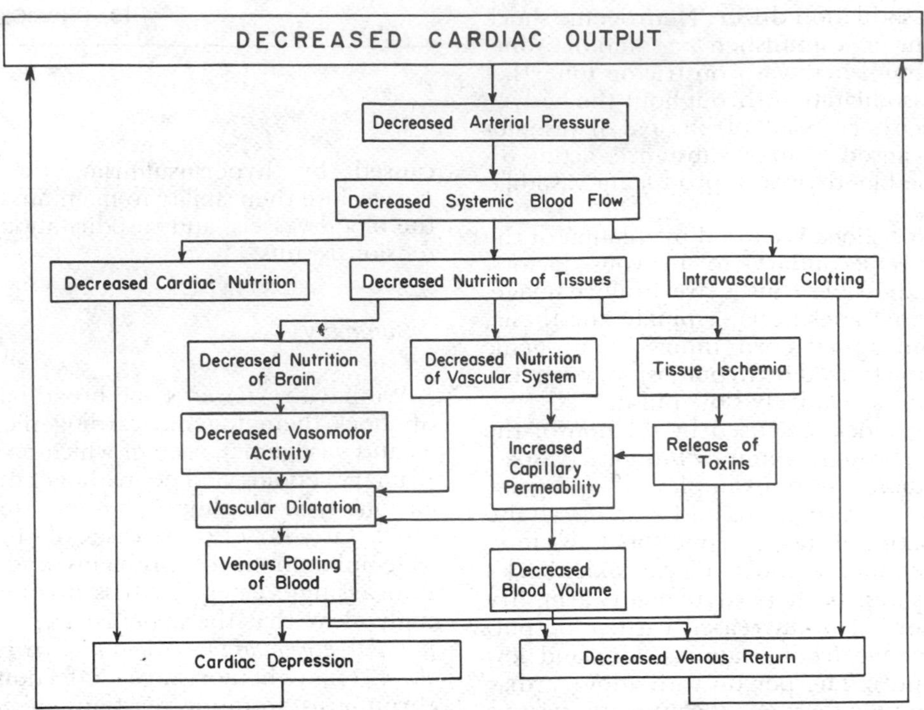

Figure 13–3. Different types of feedback that can lead to progression of shock. (From Guyton, A. C.: *Textbook of Medical Physiology,* 5th ed. Philadelphia: W. B. Saunders Co., 1976.)

STAGES OF SHOCK

Shock is a dynamic condition in which a patient's status is constantly changing; its progression can be divided into stages for easier discussion.

Initial/Compensatory Stage. The cardiac output may be insufficient to supply the normal nutritional needs of the body's tissues, but it is not low enough to cause serious symptoms. Even as cardiac output is reduced further, blood pressure tends to remain within a normal range or may, in fact, be elevated, because of compensatory vasoconstriction. Blood flow to the skin and kidneys decreases, while blood flow to the central nervous system and the myocardium tends to be maintained. A decrease occurs in the blood reservoirs.

Progressive Stage. The unfavorable changes become increasingly apparent: falling blood pressure, increasing vasoconstriction, increased heart rate, oliguria. Because compensatory mechanisms are unable to cope with the reduced cardiac output, the status quo is not maintained. During this stage, shock becomes progressively more severe, even though the initial cause of the shock is not itself becoming more severe. In other words, intrinsic factors in the person, aside from the original cause of the shock, are causing deterioration in physical condition.

Irreversible Stage. In the final stage of shock, no type of therapy can save the patient's life. There is myocardial depression and a loss of arteriolar tonus, and infused blood tends to remain in the dilated capillary bed.

TABLE 13–2. RECOGNITION OF SHOCK STAGES BY CLINICAL EVALUATION OF SIGNS AND SYMPTOMS*

Initial Compensatory Shock	Progressive Shock	Irreversible Shock
Restlessness and apprehension ⟶	Apathy and impaired sensory perception ⟶	Coma
"Warm hypotension" tachypnea ⟶	"Cold hypotension" syncope ⟶	Respiratory distress Acidosis Failure of microcirculation
Good urine volume ⟶	Oliguria ⟶	Anuria
Pulse rapid ⟶	Pulse rapid, weak and thready ⟶	Cardiac arrest

Cardinal Points to Remember
1. Shock is a dynamic condition
2. The patient is either improving or deteriorating

*Modified from Mitty, W. F., Jr., et al.: The role of the emergency room in management of shock. *Hospital Medicine,* 8:7, Jan. 1972, by permission © 1972 by Hospital Publications, Inc.

A variety of physiologic events occur in shock that set up various feedback patterns that can lead to progression of shock (Fig. 13–3).

Treatment of a patient *before progressive shock begins* is crucial for survival. Early recognition and treatment are thus essential. Table 13–2 presents some guidelines for recognition of early shock.

PHYSIOLOGIC EFFECTS OF SHOCK

The reduced blood flow through the tissues during the shock syndrome, by its very nature, impinges on almost every facet of homeostasis.[180]

Some of the physiologic mechanisms believed

to be responsible for the development of irreversible shock leading to death are:

- ▶ Respiratory failure (Adult Respiratory Distress Syndrome)
- ▶ Cardiac failure
- ▶ Failure of the microcirculation and pooling of blood
- ▶ Sludging of the blood, resulting in disseminated intravascular coagulation (DIC)*
- ▶ The release of toxic products and/or bacteria from the liver, muscle, and/or intestine
- ▶ Metabolic derangements; loss of the liver's detoxifying abilities; depression of the reticuloendothelial system
- ▶ Prolonged vasoconstriction, causing visceral damage due to mechanical limitation of blood flow and attendant stagnant anoxia, tissue necrosis and cellular death

Neuroendocrine and Other Types of Defenses During Shock[18]

The neuroendocrine responses during shock are bodily defensive reactions that occur during the stage of resistance of the general adaptation syndrome (GAS), discussed in Chapter 4. Remember that the length of the stage of resistance varies from one individual to another and is determined by the individual body's ability to compensate for its deficiencies. Therefore, one patient may be able to combat shock longer than another. For example, a previously healthy person will have a longer stage of resistance against shock than a previously debilitated person.

Keep in mind that:

> *The main purposes of the body's defenses in shock are to: (1) establish a depot of readily available energy and (2) to maintain a state of circulatory balance so that the vital organs will have the blood needed for life.*

Some basic features of the neuroendocrine responses to shock follow:

- ▶ The body is prepared for "fight or flight" and, economically, *supports vital body functions.*
- ▶ Under the control of the sympathetic nervous system, the adrenal medulla releases two hormones (norepinephrine and epinephrine) that produce effects similar to those caused by direct sympathetic stimulation (e.g., *vasoconstriction* and *increased heart rate*).
- ▶ The anterior pituitary secretes ACTH, which stimulates the adrenal cortex to produce mineralocorticoids (which act generally to *control fluid and electrolyte balance*), and glucocorticoids (which mainly *affect energy and tissue resistance*). The antidiuretic hormone (ADH) is secreted by the posterior pituitary.

Generally the hormonal response to stress results in the rapid provision of fuel for the body's various tissues, organs, and systems. These fuels (e.g., amino acids, fatty acids, glucose, sodium, and water) are produced by breaking food down into sugars, fatty acids, and amino acids that are converted into energy by a chemical process, resulting in the formation of adenosine triphosphate (ATP), the main source of energy produced and used inside the body's cells.

The glucocorticoids, particularly hydrocortisone, *mobilize energy stores.* During the initial period of shock the small stores of available carbohydrate are rapidly depleted and it becomes necessary to mobilize protein and fat stores to meet the body's energy requirements. Protein catabolism and negative nitrogen balance occur as a part of the metabolic response, as a result of gluconeogenesis (resulting from glucocorticoid action) and starvation.

The *sympathetic nervous system* and the hormones of the *adrenal medulla* initially help to maintain the arterial blood pressure. The adrenal medulla secretes epinephrine in copious amounts in response to stress; this substance accelerates the heart rate. This *increased heart rate* works together initially with *increased peripheral vascular resistance* (caused by vasoconstriction resulting from stimulation by the sympathetic nervous system) to maintain the body's blood pressure (Fig. 13–4).

The veins are a reservoir for blood; thus, the initial constriction of the veins in shock remedies the slack in the circulating blood volume by squeezing blood into the circulation from the venous reservoir. The resultant *increase in venous return* to the heart may be as great as two-and-a-half-fold. Consequently, the heart has more blood to pump back out into the circulation since it can pump only the amount of blood that it receives from the venous circuit.

With the development of shock, the blood pressure generally tends to drop, owing to an inadequate circulating volume of blood and decreased cardiac output. As a result of the decline in blood pressure, a reflex *compensatory vasoconstriction* occurs that is initially helpful but dangerous if prolonged. Vasoconstriction does provide some protection for such "high priority" organs as the brain and the heart. Also, the increased heart rate, increased peripheral resistance, and the addition of blood volume from reservoirs all help initially to maintain the blood pressure in shock.

The *vasoconstrictive activity that is triggered by the sympathoadrenal system is harmful if it is sustained,* for it further decreases the microcirculation through most tissues and organs of the body. "While it is of immediate survival value, this

*Sludging of the blood refers to a situation occurring in the smaller blood vessels in which the red cells aggregate into masses, thereby slowing the blood flow.

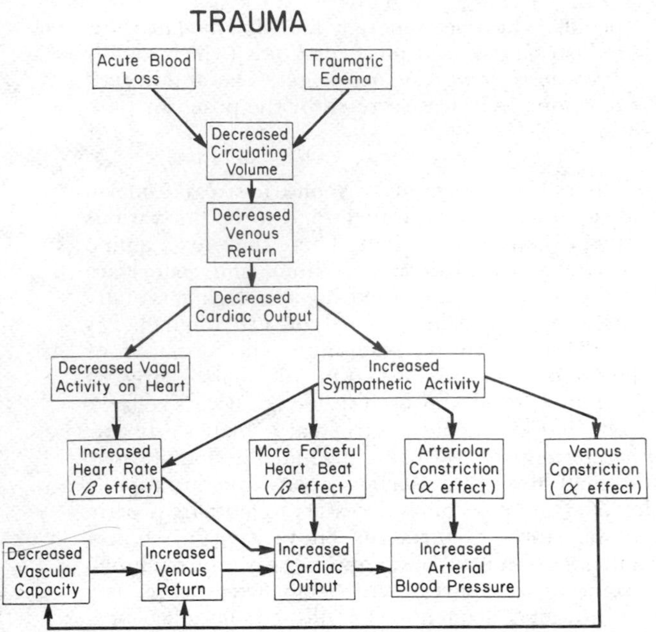

Figure 13–4. In early shock following trauma, acute blood loss and edema into traumatized tissue result in decreased venous return, which is compensated for primarily by increased sympathetic stimulation of the heart and blood vessels. (From Wilson, R. F., L. P. Leblanc, and A. J. Walt: Shock due to trauma. *In* Walt, A. J., and R. F. Wilson: *Management of Trauma: Pitfalls and Practice.* Philadelphia: Lea & Febiger, 1975, p. 58.)

reaction cannot continue for longer than a few minutes because of the resulting metabolic derangement."[142] It can be seen that if the shock state is prolonged, serious problems ensue, and reactions that are initially helpful, such as vasoconstriction, may actually become life-threatening.

Increased production of the adrenocortical and mineralocorticoid hormones occurs. The main mineralocorticoids, aldosterone and desoxycorticosterone (DOCA), help to increase the volume of the circulating fluid in the vascular compartment through their ability to retain sodium and, hence, water. *Increasing the blood's volume* increases venous return, cardiac output, and blood pressure.

The renal tubular conservation of sodium occurs with any type of fluid loss or blood volume depletion. An essential factor in this conservation of sodium is aldosterone. Because water is retained in the body along with sodium, we find that urine excretion from the kidneys is diminished during shock. This fluid is retained in the blood stream in an effort to increase the blood volume. Often the earliest sign of hypovolemia is a decreased urine volume.

Of major importance in the regulation of water and sodium balance are the antidiuretic hormone (ADH), which is produced by the *posterior pituitary gland,* and aldosterone. The osmolality of the blood increases in dehydration states, causing stimulation of the osmoreceptors in the hypothalamus to release the ADH from the posterior pituitary gland. Via the blood, the ADH is carried to the kidneys where it causes the body to retain water. The various components of the sympathoadrenal response are reviewed in Figure 13–5.

OTHER COMPENSATORY MECHANISMS

In addition to the responses of the sympathetic nervous system and the adrenal glands to shock, many other compensatory factors operate initially in shock in an attempt to maintain the blood volume. Some of these mechanisms and their actions in hemorrhagic shock are outlined below.[18]

Bone Marrow. Stimulated by the hypoxic effects produced by a decreased blood volume, the red bone marrow produces and *releases additional red blood cells into the circulation.* An increased oxygen-carrying power is made available with the increased number of red cells. Because the red cell formation takes place at an abnormally rapid speed, immature red cells are passed into the blood stream. Immature red cells have less oxygen-carrying power than mature red cells, however, for the hemoglobin content of red blood cells increases with the cells' maturity.

Immature leukocytes (white blood cells) may also be released as a result of drugs, e.g., epinephrine, crush injuries, infarctions, burns, fear, anxiety and a variety of other conditions.[16]

Liver and Spleen. *Extra red cells* are squeezed into the circulation by the liver and spleen.

Interstitial Compartment. Fluid passes from the interstitial compartment into the vascular compartment. Fluid shifts are discussed in the next section.

Carbon Dioxide. Increased carbon dioxide *dilates the arterioles located in active tissues and constricts those in nonactive tissues.* Because the heart is the most active tissue at this time, excessive CO_2 is produced in the myocardium. This directly dilates the coronary arteries leading to the myocardium and thereby allows this tissue to receive more arterial blood (with its oxygen and nutrients). CO_2 is also a powerful stimulant of the vasoconstrictor center in the sympathetic nervous system. With vasoconstriction of nonactive tissues, the blood is shunted to the more active tissues which have a greater immediate need of it.

Kidneys. A renal pressor substance (RPS) is released by the kidneys into the blood stream as a result of renal arteriolar vasoconstriction, regulated by sympathoadrenal medullary mechanisms. RPS increases the tone of arterioles and thus *aids in arteriolar constriction.* RPS is also known as vasoexcitor mechanism (VEM). The ischemic kidney produces an enzyme, renin, which acts upon a plasma protein to form a pressor substance referred to as *angiotensin.* This substance, in addition to having vasoconstrictor properties, also stimulates aldosterone secretion from the adrenal cortex and release of ADH by the posterior pituitary. The roles of aldosterone and ADH have been previously discussed.

Fluid Shifts During Shock

As we have indicated, *early* in shock, sympathoadrenal medullary mechanisms are responsible for shifting blood from the peripheral vessels of tissues that have less need for it to internal visceral vessels, whose tissues have a more urgent need for the blood. This action is accomplished by the vasoconstrictive action of norepinephrine.[18] Also, fluid is pulled from the interstitial spaces into the vascular space.

Some of the results of the shift of excessive amounts of fluid from the interstitial to the vascular compartments are:[18]

- Fluid is added to the blood volume, thereby increasing the venous return to the heart which, in turn, causes an increased cardiac output.
- Although the fluid from the interstitial compartment expands the volume of blood, it also causes a hemodilution of the blood.
- Also, the interstitial compartment becomes markedly depleted of fluid, producing tissue dehydration.
- Laboratory findings at the time of this hemodilution and tissue dehydration are: decreased red blood cells, decreased hematocrit, decreased plasma proteins, hyperglycemia, acidosis, hypochloremia, elevated blood urea nitrogen, increased polymorphonuclear leukocytes.
- The patient experiences the signs and symptoms of dehydration, e.g., thirst, dry and cracked lips, and dry mucous membranes.

Figure 13–6 demonstrates how during *early* hypovolemic shock, fluid rapidly moves out of the cells and interstitial space into the constricted vascular space. As can be seen, in *late* shock

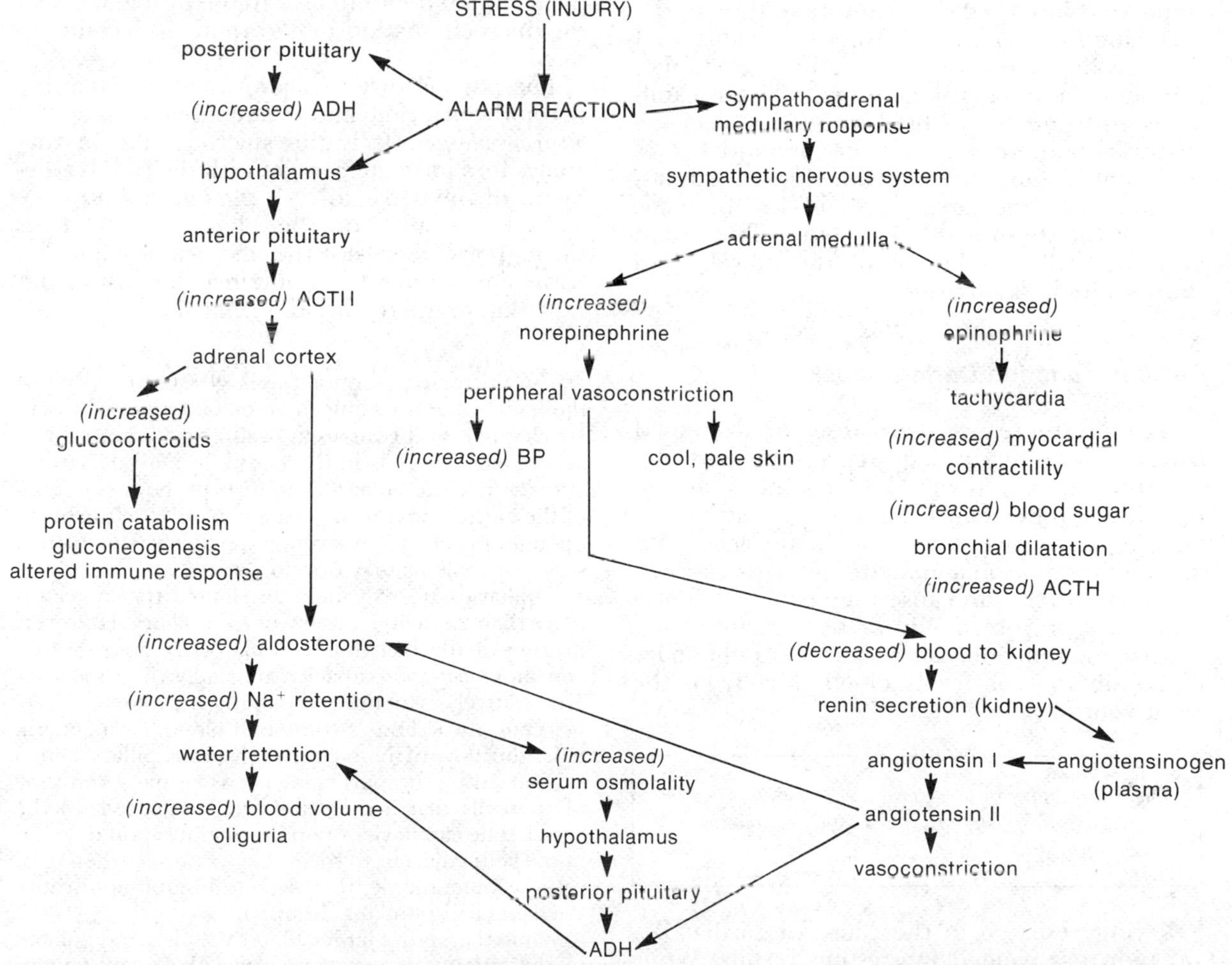

Figure 13–5. The components of the sympathoadrenal response to a major stressor. (Modified from Marcinek, M. B.: Stress in the surgical patient. *American Journal of Nursing,* 77:1809, Nov. 1977.)

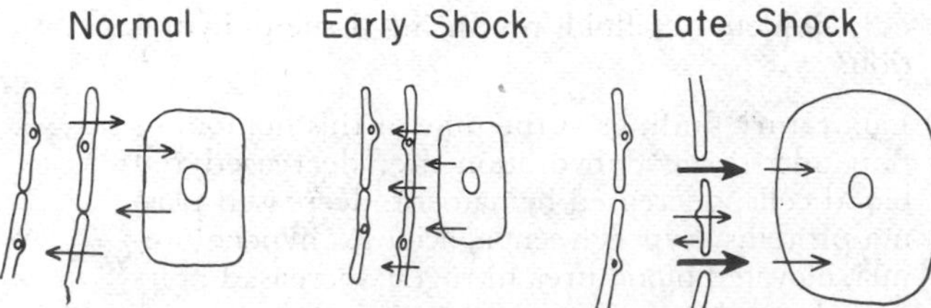

Figure 13–6. Normally there is a fairly equal movement of fluid back and forth between the vascular space and the interstitial and cellular spaces. In early hypovolemic shock, fluid moves rapidly out of the cells and interstitial space into the constricted vascular space. In late shock, increased capillary permeability and impaired cell-membrane function result in a movement of fluid into the interstitial and cellular spaces. (From Wilson, R. F., L. P. Leblanc, and A. J. Walt: Shock due to trauma. *In* Walt, A. J., and R. F. Wilson: *Management of Trauma: Pitfalls and Practice.* Philadelphia: Lea & Febiger, 1975, p. 61.)

fluid moves into the interstitial and cellular spaces as a result of increased capillary permeability and impaired cell membrane function.

During the *later* stages of shock a serious fluid shift problem can occur. If vasoconstriction is prolonged, it increases the pressure in the capillaries and thus forces fluid to be lost from the vascular compartment into the interstitial compartment.[109] One phenomenon consistently associated with the later stages of hemorrhagic shock is the presumed loss of extracellular fluid into the wall and lumen of the bowel. This causes liquid, bloody stools.

Cardiac Function During Shock

Basically there are two causes of decreased cardiac output: cardiac depression and decreased venous return. Any circulatory change that initially decreases the cardiac output can lead to progressive shock, e.g., hemorrhage, anaphylaxis, septicemia, dehydration. Also, a variety of disorders can cause the heart to fail as a pump, e.g., myocardial infarction, arrhythmias, cardiac tamponade, or a massive pulmonary embolism that obstructs blood flow from the right ventricle.

> *The heart appears to deteriorate severely as shock progresses; this deterioration is one of the major causes of death.*

Recent research in the cause of cardiac depression has yielded interesting results. While the exact cause of myocardial depression is unclear, much attention has been directed at myocardial depressant factor (MDF), a polypeptide felt to have vasoactive properties. Some researchers have identified plasma MDF in patients with shock.[6, 35] Other researchers have isolated lesions in the myocardium of animals and humans following hypovolemic shock. The role of these "myocardial zonal lesions" in the loss of ventricular contraction and resultant cardiac failure remains to be determined.[123]

Once the heart has deteriorated beyond a certain level, irreversible shock occurs and the patient's life cannot be saved. Cardiac deterioration may not be detected until almost terminal conditions have developed, because cardiac depression is frequently masked by the tremendous cardiac reserve of the normal individual. Because of this reserve, the heart can deteriorate to less than one third, or sometimes less than one fifth, of its normal pumping strength without any measurable evidence of cardiac failure.

The Microcirculation During Shock

Shock does not develop because the circulation is impaired in one specific organ; rather, the common denominator in the problem is that the microcirculation in *all* organs is decompensated.

The portion of the cardiovascular system between the arteriole and the venule is termed the *microcirculation.* It is this microcirculation that comes into intimate contact with the cellular elements of the body, for it is the end point of the transport system of the blood vessels. It is through the vessels of the microcirculation that tissue environment is mantained, since it brings nutrition to the tissues and removes waste products.

The microcirculation is the largest organic unit of the body, encompassing some 60,000 miles of vascular channels and containing well over 90 per cent of all the blood vessels in the body. Because of its very size, the microcirculation can disrupt the functioning of the entire body; if these small vessels are unable to operate properly, in even a relatively small area, serious problems may develop.

Capillaries are so widely distributed that no cell is more than 25 to 50 μ away from a capillary. However, in spite of the fact that the microcirculation has an enormous *potential* capacity, normally the capillaries are relatively ischemic, containing only some 6 to 7 per cent of the body's volume of blood. As a general rule, the flow of blood through the capillary bed is influenced by the particular needs at any given time of the cells that are located by (juxtaposed to) the vessel. The capillaries open in rotation upon demand of the cells adjacent to them. For example, when mast cells become anoxic, they secrete histamine to cause the capillary sphincters to open.

While the body's larger blood vessels are regulated by the autonomic nervous system, this is not true of the microcirculation. Arteriole and capillary sphincters are separate mechanisms that are governed by different controls. The muscle located in the microcirculation is highly sensitive and is capable of producing behavior that is precise and well coordinated and that governs the various pathways of blood flow through the capillary bed.

Microcirculatory insufficiency is the final sequence of events that results from all the basic etiologic mechanisms that precipitate shock. Peripheral vascular failure, or microcirculatory failure is, therefore, a phenomenon common to all the etiologic factors in various forms of shock. Microcirculatory failure consists physiologically of two sets of factors: microvessel dysfunction, and dysfunction of the tissues that lie closest to these vessels. These two components are functionally inseparable and act in an interdependent manner.

Regardless of the initiating circumstances, or the level of impact, an identical sequence of events occurs within the microcirculation. These events are shown diagrammatically in Figure 13–7.

One of the most striking characteristics of the microcirculation is its autonomy as a functional entity. The microcirculation's patterns of behavior, in both normal and abnormal environmental situations, are notably independent of those vasomotor influences that affect the major divisions of the circulatory system lying next to it (i.e., the systemic circulation). It is noteworthy that the systemic circulatory bed and the microcirculatory bed do not appear to have developed sensing devices; thus, events taking place within one bed do not effectively modulate or influence the events in the other. As we see next: *the relative autonomy of the microcirculation and the lack of modulation between the systemic circulation and the microcirculation are critical factors in determining the ultimate course of events in shock.*[65]

With the *onset* of shock, during the compensatory phase, the systemic circulation and the microcirculation work together. Both undergo an overall readjustment in which their activities are *coordinated* and are operating to preserve the entire system. The heart and the large vessels accomplish their part in this coordinated effort by *cardioacceleration* (increased heart rate) and *vasoconstriction;* the microcirculation alters its patterns of vasomotion and passes the blood through as rapidly as possible so that it can be returned more efficiently to the venous reservoir.

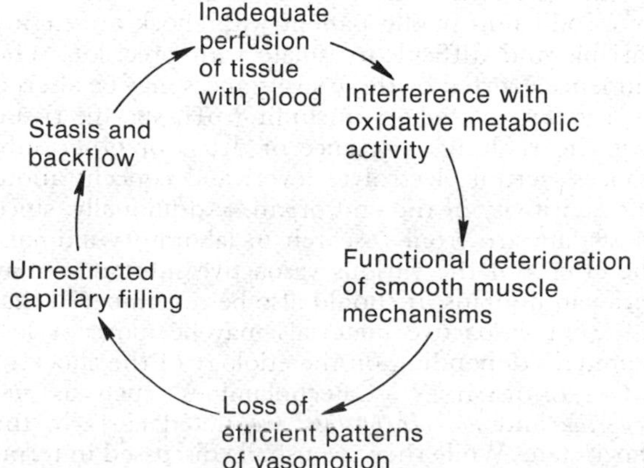

Figure 13–7. Microcirculatory hemodynamic events in shock.

As the state of shock *progresses,* however, the compensatory phase cannot be maintained, and the blood flow becomes inadequate to meet the tissues' minimal needs. The systemic circulation and the microcirculation begin to function in *opposite directions,* opposing one another in an *uncoordinated* manner. The systemic circulation sustains its initial compensatory readjustment (vasoconstriction) while the microbed does not. Thus, the response of the circulation as a whole is no longer coordinated. Specifically, the microcirculation dilates and reverses its adjustment from that of an effort to curtail blood flow toward actually trying to secure more of the limited supply of available blood for itself. The blood supply is thereby progressively sequestered in the capillary beds, i.e., the blood is said to "pool" in the microcirculation. Because the cells demand greater perfusion time, many or most of the capillaries remain open at any one time, thus increasing the vascular space.

"An increase in the vascular capacity, a decrease in the blood volume, or decreased heart action will reduce the mean circulatory pressure.* In turn, the pressure gradient for the venous return of blood is decreased, which results in a venous 'pooling' of blood, a decreased venous return to the heart, and decreased cardiac output.[18]

In the absence of modulating feedback mechanisms, the process described becomes progressively more severe, resulting in total circulatory disruption. Once the vascular space is enlarged, as a result of vasodilatation of the microcirculation, even a normal blood volume is insufficient to fill all these small vessels and also leave enough remaining volume to fill the veins. A low central venous pressure and inadequate venous return to the right side of the heart result, with a further decrease in cardiac output.

Blood Factors During Shock

Relationships have been established between the degree of hemorrhagic shock and derangements in various blood factors. (See Table 13–3) For example, the degree of shock is more than slight when a third of the blood volume is lost; a severe degree of shock exists when one half of the blood volume has been lost. The loss of hemoglobin also parallels the degree of shock; however, the percentage of hemoglobin loss is typically greater than the volume loss.

Some of the more important alterations in blood composition during shock include:

$$\text{*Mean blood pressure} = \frac{\text{systolic} + \text{diastolic}}{2}$$

TABLE 13–3. DATA INDICATING RELATIONSHIP BETWEEN DEGREES OF SHOCK AND DERANGEMENT IN BLOOD FACTORS

Degree of Shock	Blood Loss Volume (% of normal)	Hemoglobin (% of normal)	Hematocrit (% cells)	Plasma Protein (Gm. %)
None	14.4 + 3.9	20.0 + 5.2	42.5 + 1.7	6.6 + 0.1
Slight	20.7 + 4.3	29.7 + 4.1	38.4 + 1.5	6.4 + 0.1
Moderate	34.3 + 3.5	46.1 + 3.4	34.6 + 1.0	6.2 + 0.1
Severe	45.9 + 4.7	54.4 + 4.3	31.5 + 1.5	6.0 + 0.1

Data summarized from Beecher, H. K.: *Resuscitation and Anesthesia for Wounded Men.* Springfield, Illinois. Charles C Thomas, 1949, by Gladish, J. T., Winnie, A. P., and Collins, V. J.: *Postgraduate Medicine,* July, 1967, p. 44.

- Changes in hemostatic mechanisms (blood *coagulation*)
- Effects of the various *vasoactive substances*
- Changes in levels of *certain hormones*
- Changes in *immunologic mechanisms*

Coagulation. During shock, hypoxia of tissues results from the slow movement of blood in the capillaries, and anaerobic metabolism (see later) begins, causing an increase in the production of lactic acid. The slow-moving, acid blood is *hypercoagulable.* The blood, however, will not actually coagulate unless some clot-initiating factor is present. Such factors include bacterial toxins and thromboplastin of red blood cells liberated by hemolysis. Hemolysis accompanies trauma, especially trauma that causes massive crushing. When any of these factors is present, along with the stagnant acid blood of shock, widespread clotting occurs in the vessels. This disorder is called *disseminated intravascular clotting* (DIC). In DIC, circulating prothrombin is converted to thrombin, which further results in the activation of fibrinogen into fibrin. The presence of fibrin stimulates intravascular clotting. During the clotting process, there is consumption of platelets and plasma clotting factors, e.g., prothrombin, fibrinogen, proaccelerin,[179] and the antihemophilic factor.

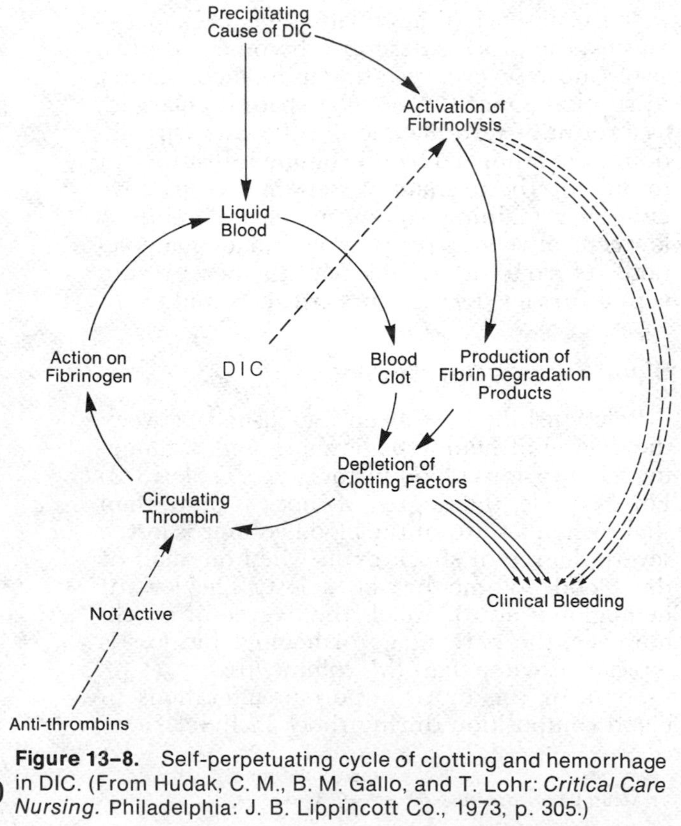

Figure 13–8. Self-perpetuating cycle of clotting and hemorrhage in DIC. (From Hudak, C. M., B. M. Gallo, and T. Lohr: *Critical Care Nursing.* Philadelphia: J. B. Lippincott Co., 1973, p. 305.)

Since the clotting factors have been consumed (consumption coagulopathy), the patient then experiences a *hypocoagulable* state. This results from the action of fibrinolysins on fibrin, splitting the fibrin into products that are anticoagulants. Although the patient may demonstrate signs of organ failure due to obstruction and ischemia, there is also oozing of serous or serosanguineous fluid wherever there is a break in the skin (e.g., from wounds, around IV catheters), and large amounts of fluid may be lost in this manner. Multiple petechiae (pinpoint hemorrhagic lesions) or purpura (confluent petechiae forming large hemorrhagic lesions) may also be noted.

In summary then, the patient with DIC may have multiple thrombi or emboli that obstruct organs and increase tissue ischemia. Clotting factors are depleted, and there is widespread hemolysis, causing anemia. Although fibrinolysins aid in the lysing of clots, tissue necrosis and organ failure result if the clots have been in place for a sustained period. Treatment of the precipitating cause and anticoagulant therapy (heparin) may be ineffective in reversing the process at this late stage, and death may ensue. The steps in the process of DIC are illustrated in Figure 13–8, and the laboratory findings associated with "classic" DIC are listed in Table 13–4.

Vasoactive Substances. The effects of the various vasoactive substances in promoting vasoconstriction or vasodilation in the patient with shock are highly variable and difficult to isolate with precision. The influence exerted by these susbstances may be altered by a variety of factors, including pH, specific tissue (e.g., heart, lung), presence of drugs or other substances, serum electrolyte levels and concentration, and sensitivity of the end organ.[6] Additionally, since most data are from research in laboratory animals, the effects of the various vasoactive substances may differ in humans. It should also be remembered that different vasoactive materials may be more or less dominant depending on the etiology of the shock.

CATECHOLAMINES. Catecholamines, such as *epinephrine* and *norepinephrine,* are noted early in the shock state. While they are usually discussed in terms of their specific effect on the alpha and beta receptors in various tissues, the general effects are to (1) increase the blood flow to the brain, heart, and striated (skeletal) muscle and (2) decrease the blood flow to the skin, splanchnic bed (which perfuses the gastrointestinal tract), and the kidney. Although the initial effect of vasoconstriction serves to increase the intravascular volume, sustained vasoconstriction contributes to stagnant hypoxia and cellular death.

HISTAMINE. Histamine is a vasodilator and increases capillary permeability. Although the precise role of histamine in shock is unclear, it is felt that the decreased arteriolar resistance and increased capillary permeability associated with late stages of shock may be due to histamine.[6] The effects of histamine are especially obvious in anaphylactic and septic shock.

VASOACTIVE POLYPEPTIDES. *Bradykinin, myocardial depressant factor,* and *angiotensin* are among the more important vasoactive polypeptides thought to play a significant role in the pathogenesis of shock. *Bradykinin* is a kinin peptide known to produce vasodilation, increased capillary permeability, relaxation of smooth muscle, pain, and infiltration of an area with leukocytes. It is believed that kinins are most active in late shock and may be a factor in the development of pulmonary insufficiency associated with shock.[6, 35]

Angiotensin, mentioned previously, results from the action of renal renin on angiotensinogen and is a very potent substance which causes vasoconstriction and increased vascular resistance.[179] Although similar to norepinephrine in effect, the action of angiotensin is considered by some to be more physiologic and its use as a therapeutic agent in the management of shock is being evaluated.[6] The role of angiotensin in sodium and water retention through the stimulation of aldosterone secretion is discussed under the sympathoadrenal response.

The *myocardial depressant factor* (MDF) is believed to be a vasoactive polypeptide that contributes to cardiac failure in patients in shock through its depressive effect on cardiac muscle contraction. Although some researchers have reported finding elevated levels of MDF in patients with shock, the actual presence of this substance is controversial.[6, 35]

PROSTAGLANDINS. Prostaglandins are substances believed to be released into the blood during ischemic, anoxic, and shock states. Possible effects of prostaglandins include hypotension, pulmonary vasoconstriction, and portal hypertension. Prostaglandins are similar in structure to hormones, and because they exert a variety of influences in different tissues, their precise role in shock states is not clear. Research efforts are currently being directed at investigating substances that inhibit prostaglandin synthesis. Two agents being studied are indomethacin (Indocin) and aspirin; however, they are not being used clinically in the management of patients with shock at this time.[6, 61, 67]

Although some of the substances discussed above may, in the long run, be more of academic interest than physiologic significance, it behooves the nurse caring for the critically ill or injured to be aware of current research in vasoactive substances that may play a role in the pathophysiology of shock.

Hormones. During shock the endocrine glands secrete increased quantities of hormones, notably catecholamines, vasopressin, and adrenocortical hormones. Increased blood catecholamine levels are found in several types of shock, e.g., hemorrhagic, toxic, traumatic, and anaphylactic forms. (See previous discussion.)

Immunologic Factors. All forms of shock produce a severe depression of the reticuloendothelial system (RES) and of antibacterial defense mechanisms. Alterations occur in the immunologic factors circulating in the blood stream.

The disturbances in the blood proper are partially due to tissue hypoxia as well as to an impairment of the monitoring activities of the RES. Indeed, the stasis, sludging, tendency to venular thrombosis, impaired capillary permeability, and subnormal vascular reactivity that occur during shock can all be traced back to dysfunction of the RES. The capacity of the RES to remove bacteria and the constantly formed endotoxins from the blood stream is greatly reduced during shock.

The impaired ability of the RES to ward off toxic agents is critical, since the reduced blood flow through the intestines during shock impairs the vitality of intestinal tissue so extensively that bacterial products from the intestine gain access to the blood stream. To further compound the problem, the individual in a state of shock is more susceptible than normal to bacterial products, particularly bacterial endotoxins, since interference with the RES leads to a reduced capacity to withstand stress.

TABLE 13-4. LABORATORY FINDINGS IN CLASSIC DIC

Test	Direction of Abnormal Values	Rationale
Prothrombin time	Prolonged	Factor V and prothrombin are measured.
Partial thromboplastin time (PTT)	Prolonged	Factors V and VIII are measured and to a lesser degree–fibrinogen.
Platelet count	Low	Thrombocytopenia present.
Fibrinogen level	Low	Patient with DIC has reduced fibrinogen.
Euglobulin lysis time (ELT)	Shortened	ELT measures fibrinolytic activity.
Antithrombin III level	Low	Antithrombin III is absent in patient with DIC.
Thrombin time	Prlonged	Fibrinogen is indirectly measured by thrombin time.
Fibrin degradation products	Elevated	These products are increased in DIC.

From C. M. Hudak, B. M. Gallo, and T. Lohr: *Critical Care Nursing.* Philadelphia: J. B. Lippincott Co., 1973, p. 306.

Inadequate Tissue Perfusion During Shock

> *In* any *type of shock, regardless of etiology, the fundamental problem is* inadequate tissue perfusion *owing to a marked reduction of blood flow through the tissues.*

Any tissue that is deprived of an adequate blood supply will suffer progressive damage and will ultimately be destroyed. Some tissues may be so damaged that their ultimate recovery is not possible, and consequently, death results if the tissue involved performs a vital function. Since various tissues have differing oxygen requirements, some organs will be irreversibly damaged before other tissues have reached this stage of destruction.

In shock, inadequate tissue perfusion does not occur uniformly in all tissues. This failure, for example, does not appear to develop to any recognizable extent in musculoskeletal areas; on the other hand, the liver and small intestine suffer marked damage. Microcirculatory failure appears to have a predilection for the abdominal visceral tissues; however, even there the changes are not uniform. For example, the *spleen* and *adrenals* demonstrate considerable changes, which are typical of vascular insufficiency; however they *do not* develop serious cellular metabolic derangements during the lethal stages of the syndrome.[65]

LIVER AND INTESTINE FUNCTION DURING SHOCK

Shock states are believed to cause important changes in the functions of the liver and the intestines. Because some aspects of these changes are interrelated, the liver and intestines are discussed together.

During shock both the liver and the intestines suffer from impaired circulation and both are believed to be possible sources of toxic materials.

The splanchnic area blood vessels are those most strongly constricted by reflex sympathetic nervous system activity and by vasopressor agents. Thus, splanchnic circulation is highly susceptible to the deleterious effects of prolonged vasoconstriction during the development of shock.

The liver has an important role in the metabolism of carbohydrate, protein, and fat. It is also a major detoxifying organ. Under normal circumstances the liver is believed to protectively trap and dispose of toxic materials (released from the bowel contents) that are the products of the action of bacterial enzymes. During shock the anoxic liver develops metabolic deficiencies and probably an impaired ability to detoxify.

With shock, enhanced bacterial invasion of the liver from the intestine appears to occur. In addition, the anoxic liver may itself release vasotoxic substances. The depressed protective action of the reticuloendothelial system (previously discussed) also allows the release of bacterial endotoxins *(Escherichia coli, Brucella melitensis),* which appear to destroy the integrity of the microcirculation.

The liver plays a key role in the splanchnic circulation. With shock, pooling of blood occurs in the splanchnic area. Pooling of blood in the liver and portal bed may be caused by the plugging of large numbers of small hepatic vessels, sinusoids, and intrahepatic radicles of the portal vein and hepatic artery with masses of agglutinated blood. The persistence of an extreme state of resistance to portal blood flow may lead to stagnation of the blood in the portal system. This presumably results in blood backing up into the vessels of the intestines, adding to mucosal congestion and pooling of blood that is present in the intestinal capillaries.

Intestinal changes seem to play a significant role in irreversible hemorrhagic and bacteremic shock. It should be emphasized that ischemic changes within the intestine are not believed to be responsible for the death of all patients suffering from prolonged hemorrhagic or bacteremic shock; gastrointestinal changes are now believed to have a more vital role in the progression of shock than was previously thought. In the human the submucosa of the bowel is the layer that becomes ischemic early in shock states. As the period of congestion and subsequent stagnant anoxia becomes prolonged, actual tissue necrosis and loss of integrity of the mucosa of the bowel occurs. Bacteria and their toxins are believed to contribute to irreversible shock by escaping into the systemic circulation as a result of destruction of the intestinal mucosal barrier.

The arterioles and venules of the intestine are evidently highly susceptible to the extensive vasoconstriction that occurs during shock. The massive amounts of tissue destruction that result from vasoconstriction and tissue anoxia are sufficient to produce death even in the absence of bacteria. Drugs that decrease peripheral vascular tone (e.g., vasodilators) are productive of more normal blood flows to organs and thereby preserve visceral integrity and improve survival rates. Of course, the circulating blood volume that has already been lost must be restored prior to the administration of such drugs. (This point will be discussed further in the section on treatment.)

KIDNEY FUNCTION DURING SHOCK

The rate of urine production reflects visceral blood flow and body fluid balance. Thus, urinary output indicates the status of the circulation through the vital organs; a good urine output indicates adequate circulation, even if the arterial blood pressure is lower than normal.[18] During shock the urine output is measured and compared with normal urine production. One ml. (or cc.) of urine per minute, or 60 ml. per hour, is the normal excretion of urine from the kidney. The patient who becomes acutely hypovolemic cannot maintain an hourly output of 40 to 60 ml. of urine. A decreased urine output (*oliguria*) typically occurs in shock. In many instances during shock the urine output may stop completely (*anuria*); when this occurs, the patient is said to be in "renal shutdown."

Glomerular filtration within the kidney depends upon the pressure at which the blood is circulated through the glomerular capillaries. As a general rule, the average capillary pressure of blood is much higher in the glomeruli than it is in the other capillaries. Interestingly enough, under usual circumstances the kidney is able to maintain this heightened capillary pressure in the glomeruli in spite of changes in the systemic blood pressure. It is not clear exactly how this is accomplished; however, it is known that the afferent arterioles supplying the glomeruli dilate as the blood pressure falls, and constrict as it rises. However, there are limits beyond which this adaptive mechanism can no longer protect the kidney against the hazards of a falling systemic blood pressure. Thus, shock produces oliguria and anuria.

We should remember that the reduction of urinary volume in itself is not of significance; the importance lies in the fact that the oligemia is due to inadequacy of the *general circulation* which, in turn, causes poor renal perfusion. Thus, oligemia reflects inadequate circulation to the kidneys and to the body as a whole. Obviously a patient in such a state is threatened with the progressive deterioration of the general circulatory function unless adequate treatment is provided immediately.

During shock, when there is a steady decline of blood volume and blood pressure, the glomerular filtrate is progressively reduced. Because it cannot be excreted by the kidneys, sodium, along with the water, leaves the body through the sweat glands. (In uremia, the frost that forms on the skin is actually sodium chloride.)[18] The damaged kidney loses its crucial ability to regulate electrolyte and acid-base balance.

Inadequate perfusion of the renal capillaries with blood is believed to be the cause of *early* renal failure in shock. The afferent and efferent arterioles constrict, and blood is shunted away from the glomeruli. *Later,* if shock persists, actual renal shutdown is caused by focal tubular necrosis. It should also be remembered that patients with large amounts of tissue damage, e.g., crush injuries, may have myoglobinuria and since the myoglobin molecule is quite large, there may be a type of mechanical renal failure.

We have indicated previously that the kidney may suffer from renal ischemia during shock because the microcirculatory failure has a predilection for the abdominal visceral tissues. Because the kidney has a high rate of metabolism, it is highly susceptible to injury of the tubule cells when the blood supply is deficient. Vasoconstriction in the kidney may unfortunately continue for a long time after the blood pressure has been restored to normal levels. When injury to the kidney is extensive and renal failure ensues, tubular necrosis occurs. The kidney can repair this condition, so that normal function will return in 10 to 14 days if the patient can be given appropriate therapy during this time and is not overloaded with fluids.

Oliguria does not contraindicate the administration of large volumes of fluid in treating shock. In fact, the restoration of renal capillary perfusion along with that of other vital capillaries restores urine volume production as long as tubular necrosis is not already present. Indeed, fluid administration may prevent renal tubular necrosis.

LUNG FUNCTION DURING SHOCK

> *Despite many advances in the prevention, early recognition, and management of shock, respiratory failure continues to be a major cause of death associated with shock states.*

The magnitude of the problem surfaced during the Viet Nam conflict when patients sustaining massive injuries and profound blood loss were successfully resuscitated only to die several days later from "shock lung." As a result, both military and civilian "shock units" were developed to study the pathophysiology and management of the pulmonary insufficiency of shock. Although the research efforts have yielded a great deal of information that has resulted in decreased mortality, many questions remain unanswered.

Adult Respiratory Distress Syndrome. Respiratory insufficiency is associated with a variety of disorders besides shock (Table 13–5) and has been given many names (Table 13–6). For purposes of clarity and consistency,[116] the term *Adult Respiratory Distress Syndrome* (ARDS) is used throughout the chapter to cover all of the terms in Table 13–6. In all cases, ARDS refers to respiratory insufficiency characterized by:

- Hypoxia that does not respond to increasing inspired oxygen concentrations, with the hypoxia

TABLE 13–5. CONDITIONS ASSOCIATED WITH ADULT RESPIRATORY DISTRESS SYNDROME

Amniotic fluid embolism	Heat stroke
Arterial emboli	High altitude pulmonary edema
Bowel infarction	Hypothermia injury
Burns	Major surgery
Carcinomatosis	Malaria
Cardiopulmonary bypass	Multiple transfusion
Clostridial sepsis	Peripheral vascular disease
Dead fetus	Ruptured aneurysm
Drug abuse	Shock
Eclampsia	Transfusion reaction
Fractures	Transplantation
Gram-negative sepsis	Trauma

Modified from F. W. Blaisdell, and F. R. Lewis: *Respiratory Distress Syndrome of Shock and Trauma: Post-traumatic Respiratory Failure.* Philadelphia: W. B. Saunders Co., 1977.

resulting from increased pulmonary arteriovenous shunting (perfusion of nonventilated segments)

- Decreased pulmonary compliance, or "stiff lung," requiring increasing pressures to maintain adequate ventilation
- Chest X-ray findings compatible with interstitial edema

Moore et al.[103] have divided the progression of ARDS following trauma into four phases: (1) injury, resuscitation, and alkalosis, (2) circulatory stabilization and beginning respiratory difficulty, (3) progressive pulmonary insufficiency, and (4) terminal hypoxia and hypercarbia with asystole.

Phase I. Injury, Resuscitation and Alkalosis

During this phase, which follows injury, blood loss, etc., the patient is adequately resuscitated and stabilized through the use of IV crystalloids, colloids, surgery, and other means, and has both respiratory and metabolic alkalosis. The respiratory alkalosis results from hyperventilation, whereas the metabolic alkalosis is due to infused citrate from whole blood, or due to bicarbonate or bicarbonate precursors, e.g., Ringer's lactate. The chest film is normal, and the patient may recover without any further problems.

Phase II. Circulatory Stabilization and Beginning Respiratory Difficulty

Characteristics of this phase include stable vital signs, adequate tissue perfusion, elevated cardiac output, and hyperventilation with hypercarbia. The pO_2 may be decreased on room air but responds only partially to 100 per cent oxygen. As noted previously, this is characteristic of increased physiologic shunting of blood through the lungs.[140] The patient does not appear acutely ill at this time.

Phase III. Progressive Pulmonary Insufficiency

Clinical signs of respiratory failure become evident during this phase. The patient has dyspnea, tachypnea, hypocarbia, and hypoxemia. The tidal volume may be large; however, the compliance of the lungs decreases. Increasing oxygen concentrations become less effective in decreasing the hypoxemia. The chest film is often characterized by increasing infiltrates and by diffuse consolidation. Figure 13–9 is a typical chest film seen in this stage. Rales and rhonchi may now be auscultated. Pulmonary infections often develop. As the patient becomes more fatigued, the respiratory drive decreases and the pCO_2 begins to rise. Endotracheal intubation and mechanical ventilation, if not initiated previously, are mandatory at this time.

Phase IV. Terminal Hypoxia and Hypercarbia with Asystole

Inability to obtain and maintain an adequate arterial pO_2, hypoxemia, and metabolic acidosis are characteristics of the final phase of ARDS. Inadequate organ perfusion is manifest by oliguria, coma, convulsions, bradycardia, and, ultimately, asystole.

Although extensive research has been conducted in attempts to precisely identify the cause(s) of ARDS, a great deal of controversy continues. Since a detailed discussion of the various factors under consideration in the pathogenesis of ARDS is beyond the scope of this

TABLE 13–6. SYNONYMS FOR ADULT RESPIRATORY DISTRESS SYNDROME

Adult hyaline membrane disease
Adult respiratory insufficiency syndrome
Bronchopulmonary dysplasia
Congestive atelectasis
Da Nang lung
Fat embolism
Hemorrhagic atelectasis
Hemorrhagic lung syndrome
Hypoxic hyperventilation
Oxygen toxicity
Post-perfusion lung
Post-transfusion lung
Post-traumatic atelectasis
Post-traumatic pulmonary insufficiency
Progressive pulmonary consolidation
Progressive respiratory distress
Pulmonary edema
Pulmonary hyaline membrane disease
Pulmonary microembolism
Pump lung
Respirator lung
Respiratory insufficiency syndrome
Shock lung
Stiff lung syndrome
Traumatic wet lung
Transplant lung
Wet lung
White lung syndrome

Modified from F. W. Blaisdell, and F. R. Lewis: *Respiratory Distress Syndrome of Shock and Trauma: Post-traumatic Respiratory Failure.* Philadelphia: W. B. Saunders Co., 1977, p. 29.

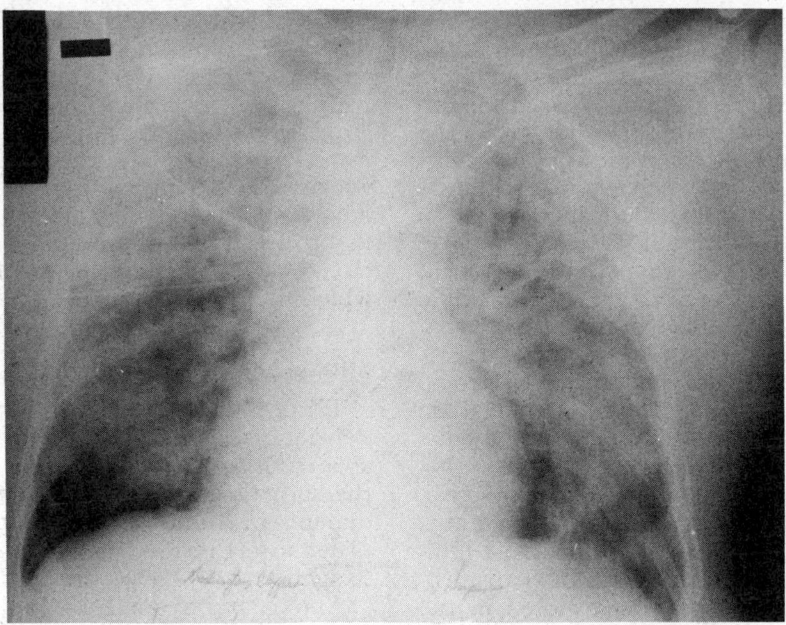

Figure 13–9. A characteristic chest x-ray in a patient with ARDS following trauma. X-ray abnormalities may not develop until 48 to 72 hours after the shock episode. (From Blaisdell, F. W., and F. R. Lewis: *Respiratory Distress Syndrome of Shock and Trauma: Post-traumatic Respiratory Failure*. Philadelphia: W. B. Saunders Co., 1977, p. 33.)

chapter, the reader is referred to the bibliography for more information. Despite the controversy, the most commonly studied etiologies are:

IV fluid overload—both colloid and crystalloid
Oxygen toxicity
Central nervous system injury
Microembolism resulting from: soft tissue trauma, multiple transfusions, and intravascular clotting.
Sepsis*
Aspiration
Ischemic pulmonary injury
Humoral factors (see Table 13–7)
Respirators

Tissue changes in the lung are variable depending upon the progression of the disorder. The lungs may appear heavy, firm, hemorrhagic, or grey. Arteriolar and interstitial hemorrhage may be noted. Surfactant production is decreased. Since surfactant plays a major role in the functioning of the alveoli, inadequate amounts of surfactant contribute to the collapse of the alveoli and, therefore, to the arteriovenous shunting associated with ARDS. Arteriolar and capillary thrombosis becomes evident within 48 hours after the onset of shock. Gradually there is consolidation of the segments and lobes, and hyaline membranes are noted. Bronchopneumonia is commonly seen after the first week. If the patient survives, collagen deposits and fibrous tissue develop. There is degeneration of the alveoli, and pneumatoceles may be identified after several weeks or months.†

In addition to direct structural and functional changes during shock, pulmonary function may also be impaired as a result of pulmonary edema developing secondary to heart failure.

Fat Embolism Syndrome. Fat embolism syndrome is another complication of shock that affects the lung as well as other systems. Fat emboli have been reported frequently in patients with long bone fractures and in patients with massive soft tissue damage and shock. Fat embolism syndrome, however, is a relatively rare, but often fatal, disorder.

*"The greatest incidence of pulmonary dysfunction or 'shock lung' is noted in the patients with sepsis *irrespective of the presence or absence of shock*."[140]

†Further information can be found in references 6, 14, 15, 27, 63, 91, 103, 116, 124, 140, and 170.

TABLE 13–7. HUMORAL FACTORS IN ADULT RESPIRATORY DISTRESS SYNDROME

Complement
Endotoxin
Fatty acids
Fibrino peptides
Histamine
Kinins
Lysosomes
Microemboli
Myocardial depressant factor
Prostaglandins
Proteolytic enzymes
Serotonin

From F. W. Blaisdell, and F. R. Lewis: *Respiratory Distress Syndrome of Shock and Trauma: Post-traumatic Respiratory Failure*. Philadelphia: W. B. Saunders Co., 1977, p. 73.

It has long been believed that the pathogenesis of fat embolism syndrome was related to the release of bone marrow in association with fractures and that the primary effect was a mechanical one. This hypothesis does not explain the fact that fat embolism syndrome is also seen in patients without trauma, such as those with diabetes, sepsis, neoplasms, sickle cell crisis, and a variety of other medical disorders. Some researchers believe that elevated free fatty acid levels are due to increased growth hormone during shock,[179] while others describe a "lipid mobilizing hormone."[45]

The symptoms of fat embolism syndrome usually develop within 72 hours of the trauma or other insult and may include tachycardia, tachypnea, cyanosis, fever, petechial rash with a characteristic pattern (involving the conjunctiva, neck, chest, and axilla), progressive hypoxemia, a sudden drop in the hematocrit, a diffuse infiltrate seen on chest radiograph, CNS disturbances, oliguria, and fat globules noted in the blood vessels of the retina. The serum lipase is elevated, and fat may be detected in the urine.[83]

The pathophysiology of the pulmonary damage is believed to result from the breakdown of large fat particles (too large to pass through the pulmonary microcirculation) into free fatty acids, thereby creating a form of chemical pneumonitis.[83]

The management may include: immobilization of any fractures, respiratory support with oxygen, volume replacement with Dextran[45] (Dextran is recommended because of its effect on reducing intravascular aggregation of erythrocytes), and steroids (hydrocortisone in doses of 100 mg. IV every 4 hours for 4 days). Recent work by Lahiri and ZuWallack[83] indicates that the presence of neutral fat in the blood can be detected by a simple analysis of rapidly frozen clotted blood. They have used the test to determine which patients were at risk for developing fat embolism syndrome and used steroids to treat some patients who had positive findings. None of the patients with positive findings who were treated developed fat embolism syndrome, while two out of three patients with positive findings, who were untreated, went on to develop the syndrome. Whether this test will be used routinely as a screening aid for high risk patients remains to be seen.

Metabolic Changes During Shock

As we have previously emphasized, shock produces prolonged circulatory insufficiency, which leads to variable and inadequate perfusion of certain organs and tissues, particularly at the microcirculation level. Such circulatory deprivation results in tissue hypoxia; many of the biochemical effects of shock are largely due to this. In addition, a variety of metabolites accumulate because of diminished venous blood flow and diminished lymphatic flow (except from areas that are traumatized directly, where lymph flow is usually increased). Widespread "toxic" effects may be produced owing to the escape of certain intracellular metabolites, which results in profound metabolic changes. The accumulated metabolites may affect local tissue circulation and metabolism as well as the circulation and metabolism of other areas to which they are eventually transported.

ANOXIA; HYPOXIA

Tissue anoxia (or most usually "hypoxia," a deficiency of oxygen) occurs in all types of shock as a result of decreased circulation of blood to the body tissues. To function properly, cells are dependent upon an adequate circulation in order to (1) receive nutrients, electrolytes, and oxygen and (2) have waste products removed.

Anoxia and hypoxia can both be tolerated for a short time. However, as the time lengthens, the chances of recovery diminish because oxygen lack appears to be a stimulus for the development of irreversible shock. If the available oxygen is sufficient to meet body need, irreversible shock should not occur. Conversely, the greater the disparity between oxygen need and available oxygen, the more rapidly irreversible shock will develop.

In view of these facts, those factors that increase the body's need for oxygen would be detrimental to the person in shock (e.g., increased metabolic rate, high temperature, physical activity); beneficial factors would be those that decrease the need for oxygen (e.g., hypothermia or low metabolic rate). Factors that increase the available oxygen (e.g., increased cardiac output or vasodilators with the arterial pressure remaining constant) would be helpful.

The flow of blood through the microcirculation of organs and tissues is so diminished in shock that there is *inadequate or no delivery of the oxygen and substrates* that are necessary for living cells to maintain normal metabolism and energy production.

Oxygen and substrates are essential to life because they make possible a series of complex chemical transformations that result in the synthesis of adenosine triphosphate (ATP), which is the ultimate source of energy for life processes.

ANAEROBIC METABOLISM; METABOLIC ACIDOSIS

When oxygen is not present, ATP is produced through a different set of reactions, referred to as *anaerobic metabolism* or "fermentation." Production of ATP in this manner is a useful emergency measure; however, it is inefficient compared with the normal process of aero-

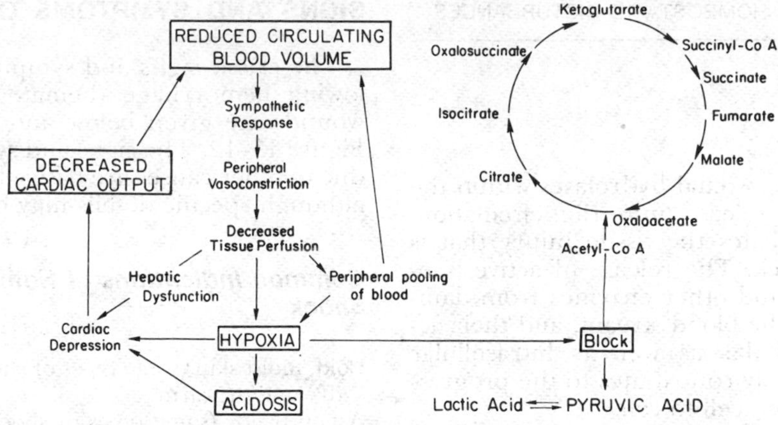

Figure 13–10. Shock leads to tissue hypoxia, with blockage of normal aerobic metabolism. Lactic acid accumulates, resulting in tissue acidosis. (From Condon, R. E., and L. M. Nyhus: *Manual of Surgical Therapeutics.* © 1978 by Robert E. Condon and Lloyd M. Nyhus.)

bic (oxidative) metabolism. Anaerobic metabolism produces anaerobic metabolites such as lactic acid (which causes intracellular acidity with consequent cellular damage) and substrates of the adenylic acid system (which depress the heart) (Fig. 13–10).

Because lactic acid is nonvolatile, it accumulates in the tissue fluids, causing them to become increasingly acid and ultimately producing a *metabolic acidosis.* During metabolic acidosis we find that blood pH, Pco_2 and bicarbonate fall, while a rise occurs in pyruvate, lactate, phosphate, and sulfate. *Respiratory alkalosis* or *respiratory acidosis* (induced by pulmonary ventilatory or diffusion changes) may be superimposed on the metabolic acidosis. This situation will become progressively worse the longer the living cells are deprived of necessary blood. (Fig. 13–11).

Unless the circulation is restored, the acidotic reaction, resulting from metabolic acidosis, will ultimately kill the cells. The build-up of lactic acid causes such a severe local acidosis that cellular enzymes become inactivated and, as a result, the cells soon die.

INTRACELLULAR OR LYSOSOMAL ENZYMES

It now appears that lysosomal enzymes are not only released in dead cells that are undergoing autolysis, but are also released just prior to cell death as a result of cellular anoxia or some other form of injury; e.g., these enzymes may be liberated as a result of trauma and endotoxins. Research on shock suggests that disruption of lysosomes and the release of their contained enzymes in free, active form occurs in the liver during shock, and that this is one mechanism of cell destruction that results from prolonged shock.

Lysosomal enzymes become most active in an acid pH range. Thus, as long as physiologic acid-base balance is maintained within the body, these enzymes are repressed within normal cells. However, in hypoxic tissues during shock states, the accompanying metabolic acidosis accelerates the solubilization and activation of these enzymes.

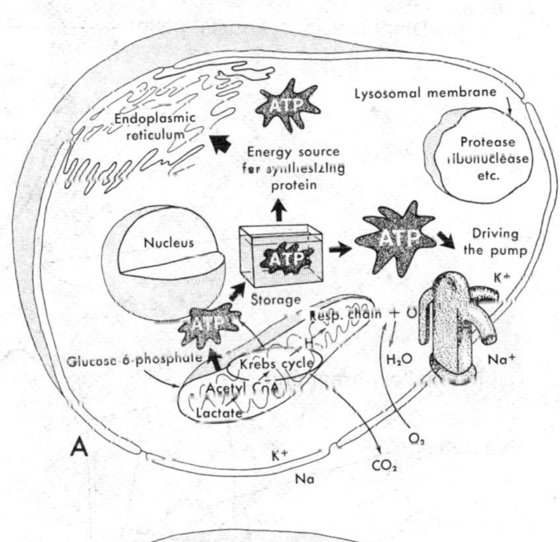

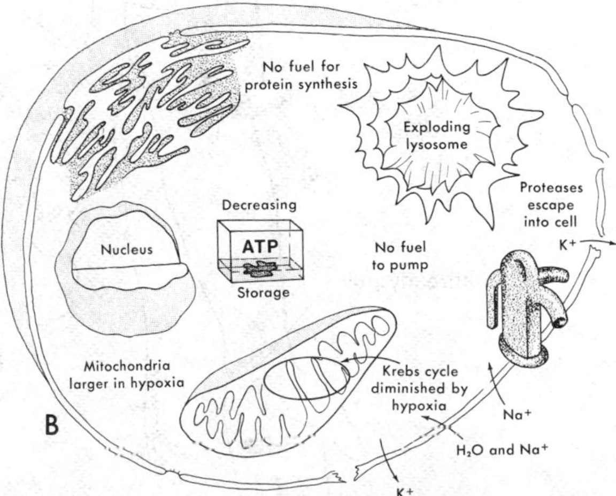

Figure 13–11. **A.** Normal cell. **B.** Cell in shock. (From Zschoche, D. A. (Ed.): *Mosby's Comprehensive Review of Critical Care.* St. Louis: C. V. Mosby Co., 1976, p. 491.)

Activation of lysosomal hydrolases within the cells, and their release into the circulation, markedly exacerbates the tissue injury that is produced in shock. The release of active lysosomal proteases and other enzymes from damaged tissue into the blood stream, and their action on extracellular as well as intracellular structures, probably contributes to the progression of injury from cell to cell.

The presence of hepatic lysosomal active enzymes in the blood stream, along with blocking of the reticuloendothelial system, is a potential factor in the lethal outcome of shock. As previously indicated, blockade of the reticuloendothelial system drastically reduces its capacity to clear bacteria from the blood stream.

SIGNS AND SYMPTOMS OF SHOCK

The classic signs and symptoms of shock following hemorrhage (hematogenic shock) and wounds are given below and are illustrated in Figure 13–12. The signs and symptoms of shock due to other causes are basically similar to these, although specific details may be different.

Common Indications of Hematogenic Shock

Cold, moist skin (some types of shock cause skin to be dry and/or warm)
Ashen pallor (some types of shock cause cyanosis or rubor)
Dryness of mucous membranes
Decreased body temperature
Low systolic and diastolic blood pressure (hypotension is usual, but normotension or hypertension occurs with some types of shock) with postural changes

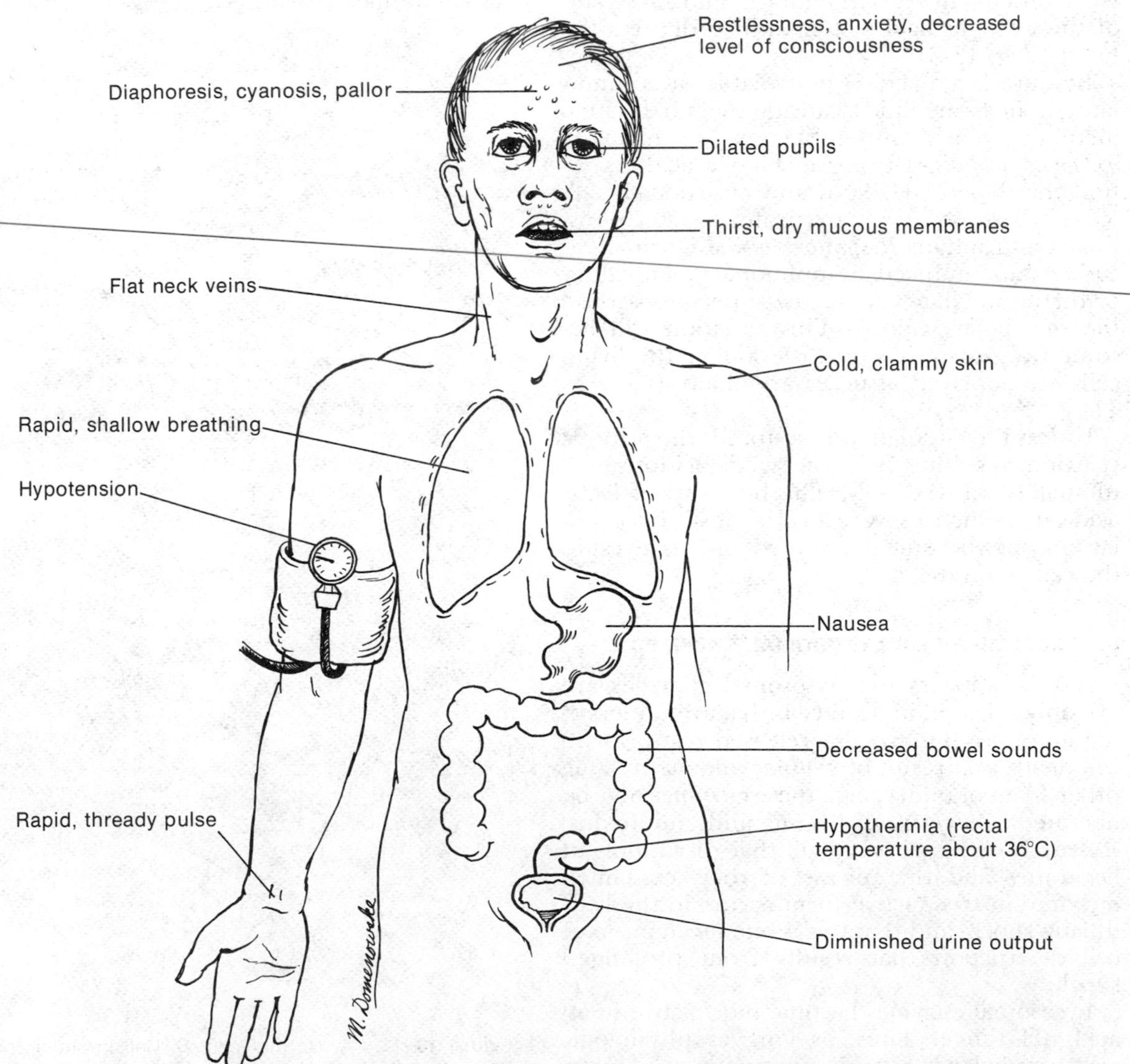

Figure 13–12. Appearance of the patient with hemorrhagic shock.

Slow capillary filling; collapse of superficial veins of extremities
Oliguria; anuria
Pilomotor and sudomotor activity
Thirst
Cold
Restlessness, nervousness, apprehension, irritability, drowsiness, stupor
Weakness
Rapid, shallow respirations; air hunger
Rapid, weak ("thready") pulse
Nausea, vomiting
Metabolic acidosis
Patient steadily progresses toward a so-called irreversible phase

> *Recognition of* early *or* impending *shock is vitally important. Treatment may become very difficult if shock is not suspected or recognized until the patient develops overt hypotension, cyanosis and a clammy, cold skin.*

Respiratory Rate in Shock

Rapid, shallow respirations typically result from decreased tissue perfusion. The respiratory rate increases as the oxygen-carrying power of the blood decreases. Also, the respiratory rate is increased because the accumulation of excessive amounts of carbon dioxide (due to metabolic acidosis) serves as a stimulus to the respiratory center.

Pulse Rate in Shock

As a general rule, the pulse rate *increases* in shock as a result of increased sympathetic stimulation. The body's compensatory mechanisms further accelerate the pulse rate by increasing the number of contractions of the heart per minute. This occurs in an attempt to maintain adequate circulation of the blood when the circulating volume of blood is not adequate. This sequence of events is particularly true in shock states caused by fluid loss or acute myocardial infarction.[19]

In addition to being more rapid, the pulse is typically weak and thready. At the onset of shock, the pulse rate is not so directly related to the severity of the pathology as is the blood pressure. This is because, in shock's early stage, worry, excitement, and fear may influence the heart rate out of proportion to the underlying conditions. However, when emotional factors are no longer significant, serial observations of the pulse rate over a period of time may be highly useful in evaluating the patient's condition and the direction of the shock state. Simeone[142] notes that elderly patients (with and without various degrees of heart block) are an exception to this. These patients may show little change in their heart rates in spite of the presence of conditions that cause circulatory failure (e.g., hemorrhage).

The pulse rate may become extremely slow in the terminal stages of irreversible shock. If the radial pulse is irregular, you should simultaneously check the apical pulse. The difference between the count of the apical pulse and the count of the radial pulse is known as the *pulse deficit.*

Blood Pressure in Shock

> *The blood pressure is inversely related to the heart rate, so that a decreased blood pressure is accompanied by an increased heart rate.*

The systolic blood pressure indicates the integrity of the cardiac mechanism, the arteries and the arterioles, while the diastolic blood pressure indicates the resistance of blood vessels.

The amount of peripheral resistance (or vasoconstriction) is indicated by the level of the diastolic blood pressure. For example, an increasing diastolic pressure indicates increasing resistance of the peripheral blood vessels; conversely, a declining diastolic pressure is indicative of decreasing peripheral resistance. When the diastolic pressure falls significantly, we know that vasoconstriction is being lost as a compensatory mechanism. When vasoconstriction is replaced by marked vasodilatation there is no resistance to blood flow and, thus, blood pressure cannot be maintained.

It is usual for the blood pressure to begin to fall when the total blood volume is decreased by about 15 to 20 per cent of normal; however, it is not unusual for some persons to lose as much as 25 per cent of their total blood volume without showing signs of shock.[18]

Typically, through the progressive stages of shock the systolic and diastolic arterial pressures drop, the systolic pressure usually dropping more than the diastolic. The pulse pressure* also falls, since pulse pressure is equal to the difference between the systolic and diastolic pressures. Actually *evaluation of the pulse pressure is more significant than evaluation of blood pressure,* since it tends to parallel the cardiac stroke volume.[109]

It should be remembered that the significance of the blood pressure in an individual patient

*Pulse pressure is often less than 20 mm. of mercury.

depends to some extent upon the *usual* blood pressure.

While some persons normally have a systolic blood pressure of about 100 mm. Hg, others may have high blood pressure, with a usual systolic pressure of 210 mm. Hg. Obviously a blood pressure of 100 mm. Hg would mean two vastly different things for these two groups of persons. A blood pressure of 100 mm. Hg or less is significant for persons whose systolic pressure usually ranges from 110 to 140 mm. Hg.

In order to maintain the coronary circulation, it is necessary to have a minimal systolic pressure of from 60 to 70 mm. Hg. In interpreting blood pressure readings it is always helpful to know what the individual's usual blood pressure has been. Also, remember that when the patient is in a supine position, a decline in blood pressure may be a late finding. Brand and Thal present the following words of caution concerning the clinical interpretation of hypotension:

It is important to realize that hypotension, by itself, is not shock, and that unless other clinical manifestations are present, a low systolic pressure should not be construed as shock. In many instances a systolic pressure of only 70 to 80 mm. of mercury may be of sufficient magnitude to permit adequate tissue perfusion in vasodilated patients.[19]

While the auscultatory blood pressure and pulse pressure are *usually* reduced in shock, some patients with all the peripheral manifestations of shock may have normal intra-arterial pressure despite markedly reduced or absent

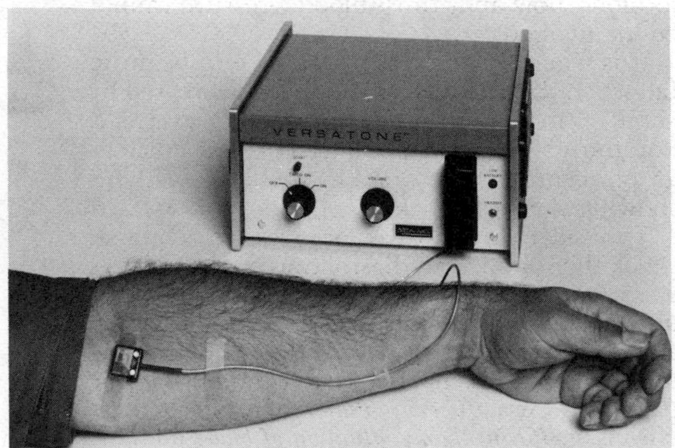

Figure 13–13. Doppler probe secured in proper position for obtaining a peripheral blood pressure. The amplifier (box) contains a loudspeaker, and the device is portable and battery operated. *Note*: It would be more comfortable for the patient if the area of skin which will be in contact with tape is shaved prior to application of the Doppler. (Courtesy of Medsonics, Incorporated. 340 Pioneer Way, P.O. Box M, Mountain View, Cal. 94042.)

cuff pressure and upper extremity pulses. Such a discrepancy between intra-arterial and cuff pressures in patients in shock can have important clinical implications.

Failure to recognize that low cuff pressure does not necessarily indicate arterial hypotension can lead to dangerous errors in therapy.

For example, should vasopressor medications be administered (as they might be because of a false impression of hypotension), they could produce hypertension and acute heart failure. Valuable information about the level of arterial pressure in vasoconstricted patients can be gained by evaluation of the strength of femoral pulsations. It may also be appropriate to use a Doppler device to obtain an accurate *peripheral blood pressure*. The Doppler is an instrument that amplifies arterial and venous pulsations through the use of ultrasound. There are a variety of probes available; the probe pictured in Figure 13–13 is especially convenient since it can be secured in position with adhesive tape. When using the Doppler, the blood pressure is measured the same way it is normally, but the Doppler probe takes the place of the stethoscope. The systolic blood pressure is easily heard if the probe is placed over the brachial artery and an adequate amount of transmission gel is used. The diastolic blood pressure is not readily obtainable when the Doppler is used.

Direct measurement of the arterial pressure may be the only accurate way to assess the status of the patient in some situations. This will be discussed again later.

There are additional problems that need to be considered in evaluating blood pressure during shock. The following facts make blood pressure per se (and particularly the systolic pressure) an unreliable criterion for determining the presence and severity of shock:

1. In the early stages of shock, blood pressure changes are generally unreliable because the arterial pressure may actually be normal or even high even though the factors that are initiating the shock are present. In fact, blood volume deficits of a liter or more may occur even though arterial and venous pressures are normal or elevated.
2. When severe vasoconstriction is present the blood pressure may be normal even though the circulation is actually highly inadequate. Also, conversely, the blood flow may not be inadequate even though the blood pressure is decreased, e.g., owing to mechanisms such as vasodilatation.
3. An unobtainable blood pressure generally indicates a very low pulse pressure and cardiac output; it does not necessarily indicate a low blood pressure.[109]

As indicated, while shock is usually associated with systemic hypotension, there are situations in which it may be associated with normal or even high blood pressures in spite of serious injury or blood loss. Such cases are referred to as "compensated shock," because vigorous sympathicoadrenal activity is "compensating" for the oligemia by precariously sustaining the blood pressure through neuroendocrine defenses. In such situations, relatively small additional blood losses, anesthesia, or even a change in the patient's position can lead to "decompensation and catastrophe."[142]

Hardaway and his associates clinically classify hypotensive, and normotensive or hypertensive shock as follows.[62]

I. Hypotensive shock
  A. Cold skin (arterioles constricted, low central venous pressure, low cardiac output)
    1. Low blood volume (responds well to transfusion)
      (a) Hemorrhage
      (b) Fluid loss (burns, massive wounds, infection, dehydration, etc.)
    a. Normal blood volume (poor response to transfusion)
      (a) Septic shock
  B. Warm skin (arterioles dilated, not real shock as capillaries are often well perfused. Increased cardiac output)
    1. Arsenic poisoning
    2. Spinal shock
    3. Shock due to any anesthesia
    4. Shock due to vasodilators
  C. Heart failure (arterioles constricted, decreased cardiac output, high central venous pressure)
II. Normotensive or hypertensive shock (arterioles constricted, decreased cardiac output, low vena cava pressure)
  A. Compensated shock
  B. Epinephrine shock
  C. "Overcompensation" shock
  D. Pheochromocytoma

Skin Appearance in Shock

As you can see from the preceding outline, the status of the skin during shock varies, depending on the etiologic basis of the shock state. Thus, you will notice clinically a striking contrast between the pallor and collapsed veins of a patient suffering from shock due to hemorrhage and/or trauma, and the cyanosis and venous distention of a patient in shock caused by pulmonary embolus or heart failure.

Generally during shock decreased tissue perfusion causes the skin to feel *"cool and clammy"* and to appear *pale*. Since blood provides warmth and color to the skin, a decreased blood volume and vasoconstriction of the blood vessels in the skin (as in hemorrhage) cause the blood supply to the skin to be deficient, and pallor results. Coolness and a clammy feel to a patient's skin during shock result from constriction of the peripheral blood vessels, caused by increased activity of the sympathetic nervous system (an early sign of shock). Clamminess also suggests an acute deficit of vascular fluid (e.g., blood and plasma) and an extensive sodium and chloride deficit.

Diaphoresis occurs in the late, severe stages of hemorrhagic shock because aldosterone secretion is decreased. As a result, sodium can no longer be retained in the body; in turn, water cannot be retained either and it leaves the body via the sweat glands.

"Clammy" skin is especially common in shock associated with overwhelming infection, with nervous reaction, or in wound shock following medication with opiates. Prior to the administration of opiates in wound shock the skin is often *cold and dry*. Also, it should be noted that in some cases of infection and hypotension the characteristic signs are *warm dry skin with rubor* (redness) and *plethora* (florid complexion) of the face.

As we have indicated, *cyanosis** may also be present during some forms of shock. Cyanosis typically occurs with pulmonary embolus or heart failure. Also, late in hemorrhagic shock the blood within the vessels is insufficient in both quantity and quality to give the skin a normal hue; the low volume of arterial blood has a proportionately low volume of hemoglobin and, thus, a decreased oxygen content. Cyanosis that appears late in hemorrhagic shock is usually caused by the presence of excessive amounts of deoxygenated blood in the skin capillaries. Also, blood flow in these vessels is very sluggish. In the old and the very young the fingernail beds and the lips will often become cyanotic before the rest of the body begins to appear blue. Cyanosis or pallor may be difficult to assess in the dark-skinned person, and subtle changes may be detected more accurately by observing the buccal mucosa or the conjunctiva.[126]

One means of evaluating peripheral circulation is to observe the effects of circulation in the nail beds. This is done by pushing down with the thumb nail on one of the patient's fingernails and then releasing the pressure and observing the return of color to the nail bed. Normally, a compressed nail bed fills within a fraction of a second after the pressure is released. Capillary filling, after compression of the skin and particularly the nail bed, is slow in shock and may take several seconds. Another means of evaluating peripheral circulation is to apply digital pressure to a peripheral vein (i.e., to "stroke" the vein) and see if it collapses. Venous collapse with digital pressure indicates that very little blood is within the vein.

*Cyanosis is discussed further in Unit XII.

Level of Consciousness in Shock

Early in shock hyperactivity of the sympathetic nervous system, with increased secretion of epinephrine, usually causes the patient to feel anxious, nervous, and irritable, and to have an anxious, worried expression.

Those signs and symptoms that are associated with a lack of blood supply to the brain are determined by the *suddenness* with which the shock develops and the *severity* of the insult. If the onset of the shock is sudden and the degree of shock is severe, the body may not have time to initiate its compensatory mechanisms of adjustment and, consequently, the brain is deprived of its blood supply, and fainting and unconsciousness result. The patient in a horizontal position may feel dizzy and faint if an upright position is assumed. If shock develops more gradually, over a period of several hours, some of the early signs may be apathy, lethargy, and confusion. On the other hand, the patient may be restless and unusually alert. Thus, changes in the degree of alertness in either direction are of importance in evaluating shock.

With shock, the amount of blood flowing to the brain may become insufficient to maintain normal mental functioning and a normal level of consciousness. When the supply of blood is limited, a decreased supply of oxygen and glucose to the brain results. The primary source of energy for the nerve cells is the oxidation of glucose. The brain cells are highly sensitive to a shortage of oxygen. Because the functioning brain cell depends on carbohydrate metabolism, and because the metabolic process depends on oxygen, metabolism within the brain is decreased in the presence of an oxygen shortage. The systolic blood pressure is an important factor in maintaining cerebral blood flow, since at least 40 mm. Hg of pressure is required to deliver blood to the brain. Usually a decrease in the systolic pressure is accompanied by a decrease in the flow of blood to the brain. However, the vessels of the brain, like those of the heart, are not constricted by the vasoconstrictor center and, thus, blood from the peripheral vessels can be shifted to the brain as an emergency compensatory measure.

The level of consciousness decreases as the circulation to the brain tissues becomes increasingly impaired, and the patient may then become confused, agitated, and restless. In patients experiencing trauma, restlessness is often mistaken for pain and the patients therefore given narcotics, which may further compound the problem. In severe and late shock, apathy may ensue. Drowsiness and stupor are more likely to occur in shock related to severe infection than in shock caused by trauma and hemorrhage. A comatose condition may ultimately be reached terminally. Because coma is unusual, except terminally, the possibility of intracranial damage must be ruled out when it does occur.[19, 142]

Kidney Function in Shock

The urine output is one of the most sensitive indices in shock. A decreased urine volume often is the earliest sign of hypovolemia and may occur even while the arterial blood pressure and pulse remain stable.

An indwelling urinary catheter, which allows measurement of urine produced, is useful in determining the status of the patient and the effectiveness of therapy. Because an indwelling catheter predisposes the patient to the danger of ascending urinary tract infection, *extreme* caution and careful technique must be used to prevent this from happening. *Remember, the patient in shock has a lowered resistance to infections!*

Urine flow should be kept above 50 ml. per hour. If the hourly output of urine diminishes significantly, treatment must be instituted to prevent renal shutdown. It is recommended that a urine output of less than 30 ml. per hour be reported to the attending physician at once; urine flow less than 20 ml. per hour can cause renal tubular necrosis, which results from inadequate renal circulation. Actually, the nurse should strive to recognize impending renal failure prior to the appearance of oliguria. Some of the changes that indicate nonoliguric renal failure are: (1) reduced specific gravity and osmolarity of the urine, (2) reduced urine creatinine clearance, (3) a rise in sodium urine concentration relative to the amount in the serum, and (4) a progressive rise in the blood's urea nitrogen, creatinine, and potassium.

Although it is much less common, a renal problem known as *high-output renal failure* is seen in selected patients with head injury, burns and soft tissue trauma. It is thought that this type of renal failure is a "renal response to a less severe or modified episode of renal injury than that required to produce classic renal failure."[140] While the creatinine and the blood urea nitrogen (BUN) may be elevated, and a mild metabolic acidosis is often noted, the patient has a normal or elevated urine output. Hyperkalemia may develop if the patient is given potassium supplements; therefore, patients on nasogastric suction, who would normally receive parenteral potassium, should not be given additional potassium if high-output renal failure is suspected. Treatment includes fluid replacement with a solution containing lactate (to treat the acidosis) and maintenance of normal serum sodium levels.[137, 140]

Metabolic Acidosis in Shock

In shock the metabolic products of cellular metabolism accumulate and produce a state of acidosis as a result of the stasis of blood and inadequate circulation. Although the body tries to compensate for this acidosis by using its many buffer systems, these compensatory mechanisms may fail. Such failure allows a dangerous state of overt acidosis to develop. For a discussion of acidosis and its signs and symptoms, see the preceding chapter.

Body Temperature in Shock

In severe shock the thermoregulatory mechanism is disturbed, causing the body temperature to fall. While the body metabolism normally produces heat, in severe shock metabolism is extremely low.

Summary of Signs and Symptoms of Shock

In summary, some major manifestations of decreased tissue perfusion are: cold and "clammy" skin; anxiety progressing to a declining level of consciousness, oliguria or anuria, hypotension, increased pulse rate, rapid and shallow respirations, and metabolic acidosis. In addition to the above, some other findings are: peripheral cyanosis, collapsed peripheral veins, elevated or reduced body temperatures, and (in cardiogenic shock) distended neck veins. These signs vary according to the etiology of the shock and are thus not present in all patients.

In Table 13–8 the clinical signs and symptoms of various degrees of shock are listed, both for conditions involving blood volume loss and those in which there is no blood loss.

As you realize, it is difficult to know when shock actually exists and when therapy should begin. Because of this difficulty it has been established that in clinical shock, as a general rule, treatment should be instituted whenever at least two of the following conditions prevail: (1) systolic blood pressure of 80 mm. Hg or less; (2) pulse pressure of 20 mm. Hg or less; and (3) pulse rate of 100 or more.[57]

CLINICAL CARE OF THE PATIENT EXPERIENCING SHOCK

The primary aim of the treatment of shock is to increase tissue perfusion. Unless this is accomplished early after onset, subsequent therapeutic measures are of no avail and death can be anticipated.[26]

Let us consider Mr. Wilson, who lies in a state of shock. In addition to a urinary catheter, he has catheters placed in the radial artery, the right atrium of the heart, and the pulmonary artery. He is being attended by senior physicians and nurses, who will remain with him until he is out of danger. Mr. Wilson's bed is custom-made, so that it is a little narrower and higher than the usual hospital bed. This makes it suitable for use as an operating table for minor surgeries, such as tracheotomy or cutdown procedures. The head and foot of the bed easily lift off so that tracheal intubation and other therapeutic maneuvers can be readily performed. Special holders for transducers, etc., are also present on the bed. A portable image intensifier can be used (e.g., to place a pulmonary artery catheter) at the bedside because the mattress and springs are made of a plastic material, so that x-rays can penetrate the bed. Mr. Wilson's radial artery pressure, central venous pressure, pulmonary artery pressure, electrocardiogram, and rectal and skin temperature are continuously monitored on a multichannel recorder and screen. A device regulates body temperature by warming or cooling him. Cardiac output is measured by the cardiac green dye method, and a computer calculates the curve. To help in monitoring fluid intake, output, and retention, the bed sits on a metabolic scale that is accurate to the nearest gram. Many hemodynamic monitoring measurements are constantly being obtained, evaluated and reported on permanent records by computers. Such a report, or *printout*, is illustrated in Figure 13–14.

Adjoining Mr. Wilson's room is a nursing station that serves as a supply center (i.e., for drugs, intravenous solutions, emergency resuscitation equipment, respirator, tracheotomy, and cutdown trays) and a data recording and processing center. A laboratory is only a few steps from the bed. It is equipped for a wide variety of blood coagulation tests, including factor assays. A diagram of the clotting process is drawn by a thromboelastograph. From the same blood sample the red blood cell mass and plasma volume are measured (with a Hemolitre). Other equipment is available for the performance of an average of more than 300 laboratory determinations per patient per day. The following is a list of some of the indices that can be determined:

1. Hemodynamic measurements
   a. Arterial blood pressure
   b. Central venous pressure
   c. Pulmonary artery and pulmonary wedge pressures
   d. Cardiac index
   e. Peripheral resistance
   f. Mean transit time
   g. Blood volume
   h. Oxygen saturation by oximetry
2. Hematologic measurements
   a. Hemoglobin and hematocrit

TABLE 13–8. CORRELATION OF CLINICAL SIGNS AND SYMPTOMS OF SHOCK WITH BLOOD VOLUME LOSS*

A. LOSS OF BLOOD VOLUME—TRAUMA AND HEMORRHAGE

Degree of Shock	Blood Pressure	Skin: *Temperature*	Skin: *Color*	Skin: *Response to Pressure Blanching*	Thirst	Mental Status	Blood Loss (% of normal volume)	Blood Loss (cc., approx. quantity)
None	126/75	Normal	Normal	Normal	Normal	Clear	14.4	750
Slight	109/66	Cool	Pale	Definite slowing	Normal	Clear, distressed	20.7	1000
Moderate	95/58	Cool	Pale	Definite slowing	Marked	Clear, some apathy	34.3	1750
Marked	49/25	Cold	Ashen to cyanotic	Very sluggish	Severe	Apathetic to comatose; little distress except thirst	45.9	2250

B. NO BLOOD LOSS—MEDICAL CONDITIONS: INFECTIONS, PERICARDITIS, MESENTERIC THROMBOSIS, ETC.

Degree of Shock	Blood Pressure	Skin: *Extremities*	Skin: *Cyanosis*	Respirations	Pulse	Mental Status	Average Blood Lactic Acid (mEq. per L.)
Minimal	Slight fall	Pale and cool	Lips, extremities or both	Normal	Thready and rapid	Restless and apprehensive	5
Moderate	80/60 to 60/40	Cold and clammy	Lips, extremities or both	Rapid and shallow	Thready and rapid	Apprehensive and confused	6
Marked	60/40 to 40/20	Cold and clammy	Lips, extremities or both	Often Cheyne-Stokes or sighing	Thready and rapid	Confused to stuporous	11
Extremely marked	20/1 to 20/0	Cold and clammy	Lips, extremities or both	Often Cheyne-Stokes or sighing	Rapid, slow or unobtainable	Stuporous to comatose	17

*Breed, E. S.: The diagnosis and management of shock. *Medical Clinics of North America* 41:669–683, May. 1957.

b. Red blood cell mass (determined with sodium chromate ^{51}Cr)
c. Plasma volume (determined with iodinated ^{131}I serum albumin)
d. White blood cell count
e. Platelet count
f. Fibrinogen concentration
g. Prothrombin time
h. Partial thromboplastin time
i. Thromboelastograph clotting time
j. Assays of proteolytic enzyme activity
k. Individual clotting factor assays (I, II, IV, V, VII, VIII, IX, X, XI, XII)

3. Metabolic measurements
   a. Frequent precise weighing
   b. Serum and urine electrolyte concentration
   c. Lactate and pyruvate concentration
   d. Blood urea nitrogen, creatinine, and liver function studies
   e. Catecholamine assay
   f. Oxygen consumption study
   g. Core and skin temperature
4. Respiratory system studies
   a. Blood pH
   b. Blood gas studies
   c. Minute volume
   d. Tidal volume
   e. Alveolar ventilation
   f. Dead space–tidal volume ratio
   g. Vital capacity
   h. Alveolar-arterial oxygen tension difference
   i. Venous-arterial shunts
5. Others
   a. X-ray studies as indicated
   b. Electrocardiographic monitoring

The situation that we have just described concerning Mr. Wilson approaches being an ideal treatment and research clinic for shock. Probably the area in which you will work will not have

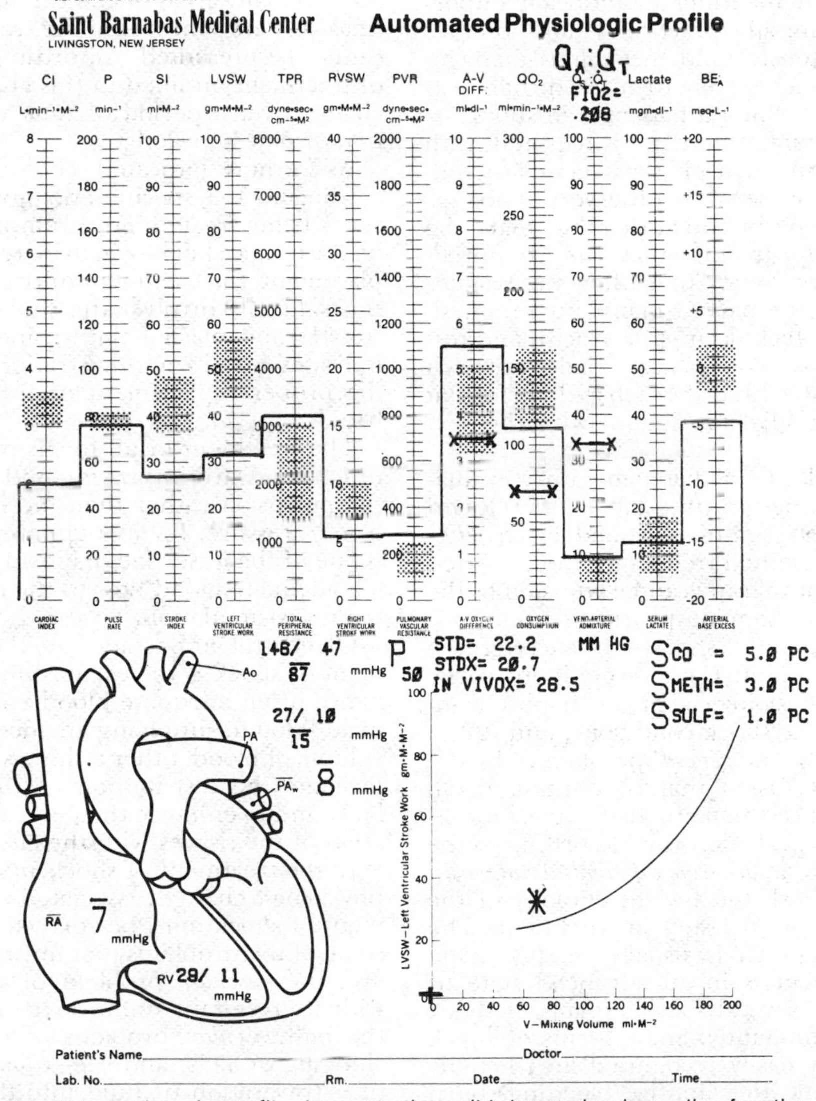

Figure 13–14. Automated physiologic profile demonstrating mild depression in cardiac function. Stippled areas indicate normal range values for young adults. (From Cohn, J. D. et al.: Physiologic profiles in circulatory support and management of the critically ill. *Journal of the American College of Emergency Physicians*, 6:479, Nov. 1977.)

all the features mentioned; however, you will undoubtedly be involved with many of these aspects of care. Regardless of where you are practicing you will undoubtedly care for patients in shock, for shock is a common condition.

> Shock can occur in any hospital area — medical, surgical, orthopedic, obstetric, operating and recovery rooms, psychiatry, dermatology, metabolic, etc. Shock can occur in any home, on any street, in any doctor's or dentist's office. In a word, shock can occur anywhere. Sometimes shock occurs when it could and should have been prevented.[18]

Caring for a patient in shock is one of the most complex, demanding and critically important areas of nursing practice. Frank observes that, "Early intensive and meticulous management is much more likely to succeed than last-ditch heroics."[49] When a patient is in shock, or close to it, constant attendance is required, with a senior, well informed physician close at hand. Physician and nurse must observe physiologic changes as they occur and at that time make the therapeutic adjustments that are required. Shock is an emergency that often necessitates team action on the part of many: nurse, physician, laboratory technician, pharmacist, and respiratory therapist — each has a vital role. Each person must know his or her job and perform it skillfully and rapidly, anticipating what the next action might be.

At the bedside, immediate laboratory evaluations are essential in treating shock. Blood chemistries, blood gases, pH, and electrolytes need to be determined frequently and reported promptly so that therapy can be adjusted to the patient's rapidly changing physiologic status.

For the treatment of shock to be successful, it must be based upon: (1) a recognition of the various pathophysiologic changes that are associated with *specific* shock conditions, and (2) an understanding of the *general* problem of inadequate tissue perfusion that is common to all shock states. Since the methods for treating inadequate tissue perfusion vary according to the specific etiology, an *accurate differential diagnosis*, which will establish the specific etiology of the shock state, is the *first* step in treatment. The differential diagnosis is usually readily made unless the patient is in an advanced state of shock, in which several specific forms of shock may exist concomitantly. Some forms of shock that are usually easily recognized are: hemorrhagic shock due to extensive bleeding, burn shock caused by extensive burns, and cardiogenic shock typified by severe chest pains and ECG readings indicative of acute myocardial infarction. Probably the least obvious diagnosis is that of toxic (i.e., septic) shock.[39, 150] Identification of toxic shock requires "astute clinical suspicion which is later confirmed by laboratory identification of the bacterial agent."[19]

Overview of Modes of Treatment

The treatment of shock, in a general sense, has changed markedly during the past few years.

> Lower his head, keep him warm, and use vasopressor drugs to elevate his blood pressure were once traditional practices in the care of the patient in shock. Now, as a result of new knowledge, all of these measures are being seriously questioned, and principal emphasis is being placed on maintenance of adequate capillary blood flow throughout the body tissues and organs.[142]

As with many areas of clinical care, clear-cut and final answers concerning the treatment of shock cannot be presented. Accordingly, the concepts of treatment outlined in this chapter will surely change over a period of time with the acquisition of new knowledge.

As we have indicated, clinical care varies according to the specific etiology of the type of shock being treated. For example, the patient in hemorrhagic shock primarily requires blood replacement; the treatment of traumatic and burn shock mainly involves the replacement of electrolytes and plasma fluids; and diabetic shock indicates insulin administration in addition to the proper replacement of fluids and electrolytes.

The treatment of all forms of shock must be directed toward improving and maintaining tissue perfusion rather than merely elevating the blood pressure, for it is apparent that pressure is one of the lesser factors involved in maintaining adequate blood flow to the tissues served by the microcirculation.

Of central importance in the current treatment of shock is the establishment and maintenance of an adequate blood volume. However, in addition to supplying an adequate circulating volume of blood, other adjuncts are necessary to facilitate the distribution of this blood to the body and to enhance the perfusion and oxygenation of the tissues with the circulating blood.

In the treatment of shock, *all* the basic pathophysiologic changes associated with the development of shock must be corrected. For example, some of the problems that must often be treated are: the *vascular* problem of vasoconstriction, with its resultant diminished tissue perfusion; the *intravascular* problem of coagulation and sludging of cells; and the *extravascular* problem of extravasation of fluid into the extravascular space.

Characteristically, impairment of tissue function is correctable at an early stage, but it may lead to death if treatment is inadequate or if the condition goes untreated. It is generally held that in the later stages of shock the condition becomes "irreversible," leading inexorably to death in spite of treatment. Before it may be concluded that shock has become irreversible the following possible causes for failure of therapy must be excluded:[142]

- Inadequate restoration of circulating blood volume.
- Failure to recognize occult bleeding (into the abdominal or thoracic cavity or into the extremities)
- Failure to recognize interference with cardiopulmonary function (cardiac tamponade, pulmonary embolism, fat embolism, coronary thrombosis, tension pneumothorax, massive atelectasis)
- Failure to recognize overwhelming infection

Let us hasten to point out that clinical treatment for "irreversible" shock is never abandoned while the patient remains alive.[86]

> The term "irreversible shock" has no meaning in the clinic and can only be justified after the fight has been lost.[49]

Assessment of the Patient in Shock

A variety of different techniques, both *invasive* and *noninvasive*, are used to determine the patient's status and the effectiveness of treatment of shock. The condition of patients can change rapidly in shock, and frequent nursing evaluation is essential. Recording of patients' progress and response to therapy should be concise yet convey their status minute by minute. A flow sheet containing all the pertinent data in an easily read format should be initiated regardless where the patient is physically located, e.g., in the field, an emergency department, or on a regular nursing unit, and should accompany the patient at all times. An example of a flow sheet designed specifically for the patient with shock is pictured in Figure 13–15.

NONINVASIVE ASSESSMENT TECHNIQUES

Since nurses frequently function as health care providers in settings other than the hospital, it is helpful to have knowledge of assessment and monitoring techniques that do not require sophisticated machinery or involve invading body tissues or cavities. These noninvasive techniques can be done rapidly, require little equipment, are relatively easy to perform, and are readily observable.

The first step in the assessment of a patient with suspected shock is a general overview with attention to the *ABC's — airway, breathing,* and *circulation*. Once it has been ascertained that the airway is patent, that air exchange is adequate, and that the patient has a pulse, a head-to-toe physical assessment should be done. This is done rapidly and is cursory at best. The goal is to identify major problems and gross abnormalities; more attention will be given to specific injuries or problems after the patient's condition has been stabilized. The *physical assessment* skills presented in Chapter 15 can be used in this situation, to help make the following observations:

Level of consciousness, orientation × 3, range of motion and sensation in all extremities, hand grasps, response to verbal and painful stimuli, posturing, pupil size, and reaction to light

State of hydration and perfusion of the skin, mucous membranes, sclera, conjunctiva, presence of pallor or cyanosis

Fullness of neck veins

Position of the trachea*

Respiratory pattern, chest wall expansion, bulges or defects of the chest wall

Presence of pain and location

Girth of abdomen and/or extremities

Peripheral pulses

Presence of lacerations, contusions, ecchymosis, petechiae, purpura

Bony deformities

Presence of medical alert tags or bracelets

After potentially life-threatening problems (e.g., airway obstruction, hemorrhage) have been dealt with, complete vital signs are taken. It is important that *postural vital signs* be taken, if it can be done safely. Postural or orthostatic vital signs are measured by taking the patient's blood pressure and pulse: first, with the patient supine; then sitting (with the legs dangling); and, finally, standing. The findings are recorded pictorially in this manner:

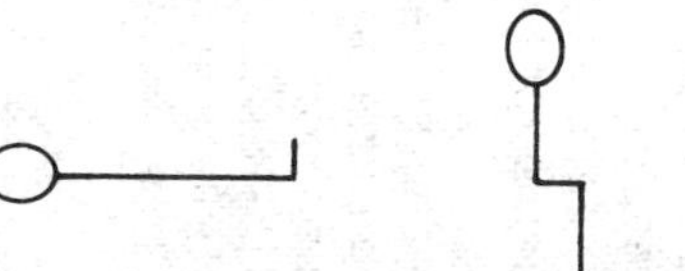
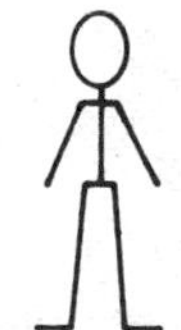

120/80 P. 84 110/60 P. 100 110/50 P. 124

If the patient has volume depletion, there is usually a drop in the systolic and diastolic blood pressures with a rise in the pulse rate. A fall in the diastolic pressure of 20 mm. Hg or greater and a rise in the pulse of 20 beats or more is

*Tracheal deviation may indicate the presence of a tension pneumothorax, which is a life-threatening problem requiring immediate relief by needle aspiration (see Chapter 57).

A guide to the initial therapy of SHOCK

DO

Start flow sheet and record vital signs.
Use a pressure dressing on major bleeding.
Maintain an adequate airway.
Obtain venous sample for hematocrit, type and cross-match.
Aid venous return and prevent air embolism *during subclavian catheterization* by placing the patient in the Trendelenburg position.
Insert large bore (15-18) central venous catheter and start infusion of electrolyte solution or plasma expander. Record CVP on flow sheet Q 30-60 minutes.
Obtain arterial blood sample for pH, pO_2 and pCO_2 in all patients with severe chest trauma, respiratory distress, or profound shock.
Splint fractures, as soon as possible.
Treat the underlying disorder resulting from the injury.
Get a chest x-ray.
Consider cardiac contusion with chest injury.
Get an IVP with hematuria.
A systematic history and physical examination.
Obtain information regarding accident.

FLOW SHEET

DATE ____________

MONTH___DAY___YEAR___

TIME OF INJURY______ (hour) ☐ am ☐ pm

HISTORY:

MAJOR PROBLEMS OR PARAMETERS:

VITAL SIGNS						INTAKE			OUTPUT					MINOR PROBLEMS NOTES AND MEDICATIONS
TIME	BP	P	R			IV#1	IV#2	ACC. TOTAL	URINE	ACC. TOTAL	PROBLEM NO.	PROBLEM NO.	PROBLEM NO.	

RESIDENT ________ ACC. TTL: ________

INTERN ________ RN: ________

ATTDG. M.D. ________ ________

SUMMARY:

FROM THE COMMITTEE ON TRAUMA
AMERICAN COLLEGE OF SURGEONS

AMERICAN COLLEGE OF SVRGEONS
FOVNDED IN 1913
OMNIBVS PER ARTEM FIDEMQVE PRODESSE

DON'T

Use vasopressors.
Move patient until vital signs are stable.
Use uncross-matched blood.
Move until spine has been evaluated.
Fail to obtain a history of associated diseases and drugs.
Forget tetanus prophylaxis.
Use a tourniquet except in traumatic amputations.
Blame head injury as a cause of shock.

Figure 13–15. A typical flow sheet to be used during the assessment and management of patients with shock and trauma. (From American College of Surgeons Committee on Trauma: A guide to the initial therapy of shock. *Consultant,* 18:94, Jan. 1978.)

considered a postural drop or a postural change. Since postural hypotension may be associated with a variety of disorders (see Table 13–9), a positive result must be related to the history and physical findings. In most emergency settings, however, a postural drop is interpreted as due to hypovolemia until proven otherwise.

Measurement of postural vital signs is indicated under the following circumstances:[17]

- History of, or presence of significant blood loss
- Unexplained tachycardia
- History of fluid loss, e.g., diarrhea, vomiting, diuretic therapy, third space loss (e.g., bowel obstruction, crush injury)
- Unexplained syncope
- Blunt chest or abdominal trauma
- Abdominal pain
- Unexplained hypotension

> Caution:
> *Postural vital signs should not be done in patients with multiple trauma if there is evidence of vertebral, pelvic, or femoral fracture, or in patients who are already hypotensive. Patients with postural hypotension should not be sent to the x-ray department for upright films (e.g., chest, abdomen) unless they are attended constantly by a nurse.*

An accurate *temperature measurement*, preferably rectal, is important in the assessment of the patient in shock. In selected patients, an indwelling flexible rectal probe connected to a continuous display monitor may be more accurate. In any case, oral temperature measurement in the shock patient is not accurate or safe. The buccal mucosa of the shock patient is poorly perfused, and the shock patient should be receiving oxygen by mask or nasal prongs. (Since these patients are hypoxemic, the procedure of removing the oxygen long enough to obtain an oral temperature is not good nursing practice.)

Other noninvasive assessment and monitoring tools are the *cardiac monitor* and the *twelve lead electrocardiogram.* We have discussed the effect of shock on cardiac function; it is appropriate to monitor the electrical activity of the heart continuously in all patients with shock, regardless of age. The decision to initiate cardiac monitoring should be a nursing decision since the information to be gained is needed in making decisions

TABLE 13–9. CAUSES OF POSTURAL HYPOTENSION

Decreased Cardiac Output
- Poor muscular pumping mechanism (muscular atrophy)
- Venous disease (incompetent valves, varicose veins or obstruction – as a late pregnancy)
- Cardiac (tamponade, constrictive pericarditis, atrial myxoma, or ball-valve thrombus)

Absolute or Relative Hypovolemia
- Relative dilatation of capacitance vessels (drug – nitrites or disease – angiomatosis)
- Absolute (hemorrhage, fluid loss, hypoaldosteronism or third spacing)

Neurologic Dysfunction
- Afferent limb (tabes dorsalis or polyneuritis)
- CNS (arteriosclerosis, syringomyelia, various myelopathies, Wernicke's Syndrome, tumors or drugs)

Sympathetic Dysfunction
- Polyneuritis (diabetic)
- Iatrogenic (postsympathectomy or neural blocking drugs)

Undetermined
- Adrenocortical insufficiency
- Diabetic acidosis
- Pheochromocytoma

From Bookman, L. B., and J. K. Simoneau: The early assessment of hypovolemia: postural vital signs. *Journal of Emergency Nursing,* 3:43, Sept.–Oct. 1977, p. 44.

about nursing care. In the initial care of patients with shock, it may be more appropriate to place the monitor electrodes on the shoulders rather than on the chest. This placement does not interfere with chest film findings and allows better access to the chest in the event that procedures need to be done in the thoracic area, e.g., insertion of chest tubes, periocardiocentesis, CVP placement. When the patient has been stabilized, the monitor electrodes may be moved to the chest.

The ability to take and interpret a twelve lead electrocardiogram is a skill that nurses caring for shock patients should develop. Time is a crucial factor for these patients, and it may be to the patient's disadvantage to wait for an ECG technician. More importantly, the information is needed to establish priorities of nursing care.

Assessment of *respiratory status* can be accomplished, to some degree by noninvasive procedures, including *spirometry* to measure tidal volume and minute volume. Another aid in assessing arterial oxygen saturation is the *ear oximeter.* This device utilizes a fiberoptic probe that is placed on the pinna of the ear. Oxygen saturation of the arterial blood is determined by the amount of light transmitted through the pinna. Studies comparing the accuracy of this method with the standard arterial blood gas measurements indicate that the ear oximeter is reliable in determining arterial oxygen saturation. While it is not expected that the ear oximeter will replace arterial blood gas analysis, it is felt that it may be a valuable tool in determining when arterial blood gases are needed.[47]

Although several noninvasive assessment and monitoring techniques have been reviewed, the most important consideration is that the patient must be observed and assessed continuously by the nurse.

INVASIVE ASSESSMENT TECHNIQUES

Invasive assessment and monitoring techniques include all the hemodynamic measurements that involve penetration of tissue or entry into body cavities. The list of devices available for invasive hemodynamic monitoring is long, and more devices are available each day. In this section we review briefly some of the hemodynamic measurements employed in the management of patients with shock. This aspect of care is covered in detail by Schroeder and Daily.[133]

Central Venous Pressure. Measurement of the *central venous pressure (CVP)* is one of the most common hemodynamic measurement techniques used in the initial management of patients with shock, especially those with hemorrhagic shock. The CVP is an estimate of the pressure in the right atrium and provides information concerning the function of the right side of the heart. While it may also provide information about left heart pressures, the CVP is not as accurate as other methods in reflecting subtle changes in left heart function. Changes in the CVP represent changes in the blood volume and in the venous return to the right side of the heart.

A CVP catheter may be inserted peripherally through a percutaneous puncture or through a cutdown, often in the antecubital fossa. Peripheral CVP catheters are usually 24 inches long; the standard size is a 14 or 16 gauge needle (the catheter size, then, since it is threaded through the needle, is 16 or 18 gauge). Central CVP lines may be inserted via the subclavian or the internal or external jugular veins. The catheter is attached to a manometer, which is connected on the opposite side to the IV fluid. The catheter may be sutured in place to prevent accidental removal.

In order to measure the CVP, the bottom of the manometer is held at the level of the right atrium in the midaxillary line. The stopcock on the manometer is turned so that the IV fluid enters the manometer. The stopcock is then turned so that the fluid will enter the patient. The fluid level in the manometer is observed, and the point at which the fluid stops in the manometer is recorded as the CVP. Respiratory motion will cause the meniscus to fluctuate, so the value may have to be approximated. The CVP should be measured with the patient supine and with the manometer placed at the same point for each reading. It is appropriate to mark the patient's chest at the correct point so that readings will be measured consistently.

When the catheter is being connected to IV tubing, the patient should be instructed to hold his or her breath to prevent an air embolism. A sterile gloved finger may also be used to occlude the hub of the catheter. *If air does inadvertently enter the catheter, immediately turn the patient onto his or her left side and adjust the bed to a Trendelenburg position.* This should cause the air to be trapped in the right atrium and allow it to be absorbed. Symptoms that may indicate that an air embolism has occurred include: sudden onset of dyspnea, tachypnea, cough, cyanosis, and respiratory arrest.[179] If the patient is symptomatic, treatment with hyperbaric oxygenation (discussed later) should be initiated without delay. High-flow oxygen should be administered, and ventilatory assist may be required.

Since the CVP catheter is large, disconnection of the tubing may result in *exsanguination.* Therefore, all connections must be secured and checked frequently. There are a variety of problems encountered when CVP catheters are in use; some of the more common ones are summarized in Table 13–10.

Although there is a wide range of normal in CVP measurement, values of 5 to 15 cm. H_2O are acceptable. It is important to understand, however, that a *change* in the CVP is more significant than the actual value. For example, a change in the CVP from 10 cm. to 5 cm. in a 5-minute period in a patient with multiple trauma is a significant finding and requires attention, even though both values are within normal limits. A CVP that is extremely low usually indicates inadequate volume, while a high CVP, i.e., above 15 cm., may be due to fluid overload, pericardial tamponade, or improper placement of the catheter. A chest x-ray film is obtained as soon as possible after insertion of a CVP line in order to insure that it is positioned properly. (When a patient with a CVP catheter and a chest tube on the same side begins to drain large amounts of fluid from the chest tube, the possibility that the catheter is in the pleural space should be considered. A hematocrit evaluation of the chest drainage may be done. If the fluid is IV solution rather than blood, the hematocrit will be significantly lower than the patient's venous hematocrit.) The IV tubing from the CVP line should be labeled clearly, and the location of the CVP recorded on the flow sheet. Additionally, since the possibility of the development of a pneumothorax always exists after a subclavian CVP attempt, the patient's respiratory rate and chest sounds should be assessed frequently.

Intra-arterial Blood Pressure Monitoring. Peripheral arterial catheters are commonly used in patients with shock in order to measure arterial blood pressure more accurately, espe-

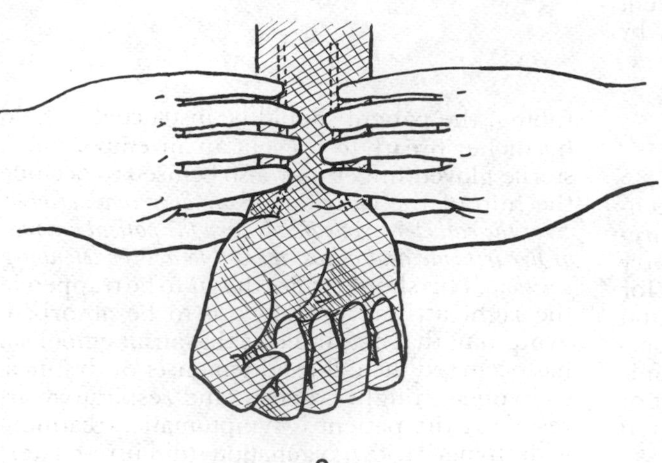

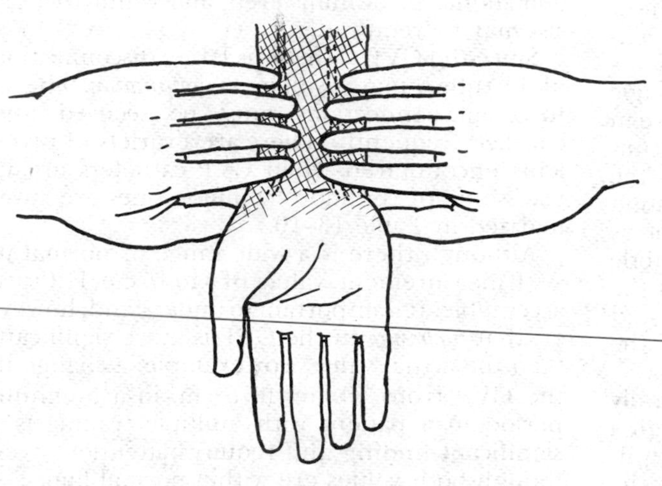

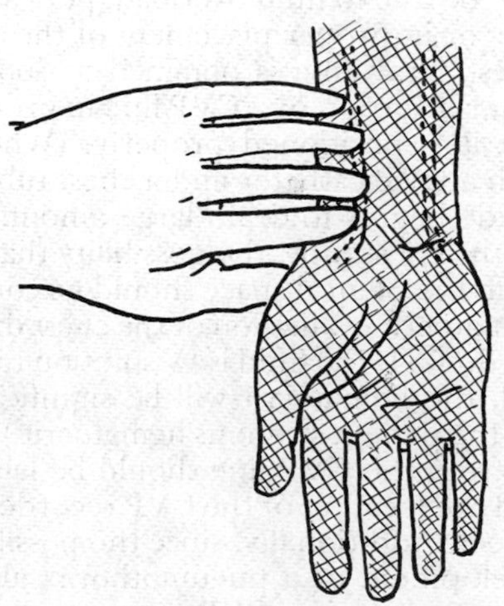

Figure 13–16. The Allen test. Before instrumenting the radial artery it is important to be sure that a competent ulnar artery is present. This can be done as follows:

1. The examiner compresses both arteries and the patient makes a tight fist to squeeze all the blood out of the hand.
2. The patient then extends the fingers, and the examiner observes the blanched hand.
3. Compression of the ulnar artery is released, and the examiner observes the hand fill with blood. If filling does not occur, the ulnar artery is presumed to be nonfunctional.

This sequence of events may be varied to test the adequacy of the radial artery as well. (From Rhoads, J. E.: Vascular Procedures. *In* Schwartz, G. et al.: *Principles and Practice of Emergency Medicine.* Philadelphia: W. B. Saunders Co., 1978.)

cially if the Korotkoff sounds cannot be detected, and to obtain samples for chemical and blood gas analysis. The catheter patency is maintained through the use of a heparinized IV solution administered either by continuous drip (under pressure) or by flush. If the latter technique is used, flushing should be limited to a 3 ml. or less bolus and administered slowly. Rapid infusion of

6 ml. or more may result in retrograde flushing to the subclavian arteries. If this occurs, cerebral embolization may result.[179]

Arterial lines may be placed in a variety of arteries; however, the radial and brachial arteries are most commonly used. *If the radial artery is selected, it is essential that the patency of the ulnar artery be assessed beforehand.* Although uncommon, gangrene of the hand following radial artery cannulation has been reported.[46] Assessment of ulnar artery patency is done by performing an *Allen test.* This involves raising the patient's hand and occluding the radial and ulnar arteries until pallor is noted. The ulnar arterial compression is released and the hand lowered. Normal color and sensation should return immediately to the hand. If this does not occur, another site should be selected. (The Allen test should also be performed before arterial puncture for blood gas analysis is carried out.)[22, 64, 133] (Fig. 13–16).

Normally, an arterial catheter is attached to a transducer so that the pressures can be monitored by use of an oscilloscope. The components of a typical system are pictured in Figure 13–17. On the oscilloscope, the wave forms appear as pictured in Figure 13–18. During systole there is a sharp upstroke which correlates with the QRS complex of the EKG. On the downstroke of the wave, there is a notch (the dicrotic notch), which is related to closure of the aortic valve. The continued fall of the wave is due to the continued fall in pressure during diastole. "The highest point of the pressure wave form is termed the systolic pressure. The lowest point just before the next systole is the diastolic pressure."[133]

If transducers are not available, it is possible to obtain continuous arterial pressures by using a system similar to that used for CVP measurement, with the exception that the manometer or extension tubing used to contain the fluid column must be longer. The setup is pictured in Figure 13–19; the procedure is as follows:*

Materials Required

1. An intravenous pole
2. Adhesive tape, 65–70" in length, 1½" wide

*This method was devised by Robert F. Wilson, M.D., Assistant Professor of Surgery, Wayne State University, College of Medicine. (From Brand, L., and Thal, A. P.: Shock. *In* Meltzer, L. E., Abdellah F. G., and Kitchell, J. R. (eds.): *Concepts and Practices of Intensive Care for Nurse Specialists.* Philadelphia, Charles Press Publishers, Inc., 1969.)

TABLE 13–10. PROBLEMS ENCOUNTERED WITH CVP CATHETERS

Problem	Cause	Prevention	Treatment
Pain and inflammation above insertion site	Mechanical irritation of catheter leading to sterile thrombophlebitis Bacterial infection ascending along catheter at insertion site	Prepare skin properly Use sterile technique during insertion and dressing change Insert catheter smoothly Change dressing, stopcocks, and connecting tubing daily Rotate insertion site every 48 to 72 hr	Remove catheter (mandatory if infection is at insertion site) Apply warm compresses Give pain medication as necessary
Poor infusion of IV fluid	Partial clotting at catheter tip	Use continuous drip Heparin 250 units/250 ml IV fluid may help Occasionally flush or use rapid drip Flush with large volume after blood withdrawal	Attach syringe to catheter and attempt to aspirate clot Irrigate gently; *do not* forcibly flush catheter without consulting physician; remove catheter and reinsert at another site if it cannot be irrigated easily
	External kinking of catheter	Coil and tape catheter carefully after insertion	Remove dressing and check for possible kinking of catheter Straighten catheter, retape, and apply new sterile dressing
Catheter tip missing when catheter is removed	Catheter cut or sheared during insertion	Never pull back catheter and readvance	Locate by palpation if in arm or by chest x-ray film; may require venous cutdown if proximal end is in arm or cardiac catheterization if proximal end is in thorax Place tourniquet on arm above catheter

Modified from Schroeder, J. S., and E. K. Daily: *Techniques in Bedside Hemodynamic Monitoring.* St. Louis: C. V. Mosby Co., 1976, p. 72.

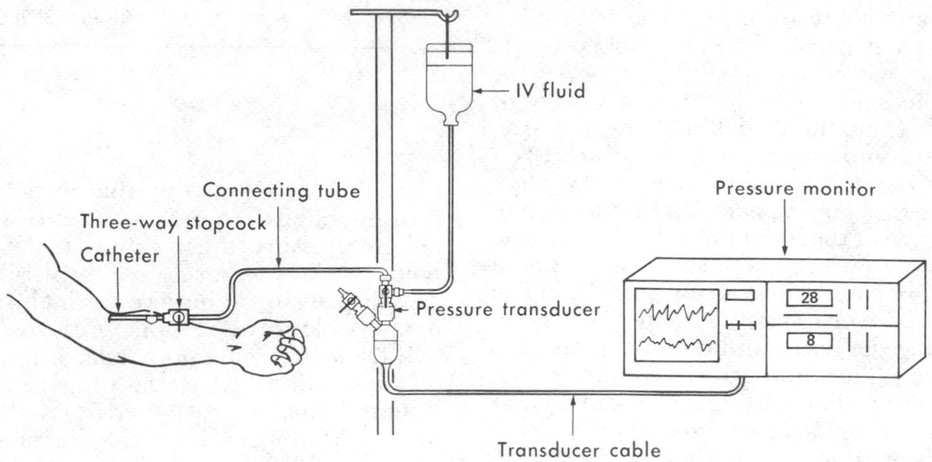

Figure 13–17. Equipment and connections used for intra-arterial monitoring using transducer and oscilloscope. (From Schroeder, J. S., and E. K. Daily: *Techniques in Bedside Hemodynamic Monitoring.* St. Louis: C. V. Mosby Co., 1976, p. 98.)

3. Extensive tubing (Bardic 1750), 30" long with a capacity of 5.8 ml. (4 tubes)
4. Three-way stopcock
5. An arterial catheter
6. Venesection tray
7. An empty sterile bottle
8. A 500 ml. flask (containing saline with heparin) along with intravenous tubing for flush purposes (flush solution)

Procedure (See Fig. 13–19)

1. Extend the intravenous pole to its maximum height.
2. The adhesive tape is marked at successive intervals of 5.4". The bottom line is labeled as zero and each successive interval as 10, 20, 30, etc. Since each 5.4" represents 10 mm. Hg, a reading scale for pressure measurement is available.
3. Secure the calibrated adhesive tape to the length of the intravenous pole with the zero point at the level of the patient's midaxillary line.
4. Connect three extension tubes together and fasten adjoining tubing to the intravenous pole so that one end extends over the top and into an empty sterile bottle and the other end (the male tip) extends free below the zero point for subsequent attachment.
5. The free end of the extension tube and the end of the intravenous tubing from the flush bottle are connected to two of the arms of a 3-way stopcock.
6. The fourth extension tube is attached to the third arm of the stopcock.
7. The entire system is filled with flush solution (the sterile bottle at the top of the tubing will catch the overflow when filling and washing out the tubing).
8. The fourth extension tube (Step 6) is then connected to an arterial catheter that has been placed in the radial artery.
9. The stopcock is turned so that the fluid in the extension tube on the intravenous pole is in continuity with the arterial system.
10. The level of fluid in the long extension tube represents the *mean* arterial blood pressure.
11. When the system is functioning correctly, the fluid level in the extension tube should fluctuate with each heart beat. If this does not occur, the arterial line is partially occluded and flushing is required.

Monitoring Pulmonary Artery Pressures. *Pulmonary artery* (PA) and *pulmonary capillary wedge* (PCW) pressure measurements are obtained in order to assess left heart function and to guide fluid administration. These pressures are measured by the used of a *Swan-Ganz catheter.* This is a flow-directed, balloon-tipped pulmonary artery catheter, which is often inserted through a cutdown in an antecubital vein. The

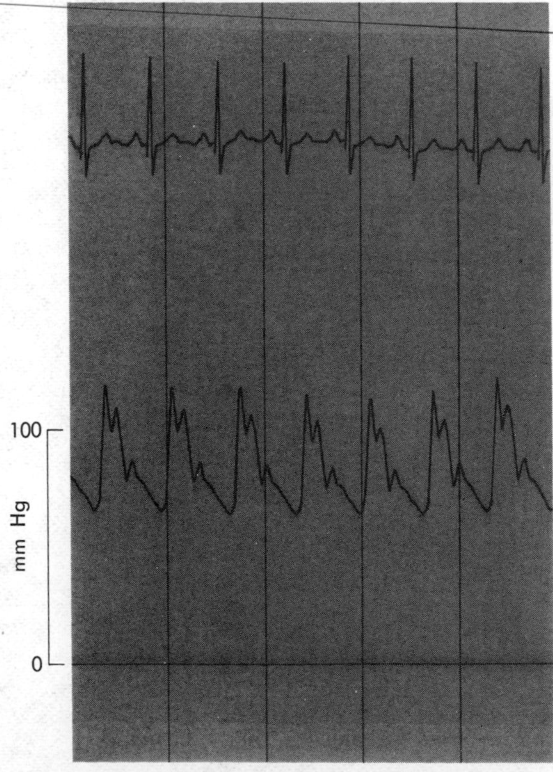

Figure 13–18. Normal peripheral arterial pressure tracing, showing sharp upstroke and clear dicrotic notch. (From Schroeder, J. S., and E. K. Daily: *Techniques in Bedside Hemodynamic Monitoring.* St. Louis: C. V. Mosby Co., 1976, p. 93.)

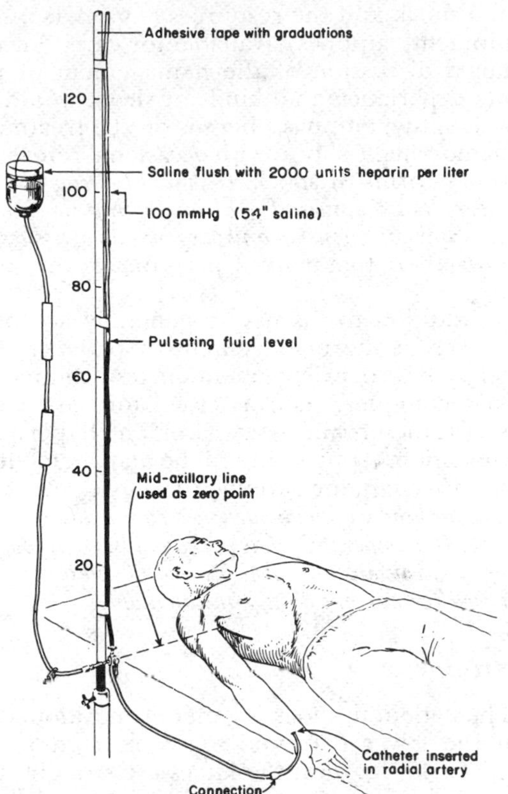

Figure 13–19. Direct measurement of arterial blood pressure. (Modified from Brand, L., and A. P. Thal: Shock. *In* Meltzer, Abdellah and Kitchell: *Concepts and Practices of Intensive Care for Nurse Specialists.* Philadelphia, The Charles Press. 1969.)

catheter is flushed with a heparinized solution and attached to a transducer. The catheter is advanced until the oscilloscope shows a wave pattern typical of the right atrium. The balloon is then inflated, and the catheter flows through the tricuspid valve to the right ventricle and into the pulmonary artery. The catheter then flows into either the left or right branch of the pulmonary artery and stops when it reaches a vessel smaller than the balloon. The progression of the catheter is noted on the oscilloscope. A pulmonary capillary wedge pressure measurement may then be taken, and the balloon is deflated to prevent necrosis.

> Caution:
> *The balloon is inflated only during passage of the catheter into the pulmonary artery and while PCW pressure measurements are being obtained.*

The catheter usually flows back into the pulmonary artery after the balloon is deflated. The PCW pressure corresponds to the left ventricular–end diastolic pressure (LVEDP), which is the pressure in the left ventricle just before contraction. A rise in the end-diastolic pressure in a patient with cardiogenic shock may be indicative of left-sided heart failure. A low value in a patient with hemorrhagic shock may indicate that volume replacement is needed.

> *It is important to remember that hemodynamic changes can be detected through the use of a pulmonary artery catheter, before the patient becomes symptomatic.*

Depending on the catheter used, it is possible to obtain other measurements besides PA and PCW pressures. Some catheters have a thermistor bead just proximal to the balloon. This is used to determine cardiac output by the thermodilution technique. A fourth lumen opens at the level of the right atrium, and CVP measurements can be obtained. A catheter with all four lumens is pictured in Figure 13–20.

Patency of the catheter is obtained either by the use of continuous flush, with a small amount of fluid delivered by a special device attached to the system, or by intermittent flushing.

Some of the *hazards of long-term use of pulmonary artery catheters* include: infection, rupture of the pulmonary artery, pulmonary thrombosis and infarction, knotting of the catheter, and cardiac arrhythmias.[165] Since the catheter is connected to a high-pressure system, special care to prevent

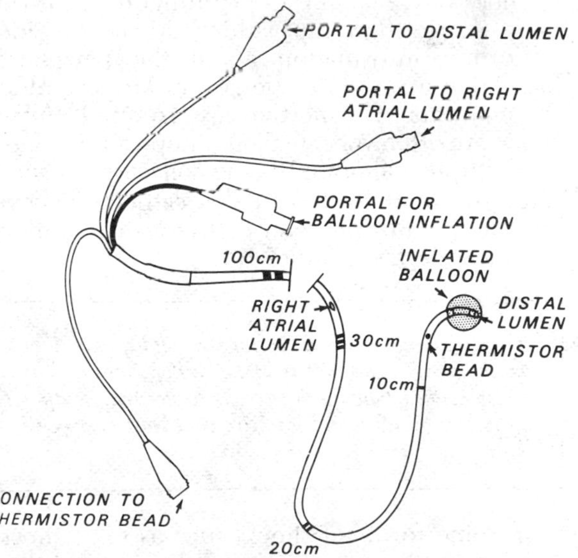

Figure 13–20. Acute hemodynamic monitoring. The features of the Swan-Ganz flow-directed catheter are diagrammed. The distal balloon can be inflated to allow advancement into the pulmonary artery under pressure monitoring alone. The right atrial and distal lumina are utilized for pressure monitoring. The thermistor bead is utilized to determine cardiac output by the thermodilution method. (From Walinsky, P.: Acute hemodynamic monitoring. *Heart and Lung,* 6:838, Sept.–Oct. 1977.)

exsanguination is needed. The reader is referred to the article by Woods for a more thorough discussion of the use of pulmonary artery catheters.[177]

Measuring Cardiac Output.[133, 165] Cardiac output measurements are obtained in order to evaluate the overall cardiac function and the function of the left ventricle. *Cardiac output,* measured in liters per minute, is the amount of blood pumped by the left ventricle into the aorta each minute. Factors that may alter the cardiac output include heart rate, peripheral resistance, age, body size, exercise, and, in patients with cardiac problems, decreased filling or emptying of the left ventricle. In shock patients, the cardiac output may be decreased because of myocardial damage resulting from a myocardial infarction or, in the patient with hypovolemic shock, from inadequate volume replacement.

Cardiac output is determined by either the Fick, indicator-dilution, or the thermodilution methods. These methods are detailed in Chapter 33 (p. 783).

The *thermodilution method* is commonly used when a Swan-Ganz catheter with a thermistor is in place. Because of the widespread use of Swan-Ganz catheters and the ease of performing the measurements, cardiac outputs are being obtained more frequently in patients with all kinds of shock.

Monitoring Urine Output. A bladder catheter is a simple means of monitoring the patient in shock. By enabling the continuous measurement of urine flow, the bladder catheter provides important information about the peripheral blood flow and the function of the kidneys. Since the amounts of urine that are excreted during shock are often very small, it is important to have an accurate, calibrated urine collector. In some settings, the indwelling Foley catheter may be attached to a urinometer collector or to a more complex electric urinometer.

Because changes in urine volume are highly important as an index of the success or failure of therapy, it is recommended that the nurse check the urine output every few minutes and measure it at least every half hour.

In some forms of shock, such as toxic shock, renal shutdown is common and may produce a rapidly increasing state of metabolic acidosis.

Management of Patients in Shock

The nursing and medical management of patients in shock largely depends upon the etiology of the shock and the resources (e.g., personnel, equipment, supplies) available for care. Since a detailed discussion of the management of patients experiencing all kinds of shock would be very lengthy, emphasis here is on the treatment of hemorrhagic shock, with occasional reference to other forms of shock. *It should be remembered, however, that the overall goal in treating shock is to achieve optimal perfusion and oxygenation of tissues.* It follows, then, that many aspects of care are similar.

In addition to discussing generally accepted therapies in the management of patients with shock, we also briefly mention less commonly used techniques, such as circulatory assist devices, the membrane oxygenator, and hyperbaric oxygenation. Approaches to the management of shock are changing rapidly; therefore, *the reader is cautioned that recommended medication dosages may change. It is imperative that package inserts accompanying medications, as well as recent literature, be reviewed for current dosage information.*

POSITIONING

The patient in shock is generally positioned so that the lower extremities are elevated to an angle of 45 degrees; the knees are straight, the trunk is horizontal or very slightly inclined, so that the thorax is lower than the pelvis; and the neck is comfortably positioned, with the head on a level with the chest or slightly higher[142] (Fig. 13–21). The advantage of this position is that it promotes increased venous return from the lower extremities without affecting blood flow through the brain. Elevation of the legs mobilizes the blood pooled in the lower extremities and, by the force of gravity, this additional circulating blood increases venous return to the heart, thereby improving the cardiac output. While this position is of temporary value in moderate oligemia, it is without value in severe oligemia because the extremities would have very little blood in them.

Until recently the Trendelenburg position was recommended in the treatment of shock. The patient was placed in a head-down position with the feet at least 30 cm. higher than the head, in the belief that this position would effectively increase cardiac output by facilitating venous return from the lower extremities and would also improve circulation to the brain. However, the Trendelenburg position is now known to *impair* cardiac output, *decrease* the effectiveness of respiration and, at times, actually *decrease* the circulation to the brain, for three reasons:

1. Trendelenburg position does not facilitate the flow of venous blood from the brain to the right atrium, or the flow of oxygenated blood from the pulmonary blood stream to the left atrium.[18]

2. If too steep, the Trendelenburg position causes the abdominal organs to push against the diaphragm, thereby decreasing the area for pulmonary expansion and decreasing the respiratory pump's effectiveness.[18]

3. Trendelenburg position may initiate aortic and carotid sinus reflexes, causing constriction of the blood vessels supplying the brain and, thus, decrease in blood flow to the brain.[11]

Another point to remember is that the patient with shock is also at risk of developing decubitus ulcers and other problems of immobility at a faster rate, since tissue perfusion is already significantly decreased. *Therefore, attention to turning and positioning the patient is mandatory. However, since these patients also have unstable cardiovascular systems, it is important that the effects of position changes on measurements such as blood pressure, CVP, cardiac rate, and rhythm be observed carefully.* Additionally, although perhaps more difficult to implement, range-of-motion exercises and appropriate positioning devices should be incorporated into the nursing care plan of patients with shock.

It is all too common that patients with life-threatening problems such as shock are adequately resuscitated only to be left with serious deformities that could have been prevented if attention had been given to this aspect of care.

TEMPERATURE

Heat, in any form, should not be applied to the patient in shock.

Heat application causes the peripheral blood vessels to dilate and draws blood back from the vital organs into the vessels of the skin, thus interfering with the body's initial compensatory mechanism of peripheral vasoconstriction. Also, heat increases the body's metabolism, thus increasing the need for oxygen and substrates and thereby putting an added strain on the heart. However, the patient should be kept comfortably warm and never allowed to become chilled.

Elevated body temperatures should be returned to nearly normal if the elevation is serious in degree; however, *hypothermia for the treatment of shock is generally not advisable, since it increases the blood's viscosity and slows the flow of blood through the microcirculation.* Also, hypothermia slows the heart, increases the possibility of ventricular fibrillation, and inhibits the body's reparative processes.

VASOCONSTRICTION AND VASODILATION

For some time a dichotomy of opinion has existed in the treatment of shock concerning the use of *vasopressors,* to *increase* peripheral resistance and systemic blood pressure, and the use of *vasodilators,* to *decrease* peripheral resistance and blood flow. Generally the cardiovascular effects of these two procedures are diametrically opposite. While pressor drugs, e.g., adrenergic drugs (sympathomimetic amines), have been used to elevate the systemic blood pressure, physicians now realize that excessive vasoconstriction may impede, rather than enhance, tissue perfusion.

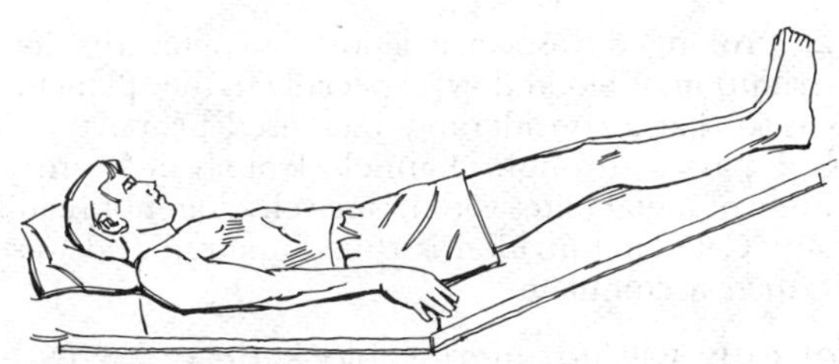

Figure 13–21. Recommended position for the treatment of shock. Legs should be elevated with the knees kept straight and the head should be on a level with, or slightly higher than, the chest. (Modified from Simeone: *American Journal of Nursing,* June, 1966.)

> Mounting laboratory and clinical evidence suggests that pressor drugs are not an unmixed blessing in shock. Their ability to produce an increase in systemic arterial pressure, largely as a result of increased peripheral resistance, offers . . . a sense of security that is often false because the response is unsustained and diverts attention from the lethal mechanisms that are in progress.[49]

As previously indicated, vasoconstriction in various vascular beds (the major effect of pressor drugs) is now accepted as a central feature of the shock syndrome. Interestingly, all the classic signs of shock are also signs of increased sympathetic nervous activity and/or vasoconstriction: pallor; cold, sweating extremities; oliguria; collapsed veins; and slow capillary filling. Physicians and nurses frequently observe, while at the bedside, that *factors that promote vasoconstriction* (e.g., pain, fear, hypoxia) *tend to accentuate the development of shock.* Studies also demonstrate that the infusion of relatively small amounts of epinephrine or norepinephrine causes vasoconstriction, which hastens circulatory failure in shock due to hemorrhage.

On the other hand, controlled experiments show that certain *agents that induce vasodilatation, or inhibit vasoconstriction, significantly increase the survival rate or survival time in shock.* Included in this group of helpful agents are adrenergic blocking agents, ganglionic blocking agents, and direct-acting peripheral vasodilators.

Adrenergic blockade will *prevent* the following harmful effects of prolonged vasoconstriction in shock:

1. Prolonged vasoconstriction increases the pressure in capillaries and thereby promotes a loss of fluid from the vascular to the interstitial compartment.

2. Prolonged vasoconstriction can alter the local distribution of blood flow, especially in the splanchnic area, so that a considerably increased proportion of blood passes through channels from which an exchange of metabolites with tissue cells does not readily occur. Cellular nutrition is thus impaired and waste products accumulate.

Not only will adrenergic blockade prevent the above changes in circulation, it may helpfully induce changes in the opposite direction. As various workers have commented, in the treatment of shock it is easy to lapse into the treatment of the patient's blood pressure per se, rather than focusing therapy on promoting the perfusion of tissues with blood.

In sum, while vasopressor drugs were once believed to be of great value in treating shock, today many practitioners and researchers believe that the basic treatment for many forms of shock is to dilate the peripheral blood vessels (and spare visceral organs from the devastating effects of prolonged vasoconstriction) instead of contributing to the vasoconstriction already present. At present, the value of vasodilators is being carefully considered. However, investigators are optimistic about this form of treatment and believe that it should be included in the armamentarium of shock therapies.

Present Role of Vasopressor Drugs. Although pressor therapy is being critically evaluated at present, it is also cited as having some *favorable effects.* For example, *increased blood flow to the brain and heart* is believed by many to be a desirable outcome of pressor therapy. Such increased blood flow may be particularly beneficial in elderly patients who cannot tolerate prolonged severe hypotension because they have arteriosclerotic narrowing of the coronary or cerebral arteries. The reduced perfusion of tissues with blood, when arterial pressures are below 60 to 70 mm. Hg, may result in myocardial infarction or a cerebral vascular accident.[49]

Perfusion of vital organs is impossible if the systolic blood pressure is below 50 mg. of Hg.

The physician may prescribe a vasopressor agent for brief use if the degree of vasoconstriction in shock is not sufficient to maintain blood flow to vital organs. Pressor drugs may also be used to *correct hypotension that is secondary to paralysis of vasoconstrictor nerves,* e.g., in spinal anesthesia.

Usually the goal of vasopressor therapy is to achieve and maintain a mean blood pressure of 70 to 80 mm. Hg, thus maintaining a blood pressure level that is sufficient to insure perfusion of tissues, rather than to attain normal blood pressures. Generally attempts to increase the blood pressure beyond the recommended level are inadvisable, since these drugs increase the oxygen demand of the heart and may thereby cause death-producing arrhythmias.[19]

Pressor therapy is used for as short a time as possible, for while drugs that cause vasoconstriction may initially be helpful in supplying improved circulation to the heart and brain, prolonged used of these drugs may cause irreversible damage in the tissues of the kidney, liver, lungs, and gastrointestinal tract. Some of the *major adverse effects* of pressor therapy are:[19, 49, 98]

1. Pressor drugs *potentiate the action of endotoxin* (or vice versa).
2. These drugs appear to *cause a further reduction of the blood flow* to the kidneys and *to the entire splanchnic area.*
3. An excessive and/or sudden rise in the arterial blood pressure, which vasopressors could cause, may precipitate *heart failure.*
4. *Overloading of the vascular system* can occur, because pressor drugs must be diluted in rather large volumes of fluid before they are administered. The use of an infusion pump, which enables the controlled delivery of minute amounts of the undiluted drug, is one solution to this problem.
5. *Ventricular arrhythmias* may develop during the administration of pressor drugs. EKG monitoring should be used and the physician notified at once if frequent premature ventricular contractions* are observed.
6. *Pulmonary edema or left ventricular decompensation* can occur. Vasopressors cause a rise in blood pressure as a result of peripheral vessel constriction. This promotes a possibly dangerous overloading of the pulmonary circulation because blood is diverted to the central circulation from peripheral areas. When such problems appear, the IV flow should be slowed to a minimum, the physician should be notified at once, and the head of the bed elevated to reduce respiratory distress.
7. *Tissue sloughing* can result from the extravasation of some vasopressors, e.g., Levophed.

Some of the most commonly used vasopressors are: levarterenol bitartrate (Levophed); metaraminol bitartrate (Aramine); mephentermine sulfate (Wyamine); phenylephrine hydrochloride (Neo-Synephrine); and isoproterenol (Isuprel). Whereas Aramine and Wyamine can be administered either intravenously or intramuscularly, Levophed (probably the most frequently used vasopressor) can be given only intravenously. Levophed should be injected into large and central veins after it has been previously diluted in an intravenous dextrose solution. The intravenous drip should be stopped at once if tissue infiltration occurs. *Since Levophed is so po-*

*See Unit XII for additional information about heart beats.

tent a vasoconstrictor, extravasation into the tissues may cause sloughing and necrosis of the area. If infiltration does occur, the area should be injected with Regitine (phentolamine), a potent vasodilator.

A combination of Levophed and Regitine has recently been proposed by Wilson et al.[172] A solution containing four ampules of Levophed and two ampules of Regitine added to 500 ml. of 5 percent dextrose in water may be administered to patients who are refractory to other vasopressors. The Regitine is used to counteract the profound vasoconstriction caused by Levophed. It also may be effective in preventing tissue necrosis if the IV fluid infiltrates the area. Two ampules of Regitine for each one ampule of Levophed may be used if the patient is profoundly vasoconstricted.[172]

When any vasopressor is administered, the arterial blood pressure should be carefully monitored to watch for undesirable elevations in blood pressure. Flow of the intravenous solution is carefully adjusted to establish and maintain the desired blood pressure.

Remember as you administer these drugs (and other intravenous infusions) that when a patient who is receiving intravenous infusions changes position, the rate of flow of the solution may be altered, causing an undesirable change in the amount of medication being delivered.

Present Role of Vasodilator Drugs. When vasoconstriction is severe and persists despite the infusion of what should be adequate fluid replacement, vasodilators may be helpful. Vasodilators are used on the premise that the peripheral blood vessels are fully constricted during shock owing to the large output of norepinephrine (which occurs as a compensatory action on the part of the body) and that *if this vasoconstriction were inhibited* a beneficial redistribution of blood would occur. The blood trapped peripherally would become available for enhancing tissue perfusion and the vascular volume should be increased.

Peripheral vasoconstriction decreases capillary blood flow and is deleterious in many hypotensive states; conversely, vasodilatation, *after adequate volume addition,* may improve capillary flow, tissue perfusion, and cellular metabolism and thus increase survival rates.

When shock is caused by hypovolemia, rapid and adequate fluid replacement must be achieved before vasodilators are used. Vasodilators are dangerous because they will result in a fall in the arterial blood pressure *if* they are given while circulating blood volume is deficient and the body is depending upon vasoconstriction for arterial pressure. However, if the vascular space is full and the cardiac venous return is adequate, then vasodilatation should result in the opening of arterioles in the lungs and elsewhere, letting the blood through and increasing the cardiac output and capillary perfusion. When a vasodilator is administered *after* adequate filling of the expanded vascular space, the resultant vasodilatation should not cause a systemic blood pressure drop. Indeed, at times a vasodilator may produce a dramatic and sustained rise in the systemic arterial pressure. *It should be remembered that patients with cardiogenic shock following myocardial infarction may also be volume depleted.*[179] If the volume status is unclear, a "fluid challenge" (discussed later) may be administered before vasodilators are given.

Blood pressure and central venous pressure or arterial pressure, if available, should be monitored continuously when vasodilator drugs are being used. Usually a mean blood pressure of 70 is considered acceptable; however, if abrupt severe hypotension should occur, administration of the drug is generally stopped and fluid administration increased.

The CVP will drop substantially if there is a marked decrease in peripheral resistance. The blood volume needs to be expanded as the vascular space enlarges, and CVP measurements are used to gauge the amount of fluid needed to fill the enlarging vascular space. The rate of fluid replacement is adjusted to maintain the desired CVP. If the CVP continues to fall in spite of fluid replacement the situation is *critical,* for this means that the rate and volume of fluid replacement are insufficient to meet the physiologic needs of the patient.

It is important to realize that with vasodilators the tissue perfusion may be improved even though the arterial blood pressure may be lower than normal. Patients receiving vasodilators should be kept in a flat position in bed; elevation of the head could produce a dangerous orthostatic hypotension.

Because of the presence of sclerotic vessels, older patients may not be able to tolerate the hypotension that may accompany treatment of shock with vasodilator drugs. When this is the situation, a cardiogenic drug may be given in combination with the vasodilator to increase the cardiac output and thus help to maintain or raise the blood pressure.

Antiadrenergic drugs appear to have prophylactic value in several types of shock. However, such drugs are potentially dangerous in that they can precipitate lethal complications. Some investigators[49] are evaluating splanchnic autonomic blockade accomplished by the introduction of longacting local anesthetic agents (lidocaine and others) into the retroperitoneal space via paravertebral needle or catheter. This procedure is done in an effort to limit the site of antiadrenergic action to the area of greatest apparent need (the splanchnic area) and thus minimize or avoid the hypotensive effect of total body adrenergic blockade.

Some examples of drugs used to produce vasodilatation and reduce peripheral resistance are: dopamine (Intropin), sodium nitroprusside (Nipride), phentolamine (Regitine), phenoxybenzamine (Dibenzyline) and chlorpromazine (Thorazine).

Dopamine, a fairly new drug used initially for the treatment of cardiogenic shock, has both vasodilator and vasoconstrictor properties. It selectively constricts vessels in skeletal muscles but improves the blood flow to the splanchnic bed and the kidney. It increases cardiac output when administered in doses of 5 to 15 micrograms per kg of body weight per minute. Higher doses (30 to 40 micrograms/kg./min.) result in more profound vasoconstriction.[102] Another advantage of dopamine over agents like isoproterenol is that it produces fewer cardiac arrhythmias.[14] It is essential that a patient have adequate circulating volume before dopamine is administered. Complications associated with dopamine use include: nausea, vomiting, and occasionally, gangrene in patients with pre-existing peripheral vascular disease.[2]

Dobutamine is an agent similar in structure to dopamine; it is currently being evaluated for clinical use.[88]

Sodium nitroprusside is also a new addition to the group of pharmacologic agents used in the management of shock. Its vasodilator properties result from relaxation of vascular smooth muscle, which decreases peripheral resistance and heart work while increasing cardiac output. It is being used in selected patients with cardiogenic shock following myocardial infarction. Although it is not used for patients with shock following trauma, it may be appropriate in the care of patients with myocardial damage following blunt injury to the chest. In general, sodium nitroprusside is used for the shock patient with low cardiac output, high atrial pressure, and increased peripheral resistance.[14, 117]

Sodium nitroprusside is commonly employed as an antihypertensive agent in patients with hypertensive emergencies (e.g., dissecting aortic aneurysm, hypertensive encephalopathy) and in producing controlled hypotension in order to decrease bleeding from wounds and traumatized tissue. This drug is administered by IV drip in *5 percent dextrose/water only.* The solution is light sensitive and must be covered (foil is included in the package). Even when covered, the solution is considered unstable after 4 hours and should be replaced. As with dopamine, patients receiving sodium nitroprusside should have continuous monitoring of the blood pressure and the PA and PCW pressures. Whenever this, or any other vasoactive medication, is administered, there should be an IV flow rate monitor with an alarm attached to the IV tubing to insure constant flow rate. To insure continuous flow, these agents should be administered through a peripheral IV line rather than a CVP line, since the CVP line flow is interrupted frequently during CVP measurements.

Phenoxybenzamine (Dibenzyline) is one of the more powerful antiadrenergic drugs. This medication reduces peripheral resistance by blocking the alpha adrenergic receptors in the walls of the blood vessels so that the blood vessels do not respond to the norepinephrine that is produced during shock. Dibenzyline also reduces the small vessels' responses to histamine and serotonin. The heart's effectiveness is increased when this vasodilator is given because it does not change the cardiac catecholamines, e.g., epinephrine and norepinephrine.

Interest has developed in the use of phenoxybenzamine as a pretreatment for surgical procedures (e.g., open-heart surgery) that are often associated with a postoperative shock-like pattern as a result of poor perfusion of vital tissues during surgery.

As we have indicated, Dibenzyline is likely to cause a further fall in blood pressure if it is given in the presence of hypovolemia, because the adrenergic blockade that it produces will increase the size of the vascular space. However, this can be remedied by giving the medication as a slow drip at the same time that plasma or blood is being given to fill up the increasing vascular space. It is important to remember that the volume of plasma needed to treat shock in such a situation is far in excess of measured losses. In other words, the best clinical results are not obtained by merely replacing estimated plasma losses. If adequate fluid replacement is not given and the Dibenzyline is administered by itself, death will rapidly follow because the blood pressure will drop to disastrously low levels, resulting in respiratory arrest. Dibenzyline may be administered in a dose of 1 mg. per kg. of body weight given intravenously over a 1- to 2-hour period, combined with plasma and blood administration.

Chlorpromazine also antagonizes vasoconstriction during shock. Small doses of chlorpromazine (0.1 to 0.2 mg. per kg. of body weight) have been found to adequately produce the desired alpha adrenergic blockade without the excessive sedation produced by higher doses. As with phenoxybenzamine, chlorpromazine should not be given unless suitable fluid can be administered to fill the expanded space in the vascular compartment that results from adrenergic blockade.[57]

GLUCAGON

Glucagon is a protein secreted by the alpha cells of the islets of Langerhans in the pancreas. It is believed that glucagon raises the blood sugar by stimulating the breakdown of glycogen stores in the liver to form glucose. Glucagon may also play a role in the conversion of amino, fatty, and lactic acids into glucose.[179] Glucagon is sometimes used in the management of diabetic patients with insulin-induced hypoglycemia. Unlike 50% glucose, which must be administered intravenously, glucagon may be given intramuscularly, subcutaneously, or intravenously. While 50% glucose is the preferred agent in the management of insulin shock, it is sometimes difficult to find a vein in which to give the glucose because patients are often profoundly vasoconstricted. Therefore, glucagon may be used as a temporary measure to raise the blood sugar until hypertonic glucose can be administered.

Glucagon may also be used in patients with other types of shock. We have mentioned that the energy stores are depleted in the shock patient. The depletion is a result of both increased cellular need for glucose (because of increased activity) and decreased production of glucose during anaerobic metabolism. It seems reasonable that agents which mobilize stored glucose would be helpful. Additionally, glucagon has been found to be of value in increasing cardiac output and stroke volume while decreasing peripheral and splanchnic bed resistance in experimental animals.[179] When used for improving cardiovascular function, glucagon may be used alone or in combination with various pressor agents discussed previously. Although there appears to be theoretical basis for its use, glucagon is employed primarily when there has been no response to other therapies and the prognosis is grave.

GLUCOSE

The use of hypertonic (50%) glucose in the management of patients with shock other than insulin shock has gained much interest in the past several years. The rationale is based on the increased demand for glucose during shock, as discussed above. Although hypertonic glucose is not routinely used in the management of shock at this time, clinical and research studies indicate that it may be of value when combined with an appropriate fluid regimen in patients with hemorrhagic shock.[31] It appears that the effectiveness of hypertonic glucose administration in the management of patients with shock warrants further investigation.

ADRENOCORTICOIDS

The early use of adrenocortical hormones in the treatment of shock was based on pioneer demonstrations that, under stress, the adrenocortical function increases. However, as yet the precise mechanisms that underlie the action of these hormones remain unidentified.[131]

Today many investigators recommend the administration of large doses of adrenocorticoids in the treatment of shock. However, while glucocorticoids (e.g., cortisone, hydrocortisone)* have an established place in the treatment of some types of shock, the therapeutic indications for use of the mineralocorticoids (e.g., aldosterone and desoxycorticosterone) have *not* been satisfactorily established.[131]

*Examples of synthetic glucocorticoids are prednisone, prednisolone, methylprednisolone, triamcinolone, and dexamethasone.

Experimental evidence indicates that adrenocorticoids may exert cardiotonic (e.g., increased cardiac output) as well as vascular effects. Glucocorticoids may counteract the reduced cardiac output and the accompanying increased total resistance to blood flow that are the two basic hemodynamic inadequacies of shock. Thus, corticosteroids may be administered in the treatment of shock on the basis that they increase blood flow and decrease blood resistance, thereby augmenting the beneficial effects of vasopressor agents. When given large doses of glucocorticoids, patients in shock may maintain a more adequate blood pressure level owing to improved systemic blood flow. Inactive pools of venous blood evidently cause reduced cardiac output in toxic shock; adrenocorticoids seem to contribute toward mobilizing such pools.[131]

The *antitoxic effect* of the adrenocorticoids is another reason for their use in the treatment of shock.[131] In addition, it is known that steroids *stabilize the lysosomal membrane* and prevent the intracellular release of enzymes. Also, they *increase blood volume* by increasing sodium retention.

When steroid therapy is used in managing shock, it is agreed that the dosages should be in pharmacologic quantities rather than merely in the range of replacement therapy. At least 3000 mg. of hydrocortisone per day is recommended by some.[19] Some typical dosage schedules of corticoids in treating shock follow.[131]

1. Intravenous doses of 500 mg. hydrocortisone (Solu-Cortef), and 100 mg. prednisolone or methylprednisolone (Hydeltrasol, Solu-Medrol), or 20 mg. dexamethasone (Decadron) may be used every 4 to 6 hours for a period usually not exceeding 3 to 5 days.
2. The initial injection is twice the amount listed above, i.e., 1 Gm. of cortisol, 200 mg. of prednisolone, or 40 mg. of dexamethasone.
3. Some physicians prefer direct, slow, intravenous injection to a more prolonged infusion by intravenous drip.
4. A gradual reduction of dosage is not necessary for corticoid treatment of such short duration, it may be stopped abruptly.
5. Doses of corticoids smaller than those listed above may prove inadequate in treating shock.

Adrenocortical hormones provide *specific* treatment for those rare instances of shock that are due to adrenal insufficiency, e.g., addisonian crisis.

Some *general* situations in which adrenocortical therapy might prove helpful include: (1) the treatment of cases of protracted hypotension associated with severe allergic (hypersensitivity) reactions, and (2) counteracting the detrimental effects of gram-negative endotoxins. Steroids improve the survival rate of patients in shock from gram-negative bacterial infection of the blood stream. In such circumstances the drug must be given in very high doses.

In spite of advances in treatment, the mortality rate in gram-negative shock remains at about 50 per cent.

Considerable interest is being expressed in the role of corticoids in combination with vasopressor agents in treating shock. Some believe that the efficiency of the hormones appears to be much greater if they are given in combination with various pressor agents.

There is some evidence that steroids may be helpful in minimizing pulmonary damage associated with shock because of their antiplatelet aggregating effect.

The conventional clinical practice of administering corticosteroids only as a final and desperate measure after vasopressor therapy has failed is not recommended.[131] When used, corticosteroids should be administered early in the course of shock, rather than as a last resort after other medications have proved unsuccessful.[19]

Several theoretical dangers to the patient may accompany steroid therapy in the high dosage ranges used in treating shock: acute gastrointestinal bleeding; the aggravation of diabetes; and inhibition of the antibody response, thereby making possible uncontrollable infection. Since patients receiving high doses of steroids are susceptible to infection, they should be protected in every way from potential sources of infection. The prevention of pneumonia, wound infection, and bacteremia should be kept in mind. Also, excretions (e.g., vomitus, urine, feces) from patients receiving large steroid doses should be examined for blood, since steroids can induce internal bleeding.

HEPARIN*

The anticoagulant effect of heparin may be desirable in either the prevention or the treatment of some of the complications of shock. Heparin is commonly employed in the treatment of patients with myocardial infarction because there is a tendency for small thrombi to form on or near large areas of infarct, and these can mobilize, resulting in systemic emboli. Heparin is also used because of the prolonged immobility that is often associated with shock. The treatment of disseminated intravascular clotting (DIC) may include heparin in an effort to minimize consumption of clotting factors, and heparin may be appropriate in the management of patients with ARDS if the primary cause of the respiratory insufficiency is believed to be the result of massive microembolism or DIC.

There is no specific dosage appropriate for the management of all the problems discussed above, and the dosage is usually adjusted according to the clotting studies. It is important, however, that the patient receiving heparin be assessed frequently for signs of excessive anticoagulation. The patient's skin should be observed for evidence of petechiae or purpura, and gastric contents, urine, and stool should be tested for occult blood.

*Further information can be found in references 14, 21, 36, 45, 62, 172, and 179.

CALCIUM

It has been a fairly common belief in the past several years that patients with hemorrhagic shock and massive blood loss are at great risk of developing hypocalcemia as a result of receiving large amounts of banked whole blood, administered rapidly. This is because the citrate in stored blood binds with the calcium in that blood. For this reason, it has been common practice to administer 1 Gm. of 10% calcium chloride slowly for every two to four units of whole blood received.[172] Recent research findings, however, indicate that the calcium levels obtained through current laboratory procedures may not be a true reflection of the amount of calcium available for use, and the need for calcium replacement in such doses is being seriously re-evaluated. It is believed that calcium replacement may be appropriate in the patient being massively transfused at a rate of one unit of blood every 5 minutes.[23] In addition, calcium may be administered to patients who demonstrate impaired cardiovascular function in other forms of shock. (Calcium should be given with extreme caution in patients who have been given digitalis, as it may precipitate digitalis toxicity.)

The nurse should be aware that *calcium chloride should be given IV only, whereas calcium gluconate may be given IM.* It is, however, very irritating to tissues. Although calcium chloride and calcium gluconate are both available as 10 per cent solutions, they are not identical in concentration and should not be used as equivalents; calcium gluconate contains fewer calcium ions than calcium chloride.

Signs of hypocalcemia may be subtle, and careful assessment of the patient is essential. Calcium is needed for normal function of the cardiovascular and nervous systems and for clotting. Indicators of hypocalcemia may include alterations in level of consciousness, irritability, increased (hyperactive) deep tendon reflexes, difficulty speaking, hypotension, and cardiac arrhythmias. The presence of *Trousseau's sign* (evidenced by flexion of the forearm when a BP cuff has been inflated on the upper arm for 5 minutes at a pressure halfway between the systolic and diastolic blood pressures) or a positive *Chvostek's sign* (spasm of the facial muscles as a result of tapping the facial nerve in front of the ear) is usually indicative of a significant hypocalcemia. Clotting disorders are usually not apparent until the calcium level is extremely low.

NARCOTICS

While a need for pain relief may be evident in patients with different types of shock, the use of narcotics for pain management is not without hazard. Narcotics interfere with vasoconstriction, which may be the only way the patient is able to sustain adequate blood pressure.

> *Administration of narcotics (e.g., morphine, meperidine) to a patient suffering from acute, multiple trauma prior to ascertaining that blood volume is adequate may cause an increased vascular capacitance, resulting in severe hypotension or shock.*[173]

Also, when narcotics are administered intramuscularly in the patient with shock, absorption may be incomplete because of vasoconstriction. Since the patient has experienced little or no pain relief a second injection may be given. After fluid restitution and restoration of circulating volume, both doses of narcotics may be absorbed and the patient may go back into shock.

It is all too common that patients who are restless, especially trauma victims, are given narcotics because their behavior is interpreted as resulting from pain. In many patients, however, the restlessness is actually due to hypoxia, and narcotics serve only to compound the problem. Since the decision to administer narcotics is often a nursing one, it is important that the need for these drugs be carefully assessed. *Attention to positioning, splinting of injured areas, breathing techniques,*[145] *and comfort measures may be safer and more effective than narcotics.*

If narcotics are appropriate for the shock patient, they should be administered intravenously in small doses. When caring for trauma patients, especially those with massive injury, the nurse is cautioned about equating tissue damage with pain. At times, observers may think injuries are causing pain, whereas, in fact, the patient's perception is of only discomfort. When narcotics are believed to be medically prudent the patient should be consulted before pain relief is administered, e.g., asked if he needs pain relief. The blood pressure should be monitored more closely immediately after IV administration of narcotics.

When surgery is imminent, the anesthesiologist or anesthetist should be involved in decisions about narcotic administration. It is not uncommon to combine preoperative medications with narcotics in order to achieve adequate pain relief and optimal preoperative sedation. *When patients are medicated with narcotics prior to being transported to another facility, it is important that the kind, dose, and route of administration of narcotics be clearly communicated to the receiving personnel and noted on the transfer sheet.* It is advisable to circle this information with red ink so that it is readily visible. For legal reasons, the patient should sign an operative permit before a narcotic is administered; many states consider the permit to be invalid if signed by a patient under the influence of a narcotic or mind-altering drug.

> *In summary, narcotics may be appropriate in relieving pain in patients with shock; however, the need for these agents should be considered carefully. In general, narcotics should be given IV in small doses, and the fact that they have been received by the patient noted clearly.*

ANTIBIOTICS

When shock is due to an infection, antibiotic therapy is highly important and must be instituted immediately. When bacteremic shock is suspected, a blood specimen for culture and sensitivity is taken at once, and then antibiotics are started even though the infecting organism has not been identified. At the same time that the blood sample is drawn, samples of urine, sputum, and any fluid from draining wounds, sinuses, and so forth, should be taken for culture. Since toxic shock is often caused by gram-negative enteric bacteria, a combination of ampicillin, polymyxin, and cephalothin may be used until the findings of the cultures and sensitivities are available.[19]

Shires et al. advocate the use of antibiotics, along with appropriate surgical management, in hypovolemic shock patients with open or potentially contaminated wounds. They recommend 1 to 5 million units of penicillin per 24 hours and parenteral tetracycline in doses of 1 to 2 Gm. for the first 24 hours. Antibiotic therapy is initiated in the emergency department.[140]

CARDIAC SUPPORT

Medications that will improve myocardial contraction are basic in treating those forms of shock that cause a decreased cardiac output, e.g., hypovolemic shock and cardiogenic shock. (See also Unit XII). Various medications may be employed to improve cardiac efficiency:

Digitalis is frequently used if there is evidence of cardiac failure. By strengthening and slowing the heart beat, digitalis gives support to a weakened heart and may reduce the rate of heart beats to a more normal level. *Ouabain* and *deslanoside (Cedilanid D)* are examples of rapidly acting digitalis preparations that may be given intravenously early in the course of shock. These medications are not given to patients who are already digitalized. In addition to being given to treat patients with pre-existing or present evidence of cardiac failure, digitalis is indicated for patients with increased central venous pressure, digitalis-responsive arrhythmias, and, controversially, in myocardial infarction.

Isoproterenol (Isuprel) is more effective than digitalis in strengthening the force of myocardial contraction and thus improving cardiac output, however, it also increases the oxygen needs of the heart and an increase in the size of a myocardial infarct may result. Because of this, isoproterenol is not routinely used in the management of patients with cardiogenic shock secondary to an MI. Isoproterenol may be employed to increase the heart rate if a bradycardia is present. This agent also is a peripheral vasodilator so it is important that the patient have an adequate circulating volume in order to prevent a worsening of the hypotension.

Quinidine and *procainamide* may be given to treat arrhythmias that tend to reduce cardiac efficiency. These medications, however, do reduce myocardial contractility.

Atropine may be used for bradycardias, which predispose to cardiogenic shock.

For a further discussion of medications used to improve cardiac efficiency see Unit XII, on the heart. The precautions necessary in using such medications should be observed as detailed in that unit.

Continuous cardiac monitoring is desirable, particularly if beta-mimetic adrenergic drugs are being administered. The use of vasopressor drugs in treating myocardial infarction is controversial. Phlebotomy may be employed to treat cardiac failure.

Cardiac support through the use of circulatory assist devices is discussed later.

RENAL SUPPORT

Impaired kidney function and acute renal tubular necrosis may result from shock, as we have discussed earlier. Thus, oliguria is often a concomitant of shock. Simeone comments:

> In the early phase of the shock immediately subsequent to severe burns, trauma, and hemorrhage, the subnormal urinary output can be corrected by restoring the circulating blood volume to normal and by providing the normal daily requirements of water and electrolytes. However, in other forms of shock (septic shock, in particular), late in severe burns, and in oligemic shock which has progressed into the late phase, restoration of normal circulating blood volume and composition may not correct the oliguria or anuria. Indeed, the cardiovascular failure may no longer exist, while the oliguria progresses to a lethal anuria.[142]

In an attempt to prevent acute renal damage the urine output is monitored with an indwelling catheter and osmotic diuretics, e.g., urea and mannitol, may be given. The correction of metabolic acidosis and the utilization of other measures to increase blood volume and improve cardiac output will also benefit the kidney as well as other tissues. If tubular necrosis is present, peritoneal or hemodialysis may be needed until the regeneration of functioning renal tubular epithelium can take place.

Mannitol is the reduced form of the 6-carbon sugar mannose; it is filtered in the urine and is neither reabsorbed nor metabolized. Mannitol acts as an osmotic diuretic and, thus, helps to rid the body of hemolyzed cells and other wastes that accumulate in the renal tubules. By restoring to active circulation the fluid that was lost (due to the block of the microcirculation), mannitol helps to alleviate the microcirculatory block in shock. Large amounts of hemoglobin or myoglobin may be in the circulation during shock. At the glomerular level these substances are filtered, and if the urinary flow is inadequate (because of the pronounced water reabsorption that occurs during shock) these substances will precipitate in the tubule. By maintaining an adequate output of urine, mannitol helps to prevent tubular damage.

Furosemide (Lasix) has also been recommended for similar use (instead of mannitol) in patients with oliguria or in whom oliguria is anticipated.

RESPIRATORY SUPPORT

The patient in shock must be checked immediately to be certain that the airway is open and functioning. If necessary, ensure ventilation by mouth-to-mouth breathing. Circulatory improvement depends on adequate respiratory function, for the arterial blood must be oxygenated by the lung and carbon dioxide must be exchanged into the atmosphere in order to help to correct the metabolic acidosis that develops with shock. By increasing the rate of pulmonary ventilation (by spontaneous or mechanical hyperventilation) it is possible to correct *minor* degrees of metabolic acidosis. The "blowing off" of carbon dioxide into the expired air results in a return of the blood pH to normal.[142]

The pCO_2 is measured to determine whether the metabolic acidosis is being effectively combated by hyperventilation: a low pCO_2 along with low pH and bicarbonate levels (metabolic acidosis) indicates that hyperventilation is compensating; a rising pCO_2 in the presence of a persistently low pH indicates that respiratory assistance will be needed because hyperventilation is failing. As hyperventilation fails, the patient's rate and depth of respiration decline and cyanosis appears. In this situation the accumulated carbon dioxide can be removed only with a respirator to assist ventilation; oxygen administration is valueless.

Brand and Thal observe that some powerful respirators can convert respiratory acidosis to respiratory alkalosis in 10 to 30 minutes.[19]

The most commonly used ventilators in the management of patients with respiratory failure are the volume respirators with alarm devices. It may be necessary to suppress the patient's respiratory effort in order to achieve maximum ventilation. Suppression is done by giving the patient paralyzing agents. At this point the patient may be completely awake but dependent upon the nursing staff for all activities.

Some of the causes of respiratory failure in shock besides those discussed earlier are:[49]

- Respiratory overload due to fever, infection and/or metabolic acidosis.
- Cerebral arterial insufficiency which obtunds the gag and cough reflexes as well as the respiratory center's sensitivity.
- Stupor, coma or aspiration of gastric contents, causing airway obstruction.
- Physical exhaustion from long, severe illness existing before the onset of shock or resulting from the shock episode itself. The patient in shock works hard to move air in and out of the lungs.

To relax the exhausted patient in severe or prolonged shock, and to correct respiratory failure, treatment often needs to include tracheal intubation or tracheostomy. An endotracheal tube may be used or a cuffed tracheostomy tube may be inserted following tracheostomy. The ventilatory dead space is reduced by a tracheostomy, and more thorough tracheobronchial hygiene can be performed. Intubation or tracheostomy may be followed promptly by an increase in blood pressure.

In all cases of shock, regardless of cause, the patient must receive supplemental oxygen for protection against hypoxemia. Oxygen concentrations above 30 per cent appear adequate to protect against hypoxemia. The prolonged administration of 100 per cent oxygen is contraindicated because of the danger of inducing oxygen toxicity. Usually the lowest concentration of oxygen that will maintain a pO_2 of 60 mm. Hg or higher is prescribed, since high oxygen concentrations are known to be damaging to the lung.

In treating shock, oxygen may be indicated to correct hypoxia caused by disorders such as pneumonia and cardiac failure.

In patients who are developing Adult Respiratory Distress Syndrome (ARDS) following shock, it may be necessary to add continuous positive end-expiratory pressure (PEEP) ventilation to the other respiratory support measures. As you may remember, ARDS is associated with collapse of the alveoli. One of the causes of alveolar collapse is damage to the type II alveolar cells which produce surfactant. Since surfactant production is decreased or absent, the alveoli collapse. This collapse contributes to the hypoxemia because nonventilated lung segments are perfused and arteriovenous shunts develop.

In an effort to open up the alveoli and keep them open, PEEP has been included in the ventilator system. The amount of PEEP required to achieve and maintain an adequate arterial oxygen tension varies with the patient; however, 5 to 15 cm. of water is commonly used. Sugerman et al. have reported that "improvement in arterial oxygen tension with continuous positive end-expiratory pressure ventilation occurs within 5 minutes and approaches an early maximum within 15 minutes. A subsequent progressive improvement then occurs over hours and days, permitting a further reduction in inspired oxygen tension and the level of PEEP."[117]

There may be a fall in blood pressure and cardiac output when PEEP is used, so it is recommended that arterial monitoring be utilized. Pneumothorax has also been reported. PEEP may increase intracranial pressure, which may be dangerous. It is essential that patients receiving PEEP have constant nursing supervision, as well as a ventilator with a fail-safe alarm system.

In addition to the respiratory support measures mentioned above, the patient should also receive vigorous pulmonary toilet and chest physical therapy including vibration, percussion, and clapping. These aspects of care are discussed in Unit XVI.

FLUID REPLACEMENT

Most forms of shock (including cardiogenic shock in some instances) involve a decreased effective circulating blood volume, owing to the external or internal loss of whole blood, plasma, and/or relatively protein-free plasma water. Recognizing this fact, the mainstay of shock therapy has been established as the expansion of the circulating blood volume by the intravenous administration of blood or other appropriate fluids.

Various fluids are given to correct specific problems, such as electrolyte or protein deficiencies or other defects of the blood, including acidosis and hyponatremia. However, in treating shock, the *immediate* results of therapy seem to depend less on the type of fluid used for fluid replacement than upon the *amount* of fluid administered. Generally enough fluid is given so that the normal blood volume is exceeded. In part, this "extra" fluid is required because of the expanded vascular space caused by the dilation of the microcirculation. Therapy must be monitored to prevent circulatory overload. Hypervolemia can be lethal.

In replacing fluids, enough volume must be added to fill the capillaries and run through into the veins. Such fluid replacement maintains the central venous pressure and provides an adequate venous return to the heart, which, in turn, promotes additional cardiac output. In addition, adequate fluid replacement will decrease the blood catecholamine level and thus produce a physiologic vasodilatation that promotes capillary flow. This adequate flow of fluids in the capillaries, in turn, perfuses tissues and prevents sludging and coagulation within the vessels.

As we have indicated earlier, a phase of *hypercoagulability* occurs in several forms of shock, producing intravascular thrombosis. Indeed, such clotting of the blood within the capillaries may begin quite early in the hypotensive period. It has been observed in experimentally produced ventricular fibrillation that minute clots appear in the circulating blood and pulmonary capillaries if resuscitation is delayed beyond 5 minutes. In traumatic shock, thrombi occur in the region of the crushed tissue; in hemorrhagic shock, thrombi appear in the vascular beds of the lungs, liver, intestines, kidneys, and other tissues.[87]

Thus, an important aspect in preventing irreversible shock is treatment that prevents hypercoagulability in the blood or that promotes the lysis of thrombi that have already formed. Heparin has been observed to prolong survival time or to reduce the mortality rate in toxic shock, acute circulatory arrest, and hemorrhagic shock, as well as in those forms of shock resulting from the administration of incompatible blood or amniotic fluid. In hemorrhagic shock the dissolution of clots by fibrinolysin therapy may at times avert irreversibility even though intravascular coagulation has occurred.[87]

Patients in shock may have multiple clotting defects involving deficiencies of several clotting factors. Fibrinogen often is high, indicating that an increase in the manufacturing of this element has exceeded the increase in its utilization. Other factors are typically decreased and may become extremely low, resulting in a tendency to hemorrhage and serious capillary bleeding. Platelet defects are also common in shock. The *rapid* administration of fresh whole blood or fresh frozen plasma may quickly and effectively treat the coagulation and platelet defects.

Whole Blood Replacement.* If hemorrhage is the primary cause of shock, the rapid administration of large volumes of whole blood may be necessary. The blood will act as a hypothermic agent unless it is warmed to body temperature. This can be hazardous in the presence of shock, because slowing of cardiac action, with decreased cardiac output or ventricular fibrillation, may result if body temperatures fall below 32° C.[19] In addition, it has been recognized that there is platelet and other particle aggregation in stored blood. Special blood filters, in addition to the standard blood filters, are usually added to the IV tubing in hopes of minimizing multiple thrombi and their possible contribution to ARDS. These filters may have to be changed every one or two units of whole blood. It becomes more difficult to pump blood at a rapid rate when special filters are in-line; therefore, the advantages of the filters must be weighed against the disadvantages. The problem of platelet aggregation does not appear to be as significant when fresh blood (less than 24 hours old) is used.[43, 93, 123]

When treating shock resulting from hemorrhage, crystalloid, e.g., Ringer's lactate, normal saline, is usually given as an initial emergency treatment to sustain blood pressure. The acute anemia, resulting from the hemorrhage, must then be corrected by replacement with whole blood to prevent hypoxemia. The physician determines the amount of blood to be given by evaluating the patient's clinical response and hematocrit. A helpful guide in determining the amount of blood to order initially is that one unit of blood is needed to raise the hematocrit by three points. For example, if the normal Hct. is 40 and the patient's Hct. is 31, then three units of blood should be ordered. Blood volume studies are also evaluated when they are available.

In fluid replacement a normal red blood cell mass should be maintained; however, fluids that are given in excess of normal volume should be fluids other than blood to allow for their easy removal from the circulation once shock is over. If the normal red blood cell mass is exceeded, it is difficult for the body to get rid of the excess when the vascular volume contracts back to normal after adequate perfusion of the tissues is achieved. Also, since there are dangers involved in blood transfusions, blood should not be used as long as another fluid can satisfactorily maintain an adequate oxygen-carrying capacity and sufficiently increase blood volume. Ringer's lactate or other fluids can be as effective as blood in increasing blood volume.

In the past it has been presumed that colloids (e.g., albumin or plasma) remain in the vascular

*For additional information on the administration of whole blood see Unit XIV and Chapter 39 of Sorensen and Luckmann, *Basic Nursing: A Psychophysiologic Approach.*

tree longer than crystalloids and are therefore preferable. Recent research, however, indicates that colloids are rapidly equilibrated into the total extracellular fluid and their effectiveness as blood volume substitutes is transient at best.[140]

Plasma Expanders. Fluids that contain molecules large enough to be retained in the blood vessels are necessary in the treatment of shock in which plasma loss is excessive, e.g., burns, acute pancreatitis, and peritonitis. Plasma, electrolyte solutions containing albumin, or dextran of high or low molecular weight may be administered.

Plasma is sometimes used in the management of patients with low serum protein levels in an effort to control fluid escape from the vascular system; however, the risk of hepatitis is significant, since the plasma is pooled. Fresh frozen plasma, which does not involve the same risk of hepatitis, is also used to improve serum protein levels. It may be administered after massive transfusions, in order to restore some of the clotting factors that are deficient in "banked" blood. Because fresh frozen plasma requires time to thaw (15 to 30 minutes), it is not used in the initial resuscitation of patients with hemorrhagic shock.

Albumin (Plasmanate) may also be used to achieve adequate osmotic pressure. Occasionally, it is administered when sufficient amounts of Ringer's lactate are unsuccessful in restoring circulating volume. The use of albumin is controversial in that the albumin may move into the pulmonary interstitial space, drawing water along with it, thereby contributing to the development of ARDS.

The once popular high and low molecular weight dextrans are also very controversial at present. Since they are large sized molecules, it seems logical that they would be effective in rapidly expanding the intravascular volume and thus would be desirable. There are, however, several significant problems associated with both high and low molecular weight dextrans, including severe allergic (antigen-antibody) reactions,[140] interference with blood type and crossmatch procedures, and interference with clotting mechanisms. Because of these problems, dextran is used infrequently in the acute management of hemorrhagic shock. If dextran must be used, because of the patient's religious beliefs regarding blood transfusions or because of the unavailability of blood, it is suggested that no more than 1.5 liters be administered in a 24 hour period.[6] If it is anticipated that blood will be administered, blood samples for type and crossmatch *must be obtained before the dextran is administered.*

Balanced Electrolyte Solutions. During oligemic shock the loss of circulating blood volume is associated with a redistribution of extravascular fluid. Thus, a sizable amount* of fluid leaves the extravascular, extracellular space *in addition* to the fluid lost from the circulating volume as a result of hemorrhage. In fluid replacement therapy, therefore, *both* the deficit of whole blood lost from the circulation and the additional fluid lost from the extravascular space must be replaced in the form of lactated Ringer's solution or other balanced saline solutions.[142] When the loss of free water has been great (as in burns) 5% dextrose in water may be given, since fluid replacement with dextrose solution is preferable to salt solutions in order to avoid electrolyte overloading.[19]

*This extravascular loss can amount to some 4 liters in moderately severe shock.

When severe metabolic acidosis is present, a buffer often needs to be added to the circulating blood, e.g., tris-(hydroxymethyl)aminomethane (THAM), or sodium bicarbonate.[142] (THAM is a complex organic agent.) It should be remembered that solutions containing sodium are frequently contraindicated in cardiac disorders. Sometimes large quantities of normal saline may be administered in treating shock.

Electrolyte solutions such as Ringer's lactate or saline buffered with bicarbonate help expand extracellular volume, reduce viscosity and prevent sludging.[19] In the past it has been felt that a solution containing lactate, e.g., Ringer's lactate, would further compound the problem of lactic acidosis. The results of many research efforts now reveal that Ringer's lactate *does not* increase serum lactate levels and does not contribute to metabolic acidosis.[6, 140, 179] In fact, lactated Ringer's solution has recently been advocated for the initial treatment of shock because it contains the electrolyte content that the kidney requires to function adequately.[6, 140, 163, 179] This solution is frequently given by intravenous infusion, for rapid expansion of the vascular volume.[19]

Specific abnormalities of electrolyte and acid-base balance are corrected as they are identified. Therapy is gauged by serial arterial pH determinations (see Chapter 12).

Care of the Patient Receiving Fluid Replacement for Shock. In a majority of cases of shock, fluid replacement is the only treatment required. In some instances up to 8 to 12 liters of fluid may be administered in only a few hours. As mentioned earlier, the volume of fluid given generally exceeds estimates of blood or fluid loss or volume deficit.

Often it is difficult to evaluate whether the fluid replacement is adequate. Internal losses of circulating fluid volume, including whole blood, into areas of trauma, infection, and so forth, are most difficult to estimate and, if a vasoconstrictor drug has been administered or if vasoconstriction has persisted for a considerable length of time, an additional considerable loss of circulating volume may have occurred as a result of the vasoconstriction.[109] The volume of fluid administered may be pushed until either (1) systemic blood pressure, urine volume, and lactate levels return to a relatively normal level or (2) central venous or pulmonary artery pressures, or both, become elevated. In patients with hemorrhagic shock it is quite common to infuse 1 to 2 liters of Ringer's lactate in the first 30 to 45 minutes.

Central venous pressure (CVP) measurement is one of the first steps in the treatment of shock since it is an important means of estimating fluid loss. The infusion of blood or other fluids is usually continued only as long as the CVP is low, below 10 cm.; when the CVP is higher than normal (e.g., above 15 cm.), benefit cannot be expected from the continued infusion of fluids or blood. When the CVP is low and the patient's lungs are clear, with no signs of cardiac asthma or left ventricular failure, fluids are administered to improve the return of blood to the heart. However, there are patients who have a normal or low CVP in spite of faulty left ventricular function; these patients readily develop pulmonary edema or cardiac asthma. Thus, a low or normal CVP does not always mean that fluid administration is advisable.[142]

The administration of fluids should be stopped prior to extremely high elevations of *pulmonary artery pressure* if an adequate systemic response has been achieved. An adequate volume of fluid causes an adequate venous return to the right heart with the result that the output of the right heart will be increased. If there is continued pulmonary obstruction due to coagulation in the microcirculation and vasoconstriction, then pulmonary artery hypertension may result; this would be reflected in the pulmonary artery pressure. In the presence of right heart failure this increase in pressure may back up through the right heart, causing an abnormal elevation in the central venous pressure. Vasodilators may be helpful in opening this partially blocked pulmonary microcirculation.

It is obvious from these discussions that an important nursing responsibility is the maintenance of a reliable IV line. Since you, as a nurse, may be the first person to recognize impending shock and begin treatment, you need to know certain considerations in the selection and placement of IV catheters. They include:

- Use the largest around-the-needle catheter available; a 16 gauge is the smallest size acceptable in adult patients with hemorrhagic shock.
- The length of time required to rapidly infuse IV fluids is directly related to the length and diameter of the catheter (see Table 13–11).
- Use around-the-needle catheters rather than through-the-needle catheters. When through-the-needle catheters are used, leakage around the catheter may occur since the hole in the vein is larger than the outside diameter of the catheter. The problem becomes especially great when fluids are being infused under pressure.
- At least two IV lines should be started in patients in shock. Place IV's as far distal as possible (the hand may be used) in order to allow room for placement of future IV and intra-arterial (IA) lines.
- Use local anesthesia (lidocaine) when inserting large catheters.
- IV placement in the lower extremities is to be avoided unless no arm veins are accessible or the patient has massive chest injury with probable damage to the superior vena cava.
- Avoid inserting IV catheters over joints.
- Use excellent aseptic technique when inserting and caring for IV catheters; don't assume that "antibiotics will take care of the infection."
- Label all IV sites with the size catheter, date, and time.
- Label all tubing, especially CVP and arterial lines.

> Caution:
> *Never use scalp vein or straight needles in a patient with shock because needles are unstable and penetrate vein walls. It is critical that a reliable avenue for IV fluid administration be maintained.*

NASOGASTRIC SUCTION

You may remember that one of the early physiologic responses in the shock state is a de-

TABLE 13–11. INFUSION TIME FOR 1 LITER OF LACTATED RINGER's OR WHOLE BLOOD THROUGH VARIOUS-SIZED CATHETERS

	Lactated Ringer's (3½ ft elevation)	Whole Blood (300 mm. Hg pressure)
24″ large (14-gauge needle) catheter (as for CVP line)	38 min.	25 min.
8″ large (14-gauge needle) catheter (as for subclavian)	19 min.	14 min.
2½″ 14-gauge plastic catheter (catheter of choice)	7½ min.	7 min.

From Iversen, L. D., and D. K. Clawson: *Manual of Acute Orthopaedic Therapeutics.* Boston: Little, Brown and Co., 1976, p. 2. (Based on Horton, W. G., unpublished data, 1972.)

crease in splanchnic circulation, with the result that the blood supply to the stomach and bowel is diminished. As a result, gastric empyting is delayed, and vomiting and aspiration of gastric contents into the lung may develop. For this reason, and for diagnostic purposes in trauma patients, it is common practice to initiate nasogastric suction on many patients with shock. In patients with trauma and hemorrhagic shock, it is usual to use a double-lumen, 18 French nasogastric tube (Salem sump tube). When a double-lumen tube is used, it is connected to *straight* or *continuous* suction rather than to intermittent suction. The gastric aspirate should be tested periodically for blood. Antacids are commonly instilled through the tube in hopes of minimizing the incidence of stress ulcer. The nasogastric tube is usually removed when bowel sounds are normal.

When shock is caused by GI bleeding, other nasogastric tubes may be used. If the suspected cause of bleeding is a gastric ulcer, a 36 French *Ewald* tube may be used. This tube has many large holes that facilitate iced saline lavage and removal of blood clots. In patients with suspected esophageal varices, a *Blakemore-Sengstaken* tube is often used. This tube is a triple-lumen tube designed to exert pressure on the lower portion of the esophagus and the upper portion of the stomach, where varices are most prominent. Pressure is provided through the use of esophageal and gastric balloons that are inflated with air. Gentle traction is applied to keep the balloons in proper position. (See Unit XVII.)

It is a nursing responsibility to insure that nasogastric suction is functioning properly and that irrigation is performed routinely as ordered by the attending physician. It is important to remember that patients may aspirate gastric contents into their lungs even though the system is operating properly, so that periodic assessment of the patient's pulmonary system is an essential aspect of nursing care.

CIRCULATORY ASSIST DEVICES*

Mechanical devices that assist circulation and decrease the workload of the heart are commonly employed as temporary measures in the management of patients with shock. We briefly discuss three devices here: (1) the intra-aortic balloon pump (IABP), (2) the external counterpulsation device, and (3) the antishock trouser.

The *intra-aortic balloon pump* is commonly used in patients with cardiogenic shock who are not responding to conventional drug therapy, following open-heart surgery, and in patients with ARDS. When the IABP is used, a balloon-tipped catheter is inserted through a femoral graft (see Fig. 13–22) and is positioned in the descending thoracic aorta just distal to the left subclavian artery. The catheter is connected to a gas-driving unit containing either helium or CO_2. In diastolic augmentation, the balloon is inflated during diastole and deflated just before systole. This counter-pulsation results in the displacement of blood back into the aorta and improves perfusion of the coronary arteries without increasing heart work or increasing oxygen consumption. There is also an increase in the mean arterial blood pressure and, therefore, enhanced perfusion of other vital organs.[133, 179]

The IABP is also beneficial because of its effect on reducing afterload of the heart. Afterload is the resistance to left ventricular ejection and is determined by the residual volume of blood in the aorta and the pressure encountered during left ventricular systole. The IABP decreases the amount of blood in the aorta (arch) and decreases the amount of resistance to blood flow from the left ventricle. The net effects of afterload reduction are: (1) decreased myocardial oxygen consumption, (2) improved coronary artery perfusion (since the period of diastole, during which the coronary arteries fill, is increased), and (3) improved cardiac output as a result of decreased resistance. An additional effect of the IABP is that improved myocardial oxygenation may result in the reversal of myocardial ischemic damage and the size of the myocardial infarction may be minimized.[44]

Whitman[168] has written a helpful programmed instruction on intra-aortic balloon pumping and cardiac mechanisms. The reader is referred to this for additional information.

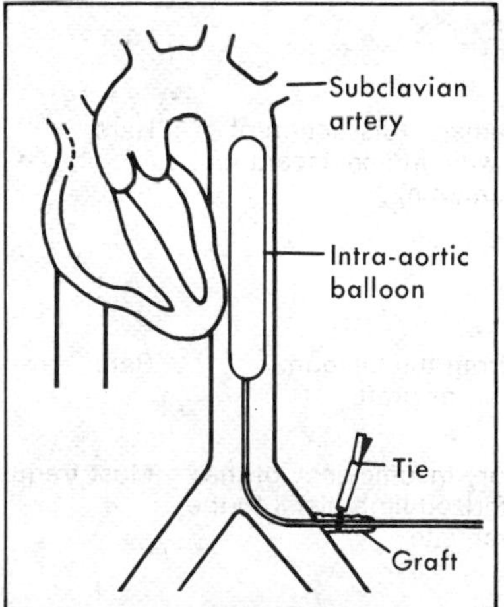

Figure 13–22. Placement of the intra-aortic balloon. Insertion is made through a side arm graft via a cutdown on the common femoral artery. The balloon position is just distal to the left subclavian artery. Ties around the graft secure the catheter in place without jeopardizing perfusion to the leg distal to the insertion site. (From Schroeder, J. S., and E. K. Daily: *Techniques in Bedside Hemodynamic Monitoring.* St. Louis: C. V. Mosby Co., 1976, p. 182.)

*Further information may be found in references 20, 40, 44, 56, 76, 96, 133, 149, 179.

Although the IABP has value in the management of patients with many different problems, it is not without hazard. Some of the complications associated with the use of the IABP are listed in Table 13–12. The mortality rate associated with cardiogenic shock approaches 80 per cent in most studies,[179] and it appears that to be effective in reducing this rate the IABP should be initiated as soon as the diagnosis of cardiogenic shock is made.

The *external counter-pulsation device* utilizes the same general principles as the IABP; however, the effects are achieved by applying pressure to the patient's legs. The legs are encased in rigid, tubular bags that are filled with air or water and connected to a pumping unit. Pressure is applied against the legs during diastole and relaxed in systole. This results in increased venous return and diastolic pressure during compression and systolic unloading when the pressure on the legs is relaxed.

While this device (Fig. 13–23) is less effective than the IABP, it is easy to apply and use and therefore may be more appealing to facilities that do not have IABP capability.

The *anti-shock trouser* is included in this discussion because it assists circulation by increasing venous return; however, the pressure exerted with the anti-shock trouser is sustained rather than intermittent, so it is not to be considered the same as the external counter-pulsation device.

The *anti-shock trouser,* commonly known as the MAST (military anti-shock trouser) suit or the "G" suit, is used primarily for the emergency management of patients with volume loss, usually hemorrhage. The patient's body is encased in the one-piece, three chambered, nylon or polyvinyl suit from the lower costal margin to the ankles; the perineal area is accessible for urinary catheter insertion. When all valves are closed, the suit is capable of sustaining an internal air pressure up to 104 pounds per square inch.

The leg and abdominal chambers are connected to a foot pump and gauges. All or some of the chambers are inflated until the pressure valve is activated or until the patient's blood pressure improves. The pressure exerted against the patient's legs and abdomen forces blood out of these areas and returns it to the heart. This autotransfusion of pooled blood may amount to 750 ml. The pressure also causes increased peripheral resistance, with the result that the patient's cardiac output and mean arterial blood pressure are increased.

The anti-shock trouser has been extremely valuable in the management of patients with

TABLE 13–12. COMPLICATIONS OF THE INTRA-AORTIC BALLOON PUMP

Complication	Incidence	Prevention
Balloon rupture with gas embolism	Rare	Use a careful insertion technique to prevent damage to the balloon Use carbon dioxide as the inflation gas; it is more soluble in blood Choose the largest femoral artery for insertion
Aortic damage (dissection of aortic wall, intimal laceration, or hematoma)	Rare	Position the balloon catheter in the descending aorta just distal to the left subclavian artery Select the correct balloon size, so that the inflated balloon does not occlude the aorta Limit patient movement; leg flexion can move the balloon tip up in the aorta, resulting in possible puncture of the arch
Emboli from the balloon, catheter, or graft	Rare	Administer heparin therapy Do not leave the balloon in place if it is collapsed and motionless
Circulatory insufficiency of the catheterized limb distal to the insertion site	Most frequent	Use the largest femoral artery with the best pulse for balloon insertion Administer heparin for anticoagulation Frequently check the limb for signs of decreased circulation When the balloon is removed, explore the femoral artery with a Fogarty catheter to remove clots
Hemolysis	Minimal	Select the correct balloon size, so that the inflated balloon does not occlude aorta
Platelet reduction	Frequent	Unknown; heparin may help

From Schroeder, J. S., and E. K. Daily: *Techniques in Bedside Hemodynamic Monitoring.* St. Louis: C. V. Mosby Company, 1976, p. 184.

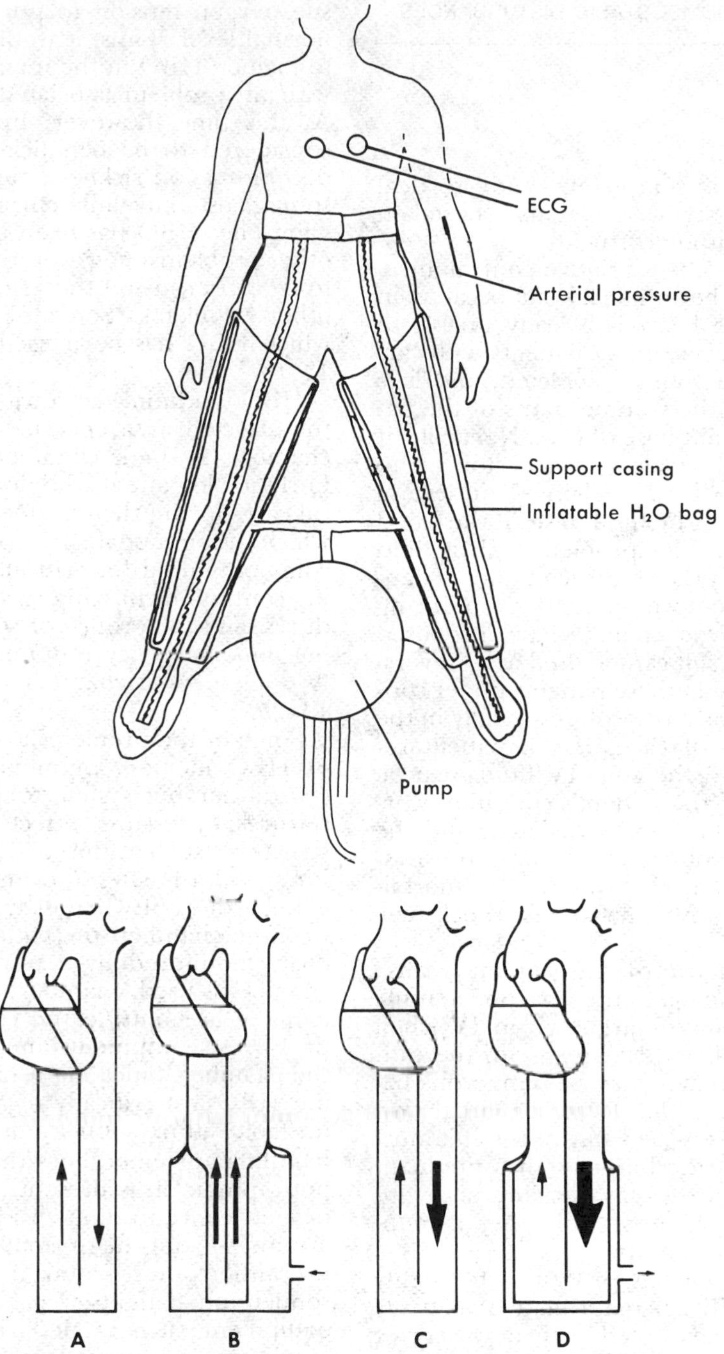

Figure 13–23. Noninvasive external circulatory assist and its method of applying counterpulsation to the peripheral vasculature: **A.** Normal unassisted volume flow during systole. **B.** Application of positive pressure at the beginning of diastole, increasing central venous return *and* retrograde arterial flow into the aorta from the legs. **C.** Release of positive pressure at the beginning of systole, producing systolic unloading by refilling the peripheral vasculature. **D.** Negative pressure during systole, accentuating the systolic unloading by increasing the peripheral vascular capacitance. (From Schroeder, J. S., and E. K. Daily: *Techniques in Bedside Hemodynamic Monitoring.* St. Louis: C. V. Mosby Co., 1976, p. 186.)

massive blood loss and no obtainable blood pressure, in fluid loss other than hemorrhage, and in cardiac arrest. Additionally, it is helpful in further decreasing bleeding in the areas it is compressing. The anti-shock suit is also of value in immobilizing fractures of the femur and pelvis.

The suit is deflated gradually over a period of several minutes, 5 mm. Hg at a time. During this period the patient's blood pressure is closely monitored and IV fluids are given to raise the patient's blood pressure to the original predeflation blood pressure. *Deflating the suit too fast will cause the patient to rapidly go back into shock.* In trauma patients, it is common that the suit is not deflated until the patient is in the operating room and the surgical team is completely ready to deal with the bleeding areas. X-rays may be taken through the suit without difficulty.

Cardiogenic shock is a relative contraindication for the use of the anti-shock suit because, in most instances, the heart is already unable to handle fluid. However, many patients with cardiogenic shock are volume depleted, and it is difficult to discern the volume status of the patient in the emergent phase of care. Normally, if the volume status is unclear, it is customary to give the patient a "fluid challenge" of several hundred milliliters of IV fluid to see if the blood pressure responds. The problem with a fluid challenge is that it may be difficult and/or dangerous to quickly remove the fluid given during the challenge. Wayne et al.[166] have proposed that the anti-shock suit can be used as a "reversible" fluid challenge in these patients under controlled situations and protocols, especially in the pre-hospital phase of care. If the patient responds favorably to the suit, IV fluids can be given. If, however, the patient's condition worsens, the suit can be rapidly deflated, and the patient will not be volume overloaded. It is possible that by using the suit in this way the mortality rate associated with cardiogenic shock may be decreased.

Since prolonged use of the suit may cause acidosis due to ischemia to the legs, one ampule of sodium bicarbonate may be given IV when the suit is being deflated.[166] The use of the anti-shock suit in pregnancy may be dangerous because of the pressure and decreased circulation to the fetus. However, the value of the suit must be weighed against the hazards. In a pregnant patient, adequate effect may be achieved by inflating the leg compartments only, thereby minimizing danger to the fetus.

The anti-shock suit has proven to be highly effective in the initial management of patients with hypotension associated with a variety of clinical problems, particularly in the pre-hospital and emergency phases of care. When used properly it is a safe, rapid, and efficient means of restoring volume and increasing mean arterial pressure. The anti-shock suit is pictured in Figure 13–24.

HYPERBARIC OXYGENATION*

Hyperbaric oxygenation (HBO) involves the use of 100 per cent oxygen administered at 2 to 3 atmospheres of pressure in order to raise tissue oxygen tension to normal levels or above normal level. Thus, it would seem appropriate to include HBO in the management of patients with any problem associated with tissue hypoxia. At this time, however, hyperbaric therapy is considered to be beneficial for air embolism, decompression sickness, carbon monoxide poisoning, osteomyelitis, chronic ulcerations, and gangrene. HBO has been used for a variety of other problems; however, there does not appear to be consensus on the value of HBO for these other problems. Some of the conditions for which HBO has been used are listed in Table 13–13.

HBO is administered with the patient or only the affected area enclosed in a rigid, air-tight chamber. A single chamber may be used for a fairly stable patient who does not require physical care during the treatment. Large chambers, which accommodate two or more people, are commonly used for critically ill patients requiring continuous nursing care, for surgical procedures, and for groups of stable patients requiring nonemergency HBO at the same pressure. A single-person chamber is pictured in Figure 13–25.

Some of the problems associated with the use of HBO include: pulmonary oxygen toxicity; central nervous system toxicity with grand mal seizures; pressure effects on air-containing structures such as the ears, sinuses, GI tract and lung; and a feeling of claustrophobia.

Regardless of whether treatment is in a small or large chamber, the patient must be continuously monitored by a nurse. When the large chamber is used, chamber technicians and often a nurse are outside the chamber, monitoring pressures, equipment, and the activities inside the chamber. Since many of the patients receiving HBO are critically ill and cardiovascularly unstable, all personnel must be fully capable of handling any emergency that arises, whether or not a physician is present. Because of the high oxygen concentration inside the chamber and around the outside of smaller chambers, special precautions must be taken to prevent fire. Personnel and patients wear special clothing, and equipment such as defibrillators may require special energy sources.

The patient undergoing HBO can, and often does, receive intensive nursing care even though the chamber is usually physically distant from the intensive care unit. Hyperbaric therapy nurses are carefully screened and selected and thoroughly trained in intensive nursing care as well as in hyperbaric nursing.

Although hyperbaric therapy may be used in the management of many different problems, it is stressed that it is used to augment standard medical-surgical therapy, not to replace it. HBO seems to be used much more extensively in countries other than the United States and the frequency of use seems dependent upon physician awareness of the indications for HBO and

*Further information may be found in references 34, 53, 97, 114, 118, 155, 161, and 164.

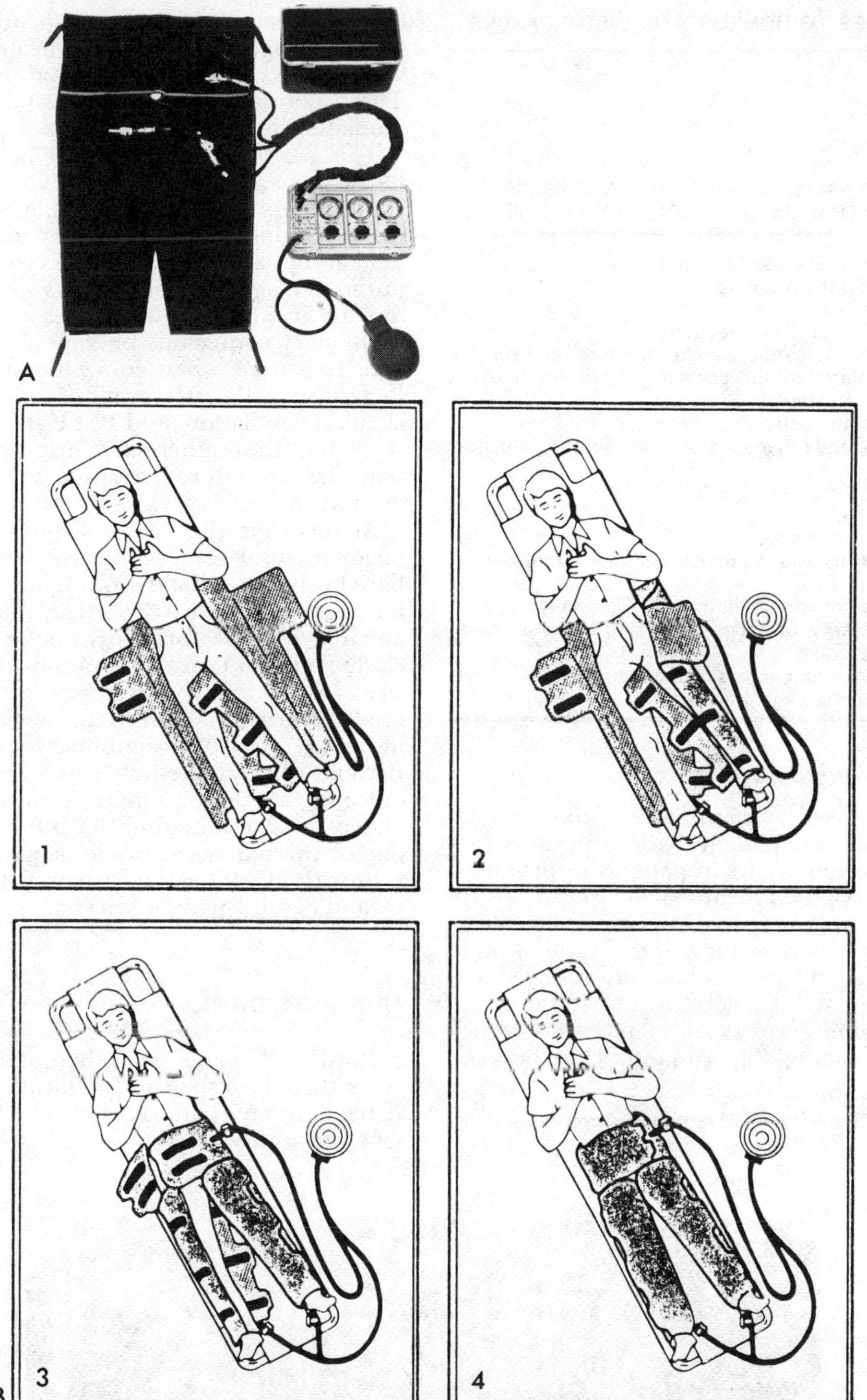

Figure 13–24. **A.** Anti-shock suit with gauges. **B.** Application of anti-shock trousers. (*A* from Section 32, Jobst Condensed Catalog No. 889 for Emergency Medical Products. *B* from Dillman, P. A.: The biophysical response to shock trousers. *Journal of Emergency Nursing.* 3:21, Nov.–Dec. 1977.)

accessibility of a chamber. Medical chambers (as opposed to research and diving chambers) may not be available in every community, because they are very costly and require a fair amount of space.

Since the need for rapid initiation of HBO is great in emergencies such as air embolism, it is important that all nurses know the logistics of notifying the hyperbaric team and transporting the patient to the chamber promptly. This information should be written in a well-developed plan and should be readily accessible.

TABLE 13–13. CONDITIONS FOR WHICH HYPERBARIC OXYGENATION MAY BE USED

Decompression sickness (the "bends")
Carbon monoxide poisoning
Air embolism
Chronic ulcers–stasis or decubitus
Before and during cardiovascular or neurologic surgery
Myocardial infarction and coronary artery thrombosis[155]
Pulmonary contusion[34]
Osteomyelitis and osteonecrosis
Gas gangrene and other anaerobic and aerobic infections
Burns
Thromboembolic conditions[53]
Cerebral edema
Hyaline membrane disease
CNS injury or disease in order to improve cognitive function
Malignancies–in conjunction with radiation therapy
Blood loss anemia in patients refusing transfusions for religious reasons
Congenital disorders, e.g., sickle cell trait
Organ or tissue storage.

MEMBRANE OXYGENATOR*

Extracorporeal membrane oxygenation (ECMO) is used in patients with respiratory failure, which often occurs in patients in profound shock (ARDS), as a means of temporarily supporting gas exchange by the use of partial cardiopulmonary bypass and a membrane oxygenator. Arterial and venous lines are inserted and some of the patient's blood is diverted to a machine containing layers of membranes (which contain the patient's blood) sandwiched between oxygen-bearing passages suspended between water passages. The water is heated, thus preventing the return of cool blood to the patient. The membrane oxygenator is similar to the hemodialysis machine in concept.

The goal of ECMO is to allow the patient's lungs to heal by minimizing ventilatory barotrauma (e.g., high flow oxygen, mechanical ventilation), while adequately oxygenating the patient at the same time. ECMO is commonly used in the management of patients with major pulmonary insults such as ARDS; near drowning; pulmonary contusion; pneumonia, and fat emboli. It is used when conventional methods of high inspired concentrations of oxygen, mechanical ventilation, and PEEP are ineffective in reversing the pulmonary insufficiency. It is, however, considered a last resort measure in most agencies.

At this time the use of ECMO is limited to major medical centers and the results thus far have been somewhat discouraging. This therapy is extremely expensive, partially due to the large amount of laboratory work required, and may easily run into tens of thousands of dollars per week. Since this therapy is sometimes considered experimental, third party payers (health insurance) may not reimburse for the expense. Because of the incredible cost and questionable outcome, the family's permission is usually obtained prior to initiating ECMO. It appears that one of the major factors in achieving good results with ECMO is the early initiation of therapy and careful patient selection.

*Further information may be found in references 21, 78, and 49.

NURSING CARE

Bordicks[18] states that there are two prime roles that the nurse must fulfull in caring for patients in any pattern of shock. These important functions are:

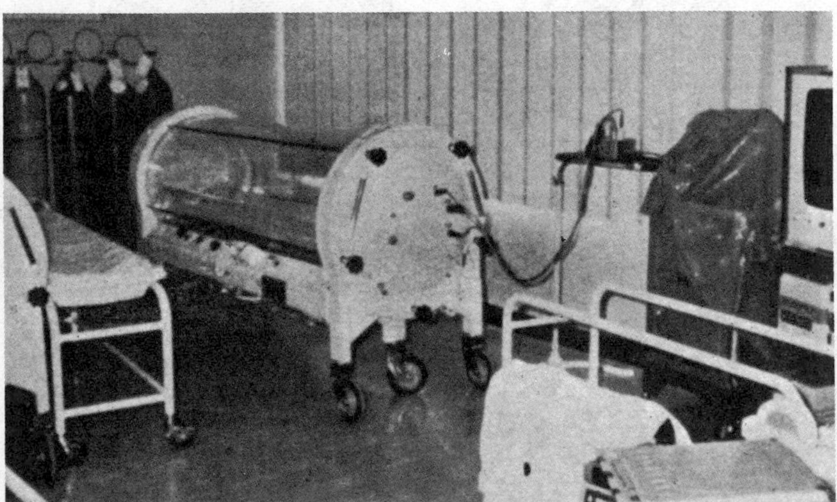

Figure 13–25. Single-person hyperbaric chamber. (From Gaul, A. L. et al.: Hyperbaric Oxygen Therapy. *American Journal of Nursing*, 72:892, May 1972.

1. The nurse must *expedite therapeutic orders* that will help the body *to obtain homeostatic balance,* without the need for compensatory mechanisms.

2. The nurse must also *understand* the compensatory mechanisms that are operative at the time and *support* them.

In other words, the responsibility of the nurse in caring for a person in shock is to *apply the nursing process.* A thorough understanding of the signs and symptoms (especially early ones) and the physiologic processes of shock is important. Careful, ongoing *observation* by a a nurse who can interpret information quickly and accurately is essential so that appropriate intervention can be made and irreversible shock prevented.

Some general points to keep in mind in caring for patients in shock are:

- Continuous monitoring and observation of the patient is imperative, since changes in cardiovascular and respiratory functions can occur rapidly, and treatment must be adjusted accordingly. Record observations clearly and concisely.
- Help the patient to feel at rest physically and emotionally. This helps reduce the physical need for oxygen and nutrients.
- Strive to reduce the patient's fears and anxieties about what is happening and about the equipment being used.
- Have all equipment and supplies (e.g., suction, emergency drugs) available and in working order.
- Use nursing interventions to prevent the complications that can develop from enforced immobilization.
- Provide adequate pain relief, since pain intensifies shock. However, do not give unnecessary narcotics or sedatives. Remember that restlessness may be due to a lack of oxygen to the brain rather than pain. Since impaired circulation can cause the delayed absorption of drugs, hypodermic injection is not advisable. Analgesics or narcotics should be given intravenously to patients in shock, the usual dose being one half to two thirds the customary intramuscular dosage.[19]
- Keep the room temperature somewhat cool (65 to 68° F.) to reduce the patient's metabolic rate.

It is clear from the material presented in this chapter that a person in shock is a person who is extremely ill; a person who may die. In addition to this serious fact, the stress of the situation is compounded by emergency medical treatment with all the people, equipment, and movement that entails. Nurses in this situation have enormous amounts of delegated medical care to attend to, as shown in this chapter. *There must be enough nursing resources at such times, however, to provide for the reassurance and emotional support of the patient and the patient's significant others.* All of the persons involved may be frightened, anxious, perhaps confused, and certainly very dependent.

The patient's significant others should be kept informed of what is happening. They need information upon which to base the decisions they have to make. The same information may need to be given to them several times. The calm repetition of information is often necessary, because anxiety narrows the perceptual field, making forgetting common. The anxious person may be unable at first to "take in" the information being given. Remember that the patient and significant others may be suffering from "psychologic shock." They are commonly in need of opportunities to discuss with professional persons the concerns that are most important to them.

Those persons dearest to a patient should not be kept away from their loved one unnecessarily. There may be times when, because of limited space, they may have to wait in another room for a while. They should not be kept away long, however; and they should not be required to leave their loved one without being given *a reason* why it is necessary.

The patient also requires emotional support. When caught up in the sudden drama of an emergency or critical care, health professionals can sometimes forget that it is all very new and *very frightening* for the patient. Unfortunately, "dehumanization" of the patient may occur during the rush of treatment. Whether the patient appears to be conscious or not, explanations should be given about what is happening. The atmosphere should be kept as quiet and orderly as possible. Unnecessary chatter and noise *must* be eliminated. It is not uncommon to learn from recovered patients that they heard what was being said even though they appeared to be unable to hear.

Health professionals working with the critically ill experience a great deal of strain. Sometimes they release nervous energy through laughter, chatter, or jokes among themselves. This can be quite helpful, of course; however, it should *never* be done in front of patients or their significant others.

Among the greatest of nurses' responsibilities are those of support, comfort, and advocacy to patients and their significant others. This is never more true than in the nursing of those people who are critically ill and in shock.

BIBLIOGRAPHY

1. Abrams, J., R. Deane, and J. Davis: Pulmonary function in patients with multiple trauma and associated severe head injury. *Journal of Trauma,* 16:543, July 1976.

2. Anderson, C. S., Y. Saks, and E. Mikulic: Pedal gan-

grene associated with the use of dopamine. *New England Journal of Medicine,* 293:591, 1975.
3. Arbitman, M., and B. H. Kart: Hydromediastinum after aberrant central venous catheter placement. *Critical Care Medicine,* 7:27, Jan. 1979.
4. Artz, C. P.: Electrical shock: Clinical features and management. *Hospital Medicine,* 14:23, Jan. 1978.
5. Artz, C. P.: Guide to Assessment and Management of Burns. *Hospital Medicine,* 13:105, Mar. 1977.
6. Ballinger, W. F. II, R. B. Rutherford, and G. D. Zuidema: *The Management of Trauma,* 2nd ed. Philadelphia: W. B. Saunders Co., 1973.
7. Barrocas, A.: Disseminated intravascular coagulation. *Military Medicine,* 138:9, Jan. 1973.
8. Beaumont, E.: Blood pressure equipment. *Nursing '75,* 5:56, Jan. 1975.
9. Beeson, P. B., and W. McDermott (Eds.): *Textbook of Medicine,* 14th ed. Philadelphia: W.B. Saunders Co., 1975.
10. Begley, L. A.: External counterpulsation for shock. *American Journal of Nursing,* 75:967, June 1975.
11. Beland, I. L., and J. Y. Passos: *Clinical Nursing,* 3rd ed. New York: The Macmillan Co., 1975.
12. Berry, M. A., and H. L. Brammell: Anatomy, physiology and pathophysiology of the cardiovascular system. *In* Hudak, C. M., B. M. Gallo, and T. L. Lohr: *Critical Care Nursing.* Philadelphia: J. B. Lippincott Co., 1973.
13. Birnbaum, M. L.: Multisystem failure: How almost everything can go wrong quickly. *Nursing '78,* 8:30, Nov. 1978.
14. Blaisdell, F. W., and F. R. Lewis, Jr.: *Respiratory Distress Syndrome of Shock and Trauma: Post-traumatic Respiratory Failure.* Philadelphia: W. B. Saunders Co., 1977.
15. Blaisdell, F. W., et al.: The mechanism of pulmonary damage following traumatic shock. *Surgery, Gynecology and Obstetrics,* 130:15, Jan. 1970.
16. Boggs, D. R., and A. Winkelstein: *White Cell Manual,* 3rd ed. Philadelphia: F. A Davis Co., 1975.
17. Bookman, L. B., and J. K. Simoneau: The early assessment of hypovolemia: postural vital signs. *Journal of Emergency Nursing,* 3:43, Sept.-Oct. 1977.
18. Bordicks, K. J.: *Patterns of Shock: Implications for Nursing Care.* New York: The Macmillan Co., 1965.
19. Brand, L., and A. P. Thal: Shock. *In* Meltzer, L. E., F. G. Abdellah, and J. R. Kitchell (Eds.): *Concepts and Practices of Intensive Care for Nurse Specialists.* Philadelphia: Charles Press Publishers, Inc., 1969.
20. Bregman, D.: Management of patients undergoing intra-aortic balloon pumping. *Heart and Lung,* 3:916, Nov.-Dec. 1974.
21. Browdie, D. A., et al.: Adult respiratory distress syndrome (ARDS), sepsis, and extracorporeal membrane oxygenation (ECMO). *Journal of Trauma,* 17:579, Aug. 1977.
22. Budassi, S. A.: An emergency nurse's guide to drawing arterial blood gases. *Journal of Emergency Nursing,* 3:29, Jan.-Feb. 1977.
23. Carrico, C. J.: Personal communication. March 1978.
24. Cauthorne, C. V.: Coping with death in the Emergency Department. *Journal of Emergency Nursing,* 1:24, Nov.-Dec. 1975.
25. Cavanaugh, D.: Septic shock in a pregnant or recently pregnant woman. *Postgraduate Medicine,* 62:62, Oct. 1977.
26. Chandler, J. G.: The physiology and treatment of shock. *RN,* 34:42, June 1971.
27. Clowes, G. H., et al.: The nonspecific pulmonary inflammatory reactions leading to respiratory failure after shock, gangrene and sepsis. *Journal of Trauma,* 8:899, May 1968.
28. Committee on Trauma, American College of Surgeons. A guide to the initial therapy of shock. *Consultant,* 18:94, Jan. 1978.
29. *Consultant* in cooperation with the Committee on Trauma, American College of Surgeons. "A Guide to the Initial Therapy of Shock," (reference chart). *Consultant,* 18:94, Jan. 1978.
30. Coodley, E. L. (Ed.): Therapeutic conference: Problem: cardiac and respiratory arrest. *Emergency Medicine,* 10:166, May 1978.
31. Cooper, C.: The waiting room. *American Journal of Nursing,* 76:273, Feb. 1970.
32. Critical care, family style: A life threatened by peritonitis. *Nursing '76,* 6:52, May 1976.
33. Crowell, J. W., and A. C. Guyton: Cardiac deterioration in shock. II. The irreversible stage. *In* Hershey, S. G. (Ed.): *Shock. International Anesthesiology Clinics.* Vol. 2. No. 2. Boston: Little, Brown and Co., 1964.
34. Damon, E. G., and R. K. Jones: Hyperbaric treatment for air embolism and pulmonary contusion resulting from primary blast injury. *In* Trapp, W. G., et al. (Eds.); *5th International Hyperbaric Conference.* Vol. 1. Burnaby 2, British Columbia, Canada: Simon Fraser University, 1974.
35. David D. and S. Rogel: Mechanical and humoral factors affecting cardiac function in shock. *Circulatory Shock,* 3:65, Mar. 1976.
36. Deadly DIC. *Emergency Medicine,* 4:17, Sept. 1972.
37. DeLaurentis, D. A.: Resuscitation in the injured patient: Do's and Dont's. *Hospital Medicine,* 14:82, June 1978.
38. Deliee, Sr. S., and A. Cardoni: Antimicrobials: Team effort keeps wonder drugs wonderful. *Nursing '75,* 5:22, Jan. 1975.
39. Denny, M. P.: Septic shock. *Journal of Emergency Nursing,* 3:19, Jan.-Feb. 1977.
40. Dillman, P. A.: The biophysical response to shock trousers. *Journal of Emergency Nursing,* 3:21, Nov.-Dec. 1977.
41. Dorr, K. S.: The intra-aortic balloon pump. *American Journal of Nursing,* 75:52, Jan. 1975.
42. Downey, J. M., et al.: The adequacy of coronary blood flow during acute hypovolemia. *Circulatory Shock,* 3:83, June 1976.
43. Dunbar, R. W., K. A. Price, and C. F. Cannarilla: Microaggregate blood filters: Effect on filtration time, plasma hemoglobin, and fresh blood platelet counts. *Anesthesia and analgesia . . . Current Researches,* 53:577, July-Aug. 1974.
44. Eckhardt, E.: Intra-aortic balloon counterpulsation in cardiogenic shock. *Heart and Lung,* 6:93, Jan.-Feb. 1977.
45. Evarts, C. M.: Fat embolism syndrome. *American Family Physician,* 1:78, Apr. 1970.
46. Fallon, W. H., J. R. Hansel, and G. Williams: Gangrene of the hand: A complication of radial artery cannulation. *Journal of Trauma,* 16:713, Sept. 1976.
47. Flick, M. R., and A. J. Block: Continous in vivo measurement of arterial saturation by oximetry. *Heart and Lung,* 6:990, Nov.-Dec. 1977.
48. Foster, S. B.: Pump Failure. *American Journal of Nursing,* 74:1830, Oct. 1974.
49. Frank, E. D.: Septic shock. *In* Hershey, S. G. (Ed.): *Shock. International Anesthesiology Clinics.* Vol. 2. No. 2. Boston: Little, Brown and Co. 1964.
50. Frazier, C. A.: The hazards of hymenoptera. *American Family Physician.* 15:91, Apr. 1977.
51. Fritz, S. D., C. T. Fitts, and D. Lurie: The effect of hypertonic glucose upon survival in hemorrhagic shock utilizing a re-stress model in sheep. *Journal of Trauma,* 16:284, Apr. 1976.

52. Fromm, D.: Stress ulcer. *Hospital Medicine,* 14:58, Nov. 1978.
53. Gaul, A. L., et al.: Hyperbaric oxygen therapy. *American Journal of Nursing,* 72:892, May 1972.
54. Geolot, D., et al.: Cardiopulmonary resuscitation. *Nurse Practitioner,* 3:24, May-June 1978.
55. Gephardt, D.: Anaphylaxis from insect stings. *Journal of Emergency Nursing,* 4:19, May-June 1978.
56. Gewertz, B., C. O'Brien, and M. Kirsh: Use of the intra-aortic balloon support for refractory low cardiac output in myocardial contusion. *Journal of Trauma,* 17:325, Apr. 1977.
57. Gladish, J. T., A. P. Winnie, and V. J. Collins: Shock: Recognition and modern management. *Postgraduate Medicine,* 42:41, July 1967.
58. Graber, I. G., and S. Sevitt: Renal function in burned patients and its relationship to morphological changes. *Journal of Clinical Pathology,* 12:25, 1959.
59. Guyton, A.: *Textbook of Medical Physiology,* 3rd ed. Philadelphia: W. B. Saunders Co. 1968.
60. Haerer, A. F.: Coma: Some differential considerations in the diagnosis and management. *Hospital Medicine,* 12:68, Apr. 1976.
61. Halevy, S., and B. Altura: Indomethacin protection in traumatic shock. *Circulatory Shock,* 3:299, Dec. 1976.
62. Hardaway, R. M., et al.: *Syndromes of Disseminated Intra vascular Coagulation: With Special Reference to Shock and Hemorrhage.* Springfield, Ill.: Charles C Thomas, 1966.
63. Harrison, L. H., et al.: Effects of endotoxin on pulmonary capillary permeability, ultrastructure, and surfactant. *Surgery, Gynecology and Obstetrics,* 129:723, Oct. 1969.
64. Hathaway, R.: Hemodynamic monitoring in shock. *Journal of Emergency Nursing,* 3:37, Sept.-Oct. 1977.
65. Hershey, S. G. (Ed.): *Shock. International Anesthesiology Clinics.* Vol. 2, No. 2. Boston: Little, Brown and Company, 1964.
66. Hillman, R. S., and C. A. Finch: *Red Cell Manual,* 4th ed. Philadelphia: F. A. Davis Co., 1974.
67. Hilton, J. G., and C. H. Wells: Effect of indomethacin and nicotinic acid on *E. coli* endotoxin shock in anesthetized dogs. *Journal of Trauma,* 16:96, Dec. 1976.
68. Hinterbuchner, L. P.: Evaluation of the Unconscious Patient. *Hospital Medicine,* 13:83, Feb. 1977.
69. Hudak, C. M., B. M. Gallo, and T. Lohr: *Critical Care Nursing.* Philadelphia: J. B. Lippincott Co., 1973.
70. In cardiac arrest, resuscitate with care. *Emergency Medicine,* 10:219, Nov. 1978.
71. Itkin, I.: Bee sting. *American Family Physician,* 13:124, May 1976.
72. Iversen, L. D., and D. K. Clawson: *Manual of Acute Orthopaedic Therapeutics.* Boston: Little, Brown and Co., 1977.
73. Janoff, A.: Alterations in lysosomes (intracellular enzymes) during shock: Effect of pre-conditioning (tolerance) and protective drugs. *In* Hershey, S. G. (Ed.): *Shock. International Anesthesiology Clinics.* Vol. 2. No. 2. Boston: Little, Brown and Co., 1964.
74. Jarvis, C. M.: Vital signs: How to take them accurately . . . and understand them fully. *Nursing '76,* 6:31, Apr. 1976.
75. Juliani, L.: Assessing renal function. *Nursing '78,* 8:34, Jan. 1978.
76. Kaplan, B. C., et al.: The military anti-shock trouser in civilian pre-hospital care. *Journal of Trauma,* 13:843, Oct. 1973.
77. Katsaros, C., and J. Bobb: Shock — the Critical Hour. *Journal of Emergency Nursing,* 4:45, Sept.-Oct. 1978.
78. Kirby, R. R.: Membrane oxygenators: What role (if any) in acute ventilatory insufficiency? *Critical Care Medicine,* 6:19, Jan.-Feb. 1978.
79. Knopp, R., and R. H. Dailey:Central venous cannulations and pressure monitoring. *Journal of American College of Emergency Physicians,* 6:358, Aug. 1977.
80. Krausz, M. M., et al.: Aberrant position of a central venous catheter: A cause for inadequate fluid replacement in septic shock. *Critical Care Medicine,* 6:337, Sept.-Oct. 1978.
81. Kuenzi, S. H., and M. V. Fenton: Crisis Intervention in acute care areas. *American Journal of Nursing,* 75:830, May 1975.
82. Kunz, F., et al.: Plasma lipids, coagulation factors, and fibrin formation after severe multiple trauma, and in adult respiratory distress syndrome. *Journal of Trauma,* 18:115, Feb. 1978.
83. Lahiri, B., and R. Z. Wallack: The early diagnosis and treatment of fat embolism syndrome. *Journal of Trauma,* 17:956, Dec. 1977.
84. Lamb, J.: Intra-arterial monitoring: rescinding the risks. *Nursing '77,* 7:65, Nov. 1977.
85. Leaf, A., and R. Cotran: *Renal Pathophysiology.* New York: Oxford University Press, 1976.
86. Levenson, S. M., A. L. Nagler, and A. Einheber: Some metabolic consequences of shock. *In* Hershey, S. G. (Ed.): *Shock: International Anesthesiology Clinics.* Vol. 2. No. 2. Boston: Little, Brown and Co., 1964.
87. Levy, M. N., and B. Blattberg: Blood factors in shock. *In* Hershey, S. G. (Ed.): *Shock. International Anesthesiology* Clinics. Vol. 2. No. 2. Boston: Little, Brown and Co., 1964.
88. Loeb, H. S., et al.: Acute hemodynamic effects of dobutamine and isoproterenol in patients with low output cardiac failure. *Circulatory Shock,* 3:55, Mar. 1976.
89. Lucas, C.: Early care of critically injured patients: Part 1. *Hospital Medicine,* 13:31, Aug. 1977.
90. Lucas, C.: Early care of critically injured patients: Part 2. *Hospital Medicine,* 13:44, Sept. 1977.
91. Lucas, C., et al.: The renal factor in post-traumatic fluid overload syndrome. *Journal of Trauma,* 17:667, Sept. 1977.
92. Marcinek, M. B.: Stress in the surgical patient. *American Journal of Nursing,* 77:1809, Nov. 1977.
93. Marshall, B. E. et al.: Microaggregate formation in stored blood. IV. Influence of fibrin on screen filtration pressure and its removal by micropore filters. *Circulatory Shock,* 3:303, Dec. 1976.
94. Martell, R., et al.: The effect of blood pH on the electrocardiogram. *Critical Care Medicine,* 7:24, Jan. 1979.
95. McFarland, M.: Fat embolism syndrome. *American Journal of Nursing,* 76:1942, Dec. 1976.
96. McSwain, N. E.: Pneumatic trousers and the management of shock. *Journal of Trauma,* 17:719, Sept. 1977.
97. Meijne, N. G.: *Hyperbaric Oxygenation.* Springfield, Ill.: Charles C Thomas, 1970.
98. Meltzer, L. E., Pinneo, R., and Kitchell, J. R.: Acute myocardial infarction. *In* Meltzer, L. E., F. G. Abdellah, and J. R. Kitchell (Eds.): *Concepts and Practices of Intensive Care for Nurse Specialists.* Philadelphia: Charles Press Publishers, Inc., 1969.
99. Miller, M. K., and L. A. Lazure: 4 Steps For Better Cardiac Care in the E.R. *Nursing '78,* 8:40, Aug. 1978
100. Mitty, W. F., Jr., et al.: The role of the emergency room in management of shock. *Hospital Medicine,* 8:7, Jan. 1972.

101. Molyneux-Luick, M.: The ABC's of multiple trauma. *Nursing '77*, 7:30, Oct. 1977.
102. Molyneux-Luick, M., and J. W. Knecht,: The emergency that supersedes all other duties: hypovolemic shock. *Nursing '77*, 7:32, Nov. 1977.
103. Moore, F. D., et al.: *Post-traumatic Pulmonary Insufficiency.* Philadelphia: W. B. Saunders Co., 1969.
104. Moss, A. J.: Classifying and evaluating syncope. *Geriatrics,* 33:103, Feb. 1978.
105. Moss, G., and A. Stein: The centrineurogenic etiology of the respiratory distress syndrome: protection by unilateral chronic pulmonary denervation in hemorrhagic shock. *Journal of Trauma,* 16:361, May 1976.
106. Moyer, J. H., and L. C. Mills: Vasopressor agents in shock. *American Journal of Nursing,* 75:620, Apr. 1975.
107. Moylan, J. A., et al.: Fat emboli syndrome. *Journal of Trauma,* 16:341, May 1976.
108. Murray, J., and J. Smallwood: CVP monitoring: Sidestepping potential perils. *Nursing '77,* 7:41, Jan. 1977.
109. Nickerson, M.: Vasoconstriction and vasodilation in shock. *In* Hershey, S. G. (Ed.): *Shock. International Anesthesiology Clinics.* Vol. 2. No. 2. Boston: Little, Brown and Co., 1964.
110. Nixon, J. R., and J. G. Brock-Utne.: Free Fatty Acids and Arterial Oxygen Changes Following Major Injury. *Journal of Trauma,* 18:23, Jan. 1978.
111. *Nursing '77* and K. Emkey: Tempering the turmoil of an office emergency. *Nursing 77,* 7:16, May 1977.
112. Nussbaum, G. B., and J. G. Hisher: A crash cart that works. *American Journal of Nursing,* 78:45, Jan. 1978.
113. O'Brian, B. S., and S. Woods: The paradox of DIC. *American Journal of Nursing,* 78:1878, Nov. 1978.
114. Onda, M., et al.: Therapeutic effect of hyperbaric oxygenation against severe bleeding. *In* Trapp, W. G., et al. (Eds.): *5th International Hyperbaric Conference. Vol. 1.* Burnaby 2, British Columbia, Canada: Simon Fraser University, 1974.
115. Ornstein, H., and R. Michaels: How to use intravenous antibiotics. *Nurses Drug Alert,* 1:89, June 1977.
116. Owen, J.: Respiratory failure after injury: a review and plea for accuracy. *Heart and Lung,* 6:303, Mar.-Apr. 1977.
117. Palmer, R. F., and K. C. Lasseter: Sodium nitroprusside. *New England Journal of Medicine,* 292:294, 1975.
118. Pelled, B., et al.: Effects of hyperoxia on the coronary circulation and myocardial function. *In* Trapp, W. G., et al. (Eds.): *5th International Hyperbaric Conference. Vol. 2.* Burnaby 2, British Columbia, Canada: Simon Fraser University, 1974.
119. Perel, A.: The variable effect of PEEP in acute respiratory failure associated with multiple trauma. *Journal of Trauma,* 18:218, Mar. 1978.
120. Peters, R. M., and J. S. Hogan: Fluid overload and post-traumatic respiratory distress syndrome. *Journal of Trauma,* 18:83, Feb. 1978.
121. Pirkle, J. C., and D. S. Gann: Expansion of interstitial fluid is required for full restitution of blood volume after hemorrhage. *Journal of Trauma,* 16:937, Dec. 1976.
122. Pollak, R., and R. A. M. Myers: Early diagnosis of fat embolism syndrome. *Journal of Trauma,* 18:121, Feb. 1978.
123. Ratliff, N. B., D. B. Hackel, and E. Mikat: Myocardial zonal lesions. *Circulatory Shock,* 3:77, June 1976.
124. Ratliff, N. B., et al.: The lung in hemorrhagic shock. *American Journal of Pathology,* 58:353, Feb. 1970.
125. Reul, G. J., A. C. Beall, and S. D. Greenberg: Protection of the pulmonary microvasculature by fine screen blood filtration. *Chest,* 66:4, July 1974.
126. Roach, L. B.: Color changes in dark skin.: *Nursing '77,* 7:48, Jan. 1977.
127. Rodman, M. J.: Drugs for treating shock. *RN,* 39:77, Mar. 1976.
128. Rosario, M. D., et al.: Blood microaggregates and ultrafilters. *Journal of Trauma,* 18:498, July 1978.
129. Rose, M.: Shock: Fluids restore circulation. *Nursing Skillbook: Monitoring Fluid and Electrolytes Precisely.* Horsham, Penn.: Intermed Communciations, Inc. (Nursing 78 Books), 1978. (Chapter 18.)
130. Russell, R. O., et al.: Acute myocardial infarction: Diagnosis, pitfalls, management. *Hospital Medicine,* 14:6, Dec. 1978.
131. Sambhi, M. P., et al.: Adrenocorticoids in the management of shock. *In* Hershey, S. G. (Ed.): *Shock. International Anesthesiology Clinics.* Vol. 2. No. 2. Boston: Little, Brown and Co. 1964.
132. Schoonmaker, F. W.: Axioms on cardiac arrest. *Hospital Medicine,* 14:24, Oct. 1978.
133. Schroeder, J. S., and E. K. Daily: *Techniques in Bedside Hemodynamic Monitoring.* St. Louis: C. V. Mosby Co., 1976.
134. Schultz, C.: Developing foundations for healing grief. *Journal of Emergency Nursing,* 3:29, Jan.-Feb. 1977.
135. Schwartz, G., et al.: Psychic numbing in the Emergency Department. *Emergency Medical Services,* 4:31, Jan.-Feb. 1975.
136. Scoggin, C., L. Nett, and T. L. Petty: Clinical evaluation of a new ear oximeter. *Heart and Lung,* 6:121, Jan-Feb. 1977.
137. Sevitt, S.: Distal tubular necrosis with little or no oliguria. *Journal of Clinical Pathology,* 9:12, 1956.
138. Sheffer, A. L.: Treatment of Anaphylaxis. *Postgraduate Medicine,* 53:62, Apr. 1973.
139. Shier, M. R., et al.: Fat embolism prophylaxis: a study of four treatment modalities. *Journal of Trauma,* 17:621, Aug. 1977.
140. Shires, G. T., et al.: *Shock.* Philadelphia: W. B. Saunders Co., 1973.
141. Sibbald, W. J., V. Sardesai, and R. F. Wilson: Hypocalcemia and nephrogenous cyclic AMP production in critically ill or injured patients. *Journal of Trauma,* 17:677, Sept. 1977.
142. Simeone, F. A.: The nature and treatment of shock. *American Journal of Nursing,* 66:1289, 1966.
143. Soroff, H. S., et al. External counterpulsation. Management of cardiogenic shock after myocardial infarction, *JAMA,* 229:1441, Sept. 1974.
144. Stephenson, C. A.: Stress in critically ill patients. *American Journal of Nursing,* 77:1806, Nov. 1977.
145. Stewart, E.: To lessen pain: Relaxation and rhythmic breathing. *American Journal of Nursing,* 76:958, June 1976.
146. Stude, C.: Cardiogenic shock. *American Journal of Nursing,* 74:1636, Sept. 1974.
147. Sugarman, H. J., et al.: Continuous positive and expiratory pressure ventilation (PEEP) for the treatment of diffuse interstitial pulmonary edema. *Journal of Trauma,* 12:263, Apr. 1972.
148. Sun, R. L.: Trendelenburg's position in hypovolemic shock. *American Journal of Nursing,* 71:1758, Sept. 1971.
149. Tarter, G.: Personal communication, Jan. 1978.
150. Taylor, C. M.: When to anticipate septic shock. *Nursing '75,* 5:34, Apr. 1975.
151. Tharp, G. D.: Shock: The overall mechanisms. *American Journal of Nursing,* 74:2208, Dec. 1974.

152. The multiply injured child. *Emergency Medicine,* 10:43, May 1978.
153. The well-dressed emergency room. *Emergency Medicine,* 11:49, Jan. 15, 1979.
154. *Therapeutic considerations in critical care medicine: Hemodynamic and respiratory aspects of shock.* The Upjohn Company, 1975. (H-4770-4).
155. Thurston, J., and T. Greenwood: Results of a controlled study of hyperbaric oxygen in acute myocardial infarction. *In*
156. Trapp, W. G., et al. (Eds.): *5th International Hyperbaric Conference. Vol. 2.* Burnaby 2, British Columbia, Canada: Simon Fraser University, 1974.
157. Tilkian, S., and M. H. Conover: *Clinical Implications of Laboratory Tests.* St. Louis: C. V. Mosby Co., 1975.
158. Tinker, J. H.: Understanding chest x-rays. *American Journal of Nursing,* 76:54, Jan. 1976.
159. Trapp, W. G., et al. (Eds.): *5th International Hyperbaric Conference.* Vol. 1. Burnaby 2, British Columbia, Canada: Simon Fraser University, 1974.
160. Trapp, W. G., et al. (Eds.): *5th International Hyperbaric Conference.* Vol. 2. Burnaby 2, British Columbia, Canada: Simon Fraser University, 1974.
161. Trimble, V. H.: *Hyperbaric Oxygenation: The Uncertain Miracle.* Garden City, New York: Doubleday and Co., Inc., 1974.
162. Trunkey, D. D.: The critically injured patient. *Consultant,* 17:81, Aug. 1977.
163. Vandermeer, B. L.: Shock, blood pressure and anesthesia. *Journal of the American Association of Nurse Anesthetists,* Apr. 1965.
164. Wada, J., et al.: Extended survival of the anoxic heart with hyperbaric oxygenation, metabolic inhibitors and hypothermia. *In* Trapp, W. G., et al. (Eds.): *5th International Hyperbaric Conference.* Vol. 1. Burnaby 2, British Columbia, Canada: Simon Fraser University, 1974.
165. Walinski, P.: Acute hemodynamic monitoring. *Heart and Lung,* 6:838, Sept.-Oct. 1977.
166. Wayne, M. A.: The M.A.S.T. suit in cardiogenic shock. *Journal of American College of Emergency Physicians,* 7:107, Mar. 1978.
167. Weil, M. H., and H. Shubin: *Diagnosis and Treatment of Shock.* Baltimore: Williams & Wilkins Co., 1967.
168. Whitman, G.: Intra-aortic balloon pumping and cardiac mechanisms: A programmed instruction. *Heart and Lung,* 7:1034, Nov.-Dec. 1978.
169. Whitman, G.: Treatment of acute myocardial infarction by external pressure circulatory assist. Study Steering Committee Interim Report, Feb. 1975.
170. Wilson, J. W., et al.: The lung in shock. *American Journal of Pathology,* 58:337, Feb. 1970.
171. Wilson, R. F.: Diagnosis and Treatment of Shock. *Consultant,* 18:109, Dec. 1978.
172. Wilson, R. F., and J. A. Wilson: Pathophysiology, diagnosis and treatment of shock. *Journal of Emergency Nursing,* 3:11, Sept-Oct. 1977.
173. Wilson, R. F., L. P. Leblanc, and A. J. Walt: Shock due to trauma. *In* Walt, A. J. and R. F. Wilson: *Management of Trauma: Pitfalls and Practice.* Philadelphia: Lea & Febiger, 1975. (Ch. 5).
174. Wilson, R. F., et al.: Central venous pressure and blood volume in clinical shock. *Surgery, Gynecology and Obstetrics,* 132:631, Apr. 1971.
175. Wilson, R. F., et al.: Factors affecting prognosis in clinical shock. *Annals of Surgery,* 169:93, Jan. 1969.
176. Wilson, R. F., et al.: Hemodynamic changes, treatment and prognosis in clinical shock. *Archives of Surgery,* 102:21, Jan. 1971.
177. Woods, S. L.: Monitoring pulmonary artery pressures. *American Journal of Nursing,* 76:1765, Nov. 1976.
178. Ziesche, S., and J. Franciosa: Clinical application of sodium nitroprusside in cardiogenic shock. *Heart and Lung,* 6:99, Jan.-Feb. 1977.
179. Zschoche, D. A. (Ed.): *Mosby's Comprehensive Review of Critical Care.* St. Louis: C. V. Mosby Co., 1976.
180. Zweifach, B. W.: Relation of the reticulo-endothelial system to natural and acquired resistance in shock. *In* Hershey, S. G. (Ed.): *Shock. International Anesthesiology Clinics.* Vol. 2. Boston: Little, Brown and Co., 1964.

SECTION TWO

PSYCHOSOCIAL AND PHYSICAL ASSESSMENT

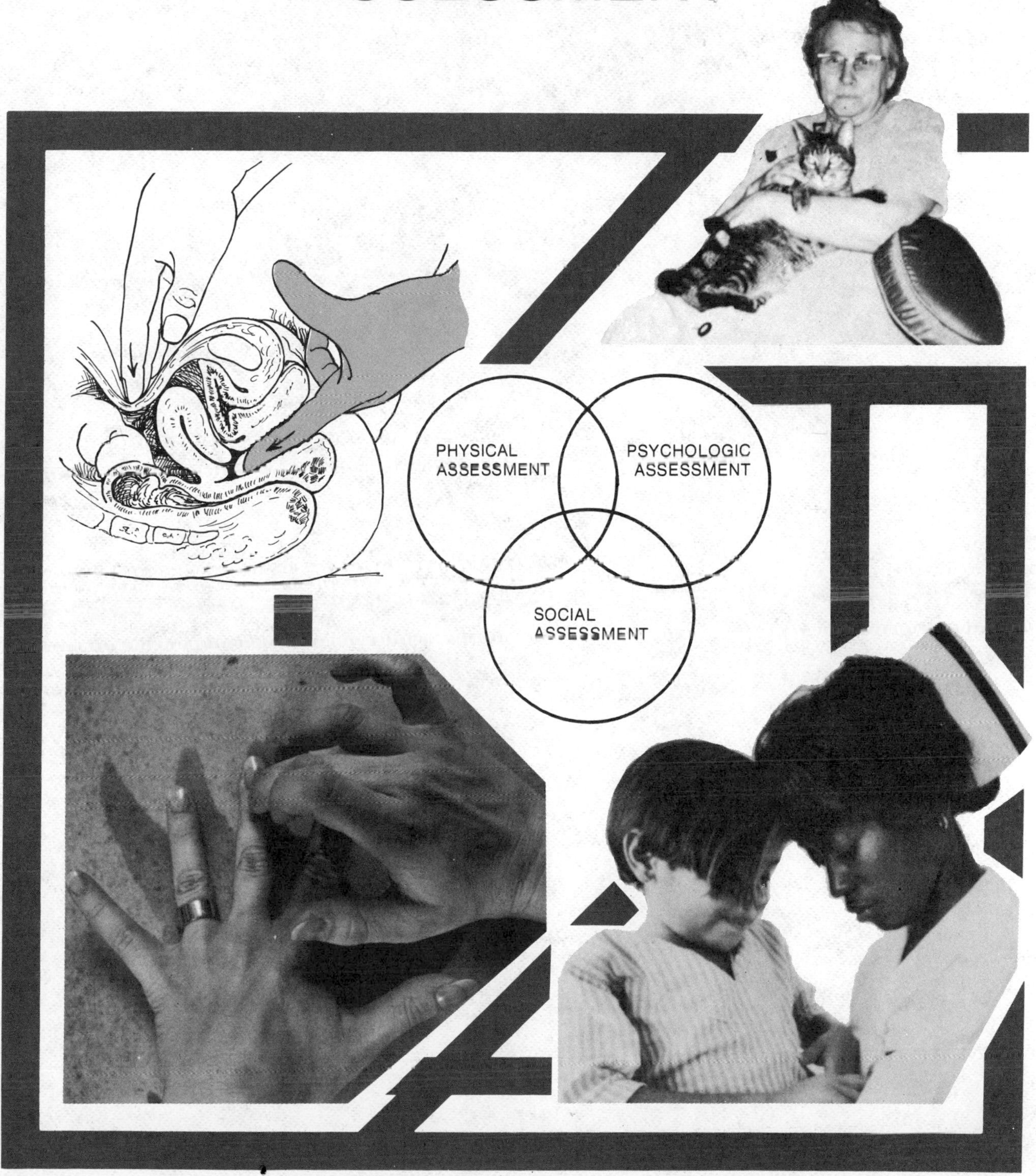

UNIT VI

PSYCHOSOCIAL ASSESSMENT

by Margaret Helen Parkinson, R.N., R.M.N., Dip. N., B. Soc. Sc., M.N.

It is only when my attention becomes fixated that I act like a part rather than a whole. When I favor my conscious perception over my total awareness, I can no longer hear the rhythm of the whole.

HUGH PRATHER[73]

INTRODUCTION AND STUDY GUIDE

People who enter the health care system to get help with medical or surgical problems are all too often viewed narrowly by health professionals. Most often this view is based on the particular physical diagnostic label that has been applied to them. Extreme, unfortunate examples of labeling occur when, for example, a person is referred to as an "appendix case" or the "coronary in Room 507." If, as sometimes happens, the symptoms a patient experiences are not easily connected with physiologic phenomena, it can be tempting for health professionals to discount this person's problem by calling it "functional" or "psychosomatic" or by describing the patient as a "hypochondriac."

While diagnostic labeling is useful for planning treatment, labels can produce negative effects if a perceptual set is established in the minds of health professionals (or even, for that matter, in the minds of patients themselves and their significant others).

> *If health professionals view patients through a narrowed perceptual field created by overattention to diagnostic labels, they will have difficulty understanding individual patients as unique, whole persons.*

In such a situation, health professionals are also likely to disregard information that does not seem consistent with the framework that a specific diagnosis creates. For these reasons, deliberate assessment of and attention to the psychosocial aspects of human experience is important for any patient — regardless of the presenting problem or the eventual diagnosis.

A holistic approach toward human beings is inherent in nursing practice. A nurse, therefore, may be more aware than other health professionals of the need to view a patient as a whole person. The excellent nurse knows that physical assessment of a patient, by itself, is not enough to provide an understanding of the *present experience* that the person is having. The excellent nurse also knows that unless the whole experience of a patient is considered it is difficult to discover what the patient's needs are and difficult to plan ways to meet the needs. These activities are, of course, what nursing is all about!

In this book we continually emphasize the indivisible nature of human beings. In Chapter 1 the interconnections between physical, intellectual, emotional, and social basic human needs were illustrated. The unity of the human mind and body was discussed in Chapters 3, 7, and 8. The effects of stress on the whole person — mind, body, and social network — were emphasized in Chapters 5 and 6. In this chapter we present the theories and techniques of psychosocial assessment, to help you incorporate into *your behavior* the knowledge, understandings, and, possibly, the attitude changes that you gained through the previous discussions.

This unit (Chapter 14) focuses on the nature and usefulness of psychosocial assessment in a nonpsychiatric health care setting. A bibliography is provided, and you are encouraged to seek further details. Extensive additional reading is possible if desired, beginning with the specific references given throughout the chapter.

After mastering the content of this unit, it can be expected that you will be able to:

- ► Appreciate the purposes and values of psychosocial assessment for the nonpsychiatric patient
- ► Identify components of your personal value and belief systems that could hamper your ability to make valid professional psychosocial assessments
- ► Discuss psychologic and social areas that are important when making appropriate psychosocial assessments
- ► List some formal psychosocial assessments tools
- ► Describe factors that can influence the validity of psychosocial assessment
- ► Use appropriately the information gathered through psychosocial assessment

As you work toward achievement of these objectives, you may find the following study guide suggestions helpful.

1. Write in your own words what you understand by the following terms:

psychosocial	psychological rape
sociologic	self-disclosure
psychologic	objective psychologic tests
psychosocial assessment	projective psychologic tests
social network	mental status exam
significant others	behavior
psychopests	socioeconomic status

2. Discuss with a group of colleagues how you think each of the following attitudes, if held by nurses, could affect their psychosocial assessments of patients:
   a. Distrust of foreigners
   b. Impatience with "noisy" children
   c. Awe of highly educated people
   d. Envy of "happily married" people
   e. Intimidation by very articulate people
   f. Discounting of strongly religious people
   g. Fear of criticism from others — especially superiors

h. Intolerance of people who do not "take care" of their own apparent health needs.
i. Self-consciousness with a patient who is, by profession, a nurse or a doctor

3. Review the amount of psychosocial information you have gathered about people you have cared for in your clinical experiences by doing the following:

a. Write down the names of three people you have taken care of recently.
b. Write down the physical diagnosis assigned each person along with pertinent information about this diagnosis.
c. Write down all you *know* about each person that does not directly involve their physical condition. (Be careful not to guess or make assumptions.)
d. Review what you have just written. Can you answer such questions as:

   Where does the person live and work?
   Who is the most significant other in the life of each person?
   What kinds of experiences has the person had with health care systems in the past?
   How does the person behave when anxious, afraid or impatient?

e. Compare the amount of information you had about each person's physical condition with the amount of information you had about each person as an individual. Do your findings tell you anything about yourself and where you have placed your priorities?

CHAPTER 14

PSYCHOSOCIAL ASSESSMENT

THE NATURE OF PSYCHOSOCIAL ASSESSMENT

> *Psychosocial assessment is the gathering of information about patients that has to do with their psychologic patterns and their social experiences.*

Psychologic patterns are those nonphysical components of a human being that are individual, e.g., thoughts, feelings, motivations, mental status, and personal strengths and weaknesses. *Social experiences* are those parts of an individual's life that are affected by or are dependent on other people. Because psychologic and social factors are not entirely separate, the term "psychosocial" is used. The psychosocial components of an individual, in turn, are not separate from the *physiologic* components. All components fuse to form the individual.

The "psyche" (mind) and the "soma" (body) we recognize as functionally indivisible (see Chapters 3, 7, and 8). There is a third component, however, that must be considered in attempting to understand the complexities of human beings. This component consists of the "social factors" of human life, that is, the circumstances and events that exist because of the interactions and interconnections that we all have with other people.

No one lives entirely without some contact (direct or indirect) with other people. Even the conception of a human being requires the social contacts of two people during sexual intercourse. (The once-fanciful notion of "test tube babies" — perhaps more real today — requires the contribution and cooperation of a laboratory staff.) An infant will not survive without the nurture and care of other people over the long human dependency period. Throughout our lives, many of our decisions are made in relation to other people. Our feelings about our life events and circumstances are influenced by others. Some authors suggest that our personalities, maybe even our physical and mental health, are at least in part determined by the nature and quality of our relationships with other people.[16, 37]

To understand the needs of people, then, the nurse must think of people not only as individuals but also as people within a unique and personal social network. For nursing assessment to be most useful, it must gather data from the physical, psychologic, and social realms of the person. Since each realm affects the other two, it is ideal for the physical and psychosocial assessments of patients to be made at the same time, by the same person. In this book we have found it convenient to discuss psychosocial assessment and physical assessment in separate chapters. Be wary of separating assessment modes in your own mind or practice, however. Such separation may cause you to make erroneous conclusions from the data you collect.

When you study physical assessment in Chapter 15, you will notice that it consists of rather specific procedures. Systematic examinations of the physical body systems are recommended and exact techniques, frequently involving precise measuring instruments, are described. Much of your learning about physical assessment involves the mastery of specific tasks and the recognition of deviations from normal in the results.

Psychosocial assessment is not as objective as physical assessment, and this, in many ways, makes it difficult to do. There are some "tools" available for measuring psychosocial variables, which you may at times use in your nursing practice. The tools are few, however. The quality (and therefore the usefulness) of the information you gather about patients' psychologic and social existence depends more on the quality of the interpersonal relationship you establish with the patient than on the tools you use.

Whether a patient shares personal, psychosocial information with you will depend upon such things as:

- The amount of *trust* the patient has in you as a person and as a professional
- How *genuine* you are within the nurse-patient relationship
- Your mastery and use of effective *listening skills*
- Your ability to make *accurate observations* and

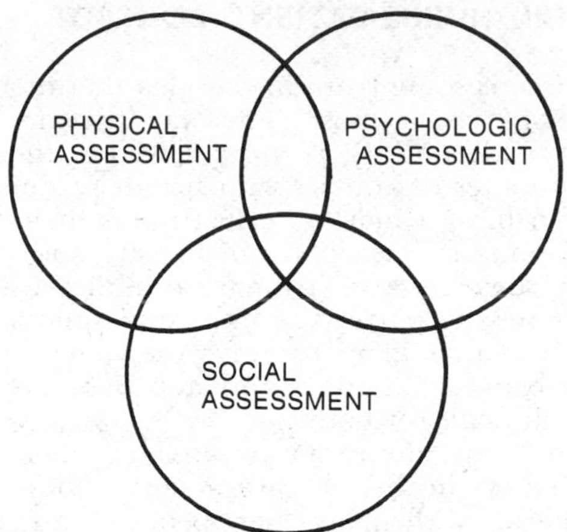

Figure 14–1. Physical and psychosocial (psychologic and social) assessments are best made relative to each other. The mind cannot be separated from the body, nor can the individual be separated from other people. Inadequate information is gathered unless the interactions within the assessment areas are considered.

have them *validated* by the patient, i.e., accurate empathy

It is clear, then, that the skills required of a professional nurse making psychosocial assessments overlap considerably with the components of a successful professional therapeutic relationship. You may find it useful to review material concerning the therapeutic nurse-patient relationship.*

THE PURPOSE OF PSYCHOSOCIAL ASSESSMENT

In Chapter 2, assessment was discussed as a major component of the nursing process. Physical assessment is concerned with gathering information about the physical needs of a patient, whereas psychosocial assessment focuses on information concerning intellectual, social, and emotional needs of a patient. The principle purpose of any kind of nursing assessment, whether physical or psychosocial, is to facilitate the accurate identification of nursing problems and the establishment of a nursing diagnosis so that appropriate nursing care can be planned.

Nurses also make patient assessments in order to recognize deviations from the normal. This is particularly true when making physical assessments. It is much less true when making psychosocial assessments of the nonpsychiatric patient. While there are fairly clear guidelines for differentiating between normal and abnormal anatomy or physiologic processes, psychosocial factors fall much less precisely into "normal" and "abnormal" categories. *Nursing psychosocial assessment seeks to understand, value, and appreciate the life experiences of an individual rather than to make judgments about them.*

Information of a psychosocial nature is often perceived by patients as being far more personal and private than physiologic data. Patients, therefore, may find it more difficult and, indeed, more threatening to disclose psychosocial information. This is particularly true if they believe they are going to be "judged." Nurses must remember that it is not appropriate professional behavior to make moral judgments about patients.

> *The excellent nurse seeks to develop a nonjudgmental attitude toward others and to communicate this attitude to patients and their significant others.*

Information should never be gathered from a patient because of personal curiosity or because of institutional routines. Nurses, or any health professionals for that matter, have no right to patient information that they do not anticipate using in a meaningful, helpful manner. This is particularly important to remember as you make psychosocial assessments. As has already been pointed out, it is very important to consider a patient's psychologic and social functioning. It is equally important not to pry. The balance in information gathering is very delicate.

Nurses are professionally inadequate if they ignore psychosocial factors concerning patients. On the other hand, nurses do patients a severe injustice if they use the power of their professional position to pressure patients into unwillingly self-disclosing information. Luft describes such people as "psychopests" and their inappropriate behavior as "psychological rape."[51] Pause for a moment and recall whether you have ever felt pressured to disclose information about yourself that you would rather not have shared. If you have been in such a position and the "psychopest" was in a position of power, you may remember the unfairness of the situation and how it caused you to feel. Clearly, as a professional, you would not want to evoke such feelings in others.

Consideration of the following questions may be helpful when deciding whether to seek specific psychosocial information from a patient.

*A good source is Parkinson, M. H.: Therapeutic nurse-patient relationship. *In* Sorensen and Luckmann: *Basic Nursing: A Psychophysiologic Approach* (Chapter 3).

- Will the information help me more accurately understand this person's present experience?
- Will disclosure of this information have therapeutic effects for this person at this time?
- Will the information enable me to offer more complete and appropriate care to this person?
- Is this person communicating either verbally or nonverbally a desire to share this information with me at this time?
- Considering that self-disclosure requires personal integration, does this person have the energy to deal with self-disclosing?

Sometimes you will gather psychosocial information that leads you to believe that a person may benefit from psychiatric help. At these times, an appropriate referral may be indicated. However, in making a psychosocial assessment, you are not primarily looking for evidence of psychiatric pathology. Remember that assessment of behavior is difficult and must be done cautiously. Keep in mind that some part of anyone's behavior might appear strange if the person were under the kind of constant observation that often happens to hospitalized people.

> *The primary purpose of psychosocial assessment of "medical-surgical patients" is to enable nurses to understand patients' experiences accurately and to offer comprehensive care to patients and their significant others.*

INITIAL NURSE-PATIENT CONTACT

There is some truth in the idea that first impressions count most. The way patients and their significant others are received in the first few minutes of contact with health professionals can have a marked effect upon their feelings about and reactions to the care and treatment they receive. It may also affect their willingness to participate in care planning. It is also true that in many ways the first interactions between a nurse and a patient are the most difficult for both.

People are almost always anxious when they first enter the health care system. They have to interact with many "new people" and share information about themselves with strangers. They are asking for help from people they do not know. Often, they have a health problem that they do not fully understand. They are unsure about how they are going to be accepted or understood by the "professional strangers" they need to depend on and trust. They may expect to have to submit themselves to embarrassing procedures and take on a dependent role. All of these kinds of factors may contribute to making the first interactions with a nurse anxiety-producing and difficult for patients and their significant others.

Initial nurse-patient contacts may also be difficult for nurses. They are meeting strangers whom they are expected to help. Because they have limited information about the patient, it is more difficult to predict patients' behavioral responses. Each of us knows that we

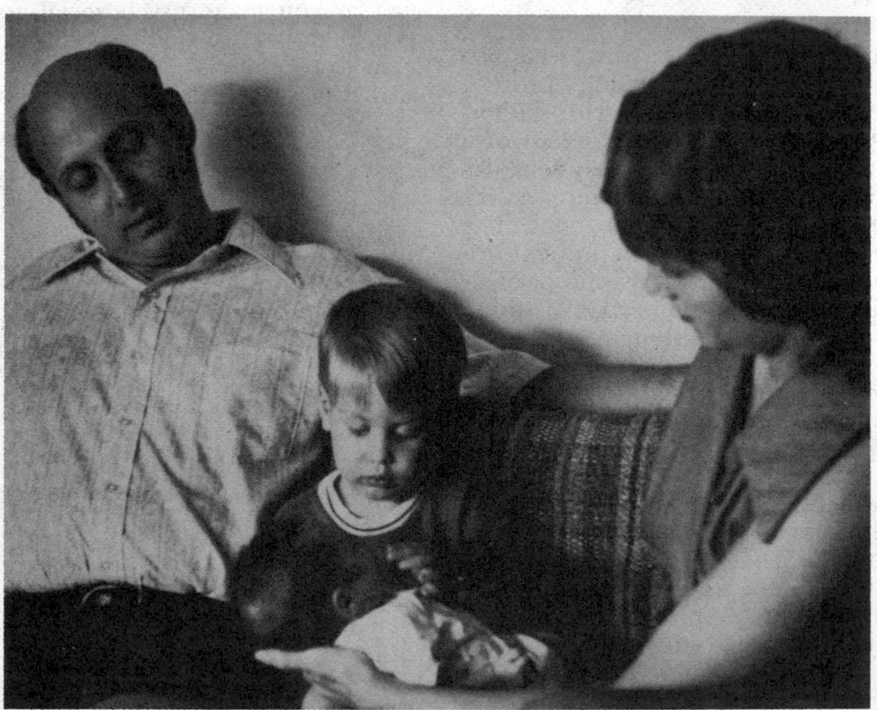

Figure 14–2. The Traditional Family Group. Some people function within this kind of social network—other people do not. (From Lugo, J. O., and G. L. Hershey: *Human Development. A Multidisciplinary Approach to the Psychology of Individual Growth.* New York: Macmillan Publishing Co., Inc., 1974, page 75.)

become nervous ourselves when we cannot predict how others will behave.

Yes, the initial nurse-patient contact is frequently difficult for both patient and nurse; yet, it is a highly important time! It is the nurse's responsibility to create an environment that is likely to reduce the anxieties and difficulties of everyone concerned. This can be facilitated if the nurse recognizes the psychosocial information that is initially available and uses it to assist the people seeking help to feel *known, accepted,* and *understood.*

What kind of information are we referring to? Let us consider a situation with which you are probably familiar. Suppose you are a nurse working in a health care facility and you are expecting a person to arrive shortly for help. You may well have some relevant information before the person does arrive. If you do not, you can get it within seconds of the person's arrival. Table 14–1 lists the kinds of psychosocial information you can obtain readily when you meet a patient for the first time. It also discusses some of the ways you could use such data in nursing intervention. *Nurses do not have to know patients or their significant others for a long period of time before they can perceive them as individual people.* Awareness of the common psychosocial information readily available and the thoughtful use of this information is all that is needed.

FACTORS THAT COMMONLY INFLUENCE PSYCHOSOCIAL ASSESSMENT

When you are making psychosocial assessments, keep in mind that the kind of information being considered is highly prone to distortion and interpretation. A number of factors — arising from the patient, the nurse, and the assessment setting — can minimize the accuracy and thus the usefulness of the information gathered.

The Patient. Myriads of individual factors make each patient different from every other patient. You will collect highly inaccurate information if you assume that the *same* situations have the *same* meanings for and the *same* effects upon *different* persons. Some factors making each patient's experiences unique are:

- *Anxiety.* Most people receiving health care services are anxious. Anxiety can cause people to behave in atypical, possibly "strange," ways. For example, as anxiety increases, perception can be narrowed, memory hampered, and verbal expression retarded. *Unless anxiety is reduced, data collected from a patient can be distorted.*
- *Fear.* Some patients are afraid of something that is happening to them — or something they imagine might happen to them. *If a patient's specific fears are not recognized and attended to, data collected from that patient can be distorted.*
- *Pain or discomfort.* Pain can absorb so much of a person's awareness that attention to anything else — including your questions — is difficult or impossible. *If pain or discomfort is not appreciated and reduced, a nurse may misinterpret information gathered from a patient.*
- *Culture.* Our cultural backgrounds may affect our behavior patterns in ways we are not even aware of. There are vast differences between cultures and between subcultures within the same society. *Unless nurses recognize when cultural differences exist between themselves and their patients, the data they collect may be misinterpreted and misunderstood.*
- *Stigma.* Patients may be in a position of being stigmatized or believing they are stigmatized. Whenever people perceive themselves as stigmatized (and therefore "judged") by others, they are likely to try to conceal information and be anxious that such information may be discovered by others. *A nonjudgmental and confidential attitude must be communicated by a nurse to overcome the barrier of stigma, even minimally.*
- *Regression and egocentricity.* Stressed and ill people often regress (use patterns of behavior that were appropriate to a previous age and developmental stage) and are frequently egocentric (experience difficulty in considering people and things outside themselves). *Unless nurses are understanding and accepting of regression and egocentricity in patients, information gathered from patients can be interpreted inaccurately.*

The Setting. People may be reluctant to share personal information with strangers, especially if the setting in which the information is being sought seems inappropriate. If the environment is stressful, the patient's verbal and nonverbal behavior will be affected. Psychosocial data can therefore be distorted. Factors to consider when trying to reduce environmental stress include:

- *Orientation.* Explain the physical surroundings, e.g., indicate where the patient may and may not go. Indicate the location of facilities the patient may need, e.g., bathroom, telephone. Briefly explain the presence of equipment or personnel that may seem "strange" and thus be anxiety provoking.
- *Privacy.* People may be hesitant to disclose personal information if they fear that they may be observed or overheard by others. More relevant information will probably be obtained if privacy is assured.
- *Belonging.* If people feel they are somewhere they ought not to be, they typically feel uncomfortable and anxious. Explanations can be reas-

> *Nurses can make more accurate psychosocial assessments if they reduce the amount of environmental stress experienced by patients and their significant others.*

suring. Also, allow the patient to comfortably ask questions.

- *Noise.* Unpredictable, unexplained noises can be annoying or even distressing to patients and their significant others, and can affect their behavior. Noise reduction is an important nursing intervention.

The Nurse. The collection of psychosocial information can be hindered or the information distorted by (1) factors hindering the creation of a therapeutic nurse-patient relationship and (2) factors tending to narrow the nurse's own perception.

TABLE 14–1. PSYCHOSOCIAL DATA READILY AVAILABLE DURING INITIAL NURSE-PATIENT CONTACT AND ITS POSSIBLE USES IN NURSING INTERVENTIONS

Data Obtainable	Possible Uses and Rationale for Obtaining Data
Name Use the patient's name, with Mr. or Ms. Ask the names of people who are with the patient: write them down if you may forget. Ask what each person prefers to be called; e.g., Ms., Mrs., first name, abbreviated name. Introduce *yourself* by name. State your role and how often the person may expect to be in touch with you.	In our society, being acknowledged by name and title is a courtesy that indicates respect. It also "feels good" psychologically. Finding out the names of significant others can be done quickly; using their names and the patient's name can reduce the patient's initial anxiety considerably. Be careful in using titles that designate marital status and gender; if you are wrong, you may reduce the patient's feeling of being treated as an individual. Stating your name and role can also reduce the patient's initial anxiety.
Gender Whether a patient is male or female is usually apparent, except with infants and occasionally older children. You may need to ask.	A person's gender may have little bearing in this situation, since human psychosocial responses are more similar than different between the sexes. Gender may matter in assigning a bed and room for a person being admitted to a health care facility. Be careful not to make assumptions or have expectations about a person's roles or behavior on the basis of gender.
Age The exact number of years (usually asked) is possibly less important than the developmental stage, e.g., infant, toddler, adolescent, adult, older adult.	Your knowledge of human growth and development will help you anticipate some needs of patients. Always remember that such theoretical knowledge describes the "average" person. Individual differences occur in everyone.
Where the person has come from The usual residence and the place from which the patient has just come may not be the same. You can use information about *both* to learn:	This information can be used in conversation. It can help individualize care and reduce anxiety.
a. How far and how long the person has traveled to reach the health care facility. b. When the person last left home. c. Whether the patient has had to depend on others to get to the health care facility. d. Whether the patient is likely to have personal items (toothbrush, nightclothes), if being admitted.	This information can help you understand some of the psychosocial stresses the patient and those accompanying the patient may have had and possibly are still experiencing. The person's ability to give such information and information about the health problem may help you in making a beginning assessment of the patient's mental status.
Reason the person is seeking help General information about the patient's health problem can give you psychosocial information as well.	This kind of information can indicate the *possible* anxieties the patient and concerned others may be having.
a. Is this a planned, elective visit, or is it an emergency situation that has taken everyone by surprise?	a. A person who has not expected to come to the health care facility may be worried about things that need attention at home or on the job. Also, other people may need to be notified about what is happening.

Trust building is very important. If a patient or the people primary to a patient do not perceive a nurse as trustworthy, they will attempt to protect themselves. For example, they may withhold information that they fear may be judged or denigrated by the nurse. The creation of a therapeutic nurse-patient relationship is vital to successful psychosocial assessment. Let us briefly review the core concept of such a relationship — self-disclosure.

Self-disclosure is often threatening and difficult, especially self-disclosure to strangers. Yet health professionals depend upon self-disclosure from patients. Unless patients share at least minimal amounts of information about themselves, health professionals have difficulty in helping. Jourard[37] suggests that the self-disclosure by patients can be facilitated by nurses who first self-disclose about themselves. This is the basis of genuine behavior. Stated in

TABLE 14–1. PSYCHOSOCIAL DATA READILY AVAILABLE DURING INITIAL NURSE-PATIENT CONTACT AND ITS POSSIBLE USES IN NURSING INTERVENTIONS (*Continued*)

Data Obtainable	Possible Uses and Rationale for Obtaining Data
Reason the person is seeking help (Continued)	
b. Is the patient experiencing pain or discomfort? How severe?	b. A person consumed with pain, discomfort, or anxiety may have little energy for anything else, e.g., history giving.
c. Is the patient's present health problem self-limiting or is it part of a progressive or on-going problem?	c. A person with a long-term health concern may understand more about it than a person who has just developed a health problem.
Significant others	
a. Notice and acknowledge persons accompanying the patient. Find out if they have questions for you.	a. Whoever the people with the patient are, they are present at a stressful and possibly a critical time. They need and deserve attention, too. It also helps the patient relax if the significant others are cared for.
b. If the patient wants a significant other to stay close by, this should be allowed if at all possible, even if that person is not "family." Ask the patient.	b. This information helps you to begin developing knowledge about the patient's social network and possible support system.
c. Find out from the patient those persons with whom the facility should stay in contact, e.g., in case of an emergency. These persons may or may not be the patient's legal next of kin.	c. Your job is to reduce patient anxiety as much as possible. Do not make assumptions about who is and who is not important to the patient. Do as the patient requests; recognize the fact that the patient may change these requests, also. If a patient has a sense of control, anxiety is reduced.
Nonverbal communication With experience, you will find you can learn much from a patient's nonverbal communication. Observe the patient and significant others for: a. Body language – posture, gestures, eye movements, use of touch b. Interactions among themselves	Often you will find evidence of anxiety in nonverbal communication during initial contact with the health care system. You may notice other things as well that can guide your behavior, e.g., does the patient rely on gesturing or touching during communication. Remember that information from nonverbal sources must be considered tentative until validated by the person or persons concerned. Nonverbal information can be used – but carefully.
Speech Listen closely not only to what people say but also to how they speak. Notice such things as: a. Choice of words b. Volume, tone, accent c. Repetition in speech d. Speech disorders	You may find evidence of anxiety in verbal communication, e.g., rapid speech, repetition, inappropriate laughter. If the person is talking very fast because of anxiety, you may be able to help by speaking slowly and clearly yourself and by repeating information as necessary. A person's accent, choice of words, or speech disorder can give you information about ability to comprehend and possible language barriers or neurologic problems.

practical terms: you are more likely to gather useful information from others if you share with them information such as:

- your name and role
- what you intend to do at this time with the patient
- your concern for the person
- what you anticipate doing with information the patient gives you
- how often and when the patient can expect to see you

> *You are more likely to get to know patients and their friends and family as* real *people if you are able to be a* real *person in your interactions with them.*

To a large extent, the amount and quality of psychosocial information you are able to gather will depend on your use of listening skills, especially those that communicate accurate empathy (e.g., reflection, clarification, and paraphrasing). Patients and their significant others will often give you a lot of information about their needs and wants. They will stop giving such information if they feel that you do not care about them, are not listening to them, or dislike them.

The personal *value systems* of nurses can greatly influence the ways they interpret and evaluate the behaviors and experiences of other people. We each have a value system, of course. That is part of being human. Professional helpers must, as individuals, develop awareness of what their values are. In fact, it is a professional responsibility to be continually striving for a heightened self-consciousness. There are many factors to consider, as demonstrated by the exercise in the box below. Take time to do the exercise, but read the directions first. It is important that your responses be quick and spontaneous.

Working to increase self-awareness helps you avoid the often harmful effects of trying to impose your own value system on other people. It also helps you to collect information from patients' and their significant others without making judgments about the information you are given. Thus, you are more likely to receive more accurate, more abundant, and more helpful information for your professional use.

COMPONENTS OF PSYCHOSOCIAL ASSESSMENT

It has been emphasized throughout this chapter that physical, psychologic, and sociologic assessments belong together. The three areas overlap and interact so greatly that significant information is lost if they are not considered in relation to each other. As we analyze each component, keep uppermost in your mind that in practice the components are inextricably intertwined.

IDENTIFICATION OF PERSONAL VALUES

Complete the first step of the exercise quickly, taking three minutes at the longest. Consider the following list privately. Beside each item on the list, *write down* "OK" if your *immediate* response is that the item is acceptable to you. Write "NOK" if your *immediate* response is that the item is not acceptable to you. Rate *every item.* Write the *first* response that comes to your mind.

___	marriage	___	nuclear power	___	suicide
___	abortion	___	interracial marriages	___	venereal disease
___	contraception	___	illegal drug use	___	mental illness
___	monogamy	___	domestic pets	___	smoking
___	feminism	___	capital punishment	___	vegetarianism
___	premarital sex	___	homosexuality	___	obesity
___	labor unions	___	religion	___	child abuse
___	pacifism	___	same sex marriages	___	divorce
___	wealthy people	___	atheism	___	illegal immigrants

Notice those items for which your response was clear and immediate, and those for which your initial response seemed to be unclear and/or a bit hesitant.

If you responded to each item quickly, you probably responded in the way you *really* believe, i.e., before you had time to think about how you "*should*" respond. Consider carefully how your values about these subjects could affect your reactions to people and your professional behavior.

Psychologic assessment involves the collection of information about variables that affect an individual's mind (or psyche) and the ways such influence is shown through behavior.[26] Let us consider some of these variables.

Behavior. Psychologists disagree over definitions of behavior. We find it useful to think of behavior as *all those activities of an organism that can be observed by someone else.* There are, of course, other processes occurring in human beings that cannot be observed directly by another person, e.g., thoughts, emotions, internal physiologic processes. How do we know that these "nonobservable" things happen? First, because we experience them ourselves and, second, because others tell us such things happen to them. Figure 14–3 illustrates the relationship between behavior and other activity (physiologic and psychologic). Behavior is, in a sense, the "keyhole" to the organism. We known that *all behavior has meaning.* What we do not always know, however, is what that meaning is, because we frequently have limited information about the physiologic and psychologic activity contributing to behavior.

It is more useful for nurses to describe behavior than to express what they think *behavior might mean.*

By describing a patient's behavior, the likelihood of making unvalidated and inaccurate assumptions is reduced. For example, a behavioral description might be: "Mr. Jones did not eat all his breakfast. He ate one piece of toast and a half a glass of orange juice. He left this cereal and coffee." This is more accurate information than: "Mr. Jones has lost his appetite," or "Mr. Jones is not hungry." These last two statements are highly subjective and, standing alone, represent mere "guesswork." They may be true or they may not be. Further validation is required.

Two general categories of behavior occur: (a) verbal behavior and (b) nonverbal behavior. *Verbal behavior* comprises the things a person says. *Nonverbal behavior* includes everything else a person does, e.g., posture, movement, facial expression, tone of voice.

The excellent nurse observes and reports both verbal and nonverbal behavior. Such a nurse recognizes that being observant is a major way of understanding another person. The excellent nurse also realizes that behavior is only a small part of a person's activity (Fig. 14–3) and recognizes that many unknown factors typically contribute to a person's behavior. A nurse might *suggest* what some of the unobserved contributing factors may be (e.g., Mr Jones *appears* unhappy, *perhaps* he is lonely) and then seeks more information (often by talking with the patient and the people close to the patient) that may validate the suggestions.

Consideration of behavior is central to all the other components of psychosocial assessment.

Mental Status. Assessment through a mental status examination was first suggested by Adolf Meyer in 1918.[68] Since then, systematic assessment of a person's mental status has become well established in both psychiatric and physical health care settings. It involves: (a) informal observation of a person's verbal and nonverbal behavior and (b) questioning directed toward assessment of the person's sensorium, i.e., consciousness. The principal areas

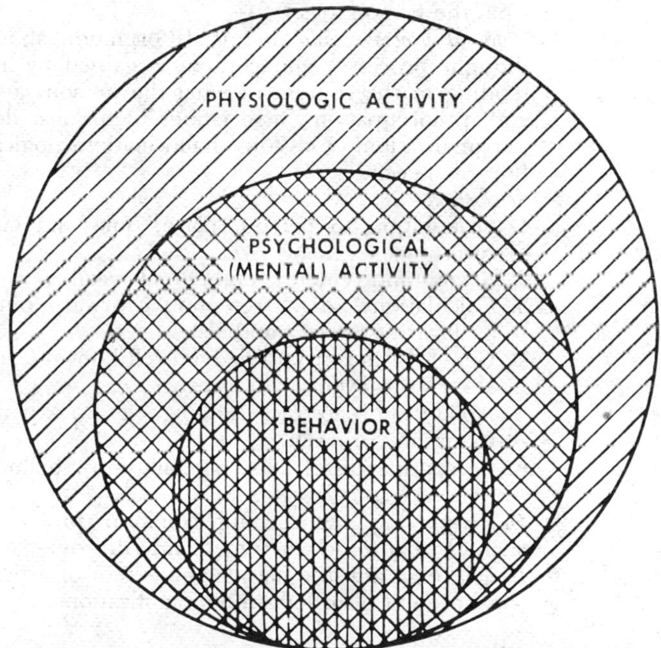

Figure 14–3. An abstract diagram to illustrate the relationships of various types of activity of the human organism. All activity, whether of the whole or of any of its parts, has a physiologic basis and, theoretically, may be studied from the standpoint of physiology. Thus all activity is shown encompassed within the large circle. Activity of the organism as a whole theoretically may be studied from either or both of two standpoints: physiology and psychology. Activity of this type is shown encompassed by the intermediate circle. A certain portion of psychological activity is accessible to the direct observation of other persons; this activity is termed behavior and, theoretically, it may be studied from three standpoints: physiologic, psychological and behavioral. It is shown here encompassed by the smallest circle. (From Hofling, C. K., and M. M. Leininger: *Basic Psychiatric Concepts in Nursing.* Philadelphia: J. B. Lippincott Co., 1960, page 99.)

and the usual reporting format for mental status examination are given below.[43, 68]

- *General appearance,* e.g., posture, facial expression, dress, grooming, any idiosyncratic and/or distinctive features.
- *Motor behavior,* e.g., gestures, gait, co-ordination of body movements, tics, tremors, grimaces, nail biting, wringing of hands, tapping of foot, involuntary movements, psychomotor retardation.
- *Affect,* e.g., lack of emotional response or presence of outward manifestations that may suggest emotion such as fear, anger, depression, elation, resentment. (Note and record the apparent *appropriateness* of a patient's affect.)
- *Mood,* i.e., the subjective description patients give of their own feeling tone.
- *Speech,* e.g., voice tone and pitch, rate of speech, spontaneity, coherence, articulation, duration of utterance, latency of response (i.e., the pause before answering), affectations, mutism. (The concern here is with *how* the person speaks, not with what the person says.)
- *Thought processes and content.* Information about thought processes and content is gained by attending to the content of what the person says, e.g., preoccupations, associations, delusions, depersonalization, obsessions, hallucinations, logical flow of speech.
- *Sensorium*
  1. Orientation to person, place, time and circumstance
  2. Recent and remote memory and recall
  3. Calculations, digit retention (forward and backward, serial 7's and 3's)
  4. General fund of knowledge (well known leaders, places, events, distances)
  5. Ability to do abstract thinking, e.g., to explain a common proverb
  6. Perceptual distortions, e.g., illusions, hallucinations
- *Judgment,* e.g., concerning common problems such as what to do when medicine runs out
- *Insight,* e.g., into the nature and extent of a person's present disorder and its ramifications.

Practice, along with the constructive feedback of others, is necessary to become skilled in doing useful mental status examinations. Extreme care is needed to avoid making invalidated assumptions and inappropriate judgments about a patient's mental status. You can help to avoid these dangers by (a) being aware of the ever present possibility of such difficulties, (b) reporting and recording the examination in terms of patient behavior as much as possible, (c) whenever possible (especially while you are learning and gaining experience), having someone else help you with the examination so that you can check out your observations and conclusions together, and (d) always striving to increase your own level of self-awareness so that you can counter the effects of your own values, beliefs, and prejudices—realizing that these could lead you to inaccurate conclusions about patients.

Remember also that your assessment of a patient's mental status is influenced by your own mental status. Practice the mental status exam with your colleagues. Take turns at being the patient. Give each other feedback and seek the critique of your teachers.

Other Psychologic Variables. While interacting with patients and their significant others, the astute and caring nurse gathers additional psychosocial information that enables nursing care to be planned in an individualized fashion. Although this is especially true when a nurse has the opportunity to know a patient over a period of time, it is also possible when the nurse-patient relationship is brief. Such information may indicate the patient's:

- *Motivations.* Does a patient give any information about personal wants, desires, goals, hopes—either in a general way or concerning current health concerns, treatment, and care?
- *Personal strengths.* Can you discern patient strengths or assets that can be used in planning individualized nursing care, e.g., verbal ability, self-awareness, creativity, special interests, ability to communicate with others. It is almost always more productive to encourage and build on a patient's strengths than to concentrate on apparent weaknesses.
- *Values and beliefs.* If you can collect data about the opinions, values and beliefs a person holds, and if you are able to accept these as valid (even though they may differ from your own), you will be able to understand the person better.
- *Lifestyle.* If you can seek information about a patient's day-to-day lifestyle preferences, along with wishes and goals the person has for future lifestyle changes, you will be in a better position to plan appropriate nursing care.

Formalized Psychologic Test. There are various formal psychologic tests that you may use or see others use, or from which you may receive results. Some of these tests require a qualified psychologist for their administration and interpretation. Common uses of formalized tests include (a) differentiation between organic and psychic disorders, (b) measurement of intelligence, and (c) assessment of psychopathology, psychodynamics, personality, and feelings.

For nursing purposes, psychosocial data gathered through interaction between the patient and the nurse are probably more useful than data from formal testing. Nursing assessment is more concerned with understanding a patient as an individual than with making diagnostic judgments.

Psychologic tests are generally classified as either objective or projective. *Objective psychologic tests* are qualitative assessments in which a person's responses are compared with established and standardized norms. Examples of such procedures include (a) vocational aptitude and interests tests, (b) intelligence tests (e.g., Wechsler Adult Intelligence Scale — WAIS), and (c) Minnesota Multiphasic Personality Inventory (MMPI). When taking an objective psychologic test, a person is required to respond in a fairly structured manner.

Projective psychologic tests give the person taking the test an opportunity to respond to stimuli in an unstructured way. These tests are designed to reflect a person's fantasies and individual modes of adaptation. Examples include (a) sentence completion tests, (b) Draw-a-Person tests, (c) Rorschach Psychodiagnosis (interpretation of inkblots), and (d) Thermatic Apperception Tests (TAT).

Sociologic Assessment

Sociologic assessment involves the collection of information about variables that influence an individual's performance of social roles and the person's positions within social systems.[26] As discussed earlier in this chapter, it is impossible to understand a person in a meaningful way without considering the social network within which the individual's life is led.

Social Network. You will recall that everyone has a basic human need for *love and belonging*. To fulfill this need, we all establish around ourselves a social network, or a group of people among whom we live our lives. Our social networks have for each of us the potential for fulfilling important functions,[53, 91] including:

- *Intimacy*, i.e., a closeness with others in which one can be warm, safe, and expressive. Intimacy is usually found with those others most personally significant or primary to an individual.
- *Social integration*, i.e., cooperative experiences occurring among people sharing similar situations and goals. Often found between friends and colleagues.
- *Nurturing behavior*, i.e., typically the care and responsibility a person has for a child. Also occurs and is important between adults.
- *Reassurance*, i.e., recognition and affirmation of worth and competence.
- *Assistance*, i.e., help and resources from others.

It is true that when people enter the health care system, nurses become temporarily a part of the patient's social network. It must be remembered, however, that patients still have the right to use their ongoing social networks that are part of their established lifestyles in the community. In addition, nurses have an obligation to provide care and support for those significant others who are experiencing stress along with a patient.

Information must be sought, therefore, concerning a patient's social network. A nurse needs to know something of the social network structure, along with the patient's wishes concerning this structure at the time. Initial information about a patient's social network may be gathered by:

- Observing who accompanies a patient to and from a health care facility and noting which persons telephone or seek to visit the patients
- Asking the patient questions:

  Who are the people most significant to the patient?

  What are the names of the persons the health care facility should keep in contact with and notify in case of an emergency?

  Does the patient want any restrictions placed on visitors or telephone calls? If so, what people are to be permitted to contact the patient? (Remember that patients may change their minds about any of these matters.)

It is a common tendency to assume that family members are the most primary people for an individual. *This is not always the case*. Social networks and significant others are very personalized, and we can make neither assumptions nor judgments about them.

MacElveen suggests the following areas for social network assessment.[53]

1. Nature of the patient's available network
   a. Kinship and nonkinship members
   b. Members nearby and at a distance
   c. Connectedness (loose or close-knit)
2. The patient's dominant network style
   a. Kinship (i.e., biological and legal family)
   b. Friendship (i.e., non-biological and non-legal relationships)
   c. Associate (i.e., organizational relationships)
   d. Restricted (i.e., limited relationships in quality and/or relationships)
3. The patient's relationships that fulfill the following needs:
   a. Intimacy
   b. Social integration
   c. Opportunities for nurturing behavior
   d. Reassurance of worth
   e. Assistance
4. The network potential to assist with current patient goals
   a. Strengths, resources, and supports
   b. Patient's history of use of network at previous times of trouble

You will notice that throughout this book we use terms such as *significant others, support systems, concerned others,* and *primary people* instead of "family." This is done to encourage you to seek information about each person's social network rather than make the assumption that everyone functions within a traditional family.

Socioeconomic Status. This refers to a person's economic position in a social system.[26]

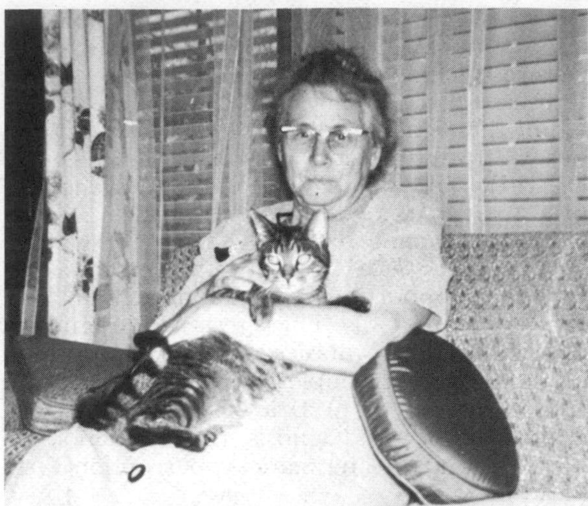

Figure 14–5. Animals can be significant others.

There is a tendency in Western society to evaluate people's worth or prestige according to their socioeconomic position. This is obviously not the reason nurses seek information of this nature. However, nurses are people and, thus, need to be aware of tendencies they may have to judge people on the basis of their material wealth and social standing.

To understand a patient better and to appreciate the concerns and stresses the patient may have, it may be appropriate for a nurse to seek information concerning:

a. The patient's occupation, current job, and any work-related concerns
b. The patient's financial concerns
c. Effects of the patient's current health status on work and finances
d. Beliefs held by the patient that socioeconomic factors have an effect upon his or her current health status
e. The patient's educational background, hopes, and goals

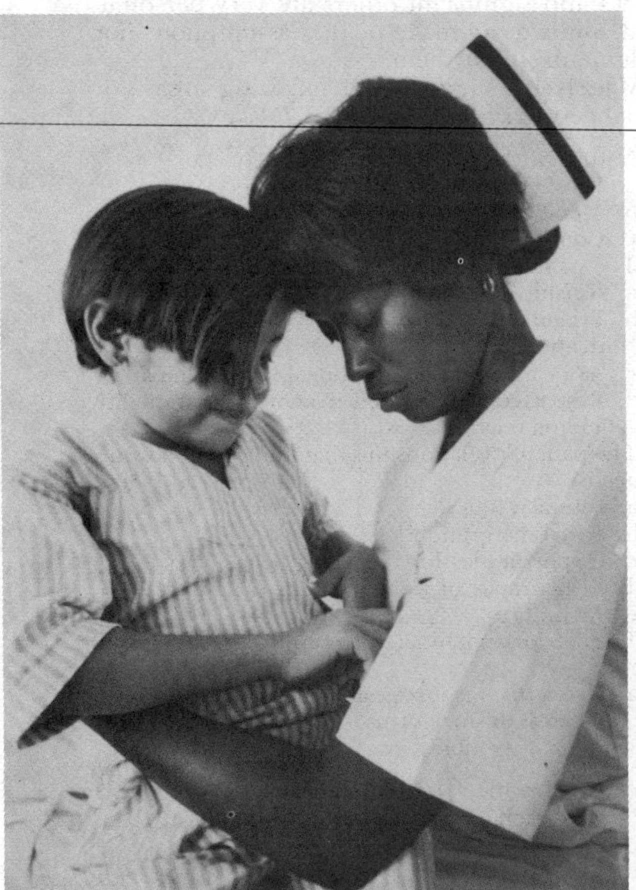

Figure 14–4. A nurse becomes a temporary member of a patient's social network. A nurse is a significant other for a patient for a time. (From Lugo, J. O., and G. L. Hershey: *Human Development. A Multidisciplinary Approach to the Psychology of Individual Growth.* New York: Macmillan Publishing Co. Inc., 1974, page 168.)

Lifestyle. Lifestyle is a term meaning "a person's typical patterns of living." Again, a nurse may understand a patient better through this kind of information. For example, it may be useful to discuss with the patient:

a. Usual roles and statuses
b. Work patterns
c. Desired leisure activities: actual leisure activities
d. Location and type of residence
e. Living arrangements
f. Where closest friends live
g. Predominant culture influencing patient's lifestyle

Sexuality. The term "sexuality" refers to actual sexual behavior and also to the perception people have of themselves as male or female. There are a number of ways in which issues relating to a person's sexuality may become important in nursing practice. These include:

a. Physical health problems that may affect a person's sexual behavior, e.g., mastectomy, colostomy, paralysis, venereal disease
b. Issues concerning reproduction, e.g., contraception, abortion, infertility
c. Patient's concerns about sexual performance, e.g., difficulty reaching orgasm, premature ejaculation, specific methods of sexual pleasuring
d. Issues or procedures relating to sex role function, e.g., feminism, equal rights for men and women, rights to privacy, transsexual surgery
e. Sexual activity for the disabled person or the long-term institutionalized person, e.g., ways for the physically disabled person to achieve sexual satisfaction; opportunity for an institutionalized person to have sexual expression

Although sexuality is increasingly discussed, it remains a difficult and delicate topic for many individuals. This is especially true for persons who think their sexuality may be judged or criticized by others. For example, persons with same-sex sexual orientation (gay persons) may be sensitive to such criticism. This group makes up an estimated 10 per cent of the population.[11]

In assessing sexuality, as in all areas of psychosocial assessment, it is important to minimize the extent to which your own values and beliefs interfere with your ability to accept and interact with other people and your ability to provide a professional level of care.

Psychosocial Development. An individual's age and stage of maturational development have a marked effect upon the data collected during psychosocial assessment and the interpretation of that data. This includes both physical and psychosocial development.

There are a number of theories of psychosocial development that can be useful in nursing practice. Always remember, however, that theoretical frameworks describe the "typical." *No one is typical in all respects*. Each person must be considered as a unique individual.

You may find it useful to seek information concerning the following theoretical approaches to psychosocial development:

- Freud's psychosexual theory of development
- Role theory concerning socialization
- Kohlberg's cognitive-developmental theory
- Social-learning theory of development
- Havinghurst's theory of developmental tasks
- Piaget's theory of cognitive development
- Erikson's psychosocial theory of development

Let us briefly consider *Erikson's*[24] popular theory of psychosocial development. As is shown in Table 14-2, Erikson believes that psychosocial development occurs over *eight stages*. At each stage the individual faces a particular crisis. For example, during the first year of life a person learns to *trust*. If this does not occur satisfactorily, then the person's personality tends to be characterized by mistrust. Likewise, in the second year a struggle typically occurs as the child strives to gain a sense of *autonomy*. Failure to achieve this task satisfactorily may result in a personality characterized by shame and doubt. Further study of Table 14-2 provides information concerning the relationship typical of each stage, the psychosocial modalities that focus at each stage, and the outcomes that occur if the individual is successful at each stage.

A sound understanding of human growth and development can give you a baseline for making assessments (being careful not to overemphasize the "normal"). It can also give you a knowledge base from which to approach each individual you meet.

WHAT TO DO WITH PSYCHOSOCIAL DATA

Be reminded again that the major reason nurses collect psychosocial data about patients is to enable them to *understand* patients better. By considering a patient's psychologic and sociologic patterns along with physiologic processes, you will be in a good position to identify nursing problems and plan comprehensive nursing care. Psychosocial data is often viewed as very private by the person concerned. Nurses must handle such information with professional confidentiality. Unless information is relevant to the patient's needs and will be *used* in providing nursing care, we have no right to it.

Occasionally you will collect psychosocial information that you consider indicative of psychiatric illness in a person. When this occurs, it would probably be helpful to discuss your observations with another health professional. Some facilities employ nurse psychiatric clinical specialists who may be used as consultants. It would also be appropriate to discuss your observations with the physician attending the patient. The decision to suggest psychiatric help for a patient will be based on several factors:

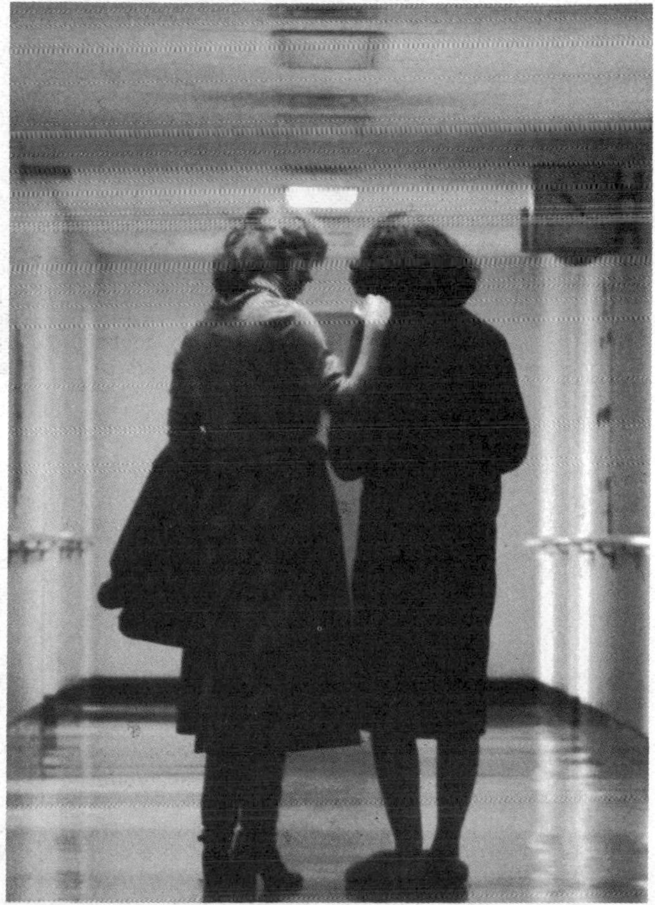

Figure 14–6. For some people, the most significant other in their lives is a person of the same sex as themselves. (From *RN*, 42(No. 4):47, 1979.)

- Amount of psychosocial discomfort the patient and/or significant others are experiencing
- Duration of the indications of possible psychiatric illness
- Evidence of psychiatric disorders in the patient's history
- The patient's wishes and desires and possibly those of the patient's significant others

SPECIFIC PSYCHOSOCIAL ASSESSMENTS

We cannot here discuss in detail all the areas of psychosocial assessment in which a nurse may be involved. There will be times when a nurse needs to make skillful, thorough assessments concerning patient situations such as loss, bereavement, crisis, potential for suicide, potential violent behavior, adjustment to long-term illness or disability, rehabilitation potential, and drug or alcohol dependency.

We have presented a brief account — only an overview really — of psychosocial assessment that may be undertaken by a nurse in a nonpsychiatric setting. An extensive bibliography is provided for more detailed study, for this surely is an area in which further study will help you develop your skills in "the caring art."

CONCLUSION

The first step of the nursing process is assessment, for the purpose of gathering information that will provide an accurate nursing diagnosis. Psychosocial assessment involves gathering information about a patient's psychosocial needs. In Maslow's terms, these are the higher needs of love and belonging, self-esteem, and self-actualization. The extent and depth of psychosocial data gathering is variable. Every patient has different circumstances, and the kind and depth of psychosocial information required to provide excellent nursing care differs greatly.

Look back now to the quote at the beginning of this unit (p. 293). Are you now in the process of focusing on the "whole" more than the "part"? Are you now more fully aware that a person cannot be understood by considering some "parts" without reference to the total person? Such is the life-long striving of excellent nurses.

BIBLIOGRAPHY

1. Aguilera, D. C.: *Review of Psychiatric Nursing*. St. Louis: C. V. Mosby Co., 1977.

TABLE 14–2. EIGHT STAGES OF PSYCHOSOCIAL DEVELOPMENT

Stages (Ages Are Approximate)	Psychosocial Crises	Radius of Significant Relations	Psychosocial Modalities	Favorable Outcome
1. Birth through first year	Trust versus mistrust	Maternal person	To get To give in return	Drive and hope
2. Second year	Autonomy versus shame, doubt	Parental persons	To hold (on) To let (go)	Self-control and willpower
3. Third year through fifth year	Initiative versus guilt	Basic family	To make (going after) To "make like" (playing)	Direction and purpose
4. Sixth year to onset of puberty	Industry versus inferiority	Neighborhood; school	To make things (competing) To make things together	Method and competence
5. Adolescence	Identity and repudiation versus identity diffusion	Peer groups and outgroups; models of leadership	To be oneself (or not to be) To share being oneself	Devotion and fidelity
6. Early adulthood	Intimacy and solidarity versus isolation	Partners in friendship, sex, competition, cooperation	To lose and find oneself in another	Affiliation and love
7. Young and middle adulthood	Generativity versus self-absorption	Divided labor and shared household	To make be To take care of	Production and care
8. Later adulthood	Integrity versus despair	"Mankind" "My kind"	To be, through having been To face not being	Renunciation and wisdom

From Kaluger, G., and M. F. Kaluger: *Human Development, The Span of Life.* St. Louis: C. V. Mosby Co., 1974, p. 89. (As modified from Erikson, E. H.: *Childhood and Society,* ed. 2. New York: W. W. Norton & Co., Inc. 1963.)

2. Alston, J. F., and J. M. Levet: What's happening: Practical applications of the mental status exam. *Nurse Practitioner*, 2:37, July-Aug. 1977.
3. American Nurses' Association Standards of Psychiatric and Mental Health Nursing Practice. American Nurses Association, 1973.
4. Arangio, A. J.: An assessment model: A systemic examination of the psychosocial needs of patients with epilepsy. *Patients Counselling and Health Education*, 1:75, Fall 1978.
5. Ashton, H.: Study of a hospitalised adolescent. *The New Zealand Nursing Journal*, 72:15, Jan. 1979.
6. Baer, E. D., et al.: How to take a health history. *American Journal of Nursing*, 77:1190, July 1977.
7. Baker, J. M., and L. K. Kelley: Loss: Some origins and nursing implications. *In* Longo D. C., and R. A. Williams (Eds.): *Clinical Practice in Psychosocial Nursing: Assessment and Intervention*. New York: Appleton-Century-Crofts, 1978.
8. Baldwin, C. A.: Mental health consultation in intensive care unit: Toward greater balance and precision of attribution. *Journal of Psychiatric Nursing and Mental Health Services*, 16:17, Feb. 1978.
9. Beckingham, C. R.: Bonds in family of origin. *The New Zealand Nursing Journal*, 72:10, Jan. 1979.
10. Bishop, B.: A guide to assessing parenting capabilities. *American Journal of Nursing*, 76:1784, Nov. 1976.
11. Brossart, J.: The gay patient. What you should be doing. *RN*, 42:50, Apr. 1979.
12. Brown, M. A.: Human sexuality. *In* Longo, D. C., and R. A. Williams (Eds.): *Clinical Practice in Psychosocial Nursing: Assessment and Intervention*. New York: Appleton-Century-Crofts, 1978.
13. Bush, M. T., and K. S. Babich: Cultural variation. *In* Longo, D. C., and R. A. Williams (Eds.): *Clinical Practice in Psychosocial Nursing: Assessment and Intervention*. New York: Appleton-Century-Crofts, 1978.
14. Byrne, M. L., and L. F. Thompson: *Key Concepts for the Study and Practice of Nursing*, 2nd ed. St. Louis: C. V. Mosby Co., 1978.
15. Caplan, G.: *Support Systems and Community Mental Health*. New York: Behavioral Publications, 1974.
16. Carkhuff, R. R.: *Helping and Human Relations. Vol. 1*. New York: Holt, Rinehart and Winston, Inc., 1969.
17. Chard, M.: An approach to examining the adolescent male. *Maternal Child Nursing*, 1:41, Jan.-Feb. 1976.
18. Chase-Marshall, J.: Virginia Satir, Everybody's family therapist. *Human Behavior*, 5:25, Sept. 1976.
19. Coombes, A. W., D. L. Avila, and W. W. Purkey: *Helping Relationships, Basic Concepts for Helping Professions*. Boston: Allyn and Bacon, 1971.
20. Dossey, B.: Perfecting your skills for systematic patient assessments. *Nursing '79*, 9:42, Feb. 1979.
21. Eggland, E. T.: How to take a meaningful nursing history. *Nursing '77*, 7:22, July 1977.
22. Eichel, E.: Assessment with a family focus. *Journal of Psychiatric Nursing and Mental Health Services*, 16:11, Jan. 1978.
23. Eisenman, E. J. P., and P.M. Dubbert: The mental health assessment interview. *In* Backer, B. A., P. M. Dubbert, and E. J. P. Eiseman: *Psychiatric/Mental Health Nursing: Contemporary Readings*. New York: D. Van Nostrand Co., Inc., 1978.
24. Erikson, E. H.: *Childhood and Society*, 2nd ed. New York: W. W. Norton and Co., 1963.
25. Fast, J.: *Body Language*. New York: J. B. Lippincott Co., 1970.
26. Francis, G. M., and B. A. Munjas: *Manual of Social-Psychologic Assessment*. New York: Appleton-Century-Crofts, 1976.
27. Gillies, D. A., and I. B. Alyn: *Patient Assessment and Management by the Nurse Practitioner*. Philadelphia: W. B. Saunders Co., 1976.
28. Goffman, E.: *Stigma*. Englewood Cliffs, N.J.: Prentice Hall, Inc., 1963.
29. Graves, H. H., and E. A. Thompson: Anxiety: A mental health vital sign. *In* Longo, D. C., and R. A. Williams (Eds.): *Clinical Practice in Psychosocial Nursing: Assessment and Intervention*. New York: Appleton-Century-Crofts, 1978.
30. Gregory, I., and D. J. Smelter: *Psychiatry Essentials of Clinical Practice*. Boston: Little, Brown and Co., 1977.
31. Gurgold, G. D., and D. H. Harden: Assessing the driving potential of the handicapped. *The American Journal of Occupational Therapy*, 32:41, Jan. 1978.
32. Hauser, M. J.: Assessment: Determining the problem and the treatment provider. *Occupational Health Nursing*, 26:15, Sept. 1978.
33. Havinghurst, R. J.: *Developmental Tasks and Education*. New York: David McKay Co., Inc., 1942.
34. Hinsie, L. E., and R. J. Campbell: *Psychiatric Dictionary*, 4th ed. New York: Oxford University Press, 1970.
35. Hofling, C. K., and M. M. Leininger: *Basic Psychiatric Concepts in Nursing*. Philadelphia: J. B. Lippincott Co., 1960.
36. Holmes, T. H., and R. H. Rahe: The social readjustment rating scale. *Journal of Psychosomatic Research*, 11:213, 1967.
37. Jourard, S.: *The Transparent Self*, revised ed. New York: D. Van Nostrand Co., 1971.
38. Kaluger, G., and M. F. Kaluger: *Human Development. The Span of Life*. St. Louis: C. V. Mosby Co., 1974.
39. Katachadorian, H., and D. Lunde: *Fundamentals of Human Sexuality*. New York: Holt, Rinehart and Winston, 1972.
40. Kohlberg, L.: Stage and sequence: The cognitive-developmental approach to socialization. *In* Goslin, D. A. (Ed.): *Handbook of Socialization Theory and Research*. Chicago: Rand McNally, 1969.
41. Kraegal, J. M., et al.: *Patient Care System*. Philadelphia: J. B. Lippincott Co., 1974.
42. Krug, S. E. (Ed.): *Psychological Assessment in Medicine*. Champaign, Ill: Institute for Personality and Ability Testing, 1977.
43. Krupp, M. A., and M. J. Chatton: *Current Medical Diagnosis and Treatment*, 16th annual revision. Los Altos, Calif.: Lange Medical Publications, 1977.
44. Lewis, J. M., W. R. Beavers, and J. T. Gossett et al.: *No Single Thread: Psychological Health in Family Systems*. New York: Brunner/Mazel Inc., 1976.
45. Lindsay, J. S. B., and D. Natham: Families. *New Zealand Medical Journal*, Sept. 25, 1974, pp. 258–263.
46. Lezak, M. D.: *Neuropsychological Assessment*. New York: Oxford University Press, 1976.
47. Lickorish, J. R.: The psychometric assessment of the family. *In* Howells, J. G. (Ed.): *Theory and Practice of Family Psychiatry*. New York: Brunner/Mazel Publishers, 1968.
48. Longo, D. C., and R. A. Williams (Ed.): *Clinical Practice in Psychosocial Nursing: Assessment and Intervention*. New York: Appleton-Century-Crofts, 1978.
49. Longo, D. C.: Communications and human behavior. *In* Longo, D. C., and R. A. Williams (Eds.) *Clinical Practice in Psychosocial Nursing: Assessment and Intervention*. New York: Appleton-Century-Crofts, 1978.
50. Lugo, J. O., and G. L. Hershey: *Human Development: A Multidisciplinary Approach to the Psychology of Individual Growth*. New York: Macmillan Publishing Co., Inc., 1974.
51. Luft, J.: *On Human Interaction*. Palo Alto, Calif.: National Press Books, 1969.
52. Lynaugh, J. E., and B. Bates: Physical diagnosis: A skill for all nurses? *American Journal of Nursing*, 74:58, Jan. 1974.
53. MacElveen, P. M.: Social networks. *In* Longo, D. C., and

R. A. Williams (Eds.): *Clinical Practice in Psychosocial Nursing: Assessment and Intervention*. New York: Appleton-Century-Crofts, 1978.
54. Malasanos, L., et al.: *Health Assessment*. St. Louis: C. V. Mosby Co., 1977.
55. Manaser, J. C., and A. M. Werner: *Instruments for Study of Nurse-Patient Interaction*. New York: Macmillan Co., 1964.
56. Mancini, J. A.: Leisure satisfaction and psychologic well-being in Old Age. *Journal of the American Geriatrics Society*, XXVI:550 Dec. 1978.
57. Marsden, A., and J. M. Sana: Nurse-patient communication and relationship in the physical appraisal process. *In* Sana, J. M., and R. D. Judge (Eds.): *Physical Appraisal Methods in Nursing Practice*. Boston: Little, Brown and Co., 1975.
58. Maslow, A. H.: *Motivation and Personality*. New York: Harper and Row, 1954.
59. Masters, W., and V. Johnson: *Pleasure Bond*. New York: Bantam Books, 1974.
60. McBride, A. B.: Can family life survive? *American Journal of Nursing* 75:1648, Oct. 1975.
61. Mechner, F.: Taking a patient's history–A programmed unit. *American Journal of Nursing*, 74:293, Feb. 1974.
62. Milton, J. E., M. D. Senn, and A. J. Solnit: *Problems in Child Behavior and Development*. Philadelphia: Lea & Febiger, 1968.
63. Mitchell, P. H., et al.: Neurological examination: Nursing assessment for nursing purposes. *Journal of Neurosurgical Nursing*, 9:23, Mar. 1977.
64. Moos, R., P. Insel, and B. Humphrey: *Preliminary Manual for Family Environment Scale*. Palo Alto, Calif.: Consulting Psychologists Press Inc., 1974.
65. Morgan, S. A., and M. J. Macy: Three assessment tools for family therapy. *Journal of Psychiatric Nursing and Mental Health Services*, 16:39, Mar. 1978.
66. Murray, R. L. E. (Ed.): The concept of body language. *Nursing Clinics of North America*, 7:617, 1972.
67. Murray, R., and J. Zentner: *Nursing Assessment and Health Promotion Through the Life Span*. Englewood Cliffs, N.J.: Prentice Hall Inc., 1975.
68. Nicholi, A. M. (Ed.): *The Harvard Guide to Modern Psychiatry*. Cambridge, Mass.: The Belknap Press of Harvard University Press, 1978.
69. Oehrtman, S. E.: Assessment and crisis intervention: A model for the family. *In* Hall, J. E., and B. R. Weaver (Eds.): *Nursing of Families in Crisis*. Philadelphia: J. B. Lippincott Co., 1974.
70. Phippen, M. L.: Intraoperative nursing assessment. *AORN*, 28:160, July 1978.
71. Piaget, J.: *The Origins of Intelligence in Children*. New York: W. W. Norton and Co., Inc., 1963.
72. Pogoncheff, E.: The gay patient. What *not* to do. *RN*, 42:46, Apr. 1979.
73. Prather, H.: *Notes to Myself*. London: Lyrebird Press Limited, 1972.
74. Quinn, J. L., and N. E. Ryan: OR nursing assessment of the older adult. *AORN* 29:235, Feb. 1979.
75. Rappaport, M.: Psychological Nursing in Industry. *Occupational Health Nursing*, 26:26, May 1978.
76. Rice, A. S.: An economic framework for viewing the family. *In* Ivan, F. N., and F. M. Bernado (Eds.): *Emerging Conceptual Frameworks in Family Analysis*. New York: Macmillan Co., 1966.
77. Robinson, L.: *Liaison Nursing: Psychological Approach to Patient Care*. Philadelphia: F. A. Davis Co., 1974.
78. Robinson, L.: *Psychological Aspects of the Care of Hospitalized Patients*, 2nd ed. Philadelphia: F. A. Davis Co., 1974.
79. Rogers, J. C., J. M. Weinstein, and J. J. Figone: The interest check list: An empirical assessment. *The American Journal of Occupational Therapy*, 32:628, Nov.-Dec. 1978.
80. Rose, M. A.: Problems families face in home care. *American Journal of Nursing*, 76:416, Mar. 1976.
81. Rostron, J., and P. M. Rostron: Assessment techniques for rehousing or adaptations for severely physically disabled adults. *International Journal Nursing Studies*, 15:203, 1978.
82. Sarason, I. G., et al.: Assessing the impact of life changes: Development of the life experiences survey. *Journal of Consulting and Clinical Psychology*, 46:932, Oct. 1978.
83. Satir, V.: *Conjoint Family Therapy*, revised edition. Palo Alto, Calif.: Science and Behavior Books, 1967.
84. Satir, V.: *Peoplemaking*. Palo Alto, Calif.: Science and Behavior Books, 1972.
85. Schaffer, H. R.: *The Growth of Sociability*, Baltimore, Md.: Penguin Books Inc., 1971.
86. Schneggenberger, C.: History taking skills: How do you rate? *Nursing '79*, 9:97, Mar. 1979.
87. Schwartz, L. H., and J. L. Schwartz: *The Psychodynamics of Patient Care*. Englewood Cliffs, N.J.: Prentice-Hall Inc., 1972.
88. Sorensen, K. C., and J. Luckmann: *Basic Nursing: A Psychophysiologic Approach*. Philadelphia: W. B. Saunders Co., 1979.
89. Speck, R. V., and C. L. Attneave: Social networks intervention. *In* Haley, J. (Ed.): *Changing Families*. New York: Grune and Stratton, 1971.
90. Storlie, F.: The family: Thirteen years of observation. *Supervisor Nurse*, 7:10, Feb. 1976.
91. Weiss, R. S.: The fund of sociability. *Trans-Action*, 6:36, July-Aug. 1969.
92. Westley, W. A., and N. B. Epstein: *Silent Majority*. San Francisco: Jossey-Bass Inc., 1970.
93. Whitley, M. P., and L. Madden: Encountering Dysfunction in the Family System. *In* Longo, D. C., and R. A. Williams (Eds.): *Clinical Practice in Psychosocial Nursing: Assessment and Intervention*. New York: Appleton-Century-Crofts, 1978.
94. Whitley, M. P., and D. Willingham: Adding a sexual assessment to the health interview. *Journal of Psychiatric Nursing and Mental Health Services*, 16:17, April 1978.
95. Williams, C. C., and T. H. Holmes: Life change, human adaptation and onset of illness. *In* Longo, D. C., and R. A. Williams (Eds.): *Clinical Practice in Psychosocial Nursing: Assessment and Intervention*. New York: Appleton-Century-Crofts, 1978.
96. Williams, R. A.: Crisis intervention. *In* Longo, D. C., and R. A. Williams (Eds.): *Clinical Practice in Psychosocial Nursing: Assessment and Intervention*. New York: Appleton-Century-Crofts, 1978.
97. Wood, N. F.: *Human Sexuality in Health and Illness*, St. Louis: C. V. Mosby Co., 1974.

UNIT VII

PHYSICAL ASSESSMENT

by Carolyn Mueller Jarvis, R.N., M.S.N.

INTRODUCTION AND STUDY GUIDE

Nurses have long been involved in the continuous observation and description of their patients' physical and emotional conditions; this data determines nursing interventions. The tools and skills used to gather this data have become increasingly sophisticated and technical. Systematic physical assessment has replaced hunches and intuition about a client's physical status. An avalanche of books and articles has been published to meet motivated nurses' growing demand for more knowledge of physical assessment skills. Additional articles address legal ramifications[14, 66] and how nursing's changing role would affect traditional relationships with other health professionals.[8, 35, 75] Many nursing leaders welcome the emphasis on physical assessment skills and the expanded role of the nurse because it shows that nursing is keeping pace with trends in health care. Proponents see the expanded role as a means to deliver better health care to more people and as a way to increase responsibility, accountability, and self-actualization for the nurse. Other nursing leaders, however, express concern that nursing is being gulled into inheriting one more task from physicians, i.e., physical assessment activities. They fear the acceptance of one more "delegated" task without concurrent grounding of that task in nursing theory.[51]

Physical assessment skills *do* have a place in expanding nursing practice. Performance of the physical examination *per se* is not a "prize" nurses should covet; that indeed would be "junior doctoring" and empty avant garde-ism. Instead:

> *Physical assessment skills should be incorporated into* nursing's *conceptual base and practiced with the focus upon the* nursing *needs of clients, families, and communities.*

Only nurses can deliver and monitor their unique product — comprehensive, high quality nursing care. To do this well, the professional nurse scientifically plans interventions by the use of the nursing process. This process (assessment, planning, implementing, evaluating) is a deliberate problem-solving approach to patient care.* The first step, assessment, is a systematic way of collecting and interpreting subjective and objective data about clients, their individual support systems, and their personal environments. Assessment includes the activities of data collection, data analysis, problem identification, and nursing diagnosis.

You already have developed many skills to aid in collecting data from and about your clients. The addition of the physical examination skills presented in this unit will *broaden and enrich your data base,* from which you develop your nursing diagnosis. Physical assessment skills can be utilized by nurses in acute, chronic, or community settings, and by independent nurse practitioners delivering primary health care.

*Refer to Chapter 2 of this text and Chapter 17 of Sorensen and Luckmann, *Basic Nursing: A Psychophysiologic Approach* for discussions of the nursing process.

Physical assessment skills do not stand on their own; rather they are best incorporated by every nurse into his or her existing nursing practice. As a systematic way of collecting data, physical assessment skills provide some *consistency in patient evaluation* among various nurses caring for the same patient. When used consistently with the same patient, physical assessment skills *establish a baseline,* identify any *change in physical health state,* and assist in the evaluation of the *effectiveness of nursing interventions.* Lynaugh and Bates list further uses of assessment skills in nursing practice, noting these skills can:

- Help confirm hypotheses growing out of the nurse's interview
- Enhance the investigation of nursing problems
- Increase the nurse's capacity to make good decisions about patients
- Enable the nurse to manage a greater range of patient care problems.[42]

You can use data gathered from physical examinations every clinical day to develop nursing judgments. For example, when postoperative patients cough or sound congested, you would auscultate the chest to search for evidence of rales. The presence and location of these adventitious breath sounds (rales) would help you determine such nursing activities as how to position the patient, how vigorously to encourage coughing and deep breathing, what other signs to look for (e.g., fever), and whether the physician should be notified. Knowledge of cardiovascular assessment skills would allow you to monitor changes in patients following myocardial infarctions, judge how well activity is tolerated, and assess patients' responses to specific medications or treatments. Assessment skills help you to make countless other clinical decisions, such as deciding when an anesthetized patient has reacted sufficiently to be discharged from the recovery room or deciding when to "advance diet as tolerated" by listening for the presence of bowel sounds in a patient's abdomen.

Physical assessment skills are used by nurses practicing in the community as well as in hospitals or other care facilities. For example, a complete health history and physical exam is performed by a *nurse practitioner* in many settings for the purposes of reinforcing health maintenance, screening for health problems, and identifying the need for health teaching. Nurse practitioners are providing entry-level care for many people. Some professionals are concerned that in performing a screening physical exam, a nurse is merely taking over the physician's task of physical diagnosis. One independent nurse practitioner, M. Lucille Kinlein, clarifies that the physical exam is merely a *tool* to gather data, and may be used by many different professionals.[36] The *goal* is what differs. A physician uses the physical exam to make a differential diagnosis and to treat specific illnesses by prescribing medications and or treatments. On the other hand:

- A nurse practitioner uses the physical examination for the goal of *health maintenance,* to identify what clients are doing to help them stay healthy. The nurse reinforces such positive aspects of the health state to increase the chances of clients' staying well.[36]
- Second, a nurse practitioner uses the physical exam to identify *actual* and *impending illness states* by comparing any detected abnormal signs and symptoms with knowledge of the range of normal physical characteristics for the client's age, sex, and race. Significant findings are referred to the appropriate health care professional. The nurse also gives professional judgment about the significance of a client's particular symptoms and helps the client make health care decisions.[36]
- Third, the nurse uses the physical exam to assess clients' needs for *health teaching* so that the clients understand their own body and can monitor their own health state. For example, health teaching may include teaching breast self-examination techniques to a woman, or discussing the importance of regular tonometry with a 42-year-old man who has a

family history of glaucoma. Teaching also would be offered to patients with chronic diseases to help them cope with disabilities and to help them recognize changes in their condition that warrant consultation with a physician or other health professional to avoid serious sequelae.

Study Guide

This unit consists of one detailed chapter (Chapter 15), including an extensive bibliography. Throughout, you are encouraged to read further about physical assessment, and specific references are mentioned in the text for this purpose. An introduction to physical assessment and health history is presented in Sorensen and Luckmann, *Basic Nursing: A Psychophysiologic Approach* (Chapter 16), including discussion of the basic techniques — inspection, auscultation, palpation, and percussion.

The preceding chapter, "Psychosocial Assessment," stresses the interrelatedness of psychosocial and physical assessment. As you study and practice physical assessment skills, try to be aware of the opportunities for integration of physical and psychosocial assessment.

After working carefully with the content of this unit you may expect to be able to:

1. Formulate and defend your personal position relative to the need for physical assessment skills in nursing practice.
2. Describe the usual sequence of a physical assessment.
3. Assist a client to be relaxed and comfortable during a physical examination.
4. Demonstrate, with supervision, the four basic techniques of physical assessment: inspection, palpation, percussion, and auscultation.
5. Incorporate interviewing and physical assessment skills in data collection for the assessment phase of the nursing process.
6. Describe the range of variation of normal physical findings.
7. Begin to identify physical deviations from "normal" and their possible significance for the client.
8. Make accurate reports of areas requiring further assessment or requiring treatment.
9. Recognize opportunities during the physical examination when it would be appropriate to teach the individual to monitor his or her own health status.
10. Appreciate your need for continuing tutored practice in order to develop and maintain competent physical assessment skills.

Take the time to review your anatomy and physiology texts and notes before studying each regional exam. This will help you recall normal findings and compare them to abnormal or pathologic ones. It also will help you to understand the principles that underlie each examination technique. You may encounter many unfamiliar terms in this chapter. We encourage you to compile your own glossary, seeking out explanations of terms you do not understand — from dictionaries, texts, and instructors — and writing down definitions in your own words.

Monitor your comprehension of the material in this chapter by answering the following questions as you study. Note that this is a *selected* list and covers only highlights of the physical examination.

1. Skills
   a. Define the terms *inspection, palpation, percussion,* and *auscultation*
   b. Define the following percussion notes considering intensity, pitch or frequency, quality, and duration: resonance, hyperresonance, tympany, dull, and flat
2. The health history: list and define the components of a complete health history
3. Overview of the examination
   a. List the basic equipment necessary to conduct a screening physical examination
   b. List environmental conditions that enhance the physical examination
   c. Describe significant aspects of the client's general appearance and behavior that should be noted during the initial contact
4. Eye
   a. Describe two ways to assess visual acuity

b. Explain these maneuvers: visual fields testing, corneal light reflex, cover-uncover test, alternating cover test, diagnostic positions test, direct and consensual light reflex, accommodation
c. List and interpret normal and abnormal signs relating to the external ocular structures
d. Describe the use of the ophthalmoscope, including proper positioning of yourself and the client
e. Systematically describe the characteristics of the normal ocular fundus: disc, vessels, general background, macula

5. Ear, nose, and throat
   a. Describe the appearance of a normal outer ear and external ear canal
   b. Describe the correct technique of otoscopic examination, including proper positioning of yourself and the client
   c. Systematically describe the normal tympanic membrane, including position, color, and landmarks
   d. Observe tonsils and grade on a scale of 1+ to 4+
6. Neck
   a. List the palpable characteristics that indicate normal, infected, or cancerous lymph nodes
   b. Describe the normal thyroid gland
7. Thorax and lungs
   a. Interpret the significance of a "barrel chest"
   b. List and describe the three types of normal breath sounds
   c. Define these adventitious sounds: rales and rhonchi
8. Breast
   a. Describe the components of the breast examination
   b. List and describe the characteristics to consider when a mass is noted in the breast
9. Cardiovascular system
   a. Define systole and diastole
   b. Explain the position of the valves of the heart during the cardiac cycle
   c. Define venous pressure and jugular venous pulse.
   d. Differentiate carotid artery pulsation from jugular venous pulsation
   e. State four guidelines to differentiate the first heart sound (S_1) from the second heart sound (S_2)
10. Abdomen
    a. Discuss inspection of the abdomen, including findings that should be noted
    b. Describe the procedure for auscultation of bowel sounds
    c. Name the organs that are normally palpable in the abdomen
11. Neurological system
    a. Define a dermatome
    b. Define the grade levels of a deep tendon reflex
    c. Describe the procedure to elicit the Babinski reflex and discuss the significance of the reflex
12. Genitalia
    a. List measures to achieve patient comfort during the genitalia exam
    b. Describe the technique for insertion of the vaginal speculum
    c. Distinguish direct and indirect inguinal hernia in the male, and describe the procedure for eliciting a possible hernia.

As you study succeeding chapters in this text, return to review related material in this chapter. For example, review "Examination of the Ear" before studying Chapter 90, "Disorders of the Ear and Related Structures." This will help you incorporate the data collection techniques from this chapter into the entire nursing process.

Consider ways assessment skills may be incorporated into nursing practice. Which assessment techniques are nurses in your clinical facility already performing while caring for patients? Which additional assessment skills could be added to enhance their nursing care?

Finally, it is important to stress that physical assessment *cannot* be learned in a "do-it-yourself" approach. Rather, tutored practice with an experienced clinician is essential to help you use proper manual techniques, to learn the wide variation of normal physical findings, and to identify and confirm abnormal ones. While manual techniques are described here, *supervised* practice sessions are essential to assure accuracy in positioning of yourself and the client and proficiency in handling of equipment.

CHAPTER 15

PHYSICAL ASSESSMENT

As you read and study this chapter, think about how *you* will incorporate skills in each regional examination into *your* nursing practice. The chapter is presented in the actual sequence of a routine screening physical examination. Components of the physical exam are integrated and are presented by anatomical area in the order that they are actually performed. Throughout the chapter, checklists are presented to review the basic components of the examination of individual body areas.

SKILLS REQUISITE FOR PHYSICAL ASSESSMENT

The physical examination calls upon the human senses of sight, hearing, touch, and smell to perceive the client's symptoms and physical signs and to relate them to knowledge of the variation of normal findings. Skills necessary for physical assessment are *interviewing, inspection, palpation, percussion,* and *auscultation.* Each body region is assessed in an orderly fashion, by the use of these skills. Inspection, palpation, percussion, and auscultation are introduced here and developed further throughout the chapter as they apply to particular body regions. Interviewing is discussed as part of obtaining the health history.

INSPECTION

Inspection is the act of visually observing the client. The purpose of inspection is to note any significant physical characteristics. This is an active process. It is *point-specific scrutiny* of the client as a whole and of each body system. Inspection yields much information, but occasionally is short-changed by the hurried or anxious examiner. That is, the nurse may be too eager to "lay on" the hands or may be embarrassed just looking at the client, without performing some manual act. Inspection should be purposeful, focused, and unhurried. If you find yourself rushing through the inspection period, try holding your hands behind your back a few moments or putting them in your pockets.

Begin physical assessment by greeting the client, introducing yourself, and shaking the client's hand. (A handshake is friendly and also provides initial information about physical status, e.g., strength of grip). Start the inspection process from the moment you first meet the client. As your inspection continues, attend specifically to the details described in this chapter, in the "Overview" and in the discussions about each body system. Concentrate also on any odors or sounds from the client. Compare your observations with established standards for the wide range of normal findings and for abnormal findings that require intervention.

PALPATION

Palpation makes use of your sense of touch to assess such factors as texture, crepitance, temperature, moisture, vibration or pulsation, swelling, rigidity or spasticity, organ location and size, presence of lumps or masses, and presence of tenderness or pain. Palpation frequently confirms observations made during inspection.

You use different parts of your hands for palpation, depending on the information you want. For example, the dorsa, or backs of the hands and fingers, are most suited for temperature assessment, because the skin there is thinner. The base of the fingers (the metacarpophalangeal joints), or the ulnar surface of the hand, is used for vibration. By placing your palm on the client's chest, you can assess the vibration of voice sounds (known as *tactile fremitus*). The tips of the fingers are the most sensitive for fine tactile discrimination and are used for such measures as skin texture, swelling, pulsatility, or to detect lumps. To determine the shape, position, and consistency of an organ or mass, use a grasping action of the fingers.

Palpation should be systematic and include bilateral comparison of body parts. Use a slow, gentle approach and be sure your hands are warm when you touch a person. Light palpation is done first; then deeper palpation is performed, while the client is encouraged to use relaxation techniques, such as deep breathing. Palpate any identified tender areas last. Finally, remember that many structures you palpate will not be visible; *you must know normal anatomy well to interpret the significance of your findings.*

PERCUSSION

Percussion involves striking the client's skin to determine the density, size, and location of an underlying structure. A brisk tap sets the body wall in motion; the quality of the sound produced describes the organ below. Each percussion "note" reflects the density (air versus solid matter) of the structure. Further, an organ can be "mapped out" by systematically percussing around its borders and noting where the percussion note changes between the organ and its neighboring tissues. The location and the size of the heart and liver, for example, are outlined this way. Percussion may identify an abnormal mass in an organ if it lies close to body surface. For example, a lung tumor that is close to the skin gives a dull percussion note instead of the normal resonance. A deeper tumor (4 to 6 cm. below the surface) would be undetected by percussion.

The method used most often is *indirect percussion* (Fig. 15–1).* The following procedure is for right-handed examiners: Place the distal portion of the left middle finger *firmly* against the client so that the skin blanches slightly. Avoid the areas over the ribs or scapulae, as percussing over a bone yields no useful information. Keep the rest of the left (or *stationary*) hand cocked up off the chest wall (see Fig. 15–1) so that the produced sound will not be damped. The middle finger of the right hand is the *striking* finger. Hold your right forearm steady; the action is all in the wrist. Cock your right hand back, and swiftly strike your right middle finger on the distal phalanx of the left middle finger just behind the nail bed. Withdraw the right hand quickly, or the sound will be muffled. Use even, staccato blows with equal force in each — no more than two or three in each body location. The amplitude of the sound is determined by the strength of the blow; use just enough force to achieve the desired sound, as very loud notes may sound distorted. You will need a heavier percussion note, however, for clients with very fat or very muscular body walls.

Each of the notes is assessed by the following characteristics:

- ▶ *Intensity* (or amplitude) — how loud or soft the sound is
- ▶ *Pitch* (or frequency) — the number of vibrations per second of a tone that yields a high, medium, or low pitch
- ▶ *Quality* — a sound's distinctive characteristics
- ▶ *Duration* — the length of time the sound lasts

In general, structures with relatively more air give a deeper, louder, and longer sound, while denser structures have a higher, softer, shorter sound.

Resonance is the tone produced over normal lung tissue. It has a clear, hollow quality, low-pitched, moderately sustained, and not very loud.

Hyperresonance is heard over lungs with an abnormal amount of air in them, such as the emphysematous or overinflated lung. This booming tone is lower and louder than resonance, moderately long, and slightly musical. It is normally heard in children, as their chest walls are thinner.

Tympany (like the kettle drum) is the higher-pitched musical sound heard over the stomach and intestines. It is loud and is the longest-sustained sound.

A *dull* sound is heard over a relatively dense organ such as the liver or spleen. It is a high-pitched, soft, short, muffled thud. It is heard pathologically when there is consolidation of lung tissue, as in pneumonia.

The *flat* sound (also called "absolute dullness") occurs when no air is present, as over thigh muscles or a large tumor. It is very soft, short, and high pitched.

Although five "normal" percussion notes are described here, there are wide variations in normal, and the "note" obtained will depend upon both the thickness of the body wall and the nature of the underlying structure. It is difficult to appreciate these various notes from written descriptions. "Live" demonstrations are, of course, necessary.

AUSCULTATION

This is the most complex of the appraisal techniques. *Auscultation is used to assess sounds produced by the heart, lungs, and abdomen and to note the presence of bruits or murmurs in the cardiovascular network.* It is a difficult skill because there are wide variations among the "normal" sounds of the body. After learning to recognize normal sounds, you can begin to distinguish normal from "abnormal" and "extra" sounds. Finally, you can begin to make discriminations about the significance of abnormal or extra ausculatory findings.

Some body sounds are heard with the unaided ear, e.g., the harsh rattling of congested breathing. However, most sounds are subtler and need to be channeled by a stethoscope to be evaluated. The stethoscope is a personal instrument, and many nurses want to purchase their own after reviewing its specifications.[9, 71]

The stethoscope must have two endpieces: diaphragm and bell (Fig. 15–2). The *diaphragm*

---

*Photographs in this chapter are reprinted with permission from the May, June, July 1977 issues of *Nursing 77*, Intermed Communications, Inc., 132 Welsh Road, Horsham, Pa. 19044. Further reproduction in whole or part expressly prohibited by law.

is used most often since it is for high-pitched sounds such as breath, bowel, and heart sounds. The diaphragm is held firmly against the client's skin. The *bell* endpiece has a concave shape and is used for soft, low-pitched sounds like murmurs or gallop rhythm. It is held lightly against the skin so that it forms a perfect seal. If you press too tightly, the skin will act as a diaphragm and filter out the low-frequency sounds. The earpieces should fit snugly in the ear canals, with the slope pointing forward toward your nose. Stethoscope tubing should be no longer than 30 cm. (12 inches) or sound may be distorted. Some clinicians think dual tubing transmits sound with less distortion than does single tubing.

You can manipulate the setting to maximize your efficiency with the stethoscope. Keep the room and the stethoscope endpiece warm for the client's comfort and to prevent shivering or involuntary muscle contractions that could drown out your findings. The room must be quiet; any extraneous room noise sounds like a roaring through the stethoscope. Be careful not to misinterpret sounds that are actually caused by bumping the tubing or from friction on the endpiece from, for example, a hairy

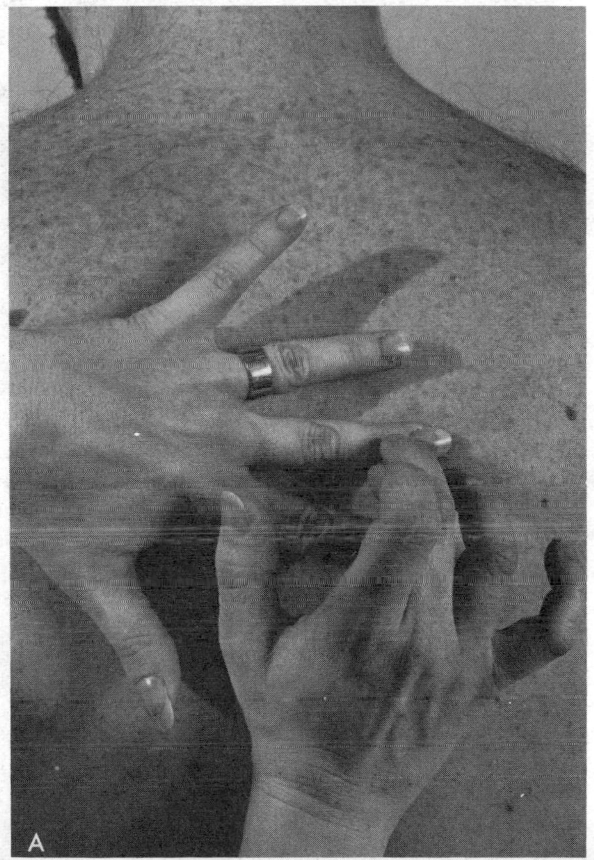

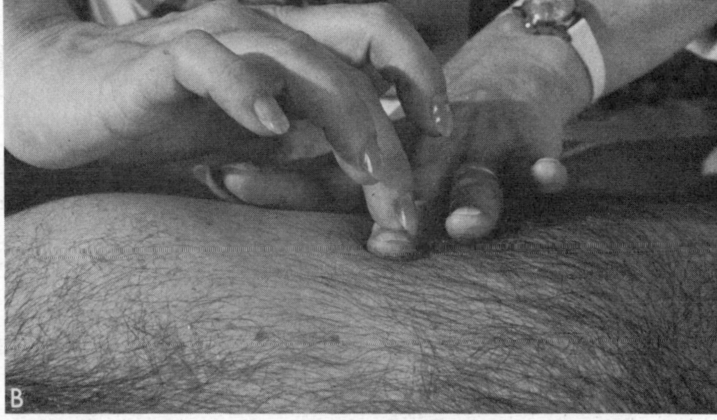

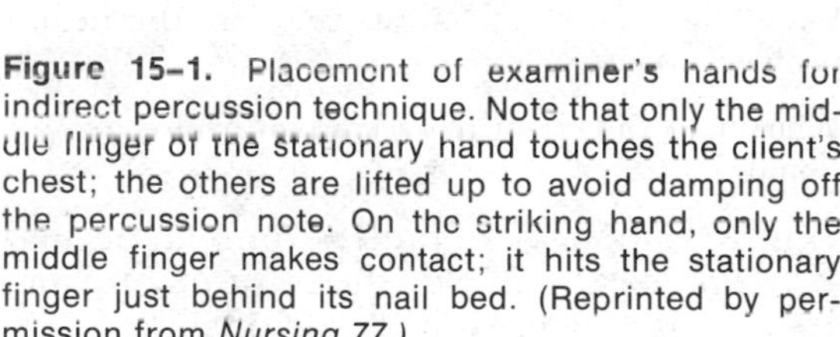
Figure 15–1. Placement of examiner's hands for indirect percussion technique. Note that only the middle finger of the stationary hand touches the client's chest; the others are lifted up to avoid damping off the percussion note. On the striking hand, only the middle finger makes contact; it hits the stationary finger just behind its nail bed. (Reprinted by permission from *Nursing 77.*)

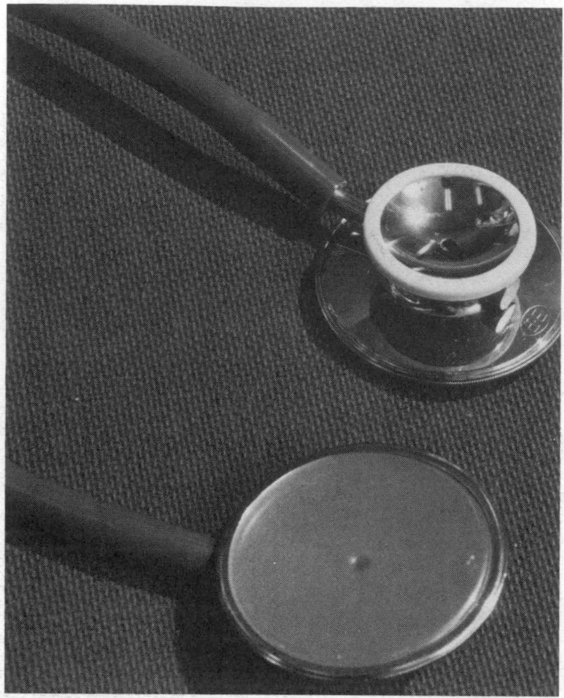

Figure 15–2. Bell (top) and diaphragm endpieces of stethoscope. (Reprinted by permission from *Nursing 77.*)

chest. (Wetting the hair before auscultating helps to decrease that sound.) In some body locations, it is possible to hear more than one sound. However, you must concentrate on only one thing at a time, and proceed slowly. As you listen, think: what *should* I hear over this organ; what do I *really* hear?

Summary

With all the assessment techniques, tutored practice with an experienced clinician is essential. With practice, you will learn to:

- ▶ Use proper manual techniques
- ▶ Recognize the wide variation of normal physical findings
- ▶ Identify and confirm abnormal findings

Study specific physical assessment texts and articles to increase your knowledge of normal anatomy and physiology and the relation of physical findings to pathology. Many appropriate references are included in the bibliography at the end of this chapter; note those cited in discussions of each regional exam. As your experience increases, you will become more confident in your skills and more independent in their use.

THE HEALTH HISTORY

The health history is an organized body of data used to assess a client's current and future health needs. (Note that a nursing history can be part of a health history.) The health history is an important clinical tool; obtaining it is the initial act of data collection, which sets the stage for subsequent gathering of information. *The interview is a means to establish rapport with the client and to develop mutual trust and respect.* The nurse strives to communicate warmth and to practice accurate empathy so that the client may feel free to offer information without fear of embarrassment, rejection, or loss of approval. Both the physical setting and skillful communication techniques can contribute to a successful interview. You would do well to review material about successful interviewing in conjunction with this chapter.*[1a, 6, 24, 44, 64]

The reasons for taking a health history are twofold. First, the history identifies what clients are doing that is helping them stay well. Second, it elicits physiologic, psychologic, and social information to assess any apparent or occult health problems. During the interview the nurse gathers data from the client and, in turn, provides the client with information. The nurse gathers data concerning:

- ▶ Identification of the areas that are health assets to the client
- ▶ A chronological development of the client's symptoms and problems
- ▶ The meaning of health problems to the client and significant others
- ▶ What the client has done to alleviate the health problem
- ▶ What help the client expects from health professionals

The information is organized into a permanent data base. While the written format varies among agencies, it usually includes: biographical data, chief "complaint," or reason for seeking care, history of present illness, past history, social history, family history, and review of body systems. In all areas, the health history must provide a profile of the client as an *individual*. Physical assessment texts can give you further descriptions of these categories.[26, 44, 55]

During the interview the nurse provides the client with information. First, during the history taking it may be helpful to explain your reasons for asking questions. For example, you might say, "I would like to ask you about your family's health. I do not mean that you have inherited or will have those health problems

*A good source of such information is Sorensen, K. C., and Luckmann, J., *Basic Nursing: A Psychophysiologic Approach,* Chapters 3 and 17.

that members of your family have. However, sometimes there is a tendency for some health problems to run in families. If your family members have any of these kinds of problems, we can discuss ways you can maintain your own health in view of your family's history."

Second, during the process of taking the health history, the nurse identifies areas where detailed client teaching will be needed during the physical exam or at a later time. For example, suppose that during the review of systems a female client tells you she does not do a monthly self-examination of her breasts. While it would not be appropriate to pursue detailed teaching of the breast exam during the health history, the need has been identified and can be met during the physical examination or at another appropriate time.

In addition to the gathering and disseminating of information, the health history is an introduction for the physical examination that follows. Many clients who enter a hospital or a clinic are anxious and embarrassed that a relative stranger will be examining their body and "invading" their privacy. By developing a warm, empathetic relationship with the client during the health history, you can alleviate much of this anxiety.

The client's history also provides cues about areas of the body that require closer scrutiny. For example, if during the history a woman client tells you she had rheumatic fever as a child and is now experiencing increasing dyspnea and swelling of the feet, you will want to evaluate her cardiovascular system very carefully. Be careful, however, not to jump to conclusions about the significance of data collected in the health history. For example, with this woman you may think you hear a heart murmur because you are certain there *ought* to be one.

OVERVIEW OF THE PHYSICAL EXAMINATION

Equipment

The following equipment is generally necessary for a screening physical examination. It should be laid out in an organized way and within easy reach:

- flashlight or penlight
- otoscope and ophthalmoscope
- nasal speculum (if a short, broad speculum is not included with the otoscope)
- tongue depressor
- sphygmomanometer
- stethoscope with bell and diaphragm endpieces
- flexible tape measure and ruler, marked in centimeters
- reflex hammer
- tuning fork
- sharp object (pin)
- cotton balls
- bivalve vaginal speculum
- clean gloves
- lubricant
- materials for cytologic study
- guaiac test reagents
- skin marking pen

Setting

The examination room should be quiet, warm, private, and well lighted. Natural daylight is preferable, but artificial light from two sources is adequate. A gooseneck lamp should be available for bright light. The examining room should be free from distracting noises that could mask body sounds and also be secure from interruptions. Place the examining table so that the client is not in shadow and so that you have easy access to both sides of the client.

Approach to the Client

The client will almost certainly be anxious. The anxiety may arise from several sources, including the physical examination itself. The nurse may be most helpful by conducting the examination in a confident and assured manner and by being considerate and empathetic. Explain each part of the exam, and encourage the client to ask questions. If the client can relax, the data gathered will more accurately reflect the person's normal state.

Ask the client to disrobe and put on an examining gown. Explain how to put on the gown, and leave the room as the client changes clothing (unless, of course, your assistance is needed). Ask the client to urinate (saving a urine specimen, if needed) before you begin the examination. Explain that an empty bladder will help the client feel more comfortable and will facilitate examination of the abdomen. Use drapes during the examination to avoid unnecessary exposure and to prevent chilling.

Before starting the examination, *wash your hands in the client's presence* — even if they are already clean. Begin by measuring the client's height, weight, blood pressure, pulse, and respirations. You may also measure visual acuity, using the Snellen eye chart. These are familiar, relatively nonthreatening maneuvers that help to gradually accustom the client to being examined by another person.

As mentioned earlier, while doing a physical examination you will use your senses of sight, hearing, touch, and smell to identify any symptoms and signs a client may have. You then relate your findings to your knowledge of variations among normal findings.

Oversights in physical examination can easily occur. The nurse needs to avoid distractions while performing an examination and concentrate on one thing at a time. While the sequence of the physical examination can vary slightly among practitioners, to avoid omissions, you should set up a system that works for you and not stray from it. It is a good idea to use a printed checklist to ensure consistency. Make sure the signs you perceive are really there. The health history can give you important background and clues, but be aware of the human tendency to distort findings to fit preconceptions.

The General Survey

While taking a health history and recording vital signs, the nurse also assesses the client in the following general areas: health state, age, sex, skin, breath and body odor, stature, nutritional state, posture, position, gait, body movement, mental status, and speech.

The general survey may show that the client's state of health is generally good with no signs of acute distress. However, if the client appears acutely or chronically ill, note the signs, e.g., difficult breathing, wheezing, tense facial expression, diaphoresis, fidgety movements. Notice any gross deformities or sensory impairment. Does the client appear the stated age? Notice the appearance of the skin. Does it feel warm and dry during the taking of the vital signs? Notice the skin color, presence of any lesions, and skin turgor.

Breath and body odor may be significant for some disease states.[43] Notice, for example, the odor of alcohol but avoid assuming that all sensory impairments are due to alcohol intoxication. The breath has a sweetish, acetone smell in persons with diabetic acidosis, and it smells like ammonia or stale urine in patients with uremia.

Notice the *stature* of the client, including height, weight, and overall body proportions. Excessively tall persons are termed *giants* if the excess growth hormone occurs before the bones unite. Such a client shows evidence of increased growth; however, body proportions are "normal." *Acromegaly* results from increased amount of growth hormone after union of the bone epiphyses. A person with this disorder has enlarged hands and feet, prominent forehead, long mandibles, and kyphosis of the dorsal spine. A person whose height is below normal for age and race is termed a *dwarf*. A *midget* is below normal height but has perfect body proportions.

As part of the general survey, the *nutritional state* is assessed, including the client's weight, amount of subcutaneous fat, and muscular development. In *exogenous* obesity (from overeating), the distribution of fat is generalized over the body. With *endogenous* obesity (due to internal endocrine abnormalities) fat is distributed about the trunk, but the arms and legs are relatively thin, as in Cushing's syndrome. The skin also gives clues to the nutritional state. With chronic disease the skin may be pale, dry, or rough, and the person may be dehydrated and have a loss of subcutaneous tissue. Such a person looks different from the healthy but very thin person.

Notice the client's *posture, position, and gait.* For example, with arthritis, the spine may be fixed and the neck rigid, and the person may move all as one unit. With meningitis or tetanus, the back may be arched. A depressed person may have a slumped sitting position and slow, lethargic movements. A person with chronic obstructive pulmonary disease may sit braced in a tripod position to aid breathing. Note the gait as the client walks. A normal gait is of appropriate speed, is smooth and even, and is accompanied by fluid arm movements. Notice any abnormal or involuntary body movements. For example, a *tic* is a muscle spasm in a small area, e.g., around the eye or in the face. A *tremor* is a rhythmic movement. Tremors may occur at rest, as in Parkinson's disease, or during voluntary activity, as with cerebellar ataxia. Some tremors are continuous, e.g., in delirium tremens in the client with alcoholism. *Convulsions* are a series of violent, involuntary contractions. Also notice any *spasticity* or increased muscle tonus. Finally, notice any incoordination or asymmetry of movement. This may be seen in the face or may be found by comparing body movements on the right and left sides.

Begin to assess the client's *mental status.* Notice facial expressions at rest and while talking, and try to assess mood. Is the client's mood appropriate or does it seem anxious, depressed, apathetic, angry, exhausted, or hostile? Notice the client's manner of thinking. It should be clear, logical, and not confused. Normally a person is oriented to date, location, and surroundings. While taking the health history, assess the client's memory for recent events (e.g., ask what was eaten for breakfast that day) and for remote events (e.g., ask about specific things in the past). Also note the state of awareness and whether the client's general knowledge seems appropriate for the stated educational level, age, occupation, and socioeconomic status.

Notice the client's articulation, or how words are formed. *Dysarthria,* or difficulty in articulating distinctly, may be due to damage of cranial nerves rather than cerebral cortex dysfunction. Stream of talking should be fluent. Any halting or interruption in flow should be noted. This may occur with a central nervous system (CNS) disorder, e.g., multiple sclerosis. Finally, notice any expressive or receptive defects, or *aphasia.* This is a loss of comprehension of verbal or written language due to pathology of corresponding cerebral cortex areas. (Neurologic assessment is discussed further in Unit X; musculoskeletal examination is presented in Unit XX.)

EXAMINATION OF THE UPPER EXTREMITIES

Detailed examination of specific regions requires touching the client's body. This can be distressing for the client if it is not performed comfortably and professionally by the nurse. Most people are accustomed to being touched on the hands by strangers (e.g., the handshake). The client's upper extremities are thus the most nonthreatening areas to touch when beginning the physical examination.

Begin by having the client sit upright on the examining table. Then explain what is going to happen. For example you might address the client by name and say, "Mr. Turner, this examination will take about 30 to 40 minutes. I will tell you everything I do as I go along, and if you have any questions I will try to answer them. First, I will look at your hands and arms."

The skills used to examine the client's hands and arms are inspection and palpation. Lift both the client's hands to your chest level and note color of skin and nailbeds, temperature, texture, thickness, turgor, and the presence of any lesions, vascularity, edema, contractures, or clubbing. The profile sign (viewing the finger from the side) is used to detect early *clubbing*.[80] In early clubbing, the normal obtuse 160 degree angle of the nailbed flattens to a straight 180 degrees. As clubbing advances, the distal phalanges take on a rounded "drumstick" appearance. Clubbing is seen in some chronic diseases, e.g., congenital cyanotic heart disease, chronic obstructive pulmonary disease (COPD), cor pulmonale, and subacute bacterial endocarditis (SBE). (Assessment of skin and nails is discussed further in Chapter 79.)

With the client's hands near heart level, check *capillary refill* by pushing the free end of the client's fingernail until the skin beneath blanches, then release. Color should return immediately. With vasodilatation, you will see capillary pulsation in the nailbeds during this maneuver, and the skin will be warm and flushed. With vasoconstriction or impaired circulation, capillary filling time is prolonged (more than one second) and the hands are cool, moist, and pale.

Next, the hands and arms are palpated. Palpate the radial pulse bilaterally, noting rate, rhythm, force (amplitude), and elasticity of the vessel wall. Practice is necessary to assess elasticity, or the "springy" property of the normal arterial wall. However, the flexible, straight, normal artery can easily be distinguished from the hard, cord-like tortuous artery present with atherosclerosis. (Cardiovascular assessment is discussed further in Units XII and XV.)

Next, gently feel the interphalangeal, metacarpophalangeal, and wrist joints between your thumb and fingers, noting any swelling, bogginess, or tenderness. Notice any nodule formation, which accompanies rheumatoid arthritis, gout, rheumatic fever, and osteoarthritis. Palpate the brachial pulse and check for an enlarged epitrochlear lymph node in the depression above and behind the medial condyle of the humerus. This is done by "shaking hands" with the client and reaching your other hand under the client's elbow to the groove between the biceps and triceps muscles. Epitrochlear nodes may be enlarged with infection of the hand or forearm.

Palpate the forearm and upper arm muscles, noting size, tone, tenderness, and symmetry between upper extremities. Note both localized atrophy, which may be congenital or have a neurologic cause, and the generalized atrophy that comes with weight loss, chronic disease, chronic disuse, or aging.

Assess range of motion (ROM) by flexing the client's hand, wrist, and forearm onto the chest, and then extending them. (Check a physical assessment text for numerical degrees of normal flexion and extension of each joint.[7, 44]) Also note any bogginess or tenderness around the joint, which suggests fluid in the joint capsule (*effusion*). During passive ROM, listen for an abnormal crunchy crackling sound called *crepitance*.

Checklist: Upper Extremities Examination

1. *Inspect hands and nails*
2. *Palpate brachial pulse and epitrochlear area*
3. *Palpate forearm and upper arm*
4. *Observe ROM of hand, wrist, arm*

EXAMINATION OF THE HEAD

Continue your examination with an assessment of the *scalp, hair, skull,* and *face.* Inspection and palpation are the skills used. A number of systemic diseases have specific characteristics that are visible on the head.

Because the *hair* can easily disguise abnormalities, ask the client about anything unusual about the hair or scalp or if there is a history of head trauma. Part the hair in several places and note the hair's quantity, thickness, texture, distribution, and also the presence of any pest inhabitants or skin lesions. The texture of hair changes with altered thyroid metabolism, becoming fine, soft, and silky with hyperthyroidism and coarse, dry, and brittle in hypothyroidism. Loss or thinning of hair is termed *alopecia.* Bilaterally symmetrical alopecia is common in men and is due to a hereditary predisposition. A transient hair loss may occur with serious emotional upsets, chronic wasting diseases that cause a protein loss (e.g., cancer), secondary syphilis, or treatment with chemotherapeutic agents. In these cases the alopecia is patchy and irregular, and any remaining hair is sparse.

Observe the scalp for scaliness, parasites, lumps, or lesions. Identify the presence of *nits* (the eggs of lice), and differentiate them from *seborrhea,* or dandruff. Nits are tiny, white, and egg-shaped and adhere to the hairs, whereas seborrhea shows as loose white flakes. Occasionally sebaceous cysts (called *wens*) occur on the scalp. These are smooth rounded growths.

Observe the general size and contour of the skull, and note any deformities, lumps, or tenderness. *Normocephalic* describes a round skull that is appropriately related to body size. An enlarged cranium may be due to *hydrocephalus* (large amount of cerebrospinal fluid), *acromegaly* (excessive growth hormone that leads to an enlarged mandible, forehead, and nose), or Paget's disease or *osteitis deformans* (an increase in bone thickness).

Place your fingers in the client's hair and palpate the scalp. The cranial bones that have normal protrusions are the frontal, parietal, occipital, and the mastoid process behind the ear. Note any other lumps or lesions. Palpate the temporal artery above the zygomatic (cheek) bone between the eye and the top of the ear. The temporomandibular joint is just below the temporal artery and anterior to the tragus. Palpate the joint as the client's mouth opens, noting any tenderness, crepitation, or limitation in range of motion. Using your thumbs, press over the maxillary sinuses below the cheekbones and over the frontal sinuses below the eyebrows. (Take care not to press over the eyeballs.) These areas become tender in clients with chronic allergies.

Inspect the face, noting the facial expression and its appropriateness to behavior or reported mood. Note symmetry of the facial structures. Facial movements are mediated by cranial nerve VII (intermediofacial) and are elicited by asking the client to wrinkle the forehead, puff out the cheeks, smile, and grimace. The face appears markedly asymmetrical if cranial nerve VII has been damaged by central cortical pathology (e.g., cerebrovascular accident [CVA]) or peripheral pathology such as Bell's palsy. Note any *tics* in the facial muscles. Edema in the face is noted first around the eyes (periorbital) and the cheeks, where the subcutaneous tissue is relatively loose. This may be caused by congestive heart failure (CHF), renal failure, or the myxedema of hypothyroidism. With Cushing's syndrome and corticosteroid therapy, the entire face appears rounded or "moon-like." The face looks sunken-in or *cachectic* in terminal cancer, dehydration, or starvation. An anxious "startled" face is seen in hyperthyroidism; the eyes look wide-open and protruding.

Alterations in skin color, including cyanosis, pallor, and jaundice, may be noted in the face and mucous membranes. Notice any patchy color change, e.g., the red "butterfly" rash that sometimes occurs across the cheeks and nose with lupus erythematosus or the yellowish-brown patch (chloasma) that sometimes appears on the forehead and cheeks during pregnancy. Any skin lesions should be noted. (Skin assessment, including lesions and color changes, is detailed later in this chapter.)

Sensation on the face is mediated by cranial nerve V (trigeminal). This nerve is tested by touching the client's face with a wisp of cotton while the client's eyes are closed and asking the client to report when the sensation is felt.

Checklist: Head Examination

1. *Inspect hair and scalp*
   A. *Quantity, thickness, texture*
   B. *Distribution, pattern of loss if any*
   C. *Nits, seborrhea*
   D. *Lesions*
2. *Inspect and palpate skull*
   A. *General size and contour*
   B. *Note any deformities, lumps, tenderness*
   C. *Palpate temporal artery and temporomandibular joint*
   D. *Palpate sinus areas for tenderness*
3. *Inspect face*
   A. *Note facial expression*
   B. *Symmetry of movement (c.n. VII)*
   C. *Any involuntary movements*
   D. *Note skin color, any edema or lesions*
   E. *Test skin sensation (c.n. V)*

EXAMINATION OF THE EYE

The eye examination is important for two major reasons: (1) to *assess visual function* and (2) to *detect ocular signs of systemic diseases,* e.g., hypertension and diabetes mellitus. A thorough assessment of the eye includes measuring visual acuity, testing visual fields and extraocular muscles, inspecting the external ocular structures, pupils and cornea, and examining the ocular fundus. Clients over 40 years old should have intraocular pressure measured by tonometry.[44] The eye is a complex organ. A review of basic anatomy and physiology of the eye (Chapter 89) will make the description of the following tests more meaningful.

Visual Acuity

Measurement of vision is done by asking the client to read the various sizes of print on the

Snellen eye chart. Position the client 20 feet away from the chart, and cover one eye at a time with an opaque card (*not* the client's fingers). Ask the client to read the smallest line of print possible. Clients who wear corrective lenses should be tested both with and without them (unless they are for reading only).

The numerical fraction located at the end of every line on the chart reflects the visual acuity, e.g., 20/30. This ratio is *not* a percentage of normal vision. Rather, the top number (numerator) is the distance the client is from the chart, and the bottom number (denominator) is the distance at which a normal eye can read those letters. Thus "20/30" visual acuity means that this client can read at 20 feet what the "normal eye" can read at 30 feet. The larger the denominator is, the poorer the client's visual acuity.

> *Normal visual acuity is 20/20. Anyone whose visual acuity is less than this (with glasses on if the person normally wears them) should be referred to an ophthalmologist.*

Vision may be impaired by opacity of the media (cornea, aqueous humor, lens, vitreous humor); a refractive error; or by pathology of the nervous tissue in the retina or optic pathway. Clients who are unable to see the largest letter on the chart (20/200) are moved closer to the chart until they can see it and *that* distance is recorded, e.g., 6/200. Ask clients who are unable to see *any* letters to count your upraised fingers in front of their eyes. If they cannot count your fingers, ask if they can perceive your hand movements (HM), or finally, check if they can distinguish light, i.e., have light perception (LP).

Near vision is normally tested only in clients over 40 years old or in persons who state that they have difficulty reading.[44] Ask the client to read from a "pocket visual screener" (a small card with various sizes of print) or some other print, e.g., a magazine. In older persons, the lens of the eye becomes harder and, thus, less flexible in accommodating to near vision. This condition is *presbyopia,* and such a client needs bifocals or reading glasses.

Visual Fields

Whereas the above tests are used to assess central vision, peripheral vision is assessed by the visual field confrontation test. Position yourself about 2 feet in front of the client and ask the person to look directly into your eyes. Cover one of the client's eyes at a time with an opaque card, and bring a pencil or your wagging finger into the client's peripheral vision from several directions. Have the client indicate when the pencil or finger can be seen.

> *When a person stares directly ahead, a moving object should be perceived within 50 degrees superiorly, 60 degrees nasally, 70 degrees inferiorly, and 90 degrees temporally.*

A blind area is a *scotoma,* and loss of an entire half of the visual field is *hemianopsia.* Such disorders may occur with problems such as CVA, pituitary tumor, or carotid artery pathology. The visual fields test is a gross measure and detects only large field losses. The client should be referred to an ophthalmologist for more specific diagnostic measures if you suspect a subtler loss of peripheral vision, e.g., with glaucoma or retinal detachment.

Extraocular Muscles

While some animals can move their eyes independently of each other, humans cannot. Human beings have a *binocular single-image visual system.* Furthermore, our retinas have an area of central (or keenest) vision, which is the *fovea centralis* within the *macula lutea.* When an object attracts our attention, there is a reflex fixation of *both* fovea on the object. Because our eyes move as a pair, our brain perceives only one image. This parallel movement of both eyes is accomplished by the synergistic action of six sets of muscles. Each eye has a superior, inferior, lateral, and medial rectus muscle, and a superior and inferior oblique muscle. They are innervated by cranial nerves III, IV, and VI. Each muscle is coordinated (yoked) with one in the other eye, so that the two eyes move together. Deviation of the axis of the eye is called a *strabismus* or *squint;* deviation to the temporal side of the head is *external strabismus* (also called *exotropia*), and deviation to the nasal side is *internal strabismus* (or *esotropia*).

Sometimes the axis deviation is obvious, and the client looks "cross-eyed." Smaller degrees of deviation (*phoria*) may be compensated by the good eye and will only be apparent in the corneal light reflex, cover test, and alternating cover test.

The *corneal light reflex* is an easy check for parallel alignment of the eye axes. Ask the client to stare straight ahead while you shine a penlight directly into the eyes from a distance of about 8 inches. The light, reflected off the cornea, should appear in exactly the same spot in each pupil. Asymmetry of the light reflex indicates eye muscle weakness or paralysis.

The *cover-uncover test* detects small degrees of eye

muscle weakness by interrupting the fusion reflex that normally keeps the eyes parallel. Ask the client to stare at a stationary object while you cover the eye with an opaque card. Watch the uncovered eye; if it jumps to fix on the object, it was not aligned before. The covered eye now has its macular image suppressed; if there is muscle weakness, the eye will drift toward its relaxed position. Quickly uncover the eye and watch for a definite jerk as the client fixes macular gaze of that eye on the object again. This test elicits mild weakness, called a *phoria.* Drift of the covered eye to the temporal side is *exophoria;* drift to the nasal side is *esophoria.*

The *alternating cover test* involves shifting the cover back and forth between eyes while the client fixes on a stationary object. The nurse watches the eye just uncovered for a jerk back to re-establish fixation. This test elicits a greater muscle imbalance called a *tropia,* which is a constant disparity of the visual axes.

The *diagnostic positions* test detects eye muscle weakness or paralysis by moving the eyes through the six cardinal positions of gaze. Ask the client to follow your moving finger or pen to each side and to the four "corners" of gaze in a clockwise pattern:[44]

```
      SR ⟶ IO                 IO ⟶ SR
    ↗ 6     1 ↘             ↗ 6     1 ↘
LR 5            2 MR 5                  2 LR
    ↖ 4     3 ↙             ↖ 4     3 ↙
      IR ⟵ SO                 SO ⟵ IR

     Right Eye                Left Eye
```

Each position of gaze involves the function of one of the six eye muscles. Failure of the eye to turn in one position indicates muscle weakness or damage to the cranial nerve innervating that muscle.

In addition to parallel movements of the eyes in each direction, you should inspect for *nystagmus,* a rhythmic oscillation of the eyes. A slight nystagmus during extreme lateral gaze is normal; in other positions, it is an abnormal finding. Finally, note the relation of the upper eyelid to the iris as the eyes move to the downward positions. Normally the eyelid overlaps the iris somewhat. A *lid lag,* or a rim of white sclera seen between the lid and the iris, is noted in hyperthyroidism.

External Ocular Structures

The client's general facial expression may cue whether visual ability is relaxed or difficult, e.g., note squinting. Also note the precision with which the client moves about the examining room and avoids obstacles. Inspect the eyebrows, noting any loss of movement (damage to cranial nerve VII).

Note the position of the eyelids in relation to the eyeballs. The lids normally cover the upper part of the iris. *Ptosis* is a drooping of the upper eyelid, which may be caused by eye muscle weakness or cranial nerve III damage, as in myasthenia gravis. As mentioned above, lid lag occurs in hyperthyroidism. Note any edema of the lids (periorbital edema occurs in hypothyroidism, CHF, renal failure, and allergy). Also note any lesions.

Xanthelasma are raised yellowish circumscribed plaques around the inner corners of the eyes, which are normal with aging.

A *chalazion* is a small painless beady nodule in the eyelid, caused by a cyst in a sebaceous gland.

A *hordeolum* (sty) is a painful reddened area around a hair follicle on the lid margin, caused by inflammation of a sebaceous gland.

Basal cell *cancer* may show as a papule with a pearly border and a depressed or punched-out center; it is more common on the lower lid.

The eyelashes normally are distributed evenly along the lid margins and curve outward. In *entropion* the lower lid is inverted due to lid spasm or contracture of scar tissue, and the inward lashes can irritate the cornea. *Ectropion* is an eversion of the lower lid from loss of muscle tone, cranial nerve VII damage, or scarring of the skin. Here the punctum on the inner canthus is turned out, making it unable to drain the tears and resulting in constant watering.

Note the position of the eyeballs within their sockets. Sunken eyeballs *(enophthalmos)* are seen in chronic wasting diseases, and protruding eyeballs *(exophthalmos)* are noted in hyperthyroidism.

The conjunctiva is the clear mucosal lining of the eyelids (palpebral conjunctiva), which is enveloped back over the sclera (bulbar conjunctiva). It does not extend over the iris. Instead, the conjunctiva joins the cornea at the edge of the iris, known as the *limbus.* Use your thumbs to slide the lids open against the bony orbit rims around the eye. Take care *not* to exert pressure on the eyeball itself. It is normal to see many small blood vessels through the transparent conjunctiva, but the overall color should reflect the structure below; i.e., deep pink over the lids, and white over the sclera. In dark-skinned clients, it is normal to see small dots of dark pigmentation on the sclera and some yellow fatty deposits under the lids away from the cornea.[57, 58]

The conjunctiva may reflect local or systemic disease. *Conjunctivitis* is manifested by a generalized reddened (injected) conjunctiva, particularly in the periphery away from the cornea. *Iritis* also appears as a red eye, but the injected color is closer to the limbus. The palpebral conjunctiva may reflect the systemic conditions of jaundice (called *icterus* in the eye), cyanosis, or pallor from anemia. Scleral icterus is a yellow color that extends to the edges of the cornea. Pallor is more accurately assessed near the outer canthus of the lower lid, because the skin pigment may be naturally lighter in the inner corner.

The lacrimal gland produces the tears that bathe the eyeball. It may be seen in the upper outer corner under the lid. This small pinkish tissue should be inspected for redness, swelling, or pain.

Pupils

The pupils should be round, regular, of equal size, and react equally to light. A small percentage (about 5 per cent) of the normal population has an unequal pupil size.[44, 55] However, a difference in pupil size may be caused by CNS disease. The pupils normally constrict when exposed to light. This is a subcortical reflex; the afferent link is the optic nerve (c.n. II) and the efferent link is the oculomotor nerve (c.n. III). As you bring a penlight beam in from the side, you should notice a *direct light reflex* (constriction of that pupil) and a *consensual light reflex* (simultaneous constriction of the other pupil). This occurs because the sensory afferent impulse in the optic nerve synapses with both sides of the brain. A client who is blind in one eye will have a direct and a consensual light reflex when the *normal* eye is illuminated but will have neither response when the blind eye is illuminated.

The pupils also are tested for *accommodation,* i.e., the adaptation of the eye for near vision. Accommodation is accomplished by increasing the curvature of the lens. Other components of accommodation are pupillary constriction and convergence of the axes of the eyeballs. Accommodation is tested by asking the client to focus on a distant object (this dilates the pupil) and then to shift his or her focus on a near object (e.g., a pen held 4 to 6 inches from the client's nose). You should note pupillary constriction and convergence of the axes. (This test shows why you always bring the light in from the *side* when testing the direct light reflex. If you bring it in from the front, the pupil constriction may indicate accommodation and not necessarily the light reflex.) In CNS syphilis, the pupil constricts with accommodation but does not react to light. This is called an *Argyll Robertson pupil.*

The pupils may be constricted owing to narcotic use or owing to treatment of glaucoma with pilocarpine eyedrops. They may be dilated by stimulation of the sympathetic nervous system, acute glaucoma, or dilating eyedrops. One pupil that is dilated and fixed may be due to trauma. Both pupils that are dilated and fixed may be seen in severe CNS disease and cardiopulmonary arrest.

If none of these abnormalities is present, pupillary function is recorded as "PERRLA," or Pupils Equal, Round, React to Light and Accommodation.

Cornea and Lens

Direct a light beam from a penlight across the cornea from the side and observe the cornea for smoothness and clarity. Although *corneal abrasions* cause intense pain and photophobia, they are difficult to detect unless fluorescein dye is instilled onto the eye surface. This is not done routinely in a screening exam. Occasionally, an abrasion may be detected without dye, as it causes irregular ridges on the cornea. A client with a suspected corneal abrasion should be referred to an ophthalmologist for prompt treatment. In older persons it is normal to see a thin gray-white ring around the edge of the cornea, called an *arcus senilus.* This condition has no pathological significance. Look for any opacities in the lens that may be visible through the pupil. A *cataract* shows as a cloudiness in the lens.

Examination of the Ocular Fundus

The ophthalmoscope is used to examine the transparent media (anterior chamber, lens, vitreous body) and the ocular fundus (the retinal structures). The room should be darkened so that the client's pupils will dilate. In some instances, dilating eyedrops may be ordered for the client, but only if glaucoma has been absolutely ruled out. It can be dangerous to dilate the pupil in the presence of glaucoma. The client's contact lenses may be left in place; if they are clean, they do not interfere. Eyeglasses should be removed by both client and examiner.

Looking through the pupil at the ocular fundus is like peering through a keyhole into an exciting room beyond. The ophthalmoscope directs a beam of light into the eye that illuminates the retinal structures. The ophthalmoscope has a series of lenses that can alter the focus. The "*O*" *lens* should bring the retina into sharp focus if both examiner and client have normal vision. The *black* or *positive numbers* focus closer in space to the ophthalmoscope. They are used to explore the media and for visualizing the retina in a farsighted client. The *negative* or *red diopter settings* focus farther away in space and are used to visualize the fundus on a nearsighted client who has longer-than-normal eyeballs. You will need to change diopter settings throughout the exam in order to visualize different levels of structures. The standard ophthalmoscope has different shaped and colored apertures, but the small round one with white light is used for routine examination.

Direct the client to stare at a distant fixed object throughout the examination, even though your head will get in the way. This helps to dilate the pupils and to hold the retinal structures still. Hold the ophthalmoscope close to your eye, braced firmly against your brow and cheek. Keep your index finger extended on the lens wheel so that you can change the diopter setting without taking the instrument away from your head. Hold the ophthalmoscope in your *right* hand to your *right* eye to visualize the client's *right* eye (Fig. 15–3). This must be done so that you will not bump noses during the exam! Similarly use the left hand and left eye for the client's left eye. Keep your free hand touching the client's shoulder or head; this helps to orient you in space.

Start at a distance of 10 to 12 inches from the client. As you look through the aperture, you will see the client's pupil glow red. This is the *red reflex* and results from the ophthalmoscopic light being reflected off the retina. Once you see this, keep on it and move slowly in toward the client until your foreheads touch. Losing the red reflex means the ophthalmoscope light has aimed off the pupil onto the iris or sclera. Redirect the light until the red reflex comes back into view.

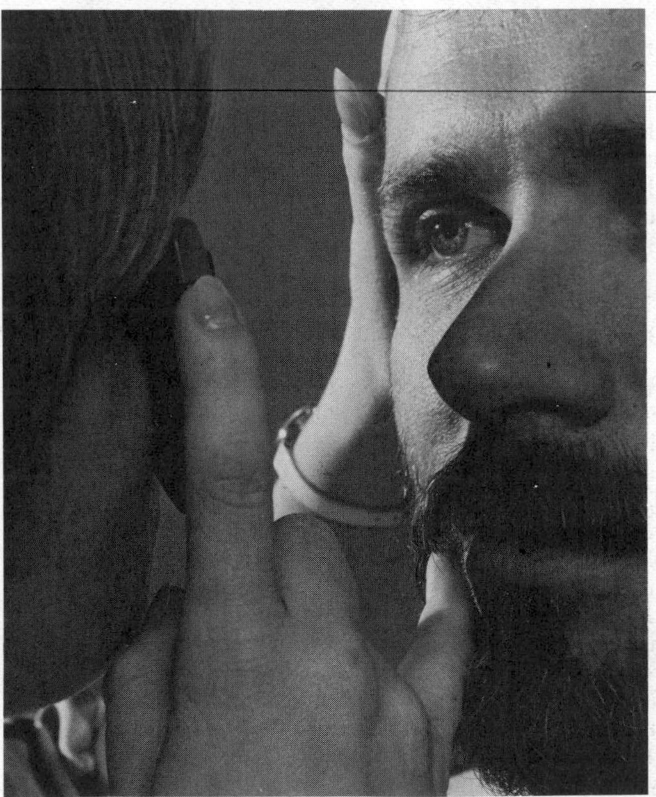

Figure 15–3. Positioning of examiner and client for the ophthalmoscopic examination. Note the examiner holds the ophthalmoscope in her *right* hand to her *right* eye to examine the client's *right* eye. The little finger extends to the client's face and the left hand rests on the client's head (or shoulder)—both maneuvers serve to orient the examiner spatially during the procedure. (Reprinted by permission from *Nursing 77.)*

As you get close to the client, use the positive numbers to visualize the nearer media—the anterior chamber, lens, and the vitreous. There should be no cloudiness or opacities. An opacity shows as a dark spot in the red reflex because it interferes with light reflection.

Slowly move the diopter setting down to "0" to bring the fundus into precise focus. Locate a blood vessel and follow it slowly in the direction in which it gets larger. This will lead you to the optic disc. Systematically explore the retinal structures in this order: (1) optic disc, (2) retinal vessels, (3) general background, and (4) macula (Fig. 15–4).

Optic Disc. The optic disc (also called optic nerve head or optic papilla) is examined for color, shape, margins, and cup-disc ratio. The disc is located toward the nasal side of the retina. Its color is creamy orange-yellow to pink. The shape is round or oval. The margins of the optic disc normally are distinct and sharply demarcated from the rest of the fundus, though this is more apparent on the temporal side.

Two variations in the optic disc may be seen in normal clients, i.e., a pigment crescent or a scleral crescent. A *pigment crescent* is a dark color extending along part of the disc margin; it is caused by a larger amount of pigment deposited in the choroid layer. A *scleral crescent* is less common and is a whitish line around a portion of the disc margin. It is due to absence of pigment in the choroid. Thus, the examiner looks directly at the sclera in the back of the eye.

The physiologic cup is the small circular area within the disc where the blood vessels exit and enter. It may be difficult to see but usually appears as a brighter yellow-white and does not extend beyond one half of the diameter of the entire disc.

Major pathologic changes of the optic disc include glaucoma, optic atrophy, and papilledema.

Glaucoma is an increased intraocular pressure that pushes both forward against the iris and backward against the optic disc. During ophthalmoscopic examination, glaucoma appears as an increased cup-disc ratio (the physiologic cup is more than one half the diameter of the disc) and by the presence of blood vessels that seem to plunge over the rim of the disc and disappear.

Optic atrophy also results from late glaucoma and appears as a very pale white disc.

Papilledema (also called choked disc) is caused by increased intracranial pressure that pushes the cranial contents out toward the eye sockets. The disc color becomes hyperemic (reddened), the shape is blurred, and the margins are fuzzy and indistinct. The retinal veins look engorged because they cannot drain effec-

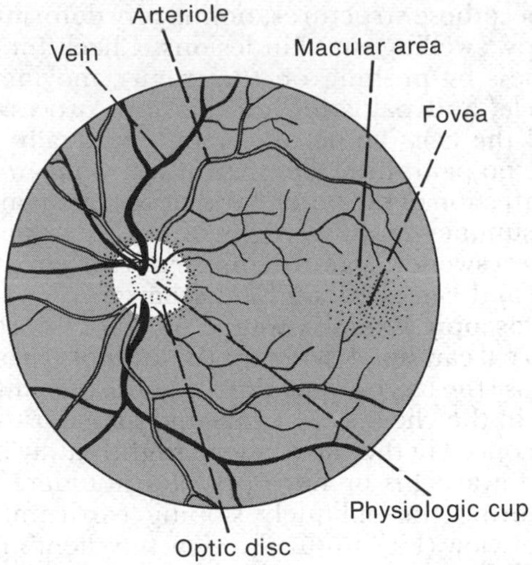

Figure 15–4. Landmarks of the ocular fundus.

tively against the increased pressure, and the blood vessels look "choked off" at the disc. There also may be dark red hemorrhages fanning out from the area of the disc.

Retinal Vessels. Inspect the blood vessels throughout the fundus. This is the only place in the body where the vascular bed can be viewed *directly.* Many systemic diseases can be assessed by observing the characteristic changes they cause in the retinal vessels. A paired artery and vein should normally extend to each quadrant. The arteries are brighter red and narrower than the veins and normally have a thin sliver of light in the middle (the arterial light reflex). The width of the artery-to-vein (A:V) ratio can be estimated; normal is 2:3 or 4:5. Change in this ratio indicates pathology. Arteries may become narrowed, as in occlusion or hypertension, or the veins may become abnormally wide, as in diabetes. The vessels should regularly decrease in caliber as they extend to the periphery. Note any focal constriction (pinching off) of a vessel that may be due to hypertension or emboli from atherosclerosis. The arterial light reflex is normally one fourth to one third the width of the blood column and looks abnormally wide in hypertension and atherosclerosis.

Arteries and veins may cross each other's paths. This is not significant if the crossing is close to the disc and if the blood flow is not interrupted in either vessel. Significant crossing phenomena (also called nicking) occur in atherosclerosis and hypertension. Here the nicking is seen more than two disc diameters from the optic disc, the vessels may change course abruptly, and the vein looks distended distal to the crossing, because its blood drainage is impeded.

Note any unusual tortuosity (twistedness) of the vessels. This is usually congenital and insignificant. However, it may reflect vascular disease if the tortuosity is greatly asymmetrical in the two eyes. Finally, you may be able to see the normal pulsations of the veins near the optic disc as they drain blood against the intermittent pressure of arterial systole. This normal pulsation disappears with the increased intracranial pressure that causes papilledema.

General Background of the Fundus. The color of the retinal background varies widely and generally corresponds to the client's skin color. Normally nothing should obscure your view of the retinal structures. Common abnormalities include hemorrhages, exudates, and microaneurysms.

Hemorrhages may be: (1) preretinal (dark red with a fluid level), (2) superficial retinal (linear or flame-shaped, as in hypertension), and (3) deep intraretinal, or dot-shaped and "splattered-on" in appearance, as in diabetes.

Exudates are yellow-white in color and may look like a soft fluffy cloud (called a cotton-wool area). This soft exudate is due to arterial microinfarction and gradually may be absorbed and disappear. Hard exudates are due to venous stasis and are usually round, discrete, and numerous. Exudates are seen with many systemic diseases, such as diabetes mellitus, hypertension, and collagen diseases, and with degeneration or inflammation of the retina.[55]

Microaneurysms are seen as very small, round dots. They are actually tiny bulges of vessel walls and characteristically accompany diabetes. Any retinal abnormality should be described by color, shape, size, and distance from the optic disc.

Macula. The macula lutea is a circular area on the temporal side of the retina. Its pigment is slightly darker than the rest of the fundus, and it appears to have no blood vessels coursing through it. In its center is a small depression called the fovea centralis, which has all cones (end-organs of vision thought to mediate color and objects in bright light) and is the area of central or keenest vision. The macular area should be inspected last in the ophthalmoscopic exam because the client will be light-dazzled and very uncomfortable and her or his eyes will water. The color of the macula should be even and homogenous. Clumped pigment is abnormal and is seen in aging, trauma, or retinal detachment.

Summary

The ophthalmoscopic exam is a difficult skill to master and requires much practice. To properly understand the normal landmarks and abnormal findings described above, review sources that have drawings and color slides of the fundus.[1c, 53e, 55]

Checklist: Eye Examination

1. *Test visual acuity*
   - A. *Snellen eye chart*
   - B. *Pocket visual screener for near vision*
2. *Test visual fields*
3. *Extraocular muscles – observe movement*
   - A. *Corneal light reflex*
   - B. *Cover-uncover test*
   - C. *Alternating cover test*
   - D. *Diagnostic positions test*
4. *Observe external ocular structures*
   - A. *General*
   - B. *Eyebrows*
   - C. *Eyelids and lashes*
   - D. *Eyeballs*
   - E. *Conjunctiva and sclera*
   - F. *Lacrimal gland*
5. *Inspect pupils*
   - A. *Size*
   - B. *Direct and consensual light reflex*
   - C. *Accommodation*
6. *Inspect cornea*
7. *Inspect ocular fundus with ophthalmoscope*
   - A. *Optic disc*
     - (1) *Shape*
     - (2) *Margins*
     - (3) *Color*
     - (4) *Cup-disc ratio*
   - B. *Vessels*
     - (1) *Number and direction*
     - (2) *Artery:vein ratio*
     - (3) *Regularity of vessel caliber*
     - (4) *Arterial light reflex*
     - (5) *Crossing phenomena*
     - (6) *Tortuosity*
     - (7) *Venous pulsations at disc*
   - C. *General background of fundus*
     - (1) *General pigmentation*
     - (2) *Retinal translucency and integrity*
   - D. *Inspect macula*

EXAMINATION OF THE EAR, NOSE, AND THROAT

The Ear

Assessment of the ear includes inspection of the external auricle, inspection of the auditory canal and eardrum, and testing of hearing acuity. These techniques, as well as management of related disorders, are discussed further in Chapter 90.

Inspection of the External Ear. The outer ear is termed the *auricle* (or *pinna*) and consists of movable cartilage. A triangular fold of cartilage, the *tragus,* lies anterior to the auditory meatus. Inspect these structures, noting any deformities, lumps, swelling, or skin lesions. Check for tenderness by pushing on the tragus, moving the auricle, and palpating the mastoid process behind the ear. These movements normally produce no pain; they are painful with *otitis externa,* an infection of the outer ear that occurs mainly in the summer months. Signs of otitis externa include a swollen, painful, injected (reddened) auricle and ear canal, and a discharge.

Otoscopic Examination. As you inspect the external ear, note the size of the auditory meatus. Choose the largest speculum that will fit comfortably in the client's ear canal and attach it to the otoscope. Tilt the client's head slightly away from you toward his or her opposite shoulder. This will bring the obliquely sloping eardrum into better view (Fig. 15–5). To view the client's right ear, hold the otoscope in your right hand, braced against the client's right cheek (Fig. 15–6). Your right hand helps steady the otoscope and prevents insertion too far into the canal, which could be painful. Use your left hand to pull the auricle up and back. This helps to straighten the anteriorly curving ear canal. The speculum itself also helps to straighten and dilate the ear canal. Insert the otoscope *gently*; the ear canal has an outer cartilaginous part followed by a "bony" section that has a very thin epithelial lining and is very sensitive to touch. Reverse the procedure for the client's left ear.

Occasionally the ear canal is partially filled with *cerumen* (yellowish-brown earwax) that makes visualization of the tympanic membrane difficult. Impacted cerumen is a common cause of conductive hearing loss. Cerumen may be removed by a number of methods.[13b] A cerumen spoon can be inserted, and the wax curetted out. This method can injure the canal, so it should be used only by a person skilled and comfortable with the procedure. The canal can be irrigated with warm water, mineral oil or half-strength hydrogen peroxide. Irrigation can be performed only if perforation of the eardrum can be absolutely ruled out, i.e., it is *not* present. Larsen recommends irrigating the canal with a dental Water-Pik device, because it has a fine pulsatile water stream that works quickly and effectively.[37]

Inspect the external canal through the otoscope, noting any foreign bodies, discharge, redness, or swelling. Inspect the *tympanic membrane* (eardrum) and systematically explore its landmarks (Fig. 15–7). The normal eardrum is a translucent membrane that has a pearly-gray color. You should notice the prominent *light reflex* in the anteroinferior quadrant. This is a conical brightness and is the reflection of your otoscope light. Its shape is distorted when the eardrum is thickened, as in chronic middle ear disease; and it is missing completely in acute otitis media.

Of the three ossicles in the middle ear, the *malleus* is the one attached directly to the eardrum. The sections of the malleus show through the translucent drum; these are the *umbo, manubrium* (handle), and the *short process.* The small superior section of the tympanic membrane is called the *pars flaccida* and the remainder of the drum is the *pars tensa.* The *annulus* is the outer fibrous rim of the drum. Normally the tympanic membrane looks concave externally and will move when the client increases middle ear pressure by performing a Valsalva maneuver.*

The tympanic membrane may show characteristic alterations to a number of middle ear pathologies (Fig. 15–8).

1. The drum may be *retracted,* making the malleus look prominent and well defined. Also, the drum will not move normally. Retraction occurs when an *obstructed eustachian tube* (auditory tube) creates a vacuum in the middle ear.
2. Because "nature abhors a vacuum," serum fills the middle ear. This is *serous otitis media;* the drum looks amber-yellow, the light reflex is absent and you may see an air-fluid level or air bubbles behind the drum. (Otitis media may be abbreviated as o.m.)
3. *Acute purulent otitis media* results when the middle ear fluid is infected. The drum is diffusely reddened, bulges outward, and all the normal landmarks are obliterated.
4. If an acute o.m. is not treated, the tympanic membrane might rupture from the increased pressure. This is a *perforation* and looks like a round darkened area on the drum. Note if a perforation is centrally located in the membrane or if it is marginal near the annulus. A marginal perforation, especially in the superior part of the drum (called an "attic" perforation), may lead to a *cholesteatoma.* This is an overgrowth of epidermal tissue that can produce hearing loss.

Measurement of Hearing Acuity. An audio meter is used to precisely measure hearing by assessing the client's ability to hear sounds of varying frequency. While this device occasionally is used in a routine physical exam, reasonably accurate alternate measures are the use of voice tests and tuning fork tests.

The types of hearing loss include: conductive, sensorineural, and mixed.

- *Conductive* loss involves dysfunction of the external or middle ear. This is only a partial loss, and clients are able to hear if the sound amplitude is increased enough to reach the normal nerve elements in the inner ear. Causes of conductive hearing loss include impacted cerumen, a perforated eardrum, pus or serum in the middle ear, and *otosclerosis* (a decrease in mobility of the ossicles).
- *Sensorineural* (or *perceptive*) loss signifies pathology of the inner ear, the eighth cranial nerve, or auditory areas of the cerebral cortex. Even with an increase in sound amplitude, the client may not understand words. An example is *presbycusis,* a decrease in hearing acuity seen in aged persons. It is caused by nerve degeneration in the inner ear or in the auditory nerve and first shows as a high frequency loss.
- *Mixed* hearing loss is a combination of the conductive and sensorineural types.

Assess the client's ability to hear a ticking watch or whispered words. *Test only one ear at a time, while masking the hearing in the other ear,* to prevent sound transmission around the head. Do this by placing one finger on the tragus and rapidly pushing it in and out of the auditory meatus. Shield your lips so that the client

*Valsalva's maneuver occurs when one forcibly exhales against the closed glottis, e.g., as when straining to defecate or cough. Valsalva's maneuver increases intrathoracic pressure.

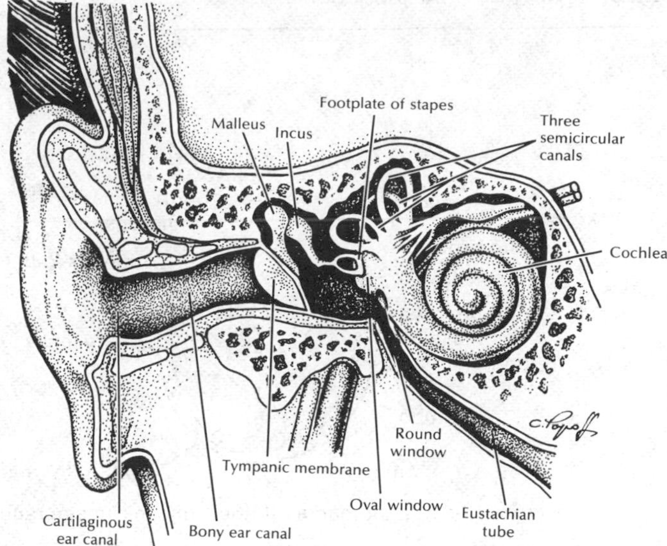

Figure 15–5. Anatomy of the ear. External auditory canal, middle ear and inner ear. (From Malasanos, L., et al.: *Health Assessment.* St. Louis: C. V. Mosby Co., 1977, p. 19.)

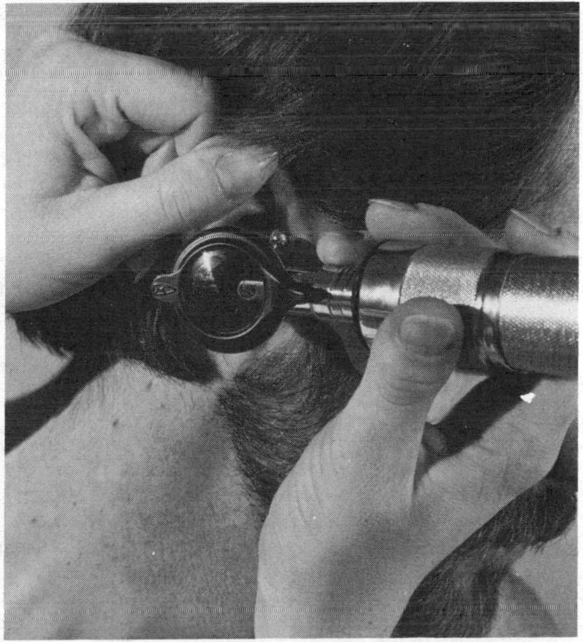

Figure 15–6. Positioning of examiner and client for insertion of the otoscope. The examiner's right hand is braced against the client's cheek to steady the otoscope. The left hand pulls the auricle up and back. (Reprinted by permission from *Nursing 77.*)

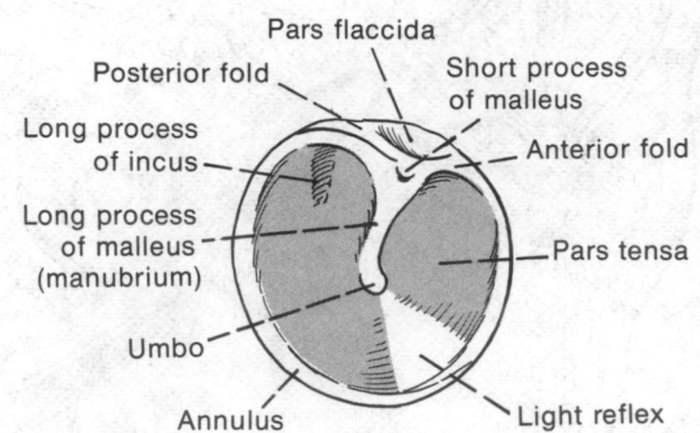

Figure 15–7. Landmarks of the tympanic membrane.

cannot lipread. Place your head 1 to 2 feet away, whisper a phrase and, ask the client to repeat it. Whispers are composed of high-frequency tones; you may have to use a normal speaking voice for a client with a sensorineural loss, which usually involves the high tones. Similarly, a watch tick is a high-frequency sound and is used to detect a high tone hearing loss.

The tuning fork tests measure hearing by *air conduction* (AC) or by *bone conduction* (BC). With BC, the sound vibrates through the cranial bones to the inner ear. The air conduction route through the ear canal and middle ear is usually the more sensitive. The *Weber test* is valuable when a client says, "I hear better with one ear than the other." Place a vibrating tuning fork in the midline of the client's skull. Normally a person hears the tone by bone conduction, and it sounds equally loud in both ears. When there is a sensorineural loss in only one ear, the sound lateralizes to the "better" (or unaffected) ear. With a conductive loss in only one ear, the sound lateralizes to the "poorer" (or affected) ear. This effect is due to the ambient background noise in the room, which masks hearing in the normal ear. The affected ear (the one with a conductive loss) does not hear this background noise and thus has a better chance to hear the bone-conducted sound than does the normal ear.

The *Rinne test* compares air-conducted and bone-conducted sound. Place the stem of the vibrating tuning fork on the client's mastoid process and ask the client to signal when the sound goes away. Quickly invert the tuning fork and hold it near the ear canal. The client should still hear a sound. Normally, sound is heard twice as long by air conduction as by bone conduction. A normal response is a "positive" Rinne, or "AC > BC." With a conductive loss, the client hears as long by bone conduction (AC = BC), or even longer by bone conduction (AC < BC, a "negative" Rinne). With a sensorineural loss the normal ratio of AC > BC is still intact, although the client hears poorly both ways.

Further hearing tests and a discussion of which types of clients warrant a more complete hearing exam are presented in the assessment literature.[15] Also look at sources with color photos of tympanic membrane disorders.[53d] Children may require modified and additional assessment techniques.[13c] Children themselves may be unaware of a hearing loss because they do not know how well they should hear. Yet they may show behaviors typical of decreased hearing, e.g., disinterest in casual conversation, social withdrawal, on accompanying speech defect.[13c, 54]

FINDING	INTERPRETATION	EXAMPLES
Bright red drum	Inflammation	Acute middle ear infection (otitis media)
Yellowish drum	Pus or serum behind drum	Acute or chronic otitis media
Bluish drum	Blood behind drum	Skull fracture
Bubbles behind drum	Serous fluid in middle ear	Chronic otitis media
Absent light reflex	Bulging of drum	Acute otitis media
Absent or diminished landmarks	Thickening of drum	Chronic otitis media or otitis externa
Oval dark areas	Perforation	Recent or old rupture of drum
Malleus very promient	Retraction of drum	Obstruction of Eustachian tube

Figure 15–8. Selected abnormalities on otoscopy. (From Sherman, Jacques L., and Sylvia Fields Kleinman: *Guide to Patient Evaluation.* © 1978 by the Medical Examination Publishing Company, Inc., Garden City, New York.)

Inspect the external nose for any deformity, asymmetry, inflammation, or skin lesions. Test the patency of each nostril by pushing one nasal wing shut with your finger while asking the client to sniff inward through the other naris. The sense of smell is mediated by cranial nerve I, the olfactory nerve, and is usually not tested in a routine exam. It may be assessed by having the client close both eyes and identify familiar aromas, such as coffee, tobacco, or an orange, offered to one nostril at a time.

Attach the short wide speculum to the otoscope head and insert it into the nasal vestibule, avoiding pressure against the tender nasal septum. View the nasal cavity first with the client's head erect and then with it tilted back. Inspect the nasal mucosa, noting color (normally redder than the oral mucosa), swelling, exudate, bleeding, or any foreign body. Observe the nasal septum for deviation, perforation, or bleeding. Observe the *turbinates,* which are bony ridges extending down from the sides of the nose.

Common abnormalities are the swollen, reddened nasal mucosa of an acute infection, e.g., the common cold. A cold also produces a nasal discharge that varies from watery and copious to thick and purulent. In clients with a chronic allergy, the nasal mucosa looks swollen, boggy, pale, and gray. *Polyps* are benign growths that may develop in the nose with allergies. They may be distinguished from the normal turbinates because polyps are pale gray in color, mobile, avascular, and nontender. Disorders of the nose and paranasal sinuses are discussed further in Chapter 91.

The Mouth and Throat

Inspect the lips for color, moisture, lumps, ulcers, or cracking. Check the tongue and mucous membranes for color. Normally, the tongue's dorsal surface is roughened from the presence of papillae. Note any abnormal smoothness. Ask the client to remove any dentures. Offer a paper towel for the client's use during denture removal. While holding the cheek open with the flat side of a wooden tongue blade, check the buccal mucosa for color, pigmentation, ulcers, or nodules. Patchy pigmentation is normal in black-skinned persons. A number of common childhood diseases have characteristic changes on the mucosa and tongue.[13e] Note Stensen's duct, the opening of the parotid salivary gland. It looks like a small dimple on the buccal mucosa, opposite the upper second molar.

Check the gums for swelling, bleeding, retraction, or discoloration. Notice any absent, loose, or carious teeth, or any abnormal position or shape of the teeth. Check the roof of the mouth. The more anterior hard palate is white, whereas the soft palate is pinker. Occasionally you may notice a bony ridge in the middle of the hard palate. This benign condition is a *torus palatinus.* The uvula is muscular tissue that hangs down from the back of the soft palate. It may be bifid. As the client phonates "ahh," the soft palate and uvula should rise in the midline (tests function of cranial nerve X); note any deviation or the absence of movement.

Notice the oval, rough-surfaced tonsils behind the anterior tonsilar pillar. Tonsils are graded as: 1+ = visible; 2+ = between 1+ and 3+; 3+ = touching the uvula; and 4+ = touching each other. It is normal to see 1+ or 2+ tonsils in healthy clients, especially in children. The color of the tonsils should be the same pink as the oral mucosa, and normally there is no whitish exudate. With an acute infection, the tonsils look injected and swollen and have an exudate or white spots.

Pressing down on the middle of the tongue with a tongue blade, note the posterior pharyngeal wall for color, skin change, or exudate. Touch the posterior wall with the tongue blade to elicit the gag reflex (a test of functioning of cranial nerves IX and X, the glossopharyngeal and vagus nerves). Ask the client to stick out the tongue; it should protrude in the midline (test of cranial nerve XII, the hypoglossal). Note any deviation, tremor, or loss of movement. Inspect the entire U-shaped area under the tongue, while the client touches the tongue to the roof of the mouth. Note any white areas, nodules, or ulcerations. Remember, this is the area where oral malignancies are most likely to develop. Palpate and notice any induration. Wharton's ducts are the openings of the submaxillary glands under the tongue on either side of the frenulum. Finally, notice any breath odors, which may indicate poor oral hygiene, alcohol ingestion, or systemic diseases such as uremia or ketoacidosis.[43]

Checklist: Ear, Nose and Throat Examination

1. *Examination of the ear*
   A. *Inspect external ear*
      (1) *Size and shape of auricle*
      (2) *Deformities, lumps, skin lesions*
      (3) *Movement of auricle and tragus*
      (4) *External auditory meatus — size, swelling, redness, discharge, cerumen, lesions, foreign bodies*
   B. *Otoscopic examination*
      (1) *External canal*
         a. *Cerumen, discharge, foreign bodies, lesions*

b. Redness or swelling of canal wall
(2) Tympanic membrane
a. Position (flat, bulging, retracted)
b. Color and characteristics
c. Integrity of membrane
C. Examine hearing acuity
(1) Voice test and watch tick test
(2) Tuning fork tests — Weber and Rinne
2. Examination of the nose
A. Inspect for deformity, asymmetry, inflammation
B. Test patency of each nostril
C. Using nasal speculum, note:
(1) Color of nasal mucosa
(2) Septum — any bleeding, perforation, deviation
(3) Turbinates — color, swelling, exudate, polyps
3. Examination of the mouth and throat
A. Inspect lips, tongue, gums, teeth, buccal mucosa
B. Inspect palate and uvula as patient phonates
C. Inspect tonsils and pharyngeal wall

EXAMINATION OF THE NECK

Examination of the neck region includes inspection of the cervical muscles for range-of-motion and strength; palpation of the lymph nodes, salivary glands, trachea, and thyroid gland; and assessment of the carotid arteries and jugular veins. These vascular structures are discussed in detail in the cardiovascular assessment section later in this chapter.

Inspection

The major neck muscles are the trapezius and the sternocleidomastoid, which are innervated by cranial nerve XI, the spinal accessory nerve. The trapezius lies across the posterior part of the neck. The sternocleidomastoid muscle extends from the top of the sternum and clavicle and travels diagonally across the neck to the mastoid process (see Figs. 15–9 and 15–11). It divides the neck into the anterior triangle in front of the muscle and the posterior triangle behind it. These "triangles" are helpful guidelines when describing findings in the neck.

Observe the neck muscles, and note any limitation of movement. Ask the client to touch chin to chest, turn the head to right and left, try to touch each ear to the corresponding shoulder, and extend the head backward. Muscle strength and cranial nerve XI intactness are tested by trying to resist the client's movements with your hands as the client shrugs her or his shoulders and turns the head to each side. Pain and limitation of neck movement may indicate arthritis in the cervical spine, inflammation in the neck muscles, or irritation of the meninges.

During this neck motion, check for asymmetry and any obvious pulsations or masses. The carotid artery runs medial to the sternocleidomastoid muscle. It creates a brisk localized pulsation just below the angle of the jaw (Fig. 15–10). Any other pulsation while the client is in the sitting position is abnormal (see further discussion in cardiovascular assessment, later in this chapter). As the client moves her or his head, note enlargement of salivary glands and lymph nodes. Also note thyroid gland enlargement. This may be unilateral, or it may be diffuse and look like a doughnut lying across the lower neck.

Palpation

Using a gentle circular motion of your fingers, palpate the *salivary glands* and the *lymph nodes.* The salivary glands are the parotid in front of the ear and submandibular and sublingual under the jaw. Normally, they are not palpable. Beginning with the pre-auricular lymph nodes in front of the ear, palpate the ten groups of lymph nodes

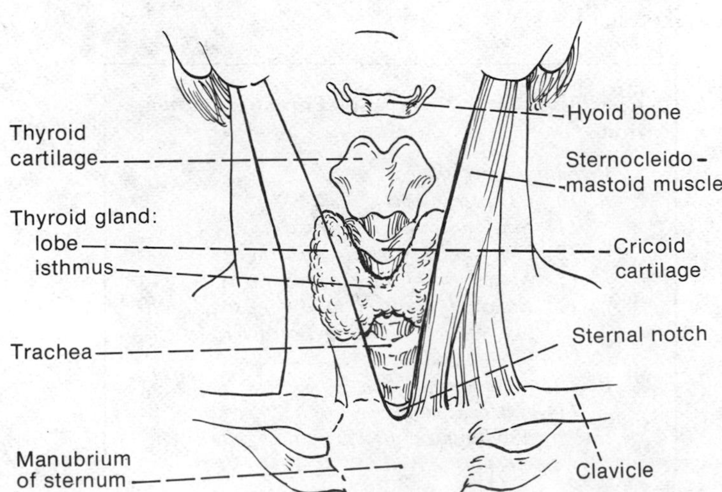

Figure 15–9. Anatomy of neck structures. (Redrawn from Malasanos, L., et al.: *Health Assessment.* St. Louis: C. V. Mosby Co., 1977.)

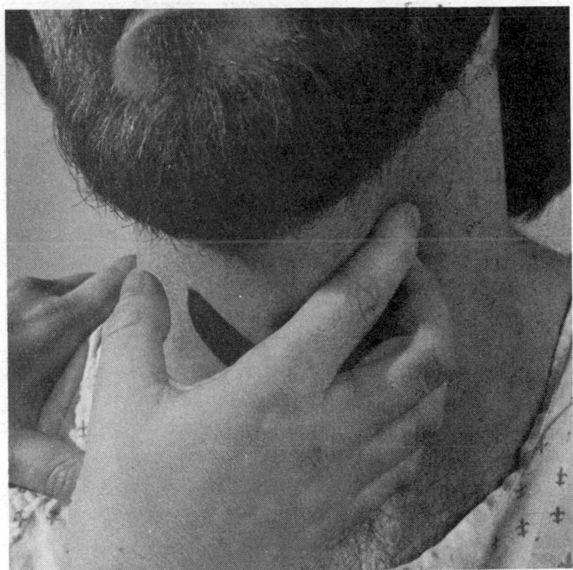

Figure 15-10. Palpating the carotid artery. The examiner gently palpates the area medial to the sternocleidomastoid muscle, and palpates only one side of the neck at a time to avoid excessive vagal stimulation. (See discussion in cardiovascular section.) (Reprinted by permission from *Nursing 77.*)

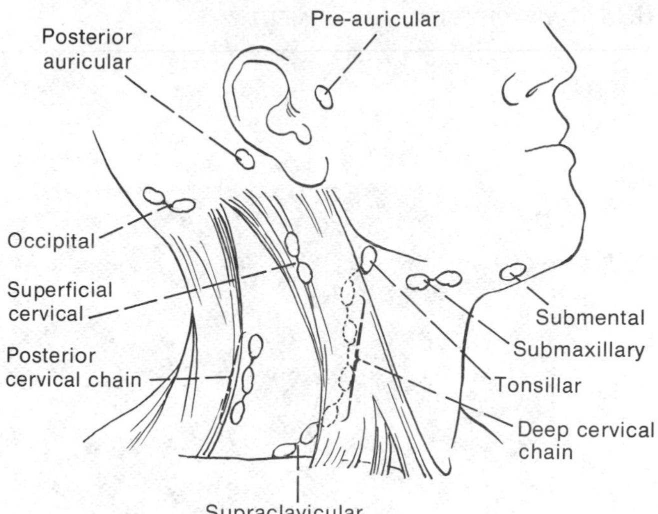

Figure 15-11. Location of lymph nodes in the neck. (Redrawn from Bates, B.: *A Guide to Physical Examination,* Philadelphia: J. B. Lippincott Co., 1974.)

(Fig. 15-11). Use gentle pressure, as too strong pressure could push the nodes into the neck muscles (Fig. 15-12). If any nodes are palpable, note their location, size, shape, delimitation (discrete or matted together), mobility, consistency, and tenderness. It is normal to find a few palpable nodes, especially in the anterior cervical triangle. They are movable, soft, and nontender. Lymph nodes in a client who has an acute infection are enlarged, tender, and firm but freely movable. Nodes are clumped with more chronic inflammations, e.g., tuberculosis. Cancerous nodes are hard, nontender, and fixed.

Palpate the *trachea* for any deviation. Place your index finger on the trachea in the sternal notch and slip it off each side (Fig. 15-13). Note any deviation from the midline. The trachea will be pushed to the unaffected side with an aortic aneurysm, tumor, unilateral thyroid lobe enlargement or pneumothorax. The trachea will be pulled toward the affected side with a large atelectasis, pleural adhesions, or fibrosis. The trachea also may be palpated for *tracheal tug.*[55] This is a rhythmic downward pull that is synchronous with ventricular systole and is noted with an aortic arch aneurysm.

Move behind the client to palpate the *thyroid gland.* It is shaped like a butterfly. Its middle part, or isthmus, lies over the trachea just below the cricoid cartilage and within 1 cm. of it (see Fig. 15-9). Each lobe curves posteriorly and lies between the trachea and the sternocleidomastoid muscle. Ask the client to sit up very straight, then to flex the neck slightly forward and to the right. This will relax the neck muscles on the side being examined. Use the fingers of your left hand to push the trachea slightly to the right (Fig. 15-14). Then curve your right fingers between the trachea and the sternocleidomastoid muscle and ask the client to swallow a sip of water. You may feel the thyroid move up under your fingers as the client swallows. Reverse the procedure for the left side. The isthmus may be palpable normally and feels like a grainy, mealy bit of tissue. The lateral lobes are usually not palpable; check them for enlargement, consistency, symmetry, and presence of nodules. In thyrotoxicosis, the gland is generally enlarged and feels soft. Tumors of the thyroid feel like solitary hard nodules.

If the thyroid gland is enlarged, it should be auscultated for the presence of a *bruit.* This is a soft whooshing blowing sound heard best with the bell of the stethoscope. Also auscultate over the carotid arteries, especially in clients over 40 years of age. A carotid artery bruit is discussed in the cardiovascular section of this chapter.

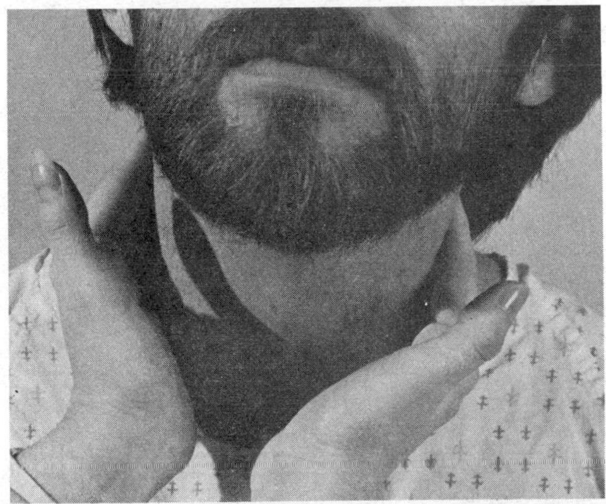

Figure 15-12. Palpating cervical lymph nodes. The examiner's hands are slightly curved; the finger pads gently rotate the client's skin in small circles to search for lymph nodes below. (Reprinted by permission from *Nursing 77.)*

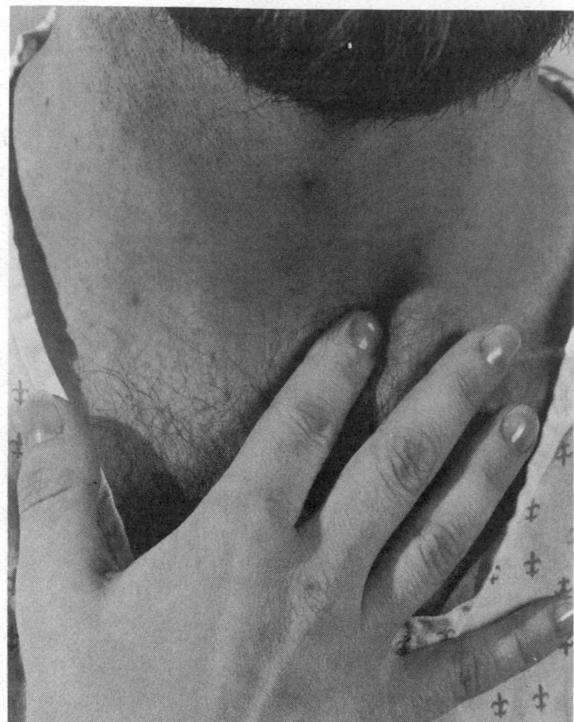

Figure 15–13. Palpating for position of trachea. In the sternal notch, the examiner's index finger gently slides next to each side of the trachea to assess its midline position. (Reprinted by permission from *Nursing 77.*)

Check the assessment literature for further discussion of the head and neck,[53g] for modifications in technique with children, and for symptom complexes of certain pathologies that are commonly seen in children.[1b, 1d]

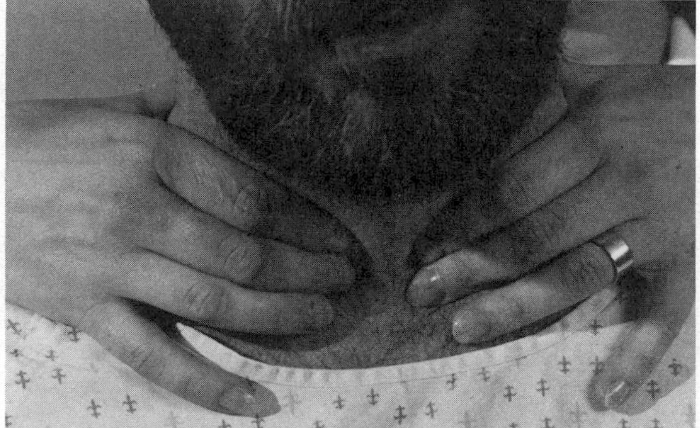

Figure 15–14. Palpating the thyroid gland. To palpate the right lobe, the client's head tilts down and to the right, and the examiner's left hand gently pushes the trachea slightly to the right. The examiner's right fingers palpate the area between the trachea and the sternocleidomastoid muscle while the client swallows. The procedure is reversed for the left lobe. (Reprinted by permission from *Nursing 77.*)

Checklist: Neck Examination

1. Inspection
- *A. Asymmetry*
  - *(1) Active range-of-motion*
  - *(2) Strength of cervical muscles*
- *B. Carotid artery pulsation*
- *C. Abnormal pulsations or masses*
- *D. Enlargement of salivary glands, lymph nodes, or thyroid gland*

2. Palpation
- *A. Salivary glands and lymph nodes*
- *B. Trachea*
- *C. Thyroid gland*

3. Auscultation
- *A. Thyroid (if enlarged) for bruit*
- *B. Carotid artery for bruit*

EXAMINATION OF THE THORAX AND LUNGS

As you complete the neck examination, you are standing behind the client to palpate the thyroid gland. Examination of the thorax is started next. The client is sitting upright and is disrobed to the waist. Equipment needed is a stethoscope, a small ruler marked in centimeters, and a marking pen. The assessment techniques (inspection, palpation, percussion, auscultation) are discussed separately below. In order to avoid repetitious front-to-back moving around the client, you should perform all four techniques on the posterior and lateral thorax while standing behind the client. Then move to face the client and repeat the four techniques on the anterior chest.

Topography and Structural Anatomy

The examiner must try to visualize underlying anatomy in order to correlate findings with specific lobes of the lungs. Respiratory findings are useless unless their position can be communicated precisely among different examiners. To facilitate communication, a standard set of landmarks and reference lines has been developed (see Fig. 15–15).

Landmarks. The following landmarks are used in the common examining language:

- ► *Angle of Louis.* Also called the *sternal* angle, this bony ridge is easily seen and felt on the anterior chest. It is the articulation of two parts of the sternum, the manubrium and the body. The angle of Louis is a useful place to start counting ribs because it is continuous with the second rib. Each intercostal space is named for the rib above it. Therefore you can run your right index finger across the angle of Louis to the client's left second rib and slide it down to the second intercostal space. If you count down each finger to the next intercostal space, your little finger ends up in the fifth intercostal space. Do this in the middle of the hemithorax, not close to the sternum, where the rib cartilages lie too close together to count. The sternal angle is also useful because it marks the site of tracheal bifurcation into the right and left bronchi, it corresponds with the upper border of the atria of the heart, and it lies above the fifth thoracic vertebra on the back.

- *Costal angle.* This is the angle (usually about 90 degrees) formed by the right and left costal margins where they meet at the xyphoid process.
- *Suprasternal notch.* This is the hollow depression above the sternum, in between the clavicles.
- *Vertebra prominens.* This bony spur protrudes on the base of the neck when the client bends the head forward; it is the seventh cervical vertebra. If two bumps seem equally prominent to you, the top one is C7 and the lower one is T1. This is a good place to begin counting thoracic vertebrae. The location of C7 marks the highest point, or apex, of lung tissue in the posterior chest; T3 or T4 marks the division between upper and lower lobes; and T10 usually corresponds to the inferior border of lung tissue in the back.

Reference Lines. On the anterior chest, the reference lines are the *midsternal* line and the *midclavicular* lines, which bisect the center of each clavicle (see Fig. 15–15). With the client's arm abducted no more than 90 degrees, the lateral chest may be divided into three lines: (1) the *anterior axillary* line extends down from the anterior axillary fold where the pectoralis major muscle inserts; (2) the *posterior axillary* line continues down from the posterior axillary fold where the latissimus dorsi muscle inserts; and (3) the *midaxillary line* runs down from the apex of the axilla and lies between and parallel to the other two. The posterior chest wall has the *vertebral* (or midspinal) line and the *scapular* line, which extends down through the inferior angle of the scapula when the client's arms are down.

With this information, you can pinpoint a thoracic finding horizontally and vertically. For example, you might find a dull percussion note at the tenth intercostal space in the left anterior axillary line. Or, a lump on a rib might be at the fifth rib, 2 cm. lateral to the right midclavicular line.

Lobes of the Lungs. (Fig. 15–16). In the anterior chest, lung tissue extends from 4 cm. above the clavicles down to the fifth intercostal space on the right and to the sixth rib in the midclavicular line on the left. Laterally, lung tissue extends from the apex of the axilla down to the seventh rib. Posteriorly, the lungs reach above the scapulae to the level of C7 and, varying with respiration, down to the tenth or twelfth thoracic vertebra.

The right lung has three lobes, and the left lung has two; the lobes are separated by fissures. The right *longitudinal* (or *diagonal*) fissure starts at T4 posteriorly, runs obliquely down through the fifth rib in the midaxillary line, and terminates at the sixth rib in the midclavicular line. It separates the upper and lower lobes posteriorly, and the middle and lower lobes on the lateral and anterior chest wall. On the left lung, the cross

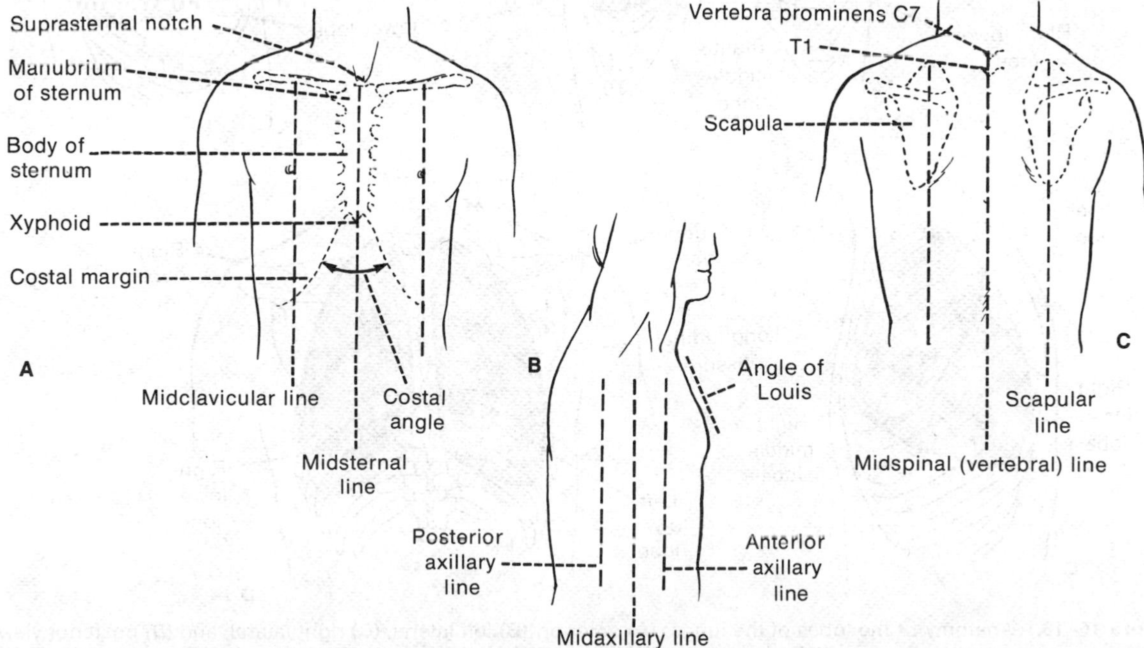

Figure 15–15. Landmarks and reference lines on **(A)** anterior, **(B)** lateral, and **(C)** posterior thorax. (Redrawn from Sana, J. S., and R. D. Judge: *Physical Appraisal Methods in Nursing Practice.* Boston: Little, Brown and Co., 1975.)

If you keep these facts in mind, the importance of turning postoperative patients to avoid pooling of secretions in the lower lobes is easily seen.

points of the longitudinal fissure are the same. There it separates the upper from the lower lobe throughout because the left lung has no middle lobe. The right lung contains one more line, the *horizontal* fissure, which divides the upper and middle lobes. It extends from the fifth rib in the right midaxillary line to the third intercostal space or to the fourth rib at the right sternal border.

With these landmarks, you can trace the outline of each lobe. Using a grease pencil, try drawing the lobes of the lungs on a fellow student before you set out to examine clients.

> *Remember:*
> 1. *The left lung has* no middle lobe
> 2. *The anterior chest is mostly upper lobe with very little lower lobe*
> 3. *The posterior chest is almost all lower lobe*

Inspection

Significant Physical Characteristics. Many factors about a client's body shape and appearance are indicative of respiratory status. For example, persons with emphysema have an anterior-posterior chest diameter as big as their transverse diameter. This is due to the hyperinflation of the lungs. Similarly, their ribs are horizontal instead of having the normal downward slope. This is called "barrel chest."

Any skeletal deformity should be noted, as it could limit excursion of the thoracic cage and thus interfere with respiration. *Scoliosis* is an S-shaped curvature of the thoracic and lumbar regions of the spine. *Lordosis* (swayback) is an anterior curvature of the lumbar spine, causing the thoracic spine to be displaced in a backward position. *Kyphosis* ("hump-back") is an exaggerated posterior curvature of the thoracic spine. A markedly sunken sternum is called *pectus excava-*

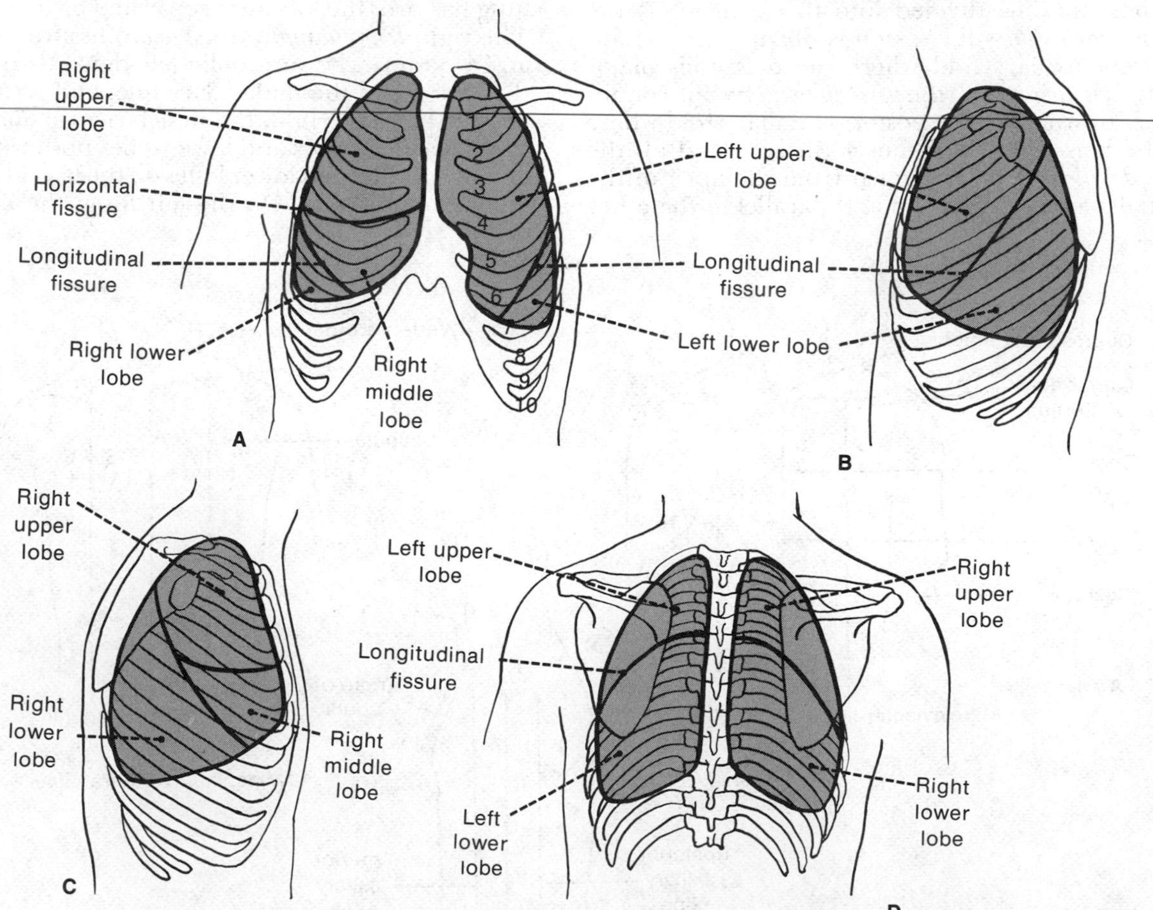

Figure 15–16. Anatomy of the lobes of the lungs: **(A)** anterior, **(B)** left lateral, **(C)** right lateral, and **(D)** posterior views. (Redrawn from Sana, J. S., and R. D. Judge: *Physical Appraisal Methods in Nursing Practice.* Boston: Little, Brown and Co., 1975.)

tum (funnel breast). This disorder occurs congenitally and with rickets, a vitamin deficiency disease. *Pectus carinatum* (pigeon breast) is a forward protrusion of the sternum, with the ribs sloping back at either side. It is often seen with active rickets.

Note the position the client takes to breathe. For example, persons with *COPD* (chronic obstructive pulmonary disease) sit leaning forward, with their arms braced against their knees, chair, or bed. This gives them leverage so that their abdominal rectus, intercostal, and accessory neck muscles all can aid to force expiration. Such persons also may purse their lips in a whistling position. By exhaling slowly and against a narrow opening, the pressure in the bronchial tree remains positive and fewer airways collapse. *Orthopnea* is the inability to breathe except when sitting in an upright position. For accuracy, record the number of pillows the client uses to sleep, e.g., "two-pillow orthopnea" or "three-pillow orthopnea."

Observe the skin and musculature of the thorax for decreased turgor or weight loss. Notice any lesions. For example, *cutaneous angiomas* (or spider nevi) are associated with liver disease or portal hypertension and may be seen on the chest. The skin also should be observed for pallor or cyanosis. Further discussion is presented in the skin section later in this chapter.

Adequate ventilation is closely related to neurologic status. *A change in the previous level of consciousness* may be the first indication of cerebral hypoxia. With progressive pulmonary decompensation, a previously alert hospitalized patient may become anxious and restless, then irritable, then excessively drowsy, and finally comatose. Or a patient who was calm and cooperative may become suddenly combative. The alert observer will pick up even subtle personality changes and can thus initiate appropriate interventions.

Quality of Respirations. Normal relaxed breathing is effortless, automatic, regular and even, and produces no noise. Notice if the client's chest expands symmetrically with each inspiration. Unequal chest expansion occurs when part of a lung is obstructed or collapsed, e.g., with pneumonia, and postoperatively when a patient "guards" the operative side to avoid incisional pain from breathing.

Notice the intercostal spaces between the ribs. Is there *retraction* of the interspaces on inspiration? This suggests obstruction of the respiratory tract or increased inspiratory effort, as is needed with atelectasis. In children, you will also note sternal retraction and nasal flaring. *Bulging* of the interspaces indicates trapped air, as in the forced expiration associated with emphysema or asthma.

Notice if the respirations are *diaphragmatic* or *costal.* While the diaphragm is the major muscle of normal breathing in both males and females, women may appear to move the chest wall more than men. The diaphragm flattens during inspiration to enlarge the size of the thoracic cage, thus the abdominal contents are pushed out. Costal respirations may be noticed on some women who have been reared to hold their stomach in and their chest out while breathing.

Also notice the use of accessory muscles to augment respiratory effort. In heavy exercise, inspiration is enhanced by the use of the accessory neck muscles (scalene, sternocleidomastoid, trapezius). Accessory muscles are used in acute airway obstruction and massive atelectasis, but they still may not improve ventilation and the extra effort may be exhausting. The abdominal rectus and internal intercostal muscles are used to force expiration in COPD. Clients with COPD have increased airway resistance from collapse of the bronchioles and have difficulty getting the air *out.* This leaves the lungs hyperinflated and flattens the diaphragm, making the diaphragm useless as a respiratory muscle. Persons with COPD forcefully contract the stomach muscles, which pushes the abdominal contents against the diaphragm and makes it dome up.

Dyspnea is difficult, labored or painful breathing. The client verbalizes a feeling of air hunger, of not getting enough air. The client's face appears anxious and tired from exertion. The nostrils flare with the increased inspiratory effort, color may be dusky, and tachycardia may be present. Recording that the client is "dyspneic" is not adequate. Include how much exertion it takes to produce the dyspnea. For example, does dyspnea occur with walking to the bathroom, or is shortness of breath present during talking, so that the client must pause every few sentences to rest?

Notice the type of respirations. The normal rate is 12 to 18 breaths per minute in adults. The depth is the volume of air moving in and out with each respiration (*tidal volume*). The pattern of breathing is normally regular and consists of inspiration, pause, longer expiration, and another pause. The following terms describe alterations in respiration (Fig. 15–17).

- *Tachypnea.* An increased respiratory rate (> 24 breaths per minute)
- *Bradypnea.* A decreased but regular rate (< 10 breaths per minute)
- *Hypoventilation.* An alteration of the pattern (irregular, or slow) and the depth (shallow)
- *Apnea.* Total cessation of breathing
- *Hyperpnea.* Increased depth of respirations (increased tidal volume)
- *Hyperventilation.* An increase in both rate and

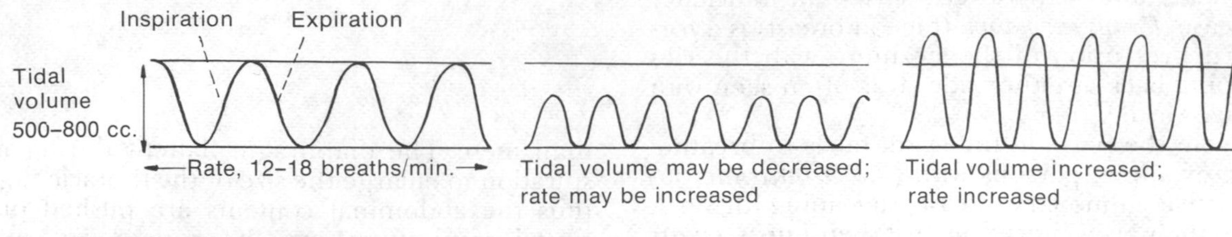

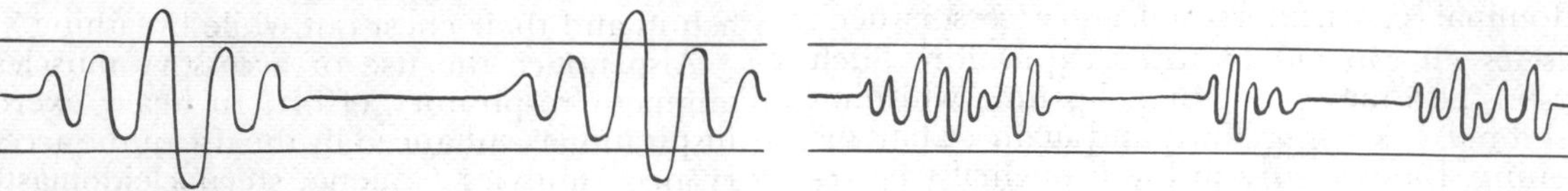

Figure 15–17. Normal and abnormal breathing patterns. (From Sorensen, K. C., and J. Luckmann,: *Basic Nursing: A Psychophysiologic Approach.* Philadelphia: W. B. Saunders Co., 1979.)

depth. An example is *Kussmaul's* respirations (air hunger), a type of dyspnea that occurs in metabolic acidosis from diabetic coma or renal failure.

- *Cheyne-Stokes.* A cycle in which respirations gradually wax and wane in a regular pattern. They increase in rate and depth and then decrease, lasting 30 to 45 seconds. Periods of apnea (20 seconds) alternate the cycles.
- *Biot's.* Similar to Cheyne-Stokes, except that each breath is of the same depth. A series of normal respirations (3 to 4 or more) is followed by a period of apnea. The cycle length is variable, lasting anywhere from 10 seconds to 1 minute.
- *Apneusis.* Prolonged, gasping inspiration, followed by extremely short, inefficient expiration.

For further discussion of these terms and related pathology, see Chapter 29 in Sorensen and Luckmann, *Basic Nursing: A Psychophysiologic Approach.* See also Unit XVI in this text.

Palpation

One major purpose in palpation of the chest wall is to verify what you saw during inspection of the chest. Check for symmetrical chest expansion by placing your warmed hands on the client's chest with your thumbs together (Fig. 15–18). On the client's anterior chest, place your hands on the anterolateral wall with your thumbs along the costal margins. On the client's back, place your hands on the posterolateral wall with your thumbs at level of T9. Your hands serve as "mechanical amplifiers." As the client inhales deeply, your thumbs should move apart symmetrically.

Next, palpate to assess *tactile* (or *vocal*) *fremitus.* Sounds generated from the client's larynx are transmitted through patent bronchi and through the lung parenchyma to the chest wall where you feel the sounds as vibrations. Using the palmar base of your fingers, touch the client's chest. Then ask the client to repeat a resonant phrase, e.g., "ninety-nine" or "blue moon." Avoid palpating over the scapulae, as bone damps out sound transmission. Start over the lung apices and palpate side-to-side. Fremitus varies among persons, but *symmetry* is most important. The vibrations should feel the same in the corresponding area on each side.

Normally, fremitus is most prominent between the scapulae and around the sternum, places where the major bronchi are closest to the chest wall. Fremitus decreases as you move downward, because more tissue impedes sound transmission. Fremitus feels greater over a thin

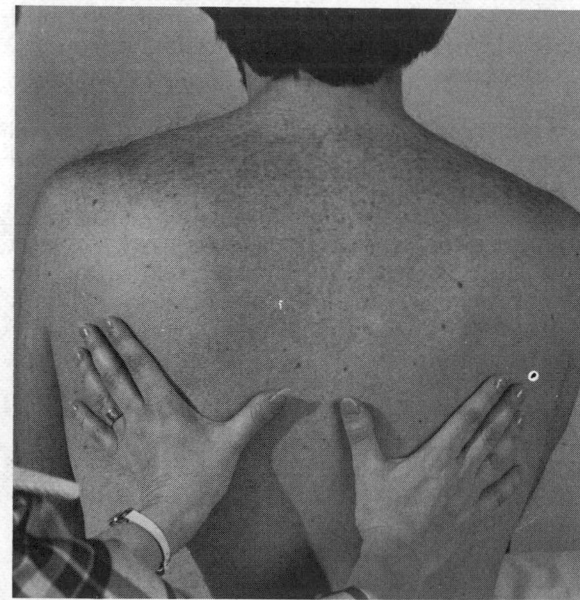

Figure 15–18. Palpating to confirm symmetrical respiratory expansion. The examiner's hands touch the client's back with the thumbs together; as the client inhales deeply, the examiner's hands should move apart symmetrically. (Reprinted by permission from *Nursing 77.)*

chest wall than over an obese or heavily muscular one, where tissue damps the vibration. Also, a low-pitched voice generates more fremitus than a soft, high-pitched one. Hence you expect more tactile fremitus over the chest wall of a thin man, than over that of a heavyset woman.

Pathologically, tactile fremitus will be *increased* with conditions that increase the density of lung tissues, thereby making a better conducting medium for vibrations. An example is pneumonia, in which the lung alveoli consolidate, or fill up with solid cellular debris and fluid. Tactile fremitus is *decreased* when anything obstructs transmission of vibrations, e.g., pleural effusion, pleural thickening, pneumothorax, emphysema, or an obstructed bronchus.

Other abnormal sounds that may be palpated include rhonchal fremitus, pleural friction rub, and crepitance.

Rhonchal fremitus is the vibration felt when inhaled air passes through thick secretions in the larger bronchi; this may decrease somewhat by coughing.

A *pleural friction rub* is produced when inflammation of the parietal or visceral pleura causes a decrease in the normal lubricating fluid. Then the opposing surfaces make a coarse grating sound when rubbed together during respiration. Though this sound is usually best *heard,* it may sometimes be felt, like two pieces of leather grating together.

Crepitance is the crackling, popping sound that occurs when feeling small air bubbles that lie in the skin planes. This condition is called "subcutaneous emphysema."

The nurse also palpates the chest wall to detect any lumps or masses, and gently palpates the ribs for tenderness. Skin turgor can be felt, as well as temperature, moisture, and edema.

Percussion

First, using the ulnar fist, directly percuss the client's vertebral spine to note any tenderness. Next use indirect percussion to determine the percussion note that predominates over the lung fields. Start percussing at the apices and make a side-to-side comparison all the way down the lungs. Avoid the damping effect of the scapulae and ribs. *Resonance* predominates in healthy lung tissue; *hyperresonance* is found when too much air is present, as in emphysema; and a *dull* note signals abnormal density in the lungs, as with pneumonia, pleural effusion, atelectasis, or tumor.

Percussion is also used to map out the lung boundaries. On the anterior chest, the location of the lungs and that of the heart can be determined by comparing lung resonance with cardiac dullness. (This is described later in the cardiovascular section of this chapter.) On the client's back, percuss down the scapular line until you notice that the sound changes from resonant to dull on each side. This locates the level of the diaphragm, separating the lungs from the abdominal viscera. It may be somewhat higher on the right (about 1 to 2 cm.) owing to the presence of the liver. Mark on the client's skin the location of the sound change, first during quiet shallow breathing and then on very deep inspiration, and measure the difference (Fig. 15–19). This difference is called the *diaphragmatic excursion.* It should be equal bilaterally and measure about 3 to 5 cm., although it may be up to 7 to 8 cm. in healthy young adult men.

Auscultation

The nurse auscultates the lungs with the diaphragm endpiece of the stethoscope to (a) assess breath sounds, (b) confirm suspicions of pathology, and (c) evaluate voice sounds. Instruct the client to breathe through the mouth a little deeper than normally as you listen to the following lung areas: *posteriorly* from the apices (at C7) to the bases (around T10); *laterally* from the axilla to the seventh rib, and *anteriorly* from the apices above the clavicles down to the sixth rib. Again, comparison between the sides is important! First evaluate normal breath sounds, then note any abnormal breath sounds, and finally any adventitious sounds.

Normal Breath Sounds. These include vesicular, bronchovesicular and tracheal breath sounds (Fig. 15–20).

Vesicular breath sounds are low-pitched, soft, and rustling — like the sound of wind in the trees. They are heard normally over the peripheral lung fields, where the air flows through the smaller bronchioles and alveoli. Inspiration sounds longer, louder, and higher-pitched than expiration.

Bronchovesicular sounds are normally heard over the major bronchi where fewer alveoli are located, anteriorly around the upper sternum in the first and second intercostal space and posteriorly between the scapulae. These sounds are of moderate pitch and loudness, and expiration is as long as inspiration.

Tracheal sounds (sometimes called *bronchial or tubular)* are the harsh, high-pitched, loud sounds heard over the largest air passageways, the trachea, and larynx. They have a hollow tubular quality with a prominent expiratory phase.

Listen to these normal sounds in their usual location on the chest walls of your fellow students and on healthy clients. You need confidence in auscultating the range of *normal* breath sounds before you can begin identifying abnormal breath sounds.

Abnormal Breath Sounds. These include

bronchial sounds, decreased or absent sounds, and voice sounds.

Bronchial sounds are much like the tracheal sounds described above, but they are heard over an abnormal location, the peripheral lung fields. They have a harsh, high-pitched, tubular quality with a prolonged expiratory phase and a distinct pause between inspiration and expiration. They sound very "close" to your stethoscope, as if they were right in the tubing close to your ear. Bronchial sounds occur when consolidation (e.g., pneumonia) or compression yields a denser lung area that *enhances* the transmission of sound from the bronchi. When inspired air reaches the alveoli, it hits solid lung tissue that conducts sound to the surface better.

Decreased or absent breath sounds are abnormal. They occur when the bronchial tree is obstructed, e.g., by a foreign body, secretions, or a mucous plug. Breath sounds also are decreased in emphysema, owing to loss of elasticity in the lung fibers and decreased force of inspired air. Furthermore, in emphysema the lungs are already hyperinflated so the inhaled air does not make as much noise. Finally, breath sounds are decreased when anything obstructs transmission of sound between the lung and your stethoscope. This may occur with disorders such as pleurisy or pleural thickening or by the presence in the pleural space of air (pneumothorax) or fluid (pleural effusion).

Voice sounds or *vocal resonance* is the third category of abnormal sounds. The spoken voice can be auscultated over the chest wall just as it can be felt in tactile fremitus, as described earlier. Ask the client to repeat "ninety-nine" while you listen over the chest wall. Normal voice transmission is soft, muffled, and indistinct; you can hear sound through the stethoscope but cannot distinguish exactly what is being said. Pathology that increases lung density (consolidation or compression) will enhance transmission of voice sounds. *Bronchophony* is present when you auscultate a loud clear voice sound. The client's words are more distinct than normal, and sound close to your ear. *Whispered pectoriloquy* is elicited by having the client whisper a phrase like "one-two-three" or "ninety-nine." The normal response is faint, muffled, and almost inaudible except over the trachea. Even with only small amounts of consolidation, however, the whispered voice is transmitted clearly and distinctly, although still somewhat faint. It sounds like the client is whispering into the endpiece of your stethoscope. *Egophony* is checked by auscultating the chest while the client phonates a long "e" sound. Normally, you should hear "e" through your stethoscope. But over areas of consolidation or compression, the spoken "e"

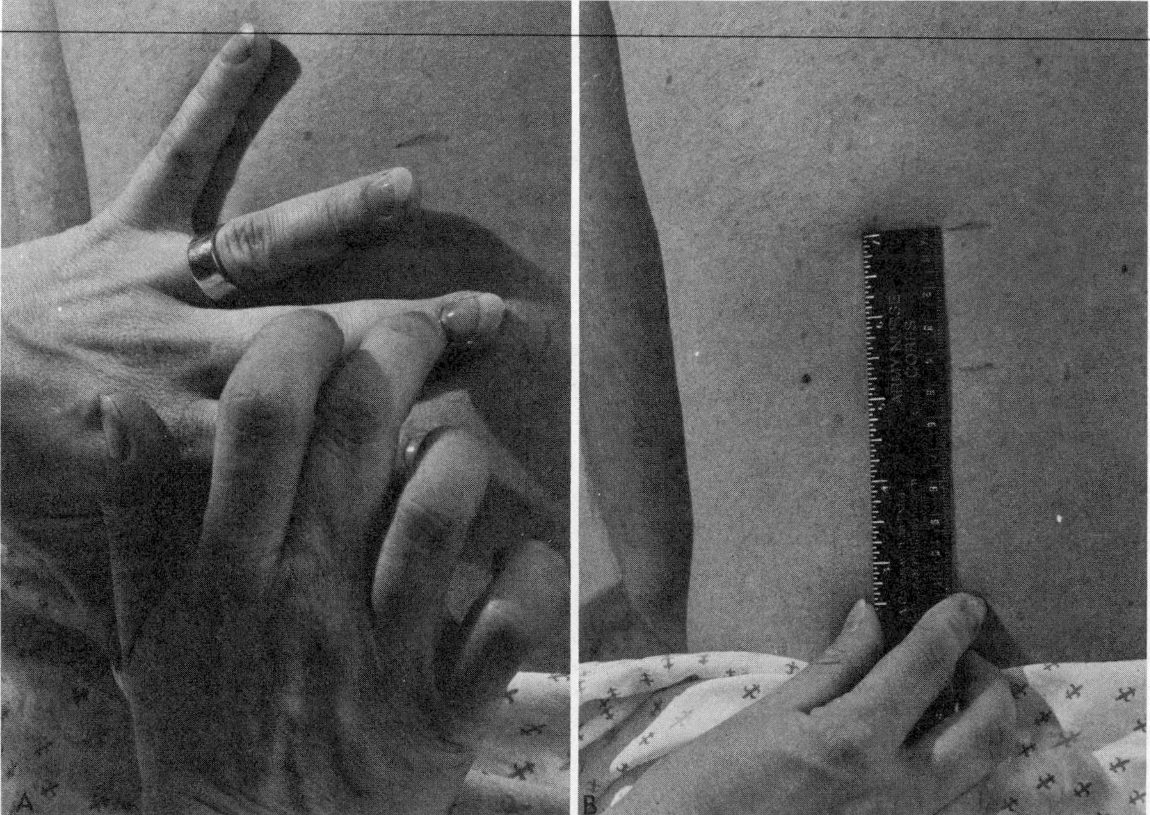

Figure 15–19. Percussing to determine diaphragmatic excursion. **A.** The examiner percusses downward in the scapular line. A mark on the skin indicates the level of the diaphragm (where the sound changes from resonant to dull) during shallow relaxed breathing, and on deep inspiration. **B.** The examiner measures between these two marks to determine diaphragmatic excursion. (Reprinted by permission from *Nursing 77*.)

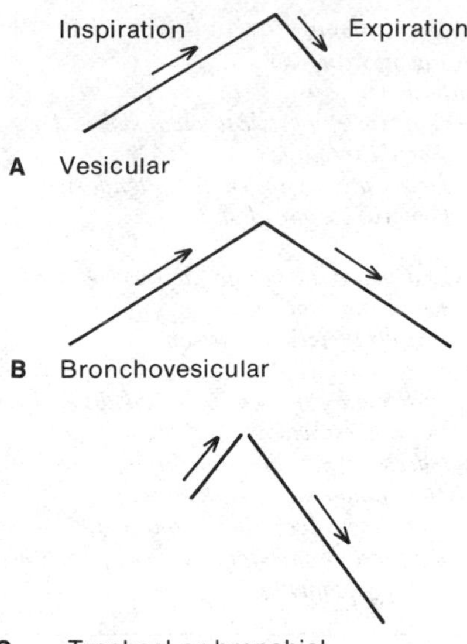

Figure 15–20. Normal breath sounds. Upstroke = inspiration; downstroke = expiration; length of line = duration of sound; angle between lines = pitch (e.g., a steep angle in *C* signifies a high pitch).

sound changes to a bleating long "a" sound. Record this as "E → A changes."

Eliciting the voice sounds is usually not done in the routine screening examination. Rather, these maneuvers are performed if the examiner suspects lung pathology from the history or from earlier parts of the physical exam. For example, if you detect increased tactile fremitus, a dull percussion note, and bronchial breathing over the posterior left lower lobe, you might suspect pneumonia and test for bronchophony.

Adventitious Sounds. These are "added-on" sounds, *not* normally heard in the lungs. They are heard superimposed on the breath sounds and are caused by the collision of moving air with secretions in the tracheobronchial passageways. Sources differ as to the clarification and nomenclature of these sounds.[33] *Rales* and *rhonchi* are terms that are commonly used by most clinicians. Rales are discontinuous, discrete, crackling sounds that are heard more on inspiration. Rhonchi are continuous, coarse, musical sounds heard all through the respiratory cycle, but more on expiration.

Rales are divided into three categories, fine, medium and coarse. Because rales are heard when inspired air reaches secretions, their pitch and timing in the inspiratory phase depend on the location of the exudate (Fig. 15–21).

- *Fine rales* (also called *crepitant*) are high-pitched, crackling, popping sounds heard at the peak of inspiration when there is moisture in the most distant alveoli. You can simulate this sound by rolling a strand of hair between your fingers near your ear, or by moistening your thumb and index finger and slowly separating them near your ear. Fine rales occur with impaired pulmonary ventilation, pneumonia, and congestive heart failure.
- *Medium rales* (also called *subcrepitant*) occur with secretions in the alveoli and small bronchioles. They are slightly louder and lower-pitched, occur in mid to late inspiration, and mimic the sound of soda fizzing. They occur with CHF, pneumonia, pulmonary edema, and bronchitis.
- *Coarse rales* are loud, low-pitched, bubbling, and gurgling sounds that start in early inspiration. They are heard when secretions are in the large

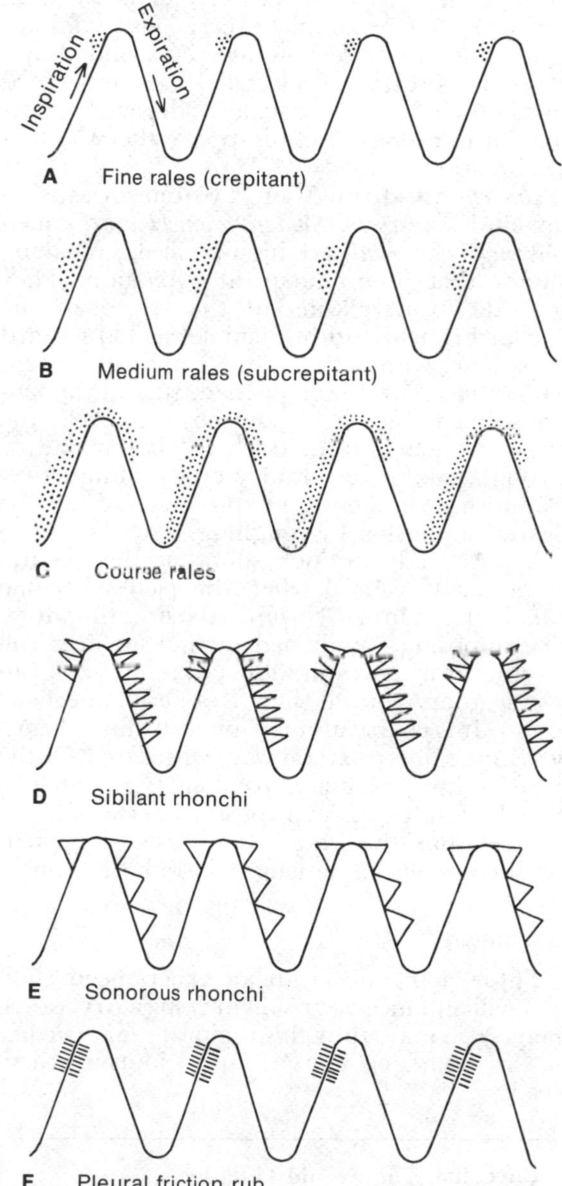

Figure 15–21. Diagram of adventitious sounds. Rales are discrete crackling sounds heard predominantly on inspiration. They occur earlier in inspiration as their severity progresses. Rhonchi are continuous coarse sounds heard more on expiration. (For further discussion, including pleural friction rub, see text.)

passageways. Coarse rales may be decreased somewhat by suctioning or coughing but will reappear shortly. They have the traditional name of "death rattle" because they occur with severe pulmonary edema or in the terminally ill who have a depressed cough reflex.

Sometimes rales are termed *atelectatic.* These sound like fine rales but do not last and are not pathological. When sections of alveoli are not fully aerated (as in the elderly or in sleeping persons), they accumulate secretions. Rales are heard when these sections are re-expanded by a few deep breaths. Atelectatic rales are heard only in the periphery, usually in dependent portions of the lungs, and disappear after the first few breaths.

Rhonchi are divided into two categories, sibilant and sonorous. *Sibilant rhonchi* (also called *wheezing* or *musical*) are high-pitched, squeaking sounds that predominate in expiration. They are due to narrowing of the lumen of the smaller bronchi and bronchioles and are heard in patients with asthma and emphysema. *Sonorous rhonchi* are lower-pitched, snoring, moaning sounds due to airflow obstruction in the larger bronchi and the trachea. They are heard throughout the respiratory cycle, though they are more prominent on expiration and may be cleared somewhat by coughing.

Another adventitious sound is the pleural friction rub, caused when the pleura become inflamed and lose their normal lubricating fluid. The opposing roughened pleural surfaces rub together during respiration and result in a grating, leathery sound. This is a very superficial sound. It is coarse and low-pitched and is heard best in the anterolateral wall, where there is the greatest lung mobility. A pleural friction rub sounds louder if you push the stethoscope harder onto the chest wall. Also, the client usually has accompanying pain with breathing.

Summary

Tutored practice with an experienced clinician will enhance your skill in respiratory assessment. You may study this regional exam further in assessment texts[23] and journal articles.[1e, 12, 33, 53c, 76]

Checklist: Thorax and Lung Examination

1. Inspection
- *A. Thoracic cage*
- *B. Client's position*
- *C. Skin*
- *D. Level of consciousness*
- *E. Respirations*
- *F. Facial expression*

2. Palpation
- *A. Confirm symmetrical expansion*
- *B. Tactile fremitus*
- *C. Detect any lumps, masses, tenderness*
- *D. General turgor of skin*

3. Percussion
- *A. Systematic survey to determine predominant percussion note*
- *B. Diaphragmatic excursion*

4. Auscultation
- *A. Systematic survey of posterior, lateral, and anterior chest wall*
- *B. Check normal breath sounds*
- *C. Note abnormal breath sounds*
- *D. Note any adventitious sounds*
- *E. Perform bronchophony, whispered pectoriloquy, egophony*

EXAMINATION OF THE BREAST

Female Breast. Inspection and palpation are the skills used to examine the female breast. Begin with the client in a sitting position, with the drape lowered to her waist. Observe the breasts and note symmetry of size and shape, and presence of any skin lesions, hyperpigmentation, focal vascular pattern, or abnormal hair distribution. It is not uncommon to have some degree of asymmetry in the shape of the breasts, but a sudden increase in the size of one breast signifies inflammation or the development of a cyst or tumor. Observe the skin over the breast and note any localized areas of redness, bulging or dimpling. Observe the nipple and note any bleeding, discharge, ulceration, or retraction. Distinguish a recently inverted nipple from one that has been inverted since puberty. Note the presence of edema. Edema exaggerates the skin pores and hair follicles and produces a "pig skin" or "orange peel" appearance (also called *peau d'orange*).

Next, change the client's position slightly to check for skin retraction. An invasive process will fibrose, or shorten, the suspensory (Cooper's) ligaments of the breast. This will be manifested by skin retraction, a lag in upward movement, or recent nipple inversion. First ask her to lift her arms slowly over her head (Fig. 15–22). Both breasts should lift up symmetrically. Note a lag in movement of one breast. Next ask her to push her hands onto her hips or to push her two palms together (Fig. 15–23). These maneuvers contract the pectoralis major muscle. Notice a dimpling or a pucker, which indicates skin retraction. Ask the client with large pendulous breasts to lean forward while you support her forearms. Note symmetrical movement of both breasts and any skin retraction.

Observe the axillary and supraclavicular regions. These sites are important lymphatic

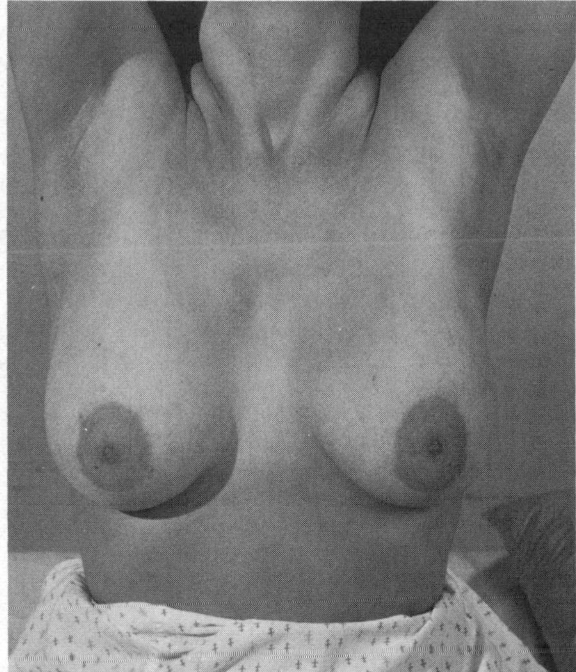

Figure 15–22. Observing the female breasts with client's arms raised. As the client slowly raises her arms, note a symmetrical rising of the breasts. A lag in upward movement of one breast is abnormal. (Reprinted by permission from *Nursing 77.*)

drainage areas and should be checked for bulging, retraction, discoloration, or edema.

Help the client to a supine position for palpation of the breasts. Tuck a small pillow under the side to be palpated and raise the client's arm over her head slightly. These maneuvers flatten the breast tissue and displace it medially. Using the pads of your first three fingers, make a gentle rotary motion on the breast. Start from the nipple and palpate out to the periphery in a pattern similar to following spokes on a wheel. You may begin at any point, but move in a clockwise direction taking care to examine each quadrant of the breast. Take care to palpate the tail of Spence, the extension of the upper lateral breast quadrant into the axilla.

The objective of breast palpation is to discover any lump or mass. If the client mentions a breast lump she has discovered herself, examine the "normal" breast first to determine normal consistency for that client. Then examine the breast containing the lump. Normally there is a firm transverse ridge of compressed tissue in the lower quadrants called the inframammary ridge. This is especially evident in large breasts and should not be confused with a tumor.

If a lump or mass is found, the following characteristics should be noted:

1. *Location.* Visualizing the breast as a clock face, describe the distance in centimeters from the nipple. For example, "3:00, 2 cm. from the nipple." Or, diagram the breast in the client's record and draw the location of the lump.

2. *Size.* Estimate in centimeters in three dimensions: width × length × thickness.

3. *Shape.* State whether round, oval, lobulated, or indistinct. Benign tumors are usually sharply demarcated with discrete margins. Malignant growths usually have irregular margins and difficult to define borders, and feel matted.

4. *Consistency.* Is it soft, firm, hard? Soft cystic lesions are usually benign; malignant ones are usually hard.

5. *Movable.* Is the lump freely movable, movable, or fixed when you try to slide it over the chestwall? Benign lumps are usually movable. With an invasive malignancy, the tumor becomes fixed to the chestwall.

6. *Number of lesions.* Note if solitary or if there is more than one, i.e., multiple.

7. *Nipple condition.* Note if displaced or retracted.

8. *Skin condition.* Note the skin over the mass. Is it retracted, dimpled, or erythematous?

9. *Tenderness.* Note any tenderness to palpation over the lump.

10. *Lymph nodes.* Are regional lymph nodes palpable?

After palpating each of the four breast quadrants, palpate the nipple and notice any induration or subareolar mass. Using your thumb and forefinger, apply gentle pressure or a stripping action to the nipple, and note the color and consistency of any discharge.

Breast Self-Examination (BSE). Breast cancer is the most common malignancy in women; one out of 13 women can expect cancer of the breast in her lifetime.[39, 77] Early detection and prompt referral are important for a good prognosis, but statistics show that a majority of

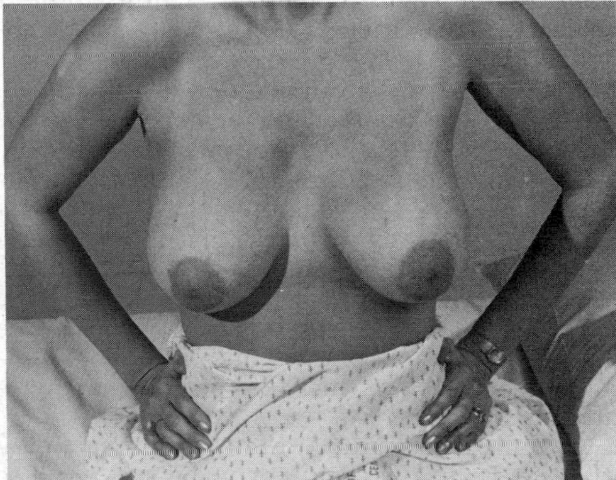

Figure 15–23. Observing female breasts as client presses her arms on her hips; a dimple or pucker is abnormal and indicates skin retraction. (Reprinted by permission from *Nursing 77.*)

women do not practice BSE regularly.[70, 81] Nurses have great opportunity and responsibility for health teaching in this area. The American Cancer Society depends on registered nurses as "specialized volunteers" for their public education program.[4]

While teaching, it is important to avoid citing frightening mortality statistics, which actually may generate excessive fear that may obstruct the woman's self-care action.[27, 70] Rather, the nurse should emphasize self-care through knowledge of risk factors, performance of the practice to increase confidence in finding abnormalities, and prompt referral for any suspicious findings.[39, 67] Harlin advocates teaching programs for the high school age population based on research that the earlier one establishes good health habits, the more likely they will be followed during adulthood.[27]

Teach the client to establish a regular schedule for her breast self-examination. The best time is immediately after the menstrual period or the fourth through seventh day of the menstrual cycle, when the breast is the smallest. Advise the menopausal or pregnant woman who is not having menstrual periods to pick a familiar date to examine her breasts each month, her birthday for example. A monthly self-examination will familiarize the client with her own breasts and their normal variation. Encourage her to report any alteration to her physician.

Teach the client about what to notice in inspection of the breast. She should inspect her breasts in front of a mirror while disrobed to the waist. Then she should lie down to palpate her breasts. After you check the client's breasts, encourage the client to palpate her own breasts while you are there to help with her technique.

Male Breast. Examination of the male breast can be abbreviated but should not be omitted. Inspect the chest wall, noting the points listed above. Palpate the nipple area for any mass. Soft, fatty enlargement of the breast will accompany obesity in the male. *Gynecomastia* is an abnormal enlargement of the breast tissue that makes it clinically distinguishable from the other tissues in the chest wall. This may be due to changes at puberty, administration of hormones, cirrhosis of the liver, leukemia or thyrotoxicosis.

Lymph Nodes and Axilla. After examining the breast, lift the client's arm and support it so that the muscles are loose and relaxed (Fig. 15–24). With the fingers of your examining hand, reach high into the axilla. Move your fingers firmly down along the chest wall in the anterior axillary line, the mid-axillary line and the posterior axillary line. Notice any enlarged and tender lymph nodes. Some tenderness is expected when palpating high in the axilla.

Disorders of the breast are discussed in Chapter 81.

Checklist: Breast Examination

1. *Observe breasts as client sits, raises arms overhead, pushes hands on hips, leans forward*
2. *Observe supraclavicular and intraclavicular areas*
3. *With client supine, palpate:*
   A. *Breast tissue, including tail of Spence*
   B. *Nipple and areola*
4. *Palplate axilla and regional lymph nodes*

EXAMINATION OF THE CARDIOVASCULAR SYSTEM

The cardiovascular exam includes assessment of the extremities, neck, and precordium. Examination of the upper and lower extremities is discussed in different sections of this chapter, as each occurs in the screening exam sequence. Examination of the neck vessels and the precordium is detailed in this section. The pulse and blood pressure, which are significant parameters of cardiovascular function, are measured at the beginning of the physical exam. Review ap-

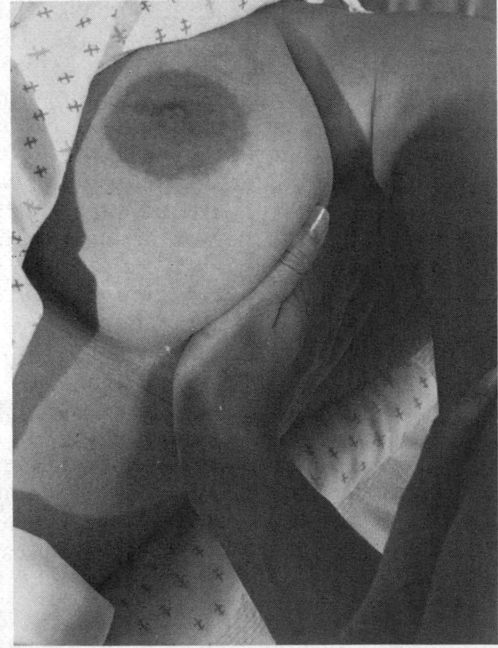

Figure 15–24. Palpating axillary lymph nodes. The examiner's nondominant hand supports the client's arm to relax the muscles, while the examining hand reaches high into the axilla. (Reprinted by permission from *Nursing 77.*)

propriate literature for correct procedure, normal parameters, and significance of abnormal findings.[28, 32] Refer also to Unit XII of this text.

Anatomy

The heart and great vessels lie in the mediastinum (the middle part) of the thoracic cage. The heart sits like an inverted triangle in the thorax: the "top" is the *base* and the "bottom" is the *apex*. Cardiac borders extend vertically from the second to the fifth intercostal space and horizontally from the right sternal border to the left midclavicular line.

The heart is two pumping systems separated by a wall, or septum. There are four chambers — an atrium and a ventricle on each side — separated by valves. These heart valves are unidirectional, so that blood can flow only one way. They open and close passively, depending on the pressure gradients in the chambers. The *atrioventricular* (AV) valves separate the atria and the ventricles; the left AV valve is the bicuspid or *mitral* and the right AV valve is the *tricuspid*. The *semilunar* valves are located between the ventricles and the great arteries. The *aortic* valve separates the left ventricle and the aorta. The *pulmonic* valve lies between the right ventricle and the pulmonary artery.

Note that there are no valves between the left atrium and the pulmonary veins, nor between the right atrium and the vena cava. That is why increasing pressure in the left heart gives symptoms of pulmonary congestion and increasing right atrial pressure is reflected in the neck veins and the abdomen.

The *precordium* is the anterior surface of the chest wall overlying the heart and great vessels. The four "valve areas" are located here, although these are *not* the actual anatomical locations of the valves themselves. Rather, the valve "areas" are the sites on the chest wall where sounds produced by the valves are best *heard* (Fig. 15–25). The sound radiates with the direction of blood flow to these areas:

- *Mitral valve area* — fifth intercostal space at the left midclavicular line
- *Tricuspid valve area* — fourth intercostal space at the left sternal border
- *Pulmonic valve area*— second intercostal space at the left sternal border
- *Aortic valve area* — second intercostal space at the right sternal border

Consult Chapter 31 for additional discussion of cardiac anatomy and physiology.

The Cardiac Cycle

The heart is a pulsatile pump that regularly ejects blood into the arteries. Sixty to 100 times a minute, specialized cells in the SA (sinoatrial) node initiate an electrical impulse. The current flows in an orderly sequence to all parts of the heart, causing it to contract. This contraction is *systole*; it is one third of the cardiac cycle. *Diastole* (or relaxation) is the resting phase and the time for the ventricles to fill with blood. This ventricular filling phase constitutes two thirds of the cardiac cycle (Fig. 15–26).

During diastole, the ventricles are relaxed and the AV valves (mitral and tricuspid) are open. Since the pressure in the atria is higher than in the ventricles, blood flows into the ventricles. Diastolic filling has three phases. The first is a passive *rapid filling phase,* also called *early* or *protodiastolic filling*. Next, filling slows down (diastasis). The third phase is atrial contraction, which pushes the last bit of blood (about 25 per cent of stroke volume) into the ventricles. This is the *active filling phase,* also called *presystole* or *atrial systole*. (Note that *atrial systole* occurs *during* ventricular diastole, a point that students often find difficult.)

Finally, so much blood has been pumped into the ventricles that ventricular pressure is greater than atrial pressure and the AV valves close (producing the first heart sound). This prevents regurgitation of blood into the atria during systole. Now all four heart valves are closed. Pressure increases greatly in the ventricles as the ventricular walls begin to contract against the four closed valves (isometric contraction). Finally ventricular pressure exceeds pressure in the aorta, the semilunar valves open, and

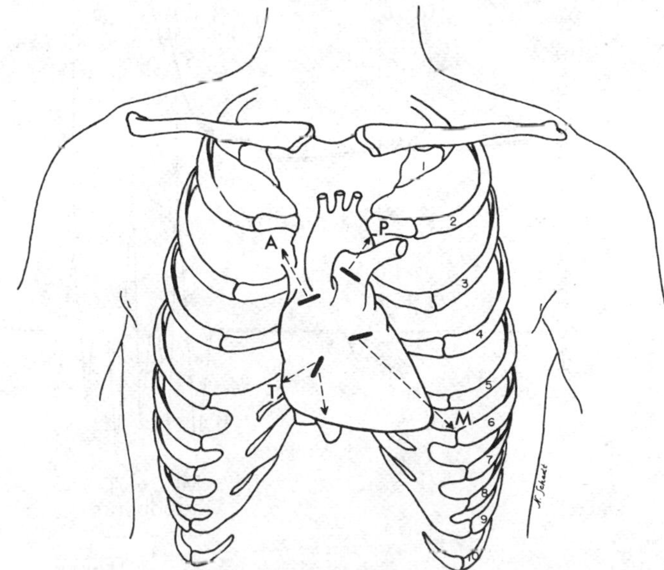

Figure 15–25. Anatomic and auscultatory valve area. Location of anatomic valve sites is represented by solid bars. The arrows designate the transmission of the valve sounds to their respective auscultatory valve areas. (From Prior, J. A., and J. S. Silberstein: *Physical Diagnosis,* 4th ed. St. Louis: C. V. Mosby Co., 1973.)

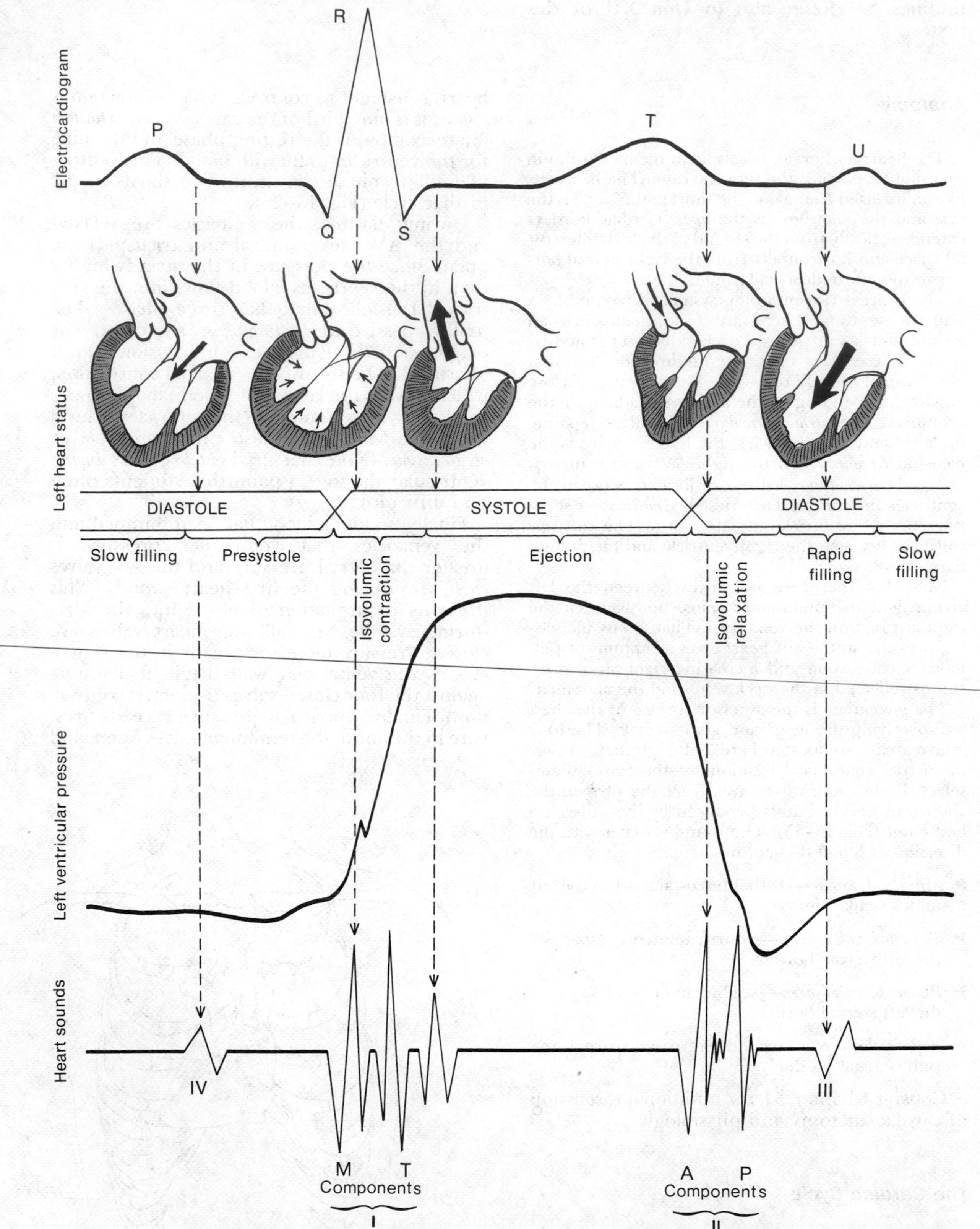

Figure 15–26. Events in the cardiac cycle. (Redrawn from F. Y. Youkman (ed.): *The Ciba Collection of Medical Illustrations.* Vol. 5, "Heart." Ciba Publications Dept., 556 Morris Ave., Summit, N.J. 07901, 1969.)

blood is ejected into the great vessels. The heart pumps blood to the pulmonary and systemic circulation simultaneously. At the end of ejection there is a slight backflow of blood, which closes the semilunar valves (the second heart sound).

Now all four valves are closed, and the ventricles relax (isometric or isovolumic relaxation). The atria have been filling with blood from the vena cava and the lungs all during systole; now atrial pressure is greater than the relaxed ventricular pressure. The AV valves open and the entire cycle repeats.

The Heart Sounds

Events in the cardiac cycle generate sounds that may be auscultated over the precordium. These include normal heart sounds, extra heart sounds, and murmurs. Every normal heartbeat has two components called the *first* and the *second heart sound,* or S_1 and S_2. These sounds are caused by events surrounding the closure of the valves. Usually the periods between S_1 and S_2 (systole) and between S_2 and the next heartbeat (diastole) are silent events. But, *extra heart sounds* may result from a ventricle resistant to filling or may result from pathology of the valves. *Murmurs* may be generated from turbulence of blood flow. All of these sound possibilities, added to the noise of breath sounds and bowel sounds that may be heard over parts of the chest, lead to a confusing cacophony! Assessment of heart sounds is a sophisticated skill, requiring study of their characteristics and much clinical practice.

Heart sounds are described by their pitch, loudness, and timing in the cardiac cycle. The first and second heart sounds are high enough in pitch and loudness to be heard with the diaphragm endpiece, but some heart sounds are very low-pitched and soft (e.g., S_4) and can be heard only with the bell. Loudness is affected by the thickness of the chest wall, too; even the normal heart sounds may sound muffled or distant in a client who is very fat, very muscular, or who has an air-filled, emphysematous lung between the heart and the chest wall. Timing of extra heart sounds in the cardiac cycle is very important; you need to be able to identify whether they occur in systole or diastole.

> *Remember that systole is the time interval between S_1 and S_2; diastole occurs between S_2 and the next S_1.*

First Heart Sound. S_1 occurs with closure of the mitral and tricuspid valves that separate the atria and the ventricles. They close right before systole so that the ventricular contraction will not cause backflow of blood into the atria. The first sound is heard over the entire precordium, though it is loudest at the apex (LUB-dup). It is heard with the diaphragm endpiece, with the client in any position. It is very important to identify S_1 accurately. This sound signals the beginning of systole and is the reference point for the timing of all other cardiac events. The following guidelines are helpful:

- The interval between S_1 and S_2 (systole) is shorter than the interval between S_2 and the next S_1 (diastole). When you hear a *pair* of sounds close together (lub-dup), S_1 is the first of the pair.
- S_1 is louder than S_2 at the apex; S_2 is louder at the base.
- S_1 corresponds with the systolic thrust of the ventricles, and thus with the carotid pulse.
- S_1 occurs with the downstroke of the R wave on the EKG monitor. (A discussion of the electrocardiogram is found in Unit XII.)

Occasionally, you may hear a normal split S_1 due to asynchronous closure of the mitral and tricuspid valves. This is best heard in the tricuspid valve area at the left sternal border. However, a split S_1 is much less common than a split S_2. A split S_1 occurs pathologically with right bundle branch block.

The first sound may be louder (more accentuated) with mitral stenosis, or with a premature ventricular contraction (PVC) that catches the left ventricle with its mitral valve wide open so that it makes more noise when it shuts. Note the assessment literature for further alterations in this and subsequent heart sounds.[38, 40, 46, 53a, 53h, 55]

Second Heart Sound. S_2 is caused by events surrounding closure of the semilunar valves — the aortic and pulmonic. At the end of systole the ventricles have ejected their contents, and the aortic and pulmonic valves close. This produces S_2 and signals the start of diastole. The second heart sound may be heard over the entire precordium, but it is loudest at the base (lub-DUP). S_2 is always louder than S_1 at the base, because the aortic and pulmonic valve areas are there, and because S_2 is higher in pitch and thus transmits better.

PHYSIOLOGIC SPLIT S_2. It is normal to hear the second heart sound split into two distinct but very close components (called A_2 and P_2) during the inspiratory phase of respiration. The physiological mechanism works this way: closure of the aortic and pulmonic valves is nearly synchronous because the timing of right and left ventricular systole is just about equal. But in some people, inspiration prolongs *right* ventricular systole, thus delaying closure of the pulmonic valve. This happens because the intrathoracic pressure is decreased during inspiration, which pushes more blood into the vena cava, increasing right heart venous return, increasing right ventricular stroke volume, prolonging right ventricular systole and delaying pulmonic closure! Meanwhile on the *left,* an increased amount of blood is trapped in the lungs during inspiration, which momentarily decreases the amount returned to the left side of the heart, decreasing left ventricular stroke volume, shortening left ventricular systole, and allowing the aortic valve to close somewhat earlier.

Thus during inspiration instead of hearing "lub-dup," you may hear "lub-T-DUP" as the aortic and pulmonic components of S_2 split apart. The two components, A_2 and P_2, are *very* close together, and the sound is like a trill or a very rapid short drum roll. Expiration collapses the lungs; blood return and ejection times of the right and left heart equalize again; and the two components merge back into a single sound — S_2. A split S_2 is heard only in the pulmonic valve area, the second left interspace.

Variations of the split S_2 that indicate pathology include wide splitting, fixed splitting, and paradoxical splitting. *Wide splitting* is due to right bundle branch block; here the split is audible on expiration and gets even wider on inspiration. *Fixed splitting* is the hallmark of atrial septal defect (ASD). Extra blood is continually being returned to the right heart through the ASD and consistently prolongs right ventricular systole. The *paradoxical split* is heard on expiration rather than inspiration. This occurs with left bundle branch block, which delays conduction and contraction of the left ventricle. Thus the pulmonic valve closes before the aortic valve, causing a split sound. Inspiration normally prolongs right ventricular systole, delaying pulmonic valve closure so that it comes at the same time as aortic valve closure.

Third Heart Sound. Diastole is normally a silent event; however, abrupt limitations to ventricular distensibility will create vibrations in the ventricular walls that may be heard over the chest. The third heart sound, S_3, occurs when the ventricles are resistant during the early rapid filling phase (protodiastole). This is just after S_2, when the AV valves open and atrial blood first rushes into the ventricles. The third heart sound is a dull, low-pitched, soft sound like "distant thunder." It is heard best at the apex with the bell endpiece, with the client in a left lateral position. In children and adolescents, the S_3 is normal and is called a *physiologic* S_3. In adults, the S_3 is abnormal and indicates decreased compliance of the ventricle, as in CHF. The abnormal S_3 is called a *ventricular gallop,* or an S_3 *gallop,* after the cadence of a galloping horse (LUB-dupp-*a*).

It may seem hard to distinguish an S_3 from a split S_2. The following guidelines are helpful:

- Location — the split S_2 is best heard at the base in the pulmonic area, and the S_3 is heard at the apex.
- The split S_2 has a respiratory variation (splits on inspiration), whereas the timing of S_3 is constant.
- The pitch of S_3 is very low, lower than a split S_2.
- Clinical picture of the patient — an abnormal S_3 may be accompanied by other symptoms of CHF.

Fourth Heart Sound. The end of diastole, or presystole, also may produce a sound when the ventricle is resistant to filling. The S_4 results when the atria contract and push blood into a noncompliant ventricle. This sound is heard just before S_1 (*da*-LUB-dup). It is a *very* low-pitched sound and is best heard at the apex, with the bell endpiece held lightly on the chest wall. This is usually an abnormal sound, but it is heard frequently in adults over 50 years who have no known heart disease.[46] The S_4 also is heard with aortic stenosis and systemic hypertension (where the ventricle is hypertrophied) and in coronary artery disease. It is also heard in conditions with increased stroke volume, such as severe anemia or hyperthyroidism.[40] Various terms for the S_4 include *atrial gallop, S_4 gallop, atrial sound,* or *presystolic extra sound.*

Opening Snap. Normally the opening of the mitral valve in diastole is a silent event. When the mitral valve becomes calcified and stenosed (e.g., from rheumatic heart disease), it takes increasingly higher left atrial pressures to open it. The rigid valve opens with a characteristic short, high-pitched *snap.* The opening snap (o.s.) occurs in diastole right after S_2 and is best heard between the apex and the lower left sternal border. It can be distinguished from an S_3 gallop at the apex because the o.s. occurs earlier in diastole than the S_3 does. Also, the o.s. is higher pitched and may radiate to the base. Because the o.s. is specific for mitral stenosis, you also may hear an accentuated S_1 and the low-pitched diastolic rumbling murmur that accompany mitral stenosis. At the base, the o.s. must be distinguished from a split S_2. The split S_2 occurs earlier than an opening snap does and has a respiratory variation, while the interval before the o.s. does not vary during respiration.

Ejection Click. Aortic stenosis produces a sound in systole just after S_1. The ventricle has to push hard against a rigid, calcified aortic valve. When the valve does open, a short high-pitched click results that may be heard at the base and at the apex.

Pericardial Friction Rub. Normally the parietal and visceral parts of the pericardium slide back and forth noiselessly. With pericarditis, these surfaces become inflamed and produce a harsh, grating, leathery, "to-and-fro" noise that is heard both in systole and diastole. It may be difficult to distinguish this sound from a murmur except that a friction rub sounds very close to your ear, as if it were *in* your stethoscope. Also, the patient may have other clinical signs suggestive of pericarditis.

Heart Murmurs. These are blowing, swooshing sounds that are produced by turbulence of blood flow in the heart or great vessels. Turbulent blood flow has various causes:

(a) The heart valves will not open properly (stenosis)
(b) The valves will not close tightly (regurgitation or insufficiency)
(c) There is increased velocity of blood flow (e.g., exercise, thyrotoxicosis)
(d) The blood has decreased viscosity (e.g., anemia)
(e) The heart chamber is dilated or there is a congenital defect in the chamber wall

When you hear a murmur over the chest wall, it should be described by the following characteristics:

- *Timing.* It is crucial to define the murmur by its occurrence in the cardiac cycle: in systole or diastole. You must be able to identify S_1 and S_2 accurately to do this. A murmur is further described as being early, mid, or late in systole or diastole, throughout the cardiac event (e.g., pansystolic or holosystolic), and whether it obscures or muffles the heart sounds.

- *Location.* The area of maximum intensity of the murmur (where it is best heard) is described by the valve areas or intercostal spaces.

- *Loudness.* The intensity is described in terms of six "grades." The conventional way to note a Grade III murmur, for example, is "III/VI."

Grade I	Barely audible, heard only in a quiet room and then with difficulty
Grade II	Clearly audible, but faint
Grade III	Moderately loud
Grade IV	Loud, associated with a thrill palpable on the chest wall
Grade V	Very loud, heard with one corner of the stethoscope lifted off the chest wall
Grade VI	Loudest, still heard with entire stethoscope lifted just off the chest wall

The intensity may follow a pattern during the cardiac phase, becoming louder (crescendo), tapering off (decrescendo), or increasing to a peak and then decreasing (crescendo-decrescendo, or diamond-shaped).

- *Pitch.* This is described as high, medium, or low and depends on the pressure and the rate of blood flow producing the murmur. For example, the murmur of mitral stenosis is low-pitched.

- *Quality.* Murmurs are described as musical, blowing, harsh, or rumbling. For example, the murmur of mitral stenosis is rumbling, while that of aortic stenosis is harsh.

- *Radiation.* The murmur sound may be transmitted downstream in the direction of blood flow and may be heard in the neck, back, axilla, or another place on the precordium.

It requires long and intense practice to describe a heart murmur accurately according to these characteristics. Consult the physical assessment texts for detailed descriptions of murmurs due to specific acquired valve pathology or congenital defects.[40, 55] Utilize tape recordings or a heart sound simulator to become familiar with the patterns before practicing on fellow students or clients. Remember that while textbooks present "pure" diseases, people often do not. A client with mitral stenosis *and* mitral insufficiency will have a combination of sounds. Also remember that some murmurs, particularly in children and adolescents, are *innocent* or *functional* and must be distinguished from pathological murmurs.[5, 13f]

The Neck Vessels

Examination of the vascular structure in the neck includes the carotid artery and the jugular veins. The carotid artery is located in the groove between the trachea and the sternocleidomastoid (SCM) muscle, medial to and alongside that muscle. It is normal to see a brisk localized pulsation in this area, but any unusually bounding pulsations should be noted. Palpate each artery just below and medial to the angle of the jaw. Take care to palpate gently. Palpate only one carotid artery at a time to avoid excessive vagal stimulation that could slow down the heart rate. Because it is central to the heart, the carotid artery yields much data about the rhythm (e.g., premature beats), quality (e.g., a full bounding "water-hammer" pulse), and amplitude (paradoxical pulse, pulsus alternans). Compare your findings bilaterally (see Figure 15–10).

Auscultate each carotid artery for the presence of a *bruit.* This indicates blood flow turbulence due to localized obstruction, such as atherosclerosis. Ask the client to hold her or his breath while you listen, so that tracheal breath sounds do not mask or mimic a carotid artery bruit.

There are two jugular veins in each side of the neck. The internal jugular lies deep and medial to the SCM muscle. It is usually not visible, although its diffuse pulsations may be seen in the sternal notch when the client is supine. The external jugular vein is more superficial and lies lateral to the SCM muscle.

You must be able to distinguish jugular pulsation from that of the carotid artery. Besides its location, the jugular vein differs from the carotid artery in the following ways:

a. The jugular pulsation is undulant and diffuse, whereas the carotid pulsation is brisk and localized.

b. The jugular vein varies with respiration, its level descending during inspiration when intrathoracic pressure is decreased, whereas the carotid artery does not vary in this way.

c. Light pressure at the base of the neck easily obliterates the jugular pulse but not the carotid.

d. The jugular pulsation flattens and disappears as the client is brought to a sitting position, whereas the carotid pulsation is unaffected.

Observe the external jugular vein while the client is supine. (The internal jugular vein is a more reliable indicator because it is larger and leads more directly to the superior vena cava; however, it is usually not visible.) Remove the pillow, turn the client's head slightly away from the examined side, and direct a strong light onto the neck. In some persons the veins are not visible at all, while in others they appear full and pulsating. Both situations are normal in the supine position. Using both of your thumbs, gently milk the external jugular vein empty of blood both up and down; then keep one thumb occluding the top of the vein and preventing venous return from the head. As you watch, the vein should fill slowly from below. Rapid filling may indicate increased central venous pressure as occurs in CHF, cor pulmonale, superior vena cava obstruction, cardiac tamponade, or constrictive pericarditis. When this rapid filling is unilateral, however, it indicates localized pressure, as from an aneurysm or kinking. (See p. 786.)

As the client is raised to a sitting position, the neck veins flatten and disappear, usually at 45 degrees. Full distended neck veins above this level signal increased central venous pressure. Think of the jugular veins as a CVP (central venous pressure) manometer attached directly to the right atrium of the heart. Because there are no valves separating the right atrium from the venous system, pathology that increases right atrial pressure (as mentioned) will be reflected in the neck veins. Methods exist to estimate the jugular venous pressure in centimeters, using the angle of Louis as a reference point.[7, 80] However, consistency in grading among examiners is difficult to achieve, so a simpler grading scale is generally used. This includes recording whether the neck veins are mildly, moderately, or markedly distended (into the angle of the jaw) and recording the client's position when the assessment is made.

Assessment of the Precordium

The precordium is examined just after assessment of the lungs and female breast. The client is supine and the nurse stands on the client's right side. This position facilitates correct hand placement by the examiner. Most of the exam is performed with the client supine, although heart sounds are also auscultated in the left lateral and sitting positions, which bring the heart closer to the chest wall. It is most important to have good lighting, a warm room, and a very quiet environment.

Inspection and Palpation. The forward thrust of the left ventricle during systole produces a normal pulsation on the chest wall. This is the *apical impulse* or *point of maximal impulse* (PMI). It is normally located at the fifth intercostal space at the left midclavicular line. The PMI may be visible in children and in thinner adults when the chest is viewed tangentially. It is palpated as a discrete, localized tapping under the examiner's fingers. Turning the client to a left lateral position brings the heart closer to the chest wall and may help locate the PMI, although it may not be felt at all in persons with thick chest walls or an increased anteroposterior diameter. The PMI indicates the position and size of the heart. With left ventricular enlargement (as in heart failure, valvular heart disease, or hypertension), the PMI is broader and more diffuse and shifts to the left of the midclavicular line, or below the fifth intercostal space. This broad abnormal pulsation has a sustained forceful quality and is known as a *heave* or *lift*.

Observe the chest wall for any other visible pulsation. It is normal to see the aorta pulsating in the epigastric area just below the xyphoid. Right ventricular enlargement produces an abnormal pulsation called a *heave* or a *lift*. This is a forceful sustained thrust seen at the left sternal border.

Using the palmar base of the fingers, palpate the precordium in each of the four valve areas to detect the presence of a *thrill*. This is a rushing vibration that signals turbulence of blood flow. It is likened to feeling the throat of a purring cat. Presence of a thrill always indicates a loud heart murmur will be heard in that area. However, its absence does not necessarily preclude a murmur, as many murmurs are too soft to produce a thrill. Thrills also may be palpated over partially obstructed blood vessels.

Percussion. Indirect percussion is used to outline the heart's borders. A chest roentgenogram yields a more accurate picture of cardiac size, but may not always be available to the nurse performing a screening exam in a clinic, office, or in the client's home. Standing on the client's right side, determine the left border of cardiac dullness (LBCD) by placing your stationary finger in the left fifth intercostal space in the anterior axillary line. Percussion here, over lung tissue, gives a resonant note. Continue to percuss while sliding your stationary hand toward yourself. Use a light percussion stroke, as this detects sound change best. Listen for the point where the note changes from resonant to dull. This should be at or medial to the midclavicular line, or about 7 to 10 cm. from the sternum. Percuss in the fourth and third intercostal spaces; the LBCD normally slopes in toward the sternum as you go up. Determine the right border of cardiac dullness (RBCD) by percussing over the right lung and sliding your stationary finger away from yourself. The RBCD normally coincides with the right sternal border.

There is a normal variation of the LBCD depending on the client's body type, e.g., tall, slender adults have narrow "skinny" hearts whereas short, heavyset persons have more horizontal hearts. The value of percussion data is also limited by a thick chest wall, breast tissue, or an abnormal amount of air in an emphysematous lung overlying the heart. However, cardiac enlargement, especially on the left, may be detected by percussion because the borders of dullness are shifted laterally, downward, or in both directions.

Auscultation. A quiet environment is essential during examination, as all heart sounds are of relatively low pitch and are easily masked by ambient noise. The client should be warm and relaxed to avoid shivering and confusing muscle noises. The examiner explores all parts of the precordium systematically, first with the diaphragm and then with the bell endpiece. Begin at the apex and "inch" your stethoscope to the left sternal border (the tricuspid valve area), up to the pulmonic valve area, and then over to the aortic valve area on the right of the sternum. (An alternate technique is to begin at the base, where S_2 is always louder than S_1, and work your way down to the apex. Use this method if S_1 and S_2 sound equally loud at the apex.)

Concentrate, and listen selectively to *one thing at a time* in the cardiac cycle. It is impossible to assess everything at once. Remember that two, three, or even up to five different sounds may be occurring in less than one second! Inch the diaphragm endpiece across the precordium, and use the following routine of auscultation:

- *Note and time the rate and rhythm.* Is the rate too fast (> 100 beats per minutes, *tachycardia*), or too slow (< 60 beats per minute, *bradycardia*)? The rate is affected by various pathologies[28, 32] or may vary normally, such as a tachycardia with exercise or anxiety, and bradycardia in the well-conditioned athlete.

  Heart rhythm should be regular. However, *sinus arrhythma* occurs normally in children and young adults. Here the rhythm varies with respiration, increasing at the peak of inspiration and decreasing with expiration. Also, notice any *premature beats.* These occur when a pacemaker other than the usual SA node fires prematurely and initiates an early systole. Finally, listen for the "irregularly-irregular" rhythm of *atrial fibrillation,* in which there are so many electrical impulses in the heart (400 to 800 per minute) that the ventricles respond and contract at random.
- Identify S_1 and S_2 and listen to each separately. Review the four techniques listed earlier to differentiate S_1 and S_2 (p. 347). Notice if each heart sound is normal, accentuated, diminished, or split.
- Focus on *systole,* and then on *diastole,* listening for any *extra heart sounds.* Review the discussion of S_3, S_4, opening snap, ejection click, and pericardial friction rub.
- Now listen for any *murmurs,* first in systole and then in diastole. Murmurs should be described by the characteristics discussed earlier.

Using the bell endpiece, repeat auscultation through all of the valve areas, noting any very low-pitched sounds. Next, ask the client to roll onto her or his left side while you hold the bell lightly on the apex, listening for any ventricular filling sounds (S_3 or S_4) or for a mitral valve murmur. Finally ask the client to sit up and lean forward while you press the diaphragm endpiece over the second left and right intercostal spaces. This position brings the base of the heart closer to the chest wall, and you may detect high-pitched murmurs of the aortic and pulmonic valves.

Checklist: Cardiovascular Examination

1. *Neck*
   - A. *Carotid pulse — observe and palpate*
   - B. *Observe jugular venous pulse*
   - C. *Estimate jugular venous pressure*
2. *Precordium*
   - A. *Inspection and palpation*
     - *(1) Describe location of PMI*
     - *(2) Note any heave (lift) or thrill*
   - B. *Percussion — outline borders of the heart*
   - C. *Auscultation*
     - *(1) Identify anatomical areas where you will listen*
     - *(2) Note rate and rhythm of heartbeat*
     - *(3) Identify S_1 and S_2 and note any variation*
     - *(4) Listen in systole and diastole for any extra heart sounds*
     - *(5) Listen in systole and diastole for any murmurs*
     - *(6) Repeat sequence with bell*
     - *(7) Listen with client in left lateral position*
     - *(8) Listen with client in sitting position*

EXAMINATION OF THE ABDOMEN

The abdominal examination follows assessment of the precordium, while the client is still

A

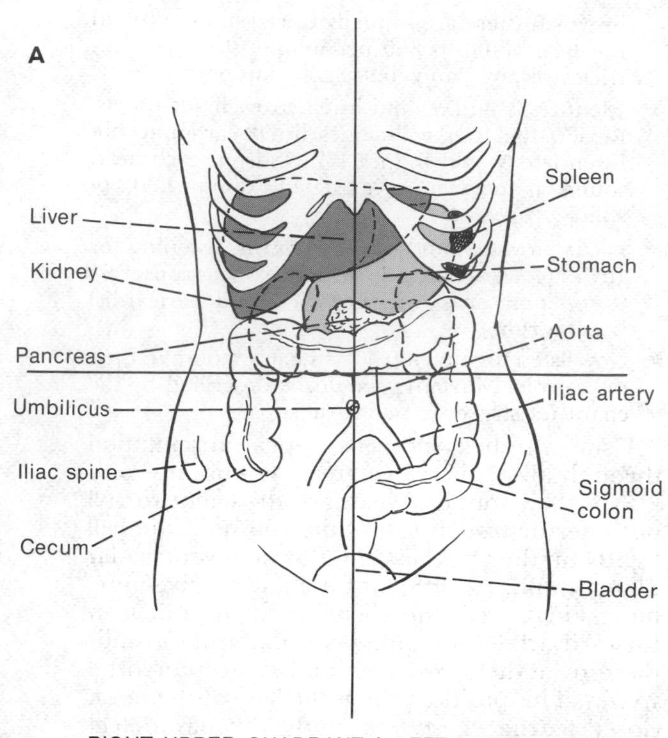

B

RIGHT UPPER QUADRANT	LEFT UPPER QUADRANT
Liver Gallbladder Duodenum Head of pancreas Right kidney and adrenal Hepatic flexure of colon Part of ascending and transverse colon	Stomach Spleen Left lobe of liver Body of pancreas Left kidney and adrenal Splenic flexure of colon Parts of transverse and descending colon
RIGHT LOWER QUADRANT	**LEFT LOWER QUADRANT**
Cecum Appendix Right ovary and tube Right ureter	Part of descending colon Sigmoid colon Left ovary and tube Left ureter

Figure 15–27. **A.** Location of the abdominal viscera. **B.** Location of the abdominal organs in the four quadrants.

supine. You will need a stethoscope, small ruler, and marking pen. All four assessment techniques are utilized, but their usual order is altered. Inspection, auscultation, and percussion are done first, with palpation last. The order is changed because palpation may alter auscultatory findings by increasing or decreasing peristalsis. Thus, it is done last.

Topography

A thorough knowledge of abdominal anatomy is essential so that you can visualize each structure that you hear or feel through the abdominal wall. To facilitate the communication of physical findings and the client's symptoms, the abdomen is subdivided into four quadrants (Fig. 15–27). These are formed by bisecting the anterior surface with a vertical line from the xyphoid process to the symphysis pubis, and a horizontal line through the umbilicus.

The small intestine is located in all four quadrants. Midline structures include the uterus, bladder, and rectum. The aorta is vertical and slightly to the left of midline in the upper quadrants; at the umbilicus the aorta bifurcates into the right and left iliac arteries. These become the femoral arteries in the inguinal region. Finally, the section of abdomen between the costal margins is also called the *epigastrium.*

Inspection

A number of environmental conditions will promote success of the abdominal exam. Strong lighting that is tangential to the abdomen will highlight any change in contour. The client's abdomen should be exposed fully, with the gown rolled up over the chest and drapes covering the symphysis. The abdominal structures lie under a thick muscular wall; complete relaxation is necessary to assess them accurately. Before starting the examination, you can promote relaxation by having the client empty the bladder, placing a pillow under the head, flexing the knees, and placing the arms at the sides rather than extended up over the head. The room must be warm to prevent shivering, and the examiner must have a warm stethoscope, warm hands, and short fingernails.

Ask the client to point to any painful area, and examine that section last. Abdominal pain may be visceral or somatic. *Visceral* pain arises from an organ; it is dull and difficult for the client to localize or characterize. *Somatic* pain arises from nerve endings in the skin, muscle wall, or peritoneum; it is sharp, bright, and easy to localize.[55]

Contour. The examiner should stand on the client's right side and view the abdomen from above, then stoop down to gaze across the level of the abdomen. Notice the general contour of the abdomen: scaphoid (concave), flat, rounded, or protuberant. The abdomen should be symmetrical contralaterally. Note any asymmetry, visible masses, or localized bulging. Even small bulges may be highlighted by shadow as the abdomen is viewed tangentially. A *hernia* is a protrusion of abdominal viscera through an abnormal opening in the body wall. A ventral hernia may occur at the umbilicus (particularly in children),[1f] through a scar from previous abdominal surgery, or in the midline through separating rectus muscles (diastasis recti abdominis). Hernias also may be in the inguinal area or in the femoral area. A hernia may be elicited by asking the client to bear down or to slowly raise up to a sitting position. These maneuvers increase the intra-abdominal pressure, thus revealing the hernia.

Skin. The skin reveals the client's overall health. Poor skin turgor reflects the dehydration that often accompanies gastrointestinal disease. Gently pinch up a fold of skin and then release. With good turgor the skin jumps back to its original position immediately. Also observe the skin for any lesions and pigment change. *Striae* (lineae albicantes) are silvery-white, jagged lines that follow prolonged stretching of the skin, as in large weight gain, ascites, or pregnancy. Notice any rashes, petechiae, or *cutaneous angiomas* (spider nevi). The latter appear with portal hypertension or liver disease. Any unusual pigmentation should be noted; for example, jaundice may show on the abdominal skin, particularly in natural sunlight. Note any surgical scars and draw their location in the client's record, with the length indicated in centimeters. If the client did not mention a past operation during the health history, ask about the scar at this time.

A fine venous network normally is seen over the abdomen. Note any prominent dilated veins, which may indicate portal hypertension or obstruction of the vena cava. These also occur with cirrhosis or *ascites* (free fluid in the peritoneum). Ascites is further characterized by tight and glistening skin, a distended abdomen, and bulging flanks due to gravitation of the fluid. The flanks will not bulge if the abdomen is distended by flatus or obesity.

Notice any pulsation or movement of the abdominal wall. It is normal to see the aorta pulsating under the skin in the epigastric area, especially in thin persons with good muscle relaxation. It also may be normal to see waves of peristalsis in very thin persons. These look like oblique ripples moving across the abdomen. However, visible peristalsis with a distended abdomen indicates intestinal obstruction.

The umbilicus should be inverted, midline, and show no sign of inflammation, discoloration, or hernia. The umbilicus becomes everted with ascites, an underlying mass, or pregnancy. The umbilicus is pushed upward in pregnancy, pushed downward with ascites, and appears deeply sunken with generalized obesity. The umbilicus has a bluish cast when there is blood in the peritoneum *(Cullen's sign)*.

Note the pattern of hair distribution in the lower abdomen. In males it has a diamond shape, and in females an inverted triangle shape. These patterns are altered with endocrine and hormone abnormalities and in chronic liver disease.

Finally, note the client's facial expression and his or her position on the examining table, as this may reveal an underlying gastrointestinal disorder. The client who is restless, constantly turning back and forth to find a comfortable position, has the characteristics of colicky pain that accompanies gastroenteritis or bowel obstruction. On the other hand, a position of absolute stillness and resistance to any movement indicates the pain of peritonitis.[34]

Auscultation

The abdomen is auscultated next before percussion and palpation, so that auscultatory findings are not altered by increased or decreased peristalsis. Because bowel sounds are relatively high-pitched, the diaphragm endpiece of the stethoscope is used. Hold it very lightly against the skin to avoid creating more bowel sounds by pressure, and listen in all four quadrants. You need to evaluate the normal, hypoactive or hyperactive *bowel sounds,* and note the presence of any *vascular bruits.*

Normal bowel sounds reflect peristalsis, or the movement of air and fluid through the small intestine. Note their character and frequency. They are normally high-pitched, gurgling, "schlurping" sounds that occur from 5 to 30 times per minute. Their frequency varies widely and depends on the time elapsed since the ingestion of food. Normally, some bowel sounds always are heard at the ileocecal valve area, which is slightly below and to the right of the umbilicus.

Bowel sounds may be hypoactive with inflammation or following abdominal surgery. However, you must listen for 5 minutes, by the clock, before stating that bowel sounds are completely absent.[79] Total absence of sounds occurs with paralytic ileus or with the immobile bowel of peritonitis.

Hyperactive bowel sounds (called *borborygmi*) are high-pitched, loud, rushing, tinkling sounds that characterize the increased motility of acute gastroenteritis and early mechanical obstruction. In the latter, the hyperactive sounds occur when the bowel proximal to the obstruction fills up with air and increases peristalsis, trying to propel its contents against the block.

A systolic bruit is heard with turbulence of blood flow through the aorta, as with atherosclerosis or aneurysm. A bruit due to stenosis or obstruction may be heard over the renal arteries or over the femoral arteries.

Percussion

Percuss the abdomen lightly in all four quadrants to assess the prevailing percussion note; tympany should predominate. Hyperresonance occurs with gaseous distention. Percussion over fluid or a tumor yields a dull note.

Percuss further to map boundaries of the liver

and the spleen. Measure the liver span in the right midclavicular line. Begin with the resonant percussion note over the right lung and percuss down each interspace until you hear a dull sound, usually between the fifth and seventh intercostal space. Mark this site. Now percuss tympany in the mid abdomen and proceed upward until the sound changes to dull. This indicates the lower border of the liver and is usually at the right costal margin. Measuring the distance between your marks yields the height of the liver span, usually between 6 and 12 cm. A distance of 12 cm. or more indicates hepatomegaly, as occurs in hepatitis, right sided CHF, cancer, or cirrhosis. In emphysema, there is a downward displacement of the liver due to the flattened diaphragm, but the total height of the liver is within normal limits.

Usually the spleen cannot be percussed because it is obscured by abdominal contents. However, it is normal to percuss a small area of dullness in the left ninth and tenth intercostal space posterior to the midaxillary line. Any dullness forward of this line is abnormal and indicates splenic enlargement, as in mononucleosis or trauma.

The presence of ascites is confirmed by percussion tests. As discussed above, ascites is suspected in a client with a distended abdomen, bulging flanks, and an umbilicus that is protruding and displaced down. The *fluid wave* test is positive with a large amount of ascites. Place the edge of the client's hand firmly on the abdomen in the midline to prevent transmission of the wave through the abdominal wall (Fig. 15–28). Stand on the right of the client and place your left hand against his or her right side. Reach across the client's abdomen with your right hand and firmly slap the left flank. With ascites, the wave will be carried through the fluid, and you will feel a distinct sharp tap on your left hand.

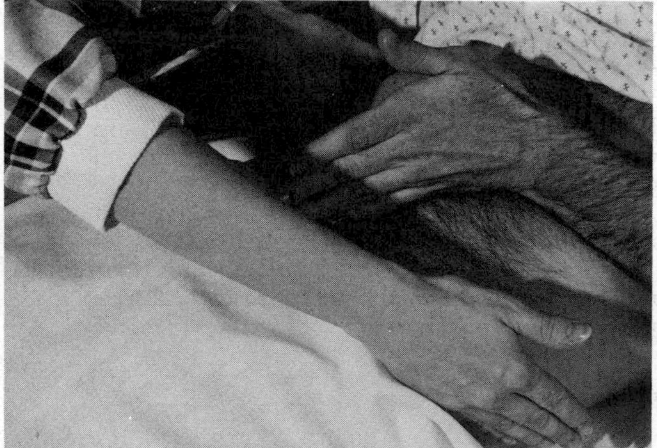

Figure 15–28. Percussing for a fluid wave. The client's hand rests on the abdominal wall to impede vibration across the skin surface. The examiner's right hand taps the client's left side; with ascites the stroke will start a fluid wave which will be felt as a tap on the examiner's left hand. (Reprinted by permission from *Nursing 77*.)

The presence of *shifting dullness* also indicates ascites. When the client is supine, the fluid gravitates to the flanks, displacing the relatively lighter bowel upward. Percussing from the midline of the abdomen down to the side gives a change in percussion note from tympany to dull *at* the level of the fluid. Next the client is rolled onto his or her side. With ascites, the fluid flows to the dependent flank and the gaseous bowel is displaced up. Percussion from the top side downward gives a *new* level of dullness, one that has shifted up toward the umbilicus. There is no change in percussion note if the abdomen is distended with gas.

Palpation

Complete muscle wall relaxation is necessary for successful palpation of the abdomen. As mentioned above, the examiner's hands should be warm and fingernails short. Many clients are fearful of having their abdomen touched, or are very ticklish. Approach these persons slowly and keep your palpating hand and forearm low and horizontal. Utilize conversation or health history questions to distract a ticklish client. Another aid is to place the client's hand under your own and feel the abdomen with your fingers curled over his or hers. This works because people are not ticklish to themselves. A similar suggestion is to palpate with your fingers curled around the stethoscope endpiece. Clients do not perceive the stethoscope as a ticklish or painful object.[55]

You must take extra care with the client who is having abdominal pain. Pressure over a painful area stimulates involuntary muscle guarding that will impede further examination. Ask the client to point out any painful spots, and examine those areas last. Watch the client's face during the exam to monitor any grimaces that indicate you are causing discomfort.

The first maneuver is *light palpation* in all four quadrants. Hold your fingers close together, keep your hand and forearm horizontal, and depress the client's skin 1 to 2 cm. Make a gentle, dipping, rotary motion with the pads of your fingers. Lift your hand to the next site; do not drag your fingers across the skin. Move around the abdomen in a clockwise pattern. Encourage the client to breathe slowly and deeply and to relax the stomach muscles as you palpate. Light palpation is a slow gentle exploration to assess the "lay of the land," and note any large masses, tenderness, or muscle guarding. Try to distinguish voluntary muscle tensing *(guarding)* due to fear or ticklishness from a true muscle rigidity. The latter is a reflex, involuntary, muscle spasm that occurs with inflammation of the peritoneum. Voluntary muscle guarding will relax somewhat during expiration, whereas the involuntary reflex stays rigid throughout respiration.

Next, perform *deep palpation.* Again, move clockwise around the abdomen, this time with the fingers pressing into the abdomen about 10 cm. (4 inches). Assess the abdominal organs as to their size, location, contour, consistency, and mobility, and note the presence of any tenderness or mass. A number of abdominal structures normally are felt during deep palpation and should not be mistaken for a mass: (a) the sigmoid colon usually contains feces and feels like a piece of rope in the left inguinal region, (b) the descending colon may also contain feces and be palpable, (c) the uterus, (d) the sacral promontory, and (e) the edges of the abdominal rectus muscles. The aorta also is palpable in thin persons, as a pulsatile tubular structure in the upper abdomen slightly left of the midline.

If a mass is noted, it should be distinguished from an enlarged organ and examined for size, contour (smooth or nodular), consistency, mobility, and tenderness. You may distinguish an abdominal wall mass from an intra-abdominal one by asking the client to slowly come to a sitting position. An abdominal wall mass will remain palpable and even be more prominent during this maneuver, while an intra-abdominal one will disappear behind the flexing muscles.

If any tenderness is present during the maneuvers described, you should check for *rebound tenderness.* Press the abdomen firmly at a point away from the tender area, and then release suddenly. Rebound tenderness is felt when the distant pressure is withdrawn, and indicates inflammation of the peritoneum.

Specific maneuvers are used to palpate the liver, spleen, and kidneys.

Liver. To palpate the liver, stand on the client's right, place your left hand behind, parallel to, and supporting the eleventh and twelfth ribs, and lift up. Place your right hand on the abdomen, below the right costal margin, with your fingers together and parallel to the midline (Fig. 15–29). Press your right hand deeply into the abdomen under the costal margin. As the client takes a deep breath, you may feel the liver edge come down and bump your fingers. The liver often is not palpable, but when it is, you will feel a firm, sharp, regular ridge with a smooth surface. The liver is enlarged if it is felt more than 1 cm. below the costal margin (except the liver in the client with emphysema, discussed earlier). If the liver is enlarged, note how many centimeters it descends below the costal margin, and note its consistency, any nodularity, and tenderness.

Spleen. The spleen usually cannot be felt; it must be enlarged three times its normal size to be palpable. Reach over the client with your left hand, place it under the left flank and lift forward (Fig. 15–30). Place your right hand obliquely under the left costal margin and press in. Ask the client to breathe in deeply; normally you feel nothing. If the spleen is enlarged, it will slide out under the costal margin and bump your fingers. It may be easier to feel an enlarged spleen by rolling the client onto her or his right side, because this brings the spleen more forward. Take care not to miss a spleen that is so large that it extends into the lower quadrants.

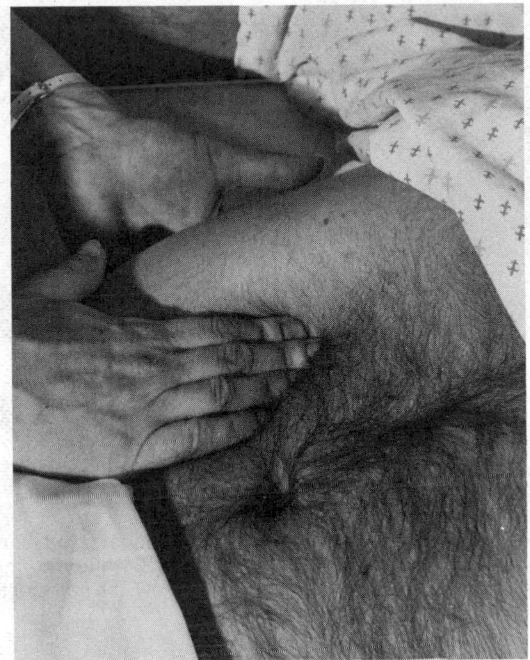

Figure 15–29. Palpating the liver. The examiner's left hand lifts up under the client's right flank. The right hand presses deep into the abdomen below the right costal margin. Then the client inhales to bring the liver edge down closer to the examiner's fingers. (Reprinted by permission from *Nursing 77.*)

> *If an enlarged spleen is palpated, make note of its location, size, and consistency, and then leave it alone. The spleen is a friable organ and can rupture with overpalpation!*

Kidneys. To palpate the right kidney, place your hands together in a "duckbill" fashion, the left hand underneath the mid abdomen and the right one on top. Press your hands together. As the client takes in a deep breath, you may feel the lower pole of the kidney slide between your fingers. It is palpable only on very thin persons. Reach across the abdomen to feel the left kidney; it is not palpable normally. The kidneys are enlarged and have cystic masses in polycystic disease. You may consult other references for additional pictures of proper positioning and placement.[31, 53b, 60]

Checklist: Abdomen Examination

1. *Inspection*
   A. *Contour and general symmetry*
   B. *Skin and umbilicus*

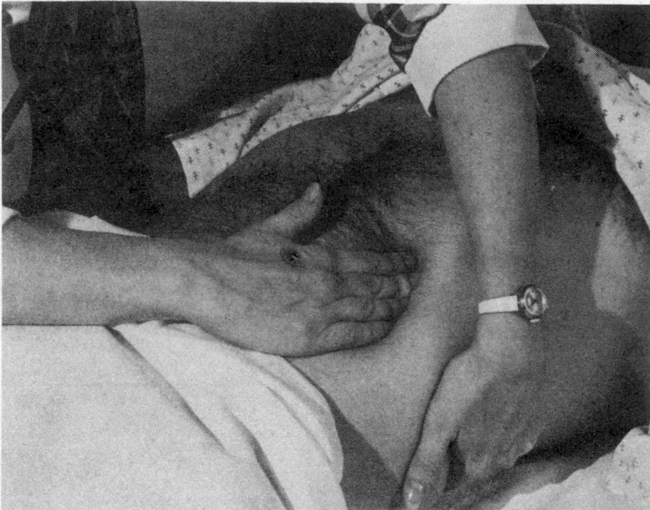

Figure 15–30. Palpating the spleen. The examiner's left hand reaches over to lift the client's left flank upward, while the right hand presses obliquely into the abdomen below the left costal margin. (Reprinted by permission from *Nursing 77.*)

- C. *Hair distribution*
- D. *Client's facial expression and body position*

2. *Auscultation*
   - A. *Describe normal bowel sounds in all four quadrants*
   - B. *Absent or hypoactive bowel sounds*
   - C. *Hyperactive bowel sounds*
   - D. *Listen for bruit over abdominal aorta, femoral arteries*
3. *Percussion*
   - A. *Percuss all four quadrants*
   - B. *Percuss borders of liver*
   - C. *Percuss for splenic dullness*
   - D. *If ascites suspected, test for fluid wave and shifting dullness*
4. *Palpation*
   - A. *Light palpation in all four quadrants*
   - B. *Deeper palpation in all four quadrants*
   - C. *Palpate for liver, spleen, kidneys*
   - D. *If tenderness is present, check for rebound tenderness*

EXAMINATION OF THE SKIN

Examination of the skin is not a separate step of the physical exam. Rather, the skin over each body part is assessed during each regional examination. The danger is one of omission. You can become so accustomed to seeing skin that you do not pay attention to its characteristics. Skills used are inspection and palpation, because some skin changes have accompanying signs that can be felt. You need strong, direct lighting (sunlight is best, though it is often not accessible in the hospital or clinic examining room) and a clear plastic ruler marked in centimeters for measuring skin lesions. Assessment of the skin is described also in Chapter 79 in this text.

Inspection. Observe the color of the skin, both its general pigmentation and any abnormal conditions such as *pallor* (white), *cyanosis* (blue), *erythema* (red), or *jaundice* (yellow). Try to control variables that could complicate your findings.[58, 64] For example, a cold examining room may give a false skin pallor, or a flushed embarrassed client may show a false erythema. Also note that edema will mask erythema, cyanosis, and jaundice because the excess fluid obscures color changes in the pigment and vascular layers below it.

Normal skin color comes mainly from the pigment melanin, and also from the condition of the vascular bed and the thickness of the skin. The amount of pigment normally present may mask color changes. Lips and nailbeds also are checked for color change, but they vary with the client's skin color and may not always be accurate parameters. Somewhat more reliable are sites with the least pigmentation: under the tongue, the buccal mucosa, the conjunctiva around the eyes, and the sclera.

The normal pink color of mucous membranes is due to oxygenated hemoglobin in the red blood cells. *Pallor,* which occurs with *anemia,* is best seen in the conjunctiva, mucous membranes, and nailbeds. The skin also looks pale with edema, and with peripheral vasoconstriction as in cigarette smoking, fear or anxiety, exposure to cold, or shock. Note any associated signs that may accompany these conditions, such as prolonged capillary filling time, cool clammy skin, decreased pulses, and changes in vital signs.

Cyanosis is a bluish mottled color that signifies a decrease in adequate tissue perfusion of oxygenated blood. It is caused by an increased amount of reduced hemoglobin in the superficial blood vessels. Check for cyanosis in the mucous membranes and nailbeds. Like pallor, cyanosis is a nonspecific sign. A client who is anemic could have hypoxemia without ever looking blue because not enough hemoglobin is present (either oxygenated *or* reduced) to color the skin. On the other hand, a client with polycythemia (increased numbers of red blood cells) will look ruddy-blue at all times and not necessarily be hypoxemic. This client just is unable to fully oxygenate the massive numbers of red blood cells.

Erythema is due to excess blood (hyperemia) in the cutaneous vessels. This may be due to fever, emotional reactions, local irritation, or polycythemia. If any red blood cells are extravascular, the resultant hemorrhagic lesions are termed:

petechiae	tiny, round, pinpoint discolorations
ecchymosis (bruise)	a larger diffuse patch of extravascular blood
hematoma	an ecchymosis that is swollen and can be palpated
purpura	confluent extensive ecchymoses, seen in generalized disorders, e.g., thrombocytopenia

The skin may be yellow *(jaundice)* with liver or biliary tract disorders or carotenemia. Jaundice also may be seen in the sclera, but it should not be confused with the normal yellow fatty deposits that are common in the outer sclera of dark-skinned clients. The scleral yellow of jaundice extends up to the edge of the iris.

Additional techniques are used to assess and interpret color changes in clients with dark skins.[57, 58] For example, pallor is better seen in the lower conjunctiva or nailbeds; cyanosis in the nailbeds, oral mucosa and conjunctiva; and jaundice on the hard palate, sclera, and conjunctiva. Check for erythema in the dark-skinned client by palpating for accompanying warmth, swelling, or tenderness in the skin. Dark skin also may mask some rashes that are specific diagnostic indices.[13a] You may need to rely on associated symptoms, such as enlarged lymph nodes and fever.[62]

Palpation. Skin areas are palpated for moisture (dry, clammy, oily), temperature, thickness, texture, and turgor. These parameters are discussed further in Chapter 79. Skin lesions should be noted and described as in Fig. 15–31. No classification is absolute (notice, for example, a

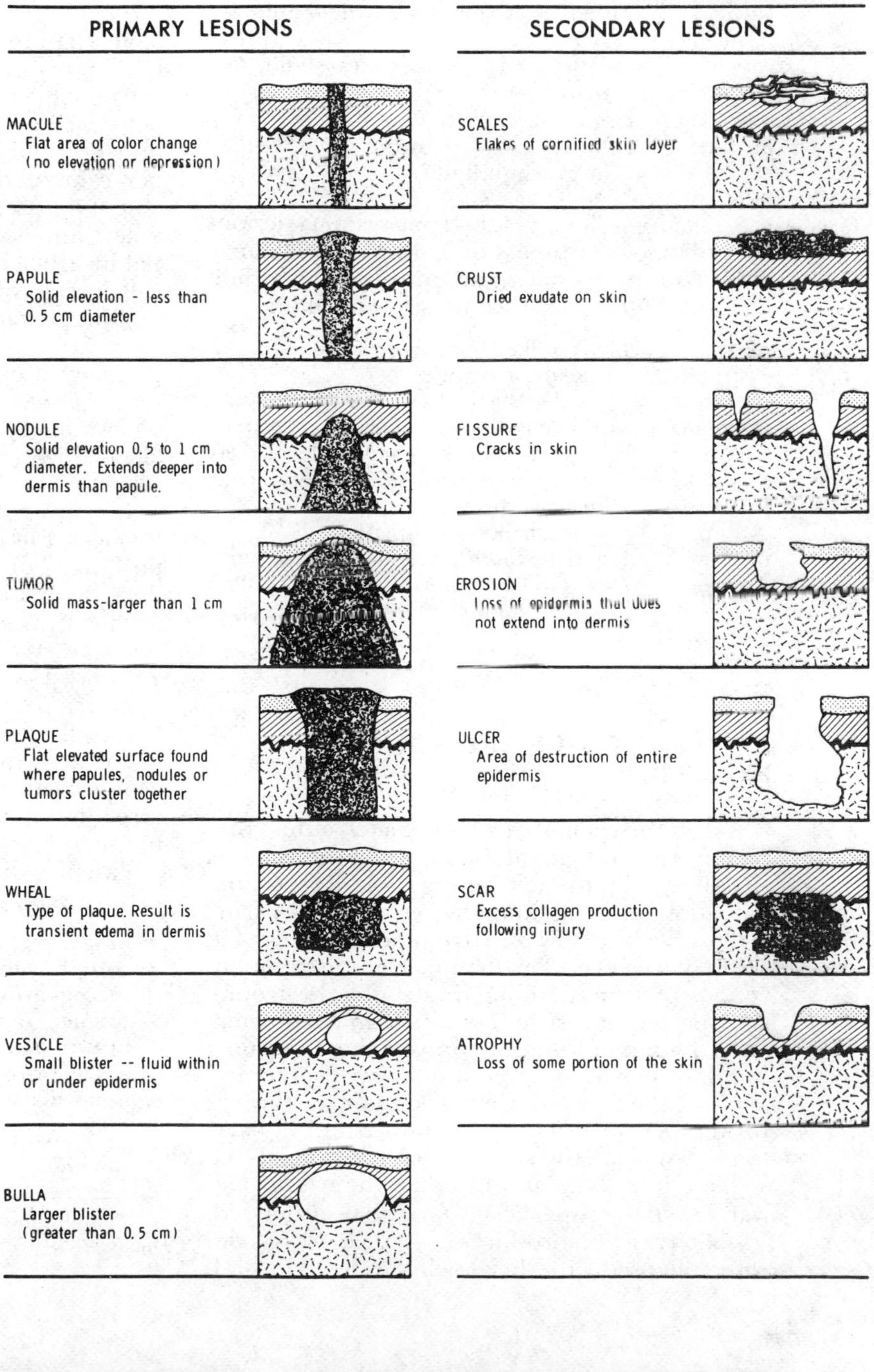

PRIMARY LESIONS

MACULE
Flat area of color change
(no elevation or depression)

PAPULE
Solid elevation - less than
0.5 cm diameter

NODULE
Solid elevation 0.5 to 1 cm
diameter. Extends deeper into
dermis than papule.

TUMOR
Solid mass-larger than 1 cm

PLAQUE
Flat elevated surface found
where papules, nodules or
tumors cluster together

WHEAL
Type of plaque. Result is
transient edema in dermis

VESICLE
Small blister -- fluid within
or under epidermis

BULLA
Larger blister
(greater than 0.5 cm)

SECONDARY LESIONS

SCALES
Flakes of cornified skin layer

CRUST
Dried exudate on skin

FISSURE
Cracks in skin

EROSION
Loss of epidermis that does
not extend into dermis

ULCER
Area of destruction of entire
epidermis

SCAR
Excess collagen production
following injury

ATROPHY
Loss of some portion of the skin

Figure 15–31. Primary and secondary skin lesions. Characteristics of common skin lesions. (From Sana, J. S., and R. D. Judge: *Physical Appraisal Methods in Nursing Practice.* Boston: Little, Brown and Co., 1975, p. 91.)

pustule can be either a primary or secondary lesion), but they help in organizing the many types of lesions.

Primary skin lesions are the immediate result of a specific causative factor. They develop without any preceding visible skin change. Primary skin lesions include:

macule	flat color change less than 1 cm.
papule	raised circumscribed area up to 0.5 cm.
nodule	solid elevation of 0.5 to 1 cm.
tumor	raised solid mass larger than a nodule
wheal (or hive)	raised lesion due to interstitial fluid
vesicle (blister)	bulging cavity of free clear fluid, less than 0.5 cm.
bulla	large vesicle, more than 0.5 cm.
pustule	elevated cavity of turbid white, yellow, or greenish fluid

Secondary lesions result from primary lesions that change over time. For example, a bulla may rupture and become a *crust,* or thickened, dried-up fluid. Other secondary lesions include:

plaque	plateau-like lesion from a confluence of wheals or papules
pustule	a vesicle that becomes infected
erythema	skin irritation from vesicles or pustules
scale	excess flakes of sloughed epidermis secondary to inflammation or erythema
fissure	a linear vertical split
erosion	a wide, shallow, scooped-out lesion
ulcer	lesion extending deep into the dermis
scar	excess collagen (fibrous tissue) deposited when skin lesions heal

EXAMINATION OF THE LOWER EXTREMITIES

Assess the client's legs immediately after completing the abdominal exam, while the client is still supine on the examining table. Inspection, palpation, and auscultation are the skills used.

Observe the lower extremities, noting skin color, pressence of clubbing, hair distribution, venous pattern, swelling, or atrophy. If atrophy is suspected, measure the muscle in centimeters and compare it with the opposite side. Also note the presence of any skin lesions or ulcerations.

Using the dorsa of your hands, palpate the legs for temperature. The temperature and vascular tone should be the same in both legs. With vasodilatation, the legs will be erythematous and warm, and the superficial veins will be distended. Vasoconstriction produces cold, pale, moist skin, with collapsed superficial veins. When bilateral, this may be due to environmental factors like smoking, room temperature, or apprehension. The presence of unilateral or localized findings indicates peripheral vascular pathology. (See also Unit XV.)

Gently compress the gastrocnemius (calf muscle) anteriorly against the tibia and note any tenderness that would indicate phlebothrombosis. This also may be elicited by sharply dorsiflexing the foot; calf pain with this maneuver is called a *positive Homan's sign.*

Palpate these arterial pulses bilaterally: femoral, popliteal, dorsalis pedis, posterior tibial.* Peripheral pulses are graded:

0	absent
1^+	weak and thready
2^+	normal
3^+	full and bounding

Note if a pulse is absent or feels unequal bilaterally. However, the dorsalis pedis pulse is absent congenitally in approximately 10 per cent[55] to 17 per cent[44] of the normal adult population. The posterior tibial pulse is absent congenitally in 9 per cent of the black adult population.[44] Any absent or decreased arterial pulse should be noted, and accompanying signs of possible arterial insufficiency checked.

Palpation of the femoral artery pulse is especially important. If this pulse feels abnormal or if there are any signs or symptoms suggestive of vascular disease, auscultate the femoral artery for a *bruit.* This is a low-pitched, blowing, swooshing sound that indicates turbulence of blood flow. (Auscultation of the femoral artery can easily be done at the time you listen to bowel sounds over the abdominal quadrants.)

Check for edema in the lower extremities by pushing your thumbs firmly on the skin over the tibia or behind the ankle. Edematous tissue usually leaves a "pit" or indentation often called "*pitting edema.*" This edema may be graded from 1^+ (mild, a slight depression) to 4^+ (severe, a deep depression). Cardiac edema (from CHF) occurs bilaterally and is dependent and pitting. Edema also can be unilateral, as in occlusion of a deep vein or artery and lymphatic obstruction. In this case it is "brawny" or non-pitting and feels hard to touch.[45]

Vascular disease in the extremities may affect the arterial system or the venous system.

- *Venous* disease is evidenced by dilated, tortuous, cordlike superficial veins and by aching pain when the legs are dependent. With chronic venous insufficiency, you will note edema, dependent cyanosis, brown skin discolorations, possible ulcers of the ankle, pruritus and paresthesia. Skin temperature is normal, and pulses are present, though they may be hard to palpate through the edema.
- *Arterial* insufficiency is hallmarked by decreased or

*For pulse location and procedure, see Sorensen and Luckmann, *Basic Nursing: A Psychophysiologic Approach* (Chapter 29).

absent arterial pulses, a possible systolic bruit over involved arteries, muscular atrophy, thin shiny hairless skin, thick ridged toenails, cool skin temperature, and ulcers on pressure points of the feet. The skin color is pale gray when the legs are elevated above heart level, and dusky red after they are dependent. Edema, if present, is mild and brawny. Related historical findings and further diagnostic techniques specific for vascular disease are described in the literature.[64, 74]

Assess ROM of the hip, knee, and ankle joints. To check muscle strength, place your hands against the lower legs and ask the client to flex or extend the knees against opposition from your hands.

Checklist: Lower Extremities Examination

1. Inspect lower extremities
2. Palpate skin temperature
3. Check for calf tenderness
4. Assess peripheral pulses
5. Check pretibial edema
6. Observe ROM and muscle strength

THE NEUROLOGIC EXAMINATION

The complete neurologic exam has five categories: mental status, cranial nerves, motor function (including cerebellar system), reflexes, and sensory function. A detailed description of these is in Chapter 25. This specialized exam is used to elicit any nervous system dysfunction when a client reports neurologic symptoms or when nervous disease is suspected. The nurse uses the neurologic exam to determine if there is any nervous system dysfunction and how it affects a client's ability to maintain self-care.[50] The physician uses information from this examination to locate the structural site of the lesion or lesions causing the abnormality. Detailed neurologic testing is not commonly done in the routine screening exam. Much of the routine neurologic testing that is done can be integrated with other parts of the general physical exam. Whenever a client's history or any physical signs arouse the examiner's suspicion, a complete neurologic exam should be performed.

Assessment literature describes the detailed neurologic exam.[2, 53j] These assessment parameters can be applied to comatose, head-injured, neurologic, or neurosurgical patients in order to monitor significant changes in status, e.g., uncal herniation, subdural hematoma.[11, 47, 48, 63, 73] The assessment parameters can be organized into a standard neurologic checklist that is scored numerically to monitor the status of hospitalized patients.[10] The neurologic exam can be modified slightly when you examine a child.[1h, 1i]

Cranial Nerves. The olfactory nerve (I) is usually not tested in the routine screening physical exam. Testing of cranial nerves II–XII may be integrated during assessment of the body part each innervates, and tests have been described throughout this chapter. Refer to Chapter 25 for an additional description of cranial nerve testing.

Mental Status. A client's current mental status is reflected in words and behavior. You judge this by assessing level of consciousness, orientation, mood, knowledge, judgment, memory and ability to calculate. Speech is assessed as an index of the ability to understand and use language, which is a higher cortical function. All these items may be assessed throughout the client history and physical exam; hence, they were described in the "Overview" section of this chapter. (The mental status examination is also discussed in Chapter 14.)

By the end of the general physical examination, you will have some data for making a generalized assessment of the client's mental status. State of consciousness is referred to as "alert" if the client is awake, makes appropriate verbal responses, and performs voluntary coordinated movements. Terms that indicate altered levels of consciousness include:

Lethargic. Person is generally drowsy, though able to communicate reasonably.

Obtunded or *stuporous.* Person is spontaneously unconscious, but can be aroused by shaking or vigorous physical stimuli. Then responds in monosyllables ("Yes," "No").

Comatose. Person is unconscious and cannot be aroused, with accompanying abnormal reflexes. May withdraw appropriately from painful stimuli.

Precise definition of these terms varies among practitioners. If there is no consensus among professionals in your facility, avoid using the terms and instead describe the client's behavior objectively.

Orientation, mood, and memory, and intelligence and speech were described in the Overview. You may test *short term memory* by asking a hospitalized patient to repeat the first five digits of his or her ID bracelet number a few minutes after reading them aloud.[50] This also gives information on visual acuity, reading, language ability, and ability to follow commands. Or ask a client to remember three things you mention at the beginning of the exam and to repeat them at the end, for example, "a cat, San Francisco, and the color blue."[3] *Judgment* can be assessed indirectly during the history or can be directly evaluated by asking a client to explain a proverb or a series of analogies. Similarly, the ability to *calculate* can be elicited through indirect questions in the history, e.g., "Let me get this straight.

Today is the 31st, and you say you have been sick for 5 days, so on what day did you first feel ill?" Direct calculation questions include asking the client to subtract 7 from 100 or to multiply simple numbers.

An abnormal response to the items listed above may indicate neurologic dysfunction or mental illness. Consult assessment literature for sets of behaviors that characterize specific psychiatric disorders.[3, 44]

Motor and Cerebellar Function. This includes assessment of muscle size and strength, tone, gait, coordination, and presence of any abnormal or involuntary movements. Muscle size and mass is assessed throughout the physical exam by observing and palpating the symmetric muscle groups (e.g., bilateral forearm, calf muscle). If muscles seem asymmetric, measure each muscle in centimeters to check for atrophy. Muscle strength can be assessed by opposing the client's flexion or extension movements. For example, beginning with the knee flexed, ask the client to try to extend a leg against your resistance. Trunk muscles are assessed by asking the client to sit up after the abdominal exam; this is normally done in the midline without deviation to one side. Assess upper extremities by asking the client to hold out both arms with the palms up. If there is weakness, one side will drift downward; if there is spasticity, the affected arm will raise and pronate. Assess muscle tone at the same time, noting:

- *Contracture* — shortening of the muscle with a decrease in ROM
- *Spasticity* — resistance to passive movement that rapidly increases and then gives way, or "clasp-knife"
- *Rigidity* — steady resistance throughout ROM or "cog-wheel"

Observation of a client's *gait* was described in the general survey. A fluid natural walk shows intactness of (a) the *extrapyramidal* motor pathway, which controls gross automatic movement, and (b) the cerebellum, which coordinates muscle activity and maintains equilibrium and posture. Some neurologic disorders cause characteristic gait patterns (e.g., ataxia, Parkinsonism, hemiplegia) and are described in Chapter 27. The other major pathway — the *corticospinal* (*pyramidal*) tract — mediates fine, discrete, voluntary movements like handwriting, and can be observed during the exam. Further tests to show cerebellar coordination are Romberg's sign, past-pointing, and the ability to do rapid successive movements. These are described in Chapter 25.

During the exam, notice any *involuntary movements* that indicate pathology of the extrapyramidal tract. These include abnormal movements, such as chorea, athetosis, tremors, and fasciculations. Also note any *muscle spasms*, such as tonic and clonic spasms, occupational spasm, and tics. These terms are discussed in Chapter 25.

Reflexes. Four categories of reflexes are outlined in Chapter 25: superficial, deep tendon, special, and pathologic. Some are not usually assessed in the routine screening exam. Others are assessed during each regional exam and have been integrated in this chapter (e.g., the pupillary light reflex). Usually, the routine exam does include assessment of the deep tendon reflexes and the Babinski.

A *deep tendon reflex* is elicited by a swift tap over a partially stretched tendon. When a client's simple reflex arc is intact, a muscle contraction will result. The examiner tests the brachioradialis, biceps, triceps, patellar (knee), and achilles (ankle) reflexes by briskly striking the tendon directly, or by striking her or his own thumb placed over the client's tendon (Fig. 15–32). The resultant muscle contraction response is graded:

0	no response
1+	diminished
2+	normal
3+	hyperactive or brisker than normal
4+	hyperactive with clonus, indicative of disease

Clonus is a repetitive jerking of the muscle while the tendon is being stretched. The grading of response may vary somewhat among examiners, but it is important that each reflex be bilaterally equal. Sustained clonus (more than two or three jerks) indicates nervous system disease.

Reflexes are increased with *upper motor neuron* lesions. These are disorders of the brain or spinal cord, e.g., cerebral palsy, multiple sclerosis, CVA, quadraplegia. *Lower motor neuron* lesions (e.g., polio or amyotrophic lateral sclerosis) are diseases of the peripheral nerves and are associated with decreased or absent reflexes.

One pathologic reflex usually tested is the *Babinski*. A normal response or negative (−) Babinski is plantar flexion of the foot and withdrawal. A pathologic, or positive (+) Babinski, is fanning of the toes and dorsiflexion of the foot. Whereas a positive Babinski is normal in newborns, in adults it indicates disease of the corticospinal (pyramidal) tract.

Sensory Function. The sensations of pain, temperature, touch, position, and vibration are conscious messages to the brain. Sensory receptors for these stimuli are located in the skin, muscles, tendons, mucous membranes, and internal organs. Sensations travel in a peripheral nerve to the spinal cord, then to the thalamus, and finally to specific sensory areas in the cerebral cortex. Each peripheral nerve collects stimuli from a segmental skin band, or *dermatome*. There is much overlap in dermatome levels.

Sensory impulses travel to the brain via two major routes: the *spinothalamic* tract mediates pain, temperature, and crude touch and the *posterior* (or *dorsal*) column tract carries fine touch, joint position, and vibration. Central lesions (such as CVA) may cause loss of all conscious sensations of one side of the body. Spinal cord transection may cause loss of one or both sensory pathways below the level of the lesion. Peripheral neuropathy produces decreased or distorted sensations at the anatomic dermatome level that the nerve innervates.

For evaluation of sensory functions, the client must be alert, cooperative, and not fatigued or highly suggestible. The examiner tests dermatome levels in a random, unpredictable order, while the client's eyes are closed. Since the spinothalamic tract mediates pain, temperature, and crude touch, just one modality is tested during a screening exam. Pain is assessed by the client's ability to perceive a gentle pin prick over different body areas. Apply both the point and blunt end of the pin, in an unpredictable sequence, and ask the client to say "sharp" or "dull" to identify the sensation being felt.

The dorsal column pathway is tested by light touch perception. Ask the client to say "yes" upon feeling a wisp of cotton or a soft brush

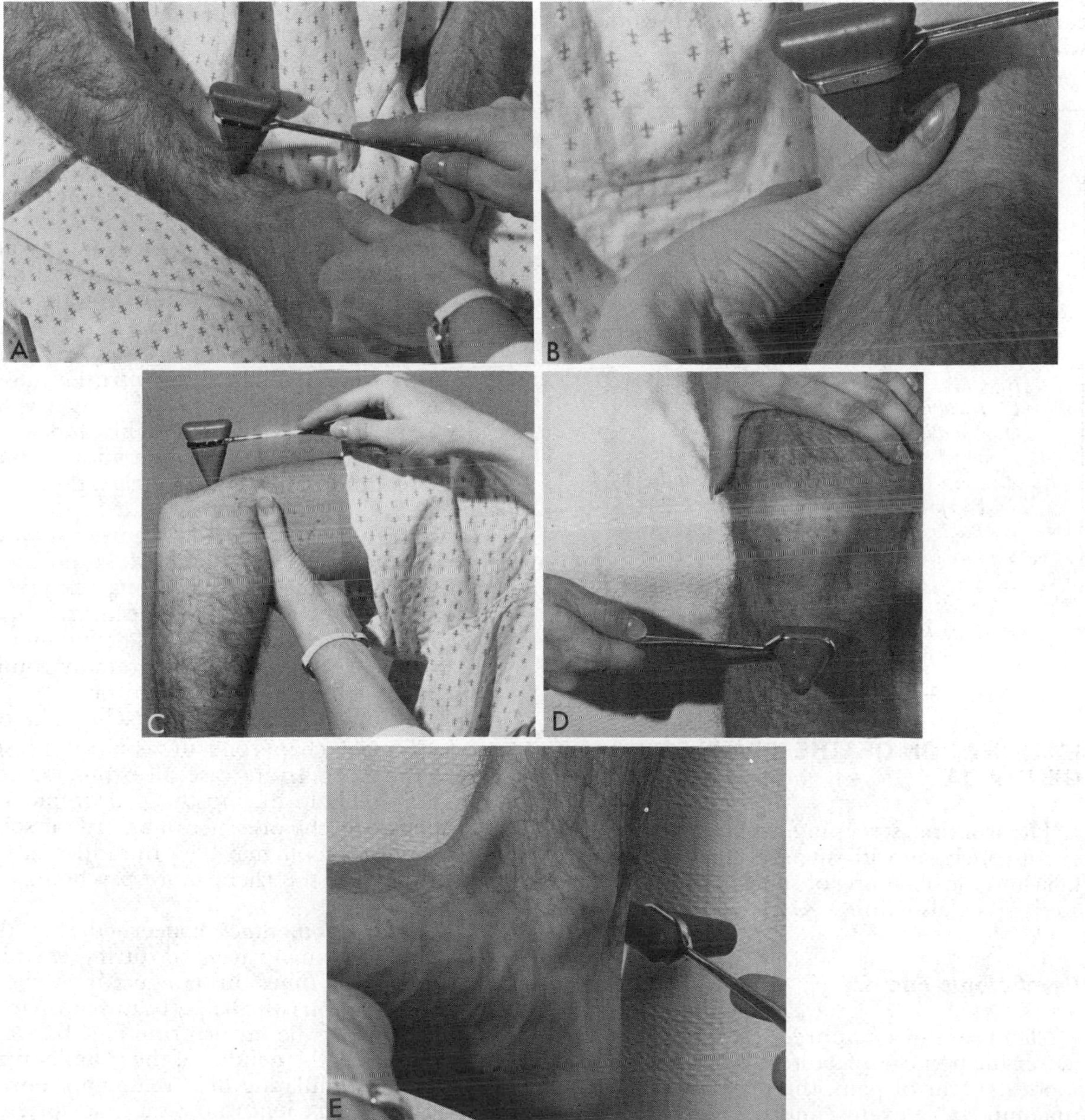

Figure 15–32. The deep tendon reflexes. **A.** brachioradialis; **B.** biceps; **C.** triceps; **D.** patellar; **E.** achilles. (Reprinted with permission from *Nursing 77*.)

lightly brushing the skin. If fine touch is intact, joint position or *kinesthesia* (ability to perceive passive movements of the digits or extremities) and *vibration* (sensation of a vibrating tuning fork over bony prominences) often are not tested in the screening exam.

Other sensory tests require cortical integration of the messages and may not be performed in the routine screening physical. These include *stereognosis* (identification of familiar objects when held in the hand), *graphesthesia* (identification of a number traced on the back or the palm by the examiner), and *two-point discrimination* (identification of one versus two skin areas being touched with pin pricks).

Checklist: Neurologic Examination

1. *Mental status and speech*
   - A. *Level of consciousness*
   - B. *Orientation, mood, and behavior*
   - C. *Intelligence, judgment, manner of speech*
   - D. *Memory*
2. *Cranial nerves, II through XII*
3. *Motor system and cerebellar function*
   - A. *Muscle size, tone, and strength*
   - B. *Gait*
   - C. *Involuntary movements*
   - D. *Coordination (cerebellar function)*
4. *Reflexes*
   - A. *Deep tendon reflexes: brachioradialis, biceps, triceps, patellar, achilles*
   - B. *Babinski reflex*
5. *Sensory function*
   - A. *Pain, temperature, crude touch (spinothalamic tract)*
   - B. *Fine touch, position, vibration (posterior column tract)*

EXAMINATION OF THE FEMALE GENITALIA

The routine screening exam of the female client concludes with an assessment of the genitalia and the obtaining of specimens for cytologic study. (See also Unit XXII.)

Psychologic Factors

Clients are often apprehensive about the pelvic exam because of culturally learned taboos, modesty, fear of pain, the memory of previous uncomfortable exams, and the fear of discovery of sexual "secrets."[44] However, it is necessary for women to understand the need for periodic pelvic examinations and to be responsible for regularly seeking out this aspect of their health care. A nurse's ability to help reduce each client's anxieties and fears concerning pelvic examination is, therefore, extremely important.

Women are seeking initial pelvic exams at younger ages, in order to acquire contraceptives and to be screened for cancer. The experience that an adolescent has in her first pelvic examination is crucial in determining how she will approach subsequent exams and how conscientious she will be in monitoring her own health care.[78]

The *teaching possibilities* at the time of pelvic examination are numerous and may include normal anatomy and physiology, vaginal self-examination, how often to seek health care check-ups, discussion of sexual behavior and intercourse, methods of contraception, and how to recognize symptoms of common pelvic conditions. The nurse is in a perfect position to establish rapport with a client, share items of health teaching, and perform the physical examination in a competent, confident way.

Nurse-client rapport is built through the examiner's warm and totally accepting manner and by environmental conditions that promote comfort and relaxation. Make sure the client has emptied her bladder before the exam; explain that this ensures a more comfortable examination. Have the room, your hands, and the speculum warm. Use adequate drapes to keep the client warm and prevent unnecessary exposure. Protect the room from sudden intrusion; possibly this will involve the use of screens. Explain every part of the exam thoroughly and in advance. Promote the client's cooperation through deep breathing and muscle relaxation techniques.

Make no unexpected movements that would surprise and tense the client. Make no movements or comments that a client may mistakenly perceive as seductive. These aspects are important, possibly more so for a male examiner, so that the client will not misinterpret any routine maneuvers as being sexually provocative. This problem may be minimized by having a helper, e.g., a female chaperone or assistant present during the exam. In any case, all examiners need an assistant's help during the procurement of specimens, and the presence of a third person in the examining room may have the added advantage of making the client more psychologically comfortable.

Clients are sometimes concerned that they may become sexually aroused during examination. Indeed, at times this may occur. A client's sexual orientation (which may be unknown to the examiner) may be a determining factor in whether or not the gender of the examiner may be sexually stimulating or threatening. For example, a woman client who is same-sex oriented *may* be more affected by a female nurse examiner than by a male nurse. Conversely, a woman who is heterosexually oriented *may* experience sexual arousal more readily when examined by a male nurse. Regardless of sexual orientation, clients generally find sexual arousal uncomfortable and distressing during physical examination, and every effort should be made by the examiner to prevent this occurrence. Remember that more important than the gender of the examiner is the examiner's ability to be professional, gentle, and accepting. These comments apply equally to the genital examination of a woman or a man. (Examination of male genitalia is discussed in the following section.)

Procedure

Assemble the following equipment: gloves, appropriately sized vaginal speculum, materials for cytologic study, lubricant, and a portable gooseneck lamp with a very strong light. Next, help the client to a *lithotomy* position: lying on her back with the buttocks close to the edge of the examining table, knees spread apart widely, and feet supported by stirrups.

External Genitalia. Inspect the client's external genitalia, noting skin color, hair distribution, and any lesions. Separate the labia majora with your gloved hand and inspect the clitoris, labia minora, urethral opening, vaginal opening, and perineum. Notice any swelling, inflammation, discharge, lesions, or ulcerations. The labia majora are normally plump and well formed. However, in the postmenopausal client the labia majora look shriveled and atrophic. In a nulliparous client (a woman who has not produced a viable child) the labia will meet in the midline; after a vaginal delivery they appear gaping.

Observe the area carefully for any skin lesions that may indicate cancer and for the chancre of primary syphilis. A chancre is oval or round, dark red, nontender, and indurated. It starts as a papule but evolves into an ulcer with an eroded center.

Skene's glands (paraurethral glands) are small multiple glands that open just behind the urethral orifice. They are usually not visible. Insert your index finger into the vagina, gently apply forward pressure and milk the urethra outward. This area is slightly sensitive, but there should be no pain or discharge. If any discharge is present, it should be cultured. Bartholin's (vulvovaginal) glands are located posterior to the vagina, above the labia, and are not palpable normally. If swelling of the labia is noted, these glands should be palpated. Palpate the posterior part of the labia between your index finger inside the vagina and your thumb outside. Check for tenderness and culture any discharge noted. Inflammation and abscess of Bartholin's gland often occur with gonococcal infection.

Separate the labia with your middle and index fingers, and assess the support of the vaginal musculature by asking the client to strain down. Any bulging of the vaginal wall is abnormal.

Cystocele is a weakening of the anterior vaginal wall, causing it and the bladder to prolapse into the vagina.

In *rectocele*, the posterior wall is weakened and the rectum bulges into the vagina.

With *uterine prolapse*, the cervix and part of the uterus may appear at the vaginal opening as the client strains.

Speculum Examination. The Graves bivalve speculum (small, medium, or large) is used with most clients. The Pedersen speculum has flat narrow blades and is used with virginal or postmenopausal clients who may have a very small or contracted vaginal opening. Select the proper size speculum and lubricate it with warm water. Lubricating jelly is not used at this point because it is bacteriostatic and would contaminate specimens to be obtained for cytology. Coach the client to take slow deep breaths and to relax her pelvic musculature.

Hold the speculum in your right hand, with your first two fingers closed over the base of the blades and your thumb under the thumbrest lever to prevent the blades from opening during insertion. Place the first two fingers of your left hand into the vaginal opening and push the perineum downward. Insert the speculum past your left fingers with the blades angled obliquely and any pressure applied downward (Fig. 15–33). Put no pressure on the sensitive anterior vaginal wall, with the urethra behind it. Remove your left fingers and point the blades down toward the small of the client's back, to follow the normal slope of the vagina. Insert the blades all the way and rotate them to a horizontal position. Open them by squeezing the speculum handles together. The round pink cervix should be in plain view. If not (as is often the case with beginning practitioners), close the blades, withdraw the speculum halfway, and reinsert in a slightly different plane. When the cervix is in full view, secure the blades in the open position by tightening the thumbscrew.

Inspect the cervix and its opening, or *os*. Note the shape of the os, color of the mucosa, and any growths or discharge. The cervical os is small and round in the nulliparous client. In the parous woman, the os is a horizontal slit and may even show lacerations off to the sides. The normal cervical mucosa is pink and smooth. It looks bluish in early pregnancy (*Chadwick's sign*). After vaginal deliveries, part of the inner cervical canal may be everted and may look like a red, beefy center inside the pink cervix. This is a cervical *erosion* and may be difficult to distinguish from a carcinoma by inspection alone.

Benign growths that are commonly seen on the cervix after childbirth are *nabothian* cysts, which are small yellow nodules that may be single or multiple. A cervical *polyp* is a growth that protrudes from the os and is bright red. *Carcinoma* begins near the os, looks like an irregular cauliflower growth, and is very friable. Finally, a normal cervical discharge may be seen. Its character varies with the menstrual cycle from clear and thin to thick, white, and stringy. It is always odorless and produces no itching. Note any discharge that is colored, irritating, or foul-smelling.

Cervical Cultures and Smears. Many hospitals and clinics perform a routine culture for *gonococcus* because gonorrhea is epidemic in the world today. Because 60 to 70 per cent of infected women are asymptomatic, they do not seek medical care, yet they can spread gonorrhea through sexual contact and will eventually have its painful sequelae. To obtain a culture, insert a sterile cotton swab into the os, rotate it completely, and leave it in place 10 to 20 seconds to ensure saturation.[44] The swab is then rolled onto a culture plate, which should be covered and incubated immediately.

Next, obtain the cervical specimens (*Papanicolaou smears*) to screen for cancer. Procedures vary among facilities, but often three smears are obtained:

1. *Endocervical swab*. Insert a sterile cotton swab into the cervix and rotate it 360 degrees. Spread the swab gently on a glass slide, and place the slide in a fixative solution or spray with a fixative.
2. *Cervical scrape*. Insert the more pointed bump of a wooden Ayre spatula into the cervical os and rotate it 360 degrees, scraping the cervix as you turn. Spread the material on a glass slide and spray with fixative.
3. *Vaginal pool*. Reverse the wooden spatula and scrape the blunt end on the vaginal floor behind the cervix. Spread the material on a slide and spray with fixative solution.

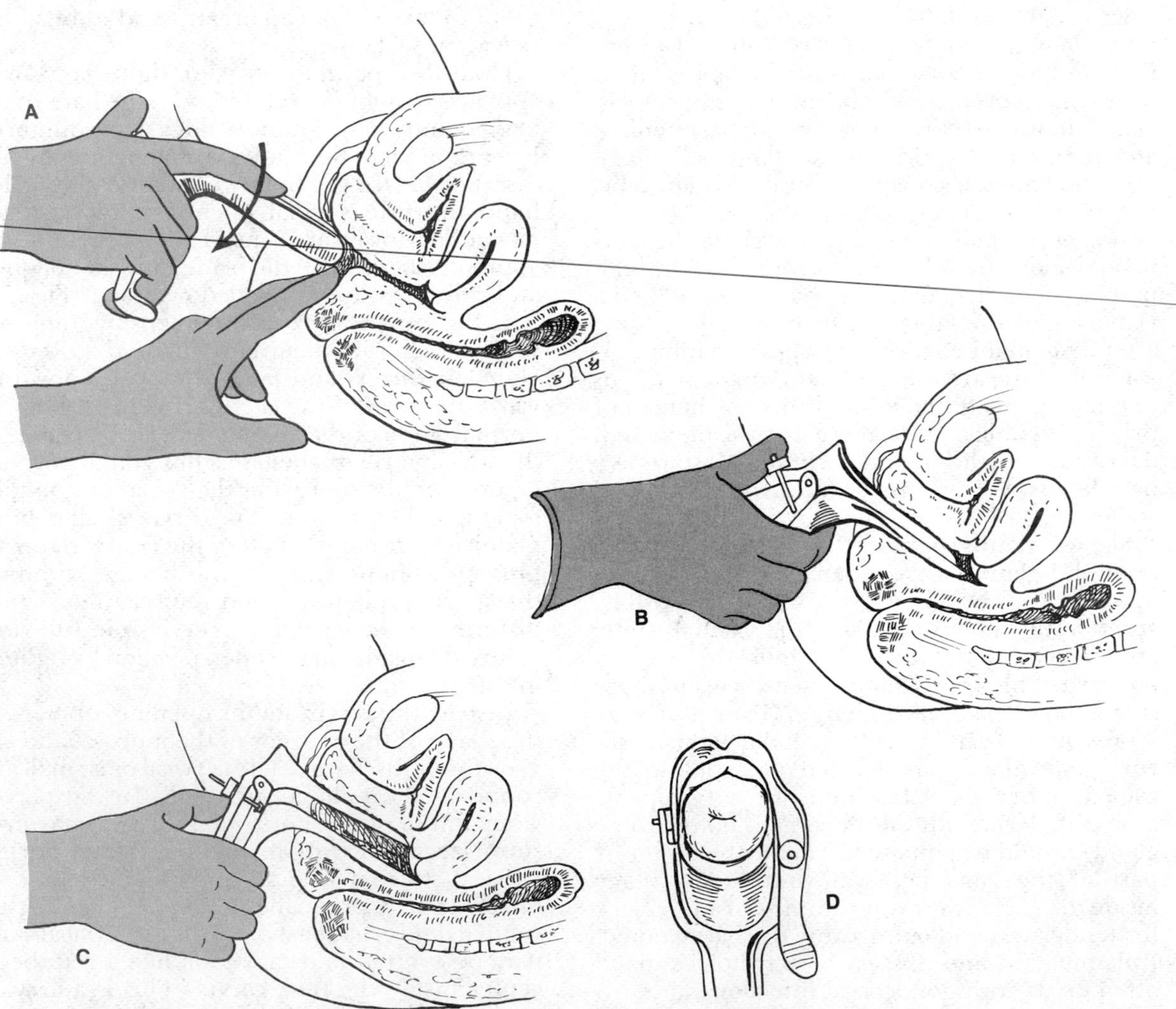

Figure 15–33. Insertion of the vaginal speculum. **A.** The speculum blades are turned obliquely and any pressure is directed downward onto the perineum. **B.** After full insertion, the blades are rotated to a horizontal position. **C.** Squeezing the speculum handles opens the blades. **D.** A full view of the cervix and cervical os.

Loosen the thumbscrew while continuing to hold the speculum blades open. Inspect the vaginal walls as you slowly withdraw and rotate the speculum. The normal vaginal walls are pink, deeply rugated, and have no inflammation or lesions. A vaginal discharge may be present with vaginitis due to gonorrhea, trichomoniasis, moniliasis, or the nonspecific or hemophilus vaginitis. If a discharge is present with gonorrhea, it is yellow and purulent. The discharge of *Trichomonas vaginalis* is yellow-green or white, frothy, thin, watery, and foul smelling. Monilial vaginitis (caused by the yeastlike organism *Candida albicans*) has a discharge that is thick, white, and curd-like. Nonspecific or hemophilus vaginitis may have a mild discharge that is yellow or gray and homogenous.

As the blades near the vaginal opening, let them close, taking care not to pinch any mucosa. Turn the blades obliquely to avoid stretching the introitus.

Bimanual Examination. The bimanual examination is done to assess the location, size, and mobility of the pelvic organs and to detect any tenderness or mass. The client remains in the lithotomy position, and the examiner stands. Practitioner preference varies as to which hand is used as the intravaginal hand. Clinically it does not matter, and each examiner should establish a routine that is best for her or him.

Lubricate the index and middle fingers of your gloved hand and insert them into the vagina. Flex the last two fingers onto your palm and have the thumb abducted up. The palmar surface should be perpendicular to the floor, and any pressure with insertion should be directed posteriorly. Palpate the vaginal wall, noting any tenderness or area of induration. Locate the cervix. A normal cervix feels firm and smooth and can be moved gently from side to side without producing pain. It should be midline and is usually on the anterior wall. The cervix usually points posteriorly, or away from the fundus of the uterus. The cervix softens with early pregnancy and feels hard with malignancy. An immobile cervix occurs with malignancy, and pain on palpation accompanies inflammation or ectopic pregnancy.

Next, use your abdominal hand to push the pelvic organs closer to the intravaginal fingers for palpation (Fig. 15–34). Begin in a position halfway between the umbilicus and the symphysis. Keep your pelvic arm horizontal and braced against your hip. In most women, the uterus is in the anterior postion and can be felt between your hands. Note its size, consistency, mobility, and any tenderness or mass.

Move both hands to the right to palpate the client's *adnexa*, or ovary and fallopian tube. The abdominal hand should be on the lower quadrant near the iliac crest, and the pelvic fingers should be in the lateral fornix of the cervix. Press the abdominal hand in toward the pelvic hand. A normal ovary is 4 to 6 cm. and feels oval, smooth, firm, and slightly sensitive to touch. The fallopian tubes are not palpable normally. Reverse the procedure for the client's other side.

In some women the uterus is positioned posteriorly (retroverted) and can be palpated only during a *recto-vaginal* examination. Withdraw your fingers from the vagina and change gloves to avoid spreading any possible infection. Lubricate your gloved fingers, and insert the index finger into the vagina and the middle finger into the rectum. Having the client bear down helps rectal insertion, but the procedure is still uncomfortable for the client and mimics the feeling of moving her bowels. Repeat the procedure described for the bimanual examination. A retroverted uterus may be palpated at this time, and its size and contour should be explored. The rectovaginal wall is palpated between the examining fingers and feels firm, smooth, and resilient. Palpate the cul-de-sac behind the cervix and note any masses. Withdraw your fingers. Any stool on your glove should be tested for occult blood.

EXAMINATION OF THE MALE GENITALIA

Psychologic Factors

Remember that male clients are often apprehensive about having their genitalia examined. Their apprehensions may stem from fears and anxieties similar to those experienced by women

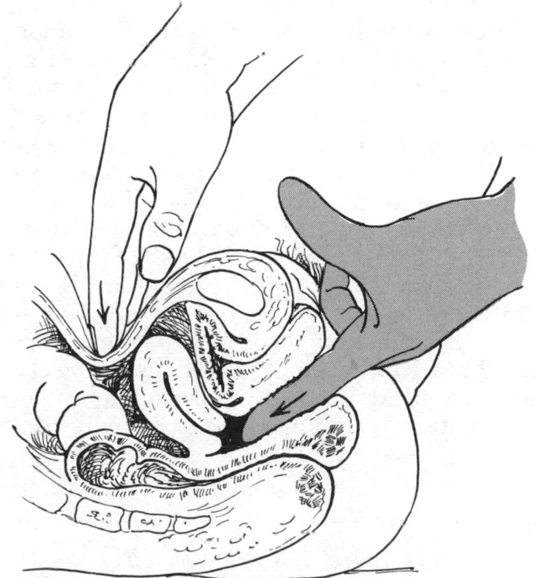

Figure 15–34. The bimanual exam. The abdominal hand presses the pelvic organs toward the intravaginal hand to be palpated.

during pelvic examination, e.g., modesty, fear of pain, the memory of previous uncomfortable exams, and the fear of discovery of sexual "secrets." Additionally, male clients may be worried that they may become sexually stimulated and that this will become obvious by an erection. (Women clients may also be concerned about sexual stimulation during examination, but their stimulation is less obvious to others.)

It is not uncommon for a male client to have an erection while his genitalia are being examined. When this happens the examiner may feel uncomfortable and perhaps even guilty for having "caused" such a reaction. The client often feels acutely embarrassed. Practitioners must critically examine their own feelings in this area of practice; any fears or uncertainties will be communicated to the client. It is helpful to approach the client's genital examination in a confident, matter-of-fact, professional way and to use firm touch rather than light, stroking touching whenever possible. When a male client does have an erection, Chard recommends assuring him that this is a "normal physiologic response to touch, just as constriction of the pupil is a normal response to light."[18] The examiner should *not* stop the procedure nor leave the room until the erection subsides; this only focuses unwanted attention on the client and increases his embarrassment. Rather the examination should continue in a matter-of-fact way, although the order of the exam may need to be altered. That is, the examiner may proceed to another area and return to palpate the shaft of the penis after the erection has subsided.

Some methods of reducing the likelihood of sexual stimulation during examination of genitalia have been previously discussed (p. 362).

Numerous *teaching possibilities* are present at the time of examination of a male client's genitalia.[19, 52] Such teaching may include normal anatomy and physiology, how often to seek health care check-ups, discussion of sexual behavior and intercourse, methods of contraception, and how to recognize common disorders. While female clients have been offered teaching in self-examination techniques for many years (e.g., breast and vaginal self-exams), male clients have received far less instruction in self-examination techniques. (See Chapters 81, 82, and 87.)

> *Remember to make teaching available to the male client in the areas of testicular self-exams and prostate self-exams.*

Procedure

Inspection and palpation are the skills used to assess the male genitalia. The client is in a standing position, with the genitalia exposed. Often no special equipment is needed, but certain techniques may require gloves, glass slides, and a penlight. Attention is given to the skin and surrounding area, the penis, and the scrotum.[53i] (See Chapter 82 also.)

Observe the skin of the genital area for color, hair distribution, and any skin lesions. The skin usually has a slightly darker pigment in the genital area than over the rest of the body. Pubic hair appears during adolescence, when the penis and testes enlarge. The hair has a diamond-shape pattern that extends up to the umbilicus. Any skin lesions should be assessed further to rule out *venereal disease*, although not all lesions have this cause. *Sebaceous cysts* are yellow, firm, nontender papules that are fairly common. Finally, observe the inguinal and femoral areas for bulges that may indicate a hernia or lymph node enlargement.

Penis. Inspect the penis, noting any inflammation, lesions, or discharge. In the circumcised male, the tip of the penis (the *glans*) is exposed and has a conical shape. If the client is uncircumcised, ask him to retract the free fold of skin covering the glans called the *prepuce* or *foreskin*. If the foreskin will not retract behind the corona of the glans, the condition is termed *phimosis*. *Paraphimosis* is a foreskin that has been constricted in the retracted position and will not move forward to cover the glans; in this condition the glans also looks edematous due to obstruction of blood flow. Inspect the glans closely for any lesions. *Carcinoma* is a nontender, indurated nodule or ulcer that may look dry and scaly. It is limited to uncircumcised men and may be hidden under the foreskin.

Note the opening of the urethral meatus; it should be centered at the tip of the penis. *Hypospadias* is a congenital displacement of the urethral meatus to the inferior (ventral) surface of the penis, with a groove extending to the normal position at the end of the penis. *Epispadias* is the location of the urethral meatus on the superior (dorsal) side of the penis.

Palpate the shaft of the penis between your thumb and first two fingers. Wear gloves if any inflammatory lesion or discharge is present. Note any tenderness or localized area of induration. Ask the client to milk the shaft of the penis from the base to the tip. If any discharge is present, it should be cultured and smeared on a glass slide.

A thick purulent penile discharge may be an early symptom of *gonorrhea*. Other symptoms are urinary frequency and painful urination. A thin mucous discharge occurs with urethritis. A *chancre* is the primary lesion of syphilis. It is oval or round, dark red, nontender, and indurated. It starts as a papule but soon looks eroded like an ulcer, and feels like a button under the skin. Usually the inguinal lymph nodes are enlarged, nontender, and hard. *Condylomata acuminata* are the papular lesions of secondary syphilis. They look like ordinary warts, soft and flat-topped, but are multiple. Another venereal disease, *herpes simplex virus type-2,* is characterized by small multiple vesicles on the penis, which are painful and cause extreme itching.

Scrotum. Inspect the scrotum, noting skin color, contour, and any nodules, ulcers, swelling or inflammation. Lift the scrotum up to inspect its posterior side as well. Check for *edema* which occurs with CHF, renal failure, or local inflammation.

It is normal for the scrotum to look somewhat asymmetrical; the left testis is lower than the right owing to its longer spermatic cord. Using your thumb and first two fingers, gently palpate each testis. A normal testis is about 4 to 6 cm. long and feels firm, smooth, freely movable, and somewhat sensitive to touch. An *atrophied* testis is small and soft. Both testes should be descended into the scrotal sac at birth. If one side of the scrotum is empty, palpate the neighboring femoral and inguinal area to try to locate the testis.[18]

Next, palpate each epididymis, located on the posterolateral side of the testis. It feels somewhat softer. Note any swelling, tenderness, or mass. Palpate each spermatic cord along its length from the epididymis to the external inguinal ring, noting any swelling or mass. If these are noted, the scrotum should be transilluminated by darkening the room and holding a lighted penlight behind the scrotum. Serous fluid will transilluminate and show as a red glow. Solid tissue and blood do not transilluminate.

A number of abnormalities may be evident in the scrotum:

A *varicocele* is a dilatation of the veins surrounding the spermatic cord, usually appearing on the left. It feels like a "bag of worms" and collapses as the scrotum is elevated when the client is supine.

A *hydrocele* is a nontender collection of fluid in the scrotum. Your examining fingers can palpate above the mass, and it transilluminates.

A *spermatocele* is a nontender, round cystic mass on the epididymis, which may feel like a third testis and will transilluminate.

A testicular *tumor* feels like a firm painless nodule on the testis.

Epididymitis is an acute inflammation in which the epididymis and vas deferens are swollen and very painful.

A scrotal *hernia* is a loop of bowel extending down through the external inguinal ring. Your fingers cannot palpate above the mass in the scrotum, and it does not transilluminate.

Not all hernias are palpated in the scrotum. A hernia may be easily reduced and appear only intermittently, with an increase in intra-abdominal pressure. Watch for such a bulge in the inguinal and femoral area as the client strains down. You also palpate for a hernia with the following maneuver: sit on a chair facing the client and ask that he shift his weight to the unexamined side. To palpate the client's right side, place your right index finger low on the right scrotal sac. Bring your finger up along the course of the spermatic cord, invaginating the scrotal skin as you go, to the external inguinal ring (Fig. 15–35). This is where the spermatic cord enters the inguinal canal; it feels like a small slit-like depression not larger than the tip of your finger. If the opening is enlarged, gently insert your finger into the inguinal canal. Ask the client to strain down in a Valsalva maneuver. You should feel nothing. If a hernia is present, you will feel a mass come down to bump your finger.

An *indirect inguinal hernia* is a loop of bowel that enters the internal inguinal ring and travels the course of the canal to the external inguinal ring.

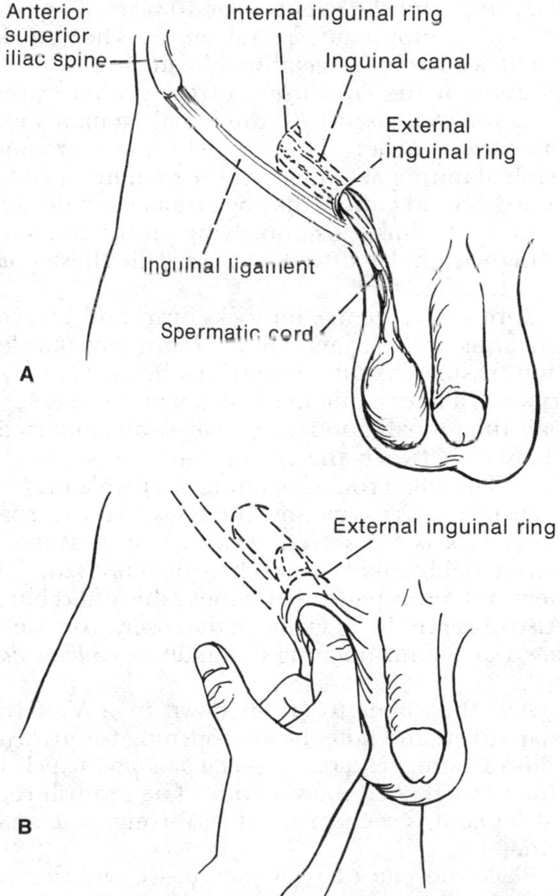

Figure 15–35. Palpating for presence of inguinal hernia. The examiner's index finger invaginates the scrotal skin and extends up along the spermatic cord to the external inguinal ring.

It is the most common type and often extends down into the scrotum. A *direct inguinal hernia* enters the inguinal canal directly through a weakness in the abdominal wall just behind the external inguinal ring. A *femoral* hernia is more common in women. It is lower and more lateral than an inguinal hernia and may look like an enlarged lymph node.

Finally, palpate the two chains of superficial inguinal lymph nodes. A *vertical* chain runs along the upper inner thigh. The *horizontal* chain lies along the groin below the inguinal ligament. Occasionally one of these nodes may be palpable normally; it feels small, soft, discrete, and movable. Notice any node that is enlarged, matted, fixed, and hard.

EXAMINATION OF THE RECTUM

The rectal exam concludes the routine screening examination of the adult client. It is particularly important in clients over 40 years of age, to screen asymptomatic rectal *cancer*. The female client is examined rectally while in the lithotomy position at the conclusion of the genital exam. This was discussed with the female genitalia examination earlier. The male client is examined while standing, leaning over the examining table. A bed-bound patient may be examined in the left lateral, or Sims, position; lying on the left side with the right leg flexed up toward the chest. (See also Unit XVII.)

Spread the client's buttocks apart and inspect the anus and perianal area. Notice any skin lesion, fissure, fistula, or external hemorrhoid. A *fissure* is a linear split in the anal canal and is very painful to palpation. A *fistula* is an abnormal channel between the rectum and the skin surface. The small round opening of a fistula may be seen in the area around the anus. An external *hemorrhoid* is a resolved varicose vein that looks like a flabby skin sac. When thrombosed, the hemorrhoid is painful and looks shiny and blue. Also observe the area above the coccyx for swelling and a sinus opening that indicates a *pilonidal cyst*.

Ask the client to strain down in a Valsalva maneuver, and note the anal opening for protrusion of hemorrhoids or rectal *prolapse*, which is due to weakened musculature. The reddish rectal mucosa is seen protruding through the anal canal.

Place the pad of your gloved, well-lubricated index finger against the anus. You will feel the anal sphincter contract, and then relax. As it relaxes, turn your finger and insert the tip into the anus directed toward the client's umbilicus. This technique is preferable to touching the anus with the tip of the finger outstretched at a right angle. The latter does not promote sphincter relaxation and is painful for the client. The whole procedure still may be somewhat uncomfortable for the client and mimics the feeling of having to move the bowels.

The anal canal is 2.5 to 4 cm. long and normally feels smooth. Note the tone of the sphincter and any tenderness or mass. Above the anal canal, the rectum turns posteriorly toward the sacrum. By inserting your finger farther, you can palpate 6 to 10 cm. of the rectum. Explore all sides of the rectal wall and note any nodularity. An internal hemorrhoid lies above the anorectal junction and is not palpable unless it is thrombosed. A *polyp* is a soft, somewhat movable mass that is difficult to distinguish from a malignant tumor by palpation. *Carcinoma* feels firm, irregular, nodular, and may have a rolled edge.

Identify the prostate gland on the anterior rectal wall of the male client. Palpate its two lateral lobes with the median sulcus in between. A normal prostate is round, heart-shaped, and about 4 cm. wide. It feels firm, smooth, resilient, and nontender and does not protrude over 1 cm. into the rectum. In *benign prostatic hypertrophy* (BPH) the gland enlarges, obliterating its median groove, but still feels firm and smooth. In acute *prostatitis* the gland is swollen and very tender to

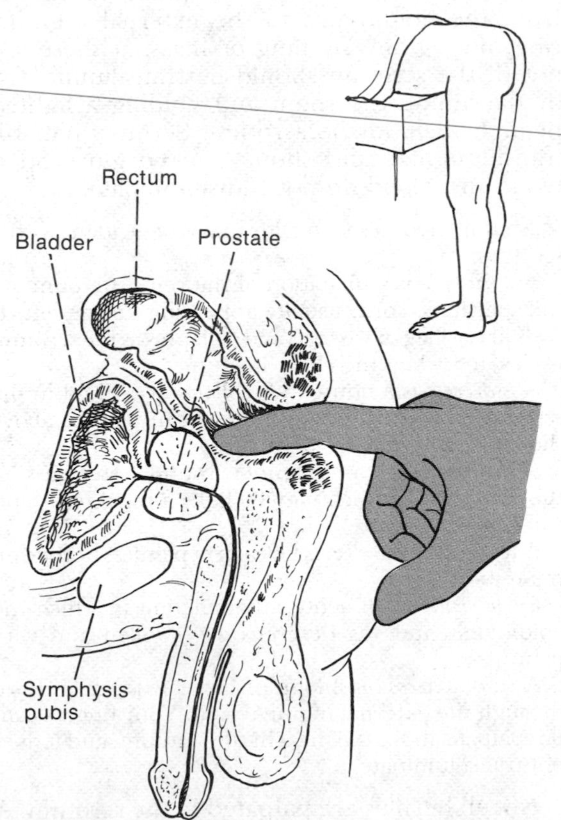

Figure 15–36. Palpating the rectum and prostate gland. (Redrawn from Morgan, W. L., and G. L. Engel: *The Clinical Approach to the Patient.* Philadelphia: W. B. Saunders Co., 1969.)

palpation. *Carcinoma* in the prostate presents as a stony-hard, irregular nodule in the gland that later becomes invasive and fixed.

In the female client, the small round cervix, palpable through the anterior rectal wall should not be mistaken for a tumor.

Gently withdraw the examining finger from the rectum. Any stool present on the glove should be tested for occult blood.

Checklist: Genital and Rectal Examinations

1. *Examination of the female genitalia*
   - A. *Inspect external genitalia*
   - B. *Using vaginal speculum, inspect cervix and vagina*
   - C. *Obtain specimens for cytologic study*
   - D. *Perform bimanual examination*
   - E. *Perform rectovaginal examination*
2. *Examination of the male genitalia*
   - A. *Inspect skin and surrounding genital area*
   - B. *Inspect and palpate penis and scrotum*
   - C. *Transilluminate scrotum if any masses are present*
   - D. *Check for presence of inguinal hernia*
   - E. *Palpate regional lymph nodes*
3. *Examination of the rectum*
   - A. *Inspect perianal area*
   - B. *Palpate anal canal, rectum*
   - C. *Palpate prostate gland*
   - D. *Test any feces for occult blood*

BIBLIOGRAPHY (Unit VII)

1. Alexander, M. M., and M. S. Brown: Physical examination. *Nursing '73–'76.*
   a. Part 2. History taking. Aug. 1973, p. 35.
   b. Part 4. The lymph system. Oct. 1973, p. 49.
   c. Part 5. Examination of the eye. Dec. 1973, p. 41.
   d. Part 6. The head, face and neck. Jan. 1974, p. 47.
   e. Part 12. Chest and lungs. Jan. 1975, p. 44.
   f. Part 13. Examining the abdomen. Jan. 1976, p. 65.
   g. Part 14. Male genitalia. Feb. 1976, p. 39.
   h. Part 17. Performing the neurologic examination. June 1976, p. 38.
   i. Part 18. Performing the neurologic examination. July 1976, p. 50.
2. Alpers, B. J., and E. L. Mancall: *Essentials of the Neurological Examination.* Philadelphia: F. A. Davis Co., 1971.
3. Alston, J. F., and J. M. Levet: What's happening: Practical applications of the mental status exam. *Nurse Practitioner,* 2:37, July-Aug. 1977.
4. American Cancer Society seeks nurses to teach breast exams. *American Nurse,* 9:11, Jan. 1977.
5. Apley, J.: *Paediatrics.* Baltimore: Williams & Wilkins Co., 1973.
6. Baer, E. D., et al.: How to take a health history. *American Journal of Nursing,* 77:1190, July 1977.
7. Bates, B.: *A Guide to Physical Examination.* Philadelphia: J. B. Lippincott Co., 1974.
8. Bates, B.: Doctor and nurse: Changing roles and relations. *New England Journal of Medicine,* 283:129, July 1970.
9. Beaumont, E.: For the latest word on stethoscopes listen here! Product survey. *Nursing '78,* 8:32, Nov. 1978.
10. Bolin, K. L.: Assessing the status of neurological patients. *American Journal of Nursing,* 77:1478, Sept. 1977.
11. Bordeaux, M.: The intensive care unit and observation of the patient acutely ill with neurologic disease. *Heart and Lung,* 2:884, Nov.-Dec. 1973.
12. Broughton, J. O.: Physical diagnosis for nurses and respiratory therapists. *Heart and Lung,* 1:200, Mar.–Apr. 1972.
13. Brown, M. S., and M. M. Alexander: Physical examination. *Nursing '74–'76.*
   a. Part 3. Examining the skin. Sept. 1973, p. 39.
   b. Part 7. Examining the ear. Feb. 1974, p. 48.
   c. Part 8. Hearing acuity. Apr. 1974, p. 61.
   d. Part 9. Examining the nose. July 1974, p. 35.
   e. Part 10. Mouth and throat. Aug. 1974, p. 57.
   f. Part 11. Examining the heart. Dec. 1974, p. 41.
   g. Part 15. Female genitalia. Mar. 1976, p. 39.
14. Bullough, B.: Influences on role expansion. *American Journal of Nursing,* 76:1476, Sept. 1976.
15. Busis, S. N., et al.: Pointers for detecting hearing loss. *Patient Care,* 11:174, Aug. 1977.
16. Castell, D. O., and B. B. Frank: Diagnostics: Abdominal examination. Role of percussion and auscultation. *Postgraduate Medicine,* 62:131, Dec. 1977.
17. Castleman, M.: A field guide to men's reproductive health. *Medical Self-Care* No. 5, 1978, p. 27.
18. Chard, M.: An approach to examining the adolescent male. *Maternal Child Nursing,* 1:41, Jan.-Feb. 1976.
19. Conklin, M., et al.: Should health teaching include self-examination of the testes? *American Journal of Nursing, 78*:2073, Dec. 1978.
20. DeJong, R. N., et al.: *Essentials of the Neurological Examination.* Philadelphia: Smith, Kline & French Laboratories, 1974.
21. Delp, M. H., and Manning, R. T.: *Major's Physical Diagnosis,* 8th ed. Philadelphia: W. B. Saunders Co., 1975.
22. Dossey, B.: Perfecting your skills for systematic patient assessment. *Nursing '79,* 9:42, Feb. 1979.
23. Druger, G.: *The Chest: Its Signs and Sounds.* Los Angeles: Humetrics Corp., 1073.
24. Eggland, E. T.: How to take a meaningful nursing history. *Nursing '77,* 7:22, July 1977.
25. Frank, M. J., and S. C. Alvarez-Mena: *Cardiovascular Physical Diagnosis.* Chicago: Year Book Medical Publishers, Inc., 1973.
26. Gillies, D. A., and I. B. Alyn: *Patient Assessment and Management by the Nurse Practitioner.* Philadelphia: W. B. Saunders Co., 1976.
27. Harlin, V.: How we do it — Teaching breast self-examination in the high school. *The Journal of School Health,* 47:243, Apr. 1977.
28. Jarvis, C. M.: Monitoring pulse, respiration and blood pressure and understanding their significance. *In* Sorensen, K. C., and J. Luckmann: *Basic Nursing: A Psychophysiologic Approach.* Philadelphia: W. B. Saunders Co., 1979.
29. Jarvis, C. M.: Perfecting physical assessment: Part 1. Hands and arms, head and neck, eye, ear, nose and throat. *Nursing '77,* 7:28, May 1977.
30. Jarvis, C. M.: Perfecting physical assessment: Part 2. Thorax and lungs, breast and heart. *Nursing '77,* 7:38, June 1977.
31. Jarvis, C. M.: Perfecting physical assessment: Part 3. Abdomen, legs, nervous system, genitalia and rectum. *Nursing '77,* 7:44, July 1977.
32. Jarvis, C. M.: Vital signs — How to take them more accurately and understand them more fully. *Nursing '76,* 6:31, April 1976.

33. Joint Committee on Pulmonary Nomenclature, American College of Chest Physicians and American Thoracic Society: Pulmonary terms and symbols. *Chest,* 67:583, May, 1975.
34. Judge, R. D., and G. D. Zuidema: *Methods of Clinical Examination: A Physiologic Approach.* Boston: Little, Brown and Company, 1974.
35. Kalisch, B. J., and P. A. Kalisch: An analysis of the sources of physician-nurse conflict. *Journal of Nursing Administration,* 7:50, Jan. 1977.
36. Kinlein, M. L.: *Independent Nursing Practice With Clients.* Philadelphia: J. B. Lippincott Co., 1977.
37. Larsen, G.: Removing cerumen with a Water Pik. *American Journal of Nursing,* 76:264, Feb. 1976.
38. Lehmann, Sr. J.: Auscultation of heart sounds. *American Journal of Nursing,* 72:1242, July 1972.
39. Leis, H. P.: The diagnosis of breast cancer. *CA — A Journal for Clinicians,* 27:209, July–Aug. 1977.
40. Leonard, J., and F. Kroetz: *Examination of the Heart, Part Four — Auscultation.* New York: American Heart Association, 1967.
41. Levene, G. M., and D. C. Calnan: *Color Atlas of Dermatology.* Chicago: Year Book Medical Publishers, Inc., 1974.
42. Lynaugh, J. E., and B. Bates: Physical diagnosis: A skill for all nurses? *American Journal of Nursing,* 74:58, Jan. 1974.
43. McVan, B.: Odors. *Nursing '77,* 7:46, Apr. 1977.
44. Malasanos, L., et al.: *Health Assessment.* St. Louis: C. V. Mosby Co., 1977.
45. Manzi, C. C.: Edema — How to tell if it's a danger sign. *Nursing '77,* 7:66, Apr. 1977.
46. Martinez-Lopez, J.: Can you recognize heart sounds in diastole? *RN,* 38:ICU-3, April 1975.
47. Megahed, M. S., and P. R. Rosendahl: Brain Tumors — An assessment for nurse practitioners. *Nurse Practitioner,* 2:9, July–Aug. 1977.
48. Meyd, C. J.: Acute brain trauma. *American Journal of Nursing,* 78:40, Jan. 1978.
49. Miller, K. M.: Assessing peripheral perfusion. *American Journal of Nursing,* 78:1673, Oct. 1978.
50. Mitchell, P. H., et al.: Neurological examination: Nursing assessment for nursing purposes. *Journal of Neurosurgical Nursing,* 9:23, Mar. 1977.
51. Murphy, J.: Role expansion or role extension? *Nursing Forum,* 4:380, No. 4, 1970.
52. Murray, B. L. S., and L. J. Wilcox: Testicular Self-Examination. *American Journal of Nursing,* 78:2074, Dec. 1978.
53. Physical Assessment: Programmed Instruction Units. *American Journal of Nursing,* 1974–1979.
    a. Auscultation of the heart. Part II, Feb. 1977.
    b. Examination of the abdomen. Sept. 1974.
    c. Examination of the chest and lungs. Sept. 1976.
    d. Examination of the ear. Mar. 1975.
    e. Examination of the eye. Part 1, Nov. 1974; Part 2, Jan. 1975.
    f. Examination of the female pelvis. Part I, Oct. 1978; Part II, Nov. 1978.
    g. Examination of the head and neck. May 1975.
    h. Examination of the heart and great vessels. Part I, Nov. 1976.
    i. Examination of the male genitalia. Apr. 1979.
    j. Neurological examination. Part I, Sept. 1975; Part II, Nov. 1975; Part III, Apr. 1976.
    k. Pulses. Jan. 1979.
54. Payne, P., and R. Payne: Behavior manifestations of children with hearing loss. *American Journal of Nursing,* 70:1718, Aug. 1970.
55. Prior, J. A., and J. S. Silberstein: *Physical Diagnosis.* St. Louis: C. V. Mosby Co., 1977.
56. Roach, L. B.: Assessing skin changes: the subtle and the obvious. *Nursing '74,* 4:65, Mar. 1974.
57. Roach, L. B.: Color changes in dark skin. *Nursing '77,* 7:48, Jan. 1977.
58. Roach, L. B.: Dark skins: Recognizing and interpreting color changes. *Critical Care Update!* 4:5, Oct. 1977.
59. Roberts, S. L.: Skin assessment for color and temperature. *American Journal of Nursing,* 75:610, Apr. 1975.
60. Robins, G. H.: *G.I. Series — Physical Examination of the Abdomen.* Richmond, Va.: A. H. Robins Co., 1971.
61. Rubin, B. A.: Black skin: Here's how to adjust your assessment and care. *RN,* 42:31, Mar. 1979.
62. Rubin, B. A.: How we do it — Black skin. *The Journal of School Health,* 47:365, June 1977.
63. Rudy, E.: Early omens of cerebral disaster. *Nursing '77,* 7:59, Feb. 1977.
64. Sana, J., and R. Judge (Eds.): *Physical Appraisal Methods in Nursing Practice.* Boston: Little, Brown and Co., 1975.
65. Schneggenberger, C.: History-taking skills: How do you rate? *Nursing '79,* 9:97, Mar. 1979.
66. Secretary's (HEW) Committee to Study Extended Roles for Nurses: Extending the scope of nursing practice. *American Journal of Nursing,* 71:2346, Dec. 1971.
67. Seidman, H.: Screening for breast cancer in younger women: Life expectancy gains and losses. *CA — A Cancer Journal for Clinicians,* 27:66, Mar.–Apr. 1977.
68. Sherman, J. L., and S. K. Fields: *Guide to Patient Evaluation.* Flushing, N.Y.: Medical Examination Publishing Co., Inc., 1974.
69. Sorensen, K. C., and J. Luckmann: *Basic Nursing: A Psychophysiologic Approach.* Philadelphia: W. B. Saunders Co., 1979.
70. Stillman, M.: Women's health beliefs about breast cancer and breast self-examination. *Nursing Research,* 26:121, Mar.–Apr. 1977.
71. Straight, P. A., and M. Soukup: How to hear it right: Evaluating and choosing a stethoscope. *American Journal of Nursing,* 77:1477, Sept. 1977.
72. Suavé, M. J., and A. Pecherer: *Concepts and Skills in Physical Assessment.* Philadelphia: W. B. Saunders Co., 1977.
73. Swift, N.: Head injury: Essentials of excellent care. *Nursing '74,* 4:27, Sept. 1974.
74. Taggart, E.: The physical assessment of the patient with arterial disease. *Nursing Clinics of North America,* 12:109, Mar. 1977.
75. Thomstad, B., et al.: Changing the rules of the doctor-nurse game. *Nursing Outlook,* 23:422, July 1975.
76. Traver, G. A.: Assessment of thorax and lungs. *American Journal of Nursing,* 73:466, March 1973.
77. Turnbull, E.: Prevention — Breast examination practices. *American Journal of Nursing,* 77:1450, Sept. 1977.
78. Wells, G. M.: Reducing the threat of a first pelvic exam. *Maternal Child Nursing,* 2:304, Sept.–Oct. 1977.
79. Willacker, J.: Bowel sounds. *American Journal of Nursing,* 73:2100, Dec. 1973.
80. Winslow, E. H.: Visual inspection of the patient with cardiopulmonary disease. *Heart and Lung,* 4:421, May–June 1975.
81. Women's attitudes regarding breast cancer. (The Gallup Organization Study.) *Occupational Health Nursing,* 22:20, Feb. 1974.
82. Wong, D. M.: Providing experience in physical assessment for students in basic programs. *American Journal of Nursing,* 75:974, June 1975.

SECTION THREE

SPECIFIC PROBLEMS IN MEDICAL-SURGICAL NURSING PRACTICE

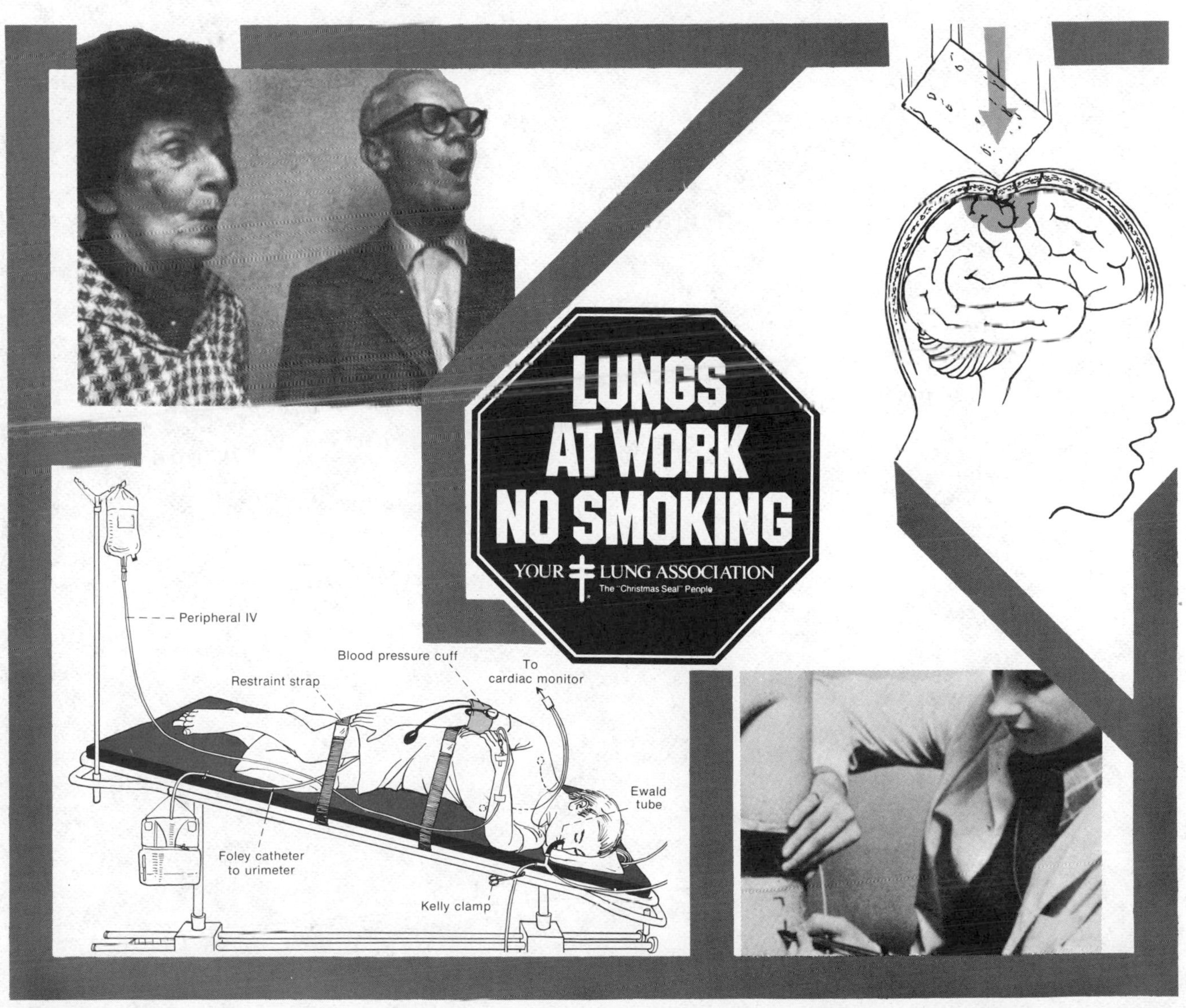

UNIT VIII*

NURSING PEOPLE EXPERIENCING SURGERY

We operate every day and an operation is but an incident in our day's work. For the patient, it is his whole life and he must and will walk through the valley of the shadow of death alone. He certainly cannot pay us a greater compliment than by putting his life into our hands and nothing but the very heart- and backbreaking best must be given back in return.[84]

INTRODUCTION AND STUDY GUIDE

The nursing of patients who are experiencing surgery is an exacting, difficult, demanding task. Yet for many nurses surgical nursing is a most challenging and gratifying specialty. The modern surgical nurse works with a wide variety of interesting patients; owing to advances in anesthesia and in surgical techniques, the nurse frequently has the pleasure of seeing patients recover quickly from their operations and return home to a productive life.

Basically, you perform your duties as a surgical nurse during the following three periods:

- ▶ The *preoperative period,* during which you admit the patient to the surgical floor and prepare the patient physically, emotionally, and legally for the operation. The emphasis, during this period, is upon (a) the correction of physiologic and psychologic problems that might increase surgical risk, (b) thorough and complete patient teaching regarding the specific surgery, and (c) instruction in and demonstration of exercises that will benefit the patient during the postoperative period.
- ▶ The *operative period,* during which you transfer the patient to the operating room where she or he is anesthetized and undergoes the scheduled surgical procedure. The emphasis, during the surgery itself, is upon asepsis, hemostasis, and the safe induction of anesthesia.
- ▶ The *postoperative period,* during which you observe and assist the patient's recovery from the anesthesia and from the stress of surgery itself. The emphasis, during this period, is upon the maintenance of body system functioning, the alleviation of pain and discomfort, the prevention of postoperative complications and adequate discharge planning and teaching.

1. As you study this unit, familiarize yourself with the following terms:

surgical risk	general anesthesia
operative permit	regional anesthesia

*Kerry E. Cavanaugh, R.N., B.S., critically reviewed and assisted with the revision of this unit. Ms. Cavanaugh expresses her gratitude to Gwen Williams, R.N., Shirley Conwell, R.N., and Dr. Murali Sivarajan for their assistance with the review.

laryngospasm
bronchospasm
hypothermia
purposeful hypotension
airway
wound dehiscence
evisceration
acute gastric dilatation
paralytic ileus
acute parotitis

2. Upon completion of this unit, you should be able to discuss the following concepts:

a. The four major types of conditions that require surgical intervention
b. The usual classification of surgical procedures
c. The estimation of surgical risk and your role in assisting the surgeon in gathering information concerning the patient
d. The typical preparation of a patient for surgery from the time of entering the hospital until the time of being transported to the operating room
e. The major differences between general and regional anesthesia
f. The complications of anesthesia — their treatment and prevention
g. Typical care of the patient in the recovery room
h. The goals of surgical care and their achievement
i. The major symptoms that herald the development of postoperative complications
j. The major postoperative complications — their prevention and treatment

3. After carefully studying this unit and relating it to your own clinical observations, you can expect to be able to:

a. Assess the patient in terms of surgical risk, i.e., help assess the patient's general health status, cardiovascular function, pulmonary function, genitourinary function, metabolic and liver function, neurologic factors, hematologic factors, prior and current use of drugs, mental outlook and occupational and economic standing
b. Conduct a purposeful interview with the patient, which will aid in the gathering of the above data
c. Plan and implement preoperative teaching sessions with the patient and significant others
d. Instruct the patient in deep breathing, coughing, turning and extremity exercises
e. Administer preoperative drugs to the patient accurately and safely
f. Give complete preoperative care on the day of surgery, e.g., obtain vital signs, give oral hygiene, remove jewelry
g. Observe the patient postoperatively and assist with postoperative patient care in the recovery room and after the patient returns to the surgical floor
h. Observe for the complications of surgery and take appropriate action should the patient develop a complication, e.g., report patient signs and symptoms to the team leader or surgeon, chart findings, give emergency care.

CHAPTER 16

THE PATIENT UNDERGOING SURGERY: GENERAL CONSIDERATIONS

Today surgery takes place in a thoroughly equipped, aseptic environment. The surgeon's task is aided by recent advances in medical technology and by knowledge of the physiologic responses of humans to stress. The anesthesiologist's responsibilities have been lightened in recent years by the development of safe yet potent anesthetic agents. The modern nurse can effectively care for surgical patients within the specialized environment of a well equipped recovery room.

However, despite such advances, for *the patient,* the decision to undergo surgery stands as a moment of crisis in life. Surgery represents a personal crisis because any operation, however minor, always carries some risk; moreover, surgery inevitably involves a certain amount of expense, discomfort, pain, and emotional stress for the patient as well as a disruption of a person's usual life pattern.

What conditions force a patient to undergo the risk of surgical procedure? What are the major types of surgeries and what are some of the general effects upon the patient? How do surgeons estimate the amount of risk that a patient will face, lying anesthetized upon the operating table? What is the role of the nurse in reducing surgical risks and in making the operation and its aftermath successful?

BASIC TYPES OF CONDITIONS REQUIRING SURGERY

Despite the large number of individual conditions that are treated by surgeons, four basic pathologic processes are the cause of almost all surgical problems.[73]

> *The four pathologic processes responsible for most surgical conditions are:*
> 1. *Obstruction*
> 2. *Perforation*
> 3. *Erosion*
> 4. *Tumors*

Obstruction or blockage mainly affects arteries (e.g., the coronary or cerebral arteries), tubes (e.g., the bronchial and eustachian tubes), and ducts (e.g., the cystic duct). For example, when the coronary arteries are blocked, a myocardial infarction results; a blockage of cerebral arteries produces a cerebral vascular accident ("stroke"). Atelectasis or lung collapse results from an obstructed bronchial tube; a middle ear infection can be caused by an obstructed eustachian tube. When a "stone" blocks the cystic duct, cholecystitis or inflammation of the gallbladder results.

Obstructions of passageways within the body are dangerous because they block the flow of such vital substances as blood, air, cerebral spinal fluid, urine, and bile.

Perforation is the rupture of an organ, artery, or bleb. Examples of perforation are: perforated duodenal ulcer, ruptured bladder, and cerebral hemorrhage due to the rupture of a major cerebral artery. Perforation is a dangerous event that usually calls for emergency surgery.

Erosion is the wearing away or eating away of the surface of a tissue as a result of continuous physical irritation, infection, ulceration, or inflammation. The process of erosion may wear away blood vessel walls, resulting in bleeding. Cancerous tumors, bladder stones, duodenal ulcers, and tuberculosis can all lead to the erosion of blood vessels and resultant bleeding.

Tumors are abnormal growths of tissue that form masses serving no physiologic function within the body, and that may be malignant. Tumors often grow very large before they are detected. A tumor may not initially produce symptoms, so a patient may unknowingly neglect the condition and fail to seek medical advice. At times such neglect may be fatal. One of the most common methods of treating tumors is by surgical excision of the mass.

MAJOR CATEGORIES OF SURGICAL PROCEDURES

Surgical procedures are categorized according to their: (1) purpose, (2) degree of risk to the patient, and (3) urgency.

Purpose. Types of surgeries categorized to

purpose are: diagnostic, exploratory, curative, (including ablative, reconstructive, and constructive) and palliative.

Diagnostic surgery enables the surgeon to make or to verify a suspected diagnosis. A common type of diagnostic surgery is the *biopsy,* in which the surgeon excises a small amount of tissue and sends it to the pathology laboratory for microscopic examination, which will establish a diagnosis. For instance, surgeons commonly take a biopsy of breast tissue if they suspect the presence of breast cancer. If the specimen of tissue is found to contain cancer cells, the surgeon then proceeds to excise the tumor and often removes the entire breast and surrounding lymph nodes.

Exploratory surgery enables the surgeon to estimate the extent of disease and, at times, to make or confirm a diagnosis. A common example is an exploratory laparotomy, during which the surgeon makes an opening in the abdomen, explores the abdominal area and organs for signs of cancer, bleeding, and so forth, hopefully diagnoses the patient's condition, and determines the need for more extensive surgery.

Curative surgery (ablative, reconstructive, and constructive) is performed to remove or to repair damaged, diseased, or congenitally malformed organs or tissues. *Ablative* surgery involves the removal of diseased organs (e.g., nephrectomy, or the removal of a kidney; *reconstructive* surgery is the partial or complete restoration of a damaged organ or tissue to a resemblance of its normal appearance and function (e.g., plastic surgery of the facial structures following a severe burn); *constructive* surgery is the repair of a congenitally defective organ to improve its function and appearance (e.g., plastic surgery of a congenital cleft palate); and *palliative* surgery relieves symptoms, although it does not cure the disease causing the symptoms. For example, nerves supplying a diseased organ may be cut to alleviate severe pain; infected necrotic tissues may be removed to reduce pain and for esthetic purposes; an intestinal bypass operation is sometimes performed to relieve symptoms of intestinal obstruction from an inoperable bowel cancer. Table 16–1 gives examples of surgeries categorized by purpose.

TABLE 16–1. SURGERIES CATEGORIZED BY PURPOSE

Type	Example
I Diagnostic	Biopsy D & C Myelogram
II Exploratory	Exploratory laparotomy
III Curative	
Ablative	Nephrectomy
Reconstructive	Plastic surgery after burns
Constructive	Plastic surgery on cleft palate
IV Palliative	Rhizotomy

Degree of Risk to Patient. Types of surgeries classified according to magnitude and degree of risk for the patient are: *major* surgery and *minor* surgery.

Major surgery involves high risk because the patient may be on the operating table for a prolonged period of time; a large amount of blood may be lost; vital organs will be handled and may be removed; and postoperative complications may develop.

Minor surgery, on the other hand, is generally not prolonged, engenders few serious complications, and involves little patient risk. Table 16–2 categorizes surgeries according to magnitude and degree of risk.

Urgency. Surgical procedures may also be classified according to *urgency.* Principal categories are emergency surgery, imperative or urgent surgery, planned required surgery, elective surgery, and optional surgery. Table 16–3 gives examples of each of the following types of surgery.

Emergency surgery must be performed *immediately* in order to: (1) save the life of the patient, (2) save the function of an organ or limb, (3) remove a damaged organ or limb as necessary, or (4) stop hemorrhage.

Imperative or urgent surgery must be performed as soon as possible, within 24 to 48 hours.

Planned required surgery is *necessary* for the patient's well-being but is *not* urgent. This required surgery may be scheduled weeks or months ahead of the proposed operation.

Elective surgery is surgery which should be performed for the patient's well-being but which is not absolutely necessary.

Optional surgery is surgery that the patient requests, generally for esthetic or psychologic reasons.

TABLE 16–2. SURGERIES CATEGORIZED ACCORDING TO MAGNITUDE AND DEGREE OF RISK

	Discussion	Example
I Major Surgery	Involves significant risk including possible large blood loss Possible postoperative complications Duration of procedure may be prolonged, increasing risk	Open heart surgery Abdominal-perineal resection Nephrectomy Kidney transplant Craniotomy Radical neck dissection
II Minor Surgery	Does not involve significant risk Procedure time is brief	Skin biopsy Excision of digital cystic neuroma

TABLE 16–3. SURGERIES CATEGORIZED ACCORDING TO URGENCY

Category	Surgical Significance	Example
1. Emergency	Immediate surgery required	Severe trauma Intestinal obstruction Extensive burns Gunshot and stab wounds Perforated ulcer
2. Imperative	Requires surgical intervention within 24–48 hours	Severe, bleeding hemorrhoids Kidney stones Eroding, bleeding cancerous tumors Bleeding of duodenal ulcer
3. Planned, Required	Surgical intervention scheduled weeks or months in advance	Cataract removal Tonsillectomy Laminectomy Gall bladder removal—when acute inflammation is not present
4. Elective	Delay or omission of surgery has no adverse effect	Simple hernia repair Scar repair Hemorrhoids that are not bleeding
5. Optional	Simple intervention for individual preference	Face lift Mammoplasty

THE EFFECT OF SURGERY UPON THE PATIENT

A surgical procedure, whether major or minor, emergency or optional, *always* affects the patient, physically and emotionally. Although each type of operation creates its own specific problems, some *general* effects of surgery upon the patient are listed and discussed below.

1. *The stress response is elicited.*
2. *The defense against infection is lowered.*
3. *The vascular system is disrupted.*
4. *Organ functions are disturbed.*
5. *The body image may be disturbed.*
6. *Lifestyles may change.*

Stress Response Is Elicited

As you recall, stress is a collective term for the many psychologic and physiologic factors that cause neurochemical changes within the body. Some of these factors include: anxiety, pain, tissue damage, blood loss, anesthesia, fever, sepsis, immobilization, and food deprivation. The stressful stimuli imposed by surgery combine both psychologic factors (anxiety, fear of the unknown) and physiologic factors (blood loss, anesthesia, pain, immobilization) in instituting the neuroendocrine response.

The severity of a stressful stimulus directly determines the degree of neuroendocrine response: *the greater the stress, the greater the degree of response.* For example, hospital admission for surgery poses a moderately stressful stimulus; it provokes a neuroendocrine response which the patient may display (a) *physiologically,* by an increased heart rate and elevated blood pressure, or (b) *psychologically,* by alterations in usual behavior. An example of a severely stressful stimulus is postoperative hemorrhage. The response in this case involves hypovolemia, profound shock, and potential death if the profuse bleeding is not immediately stopped.

Patients experience an activation of the stress response as a consequence of the surgical procedure itself. Initially the sympathetic nervous system stimulates the adrenal medulla, resulting in an increased production of *norepinephrine* and *epinephrine.* Recall that these two neuroendocrine hormones are partially responsible for a chain reaction of events involved in the stress response. A wide assortment of cardiovascular and metabolic changes are triggered biologically by stress. Some of the physiologic events accompanying the release of epinephrine are (1) increased heart rate, (2) increased blood sugar, and (3) bronchial dilation. The release of norepinephrine causes peripheral vasoconstriction, which manifests itself initially by an increased blood pressure and cool, pale, skin. (Epinephrine and norepinephrine are discussed in detail in Chapters 6 and 74.)

The success of the stress response in maintaining homeostatic balance is determined, to a large degree, by the age and physical condition of the patient as well as by the duration of the stress. In the aged or debilitated person, the ability to withstand stress and to tolerate surgery and anesthesia is often markedly reduced. One reason that the aged and debilitated respond poorly to stress is that their adrenal glands are often atrophied and reduced in size. As a result, less epinephrine is released.

Specific disorders that decrease the body's adaptive mechanisms and that should be treated prior to surgery are: liver disease, shock, hemorrhage, dehydration, electrolyte imbalance, acidosis, alkalosis, hypoproteinemia, vitamin deficiency, anemia, adrenal insufficiency, alcoholism, pulmonary disorders, heart ailments, vascular insufficiency, renal insufficiency, obesity, hyperthyroidism, diabetes mellitus, and emotional instability.

In any person, young or old, healthy or sick, prolonged stress eventually depletes the "stress hormones" as well as the substances composing them.

The need for a powerful stress response can be minimized by careful, thoughtful medical preparation and nursing care. The well prepared, calm preoperative patient and the comfortable postoperative patient rely far less on the stress response for survival than do frightened, uncomfortable patients who are left alone in pain and uncertainty.

Defense Against Infection Is Lowered

The patient's initial defense against bacterial invasion and the establishment of a clinical infection is the *skin.* The skin, when intact, cannot be penetrated and has nearly infallible protective abilities.

However, when the surgeon's scalpel incises the patient's skin, the first line of defense against bacterial invasion is destroyed. Despite sterile equipment and meticulous technique on the part of all members of the surgical team, infection remains as an ever-present potential danger for the surgical patient.

Vascular System Is Disrupted

Surgical incisions interrupt the vascular system by severing blood vessels. These severed blood vessels are clamped immediately so that blood loss may be minimized and/or controlled. However, despite the quick response of surgeons in clamping these bleeding vessels (known as "bleeders"), some blood loss always occurs during surgery. Minimizing or controlling blood loss is known as "hemostasis." An excessive blood loss can lead to hemorrhage and shock intra- or postoperatively.

Organ Functions Are Disturbed

During surgery, organs are often manipulated, causing the organ function to be temporarily disrupted during the postoperative period. Also, some operative procedures involve the removal of organ tissues or total organs. As a result of more radical surgeries, the physiologic functioning of the entire body may be seriously affected. For example, a patient with a brain tumor usually requires a craniotomy. Depending upon the type of brain tumor, residual results of brain tissue removal may be (1) arm or leg weakness, (2) impaired vision, and (3) expressive or receptive aphasia.

Body Image May Be Disturbed

Formation of body image begins in early childhood and evolves throughout life. Body image is a unique sense of identity, which is based on several factors:

- outward appearance
- inner somatic sensations
- reactions of significant others
- individualized meaning and value attached to certain parts of the body more than other parts (e.g., the breasts are more important to some women than are the legs)

Disturbances of body image may occur as the result of (1) amputations of a limb or breast, (2) disfiguring operations, e.g., radical neck surgery, and (3) operations in which organs of symbolic or emotional importance are removed. For example, a hysterectomy may make a woman feel less feminine or irreversibly changed, even though the removal of her uterus is not outwardly apparent.

Life Styles May Change

Certain types of operations may force radical alteration in a patient's whole way of life, at least during a postoperative period of learning and retraining. For example, the amputee has to learn to use an artificial limb; this can require considerable time and effort. Surgical expense and loss of work time may significantly alter the patient's financial status. Job retraining may be needed, as well as modification of recreational activities.

Summary

In sum, surgery solves certain problems only to create others. To face surgery requires courage on the patient's part as well as the ability to adapt to stress. An important role of the surgeon and the nurse is to prepare the

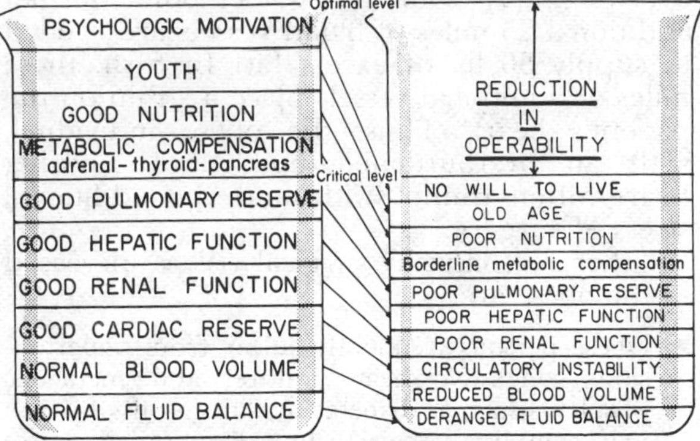

Figure 16–1. Volume of operability. (From Hardy, J. D.: *Rhoads Textbook of Surgery: Principles and Practice.* Philadelphia: J. B. Lippincott Co., 1977, p. 5.)

patient for the stresses and problems that will inevitably arise. The preparation of the patient before the operation is discussed in Chapter 17.

THE ESTIMATION OF SURGICAL RISK

The degree of surgical risk is based upon four factors: (1) the physical and mental condition of the patient, (2) the extent of the disease, (3) the magnitude of the required operation, and (4) the resources and preparation of the surgeon, nurses, and hospital.

> *These important factors can be summed up:*
>
> *The patient + the disease + the treatment = the surgical risk.*

Figure 16–1 lists some considerations in assessing a patient's ability to tolerate an operation.

Assessing the Patient's Physical and Mental Condition

The degree of surgical risk is affected profoundly by the following characteristics of the patient: (1) age, (2) nutritional state, (3) state of fluid and electrolyte balance, (4) general health, (5) types of drugs taken regularly, (6) mental health, and (7) economic and occupational outlook.

AGE

Children and young and middle-aged adults generally tolerate surgery well, while the risk of surgery increases significantly for the premature baby and the elderly person. Operating on elderly persons is risky for the following reasons.

1. The aged are highly sensitive to stress, to anesthetics, and to certain drugs that are used pre- and postoperatively, e.g., scopolamine, morphine sulfate, and barbiturates.
2. The elderly are often dehydrated and malnourished, making them prone to shock and retarded tissue healing. Senescent patients frequently are victims of degenerative diseases (e.g., congestive heart failure and arteriosclerosis) as well as chronic respiratory diseases (e.g., emphysema). Moreover, many elderly male patients have prostatic hypertrophy, which can lead to postoperative urinary and renal problems.
3. The aging process itself produces pathophysiologic organ changes. Figure 16–2 illustrates some of these changes.
4. One authority states that the most common problem seen in the aged preoperatively is a lower than normal total blood volume.[127] Patients with a lowered blood volume prior to surgery are unable to tolerate even a small amount of bleeding and go rapidly into shock. Thus, many older persons require blood transfusion *before* their operation in order to decrease risk.

In general, operative risk for older patients is lower in those operations that are brief in duration, are elective, cause little blood loss, and statistically incur a low percentage of postoperative complications. On the other hand, operations that cause the elderly patient to hemorrhage, which are lengthy or emergency in nature, or which carry a high percentage of postoperative complications all increase surgical risk.

NUTRITIONAL STATUS

The preoperative nutritional status of the patient is an important consideration in estimating the risks of surgery. Nutritional status has a direct correlation with intraoperative success and postoperative recovery. The patient who is physiologically homeostatic preoperatively is well prepared to handle the stress of actual surgery and returns to optimum health more rapidly after surgery.

Major preoperative nutritional problems are (1) debilitation and malnourishment due to protein, iron, and vitamin deficiencies and (2) obesity.

Nutritional deficiencies mainly affect the aged, the chronically ill, persons with cancer, and patients with gastrointestinal conditions that cause severe diarrhea and/or vomiting, e.g., ulcerative colitis and pyloric stenosis.

To treat preoperative patients who are *malnourished,* encourage a high intake of carbohydrates (needed for energy); protein (needed for wound healing); and vitamins (also needed for healing), especially vitamin K (necessary for proper blood coagulation). Also, parenteral hyperalimentation may be used for several days to a week prior to surgery. This method of augmenting nutritional intake involves intravenous administration of nutritional supplements to build up body tissues. Parenteral hyperalimentation is often continued postoperatively until satisfactory gastrointestinal function returns. (Parenteral hyperalimentation is discussed in Unit XVII.)

Obesity must be corrected by weight loss prior to an operation that is not of an emergency nature. The severely obese patient faces an increase in surgical risk for every pound of overweight. As some authorities point out, an additional 25 miles of blood vessels are needed to supply 30 lb. of excess fat! In turn, these miles of additional vessels place a strain on the patient's heart. Thus, the obese individual, with an overburdened body and laboring heart, often cannot withstand the additional stress of surgery.

Other reasons why surgical risk is increased in the obese are:

- Obese persons frequently suffer from hypertension, congestive heart failure, and metabolic problems such as diabetes mellitus — all of which may complicate their technical operative course and postoperative course.
- Adipose tissue increases the technical difficulty of surgery. Incisions are usually larger than normal, and after suturing, larger dead spaces are left, thereby increasing the risk of postoperative infection. In addition, obese patients are more likely to develop incisional hernias or wound dehiscence.

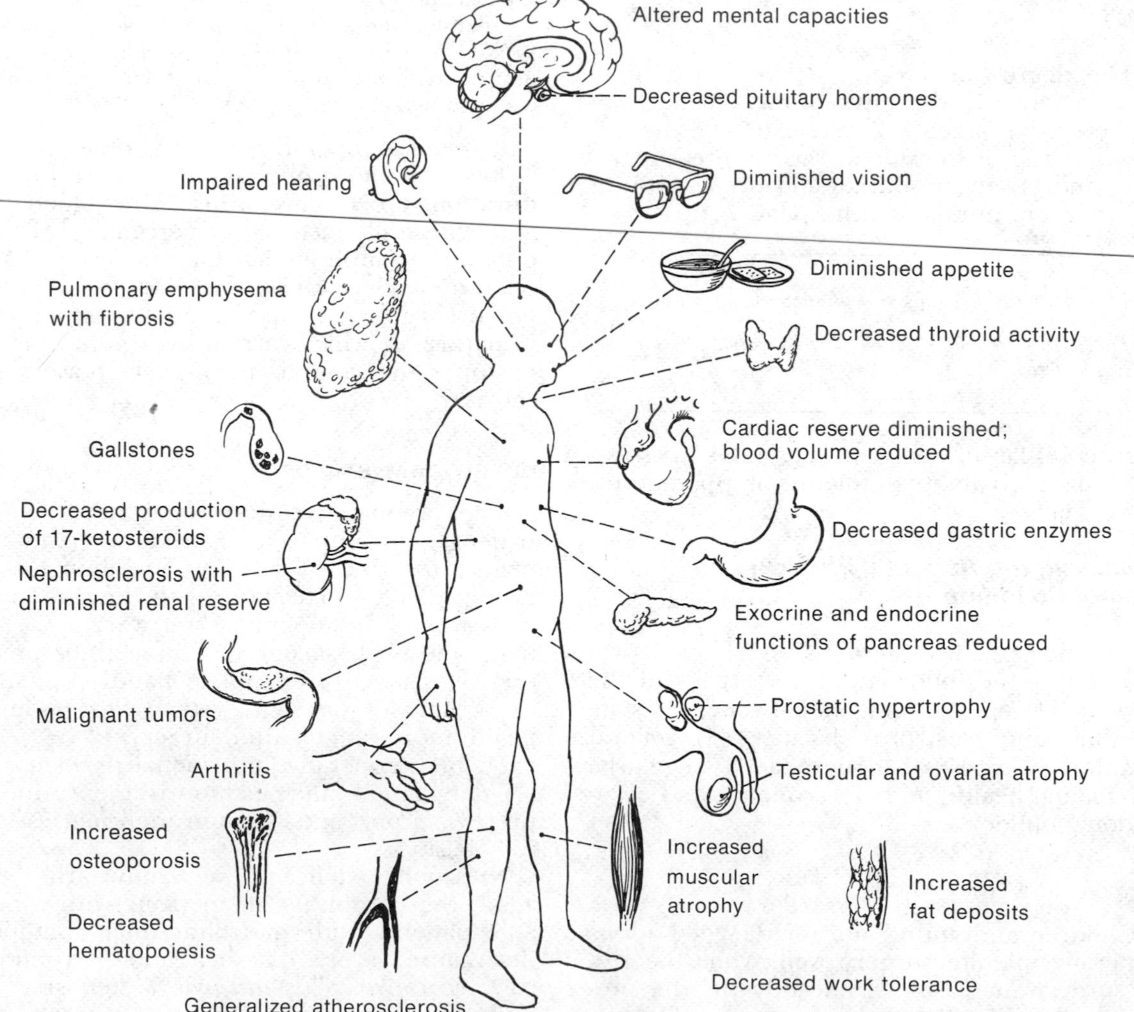

Figure 16–2. Potential pathophysiologic changes with aging. The risk of surgery increases for the elderly person because the functional reserve of body organs may have been diminished by degenerative processes or by diseases developed over the years.

▶ The obese patient is also more susceptible to postoperative pulmonary complications. Because the efficiency of respiratory muscles is decreased by obesity, coughing and deep breathing exercises may be considerably more difficult for obese patients. This difficulty with lung expansion may lead to hypoventilation and oxygen deficiency.

Treatment of the obese patient prior to surgery requires a strict reducing diet and evaluation and care of conditions such as hypertension and diabetes mellitus.

FLUID AND ELECTROLYTE BALANCE

Dehydration and hypovolemia predispose the patient to complications both during and after surgery. Dehydration may result from prolonged vomiting, diarrhea, and bleeding, coupled with inadequate fluid intake. To correct dehydration, fluids are usually administered intravenously or by hypodermoclysis during the preoperative period.

Electrolyte imbalances, like water imbalances, also increase operative risk. It is particularly important to correct K^+, Mg^{++}, and Ca^{++} deficiencies and H^+ imbalances prior to surgery by means of proper diet, IV infusions, and so forth. (See Chapter 12.)

GENERAL HEALTH

The presence of any *infectious* process or any serious *physiologic malfunctioning* increases the operative risk. Thus the surgeon, aided by the nurse and laboratory personnel, examines the surgical candidate for the presence of infection and to determine the adequacy of cardiovascular function, pulmonary function, genitourinary function, metabolic function, neurologic function, and hematologic factors.

Infection. *Any* infection, even a minor cold on the day of surgery, can affect the course of surgery adversely. In addition, when the surgical site is near the region of the lymphatics draining an infection, the likelihood of a postoperative wound infection becomes greater. Thus, physicians and nurses must be alert to the presence of such symptoms as sneezing, coughing, a sore throat, an elevated temperature, and the appearance of skin lesions, boils, or rashes. An elevated white count should also be reported to the surgeon. Any of these findings may result in the cancellation or postponement of surgery.

Cardiovascular Function. The presence of minor or well controlled heart ailments generally has little effect upon operative risk. Heart conditions that *do* increase risk are angina pectoris, a recent myocardial infarction (within the previous 6 months), malignant hypertension, and severe uncompensated congestive heart failure. In the elderly, risk is also increased by hypovolemia and anemia. Also, the presence of peripheral vascular disease can result in impaired tissue healing if the operation involves the extremities.

Patients suspected of having cardiovascular disease should be carefully observed for an elevated blood pressure; slow or rapid, irregular pulse; edema; cold, blue extremities; weakness; and shortness of breath. Typical *laboratory* and *diagnostic studies* of cardiovascular function ordered preoperatively are electrocardiogram, central venous pressure, red blood count, hematocrit, hemoglobin, and serum Na^+.

Preoperative *treatment* of patients with cardiovascular disease includes rest, a low sodium or low cholesterol diet, heart medications such as digitalis, and the judicious administration of fluids.

Pulmonary Function. Crippling pulmonary conditions, such as emphysema and bronchiectasis, increase operative risk because they impair the patient's ability to exchange CO_2 and O_2. These conditions also predispose the patient to severe pulmonary infections.

In determining the presence of hazardous pulmonary malfunction, observe patients for shortness of breath, wheezing, clubbed fingers, chest pain, and coughing with the expectoration of copious and/or purulent mucus. Question the patient carefully concerning smoking habits; also obtain a history of respiratory allergies and infections. The doctor will order a chest x-ray for diagnostic purposes.

Patients with severe respiratory disease are usually treated preoperatively with aerosol treatments, postural drainage, antibiotics, and restricted smoking. A baseline arterial blood gas to evaluate pulmonary functioning may also be obtained from a patient with known respiratory disease. To help prevent postoperative respiratory complications, these individuals need preoperative instruction in the deep breathing and coughing exercises that they will practice following surgery (see p. 388).

Genitourinary Function. The surgical patient needs adequate renal function to eliminate protein wastes and to preserve fluid and electrolyte balance. Genitourinary conditions that increase operative risk are advanced renal insufficiency, acute nephritis, and prostatic hypertrophy. As stated earlier, in the elderly male patient, prostatic hypertrophy obstructs the normal flow of urine and predisposes the patient to urinary infection.

To assess genitourinary function, observe the preoperative patient carefully for the serious symptoms of frequent urination, dysuria, and anuria. Also, check the appearance of the patient's urine; if it is cloudy or bloody rather than clear amber in color, renal disease may be present. Any abnormal findings are reported to the surgeon.

The most commonly ordered preoperative tests of renal function are:

Urinalysis. Urinalysis is performed on either a clear voided specimen or a catheterized specimen to check the urine for red or white blood cells (may indicate an infection or tumor), casts (may indicate renal disease), protein (may indicate renal disease), sugar (usually indicates diabetes), and specific gravity (if low, i.e., under 1.010, the kidney is evidently unable to concentrate urine; if elevated, i.e., over 1.025, the patient is dehydrated).

Blood Urea Nitrogen (BUN) or Non-Protein Nitrogen (NPN). These laboratory studies test the ability of the kidney to excrete urea and protein wastes. If the findings are seriously abnormal, the patient is a poor surgical risk since postoperative renal failure may develop. To decrease risk, serious kidney diseases and urinary infections must be treated with appropriate measures *prior* to surgery. (Renal function tests are covered in Unit XIII).

Metabolic and Liver Function. Untreated *diabetes mellitus* greatly magnifies surgical risks, as it predisposes the patient to infection and to poor tissue healing. As you will see in Chapter 72, diabetes is diagnosed by means of urine and blood tests and is generally treated by proper diet, proper exercise, and insulin injections.

Liver disease, such as Laennec's cirrhosis, also increases risk because an impaired liver is unable to detoxify dangerous drugs, to produce and excrete bile, and to metabolize carbohydrates, fats, and amino acids. In addition, poor liver function is associated with poor wound healing and a higher rate of infection. Patients with a history of alcoholism and with signs of jaundice and ascites require a careful examination for liver disease prior to surgery. Since these persons are usually malnourished and debilitated, the doctor will generally order a high caloric diet, IV solutions, and vitamins as a part of their preoperative regimen.

Neurologic Factors. The preoperative patient should receive a thorough neurologic physical examination that includes assessment and evaluation of the cranial nerves, reflex response of the upper and lower extremities, sensory reflexes, and cerebellar response (see Chapter 25).

The neurologic examination is important for these reasons:

a. To assess the preoperative patient's general health.

b. To assess the patient's possible reactions to the anesthetics and analgesics used during surgery—both of which have a depressant effect upon the central nervous system.

c. To develop a preoperative neurologic baseline evaluation against which to compare the patient's postoperative neurologic status—especially if the patient has suffered some disturbance in neurologic functioning during surgery.

Serious neurologic conditions, such as uncontrolled epilepsy or severe Parkinson's disease, increase surgical risk. Important neurologic findings in preoperative patients are: severe headaches, frequent dizziness, lightheadedness, ringing in the ears, unsteady gait, unequal pupils, and a history of convulsions.

Hematologic Factors. Most surgical procedures result in some blood loss, even in persons whose blood coagulates normally. Thus, patients with missing or abnormal coagulation factors face the complications of severe bleeding, hemorrhage, and shock coincident with surgery. Findings of importance that point to abnormal hematologic factors are:

a. A history of bleeding tendencies

b. Symptoms such as easy bruising, excessive bleeding following dental extractions and shaving, severe nosebleeds

c. The presence of hepatic or renal disease

d. Prior use of anticoagulants

e. Abnormal bleeding time, prothrombin time, or platelet counts (discussed in Unit XIV)

Patients with the above findings are given blood transfusions prior to surgery to correct blood volume deficits or anemia. Additional blood is always on hand for patients with coagulation problems in event of hemorrhage during surgery or during the postoperative period.

USE OF DRUGS

Many preoperative patients take prescribed or nonprescription drugs that can increase operative risk by (1) increasing coagulation time or (2) interacting unfavorably with the anesthetic. Drugs that may result in complications for the surgical patient are:

- *Anticoagulants.* Can cause hemorrhage during surgery.
- *Antibiotics.* Can combine unfavorably with the anesthetic agent, thereby causing untoward effects.
- *Tranquilizers.* Increase hypotension and, thus, can cause shock.
- *Thiazide diuretics.* Can create potassium imbalances.
- *Steroids.* Prolonged use can cause hypofunction of the adrenal cortex and thus impair physiologic responses to the stress of anesthesia and surgery.

Other drugs and their significant effects during anesthesia and surgery are listed in Table 16–4.

MENTAL OUTLOOK

The patient who greatly fears an impending operation, the anesthetic, and postoperative pain and discomforts significantly increases the surgical risk. Fears of surgery are not always in proportion to the seriousness of the surgery; therefore, the fact that a contemplated operation is minor in nature does *not* mean that a patient will be free from fear. Indeed, apprehensive patients undergoing a minor orthopedic operation or tonsillectomy have been known to die in surgery from a cardiac arrest, possibly triggered by their extreme anxiety.

A patient who feels and states that death is imminent in surgery or who is otherwise greatly afraid of surgery needs opportunities to talk about these fears with concerned staff members. Do not give false reassurance to such a patient or dismiss such fears. An extreme fear of surgery is a dangerous problem; it must be taken seriously by the staff responsible for the patient's operative course. The attending physician should be alerted when such fears are detected in preoperative patients. The physician may then be able to give the patient more information regarding the surgery.

Maladjusted patients with a past history of severe depression, paranoia, and other mental illnesses may also adapt poorly to the stress of surgery. Sometimes mentally disturbed persons, who are generally able to function at home and at work despite their emotional problems, develop full-blown psychoses or neuroses postoperatively.

The *will to live* is an important aspect of the patient's mental outlook. A patient who wants to get well will vigorously cooperate in every way possible in treatments designed to reduce postoperative complications. By turning, coughing, and deep breathing after surgery, the patient contributes to reducing the possibility of thromboembolus, pneumonia, or atelectasis. Patients who have "lost the will to live" frequently do little or nothing to help themselves, thereby prolonging their recovery from surgery.

TABLE 16–4. COMMONLY USED DRUGS WITH SIGNIFICANT EFFECTS DURING ANESTHESIA AND SURGERY

Drug	Comment
Anticoagulants	Usually should be discontinued or dosage reduced before surgery
Tetracycline	Predisposes to renal insufficiency when given with methoxyflurane anesthesia
Aminoglycoside antibiotics (kanamycin, gentamicin, streptomycin, neomycin)	May enhance neuromuscular blockage following tubocurarine, etc.
Propranolol	During anesthesia may enhance myocardial depression, induce bronchospasm, and inhibit circulatory response to blood loss
Quinidine, procainamide, lidocaine	May enhance myocardial depression, impair conduction, cause peripheral vasodilatation, and potentiate neuromuscular blockade
Antihypertensives	May aggravate hypotension
Corticosteroids	Increased demand during surgery usually requires increased dosage
Anticonvulsants (e.g., phenobarbital, phenytoin)	By inducing hepatic microsomal enzymes, may increase metabolism of anesthetic drugs
MAO inhibitors (e.g., tranylcypromine, pargyline)	May cause hypertensive crises when given in conjunction with sympathomimetic agents
Phenothiazines	May enhance hypotensive effects of other drugs
Neostigmine	May predispose to respiratory failure postoperatively in patients with myasthenia gravis
Levodopa	May cause hypotension and occasionally arrhythmias
Glaucoma medication	These drugs should usually be discontinued preoperatively
Insulin	Dosage should be reduced during surgery

From Dunphy, J. E., et al.: *Current Surgical Diagnosis and Treatment,* 3rd ed. Los Altos, Calif.: Lange Medical Publications, 1977, p. 184.

ECONOMIC AND OCCUPATIONAL STATUS

Minor surgery may entail little expense for the patient and may result in the loss of only a few days from work or school. However, major surgery, even if most medical and hospital costs are covered by insurance, often creates tremendous financial problems for the patient and significant others because the patient may have no income for weeks or even months. In addition, some surgeries may force the patient to undergo an unwanted job change. For example, a heavy construction worker who undergoes amputation of a limb will need to seek a more sedentary job following surgery.

The Extent of the Disease

Although surgical risk clearly rests upon the physical and mental condition of the patient, the degree of risk also depends upon the *disease* being treated, more specifically the *nature* of the disease, the *site* of the disease, and the *length of time* the patient has been ill with the disease.

Nature of the Disease. Is the disease *benign*

or *malignant?* This is one of the gravest questions a surgeon must answer, for malignancy greatly increases risk, even though at the same time it often makes surgery the treatment of choice for removal of the cancerous cells. When the surgeon must partially or totally remove an organ because of cancer or another disease, the extent of risk depends upon the *importance of function* of the excised organ. For example, removal of the gallbladder is not as serious as removal of the stomach.

Location of the Disease. Operative risk depends upon the location of the disease and of the organ or organs requiring surgery. Surgical risk decreases in descending order in the following sites: heart, thorax, esophagus, brain, rectum, colon, stomach, lung.[72]

Duration of the Disease. The longer a patient has had a disease, the greater the surgical risk involved in correcting the disorder. Risk increases with chronicity because chronic diseases such as cancer are severely debilitating, thereby lowering the patient's resistance to stress and infection.

Extent of the Surgical Procedure

Operative risk increases proportionately to the magnitude of the operation. Thus, the risk involved in minor surgery, e.g., a D and C (dilatation and curettage), is far less than in extensive major surgery such as colon resection. In major surgery, factors such as blood loss, tissue and organ trauma, and prolonged operating time all increase risk.

Caliber of the Professional Staff

Risk decreases for the surgical patient when the hospital staff is adequate in number, competent and well trained, and when the hospital is well equipped. Even very sick patients with prolonged illnesses who are facing lengthy operations have a greater chance of survival among interested, highly knowledgeable physicians and nurses working efficiently in a fully equipped setting.

CHAPTER 17

PREPARING THE PATIENT FOR SURGERY

In this chapter we discuss preparing patients for operations that are either required or elective and that have been scheduled by the surgeon a few days or weeks prior to the patient's admission to the hospital. In the case of emergency surgery and certain urgent procedures, some of the preparations cannot be carried out fully owing to lack of time. However, it is the responsibility of the nurse and of the surgeon to prepare every patient *as fully as possible,* despite intervening circumstances, in order to decrease operative risk and to ensure the patient's postoperative safety.

Generally, the specific preparation of a patient for a planned operation takes place during three time periods: (1) upon admission and during the day or days prior to the operation, (2) the night before surgery, and (3) on the morning or day of surgery.

GENERAL PREPARATION OF THE PATIENT PRIOR TO SURGERY

The preoperative patient may be admitted to the surgical floor the day before or several days prior to the planned surgery, depending upon the extent of preoperative treatment required. For example, alcoholic patients or cachectic patients suffering from cancer may be admitted a week or more before their scheduled operation in order to correct nutritional and fluid-electrolyte deficiencies.

During the admission of a preoperative patient, important data can be collected. A thorough assessment of patient systems enables the nurse to establish a baseline of preoperative patient functioning pertinent to nursing care. This information will aid in planning and carrying out pre- and postoperative care.

Preoperative admission of a patient includes the following:

1. Introduction of the patient and significant others to the hospital environment
2. Obtaining vital signs
3. Weighing the patient
4. Ordering necessary laboratory tests
5. Interviewing the patient

Information gathered during a *purposeful* interview will aid in detecting problems that may arise both pre- and postoperatively. The *manner* in which the interview is carried out plays a large part in determining the extent of pre- and postoperative anxiety experienced by the patient.

The nurse-patient interview has several purposes:

1. The interview allows the nurse to establish rapport with the patient and significant others.
2. The patient explains to the nurse his or her understanding of the impending surgery and from that information the nurse may evaluate the need for further teaching.
3. The patient's personality may be evaluated at this time. This information will prove useful during development of the pre- and postoperative teaching care plan (e.g., an apprehensive preoperative patient may need more frequent repetition of instruction and more reinforcement than a less anxious patient.)
4. The interview allows the nurse to reassure the patient and answer general questions.

Specific information obtained during the preoperative interview includes:

- ▶ Has the patient had any serious illnesses or previous operations?
- ▶ Which drugs has the patient taken in the past; what drugs are currently being taken?
- ▶ Does the patient have any allergies or dietary restrictions?
- ▶ Is the patient experiencing any symptoms or discomforts at this time?
- ▶ What is the patient's occupation?
- ▶ Does the patient have a religious affiliation?
- ▶ Who are the patient's significant others? For instance, is the patient married? How many dependents does the patient have?
- ▶ Does the patient have health insurance?
- ▶ Does the patient have any questions about the impending operation?

This information will help to uncover the need for support services — i.e., financial aid if the patient has no insurance, a clergyman for a pre- and postoperative visit.

After completion of the preliminary admissions procedure (including interview, documentation on the patient's chart, and preparation of a preoperative patient care plan), the following aspects of preoperative care may then be considered in detail: psychologic, legal, physiologic, instructional and preventive.

Psychologic Aspects

As we emphasized in the first chapter of this unit, all patients are somewhat fearful of surgery — some more so than others. The *extent* to which people are afraid of surgery depends upon their basic personalities, habitual reactions to stress over the years, general state of mental health, and the preconceptions that they have concerning surgery and anesthesia.

Fear of the unknown is one of the most important causes of preoperative anxiety in patients who are otherwise mentally stable. Other fears harbored by preoperative patients center on postoperative pain, the discovery of cancer, the loss of organs that have special meaning for them, the hazard of death, anesthesia hazards, vulnerability while unconscious, threat of loss of job and financial security, loss of social and familial roles, and the problem of being separated from loved ones and former activities.

Patients react in many ways to fear. When facing an operation, patients may express their fears through a variety of behavior, e.g., by becoming silent and withdrawn, hopeless and helpless, childish, belligerent, evasive, tearful, or clinging. Almost all patients, regardless of diagnosis, regress to some degree when hospitalized and feel helpless when first admitted into the hospital environment.

At times, hospital personnel may inadvertently be insensitive to the fears of a preoperative patient. Because of their familiarity with the risks and other aspects of surgical treatment, physicians and nurses may forget that the experience of surgery is *unique* to each patient.

What can you do to help the preoperative patient adjust to the hospital and overcome the fear of surgery?

- ▶ Give the patient explanations or printed information about hospital routines, visiting hours, mealtimes, the location of the chapel, and so forth.
- ▶ Giving full explanations of all procedures the patient may undergo will help to reduce anxiety and fear. The patient should have an idea of what the pre-, intra-, and postoperative course will entail. Prior consultation between the nurse and physician is important in maintaining uniformity and accuracy of content. The patient should be made aware of the reasons for x-ray and laboratory procedures; how they will be performed, and what discomfort may be experienced. Likewise, the reasons for all nursing measures are explained, and possible discomfort involved is discussed. If the physician plans to transfer the patient to the intensive care unit following surgery, answer the patient's questions concerning intensive care.
- ▶ Allow the *patient* to take the lead in asking questions concerning the operation and the postoperative period; give only as much information as the patient wishes to know. However, if the patient is very withdrawn or aggressive, use your communication skills to encourage expression of fears and concerns.
- ▶ Patients undergoing major procedures such as a mastectomy, laryngectomy, or colostomy frequently profit from being introduced to people who have successfully recovered from these operations. For example, you may wish to contact the local laryngectomy or colostomy club and arrange for a club member to visit the patient.
- ▶ Occupational therapy can be arranged for patients who are facing an extended preoperative period. Games, handicrafts, and television all serve to distract the patient and ease fear and loneliness.
- ▶ Ascertain the patient's religious preference and arrange for a priest, minister, or rabbi to visit *if the patient so desires.*

Handling fears in these ways can smooth the patient's operative course. Studies show that the calm, emotionally prepared preoperative patient is able to withstand the induction of anesthesia better and also experiences less postoperative nausea and vomiting and fewer postoperative complications.

Legal Aspects

Any patient undergoing a surgical procedure, however minor, *must* sign an operative permit. The operative permit guards the *patient* against submitting to operations that she or he does not know about or does not want; it also protects the *hospital staff* and the *surgeon* from legal action in which the patient or the family claim that an operation was performed without the patient's permission or knowledge.

> *Signed permission is needed for* each *procedure, however minor, if the surgeon plans to enter a body cavity.*

The patient must have a full explanation of the operation *before* signing the permit; pictures and diagrams may be necessary. Moreover, the patient *must* be told about possible complications and disfigurements that may result from the surgery. The patient needs to know if any organs or body parts may be removed. Explanations must be given in terms which the *patient* readily understands. In sum, the patient needs an honest and fair statement of what may be faced both in surgery and following the operation.

Adults sign their own operative permits unless they are unconscious or mentally incompetent; in these instances a relative or guardian will sign the form. Children under 18 must be signed for by an adult, preferably a relative. If the child's family cannot be present to sign the permit, permission can be obtained from a parent by telephone, wire, or letter. When the minor's relatives cannot be located at all, the surgeon may sign the permit personally, depending on the laws in the state, or a court order may have to be obtained permitting the operation.

Once the permit has been signed, it becomes a permanent part of the chart. Make certain that the operative permit accompanies the patient's chart to the operating room.

Physiologic Aspects

As we emphasized in Chapter 16, the patient should be in as optimum a state of health as possible if surgical risk is to be kept a minimum. Thus, the patient's past medical history will need to be explored carefully as well as any current medical problems. Prior to the date of surgery, the staff must make every effort to (1) correct dietary deficiencies if they exist, (2) reduce the obese paient's weight, (3) correct fluid and electrolyte imbalances, (4) restore an inadequate blood volume with blood transfusions, (5) treat any specific ailments, e.g., diabetes, heart disease, renal insufficiency, (6) halt or cure any infectious process, and (7) treat the alcoholic patient with vitamin supplementation and intravenous infusions or oral fluids if the patient is dehydrated.

Instructional and Preventive Aspects

Teaching is an important aspect of the patient's surgical preparation. Studies have shown that well-prepared patients have less difficulty undergoing anesthesia and have a shorter, less complicated postoperative hospital stay than those who are given minimal information. Basic principles of teaching should be kept in mind during preoperative patient teaching sessions.

PRINCIPLES OF TEACHING

1. Consult and confer with the physician to ascertain what information has already been given to the patient, in order to maintain uniformity and accuracy of content.
2. Increased preoperative anxiety may be caused by offering excessive information to the patient. What the patient wants and needs to know may be determined by the nurse-patient interview and by conferring with the physician.
3. Speak clearly and use terminology that the patient will understand.
4. Plan short, frequent teaching sessions rather than overwhelming the patient with large amounts of information at a single sitting.
5. *Always* allow adequate time for the patient to ask questions regarding any of the informational materials that have been given.
6. Question the patient to determine whether the material has been comprehended.
7. Require the patient to give a return demonstration of procedures and skills that have been taught, as this further shows understanding.
8. Repeat information as necessary; preoperative anxiety often interferes with the learning and retention of new information.
9. *Remember*—Each patient is a unique individual. Alter teaching methods to suit individual patient needs.
10. Involve the patient's significant others in the preoperative preparation activities and include them during preoperative teaching. Keep concerned others informed of the patient's daily postoperative progress.

Patient teaching can be achieved on an individual basis, nurse-to-patient, or in a group setting. Many times patients experience decreased postoperative complications when they are able to share their preoperative fears and anxieties with fellow patients in a group.

PREOPERATIVE INSTRUCTION

Specifically, patients need to be instructed preoperatively concerning the proper way to cough, deep breathe, turn, and move their extremities during the postoperative period. Such instruction, given in sufficient detail and at the correct time, greatly reduces operative and postoperative complications.

The best *time* to instruct patients concerning their role in preventive techniques is relatively close to the time of the surgery, e.g., the afternoon or evening prior to their operation. If instruction is given several days in advance, the patient may forget the instructions; on the other hand, the patient who is taught preventive measures an hour or so before surgery may be too apprehensive to listen or too heavily sedated to comprehend.

Unfortunately, there are times when the patient may not be adequately prepared for surgery. Such instances occur when the patient arrives late the evening before surgery and undergoes several tests in a short period of time. Emergency surgery poses a similar problem. However, always make an effort to give the patient and significant others some preoperative preparation.

Preoperative instruction must, first of all, include the practice of proper deep breathing and coughing maneuvers. These exercises are particularly valuable for patients over 50 years old, as well as for any patient experiencing shortness of breath, severe coughing, large amounts of mucus, and other respiratory problems.

Deep Breathing Exercises. The correct form of *breathing* for postoperative patients is *diaphragmatic-abdominal* breathing. This method may be demonstrated by inhaling slowly through the nose, distending the abdomen and exhaling slowly through the mouth, pulling the abdomen in until all air has been expelled. After you have demonstrated the method, ask the patient to perform it. Have the patient:

- ▶ Sit on the edge of the bed or lie back, with knees flexed to relax the abdominal musculature (the patient may lie on either side if lying on the back is impossible)
- ▶ Place hands on the lateral mid-abdomen
- ▶ Inhale through the nose until the upper abdomen balloons outward
- ▶ Exhale through the mouth while contracting the abdominal muscles and squeezing the air out

The patient should be instructed to use this breathing method five to ten times every hour during the postoperative period.

Coughing Exercises. *Coughing* exercises may be taught by using the nursing demonstration method, accompanied by an explanation to increase the patient's understanding of the rationale. The patient may be in a sitting or lying position. Have the patient take a deep breath, exhaling through the mouth, and then follow with a short breath while coughing from deep in the lungs. Deep breathing exercises should be done before coughing to stimulate the cough reflex. Patients who will have thoracic or abdominal incisions may be shown how to "splint" their incision in order to minimize pressure and control pain. To "splint" the incision, the patient will lace the fingers and hold them tightly across the incision before coughing. A small pillow or folded towel held over the incision may also be used to facilitate splinting. These breathing and coughing exercises help expand collapsed lungs and prevent postoperative pneumonia and atelectasis.

Turning Exercises. The patient will need to practice *turning* from side to side using the side rails to assist movements. Turning will help prevent venous stasis and respiratory problems. The patient should be instructed to turn every 1 to 2 hours during the postoperative period.

Extremity Exercises. Finally, the patient should practice *extremity exercises.* Ask the patient to flex and exend the hip, knee, and ankle joints and to move each foot in a circular motion. These exercises will help to prevent circulatory problems, such as thrombophlebitis, by facilitating venous return to the heart. Postoperative "gas pains" or flatus may also be decreased.

Figure 17–1 illustrates the various exercises that can be taught preoperatively.

PREPARING THE PATIENT ON THE EVE OF SURGERY

Major considerations on the evening before surgery are: (1) preparing the patient's skin, (2) preparing the patient's gastrointestinal tract, (3) preparing for anesthesia, and (4) promoting rest and sleep.

Preparing the Patient's Skin

The object of a thorough bath and a skin "prep" of the operative area is to reduce to a minimum the bacteria on the patient's skin. Such preparation reduces the number of bacteria that will be carried into the deeper tissues from the skin when the surgeon makes the incision.

"Prep" procedures are done by different staff members in different hospitals. Some institutions have a prep orderly or prep nurse who does all the skin preparation of preoperative patients. In other hospitals, nurses in charge of preoperative patients do the prep for them the evening before surgery.

The actual prep procedure also differs according to the specific hospital's policy. In most institutions an antiseptic soap is used to gently scrub the skin. This type of soap may be applied to the operative site repeatedly several days before surgery; it may also be left on the skin for 5 to 10 minutes following application. These soaps are valuable in that their repeated use leads to a substantial reduction in the number of bacteria on the skin.

No matter which cleansing agents or what prep procedure you use, you will find the following principles useful:

- ▶ The areas of the prep should always be wider and longer than the area of the proposed incision, because the surgeon may unexpectedly need to make a larger incision.
- ▶ Use a strong light, well focused, and a sterile safety razor with a new blade.
- ▶ Shave *against* the grain of the hair shaft to insure a clean, close shave.
- ▶ While doing the prep, check the skin for nicks, irritations, and cuts; all these are potential sites for infection. Chart the presence of these.

In some hospitals, a *depilatory* cream is used instead of the customary shave. Depilatory cream is a chemical compound that is applied to the surgical site, left on for 10 minutes, and then removed along with the hair. Occasionally, transient rashes result from the depilatory cream. Figure 17–2 illustrates preoperative skin preparation.

Preparing the Gastrointestinal Tract

The patient's gastrointestinal tract needs special preparation on the evening before surgery to: (1) reduce the possibility of vomiting and aspiration during anesthesia and (2) prevent contamination from fecal material during intestinal tract or bowel surgery.

Preparation of the gastrointestinal tract involves: food and fluid restriction, the administration of enemas, and sometimes the insertion of a gastric or intestinal tube.

The *restriction of foods and oral fluids* is essential to prevent vomiting during surgery, the aspiration of any vomitus, and the resultant development of aspiration pneumonia. Because solid food must be withheld 7 to 10 hours before the operation, most patients receive nothing by mouth (NPO) after midnight; however, water can usually be given up to 4 hours before surgery, depending upon the hospital policy. When surgery is not scheduled until late afternoon, the patient may eat a light breakfast in the morning.

When a patient is NPO, the staff usually (1) tells the patient not to eat or drink and why; (2) removes food and water from the patient's bedside stand; (3) places an "NPO" sign on the door and on the bed; (4) marks the patient's Kardex "NPO" (5) informs the diet kitchen that the patient is awaiting surgery, and (6) informs the oncoming staff that the patient is to receive nothing by mouth. Patients who are extremely debilitated or malnourished may receive intravenous infusions of glucose, amino acids, or plasma up to the moment of surgery.

Enemas are not routinely ordered preoperatively in most hospitals, because enemas are upsetting both psychologically and physiologically. However, two or three enemas are generally given the evening prior to *operations on the intestinal tract or colon* in order to prevent contamination of the peritoneal cavity from the spillage of fecal matter during surgery. In some cases the surgeon may order laxatives and enemas to be given over the 2 to 3 days before colonic surgery.

Tubes for gastric or intestinal suction are sometimes inserted the evening before or the morning of surgery in order to remove gastric

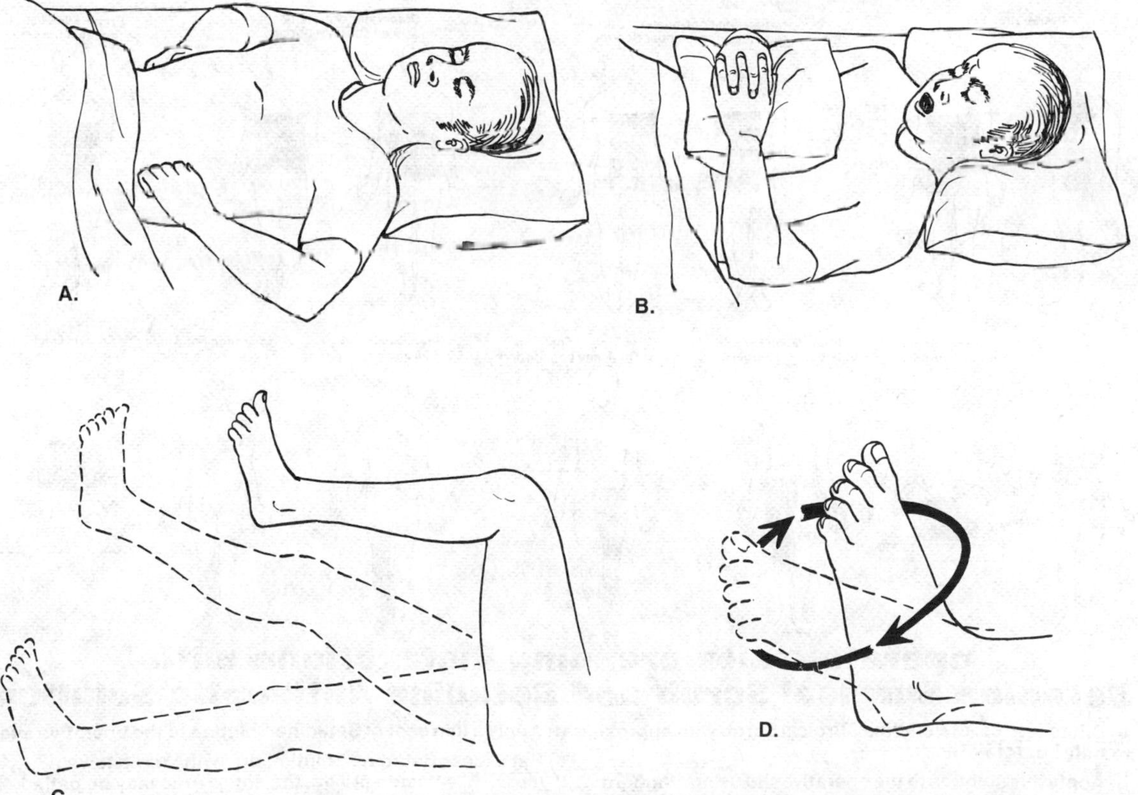

Figure 17–1. Exercises taught during the preoperative period to be done by the surgical patient postoperatively. **A.** Deep breathing exercise. **B.** Coughing exercise, with pillow to "splint" incision. **C** and **D.** Extremity exercises.

PATI I'T PR O ATIV PR PA ATION SH ET

Patient's Name______________________________

Date and Time of Operation______________________________

DATE TIME

Note: Circle the Skin Areas to be Prepared for Surgery as Determined by the Type of Operation

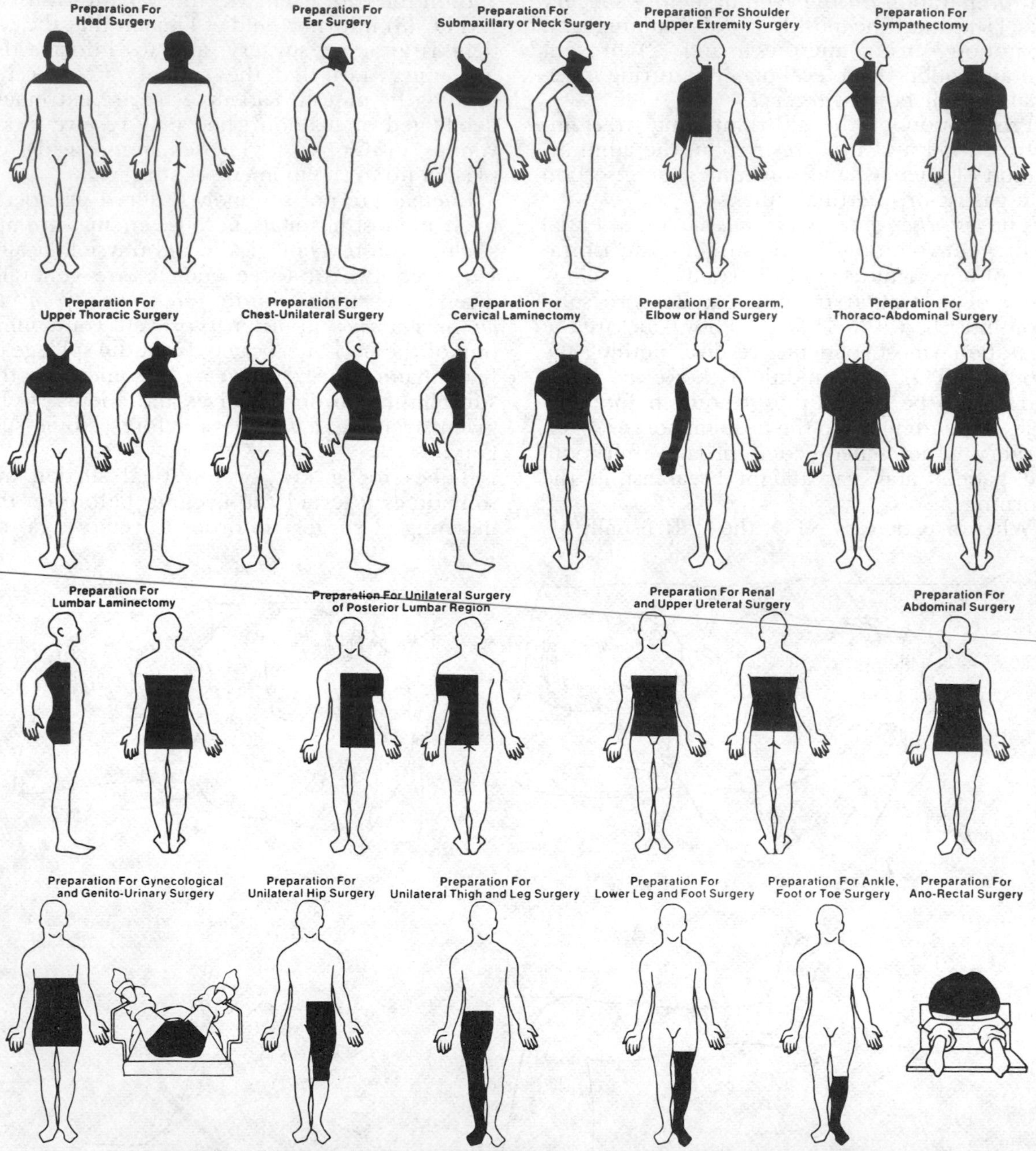

Preparation For Head Surgery

Preparation For Ear Surgery

Preparation For Submaxillary or Neck Surgery

Preparation For Shoulder and Upper Extremity Surgery

Preparation For Sympathectomy

Preparation For Upper Thoracic Surgery

Preparation For Chest-Unilateral Surgery

Preparation For Cervical Laminectomy

Preparation For Forearm, Elbow or Hand Surgery

Preparation For Thoraco-Abdominal Surgery

Preparation For Lumbar Laminectomy

Preparation For Unilateral Surgery of Posterior Lumbar Region

Preparation For Renal and Upper Ureteral Surgery

Preparation For Abdominal Surgery

Preparation For Gynecological and Genito-Urinary Surgery

Preparation For Unilateral Hip Surgery

Preparation For Unilateral Thigh and Leg Surgery

Preparation For Lower Leg and Foot Surgery

Preparation For Ankle, Foot or Toe Surgery

Preparation For Ano-Rectal Surgery

operative site prepping instructions with Betadine Surgical Scrub and Betadine Antiseptic Solution

a) Dilute 5-10 cc. of Betadine Surgical Scrub with approximately 2 oz. of water.

b) Apply this solution to the operative site using standard surgical prepping techniques and rub thoroughly for approximately 5 minutes.

c) Wipe off all Betadine Surgical Scrub with a sterile towel.

d) Apply a thin coat of Betadine Solution to the operative site.

e) Pat excess Betadine Solution dry with sterile towel. If you wish to hasten drying, the entire area may be patted dry so that some brown coloration remains on the skin.

f) If self-adhering plastic drapes are to be used, you may apply these directly over the dried Betadine Solution.

Figure 17–2. Preoperative preparation sheet. (Courtesy of Purdue Frederick Co.)

or intestinal contents. This procedure is usually performed on patients about to undergo major abdominal surgery or intestinal tract surgery. Many types of surgeries require specific preparations; the specific protocol is usually available on the hospital unit.

Preparing for Anesthesia

The anesthesiologist usually visits the preoperative patient the evening before the surgery. During this visit, the anesthesiologist generally examines the patient for evidence of pulmonary problems or upper respiratory infections and investigates the patient's smoking habits. Usually the topics discussed with the patient include the type of anesthetic that is planned, the sensations the patient will experience when undergoing anesthesia, and any fears the patient has concerning anesthesia.

At times, patients are reluctant to disclose their anxieties to the anesthesiologist but may feel comfortable in talking about them with the nurse. The nurse can then tell the anesthesiologist what the patient's anxieties appear to be and ask that these areas be explored further. As we have emphasized, a calm confident patient undergoes the induction of anesthesia more smoothly than the nervous, frightened individual.

Promoting Rest and Sleep

The preoperative patient will rest more completely on the night before surgery if physically comfortable, mentally at ease, and adequately sedated. The patient will sleep better in a freshly made bed and in a well ventilated room. In preparing the patient for rest, give a soothing backrub, and perhaps a glass of warm milk or weak tea, if fluids are not contraindicated. Talk with the patient as you give this care, and listen to any last moment doubts or fears that the patient may have concerning surgery. Try to express a positive attitude toward the surgery.

On the night before surgery, the surgeon will undoubtedly leave an order for a sleeping medication. Encourage patients (especially apprehensive persons) to take their h.s. (hour of sleep) medications so that they will have a good night's sleep to start the operative day.

PREPARING THE PATIENT ON THE DAY OF SURGERY

Early Morning Care

On the morning of surgery, the nurse usually awakens the patient about an hour before preoperative medications are scheduled. During that hour, the nurse generally performs the following tasks:

- ▶ Records the patient's *blood pressure* upon awakening so that the anesthesiologist and recovery room personnel will have a baseline blood pressure reading against which to compare later readings.
- ▶ Records the patient's *temperature, pulse,* and *respiration.*

> *Report to the surgeon any elevation of temperature, because surgery may need to be cancelled due to infection.*

- ▶ Checks to make certain that the skin prep has been completed in a thorough manner.
- ▶ Asks the patient to void and then measures and records the amount of urine.
- ▶ Gives the patient *oral hygiene* and removes any dentures or removable bridge work. (Be certain to store these valuable items according to hospital procedure.)
- ▶ Removes and stores the patient's *jewelry.* Usually patients are allowed to wear their wedding rings (which are taped on). Pierced-ear earrings are removed.
- ▶ Dresses the patient in a clean gown and perhaps ace wraps or support stockings. If the patient has very long hair, braids the hair into two braids. All hair pins are removed to prevent accidental injury, and the head is covered with a protective cap.
- ▶ *Removes colored nail polish,* because the operating room personnel frequently check the patient's nail beds for cyanosis.
- ▶ *Questions the patient* to make certain that food has not been eaten for the last 10 hours nor fluids taken during the preceding 4 hours.
- ▶ *Carries out any special orders* for the administration of enemas, insertion of a Levin tube, or the starting of an intravenous infusion.
- ▶ *Checks the patient's identification band* for accuracy and to make certain that it is secure.

To prevent errors or omissions in the performance of these many preoperation tasks, most hospitals supply nurses with a checklist, like that in Figure 17–3. As each task is completed, it is checked off.

Following these procedures, the patient is given the *preoperative medications.*

The Preoperative Medications

The pharmacologic preparation of the patient for anesthesia varies with the age and condition of the patient and the specific anesthesia which will be given. For this reason, it is important for the anesthesiologist to order the preoperative medications after conferring with the physician.

Preoperative medications are given to allay anxiety, decrease the flow of pharyngeal secretions, reduce the amount of anesthesia to be given, and create amnesia for the events that precede surgery. The four major types of preoperative medications are: sedatives, tranquiliz-

UNIVERSITY HOSPITAL
UNIVERSITY OF WASHINGTON

PRE-OPERATIVE CHECK LIST

ALLERGIES________
WHOLE BLOOD: UNITS ORDERED________
ARRIVED ☐
SKIN PREP ☐ YES ☐ NO
NAME BAND ☐
NAME ON BED ☐
TPR________
BP________
WT________
VOIDED ☐ FOLEY CATH ☐
NPO AFTER MIDNIGHT ☐

ON CHART
ADDRESSOGRAPH ☐
OPERATIVE PERMIT ☐
HISTORY AND PHYSICAL ☐
OLD CHART ☐
DOCTOR'S ORDERS ☐

GOWN ON ☐
JEWELRY: REMOVED ☐
SECURED ☐
DENTURES REMOVED ☐
PROSTHESIS
CONTACTS
GLASSES REMOVED ☐
MAKEUP
NAIL POLISH
HAIRPINS REMOVED ☐

LAB REPORTS
HCT IN CHART ☐
SENT-NO RESULTS ☐
DATE SENT________
UA IN CHART ☐
SENT-NO RESULTS ☐
DATE SENT________
EKG IN CHART ☐
DATE DONE________
MISC. LAB VALUES IF INDICATED________

HS SEDATION________ TIME________
AM SEDATION________ TIME________
HYPO________ TIME________
REMARKS________

UH Form A–293, Rev. 4/74 1-74-805 NURSE'S SIGNATURE

Figure 17–3. Preoperative check list. (Courtesy University Hospital, University of Washington, Seattle.)

ers, narcotic analgesics, and vagolytic or drying agents.

SEDATIVES

Sedatives are given to decrease the patient's anxiety, to lower blood pressure and pulse, and to reduce the amount of general anesthetic to be given in surgery. An overdose of any sedative can lead to respiratory depression. Examples of preoperative sedatives are:

- ► Pentobarbital sodium (Nembutal Sodium) 100 to 150 mg. IM 60 to 90 minutes before surgery.
- ► Secobarbital sodium (Secona Sodium) 100 mg. IM 90 minutes before surgery.

TRANQUILIZERS

Tranquilizers are useful drugs for lowering a patient's anxiety level. Examples of tranquilizers that are given preoperatively are:

- ► Thorazine 12.5 to 25 mg. IM 1 to 2 hours before surgery.
- ► Phenergan 12.5 to 25 mg. IM 1 to 2 hours before surgery.

Tranquilizers can cause a dangerous hypotension both during and after surgery. Nevertheless, one geriatrics specialist recommends using tranquilizers as a premedication for elderly patients in place of opiates. He points out that while tranquilizers cause hypotension, opiates can lead to severe respiratory depression in older patients – a potentially more dangerous situation.

NARCOTIC ANALGESICS

Narcotic analgesics are given preoperatively to relax the patient, to decrease anxiety; and to reduce the amount of narcotics given during surgery. Typical preoperative analgesic agents are:

- ► Morphine sulfate 8 to 15 mg. SQ 1 hour preoperatively.
- ► Demerol 50 to 100 mg. IM 1 hour preoperatively.

Narcotic analgesics such as these are dangerous drugs because of their tendency to cause vomiting, respiratory depression and postural hypotension. Thus, some surgeons do not use narcotic analgesics preoperatively unless the patient is in pain; instead, they order barbiturates and tranquilizers to relax the patient.

VAGOLYTIC OR DRYING AGENTS

Vagolytic or drying agents are given for the following reasons: (1) to reduce the amount of *tracheobronchial secretions,* which can clog the pulmonary tree and result in atelectasis or pneumonia; and (2) to *interrupt vagal nerve impulses,* which act to slow the heart. Tracheobronchial secretions increase during surgery because the mucus-secreting cells of the pharynx, larynx, and tracheobronchial tree are irritated by some general anesthetics, whereas vagal impulses are stimulated by procedures such as intubation during surgery.

Typical vagolytic and drying agents are:

- ► Atropine sulfate 0.3 to 0.6 mg. IM given about 45 minutes before surgery.

Atropine sulfate reduces tracheobronchial secretions and dries the mucous membranes. An overdose of atropine sulfate can cause severe tachycardia.

- ► Scopolamine (Hyoscine) 0.3 to 0.6 mg. SQ 45 minutes before surgery.

Along with drying the mucous membranes, scopolamine causes sedation, amnesia, and euphoria. Unfortunately scopolamine can cause confusion, restlessness, and even hallucinations, especially in the elderly. Elderly patients should be given a smaller than usual dose. Overdoses of scopolamine can result in severe respiratory depression.

PROCEDURE FOR ADMINISTRATION

Remember the following important items when administering preoperative medications:

1. *Give the medication to* the correct patient; *always check the patient's nameband before administering the medication.*
2. *Administer* the correct drug *to the patient; double check the preoperative orders and medication container prior to giving the medication.*

3. *Give* the correct dosage, *double check preoperative medication orders.*

4. *Use* the correct route *for administration, i.e., IM, IV, or SQ.*

5. *Give the medication at* the correct time; *preoperative medications are given at a specific time so that the peak effect occurs before the patient receives anesthesia.*

6. Chart *the pre-op medication, including the dosage, route and site of administration, time given, and the patient's reaction.*

If preoperative medications are administered too early or too late, the induction of anesthesia may be more difficult. Before giving the medication, note whether the blood pressure has been taken and recorded. If the blood pressure has not been taken, obtain a reading *before* giving the medication.

After administering the preoperative medication, put the bed siderails up, lower the shades, turn off bright lights, and tell the patient not to get up without assistance, explaining that medications may cause drowsiness or dizziness. Once the patient has slipped into a peaceful, drowsy state, speak to him or her only when necessary and then briefly and quietly.

Sometimes preoperative medications are not given according to a prepared schedule, but instead are administered "on call" just before the patient goes to surgery. Medications are usually given in this manner when the surgery schedule is tentative or is irregular. Some surgeons question whether preoperative medications given "on call" are of any value. Certainly it is a practice to be avoided whenever possible.

Transporting the Patient to Surgery

When the surgical personnel call for the patient to be transported to surgery, you as a floor nurse must carry out a number of tasks.

The sedated patient should be gently moved to a stretcher, covered with blankets for protection from drafts, and secured with a restraining belt. The nurse checks that the chart accompanies the patient to the operating room. The person responsible for wheeling the patient to surgery must be cautious not to "swing" the cart roughly or walk too rapidly, as this type of movement can cause nausea and dizziness. The physician should be notified of any significant observations made of the patient (e.g., possible allergic reaction to medication, an increased heart rate, or decreased blood pressure).

After the patient has left the floor, you will need to prepare the patient's room, especially if the hospital does not have a recovery room. Setting up the patient's room for postoperative care includes:

- Arranging furniture so the stretcher can easily be brought to the bedside
- Making a surgical bed
- Setting out an emesis basin in event of vomiting
- Bringing in additional equipment, such as blood pressure equipment, IV standards, suction machine and oxygen equipment
- Checking all equipment to make certain it is in working condition

The Patient's Significant Others

During surgery the patient's relatives or friends usually wait in a lounge on the surgical unit. If they must leave the hospital for any reason, ask them for a phone number where they can be reached; also give them the phone number of the hospital and the extension of the surgical floor.

It is important to explain to the patient's family and friends what they may see after the surgery. They should be prepared for the possibility of viewing nasogastric tubes, chest tubes with suction setup, oxygen-supplying equipment, intravenous infusions, bandages, and whatever else may be necessary for the particular patient.

Inform the patient's significant others when you receive word that the surgery is completed, and make certain that the doctor receives word that these persons are waiting to see him or her. Clarify with significant others that the gravity of the operation cannot be judged by the length of time the patient is in the operating room.

There are several reasons why the patient may be in the operating room longer than expected. Surgical patients are usually taken to the operating room in advance of the actual surgical starting time. Often the beginning of the surgery is delayed by a preceding case; the anesthesiologist may also take longer than anticipated in making preparations. The actual induction of the patient may require more time than expected and so delay the start of the surgery.

In discussing the surgery with the patient's significant others, the nurse needs to be aware of information previously given by the physician regarding the immediate surgical outcome and eventual prognosis. The nurse can then answer their questions, confident that this information is in agreement with previous statements. Everyone concerned should be aware, however, that the exact outcome of the surgery cannot be known by anyone before or during the procedure. A positive, realistic attitude should be used in all discussions. Family and friends need to be made aware of the events and issues of the surgery — this should be done by the physician. In addition to an awareness of the issues, many times these people need further interpretation of information they have been given. Thus, the nurse may need to set aside time to relay, and further explain, the information given by the physician.

CHAPTER 18

THE PATIENT IN SURGERY

ADMITTING THE PATIENT TO SURGERY

When the preoperative patient leaves the surgical floor and is wheeled to the operating room, responsibility for care is transferred to the surgical team. This is a highly anxious time for the patient: an introduction, smile, and a warm touch are helpful in allaying fears in a threatening and strange environment. Someone always remains with the premedicated patient, as the possibility of falling from the stretcher — in spite of the safety straps — is always present. The patient's nameband is always to be worn, and the nurse should check to see that all is in order. Keep the patient comfortably covered and respect the patient's modesty by avoiding unnecessary exposure. Staff conversation and noise is kept to a minimum; the patient's drowsy, premedicated state may lead to confusion and misinterpretation of conversations. A calm, assured patient undergoes anesthetic induction with greater ease than a patient who is apprehensive. Answer any questions the patient may have at this time and give reassurance as needed.

Procedures vary among institutions, but usually after admission to the operating room the patient is moved to the operating room table and prepped by the circulating nurse. (In some hospitals the prep is done on the nursing unit.) The patient is then anesthetized, positioned, and sterilely draped.

The Surgical Team

The surgical team is a group of highly trained individuals who must work together as a coordinated team for the welfare and safety of the patient. The team is composed of the surgeon, the assistants, the anesthesiologist or nurse anesthetist, the scrub nurse, and the circulating nurse (Fig. 18–1). Nurses and certain

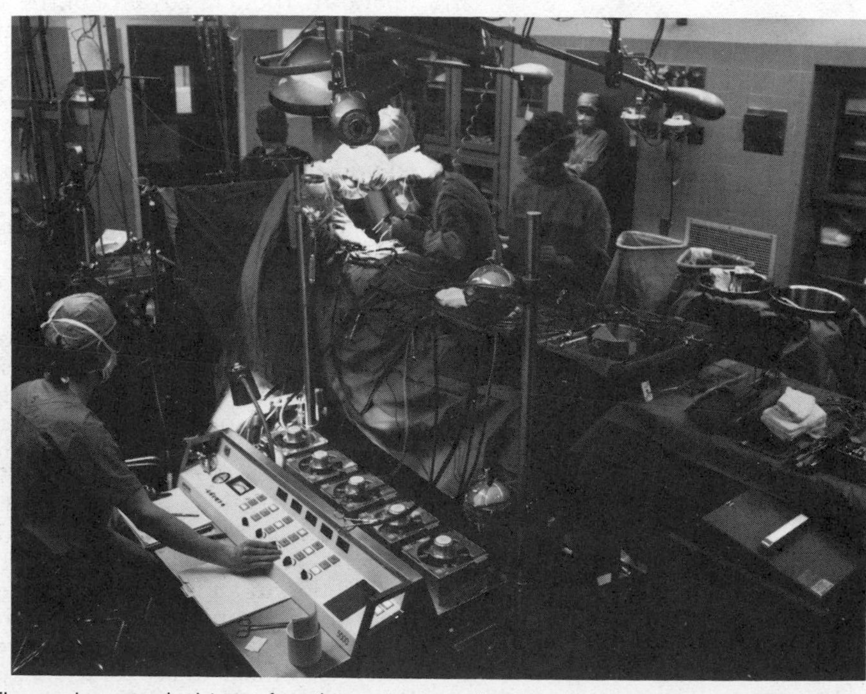

Figure 18–1. The modern surgical team functions as a coordinated unit. (Courtesy University Hospital, University of Washington, Seattle.)

experienced paraprofessionals sometimes also act as the surgeon's assistant.

The *surgeon* heads the surgical team and carries, along with the anesthesiologist, the major responsibility for the patient's life and welfare. It is the surgeon who must make the major decisions as to the course of the surgery, e.g., whether to remove an organ, amputate a limb, or make radical or extensive repairs. The surgeon must be constantly alert to the changing physiologic needs of the patient as the patient strives to adjust to the stress of surgery.

The *assistants* to the surgeon are usually other surgeons or surgical residents who plan to make surgery their career. The assistants expose the operative site by retracting tissues away from the site and by sponging and suctioning blood and serum obscuring the surgeon's vision of the site.

The *anesthesiologist* anesthetizes the patient in order to alleviate pain and induce relaxation. In addition to this major task, the anesthesiologist must maintain the patient's airway; ensure the patient an adequate $O_2 = CO_2$ exchange; infuse blood, fluids, and drugs as necessary; monitor the patient's circulation and respiration; and alert the surgeon immediately in the event of complications. The anesthesiologist carries a heavy responsibility, for it is this person's role to maintain the patient safely in a state that lies somewhere between deep sleep and death.

The *scrub nurse* stands beside the surgeon throughout the operation and supplies the surgeon with instruments and so forth. The surgeon and surgical assistants also scrub; the anesthesiologist does not.

The *circulating nurse* does not "scrub in" or wear sterile gowns or gloves. This nurse is the manager of the operating room — a taxing job indeed! The circulating nurse must make certain that all equipment is working properly before the surgery; must prepare and autoclave instruments for the surgery; alert team members of any breaks in sterile technique; label specimens; and contact the x-ray and pathology departments at the surgeon's request. The circulating nurse's job is to keep the operating room running smoothly and safely by "circulating" around the operating suite bringing needed supplies and drugs to the table and taking away unneeded items or specimens. The Joint Committee on Hospital Accreditation recommends that this role be filled only by a registered nurse.

Other members are added to the surgical team as dictated by the needs of the procedure being performed. A cardiac perfusionist may be present; a pathologist may be called upon to identify the pathologic process discovered; or an x-ray technician may be needed to perform various x-ray procedures while the patient is on the operating table.

Positioning the Surgical Patient

There are several essential factors to be considered in positioning the patient on the operating table. These include site of operation, age and size of patient, type of anesthetic used, and pain experienced by the patient upon movement. The patient's position must be consistent with the maintenance of the vital functions of respiration and circulation. The following surgical positions are shown in Figure 18–2:

1. *Dorsal recumbent position:* This position is customarily used for patients undergoing abdominal surgery.
2. *Trendelenburg position:* This position, which permits the displacement of the intestines into the upper abdomen, is often used during surgery of the lower abdomen and pelvis.
3. *Lithotomy position:* The patient's legs and thighs are flexed at right angles, exposing the perineal and rectal areas. This position facilitates vaginal repairs and dilation and curettage.
4. *Kidney position:* This position is used for the patient donating a kidney or receiving a kidney transplant.
5. *Laminectomy position:* This position is used during laminectomy procedures.
6. *Lateral or chest position:* This position is used for patients undergoing a thoracotomy.

Whatever the patient's position upon the operating table, there are certain general considerations and rules of safety to observe:

When positioning a patient on the operating room table, remember:

1. *Explain to the patient why the measures you are taking are necessary – in simple, understandable terms.*
2. *The patient's dignity must be preserved. Avoid undue exposure.*
3. *Strap the patient to the table with well-padded straps. Nerves, muscles, and bony prominences are padded to prevent nerve and tissue damage.*
4. *Adequate respiratory exchange and vascular circulation must be maintained in order to permit free exchange of gases or pressure on the chest. Pressure on body parts results in impaired and slowed circulation: this can result in sludging of blood and can predispose the patient to thrombus formation.*
5. *Do not allow the patient's extremities to dangle over the sides of the table. This may cause impaired circulation, nerve, or muscle damage.*
6. *Excessive strain on all muscles should be avoided.*
7. *Be certain that the patient's body does not rest upon the hands or fingers.*

Remember that the patient will remain immobile in one position for a long period of time, in some cases for hours! Even with careful positioning, most patients are stiff and sore postoperatively if they spend a prolonged period on the operating table. It is the responsibility of the operating room nurse to ensure that the patient is properly positioned prior to the beginning of surgery. The nurse, in addition, observes the patient throughout the surgery and adjusts any unprotected bony prominences or pressure points.

Because all surgical patients — regardless of diagnosis and type of surgery — undergo anesthesia, we discuss in some detail the purpose of anesthesia, the types of anesthesia, and the dangers and complications of anesthesia.

ANESTHESIA

In the past, a blow on the head or a heavy draft of liquor sufficed to produce an anesthetized state. Today we have many new and sophisticated means. However, despite improvements, anesthesia remains difficult to control and regulate precisely. As one authority observes:

> It [the anesthetized state] must be considered as a comatose state produced by severe drug poisoning during which the patient is subjected to trauma, hemorrhage, starvation, and other abnormal conditions.[47]

If the anesthetized state is so filled with dangers, what then are its benefits and what, more precisely, are its complications?

The Benefits of Anesthesia

Anesthetics are given primarily to completely eradicate the pain of surgery during the operative period. They are also given to relieve fear and anxiety and to relax tissues. Because of new and sophisticated types and methods of anesthesia, severely ill patients can now be operated upon and be expected to survive the operation.

General Dangers and Complications of Anesthesia

The major complications of anesthesia affect the circulatory and respiratory systems, al-

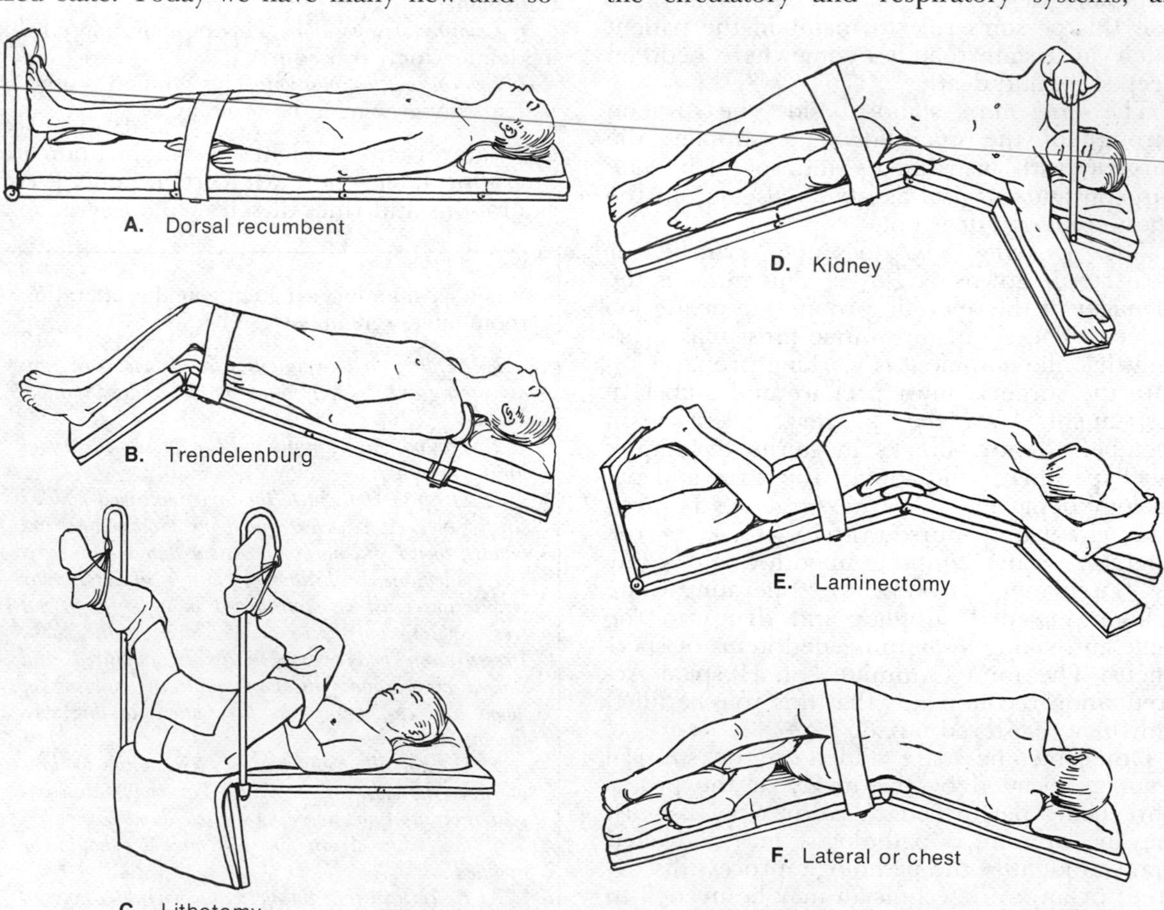

Figure 18–2. Six surgical positions.

though all physiologic functions are somewhat disturbed or suppressed by anesthesia.

Cardiac Arrhythmia and Arrest. The electrochemical process sustaining the normal rhythm of the heart is quite sensitive to many disturbing stimuli, including hypercarbia, acidosis, and others. Anesthetics depress the myocardium and result in CO_2 retention or respiratory acidosis, both of which may lead to a serious cardiac arrhythmia or cardiac arrest.

Diminished Circulation. The circulation may be impaired and diminished, mainly because of the following four problems:

1. The *venous system may fail* to return blood to the heart so that it can be pumped out to the arterial system. Certain anesthetic agents interfere with autonomic nervous system control of the vein walls: the walls become dilated and blood that should be returning to the heart pools within the relaxed veins. Thus, circulation to the heart and tissues is decreased.

2. The *contractility of cardiac muscle* may be diminished by the action of anesthetic agents and may, in turn, decrease cardiac output.

3. *Blood may be poorly distributed* throughout the body, failing to reach vital organs such as the heart, liver, and kidney in sufficient amounts. Anesthesia can upset the delicate mechanisms that control blood distribution and assure adequate circulation to vital organs.

4. *Preoperative medications, potent anesthetics, surgical trauma, anoxia,* and *blood loss* interfere with the complex physiologic mechanisms that support blood pressure. Combined, these items can all lead to *surgical hypotension* and *shock.* In addition, the use of anesthetics lowers the body's adaptive responses to shock, thereby compounding the problem.

Respiratory Depression. Respiratory complications during anesthesia may result from one of the following problems:

1. *Airway obstruction* may occur as a result of the irritation of the respiratory passages by the anesthetic agent. The excess mucus produced by this irritation causes airway obstruction and anoxia.

2. *Central nervous system depression* caused by the use of depressant drugs may lead to hypoxia, hypercarbia, and respiratory failure.

3. Peripheral *neuromuscular conduction* may be disturbed by the use of muscle relaxants. Drugs such as curare and Anectine interrupt the transmission of nervous impulses from nerves to muscles. When the respiratory muscles are affected, respiratory depression results.

4. *Severe spasm* of the bronchial smooth muscle and vocal cords produces a deadly airway obstruction. Both bronchospasm and laryngospasm can result from the irritating or allergenic effects of anesthetics on the bronchial-laryngeal mucosa. Untreated, these spasms may cause anoxia leading to cerebral edema and cardiac arrest.

Vomiting and Aspiration. Some anesthetics abolish certain protective reflexes surrounding the opening of the laryngotracheal area and irritate the gastrointestinal tract. This combination of reduced reflexes and irritation of the gastrointestinal tract may lead to vomiting of gastric content and aspiration into the respiratory tract.

Vomiting and aspiration of vomitus into the respiratory tract sometimes occur during the second, or excitement, stage of anesthesia induction. Also, patients admitted for emergency surgery may have a full stomach and will vomit and aspirate unless an endotracheal tube is inserted immediately upon induction of anesthesia.

Loss of Protective Responses to Pain. A person properly anesthetized cannot feel pain and thus fails to respond normally to painful stimuli. Because this defensive reaction is lost, patients may be accidentally injured during surgery. For example, they may be burned from cauterizing instruments, may suffer circulatory impairment from being too tightly strapped to the operating room table, or may undergo nerve trauma or paralysis as a result of careless or improper positioning during the operation.

Malignant Hyperpyrexia. *Malignant hyperpyrexia* is an unusual phenomenon that occurs while a patient is under general anesthesia. Halothane and succinylcholine are often the anesthetics involved, but cases have occurred with other anesthetics. Malignant hyperpyrexia is characterized by a significant increase in body temperature (at times the temperature may rise to 43.3°C. [110°F.]), increase in heart and respiration rates, and cyanosis.

The mortality rate of malignant hyperpyrexia is high if it is not diagnosed and treated rapidly. Treatment for excessively increased body temperature includes iced intravenous fluids, cessation of anesthesia, hyperventilation with 100% O_2, administration of sodium bicarbonate to fight metabolic acidosis, and immersion in ice.

Other Complications. While the respiratory and circulatory systems are most vulnerable to complications from anesthesia, all systems of the body are disturbed. Gastrointestinal motility and renal function decrease and may fail entirely; metabolic activities are slowed and become disturbed; and often dangerous neurologic changes occur. For example, elderly persons may suffer from a cerebral vascular accident (CVA) due to severe hypotension produced by anesthesia. Anoxia due to airway obstruction may lead to convulsions.

The complications listed above are most likely to occur during the *induction* of the anesthesia. At this critical time, overdoses of the

TABLE 18–1. TYPES OF ANESTHESIA COMPARED

General Anesthesia	Regional Anesthesia
1. *Purpose*: To cause total loss of sensation and complete loss of consciousness by blocking the "awareness areas" within the brain that control consciousness.	1. *Purpose*: To reduce all painful sensation in one region of the body without inducing unconsciousness. Produced by blocking sensory impulses to the brain.
2. *Methods employed*: a. Inhalation of gases or volatile liquids b. Intravenous infusion of anesthetic agent c. Rectal administration of agent	2. *Methods employed*: a. Topical anesthesia b. Local infiltration block c. Nerve block d. Field block e. Spinal anesthesia f. Epidural block
3. *Advantages*: a. *Flexibility*: General anesthesia can be used and modified for any type of surgery. b. *Adequate time factor*: Can be employed during lengthy procedures with maximum comfort for the patient. c. *Better monitoring*: When caring for an extremely anxious patient, the anesthesiologist is often able to better control respiratory and circulatory functions when the patient is unconscious rather than awake and fearful.	3. *Advantages*: a. *Better airway control*: The patient who is awake is better able to maintain an airway and to control mucous secretions and vomitus should vomiting occur. b. *Fewer respiratory complications*: Being awake, the patient is able to cough and breathe normally, which prevents a dangerous pooling of mucus in the bronchi. c. *Less circulatory depression*: The drugs and methods used do not have as dramatic an effect on the circulatory system as do general anesthetics.
4. *Disadvantages*: a. *Respiratory and circulatory depression*: Most anesthesia deaths result from such depressions of function. b. *Explosion hazards*: Explosions occur infrequently with the use of inhalation anesthesia as flammable anesthetics are rarely used.	4. *Disadvantages*: a. Anxiety and fear are not allayed. Patient continues to see and hear throughout operation. b. *Lack of flexibility*: Difficult to use with small children, elderly senile persons, and uncooperative persons. c. *Short time period*: Generally cannot be used for lengthy operations. d. Drugs employed can cause systemic depression. e. "*False security*": It is incorrectly believed that regional anesthesia will not cause respiratory or circulatory problems.

gas or drug can result in severe respiratory and circulatory problems. Additional complications which may occur during induction or emergence or while the patient is under anesthesia include:

1. Corneal abrasions
2. Lip and tongue injuries
3. Vocal cord damage (mainly with endotracheal intubations)
4. Damage to teeth (mainly with endotracheal intubations)
5. Peripheral nerve injury from improper positioning

It is important that all operating room personnel be aware of potential complications and try to avoid them through close observation of the patient.

TYPES OF ANESTHESIA

The types of anesthesia used vary with the age, size, physical condition, personality, and preference of the patient. Other considerations are the site and duration of the operation and the degree of technical intricacy of the procedure.

There are two major classifications of anesthesia: general and regional. *General* anesthesia is a drug-induced depression of the central nervous system which may be reversed either through elimination of the chemical agent from the body or the metabolic breakdown of the agent. It is a state of analgesia, amnesia, and unconsciousness, characterized by the loss of reflexes and muscle tone. *Regional* anesthesia, on the other hand, produces a loss of painful sensation in one region of the body only and does not result in unconsciousness. Table 18–1 compares the purpose, method of administration, advantages and disadvantages of these two major types of anesthesia.

Types of General Anesthesia

As is pointed out in Table 18–1, general anesthesia can be administered in three ways: (1) by inhalation, (2) intravenously, and (3) rectally.

INHALATION ANESTHESIA

This type of anesthesia is administered by giving the patient gases or liquids in volatilized form which are inhaled through a mask or endotracheal tube directly into the lungs. Inhalation anesthesia is the standard anesthesia used in most major surgeries involving the upper abdomen, head, neck, and thorax.

Advantages. The *advantages* of inhalation anesthesia are the prevention of pain, the relaxation of tissues, and the abolition of anxiety through the production of a state of total unconsciousness.

Disadvantages. The major *disadvantages* of this type of anesthesia are circulatory and respiratory depression. Also, certain of the gases and liquids used in inhalation anesthesia are highly *flammable* and *explosive* when they are mixed with air or oxygen, e.g., ether.

When flammable and explosive anesthetic agents are being used, observe the following rules:

Safety Rules

1. *Do not wear slips or uniforms of nylon or rayon and do not use wool blankets; these materials can set off a static spark.*
2. *Do not allow smoking in the vicinity of the operating room.*
3. *Do not allow the use of electrocautery.*
4. *Do not touch the patient in the vicinity of the breathing mask; this may cause an electric spark.*
5. *Do not allow the patient to smoke for 12 hours after the operation or visitors to smoke for 6 hours afterwards.*
6. *Do not wear shoes that are not conductive; test them daily to ensure proper grounding.*
7. *Do not use mattresses, pillows, or covering materials that are not conductive.*

Methods. The major ways to administer inhalation anesthesia are: by the open drop method, by mask, and by endotracheal tube. When the *open drop method* is used, the anesthetic liquid is dropped directly onto layers of gauze or an absorbent face mask that is held over the patient's mouth and nose. When a *mask* is used, the gases generally flow into the mask via a tube from a supply tank where the gases are held under pressure. Finally, when an endotracheal tube is used, the gases flow from a supply tank directly into the patient's tracheobronchial tree (Fig. 18–3).

The induction of inhalation anesthesia takes place in four distinct stages:

Stage I — the beginning of induction.
Stage II — loss of consciousness.
Stage III — surgical anesthesia and relaxation.
Stage IV — the danger stage.

These stages and appropriate nursing actions are described in Table 18–2.

There are many different liquids and gases used in inhalation anesthesia. Two of the most commonly used volatile liquid anesthetics are enflurane (Ethrane) and halothane (Flouthane); a commonly used gas anesthetic is nitrous oxide. These specific agents — their advantages and disadvantages — are presented in Table 18–3.

Although ether is rarely used today, it merits mention because of its historical importance as one of the oldest known anesthetics. It is an explosive anesthetic that produces a deep and prolonged anesthesia. Ether rarely produces cardiovascular complications and is therefore sometimes used for high risk patients.

INTRAVENOUS ANESTHESIA

When general anesthesia is administered intravenously, the patient experiences a simple, pleasant, and extremely rapid induction; unconsciousness generally occurs in only 30 sec-

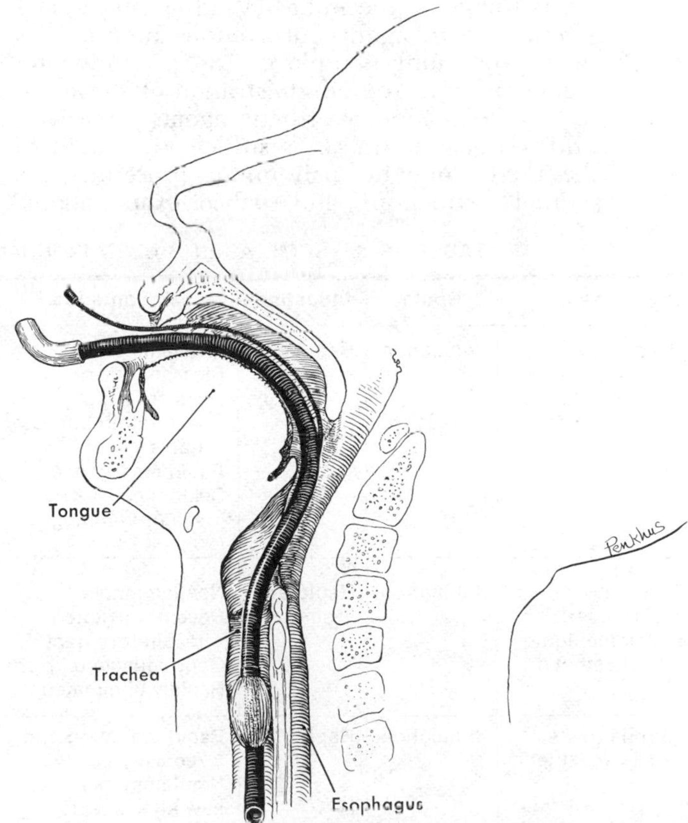

Figure 18–3. Placement of endotracheal tube for the administration of anesthesia (note inflation of cuff). (From Gruendemann, B., et al.: *The Surgical Patient: Behavioral Concepts for the Operating Room Nurse.* St. Louis: C. V. Mosby Co., 1977, p. 120.)

TABLE 18-2. FOUR STAGES OF ANESTHESIA*

	From	To	Patient Status	Nursing Action
STAGE I	Beginning administration of gas or drug	Loss of consciousness	May appear inebriated, drowsy, dizzy	Close OR doors; keep room quiet; stand by patient to assist, if necessary
STAGE II	Loss of consciousness	Relaxation	May appear excited; may breathe irregularly; may move arms and legs or body; patient very susceptible to external stimuli (noise, being touched suddenly)	Be ready to restrain patient if needed; remain at patient's side, quiet and alert; assist anesthesiologist, if needed
STAGE III	(Surgical anesthesia stage) relaxation	Loss of reflexes; depression of vital functions	Regular respiration, contracted pupils, eyelid reflexes disappear, jaw relaxed; auditory sensation lost during this stage	Begin prep only when anesthesiologist indicates Stage III has been reached and patient is under good control
STAGE IV	(Danger stage) vital functions too depressed	Respiratory failure; possible cardiac arrest	Not breathing; little or no heartbeat or pulse	If arrest occurs, react immediately to assist in establishing airway; provide cardiac arrest tray, drugs, syringes, long needles; assist surgeon with closed or open cardiac massage

*Modified from *Nursing Care of the Patient in the O.R.* Ethicon Division, Inc., Somerville, N.J.

onds following the initial IV administration of the anesthetic agent. Intravenous anesthesia is most commonly employed as an induction agent prior to the administration of the more potent inhalation anesthetic agents. However, intravenous anesthesia is sufficiently potent to be used alone in such minor procedures as dental extractions and pelvic examinations. Thiopental sodium (Pentothal sodium) is the most commonly used intravenous anesthetic.

The major *advantages* of IV anesthesia are: (1) rapid pleasant induction; (2) absence of explosive hazards; and (3) a low incidence of postoperative nausea and vomiting.

Major *dangers* are: (1) *laryngospasm* and *bronchospasm,* owing to excitement of laryngeal re-

TABLE 18-3. SOME AGENTS USED IN INHALATION ANESTHESIA ADMINISTRATION

Agent	Route	Induction	Advantages	Disadvantages	Nursing Precaution
Halothane (Fluothane): Volatile liquid anesthetic.	Inhalation	Rapid and smooth	Nonflammable Pleasant odor Does not irritate respiratory and GI tracts Rapid emergence Seldom causes nausea or vomiting	Requires special vaporizer May depress cardiovascular system Limited relaxation Expensive May cause liver damage	Watch for bradycardia and hypotension. Use of epinephrine with this agent may cause cardiac arrhythmias, including ventricular fibrillation. Body temperature may fall and patient may shiver following prolonged use.
Enflurane (Ethrane): Volatile liquid anesthetic	Inhalation	Rapid and smooth	Nonflammable Does not irritate respiratory tract Good muscle relaxant Rapidly eliminated	Potent myocardial and respiratory depressant	Watch for hypotension, respiratory depression, arrhythmias, nausea, and vomiting.
Nitrous oxide: Gas anesthetic	Inhalation	Rapid	Rapid induction and recovery Nonflammable Few after effects	Poor relaxation May produce hypoxia Must be used with other agents except for short procedures	When used with other agents, follow the precautions applying to those agents.

From Gruendemann, B., et al.: *The Surgical Patient: Behavioral Concepts for the Operating Room Nurse,* 2nd ed. St. Louis: C. V. Mosby Co., 1977, pp. 122 and 123.

flexes by the drug, (2) *hypotension,* owing to depression of the vasomotor center in the brain, and (3) *respiratory arrest,* owing to drug overdosage, which may also result in cardiac arrest. Be prepared for the above complications of intravenous anesthesia by having on hand: oxygen; an endotracheal tube; emergency drugs to stimulate the heart and respirations; and vasopressor drugs to counteract hypotension and shock should they occur. Table 18–4 discusses drugs used for intravenous anesthesia.

RECTAL ANESTHESIA

This form of general anesthesia is administered via a rectal tube. It is rarely used today, although it is useful during the induction of anesthesia of pediatric patients. Sodium pentothal is one anesthetic agent that may be administered rectally. The agent is absorbed by the rectal mucosa and delivered to the central nervous system via the circulatory system. Since rectal anesthesia is only used during induction, it must always be supplemented with other types of anesthetic agents. (See Table 18–4.)

Types of Regional Anesthesia

As shown in Table 18–1, regional anesthesia is used to anesthetize one region of the body only. Regional anesthesia is adequate for many of the procedures performed in outpatient clinics, doctors' offices, and hospitals. Examples of procedures utilizing regional anesthetics are:

1. Biopsies
2. Excision of moles and cysts
3. Hernia repairs
4. Some eye, ear, nose and throat procedures
5. Endoscopies of the gastrointestinal, respiratory, and urinary tracts
6. Operations on extremities

When regional anesthesia is being administered, the anesthetic agent is deposited either upon the surface to be anesthetized or upon a particular nerve or nerve pathway that lies between the area to be incised and operated upon and receptors of painful stimuli located within the central nervous system. This procedure, then, blocks the transmission of painful stimuli to the brain.

Types of regional anesthesia are (1) topical anesthesia, (2) local infiltration block, (3) field block, (4) nerve block, (5) spinal anesthesia, and (6) epidural block. Figure 18–4 illustrates anatomical areas used during administration of regional anesthesia.

The major differences between these various types of regional anesthesia are the *rate* at which the anesthetic agent diffuses from the site of application or injection, and the *size* of the region that is anesthetized. Topical and local anesthesia block only peripheral nerves where the incision or examination will occur; field anesthesia blocks the area *around* the incision; spinal anesthesia and epidural blocks anesthetize areas that are even further removed from the operative site. Table 18–5 discusses various agents used for regional anesthesia.

TABLE 18–4. SOME AGENTS USED IN ANESTHESIA ADMINISTRATION PER IV AND RECTAL ROUTES

Agent	Route	Induction	Advantages	Disadvantages	Nursing Precautions
Thiopental sodium (Pentothal sodium)	Intravenous Rectal	Rapid and pleasant	Rapid, pleasant induction and recovery Nonirritating Nonflammable Easy administration Good for short procedures and hypnosis during regional anesthesia	Large doses cause respiratory and circulatory depression Wide variance in tolerance Poor relaxation	Watch for circulatory and respiratory depression Be prepared for possible laryngospasm
Ketamine (Ketalar)	Intravenous	Rapid	Short action Excellent for diagnostic and short topical surgical procedures May be used to supplement weaker agents; nitrous oxide	Large doses cause respiratory and circulatory depression Wide variance in tolerance Poor relaxation Causes hallucinations and nightmares during recovery Induces blood pressure rise	Watch for circulatory and respiratory depression Maintain a quiet environment; minimize touch and speaking to patient Resuscitative equipment must be available.

Modified from Gruendemann, B., et al.: *The Surgical Patient: Behavioral Concepts for the Operating Room Nurse,* 2nd ed. St. Louis: C. V. Mosby Co., 1977, pp. 122 and 123.

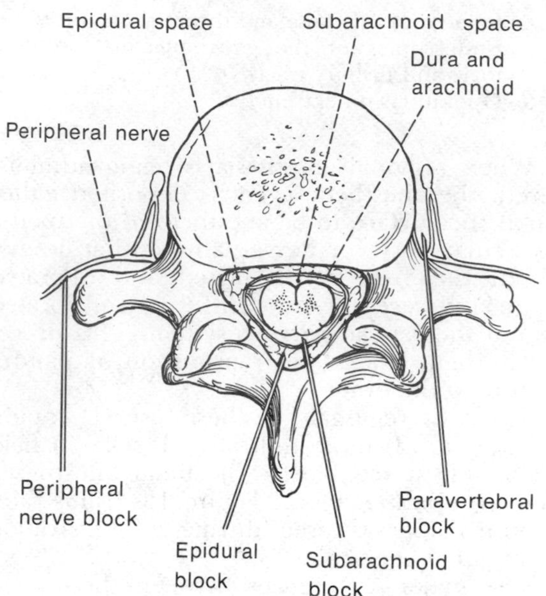

Figure 18–4. Cross section of spinal cord. Note spinal anatomy important for needle placement during administration of regional anesthesia.

TOPICAL ANESTHESIA

When an anesthetizing drug is sprayed or dropped onto an area to be desensitized, topical anesthesia is achieved. This short-acting form of anesthesia can block peripheral nerve endings in the mucous membranes of the vagina, rectum, nasopharynx, and mouth. Topical anesthesia is employed in minor procedures, e.g., rectal examinations when painful hemorrhoids are present, or to densensitize the bronchi prior to a bronchoscopic examination.

Advantages of topical anesthesia are: (1) speed of action, and (2) general nontoxicity. *Disadvantages* are that the patient's tissues are not relaxed nor is anxiety reduced.

> *To avoid an anaphylactic reaction from prior sensitization to the anesthetic drug, investigate patient drug allergies* before *topical anesthesia is used.*

One drug commonly used for topical anesthesia is *cocaine* in a 4 to 10 per cent solution. This drug is for topical use *only,* and is mainly used to anesthetize the eye and the mucous membranes of the nose, mouth, and urethra. Cocaine is a highly toxic drug if it enters the circulatory system. If accidentally injected, cocaine may cause severe excitement followed by shock, respiratory failure, and cardiac arrest. Oxygen and artificial respiration will be required to save the patient's life in event of such a severe reaction.

Other drugs used for topical anesthesia are butacaine, Pontocaine, and lidocaine (Xylocaine).

LOCAL INFILTRATION BLOCK

In contrast to topical or surface application of an anesthetic agent, local anesthesia is de-

TABLE 18–5. SOME AGENTS USED FOR REGIONAL ANESTHESIA

Agent.	Route	Induction	Advantages	Disadvantages	Nursing Precautions
Procaine hydrochloride (Novocaine; Ethocaine)	Infiltration Topical Spinal	Rapid	Low toxicity Inexpensive	Slow acting	May involve central nervous and cardiovascular systems Watch for reactions, hypotension, bradycardia, thready pulse, convulsions, irregular respirations. Have resuscitation equipment nearby. Initial effect of overdose is depression rather than excitement. Watch for drowsiness, respiratory arrest, cardiovascular collapse, and cardiac arrest.
Lidocaine hydrochloride (Xylocaine)	Infiltration Topical Block or spinal Epidural	Slow	Action is more rapid, longer acting than Procaine. Is a local vasodilator. Used to treat arrhythmias during heart surgery or general anesthesia. Suppresses laryngeal or pharyngeal reflexes.	Few; well tolerated. Untoward events may occur with overdose or faulty injection.	
Tetracaine (Pontocaine)	Spinal	Rapid	Provides adequate prolonged anesthesia (2–2½ hours or longer)	Few real disadvantages Untoward effects may occur from overdose or faulty injection	
Bupivacaine (Marcaine)	Epidural Infiltration block Nerve block	Slow	Prolonged duration (3½–4 hours) Ideal for obstetric use; little effect on fetus	Same as tetracaine	

From Gruendemann, B., et al.: *The Surgical Patient: Behavioral Concepts for the Operating Room Nurse,* 2nd ed. St. Louis: C. V. Mosby Co., 1977, pp. 122 and 123.

pendent upon the *injection* of an anesthetic agent such as procaine by needle and syringe into the skin and subcutaneous tissues of the area to be incised. As a result of local anesthesia, only the peripheral nerves around the area of the incision are blocked. Local blocks are used in short minor operations and prior to the administration of spinal anesthesia.

When a local anesthetic is administered, it is important that the doctor not allow the needle to slip into one of the patient's veins. If a local anesthetic agent is accidentally given intravenously, dangerous *cardiovascular collapse* or *convulsions* may result. For this reason, the doctor should always withdraw the plunger of the syringe before injection to make certain that the needle is not in a vein.

FIELD BLOCK

In a field block, the area *surrounding* the incision is injected and infiltrated with local anesthetics; this is in contrast to local anesthesia, in which only the area of the incision is injected. Thus, a field block actually "walls in" the area around the incision and, thereby, prevents the transmission of sensory impulses to the brain from that area. The same precautions must be taken in performing field blocks as in local infiltration blocks.

NERVE BLOCK

A nerve block acts to anesthetize nerves or individual plexuses of nerves that are further removed from the operative site than those nerves that are anesthetized by a field block.

Nerve blocks may be employed to anesthetize: an entire finger (digital nerve block), the entire upper arm (brachial plexus block), or the chest or abdominal wall (intercostal nerve block). Nerves most commonly blocked are the brachial, intercostal, sciatic, and femoral. Drugs generally used for nerve blocks are lidocaine (Xylocaine) and bupivacaine (Marcaine). Once the drug has been injected, the area is generally anesthetized within several minutes; this effect will last longer than that produced with local or topical anesthesia.

Nerve blocks, like local infiltration blocks, can produce severe systemic responses if the drug is accidentally injected into a blood vessel. Vasoconstriction produced by epinephrine may cause *ischemic necrosis* of an extremity, particularly a digit. Sometimes epinephrine is added to the local anesthetic agent in order to give a more prolonged anesthetic effect. Epinephrine causes local blood vessels to constrict: this action prevents rapid absorption of the anesthetic agent.

SPINAL ANESTHESIA

Spinal anesthesia blocks impulses from the spinal cord and nerve roots, just as local anesthesia blocks peripheral nerve fiber impulses. Spinal nerves are blocked between their emergence from the spinal cord and their exit from the spinal canal through the intervertebral foramen. When in the spinal canal, the spinal nerves course through the subarachnoid space, where they are bathed in spinal fluid, and then transverse the epidural space. Nerve blockage may occur in either the subarachnoid or the epidural space.

Autonomic nerve fibers are the first to be affected by spinal anesthesia and the last to recover. Following autonomic blockage, touch, pain, motor, pressure, and proprioceptive fibers are blocked — in that order.

Spinal anesthesia can be employed for almost any type of major procedure that is performed below the level of the diaphragm, e.g., hysterectomy, appendectomy.

Spinal anesthesia is administered by the anesthesiologist in the following steps:

Step 1. Positioning

The patient is placed on the side in a flexed position. The nurse holds the patient and instructs the patient not to move. As you can see in Figure 18–5 the patient's neck is sharply flexed, the upper arm is placed across the body and the lower arm is placed at right angles to the body.

Step 2. Lumbar puncture and spinal tap

A lumbar puncture is performed in the lower back between the levels of the third and fourth

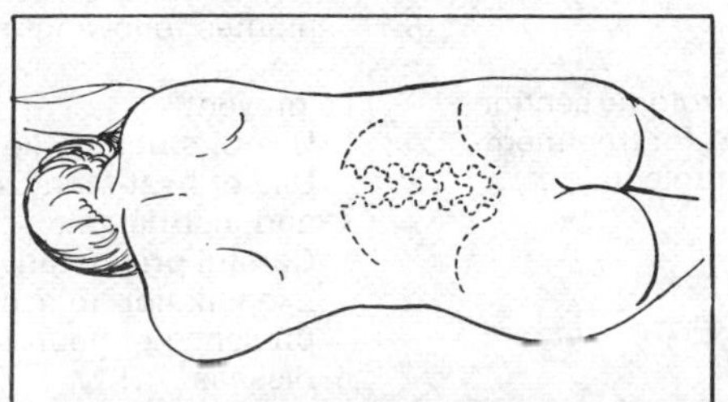

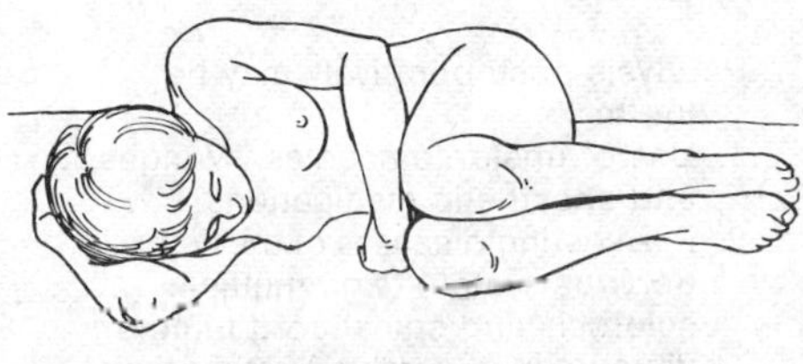

Figure 18–5. The proper position for the administration of spinal anesthesia.

lumbar vertebrae (L3–4) or the fourth and fifth lumbar vertebrae (L4–L5). There is no danger of piercing the spinal cord during this procedure, as the spinal cord stops at L2.

1. The anesthesiologist, wearing sterile gloves, first preps the patient's skin in the vicinity of the puncture with a skin antiseptic and then drapes the patient with a sterile towel.

2. Next the doctor draws an imaginary line between the patient's iliac crests in order to approximate the exact site for the puncture.

3. The area over the site of the puncture is infiltrated with a local anesthetic, producing a local block.

4. Once the area is anesthetized, the doctor inserts a spinal needle into the subarachnoid space, at the proper level and then observes the spinal fluid, which should be clear in color and flowing freely.

Step 3. Injection of the anesthetic agent

1. If the spinal fluid appears bloody or is obstructed in its flow, the anesthetic medication is not injected through the spinal needle.

2. If the spinal fluid is clear and flows freely, a local anesthetic agent is injected through the spinal needle into the subarachnoid space (i.e., between the pia mater and the arachnoid membrane). Thus, the anesthetic agent passes into the spinal fluid.

3. Almost any local anesthetic agent can be used for spinal anesthesia with or without epinephrine. Refer to Table 18–5 on regional anesthesia.

Sometimes epinephrine is added to the local anesthetic agent in order to give a more prolonged anesthetic effect, e.g., Pontocaine mixed with epinephrine provides adequate anesthesia for up to 3 or 4 hours. Epinephrine causes local blood vessels to constrict; this prevents rapid absorption of the anesthetic agent.

4. If the anesthesiologist wishes to prolong the spinal anesthesia even more, the patient may be given a "continuous spinal." To administer continuous spinal anesthesia, the anesthesiologist inserts a semirigid catheter, usually into the epidural space

TABLE 18–6. COMPLICATIONS AND DISCOMFORTS OF SPINAL ANESTHESIA

Complications and Discomforts	Causes	Clinical Care	Prevention
Hypotension	Paralysis of vasomotor nerves; usually occurs shortly after induction of anesthesia	Administer: 1. Oxygen by inhalation 2. Vasoactive drugs, ephedrine or methoxamine (Vasoxyl) IV 3. Trendelenburg position if level of anesthesia is fixed, 10 to 20 minutes after induction	In patients who are not prone to CHF, administer 500–800 ml. of IV fluids rapidly prior to block
Nausea and vomiting	Occurs mainly during abdominal surgery, due to traction placed on various structures within abdomen or at times due to hypotension	1. Ephedrine 2. Antiemetics 3. Oxygen 4. Fluids	
Headache (can be extremely painful and may last days or weeks)	Cerebral spinal fluid (which cushions the brain) is lost through dural hole; Leakage of fluid and loss of cushioning effect increased by: 1. Use of a large spinal needle 2. Poor hydration	To treat: 1. Apply tight abdominal binder 2. Administer fluids 3. Administer analgesics 4. In severe cases, inject 10 ml of patient's blood to plug hole	To prevent: 1. Use of very small spinal needle reduces incidence of spinal headache to 0.9 per cent 2. Administer IV and oral fluids before and after induction of spinal anesthesia 3. Keep patient flat and quiet
Respiratory paralysis	Occurs if drug reaches upper thoracic and cervical cord in large amounts or in heavy concentrations	Give artificial respiration by anesthesia machine or hand-held resuscitator	Avoid extreme Trendelenburg position before level of spinal anesthesia set, i.e., 10 to 20 minutes following induction
Neurologic complications (e.g., paraplegia, severe muscle weakness in legs)	Paralysis postoperatively may be due to 1. Use of unsterile needles, syringes, and anesthetic medications 2. Preexisting diseases of the central nervous system (e.g., multiple sclerosis and spinal cord tumors), which cause paralysis rather than the spinal anesthesia itself	See neurologic section, Unit X, for treatment of paraplegia	To prevent: 1. Use of strict sterile technique 2. Use of heat-sterilized drugs and instruments 3. Careful preoperative neurologic examination to ascertain the presence of neurologic disease

or, at times, into the subarachnoid space and then injects the anesthetic agent intermittently as necessary. The catheter remains in place throughout the operation.

Step 4. Positioning the patient following the administration of spinal anesthesia

1. Place the patient on his or her back following the injection of the anesthetic agent, and on his or her side if the patient is receiving a continuous spinal.
2. For a high level of anesthesia, lower the patient's head and shoulders to degree ordered by the anesthesiologist.
3. After 10 to 20 minutes the anesthesia level is set and the patient may be placed in any position desired without disturbing the anesthesia level.

Effects of Spinal Anesthesia. Within a few minutes after induction of spinal anesthesia, the patient experiences a loss of sensation and a paralysis of the toes, then feet, then legs, and finally the abdomen.

Spinal anesthesia offers many *advantages* for patients undergoing surgical procedures involving the lower half of their bodies. Major benefits are:

1. Ease of administration.
2. Expensive equipment and drugs not necessary.
3. Relative safety of method.
4. Excellent muscle relaxation provided.
5. Does not cause fetal depression, and thus can be used for cesarean sections.
6. Does not cloud patient's consciousness or alertness. However, anxious patients can be given a small dose of barbiturate, which will enable them to rest and even to sleep throughout their operation.
7. Can be used for patients with a full stomach since the patient will awake to maintain airway in event of vomiting.

Complications of spinal anesthesia are listed in Table 18–6, along with their causes, prevention, and treatment.

Remember that a patient who has undergone spinal anesthesia is a candidate for serious respiratory or cardiovascular problems. Check the patient's blood pressure and the rate and depth of breathing every 10 to 15 minutes during the recovery period. If the blood pressure begins to fall rapidly and breathing becomes difficult, notify the surgeon or anesthesiologist at once so that treatment measures can be started promptly.

As the anesthesia wears off, observe the patient carefully. The usual check on the return of motion to the extremities is to ask patients to move their toes. However, as one anesthesiologist warns, patients who can wiggle their toes has *not* necessarily recovered completely from the "spinal." A patient's ability to move the toes simply means that the motor blockade is wearing off, although *autonomic blockade is still present.* Patients who are still experiencing autonomic blockade are prone to *hypotension* despite their ability to move their toes and extremities.[20] Therefore, patients who have undergone spinal anesthesia and who are discharged from the recovery room to the surgical floor still require careful monitoring of their blood pressure. Watch these patients carefully for sudden drops in blood pressure and for other signs of shock.

A variation of spinal anesthesia commonly used in obstetrics is sometimes referred to as a "saddle block" because it chiefly produces anesthesia of the perineal or "saddle" region. Its physiologic effects are generally like those of spinal anesthesia.

EPIDURAL BLOCK

Epidural block is achieved by introducing an anesthetic agent into the epidural space (see Fig. 18–4). The epidural space is entered by a needle either at the lumbar interspace or the sacral region. The needle is carefully positioned in the epidural space, without penetrating the dura and entering the subarachnoid space. With proper positioning of the needle, the cerebral spinal fluid cannot be aspirated.

The caudal block is a variation of the epidural block. Like the saddle block, caudal anesthesia is most commonly used in obstetrics.

Since like spinal anesthesia, the epidural block also produces autonomic blockage, *hypotension* can result. Respiratory depression or paralysis may also occur if the level of the block is too high and affects respiratory muscles. Properly performed, epidural anesthesia produces no headache postoperatively.

Specialized Methods of Producing Anesthesia

Specialized anesthesia techniques are used for certain types of operations, e.g., open heart surgery. These techniques may be used alone to provide anesthesia, or they may be used to supplement other types of anesthesia.

MUSCLE RELAXANTS

Muscle relaxants are given mainly to supplement other more powerful general anesthetic agents. When given in combination with muscle relaxants, potent general anesthetic drugs can be administered in a smaller dose. This provides greater patient safety.

Muscle relaxants produce their physiologic effects by blocking the transmission of nervous impulses to the muscle fibers. This blockade produces temporary paralysis of all voluntary muscles, including the muscles that control respiration. Hence, respirations must be supported mechanically when muscle relaxants are employed.

Major drugs that act as muscle relaxants are:

- *Curare,* which is capable of producing muscle relaxation in 1 to 3 minutes. Muscles are blocked by curare in the following order: eyelids, eyeballs, the muscles of the extremities, and finally abdominal muscles and the diaphragm. Within one-half hour the effects of curare wear off and the muscles become activated again, but in the reverse order. Hypotension is a side effect of curare and must be watched for soon after administration.
- *Pancuronium,* a muscle relaxant similar to curare but having slightly longer duration of action (45 minutes to 1 hour). Pancuronium does not produce hypotension like curare and hence can be used even in patients with cardiovascular problems.
- *Succinylcholine* is a more rapidly acting muscle relaxant than curare; its action takes place in 60 to 90 seconds. In addition, succinylcholine is rapidly eliminated, usually within 3 to 5 minutes.

Respirations in patients who have received muscle relaxants should be closely watched for at least 1 hour after the relaxants appear to have worn off. Paralysis may occur again, for reasons that are not clear.

HYPOTHERMIA

A highly specialized method of anesthesia, hypothermia is the deliberate reduction of the patient's body temperature to between 28 and 30° C. (82 and 86° F.). The purpose of hypothermia is to reduce the rate of tissue metabolism and consequently, the oxygen requirement of the body and tissues. Situations in which hypothermia is employed are: heart surgery, brain surgery, surgery on large vessels supplying major organs (e.g., renal and carotid arteries and the aorta), and treatment of severely injured persons with an impaired blood supply to their vital organs.

Methods and apparatus for producing hypothermia are: ice water immersion, molding of partially filled ice bags over the patient's extremities, cooling blanket, and extracorporeal cooling devices that cool the blood outside of the body and then reinfuse the cooled blood into the patient.

Major complications of hypothermia are respiratory depression and cardiac arrest. Additional complications may be ice burns, hemorrhage, and disturbance of fluid balance. Ice burns occur if the solutions used are colder than 0° C. and are permitted to remain in contact with the patient's skin for a prolonged time. Hypothermia prolongs coagulation time and often contributing to postoperative hemorrhage. It is important that all bleeding be arrested before the patient's wound is closed.

Following surgery in which hypothermia has been employed, the patient may be rewarmed mechanically with a heating blanket until the body temperature has reached 34° C. (93.2° F.). Then the device is usually withdrawn, and the patient permitted to rewarm slowly. Excessive shivering is a complication that may occur during this period. Shivering could lead to circulatory failure because of the extra burden it places on the myocardium. Another possible complication is heat burns. These can easily occur when a rewarming device is used on a hypothermic patient whose skin blood flow is extremely slow.

> *While the warming blanket is in use, check the patient's skin periodically for evidence of potential burn areas.*

PURPOSEFUL HYPOTENSION

Anesthesiologists use this unusual technique in operations in which a reduction of bleeding at the operative site is particularly advantageous, e.g., brain surgery, radical neck surgery, and radical pelvic surgery. Purposeful hypotension is produced by either administering drugs that paralyze the patient's autonomic nervous system, or inducing a deep level of general anesthesia. One general anesthetic agent commonly employed in purposeful hypotension is halothane.

CONCLUSION

As the surgeon places the last suture and the operation ends, the patient enters the third and final phase of the operative odyssey — the postoperative period. It is during this last period that the nurse's observations and actions must be particularly skillful if the patient is to recover safely from the anesthesia and the operation itself.

CHAPTER 19

GENERAL CARE OF THE PATIENT FOLLOWING SURGERY

IMMEDIATE CARE OF THE PATIENT RECOVERING FROM ANESTHESIA

Transporting the Patient from the Operating Room

Following the completion of the operation, the operating room staff generally dress the patient in a clean gown and move the patient to a stretcher. In moving the patient from the operating table to the stretcher, the operating room personnel strive to avoid the following three problems:

1. *Exposure*, which predisposes the patient to respiratory infections and shock.
2. *Rough handling*, which may place a strain upon the patient's sutures.
3. *Hurried movements and rapid changes in position*, which predispose the patient to hypotension. In particular, the patients should be moved gradually from the lithotomy to the horizontal position and from the prone to the supine position. When moving or transferring a postoperative patient, it is important to have adequate help in order to prevent injuries to staff or patient.

After being moved to the stretcher, the patient should be covered with blankets and secured with safety belts or restraints over the knees and elbows. The side rails of the stretcher should be up to ensure patient safety in case the patient begins to awaken from anesthesia during the trip from the operating room. The anesthesiologist and sometimes the surgeon accompany the patient to the recovery room.

Some patients may be transferred directly from the operating room (OR) to the intensive care unit (ICU) for continued specialized care, with constant nursing supervision. Patients who are transferred to the ICU are usually patients who:

1. Have been identified as poor surgical risks and/or will probably have a complicated postoperative course.
2. Have undergone major surgery (e.g., resection of aortic aneurysm, open heart surgery, kidney transplant).
3. Have sufferred a cardiac or respiratory arrest during or immediately following surgery.

The Recovery Room

Because the immediate postanesthesia period is a critical time for the patient, close observation is important. The patient's physical and psychologic functioning must be supported until the effects of the anesthesia have worn off. Until then, the patient is not easily aroused and cannot call for assistance. Most hospitals are equipped with a PAR (postanesthesia recovery) room: it is here that specially trained nurses assist the patient in recovery from the immediate effects of surgery — most importantly anesthesia.

Admission of the Patient to the Recovery Room. In the morning the recovery room nurse (a specially trained person) usually receives a list of the patients who are scheduled that day. Before the arrival of each patient from surgery, the nurse generally checks each individual patient cubicle for the following equipment: a sphygmomanometer and stethoscope, IV equipment, suction apparatus, tongue depressors, an airway, an emesis basin, mouth wipes, a thermometer, and a cardiac monitor. Other supplies that should be close at hand and ready for use if needed are: emergency drugs, narcotics, tracheostomy set, airway, oxygen, cutdown tray, universal donor blood, plasma expanders, endotracheal tube, catheterization sets, defibrillator, a ventilator, gastric suction equipment, syringes, and needles.

Shock, respiratory obstruction, and *hemorrhage* are the chief immediate postoperative complications. It is imperative that nursing personnel, both in the recovery room and on the unit, remain aware of the signs and symptoms of these complications and are prepared to intervene appropriately. These complications are discussed later in this chapter and in Chapter 20.

After arriving from surgery, the patient is either moved from the stretcher to a bed or is left on the stretcher while in the recovery room. Proper positioning of an unconscious or semiconscious patient is very important to avoid respiratory complications such as airway obstruction caused by a patient's relaxed tongue falling back into the throat or by aspiration of mucus and/or vomitus. Care must be taken at all times to keep the patient's head to the side and chin extended forward (Fig. 19–1). A lateral Sims position is most often used as it allows the patient's tongue to fall forward and allows mucus and vomitus to drain out or be suctioned out. Occasionally there may be specific surgical or anatomical reasons for orders to keep some patients lying flat on their backs while in the recovery room. When this occurs, careful observation of the patient's respiratory status must be made.

At this time, the nurse begins to make a baseline assessment of the patient. The patient's vital signs are registered, including: blood pressure, pulse rate (volume and regularity), respiratory rate, airway patency, depth of respirations, chest expansion, and color of skin. The nurse also performs a brief visual assessment of the patient, noting the patient's general color, presence of IV infusions, drains, or special equipment. This will enable the nurse to address these items specifically when receiving a verbal report from the OR team.

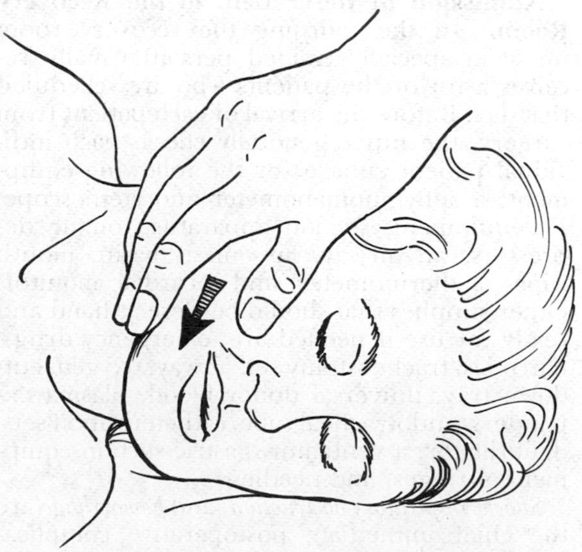

Figure 19–1. Position of hand to hold the jaw forward after inhalation of anesthesia. Note that the fingers are placed behind the angle of the jaw, and the direction of the arrow shows the direction of pressure being exerted on the jaw. As the jaw is pushed forward the tongue is brought forward so as to keep an open airway. This is important, especially after operation under general anesthesia in children, for instance, in tonsillectomy.

After the patient has been safely positioned and the baseline vital signs status ascertained, the nurse receives a verbal report from a member of the OR team usually the anesthesiologist. The following questions should be answered at this time:

- What is the patient's general condition?
- What type of operation was performed and why?
- What type of anesthetic agent, narcotic, muscle relaxant, etc., has the patient received?
- Did the patient suffer from any problems or complications during surgery that will affect the postoperative course?
- What pathologic disorders were encountered during surgery? Was cancer discovered? If so, has the family or anyone been informed? Will the patient be told that cancer is present?
- Are there any particular symptoms or complications to observe for? Are there any symptoms that should be reported immediately?
- Are there any orders that must be carried out immediately?

With the physician, the recovery room nurse next reviews the patient's chart in terms of the anesthesia record; IV's and blood received during surgery; and the length of time the patient was in surgery. A preoperative nursing assessment and history may have already been obtained if the recovery room nurse visited the patient prior to surgery.

Typical Observations and Orders

After the patient has been safely positioned, baseline nursing assessments obtained, and a postoperative report given, routine observations are made and recorded. These observations complete the immediate overall postoperative assessment of the patient. They are frequently carried out while the patient is in the recovery room.

- The *time* of admission to the recovery room.
- The *absence of reflexes*, e.g., the pharangeal reflex. Patients admitted to the PAR room without a pharangeal reflex are positioned on their side. The nurse stays at the bedside until the patient is swallowing.
- The patient's *level of responsiveness* upon admission, e.g., is there any response at all to stimuli such as light or touch? Does saying the patient's name or giving simple commands bring a response? Is the patient moving voluntarily or making audible or intelligible sounds?
- The *temperature and vital signs*. The vital signs are taken every 15 minutes until they are stable, and

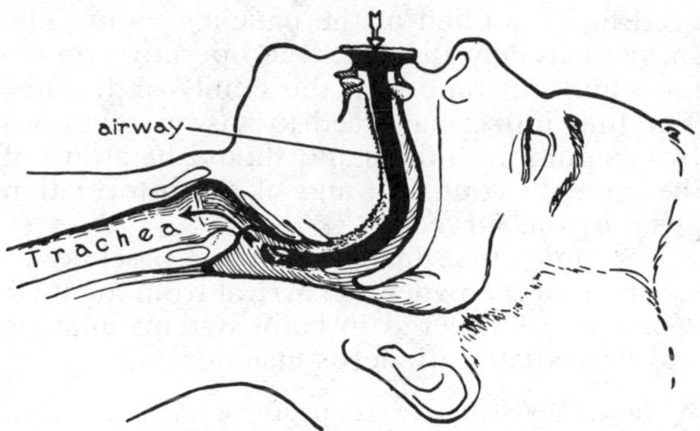

Figure 19–2. An airway functions by preventing the tongue from falling back to obstruct the patient's airway. (From Sutton, A. L.: *Bedside Nursing Techniques in Medicine and Surgery.* 1969.)

the temperature is taken every 2 to 4 hours, depending upon recovery room policy.

- The *quality and rate of respirations*. If the patient has respiratory distress, initiate oxygen therapy. The nurse notifies the anesthesiologist of any depressed respirations or change in the ventilatory pattern so that appropriate medications may be administered and/or arterial blood gas drawn. Make certain that mechanical breathing aids are available to assist ventilation if necessary.
- The *presence of an airway* in the patient's oropharynx. An airway is a hollow rubber or plastic tube that passes over the base of the tongue and acts to keep the tongue from falling back and obstructing the natural airway. The artificial air way is normally pushed out by the patient as consciousness returns.
- *Skin color and dryness*. A dusky, pale, cold, wet skin is one important sign of shock and should be reported. Also note the lips and nail beds for paleness and cyanosis.
- The *condition of the dressing*, e.g., dry or soiled. If soiled, note the color, type, and amount of drainage.
- The *presence of drainage tubes*, e.g., a T-tube or gastric tube. Is the T-tube unclamped and attached to a bottle? Are gastric tubes and intestinal tubes hooked up to suction as ordered? Make sure there are no kinks in the tubes and that the patient is not lying on them.
- *The IV infusion*. Note the type of IV solutions that are running. Also check the amount of IV solution left in the bottle, the rate of drip, whether the solution has infiltrated, and orders for any IV solutions to follow. Check to see if any medications have been added to the IV or if there are orders for any to be added.
- The presence of a *blood transfusion*. Note if a blood transfusion is running or if one is ordered. Check the rate of drip. Watch carefully for signs of a reaction.
- The presence of a bladder *catheter*. If a catheter is in place, make certain that it is unclamped, is hooked to a drainage bag or bottle, and is freely draining. Note any abnormalities in the appearance of the urine.
- *Any unusual symptoms*. Constantly observe for airway obstruction, arrhythmias, signs of shock, hemorrhage, marked elevation of temperature, and signs of circulatory overload from excess IV fluids.

Common Postoperative Orders for a Patient in Recovery Room

1. NPO until fully alert, then ice chips as tolerated. Advance diet as tolerated.
2. Vital signs every 15 minutes until stable, then every ½ hour for the next 2 hours.
3. Oropharyngeal suctioning prn.
4. Complete current IV solution, then discontinue IV if patient is tolerating fluids.
5. Phenergan 12.5 mg. IM prn nausea and vomiting when vital signs have stabilized.
6. Demerol 75 mg. IM every 3–4 hours prn pain.
7. Accurate intake and output.
8. Help patient turn, cough, and have patient deep breathe and exercise legs every 2 hours.
9. Hematocrit and electrolyte studies in AM.
10. Catheterize if patient does not void in 10 hours.
11. Reinforce dressings prn.

Most physicians also include a list of potential crisis situations for which they are to be called. A sample set of parameters is given below:

Call M.D. for:

1. B.P. systolic $<$ 90–100 or $>$ 150–160
   diastolic $<$ 50 or $>$ 90
2. H.R. $>$ 120 or $<$ 60
3. Temp. $>$ 38.3°C. (101°F.)
4. No void within 8 hrs. post-surgery
5. Increased agitation and restlessness.

In addition to routine orders, the surgeon will also write special orders that apply only to specific types of operations, e.g., neurosurgery, eye surgery, or which apply to an individual patient's problem, e.g., diabetes.

Discharge from the Recovery Room

The physician — either the surgeon or the anesthesiologist — generally discharges the patient from the recovery room. Common criteria used in the evaluation of patient discharge readiness are:

1. The patient must have recovered from the effects of general anesthesia. This usually requires a 2-hour stay in the recovery room.
2. The vital signs must be stabilized.
3. There must be no excessive drainage from any site or body cavity.
4. The physiologic effects of any narcotic medication must have stabilized. (This requires about one-half hour from the time of administration.)
5. The patient must have regained consciousness, and the level of consciousness must be satisfactory.
6. All essential orders must have been carried out and completed by the recovery room personnel.
7. Should the situation arise, provisions must be made for attendance by a private duty nurse on the clinical unit where the patient is to be moved.
8. The urine output must be adequate (30 cc. per hour). The amount must be noted and recorded.
9. The staff of the clinical unit to which the patient is to be transferred must be alerted and must be prepared for receiving the patient.

Thorough documentation of the patient's progress in the recovery room is included in the chart.

Return of the Postoperative Patient to the Clinical Unit

After meeting the PAR discharge criteria listed, the patient is returned to the clinical unit to complete recovery from surgery. Patients who have experienced complications in the recovery room are generally transferred to the intensive care unit for continued close observation.

In order to facilitate postoperative care, certain preparations need to be made on the clinical unit. These arrangements include:

1. A clear passageway to the patient's bed to assure easy transfer.
2. Clean bed linen, with pads if excessive drainage is anticipated. Additional blankets available.
3. Equipment needed (contingent upon the type of surgery), emesis basin, IV pole, tissues, suction apparatus, oxygen supplying equipment.

The recovery room generally calls the unit to notify the staff that the patient is ready for discharge. The unit nurse receives a verbal report from the recovery room nurse regarding the patient's general condition and PAR course. The patient is transferred to the unit, accompanied by a nurse.

As discussed in Chapter 17, significant others need to be notified of the patient's status. The surgeon usually discusses the operative procedure and outcome with the family or friends. The unit nurse may need to answer questions from significant others and should be aware of the patient's condition and of the information given by the surgeon.

The unit nurse makes an initial baseline assessment of the patient on arrival from the PAR room. Areas covered in body systems analysis and immediate care needs include:

- *Respiratory status*. Assess quality, depth, and rate of respirations. Skin color and temperature are also indicative of adequate oxygen exchange.
- *Neurologic status*. Is the patient alert and oriented? For laminectomy and regional anesthesia patients: Is movement possible and what are the sensations of affected extremities?
- *Cardiovascular status*. Obtain vital signs, and color and temperature of skin.
- *Wound*. Check for drainage. If drainage is present, has it increased since the patient left the PAR room?
- *Tubes — intravenous*. Note rate, patency, and amount left in bottle.
- *Tubes — drainage*. Connect any drainage tubes to appropriate outlets (e.g., nasogastric tube to low Gomco suction, chest tubes to suction, Hemovac to suction and note amount of drainage.
- *Position*. The patient's position should combine good body alignment and comfort to promote adequate ventilation and decrease pain.

After the data are recorded, a plan of postoperative care, including patient needs, nursing intervention, and patient goals should be initiated.

GOALS OF CARE THROUGHOUT THE POSTOPERATIVE PERIOD

From the moment the patient is admitted to the recovery room to the time of complete recovery from the operation, certain goals guide the care given to the patient. Typical postoperative goals are outlined below. Many of their outcomes are interrelated.

Goal 1: Maintenance of adequate cardiovascular function and tissue perfusion.
Goal 2: Maintenance of adequate respiratory function.
Goal 3: Maintenance of adequate nutrition and elimination.
Goal 4: Maintenance of adequate fluid and electrolyte balance.
Goal 5: Maintenance of adequate renal function.

Goal 6: Promotion of adequate rest, comfort, and safety.
Goal 7: Promotion of and maintenance of adequate wound healing.
Goal 8: Promotion of and maintenance of early movement and ambulation.
Goal 9: Provision of adequate psychologic support for the patient and significant others.
Goal 10: Provision of adequate discharge teaching and planning for patient and significant others.
Goal 11: Recognition of and prevention of postoperative complications.

A return to normal body system functioning is the nurse's overall goal for the patient during the postoperative period. The nurse's most valuable tool during this stage is a continual and accurate patient assessment. The nurse should also be prepared to intervene when necessary to secure the goal of a normal body function for the patient.

Goal 1: Maintenance of Adequate Cardiovascular Function and Tissue Perfusion

A satisfactory cardiac output is the basis for good tissue perfusion. Measures of cardiac output and, consequently, tissue perfusion are:

A. Arterial blood pressure
 1. Normal findings: Whether a blood pressure reading is high or low depends upon the baseline blood pressures taken *before* surgery.
 2. Abnormal readings that are reportable:
  a. Fall in systolic pressure of more than 20 mm. Hg
  b. Systolic blood pressure below 80 mm. Hg
  c. Blood pressure that is continually dropping by 5 to 10 mm. Hg over several readings.
 3. Causes of abnormal postoperative blood pressure include:
  a. Muscle relaxants.
  b. Overdose of premedications.
  c. Spinal anesthesia.
  d. Changes in patient position.
  e. Blood loss.
  f. Poor lung ventilation.
  g. Peripheral pooling of blood.

It is important for the nurse to be aware of these factors and to monitor closely the patient whose blood pressure is low, intervening appropriately. The effects of muscle relaxants, spinal anesthesia, and preoperative medications overdose usually wear off after time, thus rectifying the blood pressure problem. A change in position or coughing and deep breathing may help ventilatory problems and peripheral pooling of blood. Notify the physician in case of continued blood loss or signs of increased respiratory depression.

B. Pulse
 1. Normal finding: The pulse is usually slightly rapid immediately following surgery.
 2. Abnormal findings that are reportable:
  a. Bradycardia. Pulse below 60 beats per minute. Bradycardia results from the use of anesthetic agents and is generally of little consequence if the patient has no other symptoms.
  b. Tachycardia. Pulse above 110 beats per minute. Tachycardia may be caused by:
   (1) Blood loss during or following surgery.
   (2) Cardiac arrhythmias.
   (3) High fever.
   (4) Atelectasis.
   (5) Pneumonia.
   (6) Anxiety.
   (7) Nitrous oxide anesthesia.
   (8) Poor ventilation resulting in a decreased oxygen level
   (9) Pneumothorax
  c. Irregular pulse. May be regular irregularity, an irregular irregularity, or a skipped beat. Tachycardia and irregular pulse rate must be closely monitored and their causes investigated. Appropriate nursing intervention is dictated by the cause. Examples include: intravenous or oral agents for treatment of arrhythmias; coughing, deep breathing; ambulation; and administration of antibiotics for treatment of pneumonia.

C. Respiration
 1. Normal finding. Respirations usually slow and deep when patient is anesthetized.
 2. Abnormal findings: In certain cases, abnormal respirations represent a cardiovascular problem rather than a pulmonary problem.
 3. Abnormal findings that signify a cardiovascular problem and should be reported:
  a. Rapid difficult respirations may indicate anoxia, shock, and oxygen lack.
  b. Shallow, quiet, slow respirations may indicate depression of the respiratory tract.
  c. Shallow difficult respirations, in which the patient is using neck and diaphragmatic muscles, may indicate paralysis of the intercostal muscles from anesthesia. In this case, artificial respiration may be needed.
 4. In addition to the above, the patient may be consciously or unconsciously restricting respiratory movement to avoid further pain. Analgesics, given to keep the patient as pain free as possible, are important in the promotion of deep breathing and the circumvention of respiratory problems.

Early ambulation, in accordance with the physician's orders and the patient's ability, helps to maintain cardiac output and tissue perfusion.

Turning in bed, coughing, deep breathing, and adequate fluid and nutritional intake lend additional assistance in maintaining good cardiac output and tissue perfusion.

Goal 2: Maintenance of Adequate Respiratory Function

Normal respiratory function depends upon the maintenance of an open and clear airway during and following surgery. Nursing assessment of the patient's respiratory status begins upon admission to the recovery room and continues throughout the postoperative recovery period.

A. Causes of a *closed* airway:
   1. Obstruction due to:
      a. Mucus collection in the throat.
      b. Aspiration of mucus or vomitus.
      c. Loss of the swallowing reflex.
      d. Loss of control of the muscles of the jaw and tongue. As a result, the tongue slips back against the pharynx and blocks the airway.
   2. Laryngospasm due to:
      a. Intubation.
      b. Irritating effects of anesthetics.
   3. Bronchospasm due to:
      a. Prior respiratory diseases, e.g., chronic bronchitis, emphysema, asthma.
      b. Inhalation of gastric juices during surgery.

B. Signs of poor respiratory function
   1. Restlessness and attempts to obtain an upright position in bed (an early sign).
   2. Fast, thready pulse (an early sign).
   3. Confusion.
   4. Rapid, shallow breathing (indicative of air hunger).
   5. Nausea.
   6. Apprehension.
   7. Cyanosis (a late sign).
   8. Snoring (appears when tongue causes airway blockage).
   9. Respiratory stridor (seen in larygospasm).
   10. Wheezing (may appear in bronchospasm).

C. Results of untreated hypoventilation and respiratory obstruction are atelectasis and pneumonia.

D. Methods of promoting adequate respiratory function
   1. Methods useful in early postoperative period
      a. Whenever, possible, position patient on side with a pillow at the back, knees flexed, and chin extended. This position prevents the patient's tongue from falling back into the throat and occluding the airway.
      b. Suction mouth and pharynx gently to remove mucus.
      c. Leave airway in place until it is pushed out by the patient.
      d. Use of a mechanical respirator, such as Bird or Monaghan, beneficially controls rate and depth of respirations; also, prescribed mixtures of air and oxygen can be forced into the respiratory system.
      e. Use of the Triflo II Incentive Deep Breathing Exerciser (Fig. 19–3) provides physiologically correct exercise that encourages deep, prolonged, voluntary inspiration. It also promotes maximal alveolar inflation,

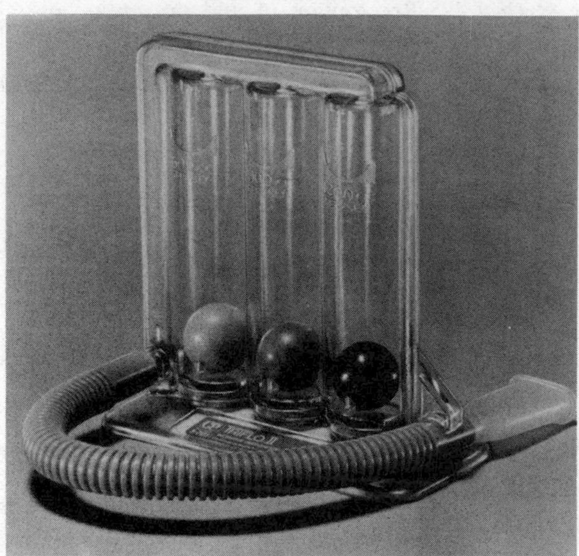

A

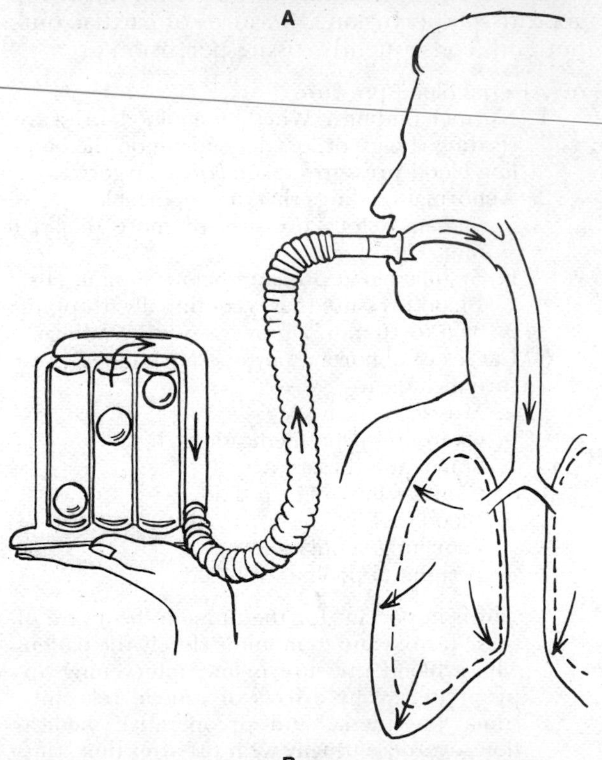

B

Figure 19–3. A. The Triflo II Incentive Deep-Breathing Exerciser. **B.** Patient using incentive deep breathing exerciser to promote maximal alveolar inflation, help restore and maintain lung capacity, and strengthen respiratory muscles. (**A,** Courtesy of Chesebrough-Ponds' Inc. Hospital Products Division, Greenwich, Conn. 06830.)

helps restore and maintain lung capacity and strengthens respiratory muscles.

2. Methods useful throughout postoperative period.
   a. Encourage the patient to breathe deeply every 2 hours in the manner described on p. 388.
   b. Encourage the patient to cough every 2 hours.
      (1) Splint the patient's incision so that coughing will be less painful and less likely to cause the incision to rupture.
      (2) Check the color and consistency of mucus expectorated. If a respiratory infection is present, the mucus may be thick, greenish, and foul smelling.
   c. Encourage and assist the patient with ambulation.

E. Emergency care of respiratory complications
   1. Oral airway insertion to prevent tongue from occluding airway.
   2. Endotracheal intubation to provide clear airway. Endotracheal tube can be attached to a mechanical respirator.
   3. Oxygen administration by means of mask catheter or endotracheal tube.
   4. Intermittent positive pressure breathing (IPPB) to give continuous ventilation to patients with airway obstruction, although many authorities question the value of this procedure.
   5. Drugs commonly used in respiratory emergencies are:
      a. Antibiotics (for infection).
      b. Bronchodilators (e.g., aminophylline, Bronchosol).
      c. Expectorants (e.g. potassium iodide and ammonium chloride).
      d. Liquefying agents (e.g., Alevaire, Mucomyst).
      e. Respiratory stimulants (e.g., Coramine, caffeine sodium benzoate).
   6. Tracheostomy for patients with complete or prolonged partial airway occlusion and for patients who cannot tolerate endotracheal intubation.

Goal 3: Maintenance of Adequate Nutrition and Elimination

An early return to a normal diet is beneficial in many ways. It promotes an early return of gastrointestinal function and is psychologically encouraging for the patient. Factors determining immediate postoperative dietary intake are physician preference, patient readiness, nature of surgery, and the type of anesthesia used.

The surgical procedure (e.g., abdominal exploration, cholecystectomy, etc.) may require that the patient abstain from oral fluids and food for a period of usually 24 to 48 hours postoperatively. Patients unable to eat usually have a nasogastric tube, which because of its decompressive properties, removes flatus and stomach secretions. Some patients who are unable to eat postoperatively may be nutritionally supplemented with intravenous fluids: blood, amino acids, or hyperalimentation if oral intake is excessively postponed.

For the first 24 to 36 hours following surgery many patients may be nauseated and experience episodes of vomiting. They do not experience an appetite, and gastrointestinal peristalsis is reduced. Liquids, as tolerated, are usually given during this period. These include: broth, tea with lemon and sugar, fruit juices, jello, and soups. Early solid foods may include: toast, light cornstarch puddings, and easily digested meats and vegetables. As the patient regains an appetite and begins to eat well, a full diet is given to promote vitamin and mineral balance and proper nitrogen balance. Muscle substance and strength then begin to be restored and a slight weight gain may be noticed.

Bowel movements are recorded. If the patient's bowels are not moving spontaneously by the second or third postoperative day (providing the patient is eating properly), the physician may order an oral stool softener or a cleansing enema.

Goal 4: Maintenance of Adequate Fluid and Electrolyte Balance

Following surgery, promotion of proper fluid and electrolyte intake and electrolyte output is crucial. Imbalances postoperatively can lead to retention of metabolic wastes, neurologic and cardiac problems, and problems of over- or underhydration.

A. The goals of postoperative fluid and electrolyte therapy are twofold:
   1. To give sufficient fluids to maintain extracellular fluid volume and blood volume. Proper fluid volume ensures:
      a. Adequate blood pressure.
      b. Adequate cardiac output.
      c. Adequate urinary flow.
   2. To prevent fluid overload with resultant congestive heart failure and pulmonary edema.

B. Normal fluid and electrolyte adjustment during the first 3 to 4 days following surgery:
   1. Renal retention of H_2O and Na^+.
   2. Expansion of ECF in excess of Na^+ and Cl^-.
   3. Transient decrease in ECF Na^+ and Cl^-.
   4. Increase in K^+ excretion.
   5. Decrease in hematocrit as a result of the expansion of ECF.

C. Normal fluid and electrolyte adjustments during the fifth through seventh day following surgery:
   1. Diuresis.
   2. Return of ECF volume to normal.

3. Serum Na^+ returns to normal.
4. Reduction of K^+ concentration in urine.

D. *Abnormal* fluid and electrolyte changes as a result of surgery are presented in Chapter 12.

E. Principal causes of postoperative *dehydration* and *electrolyte deficits*:
1. Failure to replace deficits existing prior to surgery.
2. Inadequate replacement of *normal* postoperative losses.
3. Excessive postoperative losses as a result of sweating, hyperventilation, wound drainage, gastrointestinal tract drainage, diarrhea, and vomiting.

F. Principal causes of *fluid overload* are:
1. Excessive administration of fluids.
2. Inadequate renal function.

G. Principal causes of *respiratory acidosis* (a common postoperative H^+ imbalance):
1. *Anesthesia* can cause an excessive intake of CO_2 and a reduction in respiratory rate.
2. *Narcotics* (especially in the elderly) reduce respiratory efficiency.
3. *Postoperative pain* and *bulky, uncomfortable dressings* make most patients reluctant to cough and deep breathe.
4. *Abdominal distention* (a common postoperative problem) crowds diaphragm and makes deep breathing difficult.
5. *Surgery with a high incision* involving the diaphragm reduces ventilation, e.g., hiatus hernia repair and gallbladder surgery.
6. *Postoperative complications*, e.g., *atelectasis, pneumonia*, and *bronchitis*, cause respiratory obstruction and poor ventilation.

H. Ways in which nurses can help to prevent postoperative fluid and electrolyte imbalances:
1. Record I and O accurately.
2. Report abnormal laboratory findings to surgeon immediately.
3. Administer intravenous infusions on time and at the proper rate.
4. Obtain an order for an antiemetic (e.g., Phenergan) for patients with severe, prolonged vomiting.
5. Irrigate gastric suction tubes properly (Chapter 12).
6. Instruct patient to cough and to deep breathe to prevent respiratory acidosis.

Goal 5: Maintenance of Adequate Renal Function

The patient is generally able to void 8 to 16 hours after surgery. Voiding is especially important for those patients who have undergone abdominal or gynecological procedures. Causes of an inability to void postoperatively include:

1. Effects of anesthesia
2. Pain
3. Fear and tension
4. Unfamiliar surroundings
5. Catheter obstruction

Signs of bladder distention are:

1. A fullness above the symphysis pubis that can be palpated
2. Voiding 30 to 60 ml. (1 to 2 oz.) of urine every 15 to 20 minutes (retention with overflow)

The nurse may aid the patient who is having difficulty voiding by several methods. These include: running tap water so that the patient hears it; pouring warm water over the female perineal area; assisting the male to stand at the bedside (if not contraindicated), and administering pain medication.

When permissible, encourage fluids to help promote and maintain renal function. Before administering fluids, check the fluid limits set by the physician.

Remember to administer fluids cautiously during the early postoperative period while antidiuretic hormone (ADH) is being released. "Forcing" fluids too soon can result in dangerous overhydration.

Accurately record intake and output on the I and O sheet for at least the first 48 postoperative hours. Patients on fluid limits or those whose fluid limits are being closely monitored, require a longer period of I and O observation. This record keeping may be prompted either by a physician's order or by nursing judgment.

Goal 6: Promotion of Adequate Rest, Comfort, and Safety

An environment of optimum comfort enables the patient to progress more quickly and more easily through the postoperative period. Pain, restlessnes, and nausea and vomiting may hinder a restful and comfortable postoperative period. Nursing interventions for these problems are as follows:

Pain. Factors related to a high incidence and intensity of postoperative pain include:

Type of anesthesia used. Nitrous oxide is a soluble agent that is rapidly eliminated from the body. Consequently, patients are restless and may experience pain earlier in the postoperative period when nitrous oxide is used. Halothane, also a soluble agent, causes central nervous system depression. However, because it is not excreted as rapidly as nitrous oxide its anesthetizing effects continue for hours following surgery.

High level of anxiety.

Extensive and lengthy surgical procedure.

Poor state of mental health.

Nursing intervention to help alleviate pain includes: comfort measures such as changing the patient's position, straightening bed linen, giving a backrub with lotion, cool cloth to the hands and face, and administration of ordered postoperative narcotics. Postoperative pain occurring within the first 24 hours after surgery is usually relieved by the administration of a narcotic. Drugs commonly used are morphine, Demerol, and codeine. Although these narcotic agents are given routinely during the first 24 hours after surgery, care should be taken that the patient is not overmedicated. Complications arising from a narcotic overdose may include respiratory depression, nausea, and vomiting. A thorough assessment of the patient should be made before narcotics are given. Carefully check for the following:

1. Abnormal blood pressure (if low, decrease the amount of the narcotic).
2. The presence of pressure points if the patient has a cast or splint. Relieving the pressure, by splitting the cast or cutting a window (done by a physician), may decrease pain and the need for a narcotic.
3. A distended bladder; if present, obtain an order for catheterization if the patient is unable to void.
4. Abdominal distension and flatulence; a rectal tube, obtained per order, may decrease gas pain — a common postoperative complaint.

As convalescence progresses, pain medications are administered in decreasing dosages and strengths; the nurse should discourage an overreliance by the patient upon narcotics. Comfort measures and reassurance of the patient concerning the operation often relieve pain-producing anxiety. Notify the surgeon if the patient asks for narcotics at frequent intervals several days after the operation — the patient may be developing a postoperative complication or an overreliance upon narcotics (see also Unit XI).

Restlessness. Restlessness may be caused by: (1) pain, (2) bladder distention, (3) abdominal distention, (4) fear, (5) anxiety, (6) oxygen lack, (7) wet, tight, dressings, or (8) hemorrhage.

Changing the patient's position and bed linen and giving a back massage may reduce restlessness. The patient may need pain medication or specific intervention for the causes listed (e.g., administer oxygen, loosen dressings, assist with voiding).

Nausea and Vomiting. Recent methods and types of anesthesia have helped to reduce postoperative vomiting. Vomiting and nausea still occur in some patients postoperatively and may be related to: (1) premedication, (2) type of anesthesia, (3) type of surgery, (4) an accumulation of fluid in the stomach, (5) inflation of the stomach, (6) food and fluid ingestion prior to the return of peristalsis, and (7) psychological factors such as anxiety and fear.

> *The most important nursing intervention when a patient is vomiting is preventing aspiration of vomitus into the lungs.*

Position the patient on her or his side so that the contents will be evacuated orally. Additional nursing measures include the administration of an antiemetic drug (Compazine or Phenergan) and comfort measures (e.g., cool cloth to face, mouthwash, repositioning in bed). Prolonged nausea and vomiting may indicate a postoperative complication. Notify the surgeon if the condition persists.

Goal 7: Promotion of and Maintenance of Adequate Wound Healing

> *Maintenance of* strict *asepsis both during surgery and during the postoperative period is the single most important factor in the promotion and maintenance of wound healing.*

Contamination and infection disrupt the process of wound repair. Promotion of wound healing and prevention of infection is achieved in the following ways:

Covering wounds with sterile dressings

Dressings may or may not be ordered, depending upon the surgeon's policy. They are usually ordered for:

1. Wounds that are bleeding, oozing, or have heavy drainage.
2. Wounds that can be contaminated by urine or feces.
3. Wounds requiring immobilization.

Inserting drains

Drains (e.g., Penrose drain) may be inserted into wounds that are filled with fluids. These fluid collections are harmful because fluid puts pressure on the surrounding organs. Collections of bile, urine, pus, or pancreatic juice cause tissue irritation and necrosis. As stagnant fluids, these collections also act as a bacterial culture media.

When a large amount of fluid drainage is present, the drainage tube is often attached to tubing and to low suction. A hollow tube may be inserted into an internal organ to carry drainage from the organ to the outside of the body. These tubes are sometimes called "fistula-forming" tubes; they make a hollow connection between the internal organ and the outside of the body. Examples include T-tubes, gastrostomy tubes, cecostomy tubes, and cystostomy tubes.

These tubes are usually surrounded and walled off by fibrous tissue within 7 to 10 days.

Nursing intervention to assure maintenance and promotion of wound healing includes direct wound care and continuous observation. Aseptic technique should always be used when changing dressings. The type of wound and the orders of the physician dictate the protocol used for cleaning the wound and the surrounding area. Remember to keep the area surrounding any tubing clean, since infection may be introduced from outside the body into the wound via the tubing. Also observe the dressing for signs of drainage. Report to the physician if you observe any redness around the wound, increased drainage, or elevation in temperature; these signs indicate an infection.

Types of wounds and the physiology of wound healing are discussed in Chapter 10.

Goal 8: Promotion of and Maintenance of Early Movement and Ambulation

Patients who are immobilized for long periods develop weakness, respiratory diseases such as pneumonia and atelectasis, circulatory problems such as thrombophlebitis, osteoporosis, urinary retention, bladder stones, and a negative nitrogen balance. These problems apply to the surgical patient as well as to the medical patient.

Complications of immobilization following surgery may be prevented by encouraging the patient to move, cough and deep breathe, and flex ankles and legs upon awakening from anesthesia. Patients should be encouraged and assisted to perform these activities throughout their postoperative course. Allowing patients to bathe themselves and to assume their own personal care as soon as possible is a good way to promote early movement. Patients are assisted with, and encouraged to ambulate as early as 24 hours postoperatively, if not contraindicated by physician order. Remember that each patient is a unique individual and that programs of ambulation may vary. Return to normal activity soon after surgery facilitates a shorter hospital stay and thus a decreased expense to the patient.

Goal 9: Provision of Adequate Psychologic Support for the Patient and Significant Others

The concept of surgery is different in its meanings and implications for every individual. It is important that the nurse recognize these differences and provide individualized support to the patient and significant others throughout the experience of surgery. The degree of support will vary within the individual social network. Some patients may recover quickly and in an uncomplicated manner. A patient whose postoperative course is complicated will need much more psychologic support. Beneficial support measures may come from nursing intervention (e.g., spending time listening and talking to the patient and family), comfort measures, and explanations of the treatment procedures and complications.

Intervention from a clergyman may also be helpful. Again, it is important to remember the uniqueness of each individual and to alter your care accordingly.

Goal 10: Provision of Adequate Discharge Teaching and Planning for Patient and Significant Others

The length of time needed for a patient to recuperate from surgery depends upon the patient's physical and mental condition prior to the surgery, the magnitude of the surgery, and the development of any postoperative complications.

Providing discharge teaching and planning for the patient and those who may be involved in home care is an important nursing function. The type of planning and instruction needed varies with the individual and the type of surgical procedure. Ideally, teaching and discharge planning begin preoperatively. The patient and significant others may need information about (a) diet, (b) elimination, (c) exercises that the patient should perform, (d) activities that may need to be limited, and (e) possible complications.

Teaching may take place both through verbal instructions and by various audiovisual materials (e.g., pamphlets, films). Teaching plans and results are documented on the patient care plan and chart. Special patient instructions for specific operations are discussed in appropriate sections throughout this textbook.

Goal 11: Recognition of and Prevention of Postoperative Complications

The patient should be closely observed for the following complications:

Shock	*Emotional disturbances*
Hemorrhage	*Gastric dilatation*
Pneumonia	*Fecal impaction*
Pulmonary emboli	*Postoperative bowel obstruction*
Atelectasis	*Urinary retention*
Wound dehiscence	*Renal failure*
Wound infection	*Paralytic ileus*
Thrombophlebitis	*Acute parotitis*
Decubitus ulcers	*Hiccoughs*

CHAPTER 20

PREVENTING AND TREATING POSTOPERATIVE COMPLICATIONS

One of the nurse's primary goals in caring for surgical patients is preventing the development of postoperative complications.

> *No matter how seemingly minor the surgery, the danger of postoperative complications is* always *present.*

Patients have died from hemorrhage following a tonsillectomy or have gone into severe shock following a simple hernia repair.

Postoperative complications can develop directly in the wound, in organs bordering on the operative site or far from it, or in body cavities. Complications may arise immediately following the surgery, or they may be delayed. Some authorities arbitrarily define a postoperative complication as *any untoward event arising within 30 days after surgery*. Complications may be a direct result of the operative procedure, or they may result from the processes of the disease being treated (e.g., intra-abdominal infection from an abdominal-peritoneal abscess after abdominal surgery).

The most common complications are atelectasis, wound infection, paralytic ileus, urinary retention and infection, and lower extremity venous thrombosis. Certain complications are particularly common after a devastating illness or secondary to other postoperative complications. These include respiratory distress syndrome, stress ulcer, gastric dilation, renal failure, and hepatic failure. Most cardiovascular complications (e.g., cerebral vascular accident, myocardial infarction, pulmonary embolism) and generally all serious infections (e.g., peritonitis) follow some critical event such as postoperative shock or hemorrhage.

The prevention of postoperative complications promotes rapid convalescence, saving the patient time, expense, worry, and pain, perhaps even saving life itself. Once postoperative problems develop, they are difficult to treat. Often one complication leads to other complications, greatly prolonging the patient's hospitalization.

For example, the patient who develops pneumonia following surgery will be placed on bed rest. Immobilization in bed can lead to further problems such as thrombophlebitis, osteoporosis, and the formation of renal stones. With pneumonia, appetite frequently fails and the patient may develop a negative nitrogen balance which, in turn, affects the rate of wound healing. The patient, if very ill with postoperative pneumonia, will experience fever and diaphoresis, which can result in fluid and electrolyte imbalances. Intravenous fluids will probably be ordered, and the patient then suffers additional discomforts and is even more immobilized. Finally, these many problems cause mental anguish for the patient and significant others.

In this chapter we discuss these various complications and nursing interventions to prevent them.

OBSERVING FOR POSTOPERATIVE COMPLICATIONS

To prevent postoperative complications, you must know the significant symptoms that herald the onset of a complication and be able to recognize them quickly should they develop. What are some important symptoms that you must be able to recognize? One authority states:

> Fever *is the commonest evidence of postoperative complications.* Cardiovascular collapse, *although less common, is more dramatic and emergent. Together these two signs forecast at least 90 per cent of postoperative complications.*[75]

Because recognition of these two signs will enable you to recognize the majority of postoperative complications, we shall briefly discuss their significance during the postoperative phase.

Fever

You should expect the average postoperative patient to have a slight elevation of temperature during the first day or so following surgery. However, a marked elevation of temperature (above 37.7°C [100°F] or a *persistent* fever needs to be investigated.

A sustained temperature elevation following surgery usually signals the onset of one of the following problems: (1) pulmonary complications; (2) wound infection or dehiscence; (3) urinary infections; or (4) thrombophlebitis. To remember these four complications seen in connection with fever, Liechty offers the following helpful advice:

> These causes of fever occur so frequently that they should be committed to memory as the 4 W's: "wind, wound, water, and walk." When fever occurs, these common sources should be systematically and repeatedly evaluated.[75]

PULMONARY COMPLICATIONS

Pulmonary problems generally develop within the *first* 48 hours after surgery. Postoperative respiratory complications may be caused by one or several of the following factors:

- Colds, flu, and sore throats that were not brought under control during the preoperative period.
- Exposure to respiratory infections following surgery.
- Use of anesthetics, endotracheal tubes, and oxygen — all of which irritate the tracheobronchial tree and cause increased mucous secretions.
- Aspiration of vomitus.
- Prolonged immobilization of patients upon the operating table during lengthy operations.
- History of smoking.
- Respiratory disease prior to surgery (e.g., chronic bronchitis, COPD).
- Inability of the anesthetized patient to cough, expectorate mucus, and maintain an open airway.
- Depressing effects of many narcotics upon the coughing reflex.
- Collapse of the lung during surgery and inadequate reexpansion of lung tissue following surgery.
- Severe postoperative pain, which makes the patient reluctant to turn, cough, and deep breathe.
- Surgery with a high abdominal or chest incision that causes the patient to neglect deep breathing exercises because of pain.
- Extreme debilitation and old age, which lower the patient's resistance to pulmonary infections.
- Prolonged postoperative immobilization, which leads to decreased chest expansion, the pooling of mucus in the bronchi, and hypostatic pneumonia.

The most common lung problems seen postoperatively are atelectasis, pneumonitis, bronchitis, pneumonias (bronchial, lobar, and hypostatic), pleurisy, and pulmonary emboli. These pulmonary conditions are discussed in Unit XVI.

As emphasized earlier these conditions can be *prevented* by preoperative instruction concerning moving, coughing, and breathing exercises and by vigilant and repeated postoperative coaching on a planned basis (e.g., every 2 hours) in all these areas. The maintenance of an open airway, adequate hydration (which thins mucous secretions), and early ambulation are also vital in maintaining adequate respiratory function.

Should respiratory complications develop, the patient may need to undergo uncomfortable procedures, e.g., bronchoscopy (to remove mucous plugs) and postural drainage (to move secretions in the lung). Also, antibiotic therapy may be started. If respiratory problems are severe, the patient will need oxygen and may even require the aid of a mechanical respirator to breathe.

WOUND INFECTION

Wound infections generally occur around the fifth postoperative day, although the initial inflammatory process is often evident within 36 to 48 hours after surgery. Important factors that predispose the patient to wound infections are:

- *Obesity*. Fatty tissues do not heal readily and are difficult for the surgeon to approximate and suture.
- *Debilitation*. Persons debilitated by cancer, malnutrition, ulcerative colitis, and so forth, have a lowered resistance to *all* infection.
- *Old age*. Elderly individuals with arteriosclerosis and poor circulation have lowered defenses against infection.
- *Lengthy, complicated operations*. Complex operations place an increased stress upon the patient, which lowers resistance.
- *Therapy with steroids, irradiation, and anticancer drugs*. These drugs and treatments can reduce the body's leukocyte count drastically.
- *The presence of other diseases*, in particular hypogammaglobulinemia, diabetes mellitus, obstructive jaundice, ulcerative colitis, uremia, leukemia, aplastic anemia, and malignant neoplasms greatly lowers the patient's resistance to wound infection.
- *Failure to maintain asepsis* in the operating room or during wound dressings.

Studies show that the general attitude of a

hospital staff toward infection control is an important factor in the prevention or promotion of infection. For example, some surgeons and nurses have a false confidence about infection control, fostered by the availability of multiple antibiotics. The attitude of, "Oh, well, if a wound infection develops, we can always clear it up with antibiotics" is unfortunately common. Also, hospital personnel are sometimes careless in their aseptic technique because they fail to recognize the importance of asepsis; as a result, pick-up forceps, dressing trays, bandage scissors, and adhesive tape may often be grossly contaminated. Some people almost seem to think that "bugs just aren't there if you can't see them." Thus, education of hospital staff members in various positions (nurse, aide, orderly, maid) about the principles of asepsis is one important way to prevent wound infections.

The organism most commonly responsible for wound infections is *Staphylococcus aureus*, a gram-positive, nonmotile organism. Staphylococci produce *pyogenic* infections; their presence in a wound is usually diagnosed by laboratory examination of a specimen of wound drainage. This organism can be transmitted to the surgical patient from contaminated dressing cart equipment and from staff members and patients who are carriers harboring the organism in their noses and throats. Failure to isolate patients with infections from patients with clean wounds is another common factor in the transmission of "Staph" infections.

Other organisms responsible for wound infections are *Escherichia coli, Proteus vulgaris, Aerobacter aerogenes,* and *Pseudomonas aeruginosa*.

Major symptoms of wound infections are redness, tenderness, and heat in the area of the wound or incision, coupled with the appearance of wound drainage. Obese patients should be checked carefully for signs of wound infection; surplus fatty tissue often obscures the presence of infection.

To *treat* wound infections, the surgeon generally irrigates and cleanses the wound with sterile normal saline solution, inserts a drain into the incision, cultures the infected drainage, and, on the basis of the findings of the culture, orders appropriate antibiotic therapy.

WOUND DEHISCENCE AND EVISCERATION

Wound *dehiscence* is an opening of the wound edges, whereas wound *evisceration* is characterized by the protrusion of loops of bowel through the incision. Malnourished, chronically ill, or obese patients are most prone to wound dehiscence. Related causative factors are:

- ▶ The presence of wound infections.
- ▶ Faulty closure of the wound in surgery.
- ▶ Severe stretching of the abdominal wall as a result of coughing and retching.

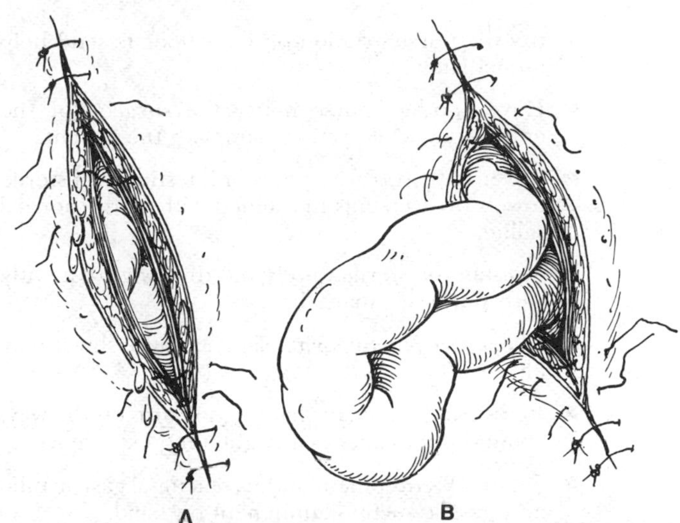

Figure 20–1. **A.** Wound dehiscence. **B.** Evisceration.

Although wound dehiscence and evisceration can occur at any time, they generally occur on the sixth to seventh postoperative day. At this time, the patient's suture line is weaker (sutures may have been removed) than it was on the first 3 days after surgery. Pulmonary complications may cause excessive coughing during the fifth, sixth, and seventh postoperative days when the suture line is the weakest and may lead to wound dehiscence or evisceration. Prevention of these complications, through the measures described previously, is crucial.

Any wound can rupture. However *midline abdominal incisions* are most prone to dehiscence and evisceration.

Typical *symptoms* of wound dehiscence are often dramatic. When an abdominal wound ruptures suddenly and evisceration occurs, coils of intestine protrude from the incision. When the wound edges part slowly, a gush of pinkish serous drainage is usually the major symptom.

> *In any postoperative patient, the sudden escape of a profuse, pink serous drainage from the wound is an ominous sign and must be investigated immediately.*

To *treat* wound dehiscence, the surgeon generally orders the patient back to surgery, where the wound is resutured.

The nurse's role in event of wound dehiscence is:

- ▶ Remain calm.
- ▶ Ring the emergency bell, put on the call light, or use the phone and have the hospital operator no-

tify the nurse's station on your floor to send help immediately.

- Have another nurse notify the surgeon of the emergency while you remain with the patient.
- Cover any protruding coils of intestine with sterile towels or dressings moistened with sterile normal saline.
- Moisten the sterile towels and dressing frequently with sterile normal saline.
- Check the patient's vital signs because shock may ensue.
- Reassure the patient that the doctor is on the way. Wound dehiscence is a frightening experience!
- Set up IV equipment and have a nasal gastric tube and gastric suction equipment on hand.
- Notify surgery that the patient will be returning to the operating room.

Wound dehiscence can often be *prevented* by the proper application of a scultetus binder. However, some surgeons object to use of scultetus binders on the grounds that a binder tends to weaken the patient's muscles. Other preventive measures are the correction of nutritional deficiencies and of obesity prior to surgery.

URINARY INFECTIONS*

Postoperative patients often have difficulty voiding and may require catheterization. The most common cause of urinary infection postoperatively is catheterization. Typical symptoms of urinary tract infection generally occur between the fifth and eighth postoperative days. Symptoms include dysuria, frequency, and fever. Treatment of urinary infections involves sending a specimen of the urine to the laboratory for culture and sensitivity testing. The *culture* results indicate which *organism* or type of organism is causing the infection; the *sensitivity* results indicate which *antibiotic* is most effective in the treatment of the infection. Appropriate antibiotics are ordered on the basis of the laboratory results.

To prevent bladder infections, *avoid catheterization* if at all possible. Various techniques for helping the patient to void are discussed in Chapter 41.

THROMBOPHLEBITIS†

Postoperative thrombophlebitis generally occurs 7 to 14 days following surgery. Thrombophlebitis is sometimes caused by injury to the vein wall from the use of tight leg straps and leg holders during gynecologic surgery. Also, stasis and an increased blood coagulability (etiologic factors in thrombophlebitis) may develop postoperatively because of dehydration and an inadequate circulation resulting from hemorrhage. Obesity, prolonged immobilization, and senility are also associated with this complication.

Thrombophlebitis can be *prevented* by the use of leg exercises postoperatively, early ambulation, and *TED* support hose while the patient is in bed and prior to the first time the patient ambulates. *Treatment* includes rest and the administration of anticoagulant drugs.

The greatest danger with thrombophlebitis is that the clot will break loose from the vein wall in the leg and will travel as an embolism to the patient's lungs, heart, or brain.

Cardiovascular Collapse (Shock)

The commonest causes of postoperative shock are:

- Bleeding and hemorrhage (hypovolemic shock)
- Sepsis (septic shock)
- Cardiac arrest and myocardial infarction (cardiogenic shock)
- Drug sensitivity (anaphylactic shock)
- Transfusion reactions
- Pulmonary embolism
- Adrenal failure

Table 20–1 discusses in brief the cause, diagnosis, and treatment of these types of shock.

With the exception of septic shock, these specific forms of shock are discussed in appropriate sections of the text. (Chapter 13 discusses physiologic shock in depth). Because sepsis is one of the most important causes of postoperative shock (indeed, some authorities state that it is the *most* common cause), we shall briefly discuss this complication.

The causes of *septic shock* are twofold. As one authority states:

> Septic shock has at least two distinctly different mechanisms for producing shock: (1) extensive cellulitis or diffuse infections of body cavities (peritonitis) cause sequestration of large amounts of plasma-like fluid into the injured tissue to produce hypovolemia and (2) toxins produced by the infecting organisms exert profound effects upon circulation.[112]

Shock produced by gram-negative organisms is more profound than that produced by gram-positive organisms. Characteristics of shock produced by gram-negative organisms are: profound vasoconstriction, toxemia, acidosis, tissue anoxia, oliguria, heart failure, and hypotension.

*Urinary infections are discussed in Unit XIII.
†Thrombophlebitis is discussed in Chapter 49.

Gram-positive organisms, on the other hand, produce vasodilatation; acidosis and anoxia do *not* occur.

Septic shock is treated by administering massive doses of antibiotics IV, fluids, corticosteroids and, as with other shock conditions, by providing support for additional failing body systems.

OTHER POSTOPERATIVE COMPLICATIONS

Other important postoperative complications include gastrointestinal (gastric dilatation, paralytic ileus, fecal impaction and postoperative bowel obstruction), urinary (renal failure and urinary retention), and miscellaneous (hiccoughs, acute parotitis, decubitus ulcers and emotional disturbances).

Gastrointestinal

Acute Gastric Dilatation

This is an uncommon postoperative complication that may follow abdominal, chest, spine, or central nervous system procedures; it may also follow untreated postoperative gastric distention. It is usually relieved within 48 hours by gastric intubation. Death from shock, however, may occur within a few hours.

A. Etiology
   1. Exact etiology unknown.
   2. Several liters of air and dark-colored, foul-smelling material collect in the stomach.
B. Symptoms
   1. Abdominal distention.
   2. Overflow type vomiting.
      a. No retching present.
      b. Nausea may not be present.
      c. Vomitus tends to pour from the mouth.
C. Clinical Care
   1. Immediate gastric intubation and suction.
   2. Replacement of fluids and electrolytes lost through vomitus and resultant hypovolemia.

Adynamic or Paralytic Ileus

This condition is manifested by a paralysis of intestinal peristalsis or lack of effective coordinated peristalsis. X-ray films reveal a dilated bowel, with gas distributed throughout the digestive tract.

TABLE 20–1. POSTOPERATIVE SHOCK

Cause	Diagnosis	Treatment
1. *Bleeding* Usually in peritoneal or pleural cavities or retroperitoneal areas	Check wounds, drain sites, open wounds, or use diagnostic aspiration if necessary; central venous pressure is low	Blood and immediate ligation of bleeding vessel
2. *Cardiac shock* Myocardial infarction or arrhythmias, arrest	Check for pulse irregularities, electrocardiogram, absence of pulse and cyanosis suggest cardiac arrest; SGOT aids diagnosis of infarction; central venous pressure is high	Dependent on diagnosis: general measures, oxygen, sedation, cardiopulmonary resuscitation
3. *Pulmonary embolus*	No specific signs; chest pain, hemoptysis suggest diagnosis; angiography can make diagnosis; obesity, previous cardiac difficulties, cancer and pelvic operations, immobility, and increased age are associated factors	Embolectomy; fibrinolytic agents to dissolve clots are promising
4. *Transfusion reaction* (contaminated blood)	Smears of blood show gram-negative organisms; shock rapidly follows blood administration	Discontinue blood; corticosteroids, massive doses of antibiotics intravenously
5. *Sepsis*	Culture of blood or suspicion of gram-negative bacterial source of septicemia	Massive intravenous antibiotics, fluids, corticosteroids
6. *Adrenal failure*	Must be diagnosed by suspicion or history of steroid therapy, lack of other causes	Intravenous corticosteroids (100 to 300 mg. of hydrocortisone)
7. *Anaphylactic shock*	Obscure clinical picture; history of drug sensitivities is vitally important; urticaria and edema may aid diagnosis	Epinephrine, antihistamines corticosteroids

From Liechty, R. D.: Postoperative care. *In* Liechty, R. D., and R. T. Soper (Eds.): *Synopsis of Surgery,* 3rd ed. St. Louis: C. V. Mosby Co. 1976, p. 127.

A. Etiology
   1. *Temporary ileus.* May be a reaction to anesthesia, trauma, or abdominal operations.
   2. *Prolonged ileus*
      a. Electrolyte imbalance.
      b. Wound infection.
      c. Metabolic diseases.
B. Symptoms
   1. Peristaltic activity of the gastrointestinal tract stops temporarily.
   2. Bowel sounds are absent.
   3. Neither gas nor feces are passed by rectum.
   4. Gastric and abdominal distention (because of air swallowed by reflex).
C. Clinical Care
   1. Nasogastric suction.
   2. IV fluid administration.
   3. Miller-Abbott intestinal tube is sometimes used.
   4. A rectal tube is used to relieve flatus.

Fecal Impaction

A. Etiology
   1. Limitation of oral fluids.
   2. Immobilization.
   3. Some narcotic analgesics.
   4. Can be aggravated by barium enema, followed by the accumulation of barium in the colon.
B. Symptoms
   1. Diarrhea.
   2. Hard stool felt upon digital rectal examination.
C. Clinical Care
   1. Digital disimpaction after giving an oil retention enema.

Postoperative Bowel Obstruction

Bowel obstruction may occur as a complication of any abdominal surgical procedure.

A. Etiology
   1. Occurs as a result of either *peritonitis* or *generalized irritation of peritoneal surface*.
   2. These conditions produce varying degrees of intestinal adhesions. When the adhesions kink or trap a segment of the intestine, an obstruction results.
B. Symptoms
   1. Constipation.
   2. Abdominal distention and, occasionally, tenderness.
   3. Abdominal pain.
   4. Nausea and vomiting (a late sign).
   5. Characteristic diagnostic x-ray findings.
C. Clinical Care
   1. Nasogastric tube.
   2. Miller-Abbott tube. Decompression via a tube will often result in the realignment of the bowel and relief of the obstruction. Adhesions may "give" enough to allow spontaneous decompression.
   3. Surgery for correction of obstruction if conservative care is not successful.

Urinary Complications

Urinary Retention

This is a common postoperative occurrence.

A. Etiology
   1. Anesthesia.
   2. Narcotics.
   3. Anticholinergic drugs (atropine).
   4. Operative trauma.
   5. Advanced age.
   6. Diseases of urinary system (e.g., enlarged prostate).
B. Symptoms
   1. Patient experiences a feeling of "fullness."
   2. Bladder distended upon palpation.
C. Clinical Care
   1. Assist patient with voiding (as discussed in Chapter 41).
   2. If patient is unable to void, insert sterile catheter.

Renal Failure

This is a rare postoperative complication, but carries a high mortality rate. It is discussed in more detail in Unit XIII.

A. Etiology
   1. Prolonged preoperative or postoperative hypotension.
   2. Postoperative septicemia.
   3. Preexisting renal disease that was not corrected prior to surgery.
B. Symptoms
   1. Oliguria or anuria despite adequate fluid intake.
   2. Low urinary specific gravity.
   3. Increased urinary sodium output.
C. Clinical Care
   1. Early peritoneal or renal dialysis.
   2. Strict fluid restriction.
   3. Protective isolation to prevent infection.

Miscellaneous Complications

Hiccoughs

Hiccoughs are usually no more than an uncomfortable nuisance that disappears after a short period. However, they may persist for weeks and, in this case, indicate a serious underlying condition. They are most likely to develop following abdominal surgery.

A. Etiology
   1. Irritation of the phrenic nerve due to:
      a. A distended abdomen.
      b. Abscesses close to the diaphragm.
      c. Gastric dilatation.
      d. Peritonitis.

2. Anxiety.
3. Acidosis.
4. Surgical procedure performed close to the diaphragm.

B. Symptoms
1. Intermittent spasms of the diaphragm produce the typical "hic" sound.
2. Hiccoughs can result in:
a. Exhaustion.
b. Vomiting.
c. Fluid and electrolyte imbalances.
d. Malnutrition.
e. Wound dehiscence.

C. Clinical Care
1. Rebreathing own air from a paper bag.
2. Whiffs of carbon dioxide.
3. Gastric lavage or suction.
4. Sedatives.
5. Tranquilizers.
6. In extreme cases:
a. Phrenic nerve block.
b. Phrenic nerve crush.

Acute Parotitis ("Surgical Mumps")

This is a rare complication of surgery. It should be given prompt attention because a secondary staphylococcal infection may develop.

A. Etiology
1. Poor oral hygiene following surgery.
2. Extreme debilitation.

B. Symptoms
1. Moderate or high fever.
2. Inflammation of the parotid gland that produces:
a. Pain.
b. Swelling.
c. Redness.

C. Clinical Care
1. X-ray therapy during the early stages.
2. Surgical incision and drainage.
3. Antibiotics.
4. Prevent by:
a. Frequent oral hygiene.
b. Giving fluids when allowed.
c. Giving the patient pieces of hard candy to suck to stimulate parotid secretions.

Decubitus Ulcers

A. Etiology
1. Immobility.
2. Extreme debilitation.
3. Prolonged pressure over bony areas.
4. Preexisting arteriosclerosis

B. Symptoms
1. Early sign — redness over bony area or pressure points (hips, ankles, sacrum)
2. Necrosis and ulceration of tissues overlying bony prominences.

C. Clinical Care
1. To *prevent*:
a. Frequent movement,
b. Early ambulation.
c. Cleanliness.
2. For treatment, see a basic nursing text.

Emotional Disturbances

These may manifest themselves through neuroses or psychoses.

A. Etiology
1. Grief over loss of a body organ or part.
2. Disturbances of body image.
3. Prior emotional problems.
4. Exhaustion and extreme debilitation, which lower resistance to stress.

B. Symptoms
1. Insomnia.
2. Restlessness.
3. Expression of hopelessness.
4. Agitation.
5. Delusions.
6. Suicidal thoughts.
7. Confusion

C. Clinical Care
1. Report these symptoms to the surgeon.
2. Determine cause. If physiologic, it may be corrected with appropriate therapy (e.g., intravenous supplementation of fluid and electrolytes). Spend time with the patient, giving reassurance and emotional support. A psychiatrist may be involved if appropriate. Involvement with a community support group composed of people who have undergone the same type of surgery often helps the patient during this adjustment period.
3. Use precautions against suicide in patients who verbalize suicidal thoughts:
a. Do not leave knives or razors with the patient
b. Observe continuously.
c. Make certain that patient swallows sleeping medications and does not hoard them.
d. Do not allow near unprotected windows, especially if high, or by fire escapes.

BIBLIOGRAPHY (Unit VIII)

1. Adair, L. P.: Patient education. *Nursing Care*, 9:29—31, Apr. 1976.
2. Anderson, D. M., and J. H. Cosgriff: Partners in practice. *Supervisor Nurse*, 5:8, July 1974.
3. Baker, P. J.: Postoperative atelectasis. *Nursing Digest*, 5:42, Spring 1977.
4. Bakutis, A. R.: Assessing the anesthesia patient. *AANA Journal*, 43:255, June 1975.
5. Barach, A. L., and M. S. Segal: The indiscriminate use of IPPB. *JAMA*, 231:1141, Mar. 1975.
6. Barnard, J. D. W., et al.: Cryoanalgesia. *Nursing Times*, 73:897–8; June 16, 1977.
7. Bartlett, R. H., et al.: Respiratory maneuvers to prevent postoperative pulmonary complications. *JAMA*, 224:1017, May 1973.
8. Biebuyck, J. F.: Role of the nurse in modern anaesthesia. *S. A. Nursing Journal*, 44: 27–9, Feb. 1977.
9. Billie, D. A.: The role of body image in patient compli-

ance and education. *Heart and Lung*, 6:143, Jan.-Feb. 1977.
10. Boore, J.: Preoperative care of patients. *Nursing Times*, 73:409, Mar. 1977.
11. Boykin, L.: Nourishing the surgical patient. *Nursing Care*, 9:16, Aug. 1976.
12. Breckon, D. J.: Highlights in the evolution of hospital based patient education programs. *Journal of Allied Health*, 5:35–9, Summer 1976.
13. Breitung, J.: Are you fudging on handwashing routines? *RN*, 40:71, June 1977.
14. Buckwalter, J. A.: Blood, coagulation, and transfusion. *In* Liechty, R. D., and R. T. Soper (Eds.): *Synopsis of Surgery*, 3rd ed. St. Louis: C. V. Mosby Co., 1976.
15. Buckwalter, J. A., and I. M. Smith: Surgical Infections. *In* Liechty, R. D. and R. T. Soper (Eds.): *Synopsis of Surgery*, 3rd ed. St. Louis: C. V. Mosby Co., 1976.
16. Bututis, A.: Anesthetic reactions. *Nursing '72*, 2:16, Sept. 1972.
17. Cap, A. G.: Pre-op classes produce more relaxed patients. *Inservice Training Education* 4:9, Aug. 1975.
18. Che-Lu, T.: The fine points of acupuncture. *AORN Journal*, 17:59, Jan 1973.
19. Clark, R. B.: The case for spinal anesthesia. *AAJN* 67:294, Feb. 1967.
20. Communication: Nursing instructions to patients. *Regan Report on Nursing Law, 16*:2, Aug. 1975.
21. Condon, R. E., and L. M. Nyhus, (Eds.): *Manual of Surgical Therapeutics*, 3rd ed. Boston: Little, Brown and Co., 1975.
22. Costello, J.: Adult respiratory distress syndrome. *Consultant*, 17(3):118, Mar. 1977.
22a. Croushore, T. M.: Postoperative assessment: The key to avoiding the most common nursing mistakes. *Nursing 79*, 9:46, Apr. 1979.
23. Cullen, D. J., et al.: Postanesthetic complications. *Surgical Clinics of North America*, 55(4):987, Aug. 1975.
24. Davison, L. A., et al.: Psychological effects of halothane and isoflurane anesthesia. *Anesthesiology*, 43(3):313, Sept. 1975.
25. Dennings, C. P.: Discharge planning and the government . . . United States. *Supervisor Nurse*, 8:48, Mar. 1977.
26. Donn. M.: Communication — The key to preparation for surgery. *Nursing Mirror*, 143:46, Oct. 1976.
27. Dripps, R. D., et al.: *Introduction to Anesthesia: The Principles of Safe Practice*, 4th ed. Philadelphia: W. B. Saunders Co., 1972.
28. Dunphy, J. E., and L. W. Way et al.: *Current Surgical Diagnosis and Treatment*, 3rd ed. Los Altos, Calif: Lange Medical Publications, 1977.
29. Dziurbejko, M. M., and J. C. Larkin: Including the family in preoperative teaching. *American Journal of Nursing*, 78:1892, Nov. 1978.
30. Eisler, J., et al.: Relationship between need for social approval and postoperative recovery and welfare. *Nursing Research*, 21:520, Nov. Dec. 1972.
31. Ellison, P. V.: The pre- and postoperative visit concept. *Nursing Times*, 71:NATN (suppl.) iv-vi, Oct. 1975.
32. Engle, S.: Things to know about postoperative care. *Consultant*, 15:59, April, 1975.
33. Epstein, L. I., et al.: A nomogram for the use of sevoflurane. *AANAJ*, 45:67, Feb. 1977.
34. Fay, M. R.: Nursing process in the recovery room. *AORN Journal*, 24:1069, Dec. 1976.
35. Fox, J. D.: What's new in surgery? *Life, Health*, 91:26, July 1976.
36. Fralic, M. F.: Developing a viable inpatient education program . . . a nursing director's perspective. *Journal of Nursing Administration*, 6:30, Sept. 1976.
37. Fried, J. L.: An evaluation of therapy to prevent postoperative atelectasis. *Respiratory Therapy*, 7:55, May-June 1977.
38. Fry, E. N.: Postoperative analgesia. *Nursing Times*, 73:655–6; May 5, 1977.
39. Furnas, D. W., and R. D. Leichty: Wounds, wound healing, and drains. *In* Liechty, R. D., and R. T. Soper (Eds.): *Synopsis of Surgery*. 3rd ed. St. Louis: C. V. Mosby Co., 1976, p. 4.
40. Giese, H. A., Jr.: Comparison of three agents used in surgical scrubs. *Ohio State Medical Journal*, 68:855, Sept. 1972.
41. Goegli, E. H., et al.: Can postoperative learning be improved? *AORN Journal*, 16:43, Nov, 1972.
42. Gold, M. I.: Stop IPPB therapy! *Respiratory Care*, 41: 712, Aug. 1976.
43. Gruber, U. F., et al.: The present state of prevention of postoperative thromboembolic complications. *Bibl. Haematol.*, 41:98, 1975.
44. Gruendemann, B., et al.: *The Surgical Patient: Behavioral Concepts for the Operating Room Nurse*, 2nd ed. St. Louis: C. V. Mosby Co., 1977.
45. Gruendemann, B.: The impact of surgery on body image. *Nursing Clinics of North America*, 10:635, Dec. 1975.
46. Gusfa, A., et al.: Patient teaching: one approach. *Supervisor Nurse*, 6:17, Dec. 1975.
47. Hamilton, W. K.: Anesthesia. *In* Liechty, R. D., and R. T. Soper, (Eds.) *Synopsis of Surgery*, 3rd ed. St. Louis: C. V. Mosby Co., 1976, p. 111.
48. Hardy, J. D.: *Rhoads Textbook of Surgery: Principles and Practice*. Philadelphia, J. P. Lippincott Co., 1977.
49. Harrington, J. D. (Ed.): Intensive care of the surgical patient. *Nursing Clinics of North America*, 10:1, Mar. 1975.
50. Haven, L. C., et al.: Reducing the patient's fear of the recovery room. *RN*, 38:28, Jan. 1975.
51. Hayward, J.: Information — a prescription against pain. *Nursing Times*, 73:8, Jan. 1977.
52. Hellawell, J.: The nurse's role in anesthesia: Preoperative preparation. Part 1. *Nursing Times*, 68:400, Apr. 1972.
53. Hellawell, J.: Postoperative care. Part 2. *Nursing Times*, 68:443, Apr. 1972.
54. Hellawell, J.: Respiratory failure. Part 3. *Nursing Times*, 68:467, Apr. 1972.
55. Hellawell, J.: Cardiac arrest and resuscitation. Part 4. *Nursing Times*, 68:512, Apr. 1972.
56. Holley, H. S.: Anesthesia, methods to recovery. *AORN Journal*, 21:822, Apr. 1975.
57. Hudson, S.: Teach breath control to ease your patient's post-op pains. *RN*, 40:37, Jan. 1977.
58. Hunt, T. E.: Rehabilitation of the elderly. *Hospital Practice*, 12:89, Jan. 1977.
59. Ionescu, M. I., and G. H. Wooler (Eds.): *Current Techniques in Extracorporeal Circulation*. London, Butterworth's, 1976.
60. Johnson, J. E., et al.: A better way to calm the patient who fears the worst. *RN*, 40:47, Apr. 1977.
61. Johnson, J. E., et al.: Psychosocial factors in the welfare of surgical patients. *Nursing Research*, 19:18, Jan.-Feb. 1970.
62. Johnson, M.: Outcome criteria to evaluate postoperative respiratory status. *American Journal of Nursing*, 75:1474, Sept. 1975.
63. Kelly, L. Y.: The patient's right to know. *Nursing Outlook*, 24:26, Jan. 1976.
64. Kirkwood, M. O., and P. P. Kaspar: The preoperative

visit — O. R. nurses and patients interact. *Hospitals*, 50:87, Apr. 1976.
65. Korten, K.: Anesthesia for diagnostic procedures. *American Family Practitioner*, 15:103, Mar. 1977.
66. Laird, M.: Techniques for teaching pre- and postoperative patients. *American Journal of Nursing*, 75:1338, Aug. 1975.
67. Lake, G. M.: Hospitalization and personality change: Recognition vital to nursing care. *Canadian Nurse*, 73:44, Jan. 1975.
68. Lamb, D. H.: On the distinction between psychological and physical stressors. *Psychological Reports*, June 1976.
69. Leighton, A. O.: 10 steps to better patient teaching. *RN*, 39:76, Oct. 1976.
70. LeMaitre, G., and J. Finnegan: *The Patient in Surgery: A Guide for Nurses*, 3rd ed. Philadelphia: W. B. Saunders Co., 1975.
71. Levine, E. C., and J. P. Fielder: Fears, facts, and fantasies about pre- and postoperative care. *Nursing Outlook*, 18:26, Feb. 1970.
72. Libman, R. H., et al.: Relieving airway obstruction in the recovery room. *American Journal of Nursing*, 75:1492, Sept. 1975.
73. Liechty, R. D.: Origins of surgical disease. *In* Liechty, R. D., and R. T. Soper (Eds.): *Synopsis of Surgery*, 3rd ed. St. Louis: C. V. Mosby Co., 1976, p. 1.
74. Liechty, R. D.: Preoperative care. *In* Liechty, R. D., and R. T. Soper (Ed.): *Synopsis of Surgery*, 3rd ed. St. Louis: C. V. Mosby Co., 1976, p. 106.
75. Liechty, R. D.: Postoperative care. *In* Liechty, R. D., and R. T. Soper (Eds.): *Synopsis of Surgery*, 3rd ed. St. Louis: C. V. Mosby Co., 1976, p. 127.
76. Lyons, M. L.: What priority do you give preop teaching? *Nursing 77*, 7:12; Jan. 1977.
77. Marcinek, M.: Stress in the surgical patient. *American Journal of Nursing*, 77:1809; Nov. 1977.
78. Metheny, N., and Snively, W. D.: *Nurse's Handbook of Fluid Balance*, 2nd ed. Philadelphia: J. B. Lippincott Co., 1974.
79. McCloskey, J.: How to make the most of the body image theory in nursing practice. *Nursing 76*, 4:68; May 1976.
80. McConnell, E.: After surgery: How you can avert the obvious hazards . . . and the not-so-obvious ones, too. *Nursing 77*, 7:32; Mar. 1977.
81. McCormick, P. W.: Immediate care of the aspiration of vomit. *Anesthesia*, 30(5):658; Sept. 1975.
82. McGown, R. G.: A technique of anaesthesia in haemorrhagic shock: Illustrative case histories and a discussion. *Anaesthesia*, 30(5):616, Sept. 1975.
83. Mitchell, M.: Routine postoperative management and immediate recovery room care. *Nursing Care*, 9:30, June 1976.
84. Moynihan, B. G.: *Abdominal Operations*. Philadelphia: W. B. Saunders Co., 1905.
85. Myer, E. M.: How far should patients decide on their own treatment? *Nursing Times*, 72:1818, Nov. 1976.
86. Newman, B.: The hex on hexachlorophene. *Medical Times*, 101:33, Feb. 1973.
87. Neff, T. A.: Meeting the challenge of pulmonary embolism. *Consultant*, 17(4):50, Apr. 1977.
88. Obese patients breathe better postop while semirecumbent. *RN*, 39:12, June 1976.
89. Organ, C. H.: OR nurse, surgeon common areas of concern. *AORN Journal* 22:898, December, 1975.
90. Paige, R. L., and J. F. Looney: Hospice care for the adult. *American Journal of Nursing*, 77:1812, Nov. 1977.
91. Parsons, M.: Postoperative complications: Assessment and intervention. *American Journal of Nursing*, 74: 240, Feb. 1974.
92. Pearson, B.: Learning tool selection. *Supervisor Nurse*, 6:30, Mar. 1975.
93. Pflug, E. A., et al.: Spinal anesthesia: bupivacaine versus tetracaine. *Anesthesia and Analgesia*, 55(4):489, July-Aug. 1976.
94. Pleitz, J. A.: Psychological complications of the surgical patient. *AORN Journal*, 16:137, Aug. 1972.
95. Polenz, J. M.: Psychological aspects of patient care. *Nursing Care*, 8:16, Oct. 1975.
96. Pomarski, M. E.: The alcoholic as a surgical patient. *AORN Journal*, 16:137, Aug. 1972.
97. Rao, D. B.: The team approach to integrated care of the elderly. *Geriatrics*, 32:88, Feb. 1977.
98. Redman, B. R.: Guidelines for quality care in patient education. *Nursing Digest*, 4:25, Sept.-Oct. 1976.
99. Rhodes, M. J., Gruendemann, B. J., and Ballinger, W. F.: *Alexander's Care of the Patient in Surgery*, 6th ed. St. Louis: C. V. Mosby Co., 1978.
100. Ridgeway, M.: Preop interviews assure quality care. *AORN Journal*, 24:1083, Dec. 1976.
101. Robinson, L. A.: Patients' information base: a key to care. *Canadian Nurse*, 70:34, Dec. 1974.
102. Role of stress in disease. *Ranf. Review*, 6:6, Feb. 1975.
103. Roy, U. T., and G. E. Goodell: Family involved in patient's care. *Hospitals*, 49:96, Mar. 1975.
104. Russell, R.: Use mind control to ease your patients' ills. *RN*, 39:32, May 1976.
105. Sabiston, D. C., and J. B. Duke (Eds.): *Davis Christopher Textbook of Surgery: The Biological Basis of Modern Surgical Practice*. Philadelphia: W. B. Saunders Co., 1977.
106. Saylor, D. E.: Understanding presurgical anxiety. *AORN Journal*, 22:624, Oct. 1975.
107. Schwartz, S. F., et al.: *Principles of Surgery*, 2nd ed. New York: McGraw-Hill, 1974.
108. Shafer, N.: Preparing the asthmatic patient for surgery. *Consultant*, 17(5):84, May 1977.
109. Shilling, J. A.: Wound healing and the inflammatory response in the aged. *Major Problems in Clinical Surgery*, 17:62, 1975.
110. Smith, B. J.: After anesthesia. *Nursing 74*, 4:28, Dec. 1974.
111. Smith, B. J.: Safeguarding your patient after anesthesia. *Nursing 78*, 8:53, Oct. 1978.
112. Soper, R. T., and R. J. Corry: Shock. *In* Liechty, R. D., and R. T. Soper (Eds.): *Synopsis of Surgery*, 3rd ed. St. Louis: C. V. Mosby Co., 1976, p. 70.
112a. Sorensen, K. C., and J. Luckmann, *Basic Nursing: A Psychophysiologic Approach*, Philadelphia: W. B. Saunders Company, 1978.
113. Statement on patient education. *Health Education* 7:22, July-Aug. 1976.
114. Steere, A., and G. Mallison: Handwashing practices for the prevention of nosocomial infection. *Annals of Internal Medicine*, 83:683, Nov. 1975.
115. Strauss, R. J., et al.: Operative risks of obese patients: nursing care. *AORN Journal*, 25:1053, May 1977.
116. Storlie, F.: *Patient Teaching in Critical Care*. New York: Appleton-Century-Crofts, 1975.
117. Sturdevant, B., et al.: Helping patients do their homework. *Supervisor Nurse*, 8:72, April 1977.
118. Tennant, C., et al.: A scale to measure the stress of life events. *Australian-New Zealand Journal of Psychiatry* March 1976.

119. The evolution of antiseptic surgery. *OR Tech,* 9:17, Jan.-Feb. 1977.
120. Tucker, S. M., et al.: *Patient Care Standards.* St. Louis: C. V. Mosby Co., 1975.
121. Vain, E. H.: Obesity in surgery. *AORN Journal* 16:85, Sept, 1972.
122. Vaughn, M.: Surgery for the morbidly obese. *Nursing Digest,* 9:60, Summer 1976.
123. Weber, C. E., et al.: Discharge medication counseling. *Hospital Topics,* 54:39, Nov.-Dec. 1976.
124. What's new in surgery. *Emergency Medicine,* 9:51, Apr. 1977.
125. What's new in surgery. *Emergency Medicine* 10:107, June 1978.
126. Wylie, W. D., and Churchill-Davidson, H. C. (eds.): *A Practice of Anaesthesia,* 3rd ed. Chicago: Year Book Medical Publishers, Inc., 1972.
127. Ziffren, S. E.: Geriatric Surgery. *In* Liechty, R. D. and R. T. Soper (Eds.): *Synopsis of Surgery,* 3rd ed. St. Louis: C. V. Mosby Co., 1976, p. 474.

UNIT IX*

NURSING PEOPLE EXPERIENCING NEOPLASTIC DISORDERS

Vast resources must indeed be mustered in the search for cancer's Achilles heel. Each advance has been hard fought, yet scientists are more hopeful than ever before. They are confident that they will come up with the answers. At stake is triumph in a human adventure of the highest drama. And with this triumph will come the prize of lessening of human suffering and of premature death throughout the world.

ORLANDO A. BATTISTA

INTRODUCTION AND STUDY GUIDE

Caring for people with cancer is one of the largest and most significant tasks facing health professionals today. Currently, cancer ranks second as a cause of death in the United States, preceded only by the cardiovascular disorders. Cancer claims over 350,000 lives per year and brings disruption into the lifestyles of many thousands more.[31] Cancer affects one of every four persons and two out of every three families. Thus, within this country and throughout the world, cancer has a tremendous psychologic, social, and economic impact.

However, despite the grim statistics that still characterize cancer, it gives one considerable hope to look closely at the work of researchers in recent years. Indeed, Donovan and Pierce have referred to the 1970's as "the decade of the crab" in American medicine. It was during this decade that cancer research made truly great strides in the direction of solving the mysteries of cancer causation and the problems of cancer therapy.[30]

Based upon the ever-changing nature of cancer research and treatment, this unit has four basic purposes. One purpose is to *inform the student about the nature of cancer* and to present relevant facts and theories concerning its prevalence, etiology, pathogenesis, diagnosis, and treatment.

A second purpose is to *examine the fear of cancer* that is so prevalent in our society. Fear can prevent a patient with a suspicious lump from seeking medical advice; fear can make a physician feel too uncomfortable to speak frankly with a patient who has cancer; fear can cause a nurse to view cancer nursing as a depressing and hopeless field of work, and to either resent or avoid the cancer patient. In this unit, we attempt to examine the roots of this fear both in our society and in ourselves.

A third purpose of the unit is to *present the challenge of cancer nursing.* For too many years the care of patients with cancer has been depreciated and devalued. Fortunately, today, nurses are becoming more aware of the rewarding aspects of cancer nursing. Indeed, the nurse plays a vital role in both the prevention and treatment of malignant tumors.

---

*Beatrice Kastenbaum, R.N., B.S.N., M.S.N., critically reviewed and assisted with the revision of this unit.

The fourth and final goal of this unit is to enable you to be able to do the following:

1. Educate the public concerning the warning signals of cancer and the need for regular physical examination.
2. Promote the physical and psychologic well-being of the patient experiencing a life-threatening disease that may require radical changes in lifestyle.
3. Give the patient needed information to cope with the disease and its treatment and prognosis.
4. Keep informed and current concerning cancer research projects.
5. Administer chemotherapeutic drugs safely.
6. Safeguard the patient, yourself, and others during the administration of radiotherapy.
7. Maintain a positive attitude toward the care of patients with far advanced or terminal cancer.

As Donovan and Pierce state, "Something can be done for all cancer patients. We should not feel useless or hopeless just because every patient is not cured."[30]

Cancer patients experiencing emotional distress need a nurse who uses all of her or his skills and knowledge while providing physical care. Thus, you may find it essential to come to terms with your own feelings about life and death. Only then can you give your patients the care they truly require and in return reap the rewards of self-growth from your work.

Study Guide

1. Before you begin your reading, ask yourself the following questions:

What does the word "cancer" mean to me?
What have I already read and heard about cancer?
What would I do if I discovered a suspicious lump or developed a symptom suggestive of cancer?
How would I react if my doctor told me I had cancer, and that it was far advanced?
How do I feel about radical surgery as a treatment for cancer?
What have I read or heard about radiation therapy?

2. As you read the unit, familiarize yourself with the following terms:

cancer cure
neoplasia
benign neoplasm
malignant neoplasm
carcinoma in situ
spontaneous remission
cell cycle
doubling time
anaplastic cells
differentiation
metastasis
cachexia
carcinoma
sarcoma
carcinogen
precancerous lesion
Papanicolaou test
exfoliative cytology
biopsy
sentinel metastasis
intra-arterial infusion
intra-arterial perfusion
radiation
isotope
radioisotope
half-life
alpha particles
beta particles
gamma rays
sealed radioisotopes
unsealed radioisotopes
tracers
curie
roentgen
rad
scintillation counter
scintillation scanner
radiosensitivity

radioresistance
external radiotherapy
x-ray therapy
teletherapy
internal radiotherapy
interstitial therapy
intracavitary therapy
distance
time
shielding
external hazard
internal hazard
anergy
blocking agents
deblocking agents
active specific immunotherapy
active nonspecific immunotherapy
passive immunotherapy
adoptive immunotherapy

3. Following your reading, attempt to answer the following questions:

a. What is the difference between a benign and a malignant neoplasm?
b. What are the major pathophysiologic problems and resultant manifestations of cancer?
c. What are the seven warning signs of cancer?
d. What are the seven safeguards against cancer?
e. What is the purpose and value of the Papanicolaou test?
f. What is the purpose of a biopsy?
g. What is the procedure for an organ scan?
h. What is the purpose of the DNCB skin test?
i. What are the four major types of surgery performed in the management of cancer?
j. What are the major classes of agents used in cancer chemotherapy?
k. What are the toxic effects of cancer chemotherapy? How can these effects be prevented or treated?
l. What are the two *regional* methods of drug administration?
m. What precautions must the nurse observe during external radiotherapy?
n. What precautions must the nurse observe during internal radiotherapy? with sealed sources? with unsealed sources?
o. What are the toxic effects of radiotherapy?
p. What is the purpose of BCG immunotherapy? procedure? benefits? problems?
q. What problems may the patient with terminal cancer face? How can you alleviate or lessen the severity of these problems?

4. When caring for a patient with a neoplastic disorder, answer the following questions:

a. What cell type is neoplastic?
b. What is the stage of the growth?
c. What is the natural history of this tumor?
d. What treatment modalities are being used?
e. What are the chances for cure, for arrest of the disease, for palliation, or for supportive-nontherapeutic care?
f. How is the person coping? What does the person know about the illness? What coping strategies work for *this individual*?
g. What preparations has the individual made for the future?
h. What family and other support systems are available and utilized by the patient?
i. What other physical, social and psychologic problems does the patient face?

CHAPTER 21

NEOPLASTIC DISEASE: TUMOR GROWTH AND THEORIES OF CAUSATION

NEOPLASTIC DISEASE: DEFINITIONS AND CONNOTATIONS

Study of neoplastic disease begins with an understanding of definitions. The word "cancer" is synonymous with the term *malignant neoplasm.* Other words connoting neoplastic disease include tumor, malignancy, carcinoma, aberrant cellular growth, and the abbreviation "ca." These terms are not interchangeable. Each requires a specific context for its respective connotion, as you will see below.

The word *neoplasm* is derived from the Greek *neos,* which means "new," and *plasia,* "growth of new tissues."

> *Defined medically, a neoplasm is an abnormal new growth of tissue, which serves no purpose and which can be highly damaging.*

A neoplasm may be either benign or malignant. A *benign* neoplasm is an abnormal growth of tissue that is relatively harmless and does not spread to and infiltrate other tissues. A *malignant* neoplasm is an abnormal growth that is always harmful to the body and that may spread, or metastasize, to other tissues far removed from the site of origin.

The terms "tumor" and "neoplasm" are not truly synonymous. Strictly defined, a *tumor* is simply an abnormal swelling or enlargment and is one of the four signs of inflammation — redness, heat, swelling (or tumor), and pain. Thus, even though the proliferation of neoplastic cells results in a tumor, tumorous swellings can also develop as a result of fluid or blood within a limited area of tissue, e.g., a hematoma. However, patients and medical personnel often use the term "tumor" in place of other terms for neoplastic disease, particularly "cancer," perhaps because it seems less frightening.

The term *malignancy,* according to one dictionary, means "a condition that, if uncorrected, tends to worsen so as to cause serious illness or death." While the word "malignant" usually is applied to neoplasms, it is also used to describe a particularly deadly form of high blood pressure, i.e., malignant hypertension. *Carcinoma* is a form of cancer that is composed of epithelial cells that tend to infiltrate surrounding tissues and that may eventually metastasize. *Aberrant cellular growth* is cellular growth that is deviating from the normal. It may or may not give rise to cancer.

Historically, Hippocrates is said to have assigned the name "cancer," meaning crab, to neoplastic diseases. The reasons for the choice are lost in antiquity, but perhaps it is because certain cancers of the breast resemble a crab, with claw-like processes buried in the normal tissue. The term may have portrayed the pain as similar to that experienced from the pinch of a crab. No evidence exists that the ancient Greeks and Romans connected the advent of malignancy with the influence of the crab, one of the constellations of the zodiac.

Basically, "cancer" is presently used as a collective term describing a "large group of diseases characterized by uncontrolled growth and spread of abnormal cells."[24] This group of diseases:

- Arise in different tissues and organs
- Differ greatly from one another in appearance and growth habits
- May follow different courses of development in their hosts
- Often show different sensitivities to the various types of therapy applied to them

For the lay public and perhaps for student nurses, "cancer" has a different connotation from the textbook definition and description above. To many, cancer means a death warrant. It means pain, suffering, disfigurement, hopelessness, and helplessness. This picture of cancer has a historical basis. Early in this century, most people who developed cancer died.

Today, the cure rate has risen to a ratio of *one cancer cure to every three deaths,* and the cure rate would be far higher if individuals were diagnosed and treated early in the course of the disease (see Chapter 22). Thus, while the term "cancer" still connotes a dread disease, it no longer means a death sentence.

While the meaning of cancer is undergoing change in the minds of the public, its meaning is also evolving in the minds of researchers. Indeed, despite research advances, investigators still remain undecided about definitions involving cancer.

The problem is our inability to define the malignant cell. A vast amount of information exists that describes what this cell does and how it does what it does; but the *why* evades us. Until now the malignant cell has been defined only in comparison with its normal version. We will be able to describe the malignant cell only in the most general terms, as a cell whose sense of order is defective — a cell which has lost its sense of belonging to a larger community.[4]

With this hazy definition of the malignant cell, we begin the study of neoplastic growth by first examining the mechanics of the *normal cell.* As researchers are discovering, the more we understand about the normal cell, (specifically the regulatory mechanisms at the gene level of the cell), the better prepared we are to understand the *abnormal* cell and its adverse effects on plants and animals as well as on humans.

TUMOR GROWTH AND CHARACTERISTICS

Characteristics of Normal Cells

What is a cancer cell? How does it differ from a normal cell and what are the factors that cause cancer cells to develop?

You will recall from Chapter 9 that the cell is the basic unit or building block of structure for all forms of plant and animal life, and that within the human body there are approximately 60,000 billion cells. Each of these cells carries out precise and highly specialized functions that are harmoniously interlocked with the activities and functions of other cells; as a result of coordinated cellular activities, the body grows and performs as an integrated whole.

The following review of certain specific characteristics of normal cells will assist us in understanding the changes that take place in neoplastic cells.

The Cell Cycle. The concept of the *cell cycle* has increased researchers' understanding of reproduction of both normal and neoplastic cells.[2] (See Fig. 21–1.) The cell cycle may be defined as "the interval between the midpoint of mitosis in a cell and the midpoint of the subsequent mitosis in one or both daughter cells."[2] It can be divided experimentally into the following intervals, or steps, with the letter "G" standing for "gap" — the interval separating mitosis and synthesis:

Step 1a: G_0

The interval in which the cell is *at rest* until a trigger in the immediate environment signals the beginning of the G_1 interval. Some cells do not replicate, or they replicate so infrequently that they are always said to be in G_0 state.

Step 1b: G_1

The interval in which *RNA and protein are synthesized.* The period of time the cell is in G_1 varies, depending on the type of cell and the proliferative activity of the tissue. With high activity, G_1 interval is short; the interval lengthens when activity is low. The acquisition of the ability to begin DNA synthesis marks the termination of G_1.

Step 2: S

Synthesis of both the DNA and proteins of new chromosomes occurs. The interval of time is usually thought to be 6 to 8 hours. It can vary in certain cell populations and under different circumstances.

Step 3: G_2

Biochemical processes, including synthesis of some RNA, occurs in preparation of mitosis. Little is known of this phase, which may only last a few hours.

Step 4: M

Actual division of the cell — mitosis — occurs, producing two daughter cells. The duration of this phase

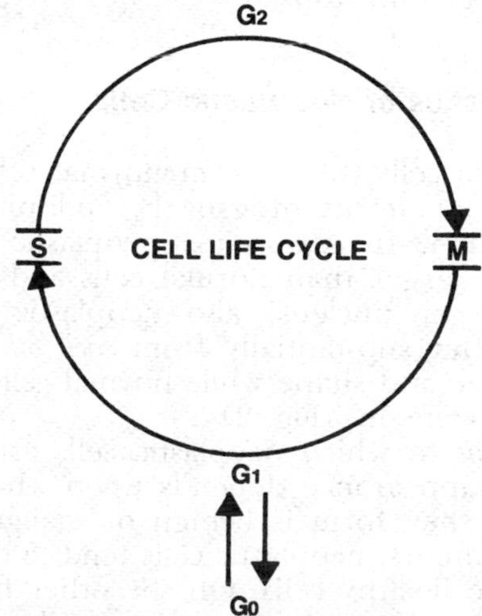

Figure 21–1. Cell life cycle. (From Marino, E. B., and LeBlanc, D. H.: Cancer chemotherapy. *Nursing '75,* 5:22, Nov. 1975.)

usually ranges from less than an hour to a few hours.

In the normal, mature organ, *cell cycling is carefully controlled* so that the function of the organ is maintained. Cells that die are replaced, but no extra cells produced. The mechanisms of this control are being researched and are not fully understood at this time.

Differentiation. A second characteristic of normal cells is *differentiation.* In the embryo, cells become different from each other as they assume the special functions of the various organs. One muscle cell looks like all the other muscle cells, but not much like kidney or liver cells. This process is called differentiation. Two points to keep in mind about differentiation are: (1) the more highly differentiated cells become, the less likely they are to divide and (2) it is believed that even a highly differentiated cell retains the same genetic potentials of every other cell. In other words, a muscle cell's potential to be a liver cell is repressed, but the genetic potential is still present in the muscle cell. There is still much to learn about the mechanisms that allow expression of some but not all the genetic material.

Contact Inhibition. Third, when normal cells are grown outside of the body on culture plates, they exhibit a characteristic of particular interest, called *contact inhibition.* Normal cells move freely about the culture medium until they contact another cell. Then they tend to adhere to each other and line up in parallel fashion. The cells grow until they reach the edges of the surface in a single layer, at which time active growth stops.

Characteristics of Neoplastic Cells

Neoplastic cells differ from normal cells in appearance, patterns of growth, and physiologic function. In *appearance,* neoplastic cells are usually larger than normal cells and they have a bigger nucleus; also neoplastic cells tend to differ substantially from *each other* in terms of size and shape while normal cells are more homogeneous (Fig. 21–2).

The *extent* to which neoplastic cells are abnormal in appearance depends upon whether the tumor they form is benign or malignant. In *benign* tumors, neoplastic cells tend to closely resemble healthy cells. On the other hand, *malignant* tumors are characterized by cells that may bear little resemblance to those cells that normally compose the afflicted tissue. Neoplastic cells that are strikingly deviant from normal cells are called *anaplastic cells.* Anaplastic cells tend to be primitive and embryonic in type, and they characteristically grow into disorganized, irregular cellular nests or sheets.

In terms of *growth,* one author has noted that "the biological characteristics of cancer cells would seem to indicate that they are specialized for growth and survival under adverse conditions."[20] Indeed, neoplastic cells seem to proliferate in response to abnormal stimuli (physical, chemical, hormonal, and viral agents). Also, neoplastic cells may demonstrate multiple mitotic spindles, resulting in more than the normal two daughter cells at the end of mitoses. Furthermore, the rules of growth that normally govern healthy cellular reproduction seem unable to halt or restrict the proliferation of neoplastic cells. Possible changes in the cell wall may be related to the loss of contact inhibition demonstrated in cancer cells — and consequently their continued uncontrollable replication. Thus Robbins raises the possibility that "the fundamental nature of cancer might be the loss of cell control, as a consequence of membrane changes."[75]

In reference to *function,* malignant cells, unlike normal cells, serve no purpose. The end result of neoplastic cellular growth is an abnormal tissue mass that does not function in any useful way and, consequently, cannot contribute to the well-being of the host.

In addition to differences in appearance, growth patterns, and function, cancer cells differ from normal cells in these ways:[75]

- development of antigens completely different from a normal cell
- chromosomal aberrations that occur as the cancer cell matures
- the return to more primitive and simplified metabolic and enzyme patterns
- the ability to invade, erode, and metastasize

In sum, neoplastic cells are the anarchists of the body. They are primitive in appearance, and they divide and multiply endlessly without regard for the normal physiologic rules of growth that dominate normal cells. Moreover, neoplastic cells exist as parasites, occupying space and drawing nutrition and sustenance from the host's body while contributing nothing in return.

Description of Neoplastic Tumors

GROWTH OF NEOPLASTIC TUMORS

Neoplastic cells mass together to form neoplastic tissue growths or tumors. What seems to account for the growth of tumors?

First, tumor growth is related to *increased*

numbers of cells. Cells may increase in number by: (1) shortening the length of the cell cycle, (2) increasing the fraction of cells going through the cell cycle, or (3) decreasing cell loss. At one time, researchers believed that neoplastic cells divided much more rapidly than other cells in the body. This rapid division was thought to account for the mass of cells that developed. Later, it was discovered that some normal cells proceed through the cell cycle faster than neoplastic cells. The current belief is that the *fraction* of proliferating cells in a tumor is higher, thus accounting for the tumor mass.

Second, the concept of "doubling time" is central to the study of tumor growth. Theoretically, cancer could start as a single abnormal cell that divides to form two cells, then four cells, and so on. Provided that the amount of time for the cell cycle remains constant, the tumor mass would double each time the cell cycle went from mitosis to mitosis.

While some tumor masses seem to steadily multiply themselves, most observations indicate this does not entirely account for the growth of tumors. For instance, there is some indication that tumors may cycle faster early in their growth. Also, there are great variations

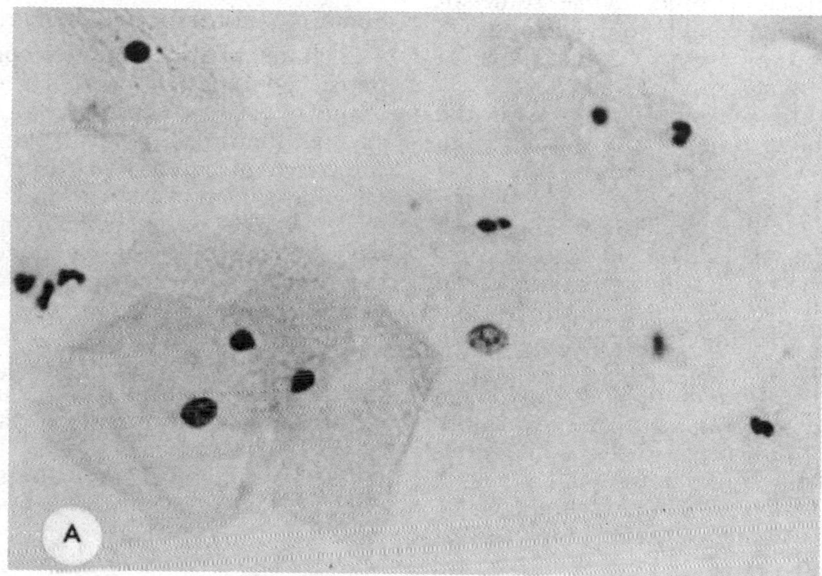

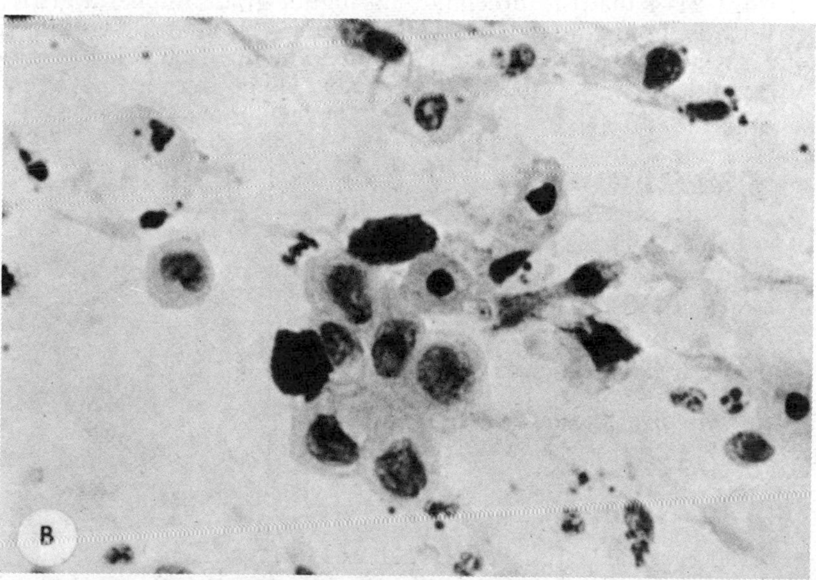

Figure 21–2. Benign (*A*) and malignant (*B*) cells. (From Price, S. A., and L. M. Wilson: *Pathophysiology: Clinical Concepts of Disease Processes.* New York: McGraw-Hill Book Co., 1978, p. 99.)

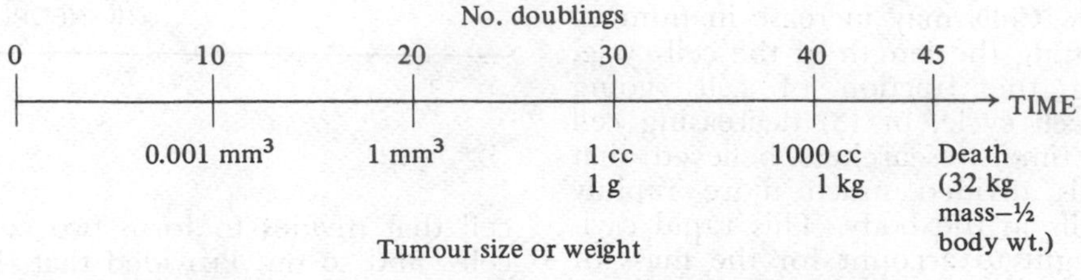

Figure 21-3. "Doubling." (From Walter, J. *Cancer and Radiotherapy*. London: J. & A. Churchill, 1971.)

in cycling times, based on the type of tumor. Furthermore, cell losses are considerable in all tumors and may counterbalance new cell output in some tumor populations. Then, too, there is a percentage of cells which is not dividing at a particular time. While some of these cells may never be able to divide and will eventually die, others are probably capable of reproduction at some point.

While there are many problems with the concept of doubling time, it is a useful way to look at the *natural history of a tumor* (Figs. 21-3 and 21-4.) Note in Figure 21-3 that approximately twenty doublings will occur before a tumor one cubic millimeter in size is produced. This is the smallest mass that one could ever hope to detect clinically. At thirty doublings, the mass would be about one cubic centimeter, weighing one gram, still a small lesion by any standards. Ten more doublings bring the mass to one kilogram, but only five more doublings brings the mass to thirty kilograms or half of body weight. It is unlikely that a person would be alive with such a tumor.

Clearly, the cell cycle of a tumor is of great clinical significance. First, the slower the cell cycle of the tumor, the longer it is before the tumor can be identified. Second, you may have noticed in Figure 21-4 that the preclinical period of growth is approximately two-thirds of the total growth period. This fact helps us to understand how metastasis, or spread, of a tumor occurs, even when the original tumor is quite small. It also explains the long period of time needed for follow-up after removal of the tumor before assurances can be given that the person is cancer-free.

COMPOSITION OF NEOPLASTIC TUMORS

Each neoplastic tumor is composed of two parts: (1) the *parenchyma* of the tumor, which is the major part and is composed of parenchymal tumor cells, and (2) the *stroma*, which is composed of connective tissue and blood vessels and which supports and provides structure for the parenchymal tumor cells. The blood vessels of the stroma feed and nourish the tumor, especially when it first forms and begins to grow.

The parenchymal tissue of neoplastic cells is graded on the basis of its *dedifferentiation,* i.e., the loss of resemblance to normal differentiated cells. The cancer may be classified as grade I, II, III or IV, each grade signifying an increase in anaplasia. For example, *Grade I indicates that tumor cells closely resemble normal cells, i.e., are well differentiated, whereas Grade IV indicates tumor cells that deviate widely from normal.* These cells may be referred to as poorly differentiated or anaplastic by the pathologist. Thus, a higher grade implies a greater degree of malignancy. Standards for individual grades are different for each form of cancer and will not be explained here.

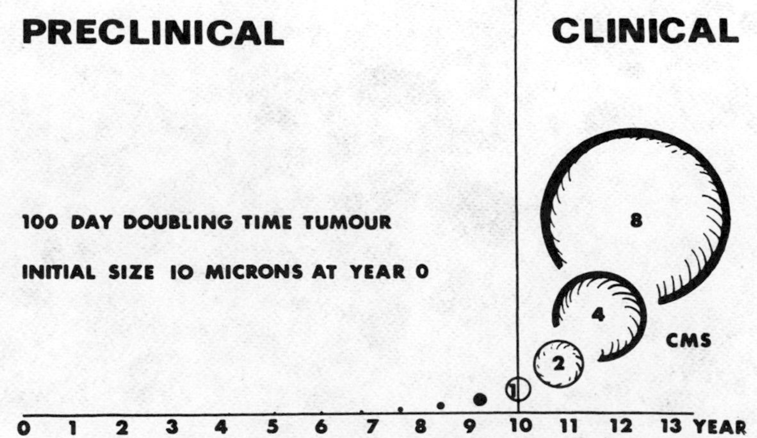

Figure 21-4. "Doubling." (From Walter, J., *Cancer and Radiotherapy*, London: J. & A. Churchill, 1971.)

Just as the grade of cancer cell anaplasia generally indicates its degree of malignancy, cancer *staging* classifies its biological behavior within the patient. The staging of cancers is based on the following:

- ▶ the size of the main tumor
- ▶ the presence or absence of metastases
- ▶ the extent or spread to nearby lymph nodes

Presence of metastases is the most difficult of these criteria to assess accurately. (Staging is discussed in more detail in Chapter 22.)

METASTASIS

Some neoplastic cells have the ability to spread from the original site of the tumor to distant organs of the body. This characteristic is called *metastasis*. The word is derived from the Greek word "meta" meaning "beyond" and "stasis" meaning "standing." The capacity of a neoplastic tumor to metastasize to other sites is a major characteristic of malignancy, and it distinguishes malignant from benign growths.

The mechanisms of tumor spread are not fully understood at this time. It is known that the walls of tumor cells are different from their normal counterparts. Furthermore, the "contact inhibition" noted in normal cells is extremely variable in tumor cells.

For the purposes of study, the metastatic process may be divided into three stages:

1. *Invasion of cells* from the primary tumor into surrounding tissue and penetration of blood and/or lymph vessels (Fig. 21–5). Tumor invasion may be caused by any of the following:
   a. increasing tumor size leading to tissue pressure and mechanical expansion
   b. loss of tumor cell cohesiveness with increasing motility
   c. destruction of the host stroma by tumor cell products
   d. factors in the host response to tumor cell invasion

2. *Spread of tumor cells* via the lymph or blood circulation, or by direct expansion.

- ▶ The *lymphatic system* provides the most common pathway for initial spread of cancer cells. The spread may be to the lymph nodes draining the region of the primary site. Distant lymph nodes may be affected later in the disease, or if the regional lymph nodes are obstructed by inflammation or other processes.
- ▶ The *blood vessels* (including both veins and arteries) carry cancer cells from the primary tumor to the capillary beds of the lungs, liver, and bones.
- ▶ *Direct expansion of tumors in body cavities* occurs as cells travel throughout the cavity to develop new growth on other serosal surfaces. Cancers of the ovary are often said to "seed" the entire peritoneal cavity. Primary tumors of the central nervous system appear to spread by direct extension, or via gravity, in the cerebral fluid.

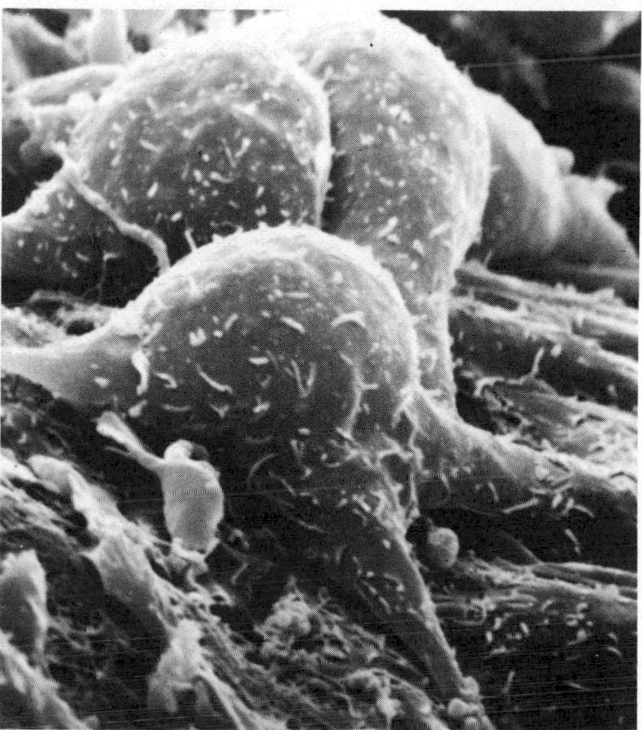

Figure 21–5. Invasion of blood vessel walls by metastatic melanoma cells. (From Nicholson, G. L.: Cancer metastasis. *Scientific American,* March, 1979; p. 66.)

3. *Establishment and growth of tumor cells at the secondary site.* The tumor develops its own vascularization in the new site and has the ability to infiltrate the adjacent tissue. Researchers have observed that certain tumor cells have an affinity for certain sites, although the reasons for this affinity are not well understood. Knowing the natural history of the tumor includes knowing the sites where it will most likely be found if it metastasizes.

As previously mentioned, the cell cycle time and host factors control the length of time it takes for the metastatic growth to be detectable. If the cells reproduce rapidly, the metastatic growth may obtain a size of 1 cm. within months; if the cells proliferate slowly, it may be many years before the metastatic lesion is large enough for detection.

The growth of metastatic tumors puts severe stress on the patient both physiologically and psychologically. As the *tumor burden* (the amount of tumor in the body) increases, it uses more and more of the metabolic resources needed by the normal cells.

TABLE 21–1. A COMPARISON OF THE CHARACTERISTICS OF BENIGN AND MALIGNANT NEOPLASMS

Characteristic	Benign Neoplasm	Malignant Neoplasm
Speed of growth	Grows slowly usually continues to grow throughout life unless surgically removed; may have periods of remission during which growth stops for a time	Grows usually rapidly, tends to grow relentlessly throughout life; rarely, neoplasm may *regress spontaneously*
Mode of growth	Grows by enlarging and expanding; always remains localized; never infiltrates surrounding tissues	Grows by infiltrating surrounding tissues; may remain localized (in situ) but usually spreads out to infiltrate other tissues
Presence of capsule	Almost always contained and confined within a fibrous capsule; capsule does not prevent expansion of neoplasm but does prevent growth by infiltration; capsule advantageous because it and enclosed tumor cells can be easily removed surgically	Never contained and confined within a capsule; absence of capsule allows neoplastic cells to invade surrounding tissues; absence of capsule makes surgical removal of tumor more difficult
Characteristics of cells composing tumor	Usually well differentiated; mitotic figures absent or scanty; cells appear adult; anaplastic cells absent; cells function poorly in comparison with normal cells from which they arise; if neoplasm arises in glandular tissue, cells may be capable of secreting hormones	Usually poorly differentiated; large numbers of normal and abnormal mitotic figures present; cells tend to be anaplastic, i.e., young, embryonic type cells; cells too abnormal to perform any physiologic functions; occasionally a malignant tumor arising in glandular tissue may secrete hormones
Recurrence	Recurrence extremely unusual when surgically removed	Recurrence common following surgery because of spread of tumor cells into surrounding tissues
Metastasis or spread of tumor from original site to other organs of body	Metastases never occur	Metastases very common; most dangerous and deadly aspect of neoplastic disease (see discussion below)
Effect of neoplasm on tissues and body as a whole	Not harmful to host unless neoplasm located in area where it causes compression of tissues or obstruction of vital organs; does not produce *cachexia* (weight loss, debilitation, anemia, weakness, wasting); neoplasm located in glandular tissue may secrete the hormone normally produced, resulting in *excess* of hormone in blood	Always harmful to the host; will result in death unless removed surgically or destroyed by radiation or chemotherapy; causes disfigurement of the body, disrupted organ functions, and nutritional imbalances; may result in ulcerations, sepsis, perforations, hemorrhage, and tissue slough; almost always produces cachexia, which leaves patient prone to pneumonia, anemia, etc.; infrequently malignant tumors secrete hormones, causing a hormonal imbalance; usually cells too poorly differentiated to produce normal body secretions
Prognosis	Very good; tumor generally removed surgically	Depends upon speed with which cancer diagnosed; poor prognosis indicated if cells are poorly differentiated and evidence exists of metastatic spread; good prognosis indicated if cells still resemble normal and there is no evidence of metastasis

Characteristics of Benign and Malignant Neoplasms

As we have said, neoplastic tumors are classified as either benign neoplasms or malignant neoplasms.

> *Deciding whether a tumor is benign or malignant is probably the most important decision a physician must make when treating a patient with a tumorous growth.*

Let us first consider the *benign tumor.* The word *benign* comes from the Latin *bene* meaning "good" and *genus* which means "sort." Thus a benign tumor is a "good sort of tumor," or at least it is a tumor of limited growth that will not radically harm or kill the host. But the benign tumor, however harmless, does *occupy space.* Consequently, if a benign neoplasm is located in a strategic position, it can obstruct tubes and compress vital tissues. As a rule, however, if a tumor is benign, the patient will generally have a good prognosis because the tumor can be readily excised.

Malignant tumors, on the other hand, represent a serious threat to the life and well-being of the host. The word *malignant* comes from the Latin word *malus* which means "bad." Thus a malignant tumor is a "bad sort of tumor." Malignant neoplasms are dangerous not only because they occupy space but also because they grow in a radical and disorganized fashion. Also, they release their cancerous cells for dissemination throughout the body. Moreover, they sap and drain the metabolic and nutritional resources of the host, leaving the patient weak, anemic, and subject to fatal infections. Malignant neoplasms, because of their invasive and metastatic nature, cannot be as readily excised or cured as can the benign tumor. Table 21–1 compares the characteristics of these two major types of neoplasms. Figure 21–6 also compares benign versus malignant growth.

Classification of Benign and Malignant Neoplasms

Neoplasms are classified not only in terms of whether they are benign or malignant; they are also grouped according to the tissue from which they arise (Table 21–2).

As you study Table 21–2, note that almost all names for tumors end in the suffix "oma," meaning "tumor." In turn, the suffix "oma" is usually attached to a term for the parent tissue of the tumors; thus adenoma comes from the Greek *aden*, "gland" plus "oma." When more than one parent tissue enters into the formation of a neoplasm, the names of the tumors are even more descriptive. For example, an adenomyoma is a benign neoplasm that contains both glandular and muscle cells; a leiomyofibroma is a fibroid tumor of the uterus that contains both smooth muscle and fibrous connective tissue.

Benign tumors of *epithelial origin* are not so easily classified and named as are tumors arising from mesenchymal origin, i.e., fibrous tissue, bone, muscle, blood vessels, lymphatics, and nerves; this is because epithelial tissues are of many different varieties. For this reason, benign tumors of epithelial origin are classified according to either their microscopic appearance (e.g., an adenoma is a tumor with glandular elements) or their gross structure; e.g., a polyp (from the Greek *polys* [many] × *pous* [foot]) is a benign tumor of epithelial origin with a pedicle or stem that attaches the growth to a mucous membrane.

Three of the most common benign tumors listed in Table 21–2 are the fibroma, lipoma, and leiomyoma.

The *fibroma* may grow anywhere in the body, but it very frequently makes its home in the uterus. Fibromas are generally small, but occasionally they grow to great size. These encapsulated, relatively harmless tumors do not cause symptoms unless, owing to location, they place pressure on a bone or nerve. Fibromas are easily removed surgically.

The *lipoma*, which is a very common benign tumor, arises in adipose tissue. Lipomas rarely cause symptoms; however, they are poorly encapsulated and they may put pressure on surrounding tissues as they expand.

The *leiomyoma*, a benign neoplasm of smooth muscle origin, is the most common benign tumor in women. Leiomyomas may develop anywhere in the body, but they most commonly grow in the uterus. Rarely (in approximately 1 per cent of cases), these tumors become malignant.

Let us consider the classification of malignant tumors. A malignant tumor that arises

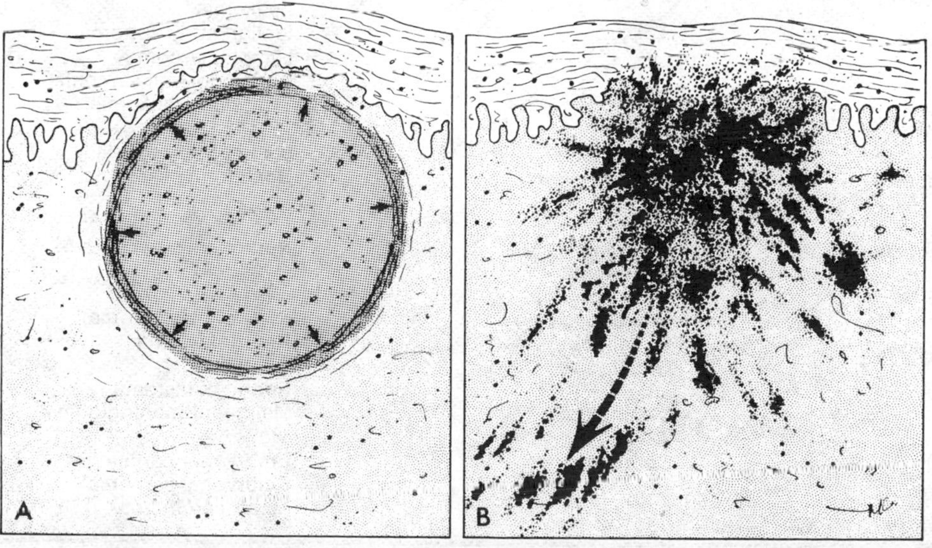

Figure 21–6. Diagram of benign versus malignant growth. (From Price, S. A., and L. M. Wilson: *Pathophysiology: Clinical Concepts of Disease Processes*. New York: McGraw-Hill Book Co., 1978, p. 93.)

from *epithelial* tissue is called a *carcinoma,* whereas a malignant neoplasm that arises from *mesenchymal* origins (i.e., blood vessels, lymphatics, nerve tissue) is called a *sarcoma* (Greek *sarc* means flesh).

Three representative examples of malignant neoplasms are carcinoma in situ, fibrosarcoma, and bronchogenic carcinoma.

Carcinoma in situ is a neoplasm of epithelial tissue that remains *confined* to the site of origin. In situ carcinoma typically affects the cervix, and it may occur in squamous epithelium in other parts of the body. This form of cancer is, by definition, localized and thus can be removed surgically. However, it is well to remember that in situ carcinoma can become invasive, eroding into surrounding tissues.

The malignant fibrosarcomas are similar to benign fibromas. Fibrosarcomas tend to grow in the same sites and may originate as benign fibromas, later becoming malignant. These bulky, well differentiated tumor masses are usually responsive to surgery. Fortunately, fibrosarcomas rarely metastasize.

Bronchogenic carcinoma is the cause of 90 per cent of all cases of lung cancer. Bronchogenic carcinoma usually develops in the lower trachea and lower bronchi. Surgical excision of the tumor is the treatment of choice. However, this type of cancer readily gives rise to metastases, and if this occurs, surgery is contraindicated.

TABLE 21–2. CLASSIFICATION OF NEOPLASMS*

Tissue of Origin	Benign	Malignant
Connective tissues		Sarcoma
Embryonic fibrous tissue	Myxoma	Myxosarcoma
Fibrous tissue	Fibroma	Fibrosarcoma
Adipose tissue	Lipoma	Liposarcoma
Cartilage	Chondroma	Chondrosarcoma
Bone	Osteoma	Osteogenic sarcoma
Epithelium		Carcinoma
Skin and mucous membrane	Papilloma	Squamous cell carcinoma
Glands	Polyp	Basal cell carcinoma
		Transitional cell carcinoma
	Adenoma	Adenocarcinoma
	Cystadenoma	
Pigmented cells (melanoblasts)	Nevus	Malignant melanoma
Endothelium		Endothelioma
Blood vessels	Hemangioma	Hemangioendothelioma
		Hemangiosarcoma
Lymph vessels	Lymphangioma	Lymphangiosarcoma
		Lymphangioendothelioma
Bone marrow		Multiple myeloma
		Ewing's sarcoma
		Leukemia
Lymphoid tissue		Malignant lymphoma
		Lymphosarcoma
		Reticulum cell sarcoma
		Lymphatic leukemia
Muscle tissue		
Smooth muscle	Leiomyoma	Leiomyosarcoma
Striated muscle	Rhabdomyoma	Rhabdomyosarcoma
Nerve tissue		
Nerve fibers and sheaths	Neuroma	Neurogenic sarcoma
	Neurinoma	
	(Neurilemoma)	
	Neurofibroma	(Neurofibrosarcoma)
Ganglion cells	Ganglioneuroma	Neuroblastoma
Glia cells	Glioma	Glioblastoma
		Spongioblastoma
Meninges	Meningioma	Malignant meningioma
Gonads	Dermoid cyst	Embryonal carcinoma
		Embryonal sarcoma
		Teratocarcinoma

*Adapted from Bouchard, R.: *Nursing Care of the Cancer Patient,* 2nd ed. St. Louis: C. V. Mosby Co., 1972.

PATHOPHYSIOLOGY OF CANCER AND ITS MANIFESTATIONS

When a malignant growth is in its early stages, it often fails to produce symptoms. Manifestations generally appear once the neoplasm has grown to a sufficiently large size to cause one or several of the following problems:

- Pressure upon surrounding organs
- Distortion of surrounding tissues
- Obstruction of lumens of tubes
- Interference with the blood supply of surrounding tissues
- Interference with organ function
- Disturbance of body metabolism
- Parasitic use of the body's nutritional supplies
- Mobilization of the body's defensive responses, resulting in inflammatory changes

These pathophysiologic changes may give rise to the manifestations listed below.*

Anemia. Anemia is a common problem for patients with cancer. Some causes for anemia are:

1. Bleeding from ulcerated lesions or erosion of a blood vessel
2. Infection
3. Bone metastases that prevent bone marrow from replacing worn-out or damaged erythrocytes
4. Bone marrow depression caused by chemotherapy or radiation therapy

Infection of Surface of Tumor. The most common site for the development of infected ulcerated cancer lesions is the breast. This results from necrosis and death of the tissues covering the neoplasm.

Serous Effusions. Serous effusions often accompany breast, lung, and ovarian cancers. They frequently result from the metastasis of tumor cells.

Pain. Pain is one of the late developments of cancer, but its appearance depends on the organ system involved. It is most likely to occur when there is obstruction or destruction of a vital organ, pressure on sensitive tissues or bone, or involvement of nerves. Bone cancer is particularly painful because the rigidity of the bone allows for little or no expansion as the tumor cells proliferate. Specific causes of pain in cancer are discussed in Chapter 23.

Syndrome of Cancer Cachexia. Cachexia is a state of profound poor health and malnutrition. It is characterized by weight loss, muscular weakness, anorexia, severe depression, acidosis, and toxemia. Furthermore, cachexia weakens patients and predisposes them to other problems, such as pneumonia. The etiology of cachexia is obscure. Some causes of this syndrome in cancer patients include the following:

1. In some cases, ulceration and infection predispose patient to a "wasting" syndrome.
2. Possibly toxic products released by the tumor promote wasting.
3. Impaired food ingestion due to obstructions of the GI tract by the tumor, or perhaps stenosis or adhesions within the tract, resulting from surgery or radiotherapy.
4. High-dosage chemotherapy may cause anorexia, nausea and toxicity, owing to the mass destruction of cells.
5. Malabsorption of food may result from surgery, chemotherapy, or radiation as well as from the tumor itself.

Causes of Death. Malignant disease that remains untreated or that is in a far-advanced metastatic stage when diagnosed is ultimately fatal. Death results from the widespread biochemical and metabolic disturbances caused by the growth and spread of the malignancy. More specifically, death typically follows the development of one of the following complications:

- Metastasis to the brain
- Uremia resulting from obstruction of ureters
- Uncontrolled hemorrhage
- Intestinal obstruction
- Obstruction of a bronchus

PATHOGENESIS AND ETIOLOGY OF CANCER

Scientists are currently looking at the pathogenesis of cancer in two basic ways:

- Healthy cells, due to some unknown mechanism, are being transformed into malignant cells upon exposure to certain etiologic agents
- Malignant cells (which are always developing within the body) are not being destroyed (as they normally should be) due to failure of the immune response.

Let us consider each of these viewpoints.

*Symptoms and treatment of anemia are discussed in Chapter 45, serous infusions in Chapter 55, and pain in Chapters 23, 29 and 30.

Cellular Transformation and Derangement

Although scientists have learned a great deal about the etiologic agents responsible for cancer (viruses, chemicals, radiation), the *exact mechanism* by which these agents transform healthy cells into neoplastic cells still remains obscure. One premise that most scientists accept today is that cancer develops as a result of alteration at the molecular level that is caused by the action of one or more etiologic agents and that results in uncontrolled cellular reproduction and growth. These inherited changes evidently develop within the cell's nucleus. Deoxyribonucleic acid (DNA), a basic constituent of the nucleus, is in some way altered so that its structure becomes abnormal. As a result, the cell changes into a cancerous cell. When this defective cell divides, the daughter cells are modeled upon the defective molecular code contained within the DNA of the mother cell. Over time, the defective daughter cells divide and multiply, and the malignancy develops and grows.

Theories attempting to explain this cellular alteration are constantly being proposed.

Concepts relating to the genetics of the origin of cancer cells include:

1. All cells may contain cancer genes. In noncancer cells, these genes are repressed.
2. Gene breakdown, with incorporation of parts of viruses into the gene, may result in abnormal cell growth.
3. Cancer may result from one or more "somatic mutations." This is unlikely because of the relatively low frequency of such mutations and the high frequency of cancer in humans.
4. Cancer may result from changes in the cell that do not involve the genes.
5. Precancerous cells that may be present in many tissues are activated by oncogenic stimuli, i.e., stimuli which give rise to tumors.[20]

It is still not known whether the cellular derangements that result in cancer are caused by a single agent or by multiple agents acting together. Laboratory experiments tend to support the *multifactoral theory of pathogenesis,* which holds that cancer develops in response to the combined action of several etiologic factors.

There are approximately 150 different types of cancer found in humans, and there are probably at least 500 different agents that can act as causative factors. In addition to etiologic agents, there are also *predisposing factors,* such as age, sex, and occupation, that can influence the *host's susceptibility* to various etiologic agents.

ETIOLOGIC FACTORS

Agents that are chiefly responsible for the development of cancer in human beings and animals can be categorized as follows:

- Viruses
- Chemical agents
- Physical agents
- Hormones

Such agents are often referred to as *carcinogens;* i.e., these agents can cause malignant changes in normal cells provided the cells are exposed to the agent over a sufficient period of time.

Carcinogens are everywhere in our environment, but not all persons are equally susceptible to the same carcinogens; for example, smokers have a higher incidence of lung cancer than nonsmokers, but not all smokers develop cancer; radiologists have a higher incidence of leukemia than do physicians in other fields, but not all radiologists develop leukemia. Exactly what causes different individuals to respond differently to the same carcinogen is not yet known.

Viruses. The study of viruses as carcinogens is one of the most promising areas in cancer research today. In spite of earlier doubts as to the validity of the theory of viral causation, there is now abundant proof that viruses cause cancer in animals. Viruses have been identified and photographed within cancerous lesions. Also scientists have injected filtrates taken from virus-infected cancerous tissue into healthy animals, and these animals have later developed cancer. Since scientists cannot experiment on human beings as they do on laboratory animals, it is difficult to obtain evidence that viruses cause human cancer. Viruses probably do not act as a single agent to cause cancer, but may be one of multiple agents required to initiate carcinogenesis.[98]

Chemical Agents. Some of the most common chemical carcinogens are: chromium, cobalt, tar, soot, asphalt, the nitrogen mustards, certain plastics, aniline dyes, the hydrocarbons in cigarette smoke, air pollutants from industry, crude paraffin oil, fuel oils, nickel, asbestos, and arsenicals. Most of these cause cancer only after close and prolonged contact, and those affected are usually workers in industries where these chemicals are employed or occur as byproducts.

Approximately 1000 different chemical substances have been identified as being cancer-producing. Many other chemicals have not been tested. In fact, validation of testing procedures itself presents a difficult problem. The controversy about the safety of saccharin use is an example of this problem.

On the other hand, it has been estimated that environmental factors contribute to 70 per cent of all cancers.[11] Since prevention of cancer is at present the best treatment available, identification and control of carcinogens in our environment is essential.

Physical Agents. The major physical agents believed to be associated with the causation of cancer are as follows:

Ionizing radiation, whether from x-rays or radioactive isotopes. Persons who work with radiant energy face the threat of developing leukemia. For example, as stated earlier, radiologists suffer a substantially higher rate of death from leukemia than do doctors in other fields. Also, there has been a substantial increase in the incidence of leukemia among victims of atomic fission and fallout (for example, the Hiroshima and Nagasaki survivors).

Sunlight and ultraviolet radiation may cause skin cancer in persons whose skins are exposed to strong sunlight over a substantial period of time. The degree to which persons expose themselves to sunlight depends, to some extent, on their *location.* For example, skin cancer is more prominent among sunbathing Californians than it is among persons who live in cloudier northern areas; also, it is more common among rural inhabitants than among urban dwellers. Furthermore, skin coloring affects the degree to which the sun can damage the skin. For example, dark-skinned persons (blacks, Puerto Ricans) are less likely to develop skin cancer upon exposure to the sun than are fair-skinned Nordic populations. Evidently, the greater pigmentation of the dark person's skin provides protection from the carcinogenic effects of strong sunlight.

Physical trauma such as mechanical blows to the body or chronic irritations may possibly cause cancer. Whether a *single physical blow* can cause cancer is a controversial question. It is true that neoplasms are sometimes discovered at the site of an injury following an accident or beating. However, one can argue that the neoplasm was located at that site already and that the physical blow or accident simply called attention to its presence.

While a single blow is a questionable carcinogen, there is more likelihood that *repeated minor trauma* associated with *infection* may give rise to malignancy. For example, pipe smoking is linked with cancer of the lip; a jagged tooth may be a causative factor in cancer of the tongue; women who have borne many children may have a higher incidence of cancer of the cervix.

Hormones. There is much to learn about the role of hormones in the causation of cancer. In animal experiments scientists have demonstrated that a relationship exists between hormonal secretion and action and tumor development and growth. Exactly what the relationship is remains obscure. Do hormones actually cause normal cells to change into cancer cells? Do hormones affect the fraction of cells in a cell population that will join the cell cycle and begin dividing? Or do hormones simply lower the host's resistance to other carcinogens? Do hormones act only to promote the growth of tumors caused by other factors? The answers to these questions lie in the future.

PREDISPOSING FACTORS*

What factors cause some individuals to be more sensitive to the carcinogens than other individuals?

Age. Cancer affects persons of all ages — children, youths, adults, and the aged. However, as we stated earlier, older persons develop cancer more readily than do younger individuals. For example, three-fourths of the persons who died from cancer in 1974 were over 55.[24] Older persons may be susceptible to cancer simply because they have been exposed to carcinogens longer than younger persons.

Sex. Women are more susceptible to *certain types* of cancer than men and vice versa. For instance, females are more susceptible to breast cancer and cancer of the intestines, whereas males are more susceptible to cancer of the lung and stomach. However, since 1949 more men have died from cancer of *all types* than women. For example, during 1978, researchers estimated that 213,500 men would die of cancer in comparison to 176,500 deaths among women.[24] The increased incidence of cancer deaths among males is apparently related to the higher incidence of lung cancer. With the current increase in women smokers, statistical differences between men and women may eventually even out.

Urban Versus Rural Residence. Cancer is more common among urban dwellers than among inhabitants of rural communities. The greater susceptibility of urbanites to cancer is probably related to their greater exposure to air pollutants.

Geographic Distribution. The susceptibility of individuals to different types of cancer varies on a national basis. For example, the incidence of cancer of the stomach is higher in Japan than it is in the United States, whereas cancer of the breast is rare in Japan but has a

*Statistics in this section refer to the United States.

high incidence in the United States. Breast cancer is also common in Europe. These differences in susceptibility to different forms of cancer probably result from environmental factors (e.g., national diet, ethnic customs, types of pollutants found in environment) rather than from genetic differences between races and nationalities.

Occupation. Persons in some occupations are more susceptible to cancer because of their greater contact with certain carcinogens, e.g., workers in chemical factories suffer from a heavy exposure to chemical carcinogens; persons who handle radioisotopes are exposed to heavy doses of radiant energy.

Familial Susceptibility. The tendency of inbred strains of mice to develop cancer of one particular site has been definitely demonstrated in the laboratory. However, there is no conclusive evidence that heredity plays a vital role in the development of most human cancers. Nonetheless, a hereditary predisposition toward malignancy of a particular organ or site is sometimes apparent in the family histories of patients with cancer.

Cancerous and Precancerous Lesions. The presence of malignancy in one tissue appears to increase the patient's susceptibility to the development of cancer in other tissues. Also, *precancerous* lesions and some benign tumors are dangerous because they may later undergo transformation into cancerous lesions and tumors. Some common precancerous lesions are pigmented moles, burn scars, senile keratosis (brown scaly patches on the epidermis), leukoplakia (whitish areas in the mouth), and benign adenomas or polyps of the colon or stomach. All these lesions need to be carefully and periodically observed for malignant changes.

*Failure of the Immune Response**

The role of *immunity* in preventing and controlling the growth and spread of cancer cells is an area of great interest for cancer researchers. As you recall from Chapter 11, the immune system protects the body against the invasion of foreign substances (chemical, protein, virus, or bacterium) in two ways: (1) by the production and release of antibodies that act to destroy the foreign antigen (humoral immunity) and (2) by the production of sensitized lymphocytes, which attack and destroy the invading antigens (cell mediated immunity). According to the immune theory of cancer control, cancer cells are always being formed within the body. The immune system perceives these cancer cells as foreign and destroys them (Recall from Chapter 11 that B lymphocytes are involved in the destruction of bacterial pathogens while *T lymphocytes* are involved with development of immunity to tumor cells, viruses, and mycobacterial pathogens; they also play a role in hypersensitivity reactions.) Apparently, a healthy immune system is able to destroy up to 10 million tumor cells. However, by the time a tumor has grown large enough to be demonstrated clinically (possibly owing to an inadequate immune response), it contains about one billion tumor cells, which act to further overwhelm the immune system.[27, 29]

Supporting evidence for this immune theory has been obtained from the postoperative experiences of heart and kidney transplant patients.[37] Because the immune response causes rejection of newly transplanted organs, patients undergoing transplants are given large doses of immunosuppressive drugs such as cortisone. The risk of developing cancer is at least 80 times greater among persons who have undergone transplantation surgery than among the population as a whole.

More data come from the histories of patients with congenital or acquired immunologic deficiencies. These persons have a far greater incidence of cancer than do persons with an intact immune system.[37]

Also, evidence is accumulating that the immune system can be "blocked" in its effort to destroy tumor-associated antigens. Researchers now know that human tumors release antigens that stimulate the patient's immune system to produce antibodies; these antibodies, in turn, act to destroy the cancerous cells. However, in some cases the tumor is not destroyed. Why is this so?[27, 29, 37]

Apparently, malignant tumor cells are capable of releasing "blocking agents" that interfere with the action of the host's own antibodies or sensitized lymphocytes, or both, thereby preventing tumor destruction. Laboratory experiments demonstrate that the immune systems of mice can thwart the action of "blocking" agents by releasing "deblocking" agents. These deblocking agents upset the action of the blocking agents which, in turn, allows the host's antibodies to act against the tumor cells. This knowledge of blocking and unblocking agents is the basis for one experimental form of immunotherapy (see Chapter 23).

Finally, whether the *spontaneous regression* of tumors is controlled by the immune system is another phenomenon under investigation. Spontaneous regressions of cancers occur in about one of every 100,000 cases. The role of

*Skin testing for immunocompetency is described in Chapter 22. Immunotherapy is discussed in Chapter 23.

the immune response in bringing about this seemingly miraculous change remains a provocative and unanswered question.

THE PATIENT'S PROGNOSIS: CANCER GROWTH VERSUS HOST RESPONSE

Two major factors influence prognosis in cancer:

1. *The rate of tumor growth and spread*
2. *The host's physiologic reaction*

As we said earlier, *tumor growth* depends upon the cell cycle of the tumor, and the fraction of proliferating cells within the tumor. Likewise, the speed at which a cancer metastasizes depends upon cell cycle time and whether the cells reproduce rapidly or slowly.

On the other hand, both the growth and metastatic potential of the tumor are also influenced by the individual *patient's reaction* to the cancer. Some individuals are more vulnerable to the development and spread of cancer than are others. The host's (patient's) degree of vulnerability may depend, to a large extent, upon heredity and the efficiency of immune defenses.

Heredity possibly plays a role in (1) the initial response of the host to a carcinogen, (2) the competency of the host's defense mechanism against cancer and (3) the manner in which the body metabolizes or disposes of carcinogenic agents.

As we have said, the host's *immune response* apparently plays a vital role in protection against cancer. The immune response can be repressed by immunosuppressive drugs, stress (which stimulates the release of plasma cortisol), and pregnancy. Cigarettes and alcohol may also act to destroy lymphocytes.[29] Finally, the immune response can be disrupted by blocking agents released by the tumor. Repression of the immune response definitely worsens the patient's prognosis and tips the scales in favor of tumor growth.

CHAPTER 22

CANCER INCIDENCE, PREVENTION, DETECTION, AND DIAGNOSIS

CANCER INCIDENCE AND MORTALITY RATES WITHIN THE UNITED STATES

According to the 1978 *Cancer Facts and Figures*, there are over 3 million Americans alive who have a history of cancer, 2 million of whom were diagnosed over 5 years ago. It was estimated that during 1978 700,000 people would be diagnosed as having cancer.[24] Furthermore, 675,000 Americans would possibly develop some form of cancer during 1979. According to another estimate, 25 per cent of today's healthy population will develop cancer in some form during their lifetime.[89]

The incidence of reported cases of cancer (i.e., the number of new cases of cancer diagnosed within a specific time span) has been steadily increasing since 1900. There are at least five reasons for this apparent increase. First of all, *diagnostic methods* are far more precise today than in the past. Thus, many more persons are now being diagnosed who would have died from "unknown causes" years ago. Second, the gathering, analysis, and publication of *statistics* concerning cancer has become more sophisticated over the years. In the past many persons with cancer were undoubtedly overlooked in the gathering of information and were not included in the yearly reports on cancer morbidity and mortality. Third, the *classification* of cancer disorders has grown to include Hodgkin's disease and leukemia. Finally, due to advances in medical science, people are *living longer* today than even a few decades ago. Because older persons are more vulnerable to cancer than young persons, the incidence of cancer is higher now than when more people died at an early age. In sum, the apparent rise in the incidence of cancer is somewhat misleading; it may simply reflect more precise diagnostic and statistical methods as well as alterations in age span of the population.

Like the incidence rate, the mortality rate (i.e., deaths due to cancer within a specified population) for cancer is also rising. In 1900 cancer ranked seventh as a cause of death in the United States; today it ranks second, preceded only by cardiovascular disorders. Today one person dies of cancer for every five persons who die from all other causes, including accidents.

While the *overall* incidence and mortality rates for cancer are on the increase, the incidence and mortality rates of the *various types* of cancer vary. Below we have briefly summarized the relative incidence of the principal types of cancer.

Breast cancer is the leading cause of cancer deaths in American women. Statistically, of every 100 women, 7 will some day suffer from breast cancer.

Lung cancer is the leading cause of cancer death in American men. Among both sexes the incidence of lung cancer is rising rapidly. The death rate for men has increased more than 25 fold in 45 years. The death rate for women is going up steadily. Researchers believe that the risk of developing lung cancer is definitely increased by habitual cigarette smoking.

Colon-rectal cancer has a higher incidence in the United States than any other form of cancer with the exception of skin cancer. Both sexes are equally susceptible to this form of malignancy.

The death rate from *uterine cancer* is fortunately decreasing; indeed, the rate is down one third from what it was 40 years ago. This decline in deaths from uterine cancer probably reflects more precise diagnostic and treament methods as well as the widespread schooling of women concerning the necessity for a "pap" smear.

Skin cancer has the highest incidence of all forms of cancer; fortunately, however, skin malignancy is also the most preventable form of cancer and has the highest cure rate.

Oral cancer and *cancer of the prostate* also affect considerable numbers of persons in the United States and elsewhere. Prostatic cancer predominantly affects men over 60.

Finally, between 1959 and 1970, *mortality rates* per 100,000 persons decreased for the following cancers:[85]

1978 ESTIMATES CANCER INCIDENCE BY SITE AND SEX†

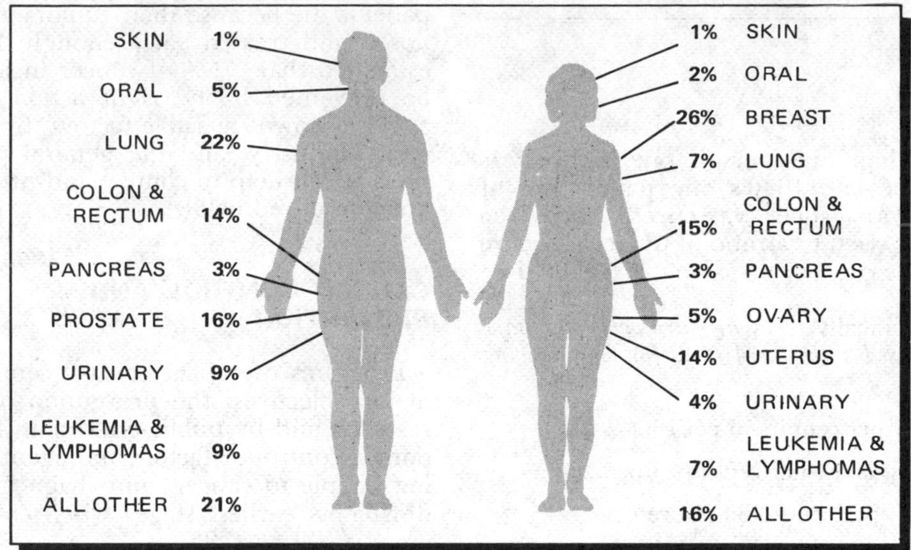

†Excluding non-melanoma skin cancer and carcinoma in situ of uterine cervix.

CANCER DEATHS BY SITE AND SEX

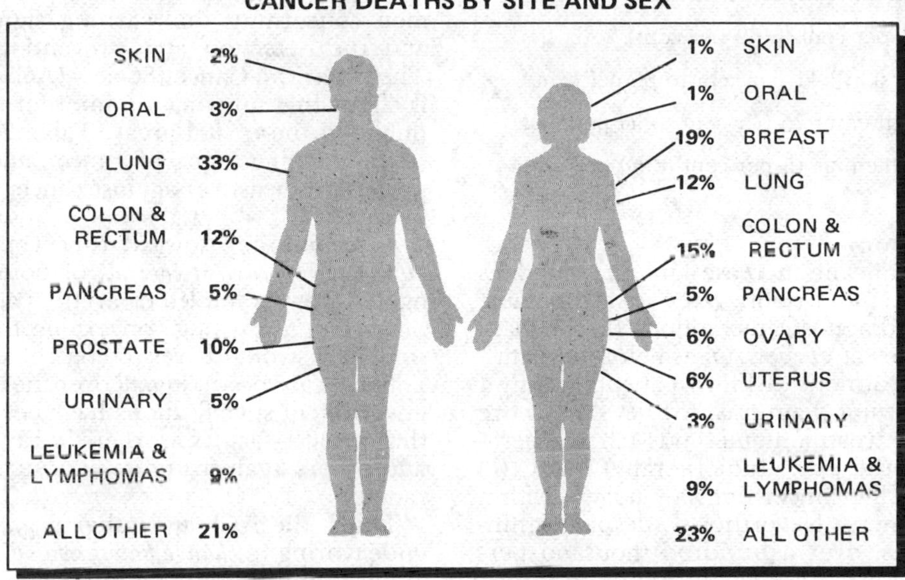

Figure 22–1. Cancer statistics, 1978. (From *CA-A Cancer Journal for Clinicians*, 28:17, Jan.–Feb. 1978.)

Uterine: 19.0 to 9.0

Rectum: 8.4 to 5.7 in males and from 5.6 to 3.3 in females

Stomach: 20.4 to 8.8 in males and from 11.1 to 4.3 in females

Bladder: 2.6 to 1.8 in females

Lip: 0.6 to 0.1 in males

Cancer deaths in *children* under 15 years of age have declined from 8.4 per 100,000 population in 1950 to 6.2 in 1970.

CANCER CURE RATES

The lay public is often concerned with the issue of cure.

> *In general, the definition of cure of cancer is that the patient be without evidence of disease for at least 5 years after diagnosis.*

The waiting period is meant to assure that there are no metastases. The 5-year period of time is arbitrary. If the cell cycle time is very short, the metastatic tumor will be quickly apparent. On the other hand, if the cell cycle is long, a metastasis may not appear for 5 years or longer.

Fortunately, cancer cure rates are accelerating more rapidly than are cancer incidence and mortality rates. Early in this century, most patients who developed cancer died. By the late

1930's less than one person out of five was cured; by the late 1940's one patient out of every four with cancer was cured. Today the cure rate has risen to a ratio of one cancer cure to every three deaths — a saving of 55,000 lives per year.

More specifically, *5 year survival rates have steadily increased since the 1940's for the following cancers:*[85]

- Prostate: 37 per cent to 56 per cent
- Uterine corpus: 61 per cent to 74 per cent
- Thyroid: 64 per cent to 85 per cent
- Kidney: 26 per cent to 42 per cent
- Bladder: 42 per cent to 61 per cent
- Larynx: 41 per cent to 62 per cent
- Melanoma (skin): 41 per cent to 66 per cent
- Hodgkin's disease: 25 per cent to 54 per cent
- Chronic leukemia: 15 per cent to 30 per cent

Summary

These significant increases in survival rates and decreases in mortality rates are attributable to: (a) better diagnostic techniques, (b) the diagnosis of cancer at earlier stages before it metastasizes, (c) treatment of more patients within 4 months following diagnosis, (d) new and more sophisticated treatment methods (chemotherapy, immunotherapy, radiotherapy), and (e) more knowledge concerning carcinogens within our environment. Nevertheless, despite significant advances, over a hundred thousand persons per year die needlessly of cancer. These patients die because their tumors are not diagnosed and treated early enough. Finally, it is estimated that "75% of cancer incidence could be prevented if the right action were taken against known causative factors" by the government, industry, and the general public.[89] Actions which help to control and prevent cancer are considered below.

CANCER CONTROL AND PREVENTION

Programs of cancer control center on three major objectives: the prevention of cancer by research and by public education, the elimination or control of factors and agents predisposing people to cancer, and diagnosis of cancer during its earliest stages when curative treatment is still possible.

The first step toward the control of cancer is *education* of both professional persons and laymen concerning the warning signs of cancer and the detection and prevention of cancer. The American Cancer Society (ACS) is constantly circulating information in order to school the public in these vital areas. Table 22–1 lists the seven warning signs of cancer and the seven protective measures against cancer emphasized by the ACS.

A second step toward cancer prevention is *increased government controls* of potential carcinogens. For example, cigarette packages must now carry a warning concerning the danger of smoking; strong drives to control air and water pollution are occurring all over the country; also government specifications have been developed that protect factory workers, x-ray technicians, and others against undue exposure to ionizing radiation.

Third, the ACS and other organizations are endeavoring to *change habits and customs* that are

TABLE 22–1. SEVEN WARNING SIGNS OF CANCER AND SEVEN SAFEGUARDS AGAINST CANCER

Cancer's Seven Warning Signs *(American Cancer Society)*	**Seven Safeguards Against Cancer**
1. Change in bowel or bladder habits	1. *Breast:* Regular monthly self-examination of breasts for lumps, nodules, or changes in contour
2. A sore that does not heal	2. *Colon-Rectum:* Annual proctoscopic examination in persons over 40
3. Unusual bleeding or discharge	3. *Lung:* Control and preferably elimination of the cigarette smoking habit; annual chest x-ray
4. Thickening or lumps in breast or elsewhere	4. *Oral:* Annual examinations of the mouth and teeth
5. Indigestion or difficulty in swallowing	5. *Skin:* Avoidance of undue exposure to sunlight
6. Obvious change in wart or mole	6. *Uterus:* Annual Papanicolaou smear for all female adults
7. Nagging cough or hoarseness	7. *Basic:* Yearly complete physical examination for all adult men and women; annual urinalysis and blood work

known to predispose Americans to cancer. For example, persons are urged, via short television presentations, to "kick the habit," i.e., to stop smoking, sunbathers are cautioned about the danger of overexposure to strong sunlight.

CANCER DETECTION TECHNIQUES

Although prevention is the ideal method of cancer control, the second best method involves early diagnosis of malignant diseases and the removal of precancerous lesions. Nurses and physicians must emphasize to their patients and to the general public the importance of discovering and eradicating cancerous lesions *early, before* they begin to metastasize from the primary site. Nurses can help in this educational process by emphasizing the need for an annual physical examination, by stressing the importance of a yearly Papanicolaou test for women, and by teaching women the technique for the monthly breast self-examination. (See Chapters 15 and 81.)

What specifically is involved in the cancer detection examination? The physician employs both general and special techniques in a complete cancer detection examination. General techniques include obtaining the patient's familial and environmental histories, performing a thorough physical examination, and ordering and evaluating laboratory examinations of the patient's blood and urine. The more specialized techniques used for cancer detection are discussed in the following sections.

Cytologic Examination or Papanicolaou Test ("Pap" Smear)

This valuable diagnostic test was developed by George N. Papanicolaou in 1943. Its original purpose was to discover cancer of the cervix during the early, noninvasive, asymptomatic stage. Today, the test is also used to detect early cancers of the digestive, respiratory, and renal tracts, and occasionally of the breast. Also the Pap smear is currently employed to evaluate the patient's response to chemotherapy and radiation therapy, as well as to detect malignant disease when it recurs postoperatively.

Materials that can be examined by Pap smears include: (1) cervical scrapings, (2) bronchial secretions and washings obtained by bronchoscopy, (3) urine sediment, (4) coughed up sputum, (5) aspirated gastric secretions, and (6) mammary gland discharge fluid.

The method for obtaining a Pap smear is fairly simple. First, the examiner either scrapes cells from a tissue (e.g., the cervix) or obtains cells by aspirating fluid or sediment from an organ (e.g., the stomach or bronchi). Next, the examiner fixes the smear by immersing it in a chemical solution of equal parts of ether and 95 per cent ethyl alcohol. Finally, the fixed slide is allowed to dry and then is sent to a cytotechnologist or pathologist for staining and evaluation.

The laboratory technique used to analyze the Pap smear is called *exfoliative cytology*, which means the examination of desquamated or sloughed-off cells. Under the microscope, the cells may have either a normal or an anaplastic appearance. The appearance of the cells is graded on the following five-point scale:

Class I – Normal
Class II – Probably normal
Class III – Doubtful (may be malignant)
Class IV – Probably malignant
Class V – Malignant

The examiner will repeat the Pap smear if the desquamated cells being examined are classified as "doubtful" (Class III). If the cells are "probably malignant" (Class IV), the physician will perform a biopsy in order to further evaluate the patient's condition.

Biopsy

A biopsy is the surgical excision of a small piece of tissue for microscopic examination; this is the method most commonly used to either rule out or confirm a diagnosis of malignancy.

The patient is usually scheduled for minor surgery. If the site for biopsy is easily accessible (e.g., cervix, breast), the patient is appropriately draped, a local anesthetic is administered, and a piece of the suspicious tissue is removed by the surgeon. Additional procedures (e.g., bronchoscopy, cystoscopy, and sigmoidoscopy) are necessary if the tumor is internal.

There are two types of biopsy procedures; the type used depends upon the *size* of the tumor. If the suspicious tumor is *small*, the entire tumor is excised for examination; this is called a *total* or *excisional* type biopsy. If the tumor is *large*, only a part of the neoplasm is excised; this is called a *subtotal* or *incisional* type biopsy. There is some question as to the safety of the subtotal biopsy. Some surgeons believe that this procedure opens vascular channels and releases tumor cells that may then metastasize to other sites during the time when the excised tissue is being examined. However, there are no studies to date that definitely confirm this fear.

Following the excision, the material obtained by the biopsy goes to the pathologist, who generally uses one of two methods for examining the specimen: the frozen section or the permanent paraffin section. To prepare a *frozen* (or *rapid*) section, the tissue is immediately frozen. Then the pathologist cuts the tissue into thin sections and examines the tissue slices under the microscope. The main advantage of the frozen section is the *speed* with which the section can be prepared and the diagnosis made — only minutes are required. In contrast, the slower more classic method of embedding the tissue in paraffin takes about 24 hours; however, the paraffin section provides the pathologist with clearer detail than does the frozen section.

Needle Biopsy. In this method of biopsy, tissue is aspirated from a suspicious nodule or mass, rather than excised. Needle or aspiration biopsy is used mainly to obtain tissue samples from the liver, kidney, spleen, and lung.

X-ray Examinations

X-ray techniques are particularly useful in the diagnosis of obstructive tumors and of the gastrointestinal, respiratory, and renal tracts. They are also valuable in the identification of bone malignancies. In addition, radiographic procedures aided by computers are helpful in pinpointing the location of brain tumors and the degree to which the tumors are compressing surrounding tissues.

Sometimes the suspicious lesion that brings a person to the doctor for a cancer detection examination is not the primary lesion, but a *metastatic* or secondary lesion. A metastatic lesion that becomes evident *before* the primary lesion appears is called a *sentinel metastasis*. Of first priority in the examination of patients with sentinel metastases is a thorough search for the hidden primary site so that treatment can be started at once.

Ultrasound Procedures

High-frequency ultrasound can be used to demonstrate the interfaces around organs, and within pathologic masses. Special equipment is used to detect and map echoes of varying density from various organs and tumors. At present, the technique is used to detect lesions in the female pelvis, abdominal lymph nodes, and other areas of the body. One advantage of this procedure is that it is a noninvasive way to demonstrate and follow the growth of neoplasms.

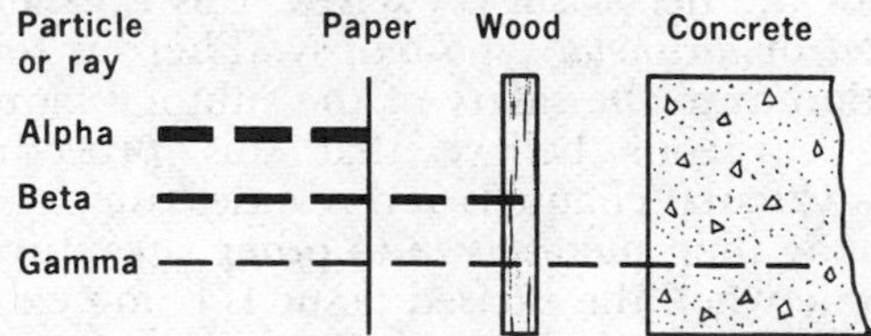

Figure 22–2. Relative penetration of alpha, beta, and gamma radiation. (From Phelan, E. W.: Radioisotopes in Medicine Booklet. *In Understanding the Atom Series.* U.S. Atomic Energy Commission, Division of Technical Information, 1966, p. 8.)

Radiodiagnostic Techniques

Radiation can be employed both as a diagnostic tool and as a therapeutic agent. (Radiotherapy is discussed in Chapter 23.) Because the use of radiation is a complex and important subject, let us pause here and review some of the definitions and concepts basic to the study of radiation.

BASIC CONCEPTS IN RADIODIAGNOSIS AND RADIOTHERAPY

Radiation is the emission of waves or particles of radiant energy. Examples of radiation are radio waves, infrared red waves, ultraviolet light, x-rays alpha particles, beta particles, and gamma rays. A substance that is *radioactive* has the property of spontaneously emitting some form of radiant energy, e.g., a radioisotope.

You will recall that an isotope is a chemical element having the same atomic number as another (i.e., the same number of nuclear protons), but having a different atomic mass (i.e., a different number of nuclear neutrons). The chemical properties of the two forms are the same. For example, the element hydrogen has three isotopes: common hydrogen (H), deuterium (H^2) and tritium (H^3).

Isotopes are either stable or unstable. A *radioisotope* or *radionuclide* is an unstable isotope that spontaneously gives off radiant energy as the unstable nuclei of its atoms decompose. A limited number of radioisotopes occur naturally; however, today the majority of radioisotopes are produced artifically in an atomic reactor by bombarding a stable isotope with neutrons. For example, radioactive cobalt can be produced by bombarding the stable isotope of cobalt with neutrons in an atomic reactor. The radioactive cobalt produced will eventually disintegrate. The resulting product will be nickel, plus the emission of a beta particle and a gamma ray from the nucleus.

Radioisotopes emit three types of radiation: alpha particles (helium nuclei), beta particles (electrons), and gamma rays (electromagnetic radiation). *Alpha particles* have a low penetrating power and are unable to penetrate even a piece of paper; *beta particles* can penetrate a few millimeters of skin, but are unable to penetrate a piece of wood; *gamma rays* have an intense penetrating power; however, they cannot penetrate a thick piece of concrete (Fig. 22–2). Beta particles and gamma rays are used in cancer detection and therapy.

The *half-life* of a radioisotope is the time it takes for one half of the atoms composing the radioisotope to decay (i.e., the time required for the radioisotope to lose one half its original energy). Some radioisotopes have a half-life of a few days, whereas others have a half-life of many years. For example, iodine-131 has a half-life of about eight days, cobalt-60 has a half-life of five years, and radium-226 has a half-life of 1620 years.

The length of the half-life is an important consideration in the choice of radioisotopes for medical use. Radioisotopes with short half-lives can be used in an *unsealed* form; for example, iodine-131 is usually administered by mouth; gold-198, which has a half-life of 2.7 days, is administered by injection. These radioisotopes expend their energy rapidly and are excreted readily by the body. On the other hand, radioisotopes with longer half-lives must be administered to the patient *sealed* in some type of metal container so that they can be removed upon discontinuation of radiotherapy. For example, radium (with a half-life of 1620 years) is administered encased in metal seeds or needles that can be removed when the course of therapy is completed.

Radiation is *measured* in several ways.

- The activity of a radioactive substance or its rate of disintegration is measured by the *curie*. One curie (Ci) is equivalent to the amount of any radioisotope that undergoes 3.7×10^{10} disintegrations per second (i.e., a curie measures the number of atoms in a particular radioisotope that disintegrate in one second). One millicurie (mCi.) equals one thousandth of a curie; one microcurie (μCi.) equals one millionth of a curie.
- The *roentgen* is the international unit of measurement of x-rays and gamma rays. The *milliroentgen* (mr.) is one thousandth of a roentgen.
- The *rad* is the measure of radiation dosage used for diagnosis and therapy. *Dosages* of radiation used to *destroy malignant growths* are measured in hundreds or thousands of *rads*, whereas *tracer doses* of radioisotopes used for *diagnostic purposes* are measured in *millirads*.

Radiation cannot be detected by ordinary methods; i.e., we cannot see, hear, smell, taste, touch or feel radiation. Consequently, sensitive instruments have been designed to detect and measure radioactivity; these instruments measure and record the physical, chemical, and electrical effects of radioactive substances upon materials. Examples of measuring instruments that are used in medicine are Geiger-Muller counters, scintillation counters, specimen counters, scanners, gamma cameras, and whole body counters.

THE ROLE OF RADIOISOTOPES IN DIAGNOSIS

Why are radioisotopes useful in the diagnosis of cancer? Isotopes are capable of entering into the same chemical reactions and the same metabolic processes in the body as are stable elements. When a radioactive isotope enters a person's body, the fate of the element can be followed, or *traced*, by *scanning machines*. Abnormal tissue shows up differently on the scan because the isotope is metabolized differently by this tissue.

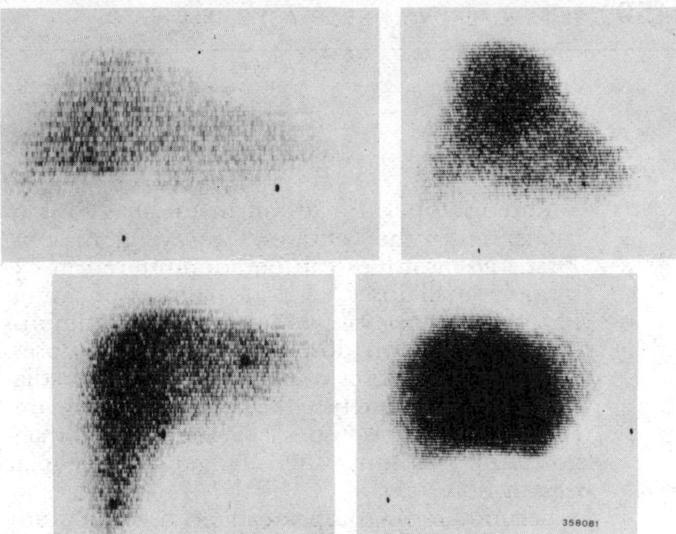

Figure 22–3. Normal liver scan. (From DeLand, F., and H. W. Wagner: *Atlas of Nuclear Medicine, Vol. 3, Reticuloendothelial System, Liver, Spleen and Thyroid.* Philadelphia: W. B. Saunders Co., 1972.)

Thyroid, bone, brain, liver, lung, and spleen are areas of the body most frequently scanned for diagnostic purposes.

Thus, when diagnostically employed, radioisotopes are used as tracers. A tracer is a material that can be administered to the patient, either orally or by injection, and then identified, located, and traced by sensitive apparatus as the radioactive material circulates through the body and concentrates in particular organs and tissues.

The *scintillation counter* is the most popular instrument used to measure radioactivity for diagnostic purposes. A photoelectric cell within the counter is able to detect radiant energy; flashes of light occur whenever particles or rays of radiant energy strike certain phosphors, such as sodium iodide crystals, and that are located within the apparatus. Each light flash represents a radioactive signal, and the intensity of the flash measures the intensity of the signal. The light flashes are converted within a photomultiplier tube into electrical impulses, amplified, and then recorded on sensitized paper by a synchronously moving pen. This type of recording is similar to the recording of electrical impulses within the heart (electrocardiogram) or electrical impulses within the brain (electroencephalogram).

The *scintillation scanner* is a device for locating and pinpointing malignant growths by measuring the uptake of a radioisotope. An important part of this apparatus is the *probe*, a container that houses the phosphor crystals and photomultiplier tube. To examine the patient, the scintillation scanner is passed back and forth over the area of the body that is being studied. If the liver is being examined, the probe will be passed back and forth over the right hypochondrium and epigastrium (Fig. 22–3).

Brain scan may be done by a *scintillation camera* that produces many images in rapid sequence, showing the transit of an isotope through cerebral vessels (Fig. 22–4).

Radioisotopes are useful in the diagnosis of cancer and other entities for several reasons. First, radioisotopes can be administered in extremely small doses, e.g., one billionth of a gram of a radioisotope can be measured for administration as a tracer dose. With such small doses, the body absorbs a minimal amount of radiation, and consequently the cells suffer no damage. Thus, radioisotopes can be employed diagnostically without the danger of cellular destruction.

Second, radioisotopes can be used to study the functions of specific organs and tissues. A classic example of this type of study is the ^{131}I uptake test that is used to evaluate thyroid function. If the presence of thyroid disease is suspected, the patient receives a tracer dose of radioactive iodine (^{131}I). The radioactive iodine will circulate to the thyroid gland and there be converted into thyroxine in precisely the same manner as regular (nonradioactive) iodine. In other words, the body cannot distinguish between radioactive or "tagged" atoms of iodine and regular iodine; it processes both types of atoms in exactly the same way. However, tagged atoms of iodine and other substances (iron [Fe], gold [Au], sodium [Na], phosphorus [P]) differ from regular atoms in one important respect: the doctor can trace, locate, and measure the tagged atoms by means of scintillation counters or scanners. Consequently, by tracing and measuring the number of tagged atoms of iodine that pass into the thyroid and the number that are secreted, the doctor can determine whether the thyroid gland is diseased. For instance, the normal thyroid picks up 30 per cent of a tracer dose of iodine and excretes 60 per cent in the urine. However, if the patient has hyperthyroidism, the thyroid will take up 70 per cent of the tracer dose and excrete 10 per cent in the urine.

Radioisotopes are also employed to measure blood volume, blood circulation rate, red blood cell turnover, cardiac output, and lung blood flow, using the same types of procedures.

Finally, radioisotopes are used to locate tumors and lesions within the brain, kidneys, liver, lungs, pericardium, and bones. Certain radioisotopes have an affinity for particular organs or tissues; e.g., ^{131}I has an affinity for thyroid tissue, ^{198}Au has an affinity for the liver, and so forth. In some cases, if the organ harbors a malignant tumor, the tagged atoms will tend to *concentrate* in the area of tumor growth; consequently a scan of the organ will reveal a high uptake of the radioisotope at the site of the tumor. For example, ^{131}I is used to locate cancerous tissues that have metastasized from the thyroid gland to other parts of the body (Fig. 22–5). An area in which the concentration of a radioisotope is unusually high is called a "hot spot." In other cases, the tagged atoms tend to concentrate *less* densely in the diseased portion of the organ than in the normal portion. For example, examine the lung scan shown in Figure 22–6. Note that the tumor growth that has involved the right upper lobe has failed to concentrate the radioisotope, and it appears as a blank area or "cold spot" on the scan.

For the patient, undergoing an organ scan is a

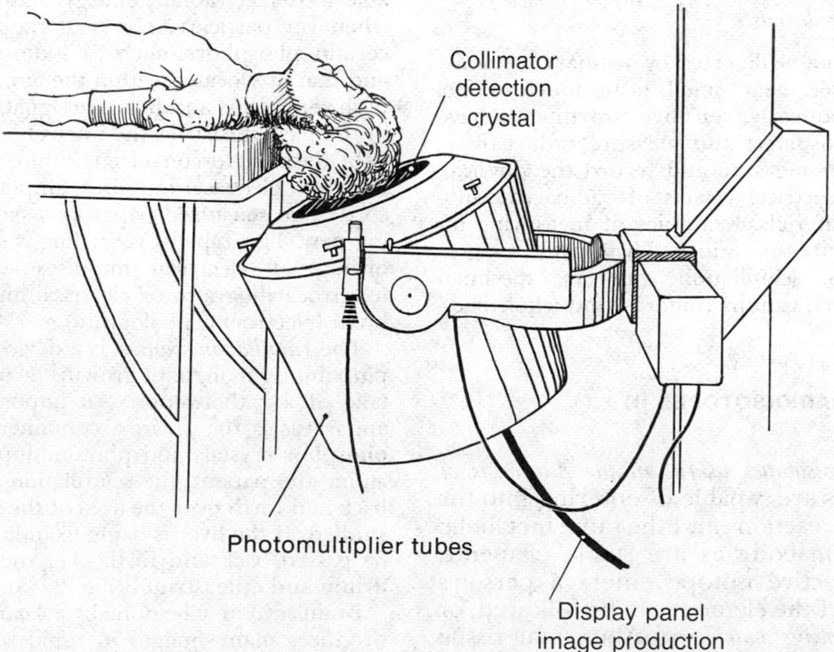

Figure 22–4. Scintillation camera. (From James, A. E., Jr., and L. F. Squire: *Exercises in Diagnostic Radiology. Nuclear Radiology,* Philadelphia: W. B. Saunders Co., 1973.)

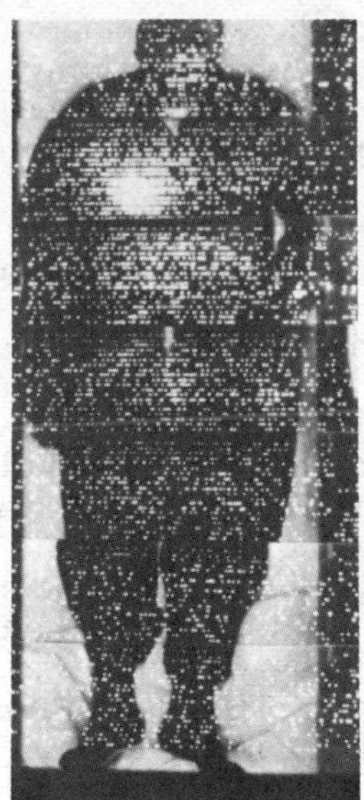

Figure 22–5. ^{131}I is used to locate tumors which have metastasized from the thyroid gland. (From Phelan, E. W.: Radioisotopes in Medicine Booklet. *In Understanding the Atom Series.* U.S. Atomic Energy Commission, Division of Technical Information, 1966.)

simple and completely painless procedure. There are three steps involved.

Step 1: Administration of the Radioisotope. The patient is given a tracer dose of the appropriate radioisotope either orally or by injection.

Step 2: Waiting Period. Before the scanning procedure can be performed, the radioisotope must be assimilated by the organ under study. The length of time required for assimilation varies; for example, it takes one hour for radioactive gold to be assimilated by the liver; therefore, the patient must wait for one hour following an IV injection of ^{198}Au for a liver scan. For a brain scan, the patient must wait one and one half hours following an injection of radioactive mercury, and 18 to 48 hours following an injection of RIHSA (radio-iodinated human serum albumin).

Step 3: The Scanning Procedure. The patient is simply asked to lie still and breathe normally while the scintillation scanner measures the radioactive atoms concentrated in the organ under study and records its findings. Sometimes restless or agitated patients require sedation before this procedure in order to relax during the examination.

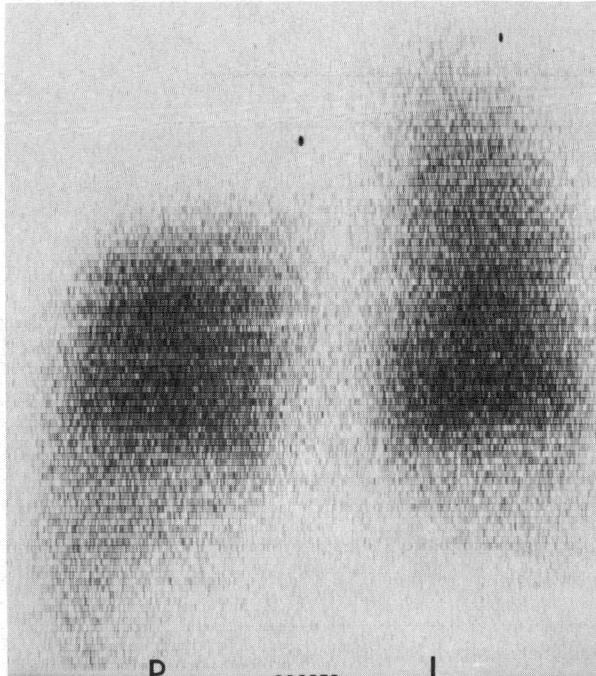

Figure 22–6. Scan showing presence of tumor in right lung. (From DeLand, F., and Wagner, H. W.: *Atlas of Nuclear Medicine. Vol. 2, Lung and Heart.* Philadelphia: W. B. Saunders Co., 1970.)

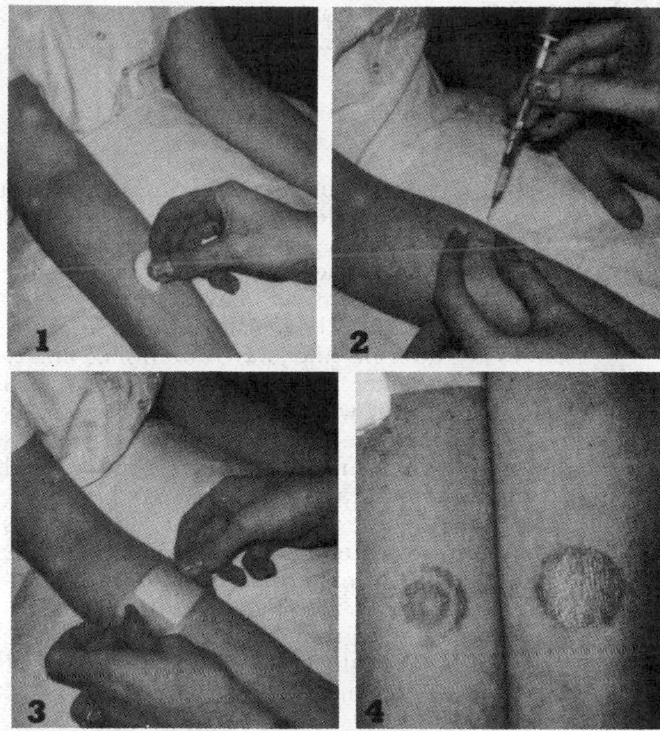

Figure 22–7. Procedure for DNCB sensitization. (From Croft, C. L.: BCG administration and nursing implications. *American Journal of Nursing,* 79:318, 1979.)

DNCB Skin Test[27, 37]

Recall from Chapter 21 that the immune system apparently plays a vital role in preventing tumor growth and in destroying those tumors that do develop. The DNCB skin test is the method currently used to assess whether or not the patient has a properly functioning immune system. Approximately 90 to 95 per cent of healthy people can be sensitized to the chemical dinitrochlorobenzene (DNCB) when it is placed on a small area of the skin. (See Figure 22–7 for the skin test procedure.) A healthy individual develops a positive response (redness, itching, and maybe blistering) within 24 to 48 hours, when given a second (challenge) dose of DNCB 14 days later, the individual then develops a delayed cutaneous hypersensitivity response (a raised red site) on the skin.

The DNCB skin test is useful in several ways. First, it acts as a diagnostic and prognostic aid. For example, patients who have a negative reaction or who cannot be sensitized to DNCB are said to be "anergic" (i.e., have diminished ability to react to specific antigens). If the person also has a rapidly growing tumor, the prognosis is likely to be poor. Second, DNCB is used to assess the patient's immunocompetence prior to and during radiotherapy and chemotherapy—both of which are modalities that can suppress the immune system. Third, the patient must be DNCB skin tested to be a candidate for immunotherapy (Chapter 23). Finally, patients in immunotherapy programs are monitored with the DNCB skin test throughout their therapeutic regimen to determine their response to therapy.

STAGING AND CLASSIFICATION

When a neoplastic growth is definitely diagnosed, it must be further defined in terms of its *extent*. This diagnostic process, called *staging*, involves a systematic search for (a) the characteristics of the primary tumor (using clinical examination and pathologic examination), (b) involvement of the lymph nodes (using clinical examination, lymphangiography, and perhaps needle biopsy), and (c) evidence of metastasis, based upon knowledge of the natural history of the disease.

Two major agencies are concerned with the classification of stages in malignant disease. They are the International Union Against Cancer (UICC) and the American Joint Committee for Cancer Staging and End Results Reporting (AJCCS). The objectives for developing and using classification of neoplastic diseases are: to aid the clinician in planning treatment, to give some indication of prognosis, to assist in the evaluation of results of treatment, to facilitate the exchange of information, and to assist in the continuing investigation of cancer.

The TNM system is the most common type of system for staging in use today. "T" stands for tumor, "T1-T4" define the increasing extent of the tumor, "N" is for the regional lymph nodes, "N1-N3" indicates advancing nodal disease, "M0" is for no metastasis, and "M1" indicates that metastasis is present. The TNM staging system is summarized in Figure 22–8. The specifications for each site are being developed and shared around the world.[44]

The stage of a neoplastic growth is determined by the patient's doctor, while the tumor classification is determined by the pathologist. Tumor *classification* involves a histologic and anatomic description of the malignant neoplasm. This staging and classification information guides the doctor in the choice of therapy and in estimating the patient's prognosis. As an exam-

Tumor	
TO	No evidence of primary tumor
TIS	Carcinoma in situ
T1 T2 T3 T4	Progressive increase in tumor size and involvement
TX	Tumor cannot be assessed.
Nodes	
NO	Regional lymph nodes not demonstrably abnormal
N1 N2 N3	Increasing degrees of demonstrable abnormality of regional lymph nodes. (For many primary sites, the subscript "a," e.g., $N1_a$, may be used to indicate that metastasis to the node is not suspected; and the subscript "b," e.g., $N1_b$, may be used to indicate that metastasis to the node is suspected or proved.)
NX	Regional lymph nodes cannot be assessed clinically.
Metastasis	
MO	No evidence of distant metastasis.
M1 M2 M3	Ascending degrees of distant metastasis, including metastasis to distant lymph nodes.

Figure 22–8. TNM Staging System. (Reprinted with permission from the American Joint Committee for Cancer Staging and End Results Reporting and from Clinical Staging System for Carcinoma of the Esophagus. *CA* 25:51, Mar.–Apr. 1975.)

Primary lesions with negative nodes:

T1 NO: Radiation and surgery are equally effective in controlling early primary lesions. Selection of method of treatment is based on cosmetic, functional, and expeditious considerations.

T2 NO: Moderate exophytic lesions are effectively irradiated with excellent results. Surgery is not precluded in event of failure.

T3 NO: Advanced lesions can be treated by irradiation, but when they invade bone or cartilage, they are better managed surgically by a composite resection. Preoperative irradiation is advisable.

T4 NO: For very extensive lesions, combination of techniques is being considered, such as radiation therapy and chemotherapy, or preoperative radiation followed by radical surgery. Preoperative chemotherapy may be used in selected cases with concept of converting an inoperable lesion into an operable one; however, this is not a general principle.

Primary lesions with positive nodes:

T1 N1: In selected cases, irradiation and surgery can be combined, i.e., primary lesion, such as tongue carcinoma or buccal carcinoma, is treated by radiation therapy followed by neck dissection.

T2-3 N2-3: The presence of cervical node metastases is generally a surgical problem and is an indication for *en bloc* dissection of both primary and neck nodes.

T4 N3: Massive lesions are most often inoperable. Palliative radiotherapy and/or chemotherapy are utilized.

Figure 22–9. A treatment protocol using the TNM Staging System. (Reprinted with permission from Bales, H. W., and J. D. Norante: Head and neck tumors. *In* Rubin, P. (Ed.): *Clinical Oncology.* New York: American Cancer Society, 1974, p. 307.)

ple, Figure 22–9 illustrates how the TNM staging system is used in developing a treatment protocol. Figure 22–10 demonstrates the use of the staging system in predicting patients' prognoses.

PSYCHOLOGIC IMPACT OF THE DIAGNOSIS OF CANCER ON THE PATIENT AND SIGNIFICANT OTHERS

We can assume that the patient who is undergoing the diagnostic process associated with a suspicious lump or other cancer symptom is afraid. The tests being experienced are unfamiliar and perhaps painful. In the past, if the diagnosis was indeed cancer, health care professionals questioned whether or not to tell the patient the truth about the diagnosis. Now, it is to be hoped, doctors and nurses respect the patient's right to know the diagnosis. Today, consequently, the difficulty of telling a person what may be very feared news must be faced. The greatest hurdle involves the feelings and fears of the health care personnel themselves.

Histologic Type	*Stage I* % *(No.)*	*Stage II* % *(No.)*	*Stage III* % *(No.)*
squamous cell	46.4 (331)	39.8 (66)	11.5 (524)
adenocarcinoma	45.9 (151)	14.3 (28)	7.9 (334)
undifferentiated, large cell	42.8 (61)	12.9 (17)	12.9 (103)
undifferentiated, small cell oat cell	6.0 (38)	5.0 (20)	3.8 (302)

**Staging according to AJCCS criteria*

Figure 22–10. Two-year survival rate for lung cancer. (Reprinted with permission from Emerson, G., and C. Phillips: Lung cancer. *In* Rubin, P. (Ed.): *Clinical Oncology.* New York: American Cancer Society, 1974, p. 159.)

We dislike being bearers of "bad tidings." Also, we fear that the patient will be so crushed by the news that "the will to live" may disappear. We fear that a person may commit suicide because *we* revealed the presence of cancer. In actuality, these responses are rare; thus they cannot be used as an excuse for avoiding our responsibility to the patient. If support is to be provided through a difficult period, health care personnel must be able to discuss the patient's condition *with the patient* — including diagnosis, treatment, care plan, and prognosis.

The following points should be considered in revealing a diagnosis to a patient:

(1) In most cases it is helpful to give the patient the information *over a period of time*. If the patient knows the alternatives that are being ruled out during the diagnostic period, the confirmation of one alternative — even if unpleasant — will not be as much of a shock. Having time to prepare for an event is part of coping successfully.

2. Explanations should be *geared to the patient's level of understanding*. It is good to use several terms or names for the diagnosis, for example, "lymphosarcoma," "tumor," "malignancy," "cancer," and even, "this thing." Patients choose whatever name is comfortable for them when they are ready to ask questions. This is especially important with children.

3. Patients need to *hear the information several times*, perhaps from several people they trust. Often patients ask the same questions over and over. Shy or fearful patients may be reluctant to take up the time of "busy doctors and nurses" with their questions. Patients need to feel that the people who may be able to provide information are willing to take time to talk with them. The nurse should communicate the patient's needs to other members of the health care team, as well.

4. At the same time that the diagnosis is confirmed, the patient needs to know *what alternatives are available for treatment*. There should be time for the patient to assimilate the information before being asked to make choices about the treatment.

As Kastenbaum[45] points out, although it is the physician's responsibility to inform the patient of the diagnosis and treatment, it is the nurse's responsibility to be informed, not only of the specific diagnosis and treatment plan for a patient, but about the disease and treatment in general.

Reactions to the diagnosis of cancer are highly variable. Certainly this time can be characterized as a period of crisis for the patient. It is marked by fear, some denial, withdrawal, anger, and other reactions to anxiety. A few patients will say that they don't want to know anything about the disease. They cope by saying, "Don't tell me anthing. Just do what you have to do." Since this probably will not be the patient's only coping strategy, it is best to remain sensitive to the patient's needs and request for information.

The goal of care at this time is to *help the patient cope* with the diagnosis, treatment, and prognosis. Coping has been defined as "The problem solving efforts made by an individual when the demands he faces are highly relevant to his welfare (that is, a situation of considerable jeopardy or promise), and when these demands tax his adaptive resources."[25] Coping successfully offers the patient the opportunity to learn new problem-solving techniques and to develop new sources of fulfillment and gratification.

It is important to remember that a person copes the best way that she or he can in a crisis situation, but that the sensitive nurse can often help the person find more successful strategies. Receiving *accurate information* about the situation is one of the keystones of coping. It is also important for the person to be *physiologically intact* enough to use the information. This implies that the person's pain is controlled, for instance. Also important is that the patient feels a *sense of control* of the situation. Nurses must be especially aware of this, because hospitalization makes most people feel helpless and not in control. This anxiety-provoking feeling can interfere with coping efforts.

If a person is helped to cope successfully during the period of diagnosis and beginning of treatment, the person will be more likely to manage during the entire course of the disease. Patients often demonstrate great strength as they learn to deal with their fears and with the difficulties of being treated for cancer. Coping with cancer is explored more fully in Chapter 23.

CHAPTER 23

MANAGEMENT OF PATIENTS WITH NEOPLASTIC DISEASE

The major objective of cancer therapy is to cure the patient and to insure that minimal functional and structural impairment results from the disease. The treatment decisions made at the time of first diagnosis are crucial, because once metastasis is discovered, the opportunity for cure is usually past. Balancing the opportunity for cure with the morbidity and mortality of a therapeutic procedure is often difficult. If cure is not possible, important alternate goals are (a) to prevent further metastasis, (b) to relieve symptoms, and (c) to maintain high-quality life for as long as possible.

The three major methods for treating patients with cancer are surgery, chemotherapy, and radiation therapy. A fourth form, which is still in experimental stages, is immunotherapy.

SURGICAL THERAPY

Four major types of surgery are performed in the management of cancer: diagnostic, radical, prophylactic, and palliative.

Diagnostic Surgery

The purpose of diagnostic surgery is to either confirm or rule out a possible diagnosis of malignancy. It establishes the type and classification of tumor. The biopsy is the procedure of choice.

Radical Surgery

Radical surgery is the most widely employed method of cancer therapy. The goal is to remove all the tumor, with minimal structural and functional impairment. Radical surgery is particularly useful in the treatment of those cancers of the skin, colon, rectum, breast, cervix, prostate, and stomach that are still in the early stages of development. Because surgery is a localized treatment, it is not curative for metastatic cancer.

One commonly employed radical procedure is the *en bloc* resection. The purpose of this procedure is to excise both the original growth and the lymph channels that drain the area around the tumor. The term "en bloc" means that the tumor and the lymph nodes are removed together; thus, the surgeon avoids slicing across lymphatic pathways. The en bloc method is employed in radical mastectomy for breast cancer and radical neck resection for cancers of the head and neck.

Unfortunately, radical surgery, if it is to be curative, often involves the sacrifice of an organ, the disruption of organ functions, or permanent disfigurement. For example, the surgeon may be forced to amputate a limb, remove the patient's breast or colon, remove a portion of the jaw, or perform other drastic surgical measures. Such extensive surgery, however necessary for survival, is difficult for patients to accept psychologically. The patient may need to learn new ways of self-care, as with a colostomy. Major changes will need to be incorporated into the patient's body image. All of this is accompanied by the fear that even with radical surgery, the cancer may still be present — a question only time can answer.

The process of rehabilitation is usually not finished by the time the patient is ready for discharge. Referral to appropriate community agencies and groups is helpful. Often, groups formed by people who have had similar radical surgery are of great benefit to the patient.

Prophylactic Surgery

You will recall that precancerous lesions (e.g., warts, polyps, senile keratosis), if left untreated, sometimes evolve into cancer later in the patient's life. The purpose of prophylactic surgery is to remove precancerous lesions while they are still harmless and nonmalignant.

Palliative Surgery

The fundamental aims of palliative surgery are: (1) to retard the growth of the tumor, and

(2) to decrease the size of the existing tumor, and (3) to relieve the distressing manifestations of cancer when a cure is no longer possible. Let us briefly consider these three aspects of treatment.

First, the *growth* of malignant tumors, in some cases, depends upon the secretion of certain hormones into the circulation, e.g., estrogens and testosterone. To slow the growth of a neoplasm, the surgeon may remove those glands (ovaries, testes, adrenal glands, pituitary gland) that secrete hormones known to stimulate the growth of cancers in certain parts of the body. For example, a bilateral oophorectomy in a premenopausal female may abate the progress of breast cancer; a hypophysectomy or bilateral adrenalectomy may further retard tumor growth in women with recurrent breast cancer following oophorectomy; removal of the testes may retard the growth of prostatic malignancies.

Second, in some situations (as with cancer of the ovary) as much of the tumor as possible is removed, even though this will not cure the patient. The rationale is that by reducing the "tumor burden" other forms of therapy may have a better chance to be effective.

Third, certain *distressing manifestations* of cancer can be relieved by palliative surgery, e.g., ulcerations, obstructions of the gastrointestinal tract, and severe or intractable pain. *Ulcerations* are removed by excision of the necrotic tissues and by antibiotic therapy. The relief of *obstructions* depends upon the site of involvement; e.g., obstruction of the gastrointestinal tract can be relieved by a gastrointestinal bypass; obstruction of the colon can be relieved by a colostomy. *Severe pain* can be relieved by the blocking of nerves with neurolytic agents or by the surgical interruption of sensory nerve pathways; in very rare instances, a cordotomy may be done (see Unit XI).

Following denervation procedures, remember that the denervated tissues are no longer sensitive to painful stimuli and that the patient needs protection against heat and pressure. These patients require special nursing care, e.g., positioning on an alternating pressure mattress, frequent position changes.

Preoperative and postoperative care for patients undergoing these four types of surgery (diagnostic, radical, prophylactic, and palliative) is essentially the same as it is for patients undergoing any other type of surgery. For discussions of specific operations (radical neck resection, mastectomy, bowel resection) and the care involved, see the appropriate unit.

CHEMOTHERAPY

Research Efforts

In July 1917, British soldiers near Ypres in Flanders were bombarded by the Germans with shells charged with an oily liquid, "sulfur mustard." The effects of this chemical were devastating to the human body. Medical attention, however, focused not only on the initial vesicant action of the chemical, but also on the systemic effects. It was noted that aplasia of the bone marrow, dissolution of the lymphoid tissue, and ulceration of the gastrointestinal tract occurred. By 1942, it was known that small doses of nitrogen mustard could cause regression of tumors in mice. The first humans were treated with the drug that year. After World War II, reports of the research were declassified, and the search for drugs to treat neoplasms began.

Even now the search continues. The National Cancer Institute in the United States screens 50,000 compounds each year. In order to be considered for further testing, the compound must increase the life span of a mouse with advanced leukemia by 50 per cent. Next, characteristics of the drug are studied, including absorption, distribution in the body, storage, and excretion. The minimum and maximum doses for mice, rats, dogs and monkeys are determined. If there is antitumor activity and an absence of prohibitive toxicity, the drug advances to human trials. Five of every 15,000 agents tested enter human trials. Of these five, only one eventually becomes commercially available.[40]

The patients who participate in these drug studies give informed consent for the doctor to use an unproved drug. They realize that while the drug may not help them, more will be learned about the drug that may assist in future treatment of cancer. The safety of the patient is protected. Data is carefully collected for analysis. The patients know that they can withdraw from the study at any time. Before a drug goes on the market, it must successfully pass three phases of research.

During *Phase I* the drug dose and schedule are established. The specific organ toxicity in humans is identified.

In *Phase II* the drug is given to groups of patients with many different types of tumors. The purpose is to identify which tumors the drug affects most.

During *Phase III,* trials are conducted to compare the drug to other forms of therapy already in use. The experimental drug must offer an advantage over the standard therapy either by having fewer or different side effects, or by being more effective against the tumor. During this phase, drugs are also tried in combination with other treatment modalities.

It usually takes years and great expense for a drug to be fully studied and ready for the commercial market, but this process cannot be bypassed, if the safety and effectiveness of cancer drugs is to be assured.

Objectives of Chemotherapy

The goal of cancer chemotherapy is to destroy all the malignant tumor cells without causing excessive destruction of the patient's normal cells. This is possible because normal cells repair the damage caused by the drugs more quickly than neoplastic cells can. Some tumors that initially respond to a drug become resistant in time. There is still much to be learned about how drugs inhibit the growth of and destroy susceptible cells.

Classification of Drugs

Agents being used today in cancer chemotherapy are classified into the following categories:

- *Antimetabolites* inhibit the biosynthesis of the nucleic acids (purine and pyrimidine bases). Interruption in the formation of these essential components of DNA and RNA, (which each cell produces in order to function and multiply), results in cell death.
- *Alkylating agents* interfere with the structure of DNA. It is believed that this occurs by the alkyl group reacting with the DNA in the cell nucleus.
- *Plant alkaloids* have the ability to disorganize the mitotic spindle, thus arresting cell division. The major toxic effect is to the central and peripheral nervous system. Death or permanent CNS damage can occur from an overdose. It is important for the patient to report any tingling, numbness, or tremors in the extremities. Constipation, ataxia, and muscle weakness may also be signs of toxicity.
- *Antibiotics* (not the same ones used to treat infections) apparently interfere with cell division by binding with DNA, thereby slowing production of DNA.
- *Steroid hormones* can be administered to alter the hormonal balance in the patient and suppress the growth of tumors arising from tissues susceptible to hormonal influences. Recently techniques have been developed to measure estrogen receptors in tumor tissue from the breast. This has made it possible to estimate the probable sensitivity (and thus success of treatment) of that tumor to estrogen deprivation.

  Estrogens are mainly used to treat carcinoma of the breast and prostate; androgens are used to treat carcinoma of the breast; adrenocortical hormones are administered in the care of leukemias, lymphomas, and multiple myeloma.
- *Radioactive isotopes* are used to selectively destroy malignant cells. Radiation therapy is discussed later in this chapter.
- *Miscellaneous drugs* are recently developed drugs that are not readily categorized (e.g., hydroxyurea, mitotane 'O,p-DDD', procarbazine, hexamethylemelamine, imidazole carboxamide dimethyltriazino, cycloleucine).[53] Some of the drugs have very selective effects (For example, O,p-DDD affects the adrenal cortex.)

See Table 23–1 for specific agents used in cancer chemotherapy and information concerning clinical usage.

Uses of Chemotherapy

Unlike surgery and radiotherapy, which affect the tumor only in the site of treatment, chemotherapy is a *systemic* treatment. Neoplastic diseases that respond to chemotherapy are listed in Table 23–2. At present, chemotherapy can be used to cure choriocarcinoma, which is a malignant tumor formed by abnormal proliferation of the placental epithelium. Also, it is now becoming possible to effect cures of Hodgkin's disease and certain forms of leukemia with drugs. Patients who have completed a course of chemotherapy must wait for a period of time to establish that no metastatic cells remain. The length of the waiting time depends upon the reproductive rate of the specific tumor.

In recent years drugs have come into use as *adjuvant therapy*. This means that after attempts at curative surgery or radiotherapy have been made, drugs are used to eliminate any potential metastatic cells. This procedure seems to be increasing the chances of certain patients for cure.

Many advances in the use of chemotherapy have been made possible, in part, by the use of *drugs in combination*. When drugs with different modes of action and side effects are combined, the effect on the tumor can be increased without increasing the severity of side effects. Researchers also utilize knowledge of the cell cycle to determine the most effective schedule for drug administration.

By far, the most important use of chemotherapy is *to control tumor growth after cure is no longer possible*. For many years, patients have been receiving the benefits of extended life and improved quality of life as a result of chemotherapy. In many ways, these patients find that for them cancer is a chronic disease and that they must learn to make necessary adjustments in lifestyle to lead a full, satisfying life.

Contraindications to Chemotherapy

Cancer chemotherapy may be withheld or postponed in a variety of conditions:[31]

- *Infection*. Because chemotherapeutic drugs are immunosuppressive and lower white blood cell counts, they are relatively contraindicated during an infection.
- *Recent surgery*. Chemotherapeutic drugs do not promote wound healing and consequently are withheld until incisions are adequately healed—approximately 5 to 7 days postoperatively.
- *Impaired renal or hepatic function*. Most chemotherapeutic agents are metabolized in the liver and excreted via the kidneys.
- *Recent radiotherapy*. Radiotherapy suppresses cell production in the bone marrow, as does chemo-

Text continued on page 462

TABLE 23–1. ANTINEOPLASTIC DRUGS

Key to Nursing Implications

A Check blood counts routinely.
B Institute bleeding precautions when indicated.
C Maintain infection control.
D Provide adequate rest periods.
E Weigh daily.
F Observe for ankle edema.
G Monitor intake and output.
H Provide low-sodium, high-potassium diet.

Drug	Route of Administration	Major Toxicities and Side Effects	Nursing Implications
		ANTIMETABOLITES	
Methotrexate (MTX, amethopterin)	IV IM po intrathecal	*Immediate* nausea, vomiting and diarrhea	1. Maintain adequate hydration 2. Include number and consistency of stools in output 3. Hydrate with IV fluids as ordered **D**
		Malaise and lethargy Skin reactions: a) rashes b) redness c) local breakdown d) burns	1. Observe for skin breakdown 2. Keep skin clean and dry 3. Instruct patient to minimize exposure to sun; wear protective clothing and sun glasses 4. Apply skin creams as ordered
		Delayed stomatitis, sore throat, GI ulceration	Maintain strict routine of oral care
		Bone marrow depression (can occur within 24 hours after administration)	**A, B, C, D**
		Impaired renal function	1. Maintain IV infusion as ordered 2. Administer $NaHCO_3$ IV or po as ordered 3. Test urine PH 4. Weigh patient daily 5. Encourage oral fluids 6. Monitor intake and output
Cytosine arabinoside (Ara-C, Cytosar)	IV sc intrathecal	Nausea and vomiting (with high doses)	Maintain adequate hydration
		Stomatitis, esophagitis	Maintain strict routine of oral care
		Bone marrow depression (occurs 5–7 days after last dose)	**A, B, C, D**
6-Thioguanine (6-Tg, Thioguanine)	po	Nausea and vomiting	Maintain adequate hydration
		Stomatitis	Maintain strict routine of oral care
		Bone marrow depression (can occur as early as 1 week after or as late as 4 weeks after beginning therapy)	**A, B, C, D**
5-Fluorouracil (5-Fu, Fluorouracil)	IV po topical	Nausea, vomiting and diarrhea	1. Maintain adequate hydration 2. Include number and consistency of stools in output
		Stomatitis	Maintain strict routine of oral care
		Bone marrow depression (occurs 9–14 days after last dose)	**A, B, C, D**
6-Mercaptopurine (6MP, Purinethal)	po	Nausea, vomiting and diarrhea	1. Maintain adequate hydration 2. Include number and consistency of stools in output
		Stomatitis	Maintain strict routine of oral care
		Bone marrow depression (can occur as early as 1 week or as late as 4 weeks after beginning therapy)	**A, B, C, D**
		ALKYLATING AGENTS	
Cyclophosphamide (Cytoxan, CTX, Endoxan)	po IV	Bone marrow depression (occurs 1–2 weeks after last dose)	**A, B, C, D**
		Nausea and vomiting	Maintain adequate hydration
		Alopecia	1. Inform patient of expected hair loss prior to treatment. 2. Explain regrowth after treatment. 3. Encourage patient to obtain a wig or wear hats and scarves.

TABLE 23–1. ANTINEOPLASTIC DRUGS *(Continued)*

Drug	Route of Administration	Major Toxicities and Side Effects	Nursing Implications
		ALKYLATING AGENTS *(Continued)*	
		Hemorrhagic cystitis (with high and low doses)	1. Administer intravenous fluids as ordered prior to and immediately after high dose cytoxan. 2. Instruct patient to void every ½ hour for 5 hours and at bedtime after high dose cytoxan. 3. Check urine for amount, color and presence of blood after each voiding. 4. Instruct patient to drink 2,000–3,000 cc's daily.
Mechlorethamine (HN2, nitrogen mustard, Mustargen)	IV (through a rapidly infusing solution) Intracavitary injection	Bone marrow depression (occurs 1–2 weeks after last dose)	**A, B, C, D**
		Severe and immediate nausea and vomiting	Maintain adequate hydration
		Extravasation (if IV infiltrates)	1. Observe IV site during infusion 2. Apply soaks to area of extravasation
Busulfan (Myleran)	po	Bone marrow depression (occurs 1–2 weeks after last dose)	**A, B, C, D**
Chlorambucil (Leukeran)	po	Bone marrow depression (onset 3rd week of treatment and continues for up to 10 days after the last dose)	**A, B, C, D**
		Nausea and vomiting (with high doses)	Maintain adequate hydration
Melphalan (Alkeran)	po	Bone marrow depression (occurs 5–30 days after last dose)	**A, B, C, D**
Triethylene thiophosphoramide (thiotepa)	IV Intracavitary Injection	Bone marrow depression (occurs 5–30 days after last dose)	**A, B, C, D**
Cis platinum diammine dichloride (CPDD)	IV	Bone marrow depression (may be long lasting)	**A, B, C, D**
		Severe and immediate nausea, vomiting and diarrhea	Maintain adequate hydration *Also* 1. Administer the antiemetic prior to treatment. 2. Hydrate with IV fluids as ordered. 3. Include number and consistency of stools in output.
		Mucositis	
		Renal toxicity	1. Assess condition of oral cavity every shift. 2. Begin routine of oral hygiene prior to therapy. 3. Encourage frequent oral hygiene especially after meals. 4. Provide nonirritating, nutritional diet.
		Ototoxicity	1. Maintain intravenous and mannitol infusions as ordered. 2. Instruct patient to void every hour and measure output (if necessary insert foley) for 24 hours. Observe for signs of hearing difficulty.
		PLANT ALKALOIDS	
Vinblastine (Velban)	IV	Bone marrow depression	**A, B, C, D**
		Extravasation (if IV infiltrates)	Insure administration through a full flowing line
Vincristine (Oncovin)	IV	Neurotoxicity (dose related)	
		a. Acute jaw pain	Report this symptom immediately
		b. Paralytic ileus	1. Prevent constipation by: a) checking for bowel movement daily b) encouraging high fluid intake, especially fruit juices c) offering laxative and stool softeners as ordered d) encouraging ambulation 2. Observe for abdominal pain and distention 3. Palpate and ausculate abdomen daily 4. Record quality of bowel sounds daily

Table continues on following page.

TABLE 23–1. ANTINEOPLASTIC DRUGS *(Continued)*

Drug	Route of Administration	Major Toxicities and Side Effects	Nursing Implications
		PLANT ALKALOIDS *(Continued)*	
		c. Peripheral neuropathy	Evaluate patient for: 1. numbness and tingling in extremities 2. loss of deep tendon reflexes in lower extremities
		Extravasation (if IV infiltrates)	Insure administration through a free flowing line
		ANTITUMOR ANTIBIOTICS	
Doxorubicin (Adriamycin)	IV	Bone marrow depression (occurs 10–15 days after administration)	**A, B, C, D**
		Stomatitis	Maintain strict routine of oral care
		Nausea and vomiting	Maintain adequate hydration
		Alopecia	Warn patient beforehand
		Extravasation (if IV infiltrates)	Insure administration through a free flowing line
		Red Urine (occurs 1–2 days after administration)	Inform patient this side effect is *not* hematuria
		Cardiac toxicities (dose related)	Evaluate for signs and symptoms of congestive heart failure
Actinomycin-D (Dactinomycin-D)	IV	Nausea and vomiting	Maintain adequate hydration
		Skin breakdown (if patient had received radiation therapy)	If patient had received prior radiation therapy: 1. assess this site daily 2. keep site clean and dry
		Bone marrow depression (occurs 1–7 days after completion of therapy)	**A, B, C, D**
		Stomatitis	Maintain strict routine of oral care
Bleomycin (Blenoxane)	IV sc IM	Chemically induced fever	1. Monitor temperature every 4 hours during administration 2. Encourage fluid intake
		Skin changes	1. Observe (especially hands and feet) for changes such as: hyperpigmentation, hyperkeratosis, pruritus, ulcerations, vesiculations 2. Treat as ordered
		Nausea, vomiting and diarrhea	1. Maintain adequate hydration 2. Include number and consistency of stools in output
		Pulmonary fibrosis (dose related)	1. Asculate the lungs daily 2. Evaluate patient for any dyspnea 3. Encourage patient to cough, turn and perform diaphragmatic breathing every 2 hours
		Alopecia	Warn patient beforehand
Mithramycin (Mithracin)	IV	Nausea and vomiting	Maintain adequate hydration
		Hypocalcemia	Observe and report signs and symptoms such as: (a) muscle cramps, (b) tingling sensation of fingertips, (c) abdominal cramps, (d) carpopedal spasms, and (e) convulsions
		Stomatitis	Maintain strict routine of oral care
		Bone marrow depression	**A, B, C, D**
Daunorubicin (Daunomycin)	IV	Nausea and vomiting	Maintain adequate hydration
		Bone marrow depression	***A, B, C, D**
		Cardiac toxicities (dose related)	Evaluate for signs and symptoms of congestive heart failure
		STEROID HORMONES	
Androgens		Nausea and vomiting	Maintain adequate hydration
Testosterone	IM	Fluid retention	**E, F, G, H**
Fluoxymesterone (Halotestin)	po	Virilization (in females)	1. Warn patient beforehand 2. Explain usually temporary
Estrogens		Nausea and vomiting	Maintain adequate hydration
Diethylstilbestrol	po	Fluid retention	**E, F, G, H**
Ethinyl estradiol	po	Feminization (in males)	1. Warn patient beforehand 2. Explain usually temporary
		Uterine bleeding	1. Observe for vaginal bleeding 2. Report to physician immediately
Progestins			
Delalutin	IM	*Rare*	
Provera	IM, po		

TABLE 23–1. ANTINEOPLASTIC DRUGS *(Continued)*

Drug	Route of Administration	Major Toxicities and Side Effects	Nursing Implications
		STEROID HORMONES *(Continued)*	
Corticosteroids			
Cortisone Acetate	po	Fluid retention	E, F, G, H
Prednisone (Meticorten)	po	Gastric irritation	1. Administer drug with an antacid, milk, or at mealtime
Dexamethasone (Decadron)	po, IM, IV		2. Test stool and emesis for blood if patient on long-term therapy 3. Check blood counts routinely
Methylprednisolone sodium succinate (Solu-medrol)	IM, IV	Increased susceptibility to infection	1. Maintain infection control 2. Check blood counts routinely
Hydrocortisone sodium succinate (Solu-cortef)	IV		

Modified from Pilapil, F., and K. V. Studva: Cancer chemotherapy. Programmed instruction: Cancer care. *Cancer Nursing,* Vol. 1 (Numbers 3, 4, 5, and 6), June through Dec. 1978.

TABLE 23–2. NEOPLASTIC DISEASES THAT RESPOND TO CHEMOTHERAPY

Type of Cancer	Useful Drugs (Generic Name)	Results Expected
Prolonged survival or cure possible		
Gestational trophoblastic tumors	methotrexate, dactinomycin, vinblastine	70% cured
Burkitt's tumor	cyclophosphamide	50% cured
Testicular tumors (seminoma)	cyclophosphamide with radiotherapy	90-95% respond, 50-60% cured
Wilms' tumor	dactinomycin with surgery and radiotherapy, vincristine	30-40% cured (advanced stage) 80-90% cured (early stage)
Neuroblastoma	cyclophosphamide, doxorubicin procarbazine, vincristine with surgery and/or with radiotherapy	Over 50% response (advanced stage) Up to 80% long term survival depending on stage
Acute lymphoblastic leukemia	daunorubicin†, prednisone†, vincristine†, 6-mercaptopurine†, methotrexate†, carmustine*, L-asparaginase	90% remission; 70% survive beyond 5 years
Hodgkin's disease Stage IIB, IIIB & IV	mechlorethamine†, vincristine†, prednisone†, doxorubicin, dacarbazine, procarbazine†, vinblastine	70% respond, 40% survive beyond 5 years
Palliation and prolongation of life possible		
Prostate carcinoma	estrogens, castration	70% respond with some prolongation of life
Breast carcinoma	androgens, estrogens, alkylating agent†, 5-fluorouracil†, vincristine†, prednisone†, methotrexate†, doxorubicin	60-80% respond with probable prolongation of life
Chronic lymphocytic leukemia and lymphosarcoma	prednisone, alkylating agents	50% respond with probable prolongation of life
Acute myeloblastic leukemia	cytarabine, thioguanine, prednisone, daunorubicin	65% remission with prolongation of life
Soft tissue and osteogenic sarcoma	doxorubicin, methotrexate-CF	20% respond
Palliation possible, but uncertain prolongation of life		
Chronic granulocytic leukemia	alkylating agents, 6-mercaptopurine, hydroxyurea*	90% respond with good control during most of course
Multiple myeloma	alkylating agents, prednisone, carmustine, vincristine	60% respond
Ovary	alkylating agents, cis-Platinum	30-40% respond
Endometrium	progestins	25% respond
Palliation possible, but not usual		
Lung	alkylating agents	30-40% respond briefly
Head and neck	alkylating agents, methotrexate, bleomycin cis-Platinum*	20-30% respond briefly
Large bowel	5-fluorouracil, cytarabine, mitomycin C, MeCCNU	30-50% respond
Stomach	5-fluorouracil, cytarabine, mitomycin C	30% respond
Pancreas and liver	5-fluorouracil	Less than 10% respond
Cervix	alkylating agents, bleomycin	20% respond
Melanoma	alkylating agents, vinblastine, dacarbazine	20% respond

†May be used in combination
*Not available in Canada
From Burns, N.: Cancer chemotherapy: a systemic approach. *Nursing 78*, Feb. 1978, p. 56–63. Adapted from the American Cancer Society.

therapy. To avoid an additive effect, chemotherapeutic drugs are usually withheld for 3 to 4 weeks following radiotherapy to marrow-producing areas.

- *Pregnancy*. Most antineoplastic drugs produce physical defects in the offspring of laboratory animals. The risk is especially high during the first 3 months of pregnancy and must be considered before starting or continuing these drugs.
- *Bone marrow depression*. As chemotherapeutic drugs are myelosuppressive, the dosages must be reduced or therapy delayed until a normal white blood count is obtained.

Drug Administration

When neoplastic disease is widely disseminated, antineoplastic agents are administered via the systemic route (oral, IM, IV). When malignant tumors are still localized, drugs can be administered via localized or regional methods. Neoplasms treated regionally may include tumors of the head and neck, advanced pelvic tumors, metastatic tumors of the liver, and various types of tumors of the extremities.

There are two *regional* methods of drug administration: intra-arterial infusion, and intra-arterial perfusion. Both these methods enable the physician to administer large doses of potent antineoplastic drugs directly into the blood vessels supplying the tumor without introducing a toxic drug into the general circulation.

In *intra-arterial infusion* an antimetabolite is injected into an artery supplying the tumor, usually the brachial, axillary, carotid, or femoral artery. At the same time a metabolite, a substance that counteracts the effects of the antimetabolite, is injected intramuscularly in order to protect the remainder of the body from cell injury. The citrovorum factor, a bacterial derivative, is used with methotrexate for this purpose. Figure 23–1 shows the procedure. The artery is cannulated and a high dose of antimetabolite is continuously pumped at a slow rate to the tumor site by a hydraulic pump.

In *regional intra-arterial perfusion* the region of the body to be perfused is isolated from the general circulation and connected to a source of extracorporeal circulation. Large doses of the antineoplastic agent can then be directed to the tumor without entering the general circulation and damaging major organ systems. Figure 23–2 shows the circuit employed in the treatment of a melanoma of the knee area. The isolated circuit is maintained for a half hour to an hour, after which a fluid not containing the drug is run directly into the extracorporeal circuit to dilute the drug and remove it from the tumor site. Because this procedure is difficult and dangerous, it is performed only in centers where skilled personnel and appropriate equipment are available.

Both regional techniques may produce the toxic effects of the drugs used, in spite of precautions.

Toxic Effects of Antineoplastic Drugs

> *All antineoplastic drugs are potentially dangerous agents. Patients receiving antineoplastic drugs must be vigilantly observed for signs of toxicity.*

Even following discontinuation of a drug, patients require careful observation, because *maximum toxicity tends to develop 5 to 7 days following cessation of chemotherapy*.

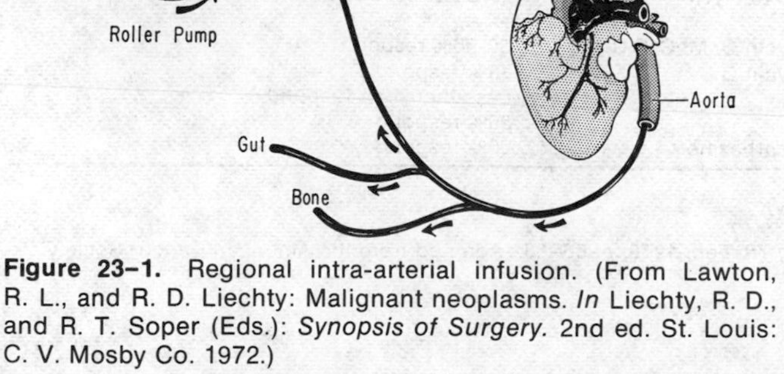

Figure 23–1. Regional intra-arterial infusion. (From Lawton, R. L., and R. D. Liechty: Malignant neoplasms. *In* Liechty, R. D., and R. T. Soper (Eds.): *Synopsis of Surgery.* 2nd ed. St. Louis: C. V. Mosby Co. 1972.)

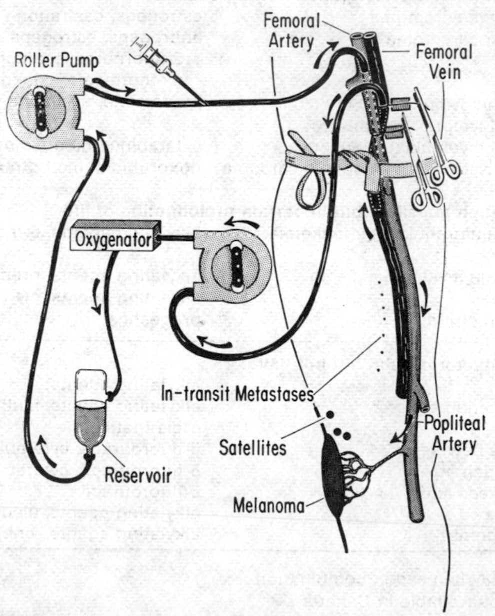

Figure 23–2. Regional intra-arterial perfusion. (From Lawton, R. L., and R. D. Liechty: Malignant neoplasms. *In* Liechty, R. L., and R. T. Soper, (Eds.): *Synopsis of Surgery.* 2nd ed. St. Louis: C. V. Mosby Co., 1972.)

Why are these therapeutic agents so toxic? Antineoplastic drugs are dangerous because they are capable of damaging and destroying not only malignant cells but also certain normal cells. *Normal* cells that are vulnerable to the antineoplastic drugs are those that are characterized (as are cancer cells) by rapid cell division and proliferation. Such cells are principally located in the blood-forming organs (e.g., the bone marrow), the lining of the gastrointestinal tract, and the hair follicles. Thus, the three major forms of drug toxicity are bone marrow depression, alopecia, and gastrointestinal tract disorders.

Bone Marrow Depression. Specific nursing care for patients who suffer these toxic affects is discussed later in this chapter. This is the most severe and dangerous complication of cancer chemotherapy; it can be caused by most of the antineoplastic drugs. When the bone marrow becomes depressed, it is unable to produce thrombocytes (platelets), leukocytes (white blood cells), and erythrocytes (red blood cells); thrombocytopenia, leukopenia, and anemia result. Symptoms accompanying each of these blood dyscrasias are:

- *Thrombocytopenia:* petechiae, ecchymosis, epistaxis
- *Leukopenia:* easy susceptibility to infection
- *Anemia:* weakness, easy fatigability, pallor

To continuously evaluate the effect of antineoplastic drugs upon the bone marrow, the physician generally orders frequent complete blood counts and platelet examinations. If the white blood count falls below 1.000 per cu. mm., the doctor may order reverse isolation to protect the patient from infection.

Alopecia. Because the hair follicles are rapidly dividing cells, they are especially susceptible to systemic chemotherapy, and temporary hair loss is common.

Gastrointestinal Tract Disorders. The four gastrointestinal tract disorders that can result from cancer chemotherapy are:

1. *Sloughing of the Colonic Mucosa.* This is the most severe form of drug toxicity; it is associated with bleeding and infection.
2. *Nausea and Vomiting.* When prolonged, nausea and vomiting result in dehydration. Also, vomiting causes a loss of H^+ and Cl^- which, in turn, leads to hypochloremic alkalosis. For care of the vomiting patient with fluid and electrolyte imbalances, see Chapter 12.
3. *Diarrhea.* Prolonged diarrhea also causes fluid and electrolyte imbalances. When uncontrolled, diarrhea results in dehydration, hypokalemia (loss of K^+), hyponatremia (loss of Na^+), hypochloremia (loss of Cl^-), and acidosis (loss of HCO^{3-}).
4. *Stomatitis.* This condition is characterized by inflammation of the oral mucosa. Early symptoms are dry mouth and burning of the lips; sometimes both painful ulcerations and secondary infections of the oral mucosa develop.

RADIOTHERAPY

Like the use of chemotherapy, the use of radiation for treatment of cancer is a relatively recent development. Since the discovery of the effects of radiation by Roentgen and the Curies near the end of the nineteenth century, much has been learned about the lethal qualities of radiation and about the opportunities to use it for treatment. The ability to produce radioactive elements by artificial methods increased our control over radiation and its potential uses in medicine. When unstable nuclei disintegrate, emitting ionizing radiation, cells are destroyed by disruption of their chemical actions — especially in the nucleus. There may also be effects on enzyme activity or breaks in chromosomes that will limit the cell's ability to divide.

As does chemotherapy, radiation affects the rapidly dividing systems of the body more than other cells. Of great concern during radiotherapy are the bone marrow tissues, the gastrointestinal tract, and the gonads. The possibility of genetic mutations, from even low doses of radiation, cannot be overlooked.

Recall that radiation has several specific medical uses:

- It is used as a *diagnostic tool*, to locate malignant tissue as well as to measure blood volume, blood circulation time, red blood cell turnover, glandular activity, and the rate of red blood cell formation.
- It is used therapeutically to *destroy tumor growths*; it can be prescribed alone or in combination with either surgery or chemotherapy.
- It is used as a *palliative measure*. In patients in whom malignancy is advanced, radiation of the tumor can relieve pain for sustained periods, ranging from months to years. For example, radiation is frequently used to relieve pain in metastatic cancer of the breast to the bone.

Radiation is a vital area in today's medical research. Many experimental radioisotope compounds are being tested currently, with the hope that some of them will lead to cancer cures.

The Role of Radiation in Therapy

Radiation, even in small doses, is somewhat injurious to all cells. However, it exerts its most destructive effects upon cells that are in rapid mitosis. Because cancer cells are characterized by *rapid cellular division*, they are vulnerable to the destructive aspects of radiation; thus, the rationale for radiotherapy in the treatment of cancer. The goal of radiotherapy is to destroy the malignant tumor without unduly harming surrounding tissues. Furthermore, the usefulness of radiation in treating neoplastic disease depends upon the fact that normal cells have a far greater ability to repair damage from radiation than do cancer cells.

Neoplastic tumors differ in their susceptibility to radiotherapy. A tumor that is *radiosensitive* is composed of cells that can be destroyed by radiation, whereas a tumor that is *radioresistant* is composed of cells that resist the destructive effects of radiant energy. Cells that are most radiosensitive are (1) rapidly dividing, (2) poorly differentiated, embryonic, and immature, (3) highly vascular with high oxygen content.

To take advantage of these aspects of radiosensitivity, radiation is often given in many small doses, *fractionation*. A common dosage schedule is 200 rads for 5 days a week for 4 to 6 weeks until the desired dose is reached, or until unacceptable side effects occur. Fractionation makes it more likely that tumor cells will be in mitosis when irradiated. It also allows time for normal cells to repair themselves.

Another way in which normal cells are spared has been to *alternate the sites of entry* (ports) of radiation. If cancer of the cervix is being treated, for example, radiation can be directed at the cervix through the patient's front, back, or sides. The maximum effect of the radiation beam will be on the cervix; the normal tissue would individually receive only a portion of the total dose.

Generally, radiotherapy produces the most favorable results in medulloblastoma (tumors of the cerebellum), lymphomas, metastatic breast cancer, and tumors of the skin, lip, mouth, tongue, uterine cervix, urinary bladder, larynx, tonsils, nasopharynx, and sinuses. Tumors that are located on the skin or mucous membranes are *most* successfully treated by radiotherapy because they can be directly subjected to large doses of radiation without great harm to adjacent structures. Radiation is *less* successful in the treatment of malignant melanoma, metastatic lung cancer, fibrosarcoma, myosarcoma, osteogenic sarcomas, and tumors of the stomach, pancreas, liver, and prostate.

Administering Radiotherapy

Radiotherapy can be administered in a variety of ways. It is useful to divide the sources into those that are outside the body (external radiotherapy) and those that emit their radiation inside the body (internal radiotherapy).

EXTERNAL RADIOTHERAPY

External radiotherapy is administered either by *x-ray machines* or by *radioisotopic sources*.

X-ray Machines. These are further classified by the penetrating power of the radiation produced. Common *x-ray tubes*, such as those used in most radiology departments, produce 200 to 250 kilovolts. Most of this radiation is absorbed at the skin level. This is a serious drawback and makes the use of this machine very uncommon today. *Supervoltage* (measured in million electron volts) is produced by *machines* (such as the betatron or linear accelerator—see Fig. 23–3) or by *radioisotopic sources* (such as cobalt-60 or cesium-137). The advantage of these sources is that the maximum absorption of radiation occurs below the level of the skin. Often the maximum effect can be made to occur in the deep seated tumor itself. The supervoltage sources are used to irradiate deep internal cancers, such as those of the brain, head, neck, esophagus, lung, and bladder.

The machinery capable of supervoltage is expensive. It has been a recent goal to make such equipment available to all citizens who need it.

Radioisotopes. Radioisotopes can also be incorporated into *external molds* and applied topically to the skin and the eye. For example, cobalt-60 can be encased within a protective mold or container and then applied to carcinomas of the ears, lips, scalp, mouth, larynx, and penis. Radioactive tantalum (^{182}Ta) can be enclosed in a flexible wire that is then bent to fit to various anatomic structures. For example, in cases of retinoblastoma (a malignancy of the retina), a wire containing ^{182}Ta can be molded into a circle and then placed directly over the tumor.

INTERNAL RADIOTHERAPY

Internal radiotherapy involves placement of specially prepared radioisotopes directly into the tumor itself or into the systemic circulation. The three major types of internal radiotherapy are:

Interstitial Therapy. In this method, the radioisotope of choice (e.g., cobalt-60, iodine-125, tantalum-182, cesium-137, iridium-192, gold-198, radon-222, or yttrium-90) is packed into needles, beads, seeds, ribbons, or catheters and then implanted directly into the malignant tumor. For example, implantations of cobalt-60, encased in gold or silver needles, are used to treat cancer of the cervix or other sites. In some cases the needles are bent so that they correspond to the shape of the tumor. In other cases the needles are spaced along a plastic ribbon that can easily be molded to the structure of the organ being irradiated. Also, implantations of ceramic beads containing yttrium-90 are sometimes used to destroy the pituitary gland, thereby slowing down tumor growth in other parts of the body.

Because accurate placement of the radioactive needles or beads is absolutely necessary, radioisotopes are implanted surgically. Implants may be left in the tumor either temporarily or permanently depending on the half-life of the source being used.

Intracavitary Isotope Therapy. The two types of malignant disease that are most amenable to intracavitary therapy are cancer of the uterus and cancer of the bladder. The radioisotopes used in intracavitary therapy can be encapsulated into needles that are inserted into the uterine tumor; placed in plastic tubes that are sutured into the cancerous tissues; or poured, in liquid form, into balloons that are positioned inside the bladder. Implants may be removable or permanent. Radium, cobalt-60, iridium-192, and tantalum-182 are used for removable implants, whereas radon-222, gold-198, and iridium-192 are used for permanent implants.

Systemic Therapy. Radioisotopes are sometimes administered intravenously. For example, sodium phosphate (^{32}P) is used in the treatment of polycythemia vera and myelogenous leukemia.

Toxic Effects of Radiation Therapy

Although radiation is beneficial because it destroys malignant cells, it also is dangerous because it damages and destroys *normal* cells at the same time. The extent to which cells and tissues can be damaged by radiation depends on the following four factors:

- *Intensity of prescribed dose*. The patient who receives one large dose of radiation is more likely to develop tissue damage than the patient who receives multiple small doses over several treatment sessions.
- *Degree of exposure*. Irradiation of a large portion of the body produces more tissue damage than irradiation of a small area.
- *Radiosensitivity of the cells*. Cells that are dividing rapidly and that are poorly differentiated are more vulnerable to radiation than are highly differentiated cells that are not dividing.
- *Individual differences*. Apparently some persons are inherently more susceptible to irradiation than are other individuals.

Important toxic effects resulting from radiotherapy include radiation sickness, skin reactions, bone marrow depression, increased chance on cancer in the irradiated area, and birth defects.

Radiation Sickness. This systemic effect of radiation is not commonly seen today. It is related to the dose of radiation received and to the amount of the body being affected by the treatments. In its early stages, this systemic reaction is characterized by nausea, vomiting, and malaise; later the patient may develop purpura, petechiae, diarrhea, and inflammation of the mouth or throat. In its most severe form, this condition can be fatal.

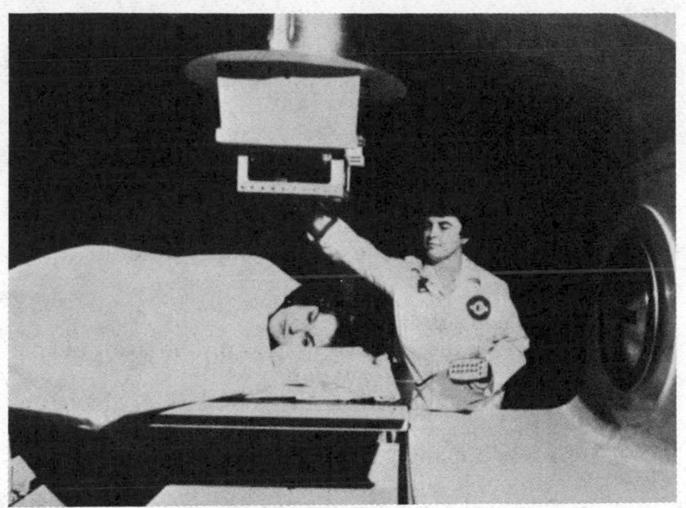

Figure 23–3. Nurse therapist operating controls of linear accelerator. (From Burgess, M. L., and H. Mangan: *The Challenge of Cancer Nursing.* USDHEW Publication No. 76-760, p. 7.)

Treatment of the patient includes: (1) bed rest, (2) small frequent feedings of a high caloric, high protein diet, (3) adequate fluid intake, and (4) the administration of vitamin B_{12}, sedatives, antihistamines, and antiemetics. It is important to maintain accurate records of the patient's intake and output. A patient who continues to vomit will require intravenous feedings.

Skin Reaction. When any part of the body is irradiated, the skin, because it is the body's outer protective covering, is also irradiated; consequently, the skin is always affected to some extent by radiation. The amount of damage depends on the dose and type of radiation. Once damage occurs, the skin tends to heal slowly and scar easily. Healing is retarded because radiation primarily damages those rapidly proliferating cells that are needed for tissue repair. Erythema (most common), desquamation, and abnormal pigmentation of the skin may develop during or soon after radiation therapy. Rarely, more serious problems such as atrophy or shrinking of the epidermal layer, telangiectasis (dilatation of capillaries due to vessel damage), depigmentation of the skin, and subcutaneous fibrosis occur months or years following discontinuation of radiotherapy. The most severe late manifestations of skin damage are skin cancer and necrotic and ulcerative lesions of the skin.

When you are caring for patients receiving radiotherapy, examine the skin frequently for redness, desquamation, and telangiectasis. If signs of a skin reaction appear, immediately notify the radiotherapist.

At the beginning of radiotherapy, the patient should be given the following instructions in order to keep the skin healthy and to avoid problems in the future.

1. Keep the area dry.
2. Wash the area with water only, no soap, and pat the skin gently. Do not rub.
3. Do not apply ointments, powders, or lotions unless prescribed by the radiotherapist.
4. Do not apply heat to the area, either during the treatment or afterwards.
5. Avoid direct sunshine or cold (wind, etc.) on the part.
6. Do not wash off the marks placed on the skin by the radiotherapist.
7. Shaving is to be done with an electric razor only. The area should not be shaved if the skin is reddened and painful.
8. Avoid clothes that rub or chafe the skin.

Skin reactions are reversible and will heal slowly, but the skin will remain somewhat vulnerable. Mucous membranes included in the radiation site are also affected.

Bone Marrow Depression. Bone marrow and lymphoid tissue are highly radiosensitive. Red blood cells are somewhat protected by their longer life span. White blood cells and platelets are affected markedly when the part of the body under treatment is large and includes the major bone marrow areas — especially the pelvis.

When the white cell and platelet counts fall, treatment may be interrupted or discontinued.

Thus white cell count must be ascertained regularly. Instruct patients with low blood counts to avoid exposure to infection and trauma. Also inform the patient about the various degrees of hemorrhage, e.g., purpura to petechiae to widespread ecchymosis. The patient should continue vigilance after radiation is finished until counts return to normal.

Increased Susceptibility to Cancer in Irradiated Areas. Cancer sometimes develops at the site of irradiation 20 or more years following the administration of radiotherapy; sites that are particularly vulnerable to this long-term effect of radiotherapy are the skin, lungs, and bones.

Birth Defects Due to Irradiation. If a pregnant woman's reproductive organs are exposed to radiation during the second to sixth weeks of gestation, the offspring may be born with congenital defects.

Alopecia. Radiation affects the epithelial cells that surround the follicles from which hair grows. Hair follicles in different parts of the body vary in their sensitivity to radiation. Sensitivity to radiation is greater where hair grows rapidly. Thus, the scalp is most sensitive to radiation — and to alopecia — followed by the male beard, the eyebrows, the axillae, the pubis, and body hair. Hair usually regrows following cessation of radiation treatments, but it grows more slowly and is thinner.

Other Toxic Effects. Leukemia, radiation cataracts due to excessive irradiation of the eye, and lung fibrosis due to excessive irradiation of the thorax may also develop.

Protecting Oneself From Radiation

Protecting yourself and others from exposure to excessive radiation depends upon three basic factors: distance, time, and *shielding.*

Distance. The greater distance you maintain from a source of x-rays or gamma rays, the less you will be exposed to radiation. To compute the amount of radiation that a person receives at varying distances from a radiating source, employ the *inverse square law*. According to this law, by simply doubling your distance from a source of x-ray or gamma radiation, you can reduce your exposure by one fourth. For example, if you stand four feet away from a source of radiation, you will be exposed to approximately one fourth the intensity of radiation received at two feet; two feet from the source, the intensity of radiation will be one fourth of that received at a distance of one foot, and so forth.

In sum, to protect yourself from x-rays or gamma rays, do not work any closer to the source of radiation than is absolutely necessary.

Time. The *less time* you spend close to a radiating source, the less you will be exposed to radiation. For example, if you remain near a source of radiation for 5 minutes instead of 10 minutes, you will reduce your exposure by one half.

Shielding. The best protection for a doctor, nurse, or technician who must work close to a source of radiation over a period of time is *shielding*, or the use of appropriate materials to halt and absorb rays from radiant energy. The type of shielding used depends upon the type of rays emitted by the source of radiation. Lead shields are needed to halt x-rays and gamma rays; consequently, persons working in the radiotherapy department wear leaded gloves and aprons. If the source is a gamma ram emitter, such as radium, a lead shield would need to be 30 cm. (about 1 foot) thick in order to absorb the rays.[74] Under these circumstances, the nurse must depend on distance and time, rather than shielding. Also, radioisotopes emitting gamma rays must be kept in leaded containers. Glass, lucite, and aluminum shields are used to screen beta rays. No shield is needed for alpha particles, because these are incapable of penetrating even a piece of paper.

Nurse's Role in Radiotherapy

The nurse plays a key role in radiotherapy, performing the following three functions: (1) preparing the patient for therapy, (2) promoting radiation safety by observing radiation precautions, and (3) psychologically supporting the patient before and throughout the administration of radiotherapy. These three aspects of the nurse's role differ, depending upon whether the patient is receiving external or internal radiotherapy. Let us briefly examine the preparatory measures, precautionary measures, and psychologic considerations involved in caring for patients undergoing each form of radiotherapy.

NURSE'S ROLE IN EXTERNAL RADIOTHERAPY

Preparing the patient for external radiation typically involves the following steps:

1. Familiarize yourself with the patient's chart. Learn (a) the type of external radiotherapy prescribed, (b) the site of the tumor undergoing radiation, (c) the purpose of the therapy (palliation or cure), (d) the number of treatments finished and planned.
2. Ascertain what the patient understands about the therapy.
3. Be sure the patient understands not to remove or wash away any skin markings that the radiotherapist makes. These marks, made with ink before the first treatment, delineate the exact area of the patient's body that is to be irradiated. The technician will reinforce the marks when needed during the weeks of treatment. The marks can be removed when the course of radiotherapy is completed.
4. If the patient is having nausea as a result of therapy, be sure antinausea medication is given before the treatment. The radiotherapist can usually arrange to give treatments when the patient is least susceptible to nausea, e.g., before lunch rather than right after breakfast or lunch.
5. Because the patient will be asked to lie still for several minutes, it is important that pain medication be given beforehand, if needed. Since radiotherapy departments are usually cool (to protect the machinery), be sure the patient has warm clothing and blankets.

The most important part of preparing a patient for radiotherapy is answering questions. Questions that patients often ask about external radiotherapy and some appropriate answers are listed here.

Q. Is radiotherapy painful?
A. Radiotherapy is absolutely painless; you will not experience any sensation during treatment.

Q. What will I be asked to do during my treatment?
A. You will simply be asked to lie very still on a special table while the treatment is being given. If you find it difficult to remain in one position for long, we will support you with pillows or sandbags.

Q. Will I be left alone during treatment?
A. Yes, as a safety precaution, you will remain alone in the treatment room while the x-ray or teletherapy units are in operation. Although the radiation coming from the treatment apparatus is benefiting you, scattered radiation within the room can harm personnel who are exposed to it.

Q. What if I should become sick during my treatment and need a nurse? What should I do?
A. Although you will be alone in the room, you will be able to talk at any time to the technician via an intercom system. Also, the technician will be right outside your room and will be observing you constantly through a window or by television. Should you need help, the therapy can be discontinued and the technician or nurse will enter the room to assist you.

Q. Will I be radioactive after my treatment? Will I have to be isolated in a room away from everyone?
A. Safety precautions are necessary only during that time you are actually undergoing radiotherapy. Once your treatment is completed, you will be transported from the radiotherapy department to your own room, and special safety precautions and isolation policies will be unnecessary.

Personnel in the radiotherapy department are protected from radiation by environmental design and rules of activity and location which assure shielding and distance from the radiation source. This department is usually found in the basement of the building, allowing radiation to be beamed into the ground. The walls of the therapy rooms are thick concrete, sometimes shielded with lead. Often the doors are lead.

The amount of radiation received by personnel is constantly monitored by film badges or other devices. Visitors to the department are instructed in safe actions while there.

NURSE'S ROLE IN INTERNAL RADIOTHERAPY

Preparation of the patient for internal radiotherapy differs, depending upon whether the radioisotope is to be implanted or administered systemically. If the radioisotope (sealed in needles, beads, or wires) is to be implanted into either a tissue or organ cavity, the patient is prepared for surgery. No special preparation is required when the radioisotope is unsealed and is to be administered either systemically (orally or intravenously) or injected directly into a body cavity.

Following administration or implantation of a radioisotope, the patient requires special care. Once the radioisotope is within the patient's body, the patient must be isolated. Isolation is necessary because *the patient is a source of radioactivity* as long as the implanted or injected radioisotope remains within the body and continues to emanate rays of radiant energy.

Key points that will help you to care for the patient receiving internal radiotherapy with either sealed or unsealed radioisotopes are as follows:

1. Familiarize yourself with the patient's chart, learn: (a) what radioisotope is being used; (b) the type of source (i.e., is the radioisotope sealed in an applicator, seeds, beads, needles, or in unsealed form); (c) the mode of administration (interstitial implantation, intracavitary insertion or implantation, or systemic administration); (d) the date when treatment started; (e) the site of implantation (if a sealed source); and (f) the number of days during which the patient must be isolated.

2. Familiarize yourself with the *radioisotope* being used; learn (a) its half-life, (b) the type of radiation emitted (gamma rays or beta particles), and (c) if an unsealed source, the manner in which it is metabolized and excreted.

3. Familiarize yourself with the *hospital's policy* concerning radiation safety. Study the radiation instruction sheet that should be in the patient's chart. Learn where you can contact the radiation officer should radioactive contamination occur.*

4. *Isolate* the patient receiving internal radiotherapy. The patient should be assigned a private room that has a phone, an intercom system linked to the nurse's desk, and an observation window through which the patient can be observed by the staff. Instruct visitors not to enter the room but to stand outside the observation window or at the door. Wear a gown and gloves when caring for the patient, and discard these items into special hampers and containers before leaving the room.

5. *Identify* the patient receiving internal radiotherapy. Note the necessity for radiation precautions on the patient's chart and Kardex; place a sign that displays the radioactive symbol on the patient's door (Fig. 23–4).

6. Maintain *distance* from the patient; stand within 3 feet of the patient only long enough to give basic care.

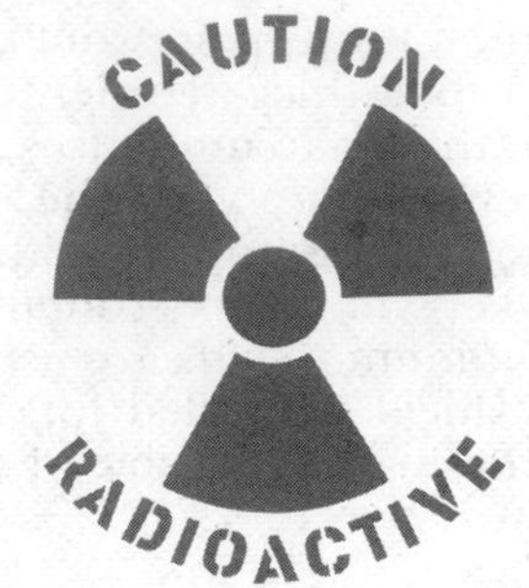

Figure 23–4. Radiation symbol.

7. Recognize the *time* factor: give necessary care as rapidly as possible. Time limits may be stated by the radiation officer.

8. *Protect yourself.* Wear an exposure meter (film badge) on your pocket if you are working daily near radioactive sources. If the badge indicates that you are receiving more than the maximum permissible dose (MPD) advocated by the National Committee for Radiation Safety (NCRS), make certain that you are temporarily relieved from the care of patients undergoing radiotherapy.

9. Give *psychologic support* to the patient and significant others during this trying period of physical and social isolation. Explain the rationale for radiation precautions. Emphasize that isolation is a temporary measure and that it will be discontinued as soon as the radioisotope is either excreted (if an unsealed source) or removed (if a sealed source). The patient's sense of loneliness can be somewhat abated by listening to the radio, watching television, and talking with family and friends on the telephone.

10. Immediately notify the *radiation officer* should a radioactive source be spilled, dropped on the floor, lost, or accidentally discarded; if there is any question of radioactive contamination, the room will need to be monitored with special apparatus designed to detect the presence of radioactivity.

ADDITIONAL PRECAUTIONS

The general points of care and the precautions listed above apply to *all* forms of internal radiotherapy as well as to both sealed and unsealed sources of radioactivity. However, because sealed and unsealed sources differ from each other in certain respects, each type requires the employment of *additional* precautionary measures for safe use.

Sealed Sources. Sealed sources of internal radiation differ from unsealed sources in that the radioisotope is completely enclosed by a nonradioactive material. Thus, the radioisotope cannot circulate through the patient's body nor can it contaminate the patient's urine, sweat, blood, or vomitus. Consequently, you can dispose of the patient's body discharges and excretions without exposing yourself to radiation.

Contamination from sealed sources can result from the following *external* forms of exposure: (1) direct (external) contact with the sealed ra-

*Radiation officers are persons who have been specially trained and licensed by the U.S. Atomic Energy Commission to work with radioactive sources.

dioisotope, i.e., touching a sealed source with bare hands and (2) lengthy exposure to the gamma rays that emanate from the tumor site where the radioisotope is implanted.

To prevent external hazards arising from contact with sealed sources of radioactivity, remember the following rules:

> 1. *Limit your* time *with the patient in order to decrease exposure to gamma rays.*
> 2. *Maintain* distance *from the source; e.g., if the sealed source is implanted in the pituitary gland, as often as possible stand at the foot of the bed rather than at the head of the bed.*
> 3. *Use* shielding. *If a sealed source is dislodged and falls into the bed or onto the floor, pick it up with long-handled forceps and place it into a leaded container.* Never touch a radioactive source with your bare hands!
> 4. *Before discarding used dressings, always check the dressing thoroughly for sealed sources that may have become dislodged. Transfer a dislodged source with forceps from the dressing to a leaded container. Report the incident to the radiotherapist and radiation officer.*

Unsealed Sources. Unsealed sources used for internal radiotherapy are given by intravenous injection, by mouth, or by instillation directly into a body cavity. Unlike sealed sources, unsealed radioisotopes are not encased in nonradioactive protective containers. Consequently, unsealed sources can result in two types of contamination hazards: (1) an *external* hazard due to the emission of gamma rays or beta rays from the patient's body and (2) an *internal* hazard due to radioactive contamination of one or all of the patient's body fluids and products, e.g., feces, urine, sweat, vomitus, cavity drainage. Thus, when you care for patients receiving unsealed internal radiation, remember these rules:

> 1. *Maintain* distance *and observe the* time *factor in order to avoid (external) exposure to the rays of radiant energy emanating from the patient.*
> 2. *Avoid contact with and properly dispose of all contaminated body discharges.*

The three principal radioisotopes used for unsealed internal radiotherapy are iodine-131, phosphorus-32 and gold-198. No special precautions are required when the patient receives tiny tracer doses of these substances; however, strict precautionary measures are needed when the patient is receiving therapeutic dosages. Below are summarized the precautions that you should observe when caring for patients receiving unsealed radiotherapy with ^{131}I, ^{32}P, or ^{198}Au.

Iodine-131 (^{131}I). Half-life of this radioisotope is 8 days. The patient's body will emit gamma rays. The medication is administered orally and the major source of radioactive contamination will be the urine, with lesser hazard from sputum, vomitus, sweat, feces, and blood.

> *Precautionary Measures*
>
> 1. *Observe principles of distance, time, and shielding.*
> 2. *Mark bedpans for patient's use only.*
> 3. *Pour urine into leaded container and transfer to radiotherapy department for safe disposal.*
> 4. *Wear gloves when touching bedpans, bedclothes, or patient's linens.*
> 5. *Wash patient's dishes within the room and then monitor them for radioactivity, or use paper plates.*
> 6. *Following removal of isolation precautions, thoroughly scrub and air the room until monitoring equipment indicates that the environment is safe.*

Phosphorus-32 (^{32}P). ^{32}P may be administered orally, intravenously, and by intracavitary insertion. Its half-life is 14 days, and the patient's body is not a hazard, as the beta rays emitted are not considered dangerous. Vomitus, wound seepage, and feces should be handled with special care.

> *Precautionary Measures*
>
> 1. *Remove dressings with long-handled forceps.*
> 2. *Place used dressing in leaded container; carry to radiotherapy department for disposal.*
> 3. *Wash hands carefully with soap and water following patient care.*

Gold-198 (^{198}Au). Gamma rays may be emitted by the body of the patient who has had ^{198}Au inserted into a body cavity. Half-life of the isotope is 2.7 days. Wound seepage and cavity drainage will require special care.

> *Precautionary Measures*
>
> 1. *Observe principles of distance, time, and shielding.*
> 2. *Remove dressings with long-handled forceps, place in leaded containers, and transport to proper area for disposal.*

IMMUNOTHERAPY[27, 29, 37, 54, 88]

Immunotherapy is a new method for treating cancer that is still under investigation. Immunotherapy rests upon the theory that cancer seems to develop with greater frequency in the person whose immunologic system is depressed or malfunctioning. Thus the major goal of immunotherapy is to *strengthen the immunole response* of the patient to tumor cells. This, in turn, leads to destruction of the cancer. An ultimate future goal of immunotherapy is to *prevent cancer* by immunizing individuals against tumor cells.

Several immunotherapeutic modalities are currently under investigation. These include (1) active immunotherapy, which may be either specific or nonspecific, (2) passive immunotherapy, (3) adoptive immunotherapy, and (4) augmentative measures.

Active Immunotherapy

In active immunotherapy, the patient is injected with an antigen that stimulates the subsequent development of antibody by the patient. Thus the individual's own immune response against tumor cells is enhanced and immune system is stimulated into action. This type of cancer therapy is similar to giving people vaccine to protect them from measles or mumps.

Active immunotherapy may be either specific or nonspecific in nature. Active specific immunotherapy involves vaccinating the patient with a *tumor-associated antigen* in order to stimulate an immune response. Active nonspecific immunotherapy involves injecting the patient with materials that have *no relationship to the tumor* but that can increase the general immune capacity of the individual.

Active Specific Immunotherapy. This form of immunotherapy includes injecting the patient with one of the following:

1. An *autologous* vaccine, which is prepared from the patient's own tumor.
2. An *allogeneic* vaccine, which is prepared from the tumor cells of a donor and which acts to introduce new antigens into the patient's body, which will, it is hoped, stimulate the patient's immune system.
3. A vaccine composed of *living tumor cells* that have been modified and attenuated by irradiation and exposure to certain chemicals. These modified cells will stimulate an immune response without the danger of their multiplying within the patient.

Tumor cell vaccines are administered in small dosages intradermally. The site of injection may become inflamed and irritated and in some cases ulcerated. Also, the patient may suffer a systemic reaction to the injection, with fever, chills, and malaise. Instruct patients to wash injection sites twice daily. Aspirin or acetaminophen (Tylenol) (2 tablets q 4–6 hours) usually controls the systemic reaction.

Active Nonspecific Immunotherapy. The most publicized and widely used nonspecific agent is BCG (bacillus Calmette-Guerin) vaccine. A live, attenuated organism derived from the bovine tubercle bacillus, BCG is capable of stimulating the reticulendothelial system to activate macrophages and attract lymphocytes to tumors. BCG injections enhance both humoral and cell-mediated immunity. While BCG therapy is not a cure for cancer, it does destroy tumor cells. Although experimental, BCG therapy shows promise in the treatment of some types of cancer, notably malignant melanoma. How BCG stimulates a nonspecific cell-mediated immune response that kills tumor cells is delineated in Figure 23–5.

BCG therapy is most successful under these conditions: (a) the patient has been skin tested and is immunocompetent; (b) the tumor is clearly capable of inducing the formation of antibodies (antigenic); (c) the tumor volume has been reduced to a minimum by conventional therapies; and (d) the BCG vaccine is injected as close to the tumor as possible.

There are many ways to administer BCG. Among the methods are: (a) scarification (producing many superficial scratches on the skin into which the vaccine is introduced); (b) multiple puncture tine technique, (c) by interdermal injection, (d) by mouth, (e) into the thoracic or abdominal cavities via thoracentesis or paracentesis, and (f) into the lungs by aerosol. When BCG is given by injection, the patient typically develops an inflammatory reaction at the injection site.

The most common major side effects of BCG therapy include immediate or delayed *allergic reactions,* which vary from mild to life threatening. Symptoms include swelling of lymph nodes, local abscesses, fever, and malaise. Furthermore, *liver dysfunction,* primarily hepatomegaly (enlarged liver) may develop. Finally the most potentially frightening complication of BCG therapy is the possibility that BCG may *enhance* rather than retard tumor growth. For this reason, patients on BCG therapy should be skin tested frequently; BCG therapy must be discontinued if skin tests demonstrate suppression of the patient's immune system.

Passive Immunotherapy

Passive immunotherapy involves the direct transfer of antitumor antibodies, immunologically competent lymphocytes, or immune lymphoid cells from the donor (usually a person cured of cancer or in remission) to the patient with an active neoplasm. Unlike active immunotherapy, passive immunotherapy confers immunity upon the patient for a *short* period of time — only weeks to months. Compatible donors of lymphocytes are identified by means of human leukocyte antigen typing (HLA) typ-

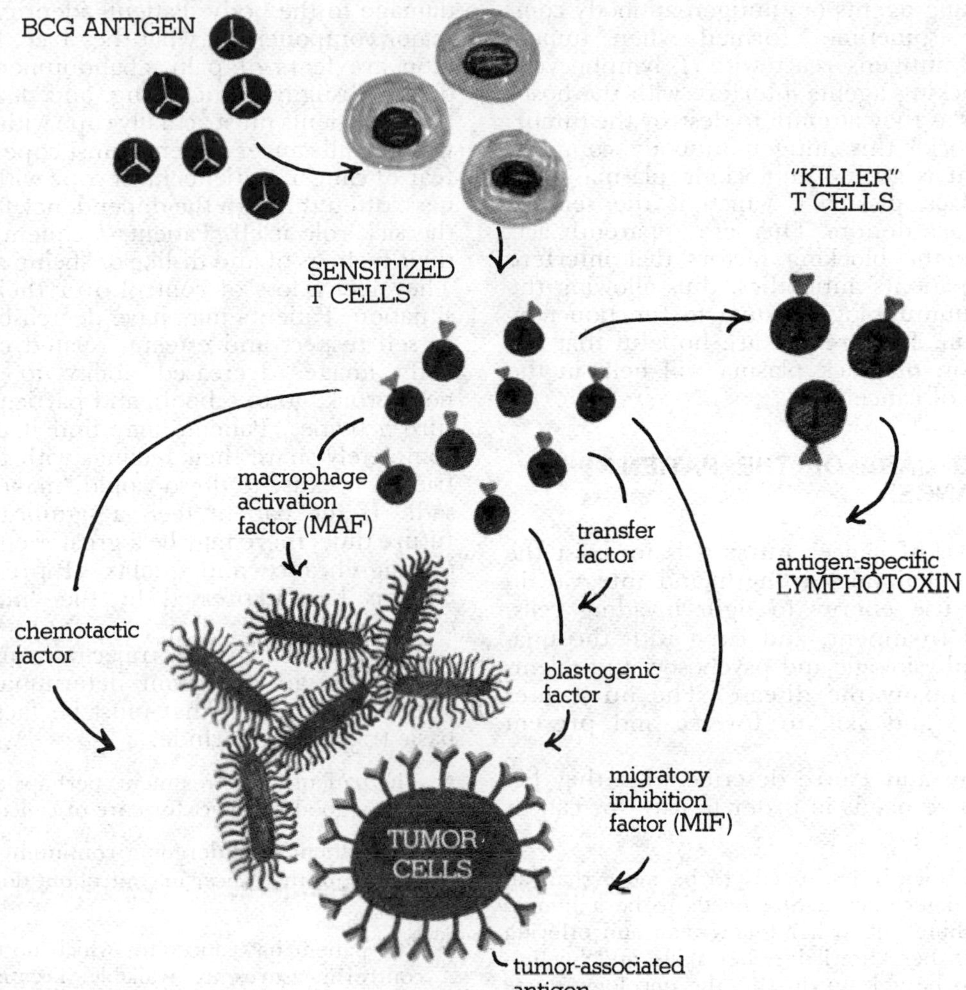

Figure 23–5. Role of BCG and transfer factor as used in immunotherapy. (From Dodd, M. J.: Theoretical bases of immunotherapy. *American Journal of Nursing*, 79:310, Feb. 1979.)

ing). Also, researchers are attempting to isolate *tumor-associated* antibodies in the sera of donors from other nontumor associated antibodies. Administering only tumor-associated antibodies to the patient reduces the risk of the donor's non-tumor-associated antibodies attacking the patient's normal tissues.

Adoptive Immunotherapy

Adoptive immunotherapy involves the *transfer of passive immunity* to the patient, with the *later development and maintenance of active immunity* by the patient. The major advantage of adoptive immunotherapy is that the patient adopts the immunity that has been passively received and incorporates it into his or her own immune system.

One form of adoptive immunotherapy involves *stimulating the patient's own lymphocytes* by incubating them with tumor cells in the laboratory and then reinfusing them into the patient. Another method used is the transference of immunity at the *informational level.* The patient is given extracts of human white cells called *transfer factor* or animal lymphoid extracts called *immune RNA*. These substances carry an immune message to the recipient's immune system (see Figure 23–5). Also, these extracts have the advantage that they are not rejected by the patient's immunologic system as would be the lymphocytes of another person. Thus the problem of donor-recipient incompatibility is eliminated.

Augmentative Therapies

The goal of augmentative therapies is to help the patient's existing immunologic system function at its highest capacity and thus destroy cancer cells. One major method is to *reduce the patient's tumor load* by such means as chemotherapy, radiation, and surgery. The smaller the patient's tumor, the fewer lymphocytes will be required to destroy the tumor.

A second method is to "*unblock*" the patient's immunologic system. Recall from Chapter 21 that blocking agents (an antigen-antibody complex) are sometimes formed when tumor-associated antigens react with T lymphocytes. These blocking agents interfere with the host's antibodies as they attempt to destroy the tumor. To "unblock" this antigen-antibody complex, the patient is given "unblocking plasma" (also called "black plasma"), which is the sera of healthy black donors. This sera apparently acts to reverse the blocking factors that interfere with the patients antibodies, thus allowing the patient's immunologic system to function normally again. Researchers are hopeful that administration of black plasma will help in the treatment of cancer.[27, 29]

NURSING CARE OF THE PATIENT WITH CANCER

The goal of cancer nursing is to assist the patient to maintain strength and integrity in order to use energy to fight invading cells, withstand treatment, and cope with the unavoidable physiologic and psychosocial problems that accompany the disease. The nurse uses knowledge and skill to foresee and prevent problems.

Donovan and Pierce describe what they believe a nurse needs in order to care for cancer patients:

> The oncologic nurse needs to be more than an experienced technician. She needs to be a human being reaching out to her fellow man and offering herself with her knowledge, her skills, and her humanity. To be able to do this the oncologic nurse needs four things: (1) knowledge, (2) a philosophy of life compatible with cancer nursing, (3) satisfaction (positive reinforcement), and (4) supportive guidance (peer support). The philosophy of life compatible with cancer nursing includes valuing life and confronting the inevitability of death. Most important is the belief that, "I, all that I am, all that I know, and all that I can do, can be of help to this other person."[30]

In this section we discuss the special problems that the cancer patient faces. As for other patients, thorough data collection and assessment is the basis of care for the cancer patient. Age, cultural background, support system, and past experiences affect a person's ability to cope with cancer. Also, the patient experiences different problems depending upon the stage of the disease and the type of treatment prescribed. How patients cope with cancer and how *we* can help them cope more successfully are considered here.

Coping with Cancer

What must cancer patients cope with in addition to the physical manifestations of the disease? It is true that fighting cancer is as much an emotional battle as a physical one. The effects of the disease extend much beyond the physical damage to the body. Patients identify fear as a major component of what they face. Most common are fears of pain, abandonment, dependency, disfigurement, dying, and death. While not all patients must actually cope with the dying process, all cancer patients must cope with their fear of cancer. Patients must cope with helplessness, often through the dependency fostered by the sick role itself. Patients frequently express their feelings of and dislike of "being a burden." They feel a loss of control over their life and situation. Patients may have decreased feelings of self-respect and esteem, related changes in body image, decreased ability to work (do housework, go to school), and participate in leisure activities. Patients may find it difficult to completely share their feelings with family and friends because to do so would "make them too sad." If the patient feels a significant loss of future time, there may be a greater emphasis on the significance and quality of present time. This is best expressed by the "make today count" approach.

The patient's disease trajectory, or probable outlook, is an important determinant of the stresses and reality that must be faced. Three basic trajectories include:

- The patient faces treatment, perhaps disfiguring, with a good prospect for cure of cancer.
- The patient is undergoing continuing treatment that keeps the cancer in control but does not cure it.
- The patient has cancer for which no curative or control measures are available. Treatment incorporates comfort measures for the relatively short period of time remaining.

Strategies for coping with problems are as varied as all of human kind. In assessing an individual patient's coping, the nurse must remember that each patient's needs and abilities to cope are different. Most coping strategies are two-edged swords, i.e., they help us cope with a problem, but they may also prevent use from finding better ways to cope. An individual's repertoire of strategies has been learned as problems have been met throughout life. Some common coping strategies used by cancer patients are considered here.

Denial. Denial is the patient's refusal (not conscious) to believe the truth about the situation. Denying would not be needed unless the patient knows at some level that there is something to deny. Denial allows the patient time to take the reality of the situation into conscious awareness, and to make necessary adjustments in thinking and in dealing with life. If denial is the only coping strategy in a person's repertoire, it will be held tenaciously. Unfortunately, denial can interfere with acceptance of and cooperation in treatment. While denial is common in cancer patients, extreme denial (like any extreme) is uncommon.

Occasionally denial seems to offer the cancer patient a vacation from the reality of the disease. This is sometimes seen in patients who have been coping with the disease for a length of time. This retreat from the situation is usually short-lived. It seems to help the patient conserve energy.

Depression, Grief, and Withdrawal. These strategies are often difficult to identify separately. It is well to save the term "depression" for a diagnostic category of specific, well-documented symptoms. Grief is a normal feeling related to the many losses cancer patients face. Withdrawal sometimes can assist the patient to conserve energy. Understanding the positive as well as negative aspects of these strategies will guide appropriate care.

Anger. The cancer patient has much to be angry about — and nothing at all to be angry about. The patient must face significant losses, including health, income, self-esteem, freedom of movement, privacy, and perhaps life. But no one thing can be blamed. In most cases, no one person or cause can be identified that is responsible for the anger. For instance, we do not know why one smoker gets lung cancer and another does not. We do not know why some early radiologists developed leukemia and others did not. The unknowns make anger difficult to focus. Consequently, it is important for the patient, significant others, and nurse to remember not to take anger too personally when the patient lashes out at a safe person or object, or grumps at the world in general. These outbursts relieve tension. On the other hand, awareness that an angry patient may have a bona fide reason for the anger must be maintained.

Hope. There is much myth and not much knowledge surrounding the function of hope. Some believe that if hope is lost the patient will die. Others realize that hope is very changeable, that hoping for a visit home for the weekend can be as salient as hoping for a cure. Hoping becomes detrimental when it leads the patient to expensive, unproven forms of medicine. When the doctors must say truthfully. "We cannot cure you," some patients turn to the "quacks" who will promise anything the patient wants to hear. This is particularly unfortunate when it costs the patient months or years of comfortable life.

Controlling Maneuvers and Manipulation. The effort to retain control of one's own life and body is a major coping strategy. The strength and self-esteem that comes from feeling "in control" may help the patient to continue with an unpleasant therapeutic program. However, the need of some patients to be "in control" can be dangerous to their well-being, e.g., the patient who refuses medications or treatments or alienates family and other supportive persons.

Giving Away Responsibility. Responsibility for decisions and, thus, outcomes may be given over to the doctor, nurse, spouse, God, or any other entity that the patient thinks will take on the burden. Adult patients who are frightened and bewildered by the diagnosis of cancer may need to regress to a childlike role — at least for a time and until they have adjusted to their situation.

Information Seeking. Understanding their situation as fully as possible helps patients make necessary life adjustments and helps them actively continue treatments. Lack of understanding can lead to anxiety, fear, and irrational actions. For example, it helps patients to know about the expected side effects of treatment and to know that measures are available for comfort and relief. On the other hand, it is important for a patient not to over-intellectualize the diagnosis of cancer. By over-intellectualizing, the patient is attempting to submerge real feelings and fears about cancer and the adverse changes that it may bring. The energy that is used to submerge emotional tensions and conflicts could be put to better use by the patient, e.g., in adjusting to a therapy program or coming to terms with reality.

Helping Patients Cope with Cancer

What can we, as nurses, do to help a patient cope with cancer? First, it is important to *listen* to the patient. Too often we assume that patients are coping with the problems *we* think they should have, in the ways *we* would cope if *we* had cancer. The best antidote is to listen carefully to what pateints say about themselves. Most cancer patients view our interest and concern as helpful. They want and need to talk. The following questions help us to learn about the patient's coping: (1) What does having cancer mean to the patient and to significant others? (2) What lifestyle changes must the patient make because of the disease? (3) What resources does the patient feel are available and for what purposes? (4) What does the patient feel the future holds? (5) What do the patient and significant others say about the way they are coping at present?

Second, it is essential *to teach* the patient and close associates about the condition. No matter what combination of coping strategies the patient is using, information about the disease, treatments, hospital, nursing care, and community resources can enhance the range of choices available.

Finally, help the patient and significant others to *understand the coping strategies* that are in use, and to remember and utilize coping methods that have worked in the past. Assist the patient to use the social network and community resources available. In sum, help the patient focus on what is possible rather than on what is lost.

Helping Patients Cope with Specific Problems

Change in Body Image. Change in body image is a common problem that challenges the cancer patient's coping skills. Mutilating surgery, radiation therapy, chemotherapy, alopecia, cachexia, loss of sexual functioning, and presence of odors all affect patients' sense of "feeling good" about their bodies. Nurses are often the first sounding board as patients try to integrate, accept, and learn to live with changes in their bodies. Nurses' reactions to the changes, information given to the patients about the changes, and instruction in new self-care procedures give patients their first reflection of a new image. Patients will integrate changes in body image as they experience the honest reactions of family and friends and as they provide their own self-care. This process takes time and may require use of community resources. Maintenance of normal hygiene routines, attractive clothing, and satisfactory functioning in the environment all assist the patient to retain a positive body image.

Nutrition, Hydration, and Elimination. Maintenance of nutrition and hydration becomes a problem for most cancer patients at some time during the course of their disease. Nurses have the opportunity to assess the patient's nutritional status regularly. When interference with the intake or absorption of nutrients occurs, the body draws from its own reserves, resulting in weight loss. All cancer patients should become aware of their own weight gain or loss patterns. The hospitalized patient in active treatment should be weighed daily. A record of intake and calorie count may be indicated for some patients. *A weight loss may signal a need for nutritional intervention.*

Concern about and attention to food intake can serve to demonstrate the nurse's "caring" to the patient in a nonhurtful, "normal" way, while assuring adequate nutritional intake. It remains true, even in these days of weight-consciousness, that food symbolizes love to many people.

The role of nutrition in the treatment of cancer is receiving increasing attention. Both host and tumor are dependent on intake of nutrients for cell growth and division. Restriction of vitamins and minerals is being studied in the hope that tumor growth can be affected. In general, however, the goal is to maintain the best possible nutritional therapy. *Parenteral hyperalimentation* may be utilized when the gastrointestinal tract is severely affected by tumor or treatment (see Unit XVII).

Various nutrition-related problems occur for the cancer patient. It is thought that tumor growth itself can affect the patient's appetite, causing anorexia. Obstruction can become a problem with gastrointestinal and some genitourinary tumors. Observation for symptoms of obstruction should be included in nursing care. Extreme malnutrition, weight loss, and cachexia occur as a result of inadequate intake, increased energy use by the tumor, and the body's attempts to repair normal cells after treatment. Other problems that nursing care is directed toward include nausea and vomiting, stomatitis, diarrhea, and constipation.

Nausea and Vomiting. Nursing care of the patient with nausea and vomiting includes appropriate use of antiemetics before the patient is to receive chemotherapy or radiotherapy. The patient should continue the use of antiemetics, particularly before meals. Use of prolonged action (timed-release) medications may be helpful. The patient may be able to avoid nausea if administration of chemotherapy is arranged so that peak side effects occur during the hours of sleep.

With the help of the dietician, the nurse and patient can plan small, frequent meals to keep the stomach full during times of freedom from nausea. The diet should be high in protein and calories. (The active treatment period is not an appropriate time for an obese patient to attempt a weight-reduction regimen.) Cold foods may be better tolerated if odors are triggering nausea. As nausea ends, it is important to discuss with the patient what foods are liked. The patient may choose tea and toast, ginger ale, or other family favorites.

Appropriate care for the weakened patient who is vomiting includes easy access to a basin, cool water or mouth wash for rinsing, frequent emptying of the basin, and use of suggestion to limit or prevent actual vomiting, (for example, a firm swallow or concentration on even, deep breathing may help the sensation of nausea to pass.) A calm environment is helpful, but also gentle distraction may limit the unpleasant sensation of nausea.

Stomatitis. There are almost as many treatments for stomatitis as for decubitus ulcers. The first indication of stomatitis may be a burning sensation near the lips when the patient drinks orange juice in the morning. Erythema, small vesicles, or shallow ulcers may be observed on the cheeks, lips, and tongue as the stomatitis develops. Teach the patient to avoid trauma to the mouth and to use *soft* toothbrush or sponge to maintain oral hygiene. Frequent rinsing with saline and hydrogen peroxide can maintain hygiene when symptoms are severe. Hard foods, hot, spicy foods, alcoholic beverages, and cigarette smoking should be avoided. Adequate humidification of the environment is essential. Pain may be relieved by rinses with lidocaine or other medication before meals. Unit XVII contains a more complete discussion of stomatitis.

Diarrhea. Serious diarrhea can be life-threatening. Observations that help determine the seriousness of the episode include: (a) noting the day of onset in relation to the administration of chemotherapy or radiotherapy, (b) the amount, frequency, and consistency of the stool, and (c) the presence of blood in the stools. It is important to ascertain this information as specifically as possible. Antidiarrhea medications are useful. Observation should continue as long as the irritation to the gastrointestinal tract continues. Gentle wiping protects the perineum from trauma. Sitz baths may be comforting. Low roughage together with constipating foods may be added to the diet. If diarrhea is severe, observe the patient for dehydration and electrolyte imbalance. Replacement therapy may be needed.

Constipation. While most anticancer drugs cause diarrhea, the plant alkaloids can cause constipation, as can most pain medications. With a decrease in mobility caused by weakness, constipation becomes a problem for most patients with advanced cancer. Assessment of activity, fluid intake, drug use, roughage intake, and privacy for evacuation assist the nurse to identify appropriate actions to maintain normal function. Prevention is the single best approach to this problem. Use of laxatives may be ineffective and painful unless fluid intake, roughage, privacy and other factors are considered. Patients must understand the seriousness of constipation so that they will cooperate in prevention. The possibility that obstruction is causing the constipation should be kept in the mind with certain types of tumors.

Activity, Mobility, and Rest. Being able to freely move around in the environment underlies much of our emotional health and coping success. The cancer patient faces several potential impediments to mobility. The most serious of these is *pathological fractures,* which can affect patients with breast cancer and those with other tumors that affect the bones. Nurses should be aware of the patient's discomforts so that bony metastasis can be identified before fracture occurs. In many cases, fractures can be prevented by radiation therapy.

Generalized weakness that accompanies inadequate nutrition and anemia caused by treatment is also a limiting factor. *Neurotoxicities* caused by the plant alkaloids also interfere with the patient's mobility. As mobility decreases, *sensory deprivation* can occur. They may both cause and be a result of depression.

The nurse's goal is to maintain the patient's mobility at the highest level possible. For the patient at home this may mean contact with community groups and services that can assist with appropriate forms of transportation. The patient may need assistance in spacing activities and planning projects that will not overtire, but will allow continued activity. Some patients benefit by learning gentle toning and tension reducing exercises.

Sleep and rest can become difficult when discomfort and unfamiliar surroundings affect sleep time. Before medications become a crutch, encourage the patient to do relaxing exercises, take warm milk, or drink a small amount of wine. Establishing regular rest hours, maintaining a quiet environment, or taking a pain medication at bedtime also may help.

Alopecia. The loss of hair, while not a dangerous side effect of cancer therapy, can markedly affect the patient's body image. It can be an especially traumatic experience for the female patient because of the emphasis upon beautiful hair as a prerequisite for femininity in our society. The woman who is losing her hair may also fear that she is losing her desirability as a woman. The feeling of loss can add to the sense of despair that patients with cancer frequently feel. Use your communication skills to encourage patients to express their feelings about their condition. Emphasize that their baldness is a temporary side effect of the radiotherapy or chemotherapy they are receiving and that their hair will grow out again once the therapy is discontinued. In the meanwhile, the patient's morale can be greatly bolstered by the wearing of an attractive wig or some bright scarves. Male patients, too may feel in better spirits if you encourage them to wear a hair piece or colorful cap. Wearing a scarf or cap to sleep when hair loss is imminent can prevent the discomfort of waking to a pillow full of hair.

Ascites and Pleural Effusions. Cancer cells can cause irritation to membranes lining the peritoneum and pleura. Fluid containing *protein* is produced in response and will continue to be produced as long as the cancer cells are present. Production of fluid is decreased when the pressure gradient around the cells is equalized. If fluid is removed (to increase lung capacity or relieve abdominal discomfort) the pressure gradient falls and thus production of protein-containing fluid increases. The patient's total protein can be markedly reduced in this way. Under these circumstances, the doctor may be reluctant to remove fluid. Careful attention to adequate protein in the diet is essential.

Pain. The lay public and professionals fear cancer. The reason for this fear is the pain and suffering thought to be associated with cancer. A closer look at cancer pain and the myths that surround it will assist the health professional to provide reassurance and comfort for the cancer patient.

Myth 1: Pain invariably accompanies cancer. Twycross found that "as many as 50% of all cancer patients have no pain or negligible discomfort, that 40% experience severe pain, and that the remainder have less intense pain."[6]

Myth 2: Pain gets worse and worse as cancer progresses until it is unbearable. Pain is a relatively *late* symptom in most types of cancer. It is related to: (a) infiltration of nerves, blood vessels, and the lymphatic system by tumor cells, (b) mechanical pressure of the tumor or metastases on blood or lymph vessels, (c) invasion of the periosteum or relatively inelastic connective tissue, or (d) inflammatory and necrotic tissue change in any pain-sensitive area of the body.

The distinguishing feature about most cancer pain (85 per cent) is its *continuous nature.* When tumor cells have infiltrated an area and are causing pain, the pain will disappear only if the tumor size is decreased or eliminated through therapy or spontaneous remission. Unlike postoperative pain or other types of episodic pain, cancer pain tends to be chronic, continuous, and long term. This chronic nature does not mean that the pain must become worse and worse inexorably. Other factors markedly affect the degree to which pain is "bearable" or "unbearable." These include: the meaning of the pain to the patient, cultural and ethnic background, and past experience with pain. High anxiety can make the pain less bearable.

Myth 3: *Cancer pain cannot be controlled even by drugs.* Also *drugs must be used conservatively so that patient will not become addicted or relief will not be possible when really needed near the time of death.* In fact, the key to the control of the cancer patient's pain lies *with the patient,* not with drugs. Melzack states, "We should not aim at abolishing the pain, but, rather reducing it to bearable levels."[57] The patient needs to feel in control of the pain and to understand what it means. Drugs can help the patient gain control, but they are not the sole modality available.

The nurse's role is to give the patient information about pain control techniques and about the actions of drugs. The nurse maintains as nonhurtful an environment for the patient as possible and helps the patient function at the highest level possible in view of the extent of disease.

The primary treatment for cancer pain is to remove, destroy, or diminish the tumor. Even when cure is not possible, life can be improved and lengthened, and pain reduced through palliative use of surgery, radition, and cancer chemotherapy.

The nurse has a much larger responsibility in helping a patient control pain than just medicating. Comforting involves thoughtfulness and consistency of approach. The following are suggestions which can guide your nursing interventions:

1. Decrease the factors in the environment that are stressful to the patient.
2. Prevent the side effects of immobility. Cancer patients suffer all too often from the preventable discomfort of decubiti, urinary tract infections, constipation, and even contractures. Prevention starts early.
3. Prevent the depressing effects of sensory deprivation associated with immobility, protective isolation, or radiation isolation.
4. Assist the patient to maintain personal cleanliness, including control of odor.
5. Use gentle touch and voice with the patient.
6. Always approach the patient courteously.
7. Teach the patient to avoid trauma and infection.

The nurse's attitude about the patient's pain can affect the patient's stress and anxiety level. Nurses need to remain confident that they are helping the patient, that what they do is meaningful to themselves as well as to the patient. Pain becomes unbearable when hope, understanding, and personal interest are withheld.

Neurosurgical intervention, group therapy, hypnosis, distraction, behavior modification, and stimulus control devices all provide pain control for some patients.

Although it is clear that there is much more to pain control than medication, medications do have a role in pain control. Because cancer pain is chronic, medications that have short periods of action are not very useful. Oral medications, particularly those with anti-inflammatory effects, can be useful because they can be taken by the patient on a regular basis. Long-acting oral narcotics, such as methadone, are very useful. When injectable narcotics are used, great care must be exercised to assure that the patient remains in control of the pain, and the medication. Too often the patients feel that the only time they see a nurse is when medication is given. If this occurs, anxiety surely increases.

An oral liquid mixture often called *Brompton Cocktail,* used in Great Britain and Canada, has recently gained acceptance in the United States. The mixture contains morphine, cocaine, alcohol, and flavoring syrup. A phenothiazine, such as Compazine or Thorazine, is felt to potentiate the effects of the narcotics and alcohol. The mixture and a phenothiazine are given around the clock on a regular schedule. The major side effects are respiratory depression, constipation, and drowsiness.

> *It is important to remember that any medication is only part of pain control. Thorough assessment and use of all appropriate approaches can mean that no cancer patient need have unbearable pain.*

Family and Social Integrity

The diagnosis of cancer in a member of a family is an assault on the integrity of the whole family. The stability of a family may be markedly affected as it deals with serious disease in one member, potential loss of income, and costs of illness. The social network and support system that surround a person may be seriously affected by the strains of cancer. Transportation for the patient to and from medical appointments can present difficulties. Child care may be a concern.

The family members and close friends can be a major source of support for the patient, but it is well to recognize the stress of the situation for them. Too often family members and those closest to the patient neglect their own health during the illness. There is stress of an uncertain certainty when the patient has uncured cancer. Anticipatory grieving may occur. In addition to the emotional stress, physical stress comes from providing physical care for the patient, lack of sleep, and perhaps inadequate nutrition and neglect of regular exercise.

More and more it is realized that the cancer patient's significant others deserve care along with the patient. Preventive care during the patient's illness can be a major determinant of the health of the people involved for many years in the future. Careful assessment of the stresses is the basis of appropriate family care. Teaching about nursing care measures and conservation of energy in care may be useful for the patient who cannot provide for self-care. Encourage use of community resources. Transportation and other services may be offered by the American Cancer Society and other cancer organizations. The Visiting Nurse Association can provide assistance and teaching in the home.

In addition to being concerned about loved ones, the cancer patient may be concerned about loss of income and employment. There is interruption of the patient's ability to fulfill developmental tasks. The patient's role in community activities may be limited. As the disease becomes chronic, this creates a loss of self-esteem for the patient.

The Future of Cancer Nursing

Care of cancer patients has become a specialty within nursing in recent years. It has been recognized that acutely ill cancer patients benefit most when the nurses are knowledgeable and experienced in the care of the illness presented. Nurses are playing a larger role in prevention and early detection of cancer. More and more of our attention is being directed to the care of the patient living with controlled cancer. There is a need for nurses who can follow patients through stays in the hospital to their homes. The nurse provides support, information as it is needed, and continuity of care for patient and significant others.

The needs of cancer nurses have led to the formation of the Oncology Nursing Society and local cancer nursing groups for the purpose of sharing information and supporting each other. The journal *Cancer Nursing: An International Journal for Cancer Care* came into publication in 1978. There is more research and development of creative nursing care for the cancer patient being published. Not every patient will be cared for by a cancer nurse. It is important for *all* nurses to keep abreast of new developments in the nursing care of the cancer patient.

BIBLIOGRAPHY (Unit IX)

1. Andrews, H. L.: *Radiation Biophysics.* Englewood Cliffs, N. J.: Prentice-Hall, Inc., 1974.
2. Baserga, R.: *The Cell Cycle and Cancer.* New York: Marcel Dekker, Inc., 1971.
3. BCG in cancer therapy. *American Journal of Nursing,* 79:309, Feb. 1979.
4. Becker, F.: *Cancer: A Comprehensive Treatise.* New York: Plenum Press, 1975.
5. Behnke, H.: *Guidelines for Comprehensive Nursing Care in Cancer.* New York: Springer Publishing Company, Inc., 1973.
6. Benoliel, J. Q., and D. Crowley: The patient in pain: New concepts. *Proceedings of the National Conference on Cancer Nursing.* American Cancer Society, 1974.
7. Benoliel, J. Q., and R. McCorkle: A holistic approach to terminal illness. *Cancer Nursing,* 1:2, Apr. 1978.
8. Benton, B.: Stilbestrol and vaginal cancer. *American Journal of Nursing,* 74:900, May 1974.
9. Bingham, C. A.: The cell cycle and cancer chemotherapy. *American Journal of Nursing,* 78:1201, July 1978.
10. Bourchard, R., and N. Owens: *Nursing care of the cancer patient.* St. Louis: C. V. Mosby Company, 1976.
11. Braun, A. C.: *The Cancer Problem: A Critical Analysis and Modern Synthesis.* New York: Columbia University Press, 1969.
12. Breeding, M. A., and M. Wollin: Working safely around implanted radiation sources. *Nursing 76,* 6:58, May 1976.
13. Bruya, M. A.: Stomatitis after chemotherapy. *American Journal of Nursing,* 75:1349, Aug. 1975.
14. Buehler, J.: What contributes to hope in the cancer patient? *American Journal of Nursing,* 75:1353, Aug. 1975.
15. Bunch, B., and D. Zahra: Dealing with death: The unlearned role. *American Journal of Nursing* 76:1486, Sept. 1976.
16. Burgess, M. L., and H. Mangan: *The Challenge of Cancer Nursing.* USDHEW Publication No. 76–760.
17. Burkhalter, P.: Cancer quackery. *American Journal of Nursing,* 77:451, Mar. 1977.
18. Burkhalter, P., and D. Donley: *Dynamics of Oncology Nursing.* New York: McGraw-Hill Book Company, 1978.
19. Burns, N.: Cancer chemotherapy: A systemic approach. *Nursing 78,* 8:56, Feb. 1978.
20. Busch, H.: *The Molecular Biology of Cancer.* New York: Academic Press, 1974.
21. Butler, J.: A tool for assessing the nutritional status of cancer patients. *Oncology Nursing Forum,* 5:1, Winter-Spring 1978.
22. Cain, M., and C. Henke: Living with cancer: A random sample of 50 patients in a hematology oncology clinic. *Oncology Nursing Forum,* 5:4, July 1978.
23. *Cancer: A Manual for Practitioners,* 5th ed., Boston: American Cancer Society, Massachusetts Division, Inc.
24. *'78 Cancer Facts and Figures.* New York: American Cancer Society, Inc., 1977.
25. Coelho, G., *et al.: Coping and Adaptation.* New York: Basic Books, Inc., 1974.
26. Costello, A.: Supporting the patient with problems related to body image. *Proceedings of the National Conference on Cancer Nursing.* American Cancer Society, 1974.

26a. Crises in cancer. *Emergency Medicine,* 11:75, Apr. 1979.

27. Croft, C. L.: BCG administration and nursing implications. *American Journal of Nursing,* 79:315, Feb. 1979.
28. Davitz, L., Y. Sameshima, and J. Davitz. Suffering as viewed in six different cultures. *American Journal of Nursing,* 76:1296, Aug. 1976.
29. Dodd, M.J.: Theoretical bases of immunotherapy. *American Journal of Nursing,* 79:310, Feb. 1979.
30. Donovan, M. K., and S. G. Pierce: *Cancer Care Nursing.* New York: Appleton-Century-Crofts, 1976.
31. Einhorn, L. H.: Cancer chemotherapy. *American Family Physician,* 15:186, Mar. 1977.
32. Fuller, A.: The DES syndrome and clear cell adenocarcinoma in young women. *Cancer Nursing,* 1:3, 1978.
33. George, F. W. III: Particle therapy for uncontrolled cancer. *Consultant,* 17:158, Aug. 1977.
34. Giacquinta, B.: Helping families face the crisis of cancer. *American Journal of Nursing,* 77:1585, Oct. 1977.
35. Golden, S.: Cancer chemotherapy and management of patient problems. *Nursing Forum,* 14:3, 1975.
36. Halman, M., and J. Suttinger: Family-centered care for cancer patients. *Nursing 78,* Mar. 1978.
37. Helping cancer patients — effectively. *Nursing 77 Books,* Horsham, Pa.: Intermed Communications, 1977.
38. Heusinkveld, E.: Cues to communication with the terminal cancer patient. *Nursing Forum,* 11:1, 1972.

39. Hildebrand, B. F.: Symposium on the nursing management of the cancer patient receiving chemotherapy. *Nursing Clinics of North America,* 13:267, June 1978.
40. Hubbard, S., and V. DeVita: Chemotherapy research nurse. *American Journal of Nursing,* 76:560, Apr. 1976.
41. The immune system. *American Journal of Nursing,* 76:1613, Oct. 1976.
42. Isler, C.: Delivering total care — everywhere. *RN,* 41:59, Apr. 1978.
43. Isler, C.: Approaching the final days. *RN,* 41:63, Apr. 1978.
44. Jackson, B. A.: A tumor classification system. *American Journal of Nursing,* 76:1320, Aug. 1976.
45. Kastenbaum, B., and R. Spector: What should a nurse tell a cancer patient? *American Journal of Nursing,* 78:640, Apr. 1978.
46. Kennedy, P. S., and D. W. Luedke: Adenocarcinoma of unknown origin. *Postgraduate Medicine,* 65: Jan. 1979.
47. Koons, S.: The future of cancer nursing. *RN,* 39:23, Aug. 1976.
48. Krant, M.: Rights of the cancer patient. *Ca – A Cancer Journal for Clinicians,* 25:2, Mar.-Apr. 1975.
49. Lawison, E.: *Conference on Spontaneous Regression of Cancer.* USDHEW Publication No. 76–1038, 1976.
50. Levin, D., et al. Cancer Rates and Risks. USDHEW-NCI Publication No. 75–691, 1975.
51. Madden, B.: Rehabilitation: Principles, Philosophy, practice. *Proceedings of the National Conference on Cancer Nursing.* American Cancer Society, 1974.
52. Maher, R. M.: Cancer pain in relation to nursing care. *Nursing Times,* 71:344, Feb. 1975.
53. Marino, E., and D. LeBlanc: Cancer chemotherapy. *Nursing 75,* 5:22, Nov. 1975.
54. McCalla, J.: Immunotherapy: Concepts and nursing implications. *Nursing Clinics of North America,* 11:59, Mar. 1976.
55. McCorkle, M. R.: Coping with physical symptoms in metastatic breast cancer. *American Journal of Nursing,* 73:1034, June 1973.
56. McCorkle, M. R., and K. Young: Development of a symptom distress scale. *Cancer Nursing,* 1:5, Oct. 1978.
57. Melzack, R.: *The Puzzle of Pain.* New York: Basic Books, Inc. 1973.
58. Miller, M., and C. Nygren: Living with cancer — coping behaviors. *Cancer Nursing,* 1:4, Aug. 1978.
59. Miller, S.: Oncology nurse and chemotherapy. *American Journal of Nursing,* 77:989, June 1977.
60. Mount, B., et al.: Use of the Brompton mixture in treating the chronic pain of malignant disease. *Canadian Medical Association Journal,* 115:122, July 1976.
61. Mundinger, M.: Nursing diagnosis for cancer patients. *Cancer Nursing,* 1:3, June 1978.
62. Murawski, J., D. Perman, and M. Schmitt: Social support in health and illness: The concept and its measurement. *Cancer Nursing,* 1:365, Oct. 1978.
63. Nicolson, G. L.: Cancer metastasis. *Scientific American,* Mar. 1979, p. 66.
64. Nirenberg, A.: High-dose methotrexate for the patient with osteogenic sarcoma. *American Journal of Nursing,* 76:1776, Nov. 1976.
65. Pace, J.: *Pain: A Personal Experience.* Chicago: Nelson-Hall, 1976.
66. Pain and Suffering. *American Journal of Nursing,* 74:489, Mar. 1974.
67. Parsell, S., and E. Tagliareni: Cancer patients help each other. *American Journal of Nursing,* 74:650, Apr. 1974.
68. Paulen, A., and T. Kuenstler: Learning to discuss the unmentionable. *Cancer Nursing,* 1:197, June 1978.
69. Paulen, A., and S. Sylvester: Caring for the patient who's well. *RN,* 41:56, April, 1978.
70. Peterson, B., and C. Kellogg: *Current Practice in Oncologic Nursing.* St. Louis: C. V. Mosby Co., 1976.
71. Plumb, M. M., and J. Holland: Cancer in adolescents: the symptom is the thing. *Nursing Digest,* Summer 1977, p. 56.
72. Pohutsky, L., and K. Pohutsky: Computerized axial tomography of the brain: A new diagnostic tool. *American Journal of Nursing,* 75:1341, Aug. 1975.
73. Price, S. A., and L. M. Wilson: *Pathophysiology: Clinical Concepts of Disease Processes.* New York: McGraw-Hill Book Co., 1978.
74. Rees, D. J.: *Health Physics: Principles of Radiation Protection.* Cambridge, Ma.: The M. I. T. Press, 1967.
75. Robbins, S. L., and M. Angell: *Basic Pathology,* 2nd ed. Philadelphia: W. B. Saunders Co., 1976.
76. Robbins, S., and D. Crawford: Nursing and the pion irradiation project. *American Journal of Nursing,* 76:1445, Sept. 1976.
77. Rose, J.: Nutritional problems in radiotherapy patients. *American Journal of Nursing,* 78:1194, July 1978.,
78. Rose, M. A.: Problems families face in home care. *American Journal of Nursing,* 76:416, Mar. 1976.
79. Rowlingson, J. C.: Management of cancer pain. *Cancer Nursing,* 1:317, Aug. 1978.
80. Rubin, P.: *Clinical Oncology for Medical Students and Physicians.* Rochester, N. Y.: American Cancer Society, 1974.
81. Schwind, J. V.: Cancer: Regressive evolution? *Oncology,* 29:172, 1974.
82. Seybolt, J. F.: Expanding the scope of the pap test. Consultant, 17:85, Nov. 1977.
83. Shubin, S.: Cancer widows: A special challenge. *Nursing 78, 8:56, Apr. 1978.*
84. *Siegele, D.: The gate control theory. American Journal of Nursing,* 74:498, Mar. 1974.
85. Silverberg, D., and I. H. Arthur: The cancer survival race: Dramatic gains charted. *Seattle Post Intelligencer,* Feb. 16, 1975.
86. Silverstein, M., and D. Morton: Cancer immunotherapy. *American Journal of Nursing,* 73:1178, July 1973.
87. Solzhenitsyn, A. I.: *The Cancer Ward.* New York: The Dial Press, Inc., 1968.
88. Sullivan, B. P.: Patient responses to BCG therapy for malignant melanoma. *American Journal of Nursing,* Feb. 1979.
89. Stromberg, M. F., and N. Bourque: A Cancer detection clinic: Patient motivation and satisfaction. *Nurse Practitioner,* 4:10, Jan.-Feb. 1979.
90. Theologides, A.: Why cancer patients have anorexia. *Geriatrics,* 31:69, June 1976.
91. Tiedt, E.: The psychodynamic process of the oncological experience. *Nursing Forum,* 14:264, 1975.
92. Valentine, A., S. Steckel, and M. Weintraub: Pain relief for cancer patients. *American Journal of Nursing,* 78:2054, Dec. 1978.
93. Van Scoy-Mosher, C.: The oncology nurse in independent professional practice. *Cancer Nursing,* 1:21, Feb. 1978.
94. Van Scoy-Mosher, M.: Chemotherapy: A manual for patients and their families. *Cancer Nursing,* 1:234, June 1978.
95. Varricchio, C.: Nursing care during total body irradiation. *American Journal of Nursing,* 77:1314, Aug. 1977.
96. Walter, J.: *Cancer and Radiotherapy.* London: J. and A. Churchill, 1971.
97. Weisenberg, M.: *Pain: Clinical and Experimental Perspectives.* St. Louis: C. V. Mosby Co., 1975.
98. Winters, W.: Viruses and cancer. *American Journal of Nursing,* 78:249, Feb. 1978.
99. White, L., et. al.: Screening of cancer by nurses. *Cancer Nursing,* 1:15, Feb. 1978.
100. Zimmerman, S., et al.: Bone marrow transplantation. *American Journal of Nursing,* 77:1311, Aug. 1977.

UNIT X*

NURSING PEOPLE EXPERIENCING DISTURBANCES OF NEUROLOGIC FUNCTION

INTRODUCTION AND STUDY GUIDE

The nervous system is the body's most highly organized system. The nervous system is highly valued, having both structural (i.e., anatomic) and functional (i.e., physiologic) preference among body systems. This unit discusses why the nervous system is of such vital importance to human life and what the major consequences are from neural† disorders. The onset of neurologic disorders may be sudden, e.g., traumatic severance of the spinal cord or rupture of a cerebral aneurysm, or insidious, e.g., Parkinson's disease or multiple sclerosis. We are able to discuss in detail only the most common neurologic disorders and their clinical management. Some less common disorders are briefly mentioned to give a more complete picture of neurologic problems. Of necessity our discussion of neurosurgical procedures is brief.

Neurologic nursing is an intriguing area of practice that is both highly demanding and highly rewarding for nurses. Understanding of neurologic and neurosurgical problems is based upon a discernment of the interrelated aspects of neurologic functioning. Such an understanding requires a sound basic knowledge of the anatomy and physiology of the nervous system. With such knowledge, you, as a nurse, can *logically* understand how a specific neurologic disorder causes the resulting symptoms that a patient experiences—the symptoms that you will try to alleviate and with which you will help a patient to cope. The nurse's ability to make precise clinical observations of neurologic symptoms (e.g., perform "neuro checks") is also highly important and often ultimately helps to establish an accurate diagnosis that correctly localizes the area of disturbance.

Most important, sound knowledge and understanding of nervous system anatomy and physiology, pathology, symptomatology, diagnostic procedures, and treatment regimens are essential for a skillful nursing approach to patient care. Such information, along with a nurse's sensitive ability to find out the individual experience of each person, forms a baseline for problem solving (nursing process) that helps a patient and significant others adapt to the changes that are occurring in their lives.

Neurologic disorders are often frightening for people to experience. They may interfere with an individual's means of keeping in touch with the

---

*This unit has been critically reviewed and revised by Judith Atwood, R.N., M.N., and Helen K. Schnell Braun, R.N. Allan S. Troupin, M.D., assisted in this process.

†Neural is frequently used as the adjective for nerve or central nervous system (CNS).

environment, e.g., by blinding or numbing him or her, they may rob a person of the vital need to move, e.g., through paralysis; or they may prevent communication, e.g., through loss of the ability to speak or to understand the spoken or written word. Diagnostic tests pertaining to neurologic disorders are also frequently frightening, and disturbances of the brain are viewed by many people as shrouded with mystery. Also, surgery on the brain or spinal cord may be a terrifying experience for the people concerned. Certainly such procedures have hazardous potential postoperative sequelae and require skilled management. The patient with a neurologic problem is often forced to become heavily dependent upon others; indeed, sometimes *totally* dependent—unconscious and relying on a respirator for every breath.

Nursing people experiencing disturbances of neurologic function requires an abundance of patience on the nurse's part. For example, patients' movements are frequently slow and inaccurate. However, remember that the patience required of *you*, the nurse, is nominal when compared with the infinite patience required by the victim of neurologic disease. Patients and their significant others must adjust to the changes imposed by the illness; often a patient has to work to relearn skills that most adults take for granted. For example, patients may be incontinent and have to relearn bowel and bladder control; some may have to relearn how to feed and dress themselves or how to talk, write, and walk. The frustrations are many, and a nurse's encouragement and enthusiasm are needed many times each day.

Along with assisting neurologic patients with tasks they cannot perform for themselves, nurses work to find ways to *rehabilitate* patients so that they may eventually regain functions, if possible, and adapt to the loss of those that cannot be regained. *Rehabilitative care is an integral part of nursing care for people with temporary, progressive, or permanent neurologic disturbances.* Through imaginative and creative care, nurses can inspire patients to become a part of the rehabilitation process. Without the effort and determination of everyone concerned, particularly the patient, rehabilitative procedures are usually doomed to failure.

Preserving and restoring function are everpresent goals for nurse and patient, even though ultimate complete restoration of function may be impossible.

Muscle tone, range of motion, and proper positioning need to be constantly maintained in a paralyzed limb, in hopes that a patient may be able to again use that limb. Nothing is more tragic than for a patient to survive the initial insult of a "stroke" (cerebrovascular accident), for example, only to face living with a withered, contractured arm or leg that is useless because it was not properly cared for during the acute phases of the illness. Possibly such neglect occurred because a health professional falsely believed that any return of function was "hopeless."

Recent advances in the control of neurologic disorders are impressive. New medications, improved surgical techniques, and advances in knowledge of neuroanatomy and neurophysiology are today bringing relief and hope to many people for whom any kind of "normal" life was once thought impossible. For example, the medication L-dopa has provided relief for many persons from the confining rigidity and stiffness associated with Parkinson's disease; improved neurosurgery has provided relief from many excruciating pain syndromes once considered to be "intractable," and recent research indicates that even the problem of neural regeneration in human beings should no longer be viewed as insolvable.

The functional interrelationship between mind and body expresses itself constantly in people experiencing neurologic problems.

Neurologic nursing is truly psychophysiologic nursing, for in the nervous system, perhaps more than any other system of the body, psyche and soma are one. Because mental experience is housed in the brain, it is natural that disorders of the brain often cause disturbed mental experiences. Thus, patients with various neurologic disorders may experience personality or behavioral changes; some patients with neurologic problems may hallucinate or experience illusions as a result of organic brain changes. Excellent nursing care of patients with neurologic conditions therefore requires implementation of a plan of care designed to meet both the physical and mental needs of individual patients.

Neurology and psychiatry are both therapeutic disciplines applying to mental processes in some way. Let us clarify that *neurology* is basically concerned with disorders of the nervous system in which *organic* disorders are apparent, whereas *psychiatry* is fundamentally concerned with *functional* disorders lacking a demonstrable physical basis. Of course such distinctions are not clear-cut in practice, since much is unknown about the physical basis of the psyche and also since it is sometimes impossible to demonstrate physical disorders of the nervous system even though it is known that something is organically wrong.

Objectives

After studying this unit carefully and relating it to your experiences in clinical practice you should be able to:

1. Demonstrate a thorough and accurate understanding of the anatomy and physiology of the nervous system.
2. Understand the basic elements of patient history, physical examination, diagnostic procedures, and nursing assessment of people experiencing neurologic problems.
3. Offer competent and supportive care to patients before, during, and after neurologic assessment and treatment procedures.
4. Understand in detail common clinical problems that can happen to people experiencing neurologic pathology.
5. Skillfully observe patients for signs and symptoms of neurologic complications, and interpret such observations accurately and appropriately.
6. Perform emergency measures safely and responsibly during a neurologic crisis.
7. Appreciate the profound physical, psychologic, social, and sexual adjustments people who experience permanent or progressive neurologic problems must often make.
8. Know the usual clinical care and neurosurgical procedures of pathologic neurologic conditions and be able to understand the principles involved when such care varies from the usual.
9. Communicate relevant and accurate information concerning neurologic anatomy and physiology, pathology, diagnostic procedures, treatment regimens, and rehabilitative processes to patients and their significant others.
10. Competently plan personalized nursing care with people experiencing neurologic problems on a short- and long-term basis.

Study Guide

The following guides may help you as you work to achieve the objectives of this unit.

1. Chapter 24 outlines basic anatomy and physiology of the nervous system. You can understand neurologic disorders only if you understand

how these disorders affect the *normal* structure (anatomy) and function (physiology) of the nervous system. Do not skim over the outline in Chapter 24, but rather read it slowly, pausing to ask yourself if you are really familiar with the points included. Review those you are not familiar with *before* reading subsequent chapters. Do the following as part of your review.

- ▶ Name the general functions of the nervous system and identify and discuss the three divisions of the nervous system.
- ▶ Describe the autonomic nervous system. What are the two main parts of the autonomic nervous system and how do they function?
- ▶ Describe a neuron, how it functions, and its basic parts.
- ▶ Locate and name the brain's main parts and the major functions of each area. State the functions of the cerebrospinal fluid.
- ▶ Locate and describe the spinal cord and its major functions.
- ▶ Review the names and functions of the cranial nerves. Describe a plexus. Locate and name the three major plexuses of the spinal nerves.
- ▶ Name the covering of the brain and spinal cord and its layers. What are the functions of the layers?

2. Chapter 25 discusses how the nervous system is clinically examined and assessed. Some aspects of the neurologic examination are performed by a nurse during "routine" care to selected patients; for example, a nurse often tests certain reflexes and sensations. Study carefully those aspects of the neurologic examination that you will perform (they are identified throughout the Unit). Chapter 25 also discusses diagnostic tests and procedures commonly used in evaluating the status of a patient's nervous system. Nurses prepare patients for these tests (physically and emotionally); assist with the performance of some of these tests, e.g., the lumbar puncture; and give care to the patient following the tests. The care given following some neurologic diagnostic tests, e.g., pneumoencephalogram and myelogram, is extremely important both to decrease a patient's discomfort and to prevent complications. Nurses knowledgeably assess the condition of patients following the various neurologic tests and procedures and alert the physician when symptoms of impending complications appear. Study with special attention the section of Chapter 25 that discusses neurologic diagnostic tests and procedures.

3. Chapter 26 discusses common clinical problems that occur as a result of altered neuroanatomy or neurophysiology. Such clinical problems include: altered states of consciousness, increased intracranial pressure, abnormal body temperature elevations, seizures and convulsions, neurogenic shock, respiratory failure, infection, problems related to spinal disorders, hemiplegia, language disorders, and emotional and behavioral changes. The clinical care discussed in Chapter 26 is of central importance not only in the nursing care of patients with primarily neurologic disorders but also in caring for patients with numerous other primary disorders. For example, patients may be unconscious for various reasons. Because the care discussed in Chapter 26 is of importance in many of your responsibilities as a nurse, you will want to be thoroughly familiar with its content. We have emphasized in Chapter 26 the *reasons why* the various aspects of clinical care are important. Focus on those reasons in your studying so you will know why you perform certain actions and will not simply perform them automatically.

4. Chapter 27 discusses specific neurologic disorders. Limited space requires that we discuss only the more common disorders and makes it necessary for even those discussions to be brief. Of the conditions discussed in Chapter 27, some occur with greater frequency than others and should therefore receive greater consideration in your studies, e.g., meningitis, intracranial tumors, transient cerebral attacks, intracranial aneurysms and primary (spontaneous) subarachnoid hemorrhage, cerebrovascular accidents (CVA's strokes), Parkinson's disease, myasthenia gravis, multiple scle-

rosis, epilepsy, vascular headaches (e.g., migraine), muscle contraction headaches, head injury, spinal injury, sciatic nerve injury, and trigeminal neuralgia. The discussions of clinical care are generally brief in this chapter; only points that specifically and commonly apply to a given condition are discussed, since general clinical problems were discussed in detail in Chapter 26. Refer back to Chapter 26 as necessary.

5. The discussions of head injuries and spinal injuries presented in Chapter 27 form a basis for discussion in Chapter 28 of clinical care of patients undergoing neurosurgery; therefore, you may need to refer back to these discussions as you study Chapter 28. You may also need to refer back to Chapter 26, e.g., for discussions of increased intracranial pressure, paralysis, and so forth.

In conclusion, if you study this unit carefully and in the manner just outlined you will obtain a firm foundation of knowledge upon which to base your nursing actions. The study of neurologic disorders is *complex*, because the nervous system affects all the other systems of the body. However, the study of the nervous system is *difficult* only if it is approached illogically or haphazardly. As you can see, the chapters of this unit logically build upon one another. Appropriate medications are discussed throughout the unit; however, you should consult a textbook of pharmacology for details, particularly of dosages.

Overview of Basic Types of Neurologic Disorders

Neurologic disorders are complex because of the anatomic variability of the nervous system. Moreover, almost all diseases use the nervous system to express themselves. For example, while such symptoms as pain, weakness, sensory loss, disturbed thinking, and impaired mood or alertness may be symptoms of *primary* disease of the nervous system, even more often they are of a *secondary* nature, reflecting disease in some other bodily organ or system. Also, such symptoms are most frequently expressions of faulty

TYPICAL EXAMPLES OF NEUROLOGIC DISORDERS

Causative Factor	Examples of Disorders
Infection	Acute (Sydenham's) chorea; brain abscess; infections of meninges; subdural and epidural infections, e.g., empyema and abscess; virus infections, e.g., acute anterior poliomyelitis and herpes zoster; rickettsial infections, e.g., spotted fever and typhus fever; syphilis; infections from other microorganisms
Tumors	Intracranial tumors, e.g., tumors of meninges, cranial nerves, supportive tissue, ductless glands, congenital tumors, granulomas; spinal tumors; tumors of peripheral nerves
Vascular lesions	Vascular lesions of brain, e.g., cerebral infarction (embolism and thrombus), cerebral hemorrhage, hypertensive encephalopathy, subarachnoid hemorrhage, intracranial aneurysms; vascular lesions of spinal cord
Developmental defects	Developmental defects of brain, e.g., congenital hydrocephalus; developmental defects of spinal cord, e.g., spina bifida
Degenerative diseases	Presenile dementia (Pick's disease, Alzheimer's disease); cerebral palsy; chronic (Huntington's) chorea; Parkinson's syndrome; spasmodic torticollis; amyotrophic lateral sclerosis (ALS); syringomyelia and syringobulbia; progressive muscular dystrophy; myasthenia gravis
Demyelinating disease	Multiple sclerosis
Paroxysmal disorders	Epilepsy (convulsive disorders); syncope (fainting); Meniere's syndrome; migraine, and other forms of headache
Nutritional disorders	Deficiencies of vitamins, trace minerals, and amino acids
Trauma, e.g., puncture, blows, fracture, crush, chemicals, ionizing radiation, electrical injuries, decompression sickness	Injuries to head (craniocerebral trauma); injuries to spinal cord or its roots; injuries to cranial and peripheral nerves

adjustments to the environment. Possible *psychophysiologic* bases for symptoms must be carefully evaluated since the nervous system expresses psychologic and somatic symptoms in response to both real and symbolic threat or injury.

There are many different ways to classify neurologic disorders. We have chosen to follow the classification below, which lists typical examples of neurologic disorders. In Chapter 27 we shall discuss the various disorders listed.

As indicated previously, the nervous system may become involved in a wide variety of diseases that are not neurologic diseases per se, i.e., not primary neurologic diseases. For example, pernicious anemia can cause subacute combined degeneration of the spinal cord (which selectively affects the long tracts of the posterior, lateral, or anterolateral areas of the cord), and diabetes may cause neuritis (involvement of the peripheral nerves) or central nervous system symptoms. Such secondary causes of neurologic disorders are discussed in appropriate sections elsewhere in the text.

CHAPTER 24

BASIC ANATOMY AND PHYSIOLOGY OF THE NERVOUS SYSTEM

Although various aspects of the anatomy and physiology of the nervous system will be referred to in greater detail throughout this unit, the following basic outline is presented to help you orient yourself to the nervous system as a whole. Refer as necessary to a good textbook of anatomy and physiology.

The general functions of the nervous system can be summed up as follows:

- Controls and coordinates all parts of the body (each structure of the body communicates directly with the brain)
- Receives stimuli from the body's interior and from external environments, through the sensory system
- Largely determines the body's responses to these impulse-messages, through the motor system
- Contains the human higher functions, e.g., memory, reasoning

For convenience in discussion, we consider the nervous system as three divisions (Fig. 24–1):

1. The *central nervous system*, made up of the brain and spinal cord.
2. The *peripheral nervous system*, composed of the cranial nerves and spinal nerves.
3. The *autonomic nervous system*, consisting of the sympathetic nervous system and the parasympathetic nervous system.

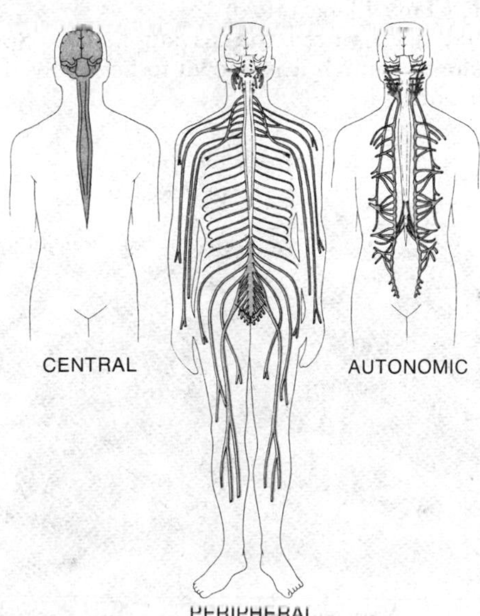

Figure 24–1. Divisions of the nervous system. (From Schifferes, J. J.: *Essentials of Healthier Living,* 4th ed. New York: John Wiley & Sons, Inc., 1972.)

I. Central Nervous System

Brain and spinal cord. Cranial cavity (containing brain) and spinal canal (containing spinal cord) from body's dorsal cavities; these cavities join, forming a continuous space.

A. Brain (Fig. 24–2)

1. Cerebral hemispheres (cerebrum)

Two hemispheres — right and left. Make up 80 per cent of total weight of brain.

Gray matter — cortex, made up of nerve cell bodies.

White matter — made up of processes coming off cell bodies.

Convolutions — called *gyri* (gyrus).

Identations — *fissures* or *sulci* (sulcus).

a. Lobes. Each hemisphere is made up of four lobes.

(1) Frontal lobe (two)

Contains "motor cortex" (in precentral gyrus), which controls motor function.

> *Right side of brain controls left side of body; left side of brain controls right side of body.*

Also contains motor aspects of speech and written speech center, which governs ability to write words. Farther forward are the frontal association areas, where mental activity goes on and where primitive reflexes are inhibited.

(2) Parietal lobe (two)

Contains principal sensory areas for appreciation and discrimination of sensory impulses (e.g., pain, touch, temperature) in right parietal lobe from left side of body, and vice versa. Also contains association sensory areas and the sensory speech center.

(3) Temporal lobe (two)

Contains the auditory center, where sound is interpreted. Also the auditory speech center, which make possible the understanding of spoken words. Equally important are the vital centers that control behavior and emotions.

(4) Occipital lobe (two)

Contains primarily the visual center, where vision is interpreted. Also located here is the visual speech center, which governs ability to understand written words.

Two additional areas are sometimes referred to as lobes:

(5) Insula (central lobes) (two)

Located deep within the sylvian fissure. Specific functions are not known, though it is known to be involved with various visceral functions.

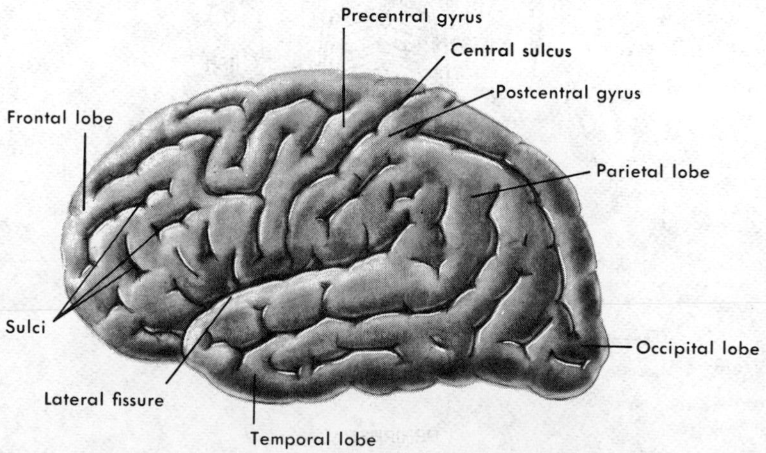

Figure 24–2. The external surface of the brain. (From Dienhart, C. M.: *Basic Human Anatomy and Physiology,* 3rd ed. Philadelphia, W. B. Saunders Co., 1979, p. 104.)

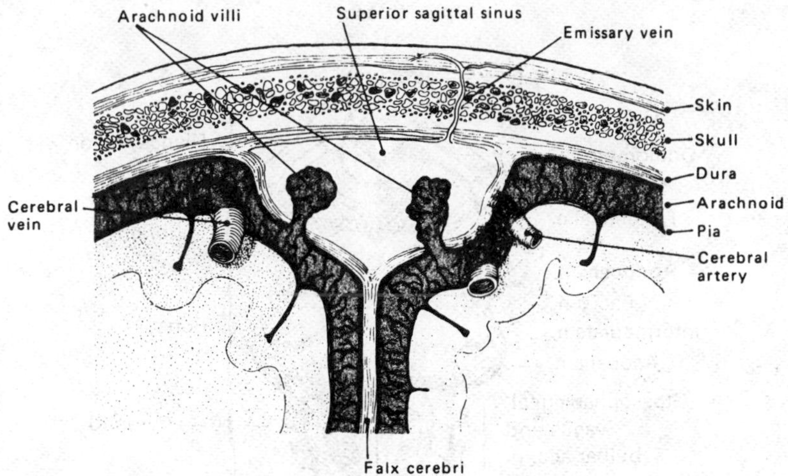

Figure 24–3. Meninges in greater detail. Coronal section through the superior sagittal sinus. Emissary vein shown connecting scalp with superior sagittal sinus. The subarachnoid space is filled with cerebrospinal fluid. It enters the sinus through the arachnoid villi. (From L. L. Langley, I. R. Telford, and J. B. Christensen: *Dynamic Anatomy and Physiology,* 4th ed. McGraw-Hill Book Co., New York, 1974, p. 508.)

(6) Limbic lobe (rhinencephalon)
Has to do with interpretation of smell, emotional responses, and some visceral reflexes.

b. Basal ganglia
These are areas of gray matter, or groups of nerve cell bodies, located at the base of each hemisphere. Three major components are the caudate nucleus, the putamen, and the globus pallidus. Together they regulate and integrate motor activity that originates in the cerebral cortex.

c. Internal capsule
Vital area in the region of the basal ganglia, where nerve fibers from the cerebral cortex (primarily motor fibers) converge as they pass to other parts of the nervous system and to the entire body.

d. Meninges (Fig. 24–3)
A special covering of fibrous connective tissue, over the cerebral hemispheres and continuing on (in essentially the same form) to cover the entire spinal cord. These meninges serve to provide support and protection for the brain, provide nourishment, and in part carry blood supply. There are three separate layers:

(1) Dura mater — "hard mother"
This thick, tough outermost membrane is the main support layer. Its outer layer attaches to the periosteum of the skull. The two layers of the dura separate in places to form large venous channels draining blood from the brain. Its inner layer connects in various areas, forming compartments. One such fold is the *tentorium,* where the dura mater is tautly connected to separate between the occipital lobes of the cerebrum and the cerebellum (part of the brain stem). An opening in the tentorium allows for passage of the brain stem.

(2) Arachnoid — "spider-web-like"
A more delicate layer, separated from the dura mater by a potential space known as the subdural space. It is closely attached to the surface of the hemisphere and helps to cushion and protect the brain. Along the upper surface of the hemispheres, the arachnoid sends tiny fingerlike projections (arachnoid villi) through the inner layer of the dura mater, into the venous sinuses, to aid in reabsorption of cerebrospinal fluid into the blood stream. Immediately below the arachnoid is the subarachnoid space, in which CSF circulates. In several areas, especially at the base of the brain, the arachnoid is farther removed from the surface of the brain, forming cisterns, or collections of CSF. The larger blood vessels of the brain lie in the subarachnoid space, branches of which pass through the pia mater into the brain substance to provide a majority of the brain's blood supply.

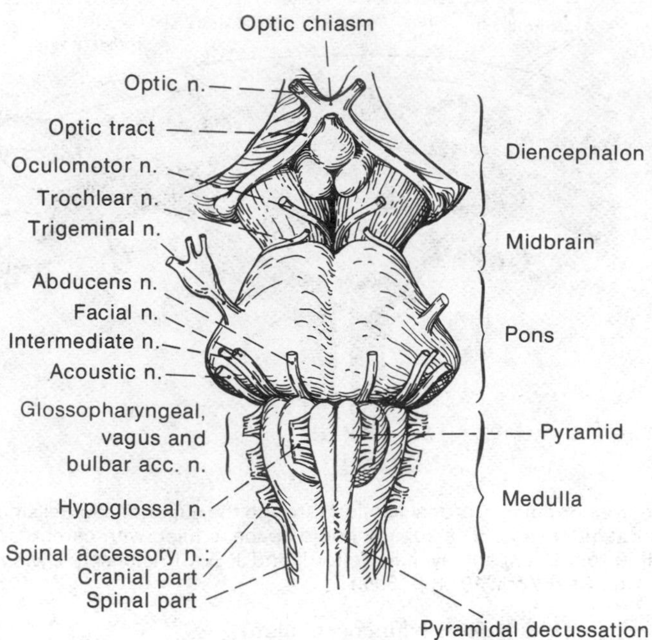

Figure 24–4. Ventral view of the brain stem.

(3) Pia mater — "gentle mother"
The innermost layer of the meninges. Adheres closely to the cortex, following the dips and curves of the brain's surface. It is a delicate, vascular membrane. The pia is also one of the components of the choroid plexus, which manufactures CSF.

2. Diencephalon
The area deep within the brain that comprises several small vital areas, the two most important of which are the thalamus and the hypothalamus.
   a. Thalamus
   Located on either side of the third ventricle. Composed of many separate nuclei. Monitors sensory input and acts as a relay station for sensation.
   b. Hypothalamus
   Small area making up the anterior wall of the third ventricle. Controls such vital functions as water balance, blood pressure, sleep, appetite, and body temperature. Also affects some emotional responses (e.g., pleasure, fear). It is the control center for the pituitary and affects both divisions of the autonomic nervous system.
3. Midbrain (mesencephalon)
A very small area between the diencephalon and the pons, where the third and fourth cranial nerves originate. Sometimes considered the upper part of the brain stem. Composed of the tectum (posteriorly), the tegmentum (centrally), and the cerebral peduncles (anteriorly). Conducts impulses from the lower centers of the brain to the cortex via ascending tracts in the tegmentum. Is also a relay center for sight and hearing. The cerebral peduncles contain the descending motor tracts.
4. Brain stem (Fig. 24–4)
   a. Pons (bridge)
   Located between the midbrain and the medulla oblongata. The nuclei of the 5th, 6th, 7th, and 8th cranial nerves are in the pons.
   It contains many ascending and descending tracts, some having to do especially with eye movement. The reticular formation, which has to do with keeping us awake, is located diffusely deep within the pons and midbrain.
   b. Medulla oblongata
   An area approximately one inch in length; connects the brain with the spinal cord. Cranial nerves IX, X, XI, and XII originate from their nuclei here.

The motor tracts running from the cortex to the spinal cord and the rest of the body cross over at the lower edge of the medulla — explaining the fact that the right side of the brain controls the left side of the body, and vice versa.

The medulla contains several vital centers, such as those for respiration, vomiting, and hiccoughing.

5. Cerebellum — "lesser brain"

Located posterior to the pons and connected to it by the cerebral peduncles.

It is a complex feedback system. Is interconnected with the thalamus and the cerebral cortex to control and coordinate motor movement.

6. Ventricular system (Fig. 24–5)

A system of four irregularly shaped spaces within the brain, all interconnected, for the production and circulation of CSF.

a. Structure

(1) Lateral ventricles (two)

One in each cerebral hemisphere. Extends into each lobe. Contain the major part of the choroid plexus which produces CSF.

(2) Third ventricle

Small space deep within the brain, just posterior to the hypothalamus.

(3) Fourth ventricle

A rhomboid-shaped space located in the brain stem, posterior to the pons and anterior to the cerebellum.

b. Cerebrospinal fluid (CSF)

(1) Function

To cushion and support the brain and spinal cord within the

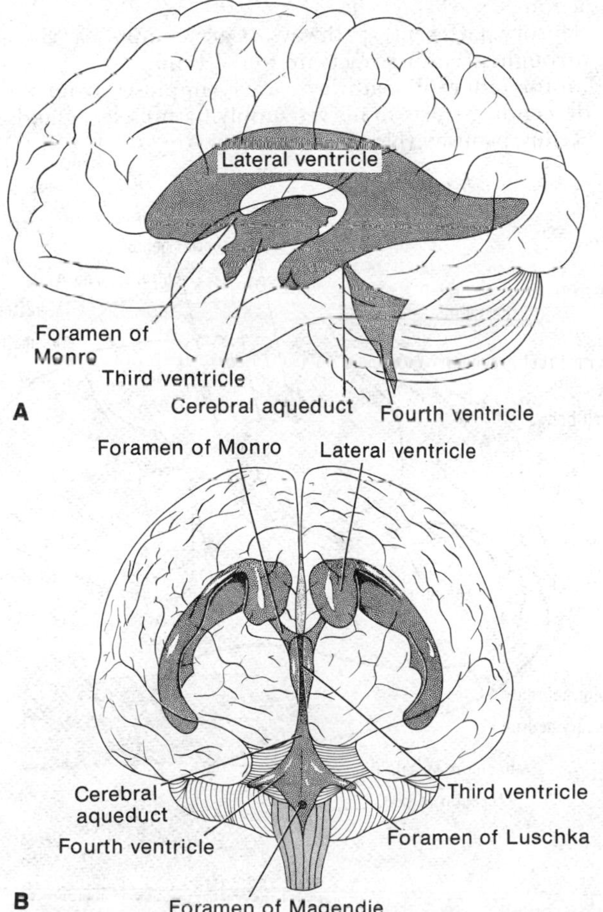

Figure 24–5. The human cerebral ventricular system shown in lateral (*A*) and anteroposterior (*B*) views. (From Curtis et al: *An Introduction to the Neurosciences.* Philadelphia: W. B. Saunders Co., 1972.)

skull and vertebral canal. To carry nutrients to various areas of the brain and spinal cord.

(2) Formation and circulation

Major part is formed by the choroid plexus in the lateral ventricles, as well as small amounts in the third and fourth ventricles.

Flows from each lateral ventricle via two foramina of Monro into the third ventricle. Flows from third ventricle via the narrow aqueduct of Sylvius (cerebral aqueduct) to the fourth ventricle. From the fourth ventricle, flows via two foramina of Luschka laterally and the caudal foramen of Magendie into the subarachnoid space. It bathes the spinal cord and flows over the surface of the hemispheres to the superior sagittal sinus, where it is reabsorbed.

7. Reticular formation

Making up the central core of the brain stem, beginning in the medulla and lower pons, is a diffuse system of fibers and nerve cells known as the *reticular formation.* Arising in this reticular formation and extending up to the thalamus and hypothalamus, with diffuse projections to the cerebral cortex, is a mechanism known as the *reticular activating system.* This system is associated with initiating and maintaining alert wakefulness.

Its actual function is still the subject of research and speculation, but it is known to be essential for arousing from sleep and remaining alert. Injury to this area produces anesthesia and coma.

B. Spinal cord

Continuous with brain stem. Contained within the vertebral canal. Extends to level of first or second lumbar vertebra.

1. Structure

H-shaped gray matter in the center (nerve cell bodies) surrounded by white matter (nerve tracts and fibers).

2. Function

a. Sensory (afferent) pathways. Carry impulses via afferent nerves through ascending tracts up to the brain.

b. Motor (efferent) pathways. Carry impulses from the brain through descending tracts to nerves supplying muscles, glands, etc.

c. Reflex pathway (Fig. 24–6)

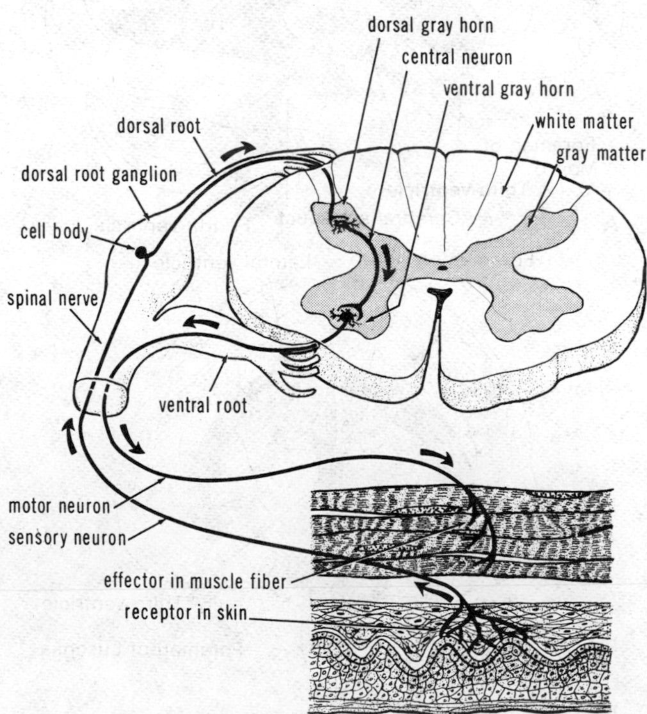

Figure 24–6. Spinal reflex arc. (From Memmler, R. L., and R. B. Rada: *The Human Body in Health and Disease,* 3rd ed. Philadelphia: J. B. Lippincott Co., 1970.)

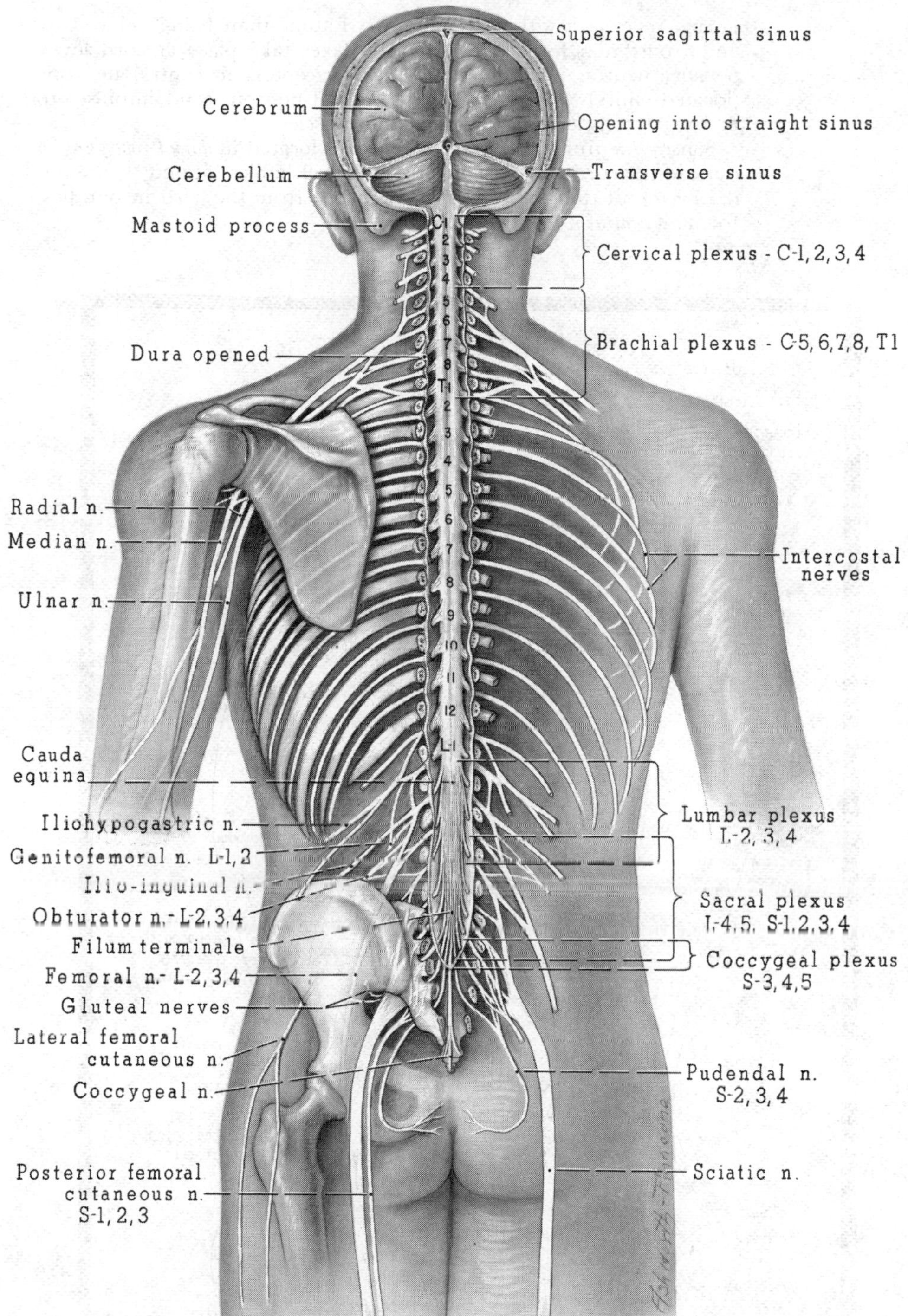

Figure 24–7. Spinal cord and nerves emerging from it. (From Jacob, S. W., C. A. Francone, and W. J. Lossow: *Structure and Function in Man,* 4th ed. Philadelphia: W. B. Saunders Co., 1978, p. 256.)

Forms reflex arc within spinal cord. Rather than being relayed to and from brain for action, spinal reflexes take place at cord level. Sensory neuron relays impulses from receptors to central neurons (located entirely within the cord); central neurons send impulses to motor neurons leading to glands and muscles.

Sensory neurons have their cell bodies located in *dorsal root ganglia* outside the cord; motor neurons have cell bodies located in the *anterior horns* of the spinal cord and emerge from the cord in bundles, forming *ventral roots*.

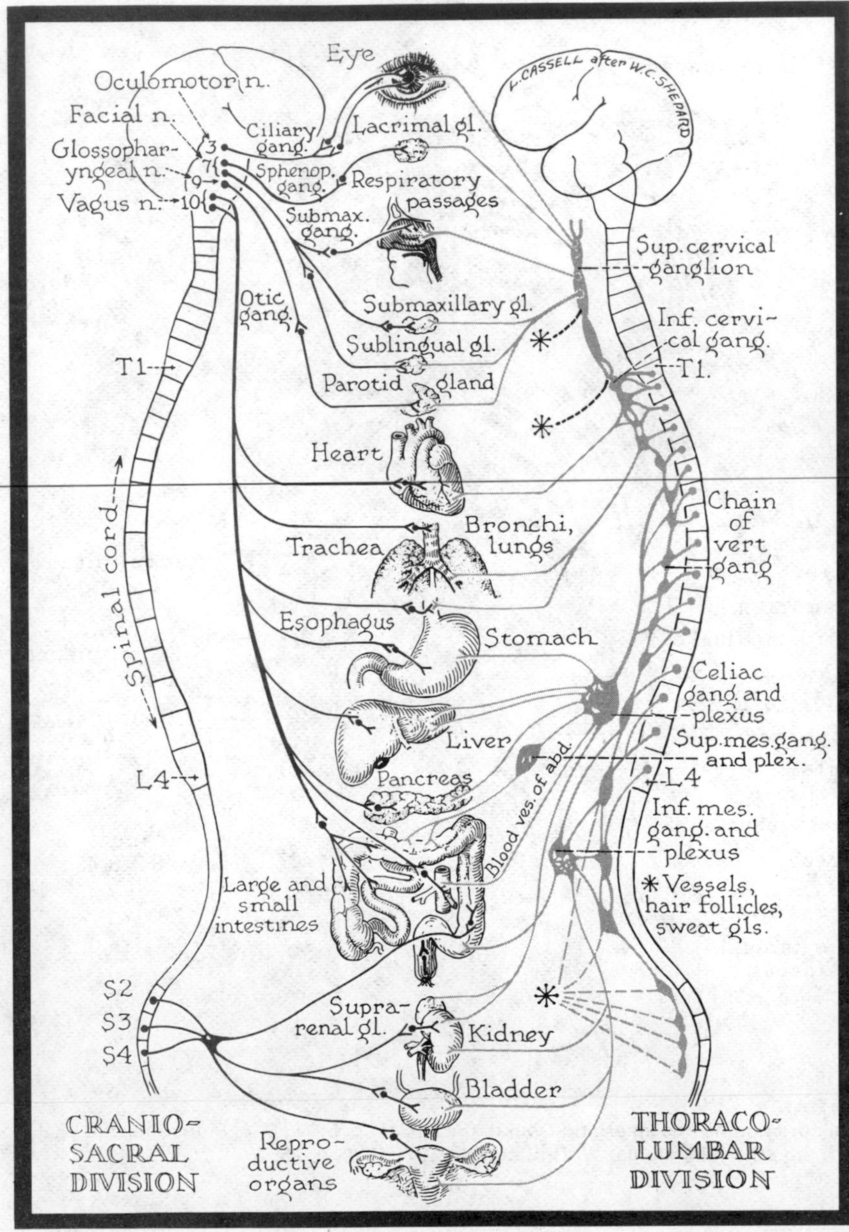

Figure 24–8. Diagram of the autonomic nervous system. (From King, B. G., and M. J. Showers: *Human Anatomy and Physiology*, 6th ed. Philadelphia: W. B. Saunders Co., 1969.)

II. Peripheral Nervous System

Made up of cranial and spinal nerves. These nerves may be afferent (carry impulses toward CNS), efferent (carry impulses from CNS to other parts of the body), or mixed (composed of both afferent and efferent fibers.)

A. Cranial nerves (12 pair) (See Fig. 24–4. Also see Table 25–1.)
   1. Olfactory — smell
   2. Optic — vision
   3. Oculomotor — movement of most eye muscles
   4. Trochlear — innervates one eye muscle
   5. Trigeminal — sensory to head and face, motor to chewing muscles
   6. Abducens — movement to one eye muscle
   7. Facial — motor to most facial muscles, sensory to tongue
   8. Acoustic — hearing and balance (also called *vestibulocochlear*)
   9. Glossopharyngeal — motor to swallowing muscles in pharynx; sensory to tongue and throat
   10. Vagus — supplies most abdominal and thoracic organs, and larynx
   11. Spinal accessory — motor to two neck muscles
   12. Hypoglossal — motor to tongue muscles

B. Spinal nerves (Fig. 24–7)
   1. 31 pairs:
      8 cervical
      12 thoracic
      5 lumbar
      5 sacral
      1 coccygeal
   2. Each nerve is attached to the spinal cord by two roots: *dorsal root* receives sensory input from sensory receptors throughout the body; *ventral root* contains a combination of motor fibers innervating glands and voluntary and involuntary muscles.
   3. *Spinal nerve plexuses.* A short distance from spinal cord, each spinal nerve branches into small posterior divisions and large anterior divisions. Anterior branches interweave, forming three major plexuses (networks) which then branch out to body parts.
      a. *Cervical plexus.* Sends motor impulses to neck muscles and sends out phrenic nerve, activating diaphragm; receives sensory impulses from neck and back of head.
      b. *Brachial plexus.* Innervates shoulder, arm, forearm, wrist, and hand.
      c. *Lumbosacral plexus.* Innervates lower extremities; sends out large sciatic nerve.

III. Autonomic Nervous System* (Fig. 24–8)

Actually a part of the peripheral nervous system.

A. Function

Regulates smooth muscles (located in walls of tubes, hollow organs, etc.), cardiac muscle, and glands. Is an involuntary system that works to keep a constant state inside the body despite changing external conditions.

B. Divisions
   1. Sympathetic nervous system

      Originates from the thoracic and lumbar areas of the spinal cord. Accelerates some body processes in response to stress.
   2. Parasympathetic nervous system

      Originates in cranial nerves III, VII, IX, and X, and in the sacral segment of the spinal cord. Balances action of sympathetic nervous system.

*The autonomic nervous system is discussed further in Chapter 6.

CHAPTER 25

EXAMINATION AND ASSESSMENT OF THE PERSON WITH A NEUROLOGIC DISORDER

INTRODUCTION*

Assessment of the health status of patients with nervous system disease or dysfunction follows the same *general* format as does examination of other patients. The obvious difference is an emphasis on *detailed* assessment of nervous system functions. The components of assessment can be divided into several categories: (1) medical history, including neurologic history; (2) physical examination, including special attention to a detailed neurologic examination; (3) general and special (neurologic) diagnostic studies; and (4) a nursing assessment with special attention to functions served by the nervous system. The first three components are performed most frequently by a physician for the primary purpose of establishing a diagnosis and treatment plan.

Findings from the history help guide some of the emphasis of the physical examination. After the history and physical examination are completed, the abnormalities are collated, and specific anatomic, pathologic, and etiologic diagnostic possibilities are established. The *anatomic diagnosis* identifies as accurately as possible where a lesion is located, e.g., the general location in the peripheral or central nervous system or, if possible, a more precise location. The *pathologic diagnosis* tells what type of lesion is present, e.g., infectious, traumatic, tumor. The *etiologic diagnosis* describes the process (or agent) responsible for the lesion, e.g., an infectious agent or arteriosclerosis, in some vascular problems,

Each component of the diagnostic assessment helps determine which special diagnostic studies may be indicated to confirm the diagnosis. Moreover, they can guide the nurse's assessment of a patient's ability to perform activities of daily living. The diagnostic assessment can be used by nurses to help them to focus on areas needing attention and also help them avoid missing subtle changes.

Nursing assessment is directed toward determining a patient's ability to live effectively with changes necessary because of actual or potential dysfunction.

First the nurse needs to find out if there is some dysfunction. If so, will it be permanent? Next, the effect of the dysfunction on the patient's self-care activities is determined. From this, a plan of care is developed. Data supporting this plan can be obtained from a variety of sources, including the patient, significant others, the medical work-up, the physician, and the nurse's knowledge base. For example, the nurse may learn that a patient has become more clumsy and drops things easily. In the medical examination record, a right homonymous hemianopsia may be noted in the visual fields section. The diagnosis is a lesion in the left parietal area of the brain. Based on this information, the care plan will take into account the fact that the patient cannot see to the right, and compensation for this must be made.

When a patient presents with a potentially life-threatening problem, both nurse and physician need to adjust their focus. In such a situation, the physician usually concentrates on rapid assessment of the presenting problem and initiation of treatment designed to prevent the patient from dying or becoming irreversibly ill. The nurse also needs to concentrate on careful observation of the progression

*Refer also as necessary to Chapters 14 and 15 (psychosocial and physical assessment) and Chapter 95 (emergency nursing).

of the presenting problem's signs and symptoms.

Nurses need to be astute observers and be knowledgeable of the meaning of subtle changes in a patient's status. They also need to be skillful at providing thoughtful, crisis-oriented support to a patient and significant others.

This chapter focuses on some elements of the neurologic history, physical examination, diagnostic studies, and nursing assessment of people with neurologic disorders. Inherent in each of these areas are the nursing roles of (a) teaching, counseling, and supporting the patient and significant others; (b) preparing them for special studies; (c) making knowledgeable, goal-directed observations; and (d) providing care related to changes in the patient's status.

The Diagnostic Process

You may recall that the purpose of a medical history and physical examination is to identify problems. The saying that "patients will tell you what is wrong with them" is largely true. However, it is also important to ask questions designed to insure that all of the available information has been obtained. Thus the *medical history* is obtained by asking (a) open questions designed to allow a patient to tell the "story" of the present condition, (b) closed questions to screen for other problems, and (c) "branching logic" questions to obtain more information about the identified problems.

The *physical examination* has some of the same characteristics. It is also divided into three general areas. These are (a) general observations of a patient, (b) a "screening" physical examination, and (c) more detailed physical examination to acquire further information about problems identified in the screening examination or history.

The basic kinds of information gathered from the history and physical examination vary little from patient to patient. Individual physicians tend to develop a style and thus gather similar information on all their patients. However, wide variations in available information occur. Hence, various professional groups are attempting to establish standards for the basic history and physical examination.

The *diagnostic studies* include (a) screening tests, (b) tests done to rule out possible (but unlikely) diagnoses, and (c) tests done to establish a specific individual diagnosis. This is also an area in which efforts are being directed toward establishing standards for what particular screening tests are indicated.

THE NEUROLOGIC HISTORY

The neurologic history is part of the general medical history. As such it generally consists of the following elements:

- *Identification data* are fairly standard and include such things as demographic, administrative, and insurance data. Frequently included in this category is a patient profile or brief description of the patient. The source of the history, e.g., patient, wife, friend, is usually stated. The mental status of the patient (and hence, reliability of the data) is frequently commented upon. It is common for neurologic illness to affect mental status. Thus considerable effort needs to be expended to obtain an accurate history.
- *History of the present disorder* requires a detailed description of the events leading the patient to seek care. The sequence of development of signs and symptoms is important in arriving at an accurate diagnosis.
- *Past history, review of systems,* and *social history* are all important in diagnosing neurologic illness. Neurologic illnesses frequently affect a person's ability to function in an integrated fashion. Their effects may be subtle. Hence it is important to acquire some understanding of factors such as a patient's educational background, level of job performance, and personality changes in order to make an accurate assessment. The *birth history* and *perinatal history* are important, as is the *history of several symptoms.* These include changes in consciousness, headaches, seizures, changes in vision including decreased vision or double vision, changes in speech or motor strength, sensory changes, dizziness or vertigo, changes in gait or body posture while standing (station) and others. The *review of systems* may yield clues as to other diseases (or disorders) that directly relate to the presenting problem, e.g., a history of angina and other cardiovascular problems in a patient presenting with a possible stroke.
- *Family history* has become an increasingly important part of the general history as it becomes more evident that many neurologic disorders have a hereditary component. Generally family history is recorded for three generations. The age and cause of death is recorded, as are major diseases of family members who are still alive.

THE NEUROLOGIC PHYSICAL EXAMINATION

The neurologic physical examination is part of the general physical examination, as is the history. The history will often indicate that parts of the physical examination need special emphasis. However, it is important to avoid becoming too focused on specific "expected" findings, in order to avoid overlooking other pertinent abnormalities. Thus, the physical examination combines screening maneuvers and maneuvers dictated by abnormal findings.

General Information. The source of information (i.e., whether the patient or someone else) is noted in the patient's record. Also, comments on the presence of obvious abnormalities and the patient's behavior, ability to communicate, and ability to cooperate with the examiner are recorded.

Mental Status. General data about the patient's mental status are usually recorded. The level of consciousness, orientation, mood, speech, content of thought, and memory are the areas most commonly tested. The level of consciousness descriptive terminology is given in Chapter 26 (p. 526). Mental status examinations are also discussed on pp. 303 and 359.

Time, place, and person are the areas of inquiry to establish a patient's orientation. Speech is evaluated to determine whether there are problems with articulation (generally motor disorders) or problems in language formation (asphasic disorders). Inquiring into thought content requires tact. Basically, determining whether reasoning, thinking, problem solving or other integrative processes are abnormal helps indicate if a major problem with content of thought exists. The way a person appears (e.g., euphoric or depressed) and reports from the patient and significant others help assess a patient's mood. Gross deficits in long- and short-term memory can be identifed with simple testing. For example, long-term memory can be tested by asking the person to recall and relate his or her own past medical history. (Of course, the examiner must have another source to validate the data.) Short-term memory can be tested by giving the person three words to remember (e.g., red, Broadway, three), asking the person to repeat the words immediately after you, and in a few minutes asking the person to repeat the words again.

Gait and Station. These functions are tested by having the patient do the following: stand still, walk, and walk in tandem (one foot in front of the other in a straight line). Walking is truly a complex function, involving several functions — motor power, sensation, and coordination. Each of these is tested separately later in the examination. The ability to stand quietly with one's feet together also requires coordination and intact proprioception. If there is a problem with standing, further testing is done to see if the patient is weak or unsteady.

Head, Neck, and Spine Examination. Inspection, palpation, auscultation, and percussion of these areas may yield useful diagnostic information. The head, neck, and spine are carefully inspected for abnormalities. Percussion of these areas may produce pain or tenderness in discrete areas, requiring further investigation. Palpation of the neck muscles and the detection of obvious masses can also yield clues for further investigation. Auscultation of the major neck vessels and other vessels is done to hear bruits or other abnormal sounds indicative of underlying pathology. Tumors, vascular disorders, traumatic disorders, and problems involving the vertebrae and surrounding muscles are common problems that may be suspected after examination of the head, neck and spine. (Head and neck examination is discussed further in Chapter 15, pp. 321–334.)

Examination of the Cranial Nerves. Cranial nerves (c.n.) may be referred to by specific name or number. Some points about cranial nerve function may help you understand the rationale of the examination:

1. Half of all the cranial nerves innervate the functions of the eyes. Therefore, careful examination of all eye functions yields a great deal of information.
2. The majority of the cranial nerves arise from the brain stem. This means that testing their functions yields a great deal of information about the brain stem.
3. Normal cranial nerve functioning means that the following two events are present: (a) The input stimulus is being appropriately received and (b) an appropriate output (response) is resulting. Failure to get a normal response when testing cranial nerves can be a result of: (a) failure to receive stimuli (*input failure*), (b) failure to respond appropriately (*output failure*), and (c) a combination of both input and output failure. Determining which of these problems exists is often difficult. For example, vision is a function of c.n. II, and the pupillary light response is a function of c.n. III. If a patient is blind, however, the pupillary light response cannot be tested, as testing this reflex requires that both c.n. II and III be intact. (See Figure 25–1 and Table 25–1.)

Olfactory (I). Smell. The patient is asked to identify an aromatic, nonpungent odor with each nostril. Although inability to smell may not be pathologic in the elderly, a cause should be looked for, e.g., basal skull fracture or a tumor of the olfactory groove.

Optic (II). Vision. Evaluation of this nerve's function involves testing visual acuity, inspecting the globe with the naked eye and with an ophthalmoscope, and testing the visual fields. Visual acuity may be grossly tested by having the patient read from a newspaper and a sign at a distance or read from a Snellen chart. Visual fields are tested to determine if the patient has lost vision in one or more directions. Such losses can be expected in patients with a wide variety of diagnoses and correlate with the area of the brain involved. Gross inspection of the eyes and examination of the fundus can yield a great deal of information about neurologic disease.

Oculomotor (III), Trochlear (IV) and Abducens (VI). Eyes and eye movement. The size and shape of the pupils are noted (III). They should be equal in size and round. The pupils are each tested for a direct and consensual response (pupillary constriction) to a light. The direct response is that which occurs in the eye being tested. The consensual response occurs in the other eye (constriction of the pupil). Accommodation is tested by having the patient look across the room (away from the light source) and then look at the examiner's fingers, held about 6 inches from the patient's nose. The shape of the lens changes and the pupils constrict if the patient's vision is able to accommodate to see objects both close and far away. The notation "PERRLA" in the chart indicates that these functions are normal. This abbreviation means *p*upils *e*qual, *r*ound, *r*eactive to *l*ight and *a*ccommodation present. Destruction of part of c.n. III can also cause ptosis (drooping) of the eyelid.

Coordination activities of cranial nerves III, IV, and VI control the movement of the eyes in all six cardinal directions of gaze. Function of these nerves can be tested in a variety of ways. The person can be asked to move the eyes in the six directions or to

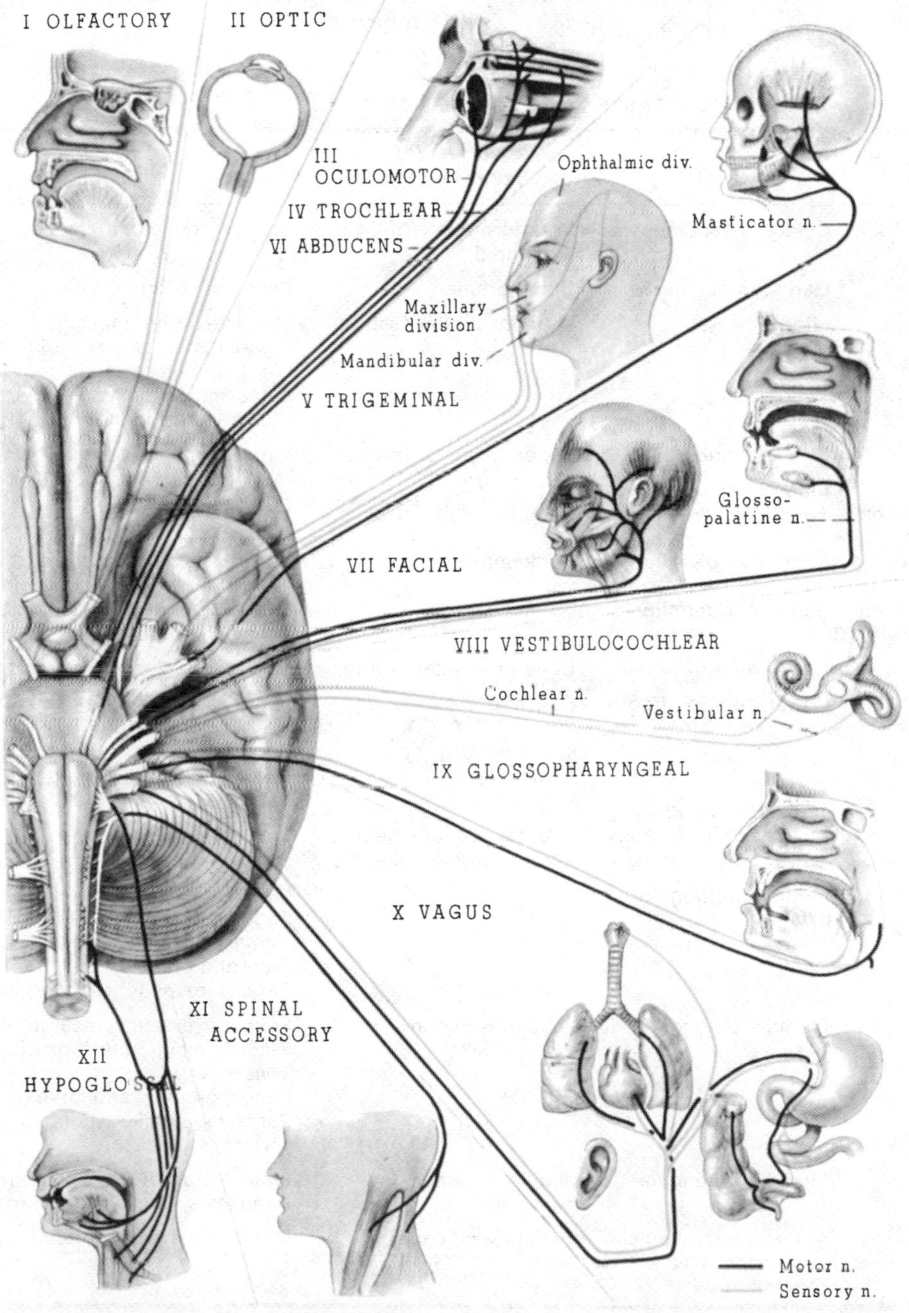

Figure 25–1. Distribution of cranial nerves. (After Netter.) (From Jacob, S. W., C. A. Francone, and W. J. Lossow: *Structure and Function in Man,* 4th ed. Philadelphia: W. B. Saunders Co., 1978, p. 265.)

follow an object with the eyes while the examiner moves it in the different directions. If a patient has diplopia (double vision) and no muscle weakness can be demonstrated, shine a light so it reflects on both eyes. The area of reflection is normally symmetrical, meaning that the patient has a conjugate gaze. A dysconjugate gaze is present if the light's reflection is asymmetrical, i.e., not the same in both eyes. If the extraocular movements are intact, the notation "EOM's intact" is recorded (See also pp. 323 and 528.)

Trigeminal (V). The fifth cranial nerve has a motor and a sensory division. The *motor division* innervates the muscles of mastication and is tested by asking the patient to clamp the jaws, open the mouth against resistance, widely open the mouth, move the jaws from side to side, and make chewing movements. The nerve's *sensory division* mediates all sensations for the entire face, for the scalp to the vertex, and for the nasal and oral cavities. Sensations such as pain (e.g., pin prick), touch (e.g., wisp of cotton or soft brush) and temperature (e.g., hot and cold bottles of water) are tested on both sides of the face in all areas from the vertex (i.e., top of the head) to the chin. The *corneal reflexes* are tested by gently touching the cornea with a wisp of cotton. The normal response is a brisk blinking of the eye lids. (See also p. 528 for discussion of corneal reflexes.)

TABLE 25–1. CRANIAL NERVES

Number	Name	Origin	Exit from Skull	Function
I	Olfactory	Cells of nasal mucosa	Cribriform plate of ethmoid	Sensory; olfactory (smell)
II	Optic	Ganglion cell in retina	Optic foramen	Sensory: vision
III	Oculomotor	Midbrain	Superior orbital fissure	Motor: external muscles of eyes except lateral rectus and superior oblique; levator palpebrae superioris Parasympathetic: sphincter of pupil and ciliary muscle of lens
IV	Trochlear	Roof of midbrain	Superior orbital fissure	Motor: superior oblique muscle
V	Trigeminal	Lateral aspect of pons		
	Ophthalmic branch	Semilunar ganglion	Superior orbital fissure	Sensory: cornea; nasal mucous membrane; skin of face
	Maxillary branch	Semilunar ganglion	Foramen rotundum	Sensory: skin of face; oral cavity; anterior two-thirds of tongue; teeth
	Mandibular branch	Semilunar ganglion	Foramen ovale	Motor: muscles of mastication Sensory: skin of face
VI	Abducens	Lower margin of pons	Superior orbital fissure	Motor: lateral rectus muscle
VII	Facial	Lower margin of pons	Stylomastoid foramen	Motor: muscles of facial expression Sensory: taste, anterior two-thirds of tongue Parasympathetic: lacrimal, submandibular, and sublingual glands
VIII	Vestibulocochlear			
	Vestibular	Lower border of pons	Internal auditory meatus	Sensory: equilbrium
	Cochlear	Lower border of pons	Internal auditory meatus	Sensory: hearing
IX	Glossopharyngeal	Medulla oblongata	Jugular foramen	Motor: stylopharyngeus muscle Sensory: taste posterior one-third of tongue; pharynx; branch of the carotid sinus and carotid body Parasympathetic: parotid gland
X	Vagus	Medulla oblongata	Jugular foramen	Sensory: external meatus, pharynx, larynx, aortic sinus, and thoracic and abdominal viscera Motor: pharynx and larynx Parasympathetic: thoracic and abdominal viscera
XI	Accessory	Medulla oblongata	Jugular foramen	Motor: trapezius and sternocleidomastoid muscles; muscles of pharynx and larynx
XII	Hypoglossal	Anterior lateral sulcus between olive and pyramid	Hypoglossal canal	Motor: muscles of tongue

From Jacob, S. W., C. A. Francone, and W. J. Lossow: *Structure and Function in Man,* 4th ed. Philadelphia: W. B. Saunders Co., 1978, p. 276.

Facial (VII). The seventh cranial nerve also has both a *motor* and *sensory* division. It innervates the muscles that give the face expression. The face is observed for symmetry and the ability to contract facial muscles. The patient is asked to smile, frown, elevate the forehead and eyebrows, tightly close the eyes and resist attempts to open them, whistle, show the teeth, and blow out the cheeks. The sense of taste is tested with various sweet, salty, acidic (sour), or bitter substances.

Acoustic (VIII). The eighth cranial nerve has two divisions: (a) The *cochlear nerve* is tested for *auditory acuity* by having the patient listen to the whispered voice, the tick of a watch, or a tuning fork at various distances from the ear. Testing of bone and air conduction is carried out with a tuning fork. Additionally, an audiometer may be used for a precise evaluation of auditory acuity. (b) The *vestibular nerve* is concerned with reflexes that maintain equilibrium in space by coordinating muscles of the eye, neck, trunk, and extremities. Various tests may be used to evaluate vestibular function, e.g., caloric test and electronystagmography. (For detailed discussion of evaluation of hearing and equilibrium, see Unit XXIII and pp. 329 and 516.)

Glossopharyngeal (IX) and Vagus (X). Because of the overlapping *innervation of the pharynx,* the ninth and tenth cranial nerves are examined together. The patient is asked to open the mouth widely and say, "Ah." While this is done, the palate's evaluation, position, and movement are checked. The *gag reflex* is checked by gently touching the pharynx with a tongue depressor. This should elicit a brisk gag response. Also the patient's ability to swallow a small amount of water is assessed. The posterior third of the tongue is tested for taste, as with the seventh cranial nerve. The patient is asked to cough and to speak to test the vagus nerve. Damage to this nerve results in an ineffectual cough and a weak, hoarse voice.

Spinal Accessory (XI). This nerve innervates the *sternocleidomastoid muscle* and the *upper portion of the trapezius muscle.* In testing, the patient is asked to elevate the shoulders (with and without resistance) and to turn the head to one side and resist the examiner's attempt to pull the chin back toward midline.

Hypoglossal (XII). The twelfth cranial nerve provides the *tongue with motor innervation.* The patient is asked to open the mouth widely, stick out the tongue, rapidly move the tongue from side to side and in and out. Also, the strength of the tongue is tested by having the patient push the tongue against the inside of the cheek and resist pressure applied to the area externally by the examiner.

Evaluation of the Sensory System. A complete sensory examination can be performed only on a conscious patient because the patient must be able to focus attention on the stimuli and cooperate with the examiner. A stuporous patient may be tested for the presence of responses to painful stimuli (e.g., reflex withdrawal of limbs, wincing, grimacing); however, it is impossible to perform other aspects of the sensory examination. In performing the complete sensory examination, sensation is tested with the *patient's eyes closed.*

We have already discussed some aspects of the sensory examination. You will recall that we have mentioned evaluation of vision, hearing, smell and taste, as well as touch, pain, and temperature.

Various disturbances of sensation may occur. For example, *dysesthesias* are well-localized sensations that are irritative to the patient, e.g., sensations of warmth, coldness, itching, tickling, crawling, prickling, and tingling. *Paresthesias* are distortions of sensory stimuli, e.g., light touch may be experienced as a burning or painful sensation. Absence of the sense of touch is called *anesthesia,* while reduced sense of touch is *hypesthesia* and a pathologic over-perception of touch is *hyperesthesia.* An area of reduced sensation of pain is termed *hypalgesic,* increased is *hyperalgesic,* and absence of pain is *analgesic.* Other disturbances of sensation are discussed throughout the unit.

Routinely during the sensory examination, tests are carried out for touch, pressure, movement, position (proprioception), vibration, and pain. When there is a loss of the sense of pain, tests for temperature awareness are performed. In the sensory examination *stereognosis* (i.e., the form and configuration of felt objects, or three-dimensional discrimination) is also tested. The loss of this sense is called *astereognosis.*

Figure 25–2 summarizes some important patterns of sensory loss.

Evaluation of the Motor System. Evaluation of the motor system can involve a large number of complex activities and tests. Here we discuss: (a) some examinations done as screening maneuvers, (b) common abnormalities, and (c) a few activities performed when abnormal function is found.

Examination of *symmetry, size, and shape of muscles* involves careful inspection and comparison of the muscles on both sides of the body for abnormalities. The muscles are then palpated for tone, consistency, and tenderness or pain. Next the muscles are examined for "fine" and "gross" abnormal movements. Examples of fine movements include *fasiculations,* which are involuntary ripples or twitches present when the patient is relaxed. These movements may indicate the presence of lower motor neuron disease. Examples of more grossly abnormal movements, often representing extrapyramidal disease, include:

- *Chorea,* a discrete, jerky, purposeless movement seen in the distal extremities and face
- *Athetosis,* a gross, writhing, worm-like movement
- *Dystonia,* a prolonged twisting movement

- *Myoclonus*, a sudden muscle contraction of varying intensity, which may involve only a small part of one extremity or may involve the entire body and be so violent as to fling a patient to the floor
- *Tic*, frequently of psychogenic origin and often can be voluntarily inhibited; involves the same musculature each time in a stereotyped movement of varying complexity
- *Tremors* vary in direction, amplitude, rhythmicity, parts involved, speed, and timing in relation to rest or activity; types can include Parkinsonian, familial, and senile

After inspecting the muscles, all the joints are moved through a full range of passive motions. Pathology of a joint, pain, contractures, and muscle resistance are all abnormal findings.

Next, *muscle power* is tested. This has already been partially evaluated with the evaluation of gait and station. The person is (a) asked to walk on the heels and then toes and (b) to hold the arms straight out in front with palms up, and maintain that posture with eyes closed. A "drift" is said to be present if one arm moves upward or if one hand begins to pronate. Otherwise, unless indicated, the only

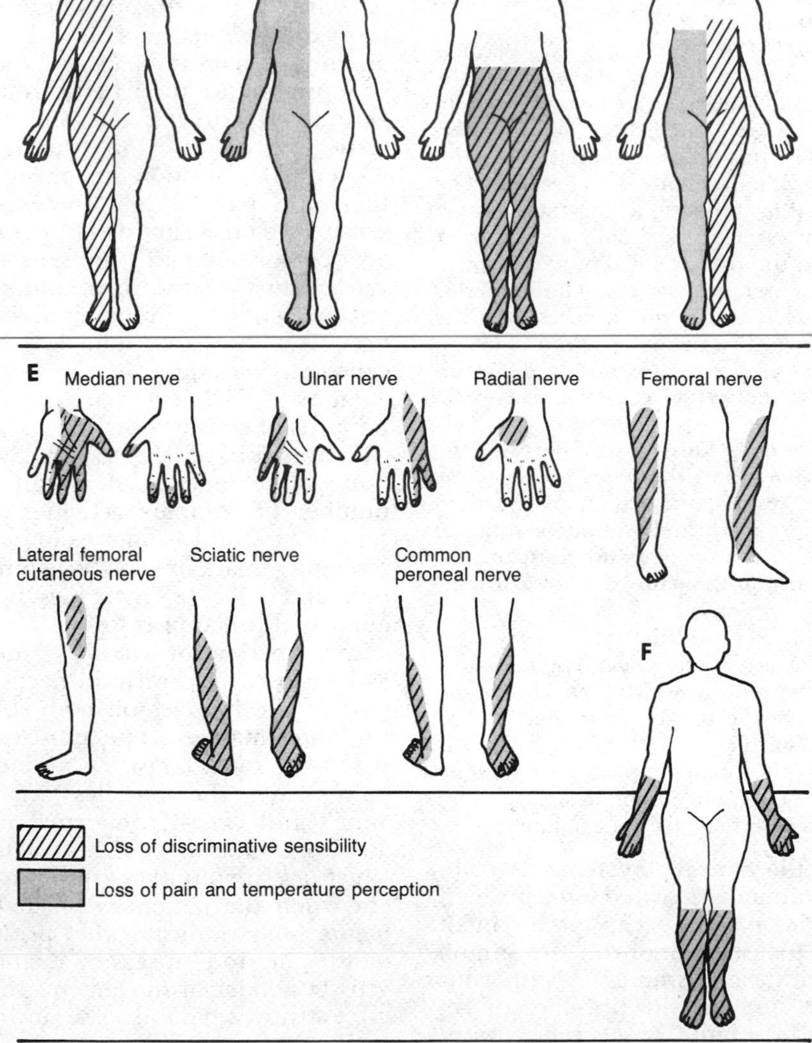

Figure 25–2. Important patterns of sensory loss. **A.** Lesion of the left cerebral hemisphere. **B.** Lesion of the left side of the brain stem. **C.** Complete transverse lesion of the spinal cord. **D.** Lesion on the left side of the spinal cord (Brown-Sequard syndrome). **E.** Lesions of important peripheral nerves. **F.** Polyneuropathy. (From Magee, R. R.: The neurologic workup by the primary care physician. *Postgraduate Medicine* 61(3):83, Mar. 1977.)

other tests frequently performed are those involving testing major muscle groups against resistance. If other abnormalities are found, there are a variety of examinations and tests that may be indicated, such as electromyography, (see p. 513).

Coordination and accuracy of muscle function are tested next. These are primarily tests of cerebellar function. *Point-to-point tests* with the eyes open and closed are performed on all extremities (e.g., the patient touches the examiner's finger and then his or her own nose. Ability to perform rapid alternating movements is tested. An example of this test is rapidly touching the thumb with each finger in sequence.

Apraxia is the inability to carry out a learned movement on command in the absence of weakness or paralysis. This can be demonstrated by asking the patient to do any of a wide variety of things, e.g., tying shoes. True apraxia can only be said to be present if a person can perform an act spontaneously but fails to do so on command.

Evaluation of Reflex Activity. Muscles normally contract and relax promptly. This response can be elicited by striking the muscle with a reflex hammer.

Assessment of a person's reflexes is part of a diagnostic neurologic examination as well as an important procedure in the ongoing clinical assessment of a person with an established neurologic disorder. Evaluation of reflex responses can provide information about the nature, location, and progression of neurologic disorders.

Two types of reflexes are normally present: (1) superficial or cutaneous reflexes and (2) deep tendon or stretch reflexes.

Superficial or cutaneous reflexes are produced by cutaneous or mucous membrane stimulation. The stimulus is produced by stroking a sensory zone. Examples of superficial reflexes: (a) the *abdominal reflex*, in which scratching of the skin of a quadrant of the abdomen normally results in contraction of the abdominal muscles of that quadrant and (b) the *plantar reflex*, in which scratching the outer aspect of the plantar surface of the foot (i.e., the outer sole of the foot), from the heel toward the toes, normally contracts or flexes the toes and sometimes the foot.

Other superficial reflexes are: the *corneal reflex*, in which gentle stroking of cornea with a wisp of cotton causes reflex blinking (to test the left eye have the patient look up and to the right — vice versa for the right eye — and bring the stimulus in from the side in such a manner that the patient cannot see your hand, then very gently touch the outer edge of the cornea); and the *pharyngeal reflex* or *"gag" reflex*, in which gentle stimulation of the back of the throat and the pharynx with a tongue blade produces gagging.

Deep tendon reflexes are of greater diagnostic value than are superficial or cutaneous reflexes. Such reflexes are also called *muscle stretch* or *myotatic reflexes* since the reflex contraction of a muscle results from stimulation by rapid stretching of the muscle. This is clinically achieved by sharply striking a muscle's tendon of insertion with a sudden, brief blow.

> *Reflex sites usually examined are the Achilles tendon, patella, biceps, and triceps.*

Tapping the Achilles tendon normally produces an *ankle jerk*, resulting in plantar flexion of the foot; tapping the quadriceps femoris tendon just below the patella normally produces a *knee jerk, quadriceps jerk* or *patellar reflex*, resulting in extension of the leg; tapping the biceps brachii tendon normally produces a *biceps jerk*, resulting in flexion of the forearm; and tapping the triceps brachii tendon at the elbow normally produces a *triceps jerk*, resulting in extension of the forearm.

These reflexes are graded from 0 to 4+. A 2+ is normal. While 1+ or 3+ responses are not considered normal, they may not represent significant findings. Far more significant is asymmetry of responses. Abnormal reflexes do not necessarily reflect neurologic disease, since they are also commonly present in metabolic disorders.

Table 25–2 summarizes some important reflexes.

Some other "special" reflexes normally occur which involve structures other than the skeletal muscles. For example, reflex mechanisms normally help to maintain respiration and keep blood pressure within normal limits. Reflex salivation may follow a taste of food. Flashing a light in an eye normally causes the diameter of the pupils of both eyes to lessen, thereby limiting the amount of light that can enter; this is known as the *light reflex* or *pupillary reflex*. (See also p. 528.)

Pathologic reflexes or abnormal reflexes are reflexes that do not normally occur. The presence of such reflexes may indicate neurologic disorders, frequently of the spinal cord or higher centers. The *jaw reflex* (in which the jaw contracts and closes the mouth as a result of downward tapping on the lower jaw, when the mouth is relaxed and hangs passively partially open) occurs only rarely in healthy individuals, but is noticeably present in a variety of disorders, e.g., sclerosis of the spinal cord's lateral columns. The jaw reflex is also called the "mandibular reflex" or the "jaw jerk."

The *palm-chin* (palmo-mental) reflex is another pathologic reflex produced by vigorous, rapid irritation with a blunt instrument on the mound of the palm at the thumb's base, causing the muscles of the chin to be pulled up on the same side.

Clonus refers to rapidly alternating flexions and extensions at the joint, resulting from the continuous rhythmic contractions of a muscle subjected to stretch. This is unlike the normal stretch reflex, which typically produces one reflex action. With clonus, the action continues.

Babinski reflex occurs when the sole of the foot is scratched with a blunt point, causing dorsiflexion of the big toe and frequently fanning of the other toes, instead of normal plantar flexion (Fig. 25–3). In extreme circumstances this may be accompanied by dorsiflexion of the foot at the ankle and flexion at the knee and hip. *The Babinski reflex is probably the most important single pathologic sign in neurology.* In eliciting the Babinski reflex, the stimulus is started at the midpoint of the heel and is carried upward and laterally along the sole's outer border until the ball of the foot is reached. There the stimulus is directed across the ball of the foot toward the medial side. Or the stimulus may be started at the midlateral sole and carried down toward the heel.[303] Generally if exaggerated deep reflexes are found, the superficial reflexes are found to be diminished or absent, and such pathologic reflexes as the Babinski toe sign are found.[148]

Evaluation of the Autonomic Nervous System

Many diseases that are not primarily of the nervous system have symptoms related to impaired autonomic function, e.g., postural hypotension, Raynaud's disease. Unit XIX discusses autonomic disorders related to the endocrine organs e.g., symptoms of overaction of the sympathetic system are outstanding in hyperthyroidism. In this unit we focus on disorders in which neurologic components are of

TABLE 25–2. IMPORTANT REFLEXES

Reflex	Method	Effect	Localization
TENDON REFLEXES			
Jaw reflex	Light blow on center of slightly opened lower jaw	Closure of jaw	Fifth cranial nerve
Biceps reflex	A blow on the examiner's thumb placed over the biceps tendon	Flexion of elbow	C5 and C6
Brachioradialis reflex	Styloid process of radius is tapped while forearm is in semiflexion and semipronation.	Flexion of elbow	C5 and C6
Triceps reflex	Blow on triceps tendon just above the olecranon	Extension of elbow	C7
Finger flexion reflex	Examiner taps his index and middle fingers placed across volar surfaces of phalanges of patient's four fingers	Flexion of fingers and distal portion of thumb	C6 to C8
Patellar reflex (knee jerk)	Blow on patellar tendon	Leg extends	L2 to L4
Achilles reflex (ankle jerk)	Blow on Achilles tendon	Plantar flexion of foot	S1
SUPERFICIAL REFLEXES			
Corneal reflex	Light touch at the corneoscleral junction	Closure of eyelids	Fifth and seventh cranial nerves
Palatal and pharyngeal reflexes	Light touch to soft palate and pharynx	Elevation of palate; gagging	Ninth and tenth cranial nerves
Abdominal reflexes	Stroke skin of upper, middle and lower abdomen	Contraction of abdominal wall	Upper–T7 to T9 Middle–T9 to T11 Lower–T11 to T12
Cremasteric reflex	Stroke medial surface of upper thigh	Elevation of scrotum and testicle	T12 and L1
Anal reflex	Stroke perianal region	Contraction of external anal sphincter	S5
Plantar reflex (normal)	Stroke sole of foot	Flexion of toes	S1 and S2
Plantar reflex (pathological; sign of Babinski)	Stroke sole of foot	Dorsiflexion of great toe and fanning of other toes	S1 and S2

From Vick, N. A.: *Grinker's Neurology,* 7th ed. Springfield, Ill.: Charles C Thomas, 1976, page 35.

major significance, e.g., causalgia, syringomyelia, and peripheral neuropathy.

Some general symptoms of autonomic dysfunction include: alterations in patterns of perspiration; faulty body temperature regulation (i.e., hypothermia and hyperthermia); abnormal pulse rate and pilomotor responses; as well as trophic, vasomotor, and pupillary changes. Autonomic dysfunctions in organic disease are often localized in a certain area of the body.

In examining for autonomic disturbances inquiry is made about *polyuria, abnormal motility of the gastrointestinal tract,* and possibly *urinary* or *fecal incontinence.* The abdomen is examined for evidence of *bowel* and *urinary bladder distention. Changes in thirst, energy, potency, libido, weight,* and *appetite* may also be significant.

The patient's skin, mucous membranes, hair, and nails are examined for obvious *trophic changes.* Trophic changes occur in various diseases and cause the loss of innervation incorporating the autonomic nerve supply. Trophic disturbances may be manifested by changes in the affected area's temperature, sweating, and color, e.g., pallor, cyanosis, and erythema. Paralyzed limbs may be cooler to touch than other areas of the patient's body. Also, with trophic changes the nails may become curved, brittle, broken, and thickened; the skin may be painlessly ulcerated, thickened, atrophied, pigmented, oily, scaly and rough, or tight, shiny and dry. The hair may become oily, brittle, and dry, or loss of hair or abnormal hair growth may occur. Painless ulceration may be present on the fingers, toes, or other regions. Decubitus ulcers occur in denervated regions of the skin, beginning at areas subjected to prolonged pressure. *Palpitation,* i.e., unduly rapid action of the heart which is felt by the patient, may also indicate autonomic dysfunction.

NEUROLOGIC TESTS AND DIAGNOSTIC PROCEDURES

As has been pointed out neurologic examination involves taking a careful patient and family history and giving a thorough physical examination. To these processes are added a variety of special diagnostic tests and procedures that supplement and add precision to clinical neurologic diagnosis. While some of these special tests are simple and painless, others are complex and cause pain and discomfort. Since some neurologic diagnostic procedures are actually potentially life-threatening, the health professionals in attendance must be prepared to promptly detect and correct complications. Observations of a patient's condition, made and recorded by members of the nursing staff, are an important source of information during the diagnostic process as well as later during therapy.

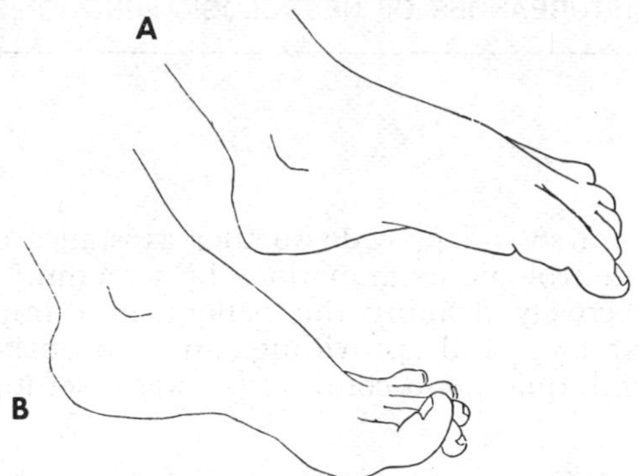

Figure 25–3. The Babinski response. **A.** The normal adult response to stimulation of the foot. **B.** The normal infant and abnormal adult response. (From Gardner, E. D.: *Fundamentals of Neurology,* 6th ed. Philadelphia: W. B. Saunders Co., 1975, p. 215.)

Remember that preparation for any diagnostic examination or test involves both physical and psychologic preparation of the patient. The supportive care a nurse gives to a patient undergoing diagnostic and evaluative procedures is extremely important. Supportive nursing care enhances a patient's sense of well-being and promotes confidence in unfamiliar people and procedures. An excellent nurse also facilitates the expression of fears and other concerns and answers requests for information by both patients and significant others.

In addition to scheduling diagnostic tests, preparing patients, and assisting the physician a nurse has the important responsibility of caring for patients after the various diagnostic procedures. Such care centers on: (1) keeping the patient comfortable physicially and psychologically; (2) observing for the onset of complications resulting from the procedure and reporting these; (3) helping the patient's significant others during this stressful time; and (4) protecting the patient from injury or complications.

Protecting the patient involves such activities as observing for special potential complications following diagnostic tests (discussed with the various tests) and keeping all staff members informed of specific orders following the tests. For example, if a patient's bed is to be kept flat following a procedure, the patient should be informed of the order and a sign should be placed on the patient's bed where it can be seen by all persons coming into the room. Keeping the patient and all persons coming to the patient's bedside informed of necessary restrictions is a highly important aspect of nursing practice. Failure to conscientiously perform this responsibility not only can delay a patient's recovery and cause discomfort, but at times may be life-threatening. Additional precautions, e.g., siderails, assistance in walking, and so forth, should be used as indicated for patient safety.

A nurse can provide further assistance during neurologic examinations by screening and protectively draping the patient, encouraging relaxation, and providing an appropriately lighted, quiet, and comfortably warm setting.

Central Nervous System X-Rays

Spine and/or skull x-rays are among the first and most common neurologic studies ordered. Changes in bone structure (destruction and healing) and calcification of structures may be demonstrated. When trauma (e.g., skull or vertebral fractures), abnormal development of bony structures (e.g., asymmetry of the skull), vascular diseases, bone diseases, or a tumor is suspected, x-rays are ordered. Because there are several common views to choose from, the physician decides precisely what view to order based on the suspected diagnosis.

The nurse is responsible for seeing that appropriate care is given while the patient is being transported to and from the x-ray department and while x-rays are being taken. Thus, a confused combative patient or one who is unstable, one requiring special therapy such as oxygen, or other patients requiring close supervision of their care may need to be accompanied to x-ray by a nurse. The physician in charge of the care assumes the responsibility for moving the patient with a spinal fracture safely to avoid damage (or further damage) to the spinal cord. Thus, while the x-ray procedures themselves require no special care, judgment must be exercised to assure that patient care remains appropriate.

When "routine" skull x-rays are ordered, the radiologist takes a series of films, often including the following projections: lateral, half axial, axial, and posteroanterior. Additional specialized views may also be ordered and/or tomograms may be taken. *Tomograms* are selected horizontal or vertical layered exposures taken at measured depths. When tomograms are sequentially reviewed it is possible to obtain some idea of the two-dimensional shape of a defect, e.g., an abscess.

Lumbar Puncture

Definition. A lumbar puncture (LP; "spinal tap"; spinal puncture) is the insertion of a needle into the lumbar region of the spine in such a manner that the needle enters the lumbar subarachnoid space of the spinal canal below the level of the spinal cord so that cerebrospinal fluid (CSF) can be withdrawn or a substance can be therapeutically or diagnostically injected.

Purposes. Lumbar puncture may be performed for a variety of therapeutic and diagnostic purposes. *Therapeutically*, lumbar puncture is commonly performed to administer spinal anesthesia (spinal anesthetics are discussed in Unit VIII) or to administer medications. The latter is rare, however, in treating neurologic illnesses. LP has also been used therapeutically to *remove* blood and pus from the subarachnoid space or to remove CSF and thereby reduce intracranial pressure if it is dangerously high.

Diagnostically, lumbar puncture enables the removal of a sample of CSF for inspection and the measurement of the CSF pressure. At the time this is done, the physician may elect to perform "spinal dynamics" (discussed later), which could indicate a block in CSF circulation. This is done to determine whether the lumbar subarachnoid space is in communication with the cerebral ventricles. Also, after some CSF is removed, air, oxygen, or radiopaque substances may be injected and diagnostic x-rays taken (e.g., encephalograms), which may help to locate tumors or other brain disorders. Such x-rays are discussed later in this chapter.

Hazards. Lumbar punctures are done quite commonly. However, they are not "routine," since they are uncomfortable for the patient and they carry a risk of potential morbidity and mortality. Potential hazards with LP include leakage of CSF, infection, damage to intervertebral discs, respiratory failure, and postpuncture headache. The necessity for the procedure is carefully evaluated before it is carried out.

The procedure is performed by a physician, using strict aseptic technique. Strict aseptic technique is important in all procedures in which the CNS is directly penetrated since the introduction of an infectious agent could produce a serious, perhaps fatal, infection.

> *Lumbar puncture is risky in the presence of increased intracranial pressure and may produce a herniation syndrome (see Chapter 26). Usually only patients with suspected meningitis and subarachnoid hemorrhage are tapped in the presence of increased intracranial pressure. Lumbar puncture is also avoided in the presence of the lumbar skin infection.*

The presence of a space-occupying lesion within the cranium, e.g., tumor, may greatly increase the CSF pressure, producing papilledema. In such conditions, LP is generally contraindicated because the rapid reduction in pressure caused by the removal of CSF can cause herniation of the brain structures into the foramen magnum. This, in turn, puts pressure on the vital centers in the medulla, e.g., the respiratory center, and could cause sudden death.

Should displacement of the brain cause sudden collapse, the emergency treatment consists of the establishment and maintenance of a patent airway, and resuscitation. Removal of CSF from the lateral ventricles may also be indicated.

Preparation of the Patient. Prior to the procedure, discuss it with the patient. *Even though a patient appears confused or stuporous, always give information about what is going to happen and what to expect next as the procedure is being performed.* The patient may want to know only that the doctor is going to take a small sample of spinal fluid from the lower spine. If the patient wants to know and is able to understand more details, before the procedure explain the following:

1. The patient's position will be side-lying with legs pulled close to the chin.
2. Movement by the patient during the procedure may cause injury; hence it is important to lie very still. (A restless patient may need to be held to prevent movement during the procedure.)
3. The procedure may be a little painful, but mostly there will be a feeling of pressure from the needle.
4. Brief, shooting pains may occur in the legs or hips if the needle touches nerves that run to these areas.
5. The doctor will give a little local anesthetic (usually 1 per cent xylocaine) in the area to help to reduce the discomfort caused by the needle.
6. The procedure takes only a few minutes to perform.
7. The needle is inserted well below the end of the spinal cord so there is no danger of the needle entering the spinal cord and causing damage.

If a signed permit is necessary for lumbar puncture in your facility, see that one has been obtained. Next assemble the equipment that will be needed. Clear a clean working area beside the treatment table or at the bedside and have the area well lighted. Usually hospitals have preassembled sterile spinal trays that contain most of the necessary equipment, e.g., needles, syringes, manometer, test tubes, and sponges. You may need to obtain local anesthetic, sterile gloves, the materials to surgically clean the puncture site, and a band aid to place over the puncture area after the procedure. Also you may need a laboratory slip and a marking pencil to number the specimens.

Just prior to the procedure, have the patient empty the bladder and bowels if possible.

Procedure. The patient is placed in a side-lying (lateral recumbent) position at the edge of the bed, with a pillow under the flank so that the spinous processes are horizontal. Placing the patient's back close to the edge of the bed makes the back readily accessible to the physician. Additional pillows may be placed between the patient's knees and under the head to keep the spine on a horizontal plane and facilitate patient comfort. The patient assumes a curved position to separate the vertebrae and increase the space between them so that the needle can be inserted more easily. (See Fig. 18–5, p. 403.)

The nurse often needs to assist the patient into a curled position. Ask the patient to draw the knees up to the chin. It may be necessary to hold a patient if the person finds it to difficult to maintain this position without help. The nurse usually stands in front of the patient and places one hand behind the patient's knees and the other on the upper shoulder, either as a reminder or as an aid to the patient in keeping the desired position. The nurse helps keep the patient's upper shoulder from falling forward, thus preventing rotation of the spine. It is important to remember that the patient may well be uncomfortable, tense, and frightened during a lumbar puncture. Keeping the patient's feelings in mind, the helpful nurse speaks to the patient throughout the procedure, acknowledging the patient's situation and promoting relaxation when possible, e.g., "breathe normally" or "breathe slowly through your mouth." Also, the nurse reminds the patient not to make sudden movements. Remember you will also be communicating with the patient nonverbally, e.g., through touch, facial expression, and tone of voice.

The physician wears sterile gloves when performing a spinal tap. The doctor may prepare the skin of the patient's back over the site to be punctured, or a nurse may be asked to do it. A sterile drape may or may not be used, depending upon the preference of the doctor. All equipment, including a spinal manometer for measuring the CSF pressure, is sterile.

With a small needle, syringe, and local anesthetic agent, the doctor anesthetizes the area and then introduces the large spinal needle with a stylus. The needle is inserted in adults about level with the top of the iliac crests (hip bones) or at the next level below (usually between the 3rd and 4th or 4th and 5th lumbar vertebrae). The spinal cord generally ends at the lower border of the 1st lumbar vertebra in adults. Thus the puncture site is low enough to avoid danger of injury to the spinal cord. A lumbar puncture for removal of a sample of cerebrospinal fluid (CSF) is described here;

the general principles apply to any LP procedure.

When the end of the needle has entered the subarachnoid space, the doctor removes the stylus and attaches a stopcock and manometer. The latter is used to measure "opening" CSF pressure before any fluid is removed.

In measuring the CSF pressure, the doctor watches how high the spinal fluid rises within the manometer's column. The doctor may say the pressure reading out loud so you can help to remember the figure. The doctor may ask you to steady the manometer or to help hold it straight. If you are not wearing sterile gloves, hold only the very top of the manometer with your fingers to steady it.

The first stabilized CFS pressure reading is called the *opening pressure.* (Normal opening CSF pressure with the patient in a horizontal position is 6 to 13 mm. Hg or 80 to 180 mm. of H_2O. Pressures over 200 mm. of H_2O are considered abnormal.) Normally the CSF oscillates in the manometer, readily responding to coughing, straining, and changes in the patient's breathing.

In collecting *specimens of CSF* the doctor allows the fluid to drip into a series of small sterile test tubes, numbered in sequence of col-

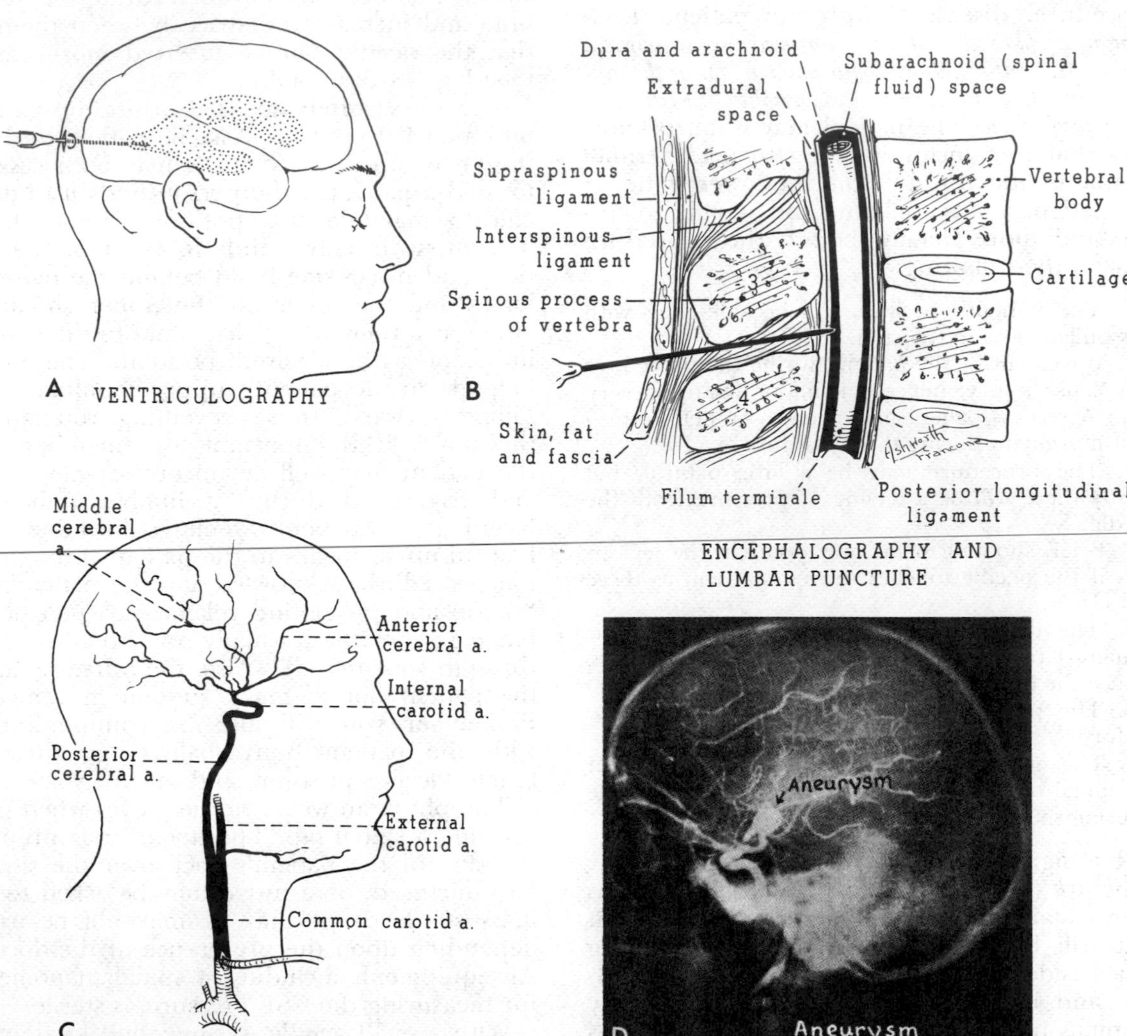

Figure 25-4. A. *Ventriculography:* An opening is made in the skull in the parieto-occipital region and a needle is introduced into the lateral ventricle. The cerebrospinal fluid is slowly withdrawn and replaced by air and x-ray examinations are made.

B. *Encephalography:* X-ray examination of the brain is made following replacement of cerebrospinal fluid by air via the lumbar puncture route. *Lumbar puncture:* Tapping of the subarachnoid space in the lumbar region, usually between the third and fourth lumbar vertebrae.

C. *Cerebral angiography:* X-ray examination of the vascular system of the brain is made after the injection of radiopaque material into the common carotid artery.

D. *Lateral angiogram,* to illustrate aneurysms of the internal carotid artery in the neck and of the middle cerebral artery. (**A, B,** and **C** from Jacob, S. W., C. A. Francone, and W. J. Lossow: *Structure and Function in Man,* Philadelphia: W. B. Saunders Company, 4th ed. 1978, p. 249. **D** from Vick, N. A.: *Grinker's Neurology,* 7th ed. Springfield, Ill.: Charles C Thomas, 1976, p. 71.)

lection, e.g., No. 1, No. 2, and No. 3. Two to three ml. of fluid is collected in each tube. A total of 8 to 10 ml. may be removed. If you are handed filled tubes, take care not to contaminate the doctor's gloves or the sterile field. Since CSF may contain highly virulent organisms, e.g., those causing meningitis, handle the specimens carefully, taking care not to contaminate yourself or other patients. Wash thoroughly immediately after handling specimen tubes.

Post-Procedure Activities. Following the LP, chart that the procedure was performed, the time, the doctor's name, and how the patient tolerated the procedure. In addition, chart the amount and character of fluid removed and the specimens sent to the laboratory. Record any significant reactions to the procedure relative to the patient's pulse, coloring, and respirations. Also note the presence of such reactions as nausea, vomiting, urinary retention, and headache. If the patient has a known intracranial disorder, carefully follow the vital signs and observe for changes in the level of consciousness.

Specimens of CSF should be taken *directly* to a clinical laboratory so they can be examined as quickly as possible. If allowed to stand, changes take place in the fluid that alter the findings.

When it is necessary to perform an LP on a patient with known or possible increased intracranial pressure, the manometer is connected to a stopcock and filled with saline to prevent rapid loss of large amounts of CSF. As mentioned, one of the herniation syndromes may occur in the presence of increased intracranial pressures (see Chapter 26). Herniation does not always occur immediately during or after lumbar puncture. Therefore, *patients at risk need to be watched closely for several hours.* Progression of existing neurologic symptoms or development of new ones is reported to the physician immediately. Should a problem occur, it is generally treated with dehydrating agents (see discussion of increased intracranial pressure).

> *Various problems may occur after LP. The sudden collapse of vital centers, due to herniation syndrome, is the most crucial.*

It has been estimated that one out of four patients suffers some kind of sequelae from LP, including the following: transient difficulty in voiding; temperature elevation preceded by meningeal irritation; local pain, edema, or hematoma resulting from trauma at the puncture site; and pain radiating to the thigh, caused by nerve root irritation. An additional problem following LP is headache.

POSTPUNCTURE HEADACHE. Postlumbar-puncture headache (*spinal-puncture headache; spinal headache*), typically bifrontal and suboccipital, appears a few hours to several days after the procedure. This headache is characteristically relieved when the patient is lying down but resumes when the patient sits up. Post-puncture headache is worsened by a sudden jolt of the head and by jugular compression. Usually the headache is of a throbbing nature. Although such headaches frequently disappear within 24 hours, they may last for several days. The precise etiology of postpuncture headaches is unknown. The most probable cause is thought to be related to continuing leakage of CSF through the opening in the dura made by the needle insertion.

It has been found that postpuncture headaches do not occur more often in patients who are ambulatory following the procedure than in those who are conservatively treated with bed rest. Nonetheless, while most physicians believe it unnecessary to keep a patient in bed following LP, others try various measures to prevent postpuncture headache. Some doctors order recumbency in bed for various lengths of time, e.g., 12 to 24 hours following LP. If the patient is to remain flat, immediately place a sign on the bed to inform all staff members and visitors of this order. Remember, of course, to also tell the patient.

Once a post-puncture headache begins, various treatments may be ordered. Commonly the patient is placed on bed rest in a quiet darkened room, and analgesic medications are administered as ordered. Increasing oral fluid intake may also help to reestablish the CSF level.

Queckenstedt Test (Spinal Dynamics; CSF Pressure Readings; Manometric Tests). This procedure is carried out when the physician suspects compression of the spinal cord, e.g., due to the presence of a spinal tumor, or following dislocation or fracture of vertebrae. These disorders may produce partial or complete blockage of CSF circulation in the spinal subarachnoid space. The physician looks for indications of such obstruction by noting the manner in which CSF pressure readings vary following timed compression of the jugular veins on each side of the neck. (Consult a textbook of neurologic nursing for details concerning this test.) Performance of the Queckenstedt test is contraindicated in the presence of intracranial disease, particularly in the presence of indications of hemorrhage or increased intracranial pressure.

Cisternal Puncture

Cisternal puncture is puncture of the cisterna magna (the small reservoir of CSF between the cerebellum and the medulla). It is done by the introduction of a short-beveled needle below the occipital bone and between the first cervical lamina and the rim of the foramen magnum. The CSF may be tapped in this manner to drain CSF or to obtain a CSF specimen if there is a block in the spinal subarachnoid space or if lumbar puncture is contraindicated. Cisternal punture may also be done to perform encephalography, to inject air or dye for myelography or for other reasons.

Preparation of a patient for cisternal puncture includes explaining the procedure and obtaining an informed consent. The nape of the patient's neck may be ordered shaved up to the external occipital protuberance in the midline. Because this puncture is closer to the brain than a lumbar puncture, patients are frequently even more fearful. Individualized supportive and anxiety-reducing measures are very important. The patient's cooperation is necessary. Thus, along with offering other appropriate teaching, the nurse instructs the patient not to move during the procedure.

The patient is positioned at the edge of the treatment table or the bed, in a side-long position. A sandbag is slipped under the patient's head to keept the cervical spine and head in a straight line with the thoracic spine. The patient's head is flexed forward and held firmly in position by the nurse. Following skin preparation, as for lumbar puncture, a local anesthetic may or may not be injected. Then a cisternal needle with stylet in place is inserted to a depth of about 5 cm. (Fig. 25–5). The subsequent procedures are essentially the same as with lumbar puncture.

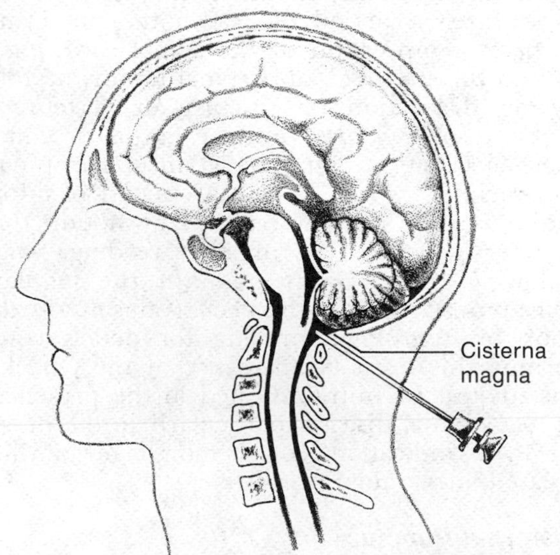

Figure 25–5. Position of needle for cisternal puncture. Note short bevel and length of needle.

Usually post-puncture headache does not follow cisternal puncture. However, *immediately following the procedure the patient should be observed for apnea, cyanosis, and dyspnea*. These complications are rare; typically the patient is able to assume prepuncture activities soon after the cisternal puncture is completed.

Laboratory Examination of Cerebrospinal Fluid

A few helpful "rules of thumb" concerning cerebrospinal fluid (CSF) laboratory findings are as follows:

- *Blood.* Many red blood cells (RBC) in the CSF indicate hemorrhage somewhere in the central nervous system, e.g., torn or ruptured blood vessels from injury or a ruptured aneurysm. *Xanthochromia* (a yellow color from old blood) of the spinal fluid implies bleeding unless there is a high serum bilirubin.
- *Increased white blood cells (WBC)* may indicate infection somewhere in the CNS. For example, polymorphonuclear leukocytes may be increased as a result of pyogenic infection; increased lymphocytes may occur with viral infections and tuberculosis. If extremely large numbers of cells are present, the CSF may actually appear cloudy.
- *Lowered blood sugar* often results from bacterial infections of the CNS.
- *Lowered chloride level* also often results from bacterial infections of the CNS.
- *Increased protein level* occurs in the presence of many neurologic disorders, e.g., brain tumors.

Cerebral Angiography, Pneumoencephalography, Ventriculography, and Ventricular Puncture

Cerebral angiography, pneumoencephalography, and ventriculography are all *contrast studies* used in neuroradiology.

1. *Cerebral angiography* is visualization of the brain's vascular system by injection of a contrast dye into the circulating blood.
2. *Pneumoencephalography* is visualization of the brain's ventricles and subarachnoid spaces (i.e., the CSF spaces in and around the brain) by withdrawal of CSF and the injection of air or oxygen into the spinal subarachnoid space through a lumbar puncture.
3. *Ventriculography* is the visualization of the brain's ventricles by removal of CSF and injection of air or oxygen directly into the ventricles through burr holes in the skull.

Certain guidelines typically apply to all of these diagnostic tests:

- The procedure is discussed with the patient and significant others as appropriate. The physician discusses the purpose for the procedure and any risks involved with the patient's significant others and the patient.
- A signed permit is required.
- Prior to these procedures, vital signs are taken and recorded to establish a baseline of information. Additionally, the size and reaction of the patient's pupils, facial symmetry, level of consciousness, and the motion and strength of the extremities should be ascertained and the observations charted for similar control purposes. These same points are evaluated periodically by the nurse following the procedure.
- A general anesthetic is usually not given for these procedures unless the patient is a child or a very restless adult. (For discussion of the care of patients following general anesthesia see Unit VIII.).
- For some of these procedures the patient is prepared as for surgery, e.g., food and fluids are withheld for 6 hours, and premedication, such as atropine sulfate and an analgesic, is administered. (See Unit VIII.) Indeed, surgery sometimes does immediately follow the diagnostic procedure, especially a pneumoencephalogram.
- Emergency equipment and drugs must be readily available because these diagnostic tests may produce respiratory distress and shock.

Cerebral angiography, pneumoencephalography, and ventriculography are all potentially hazardous procedures. The contrast dyes used in angiography may be irritating to the vessels, and since the dye is a foreign substance, some patients may experience allergic reactions and possibly go into anaphylactic shock as a result of sensitivity to the dye. Likewise, the gases (air or oxygen) injected during pneumoencephalography or ventriculography are foreign substances and can cause irritative cellular reactions.

Cerebral Angiography. A cerebral angiogram allows x-ray visualization of the brain's vascular system during the injection of a radiopaque material into the arterial system. Complete angiograms include the arterial, capillary, and venous phases. Sometimes, however, only the arteries are visualized (see Fig. 25–4).

Angiography is preferred to air studies (i.e., pneumoencephalography and ventriculography) because it has a lower mortality rate and is less traumatizing. In an attempt to prevent an anaphylactic shock reaction (as a result of sensitivity to the radiopaque material), a sensitivity test may be performed the day prior to the angiogram.

There are several ways to inject the arterial system in order to perform cerebral angiography via a closed method. Direct injection of the common carotid (a *percutaneous carotid arteriogram*) or injection of the brachial artery (*retrograde brachial approach*) with insertion of a catheter into the artery are commonly done. More frequently, however, insertion of a catheter through a needle into the *femoral artery* yields a more satisfactory study. The catheter is passed under fluoroscopic control into the descending aorta and from there into the desired vessels in the head.

Once the appropriate vessel has been reached, the contrast material is injected and a series of films are rapidly taken from both lateral (Lat) and anterior-posterior (AP) approaches. The sequential films are helpful in diagnosing such disorders as aneurysms, arteriovenous malformations, blood vessel tumors, and occlusive vascular diseases, among others. The location, size, and distribution of the blood supply to a brain tumor can also often be seen. Subdural and epidural hematomas are commonly diagnosed with arteriograms.

Upon completion of angiography, after the needle is removed, a sterile sponge is placed over the puncture site and firm pressure is kept on the area for 10 minutes in an attempt to prevent hematoma formation. Later an ice bag may be ordered for the injection site to minimize swelling and discomfort. The injection site may be tender and slightly swollen.

Angiography is generally well tolerated although it may be frightening and painful. Untoward reactions rarely occur, but when they do they usually take place during the procedure or immediately following it.

Untoward reactions can include local and/or systemic allergic reactions to the contrast material; spasm or occlusion of the vessel by a clot; hemorrhage; and obstructive clot formation above a femoral injection site. Reactions to the contrast material vary from unpleasant warmth and flushing during injection to an allergic reaction requiring that the study be discontinued and the patient immediately treated. (Anaphylactic reactions are discussed in Chapter 11.) Spasm or occlusion of the target vessel(s) causes symptoms similar to those seen with a stroke (see discussion of strokes, p. 610). Clot formation at the injection site also causes ischemic signs and symptoms of the affected area. All of these adverse reactions are usually reversible, however they may rarely cause a patient to have permanent damage.

Symptoms of untoward reactions vary depending on their cause or causes. For example, indications of centrally located reactions may include: changes in level of consciousness (LOC), aphasia, hemiplegia, hemiparesis, convulsive seizures, or an increase in focal symptoms. A local hematoma in the neck may cause difficulty in breathing or swallowing. If such a hematoma is large, it may compress the trachea and esophagus. Emergency tracheostomy may be necessary. Nausea, vomiting, numbness or weakness of the extremities, speech disturbances, profuse sweating, and alterations in LOC may indicate delayed reaction to the contrast material.

Following angiography, the patient is positioned safely and comfortably and is kept at bed rest for as long as the physician deems necessary (often about 12 hours). The injection site is checked frequently for bleeding and/or formation of a hematoma. The affected extremity (arm or leg) or neck is kept straight to prevent kinking of the vessel, with clot formation. Vital signs, the pulses distal to the injection, the color, temperature, and ability to move the distal extremity are all checked frequently at first and less frequently over the next day or so. A regular diet can usually be resumed immediately, and activity is resumed after the prescribed period of bed rest.

Pneumoencephalogram. With the advent of newer technology (e.g., computerized axial tomography), the pneumoencephalography (PEG, "pneumo") is infrequently performed. This is fortunate indeed since the newer studies are safe and less traumatic for the patient. PEG is usually a painful, frightening experience for patients and it may be hazardous.

A pneumoencephalogram is a special contrast study which allows visualization of the brain's subarachnoid space and ventricles. A lumbar puncture is performed with the patient sitting up and then air or oxygen is injected into the spinal subarachnoid space. The air rises, allowing x-ray visualization of the ventricles and intracranial subarachnoid space. As air is injected, the patient feels it rising up the spine into the head. During the procedure the blood pressure of the patient is closely monitored. As the patient's head is frequently repositioned, the patient hears the "sloshing" sounds of air moving in the ventricles.

Pneumoencephalography is useful in diagnosing tumors adjacent to the ventricular system and congenital malformations of the brain such as cysts and in detecting atrophy of the cerebral and cerebellar cortex.

In the presence of an intracranial mass, the pneumoencephalogram can have the same untoward complication as can lumbar puncture. Withdrawal of a large amount of CSF can cause downward dislocation of the medulla into the foramen magnum (one of the herniation syndromes). This can result in severe depression of respiration, and possibly death.

If an intracranial mass lesion is found or if the PEG causes dangerous pressure shifts intracranially, immediate surgey is performed to avoid the possibility of herniation. Preoperative permission is thus routinely obtained for both PEG and craniotomy.

While herniation is uncommon, a headache following PEG is very common. It varies from mild to severe and may last for several days. Headache may be accompanied by signs of meningeal irritation, such as a stiff neck, photophobia, and by nausea, vomiting, and lightheadedness. Blood pressure changes are common, and the patient needs careful monitoring. Mild chills and a low-grade fever may occur.

Post-procedure care includes the following: careful, frequent monitoring of the vital and neurologic signs, bedrest for about 48 hours, increasing oral fluids (the patient often receives intravenous fluids during the early stages), and the use of analgesics and antiemetics as appropriate. It is a challenge to a nurse to keep a patient comfortable in the post-procedure phase of care following PEG. A quiet, darkened environment may give some comfort.

Special positioning measures may be advisable following PEG. It is commonly recommended that the patient be kept flat in bed without a pillow for 12 to 24 hours following the procedure. Of course, items the patient may need should be placed within reach. Because the injected air is light, it tends to pocket in the uppermost ventricle. The ventricle has no method for absorption. Thus, to hasten the passage of the air from the ventricles into the CSF circulation, the patient should turn from side to side (while flat) at least every 2 hours. Because rolling over is painful, especially during the first few post-procedure hours, you will need to encourage the patient and assist in rolling smoothly. Naturally, sudden, jarring movements increase discomfort. It may be helpful to explain to the patient that the rolling over speeds up recovery from the procedure. Once the intracranial air is absorbed and is replaced with CSF, the post-procedure headache subsides. Generally this takes 24 to 36 hours. When air is present in the ventricles, the patient temporarily hears "noises" in the head. This symptom may be increased during movement. Although aggravating, these swooshing noises gradually disappear as the gas is absorbed and replaced with CSF.

Once it is time to begin elevating the patient's head, the head of the bed is generally elevated *slowly* and progressively, a little every few hours. If nausea and headache increase when the patient is up, they are generally relieved by resumption of a flat position.

Initial care may involve prevention of aspiration of vomitus. Also, during the initial period following the procedure, the nurse observes the patient carefully for indications of increased intracranial pressure and other indications of possible untoward reactions such as seizures, shock, sustained vomiting, respiratory difficulty, chills, or fever.

Ventriculogram and Ventricular Puncture. This is another contrast study in which air is injected. With this procedure, air is injected directly into the ventricles of the brain. A needle is passed through a small twist drill hole in the skull, through the brain substance and into one of the lateral ventricles (see Fig. 25–4).

The term *ventricular puncture* refers to the insertion of a special short-beveled ventricular needle directly into the lateral ventricle. In adults it is necessary to make a small scalp incision and a small twist drill hole in the skull through which the needle may be inserted. This drilling is not necessary in infants; the needle with stylet is pushed through the infant's scalp and anterior fontanel. A ventricular puncture is required for a ventriculogram.

This study is also not commonly done. The indications include cases where pneumoencephalogram is contraindicated (and the more modern studies are not useful), such as in the case of a mass lesion with increased intracranial pressure or blockage of the CSF circulation above the lumbar area.

Complications can include hemorrhage from an injured blood vessel, ventriculitis from the introduction of an organism, and transient blindness from damage to the optic radiations.

After the procedure, the patient's head is elevated 15 to 20 degrees, and bedrest is prescribed for about 24 hours. The vital signs are monitored frequently, and the needle entry site if covered with a sterile dressing. Prevention of infection in the area of insertion is imperative, since the route of infection leads directly into the brain.

Some of the serious complications that may occur following ventriculography are shock, respiratory collapse, hemorrhage, and increasing intracranial pressure. A lumbar puncture tray may be kept at the patient's bedside so the doctor can immediately perform a spinal tap if the CSF pressure suddenly increases.

Analgesics and an ice bag may be ordered to relieve headache. Fluids and food are given as tolerated. The head of the bed is elevated further as tolerated on the day following the procedure.

A variation of this procedure is the insertion of a tube (a pediatric feeding tube may be used) to allow intracranial pressure to be monitored, and in the face of increased intracranial pressure (in specific instances), to establish a continuous opportunity for excess CSF to drain. This procedure can be done in a variety of ways, and care of the patient requires detailed understanding of the particular system used to lower the intracranial pressure. In any event, *continuous drainage* puts the patient at risk for developing an infection, so meticulous aseptic principles must be followed. Moreover, blockage of the system or malfunction allowing too much fluid to drain rapidly or allowing fluid to return to the ventricles must be avoided. *If you encounter a continuous drainage system, it is essential that you learn how it works before undertaking the care of the patient.*

Myelography

Myelography is the x-ray examination of the spinal cord and vertebral canal following introduction of contrast media into the spinal subarachnoid space. It is used to study the spinal canal and subarachnoid space. This is a particularly valuable diagnostic procedure when the spinal cord is believed to be compressed, e.g., by herniated intervertebral disk or tumor encroaching on the spinal subarachnoid space. It is also useful in diagnosing such spinal cord pathology as intramedullary tumors, syringomyelia, and arteriovenous malformations. Arachnoiditis, an inflammation of arachnoidal tissue which often produces symptoms similar to those seen with herniated disks, can be detected by myelography. Myelography is rarely used to identify traumatic lesions of the vertebra or spinal cord, since the procedure could aggravate the injury.

Discography may be performed as a diagnostic procedure in a suspected rupture of an intervertebral disk. This is radiographic visualization of a disk by injection of an absorbable contrast medium directly into the disk.

Special preparation is not usually necessary for a myelogram. The patient is given a clear explanation of the procedure and is asked to sign a consent form.

In a radiology department, a lumbar puncture is performed, a small amount of cerebrospinal fluid is withdrawn, and the contrast material is injected. While the needle is left in place, and the patient is placed on the abdomen. The patient is secured to the radiology table by foot and shoulder supports. While the radiologist follows carefully with fluoroscopy, the table is slowly tilted to allow the column of dye to move up or down within the subarachnoid space, permitting visualization of the desired areas. Standard films are taken of these areas. If pathology of the posterior fossa is suspected, the dye is allowed to enter the posterior fossa to outline that area also. When the necessary information has been obtained, the contrast material is pooled into the area of the needle and as much as possible of it is aspirated under fluoroscopy. Some of the most recently developed types of contrast media can be absorbed by the body and so do not have to be removed. Irritation of nerve roots during the withdrawal of the contrast media is often painful.

After a myelogram, the patient is usually kept flat in bed for 6 to 8 hours and then gradually resumes normal activity. Back pain in the area of the needle insertion may occur, lasting only a few days. Particularly if the contrast material has been allowed to rise to high thoracic or cervical levels, the patient may experience stiff neck and headache for a few days. This is much less severe than with a PEG and is usually relieved by mild analgesics.

Electroencephalogram (EEG)

Simply stated, the EEG is a measurement of the brain's electrical activity. It "provides a visible record, in the form of wave patterns, of the electrical potentials generated from neuronal activity within the brain."[291a] This is done by attaching a varying number of electrodes to standard locations on the scalp (Fig. 25–6). These electrodes are attached to a recording machine, which amplifies the electrical activity and records it on moving paper.

Electroencephalograms can be taken in the office or laboratory or at the patient's bedside, if necessary, with lightweight, compact, wheeled instruments. Once a record of brain wave activity is obtained, specialists interpret the record according to the brain wave's characteristics, frequency, and amplitude.

The patient should be given a careful explanation of the procedure, with special attention to allaying fears and apprehensions. Assure the

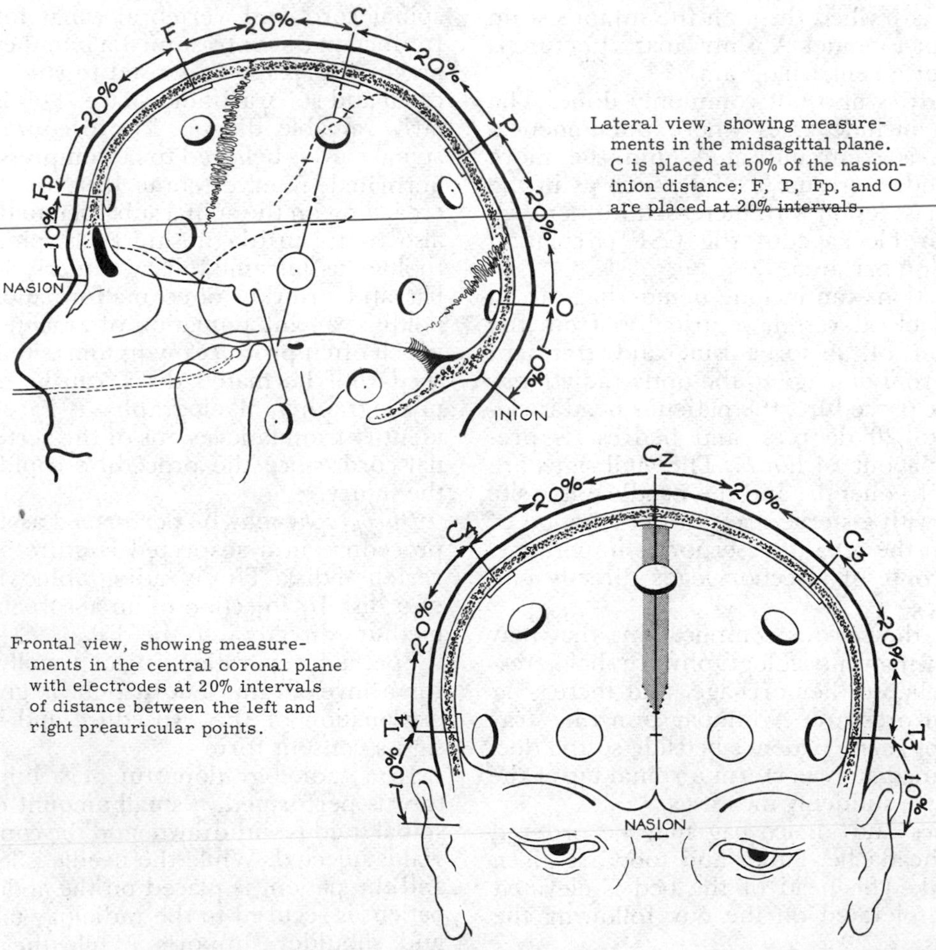

Figure 25–6. Electrode placements in the "ten twenty" electrode system. (Fp = frontal pole. F = frontal. C = central. P = parietal. O = occipital.) (From Chusid, J. G., and J. J. McDonald: *Correlative Neuroanatomy and Functional Neurology*, 13th ed. Los Altos, Calif.: Lange Medical Publications, 1967, p. 228.)

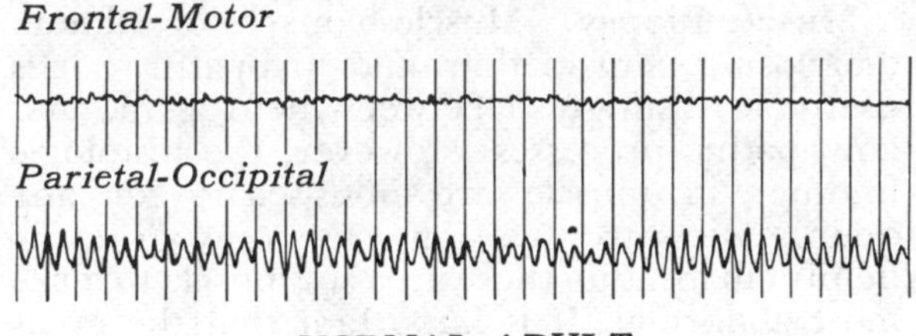

NORMAL ADULT
10/sec. activity in occipital area

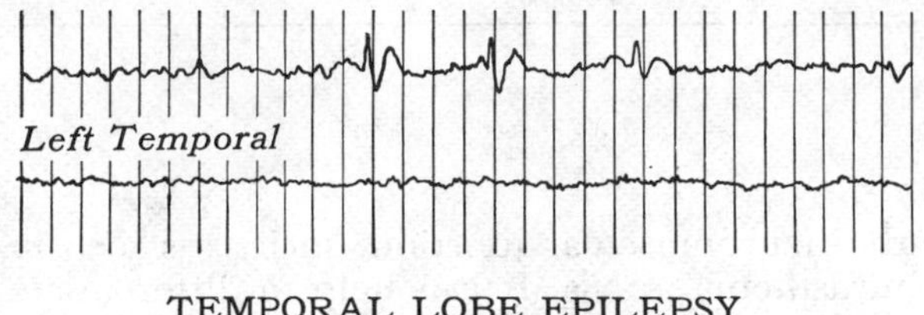

TEMPORAL LOBE EPILEPSY
Right temporal spike focus

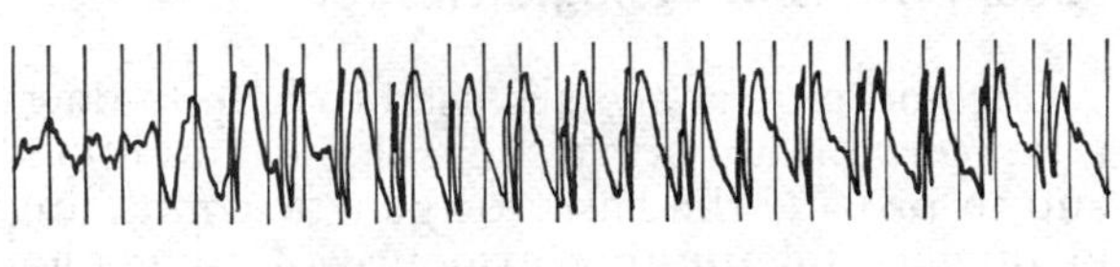

PETIT MAL SEIZURE
Synchronous 3/sec. spikes & waves

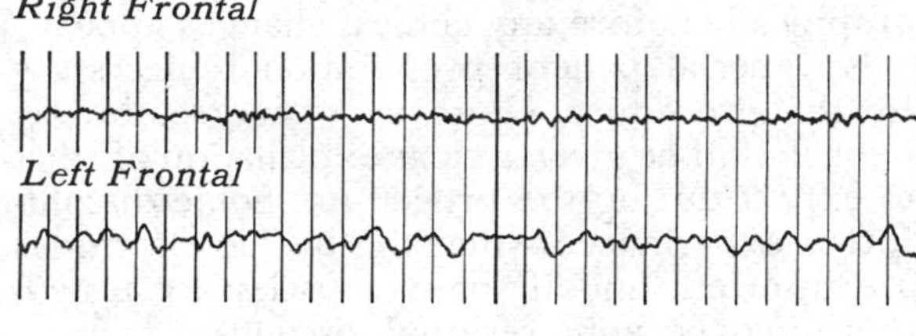

BRAIN TUMOR
Left frontal slow wave focus

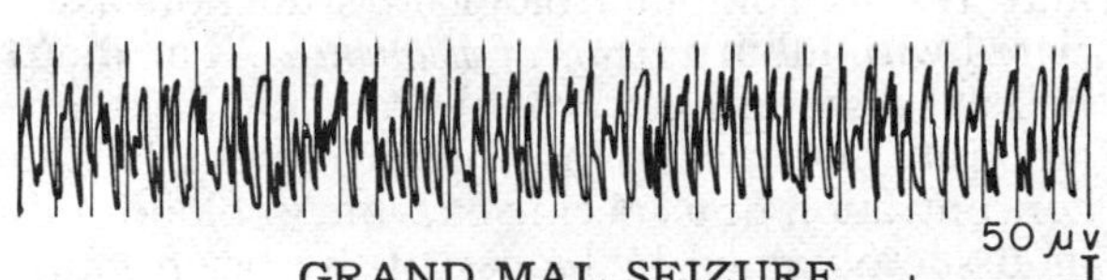

50 μv
1 sec.

GRAND MAL SEIZURE
High voltage spikes, generalized

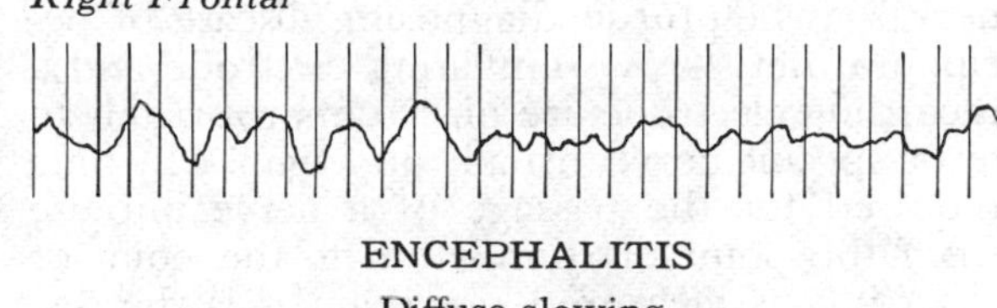

ENCEPHALITIS
Diffuse slowing

Figure 25–7. Examples of normal and abnormal EEG's. (From Berkow, R., et al. (Eds.): *The Merck Manual,* Rahway, N.J.: Merck Sharp and Dohme, 13th edition, 1977.)

patient that an electric shock will not occur during the procedure and that the machine is not able to "read the mind."

Prior to the procedure the technician cleans the scalp and applies the electrodes to the scalp with collodion or tiny pins inserted into the scalp. Some discomfort is experienced with pin insertion. The procedure is performed with the patient lying on a bed in a quiet room with subdued lighting. During the recording the patient rests and relaxes. At certain times, the patient may be asked to hyperventilate, or the technician may rhythmically flash a bright light in front of the eyes—both of these stimuli can evoke or accentuate certain abnormal wave patterns.

Often the doctor also requests a sleep recording. For this the patient is given a sedative, such as chloral hydrate, and the recording continues: (a) while the patient is falling asleep, (b) while asleep, and (c) while waking up. Some abnormalities that are not seen when the patient is awake become evident during sleep.

After an EEG, which takes approximately 1 hour, the patient can return to previous normal activity. Assist the patient in using acetone to remove the collodian from the hair and scalp. The scalp may remain sore for several days if pins were inserted.

EEG is particularly useful in evaluating patients with any type of seizure disorder. It can also be helpful in localizing tumors. The EEG is diffusely abnormal in various metabolic disturbances, toxic conditions (i.e., drug overdose), and infections such as meningitis and encephalitis. Normal and abnormal EEG's are shown in Figure 25–7.

Electromyography (EMG)

Electromyography is a diagnostic procedure that measures and records the electric currents produced by skeletal muscles, called "muscle action potentials." The instrument used is the *electromyograph.* The procedure involves insertion of a small needle electrode into a muscle. The electric potentials of that muscle are recorded, amplified, transmitted to an oscilloscope, and displayed on a screen. The recording can also be made audible at the same time and can be recorded on paper (Fig. 25–8).

EMG can give objective information especially valuable in diagnosing various neuromuscular diseases. It is helpful in differentiating between primary muscle disease and that which is secondary to denervation. EMG aids in determining specific types of primary muscle disease. It may give evidence of a defect in transmission at the neuromuscular junction, such as is seen in myasthenia gravis. It can help to differentiate diseases of the anterior horn cells from those primarily of the peripheral nerves. Frequently, the processes of peripheral nerve degeneration and regeneration can be monitored electromyographically before any clinical changes appear.

No special patient preparation is necessary for this procedure. However, of course, the patient should be given a clear explanation of what to expect during the procedure. Some discomfort is experienced when the needle electrodes are inserted, and if many muscles are tested, there may be some residual discomfort.

A procedure frequently done in conjunction with the EMG is the *nerve conduction study*. This procedure, which studies the excitability and conduction velocities of motor and sensory nerves, is helpful in diagnosing disease of peripheral nerves. A stimulating electrode and a recording electrode are placed appropriately to test a specific nerve, usually on a limb. The time required for the passage of a nerve impulse from the point of stimulation to the point of recording is measured precisely, as is the distance from stimulation to recording on the patient's limb. From this information, the conduction velocity is calculated. Both motor and sensory modalities are altered in disorders of the peripheral nervous system such as the carpal tunnel syndrome, whereas only motor fibers are affected in chronic diseases of the anterior horn cell or motor nerve roots.

The patient will experience the discomfort of mild electric shock during the procedure, but there should be no sequelae.

Muscle Biopsy. Muscle biopsy is of value in diagnosing neuropathies and myopathies. It is useful to distinguish between neurogenic and amyopathic processes. However, the histologic findings in muscle are nonspecific for any neurogenic atrophy. An electromyogram is helpful in locating those areas of muscle that are most abnormal. It is important that the areas that have actually been traumatized by the needle electrodes be avoided when tissue is taken for biopsy.

Special Tests of Biologic Tissues

Chromosome analysis is used to help to diagnose certain abnormal neurologic conditions and to provide the basis for genetic counseling in families manifesting evidence of congenital neurologic malformations. Chromosomes can be prepared for microscopic examination from the tissue culture of cells obtained from peripheral blood, bone marrow, or skin.

Mental retardation and/or *convulsive seizures* may result from neurologic dysfunction associated with inborn *errors of metabolism*. The diagnosis of disorders of carbohydrate and lipid metabolism may necessitate measurement of the concentration of a specific enzyme in blood cells or tissue obtained by biopsy of the brain, muscle, liver, or peripheral nerve. Usually disorders of protein metabolism are indicated by increased amounts of particular amino acids in the urine or blood.

Echoencephalography

Echoencephalography is a diagnostic technique that utilizes sound. In 1956 it was first demonstrated that by passing a beam of pulsed ultrasound through the head in the temporo-

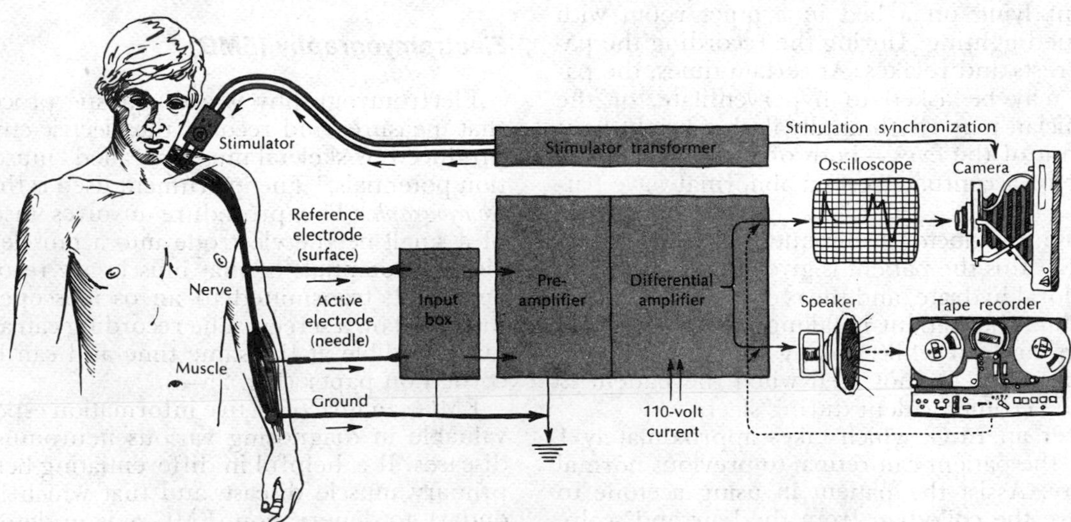

Figure 25–8. The instrument and attachments for recording neuromuscular electrophysiology. (From Spiegel, M. B.: Electromyoneurography. *American Family Physician,* 18:119, Nov. 1978.)

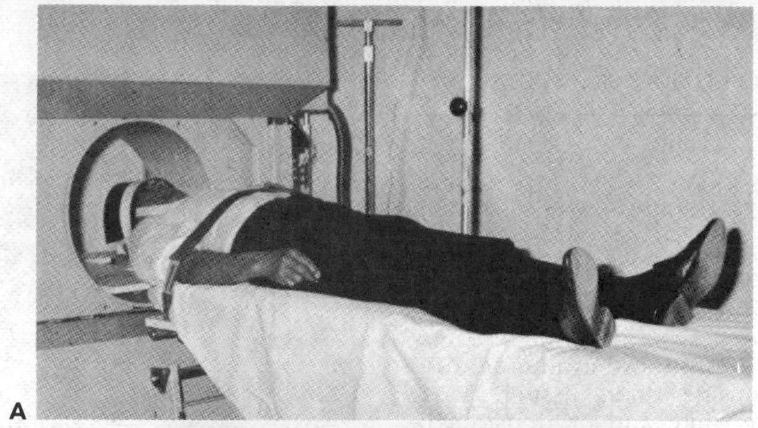

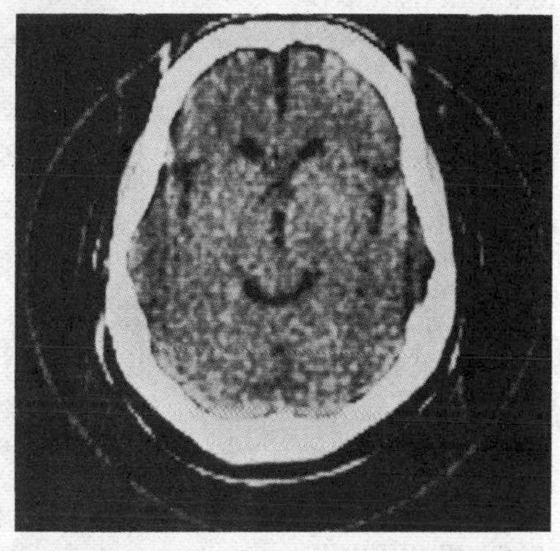

Figure 25–9. Computerized tomography of the brain. **A.** Because the equipment looks formidable, the person undergoing a CT examination may be anxious or frightened. The nurse can give reassurance that other than the need to be perfectly still, the patient will experience no pain or discomfort. **B.** Polaroid photograph of an EMI scan. (*A* from Korten, K.: Anesthesia for diagnostic purposes. American Family Physician, 15:3, Mar. 1977. *B* from Reeves, K. R.: This CAT is a revolutionary scanner. *RN*, 39:41, Aug. 1976.)

parietal region, and recording the returning echoes, it was possible to measure the position of structures in the cerebral midline and to determine whether these had been displaced to one or the other side of the midline by deforming intracranial disease. The midline structures, especially the lateral walls of the third ventricle but also some other structures, send back echoes that can be used to determine the presence or absence of displacement of these structures.

Computerized Tomography

Computerized tomography (CT scan, also termed *computerized axial tomography* or *CAT scan*) is a unique relatively new radiologic method that has drastically changed neurodiagnosis. It provides three-dimensional views of the cranial contents. In many institutions, it has appreciably decreased the use of brain scanning and has caused a dramatic reduction in the use of the pneumoencephalogram (Fig. 25–9).

Several types of equipment are now available, but the first available commercially was the EMI scanner (EMI, Ltd., Hayes Middlesex, England). This scanner, still the most widely used across the United States, is discussed here, although the general principles are the same with all equipment.

No special preparation of the patient is necessary except that wigs and any clips and pins are removed from the patient's head. No food or fluid for 4 to 6 hours prior to the scan is sometimes ordered because the contrast medium can cause nausea. A clear explanation of the procedure to the patient is particularly vital. While a CT scan is a noninvasive procedure and is safe for the patient, it can be frightening because of the complexity of the machine and the position required during the procedure. The person should be asked about any known allergy to iodine.

The patient is asked to lie on a table in front of the scanner. A wide rubberized band is wrapped very snugly around the head, from the forehead to the occipital area. The patient's head is then placed into an opening in the scanner, which is adjusted to fit snugly around the rubberized band. The patient is made comfortable in this position and reminded to *lie very still* during the scanning. Even slight movement of the head can cause distortion in the EEG recording. The patient is in a room alone during the examination and is observed by a technician from a control room. The patient can speak to the technician through an intercom system.

The scanner takes cross-sectional pictures of the brain in a modified coronal plane. When the scanner is in position, a small beam of x-ray is passed through the brain from one side to the other. The image is recorded on a detector on the opposite side. The computer calculates the amount of x-ray absorbed in the various brain tissues and produces a printout of the information, which is then reproduced as photographs showing varying densities of the tissues. Dense substances appear as white, and low-density substances show as dark, with varying shades of gray in between. The machine then rotates 1 degree, and the procedure is repeated. This is done at each degree through an entire 180-degree arc. One complete rotation takes about 5 minutes.

The machine is then moved down about 2 cm. and the whole procedure is repeated, to a total of five "cuts." The computer images can be seen immediately on a viewing screen, and the pictures are available within minutes for a permanent record. The computer is able to detect differences in radiation absorption, and hence differences in tissue densities, that are too subtle to be picked up by conventional x-ray examination.

Usually the patient is then given an intravenous injection of an iodine-containing contrast material and the entire scan is repeated, with "*contrast enhancement*." An entire scan, with and without enhancement, takes about 1 hour. Following the procedure, the patient may return to all previous activities.

The CT scan is especially helpful in detecting brain tumors, both primary and metastatic, except those of the posterior fossa. In diagnosing vascular lesions, it is particularly helpful in detecting large aneurysms, infarctions, intracranial hemorrhage and hematomas, subarachnoid hemorrhage, acute subdural hematomas, and arteriovenous malformations (after enhancement). It is also of great value in demonstrating hydrocephalus and cerebral atrophy.

Essentially the only risk involved is the possibility of allergic reaction to the iodine dye. The amount of radiation received by the patient during the procedure is approximately equivalent to that with a conventional skull x-ray examination.

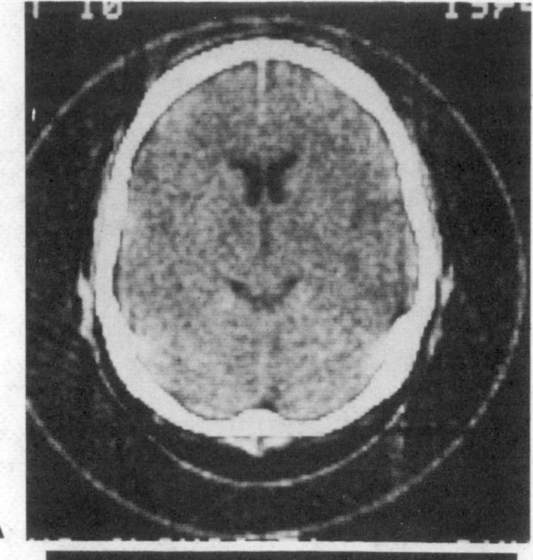

A

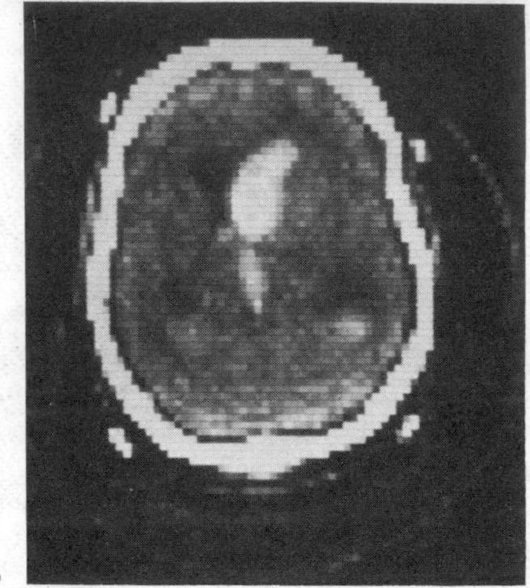

B

Figure 25–10. **A.** Normal scan at the level of the quadrigeminal cistern. **B.** Scan showing a hematoma in the right hemisphere with extension into the lateral ventricle. (From Mayo Clinic and Mayo Foundation: *Clinical Examinations in Neurology.* Philadelphia: W. B. Saunders Co., 1976, p. 272.)

Brain Scan

A brain scan is a useful ancillary test frequently used early in the diagnostic process in patients suspected of having a brain tumor, brain abscess or such cerebrovascular problems as subdural hematoma, arteriovenous malformation, or intracerebral hemorrhage (Fig. 25–10).

In the nuclear medicine department the patient is given an intravenous injection of a radioactive isotope. After a suitable delay, the patient is positioned on a table with the head directly beneath a scintillation scanner. The isotope accumulates in areas of abnormal or damaged brain tissue, and the radiation emitted is recorded by the scanner. Recording is done in anteroposterior (AP) and lateral positions and the areas of pathology show up as well-defined areas of abnormal uptake. The total scanning procedure requires 1 to 2 hours.

Brain scanning is an innocuous procedure. Apart from a clear explanation of the procedure, no special patient preparation is necessary. Assure the patient that the radioactive substance will be excreted from the body within 24 hours and that the amount of radiation received during a brain scan is less than that received with a regular skull x-ray examination.

Caloric Tests

The *oculovestibular* reflex or "caloric test"[63] is a diagnostic examination that provides information about the function of the vestibular portion of the eighth cranial nerve. Its purpose is to aid in the differential diagnosis of lesions in the cerebellum and brain stem.

The test is done by introducing either cold or hot water into the external auditory canal. A current then flows through the endolymphatic fluid. Typically, when the vestibular eighth cranial nerve is normal, stimulation of the auditory canal with *hot* water produces a rotary nystagmus *toward* the side of the irrigated ear. When *cold* water is used, the normal response is rotary nystagmus *away* from the irrigated ear. (Nystagmus is involuntary, rapid eyeball movement.) As with Doll's eye test, a number of variations of response can occur.

If pathology exists, nystagmus does not occur. Sometimes rather unpleasant symptoms such as vertigo, dizziness, nausea, and vomiting occur. The patient needs to be warned of the possibility of such symptoms and needs supportive nursing care if they do occur. Caloric tests are contraindicated in people with perforated ear drums or with *acute* labyrinth disease.

As with pupil signs, abnormalities in eye movements help to localize the area of a disorder. They also help to differentiate between structural and metabolic causes of coma.

Bithermal caloric tests are a recent development to evaluate vestibular function. Alternate ear irrigations of hot and cold water are done. Similiar, although more specific, findings are obtained. The nystagmus is measured by an *electronystagmography* (ENG). (See also Chapter 90.)

Other Tests

Numerous other diagnostic tests may be used in assessing persons with neurologic disorders. Among these are the following noninvasive tests used to search for specific evidence of vascular disease:

- *Ophthalmodynamometry (ODM)*. This test compares the retinal artery pressures in both eyes and may help diagnose extracranial vascular disease. While the retina is observed through an ophthalmoscope, pressure (or suction) is applied to the eyeball by a dynamometer. Pressure is read on the dynamometer.
- *Thermography*. Facial thermography photographically measures facial skin temperatures. In this test the patient sits in a chair and the face is "photographed" with a special scanning camera. Skin temperatures fluctuate in relation to variations in blood flow. Thus, for example, reduced skin temperatures may be identified in the medial supraorbital area of the forehead in the presence of occlusion or severe stenosis of the internal carotid artery.
- *Doppler Ultrasonography*. The Doppler effect may be used to measure blood flow in the supraorbital region. In occlusion or stenosis of the internal carotid artery the direction of blood flow is altered (reversed) in the supraorbital artery. This change may be detected by ultrasonography.

NEUROPSYCHOLOGIC TESTING*

In addition to the other procedures used to evaluate the integrity of brain functions, neuropsychologic testing is an approach that is becoming increasingly popular. Batteries of tests have been developed which are both sensitive to brain functions and which span many types of abilities (motor, perceptual, language, visual-spatial, cognitive, etc.). By employing carefully worked out methods of test interpretation, inferences can be made about the extent of impairment in brain functions.

The outstanding advantage of the approach appears to be that inferences can be made from the tests concerning the actual effect that any brain lesion is likely to have upon a person's ability to function. The other neurodiagnostic methods provide information that is only indirectly relevant to this issue. A person may be referred for a neuropsychologic evaluation some months following a head injury, for example, when the physical neurologic examination is entirely normal and when the EEG reveals only mild generalized abnormalities. The neuropsychologic tests may point to specific areas of deficit, however, and may result in recommendations concerning educational and vocational placement. Thus, these tests measure deficits in coping skills by evaluating these skills directly, and referral for neuropsychologic testing is suggested when deficits in adaptive abilities are suspected. The tests typically require several hours for administration and are often supplemented by general measures of intelligence (such as the Wechsler Adult Intelligence Scale or the Wechsler Intelligence Scale for Children — Revised) as well as tests of emotional and personal adjustment (such as the Minnesota Multiphasic Personality Inventory).

NURSING ASSESSMENT OF PEOPLE WITH NEUROLOGIC DISORDERS

Nursing assessment of a person with a neurologic disorder is similar to that done for any patient. Information is gathered about the total health status of the individual. However, the process of gathering some of the assessment data may vary in focus from that used with patients presenting for care for other types of illnesses. This is because a patient with a neuro-

*This section was written by Carl B. Dodrill, Ph.D., Neuropsychologist, Research Assistant Professor, Department of Neurological Surgery, University of Washington, Seattle.

logic disorder is usually experiencing a problem or problems which disrupt basic functional abilities either permanently or temporarily. Thus the patient's ability to cope effectively with daily living activities (i.e., ability to meet basic human needs) is often altered, perhaps permanently. For example, a patient's disorder may cause problems seeing, hearing, breathing, walking, talking, or eating. A patient with a neurologic disorder may be frustrated daily just trying to do the things we all take for granted!

Mitchell and Irvin developed a useful tool for nursing neurologic assessment. The tool is based on the principle that "the primary purpose of nursing is to assist people to *cope effectively with daily living in response to actual or potential disease*."[223] The tool provides a system for assessing a patient for the presence of *functional disabilities*.

Study Table 25–3 carefully. Note, for example, that when assessing a patient's mentation, you can gain information about human functions such as thinking, feeling, language, and remembering. The results of your assessment can then be directed toward assisting the person with any functions of mentation which you identify as impaired. Such is the purpose of neurologic *nursing* assessment. Neurologic medical assessment, on the other hand, is directed toward identifying the causative pathologic state of the patient. (Refer to Chapter 2 for a discussion of the difference between nursing and medical diagnoses.)

Consider Ms. Wix, a middle-aged woman whose medical history describes her as dysphasic. Cranial nerve examination describes her visual field cut, and motor examination reveals apraxia. The nursing assessment of Ms. Wix identifies three functional prob-

TABLE 25–3. ORGANIZATION OF A FUNCTIONALLY ORIENTED NURSING NEUROLOGIC EVALUATION

General Category	Functional Category	Examples of Specific Function Which May be Tested
Consciousness	Arousing (reticular activating system)	Arousability, response to verbal, tactile stimuli
Mentation	Thinking (general cortical function plus specific regional functions)	Educational level Content of conversation Orientation Fund of information Insight, judgment, planning
	Feeling (affective)	Mood and affect Perception and reaction to ability, disability
	Language	Content and quantity of speech Ability to name objects Ability to repeat phrases Ability to read, write, copy
	Remembering	Attention span Recent and remote memory
Motor function	Seeing (cranial nerves, II, III, IV, VI))	Acuity Visual fields Extraocular movement Pupil size, shape, reactivity Presence or absence of diplopia, nystagmus
	Eating (cranial nerves V, IX, X, XII)	Chewing Swallowing Gag (if swallowing impaired)
	Expressing (facially) (cranial nerve VII)	Symmetry of smile, frown
	Speaking (cranial nerves VII, IX, X, XII)	Clarity, presence or absence of nasality
	Moving (Motor and cerebellar systems)	Muscle tone, mass, strength Presence or absence of involuntary movements Coordination: heel-to-toe walk, observe during dressing Posture, gait, position
Sensory function	Smelling (cranial nerve I)	Ability to detect odors
	Blinking (cranial nerve V)	Corneal reflex
	Hearing (cranial nerve VII)	Acuity, presence or absence of unusual sounds
	Feeling (sensory pathways)	Pain-pinprick Touch, stereognosis Temperature-warm, cold

Note: *Examples of specific functions that may be tested in each functional category are shown. The structures involved in each of the functions categorized are indicated in parentheses.*

From Mitchell, P. H., and N. J. Irvin: Neurological examination for nursing purposes. *Journal of Neurosurgical Nursing*, 9:25, Mar. 1977.

TABLE 25–4. NURSING INTERPRETATION OF THE SIGNIFICANCE OF SELECTED ABNORMALITIES IN SELECTED FUNCTIONAL CATEGORIES

Functional Category	Abnormality	Interpertation
Arousing	Coma	Complete interruption in self-care; nurse must compensate totally for patient.
Language	Fluent aphasia	Major difficulty in interpreting verbal language; patient may respond best to pantomimed and symbolic instructions.
Remembering	Loss of short-term memory	Cannot learn new material; instructions will need to be repeated each time.
Seeing	Diplopia	Cannot read or watch television comfortably, may become nauseated. Eye patch will alleviate.
Eating	Bulbar weakness	High risk of aspiration; may tolerate substances of thick consistency if some swallowing ability present.
Moving	Tremor	Partial loss of self-care abilities in activities requiring fine movement.

From Mitchell, P. H., and N. J. Irvin: Neurological examination for nursing purposes. *Journal of Neurosurgical Nursing*, 9:25, Mar. 1977.

lems: (1) difficulty in seeing the periphery to the left, (2) difficulty talking and expressing her thoughts and feelings, and (3) difficulty moving, especially coordinating her movements to perform activities skillfully. The nursing care planned for Ms. Wix focuses heavily on these functional problems. Such a plan includes such things as: (a) approaching Ms. Wix from the right side and making sure that the furniture and equipment she needs (e.g., bedside table) is conveniently placed on her right side; (b) providing assistance for Ms. Wix with dressing, bathing and moving, and (c) giving attention to protecting the left side of Ms. Wix's body. The plan for this patient's medical care, on the other hand, is concerned with diagnosing the causes of her signs and symptoms by such measures as brain scan, CT scan, or arteriogram.

Table 25–4 gives further examples of how medical diagnoses (abnormalities) can be interpreted in terms of the functional effects they have for a patient. Consider various *nursing* approaches you may make for each of the examples given in Table 25–4.

Neurologic information can be obtained from a number of sources, as has been shown throughout this chapter. A careful and observant nurse has many opportunities to collect data during day-to-day nurse-patient interactions. Watching a patient attend to ordinary activities (e.g., getting dressed, eating a meal) can provide a nurse with information concerning the neurologic functions the person may require help with as well as the functions that require more detailed testing.

A creative nurse devises ways of assessing various neurologic functions during normal interaction with the patient. Mitchell and Irvin[223] suggest some simple procedures that may be useful. Consider the following example, which is based on Mitchell and Irvin's suggestions.

Robert Parley is an elderly gentleman admitted to the hospital for a neurologic investigation. Imagine you are to be his nurse. In addition to observing Mr. Parley's general behavior you could carry out the following assessment procedures:

- ▶ Ask Mr. Parley to describe the reasons he has come to the hospital and what he considers to be his major problem. As you listen to what this patient says you may get some indication of his memory, orientation, thought processes, and language skills.
- ▶ Ask Mr. Parley to read the information on his hospital identification bracelet out loud. Observe how close to his eyes he holds the bracelet. This will give you a rough estimation of his visual acuity. You may notice, too, something of his reading language ability. Ask Mr. Parley to remember the first five digits of his identification number. His short-term memory can be tested by asking him to recall these numbers a few minutes later. (Remember, of course, that these activities can be carried out only if the patient can read English and if he has any necessary reading aids, e.g., eyeglasses. Thus, these assessments must be made first.
- ▶ Ask Mr. Parley to stand up and walk across the room and back. Observe his gait and coordination. Sometimes patients may be confined to bed and so be unable to do this. You could test for resistance and notice any drift. You could test Mr. Parley's coordination by asking him to run the heel of one foot down the shin of the opposite leg.
- ▶ Take a glass of water in your right hand and ask Mr. Parley to take it in his left hand, drink from it, and pass the glass back to you. This simple test can give you information concerning Mr. Parley's ability to: (a) follow instructions; (b) identify right from left; (c) cross the midline; and (d) swallow. Difficulties with any of these things suggest a need for more detailed testing of parietal lobe function, visual fields, and ability to follow commands. Learn from the patient whether he is normally right-handed or left-handed.

► Ask Mr. Parley to take off his shirt without looking at it and to then put on a hospital gown. Watch his fine motor coordination. Note especially the way he handles any buttons and zippers. Normally people will feel buttons and zippers with their fingertips when they cannot see them. If Mr. Parley has sensory loss, he may feel buttons or zippers with his palms rather than fingertips. He may even have difficulty grasping the buttons or zipper with his fingertips. If this happens, more detailed testing of coordination and sensation is needed.

It is clear that simple procedures such as those above can provide indications for further testing. They also provide significant information for planning nursing care. For example, if you find that Mr. Parley has sensory loss and cannot make fine hand movements, you might expect that he may need help with such activities as writing, eating, and dressing.

During the diagnostic phase of care, two other areas of assessment are especially prominent for nurses. These are (1) assessment of the patient and significant others and (2) identification of particular signs and symptoms that a nurse needs to watch for because they herald progression (worsening) of a patient's illness or the onset of complications from diagnostic studies or the treatment regimen. These signs and symptoms are discussed throughout this unit, along with specific illnesses and therapy.

The *learning needs* of a patient and significant others, while usually not difficult to identify, are frequently difficult to meet. Especially during the diagnostic phase of an illness, patients and their significant others are frequently in a state of crisis. A state of crisis, with attendant protective mechanisms in operation, makes learning difficult. Moreover, the physical condition of the patient is frequently less than optimal and much of the patient's energy is directed toward regaining physical health. Typically a physician explains the diagnostic studies, thoughts about probable diagnosis and possible outcome, and the treatment plan. While such explanations may be given several times, it is still common for patients or significant others to be unable to remember or understand what they were told. Clearly, nursing intervention, is also needed. Making a sensible care plan to meet a patient's *learning needs* is a challenge for a nurse, and it is part of nursing responsibilities.

One approach is as follows:

1. Assess the patient's functional ability to learn, e.g., memory, emotional state, ability to reason.

2. Assess the patient's readiness to learn, e.g., is the patient in a state of crisis?

3. Assess what the patient perceives a need to know.

4. Identify additional information the patient needs to know.

5. Design and implement a plan to teach the patient, based on numbers 1, 2, 3.

6. Evaluate the patient's learning and repeat the teaching as necessary.

7. Design a plan to help broaden the patient's perception of what he or she needs to know based on number 4.

8. Arrange for post-discharge care to include teaching as needed.

Naturally the teaching of a patient's significant others could proceed along similar guidelines. In many cases the patient and significant others will be learning together.

Nursing assessment and care of the patient with neurologic dysfunction provides a great challenge for nurses. Because the dysfunction can be widespread and may involve many of the basic activities of daily living, the nurse needs a sound basic understanding of neurologic illnesses and their sequelae and great ingenuity to offer excellent care to such patients.

As you assess patients with neurologic disorders and plan their care, refer as necessary to Units I, VI, and VII.

CHAPTER 26

CLINICAL PROBLEMS RESULTING FROM ALTERED NEUROLOGIC STRUCTURE AND FUNCTION

The nervous system functions basically to transmit information in the body. Therefore, when disorders occur within the nervous system a patient may experience various clinical problems that are manifestations of bodily "communication problems." For example, disorders of the nervous system may cause a patient to experience *distorted* mental activities (e.g., hallucinations, memory difficulties, or perceptual distortions) or perhaps to *lose* entirely some mental activities (e.g., coma may occur). Disorders of the nervous system may also result in the distortion or loss of regulation of body movements; e.g., reflexes may be exaggerated or paralysis may develop. Additionally, autonomic and trophic activities may be altered by disorders of the nervous system; e.g., muscle atrophy may occur or changes may develop in the temperature or sweating pattern of an affected area.

Numerous clinical problems, such as the above examples, can result from altered neurologic structure and/or function. In this chapter we focus on some of the more common clinical problems associated with neurologic disorders.

THE PERSONAL IMPACT OF NEUROLOGIC PROBLEMS*

Introduction

Good health and problem-free physiologic and mental functioning are taken for granted by most of us. Often it is only when changes occur that we become "aware" of our body functions and realize how inconvenient and difficult life can become when some physical and mental functions no longer occur smoothly. Such inconveniences and difficulties may be annoying when brought about by a *temporary* health problem (i.e., a problem of relatively short duration from which a person can expect complete return to the premorbid health status). When a health problem is either *progressive* or *permanent,* what was merely annoying may become devastating. (A progressive health problem is one that exists in a dynamic form throughout a person's life, and a permanent health problem is one that may not change, but cannot be reversed. For example, multiple sclerosis is a progressive health problem, and paraplegia from a spinal cord injury is a permanent health problem.)

Neurologic health problems are frequently progressive or permanent, and people experiencing them may face long-term, irreversible and often radical life style changes. Helping patients and their significant others cope with such changes is a major nursing challenge.

In your imagination, place yourself in the position so many people find themselves in and consider how your feelings about yourself, your interactions with others, your ability to perform usual activities of daily living, and your ability to function within society would be affected by the following:

- *Changes in perception,* e.g., visual changes, hearing changes, altered perception of hot and cold, difficulty or inability to accurately interpret the meaning of sight or sound, inaccurate tactile perception, hallucinations, loss of a sense of smell, impairment of distance and depth judgment.
- *Loss of motor facility,* e.g., paralysis — paraplegia, quadriplegia, hemiplegia, facial paralysis; loss of manual dexterity; acute and unpredictable muscle fatigue; muscle tics; difficulty walking or inability to walk at all.
- *Changes in communication processes,* e.g., inability to speak, difficulty speaking, loss of facial expression, loss of voice tone and/or volume, changes in usual patterns of sexual expression, inability to write or read, loss of memory.
- *Changes in state of consciousness,* e.g., persistent leth-

*This section was written by Margaret Helen Parkinson, R.N., M.N.

argy, stupor, drowsiness, unconsciousness, unpredictable seizures.

- *Sudden, unexpected change in health status,* e.g., trauma producing head injury or spinal cord injury, stroke, infections such as meningitis, brain abscess.
- *Pain,* e.g., headaches, muscular spasm, joint pain, back pain, pain along nerve pathways, trigeminal neuralgia.
- *Painful or uncomfortable diagnostic or treatment procedures,* e.g., surgical procedures requiring a conscious patient, spinal punctures.
- *Behavioral changes,* e.g., crying when you don't feel sad, unpredictable emotional outbursts, disorganized behavior, undirected behavior.
- *Emotional and mental changes,* e.g., difficulty in concentration, difficulty in focusing thoughts, inappropriate euphoria, depression, scattered thought processes.
- *Specific body function changes,* e.g., loss of bowel and bladder control, skin breakdown, increased susceptibility to respiratory infections, muscle wasting.

These, and many other disturbing experiences, are common to people with neurologic problems. The consequences and ramifications are enormous, especially since in many instances such conditions will exist throughout a person's life — they will not "get better." As you study the problems, diseases, and disorders of the nervous system, try to think about the long-term effects of each on the individual.

While every individual experiences life events in unique ways, certain typical response patterns seem to develop. A person's reaction to a health problem of a progressive or permanent kind is often similar to a typical *grief reaction.* This may be expected, of course, as the crises such a person is experiencing are crises of loss, e.g., losses of physical structure and function; loss of social role and identity; loss of control; loss of familiar environment. Such people and their significant others require the same kind of supportive caring attention as do people who are grieving through bereavement.

Effect of Crises

Stephen Fink[90] has developed a model to describe the typical reactions of people experiencing a crisis (Table 26–1). Notice that the phases Fink describes are similar to the phases of grief. A person moves from *shock* through *defensive retreat* to *acknowledgment* and then *adaptation.* The time taken to move through the four phases varies with each individual and depends on the way the person perceives present circumstances (i.e., reality perceptions). When, for example, an injured person changes from perceiving his or her situation as overwhelming and instead tries to "block out" or deny the problems, then the person moves from the "shock" stage to "defensive retreat." Likewise, when a person starts to look for new ways of coping with life to accommodate residual and permanent disability, the person has begun "adaptation." A patient may even say "I see things this way now," indicating a change in reality perception. Of course, a person may fluctuate between phases and may, at times, even move backwards. Sometimes a person will become fixed at one phase and be unable to move beyond it.

Table 26–1 provides descriptive information about each phase: how people will see them-

TABLE 26–1. PSYCHOLOGIC PHASES OF CRISIS

TIME	Phase	Self-Experience	Reality Perceptions	Emotional Experience	Cognitive Structure	Physical Disability
↓	Shock (stress)	Threat to existing structures	Perceived as overwhelming	Panic; anxiety; helplessness	Disorganization; inability to plan or to reason or to understand situation	Acute somatic damage requiring full medical care
	Defensive retreat	Attempt to maintain old structures	Avoidance of reality; "wishful thinking": denial; repression	Indifference or euphoria (except when challenged, in which case anger): (low anxiety)	Defensive reorganization; resistance to change	Physical recovery from acute phase; functional return to maximum possible level
	Acknowledgment (renewed stress)	Giving up existing structure; self depreciation	Facing reality; facts "impose" themselves	Depression with apathy or agitation; bitterness; mourning; high anxiety; if overwhelming, suicide	Defensive breakdown; (1) disorganization; (2) reorganization in terms of altered reality perceptions	Physical plateau; gradual slowing of improvement until no change is experienced
	Adaptation and change	Establishing new structure; sense of worth	New reality testing	Gradual increase in satisfying experiences; (gradual lowering of anxiety)	Reorganization in terms of present resources and abilities	No change in physical disability status

From Fink, S.: Crisis motivation: A theoretical model. *Archives of Physical Medicine and Rehabilitation,* November 1967, p. 592.

selves, perceive reality, react emotionally, think and reason (i.e., cognitive structure), and the typical status of physical disability at each stage. Studying Fink's work will help you to understand and accept the behavior and experience of people undergoing the often "life-shattering" crises of neurologic problems.

> Remember:
> *Those people significant to the patient often experience the same crisis reaction as does the patient.*

Guidelines to Therapeutic Approach. It is important to remember that each stage represents necessary responses for the people involved. *It is not helpful to attempt to hurry a person to the adaptation stage.* The therapeutic approach is "present-oriented" and focuses around the needs that dominate each stage. Supportive empathetic care is helpful during the first three stages. Such care is often directed toward the satisfaction of safety needs — physical and psychologic. People can be encouraged to express feelings. They should be given truthful information and should never be judged for their behavior.

Intervention directed toward long-term planning and the construction of a new life style is probably not useful until adaptation has begun. Until then, people experiencing crises do not perceive their situation as permanent.

Psychosocial Care During the Shock Phase. Emotional and psychologic support of the patient and significant others is extremely important and must never be overlooked. In essence, providing emotional and psychologic support means communicating to all the people personally concerned that (a) you care about them as individuals in the crises they are experiencing and (b) you accept them and can tolerate their behavior as shocked and grieving people. (Remember some quite atypical behavior may occur in people at this time, e.g., anger, hostility, crying, shouting.)

It is often extremely important that you give orienting information. The patient will need to be told what has happened, where he or she is, and what is presently taking place. For example, you may say to an injured person, "Mr. Jones, you have had an accident in your car and you are in a hospital. I am your nurse. My name is Pam Smith. We found your mother's name in your wallet and called her. She will be here in a half hour." This information may need to be repeated several times. Tell the person what is going to happen *before* it occurs. Use simple, straightforward language. Even if the person is apparently unconscious, such orienting information should be offered, as we never really know how aware of the environment the person is.

The significant others of an injured person need to be given information concerning what has happened and what treatment and care the person is receiving. Remember these people are often shocked, and everything around them may seem strange and frightening. They need someone to acknowledge their presence and watch out for them. If at all possible, they should be allowed to stay with the patient.

A patient's significant others may feel impotent, guilty (often without cause), angry, and uncertain and may experience a variety of conflicting emotions. In their initial overloaded emotional state, they frequently do not comprehend the explanations given to them. Their actions may not reflect their inner turmoil. Gradually as they cope with the shock, they have many voiced and unvoiced questions. Generally the most important one to them is "What will happen to the patient?" It is often very difficult to give an answer and most often no one knows. We can never say that "everything will be all right" — we do not know that. Generally, it is best to say that we do not know and to keep the significant others informed of the patient's condition and comfort. It is often helpful to be told, for example, "Your friend slept well last night. We washed her face and her back at about 9 PM and that seemed to settle her a lot. She asked if you were coming to see her today." Sometimes this is the kind of information people want to know. They certainly need someone who lets them express their concerns and who is willing to go over the same issues time and time again.

Psychosocial Care After Shock Has Subsided. After the extreme stress (and, in some ways, excitement) of the shock stage is over, long-term supportive care for the patient and significant others is needed. Such care is discussed in relation to specific problems throughout the text. The following principles may guide therapeutic approaches:

- The person must be treated as a unique human being and not as a member of a disabled group of people.
- Significant others must be treated as individuals and not as "the patient's friend."
- Allowances must be made for variations in behavior — everyone has mood fluctuations, even people with disabilities!
- The opinions, needs, and wishes of the people personally involved must be considered. Patients and their significant others must retain control in decision making.
- Plans should build on the patient's strengths and capabilities rather than centering on the weaknesses and disabilities.

Many people experiencing progressive or permanent disabilities find helpful the kind of *peer support* that can be obtained through membership in organizations and groups. Most such groups are *self-help* in nature, although they may seek professional support and consultation from time to time. There are, for example, groups for people with epilepsy, Parkinson's disease, multiple sclerosis, muscular dystrophy, and paralysis. Spend some time finding out what groups of this kind are available in your community. (Remember, of course, that some people you care for will not want to be involved with such organizations — at least not at that particular time. Give information, and do not try to force anyone to do something they do not want to do.)

Various community agencies exist that can provide some service to the people involved in a long-term health problem, e.g., Meals-on-Wheels, Visiting Nurses Association. Find out which agencies are available in your community and identify what services they offer to whom.

It is prudent for the person with an ongoing health problem to wear an identification bracelet or medallion or carry some other form of ID that states the health problem and who to contact (i.e., doctor and significant other) in an emergency that renders the person out of control.

It cannot be emphasized enough that control should always be available to the people to whom the problem belongs. This includes, for example, control in decision making — from small issues ("*This is the best way to move me*") to larger issues ("*Yes, I would like to try this kind of treatment procedure*").

For further consideration of the issues in this section, refer to Sorensen and Luckmann, *Basic Nursing: A Psychophysiologic Approach.* Look especially at discussions on the therapeutic relationship, understanding the existence of the ill, rehabilitation, and caring for grieving persons.

ALTERED STATES OF CONSCIOUSNESS

Introduction and Definitions

"Consciousness means awareness of self and the environment."[249] Consciousness is an extremely complex entity, requiring that many of the brain's functions be in working order. Thus, *altered states of consciousness* indicate some degree of *brain failure.* Evaluation of the state of the brain's function or consciousness is difficult because of the rich range of behaviors possible in any human being. As with any other complex activity, attempts have been made to categorize the *conscious to unconscious continuum.* Since none of these attempts has been satisfactory, many systems continue to exist. Each system is helpful, however, in that each helps to *diagnose* the cause of an altered state of consciousness and to *treat* it or at least avoid having the problem make the patient worse.

Plum and Posner have defined consciousness as having two aspects. These are the *content of consciousness,* which they define as ". . . the sum of mental functions"; the other is *arousal,* which they define as ". . . closely linked to the appearance of wakefulness."[249] They further note that the type of disease present tends to affect these two aspects of consciousness differently. The arousal system is principally a function of the brain stem reticular activating system, while the content of consciousness is mostly a function of the structures of the cerebral hemispheres. Thus, a patient with failure of the arousal system often has brain stem disease, although diffuse bilateral disease of the cerebral hemispheres may also be present. Conversely, a patient with content problems generally has cerebral hemisphere disease. While these concepts help clarify altered states of consciousness, they are not foolproof. Content and arousal do not always vary independently from one another. Also, consciousness is evaluated in relation to a patient's *behavior,* which is the sum of these as well as other systems. Thus, a patient with aphasia has a content disorder. However, since speech is one way of testing the awakeness (arousal) of the patient, if the person is aphasic it becomes difficult to establish whether an arousal disorder is present as well.[249]

Problems causing alterations of a person's state of consciousness can be *generally* considered in these classifications: structural, metabolic, or psychogenic (Fig. 26–1). *Structural* brain lesions are often divided into (a) *supratentorial* lesions, which can cause coma secondarily by compressing brainstem structures, and (b) *subtentorial* lesions, which damage the brainstem itself. *Metabolic* disorders can cause an altered state of consciousness by widely depressing brain function (Fig. 26–1).

In the following discussion, people experiencing altered states of consciousness are considered. The emphasis is on the care of patients with severe brain dysfunctions, e.g., those with stupor and coma, since such people require intensive nursing care and medical treatment.

Neuro Checks

The first aspect of professional attention to people with altered states of consciousness is thorough and ongoing evaluation. Expressed simply, it is important to be constantly aware of whether the patient is *better, worse,* or *the same.*

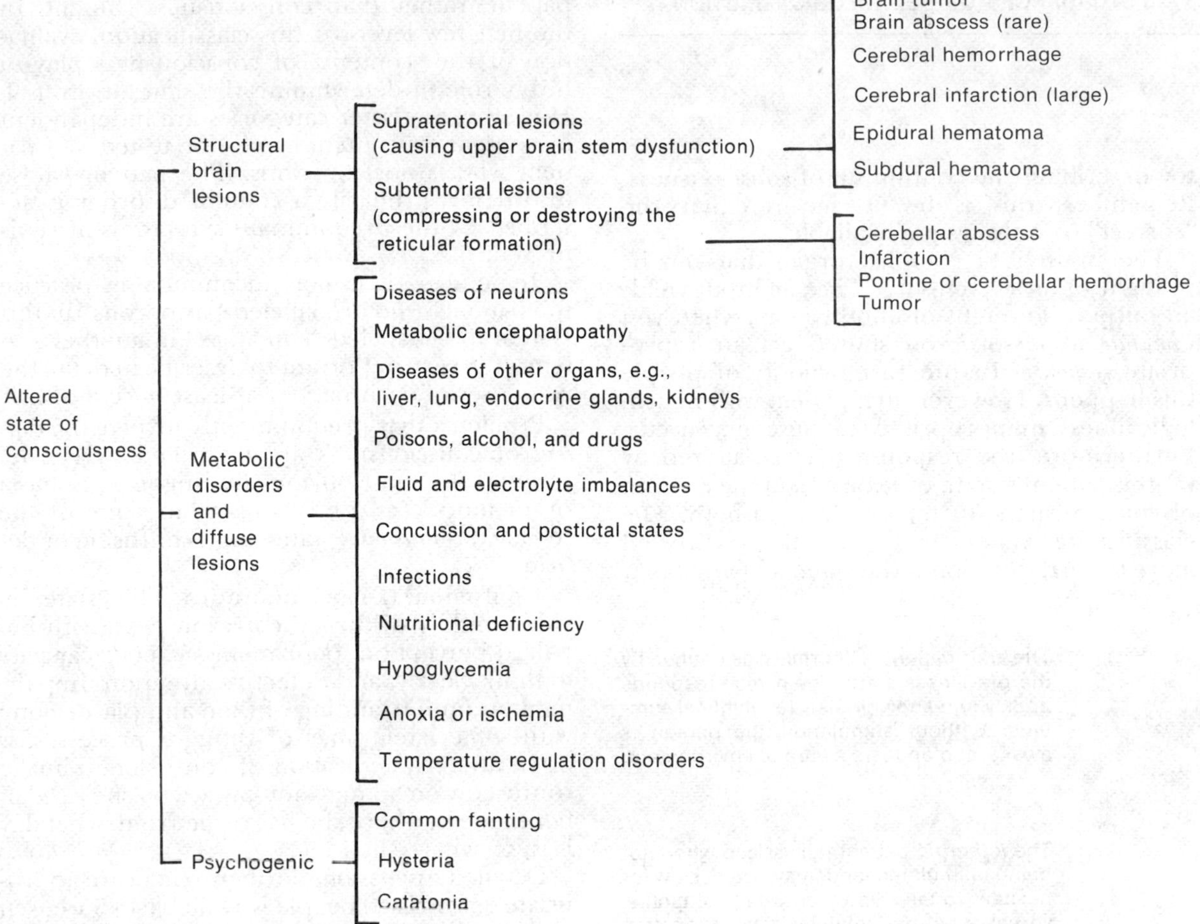

Figure 26–1. Some causes of altered states of consciousness. (Note that *supratentorial* lesions are located *above* the dura roofing in the cerebellum, which separates the cerebellum from the cerebrum. *Subtentorial* lesions lie *beneath* the dura roofing in the cerebellum.)

This is determined through several areas of assessment, often called "neuro checks."

> *The usual ongoing assessment areas for patients experiencing altered states of consciousness ("the neuro checks") include:*
>
> *Level of consciousness (LOC)*
> *Respiratory patterns*
> *Pupillary signs*
> *Eye movements*
> *Motor responses*
> *Vital signs*

The exact meaning of the order for "neuro checks" must be determined within the institution where a patient is receiving care, as established standards vary. Also, as nurses become more sophisticated in neurologic examination, the types of observations they record tend to increase. In any event, several observations are standard and virtually always done when "neuro checks" are ordered. From these raw data, the nurse analyzes whether the patient's condition is the same, improving, or deteriorating.

Levels of Consciousness (LOC). Assessment of the *level of consciousness* (LOC) is usually the first and most important of the numerous observations made on a patient with a neurologic disorder. Since consciousness is a complex expression of the state of the brain, it is frequently described as a continuum ranging from alert to coma. Between the states of alertness and coma, arbitrary subdivisions are often assigned, and various terms are used to describe a patient's status. However, as with many continuums, these divisions are artificial and authorities rarely agree on either the terms used or the meaning of terms.

For this reason, it is extremely important for a nurse observer to initially *describe* a patient's *state of consciousness* in detail rather than merely using a term, e.g., stupor. It would be ideal for each subsequent description of a patient to also be a full description. However, when frequent observations are being made, this is not practical. Terms (labels) may then be used. However, if the patient's condition changes, and hence the necessary descriptive term changes, a full description is again necessary.

Each nurse must learn and accurately use the "labeling system" used in the practice environment. Figure 26–2 presents one labeling system for describing the continuum of consciousness. Remember, this is by no means either the "correct" or only system available.

The brain is a complex organ that can be thought of as a "computer," i.e., an input yields an output. Thought of another way, when you *stimulate* a person, you should get an appropriate *response.* In the vast majority of people this happens. However, in a patient with neurologic illness, inappropriate responses may occur. Furthermore, the response may be altered by (a) the patient's state of arousal, (b) the content of consciousness, or (c) a mixture of both. The classification system in Figure 26–2 is directed more toward describing the state of arousal of a patient, rather than consciousness content. In the first few levels of this classification, evaluation of the "content" of consciousness plays a heavy role in determining the state of arousal. However, the latter categories are independent of content, as content cannot be tested in a patient who is not conscious. The patient whose disorder is primarily a content disorder is described by the predominant symptoms or signs present.

Remember, it is not uncommon in practice for patients who are labeled "stuporous" in this system to be labeled "comatose" in another system. It is very important to describe in detail the responses of each patient at least once a day.

Problems that predominantly involve the *content* of consciousness are described by (1) describing the most obvious finding, e.g., aphasia or memory loss, or (2) describing one of the so-called *confusional* states, e.g., confusion or delirium.

Alert	The *alert* patient is "normal," as defined by the pre-illness state. The person responds briskly and appropriately to a minimal stimulus. Without stimulation, the person is awake and appears aware of environment.
Lethargic	The *lethargic* patient falls asleep when not being stimulated and may seem slow or hesitant to talk. However, with light tactile, verbal, or other minimal stimulation, the patient responds appropriately and becomes almost alert. The patient may be somewhat confused by complex problems and may move like an intoxicated person.
Obtunded	The *obtunded* patient requires increased sensory input to produce an output. The patient must be shaken or given a painful stimulus to produce any response. Response may be verbal but usually does not make sense and is confined to a few words. Patient may make purposeful attempt to remove painful stimuli, but such attempts are very slow.
Stuporous	The *stuporous* patient makes no verbal response, even to forceful, painful stimulation. Movement occurs, but is a patterned response that is not meaningful in relation to the stimulus.
Coma	The patient in *coma* gives no output when maximally stimulated. Vital functions (such as respirations) may or may not be maintained independently. In any event, the respirations and other functions are not normal.

Figure 26–2. The continuum of consciousness.

Confusion (Disorientation). This state involves mildly disturbed consciousness, with impaired perception, poor memory, poor capacity to think clearly, and defective attention. Impairment in understanding of time and place, along with some irrelevancy of thought processes, is often an early indication of confusion. Thus, a confused woman may not know who she is, what her name is, where she has come from, what day it is, or where she is.

Detailed discussion of the nursing care appropriate to confused people is available in Sorensen and Luckmann: *Basic Nursing: A Psychophysiologic Approach,* Chapter 14.

Hallucinations, Illusions, and Delusional Thinking. Hallucinations, illusions, and delusional thinking are all examples of disordered behavior and thought disturbances.

Hallucinations are sensory impressions occurring in the absence of external stimuli. The patient may or may not be aware that the impressions experienced are "unreal." A hallucinating person may see, hear, feel, smell, or taste things that are not actually present in the environment. The hallucinations are sensations arising from within the person.

Illusions differ from hallucinations in that illusions do have a real stimulus in the environment, but the patient *misinterprets* the stimulus. For example, it is an illusion when a person sees a shadow on a wall and believes that the shadow is actually a person standing there.

Delusional thinking refers to thought or beliefs that are false, i.e., the thoughts or beliefs are quite contrary to the facts. For example, a man may believe a friend is stealing from him when this is in fact not true.

Delirium. A delirious person is typically loud, suspicious, fearful, irritable, disoriented, and hyperactive and frequently has visual hallucinations. Lucid and delirious intervals may alternate. A delirious state is very frightening to the patient. A delirious patient is frequently agitated and out of contact with the environment and presents a real nursing management challenge.

Delirium often develops suddenly and may disappear with equal rapidity. The symptoms may be most prominent at night. Delirium basically results from metabolic and toxic disorders of the brain. The physician's efforts are primarily directed toward treating the underlying disorder causing the delirium, e.g., infection, fever, drug toxicity. The nurse attempts to reduce the patient's distressing symptoms, promotes patient comfort, and safety and carries out prescribed treatments. Some of the nurse's efforts are also directed at reducing fever in the hyperthermic patient.

The following points are important in caring for a delirious patient:

- The patient cannot control his or her behavior — it is unpredictable, irrational, and impulsive.
- Protect the patient from injury. Accidents happen easily. Keep side rails up, closely supervise the patient, and try to avoid the use of restraints. (Obtain a doctor's order if that is the appropriate policy.) Position changes (e.g., sitting up) may help reduce restlessness. Keep away potentially dangerous objects from the patient. Reassure the patient frequently and try to maintain a calm and nonaggressive manner. Speak quietly, slowly, and repetitively to help to orient the patient, e.g., "You are in the hospital. I am David, your nurse." Give simple, brief explanations of your actions.
- Supervise and assist with eating and drinking. Usually a delirious patient cannot "calm down" enough to pause to eat or drink without help. Sometimes extra fluids and between-meal feedings are indicated.
- Reduce sensory stimuli to a minimum to prevent increasing confusion and hyperactivity. Maintain a patient environment that is quiet and softly lighted (keep some light on at night). Conversation at the bedside should be minimal and appropriate.
- Keep in mind that this patient is often frightened and suspicious. Be calm and reassuring in your approach.

Although the dramatic examples of altered states of consciousness are more easily recognized (e.g., deep coma following head injury) the skillful nurse is also alert to some of the more common subtly altered states of consciousness present in patients. For example, when a patient is given a tranquilizer or sedative this imposes an organic disorder of brain function that alters that patient's state of consciousness.

Other Standard Neurologic Observations (Neuro Checks)

In addition to level of consciousness, four other areas are routinely assessed in the patient with an altered state of consciousness. Each area has potential diagnostic implications and is instrumental in determining if a patient's condition is improving, deteriorating, or staying the same. The areas are *pattern of respirations, pupillary signs, ocular movements,* and *motor responses.* Of course, *vital signs* are also monitored. Once the diagnosis has been established and the condition of the patient stabilized, the frequency of making the observations decreases.

Respiratory Patterns. Breathing is an integrated act that is influenced at almost all levels of the brain. Therefore, observations of respiratory signs yield useful information. Various *respiratory patterns,* some discussed below, may accompany neurologic problems as well as problems of other body organs, e.g., pneumonia. Therefore, a nurse who notes a breathing abnormality does not assume it is purely related to the neurologic illness.

Assessing respiratory status includes all of the conventional observations such as rate and depth (see also Chapter 15, p. 337).* It also includes *describing the current respiratory pattern and watching for pattern changes.* Periodic arterial blood gas determinations are indicated. Several abnormal patterns are described below.

- *Posthyperventilation apnea.* Seen in patients with widespread forebrain disease, this is an abnormality that requires the cooperation of the patient to elicit. It is usually seen in patients with metabolic disorders. The patient is asked to take five deep breaths, which results in lowering the CO_2 tension. The "normal" response is apnea for a period of less than 10 seconds. An abnormal response is apnea lasting longer, e.g., 12 to 30 seconds.
- *Cheyne-Stokes respirations (CSR).* This is a pattern of breathing in which periods of hyperpnea regularly alternate with periods of apnea. The hyperpneic periods build up from breath to breath until a peak is reached; then they diminish in an equally smooth fashion. This pattern is caused by both structural and metabolic problems. Blood gases usually show a lowered CO_2 and the O_2 may be decreased slightly.
- *Central neurogenic hyperventilation (CNH).* This pattern is one of sustained hyperpnea. It is regular and rapid, and blood gases reveal respiratory alkalosis. The arterial oxygen tension helps to differentiate between hyperventilation related to brain dysfunction and that seen with heart failure or other systemic problems. With the former it is normal, while with the latter, decreased. The area of brain dysfunction in a patient with CNH is (often) within the brain stem.

---

*For a more complete discussion of respiratory assessment, see Unit XVI of this text and Sorensen and Luckmann, *Basic Nursing: A Psychophysiologic Approach,* Chapters 29 and 36.

- *Apneustic breathing.* This is a rare finding, in which the patient pauses at full inspiration. In some patients a pause at the end of inspiration and/or expiratory pauses may be present. The presence of apneustic breathing indicates dysfunction of the respiratory center in the pons. It may be seen in structural lesions of the pons and in some metabolic problems.

- *Ataxic breathing.* This is a sign of dysfunction of the respiratory centers of the medulla — specifically, the centers controlling the reciprocal inspiratory/expiratory neurons. The breathing pattern is completely irregular. Structural lesions, particularly of the posterior fossa, cause this sign. Other problems that cause compression of the medulla also can cause this pattern. Ataxic breathing is often seen just before a patient's death.

Pupillary Reaction. Fifty per cent of the cranial nerves innervate the eyes and eye movements (see Chapter 24). Thus, checking (a) the *responsiveness of the pupils,* (b) the *placement of the eyes at rest and with stimulation,* and (c) the *corneal reflex* yields a great deal of information about the functioning of the brain stem. Testing the various cranial nerves is discussed in Chapter 25 and can be reviewed there. (See also Chapters 15 and 89 for additional discussion of the eyes and Chapter 95 for discussion of pupillary reaction during emergency care.)

The "pupil check" is a test commonly done by nurses and is an important "neuro check." Checking the pupil involves observing the size of the pupil and its size in relation to the other one. (Note that pupil checks *do not* refer to testing the size of the eye in general, e.g., whether the eyes are open or not.) Obviously, it is important to be certain that the patient does not have an artificial eye before carrying out pupil checks. (This mistake has occurred, and the pupil in the prosthesis was reported as "fixed"!)

It is not sufficient to check only the direct light reflex in each eye and note the equality (or lack of same) of the pupils. A pupil check involves more than this. Questions to be answered in a pupil check:

Are both pupils *equal* in size? (Chart by making a labeled drawing of the relative size of both pupils, e.g., R • L ●.)

What is the *specific size* of each pupil measured in millimeters?

What is the *general appearance* of each pupil? For example, dilated or pinpoint.

Are the pupils *positioned* in midline, or are they deviated from midline?

When a light is shined in one eye, does the pupil in that eye *constrict*? This is called *"direct response."* Does the pupil react sluggishly or briskly or is there no reaction to light?

Does the pupil in the *other* eye *also respond* when a light is shined into one eye? (The light should be brought in toward the eye from the side of the head [by the ear] and not straight in from the front of the eye.) Response of the "other" pupil is called a *consensual response.*

What is the *shape* of each pupil? Is each pupil round? If not, describe the shape, e.g., oval.

Is each pupil *regular* in the shape of its borders? Irregular pupils may mean midbrain damage.

Do the pupils *accommodate?* (See Chapter 15, p. 325.)

Some abbreviations used for recording pupillary findings are:

RB "reacting briskly," the normal reaction
R "reacting," the constriction is both less and slower than in the opposite eye
RS "reacting slowly," the response is markedly slower
F "fixed," the pupil fails to constrict when the retina is stimulated with light

BLINK REFLEX AND CORNEAL REFLEX. The *blink reflex* occurs normally in response to threat. Test this by moving your hand quickly toward the eyes. Protective blinking should occur. The *corneal reflex* is tested by gently stroking the patient's cornea with a wisp of cotton. Normally, reflex blinking should occur. Have the patient look up to the right to test the left eye (vice versa for the right eye) and bring the cotton in from the side so that the patient cannot see your hand. Very gently touch the outer corner of the cornea (see Chapters 24 and 25). Impairment of the corneal reflex is important neurologic information. It is also very important nursing information. If the corneal reflex is absent, special care is necessary to protect the eye from damage. This care is discussed on p. 536.

A complete listing of the abnormalities found when checking the pupils is beyond the scope of this discussion. Basically, the pupillary light response is subserved by brain stem areas that are adjacent to the midbrain, which contains areas controlling consciousness. Abnormal pupillary signs are quite helpful in differentiating structural from metabolic causes of coma. In metabolic coma, the pupils are generally small, equal and reactive. A variety of sometimes dramatic findings may occur with structural damage (Fig. 26–3).

Eye Movements. As mentioned, eye movements are frequently checked at the same time as the pupils. Changes in eye movements should be recorded. Without special training and knowledge a nurse should not test the oculocephalic and oculovestibular responses (discussed below). However, the nurse should note the position of the eyes when checking the pupils and may also note involuntary eye movements.

At rest, the eyes normally gaze straight ahead in an awake and alert patient. They track togeth-

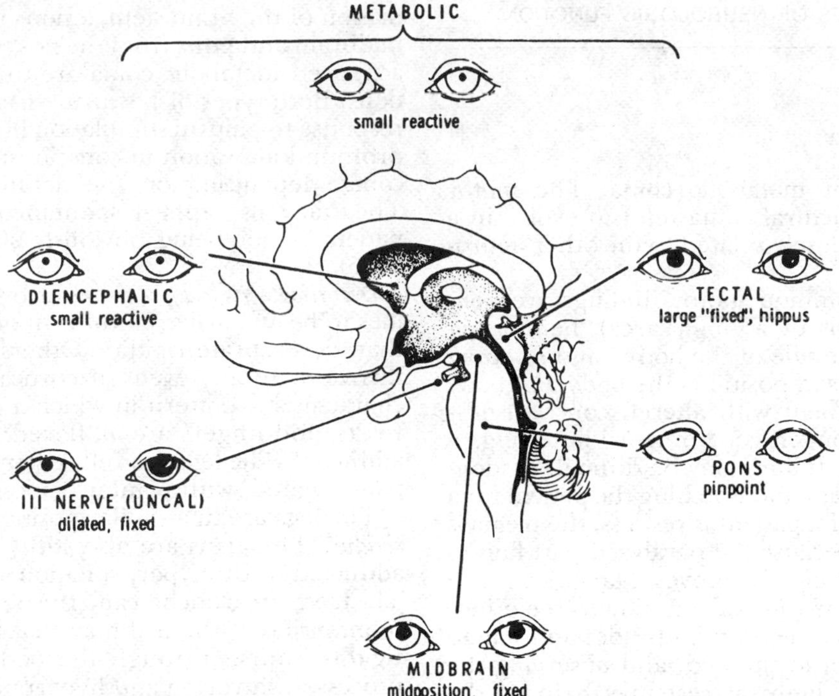

Figure 26–3. Pupils in comatose patients. (From Plum, F., and J. B. Posner: *Diagnosis of Stupor and Coma,* 2nd ed. Philadelphia: F. A. Davis Company, 1972, p. 36.)

er to look at something. "Tracking together" means that the gaze is *conjugate.* When one eye continues to gaze straight ahead while the other deviates to the side (or downward), the gaze is said to be *dysconjugate.* The presence of a *dysconjugate gaze* or a *conjugate deviation* of both eyes at rest implies failure of function of one or more of the muscles serving the eyes. To detect subtle abnormalities, shine a flashlight from the front to a spot between the patient's eyes. The light should be reflected at the same position on each of the eyes. If it is not, the patient's gaze is dysconjugate.

Normally there are no involuntary movements of the eyes. Several types of *abnormal involuntary eye movements* may occur. Two examples are *ocular bobbing* (when the eyes appear to be slowly "jumping up and down") and *roving eye movements* (when the eyes slowly wander or rove around). These are significant findings.

The *oculocephalic response* (also called the *doll's head eye phenomenon*) is commonly tested by a physician. Basically, with the eyes open, the patient's head is moved rapidly from side to side or up and down. Doll's eyes are said to be present if, when the head is rotated to the left, the eyes deviate to the right, and vice versa (Fig. 26–4). The same principle applies with up and down movement. The eyes normally should rapidly return to the resting position after the maneuver. "Doll's eyes" do not occur in normal, awake, alert people. The abnormal doll's eyes phenomenon appears as the level of consciousness diminishes and disappears again with deep loss of consciousness (coma). A number of variations of the response may occur, e.g., the eyes may fail to go past the midline on one side.

Motor Responses. Evaluating motor responses gives information about almost all levels of the nervous system. Classically, motor findings at one level and respiratory, pupillary, and ocular movement findings at a different level are

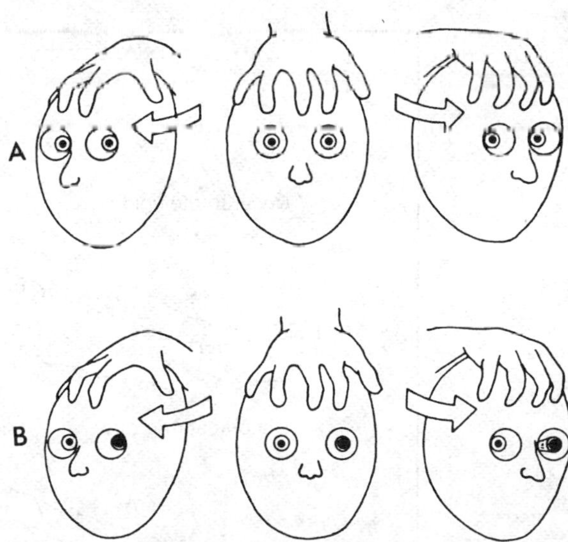

Figure 26–4. Doll's eye maneuver (diagrammatic). **A.** On initial examination, the eyes moved normally with head rotation. **B.** Change, on examination an hour later, indicates the development of a life-threatening hematoma in the left middle fossa. (From Miller, R. H., and J. R. Cantrell: *Textbook of Emergency Medicine.* St. Louis: C. V. Mosby Co., 1975, p. 112.)

characteristic of metabolic coma. The motor findings in structural coma tend to evolve in a manner more closely related to the other neurologic signs.

The most common motor findings are *monoplegia* (paralysis of a single area), hemiplegia (paralysis of one side of the body), and *posturing* (the ways a person positions the body and body parts). In a patient with altered consciousness who can no longer cooperate with testing, a plegic (paralyzed) limb may be difficult to identify. Standing back and watching the patient for a time is useful. If a patient is restless, the plegia is often obvious because the paralyzed part fails to move as everything else moves. Maneuvers such as comparing the tone of one side to the other, lifting the arms or legs on both sides and watching them return to the bed, and observing the position of the limbs at rest may help. If the patient can cooperate, testing the "drift" may show subtle alterations in tone. To do this, have the patient hold both arms up in front of the body with the hands upward and the eyes closed. If one arm "drifts" — moves upward or down toward the bed and the hand turns over — the muscles are weak. This provides a far more objective test of motor strength than checking bilateral hand grasps.

Posturing refers to the presence of *decerebrate rigidity* or *decorticate rigidity*. Both are seen in situations of *severe* dysfunction of the brain. Herniation of the brain stem, lesions pushing on the midbrain and pons from the posterior fossa, and advanced metabolic coma are three such situations. Both types of posturing usually appear in response to painful stimulation in patients with a profound alteration in consciousness (stupor or coma, depending on the definition of each). They may also appear spontaneously when the patient is not being obviously stimulated (Fig. 26–5).

Decorticate rigidity is thought by some authorities to be an earlier motor sign of deterioration than decerebrate rigidity. Others disagree with this view. In any event, decorticate rigidity is a characteristic pattern in which a patient's arms, wrists, and fingers are all flexed. The arms are adducted. The legs are fully extended and internally rotated, with plantar flexion of the feet.

The legs are in a similar position in *decerebrate rigidity*. The arms are also stiffly extended and adducted with hyperpronation of the hands. The teeth are clenched and the posturing may be so intense that the bed may shake, as spasms of rigidity course through the body. With acute processes, shivering and hyperpnea may accompany the posturing. The shivering may further elevate the temperature. A patient with decerebrate rigidity appears extremely ill!

Decerebrate posturing in the upper extremities with flaccidity in the lower extremities is a more serious sign than classical decerebrate rigidity. Total flaccidity is also a poor prognostic sign. The patient with a poor prognosis may also show various spinal reflex activities.

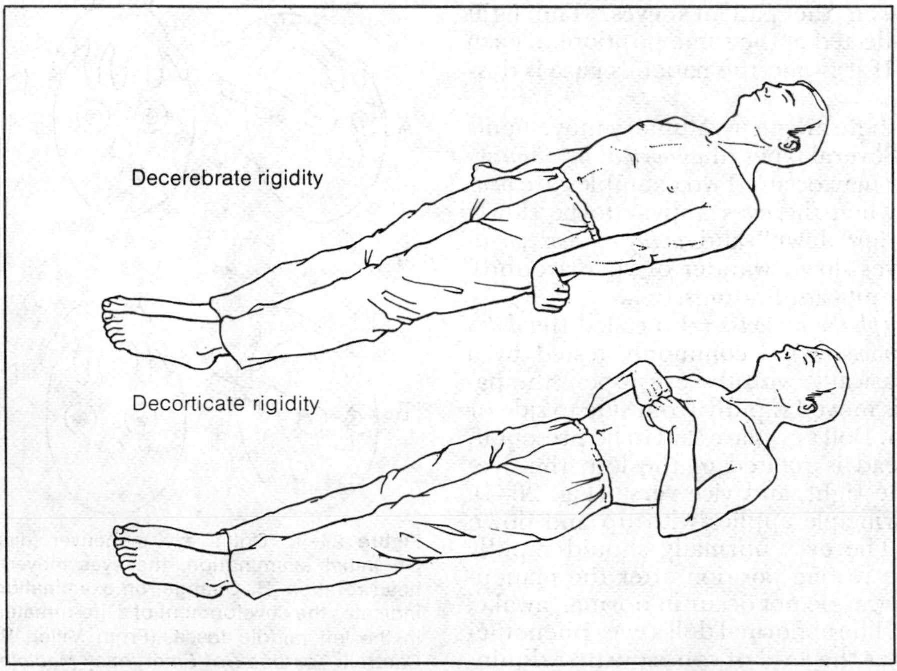

Figure 26–5. Pathologic posturings. (From: To diagnose the comatose. *Emergency Medicine*, 9:131, Oct. 1977, p. 135.)

Other motor signs may be present in a patient with cerebral hemisphere damage. Primitive reflexes such as sucking or the snout reflex may be present. The patient may have a strong reflex grasp. Restlessness, picking movements with the hands, resistance to passive movement, grasping, and focal motor seizures may be seen. Various patterned movements such as chorea are sometimes present; also hemiplegia or hemiparesis may occur.

The motor problems seen with patients with altered states of consciousness are varied. Careful assessment in a systematic fashion is essential to note all of the potential findings.

Vital Signs. Widely varying changes in the vital signs may be present in a patient experiencing altered states of consciousness. Some of these changes may be related directly to the *cause* (disease or problem) of the consciousness alteration, while others may be related to complications of the initial problem, therapies, or the patient's general immobility. *Serial* recorded observations of blood pressure, pulse, and respiration are necessary because *serial* changes in vital signs may be critical in identifying a wide variety of problems, including late developing shock (decreased blood pressure and increased pulse), various cardiac rhythm abnormalities, fluid balance problems, and increasing hypertension.*

The temperature is also monitored frequently, usually every 2 hours initially. If serious hypothermia or hyperthermia is present, continuous monitoring with a rectal probe is indicated. Treatment of these problems is discussed later in this chapter (p. 549).

Some conditions causing stupor and coma may also cause autonomic nervous system instability because of impairment of hypothalamic regulatory mechanisms. These disorders often cause the blood pressure and pulse to vary widely. The temperature may also be altered by this entity. Patients with instability of the autonomic nervous system appear very unstable.

Finally, classic *Cushing changes* may develop with increasing intracranial pressure. These changes are a decreased pulse and increased blood pressure with a widening pulse pressure. Cushing changes are not a reliable warning of intracranial pressure increase because they do *not always* occur and, when they do occur, they often occur *late* in the course of rising pressure. Also, they are sometimes difficult to differentiate from other causes of hypertension and/or a slow pulse. However, you should continue to watch for these classic signs and report them if they occur.

Other Observations. Various other reflexes also need to be tested. Among these are the *corneal reflex* (p. 528) and the *gag reflex* (p. 501). Absence of either of these reflexes has implications for nursing care, described in the subsequent section.

*For a complete discussion of vital signs see Sorensen and Luckmann, *Basic Nursing: A Psychophysiologic Approach,* Chapters 28 and 29.

Nursing implications of neurologic observations

You will notice that many of the assessment findings can be used for both medical and nursing purposes. For example, knowing that a patient does not have corneal reflexes tells the doctor something about the patient's pathophysiologic state. *The same information tells the nurse that during the time the corneal reflex is absent the patient requires very careful protective eye hygiene care in order to avoid serious eye damage.* Finding that a person's level of consciousness is low and that the person is very slow to respond to external stimuli tells the doctor that something is neurologically wrong with the person. *The same information tells the nurse that the patient may well need constant attention if dangers in the environment are to be avoided.*

Figure 26–6 presents one sample neurologic flow sheet, designed to simplify patient monitoring.

CLINICAL CARE OF AN UNCONSCIOUS PERSON

Unconsciousness is a common clinical situation. Patients are frequently brought to hospitals in an unconscious state, or they may suddenly or gradually become unconscious while hospitalized. It is thus imperative to know how to care properly for such totally dependent persons. *Indeed, one of the most important functions you may perform as a nurse is the care of an unconscious person.* Your actions in caring for such a patient and the thoroughness of your care may mean the difference between the patient's life or death. For the enthusiastic, competent nurse this area of clinical care can be one of challenge and reward.

Because *protective reflexes are impaired,* the unconscious patient is helpless and totally dependent upon others. The nurse takes the place of the unconscious patient's lost protective reflexes until the patient regains them or until the patient dies. By recalling what some of the protective reflexes are, you can identify some important nursing functions in the care of the comatose patient.† For example, because of the loss of normal spontaneous movements, the patient needs protection from skin breakdown due to prolonged pressure on bony prominences, and protection from the pooling of secretions in

†For a complete discussion of the problems and potential complications associated with prolonged bed rest and the clinical care of the patient immobilized for prolonged periods of time, see a fundamental nursing text. A good source is Sorensen and Luckmann, *Basic Nursing: A Psychophysiologic Approach,* Chapter 33.

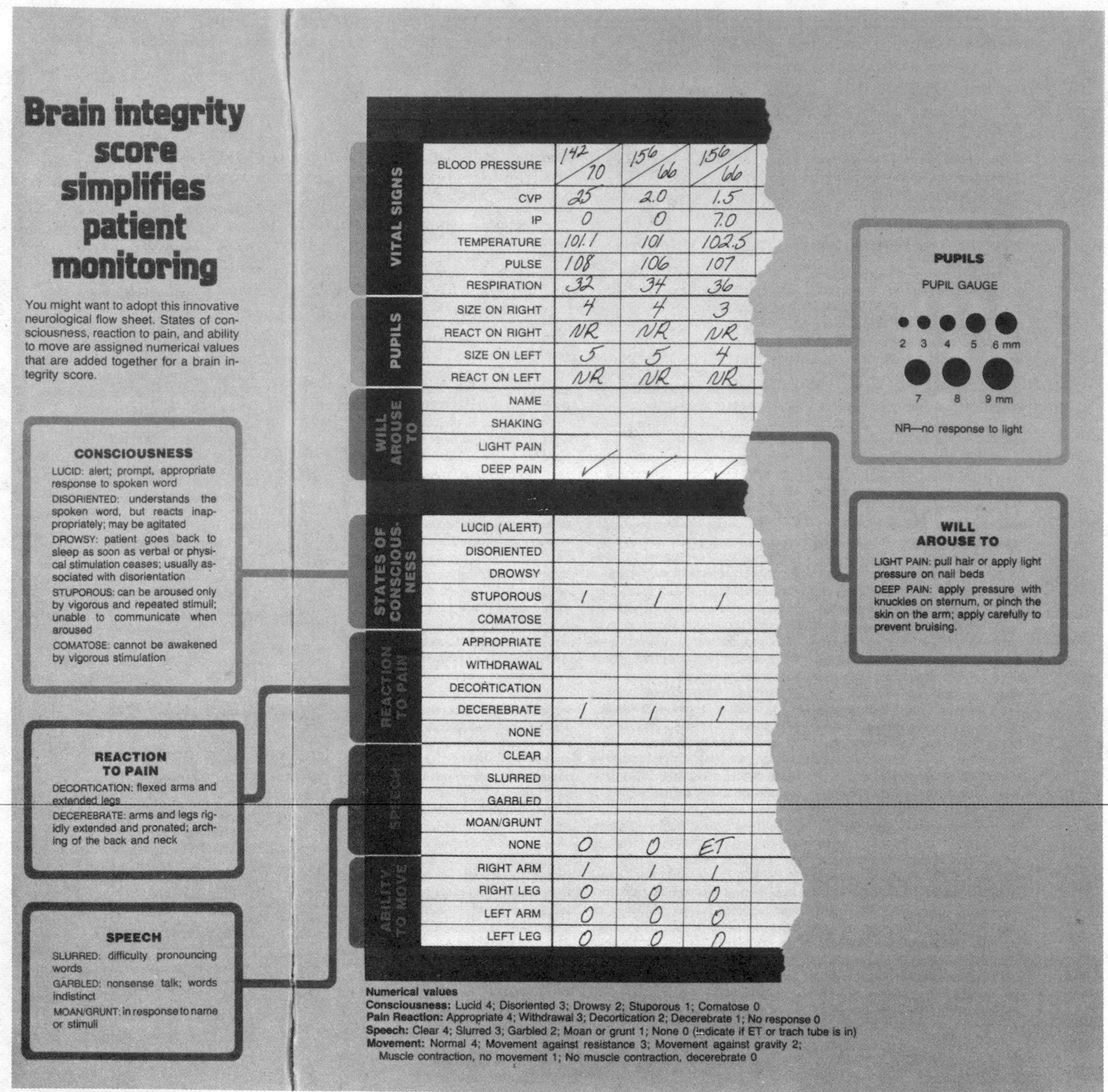

Brain integrity score simplifies patient monitoring

You might want to adopt this innovative neurological flow sheet. States of consciousness, reaction to pain, and ability to move are assigned numerical values that are added together for a brain integrity score.

VITAL SIGNS	BLOOD PRESSURE	142/70	156/66	156/66	
	CVP	25	2.0	1.5	
	IP	0	0	7.0	
	TEMPERATURE	101.1	101	102.5	
	PULSE	108	106	107	
	RESPIRATION	32	34	36	
PUPILS	SIZE ON RIGHT	4	4	3	
	REACT ON RIGHT	NR	NR	NR	
	SIZE ON LEFT	5	5	4	
	REACT ON LEFT	NR	NR	NR	
WILL AROUSE TO	NAME				
	SHAKING				
	LIGHT PAIN				
	DEEP PAIN	✓	✓	✓	
STATES OF CONSCIOUSNESS	LUCID (ALERT)				
	DISORIENTED				
	DROWSY				
	STUPOROUS	1	1	1	
	COMATOSE				
REACTION TO PAIN	APPROPRIATE				
	WITHDRAWAL				
	DECORTICATION				
	DECEREBRATE	1	1	1	
	NONE				
SPEECH	CLEAR				
	SLURRED				
	GARBLED				
	MOAN/GRUNT				
	NONE	0	0	ET	
ABILITY TO MOVE	RIGHT ARM	1	1	1	
	RIGHT LEG	0	0	0	
	LEFT ARM	0	0	0	
	LEFT LEG	0	0	0	

PUPILS

PUPIL GAUGE

2 3 4 5 6 mm

7 8 9 mm

NR—no response to light

CONSCIOUSNESS

LUCID: alert; prompt, appropriate response to spoken word

DISORIENTED: understands the spoken word, but reacts inappropriately; may be agitated

DROWSY: patient goes back to sleep as soon as verbal or physical stimulation ceases; usually associated with disorientation

STUPOROUS: can be aroused only by vigorous and repeated stimuli; unable to communicate when aroused

COMATOSE: cannot be awakened by vigorous stimulation

WILL AROUSE TO

LIGHT PAIN: pull hair or apply light pressure on nail beds

DEEP PAIN: apply pressure with knuckles on sternum, or pinch the skin on the arm; apply carefully to prevent bruising.

REACTION TO PAIN

DECORTICATION: flexed arms and extended legs

DECEREBRATE: arms and legs rigidly extended and pronated; arching of the back and neck

SPEECH

SLURRED: difficulty pronouncing words

GARBLED: nonsense talk; words indistinct

MOAN/GRUNT: in response to name or stimuli

Numerical values
Consciousness: Lucid 4; Disoriented 3; Drowsy 2; Stuporous 1; Comatose 0
Pain Reaction: Appropriate 4; Withdrawal 3; Decortication 2; Decerebrate 1; No response 0
Speech: Clear 4; Slurred 3; Garbled 2; Moan or grunt 1; None 0 (indicate if ET or trach tube is in)
Movement: Normal 4; Movement against resistance 3; Movement against gravity 2; Muscle contraction, no movement 1; No muscle contraction, decerebrate 0

Figure 26–6 Sample neurologic monitoring sheet. (From Ranirez, B.: When you're faced with a neuro patient. *RN,* 42:67, Jan. 1979, p. 75.)

the lungs. Likewise, because of an inability to swallow or cough, the unconscious patient needs protection from choking and needs to have alternative ways of maintaining fluid and electrolyte balance established. Because the blink reflex is lost, the eyes of an unconscious patient must be protected, especially if they are open. In fact, all the person's hygiene needs must be attended to by others. Protection from environmental changes is needed since the person may well be unaware of the environment or at least be unable to respond to environmental stimuli. Because of a lack of awareness of body position, the patient needs to be positioned correctly so that limbs will not be injured from the weight of the body on them or from being left in awkward positions for long periods of time. Because the person cannot move about and keep joints lubricated and mobile, the dependent patient needs to have limbs exercised passively. In fact, an unconscious patient requires help with the whole range of basic human needs. Remembering that a nurse is an expert in assisting people with their basic human needs, it is clear that an unconscious person is in *acute* need of very good nursing care.

Coma results from numerous causes. Our emphasis in this section is on therapeutic measures that are common to the care of all unconscious patients regardless of the etiology of the coma. Special care required by the specific causes of the state of unconsciousness is discussed in other sections of this text. Care of the postoperative patient who is unconscious from anesthesia is discussed in Unit VIII.

Unconsciousness is frequently a *medical emergency*. Often specific therapy, requiring intensive treatment, is needed to save the unconscious patient's life. While the physician is busy trying to establish the specific diagnosis, nursing personnel institute necessary measures to maintain the patient and to prevent complications during the time diagnostic examinations are being performed. *Preventive measures begin immediately.* Once life-saving preventive measures are completed, e.g., prevention of airway obstruction and prevention of shock, the nurse then concentrates on less urgent but highly important measures such as prevention of deformity.

> *Because many causes of coma are actually reversible processes, unconscious patients may often fully recover if they receive proper care during the critical phase of their illness.*

Objectives and Clinical Approach

Basic *objectives* in the care of an unconscious patient are to: (1) maintain and support normal body activities and functions; (2) prevent the development of complications that may retard the patient's recovery or that could cause residual problems once consciousness returns; (3) treat the trauma or disorder that produced the unconsciousness; and (4) treat the unconscious state itself.

Lifesaving measures may be necessary in treating an unconscious patient before a specific etiologic diagnosis can be established. Once immediate lifesaving treatment is given, the physician pauses to evaluate the cause of coma carefully; additional actions, without such specific knowledge, are potentially dangerous.

The *initial clinical approach to an unconscious patient* is generally as follows:

- First, treat life-threatening emergencies such as pulmonary obstruction or shock. Find cause if present.
- Ensure maintenance of adequate circulation and ventilation after emergency treatment.
- Quickly assess the patient for other potential major problems, e.g., spinal cord injury or status epilepticus. Treat these. Check the extremities for tourniquets if the person has been injured and received first aid.
- Initiate measures to prevent further injury to the brain and other vital organs.
- Examine the patient more thoroughly and obtain a history if possible.
- *Start an intravenous infusion* (with a large bore needle) on all patients in coma. When starting IV, obtain blood samples for various studies.
- *Evaluate depth of consciousness* by observing responses to stimuli and *determine presence of localizing neurologic symptoms* pointing to focal intracranial disease.
- *Examine the pupil sizes and reactivity to light for indications of increased intracranial pressure* or other indications of the cause of the coma.
- *Examine deep and superficial reflexes* (e.g., determine if they are overactive, underactive, absent, unequal on the body's two sides, or unaltered). Examination of reflexes is particularly valuable in a comatose patient because they give objective indications of the patient's condition without requiring the patient's conscious participation. Check corneal reflex.
- *Examine for response to painful stimuli.* Other aspects of the sensory examination are not possible or are unreliable in patients with reduced consciousness.
- *Examine for evidence of trauma.* Remember that trauma may be the *result* of some causes of coma rather than the *initial cause* itself of the coma, e.g., a bitten tongue may result from a convulsion. Examine ears for ruptured tympanic membranes.
- *Obtain blood sample* for sugar determination. Glucose may be administered when symptoms indicate a metabolic disease (other than *hyper*glycemia) or if the cause of coma is not clear. Prompt IV administration of glucose prevents further cerebral damage during the time laboratory tests are being performed if the cause of coma is hypoglycemic encephalopathy. Even if the coma later is proved to have some other cause, the IV sugar does no harm.[309]

Nursing Observation and Reporting

Nursing care of the unconscious patient includes making frequent, objective observations, followed by evaluation of the observations and detailed, accurate recording and reporting. Physicians rely heavily upon nurses to observe, assess, and record an unconscious patient's neurologic status and to report significant changes.

A set of *serial observations* is valuable for comparison when a change occurs or a new sign appears. Even though the findings may seem unremarkable for long periods of time, a record or pattern is being established as a baseline for future observations.

Neuro checks are made, often every 15 minutes for the first few hours of unconsciousness. As the patient's condition improves, the intervals between observations may be lengthened. (See the preceding discussion of "neuro signs" on pp. 524–531.)

In order to properly care for an unconscious person, the nurse periodically does a complete body examination. This includes checking for lacerations, bruises, ulcerations, fractures, dislocations, and contractures, as well as observing the color, texture, and temperature of the skin. Any dressings present are inspected frequently for bloody drainage, or if on the head, for indications of possible leakage of CSF.

The following questions may guide a nurse's observations of an unconscious person:

- Are the circulation and respirations effective? Is the pulse slowing and BP widening? (If so, report to the physician at once, for these are indications of possible increasing intracranial pressure.) Does the person appear to be going into shock?
- Is the person's airway patent? Is the color of nail beds and mucous membranes normal?
- Are the pupillary responses normal and are corneal responses present? Are the pupils of equal size? Are abnormal eye movements or position present?
- Are some normal reflexes absent? Are some abnormal reflexes present?
- In what position are the patient's head, limbs, and trunk? Does the patient change these positions? Is the neck rigid or stiff? Are there other indications of meningeal irritation? Are there changes in muscle tone? Is paralysis evident? Is the patient making any voluntary movements?
- Are any seizures occurring? (Give detailed report of the onset and progression of any convulsions — focal or generalized.)
- Is the patient incontinent? Is the abdomen distended?
- Are there any indications of fluid and electrolyte imbalances present?
- If the patient had head injuries or cranial surgery, is there any periocular or facial edema present?
- Does the patient respond to noxious stimuli? Is the person resistive to care? Is spontaneous behavior occurring? What is the person's level of consciousness?

Maintaining Circulation and Respiration*

Partial airway obstruction is the commonest source of harm to patients with depressed consciousness.

Support the unconscious patient's circulation; establish and maintain the airway; and prevent aspiration of secretions and vomitus. When a person is found unconscious *loosen all tight clothing,* particularly around the neck, and *clear the airway immediately.* (See Chapter 95.)

Partial airway obstruction is manifest through noisy respirations and/or obvious efforts in breathing. *Remember: a noisy airway is an obstructed airway.* Measures must be taken to protect the patient against partial airway obstruction even though obstruction is not obvious. The simplest measure is keeping the patient properly positioned. The *lateral* or *semiprone* position facilitates drainage of respiratory secretions and prevents the tongue from falling backward and obstructing the airway. In positioning the patient to facilitate easy respiration do not acutely flex the patient's neck by placing a large pillow under the head; such flexion could compress the airway. *Frequently* check the patient's position. Be certain that comatose patients are kept in the lateral position if they are not intubated.

However:

CAUTION: Do not change the position of a recently injured patient until you have assurance that the cervical spine has not been injured.

An intubated patient must not be placed in a prone position. Carefully check this patient after positioning to be sure that the endotracheal tube or tracheostomy is not occluded. If the patient is connected to a ventilator, patency of the equipment must be assured.

Never allow an unconscious patient who is not intubated to remain unattended on his or her back *because the tongue may fall back, occluding the airway; also, secretions pool in the pharynx.* Aspiration is a serious threat to the unconscious patient *because it may cause blockage of the airway, leading to respiratory failure or other pulmonary complications, e.g., infection.*

Inadequate respiratory exchange may cause (1) CO_2 retention, which contributes to cerebral edema and increased intracranial pressure, or (2) decreased arterial O_2 level, resulting in lack of oxygen to brain tissue. Obviously, the balance of O_2 and CO_2 in the blood stream must be maintained at proper levels if respiration is to be adequate. Respiratory failure will occur if a patient has insufficient lung ventilation and inadequate gas exchange (as revealed by arterial

*Refer as necessary to Unit XII: Nursing Patients Experiencing Disturbances of Cardiovascular Function and Blood Flow and Unit XVI: Nursing Patients Experiencing Disturbances of Respiratory Function.

blood gas measurements). To prevent respiratory failure in such a situation, O_2 therapy, positive pressure–assisted breathing techniques, or a ventilator is indicated.

When observing the status of a patient's airway, also observe the rate and rhythm of respiration. Cyclic or slowed respirations may indicated increased intracranial pressure. These findings should be reported at once, so that proper treatment can be instituted.

A nasal or oral airway may be used for a short period of time. Then, if necessary, a cuffed endotracheal tube is inserted to: (1) allow long-term ventilation; (2) permit removal of tracheobronchial secretions; and (3) seal off the digestive tract from the air passages and prevent aspiration. Many semiconscious or unconscious patients have food in their stomachs. A cuffed endotracheal tube helps prevent aspiration of vomitus because the inflated cuff decreases regurgitation into the tracheobronchial tree. The tube is kept in place until the patient's ventilation is assessed as adequate and the person is sufficiently awake so that secretions or vomitus will not be aspirated or until the decision is made to insert a cuffed tracheostomy tube. Often, an open route for suction of the trachea in a comatose patient is lifesaving. Significant respiratory changes or hypoxia should be reported at once. Suction equipment should constantly be available at the bedside of the comatose patient, ready for instant use. Frequent suctioning of the tracheobronchial tree is often necessary to prevent or decrease the effects of immobility, e.g., hypostatic pneumonia. The nurse assesses the breath sounds and arterial blood gases to determine the frequency of need for suctioning. Even though suctioning may increase intracranial pressure, the deleterious effects of hypoxemia and hypercarbia make the removal of lung secretions essential.

Because the comatose patient lacks pharyngeal reflexes and is unable to swallow, the accumulation of secretions in the pharynx creates the potential danger of aspiration. Suctioning of the posterior pharynx and upper trachea should therefore also be performed as indicated.

In addition to suctioning, frequent turning is employed with comatose people to facilitate proper drainage of secretions and thus to prevent atelectasis and hypostatic pneumonia.

> *Never place an unconscious patient with the head down below the heart without an order. This position increases intracranial pressure.*

Evaluation of "Neuro Signs"*

The level of consciousness, respiratory patterns, pupillary signs, eye movements, motor responses and vital signs (i.e., "neuro signs") are evaluated as frequently as every 15 minutes initially in unconscious patients. After they are stable, the frequency of observation may be decreased to hourly. Hourly observations are often continued for several days. An exception to the above regimen is the temperature, which is monitored either every 2 hours or continuously with a rectal probe if a patient is seriously hyper- or hypothermic.

Trends indicating deteriorating neuro signs are reported immediately.

One of the most significant changes in any patient is the level of consciousness—the measure of cerebral function. Localizing signs, particularly a change in the size and reactivity of one pupil, are also important to report immediately.

Seizures. Observing an unconscious patient for seizure activity is also important. Both focal motor (partial) and generalized seizures may occur, especially in the patient with irritative lesions. Seizures and the care of people experiencing seizures are discussed on pp. 554 and 640.

Reflexes. The nurse may be asked to check the *Babinski reflex* (see Chapter 25, Fig. 25–3). Two other important reflexes that the nurse checks are the *corneal reflex* and the *gag reflex* (see Chapter 25). Absence of the corneal reflex usually indicates upper pontive failure (at the level of the nucleus of V). When this reflex is absent, the nurse gives appropriate eye care (p. 536). Absence of the gag reflex means danger of aspiration and requires special preventive nursing measures, e.g., positioning, suctioning.

Hygiene, Environment, and Preventive Measures

The unconscious patient should be *bathed,* have *hair combed,* and *receive skin and nail care* the same as any other patient receiving total care. Patients often tend to scratch themselves as the depth of their consciousness lessens; thus, their nails should be trimmed. Patients who are comatose for long periods may be lifted occasionally into a bathtub half filled with warm water. For unconscious patients (or any patient with long-term debilitating disorders) application of superfatted solutions, e.g., castile, baby oil, cold cream, may be substituted for a bath every fourth or fifth day. This prevents loss of cutaneous oils and the subsequent development of skin irritations or dryness. When unconsciousness persists for long periods, the physician usually allows a *shampoo.*

*See also pp. 524–531.

Environmental room temperature is determined according to the patient's condition, e.g., a hyperthermic patient may be covered with only a sheet or loin cloth.

Safety and Preventive Measures. *Side rails should be kept up at all times when a comatose patient is not receiving direct care or is unattended.* Observe seizure precautions for persons with seizure histories and for those patients who could possibly have a seizure for the first time.

When moving or turning an unconscious patient, give adequate support to the limbs and head. A limb without tone may dislocate if allowed to fall unsupported. Also, always turn an unconscious patient toward you or toward another person, to protect the patient from rolling off the bed. In addition, protect an unconscious patient from external sources of heat, e.g., hot water bottles, heating pads, radiators, exposed light bulbs, and heat lamps.

Remove and safely store an unconscious patient's dentures and dental bridges. They could cause airway obstruction or could be swallowed or broken. Also, examine the patient for contact lenses and remove and store them if they are present.

Protect the patient from injury during seizures or periods of hyperexcitability. Such protection may be provided by physical measures, e.g., padded side rails and keeping the patient's nails short and clean, or by pharmacologic means. Caution must be taken so that the unconscious patient is not overly sedated because *excessive sedation impedes evaluation of the level of consciousness.*

Avoid restraining the patient unless absolutely necessary. Remember that a restrained patient is likely to become increasingly confused and combative.

Unstable patients ideally *should not be left unattended.* Because emergencies can develop rapidly in the unconscious patient, routine *emergency equipment* is kept readily available, e.g., endotracheal tubes, airways, suction, oxygen, respirators, IV standard, cutdown tray, IV solutions, and emergency medications.

The use of *prophylactic antibiotics* is *not* recommended in the long-term management of unconscious patients because of the danger of superinfection from resistant organisms. When infections occur, they are treated vigorously with an appropriate course of a suitable antibiotic.

The judicious use of *elastic stockings* may forstall thrombophlebitis (a frequent complication of bed rest). These should be removed several times each day.

Positioning and Exercises. By keeping an unconscious patient properly positioned at all times and by moving the patient about periodically and passively exercising extremities, a nurse can prevent the development of numerous complications.

Remember that devitalized, i.e., denervated, tissue in a paralyzed area easily breaks down, forming decubitus ulcers. *The prevention of decubitus ulcer formation is thus highly important in unconscious and paralyzed patients.* Because these patients may remain absolutely still in any position in which you place them make certain that the position is a safe one. A comprehensive program of decubitus ulcer prevention and management must be instituted. This may include an alternating air pressure mattress, in conjunction with turning and passive exercises, to prevent tissue ischemia, which predisposes to decubitus ulcer formation. Patients with neurologic disorders are also particularly prone to the development of *deformities and contractures.* See Sorensen and Luckmann, *Basic Nursing: A Psychophysiologic Approach,* Chapter 33, for a full discussion of decubitus ulcer care.

A hand roll may be used to maintain the hand in a position of function. If the patient's thumb tends to fall forward so that it does not grip the roll, gauze may be placed over the thumb and then loosely taped to the hand roll to keep the thumb in a position of function. Of course, such supportive bandages must be removed to exercise the hand, wrist, and fingers properly. The hand roll prevents *flexion contractures of the fingers* (Fig. 26–7*B*, *C*). "Cock-up" arm splints may be used to prevent *wristdrop* (Fig. 26–7*A*).

Some sources[70] suggest using a hard palmar hand-positioning device (Fig. 26–7*D*) to decrease flexor activity and increase hand function. Persons who recommend *hard* hand-positioning devices believe that soft devices may actually contribute to flexion of the hand.

Eye Care. The cornea may be kept moist by the use of commercially available eye drops, e.g., methyl cellulose (0.5 to 1 per cent solution).

A protective *eye shield* should be applied if the corneal reflex is absent and if the eyes are open and/or appear irritated. This prevents the cornea from being scratched or otherwise irritated. Or it may be desirable to close the eyelids of the unconscious patient with small carefully applied adhesive strips. Unless properly applied, such dressings may irritate the eye rather than protect it. When patients are unconscious for long periods, their eyelids may be sutured shut (*temporary tarsorrhaphy*) by a physician. (Additional discussion of eye care is given in Chapter 89.)

Nose and Ear Care. Nasal passages may become occluded because an unconscious patient is unable to sniff, blow, or normally clean the nose. To clear the nasal passages of mucus and crust formations, first gently swab the nose with an applicator moistened with water or normal saline. Next, use one lightly lubricated with mineral oil. Various types of room humidification may be used with these patients to relieve excessive dryness of the mucous membranes of the nose and mouth.

> Never *clean or suction the nasal passages or ears of patients who have had brain surgery or suffered a head injury without a specific doctor's order. If* bleeding *is noted from the patient's ears or nose, or if* cerebrospinal fluid *(looking like a watery discharge) appears to be draining from these areas,* notify the physician at once!

Mouth Care. Mouth care is conscientiously given to unconscious persons *every 2 hours* (as a *scheduled* treatment) to: (1) provide oral hygiene; (2) prevent excessive drying of the oral mucous membranes; and (3) prevent other complications such as parotitis, aspiration, and respiratory tract infection.

> *Aspiration and respiratory tract infections are common causes of death in unconscious patients.*

Mouth care is performed gently but thoroughly. Place the unconscious patient well over onto one side to prevent possible aspiration. The affected side should be uppermost in patients with

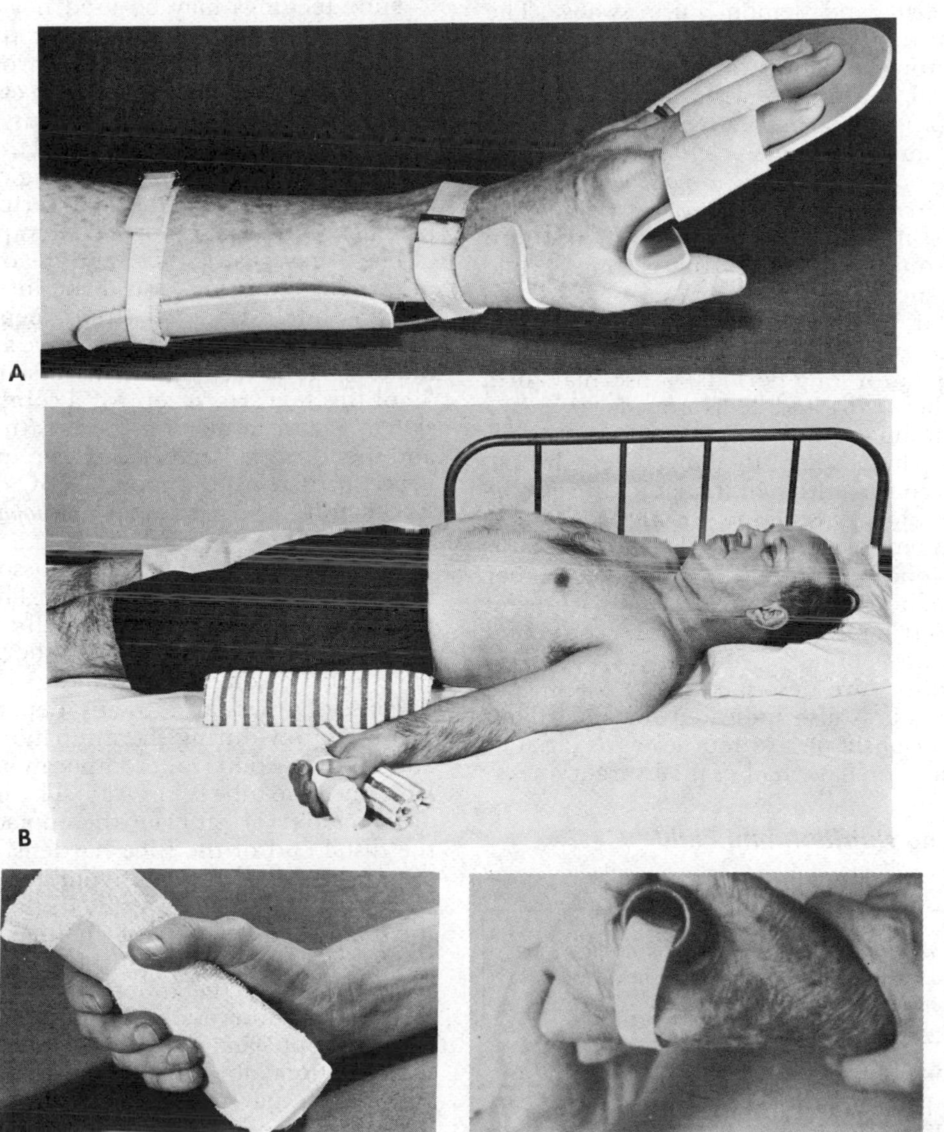

Figure 26–7. Wrist and hand positioning. **A.** Cock-up arm splint. **B** and **C.** Soft hand roll. **D.** Hard hand-positioning device. (*A, B,* and *C* from Krusen, F. H., F. J. Kottke, and P. M. Ellwood, Jr.: *Handbook of Physical Medicine and Rehabilitation*, 2nd ed., 1971. *D* from Dayoff, N.: Re-thinking stroke. Soft or hard devices to position hands? *American Journal of Nursing*, 75:1142, July 1975.)

facial paralysis. Have the bottom sheet protectively covered and place a towel under the patient's chin and over the upper shoulder. Place an emesis basin beside the mouth. Prop the mouth open by placing a padded tongue blade or soft roll between the patient's jaws. Do not put your fingers in an unconscious patient's mouth when giving mouth care. If the prop slips, you could be bitten accidentally. A human bite is potentially very dangerous.

An unconscious patient's teeth are carefully brushed with a small toothbrush at least twice daily. The mouth's mucous membranes, tongue, and gums are cleaned with various preparations, e.g., glycerin and lemon juice swabs. The mouth is then rinsed out. Gauze wrapped around a tongue depressor or around a toothbrush (and saturated with an appropriate preparation) may be useful in carrying out some aspects of mouth care. *During mouth care of the unconscious patient aspiration must be prevented and excess secretions should be removed with suction.* It is easiest if two persons perform mouth care together; one person does the cleaning while the other suctions as necessary.

Particular care must be given to the area around the uvula in patients breathing with their mouths open for long periods. Crusts may form that may break off and be aspirated.

Use a flashlight and tongue depressor to inspect the patient's mouth daily. Keep the patient's lips coated with a lubricant to prevent the formation of encrustations, drying, and cracking. Always inspect a paralyzed cheek for crusts or other conditions requiring care. Remember to have good light when giving mouth care and to wash your hands prior to the procedure and upon its completion.

The mouth care described above for unconscious patients is also indicated for all patients who are seriously ill, are febrile, have facial or bulbar palsy, or have had cranial surgery.

Maintaining Nutrition and Fluid Balance

> *Because an unconscious person cannot swallow normally and would thus aspirate, food or liquids are not given by mouth.*

Nutritional and fluid-electrolyte needs of unconscious persons are met in other ways, e.g., through nasogastric tube feedings, intravenous infusion, or hyperalimentation (see Chapter 59).

Fluid balance is generally maintained by intravenous infusion for the initial 2 to 5 days (sometimes longer) of unconsciousness; then, if coma continues, hyperalimentation or nasogastric tube feedings are started. The latter may be started earlier if the patient's veins are poor or to facilitate frequent position change.

Tube Feedings. Tube feedings are one desirable method of providing prolonged nourishment for an unconscious person because, while protein and carbohydrates can be administered parenterally, intravenous fats in the form of intralipid therapy have only recently begun to be used in major treatment centers. *Paralytic ileus occurs fairly often in unconscious persons, and a nasogastric tube used for gastric decompression can be subsequently used for feeding after the ileus is resolved.* Tube feeding may also be more convenient and safe than long-term intravenous therapy in settings where skilled nursing is limited.

Tube feedings may be used not only for an unconscious patient but also for patients with such disorders as: paralysis of throat musculature; senility with loss of desire to eat; cancer of the lip, tongue, pharynx, esophagus, or stomach; fistula of the gastrointestinal tract, or multiple sclerosis. More commonly, feeding ostomies are surgically created for the long-term feeding of patients requiring prolonged therapy.

The use of gastric tubes and the ongoing care of persons requiring gastric and intestinal tubes are absolutely essential, fundamental nursing skills. Many aspects of nursing care and the techniques of tube feeding are discussed in Chapter 59 of this text. However, for a complete discussion of gastric intubation, gavage (tube feeding), and the nursing care of persons requiring these procedures, consult Chapter 41 of Sorensen and Luckmann, *Basic Nursing: A Psychophysiologic Approach.*

The nursing responsibilities associated with tube feedings are especially critical in caring for the unconscious patient, because the person cannot communicate and because the person may have lost the cough reflex and gag reflex. The unconscious person is totally dependent upon you for safety during the intubation procedure and for protection from complications and problems once the tube is inserted. The possible hazards include: (1) trauma to the stomach mucosa if the distal end of the tube hardens, as happens after a period of time; (2) vomiting and aspiration if the stomach is overfilled; (3) plugging of the tube; (4) dislocation of the tube into trachea or lungs, thereby causing aspiration of anything passed through the tube; (5) development of ulcerations and crustations in the nares; and (6) tracheoesophageal fistula. (Tracheoesophageal fistula is breakdown of the anterior esophageal wall, which may result from prolonged contact between the nasogastric tube and a tracheostomy tube [if present]. Tracheoesophageal fistula becomes apparent when gastric contents appear in tracheal excretions; it requires immediate treatment.)

The unconscious patient is often restless. Watch that the patient does not pull out the tube. Aspiration may result if a feeding tube is pulled out during a feeding session or at any time it is unclamped. During feeding sessions, cloth wristlets or wrist restraints may be needed.

Aspiration pneumonia is always a hazard for a tube-fed patient, especially the unconscious patient. If the patient's head is elevated to a 45 degree angle during feeding, this hazard is reduced because, if the tube is displaced, there is less possibility of food entering the trachea. A patient should not be fed in the supine position unless other positions are impossible.

Maintaining Fluid and Electrolyte Balance. Important aspects in maintaining fluid balance in the unconscious patient are: maintaining accurate intake and output records; weighing the patient daily; and staying aware of the significance of such symptoms as excessive sweating, diarrhea, or vomiting.

Before fluid and electrolyte therapy can be planned for a comatose patient it must be determined if the coma itself is related to a disturbance in the patient's fluid or electrolyte state, or if the patient has a normal electrolyte state that must be maintained during the period of coma. In order to detect electrolyte imbalances various tests are made, e.g., blood sugar, blood urea nitrogen or creatinine, serum sodium, potassium, chloride, and carbon dioxide. Dehydration and water intoxication (true hyponatremia) are two common causes of electrolyte imbalance associated with coma.

Fluid and electrolyte therapy in treating comatose patients is controversial, particularly if cerebral swelling or edema is a problem. Basically, the controversy is over whether a patient should be kept "dry" (dehydrated) or normovolemic. Overhydration, however, is always avoided. The rates of IV infusion and administration and the types of solutions prescribed vary according to physician philosophy and patient need. A nurse needs to understand the prevailing philosophy of the institution and attending physicians.

> Remember:
> *Rapid infusion of large amounts of fluids to an unconscious person must be avoided. Careful monitoring of infusion rates and the neurologic status of the patient are essential.*

Returning to Oral Feedings. When a previously comatose patient begins to respond to verbal stimuli and has a gag reflex, test the patient's ability to suck and swallow water. Prior to the test the patient is placed well over onto one side and suction is started, to be used if needed. Water is used in testing the ability to swallow to reduce the dangers in case of aspiration. The patient is given water to suck through a straw, or on a wet swab, or a small amount is introduced into the back of the mouth.

Once it is established that a patient can safely swallow, small oral feedings may be started. Tube feedings are ended when the patient is able to take sufficient nutrition orally. Initially, for patients who cannot suck through a straw or drink from a glass due to facial paralysis, fluids may be placed into the unaffected side of the patient's mouth with an Asepto syringe. A small piece of rubber tubing may be placed on the end of a syringe if it is made of glass. This helps protect the patient if the glass tip is accidentally broken.

During the first attempts to eat independently again, a patient needs the nurse's quiet reassurance, calm advice and reminders, e.g., to eat slowly, to swallow, and so forth. The patient should not be hurried or feel rushed. Gradually progression occurs to a soft diet. Positioning is important as the patient begins to eat and swallow. Food and fluids should be taken into the unaffected side of the mouth if the patient has residual facial paralysis. This makes chewing easier and reduces drooling. In bed the patient with residual facial paralysis should be positioned with the affected side up before feeding.

Maintaining Elimination

An unconscious person cannot control urinary or bowel elimination. For esthetic reasons, as well as to prevent skin maceration, infections, and decubitus ulcer formation, the patient's skin is kept clean and dry. Elimination is always recorded, and the amount excreted is estimated as accurately as possible. It is important to record what time elimination occurred so some idea of the patient's pattern can be established. This can be helpful in retraining the patient during recovery. Even while a patient remains unconscious a urinal may be placed or the patient put on the bedpan at times when the patient's elimination "pattern" shows that elimination from bowels or bladder may be expected. Of course, a urinal or bedpan cannot be left in place for long or skin damage may occur.

Urinary elimination may be contained by the use of an indwelling catheter (Foley) or an external drainage apparatus (e.g., condom catheter). Occasionally a form of tidal drainage may be employed to maintain bladder capacity and muscle tone and to try to prevent bladder infection. The physician decides whether a catheter should be inserted. Because catheters are possible sources of infection and are "foreign bodies," they should be removed as soon as possible and bladder training started. Careful observations and cystometrogram studies aid in determining when the catheter can be removed. Bladder retraining is often possible during recovery by encouraging the patient to maintain a regulated fluid intake and to develop a pattern of habitually emptying the bladder.

The abdomen of an unconscious patient should frequently be checked for indications of bladder or bowel distention. A full bladder may be an overlooked cause of incontinence; i.e., dribbling may indicate retention with overflow. (See Unit XIII.) Also, constipation and fecal impaction may occur; small, frequent liquid stools may indicate impaction. (See Unit XVII.)

An unconscious patient requires a program of bowel care planned to control bowel movements and keep them on a fairly normal schedule and to prevent fecal impaction or constipation.

As soon as the patient is able, a program of bowel training should be instituted. Maintenance of a *regular* schedule is important in establishing a bowel control program. Thus, bowel care, e.g., stool softeners, suppositories, and digital removal, are administered at approximately the *same time* each day. Unit XVII of this text discusses specific problems with elimination, and Unit XIII discusses catheters.*

If a vaginal discharge or odor is noted, the physician may order cleansing douches. Unconscious female patients also need hygienic menstrual care.

The Significant Others of the Unconscious Patient

Unconsciousness is upsetting for a patient's loved ones to witness. They cannot communicate with the patient. They fear for irreversible brain damage. They may worry that the patient's condition will remain the same for a time. Or, they may be anxious about necessary treatments or possible death. The expense of highly specialized, long-term care is an additional concern for many. Family members and friends receive comfort from seeing their loved one receive concerned, quality care. Thus, it may be helpful for them to see the unconscious patient kept clean and attractive in appearance. Remember that although the patient appears unable to hear, he or she may actually hear everything that is said nearby. Discuss this fact with the patient's significant others and remember yourself to keep conversation appropriate in the presence of the patient.

*Consult Sorensen and Luckmann, *Basic Nursing: A Psychophysiologic Approach,* Chapters 30 and 40, for the fundamentals of maintaining elimination and caring for persons requiring urinary catheters.

INCREASED INTRACRANIAL PRESSURE

Introduction

Increased intracranial pressure (*intracranial hypertension*) is a frequent clinical problem that is commonly associated with altered states of consciousness. For many years, understanding increased intracranial pressure — the signs and symptoms attributed to it, and the treatment and prognosis — seemed fairly straightforward. Nurses took the limited available information and used what they could in planning and giving nursing care. Recently, however, the advent of new technologies such as continuous intracranial pressure monitoring has opened up new avenues of research and clinical care. Many previously learned "facts" have been challenged, and a "new" understanding of intracranial pressure dynamics is gradually developing. Even terms such as "cerebral edema" must be redefined in the face of newer information. As often happens, "old" and "new" facts must be put together and suddenly what was once viewed as relatively "simple" becomes quite complex. It is exciting to follow the expanding knowledge of intracranial dynamics and the promising related therapeutic changes. Because information about increased intracranial pressure is rapidly changing, the nurse is encouraged to continue to read current literature to update information in this discussion.

Increases in intracranial pressure have long been recognized as the cause of death and/or significant morbidity in a large portion of patients seen by neurosurgeons and neurologists. In the past, a *diagnosis* of increased intracranial pressure could be established by various noncontinuous methods, most commonly, the measurement of cerebrospinal fluid pressure by lumbar puncture. The patient's *progress,* however, had to be inferred from the signs and symptoms. Recently, however, various methods for continuously monitoring intracranial pressure readings have become available. This technology has reopened a broad interest in understanding intracranial pressure dynamics and devising more effective treatment regimens.

Causes and Mechanisms

Increased intracranial pressure is caused by various basic problems including: (1) increases in the intracranial blood volume, (2) increases in the cerebrospinal fluid (CSF) volume, and (3) increases in the bulk of the brain tissue. These increases occur with a *variety of conditions* and can occur (a) *rapidly* or *slowly* and (b) *diffusely* or *locally*. The rapidity and diffuseness of the changes appear to have an effect on the brain's ability to compensate for the changes. In other words, rapid and/or diffuse processes tend to overwhelm the brain's compensatory mechanisms quickly and produce the evolving, devastating signs and symptoms commonly associated with increased intracranial pressure.

The *basic compensatory mechanisms* appear to be: (1) displacement and reduction of the volume of the cerebrospinal fluid, (2) reduction of the volume of blood (with eventual critical decreases in cerebral metabolism), and (3) displacement of the tissues of the brain (e.g., herniation).

Basic to understanding these compensatory mechanisms is an understanding of the *Monro-Kellie hypothesis,* which in essence states that the skull is a "closed container" with a fixed volume of blood, CSF, and brain tissue (Fig. 26–8). Thus,

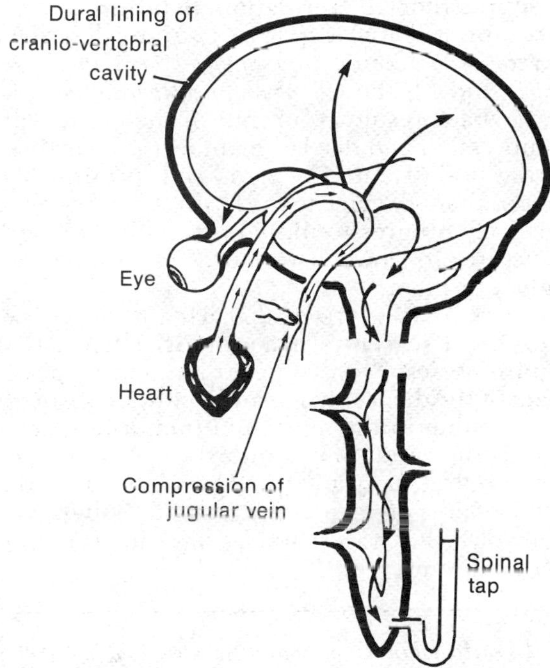

Figure 26–8. The Monro-Kellie doctrine. The craniovertebral cavity and its dural lining (represented by heavy contour) is a tightly closed space. Nerves and vessels penetrating the wall are sealed to the meninges and bone by dense connective tissue. Increase of any labile element of the contents — nervous tissue, CSF, blood — can take place only at the expense of others, or by increase of pressure.

Thus, compression of, say, the jugular veins, damming blood back into the skull, causes a rise of intracranial pressure. And since the cranial and vertebral cavities are continuous, this rise can be recorded from the lumbar cistern, unless passage is blocked.

The optic nerve, ensheathed in a continuation of the meninges and subarachnoid space, is compressed by any rise in intracranial pressure, with constriction of its central vessels, particularly the veins. Thus, engorgement of the retinal vessels is a readily accessible sign of heightened intracranial pressure. (From Elliott, H. C.: *Textbook of Neuroanatomy,* 2nd ed. Philadelphia: J. B. Lippincott Company, 1969, p. 420.)

an increase in the volume of any one of the contents results in a reciprocal change in the volume of one of the other contents. This hypothesis is valid because the skull is a rigid sphere with little room (or slack) for expansion of the contents. The various volumes *almost* fill the sphere, and the total volume remains *nearly* constant. Thus, the compensatory mechanisms may be quickly overwhelmed with resultant significant damage to the brain.

Two events thought to be responsible for brain tissue damage when the compensatory mechanisms fail are *tissue ischemia* and *compression.* Ischemia results in inadequate tissue metabolism; however, exactly how this occurs is not clear. Compression is seen with the so-called "mass lesions," e.g., tumors, hematomas.

Mass lesions displace brain tissue or cause *herniation.* Direct destruction of tissues can also occur. *Herniation can basically occur in two ways: across the tentorium* or *through the foramen magnum.*

The *tentorium* is a thick membrane that divides the brain into two compartments: the anterior (supratentorial) and the posterior (subtentorial). The contents of the anterior fossa and posterior fossa connect through an opening in the tentorium that is present in the midline. This is called the *tentorial incisura.* A variety of brain contents are adjacent to this opening, including the midbrain (posterior fossa contents) and the temporal lobes (supratentorial). The *foramen magnum* is another opening; it allows the brain stem to connect to the spinal cord. While the brain substance can move across the tentorium or through the foramen magnum, such movement does not happen without a cost. The cost is compression of tissues and, ultimately, their destruction. Moreover, enough brain tissue can be damaged to cause death.

Identification of impending or early herniation is one principal goal in caring for patients with raised intracranial pressure.

Increased blood flow because of dilatation of blood vessels, increases in the CSF for a variety of reasons, and increases in brain tissue mass from mass lesions can all cause increased intracranial pressure. *Cerebral edema* and increased intracranial pressure are sometimes spoken of as interchangeable entities. However, they are not the same. Cerebral edema, which increases the bulk of brain tissues, is only one cause of increased intracranial pressure. Moreover, cerebral edema and brain swelling are not the same thing. Rather, cerebral edema is *one type* of brain swelling.

Differentiating between brain swelling and cerebral edema is important because the treatment of the two is different.

> *Cerebral edema is an increase in the water content in the white matter of the brain, which leads to an increase in tissue volume.*

Vascular congestion, petechial hemorrhages, contusions, and other changes in the brain all can contribute to an increase in brain volume — yet they cannot correctly be called edema. Thus, the term *brain swelling* is used to denote a variety of changes (including cerebral edema) that increase the volume of the intracranial contents and lead to increased intracranial pressure. These other changes *may lead* to cerebral edema.

Cerebral edema is most commonly seen as a result of cerebral trauma or mass lesions. There are several theories as to the cause or causes of cerebral edema. Recent research has attempted to further clarify the pathophysiology of this entity in order to develop rational therapeutic approaches. At the present, however, although therapy is guided by various principles, it is largely empirical or based upon an incomplete understanding of the process of cerebral edema.

SIGNS AND SYMPTOMS OF INCREASED INTRACRANIAL PRESSURE

Increased intracranial pressure is best thought of as *several* entities rather than one in order to understand that no clinical sign or symptom is *always* present due to increased intracranial pressure.

> *The signs and symptoms of increased intracranial pressure tend to be related to the location and cause of the raised pressure and to the speed and extent of its development.*

Thus the identification of increased intracranial pressure is difficult *clinically* until overt signs and symptoms of compromise of the brain's function are present. Moreover, clinical signs and symptoms may not appear or may fail to be recognized until after significant damage has been done. Hence the advent of continuous intracranial pressure monitoring and other modalities discussed in the subsequent section on monitoring.

Signs and symptoms not necessarily caused by increased pressure but which may be present include headache, nausea, vomiting, and — as discussed before in this chapter — changes in level of consciousness, motor function, respirations, pupils, ocular movements and/or vital signs. Signs of the various herniation syndromes may also be evident.

HERNIATION SYNDROMES

As previously stated, there are several ways increased intracranial pressure can occur. One of these ways seems to be generally associated with brain shift, resulting in several recognizable patterns of findings. These patterns, named by their end-stage, can occur in the supratentorial compartment or the subtentorial (infratentorial) one (Fig. 26–9*A*).

Supratentorial Herniation Syndromes. Of the supratentorial patterns, two are described here: (1) *the central transtentorial herniation syndrome* and (2) the *lateral or uncal herniation syndrome.* Each results from shift of the brain, with compression and displacement of the structures of the brain stem. The signs and, presumably, the resultant damage to the brain stem occur in a relatively progressive fashion from the "higher" structures to "lower" structures or in a rostral-caudal fashion.

CENTRAL TRANSTENTORIAL HERNIATION SYNDROME. The central transtentorial herniation syndrome results in compression and displacement of the diencephalon and midbrain through the opening in the tentorium (tentorial notch). This is the result of downward displacement of the cerebral hemispheres. Mass lesions of the hemispheres are common causes, although centrally placed extracerebral lesions can also cause this syndrome.

> *An early indication of central transtentorial herniation is a change in the level of consciousness.*

- ▶ Impairment of the *diencephalon* (see Chapter 24) causes the first symptom, a change in the level of consciousness (LOC). The patient becomes less alert or has subtle behavior changes, e.g., agitation or apathy. If tissue displacement continues, the patient eventually progresses to a state of stupor and coma. Pauses, signs, or yawns may interrupt respirations, and gradually Cheyne-Stokes respirations occur. The pupils are small but react to light, although the reaction may appear to be absent without careful scrutiny. The ocular movements may be roving. They may also be conjugate, with the presence of the doll's eyes phenomenon (remember that "doll's eyes" are *absent* in a normal individual and *disappear* with deep coma) and characteristic findings in the caloric test (see p.

516). The motor signs usually are a generalized increased tone and a bilateral positive Babinski response. With progression, the grasp reflex may emerge, and finally decorticate posturing to painful stimuli appears on one side. If a preexisting hemiplegia is present, that side may decerebrate while the other side decorticates.

► The *midbrain–upper pons* stage of deterioration is characterized by progressive signs of brain stem failure. These patients classically look "sick." Cheyne-Stokes respirations change to central neurogenic hyperventilation, and the pupils dilate and fix at midposition. Eye movement responses to oculovestibular or oculocephalic testing become more difficult to elicit. When a response appears, although both eyes move, they are frequently dysconjugate (do not move together). Decorticate posturing changes to bilateral decerebrate rigidity in response to painful stimulation. The patient may also decerebrate spontaneously. During this stage, signs of disruption of the function of the pituitary and hypothalamus may appear. These can include the onset of diabetes insipidus and wide swings in body temperature. The hyperthermia present earlier frequently changes to hypothermia. Wide swings in the other vital signs are often present.

► The next stage, the *lower pontine–upper medullary* stage, is quieter and the patient appears calmer. The prognosis is very poor. The breathing pattern changes and appears superficially normal, but the rate is faster and depth is shallow. The pupils do not change, but the eye movements can no longer

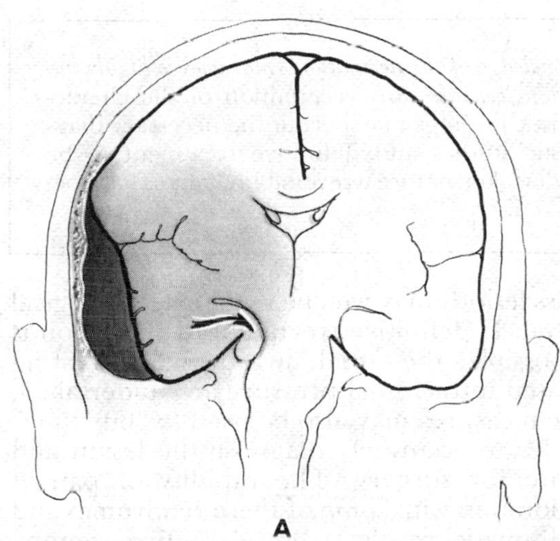

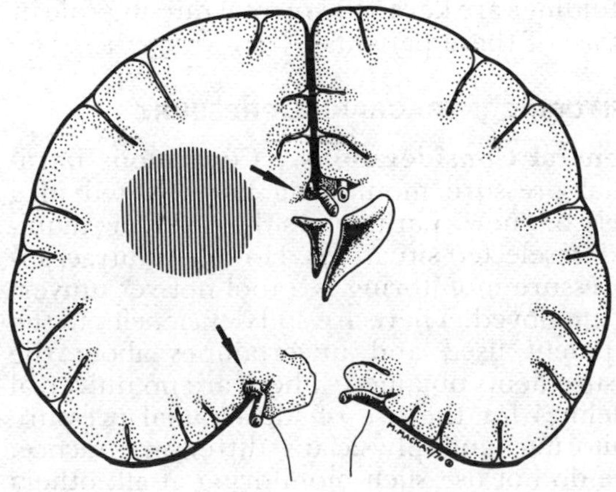

Figure 26–9. A. Mechanism of tontorial herniation. As the tissue mass increases, the brain is pushed toward and ultimately through the incisural notch (arrow). **B.** Uncal herniation compresses the midbrain laterally. (From Youmans, J. (Ed.); *Neurological Surgery.* Philadelphia: W. B. Saunders Co., 1973.)

be stimulated by the caloric test. The patient is flaccid.

- The *medullary stage* is terminal. The respirations become slower and irregular, the pulse may be either slow or fast, and the blood pressure drops. Finally breathing stops, the pupils dilate widely and death occurs.

LATERAL OR UNCAL HERNIATION SYNDROME. The lateral or uncal herniation syndrome (Fig. 26–9*B*) is often caused by lesions in the temporal lobe or by lateral extracerebral lesions. Characteristically, the lateral pressure cone first impinges on the midbrain structures, causing third nerve signs to occur first. Thus, a change in the level of consciousness is not usually the first sign of lateral or uncal herniation.

> *The most reliable early sign of lateral herniation is dilatation of one of the pupils.*

- The first stage in this syndrome is called the *early third nerve stage* because of the characteristic dilatation of one of the pupils. The light reaction in the dilated pupil is usually still present but is sluggish. This sign, which may last for several hours, is usually the *only* early sign seen. Other changes in the "neuro signs" occur later. However:

> *Lateral or uncal herniation usually progresses very rapidly once the patient begins to show signs of deterioration.*

- The *late third nerve stage* progresses very rapidly. The patient becomes stuporous, then comatose. The affected pupil fully dilates; the extraocular movements are at first abnormal to testing, then disappear. Ipsilateral hemiplegia appears, followed by decerebration. *The need for treatment is urgent.*

- Failing treatment, the patient progresses to the *midbrain–upper pons stage.* The other (not dilated) pupil dilates either to midposition or widely and becomes fixed. Neurogenic hyperventilation and bilateral decerebrate posturing are present. Eye movements are impaired or absent to testing. Further deteriorations at this point cannot be differentiated from those seen with the central transtentorial herniation syndrome.

Subtentorial or Posterior Fossa Herniation Syndromes. The *subtentorial or posterior fossa herniation syndromes* present less clearcut patterns of deterioration of the affected patient. The findings of the two syndromes, *upward herniation* and *downward herniation,* are difficult to distinguish from those caused by direct compression of the brain stem. Coma, severe respiratory abnormalities, severe motor changes, pupil and ocular movement changes, and the Cushing reflex may be present in differing combinations.

The upward syndrome, which is rarely seen, may present with loss of upward gaze and acute hydrocephalus. The downward herniation, because of lateral pressure on the vital centers of the pons and medulla, may present very rapidly. The Cushing reflex (increased blood pressure, decreased pulse, and widened pulse pressure), accompanied by a temperature increase and severely depressed respirations (even apnea), may be the findings. These patients do not always lose consciousness early. The signs develop rapidly, making emergency treatment essential to prevent death.

> *Knowledge of the herniation syndromes is highly important because early* recognition of the characteristic findings may permit the necessary diagnostic studies and definitive treatment to be undertaken before irreversible changes have occurred.

Mass lesions may well be amenable to surgical removal. If definitive treatment of the lesion is not possible, the usual measures for treating increased intracranial pressure are undertaken. These measures may also be used to "buy time" in order to accurately diagnose the lesion and prepare for surgery. The rapidity of patient deterioration with some of these syndromes and the dramatic results from definitive therapy make patients experiencing brain herniation syndromes a challenge for nursing care. Well developed neurologic observation skills and a high index of suspicion in the presence of abnormal findings are key to the pivotal nursing role in the care of these patients.[249]

MONITORING INTRACRANIAL PRESSURE

General Considerations. Continuous intracranial pressure monitoring has resulted in a variety of "new" parameters that are now monitored in selected situations. However, intracranial pressure monitoring is a tool not yet universally employed. There are still deficiencies in the equipment used and uncertainties about the measurements obtained. There are no universal guidelines for the use of intracranial pressure monitoring, and physicians differ in practice. Some do not use such monitoring at all; others use it liberally in a variety of conditions associated with elevated intracranial pressure, including head trauma (especially with associated chest trauma that requires mechanical ventilation) and in pre- and postoperative situations with tumors, aneurysms and posterior fossa lesions. No matter what the indications are, monitoring supplements rather than replaces careful, serial observations of the patient's condition.

> *Clinical monitoring of a patient's "neuro signs" is essential and is not replaced by intracranial pressure monitoring.*

Monitoring devices for intracranial pressure are many, varied, and complex. Intraventricular, subarachnoid, subdural, and direct intracerebral monitors are available. Each works differently, each has very important nursing considerations, and the technology is complex (Fig. 26–10). A nurse *must* learn about the specific characteristics of the particular monitoring device in the setting in which it is used. Moreover, as different areas are monitored, it is also important to learn about the advantages and disadvantages of the site used and the "meaning" of the values obtained in particular types of patients. The pressure in one compartment of the brain is not necessarily the same as that in another one. This is especially true in the presence of a mass lesion. Hence, intracranial pressure is really intracranial pressure*s*.

Despite all of the obstacles, continuous intracranial pressure monitoring is a valuable tool in caring for patients. Some advantages of this technique are:

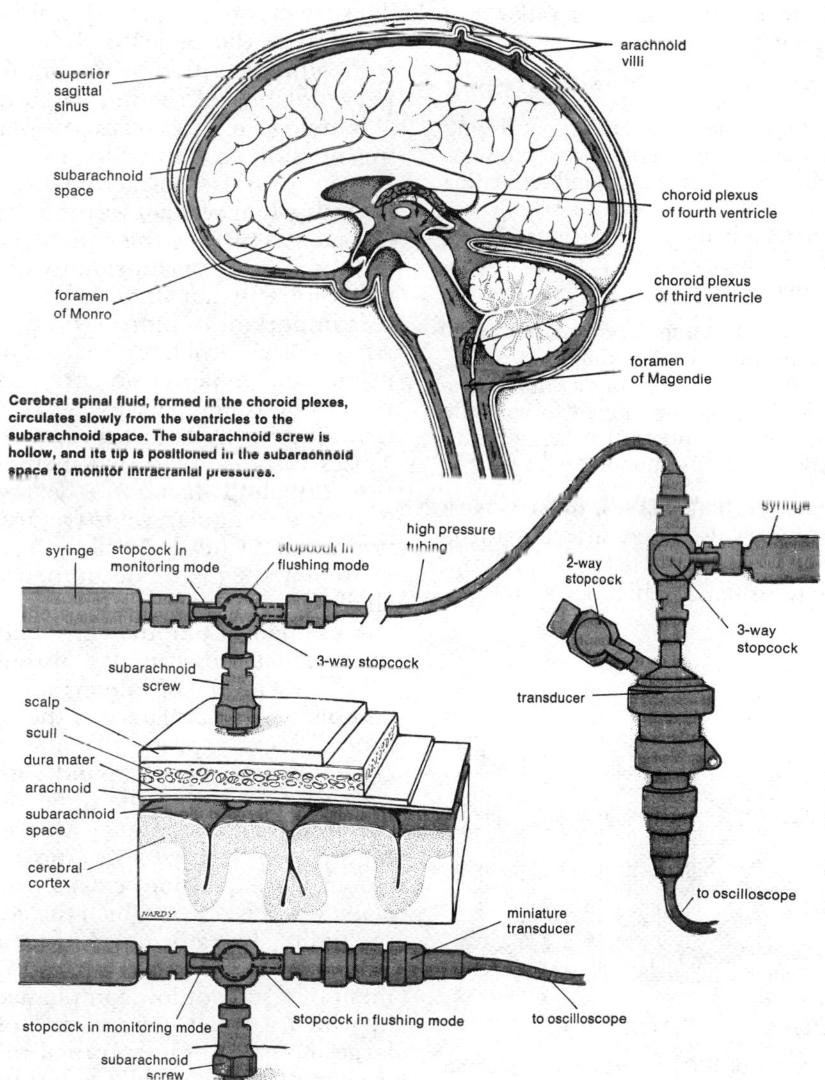

Figure 26–10. The subarachnoid screw is inserted through a burr hole in the skull, and connects to a transducer and oscilloscope for continuous monitoring. Standard size transducer (top) connects to screw via pressure tubing and is secured to I.V. pole. Miniature transducer (bottom) attaches directly to threeway stopcock. Tail of stopcock is the closed side. (From Johnson, M., and J. Quinn: The subarachnoid screw. *American Journal of Nursing,* 77:448, Mar. 1977.)

- Pressure increase may be recognized and treated *prior* to the onset of signs and symptoms.
- Some systems allow drainage of ventricular fluid above a set pressure, thus allowing the system to be used as part of the therapy.
- Delays in bringing the patient to definitive therapy, e.g., surgery, can, at times, be avoided.
- Various other types of treatments can be monitored for their effectiveness.
- The presence of sustained pressure waves (plateau waves) can be detected (see discussion below).
- Intracranial compliance can be measured (see below).
- The level of intracranial pressure elevation can provide prognostic information.
- Cerebral perfusion can be calculated (see below).
- Some patients (e.g., those requiring paralyzing drugs such as curare for mechanical ventilation or those being treated with barbiturate-induced coma or induced hypothermia) cannot be readily assessed for key changes in their "neuro signs." Intracranial pressure monitoring is of particular value with these patients.
- Finally, the effect of nursing care on intracranial pressure can be monitored. The timing of procedures that are known to raise intracranial pressure, e.g., suctioning, can be altered to coincide with periods of "lower" pressure when plateau waves are not occurring in patients.

Plateau Waves. Plateau waves, or A waves, occur at varying intervals. They are said to be present when intracranial pressure rises from a patient's baseline to unusually high levels and remains elevated for from 5 to 20 minutes. These periods of sustained pressure elevation may be followed or accompanied by signs and symptoms such as decerebrate posturing and disorientation. The waves occur "spontaneously" and paroxysmally. They also may occur when the treatment of the patient is causing the pressure to rise. For example, suctioning can cause a marked elevation in intracranial pressure and plateau waves may appear. Figure 26–11 shows an example of plateau waves.

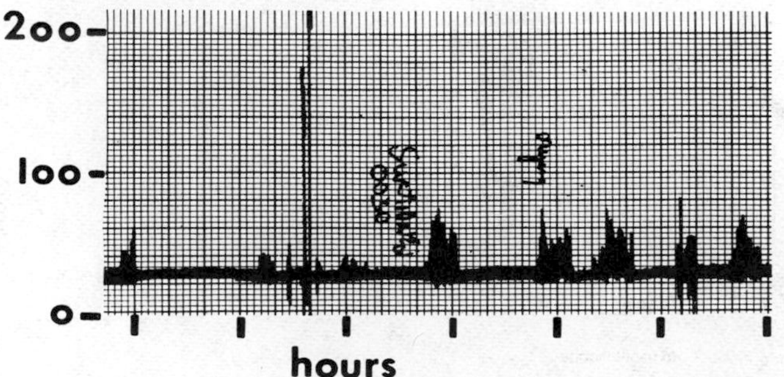

Figure 26–11. Actual recording of ICP. In this patient, plateau waves and pressure wave symptoms were observed (arrows). (From Taylor, F., and H. Schutz: Symptoms caused by intracranial pressure waves. *Journal of Neurological Nursing*, 9:144, Dec. 1977.)

> *It is generally thought that plateau waves and/or their related signs and symptoms are signs of impending decompensation.*

Recognition of plateau waves allows a nurse to note that a patient's intracranial compliance (see discussion below) is poor. Treatment to lower intracranial pressure needs to be undertaken. This treatment could be definitive (e.g., surgical removal of the cause) or treatment of the sign (e.g., administration of mannitol or manual hyperventilation of the intubated patient).

Nursing therapy consists of planning and timing nursing care in order to avoid giving care known to raise intracranial pressure during periods when plateau waves are present. Activities such as turning the patient, suctioning, moving the patient's head side to side, or removing the respirator can all raise intracranial pressure. It is important to thoroughly assess the patient. Among the problems that may contribute to intracranial hypertension are excess water in the respirator tubing; excess secretions in the patient, causing a rise in arterial pCO_2 (hypercarbia causes vasodilatation that increases intracranial pressure); and an endotracheal tube taped tightly over the jugular veins (retarding venous return from the head). In sum, the care of a patient who shows signs of decompensating is indeed challenging.

Measuring Compliance. The monitoring of intracranial pressure may also allow use of another method of determining intracranial compliance. Compliance is the measure of how much "slack" is present — how much the intracranial contents can expand within the nondistensible skull before the fit becomes "tight" and the intracranial contents are compromised. A highly *compliant system* is one in which "slack" (room for expansion) exists, whereas a *noncompliant system* is one in which the compliance is low or "tight." The advantage of measuring compliance is the early identification of the development of a state of low compliance, i.e., that state in which a small increase in volume produces large increases in intracranial pressure.

Compliance is usually tested by introducing a known volume of fluid into the ventricle and measuring its effect on intracranial pressure. Detecting a change in the critical relationship between volume and pressure allows early treatment of the problem *before* the onset of signs and symptoms or sustained elevation of the intracranial pressure. The treatment and related care is similar to that discussed before with plateau waves.

Measurements of cerebral blood flow, cerebral perfusion pressure, and *cerebral metabolism* are all relatively new applications of techniques discussed previously. Use of these techniques is mainly in medical centers involved in research on intracranial pressure dynamics. Measurement of the intracranial pressure and arterial pressure allows calculation of the cerebral perfusion pressure and direct measurement of the total and regional blood flow. Cerebral metabolism is calculated. These techniques for more exact appraisal of the brain's function are in early stages of development and many questions about intracranial dynamics and the value of these parameters remain to be answered. Continuous monitoring of the EEG is in a similar stage of development.

Treatment and Related Care

The treatment of a patient with increased intracranial pressure includes the activities previously discussed for patients with altered states of consciousness. Treatment of increased intracranial pressure is basically (a) *direct* by removing the cause or (b) *indirect* by using osmotic diuretics (e.g., mannitol, urea), steroids, and possibly induced hyperventilation (on a mechanical respirator).

The most commonly used *diuretic* is mannitol. It removes water from the *normal* brain tissue, not from edematous tissue. A number of problems may occur with the use of mannitol, including: (1) a "rebound" effect, in which after an initial decrease, the intracranial pressure becomes high again, (2) production of hyperosmolar states, (3) decreased effectiveness with repeated use, and (4) aggravation of edema in some patients.[340]

Steroids, frequently dexamethasone in conventional doses, are used; recently some investigators are using large doses.[107] The mechanisms by which steroids work is unknown, so their use is empirical. Recently, steroids have been noted to decrease the frequency of plateau waves but not the absolute intracranial pressure.[226] Because of the risk of gastrointestinal hemorrhage, prophylaxis, often with antacids, is done (see discussion of head injuries, Chapter 27, p. 656).

Finally, *hyperventilation* induced by a respirator or by bagging a patient is used, despite the many problems with this technique. Since hypocapnia reduces cerebral blood volume and intracranial pressure, the use of hyperventilation to induce hypocapnia is a well-recognized form of therapy. This maneuver may be lifesaving while readying the patient for other forms of therapy. Manual hyperventilation is also sometimes done during plateau waves or when sudden clinical signs of deterioration appear. Continuous controlled hyperventilation is more controversial, because its effect on the blood vessels and blood volume seems to be attenuated over time.[251]

Whether hyperventilation is used or not, meticulous *respiratory care* is essential. Frequent arterial blood gas analysis is usually done. Acid-base imbalances are corrected, and oxygenation is kept adequate. (Exceptions in correction occur and may include patients who have a self-induced respiratory alkalosis because they have central hyperventilation.)

Respiratory toilet measures are used, but used with caution in patients with low intracranial compliance since coughing and suctioning may markedly elevate intracranial pressure (Fig. 26–12). However, retained secretions may cause a patient to retain carbon dioxide and thus elevate the intracranial pressure. Therefore, removing the secretions is essential. A minimum-trauma suctioning technique should be used.[276] These patients are usually intubated, and current suctioning techniques often require the use of hyperinflation of the lungs with an anesthesia bag between each passage of the suction catheter. This hyperinflation, if done too vigorously, may have a PEEP-like effect and markedly raise intracranial pressure.

PEEP or positive end-expiratory pressure is a method of increasing the oxygenation of a patient experiencing severe respiratory insufficiency. (See Unit XVI.) PEEP's effect on intracranial pressure is inconsistent; in some patients the pressure markedly rises, in others the pressure remains unchanged or drops. Since PEEP is used in patients in whom adequate oxygenation cannot otherwise be maintained, it may occasionally be used in patients with increased intracranial pressure. Never suction through the nose, as nasal drainage may have diagnostic significance.

Keeping respiratory secretions loose is often a problem in caring for people with increased intracranial pressure. Prescribed fluid therapy may aggravate this problem. Moreover, postural drainage, especially in the head-down position, is contraindicated, as is chest physiotherapy. (The patient's head is typically ordered to be elevated 15 to 20 degrees.) Also, turning the patient's head far to the side, as is done with suctioning, may cause intracranial pressure to rise suddenly.[139] (See Unit XVI.)

Fluid therapy in the presence of increased intracranial pressure has long been the subject of controversy. Currently, opinion seems to be favoring the use of a balanced salt solution such as isotonic saline or Ringer's lactate solution for persons with increased intracranial pressure.[340] The rationale is that these fluids remain in the vascular space longer and, hence, contribute less to cerebral edema. However, while balanced salt solutions are generally used, other solutions may be necessary should complications or other problems be present, e.g., shock. A common error to be avoided in fluid administration is using the wrong solution for intravenous medication administration and for the maintenance of various monitoring devices, e.g., indwelling arterial lines. A considerable amount of fluid can be administered by these routes and yet not be calculated as part of the patient's intake. The *type* and *amount* of such fluids must be taken into account.

Fluids are carefully monitored so that they are not infused too rapidly.

The actual amount of fluid to infuse per hour is determined by a variety of factors related to a patient's overall condition. You should not infuse more than the ordered amount; if fluid therapy falls behind, consult the physician. This is especially important for a patient with low intracranial compliance. It is also important to remember that mechanical ventilation causes the patient to retain water.

The use of induced hypothermia to decrease cerebral metabolism and, hence, treat intracranial hypertension is currently not popular.[340] Methods of inducing hypothermia are discussed briefly in the next section. Although induction of hypothermia is rare, control of an elevated temperature is a common problem in these patients. A lowered temperature may also be a problem. The *cooling and warming of patients for temperature control* are discussed in the following section.

Seizures also cause a marked increase in intracranial pressure. Patients with irritative lesions are particularly prone to developing seizures. (See the brief section in this chapter on p. 554 and the section on epilepsy in the next chapter for a more extensive discussion of seizures.)

Various *surgical techniques* are used to treat patients with increased intracranial pressure. Optimally, the cause of the intracranial hypertension can be located and removed. Other techniques include placing a shunt to allow drainage if CSF is blocked, and decompressive surgery. The latter is done by removing part of the brain tissues, e.g., part of the temporal lobe, to give the remaining structures room to expand. Also, if compliance is low at surgery, the bone flap removed to gain access to the brain is not replaced and/or the dura may not be closed. Subsequent surgery is required to repair the defect. (Neurosurgery is discussed in Chapter 28.)

New therapies are continuously being tried. One of these is the *induction of barbiturate coma.* Early experience with this technique looks promising, but assessment of its real effectiveness awaits further investigation.[205] Currently, research efforts in managing the patient with intracranial hypertension are numerous. It is hoped that new techniques of management will improve the survival rate and the later quality of life for persons with this problem.

ABNORMAL BODY TEMPERATURE ALTERATIONS

The normal range of oral temperature in a resting person is from 36° to 38° C. (96.8 to 100.4° F.). Body heat must be regulated within a relatively small range in order for various physiologic processes to operate successfully. CNS function is impaired when body temperature varies 4° C. (9° F.) either above or below the normal range, and convulsions frequently occur

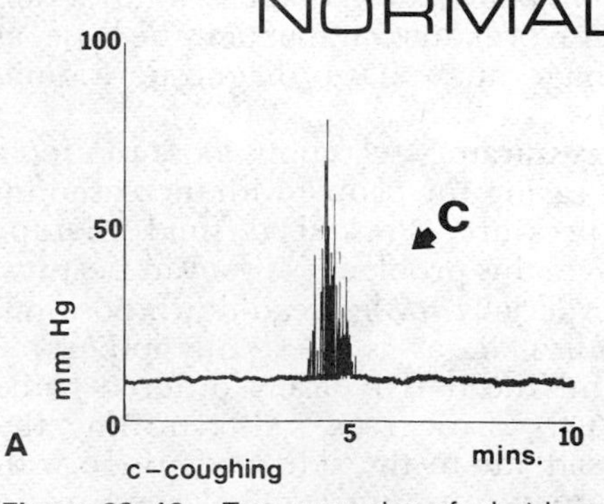

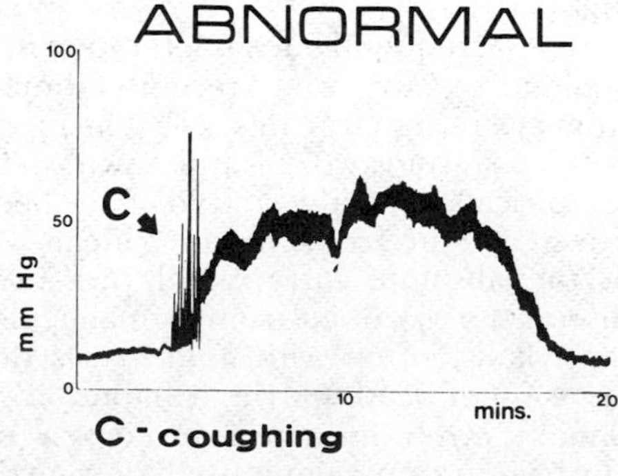

Figure 26–12. Two examples of what happens when intracranial volume is increased by coughing, vomiting, suctioning, straining, etc. *A* demonstrates a sudden momentary rise in ICP. However, because compliance is normal, the increased intracranial pressure dissipates rapidly. *B* demonstrates what happens during coughing when compliance is low. (From Hanlon, K.: Intracranial compliance interpretation and clinical application. *Journal of Neurosurgical Nursing,* 9:35, Mar. 1977.)

when body temperature exceeds 41° C. (105.8° F.). Thermal death results from irreversible changes that occur if body temperature rises above 44 to 45° C. Unassisted survival is generally impossible if body temperature exceeds 8° C. above normal or drops 10° C. below normal. The body protects itself more vigorously against overheating than against excessive cooling.

Hyperthermia

Hyperthermia (hyperpyrexia) is a body *temperature elevation* to 41° C. (106° F.) or above. During hyperthermia body metabolism continues to produce heat; however, little heat is dissipated from the body. Because the patient does not perspire and because the superficial blood vessels fail to dilate, the fever continues to rise. Typically a hyperthermic patient's skin appears pale and is perhaps mottled instead of red. While the trunk feels hot and dry, the limbs may feel cold. A shaking chill or quivering of the arms and legs may occur.

At temperatures above 41° C. (106° F.) the rate of cellular metabolism is so greatly increased that physiologic regulation can no longer overcome the rapid rate at which heat is produced. Because the patient's own cooling mechanisms are inadequate, death will occur unless intensive treatment is instituted immediately.

For each centigrade degree of rise in body temperature the body tissues' oxygen requirements increase by approximately 13 per cent (or 7 per cent for each Fahrenheit degree).

> *Brain tissue is highly susceptible to hypoxia. To prevent brain tissue damage from the hypoxia which occurs with hyperthermia, prompt therapy is needed to reduce the body temperature to safe levels.*

Causes of Hyperthermia. Hyperthermia may result from various causes, e.g., infection, malfunction of the body's thermoregulatory center, prolonged exposure to excessively high environmental temperatures.

The body's thermoregulatory center may malfunction, producing hyperthermia, in the following instances:

- As a result of cerebral edema
- Following cerebrovascular accidents
- Following intracranial surgery
- Following head injury
- As a result of brain tumors or other lesions
- In association with one of the herniation syndromes

As stated, hyperthermia also occurs as a result of excessive exposure to high environmental temperatures. This condition, called *"heatstroke"* or *"sunstroke,"* develops because the body cannot dissipate heat faster than it is being received externally. Hence, environmental heat gain occurs and the body's temperature increases. Additionally, another source of heat is produced within the body because this increased tissue temperature increases cellular metabolism. For example, at 42° C. (107.6° F.) cellular metabolism is increased to a rate 50 per cent higher than that of tissues at normal temperatures.

Early symptoms of heatstroke include visual disturbances, headache, nausea, and vomiting. Additional symptoms include: rapid respirations, rapid bounding pulse, weakness and muscle flaccidity. As the condition progresses, the patient becomes delirious and eventually lapses into coma. The thermoregulatory center appears to fail when body temperature exceeds 41° C. (106° F.). At this time, in addition to the presence of a high temperature, the patient typically collapses and there is a noticeable *absence* of sweating. Sweating normally is a protective mechanism which cools the overly heated body. However, in this instance sweating fails to occur (even though desperately needed) because of CNS damage. Without proper therapy, death results within a few hours. (*Note:* Heatstroke differs from *heat cramps* or *heat exhaustion* [heat prostration], in which a marked body temperature rise does not occur.)

Clinical Care of the Febrile or Hyperthermic Patient. Clinical care focuses on reducing the elevated body temperature. When a patient's temperature is moderately elevated, e.g., 38.1° C. (101° F.), the room temperature should be maintained at 70° F. and blankets and excess clothing removed. The patient may be covered only by a sheet or occasionally both sheet and gown are removed and only a breast covering and loin cloth are used. Various methods of cooling (discussed on p. 551) may be prescribed by the physician if the patient's temperature continues to rise.

Unless contraindicated, fluid intake is increased to 3000 ml. every 24 hours. In the presence of increased intracranial pressure, the fluid intake may not be increased.

Antipyretics are frequently ordered. Antipyretic drugs appear to act on hypothalamic centers and obtain their effects through normal physiologic processes, e.g., by reducing the thermoregulatory center's sensitivity and producing diaphoresis. They are often given on a scheduled basis (e.g., every 4 hours) rather than as necessary for temperature elevations over a specified level. Cooling measures such as putting wet sheets over the patient or applying packs of chipped ice in selected areas may be used. Generally, however, the patient is cooled by a hypothermia blanket.

> *It is extremely important to avoid cooling a patient too rapidly or too much.*

Rapid cooling not only may induce serious arrhythmias but also may cause the patient to shiver. Shivering increases the metabolic rate. It can also raise intracranial pressure. Shivering can be treated with a variety of drugs, e.g., chlorpromazine, and prevented in some patients by using muscle relaxants.[341] A cooling blanket can also quickly damage the skin. Extremely careful skin care must be given. The blanket should be covered with bath blankets and the patient's skin should be inspected at least hourly. Lanolin, cold cream, or mineral oil should be applied to the skin to prevent drying. The patient should be turned at least every 2 hours.

During treatment of hyperthermia, especially with a cooling blanket, the patient's temperature is usually monitored continuously with a rectal probe. (The temperature can also be continuously monitored in the esophagus.) When a predetermined, stable, acceptable level of temperature elevation has been reached, taking rectal temperatures with a thermometer may be resumed. As long as the cooling blanket is being used, continuous monitoring of temperature is advisable to avoid inducing hypothermia.

General comfort measures are important in the care of any patient with an elevated body temperature. For example, the patient should be kept dry and clean (this is especially important if perspiring heavily) and frequent skin, mouth, and nose care should be given.

Induced hypothermia (discussed below) may be necessary to protect the patient from the hazards of excessively high body temperatures.

Hypothermia

Induced hypothermia is deliberate cooling of a patient to below a normal temperature. It can be done by a variety of techniques including using the hypothermia blanket, packing the patient in ice, and various maneuvers used principally in the operating room. Currently, it is infrequently used in the treatment of patients with neurologic disorders.[432] The body can also become hypothermic *accidentally,* e.g., from prolonged exposure to an excessively cold environment. This discussion focuses on general hypothermia induced for therapeutic purposes.

By definition, *"induced hypothermia"* is the controlled reduction of body temperature to a level considerably below normal and the maintenance of the temperature at that level. Given proper care it is possible for an individual to survive induced hypothermia that reduces body temperature to below 24°C. In practice generally, however, body temperature is not allowed to reach such a low level. The level of hypothermia desired for a given patient varies, depending upon the reasons for the procedure. A physician determines the level of hypothermia to be maintained and the length of time a patient will be maintained at that subnormal temperature. Hypothermia may be described as mild (30 to 35°C; 86 to 95°F.), moderate (24 to 30°C; 75.2 to 86°F.) and deep (below 24°C; 75.2°F.).

Uses of Hypothermia. Hypothermia may be used for either medical or surgical purposes, although its use is controversial.

In *surgery* hypothermia has several uses: to facilitate selected procedures by reducing blood flow; to lower the operative risk in severely debilitated "poor risk" patients; to relieve intractable pain (e.g., in terminal cancer); and to reduce the amount of anesthesia necessary during surgery. Surgical procedures for which hypothermia may be utilized include amputations, cardiac surgery, vascular surgery, and lengthy brain operations, although this is infrequent. By reducing cerebral blood flow, hypothermia is useful in intracranial operations for aneurysms and highly vascular tumors.

During some surgery, hypothermia may be used in conjunction with general anesthesia to decrease metabolic demands and thereby reduce blood flow. The use of hypothermia influences the amount of anesthetic needed and the speed with which the anesthetic agent is eliminated from the body. (Anesthesia is discussed generally in Unit VIII.)

In *medical* situations hypothermia may be employed to treat or prevent extreme temperature elevations. Hypothermia may be used occasionally in the treatment of shock, cardiac arrest, and gastrointestinal hemorrhage.

Responses to General Hypothermia. Among the physiologic changes that take place as body temperature is lowered are the following:

Rate of metabolism decreases. Body metabolism is reduced by almost 50 per cent when body temperature is reduced to 30°C. (86°F.), and is reduced to 25 per cent of normal if temperature reaches 20°C. (68°F.). Death may then occur suddenly.

Endocrine, liver, and kidney functions decrease as the rate of metabolism decreases.

Heart tissue is affected. The critical level below which arrhythmia occurs (due to altered myocardial irritability) varies with the level of hypothermia used and the patient's age and condition.

Circulation slows. The volume of circulating blood is reduced as plasma pools in peripheral capillary beds. Slowing occurs as the heart's neuromuscular tissue is affected by the reduced temperature.

Oxygen consumption is reduced.
Pulse and respiration rates are reduced, and blood pressure falls.
Venous and cerebral spinal fluid pressures decrease.
Cerebral function is reduced. Cerebral blood flow is reduced about 6 per cent for every degree the centigrade temperature is reduced below normal; brain bulk is reduced.

When observing and caring for a patient as the body temperature is being reduced, the nurse keeps in mind the expected responses to hypothermia in order to quickly identify responses that indicate the development of complications. Typical responses to reduced body temperature occur in the following sequence: (1) rate of metabolism decreases and heart rate and respiratory rate begin to fall; (2) impairment of higher mental processes occurs, and the patient responds to verbal commands but has difficulty performing complicated acts; (3) patient becomes stuporous and has reduced responses to external stimulation; (4) unconsciousness ensues, although heart action is usually not disturbed; and (5) finally, the heart rate, blood pressure, and respiratory rate continue to fall and ventricular fibrillation may occur. At this final level the patient is comatose; pupillary reaction to light and corneal and gag reflexes are absent.

Methods of Inducing General Hypothermia

- *Chemical hypothermia.* A combination of drugs known as a *"lytic cocktail"* may be given to suppress the brain's heat regulatory center, reduce temperature to a subnormal level, sedate the patient, and prevent shivering. The medications most commonly used in such combinations are chlorpromazine hydrochloride (Thorazine) and meperidine hydrochloride (Demerol) or promethazine hydrochloride (Phenergan). Body temperature may be reduced about 4° by this method.
- *Internal surface cooling.* Various body surfaces may be cooled internally. For example, a nurse may give ice water enemas or a surgeon may pour cold saline solutions into a patient's abdominal or thoracic cavities. Gastrointestinal bleeding may be treated by circulating ice water in a balloon inflated in the stomach. The latter procedure is called "intragastric cooling."
- *Extracorporeal cooling.* Blood stream cooling is accomplished by removing blood from a large vessel, cooling it, and returning it to the body's circulation. Extracorporeal cooling is performed with special apparatus, a heart-lung machine. The blood is cooled as it passes through coils within the machine. During the procedure heparin is given to prevent blood clotting. Extracorporeal cooling rapidly produces hypothermia and is mainly used during cardiac and vascular surgery. At the end of surgery the blood may be rewarmed by changing the machine's settings. (Heart surgery is discussed in Chapter 39.)
- *External surface cooling.* The body's external surface may be cooled by several methods: immersion in ice water; covering with electrically refrigerating (hypothermia) blankets; exposure to cool air (e.g., from an electric fan); or application of ice bags in selected locations.

Because the nurse is most often involved in methods of external surface cooling, let us discuss these procedures further and the general clinical care given a hypothermic patient.

Surface cooling may reduce body temperature to as low as 25°C. (77°F.). However, surface cooling to such a low temperature is used only in surgery. More commonly, body temperature is reduced by only a few degrees. As a general rule, surface hypothermia is maintained above 27.8°C. (82°F.) to prevent irreversible complications, e.g., irreversible ventricular fibrillation.

When surface cooling is used, treatment is directed at not only cooling the body, but also at *preventing shivering,* e.g., by the intravenous administration of such medications as chlorpromazine and sodium phenobarbital. Shivering must be prevented because it increases metabolic activity, produces heat, markedly increases oxygen usage, increases circulation, may produce hypoglycemia (by using up muscle and liver glycogen), and may cause hyperventilation and respiratory alkalosis. Also, it takes a longer time to reduce body temperature in a shivering patient.

As previously indicated, body temperature can be reduced by various methods of surface cooling. An *electric fan* may be directed toward the patient to cool the body by evaporation. A loin cloth may be placed over the patient and a *bath towel or sheet saturated with cold water* placed over the trunk. The towel is periodically resaturated and an electric fan is directed toward the towel. Also, *ice caps* may be placed at the patient's groins and axillas.

Occasionally, in emergency situations, a hyperthermic patient may be placed in a *tub of ice water* to halt a rapidly rising fever. However, *tepid sponges* are tolerated better than such cold baths. Also, because they are less likely to cause shivering, tepid sponges are often more effective. Solutions used for tepid sponges include water, alcohol, or a mixture of both.

A cold sponge bath or tub bath causes heat loss by conduction and by evaporation, i.e., some of the body's heat is transferred from the skin surface into the bathing solution and other body heat is lost as the heat of vaporization. With a tepid sponge, heat loss occurs by evaporative cooling. Because cooling results from continuous evaporization, an electric fan is frequently used to keep the air in motion over cooling sponges.

Sponge friction massage may be employed if the patient's skin is cold during a temperature elevation. After the patient is packed in ice for 15 minutes, the skin is rubbed with a towel. By improving cutaneous vasodilation, this procedure draws more warm blood to the body's surface, where the heat is dissipated.

Remember, if a cooling sponge bath is not properly

administered or is too brief, the procedure may stimulate shivering and thereby increase heat production rather than contribute to heat loss.

If cooling sponges fail to reduce body temperature, the physician may order *cool* to *ice-cold lavages* or *enemas,* although this is uncommon. A persistent fever may require that the patient be packed in ice, put in a tub of cold water, or placed on a *hypothermic mattress.*

Most hospitals have *hypothermic mattresses,* i.e., a refrigerating machine and cooling blankets made of rubber or vinyl. A cooled solution of alcohol and water is circulated through coils in the blanket (Fig. 26–13). Several different hypothermic units are on the market. The *hypothermic blanket* causes heat loss by conduction and convection, i.e., heat is transferred from the body surface to the cooling blanket. Use of a hypothermic unit is the procedure of choice for treating hyperthermia related to hypothalamic damage. For details of the operation of hypothermic units consult manufacturers' information booklets.

Hypothermic mattresses are the simplest, most efficient, and most precise method of inducing general hypothermia. By the setting of a gauge at the desired level of coolness, the fluid flowing through the coils is maintained at the desired temperature.

Hypothermic mattresses may also be used to rewarm patients. However, this is rarely done. In carefully controlled situations where patients with serious side effects (such as cardiac arrhythmias) require rewarming, the mattress may be used. Most generally, however, patients are rewarmed with blankets.

Because nurses practice in a variety of settings, they need to be familiar with different methods of external surface cooling. While hypothermic units may be the most desirable method, they are not always available.

Clinical Care Associated with Hypothermia. Skilled nursing care is necessary with induced hypothermia. Such patients are usually cared for in an intensive care setting.

The following activities are typically of importance *prior to* prolonged hypothermia (i.e., maintained possibly for several days): (1) bathe the patient, inspect the skin for discolorations or lesions, and apply a thin

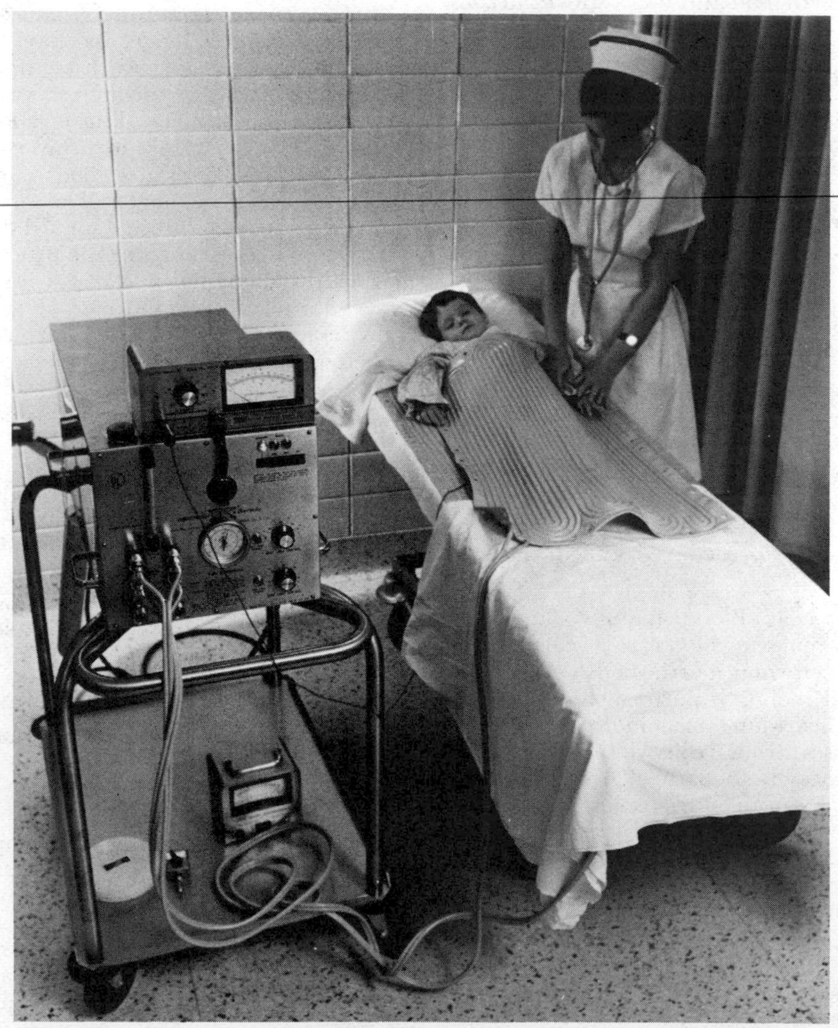

Figure 26–13. Hypothermic blanket. (Courtesy of Gorman-Rupp, Inc., Belleville, Ohio.)

coating of lanolin, oil, or cream to the entire body; (2) administer a cleansing enema; (3) insert a retention urinary catheter (to evaluate renal function and renal output); (4) start an intravenous infusion or assist with an intravenous cutdown (to maintain fluid-electrolyte balance); (5) administer preinduction medications such as meperidine hydrochloride (Demerol), chlorpromazine (Thorazine), or promethazine hydrochloride (Phenergan) to depress the heat-regulating center of the brain, prevent shivering, and help the conscious patient to relax during the cooling procedure; (6) make baseline observations and recordings of the patient's vital signs, level of consciousness, and responsiveness; and (7) assemble emergency equipment and medications, e.g., vasopressors, cardiac stimulants, respiratory stimulants, respirators, and tracheostomy tray. Intravenous infusions must be started prior to the procedure, since the peripheral veins collapse in the hypothermic state.

Prior to any hypothermic procedure, explain the procedure to the conscious patient and give reassurance that someone will be in constant attendance. Hypothermia is quite uncomfortable for patients who are conscious. They need constant support and attention. Give appropriate explanations and reassurance to significant others.

During prolonged hypothermic therapy the following activities are of importance:

- *Take, record, and evaluate vital signs frequently.* During hypothermic therapy, an electric thermometer (with a probe inserted into the patient's rectum) is commonly used to check the patient's temperature. By this device the body temperature is continually monitored when attached to a recording device. The most accurate indication of body temperature may be obtained if the rectal temperature probe is inserted at least three inches and is angled anteriorly. An electric thermometer (Thermisto probe) may also be placed in the patient's esophagus (e.g., in the anesthetized patient). The goal of therapy is to maintain the desired level of hypothermia. Because a downward drift of 1 or 2 degrees typically occurs after the cooling devices are removed, it is customary to stop the procedure, or to reduce it, when the patient's body temperature is within 1 or 2 degrees of the desired temperature. An electrocardiograph and electroencephalograph may be used during hypothermia to detect cardiac arrhythmias and cerebral anoxia. It is expected that vital signs will gradually be reduced as body temperature is being lowered. *Report immediately* undesired levels of body temperature, shivering, marked changes in cardiac rate, irregular cardiac rhythms, or other fluctuations or abnormalities in vital signs. If the temperature is undesirably low, cardiac arrest may occur.
- *Administer medications as ordered to prevent shivering.* Shivering typically occurs when body temperature reaches 30°C. (86°F.).
- *Make certain the patient is attended constantly.*
- *Maintain a patent airway,* e.g., by suctioning and correct positioning. Because the gag reflex may be absent, the patient must be protected from aspiration. If indicated, use a respirator to support ventilation.

- *Protect the patient's eyes* in the absence of the corneal reflex and when protective eye secretions are reduced. (See Chapter 89 and also p. 536 of this chapter.)
- *Prevent complications of immobility.* For example, correctly position the patient, turn every 2 hours, and carry out range-of-motion exercises passively. Turn the patient frequently if cooling blankets are used. Sometimes patients undergoing hypothermia are placed on CircOlectric beds so they can be turned more easily.
- *Observe the patient's skin* every 1 or 2 hours for indications of pressure, discoloration, edema, or frostbite (e.g., immovable firm areas of skin caused by fat necrosis or crystallization of tissue).
- *Give frequent oral hygiene* and *remove crusts from the nares.* (See pp. 536 and 537.)
- *Measure and evaluate urinary output periodically.* It is expected that urinary output will decrease when the temperature is lowered to 32°C. (89°F.). Urine specimens for analysis may be collected frequently.
- *Provide intake as ordered,* e.g., intravenously and/or via nasogastric tube. Oral intake is not permitted because hypothermia may depress or remove the gag reflex. (Other reflexes are also altered.)

Clinical care *during and immediately after rewarming* of the patient continues to be intensive. The physician decides when to terminate hypothermia and rewarm the patient to a normal body temperature. Rewarming may be accomplished by: (1) changing the setting on a warming-cooling blanket so that warm liquid is circulated through the blanket; (2) removing the cooling blanket, covering the patient with regular blankets, and allowing rewarming by exposure to a warmer environment; or (3) partially immersing the patient in warm or tepid water. In practice, the second option is the usual choice.

During the rewarming procedure, be careful not to burn the patient or to permit exposure to excessively warm temperatures. Attend the patient constantly and evaluate vital signs. Report immediately any abnormalities. Usually the rewarming procedures are ended when the patient's temperature reaches a level that is 1 to 2 degrees below normal. The procedure is terminated at this time because some upward temperature drift usually occurs. Consciousness is usually regained when body temperature reaches around 32°C. (89°F.).

Following hypothermia the patient's temperature is closely observed (e.g., every 3 or 4 hours for several days). Excessive temperature elevations may occur, because the temperature-regulating mechanism is often unstable for a while. Also, because cardiac irregularity and fibrillations can occur after rewarming, the patient may be monitored with a cardiac monitor.

SEIZURES AND CONVULSIONS*

Seizures are sudden episodes of varying severity precipitated by abnormal, excessive neuronal discharges within the brain. Seizures may be manifestations of numerous diverse disorders. Here we focus on the clinical care of any patient experiencing a seizure from any cause. In its broadest sense, the term "epilepsy" is synonymous with "seizure." Occasionally lay persons refer to a seizure or convulsion as a "fit" or "attack." A seizure is a phenomenon or symptom, not a disease. We do not in this chapter discuss in detail the causes of seizures. Let us simply say here that seizures may be symptomatic of any condition that interferes with neuronal metabolism or that injures neurons. Actually at least 50 various conditions are *known* to induce seizures. However, *the causes of most seizures remain unknown.*

Clinical Care During Seizures

Seizures range in intensity from imperceptible impulse changes within the brain to the rather dramatic "grand mal" seizures (generalized tonic-clonic), in which a person suddenly loses consciousness, falls to the floor, becomes cyanotic, and experiences rhythmic contractions of all extremities.

Witnessing a seizure for the first time can be a frightening experience. If you have not seen a person having a seizure before, try to remember — when it does occur — that you are observing *exaggerations* of normal actions, e.g., exaggerated movements and exaggerated salivation. It may be helpful to also remember that once a seizure has started, there is nothing one can do to stop it. A nurse's responsibility is to *protect* the patient during a generalized convulsive seizure and to make careful, pertinent *observations.*

Protective Measures

1. Remain calm and stay with the person.
2. *Do not attempt to restrain the person's movements.* To do so could cause injury. If the person has not already fallen, ease him or her carefully to the floor. Place a folded blanket or towel (or anything soft that is readily available) under the person's head to protect it from striking the floor. *Do not attempt to lift a person during a seizure.* To do so could cause injury to both the patient and yourself. Instead of moving a person during a seizure, move away things in the environment that could cause injury if the person banged into them.
3. Insure a *patent airway* and *adequate ventilation.* Loosen tight clothing if possible. Turn the person to one side with head turned to the same side to (a) allow secretions to drain from the mouth and prevent aspiration and (b) keep the tongue from falling back to obstruct the airway.
4. *Do not attempt to force anything between the person's teeth.* To do so could break or loosen a tooth or injure the lips.

If the patient has an aura at the beginning of a grand mal seizure, there may be time for the person to lie down and place something between the teeth before the seizure begins.

5. After the convulsive movements have stopped, the person will relax and be unresponsive. The duration of this state varies. Be sure that he or she is turned well onto one side and is safe and comfortable, and covered if necessary to keep warm. Let the person remain in this position until a state of responsiveness and alertness returns. During this time remain with or check the person frequently.

Observations

1. Were there any warning signs? What was the position of the patient's head, body, and extremities before and after the onset of the seizure?
2. Where did the seizure begin? What was the *initial activity*? Did the seizure begin in the hand? face? foot? Did the head turn to one side or the other? Did the person fall at the beginning of the seizure? How did the person attract your attention?
3. What was the *progression of seizure activity*? (Observe the patient's whole body during the seizure.) What parts of the body were involved? Was the muscular movement tonic, clonic, localized (focal), or generalized? Did the muscular movements change in character during the seizure?
4. Did the *eyes* deviate? To what side? Did the pupils change in size? React to light? Were the pupils equal? Was the patient unresponsive during the seizure? What was the person's *level of consciousness* prior to the seizure?
5. Was there any *incontinence* of urine or feces? Was there any thick salivation or mucus, vomiting, or bleeding? Describe the person's *respiratory character*, e.g., apnea, stertor. What was the res-

*Refer also to the discussion of epilepsy in Chapter 27, p. 640.

piratory rate? Describe the skin color of face and lips, e.g., cyanosis.

6. How long did the seizure last? How long was the period of unconsciousness? How long was the tonic stage? the clonic stage? Were there multiple seizures? What was the frequency and number of seizures?

7. What was the patient's condition after the seizure activity stopped (*postictal*)? Was there any evidence of muscle weakness? Did the person have any headache? Was there any injury or apparent injury as a result of falling or other activity during the seizure? Was there any pain, discomfort, paralysis or aphasia following the seizure? Does the patient report noticing any disturbances in coordination; impaired speech or thought processes; changes in vision, hearing, motor power; or paresthesias or any other symptom before or after the seizure?

After the seizure, check and record the patient's vital signs. Ask if an aura was experienced prior to the seizure. If awake and comfortable, the patient may be left to rest and fully recover. Reassure the patient and reorient if necessary.

The nurse's observations help the physician (1) to identify which area of the brain is involved, (2) to plan appropriate medical and surgical treatment, and (3) to plan appropriate teaching and counseling.

In planning care for the seizure-prone patient, plan individualized care that does not impose unnecessary limitations on the patient's activities. It is best, of course, for the patient to be ambulatory if possible.

NEUROGENIC SHOCK

Shock is discussed generally in Chapter 13. You will recall that most shock results from a disproportion between the circulating blood volume and the size of the vascular bed. During health an adequate blood supply is maintained to all the body's tissues because a dynamic equilibrium is maintained between the blood volume, the heart pump mechanisms, and the size of the vascular bed.

With neurogenic shock the volume of blood in the body is normal, but the *vascular bed is greatly increased in size.* This increased vascular capacity means that the normal blood volume is incapable of adequately filling the blood vessels. This disproportion reduces the mean circulatory pressure. The pressure gradient for the return of venous blood is, in turn, decreased, resulting in: (1) venous "pooling" of blood; (2) decreased venous return to the heart; and (3) decreased cardiac output. Following this, generalized tissue anoxia occurs along with other signs and symptoms of oxygen deficiency. Cyanosis, however, rarely occurs in neurogenic shock.

Neurogenic shock may occur from spinal injury, deep general anesthesia, fainting, and spinal anesthesia (common cause). It is important that a nurse be able to differentiate neurogenic shock (due to peripheral vasodilatation) from hemorrhagic shock (due to reduced blood volume). Failure to make this differentiation could cause a nurse to make the possibly fatal mistake of increasing the rate of flow in a blood transfusion being received by a patient in neurogenic shock, because of incorrectly thinking the cause of the shock was decreased blood volume. Such an overloading of circulating blood volume would place a burden on the patient's heart once vasomotor tone has been restored or stimulated, e.g., with pressor drugs. If this added burden to the heart occurred in a patient with any cardiac weakness, congestive heart failure and pulmonary edema could develop.

The *treatment* of neurogenic shock centers around *administration of a vasopressor,* i.e., vasoconstrictor usually given intravenously in solution. Once the immediate danger of shock has passed, the vasopressor therapy is stopped to prevent pulmonary and renal problems. Severe *ischemic nephrosis,* causing oliguria or anuria as a result of intense, prolonged renal vasoconstriction, can be caused by the indiscriminate administration of vasopressors. For several days following vasopressor treatment of neurogenic shock the patient's urine volume is measured hourly. An indication of the development of ischemic nephrosis is the presence of a *sharp decline in renal output,* in the absence of symptoms of shock. When this happens, the doctor usually limits fluid intake and potassium.

RESPIRATORY FAILURE FROM NEUROLOGIC DISORDERS

Neurologic disorders frequently cause respiratory failure by: (1) depressing or destroying the cells in the lower brain stem that integrate respiration; (2) damaging the spinal motor pathways for breathing, their nerves, or respiratory muscular structures; or (3) producing paralysis or sensory loss that results in airway obstruction. Providing appropriate respiratory assistance is therefore an important aspect of the clinical care of many patients with neurologic disorders. (Respiratory failure is discussed in detail in Unit XVI. See also the discussion of neurogenic pulmonary edema in the next chapter, p. 666.)

INFECTION COMPLICATING NEUROLOGIC DISORDERS

Neurologic disorders mainly predispose to infections as a result of the depressed levels of consciousness, the immobility, and the paralysis that they may cause. Some of the major potential infections that may occur are respiratory infections (e.g., pneumonia), skin infections (e.g., decubitus ulcers), and infections of the genitourinary tract.

The use of antibiotics is generally reserved for the specific, vigorous treatment of bacteriologically identified infections *after* the infection has appeared and findings from a culture or smear have been reported. However, chemoprophylaxis does reduce the incidence of pneumonia during convalescence from short episodes of coma, e.g., those resulting from drug poisoning. The use of chemoprophylaxis in such circumstances is the exception rather than the general practice with unconscious or immobilized patients.

PROBLEMS RELATED TO SPINAL DISORDERS

This section focuses on a variety of problems that result from impaired functioning or altered structure of the spinal cord. Although the discussion emphasizes the more extreme degrees of clinical problems, remember that spinal disorders may also cause similar problems of lesser degree.

Causes of Spinal Disorders

Because of the many unique anatomic and physiologic features of the spinal cord, disorders of the cord produce a number of distinctive and debilitating syndromes. In no other part of the body can a local insult result in such extensive clinical devastation in proportion to the extent of tissue involvement. Some of the common disease processes that affect the spinal cord and produce significant symptomatology are:

- *Myelitis* — infective or noninfective inflammatory processes.
- *Vascular diseases* — usually infarction or hemorrhage (hematomyelia).
- *Cervical spondylosis* with myelopathy — producing narrowing of the spinal canal and causing progressive injury to the cord and roots.
- *Syringomyelia* — central cavitation of the cord.

TABLE 26–2. FUNCTIONAL GOALS IN SPINAL CORD LESIONS

Spinal Cord Level	Muscle Function	Functional Goals
C3–4	Neck control Scapular elevators	Manipulate electric wheelchair with mouth stick Limited self-feeding with ball-bearing feeders.
C5	Fair to good shoulder control Good elbow flexion	Dress upper trunk. Turn self in bed with arm slings. Propel wheelchair with handrim projections. Self-feeding with handsplints. Assist getting to and from bed.
C6	Good shoulder control Wrist extension Supinators	Dress upper trunk. Turn self in bed with arm slings. Propel wheelchair with handrim projections. Self-feeding with handsplints. Transfer from wheelchair to bed with or without minimal assistance. Self feeding with tenodesis hands. Assist getting to and from commode chair.
C7	Weak shoulder depression Weak elbow extension Some hand function	Independent in transfer to bed, car and toilet. Total dressing independence. Wheelchair without handrim projections. Self-feeding with no assistive devices
T1 to T4	Good to normal upper extremity muscle function	Independent in transfer to bed; car; and toilet. Total dressing independence. Wheelchair without handrim projections. Self-feeding with no assistive devices. Wheelchair to floor and return. Wheelchair up and down curb. Wheelchair to tub and return.
T5 to L2	Partial to good trunk stability	Total wheelchair independence. Limited ambulation with bilateral long leg braces and crutches.
L3 to L4	All trunk-pelvic stabilizers intact Hip flexors Adductors Quadriceps	Ambulation with short leg braces with or without crutches depending on level.
L5 to S3	Hip extensors Abductors, knee flexors, ankle control	No equipment needed if plantar flexion strong enough for push off at end of stance.

Modified from Rancho Los Amigos Hospital, Physical Therapy Department, Downey, California.

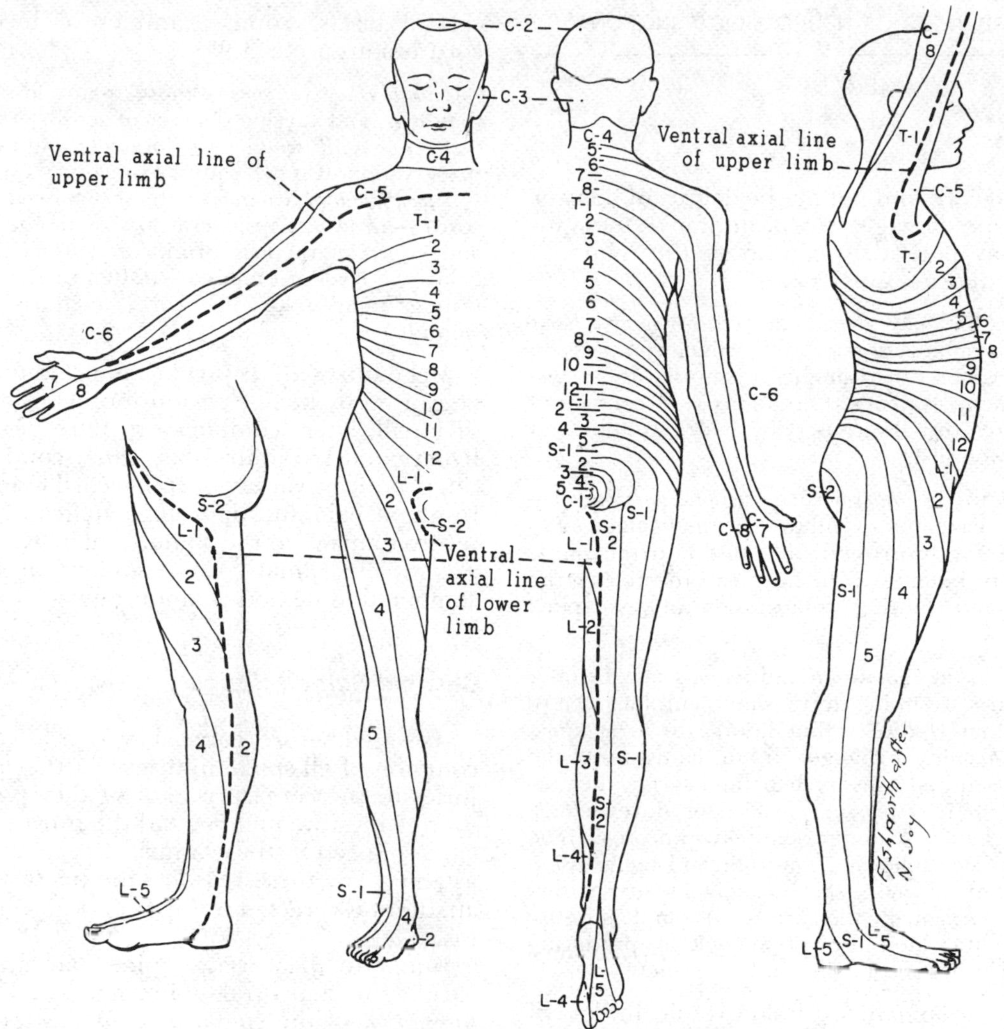

Figure 26–14. Cutaneous distribution of spinal nerves and dermatomes. Knowledge of the cutaneous distribution of the nerve roots makes it possible to locate level of a spinal cord injury by noting a lack of sensation in the appropriate area. From a nursing viewpoint, knowledge of dermatomes can give information concerning the expected functional impairments of people with spinal cord injuries at various levels. (From Jacob, S. W., C. A. Francone, and W. J. Lossow: *Structure and Function in Man*, 4th ed. Philadelphia: W. B. Saunders Co., 1978, p. 263.)

- *Trauma* — direct or indirect to the cord, or to the surrounding vertebral column.

Of these causes of spinal cord disorders, trauma is the most common. Thus, spinal cord injury (SCI) is the major consideration in this section. Any of the other disease processes, however, may produce similar symptoms of varying degrees of severity.

Spinal Cord Injury

The symptoms related to spinal cord damage vary, depending on the level, extent, and mechanisms of the lesion.

Level of Injury. Damage to the spinal cord may cause loss of function of the areas of the body innervated by nerves leaving the cord *below* the level of the disorder (see Table 26–2 and Fig. 26–14).

- *Cervical injuries* are the most common of all spinal injuries. These may occur at any cervical level, but the fifth and sixth cervical vertebrae (C5 and C6) are most frequently involved.
- *Thoracic injury* occurs much less frequently, since that area of the spine is well protected and more structurally stable. T12 is the area most often injured.
- *Lumbar injury* occurs next to cervical injury in frequency. L1 and L5 are the most common levels of injury.

Later in this section we deal in greater detail with each of these various levels of injury and the specific symptoms they produce.

Extent of Injury. Trauma to the spine may result in damage to the bony vertebral column only, to the surrounding ligaments, or to the spinal cord. Rarely does a serious injury involve only one or two of these components. The seriousness of a spinal injury depends upon the extent and level of segmented involvement of the spinal cord and not on the degree of bony or other tissue damage, except insofar as these injuries may potentially aggravate the injury to the cord and its roots.

- Injury that may affect only the *vertebral column* include subluxation or dislocation, compression fractures or other simple fractures without displacement, fracture dislocations, and compound fractures (usually caused by bullet wounds and knife wounds).
- Injury to the *anterior* or *posterior ligaments* may cause weakening or rupture of the ligaments (allowing for protrusion of a disc into the spinal canal) or bulging of the ligaments (narrowing the canal and causing compression of the spinal cord).
- Injury to the *spinal cord* and its *roots* may be (a) a *concussion,* resulting in transient neurologic symptoms that resolve within hours, (b) a *contusion,* which results in changes within the tissues of the cord itself and causes edema and surface hemorrhage, or (c) *compression,* which produces edema and ischemia, leading eventually to necrosis. The deficits seen following contusion and compression resolve much more slowly, and some are permanent. Occasionally the cord is (d) completely *transected,* either literally or physiologically, producing a deficit that is complete and permanent.

A *complete* spinal cord lesion results in: loss of all voluntary movements in the parts of the body below the lesion; loss of all sensation from the parts of the body below the lesion, and loss of reflex function in the isolated segment of the cord. An *incomplete* lesion results in varying degrees of loss of motor and sensory functions below the level of the lesion, with sparing of

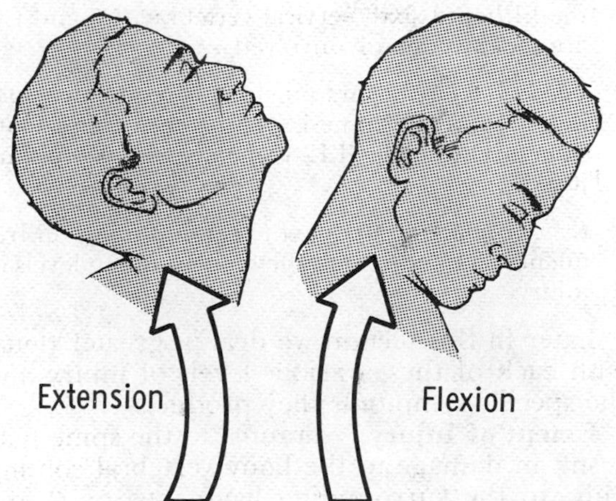

Figure 26–15. Mechanics of a whiplash injury. (From Chusid, J. G., and J. J. McDonald: *Correlative Neuroanatomy and Functional Neurology,* 13th ed. Los Altos, Calif.: Lange Medical Publications, 1967, p. 330.)

certain tracts. Some examples of incomplete cord lesions are as follows:

Central cord syndrome — more motor loss in arms than legs, and varying degrees of sensory loss.

Anterior cord syndrome — complete paralysis with preservation of much sensory function.

Brown-Sequard Syndrome (lateral hemisection of the cord) — produces ipsilateral loss of motor function and contralateral loss of major sensory function, below the level of the lesion. (Often seen with penetrating injuries of the cord, such as gunshot wounds.)

Mechanism of Injury. Spinal injuries may be caused by flexion, extension, or rotation, individually or in combination. Pure flexion and hyperextension injuries are fairly common and can produce a variety of spinal cord lesions, with resultant pain and neurologic deficit. The most severe damage to the spine, usually resulting in a complete spinal cord lesion, is caused by a combination flexion-rotation injury.

Cervical Spine Injuries

As stated before, cervical injuries are the most common of all spinal injuries. Furthermore, injuries to the cervical region of the spinal cord may be life-threatening, and the functional deficits produced by these injuries are the most devastating. For these reasons, the majority of our attention is directed toward cervical spinal trauma.

Injury to the cervical spine may result in a variety of structural abnormalities. Complete *transection* of the spinal cord in the cervical region essentially produces *quadriplegia.*

> *Quadriplegia consists of paralysis of the lower extremities and trunk, and varying degrees of paresis or paralysis of the upper extremities, depending on the specific level of injury.*

Loss of sensory function affects essentially the same areas. For instance, an injury to C2 or C3 produces complete respiratory paralysis, complete flaccidity and loss of reflexes, and the person is usually dead within a few minutes unless immediate respiratory assistance is available. If the injury is to C5 or C6 (which is the most common level for cervical cord injury), the person has use of the shoulder girdle, deltoids and biceps, with loss of deep tendon reflexes, and loss of sensation below the clavicles. With each descending level of lesion, further functions are retained.

More often than complete transection of the cervical cord, varying degrees of incomplete involvement are seen. The *central cord syndrome,* which occurs most frequently in hyperextension-hyperflexion injuries, is characterized

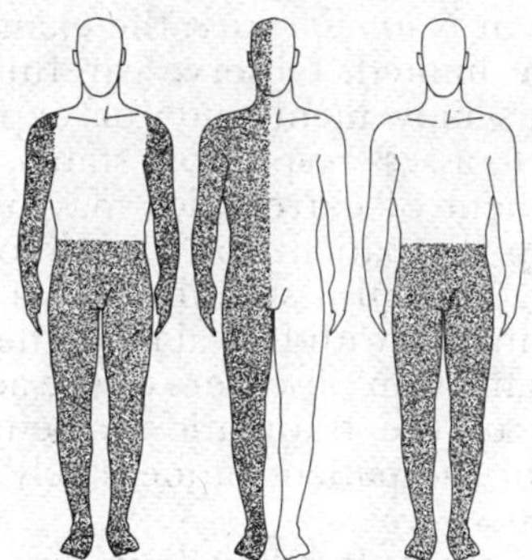

Figure 26-16. Areas of paralysis. Left, quadriplegia; center, hemiplegia; right, paraplegia. Note that this is a generalized diagram. Specific areas of paralysis typically vary from individual to individual. (From Culver, V. M.: *Modern Bedside Nursing,* 8th ed. 1974.)

by more weakness in the upper extremities than in the lower. This is thought to be caused by edema and hemorrhage in the central area of the cord, predominantly occupied by tracts to the hands and arms. A lesion to the anterior spinal cord results in the *anterior cord syndrome,* in which there is complete loss of motor function, decreased pain sensation, and preservation of such other sensations as touch, position, and vibration. *Concussion* of the cervical cord may produce varying degrees of motor and sensory deficit, which completely resolve within hours. Occasionally, trauma to the cervical cord results in only root injuries, which may cause paralysis of isolated muscles or muscle groups in the arms and shoulders. These deficits are usually permanent.

The *Brown-Sequard Syndrome* is caused by lateral hemisection of the cord (hemisection occurs when a lesion cuts or affects one-half of the cord), as with a bullet wound or knife wound. This results in an ipsilateral motor paralysis and loss of vibratory and position sense and in a contralateral loss of pain and temperature sensation.

Spinal Shock. Following a complete cord transection (and occasionally accompanying an incomplete lesion), the patient often experiences *spinal shock.* This is a condition characterized by a complete and immediate loss of motor, sensory, autonomic, and reflex activity below the level of the lesion. Spinal shock may subside within a few weeks or a few months after injury. The initial indication of recovery is minimal reflex activity. The flaccid paralysis becomes spastic. Autonomic functions are gradually restored, and the bowel and urinary bladder (which were initially atonic) begin to contract reflexly.

TREATMENT AND NURSING CARE

The care that a spinal cord injured person receives, especially during the first hour after trauma and also on a long-term basis, to a great degree determines: (a) the extent of the injury and associated deficits, (b) how well the acute phase of injury is survived, and (c) how completely the person can recover and be rehabilitated. It is therefore important for nurses to understand and practice the essential concepts of care and rehabilitation for patients following spinal cord injury.

Acute Care. Spinal trauma is most often associated with other injuries (frequently a head injury). Any person found at the scene of an accident or brought to a hospital emergency room with evidence of multiple trauma should be suspected of having a spinal injury until adequate assessment and diagnostic procedures have proven otherwise. Every precaution must be taken to insure that a possible vertebral column injury is not complicated by improper management to become a spinal cord injury. (See also discussion of emergency care in Chapter 95.)

In handling a person suspected of having a cervical spinal injury, the spine must be kept in neutral alignment, with particular emphasis on preventing flexion.[127] If the patient must be turned, it should be done in a log-rolling manner. The patient should be placed in a supine position on a firm surface, e.g., a board or solid stretcher. If a cervical injury is suspected, the head must be supported in alignment with the body and immobilized by placing sand bags on either side or by applying a firm padded cervical collar (Fig. 26-17). If halter traction is available,

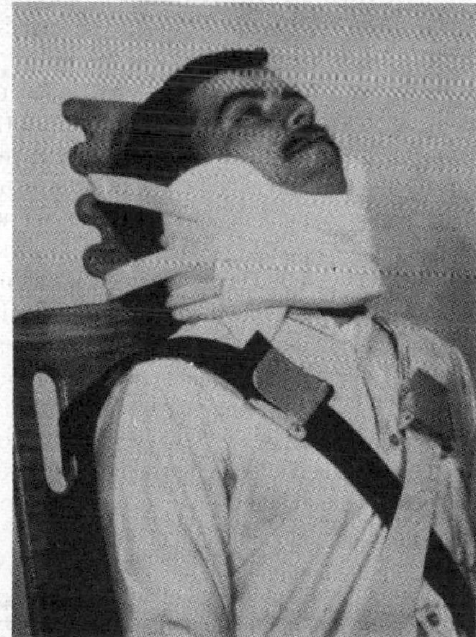

Figure 26-17. Every patient with a suspected spinal injury should have the cervical spine immobilized — here, with a spine board and Hare extrication collar. Some authorities recommend cervical spine immobilization that has *less* neck extension than shown in this figure. (From Jackson. F. E.: Vulnerable vertebrae. *Emergency Medicine,* 11:33, Mar. 1979, p. 34.)

some physicians prefer to use it immediately to keep the cervical spine in good alignment and prevent movement. No attempt should be made to remove the patient's clothing, until a definite diagnosis has been made.

Death or permanent disabilities result more frequently from improper transportation of a patient with a fracture of the spine, sometimes unrecognized, than from any initial injury.

As in all emergency situations, make sure that the patient has an *adequate airway.* Suction equipment should be immediately available. If the patient has sustained a cervical injury, respiratory distress may occur and immediate action must be taken to maintain the airway and provide adequate oxygenation. Damage at the C3 to C5 cord levels can involve the phrenic nerve, causing diaphragmatic paralysis and respiratory failure. If intubation is immediately necessary, care must be taken not to hyperextend the neck before complete assessment can be made.

Equipment should be available to suction, perform intubation, and mechanically assist respiration. Mechanical respiratory assistance is required when a definite loss or impairment of respiratory muscle function occurs. Respiratory failure resulting from neurologic disorders is discussed in Unit XVI. Careful preventive care, e.g., coughing and deep breathing, is established to *prevent pulmonary infection.*

While the patient is being prepared for x-ray examination, the nurse and/or physician must do a brief but thorough *neurologic examination* to assess the extent of injury. If the patient is conscious, ask where any pain is occurring. Then test sensation by determining if the patient can feel your touch or a pin prick in the feet, legs, trunk, hands, and arms. Make a careful note of the levels of sensation. Repeat the same testing for motor function. Ask the patient to wiggle the toes, move the ankles, flex the knees, and move the hands and arms. Carefully note the location, symmetry, and strength of muscle movement. Briefly test the major reflexes, i.e., ankle, knee, biceps, and triceps. Be especially careful to look for any areas of sensory sparing, such as sacral sparing.* This examination establishes a baseline of function and involvement by which later improvements or regression can be determined.

If a patient is *unresponsive,* the examination is much more limited. Observe carefully for any spontaneous movement and for expansion of the thorax to assess respiratory status. Sensation and movement of extremities may be assessed by watching the patient for a few moments, or by applying a painful stimulus like a pin prick and observing for withdrawal from the stimulus. Try to obtain from observers of the accident all the details of the traumatic incident and the condition of the patient immediately following the accident.

As a rule, the only other diagnostic measures are x-rays to determine the type of lesion. The patient is transported on a flat firm stretcher, usually with halter traction. A physician should remain with the patient while films are taken to insure that the cervical spine is not moved. Usually standard lateral and anteroposterior projections are not sufficient. Lower cervical fractures are difficult to visualize and necessitate applying downward traction to arms or having the arms in swimmer's position during the x-ray examination. If a high cervical lesion is suspected, a special view through the open mouth may be necessary.

Treatment. The patient who has sustained a severe cervical injury, such as a fracture and dislocation, should be placed immediately in *skeletal traction* to immobilize the cervical spine and to reduce the fracture and dislocation. Various types of tongs may be used, depending on the preference of the particular neurosurgeon. Crutchfield tongs, Barton tongs and Gardner-Wells tongs are some examples. These tongs are inserted via prepared areas of the scalp and extend through the outer table of the skull. (See Fig. 26–18.) Traction is applied to the tongs via rope and pulleys. Weights are added to the traction, beginning with 10 to 20 pounds (4.5 to 9.1 kg.) and gradually increasing as necessary to accomplish the bony reduction. When proper alignment has been obtained, the amount of traction may be reduced to that sufficient to maintain the position. If skeletal traction is to be the only means of immobilization and stabilization, the tongs are generally left in place for several weeks.

Another form of treatment sometimes introduced during the acute stage is the use of *steroids* to reduce edema of the injured cord. This form of treatment has not been widely accepted since there are no studies that give conclusive evidence of its effectiveness.

There has been much interest and research within the past 10 years regarding the possible benefits of *spinal cord cooling* in reducing cord edema and decreasing the severity of permanent damage. The use of hypothermic perfusion of the cord is advocated on the same basis as the use of hypothermia for the control of brain edema. There is some evidence that this procedure may be partially effective for the minimal or threshold degree of injury. Howev-

---

**Sacral sparing* is often seen following cervical spine injuries in which the spinal cord is contused but not transected. Damage to the central part of the cord results, but the lateral aspects of the cord (which contain the sensory fibers from the lower extremities and sacral area) are spared. Sparing of these sensory fibers is detected by applying a mild painful stimulus (pin prick) to the anal or perineal area. Sacral sparing is believed by some doctors to indicate that return of some sensory and motor function is possible.

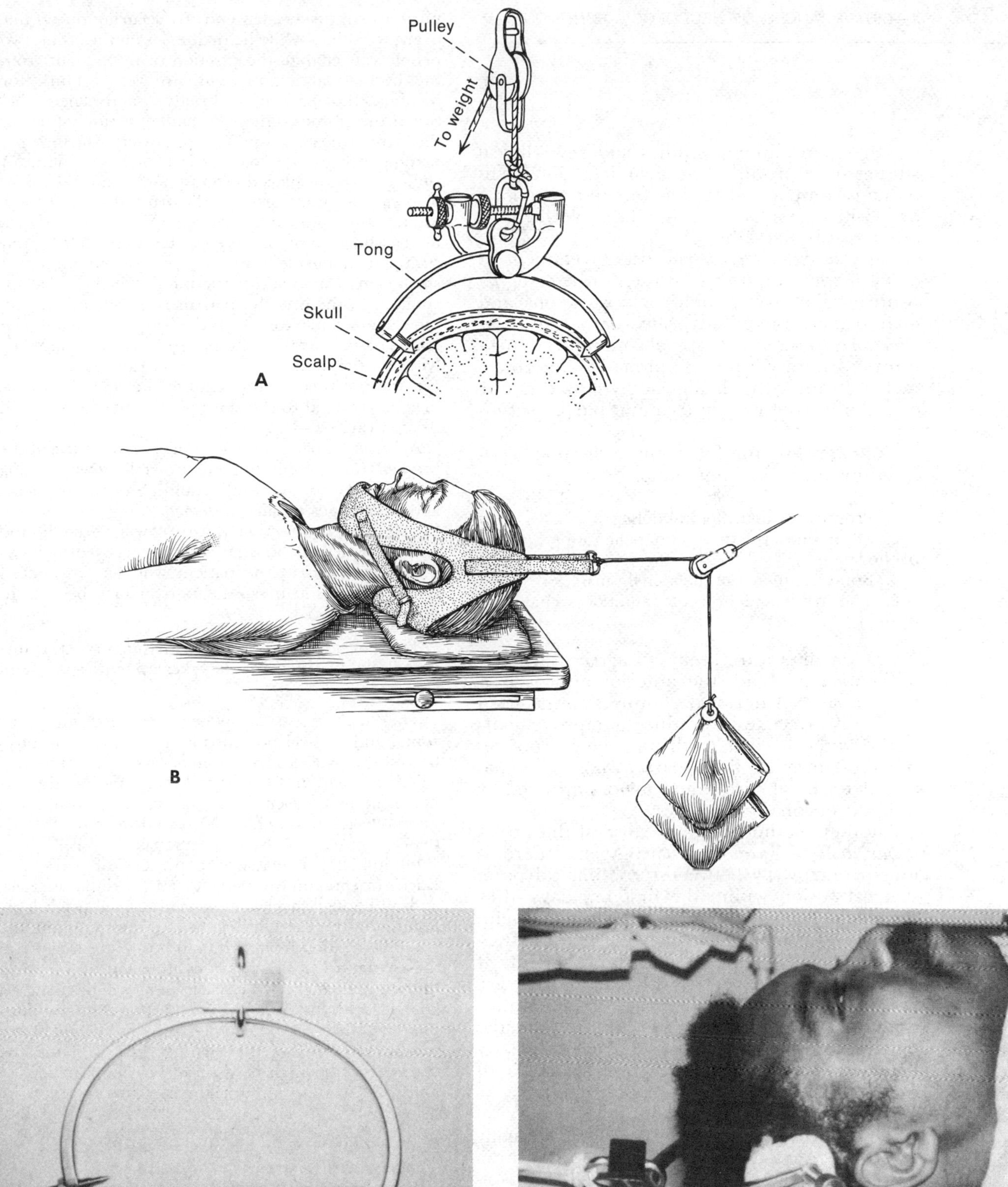

Figure 26–18. **A.** Attachment of tongs to skull. **B.** Halter traction in place. Note that direction of pull is in line with the vertebral column. **C** and **D.** Gardner-Wells tongs are attached to the patient just above the tip of each ear. (*B* from Committee on Trauma, American College of Surgeons. *Early Care of the Injured Patient.* Philadelphia: W. B. Saunders Co., 1972, p. 101. *C* and *D* from Jackson, F. E.: Vulnerable vertebrae. *Emergency Medicine,* 11:33, March 15, 1979, p. 56.)

er, the many animal studies and few clinical studies have produced no firm data. The technique is complicated, and as yet the few reports of positive results have not been verified by other researchers.[226]

Early *surgical intervention* in the treatment of cervical spine injuries continues to be a highly controversial issue. Some neurosurgeons and orthopedic surgeons advocate a *decompressive laminectomy* for complete spinal cord injuries in an effort to improve the symptoms. Many others feel as strongly that laminectomy should not be considered routinely in treating spinal cord injury.[226]

Youmans lists the following as the major criteria for operative intervention:[340]

1. Progressive neurological deficit
2. Compound fractures and penetrating wounds of the spine
3. Bone fragments in the spinal canal
4. The syndrome of acute anterior spinal cord trauma

Current literature seems to agree that if *decompression* is done, the anterior approach is preferable.[340] Anterior decompression has been especially effective in producing improvements in the anterior cord syndrome and in root recovery. However, it appears at this time that complete spinal cord injury is not improved by decompression.

Another method of early surgical therapy is *stabilization by surgical fusion.* Again, there is much controversy between those who advocate surgical fusion within the first few days after trauma and those who believe it is of no benefit. Some neurosurgeons believe that cervical fractures generally heal well with bony stability if immobilized in a *brace* or *halo jacket.* However, very often after several weeks of conservative treatment, the spine remains unstable and the only resort is fusion. Those who advocate early fusion do so on the basis that it insures both early mobilization and permanent rigidity.

Nursing Care. A patient with a cervical spine fracture who has tongs in place is usually cared for on a Stryker or Foster frame or a CircOlectric bed rather than on a regular hospital bed. Each type of bed has advantages and disadvantages, and the choice is made according to the physician's preference. The specialized beds aid in turning the patient and maintaining proper position, and they facilitate good nursing care and biomechanics.

The *Stryker frame* has two metal frames (an anterior frame and a posterior frame) with taut canvas covers and a thin protective padding over each frame. These frames are supported on a movable cart that has a pivot apparatus at each end. By securing one frame over the patient while he or she lies on the other, two people can change the position of the patient from the back to abdomen, and vice versa. Thus, for turning, the patient is briefly "sandwiched" between the frames. Once the patient is safely turned, the uppermost frame is removed. During the turning process the patient is kept from falling or sliding by straps placed around both frames. Patients who can use their arms are instructed to fold them around the anterior frame while being turned. Patients who cannot use their arms have them safely strapped alongside the body to prevent injury. A small canvas strip across the middle of the posterior frame, i.e., the one the patient is on when lying supine is removable for use of the bedpan. The anterior frame has a space for the patient's face so that when lying on the abdomen the person can rest, read, or eat, without turning the head to the side. Arm rests may be fastened to the sides of the anterior frame if desired (Fig. 26–19).

A conscious patient must be prepared for use of the Stryker frame to eliminate fear of falling while being turned and promote understanding of the purposes and advantages of such a device. Always tell the patient in which direction the turn will be made and always say when the turn is to begin. Give such explanations even to the patient who has an altered state of consciousness; the person may be able to hear you.

The *Foster frame* is similar to the Stryker frame except that it is more stable, takes up more space, and is heavier.

The *CircOlectric* bed may be placed in various horizontal and vertical positions and also in sitting positions if the patient's condition allows. Levers are provided for head and knee gatches. As indicated by its name the bed is electrically operated. A pushbutton on an electrical switch is depressed to move the patient to "face" and "back" positions.

Equipment is available to set up cervical, pelvic, and Buck's traction on this bed. A transfer sling, siderails, and additional special equipment are also available for use on the CircOlectric bed. When changing the patient's position from prone to supine (or vice versa) the change of position is accomplished by vertically turning the patient in a circle as he or she lies between anterior and posterior frames (Fig. 26–20). The position of the bed can be stopped and maintained at any specific level during the turning process. Thus, the CircOlectric bed can be used in helping a patient to gradually assume an upright standing position by using it like a tilt table (Fig. 26–21). It is good safety practice to have two people operate the CircOlectric bed.

For details concerning the actual manipulation and set-ups for Stryker and Foster frames or the CircOlectric bed, consult procedure books and the manufacturers' product information. Of course, you should be thoroughly familiar with how this equipment operates and what it feels like to have it used on you before you use it on a patient.

NURSING CARE PLAN. Caring for patients following a cervical spinal cord injury presents a nurse with a particular challenge. These pa-

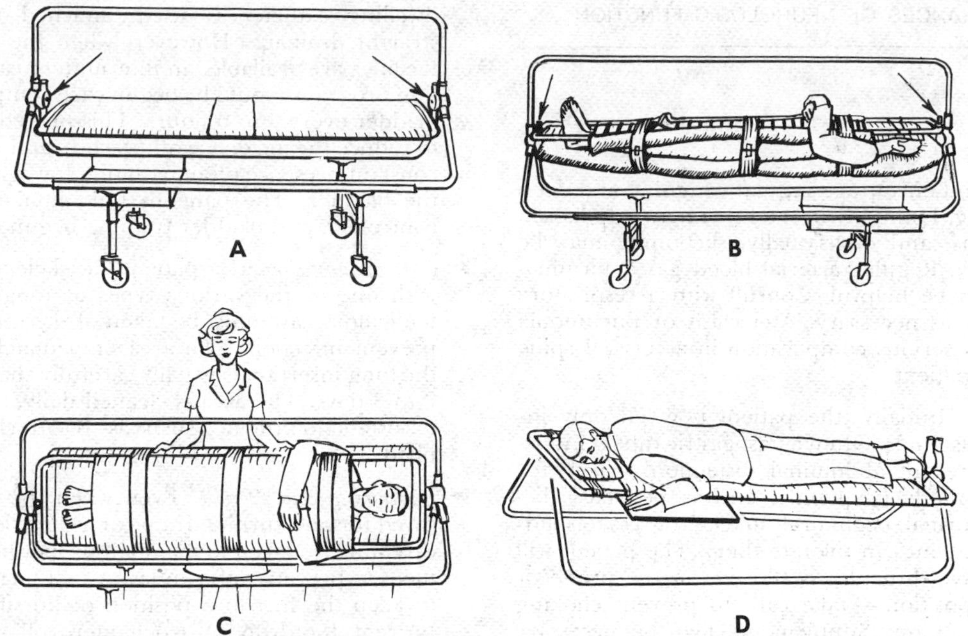

Figure 26–19. **A.** Stryker frame, unoccupied. **B.** Patient positioned for turning between anterior and posterior frames (note protective straps). **C.** Patient being turned by one nurse. **D.** Patient prone on anterior frame with arm rest fastened to side of frame. Note: Two people are needed to turn a patient in a Stryker frame safely. (From Sutton, A.: *Bedside Nursing Techniques*, 2nd ed. Philadelphia: W. B. Saunders, 1969.)

tients are often totally helpless and dependent. Their survival, and the quality of it, very often depend on the quality of nursing care received during the first few weeks after injury. During the *acute phase,* a comprehensive nursing care plan includes attention to the following:

▶ *Respiratory care.* Even after the patient has survived that critical period in the emergency room, close attention must be given to the respiratory status, especially if the injury is high cervical. Watch for decreased lung expansion. The patient will have difficulty in coughing and in clearing secretions.

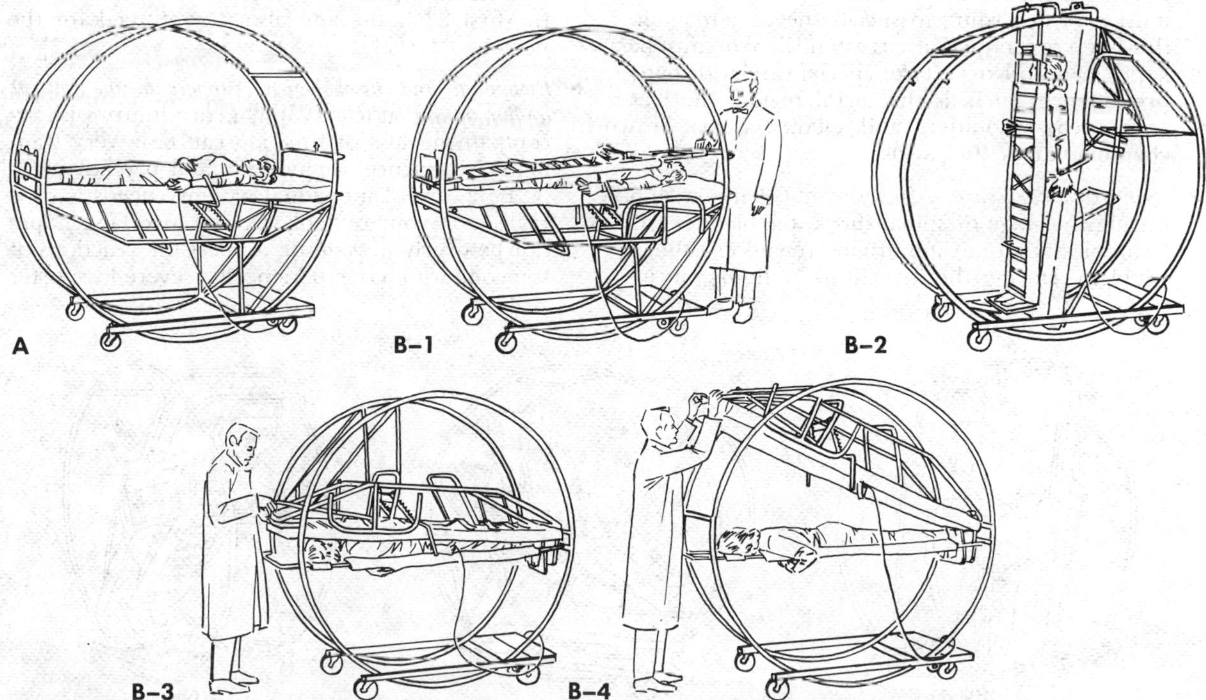

Figure 26–20. *A,* The CircOlectric bed "back" position. *B-1, B-2, B-3,* and *B-4,* Sequence of changing patient's position from supine to prone. Note: Two people are needed to turn a person in a CircOlectric bed safely. (From Sutton, A.: *Bedside Nursing Techniques*, 2nd ed. Philadelphia: W. B. Saunders, 1969.)

Teach and encourage regular coughing and deep breathing. Humidity in the room may help loosen secretions, and occasionally, suctioning may be necessary. Regular arterial blood gas determinations can be helpful. Consult with a respiratory therapist as necessary. Atelectasis or pneumonia can be a serious complication in a cervical spine injured patient.

- *Nutrition.* Initially, the patient is given only intravenous fluids. Often a nasogastric tube is inserted to prevent abdominal distention. Check for bowel sounds frequently, and as peristalsis becomes normal, begin oral fluids. Progress to solids as the patient can tolerate them. The patient will often have difficulty swallowing in the prone or supine position — take care to prevent choking and aspiration. Supplements may be necessary until the patient can take an adequate diet. Meals may be eaten prone or supine; adapt meal times to the patient's most comfortable position. When feeding a patient, do so in an unhurried manner. This is a good opportunity for you to establish a relationship with the patient, to discuss concerns, answer questions, and begin appropriate teaching.
- *Skin care.* This is of utmost importance since decubitus ulcers are one of the most frequent and distressing complications of the spinal cord injured patient. Patients on turning frames are usually turned to their abdomens for 1 hour and to their backs for 2 hours; however, the schedule must vary according to specific needs. Frequent, thorough preventive care is essential. Skin must be kept clean and dry. Take special care with bony prominences such as the sacral region, the iliac crest areas, shoulders and elbows, ischia, trochanters, knees, and heels.
- *Urinary bladder care.* After the initial injury and during the stage of spinal shock, the bladder will be atonic (lack tone) and urinary retention is thus a problem. During the first 48 to 72 hours, an indwelling catheter is used, attached to closed straight drainage. However, when the necessary facilities are available, an intermittent catheterization program should be begun early, emptying the bladder every 4 to 6 hours. This procedure helps to reduce the incidence of infection and avoids the constant presence of an irritating foreign object in the bladder. The patient's fluid intake must be controlled, and bladder training begun early.
- *Care of tong sites.* If a patient has skeletal traction with one of the various types of tongs, regular meticulous care must be taken of the tong sites to prevent infection. The area immediately around the tong insertion is usually carefully shaved every 2 to 3 days. The area is cleaned daily, and a bacteriostatic ointment (such as Bacitracin) is applied.
- *Positioning and exercise.* Even when the patient is cared for on a turning frame or a CircOlectric bed, care must be taken to maintain proper body alignment to prevent deformities. A foot board is used to keep the feet in a position of dorsiflexion, to prevent footdrop. A trochanter roll should be used when the patient is supine to prevent outward rotation at the hip joints. As soon as the injury has been stabilized with traction, passive range-of-motion exercises are started on *all* joints and extremities to prevent contractures and deformities. These should be done each time the patient is turned.
- *Regular assessment of status.* Using the initial assessment of motor and sensory function done in the emergency room as a baseline, the nurse performs a regular (every 2 to 4 hours) brief assessment of the patient's status. This permits early detection of any progression of symptoms or return of function. This is especially important in the first 24 hours and also is continued for the next 1 to 2 weeks.
- *Emotional and psychological support to the patient and/or significant others.* Spinal cord injury with accompanying loss of function can be a very traumatic experience — physically and psychologically. Be aware of individual patients' needs and be realistic in your outlook. Do not give false hopes nor be overly pessimistic. Expect the reactions of someone who has experienced a severe loss; offer

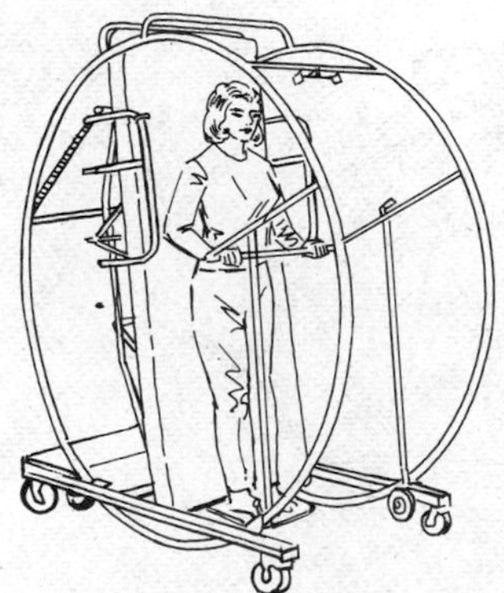
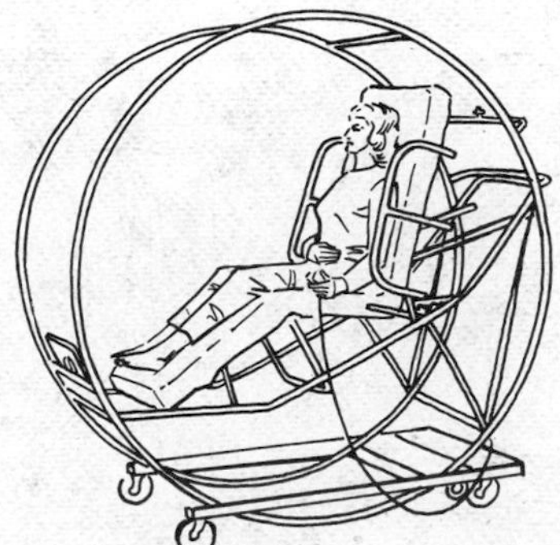
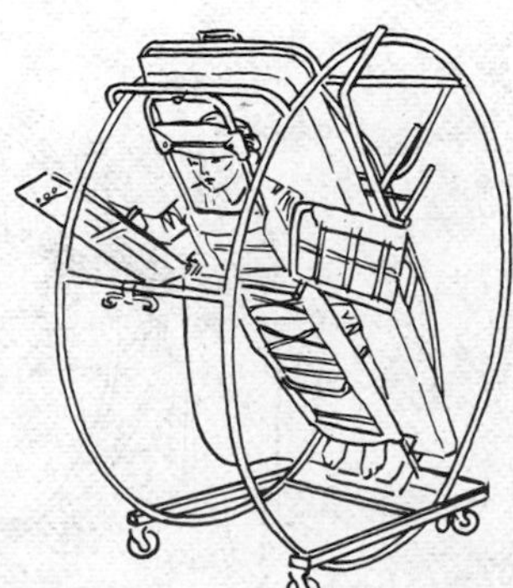

Figure 26–21. Various positions possible with CircOlectric bed. (From Sutton, A. *Bedside Nursing Techniques,* 2nd ed. Philadelphia: W. B. Saunders, 1969.)

the support needed by grieving people, as discussed earlier in this chapter (p. 521).

LONG-TERM CARE AND REHABILITATION

The long-term needs of a patient with a cervical spinal cord injury depend on the degree of the lesion and the accompanying prognosis. According to Stauffer, a patient who has sustained an immediate and complete motor and sensory paralysis that persists for 24 hours can be considered to have a complete and permanent lesion.[226] However, this diagnosis can be confirmed only when the *bulbocavernous reflex* returns. Immediately following the injury, the patient is in *spinal shock* and all reflexes below the level of the lesion are absent. Thus when the bulbocavernous and anal reflexes return, the period of spinal shock is over and the residual loss of function is generally said to be permanent. It is probably wise for a physician to wait 6 weeks before making the firm prognosis of a total and permanent lesion.

Rehabilitation must begin upon a patient's admission to the hospital. Although attention centers on the immediate nursing care measures described, consideration can be given to the patient's long-term needs, to prevention of complications, and to rehabilitative measures that can be started before a patient is transferred to a rehabilitation unit. It is important for nurses to remember that they work as important members of a multidisciplinary care team, along with physicians, physical therapists, occupational therapists, and many others. (Consult a current textbook on rehabilitation nursing for a more in-depth discussion as necessary.)

Bowel and Urinary Bladder Function. Disorders of both the brain and the spinal cord can alter *urinary bladder function.* Patients with CNS disorders therefore need to be observed for incontinence, retention, urgency, dribbling, frequency, enuresis, precipitate micturition, and other indications of faulty bladder control. Such observations should be recorded. Possible bladder infections are diagnostically investigated when symptoms appear.

Central nervous system disorders may also *impair* the *bowel's* sphincter control. Therefore, observe and report constipation, diarrhea, and tenesmus, i.e., ineffectual, painful straining at stool. (For detailed discussion of significant observations and nursing care of patients with intestinal disorders, see Unit XIII.)

In planning care of the paralyzed patient's urinary bladder and bowels, keep several objectives in mind. Among these are: (1) prevention of urinary tract infection; (2) preservation of normal bladder and bowel capacity and normal muscle tone in these areas; (3) preservation of a normal, routine pattern of elimination which requires a minimum of artificial assistance; and (4) teaching the patient to regain bladder and bowel control (by means of governing reflex functioning) when this is possible, and when this is not possible teaching self-help measures to maintain regularity and to prevent complications.

Urinary Tract Problems. The period of urinary bladder atony after spinal cord injury may last several weeks or months. Upon recovery from spinal shock, and the return of the reflex arc, the bladder may become *automatic,* i.e., it may empty reflexively as in the infant. During the period of atony, a retention catheter may be inserted to prevent bladder distention, and to keep the patient dry and comfortable. *Overdistention* of the bladder causes stretching and fissure formation, which can predispose to *infection.* Prolonged use of a catheter also predisposes to infection.

Remember, when sensory pathways are affected, the patient may be unable to feel the discomfort of bladder distention. Nursing responsibilities include: periodically checking the patient for distention; maintaining an accurate record of intake and output; maintaining aseptic technique when giving care related to indwelling catheters (because of the possibility of urinary tract infections); and observing for signs of bladder infection, e.g., malodorous, cloudy urine or more frequent reflex emptying.

Renal complications begin as a result of incomplete emptying of the bladder, which initially necessitates catheterization; catheterization may then be followed by secondary infection and vesicoureteral reflux. Thus, everything possible must be done to prevent these complications. (See Units V and XIII.)

> *Renal calculi, pyelonephritis, and hydronephrosis are major causes of death in paraplegic persons and cause considerable disability in persons with less extensive paralysis. Regardless of the extent of paralysis, complications are an additional source of stress – psychologic and physical.*

Along with preventing *infections of the genitourinary tract,* efforts are made to prevent the formation of *renal calculi* (kidney stones). The prevention of calculi formation partially depends on the patient drinking substantial amounts of water. While for some incontinent patients this increases the problems of keeping dry, it is nonetheless a necessary measure. It is recommended that adequate fluid balance be maintained with a minimal output of 2000 ml. every 24 hours; this generally requires a minimal 24-hour fluid intake of 4000 ml. (See Chapter 12.)

As previously mentioned, an *intermittent catheterization* program is the preferred procedure for bladder drainage during the early weeks after injury. However, the patient must then be taught other methods of emptying the bladder, with the objective being a catheter-free state. Such methods include *rectal stretch, Credé maneuver, Valsalva maneuver,* or any of a number of other *methods to increase intra-abdominal pressure on the bladder* to promote emptying.

- *Credé maneuver:* The nurse makes a fist with a hand and presses directly over the bladder and down toward the pubic bone, with a kneading motion.
- *Valsalva maneuver:* The nurse asks the patient to gently inhale a deep breath, hold it, and push down as hard as possible, as in bearing down for a bowel movement.
- *Rectal stretch:* The nurse or patient inserts a finger into the rectum. When the anal sphincter is relaxed, the patient maintains the relaxation by gently pulling on the sphincter, which relaxes the perineal floor. At the same time, the patient is instructed to perform the Valsalva maneuver.

Occasionally, a surgical procedure such as a *sphincterotomy* may be necessary. The bladder then empties continually. In male patients condoms may be used for drainage, connected to a straight closed drainage system. Appliances for female patients are less satisfactory.

Medications such as *ascorbic acid* and *Mandelamine* are usually given in an effort to maintain acidified urine. Prophylactic antibiotics should *not* be used.

Autonomic Dysreflexia (Hyperreflexia). Autonomic dysreflexia is a pathologic reflex condition characterized by exaggerated autonomic responses to stimuli, primarily seen in patients with cervical and high thoracic cord lesions.[310] (See Fig. 26–22.)

Usually, a distended bladder or bowel acts as the stimulus, which initiates an exaggerated sympathetic discharge. Because of the cord lesion, there is no control from the higher centers in the brain. The patient suddenly develops symptoms: severe hypertension (often as high as 300/160), a severe throbbing headache, profuse diaphoresis, flushing of the skin above the level of the lesion, nasal stuffiness, pilomotor spasm, blurred vision, nausea, and bradycardia.

Autonomic dysreflexia is an emergency situation with the greatest danger being intraocular or intracerebral hemorrhage. Immediate treatment is necessary.

While one nurse monitors the patient's blood pressure closely, another nurse elevates the head of the bed to a sitting position and checks for the possible source of irritation. The catheter may be kinked or otherwise obstructed, or the bladder or lower bowel may be distended. In the meantime, the physician should have been notified. Once the source of irritation has been removed, the symptoms usually begin to subside. If the blood pressure remains elevated, it may be necessary to give some medication such as hydralazine (Apresoline) to aid in lowering the blood pressure.

Once the symptoms have subsided, nurses must closely monitor the patient for a period of 3 to 4 hours, since the blood pressure may drop severely, or the problem of dysreflexia may recur.

Most quadriplegic patients experience autonomic dysreflexia at some time or another. The overall incidence of this complication has decreased markedly in recent years with the decrease in long-term use of indwelling catheters. If it recurs frequently, a surgical procedure such as *chordotomy* or *pudendal nerve resection* may be necessary to effect permanent relief.

Patients and significant others must be given careful instruction about how to manage this complication should it occur following hospital discharge.

Bowel Function. During the acute phase after cervical cord injury, the bowel is *atonic* and the patient usually also has a *paralytic ileus.* As previously stated, a nasogastric tube may be inserted for a few days, until bowel activity returns, to prevent or alleviate distention. When peristalsis returns, oral feeding is started, and attention must be given to bowel function.

If a patient becomes impacted, a cleansing enema may be necessary initially to empty the lower bowel. On a long-term basis, however, enemas should be avoided if possible. When giving an enema or lavage to the paraplegic or quadriplegic person, remember that the patient cannot retain the solution. Protectively cover your clothes and drape the patient's bed.

CAUTION: *Because the paralyzed person's intestine distends easily, enemas should be given carefully, with care not to administer excessive amounts of fluid.*

Specifically, nursing care is directed at: (1) prevention of constipation, distention and impaction; (2) early detection and treatment of these conditions if they do occur; and (3) reestablishment of habitual, controlled bowel movements by conditioned reflex activity.

A bowel program should be instituted as early as possible, since bowel training is possible in most patients who have paraplegia or quadriplegia.

Bowel retraining is accomplished (as with bladder retraining) by (1) keeping a careful record of the patient's individual pattern of intake and elimination, and then (2) by establishing routine patterns of bowel elimination through the use of suppositories and other means of stimulating evacuation until (3) reflex evacuation at desirable times is possible.

A bowel program should be carried out *regularly* (daily at first) at the *same time each day.* A sample of an effective bowel program is as fol lows:

- ▶ Upon awakening for the day, the patient drinks a warm beverage.
- ▶ About 30 minutes later the patient has a rectal suppository, followed with rectal stimulation every 10 to 15 minutes until a bowel movement occurs. (See Fig. 26–23.)

In addition, the patient must have an adequate daily fluid intake (3000 to 4000 ml. per day), a diet adequate in bulk and roughage, and may take a stool softener (such as Colace) daily. Laxatives should be avoided.

Training the patient to have habitual, controlled bowel movements (by conditioned reflex activity) is started as soon as the patient is able to sit up in a chair. It is easier if a patient is able to sit on the toilet (or a commode if necessary) since the bedpan impedes normal bowel evacuation. The thoughtful nurse assures privacy for a patient during the daily bowel routine.

With an effective bowel program, a patient will have a bowel movement once every day or every other day, and then will not be incontinent at other times during the day. In addition to working closely with the patient, the nurse may include the significant others in the program, since they may be involved in this aspect of the patient's long term care.

Attaining continence once more may determine a patient's vocational future and may make a difference in the person's ability to continue satisfying family and social relationships. In addition, bowel and bladder training may give a patient the self-confidence and psychologic boost necessary to withstand the other problems created by paralysis.

Spinal Automatisms. Following transection of the spinal cord the lower part of the cord eventually works automatically on its own; the brain can no longer influence the segmental spinal cord reflex movements, i.e., those reflex movements that are "built into" the spinal cord. Spinal reflex activities which *automatically occur* following severance of the cord are called *"spinal automatisms,"* e.g., the flexor withdrawal reflex, and the reflex emptying of the urinary bladder and bowel.

Spinal automatisms are primitive spinal mechanisms normally kept inactive by higher centers. However, when these normal inhibitions of the higher centers are destroyed by severe spinal cord disease or decerebrate states at the midbrain level, the spinal automatisms are "released." (*Decerebration* refers to interruption or sectioning of the nervous system below the level of the cerebral hemispheres. Do not mix the terms *decerebration* and *decortication* in your thinking. Decortication refers to destruction of the cerebral cortex.)

When the spinal cord is severed, the blood

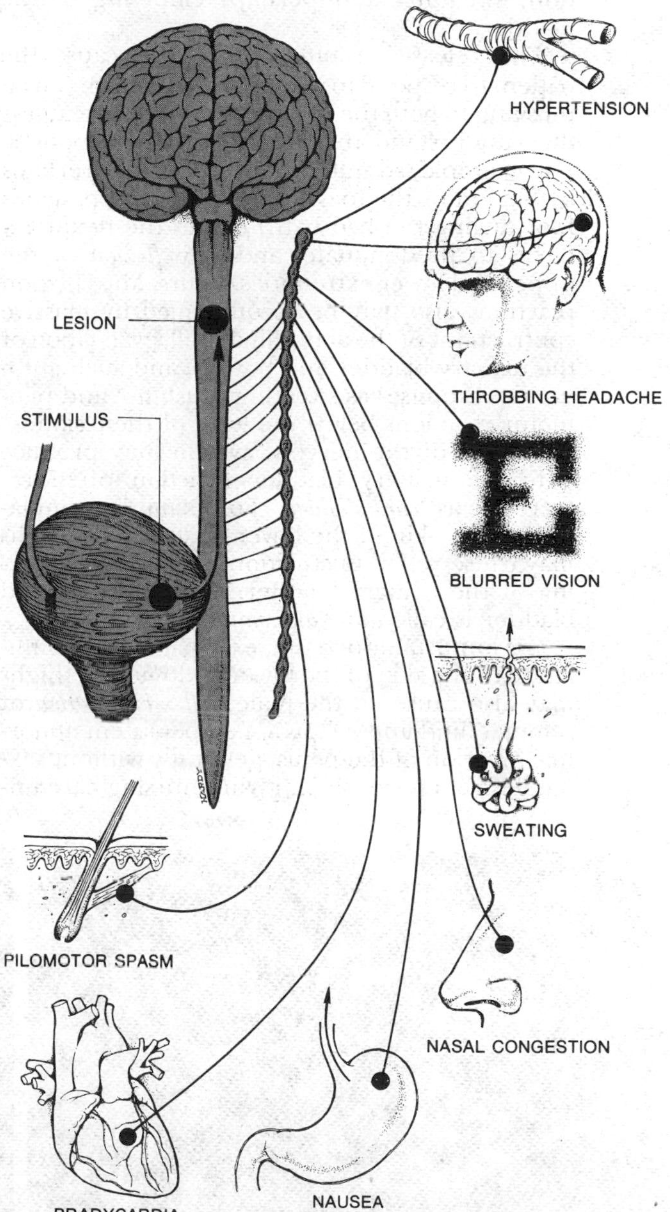

Figure 26–22. The symptoms of autonomic hyperreflexia, a dire threat to some patients with spinal cord injury, are triggered by distention or contraction of the bladder or rectum, stimulation of pain receptors, and stimulation of the skin. Immediate removal of the triggering factor is the essential treatment. (From Feustel, D.: Autonomic hyperreflexia. *American Journal of Nursing,* 76:228, Feb. 1976.)

pressure and temperature in the part of the body supplied by the isolated spinal cord fall markedly and respond poorly to reflex stimuli. Other functions may occur reflexly, e.g., control of the urinary bladder, but lack integration with other visceral activities. Visceral activities may be initiated by stimuli which are normally ineffective, e.g., scratching of the skin may cause vasodilatation, sweating, and perhaps emptying of the bladder.

The "release" of spinal automatisms causes the patient to respond to stimuli in ways which can be puzzling to both the patient and the nurse unless they understand the origin of such responses. For example, stimulation of the limbs (perhaps by flexion of the toes while drying the patient's foot during the bed bath) causes the flexor reflexes to predominate, and *mass flexion* of the upper and lower extremities occurs. Mass flexion reactions also may be accompanied by massive contractions of the abdominal wall, evacuation of the urinary bladder and bowels, and such autonomic responses as sweating, flushing, and pilomotor reactions below the level of the lesion.

Lesions of the nervous system may produce defective urinary bladder function often referred to as "*cord bladder.*" For example, stimulation of the skin of the lower abdomen or thighs may cause reflex micturition, i.e., reflex emptying of the urinary bladder. This form of cord bladder is called an "*automatic bladder.*"

It is important for a nurse to realize that stimulation of the skin of the lower abdomen or thighs may also cause, in the male, *reflex ejaculation* of seminal fluid and *priapism,* i.e., persistent abnormal erection of the penis, generally without sexual desire. Obviously in giving nursing care unnecessary stimulation of those areas that elicit such reflex spinal automatisms should be avoided. When such reactions do occur, the nurse's unembarrassed, accepting response to the situation helps to relieve the patient's anxiety and embarrassment. An explanation of the cause of some of these spinal patterns of movement may help uninformed patients to understand why their bodies react as they do.

Spasticity; Muscle Spasms. Spasticity may result from various CNS injuries or diseases, e.g., cerebrovascular accidents, spinal cord injuries, cerebral palsy. Spasticity may develop 2 weeks to several months following injury to the spinal cord. Flaccidity occurs first (*spinal shock*), and spasticity begins to appear some time during the first few months. It increases to a maximum for that individual, and then may continue indefinitely or gradually decrease over many months.

Spastic movements may be initiated by such emotions as apprehension, crying, anger, or laughing, or from cutaneous stimulation, e.g., tickling, stroking, or pinching. While spastic movements may be annoying to experience, a patient may also learn to recognize events that trigger such movements and then use some of these triggering activities to assist with various activities such as emptying the bladder.

Following traumatic complete transverse lesion of the spinal cord, painful intense *spasms of the muscles* of the lower extremities occur. (Such spasms may also occur with other severe neurologic disorders.) A paralyzed patient must tactfully be told that the occurrence of muscle spasms does not mean that voluntary movement is returning, but rather that these spasms occur involuntarily. This may be very disappointing and discouraging for the person to hear.

Muscle spasms vary, according to the patient's posture, from mild muscular twitchings to vigorous mass reflex states. Because violent involuntary muscle spasms can actually throw a paralyzed patient off a bed or frame, it is important to

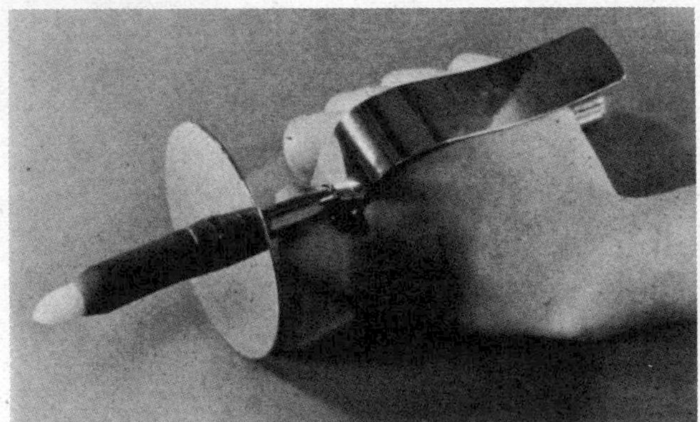

A

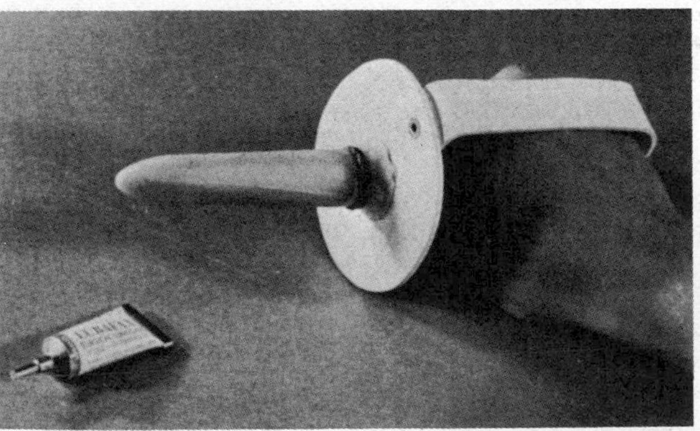

B

Figure 26–23. **A.** Rectal suppository inserter. A spring plunger enables a quadriplegic person to insert a suppository. Suppository is lubricated before insertion. A suspended mirror is necessary for visibility for self-insertion. (The inserter shown above can be obtained from the G. F. Strong Rehabilitation Centre, 900 W. 27th Ave., Vancouver, British Columbia.) **B.** Artificial finger extension for rectal massage. Note large handle for use by quadriplegic patients. (Developed by Marilyn Wittmeyer, chief occupational therapist, Department of Rehabilitation Medicine, University of Washington School of Medicine.) (From Taylor, N., R. Berni, and M. R. Horning: Neurogenic bowel management. *American Family Physician,* 7:126, May 1973.)

keep bed siderails up and to always have restraining straps comfortably secured over the patient's body when he or she is lying on a frame or being transported on a stretcher. Muscle spasms are typically aggravated by cold weather, by sitting for prolonged periods of time, and by emotionally upsetting events.

Reflex spasms may become intolerable and may be triggered by extrinsic or visceral stimuli, e.g., a distended bladder.

A certain amount of muscle spasm may actually help a paraplegic person to support the trunk or to position an extremity. However, painful or recurrent spasms that forcibly flex or adduct the lower limbs prevent rehabilitation by interfering with sitting and ambulation. These flexor spasms are reflex responses. Thus, to try to prevent their occurrence it is necessary to remove sources of noxious stimulation that could trigger the reflex spasms, e.g., treat bladder infections and decubitus ulcers if present.

Medications employed in treating muscle spasms include: methocarbamol, meprobamate, diazepam (Valium), dantraline sodium (Dantrium), and chlordiazepoxide hydrochloride. Side effects of such medications include drowsiness and muscle weakness. Muscle spasms may also be treated with such physical therapy practices as stretching exercises and warm tub baths. Exercises under water and Hubbard baths may not only relieve muscle spasm, but may also relieve pain, improve muscle tone, and stimulate circulation.

When painful, severe muscle spasms or spasticity cannot be controlled by conservative measures, e.g., with specific pharmacologic agents or physical therapy, it may be necessary to employ more drastic measures. Various *surgical procedures* have been useful in individual circumstances, including chordotomies, rhizotomies, peripheral neurotomies, and tendon releases. (Pain is discussed in Unit XI.) Recently, attempts have been made to correct spastic deformities with *neuroelectric stimulation.*

Pain. Often patients with spinal injuries have pain at the level of the injury, which radiates along the spinal nerves originating in that area. For example, chest pain may occur following a thoracic injury, while leg pain may follow an injury at the lumbar level. Analgesics (acetylsalicylic acid, narcotics) may be prescribed and should be given as indicated for pain relief. However, remember:

Narcotics are not *administered in the presence of high cervical injuries because they tend to add to respiratory depression.*

Patients with thoracic level injuries often tend to splint their chests and to breathe shallowly to avoid pain. Of course, these actions set the stage for the development of respiratory complications. To prevent this, narcotics may be given for pain control and then deep breathing and coughing (unless contraindicated) are encouraged to aerate the lungs and to move secretions in the respiratory passages. Thoracic pain may also be relieved by paravertebral nerve blocks.

Usually pain occurs later than muscular spasms. Some paraplegic and quadriplegic patients have both pain and muscle spasms. Pain most frequently occurs in the lower extremities.

Pain associated with spasticity may be treated with such drugs as opiates, sedatives, antispasmodics, anticonvulsants, or ataractics. When medical pain relief cannot be obtained, neurosurgery may be considered, e.g., neurectomy, chordotomy. (Pain is discussed further in Unit XI.)

Tendon Contractures; Ankylosis of Joints; Muscle Shortening. Other complications of paralyzed limbs are muscle shortening, tendon contractures, and ankylosis of joints. These problems are caused by improper positioning of a patient in bed or chair and by lack of joint movements, e.g., because of spasticity or immobility. Measures that can prevent such complications are: position changes; proper positioning of joints at all times; use of footboard in supine position; draping bedding over frames to keep pressure from the pull of bed linens off feet; maintenance of 15 degree flexion of knee joints in supine position; conditioning exercises (active and passive); and other physiotherapeutic measures *performed regularly.*

Passive exercises prevent contractures as well as future painful reflex dystrophies of the hand and shoulder. Passive exercises may be started 48 to 72 hours after spinal injury if ordered. Passive exercises should be performed as early as prescribed by the physician; check to determine when exercises may be started. When a patient's condition permits, *active exercises, massage,* and *electrical stimulation* may also be prescribed.

Muscle Weakness; Fatigue. Wristdrop and footdrop *will* develop following paralysis of the extremities unless proper preventive measures are carefully taken. These problems and contractures may take months to overcome once they develop and may prevent some patients from ever walking, even with crutches and braces.

Provide continual support for paretic or paralyzed extremities.

To counteract the force of gravity on weakened muscles and thereby prevent footdrop, keep the patient's feet firmly supported in dorsiflexion at right angles to the hips. A paralyzed upper extremity is supported in a sling when the patient is out of bed and with cock-up splints while in bed. Usually the hand end of the splint is elevated 2 inches to support the wrist, and the fingers are maintained in a position of function. Posterior molded casts may be used instead of splints to support a paralyzed wrist while the patient is in bed. For some patients, pillows and a hand roll suffice.

Rehabilitative programs often require strength and endurance on the part of the patient. To prepare for ambulation, the unaffected parts of a patient's body are strengthened, and suitable exercises are started early. The patient's tolerance for activity is gradually increased; take care not to *fatigue* the patient. Periods of planned rest and recreation are important.

Weight Bearing; Assuming an Upright Position. Following cord injury, weight bearing is started as early as possible, to stimulate osteoblastic activity and thus decrease the demineralization of bone, or osteoporosis, that develops with prolonged immobilization. If a CircOlectric bed is not available to gradually assist a patient to a standing position, standing boards or tilt tables can be used (Fig. 26–24). Having the patient assume a standing position for at least a few minutes each day may also help prevent contractures. For example, contractures could develop in the hips from prolonged periods of sitting.

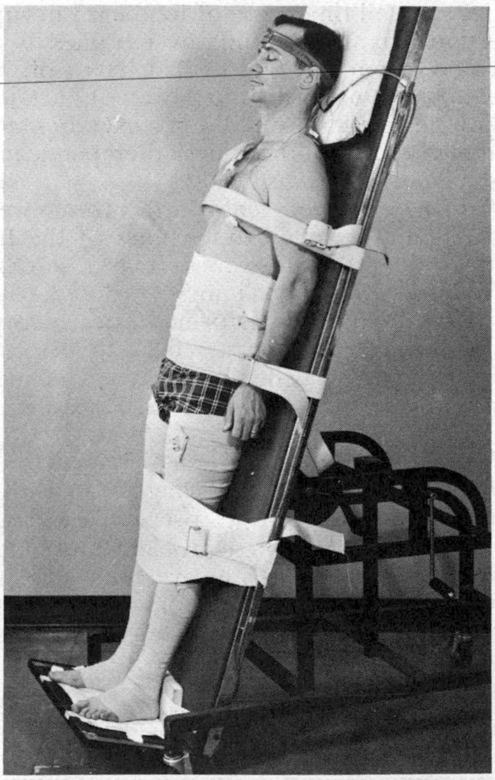

Figure 26–24. The tilt table may be used to provide security for a patient while developing tolerance to the upright position. (From Krusen, F. H., F. J. Kottke, and P. M. Ellwood, Jr: *Handbook of Physical Medicine and Rehabilitation,* 2nd ed. Philadelphia: W. B. Saunders Co., 1971, p. 411.)

Wheelchairs. Many patients are mobilized by modern, folding *wheelchairs.* Wheelchair selection needs to be tailored to meet the needs of individual patients because the wheelchair is the most important orthopedic appliance for persons whose normal means of locomotion is either completely abolished or impaired due to limb paralysis.

Let us emphasize that:

> Prolonged, unrelieved *periods of sitting in a wheelchair can lead to various complications, e.g., flexion contractures, decubitus ulcers, bone atrophy, loss of calcium from bones, pathologic fractures, and renal calculi.*

When sitting up, e.g., in a wheelchair, the paralyzed person needs to periodically shift body weight and lift this weight (by pushing with the arms and hands against the chair arms or seat). This relieves the constant pressure on the buttocks. Failure to perform these pushups, either through neglect or forgetfulness, may be one cause of skin breakdown.

Impaired Circulation; Decubitus Ulcers; Absence of Sensations

> *Decubitus ulcers (pressure sores) are a serious potential complication of paralysis since* circulation is poor *in denervated tissue because of lack of muscle activity.*

Because of loss of sensation in an anesthetic area, pain and pressure that normally prompt a change in position are not felt. Sometimes merely the weight of bedding can cause the tips of a patient's toes to break down. Skin breakdown may also occur when plaster casts are applied over anesthetic areas. Decubitus ulcers have been known to develop within a period of 2 to 3 hours. This complication can be prevented, however, by frequent, knowledgeable skin assessment, careful nursing care, and by teaching the patient self-help measures.*

Like renal calculi, decubitus ulcers can be partially prevented if a patient is able to stand in braces in an upright position. Range-of-motion exercise and gentle total body massage improve a paralyzed person's circulation. Elastic stockings may improve circulation in the legs.

Paralyzed persons and their significant others or attendants are taught to frequently and regularly inspect the skin for red spots or other signs of pressure, rubbing, chafing, or irritation that could progress to ulcer formation. The paralyzed person's entire body is inspected daily for

*The care of people experiencing or at risk of decubitus ulcers is discussed in Sorensen and Luckmann, *Basic Nursing: A Psychophysiologic Approach,* Chapter 33.

skin breakdown; specific areas prone to pressure damage are, of course, inspected more frequently. The skin is kept clean and dry; special attention is given to the perineal area. When the patient is confined to bed, skin care is given at least every 2 hours, immediately after the patient is turned. Let us reemphasize that the paralyzed patient must be turned at least every 2 hours — *day and night* — to compensate for the loss of spontaneous movements.

Sensory loss poses serious problems for paralyzed persons because they cannot feel the pain or pressure that normally signals tissue damage. A paralyzed patient (or any person with impaired sensation) should thus avoid wearing tight, restrictive clothing or ill-fitting shoes or braces. Since patients with impaired sensation cannot *feel* injury occurring, they must learn and practice *preventive thinking* — avoiding potential sources of danger. This includes avoiding close proximity to heaters, radiators, and fireplaces and avoiding the use of heating pads and hot water bottles. *Burns can pose serious problems because of impaired circulation.*

> *Do not apply external heat if there has been a loss of sensation. Be careful that bath water is not too warm.*

Regular *foot* and *nail care* is needed to prevent nails from rubbing or cutting the skin and to prevent ingrown nails. Foot infections must be prevented, e.g., the patient is instructed not to cut corns or calluses. (Foot care is discussed further in Units XV and XIX.)

It is best to give *injections of medications* above the level of a patient's cord lesion whenever possible. Adequate absorption of injectable medication is not likely to occur in denervated areas of the body, which have impaired capillary and precapillary circulation.

Thoracic and Lumbar Spine Injuries

Much of the previous discussion about cervical spine injuries also pertains to the care and treatment of persons with thoracic and lumbar spine injuries. However, injuries at the thoracic and lumbar levels are not as acutely life-threatening and do not cause such devastating losses of neurologic function.

Injury to the cord in the thoracic region occurs only after violent trauma, since the unique architecture of the thoracic spine and thorax provide considerable structural stability. T12 is the most common level of injury. Because the spinal canal is narrow in the thoracic region and the cord lies in close proximity to the vertebral column, a fracture-dislocation in this area usually produces complete physiological transection of the cord, with resultant paraplegia.

> *Paraplegia is characterized by loss of motor and sensory function in the lower extremities, and some portion of the lower trunk, depending on the specific level of injury. (Refer to Fig. 26–16.)*

Anterior cord syndrome is rarely seen in this area. (Refer to p. 559 for discussion of anterior cord syndrome).

Lumbar spinal cord injuries usually result from a compression fracture of the vertebral body with forward displacement. Level T12 to L1 is a frequent location of injury, as is L4 to L5. Injuries to the lumbar spine result in injury to the cauda equina, since the spinal cord usually ends at the upper border of the first lumbar vertebra. This damage to the lumbar and sacral spinal roots presents the following *symptom picture:* flaccid paralysis of the lower extremities, loss of deep tendon reflexes, urinary retention, fecal incontinence, loss of sensation in the areas of lumbar and sacral segments and usually severe low back pain. The functional loss of bowel and bladder control is usually permanent.

TREATMENT AND NURSING CARE

First aid to a person with a thoracic or lumbar spine injury is as important as with the cervical injury. *The spine must be kept in neutral alignment.* The patient should be placed supine on a firm surface (a board or stretcher), with possibly a small folded blanket under the lumbar area to maintain the normal curvature.

Since injury to the thoracic and lumbar spine does not usually affect the muscles of respiration, the incidence of life-threatening respiratory emergencies is much less frequent. Rather, attention must be directed toward the possibility of concomitant intrathoracic or intra-abdominal injury. The examination in the emergency room must also include a brief neurological evaluation to determine the baseline of neurologic deficit. Diagnosis of the extent and type of injury is established by x-ray. (Emergency care is discussed further in Chapter 95.)

Treatment. General principles of treatment used with cervical cord injuries pertain also to injuries of the thoracic and lumbar spine, with a few modifications. *Traction is not used* to stabilize and immobilize fractures and fracture-dislocations of these two areas, because there is no effective way to provide traction.

With *thoracic spine trauma,* when the transection is complete, surgery is usually not indicated, unless it is possible within a few hours of the trauma. In the rare instance of thoracic anterior cord syndrome, it is generally accepted that immediate *laminectomy* is indicated, but surgical *fusion* is rarely done because of the stability of the thoracic spine. If the lesion is incomplete and there is evidence of progressive neurologic deficit, decompression is indicated to preserve what function remains and to prevent further damage.

With *lumbar injuries,* indications for decompressive laminectomy are again controversial. Some physicians feel that for any neurological deficit, decompression by *laminectomy* is advisable. Others maintain that *exploratory surgery* should always be done to open the dura and inspect the conus medullaries and cauda equina, since there is considerable potential for regeneration with certain elements of the cauda equina.[340]

The matter of *spinal fusion* in lumbar injuries is also controversial. In past years, fusion was frequently done, but more recently, surgeons are less quick to fuse unless there is evidence of instability of the fracture. Fusion allows for early ambulation and aids in preventing many complications of bedrest.

Nursing Care. Patients with thoracic and lumbar spine injuries are usually cared for on a Stryker frame or Foster frame or — less likely — on a CircOlectric bed. Essentially all the nursing care measures outlined for cervical spine injuries pertain to these injuries also. Exercise of the shoulders and upper extremities is important to begin early. Strong musculature in these areas and the chest and back will be necessary for effective self-transfers and ambulation when the lower spine is stable enough to permit mobilization.

Lumbar spine injured patients can usually be rehabilitated to ambulate with the use of some appliance such as long or short leg *braces.* They may become completely independent in all activities of daily living. Many can drive and attend outside jobs. Since lower lumbar injuries affect the cauda equina, there is no recovery of reflex function of the bladder, and it becomes large and atonic. Some procedure is necessary by which continuous urine drainage is possible, i.e., *sphincterotomy* or *ileal loop drainage.*

Braces; Corsets; Orthopedic Shoes. A back brace or corset is often prescribed and custom fitted to a patient following ruptured lumbar intervertebral disks or other spinal injuries. (*Casts* are also used in supportive treatment after an injury is stabilized. See Unit XX.) The appliance, e.g., a *Taylor back brace* or splint (Fig. 26–25) or a heavy muslin corset with stays, may initially be prescribed to be worn for periods of time while the patient is in bed and turning. Later it may be worn only when the patient plans to get up. The patient is turned to one side, the brace or corset is then placed up against the back. The person is then rolled back into the appliance. Finally, the brace or corset is secured with straps while the patient lies supine in bed. It is desirable for a thin knitted undershirt to be worn next to the skin under a brace, to protect the skin and also to keep the brace clean. The brace or corset is applied *before* the patient is helped out of bed. As improvement occurs, and with teaching, some patients learn to apply their own braces and corsets while in bed. Other patients continue to need help even after discharge. The degree of arm and hand function the person has determines the person's ability to put on braces and corsets alone. People who can use their arms and hands can almost always put on their own appliances.

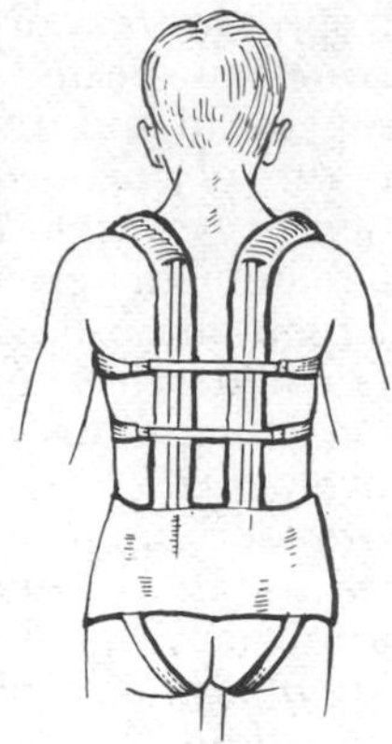

Figure 26–25. Taylor splint. (From *Dorland's Illustrated Medical Dictionary.* 25th ed. Philadelphia: W. B. Saunders, 1974.)

A *neck brace* (fitted so the patient's chin rests on a cup and the neck is kept hyperextended), a *Thomas collar* (which extends up under the chin and prevents flexion of the neck) or a *Chandler felt collar splint* may be necessary following fracture of a cervical vertebra or rupture of a cervical disk. Such appliances may be worn following "whiplash" injuries resulting from automobile accidents.

The patient wearing a brace must learn to be careful not to fall or otherwise lose balance because of the brace. The weight of a brace may be surprisingly heavy at first to a patient who is weak from lying in bed and from being ill. Neck braces tend to limit vision, since people wearing them cannot look down at their feet.

Shoes should be worn, rather than slippers, by all patients who have had spinal injuries, and indeed by any patient learning how to walk again after any injury or prolonged illness. Preferably the shoes should tie (so firm support is possible), and they should have a low heel. Of course, slick soles and slick heels are hazardous. Orthopedic shoes may be advisable. Wearing shoes also helps to prevent footdrop when the patient lies down.

The *appearance* of braces, corsets, and shoes is important — at least the person wearing them may well think so! There has been a tendency for the professional who is not disabled to believe that people should be concerned only about the function and not the appearance of such appliances. Nurses need to be understanding of and helpful to the person who wishes to be stylish as well as wants the benefits of these therapeutic garments. A good designer of supportive devices takes time to find out what the patient's hopes and wants are concerning appearance. People who wear such appliances can be helped if they are allowed to discuss their feelings concerning their self-image and to have these feelings taken into consideration.

It is also important to achieve a really good, comfortable fit in braces, corsets, and shoes. Such appliances can be quite painful when they are first worn, and this is increased unnecessarily if they do not fit well. Very careful and frequent skin checks must be made — especially at first — as pressure can occur and decubitus ulcers develop very quickly.

Some modern braces are made from plastic, which makes them much lighter and often gives a more attractive appearance to the person.

Transfers. The paraplegic patient must learn a variety of transfers to become self-sufficient. A few of these are pictured in Figures 26–26, 26–27 and 26–28. Learning to sit up, of course, always precedes learning to transfer.

Nutrition

> *It is best not to feed patients who have neurologic disorders until they have been examined to be certain that their condition has not impaired the mechanics of swallowing and that their stomachs are not distended.*

The paralyzed patient or the immobilized patient often must be fed by others for a period of time. With special devices paralyzed patients can often learn eventually to feed themselves. As discussed, patients in hyperextension may have difficulty swallowing. Take care in feeding such patients or giving them liquids. Always have suction apparatus ready to use if the patient chokes.

Numerous problems can lead to nutritional difficulties in paralyzed patients, e.g., inactivity, anorexia, decubitus ulcers, paralytic ileus. Osteoporosis causes excessive calcium loss; the alkalinization of urine by citrus fruits can contribute to urinary sepsis and the formation of renal calculi; and decubitus ulcers contribute to hypoproteinemia. A protein loss over a period of time can lower tissue resistance and lower resistance to infection, in addition to causing weight loss and malnutrition.

It is essential that the paraplegic or quadriplegic patient's diet have an average daily protein intake of 150 to 300 grams and that it is also high in vitamins and calories. Since B vitamins occur in high protein foods, a deficiency of these vitamins generally accompanies an inadequate intake of protein. A high protein, high caloric diet helps to heal injured tissue and to prevent decubitus ulcer formation. At first 2000 to 3500 calories may be given daily. However, in order to

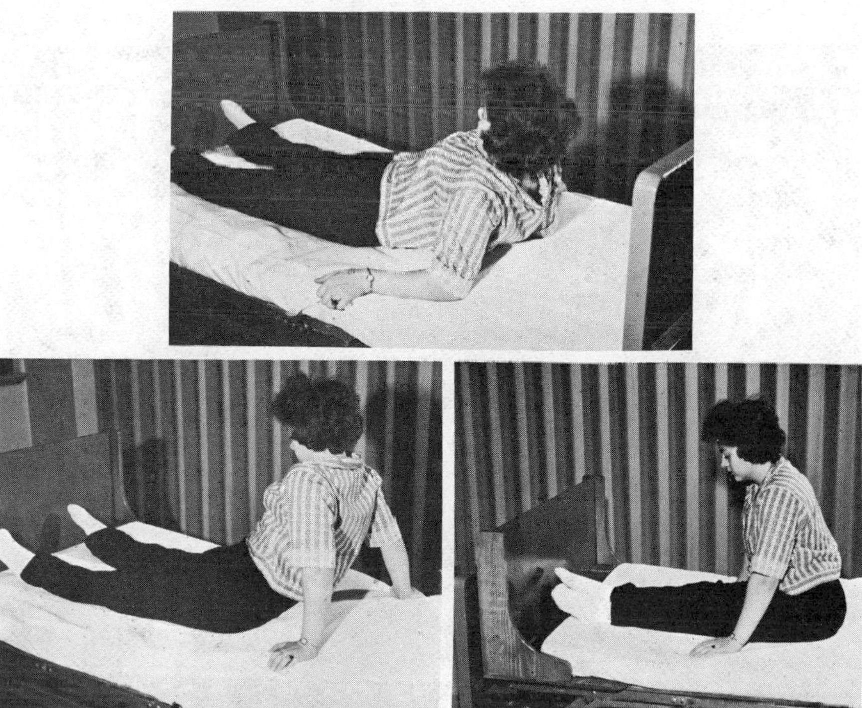

Figure 26–26. Paraplegic patient coming to sitting position. (From Krusen, F. H., F. J. Kottke, and P. M. Ellwood, Jr.: *Handbook of Physical Medicine and Rehabilitation,* 2nd ed. Philadelphia: W. B. Saunders Co., 1971.)

avoid obesity, this may need to be lowered later on. Obesity greatly complicates the problems of a paralyzed person and increases the possibilities of complications. To minimize the possibility of urinary calculi formation, the calcium intake is reduced during the first few months.

SEXUALITY*

A person who has experienced a spinal cord injury very often has concerns about sexuality and about his or her ability to achieve sexual fulfillment. It is likely that such concerns will be present long before the person expresses them to anyone. It is also likely that the first professional a person speaks to will be a nurse. Maybe this is because people who incur severe physical disabilities do, by necessity, allow nurses to tend to them in quite intimate ways. If this care is offered well, a high degree of trust between a patient and a nurse is likely to develop.

Some people will bring up the issue of their own sexual potential quite directly. Others will refer to it in oblique ways. Sometimes patients may seem to be crude in the way they introduce the topic. A patient may make an apparently inappropriate sexual comment or may make a "pass" at a nurse or some other person. If you understand such behavior as the person's attempt to receive acknowledgment as a sexual being, you can avoid being offended and causing the patient to feel reprimanded and put down. However the person brings up the topic, you can matter-of-factly acknowledge the person's concern and indicate your willingness to discuss it. You might say something like "You seem to be concerned about your own sexuality, Janet. I can understand that and I would really like to talk with you about it if that is what you want."

Nurses have a good opportunity to facilitate straightforward communication when a patient and significant others seek to reexamine the injured person's sexuality. Unfortunately this natural and common concern is often inadequately dealt with by nurses and other health professionals. Too often, questions about sexual function are met with embarrassment or misinformation, or a brisk referral is made.

If individual nurses are to be helpful to disabled people, they need to be able to talk about sexual issues without embarrassment. They also need accurate information about "normal" sexuality and the kinds of physiologic changes that may occur as a result of injury. It may be appropriate to refer the patient to another person or agency if you and the patient believe that more help can be gained that way. Do not make such a referral too quickly, however. Remember that if a person brings up such an emotionally laden subject as "sex" with you, it is probably because *at this time* the person feels most comfort-

*This section was written by Margaret Helen Parkinson, R.N., M.N., in consultation with Jane Elder Bogle, B.A., M.P.A., Family Planning and Sexuality Consultant, Seattle, Washington.

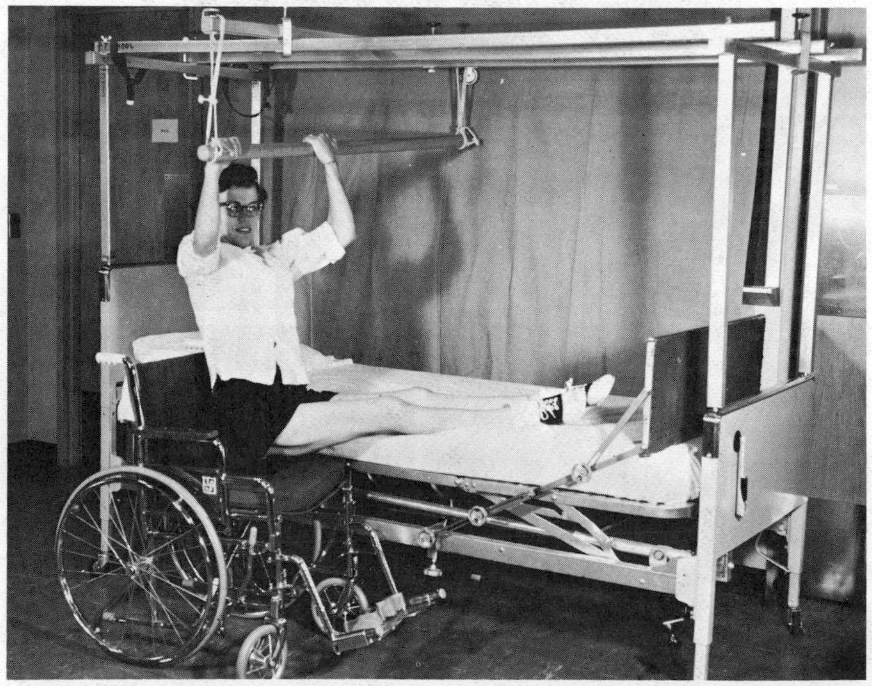

Figure 26–27. Paraplegic patient transferring from bed to wheelchair using a 4-foot trapeze bar. (From Krusen, F. H., F. J. Kottke, and P. M. Ellwood, Jr.: *Handbook of Physical Medicine and Rehabilitation,* 2nd ed. 1971.)

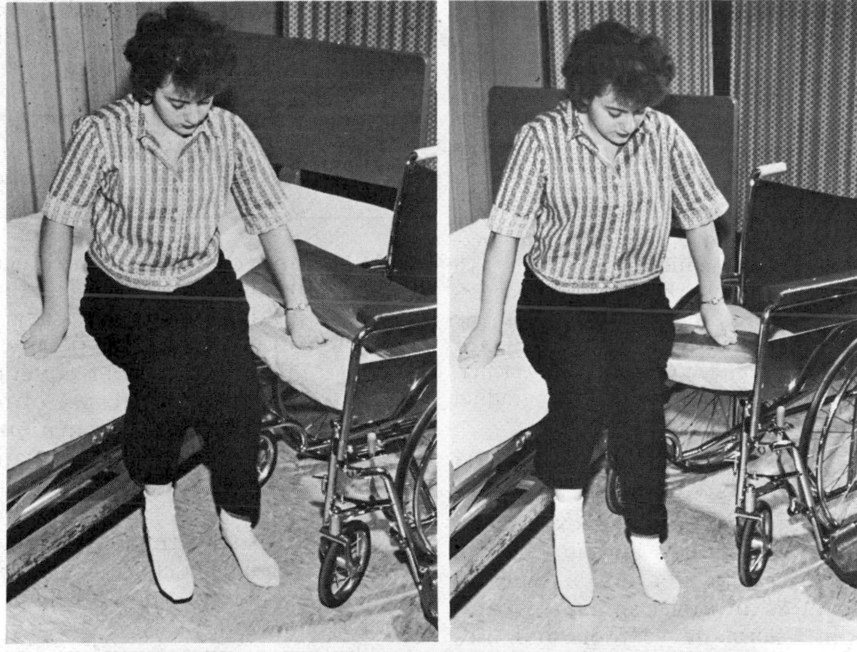

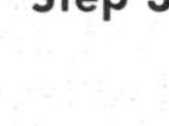

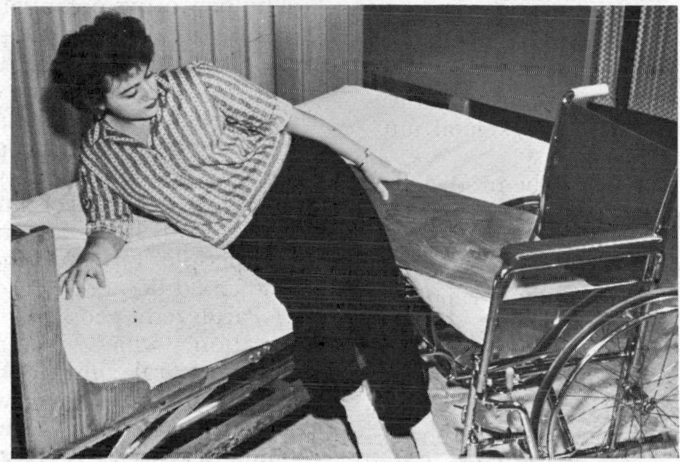

Figure 26–28. Paraplegic bed to wheelchair lateral transfer using a sliding board. (From Krusen, F. H., F. J. Kottke, and P. M. Ellwood, Jr.: *Handbook of Physical Medicine and Rehabilitation,* 2nd ed. 1971.)

able speaking to *you* about it. Allow the person to take the lead in the conversation. In other words, talk about the issues he or she wishes to discuss. This is not as easy as it sounds! Professionals can easily feel they know what the patient needs and wants, without listening to the *patient.*

Although you may not directly "teach" it to a patient, knowledge of female and male sexual physiology is important if a nurse is to be helpful. In the past 15 years, scientific study has led to greater understanding of sexual function in both the nondisabled and the disabled person. Remember, of course, that much more is involved in sexual expression than the physiologic response.

Female Sexual Response

The female physiologic sexual response involves four phases: (1) The *excitement phase,* in which genital vasocongestion begins: the vagina becomes lubricated, lengthens, and distends; blood pressure, heart rate, and respirations increase, and muscles become tense (myotonia). Sexual excitement gradually builds. (2) In the *plateau phase,* sexual excitement reaches a height and remains there; lubrication and vasocongestion increase. The "orgasmic platform" develops (the outer congested third of the vagina and the area of congested tissue that surrounds the vaginal entrance), and the inner two thirds of the vagina balloons. (3) When *pelvic* congestion reaches a critical point, a reflex mechanism occurs that causes the muscles of the orgasmic platform to contract strongly. These contractions (along with uterine contractions) constitute *orgasm.* (4) The *resolution phase* is the return to a relaxed body state after orgasm. The orgasmic platform becomes disengorged; the vagina returns to normal size; and heart rate, blood pressure, and respirations return gradually to normal.

Male Sexual Response

The male physiologic sexual response occurs in the same phases as described for a woman. Chiefly because of vasocongestion, the penis becomes erect (excitement phase) and increases to a maximum size (plateau phase). Erection may be of two kinds, *psychogenic erection* and *reflex erection.* Psychogenic erection occurs as a response to stimulating sight or thoughts. Reflex erection occurs as a response to stimulation by touch to the external genitalia or perineal area. Orgasm consists of strong penile muscular contractions, causing ejaculation of seminal fluid, and resolution is the gradual return of the body to a nonaroused state.

Generally, an intact nervous system is needed for physiologic sexual response as described above in both men and women. For example, a psychogenic erection requires an intact spinal cord and parasympathetic nervous system; reflex erection requires an intact spinal cord and 2nd, 3rd and 4th sacral nerve roots and uses spinal reflexes; ejaculation is a function of skeletal muscle and is controlled by the somatic center in the pudendal nerve originating from the 2nd, 3rd and 4th sacral roots; and orgasm involves contraction of both smooth and skeletal muscle.

Objectively, sexual function can be predicted to some extent according to the level of spinal cord lesion. For example, psychogenic erection is often difficult or even impossible following most spinal cord injury, but reflex erection is possible after cervical cord injuries. However, although physical limitations certainly occur, *every individual is different.* Many men report erections after having experienced spinal cord injury. (The kind of erection often matters little to the person.) Likewise, many such people (women and men) do enjoy "paraorgasm" (literally meaning *phantom orgasm*) through the development of alternative erogenous zones. Such orgasms can be very pleasurable.

The genitals are not the only body area that can be sexually excited, and intercourse is not the only means of sexual expression.

While it may be disappointing — devastating at times — for individuals to find they can no longer function in the same ways sexually as they did before an injury, they can be helped to learn new ways of giving and receiving pleasure through their bodies and the bodies of their sexual partners. Sometimes sexual and relationship counseling is needed for patients and their partners; sometimes it is not.

The important thing for a nurse to do is to facilitate the expression of feelings and concerns in a straightforward manner and to always convey hope — not the hope that previous sexual enjoyments may become possible, but rather the hope that new, real enjoyments can be found.

Some form of sexual expression is possible for, and the right of, anyone regardless of disability.

Questions concerning reproduction may arise during discussions about sexuality. Thorough physical evaluation is necessary to determine whether an individual will be able to reproduce or not. Male infertility is a frequent complication of spinal cord injury because of testicular atrophy, decreased sperm formation, and the infrequency of ejaculation. Ejaculation is possible in only a small percentage of spinal cord injured men.

Women usually remain fertile and can conceive and deliver a child. Pregnancy, labor, and delivery usually proceed normally, with few adaptations needed.

The parenting potential of disabled people is currently receiving serious attention — more so than it has in the past. Adoption is becoming a viable option and some consideration is currently being given to artificial insemination as a means of achieving conception.

Successful contraception can be a concern for disabled people. Little is known about the effects of the various kinds of contraceptives upon disabled people. Oral contraceptives may be contraindicated because of the danger of thrombosis. Paralyzed people often have a slowed circulation, which increases the circulatory dangers of oral contraceptives. Intrauterine devices (IUD) require that a woman have feeling in her pelvic area so that early signs of pelvic inflammatory disease (PID) can be detected. Many paralyzed women do not have such feeling. Barrier devices such as the diaphragm, condom, or foam can be used if at least one partner has sufficient manual dexterity to insert the diaphragm or foam or put on the condom, as well as the desire and motivation to use such devices.

Sexuality is a concern for the person with nervous system problems other than spinal cord injury, too. Table 26–3 considers in detail the effects of various disorders on female reproductive functioning, contraception methods, and sexual activity.

For further information concerning this subject, refer especially to Chipouras[52] and Shaul.[287]

PSYCHOLOGIC ADJUSTMENTS TO THE EFFECTS OF SPINAL CORD INJURY

Adjustments to paralysis are often difficult both physically and psychologically for patients and their significant others. Sudden paralysis of a previously healthy, active individual can be devastating and may produce psychologic problems for all concerned. (It *may not* pose such difficulties, however. If we assume certain problems will occur, we may, in fact, "see" psychologic conflicts that do not exist for the people involved.)

Typically, people faced with a sudden life change brought about by serious spinal cord injury experience a series of reactions similar to a *grief reaction.* This may involve initial shock and a denial of the disability. The person may become depressed (possibly deeply depressed) or angry or both. The person may need to cry, or to talk a lot about the injury and what caused it and go over and over the same things (see p. 521).

The process of adaptation may take time and requires that the person be able to accept the fact of the disability and gradually develop the ability to cope with that fact. Psychologic adjustment and recovery is, in essence, the patient's ability to accept and deal with reality.

The people who share life with the patient (significant others) may experience the same reactions and may need the same kind of help as the patient does.

A person may use some psychologic defense mechanisms while attempting to adjust to paralysis. When you are caring for such a person, try to evaluate the possible reasons for the patient's behavior. A patient's hostility, depression, anger, or withdrawal can be very upsetting personally if you fail to remember that the patient's behavior is not necessarily directed toward you.

Paralysis may cause complex changes in a person's self-concept and body image. In the acute phase, immobilization (e.g., confinement to bed in splints and casts) can contribute to sensory deprivation and its effects, e.g., hallucinations. Sensory deprivation can be minimized for example, by providing visual, auditory, and tactile stimulation as desired by the patient. It is important to make every effort to reduce the patient's boredom.

Paralyzed persons often do best initially in an environment in which there are others who face and must overcome similar problems. Patients should be dressed in their own clothing as soon as possible and encouraged to be out of bed and out of their rooms. Planned social activities can reduce feelings of social isolation and help patients regain self-confidence. Some success is being achieved by the use of "peer counseling," through which a newly disabled person can talk with someone who has adjusted to a similar disability.

A sense of security is important for everyone. It is particularly important for a newly paralyzed person to feel secure while adjusting to any necessary aspects of dependency that accompany a state of paralysis. Regular visits by an interested nurse can help create a feeling of security. A patient should always have available a means of summoning help; a paralyzed person also needs to learn that it is safe to be alone for periods of time. Gradually, newly paralyzed people learn to trust their own abilities and resources and learn to relinquish their reliance on others as much as possible. Such feelings and attitudes develop slowly. They are not things a paralyzed person can be told — they are things that are learned through experiencing the environment as truly trustworthy, including the people within it.

To avoid creating unnecessary frustrations, a sensitive nurse tries to keep each patient's environment comfortable, with all necessary items conveniently placed, e.g., telephone, call bell, television controls. It is difficult for the patient and perhaps depressing, to need to ask for help repeatedly.

While a great change has occurred in the past half century regarding the rehabilitative prognosis of paraplegic and quadriplegic people, the wise nurse assumes a *realistic* as well as optimistic viewpoint and tries to understand the tremendous change in life style that the patient is experiencing. Some people can be rehabilitated to a level of near-independence: they are able to walk (maybe with braces or other appliances), to drive a car, and to cope with full-time employment outside their home. People who are quadriplegic usually rely on a wheelchair for mobility, and with the many other devices and appliances currently available, some can become productive and happy members of society. Even if some are unable to be "productive," all disabled people have a right to a satisfying and happy life as defined by themselves.

Although some paralyzed people happily progress to achieve complete rehabilitation, many lead lives that are difficult, frustrating, and physiologically complex. Indeed, so great are the trials faced by paraplegic people that suicide frequently occurs. At times, a severe mental depression may appear as the patient realizes that paralysis and the need to be partially (or perhaps even completely) dependent are permanent. Depth of depression must be carefully and sensitively evaluated, and psychiatric help offered if indicated.

The things you can do for a disabled person and significant others are the same as the things you would do to support anyone who is experiencing stress. If you can enter into an effective therapeutic relationship with the people concerned; if you can be genuine, warm, nonjudgmental and empathetic; if you can help the people involved to feel accepted and valued and able to express their real feelings, and if you can skillfully help everyone concerned to problem-solve effectively, then you will be offering truly excellent care.

TABLE 26–3. IMPLICATIONS OF CERTAIN NEUROLOGIC DISABILITIES FOR FEMALE SEXUALITY

Female Sexuality	Reproductive Functioning	Special Considerations for Contraceptive Methods
	SPINAL CORD INJURY	
Lesions above conus medullaris: with genital stimulation there is reflex sexual response Lesions transecting conus medullaris and below: with genital stimulation there is no reflex sexual response. When both sensory and motor pathways are transected: no sensation of orgasm Other parts of body above lesion may become erogenous zones Coitus in some positions may be difficult because of hip and leg muscle spasms Increased risk of urinary and bowel incontinence during masturbation and coitus Danger of autonomic hyperreflexia in quadriplegic women during sexual arousal Increased risk of decubitus ulcers (skin breakdown) on weight bearing areas Masturbation for quad women difficult or impossible without assistance	Menstruation, fertility are unaffected Pregnancy not affected Increased incidence of bladder infection during pregnancy Increased risk of autonomic hyperreflexia during delivery and labor	BCP (birth control pills) are contraindicated when circulatory problems present: thrombophlebitis could go undetected due to lack of sensation in extremities IUD may be contraindicated because PID (pelvic inflammatory disease) and other problems could remain undetected due to lack of sensation.
	MULTIPLE SCLEROSIS	
Sex drive may decrease during periods of extreme fatigue Orgasm may be difficult because of impaired sensation Adductor spasms of hip and legs may make coitus in certain positions difficult Increased frequency of urinary incontinence during coitus and masturbation	Menstruation, fertility are unaffected Pregnancy possible, but may not be recommended because some evidence suggests that MS symptoms may be exacerbated Delivery may be complicated by hip adductor spasms	BCP may aggravate symptoms of MS (Heslinga) IUD may be contraindicated because PID and other problems could remain undetected due to lack of sensation
	POLIO	
Back and hip deformities may interfere with coitus in certain positions Sexual response cycle unaffected Flaccid paralysis and deformity of hands may make masturbation difficult to impossible Energy limitations of bulbo-spinal polio may seriously limit masturbation and coitus Iron-lung or mechanical respirator may present absolute barrier to sexual contact except for face	Fertility, menstruation are unaffected Pregnancy and delivery may be difficult for women with back deformity; for women with bulbospinal polio because of respiratory insufficiency and energy limitations Women with bulbo-spinal polio may experience respiratory problems with pregnancy and delivery because of respiratory insufficiency and energy limitations. Chronic respiratory insufficiency may compromise fetal development	BCP: poor circulation may increase the risk of thromboembolism

*The Use of Language and the Disabled Person**

The way we use language has a powerful effect on the way we view the world. It molds our attitudes to a considerable extent. The language we choose in speaking about or in speaking to people with disabilities has great implications — personally, interpersonally, and within a wider social context. Imagine, for example, that you have a spinal cord injury and you find yourself labeled a "paraplegic" or a "quad." After a time you may feel that you *are only* a paraplegic or quad — not a whole person! Consider the impact of such words as *invalid,* which literally means "not valid," or *handicapped,* which arises from the time when people with disabilities were forced to beg for a living and so had "cap in hand." It is helpful to think of disabilities as what people *have,* and handicaps as what other people *attribute to them.*

*This section was written by Margaret Helen Parkinson, R.N., M.N., in consultation with Jane Elder Bogle B.A., M.P.A.

Language Guidelines

- Avoid terms such as "handicapped," "cripple," and "invalid." "Disabled" is the best, nonjudgmental word.
- Avoid labels. Use words such as disabled, paraplegia, and quadriplegia as *adjectives* rather than nouns. For example, speak of a "disabled person"

TABLE 26–3. IMPLICATIONS OF CERTAIN NEUROLOGIC DISABILITIES FOR FEMALE SEXUALITY (*Continued*)

Female Sexuality	Reproductive Functioning	Special Considerations for Contraceptive Methods
	CVA	
Brief period of lack of interest following CVA disappearing after a few months Severe adductor spasms and internal rotation of affected leg complicate coitus in some positions Urinary incontinence possible Orgasm possible: may require more time and attention	Menstruation, fertility are unaffected Pregnancy may increase incidence of urinary incontinence	BCP absolutely contraindicated if CVA resultant from diabetes, thrombophlebitis, hypertension or heart disease IUD requires alertness to increased bleeding
	CEREBRAL PALSY	
Increased spasms and athetoid movements from stimulation and arousal Spasticity and flexion contractures of hips and knees may make coitus in certain positions painful and difficult Spasticity, deformity of arms and hands, may make masturbation difficult or impossible Genital sensation is unaffected	Menstruation, fertility are unaffected Pregnancy possible Delivery may be complicated by muscle spasms and inability of mother to bear down No data on pregnancy and delivery in severe forms of CP	
	MUSCULAR DISEASES	
Deformity of back and lower extremities may interfere with coitus in some positions Sexual response cycle unaffected No loss of sensation Masturbation may be difficult due to hand and upper extremity involvement	Menstruation, fertility, pregnancy not affected Genetic counseling essential for women who have dystrophies of genetic origin Delivery may be complicated by back and hip deformities and inability to bear down with atrophied muscles	BCP: poor circulation may increase the risk of thromboembolism
	SPINA BIFIDA APERTA	
Increased risk of urinary and bowel incontinence during sexual arousal Genital sensation may be limited or absent Deformities, weakness or paralysis may interfere with coitus in certain positions	Fertility, menstruation unaffected Pregnancy may increase urinary tract infections and incontinence Pregnancy and delivery may exacerbate back problems Genetic counseling essential Prenatal diagnosis may be indicated	BCP used with special caution if circulatory problems exist Diaphragm and IUD may be difficult to insert or fit due to pelvic deformity

Note: *Contraceptive Technology, 1976–1977* (Hatcher, Stewart et. al.) lists the following absolute contraindications to the use of oral contraceptives: (partial list) Thromboembolic disorders (or history thereof), CVA (or history thereof), impaired liver function . . . And the following Strong Relative Contraindications: (partial list) Migraine headaches, hypertension, active or postcholecystectomy, sickle cell disease . . . and Other Relative Contraindications: (partial list) Cardiac or renal disease, epilepsy and depression.

Adapted from Shaul, S., J. Bogle, J. Hale-Harbaugh, and A. D. Norman: *Toward Intimacy: Family Planning and Sexuality Concerns of Physically Disabled Women.* New York: Human Sciences Press, 1978.

or "people who have disabilities" rather than "the disabled."

- Avoid using the subculture slang that may be appropriate for disabled people to use among themselves, e.g., "para," "quad," "gimp," "crip," "supercrip." A person must really be accepted by a group before it is "OK" to use in-group terms. It would be very offensive for you to use such terms inappropriately or without the permission of disabled people themselves.

BULBAR DYSFUNCTION

Various neurologic diseases involve the lower brain stem, producing difficulties in respiration, talking, swallowing, and coughing, e.g., tetanus, myasthenia gravis, bulbar poliomyelitis.

Bulbar involvement in such conditions manifests itself by the following *symptoms:* pooling of food and saliva in pharynx and increased accumulation of secretions in the oropharynx; inability or difficulty in swallowing (dysphagia); hypoxia; hoarseness; and perhaps laryngeal stridor.

> *Accumulations of food or secretions cause airway obstruction; pulmonary aspiration, and asphyxia. Mortality is high in bulbar disorders.*

In caring for patients with bulbar dysfunction, stay alert for early evidence of hypoxia, e.g., anxiety, restlessness, apprehension, sleeplessness, increasing respiratory effort, and increasing pulse rate. The onset of hypoxia may be only subtly indicated (e.g., small, apparently insignificant requests by the patient), and early detection requires careful observation.

Indications of hypoxia in a patient with bulbar dysfunction require investigation by the nurse for possible causes of airway obstruction. Frequently, a tracheotomy is performed on patients with embarrassment of bulbar function, and mechanical ventilatory help may be necessary. (See Unit XVI.) Since many patients with bulbar problems are conscious but immobile and have difficulty speaking, the impending or progressing loss of respiratory function is terrifying to them. Diligence in observation and sensitivity in communicating with the patient help to reduce the patient's distress. Technical skills help reassure the patient that respiration will be maintained.

The nursing care of patients with bulbar involvement is similar to that previously described for patients with altered states of consciousness, in regard to observation of vital signs, deformity prevention, maintenance of airway, and maintenance of fluid balance.

The nurse may test a patient's ability to swallow before offering food or fluids. First turn the patient well over onto one side. Next, while you hold a suction catheter in one hand, give the patient a teaspoon of water with the other hand. If the patient cannot swallow the water, quickly suction it back.

A diet that eliminates milk products and many sticky carbohydrate foods is ordered in small, frequent feedings for patients with dysphagia. A calorie count may be needed to be certain of adequate caloric intake. Such a diet is often tolerated better than a puréed or full liquid diet. A small glass or cup is desirable in administering liquids because the patient may be unable to suck and swallow if a straw is used. With progressive dysphagia it may be necessary to maintain nutrition with tube feedings or a gastrostomy. (Tube feedings are discussed on p. 538.)

The extent of bulbar paralysis and the return of muscle function vary. The patient with persisting partial bulbar paralysis is particularly handi-

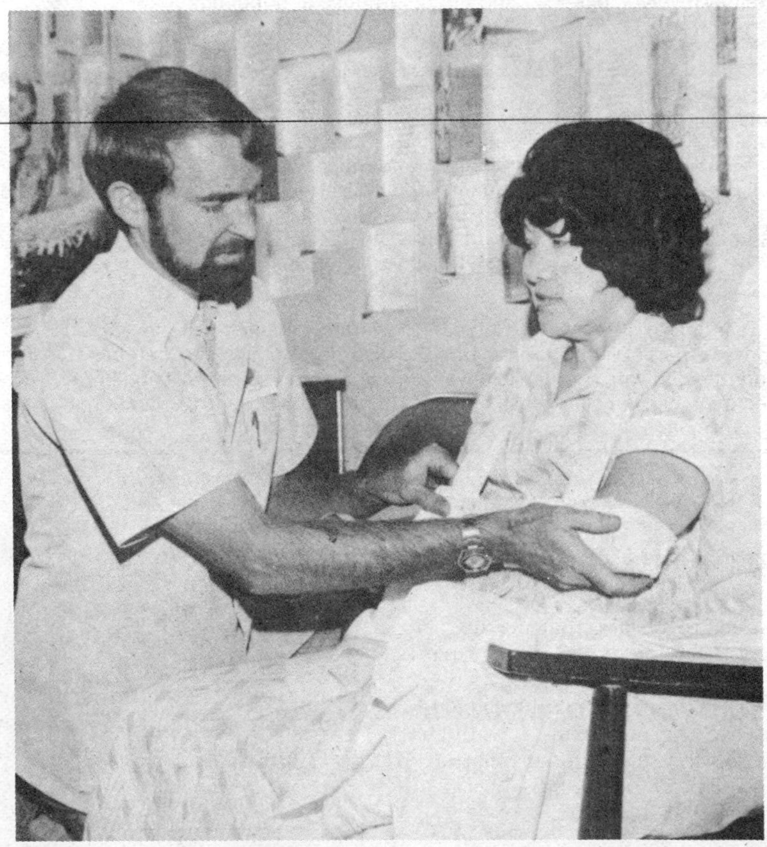

Close and personal interaction is needed to support—physically, socially, and emotionally—people experiencing neurologic problems. Note that in this instance the nurse is sitting down beside the patient so that he can work at eye level with her as well as maintain good biomechanics. (From: The stroke clinician. *Washington State Journal of Nursing*, Winter 1975.)

capped and may need to wear a permanent tracheostomy tube (which must be periodically removed and cleansed. (See Unit XXIV.) Often, expensive suction equipment is necessary in the home (and a person skilled in its use.) Eating, drinking, and common colds are all potentially hazardous.

HEMIPLEGIA

Hemiplegia is paralysis of one-half of the body. (Refer again to Fig. 26–16.) A complete hemiplegia thus involves one-half of the face and tongue and the arm and the leg of the same side.

The paralysis of hemiplegia results from destruction in the *motor area of the cortex* or the fibers in the *pyramidal tract.* A disorder, e.g., hemorrhage or clot, in the brain's right side causes a left-sided hemiplegia, and vice versa. This is because there is a crossover of nerve fibers in the pyramidal tract as they course down from the brain to the spinal cord. *Other cortical areas* may be affected also, producing additional localized symptoms, e.g., hemianesthesia, hemianopia, apraxia, agnosia, aphasia.

The muscles of the thorax and abdomen are usually not paralyzed, because they receive innervation from both cerebral hemispheres. Hemiplegia of sudden onset *typically* results from a cerebral thrombosis—the occlusion of an artery supplying a portion of one side of the brain, leading to impairment of the functions residing in that area. This is sometimes referred to as cerebral vascular accident (CVA, also called "stroke" or "apoplexy"). The specific causes of cerebral vascular disease and its immediate treatment are discussed more completely in Chapter 27.

The *clinical assessment* of a hemiplegic patient includes evaluation of motor function, reflex activity, and mental functions, e.g., perception, cognition, comprehension, communication, memory, and orientation. The patient's mental attitudes, personality pattern, and awareness of the disability are also evaluated, and the potential for recovery is estimated. It is, of course, necessary for the nurse to be aware of a patient's specific, individual defects in order to plan and give appropriate care.

Many problems associated with paralysis have been discussed in the preceding section on spinal disorders. A hemiplegic patient may have many of the same problems, e.g., spasticity, muscle spasms, rigidity, pain, tendon contractures, ankylosis of joints, muscle shortening, muscle weakness, fatigue, paralysis, impaired circulation, decubitus ulcers, absence of sensations, and psychologic adjustments to paralysis. Additionally, a person who is hemiplegic (typically, but not always, an older person) is likely to have impaired rather than absent bowel and urinary bladder functions.

As with paraplegia and quadriplegia, the rehabilitation program for patients with complicated hemiplegia is most effective when it involves a comprehensive approach supported by a variety of trained paramedical personnel. A highly optimistic morale and a high level of motivation are important for successful rehabilitation. Staff members set this tone.

Return of Function

The degree of paralysis in hemiplegia of vascular origin is usually greater, i.e., more complete, early in the illness than it will be later on. This is because edema and pressure from other sources may be impairing brain function in some areas only temporarily. False hopes are never raised, but the patient is given realistic encouragement, and every attempt is made to prevent the development of complications that will add to the patient's confinement or impede or prevent optimum recovery.

Examination of the Comatose Hemiplegic Person

In a comatose patient hemiplegia may be identified by *flaccidity of the limbs* on the paralyzed side. This is analogous to spinal shock. The unsupported paralyzed leg of the hemiplegic patient typically lies with the foot everted. The leg must be supported to keep a position of normal alignment and function. You will also notice in a hemiplegic patient that if both eyelids are lifted together, then suddenly released, the *eyelid* on the affected side may *not close completely,* or it will close more slowly than the lid on the unaffected side. Indications of *lower facial weakness* are also frequently apparent in the comatose hemiplegic patient. For example, you may observe ballooning of the cheek on the paralyzed side during expiration; weakness of the muscles around the mouth; and asymmetry or drooping of the mouth on the affected side. These lower facial weaknesses are clearly apparent from observation of the patient's facial response to painful stimuli, such as pressure over the supraorbital notch. The facial grimacing in response to the pain is asymmetrical.

Rehabilitation Potential, Goals, and Techniques

After the nurse has helped a hemiplegic patient to survive the acute phase of illness with a minimum of complications and deformities, the next challenge is of helping the patient achieve rehabilitation to a level at which life is meaningful. This challenge requires patience, ingenuity, and knowledge of the rehabilitative process. *Successful rehabilitation is not achieved without detailed planning.* All members of the rehabilitation team work together to help a patient to regain lost abilities and to gain new abilities. For the aphasic hemiplegic the special skills of a speech therapist are needed in addition to those of other specialists.

Among the *goals of a rehabilitation program* for the hemiplegic are: (1) prevention of complications during the acute phase; (2) correction of any deformities that have developed; (3) retraining of the patient to achieve maximum independence, e.g., to walk, to use the affected upper extremity to the maximum, to perform self-care activities, to be employable (if of employable age); and (4) helping the patient make the necessary psychologic and social adjustments. *Remember: rehabilitation begins with admission to the hospital!*

Although it may be difficult, hemiplegic patients do better if they are able to realize early in their illness that doing certain things for themselves is beneficial. Activity is an important part of treatment. Encouragement is frequently needed to get a patient to use the paretic limb to its maximum potential; there is a tendency to do everything with the unaffected limb.

As soon as the person can sit up in bed, hemiplegic patients are encouraged to perform all the *self-care activities* they can using the unaffected hand, e.g., brush teeth, eat, comb hair, shave, and bathe. This helps to preserve the adult pattern of independent self-care. The nurse assists as necessary but does not needlessly "rush in." A method by which a hemiplegic patient can move from bed to wheelchair independently is illustrated in Figure 26–29.

Positioning and Exercising the Hemiplegic Person. *Proper positioning, exercising, and turning of the hemiplegic patient can prevent the development of many deformities and complications.*

Frequently the hemiplegic patient prefers to lie on the involved side and may not want to turn over onto the unaffected side. However, lying on either side too long may cause skin breakdown over the external malleoli and greater trochanters. The sacral and heel areas are particularly vulnerable to breakdown if the patient lies supine (on the back) too long.

The hemiplegic patient is turned mainly onto the unaffected side. Brief positioning on the affected side (taking care that body weight is not causing harm to paralyzed extremities) or on the back is necessary to relieve pressure. The person should not be allowed to sit upright in bed for extended periods of time because this position may contribute to *hip flexion deformity.* The flat position is best. When on the side, the patient should not flex the upper thigh acutely. The patient's *position should be changed every 2 hours.*

When the patient is turned prone (as is desirable for 15 to 30 minutes several times daily), hyperextension of the hip joints may be obtained by placing a small pillow under the pelvis from the umbilicus down to the thighs' upper third.

A pillow should not be placed under the affected knee because this encourages a flexion deformity and impedes circulation. However, if there is a tendency to develop *hyperextension of the knee,* a folded towel may be placed under the knee for short periods of time while the patient is lying supine.

Place a *footboard* to prevent *footdrop and heel cord shortening* and to prevent plantar flexion caused by the weight of bed linens. The best ways to prevent footdrop are avoidance of pressure, frequent passive range-of-motion (ROM) exercises, and early sitting up with the feet flat on the floor.

A *padded posterior splint* may be applied to the affected leg at night to maintain correct positioning and prevent *flexion of the leg.*

A *trochanter roll,* extending from the crest of the ilium to mid-thigh, prevents *external rotation at the hip* by wedging under the projection of the greater trochanter and preventing the femur from rolling.

Support the affected leg when turning and positioning the hemiplegic patient. If the flaccid leg falls forward and downward when the patient is turned onto the unaffected side, a *complete dislocation of the hip joint* may occur as the head of the femur slips out of its socket. A pillow placed between the patient's legs provides adequate support.

The return of motor impulses usually begins sometime between 2 to 14 days after a stroke. When these impulses begin to return, the affected part (which was initially flaccid) becomes spastic as the spinal cord motor systems establish their autonomy. With spasticity comes the problem of contractures, although some contractures are the result of fibrosis in inactive muscles and joints. Therefore, even before spasticity sets in, passive exercises are started to prevent contractures and "frozen" joints. Passive exercises are more difficult to perform once the affected muscles begin to tighten. In exercising the extremities, do not force them beyond the point of initiating pain. Passive exercises also stimulate circulation and help to reestablish neuromuscular pathways.

Frequent ROM *passive exercises* are employed to prevent joint immobility, tendon contractures, and muscle atrophy and weakness. Once some voluntary movement returns, assisted movements are performed; the force of gravity can be eliminated during such movements by utilizing *sling-suspensions.* When the strength of movements is increased, then *resisted movements* may be used to strengthen the weakened muscle and to restore muscle bulk. ROM exercises are given q.i.d. daily for stroke patients after the first 24 hours unless otherwise ordered. No order is necessary to perform ROM passive exercises this often; it is good nursing care to do so.

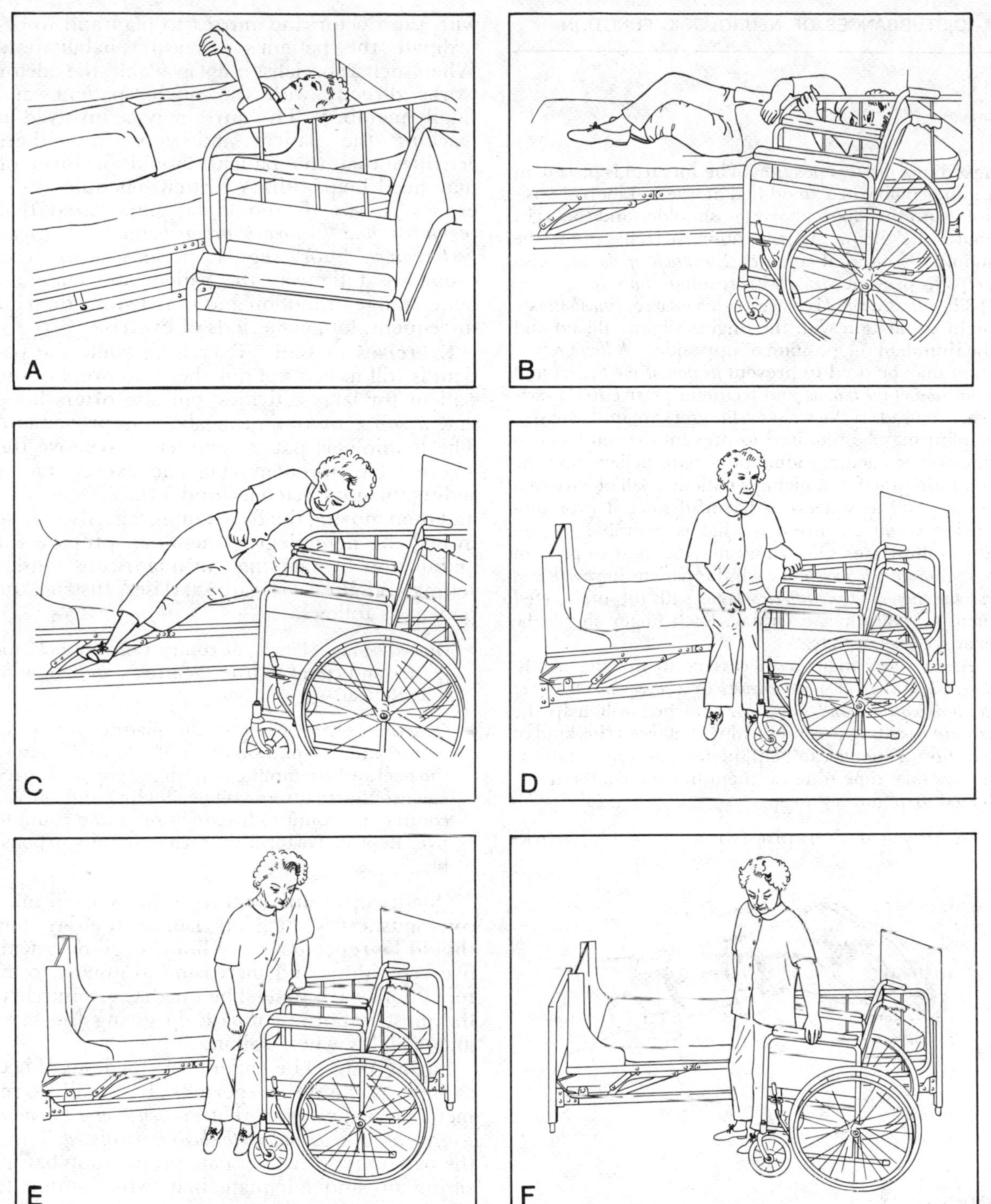

Figure 26–29. The standing (hemiplegic) transfer from bed to wheelchair. (From Krusen, F. H., F. J. Kottke, and P. M. Ellwood, Jr.: *Handbook of Physical Medicine and Rehabilitation,* 2nd ed. Philadelphia: W. B. Saunders Co., 1971.)

The *weight of the immobile arm* may cause (1) pain and limitation of movement ("frozen shoulder") owing to fibrositis of the shoulder joint, or (2) *subluxation,* i.e., incomplete dislocation, of the arm at the shoulder joint. To prevent these problems the *completely paralyzed flaccid arm must be supported in a sling when the patient is walking,* and supported on a pillow when the patient is in bed or seated in an arm chair. If a sling is used, the patient is taught to periodically take the arm from the sling (by using unaffected arm) and to then put the paralyzed arm through ROM exercises. Even while in bed the patient should exercise the affected arm by grasping it at the wrist with the unaffected hand and raising the affected arm over the head.

While in bed, *adduction of the affected shoulder* is prevented by placing a pillow in the axilla, between the upper arm and chest wall, to keep the arm in abduction at an angle of about 60 degrees. The arm is slightly flexed in a neutral position. The forearm is placed on another pillow in a "modified Statue of Liberty" position, with the elbow above the shoulder and the wrist above the elbow. This position stretches tight the shoulder's internal rotators. *Elevation of the arm* also helps to prevent *edema* with resultant *fibrosis.*

The *affected hand* is placed in a *position of function,* i.e., slight supination with the fingers slightly flexed and the thumb in the position of opposition. A *hand roll* or *splint* may be used to prevent *flexion of the fingers* and *adduction of the thumb,* and frequent passive *ROM exercises* are used. If the wrist and fingers are quite spastic, a splint may be required to prevent the tendency to flexion contracture. Some physicians believe that the common practice of giving a patient a ball of yarn or a rubber ball to squeeze is harmful since it promotes flexion when extension is what is desirable. Figure 26–30 illustrates splints that may be used to prevent *wristdrop* and *footdrop.* Teach the patient to *stretch and rub the fingers of the affected hand* with the unaffected hand several times each day. Each finger should be exercised separately.

Assist the patient as necessary in moving about. *Siderails* and an *overhead trapeze* or a *rope from the foot of the bed with a hand grasp bar* attached will help the patient in sitting up and turning if allowed this kind of exertion. Patients can help themselves considerably if nurses take time to teach them how to use the unaffected arm and leg properly.

A physical therapist (when available) works with the doctor and nurses to plan and to coordinate the patient's physical rehabilitation. When such a specialist is not available, the doctor works directly with the nurse, patient, and family members. The nurse may be involved in teaching the patient and significant others activities that the patient should perform or may need help with. A written schedule of exercises is best. It should be emphasized that *regularity and frequency are important in exercise performance.* Short regular periods of exercise cause less fatigue to the patient and maintain better range of motion and muscle tone than do infrequent, longer periods of exercise.

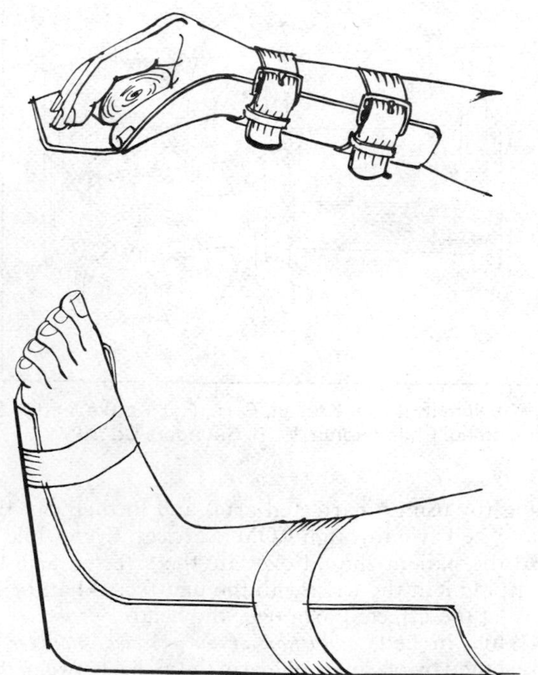

Figure 26–30. Splints used to prevent wristdrop and footdrop. (From Sutton, A.: *Bedside Nursing Techniques,* 2nd ed. Philadelphia: W. B. Saunders, 1969.)

Exercises in Bed. Exercising while the patient is still in bed not only helps to prepare the patient for later activities, but also offers hope and a sense of optimism about improvement. The hemiplegic patient can learn to move the affected leg, when moving and exercising, by sliding the unaffected leg under the affected one and then moving the functioning leg. Also, while in bed the hemiplegic patient can prepare for ambulation by carrying out quadriceps muscle setting and gluteal setting exercises. Instruct the patient as follows:

- *Gluteal setting.* "Pinch" or contract the buttocks together and count to five; then relax and count to five. Repeat.
- *Quadriceps setting.* Contract the quadriceps muscle, on the anterior portion of the thigh, while raising the heel and attempting to push the popliteal space against the mattress. While holding the muscle contracture count to five, then relax and count to five. Repeat. Perform on each extremity if possible.

Quadriceps setting exercises are started once consciousness is regained. During the day they should be repeated every hour, beginning with five repetitions and increasing gradually to 20 repetitions each time. The quadriceps muscle is the most important muscle in giving the knee joint stability when walking.

Sitting Up. The patient is helped out of bed as soon as the doctor permits. It should be remembered, however, that *the sense of balance is severely affected when half the body is paralyzed.* Thus, the patient is given adequate preparation before sitting up and adequate help while sitting to prevent a sense of insecurity.

The patient's head is *slowly* raised in bed, and time is allowed for the person to become accustomed to having the head elevated after lying flat. Often the hemiplegic patient tends to lean toward the paralyzed side and to lose balance when sitting up for the first few times. To correct this the person is taught to lean toward the uninvolved side. Initially the nurse supports a patient on the paralyzed side. The patient must also be taught how to balance the head. Back and head must be supported when the patient first sits up. Gradually the person learns to sit alone with the head of the bed elevated. The next step is to learn to sit on the edge of the bed, with feet on a firm surface. The patient can help to maintain balance by extending the affected arm and placing the hand palm down on the bed. Be patient and encouraging as the patient regains balance.

Eventually the patient learns to raise the paralyzed leg with the unaffected leg and to then swing both legs laterally over the side of the bed onto the floor. The hemiplegic patient can get up most easily by getting out of bed on the side *away* from the paralyzed side.

Wheelchair. The hemiplegic patient is taught safe techniques for transfer from bed into a chair, onto a commode, or into a wheelchair. The patient can propel a wheelchair with the unaffected arm and leg. One-arm drive wheelchairs are available for patients with unilateral paralysis. Once in a wheelchair, the patient's level of independence increases greatly.

Standing and Walking

> *In preparation for walking, the patient is helped out of bed and into a standing position as soon as possible. This helps the person to maintain a sense of balance and prevents disuse atrophy.*

In spite of weakness in the affected limb, the hemiplegic often develops an extensor reflex, i.e., reflex patterns of extension, which facilitate standing. A tilt table may be used if the patient has difficulty in achieving standing balance.

Using a wheelchair is helpful, but walking is best for the patient. As soon as the quadriceps muscle on the unaffected side has regained its normal strength, practice in standing begins. The patient may be seated at the foot of the bed and instructed to rise, using the muscle power of the unaffected leg. Balance can be maintained with the unaffected hand. There may be a tendency to swing round toward the affected side. The patient gradually learns to take an increasing amount of weight on the weaker side. Most hemiplegic patients can be taught to walk. The patient is frequently reminded to keep the weight of the body forward over the feet.

It is important that the patient practice and learn to walk correctly. If incorrect habits develop, they may be extremely difficult to overcome later. The nurse supervises carefully until the person is capable of walking alone without fear of falling. Heel-toe walking with a reciprocal gait pattern is the goal of ambulation. The patient who has been properly trained to walk should not show circumduction, scraping of the toes, or any other characteristics of the hemiplegic gait.

Bracing. Usually the decision regarding the need for *leg bracing* is deterred until after training for standing and ambulation has started. This is because the hemiplegic person frequently does not need any leg bracing for ambulation. The most commonly used *short leg brace* for a hemiplegic patient is the double-bar 90 degree ankle stop with a posterior metal calf band. An orthopedic type oxford shoe, properly fitted to the patient, is used as a basis and support for the brace.

Any patient with a brace must be taught to properly apply and remove the brace, give proper skin care, observe for skin breakdown, and properly care for the brace itself.

Safety. *Siderails* are kept up while the patient with a recent onset of hemiplegia is in bed because the person has a poor sense of balance and can easily roll out of bed. As the patient's condition improves siderails may be used to pull against when sitting up or turning. Once the patient is able to get out of bed unassisted, full siderails may hinder ambulation so at this stage half siderails may be more useful. The patient who has *impaired sensation* must take care to avoid injury and should check frequently for signs of skin lesions. *Visual disturbances* may also increase the hazards to a hemiplegic's safety.

Hemiplegic patients are more likely to *fall* than other persons. To prevent a fall patients must be taught to stand and walk slowly, rest adequately between intervals of walking, have adequate light, and watch carefully where they are going.

Feeding the Hemiplegic Person. Feeding the patient who has partial paralysis of tongue, mouth, and throat must be done carefully to prevent choking and aspiration. The patient is often fearful of choking and is frustrated by the difficulties in eating. The person feeding the patient must be unhurried and encourage the patient to persist in attempts to swallow. Unless there is some reason why the patient is not permitted to be in a sitting position, most patients swallow best sitting up. Place the food into the *unparalyzed side of the mouth.* It is often best to begin the feeding by letting the patient take some water. This tests swallowing ability and gives practice swallowing. Then food is given in small bites. Foods that can easily cause choking are best eliminated from the diet, e.g., stringy meats, unboned fish, semicooked vegetables.

The patient's nutritional status is carefully evaluated to ensure adequate nutrition. Intake is recorded, and supplemental feedings are given as indicated. If the patient is incapable of swallowing, tube feedings may be given.

It is desirable for hemiplegic people to learn to feed themselves and thus regain independence. Numerous devices are available to help (Fig. 26–31). Patient help and encouragement are required.

Food may need to be cut into bite size pieces,

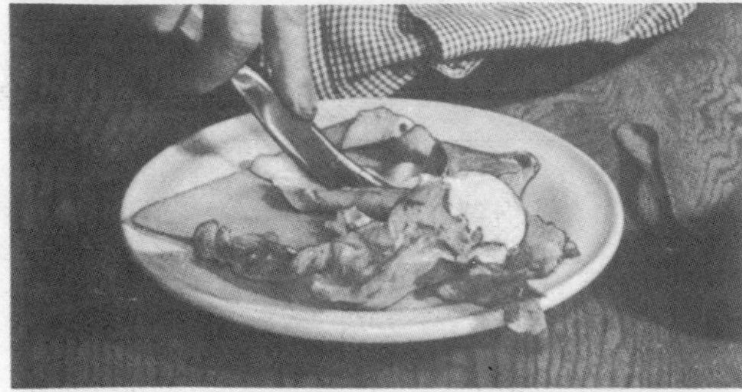

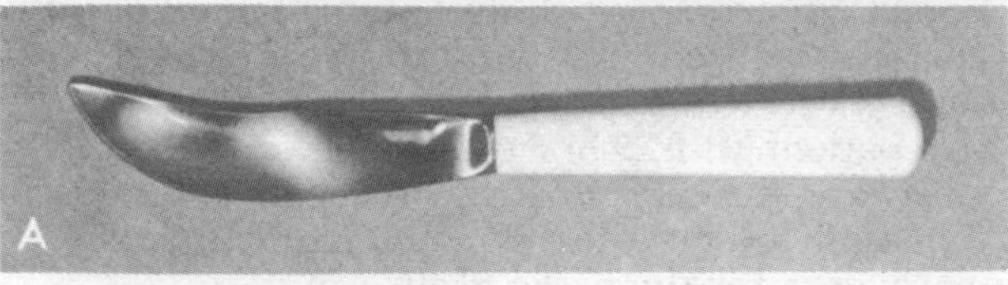

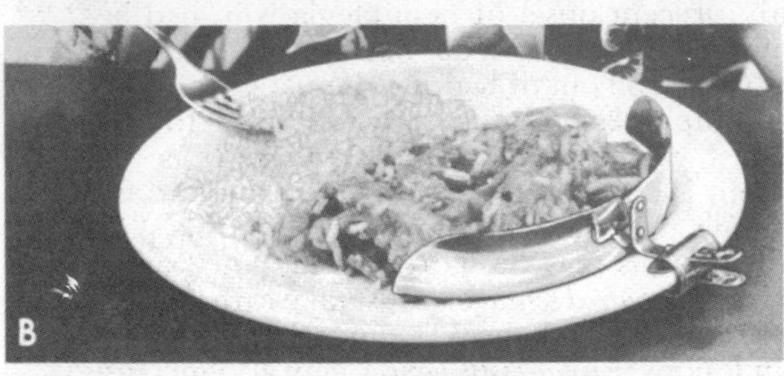

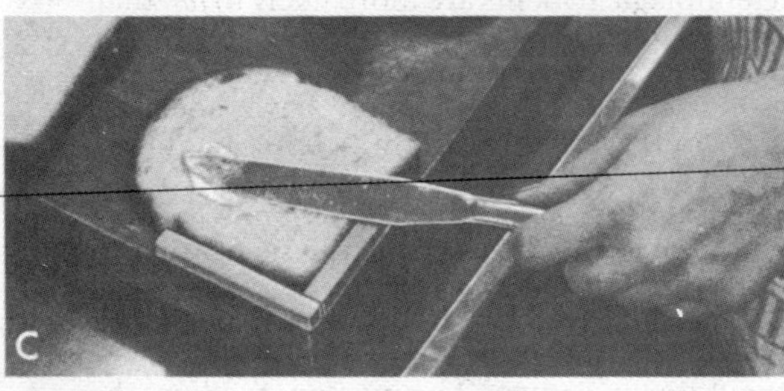

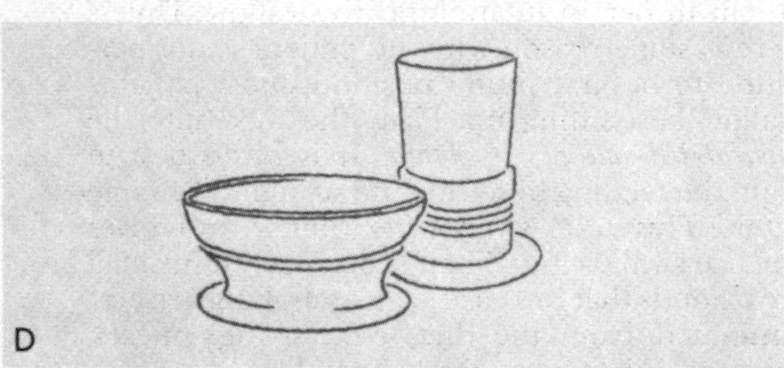

Figure 26–31. Self-help devices, making self-feeding easier for hemiplegic persons. **A.** This rocker knife enables food to be cut with one hand. The motion used is like that of a rocking chair, and the blade must be kept sharp. **B.** This "food guard" keeps food from falling off the plate, and can be easily removed for cleaning. **C.** A right-angled ledge mounted on one corner of a bread board — a simple device that can be made at home — holds the bread slice in place, enabling a person to butter the bread using only one hand. **D.** Rubber suction cups will steady dishes and glasses, making eating easier. (From Do it Yourself Again: Self-Help Devices for the Stroke Patient. New York: American Heart Association, 1969.)

but patients should be helped to feed themselves; this improves appetite and the person's self-image. Patients may need to be protected from spillage while eating, and if spills should occur a clean gown or shirt should be provided immediately. Bed linens soiled during a meal should also be changed promptly. Following the meal, the patient's face and hands are washed and oral hygiene is given; food tends to accumulate in the paralyzed side of the mouth, and this area is given special attention to make sure it is cleansed thoroughly.

Helping a dysphagic person eat is an important nursing function. The following factors can make all the difference between a happy, successful meal and a frustrating and embarrassing experience for both patient and nurse.[104]

- *Head control.* If the person has limited or no voluntary head control, a hand on the forehead may help. The patient should be facing forward rather than to the side. Remind the person to avoid throwing the head back to aid propulsion of food, as this can lead to aspiration.
- *Position.* A semi-reclining position in either bed or chair is best. Support the head to counteract hyperextension.
- *Mouth opening.* If a person cannot open his or her mouth, lightly touch both lips with the tip of a spoon. If this does not work, apply light pressure with a finger to the chin just below the lower lip. Ask the patient to open at the same time. Stroking the muscle under the chin (digastric muscle), without crossing the midline, also stimulates mouth opening.
- *Mouth closing.* Eating can be inhibited if the person cannot close the lips, as swallowing is more difficult. Lip closure may be stimulated by (a) stroking the lips with a finger or ice several times or (b) applying gentle pressure just above the upper lip with thumb or forefinger.
- *Sucking.* A person needs help to strengthen sucking if he or she cannot remove food from a spoon. This can be helped by placing a small disc at the end of a short straw and having the person drink through it. Gradually lengthen the straw and use thicker liquids.
- *Tongue movement.* Tongue movement on all planes can be improved by a number of methods: (a) Lightly touch various parts of the mouth with a tongue blade. This encourages the tongue to move to that place. (b) Icing weak tongue muscles. (c) Applying pressure to the soft tissue under the mandible helps correct tongue protrusion. (d) Walking a tongue blade from the tip of the tongue to the back will inhibit tongue thrust and also stifle the gag reflex.
- *Saliva secretion.* Ice (either plain or a Popsicle) stimulates saliva secretion.
- *Swallowing.* Concentration is needed for a dysphagic person to swallow. A quiet environment, free from distractions, is therefore helpful. Swallowing

is helped by icing the sternal notch and briskly rubbing the back of the neck near the occiput with a terrycloth washcloth.

Meal times should be pleasant and unhurried occasions. The food should be served well, at the appropriate temperature. People who are dysphagic are often afraid to eat and embarrassed about their difficulty in eating. The excellent nurse uses manual and interpersonal skills to reduce both fear and embarrassment.

Hemiplegic Deformities and Other Complications

Needless to say, all the previously described activities are more difficult (sometimes impossible) for the hemiplegic patient to perform if deformities or other complications have developed.

> *The* flexor muscles *are the body muscles that will cause hemiplegic deformities and contractures unless the patient is properly positioned and exercised.*

When control of voluntary muscles is destroyed, the strong flexor muscles overbalance the extensors. This natural tendency can cause serious deformities. For example, in the patient with hemiplegia the affected arm tends to adduct, since the adductor muscles are stronger than the abductors, and to rotate internally. The elbow, wrist, and fingers tend to flex on the affected arm. The affected leg tends to rotate externally at the hip joint, flex at the knee, and plantar flex and supinate at the ankle joint (Fig. 26–32).

> *The two most common complications associated with hemiplegia are: (1) a frozen shoulder; and (2) a shortened heel cord, with plantar flexion of the foot. Both these complications are* preventable *if proper care is given during the acute phase of paralysis.*

Incontinence. Incontinence of urine in the hemiplegic patient is not the result of brain damage following stroke unless there is extensive encephalomalacia. Research has demonstrated that there is no physiologic reason for the patient with a unilateral hemisphere lesion to be incontinent. Rather, much of the incontinence that occurs in this group of patients, or other hemiplegic patients, results from inattention, memory lapses, emotional factors, use as an attention-getting mechanism, and inability to make needs known. The patient is thus often dependent on the nurse to anticipate elimination needs, make provisions for them, and to provide a program of bowel and bladder rehabilitation.

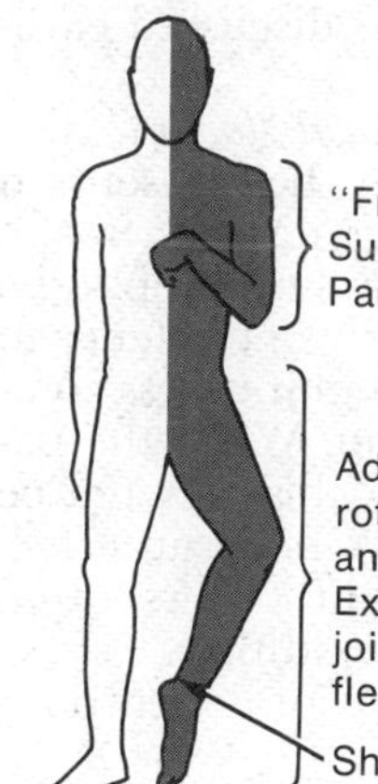

Figure 26–32. Hemiplegic deformities to be prevented. Note that the elbow is bent, the wrist is flexed and the fingers are curled into palmar flexion; the knee is bent and the heel cord shortened.

Facial Paralysis. *Paralysis* of the lower two-thirds of the face may occur with hemiplegia. There is often good return of function. However, until it does, a *facial sling* (Fig. 26–33) may be used, and massage and electrical stimulation of the facial nerve will help to retain the tonus of the facial musculature. A flacial sling on the affected side gives support to the drooping mouth and lessens drooling. Facial paralysis occurs on the same side as the hemiplegia in cerebral lesions, on the opposite side in pontine lesions. When facial paralysis is present it may be helpful at first to give liquids through a rubber tipped Asepto syringe. Special care must be

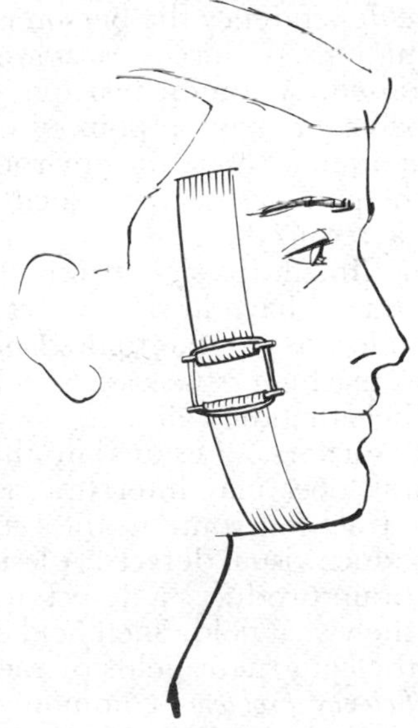

Figure 26–33. Facial sling; used with facial paralysis. (From Sutton, A.: *Bedside Nursing Techniques,* 2nd ed. Philadelphia: W. B. Saunders, 1969.)

taken in feeding the patient, as discussed earlier.

Emotional Lability. *Emotional lability,* i.e., "emotional incontinence," may be present in cerebrovascular disease. It is generally a result of bilateral disease and not a single episode. This condition is characterized by a tendency to burst into tears or burst out laughing (less commonly) without any provocation. While the patient appears highly distressed, this may not be the case. This condition differs from an affective depressed state. Significant others often need help to understand this condition.

Other emotional and behavioral reactions may occur. These include:

- Severe mood swings
- Withdrawal from others (especially in aphasic and dysphasic people)
- Inappropriate sexual behavior
- Outbursts of frustration and anger
- Regression to earlier behavior, perhaps childlike

Each of these reactions (and others) can be understood when the extent of the change and dysfunction that has occurred in the person's life is appreciated. Kindness and understanding is called for. Supportive statements are often helpful, e.g., "I am sure it is very hard for you not to be able to dress alone any more. I will try to help you in a way that makes it as easy for you as possible."

Nurses need to care for the person in such a way that the dependency the person is forced to take on is minimized. Successes (however small) must be praised. At times, disruptive or inappropriate behavior may be pointed out kindly. A nurse can often arrange the environment and anticipate the patient's needs in such a way that frustration is reduced.

It is often difficult for significant others to see their loved one behave in these ways, and they may feel at a loss as to what to do. Considerable support and teaching is necessary to help them cope with the situation well.

Visual Disorders. Lesions in the parietal and temporal lobes may interrupt visual fibers of the optic tract (en route to the occipital cortex) and produce visual defects. A lesion on one side of the brain produces a defect in the opposite half of the visual field. Such field defects are present in the congruent fields of each eye.

Visual deficiency problems commonly occur in association with hemiplegia and may prevent the patient from seeing recognizable cues. Also, visual disorders may interfere with the patient's ability to relearn motor skills and may increase susceptibility to accidents and physical hazards.

Homonymous hemianopia refers to defective vision or the loss of vision in the same half of the visual field of each eye, such that the affected patient sees only one-half of what a person with normal vision sees in any position (Fig. 26–34). The patient may see clearly on one side of the midline but nothing on the other side. The patient with homonymous hemianopia cannot see past the midline toward the side opposite the lesion without turning the head toward that side.

The hemiplegic patient who is able to ambulate needs warning to be particularly careful when crossing streets because of the danger of not seeing traffic approaching from the affected side. A patient with hemianopia is taught to position the head to increase the visual field and to help to reestablish good body image.

Depth perception and *visual perception in the horizontal and vertical planes* may also be impaired in the hemiplegic, causing problems in the patient's motor performance, both in gait and posture (Fig. 26–35). The patient may or may not be aware of any perceptual difficulty. Perceptual defects may cause the patient's behavior to appear bizarre and may increase vulnerability to accidents.

The patient with perceptual defects benefits from simplicity. A busy or noisy environment may be confusing. Clothing that is simply designed and easy to put on, directions that are simply given in a brief, concise manner, and food trays that are set with a minimum number of utensils, dishes, and foods are easiest for the patient to cope with, because decision making and complexity are thereby reduced.

Hemianesthesia; Paresthesia; Loss of Muscle-Joint Sense. The *hemianesthesia* that may accompany hemiplegia is generally incomplete. It may be unnoticed by the patient, or *paresthesia* may be experienced on the affected side. Some patients experience unpleasant sensations of numbness or heaviness. Occasionally the hemiplegic suffers with persistent, boring pain, i.e., thalamic pain. An additional problem that may accompany hemianesthesia (or may occur alone) is a *disturbance of proprioception* and *postural sense* with *loss of muscle-joint sense.* This disability may interfere seriously with the patient's ability to ambulate, because of lack of balance control and inappropriate movements. A patient with this impairment must learn to watch his or her feet very carefully while walking. The risk of falling is high because of the tendency to misplace the feet when walking.

Agnosia. Loss of muscle-joint sensation may be accompanied by *agnosia;* i.e., a disturbance in the interpretation of visual, tactile, or other sensory information in the brain. With agnosia there is a *loss of the ability to recognize objects.* Whether the patient has visual, auditory or tactile agnosia, an impairment in the transmission

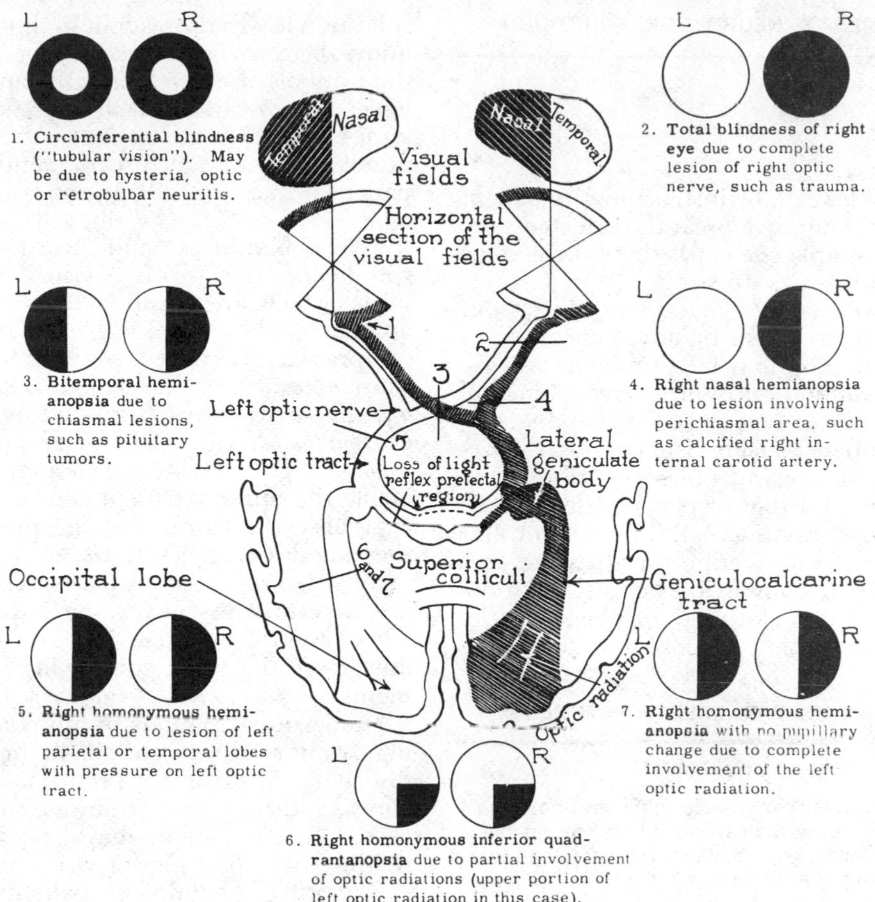

Figure 26–34. Visual field defects associated with lesions of visual system. (From Chusid, J. G., and J. J. McDonald: *Correlative Neuroanatomy and Functional Neurology,* Los Altos, Calif.: Lange Medical Publications, 1967, p. 85.)

of sensory signals to the conceptual level is occurring. *Agnosia* does not refer to deafness, blindness, or loss of touch.

As indicated, agnosias of various kinds may occur. For example, loss of muscle-joint sensation may be accompanied by *delusional beliefs about the position of a limb in space or its existence or ownership.* In such conditions a man may not feel that his arm is actually a part of his own body; he may not be aware of the position of his arm; or he may deny that a limb is paralyzed when it obviously is.

Another type of agnosia affects only one-half of external space, and objects on one side are correctly interpreted while those on the other side are ignored, e.g., a woman may be able to tell time only if it is between 12 and 6 o'clock and not if it is between 7 and 12 o'clock. A patient with this condition, of *neglecting the left half of space,* generally has left hemiplegia and may tend to avert the head and eyes to the right.

Naturally a nurse needs to be aware of these conditions and needs to plan accordingly. The patient can be helped to avoid overlooking objects or activities on the left side (if that is the affected side): eating food on the left side of the plate; grooming the left side of the head and body. Also, the patient needs protection from injury by objects close to or approaching on the left side.

When the patient neglects the affected side, the nurse can either arrange the patient's environment so that important items are on the involved side or train the patient to take care of

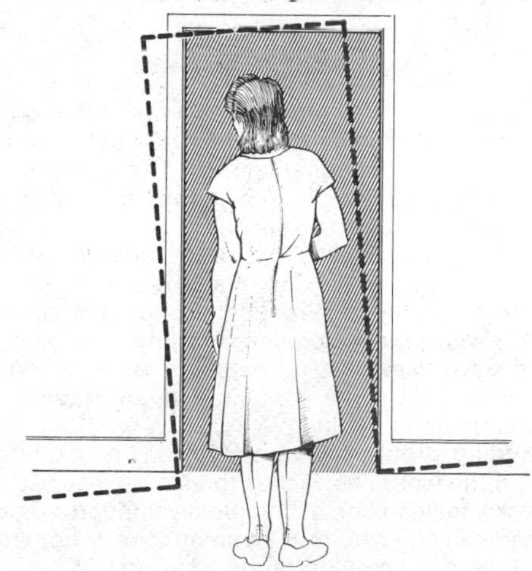

Figure 26–35. Perceptual disturbance in hemiplegia. (From Krusen, F. H., F. J. Kottke, and P. M. Ellwood, Jr.: *Handbook of Physical Medicine and Rehabilitation,* 2nd ed. Philadelphia: W. B. Saunders Co., 1971.)

the affected side, e.g., by instructing the patient to turn and frequently look at the affected side, and to follow simple cue cards that list the steps of such procedures as dressing.

A patient with *visual agnosia* sees objects but does not recognize them or attach meaning to them. Disorientation may be a problem because the person cannot recognize environmental cues or may fail to recognize familiar faces or symbols. The patient with visual agnosia is frequently seen picking up objects, curiously examining them, and then replacing them — still puzzled about their function. The patient may need assistance with eating or dressing and other activities of daily living because such objects as silverware, clothing, or toilet articles seem strange and their purpose unknown. This condition leaves the patient highly vulnerable to injury, because of failure to recognize danger or the symbols used to warn of danger. *Extensive visual agnosia* can result in such extreme behavioral effects that the patient is frequently diagnosed as having diffuse dementia. In such a patient an accurate diagnosis is difficult to establish.

"Word blindness" and "word deafness" are specific localized forms of visual or auditory agnosia, which are mentioned in the section on aphasia.

Apraxia. Localized brain injury may also cause *apraxia;* i.e., the patient is *able to move the affected part* (it is *not* paralyzed or uncoordinated), *but the part cannot be used for specific purposeful actions,* e.g., walking, speaking, or dressing. While the apraxic patient can conceive or conceptualize the content of the message to send the muscles (e.g., "stand"), it is impossible to reconstruct those motor patterns or schema that are necessary to convey the impulse message. Thus, accurate "instructions" do not reach the limb from the brain concerning specific movements.

Numerous variations of apraxia occur, ranging from relatively simple to highly complex disorders. Apraxia may occur in any or all modalities, and may vary from one modality to another; e.g., a patient may have less difficulty writing than speaking, or vice versa.

Generally in hemiplegic patients, apraxic and agnosic states occur along with other clinical signs and such people have a poor prognosis for functional recovery. The disorders of cortical function, which we have been discussing, make rehabilitation difficult unless spontaneous recovery of the affected cortical functions returns.

SOME TERMS USED IN SPEECH PATHOLOGY

Types of aphasia*

Receptive. The patient experiences difficulty *understanding* the spoken or written word. He may be unable to comprehend gestures. His ability to understand number relationships and time concepts is frequently affected.

Expressive. The patient has difficulty *communicating* through spoken words, gestures, or writing. His difficulty is with symbols and their meanings, not with the muscles of speech.

Jargon. The patient speaks recognizable words with inflection and meaning, but the words are linked in meaningless fashion. He may appear unaware that he is not communicating sensibly. Some brief indications of meaning appear occasionally, but they are lost again in a flow of nonsense.

Global. The patient neither understands nor communicates in any fashion due to severe, generalized brain dysfunction.

Concomitant problems

Apraxia. Difficulty imitating oral movements required in speaking, and problems with motor planning (initiating movements in accurate fashion). This problem may exist independently of or in addition to disability in moving the muscles of speech.

Dysarthria. Physical weakness of the muscles of the lips, tongue, velum, pharynx, and larynx, ranging from mild paresis to paralysis. Frequently encountered in connection with swallowing and drooling problems.

Graphic performance. The patient's ability to copy another's writing, write to dictation, or spontaneously communicate in writing.

Word-finding problem. The patient has difficulty calling to mind the words he wishes to use. He may use a similar word instead, or a completely inappropriate one. Occasionally he can think of an unusual synonym more readily than a simple, often-used word.

*Four of the more common types. *Dorland's Illustrated Medical Dictionary* lists some 50 classifications.

From Behringer, S. M.: Speech pathologist's view: How the nurse can help. RN, 37:43, Mar. 1974.

LANGUAGE DISORDERS

Many neurologic patients may have language disorders of various kinds that may be related to their neurologic disorders. The nurse assists with the identification and evaluation of these language disorders as well as with language rehabilitation.

Many hospitals today have available a *speech doctor* and/or speech therapist. A nurse may work with a patient who has a language disorder under the direction of these speech specialists, or with a physician. In some areas speech therapy consultation can be arranged by contacting a voluntary or governmental service agency.

A nurse can help patients with speech disorders in a variety of ways, depending on the specific problem. When a patient is not speaking loudly enough, the nurse can suggest stopping and taking a deeper breath; this will enable the person to use more energy when speaking. If the quality of a patient's speech is too nasal, the nurse can help correct this by having the patient open the mouth wider while speaking; this allows more sounds to come through the mouth instead of being diverted through the nose. A patient who speaks too rapidly can be reminded to slow the speech pattern down.

Aphasia

Definition of the Problem. Aphasia is a defect in the utilization and interpretation of the symbols of language, caused by a disorder of the cerebral cortex. The defect is a symptom complex that may involve any or all aspects of the use of language, e.g., speaking, reading, writing, and understanding spoken language. It is estimated that there are over one million aphasic persons in the United States.

Types of Aphasia and Speech Patterns. An aphasia may be of a *sensory* nature (receptive aphasia), which affects the comprehension of speech, or it may be of a *motor* nature (expressive aphasia or executive aphasia), which affects the production of speech.

Sensory aphasias involve loss of the ability to comprehend written (or printed) or spoken words. For example, with *auditory* or *acoustic aphasia* ("word deafness") patients have difficulty understanding what is being said. They are not deaf; they hear sounds which fail to make sense because they cannot understand the symbolic communication associated with the sounds. *Visual aphasia* ("word blindness") is similar, except that patients cannot read words even though they can see them. They have lost the ability to understand the symbolic content of the printed or written figures.

Motor aphasias encompass any of the varieties of aphasia in which the power of expression by writing, making signs, or speaking is lost. For example, with motor aphasia a patient may find that even though words can be recalled the ability to combine speech sounds into words and syllables is lost.

Pure motor or pure sensory aphasias rarely occur. Thus, the most common aphasias are of a *mixed* nature (expressive-receptive aphasia) in which both expressive and receptive elements are affected. Also, most aphasias are partial rather than complete. *Global aphasia* (total aphasia) is of such a degree that neither expressive nor receptive language abilities are retained.

Causes. The pathology of aphasia depends more on the lesion's location than its histologic abnormality, since a wide variety of pathologic lesions can cause aphasia. However, *the most common cause of aphasia is vascular disease of the brain. The middle cerebral artery is the most common major vessel to be associated with aphasia.* Aphasia may result when circulation to the patient's speech center is cut off. It is associated with hemiplegia involving the patient's dominant hemisphere, and within that area a lesion involving the posterior aspect of the inferior frontal gyrus. The speech center for a right-handed person is located in the left cerebral hemisphere, while the speech center for a left-handed person may lie on the right side of the brain. Thus, a right-handed person with a right-sided hemiplegia may have aphasia, since the speech center is in the affected left hemisphere.

Severity of Aphasia. The severity of aphasia varies with the area and the extent of cerebral damage (Fig. 26–36). Severe damage may deprive the patient of any meaningful relationship with the environment.

Communication involves the dual processes of sending and receiving language. While either dimension can be equally affected, the more common pattern, following initial recovery, is for the expressive defect to be greater than the receptive.

Occasionally the residual brain function is not adequate for the aphasic person to relearn the complicated processes of communication. Many

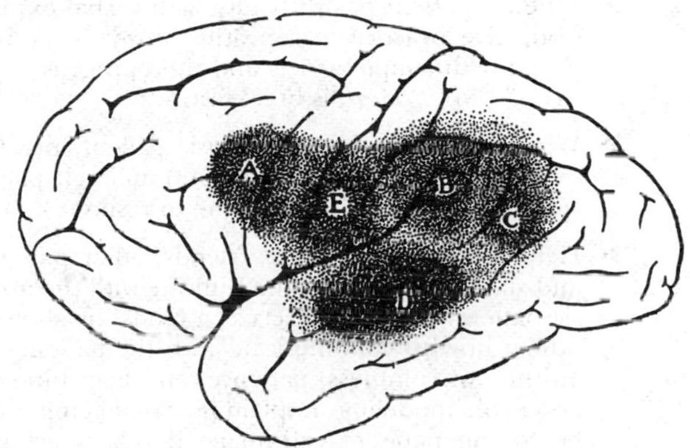

Figure 26–36. The "Aphasic Zone" of the left cerebral hemisphere (after Bailey). Area A includes the posterior portion of the middle and inferior frontal convolutions and the lower end of the precentral gyrus. Involvement of it leads to anarthria. This is primarily a motor or expressive defect. However, it is often associated with an alexia, as well as a contralateral facial weakness. Area B includes the supramarginal gyrus. A lesion here results in a severe generalized aphasia. It may be associated with a hemianesthesia and a hemianopsia. Area C includes the angular gyrus. Its destruction results in an aphasia with a disturbance in reading as the outstanding manifestation. There may be an inferior homonymous quadrantic defect in the visual fields, a hemiplegia and hemianesthesia. When area D in the posterior part of the superior and middle temporal gyri is involved the aphasia is principally a comprehensive or sensory one. There may also be *a paraphasia* (the misuse of words, or loss of the ability to formulate words into language), *jargon aphasia* (the use of unintelligible sounds and syllables), and *perseveration* (the repetition of the same sounds or words). There is commonly a hemianopsia or an inferior quadrantanopsia. Area E includes the island of Reil. A deep-seated lesion here produces a severe aphasia, anarthria, and a right hemiplegia. (From Vick, N. A.: *Grinker's Neurology,* 7th ed. Springfield, Ill.: Charles C Thomas, 1976, p. 375.)

aphasic persons do well with speech therapy or show a tendency to spontaneous recovery. Because it cannot be assumed that spontaneous recovery will occur, speech therapy should ideally be started early. However, some benefit from speech therapy may be derived even 2 or more years following the origin of the speech disorder.

Clinical Care. A nurse can frequently continue and reinforce lessons that the speech therapist has initiated. In the absence of a therapist, a nurse may conduct language rehabilitation sessions with the physician's approval. During such sessions the nurse takes care not to fatigue the patient and to remember that the patient may have a short attention span. *Every encounter* with a patient can be used to encourage and support communication.

The following ideas may be useful in taking care of an aphasic patient:

- ▶ When a patient cannot understand the spoken word, repeat simple directions until they are understood, e.g., "Drink this juice." Also use nonverbal techniques of communication.
- ▶ When a patient cannot identify objects by name, give practice in receiving word images. For example, point to an object and clearly enunciate its name, e.g., "hand," "glass."
- ▶ When a patient has difficulty with verbal expression, give practice in repeating words after you. Begin with simple words and then progress, e.g., "Yes," "No," "Here is breakfast."
- ▶ When working with the aphasic patient, practice expanded speech (a slower rate) and self-pacing (permitting the individual time to respond).
- ▶ Help the patient's family, friends, other patients, and staff members to communicate with the aphasic patient. The nurse acts as a model by showing others how to communicate with the patient. An attitude of calmness, patience, and helpfulness is good role modeling. Explain how damaging it can be to the patient's self-image if others act embarassed or amused by his or her attempts to communicate.
- ▶ Listen and watch carefully when the aphasic patient attempts to communicate and try especially hard to understand. This reduces the patient's frustration.
- ▶ Anticipate the aphasic patient's need to reduce feelings of helplessness because of the communication handicap.
- ▶ Gradually shift topics of conversation when talking to the patient who has receptive difficulty. It may be necessary to tell the patient that you are going to change the topic.
- ▶ Sometimes it is helpful, when talking to an aphasic patient who has receptive difficulty, to be within 6 feet or less of the patient and to face the person directly.
- ▶ If the patient has *word deafness,* give simple directions. Repeat directions until they are understood.
- ▶ If the patient has *naming aphasia,* encourage practice in naming objects frequently used. This gives practice in recalling word images.
- ▶ If the patient has *motor aphasia,* encourage practice in trying to repeat words and sounds after you.

Initial care involves trying to put aphasic patients at ease and reduce the feelings of panic that may occur when they first realize that they cannot communicate as well as they did formerly. It is important for the nurse to speak slowly and clearly and to offer calm reassurance. The fact that the nurse understands the problem will help.

An excellent nurse shows patients the call bell and has them practice using it. Tell such patients that they will be watched closely and that they can indicate their needs by use of sign language. It is important to talk to aphasic patients without exerting pressure for verbal response. When an individual patient appears ready, a nurse may introduce picture or word cards or picture books to temporarily facilitate communication.

Aphasic patients often express their emotional state by irritability and periods of "moodiness." Often these frustrated people are anxious, bewildered, and depressed. Emotional lability may be an additional result of cerebral damage. Such behavior is accepted matter-of-factly but kindly and without embarrassment. Every attempt is made to reduce the patient's frustrations and to teach effective communication patterns.

Dysarthria

Dysarthria (anarthria) is a difficulty in speaking that *results from imperfect articulation.* It is important to differentiate between dysarthric and aphasic speech. With dysarthria the patient understands and comprehends language but has difficulty pronouncing words and may slur them, enunciating poorly. No disturbance occurs with grammar or in the construction of a phrase or sentence. The dysarthric patient can understand verbal speech, can read, and can write (unless the writing hand is paralyzed, absent, or injured).

Dysarthria may result from a weakness or paralysis of the muscles of the lips, tongue, and larynx or a loss of sensation. In addition to speaking problems, patients with dysarthria often have difficulty chewing and swallowing food because of lack of muscle control.

Generally the *evaluation* of dysarthria includes: examination of the peripheral speech mechanism, tests for specific speech skills, otolaryngologic consultation, and assessment of the patient's functional ability based on the clarity of speech in conversation. *Speech therapy* is of benefit to many dysarthric patients.

CHAPTER 27

SPECIFIC NEUROLOGIC DISORDERS

This chapter focuses on specific neurologic disorders. Major topics are infections, tumors, vascular lesions, developmental defects, degenerative disease, demyelinating diseases, paroxysmal disorders, trauma, and diseases of the cranial and peripheral nerves. Because the major areas of clinical care of neurologic patients have been discussed in Chapter 26, only details of care that are highly specific to a given disorder are presented. The personal, psychosocial impact of neurologic disorders on patients and their significant others is discussed in Chapter 26, specifically in terms of reaction to crises (p. 521), in relation to sexuality (p. 574), and in relation to the disabled person (p. 576). The need for understanding and supportive nursing care applies also to person's experiencing the neurologic disorders discussed in this chapter.

As you study this chapter, you may find that your understanding of specific neurologic disorders and the care needed in individual situations is enhanced by referring frequently to other sections of this book. The following areas may be especially helpful:

Diagnostic neurologic examinations	Chapter 25
Review of neuroanatomy and physiology	Chapter 24
Neurosurgery	Chapter 28
Care of persons undergoing surgery	Unit VIII
Care of persons with neoplastic disorders	Unit IX
Care of persons experiencing pain	Unit XI
Emergency care	Chapter 95

INFECTIONS OF THE NERVOUS SYSTEM

Classification of Infections of the Nervous System

A. Bacterial or pyogenic infections
  1. Bacterial meningitis
  2. Brain abscess
  3. Other bacterial infections

B. Viral infections
  1. Viral meningitis
  2. Viral encephalitis
    a. Arbovirus encephalitides
    b. Herpes simplex virus encephalitis
    c. Acute anterior poliomyelitis (polio)
    d. Herpes zoster (shingles, zona)

C. Other infections
  1. Fungal infections
  2. Neurosyphilis
  3. Disorders due to bacterial toxins
    a. Tetanus
    b. Diphtheria
    c. Botulism

Practically all the pathogenic microorganisms may invade the parenchyma, coverings, and blood vessels of the nervous system. In order to clarify discussion, the various infectious syndromes are sometimes divided according to the main area of involvement, e.g., infections of the meninges, subdural and epidural infections, and so forth. For this discussion, infections are divided into three major categories: (1) bacterial or pyogenic infections, (2) viral infections, and (3) other infections. Before discussing specific infections, let us first briefly review appropriate general care.

General Care in Infections

The treatment and clinical care of patients with infections that affect the nervous system consist basically of : (1) administering antibiotics that are specific for the causative organism; (2) treating increased intracranial pressure and/or hyperthermia if they occur; (3) protecting the delirious patient (see Chapter 26); (4) providing symptomatic care, e.g., keeping linens dry if the patient is perspiring excessively, keeping the room quiet and darkened if the patient has a headache or is photophobic; offering oral hygiene if emesis occurs, handling the patient gently and unhurriedly if nausea occurs or if the patient's skin and muscles are unusually sensitive, placing a cool cloth over the patient's forehead and eyes if desired; (5) maintaining fluid-electrolyte balance; (6) enforcing isolation as necessary; (7) preventing complications of bed rest; and (8) making frequent observations of the patient, because rapid worsening of the condition may occur. Observations include looking for symptoms of meningeal irritation, increased intracranial pressure, changes in level of consciousness, and hyperthermia. Systematic "neuro checks" (see p. 524) are frequently part of the observation process when providing acute care. The nurse makes detailed notes concerning how patients appear and how they say they are feeling.

Bacterial or Pyogenic Infections

In bacterial infections the invading organism may reach the central nervous system in one of two major ways: (1) via the *vascular system,* following a systemic or blood stream infection, or (2) by *direct extension* from an adjacent cranial structure.

For example, pathogenic microorganisms may accidentally be introduced to the CNS during a lumbar puncture, or they may enter the subarachnoid space through a compound skull fracture or fractures through the mastoid or nasal sinuses. Organisms may also invade the meninges by the direct extension of an infected area in the skull, spine, or parenchyma of the nervous system. Similarly, pathogenic microorganisms may metastasize from infections of the viscera (e.g., heart, lung), or they may migrate through the blood stream.

Major categories of discussion below are bacterial meningitis, brain abscess, and other bacterial infections.

BACTERIAL MENINGITIS*

This condition involves essentially the arachnoid, the pia, and the subarachnoid space. It is frequently referred to as *leptomeningitis.* Since the subarachnoid space is continuous around the brain and spinal cord, *bacterial meningitis is always cerebral and spinal.*

When a pathogenic organism gains access to the subarachnoid space, an inflammatory reaction begins, resulting in clouding of the CSF, formation of an exudate, changes in the subarachnoid arteries, and congestion of adjacent tissues. The pia-arachnoid becomes thickened and adhesions form, especially in the area of the basal cisterns. In the early stages of meningitis, very little change in the substance of the brain itself is evident.

Almost any bacteria gaining entrance to the body can cause meningitis, but the most common are the meningococcus (*Neisseria meningitidis*), the pneumococcus (*Diplococcus pneumoniae*), and *Hemophilus influenzae*. All three are commonly found in the nasopharynx, but the mechanism by which they gain access to the bloodstream and then to the subarachnoid space is still unknown.

Bacterial meningitis is found worldwide, in all seasons of the year, and in all ages. *Hemophilus influenzae* meningitis is encountered almost exclusively in children; meningococcal meningitis occurs in children, adolescents, and adults; and pneumococcal meningitis occurs in the very young and in adults over 40 years of age. Males are affected slightly more often than females.

The *onset of meningitis* is typically manifested by headache, prostration, nausea and vomiting, back pain, stiff neck, and chills and fever. Although the patient is usually irritable at the onset of the illness, as the infection progresses the sensorium often becomes gradually clouded, and stupor or coma may develop. Generally persons with meningitis appear acutely ill and confused, stuporous or semicomatose. Focal neurologic signs rarely occur; however, generalized convulsive seizures are often an early symptom and frequently are seen. A petechial or hemorrhagic rash often accompanies meningococcal infection. The patient appears acutely ill. Temperature is elevated moderately, and pulse and respiratory rate are increased. Blood pressure is usually normal.

> *Persons with meningitis typically demonstrate the following classic* signs of meningeal irritation: nuchal rigidity *(rigidity of the neck);* positive Kernig's sign *(inability to straighten knee when hip is flexed); and* positive Brudzinski's sign *(flexion at the hip and knee in response to forward flexion of the neck).*

The Kernig and Brudzinski signs are elicited in the following manner:

Brudzinski's sign. The patient's chest is held down as the head is rapidly elevated from the bed. In meningeal irritation such passive flexion of the neck produces flexion of both thighs at the hips, as well as flexure movements of the ankle and knee (Fig. 27–1).

Kernig's sign. The patient is recumbent and the thigh is flexed to a right angle, i.e., toward the abdomen, keeping the knee flexed at a 90 degree angle to the thigh. Extension of the leg upward then causes spasm of the hamstring muscles, resistance to additional extension of the leg at the knee, and pain.

Diagnosis and therapy of bacterial meningitis depend upon isolating and identifying the *specific* microorganism and determining the source of the infection.

*Viral meningitis is discussed on p. 597.

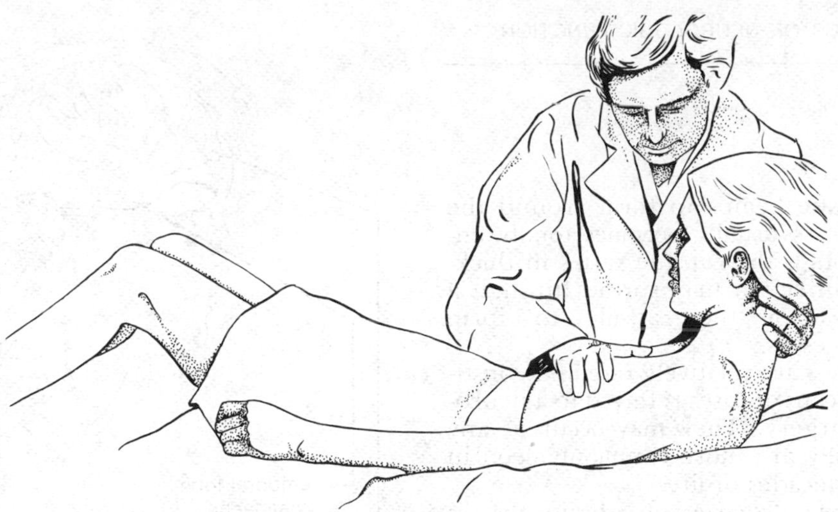

Figure 27–1. Brudzinski's sign.

Diagnosis is usually made on the basis of the clinical signs and symptoms but is definitely confirmed only by isolating the organism from the CSF. Speed is essential in diagnosing and treating bacterial meningitis. A lumbar puncture is an essential part of the work-up. Cultures are promptly done on CSF and blood. Patients with bacterial pneumomeningitis show the following: CSF pressure is elevated, protein is elevated, glucose is decreased, and the cell count is markedly increased with predominantly polymorphonuclear leukocytes.

> *Bacterial meningitis must be treated as a medical emergency.*

Therapy for bacterial meningitis is mainly concerned with early administration of large doses of the appropriate antibiotic, given four to six times daily over a 10-day period. Other treatment is symptomatic. Maintenance of adequate fluid and electrolyte balance is important. Frequent assessment of neurologic status is essential to detect early signs of increasing intracranial pressure, so that treatment can begin promptly. Seizures are treated with anticonvulsants. An effort is made to identify the primary focus of infection; it is then eradicated surgically if necessary.

Nursing care of the patient with meningitis focuses on the measures mentioned earlier in this section, in addition to the general care of the comatose and debilitated patient, discussed in Chapter 26.

Antibiotics have been highly successful in reducing the mortality rate of all forms of bacterial meningitis. Complications and sequelae of meningeal infection rarely occur with modern treatment, and those complications caused by involvement of other parts of the body by meningococci or other intercurrent infections are more easily controlled than in the past.

The *prognosis* in cases of bacterial meningitis varies according to the specific causative organism. In general, the mortality rate is less than 5 percent; it is highest in the newborn infant and the elderly patient.

Common *complications* of bacterial meningitis are septic shock, vasomotor collapse, hydrocephalus, and persisting convulsive seizures. With meningococcal meningitis, residual neurologic deficits are rare. Such deficits are seen more frequently with *Hemophilus influenzae* meningitis and in almost one-third of patients with pneumococcal meningitis.

BRAIN ABSCESS

A brain abscess is a collection of encapsulated or free pus within the substance of the brain tissue, usually following an acute purulent infection elsewhere in the body.

The primary source of infection is usually the ear and mastoid sinuses or the nasal sinuses, with the brain abscess arising from direct extension of such infection. A smaller percentage of cases follow open head injury or intracranial surgery. Even less frequently, abscesses are due to metastasis from suppurative processes elsewhere in the body, especially the lungs. Subacute bacterial endocarditis seldom gives rise to brain abscess, though the more fulminant acute bacterial endocarditis frequently causes many small abscesses. The *most common organisms* causing brain abscess are *streptococci and staphylococci.* Abscesses vary in size, from an area of purulent necrosis involving the major part of one hemisphere of the brain, down to lesions of microscopic size.

In its early stages, an abscess is characterized by inflammation, necrotic tissue, and surrounding edema. Within several days, the center of the abscess begins to look like pus and a wall of granulation tissue begins to form around the edge. The abscess usually becomes totally encapsulated, though the capsule varies in thickness, and the infection may spread through a weakened area of the capsule to form "daughter" abscesses.

Brain abscesses are relatively rare and constitute only 2 per cent of cases referred to a neurosurgeon for surgery. They may occur at any age, though they are more commonly seen in the first three decades of life.

The *clinical manifestations* of a brain abscess are essentially the same as those of any space-occupying lesion of the brain. Headache is the most frequent early symptom. Symptoms of infection (e.g., fever, chills) are usually not present. Other early symptoms may include drowsiness and confusion or some transient focal neurologic disorder. These early signs may improve or subside. Within a few days or weeks, signs of increasing intracranial pressure develop, e.g., recurrent headaches, changes in level of consciousness, and focal or generalized seizures (Fig. 27–2).

Specific neurologic signs develop according to the *location of the abscess:*

Temporal lobe abscesses may present with headache, aphasia (if in dominant hemisphere), and visual field deficits.

In *frontal lobe* abscesses, headache, drowsiness, and general impairment of mental function are prominent. However, the most frequent neurologic signs are hemiparesis, focal motor seizures, and motor dysphasia.

Parietal lobe abscesses will present with any of a variety of focal sensory abnormalities.

An abscess of the *occipital lobe* usually presents with homonymous hemianopia.

In *cerebellar* abscesses, the headache is posterior, and other manifestations include nystagmus, cerebellar ataxia, and early presentation of signs of increased intracranial pressure.

Brain stem abscesses are rare and are usually found only at autopsy.

Diagnosis of brain abscess is easily made when seizures, focal neurologic signs, and increased intracranial pressure develop in a patient with an infection in one of the usual contributing areas. The diagnosis may be confirmed by a CT scan. In the absence of any obvious focus of infection, the diagnostic work-up is the same as that for any space-occupying lesion, including skull x-rays, EEG, and CT scan. Cerebral angiography may be ordered; however, with the advent of the CT scan, the angiography will probably not be necessary. When an abscess has been diagnosed, the work-up should extend to include a search for the focus of infection.

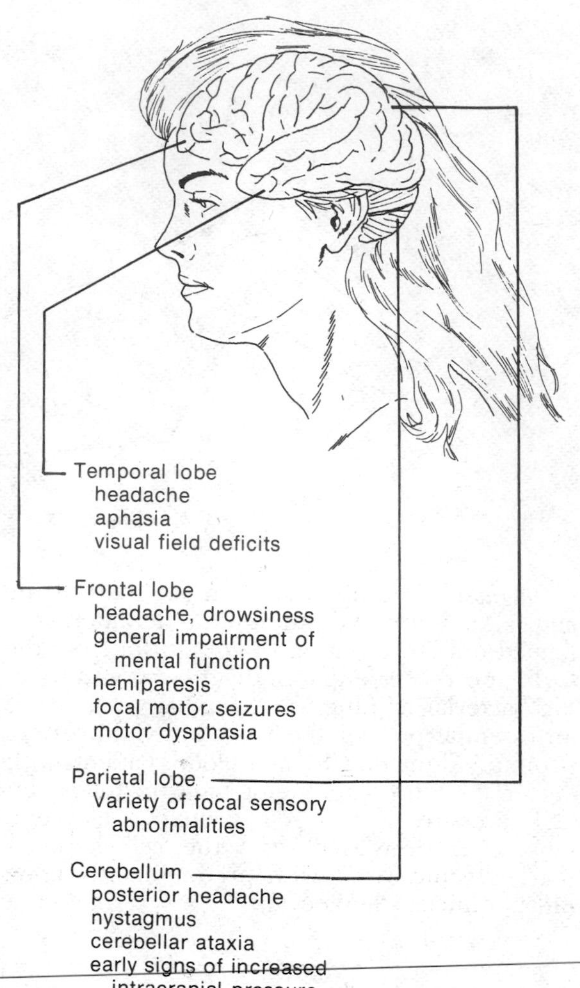

Figure 27–2. General focal findings of brain abscess in various locations.

The only successful form of *treatment* for a brain abscess is *surgical.* Surgery is not attempted early in the abscess formation unless increasing intracranial pressure and the threat of herniation make some surgical intervention necessary. Early surgery accomplishes little and could disseminate the infection. It should be delayed until the abscess is firmly encapsulated. Occasionally a needle aspiration of the suspected abscess is done for diagnostic purposes.

The ideal treatment is total removal of the abscess within its capsule, but this is not always possible. Alternate methods include aspiration of the abscess, followed by repeated injections of antimicrobial agents (used particularly if the abscess is deep within the brain substance) and packing of the cavity. All surgical procedures should be combined with administration of large doses of antibiotics, both pre- and postoperatively.

Untreated brain abscesses are almost invariably

fatal. With surgical treatment, mortality is between 20 and 75 per cent. Neurologic residua occur in about 30 per cent of patients who survive, with focal seizures being the most frequent and refractory to treatment. (Epilepsy is discussed on p. 640.) The patient with a brain abscess may expect a long and frustrating course.

OTHER BACTERIAL INFECTIONS

Other bacterial infections, which are seen less frequently, are mentioned briefly below:

- *Subdural empyema* — suppurative process in the cranial subdural space
- *Epidural abscess* — usually associated with osteomyelitis of the cranial bones
- *Spinal epidural abscess*
- *Thrombophlebitis* (or infective thrombosis) *of the large dural sinuses,* especially the lateral sinus, cavernous sinus, and superior sagittal sinus

Viral Infections

Viral infections of the nervous system, with few exceptions, are complications of generalized systemic viral infections. However, the neurologic aspect of the infection tends to be clinically more devastating than the systemic illness.

Viruses can enter the body by various pathways. The most common viruses enter via the respiratory system. Others enter via the oral route, the genital route, or via inoculation by an insect or animal bite. Once in the body, they multiply and cause a viremia. They may then invade the central nervous system via cerebral capillaries and choroid plexus or along peripheral nerves. Once inside the CNS, various viruses appear to have an affinity for specific cell types.

Rabies, potentially the most dangerous viral infection of the nervous system, is rarely seen. Of the various clinical syndromes associated with known viral infections, we discuss only those most commonly seen — a representative group. These are: viral "aseptic" meningitis, viral encephalitis, acute anterior poliomyelitis, and herpes zoster. (Some diseases of the nervous system the etiologies of which are unknown at present may eventually prove to be caused by viruses.)

While *immunization procedures* are available for rabies, poliomyelitis and some of the encephalitides, they are not available against most of the viral encephalitides. *At present, mass immunization has proved to be practical only for acute anterior poliomyelitis.* The greatest hope for the control of other viral diseases is believed to lie in the identification and elimination of the vectors responsible for their transmission. *No adequate treatment exists for the majority of the CNS viral infections.*

VIRAL MENINGITIS

Most cases of *acute viral meningitis* ("aseptic" meningitis) are due to *mumps virus* or one of the *picornaviruses.* Although most of these agents can cause severe encephalitis, the course of aseptic meningitis is self-limited and benign.

The *clinical syndrome* consists of fever, headache, and other signs of meningeal irritation. There may be some degree of drowsiness. The patient experiences distressing photophobia (abnormal intolerance to light) and pain on moving the eyes. Stiffness of the neck and spine on flexion are additional evidence of the presence of meningeal irritation. There may be other generalized symptoms, such as weakness and pain in the extremities, but in general all symptoms are mild.

Treatment of the patient with aseptic meningitis is mainly symptomatic and consists of supportive measures. The patient is kept at bedrest during the acute phase, and measures are taken to relieve headache, control fever, and otherwise keep the patient comfortable. If seizures occur, they are treated with appropriate anticonvulsants. Attempts should be made to identify the specific virus, using acute and convalescent serologic testing and appropriate viral cultures.

VIRAL ENCEPHALITIS

Many of the same viruses that are present in a benign viral meningitis may become much more destructive when they invade the substance of the brain itself and cause acute *viral encephalitis.*

Basically, the encephalitis consists of an acute febrile illness with signs of meningeal involvement and accompanied by various combinations of *symptoms:* convulsive seizures; confusion and delirium; stupor or coma; aphasia; motor involvement such as hemiparesis or asymmetrical reflexes; and involuntary movements. The course of the illness is unpredictable. Generally death occurs in 5 to 20 per cent of patients, with a much higher mortality rate with herpes simplex encephalitis. Such residual signs as mental deterioration, personality changes, and hemiparesis are seen in 20 per cent of patients, with a much higher incidence with eastern equine encephalitis.

As previously stated, any of a large number of viruses can cause encephalitis. We discuss only the two seen most commonly: *arthropod-borne (arbo) virus encephalitis* and *herpes simplex, type I virus encephalitis.*

Arbovirus Encephalitides. *Arboviruses* are

those capable of multiplying in a blood-sucking vector, usually a mosquito or tick, and are transmitted to humans by the bite of the insect. Diseases due to arboviruses usually have a characteristic seasonal and geographic incidence. Those in the United States typically occur in late summer and early fall; most frequently encountered are St. Louis encephalitis and eastern and western equine encephalitis.

In all but eastern equine encephalitis, the sites of infection are microscopic and scattered throughout the grey and white matter of the cerebral hemispheres. Eastern equine encephalitis can destroy major portions of a lobe or hemisphere.

The *clinical manifestations* of all arbovirus encephalitides are similar. In adults and older children, the onset is gradual, with headache, nausea and vomiting, listlessness, and fever. The disease progresses in a few days to seizures, stiff neck, and stupor and coma. Other symptoms that may be seen include photophobia, hemiparesis and asymmetrical reflexes. Unless the patient dies or has irreversible CNS changes, the fever and neurologic signs subside within 2 weeks.

Eastern equine encephalitis is the most devastating of the arboviruses. Two-thirds of those persons stricken die or are left with severe residuals, e.g., mental retardation, emotional disorders, recurrent seizures, blindness, deafness or speech disorders, and hemiplegia.

Herpes Simplex Virus Encephalitis. Herpes simplex virus encephalitis can occur throughout the year, in all parts of the world, in persons of all ages. The gradually evolving initial *symptoms* are similar to those of other acute encephalitides. However, since this virus has a special affinity for the inferomedial portions of the frontal and temporal lobes, other serious symptoms soon develop. These include olfactory and gustatory hallucinations, temporal lobe seizures, aphasia, bizarre or psychotic behavior, and occasionally hemiparesis. Swelling of the temporal lobe can cause transtentorial herniation and rapidly lead to deep coma and death, if not treated immediately.

Diagnosis of herpes simplex virus encephalitis is difficult. CSF studies are of little help except to rule out other causes. The only certain way to establish the diagnosis is by brain biopsy. Unfortunately, the diagnosis is often made only at autopsy.

The *prognosis* is grave, but not hopeless. The mortality rate is estimated to be from 30 to 70 per cent.[6] Of those who survive, many are left with severe neurologic and mental sequelae, such as global dementia, seizures, and aphasia. Some, however, are able to recover and resume an independent life.

There is no specific *treatment* for herpes simplex encephalitis. Several antiviral agents have been tried experimentally, but the results have not been promising and the toxic side effects have been substantial. One recent study, however, has shown a new antiviral agent, adenine arabinoside, to be significant in decreasing mortality and morbidity. It can be given in biopsy-confirmed cases and must be given early in the course of the disease to be most effective. The control of cerebral edema is another important consideration in the treatment regimen. The use of corticosteroids appears to be helpful. In an acute situation, with impending herniation, osmotic diuretics may be used. Some neurosurgeons recommend early surgical decompression, which serves both to alleviate intracranial pressure and to provide a definitive diagnosis.

Nursing care of the patient with a viral encephalitis presents an unusual challenge to the nurse. The patient is initially acutely ill, and all the nurse's knowledge and expertise are needed to help the patient return to a normal physiologic state. More frustrating and demanding for a nurse can be the attempts to cope with the patient's changes in behavior and mental status. The patient often becomes restless and combative and exhibits bizarre behavior. The nurse must protect patients from inflicting injury on themselves and others. When these behavioral changes and mental deterioration become part of the long-term residua, the nurse must work with other members of the rehabilitation team to help the patient function as fully as possible within the limitations of her or his deficits.

ACUTE ANTERIOR POLIOMYELITIS

Acute anterior poliomyelitis (infantile paralysis, "polio") is a generalized disease characterized by (a) the destruction of the motor cells (particularly the anterior horn cells in the spinal cord and the brain stem, especially the medulla) and (b) the appearance of a flaccid paralysis of those muscles innervated by the affected neurons. This disease is caused by one of the three types of poliovirus and spreads from the gastrointestinal tract to the nervous system.

Cases of poliomyelitis are divided into two groups, depending upon whether paralysis is present. Paralytic cases are subdivided into spinal forms and bulbar forms.

In the *spinal form* paralysis is restricted to the spinal segments. Such paralysis is flaccid in nature, usually is asymmetrical, and is scattered in distribution, although it tends to be more severe in one extremity (most frequently the legs are involved). Involvement of the diaphragm and intercostal muscles or damage to the medulla oblongata's respiratory centers may produce respiratory paralysis. Occasionally a transient bladder paralysis may occur.

In the *bulbar form of paralytic acute anterior poliomyelitis* there is involvement of the muscles supplied by the cranial nerves, because the bulbar nuclei are involved. These muscles may be affected alone or in combination with spinal musculature. The disorder is commonly unilateral. Respiratory paralysis results from lesions in the reticular formation.

Patients with paralysis of the respiratory muscles require prompt, intensive care. At the first indication of respiratory embarrassment, the patient should immediately be placed on a ventilator and given frequent reassurance that breathing will be supported. Such treatment, *before* serious respiratory paralysis develops, greatly increases chances of recovery. Some physicians routinely perform a tracheotomy on all patients receiving ventilator care. Tracheotomy is always indicated in the presence of spasm of the laryngeal muscles or when mucus occludes the air passages.

Since the 1950's, mass *immunization programs* using either killed (inactivated) virus (*Salk*) injected parenterally, or the liver attenuated virus (*Sabin*) by mouth have caused remarkable reductions in the number of cases of paralytic acute anterior poliomyelitis worldwide. However, *carelessness with respect to keeping up immunizations has recently caused some increase in the number of reported cases of "polio."* This is indeed unfortunate, since this devastating disease can be prevented with proper immunization.

Infancy is the most desirable time to immunize against poliomyelitis. Trivalent oral poliomyelitis vaccine has almost completely replaced both the inactivated and monovalent vaccines in some countries because of the ease of administration and supervision.

HERPES ZOSTER

Herpes zoster ("shingles," zona) is a common, acute viral infection of the nervous system caused by the *varicella* or *varicella-zoster virus* (similar in structure to the herpes simplex virus). The virus causing herpes zoster is the same virus that causes chickenpox (varicella). The virus causes an inflammatory reaction in isolated spinal and cranial sensory ganglia and in the posterior gray matter of the spinal cord (Fig. 27–3).

Cross-immunization studies have demonstrated that exposure to herpes zoster may cause chickenpox; however, the reverse is far less common. Recurrence is uncommon. Generally, a lasting immunity follows an attack.

> *Herpes zoster is characterized by radicular pain, a vesicular skin eruption, and sometimes segmental motor and sensory loss.*

In herpes zoster a nodular or vesicular eruption of the skin (*herpes*) occurs in conjunction with acute segmental neuralgia (*zoster*). The zoster or neuralgia occurs first, and is followed in 3 to 4 days by the development of the skin lesions in the same area. Malaise and fever may also precede the skin eruption. During the acute stage of the illness a meningitis with fever, stiff neck, malaise, and headache may occur, preceding or accompanying the selective nerve root involvement.

Typically, herpes zoster is characterized by a grouping of painful nodules or vesicles that are arranged along the course of a nerve or group of nerves, usually on only one side of the body. The intercostal nerves (branches of the thoracic spinal nerves in the area of the waist) are most commonly affected. The thoracic dermatomes T_5 to T_{10} are the most common sites. Another relatively common site is the first branch (ophthalmic division) of the fifth cranial nerve, causing pain in the eyeball and surrounding tissues (*ophthalmic herpes zoster*). Lesions may appear on the face, along the area of nerve distribution, and at times keratoconjunctivitis develops. Oculomotor function may also be impaired.

There is no medication available to specifically treat herpes zoster, as is true of nearly all other virus infections. Attention is thus directed toward *symptomatic treatment. Nursing care centers on prevention of infection of the skin lesions and keeping the patient as comfortable and pain-free as possible.* Wet dressings may be recommended for acute and extensive inflammatory lesions. Some physi-

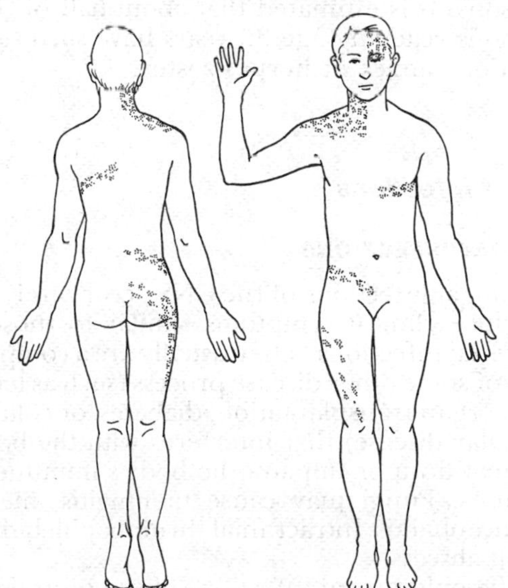

Figure 27–3. Herpes zoster. (Redrawn from Fitzpatrick, T. B. et al.: *Dermatology in General Medicine*. New York, McGraw Hill Book Co., 1971.)

cians order lotions (e.g., calamine lotion) that are cooling, drying, and antipruritic. These lotions are applied liberally and covered with a layer of cotton batting to protect the lesions from trauma. Some sources recommend that unbroken lesions on the trunk be painted with tincture of benzoin or collodion. During the acute phase of the illness, bed rest and symptomatic care are given as indicated. Nonaddicting analgesics may be ordered for pain relief. If bacterial infection of the rash develops, local or systemic treatment with antimicrobial medications is indicated. Some physicians believe that the administration of corticosteroids may shorten the duration of the disease. If trigeminal herpes involves the cornea, local antimicrobials and adrenocorticosteroids may be instilled into the eye. Mild sedatives may help to control the tension and nervousness that may be associated with the neuralgia.

The patient with *uncomplicated* herpes zoster makes an uneventful recovery as the lesions dry and disappear along with the pain. While the skin eruption usually clears within 2 to 3 weeks, a scar may remain. The accompanying pain may persist longer than the lesions. With *complicated* herpes zoster, the patient may develop a *postherpetic neuralgia* that causes pain of varying severity and intractability. This develops because the sensory ganglia located on the posterior nerve roots are affected. Postherpetic neuralgia may cause pain lasting for years and may present a difficult management problem for both patient and physician. (See Chapter 30 for discussion of the treatment of pain.)

Herpes zoster occurs more commonly in older persons. It is estimated that about half of those persons reaching age 85 years have suffered at least one attack of herpes zoster.

Other Infections

FUNGAL INFECTIONS

Fungal infections of the CNS occur rarely and produce clinical symptoms similar to those of bacterial infections. They usually are a complication of some other disease process (such as leukemia, organ transplantation, diabetes, or collagen vascular disease) that interferes with the body's normal flora or impairs the body's immune responses. Fungi may cause meningitis, meningoencephalitis, intracranial thrombophlebitis, or brain abscess.

The only fungal infections of the central nervous system seen frequently enough to be mentioned here are coccidioidomycosis, cryptococcosis, and mucormycosis.

- *Coccidioidomycosis* involves mostly the lungs but occasionally spreads to involve the meninges. Despite diligent treatment with amphotericin B, intravenously and intraventricularly, only half of those patients with meningeal involvement survive.
- *Cryptococcosis* is the most frequent CNS fungal infection. The cryptococcus, a common soil fungus, can cause granulomatous meningitis, small granulomas and cysts within the cortex, and large granulomas and cystic nodules deep within the brain. Symptoms may vary, and diagnosis is confirmed only on finding *Cryptococcus neoformans* in the CSF. If untreated, this infection will be fatal within a few weeks. Again, treatment consists of intravenous and intrathecal injection of amphotericin B. Even with treatment, the mortality rate is about 40 per cent.
- *Mucormycosis* is a malignant infection of cerebral vessels, occurring as a rare complication of diabetic acidosis. Beginning in the nose and paranasal sinuses and spreading to the brain, this condition is usually rapidly fatal.

NEUROSYPHILIS

Neurosyphilis (syphilis affecting the nervous system) is due to the invasion of the CNS by the *Treponema pallidum,* the spirochete that causes general syphilis (see Chapter 84). Neurosyphilis does not develop in all persons with syphilis. The organism invades the nervous system within 3 to 18 months of the original infection in approximately 25 per cent of all cases of syphilis. The incidence of neurosyphilis has declined dramatically in recent decades, probably because early syphilis is treated with penicillin or other antibiotic.

The *clinical manifestations* of neurosyphilis vary greatly, depending on the extent of involvement of the meninges, the blood vessels, and the brain parenchyma. In the first few years after infection, neurosyphilis is asymptomatic, producing only an abnormality of the CSF (increased white cells, with or without a protein increase, a positive serologic reaction), with no other symptoms. This stage usually goes unnoticed and untreated for a number of years, unless a lumbar puncture is performed for some other reason and the abnormality is found.

Meningovascular neurosyphilis may develop any time after the primary infection. Generally, however, meningeal involvement appears 6 to 7 years after the initial infection. Meningeal involvement may be diffuse or focal and can produce symptoms of increased intracranial pressure due to hydrocephalus, symptoms of cranial nerve involvement due to cranial nerve damage, or symptoms of invasion of the brain substance by focal growth of granulation tissue. The cerebral vascular component produces inflammation of the arteries, which leads first to fibrosis and then to occlusion of the vessel. The symptoms are those produced by any cerebral vascular lesions, e.g., aphasia, hemiplegia. Treatment with penicillin arrests the disease, but the neurologic deficits are not reversible.

Appropriate surgical intervention is sometimes necessary. For example, when the meningitis is focal, *granuloma formation* (*gumma*) occurs. A gumma is a circumscribed mass of granulation tissue. When they occur, gummata typically grow from the pia mater, compressing and invading the brain's parenchyma. Although the symptoms of diffuse syphilitic meningitis typically respond readily to treatment with penicillin, intracranial gummata are not responsive to such therapy and must be surgically removed.

Two *late forms of neurosyphilis,* which develop from 10 to 20 years after the original infection, are *tabes dorsalis* and *dementia paralytica* (also called *general paresis* or *paretic neurosyphilis*). Both are associated with invasion of the parenchyma of the brain or spinal cord (hence are sometimes called parenchymatous neurosyphilis). Fortunately, with the general decline in neurosyphilis and improved early treatment, both of these conditions are now rarely seen.

- *Tabes dorsalis* is also called "progressive locomotor ataxia", because ambulation disorders predominate. Tabes dorsalis results from degenerative changes in the brain stem and the posterior columns of the spinal cord. Clinically, it is characterized by: lightning pains (usually in the legs); ataxia due to sensory defects; a peculiar slapping gait; urinary overflow incontinence; *Argyll Robertson pupils*;* absent deep tendon reflexes and loss of proprioception; and various scattered paresthesias, e.g., zones of hyperesthesia (diminished sensitivity) and hypalgesia (excessive pain sensitivity). As the condition becomes established, *Charcot joints* develop. These arthropathies are characterized by enlargment of the joint, hypermobility and deformity, but a characteristic absence of pain. The deformity results from dislocations, deposition of new bone, fractures and erosions. *Visceral crises* such as severe thoracic or epigastric pain, are another manifestation. Treatment with penicillin will arrest the disease and produce minimal improvement in some symptoms.

- *Dementia paralytica* was formerly a common cause of admission to mental hospitals. This disorder is a chronic meningoencephalitis, which destroys cerebral cortex. This serious destruction is characterized by progressive mental and physical degeneration. Clinically the symptoms of both the major and minor psychoses occur; dementia paralytica may simulate any type of mental disturbance with either a functional or organic basis. The onset is insidious, with memory deficits, diminishing powers of reasoning and judgment, and gradual loss of interest in personal appearance and behavior. This progresses to total dilapidation of intellectual function, accompanied by psychosis with elaborate delusional systems. Physical deterioration progresses to include general debility, muscular hypotonia, tremors, hemiplegia, cranial nerve palsies and seizures — leading eventually to a bedridden state. The disease may be arrested by treatment with penicillin, but the deficits remain. Without treatment, death usually occurs in 3 to 4 years.

*Argyll Robertson pupils may be seen in disorders other than neurosyphilis, e.g., multiple sclerosis, epidemic encephalitis, diabetes mellitus, midbrain and pineal tumors, and chronic alcoholism.

DISORDERS DUE TO BACTERIAL TOXINS

The toxins produced by several pathogenic bacteria have a special affinity for the nervous system. We briefly consider three diseases that in recent years have been seen with increasing frequency in major medical centers: tetanus, diphtheria, and botulism.

Tetanus. Tetanus is caused by the anaerobic spore-forming rod *Clostridium tetani,* whose spores produce an exotoxin when they are introduced into a wound. The exact mode of action of the tetanus toxin is unknown, but it suppresses spinal and brain stem inhibitory neurons and may also act directly on the skeletal muscle at the point of entrance.

Symptoms may be localized or generalized. Locally, it causes painful muscular spasms and contractions in the affected extremity. In the more common generalized form, spasm begins with trismus of the jaw muscles and progresses to involve muscles of the neck, trunk, and limbs. The affected muscles become constantly rigid, with painful paroxysms of tonic contractions in response to the slightest external stimulus.

Treatment of tetanus consists of several measures:

- A single dose of *antitoxin* (hyperimmune serum [Hyper-Tet])
- A 10-day course of *antibiotic* to combat the *Clostridium tetani.*
- *Intensive nursing care* in a quiet, dark isolation room.
- *Respiratory support.* Tracheostomy may be necessary.
- *Medications* as necessary to control muscle spasms. Short-acting barbiturates along with chlorpromazine (Thorazine) are most useful. If all other measures fail, a tubocurarine may be used to abolish all muscle activity and essentially paralyze the patient for as long as necessary. If this is done, meticulous attention to nursing care measures is essential.

*Prevention of tetanus with immunization and regular booster doses of toxoid is the best approach! An injured person who has not had adequate immunization should receive both toxoid and antitoxin (Hyper-Tet).**

*See Chapters 11 and 95 for immunization schedules.

Diphtheria. *Diphtheria* is an acute inflammatory disease of the throat and trachea caused by the *Corynebacterium diphtheriae.* In approximately 20 per cent of the cases, this bacteria produces an exotoxin that affects the nervous system.

The CNS involvement usually begins with paralysis of the palate and progresses to involve other cranial nerves, especially the trigeminal, facial, vagus, and hypoglossal. Signs of CNS involvement may clear without further involvement, or the disease may progress to a polyneuropathy involving both motor and sensory systems. These *symptoms* progress for a week or two. If a patient survives respiratory and cardiac crises, the condition typically stabilizes and then improves slowly and completely.

There is no specific *treatment* for the condition, although some physicians feel that administration of antitoxin within 48 hours of the earliest symptoms lessens the severity of complications. Again *prophylactic immunization is essential*!

Botulism. *Botulism* is a food-borne illness caused by the exotoxin of *Clostridium botulinum.* The source of the poisoning is usually inadequately preserved food, very often home-preserved. The toxin acts at the neuromuscular junction when it affects the release of acetylcholine.

Symptoms begin within 12 to 48 hours after eating contaminated food, beginning with nausea, vomiting, and diarrhea. Then the ocular muscles become involved, leading to ptosis and paralysis of extraocular muscles. The weakness spreads to involve jaw muscles and muscles of the trunk and extremities. Sensation and consciousness remain intact. The severity of the symptoms and the course of the disease depend on the amount of toxin ingested. Many patients die because of respiratory failure. Survivors begin to show improvement within a few weeks, beginning with the eye muscles. Complete recovery is possible but may take many months.

As soon as the diagnosis is made, the patient should receive antitoxin in daily doses until improvement begins. However, the degree of recovery depends entirely on the quality of care given during the acute debilitated state, i.e., good respiratory care, prevention of infection. Excellent nursing can thus make an important difference in the outcome of this illness.

TUMORS OF THE NERVOUS SYSTEM

Various tumors affect the nervous system. Some originate within the nervous system (*primary tumors*) and others (*secondary tumors*) are implanted there as a result of metastases from different regions of the body. The large majority are primary tumors. Tumors may be malignant or benign. (Nursing people experiencing neoplastic disorders is discussed in the preceding unit, Unit IX).

Nervous system tumors may be classified into two groups: (1) those of the *central nervous system* and (2) those of the *peripheral nervous system.* Tumors of the peripheral nervous system are mentioned only briefly at the end of this section. Our discussion focuses mainly on central nervous system tumors, which we further divide into two subgroups: (a) *intracranial tumors* and (b) *tumors causing spinal root and cord compression.*

Classification of Tumors of the Nervous System

A. *Intracranial tumors*
   1. *Primary intracranial tumors*
   2. *Metastatic intracranial tumors*
   3. *Granulomas*
B. *Spinal tumors*
C. *Tumors of peripheral nerves*

Intracranial Tumors

Intracranial tumors are among the most *common* of all disorders affecting the nervous system and thus account for many admissions to neurologic care units. Intracranial tumors are second only to cerebrovascular disease as the most common endogenous neurologic problem, i.e., produced within the body as opposed to that originating externally (exogenous).

All intracranial tumors, whether histologically benign or malignant, are potentially fatal. The skull is rigid, with little room for expansion of any of its contents. Untreated brain tumors cause death by (a) local destruction and compression of brain tissue and (b) progressively increasing intracranial pressure, causing herniation and death.

Brain tumors are not inevitably fatal. However, even though some progress has been made because of improved diagnostic procedures and neurosurgical management, a good treatment outcome is not always possible; and the prognosis is guarded for most persons with a brain tumor. In individual cases the outcome depends on such factors as the location, size, and type of tumor. Benign tumors (neurinomas, meningiomas) and some gliomas (particularly those in frontal and occipital locations) may be cured, with early diagnosis and successful neurosurgery. On the other hand, the high incidence of invasive malignant glioblastomas and metastatic intracranial tumors account for many treatment failures.

Generally, surgery is the treatment of choice for intracranial tumors. In some treatment centers, combination therapy is employed with brain tumors, e.g., operative resection, radiation therapy, and chemotherapy. Treatment results are generally not good except for tumors that are clearly demarcated from brain tissue itself (e.g., meningiomas) or are well encapsulated. For example, often meningiomas can be completely resected surgically, while gliomas tend to be more invasive and thus make total surgical resection virtually impossible.

The *clinical course* of persons with intracranial tumors is closely related to the type of tumor. *Typically, indications of intracranial tumors are of slow onset and then progress until the person dies or is successfully treated.* Remissions are infrequent but do occur occasionally.

TYPES OF INTRACRANIAL TUMORS

Primary Intracranial Tumors. Primary intracranial tumors may be classified as follows:

- *Gliomas* — composed of malignant glial cells and arising from the various support tissues within the brain
- *Neuromas or neurofibromas* — arising from nerve cells
- *Meningiomas* — arising from the meninges
- *Various blood vessel tumors* — e.g., hemangiomas
- *Developmental tumors* — usually cysts, such as colloid cysts or dermoid cysts
- *Miscellaneous tumors* — e.g., pineal tumors and pituitary tumors

It may be helpful to realize that there are two basically different categories of brain tumors: (1) those intracranial tumors that are *inside the brain substance,* e.g., tumors of the supportive tissue (gliomas) and tumors of the blood vessels; and (2) those intracranial tumors that are *outside the brain substance,* e.g., tumors of the meninges (such as meningiomas), tumors of the cranial nerves (such as acoustic neuromas), and tumors of the pituitary region. Metastatic tumors (discussed below) may occur either inside or outside the brain substance, or in both areas. *Primary brain tumors occur more frequently within the brain than outside it, and more than 50 per cent of all primary tumors within the brain are gliomas.*

Gliomas are subdivided into various types, depending upon the principal cell types and morphology, e.g., glioblastoma multiforme, (the most malignant gliomas), astrocytoma, ependymoma, medulloblastoma, oligodendroglioma.

Table 27–1 illustrates the frequency of major types of brain tumors.

The *cranial nerves* may be compressed or invaded by benign or malignant tumors or they may be the primary site of tumors. Here we consider the latter. While any of the cranial nerves may be the site of origin of a tumor, those most commonly affected are the optic nerve (by glioma), the eighth cranial (acoustic) nerve (by neurofibroma), and the fifth cranial nerve (by neurofibroma). Of these, the eighth cranial nerve is most commonly affected. *Neurofibromas of the eighth cranial nerve,* i.e., *acoustic nerve,* are acoustic neuroma, acoustic neurinoma, cerebellopontine angle tumor, and perineural fibroblastoma of the eighth nerve.

Numerous *malformations of blood vessels* are sometimes included in the literature under tumors. There are a number of different classifications of these vascular anomalies and malformations. Generally there are two main groups: (1) *angiomas,* which are malformations composed of blood vessels of adult structure; and (2) *angioblastomas* (also called hemangioblastomas), which are tumors comprised of embryonic vascular channels and blood vessel-forming cells. The latter are the only true tumors of blood vessels in the brain. These tumors are cystic lesions (often red and hemorrhagic) that are quite rare and generally occur in early middle life in the area of the cerebellum.

Metastatic Intracranial Tumors. Metastatic tumors comprise 10 to 20 per cent of intracranial tumors. Metastatic brain tumors are generally a manifestation of generalized metastases. (See also Unit IX). Almost all carcinomas or sarcomas located elsewhere in the body may metastasize to the brain or its coverings. Carcinomas metastasize intracranially more often than sarcomas. *In many persons the primary sites of intracranial metastatic tumors are the lung (bronchus) or breast.* Carcinoma of the intestine, thyroid, and bladder also spread to the brain. Carcinomas of the prostate and cervix uteri may involve the brain's dura or

TABLE 27–1. FREQUENCY OF MAJOR TYPES OF BRAIN TUMORS

Intracranial Tumors*		Frequency of Occurrence
Gliomas		50%
Glioblastoma multiforme	50%	
Astrocytoma	20%	
Ependymoma	10%	
Medulloblastoma	10%	
Oligodendroglioma	5%	
Mixed	5%	
Meningiomas		20%
Nerve sheath tumors		10%
Metastatic tumors		10%
Congenital tumors		5%
Miscellaneous tumors		5%

*Exclusive of pituitary tumors.

From Dunphy, J. E., and L. W. Way: *Current Surgical Diagnosis and Treatment,* 3rd ed. Los Altos, Calif.: Lange Medical Publications, 1977, p. 766.

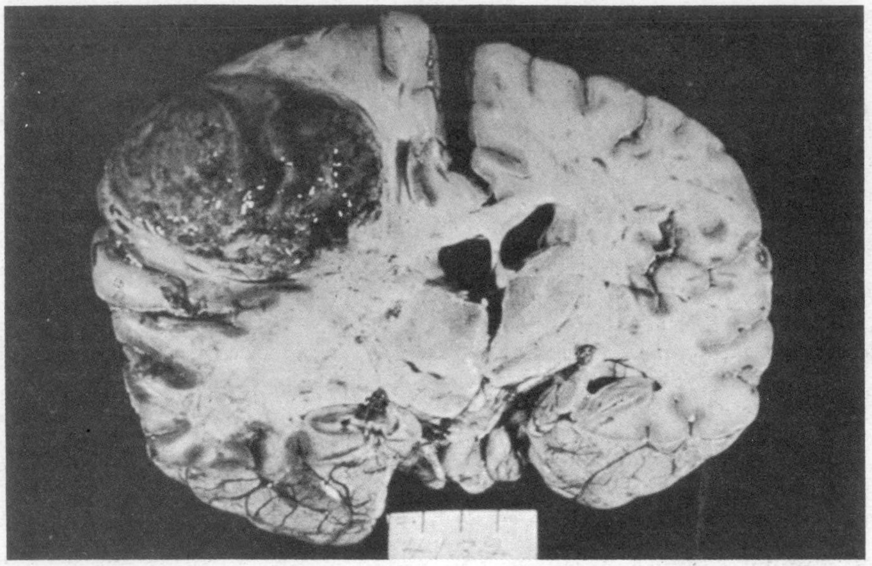

Figure 27–4. Glioblastoma multiforme. Infiltration of parietal lobe by hemorrhagic glioblastoma. (Courtesy Dr. J. Kepes.) (From Merritt, H. H.: *A Textbook of Neurology*, 5th ed. Philadelphia: Lea & Febiger, 1973, p. 260.)

the skull, but they rarely involve the brain substance itself. While metastatic tumors of the brain may develop at any age, they typically parallel the age incidence of malignant tumors in general, thus occurring most often between the ages of 40 and 70.

The brain tissue reacts severely to the presence of metastatic tumors. Profound swelling and an outpouring of phagocytic cells occurs. The individual metastatic nodules are usually well circumscribed; and, as they enlarge, their centers degenerate and they become cystic.

Usually metastatic tumors are characterized by a rapid onset and progression of symptoms; death may occur within a few months of appearance of the first symptoms. Many metastatic nodules are found throughout the CNS at autopsy. However, sometimes a solitary nodule occurs in the brain. When a single metastasis does occur it can be removed, if it is in a suitable area of the brain, and the patient experiences temporary relief of symptoms and may gain several useful months (possibly years) of life. However, generally the metastases are multiple, as mentioned, and operation is rarely advisable.

While metastasis occurs fairly commonly to the brain, the opposite is seldom true. Primary brain tumors only rarely metastasize out of the CNS. This is true even of highly anaplastic gliomas.

TABLE 27–2. BRAIN TUMOR TYPES ACCORDING TO AGE AND SITE

Age	Cerebral Hemisphere	Intrasellar and Parasellar	Posterior Fossa
Childhood and adolescence	Ependymomas; less commonly, astrocytomas.	Astrocytomas, mixed gliomas, ependymomas.	Astrocytomas, medulloblastomas, ependymomas.
Age 20–40	Meningiomas, astrocytomas; less commonly, metastatic tumors.	Pituitary adenomas; less commonly, meningiomas.	Acoustic neuromas, meningiomas, hemangioblastomas; less commonly, metastatic tumors.
Over age 40	Glioblastoma multiforme, meningiomas, metastatic tumors.	Pituitary adenomas; less commonly, meningiomas.	Metastatic tumors, acoustic neuromas, meningiomas.

From Dunphy, J. E., and L. W. Way: *Current Surgical Diagnosis and Treatment*, 3rd Ed. Los Altos, Calif.: Lange Medical Publications, 1977; p. 766.

Granulomas. Granulomas are tumors or neoplasms composed of granulation tissue. Granuloma formation may occur in the nervous system following infections with syphilis, the larvae of various intestinal parasites, fungi, sarcoidosis, and tuberculosis. *Tuberculomas* of the brain are always secondary to tuberculosis elsewhere in the body; however, the tuberculosis need not necessarily be active.

Intracranial tumors may be found in any age group and are generally seen equally in males and females. Heredity plays only a minor role in the occurrence of brain tumors, except for tumors of neurofibromatosis, tuberous sclerosis, and other phakomatoses.

Table 27–2 lists some types of brain tumors according to age and site.

SIGNS AND SYMPTOMS

The manifestations of intracranial tumors vary, depending upon the specific area of the brain affected (Table 27–3).

Localized signs and symptoms of intracranial tumors are those caused by destruction, irrita-

Location	Usual Clinical Manifestations
Cerebrum	Generalized convulsion Increased intracranial pressure
Frontal lobe	Changes in personality, behavior Defects in mentation Hemiparesis Aphasia (dominant hemisphere) Focal motor seizures
Parietal lobe	Hemisensory impairment Inferior quadrantic hemianopsia Focal sensory seizures
Temporal lobe	Defects in memory Nominal aphasia (dominant hemisphere) Superior quadrantic hemianopsia Psychomotor seizures, aura gustatory, déjà vu, and other visual images
Occipital lobe	Homonymous hemianopsia Seizures, aura flashes of light
Cerebellum	Increased intracranial pressure Ataxia, nystagmus, dysmetria Unsteady gait
Brain stem	Hemiparesis Nystagmus Facial paresis Vomiting
Pituitary (in relation to sella turcica)	
Intrasellar	Endocrine Hyperpituitarism
Intra- and extrasellar	Endocrine Hyperpituitarism Hypopituitarism Optic nerve Optic atrophy Decreased visual acuity Optic chiasm Peripheral visual field defects, especially bitemporal hemianopsia Hypothalamus Somnolence, diabetes insipidus Adiposity Sexual dystrophy
Cranial nerves	Dizziness, vertigo Neurogenic hearing deficit Depressed vestibular response Pain and sensory deficits in trigeminal distribution Depressed corneal reflex Peripheral facial palsy Cerebellar ataxia

From McKhann, G.: Mass Lesions. *In* Harvey, A. McGehee, et al. (Eds.): *The Principles and Practices of Medicine,* 19th ed. New York: Appleton-Century-Crofts, 1976, p. 1553.

tion, or compression by the tumor of that part of the brain in or near which the tumor lies. Blood supply is also imparied to the affected area. Localized signs and symptoms may include: focal weaknesses such as hemipareses; sensory disturbances such as anesthesia or paresthesia; language disturbances; coordination disturbances such as staggering gait, and visual disturbances such as diplopia (double vision) or visual field deficit, e.g., hemianopia.

General signs and symptoms are caused by a generalized disturbance of cerebral function resulting from edema and increased intracranial pressure.

- *Headaches* may be localized or general, but are often most severe in the frontal or occipital region. They are usually intermittent, of increasing duration, and may be increased by change in posture or straining. Recurrent, severe headaches in a person previously free of them may suggest tumor formation and should be investigated. Likewise, recurrent headaches which most commonly occur in the early morning and increase in frequency and severity without apparent cause may indicate brain tumor.
- *Nausea and vomiting* are usually not seen until late in the course of tumor progression. Vomiting may have no constant relation to meals. Nausea may be marked. Increasingly severe vomiting is especially suggestive of brain tumors in children.
- *Papilledema* (edema and hyperemia of the optic disc, *choked disc*) is commonly seen in persons with intracranial tumors, presenting with swelling of the optic nerve head, enlargement of retinal veins, and eventually hemorrhages into the nerve and adjacent retina. In some persons, papilledema may be the first sign. Although the underlying pathophysiology is not clearly understood, the cause is generally believed to be increased pressure in the central retinal vein due to obstruction of venous return from the eye. Early papilledema does not cause changes in visual acuity, but prolonged papilledema causes optic atrophy and greatly diminished visual acuity.
- *Seizures*, focal or generalized, are frequently seen in persons with intracranial tumors (especially tumors in the cerebral hemispheres). Often a seizure is the first symptom of a tumor. A tumor must be suspected in adult patients in whom seizures begin without an obvious cause such as head trauma. The characteristics and progression of a seizure can help to localize the tumor. Hence, careful observations and accurate recording of the nature and progression of seizures is important.
- *Dizziness and vertigo* may develop from intracranial circulatory impairment.
- *Changes in mental status* frequently accompany an intracranial tumor and may include lethargy and drowsiness, confusion and disorientation, personality changes, and even psychotic episodes.

As an intracranial tumor enlarges, it shifts intracranial structures and may produce herniation.

DIAGNOSIS

A complete history from the patient and/or significant others is especially important. This must be followed by a thorough physical examination, especially a neurologic examination. When these two components point toward a tumor, the following studies can be especially helpful to confirm the diagnosis: skull x-rays, echoencephalography, electroencephalography, angiography, radioisotopic brain scan and computerized tomography (CT scan).

Echoencephalography is a safe procedure, and experts recommend that it be performed on all patients believed to have brain tumors.

Electroencephalography is especially helpful in localizing tumors near the surface of the cerebral hemispheres.

Angiography is highly valuable in diagnosing and localizing brain tumors. The tumors are localized by noting the displacement of arteries and veins and by finding abnormal vascular patterns on the angiogram. Often the type of the tumor can be determined by the nature of its vasculature.

Radioactive scanning is highly valuable in localizing brain tumors (by means of their differential uptake of gamma-emitting labeled carriers).

Lumbar puncture is hazardous in the presence of increased intracranial pressure (because of danger of tentorial herniation) and hence this test is often not performed in establishing the diagnosis of brain tumor. A ventriculogram or pneumoencephalogram would be ordered only in unusual circumstances since both of these procedures are accompanied by a definite risk in persons with intracranial tumors.

Since the development of computerized tomography, the diagnostic work-up of a patient suspected of having a brain tumor has greatly changed (Fig. 27-5). The computerized tomography scan has almost completely replaced the radioisotope brain scan and the ventriculogram or pneumoencephalogram. In current practice, in a center which has an EMI scanner or other such equipment, the progression of diagnostic tests would probably be: (1) skull x-rays, (2) EEG, (3) computerized tomography scan, and (4) angiography. During the diagnostic work-up, various studies may be performed to determine the primary site of a metastatic brain tumor, e.g., chest x-ray, gastrointestinal series, urograms.

TREATMENT OF INTRACRANIAL TUMORS

Early diagnosis and treatment are of utmost importance. Intracranial tumors are treated by *surgical removal* of the tumor when possible. The usual procedure is to remove as much of the tumor as possible and follow with a course of *radiation therapy* when appropriate. *Chemotherapy* (with drugs such as methotrexate, CCNU and BCNU) is being tried experimentally. However, in general, chemotherapy has not been found to be effective. It may be partially effective in a few persons. The nitrosourea—carmustine (BCNU), lomustine (CCNU), and semustine (methyl-CCNU)—are lipid-soluble compounds that easily cross the blood-brain barrier.

When surgical consultation is not readily available, *temporary treatment measures may be necessary to reduce increased intracranial pressure.* Preoperatively and in the early postoperative phase, parenteral corticosteroids may be used to reduce cerebral edema. Mannitol or urea may be administered to help reduce increased intracranial pressure in the operative and early postoperative periods.

Increased intracranial pressure is discussed in Chapter 26; intracranial surgery is discussed in Chapter 28.

A special word must be said about *metastatic tumors.* Often a needle biopsy is done to confirm the diagnosis, but surgery to attempt excision of the tumor is not usually done. Radiation therapy is most often given to slow the growth of the tumor and improve the quality of life.

The *clinical course* of a patient with an intracranial tumor varies with the specific type of tumor present. For example, a person with a low-grade glioma, who has partial excision of the tumor followed by radiation, can often survive 5 to 15 meaningful years. In contrast, a glioblastoma multiforme is highly malignant; a person with this kind of tumor may survive only 6 months to 1 year, even with radiation.

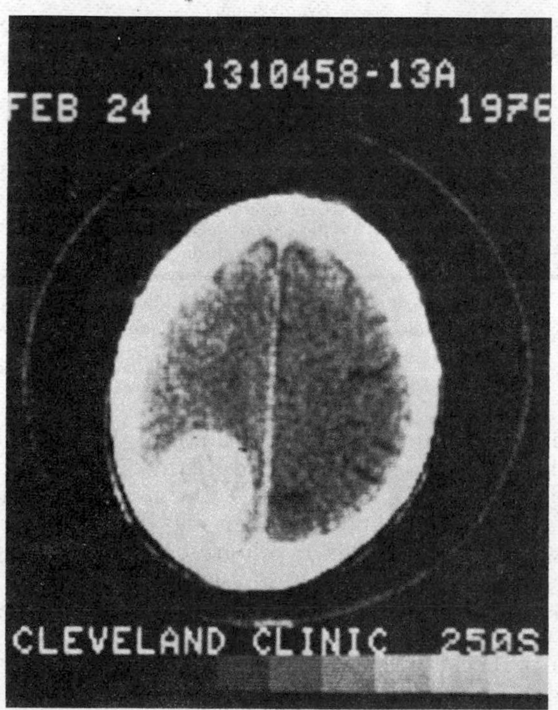

Figure 27–5. A CT scan showing a left occipital meningioma. (From Calvin, R.: Quiz Yourself on Computerized Axial Tomography. *Journal of Neurosurgical Nursing,* 9:164, Dec. 1977.)

Clinical care varies with the type and location of the tumor and the patient's symptoms. Symptomatic therapy may involve administration of sedatives, analgesics, and anticonvulsants. In Chapter 26, we have discussed care of persons who are unconscious, or have seizures, increased intracranial pressure, or other kinds of problems which may occur with some brain tumors. Care of the person receiving radiation treatment has been covered in Chapter 23. Nursing care in the presence of brain tumor may involve meeting the physiologic needs of a debilitated, possibly comatose person.

The nurse's role in caring for a person with a brain tumor is vital. Specifically, when caring for a person with a brain tumor (or suspected brain tumor) you may routinely observe for:

- *Indications of increasing intracranial pressure,* noting carefully any subtle changes in level of consciousness (LOC) and orientation. Observe changes in pupil size and reaction to light.
- Early signs of *impaired motor function.*
- Evidence of *hyperthermia, seizures, pain,* and or *vomiting.* Note the location, duration, and severity of headache (or any pain) and the position the patient assumes to obtain maximum comfort during the headache. Note the nature of vomiting, e.g., whether it is related to meals, accompanied by nausea and vomiting (often abbreviated N&V), or projectile.
- Significant alterations in *vital signs.*

Caution the conscious patient not to strain if possible (e.g., while vomiting or using the bedpan), because straining increases intracranial pressure.

People who suspect or know they have brain tumors are frightened and apprehensive. They and their significant others require the nurse's kindness, patience, and understanding. Often people have questions about the nature of brain tumors and about brain surgery. Find out from the doctor if the person with a malignant tumor has been told about the malignancy and what else has been discussed concerning the diagnosis and treatment. Answer questions as honestly and carefully as possible.

Spinal Tumors

Spinal tumors are much less common than intracranial tumors, but are similar in nature and origin to intracranial tumors. They occur most frequently in young or middle-aged adults and most often involve the thoracic region. They may occur within the substance of the spinal cord (*intramedullary*) or outside of the spinal cord (*extramedullary*). The extramedullary tumors may be *intradural, extradural,* or *extravertebral. Neurofibromas* and *meningiomas* are the two most common tumors affecting the spinal cord. Both are benign, operable, and may not produce permanent damage if removed early enough.

Signs and Symptoms. The signs and symptoms of spinal tumors vary according to their location.

> *Cord compression is the common pathologic feature of all tumors within the spinal canal, since there is little room for expansion in the canal. Compression of the spinal cord interrupts the function of nerve fibers in the cord's peripheral portions.*

Extramedullary Tumors. Extramedullary tumors cause symptoms by compressing the spinal cord or some of its nerve roots, or by occluding blood vessels supplying the cord:

- Early symptoms of cord compression include pain, sensory loss, muscle weakness and wasting.
- Symptoms indicating progressive compression of the cord include spastic weakness, below the level of the lesion, decreased sensation, and increased reflexes.
- Severe compression causes destruction of the cord and produces signs and symptoms of complete transsection of the cord--essentially paraplegia or quadriplegia.

Intramedullary Tumors. Intramedullary tumors produce signs and symptoms that are much more variable. If the high cervical cord is involved, the patient develops spastic quadriplegia with a similar level of sensory changes. Tumors in the descending areas of the cord produce motor and sensory changes appropriate with functions at that level.

Diagnosis. *Diagnosis* of spinal cord tumors is made after complete general neurologic examination confirmed by x-ray — both plain spine films and contrast myelography.

Treatment. The *treatment* of spinal tumors is more frequently effective than that of brain tumors and usually consists of surgery or radiation therapy, or both. Immediate surgery is indicated if the signs and symptoms are being caused by compression of the cord or nerve roots. In such cases, marked improvement or complete restoration of function can be expected, especially if the tumor is a meningioma, lipoma, or some other encapsulated tumor. Results of surgery tend to be poor if necrosis of the cord has occurred owing to compression or interrupted blood supply. An intramedullary tumor can rarely be completely removed, but often radiation following partial resection can improve signs and symptoms. However, the general course is gradually progressive.

Tumors of Peripheral Nerves

While solitary tumors (generally neurofibromas) may develop on any of the peripheral nerves, most often multiple tumors occur and are part of the syndrome known as *neurofibromatosis (von Recklinghausen's disease)*. This is a hereditary disorder characterized by multiple tumors of spinal and cranial nerves, along with the involvement of many other systems. The disease is usually not life threatening, and the lesions are excised only when they interfere with normal activity. Intracranial and intraspinal tumors are usually removed.

VASCULAR LESIONS OF THE NERVOUS SYSTEM

Classification of Vascular Lesions of the Nervous System

A. *Vascular lesions of the brain*
   1. *Strokes (cerebrovascular accidents)*
   2. *Transient ischemic attacks (TIA's)*
   3. *Intracranial aneurysms and primary subarachnoid hemorrhage*
B. *Vascular lesions of the spinal cord*
   1. *Myelomalacia*
   2. *Hematomyelia*
C. *Vascular lesions of the cerebral veins and sinuses*

VASCULAR LESIONS OF THE BRAIN

Cerebrovascular diseases are diseases of the brain's blood vessels. As elsewhere in the body, hypertension and arteriosclerosis are the major underlying causes of cerebrovascular diseases.[269]

Preventive measures and precrisis recognition are highly important with cerebrovascular diseases.

Diseases of the brain's vascular system are responsible for the largest proportion of the neurologic illnesses. In the United States, vascular lesions of the central nervous system rank third as a cause of death, exceeded only by heart disease and cancer. In addition to being a major cause of death, *cerebrovascular diseases are probably the number one cause of chronic disability.* The incidence of cerebrovascular disease is particularly high in persons over 65 years, and it is increasing among much younger population. It is evident, therefore, that a careful study of the blood supply to the brain and the disorders that interfere with it are of great importance to nurses.

Cerebral Circulation

In order to understand the various cerebrovascular disorders, a nurse must be familiar with cerebral circulation. It is important to know how the blood supply reaches the brain, what areas of the brain are supplied by the various major vessels, and the basics of the physiology of cerebral circulation.

Blood is carried to the cerebral hemispheres and the brainstem by two paired systems of vessels: the carotid and vertebral-basilar systems. The *internal carotid arteries* branch off the common carotid arteries in the neck, enter the cranium, and give off branches which supply most of the areas of the cerebral hemispheres. Their major branches are the middle cerebral, anterior cerebral and posterior communicating arteries. The *vertebral arteries* enter the cranium through the foramen magnum, ascend, and join to form the basilar artery. The basilar artery gives off several branches, which supply the posterior areas of the cerebral hemispheres and the brainstem.

At the base of the brain, the branches of the internal carotid system and the vertebral-basilar system join in a network of vessels called the *circle of Willis* (Fig. 27–6). The circle of Willis provides a shunting mechanism between the two systems that allows for a continual blood supply to the entire brain when one system or the other is affected by trauma or other lesions.

The blood is drained from the brain by a complex *venous system.* Both internal and external veins drain into a system of venous sinuses in the dura, which ultimately empty into the internal jugular vein (Fig. 27–7).

It is important to remember that the brain has a tremendous oxygen requirement.

Although the brain's weight is only 2 per cent that of the whole body, the adult human brain requires 20 per cent of the cardiac output, 20 per cent of the oxygen consumption, and 70 per cent of the glucose consumption (which is supplied through the blood stream). When the blood supply to a part of the brain is decreased or totally interrupted, the brain gets neither oxygen nor glucose. If the ischemia lasts more than a few minutes, the cells are irreversibly damaged and necrosis of tissue elements will occur.

Blood supply to the brain may be altered (slowly or rapidly) by such local disorders as thrombi, emboli, hemorrhage, or vascular spasms, or by

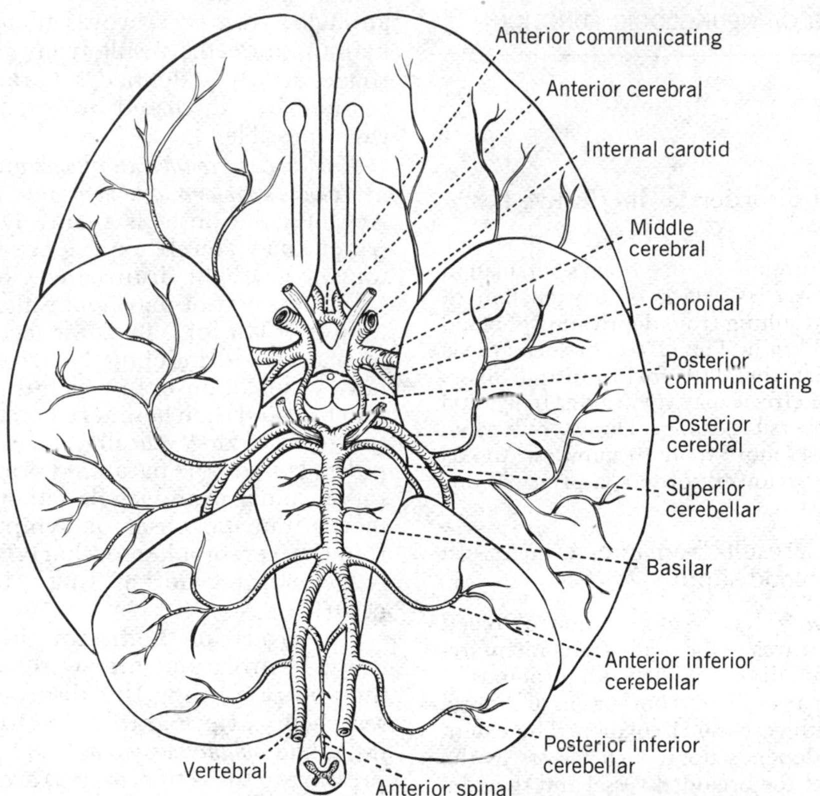

Figure 27–6. Major branches of the vertebral and internal carotid systems of arteries at the base of the brain. (From Patton, H. D., et al.: *Introduction to Basic Neurology.* Philadelphia: W. B. Saunders Co., 1976, p. 375.)

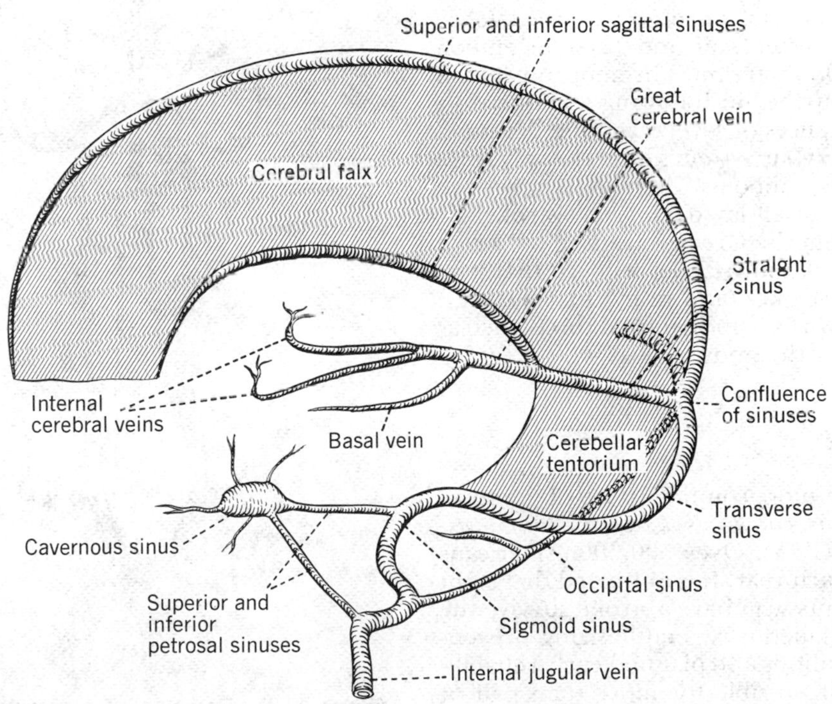

Figure 27–7. Major cerebral sinuses receiving the cerebral veins. (From Patton, H. D., et al.: *Introduction to Basic Neurology.* Philadelphia, W. B. Saunders Co., 1976, p. 381.)

such generalized disorders as ineffective heart-lung actions.

Extensive interruption of the brain's circulation causes *cerebral anoxia,* i.e., lack of oxygenation of the brain's tissues resulting from deprivation of blood supply to the total brain. The effects of such anoxia may be reversible in the adult for up to four to six minutes. While the effects may vary under individual circumstances, irreversible changes always occur when cerebral anoxia lasts more than 10 minutes. Anoxia may be caused by various disorders, a principal one being cardiac arrest.

Cerebral anoxia results from interference with the brain's total blood supply.

Cerebral infarction refers to deprivation of blood supply to a localized area of the brain. Cerebral infarction may result from disorders such as a thrombus or embolus occluding a vessel, or from spasms of a vessel which interfere with cerebral circulation. The extent of the infarction depends upon such factors as the location and size of the occluded vessel and the adequacy of collateral circulation to the area supplied by the occluded vessel.

Atherosclerotic disease frequently affects the arteries leading to the brain. Common sites of plaque formation in these arteries are shown in Figure 27–8. Thrombi may form on atherosclerotic plaques, or blood may clot in an area of stenosis where the blood stream is slowed or where eddying occurs. Thrombi can break loose from a blood vessel wall and become emboli carried in the blood stream. Thrombi and emboli are discussed further in following sections.

The consequences of severe, sudden derangements in the nervous system's blood supply, e.g., from thrombus, embolus, or hemorrhage, are familiar to almost all lay persons as "stroke" or "apoplexy" (from the Greek, meaning to "strike down.") In Greek times it was believed that persons suffering strokes (and grand mal seizures) were struck down by some external force, such as an act by one of the gods.

Strokes

Probably the most common type of cerebrovascular lesion is known as a *stroke* or *cerebrovascular accident* (CVA). Over 500,000 Americans suffer a CVA each year. It is estimated that eight out of 10 patients who have a stroke survive the initial phase. Skilled care, emphasizing prevention of complications and planned early rehabilitation, makes it possible for more than half of those persons who survive a stroke to return to productive work. Nevertheless, more than 200,000 persons die in the United States alone annually from cerebrovascular disease. Over half these deaths result from cerebral hemorrhage, which is defined separately in this discussion but discussed with occlusive disease when possible.

Strokes may produce an almost unlimited variety of neurologic symptoms, and their onset is highly variable. At times the onset is relatively mild, and the patient may merely experience transient symptoms, e.g., slight disturbances of speech. Consciousness may or may not be altered, and symptoms may last for only a few seconds or minutes or may persist indefinitely. Larger strokes may have a violent onset in which the patient falls to the floor and then lies inert, comatose, breathing stertorously or cyclically, face flushed, cheek puffing out on the paralyzed side with each expiration, and arm and leg flaccid on that side. (The more dramatic onset of symptoms is usually found in cerebral hemorrhage.) Seizures (usually generalized but at times focal) may also occur.

Numerous methods for investigating the causes of stroke and improved means of diagnosing and preventing this disorder are being researched. Arteriography, isotope brain scanning, and *ophthalmodynamometry* (to measure the pressure in the retinal artery) are used in diagnosis. Anticoagulation is selectively used to prevent repetition of arterial occlusion. This is a controversial therapy.

Research is underway to try to predict when a likely candidate for a stroke will actually suffer

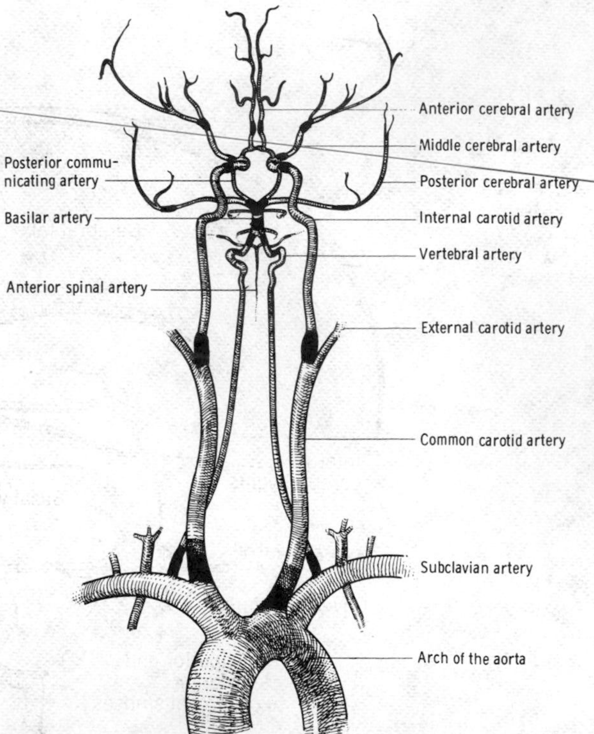

Figure 27–8. Common sites of extracranial atheroma formation. (From McDowell, F. H.: *In* Beeson, P. B., W. McDermott and J. B. Wyngaarden (Eds.): *Cecil Textbook of Medicine.* 15th ed., 1979.)

the attack. By identifying various risk factors, it is possible to identify persons who are particularly prone to developing ischemic thrombotic cerebrovascular disease.

Several *risk factors* related to stroke have been identified, including presence of the following: (1) hypertension (found in 80 per cent of patients with occlusive disease); (2) heart disease, such as previous myocardial infarction, arrhythmias, or cardiac enlargement; (3) diabetes mellitus, or other disorders of glucose tolerance; (4) hypercholesterolemia; (5) oral contraceptive use; and (6) obesity and family history of stroke.

ETIOLOGY OF STROKES

As stated earlier, a common cause of stroke is a narrowing or complete closing of one of the blood vessels supplying the brain, i.e., occlusive vascular disease. Several events that impair brain function can occur in the cerebral circulation. These events are briefly defined next, then discussed in following sections. These include *thrombosis* (blood clot formation), *embolism* (blocking of a vessel by a blood clot floating in the blood stream), *hemorrhage* (bleeding), *compression* (pressure), and *spasm* (tightening and closing down of the walls of an artery due to vasoconstriction). These latter two are relatively infrequent.

Spasm. Arterial spasm, which is due to some irritation of the outer portion of the arterial wall, reduces blood flow to the area of the brain supplied by the constricted vessel. Spasm of short duration does not necessarily cause permanent brain damage.

Compression. Compression of cerebral vessels may result from a tumor, a large blood clot, swollen brain tissue, or other disorders.

> *The three most common causes of stroke are thrombosis, embolism and hemorrhage, although compression or arterial spasm can cause infarction of the brain.*

Thrombosis. *Thrombosis is the commonest cause of* cerebral infarction and is most often due to atherosclerosis. Rarely, occlusion may also be secondary to an inflammatory reaction in vessel walls.

The vessel affected by thrombosis may be intracerebral; however, *the main site of obstruction usually is not within the brain but is in the extracerebral vessels.* Formerly it was thought that most cases of cerebral infarction resulted from thrombosis within the three main cerebral arteries (or their branches) intracranially. However, the importance of the vessels in the neck and their points of origin from the aorta is now established. The presence or absence of symptoms in patients with occlusive lesions in the neck depends on the adequacy of the collateral circulation.

Thrombosis produces an *ischemia* of the brain tissue that is supplied by the affected vessel, and edema and congestion in the surrounding areas. The area of *edema* may cause greater dysfunction than that caused by the infarct itself. The edema subsides after a few hours in some patients, although it may take several days in others. *As the edema subsides, the patient begins to show improvement and may regain some functions that were impaired by the edema.*

A stroke caused by thrombus formation tends to develop while the patient is asleep or within an hour after arising. This differs from a stroke caused by cerebral hemorrhage, which most often occurs during active waking hours. (Strokes resulting from embolism have no apparent time pattern.) Cerebral thrombosis may also occur during vascular collapse in myocardial infarctions in relation to surgery.

The *symptoms* of thrombosis are highly variable, depending on the site of the vessel occluded and the size of the area affected in the brain. The symptoms of thrombosis may occasionally take several days to develop. This clinical picture is strikingly different from a stroke caused by cerebral hemorrhage (in which symptoms occur within minutes, or hours at the longest) and that caused by cerebral embolism (in which the symptoms follow even more rapidly). Symptoms appear more slowly with a thrombus than with an embolus because a thrombus more gradually produces ischemia.

Embolism. The incidence of cerebral embolism increases after age 40. *"Cerebral embolism"* refers to the occlusion of a cerebral vessel by such substances as a fragment of clotted blood, tumor, fat, bacteria, or air. Typically, cerebral embolism is associated with heart diseases in which fragments of clotted blood or bacterial vegetations are released from the heart's walls or valves and then lodge in the cerebral arterial system.

Occlusion of cerebral vessels by an embolus causes necrosis and edema similar to that following thrombosis, unless the embolus contains bacteria. If it is septic, and the infection extends beyond the walls of the vessel, an abscess forms or encephalitis develops. If the infection remains contained within the occluded vessel, an aneurysmal dilation of the vessel, called a *mycotic aneurysm,* may develop. This is dangerous because cerebral hemorrhage may occur later if the aneurysm ruptures.

As indicated earlier, the onset of cerebral embolism typically occurs rapidly. Symptoms may develop, without warning, within from 10 to 30 seconds. The embolus most often lodges at the bifurcation of the middle cerebral artery. *The extent of damage is often less severe and the recovery more rapid following embolism than following thrombosis or cerebral hemorrhage.* Not infrequently, the embolus breaks apart and moves into smaller vessels, with reduction in the volume of compromised brain and clearing of many of the early, acute symptoms.

Intracerebral Hemorrhage. Let us first clarify that hemorrhage may occur outside the dura mater (extradural hemorrhage, p. 662), beneath the dura mater (subdural hemorrhage, p. 663), in the subarachnoid space (subarachnoid hemorrhage, p. 619), or within the brain substance (cerebral or intracerebral hemorrhage). In this section we are concerned only with the last-named hemorrhage.

Intracerebral hemorrhage results from rupture of a cerebral vessel. Cerebral hemorrhage, due to arteriosclerosis and hypertension, is most common after age 50. These hemorrhages usually result in the most extensive residual functional deficits and the slowest recoveries of the various types of strokes. Large hemorrhages usually come from arteries, whereas small extravasations may come from the veins and capillaries. As with the previously discussed conditions, the effects of intracerebral hemorrhages vary, depending on the site of the hemorrhage and its extent.

The rupture of arteriosclerotic hypertensive vessels is the cause of most hemorrhages into the brain.[269] Most intracerebral hemorrhages are very large; therefore, it is not surprising that *hypertensive hemorrhage into the brain is the most common cause of death in the group of cerebrovascular diseases.*[269] While infarcts from thrombosis occur more commonly, they do not cause death unless they are massive. Although recovery is possible following hypertensive hemorrhage, it is less likely and less complete. (Intracerebral hemorrhage following head injury is discussed on page 664.)

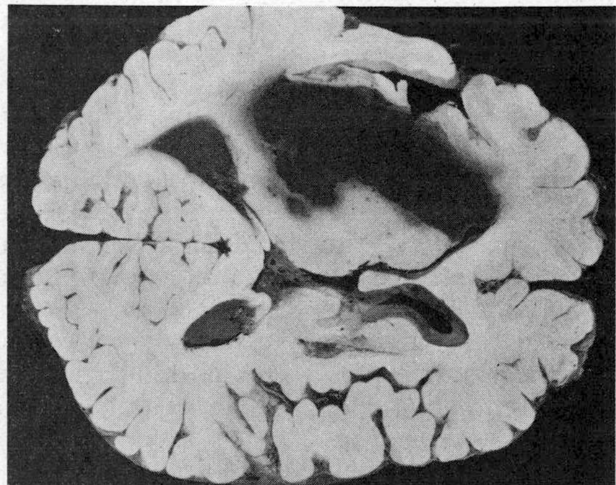

Figure 27–9. Massive hypertensive hemorrhage, rupturing into lateral ventricle. This type of hemorrhage is in general very large, occupying 25 to 80 per cent of an entire hemisphere. Most cerebral hemorrhages arise in the deep part of the cerebrum. (From Robbins, S. L., and R. S. Cotran: *Pathologic Basis of Disease,* 2nd ed. Philadelphia: W. B. Saunders Co., 1979, p. 1557.)

ONSET, SYMPTOMS AND CLINICAL COURSE OF STROKES

The nurse caring for a patient with CVA needs an understanding of the etiology of stroke and must be able to recognize its precipitating as well as its progressive symptoms. Often a patient with cerebral vascular disease first comes to the attention of nurses and physicians following the sudden, frequently dramatic, onset of coma or focal neurologic symptoms, e.g., hemiplegia, aphasia. Strokes most often occur suddenly, the symptoms reaching maximal intensity within a few minutes or few hours at most.

Premonitory symptoms ("warning" symptoms) of a focal nature occur in many patients with stenosis of the great vessels in the neck, but are infrequently recognized as such. Less frequently, generalized "warning symptoms" occur such as mental confusion, drowsiness, dizziness, and headache. A transient loss of speech, hemiplegia, or paresthesias of half of the body may precede the onset of a severe paralysis by a few hours or days. These "transient" ischemic attacks (TIA's) should not be ignored. (TIA's are discussed further on p. 619.)

Typical symptoms associated with strokes may include: *generalized symptoms* such as headache, vomiting, seizures, coma, nuchal rigidity, fever, hypertension, abnormalities of the heart, sclerosis of peripheral and retinal vessels, confusion, disorientation, memory impairment and other mental changes; and *focal neurologic symptoms* related to the site of the hemorrhage or infarct, e.g., weakness or paralysis, sensory loss, language disorders, and reflex changes.

Usually the *general symptoms* are most intense immediately after the onset of the stroke; however, sometimes there is a gradual increase in the depth of the coma. The *focal symptoms* also are typically most severe immediately following onset. However, occasionally following intracerebral hemorrhage the focal neurologic symptoms may increase in severity or extent for a few hours as the hemorrhage continues to enlarge in size. Progression of focal neurologic symptoms may sometimes occur following cerebral thrombosis or embolism. This is sometimes known as *"stroke in evolution."*

The focal symptoms that result from cerebral hemorrhage vary, depending on the site of the hemorrhage. However, *complete hemiplegia* (with or without a hemianopia or hemianesthesia) *commonly occurs, since the basal ganglia and adjacent internal capsule are affected in more than two-thirds of these patients.* It is in this region that the motor pathways to the body are gathered together into a relatively small space before they pass down into the spinal cord. Thus, the hemorrhage destroys or compresses those fibers, and motor impulses are cut off from the extremities. As a result, the side of the body, e.g., face, arm, leg, that is supplied by the side of the brain affected by the hemorrhage is paralyzed, i.e., becomes hemiplegic.

Because the motor fibers from one side of the brain cross to the opposite side before passing down the cord, hemorrhage on the brain's right side causes left-sided hemiplegia, and vice versa.

It is significant that the speech center in right-handed persons is most commonly on the brain's left side, i.e., in the dominant hemisphere. Thus, hemorrhage into the left side often produces aphasia as well as right-sided hemiplegia. The symptoms of cerebral hemorrhage vary with the areas of the hemisphere involved.

The focal symptoms produced by thrombosis or cerebral embolism within the arterial system supplying the brain are highly characteristic of the area of involvement. Thus, these symptoms are extremely helpful in establishing a precise diagnosis, and the nurse's observations of these symptoms are important.

The *thalamic syndrome* is occasionally observed following a stroke that involves the region of the thalamus. Typically this syndrome is manifested by a burning or aching dysesthesia which involves an entire half of the body. Discomfort is most intense in the extremities, especially the hand. This pain usually begins first several weeks following the stroke. Thalamic pain is intensified by emotional disturbances. Increased emotional lability, with unmotivated crying or laughing, may be associated with the thalamic syndrome.

Extensive cerebral lesions (resulting from hemorrhage more often than from thrombosis) often produce *conjugate deviation of the eyes,* or *head and eyes,* toward the side of the lesion. The comment is often heard that the patient's eyes "look toward the lesion." Usually when such deviation is present the patient also has only limited movements of the head and eyes toward the opposite direction. As the patient's condition improves generally, these symptoms tend to resolve.

Pupillary abnormalities vary in type and frequency following stroke; however, frequently inequalities of pupil size occur. Typically the larger pupil is on the same side as the cerebral lesion.

Changes in a patient's reflexes and plantar responses and other symptoms of focal brain damage, e.g., hemiplegia, aphasia, hemianopia, are related to the lesion's site.

Strokes due to occlusal disease are rarely the cause of sudden death. When sudden death does occur, it is usually due to heart failure. However, if an intracerebral hemorrhage ruptures into the ventricles, the outcome is fatal. Symptoms of increased intracranial pressure may develop.

In fatal cases of strokes of all types the duration of life varies from a few hours to several months following the original attack. Death may occur within 3 to 12 hours, but it usually is delayed for a period of 1 to 14 days.

In patients with any type of *fatal CVA* there may be a rise of temperature, pulse rate, and respiratory rate several hours or days before death. These symptoms result from impairment of vital centers. Increase in depth of coma or lapse into coma also occurs. These symptoms indicate a collapse of the vasomotor and heat-regulating centers.

There are *two primary causes of death in stroke patients:* respiratory infection and brainstem failure. Somewhat less commonly, death results from associated cardiac disease. Impairment of consciousness, altered attention, and feeding and swallowing problems all predispose to pulmonary infections which frequently lead to death due to progressive hypoxia. Increasing intracranial pressure, central herniation, and brainstem hemorrhage lead to death from depression of the vital centers in the medulla.

DIAGNOSIS OF CEREBRAL VASCULAR DISEASE

Diagnostic methods that may be employed in the evaluation of a stroke typically include: skull x-ray, blood work (particularly WBC, blood urea nitrogen, blood sugar), urinalysis (obtained by catheterization only if necessary).

Examination of CSF is ordered when subarachnoid hemorrhage is suspected, but the danger of herniation must be recognized. Angiography is indicated especially when investigating transient ischemic attacks for diagnosis of cerebral hemorrhage, or for demonstrating intracranial aneurysms. Sometimes other procedures may be necessary, such as an EEG, echoencephalogram, radioisotope brain scan, CT scan, or cerebral angiography. Of course, physical (including neurologic) examinations are done.

It is important for the specific cause of a stroke to be identified, because treatment is directed at the cause and also because the prognosis varies with the cause.

Possible intracerebral hemorrhage must be ruled out before anticoagulant therapy is administered. The administration of an anticoagulant in the presence of hemorrhage would gravely worsen the hemorrhage by preventing clotting.

TABLE 27-4. DIAGNOSIS OF CEREBROVASCULAR DISORDERS

	Intracerebral Hemorrhage	Cerebral Thrombosis	Cerebral Embolism	Subarachnoid Hemorrhage	Vascular Malformation and Intracranial Bleeding
Onset	Generally during activity. Severe headache (if patient is able to report findings).	Prodromal episode of dizziness, aphasia, etc, often with improvement between attacks. Unrelated to activity.	Onset usually within seconds or minutes. No headache. Usually no prodrome. Unrelated to activity.	Sudden onset of severe headache unrelated to activity.	Sudden "stroke" in young patient. No headache. Unrelated to activity.
Course	Rapid hemiplegia and other phenomena over minutes to 1 hour.	Gradual progression over minutes to hours. Rapid improvement at times.	Rapid improvement may occur.	Variable; apt to be at worst in initial few days after onset.	Most critical period is usually in early stages.
History and related disorders	Suspect diagnosis especially if other hemorrhagic manifestations are present and in acute leukemia, aplastic anemia, thrombocytopenic purpura, and cirrhosis of the liver.	Evidence of arteriosclerosis, especially coronary, peripheral vessels, aorta. Associated disorders: diabetes mellitus, xanthomatosis.	Evidence of recent emboli: (1) other organs (spleen, kidneys, lungs), extremities, intestines; (2) several regions of brain in different cerebrovascular areas.	History of recurrent stiff neck, headaches, subarachnoid bleeding.	History of repeated subarachnoid hemorrhages, epilepsy.
Sensorium	Rapid progression to coma.	Relative preservation of consciousness.	Relative preservation of consciousness.	Relatively brief disturbance of consciousness.	Relatively brief disturbance of consciousness.
Neurologic examination	Focal neurologic signs or special arterial syndromes; nuchal rigidity.	Focal neurologic signs or special arterial syndromes.	Focal neurologic signs or special arterial syndromes	Focal neurologic signs frequently absent; nuchal rigidity, positive Kernig and Brudzinski signs.	Focal neurologic signs; cranial bruit.
Special findings	Hypertensive retinopathy, cardiac hypertrophy, and other evidences of hypertensive cerebrovascular disease may be present.	Evidence of arteriosclerotic cardiovascular disease frequently present.	Cardiac arrhythmias or infarction (source of emboli usually in the heart).	Subhyaloid (preretinal) hemorrhages.	Subhyaloid (preretinal) hemorrhages and retinal angioma.
Blood pressure	Arterial hypertension.	Arterial hypertension frequent.	Normotensive.	Arterial hypertension frequent.	Normotensive.
CSF	Grossly bloody.	Clear.	Clear.	Grossly bloody.	Grossly bloody.
Skull x-ray	Shift of pineal to opposite side.	Calcification of internal carotid artery siphon visible; shift of pineal to opposite side may occur.	Pineal apt to show little if any displacement.	Partial calcification of walls of aneurysm sometimes noted.	Characteristic calcifications in skull x-rays may be present.
Cerebral angiography	Hemorrhagic area seen as vascular zone surrounded by stretched and displaced arteries and veins.	Arterial obstruction or narrowing of circle of Willis (internal carotid, etc).	Arterial obstruction of circle of Willis branches (internal carotid, etc).	Typical aneurysmal pattern in circle of Willis arteries (internal carotid, middle cerebral, anterior cerebral, etc).	Characteristic pattern showing cerebral arteriovenous malformation.
Brain scan	May show increased uptake in affected cerebral area. Most marked in 2–3 weeks, with diminution or clearing thereafter.			Apt to be normal.	Increased uptake may be seen in area of arteriovenous malformation.
Echoencephalography	May show shift of midline toward opposite side in those patients with a cerebral lesion acting as a mass.				
Computerized tomography (CT)	May show area of hematoma, infarct, etc with distortion or shift of ventricles.				

From Chusid, J. G.: *Correlative Neuroanatomy & Functional Neurology,* 16th ed. Los Altos, Calif.: Lange Medical Publications, 1977.

CLINICAL CARE DURING ACUTE STAGE OF STROKE

The treatment of stroke is generally divided, for purposes of discussion, into care during the acute phase and care during the stage of recovery or convalescence. In the acute stage, or the period immediately following onset of the CVA, the clinical care is directed mainly at saving the patient's life. During the convalescent stage residual defects are treated and care is directed toward helping the patient function at the maximum of his or her capacity. Here we focus on the acute stage. See the section on hemiplegia (Chap. 26) for further discussion of the rehabilitative aspects of care.

First Aid for the Stroke Victim. (See also Chapter 95.) When a stroke occurs, the first consideration is to *maintain the patient's airway.* Loosen tight clothing to facilitate respirations and circulation to the head. Position an unconscious patient on the side that facilitates drainage to prevent aspiration of saliva. Care of the unconscious patient, including airway maintenance, is discussed in Chapter 26. The conscious patient may assume a position of comfort. Elevate the patient's head slightly to avoid exacerbation of increased intracranial pressure or headache. Start oxygen inhalation if the patient is cyanotic or appears to have difficulty breathing. Blood gas analysis needs to be done quickly. Keep the patient warm. Offer reassurance even though the patient may appear unable to hear you. Remember that the ability to hear is often maintained longer than may be apparent. Send for medical help at once and keep the patient quiet.

General Care. When the patient is admitted to the hospital the head is carefully examined for indications of external injury, and presence or absence of stiffness of the neck is noted. Temperature, pulse, respirations, and blood pressure are checked, as well as the optic disks and the size and reactions of the pupils. The odor of the patient's breath is noted, and examination is made to identify paralysis (particularly hemiplegia) and other focal neurologic symptoms. Examination of the comatose hemiplegic is discussed in Chapter 26.

Skilled nursing care is essential during this acute period while the patient is at complete bed rest. The patient is handled carefully to avoid injury. If a patient is unconscious or has increased intracranial pressure, appropriate care is given as discussed in Chapter 26. Let us summarize some essential points concerning general care of the patient following stroke:

Maintain patent, adequate airway and oxygenation. An artificial airway is usually inserted if stertorous respirations occur. At times, intubation is indicated. Frequent suctioning may be necessary. Oxygen administration may be prescribed.

Make frequent observations and take vital signs. Observe for symptoms of hyperthermia, shock, increasing intracranial pressure, seizures, and changes in level of consciousness. Specifically, make frequent observations and recordings concerning: pupillary reactions, posture, motor abilities (presence or absence of voluntary or involuntary movements, grip), loss of sensation or heightened sensation, pain, bulbar symptoms, respiratory symptoms, level of consciousness, stiffness or flaccidity of neck, vital signs, skin color, skin temperature, skin moistness or dryness, input and output, vomiting, incontinence, abdominal distention, and bladder distention.

Observe closely for signs of progression of either thrombosis or hemorrhage. Be particularly aware of changes in level of consciousness, progressive loss of motor and sensory function, progressive aphasia or increasing respiratory difficulty.

Ensure adequate fluid-electrolyte balance. For a few days fluids may be restricted in an attempt to reduce intracranial pressure. (See Chapter 12.) Intravenous feedings are typically given for the first several days. Then if the patient continues to be comatose or has impaired swallowing (dysphagia), tube feedings may be given. Maintain proper nutrition.

Maintain proper positioning and alignment; turn and reposition frequently; maintain muscle tone. (See discussions in Chapter 26). *Prevent complications of bed rest,* e.g., pneumonia, urinary stasis, contractures, decubitus ulcers and so forth.

> *Frequent changing of position is necessary. As soon as the patient responds to commands, encourage deep breathing and coughing each time the patient is turned. Start range-of-motion exercises for all extremities on day of admission.*

Maintain adequate elimination. A urinary catheter may be inserted initially when the patient is unconscious or stuporous. Later, bladder and bowel training is started. However, some physicians do not think a catheter should be inserted routinely merely to keep the bed dry, since a catheter makes retraining more difficult and is a primary cause of severe urinary tract infection. Some patients regain bladder control within 3 to 5 days. Thus, rather than catheterize for incontinence alone, catheterization is avoided unless it is necessary for other reasons. If a patient is not catheterized, the urinal or bedpan is offered every 2 hours, *day and night,* for the first 48 to 72 hours. For the male patient, an external device such as a *urosheath* may be used. If a catheter is inserted, a completely closed, sterile set-up is necessary and fluids are forced, to 3000 ml. per day unless contraindicated. Following removal of the catheter watch for *urinary retention.* Bladder and bowel retraining have been discussed in Chapter 26. The patient should be reassured that bowel and bladder control will probably improve daily.

Prevent constipation and impactions. (See Chapter 26.) It is important that the stroke patient *not strain at bowel movements,* because this increases intracranial and vascular pressures, which, in turn, encourages hemorrhage, rupture of aneurysms, and so forth. Be prepared for *fecal incontinence* during the early stages. Give frequent skin care to the incontinent patient to prevent skin breakdown.

Measure and record intake and output. See Chapter 12.

Include significant others in your plan of care. Let them help when possible, if they desire to do so, and help them to understand the patient's condition.

Provide a restful, quiet atmosphere and planned periods of rest. Do not attempt to awaken the lethargic patient except for necessary care, e.g., bedpan, neurologic testing, and so forth.

Administer medications as ordered. Antibiotics, medications to control blood pressure, and occasionally anticoagulants may be ordered. Avoid sedatives and tranquilizers if at all possible. Avoid opiates because they tend to depress respiratory centers and may obscure important observations.

Observe for visual and perceptual defects. Plan care accordingly.

Protect the patient's eye on the affected side. Irrigate with physiologic saline and instill artificial tears in affected eye prn. Cover with patch as necessary. An eye patch over one eye in people with diplopia can often make them more comfortable.

Give mouth care at least every 3 to 4 hours day and night. Give special attention to the paralyzed side of the tongue and mouth.

Prevent intellectual regression and disorientation. *Reorient the patient regaining consciousness, the confused, and the aphasic patient.* Establish communication with the aphasic patient.

Cerebrovascular diseases contribute to numerous *behavioral* as well as neurologic and physiologic deviations. Some of the associated behavioral changes that may follow a stroke are confusion, loss of memory, language disorders, and emotional lability. Behavioral changes may also accompany the problems of paralysis, and there may be changes in body image, sensation, vision and perception. (See appropriate sections in Chapter 26.) Cerebral edema may contribute to a patient's confusion for a while.

> *Empathetic understanding is necessary as the patient regains consciousness following a stroke.*

Imagine what it would be like to regain consciousness following a stroke and find that your right arm and leg are paralyzed and that you cannot talk to anyone about your situation. Perhaps you cannot even understand what is said to you. This *is* the plight of many hemiplegic aphasic persons.

The length of time that a patient must remain on bed rest following a stroke varies, depending on the preference of the physician and the underlying cerebrovascular disease. Some physicians believe patients should be mobilized early, whereas others prefer a rather prolonged course of bed rest. One fairly standard practice is to begin mobilization and active rehabilitation as soon as consciousness is regained if the cause of hemiplegia is from a cerebral thrombosis. If a cerebral hemorrhage has caused the stroke, the patient cannot begin active mobilization until the danger of rebleeding has become minimal. This may take at least 3 weeks and often longer.

Many hospitals now have intensive care units (ICU) for neurologic patients. These are areas where patients with strokes may be given intensive treatment during the acute phase of illness. It is important to help the patient and significant others to realize that such an area is not just for treatment, but also is designed to try to help the patient to avoid becoming more ill. The complexity of equipment and activity within an ICU may be frightening to the patient and significant others. Provide opportunities for questions and discussion, explain carefully what is being done, and give frequent reassurance and support.

The nurse caring for a person with a stroke realizes that *cardiovascular consideratains* are important during the patient's acute care for the following reasons:[226]

- ▶ Stroke patients have a relatively high incidence of *arteriosclerosis.*
- ▶ Stroke may be a complication of *heart disease.*
- ▶ Hemorrhagic strokes are generally associated with longstanding *hypertensive cardiovascular disease.*
- ▶ *Arrhythmias* may develop from pressure being exerted on those brainstem centers of importance in heart regulation.
- ▶ *Pulmonary emboli* are a relatively common complication in immobilized patients.

Thus, the nurse must be aware of the signs and symptoms of cardiac problems and know when and how to initiate emergency measures. (Cardiac disorders are discussed in Unit XII.)

Specific Treatment. Once a specific diagnosis is established, the physician institutes treatment based on the specific etiology. Let us first discuss treatment of a patient with a cerebral infarction resulting from thrombosis and embolism, followed by consideration of appropriate treatment of a patient with a cerebral hemorrhage.

Treatment of Cerebral Infarct (Thrombosis, Embolus)

The management of a recent cerebral infarct centers basically around attempts to: (a) maintain adequate perfusion of cerebral tissues with oxygenated blood; (b) support marginal tissue around the infarct; (c) stimulate restitution of function in those neurons in which the damage is reversible; and (d) prevent further clot formation or additional cerebral impairment. Recently additional attempts have been made to surgically remove existing clots and to reconstruct partially occluded arteries.

Treatment of cerebral infarct may be directed at:

- *Maintaining cerebral blood flow.* Bed rest, with careful monitoring of the patient's blood pressure and level of consciousness. Following the physician's specific orders.
- *Maintaining blood pressure and reducing any factors that acutely reduce cardiac output.* Maintenance of circulation, prevention of shock.
- *Correcting any conditions that may have precipitated the infarct,* e.g., treatment of myocardial infarction.
- *Reducing pooling of blood in the lower extremities* by applying elastic stockings.
- *Avoiding sudden postural changes.*
- *Preventing further clot formation. Anticoagulants,* e.g., Dicumarol and heparin, may be administered.

Many strokes progress in a fluctuating or stepwise pattern. Such *progressing strokes,* due to an enlarging cerebral thrombus with downstream propagation and embolization, are often called *strokes-in-evolution* or *strokes-in-progress.* Persons with these disorders may benefit from *immediate* anticoagulant therapy. It is thus important for physician and nurse to: (a) identify *early* those strokes due to thrombo-occlusive disease that develop gradually over several hours or days in a fluctuating or stepwise progression; (b) rapidly establish a diagnosis of thrombosis (and rule out intracranial hemorrhage); and (c) immediately institute appropriate anticoagulant therapy.[318]

Agreement has not been reached concerning how long *anticoagulant therapy** should be continued. However, the *appearance of signs of bleeding anywhere in the body* (e.g., gums, urine) *indicates that treatment should be reduced or stopped.* Monitor appropriate blood parameters. Parameters vary according to medications used and specific agency policies. Thus:

> *The nurse should watch for signs of bleeding when patients are on anticoagulant therapy.*

Also attempts have been made to *surgically* reestablish circulation to the brain by: (a) *removing clots* from thrombosed carotid or vertebral arteries, (b) *reconstructing arteries* that are partially or completely occluded, or (c) *bypassing the occluded portion of an artery* with a venous graft. It is debatable whether a fresh clot can be removed from a major vessel in time to prevent necrosis in the region of infarction. Vascular supply to a compromised hemisphere can be improved by an anastomosis of the superficial temporal artery to the middle cerebral artery. (Intracranial surgery is discussed in Chapter 28.)

An ideal long-term treatment goal is the prevention and alleviation of atherosclerosis. Indications of current research are that results of diet and use of various drugs to decrease blood cholesterol have been disappointing, especially in the elderly. However, in specific patients, dietary changes and drug therapy may achieve some of the desired results. (Atherosclerosis is discussed in Chapter 36).

*Anticoagulant therapy is discussed further in Unit XII.

Treatment of Intracerebral Hemorrhage

Goals of therapy are to: (1) preserve life; (b) minimize resultant disability; and (c) prevent recurrence. The clinical care specifically centers on:

- *Control of hyperthermia.* Often, mass intracerebral hemorrhages are accompanied by a rapid increase in temperature. A hypothermia blanket or ice packs may be indicated.
- *Control of seizures.* In cases complicated by seizures, diphenylhydantoin (Dilantin) may be given IV both in a loading dose and for daily maintenance. Intravenous barbituates and other sedatives should be avoided. (Seizures are discussed on p. 640.)
- *Treatment of hypertension* with methods appropriate for the particular patient. Usually diuretics and antihypertensive agents are used, and the patient's sodium intake is limited. (Hypertension is discussed in Chapter 37.)
- *Symptomatic treatment of delirium and restlessness.* Delirium can last for as long as 2 weeks. (The clinical management of delirium is discussed in Chapter 26). *Control of restlessness.* Make certain the patient is not restless from preventable reasons, e.g., full bladder. At times it may be necessary to administer chlorpromazine (Thorazine) intravenously in small doses. The nurse must bear in mind that this medication may also sedate the patient and mask changes in neurologic status.
- *Relief of headache and stiff neck.* Relief of pain may be accomplished in a variety of ways. It is desirable to *avoid use of narcotics with heavy sedating properties* (e.g., morphine or meperidine). Therefore, acetaminophen, alone or in combination with codeine, is frequently used. Avoid medications which sedate heavily and depress respirations. Obtaining adequate pain relief may relieve restlessness. Remember to use an appropriate range of nursing activities to help prevent or relieve pain, e.g., comfortable positioning.

> Five important symptoms that may foreshadow cerebral hemorrhage in a hypertensive patient are:
> 1. *Severe occipital (back of head) or nuchal (nape of neck) headaches*
> 2. *Vertigo (dizziness) or syncope (fainting)*
> 3. *Motor or sensory disturbances (e.g., tingling, paresthesias, transient paralysis)*
> 4. *Nosebleeds*
> 5. *Retinal hemorrhages*
>
> *Report such symptoms so that prophylactic measures can be employed.*

- Prevention of straining, e.g., straining at stool, excessive coughing, vomiting, lifting, or use of arms to change position. Avoid constipation by the use of stool softeners and mild laxatives. Prevent aspiration, choking, excessive coughing, and vomiting by withholding oral fluids and food for 24 to 48 hours. When the patient is able to swallow adequately, begin with clear liquids and progress to a soft diet as the patient can tolerate.
- *Provision for rest and quiet.* During the acute phase following intracerebral hemorrhage, the patient is typically kept in bed as long as the presence of stiff neck, headache, and prostration require. Some physicians believe that moderate sedation, antihypertensive drugs, and bed rest should be continued for 10 to 14 days, or longer if indicated.
- *Reduction of increased intracranial pressure.* Measures which aid in the control of increased intracranial pressure include *elevating the head* of the bed. *Steroids* are usually administered, but their effectiveness in controlling increased intracranial pressure has not been definitely established. In selected cases, the physician may choose to establish *external ventriculostomy drainage* for 2 to 3 days for temporary relief of pressure.
- *Operative removal of blood clot.* Whether or not to operate on a patient who has had an intracerebral hemorrhage, and when to operate, are widely debated topics. In carefully selected persons this surgery may be lifesaving and may reduce the neurological deficit. Patients who have massively increased intracranial pressure are frequently not considered as operative candidates. Surgery is also not contemplated when angiography shows that severe vasospasm is still present.

Summary of Basic Treatment of Strokes During Acute Phase:

Remember that treatment hinges on a specific diagnosis of the cause of the stroke. Once this is established, proper treatment — directed at that cause — is provided. Basically, treatment may include:

- *Anticoagulants* for stroke resulting from infarction (thrombus, embolus). These are given to slow the blood's coagulation time, with the goal of preventing further clot formation. Anticoagulants are given only if hemorrhage has been ruled out.
- *Medications* may also be given to reduce dangerously high *blood pressure,* or to elevate alarmingly low blood pressure.
- *Surgery* may be employed on selected persons to remove clots, or to correct an atherosclerotic stenosis of one of the great vessels in the neck.

CARE AFTER THE ACUTE STAGE

The preceding section of this chapter has dealt primarily with the nursing and medical attention needed by people during the acute stage of stroke. As discussed earlier, the people involved face difficult tasks when the acute stages have passed and residual disabilities become obvious (see p. 610). The energy of a multidisciplinary rehabilitative team may be a helpful approach to assist and support people during this time. Assessing functional abilities of the patient and setting rehabilitative goals are part of this approach. (Always remember that goals are more likely to be met if the people involved participate in setting the goals.)

The kinds of tasks the patient and significant others face include:

- Learning to use strengths and abilities that are intact to compensate for impaired functions.
- Learning to become independent in activities of daily living, e.g., bathing, dressing, eating.
- Developing behavior patterns that are likely to prevent the recurrence of symptoms, e.g., taking prescribed medications, stopping smoking, reducing day-to-day stress, modifying diet

Considerable teaching, support, and encouragement are often needed. Specific teaching may include information about the physiologic changes that have occurred as well as the kinds of services and appliances that are available and may be helpful. (Information of this kind is available from associations and foundations, e.g., American Heart Association. See Fig. 26–31.) Support and encouragement involve allowing the patient and significant others to express their fears and disappointments and their joys and successes. Always remember that it is as important to be able to share the positive experiences of life as it is to be able to share the negative.

> *People whose lives have been affected by stroke are helped more by professionals who build on their strengths and assets rather than concentrate on weaknesses and limitations.*

Transient Cerebral Ischemic Attacks

Transient ischemic attacks ("little strokes", TIA's) are *brief, reversible* episodes of neurologic dysfunction caused by a temporary focal cerebral ischemia. TIA's are also called "intermittent cerebrovascular insufficiency." The basic abnormality common to all patients with TIA's is a *transient* decrease in delivery of blood to a focal area of the cerebrum or brainstem. Numerous factors can cause this ischemia.

Occlusive disease of the extracranial cerebral vessels is the most common cause of TIA's, as with cerebrovascular accidents, although there are other causes. The most frequent site of this occlusion is the origin of the internal carotid artery. However, lesions may also occur at the origin of the common carotid or vertebral arteries.

The *symptoms* vary, depending upon which area of the brain is ischemic. Examples of the types of symptoms produced by TIA's are: visual, auditory, or vestibular disturbances; various motor and sensory disturbances; headache; slowing of mental processes; or seizures.

Generally TIA's last only minutes (often 2 to 10 minutes) to an hour. Occasionally they may last only a few seconds or as long as 24 hours. While the attacks are frequently recurrent, some patients have only one or two TIA's. TIA's may occur for as long as 2 years prior to cerebral infarction, or clusters of TIA's may first appear only a few hours or days before cerebral infarction occurs. Between attacks a patient's neurologic examination is generally entirely normal.

> *TIA's are warning signs and must not be ignored. It is important that they be fully investigated.*

Four important investigations in the *diagnosis* of TIA's involving the internal carotid artery are: (1) stethoscopic examination for bruits; (2) ophthalmodynamometry, i.e., indirect measurement of pressure in the retinal artery; (3) angiographic studies of intracranial and extracranial blood vessels; and (4) Doppler determinations of cerebral blood flow.

Vascular surgery or anticoagulation may prevent fatal attacks in some patients who have TIA's. At the present time *surgical treatment* is available only for obstructive lesions within the extracranial vessels. The procedure most commonly performed is *endarterectomy,* i.e., surgical removal of the thickened areas of the innermost lining of the affected artery. Signs of cranial nerve injury following carotid endarterectomy are presented in Fig. 27–10. Surgery is most successfully performed before a stenotic artery has become completely occluded.

Anastomosis of the superficial temporal artery to the middle cerebral artery is also useful in certain persons. Those patients who are unable to have surgery may benefit from prolonged *anticoagulant therapy* in an attempt to: (1) reduce the incidence of emboli; (2) prevent thrombus formation; and (3) alter blood coagulation factors or reduce blood sludging. Not all persons are candidates for anticoagulant therapy. Patients are selected cautiously for this therapy to prevent hemorrhagic complications. In current practice, the patient with TIA's is often treated with a combination of *aspirin* and *Persantin,* which inhibits platelet aggregation and has been useful in preventing progression of symptoms.

Intracranial Aneurysms and Primary Subarachnoid Hemorrhage

Statistics indicate that approximately 10 per cent of all cerebrovascular lesions result from ruptured aneurysms occurring in one of the major vessels that lie within the subarachnoid space. *This serious condition is the cause of death in over 50 per cent of all fatal cerebrovascular lesions in patients under age 45.* While the symptoms resulting from bleeding in the subarachnoid space can occur at any age, they most commonly occur between the ages of 35 and 65. Thus, this condition typically affects a younger population than most strokes. (Incidence is slightly higher in women than in men.)

Etiology. Hemorrhage into the subarachnoid space has a variety of causes. Probably the most common cause is *trauma* to the head, in which meningeal vessels are ruptured. *Spontaneous hemorrhage* into the subarachnoid space may be associated with blood dyscrasias, primary or metastatic intracranial tumors, vascular anomalies (such as angiomas or arteriovenous malformations), infections of the CNS, or intracerebral hemorrhages that spread to the subarachnoid space. However, *the most common cause of spontaneous subarachnoid hemorrhage is leaking or rupture of an aneurysm in the subarachnoid space.* Therefore, the discussion to follow will focus on this problem.

The *berry aneurysm* (congenital saccular aneurysm) is the most common type of aneurysm of the brain's blood vessels. This type of aneurysm is characterized by an outpouching of the arterial wall, usually at the bifurcation of a vessel, with a "neck" or narrowed portion attaching to the vessel itself. It is a commonly accepted theory that an aneurysm *results from* the combination of (1) a congenital defect in the middle layer of the vessel wall, (2) degenerative changes in the vessel wall at the same site, and (3) the constant stress caused by the force of the flow of blood, particularly at a bifurcation. The internal carotid artery is the most common *site* for these aneurysms. The

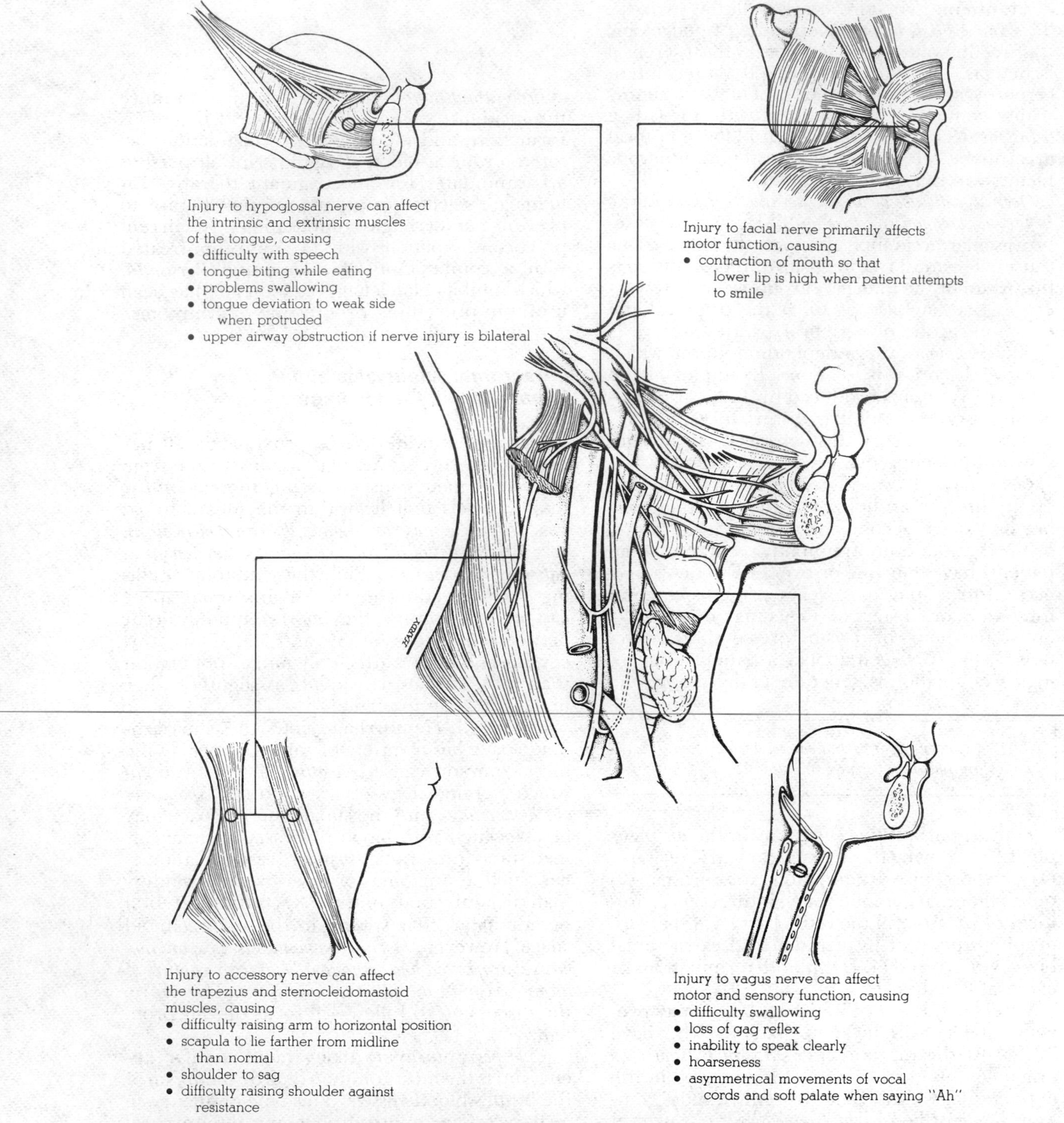

Figure 27–10. Signs of cranial nerve injury following carotid endarterectomy. (From Webb, P. H.: Neurological deficit after carotid endarterectomy. *American Journal of Nursing*, 79:655, Apr. 1979, p. 655.)

next most frequent sites are the anterior cerebral and anterior communicating arteries, followed by the middle cerebral artery. Aneurysms arising from the vertebral-basilar system make up only 10 to 15 per cent of all cerebral aneurysms.

Symptoms. Intracranial aneurysms produce symptoms in two ways. They may produce symptoms *by compression of surrounding brain tissue or cranial nerves.* For instance, an aneurysm of the anterior communicating or anterior cerebral artery may compress the optic nerve, causing unilateral impairment of vision, or an aneurysm of the posterior communicating artery may cause paralysis of the third cranial nerve, with diplopia and a dilated pupil.

However, most often an aneurysm produces no symptoms until it *ruptures, causing the classic symptom of subarachnoid hemorrhage.* Aside from the occasional premonitory signs of mild headache, confusion, fainting or vertigo, the onset of symptoms is sudden. The patient will complain of a sudden onset of severe headache ("the worst I've ever had"), usually in the occipital area and often accompanied by vomiting. The patient may lose consciousness immediately or may initially present with confusion and lethargy and progress to coma within hours of the onset of the symptoms. Generalized seizures may occur. The patient often develops signs of meningeal irritation, such as stiff neck and back and leg pain, due to irritation of the meninges by the blood in the subarachnoid space. Focal neurologic deficits include cranial nerve involvement, usually the third and sixth cranial nerves, and motor weakness, usually monoparesis or hemiparesis.

Grading. Several methods have been developed for grading aneurysmal patients. Grading has important implications when considering treatment and prognosis. One commonly used *grading system* is:

Grade I — (minimal bleeding) alert, no neurologic deficit.
Grade II — (mild bleeding) alert, minimal neurologic deficit such as third nerve palsy, stiff neck.
Grade III — (moderate bleeding) drowsy or confused, stiff neck, with or without neurologic deficit.
Grade IV — (moderate to severe bleeding) semicoma, with or without neurologic deficit.
Grade V — (severe bleeding) coma and decerebrate movements.

Patients over 50 years of age are classified one grade higher than their signs indicate.

In general, grade I and II patients are considered reasonable operative risks; grade III patients are less optimal risks; and grade IV and V patients are rarely considered suitable for surgery. Prognosis varies from good to grave as the patient progresses from grades I to IV.

Diagnosis. Diagnosis of subarachnoid hemorrhage is usually established on the basis of clinical presentation and the physical signs and symptoms present. A *lumbar puncture* is usually done to confirm the presence of blood in the subarachnoid space, although great caution must be used when the patient shows signs of increased intracranial pressure. There are great variations in the pressure, color, and cell content of the CSF, depending on the timing of the lumbar puncture in relation to the hemorrhage.

Although various other procedures such as skull x-rays and echoencephalography may be ordered, *angiography* is the definitive diagnostic test. It is important that a four-vessel study be done to provide adequate visualization of both the carotid circulation and the vertebral-basilar circulation. The angiogram will usually demonstrate: the structure and location of the aneurysm(s), what vessels are supplying it, whether there is an intracerebral clot, and whether there is vasospasm of any vessels surrounding the aneurysm or distant from it. There is controversy among physicians as to the timing of angiograms. Some feel that angiography should be done immediately, while others feel that it should be delayed until the patient's condition stabilizes. (See Chapter 25 for further information on cerebral angiography.)

When it is readily available, *computerized tomography* may also be a valuable tool in diagnosis. Because it is a safe, noninvasive procedure, it may sometimes precede angiography in the diagnostic work-up. It is of particular value in identifying large aneurysm, intracerebral clots, and large clots surrounding an aneurysm.

Complications and Clinical Care. Two common problems following subarachnoid hemorrhage may complicate the patient's condition and the subsequent treatment plan. These are vasospasm and hydrocephalus.

- ▶ *Vasospasm* is a temporary narrowing of the lumen of a vessel, the actual cause of which is still unknown and is the subject of much ongoing research. Spasm usually occurs in the vessel adjacent to the ruptured aneurysm and may spread throughout all the major vessels at the base of the brain. It produces symptoms of ischemia, and, if extensive and prolonged, results in infarction and permanent neurologic deficit. To date no effective treatment for vasospasm exists.

- ▶ *Hydrocephalus* is caused by blood in the subarachnoid space, which prevents adequate circulation of CSF. It is often seen in the acute stage and contributes to symptoms of increased intracranial pressure. It may be treated by short-term external ventriculostomy to help decrease intracranial pressure, but will often resolve spontaneously. It may develop again after several weeks, this time developing more slowly and presenting with symptoms of dementia and ataxia. Treatment for chronic hydrocephalus is usually a ventriculo-peritoneal or ventriculo-atrial shunt (see Figs. 27–11 and 27–12).

The *care* and *treatment* of the patient with subarachnoid hemorrhage from a ruptured intracranial aneurysm presents a most difficult challenge for the neurologist or neurosurgeon and for the nurse. The *goals* are to help the patient

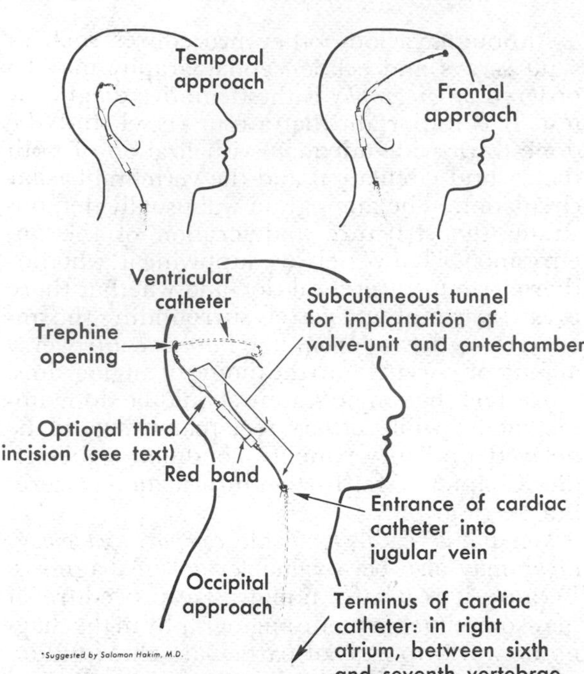

Figure 27–11. Diagram of placement of a Hakim ventriculo-atrial shunt. (From Rhodes, M. J., B. J. Gruendemann, and W. F. Ballinger: *Alexander's Care of the Patient in Surgery,* 6th ed. St. Louis: C. V. Mosby Co., 1978, p. 813.)

survive the effects of the hemorrhage and to prevent rebleeding. Generally the goals are pursued with conservative medical management, although at times early surgical intervention is indicated.

Nonoperative management is the treatment of choice for patients of grades IV and V, whose general condition is critical and who would not benefit from a surgical procedure, or for patients of grade III until their condition has stabilized sufficiently to make surgery possible. Grade I and II patients are more frequently offered *surgical intervention* at some point in their care. Whether this treatment should be offered early in the acute phase or delayed until later is a subject of controversy among neurosurgeons.

Acutely, the patient is kept at complete bed rest, with the head of the bed elevated 20 to 30 degrees, in a quiet environment for a period of 3 to 4 weeks. Vital signs are carefully checked, as frequently as the instability of the patient's condition dictates, with special attention to blood pressure. The patient's respiratory status is assessed frequently, and adequate oxygenation is provided to avoid anoxic cerebral damage or cerebral edema caused by build up of carbon dioxide. Every effort is made to avoid rectal stimulation or straining at stool, which may contribute to increased intracranial pressure. Bowels are managed with stool softeners and mild laxatives. Adequate nutrition and hydration are provided via intravenous or tube feeding. Moderate restriction of fluids is usually ordered.

Special attention is given to arterial blood pressure. An elevated pressure may contribute to further bleeding from the ruptured aneurysm, yet sufficient pressure must be maintained to assure adequate perfusion of cerebral vessels, especially in the presence of vasospasm. This is a delicate balance to maintain. It is the nurse's responsibility to monitor the pressure carefully, to administer hypotensive agents with caution, and to be alert to any changes in the status of the patient, especially decreasing level of consciousness or progressing motor weakness.

> *After an aneurysm ruptures, a clot forms at the site of the hemorrhage, and for a few days rebleeding is prevented. As the clot begins to dissolve, the chance of rebleeding increases, with the greatest risk of rebleeding occurring at about the seventh day.*

In recent years, many physicians have advocated the use of *antifibrinolytic agents* in an attempt to prevent lysis of the clot and thus reduce the risk of rebleeding. Epsilon-aminocaproic acid (EACA, Amicar) is the agent most commonly used. Early studies have shown a reduction in the incidence of rebleeding when this drug is used alone and in combination with hypotensive agents. The drug may be given orally or parenterally in carefully calculated dosages to maintain an effective level over a 2 to 3 week period. The use of the drug is contraindicated in the presence of some coagulation disorders. Careful nursing assessment of neuro signs is essential.

Increased intracranial pressure, resulting from cerebral edema, intracranial hematoma, hydrocephalus, or various other factors, accompanies subarachnoid hemorrhage. Among the nonoperative measures to help decrease this pressure are fluid restriction, administration of dexamethasone (Decadron), the cautious use of osmotic agents, and measures such as elevating the head of the bed 20 to 30 degrees, and adequate pulmonary toilet (to prevent increased pCO_2).

Other aspects of treatment in nonoperative management are mostly *symptomatic.* Prophylactic anticonvulsants are usually begun to prevent seizures; diphenylhydantoin (Dilantin) is the drug of choice. Headache and neck pain are relieved as much as possible with analgesics. Narcotics are avoided since they may depress respirations and may mask symptoms of changing status. Codeine may be prescribed if the pain is severe. An elevated temperature often follows subarachnoid hemorrhage. Every effort, including the use of the cooling mattress, should be made to return the temperature to normal.

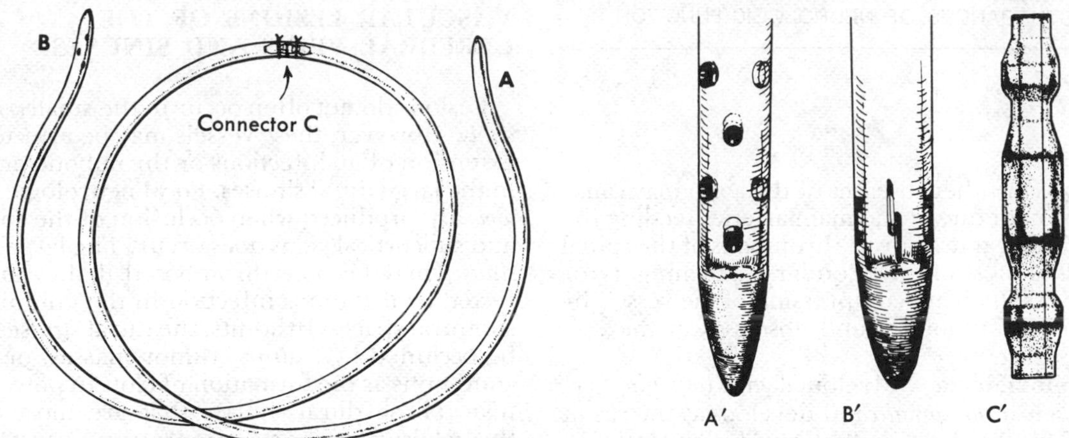

Figure 27–12. Detailed views of the Hakim ventriculo-atrial shunt. Shunt is made from silicone tubing and consists of three parts: (*A*) cardiac tube with slit valve in side wall near the tip, (*B*) ventricular tube with side perforations, and (*C*) nylon connector. Slit valve is designed to allow cerebrospinal fluid to flow freely when pressure in the tube exceeds the predetermined pressure specified by the manufacturer for the particular model used. When intraventricular pressure falls below the specified level, valve slits remain closed and prevent escape of fluid. (From Rhodes, M. J., B. J. Gruendemann, and W. F. Ballinger: *Alexander's Care of the Patient in Surgery,* 6th ed. St. Louis: C. V. Mosby Co., 1978.)

VASCULAR LESIONS OF THE SPINAL CORD

Blood is supplied to the spinal cord via three major routes: the anterior and posterior spinal arteries and the radicular arteries (Fig. 27–13). The anterior spinal artery is the major vessel supplying most of the cross-sectional area of the cord. The posterior spinal arteries nourish the posterior white columns and part of the posterior gray. The various branches of the radicular arteries supply the superficial areas of the white matter. A complex venous system drains the cord and empties into four major channels: the anterior and posterior spinal veins, located in the midline anteriorly and posteriorly, and the two lateral veins.

Vascular lesions of the spinal cord are similar to those occurring in the brain in that they may be *caused by* rupture, thrombosis, or embolism of the blood vessels supplying the spinal cord. Trauma is the usual cause of *hemorrhage* into the spinal cord or its covering. *Embolism* of the spinal vessels rarely occurs. Unlike the cerebral blood vessels, arteriosclerosis of the spinal vessels is not a common cause of *thrombosis.* Although arterio-

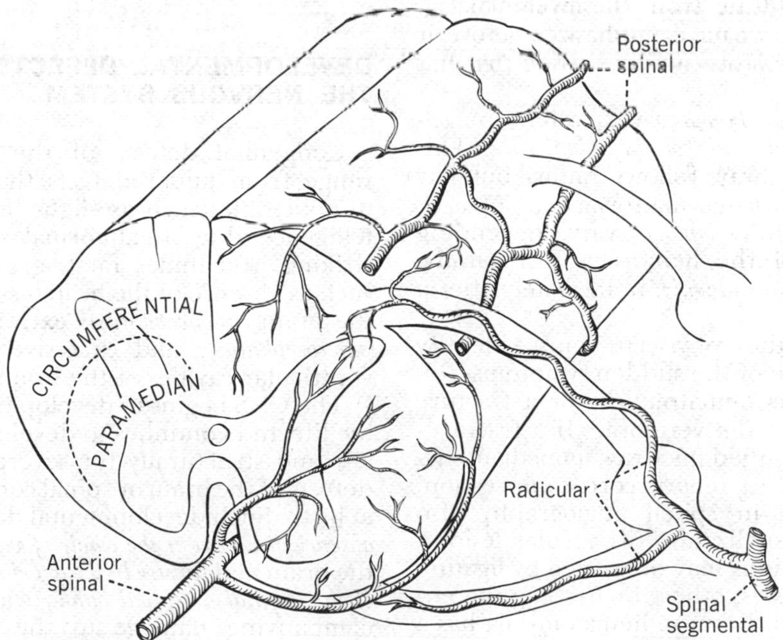

Figure 27–13. Arterial supply to the spinal cord. (From Patton, H. D., et al.: *Introduction to Basic Neurology.* Philadelphia: W. B. Saunders Co., 1976, p. 385.)

sclerosis or other diseases of the aorta may cause occlusion of one of the main arteries feeding the spinal cord at its source, thrombosis of the spinal vessels is most often secondary to meningitis, or else it results from compression of the vessels by tumors, granulomas, and abscesses in the epidural space.

Myelomalacia. Myelomalacia *(softening or infarction of the spinal cord)* develops as the result of *occlusion* of the spinal artery. Myelomalacia is a serious condition and has a poor prognosis because there is usually little or no return of function to the involved areas. The diagnosis is presumed whenever there is the *sudden* appearance of symptoms of a transverse myelitis.

The *symptoms* of myelomalacia vary, depending upon the level of the infarction. For example, a cervical level occlusion produces *sudden* quadriplegia. Occlusion at the thoracic level produces similar symptoms except that the arms are not affected. Involvement at the level of the lumbar spine results in paraplegia, disturbed bladder and bowel function, and impaired pain and temperature sensation. (See Chapter 26.)

The *treatment* of myelomalacia is two-pronged: one aspect is concerned with the symptomatic care of the problems resulting from the cord lesion, e.g., the paralysis, loss of sensation; the other is directed at treatment of the disease that caused the vascular lesion in the first place. Treatment of the cause of the condition does not produce any significant degree of improvement in symptoms resulting from the myelomalacia. This is because, as we have emphasized before, it is impossible to restore nervous tissue that has been destroyed.

Hematomyelia. *Hematomyelia* refers to *hemorrhage into the substance of the spinal cord.* This condition almost always follows trauma, but may be traceable to a vascular malformation or bleeding disorder. The *symptoms* vary, depending upon the size of the hemorrhage. Typically, symptoms develop *suddenly,* immediately after a spinal injury.

Diagnostically the physician must identify whether the cause of the sudden symptoms (following trauma) is hematomyelia or a fracture and dislocation of the vertebrae. If a fracture-dislocation is identified on x-ray, immediate surgery is indicated to relieve cord compression. Recent advances in spinal angiography also make possible visualization of vascular lesions. Some of these lesions may be treated by ligating their feeding vessels, others by excising the entire malformation. Because hematomyelia has a better prognosis for spontaneous return of function than does myelomalacia, rehabilitative care is highly important.

VASCULAR LESIONS OF THE CEREBRAL VEINS AND SINUSES

Lesions do not often occur in the small *cerebral veins.* However, these vessels may be affected by extension of an infectious or thrombotic process in the large dural sinuses. Focal neurologic *symptoms* are produced when occlusion of the cortical and subcortical veins does occur. The large *dural sinuses* may become thrombosed if they are infected or if there is infection in the epidural or subdural spaces. In adults, the dural sinuses may be occluded by trauma, tumor masses, or such conditions as the formation of clots in polycythemia. Those dural sinuses that are most often thrombosed are the superior sagittal, lateral, and cavernous.

The *superior sagittal sinus* is less commonly affected by an infective thrombosis than either the lateral or cavernous sinus. Thrombosis of the *lateral sinus* is generally secondary to otitis media and mastoiditis; however, it rarely occurs today, owing to effective antibiotic treatment of these conditions.

Cavernous sinus thrombosis typically occurs secondary to suppurative processes in the orbit, nasal sinuses, or upper half of the face. The infection commonly first involves one sinus and then rapidly spreads to the opposite side. Symptoms of a septic thrombosis occur suddenly. The patient is acutely ill, has a septic kind of febrile reaction, and has pain in the eye. Visual acuity may or may not be affected, and pupillary reactions may or may not be preserved. The pupils may be small or dilated; the corneae are cloudy and corneal ulcers may develop. Although fatal until recently, this condition may now be treated with antibiotics, and possibly anticoagulants.

DEVELOPMENTAL DEFECTS OF THE NERVOUS SYSTEM

Congenital defects of the nervous system range from minor defects that are practically unnoticeable (such as slight impairment of intelligence due to abnormal development) to striking, sometimes fatal, gross abnormalities, such as absence of the head *(acrania);* absence of the brain *(anencephalus);* extremely small brain *(microcephalus);* and excessive enlargement of ventricular cavities of the brain *(hydrocephalus).*

The CNS begins to develop early in intrauterine life and continues to develop both functionally and structurally for several years. Various defects of the brain or spinal cord may be present at birth. Such developmental defects include the *absence of a part or the whole of various structures* of the brain and *failure in the development of or closure of the cranial or spinal bones,* with or without accompanying damage to the brain or spinal cord.

Syringomyelia is believed to be a developmental disorder. The condition is discussed in the following section, "Degenerative Disorders of the Nervous System," because of its progressive, degenerative nature.

Developmental defects are discussed more completely in pediatrics and neurologic textbooks.

Hydrocephalus

Hydrocephalus refers to an abnormal accumulation of CSF in the cranial vault. This condition most frequently occurs in infants. Since the bones of the skull are not fused together in the infant, the pressure of the accumulating fluid forces the head to actually enlarge, sometimes tremendously, and the forehead to become prominent (Fig. 27–14). Adults have no cranial enlargement with hydrocephalus because the cranium is fixed in size and cannot "give." In both infants and adults, the mounting pressure caused by excess fluid within the skull squeezes the brain tissue against the skull, causing tissue atrophy and tissue death, seizures, and intellectual impairment.

Hydrocephalus present at birth is called *congenital, primary,* or *chronic hydrocephalus. Secondary* or *acute hydrocephalus* may result from meningitis (e.g., tubercular meningitis), obstruction of the brain's venous outflow, or spread of the inflammation of otitis media from the ear to the cranial cavity.

Various *surgical procedures* have been developed to treat hydrocephalus by implanting artificial drains in the brain and creating new paths of circulation for the cerebrospinal fluid. For example, silicone tubes or tubes of various other compositions may be placed from the brain ventricle, behind the ear, and down the neck under the skin. Finally, the tube is spliced into the jugular vein where the fluid can drain into the circulating blood.

Spina Bifida

Spina bifida is a term used to cover a wide range of closure defects that generally occur in the lower lumbar region. A minor defect may occur only in the bony vertebral arches; however, in a more severe defect, the meninges or the meninges along with the spinal cord are displaced backward, although the defect remains covered with skin.

A *meningocele* (protruding sac of meninges) or a *meningomyelocele* (protruding sac containing meninges, spinal cord, and roots) may occur with spina bifida, as elements in the spinal canal balloon out through the defect. In the latter unfortunate condition, the infant is generally paralyzed in both motor and sensory spheres below the level of the deformity. Neural control of bladder and bowel function is also typically absent. Additionally, the protruding sac, con-

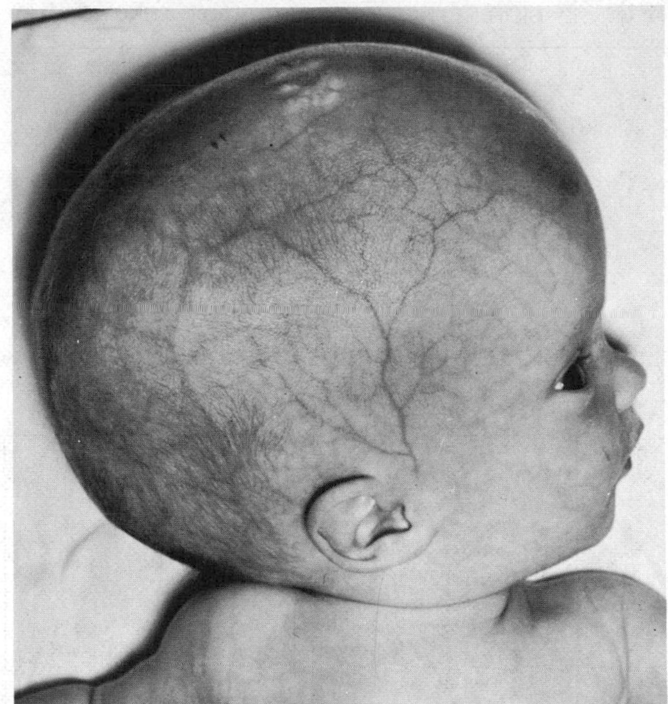

A

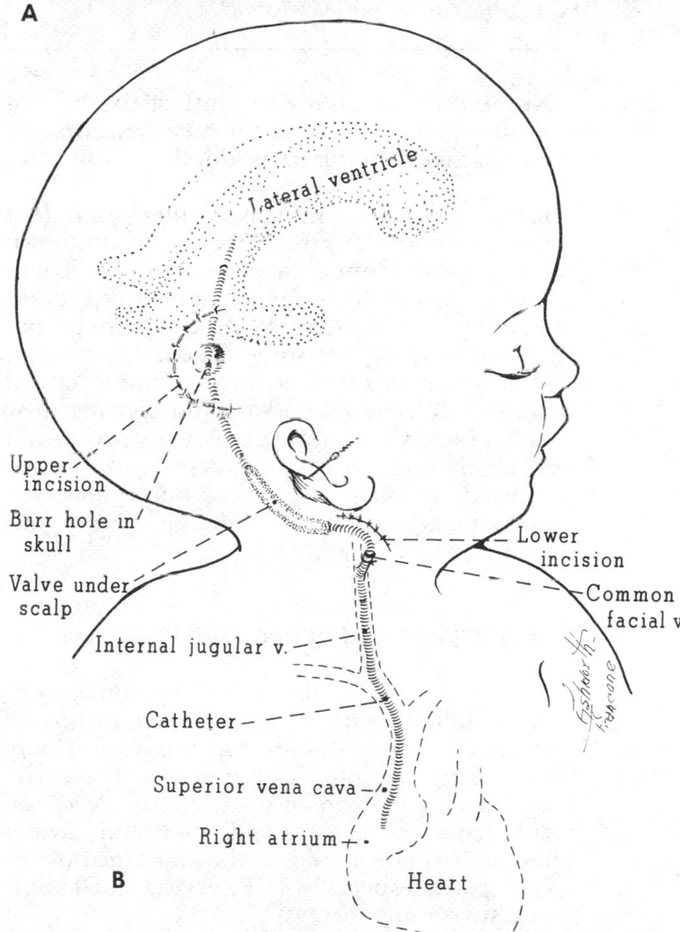

Figure 27–14. A. Child, age 4 months, with hydrocephalus. **B.** Operative procedure for hydrocephalus, in which a catheter drains the ventricular system into the right atrium. (From Jacob, S. W., C. A. Francone, and W. J. Lossow: *Structure and Function in Man,* 4th ed. Philadelphia: W. B. Saunders Co., 1978.)

taining CSF, is often dangerously fragile and infection is possible, producing fatal meningitis.

DEGENERATIVE DISORDERS OF THE NERVOUS SYSTEM

Outline of Degenerative Disorders of the Nervous System

A. *Syringomyelia and syringobulbia*
B. *Extrapyramidal disorders*
   1. *Huntington's chorea*
   2. *Parkinson's disease*
C. *Amyotrophic lateral sclerosis (ALS, motor-system disease)*
D. *Myasthenia gravis*
E. *Progressive muscular dystrophies*

Numerous conditions that affect the central nervous system have unknown causes. Most of those discussed in this section fall into this category.

Research may some day demonstrate that some disorders that are currently of unknown etiology result from damage caused by exogenous or endogenous toxins or genetically conditioned metabolic defects. Recently there has been speculation that some chronic diseases of the nervous system (e.g., amyotrophic lateral sclerosis, multiple sclerosis) could be caused by slow viruses. Currently there is no proof that any degenerative neurologic disease in humans is caused by such organisms, but research is underway which may eventually prove differently.

Syringomyelia and Syringobulbia

Syringomyelia is a disease of the spinal cord and medulla of unknown origin, characterized by muscular weakness and wasting, various sensory defects, symptoms of injury to the cord's long tracts, and trophic disturbances. *Symptoms* result from the presence of abnormal cavities filled with yellow liquid in the substance of the spinal cord, especially the cervical cord. Scar tissue surrounds the cysts.

Syringobulbia refers specifically to the presence of similar cavities in the medulla oblongata. Such cavities may occur only in the medulla (without involving the spinal cord), but they more frequently occur in combination with cervical syringomyelia. Typical symptoms of syringobulbia are atrophy and fibrillation of the tongue, loss of pain and temperature sense in one or both sides of the face, nystagmus, respiratory stridor or dysphonia.

Syringomyelia is believed to be a *developmental anomaly* since it is fairly often associated with other developmental defects. Symptoms may begin at any age but most often occur at ages 30 to 40. Symptom onset is insidious. With cervical syringomyelia the early symptoms often include: atrophy, weakness, and fibrillations of the small muscles of the hands; loss of pain sense in the fingers or forearm; weakness and atrophy of the muscles of the shoulder girdle; Horner's syndrome; nystagmus; and vasomotor and trophic disturbances of the upper extremities. Although there is segmental loss or impairment of the sensibility for pain and temperature, there is preservation of sensibility for light touch. Segments of sensory loss may be separated by zones of normal sensibility. Spasticity, ataxia, or paralysis of the lower extremities may occur as well as disturbed bladder control.

Cranial nerve involvement may introduce additional problems, e.g., impairment of pain and temperature sense in the face, loss of the corneal reflex (necessitating protection of the eye), dysphagia, dysarthria, laryngeal stridor (which may necessitate tracheotomy to enable normal respiration), nystagmus, and atrophy and fibrillation of the tongue muscles.

Kyphosis (i.e., abnormally increased convexity in curvature of the thoracic spine when viewed from the side, referred to as "humpback" by lay persons) and *scoliosis* (i.e., a noticeable lateral deviation in the normally straight vertical line of the spine) often occur in syringomyelia, along with club foot. Charcot joints occur more frequently with syringomyelia than with tabes dorsalis.

The *course* of syringomyelia is a progressive one. However, it may remain stationary for many years. Some patients live 40 years after onset. In others the disease is rapidly progressive, causing incapacitation (from paralysis or sensory defects) or death with a few years. Refer to p. 521 for discussion of the *personal impact* of neurologic problems and *supportive care.*

No effective treatment exists for syringomyelia or syringobulbia. X-ray treatment has been recommended to the affected areas of the cord, but has not been successful in preventing further damage. Surgical drainage of the cystic cavity after laminectomy (see Chapter 28) may be beneficial, especially when a complete subarachnoid block exists. In such cases, incising and evacuating the contents of the cavity may relieve pressure on the cord. Symptomatic treatment is given to Charcot joints, sores, felons, and so forth. The patient is instructed to be particularly careful of analgesic areas of the body to prevent injury, e.g., chafing of the skin, ulceration, burns.

The *extrapyramidal system* is that system which indirectly influences motor activity. It is responsible for integration and coordination of voluntary movement. Although technically incorrect, the term "extrapyramidal system" is restricted in clinical use to denote the components of the basal ganglia and related subcortical nuclei that influence motor activity. Extrapyramidal disorders are characterized by abnormal involuntary movements (dyskinesias), disturbances in bodily posture, and changes in muscle tone. We consider two extrapyramidal disorders in this section: Huntington's chorea, and Parkinson's disease.

HUNTINGTON'S CHOREA

Huntington's chorea is also called Huntington's disease or chronic progressive chorea. Huntington's chorea is a hereditary disease of the basal ganglia and cerebral cortex that typically appears in adult life. The disorder is distinguished by the triad of *dominant inheritance, choreoathetosis,* and *progressive dementia.*

In large medical centers, Huntington's chorea is one of the most frequently seen of the *hereditary diseases* of the nervous system. It is transmitted as an autosomal dominant trait. Both sexes are affected, with a slightly higher incidence in males, and the disease may be transmitted by either sex. Almost 50 per cent of offspring inherit the disorder. The usual age of onset is the fourth or fifth decade, although it may be found occasionally in younger ages, some even in childhood. Huntington's chorea is a relentlessly progressive disease, leading to inevitable debility and death.

Pathologically, Huntington's chorea is characterized by degenerative changes in the caudate nuclei and putamen, usually accompanied by cortical atrophy of the gyri of the frontal and temporal lobes. The exact *cause* of the degenerative process is not known. There has been much research recently into the biochemical changes accompanying the disease. There appears to be a deficiency in the GABA (gamma-aminobutyric acid) inhibitory system in the basal ganglia, which leads in turn to a relative excess in the dopaminergic system. It is this dopamine excess that leads to the typical movements of the disease.

Symptoms. Presenting *indications* of Huntington's disease are emotional disturbances, mental deterioration, and choreiform movements. These three components may appear in any order. The mental deterioration may be very subtle at first, with only slight changes in character, but progresses as the patient becomes negative, suspicious and irritable. Gradual loss of self-control may be evidenced by outbursts of temper and by sexual promiscuity. Intellect begins to fail, and attention and memory are poor. Severe mood swings are common. Eventually the patient may become totally demented, unkempt, incontinent, and completely helpless.

The abnormal movements, which may or may not precede the mental and emotional deterioration, are slight at first, and the person is thought to be restless or "fidgety." These gradually become more pronounced until all body muscles are involved, and the patient is seldom still for more than a few minutes. The movements are rapid and jerky. The trunk and limbs are particularly involved, though there is also grimacing of the face and shrugging of the shoulders. These abnormal movements are aggravated by stress, emotional situations, and attempts to perform voluntary movements.

Treatment. There is no known effective *treatment* for Huntington's disease. Haloperidol (Haldol) — a dopamine blocker — can be quite effective in controlling the abnormal movements and some of the behavioral manifestations. Nevertheless, the disease is inevitably fatal. Death comes as a result of intercurrent infections or suicide, on an average about 15 years after the onset of symptoms.

Genetic counseling — before having children — is highly important for persons with a family history of the disease.

Refer to p. 521 for discussion of the *personal impact* of neurologic disorders and appropriate *supportive care.*

PARKINSON'S DISEASE

Parkinson's disease (also referred to as *paralysis agitans, Parkinson's syndrome,* and *parkinsonism*) was first adequately described by James Parkinson in 1817. It is actually a complex clinical syndrome rather than a specific disease entity.

There are several forms of Parkinson's disease, but they may be *classified etiologically* as follows:

- *Idiopathic or degenerative*
- *Postencephalitic.* Formerly occurred as a sequel in a large percentage of those who suffered from epidemic encephalitis; now rarely seen.
- *Atherosclerotic.* Atherosclerosis of the CNS can produce some Parkinson-like symptoms, but not a true Parkinson's syndrome.
- *Drug induced.* Long-term therapy with large doses of medication such as reserpine, the phenothiazines, and haloperidol can produce parkinson-like symptoms. These symptoms disappear when the drugs are withdrawn.

- *Toxic.* Such toxins as carbon monoxide, mercury or manganese can cause brain damage and result in conditions resembling Parkinson's disease. This etiology is rare.
- *Trauma* and other neurologic disturbances causing *midbrain compression* may rarely produce some of the manifestations of Parkinson's disease.

Since the *idiopathic* or *degenerative type* of the disease is that seen most commonly, we focus our attention on that form.

Idiopathic Parkinson's disease is related to a degenerative process involving the basal ganglia and substantia nigra. In this disease, the concentration of the neurotransmitter dopamine and its major metabolite is greatly decreased in the caudate and putamen and also in the substantia nigra. In postmortem examinations, it has been found that the degree of this deficiency correlates with the degree of cell loss in the substantia nigra. This is the most constant finding in patients with idiopathic Parkinson's disease. The underlying cause of the dopamine deficiency and cell degeneration remains a mystery (i.e., idiopathic).

Parkinson's disease begins most often in the sixth decade of life, and affects men and women equally. It is found worldwide, and despite a few reports to the contrary, it is not a familial disease. About 1 per cent of persons over age 50 years experience Parkinson's disease.

Course and Symptoms. In well advanced cases of Parkinson's disease the *diagnosis* is easily made by finding the characteristic manifestations of the disorder. Generally the results of laboratory examinations are within normal limits. Parkinson's disease is slowly progressive. The course is often rapid for the first few years and then levels off. The advance of symptoms most often extends over several decades.

The syndrome is characterized by three cardinal features — *tremor, rigidity,* and *akinesia.* All other symptoms are in some way related to these three.

Early in the illness the patient may notice a slight *slowing* of the ability to perform usual activities. A general feeling of *stiffness* may be noticed, along with *mild diffuse muscular pains.*

Tremor is a common early symptom of Parkinson's disease. It usually occurs in one of the upper limbs. Tremor is commonly accompanied by *"pill-rolling" movements* of the thumb against the fingers. Typically the tremor is an alternating tremor (i.e., it consists of alternating movements of opposing muscles) and varies in intensity and distribution. Usually tremor is reduced or abolished by voluntary movement; however, some patients have an intention tremor (i.e., voluntary movement worsens the tremor). In such a

TABLE 27-5. MAJOR NEUROLOGIC FINDINGS IN PARKINSON'S SYNDROME

Neurological Finding	Comment
Hyperactive glabellar (blink) reflex	Exaggerated sensitivity to finger tapping over glabella (between eyebrows) causing the patient to blink with each tap. It takes effort for a normal person to blink. Early sign of Parkinson's syndrome.
Palmomental reflex	Palm of hand stroked by thumb causes ipsilateral response in mentalis muscle with resulting wrinkling of the skin of the chin. If the Parkinson's disease is unilateral, the response may only be found on the affected side. Palmomental reflex negative in normal persons.
Masklike facies	Wide-eyed, unblinking, staring expression. Blinks 2 to 3 times per minute. Normal blinking 12 to 20 times per minute.
Rest tremor	Pill-rolling movement of hands characteristic. Tremor decreased with voluntary movement and during sleep.
Cogwheel rigidity	Motion interrupted by "catches."
Postural abnormalities	Kyphosis, stooped posture, shuffling gait with short steps (festinating gait).
Micrographia, monotone	Small handwriting; expressionless speech.

Price, S. A., and L. M. C. Wilson: *Pathophysiology: Clinical Concepts of Disease Processes.* New York: McGraw-Hill Book Company, 1978.

IMPORTANT CLINICAL FEATURES OF TREMOR IN PARKINSON'S DISEASE

Static tremor of hand muscles
- Increases when person walks
- Generally disappears during sleep
- Increases with emotional stress

Action tremor
- Is present in a few patients instead of, or in addition to, static tremor
- Is faster than static tremor (has frequency of 7 to 12 contractions per second)
- Is seen when limbs are outstretched or during active movement

Tremor of the tongue
- Tongue tremor common
- Tremors of lips, jaw, and head less common

"Pill-rolling" tremor
- Common early symptom
- Characteristic movement of thumb against the fingers
- Varies among patients; in some persons, is decreased by voluntary movement, whereas in others is worsened

Modified from Clinical Highlights: Important clinical features of the tremor of parkinsonism. *Hospital Medicine,* 14(4):99, Apr. 1978.

case, the tremor may be the main cause of disability; however, more often the main cause of disability is *akinesia* (i.e., absence or poverty of movements) or *dyskinesia* (i.e., impaired voluntary activity resulting in fragmentary or incomplete movements).

Dyskinesia, another frequent early symptom, often begins by affecting one arm, or only the fingers and thumb. Complicated movements are slow and are difficult to perform. Muscular power usually becomes affected when the disease is well advanced. Failure to swing the affected arm while walking, i.e., *loss of automatic associated movements,* is one of the earliest symptoms. *Poverty* and *slowness of movements* may occur in all the normal activities of daily living, e.g., dressing, eating. *Impaired handwriting* is another early symptom. Rigidity of the arms results in *jerky, "cogwheel" motions.*

The effects on the legs appear as *various disorders of locomotion.* In the early stages there may be a slight stiffness of one leg in walking, and the corresponding arm may be held flexed at the elbow and abducted at the shoulder. Also, the patient may catch or drag one foot. Later, when both sides of the body are involved, patients begin to show a typical *shuffling gait with little steps.* Some patients begin to take quicker and quicker steps (*propulsive gait*); occasionally this occurs in the backward direction (*retropulsion*). The person with a propulsive gait is in danger of falling and at times has difficulty stopping. It helps to take hold of the person's arm to slow him or her down. Some patients have difficulty starting locomotion, and then break into a propulsive gait, whereas others merely walk with a slow, shuffling gait without swinging their arms. In advanced cases the *posture* becomes affected so that the person stands with head flexed, shoulders stooped, and spine arched forward (Fig. 27–15.)

Often a *characteristic facial appearance* occurs with Parkinson's disease, and the face appears stiff, mask-like, and staring. Sometimes *oculogyric crises* occur, and the patient's eyes are fixed upward, upward and to one side, or downward. These crises may last for several hours. *Blepharospasm* producing almost total closure of the eyelid is a symptom in some patients.

Typically the *speech* of a patient with Parkinson's disease is low pitched, monotonous, slow, lacks modulation, and is poorly articulated (dysarthric). Frequently *saliva flows involuntarily from the mouth* because it is not directed to the back of the mouth and swallowed. Various *autonomic effects* accompany Parkinson's disease, e.g., lacrimation, constipation, incontinence, and decreased sexual capacity. Excessive perspiration and undue sensitivity to heat also commonly occur.

Parkinson's disease does not usually affect the *intellectual faculties.* However, because the emotional strain of living with such a condition is great, *mood disturbances* often occur. Usually the symptoms are greatly intensified during periods of emotional tension.

Many symptoms of Parkinson's disease vary in degree, are seldom proportional to each other, and are highly individualized.

Treatment. Since the underlying cause of degenerative changes in the basal ganglia remains a mystery, there is no known treatment to halt the degenerative process. Attention is directed toward relief of symptoms. Treatment can be medical or surgical, or a combination of both. In recent years, physicians have come to depend almost entirely on various *medications,* particularly L-dopa, as well as anticholinergic drugs.

L-dihydroxyphenylalanine (*L-dopa*) was first demonstrated to be therapeutically effective in the early 1960's. A synthetic compound, *levodopa,* is commonly used. These medications are currently the most effective treatment for Parkinson's disease, giving better therapeutic results than have been obtained with other drugs.

The symptoms of Parkinson's disease are associated with depletion of dopamine in the

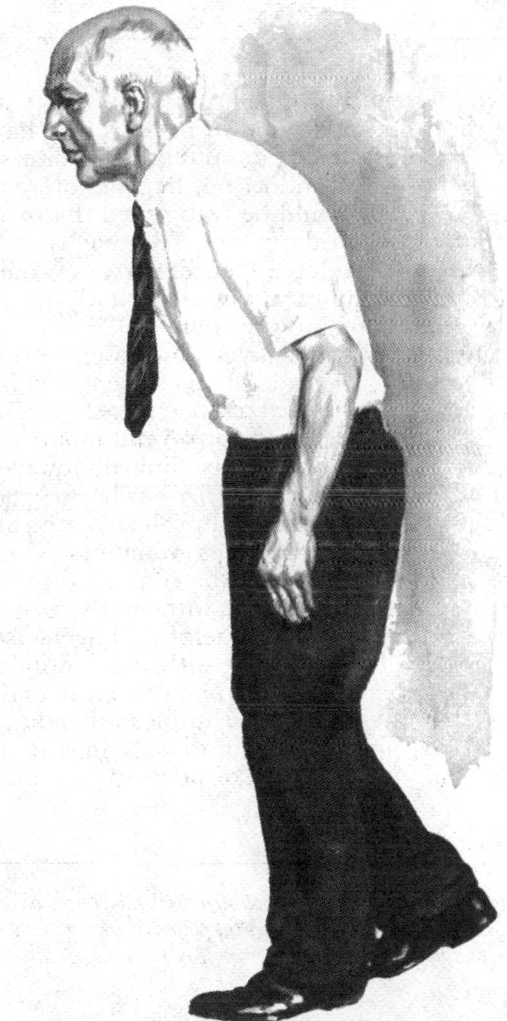

Figure 27–15. The typical rigidity and stooped posture of Parkinson's disease. (© Copyright 1976 CIBA Pharmaceutical Company, Division of CIBA-GEIGY Corporation. Reproduced, with permission, from *Clinical Symposia,* illustrated by Frank H. Netler, M.D. All rights reserved.)

brain. Dopamine itself cannot be given because, apparently, it does not cross the blood-brain barrier. Levodopa (the metabolic precursor of dopamine) does cross this barrier and is believed to convert to dopamine in the basal ganglia. Administering oral levodopa thus relieves some symptoms of Parkinson's disease, e.g., rigidity, akinesia, loss of postural reflexes and tremor.

Monoamine oxidase (MAO) inhibitors and levodopa should not be given together. These inhibitors must be stopped 2 weeks before beginning therapy with levodopa. Levodopa is contraindicated in persons with narrow angle glaucoma and known hypersensitivity to levodopa.

Levodopa must be given cautiously and treatment carefully supervised in persons who have severe cardiovascular or pulmonary disease, bronchial asthma, endocrine, hepatic, or renal disease. Also, it should be recognized that pyridoxine hydrochloride (vitamin B_6) may reverse the effects of levodopa. Hence, persons requiring levodopa may be advised to avoid vitamin preparations containing vitamin B_6.

Beginning with a relatively low dose, the dosage of levodopa is gradually increased until the desired therapeutic level has been reached. This level may not be reached for several months.

The use of levodopa may be limited, however, by rather serious *toxic side effects.* The first noticed may be gastrointestinal problems, e.g., anorexia, nausea and perhaps vomiting. These distressing experiences can be controlled somewhat by taking medication with meals. Use of antiemetic drugs may be helpful. The nausea often gradually disappears with the continued use of the drug. (Such information may help the patient tolerate these early unpleasant side effects.) Gastrointestinal hemorrhage may occur in persons with a history of active peptic ulcer disease.

Supportive nursing care coupled with thorough assessment is extremely important when working with persons beginning drug therapy for Parkinson's disease.

When the daily dose of levodopa approaches the desired level, the patient will often manifest involuntary choreoathetoid movements, especially of the face, mouth and tongue, or myoclonus, necessitating a slight decrease in dosage. Any of a variety of psychiatric symptoms may also appear, varying from anxiety, agitation, confusion, insomnia, nightmares, delusions, and nocturnal visual hallucinations, to a full blown psychotic response. Depression may also occur. Cardiac arrhythmias and myocardial infarction and urinary retention have been reported in some patients receiving levodopa. A more common problem, seen in about a third of patients taking the drug, is postural hypotension (orthostatic hypotension), but it also usually responds to decreases in dosage. Elastic stockings may help relieve postural hypotension, and the patient needs to be cautioned to make position changes slowly.

It is very evident that establishing the proper dosage for each person is an individual matter that involves finding the right balance between optimum therapeutic effect and tolerable side effects.

Persons receiving levodopa for extended periods of time require periodic assessments of their hepatic, hematopoietic, cardiovascular and renal function. Intra-ocular pressure should also be carefully monitored.

More recently a new drug, *Carbidopa,* has been introduced for use along with levodopa. The combination of these two drugs permits therapeutic control of symptoms more quickly, at lower doses, and with fewer toxic side effects.

Prior to the advent of L-dopa, the medications used in the treatment of Parkinson's disease were mostly *anticholinergic agents.* Today they are used mainly in conjunction with L-dopa or in patients who cannot tolerate L-dopa. Anticholinergic agents act by blocking muscarinic receptors at cholinergic synapses with the central nervous system. They are most effective in relieving tremor and rigidity, but the akinesia does not usually respond well. Various synthetic preparations are used, including trihexyphenidyl (Artane), procyclidine (Kemadrin), and benztropine mesylate (Cogentin). Treatment should begin with small doses, gradually increasing the dosage until toxic effects begin to appear. Toxic effects include dryness of the mouth, blurred vision, constipation and urinary retention, and mental dulling and confusion. Anticholinergic drugs should never be withdrawn suddenly. To do so could precipitate a sudden, incapacitating increase in symptoms.

Amantadine (Symmetrel) was discovered by chance to be an effective antiparkinsonism drug. It is less effective than L-dopa, but is very well tolerated. Its mechanism of action remains unknown. It is effective against all the various symptoms of the disease in about 50 per cent of patients. Its side effects, restlessness and mental and emotional changes, are reversible by withdrawing the drug.

Occasionally, patients with Parkinson's disease experience what is called a "*Parkinsonian crisis,*" as a result of sudden withdrawal of antiparkinsonism medication or some emotional trauma. The patient has a sudden severe exacerbation of tremor, rigidity and akinesia, accompanied by acute anxiety, sweating, tachycardia, and hyperpnea.

> *A Parkinsonian crisis is a medical emergency. It must be recognized quickly and appropriate action taken, or the person may die.*

A Parkinsonian crisis calls for immediate treatment, e.g., respiratory and cardiac support. The patient is placed in a quiet room with subdued light. An intramuscular or intravenous injection of sodium phenobarbital may be given, or in moderately severe cases sodium amylbarbital may be given orally. Antiparkinsonism medications are also given.

Various *surgical procedures* have been devised over the years in an attempt to relieve the symptoms of Parkinson's disease. Most recently attention was focused on various stereotactic procedures employing alcohol, freezing (cryosurgery), electric cautery, and ultrasound in an attempt to destroy discrete areas within the globus pallidus and ventrolateral thalamus. Carefully placed lesions in these areas were effective in reducing the tremor and rigidity without evidence of weakness. Best results were obtained in young patients who were in good health, with sound mentality, in whom tremor and rigidity were the predominant signs. The need for surgical intervention has greatly decreased in the past several years since the advent of L-dopa and the other effective drugs.

Clinical management of the patient with Parkinson's disease provides the nurse and physician with an unusual challenge. In spite of the discovery of highly effective drugs to ameliorate the symptoms of the disease, the length and quality of the patient's life depends on the maintenance of optimum general health. The care must include a planned program of exercise, activity and rest, as well as emotional support to the patient and significant others to help them cope with the stress of a long-term illness (see pp. 521–524).

The kinds of exercises that are recommended include:

1. *Deep diaphragmatic breathing* to improve lung capacity and volume.
2. *Holding a sound for 5 seconds.* This helps to improve the person's facial control and expression. Vowel sounds are best.
3. *Reading aloud* helps people become aware of their voice intonation, making it easier for them to modify intonation if necessary.
4. *Singing the scales.* Also helps improve tone inflection.
5. *Extending the tongue to the nose and chin and then laterally.* This develops tongue control.
6. *Range-of-motion exercises* for the entire body. Start at one part of the body and work systematically through rotation, flexion, and extension as appropriate.

Carroll[50] suggests that people with Parkinson's disease can often benefit from group exercises. This way they not only gain the benefit of the exercises, but they also enjoy group support and encouragement (Fig. 27–16).

The following are some additional important considerations:

- *Physical therapy* helps to combat the muscular rigidity that accompanies the illness and helps to prevent contractures.
- The patient must be taught to pay attention to *posture* and prevent postural deformities. Observe carefully for the tendency of the head and neck to become flexed. *Prevention* is imperative. Postural exercises are important to keep the head and neck erect. When resting, the person should lie on a firm bed without a pillow (to prevent the spine from being flexed forward); periodically the person should lie prone.
- *Gait training* is important because of the tendency for the gait to become shuffling and propulsive.
- All measures that *improve general health* are encouraged, e.g., fresh air, moderate exercise, adequate rest, and a good diet. The progress of the illness may be slowed by such measures. The person experiencing Parkinson's disease often has *difficulty maintaining weight* because of problems with eating and side effects from medications. The person should be weighed periodically. Supplementary feedings may help to keep up caloric intake. Warming trays keep the patient's food hot and yet allow time to rest while eating.
- The patient with *excessive tremor* may find that partial control of the tremor in hands and arms is possible by sitting in an arm chair and gripping the arms of the chair.
- If the person's *voice* is extremely weak, a small electric voice amplifier (such as is used following laryngectomy) may help. (See Unit XVI.)
- *Constipation* often results from the side effects of medications, lack of exercise, lack of saliva in the gastrointestinal tract (lost through drooling), and weakness of the muscles necessary for adequate defecation. If swallowing is impaired, the person may not be taking an adequate fluid intake. (See Unit XVII for discussion of constipation. Also refer to Sorensen and Luckmann, *Basic Nursing: A Psychophysiologic Approach.*)

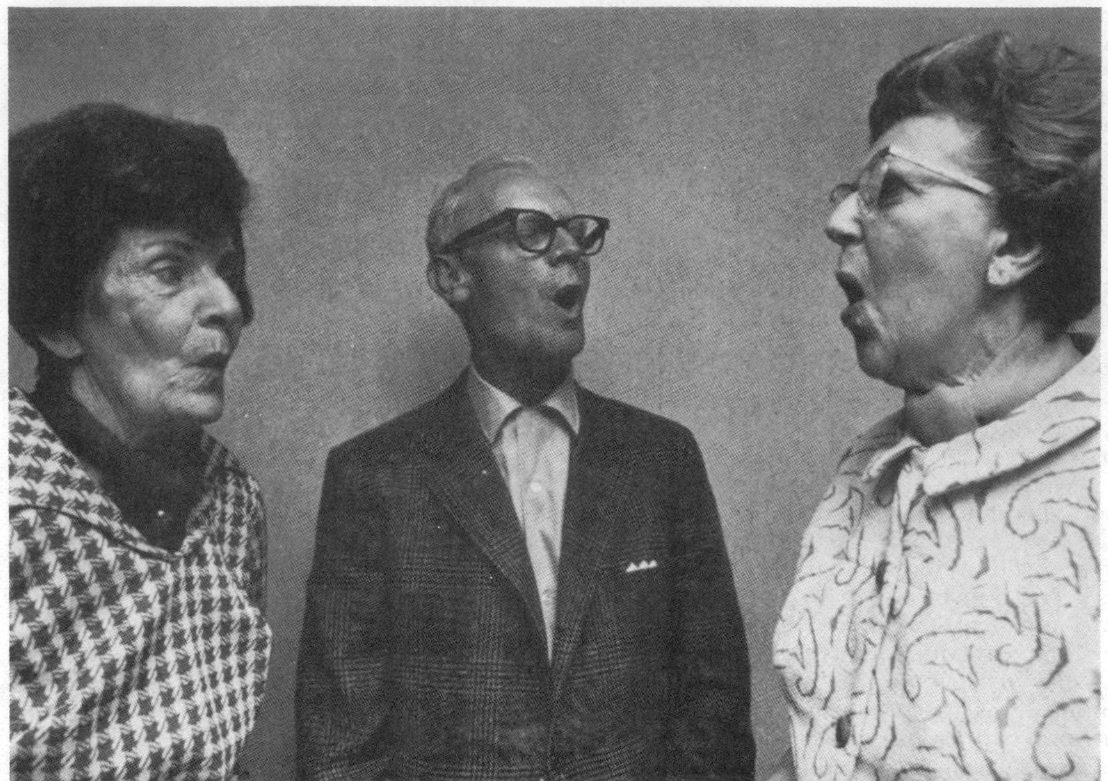

Figure 27–16. Reciting the vowels helps people with Parkinson's disease develop control of their facial muscles. (From Carroll, B.: Fingers to toes. *American Journal of Nursing,* 71:550, Mar. 1971.)

- The person experiencing far advanced disease may have extreme *difficulty in swallowing* and is in danger of choking while eating or drinking. Have suction available and do not rush the patient while eating. Aspiration pneumonia is a serious, sometimes fatal, occurrence.
- *Lassitude* is frequently present with Parkinson's disease and the person may therefore want to accept more help than is necessary or beneficial.

A cheerful mental outlook is to be encouraged, and it is helpful if the patient can live in a pleasant emotional climate. As the condition progresses the person will need increasing help, which should be given as sensitively as possible. Patient and significant others need to realize that Parkinson's disease does not impair sight or hearing, nor does it shorten life. Education about the illness should be given to both patient and significant others. It should be emphasized that the condition does *not* cause eventual paralysis and is painful only if the patient neglects to perform proper exercises and movements faithfully (or if this is neglected by others).

Amyotrophic Lateral Sclerosis (ALS, Motor-System Disease)

Amyotrophic lateral sclerosis (ALS) is the term commonly used for any of several progressive degenerative disorders of motor neurons in the spinal cord, brain stem, and motor cortex, characterized clinically by muscular weakness, atrophy, and various pyramidal tract signs. More correct terms to encompass all the syndromes are "motor-system disease" and "motor neuron disease." The etiology is unknown; the pathology is essentially a degeneration of the motor cells, along with secondary degeneration of some motor tracts. This disorder is usually sporadic but rarely familial. An estimated 3000 new cases occur annually in the United States.

The disease was first adequately described by Charcot in 1874. ALS is a disease of middle age, with the onset usually in the early 50's. Males are affected more often than females. The *course* of the disease is progressive with no remissions, and death usually follows 2 to 6 years after onset.

Motor-system disease is classified according to particular groups of signs and symptoms.

- The most frequent form is *amyotropic lateral sclerosis,* in which hyperreflexia is combined with amyotrophy.
- Another form is called *progressive muscular atrophy* and is characterized by weakness and atrophy alone, without evidence of pyramidal tract dysfunction.
- The third major form affects primarily the muscles of the jaw, face, tongue, pharynx, and larynx (those muscles innervated by cranial nerves origi-

nating in the medulla). This form is called *progressive bulbar palsy.*

- ▶ A fourth rare form is characterized by spasticity and hyperreflexia, and is called *primary lateral sclerosis.*
- ▶ A few special forms of the disease affect infants and children.

Rarely is one form seen alone. Rather, one group of signs and symptoms is usually first to appear and becomes dominant throughout the course of the disease, but various other manifestations complicate the patient's deteriorating condition.

Symptoms. In ALS, the first indications of disease are usually seen in one hand. The patient begins to drop things and becomes awkward in tasks that require fine hand movements. This is followed by weakness and wasting of the hand muscles, cramping, and slight twitching. In a matter of weeks or months, the arm is similarly affected, and the symptoms are duplicated in the other hand and arm. Soon the classic symptoms — weakness and atrophy of the hands and forearms, slight spasticity of the legs, and hyperactive reflexes — make the diagnosis definite. These symptoms progress to involve the upper arms and shoulders and, later, the muscles of the neck, pharynx, and larynx. The trunk and lower extremities are spared until very late in the course of the disease.

Throughout the disease there is *no sensory loss.* There may be some aching of involved muscles but no true paresthesias. Bowel and urinary sphincters remain intact even after the patient is totally debilitated. *Fasciculations of the involved muscles,* caused by spontaneous irregular discharges of motor neurons and reflected peripherally as irregular twitchings or contractions of individual muscle fibers or muscle bundles, are a classic feature. Fasciculations may be observed by the patient and others as the continuous movement of portions of muscles anywhere in the body. Intellect is intact to the very end. Terminally, muscular weakness and atrophy are generalized and there may be quadriplegia and bulbar paralysis.

There are many variations in the muscles involved and the order of their involvement, but the disease is always progressive and fatal. When the symptoms are primarily those of progressive muscular atrophy, patients often survive 15 years and more. However, with *progressive bulbar palsy,* or when bulbar involvement complicates the other syndromes, the progression is more rapid, and patients usually die of aspiration pneumonia within 2 to 3 years. Both flaccid bulbar and spastic bulbar paralysis occurs. However, in the late stages of the illness only true bulbar, flaccid paralysis is present. Affective outbursts, e.g., explosive uncontrollable outbursts of laughing, crying, or a mixture of both may occur with progressive bulbar palsy. Slurring dysarthria may also develop, i.e., slurring speech.

Weakness of the muscles of the palate, pharynx, and tongue pose difficult problems for some patients, e.g., swallowing is impaired, liquids are regurgitated through the nose. In the last stages of illness, complete aphagia (loss of ability to swallow) may occur, necessitating alternate routes of maintaining nutrition.

Diagnosis. The laboratory test of greatest value in diagnosis is electromyography (EMG), to demonstrate muscle denervation. Muscle biopsy may be employed to distinguish between a neurogenic and amyopathic process. Serum creatine phosphokinase activity may be elevated. A careful history and physical examination are essential. Diagnosis must be established with certainty in this disorder, as in others which hold a bleak prognosis. Typical presenting findings include: painless, diffuse, progressive muscle weakness with atrophy, fasiculations, and associated spasticity; enhanced stretch reflexes and extensor plantar responses.

Treatment. As there is no specific treatment for ALS, only *supportive* measures can be used (Fig. 27–17). The nurse practicing in a hospital usually sees persons with ALS twice in the course of their illness: first, at the time of diagnosis, and second, when they have become too debilitated to be cared for in other settings.

At the time of diagnosis, the patient and significant others need support to face the prospect of an invariably fatal disease and to cope with the progressive debilities. During the later, often lengthy, hospitalization, the patient usually becomes totally dependent. Keeping in mind that the patient's intellect and sensation are intact, the skillful nurse makes every effort to keep the patient comfortable and provide the necessary support to the patient and significant others. Refer to p. 521 for discussion of the personal impact of neurologic disorders and appropriate supportive care.

Myasthenia Gravis

Myasthenia gravis is a muscle disease characterized by fluctuating weakness of certain voluntary (striated) muscles, especially those innervated by cranial nerves originating in the brain stem. Those muscles usually involved are ocular, facial, lingual, and the muscles of mastication and deglutition. As the name implies, myasthenia gravis is "a muscular weakness of grave prognosis."[3]

This disease affects persons at any age; the

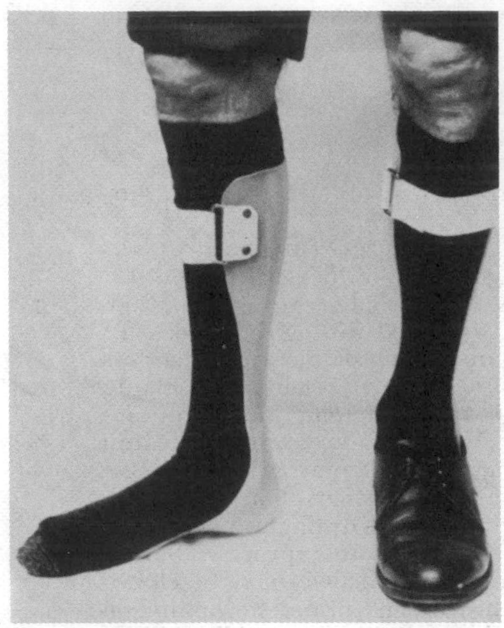

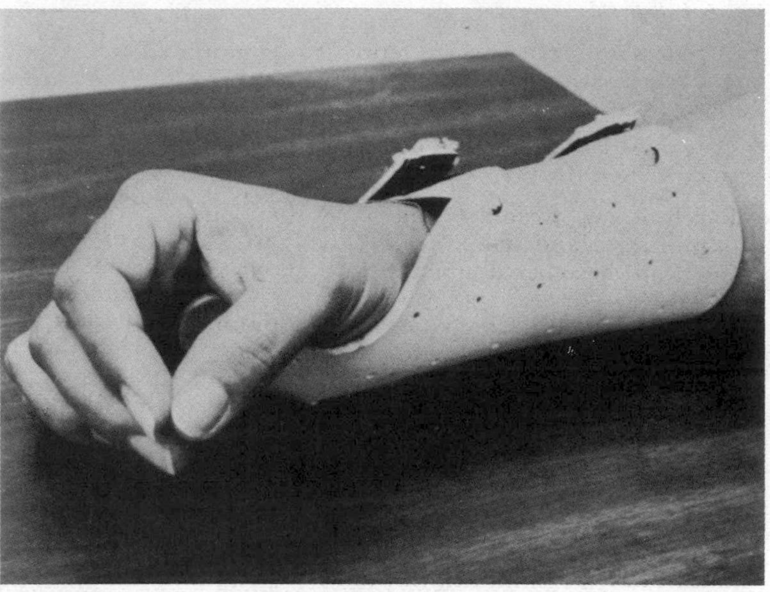

Figure 27–17. Splints used to provide support for persons with amyotrophic lateral sclerosis. **A.** Lightweight, plastic insert ankle-foot orthoses provide dorsiflexion assist and mediolateral stability to improve gait. **B.** Static resting wrist cockup orthosis provides wrist extension and improves hand function. (From DeLisa, J. A., et al.: Amyotrophic lateral sclerosis: comprehensive management. *American Family Physician,* 19:137, Mar. 1979.)

peak period of onset is between 20 and 30 years. In the younger years, women are affected more frequently. However, in patients over 50 years, males tend to be more numerous.

Etiology. Myasthenia gravis is caused by a defect in the transmission of the nerve impulse at the neuromuscular junction. Whether this defect is due to a deficiency of either acetylcholine or its enzyme, acetylcholinesterase, remains unresolved. Recent studies have shown a decrease in the number of acetylcholine receptor sites on the postsynaptic muscle membrane at the neuromuscular junction in patients with myasthenia.[3] The basic mechanism for this defect is currently accepted to be an autoimmune reaction, initially involving the thymus gland.[3] (Autoimmune diseases are discussed in Chapter 11.)

Symptoms. Myasthenia gravis produces symptoms that are essentially all due to weakness. Usually *symptom onset* is insidious and progresses slowly. The outstanding characteristic of the disease is the relationship of muscular weakness to muscular activity. The power of contraction rapidly diminishes after a few repeated activities of the muscles involved; with rest, the muscles rapidly regain their power of contraction. Not all muscles recover in this fashion, however, and certain muscles have a continually reduced function. The muscles affected by residual weakness vary somewhat in location and degree of weakness. However, the muscles of the eyes (extraocular muscles) are most often the first affected and are affected at some time during the course of myasthenia in almost all patients. *Involvement of the ocular muscles is the most common initial symptom.*

Weakness of facial and levator palpebrae muscles produces an *expressionless appearance,* characterized by droopy eyelids (ptosis), smoothed features, full lips with underlip slightly everted, and a tendency for the mouth to hang open. The person with myasthenia gravis often seems to be snarling when trying to smile. Other ocular palsies may occur, with diplopia (double vision) and nystagmus. Variability in ocular symptoms from day to day is characteristic.

With progression of the disease, other muscles become involved. Muscle of facial expression, chewing, swallowing and speaking are next most frequently involved. Involvement of the muscles of deglutition results in choking spells and nasal regurgitation. Fatalities usually result from respiratory complications. Involvement of the muscles of speech causes a nasal voice. The voice fades after much talking. Aphonia (voice loss) may develop with severe involvement. When the muscles of mastication are affected the jaw sags. Muscles of the neck, shoulders, and trunk are affected less often. However, if the flexors of the neck are involved, the patient may constantly hold a hand under the chin to support the head. The extremities are often involved. The upper are usually affected before the lower and the proximal muscles before the distal ones. Early in the disease the patient may notice difficulty in brushing teeth, shaving, and combing hair. In advanced cases, all muscles may be affected, including bowel and bladder sphincters. Characteristically, weakness of muscles is greater after exercise or at the end of the day, and muscle strength improves after rest. The affected muscles frequently undergo mild atrophy. There is usually no sensory loss. Paresthesias and aching of weakened muscles may occur.

Course. The *course* of myasthenia gravis is variable and may be characterized by *remissions* and *exacerbations.* Symptom progression may be rapid or slow. Symptoms may fluctuate in severity from day to day, and spontaneous remissions may develop that last for many years. Some patients experience a gradual extension of the involved areas, which progresses to a relatively steady state of weakness, remaining unchanged for many years except for moderate changes in severity. Others experience more rapid progression of involvement. However, with adequate treatment many persons with myasthenia gravis can live long, productive lives.

Diagnosis. Generally myasthenia gravis can be easily *diagnosed* on the basis of *symptoms* alone. The person who presents with drooping eyelids, little facial movement, a smile that looks like a snarl, and a jaw which tends to hang open, is easily diagnosed as having myasthenia gravis. Additionally, dramatic improvement in muscular strength typically occurs following the administration of neostigmine (Prostigmine) or edrophonium chloride (Tensilon). This pharmacologic test may be used for diagnostic testing and for the regulation of drug dosage.

Whenever anticholinesterase drugs are used for testing, a syringe containing atropine sulfate should be available at the bedside to be given in aliquots intravenously if needed to counteract cardiac irregularities and other muscarinic effects, i.e., severe cholinergic reactions. When *Tensilon* is injected IV, a positive test consists of objective and subjective improvement in muscle strength within 1 minute. *Neostigmine* (Prostigmine) may also be used as a diagnostic test. It may be given orally, IM, or IV; a positive test also produces improvement in muscle strength, but does it more slowly. If neither Tensilon nor neostigmine is effective diagnostically, *curare* may be given in minute doses. *Respiratory assistance must be immediately available,* since the patient with myasthenia will show immediate definite increase in weakness.

Further investigation for diagnostic purposes may include: (1) *electrical stimulation,* which demonstrates fatigability of the affected muscles *(Jolly reaction)* and (2) *electromyography,* which demonstrates a similar but less dramatic diminution of the action potentials of the muscles.

Treatment. The treatment of myasthenia gravis may be medical or surgical, or both.

MEDICAL TREATMENT. Medical treatment consists of the careful use of two groups of drugs: (1) short-acting anticholinesterase compounds and (2) corticosteroids. The first group, the *short-acting anticholinesterase drugs,* blocks the breakdown of acetylcholine at the neuromuscular junction i.e., inhibit cholinesterase. The two most effective drugs are *neostigmine* (Prostigmine) and *pyridostigmine* (Mestinon). The dose of each drug and distribution of the dosage throughout the day vary with the needs of each person. There must be flexibility in the medication program. Ideally, each patient is given thorough instruction in the use of the medication and its potential side effects, and then may be allowed to adjust the dosage to meet his or her own needs. Most patients become weakest in the late afternoon. Some experience significant weakness during the night or upon waking for the day. These people may benefit from one of the time-release forms of the drug, taken at bed time.

The optimal drug regimen is the smallest dosage that will produce the greatest strength. One drug is usually recommended rather than combinations. The nurse needs to be familiar with the actions and possible side effects of these drugs in order to assist patients in their medication programs.

Persons receiving anticholinesterase compounds may develop excessive salivation, sweating, nausea, diarrhea, abdominal cramps, and occasional vomiting. To prevent or alleviate such visceral disturbances, tincture of belladonna or atropine sulfate may be prescribed with the anticholinesterase agent.

For some patients ephedrine, guanidine or potassium chloride may produce a slight increase in strength when administered as *adjuvants* to anticholinesterase medication.

> *Cholinergic crisis is a medical emergency.*

Persons with mysathenia gravis, especially those on high doses of anticholinesterase drugs, may experience a *cholinergic crisis.* This may be secondary to an infection or to an error in medication dosage, or the cause may be unknown. The crisis is characterized by *a dramatic increase in myasthenic symptoms,* along with development of parasympathomimetic side effects (e.g., nausea, vomiting, sweating, salivation, bradycardia) and various degrees of muscular tightness and fasiculations. Generalized weakness, dysphagia, and respiratory weakness may result. This is a true emergency. Ideally the patient is intubated and given respiratory assistance, usually in an intensive care unit. All anticholinesterase medications are typically withheld for 24 to 72 hours and are then gradually reinstituted. With good respiratory and general care, the patient usually improves to the point of remission.

For patients who do not respond adequately

to the anticholinesterase drugs (or for older patients), *corticosteroids* may be used, either in place of or in addition to the anticholinesterase drugs. The patient is usually hospitalized for the initiation of this treatment. Prednisone, the form usually given, is typically begun with a rather large dose and may cause a transient worsening of symptoms, followed by gradual improvement in muscle strength. The medication is usually given on alternate days. When a peak of improvement has been reached and maintained for several weeks, the dosage of both prednisone and anticholinesterase medication may be gradually adjusted downward. A low maintenance-dose of alternate day prednisone may be effective treatment for many months or years. The usual precautions for any steroid therapy must be followed, including potassium supplements and liberal use of antacids.

SURGICAL TREATMENT. Surgical therapy for myasthenia gravis involves removal of the thymus gland. Though the relationship of the thymus gland to myasthenia has never been definitely established, marked improvement in symptoms has been reported in a high percentage of cases following *thymectomy,* i.e., removal of the thymus gland. It is presumed that removal of the thymus acts in some beneficial way on the autoimmune mechanism.[137] Some physicians recommend thymectomy for all cases of myasthenia gravis; others reserve it for those who do not respond to anticholinesterase drugs. If the surgery is done early in the course of the disease (within 2 years of onset), complete remission occurs in about 40 per cent of patients and another 40 per cent have marked improvement in symptoms.[137]

Nursing Care. Nurses most often encounter patients with myasthenia gravis in doctor's offices or outpatient clinics. However, when such patients are hospitalized, at the time of diagnosis or during a crisis, the following problems often require the nurse's special attention:

Difficulty taking nourishment. Involvement of the muscles of chewing and swallowing makes eating a difficult and slow process. A patient may be able to eat the first part of a meal without difficulty, but with each successive bite, chewing and swallowing become progressively more difficult. It is important that meals not be rushed and helpful if hot meals are served on a warming tray. Small frequent feedings may be helpful. The dysphagic patient requires a diet that can be swallowed easily, e.g., minced food. Adjust medication times so the doses are given about 1 hour before meals. Often weakness of the palate and pharyngeal muscles causes regurgitation of fluid through the nose. Suction equipment should be readily available to prevent aspiration. Tube feedings and intravenous infusions may be necessary for some persons.

Dyspnea and impaired ability to cough and swallow. Involvement of the muscles of respiration may cause weakness of cough, dyspnea on exertion, and finally dyspnea even at rest. The patient has difficulty clearing the respiratory tract of mucus and saliva. Respiratory distress and inability to swallow may necessitate intubation or tracheostomy.

Weakness. Weakness is greatest following exertion and at the end of the day. A patient's activities must be carefully planned to conserve energy. With rest, muscle strength typically improves. Sometimes a patient's muscles become weak even without exercise. Vocational rehabilitation may be advisable for some persons. Also, changes may be helpful in a patient's pattern of activities and in the arrangement of the home to prevent unnecessary expenditure of energy. Lid crutches may help to relieve ptosis. The extremely weak patient is totally dependent on others and requires total care. Occasionally the neck muscles may become so weakened that a patient is unable to lift the head from the pillow. Prevention of the complication of immobility and maintenance of patient comfort are challenging nursing considerations.

Education and support. The nurse has a responsibility to help the patient and significant others understand the nature of myasthenia gravis and the objectives of the treatment program, e.g., that the anticholinesterase compounds only ameliorate weakness — they do not produce a "cure." Education about what to do in the event of a cholinergic crisis is very important. The nurse helps the patient become familiar with prescribed medications and their possible side effects. The nurse works with patient and physician in establishing an *individualized* treatment program. Achieving proper drug dosage is important, since overtreatment can itself cause weakness. It is important for the patient to maintain good general health and avoid respiratory infections (such infections are serious because of the patient's inability to cough productively). Supportive emotional care is extremely important. (Refer to p. 521 for discussion of the personal impact of neurologic disorders and appropriate related care.)

Progressive Muscular Dystrophies

The *progressive muscular dystrophies* are a group of progressive, *hereditary degenerative* diseases of skeletal muscle. These diseases are characterized by degenerative changes in the muscle fibers themselves, rather than in the spinal motor neurons, nerves, or nerve endings. Thus, major *pathologic findings* are confined to the muscles, while the peripheral and central nervous systems remain normal. The *characteristic features* are symmetrical muscular weakness and atrophy, intact sensation, and the tendency to heredofamilial incidence. The pattern of muscle involvement helps distinguish these disorders from other muscle diseases. Mainly the muscles of the girdle, proximal limbs, and eyes are affected.

Etiology. The cause of the degenerative changes in the muscle fibers is not known. Biochemical studies have revealed disturbances in the enzyme systems concerned with muscle metabolism. However, there is no agreement as to which biochemical defect leads to the necrosis and atrophy.[3]

Classification. Many methods of classification have been proposed, but there is a total lack of agreement among authors. We consider briefly only two general types:

- *Duchenne's type,* or severe generalized muscular dystrophy of childhood. This disease begins early in childhood and progresses rapidly, usually leading to death during adolescence. It occurs predominantly in males, with the onset of symptoms usually before the age of 6 years. Early symptoms include difficulty walking, running, and climbing stairs, and a waddling gait. Calves and other muscles become enlarged (pseudohypertrophy). Weakness and atrophy spread to the muscles of the pelvic girdle, shoulders, abdomen, and later to the legs and forearms. Muscles of the face, neck, and hands may be involved later. The child eventually becomes totally debilitated and dies.
- *Facioscapulohumeral dystrophy.* This is a milder, slowly progressive muscular dystrophy restricted to the muscles of the shoulder and the face. The onset is usually in adolescence and early adult life, and the slow progression is often interrupted by long remissions. The weakness and atrophy affect all the muscles of the face, shoulders and upper arms, and scapulae. The scapulae become winged, and the upper arms become thinner than the forearms ("Popeye" effect). Pelvic muscles may become affected later.

Many other variants and subtypes have been identified, some of which are:

- Progressive external ophthalmoplegia
- Oculopharyngeal dystrophy
- Myotonic dystrophy
- Welander's distal dystrophy

Wide variation exists in the *course* of progressive muscular dystrophies. When death occurs, it may result from involvement of the bulbar, respiratory, and cardiac musculature or from intercurrent infections.

Clinical Management. There is *no specific treatment* for any of the progressive muscular dystrophies. The progression of weakness and wasting is unrelenting. Factors important in clinical care include the following:

- Encourage the patient to maintain as full and normal a life as possible. Discourage prolonged bed rest.
- Prevent contractures and deformities by a regular program of active and passive stretching exercises. Individualized exercise programs are helpful.
- Encourage the patient to avoid obesity. Provide teaching or referral to weight-control assistance as needed.
- Investigate the use of light spinal braces or long leg braces. They may permit ambulation for several years.
- Introduce the patient to self-help devices as muscle weakness progresses.
- Refer the patient for genetic counseling if he or she is considering having children.
- Encourage the patient to maintain a level of good general health and to especially try to avoid respiratory infections.
- Provide supportive emotional care. (See discussion on p. 521 of the psychologic impact of neurologic disorders and related nursing care.)

DEMYELINATING DISORDERS OF THE NERVOUS SYSTEM

Destruction of myelin *(demyelination)* is a prominent feature of numerous disorders of the brain and spinal cord. For example, demyelination or myelin breakdown may be a *secondary* aspect of infections, deficiency states, intoxications, or degenerations affecting the nervous system. In a true demyelinating disease, only the myelin sheaths of nerve fibers are destroyed, while other elements of nervous tissue are spared. Included in this category are such diseases as acute *disseminated encephalomyelitis, diffuse cerebral sclerosis,* and *necrotizing hemorrhagic encephalopathy.* The one most commonly seen, however, is *multiple sclerosis* (also called disseminated sclerosis), which will be the focus of our attention in this section.

The causes of most demyelinating disorders remain unknown. Current evidence indicates that an autoimmune basis might be present for most of the primary demyelinating disorders, with genetic and geographic factors influencing susceptibility.

Multiple Sclerosis (MS)

Multiple sclerosis is the most common cause of progressive neurologic disability in young adults in the United States, as well as in many other countries.[206] It is a disorder characterized by multifocal areas of demyelination diffusely scattered throughout the central nervous system, presenting with a history of remissions and exacerbations. Women are affected almost twice as often as men, and the usual age of onset is between 20 and 40 years. The incidence of multiple sclerosis is highest in cool and temperate climates. For instance, in Canada, the northern United States, and northern Europe, it occurs in 30 to 80 persons per 100,000; in areas close to the equator, it has a prevelance of less than 1 per 100,000.[3] There is a *familial tendency* toward multiple sclerosis, which may be due to common environmental factors as well as to hereditary factors.

The *precise cause or causes* remain unknown. As with many other neurologic diseases, a viral infection is frequently implicated as being a contributing factor. A more popular current theory maintains that an autoimmune reaction is responsible for destroying the myelin. Whatever the underlying etiology, several precipitating factors have been identified. Infection, trauma, and pregnancy are the three most important of these, frequently preceding both the initial symptoms and later exacerbations.

Signs and Symptoms. The onset of the disease varies. In some people, symptoms develop within a matter of minutes to hours. In others, symptoms develop slowly over several weeks to months, while in a few symptoms develop very slowly and insidiously over months or years.

Early *signs and symptoms* include the following:

- *Weakness and paresthesias* in one or more limbs (in approximately one-half of all cases)
- *Retrobulbar (optic) neuritis,* producing partial or total loss of vision in one eye (in about 25 per cent of all patients)
- *Unsteady gait* — cerebellar atoxia
- *Brain stem signs* — diplopia, dizziness, nystagmus, nausea and vomiting, signs of facial and trigeminal nerve involvement
- *Symptoms of bladder dysfunction* — retention and incontinence.

Pain is not an outstanding feature of the disease, although dull low back pain and sharp burning leg pains may be experienced.

However, the lesions of multiple sclerosis are diffusely scattered throughout all parts of the brain and spinal cord, and *the symptoms of multiple sclerosis are highly variable.* Hallmarks of MS are: (1) its chronic and relapsing nature punctuated by remissions and exacerbations (although as many as 30 per cent of affected patients steadily worsen from the onset) and (2) the multiplicity of the symptoms and their tendency to vary in nature and severity with the passage of time.

TABLE 27–6. FREQUENCY OF OCCURRENCE OF SYMPTOMS AND SIGNS IN COURSE OF MULTIPLE SCLEROSIS

	Carter et al. (46 Cases)	Posser (111 Cases)
	per cent	*per cent*
Weakness (symptom or sign)	89	96
Abnormal movements	67	
Abnormal reflexes (absent superficials, Babinski signs, or hyperreflexia)	99	95
Sphincter and genital difficulties	78	82
Visual disturbance (symptom or sign)	100	85
Nystagmus (any type)	85	70
Disc pallor, atrophy, decreased acuity	75	85
Third nerve impairment (and internuclear ophthalmoplegia)	67	
Tremor, ataxia	93	79
Impaired vibration and position sense	81	58
Impaired touch, pain, temperature sense	35	35
Mental changes (symptom or sign)	61	45
Paresthesias	44	65
Pain	42	19
Vertigo or dizziness	18	15

From Beeson, P. B., W. McDermott and J. B. Wyngaarden (Eds.): *Cecil Textbook of Medicine,* 15th ed., Philadelphia: W. B. Saunders Co., 1979, p. 847.

PHYSICAL FINDINGS IN MULTIPLE SCLEROSIS

Visual
- Temporal pallor of the disks
- Abnormal fields of vision
- Abnormal ocular motor function (strabismus)
- Nystagmus

Motor findings
- Motor weakness or paralysis of extremities
- Scanning speech
- Ataxia
- Muscular atrophy in late stages
- Manual dysmetria

Sensory alteration
- Decreased perception to pain, touch, temperature
- Decrease or absence of positional sense
- Decrease or absence of vibration sense

Lhermitte's sign (an "electric sensation" or "shock" down the back following passive flexion of the neck)

Reflex findings
- Exaggerated tendon reflexes
- Absent or diminished abdominal skin reflexes
- Absent or diminished cremasteric reflexes
- Babinski's sign
- Hoffmann's sign

Charcot's triad (nystagmus, intention tremor, scanning speech)

Possible mental changes
- Early
  - Apathy
  - Euphoria
  - Inattentiveness
- Late
  - Depression
  - Confusion
  - Disorientation
  - Memory defect

From Clinical Highlights: Physical findings in multiple sclerosis. *Hospital Medicine,* 13(9):108, Sept. 1977.

Weakness of the extremities is the most common symptom. There may also be generalized weakness that is out of proportion to the demonstrable muscular weakness. Usually weakness begins or is most noticeable in the lower extremities. When both lower extremities are involved, urinary disturbances (e.g., urgency, frequency) often appear. The extent of impairment ranges from minor weakness to total paralysis. Spasticity, hyperreflexia, and pathologic reflexes are often present.

Multiple sclerosis has no classic form; however, most patients who have had the illness for many years display the triad of symptoms known as *Charcot's triad:* (1) nystagmus, (2) intention tremor, and (3) scanning speech, i.e., slow enunciation with a tendency to hesitate at the beginning of a word or syllable. Loss of coordination frequently causes the MS patient to be ataxic and clumsy, and to walk with a combination spastic-ataxic gait. An impairment of pain and temperature sense occurs fairly often in one-half of the trunk and in the corresponding lower extremity. A patient with this involvement requires special attention to prevent injury to these areas of anesthesia. A common early finding in MS is deficiency of touch sensation of one hand. Complete blindness rarely occurs; however, considerable permanent visual loss is common.

Terminally, paresis or complete paralysis of the lower extremities is almost always present. The use of the arms may be severely limited as a result of ataxia or cerebellar involvement.

Accompanying the various physical manifestations are any of a number of mental abnormalities. Persons with MS have been traditionally thought of as exhibiting a euphoria, or inappropriate cheerfulness and lack of concern. This may indeed be the case if there is extensive involvement of the white matter of the frontal lobes. More commonly, however, the patient is depressed and irritable. In the late stages of the disease, a small percentage of patients exhibit a gross loss of memory or a global dementia. It is not unusual to find mild emotional disturbances in the early course of the illness. Such disturbances make diagnosis difficult; it is not uncommon for patients early in the course of MS to be viewed as neurotic because of their varied, temporary symptoms, and emotional instability.

Diagnosis. Diagnosis is usually made on the basis of clinical presentation alone. When the patient presents with a neurologic disease characterized by remissions and exacerbations and evidence of more than one discrete lesion of the central nervous system, there is rarely any doubt about the diagnosis of multiple sclerosis. When the onset is acute or when the progression of the disease is slow and steady, further investigation may be necessary. CSF examination may be helpful. In the purely spinal form of MS, a myelogram may be necessary to rule out spondylosis or some other cause of spinal cord compression.

In about two-thirds of patients the gamma globulin content in the CSF is elevated. Also there may be an abnormal colloidal gold curve which is accompanied by a negative serologic test for syphilis. During the acute disease, a mild mononuclear pleocytosis may occur. EEG findings are mildly abnormal in about two-thirds of patients. A definite diagnosis can seldom be made at the time of the first attack.

Clinical Course. The clinical course of MS is variable. The disease usually advances stepwise, with the remissions becoming progressively shorter and the exacerbations more severe. It appears that partial healing may occur in the areas of degeneration and that this accounts for the transitory character of many of the early symptoms. Over a period of years increasing neurologic deficits occur as a result of an increasing number of disseminated lesions and lesion enlargements. Some patients may experience one or two attacks and then may not experience any more symptoms for a number of years. In a small percentage of cases, the disease progresses steadily and rapidly to a spastic paraparesis and total disability. The usual duration of the disease is 20 years or more, but that also is variable. Even with the various forms of treatment, affected persons usually become totally debilitated, and death often follows as a result of intercurrent infection or other complications.

Treatment. There is no specific cure for MS; however, various forms of *treatment* have been proposed. The care of the patient with MS is basically a matter of symptomatic general care that varies with the person's current needs. Management of the patient has three aspects: (1) managing the acute episode; (2) care during remissions; and (3) managing the chronic neurologic disabilities.

During the *acute episode,* treatment is directed toward controlling the exacerbation as quickly as possible. The following measures are important:

- *Rest* and relief from fatigue and stressful situations. This does not necessarily mean strict bed rest.
- Since fever often triggers an acute episode, measures should be taken to *cool the body temperature.* Cool baths or ice packs may give temporary improvement. Underlying infections should be treated specifically.
- If the person is restricted to bed, regular *passive ROM exercises* are usually given to prevent contractures. Care must be taken not to cause fatigue.
- Various *steroid preparations* may be administered, usually in high doses for short periods of time. There is no substantial evidence that their use is

effective, except when the optic nerve is involved.

During periods of *remission,* it is important that persons with multiple sclerosis take whatever measures necessary to avoid exacerbations. Various diets have been advocated as influencing the course of the disease. While there is no evidence of any therapeutic value to any of the specific diets, it may help the patient to try a certain dietary program, provided it is not harmful. Ideally the patient should be advised to eat a well balanced diet to help maintain an optimum weight. The use of medications during the remission, such as long-term corticosteroids or immumosuppressive agents, is usually discouraged. Instead, the patient should be encouraged to exercise moderately, avoid infections and other illnesses, and maintain the highest level of activity possible within individual physical limitations.

When the neurologic problems become *chronic,* the management of the affected person becomes a greater challenge to physicians and nurses. The following problems usually require specific attention:

- *Bladder dysfunction* — may include a variety of problems, from retention and inability to completely empty the bladder, to dribbling or complete incontinence. Bladder infections are frequent. Use good technique for any catheter procedures and attempt to acidify the urine (with medication and diet).
- *Bowel problems* — constipation and impaction often occur. These distressing problems may be minimized by proper diet, adequate fluid intake, and institution of a regular bowel program, usually with a suppository every other day.
- *Spasticity and spasm* are additional difficult problems. Various medications may be used (such as diazepam) in an attempt to provide relief, but none is totally effective. Encourage the person to keep active as much as possible, with the aid of crutches or a walker if necessary. If a person is restricted to bed or chair, a program of full ROM exercises to all extremities should be carried out several times a day. The significant others may be recruited to help with this.
- *Pressure problems* — If the person spends a lot of time in bed or chair, special care must be taken to prevent decubitus ulcers and prevent contractures.

General Nursing Care Considerations. In general, the following are advocated: a *regular* daily program of activity, rest, and relaxation; avoidance of overwork and fatigue; moderate exercise and physiotherapy; warm baths; psychotherapy; a calm, relaxed environment that does not require the patient to respond rapidly (either physically or emotionally); a well-balanced diet with ample high-vitamin foods and fluids; fresh air and sunshine; and avoidance of overheating and chilling. As with all patients who have neurologic disabilities, the patient with MS is encouraged to remain active as long as possible, and every attempt is made to prevent "invalidism." The person with MS may benefit from the cultivation of hobbies and activities that can replace activities that are no longer possible. Social activities are encouraged, and the patient's normal social contacts should continue. Vocational retraining may be indicated.

If some muscles are permanently affected, it is frequently possible to train other muscles to assume the lost action. Self-help devices may be useful, enabling the person to remain independent longer. The installation of ramps and handrails and other structural adaptations may be required at home. The person may require the care discussed in the sections pertaining to hemiplegia or paraplegia in Chapter 26. Unnecessary catheterization is avoided (as with all patients) because of the possible serious consequences. Visual disturbances may pose special problems by further curtailing the person's activities. Safety measures are obviously of prime importance.

The patient's significant others often need a lot of help in understanding the patient's condition and such manifestations of the illness as emotional lability, slowness of speech, and slowness in ability to respond. The major disabilities are often spasticity, disturbances of coordination, and disturbances of bowel and bladder function.

Such problems can be difficult to deal with for the people who live day to day with a person experiencing MS. MS is a hard condition to adapt to, especially because it is so changeable. Everyone concerned needs and deserves support, understanding, and help with problem solving. Children and adolescents with a parent who has MS need special attention, too. They can sometimes be overlooked. MS can be hard for everyone. Consider again the issues discussed concerning the personal impact of neurologic disorders on pp. 521–524.

PAROXYSMAL DISORDERS OF THE NERVOUS SYSTEM

Outline of Paroxysmal Disorders of the Nervous System

A. Epilepsy
  1. Generalized seizures
    a. Grand mal seizures
    b. Petit mal seizures
    c. Minor motor seizures
  2. Partial seizures

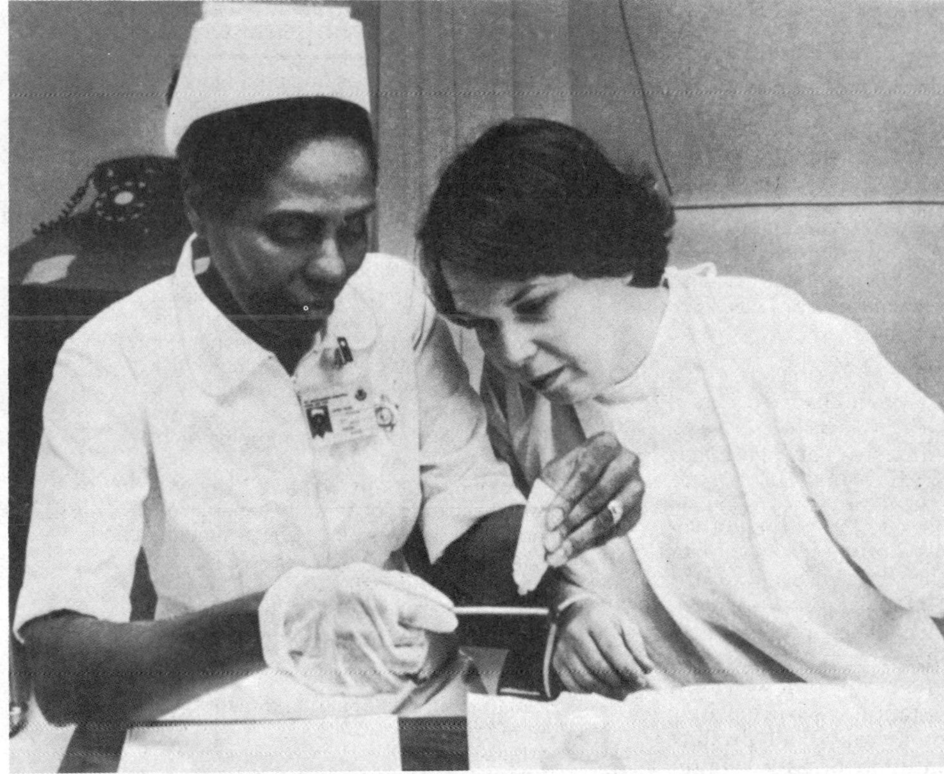

A

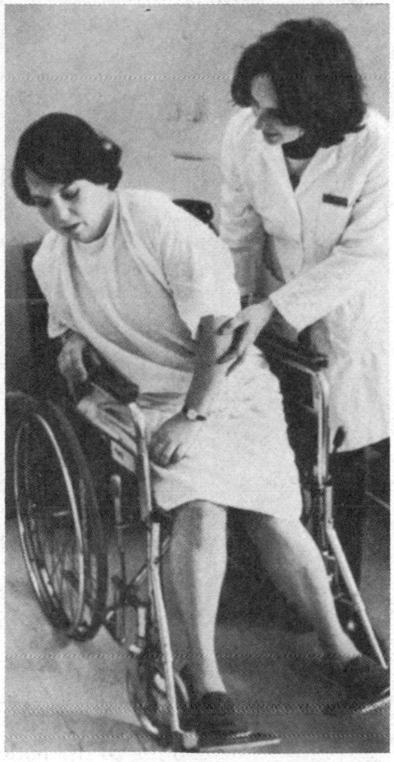

B

Figure 27–18. Nurses at St. Barnabas Hospital, Bronx, N.Y., which has a comprehensive MS treatment program, demonstrate some ways to help MS patients avoid complications. Many patients with bladder problems, for example, can learn to perform intermittent catheterization at home which helps reduce the risk of urinary-tract infection and avoids the need for a permanent catheter. *A,* a nurse demonstrates how to lubricate the catheter. *B,* a nurse-practitioner gives pointers on shifting position to prevent decubitus ulcers. Wheelchair-dependent patients should change position every 15 to 20 minutes either by pushing against the arms of the chair to lift themselves off the seat or by shifting weight from side to side, as shown here, if they cannot lift themselves. Special pads available for chair seats are often helpful. MS patients should also be taught to turn from side to side regularly while in bed, to inspect the area around the coccyx and the buttocks with a mirror for signs of skin breakdown, and to be alert for symptoms of phlebitis. (From Catanzaro, M.: Multiple sclerosis. Exploding myths that compromise patient care. *RN, 40*:42, Dec. 1977.)

a. Partial motor seizures
b. Partial sensory seizures
c. Partial seizures with complex symptomology
3. Status epilepticus
B. Syncope
C. Meniere's disease
D. Headache (cephalgia)
1. Migraine
2. Cluster
3. Muscle contraction headaches (tension)
4. Head pain related to the eyes, ears, teeth, and paranasal sinuses

Epilepsy (Seizure Disorders)

Millions of persons throughout the world experience seizure disorders. Although these nervous system disorders have been written about for 2500 years, they remain poorly understood, surrounded by myths and superstitions, and often inadequately treated. Fortunately, recent increased interest in epilepsy has been responsible for the establishment of several epilepsy centers, with comprehensive diagnostic, treatment, and rehabilitation programs.

DEFINITIONS

"Epilepsy" is derived from the Greek word *epilepsia,* meaning to "take hold of" or "seize." In early times epilepsy was viewed as being of divine origin and was called "the sacred disease" because it was believed that a person with epilepsy was "seized" by the gods. This ancient explanation has been replaced with the current concept that *epilepsies are paroxysmal disorders of the nervous system that result in recurrent attacks of loss of consciousness or other types of seizures in which convulsive movements or other motor activity, sensory phenomena, or behavioral abnormalities may occur.* The word "recurrent" is important in this definition. The occurrence of an isolated, single seizure thus does not mean that the affected person has epilepsy.

It is more appropriate to refer to "the epilepsies" rather than merely "epilepsy," since many types of *recurrent* seizures occur. These seizures result from paroxysmal excessive neuronal discharges in different parts of the brain. The acute disturbance in cerebral function that produces a seizure can usually be demonstrated on an EEG (electroencephalogram).

Below are some important definitions:

- *Seizure.* A seizure is a paroxysmal uncontrolled abnormal discharge of electrical activity in the gray matter of the brain, causing clinical signs and symptoms that interfere with normal function. A seizure is a symptom rather than a disease.
- *Prodromal phase.* Some seizures are preceded by a prodromal phase in which a vague change occurs in emotional reactivity or affective responses, e.g., increasing depression or anxiety. This phase may last minutes or even hours.
- *Aura.* An "aura" occurs at the onset of some seizures. An aura is generally a brief sensory experience directly related to the point of origin of the seizure, e.g., a feeling of weakness, dizziness, strange sensations in an arm or leg, numbness, or an unpleasant odor. An aura is often of importance in localizing the area of the brain from which the seizure originates. For instance, a seizure arising from a focus in the motor strip could produce twitching in the patient's thumb, or a focus in the temporal lobe could cause a patient to experience an unpleasant odor as the first part of the seizure. Usually the aura precedes the other manifestations of the seizure by only a few seconds. Occasionally the aura may give the patient enough time to lie down, or may not even be followed by a complete seizure.

TABLE 27–7. INTERNATIONAL CLASSIFICATION OF EPILEPTIC SEIZURES*

I. Partial seizures (seizures beginning locally)
   A. Partial seizures with elementary symptomatology (generally without impairment of consciousness)
      1. With motor symptoms (includes Jacksonian seizures)
      2. With special sensory or somatosensory symptoms
      3. With autonomic symptoms
      4. Compound forms
   B. Partial seizures with complex symptomatology; generally with impairment of consciousness (temporal lobe or psychomotor seizures)
      1. With impairment of consciousness only
      2. With cognitive symptomatology
      3. With affective symptomatology
      4. With "psychosensory" symptomatology
      5. With "psychomotor" symptomatology (automatisms)
      6. Compound forms
   C. Partial seizures secondarily generalized
II. Generalized seizures (bilaterally symmetrical and without local onset)
   A. Absences (petit mal)
   B. Bilateral massive epileptic myoclonus
   C. Infantile spasms
   D. Clonic seizures
   E. Tonic seizures
   F. Tonic-clonic seizures (grand mal)
   G. Atonic seizures
   H. Akinetic seizures
III. Unilateral seizures (or predominantly)
IV. Unclassified epileptic seizures (unclassified owing to incomplete data)

*Abstracted from Gastaut, H.: Clinical and electroencephalographic classification of epileptic seizures. *Epilepsia* (Amsterdam) 10 (Supplement):1–28, 1969.

- *"Epileptic cry."* The cry, which occurs in some seizures, is caused by a thoracic and abdominal spasm which expels air through the narrowed spastic glottis.
- *Ictus; postictal.* The word "ictus" is synonymous with "seizure." "Postictal" thus refers to that time immediately after a seizure during which a patient usually experiences some change in consciousness, behavior, or activity.

It is important to remember that convulsive seizures may be caused in "normal" persons by electrical stimulation or by administration of convulsion-causing drugs. Also, occasionally simulated convulsive attacks occur in hysterical or other psychoneurotic patients; usually persons having such simulated attacks do not injure themselves during the attack or as a result of falling from the seizure. Such attacks are not "true" seizures.

CLASSIFICATIONS

To understand epilepsy, a nurse must have an understanding of the various types. Numerous methods of classification have been used, most of which have been complex and cumbersome. The method of classification most widely accepted currently is shown in Table 27–7.

With few exceptions, seizures can be divided into two major groups: (1) *generalized seizures,* which begin bilaterally without local onset and show diffuse EEG abnormalities, and (2) *partial seizures* (or focal epilepsy), which begin in one localized area of the cortex and produce abnormalities in one area of the electroencephalogram.

Generalized Seizures. Generalized epilepsy makes up only about one-third of all classified cases. Of the various types of generalized seizures, these are the most common: (1) grand mal seizures (generalized tonic-clonic), (2) petit mal (absence) seizures, and (3) those sometimes referred to as "minor motor seizures" such as myoclonic, akinetic, and atonic.

Grand mal seizures (generalized tonic-clonic) are the type of seizures most people think of when the word "epilepsy" is mentioned. However, they actually make up only about 10 per cent of all seizures. The grand mal seizure typically proceeds as follows:

- *Sudden loss of consciousness.*
- *Tonic phase,* in which the person's entire body stiffens in a state of rigid tonic contraction. (In Figure 27–19*A*, note the stiffening of the trunk and extremities.) If standing or sitting, the person falls stiffly to the floor. A cry may be uttered. During this

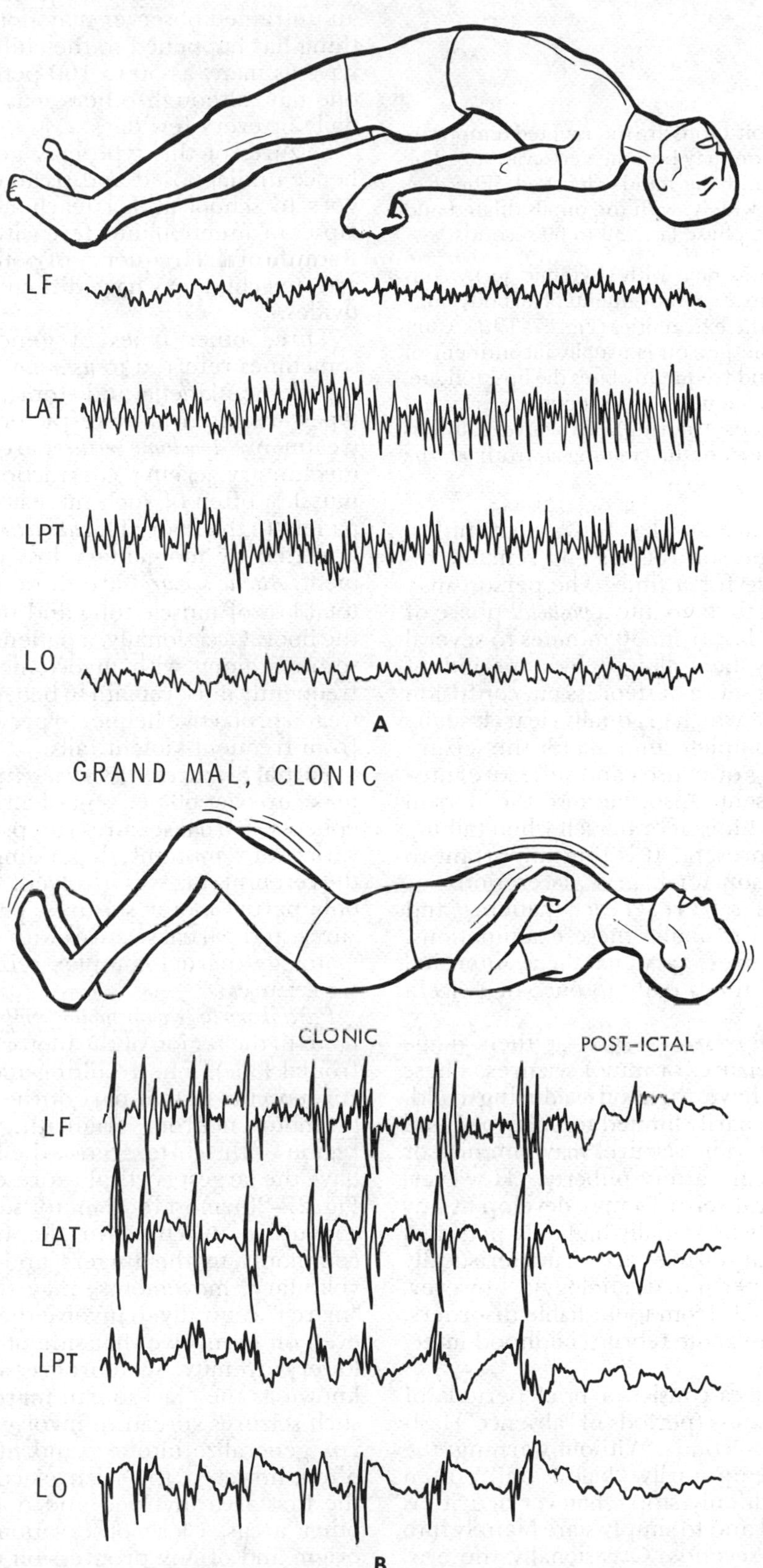

Figure 27–19. **A.** Patient and EEG tracing during *tonic phase* of grand mal seizure. **B.** Patient and EEG tracing during *clonic phase* of grand mal seizure. (Note that EEG tracings for right side of brain are not shown here. Key. LF = left frontal; LAT = left anterior temporal; LPT = left posterior temporal; LO = left occipital.) (From Solomon, G. E., and F. Plum: *Clinical Management of Seizures.* Philadelphia: W. B. Saunders Co., 1976, pp. 26, 27.)

tonic phase, respirations are interrupted temporarily and the person may become very cyanotic. The jaws are fixed and the hands clenched. The eyes may be opened widely, with the pupils dilated and fixed. The tonic phase lasts 30 to 60 seconds.

- *Clonic phase* begins next with rhythmic, jerky contraction and relaxation movements of all body muscles, especially the extremities (Fig. 27–19*B*). During this time, the person is usually incontinent of urine or feces and frequently bites the lips, tongue, and inside of the mouth. Respirations are jerky and become stertorous (snoring). Excessive saliva is blown from the mouth, creating a froth at the lips.

The entire seizure may last for 2 to 5 minutes, after which the person relaxes and remains totally unresponsive for a time. The person may rouse briefly and then go into a *postictal* phase of sleep, which may last from 30 minutes to several hours. This may be followed by a period of general fatigue, a sense of depression, confusion or headache, all of which gradually clear. Usually the person has complete amnesia for the seizure episode. A feeling of nausea and stiff, sore muscles may be present. Also, because the person could not protect himself or herself when falling, injuries may be present. It is thus important to examine the person for bruises, lacerations, or fractures after a seizure. Teach patients and significant others to make these examinations. Grand mal seizures vary in their intensity, e.g., from many times daily to once or twice a year.

Petit mal (absence) seizures are, as their name implies, "little" seizures or minor seizures. These seizures usually have their onset during childhood and are primarily limited to childhood and early adolescence. The seizures may diminish or possibly disappear after puberty. However, grand mal or focal seizures may develop at any time in a patient who initially had only petit mal seizures. Petit mal seizures are characteristically idiopathic (undetermined etiology); however, they may also result from identifiable disorders, e.g., birth injuries, acute febrile childhood infections.

Petit mal seizures consist of brief periods of altered consciousness (periods of "absence") lasting from 5 to 30 seconds. Without warning, the affected child temporarily "blacks out," often appearing to suddenly stop whatever activity is being performed and to simply stare blankly into space for a few seconds. Occasionally the eyes may blink or there may be slight rhythmic movements of the facial muscles or extremities. Since there is no loss of muscle tone, the child seldom falls. When the seizure is over, the child is alert and continues on with previous activities. Petit mal seizures may be so frequent and so brief that an untrained observer may not realize that anything has happened to the child. Some children have as many as 50 to 100 petit mal seizures in one day, although others may have only a few daily or every few days.

Seizures of this type may go unnoticed (and hence undiagnosed and treated) until the child goes to school and a teacher notices that the lapses in attention interfere with learning ability. Because of the frequency of petit mal seizures, an affected child may have difficulty with school activities.

Three other types of generalized seizures, sometimes referred to as *minor motor seizures* are myoclonic, akinetic, and atonic. Seizures of these types are often most refractory to any type of treatment. *Myoclonic seizures* are characterized by involuntary jerking contractions of the major muscles, often of such intensity as to throw the patient to the floor. The *akinetic seizures* are characterized by momentary loss of muscle movement. *Atonic seizures* are those in which there is total loss of muscle tone and the patient falls to the floor. Occasionally, a patient may have atonic seizures along with myoclonic. Such a patient frequently must remain in bed, or when up, must wear a protective helmet to prevent head injuries from frequent violent falls.

Partial Seizures. *Partial seizures (focal seizures)* make up over 60 per cent of all classified cases of epilepsy. Partial seizures can present with a wide variety of symptoms, depending on what part of the cerebral cortex is involved. We consider here only partial motor seizures, partial sensory seizures, and partial seizures with complex symptomatology (partial complex seizures, psychomotor seizures).

Partial seizures with motor symptoms arise from a focus in the region of the motor cortex (posterior frontal lobe). The resulting motor activity (seizure) occurs in that part of the body innervated by motor neurons originating in the affected region of the cortex. Since the hand and fingers have the largest cortical representation (refer to Fig. 27–20), most focal motor seizures begin with convulsive twitching in the upper extremity, commonly in the fingers and hands. The involuntary movements may then spread or "march" centrally to involve the entire limb, and even on to involve that side of the face and the lower extremity. Such progression or "spread" is known as the "Jacksonian march." Occasionally such seizures spread to involve the entire body, i.e., generalize into a grand mal seizure. More often, however, the seizure activity is limited to the first area involved and does not spread to other areas. Close observation of the area of origin and of any progression of movements in this type of seizure is important. It may help to identify the precise area in which the focal cerebral lesion is located.

Partial seizures with sensory symptoms may also

present with a variety of transient symptoms. If the seizure arises from a focus in the parietal area, the person will experience such sensory phenomena as numbness and tingling in the affected area. If the focus is in the occipital region, the person may experience bright, flashing lights in the field of vision opposite to the side of the focus. If the involvement is in the posterior temporal area of the dominant hemisphere (usually the left), the person will experience difficulty with speaking or total speech arrest.

Focal seizures that originate in the anterior temporal lobe present with a complex array of symptoms. Such seizures are variously referred to as *temporal lobe seizures, psychomotor seizures,* and *partial complex seizures.* Frequently these seizures begin with an *aura,* or recognizable sensation, that helps to localize the focus. Often the aura will consist of a sense of "rising" or "welling up" in the epigastric region, or the experiencing of an unpleasant odor. Visual distortions and such feelings as the "déjà vu" phenomenon are not uncommon. The most characteristic part of a psychomotor seizure is the "automatisms" during the seizure, i.e., the patient carries out purposeless and repetitive activities such as lip-smacking, chewing, patting a part of the body, or picking at clothes, while appearing to be in a dreamy state. Such automatic activity during an attack may include inappropriate or asocial behavior. However, in some instances, an untrained observer may not detect any abnormality.

These temporal lobe seizures usually last only 2 to 3 minutes, but may last up to 15 minutes. The patient is usually unaware of any activity during the seizure and may be confused or drowsy *postictally.* If an attempt is made to restrain the patient during a seizure, this often may prompt combative and uncooperative behavior. The unusual behavior demonstrated during a psychomotor seizures often leads to the affected person's being labeled psychotic or otherwise mentally disturbed.

Status Epilepticus. *Status epilepticus* is a state in which seizures are continuous or occur successively so rapidly that recovery between seizures is incomplete. There may be status epilepticus of focal seizures, of the generalized nonconvulsive seizures ("petit mal"), or of the generalized convulsive seizures ("grand mal"). The usual cause of "status" is the abrupt withdrawal of anticonvulsants, although other metabolic factors may be involved. (see p. 649.)

ETIOLOGY

Seizures can be divided into two broad groups according to their etiology: (1) *symptomatic* or *secondary epilepsy,* in which the probable cause of the seizures can be determined, and (2) *idiopathic* or *primary epilepsy,* in which investigation of the patient fails to reveal a definite cause for the seizures.

As will be seen later in this discussion, there is a great deal of dispute over the role of inheritance in the occurrence of idiopathic seizures. The

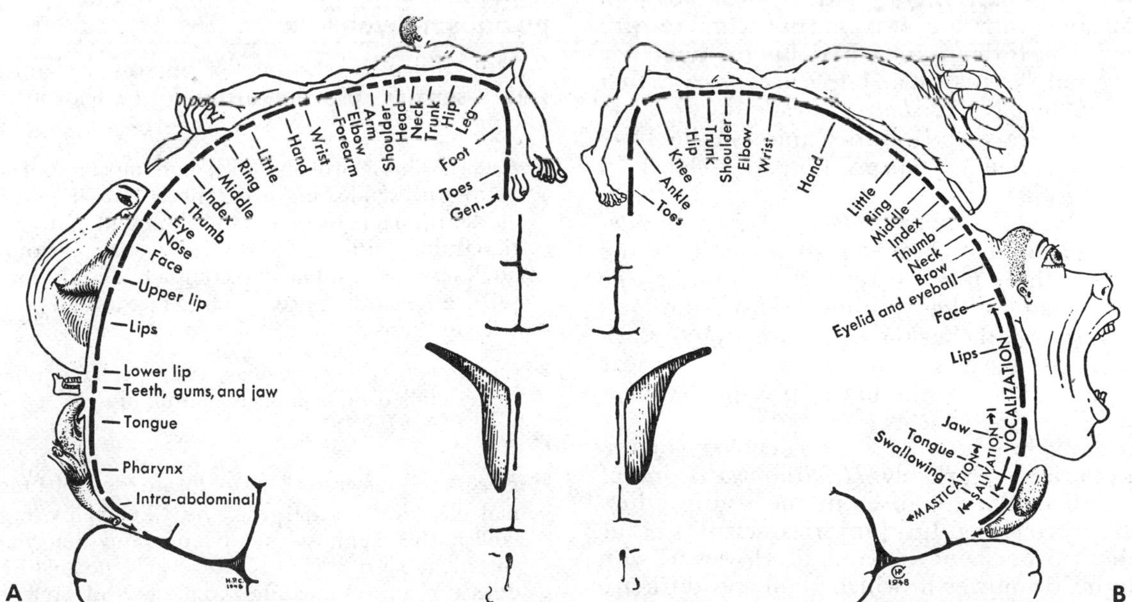

Figure 27–20. **A.** Sensory homunculus, drawn overlying a coronal section through the postcentral gyrus. **B.** Motor homunculus, drawn overlying a coronal section through the precentral gyrus. These figures represent the location of cortical representation of the various parts. The size of the various parts is proportionate to the amount of cortical area devoted to them. (From Penfield, W., and T. Rasmussen: *The Cerebral Cortex of Man: A Clinical Study of Localization of Function.* New York: Macmillan Publishing Co., Inc., 1950.)

causes of symptomatic epilepsy (due to organic or other known factors) are multiple. Among these are: hyperpyrexia, CNS infections, cerebral hypoxia, toxic agents or poisons, metabolic intoxications and disturbances, convulsive agents, cerebral trauma, brain defects, expanding brain lesions, anaphylaxis, and degenerative brain disorders. Some of these etiologic factors are discussed below.

In many of the above conditions, seizures may appear only as transient symptoms and may not recur following treatment of the basic disorder. However, recurrent seizures may persist for years or indefinitely if a permanent lesion or scar remains in the CNS.

Idiopathic epilepsy begins more commonly prior to age 20 years and rarely is initiated after age 30. Thus, beyond 20 years of age, generalized convulsions may often result from an identifiable cause. Of these causes, brain tumors are the most common. (Brain tumors are discussed on p. 602.)

Obviously the causes of seizures are many and are somewhat related to age of onset. Seizures beginning in newborns and infants are most likely due to *congenital brain defects, birth injuries,* or *metabolic problems* such as anoxia, hypoglycemia, or hypocalcemia. Keep in mind also that though the underlying cause may be perinatal, the seizures may not begin until many years later, very often during puberty.

Genetic factors are particularly important in epilepsy that begins in childhood, but decrease in importance with age. It is not the actual seizure disorder itself that is inherited, but the tendency to cerebral dysrhythmia. These are the cases that are usually labeled *idiopathic epilepsy,* since no specific causes can be found. Clinical studies have shown a genetic predisposition to epilepsy in monozygotic twins.

Most seizures occur without obvious precipitating stimuli. However, in some patients the seizure activity may be related to some *specific stimulus.* Among these stimuli are: sudden loud noises, music, flickering light, prolonged reading, coughing, drugs, and sleep. It is not clear whether emotional stimuli can precipitate an attack.

In the adult population, the etiology of seizures varies remarkably. *Head trauma* is one of the most common causes in the young adult. With severe closed head injuries, seizures occur in about 5 per cent of patients. However, with open head injuries in which skull and dura are penetrated, the incidence rises to 30 to 50 per cent.[299] Post-traumatic seizures most likely occur within the first year after injury. For this reason, many neurosurgeons prescribe prophylactic anticonvulsants for their patients with head injuries, to be continued for at least a year after the injury.

When a seizure disorder begins after the age of 20 years, in the absence of head trauma, the patient has a 10 per cent chance of having a *brain tumor.* Seizures caused by neoplasms are usually focal and are often the first symptom of an intracranial mass lesion. In patients over the age of 50 years, *arteriosclerotic cerebrovascular disease* is the most common cause of seizures. These episodes usually accompany a stroke due to infarct or intracerebral hemorrhage. *Other vascular lesions,* such as arteriovenous malformations, present with seizures as the first symptom in 20 to 30 per cent of patients with such lesions.

Infections of the central nervous system frequently result in seizures, either in the acute phase or chronically thereafter. Virus infections, which cause brain destruction, and postinfectious encephalitides can lead to persistent convulsive disorders. Likewise, meningitis, especially in childhood, and brain abscesses are often accompanied by seizures.

Any of a number of *toxic substances* that interfere with brain metabolism or with the supply of oxygen or glucose to the brain can cause seizures. Alcohol is one of the most frequently ingested toxins and can cause seizures either during ingestion or during withdrawal. Lead intoxication, usually in children, can result in lead encephalopathy and a persistent seizure disorder. Chronic drug abuse, especially of barbiturates, can lead to seizures when the drug is withdrawn.

Status epilepticus may be precipitated by the sudden withdrawal of anticonvulsant medication.

DIAGNOSTIC WORK-UP

The clinical work-up of a person presenting with a seizure disorder usually incudes the following:

- *History.* This is probably the single most important factor in establishing a diagnosis and should include: prenatal, birth and developmental information, family history, age at seizure onset, history of all illness and trauma, and complete description of seizures, including precipitating factors and postictal symptoms.
- *Complete physical examination,* with special emphasis on a detailed neurological examination.
- *Skull x-rays.*
- *Electroencephalogram* (EEG) to locate focus of abnormal electrical discharges. The EEG helps to establish the diagnosis of epilepsy and determine specific types of seizures. However, a normal EEG does not always exclude a diagnosis of epilepsy; likewise, the finding of minor abnormalities does not always confirm the diagnosis. During a seizure the EEG abnormalities involve all portions of the cortex. Between seizures patients with epilepsy may

show short bursts of abnormal EEG activity and other EEG abnormalities.

- *CT scan,* to detect congenital abnormalities or presence of mass lesions such as tumors.

Occasionally such other diagnostic tests as *lumbar puncture, cerebral angiography,* and *pneumoencephalography* may be indicated.

An observer's comments about a patient's seizures can be very helpful diagnostically. Seizures should be described in minute detail, including the sequence in which phenomena occur.

MANAGEMENT

For purposes of discussion the management of epilepsy is divided into five areas: (1) elimination of factors that may cause or precipitate seizures; (2) physical and mental health; (3) medical treatment; (4) surgical treatment; and (5) electrical stimulation. The successful management of epilepsy ultimately rests on preventing seizures.

Elimination of Causative Factors. In the process of diagnosis, hopefully the cause of a patient's seizures can be found. The next step is to remove the cause if possible. When definite factors or disorders are known to be the underlying cause of symptomatic epilepsy, every attempt is made to correct these disorders with specific medical or surgical therapy.

Physical and Mental Health. It is important that the person with epilepsy live as normal a life as possible and not be made to feel excessively "different" from others. The patient and significant others must learn to accept the patient's condition and not exaggerate it or make the patient into an invalid through overprotection. While certain dangerous activities should be avoided by the patient or should be engaged in only with special safeguards (e.g., swimming or horseback riding), there is still a wide range of activities that can be enjoyed. The driving of motor vehicles will depend on local laws and the patient's medical control. Significant others should be taught how to care for the patient during a seizure. *Care of a person during a seizure is discussed in Chapter 26, p. 554.* Persons with epilepsy should always wear or carry identification that states they have epilepsy and lists the name of their physician.

A *regular* pattern of adequate diet, fluid intake, and sleep, and moderate recreation and exercise may be helpful. Alcoholic beverages are contraindicated. A good level of general health is, of course, desireable.

Persons with epilepsy often have a *poor self-image,* feelings of inferiority, self-consciousness, guilt, anger, depression and other emotional problems that can be overcome through education and the support and understanding of persons who care about them. Naturally a patient's fears and anxieties over future seizures may be great, e.g., "Where will I be when it happens? What will I be doing? Who will be with me?" Social attitudes concerning epilepsy have changed a great deal in recent years, but more education of the public will be necessary before this illness will lose the mystery and fear with which so many lay persons continue to view it. Only when social attitudes are changed and informed legislation is enacted will persons with epilepsy be able to lead realistic, more fulfilling lives. Various organizations exist that are trying to accomplish these goals and assist persons with epilepsy with their illness-related problems, e.g., the National Epilepsy League, Inc., with headquarters at 130 North Wells St., Chicago, Ill., 60606, and the National Association to Control Epilepsy Inc., with headquarters at 22 East 67th St., New York, N.Y., 10021. Some adults may benefit from vocational rehabilitation. Selected patients may also benefit from counseling. See p. 521 for discussion of the psychologic impact of neurologic disorders and related nursing care.

Medical Therapy. The most effective method of controlling seizures is the use of anticonvulsant drugs, of which there are many.

A few general principles should be kept in mind in the use of *anticonvulsants.* The use of high doses of a single anticonvulsant is likely to be more beneficial than the use of smaller doses of several drugs. Ideally, initial treatment should begin with a single drug (primary anticonvulsant) until either seizure control is attained or unacceptable side effects appear. In the latter case, the dosage of the primary drug should be lowered and a secondary agent added. Various combinations must be tried, until one is found that provides the best possible seizure control with side effects that are tolerable.

The choice of anticonvulsants is based upon the various seizure classifications. *Primary anticonvulsants* are those drugs which, when given alone, provide complete control of the seizures of most patients in the appropriate category. *Secondary anticonvulsants* are those drugs which only rarely provide seizure control alone, but which, when given with a primary anticonvulsant, produce a significant improvement in control. *Ancillary drugs* are not anticonvulsants as such but in some way enhance the effect of an already established anticonvulsant program.

Table 27–8 is a brief summary of the major drugs in each of the three categories for the various classifications of seizures. Consult a current textbook of pharmacology for more detailed information on these drugs.

Clearly, no one anticonvulsant medication will achieve complete seizure control in all patients. Medical therapy for epilepsy thus involves various programs of drugs, which are carefully selected for each individual. This process may require weeks of trial and error and adjustment. During this period the patient and significant others (and frequently the nurse) must observe carefully any seizure activity and side effects from the medications. Also, a patient being treated for the first time should try to identify any factors that may precipitate a seizure. The decision as to which medications to administer to a given patient rests basically on correctly identifying the nature of the attack.

Anticonvulsant medications must be built up in dosage during observation to see that they do

TABLE 27–8. CHOICE OF ANTICONVULSANTS

Classification of Seizure	Primary, Secondary and Ancillary Anticonvulsants	Side Effects
Focal and generalized seizures	*Primary*	
	Phenytoin (Dilantin)	Mental dullness, ataxia, diplopia, gingival hypertrophy.
	Carbamazepine (Tegretol)	Nystagmus, ataxia, rash, *blood dyscrasia;* check WBC and hematocrit monthly.
	Mephenytoin (Mesantoin)	Drowsiness, rash, *blood dyscrasia.* Check WBC and hematocrit monthly.
	Phenacemide (Phenurone)	*Blood dyscrasia;* hepatic destruction, psychosis, Check WBC and hematocrit and test liver function monthly. Used only in most refractory seizure disorder.
	Secondary	
	Phenobarbital	Mental changes, withdrawal seizures if drug stopped abruptly.
	Primidone (Myosoline)	Emotional and mental changes including depression, irritability, impotence. Withdrawal seizures if drug not reduced very slowly at discontinuance.
	Succinimides	
	Phensuximide (Milontin)	Drowsiness, headache
	Methsuximide (Celontin)	Drowsiness, headache
	Benzodiazepines	
	Diazepam (Valium)	
	Clorazepate (Tranxene)	Few side effects; some sleepiness.
	Clonazepam (Clonopin)	Drowsiness, exacerbation of childhood hyperactivity, withdrawal seizures and status epilepticus if drug removed too quickly.
	Ancillary Drugs	
	Acetazolamide (Diamox)	Anorexia, numbness of extremities.
	Dextroamphetamine (Dexedrine)	Anorexia, irritability, insomnia.
True petit mal seizures	**Primary**	
	Ethsuximide (Zarontin)	Gastric distress, nausea, dizziness, drowsiness.
	Sodium valproate (Depakene)	Transient nausea, potential bleeding problems, liver damage.
	Clonazepam (Clonopin)	Drowsiness; exacerbation of childhood hyperactivity, withdrawal seizures and status epilepticus if drug removed too quickly.
	Secondary	
	Trimethadione (Tridione)	Hemeralopia ("glare effect"), blood dyscrasia, immune disorders
	Paramethadione (Paradione)	Anorexia, photophobia, hiccups, blood dyscrasia. Check WBC and hematocrit monthly.
Other minor motor seizures		
Akinetic-atonic seizures	Same drugs as for focal and major generalized seizures	
	Sodium valproate (Depakene)	Transient nausea, potential bleeding problems, liver damage.
Myoclonic seizures	Phenytoin (Dilantin)	(Same as listed above)
	Mephenytoin (Mesantoin)	
	Clonazepam (Clonopin)	
	Sodium Valproate (Depakene)	

not produce untoward toxic side effects. The patient must realize that *it is necessary to take anticonvulsant medicine regularly* and that the dosage should neither be increased nor decreased without consultation with the doctor. The physician will decide if and when a patient who has remained seizure-free for a prolonged period of time can stop taking medication. Frequent and rapid shifting or replacement of drugs is undesirable.

Status Epilepticus. Status epilepticus may be precipitated by the sudden withdrawal of anticonvulsant medication. Patients in status epilepticus may remain comatose and have repetitive seizures for hours.

> *Status epilepticus is a medical emergency. During a seizure, the metabolic demands on the brain are increased dramatically. If these demands continue with no opportunity for the body to recover, the supply of glucose and oxygen to the brain is inadequate and the result may be permanent brain damage.*

The treatment of status epilepticus consists of the following basic measures:

- *Maintain an adequate airway.* Prevent aspiration (e.g., by positioning and suctioning) and provide adequate oxygenation. Pulmonary edema is an occasional complication.
- *Constantly observe* the patient and *provide protection* from self-injury during seizures, e.g., pad siderails.
- *Begin an intravenous infusion* and *keep the line open.*
- Attempt to *prevent exhaustion* and to *terminate seizures* by beginning *emergency anticonvulsant therapy.* The drug of choice is usually intravenous diazepam (Valium), given *slowly* until the seizures stop. This drug may depress respirations, so emergency equipment should be at the bedside. Other medications which may be given intravenously are phenobarbital or phenytoin (Dilantin). Phenobarbital may also depress respirations and may produce a prolonged period of depressed consciousness. Dilantin given intravenously may produce cardiac arrhythmias, so it must be given *very slowly.* Necessary precautionary measures must be taken in administering the above medications. Treatment of status epilepticus is best carried out in a setting where emergency equipment and skilled personnel are available.
- After the seizures have been controlled, *maintenance anticonvulsants* must be instituted (usually Dilantin).

Because status epilepticus is a condition especially difficult for a patient's significant others to witness, they should be given special consideration and assisted in every way possible. Even after the seizures are controlled, the patient may continue to be unconscious for a time. *The development of recurrent seizures must be immediately reported.*

Surgical Treatment. When a patient's seizures do not respond to various combinations of medications, one of several forms of *surgical therapy* may be considered. The first considered, and probably most commonly performed, is *cortical resection.* The usual criteria for this surgical procedure include failure of the medical approach and localization and identification of a focus of abnormal discharge that is easily accessible and is located in dispensable cortex (Fig. 27–21). Results with this type of surgery are most favorable in seizures arising from a focus in the anterior temporal lobe.

Preoperative preparation for cortical resection requires an extensive work-up including several EEGs, extensive neuropsychologic testing, a CT scan, and a cerebral angiogram with WADA procedure to determine hemisphere dominance and location of the speech center.* It also requires that the patient be highly motivated and be prepared psychologically. The surgical procedure is quite long and the patient must be awake during most of it. Complete patient cooperation is essential to success of the surgery.

Surgical intervention is important in other aspects of the treatment of epilepsy. In some patients, epileptic foci are not identified on standard scalp EEGs. In these patients, electrodes may be implanted surgically into the deeper structures of the brain to help localize the focus. Some neurosurgeons have advocated the use of stereotaxic procedures in an effort to destroy foci, to interrupt the pathways of the spread of electrical activity, or to alter the activity of cortical neurons. Results of such procedures have not been gratifying. Other more drastic procedures such as division of the corpus callosum and anterior commissure or hemispherectomy are used on rare occasion. As mentioned earlier, some convulsive seizures are caused by lesions of the brain that can be surgically removed, e.g., operable brain tumors, cysts, or abscesses. (Neurosurgery is discussed in Chapter 28.)

Electrical Stimulation. Electrical stimulation of the anterior cerebellum has been widely publicized as a new treatment for seizures. Since that area of the cerebellum is predominantly inhibitory, it is believed that activation of that system may inhibit seizure foci. However, results of such studies are presently inconclusive.

NURSING CONSIDERATIONS

The nurse plays an important role in the care of patients with seizures. Epilepsy is not usually treated on an inpatient basis. A patient may be hospitalized at the time of diagnosis and possibly later if seizures become uncontrolled or if status

*The WADA procedure involves the intracarotid injection of sodium amytal to determine the location of the speech area.

epilepticus develops. Otherwise treatment is totally on an outpatient basis.

One of the major emphases of the nursing care of a person with epilepsy is in *patient teaching.* How well a patient copes with the disorder and adheres to the treatment program depends to a great degree on how well the nurse works with other members of the treatment team to help the patient understand the disease, understand the importance of adhering to the prescribed medication program, and learn how to live a full life in spite of the seizure disorder. Such factors as increased stress, lack of sleep, emotional upset, and use of alcohol tend to precipitate seizures in an otherwise well controlled patient. Therefore, the patient must realize the importance of trying to eliminate these factors. This task may indeed be difficult.

Many nursing considerations in the care of persons with epilepsy have been presented throughout this discussion and in earlier chapters of this unit. Refer to the discussion in Chapter 26 of the personal impact of neurologic problems, p. 521. Also in that chapter is a detailed discussion of the clinical care of persons during seizures (p. 554) and during reduced states of consciousness (pp. 531–540).

Syncope (Fainting)

Syncope (fainting) is a transient loss of consciousness, for a few seconds up to 1 or 2 minutes. Typically syncope occurs when the person is standing and has experienced prodromal symptoms for a few seconds before losing consciousness. Common prodromal symptoms are dizziness, sweating, epigastric discomfort, and lightheadedness. While unconscious the person is pale or ashen in color, perspires heavily, feels cold to the touch, and has a weak pulse and dilated pupils. Upon recovering consciousness the person is usually immediately mentally alert but may feel weak.

Most frequently syncope results from a sudden decrease in the brain's circulation. The most common type of attack is *vasovagal syncope.* In this condition, which usually occurs in normal adults, there is a sudden loss of resistance in the peripheral blood vessels. Because the blood pools in these dilated peripheral vessels, the circulation to the brain becomes inadequate, causing cerebral ischemia. This common cause of fainting is often associated with gastrointestinal disturbances, anxiety, tension states, and so forth, which may be precipitated by emotional or environmental stresses. At the immediate onset of symptoms the patient should lie down or else sit down and lower the head between the knees.

The second most common cause of syncope is *orthostatic hypotension.* Cerebral ischemia occurs when a patient whose cardiovascular reflexes are impaired assumes an erect posture and an excessive drop in blood pressure occurs. Usually orthostatic hypotension occurs without obvious organic illness other than advancing age. However, it may also be related to various organic conditions of the central or peripheral nervous system, e.g., Parkinson's disease, after sympathectomy or with diabetic neuritis. Persons affected by orthostatic hypotension are taught to exercise their extremities while lying down be-

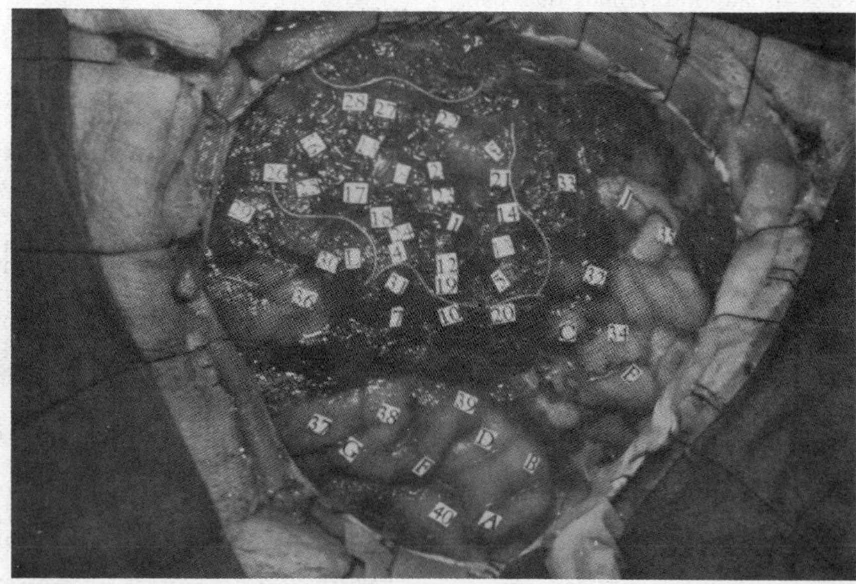

Figure 27–21. The brain is shown exposed here for EEG testing in preparation for excision of seizure focus. Area to be excised marked with piece of thread. (From Isaacs, N. M.: The surgical treatment of epilepsy. *Journal of Neurosurgical Nursing,* 8:165, Dec. 1976.)

fore they sit up, then to exercise them again while sitting on the edge of the bed, and finally to rise *slowly.* This gradual change from a recumbent posture to an erect posture often prevents syncope. Some patients require an abdominal support and leg bandages.

Meniere's Disease

Meniere's disease is a relatively common, chronic disorder of the inner ear, characterized by recurring attacks of vertigo, associated with tinnitus and deafness. It typically affects persons between 40 and 50 years of age. The exact cause is not clear, though it is associated with some process that causes degeneration of the tiny cochlear hair cells.

Symptoms. During an *acute attack,* the person experiences such severe vertigo of the rotational type (feelings of the person spinning or spinning of surrounding objects) that standing or walking may be impossible. This is accompanied by nausea and vomiting, diaphoresis, tinnitus, hearing loss and a feeling of pressure in the ear. It is important to note that true vertigo is present in this disorder, not merely "dizziness." Nystagmus may be present, and at times a brief loss of consciousness may occur. (Nystagmus is a rapid, involuntary movement of the eyeball.) An attack begins suddenly and may last for a few minutes or hours. An attack may recur several times a week or at irregular intervals of several weeks or months.

Hearing loss usually begins with the first attack of vertigo and is progressive. It is a nerve-type deafness and is unilateral in about 90 per cent of patients. Though the other symptoms often subside spontaneously or after treatment, the hearing loss is usually permanent.

Diagnosis. *Diagnostically,* caloric testing may show abnormal vestibular function and electronystagmography (ENG) may measure the nystagmus produced during testing. However, diagnosis depends upon a characteristic history and audiometric (hearing test) findings that show poor speech discrimination and possibly identify a nerve type of hearing loss. (See Chapter 90.)

Treatment. During acute attacks, bed rest is the most effective treatment. The patient will find a comfortable position, usually with the affected ear uppermost. Various medications may be used. Atropine sulfate may be given subcutaneously as soon as possible. (Some persons are taught to give their own injections of this medication.) Intravenous diazepam may also be given *slowly,* to control the vertigo. It is necessary to take appropriate precautions to cope with possible respiratory and cardiac emergencies. The symptoms should subside in one to several hours.

Long term medical management usually includes:

- *Medications.* Medications used most often include antihistaminic drugs such as dimenhydrinate (Dramamine), cyclizine (Marezine), or meclizine (Antivert). Some physicians may prescribe niacin in flushing doses, vasodilating agents, and autonomic blocking agents; but their use is not widely accepted. Diuretics such as acetazolamide (Diamox) and chlorothiazide (Diuril) are also frequently used, but their value has never been established. Mild sedative or hypnotic drugs may be prescribed to help overcome the anxiety experienced by patients between attacks.
- *Emotional support* and reassurance are highly important aspects of management.
- *Dietary management.* For many years physicians have prescribed a low-salt diet to prevent fluid retention. However, the value of this has never been established. Management may include diet therapy to correct obesity and such metabolic disorders as hypoglycemia and hyperlipoproteinemia. Food allergies must also be ruled out, since they appear to trigger attacks in some persons.
- *Changes in habits.* The patient is usually instructed to discontinue smoking to avoid vasospasm and vasoconstriction.

If a person with Meniere's disease does not respond to medical management, one of the various forms of *surgical intervention* may be necessary. Early surgical procedures include shunting or decompression of the endolymphatic sac and section of the vestibular nerve via the middle fossa approach. These procedures usually preserve what hearing is left. However, if hearing has been destroyed and the patient is incapacitated by continuous attacks, a destructive surgical procedure is indicated to remove the organs of the inner ear. This usually involves destruction of the labyrinth (labyrinthectomy) by surgical or cryosurgical means.

Nursing Care. Nursing care of a person hospitalized with Meniere's disease consists basically of:

- *Providing understanding and emotional support* to the person experiencing this incapacitating and distressing disease. The thoughtful nurse bears in mind how frustrating and uncomfortable acute attacks of this disease are for the patient.
- *Providing appropriate teaching* to the patient and significant others concerning the nature of Meniere's disease and prescribed treatments.
- *Providing a quiet, safe environment* for the patient during acute attacks. Because a patient can fall during a severe attack of vertigo, keep the environment safe (e.g., bed siderails up) and provide assistance when the patient is out of bed. Instruct the

patient about (a) the helpfulness of making slow position changes or other movements, (b) any limitations of activity, and (c) the need for these limitations. Keep a call signal convenient for the patient at all times.

- ▶ *Handling the patient gently and slowly and allowing as much self-care as possible.* Allowing a patient to pace self-care activities may minimize vertigo, nausea, and vomiting. Permitting a patient to *have control over his or her own movements* may help the person to relax.
- ▶ *Administering prescribed medications early in an attack* to provide prompt relief of symptoms. Encourage the patient to notify you at the first indication of an attack so that medication can be given.
- ▶ *Arranging for or giving dietary instructions* as prescribed.
- ▶ *Explaining and carrying out pre- and postoperative care if surgery is performed.* Major areas of postoperative nursing care may include: management of nausea, vomiting, and vertigo; prevention of infection; and provision of supportive care and a safe environment.

Headache (Cephalgia)

Headache, *the most common of pains,* may occur either in the absence of organic disease or as a manifestation of serious disease. It is estimated that some form of headache affects over 90 per cent of people at some time. While most headaches are transient and of only moderate or slight severity, a few are chronic, intense and frequently recurrent over a period of months or years. (Pain is discussed in detail in Unit XI.)

> *Headache is a symptom of an underlying disorder, rather than a disease in itself. The cause must be identified so that treatment can be provided.*

Headaches are commonly "self-treated" with over-the-counter medications, available without prescription. Nurses should encourage persons with persistent or repetitive headaches to seek medical evaluation. Excessive use of coal-tar analgesics or any habit-forming drug for relief of pain is to be discouraged.

Some serious disorders that commonly give rise to headache include: intracranial tumors and infections; bacterial or viral meningitis; acute systemic infections; head injuries; cerebral hypoxia; severe hypertension; and chronic or acute diseases of the eye, ear, nose, or throat. Fortunately, most headaches do not indicate serious disease.

The types of headaches are numerous; we discuss only those seen most frequently: (a) migraine, (b) cluster headaches, (c) tension headaches, and (d) head pain related to the eyes, ears, teeth, and paranasal structures. Certain individuals have several types of headaches, e.g., migraine and tension headaches are often associated (Table 27–9).

Diagnosis of Headache. To determine the cause of recurrent or chronic headaches, the physician takes a detailed history and thoroughly studies the patient both physically and psychologically. Special attention is given to neurologic assessment. Diagnostic tests that may be performed include skull x-rays, EEG, and lumbar puncture with CSF examination. If an intracranial lesion is suspected, the investigation may also include echoencephalography, radioisotope brain scan, angiography, and a CT scan.

The history includes asking about: (1) localization and paths of pain radiation; (2) character of the headache, e.g., sharp, dull, throbbing; (3) intensity of pain; (4) mode of onset, duration, and frequency of headache; (5) mode of cessation of headache; (6) localized tenderness; (7) associated phenomena and/or precipitating factors, and (8) familial incidence.

The *nurse's observations* of a patient's headaches can help to establish the diagnosis and thus should be detailed and precise.

MIGRAINE HEADACHES

Migraine headaches are a paroxysmal disorder characterized by recurrent throbbing headaches. The headaches typically first appear during puberty or in the second and third decades of life. They generally decrease in frequency and severity with advancing years. An estimated 5 to 10 per cent of the general population experience migraine, with females more susceptible than males. The headaches often occur during the premenstrual period and are rare during pregnancy. Migraines are most commonly experienced at irregular intervals. The frequency of the headaches varies, e.g., they recur several times weekly in some individuals and only several times a year in others.

Pathogenesis. The specific pathophysiology of migraine is not definitely known; however, the *vascular theory* has come to be accepted. The early neurologic symptoms are postulated to be due to vasoconstriction, and the later intense, throbbing headache due to dilatation of extracranial and intracranial branches of the external carotid artery. Researchers are uncertain about the underlying mechanism that causes this periodic spasm and dilatation of vessels.

The pathogenesis of migraine includes psychologic as well as physical factors. These headaches most often occur in persons who have "perfectionist" tendencies. Individual attacks of migraine may be precipitated by various conditions, often of a repetitive nature, e.g., fatigue, hunger, refractive errors, bright light, surprises, mental and emotional excitement, excessive smoking, high altitudes, drinking alcoholic beverages. Certain foods may precipitate attacks, e.g., onions, nuts, chocolate, cheese, nitrites (as in ham, hot dogs), monosodium glutamate (MSG), coffee, tea, sucrose, fermented or marinated foods, or fried foods.[262] All writers stress the hereditary and familial character of these headaches. The use of oral contraceptives is believed by many to exacerbate migraines, inducing their onset in women previously free from significant headaches.

Symptoms. The "classic" or "typical" migraine headache may be preceded by an *aura* or *prodromal phase* in which the patient may feel depressed, irritable, restless, and perhaps anorexic. During this period the person may also experience *transient neurologic disturbances,* e.g., visual disturbances (flashes of lights, bright spots, distorted vision, diplopia, transitory impaired vision), vertigo, nausea, diarrhea, abdominal pain, paresthesias (numbness or tingling of lips, face, or extremities) or transient hemiparesis. The prodromal symptoms may last only a few minutes or several hours.

A migraine headache has a "crescendo" quality, gradually increasing in severity until the pain becomes intense and all-encompassing. The

TABLE 27–9. CHARACTERISTICS OF COMMON VASCULAR HEADACHES AND TENSION HEADACHES

Type of Headache	Onset	Frequency	Duration	Nature of Pain	Location	Prodromal Signs and Symptoms	Associated Symptoms	Remarks
Vascular Classic migraine	May begin at any age, usually adolescence.	Periodic and recurrent.	Usually 4–6 hours.	Usually severe.	Unilateral, frontal, or temporal at onset, but may vary.	Transient visual field defects. Transient paresthesias, paralysis of an extremity, or confusion. These subside as pain begins.	Irritability, photophobia, nausea, vomiting, constipation or diarrhea, chills, tremors, pallor, sweating.	Hereditary incidence high. Following attack, often have feeling of well-being, unusual energy. Personality factors often contribute.
Common migraine	May begin at any age. Gradual onset.	Episodic. Increase with life crisis.	Many hours to several days.	Usually starts slowly and builds throbbing aching pain. May awaken with severe headache	Variable. May start unilaterally and spread.	No striking prodome. May have changes in fluid balance, GI symptoms, vague psychic disturbances for several hours or days before onset of headache.	Nausea, vomiting, fatigue, chills, localized or general edema and diuresis, nasal stuffiness (autonomic disturbances).	Hereditary incidence high. Often relieved by pregnancy, illness. May be correlated with "let down" activities: "Weekend, Monday, menstrual, premenstrual, relaxation headache."
Cluster migraine	May start in early adulthood. Usually precipitated by vasodilators, alcohol, nitrites, histamine. Sudden onset.	Many attacks in quick succession over few days or weeks followed by remission which lasts for months.	Few minutes to few hours; usually 30–90 minutes.	Intense pain, boring, throbbing. Starts and stops suddenly.	Usually unilateral.	Uncommon.	Profuse watering and redness of conjunctiva, nasal stuffiness, increased perspiration, swelling of temporal vessels.	May be a family history of migraine. More common in older men. During remission, usual precipitants (alcohol) do not cause attack.
Muscle contraction (Tension)	Usually in adolescence. Associated with tension or anxiety. Gradual onset.	Varies with stress. Episodic.	Variable. Can be constant without treatment.	Dull, constant, tight band pressure. Non-pulsating. Varies in intensity.	Usually bilateral, but may be poorly defined. Involves neck, shoulders, occiput. May spread to frontal region.	None.	Sustained contraction of neck and head muscles.	No familial history.

Hoskins, L. M.: Vascular and tension headaches. *American Journal of Nursing,* 74:846, May 1974.

head pain is unilateral with "classic" migraines. The pain may be localized to the front, back, or side of the head, and may begin at any point in the head. The temple and the eye area are common locations. The prodromal symptoms and the head pain rarely recur in the same location in every attack.

Pain varies in intensity, from mild discomfort to a prostrating, throbbing pain that forces the patient to seek seclusion and take to bed in a darkened room. The pain is variously described as vise-like, dull and boring, pressing, throbbing, or hammering. During the period of the attack (typically 4 to 6 hours) the patient is acutely ill and may be extremely irritable. Various somatic manifestations may accompany severe attacks: photophobia, nausea, vomiting, vertigo, tremor, diarrhea, and excessive sweating or chilliness. (The common symptoms of nausea and vomiting explain why many people commonly call migraine headaches "sick headaches.") There is usually a general hypersensitiveness of all the sensory organs, e.g., the patient withdraws from light and sound. During the attack the arteries of the head may become prominent and the amplitude of their pulsations increased. Superficially the patient's head may be very tender. Swelling, redness, and excessive tearing of the eyes and swelling of the nasal mucosa (sometimes accompanied by epistaxis) may occur with the headache. While the pain is initially often of a throbbing nature, it may later become a steady ache.

With "atypical" or "common" migraine, the headache begins suddenly, with or without prodromal symptoms, may be generalized or unilateral, and may or may not be accompanied by nausea and vomiting. There are numerous variants of the migraine syndrome, and many variations within individual patients.

Treatment. The treatment of migraine involves both prevention of attacks and treatment of acute attacks. In general, the treatment of migraine is not totally successful.

Treatment of an acute attack of migraine varies with the intensity of the attack. No treatment is given for the transient neurologic symptoms. If the headache is *mild*, such analgesics as acetaminophen or acetylsalicylic acid may provide relief. *More severe headaches* respond only to ergot preparations, and only if these are given within 30 to 60 minutes after onset of the headache. The ergot preparation may be given orally, intravenously, or rectally. Ergot must be taken *before* the vessels become rigid from edema in their walls. Once the headache has become intense, ergot is of little value, and a stronger analgesic such as codeine sulfate or meperidine should be used.

Some sources say the pain of migraine may be reduced by applying pressure on the common carotid artery and the affected superficial artery. Provision of a therapeutic environment is helpful during an attack, e.g., a quiet, darkened room. Some patients find additional relief from damp compresses.

Between attacks, the individual is usually in a normal state of health. If the migraine attacks occur as frequently as once a week or more often, an attempt should be made to *prevent* them. Methysergide (Sansert) is the medication most often used. It can be effective in reducing the frequency of attacks or abolishing them completely. However, since this drug can have serious complications if used over a long period, it should be discontinued for several weeks in every 6 months of treatment.

Some persons with migraine may benefit from relaxation techniques or counseling, directed at preventing attacks by helping the patient understand tensions and resolve major life conflicts. (You may find it helpful to refer to Chapter 3, "Mind-Body (Psyche-Soma) Interaction," and Unit III, "Stress and Illness.")

Another prophylactic measure is prescription of a restrictive diet directed at trying to avoid food substances found to predispose to migraine headaches.

CLUSTER HEADACHES

Cluster headaches (histamine headaches) are classified by some as a form of migraine, formerly believed to be caused by a sensitivity to histamine. Most persons with cluster headaches do not have a background of migraine headaches. Patients with cluster headaches have excruciatingly painful, unilateral headaches that tend to occur in clusters, i.e., numerous attacks occur within a few days, weeks, or occasionally months, and then there is a remission, with no symptoms for months or years. Following the remission, the headaches again recur in clusters. Men are affected more frequently than women with this agonizing head pain. Attacks usually begin in middle life. Recurrent attacks are dreaded because of the intense suffering they bring.

The individual attacks begin suddenly and may last only a few minutes or as long as 2 to 3 hours. Attacks often begin at night at approximately the same time. During the attack the patient typically experiences intense, throbbing or steady pain arising high in the nostril and spreading to one side of the forehead, around and behind the eye on the affected side. During the attack, on the side of the pain, the nose and eye water and the skin reddens. Nasal congestion and injection of the conjunctiva commonly occur. The cluster of attacks subsides as suddenly and inexplicably as it began.

Cluster headaches may recur at irregular intervals over many years, often related to times of stress, anxiety or emotional upset. During a "cluster," the ingestion of alcohol sometimes precipitates attacks.

Treatment of cluster headaches is ineffective because of the shortness of the attacks. The patient is acutely ill during the attack and desires to be alone and quiet. The application of cold helps bring relief to some persons. Some physicians suggest a single dose of ergot to be given at bed time every night during the cluster. The practice of "desensitizing" a patient by daily slow intravenous injections of histamine acid phosphate is no longer used. Supportive care is important, since persons with cluster headaches may become depressed over their condition and are often *very fearful of recurrent attacks.*

MUSCLE CONTRACTION HEADACHES (TENSION HEADACHES)

Muscle contraction headaches result from long-sustained contraction of skeletal muscles around the scalp, face, neck, and upper back. Vasodilatation of the associated cranial arteries also may contribute to the irritability of the involved muscles and the head pain. The long-sustained contraction causes the muscles to become tender and, as a result, the patient further restricts their motion. This prolonged muscle contraction is the primary source of many headaches that are associated with states of excessive emotional tension. These headaches often have their onset in adolescence. Tension headaches tend to occur most often in middle age and may be associated with anxiety and depression, increasing markedly with menopause. Often premenstrual headaches are of this type.

Sustained muscle contraction may also cause headaches secondary to painful stimuli from other cranial structures, e.g., brain tumor, the distended arteries of vascular headache, inflammation in the eye, ear, nose, paranasal spaces, or teeth.

Muscle contraction headaches typically cause a steady, nonpulsatile ache (unilateral or bilateral) in any region of the head. Often pain occurs in the occipital and upper cervical regions, and extends diffusely over the top of the head. The pain is variably described as feelings of tightness, fullness, drawing sensations, or pressure. The headaches may last unrelieved for weeks, months, or years. The pain may be localized or change frequently in location and intensity. Sometimes these headaches are fleeting but recurrent. The onset of tension headaches is more gradual than with migraine. Nausea and vomiting may accompany tension headache, but as a late reaction to pain. The headache may be spontaneously accompanied by dizziness, tinnitus, or lacrimation, or these symptoms may be elicited by pressing on the tender muscles. Palpation may demonstrate contracted muscles with localized painful areas or nodules. The patient may experience pain upon combing the hair or wearing a hat, and exposure to cold may precipitate or aggravate a headache.

Muscle contraction headaches are *treated* when possible by removing the primary source of stimulation, e.g., treating disease of the teeth or nose. Persons with prolonged or recurrent muscle contraction headaches of psychologic origin are treated with counseling (as discussed under migraine). The symptomatic treatment of the headaches themselves includes: massage of the affected muscles, local application of heat, rest, and the use of various relaxation techniques. Sometimes local injections of procaine are given. Tension headaches respond best to a medication which combines a non-narcotic analgesic with a drug to relieve anxiety. Occasionally a stronger analgesic is needed, such as codeine sulfate or meperidine.

HEAD PAIN RELATED TO THE EYES, EARS, TEETH, AND PARANASAL STRUCTURES

Eyes. Headaches may result from errors of refraction, glaucoma (with increased intraocular pressure), inflammation, and disturbances of ocular muscle equilibrium.

Ears. Primary ear disease which produces headache is relatively rare, but when it does occur the process is usually inflammatory or destructive.

Teeth. Painful stimuli in a tooth produce local toothache, which may be accompanied by a secondary headache resulting from prolonged muscle contraction.

Paranasal Structures. The openings to the sinuses are more highly sensitive to pain than the sinuses' walls, and thus the pain associated with sinus infection is most likely due to irritation and inflammation of these openings. The pain of the *sinus headache* is typically reduced or eliminated by the intranasal application of vasoconstrictor agents or topical anesthetics, particularly around the openings to the sinuses.

Conclusion

The care of persons with any of the various types of recurring headache requires patience and understanding. The nurse and physician need to communicate their support and caring and encourage the individual to minimize stresses and tensions and live as normal a life as possible in spite of this persistent disorder.

Headaches *are* common, but distressing nevertheless, and nurses in various settings are asked to help provide relief. There is much that a creative nurse can do to help provide comfort, e.g., establish and maintain a therapeutic environment, promptly administer medications, provide compresses and massage. Detailed discussion of the nursing role in providing pain relief is provided in Unit XI of this text and in Sorensen and Luckmann, *Basic Nursing: A Psychophysiologic Approach,* Chapter 34.

TRAUMA AFFECTING THE NERVOUS SYSTEM

Outline of Trauma Affecting the Nervous System

A. Injuries to the head
  1. Primary injuries in head trauma
    a. Injuries to the scalp
    b. Injuries to the skull
    c. Injuries to the brain
      (1) Concussions
      (2) Contusions
  2. Secondary event in head trauma
    a. Epidural hematoma (extradural hematoma)
    b. Subdural hematoma (SDH)
    c. Intracerebral hematoma
    d. Brain swelling and edema
    e. Infections
    f. Complications and sequelae
  3. Clinical care following head injury
B. Injuries to the spinal cord or its roots
  1. Ruptured intervertebral disk
C. Injuries to peripheral nerves
  1. Median nerve compression at the wrist
  2. Ulnar nerve compression at the elbow
  3. Sciatic nerve injury

The nervous system can be traumatized in many ways, e.g., through physical injuries or by chemicals, electric currents, or radiation. The primary focus of this discussion is on accidental injuries resulting in forceful puncture, blows, fractures, or crushing injuries.

*Overview of Injuries to the Head (Craniocerebral Trauma)**

Introduction. *Head injury is frequently only one aspect of the problems seen in the traumatized patient.* It is not uncommon for a person with a head injury to have other significant injuries. General trauma is known to be the single most common cause of death and significant morbidity in young people (up to about age 40). Two thirds of those who die in motor vehicle accidents have head injuries[151] which may or may not be associated with other injuries.

Although physicians and nurses have no way of preventing the *primary* brain trauma caused by the original accident (e.g., contusions and hemorrhages), prompt treatment may minimize the development of *secondary* lesions resulting from circulatory impairment and cerebral edema. Vigorous treatment of hypoxia and acid-base disturbances (which almost always occur in comatose patients) may be an effective means of reducing head injury mortality.

Many patients suffer primary, irreversible brain injury at the time of the accident, which ultimately causes death. Brain stem hemorrhage is the most common cause of death from such injuries. *Severe cerebral swelling* commonly follows brain injury and is probably the most common cause of death in those who survive an initial injury and who do not develop intracranial mass lesions. Some patients survive the initial trauma of head injury only to later develop intracranial mass lesions. Some patients survive the initial trauma of head injury only to later develop *expanding hematomas,* e.g., epidural and subdural hemorrhages, which may be fatal unless promptly diagnosed and treated.

Among other major injuries commonly seen in patients with head injury are: facial fractures, injuries to the lungs or heart, cervical neck fractures, abdominal injuries, and musculoskeletal injuries. Both facial fractures and injury to the lungs can contribute to respiratory insufficiency. Obstruction of the airway (facial fractures) and decreased ability to ventilate (e.g., from pulmonary contusion, flail chest, pneumothorax) contribute to respiratory insufficiency and poor oxygenation of brain (and other) tissues. Poor oxygenation can contribute to the death of the brain injured patient. Because of this, *establishing airway patency and adequate breathing assume top priority* in treating a head-injured person (as is true in persons with other disorders).

Maintaining appropriate circulation is the next priority. Hemorrhagic shock may be present in a patient with multiple trauma. It is rarely (possibly never) caused by the head injury itself, but rather is frequently related to (1) rupture of one of the abdominal organs and (2) musculoskeletal injuries such as a fractured femur and pelvis. Circulation may be further compromised by the presence of a cardiac contusion with associated arrhythmias. (Head injuries can also cause arrhythmias and further complicate the situation.)

Generally, prior to extensive manipulation of the patient to treat these priorities, care is taken to protect

*See also section concerning neurologic and neurosurgical emergencies in Chapter 95.

the neck. Until the presence of a cervical neck fracture can be ruled out, a neck collar is often applied. If this is not done, cervical spinal cord injury, producing quadriplegia, can be a complication of resuscitation (e.g., intubation) procedures.

> *Neck fractures are commonly associated with head injury, and although other life-saving treatments may have priority over diagnosing a neck fracture, protecting the patient from further spinal cord injury until the diagnosis can be ruled out is extremely important and can be quickly accomplished.*

Once the physical condition of a person with *multiple trauma* has been stabilized, subsequent care is usually provided in an intensive care setting. Recent attention to the scope of the problem of trauma has resulted in increased research in this area, and the development of specialized units to care for trauma victims. Even without a specialized trauma unit persons with head injury and other trauma are generally cared for by a multidisciplinary team, including nurses, social workers, and a variety of specialists. It is challenging for a nurse to be part of such a specialized team. It requires the nurse to have an extensive knowledge of pathophysiology, signs and symptoms, and treatment protocols, as a patient with multiple injuries often requires conflicting types of therapy for the various injuries. For instance, the challenge of minimizing the complications of immobility can easily be overlooked in the rush to provide care even when one-to-one nursing care is possible.

> *The nurse must be continuously alert to see that treatment of one injury does not make another one worse!*

Considerable investigative attention is being given to *identifying patients for whom the inevitable outcome is death.* Yearly this becomes a more serious problem as continued technologic advances occur. In the areas of head injury and medical coma, active research is being done to identify signs and symptoms that correlate with the eventual death of patients. Recent publications address predicting the outcomes in various types of patients with head injury. These data have already helped clarify some *predictive criteria,* signs and symptoms to be observed for and the results of various types of therapy.[153, 154, 155, 156, 312] Jannett and associates have taken the lead in the study of head injuries, while Plum and others are striving for the same type of data related to medical coma.[252]

Mechanisms of Injury. *Head injuries are the result of the sudden application of force to the head.* The results of the force are complex and not fully understood. Three mechanisms have been identified as major contributors to head trauma: acceleration, deceleration, and deformation. When a blow is struck to the head and the head is free to move, the injury produced is called an *acceleration injury.* If the head is not able to move freely, the injury is termed a *deceleration injury. Deformation* refers to injuries that result in deforming and disrupting the integrity of the impacted structure, e.g., fractures of the skull. Some mechanisms in head injuries are summarized in Figure 27–22.

Another way to categorize head trauma is by description of the injury, i.e., *blunt* or *penetrating* trauma. *Blunt trauma* results frequently in acceleration/deceleration injuries. The injury produced is complex and involves several head structures, e.g., brain substance, blood vessels. Since the skull and intracranial contents move at different rates, the brain, which is "floating in fluid," whipsaws within the skull, creating injuries at multiple points. It is important to remember that the brain is partly tethered down and also is suspended in fluid. A blow to the skull can cause swirling of the hemispheres and twisting of the brain stem (which is fixed). As the brain moves, it is raked over the prominences of the skull, which is *not* smooth on the inside. This causes bruising and laceration of the brain tissue and may cause disruption of the small surface blood vessels. Cranial nerves, nerve tracts, larger blood vessels and other tissues may be stretched, twisted, and rotated, with resulting disruption in their functions. Changes in vascular integrity may lead to fluid shifts and petechial hemorrhages. Immediately below the point of impact, the brain surface injury produced by the blow is called a *coup* injury. On the opposite side of the brain, the injury caused by the same blow is called a *contrecoup* injury. (Contrecoup is derived from a French word meaning "reverse-blow.") In addition to these two sites, there are frequently multiple areas of injury along the line of the force of the blow. The tissues around the major injured areas are often swollen. The swelling itself increases the overall effect of the injury.

Penetrating injuries include those made by foreign bodies such as knives or bullets or those made by bone fragments from a skull fracture.

> Never remove a penetrating object that is still in a head injury. *This should be done in an operating room under close medical supervision.*

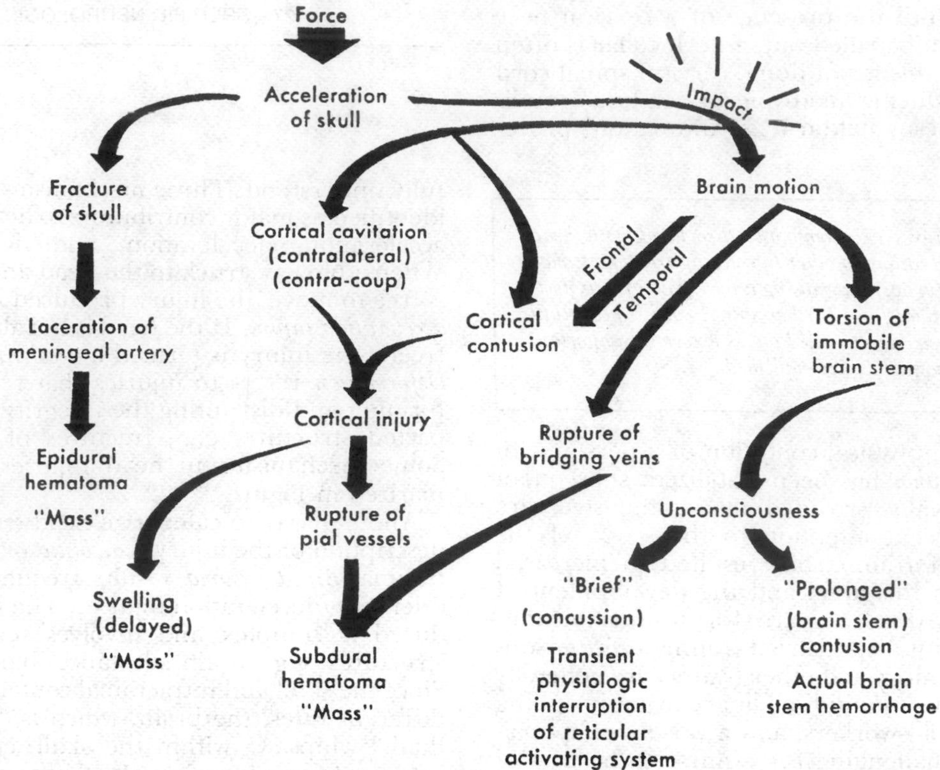

Figure 27–22. The mechanisms in head injuries. (From Sproul, C., and R. Mullanney (Eds.): *Emergency Care: Assessment and Intervention.* St. Louis: C. V. Mosby Co., 1974, p. 225.)

The velocity with which the penetrating object pierces the skull and brain is related to the amount of injury caused in many instances. For example, the bone fragments from a skull fracture may cause local injury to the brain by lacerating the tissue and causing damage to other structures such as nerves and blood vessels. If a major blood vessel ruptures, a large clot may form, causing damage to adjacent and even remote structures (e.g., compression of the brain stem from one of the herniation syndromes — see Chapter 26). In this case, the secondary effect, i.e., a hematoma will cause extensive damage to brain tissues (Fig. 27–23).

High-velocity objects such as bullets impart a shock wave to the skull and brain. The shock wave may cause significant damage to brain structures away from those in the actual path of

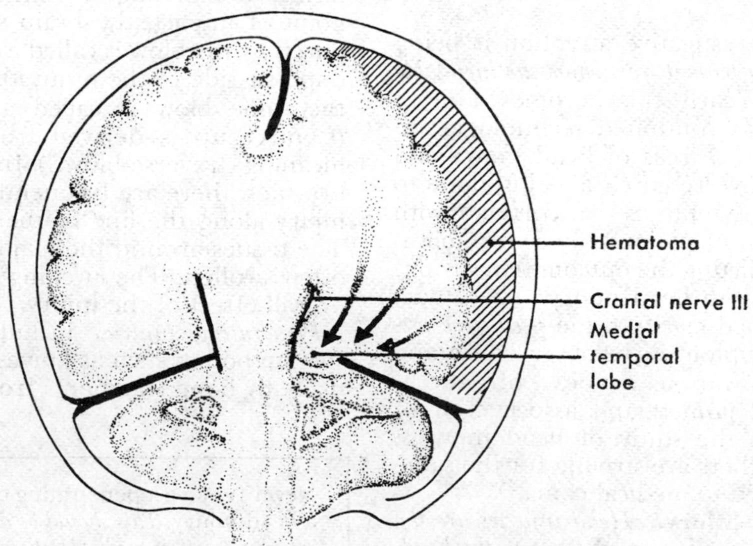

Figure 27–23. Transtentorial herniation secondary to a hematoma. (From Sproul, C., and R. Mullanney (Eds.): *Emergency Care: Assessment and Intervention.* St. Louis: C. V. Mosby Co., 1974, p. 227.)

the missile. Actual "explosion" of the brain substance occurs, although it is more common to see lacerations and maceration of the tissues. Frequently, with low- and high-velocity penetrating wounds, there is open communication between the exterior (external environment) and the cranial cavity. Thus, these injuries are a ready focus for infection. They are commonly treated surgically, with debridement of the tissues and closure of the wound.

Injuries may also be classified according to the structure damaged and according to whether they are primary or secondary. *Primary* refers to the *impact* damage, the severity of which can be estimated by the initial signs and symptoms shown by the patient. *Secondary* or *delayed* events include edema, hemorrhage, or infection. These processes can significantly impede recovery or even result in the death of a person with an otherwise mild injury. The following discussion is divided first into primary injuries and secondary events. These two sections are subdivided according to location of the injury. After the presentation of the types of head injuries, sequelae and complications are discussed. Finally, the general treatment and nursing care conclude the section on the head-injured patient.

Primary Injuries in Head Trauma

Primary injuries that may occur with head trauma include injuries to the scalp, skull, and/or brain. These injuries, which occur in various combinations, are the result of the original *impact.*

INJURIES TO THE SCALP

Injuries to the scalp can cause lacerations, hematomas, and damage to the skin (contusions or abrasions). They may bleed profusely and may be unsightly. Without accompanying damage to other areas, these are minor injuries, rarely causing a patient to be admitted to a hospital. The nurse may instruct the patient in the care of the wound as needed. Infants, small children, and hypovolemic adults are especially prone to shock.

INJURIES TO THE SKULL

Skull fractures are the principal injuries to the skull. The fractures themselves *do not* automatically mean that brain injury is also present, although skull fractures are often present in patients with serious brain injuries. Depressed fractures injure the brain by bruising it (abrasion) or by bone fragments being driven into the brain (lacerations). Moreover, fractures are commonly caused by a force that is sufficient to cause both the fracture and the brain injury. Nurses need to differentiate between these two injuries, however, because the site of the fracture and the extent of the brain injury may not correlate.

There are three basic *types of skull fractures:* linear, depressed, and basilar.

Linear fractures, seen as thin lines on x-ray, do not require any treatment. They are important only if there is significant underlying brain damage.

Depressed skull fractures are also diagnosed by x-ray. Surgical intervention may be necessary within the first 24 hours after injury. Depressed fractures may be associated with bone fragments penetrating into the substance of the brain. If such fragments are present, the area is usually surgically explored and debrided, and debris is removed.

Basilar skull fractures are those that occur along the base of the skull. Rarely are they diagnosed by x-ray. Rather, the presence of CSF draining from the ear or nose, various cranial nerve injuries, the presence of blood behind the ear drum (and later a bruise over the mastoid called a *Battle sign*), drainage from the

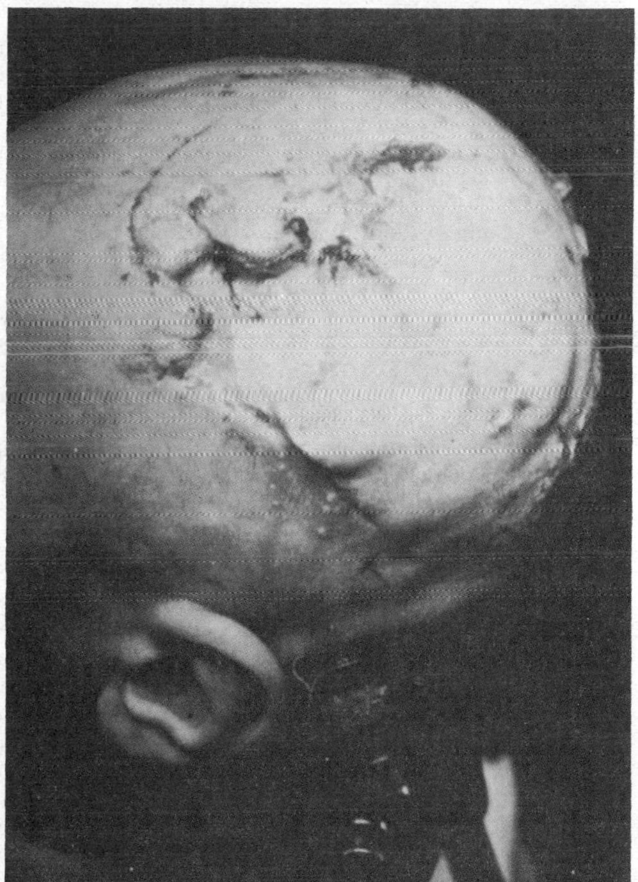

Figure 27–24. Extensive laceration and partial avulsion of scalp that required shaving of entire head before suturing. (From Javid, M.: Traumatic injuries. Office treatment of craniocerebral trauma. *Postgraduate Medicine*, 61:233, May 1977, p. 236).

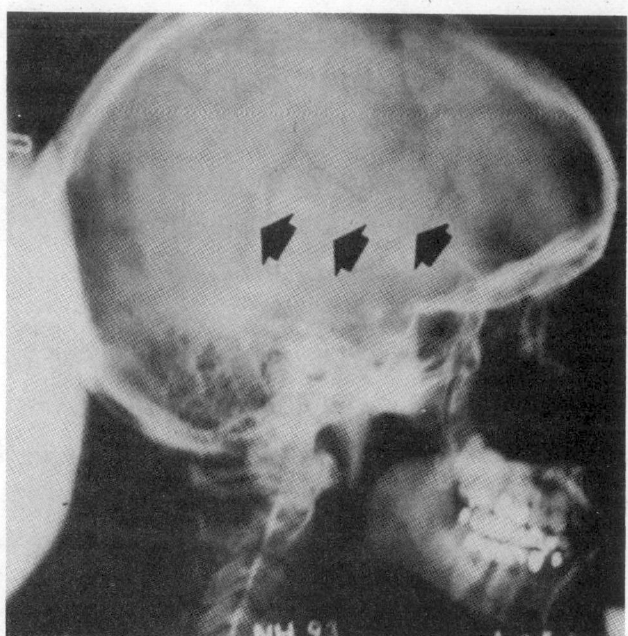

Figure 27–25. Right lateral skull x-ray demonstrating multiple linear and compound depressed skull fractures (arrows), the result of a high-speed propeller injury. (From Jackson, F. E., Back, J. V., and R. Pratt, III: Current management of acute injuries of the skull and brain. *American Family Physician,* 10:82, Aug. 1974.)

nose or ear, and periorbital ecchymosis (i.e., a bruise around the eyes) are some of the diagnostic criteria. Some of the signs of cranial nerve damage that the person may have are the following:

1. A loss of vision, i.e., blindness or blurred vision (optic nerve damage)
2. A loss of hearing, with postural vertigo and nystagmus (auditory nerve damage)
3. A loss of the sense of smell on one or both sides (olfactory nerve damage)
4. A squint and/or fixed dilated pupil, with loss of some of the eye movements (oculomotor nerve damage)
5. A facial paresis/paralysis on one side of the face (facial nerve damage)

These signs may be present at the time of the initial injury or may develop later. Sequelae of the fracture may include permanent loss of the functions mentioned or persistence of the abnormal symptoms.

Basilar skull fractures, depressed fractures, and other open (i.e., compound) fractures all allow ready communication between the exterior environment and the brain. Thus, the possibility of the patient's developing an infection is high (see brain abscess, meningitis, pp. 594 and 595). *Care is directed toward prevention of infection.* The patient may receive prophylactic antibiotics, although the use of these is controversial.

Detecting CSF leakage from the nose or ear (indicative of *intracranial cerebrospinal fluid fistula*) is a vital nursing observation after a skull injury. It is not always easy to detect CSF leakage, because it is frequently mixed with blood early after the injury. How to detect leakage, the goals of treatment, and the important nursing precautions and nursing care needed for a person who has or is suspected of having CSF leakage are discussed on p. 669. If the CSF fistula persists longer than 24 hours, tomograms are generally ordered, and the head of the bed is kept elevated. Diamox may be ordered to decrease CSF formation, and serial lumbar punctures to decrease pressure may be done. Surgery to close the fistula is rarely necessary.

INJURIES TO THE BRAIN

Because of the wide variety of injuries to the brain substance (see previous section on mechanisms of injury), a single classification system for brain injuries does not exist. Thus, the written diagnosis assigned a patient may indicate a variety of findings and various degrees of seriousness. The actual status or "picture of the patient" must be determined by further investigation! There is an increasing tendency to label head injuries as "mild," "moderate," and "severe," depending on the degree of damage (alteration in consciousness) to the brain itself. The classifications of "open" or "closed" are also commonly used. So is the classification of "concussion" and "contusion." None of these systems is totally satisfactory. Here we focus on the classification of concussion and contusion, recognizing that considerable controversy exists over the use of these terms.

Two types of brain injury are defined: *concussion* and *contusion.* Two types of contusions are presented: (1) those involving the cerebral hemispheres and (2) those involving the brain stem. These impact (primary) injuries are differentiated for purposes of discussion from secondary injuries, e.g., hematoma.

Concussions. A *concussion* may be defined as a transient cerebral paralysis. It is the least serious form of brain trauma. A concussion may be further described as head trauma leading to a brief loss of consciousness, followed immediately by a period of confusion or memory loss (i.e., amnesia). No other abnormal neurologic findings are usually present. Although it was once believed that no brain damage occurred with concussions, this has been shown to be untrue. The severity of the concussion is thought to correlate with the duration of amnesia.[275] The period of amnesia is measured by determining when the head-injured person experiences memory loss. This period is usually from before the event until after full consciousness has returned. It does not include the period of confusion after awakening.

Persons who have concussions are frequently seen in the emergency room; however, they may not need to be admitted to hospital. They do require close observation to be sure that no untoward effects of the concussion develop.

The emergency room nurse can help in arranging safe care by ensuring (1) that a reliable person is able to observe the patient closely at home, (2) that this person knows what to look for, (3) that subsequent medical intervention is readily available if needed and (4) that the patient and "observer" know how to obtain such care.

Contusions. Contusions are associated with damage to the brain substance itself. Multiple areas of petechial and punctate hemorrhage are present, as well as bruised areas. Microscopic lesions of nerve fibers can also be seen. Although the abnormalities may be predominantly in one area of the brain, the nature of the injury is such that areas outside the principal area are also often injured. This is particularly true of brain stem contusions, which in this classification system, are the more serious type of lesion. The great variety of findings in patients with contusions is partly explained by the multiple areas of damage. The damage with contusions is more extensive than that seen with concussions. Contusions are often associated with other serious injuries, e.g., cervical fractures. Secondary effects, such as brain swelling and edema, accompany serious contusions. Increased intracranial pressure and herniation syndromes may result.

We separate contusions into *cerebral contusions* and *brain stem contusions;* not everyone makes this distinction. If contusions are considered as one entity, the findings of course include a combination of those discussed below.

CEREBRAL CONTUSIONS. Cerebral contusions are diagnosed in *alert patients only,* although they may be present in patients who are comatose. The findings vary with the areas of the hemispheres that are damaged. An agitated and confused patient who remains alert, has not been drinking, and is frequently "foul-mouthed" may have a temporal lobe contusion. The presence of hemiparesis in an alert head-injured patient may indicate a frontal contusion. A frontal-temporal contusion may result in a patient being aphasic. Other findings signal contusions in other areas. It is important to remember that these findings, while correlating with cerebral contusion, *do not* rule out the presence of other abnormalities, such as developing mass lesion. Adverse changes in the patient's condition need prompt medical attention. They quite possibly indicate treatable complications.

> *One of the most important aspects of nursing care is providing systematic, frequent assessment of the patient's neurologic state. A steady worsening of the level of consciousness is significant and probably indicates the development of secondary events, as described on p. 662.*

BRAIN STEM CONTUSIONS. Brain stem contusions render a person comatose *immediately,* because of significant disruption to the brain stem and its relationship to consciousness through the reticular activating system. The patient may either improve to a state of partial consciousness within hours after injury, or he or she may remain in a coma. Thus, in diagnosing the presence of a brain stem contusion, knowing whether the person became unconscious immediately after the injury is extremely important. If this information is not available, the presence of a hematoma must always be considered.

The patient with a brain stem contusion presents as comatose or partially comatose and typically continues to have an altered level of consciousness for at least several hours and usually days or weeks. A variety of other neurologic abnormalities are present. These are usually symmetric (found on both sides of the body), but some may be lateralized (asymmetric, i.e., found only on one side of the body). If lateralizing signs are found, however, it is likely that a secondary event such as the development of a hematoma has occurred.

In addition to the altered state of consciousness that is always present with brain stem contusions, respiratory, pupillary, eye movement, and motor abnormalities may occur. Respirations may be normal, ataxic, periodic, or very rapid. The pupils are usually small, equal, and reactive; but damage to the upper brain stem (third cranial nerve) may cause pupillary abnormalities. Similarly, the pathways controlling the eye movements traverse the midbrain and pons, and loss of normal eye movements may occur. The patient may respond to light or to noxious stimuli by purposeful movements to push the offending stimulus away. In the presence of more profound alterations in level of consciousness, decerebrate or decorticate posturing may be elicited with or even without noxious stimuli. It is also possible for a patient with this injury to have no response to stimuli, i.e., to be flaccid. Moreover, the findings often vary from observation to observation (those seen signaling a developing hematoma are more consistent). This inconsistency in findings makes it very important to *identify patterns or developing trends of improvement or deterioration.*

Rarely do brain stem contusions injure only brain stem tissue. Swelling or direct injury to the hypothalamus may produce *autonomic nervous system* effects. The patient has a high temperature, rapid pulse and respirations, and perspires profusely. These effects may wax and wane, but if sustained, they can lead to serious consequences. Intervention is usually indicated to alter the symptoms before "fatigue" of the patient occurs.

Summary of Primary Events in Head Injury

- *Scalp damage,* while frequently disfiguring in appearance, is usually treated readily and may be of only "minor" importance in contributing to disability or death.
- *Skull injuries* are principally fractures and may or may not be related to damage to the brain.
- *Concussions* damage the brain, but the damage should not "disable" the patient in any way.
- *Contusions* produce significant damage to the brain and may result in permanent disability or in death.
- Other structures, including the meninges and major arteries, may be damaged.

Secondary Events in Head Trauma

Secondary events are problems that occur soon after the primary insult of the head injury. Frequently, they cause a rapid deterioration in a patient's condition. Most important among these *secondary events* are: hemorrhage, with hematoma formation (epidural, subdural, and intracerebral hematoma); infections, including meningitis and brain abscess; secondary brain swelling and edema; and carotid artery occlusion. Although the time course for the development of these problems is variable, all have the potential for turning a relatively "benign" head injury into a disastrous event.

HEMORRHAGE

Epidural Hematoma (Extradural Hematoma). An epidural hematoma occurs *between* the skull and the dura (i.e., outer meninges). They occur in about 1 to 2 per cent of all head injuries and are associated with a skull fracture about 90 per cent of the time.[151] Epidural hematomas are the result of injury to the extracerebral blood vessels, usually the middle meningeal artery and vein. Generally the signs and symptoms are acute, as the bleeding is often arterial. The bleeding is almost always continuous, with the formation of a large clot that separates the dura

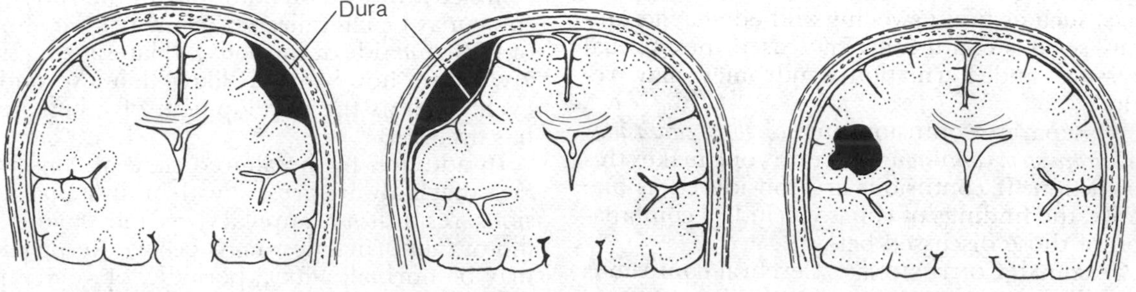

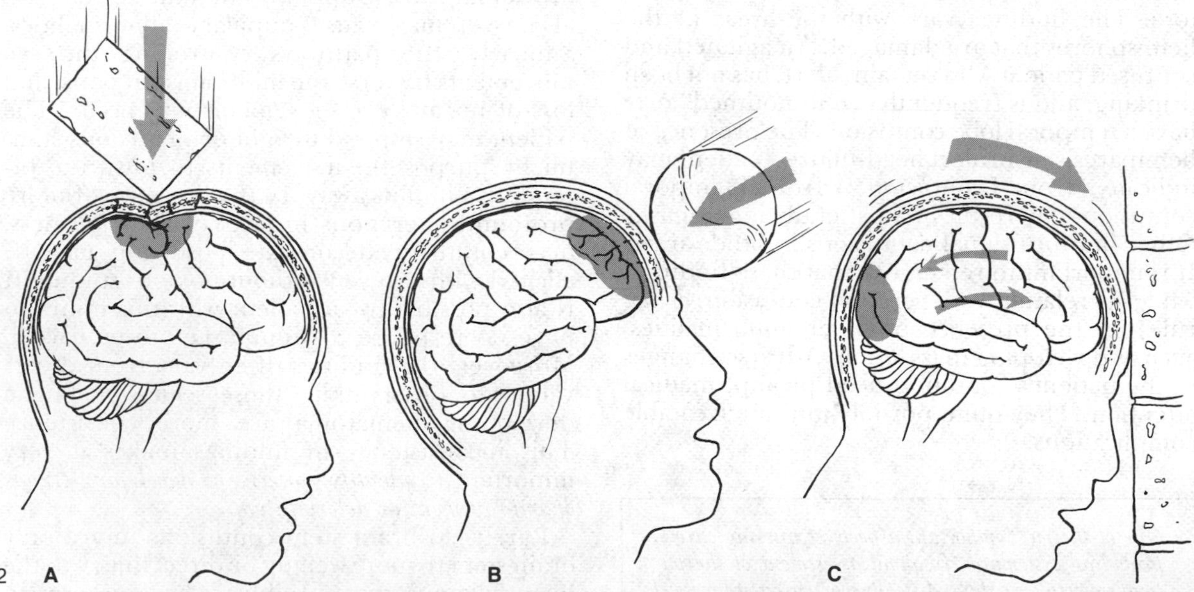

Figure 27–26. Part 1. The different types of hematoma. Part 2. Some mechanisms of head injury. Head injury results from penetration or impact. **A.** A direct injury (blow to skull) may fracture the skull. Contusion and laceration of the brain may result from fractures. Depressed portions of the skull may compress or penetrate brain tissue. **B.** In the absence of skull fracture, a blow to the skull may cause the brain to move enough to tear some of the veins going from the cortical surface to the dura. Subsequently, subdural hematoma may develop. Note areas of cerebral contusion (shaded). **C.** Rebound of the cranial contents may result in an area of injury opposite the point of impact. Such an injury is called a "contrecoup injury." In addition to the three injuries depicted, secondary phenomena may result from the injury and cause additional brain dysfunction or damage. For example, ischemia, especially cerebral edema, may occur, causing elevation of intracranial pressure.

from the skull, and ceases only with medical intervention or the death of the patient. Occasionally, the clot may develop slowly, and the patient may be asymptomatic for a week or even a month.

The "classical" picture of an epidural hematoma is seen in a patient who is unconscious immediately after head trauma, then awakens and *is lucid,* and next lapses into a coma. Focal signs generally appear first. These consist of dilatation of the pupil on the same side, paralysis of some of the eye movements on that side, and a rapid deterioration of level of consciousness. Hemiparesis of the opposite side and seizures may also occur. The patient may continue to rapidly deteriorate, showing signs of increasing intracranial pressure and tentorial herniation until death by respiratory arrest occurs. (See Chapter 26 for discussion of intracranial pressure and herniation syndrome.)

Extradural hemorrhage is the most serious complication following head injury. In untreated cases the mortality rate is nearly 100 per cent. While there may be no clinical signs of this complication immediately after the initial trauma, once the hematoma grows to a critical level in several hours, deterioration progresses rapidly, and the patient may die, especially if discharged with inadequate observation. For this reason patients are usually hospitalized for a time, even following minor head injuries. In spite of their rarity, learning to recognize extradural hemorrhages is important because they are potentially fatal and because prompt, proper treatment can mean recovery if the patient has not suffered other injuries.

The diagnosis of epidural hematoma is established by recognizing the signs and symptoms and by having available a careful history which notes that the patient had a lucid interval post trauma. Skull x-ray, CT scan, and arteriography may be used to confirm the diagnosis. *Rapid diagnosis and prompt treatment are essential,* and the nurse's observations and notification of the physician of significant changes in the patient's condition are imperative.

Treatment may include *lowering the intracranial pressure* with osmotic diuretic (e.g., mannitol). Emergency *burr holes* or *twist drills* may also be done. *Subtemporal decompression* or other surgical management appropriate to the hematoma location is the usual treatment. The objectives of surgery generally include (1) removal of the hematoma and (2) drainage and ligation of the bleeding vessel.

Subdural Hematoma (SDH). Subdural hematoma is a common complication of head injury. It is defined as a collection of blood between the dura (outer meninges) and arachnoid (middle meninges) in the subdural space between the dura and arachnoid meninges). Blood that escapes into the subdural space is not absorbed, but is organized or encapsulated by the dura. As the blood organizes into a clot, the blood cells within the clot's membrane lyse, forming a fluid of high osmotic character. Water from the surrounding subarachnoid space is drawn into the clot, producing a gradually increasing intracranial mass. Large clots may produce such high intracranial pressure that cerebral herniation occurs, and death may result. These hematomas are classified as *acute, subacute,* or *chronic,* depending on the rapidity with which the signs and symptoms develop. (Another classification recognizes only "acute" and "chronic," combining the acute and subacute designations.) *Acute* hematomas are defined as those occurring within 24 hours of injury; *subacute* as those which are symptomatic in 2–10 days; and *chronic* as those occurring several weeks later.

Acute Subdural Hematoma. Acute subdural hematomas result from laceration of the brain, with a tear in the arachnoid allowing blood (from the small pial veins bridging the subdural space) and CSF to collect in the subdural space. Occasionally acute subdural hematomas may also result from a ruptured saccular aneurysm or intracerebral hemorrhage if there has been tearing of the arachnoid over the source of the hemorrhage.

The signs and symptoms of an *acute SDH* (subdural hematoma) are basically the same as those seen with an acute epidural hematoma, as both are a type of "mass" lesion. The onset and development of the symptoms may be somewhat slower, because the bleeding is more frequently venous (rather than arterial as in most epidural hematomas). However, recognition of the symptoms may be quite difficult since subdural hematomas are often associated with moderate or severe trauma to the brain substance. Therefore, subtle changes such as progressive changes in the level of consciousness and the development of lateralizing (on one side) changes, such as hemiparesis, pupillary dilatation, extraocular eye movement paralysis, are important findings. *Careful documentation of nursing observations is important.*

The patient developing an acute subdural hematoma may remain unconscious following the injury, or the state of consciousness may be variable (depending partially upon the extent of injury). If the patient is conscious, headache is usually present. The patient may then become irritable, confused, and lapse again into coma or show fluctuating levels of consciousness. Symptoms of increasing intracranial pressure occur. A lumbar puncture is contraindicated since it may precipitate herniation (see Ch. 26). However, if CSF is obtained, it may be bloody or xanthochromic, have increased protein, and show elevated pressure. Usually patients who develop acute subdural hematoma have underlying brain damage and severe brain swelling. *Acute subdural hematomas are a serious complication requiring prompt treatment since they compress and distort an already damaged and edematous brain.*

Subacute and Chronic Subdural Hematomas. These hematomas often develop after a patient has gone home or to an extended care facility. The person may not come to treatment for many weeks or months following injury. With subacute and chronic subdural hematomas there is an interval during which the patient appears to be recovering from the initial injury or seems completely recovered, and then days, weeks, or months later develops gradually progressive neurologic symptoms. The most prominent symptoms usually relate to disturbances in consciousness; the patient may be drowsy, think incoherently, display personality changes, and be inattentive. Often headaches are another prominent symptom. These symptoms may be overlooked by the significant others or by extended care facility attendants. The symptoms are then not brought to the attention of the physician until focal or lateralizing signs appear, e.g., hemiparesis, pupil signs. Changes in the level of consciousness continue but may fluctuate widely. *It is important for the nurse to help the patient's significant others to recognize the symptoms early.*

DIAGNOSIS AND TREATMENT. The diagnostic work-up of subdural hematomas is similar to that of epidural hematomas; scans and arteriography are the definitive tools. The surgical approach is usually the placement of several *burr holes* or *craniotomy*. The treatment results vary, depending on the condition of the patient before surgery.

Intracerebral Hematoma. Intracerebral hematomas occur less commonly than epidural or subdural hematomas and are caused by bleeding *directly into* the brain tissues. They may occur in the area of injury or some distance away. The symptoms are similar to those seen with epidural or subdural hematomas, although hemiplegia is more common than hemiparesis in this type of hematoma.[3] Many of the symptoms are related to the "mass effect" of the lesion (see Chapter 26, increased intracranial pressure). A wide variety of other symptoms may also be present, related to the location of the hematoma.

The diagnosis is established as with other types of hematomas; the treatment is surgical. Operative results are poor, with a high mortality rate because of damage to brain tissue caused by the hematoma.

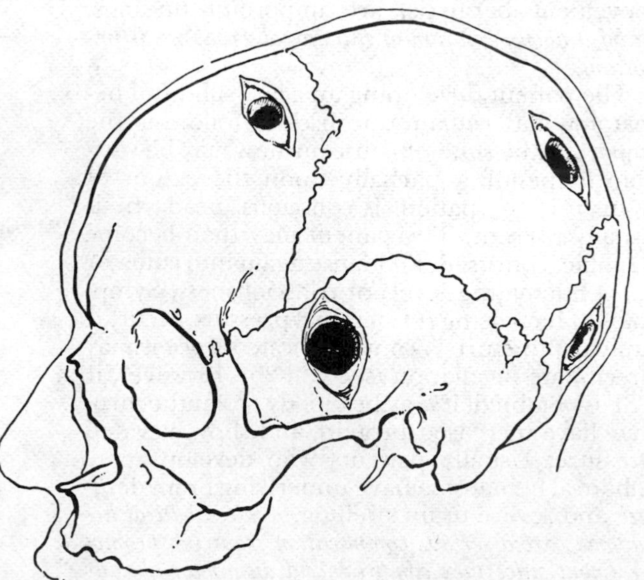

Figure 27–27. Placement of burr holes in the skull. (From American College of Surgeons Committee on Trauma: *Early Care of the Injured Patient.* Philadelphia: W. B. Saunders Co., 1972, p. 94.)

BRAIN SWELLING AND EDEMA

Serious head injuries are almost always associated with brain swelling and edema. Since the skull is essentially a "closed box," with little "spare" room, once the swelling and edema reach a critical point, a "mass effect" occurs, and intracranial pressure increases. Signs and symptoms of compromised brain function develop. These signs and symptoms and a discussion of increased intracranial pressure are discussed in Chapter 26.

INFECTIONS

The usual infections that occur after head trauma are meningitis and brain abscess. They generally occur in patients who have sustained "open" head injuries. Both types of infection are discussed earlier in this chapter.

COMPLICATIONS AND SEQUELAE

A head injured patient is prone to a variety of complications and/or sequelae. A brain injured person is at risk not only of developing problems related to the head injury itself but also of developing many of the complications seen in seriously ill patients, e.g., those complications seen in an immobilized patient. Some of these problems are addressed in the clinical care section (see p. 667).

Epilepsy. *Post-traumatic epilepsy* can develop early or late and in patients with both minor and major head injuries. It is most commonly seen associated with open injuries and is discussed earlier in this chapter (see p. 640).

The incidence of post-traumatic epilepsy following head injury varies depending upon the severity of the injury. The incidence is much higher when there has been penetration of the dura and laceration of the underlying cortex with formation of a cerebromeningeal scar.

Occasionally, post-traumatic seizures occur immediately following the injury or within the first few days after the injury. In these cases, the seizures are believed to be related to acute brain damage or to the presence of hematomas, abscesses, or meningitis. The more typical picture of post-traumatic seizures is for seizures to begin several months after the initial injury. Post-traumatic seizures are more often generalized than focal. In some cases the seizures may spontaneously cease or decrease in frequency.

Following head injury *prophylactic measures* to prevent post-traumatic epilepsy may include:

- Elevating depressed skull fractures.
- Thoroughly debriding compound skull fractures and suturing the dura to prevent infection decrease the amount of scar formation (and thus the likelihood of seizures).
- Administering anticonvulsant medications prophylactically for 1 to 2 years (1) to patients who have sustained a severe head injury and (2) to patients who have a persistent focus of abnormal activity in their EEG.

Stress Ulcers. Ulceration of the gastrointestinal tract, the so-called *stress ulcer,* is one of the major complications that can follow trauma. Although the incidence of gastrointestinal hemorrhage is not high, when it does occur the mortality rate is high.

The cause of stress ulcers is not known, although several theories have been advanced. The ulcers are seen in several major groups of patients including those with trauma (stress ulcers), burns (Curling ulcers) and head injuries (Cushing's ulcers). They are found in portions of the gastrointestinal tract innervated by the vagus nerve. Those found in the stomach and duodenum are generally the most significant clinically. (See also Chapter 62, p. 1432.)

The diagnosis is established by the presence of bleeding in gastric secretions or stool. If hemorrhage occurs, it is treated conventionally. Gastrectomy with vagotomy may be required at times but is accompanied by a mortality rate as high[340] as 80 per cent.

Because of the serious consequences with stress ulcers, it is highly important to try to *prevent* this disorder. Since most seriously head injured patients have a nasogastric tube in place, it is possible to measure the pH of gastric secretions. A variety of drugs, including antacids, anticholinergic drugs, and cimetidine, may be prescribed to alter gastric acidity. The nurse has an important role in monitoring and detection of gastrointestinal bleeding. Even microscopic bleeding (guaiac positive stool or nasogastric secretions) should be promptly reported.

Intracranial Cerebrospinal Fluid Fistula. The drainage of CSF from the nose or ear denotes the presence of a fistula from the subarachnoid space through the skull to the nose or ear. These fistulae can occur immediately or later and may be traumatic or nontraumatic in origin. In a head-injured person, they are traumatic in origin and immediate in onset in association with fractures. Occasionally, the fistuale may develop weeks or months after trauma.

The diagnosis and treatment were mentioned in the section of skull fractures (p. 659) and are detailed on p. 669. It is important to note that treatment protocols vary greatly, as there is no general agreement as to whether initial treatment should be surgical or conservative. Nor is there agreement on what the conservative treatment should be or what constitutes failure of conservative therapy and indicates surgical intervention. It is, however, generally agreed that there are two *goals of treatment*: (1) to decrease the chance of meningitis and (2) to enhance the healing of the fistula.[340]

Diabetes Insipidus and Inappropriate ADH Release. If head trauma compromises the function of the pituitary gland, the patient may develop diabetes insipidus. Its appearance is signaled by a large, clear (not concentrated) urinary output. The output may be as much as 500 ml. per hour; the specific gravity is typically very low. The ability of the kidneys to concentrate urine has been altered because of decreased pituitary secretion of ADH (antidiuretic hormone). *With the loss of a large amount of fluid, the patient can rapidly develop a hyperosmolar state,* and thus replacement of urinary losses is usually the first treatment. Aqueous pitressin (injectable) or Tegretol (oral) may be used if the condition is prolonged.

Inappropriate release of the antidiuretic hormone leads to impairment of free water clearance by the kidneys. Water retention with expansion of extracellular volume occurs, which then leads to decreased aldosterone output and loss of urinary salt (also called *cerebral salt wasting syndrome).* This syndrome is also thought to be related to injuries to and/or hypoxia of certain brain structures. The characteristic signs and symptoms are altered urinary output and specific gravity (greater than 1.020) and findings related to an expanded extracellular volume, e.g., full neck veins and pulse, decreased blood (plasma) osmolarity. (See Ch. 12 on fluid and electrolyte imbalances.) The patient will be water intoxicated, have increased cerebral edema, may have seizures, and eventually becomes hyponatremic.

Nursing care for diabetes insipidus and for inappropriate ADH release involves:

- Accurate measurement of intake and output (I&O)
- Frequent determination (i.e., every 2 hours) of I&O and specific gravity
- Assessment of the patient for indications of fluid and electrolyte imbalance
- Accurate monitoring of ordered fluid replacement
- Prompt reporting of changes in the patient's status or therapy

Acute Hydrocephalus. *Acute hydrocephalus* develops when there is increased CSF accumulated in the ventricles. This results from defective reabsorption or from blockage of the CSF flow. Traumatic or infectious blockage of flow can occur with head injuries. As the CSF pressure rises, signs of increased intracranial pressure result (see Chapter 26). Treatment includes surgical shunting and/or the placement of a ventriculostomy.

Arteriovenous Aneurysms. Common causes of arteriovenous aneurysms are trauma which lacerates the internal carotid artery (as it passes through the cavernous sinus) such as by penetrating missiles or fracture of the sphenoid bone. Immediately after the accident, the patient may notice a bruit, synchronous with the pulse. Other symptoms may include exophthalmos, distended orbital and periorbital veins, and paralysis of cranial nerves. These symptoms result from increased tension in the cavernous sinus due to the accumulation of arterial blood. It may be necessary to surgically ligate the internal carotid artery in the neck and intracranially ligate the internal carotid and ophthalmic arteries.

Carotid Artery Occlusion. Trauma either directly to the artery or to the head may produce a rapid partial or complete occlusion of the artery. Trauma to the rest of the body may also result in occlusion of the carotid or other arteries. The signs and symptoms of carotid artery occlusion are those of a stroke (see p. 612). Indications of this disorder may be difficult to diagnose in a patient with an already altered neurologic state, but they illustrate the importance of careful nursing observation of *all* changes.

Neurogenic Pulmonary Edema. Neurogenic pulmonary edema is an entity that not all authorities believe exists. However, it is agreed that some patients with head injuries and frequently other trauma develop what is termed *adult respiratory distress syndrome (ARDS),* which may not respond well to conventional therapy (See Chapter 13, p. 243). ARDS is characterized by altered pulmonary capillary permeability which leads to leakage of fluid into the interstitial and intra-alveolar spaces. This in turn, leads to hypoxemia (often profound and not responsive to high levels of inspired oxygen), pulmonary congestion, and atelectasis and failure of the ventricles. The cause of ARDS is unknown. Some of those who believe in neurogenic pulmonary edema as a type of ARDS postulate that damage to the hypothalamus leads to massive sympathetic outflow, which they then treat with a sympathetic blocking agent, e.g. Thorazine.[243] Conventional therapy with intubation, mechanical ventilation, and oxygen is generally used. PEEP (positive-end-expiratory-pressure) may be necessary to treat the extreme, unresponsive to oxygen, hypoxemia (see Unit XVI).

Mental Distubances. A variety of mental disturbances may occur as sequelae of head injuries, e.g., confusion, inability to concentrate, emotional disturbances, changes of personality, transient psychotic episodes, mental deterioration, post-traumatic personality disorders, and amnesia. The severity of the mental disturbance is variable, as well as the duration of the problem. Following head injury it is important to determine the degree and duration of any change in consciousness. *Traumatic amnesia* is divided into: (1) *retrograde amnesia,* loss of memory of events preceding the injury, and (2) *anterograde amnesia,* amnesia for events following the injury.

Post-traumatic Syndrome. Post-traumatic syndrome comprises a *set of complications* that may emerge in the recovery phase after head injury and continue for months and even years. A variety of signs and symptoms make up this loosely defined syndrome. Usually a "syndrome" is a defined set of signs and symptoms caused by a specific pathophysiologic mechanism. However, in this case, the term refers to several groups of symptoms for which the pathophysiologic mechanisms are either unknown or poorly defined. It generally occurs in people who have sustained a "minor" head injury. Such a syndrome may include headache, poor concentration (especially in reading), dizziness, and unsteadiness related to sudden head movements, irritability, sensitivity to noise, insomnia, restlessness, hyperhidrosis, depression, personality changes, nervousness, impaired memory, anxiety, alcohol intolerance, and easy fatiguability. While as many as half of the number of head-injured patients may experience these symptoms in mild form for a short time, the symptoms are not referred to as "post-traumatic" or "postconcussional syndrome" unless they persist for weeks or perhaps years and incapacitate the patient for work.

The syndrome is seen in patients (a) who characteristically get worse over time, (b) whose extent of injury does not correlate with the severity of the syndrome, and (c) who tend to have complex overlapping neurologic and psychogenic symptoms. Whether the symptoms are related to brain damage or are psychogenic is not known and is the subject of much controversy. Sometimes no organic cause can be demonstrated in examining a patient, but careful neuropsychologic testing demonstrates abnormalities in testing areas that are compatible with brain damage. Neuropsychologic testing and other research currently being done may be able to clarify this syndrome and answer the question of its prevention or reversibility.

Treatment is basically symptomatic. Counseling for the patient and significant others may be helpful. If the symptoms begin to appear while the patient is still hospitalized after experiencing a head injury, some authorities suggest avoiding early discharge.[213, 340]

Traumatic Delirium, Automatic Behavior. Once a patient begins to regain consciousness following head injury, after a period of perhaps several days of unconsciousness, it is not unusual for his or her behavior to be noisy and generally disturbed and confused. Such a patient is often experiencing *traumatic delirium* resulting from cerebral irritation.

This is a temporary phase during which the patient must be protected, reassured, and cared for as with other delirious states. Because this partially confused state may remain even after the person can clearly speak and cooperate in some respects, the nurse may incorrectly believe that the patient is being willfully uncooperative. After this phase comes a time in which the patient appears to have fully regained mental faculties. The person may be up and about, recognize visitors, cooperate, and so forth, yet memory of these activities is impaired. This is a state of *automatic behavior* during which the person has no memory of day-to-day events and yet is able to carry on activities in a seemingly normal manner.

Clinical Care Following Head Injury

After head injury, initial medical management is directed toward making the diagnosis and beginning conservative medical therapy.* For most patients, continued management is also conservative because acute surgical intervention is rarely indicated for the primary damage done on impact. Usually surgery is necessary during the acute phase of hospitalization only for treating a depressed skull fracture or removing a hematoma. Later in the hospitalization or in the course of rehabilitation, other types of surgery may be needed, e.g., repair of a CSF fistula.

Two major goals in the care of the head-injured patient are: (1) prompt recognition and treatment of hypoxia and acid-base disturbances that can contribute to cerebral edema and (2) prompt recognition and treatment of increasing intracranial pressure resulting from such factors as cerebral edema and/or expanding hematoma.

Among the most significant recent advances in the care of patients with head injuries are: (1) increasing knowledge of how to properly care for an unconscious patient and (2) recognition of the contribution of respiratory insufficiency to secondary brain swelling and neuronal dysfunction. We have previously discussed care of the unconscious patient. Let us reemphasize here that of primary importance in the care of an unconscious person is the *maintenance of a clear airway and effective respirations.* Inadequate respiratory function causes cerebral hypoxia and contributes to cerebral edema.

Few patients die immediately from head injury; however, many die within the first few minutes from associated difficulties with respiration or shock. Early death may result from damage to the brain stem. Because severe mechanical trauma to the brain is associated with a high rate of morbidity and mortality, vigorous treatment must be started immediately. Initial care is directed at saving the patient's life, preventing the development of secondary brain injury as much as possible, and preventing further injury to the entire body.

Summary of clinical care of head-injured persons

First, establish an airway and adequate respiratory exchange.

Prevent aspiration.

Check for the presence of shock; insure regular heart rate and adequate blood pressure.

Search for evidence of spinal injuries.

Observe for scalp and skull injuries.

Prevent infection.

Observe for cerebrospinal fluid leakage.

Maintain normothermia.

Establish baseline observations of the patient's neurologic status and vital signs; make frequent repeated observations.

Observe for symptoms of increasing intracranial pressure.

Prevent the patient from unnecessary straining.

Observe for nuchal rigidity.

Maintain fluid-electrolyte, acid-base balances and nutrition; record and evaluate intake and output.

Control restlessness and pain; reorient the patient as consciousness returns.

Observe for seizures and be prepared to care for the patient during seizures.

Position the patient as indicated and/or ordered.

Present stress ulcers.

Ensure rest; prevent complications of bed rest and of unconsciousness.

Obtain history of how the injury occurred and how it affected the patient, e.g., did the patient lose consciousness?

Observe for the various sequelae that can follow head injury and treat appropriately.

Airway Establishment; Maintenance of Respirations. First establish an airway and adequate respiratory exchange. The patient may be intubated with an endotracheal tube. Rarely,

*For additional discussion of the emergency management of head trauma see Chapter 95. See also some of the basic considerations of nursing people with neurologic problems in Chapter 26.

trauma other than the head injury (e.g., fractured mandible) will make immediate tracheostomy necessary. Supplemental oxygen therapy is started if needed. *Arterial blood gases* are studied to determine adequacy of respiratory exchange. *Assisted ventilation* may be necessary to make sure the patient is adequately exchanging air (e.g. mechanical ventilation). Carefully evaluate the patient's respiratory status. Prevention of respiratory complications in the comatose patient have been discussed in Chapter 26. (Respiratory care is discussed in Unit XVI.)

Cerebral anoxia from inadequate respiratory exchange is a leading cause of death in head-injured patients. In the brain-injured patient, intracranial pressure is highly sensitive to changes in the blood's O_2 and CO_2 content and pH. Therefore, relatively mild degrees of hypoxia or hypercapnia cause great increases in intracranial pressure and can rapidly result in the patient's death. Hyperventilation, hypoventilation, and impaired cellular respiration can rapidly add to the development of secondary brain injury, e.g., circulatory dysfunction and cerebral edema.

Aspiration Prevention. In patients without spinal injuries, use the side-lying position. Aspiration may also be prevented in the unconscious head-injured patient by other treatment measures, e.g., suctioning, nasogastric tube. Aspiration can occur from inhalation of vomitus, blood, secretions, and so forth. Head-injured patients often vomit; some have been drinking alcoholic beverages prior to their accidents. Hemorrhage may result from nasopharyngeal injuries. Additionally, highly anxious patients may swallow large amounts of air following an accident. The air may then acutely dilate the stomach and produce emesis. The stomach may also be acutely dilated by ileus following severe injuries. A *nasogastric tube* may be passed to prevent emesis and aspiration of the stomach's contents and help prevent or to treat stress ulcers. The tube is generally connected to intermittent or continuous nasogastric suction.

Nasopharyngeal bleeding may be a problem with damaged nasal passages. The nasal passages are packed to stop bleeding. An endotracheal tube is usually placed through the mouth to minimize aspiration of large amounts of blood. The tube's cuff seals off the airway except when large amounts of blood exert enough pressure on the cuff to permit aspiration. It is thus important to suction the mouth around the tube as well as through the tube's lumen.

Cardiovascular Complications. Check for the presence of shock; insure the presence of a regular heart rate and adequate blood pressure. Keep the patient quiet and comfortably warm. Frequently evaluate pulse and blood pressure. *If the patient appears to be in hypovolemic shock elevate the extremities; do not put the person in the head-down position,* i.e., Trendelenburg position. If the brain is damaged, the head-low position increases intracranial pressure, produces cerebral venous stasis, and produces respiratory embarrassment (by causing pressure of the abdominal contents against the diaphragm). Elevation of the extremities does not contribute to cerebral edema; it favorably increases return of blood to the heart. (Shock is discussed in Chapter 13). Some head-injured patients experience *cardiac arrest* and other cardiovascular complications. (See Unit XII.)

Spinal Injuries. The patient is carefully examined for spinal injuries. Do not allow the newly injured patient to move about even if conscious. Assume that all patients who are unconscious from head injuries may well have a spinal fracture until proved otherwise. Use extreme care in moving the patient. Unless contraindicated, turn the patient by the logrolling method every 2 hours to reduce pulmonary complications and other complications of bed rest.

Head injury is quite often associated with spinal cord damage.

Skull and Scalp Injuries. Cover *open head wounds* with the cleanest material available at the scene of the accident. Apply pressure to bleeding scalp wounds only if there does not appear to be an underlying depressed or compound skull fracture. Do not attempt to remove foreign objects, or any objects causing penetrating injuries, from the wound. In the emergency room, uncomplicated scalp wounds (which do not lie over depressed or compound skull fractures) are anesthetized locally, cleansed, and sutured.

Simple skull depressions are *electively* treated in surgery by elevation of the depressed bone fragment and repair of the dura if it is lacerated. All bone fragments are removed. *Compound depressed skull fractures* are *immediately* treated surgically; the scalp, skull, and devitalized brain are debrided and the wound cleansed thoroughly. Unless all foreign material is removed, a brain abscess develops. Debridement of a penetrating wound or depressed skull fracture frequently leaves a cranial defect that is cosmetically unsightly. Fortunately, *cranioplasty* can be performed to correct this defect. Cranioplasty has been simplified and cosmetic results improved by the current use of various synthetic materials, e.g., acrylic plastic, tantalum, and stainless steel.

Infection Prevention. The risks of infection are more serious in a head wound than elsewhere in the body. In the emergency room, antibiotics and prophylactic drugs for tetanus are administered if scalp lacerations or open fractures are present. Do not make vigorous efforts to clean the patient during the acute period following head injury; rest is important. Use meticulous aseptic technique for all dressing changes and other sterile procedures. Early surgical treatment of compound skull fractures establishes a basis for infection-free healing.

Cerebrospinal Fluid Fistulas. Observe the head-injured patient carefully for serous (or blood) drainage from the ears or nose. This drainage may indicate a cerebrospinal fluid fistula through which infection (e.g., meningitis) can be introduced into the intracranial cavity. Drainage of CSF from the nose *(cerebrospinal fluid rhinorrhea)* is usually preceded by bleeding from the nose and may not be recognized until the bleeding has stopped. Fracture through the ethmoid bone is usually the cause of CSF rhinorrhea. *Cerebrospinal fluid otorrhea* is associated with fractures of the temporal bone. Usually the drainage is self-limited, lasting a few hours or at most 2 weeks. Typically surgical repair is not necessary, unlike with CSF rhinorrhea.

> *Bring to the physician's attention any seepage of fluid from the nose or ears of head-injured patients (including patients who have undergone cranial surgery).*

Drainage may be clear, serosanguineous, or frankly bloody. It is important to distinguish between blood that is draining from local trauma (e.g., fractured nose) and blood that contains CSF coming from a meningeal tear. To determine if CSF is present in bloody discharge, a clear wet halo or watery pale ring will encircle the bloody spot on the gauze. Clear fluid draining from the nose may be either CSF or normal watery mucus. Testape is useful in distinguishing these fluids; with CSF a positive sugar reaction is often present and with mucus a negative reaction may occur.

Clinical care of a patient with a CSF fistula focuses on the following major points:

- *Administer antibiotics* as ordered.
- *Never attempt to clean the ears or nose of any head-injured patient until the doctor agrees it is time to do so.* If a CSF fistula is present, cleaning can introduce infection; therefore cleaning is done under strict sterile conditions. Irrigations are prohibited.
- *Never use nasal suction,* for to do so could cause serious additional brain damage or possibly introduce infection.
- *Instruct the patient not to cough, sneeze, or blow his or her nose.* These activities increase the likelihood of meningitis developing and may also allow air to enter the cranial cavity (forming a *pneumocele* which may further increase intracranial pressure). Remember that actions like nose blowing are almost automatic, so the patient may need to be reminded periodically.
- Gently place a sterile pad near the *outer* opening of the ear or nose for absorbency or place a loosely slung external bandage, e.g., sterile pad, over the *external* ear to absorb the discharge. Do not *pack* cotton or gauze in place, as it obstructs the fluid's free flow.
- *Replace dressings as soon as they become moist* to prevent germs from passing through the moisture of the dressing and then traveling to the brain.
- *Note color, consistency, and approximate amount of drainage.*
- *Position the patient in such a way that free drainage of the CSF is possible.* A position with the person's head elevated about 20 degrees is frequently ordered. Do not allow the patient to remain for long in a position that allows stasis of the CSF drainage.
- If the patient is conscious, considerable patient teaching is required including all of the above points. Such explanations may need to be repeated.

Some sources recommend that the patient with a CSF fistula be placed in *protective isolation.* If this is not done, the nurse should at least *practice thorough handwashing and sterile dressing technique.*

Notify the physician if the patient shows indications of possible meningitis, e.g., fever, increasing confusion, increasing headache. Prompt treatment is necessary.

Prevention of Straining. Prevent the patient from straining whenever possible, since straining increases intracranial pressure. Bowel function may not be stimulated for several days following injury in an attempt to prevent the patient from straining during a bowel movement. Occasionally gentle acting suppositories, mild bulk laxatives, colon lavages, or oil retention enemas may be ordered.

Maintenance of Normothermia. Head injuries may cause a patient to be hypothermic or hyperthermic. The aim of temperature-controlling therapeutic measures is to maintain normothermia (see pp. 548–554).

Establishment of Baseline Observations: Observation Period. As soon as possible after head injury, the patient is evaluated in terms of vital signs and neurologic status. These initial observations establish a baseline for numerous additional evaluations. Informed, regularly repeated observations are highly important. The nurse is in a key position for: (1) detecting early symptoms of complications; (2) reporting these to the physician for early treatment; and (3) carrying out appropriate actions until the physician arrives. Only through careful observations is it possible to detect the presence of a mass lesion, e.g., hematoma, requiring surgery or other treatable complications. It is particularly difficult to evaluate the condition of a head-injured patient who has ingested large amounts of alcohol or drugs prior to injury. The "drugged state" may obscure important symptoms.

Following head injury it is desirable to hospitalize the patient for a period of observation because of the danger of extradural hemorrhage. This period of observation is highly important if consciousness was lost at the time of the accident (or later). The minimal period of observation is 6 hours, and the ideal period of observation is 48 hours for all patients who have been unconscious following head injury, even though the period of unconsciousness was only minutes or seconds long. If the patient remains at home, instructions must be given to significant others: to awaken the patient hourly; how to examine the person and what to look for; and what to do in the event of seizures or other symptoms of complications. The importance of these repeated examinations following head injury are emphasized both to the conscious patient and to significant others.

In the hospital the frequency of vital sign measurements varies with the patient's condition, but usually these measurements are taken every 15 minutes until they are stable within safe limits. It may be necessary to awaken a head-injured patient hourly during the first 24 to 48 hours following injury to evaluate vital signs and neurologic status, i.e. perform neuro checks (see p. 524). The various parameters evaluated may include: level of consciousness and responsiveness; pupillary diameters and responses to light; pulse; blood pressure; respiratory rate; temperature (rectal); motor strength; speech; vision; reaction to auditory and painful stimuli; response to command; spontaneous activity; and general responsiveness to stimulation

Recall from the discussions on coma, intracranial pressure and herniation syndromes (in the preceding chapter) and from the discussion of primary versus secondary damage in relation to head injuries (in this chapter), that *trends* in changes in the neuro checks are indications of changes in the patient's condition. Moreover, *deterioration in the level of consciousness and pupillary signs are relatively early signs of the onset of secondary damage such as a developing hematoma.* Early recognition of these changes may save the patient's life or prevent further permanent neurologic damage. During the observation period sedatives and narcotics are contraindicated except when specifically ordered; they are sometimes ordered if the patient is highly restless and an intracranial hematoma has been ruled out by surgery or angiography.

Decreasing level of consciousness is the single most important criterion of increasing intracranial pressure, e.g., from an expanding hematoma or cerebral edema. However, the patient may show worsening of any or all of the following parameters during observation: (1) responsiveness; (2) focal motor ability; (3) pupillary reactions and size; and/or (4) vital signs.

Be sure to inform the physician immediately of symptoms and signs such as: deepening levels of consciousness, restlessness, bradycardia, sudden temperature alterations, increasing blood pressure, sudden drop in blood pressure, cyanosis, or worsening of focal symptoms.

The needs of the *alert patient* are sometimes overlooked. In addition to the possibility of being "overlooked" because of an apparently "stable" condition, the alert person's impairments may go unnoticed without careful nursing assessment. For example, such a patient may be experiencing "minor" symptoms such as dizziness when walking, and impaired judgment. These problems make the patient more prone to accidents and necessitate close supervision and assistance.

Nuchal Rigidity. Nuchal rigidity, i.e., involuntary stiffness of neck muscles, may indicate cervical spine injuries, meningeal irritation, or subarachnoid bleeding following head injury. In the presence of nuchal rigidity immobilize the patient's head until cervical spine injuries are ruled out.

Fluid-Electrolyte, Acid-Base Maintenance; Nutrition. Maintain fluid-electrolyte and acid-base balances and nutrition; record and evaluate intake and output. In the severely head-injured patient, continuous intravenous infusion is maintained and fluid-electrolyte and acid-base balances are carefully managed. (The administration of medications may be facilitated by intravenous fluid therapy.) The choice of fluid is often a balanced salt solution, e.g., lactated Ringer's. (See Unit V, Chapter 12, and Chapter 26 for sections of related importance.) Periodically laboratory evaluation may be made of such factors as blood electrolytes, blood urea nitrogen, blood gases, and pH.

A properly balanced fluid intake is gradually given to the patient as ordered. *Intravenous feedings* may be continued for several days. *Tube feedings* cannot be given until adequate peristalsis returns (usually about 48 hours after the accident) and cannot be used if marked abdominal distention or gastric retention develops following feedings. *Oral feedings* are avoided if they could precipitate vomiting, since vomiting increases intracranial pressure and can also result in aspiration.

As discussed previously, some physicians restrict both oral and parenteral fluids in some head-injured patients in an attempt to prevent excessive intracranial pressure. Intravenous fluids are typically administered at a minimal flow rate because of the possible danger of cerebral edema.

A retention catheter (or condom drainage apparatus for male patients) may be used to provide a means for accurately measuring urinary output, monitor urine specific gravity, and to avoid incontinence and restlessness. *Initially check urinary output regularly* to ascertain the adequacy of the circulatory system in the semiconscious or unconscious head-injured patient. Occasionally severe brain injury is associated with impaired renal function of unknown etiology. In spite of treatment the patient may die from renal failure.

Restlessness; Pain; Disorientation. Evaluate and control restlessness and pain; reorient the patient as consciousness returns.

Pain in the head-injured patient is best relieved by carefully administering codeine or other *ordered* mild analgesics. Occasionally if a major bone is fractured and the patient does not have symptoms of increased intracranial pressure, an opiate may be ordered to be given *with caution* so that pain is relieved without excessively depressing the patient.

> *Narcotics are generally contraindicated following head injury. Narcotics are not given if increased intracranial pressure is present.*

Evaluate *restlessness* in an attempt to identify its cause. Restlessness in a head-injured patient may result from: (1) brain injury; (2) returning consciousness; or (3) other causes, e.g., increasing intracranial pressure, pain, full bladder, respiratory insufficiency, uncomfortable position, tight dressing. Try to correct manageable situations that may be causing the patient's restlessness, e.g., change position. If the patient remains restless, inform the physician.

Sometimes the physician tries to relieve the patient's restlessness by prescribing *hypotensive drugs* (to reduce intracranial pressure) or by performing a *lumbar puncture* (to remove a small amount of CSF). At other times the physician prescribes *light sedation* with small initial doses of short-acting, mild medications. *Excessive sedation must be avoided in head-injured patients.* It is better to let the patient be a little noisy and a little restless rather than risk oversedation. Restraints are quite undesirable since they may increase the patient's agitation and thereby increase intracranial pressure. Protect the restless patient from injury.

As the patient gradually regains consciousness, reorientation is essential, e.g., tell the person generally what has happened where he or she is and that the person is being taken care of. (See also p. 523.)

Seizures. Be prepared to care for the head-injured patient if seizures develop. Observe the patient closely for indications of seizure activity. Seizures may worsen a head-injured patient's condition; therefore, every attempt is made to prevent them, e.g., anticonvulsants may be prescribed prophylactically. Anticonvulsants are always ordered once a seizure does occur. If appropriate orders have not been left, be certain to inform the physician immediately, if a seizure occurs.

Positioning. Position the head-injured patient as indicated and/or ordered. The patient frequently is placed in semi-Fowler's position unless contraindicated, e.g. the patient comatose, in shock, or has spinal injuries. (Positioning appropriate in treating these complications has been previously discussed).

Stress Ulcers. Stress ulcers are best prevented by frequently (initially even hourly) measuring the gastric pH and administering antacids as prescribed via a nasogastric tube. (See pp. 665 and 1432).

Rest; Complications of Inactivity. Rest is important following head injuries and therefore the patient is aroused only as often as absolutely necessary. However, it is of equal importance that the patient be kept active enough to prevent the complications associated with inactivity. The conscious head-injured patient may become very tired because hourly awakening and testing may take place for the first 24 to 48 postinjury hours. Keep the patient's environment quiet. Plan clinical care to ensure rest periods.

History. A history of how a patient was injured can be helpful to the physician. Therefore when accident witnesses accompany a newly injured patient to the hospital, ask them to wait to talk with the doctor. If they cannot wait get information from them yourself.

Observation for Sequelae. Following head injury the patient is closely observed (for as long as necessary) to detect possible disorders which may have been caused by the injury, e.g., mental changes, headache, dizziness. Possible results of head injury have been discussed.

Medication Summary. Several types of medications may be given either as a single dose or over a period of time following head injury. If lacerations, abrasions, or open injuries are present, tetanus prophylaxis is often given. Steroid therapy may be used on the theoretical basis that steroids stabilize cellular membranes and prevent cerebral edema from developing.[60] The drug dosage and choice is the subject of current controversy, although dexamethasone is a frequent choice. Anticonvulsants are also usually given to the patient for seizure prophylaxis. Should seizures occur, additional drugs are used (see section on epilepsy, p. 640). The indications for the use of an osmotic diuretic, often Mannitol, is also controversial. It is used for cerebral decompression in the face of cerebral edema/swelling. However, it works on normal tissue and is accompanied by a "rebound" phenomena. Thus, most authorities agree that it is used to "buy time" to get the patient to the operating room if operative intervention is possible. Other uses relate to the condition of the patient and the physician's philosophy. Antibiotics may be given in some situations. Finally, an antacid or some other type of medication is often given to prevent bleeding from stress ulcers, particularly if the patient is receiving steroid therapy.

Injuries to the Spinal Cord or Its Roots

Spinal cord injuries may occur in many ways, e.g., from penetrating or crushing wounds, spinal fractures, spinal dislocations, compressing spinal tumors, or ruptured disks. Symptoms that develop from trauma to the spine may result from injury to the substance of the spinal cord or injury to the nerve roots. Injury to the bony spine is in itself not of practical importance except when the injury affects the spinal cord or its roots. Damage to the spinal cord may result from disorders such as: (1) simple concussion that does not directly traumatize the cord; (2) penetrating missiles or fracture dislocations which compress, contuse, or lacerate the cord substance; (3) hemorrhage into the cord's substance, i.e., hematomyelia, and (4) compression of the cord's vascular supply. As discussed before, symptoms that result from cord injury vary, depending on the seriousness of the injury and the level of the injury. The care of patients with traumatic spinal cord injuries has been discussed earlier (see pp. 556–579).

RUPTURED INTERVERTEBRAL DISK

In about 98 per cent of cases, ruptured, prolapsed, or herniated intervertebral disks occur at the 4th and 5th intervertebral spaces in the lumbar spine. Less frequently, herniation of a disk occurs in the cervical region. Herniation of lumbar intervertebral disks is the most common cause of pain of sciatic distribution. The intervertebral disks (particularly between the 4th and 5th lumbar vertebrae and between the 5th lumbar and sacrum) are subject to tremendous forces and degenerative changes. When the surrounding ligaments are also injured and weakened, disk material (the nucleus pulposus) begins to extrude through the ligaments and compress the spinal cord and/or displace spinal nerve roots (Fig. 27–28). Ruptured disks cause an estimated 10 per cent of those backaches that prompt people to seek the help of a physician. When herniation occurs rapidly, the patient experiences *acute low back syndrome;* if it occurs gradually the resulting persisting pressure causes *chronic low back pain.* Often younger patients report a history of a flexion injury, e.g., injury caused by heavy lifting from a stooped position during which they "feel something give way" in their backs. In older persons with degenerative changes, even trivial trauma, e.g., sneezing or a misstep, may cause disk herniation.

Common *symptoms of lumbar disk herniation* include: lower back pain, radiating down the posterior thigh; muscle spasm; aggravation of pain by straining (e.g., coughing, defecation, bending, lifting, and straight leg raising); depression of deep tendon reflexes; and hypesthesia in the distribution of the affected nerve roots. Myelography may be normal or may show narrowing of one of the lower disk spaces. Rupture of a small laterally placed *cervical disk* typically causes stiff neck, shoulder pain radiating down the arm into the hand, and paresthesias and sensory disturbances in the hand. Electromyography or electrical testing of the peripheral nerves is valuable in localizing the site of ruptured disk (see Chapter 25).

Most disk herniation is *treated conservatively* with strict bed rest, at least initially. (The usual exception to this rule is the presence of progressive neurologic dysfunction). More recently, however, alternative forms of therapy including *chymopapain* injection have been used in the initial treatment phase (see p. 674).

Conservative treatment consists of strict bed rest on a firm mattress and the use of various drugs, including analgesics, sedatives, anti-inflammatory agents, and muscle relaxants. Diathermy and local heat applications are also used. It should be remembered that prolonged heat increases congestion and is thus undesirable. Morphine or other narcotics may be indicated for severe pain, but the potential danger of addiction with prolonged usage must be remembered. Corsets may be used for additional support in a person with a lumbar disk problem. With herniation of a cervical disk, a cervical collar is frequently used to keep the head in a slightly flexed position. The neck should not be hyperextended. Traction may be applied for a cervical disk herniation; however, its use in treating a similar lumbar disk disorder is controversial. With a cervical disk herniation, traction is used to relieve pressure on the nerve.

While on bed rest the patient is encouraged to systematically change position in bed (when not in traction). The patient with back pain may be most comfortable with the backrest elevated 20 to 30 degrees and the knees slightly flexed.

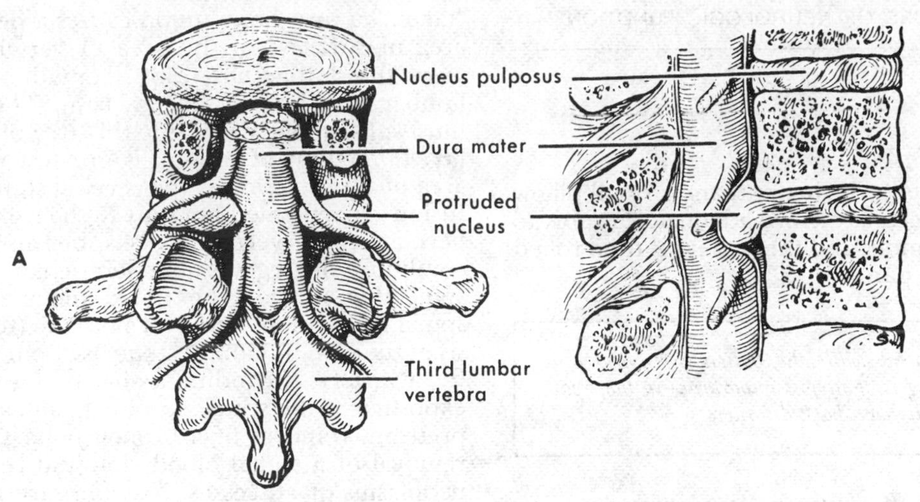

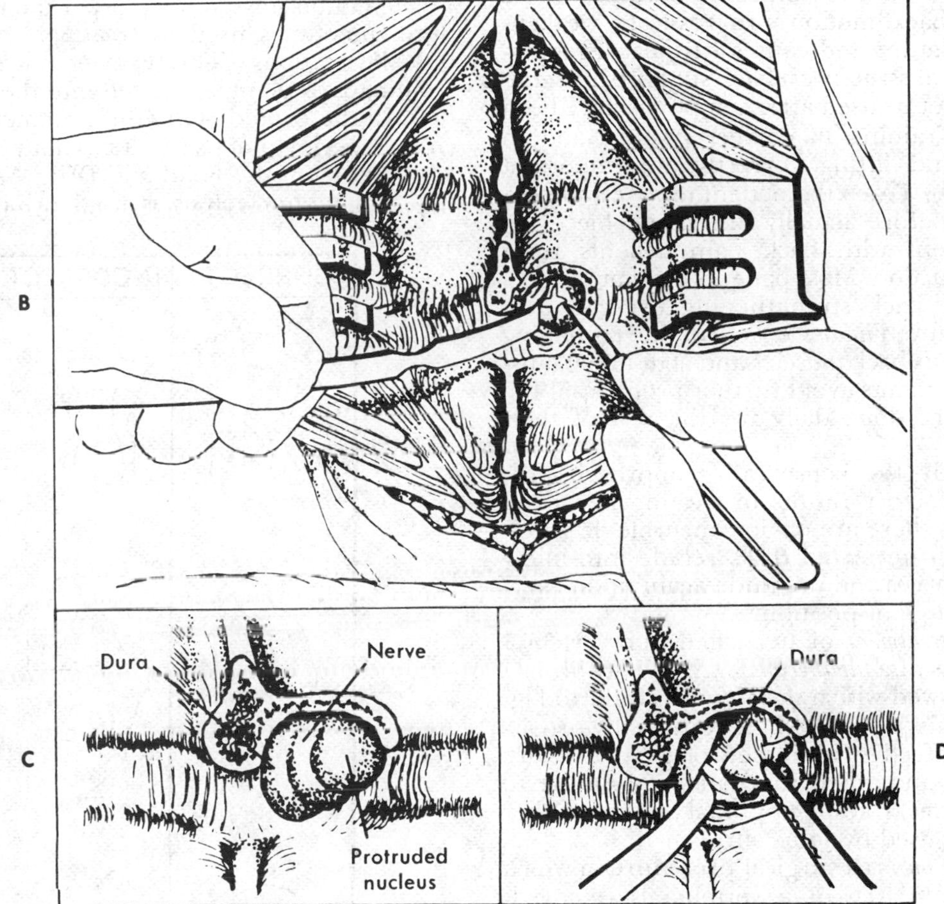

Figure 27–28. **A.** Normal and herniated nucleus pulposus (disc). **B.** Window has been made in lamina, and ligament has been incised to expose underlying dura mater and nerve root. **C.** Relationship of dura mater, nerve root, and protruded nucleus pulposus (disc). **D.** Retraction of nerve root over dura mater and removal of disc. (From Conway, B. L.: *Carini and Owens' Neurological and Neurosurgical Nursing*, 7th ed. St. Louis: C. V. Mosby Co. 1978.)

Other positions that may be comfortable are (1) supine, with pillows under the legs or (2) on either side, with a thin pillow between the knees. Physicians who prescribe the semisitting position (which encourages forward flexion of the lumbar spine and thus reduces strain on the back) do not permit the patient to lie in the prone position at any time since this causes hyperextension of the spine. Also, the patient should not use an overbed trapeze. In bed, the patient is turned in a logrolling manner and uses a fracture bedpan or child's bedpan (see Fig. 28–7). In placing the bedpan, the patient is rolled onto one side (be sure to have a turning sheet on the bed), the bedpan and a small pillow or roll are placed to ensure adequate support to the lumbar region, and the patient is then rolled back onto the pan.

> *Proper alignment while the patient is in bed and during turning is of utmost importance in the treatment of patients with back disorders.*

When first allowed out of bed, the patient usually wears a back brace or a corset. Since restricted back motion progressively weakens the musculature and causes further degeneration of spinal structures, back supports generally should not be used after symptoms have been relieved. Training in correct posture and in stooping and lifting correctly are important (Fig. 27–29). Teach the patient to *think* and plan a method before actually lifting an object. An obese patient with back pain benefits from weight reduction. Most patients are started on a progressive back strengthening exercise program (usually *Williams exercises*). Strengthening of the various back muscles and abdominal muscles helps patients avoid further problems if the exercises are done daily for the rest of their lives.

Frequently the conservative approach produces satisfactory results in treating herniated disk, unless there are obvious neurologic symptoms. Often herniated disks recede into intervertebral spaces and protrude again upon exertion or change of position.

Surgical treatment of herniated intervertebral disk consists of a *laminectomy,* which may or may not be followed with a *spinal fusion* (refer to Fig. 27–28). This is done when conservative treatment is ineffective, when neurologic deficits are increasing, and when the patient is subject to repeated attacks despite optimal therapy. Other criteria are used by some surgeons.

A *laminectomy* is a surgical procedure in which the posterior arch of a vertebra is removed. This exposes the spinal cord. In treating a herniated intervertebral disk, the surgeon removes the portion of the nucleus pulposus that is protruding or ruptured from the intervertebral disk. General agreement does not exist as to whether spinal fusion should be performed at the same time that the ruptured disk is removed.

Spinal fusion consists of removal of a piece or pieces of bone from another region of the body (e.g., iliac crest) and grafting these bone chips or pieces onto the vertebrae. Once the graft has "taken," a firm bony union causes a permanent area of stiffness in the area of vertebrae that were fused together, e.g., from the involved lumbar vertebrae to the sacrum. The patient must subsequently adjust to this area of immobility. Limitation of motion is greatest when the area of fusion involves the cervical spine. Spinal fusion is performed not only in the treatment of herniated intervertebral disks, but also in such conditions as degenerative joint changes in the spine that weaken the spine, spinal fractures, spinal dislocation, and Pott's disease (tuberculosis of the spine). Laminectomy is also performed for a variety of conditions that require surgical exposure of the spinal cord, e.g., spinal decompression, removal of a broken bone fragment, removal of a spinal blood clot, and removal of neoplasms or abscesses. Nursing care following spinal surgery is discussed in Chapter 28.

Chemonucleolysis is an experimental procedure sometimes used in treatment of lumbar disk herniations. The enzyme chymopapain from papaya plant is injected into the ruptured disk. In the United States this treatment is limited to experimental use, as it has not yet received approval from the Food and Drug Administration. Chemonucleolysis is used principally for

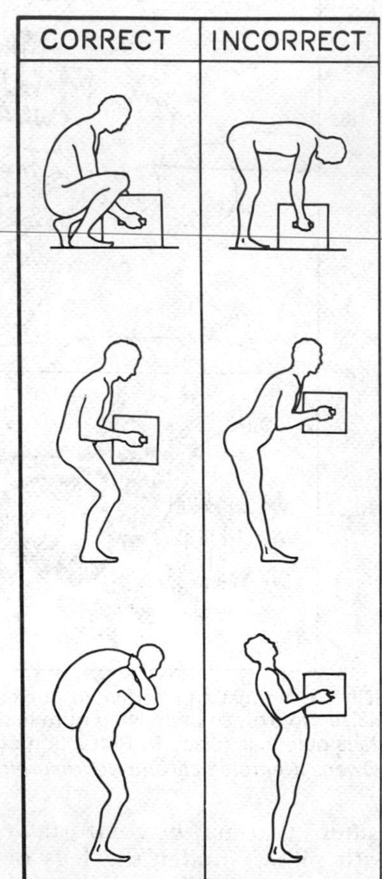

Figure 27–29. Correct and incorrect postural attitudes. (From Krussen, F. H., F. J. Kottke, and P. M. Ellwood Jr.: *Handbook of Physical Medicine and Rehabilitation,* 2nd ed. Philadelphia: W. B. Saunders Co., 1971.)

patients in whom a laminectomy has failed. However, some investigators use it as a primary method of therapy, e.g., if bed rest does not improve the patient.

Injection of chymopapain is done in the x-ray department or operating room. The person is lying in a lateral position. One or several doses may be injected. The enzyme dissolves or "chemically digests" the damaged tissue. The major side effect is anaphylactic reaction, often during the injection. Some investigators give corticosteroids prior to the injection to diminish this untoward reaction. Others give corticosteroids and epinephrine immediately should a reaction occur. Although the reaction is usually immediate, the patient is watched closely for delayed reactions.

Finally, a small but persistent number of patients with disk herniation will receive no relief from any form of therapy and will become persons experiencing *chronic pain* (see Unit XI).

Injuries to Peripheral Nerves

Only some of the most common injuries of the peripheral nerves are considered here. The peripheral nerves can be injured in numerous ways, e.g., fractures of the bones and stretching of the nerves, constriction by fascial bands, pressure, trauma associated with perforating wounds, or the injection of drugs. *The nerves most commonly subjected to external pressure are the radial, common peroneal, ulnar, and long thoracic nerves.* The *median* nerve is most often affected by constriction by fascial bands: The *axillary* nerve is commonly affected in an allergic reaction to injections of serum; and the *sciatic* is commonly injured by the direct injection of medications. Of course, any of the peripheral nerves can be injured by bone fractures or perforating wounds.

When a peripheral nerve is traumatically severed, the ends should be anastomosed surgically to enable healing. When nerves are only slightly damaged, mild edema occurs at the site of the injury. This may cause temporary symptoms that recede in a period of only a few days or possibly weeks. The nearer the site of injury occurs to the central nervous system in a completely severed peripheral nerve, the poorer the chance of regeneration occurring.

Median Nerve Compression at the Wrist (Carpal Tunnel Syndrome). *Carpal tunnel syndrome* may develop spontaneously without a known cause or may occur as a result of disease or injury. A common cause is trauma to the wrist involving the distal end of the radius and the carpal bones.

When the symptoms are mild and of short duration, or if the patient does not want surgery, the wrist may be immobilized on a splint, or temporary relief may be obtained by the injection of hydrocortisone acetate suspension into the carpal tunnel. Surgery is indicated when the symptoms are severe and of long duration, when muscle atrophy occurs, or when the sensory loss in the fingers and hand is progressive. Standard surgical treatment for carpal tunnel syndrome is decompression of the medial nerve by section of the transverse carpal ligament (Fig. 27–30).

The counterpart of the carpal tunnel syndrome in the lower extremity is the *"tarsal tunnel syndrome,"* in which the posterior tibial nerve is trapped beneath the flexor retinaculum and deep fascia along the medial border of the foot.

Ulnar Nerve Compression at the Elbow. Lying within a bony groove at the elbow, the ulnar nerve is susceptible to compression either from direct trauma to the elbow (hitting the "crazy" bone) or from changes within the groove that cause the nerve to be gradually squeezed. Repeated mild trauma (e.g., habitual leaning on the elbows upon a hard surface) can also injure the ulnar nerve. Resultant sensory changes occur in the ulnar aspect of the hand and wrist. The usual treatment for ulnar nerve compression at the elbow is transplantation of the ulnar nerve.

Sciatic Nerve Injury. The sciatic nerve is the longest nerve in the body. *The common peroneal nerve (a terminal branch of the sciatic) is more often subject to trauma than any other nerve in the body.* Because of its peculiar course and distribution, the sciatic nerve is more exposed to internal and external trauma and inflammation than any other nerve.

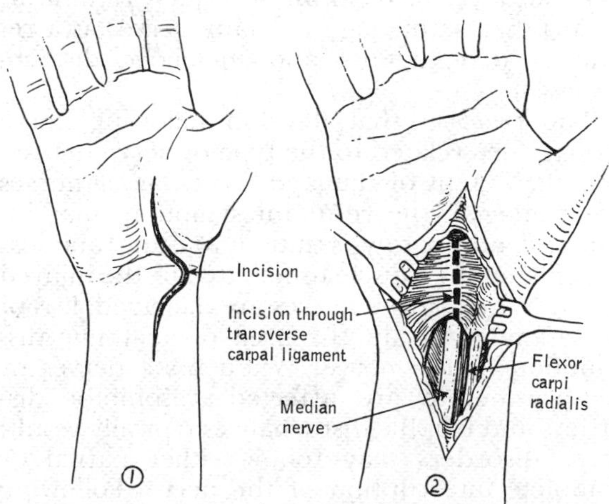

Figure 27–30. Technique of section of transverse carpal ligament. (From Finneson, B. E.: *Diagnosis and Management of Pain Syndromes,* 2nd ed. Philadelphia: W. B. Saunders Co., 1969.)

Nurses are aware that sciatic nerve injury can result from faulty injection technique.

Sciatica refers to severe pain in the lower extremity that occurs along the course of the sciatic nerve and its branches. There are numerous causes of sciatica, but in about 90 per cent of patients the causes are rupture of an intervertebral disk and osteoarthritis of the lumbosacral spine producing mechanical pressure on the nerve or its spinal roots. Typically the pain of sciatica begins in the buttocks and extends down the back of the thigh and leg to the ankle. Usually sciatic pain is constant. Any movement of the lower extremity that stretches the nerve causes pain and involuntary resistance. Straight leg raising on the affected side is limited, and complete extension of the leg is not possible when the thigh is flexed on the abdomen *(Lasègue's sign).* The treatment of sciatica is based upon treating the underlying cause when possible. (See also discussions of ruptured intervertebral disk and arthritis.)

DISEASES OF THE CRANIAL AND PERIPHERAL NERVES

The cranial and peripheral nerves may be damaged by: tumors, infections, trauma, vascular and metabolic disturbances, and toxic agents. *Neuritis* refers to nerve damage from any cause. *Mononeuritis* refers to injury to a single nerve as a result of localized injury; *polyneuritis* means diffuse damage to many nerves as a result of toxic agents and metabolic disturbances.

The *symptoms* that develop following nerve damage are related to the type of nerve injured and the extent of damage. When *motor* nerves are damaged, the resultant symptoms may include: flaccid paralysis, muscle wasting, and loss of reflex in the muscle innervated by the injured nerve. When *sensory* nerves are damaged, loss of sensation occurs in the area of anatomic distribution of the nerve. When *mixed* nerves or sensory nerves are affected, vasomotor disorders and trophic disturbances typically result; these disorders may follow either partial or complete interruption of the nerve. Following partial injury or incomplete division of a nerve the patient may experience stabbing pains, dysesthesias, e.g., pins and needles sensations, and occasionally the burning pains of causalgia.

Cranial Nerves

Outline of Diseases of the Cranial and Peripheral Nerves

A. Cranial nerves
  1. Fifth cranial nerve (trigeminal neuralgia)
  2. Seventh cranial nerve (facial paralysis; Bell's palsy)
  3. Eighth cranial nerve disorders
B. Polyneuropathies
  1. Guillain-Barré syndrome.

The cranial nerves can be affected in numerous ways in association with various disorders of the nervous system as we have seen. For example, they may be *secondarily* affected from compression resulting from increased intracranial pressure or they may be *directly* injured as a result of head injuries. In this section we discuss only *disease conditions that are specific to the cranial nerves* and do not occur in association with other disorders. Only the most common cranial nerve disorders will be considered.

It is noteworthy that regeneration of the first (olfactory) or second (optic) cranial nerves does not occur, since these nerves are actually part of the CNS.

Fifth Cranial Nerve (Trigeminal). *Trigeminal neuralgia* (also called *tic douloureux*) is a neuralgic disorder specifically affecting the fifth cranial nerve. This condition is a disorder of unknown etiology that affects function of the *sensory* division of this nerve, causing excruciating, recurrent paroxysms of sharp, stabbing pains in the distribution of one or more of the nerve's three branches. The trigeminal nerve is one of the largest of the cranial nerves and consists of the following divisions: I, ophthalmic; II, maxillary; and III, mandibular (Fig. 27–31).

Trigeminal neuralgia is possibly the most agonizing benign condition, and has been known to prompt severe depression and suicide.

This neuralgia is called "tic douloureux" because patients often wince repeatedly at the severity of the pain. The attack of pain typically begins suddenly, e.g., like a tooth fracturing. The pain is limited strictly to one or more branches of the fifth cranial nerve and does not spread beyond the nerve's distribution of innervation. The second and third divisions of the nerve are most commonly involved with the pain.

Trigeminal neuralgia attacks are characterized by the presence of sensitive *trigger zones,* the stimulation of which sets off one of the paroxysms of pain. These trigger areas are often small areas on the patient's upper or lower lips, gums, side of the nose, or cheek. A trigger zone may be triggered into producing pain if it is even mildly stimulated, e.g., by cold wind, shaving, washing, chewing, swallowing, or talking. The fearful patient may try to prevent the paroxysms of pain by going without nourishment, oral hygiene, or shaving for days, or by trying to keep the face immobile while talking. Pain may interfere with sleep. In an attempt to avoid drafts, the patient may keep the face and head covered. Often the patient is fearful of being approached by other persons who might inadvertently trigger an attack.

Trigeminal neuralgia is the *most frequent of all primary neuralgias.* It affects more women than men and most often appears in middle or late life.

Treatment. Numerous medical and surgical treatments have been tried for trigeminal neuralgia. None has proven totally successful. There is still no safe, proven treatment for this disorder. Therefore, nurses caring for persons with this agonizing disorder need to investigate the advantages and disadvantages of the therapeutic modality being used and plan care accordingly.

Various *medications* are used in treating trigeminal neuralgia. They have two principal disadvantages: (1) They fail to work at all in some patients and only for varying lengths of time in others; and (2) each of the medications has serious toxic effects. Some patients receive *pain medications,* including narcotics. However, pain relief may not be adequate and narcotics carry a risk of addiction. The narcotics particularly are avoided whenever possible. They are given only if other measures have failed and pain relief must be obtained until other therapeutic strategy can be tried.

Diphenylhydantoin (Dilantin) at times will abort an acute attack of trigeminal neuralgia if it is injected intravenously. The daily administration of this anticonvulsant may prevent recurrent attacks in some persons. Recently *carbamazepine (Tegretol),* another anticonvulsant, has been found to be more effective than Dilantin.

> *Tegretol and Dilantin both have potentially serious (sometimes fatal) untoward reactions involving the hemopoietic system.*

Hemopoietic complications occasionally reported in association with the administration of Dilantin include: thrombocytopenia, leukopenia, granulocytopenia, agranulocytosis and pan-

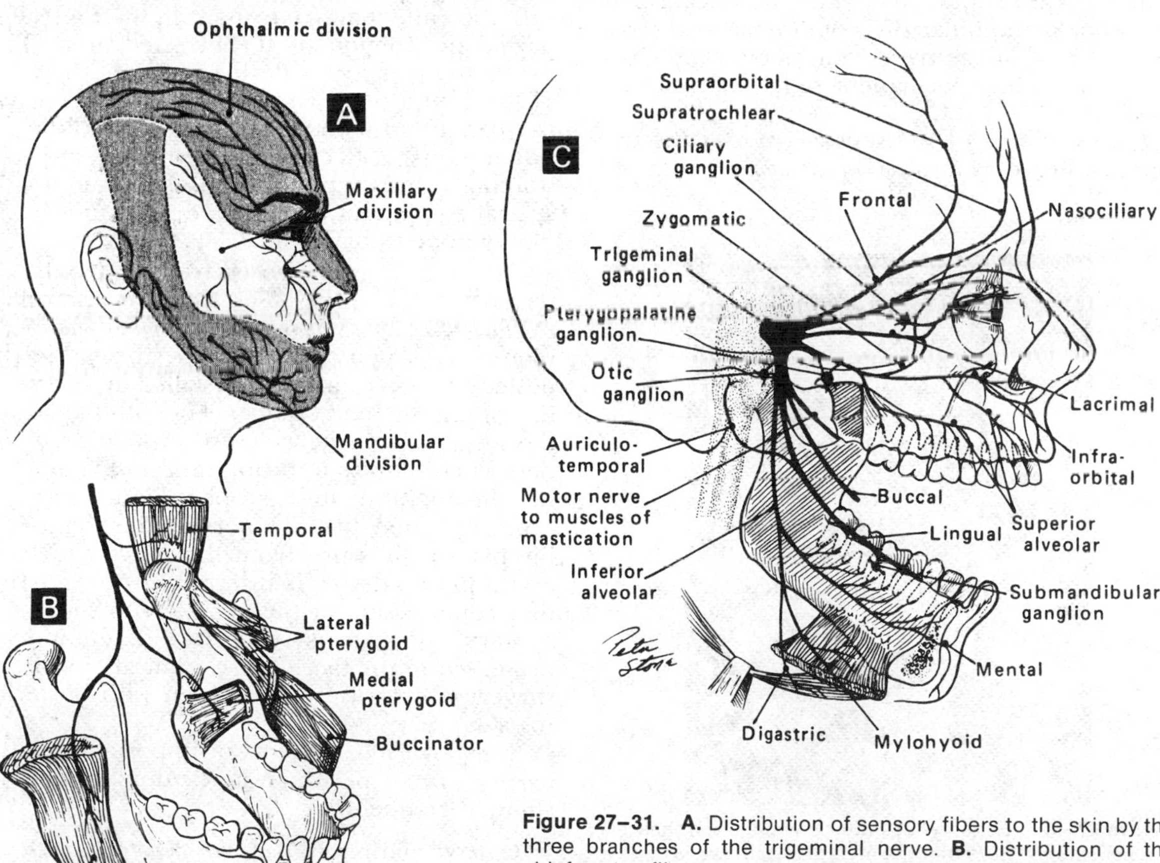

Figure 27–31. **A.** Distribution of sensory fibers to the skin by the three branches of the trigeminal nerve. **B.** Distribution of the chief motor fibers to muscles of mastication. **C.** Distribution of terminal branches. (From Langley, L. L., I. R. Telford, and J. B. Christensen: *Dynamic Anatomy and Physiology,* 4th ed. McGraw-Hill: New York, 1974, p. 254.)

cytopenia. Following treatment with Tegretol, thrombocytopenia, leukopenia, agranulocytosis and aplastic anemia have been reported. Persons receiving Tegretol must have their *blood counts monitored carefully* before and during treatment, e.g., possibly weekly during early treatment. Also, these patients must be taught the *early* toxic indications of a potential problem in their blood. These include: fever, sore throat, easy bruising, ulcers in the mouth, petechial or purpuric hemorrhage. They should be advised to immediately stop taking the drug and see their physician if such indications appear. *Early* detection of blood change is important because aplastic anemia is reversible in some persons. (Refer also to section on epilepsy [p. 640] in this chapter and to Unit XIV's discussions of blood disorders.)

Persons with tic douloureux may also be referred for *surgical treatment.* The trigeminal system may be treated surgically in a variety of ways, intracranially or peripherally. *Peripheral measures* may include alcohol injection or avulsion of the supraorbital nerve, infraorbital nerve, or mandibular division. *Intracranially* the sensory root of the trigeminal nerve can be divided, providing permanent relief from the attacks.

Total severance of the sensory root of the trigeminal nerve *(retrogasserian rhizotomy)* produces *permanent* aftereffects. (See Fig. 27–32.) Permanent anesthesia of the innervated area results and the patient may also experience various disturbing sensations, e.g., numbness, stiffness, and occasionally burning. An alcohol injection may be performed before the nerve is sectioned so the patient can *temporarily* experience the aftereffects before deciding upon the surgery. Whenever possible, *partial sectioning* of the nerve is carried out to spare the division or divisions of the nerve not affected. For example, since severance of the first section of the nerve results in corneal anesthesia, this section is not cut unless it is affected with the pain. Microsurgery has improved the precision with which the fibers can be selectively cut. For example, while eliminating the sensations of pain and temperature it is possible to preserve the corneal reflex and the sensation of touch.

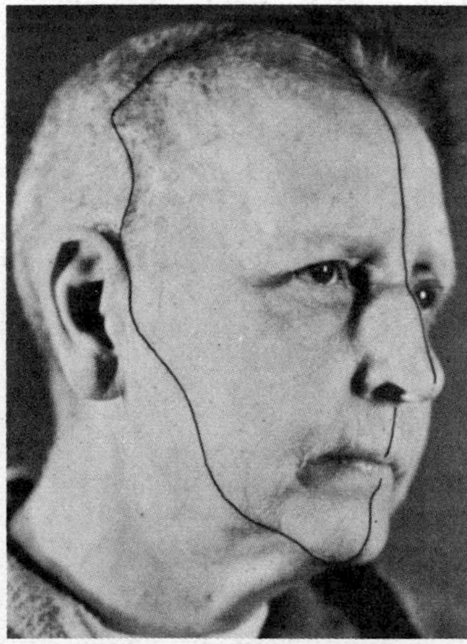

Figure 27–32. Sensory loss after complete retrogasserian neurotomy. Note that the area of anesthesia is curved upward because a portion of this area is innervated by cervical nerves. (From Vick, N. A.: *Grinker's Neurology,* 7th ed. Springfield, Ill.: Charles C Thomas Publisher, 1976, p. 284.)

Retrogasserian rhizotomy is an older procedure. Recently, two newer surgical procedures have been introduced. Both have gained acceptance in a variety of settings as they appear to produce fewer complications with acceptable results.

The *percutaneous radio-frequency rhizotomy* provides ablation of the trigeminal nerve in the area of the ganglion. This procedure does not require major surgery. A low-voltage electrical current is introduced through a spinal needle, with the patient awake to assist in the controlled partial destruction of the affected area. This procedure usually results in sparing of the sense of touch and the corneal reflex and thus leaves the patient with total pain relief and little residual damage. Because of the need for special training in this type of surgical technique and special equipment, this procedure is most commonly done in major medical centers.

The second new procedure, commonly referred to as the *Jannetta procedure,* is also called *vascular decompression of the trigeminal nerve.* It requires an open craniotomy performed in the posterior fossa by a surgeon skilled in the use of the operating microscope. The complexity of the surgery limits its wide use. Also, elderly patients may not be appropriate candidates. Under the operating microscope, a loop of artery is carefully lifted off the nerve (thus removing mechanical pressure from the nerve's surface) and a plastic device is inserted to prevent further compression of the nerve. With successful surgery, the pain is relieved and sensation is preserved in the face. The complications of this surgery are basically those seen with posterior fossa surgery.

Nursing Care. Points of importance in the *nursing care* of persons with tic douloureux are summarized below:

- Observe and record *characteristics of the attack,* including precipitating factors, location of trigger zones, description of the pain.
- Note individual ways in which patients try to *protect*

themselves from precipitating attacks, e.g., avoiding drafts, and remaining in his or her room, avoiding chewing and shaving.

- ▶ *Individualize diet and fluids,* e.g., frequent, small feedings of semiliquid foods served at room temperature may be preferred. Avoid very hot or cold foods and fluids.
- ▶ *Encourage maximum activity and self-help.* Older patients especially should be encouraged to remain active. Often persons with this disorder prefer to *care for themselves* since they know how to avoid trigger areas that another person might accidentally stimulate.
- ▶ *Avoid triggering attacks.* Protect the patient from drafts. Avoid jarring the patient or the bed. Do not force activities that may trigger pain. If it is necessary to insert a nasogastric tube for feeding, be certain to insert it in the nostril on the *unaffected* side of the face.
- ▶ *Administer medications* as ordered; record apparent effects; give appropriate teaching regarding medications.
- ▶ *Offer emotional support* both preoperatively and postoperatively.
- ▶ *Postoperatively,* know the expected aftereffects and what complications may be present. For example know which branches of the nerve have been sectioned and provide appropriate protection and patient teaching. For example, if the first (ophthalamic) branch is severed completely, the corneal reflex on that side will be absent and the patient should receive appropriate *protective eye care* and instructions about how to care for the affected eye. If the second and third branches of the nerve are cut, the patient must: (1) avoid hot beverages and foods that could burn oral mucous membranes; (2) avoid biting oral mucous membranes while chewing; and (3) routinely visit a dentist semiannually, since pain will not be felt in the areas innervated by the second and third branches of the nerve. Eating may be initially difficult if the nerve's lower branches are cut; the patient should be told to take food in on the mouth's unaffected side. Because food may accumulate in the mouth and not be felt on the affected side, frequent oral hygiene is necessary. The male patient must be especially careful not to cut himself while shaving. Often herpes simplex (cold sores) develop following section of the fifth cranial nerve, owing to injury to the gasserian ganglion, or hyperthemia or dehydration. These lesions usually heal in a week and may be treated topically.

Seventh Cranial Nerve (Facial). Our discussion here is concerned with the *motor aspects* of the facial nerve. The facial nerve is the main motor nerve of the muscles of the face. *Paralysis of the facial nerve occurs more commonly than paralysis of any other nerve, cranial or somatic.*

Facial paralysis may be central or peripheral in origin. A *central facial palsy* is an upper motor neuron paralysis or paresis. Sometimes central facial palsy produces dissociation of motor function such that a patient cannot voluntarily show the teeth on the paralyzed side of the face, but can show the teeth with emotional stimulation, which causes smiling or laughing. This phenomenon is called *"voluntary-emotional dissociation."*

BELL'S PALSY. The most common type of *peripheral facial paralysis* is called *Bell's palsy.* This is paralysis of the muscles of expression of one side of the face, when no evidence can be found of any pathologic cause.

With Bell's palsy there is typically: (1) an upward movement of the eyeball on the affected side upon closing the eye, i.e., *"Bell's phenomenon";* (2) drooping of the mouth on the affected side; (3) flattening of the nasolabial fold; (4) widening of the palpebral fissure on the affected side; and (5) a slight lag on the affected side upon closing the eyes. Note in Figure 27–33 the weakness of the face on the affected side.

Bell's palsy affects males and females about equally. While all age groups (from ages two to 85 years) have been affected, the most common age range is between ages 20 and 40. There is no known cure for Bell's palsy. Various palliative measures may be employed, including:[332a]

1. Analgesics if discomfort is present owing to herpetic involvement.
2. Cortisone drugs for the first few days (to possibly decrease nerve tissue swelling.)
3. Physiotherapy, e.g., moist heat, gentle massage, stimulation of the facial nerve with faradic current.
4. Support of sagging facial muscles with strips of adhesive or with a facial sling and

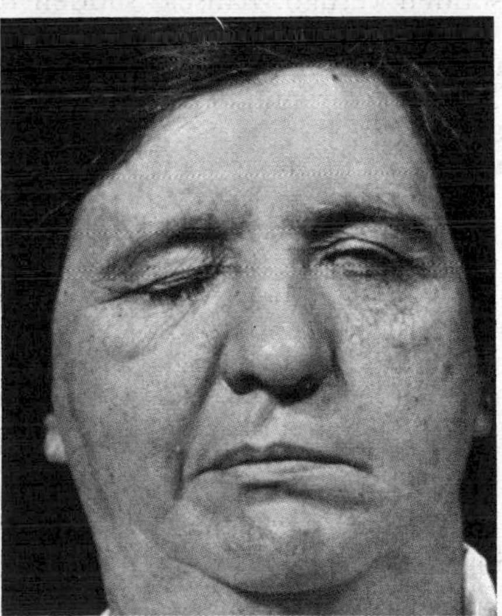

Figure 27–33. Bell's palsy. Peripheral facial paralysis on the patient's left side. (From Vick, N. A.: *Grinker's Neurology,* 7th ed. Springfield, Ill.: Charles C Thomas Publisher, 1976, p. 288.)

5. Protection of the cornea, e.g., with artificial tear solution, sunglasses, eyepatch at night, periodic gentle manual closure of the eye.

The patient with Bell's palsy needs to be reassured that a stroke has not occurred and that chances of complete recovery in a few weeks' time are good. Eating may be difficult.

A patient can participate in recovery by performing passive exercises which improve muscle tone and position. When active exercise of the facial muscles becomes possible, grimacing exercises are to be performed in front of a mirror (three times each day for five minutes each).[332a]

Most persons with Bell's palsy recover within a few weeks, without residual symptoms. When permanent complete facial paralysis results, *surgery* may be performed. Anastomosis of the peripheral end of the facial nerve with the spinal accessory or the hypoglossal nerve allows closure of the eye during sleep and restores tone to the facial musculature.

Eighth Cranial Nerve (Acoustic). Each eighth cranial nerve has *two divisions*: the auditory (cochlear), and the vestibular portions (the nerve to the semicircular canal system). *Symptoms* of involvement of the *auditory* branch include loss of hearing and tinnitus; those of involvement of the *vestibular* portion include vertigo, disturbance of equilibrium, and impaired ocular movements. Tinnitus and loss of hearing are considered in Chapter 90.

Functional disturbances of the labyrinth may occur either as recurrent attacks, i.e., Meniere's syndrome, or as an isolated event, i.e., acute labyrinthitis.

The cause of *acute labyrinthitis* is unknown. While the condition may follow a head cold, it may also occur without antecedent infection of the nasopharynx. Typical symptoms include: severe sudden vertigo, nausea, sudden disturbance of equilibrium, and sudden nystagmus. During the attack the patient typically prefers to lie in a darkened room; lies quietly in bed without turning the head; is photophobic; has a headache; has an ataxic gait; and may refuse food. No specific *treatment* exists. To relieve the vertigo the patient may be given dimenhydrinate or perphenazine. Because of severe vertigo the patient should be assisted when walking, and siderails are kept up on the bed. If the patient prefers, the room is kept darkened. Feedings are individualized in the presence of nausea and vomiting. Generally after several days or weeks the nystagmus disappears and the vertigo diminishes.

As the above symptoms indicate, acute labrynthitis is miserable to experience. A considerate nurse provides individualized supportive care which includes providing a safe, therapeutic environment.

Polyneuropathies

Polyneuritis or "multiple peripheral neuritis" refers to the clinical syndrome produced by *widespread involvement* of the peripheral nerves, with resultant sensory loss and reflex impairment. Generally a polyneuritis is related to either a toxic or metabolic condition. Examples of some polyneuropathies are: diphtheritic polyneuropathy; porphyric polyneuropathy; acute polyneuritis complicating viral hepatitis; alcohol–vitamin deficiency polyneuritis; arsenic or lead polyneuritis; polyneuritis associated with deficiency states; diabetic polyneuritis; polyneuritis complicating infectious mononucleosis; polyneuritis associated with carcinoma and other malignant neoplasms; diphtheritic polyneuritis; and acute idiopathic polyneuritis (Guillain-Barré syndrome).

Guillain-Barré Syndrome. This syndrome (also called Guillain-Barré-Strol syndrome, acute inflammatory polyradiculo-neuropathy, Landry-Guillain-Barré disease, postinfectious or infectious polyneuritis and acute idiopathic polyneuritis) is an inflammatory disease of unknown etiology characterized by widespread involvement of peripheral and cranial nerves. It is found worldwide and occurs in all seasons. Guillain-Barré syndrome usually affects young adults (ages 30-40) of both sexes. Many persons with this syndrome experience a mild respiratory or gastrointestinal infection 1 to 3 weeks before the onset of the neuritic signs and symptoms. Symptoms of the infection usually last for only a few days, and the indications of neutiric involvement appear anywhere from a few days to a few weeks after the symptoms of infection subside.

Etiology. As previously stated, the *cause* of this inflammatory disease is unknown. Much evidence supports the theory that the disorder is due to a "cell-mediated immunologic reaction directed at the peripheral nerve."[3] However, the possibility of some viral influence has not been discounted, especially in view of the frequency of a preceding respiratory infection. Whatever the underlying process, inflammatory cells (lymphocytes) enter the perivascular spaces, causing demyelination and degeneration of the nerve.

Guillain-Barré syndrome is the most rapidly developing and potentially fatal form of polyneuropathy.

Symptoms. Weakness, usually beginning in the distal muscles of the limbs, develops bilaterally over a period of a few days. In most patients, the weakness begins in the legs and ascends to the trunk, arms, and cranial muscles, producing *total motor paralysis* within a few days (usually 10 to 14 days). The motor paralysis is flaccid and typically tends to ascend the body (*Landry's ascending paralysis*). Generally, the motor weakness in the muscles of the trunk and extremities is quite severe and may result in a flaccid paraplegia and weakness of the muscles of respiration. If the weakness or paralysis involves cranial nerves also, affected persons become so debilitated that they cannot move, masticate, swallow, talk, or even close their eyes. Choked disks sometimes occur.

There is no muscle atrophy with Guillain-Barré syndrome, but decreased tone and absent reflexes occur. Paresthesias are common, but pain is rare. Sensory changes are usually minor. There may be variations of the clinical picture. For example, in milder cases, the legs may be totally affected and the arms not at all. Also, some persons experience muscle tenderness or sensitivity of the nerves to pressure.

DIAGNOSIS. Diagnosis is usually made on the basis of clinical presentation, i.e., signs, symptoms, history. Usually the only abnormal laboratory finding is a markedly elevated CSF protein content, probably due to the widespread inflammatory disease of the nerve roots.

COURSE. Progression of Guillain Barré syndrome may stop at any point in the course of the disease. A *plateau* typically occurs (lasting several days to several weeks) once weakness reaches its maximum. Improvement then begins and usually lasts several weeks. Rate of recovery is variable. In most persons, the disease remits naturally, and recovery is generally total although prolonged. With marked quadriplegia, full recovery may take over a year. While recovery from paralysis is typically good, some patients are left with varying degrees of muscle weakness and atrophy.

> *Some persons with Guillain-Barré* syndrome die of respiratory and vasomotor failure if mechanical ventilation and vasopressor agents are not available. Intercurrent infection may also result in death.

CLINICAL CARE. During the *acute stage* of the disease, the key to treatment is provision of necessary *respiratory support* and *complete nursing care* in an intensive setting if possible. Respiratory assistance is begun at the first signs of distress. (Respiratory management is discussed in Unit XVI.) Often an endotracheal tube is sufficient; but if the weakness persists, a tracheostomy may be necessary to provide adequate oxygenation and to help clear secretions from the tracheobronchial tree. Every effort should be made to control infections and maintain the patient in optimum condition. *There is no specific treatment.* Medications are usually not used, although some physicians may use a short course of steroids to counteract the inflammation.

Exercise and activity are restricted during the acute stage. The nurse must take care to maintain the patient in good body alignment to prevent deformities and injury to paralyzed limbs. (Nursing care of paralyzed persons is discussed in Chapter 26.) Once a patient's condition has stabilized, full passive range-of-motion exercise is begun and gradually increased as the patient can tolerate.

Guillain-Barré syndrome is clearly a serious, potentially life-threatening illness that may be frightening for patients to experience and for their significant others to observe.

> *As with so many disorders involving the nervous system, the nurse's expertise in performing "caring" activities and delegated medical tasks may make the important difference between a patient's survival and subsequent well being or long-term disability or death. Frequent patient assessment, thoughtful planning of individualized care, prevention of complications, and provision of sensitive emotional support are ever present in the skillful nurse's practice.*

CHAPTER 28

NEUROSURGERY

In the preceding chapters of this unit, we mention briefly the surgical intervention for a large number of disorders of the nervous system. Common procedures include: *extracerebral surgery,* such as the placement of burr holes; *extracranial surgery* on structures like the carotid artery; *intracranial surgery,* such as a craniotomy for removal of a mass lesion; *spinal surgery,* such as that done for disks or partial compression of the spinal cord; and surgery on the *peripheral nerves.* Neurosurgery encompasses:

- ▶ The brain and its related structures, such as the blood vessels
- ▶ The spinal cord and its related structures, such as the vertebrae
- ▶ Peripheral nerves

Neurosurgeons share their operative responsibilities with a variety of other specialized surgeons. For example, carotid artery surgery may be done by vascular surgeons; hand surgeons may collaborate in operations involving peripheral nerves, orthopedists in various types of spinal surgery. Ear, nose and throat surgeons, oral surgeons, and plastic surgeons are others who frequently collaborate with neurosurgeons. In addition to surgery by a team of specialists, neurosurgical patients may receive care from a variety of physician specialists. For example, general surgeons, respiratory medicine specialists, radiologists, oncologists, and hematologists may be involved in the care of persons requiring neurosurgery.

With the advent of complex new procedures and with the increasing complexity of "standard" surgery, nurses have also acquired additional knowledge and responsibilities in caring for neurosurgical patients. For example, nurses whose field is operating room nursing may specialize in assisting with neurosurgical procedures, and intensive care nurses may specialize in neurologic intensive care.

Other disciplines, e.g., physical therapy, also contribute to the team caring for the patient. Thus, the care of a patient with a neurologic disorder is frequently a multidisciplinary effort, and you may be working with a large and varied health care team. With so many specialists involved in the patient's treatment, with so many techniques being used, it may well be that the patient *as a person* is forgotten. The nurse can be especially effective in keeping the interests of the person foremost — answering questions, providing emotional support, supplying information to significant others, and in general, ensuring that the technology of neurosurgery does not overwhelm the *human beings* involved.

The modern neurosurgeon provides many basic procedures, such as intracranial surgery and spinal surgery. In addition, a number of refinements and new techniques have been developed. For example, there are various new *pain-relieving procedures* such as the ones described in relation to trigeminal neuralgia in Chapter 27. (Other pain-relieving procedures are described in Chapter 30.) *Surgery for epilepsy,* although not done on a large scale, has markedly improved the outlook for previously uncontrolled patients. It is briefly discussed in Chapter 27.

Stereotaxic instruments have permitted precise local stimulation or destruction of areas of the brain (see Fig. 28–1). Such instruments essentially are metal frames in which the patient's head can be clamped in a standard position, and on which a needle holder can be moved in three planes along graduated scales. The needle tip can be guided accurately to reach calculated areas within the brain. Probes can also be stereotactically inserted into the brain. Through the probes, a variety of agents can be used to ablate the lesion. These include heat, cold, ultrasound, and injections of corrosive or sclerosing fluids. The complications of this type of surgery are principally related to the location of the surgical approach.

Microsurgical techniques are also now applied to neurosurgery and have improved classic techniques and made possible new approaches to the cranial structures, e.g., transsphenoidal, translabyrinthine. Microsurgical techniques are also used in some spinal surgery.

Improved clinical care of unconscious patients and head-injured patients is an additional and important factor in making surgery on the nervous system more effective.

INTRACRANIAL SURGERY

A *craniotomy* is an opening into the skull. Such openings may be made in several ways, e.g.:

(1) *attached cranial section,* in which the bone flap remains attached and hinged to muscles and other structures, or (2) *detached cranial section,* in which a section of cranium is cut away from its attachments and temporarily removed for surgical exposure of the cranial contents. A "craniotomy" is done by excising part of the skull, e.g., by trephination, in which a circular piece or "button" of cranium is removed by a trephine. This bone is not replaced, at least not immediately. Rather, a *cranioplasty* may be done to repair the defect 6 to 12 months later. A *craniectomy* is sometimes done for decompression. A portion of cranium is removed and not replaced. (See Fig. 28–2.)

As with many other surgical procedures, neurosurgical procedures are often described in terms of the operative approach taken, e.g., subtemporal, suboccipital, transmastoidal, transorbital, anterior, posterior. Craniotomies may be described in relation to the tentorium, e.g., supratentorial, infratentorial.

Preoperative Care

Generally the preoperative preparation of a patient for intracranial surgery differs little from that for general surgery, particularly when the operation is not an emergency procedure, and the patient's general condition is good. There are some factors that should be emphasized concerning preoperative preparation for intracranial surgery. (See also Chapter 17 for discussion of preoperative care with general surgery.)

1. Give preoperative bowel care cautiously and *only as ordered.* The patient is instructed not to strain at defecation since the valsalva maneu-

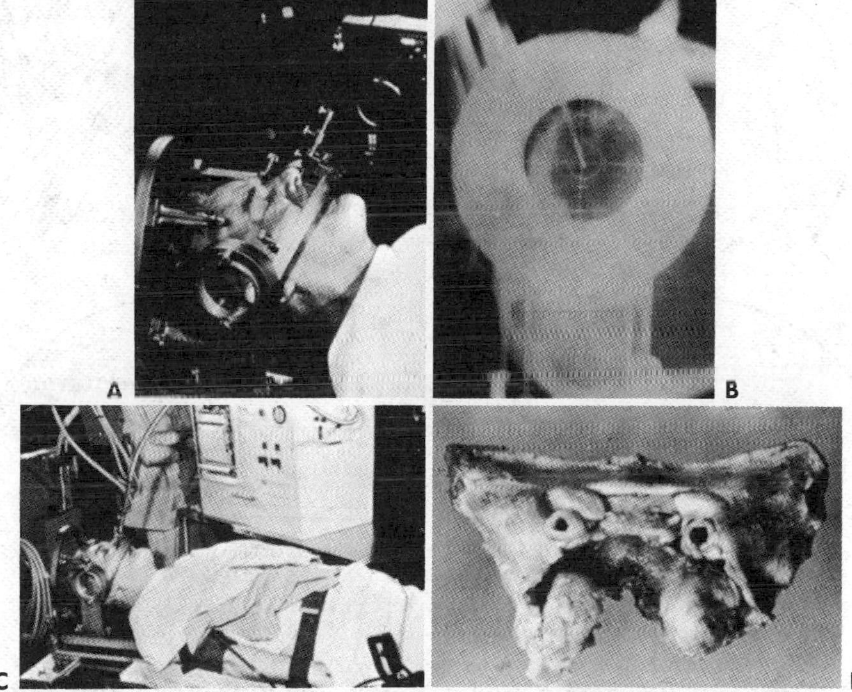

Figure 28–1. A. The patient's head is fixed to a stereotactic unit. A twist drill is inserted into the anterior wall of the sphenoid sinus by way of the left nostril into the nasopharynx. **B.** Lateral x-ray film demonstrating freezing unit properly placed in target area (pituitary gland). The circle and cross hairs are positioned at target point prior to insertion of cannula. **C.** The cannula in the patient's left nostril is attached to the freezing unit on the table. X-ray equipment is seen in the upper left background. Since the procedure is performed with the patient under local anesthesia, body straps are used to immobilize the patient. **D.** The sella turcica viewed from above, demonstrating bone perforation at base through which cannula was inserted. To either side of the sella turcica, the internal carotid arteries are seen (below, the siphon; above with open lumen, the cranial extension). Above the sectioned arteries, the optic nerves are seen passing into the orbits. (From Conway, B. L : *Carini and Owens' Neurological and Neurosurgical Nursing,* 7th ed. St. Louis: C. V. Mosby Co., 1978.)

ver (during straining) aggravates increased intracranial pressure.

2. Withhold food and fluids as ordered. Some patients may already be on restricted fluids because of cerebral swelling.

3. Explain preoperative procedures. Even though patients may be stuporous or even appear unconscious, they may still be able to hear.

4. See that operative permission has been obtained in accordance with the law and with procedures in the particular hospital. It is the physician's responsibility to obtain such permission after explaining the proposed surgery and its complications to the patient and significant others.

5. Administer preoperative medications as order (see p. 685).

6. Prepare the patient's scalp according to instructions in the individual situation. A sham-

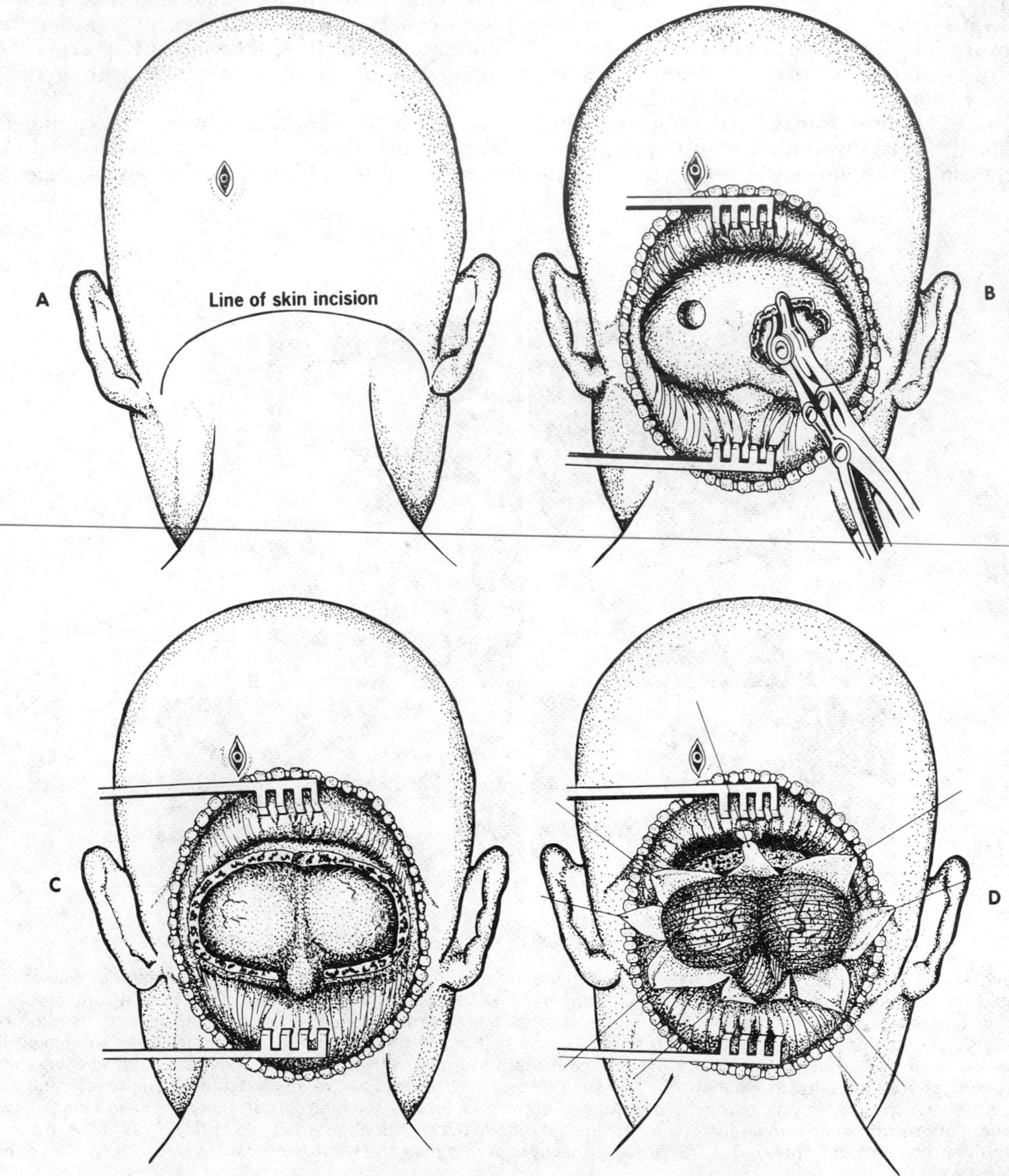

Figure 28–2. Suboccipital craniectomy. **A.** Skin incision; note signs of left ventricular puncture. **B.** Scalp retractors, bone being rongeured around right burr hole. **C.** Dura exposed. **D.** Dura incised and cerebellum exposed. (From Carini, E., and G. Owens: *Neurological and Neurosurgical Nursing*, 6th ed. St. Louis: C. V. Mosby Co., 1974.)

poo may be ordered; during the shampoo, examine the scalp closely. Report any unusual condition, e.g., dermatitis, infection. (Keeping your fingernails short can help avoid scratching the patient's scalp.) Frequently, the patient's scalp is not shaved over the operative area until an anesthetized state has been achieved in the operating room. Usually only a small area of the head is shaved, and hair is left on the patient's head, if possible, to cover the scar during convalescence. Reassure the patient that the hair will grow back in the area shaved. In some hospitals the patient's cut hair is saved; some patient's may wish to have their long hair made into hairpieces. Today the commercial availability of wigs and other hairpieces reduces the depersonalizing effects that patients often experience when their hair is cut for cranial surgery. Generally, the scalp is prepared immediately before surgery so that if it is accidentally cut, the wound will not have time to become infected. If preparation of the patient's head is done on the ward, a clean towel is pinned around the patient's head following the preparation.

7. Have the patient void. For major procedures or if the patient has intracranial hypertension, a Foley retention catheter is usually inserted.

8. Provide a relaxed, restful atmosphere in which the patient feels comfortable in expressing concerns. Direct your help and attention not only to the patient but also to significant others.

9. Evaluate and note:

a. The patient's temperature (rectal), pulse, respirations, blood pressure, level of consciousness, orientation (e.g., concerning person, place, time), awareness of what is happening and ability to follow instructions, mental status generally and mood, pupil size, pupil equality and reaction to light, limb movements, strength in extremities (e.g., grip), skin color and palpable skin temperature (e.g., cool, warm).

b. Any paresis or paralysis, limitations or exaggerations of movements, sensory abnormalities, indications of skin pressure, burns, irritations, abrasions, bruises, hematomas, or edema.

c. Any other abnormal observations, e.g., symptoms of dehydration, chest congestion, seizures, aphasia, visual or auditory disorders. (Report immediately any symptoms of increasing intracranial pressure or respiratory congestion.)

The preceding observations provide a basis for comparison with postoperative findings. It is thus possible to determine if the patient's condition is worsened, improved, or unchanged in these various parameters as a result of surgical intervention.

Special Preoperative Considerations. Preoperatively, and in the early postoperative phase, parenteral corticosteroids may be used to reduce cerebral edema. Mannitol or urea may be administered to help reduce increased intracranial pressure in the operative and early postoperative period.

The patient requiring neurosurgery often has an altered ability to tolerate the conventional *premedications.* As you will recall, the purposes of *preoperative medication* are to allay anxiety, to ready the patient for a smooth induction of anesthesia, and to provide protection from harmful reflexes. Hypoventilation and circulatory depression may cause major problems, particularly in patients with increased intracranial pressure or coma. Therefore, *narcotics* and *hypnotics* are *not* used in these patients. They may also be undesirable in other neurosurgery patients. The nurse should always reconfirm with the neurosurgeon any order for such agents, *prior* to their administration.

Atropine, which reduces tracheobronchial secretions, is commonly used as a preoperative medication. It has the additional effect of reducing the vagal influences on the heart caused by the procedure or the anesthesia. Vagal effects are common with manipulation of the carotid artery and in posterior fossa surgery.

Preoperatively, the lower extremities are placed in *antiembolic stockings.* The *eyes* are protected with a bland ophthalmic ointment and covered. The patient is usually anesthetized before these measures.

Both local and general anesthetics may be used. It is important to remember that all general anesthetics and techniques alter cerebral dynamics. However, general anesthesia does permit much greater control of the patient's vital functions. Local anesthesia, which is used when the patient's response to manipulation of the brain must be assessed, is not without its problems. Problems can include patient discomfort, nausea, vomiting, straining or coughing at the wrong time, and lack of ability to control the airway. Moreover, patients who are unable to cooperate may require excess sedation. Sometimes, for such patients, *neuroleptics* are used in combination with local anesthesia. Neuroleptics are agents that produce a sedate but arousable patient who is emotionally detached.

Operative Care

Various techniques may be used in combination with the anesthesia during surgery. These include *induced hyperventilation, induced hypothermia,* and *induced hypotension.* Hyperventilation is used in an attempt to make the "tight" brain more slack. Unfortunately, it does not always succeed. Hypothermia and induced hypotension are occasionally used for surgery on blood vessels or vascular tumors; both of these techniques are controversial.

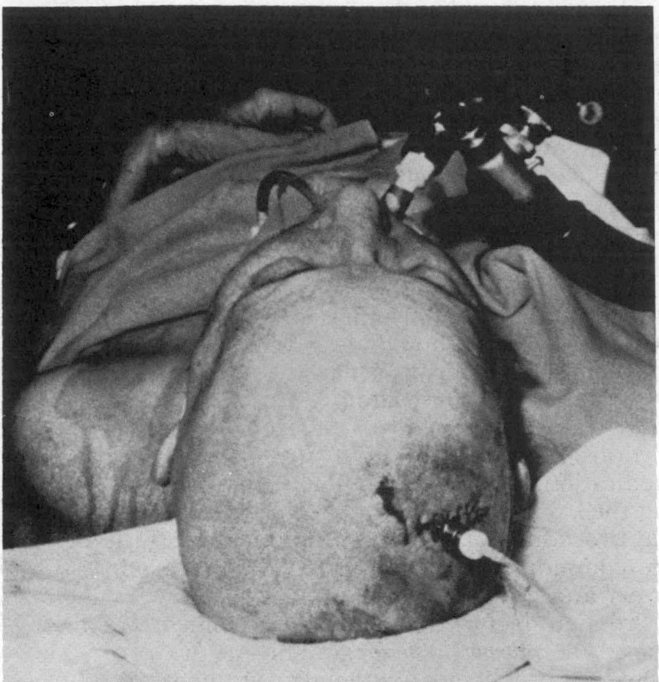

Figure 28–3. A patient with a left temporal lobe glioma, just after induction of anesthesia in the operating room. The hollow screw is connected to saline filled tubing that goes to a strain gauge transducer attached to an IV pole. (From Becker, D. P., et al.: Monitoring in patients with brain tumors. *In* Wilkins, R. H., et al. (Eds.): *Clinical Neurosurgery*. Proceedings of the Congress of Neurological Surgeons, Vancouver, B. C., 1974. Baltimore: Waverly Press, Inc., 1975.)

If any of the above techniques are used, or with most major procedures, *intraoperative monitoring* of various parameters is generally used. The cardiac rate and rhythm are monitored with a cardiac monitor. Arterial blood pressure is monitored using an indwelling arterial line; this also allows easy access for analysis of blood gases. The temperature is monitored continuously, usually in two sites.

> *Monitoring is especially indicated during posterior fossa surgery, when traction or pressure on the brain stem's vital centers may cause cardiac or ventilatory arrest.*

The patient may be *positioned* in a variety of ways during neurosurgery for the various types of surgical procedures. These can include:

- *Supine* — Venous pooling is minimized with antiembolic stockings. Pressure areas may develop if the surgery is prolonged.
- *Lateral* — The shoulders and pelvis must be supported. Excess flexion of the head must also be avoided, to allow adequate drainage from the head.
- *Prone* — This position often interferes with cardiac and respiratory function. The iliac crests and chest must be properly supported. Postoperatively, pressure areas and atelectasis may be early problems.
- *Sitting* — Posterior fossa, middle fossa, and cervical surgery may be done with the patient in this position. Venous drainage and good exposure of the operative areas are the advantages. The patient must be put into the position slowly to avoid hypotension. The legs are generally placed in antiembolic stockings and elevated. Cardiac and/or respiratory embarrassment may occur, as may venous air embolism.

In several of these positions, the head is supported in a special frame. The frame may cause significant pressure on various structures of the head, which may produce edema of the face, pressure sores, and other problems postoperatively. Moreover, improper positioning of the patient in surgery may also cause injury to the peripheral nerves (e.g., peroneal, brachial plexus) and injury to the eyes and eyelids.

Intraoperative complications may include any of the following. The more serious complications will affect the postoperative care of the patient. Complications include:[340]

- Shock or states of poor tissue perfusion
- Blood coagulation deficits, such as diffuse intravascular coagulation (DIC)
- Air embolism
- Cardiac and respiratory embarrassment, including arrest
- Acute brain swelling
- Transfusion reactions

See Chapter 18 for basic discussion about the care of a patient in surgery.

Postoperative Care

Usually after cranial surgery patients are kept in the intensive care unit until their condition is stabilized and they can safely be returned to the general care unit. The principles of care for unconscious patients and patients with intracranial hypertension (discussed in Chapter 26) also apply to care of patients following cranial surgery (see also Chapters 19 and 20). Here we summarize some points of outstanding importance regarding postoperative care of patients who have had cranial surgery:

1. Prevent aspiration and ensure adequate respiratory ventilation. Promptly treat respiratory obstruction or respiratory failure.

2. Appropriately position and turn the patient. Enforce necessary restrictions of activity and position, and encourage allowed activities.

3. Attempt to prevent postoperative complications.

4. Frequently observe and evaluate the patient, watching closely for indications of developing complications, e.g., cerebral swelling, bleeding, CSF leakage.

5. Promptly report indications of developing complications and take necessary emergency actions. (See complications below.)

6. Observe for, evaluate cause of, and provide adequate protective care when restlessness occurs.

7. Observe for and relieve periocular edema (puffing or swelling of the eyelids).

8. Observe for, report, and administer appropriate care for such postoperative residual disorders as paralysis, muscle weakness, corneal anesthesia or other sensory losses, difficulty in swallowing, visual or language disorders, and/or personality disorders. (See discussion of neuro checks pp. 524–531.)

9. Observe for indications of seizure activity. When possible, prevent seizures. Administer appropriate care in the presence of seizures or status epilepticus. (See pp. 554 and 640.)

10. Frequently inspect dressings and reinforce as necessary. Report abnormally tight dressings, abnormal bleeding, or CSF leakage. Maintain sterile technique to prevent wound infection and possible meningitis.

11. Administer medications as ordered, bearing in mind the special precautions of importance following intracranial surgery.

12. Take appropriate action to relieve headache.

13. Prevent straining by the patient, e.g., at restraints, during bowel movements, during coughing. Remember, straining increases intracranial pressure.

14. Provide a quiet, restful environment.

There are several important ***"Do not's"*** that should be remembered when caring for patients following intracranial surgery:

- *Do not* suction the patient's nose without a written order.
- *Do not* lower the patient's head. A head-low position increases intracranial pressure.
- *Do not* restrain the restless patient unless all other measures fail to control restlessness or to provide protection. If restraints seem necessary, try applying protective mittens before using wrist restraints. Follow agency policy concerning restraints.
- *Do not* take the patient's temperature orally.

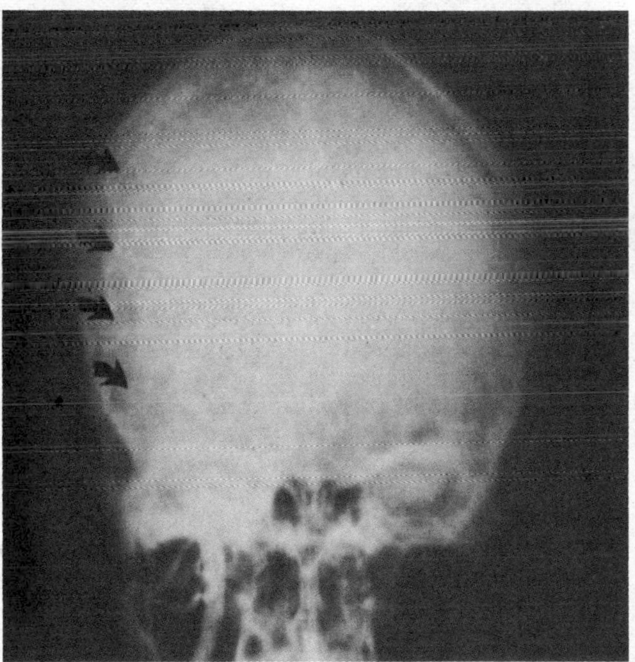

A

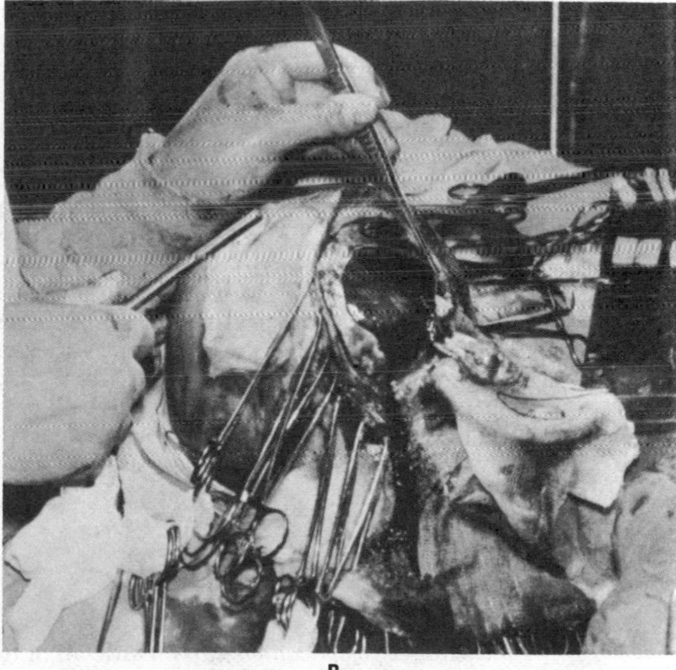

B

Figure 28–4. **A.** Right carotid angiogram, revealing a shift of the anterior cerebral artery from right to left and displacement of arteries from the inner table of the skull, owing to a large subdural hematoma over the right cerebral hemisphere. **B.** View of chronic subdural hematoma at surgery. A right parietal osteoplastic craniotomy is being performed. The dura has been opened, and the thick outer membrane of the subdural hematoma enclosing the chronic blood clot that overlies the brain is shown. The blood clot and the enveloping outer membranes are removed via osteoplastic craniotomy. (From Jackson, F. E., J. V. Back, and R. Pratt III: Current management of acute injuries of the skull and brain. *American Family Physician,* 10:82, Aug. 1974.)

- *Do not* heavily sedate the patient.
- *Do not* administer narcotics unless you have double checked an order to do so.
- *Do not* administer intravenous solutions rapidly.
- *Do not* administer fluids orally until they are ordered, and then do so only after the patient's gag and swallowing reflexes have been tested.
- *Do not* administer cathartics, enemas, and so forth, or attempt to remove impactions unless ordered.

Following surgery, the patient may have an IV running into the arm, an indwelling catheter in the urinary bladder, a Levin tube in the gastrointestinal tract, nasal prongs and/or an endotracheal tube in the throat. Breathing may be assisted by a respirator and body temperature controlled with a hypothermia blanket. Additionally, the patient may have a catheter placed in one of the cerebral ventricles, which is attached to a drainage system and/or intracranial pressure monitoring device.

The care of such a patient is complex and requires skill. Even such maneuvers as turning and positioning the patient who is attached to and probed by so much equipment is difficult. In some settings the patient's temperature, respirations, pulse, and intracranial pressure are monitored continuously and cerebral blood flow is measured. Currently these are not routine practices. However, it is not unusual to have investigations by EEG, ECG, radiography or ultrasound performed at the bedside.

The nursing staff must be prepared for such emergencies as cardiac or respiratory arrest and have appropriate equipment and drugs ready to treat such complications.

In spite of the long duration of many intracranial operations, surgical shock is not a common after-effect. However, these operations are associated with special hazards of their own, which can be prevented only by keen observation. The recognition of these hazards forms the basis of postoperative care following intracranial surgery.

POSTOPERATIVE COMPLICATIONS AND THEIR PREVENTION

Postoperative complications can include all of the usual complications seen after major surgery: *respiratory,* such as atelectasis and pneumonia; *cardiac,* such as rhythm problems, CHF and others; *fluid and electrolyte balance problems; kidney problems* and *gastrointestinal* problems. (See Unit VIII for discussions of caring for the surgical patient.)

Seizures and elevated temperature as well as the problems which started intraoperatively may complicate postoperative recovery in a patient who has undergone neurosurgery. Infection of the wound or brain can occur. A CSF leak may be present, with the possibility of an infection or meningitis developing (see Chapter 27). A CSF leak may be indicated by otorrhea, rhinorrhea, or saturation of the dressing with CSF. Postoperative brain edema, swelling, bleeding (with hematoma formation), and spasm of the blood vessels may significantly disrupt cerebral metabolism and cause the patient to be seriously ill (see Chapter 26).

Other signs of postoperative complications include: increased intracranial pressure; worsening of focal symptoms; lowering of level of consciousness; impaired motor function, e.g., paresis, paralysis (monoplegia, paraplegia); facial weakness or facial paralysis; difficulty in swallowing; loss of gag reflex; corneal anesthesia or other alterations in sensation or reflex action; pain; headache; visual or speech disturbances; changes in personality or behavior patterns; herpes simplex; sordes; parotitis.

Finally, if the patient has had surgery in the *posterior fossa,* the proximity of the surgical site to the vital centers in the brain stem increases the risk of complications. These patients may have in addition to the more common complications:

1. Dysfunction of the ninth, tenth, and eleventh cranial nerves. Examples of functional disabilities can include *loss of airway protection with aspiration, interference with swallowing,* and *cardiac arrhythmias.*
2. The potential aftereffects of air embolism.
3. The site of the incision makes it more vulnerable to tension from intracranial structures. If closure of the wound has been difficult, the wound is more vulnerable to losing its integrity. If this is anticipated to be a problem, a compression dressing is applied and the movement of the patient's neck restricted. The patient should be positioned in such a way as to avoid tension on the suture line.

Let us now discuss the major aspects of neurosurgical postoperative care and complication prevention in more detail.

Observation and Evaluation. In caring for a patient after intracranial surgery, the nurse makes frequent neurologic observations, measurements of vital signs, and evaluations of the patient's status. Periodically assessments are compared with the preoperative parameters and evaluations. If the patient is stuporous or unconscious, the nurse tests for reaction to stimuli, e.g., insertion of the rectal thermometer, mildly painful stimuli, and the patient's reflex status. These findings are compared with those recorded preoperatively. The frequency with which observations are made varies with a patient's condition and the doctor's preferences and may range from every 5 minutes to every 2 hours during the first few hours following surgery.

Airway Care. Prevention of respiratory obstruction requires special attention following intracranial surgery since the lesion itself or the operative interference may cause paralysis of swallowing muscles and the risk of inhalation of vomitus and secretions. An unconscious person with a lesion in the brain tends to have excessive secretions in the respiratory tract and cannot adequately expel them by coughing. Such a patient must be carefully positioned to promote secretion drainage. The lateral position will help keep the tongue from falling back and obstructing the oral pharynx if the patient is not intubated.

Oxygen therapy may be indicated. It can be administered through the endotracheal tube or by nasal prongs or mask. If ventilatory efforts are poor, a mechanical respirator is used. *Vigorous coughing and suctioning are dangerous following intracranial surgery because they increase intracranial pressure*. Thus, suctioning is carefully performed and the conscious patient is instructed to deep breathe periodically to clear the lungs, but not to cough strenuously. *Since even mild hypoxia increases swelling of the brain; every attempt is made to prevent hypoxia*.

Position, Turning, Activity. Sometimes in intracranial procedures bone flaps are left out postoperatively to allow expansion of inoperable tumors and/or to reduce pressure from postoperative swelling. The bone may be saved and later replaced, or cranioplasty may be performed at a later date.

There are some general guidelines to follow in *positioning patients following intracranial surgical procedures*:

- *Following infratentorial surgery* it may be necessary to keep the patient positioned *flat* on *either side* with *head properly aligned* with the spinal column, e.g., a small pillow may be necessary under the head. Keep the patient off the back for the first 24 to 48 hours; after this period of time, the physician may order the head of the bed gradually elevated over a period of several days.

- Usually *following supratentorial surgery* the patient is positioned on the side or back if intubated with the head elevated 20 degrees (unless in shock). This position is maintained in an attempt to: (1) reduce cerebral swelling; (2) minimize the possibility of hemorrhage; and (3) improve CSF circulation.

Following intracranial surgery, *do not lower the patient's head* without a written order from the neurosurgeon, since the head-low position increases the brain's blood supply and may precipitate venous bleeding. A patient in shock may be ordered to be placed flat with the extremities elevated.

As with any patient in bed, frequent *turning* (at least every 2 hours) is important following intracranial surgery, to prevent the complications of immobility. The patient who has had infratentorial surgery should be *positioned* and turned in such a manner that the head is kept properly aligned with the body at all times. In turning the patient, one nurse supports the patient's head, preventing twisting of the neck; the patient is positioned in such a manner (on the side) that the nose is in line with the breastbone.

Instruct the postoperative patient concerning any limitations of activity and position. Explain to the patient how you will help him or her move, change position, and so forth. Place a sign on the head of the bed clearly stating any restrictions regarding position. Discuss these limitations with significant others if they visit.

Usually the patient who has had intracranial surgery is kept quiet and is given total care for the first 48 hours after surgery. In some hospitals this care is given in an intensive care unit. If in bed on the ward, the patient may be positioned with head at the foot of the bed to facilitate observation, support, and positioning of the head. A turning sheet is placed on the postoperative bed; put the sheet on the bed so that it will extend well above the patient's head.

On the third postoperative day, if complications are not present, the patient is often allowed to assume some self-care. Occasionally a patient may be allowed up in a bedside chair on the day of surgery if the nature of the surgery and the patient's condition permit. Typically, following infratentorial surgery patients may not be allowed up until the tenth postoperative day; following supratentorial surgery the patient is allowed up in a chair on the third to fifth postoperative day.

Intracranial Pressure, Cerebral Swelling, Intracranial Bleeding

> *Varying degrees of cerebral swelling occur following intracranial surgery, and occasionally bleeding may also occur. Both these factors may cause increased intracranial pressure.*

The nurse observes for symptoms of increasing intracranial pressure and attempts to control postoperative swelling by following the physician's orders. The usual measures to treat elevated intracranial pressure are undertaken. Tapping of one of the ventricles (when they are large) may be done.

Continuous *ventricular catheter drainage* attached to a sterile reservoir maintained at a level that roughly equals normal CSF pressure may also be used. When *continuous ventricular drainage* is employed to drain off excess spinal fluid, the nurse takes care to: (1) prevent traction on the tubing which could displace the catheter in the

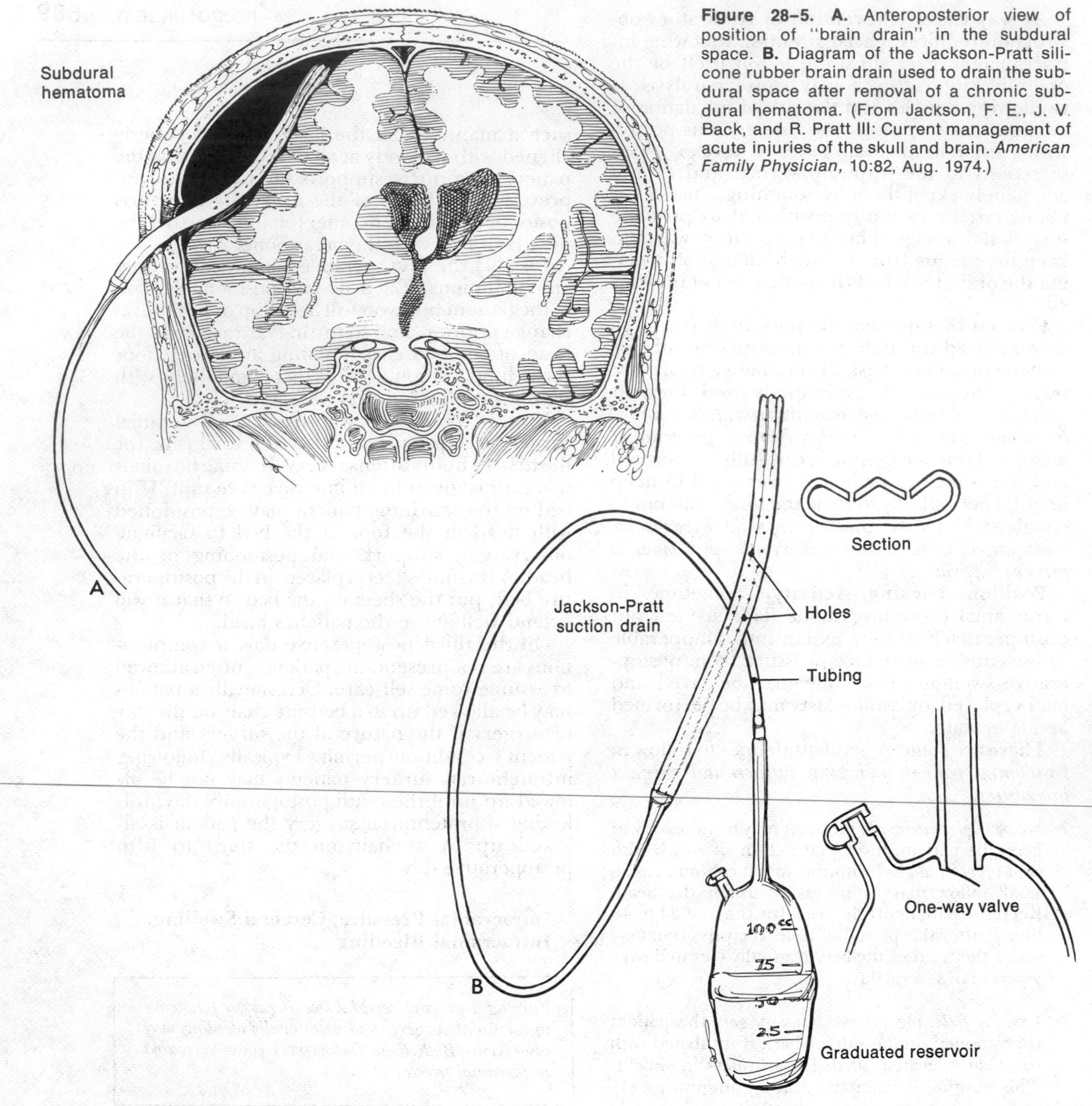

Figure 28–5. **A.** Anteroposterior view of position of "brain drain" in the subdural space. **B.** Diagram of the Jackson-Pratt silicone rubber brain drain used to drain the subdural space after removal of a chronic subdural hematoma. (From Jackson, F. E., J. V. Back, and R. Pratt III: Current management of acute injuries of the skull and brain. *American Family Physician*, 10:82, Aug. 1974.)

ventricle; (2) prevent kinks in the tubing, which could obstruct free flow of CSF; (3) keep the patient's head and drainage receptable at proper heights to maintain approximately normal CSF pressure; (4) keep the tubing and collecting bottle sterile to prevent introduction of pathogens into the brain; and (5) notify the physician if the drainage appears to stop or is excessive, so that the patient's condition can be reevaluated. Generally the doctor removes the catheter after 24 to 48 hours.

Dressing. Frequently observe the dressing. Report at once indications of hemorrhage, excessive CSF leakage, and tightness of the dressing. Clear or yellow drainage may indicate loss of CSF.

Reinforce dressings as necessary with *sterile* dressings to prevent the absorption of pathogens through the dressing to the wound by capillary action. Meningitis can result from wound infection following cranial surgery.

Sometimes a *drain* is left in place for 24 to 48 hours; if so, reinforce the dressing as necessary and cover the reinforcement with a sterile towel. Change the towel every half hour and hold it in place with tape. Observe a restless patient carefully to be sure the patient does not disturb dressings or contaminate the wound, e.g., by stretching.

The frequency with which the physician removes and changes dressings varies. Fluid may be seen to collect under the scalp, and the physician may aspirate it when the dressing is changed.

After the dressings have been removed, following suture removal, it may be noticed that the scalp has become encrusted and may have some dried blood on it. Hydrogen peroxide is used to remove the dried blood. The crusts may be softened and then removed by: (1) oiling the scalp with olive oil or mineral oil or coating it with yellow petroleum jelly; (2) covering the oiled or greased scalp overnight with a soft towel; and (3) gently washing the area the next morning with soap and water. When cleaning the scalp, rub lightly; do *not* rub over the operated area. Make the rubbing motions *toward* the suture line (do not place stress on the suture line in rubbing the scalp). After the dressings are removed, inspect the wound at least twice daily, looking for bulging (indicative of increasing intracranial pressure or fluid accumulation) or signs of injury to the wound.

While the wound is healing the patient may wear a protective stockinette cap or scarf. Warn the patient to take care not to scratch or bump her or his head. This is particularly important if a portion of the brain is unprotected because bone was removed at the time of surgery and not replaced.

Hyperthermia, Hypothermia. Surgery in the region of the hypothalamus may disturb the nerve cells responsible for temperature control. As a result, the patient's body temperature may either drop or increase until death. If temperature disturbances seem to be developing, the patient's temperature is taken frequently or monitored continuously to assess the problem and permit institution of proper treatment.

Hyperthermia may result not only from damage to the heat controlling mechanisms of the hypothalamus and brain stem, but also from excessive dehydration, thrombophlebitis, or local or general infection. Hyperpyrexia may last for 48 hours postoperatively owing to the presence of blood in the cranium.

Seizures. Patients with intracranial lesions and particularly head-injured patients, including the head injury caused by intracranial surgery, may develop epilepsy. These persons may have only a single seizure, or they may have many and even progress to the serious condition of status epilepticus. Because seizures increase cerebral metabolic demands, the physician frequently attempts to prevent their initial occurrence by prophylactically administering such medications as phenyltoin.

Restlessness. Restlessness, ranging from moderate restlessness to wild thrashing about, is generally most acute the second or third postoperative day when the patient's general condition has improved enough to move about, but mental confusion may still persist. Evaluation of restlessness and care of the restless patient have been previously discussed. Following cranial surgery, restlessness may last for several days. *The administration of barbiturates may make a patient even less manageable.* Paraldehyde is possibly the most sat-

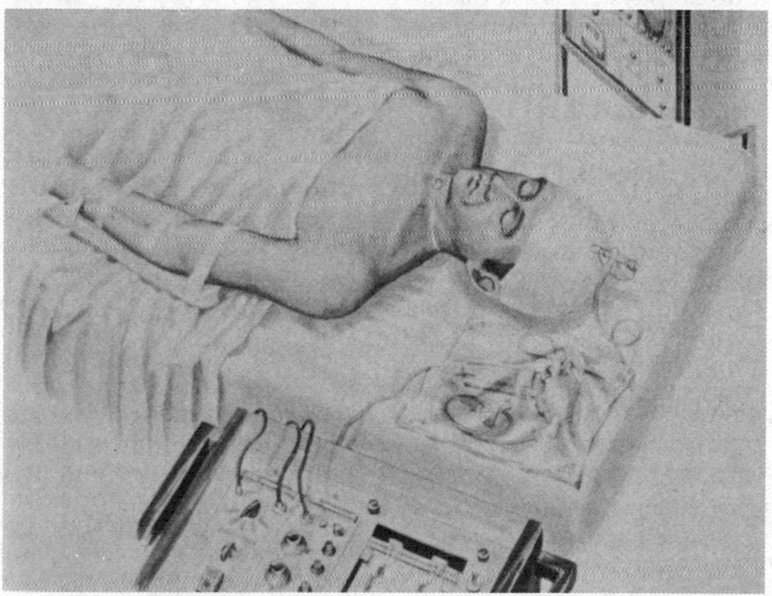

Figure 28–6. Continuous intracranial pressure monitoring. (From Pizzi, F. J., et al.: A protocol for the management of head trauma. *American Family Physician,* 10:163, Nov. 1974.)

isfactory sedative. Tranquilizers, e.g., chlorpromazine, may be ordered.

Headache. Severe headache may occur for 24 to 48 hours postoperatively. The patient may be given an ice bag to the head p.r.n. Do not jar the patient's bed or cause sudden movements. Keep the environment quiet, calm, and dimly lit. Administer appropriate medications as indicated for pain relief. Medications that may be ordered include aspirin, acetaminophen, or codeine.

> Remember:
> *Barbiturates and narcotics are generally contraindicated because of possible medullary (and hence respiratory) depression and masking of symptoms of increasing intracranial pressure.*

Bowel, Urinary Bladder. Periodically check the patient for distention of the bowel and urinary bladder (if a catheter is not in place). Often a dehydrated postoperative patient can go as long as 12 hours following intracranial surgery without voiding. The patient may or may not be catheterized, depending upon the doctor's judgment. *Metabolic disorders of CNS origin can cause an abnormal increase or decrease in urinary output.* An intake and output record is kept on all patients. The specific gravity of the urine may need to be measured periodically.

Never administer a cathartic or enema following intracranial surgery without a written order from the doctor. Straining at stool may dangerously increase intracranial pressure. Some physicians ask the patient not to try to have a bowel movement for several days. Patients often receive stool softeners. If these are not adequate, a suppository or small enema may be ordered. Report impactions to the physician for removal. The patient who was able to have adequate preoperative bowel preparation is less likely to have problems during the postoperative period. However, in some instances it is not possible to cleanse the colon prior to surgery.

Fluids, Food. Many physicians today believe it is unnecessary to restrict fluids postoperatively in an attempt to offset cerebral swelling. However, some physicians still limit fluid intake to 1500 ml. for several days.

> *Do not administer intravenous fluids rapidly following intracranial surgery; this could cause a dangerous increase in intracranial pressure or it could cause pulmonary edema.*

Following supratentorial surgery, in contrast to abdominal operations, there is no contraindication to giving fluids orally and food by mouth as soon as the patient is alert and can swallow. In such cases fluids may be ordered orally on the day of surgery. If vomiting is present, e.g., from increased intracranial pressure, oral intake may be temporarily discontinued since the strain of vomiting could cause intracranial bleeding.

Following infratentorial surgery a patient may be kept NPO for 24 hours because of impaired swallowing and gag reflexes. After 24 hours the physician may test these reflexes, and if they appear to be functioning, water may be given (with suctioning equipment at hand), followed later by other fluids. Withhold all oral feedings if any symptoms of difficulty in swallowing appear. Tube feedings may be necessary if there is paralysis of the muscles that govern swallowing. When necessary, tube feedings are usually started 48 hours postoperatively. The physician inserts the tube if there is a possibility that tube insertion may endanger the patient.

Once patients are alert, able to swallow, and have oral feedings ordered, they are usually fed by a worker during the first 48 hours, to insure adequate intake while preventing unnecessary movements and exertion.

Metabolic Disturbances. Following intracranial surgery, metabolic disturbances of various types may occur as a result of surgical trauma. These disturbances may potentially lead to coma. They must rapidly be identified, and the imbalance corrected.

Ecchymosis, Periocular Edema. Following surgery, ecchymosis and edema, e.g., periocular edema, may distort the patient's features. Significant others should be told about the patient's appearance before they are allowed to visit for the first time postoperatively. Additionally, if any noticeable defects have been detected postoperatively, e.g., facial paralysis, or aphasia, visitors should be prepared for these.

Relieve periocular edema by applying a light coating of petroleum jelly around the patient's eyes and on the eyelids, and then periodically applying light cold compresses (of crushed ice in Pliofilm taped over the affected eye).

Complications of Bed Rest. The nurse works to prevent all the complications of bed rest for the patient who is immobilized after intracranial surgery. Check with the physician concerning when to begin passive exercises and whether you can ask the patient to cough routinely. (See Sorensen and Luckmann, *Basic Nursing: A Psychophysiologic Approach*, for detailed discussion of dangers of bed rest.)

Emotional Support. Provide emotional support to the patient and significant others during the postoperative period. Support and understanding are particularly important if postoperative problems occur (e.g., paralysis, skull defects, associated complications) or if the surgery appears unsuccessful. If a defect remains in the skull owing to removal of bone, the physician should discuss with the patient plans for cranioplasty (to protect the area and improve appearance) before the patient sees the defect.

Convalescence. During convalescence the patient may have to adapt to various residual disorders. Some may be temporary (e.g., double vision), whereas others may be permanent (e.g., paralysis, aphasia). The patient's concern about double vision may be relieved by alternately covering one eye each day with an opaque eye shield. The management of many other defects and complications has been discussed previously in this unit. Eventually plans may be carried out for restyling the patient's hair and, if desired, obtaining a wig or hairpiece.

As you can imagine, considerable changes in body image can occur postoperatively. People need supportive and empathetic understanding as they attempt to reintegrate their perceptions and appreciation of themselves. This may take time. The person's own wishes and desires must be taken into consideration when any cosmetic advice is given.

SPINAL SURGERY

Laminectomy and spinal fusion have been discussed previously, in the section on herniated vertebral disk (Chapter 27). Here we discuss the pre- and postoperative care of patients undergoing these operations. Generally, postoperative restrictions are fewer following laminectomy than following spinal fusion.

Spinal fusion may be done by the anterior or posterior approach. The anterior approach is usually used only in cervical spine fusions, but may be used in thoracic and lumbar fusions when unusual circumstances make a posterior approach impossible.

Anterior fusion is performed by reaching the lumbar spine through the abdomen, or by removal of midline disks and bony spurs in the cervical spine through an anterior approach to the spinal canal in such a manner that the vertebral bodies are exposed through the anterior aspect of the neck. *Posterior fusion* is performed by reaching the spine directly through an incision in the patient's back, e.g., back of the neck or back of the lumbar spine.

> *Postoperative care and positioning vary, depending upon whether the spinal fusion was anterior or posterior. It is helpful to remember that the goal of care is to prevent strain or flexion at the surgical site.*

Since *posterior lumbar fusions* are the most common type of spinal fusion, our discussion focuses mainly on the care of patients who have undergone that procedure.

Preoperative Care

Patients are prepared for spinal surgery as ordered. (The routine preparation of a patient for surgery has been discussed in Unit VIII.) Summarized below are points that pertain specifically to preoperative preparation for spinal surgery.

- Show the patient the log rolling manner of turning that will be used postoperatively. Teach muscle conditioning exercises that may be ordered postoperatively. If her or his physical condition permits, have the patient practice turning and practice the exercises with your help and guidance. Familiarize the patient with the Stryker frame or any other special equipment that may be used postoperatively. Instruct the patient about necessary postoperative limitations of activity, and point out self-help measures, e.g., periodic deep breathing. Teach the patient how to roll onto a bedpan (rather than lifting the hips); encourage practice of this with your help. Also, teach the patient the technique to be used for getting out of bed when this is allowed postoperatively. (Various techniques may be used; the nurse must be familiar with the preferences of the particular surgeon involved.)

  Explain that the patient will be turned frequently after surgery according to the doctor's instructions, and that turning in the correct manner will not be harmful but will actually help.

  Explain to the patient that reaching for things (e.g., telephone, water, urinal) can cause a strain the first few days after surgery. Instruct the patient to ask for items to be handed to him or her instead.

- Allow the patient to express concerns and fears about the surgery. Many patients dread spinal surgery because they fear paralysis postoperatively; if the patient does not mention this fear, do not suggest it, you may possibly add new worries. Allay anxieties whenever possible and encourage patient and significant others to express their concerns.

Postoperative Care

Following spinal surgery, postoperative care is directed at preventing complications, preventing further spinal injury, and providing an opportunity for the wound (and graft if present) to heal. It is of critical importance to *be certain the patient's spine is in a position of correct alignment at all times and that the bed is flat.* Postoperative orders vary with the surgery performed and the physician's preferences. Some physicians allow greater activity than others. Check postoperative orders carefully concerning the amount of activity the pa-

VARIOUS NEURO-SURGICAL PROCEDURES

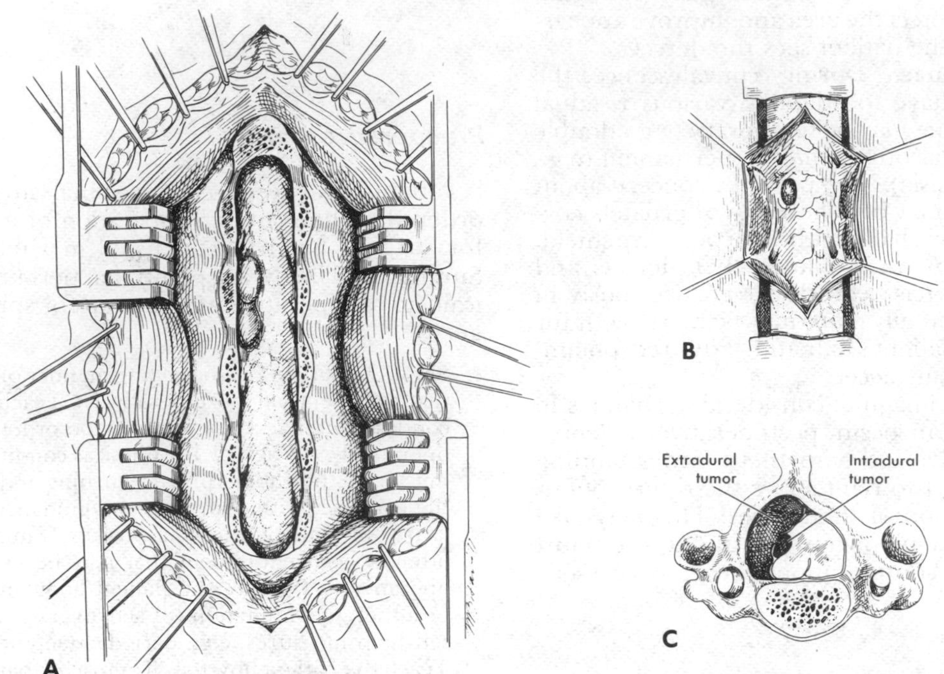

A. Laminectomy completed: dura mater and tumor exposed. **B.** Dura mater incised and retracted, revealing pia arachnoidea membrane over the spinal cord and part of tumor. **C.** Diagram showing a cross section of the tumor site and the location of the extradural and intradural pathology. (From Conway, B. L.: *Carini and Owens' Neurological and Neurosurgical Nursing*, 7th ed. St. Louis: C. V. Mosby Co., 1978.)

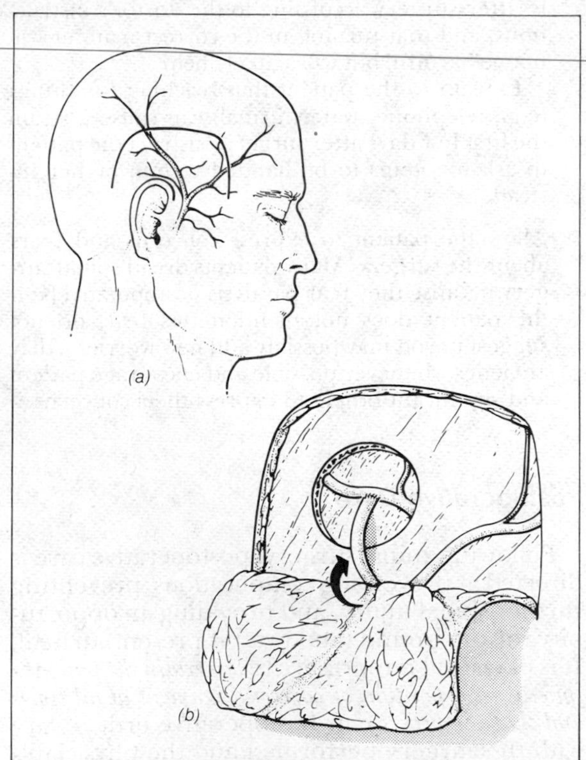

Cerebral artery bypass (From Bander, M. S. (Ed.): *MGH News,* 35:3, Massachusetts General Hospital, Boston. June–Aug. 1976. Used with permission.)

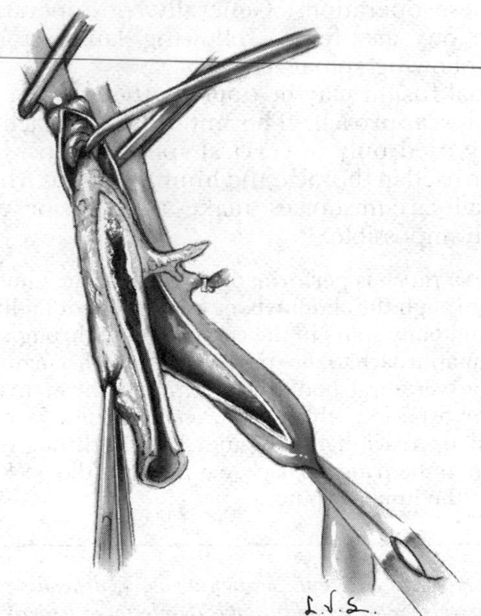

Diagram of a carotid endarterectomy. (From Sabiston, D. C., Jr., (Ed.): *Davis Christopher Textbook of Surgery,* 11th ed. Philadelphia: W. B. Saunders Co., 1977, p. 1690.)

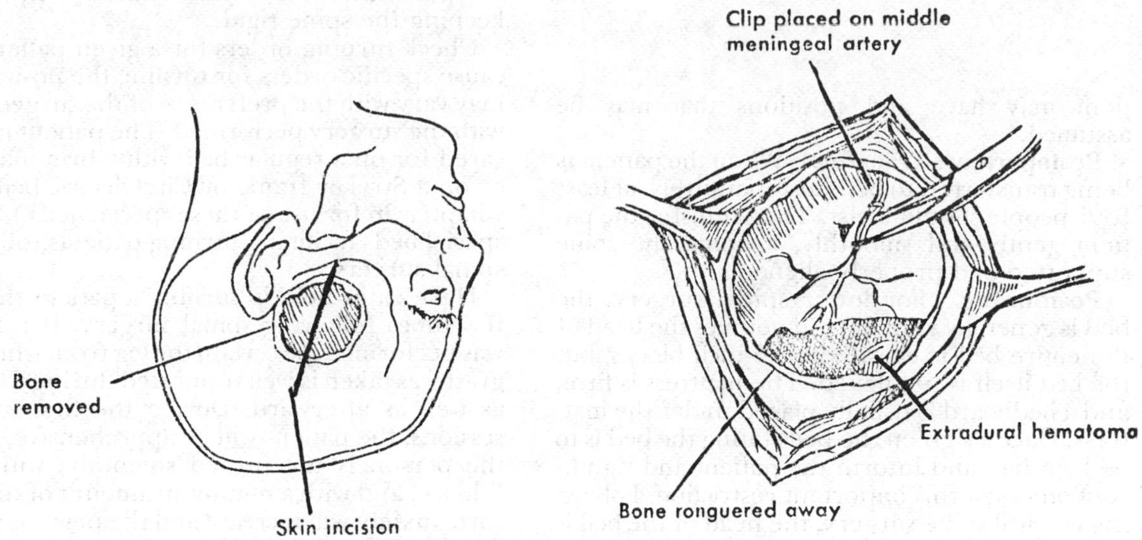

Extradural hemorrhage. (From Richards, V.: *Surgery for General Practice.* St. Louis: C. V. Mosby Co.)

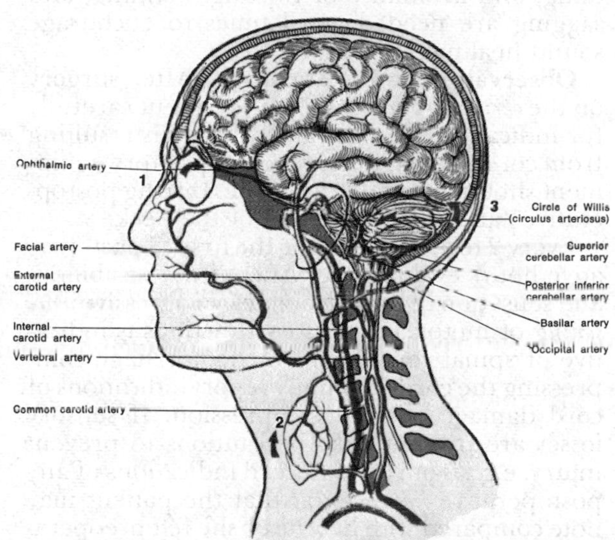

Some potential extracranial-to-intracranial and extracranial-to-extracranial arterial shunts (1) A shunt from the external carotid, via the facial artery, to the ophthalmic artery to the circle of Willis (retrograde flow) may compensate for sternal occlusion. (2) A shunt through the thyroid circulation can compensate for common carotid occlusion. (3) A shunt from the posterior inferior cerebellar artery to the superior cerebellar artery (retrograde flow) to the distal basilar artery can compensate for intracranial vertebral artery occlusion. (From Fincham, R. W., and Davenport, S. S.: Occlusive cerebrovascular disease. *American Family Physician,* 7:68, April 1973.)

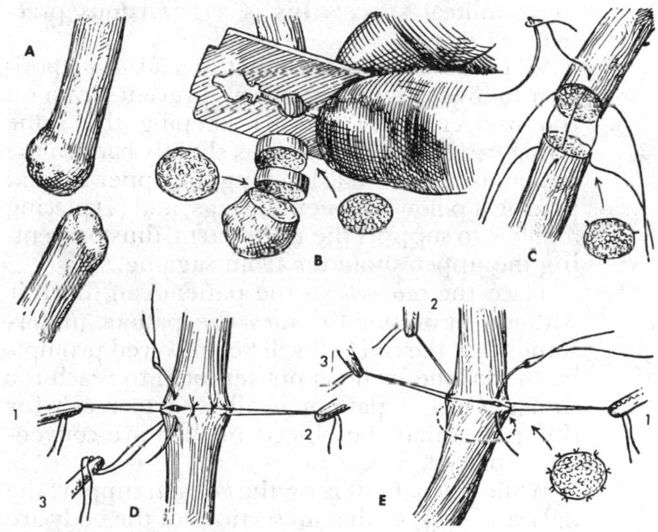

Nerve repair. **A.** Divided nerve with neuroma. **B.** Serial resection of neuroma to healthy nerve fibers. **C.** Placement of sutures in epineurium. **D** and **E.** Approximation and tying of sutures. (From Sachs, E.: *Diagnosis and Treatment of Brain Tumors and Care of the Neurosurgical Patient,* 2nd ed. St. Louis: C. V. Mosby Co.)

tient may have and positions that may be assumed.

Postoperative Transfer. When the patient is being transferred to bed postoperatively, at least four people should assist. They transfer the patient gently and smoothly, keeping the spine supported and properly aligned.

Positioning. For lower spinal surgery, the bed is generally kept flat. Sometimes the head of the entire bed is elevated on 6-inch blocks, but the bed itself is not flexed. The mattress is firm, and a bedboard is usually placed under the mattress. Place a sign on the bed stating the bed is to be kept flat, and inform the patient and significant others of this important restriction. Following cervical spine surgery, the head of the bed is often allowed to be elevated slightly for comfort.

When the patient is positioned on the *back*, the lower back muscles may be relaxed somewhat if pillows are placed under the *entire length* of the patient's legs. This may also reduce the possibility of thrombophlebitis in the femoral vessels. Take care, however, that you *do not* flex the patient's knees by placing a folded pillow under the popliteal space; this is a hazardous practice.

When positioning a patient in a *side-lying* position following spinal surgery, prevent strain on the back muscles by: (1) keeping the spine straight; (2) pulling the hips slightly back so the patient is balanced; (3) flexing the upper leg and placing a pillow between the legs; and (4) placing a pillow to support the upper arm, thus preventing the upper shoulder from sagging.

Place the *call bell* so the patient can touch it without straining. Be sure the patient understands that the call bell will be answered promptly, so that she or he is not tempted to reach for things. Once a patient is allowed to reach for things, see that the objects needed are conveniently placed.

While the patient is on the *bedpan*, support the back and legs, so that all sections of the body are on the same plane. Use a fracture bedpan or a small child's bedpan. *Stimulate circulation* in the patient's back, head, and neck following spinal surgery. Give frequent, gentle back rubs that include the scalp, neck, and thighs. Avoid the area of surgery when rubbing. When permitted, it is desirable to reestablish circulation in the dependent areas of the back and thighs by having the patient lie prone periodically.[191] Explaining the importance of the prone position helps the patient to tolerate it better.

Turning. Be sure the patient's bed has a turning sheet placed on it postoperatively. When turning the patient to the side, use a logrolling maneuver (see Fig. 28–7). Avoid twisting the patient's spine or twisting at the hips. Eventually the patient is able to turn without help, while keeping the spine rigid.

Check turning orders for a given patient, because specific orders for turning the positioning may vary with the preference of the surgeon and with the surgery performed. The patient may be cared for on a regular bed with a firm mattress, or on a Stryker frame or CircOlectric bed. (See Chapter 26 for use of these special beds.) Use of special beds facilitates turning patients following spinal surgery.

Have extra help in turning a patient the first few times following spinal surgery. If a fusion was performed, be certain the leg from which the graft was taken is well supported during the turn as well as afterward. During the first turning sessions, the patient will be apprehensive, and if the person is not turned smoothly, with confidence, and with a minimum amount of discomfort, anxiety will increase and the person may be fearful of future turning sessions.

It is equally important to keep up vigilance and continue to practice *careful turning* with adequate help even after several weeks have passed and the patient is able to help in the turning process. Particular care is needed during the fourth and fifth postoperative weeks. Spinal bone grafts are delicate and heal slowly. Gentleness, proper handling, and avoidance of twisting, bending, and sagging are needed at all times to encourage sound healing.

Observation and Evaluation. After surgery on the *cervical spine*, observe the patient carefully for indications of respiratory paralysis resulting from cord edema. Emergency respiratory equipment should be readily available. During postoperative care, prevent flexion of the neck.

Every 2 to 4 hours during the first 48 postoperative hours evaluate the patient's motor abilities and sensation in the extremities. Progressive *worsening* of motor and sensory functions is indicative of spinal cord edema or hemorrhage compressing the cord. Promptly report indications of cord damage or cord compression, If sensory losses are present, take precautions to prevent injury, e.g., from heat. Record indications of any postoperative *improvement* that the patient may note compared with how he or she felt preoperatively, e.g., "The tingling I had in my leg is gone."

Dressing. Skin incisions for laminectomies and posterior spinal fusions are made directly over the spinous processes. Observe the wound or dressing for indications of hemorrhage or CSF leakage; if present, notify the surgeon. Reinforce the dressing as necessary with *sterile* compresses. If the dressing becomes contaminated, e.g., with urine from the bedpan, it must be changed. Most physicians wish to do the first dressing change themselves. As with any wound, observe the surgical wound for indications of infection. When spinal fusion has been performed, be certain to also inspect the dressing at the site from which the bone graft was taken.

Pain, Muscle Spasms. Compression of various structures by edema may cause pain for some time postoperatively. Spasms may occur in the back and thigh muscles as a result of irritation of nerves during surgery. The area from which bone was taken for a spinal fusion may also be quite painful for several days. Provide pain relief as indicated and take appropriate nursing actions to prevent or minimize pain. (See Unit XI.) Keeping the operative leg and the spine correctly and comfortably positioned helps to reduce pain and muscle spasms.

Complications of Bed Rest. Prevent the complications that can develop from prolonged immobility. Don't forget to place a footboard on the patient's bed and to correctly position the patient against it.

Food, Fluids. Usually fluids are encouraged as soon as nausea subsides, and diet is increased as tolerated following spinal surgery.

Urinary Bladder, Bowels. Check the patient every 2 to 4 hours postoperatively for bladder or bowel distention. Bladder and bowel dysfunction may occur for several days postoperatively. Force fluids as ordered, encourage a regular time for bowel movements and bowel care, provide roughage in the diet (when allowed), and administer medications and enemas as orderd, e.g., mild bulk laxative, Dulcolax suppository. Inactivity often causes problems with bowel elimination. Instruct the patient not to strain at bowel movement. Straining increases pain and also increases CSF pressure.

Activity. Surgeons have individual preferences about activity orders for their patients. A nurse must be familiar with the specific orders and restrictions for each patient before beginning *any* activity. Check with the physician about which active and passive exercises are allowed. (Some are contraindicated because of the strain they place on the back, e.g., straight leg raising while lying flat in bed.) Supervise new activities as

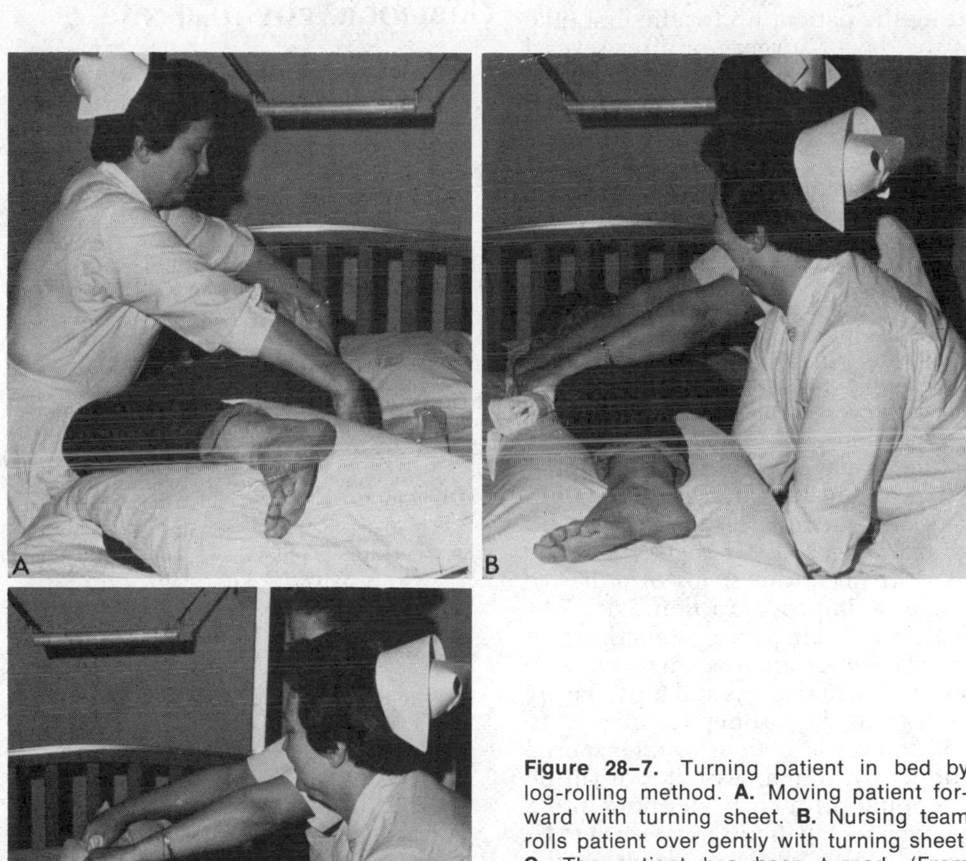

Figure 28–7. Turning patient in bed by log-rolling method. **A.** Moving patient forward with turning sheet. **B.** Nursing team rolls patient over gently with turning sheet. **C.** The patient has been turned. (From Musick, D. T., and M. MacKenzie: *Nursing Clinics of North America, 2*:437, Sept. 1967.)

they are ordered. Provide teaching as needed about exercises, proper lifting, limitations of activities (avoid straight leg raising, avoid bending at the waist). Teach the patient how to move correctly, how to hold the spine straight, and how to prevent reinjury to the spine.

Following spinal surgery, many surgeons will not allow their patients to sit for a period of 4 to 6 weeks, especially after lumbar spine surgery. The patients may only lie, stand, or walk. However, if sitting is allowed, teach the patient to select a staight, firm chair and to keep both feet flat on the floor — not on a footstool and not with the legs crossed. Teach the patient to keep her or his back straight in sitting down on a chair or standing up. Be certain the chair is held firmly; placing the chair against a wall is a good way to prevent it from slipping away as the patient sits down or gets up.

When getting the patient up for the first time (whether on the day of surgery or after several weeks of bed rest), be sure to use the technique specified by the surgeon and be certain that you and the other workers can support the patient if he or she should faint. Watch the patient for signs of dizziness, weakness, or fainting. Postural hypotension may be a problem, since the patient's bed cannot be elevated gradually because of the danger of flexing the spine. If the patient collapses, the workers providing help must be able to continue support, *maintaing proper spinal alignment* while returning the patient o bed. If there is *any* question about your ability to support the patient — to prevent a fall and reinjury to the spine — *get more help*.

Have the patient wear stockings and firm walking shoes when ambulating, not slippers. Slippers do not provide adequate support, tend to slip off, and are dangerous. If the soles of the patient's shoes are slick, put strips of adhesive tape across them to improve traction.

Teach the patient that in picking something up from the floor, it is important to squat down, with the back held straight and knees and hips sharply flexed. Demonstrate the proper techniques to the patient. Caution the patient to take special care not to suddently stretch, twist, flex or jar the back (as in stepping off a curb, stepping into a hole, or stubbing a toe). Patients must learn to be alert as they walk, keeping close watch on the terrain. Climbing stairs, lifting any weight greater than 5 pounds, and driving a car may be prohibited for a time, to prevent strain on the back. Instruct the patient not to do these things without checking first with the physician.

Braces, Body Casts. Following spinal surgery a patient may wear a body cast, brace, or corset. Initially back braces or corsets may be worn all the time whether the patient is in bed or out. Evenutally the person is allowed to be up for short periods without them. (Braces are discussed further in Unit XX.)

Sometimes body casts are applied following spinal fusion. Such casts are usually worn 6 to 8 weeks. After cast removal, the patient is fitted with a back brace, which is worn for an additional 3 to 6 months. Activities allowed for patients in body casts vary. Some patients are allowed up in the cast, whereas others are confined to bed. (Cast care is discussed in Unit XX.)

Patients who must be inactive for long periods following spinal surgery often become bored and restless during their convalescence. It is a challenge to the nurse's imagination to keep them occupied in an interesting manner. Occupational therapy, radio, television, reading material, and the company of others helps the time to pass. Such patients do best in a ward setting where they can visit with other patients and where they can be distracted by the various activities of ward living.

BIBLIOGRAPHY (Unit X)

1. Abramsky, O., and Y. Litvin: Autoimmune responses to dopamine-receptor as a possible mechanism in the pathogenesis of Parkinson's disease and schizophrenia. *Perspectives in Biology and Medicine,* 22:104, Autumn 1978.
2. Adams, N.R.: Prolonged coma: Your care makes all the difference. *Nursing 77*, 7:20, Aug. 1977.
3. Adams, R.D., and M. Victor: *Principles of Neurology.* New York: McGraw-Hill Book Co., 1977.
4. Aidinis, S.J., et al.: Intracranial responses to PEEP, *Anesthesiology,* 45:275, 1976.
5. Alter, M., and B.S. Rosenberg: Are all degenerative neurologic diseases slow virus infections? *Geriatrics,* 32:77, Nov. 1977.
6. Andriola, M.J.: When an elderly patient complains of weakness . . .. *Geriatrics,* 33:79, June 1978.
7. Andriola, M.R.: Role of the EEG in evaluating central nervous system dysfunction. *Geriatrics,* 33:59, Feb. 1978.
8. Apfelbach, H.W., et al.: Chemonucleolysis in the treatment of low back pain and sciatica. *Surgical Clinics of North America,* 55:181, 1975.
9. Appel, S.H.: The muscular dystrophies. *Postgraduate Medicine,* 64.93, Aug. 1978.
10. Arangio, A.J.: An assessment model: A systematic examination of the psychosocial needs of patients with epilepsy. *Patient Counseling and Health Education.* 1:75, Fall 1978.
11. Bailey, J.: Head trauma: A matter of life or death. *RN,* 42:44, May 1979.
12. Basmajian, J.V., E.M. Regenos, and M.P. Baker: Rehabilitating stroke patients with biofeedback. *Geriatrics* 32:85, July 1977.
13. Bates, B.: *A Guide to Physical Examination.* Philadelphia: J.B. Lippincott Co., 1974.
14. Baxter, R.T., and A. Linn: Sex counseling and the SCI patient. *Nursing 78*, 8:46, Sept. 1978.
15. Becker, D.P., et al.: Severe head injury with early diagnosis and intensive management. *Journal of Neurology,* 47:491, 1977.
16. Beks, J.W.F., D.A. Bosch, and M. Brock: *Intracranial Pressure III.* Berlin: Springer-Verlag, 1976.

17. Belt, L.H.: Working with dysphasic patients. *American Journal of Nursing,* 74:1320, July 1974.
18. Bercaw, B.L.: When loss of consciousness is not caused by epilepsy. *Geriatrics,* 31:95, July 1976.
19. Bergentz, S.E.: On bleeding and clotting problems in post-traumatic states. *Critical Care Medicine,* Vol. 4, 2:41, Mar.-Apr. 1976.
20. Berkman, A.H., et al.: Sexual adjustment of spinal cord injured veterans living in the community. *Archives of Physical Medicine and Rehabilitation,* 59:27, Jan. 1978.
21. Bianchine, J.R.: Drug therapy of Parkinsonism. *The New England Journal of Medicine,* 295:814, Oct. 1976.
22. Binzeley, V.: State: Overlooked factor in newborn nursing. *American Journal of Nursing,* 77:102, Jan. 1977.
23. Blackwell, C.A.: PEG and angiography: A patient's sensations. *American Journal of Nursing,* 75:264, Feb. 1975.
24. Blanchard, M.G.: Sex education of spinal cord injury patients and their nurses. *Supervisor Nurse,* 7:20, Feb. 1976.
25. Blount, M. and A. Kinney (Eds.): Symposium on neurologic and neurosurgical nursing. *Nursing Clinics of North America,* Dec. 1974.
26. Blount, M., et al.: What to remember about an EEG. *Nursing 74,* 4:36, Aug. 1974.
27. Bolin, K.L.: Assessing the status of neurological patients. *American Journal of Nursing,* 77:1478, Sept. 1977.
28. Boshes, L.D.: Gilles de la Tourette's syndrome. *American Journal of Nursing,* 76:1637, Oct. 1976.
29. Boyle, M.A., and R. Cuica: Amytrophic lateral sclerosis. *American Journal of Nursing,* 76:66, 1976.
30. Bracke, M., A.G. Taylor, and A. B. Kinney: External drainage of cerebrospinal fluid. *American Journal of Nursing,* 78:1355, Aug. 1978.
31. Brennan, R.W.: Rehabilitation of the patient with hemiplegia. *In* Conn, H.F. (ed.): *Current Therapy 1978.* Philadelphia: W.B. Saunders, Co., 1978.
32. Breu, C., and K. Dracup: Helping the spouses of critically ill patients. *American Journal of Nursing,* 78:50, Jan. 1978.
33. Breunig, K.A.: After the blowup . . . How to care for the patient with a ruptured cerebral aneurysm. *Nursing 76,* 6:37, Dec. 1976.
34. Brief consultation: Any help for patients with ALS? *Consultant,* 18:147, Jan. 1978.
35. Brown, M.A.: Human sexuality. *In* Longo, D.C., and R.A. Williams (Eds.): *Clinical Practice in Psychosocial Nursing: Assessment and Intervention.* New York: Appleton-Century-Crofts, 1978.
36. Brown, L.W., Valproic acid: A new antiepileptic agent. *American Family Physician:* 19:166, Feb. 1979.
37. Bruya, M.A., and R. H. Bolen: Epilepsy: A controlled disease. *American Journal of Nursing,* 76:388, Mar. 1976.
38. Buchanan, D.S.: Iatrogenic causes of neurologic disorders: Part 1. Affect, convulsions, and encephalopathies. *Geriatrics,* 33:59, Aug. 1978.
39. Buchanan, D.S.: Iatrogenic causes of neurologic disorders: Part 2. Drug-related dysfunctions. *Geriatrics,* 33:47, Sept. 1978.
40. Bunker, R. H.: Thoracic outlet compression syndrome: Diagnosis and treatment. *Hospital Medicine,* 12:46, Sept. 1976.
41. Burridge, R.: A paraplegic reflects . . .. *American Journal of Nursing,* 75:643, Apr. 1975.
42. Cannon, M.: To Sharon, with love. *American Journal of Nursing,* 79:642, Apr. 1979.
43. Cantanzaro, M.: Multiple sclerosis: Exploding myths that compromise patient care. *RN,* 40:42, Dec. 1977.
44. Canter, A.: How to do office-based screening for organic brain disorders. *Geriatrics,* 33:86, Nov. 1978.
45. Cantrell, D.: Scoliosis: Screening potential victims. *RN,* 39:56, Nov. 1976.
46. Caronna, J.J., and S. Finklestein: Neurological syndromes after cardiac arrest. *Stroke,* XIII:9, May-June 1078.
47. Caronna, J.J., et al.: The outcome of medical coma; Prediction by bedside assessment of physical signs. *Archives of Neurology,* 32:349, 1975.
48. Carrico, C.J., et al.: Fluid resuscitation following injury: Rationale for the use of balanced salt solutions. *Critical Care Medicine,* Vol. 4, 2:45, Mar.-Apr., 1976.
49. Carrico, C.J., J.H. Horovitz, and L.M. Flint, Jr.: Pulmonary responses. *In* Shires, G.T., C.J., Carrico, and P.C., Canizaro, *Shock.* Philadelphia, W.B. Saunders Co., 1973.
50. Carroll, B.: Fingers and toes. *American Journal of Nursing,* 71:550, Mar. 1971.
51. Cherlow, D.G., and E.A. Serafetinides: Speech and memory assessment in psychomotor epileptics. *Cortex,* 12:21, 1976.
52. Chipauras, S., D. Cornelius, S.M. Daniels, and E. Makas: *Who Cares? A Handbook on Sex Education and Counselling Services for Disabled People.* Sex Disability Project. George Washington University, Washington, D.C., 1979.
53. Christopherson, V.A., P.P. Coulter, amd M.O. Wolanin: *Rehabilitation Nursing. Perspectives and Applications.* New York: McGraw-Hill Book Co., 1974.
54. Clancey, J.K., and L.A. Abruzzi: Nursing intervention of patients with pituitary tumors. *Journal of Neurosurgical Nursing,* 10:24, Mar. 1978.
55. Clark, R.I.: *Manter & Gatz's Essentials of Clinical Neuroanatomy and Physiology,* 5th ed. Philadelphia: F.A. Davis Co., 1975.
56. Coleman, L.: The objectives and final goals of physical therapy. *Geriatrics,* 31:91, May 1976.
57. Coleman, P.: Trigeminal neuralgia: Diagnosis and treatment with special reference to percutaneous radiofrequency rhizotomy. *Journal of Neurosurgical Nursing,* 7:91, Dec. 1975.
58. Collins, J.: Problems associated with the massive transfusions of stored blood. *Surgery,* 75(2):274, Feb. 1974.
59. Comarr, A.E., and B.B. Gunderson: Sexual function in traumatic paraplegia and quadriplegia. *American Journal of Nursing,* 75:250, Feb. 1975.
60. Conn, H.F.: *Current Therapy 1978.* Philadelphia: W.B. Saunders Co., 1978.
61. Conomy, J.P.: Cryptic subdural hematoma: A neurologic Trojan horse. *Consultant,* 18:164, May 1978.
62. Conomy, J.P.: Long term use of the major anticonvulsant drugs. *American Family Physician,* 18:107, Oct. 1978.
63. Conway, B.L.: *Neurological and Neurosurgical Nursing,* 7th edition. St. Louis: C.V. Mosby Co., 1978.
64. Couch, J.R.: Diagnosing functional and organic headache. *Consultant,* 18:21, Jan. 1978.
65. Crawford, A.H.: Neurofibromatosis in children. *American Family Physician,* 17:163, Mar. 1978.
66. Crigler, L.: Sexual concerns of the spinal cord-injured. *In* Blount, M. and A. Kinney (Eds.): *Nursing Clinics of North America,* Dec., 1974.
67. Cushing, H.: Concerning a definite regulatory mechanism of the vasomotor centre which controls blood

pressure during cerebral compression. *Johns Hopkins Hospital Bulletin,* 12:290, 1971.

68. Dahlberg, C.C.: Stroke. *Psychology Today,* June 1977, p. 121.
69. Dalessio, D.J.: Mechanisms and biochemistry of headaches. *Nursing Digest,* III:30, May-June 1975.
70. Dayhoff, N.: Re-thinking stroke: Soft or hard devices to position hands? *American Journal of Nursing,* 75:1142, July 1975.
71. DeLisa, J.A., M.A. Mikulic, R.M. Miller, and R.R. Melnick: Amyotrophic lateral sclerosis: Comprehensive management. *American Family Physician,* 19:137, Mar. 1979.
72. DeMeyer, W.: *Technique of the Neurologic Examination,* 2nd ed. New York: McGraw-Hill Book Co., 1974.
73. Department of Health, Education and Welfare: *Handicapped Persons Rights Under the Federal Law.* Mar., 1978.
74. Digregorio, G.J.: Antivertigo and antimotion sickness drugs. *American Family Physician,* 18:130, Dec. 1978.
75. Dipalma, J.R.: Bromocriptine: Dopamine-receptor agonist. *American Family Physician,* 14:88, Dec. 1976.
76. Dolan, M.B.: Re-thinking stroke: Autumn months, autumn years. *American Journal of Nursing,* 75:1145, July 1975.
77. Domstead, D.J.: With Mr. J. we didn't know where to begin. *Nursing 77,* 7:28, Aug. 1977.
78. Donovan, L.: Low back pain: Where care is the key to recovery. *RN,* 41:71, Oct. 1978.
79. Drew, N.: How to cope with speech defects in stroke patients. *Nursing '74,* 4:20, Feb. 1974.
80. Dunphy, J. E., and L. W. Way: *Current Surgical Diagnosis and Treatment,* 3rd ed. Los Altos: Lange Medical Publishers, 1975.
81. Duvoisin, R.: *Clinical Symposia: Parkinsonism.* Summit, N.J.: Ciba-Geigy Co., 1976.
82. Eisenberg, M.G., and L.C. Rustad: Sex education and counseling program on a spinal cord injury service. *Archives of Physical Medicine and Rehabilitation,* 57:135, Mar., 1976.
83. Engler, G.L.: The many ways a back can ache. *Emergency Medicine,* 9:43, Nov., 1977.
84. Enna, S.J., and E.D. Bird: Huntington's chorea: Changes in neurotransmitter receptors in the brain. *New England Journal of Medicine,* 294:1305, 1976.
85. Epilepsy Foundation of America; *The Legal Rights of Persons with Epilepsy,* 4th ed. Washington, D.C.: Epilepsy Foundation of America, 1976.
86. Epstein, B.S.: Guide to cranial and intracranial calcifications. Part 1. *Hospital Medicine,* 15:135, Mar. 1979.
87. Falicov, R.E., and A.J. Bochna: Syncope: A clinical approach. *Hospital Medicine,* 14:8, Feb. 1978.
88. Feustel, D.: Autonomic hyperreflexia. *American Journal of Nursing,* 76:228, Feb. 1976.
89. Fincham, R.W., and H.P. Adams, Jr.: Brain tumor as a cause of epilepsy. *American Family Physician,* 16:165, Oct. 1977.
90. Fink, S.: Crisis motivation: A theoretical model. *Archives of Physical Medicine and Rehabilitation,* 90:592, Nov. 1967.
91. Fischbach, F.T.: Easing adjustment to Parkinson's disease. *American Journal of Nursing,* 78:66, Jan. 1978.
92. Fisher, C.M.: Reducing risks of cerebral embolism. *Geriatrics,* 34:59, Feb. 1979.
93. Flechsig, L.: Living with cerebral palsy. *American Journal of Nursing,* 78:1212, July 1978.
94. Flom, R.P., et al.: Biofeedback training to overcome poststroke foot-drop. *Geriatrics,* 31:47, Dec. 1976.
95. Ford, B.: Head injuries — What happens to survivors. *Medical Journal of Australia,* 1:603, 1976.
96. Ford, J.R., and B. Duckworth: *Physical Management for the Quadriplegic Patient.* Philadelphia: F.A. Davis Co., 1977.
97. Foster, J.B.: Differentiating causes of headaches. *Geriatrics,* 32:115, Sept. 1977.
98. Four aspirin a day keeps ischemia away. *Emergency Medicine,* 9:97, Aug. 1977.
99. Fox, M.J.: Patients with receptive aphasia: They really don't understand. *American Journal of Nursing,* 76:1596, Oct. 1976.
100. Fraser, R.A.R.: Brain abscess. *In* Conn, H.F. (Ed.): *Current Therapy 1978.* Philadelphia: W.B. Saunders Co., 1978.
101. Fraser, D.W.: Vaccines against bacterial meningitis. *Postgraduate Medicine,* 62:105, Aug. 1977.
102. Free, J.W., and C. McPhillips: Huntington's disease: How to solve its unique care problems. *RN,* 40:44, Aug. 1977.
103. Fromm, G.H.: The importance of the workup in epilepsy. *Consultant,* 16:187, Nov. 1976.
104. Gaffney, T.W., and R. P. Campbell: Feeding techniques for dysphagic patients. *American Journal of Nursing,* 74:2194, Dec. 1974.
105. Galdi, A.P.: Essentials in the management of myasthenia gravis. *American Family Physician,* 17:95, June 1978.
106. Gilmore, R.L.: Recognizing the remote effects of malignancy on the nervous system. *Geriatrics,* 34:102, Mar. 1979.
107. Gobiet, W., et al.: Treatment of acute cerebral edema with high dose of dexamethasone. *In* J. W. F. Beks, D. A. Bosch, M. Brock, (Eds.): *Intracranial Pressure III,* Berlin: Springer-Verlag, 232, 1976.
108. Goloskov, J.W., and P.L. LeRoy: The role of the nurse in quantitative intracranial pressure determinations. *Journal of Neurosurgical Nursing,* 10:17, Mar. 1978.
109. Gorman, R.J., and O.C. Snead: Febrile Seizures. *American Family Physician,* 19:101, Jan. 1979.
110. Gotshall, R.A., and L.A. Harker: Using antithrombotic therapy in ischemic cerebrovascular disease. *Geriatrics,* 32:101, November, 1977.
111. Graham, L.: Stroke rehabilitation–a creative process. *Nursing Digest,* 5:64, Spring 1977.
112. Greenfield, L.D., and L.R. Bennett: Brain imaging. *American Family Physician,* 13:95, Apr. 1976.
113. Greer, M.: How to achieve maximum benefit for the patient with Parkinson's disease. *Geriatrics,* 31:89, Apr. 1976.
114. Greer, M.: Uncommon causes of strokes. Part 1. Diseases of the vessel wall. *Geriatrics,* 32:28, Dec. 1977.
115. Grens, M.: For me, there's no such thing as "Another CVA" anymore. *RN,* 40:85, Sept. 1977.
116. Grynbaum, B.B., et al.: Sensory feedback therapy for stroke patients. *Geriatrics,* 31:43, June 1976.
117. Guillemin, R.: New endocrinology of the brain. *Perspectives in Biology and Medicine,* 22:S74, Winter 1979.
118. Hackler, E.S.: Expanding the role of nurses in rehabilitation. *Geriatrics,* 31:77, May 1976.
119. Hanlon, K.: Description and uses of intracranial pressure monitoring. *Heart and Lung: The Journal of Critical Care,* 5:277, Mar.-Apr. 1976.
120. Hansen, R.W., and M.R. Franklin: Sexual losses in relation to other functional losses for spinal cord injured males. *Archives of Physical Medicine and Rehabilitation,* 57:291, 1976.
121. Harkness, L.: Bringing epilepsy out of the closet. *American Journal of Nursing,* 74:875, May 1974.

122. Hass, W.K.: Acute ischemic cerebrovascular disease. *In* Conn, H.F. (Ed.): *Current Therapy 1978*. Philadelphia; W.B. Saunders Co., 1978.
123. Hastings, D.E.: Back pain. A multifaceted syndrome. *Postgraduate Medicine* 62:159, July 1977.
124. Hawken, M.: Epilepsy nurse specialist. *Nursing 78*, 78:114, Sept. 1978.
125. Hawley, D., and D.W. Reiser: Reducing muscle spasms in a child with cerebral palsy. *American Journal of Nursing*, 78:1214, July 1978.
126. Heading off posttraumatic seizures. *Emergency Medicine* 9:187, Apr. 1977.
127. Heard, L.: *Understanding Spinal Cord Injury*. Unpublished material, University Hospital, University of Washington, Seattle.
128. Heilman, K.M.: Exploring the enigmas of frontal lobe dysfunction. *Geriatrics*, 31:81, Dec. 1976.
129. Henterbuchner, L.P.: Idiopathic peripheral facial paralysis (Bell's Palsy). *In* Conn, H.F. (Ed.): *Current Therapy 1978*. Philadelphia: W.B. Saunders Co., 1978.
130. Herpes — holding it back. *Emergency Medicine*, 10:89, June 1978.
131. Hines, J.D., and G.A. Nankervis: Herpes zoster infection. *Hospital Medicine*, 13:72, Aug. 1977.
132. Hirsh, L.F.: Tardy ulnar palsy. *Hospital Medicine*, 12:67, Nov. 1976.
133. Hirschberg, G.G.: Ambulation and self-care are goals of rehabilitation after stroke. *Geriatrics*, 31:61, May 1976.
134. Hirschberg, G.G., et al.: *Rehabilitation*, 2nd ed. Philadelphia: J.B. Lippincott Co., 1976, pp. 286–288.
135. Hoff, J.T.: Intracerebral hemorrahge. *In* Conn, Howard F. (Ed.): *Current Therapy 1978*. Philadelphia: W.B. Saunders Co., 1978.
136. Hogan, L., and I. Beland: Cervical spine syndrome. *American Journal of Nursing*, 76:1104, July 1976.
137. Howard, F.M.: Myasthenia gravis. *In* Conn, H.F., (Ed.): *Current Therapy 1978*. Philadelphia: W.B. Saunders Co., 1978.
138. Howe, J.R.: *Patient Care in Neurosurgery*. Boston: Little, Brown & Co., 1977.
139. Hulme, A., and R. Cooper: The effects of head position and jugular vein compression (JVC) on intracranial pressure (ICP). A clinical study. *In* Beks, J.W.F., D.A. Bosch, and M. Brock (Eds.): *Intracranial Pressure III*. Berlin: Springer-Verlag, 1976, pp. 259–263.
140. Hunko, V.: Numidia looked like a model — But she wasn't a model patient. *Nursing 78*, 8:51, Dec. 1978.
141. Hunt, W.E., and J.E. Goodman: Acute head injuries. *In* Conn, H.F. (Ed.): *Current Therapy 1978*. Philadelphia: W.B. Saunders Co., 1978.
142. Isaacs, B.: Problems and solutions in rehabilitation of stroke patients. *Geriatrics*, 33:87, July 1978.
143. Jackson, D.W.: Low back pain in young adults: How useful are diagnostic tests? *Consultant*, 18:184, Sept. 1978.
144. Jackson, F. E.: *Clinical Symposia: The Pathophysiology of Head Injuries*. Summit: Ciba-Geigy Co., 1966.
145. Jackson, F.E.: The Achilles' neck and other vulnerable vertebrae. *Emergency Medicine*, 9:22, Mar. 1977.
146. Jackson, F.E.: Vulnerable vertebrae. *Emergency Medicine*, 11:33 Mar. 1979.
147. Jackson, L.G., P. Nimoityn, H.S. Faust, and L.R. Glazerman: Community Screening for Tay-Sachs Disease. *American Family Physician*, 13:111, Apr. 1976.
148. Jacob, S.W., C.A. Francone, and W.J. Lossow: *Structure and Function in Man*, 4th ed. Philadelphia: W.B. Saunders Co., 1978.
149. James, H.L.T.W., and V.S. Kumar: Analysis of the response to therapeutic measures to reduce intracranial pressure in head injured patients. *Journal of Trauma*, 16:437, 1976.
150. Janecki, C.J., and J.M. Lipke: Whiplash syndrome. *American Family Physician*, 17:144, Apr. 1978.
151. Javid, M.: Current concepts: Head injuries. *The New England Journal of Medicine*, 291:890, Oct. 1974.
152. Javid, M.: Traumatic injuries, office treatment of craniocerebral trauma. *Postgraduate Medicine*, 61:233, May 1977.
153. Jennett, B.: Assessment of the severity of head injury. *Journal of Neurology, Neurosrugery and Psychiatry*, 39:647, 1976.
154. Jennett, B.: Outcome after severe head injury: Definitions and predictions. *Medical Journal of Australia*, 2:475, 1976.
155. Jennett, B., and G. Teasdale: Aspects of coma after severe head injury. *Lancet*, 1:878, Apr. 1977.
156. Jennett, B., and G. Teasdale: Predicting outcome in individual patients after severe head injury. *Lancet*, 1:1031, May 1976.
157. Johnson, M.R.: Emergency management of head and spinal injury. *Nursing Clinics of North America*, 8:389, Sept. 1973.
158. Johnson, M., and J. Quinn: The subarachnoid screw. *American Journal of Nursing*, 77:448, Mar. 1977.
159. Jones, F. H.: Rehabilitation of the stroke patient. *American Family Physician*, 15:178, Jan. 1977.
160. Kannel, W.B., P. Wolf, and T.R. Dawber: Hypertension and cardiac impairments increase stroke risk. *Geriatrics*, 33:71, Sept. 1978.
161. Katzman, R., et al.: Brain edema in stroke. *Stroke*, 8:512, 1977.
162. Kavchak Keyes, M.A.: Comeback from disaster: Helping the stroke patient learn to help himself. *Nursing 79*, 9:32, Jan. 1979.
163. Kealy, S.L.: Respiratory care in Guillain-Barré syndrome. *American Journal of Nursing*, Jan. 1977.
164. Keane, J.R.: Vertigo as a vestibular symptom. *Hospital Medicine*, 14:76, Nov. 1978.
165. Keeping their heads together. *Emergency Medicine*, 9:26, May 1977.
166. Keith, R.L.: Caring for the aphasic patient. *Nursing Digest*, IV:37, Fall 1976.
167. Kelly, W.A.: Brain tumors. *In* Conn, H.F. (Ed.): *Current Therapy 1978*. Philadelphia: W.B. Saunders Co., 1978.
168. Kent, S.: Assessing function: A key to care of the aging. *Geriatrics*, 32:83, Aug. 1977.
169. Kent, S.: Classifying and treating organic brain syndrome. *Geriatrics*, 32:87, Sept. 1977.
170. Kent, S.: Neurotransmitters may be weak link in the aging brain's communication network. *Geriatrics*, 31:105, July 1976.
171. Kent, S.: Scientists count brain cells to figure theory of aging. *Geriatrics*, 31:114, Apr. 1976.
172. Kent, S.: Structural changes in the brain transfer in information. *Geriatrics*, 31:128, June 1976.
173. Kinash, R.G.: Experiences and nursing needs of spinal cord-injured patients. *Journal of Neurosurgical Nursing*, 10:29, Mar. 1978.
174. Kirkaldy-Willis, W.H.: Five common back disorders: How to diagnosis and treat them. *Geriatrics*, 33:32, Dec. 1978.
175. Klawans, H.L., and M.M. Cohen: Diseases of the extrapyramidal system. *Disease-a-Month*, Jan. 1970, pp. 3–52.

176. Klawans, H.L., and D.B. Calne: Parkinson's disease. *In* Conn, H.F. (Ed.): *Current Therapy 1978*. Philadelphia: W.B. Saunders Co., 1978.
177. Koff, S.A., A.C. Dioko, and J. Lapides: Neurogenic bladder dysfunction. *American Family Physician,* 19:100, Feb. 1979.
178. Koprowski, H., and K.G. Warren: Can a defective herpes simplex virus cause multiple sclerosis? *Perspectives in Biology and Medicine,* 22:10, Aug. 1978.
179. Kossoff, J., and J. Pais: The emergency x-ray. *Emergency Medicine,* 10:51, Nov. 1978.
180. Krasney, J.A., and R.C. Koehler: Heart rate and rhythm and intracranial pressure. *American Journal of Physiology,* 230:1695, June 1976.
181. Krupp, M.A., and M.J. Chatton: *Current Medical Diagnosis and Treatment.* Los Altos: Lange Medical Publishers, 1978.
182. Kubo, W.M., and M.M. Grant: The syndrome of inappropriate secretion of antidiuretic hormone. *Heart and Lung: The Journal of Critical Care,* 7:469, May-June 1978.
183. Kunkel, J., and J.K. Wiley: Acute head injury: What to do when . . . and why. *Nursing 79*, 9:23, Mar. 1979.
184. Kurtzke, J.F.: MS: Six criteria for diagnosis. *Consultant,* 17:85, July 1977.
185. Kurtzke, J.F.: Recognizing focal seizures early. *Consultant,* 17:29, May 1977.
186. Langan, R.J. and G.C. Cotzias: Do's and dont's for the patient on levodopa therapy. *American Journal of Nursing,* 76:917, June 1976.
187. Langan, R.J.: Parkinson's disease: Assessment procedures and guidelines for counseling. *Nurse Practitioner,* 2:13, Dec. 1976.
188. Langfitt, T.W. (Ed.): *Cerebral Circulation and Metabolism.* Berlin: Springer-Verlag, 1975.
189. Lapides, J.: Symposium on neurogenic bladder. *Urologic Clinics of North America,* Feb. 1974.
190. Large, H., et al.: In the first stroke intensive care unit. *American Journal of Nursing,* 69:76, Jan. 1969.
191. Larrabee, J.H.: The person with a spinal cord injury: Physical care during early recovery. *American Journal of Nursing,* 77:1320, Aug. 1977.
192. Lawrence, S.A., and R.M. Lawrence: A model of adaptation to the stress of chronic illness. Nursing Forum, 28(1):33, 1979.
193. Leigh, J., and D.A. Shaw: Rapid regular respiration in unconscious patients. *Archives of Neurology,* 33:356, 1976.
194. Librach, G., et al.: Stroke: Incidence and risk factors. *Geriatrics,* 32:85, Apr. 1977.
195. Lin, J.P.: Computed tomography of the head in adults. *Postgraduate Medicine,* 60:113, Aug. 1976.
196. Livingston, S.: 10 questions physicians most often ask . . . About epilepsy. *Consultant,* 18:103, Feb. 1978.
197. Loerrerle, B.C., et al.: Cerebellar stimulation; Pacing the brain. *American Journal of Nursing,* 75:958, June 1975.
198. Lowry, T.: What happens in spinal cord injury. *Nursing 78,* 8:74, Oct. 1978.
199. Luetje, C.M.: Meniere's disease. *In* Conn, H.F. (Ed.): *Current Therapy 1978*. Philadelphia: W.B. Saunders Co., 1978.
200. Macauley, C.: Eddie: A successful quad. *American Journal of Nursing,* 77:1336, Aug. 1977.
201. Mack, E.W., and W.N. Dawson, Jr.: Injury to the spine and spinal cord. *Hospital Medicine,* 12:23, July 1976.
202. Madeja, C.: Computerized tomography: An introduction. *Journal of Neurosurgical Nursing,* 9:87, June 1977.
203. Magee, K.R.: The neurologic workup by the primary care physician. *Postgraduate Medicine,* 61:77, Mar. 1977.
204. Maki, D.G.: Septic thrombophlebitis (Part 2). *Hospital Medicine,* 13:6, Jan. 1977.
205. March, M.L., et al.: Neurosurgical intensive care. *Anesthesiology.* 47:149, 1977.
206. Marcus, E.M.: Multiple sclerosis. *In* Conn, H.F. (Ed.): *Current Therapy 1978*. Philadelphia: W.B. Saunders, 1978.
207. Marks, R.L., and G.A. Bahr: How to manage neurogenic bladder after stroke. *Geriatrics,* 32:50, Dec. 1977.
208. Masland, R.L.: The diagnosis and treatment of little seizures. *Hospital Medicine,* 12:85, Jan. 1976.
209. Massanari, R.M.: Purulent meningitis in the elderly: When to suspect an unusual pathogen. *Geriatrics,* 32:55, Mar. 1977.
210. Massey, E.W.: Neuroemergencies sans coma. *Emergency Medicine,* 10:24, Dec. 1978.
211. Masters, W., and V. Johnson: *Human Sexual Response.* Boston: Little, Brown Co., 1977.
212. Mathews, N.C.: Helping a quadriplegic veteran decide to live. *American Journal of Nursing.* 76:441, Mar. 1976.
213. McLaurin, R.L., (ed.): *Head Injuries. Second Chicago Symposium on Neural Trauma.* New York: Grune and Stratton, 1976.
214. McQuillen, M.P.: Neuromuscular fatigue in middle life: What it means and how to treat it. *Geriatrics,* 34:67, May 1979.
215. Mechner, F., et al.: Patient assessment: Neurological examination, Parts I, II, III. *American Journal of Nursing,* 75:1511; 75:2037; 76:609, Sept. and Nov., 1975, 1976.
216. Megahed, M.S., and P.R. Rosendahl: Brain tumors — An assessment for nurse practitioners. *Nurse Practitioner,* 2:9, July-Aug. 1977.
217. Melen, O., S.F. Olson, and B.L. Hodes; Visual disturbances in migraine. *Postgraduate Medicine,* 64:139, July 1978.
218. Merritt, H.H.: *A Textbook of Neurology,* 5th ed. Philadelphia: Lea and Febiger, 1973.
219. Meyd, J.: Acute brain tumor. *American Journal of Nursing,* 78:40, Jan. 1978.
220. Michael, J.A.: Physiology of the nervous system: From the molecular to the behavioral. *Nursing Digest,* IV:20, Fall 1976.
221. Migraine plus. *Emergency Medicine,* 10:110, Dec. 1978.
222. Mitchell, P.H., and N. Mauss: Intracranial pressure: Fact and fancy. *Nursing 76,* 6:53, 1976.
223. Mitchell, P.H., and N. Irvin: Neurological examination: Nursing assessment for nursing purposes. *Journal of Neurosurgical Nursing,* 9:23, Mar. 1977.
224. Moe, P.G.: Headaches in children. *Postgraduate Medicine,* 63:169, Apr. 1978.
225. Mooney, T.O., T.M. Cole, and R.A. Chilgren: *Sexual Options for Paraplegics and Quadriplegics.* Boston: Little, Brown and Co., 1975.
226. Morley, T.P. (Ed.): *Current Controversies in Neurosurgery.* Philadelphia: W.B. Saunders Co., 1976.
227. Myers, M.G.: Varicella and herpes zoster: Comparisons in the old and young. *Geriatrics,* 32:77, Mar. 1977.
228. Naidich, T.P., and I.I. Kricheff: Computed tomography of the head in children. *Postgraduate Medicine,* 60:123, Aug. 1976.
229. Naiman, H.: Screening for Tay-Sachs disease. *American Journal of Nursing* 75:436, Mar. 1975.
230. New, P.F.J., and W.R. Scott: *Computed Tomography of the Brain and Orbit (EMI Scanning).* Baltimore: Williams and Wilkins Co., 1975.
231. Nikas, D., and R. Konkoly: Nursing responsibilities in arterial and intracranial pressure monitoring. *Journal of Neurosurgical Nursing,* 7:116, Dec. 1975.
232. Nugent, G.R.: Trigeminal and glossopharyngeal neu-

ralgia. *In* Conn, H.F. (Ed.): *Current Therapy 1978.* Philadelphia: W.B. Saunders Co., 1978.

233. O'Connor, A.B. (Ed.): *Nursing in Neurological Disorders.* New York: The American Journal of Nursing Co., 1976.
234. Oliveto, M.J., S. Wilson, and H.A. Mackinnon: Sara: Her rehabilitation and its cost. *American Journal of Nursing,* 77:1338, Aug. 1977.
235. Osoff, A.: Caring for the child with familial dysautonomia. *American Journal of Nursing,* 75:1158, July 1975.
236. Ostrow, L.S.: New hope for patients with trigeminal neuralgia. *American Journal of Nursing,* 76:1301, Aug. 1976.
237. Packard, R.C.: Case report. Changes in migraine headache pattern following sudden increase in ergotamine intake. *Postgraduate Medicine,* 61:255, May 1977.
238. Palkovitz, H.P.: Parkinson's disease: An update on diagnosis and treatment. *Consultant,* 18:54, Oct. 1978.
239. Panieczko, S.: Attitudes and Disability: *A Selected Annotated Bibliography.* Regional Rehabilitation Research Institute and Attitudinal, Legal, and Leisure Barriers. George Washington University, Washington, D.C.
240. Patterson, T.D.: Scoliosis. *RN,* 39:58–80, Nov. 1976.
241. Patton, H.D., et al.: *Introduction to Basic Neurology.* Philadelphia: W.B. Saunders Co., 1976.
242. Pearson, L.B.: A protocol for the chief complaint of headache. *Nurse Practitioner,* 2:12, Sept.-Oct. 1976.
243. Peirce, K., M.D.: *Personal communication,* 1978.
244. Pepper, G.A.: The person with a spinal cord injury: Psychological care. *American Journal of Nursing,* 77:1330, Aug. 1977.
245. Perez, F.I., et al.: Analysis of intellectual and cognitive performance in patients with multi-infarct dementia, vertebrobasilar insufficiency with dementia, and Alzheimer's disease. *Journal of Neurology, Neurosurgery, and Psychiatry,* 38:533, 1975.
246. Peterson, G.C.: Psychiatric aspects of chronic organic brain syndromes. *Postgraduate Medicine,* 60:162, Nov. 1976.
247. Pierce, D., and V. Nickel: *The Total Care of Spinal Cord Injuries.* Boston: Little, Brown and Co., 1977.
248. Plum, F.: Axioms on coma. *Hospital Medicine,* 4:20, May 1968.
249. Plum, F., and J. Posner: *Diagnosis of Stupor and Coma.* 2nd ed. Philadelphia: F.A. Davis Co., 1972.
250. Plum, F.; Headache. *In* Beeson, P.B., and W. McDermott (Eds.). *Cecil-Loeb Textbook of Medicine,* 13th ed. Philadelphia: W.B. Saunders Co., 1971.
251. Plum, F., and B.K. Siesjo, : Recent advances in CSF physiology. *Anesthesiology,* 42:608, 1975.
252. Plum, F.: Seminar on Medical Coma. University of Washington School of Medicine, Fall 1977.
253. Plum, F.: The pathogenesis of stupor and coma. *In* Beeson, P.B., and W. McDermott (Eds.(: *Cecil-Loeb Textbook of Medicine.* 13th ed. Philadelphia: W.B. Saunders Co., 1971.
254. Pohutsky, L.C., and K.R. Pohutsky: Cancer update. Computerized axial tomography of the brain: A new diagnostic tool. *American Journal of Nursing.* 75:1341, Aug. 1975.
255. Poser, C.M.: The types of headache that affect the elderly. *Geriatrics* 31:103, Sept. 1976.
256. Post, F.: Dementia, depression and pseudodementia. *In* Benson, D.F., and D. Blumer. (Eds.): *Psychiatric Aspects of Neurological Disease.* New York: Grune and Stratton, 1975.
257. Potter, J.F., and A.H. Fruin: Chronic subdural hematoma — The "Great imitator". *Geriatrics,* 32:61, June 1977.
258. Quencer, R.M., and M.J.D. Post: Evaluating spinal injuries from plain films. *Consultant,* 17:118, Oct. 1977.
259. Ramirez, B.: When you're faced with a neuro patient. *RN,* 42:67, Jan. 1979.
260. Ransohoff, J., and M. Koslow: Guide to the diagnosis and management of cerebral injury. *Hospital Medicine,* 14:127, May 1978.
261. Ransohoff, J.: Help for the injured head. *Emergency Medicine,* 9:35, Nov. 1977.
262. Raskin, N.H.: Headache. *In* Conn, H.F. (Ed.): *Current Therapy 1978.* Philadelphia: W.B. Saunders Co., 1978.
263. Reeves, K.R.: Beware of Reye's syndrome. *American Journal of Nursing,* 74:1621, Sept. 1974.
264. Reitan, R.M., and L.A. Davidson: *Clinical Neuropsychology: Current Status and Applications.* Washington, D.C.: V.H. Winston & Sons, 1974.
265. Rhoton, A.L., et al.: *Clinical Symposia: Congenital and Intracranial Aneurysms.* Summit, N.J.: Ciba-Geigy Corp., 1977.
266. Roberts, J.M.: Scoliosis: The clinical interview. *RN* 39:57, Nov. 1976.
267. Roberts, J.M.: Spinal fusion, Harrington instrumentation, and Dwyer instrumentation. *RN,* 39:76, Nov. 1976.
268. Roberts, J.M.: Treatment with Cotrel's traction and the Risser cast. *RN,* 39:68, Nov. 1976.
269. Robbins, S. L., and R.S. Cotran: *Pathologic Basis of Disease,* 2nd ed. Philadelphia: W. B. Saunders Co., 1979.
270. Rosell, C.: Pitfalls of emotional involvement: Sympathetic nursing care of a patient with a cervical spine injury. *Nursing 76,* 6:42 Mar. 1976.
271. Ross, R.T.: *How to Examine the Nervous System.* Springfield, Ill.: Charles C Thomas, 1978.
272. Rossier, A.: *Rehabilitation of the Spinal Cord Injury Patient.* Summit, N.J.: Ciba-Geigy Corp., 1975.
273. Roth, M., and D.H. Myers: The diagnosis of dementia. *British Journal of Psychiatry. Special Publications,* No. 9, 87, 1975.
274. Rudy, E.: Early omens of cerebral disaster. *Nursing 77,* 7:58, Feb. 1977.
275. Rutherford, W.H.: Sequelae of concussion caused by minor head injuries. *Lancet,* 1:1, Jan. 1978.
276. Sackner, M.A., et al.: Pathogenesis and prevention of tracheobronchial damage with suction procedures. *Chest,* 64:284, 1973.
277. San Luis, R.R.: Simple tests can indicate type of brain damage. *Geriatrics,* 32:115, June 1977.
278. Sarkar, T.K., and A.T. Munshi: Case report. Postical pulmonary edema. *Postgraduate Medicine,* 61:281, Jan. 1977.
279. Schutz, M.K.: What must be done when all else fails. *RN,* 42:52, May 1979.
280. Schwartz, C.J., L.A. Ehrhart, and R.G. Gerrity: Atheroma: A review. *Hospital Medicine,* 13:18, Nov. 1977.
281. Sears, E.S.: Therapeutics of disordered movement. *American Family Physician.* 16:145, Sept. 1977.
282. Sell, S.: The treatment of tic douloureux by vascular decompression of the trigeminal nerve. *Journal of Neurosurgical Nursing,* 9:19, Mar. 1977.
283. Shafer, N.: The meaning of tremors. *Consultant,* 16:68, Aug. 1976.
284. Shapiro, H.M., et al.: Barbiturate-augmented hypothermia for reduction of persistent intracranial hypertension. *Journal of Neurosurgery,* 40:90, 1974.
285. Shapiro, H.M., and S.J. Aidinis: Neurosurgical anesthesia. *Surgical Clinics of North America,* 55:913, 1975.
286. Shapiro, J.S.: Benign intracranial hypertension. *American Family Physician,* 17:155, Apr. 1978.
287. Shaul, S., J. Bogle, J. Hale, and A.D. Norman: *Toward Intimacy: Family Planning and Sexuality Concerns of*

Physically Disabled Women. 2nd ed. New York: Human Sciences Press, 1978.

288. Shearer, D., B. Collins, and D. Creel: Preparing a patient for EEG. *American Journal of Nursing,* 75:63, Jan. 1975.
289. Sheridan, J.: Restoring speech and language skills. *Geriatrics,* 31:83, May 1976.
290. Siesjo, B.K., et al.: Brain metabolism in the circtically ill. *Critical Care Medicine,* 4:283, 1976.
291. Silberberg, D.H.: Multiple sclerosis, Highlights of studies relating to nature and cause. *Postgraduate Medicine,* 64:107, Aug. 1978.

291a. Simpson, J.F., and K.R. Magee: *Clinical Evaluation of the Nervous System.* Boston: Little Brown and Company, 1973.

292. Skelly, M.: Rethinking stroke. Aphasic patients talk back. *American Journal of Nursing,* 75:1140, July 1975.
293. Smith, A.: Neuropsychological testing in neurological disorders. *In* Friedlander, W.J.: *Advances in Neurology,* Vol. 7. New York: Raven Press.
294. Smith, A.L., and J.J. Marque: Anesthetics and cerebral edema. *Anesthesiology,* 45:64, 1976.
295. Smith, A., and O. Sugar: Development of above normal language and intelligence 21 years after left hemispherectomy. *Neurology,* 25:813, 1975.
296. Smith, B.H.: Headaches: The ominous few. *Consultant,* 16:59, Aug. 1976.
297. Smith, J.L.: Optic neuritis. *In* Conn, H.F. (Ed.): *Current Therapy 1978.* Philadelphia: W.B. Saunders Co., 1978.
298. Smith, J., and B. Bullough: Sexuality and the severely disabled person. *American Journal of Nursing,* 75:2194, Dec. 1975.
299. Solomon, G.E., and F. Plum,: *Clinical Management of Seizures.* Philadelphia: W.B. Saunders Co., 1976.
300. Solomon, G.E.: Epilepsy in adolescents and adults. *In* Conn, H.F., (Ed.): *Current Therapy 1978.* Philadelphia: W.B. Saunders Co., 1978.
301. Sperling, K.: Intermittent catheterization to obtain catheter-free bladder function in spinal cord injury. *Archives of Physical Medicine and Rehabilitation,* 59:43, Jan. 1978.
302. Spiegel, M.B.: Electromyoneurography. *American Family Physician,* 18:119, Nov. 1978.
303. Steegman, A.T.: *Examination of the Nervous System,* 3rd ed. Chicago: Year Book Medical Publishers, Inc., 1970.
304. Steel, K., and R.G. Feldman: Diagnosing dementia and its treatable causes. *Geriatrics,* 34:79, Mar. 1979.
305. Stockton, V., et al.: *Core Curriculum for Neurosurgical Nursing.* Baltimore: The American Association of Neurosurgical Nurses, 1977.
306. Stone, B.H.: Computerized transaxial brain scan. *Journal of Neurosurgical Nursing,* 77:1601, Oct. 1977.
307. Suter, P.M., et al.: Optimum end-expiratory pressure in patients with acute pulmonary failure. *New England Journal of Medicine,* 292:284, 1975.
308. Swift, N., and R.M. Mabel: *Manual of Neurological Nursing,* Boston: Little, Brown and Co., 1978.
309. Tanner, P.: Relearning an old lesson from an unconscious patient. *RN,* 41:66, April 1978.
310. Taylor, A.G.: Autonomic dysreflexia in spinal cord injury. *In Nursing Clinics of North America,* Dec. 1974.
311. Taylor, F., and H. Schutz: Symptoms caused by intracranial pressure waves. *Journal of Neurosurgical Nursing,* 9:144, Dec. 1977.
312. Teasdale, G.: Assessment of head injuries. *British Journal of Anaesthesia,* 48:761, 1976.
313. Thomas, S.F.: Guide to reflexes in neurologic diagnosis. *Hospital Medicine,* 13:88, April 1977.
314. Thorn, G.W., et al.: *Harrison's Principles of Internal Medicine,* 8th ed. New York: McGraw-Hill Book Co., 1977.
315. Tindall, G.T., and A.S. Fleischer: Head injury. *Hospital Medicine,* 12:89, May 1976.
316. Tindall, G.T., and A.S. Fleischer: Intracranial pressure (ICP) monitoring and prognosis in closed head injury. *In,* McLaurin, R.L. (Ed.): *Head Injuries: Second Chicago Symposium on Neural Trauma.* New York: Grune and Stratton, 1976.
317. Tyler, H.R.: Answers to questions of stroke. *Hospital Medicine,* 13:26, June 1977.
318. Udall, J.A.: Anticoagulant therapy for progressing strokes. *Postgraduate Medicine,* 42:212, Sept. 1967.
319. Valenstein, E.: Making sense of cerebral dominance and syndromes of the nondominant hemisphere. *Geriatrics,* 31:111, Nov. 1976.
320. Valergakis, F.E.G.: Cervical spondylosis: Most common cause of position and vibratory sense loss. *Geriatrics,* 31:51, July 1976.
321. Vemireddi, N.K.: Sexual counseling for chronically disabled patients. *Geriatrics,* 33:65, July 1978.
322. Wachter-Shikara, N.: Trigeminal neuralgia: Current concepts and nursing implications. *Journal of Neurosurgical Nursing,* 9:78, June 1977.
323. Wahl, S.: Assessment. Only a concussion. *Nursing 76,* 6:44, Aug. 1976.
324. Walleck, C.: Pulmonary complications in the neurosurgical patient. *Journal of Neurosurgical Nursing,* 9:102, Sept. 1977.
325. Walsh, K.V.: *Neuropsychology: A Clinical Approach.* New York: Churchill Livingstone, 1978.
326. Watts, C., and L. Porto: Recognizing spontaneous spinal epidural hematoma. *Geriatrics,* 31:97, Sept. 1976.
327. Waxman, J.: Coping with common back problems. *Consultant,* 17:164, June 1977.
328. Webb, P.H.: Neurological deficit after cartoid endarterectomy. *American Journal of Nursing,* 79:654, Apr. 1979.
329. Wertenbaker, C., and H. Schaumburg: Peripheral Neuropathy. *In* Conn, H.F.(Ed.): *Current Therapy 1978.* Philadelphia: W.B. Saunders Co., 1978.
330. Wheeler, P.: Care of a patient with a cerebellar tumor. *American Journal of Nursing,* 77:263, Feb. 1977.
331. When the brain is injured, look to the lungs. *Emergency Medicine,* 9:163, Mar. 1977.
332. White, S.J.: An on-the-run guide to neurological drugs. *RN,* 41:59, Sept. 1978.

332a. Whiteman, M.: Bell's palsy. *American Journal of Nursing,* 71:2139, Nov. 1971.

333. Wiebe, R.A.: Bacterial meningitis. *Hospital Medicine,* 12:66, July 1976.
334. Wilkiemeyer, D.: The man who knew too much. *Nursing 78,* 8:26, Jan. 1978.
335. Wingerson, E.: The value of occupational therapy in rehabilitation. *Geriatrics,* 31:99, May 1976.
336. Winkelman, A.C.: Update on drug treatment of Parkinsonism. *American Family Physician,* 16:118, July 1977.
337. Wisser, S.H.: When the walls listened. *American Journal of Nursing,* 78:1016, June 1978.
338. Wolinsky, J.S.: Viral meningoencephalitis. *In* Conn, H.F. (Ed.): *Current Therapy 1978.* Philadelphia: W.B. Saunders Co., 1978.
339. Wright, G.N.: *Epilepsy Rehabilitation.* Boston: Little, Brown and Co., 1975.
340. Youmans, J. (Ed.): *Neurological Surgery.* Volumes 1, 2, and 3. Philadelphia: W.B. Saunders Co., 1973.
341. Zinn, W.: Hypothermia in critical-care unit. *Heart and Lung: The Journal of Critical Care,* 2:58, Jan.-Feb. 1973.

UNIT XI*

NURSING PEOPLE EXPERIENCING PAIN

Most people have been brought up in our culture to think of pain as a sensation in the form of input, like vision, or hearing. Pain is not a sensation.[111]

BENJAMIN L. CRUE, M.D.

INTRODUCTION AND STUDY GUIDE

How would you define pain? Take a pencil and paper *now* and try to write a definition that would accurately describe this very individual, yet universal phenomenon.

Perhaps your definition included what one dictionary suggests, i.e., that pain is "a feeling of distress, suffering or agony caused by stimulation of specialized nerve endings."[110] However, most likely your thoughts included some more personal words that reflect your own painful *experiences.* The pain *you* have experienced is, after all, the only pain you really *know* about!

We are all aware, of course, that pain exists in others. Yet, ultimately pain is defined by each individual introspectively, in terms of one's own personal experience. Possibly it is most helpful to simply remember, "Pain is what the subject says hurts."[108a]

Nurses are asked for help from people who are experiencing pain — and they are expected to provide relief. This is not always easy. It is to help you with this responsibility that we include this unit. Before studying the following chapters, you may benefit from reviewing related material in basic nursing texts and notes from your introductory nursing classes. (A suggested source of review is Sorensen and Luckmann, *Basic Nursing: A Psychophysiologic Approach.)*

After completing your review, studying the material in this unit, and applying it during your clinical experience, you can expect to be able to meet the following *objectives:*

- Appreciate the subjective nature of pain and thus approach each person experiencing pain as a unique individual.
- Differentiate between the different types of pain.
- Discuss the specificity theory, the pattern theories, and the gate-control theory used to explain pain.
- List and describe the various kinds of regimens currently used in the treatment of pain. Identify the kinds of pain experiences for which each approach is most useful.
- Carry out nursing responsibilities associated with the regimens used today in the treatment of pain.

---

*Ruth McCorkle, R.N., Ph.D., and T. Hongladarom, M.D., critically reviewed and assisted with the revision of this unit.

▶ Establish a therapeutic relationship with a person experiencing pain.

▶ Apply the nursing process successfully when caring for people experiencing pain.

While studying the material that will help you to achieve these objectives, you may find it helpful to use some or all of the following suggestions.

1. Spend some time writing down or talking with someone about the pains you have experienced in your own life. Include such things as: when you had pain and in what circumstances; what you did about the pain; who you told and how you told them about your pain; who helped you, if anyone, and what things actually helped relieve the pain; why you think you had the pain; how you felt about the pain experience at the time and how you feel about it now. Can you really remember exactly what the pain felt like? Discussing or writing about your own pain in this way will help you clarify your own opinions and beliefs about pain. Unless you are aware of your own opinions and beliefs, they may interfere with your nursing care of others.

2. Discuss with others some of the "unanswerable" questions about pain:

Why do people experience pain?
Is there any "purpose" in suffering?
What does pain mean?

Think about each question from a physical, social, emotional and intellectual point of view. Think about how your own moral or spiritual beliefs affect your point of view.

3. Recall some reasons why the pain experience is a complex mind-body experience. Also state in your own words what you know about the various ways that pain is described.

4. There are many different types of pain. Distinguish between the different types. In your own words state what you know about: the function of pain, acute pain, chronic pain, and the evaluation of pain.

5. Summarize in your own words the descriptions of the specificity theory of pain, the pattern theories of pain, and the gate-control theory of pain.

6. Summarize in your own words the ways each of the therapeutic approaches described in this unit contribute to comprehensive pain therapy.

7. Nurses frequently give medications for purposes of pain relief. When studying about pain-relieving medications and their administration, concentrate on how you can most safely and effectively utilize medications to relieve pain. Remember the basic rule for nurses giving medications is to be knowledgeable about the medication *before* administering it. Refer as needed to basic nursing texts, pharmacology texts, and package inserts.

8. Identify and discuss with others the unique contributions nurses can make in helping people who are experiencing or expect to experience pain.

9. Start a file of the nursing care plans you have developed and used when caring for people experiencing pain during your clinical experience. Be sure to include a written evaluation of each plan. As you collect a number of such plans, you will begin to see patterns developing. You will begin to notice similarities and differences in the approaches that were helpful and not helpful for various people at different times. Your clinical work contains extremely important learning experiences for you. The more you can record those experiences and integrate your theoretical learning with them, the more effective your learning will become.

10. Seek information about facilities available in your own community for the treatment of pain. What kinds of pain does each treat? How costly is each treatment regimen? Which treatment regimens are covered by insurance and which ones are not? How would a person gain access to each of the facilities available?

CHAPTER 29

THEORIES AND TYPES OF PAIN

THEORIES OF PAIN MECHANISMS

Concepts of pain mechanisms have changed markedly during this century and particularly during recent decades. Because some of the older theories are still taught today and still appear in books and articles about pain, we discuss them along with the most widely accepted current theory. We discuss in this chapter (1) *specificity theory,* (2) a group of theories called *pattern theories,* and (3) today's prevailing theory, the *gate control theory of pain* (which, in fact, has been built upon some aspects of the earlier theories). We also mention several psychologic theories of pain.

SPECIFICITY THEORY

The specificity theory of pain is still taught today, although one author wrote in 1967, "it is probable that it will soon become untenable."[108] This theory maintains that pain is a specific sensory modality, having its own *specific end-organs (pain receptors), specific sensory fibers in the peripheral nerves, and specific tracts in the central nervous system.* Also, the theory maintains that there is a single "pain center" in the brain. Traditionally, it has been thought that free nerve endings are "pain receptors" that generate "pain impulses," which are carried by specific fibers in peripheral nerves and by the lateral spinothalamic tract in the spinal cord to a "pain center" in the thalamus. However, while recent evidence shows us that somesthetic receptors, fibers, and pathways are specialized for the transmission of particular kinds of information, there is no evidence that allows us to assume that each pathway carries information about a single physical dimension and can give rise to only one psychological sensory dimension (e.g., pain).[105]

Moreover, the idea of "*a* pain center" or "*one* terminal pain center" in the brain has become meaningless, since the thalamus, limbic system, hypothalamus, brain stem reticular formation, parietal cortex, and frontal cortex have all been proven to be a part of pain perception (in addition to those other areas of the brain that are involved in the motor and emotional aspects of the behavior sequence). It has been demonstrated[108] that the stimulation of a single tooth results in the eventual activation of as many as five distinct brain stem pathways. Obviously pain mechanisms are far more complex than the specificity theory's explanation of them.

PATTERN THEORIES

Pattern theories of pain generally maintain that there are *no specific fibers* or specific nerve endings for pain and that the nerve impulse pattern for pain is produced by intensive stimulation of nonspecific receptors. One major type of pattern theory states that essentially all nerve fiber endings are alike, so the pattern for pain recognition by the brain is produced by intense stimulation of nonspecific receptors. Unfortunately, this theory ignores the fact that physiologic evidence has revealed a high degree of receptor-fiber specialization.

Another group of pattern theories introduced certain concepts of *central summation:* Intense pathological stimulation of the body sets up reverberating circuits between various spinal nerve cells. This reverberation intensifies the normally non-noxious nerve impulses and generates abnormal volleys of nerve impulses that are transmitted to the brain and interpreted as pain. Also the concept of a *specialized input-controlling system* was postulated. This system normally prevents summation from occurring. Pathological pain states, then, result from destruction of this system.

While the concepts of central summation and input control were able to explain many of the clinical phenomena of pain, they were criticized because they did not integrate all the diverse theoretical mechanisms into a general theory of pain. Also, these theories did not have substantial experimental verification.

GATE CONTROL THEORY

In recent decades new views of the nature of pain and neural mechanisms have accumulated; these are summarized in the gate control theory, proposed by Melzack and Wall in 1965[106] and extended in 1967 by Casey and Melzack.[25] The gate control theory of pain has been able to explain many pain phenomena that had previously been baffling. Proponents of the gate control theory maintain that the other pain theories do not adequately explain the nature of pain and that they have not been experimentally verified. Nevertheless, some aspects of the earlier theories are part of the gate control theory.

Melzack and Wall's Original Theory

In writing about their new theory of pain mechanisms, Melzack and Wall stated:

> We believe that recent physiological evidence on spinal mechanisms, together with the evidence demonstrating central control over afferent input, provides the basis for a new theory of pain mechanisms that is consistent with the concepts of physiological specialization as well as with those of central summation and input control.[106]

Thus, the gate control theory has retained (a) the concept of physiological specialization within the somesthetic system from the specificity theory, and has retained the concepts of (b) central summation and (c) patterning of input control from the pattern theories.

> *The gate control theory is based on an abundance of observational data and emphasizes that pain depends on a complex balance of various activities rather than the disturbance of a single center. Moreover, the gate control theory recognizes that, in addition to sensory input, many psychologic variables influence the amount and quality of perceived pain.*

In this discussion we refer to "input" and "output." These terms refer to various "impulses" being transmitted in and out of different areas. The impulses are varieties of *electrical activity* in the nerve fibers of the peripheral and central nervous system. There is no "pain impulse," as such; the impulses themselves are not "pain," because pain is actually a psychologic phenomenon. However, the impulses may ultimately come to be interpreted as pain in the brain.[108]

THE GATE

The gate control theory maintains that an area within the spinal cord, known as the *substantia gelatinosa,* acts as a "gating mechanism." The "gate" is controlled, that is, "opened" and "closed," by a relative balance of impulse input from small and from large peripheral nerve fibers. Increased impulse activity in the large fibers partially "closes the gate." Increased small fiber activity acts to "open the gate." This gating mechanism, in turn, influences a group of ascending neurons in the spinal cord, which are called "T cells." The wider the gate is open and the longer it stays open, the greater the number of impulses that will pass through and reach the T cells. When the activity of the T cells reaches a certain critical level, a "pain reaction system," (also called *action system)* in the brain is triggered, and the individual *experiences pain.*

The normal (usual) activity of the substantia gelatinosa is to limit activation of the T cells by keeping the gate partially closed. Thus, *activation of the substantia gelatinosa* means that its usual activity is increased, further shutting the gate through which the impulses pass. On the other hand, *inhibition of the substantia gelatinosa* means that its usual activity is slowed down; the gate then opens and a greater volley of impulses passes through.

Now, keep in mind these two sequences:

1. *Increased* activity of the *large* peripheral nerve fibers causes *activation* of the substantia gelatinosa, thus partially closing the gate and preventing the T cells from triggering or firing the brain's action system. Therefore, increased large fiber activity prevents an awareness of pain.
2. *Increased* activity of the *small* fibers causes *inhibition* of the substantia gelatinosa and facilitates an awareness of pain by opening the gate further. This allows more impulses to pass on to the T cells, where summation may ultimately occur and the brain's action system will be mobilized.

These actions are summarized in Figure 29–1.

It is important to understand that the cells of the substantia gelatinosa modulate afferent nerve impulses *before* they synapse to the T cells. Therefore, the gate control system is *presynaptic.*

CENTRAL CONTROL

It is well known that pain perception is not simply a function of the amount of physical damage done alone, but is also determined by anxiety, past experience, attention and expectation, and the meaning of the situation in which injury occurs. Brain activities such as distraction or anxiety may intervene between stimulus and sensation.[105] In the past it had been assumed that pain is a primary sensation and that these motivational and cognitive processes are secondary considerations, or *reactions to pain.*

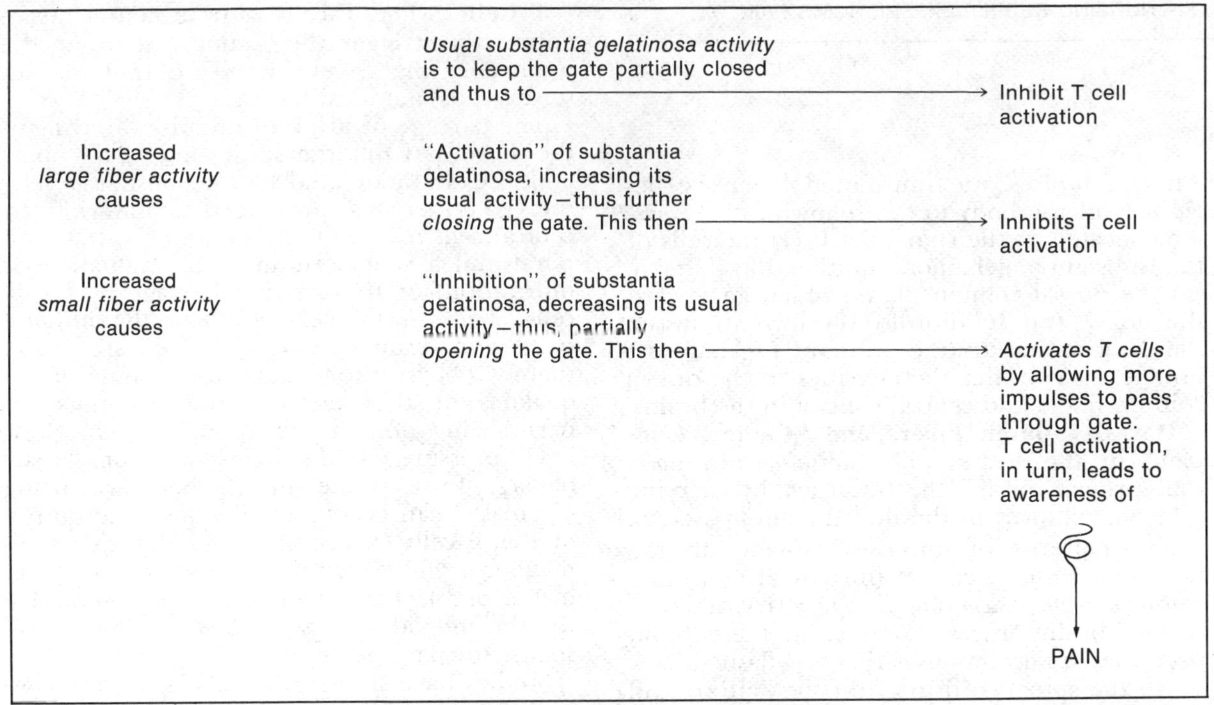

Figure 29–1. Gating mechanism

The gate control theory, however, has postulated a mechanism for the modulation of nerve impulses *before they are transmitted to the brain.* Descending impulses, coming down to the substantia gelatinosa from higher levels of the nervous system (the brain), can modify nerve impulses by influencing the gating mechanism. Thus, the presence or absence of pain is actually determined by a relative balance between the sensory (peripheral nerve) input and the central control (in the brain) input to the gate control system.

As we discuss this theory, locate the components of the gate control mechanism in Figure 29–2.

Impulses evoked by stimulation of the peripheral nerves (sensory input) are transmitted by large and small diameter nerve fibers.

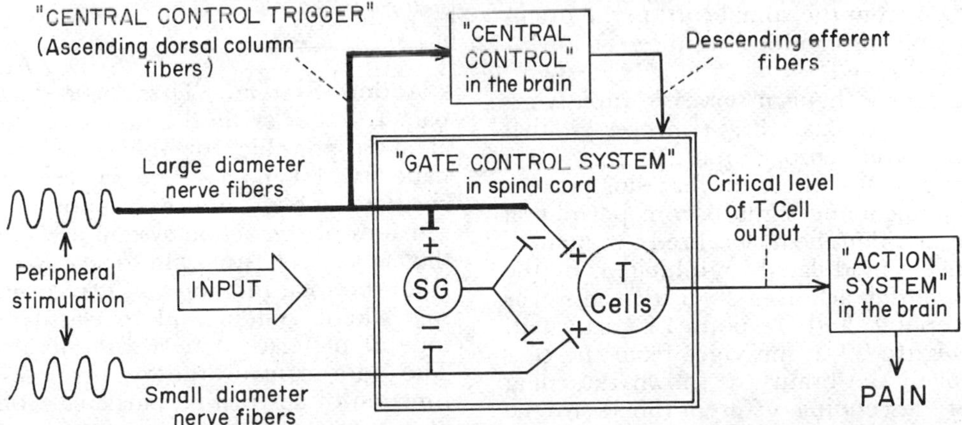

Figure 29–2. Diagram of the gate control theory of pain mechanisms: the large diameter fibers and the small diameter fibers project from the periphery, where they are stimulated, to the substantia gelatinosa (SG) and the (T cells) first transmission cells in the spinal cord. The T cells project to the entry cells of the "action system." Plus (+) equals excitation and minus (−) equals inhibition. The inhibitory effect exerted by SG on the afferent fiber terminals is increased by activity in large fibers and decreased by activity in small fibers. When the T cells are excited to the point that their output exceeds a critical level, the action system in the brain is triggered and pain responses and pain experiences are elicited. (Adapted from Melzack, R., and P. D. Wall: Pain mechanisms: A new theory. *Science*, 150:971, Nov. 1965.)

These impulses are transmitted from the periphery of the body to the following three systems located in the spinal cord: (1) the cells of the substantia gelatinosa in the dorsal horn, (2) the dorsal column fibers, which go toward the brain, and (3) T cells. We have discussed the functioning of the substantia gelatinosa; now let us consider the activities of the dorsal column fibers and central control in the brain.

Dorsal Column Fibers and "Central Control" in the Brain. The *dorsal-column fibers* that project toward the brain act by carrying afferent patterns in the dorsal column system. These patterns of impulses moving up the dorsal column system act (in part at least) as a *central nervous system control trigger* that activates certain brain processes. In turn, these brain processes set up impulses that are flashed back down the spinal cord to affect the gate control system. *This occurs prior to the synapse to the T cells.*

It has been clearly demonstrated that it is possible for stimulation of the brain to activate *descending efferent* fibers so rapidly that they can influence *afferent* conduction at its earliest synaptic levels of the somesthetic system. This means that those nervous system activities that are related to attention, emotion, and memories of prior experience may *actually exert control over sensory input!* Let us pursue this further.

Notice that coming off the large diameter fiber in Figure 29–2 is a heavy line going up to the "central control in the brain." That branch represents certain of the dorsal column fibers that go from the spinal cord to the brain, which are able to conduct impulses at an incredibly rapid speed.

This trigger mechanism serves to rapidly activate those particular brain processes that exert control over sensory input. By racing impulses to the cortex, these mechanisms make it possible for incoming signals from peripheral nerves to be identified, localized, evaluated, and selectively modulated or inhibited, by the brain, *before* the action system that governs pain perception and response is activated! Thus, in Figure 29–2, messages from the central control of the brain are shown returning by way of descending efferent fibers to the gate control system. By "alerting" portions of the brain, this rapidly-conducting system is believed to activate those selective brain processes that will influence information being transmitted up the more slowly conducting pathways or information that is still arriving over slowly conducting fibers.

T Cells. The T cells activate neural mechanisms that trigger the "action system" in the brain once the T cell impulse output reaches (or exceeds) a critical level.

The barrage of afferent impulses arriving at the T cells (from the large and small fibers and already modulated by the substantia gelatinosa) undergoes prolonged monitoring by central cells in the brain. There is both a temporal and a spatial summation (evaluation or integration) of the arriving barrage by the T cells. The central cells evaluate the impulse pattern in terms of both time and space and thereby obtain information about some of the qualities of the sensory input stimulus (or harm being done to the body). In this way, light pressure is distinguished from tissue damage, for example, and the body area being stimulated can be identified. When the output of the T cells exceeds a critical level of summation, it "fires" or triggers the action system in the brain. The action system is responsible for the individual's pain experience, pain response, or pain perception.

Studies have shown that volleys of nerve impulses in *large fibers are extremely effective in initially activating the T cells, but that their later effect is reduced by a negative feedback mechanism.* In contrast, a positive feedback mechanism is activated by volleys in small fibers; this serves to amplify the effect of the arriving impulses. The cells in the substantia gelatinosa mediate these feedback effects as activity in these cells modulates the membrane potential of the afferent fiber terminals and thereby determines the excitatory effect of arriving impulses.

The output of the T cell is centrally monitored over a prolonged period of time, and when a critical intensity is reached or exceeded, the action system is triggered.

Action System. The "action system" (or pain reaction system) consists of those neural areas responsible for the complex sequential patterns of behavior and experience that are characteristic of pain. Perception and response activities of the action system are a function of the capacity of the brain to select out impulses from the total information it receives from the somesthetic system and to classify the multitude of patterns of nerve impulses it receives. The gate control theory proposes that the function of abstracting particular constellations of events from the nerve impulse patterns is aided by certain sets of complex nerve fibers in the spinal cord.

CLINICAL IMPLICATIONS

The clinical implications of the gate control theory are numerous. Many pain phenomena that are difficult to explain in terms of the specificity or patterning theories can be readily explained by the gate control theory. All of the following "pain phenomena" have been explained by researchers by applying concepts of the interacting gate control and action systems:

- Hyperalgesia, for example, hyperalgesia following traumatic peripheral nerve lesions or in some of the neuropathies such as postherpetic neuralgia.
- Congenital insensitivity to pain; referred pain, spread of pain.
- Spontaneous pain in the absence of stimulation, e.g., the pains of anesthesia dolorosa and the 'spontaneous' pains that develop after peripheral nerve and dorsal root lesions.
- Long delays between stimulation and the perception of pain (as much as 10 seconds), which are characteristic of pathological pain syndromes.
- The relief from phantom pain obtained by some amputees by tapping the stump gently with a rubber mallet.
- Trigger points distant from the original site of body injury which may precipitate pain when stimulated.

To illustrate how the gate-control theory can explain various pain phenomena, consider the following example.

If the smaller peripheral nerve fibers are relatively intact, but there is a selective destruction of the large fibers, as in *alcoholic* or *diabetic neuropathy,* the normal presynaptic inhibition of the input by the gate-control system does not occur. The input arriving over the remaining smaller fibers is, therefore, transmitted through the unchecked, open gate and would provide the basis for intense, pathological pain. Also, since the total number of peripheral fibers is reduced, it may take a considerable time before the T cells can be "wound up" to the discharge level necessary to trigger pain. This would account for the delays often observed in pathological pain states. Similar mechanisms are believed to account for neuralgic pains.

Sensory mechanisms by themselves cannot sufficiently explain why it is that nerve lesions do not always produce pain or why, when they do, the pain is usually not continuous in nature. The gate control theory proposes that the presence or absence of pain is determined by the balance between the sensory *and* the central inputs to the gate control system. In addition to the sensory influences on the gate control systems, there is an input to the system from higher levels of the central nervous system that exerts an inhibitory affect on the sensory input. Thus, any lesion that impairs the normal downflow of impulses to the gate control system would open the gate. For example, central nervous system lesions associated with hyperalgesia and spontaneous pain could have this effect. Any central nervous system condition that increases the flow of descending impulses would tend, on the other hand, to close the gate.

THERAPEUTIC IMPLICATIONS

The therapeutic implications of the gate control therapy of pain include the following:

1. This theory suggests that the control of pain might be achieved by selectively influencing the large, rapidly conducting fibers. Decreasing the small fiber input and enhancing the large fiber input may close the gate. Also, any procedure that cuts down the sensory input lessens the opportunity for summation and pain.
2. A better understanding of the physiology and pharmacology of the substantia gelatinosa may lead to new ways of controlling pain by means of drugs that affect the excitation or inhibition of substantia gelatinosa activity.

Casey and Melzacks's Elaboration of the Gate Control Theory

A second diagram, relating the gate control system to the *sensory-discriminative, motivational-affective,* and *central control determinants* of pain, is presented in Figure 29–3. Pain has both sensory and affective components. It represents the result of at least two neuropsychologic processes: (a) A *sensory discriminative process* by which stimuli are recognized by the brain in terms of space, time, and along an intensity continuum; and (b) A *motivational-affective component* that sets the organism into activity aimed at stopping the pain as quickly as possible.

We have already discussed the *central control* processes that are activated by the dorsal column fibers ascending to the brain. Let us add here, in reference to these processes, that the neocortical (or higher central nervous system) processes that we have mentioned (i.e., evaluation of the input in terms of past experience) control activity in both the sensory-discriminative and motivational-affective systems.

Consider the effects of the T cell output at the brain level as related to the sensory and motivational aspects of pain. The output of the dorsal horn T cells is transmitted toward the brain by fibers in the spinal cord and ultimately is projected into two major brain systems:

1. The ventrobasal nuclei of the thalamus and the somatosensory cortex by way of the neospinothalamic tract
2. The reticular core of the brain stem and the medial thalamus by way of the paramedial ascending system.

- The classical neospinothalamic projecting system in the brain functions by providing information about the location of peripheral stimulation in space, in time, and along an intensity continuum. It thus provides *sensory-discriminative* information about pain.
- Those impulses that are transmitted into the reticular core of the brain stem and the medial thalamus from the spinothalamic tract by way of the paramedial ascending system, activate reticular and limbic systems which provoke the powerful *motivational* drive and unpleasant *affect* that trigger the organism into action.

It is believed that the three categories of activity just discussed (the sensory-discriminative, motivational-affective, and central control determinants of pain) interact with each other to provide *perceptual information* regarding such factors as: the location, magnitude, and spatiotemporal properties of the noxious stimulus; motivational tendency toward escape or attack; and cognitive information based on analysis of multimodal information, past experience, and probability of outcome of different kinds of response strategies. These three forms of activity are thus believed to influence the motor mechanisms that produce the complex pattern of overt responses that characterize pain.

What are some of these *overt responses which characterize pain?* Although everyone who has experienced pain is familiar with them, let us briefly list some typical responses to pain. For example, some overt responses which occur after unexpected, sudden damage to the skin are:[105]

a. A startle response
b. A withdrawal reflex
c. Postural readjustment
d. Vocalization
e. Orientation of the head and eyes to examine the damaged area
f. Autonomic responses
g. Talking about past experiences in similar situations and prediction of what the consequences of the stimulation might be, i.e., "Maybe I'll have to have stitches."
h. Many other patterns of behavior that are aimed at reducing the sensory and affective aspects of the whole experience, e.g., avoidance behavior, rubbing the damaged area.

During all of this activity, the perceptual awareness that accompanies these events changes in intensity and quality.

Clinical and Therapeutic Implications. As we have observed, the gate control theory notes that past experience, attention, emotion, and other psychologic factors influence pain perception and pain response by acting on the gate control system. Let us see how these facts

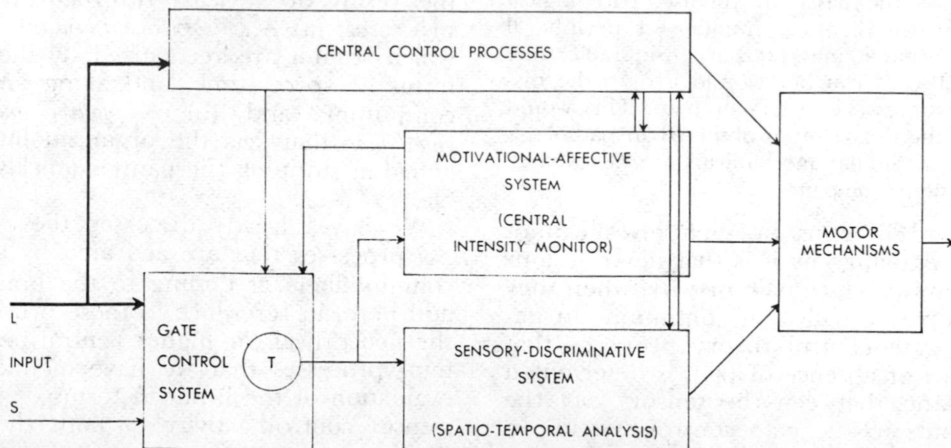

Figure 29–3. Conceptual model of the sensory, motivational, and central control determinants of pain. The output of the T cells of the gate control system projects to the sensory-discriminative system (via neospinothalamic fibers) and the motivational-affective system (via the paramedial ascending system). The central control trigger (comprising the dorsal-column and dorsolateral projection systems) is represented by the heavy line running from the large fiber input to the central control processes. These, in turn, project back to the gate control system, and to the sensory-discriminative and motivational-affective systems. All three systems interact with one another, and project to the motor system. (From Melzack, R., and K. L. Casey: *In* Kemshalo, D. (Ed.): *International Symposium on the Skin Senses.* Springfield, Ill.: Charles C Thomas, 1967.)

can be *clinically applied.* While some factors may affect both the sensory-discrimination and affective-motivational experiences, others may primarily modify the affective-motivational dimension of pain. For example, the excitement of games or that of war seems to block both dimensions of pain; suggestion and placebos appear to modulate the motivational-affective dimension while barely disturbing the sensory-discriminative system. Finally, the balance between sensory facilitation and central inhibition of the input after a peripheral-nerve lesion could account for the variability of pain even in those situations where the injury is severe. Thus, while one person may have excruciating pain following a severe injury, another may feel no pain or only slight pain.

A final *therapeutic implication* that the extended gate control theory suggests is that pain therapy should be based on more than just surgical intervention, anesthetic block, or any other measures aimed only at blocking "pain pathways or fibers." In addition to such "sensory" maneuvers, the motivational and cognitive aspects of the pain experience must be considered and treated.

The historical emphasis on sensory mechanisms has caused the motivational and cognitive processes that are part of pain perception to be neglected in pain management. It is now recognized that tranquilizers, relaxants, sedatives, placebos, and many feeling states — anxiety, suggestion, hypnosis, fear, apprehension, motivation, psychiatric disorders, and others—all influence pain. Moreover, it is realized that many of these emotional states are determined by early experience, religious beliefs, culture, prior conditioning, and other psychodynamic mechanisms. A comprehensive approach to pain therapy today, recognizing the gate control theory of pain mechanisms, will integrate motivational and cognitive considerations.

PSYCHOLOGIC THEORIES OF PAIN

In addition to main physiological theories of pain discussed, there are several psychological theories.

Merskey and Spear observe that, "As the physiological theories of pain have been developed primarily to account for situations where there is bodily dysfunction, so the psychological theories which have been elaborated are related to the need to account for situations where there is little or no bodily disturbance and the pain appears to be closely related to psychological states.[108] The three principal psychological theories that they list are:

1. That pain is a consequence of hostility, either as a substitute following the repression of hostility or as an expression of guilt for overt hostility.
2. That pain arises in patients of a certain personality type, called "pain-prone," who use the complaint of pain as a means of communication and of emotional expression.
3. That pain arises as a consequence of a threat to the integrity of the body. Here the body is regarded as an object of concern to the self. The pain will be classed as "psychogenic" when the threat is not apparent to an outside observer.

The hostility hypothesis is the most widely accepted of the psychological theories.

TYPES OF PAIN

It is important for nurses to realize that there are many different types of pain, so they can more knowledgeably participate in the specific treatment and nursing assessment and nursing care of persons experiencing pain.

Pain is one of the most common and universal experiences of human beings, and there have been numerous attempts to understand its action.

There are various ways of discussing types of pains. For example, pain may be referred to in terms of:

Onset or time of occurrence, e.g., "postoperative"* pain.

- *Duration or length of time* experienced, e.g., "chronic pain" or "acute pain," and *"intensity of pain,"* e.g., "severe pain," "mild pain."
- *Force or agent causing pain to occur,* e.g., "spontaneous pain," "self-inflicted pain," or "other-inflicted pain."
- *Mode of transmission,* e.g., "projected or referred pain."
- *Ease of transmission,* e.g., "facilitated pain" or "inhibited pain."
- *Location or source,* e.g., "pain from the gallbladder" or "superficial, deep or central pains."
- *Symptoms or manner in which pain is experienced,* e.g., "sharp pain," "burning pain."
- *Causation,* e.g., "organic pain," "pretended pain," "psychogenic pain," "psychophysiologic pain."

Here we discuss (1) acute and chronic pain, (2) source of pain, (3) deep pain syndromes, (4)

*See Unit VIII for a discussion of postoperative pain.

pretended, psychogenic, and psychophysiologic pains, and (5) facilitated and inhibited pains.

ACUTE PAIN AND CHRONIC PAIN

One useful way to consider pain is by types based upon pathology and duration. There appear to be two distinct types of pain in relation to duration — acute pain and chronic pain.

In general, *acute pain* is temporary, has immediate onset, and eventually subsides after treatment, or often without treatment. Examples of acute pain are the pains of traumatic injury, ordinary headache, and renal colic. Acute pain may be useful in that it causes the sufferer to attempt to determine its cause and to seek relief, e.g., to notice that his or her finger is on a hot stove and to pull it away.

Figure 29–4 illustrates that as pain increases so does a person's anxiety, until a certain point is reached. Then the individual does something to obtain relief, before the pain becomes even more severe.

In contrast to acute pain, *chronic pain* is continual, may begin gradually, persists or recurs for an indefinite period, and is more difficult to manage effectively. Examples of chronic pains are those caused by trigeminal neuralgia, severe rheumatoid arthritis, and advanced cancer. Chronic pain is often frustrating and difficult to live with, since it gives patients no clue as to how to lessen it. Similarly, health care providers also experience frustration and a sense of failure when their attempts to manage chronic pain are ineffective.

An individual's mental reaction to pain depends on the duration of the pain and, to a far lesser extent, its intensity.

> *Pain that is constant, continuous, and moderate is much more difficult to bear than that which is paroxysmal and intense.*

Persons who experience a continuous sensation of pain (e.g., in anesthesia dolorosa*) tend to become increasingly engrossed by their illness, fearful, tense, depressed, and may appear somewhat mentally withdrawn. On the other hand, persons experiencing *acute* attacks of intense pain may come to terms with their periods of pain; although they may have an agonized appearance at the time of an attack, they appear normal between attacks.

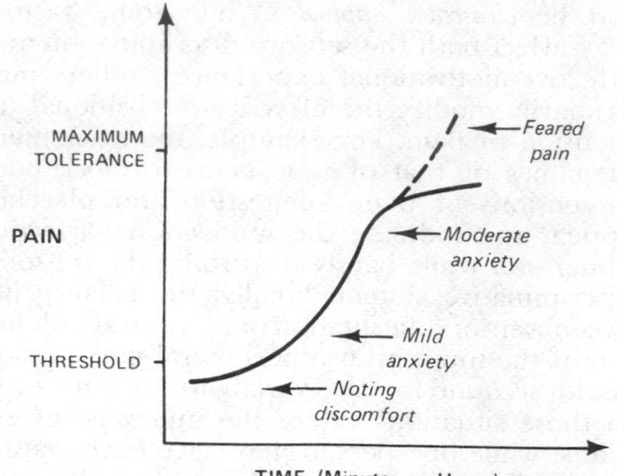

Figure 29–4. Sequence of reactions to acute pain. (From Sternbach, R. A.: *Pain Patients—Traits and Treatment.* New York: Academic Press, 1974, p. 6.)

Pains caused by cancer vary in their intensity, but they rarely, if ever, reach the *severity* of some of the other pains that humans suffer, e.g., the pains of tic douloureux or of renal colic. Thus, rather than the intensity of long-term pains, it is their *chronic and prolonged natures* which at times make them exhausting and virtually unbearable. Let us emphasize again that not all persons with cancer experience pain. However, when pain is present and is persistent, it drags the patient on a downhill course often manifested by emotional deterioration, insomnia, anorexia, weight loss, and loss of strength.

Figure 29–5 depicts the course of chronic pain — months and years of pain — not minutes or hours. Chronic pain is associated with

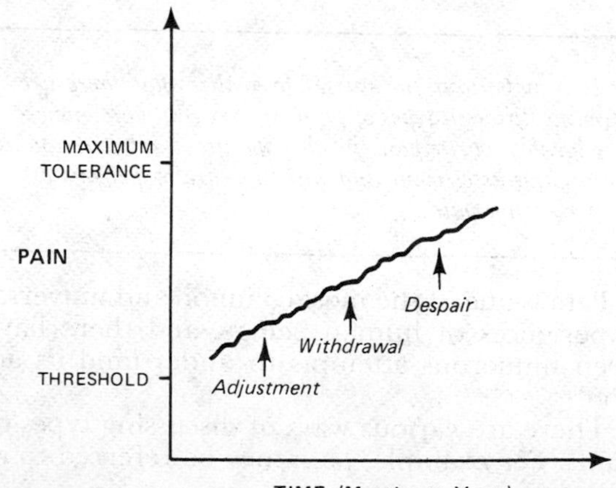

Figure 29–5. Sequence of reactions to chronic pain. (From Sternbach, R. A.: *Pain Patients—Traits and Treatment.* New York: Academic Press, 1974, p. 8.)

**Anesthesia dolorosa* is a condition occurring in paralysis or in some spinal cord diseases in which there is tactile anesthesia with severe pain in the part.

withdrawal and despair; anxiety has given way to depression.

Extremely intense pain is unlikely to be felt over a long period, because such pain usually means that the nerve endings themselves are being destroyed. Once nerve endings are destroyed, pain is likely to cease or at least diminish in intensity. However, an important exception occurs with causalgia (see p. 719), when the nerve trunk itself is damaged and intense pain is experienced over long periods.

> *Pains caused by* organic *diseases are seldom constant in nature; rather, they vary because the organic etiologic factors fluctuate and also because nerve centers periodically tire. Often, although not always, a patient's pain is diagnosed as* psychoneurotic *in origin if the patient says that the same pain is constantly present.*

Intractable, chronic pain states, producing *prolonged* and *intense* bombardment of the central nervous system, can destroy the sufferer. These pain states "may too often — and not unexpectedly — terminate in a self-dissolution of life."[71] This mental state is typified in the final entry that was made in the *Journal* of Alice James (sister to Henry James) two days before her death:

> I am being ground slowly on the grim grindstone of physical pain, and on two nights I had almost asked for K's lethal dose; but one steps hesitantly along such unaccustomed ways, and endures from second to second.

Recently most clinicians and researchers agree that psychologic and sociocultural factors influence how a person experiences pain; however, there is still little consensus about the specific ways in which these factors operate.

Pain has been defined in many ways. Sternbach, who defines pain broadly, says that pain is "an abstract concept which refers to (1) a personal, private sensation of hurt, (2) a harmful stimulus which signals current or impending tissue damage; and (3) a pattern of responses which operate to protect the organism from harm."[143] This definition is useful for our discussion because it encompasses the subjectivity of the pain experience and it also includes two components of pain - "a sensory stimulus" and "a response."

SOURCE OF PAIN

The source of pain determines the descriptive sensory characteristics of pain. Three general pain sources are considered: (1) *cutaneous,* which includes superficial somatic structures located in skin and subcutaneous tissue; (2) *deep somatic,* which includes bone, nerve, muscle, and other tissues supporting these structures, and (3) *viscera,* which includes all body organs located in the body cavities.

Cutaneous or Superficial Pain Sources. Cutaneous (superficial) pain is sometimes called "direct pain" because the pain accurately localizes the point of disturbance. Two types of cutaneous pain have been described: (1) pain with an *abrupt onset* and a burning quality and (2) pain of *slower onset,* with a burning quality. Cutaneous pain may be delineated by having the patient point to the painful area. Cutaneous pain may occur along dermatomes, each segment representing a portion of the body surface innervated by one dorsal root (refer to Figure 26–14, p. 557). The area of skin supplied by one dorsal root is a *dermatome,* or skin segment. Although the boundaries may be shown as distinct in drawings, there is actually an overlap of nerve distribution; irritation of one posterior root, e.g., T6, will give rise to pain experienced in the adjacent dermatomes, T5 and T7, as well as T6.[52]

Cutaneous pain is relatively uncomplicated, since it is directly perceived and can readily be localized. Therefore we turn our attention to the more complicated phenomena of pain in the deep somatic structures and viscera. See Table 29–1 for comparison of deep pain with cutaneous pain. The main difference between cutaneous and deep sensibility is the different nature of the pain evoked by noxious stimuli. Unlike cutaneous pain, *deep pain* (a) is poorly localized; (b) produces nausea; and (c) is frequently associated with sweating and changes in blood pressure.

Deep Somatic Pain Sources. Pain arising from deep somatic structures varies individually by degrees of pain sensitivity. Highly sensitive structures include tendons, deep fascia, ligaments, joints, bone periosteum, blood vessels, and nerves. The sensitivity of skeletal muscle is limited to stretching and ischemia. Bone and cartilage respond only to extreme pressures. In general, deep somatic pain is diffuse because the *scleratome,* or area supplied by one posterior nerve root, is less well defined than a dermatome and does not correspond with a dermal segment. Pain from deep structures frequently radiates from the primary site, e.g., pain from a lumbar disk travels along the sciatic nerve.

Visceral Pain Sources. A *viscus* (*viscera* is the plural form) is any of the large interior body organs occupying one of the body's cavities, e.g., the cranial, thoracic, abdominal, or pelvic cavity. The word *splanchnic* pertains to the viscera. Thus, *visceral pain may also be called splanchnic*

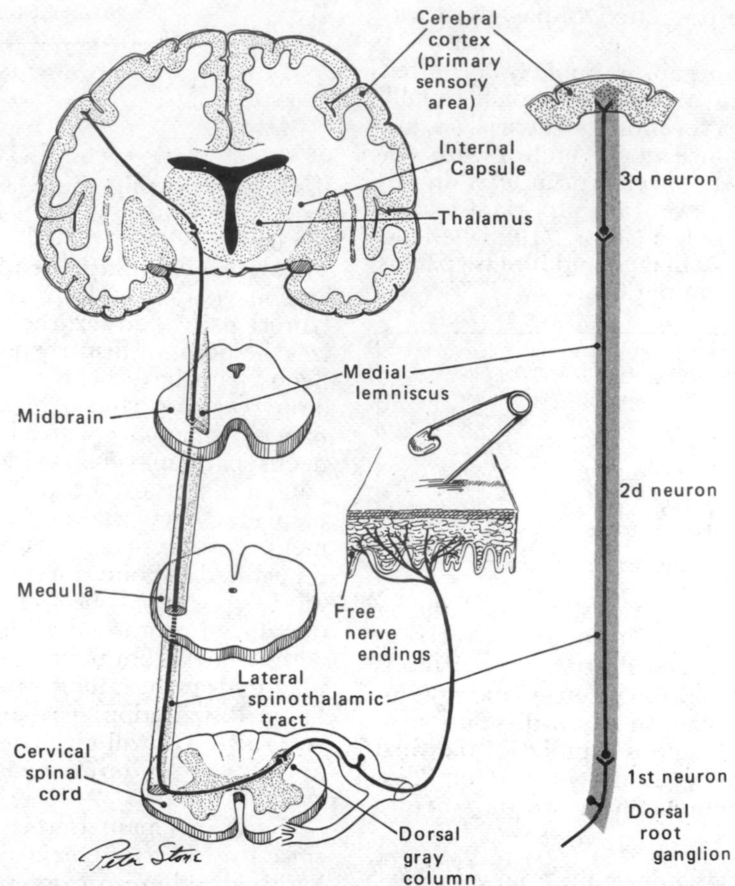

The central pathway for impulses perceived as pain, the lateral spinothalamic tract. Note that the fibers cross upon entering the spinal cord. (From: Langley, L. L., I. R. Telford, and J. B. Christensen: *Dynamic Anatomy and Physiology*, 4th ed. New York: McGraw-Hill Book Co., 1974, p. 271.)

TABLE 29–1. COMPARISON BETWEEN CUTANEOUS AND DEEP PAIN

Cutaneous Pain	Deep Pain
Associated symptoms may be hyperalgesia, paresthesia, tickling, or itching. Also associated with brisk movements, a quick pulse, and a sense of invigoration.	*Associated symptoms* due to autonomic responses include: pallor, sweating, nausea, vomiting, and, at times, bradycardia, fall in blood pressure, syncope, faintness, and perhaps even death in shock. Also associated with quiescence and sometimes local muscular rigidity of the abdominal wall.
Nausea never occurs.	*Nausea* ("sickening pain") is found only when deep structures are involved, e.g., in renal and intestinal colic, gallstones, and angina.
Quality of pain is a sharp, bright sensation felt superficially.	*Quality* of pain is primarily dull, aching. May be described as boring, crushing, throbbing, or cramping, or, if less intense, as a soreness or hurting.
Duration is typically shorter than deep pain.	*Duration* is often fairly long.
Localization tends to be more precise than with deep pain. Pain is often experienced as a point, surface, or line.	*Localization* is often diffuse and inaccurate; seems to originate in a fairly broad area. Pain frequently is felt as if it were of three dimensions and occupied space.
Hyperalgesia of a primary nature may occur with superficial pain. The hyperalgesia occurs at the site of the original noxious stimulation.	*Hyperalgesia* secondary in nature may exist with deep pain, occurring at a distance from the original noxious stimulus. Thus, in referred pain, a superficial hyperalgesia may be associated with deep pain.
	Muscle contraction and tenderness occur often.
	Segmental spread of pain is frequently noted. Pain may not remain confined to the original spinal segment but may spread into one or more adjacent segments.

pain. Usually the term *viscera* refers to the abdominal viscera.

Pain within the viscera also tends to be diffuse; however, it may become more localized if it persists. Nerve fibers innervating body organs follow the sympathetic nerves to the spinal cord. This may account for the fact that autonomic symptoms frequently accompany visceral pain. Some typical visceral pains that are discussed more completely in appropriate chapters of the book are the pains of acute appendicitis; cholecystitis; inflammations of the biliary-pancreatic tract; gastroduodenal disease; cardiovascular disease; pleurisy; and renal and ureteral colic.

Most of the viscera are not sensitive to those stimuli that excite pain in somatic structures (such as cutting, burning, or pressure). This is understandable, since the viscera are not normally exposed to such trauma, and the body does not "need" a response system.[72] Although these types of stimuli do not produce pain in most of the viscera, other stimuli, such as violent or abnormal contractions of hollow viscera (like the ureters and alimentary tract), may cause severe pain.

DEEP PAIN SYNDROMES

Pain arising from structures deeper than the surface structures is termed *deep pain.* Three varieties occur: (1) *true visceral (splanchnic)* and *deep somatic pain,* which is felt at the point of noxious stimulation and may or may not be associated with referred pain, (2) *referred pain,* which is pain experienced at a site other than the area of stimulus, and (3) pain from *secondary skeletal muscle contraction.*

At this point let us look more closely at pains of muscular origin, vascular pains, and pains due to inflammation.

Pains of Muscular and Bony Origin

The primary cause of muscle pain is believed to be not muscle tension itself, but rather the compression or constriction of blood vessels within the muscle or traction on the periosteum. The sustained clenching of muscles or their continued overwork may produce muscular pain.

Ligaments, joint capsules, fascia, tendons, and muscle all vary in the density of their innervation; the periosteum is the most sensitive.

Spontaneous pain may be induced by spasms, rupture, ischemia, inflammation, or other disturbances of the ligaments, tendons, muscles, and periosteum of bones and joints.

While chemical irritants injected into muscles may give rise to considerable pain, the usual ways in which muscular pains occur are in association with stretching, ischemia, or forceful or sustained contractile activity.

When muscle pain causes a sustained reflex contraction of the muscle, a vicious circle of pain may occur. The contraction successively increases muscular pain and the pain gradually radiates into adjacent areas.

A large proportion of headaches, especially those accompanied by stiffness or tenderness in the neck and occipital region, originate from sustained contraction of underlying neck muscles. (See p. 652, Chapter 27, for discussion of headache.)

Muscular ischemia induces pain in the extremities in intermittent claudication and occlusive vascular disease and is the basis of the pain of coronary occlusion.

Vascular Pains

The precise vascular pain mechanism is not understood, but it is believed to originate from some pathologic condition of the vessels or perivascular tissues. Also considered of importance is the participation of some pain-producing chemical substances.

The blood vessels are frequently involved with the mediation of pain. Blood vessels are believed to be associated with pain induced by cold. Also, distortion of cranial vessels by pulling, displacement, or distention is the source of a large proportion of headaches, including migraine and those headaches associated with arterial hypertension, brain tumor, and variations in the hydrodynamics of the cerebrospinal fluid.

Other Deep Pains

Inflammation induces a hyperalgesic state in the affected tissue. Inflammation is one of the commonest pathologic conditions that influence pain sensitivity.

Pain in the alimentary tract is a common medical occurrence and appears to emanate mainly from the muscular and serous coats. Such pains are believed to occur when the intestinal mucosa is inflamed, ulcerated, or otherwise abnormal, or when the visceral muscles contract strongly or pass into spasm. Thus, although the wall of the intestine itself may be insensitive to cutting, burning, or crushing, it does produce pain under other conditions.

The *parietal peritoneum,* the *mesentery,* and many *blood vessels* are sensitive to injuries such as cutting, stretching, and handling. Also, the *mucosal linings* of the urethra, bladder, ureters, and kidney pelvis are sensitive to pain.

Abdominal pain may also be caused by the *perforation of body organs,* with the result that their contents drain into the peritoneal cavity. The various kinds of intraperitoneal fluid that may accumulate are listed here, in order from the most irritating to the least irritating:[45a]

1. Pancreatic enzyme fluid
2. Gastric or duodenal fluid

3. Fecal fluid
   a. Colon
   b. Appendiceal
   c. Small bowel
4. Bile
5. Urine
6. Blood
7. Lymph

In the chest, the parietal pleura is richly supplied with pain endings through the intercostal nerves, and on the diaphragmatic surface, by the phrenic nerve as well. The visceral pleura in the chest, however, is insensitive to pain. Elsewhere and throughout their serous surfaces, both the visceral and parietal pericardia are insensitive to pain, with the exception that the lower portion of the fibrous pericardium appears to be supplied with pain fibers from the phrenic nerve.

Referred Pain

Whereas deep pain may arise from disease of the viscera or from a lesion of a deep somatic structure (such as one of the vertebrae, a muscle, or an interspinous ligament), both visceral and somatic pain may be, and in fact usually are, referred to a segment of the skin. The referral of pain to a segment of the skin is clearly illustrated in herpes zoster, in which inflammation of the ganglion of a particular posterior nerve root (lying beside the spinal column) causes lesions and sensations to appear on the surface of the body on the segment of skin that is innervated by the affected nerve (see Chapter 27, p. 599.)

Referred pain is curious because in some instances it may be intense, whereas there may be little or no pain *in situ*, i.e., at the point of noxious stimulation. In other situations, the *in situ* pain may predominate. Referred pain may occur with or without hyperalgesia (excessive sensitivity to pain), and in the presence or absence of pain or tenderness due to secondary muscle spasm.

Identification of the segment of the spinal cord that is involved in transmitting the pain is diagnostically helpful. Pain arising from a deep structure, whether a viscus or a deep somatic structure, will have a *referred segmental distribution,* or pattern of pain, that is determined according to the segment of the spinal cord supplying the structure.

> *Referred pain due to visceral disease follows dermatome patterns, whereas somatic referred pain does not.*

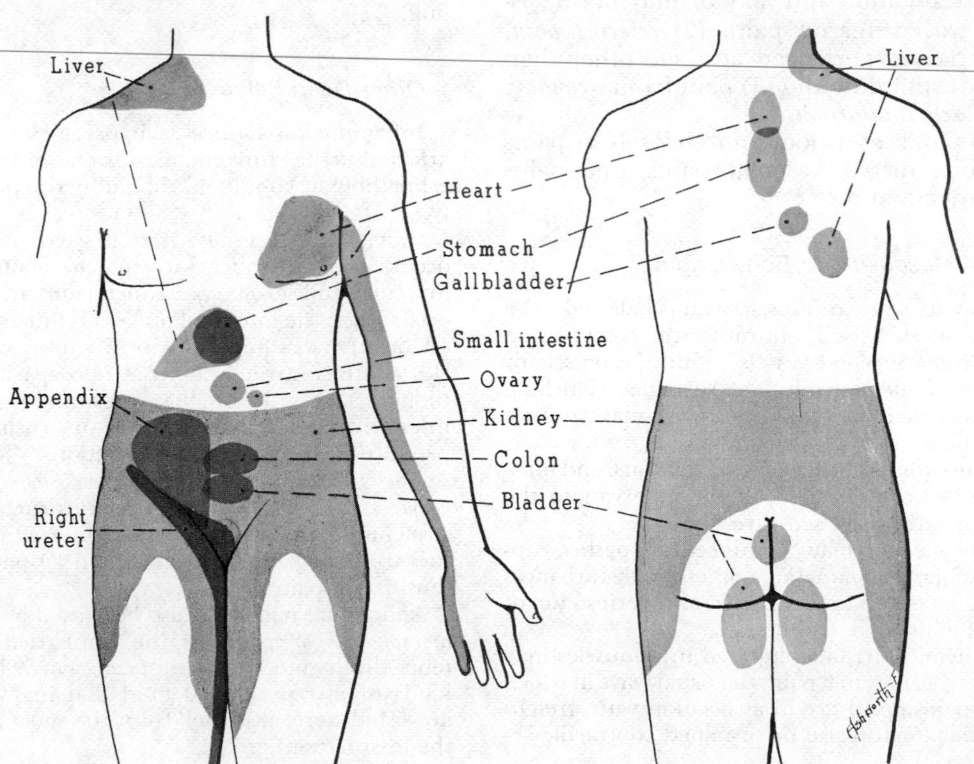

Figure 29–6. Some areas of referred pain, anterior and posterior views. (From Jacob, S. W., C. A. Francone, and W. J. Lossow: *Structure and Function in Man,* 4th ed. Philadelphia: W. B. Saunders Co., 1978, p. 290.)

Referred pains are often baffling and call for a careful differential diagnosis. Examples of common patterns include: the pain of coronary heart disease felt in the left axilla or radiating down the inside of the left arm; pleural pain of the diaphragm felt in the shoulder; and pain of cholecystitis felt in the back and in the angle of the scapula. Figure 29–6 illustrates common sites of referred pain.

It is important for nurses to be familiar with areas of referred pain not only so they themselves may more clearly understand the symptoms of given patients, but also so they can help interpret referred pains to specific patients. For example, if a patient known to have gallstones is experiencing pain in the region of the scapulae in the upper back, the nurse can explain that this is a not uncommon referred pain pattern. *Understanding* the pain may reduce a patient's anxiety and thus may help reduce the pain. Also, the nurse should know that increased pain may occur if the area of referred pain (or the organ from which the pain is referred) is stimulated.[92]

Central Pain Syndromes

Causalgias, phantom limb pains, and central pains are sometimes spoken of collectively as "central pain syndromes," even though their etiologies differ.

Causalgia is sometimes listed separately from central pain, but the fact remains that *causalgia, phantom limb pain,* and *central pain* are all related because all three have autonomic manifestations. Thus, despite having widely differing etiologies, these disorders have a striking similarity of underlying pathophysiologic mechanisms and clinical features.

Central pain syndromes have been clinically observed to have the following factors in common:[108, 119]

- All patients with central pain complain of pain that is present in the absence of peripheral stimulation or of an obvious pathologic process to account for the pain.
- Peripheral stimulation will usually change the pain in those areas in which the pain is localized.
- All types of stimuli cause pain, including those that do not evoke pain when they are applied to normal areas in the same patient.
- Although the change in cutaneous sensibility may occur in a variety of ways, the main common denominator is that there is damage to the afferent pathways.*
- There is frequently total loss of sensory communication from the part to which the pain is referred. Thus, sensations appear to arise in a part in which central afferent connections have been severed. When viewed in this manner causalgia and central pain are somewhat "phantom-like," even though they differ from true phantom limb pain in which feelings are perceived in an absent part of the body.

Syndromes with the above features are called central pain syndromes because the damage is central to the peripheral receptors.

Lesions of the peripheral somatic afferent nerves are included within this definition. "These conditions may be found with traumatic lesions of peripheral nerves such as causalgia, lesions of the spinal cord, vascular lesions of the brainstem, the thalamus syndrome, certain subcortical or even cortical lesions."[119] Another example is postherpetic neuralgia (discussed later).

Let us now proceed to examine some of the specific types of pain that we have just been referring to, namely: central pain, causalgia, and phantom limb pain. Treatment for these painful conditions is discussed.

Central Pain. In the past, central pain was believed to be primarily produced by lesions *within* the CNS that *directly* affected the pain pathways.

Recently some authors have enlarged the definition of "central pain" to include sensations of pain arising from within the nervous system itself, regardless of the location (to include "all lesions central to the nerve endings"[119]). Central pain states are often associated with diseases or injuries that directly affect the neurons, their processes, and synapses. These states seem to divide into two distinct clinical syndromes: *episodic* and *constant* (Table 29–2).

Tic douloureux, a prototype of *episodic* pain, is unique because of its responsiveness to denervating procedures. These pains usually have a trigger area which produces pain when lightly stimulated; attacks are characterized by sudden onset and rapid termination. (See p. 676, Chapter 27.)

The *constant* forms of central pain are associated with damage to the CNS, usually at the peripheral nerve level. *Thalamic pain* is the only exception to the peripheral location of disease. Lesions producing central pain may involve the spinothalamic tract at any level from the spinal

---

**Afferent* nerves transmit impulses from the periphery toward the central nervous system, i.e., sensory nerves; *efferent* nerves transmit impulses from the central nervous system toward the periphery.

TABLE 29–2. CENTRAL PAINS

Episodic
1. Tic douloureux
2. Tabes dorsalis
3. Multiple sclerosis (some)
4. Postparaplegia pains (some)
Constant
1. Postherpetic neuralgia
2. Intercostal neuralgia
3. Post-thoracotomy neuralgia
4. Atypical facial pain
5. Thalamic syndrome
6. Causalgia
7. Peripheral neuropathies (some)
8. Multiple sclerosis (some)
9. Postparaplegia pains (some)
10. Anesthesia dolorosa
11. Phantom limb pain
12. Reflex sympathetic dystrophy

Loesser, J. D.: Central pains. *Clinical Medicine,* 82:25, May 1975.

cord to the thalamus, as well as the thalamocortical radiations from the thalamus to the cerebral cortex.

Central pain is typically *experienced as*: spontaneous; variable in severity, although usually constantly present; and subject to spontaneous aggravation, although its intensity may also be increased by such specific stimuli as sudden temperature changes, anxiety, and emotional stress. Overreaction to stimuli may occur, so that normally nonpainful stimuli may be experienced as painful. Also, there may be an unusually prolonged time lag between the initiation of a painful stimulus and the feeling of pain. Moreover, the feeling of pain may then long outlast the stimulus. Frequently signs of autonomic dysfunction (such as increased perspiration, cyanosis, and lowered skin temperature) may accompany the pain. While many people with central pain find it difficult to describe the quality of their sensations, others refer to their pains as boring, cold, burning, aching, or gnawing.

The *mechanism* by which central pain occurs is not precisely known, but it is speculated that "irritation" at the lesion site and/or "reduction of central inhibition" are important factors. Also, since *psychologic stress obviously aggravates central pain,* it is believed that regardless of what the specific pain mechanism is, pain production is somehow connected (in the highest integrative levels of the brain) to those neurologic circuits relating to emotions.

POSTHERPETIC NEURALGIA. One type of central pain that presents some interesting histologic changes in nerve structure is *postherpetic neuralgia.* Following the extremely painful acute vesicular eruption of herpes zoster, and after these vesicles have subsided and disappeared, some patients experience a persistent, severe, intractable pain within the area of the original skin eruption, or postherpetic neuralgia. This pain syndrome is one of the most annoying and tormenting, with the unrelenting pain causing sleepless nights and virtually unbearable days. Patients may be willing to undergo any treatment in hopes of relief. However, the results of therapy may be poor, and the postherpetic pain may be intractable to all forms of treatment.

The cause of the persistent pain in postherpetic neuralgia is not fully understood. However, scarring and degenerative changes involving the spinal cord, ganglia, nerve trunks, and skin may be important factors in this pain problem.

SPINAL CORD LESIONS. *Spinal cord lesions,* which may produce central pain, may arise from syringomyelia, trauma to the spinal cord, and spinal cord tumors.

BRAIN STEM LESIONS. *Brain stem lesions* may produce central pain that has a crossed pain pattern such that the face is involved on the side of the lesion (i.e., "ipsilateral" facial pain) while the trunk and limbs are affected on the side opposite the lesion (because of the fact that spinothalamic fibers are involved which cross to innervate the opposite side of the body). Only a small proportion of brain stem lesions produce pain. These lesions are typically those involving the medulla and pons (which contain the descending sensory nucleus of the trigeminal nerve) rather than those in the mesencephalon (which has no sensory nuclei).

THALAMIC LESIONS. *Thalamic lesions,* the most common cause of central pain, typically produce symptoms that affect the side of the body opposite the lesion. Vascular lesions of the thalamus, which involve the lateral nucleus of the thalamus, are the most common thalamic source of central pain. However, tumor, trauma, or inflammation of this area may also produce spontaneous pain. When thalamic infarct or thrombosis occurs, the pains usually do not begin for several weeks. These pains may range from paresthesia to agonizing, boring, burning pains which are often associated with a sensation that the hand or foot is being twisted. Such thalamic pains following thalamic infarct (cerebrovascular accident or stroke) may involve an entire half of the body. The pain, following the stroke by several weeks, is generally most intense in the extremities, especially the hand. Thalamic pain may be intensified by emotional disturbances and increased emotional lability; i.e., unmotivated crying or laughing is often associated with this syndrome.

The syndrome produced by thalamic lesions is referred to as the *thalamic syndrome,* and typically consists of the following signs and symptoms (all of which appear on the side opposite the lesion): (1) transient hemiparesis or hemiplegia; (2) loss of deep sensation and impairment of superficial sensation; (3) tremor, ataxia, and choreoathetoid movements; and (4) spontaneous, excruciating pains, hyperalgesia, and excessive reaction to stimulation of involved bodily areas. Hyperpathic pain may be present in the entire contralateral half of the head and body, or smaller contiguous areas may be affected.

The nurse will want to bear in mind that patients with thalamic syndrome will overrespond to stimuli, such as pinprick, stroking, and deep pressure on the involved area of the skin. Also, bright light, sudden noises, temperature changes (cold especially), fatigue, debilitation, and apprehension will all intensify the pain. In addition, these patients may laugh or cry without apparent motivation, since extreme emotional lability is a part of their illness.

Cerebral cortex lesions, such as brain tumors and other mass lesions, as well as cortical ischemic lesions resulting from cerebrovascular occlusive disease, may involve the cerebral cortex and not the thalamus. These may produce central pain in the contralateral side of the body. A careful neurologic examination must be carried out before treating a patient for "thalamic pain," so that a possible surgical lesion is not overlooked.

Causalgia. *The pain syndrome of causalgia typically follows injury to a peripheral nerve* and is characterized by burning pain that is often severe, persistent, diffuse, spontaneous, and aggravated by motion, touch, or emotional stimuli. Generally the pain is associated with dystrophic* and vasomotor changes and may cause emotional disturbances and changes if it is prolonged. The brachial plexus and the median and sciatic nerves are involved most frequently. While peripheral nerve damage is the usual cause, other conditions may rarely precipitate the problem, for example: sprains, bruises, fractures, amputations, and arterial and venous occlusions.

Since virtually any stimulus may set off paroxysms of excruciating pain (e.g., stimuli such as drafts of air, eating, temperature changes, contact with clothing), the person with prolonged causalgia pain may develop "into a nervous recluse who adopts such elaborate precautions to prevent paroxysms of pain that they may seem absurd. Apathy associated with a haggard and woebegone expression reflecting constant, severe suffering is the typical picture of this disease. . . . The symptoms may increase in intensity and area of involvement, the intractable pain leading eventually to drug addiction, invalidism, and even suicide."[49] The patient may attempt to prevent pain by keeping the affected joints rigid and may attempt to obtain some relief by wrapping the part in a moist cloth.

> *Neuralgia differs from causalgia in that the pain of neuralgia is typically throbbing or tingling, whereas that of causalgia is burning. Also, the pain of most neuralgias is less severe and is generally restricted to the field of the affected nerve.*

Phantom Limb Pain. Patients may feel various sensations in their phantom limbs (amputated extremity). These paresthesias (abnormal sensations) may commonly be: feelings of itching in the palm of the missing hand or sole of the foot; pressure sensations, tingling feelings, or the sensation described as "pins and needles."

While phantom sensations are relatively common, phantom pain is quite uncommon. When phantom pain does occur, throbbing, burning sensation of the hand or foot is the most persistent and common pain. "Another common pain is appreciated as a cramped and twisted abnormal posturing of the limb, which is maintained immovably rigid in spite of the desire of the patient to change position. This latter type of pain does not occur when the patient has the illusion of being able to move the phantom voluntarily. The fist may be clenched tightly with the nails tearing into the palm."[49] Patients with amputated legs or feet may feel their missing toes are tightly curled and cramped. Phantom pains may be of a stabbing, boring, or vise-like nature.

Although persons affected can tolerate most phantom paresthesias, occasionally some phantom pains are intensely intolerable. Pain quality varies widely, but exacerbations may be precipitated by fatigue, excitement, sickness, weather changes, emotional stress, and other stimuli. A painless phantom limb may gradually become painful, but the more typical occurrence is for those phantoms that pose severe problems to be painful immediately postamputation. It is now clearly established that phantom limb pain affects only those who are born with a limb and lose it. Fortunately, only a small proportion of persons with a phantom limb have significant pain in it.[108]

Stump pain often is associated with phantom limb pain but is not necessarily related to it. Although patients usually experience some stump discomfort along with their phantom pain, some persons have phantom pain but have no stump problems.

*Reflex sympathetic dystrophy is a disorder of the sympathetic nervous system that may follow injury to the nerves or blood vessels, fracture, or sprain. It is characterized by rubor or pallor, sweating or dryness, edema, pain, or skin atrophy.

PRETENDED PAIN, PSYCHOGENIC PAIN, AND PSYCHOPHYSIOLOGIC PAIN

Pretended Pain. *Pretended pain* is neither psychogenic nor physiologic (organic) in origin, for pain is actually present in both these situations, whereas it is *not present* in persons who pretend to be in pain.

What are some reasons why people might pretend to have pain when pain is actually absent?

- Pretended pain may be used as a means of concentrating interest and sympathy upon oneself.
- Pretended pain may be used to escape the demands and boredom of everyday life, e.g., "I can't do the dishes, I have a headache."
- Pain may be pretended in an attempt to obtain some economic gain in the form of damages, i.e., compensation neurosis.
- Pretended pain may be used for purposes of obtaining narcotics.

In each of these situations the individuals are pretending to have pain in an attempt to control how others will act toward them. For example, "You should help me by (giving me medicine) (money) (doing my work) because I'm in pain."

It should not be assumed that pain is being pretended. A careful assessment is necessary.

Psychogenic Pain. *Psychogenic pain* can be defined as follows:[108] (1) Pain that is independent of peripheral stimulation or of damage to the nervous system and due to emotional factors; or (2) Pain in which any peripheral change, such as muscle tension, is a consequence of emotional factors.

An estimated 50 per cent of pain symptoms seen in general medicine are psychogenic in nature.[83]

Wang[152] offers some additional criteria for determining whether pain is psychogenic in origin, proposing that pain is psychogenic when no anatomic or physiologic explanation can be detected, when narcotics do not provide relief, when much relief is obtained with sedatives and placebos, and when it is possible to alleviate the pain by distracting the patient's attention.

Psychophysiologic Pain. *Psychophysiologic pain* is pain produced as a result of a chronic and exaggerated state of the normal physiologic expression of emotion, e.g., rage, fear. These long-continued visceral changes, resulting from repressed feelings, may eventually produce structural changes. While psychophysiologic leg pains, back pains, and abdominal pains are not uncommon, the most common pain of this nature is tension headache, resulting from muscle spasms secondary to anxiety.

FACILITATED AND INHIBITED PAINS

Sensitivity to pain varies widely.

> There are some patients with pain whose symptoms are difficult, if not impossible, to relieve, even by surgery that interrupts all known nervous pathways connecting the site of injury or disease with the cerebral cortex. At the other extreme are persons without any detectable development or other lesion of their nervous systems who do not experience pain as a result of any form of injury or disease.[154a]

One explanation of such wide differences in response to pain is that in some instances the perception of pain may be "facilitated," whereas, at the other extreme, the perception is "inhibited."

Facilitated pain means that various phenomena have taken place that facilitate or "make it easier" for pain to occur. For example, after repeated stimulation, the sense-perceptive areas of the brain may become hypersensitive and, thus, easily triggered. For example, because of overused pain pathways, a person who has long suffered with chronic cholecystitis may have typical gallbladder pain even *after* the removal of that organ. Also, the cortical threshold may be lowered generally as well as locally, e.g., a marked general hyperalgesia may be experienced with pneumonia. Another example of "supersensitive" pain pathways (which facilitate the transmission of stimuli producing pain) are those of the individual with chronic rheumatism who can predict weather changes by noting exacerbations of pain.

Inhibited pain responses are those which "make it harder" for pain to be experienced. It is known that *emotional attitudes* toward pain can greatly alter perception of the stimulus, and thus the learning process can influence perception.

Through training and will power some persons can inhibit and control their responses to pain.

It has been observed that during periods of excitement or hysteria, an injury may not be experienced as painful. Also, some persons with chronic schizophrenia have been observed to show no painful response to severe physical disease that might be expected to produce pain. Moreover, persons who are severely subnormal mentally have been known to harm themselves without apparent discomfort.[108]

In addition to these situations there are several other types of indifference to pain that are of importance.[108] For example, a lack or pain perception or *"nonpain"* may be *clinically produced,* e.g., by surgically severing nerves for purposes of pain control, or may occur by *accident,* e.g., traumatic injury to the spinal cord.* Other persons may be born with an abnormally weak mental reaction to pain. Some of these congenital cases are probably attributable to a developmental defect, most likely central in origin.

Rarely, one encounters a person who has an apparently normal sensibility of pain, but an absence of mental reaction to it; this is referred to as *pain asymbolia.* Asymbolia refers to loss of the ability to understand symbolic things. Thus, with "pain asymbolia" the patient loses the ability to understand the symbolism of pain. A person with such an affliction might wince upon noxious stimulation, but not withdraw from the pain-producing stimulus nor respond to other threats of damage. Since the threats are not symbolically thought of as damaging or harmful, the individual does not respond even though pain appears to be experienced. This condition has been related to cerebral lesions.

*For a further discussion see the unit on neurology, Unit X.

CHAPTER 30

THERAPEUTIC APPROACHES TO PAIN

Not only degrees of Pain, buts its existence, in any degree, must be taken upon the testimony of the patient.

PETER MERE LATHAM (1789–1875)
Diseases of the Heart, Lect. XI

Concerned human beings have tried through the ages to avoid, treat and understand pain. Even though impressive gains have been made during recent decades in knowledge of pain mechanisms and pain control, many persons experiencing pain continue to fail to obtain relief.

PATIENTS' RESPONSES WHEN ASKED WHAT NURSES AND DOCTORS COULD DO ABOUT PAIN

"Slow down, don't hurry so, you can't hurry pain."
"What is more important than talking to patients about pain?"
"Be prompt. Try to understand. Make more of an effort."
"Stop telling people they don't have pain when they actually do. Don't try to feel for people when you can't know if they hurt or not."
"Don't make judgments when you don't know and haven't hurt."
"Don't ignore patients in pain and give them the brushoff—we aren't a bunch of neurotics."
"Have confidence you can help the pain—if you had more confidence we would, too."
"Be realistic about pain. Don't be too casual or flip."
"Don't assume the shot or pill helps."
"If you had hurt just once, you wouldn't hand out this 'It won't hurt a bit' routine."
"I'd like one doctor and one nurse each shift. There isn't enough energy to describe the pain over and over again."
"See patients as individuals and not textbook pictures."
"Don't be callous. You treat patients like a garage repairman but we aren't automobiles."
"Prescribe fewer pain pills and shots and get down to the cause."

Pain prompts people to seek medical help more often than any other symptom. Often the causes of pain are disorders that can be relieved with medications or by a surgical procedure. Thus, most pains are "acute" in nature and are amenable to therapy, or they may simply be self-limiting and vanish with the passage of time. Some pains are chronic, however, and intractable.

OVERVIEW OF PAIN THERAPY

Despite the potential aid of modern medicine, it is surprising how patient morbidity is seemingly accepted. Too often the physician is unaware of the magnitude of the pain problem while the nurse and relatives, too well aware of the problem, are unaware of the potential alleviation that can be made available from sources other than drugs.[74]

The comprehensive management of persons having pain requires a multiphasic approach. This is particularly true of those pains that become severe and intractable. Several therapeutic measures may be necessary, each precisely selected for certain effects. All forms of pain therapy should consider both the physical and mental aspects of the pain experience.

Remember:
It is important to avoid overtreatment and undertreatment in pain management.

Since pain often functions as an indicator of disease, the presence of pain usually calls for an *investigation* of its *underlying cause* rather than only the relief of the patient's suffering. For example, a person suffering pain from an inflamed appendix needs an appendectomy, not aspirin. Logically, whenever possible, the treatment of pain should center on the elimination of the underlying cause of the pain rather than on palliative measures.

In approaching treatment, differentiation can be made between pains that are primarily structural, primarily psychologic, and primarily physiologic in origin. Once a diagnosis is established and the mechanism of pain determined, treatment is planned carefully considering:

1. The pain's cause, site, type, mechanism, intensity, and probable duration
2. Nature of the disorder causing the pain
3. The patient's age, mental and physical status, life expectancy and social obligations
4. Methods of treatment that are practical and are locally available
5. Possible treatment-related complications.

> *A goal of pain therapy is to lessen responses to pain or perception of pain without complications, e.g., the loss of consciousness or other sensations.*

This means that the goal of therapy in *surgical* pain-relieving procedures is to free patients of pain without causing loss of function or sensation (e.g., without producing permanent numbness of an area as a result of interruption of cutaneous sensation). *Medically,* drug therapy strives to relieve pain without creating new problems for the patient (e.g., addiction, constipation, dizziness).

A wide variety of clinical measure can be employed in pain therapy. Some of these are:

- *Specific medical and/or surgical therapy* directed at the pain-producing problem, e.g., antibiotics can relieve the pain of infection by reducing the infection; inflamed or malfunctioning organs can be removed surgically.
- *General measures,* e.g., positioning, distraction.
- *Radiology,* to relieve pain caused by pressure from neoplasms by shrinking the tumor in size.
- *Reduction of pain-producing anxiety,* e.g., hypnosis, psychotherapy, sedatives, ataractic drugs, placebos, prefrontal lobotomy.
- *Behavioral techniques,* e.g., operant conditioning, biofeedback, autogenic training, meditation.
- *Biostimulation therapy,* e.g., transcutaneous nerve stimulator, peripheral nerve and dorsal column stimulators.
- *Physical therapies,* e.g., rest, heat, cold, massage.
- *Production of analgesia or anesthesia,* e.g., analgesic medications, acupuncture, nerve blocks, general anesthesia, neurosurgery.

"Pain clinics" exist in some communities for the diagnosis and management of pain syndromes. Such clinics usually consist of a team of professionals, such as a neurologist, neurosurgeon, internist, general surgeon, orthopedist, psychiatrist, radiologist, anesthesiologist, social worker, psychologist, physiatrist and nurses. These clinics can be valuable for some patients experiencing pain because of their comprehensive approach to pain therapy.

In those painful conditions caused by medical disorders that are *self-limiting* and in those pain problems that can be solved by the specific surgical removal of an organ (e.g., appendectomy) or administration of specific medications, pain problems can be solved relatively simply, and the management is clearcut. However, in situations of *intractable* protracted pain the problem is difficult to comprehend and solve. Examples of such chronic pain syndromes are: (1) visceral pain; (2) neuralgia; (3) myofascial syndromes; (4) reflex sympathetic dystrophics; and (5) some pain syndromes associated with cancer. (Remember not all people with cancer have pain.) In those situations in which the cause of pain is not known or, if known, cannot be eliminated, then the pain itself must be treated, and the services of a pain clinic may be essential if the patient's distress is to be lessened.

Later in this chapter we describe some specific methods of relieving pain. As a nurse you will be using or assisting in the use of these methods. *It is important to remember, however, that the intimate, personal process of nursing can itself relieve pain.* Nursing skills, alone or in combination with other therapeutic approaches, are helpful in pain management.

NURSING APPROACHES TO RELIEVING PAIN: AN OVERVIEW*

> *Nurses, because of their prolonged and intimate contacts with patients, are in a unique position to aid persons in pain. Providing such help is a challenge, a responsibility, and a privilege.*

Nursing Assessment

1. *Ongoing assessment* of a person's pain experience is vital. This includes *objective* and *subjec-*

*In this discussion, basic nursing considerations are presented in overview only. Refer to Sorensen and Luckmann, *Basic Nursing: A Psychophysiologic Approach,* Chapter 34, for a more detailed presentation of nursing approaches to the relief of pain.

tive elements, i.e., a nurse's observations of a patient's behavior and a patient's verbal descriptions of the pain experience.

2. *Each person has a basic human need to be free of pain and discomfort.* (See Chapter 1, pp. 8 and 10.) Human beings are motivated to avoid pain. Pain can occur as a consequence of unsatisfactory attainment of other basic human needs. For example, if the need to eliminate urine cannot be met because urinary stones block the outlet from the bladder, pain will occur. Similarly, if a person does not experience affection and caring from someone else, (i.e., to satisfy the need for love and belonging), some form of psychogenic pain may occur. *Part of a nursing assessment is to identify any unmet needs that may be contributing to a person's pain.*

3. Pain assessment is difficult because it is an entirely *subjective experience.*
   a. Psychic and somatic factors interact indivisibly.
   b. Each person experiences and expresses pain in unique ways.
   c. Each person attaches personal "meanings" or "explanations" to their pain experiences.
   d. The personal meanings nurses attach to pain may interfere with their assessments, e.g., nurses may interpret a person's pain according to their own experiences rather than from the patient's point of view.
   e. The frequent exposure nurses have to the pain of others may lead them to make inappropriate judgments about the significance of pain for others.

> *Useful nursing assessments of people experiencing pain demand*
> *(a) that each patient be considered as an individual and*
> *(b) that every nurse clarify his or her personal concepts of pain to avoid applying them to others.*

4. *Personal meanings* attached to pain occur as a result of personal pain experiences throughout life.

5. Personal meanings attached to pain may arise from a person's (a) *individual experiences* and (b) *sociocultural experiences.* The cultural and familial role modeling a child is exposed to teaches the individual such things as:
   a. What pain is appropriate to talk about and what is not.
   b. What is appropriate behavior when one experiences pain and what is inappropriate.
   c. What circumstances are likely to produce pain and should therefore be avoided.
   d. Various methods to avoid or relieve pain.
   e. The "reasons" why one may experience pain, e.g., as punishment, as "testing" by supernatural or divine powers, or because of "bad thoughts."
   f. Possible consequences of pain, e.g., attention from others, imminent death.

Such childhood learnings may influence a person's behavior throughout life, regardless of how appropriate or valid they are in later life.

6. A pain experience is also affected by *personal factors:*
   a. Pain expectancy (the anticipation of pain)
   b. Pain acceptance (willingness to experience pain)
   c. Pain apprehension (generalized desire to avoid pain)
   d. Pain anxiety (the anxiety a pain experience provokes through its mystery, loneliness, helplessness, threat.)

7. Pain evokes *emotional responses* that have *behaviorial expressions.* Observations of behavior will provide a nurse with some understanding of a patient's feelings and what pain "means" to a particular person. By accepting behaviors (such as in Table 30–1) and trying to understand their emotional origins, nurses are helpful to patients. To do this well, a nurse must (a) *observe* a patient's behavior accurately, (b) *listen to all a patient says,* and (c) *never judge* a patient or "jump to conclusions."

8. *Remember:* Although most people experience pain as unpleasant, for a few individuals pain may be psychologically beneficial. For others, pain may actually herald physical improvement, e.g., the return of sensation to an analgesic body area.

TABLE 30–1. POSSIBLE RESPONSES TO PAIN

Possible Emotional Responses
Depression
Anger
Fear
Sadness
Excitement
Resentment
Denial
Possible Behavioral Expressions
Withdrawal
Verbal expression of emotion – direct or indirect
Irritability
Restlessness
Childlike behavior (regression)
Inability to concentrate
Difficulty in remembering
Egocentricity

9. Perception of pain is influenced by such factors as:

a. The integrity of a person's nervous system.
b. The person's state of consciousness.
c. The person's age.
d. Physical state, e.g., fatigue, debility, lack of sleep, and prolonged suffering all reduce a person's ability to tolerate pain.
e. Emotional state, e.g., worry, fear, and anxiety reduce a person's ability to tolerate pain.

10. *Systematic assessment* of pain is necessary. (See p. 746.) Whatever assessment method is used, information is gathered about:

a. History of the origin and occurrence of pain.
b. Localization of pain.
c. Extension, radiation, depth, and duration of pain.
d. Factors that increase or decrease pain.
e. Time of onset and pattern of pain.
f. Character or quality and intensity of pain.
g. Previous treatments and their effectiveness.
h. Cessation of pain, when and how the pain stops.
i. Associated symptoms, e.g., skin changes, sensory changes, vomiting, fever.
j. The patient's opinions of what causes and relieves the pain.
k. Previous assessments and findings.
l. Disability resulting from pain.

Take note of and record a patient's own words when he or she describes pain. Remember: *Not everyone is able to express pain verbally. Hence, behavioral and physiologic observations are also important.*

11. *Indications* of pain include:

a. *Sympathetic responses* — often occur with pain of low to moderate intensity or superficial pain.
   (1) Pallor
   (2) Elevated blood pressure
   (3) Dilated pupils
   (4) Skeletal muscular tension
   (5) Increased respirations
   (6) Increased heart rate
b. *Parasympathetic responses*—often occur with pain of severe intensity or deep pain.
   (1) Pallor
   (2) Decreased blood pressure
   (3) Decreased heart rate
   (4) Nausea and vomiting
   (5) Weakness and fainting
   (6) Prostration
   (7) Possible loss of consciousness
c. *Behavioral responses.* The patient experiencing pain may show the following behaviors:
   (1) Take a posture that minimizes the pain, e.g., lie rigidly, draw legs up
   (2) Moan; grimace, clench jaws or fists
   (3) Blink rapidly
   (4) Cry; appear frightened or restless
   (5) Withdraw when touched
   (6) Have a drawn facial expression
   (7) Have twitching muscles
   (8) Have diaphoresis
   (9) Hold or protect the painful area, not move.

Nursing Interventions

1. When helping a person who is experiencing pain, an *excellent nurse:*

- Works *with* a patient in seeking ways to reduce or remove pain. Listens to what the patient thinks will help and decides with the patient what should be done. *Allows* the patient a sense of control over the pain experience, rather than promoting a feeling that the patient is helpless in "the grip of pain."
- Makes *frequent reassessments* (a person's experiences of pain change, sometimes rapidly) and *adjusts nursing interventions* accordingly.
- *Realizes* that an intervention helpful at one time for one person is not necessarily helpful at another time for another person.
- Remembers that *the quality of the nurse-patient relationship may be as important as the pain-relieving skills used;* thus the nurse creates a relationship with a patient that is characterized by genuineness, warmth, accurate empathy, and respect.

2. If a person's basic human needs are met, pain or discomfort (physical and psychogenic) may be reduced or even eliminated. Careful nursing assessment, which reveals unmet basic human needs, will indicate appropriate nursing intervention.

3. *Specific therapy* should, whenever possible, be directed at the *cause* of pain. *Ancillary problems* that aggravate pain (e.g., coughing, anorexia, diarrhea, constipation) need to be treated as well. *Palliation* may be used: (a) when the primary cause of pain cannot be treated or removed, (b) temporarily, until the primary cause can be found, or (c) to supplement other therapeutic measures.

PSYCHOLOGIC ASPECTS OF CARE

1. Relieving anxiety

> *The greater a person's anxiety, the greater will be the suffering associated with pain.*

   a. Stay with the person for a while.
   b. Allow the person to talk.
   c. Communicate empathy and a willingness to listen.
   d. Allow the person to have control by having input into the nursing plan.
   e. Encourage and teach the patient to use relaxation and meditative techniques. (See Chapters 6 and 8.)
   f. Use therapeutic touch and/or other measures to relieve physical tension, promote comfort, and help the patient relax, e.g., give a backrub, apply a cool cloth.
   g. Do everything possible to relieve the pain — be sure the person really experiences that everything possible is being done.
   h. Inform the person whenever a procedure is likely to be painful.
   i. Instruct the patient to say "ouch" out loud at the moment of pain during a painful procedure, e.g., as a needle is being inserted.
   j. Establish a means for the person to contact someone if necessary when alone, e.g., telephone, call bell.

2. Using distraction and diversion

> *In general, the intensity of suffering depends upon the extent to which pain dominates the conscious mind. Pain perception can be reduced if conscious awareness of pain is reduced.*

   a. Distraction is more useful in mild pain than in severe pain.
   b. When carrying out painful procedures, a delicate balance is needed between keeping a patient informed and focusing attention on other things, i.e., using distraction. Appropriate timing and a sincere manner are necessary, or patients may feel their pain is being discounted. It may be helpful if a nurse speaks quietly to a patient during the painful moments of a procedure.
   c. Occupational therapy, conversation, reading, television, and radio may all be helpful means of distraction and diversion *provided they are interesting to the patient.* Individual preferences must be considered.
   d. Small talk (idle chatter) and excessive noise is tiring rather than helpful. Some people find barely audible noise (e.g., a radio on very softly) irritating and therefore tension-producing, while others find it relaxing.
   e. Encourage patients to use any patterns of behavior they have found helpful to them in relieving pain. Ask them what they have found helpful in the past, and facilitate their using the same methods again.
   f. Self-hypnosis and autosuggestion may be helpful. (See also Chapters 6 and 8.)
   g. Involve the patient in some self-help activities. Give specific, clear instructions as appropriate, e.g., tell the person to "concentrate on breathing through your mouth," "move your legs around," "hold on to the rail and turn to your right side."

3. Combating anticipatory fears

> *Anticipatory fears are those that occur prior to and in expectation of a pain-producing stimuli. Nurses can help prepare patients to meet pains that are inevitable by talking with them about the pains they fear.*

   a. Prior to painful procedures, talk with patients about what they can expect. This may encourage relaxation and reduce muscle resistance that could be pain-producing. Discuss the kind of pain or discomfort a person may expect to experience. ("You will feel a sharp prick." "You will probably feel some pressure which may be uncomfortable but not painful.") *Patients who are given information about the procedures and sensations they are going to experience have less anticipatory distress and are more relaxed throughout the procedure than those who are not.*[79a]
   b. Help patients assume body alignment and positioning that will help them tolerate painful procedures more comfortably.
   c. Reassure preoperative patients that they will be given adequate medication to control postoperative pain.
   d. Nurses using pain-relieving techniques should communicate a belief that the methods will, in fact, relieve pain. Suggestion is a powerful phenomenon.
   e. If patients know that they will prompt-

ly receive pain-relieving medication when they need it, they will be less likely to request medication unnecessarily or too early in anticipation of pain.

f. Anticipatory fears are reduced also by the techniques described for reducing anxiety.

PHYSICAL ASPECTS OF CARE

1. Excellent nursing care is directed at minimizing irritations that lower a person's pain tolerance. This includes protecting patients from pain-producing stimuli such as:
   a. Local irritation or inflammation, e.g., infection, thrombosis.
   b. Muscle spasm or muscle strain.
   c. Interference with local blood supply and venous and lymphatic drainage.
   d. Distention of hollow visceral organs, e.g., bowel, bladder.
   e. Further damage to traumatized tissue.
2. General principles of care include:
   a. Injured tissue should be handled carefully.
   b. Painful procedures should be done at a time when pain-relieving medications are having their maximum effect.
   c. Drainage tubes should be checked frequently to ensure they are not caught, stretched, pulled, kinked, or looped and that they are positioned correctly.
   d. Care must be taken to prevent patient fatigue. Overtiredness decreases pain tolerance.
   e. Immobilization may reduce pain caused by inflammation or the interruption of blood supply.
   f. Elevation may relieve pain in swollen body parts.
   g. A position of semiflexion may reduce the pain of joint disorders.
   h. The pain of muscle spasm may be relieved by a change in position.
   i. Frequent position changes along with a good body alignment may prevent painful muscle contractures.

> *Know exactly what you are going to do* before *moving a person who is experiencing pain. Listen to the patient's advice, and whenever possible, allow the patient to control the movement.*

   j. Gentle massage may help relieve muscle pain and prevent clot formation. However, *never vigorously massage the calf of the leg, as blood clots may form in that area and massage could break loose the clots and possibly cause a fatal embolism!*
   k. Hot and cold applications are useful in relieving some pains.

3. The administration of pain-relieving medications is an important nursing function and is discussed later in this chapter. Specific pain-relieving medications are discussed in textbooks of pharmacology.

4. *Chronic, intractable pain* (pain that cannot be relieved by physical means) presents additional difficulties for those people experiencing it. Nursing such patients is often a challenge that requires long-term support and patience. People experiencing chronic intractable pain may be treated by the psychologic and physical nursing interventions just discussed. Specific pain-relieving therapy is described later in this chapter. *It is important, however, that medical and nursing therapeutic regimens are coordinated and consistent to ensure a unified approach to the patient.*

5. People experiencing *progressive pain* (pain associated with progressive malignant diseases) may be helped by the methods described in this chapter. However, one important difference should be remembered. Pain-relieving medication may be used more routinely — as a preventive measure—as, for example, when vasodilators are taken by a person with ischemic heart disease. Some patients may hesitate to take pain-relieving medications routinely and preventively because of fear of addiction. It is important to remember, however, that a person experiencing pain because of widespread cancer has a disorder *requiring* pain-relieving medications and thus is no more addicted to narcotics than a person with heart disease is addicted to vasodilators.

Nursing Evaluation

As with all nursing measures, pain-relieving interventions have a reduced value if they are not evaluated for their effectiveness. Changes in a person's pain experiences can be assessed by asking the person to rate the pain on a scale of "one to ten." ("One" represents no pain at all, and "ten" represents so much pain that the person would rather die than continue to live with the pain.) Have patients rate their pain before and after interventions to evaluate the effectiveness of the nursing actions.

Also, notice changes in the person's behavioral responses. As pain is reduced, removed, or becomes more tolerable, the behavioral responses indicative of pain are altered. (See Table 30–1 for some possible behavioral responses to pain.) For example, a person who responds to pain by becoming irritable and restless may become more amicable and calm when nursing interventions directed toward relieving pain are successful.

Never simply assume *that your nursing interventions have been successful. Always evaluate their effects. What you have done may or may not be helpful. Plan future nursing actions on the basis of evaluation.*

SPECIFIC MEDICAL AND SURGICAL THERAPIES

Much pain therapy is conducted by administering *medications* that will act on the particular end-organ that is the source of pain, e.g., the heart. For example, medications such as nitroglycerine relieve the pain of angina pectoris by affecting the heart–the "painful end-organ." Such medications act directly on the pain-producing organ itself, rather than on the higher centers responsible for pain perception. Such medications are *not* analgesics. Analgesics act peripherally and/or centrally to modify pain perception or reaction. For example, while atropine may relieve pains caused by smooth muscle spasm by relieving the muscle spasm, and while ergotamine constricts overdistended arteries in the brain, thereby relieving the pain of some migrane headaches, neither of these medications can accurately be called an analgesic.[161]

Specific medications having direct effects upon specific pain-producing end-organs are discussed in appropriate sections of the text (e.g., medications affecting the heart are discussed in the unit on cardiovascular function). Likewise, *specific surgical procedures* that eliminate pain by removing or correcting the specific pain-producing organ are discussed in appropriate sections of the text (e.g., appendectomy is discussed in the unit on gastrointestinal function, and fractures are discussed in the muscular-skeletal unit).

GENERAL MEASURES

In pain therapy, general procedures are always employed in an attempt to interrupt the pain-producing mechanism *before* resorting to more radical procedures that could create iatrogenic problems, e.g., analgesic medications, surgical procedures, nerve blocks.

Remember:
Plan general nursing care measures to relieve pain in conjunction with a careful assessment to determine if analgesics are needed.

For example, you may find that a patient has pain because of an uncomfortable position in bed. Perhaps the person has had a leg cast applied and the leg has rolled off a pillow and is uncomfortably twisted. By correctly positioning the patient's leg, pain may be relieved so that no analgesic is required. Always evaluate a patient in pain to determine general measures of nursing care (such as those described in the first part of this chapter) that may help, and employ these measures *first*.

PHYSICAL THERAPIES

Various types of physical therapy may be used to treat pain, e.g., rest, passive and active exercise, massage, heat and cold. Such therapies may be of great value in the early stages of painful conditions. Physical therapies are often greatly appreciated by patients. In the past there was a tendency to emphasize the more *passive* forms of *physiotherapy;* today the more *active* forms of physiotherapy are also recognized. For example, while some alleviation of the pain of a sprained ankle may be obtained by rest, *active exercise* rather than passive physiotherapy is the best means of removing inflammatory exudate, which is pain-producing.

► *Rest* does have value in relieving pain. Indeed, rest, *proper positioning,* and *posture* are all extremely important in the physical treatment of many painful disorders. This is especially true immediately following trauma, as well as during any period of acute inflammation. Complete, prolonged immobilization is dangerous, however, since among other problems, muscle atrophy can occur along with the formation of painful adhesions.*

When rest is therapeutically indicated, those muscles that are guarding inflamed or injured tissues should be supported in a way that insures complete relaxation. Only with complete relaxation is physiologic rest possible for the affected part.

► The use of *heat* and *cold* can be pain relieving.* Depth of tissue penetration by heat varies with the modality used. For example, while ultrasound penetrates deeply, hot water bottles and heating pads penetrate less deeply. Both heat and

*A detailed discussion of the complications of immobility and the therapeutic use of heat and cold is available in Sorensen, and Luckmann, *Basic Nursing: A Psychophysiologic Approach.*

cold may be applied either wet (e.g., soaks) or dry (e.g., diathermy, electric pad, heat lamp, ice bag or hot water bag).

- *Massage* is most useful in the early stage of inflammatory swellings and in treating the pain of various forms of myalgia as well as fibrositis. Massage used in combination with some form of heat is useful to prepare for more active forms of remedial exercise.
- Numerous *local applications,* such as nonadherent dressings, analgesic ointments, and analgesic liniments, may be beneficial in treating the more superficial forms of pain. Such pains may be due to neuritis, ulceration, and inflammatory conditions.

RADIOLOGY

Because of multiple possible complications, it is *not* generally advisable for radiation therapy to be used in the treatment of *benign* diseases if the condition can be managed by more conservative measures. Although there are a few indications for radiation treatment of benign conditions for the symptomatic relief of pain, these indications are becoming fewer in number each year. Radiation therapy is extensively employed, however, in treating pains due to *malignant* conditions. (See Unit IX.)

REDUCTION OF PAIN-PRODUCING ANXIETY

Since heightened *anxiety* is known to increase pain, a variety of therapeutic measures may be employed to relieve and thereby *dissociate* the pain from responses to it. That is, the pain is still perceived but suffering is abolished or reduced. For example, a person may have pain (be aware of it), but not care about it. Examples of therapies that can cause such an altered reaction are: leukotomy (prefrontal lobotomy), electroshock therapy, psychotherapy, and ataractic drugs. Religious or hysterical mental states may, likewise, cause such dissociation.

Pain that is primarily *psychogenic* in nature generally is more difficult to treat than that which results from demonstrable physical pathology. Since psychogenic pain may result from an inability to cope with reality, and an unconscious escape from such an intolerable reality, the sufferer needs treatment which employs *psychotherapy* and *reeducation.* Actually, psychotherapy can be a valuable adjunct to any type of pain therapy (for both organic and psychogenic pain), since even intense pain caused by physical pathology may be partially reduced through supportive care.

Hypnosis. In the eighteenth century Mesmer introduced hypnosis as a treatment in formal medical practice. Since then the use of hypnosis in medicine has been disputed by some physicians and praised by others. One of Mesmer's followers accidentally discovered the level of trance that became classically recognized as hypnosis, i.e., the somnambulistic state of deep trance or hypnotic sleep associated with amnesia. This state was utilized for surgical anesthesia. However, once safe chemical anesthetics became available hypnosis was virtually abandoned in operative procedures. Only in recent decades has there been a reawakening of interest in the use of hypnosis in the operating room as an adjunct to chemical anesthetics.

Hypnosis has multiple uses, one of the most rewarding of which is the reduction of pain. Hypnosis is a type of pain therapy based on the power of suggestion and the process of focusing attention. *An individual's reactions to pain can be decidedly altered by hypnosis.* Hypnosis may be used as an adjunct to other pain-relieving therapies and is useful in a number of types of pain problems, e.g., dentistry, surgery, childbirth, and malignant diseases. Removal of pain with hypnosis should be done with care, only by persons aware of the diagnostic and treatment problems of organic illness.

The hypnotic trance has been divided into three stages: light, medium, and deep. Most investigators believe that 20 per cent of the general population can attain the stage of deep trance. Apparently the depth of trance is not related to the degree of success attained in pain therapy.

A variety of procedures may be employed to relieve pain following induction of the trance state, e.g., suggestion to alter the character of pain or the patient's attitude toward it; body disorientations and dissociations; anesthesia and analgesia for superficial and deep sensation.

Hypnosis cannot change organic lesions that are producing pain, but it can be used to reduce discomfort in a wide range of medical and surgical conditions. For example, hypnosis either by itself or in conjunction with other therapeutic measures has proved useful in decreasing discomfort associated with: peptic ulcer, painful conversion reactions, cervical disk disease, causalgia, postherpetic neuralgia, and trigeminal neuralgia. Moreover, along with producing analgesia, hypnosis has been helpful in the treatment of burned patients by improving their fluid balance, nutritional status, cooperation with treatment, and the will to live.

Hypnosis is not without its hazards. The procedure itself is relatively simple and innocuous compared to the administration of many anesthetic and analgesic drugs. However, the operator must be skilled and informed and the patient carefully selected to avoid untoward effects from hypnosis.

Attempts to remove symptoms by means of hypnosis must be tempered with the realization that for *some* patients, symptoms may satisfy certain needs and may perform an adaptive or defensive service. In patients with chronic organic pain, the operator must be careful to phrase suggestions in such a way that not all perception of pain is blocked. For example, the patient may be told that the pain will grow much less, but there will be some residual left. This approach is needed so that the patient will have sufficient perception of pain to detect any change in the course of the organic illness.[32] Also, *posthypnotic suggestion* must be used cautiously, even though it is a valuable reinforcing mechanism in the prolonged relief of pain.

In situations of chronic pain, posthypnotic suggestion may be used in combination with *autohypnosis* (*self-hypnosis*) to provide prolonged relief. It is possible for many hypnotic subjects to be successfully trained in deliberate spontaneous trance induction or autohypnosis. The subject must be cautioned to use this procedure with care.

Placebos. *Placebos are pharmacologically inert substances.* Placebos were formerly used primarily to "please" patients more than to help them. They are now used extensively as a control in experiments that examine the effects of drugs.[144] Their use demonstrates that the "psychologic action" of a "medication" is often of prime importance in producing analgesia. Over 30 per cent of patients display analgesic response to placebo therapy.

Whereas some persons react to placebos, others do not. Some patients are almost consistent "placebo reactors" or "nonreactors." Others may respond at some times to placebo medications, and at other times they will not. While it might seem to be desirable to be able to bring relief so easily to many patients, in fact the placebo effect makes it difficult to evaluate the patients' response to pharmacologically active substances. These inconsistencies in response have necessitated that placebo use be confined to using them as controls in experimental studies.

Examples of substances used as placebos include sodium bicarbonate, vitamins, distilled water, lactose capsules, or physiologic saline solution. With placebos, it is the power of *suggestion* that acts in relieving pain, since the patient *believes* that a pain-relieving medication is being administered. The expectations of patient, nurse, and physician thus become of importance in placebo therapy. *Remember that suggestion is a powerful tool.* Placebo therapy needs careful management and should be carried out only on order of a physician and with the patient's consent.

Placebos may be potent in producing both side effects and toxicity in many patients. They have been shown to actually cause changes in laboratory data. Once again it is demonstrated that the psyche (mind) and soma (body) cannot be separated. (Mind-body interaction is discussed in Chapter 3.)

In the past, patients were not told they were receiving a placebo, but rather they were merely told they were being given a medication "to ease the pain" or whatever the desired action was. The abuse of placebo administration caused some patients to become suspicious of all medications. Today, by law in the United States, people are protected by human right review committees which demand that patients be informed if their treatment may include the administration of placebos.

BEHAVIORAL TECHNIQUES*

Patients who experience chronic pain over long periods of time often learn to or become conditioned to display a complex set of "pain behaviors." In turn, by enacting these "pain behaviors," they reinforce their feelings of pain.

Fordyce[50] has found that learning factors play an important role in chronic pain. Physicians and other health care providers often react to indications of pain in such a fashion as to promote and strengthen pain behaviors. Changes in severity of the pain and related functional impairment have been found to occur without any change in the underlying pathologic disease when patients learn that people respond differently to their request for help.

In circumstances where patients have learned pain behaviors, modification of the patient's behavior can be helpful. There are several techniques in which the person is in control of what is happening. These self-control techniques include operant learning approaches, biofeedback, autogenic training, and various forms and styles of meditation.

Operant Conditioning. An operant conditioning program does not cure pain, but it can help reduce pain. It is a program designed for patients who are experiencing operant pain and not for patients whose pain behaviors are caused by active organic disease. The purposes

*These techniques are also discussed in Chapters 6 and 8.

of an operant conditioning program are: (a) to reduce "pain behaviors" by withdrawing positive reinforcement for such behavior; (b) to increase the person's "well behaviors" by programming positive reinforcement contingent upon increasing desirable behaviors; (c) to teach significant others to reinforce "well behaviors" and to avoid reinforcement of the person's "pain behaviors"; and (d) to refer patients to other health professionals who can help with other functional impairments when the patients are no longer limited by pain. The success of an operant conditioning program rests on fully informing the patient and significant others of every element before proceeding. (See also p. 90.)

Biofeedback. "Biofeedback" is a term that refers to a wide variety of techniques that use instrumentation to provide a patient with information about changes in bodily functions of which the person is usually not aware. The information provided to the patient is immediate and continuous; some patients learn to use the information to control previously involuntary functions. The purpose of biofeedback techniques is to teach the patient self-control of physiologic states such as pain, mood, attention, emotions, or other involuntary functions.

Patients are taught to manipulate and control their degree of relaxation and tension directly by means of biofeedback training using electroencephalogram (EEG) patterns or electromyogram (EMG) muscle potential. For example, muscle tension pain may be reduced by training the person to relax certain groups of muscles. This may be accomplished by attaching surface electrodes from an electromyograph to the site of muscle tension. The amount of electrical activity (tension level) of the muscles then is portrayed in any of several ways, such as on a dial. The patient then may be able to try different procedures and techniques to produce relaxation. Given the continuous and precise feedback information about the effectiveness of each method, the person often can find a way to bring down the tension level. Some nurses specially prepared in these techniques are currently becoming biofeedback therapists. (See Figure 8–2, p. 90.)

Autogenic Training. It was not until the end of the nineteenth century that medical and philosophical attention was paid to the physiologic phenomena of hypnotism, spiritualism, and various yogic disciplines. By 1910, a mind-body training system, eventually called *autogenic training*, had begun to be developed by Dr. Johannes Schultz in Germany. The purpose of the training was to *help patients to be self-generated or self-motivated.* This technique evolved at approximately the same time that Freud gave up the use of hypnosis as a medical tool because it was unpredictable. It occurred to Schultz that perhaps hypnosis was an erratic tool because the patient often unconsciously resisted the doctor. If the *patient was able to direct* the procedure being used with pain relief, for example, with the doctor acting as a teacher, then the control technique would come into the realm of self-regulation and perhaps be more effective. Since that time, Schultz and Luthe[137] have written a handbook on autogenic training that includes a training system of "meditative" exercises. These exercises gradually lead into a kind of self-awareness in which the person develops both physiologic and psychologic self-knowledge.

Systematized relaxation training procedures (autogenic training) have been used to treat a variety of physical and psychologic problems, including pain. Subjects are taught to passively concentrate on relaxing the muscles in various parts of their bodies. Procedures such as these and the ones used in hypnosis have been found to cause a variety of physiologic changes, including dilation of peripheral blood vessels, changes in blood sugar levels, and a reduction in muscle tension related to pains. It has been found recently that meditation procedures also result in some of the changes in physiology described above. (See also p. 29.)

PRODUCTION OF ANALGESIA OR ANESTHESIA

Analgesia and Anesthesia

An *analgesic* is defined as a substance that "reduces or abolishes suffering from pain without producing unconsciousness."[132] Thus, in *analgesia* the sensation of pain and the associated psychic reactions are abolished or reduced without impairment of consciousness; the perception of pain is altered. By changing a patient's attitude and mood toward pain, analgesics induce apathy to the pain and promote feelings of well-being and freedom from anxiety.[65] *Anesthesia* refers generally to a loss of feeling or a loss of sensation, particularly a loss of the sensation of pain. There are many different types of anesthetics, e.g., spinal anesthesia, general anesthesia, and local anesthesia.

Analgesia can be produced at any of the points in the pathway of pain. A procedure frequently used in minor surgery is the *local infiltration* of an *anesthetic agent* to produce loss of sensation; or, to produce a *local nerve block*, the sensory nerve trunk may be infiltrated. At certain critical points almost any spinal or cranial nerve can be blocked with local anesthetic agents or neurolytic agents. Temporary or reversible nerve blocks are produced by local anesthetic. *Neurolytic agents,* like phenol and alcohol, produce prolonged effects, since they are destructive of the nerve. ("Neuro" refers to "nerve", "lysis" means "destruction.")

Local anesthesia is also called "regional anesthesia." In this state a particular region of the body is rendered insensible to pain, although the patient's general state of consciousness is not otherwise affected. Local anesthetic agents, whether applied topically, by the intravenous route, or by regional nerve trunk blocks, act by blocking the sensory nerve impulses between the peripheral structures and higher centers. Local anesthetics do not cause a loss of consciousness, but there is a specific loss of pain sensation.

The *injection of anesthetic agents into the spinal fluid* anesthetizes both dorsal and ventral nerve trunks, producing loss of both motor and sensory functions. Patients under *spinal anesthesia* may not experience pain, and yet may retain tactile discrimination and motor function. Such patients may say that they can "feel the doctor working" but that they do not experience pain. They may be able to move their toes and retain some of their reflex mechanisms. This is because local anesthetics block the smaller nerve fibers before the larger ones.

A *general anesthetic agent,* acting upon central function will produce various degrees of depression of total response or the total depression of all sensation. General anesthetics render the patient unconscious and thereby prevent perception of pain anywhere in the body. Anesthetics are discussed in Unit VIII.

The pain threshold can be raised or obliterated by local anesthetization. *Analgesics* can also raise the pain threshold. Analgesics, like morphine and alcohol, tend to have a much greater effect upon the reaction to pain than they do upon the perception of pain. Thus while the pain is actually felt at almost the same intensity, the patient loses reactions such as anxiety, which usually accompany perception of pain.

Generally it is assumed that the analgesics, like the general anesthetics, produce their effects by acting on the *central* nervous system. However, some analgesics block the nerve-endings or receptors for pain and, thus act *peripherally.* This point will be discussed again.

Acupuncture

Acupuncture, folklore therapy from China, is believed to be at least 3,000 years old. However, China began publicizing the use of acupuncture to control pain as analgesia in surgery without chemical anesthetics only a few years ago. The term "acupuncture" derives its meaning from the Latin "acus," needle, and "punctura," a puncture.

> *Acupuncture is a method of preventing, diagnosing, and treating pain and disease by the skilled insertion of special metal needles into the body at designated locations and at various depths and angles.*

There are approximately one thousand known *acupuncture points,* such as "*hoku points.*" (See Figure 30–1.) These points form essentially fourteen groups. The points in each group form a pattern known as a "*meridian,*" which is directly associated with an organ. A meridian runs along one of the major organs and terminates at the tips of the toes or fingers. Meridians occur separately on each side of the body and are paired with corresponding areas.

Needle insertion is determined in part by the angle and depth of insertion to be used as well as the duration and frequency of the treatment.

Acupuncture has been used as an alternative to other forms of analgesia for most minor surgical procedures in China. Approximately 20 minutes prior to surgery, the needle or needles are inserted into the area and are rotated manually or connected to a battery operated pulsator. Major operations on the abdomen, chest,and head have been performed in fully awake and alert patients who were stimulated by placement of acupuncture needles. As anesthesia, acupuncture seems to be far superior to other types of anesthesia, since it does not lower the patient's blood pressure or create respiratory tract complications.

There are no simple explanations for the mechanisms that underlie the analgesia-producing effects of acupuncture, although the technique is seemingly simple. Within our traditional Western medical doctrine, there are no reasons to explain why somatic stimulation through acupuncture needles produces analgesia or to account for the fact that analgesia outlasts the period of stimulation by several hours. Many people find acupuncture helpful, however, despite the fact that its therapeutic mechanism cannot be readily explained.

Nerve Blocks

Essentially, *nerve blocks are injections of various substances* (for example, local anesthetics) *close to nerves*, thereby "blocking" off the conductivity of those nerves. Nerve blocking techniques may be employed to produce a complete, *reversible* interruption of nervous pathways for four different purposes.[14]

- ▶ 1. To eliminate a local focus of noxious stimulation or nervous irritation
- ▶ 2. To interrupt the perception of pain, either at the source of the pain or anywhere along the peripheral afferent neurons
- ▶ 3. To interrupt reflex mechanisms that are maintaining an abnormal activity of blood vessels, glands, skeletal or smooth muscle
- ▶ 4. To eliminate such reflex responses by direct infiltration of the skeletal muscle and other involved structures

Some *irreversible* nerve blocking procedures are also possible, as we stated previously.

Most nerve blocks are used for the purpose of providing *symptomatic relief of severe pain*; however, they may also be used for diagnosis, prognosis, and prophylaxis.[14] Blocks given for pain relief are called "analgesic blocks." The analgesia, generally produced by the injection of a local anesthetic agent, relieves pain and can make possible certain treatment that would otherwise be excessively painful, e.g., manipulation of a painful joint. Sometimes, by interrupting reflexes that operate to cause sustained pain, analgesic blocks can produce a beneficial effect which is prolonged beyond the effective duration of the agent injected.

Analgesic blocks are useful in a variety of acute and chronic disorders and often serve to reduce the amounts of narcotic agents that might otherwise be needed. Injection of procaine in the muscle or skin of an area of referred pain may greatly modify pain from visceral or other deep noxious stimulation. However, the pain cannot be eliminated unless the primary afferent impulses are terminated or blocked at their source by surgical or chemical means.

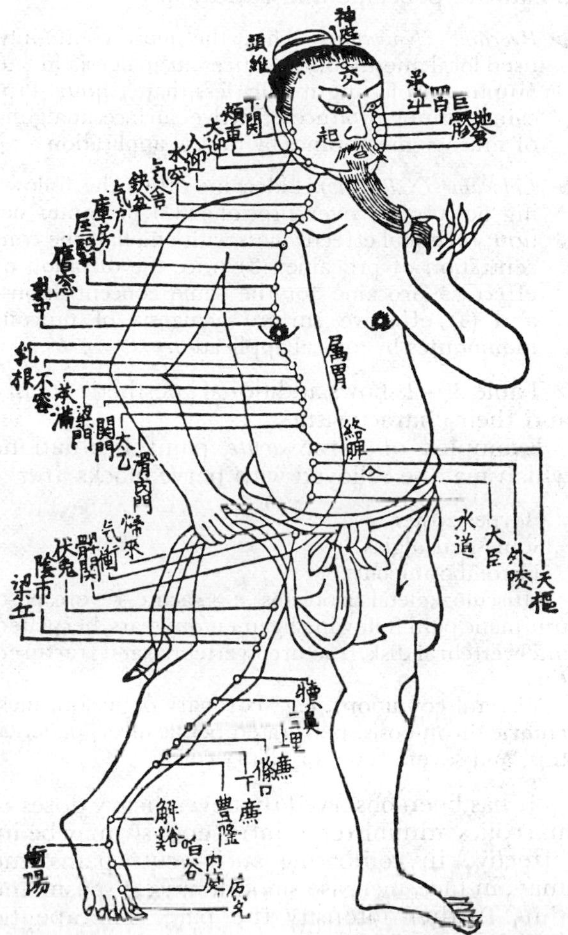

Figure 30–1. A typical acupuncture chart, showing the sites for insertion of needles along one of the major body meridians. After two or more needles are inserted, electric current is usually passed through the needles for about 20 minutes. The resulting analgesia can permit major surgery. (From Melzack, R., and M. E. Jeans: Acupuncture analgesia. *Minnesota Medicine*, Mar. 1974.)

> *Although nerve blocks may be extremely helpful, not all patients benefit from such procedures. Also, the chemical interruption of nervous pathways by nerve block techniques constitutes only one aspect of the management of any pain syndrome.*

Because all drugs used for local anesthesia are vasodilators, it is possible to potentiate the action of local anesthetic agents through the *supplementary use of epinephrine*[14, 115] which is a vasopressor or a vasoconstrictor. Adding a vasoconstrictor to the local anesthetic makes it possible to prolong the effect of anesthesia, by causing a local vasoconstriction that allows the anesthetic agent to stay in contact with the tissue for a longer time.

In addition to prolonging the effects of the anesthesia, the supplementary use of a vasopressor reduces the possibility of the anesthetic reaching a toxic blood level. The toxicity of local analgesic drugs depends upon their concentration in the blood; this, in turn, depends upon the speed of absorption. *By causing vasoconstriction, vasopressor drugs delay absorption of the local analgesic solution and thus prevent a suddenly high blood concentration.* This gives the body more time to metabolize and detoxify the medication. Also, bleeding is reduced by the vasopressor.

Two local anesthetics used for nerve blocks

with which the nurse should be particularly familiar are procaine and lidocaine.

- *Procaine (Novocain).* This, the most commonly used local anesthetic, produces an analgesia in 3 to 10 minutes, lasting usually less than 1 hour. Procaine cannot produce effective surface analgesia of mucous membranes by topical application.

- *Lidocaine (Xylocaine).* Lidocaine offers the following advantages over procaine: (1) prompter action; (2) equal effectiveness with one-half the concentration of procaine; (3) twice the duration of effect as procaine for the same concentrations; and (4) effective surface analgesia of mucous membranes by topical application

Table 30–2 shows additional anesthetic agents and their characteristics.

Examples of some *acute* painful situations which may be relieved with nerve blocks are:

Herpes zoster
Some neuralgias
Thrombophlebitis
Musculoskeletal problems, e.g., acute, severe posttraumatic pain following ligamentous tears, herniated intervertebral disk, fractured vertebrae and fractured ribs.
Visceral conditions, e.g., coronary occlusion, mesenteric thrombosis, perforated peptic ulcer, pancreatitis, and severe renal or biliary colic.

It has been observed that even heavy doses of narcotics administered intravenously may be ineffective in combating such acute pains and may, in fact, increase smooth muscle spasm and thus further intensify the pain. Therapeutic nerve blocks, which can be maintained for days if necessary, provide relief from such intense pain as that resulting from sudden, acute circulatory insufficiency created by embolus, vasospasm, thrombus, or trauma.

Sensory nerve fibers are more readily affected by local anesthetics than are motor fibers. For example, if a mixed (motor and sensory) nerve were infiltrated, a complete anesthesia could be produced in the absence of any detectable motor weakness. In addition to pain fibers, local anesthetics will also affect the small thinly myelinated or unmyelinated fibers carrying sympathetic impulses.

Some of the *major types of nerve blocks* are: (1) local blocks (infiltration and topical application); (2) paravertebral and prevertebral sympathetic (autonomic) blocks; (3) somatic nerve blocks of spinal nerves; (4) extradural blocks (caudal and segmental spinal epidural block); (5) subarachnoid blocks; and (6) blocks of cranial nerves.

Various nerve blocking procedures may be useful in managing *chronic* pains (Table 30–3). Indeed, nerve blocks can be more desirable to use in patients with non-malignant diseases than the prolonged administration of analgesics that may lead to addiction. Such blocks may provide pain relief to patients who would have developed tolerance to the analgesic action of narcotics — such that even high doses of narcotics would not alleviate the pain. Bonica observes:

> The administration of narcotics to patients with chronic pain is a frustrating, short-lived type of kindness; such a sense of mistaken humanitarianism is inevitably productive of tolerance and other phases of addiction. It is really a great disservice to the patient because with continued use of the addictive analgesics tolerance to the analgesic action develops until eventually an impasse is reached in which the patient's daily narcotic requirements are high while the alleviation of pain is inadequate.[14]

TABLE 30–2. CHARACTERISTICS OF LOCAL ANESTHETICS

Agent	Corrected toxicity ratio*	Speed of Action	Penetration	Duration
Procaine (Novocain)	1	Moderate	Moderate	Short
Chloroprocaine (Nesacaine)	0.7	Fast	High	Short
Lidocaine (Xylocaine)	1	Fast	High	Moderate
Mepivacaine (Carbocaine)	1	Fast	High	Moderate
Prilocaine (Citanest)	0.8	Fast	High	Moderate
Tetracaine (Pontocaine)	0.8	Slow	Low	Long
Dibucaine (Nupercaine)	1.2	Slow	Low	Very long
Bupivacaine (Marcaine)	?	Moderate	Moderate	Very long

*Relative toxicity to relative anesthetic potency, with procaine as standard of reference. Ratio of less than 1 indicates toxicity lower than procaine with doses that provide equal anesthetic effect.

Extracted from Black, R. G., and J. J. Bonica: Analgesic blocks. *Postgraduate Medicine,* 53:105, May 1973.

TABLE 30–3. INDICATIONS FOR THERAPEUTIC NERVE BLOCKS FOR CHRONIC PAIN

Indications	Types of nerve block
Causalgia and other reflex sympathetic dystrophies Acute herpes zoster and postherpetic syndrome	Blockade of appropriate sympathetic pathways; occasionally, epidural or subarachnoid injection of neurolytic agents (phenol or alcohol) to interrupt preganglionic pathways
Chronic pancreatitis Upper abdominal cancer	Blockade of celiac plexus (injection of neurolytic agents)
Chronic myofascial pain dysfunction syndromes	Infiltration of "trigger" areas with anesthetic agents
Chronic back pain with nerve root irritation (no myelographic evidence of acute herniated intervertebral disc)	Injection of steroids and a local anesthetic into the subarachnoid or epidural space Continuous epidural techniques (to provide profound muscle relaxation as an adjunct to bed rest and traction)
Posttraumatic and postinfectious neuralgia	Intercostal nerve blocks
Terminal stage of metastatic cancer in patients with clearly unilateral and well-circumscribed pain	Subarachnoid block with neurolytic agents
Painful spasticity	Fanwise injections of 45 percent alcohol into clonic and stretched muscle belly (to decrease muscle tone and clonus)

From Ghia, J. N., et al.: Therapeutic nerve blocks for chronic pain. *American Family Physician*, 20:74, July 1979

Disadvantages of Nerve Blocks. Lest we give the impression that nerve blocks provide a simple solution to the complex problems of disease and pain, let us consider some of their *problems, contraindications,* and *complications.*

▶ Nerve blocks may often be *unsuccessful* due to *problems* such as: (1) difficulties in identifying the pain pathways or in locating the correct nerve for injection, and (2) the complexity of pain psychophysiopathology involving, as it does, the patient's subjective reactions, central nervous system, and peripheral structures. Some additional problems are caused by the fact that only small volumes of solution can be injected at one time.

▶ Nerve blocks are *contraindicated* in patients who (1) are psychoneurotic or psychotic, (2) have an infection at the site of injection, and (3) are in shock or are debilitated, especially if extensive vasomotor paralysis will be produced or if large amounts of local anesthetic solution are required.

> *Because of potential complications, nerve blocks should be performed with resuscitative equipment and necessary drugs on hand to combat untoward reactions.*

▶ Some *complications of nerve blocks are*[14] hypotension; hypertension; mild, moderate, or severe toxic reactions to local anesthetic drugs; idiosyncratic reactions; overdosage of epinephrine or other vasoconstrictors; allergic reactions; pneumothorax; psychogenic reactions; inadvertent subarachnoid (spinal) block; hematoma; postinjection neuropathy; respiratory dysfunction and paralysis; and cardiac arrest.

Topical Applications for Pain Relief. Dilute solutions of local anesthetics may be applied topically in the form of pastes, sprays, or other preparations. This may be effective in reducing the severe pain of burns, abrasions, and necrosis of the mucous membranes and skin. However, if the condition is extensive (e.g., extensive burns or pruritus), the intravenous administration of local anesthetics such as procaine or tetracaine may be preferable to the form of topical application.

Cocaine, a highly toxic agent, is sometimes used for topical anesthesia (sometimes in an atomizer for topical spray), but *never* for infiltration anesthesia.

Toxic reactions to overdosages of topical medications can easily occur. Therefore, you should use dilute solutions of the drugs and take care not to exceed the recommended total dosage.

> Remember: *Following the application of local anesthetic drugs to burned or abraded skin or mucous membranes, the absorption of the medication is almost as rapid as following intravenous administration!*

Ethyl chloride may be used as a spray in treating some myofascial pain problems and other disorders that are caused and maintained by trigger areas located in superficial tissue. Several points to bear in mind for the successful use of this spray are: (1) have the patient comfortable, with the body area to be sprayed well supported, so that muscles are relaxed; (2) apply the spray from 12 to 24 inches above the skin at an angle to the skin; (3) maintain slow, even sweeping motions moving in one direction rather than back and forth; (4) begin the sweep of direction at trigger areas and move toward the reference zone; (5) shield the patient's face; (6) repeat in a few seconds and then wait a few seconds until the entire reference zone is sprayed; and (7) if aching develops, lengthen the interval between sweeps.[14]

Cranial Nerve Blocks. Those cranial nerves that can most easily be blocked are the 5th (trigeminal), 7th (facial), 9th (glossopharyngeal), 10th (vagus), 11th (spinal accessory), and 12th (hypoglossal).

> *Cranial nerve blocks are useful in managing the pain of idiopathic neuralgias, mechanical neuropathy, neuritis, and neoplastic lesions of the head. Also, certain autonomic disturbances involving pathways associated with these cranial nerves may be partially managed by nerve blocks.*

Post-Procedure Observations. Following a nerve block procedure these observations are made and recorded:

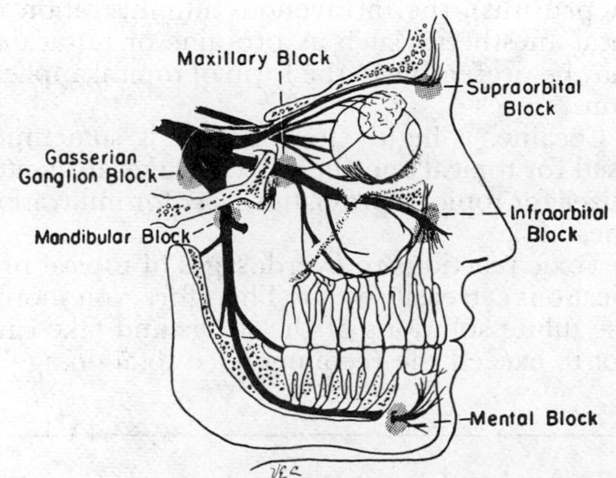

Figure 30–2. Anatomy and distribution of the trigeminal nerve and the optimal site of injecting it (stippled areas). From Bonica, J. J.: *Clinical Application of Diagnostic and Therapeutic Nerve Blocks.* Springfield, Ill.: Charles C Thomas Publisher, 1959.)

- Any complications or untoward effects
- The patient's descriptions of symptoms and relief
- The apparent amount, type and duration of relief
- Any analgesics administered

Such observations may continue for several weeks to help determine how effective the block was. It should be realized that when alcohol has been used for the block, the maximal effects do not occur for several days.

Administration of Medications for Pain Relief

> *The administration of medications for pain relief occurs only after the nurse has carefully assessed and evaluated a patient's pain.*

Kaufmann and Brown discuss the importance of knowledgeable nursing care in pain therapy:[80]

> Administering a medication, while a primary means of relieving pain, may or may not be the best means. Too often, by giving a shot or a pill, the nurse can practice "avoidism" — avoiding listening and understanding, avoiding nursing measures which might bring comfort in conjunction with or even instead of the medication. By so doing she may well withhold the support, assurance, and understanding which may relieve the patient of the necessity of having intense pain. A reverse aspect of this is the delay or withholding of a drug by the nurse, or by the patient himself. At times the nurse will put off giving a medication until the patient demonstrates marked discomfort. By the same token, the patient may fail to report pain until it becomes intense. He may do so to avoid being a nuisance, because he feels it is more courageous, because he is in one way or another opposed to taking medication, or for other reasons.[80]

> *The usual clinical practice for controlling pain is to give analgesic medications* along with other *supplementary medications or therapeutic measures, e.g., rest, proper position, and so forth.*

While analgesic medications, especially the narcotics, are the most frequently used type of therapy, they must be used judiciously because of their undesirable side effects. Generally narcotics should not be utilized in treating pain unless other methods of treatment are not feasible or have failed.

Although habituation, tolerance, and addiction can occur when potent analgesics are given, this does not mean that these medications should be withheld unnecesarily. Narcotics can be high-

TABLE 30–4. SOME TYPES OF MEDICATIONS USED FOR PAIN RELIEF*

Non-Narcotic Analgesic Agents
- I. Salicylates
- II. Para-aminophenols
- III. Pyrazolines
- IV. Other synthetic analgesics
- V. Skeletal muscle relaxant analgesics

Narcotic Analgesic Agents
- I. Opiates
  - A. Natural opiates
  - B. Synthetic opiates
- II. Nonopiate, addicting analgesics (Opioids)

Analgesic Adjuncts
- I. Barbiturates
  - A. Short-acting barbiturates
  - B. Intermediate-acting barbiturates
  - C. Long-acting barbiturates
- II. Amphetamines
- III. Opiate antagonists
- IV. Tranquilizers
  - A. Rauwolfia compounds
  - B. Phenothiazine derivatives

*Outline based on Kolodny, A. L., and McLoughlin, P. T.: *Comprehensive Approach to the Therapy of Pain.* Springfield, Ill., Charles C Thomas, 1966.

ly useful if employed wisely. Habituation, tolerance, and addiction are not likely to occur in *short-term* pain therapy. Patients should not be made to suffer by the unnecessary withholding of narcotics.

Medications used in pain therapy are many, and they are administered in a variety of ways, e.g., by mouth, by topical application, by inhalation, or by injection. Medications may be injected by the usual subcutaneous, intramuscular, and intravenous routes. Also, in some instances, certain medications may be injected spinally, paravertebrally, or into selected nerves to produce nerve blocks, as discussed in the previous section. The latter types of injections are performed by physicians, and nurses often assist with the procedures.

Some of the types of medications used in alleviating, or at least reducing, pain are outlined in Table 30–4. *Systemic analgesic drugs* are the prevalent and most frequently used means of pain control. *Analgesics include the most commonly prescribed drugs,*[132] *and therefore are the most widely used of all medications.*[65] This is not unexpected, since pain is usually the first symptom of injury and most diseases begin with or include pain at some time during their course.

> *Analgesics may well be the medications that you will administer* most frequently *in your nursing practice. Familiarize yourself with them.*

Other types of drugs are useful singly or in combination with analgesics insofar as they can decrease fear, anxiety, and apprehension; reverse depression; promote sleep; or reverse psychotic pain symptoms as summarized in Table 30–5.

THE "IDEAL" ANALGESIC

Investigators and clinicians constantly speak of the elusive search for the ideal drug for this illness or that disorder. Unfortunately, as a rule, increased potency produces increased toxicity. Nevertheless, pharmacologists indefatigably strive to reach this goal.[84]

TABLE 30–5. ANALGESICS AND OTHER DRUGS FOR RELIEF OF PAIN

Mechanisms of Interference With Pain	Drug Type
Reversal of specific pathophysiologic events, such as	
Infection	Antibiotics
Inflammation	Anti-inflammatory agents
Gout	Antihyperuricemic agents
Interference with specific chemical substance involved in pain reception peripherally	Antipyretic analgesics
Interference with conduction of pain away from affected site	Local anesthetics
Interference with central nervous system perception of pain and development of affective responses	Narcotic analgesics
Interference with anxiety, tension, or depression	Sedatives and hypnotics Phenothiazine tranquilizers Skeletal muscle relaxants Antidepressants
Interference with consciousness	Anesthetics

From Halpern, L. M.: Analgesics and other drugs for relief of pain. *Postgraduate Medicine,* 53:91, May 1973.

The task of the pharmacologist is difficult indeed: to prepare a medication that will have the desired effects while excluding the undesirable ones. Actually, pharmacologists have come a long way toward achieving the separation of clinical analgesia and dependence liability. With further research, an even more successful separation of analgesic and physical-dependence properties may be hoped for. Some of the requirements of the ideal analgesic are that it would:[65, 84]

▶ Have rapid onset and long duration of action.
▶ Obliterate pain, diminish the anxiety associated with pain, and relax muscle spasms.
▶ Be effective for all patients regardless of age or disease.
▶ Be effective orally as well as parenterally.
▶ Be well tolerated and capable of prolonged use.
▶ Be free of side effects such as respiratory depression, constipation, nausea, vomiting, and circulatory depression.
▶ Exert a minimal degree of stupefaction and narcosis, i.e., be nontoxic.
▶ Have no tendency to allow the development of tolerance, addiction, or habituation.
▶ Act not only at the chemoreceptor level but also by blockage of the peripheral transmission system within the neuraxis.
▶ Be easily sterilized and possess a long shelf life.
▶ Be relatively inexpensive.

The ideal analgesic does not exist; instead, an overwhelming number of drugs are available for pain therapy.

MECHANISMS OF ANALGESIA

Analgesics do not all act in the same way. For example, acetylsalicylic acid, acetanilid, acetophenetidin, and aminopyrine act mainly on the *threshold for pain perception* and appear to have relatively little effect on the reaction to pain. On the other hand, opiates and alcohol owe their analgesic effects to their ability to control *reaction to pain* as well as to raise the pain perception threshold. The relaxation, apathy, and freedom from anxiety that follow the administration of morphine long outlast its effects on the threshold for pain perception.

Recent evidence indicates that analgesics act *peripherally as well as centrally.* Peripheral action of analgesics is independent of any anti-inflammatory action that they may exert. Generally analgesics can be viewed as medications that modify the central reception of pain within the central nervous system, i.e., spinal cord and brain, by: "(1) blocking the facilitating reflexes and thereby elevating the pain threshold; (2) interrupting pathways for transmission of pain impulses in the brain, thereby modifying the central perception, interpretation, and reaction to the painful stimulus; and (3) modifying the central perception of pain and reducing psychogenic pain by depressing reflex activity."[65]

TYPES OF ANALGESICS

For many years analgesics have been divided into two classes on the basis of their clinical effectiveness: (1) the "strong" narcotic analgesics and (2) the "weak" non-narcotic, antipyretic analgesics. Selection of the optimal agent for a specific patient requires consideration of a variety of factors. These include the quality, intensity, duration and distribution of the patient's pain. Differences between the two classes clinically are based upon the nature of the pain condition for which each has been found to be effective rather than on analgesic potency. Generally the narcotic analgesics are administered for the relief of severe pains resulting from burns, fractures, coronary occlusion, renal colic, and so forth, whereas the non-narcotic analgesics are usually given for muscular aches, headaches, and pains of inflammatory origin.

Strong Narcotic Analgesics. These consist of morphine itself, plus various morphine-like agents differing from morphine only in certain characteristics (rate of onset, duration of action, route of administration, adverse side effects, and chemical configuration.) Drugs in this class induce drug dependence and tolerance. Since

TABLE 30–6. CHEMICAL BASES OF "STRONG" ANALGESICS

Morphine →	Codeine Heroin Pantopon
Semisynthetic compounds → Numorphan	Paracodin Dilaudid Metapon
Synthetic compounds → Meperidine	Demerol Nisentil Leritine Alvodine
Methadone →	Dolophine Pipadone Palfium
Morphinan →	Dromoran Phenazocine
Antagonists → Nalorphine	Levallorphan Pentazocine Cyclazocine

From Poswillo, D. E.: *In* Alling, C., III, et al. (Eds.): *Facial Pain.* Philadelphia: Lea & Febiger, 1968, p. 65.

these drugs have structural similarities, it is relatively easy to classify them on the basis of chemical composition (Table 30–6).

The narcotic analgesic group includes morphine and a large number of morphine-mimetic drugs, e.g., the opiates (or morphine congeners) and the opioids (nonopiate addicting analgesics). Pharmacologic actions of the congeners of morphine are similar to those of the parent compound, morphine. Differences occur in: potency; effects on respiratory depression; histamine release; and, to a lesser degree, liability to tolerance and addiction. These drugs share the "ability to act in the place of morphine, not only in producing analgesia, but also in supporting physical dependence.... They are all, with the possible exception of codeine, potent systemic pain-relieving drugs, even though their potencies relative to one another may differ.... The adjective 'strong' applied to their analgesic potential should not be confused with 'potent.'"[132] See Table 30–7 for a large and varied group of strong analgesic drugs.

Morphine is probably the most useful drug in clinical practice, when given under appropriate circumstances and with the proper indications. Codeine

TABLE 30–7. POTENT, HIGHLY ADDICTIVE ANALGESIC DRUGS

Generic Name	Proprietary Name	Duration of Action (Hours)	Abuse Liability
		Morphine and Its Congeners	
Morphine	–	4–5	Relatively high
Papaveretum	Pantopon, Omnopon	4–5	Relatively high
Hydromorphone, dihydromorphinone	Dilaudid	4–5	Similar to morphine
Oxymorphone	Numorphan	4–5	Similar to morphine
Metopon	–	4–5	Similar to morphine
Heroin	–	3–4	Similar to morphine
Nalorphine (antagonist)	Nalline	Not used for analgesia	None
Naloxone (antagonist)	Narcan	No analgesic activity	None
		Synthetic Analgesics of the Morphinan Series	
Racemorphan	Dromoran	4–5	Similar to morphine
Levorphanol	Levo-Dromoran, Levorphan	4–5	Similar to morphine
Dextromethorphan	Many cough mixtures	No analgesic activity	None
Levallorphan (antagonist)	Lorfan	Very little analgesic activity at any dose	None
		Synthetic Analgesics of the Benzomorphan Series	
Phenazocine	Prinadol	4–5	Similar to morphine
Pentazocine	Talwin	2–3	Substantially less than morphine
Cyclazocine	Not available	4–5	None
		Synthetic Analgesics of the Phenylpiperidine (Meperidine) Series	
Meperidine, pethidine	Demerol	2–4	Similar to morphine
Anileridine	Leritine, Apodol	2–3	Similar to morphine
Piminodine	Alvodine	2–4	Similar to morphine
Alphaprodine	Nisentil	Very short	Similar to morphine
		Synthetic Analgesics of the Diphenylpropylamine (Methadone) Series	
Methadone	Dolophine	4–5, single dose; longer in tolerant individuals	Similar to morphine
Dipipanone	Pipadone	4–5	Similar to morphine
Dextromoramide	Palfium, Dimorlin	4–5	Similar to morphine
Fentanyl	Sublimaze	4–5	Similar to morphine
		Phenothiazines	
Methotrimeprazine (formerly levomepromazine)	Levoprome	4–5	None

Modified from Halpern, L. M.: Analgesics and other drugs for relief of pain. *Postgraduate Medicine,* 53:91 May 1973.

is probably second only to morphine as a drug of choice for pain relief. Codeine has the advantage of being particularly useful in combination with nonaddicting analgesics. Pain that does not respond to the oral administration of codeine, with or without aspirin, should be evaluated for treatment with an opioid drug.

Narcotic analgesics are *slowly absorbed* from several sources: the gastrointestinal tract, subcutaneous tissues, muscles, and intravenously. Even when analgesics are given intravenously, the full effect is not reached for at least 20 minutes. Although the narcotic effects last only about 4 to 6 hours, the *detoxification* of the drug is only about 90 per cent completed 36 hours after administration. Thus, both detoxification and absorption are slow processes. Detoxification occurs primarily in the liver by the process of conjugation; the kidneys excrete the main by-product.

The morphine-mimetic drugs can cause many serious side effects, in addition to their potential for addiction.

> *The morphine-mimetic drugs affect every organ of the body!*

Weak Non-Narcotic Analgesics. These are a diverse group of synthetic chemical agents. The pharmacologic properties of the weak analgesics overlap, but it is possible to classify them on the basis of their chemical structures into the six subgroups presented in Table 30–8.

TABLE 30–8. CHEMICAL BASES OF "WEAK" ANALGESICS

Salicylates	→	Aspirin Salamide Salophen
Anilines	→	Phenacetin Antifebrin Tempra
Pyrazolines	→	Phenazone Pyramidon Butazolidin Tanderil
Mefenamic acid	→	Ponstan
Amphetamines	→	Benzedrine Dexedrine Apamine Preludin
Muscle relaxants and tranquilizers	→	Carisoprodol Chlorpromazine

From Poswillo, D. E.: *In* Alling, C., III, et al. (Eds.): *Facial Pain.* Philadelphia: Lea & Febiger, 1968, p. 62.

Although described as "weak," the non-narcotic analgesics are actually highly effective in relieving pain in many situations. Variables of dose and route of administration affect the potency of these medications. Non-narcotic analgesics are all readily absorbed from the gastric mucosa and rapidly hydrolyzed in the plasma; and the metabolites are excreted.[132]

Toxic reactions can be produced by all weak analgesics. Aminopyrine and phenylbutazone have adverse effects on blood-forming tissues. The phenacetin compounds have been demonstrated as toxic to the kidneys following prolonged administration. The salicylates probably are the most effective analgesics, having the least adverse reactions.[132]

"Mixed" or Combined Analgesics. A combination of drugs acting by different mechanisms may exert a synergistic additive effect. By selective mixing the effects of individual drugs (e.g., analgesic, anti-inflammatory, antipyretic, muscle-relaxant, tranquilizing) may be combined. A wide variety of mixed compounds are available for clinical therapy, "utilizing the sum of the properties of the components."[132] Examples of some analgesic combinations are:

A.P.C. Compound	aspirin, phenacetin, caffeine
Darvon Compound	aspirin, phenacetin, caffeine, propoxyphene
Fiorinal	aspirin, phenacetin, caffeine, isobutylallylbarbituric acid
Penaphen	aspirin, phenacetin, hyoscyamine, phenobarbital

Moertel[112] and associates conducted a double-blind study of analgesic drug combinations involving 100 patients with pain due to cancer. Look at Figure 30–3 and determine which drugs (in combination with aspirin) patients reported as providing the most pain relief. In this study, the side effects for a single dose of the effective combinations were found to be essentially equal and clinically tolerable.

It is clearly established that the administration of mood-changing medications along with analgesics is helpful. The use of such potentiating adjuncts, e.g., barbiturates, tranquilizers, which not only affect the emotional input but also permit lower doses of narcotic agents, can significantly reduce suffering.[84]

COMPLICATIONS AND MISUSE OF ANALGESICS

The administration of narcotics and other analgesics may produce pain relief; however, *both short-term and long-term analgesic administration is fraught with problems.* While potential complications should not prevent the use of analgesic agents, these drugs must be used with caution and with an understanding of possible side effects and how these hazards might be reversed or avoided. Although the nature and incidence of complications will vary from patient to patient, it is possible to identify some common problems.

Nausea and Vomiting. Narcotics may precipitate nausea and vomiting. It has been reported that in selected surgical patients the incidence of emesis associated with morphine may be as high as 46 per cent, and with meperidine as high as 36 per cent.[142]

Paresthesia. The subcutaneous or intramuscular injection of analgesic drugs is generally not irritating to the local tissues. However, if the drug is deposited in the region of a nerve, paresthesia and paresis may be precipitated along its course.[142] The nurse's knowledge of proper injection techniques and sites can prevent nerve injury.

Addiction. The problem of drug addiction has cast its shadow over pain therapy for centuries. A major problem in the drug therapy of pain is the development by the patient of physical and psychologic dependence on the drugs used. Persons who have pain with a considerable psychogenic overlay are particularly prone to the development of drug dependency.

Drug dependency means that the patient begins to rely or depend on the drug for escape from reality or to change reality. Such a patient asks for the drug with increasing frequency and steadily wants larger doses, to obtain the physical and psychologic feelings that the drug produces. The original need for the drug (i.e., to alleviate pain) is replaced by the acquired physical and psychologic dependence on it, so that the patient comes to feel that having the drug is essential.

Closely observe patients receiving addicting drugs for indications of drug dependency.

When a patient has developed drug addiction and is then deprived of the drugs, careful observation for withdrawal symptoms is essential. Such symptoms include: anxiety, abdominal cramps, diarrhea, sweating, restlessness, and rhinorrhea.

Circulatory Depression. Following the injection of certain narcotic drugs, hypotension may occur—at times to such a degree that cardiovascular collapse ensues. Although the exact etiologic mechanisms for these cardiovascular changes are not known, it appears that: (1) hypotension may be caused by a direct dilating action on peripheral vessels; and (2) a

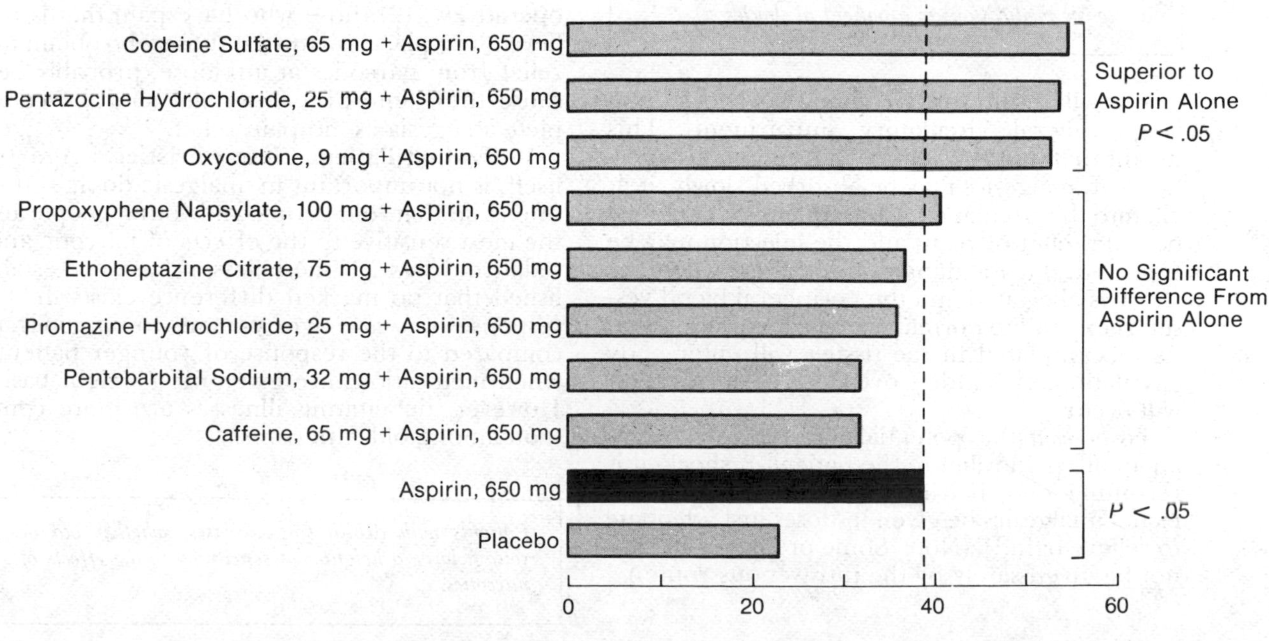

Figure 30-3. Comparative therapeutic effect of placebo, aspirin alone, and aspirin combinations according to percentage of patients achieving significant (i.e., more than 50%) relief of pain. (From Moertel, C. G., et al.: Relief of pain by oral medications. *Journal of American Medical Association,* 229:55, July 1974.)

shock-like state may also be secondary to a release of histamine.[142]

Because of potential circulatory depression with hypotension, patients under the influence of narcotic drugs should not *be allowed to walk and they should* not *be transported in a wheelchair. A stretcher should be used.*

Respiratory Depression. Respiratory depression, a common complication of analgesic therapy, is caused by the diminished sensitivity of the respiratory center to carbon dioxide. This problem is dose-related and accompanies the administration of all potent analgesic drugs, whether narcotics or narcotic antagonists. Stephen observes: "Each new potent analgesic is usually introduced with claims that it has a relative sparing effect on the respiratory center; however, up to now these claims have not withstood the test of careful investigation."[142] The potential of respiratory depression is particularly dangerous for elderly persons with respiratory impairment.

Shock

Extreme caution must be observed in administering analgesic medications to a patient in shock.

You will recall from Chapter 13 in shock there is peripheral circulatory impairment. This means that intramuscular or subcutaneous injections of analgesics may be absorbed slowly, if at all, into the circulation. Consequently, there may be little relief of pain; and the injection may be repeated. This is dangerous because when the shock is alleviated and the peripheral blood vessels reexpand to normal size, the medication that has accumulated in the tissues will enter body circulation. A sudden overdose of medication will occur.

To *prevent* this potential disaster and to give adequate pain relief to the patient in shock, it is recommended that intravenous injection of selected analgesics be given in doses just adequate to relieve pain.[142] (Note: Some preparations cannot be given safely by the intravenous route.)

ASSESSMENT OF THE PATIENT FOR PAIN RELIEF

Assume that you are at the bedside of a patient who needs a morphine-like analgesic to relieve moderate-to-severe pain. What factors about such a patient should be considered *before* drug therapy is used to relieve pain? Why, for example, isn't the patient in pain just routinely given an injection of morphine?

Assessment of a patient before initiating analgesic drug therapy is imperative, to insure safe and adequate pain relief. Factors to be assessed include:

1. Body weight
2. Individual pain experience
3. Individual patient characteristics: age, general state of health, mental status, probable duration of pain, and probable life expectancy
4. Cardiac, respiratory, renal, and nervous system status
5. Presence or absence of cross-tolerance

Body Weight. The dose of morphine considered "standard" is 10 mg. per 70 kg. of body weight, although some patients require more and others less. Both the analgesic effect and the side effects of morphine, such as vomiting and respiratory depression, are dose-related.

Individual Pain Experience. The great variation in the individual pain experience probably outweighs any effect of body size in pain and analgesia. The need for analgesic medications for the relief of postoperative pain clearly demonstrates the spectrum of individuality associated with "painfulness." Figure 30–4 represents data from several sources, all pertaining to postoperative pain, expressed in terms of the drugs and doses required to relieve the pain.

As you see, some patients have little pain, others have a great deal of pain. Note these three groups: (1) those who have no pain postoperatively, (2) those who have pain that is relieved by a placebo; and (3) those who obtain no relief from narcotics at any dose, probably because they "interpret any relief short of complete analgesia as 'no pain relief.'"[81]

Individual Patient Characteristics. Age, by itself, is not important in analgesic dosage. It is often said that "old people and young people are the most sensitive to the effects of narcotic and sedative drugs." Nonetheless, it has been established that no marked difference exists in the response of *healthy aged* persons to narcotics as compared to the response of younger patients when medications are given on a weight basis. However, debilitating illnesses are more common among older persons.

Patients with debilitating diseases, whether old or young, have a heightened sensitivity to the effects of narcotics.

A patient's *general mental status,* the *probable duration of the pain,* and the person's *probable life expectancy* should also be considered in planning drug therapy for pain relief. The mentally anxious individual may benefit from a tranquilizer or phenothiazine in addition to an analgesic. The patient whose life expectancy is short may be given narcotics more readily than the individual with a chronic pain problem that will probably continue for a long period. If a patient will require prolonged therapy for relief of chronic pains, the side effects of analgesics (especially the addicting quality of morphine) must be considered.

Body System Assessment. Since many analgesic agents depress breathing or produce hypotension, an evaluation of the patient's cardiac, respiratory, renal, and nervous system status is of importance. Hepatic function must also be assessed since the liver is important for detoxification of analgesics. The presence of increased intracranial pressure is cause for special concern.

▶ *Increased intracranial pressure.* Potent narcotic analgesics are contraindicated in patients with increased intracranial pressure because narcotics further increase cerebrospinal fluid pressure. This increase is secondary to carbon dioxide retention (increased arterial carbon dioxide tension), which always follows narcotic-induced respiratory depression. (See Ch. 26.)

A point of interest is that patients who are being artificially ventilated will not suffer from respiratory depression and carbon dioxide retention after receiving morphine, so they can receive narcotics in spite of an elevated cerebrospinal fluid pressure.

> *As a general rule, morphine is not given to patients who are suffering from* internal abdominal injuries, respiratory distress, *or head injuries.*

In all three of these conditions morphine may cause vomiting, with serious effects. Suppression of the respiratory center in patients with respiratory distress may prove fatal: *morphine should not be given to patients with respirations of 12 per minute or less.* Concerning head injuries (in addition to the danger of increasing the cerebrospinal fluid pressure) internal cerebral hemorrhage may be present, causing depression of the respiratory center, which morphine would worsen. Moreover, the fact that morphine affects pupil size* could confuse clinical observations of pupil size, which are important with head injuries.†

Cross-Tolerance. The presence of cross-tolerance can make effective drug therapy pain relief difficult to achieve.

▶ *Cross-tolerance.* The use of tranquilizers during the day, hypnotics at night, and alcohol in between has caused numerous persons in our fast-moving society to become tolerant to sedatives and narcotics. "For some persons it has brought death. A usual dose of hypnotics, which is large because of tolerance, after an extra large alcohol intake has led to asphyxia, either by simple respiratory obstruction or secondary to vomiting and aspiration."[81] (See Ch. 94.)

Tolerance develops to both the sedative and analgesic effects of narcotics, so that chronic users of tranquilizers, hypnotics, and alcohol become resistant to potent analgesics.

Before leaving the discussion of tolerance we should briefly discuss the patient with *liver disease.* Although pharmacologists classically teach that patients with liver or kidney disease should not receive medications that have to be excreted by these organs, clinical practice shows that there is no reason for withholding medications such as pentobarbital from a person with decreased liver function if the possibility of a longer effect is anticipated. The administration of drugs that are excreted through the liver or kidney to persons

*Morphine acts as a miotic; that is, it constricts the pupil of the eye.

†Head injuries are discussed in Units X and XXVI.

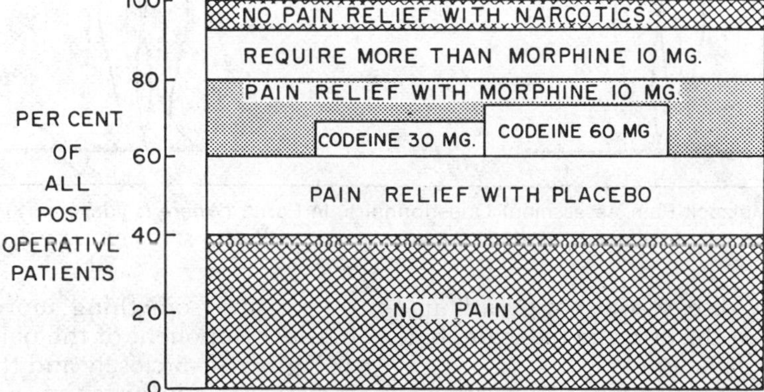

Figure 30–4. Variation in severity of postoperative pain expressed in terms of the drugs and doses required to relieve the pain. All postoperative patients were included. (From Keats, A. S., and M. Lane: The symptomatic therapy of pain. *In: Disease-A-Month* by Dowling, H. F. (Ed.). Copyright 1963 by Year Book Medical Publishers, Inc., Chicago, used by permission.)

Patient's name____________________Age________

Hospital No.____________________

Clinical category (e.g. Cardiac, Neurological, etc.):________________

Diagnosis:____________________

____

____

Analgesic (if already administered):

1. Type________________
2. Dosage________________
3. Time given in relation to this test________________

Patient's intelligence: Circle number that represents best estimate.

1 (low) 2 3 4 5 (high)

****

This questionnaire has been designed to tell us more about your pain. Four major questions we ask are:

1. Where is your pain?
2. What does it feel like?
3. How does it change with time?
4. How strong is it?

It is important that you tell us how your pain feels now. Please follow the instructions at the beginning of each part.

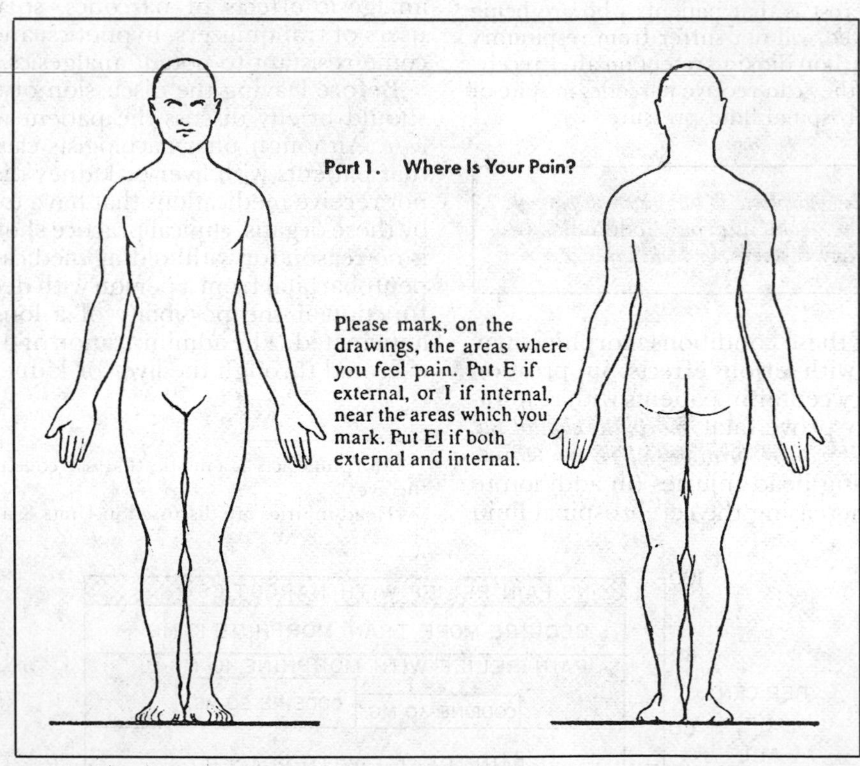

Figure 30–5. McGill-Melzack Pain Assessment Questionnaire. In Part 1 (*Where is your pain?*) the person is asked to mark the body areas where he or she is experiencing pain.

with liver or kidney disease will not greatly increase the intensity of the effect of the drug, but rather will prolong its action.[81]

McGill-Melzack[103] have developed a relatively new instrument in the quest to quantify clinical pain—a four part questionnaire that attempts to measure something more than just the intensity component of the pain experience. Look at Figure 30–5 closely and think about the ways in which this information could be used in determining the relative effectiveness of different procedures in the treatment of clinical pain.

Part 2. What Does Your Pain Feel Like?

Some of the words below describe your present pain. Circle ONLY those words that best describe it. Leave out any category that is not suitable. Use only a single word in each appropriate category--the one that applies best.

1	2	3	4	5
Flickering Quivering Pulsing Throbbing Beating	Jumping Flashing Shooting	Pricking Boring Drilling Stabbing Lancinating	Sharp Cutting Lacerating	Pinching Pressing Gnawing Cramping Crushing
6	**7**	**8**	**9**	**10**
Tugging Pulling Wrenching	Hot Burning Scalding Searing	Tingling Itchy Smarting Stinging	Dull Sore Hurting Aching Heavy	Tender Taut Rasping Splitting
11	**12**	**13**	**14**	**15**
Tiring Exhausting	Sickening Suffocating	Fearful Frightful Terrifying	Punishing Gruelling Cruel Vicious Killing	Wretched Blinding
16	**17**	**18**	**19**	**20**
Annoying Troublesome Miserable Intense Unbearable	Spreading Radiating Penetrating Piercing	Tight Numb Drawing Squeezing Tearing	Cool Cold Freezing	Nagging Nauseating Agonizing Dreadful Torturing

Part 3. How Does Your Pain Change With Time?

1. Which word or words would you use to describe the pattern of your pain?

1	2	3
Continuous Steady Constant	Rhythmic Periodic Intermittent	Brief Momentary Transient

2. What kind of things relieve your pain?

____

3. What kind of things increase your pain?

____

Part 4. How Strong Is Your Pain?

People agree that the following 5 words represent pain of increasing intensity. They are:

1	2	3	4	5
Mild	Discomforting	Distressing	Horrible	Excruciating

To answer each question below, write the number of the most appropriate word in the space beside the question.

1. Which word describes your pain right now? ____
2. Which word describes it at its worst? ____
3. Which word describes it when it is the least? ____
4. Which word describes the worst toothache you ever had? ____
5. Which word describes the worst headache you ever had? ____
6. Which word describes the worst stomach-ache you ever had? ____

Figure 30–5. *Continued.* Part 2 (*What does your pain feel like?*) consists of 20 word groupings intended to provide descriptions for the patient's present pain. Only one word per group can be chosen. These groupings include three different aspects of the pain experience: sensory (groups 1-10), affective (groups 11-15), and evaluative (group 16). Groups 17 to 20 are classified as miscellaneous. Part 3 (*How does it change with time?*) provides for a description of the pattern of pain, along with questions about its relief and aggravation. Part 4 (*How strong is it?*) provides a scale for the subject to rate intensity of pain for six separate situations. This part represents an effort to gain information on the person's general perception of pain intensity. The questionnaire is accompanied with a cover sheet that has space for patient information, such as diagnosis and analgesics administered. (From Melzack, R.: The McGill pain questionnaire: Major properties and scoring methods. *Pain,* 1:277, 1975.)

NEUROSURGICAL PROCEDURES FOR PAIN RELIEF

When there is persistent, intractable pain of high intensity, neurosurgical procedures may be used. The neurosurgeon attempts to relieve pain by interrupting parts of the paths in the nervous system that relay sensations to the brain from their point of origin. The goal of such surgery is to provide pain relief without causing the loss of other sensations, for example, the loss of all feeling in an area.

Such operations may be performed peripherally or centrally on the spinal cord and brain itself. In addition, surgery on the autonomic nervous system, *sympathectomy,* may be performed alone, or in combination with other procedures for the pains of causalgia or vascular disease.

Summarized below are a few of the various neurosurgical procedures utilized in pain therapy:

Neurectomy is the interruption of cranial or peripheral nerves by means of incision or injection. This procedure is employed when pain is localized to a small part of the body. When a cranial neurectomy is performed, a craniotomy is necessary.

▶ *Rhizotomy* is the interruption of the anterior or posterior nerve root area close to the spinal cord. Rhizotomy is performed when pain is more widely distributed than that occurring in a small area of the body. As many roots are divided as necessary to control the pain. A laminectomy is necessary for this procedure.

▶ *Chordotomy* is the surgical interruption of the pain-conducting pathways within the spinal cord. An incision a few millimeters in length is made in the anterolateral pathway opposite the side on which the pain is located. When pain is midline in nature, a bilateral chordotomy must be performed. A laminectomy is necessary for this operation.

▶ *Percutaneous cervical chordotomy* is a preferred procedure for the relief of intractable pain in patients who are poor surgical risks or who have terminal cancer. The operaioin is relatively simple, is well tolerated, and has a short convalescence and a low morbidity. By means of this procedure a nonsurgical stereotaxic destruction of the anterolateral spinothalamic tracts is possible. Percutaneous chordotomy is a simplified form of surgical chordotomy that interrupts or destroys the conduction of pain in the pain pathways of the spinal cord. The procedure is performed under local anesthesia by inserting a needle into the neck, below and behind the mastoid process. X-ray control is used in guiding the needle into the spinal cord. Some physicians believe that percutaneous chordotomy is simpler, more accurate, and safer than surgical chordotomy. A lateral cervical approach and an anterior approach have been used.

▶ *Tractotomy* is the surgical division of the anterolateral pathway in the brainstem. A craniotomy is necessary in order to accomplish this procedure.

▶ *Gyrectomy* involves the removal of the postcentral gyrus corresponding to the painful part. This is done to attempt to remove the registration of pain within the cortex of the brain. Therefore, this is a cerebral operation.

▶ *Frontal leukotomy (lobotomy)* causes the destruction of cerebral tissue in the frontal lobes of the brain.

Some neurosurgical procedures designed to alleviate pain are shown in Figure 30–6.

It should be remembered that when *sensory* nerves are cut, the tissues which are no longer supplied with sensory innervation become highly susceptible to injury. With sensory innervation gone, feelings of pain, pressure, and temperature are no longer present, and injury can occur without the patient's even being aware that it has happened. Because the interruption of sensory nerve pathways deprives body tissues of these

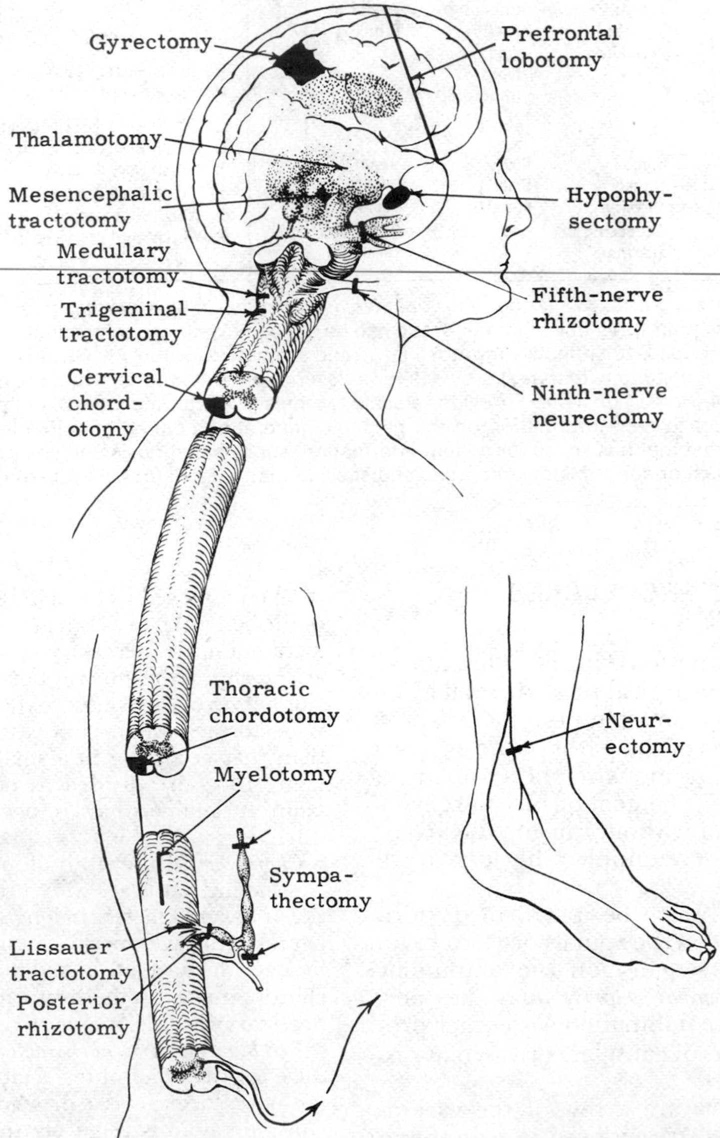

Figure 30–6. Schematic diagram illustrating various surgical procedures designed to alleviate pain. (From Chusid, J. G., and J. J. McDonald: *Correlative Neuroanatomy and Functional Neurology,* 13th ed. Los Altos, Calif.: Lange Medical Publications, 1967.)

protective mechanisms, this procedure is usually not carried out unless other less radical treatment measures have failed.

> *Interruption of sensory nerves deprives tissues of protective reflexes, such as feelings of pain, pressure, and heat.*

*Stereotaxic Pain Surgery**

In 1920 it was suggested that application of the techniques of stereotaxic surgery be used for the treatment of pain, by the section of deep fiber tracts in the brain. The first stereotaxic operations for pain were done around 1930, and the animal-perfected technique was then applied to human beings in the 1940's.

Stereotaxic brain surgery, aiming at the modification of cerebral function by the section of tracts and destruction of nuclei, may now be divided into two categories according to method of approach: (1) *open* stereotaxic surgery, using electrodes or other techniques, i.e., cryogenic surgery, radio frequency heating, implantation of radio isotopes, ultrasound; and (2) *closed,* bloodless stereotaxic *radiosurgery* with ionizing radiation, i.e., gamma rays, x-rays, protons, and other heavy particles.

Open stereotaxic techniques have been successfully developed for the treatment of intractable pain. Although the surgery is referred to as "open," it is not like conventional surgery where the area being treated is visually seen and manually felt by the surgeon. Stereotaxic operations are dependent upon technical apparatus, and the operation is precisely precalculated anatomically and technically.

With open stereotaxic pain-relieving procedures a needle or probe can be inserted into one or more specific sites in the brain, by way of a small hole drilled in the skull. When the probe is inserted the physician applies a heating current that results in coagulation of adjacent tissue; if a needle is inserted, a neurolytic agent is injected.

Many agents can be neurolytic, i.e., can destroy either nerve fibers themselves or their cells of origin. The effectiveness of injectable agents varies and is influenced by the location of the injection and the concentration and volume of the neurolytic agent. Hot water, disinfectants (e.g., phenol), and alcohol are examples of injectable neurolytic agents. Other agents that can be neurolytic include high frequency sound, radiation, and dry ice.

*"Stereotaxic" refers to precise positioning in space. In relation to surgery it connotes the location of operative sites deep within the body — frequently within the cranium — by instrumentation from outside the body.

Stereotaxic procedures can be done with a high degree of accuracy and with little discomfort to the patient. By referring to right-angle coordinates, standard charts, and special x-rays, it is possible to selectively destroy tissue in preselected sites deep within the brain.

Both the size of the lesion and the position of the target are determined preoperatively. Although it is technically possible to place an accurate stereotaxic lesion anywhere in the depth of the brain with minimal risk, the surgery is not without problems, i.e., there is often a tendency for pain to recur in time, as with the more conventional pain surgery. However, it is also possible for such minute lesions to produce a permanent cure. The clinical result often cannot be judged for several months after the operation.

With *radiosurgery,* as well, the operative effect does not appear immediately, but rather after a latent period that varies with factors such as the dose of radiation. Some of the advantages of radiosurgery over the open method are: (1) there is no operative shock and practically no mortality risk; (2) the risks of infection and bleeding are eliminated; and (3) the patient can leave the hospital the day after the procedure. Since the lesion produced by radiosurgery continues to enlarge for several months, care must be taken that the ultimate size of the lesion will not produce undesirable side effects.

For the patient suffering from longstanding pain, pain can become totally absorbing, completely dominating life. When such pain is removed, by surgical interruption of pain pathways, with resultant abolition of pain perception, the problem is not entirely solved. Because of the complicated nature of chronically painful conditions, such a patient frequently requires long-term psychotherapeutic and rehabilitative measures after surgery. Once surgical pain relief is obtained, function must be restored and new goals found. Occupational therapy may be necessary. The patient's significant others should be included in the therapeutic approaches used.

Stimulation Therapy

The relief of chronic pain by electrical stimulation became a new modality of clinical management after Melzack and Wall proposed the gate theory of pain transmission.

Recall from Chapter 29 that this theory describes a spinal cord modulating mechanism in which one type of sensation, such as vibration or light touch, can impede the transmission of another sensation such as pain. The former sensations are transmitted by larger, more rapidly conducting fibers in the peripheral nerves. These sensations reach the spinal cord sooner than the small fibers which conduct painful impulses. Because sensations such as vibration or light touch reach the spinal cord before the painful impulses, they can activate a pool of modulating neurons and block the incoming pain signal.

Electrical nerve stimulators have been developed which can activate the large fibers producing a tingling or vibratory sensation, thereby blocking painful stimuli.

Since it is known that the dorsal columns carry the majority of light touch and vibratory sense to higher centers, the idea developed that stimulation of the dorsal columns directly could achieve a wider area of stimulation and pain relief. Other techniques have involved attention directly to the thalamus, including methods of electrode implantation and chronic stimulation for pain relief. Three types of electrical nerve stimulators are discussed here.

Transcutaneous Electrical Nerve Stimulation. Transcutaneous electrical nerve stimulation (TENS) developed from the need to screen patients for dorsal column stimulator implants. The screening procedure itself was found to be effective in relieving pain in many patients. Success depends upon the patient's understanding of, interest in, and motivation for the treatment. Usually a superficial nerve close to the pain is selected for stimulation. Electrode placement depends on the site of pain. Figure 30–7 shows a nurse assisting the patient in placement of transcutaneous electrodes. Electrodes of unidirec-

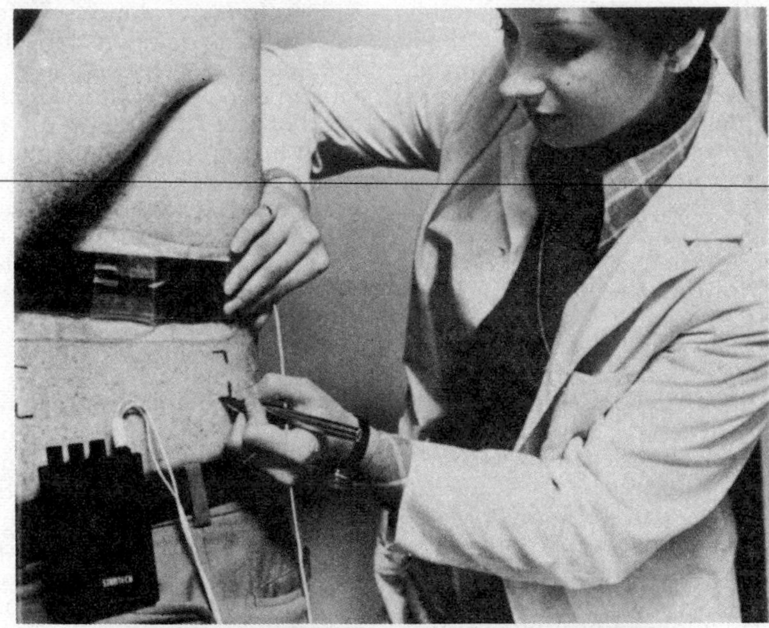

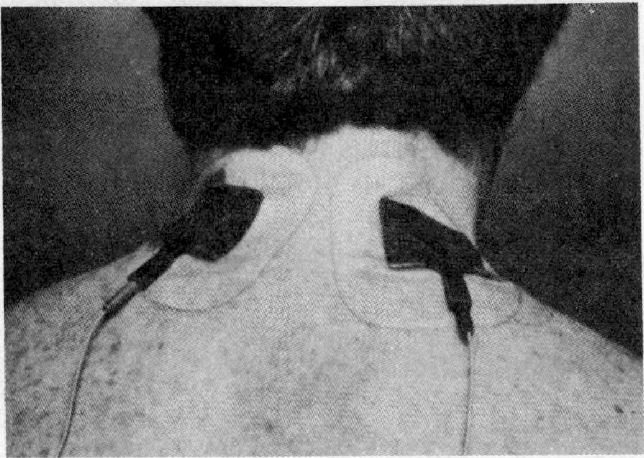

Figure 30–7. A nurse marks the electrode site with indelible ink so that the patient can find it easily. The pulse generator is often clipped to the patient's belt, as shown; although most generators are small enough to be carried in a pocket. Smaller electrodes may be used on areas such as the neck. (From Davis, A. J.: Teaching your patients to use electricity to ward off pain. *RN*, 41:43, Feb. 1978.)

tional stimulation have both positive and negative poles and are usually placed within several inches of each other. Voltage and pulsation are controlled by the patient. The electrodes are moistened with nonsaline aquaphylic electrode jelly to insure proper conduction. Both skin and electrodes are cleaned and fresh jelly applied every 8 hours. When stimulation is not effective, the entire painful area is explored for subsequent electrode placement.[94]

Percutaneous Epidural Dorsal Column Stimulation. A single (unipolar) electrode or two (bipolar) insulated-wire electrodes are placed percutaneously into the spinal epidural space. This procedure allows temporary stimulation of the dorsal column as a screening technique prior to permanent implantation of a stimulator. It is a necessary part of the evaluation of a patient to assess whether or not a stimulator would be beneficial.

Local anesthesia is injected in the tissue overlying the interspinous space. A curved needle is inserted, and the wire electrode is gently passed through the needle into the epidural space. After the electrode has been manipulated into proper position under fluoroscopy, the needle is withdrawn and the electrode left in place. This procedure is then repeated at the same place or at a different interspace for placement of the second electrode. The electrodes are then attached to an external power source, by which the patient can control the amount of dorsal column stimulation received. Figure 30–8 shows a percutaneous electrode epidural stimulation, temporary implant.[94]

Dorsal Column Spinal Cord Stimulation. Success with this type of pain therapy requires careful patient evaluation and selection. Pain must be due to a definitely diagnosed organic cause; the patients selected have undergone multiple previous therapies in an attempt to relieve their pain. Initial screening is done with a percutaneous epidural dorsal column stimulator; if the patient experiences pain relief by this temporary technique, then placement of a dorsal column stimulation implant is indicated. The implant stimulation device is a transistorized receiver. In a surgical procedure, a subcutaneous pocket is formed for the receiver. The pocket is usually in the infraclavicular region or the abdomen. The electrodes are passed subcutaneously from the receiver to a laminectomy incision. The electrode buttons are imbedded in a rectangular insulation sheet that is placed between the leaves of the dura. The laminectomy is usually done in the dorsal or cervical region, depending upon the location of pain.

Relief of chronic pain from the dorsal column stimulator has been reported to diminish with time, and results have not been as encouraging as

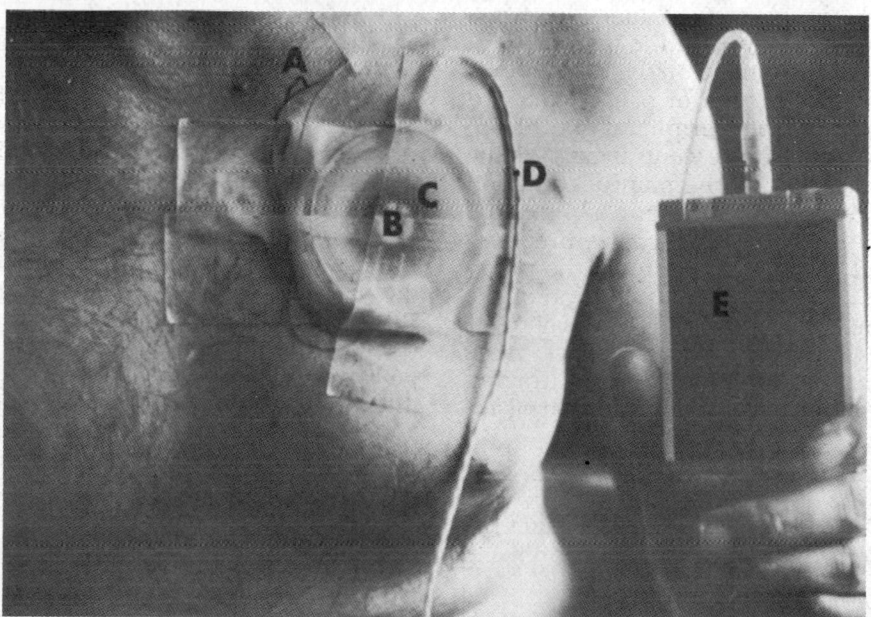

Figure 30–8. Percutaneous electrode epidural stimulation, temporary implant: (*A*) Electrode wires (external portion). (*B*) Receiver (external temporary type). (*C*) Antenna. (*D*) Antenna lead wire. (*E*) Transmitter power unit. External appliances are worn in convenient position; wires have been inserted posteriorly between the spinous processes into the epidural space (not shown). (Avery Laboratories, Inc., Farmingdale, New York.) (From McDonnell, D.: Surgical and electrical stimulation methods for relief of pain. *In* Jacob, A. K. (Ed.): *Pain: A Source Book for Nurses and Other Health Professionals.* Boston: Little, Brown and Co., 1977.)

hoped for. Implantation of the peripheral nerve stimulators is safer and easier then implanation of dorsal column stimulators.[94]

Treatment of Central Pain Syndromes

Causalgia. Treatment for causalgia should start promptly to prevent progressive incapacitation and suffering. The treatment of choice is interruption of the sympathetic chain that supplies the painful part. *Sympathetic blocks* with local anesthetics may be used both diagnostically and therapeutically. Successive blocks may produce effects of increasing duration such that the symptom may be mild and relatively undisturbing or may entirely vanish. However, a *sympathectomy* may be necessary if several blocks fail to provide satisfactory relief. A dorsal preganglionic sympathectomy is the procedure of choice for causalgias of the upper extremities; lumbar sympathectomy is the surgical approach for causalgias of the lower extremities. Once severe pain has been relieved, the patient is given immediate physical therapy, e.g. active and passive movement.

Phantom Limb Pain. Treatment for phantom limb pain poses frustrating problems, since uniform success has never been obtained from any one type of treatment. Following amputation, it is important that phantom pain is distinguished from other phantom sensations that commonly occur. The other phantom sensations require giving assurance to the patient that the sensations will not markedly increase; the presence of phantom pain may require a more aggressive medical intervention. It appears that with the passage of time there is a progressive "centralization" of the pain process. That is to say, a movement of the factors predominant in the production of pain occurs in a direction *away* from the peripheral site of the amputation and to a more central part of the nervous system. Thus, as the painful condition becomes long-term and chronic in nature, the cerebral cortex of the brain becomes predominantly involved in the projections of the phantom pain. This progressive centralization of the pain process makes it inadvisable to delay treatment in hopes of spontaneous recovery. Also, postponing treatment is mentally discouraging to the patient and invites problems with drug addiction.

The following procedures have a role in the relief or modification of phantom pain:

1. *Local, peripheral procedures performed on the amputation stump*
2. *Sympathetic nerve block and sympathectomy*
3. *Anterolateral chordotomy*
4. *Resection of the sensory cortex (cortical resection)*
5. *Prefrontal lobotomy (leukotomy)*

PERIPHERAL PROCEDURES. Procedures such as stump revison may lose their effectiveness once centralization of the pain has taken place. Therefore, these treatments should be performed as early as possible if they are necessary. Various peripheral procedures that may be performed upon the stump of the amputated limb include:

▶ *Revision of the stump,* with *reamputation* at a higher level, should seldom be performed for the relief of phantom pain, since the pain typically recurs in the new stump. Revisions of the stump may be performed, however, when it is necessary to do so to fit a prosthesis. It is essential that the patient be fitted properly with a prosthesis as soon as possible and be encouraged to wear it. Daily massage and ultrasound treatments may help the patient adjust more readily to the new artificial limb, thereby reducing pain.

▶ *Local infiltration with procaine* may be used when there is point tenderness in the stump or when a painful, adherent scar is producing the phantom pain.

▶ *Mechanical percussion* of sensitive amputation neuromas* may be employed when phantom limb pain is associated with a locally painful area in the stump. This unusual method of treatment is believed to produce progressive fibrosis of the nerve end and shrinkage of the neuroma as a result of the continued trauma.

The percussion is obtained by (1) striking the sensitive area of a *digital* stump vigorously and repeatedly against a solid object; (2) placing one end of a wooden peg which is about one inch in diameter over the sensitive area of a *lower extremity stump* and striking the other end with a wooden mallet for 10 to 20 minutes; or (3) using a mechanical vibrator for *either* a digital or lower extremity stump. While the percussion is initially performed several times per day, the duration and frequency of the percussion sessions are reduced with improvement.

▶ *Resection of a painful neuroma* may be attempted *one* time if repeated infiltrations with procaine and percussion fail to bring sustained relief and if the pain is localized and can consistently be relieved for short periods of time with procaine infiltration.

SYMPATHETIC NERVE BLOCK AND SYMPATHECTOMY. These may relieve phantom limb pain when it is associated with vasomotor and sudomotor disturbances in the stump. An amputation stump that has such disturbances may be cold, cyanotic, hyperesthetic (excessively sensitive), painful, and covered with excessive perspiration during periods of discomfort. Exposure to cold and heightened emotional stress may increase the pain. Following a successful sympathetic ganglion nerve block, which denervates the sympathetic outflow to the stump, the affected area becomes warm, nontender, and dry. If the nerve

**Neuromas* are tumors growing from a nerve. These areas of new growth or tumors are predominantly made up of nerve cells and nerve fibers. *Amputation neuromas* are those traumatic neuromas that occur following amputation. The neuroma is often sensitive to traction and pressure and, in addition, may be a source of pain referred to the phantom extremity.

block proves to be successful, it should be followed by a sympathectomy to insure more permanent results.

ANTEROLATERAL CHORDOTOMY. This may be performed if the previously discussed procedures are unsuccessful or are not indicated, and if the patient is incapacitated by a painful phantom limb.

Chordotomy is technically easier to perform, and produces greater pain relief, when the lower extremities are involved than when the upper extremities are affected. *Percutaneous high cervical radiofrequency chordotomy* has proved to be a useful procedure that enlarges the scope of the original open surgical operation. Although chordotomy may relieve stump pain and local tenderness, it is less effective in relieving the pain in the missing phantom limb. Nonetheless, chordotomy is still the best available neurosurgical approach.

RESECTION OF THE SENSORY CORTEX (CORTICAL RESECTION). In theory this is the procedure of choice for relieving phantom pain, since this pain is believed to progressively migrate to the brain and eventually be projected by the cerebral cortex. However, it has been demonstrated that the majority of patients who have had cortical resection for phantom pain have had a recurrence of their symptoms. In addition, since the operation involves scar formation adjacent to the motor strip in the brain, epilepsy is a common complication. For these reasons, cortical resection is not a standard treatment for phantom pain.

PREFRONTAL LOBOTOMY (LEUKOTOMY). This is a surgical procedure that poses many problems, although it may still be performed in managing phantom pain after careful consideration is given to its long-term effects. The primary problem is that when sufficient damage is done to the frontal lobes, so that pain appreciation is altered, then mental deterioration results. *Bilateral* destruction of the frontal lobes produces severe mental deterioration, although it does alter pain appreciation. On the other hand, unilateral frontal lobotomy does not produce prolonged pain relief.

PSYCHOLOGIC THERAPIES. Various psychologic theories have been proposed to account for phantom limb experiences and phantom limb pain. Psychiatrists have treated patients with phantom limb pain, and they report some successes and some failures from psychotherapy, hyponosis, narco-analysis, and electric shock. Clearly there is an interrelationship between attitude and the experience of pain.

The psychologic significance of phantom limb pain and similar central pains is most often considered in relation to its *effects* rather than its *causes.* At times, formal psychiatric treatment may help patients with various forms of neurogenic or central pain. In some cases an associated depressive illness may be treated with some benefit to the pain. However, more often the appropriate treatment measures involve the use of tranquilizers, local anesthesia, vibrators, and relatively minor surgical procedures.

Alternatives to surgical interventions should be explored thoroughly with patients. If a chordotomy, cortical resection, or lobotomy becomes necessary, patients must be taught to protect themselves from injury. Once surgery is done, they invariably will not be able to wear a prosthesis and use it.

BIBLIOGRAPHY (UNIT XI)

1. Adams, R. D.: General Considerations. Pain. *In* Thorn, E. W., et al.: *Harrison's Principles of Internal Medicine,* 8th ed. New York: McGraw-Hill Book Co., 1974.
2. Alexander, J. K.: Differential guide to chest pain. *Hospital Medicine, 12*:6, May 1976.
3. Analgesics: The special challenge of chronic pain. *Patient Care* 6:135, March 15, 1972.
4. Barras, A., Str.: Low back pain. We must get through. *RN,* 41.78, Oct. 1978.
5. Battista, A. F.: Subarachnoid cold saline wash for pain relief. *Archives of Surgery,* 103:672, Dec. 1971.
6. Beecher, H. K.: Relationship of wound to pain experienced. *J.A.M.A.,* 161:1609, 1956.
7. Beecher, H. K.: *Measurement of Subjective Responses.* New York, Oxford University Press, 1959, p. 158.
8. Beecher, H. K.: Anxiety and pain. *J.A.M.A.,* 209:1080, Aug. 1969.
9. Bellville, J. W., et al.: Influence of age on pain relief from analgesics. A study of postoperative patients. *J.A.M.A.,* 217:1835, 1971.
10. Berni, R., and W. E. Fordyce: *Behavior Modification and the Nursing Process.* St. Louis: C. V. Mosby Company, 1977.
11. Billars, K. S.: You have pain? I think this will help. *American Journal of Nursing,* 70:2143, Oct., 1970.
12. Black, R. G., and J. J. Bonica: Analgesic blocks. *Postgraduate Medicine,* 53:105, May 1973.
13. Bobey, M. J., et al.: Psychological factors affecting pain tolerance. *Journal of Psychosomatic Research* 14:371, Dec. 1970.
14. Bonica, J. J.: *Clinical Applications of Diagnostic and Therapeutic Nerve Blocks.* Springfield, Ill.: Charles C Thomas, 1959.
15. Botton, J. E.: Neurosurgical procedures for the management of intractable pain. *Clinical Orthopaedics and Related Research,* 73:101, Nov.–Dec. 1970.
16. Brannon, M. E.: The problem-back service. *American Journal of Nursing,* 75:1295, Aug. 1975.
17. Brewer, B. J.: Low back pain. *American Family Physician,* 19:114, June 1979.
18. Bruegel, M. A.: Relationship of preoperative anxiety to perception of postoperative pain. *Nursing Research,* 20:26, Jan.–Feb. 1970.
19. Budzynski, T. H.: Biofeedback procedures in the clinic. *Seminars in Psychiatry,* 4:5, 1973.
20. Burton, C., et al.: Treating low back pain in the elderly. *Geriatrics,* 33:61, Oct. 1978.
21. Cady, J. W.: "Dear Pain. . ." *American Journal of Nursing,* 76:960, June 1976.

22. Caghan, S. B., et al.: When adolescents complain of pain. *Nurse Practitioner,* 3:19, July-Aug. 1978.
23. Campbell, D.: The management of pain in the intensive care unit. *British Journal of Surgery,* 57:721, Oct. 1970.
24. Caperton, E. M., and P. J. Bilka: Painful shoulder. *Hospital Medicine,* 15:100, Feb. 1979.
25. Casey, K. L., and R. Melzack: Neural mechanisms of pain: A conceptual model. *In* E. L. Way (Ed.): *New Concepts of Pain and Its Clinical Management.* Philadelphia: F. A. Davis Co., 1967.
26. Catalano, R. B.: The medical approach to management of pain caused by cancer. *Seminars in Oncology,* 2:379, Dec. 1975.
27. Chambers, W. G., and G. G. Price: Influence of nurse upon effects of analgesics administered. *Nursing Research,* 16:228, Summer 1967.
28. Chapman, C. R.: The management of chronic pain in the United States and Japan: A cross cultural comparison. *Clinical Medicine,* 82:39, May 1975.
29. Copley, I. J.: No matter what you call it, it's still pain to the patient. *RN,* 41:64, Feb. 1978.
30. Copp, L. A.: The spectrum of suffering. *American Journal of Nursing, 74*:491, Mar. 1974.
31. Copple, D.: What can a nurse do to relieve pain without resort to drugs? *Nursing Times,* 68:584, May 1972.
32. Crasilneck, H. B., and J. A. Hall: Clinical hypnosis in problems of pain. *The American Journal of Clinical Hypnosis,* 15:153, Jan. 1973.
33. Crowley, D. M.: *Pain and Its Alleviation.* University of California, 1962.
34. Dalessio, D. J.: Evaluation of the patient with chronic facial pain. *American Family Physician,* 16:84, Sept. 1977.
35. Davidson, P. O.: *The Behavioral Management of Anxiety, Depression and Pain.* New York: Brunner/Mazel, 1976.
36. Davis, A. J.: Brompton's cocktail: Making goodbyes possible. *American Journal of Nursing,* 78:610, Apr. 1978.
37. Davis, A. J.: Teaching your patients to use electricity to ward off pain. *RN,* 41:43, Feb. 1978.
38. Davitz, L. J., and J. R. Davitz: How do nurses feel when patients suffer. *American Journal of Nursing,* 75:1505, Sept. 1975.
39. Davitz, L. J., Y. Sameshima, and J. Davitz: Suffering as viewed in six different cultures. *American Journal of Nursing,* 76:1296, Aug. 1976.
40. de Grood, M. P.: Stereotaxic treatment of pain. *Journal of Neurology, Neurosurgery and Psychiatry,* 34:106, Feb. 1971.
41. Dennison, A. D.: Chest pain: When to admit. *Emergency Medicine,* 11:55, Feb. 1979.
42. Derrick, W. S.: Subarachnoid alcohol block in the control of pain. *CA,* 21:249, July–Aug. 1971.
43. DiBlasi, M., and C. J. Washburn: Using analgesics effectively. *American Journal of Nursing,* 79:74, Jan. 1979.
44. Diers, D., et al.: The effect of nursing interaction on patients in pain. *Nursing Research,* 21:419, Sept.–Oct. 1972.
45. Done, A. K.: The toxic emergency. Not-so-local anesthetics. *Emergency Medicine,* 10:59, Dec. 1978.
45a. Dorsey, J. M.: Problems with pain in a general surgical practice. *Medical Clinics of North America,* 52:103, Jan. 1968.
46. Drakontides, A. B.: Drugs to treat pain. *American Journal of Nursing,* 74:508, Mar. 1974.
47. Eland, J. M.: Living with pain. *Nursing Outlook,* 26:430, July 1978.
48. Ewin, D. M.: Relieving suffering — and pain — with hypnosis. *Geriatrics,* 33:87, June 1978.
49. Finneson, B.: *Diagnosis and Management of Pain Syndromes,* 2nd ed. Philadelphia: W. B. Saunders Co., 1969.
50. Fordyce, W. E.: Operant conditioning as a treatment method in the management of selected chronic pain problems. *Northwest Medicine* 69:580, Aug. 1970.
51. Forshee, T., and B. Minckley: How to put lumbar sympathectomy patients on their own two feet. *RN,* 39:18, July 1976.
52. Ganong, W. F.: *Review of Medical Physiology,* 8th ed. Los Altos, Calif.: Lange Medical Publications, 1977.
53. Gatz, A. J.: *Manter's Essentials of Clinical Neuroanatomy and Neurophysiology.* Philadelphia: F. A. Davis Co., 1970.
54. Gaumer, W. R.: Electrical stimulation in chronic pain. *American Journal of Nursing,* 74:504, Mar. 1974.
55. Gaumer, W. C.: Psychological potentials of chronic pain. *Journal of Psychiatric Nursing and Mental Health Services,* 12:23, Sept.–Oct. 1974.
56. Gebhart, G. F.: Narcotic and non-narcotic analgesics for relief of pain. *In* Jacox, A. K. (Ed.): *Pain: A Source Book for Nurses and Other Health Professionals.* Boston: Little, Brown and Company, 1977.
57. Ghia, J. N., et al.: Therapeutic nerve blocks for chronic pain. *American Family Physician,* 20:74, July 1979.
58. Gilbertson, B.: Low back pain. . .what to look for. . .what to do. *RN,* 41:75, Oct. 1978.
59. Gillman, J.: Pain relief and other effects following barbotage. *Lancet* 1:746, April 1, 1972.
60. Goloskov, J., and P. LeRoy: Use of the dorsal column stimulator. *American Journal of Nursing,* 74:506, Mar. 1974.
61. Grad, R. K., and J. Woodside: Obstetrical analgesics and anesthesia: Methods of relief for the patient in labor. *American Journal of Nursing,* 77:242, Feb. 1977.
62. Gramse, C. A.: For control of severe pain: Dorsal column stimulation. *American Journal of Nursing,* 78:1022, June 1978.
63. Greenhoot, J. H., and R. A. Sternbach: Conjoint treatment of chronic pain. *In* Bonica, J. J. (Ed.): *Pain: Advances in Neurology,* Raven Press, 1974.
64. Griem, M. L.: The radiologist and the relief of pain. *Medical Clinics of North America,* 52:203, Jan. 1968.
65. Grollman, A.: Use of drugs in relief of pain. *In* Finneson, B.: *Diagnosis and Management of Pain Syndromes,* 2nd ed. Philadelphia: W. B. Saunders Co., 1969.
66. Guyton, A. C.: *Basic Human Physiology: Normal Function and Mechanisms of Disease.* Philadelphia: W. B. Saunders Co., 1977.
67. Hackett, T. P.: Pain and prejudice. Why do we doubt that the patient is in pain? *Medical Times,* 99:130, Feb. 1971.
68. Halpern, L. M.: Analgesics and other drugs for relief of pain. *Postgraduate Medicine,* 53:91, May 1973.
69. Halpern, L. M.: Treating pain with drugs. *Minnesota Medicine,* 3:57, Mar. 1974.
70. Harris, A. B.: Critical evaluation and the neurosurgical treatment of pain. *Northwest Medicine,* 69:576, Aug. 1970.
71. Hilgard, E. R.: A neodissociation interpretation of pain reduction in hypnosis. *Psychological Review,* 80:396, Sept. 1973.
72. Holmes, G.: Some clinical aspects of pain. *In* Ogilvie, W., and W. Thomson (Eds.): *Pain and Its Problems.* London: Eyre and Spottiswoode, 1950.
73. Houser, D.: What to do first when a patient complains of chest pain. *Nursing 76,* 6:54, Nov. 1976.

74. Hunter, J.: The mark of pain. *American Journal of Nursing,* 61:96, Oct. 1961.
75. Indeck, W.: Pain in the geriatric patient. *Geriatrics,* 32:43, Nov. 1977.
76. Jacob, S. W., C. A. Francone, and W. J. Lossow: *Structure and Function in Man,* 4th ed. Philadelphia, W. B. Saunders Co., 1978.
77. Jacox, A. K.: Assessing pain. *American Journal of Nursing,* 79:895, May 1979.
78. Jacox, A. K.: *Pain: A Source Book for Nurses and Other Health Professionals.* Boston: Little Brown and Company, 1977.
79. Johnson, J. E.: Effects of accurate expectations about sensations on the sensory and distress components of pain. *Journal of Personality and Social Psychology* 27:261, Aug. 1973.
79a. Johnson, J. E.: Effects of structuring patients' expectations on their reactions to threatening events. *Nursing Research,* 21:489, 1972.
80. Kaufman, M. A., and D. E. Brown: Pain wears many faces. *American Journal of Nursing,* 61:48, Jan. 1961.
81. Keats, A. S.: Use of analgetics at the bedside. *In* Way, E. L. (Ed.): *New Concepts in Pain and Its Clinical Management.* Philadelphia: F. A. Davis, Co., 1967.
82. Keough, G., and J. L. Fox: The neuropacemaker — relief for patients with intractable pain. *RN,* 35:OR7, July 1972.
83. Klein, R. F., and W. Brown: Pain descriptions in the medical setting. *Journal of Psychosomatic Research,* 10:367, May 1967.
84. Kolodny, A. L., and P. T. McLoughlin: *Comprehensive Approach to the Therapy of Pain.* Springfield, Ill.: Charles C Thomas, 1966.
85. Korten, K.: Anesthesia for diagnostic procedures. *American Family Physician,* 15:103, Mar. 1977.
86. Kraus, H.: Controlling hypokinetic backache: Treating the patient instead of the back. *Nursing Digest,* 5:31, Spring 1977.
87. Livingston, W. K.: *Pain Mechanisms: A Physiologic Interpretation of Causalgia and Its Related States.* New York: Plenum Press, 1976.
88. Lloyd, J. W., J. D. W. Barnard, and G. J. Glynn: Cryoanalgesia — A new approach to pain relief. *Lancet,* 2:932, Oct. 1976.
89. Loeser, J. D.: Central pains. *Clinical Medicine,* 82, May 1975.
90. Marks, R. G.: Intractable headache? Biofeedback could be a solution. *RN,* 42:73, July 1979.
91. McCaffery, M.: Intelligent approach to intractable pain. *Nursing 73,* 3:26, Nov. 1973.
92. McCaffery, M.: *Nursing Management of the Patient with Pain.* Philadelphia, J. B. Lippincott Co., 1972.
93. McCaffery, M., and L. Hart: Undertreatment of acute pain with narcotics. *American Journal of Nursing,* 76:1586, Oct. 1976.
94. McDonnell, D.: Surgical and electrical stimulation methods for relief of pain. *In* Jacox, A. K. (Ed.): *Pain: A Source Book for Nurses and Other Health Professionals.* Boston: Little, Brown and Co., 1977.
95. McHardy, G.: Acute anterior chest pain: Angina or esophagitis? *Consultant,* 16:164, Nov. 1976.
96. McLachlan, E.: Recognizing pain. *American Journal of Nursing,* 74:496, Mar. 1974.
97. McMahon, M. A., and P. Miller: Pain response: The influence of psycho-social-cultural factors. *Nursing Forum,* 17(1):58, 1978.
98. McMasters, R.: A clinical approach to pain. *Southern Medical Journal,* 67:173, Feb. 1974.
99. Mastrovito, R. C.: Psychogenic pain. *American Journal of Nursing* 74:514, Mar. 1974.
100. Meares, A.: *Relief Without Drugs: The Self-Management of Tension, Anxiety, and Pain.* Garden City, N.Y.: Doubleday, 1967.
101. Melzack, R.: *The Puzzle of Pain.* New York, Basic Books, Inc., 1973.
102. Melzack, R.: How acupuncture works — a sophisticated western theory takes the mystery out. *Psychology Today,* 7:28, June 1973.
103. Melzack, R.: The McGill pain questionnaire, major properties and scoring methods. *Pain,* 1:277, Sept. 1975.
104. Melzack, R., and P. Taenzer: Concepts of pain perception and therapy. *Geriatrics,* 32:44, Nov. 1977.
105. Melzack, R., and P. D. Wall: Gate control theory of pain. *In* Soulairac, A., J. Cahn, and J. Charpentier (Eds.): *Pain.* New York: Academic Press, 1968.
106. Melzack, R., and P. D. Wall: Pain mechanisms: A new theory. *Science,* 150:971, Nov. 1965.
107. Melzack, R., J. G. Ofiesh, and B. M. Mount: The Brompton mixture: Effects on pain in cancer patients. *Canadian Medical Association Journal,* 115:125, July 17, 1976.
108. Merskey, H., and F. G. Spear: *Pain: Psychological and Psychiatric Aspects.* London, Baillière, Tindall and Cassell, 1967.
108a. Mettler, F. A.: Pain. I.: What is it? *The Journal of the Medical Society of New Jersey,* 61:10, Jan. 1964.
109. Millard, L.: Low back pain: Guide to evaluation. *Hospital Medicine,* 14:79, Sept. 1978.
110. Miller, B. F., and C. B. Keane: *Encyclopedia and Dictionary of Medicine, Nursing, and Allied Health,* 2nd ed. Philadelphia: W. B. Saunders Co., 1978.
111. Mines, S.: *The Conquest of Pain.* New York: Grosset and Dunlap, 1974.
112. Moertel, C. G., et al.: Relief of pain by oral medications. *Journal of American Medical Association,* 229:55, July 1, 1974.
113. Moore, M. E.: Relieving chronic pain without strong analgesics. Part I — The nonsteroidal anti-inflammatories. *Consultant,* 17:95, Oct. 1977.
114. Moore, M. E.: Relieving chronic pain without strong analgesics. Part 2 — Corticosteroids, psychotropics, anticonvulsants and placebos. *Consultant,* 17:155, Nov. 1977.
115. Morch, E. T.: Pain relief for office procedures. *Medical Clinics of North America* 52:173, Jan. 1968.
116. Morgan, W. L., and G. L. Engel: *The Clinical Approach to the Patient.* Philadelphia, W. B. Saunders Co., 1969.
117. Mozingo, J. N.: Pain in labor: A conceptual model for intervention. *Journal of Obstetric, Gynecologic and Neonatal Nursing,* 7:47, July–Aug. 1978.
118. Murray, J. B.: Psychology of the pain experience. *Journal of Psychology,* 78:193, July 1971.
119. Noordenbos, W.: Physiological correlates of clinical pain syndromes. *In* Soulairac, A., J. Cahn, and J. Charpentier (Eds.): *Pain.* New York: Academic Press, Inc., 1968.
120. Noordenbos, W.: Pathologic aspects of central pain states. *In* Bonica, J. J. (Ed.): *Advances in Neurology.* New York: Raven Press, 1974.
121. Older, J.: Pain and the physician. *Postgraduate Medicine,* 62:35, Nov. 1977.
122. O'Neal, J. T.: Managing chronic pain. *American Family Physician,* 10:74, Dec. 1974.
123. Pace, J. B.: *Pain, A Personal Experience.* Chicago: Nelson-Hall Publishers, 1976.
124. Pace, J. B.: Helping patients overcome the disabling effects of chronic pain. *Nursing 77,* 7:38, July 1977.
125. Palmer, E. D.: Two causes of nonvisceral abdominal wall pain. *American Family Physician,* 17:115, Apr., 1978.
126. Parker, R. G.: Pain relief for the cancer patient through selective radiation therapy. *Northwest Medicine,* 69:665, Sept. 1970.

127. Peircey, M. L.: Assessment of low back pain. *Nurse Practitioner,* 1:18, Mar.–Apr. 1976.
128. Pichard, A. D.: Axioms on chest pain. *Hospital Medicine,* 13:8, Sept. 1977.
129. Pinto, C. M.: *Acupuncture: Science or charlatanism?* Ardmore, Pa.: Dorrance and Co., 1978.
130. Plein, J. B.: Perspectives on aspirin. Part 1: Aspirin as an analgesic. *Nurse Practitioner,* 1:34, Mar.–Apr. 1976.
131. Poulton, T. J., and G. R. Mims: Peripheral nerve Blocks. *American Family Physician,* 16:100, Nov. 1977.
132. Poswillo, D. E.: Pharmacodynamics of pain relief. *In* Alling, C. C., III, et al. (Eds.): *Facial Pain.* Philadelphia: Lea & Febiger, 1968.
133. Raney, J. O.: Pain, emotion and a rationale for therapy. *Northwest Medicine,* 69:659, Sept. 1970.
134. Ratts, T. E.: Axioms on coronary artery disease. *Hospital Medicine,* 14:36, Mar. 1978.
135. Ryan, R. E.: Common and uncommon causes of head and face pain. *Consultant,* 18:90, Nov. 1978.
136. Scheinman, M. M.: Finding the cause of chest pain. *Consultant,* 16:49, Nov. 1976.
137. Schultz, J., and W. Luthe: *Autogenic Training.* New York: Grune and Stratton, 1959.
138. Shealy, C. N.: The pain patient. *American Family Physician,* 9:130, Mar. 1974.
139. Siegele, D. S.: The gate control theory. *American Journal of Nursing,* 74:498, Mar. 1974.
140. Silman, J.: The management of pain. Reference guide to analgesics. *American Journal of Nursing,* 79:74, Jan. 1979.
141. Staub, E., B. Tursky, and G. E. Schwartz: Self-control and predictability — Their effects on reactions to anersine stimulation, *Journal of Personality and Social Psychology,* 18:157, May 1971.
142. Stephen, C. R.: Complications of analgetic therapy. *In* Way, E. L. (Ed.): *New Concepts in Pain and Its Clinical Management.* Philadelphia: F. A. Davis Co., 1967.
143. Sternbach, R. A.: *Pain: A Psychophysiological Analysis.* New York: Academic Press, Inc., 1968.
144. Sternbach, R. Z.: *Pain Patients—Traits and Treatment.* New York: Academic Press, Inc., 1974.
145. Stewart, E.: To lessen pain: Relaxation and rhythmic breathing. *American Journal of Nursing,* 76:958, June 1976.
146. Swanson, D. W.: Less obvious aspects of chronic pain. *Postgraduate Medicine,* 60:130, Nov. 1976.
147. Sweeney, S. S., M. Johnson, and J. M. Eland: Pain associated with neurological conditions. *In* Jacox, J. K.: *Pain: A Source Book for Nurses and Other Health Professionals.* Boston: Little, Brown and Co., 1977.
148. Szasz, T. S.: The nature of pain. *Archives of Neurology and Psychiatry,* (Chicago), 74:174, Aug. 1955.
149. Turnbull, F.: Pain and suffering in cancer. *Canadian Nurse,* 67:28, Aug. 1971.
150. Urban, B. J.: The current use of nerve blocks in the management of chronic pain. *Clinical Medicine,* 82:27, May 1975.
151. Valentine, A. S., S. Steckel, and M. Weintraub: Pain relief for cancer patients. *American Journal of Nursing,* 78:2055, Dec. 1978.
152. Wang, R. I. H.: Control of pain. *The American Journal of the Medical Sciences,* 246:112, Nov. 1963.
153. Waxman, J.: Diagnosis of shoulder and hip pain. *Consultant,* 18:59, Feb. 1978.
154. Way, E. L. (Ed.): *New Concepts in Pain and Its Clinical Management.* Philadelphia: F. A. Davis Co., 1967.
154a. Weddell, G.: The relationship between pain sensibility and peripheral nerve fibers. *In* Knighton, R., and P. Dumke (Eds.): *Pain.* Boston: Little, Brown and Co., 1966.
155. Weisenberg, M.: *Pain — Clinical and Experimental Perspectives.* St. Louis: C. V. Mosby Co., 1975.
156. Wiley, L.: Intractable pain: How nursing care can help you. *Nursing '74.* 4:54, Sept. 1974.
157. Wiley, L. (Ed.): Caring for the cancer patient. Delusions increase the pain. *Nursing 77,* 7:30, Aug. 1977.
158. Wiley, L. (Ed.): Waiting to plan is the same as not planning at all. *Nursing 77,* 7:66, Oct. 1977.
159. Wise, T. N.: Pain. The most common psychosomatic problem. *Medical Clinics of North America,* 61:771, July 1977.
160. Wolf, S.: Placebos: Problems and pitfalls. *Clinical Pharmacology and Therapeutics,* 3:254, 1962.
161. Wolff, H. G., and S. Wolf: *Pain.* Springfield, Ill.: Charles C Thomas, 1958.
162. Zborowski, M.: *People in Pain.* San Francisco: Jossey-Bass, Inc., 1969.

UNIT XII*

NURSING PEOPLE EXPERIENCING DISTURBANCES OF CARDIOVASCULAR FUNCTION AND BLOOD FLOW

INTRODUCTION AND STUDY GUIDE

Heart disease is currently the leading cause of death throughout the western world. This widespread problem has twice as high a mortality rate as does cancer, which ranks second to heart disease as a cause of death. Within the United States alone, more than 1 million people die every year from cardiovascular ailments; more than 30 million persons are afflicted with some type of heart problem; and more than 40 billion dollars is lost from the economy due to the death or disability of patients with cardiac disturbances.[55] Ninety five per cent of cardiac deaths result from the following disorders, ranked in order of their lethality:[199]

1. Ischemic heart disease	90 per cent
2. Hypertensive heart disease	1 to 2 per cent
3. Rheumatic heart disease	1 to 2 per cent
4. Congenital heart disease	<1 per cent
5. Infective endocarditis	<1 per cent
6. Cor pulmonale	<1 per cent
7. Syphilitic heart disease	<1 per cent

Despite these statistics, heart disease as a cause of death has been gradually declining since the early 1970's. Heart disease was the cause of only 10 per cent of deaths at the turn of the century, rising to 39 per cent of deaths in the 1960's. Since 1970, deaths from heart disease have begun to decline, primarily because ischemic heart disease is currently resulting in fewer fatalities.[199] With continued advances in medical research and clinical practice, the coming decades may see additional breakthroughs in the prevention and treatment of this worldwide problem.

Because of greater understanding of cardiovascular disease and its causes and risks, the care of patients with heart disease is one of the most progressive areas in nursing today. With each advance have come new responsibilities and challenges for nurses.

Today, nurses who work in special care units for critically ill cardiac

*This unit was critically reviewed and revised by Susan L. Zimmerman Ashburn, R.N., B.S., M.S.

patients (such as a coronary care unit or an intensive care unit for postoperative cardiac surgery patients) must have a detailed knowledge of cardiology. They must be able to swiftly identify life-threatening arrhythmias on an electrocardiogram and to perform emergency resuscitation measures, if necessary, without the aid of a doctor. The nurse specializing in the care of people experiencing cardiac problems has truly become a significant and respected figure in the total field of health care.

Our goal in this unit is to give you a basic knowledge of heart disease — its cause and treatment — which will help you give comprehensive care (under supervision) to critically ill cardiac patients. Because cardiology is a vast and complex area of medical and nursing practice, this unit is both large and complex. In the study guide below we have listed only those terms, diets, and drug groups that we feel are absolutely basic to a knowledge of cardiac nursing.

1. Chapter 31 of this unit is a review of basic material from anatomy and physiology which is pertinent to the following discussions of heart disease. Careful study of the normal cardiac structure and function presented will help you to understand the abnormalities that we discuss throughout this unit. Refer also to Chapter 15 for discussion of assessment of the cardiovascular system.

2. As you study this unit, familiarize yourself with the following terms:

cardiac reserve
cardiac output
circulatory failure
thrombosis
embolism
infarction
arrhythmia
cardiogenic shock
anastomosis
coronary care unit (CCU)
the Fick principle
fluoroscopy
angiocardiography
cardiac catheterization
electrocardiogram (ECG)
leads
ballistocardiogram
phonocardiogram
cardiac compensation
cardiac decompensation
forward failure theory
backward failure theory
low-output failure
high-output failure
cardiac arrest
cardiopulmonary resuscitation (CPR)
ectopic foci
defibrillation
cardioversion
pacemaker
cardiac index
cor pulmonale
cineangiography
Swan-Ganz catheter
pulmonary artery and pulmonary capillary wedge pressures
echocardiogram
heart block
precordial thump
precordial shock
coronary artery disease (CAD)
coronary heart disease (CHD)
stress testing
high and low density lipoproteins
hyperlipoproteinemia
aerobic exercise
coronary artery bypass graft
diastolic hypertension
systolic hypertension
primary (essential) hypertension
secondary hypertension
renin hypertension (low, medium, and high)
malignant hypertension
renin-angiotensin-aldosterone system
"stepped care" drug approach
pericardial tamponade
atherosclerosis
angina pectoris
myocardial infarction
rheumatic fever
bacterial endocarditis
valvular stenosis and regurgitation
ball-in-cage valve prosthesis
pericarditis
cardiac tamponade
open heart surgery
hypothermia
extracorporeal circulation (ECC)
heart-lung machine

3. Familiarize yourself with these diets: low sodium, low cholesterol, bland low residue, high fiber–low caloric.

4. Carefully study the following drug groups, which are used to correct heart conditions: cardiac glycosides, cardiac depressants, diuretics, coronary dilators, antihypertensive agents, vasopressors, anticoagulants, venous dilators, arterial dilators, beta-adrenergic blocking agents.

Upon completion of this unit, you should be able to apply the knowledge obtained in the clinical situation in the following ways:

- ► Assess risk factors that threaten patients with potential or actual heart disease.
- ► Develop (with the physician) a teaching program to help cardiac patients reduce such risk factors as smoking, overeating, lack of exercise, etc.
- ► Assess and evaluate signs and symptoms of heart disease in your cardiac patients. Look for the six cardinal signs of a heart disorder.
- ► Perform assessment skills accurately: take the blood pressure, examine the neck veins, listen for heart and pulmonary sounds, check pulse, read an ECG for dangerous changes.
- ► Develop imaginative ways in which to promote both the mental and physical health of heart patients in your care.
- ► Understand the drugs that treat heart disease, know the dangerous side effects before administering a cardiac drug.
- ► Assist patients in complying with their program of treatment, help them to set up their goals for long-term rehabilitation and preventive care.
- ► Assist with psychologic support of the patient and significant others during cardiac emergencies and following heart surgery.

CHAPTER 31

THE CARDIOVASCULAR SYSTEM: AN OVERVIEW OF NORMAL ANATOMY AND PHYSIOLOGY

The human heart beats approximately 72 times per minute, forcing oxygen-carrying blood into the arterial system with every stroke. Moreover, this small, powerful pump contracts between 70 and 80 times *every* minute of *every* day throughout a person's lifetime, resting only 0.4 of a second between beats. Unlike other muscles of the body, the heart cannot stop and rest when tired and worn from work. Instead, it must keep pumping regularly, continuously, and with sufficient force for blood and oxygen to circulate properly to all parts of the vascular system and, thus, to all parts of the body.

The job of carrying oxygen and nutrients to cells, and metabolic wastes from cells for excretion, is a task that the heart and circulatory system must perform whether we are asleep or awake, active or sedentary. Therefore, not only must the heart labor constantly to meet the body's basal needs for oxygen and nutrients, it must also be able to *increase* its work output four or fives times the normal if it is to sustain the body during periods of stress, e.g., hard exercise, great emotion, illness, and high fever. In sum, the heart, in addition to maintaining a steady normal workload, must also be able to quickly adjust and adapt to the various pressures of life.

One authority describes the enormity of the heart's tasks:

> The work done by the heart is out of all proportion to its size. Let us look at some figures. Even while we are asleep the heart pumps about two ounces of blood with each beat, a teacup with every three beats, nearly five quarts per minute, 75 gallons per hour. In other words, it pumps enough blood to fill an average gasoline tank almost four times every hour just to keep the machinery of the body idling. When the body is moderately active, the heart doubles this output. During strenuous muscular efforts, such as running to catch a train or playing a game of tennis, the cardiac output may go up to 14 barrels per hour. Over the 24 hours of an average day, involving not too vigorous work, it amounts to some 70 barrels, and in a lifetime of 70 years the heart pumps nearly 18 million barrels![250]

Although normally a remarkably precise, durable and efficient structure, the heart, like any machine, can unfortunately develop defects of structure and disturbances of function. What happens to the body when this mechanism, so necessary to life, begins to weaken and fail? What happens to the tissues and cells of the brain and other vital organs when oxygenated blood is no longer pumped to them in adequate amounts?

Let us first review aspects of *normal* cardiovascular structure and function basic to the discussions of pathologic conditions in the following chapters. The heart's major structures and the important mechanisms controlling the heart and circulation are presented below. As you study this outline, ask yourself these questions:

1. In what ways can each of the cardiac structures and functions listed in the outline be adversely altered?
2. What physiologic disturbances can result from these alterations?
3. What effects do major pathologic alterations in the heart and circulatory system have upon the body as a whole? (The answers to these questions are discussed in Chapter 32.)

FUNCTION OF THE CARDIOVASCULAR SYSTEM

▶ The role of the *circulation* is to:

1. Continuously deliver oxygen, nutrients, hormones, and antibodies to organs, tissues, and cells throughout the body in response to varying tissue demands.
2. Remove end products of metabolism from tissues and cells.

▶ The role of the *heart* is to:

1. Pump oxygenated blood into the arterial system, where it is carried to the capillaries supplying tissues.
2. Collect oxygen-poor blood from the venous system and pump it through the lungs to be reoxygenated.

► The role of the *blood vessels* (arteries, capillaries, veins) is to carry blood to and from the body's tissues and cells.

STRUCTURE OF THE HEART

The heart is a cone-shaped, hollow, muscular organ, weighing 300 grams, located in the *mediastinum,* a space between the lungs within the thoracic cavity. Its base is directed toward the body's right side. Its apex is directed toward the left and rests upon the diaphragm.

The heart is a double pump having two sides. The *right* side receives *deoxygenated* blood from the body and pumps it to the lungs to be oxygenated; the *left* side receives oxygenated blood from the lungs and pumps it out through the aorta to all parts of the body (Fig. 31–1).

The *pericardium,* the loose fitting covering of the heart, is composed of:

1. *Fibrous pericardium,* a tough fibrous membrane attached to the great vessels.
2. *Serous pericardium,* composed of two layers: (a) an outer parietal layer that lines fibrous pericardium, and (b) an inner visceral layer, i.e., epicardium, that adheres closely to the heart.
3. The *pericardial space,* between the visceral and parietal layers, filled with *pericardial fluid* (5 to 20 ml.) The fluid (a) lubricates the heart's surfaces as they slide over each other, and (b) alleviates friction between the heart's surfaces as the heart beats.

The *cardiac layers* are:

1. *Epicardium* — outer layer — same structure as visceral pericardium.
2. *Myocardium* — middle layer — composed of *striated* muscle fibers, interlaced together into bundles. This muscle causes the heart's contraction, which squeezes blood out of the heart into the arterial system.
3. *Endocardium* — innermost layer — composed of endothelial tissue and continuous with the blood of endothelial tissue and continuous with the blood vessels. It lines the heart's cavities and covers the heart valves.

The *cardiac chambers* are:

1. *Atria* — the two upper "receiving" chambers. (a) The *right atrium* receives deoxygenated blood from all over the body via the superior and inferior venae cavae, and pumps blood received into the right ventricle from whence it is pumped to the lungs. (b) The *left atrium* receives *oxygenated* blood from the lungs

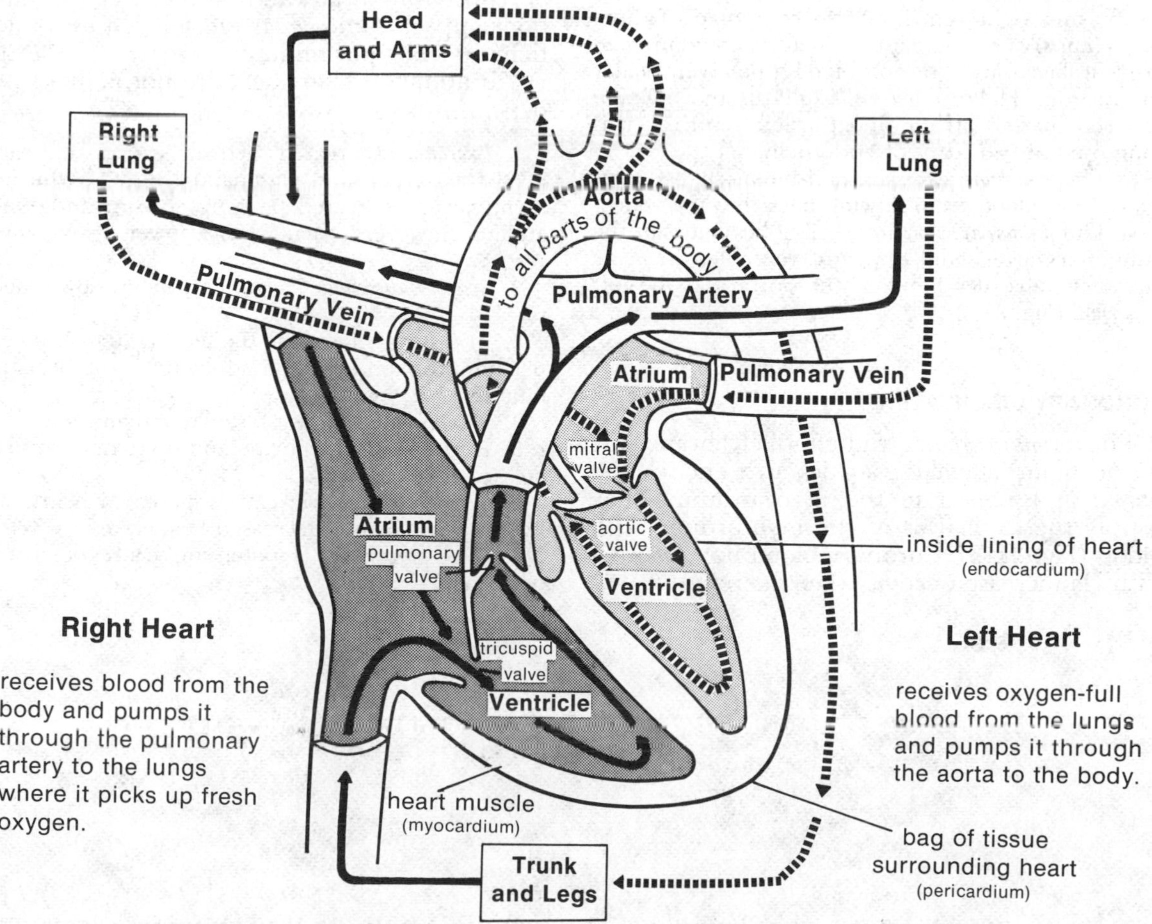

Figure 31–1. Diagram of the heart. (Courtesy of American Heart Association.)

and pumps oxygenated blood to the left ventricle, from which it is pumped out of the body. The *interatrial septum* separates the atria.

2. *Ventricles* — the two lower "distributing" chambers. The inner wall of the ventricles is characterized by *trabeculae carneae,* interlacing bundles of muscle; *papillary muscles,* finger or nipple-shaped projections; and *chordae tendineae,* cordlike structures (composed of dense fibrous connective tissue) that are attached to the valve leaflets. (a) The *right* ventricle receives blood from the right atrium, and pumps it out to the lungs via the *pulmonary artery.* (b) The *left ventricle* — the heart's largest, most muscular chamber — receives *oxygenated* blood from the lungs via the left atrium, and pumps it out to all parts of the body; the *interventricular septum* separates the ventricles.

The *cardiac valves* are:

1. The *atrioventricular valves,* i.e., the tricuspid and bicuspid (mitral) valves, which guard openings between the atria and ventricles, forcing blood to flow forward from atria to ventricles, and preventing blood from flowing backward from ventricles to atria. The *tricuspid valve* guards the opening between right atrium and right ventricle. It is composed of three cusps (flaps) of endothelium, which close and unite to prevent backward flow of blood upon ventricular contraction. The *bicuspid valve* guards the opening between the left atrium and the left ventricle; it is composed of two cusps of endothelium.

2. The *semilunar valves* are half-moon–shaped flaps preventing blood from flowing back into the ventricles. The *pulmonary semilunar* valve lies between the pulmonary artery and the right ventricle; the *aortic semilunar* valve lies between the aorta and the left ventricle (Fig. 31–2).

CORONARY CIRCULATION

The *coronary arteries* (right and left) branch off the aorta just above the aortic valve, encircle the heart, and penetrate the myocardium. They supply the capillaries of the myocardium with blood (Fig. 31–3). Coronary blood flow *increases* with (1) increased activity (i.e., exercise); (2) increased heart rate; and (3) increased stimulation of the sympathetic nervous system.

The *coronary veins* return blood from the myocardium to the right atrium via the *coronary sinus.*

The *capillaries* of the heart muscle exchange oxygen and nutrients for waste products which are later excreted via the kidneys and lungs.

> *Myocardial capillaries are the heart's most essential structures; they* must *receive an adequate blood supply or heart failure will result.*

PULMONARY CIRCULATION

The pulmonary circulation involves blood flow from heart to lungs and back to heart. Blood flows from the right ventricle, through the semilunar valve, to the pulmonary artery, to the lungs, to four pulmonary veins, and back to the left atrium.

HEART RATE

The normal heart rate is 60 to 90 beats per minute. *Sinus tachycardia* is a rate of over 100 beats per minute; it can follow exercise or emotional upset. *Sinus bradycardia* is a rate of less than 60 beats per minute.

Variations in heart beat are normally caused by:

1. *Exercise:* Increased activity causes increased need for oxygen and elimination of CO_2, which, in turn, causes increased heart rate. The conditioned athlete, however, usually has a lower heart rate at rest.
2. *Size of individual:* Larger person has slower heart rate.
3. *Age:* Beat is fastest in the fetus (120 to 160 beats per minute) and lowest in adults (65 to 80 beats per minute).
4. *Sex:* Women have a faster rate than men.
5. *Hormones:* Epinephrine and thyroxine cause increased rate.
6. *Temperature:* Fever causes increased heart rate; hypothermia causes decreased heart rate.
7. *Blood pressure:* Hypotension causes increased heart rate.

VALVES

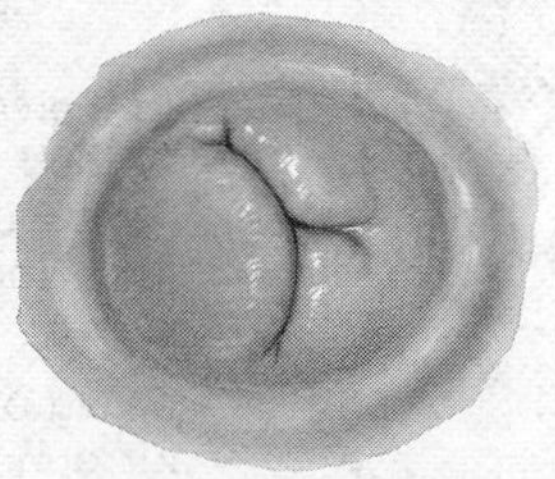

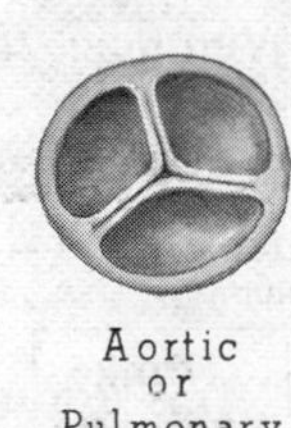

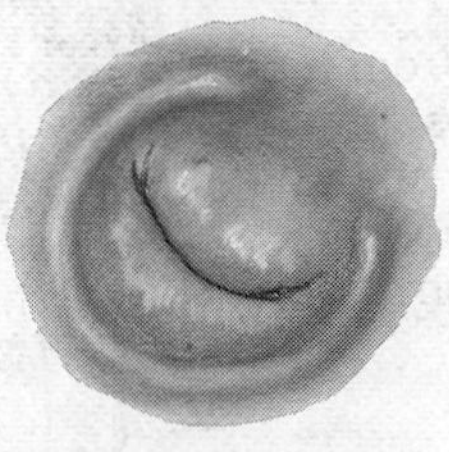

Figure 31–2. Schematic "transparent" drawing of the heart showing the relations of the various heart valves. (From Jacob, S. W., C. A. Francone, and W. J. Lossow: *Structure and Function in Man,* 4th ed. Philadelphia: W. B. Saunders Co., 1978, p. 348.)

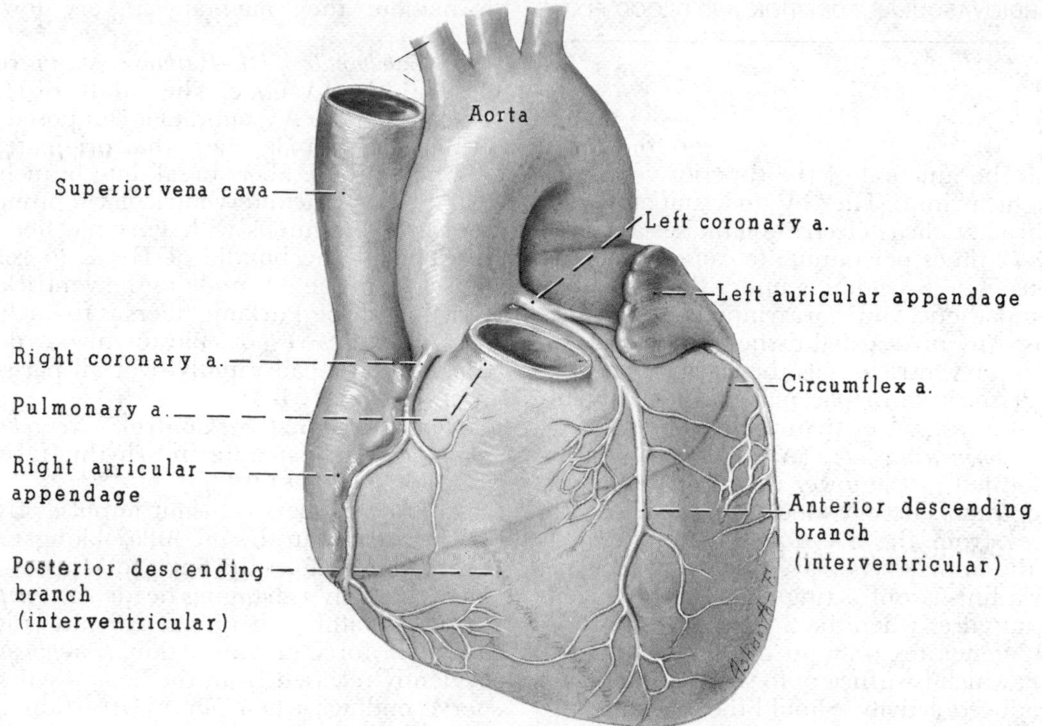

Figure 31–3. Coronary arteries supplying the heart. (From Jacob, S. W., C. A. Francone, and W. J. Lossow: *Structure and Function in Man,* 4th ed. Philadelphia: W. B. Saunders Co., 1978, p. 350.)

REGULATION OF HEART RATE AND RHYTHM*

Seven special properties of *cardiac muscle* are necessary for regulation of heart rate and rhythm:

1. *Rhythmicity:* Rhythm in both the formation and conduction of electrical impulses from atria to ventricles. The heart beats with a definite rhythm based on four phases: (a) stimulation, (b) transmission, (c) contraction, and (d) relaxation. Each contraction is accompanied by an electrical charge, thus forming the basis for electrocardiography.

2. *Irritability* (excitability): The ability of cardiac muscle cells to respond to stimuli. When irritable, heart muscle responds to stimuli with the strongest possible contraction (all-or-nothing law). Irritability is influenced by (a) neural, hormonal, and nutritional balance, (b) adequacy of oxygen supply, (c) drug therapy, and (d) products of infection.

3. *Refractoriness:* This prevents heart muscle from responding to a new stimulus while the heart is still in a state of contraction due to an earlier stimulus, and thus helps to preserve heart rhythm. Irritability is lowest during the refractory period. During the *absolute refractory period* the heart muscle will not respond to *any* stimulus, however strong; during the *relative refractory period* the heart muscle slowly regains irritability.

4. *Conductivity:* Ability of heart muscle fibers to transmit electrical impulses.

5. *Contractility:* Shortening of heart muscle fibers in response to stimuli.

6. *Automaticity:* Ability of heart to beat spontaneously and repetitively without external neurohormonal control. Given the proper laboratory conditions, the heart is able to continue beating outside of the body by means of its own intrinsic control system. The heart's automaticity is evidently linked to fluid and electrolyte balance rather than to nervous system control.

7. *Extensibility* (expansibility): Ability of heart muscle to *stretch* as the heart fills with blood between contractions.

> *Starling's "law of the heart" states: the greater the stretch of cardiac muscle, the more forceful are the heart's contraction and beat.*

However, when muscle is *overstretched,* the force of contraction may *decrease* below normal level, causing circulatory failure.

Cardiac Conduction System. The *cardiac conduction system* is composed of modified cardiac muscle cells characterized by the ability to conduct electrical impulses. The *purpose* of the conduction system is to enable atria and ventricles to contract at the *same rate,* rather than separately and at different rates. The *structures* of the conduction system are:

1. *Sinoatrial node* (SA node) or *pacemaker,* lo-

*Electrophysiology of the heart is discussed in more detail in Chapter 33.

cated at the junction of the superior vena cava and right atrium. The SA node initiates each heart beat. It elicits electrical impulses approximately 72 times per minute to cause atrial contractions. The SA node is under the control of the sympathetic and parasympathetic nervous systems. Any myocardial tissue in the atria, AV junction, or ventricles has the capability of taking over the role of pacemaker if it elicits impulses at a rate faster than the SA node.

2. *Atrioventricular node* (AV node, or AV junction), located in the lower aspect of the interatrial septum. The AV node receives electrical impulses from the SA node. Within the AV node, the impulse is delayed 0.07 second while the atria finish contracting. The AV node generates impulses when the SA node fails to function. It generates only 40 to 50 impulses per minute, which is sufficient to sustain human life with reduced activity. Should the AV node also fail, *lower pacemakers* take over the job of impulse formation; they maintain a very low heart rate.

3. The *bundle of His–Purkinje system* is continuous with the AV node. The bundle of His (now often called the AV bundle) is composed of special cardiac muscle fibers that originate in the AV node; these fibers break into branches that extend down the interventricular septum where they are continuous with Purkinje fibers. The function of the bundle of His is to relay impulses from the AV node to the ventricles. The function of the Purkinje fibers is to enable electrical impulses responsible for myocardial contraction to spread rapidly over all parts of the ventricles (Fig. 31–4).

Neurohormonal Control. *Neurohormonal control* of the heart rate and rhythm takes place as follows:

1. *Efferent* fibers transmit impulses from the cardiac center in the medulla oblongata to the heart. This enables the heart to adjust its rate to meet the body's changing needs. (a) *Sympathetic,* or accelerator, fibers *speed* heart rate and *strengthen* force of contraction. *Norepinephrine* is evidently released from the heart's sympathetic nerve endings when nerves are stimulated. It acts to increase heart rate, decrease the refracto-

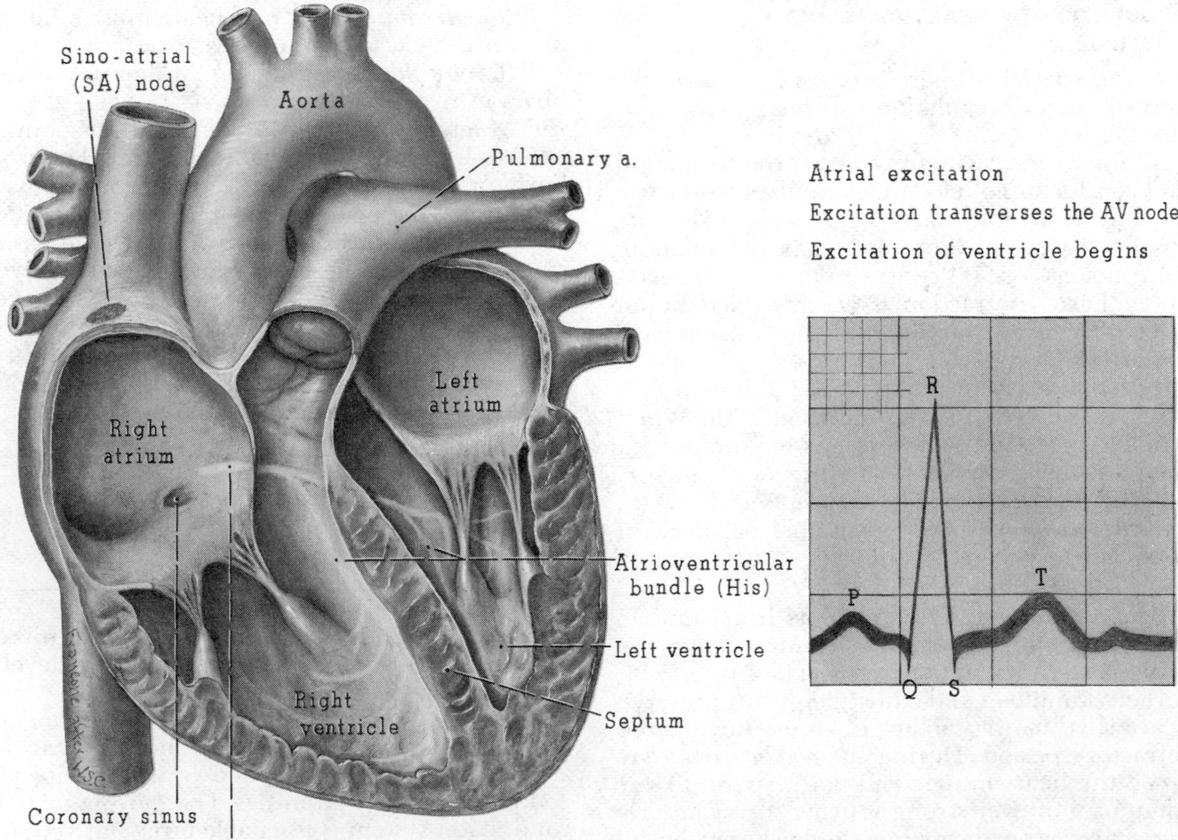

Figure 31–4. Conducting system of the heart showing source of electrical impulses produced on electrocardiogram. (From Jacob, S. W., C. A. Francone, and W. J. Lossow: *Structure and Function in Man,* 4th ed. Philadelphia: W. B. Saunders Co., 1978, p. 355.)

ry period of the A-V node, and increase cardiac workload. (b) *Parasympathetic,* or inhibitory, fibers travel in the two *vagus* nerves and act to *slow* heart rate and to *lengthen* the heart muscle's rest period. *Acetylcholine* is released by vagal nerve endings in the SA node and AV node. It acts to decrease heart rate and increase the refractory period.

2. *Afferent* fibers conduct only *pain* impulses from the heart to the brain (e.g., when the myocardium's oxygen supply is decreased).

CARDIAC CYCLE*

One cardiac cycle is equivalent to one complete heart beat; it lasts 0.8 second. It consists of two parts:

1. *Systole,* or contraction of both atria and then both ventricles; systole is initiated by release of an impulse from the SA node.
2. *Diastole,* or relaxation of both atria and then both ventricles.

HEART SOUNDS*

The *first* sound, "lubb," is of dull quality and low pitch; it signals

1. Onset of ventricular systole.
2. Abrupt closure of atrioventricular valves; closure sets up vibrations in blood and heart walls; these vibrations are transmitted to the chest wall.

The *second* sound, "dubb," has a snapping quality; it signifies

1. Onset of diastole.
2. Closure of semilunar valves, which causes vibrations in blood and heart walls.

The *third* and *fourth* heart sounds are not normally heard. The third heart sound may occur immediately after the AV valves open and the blood rushes from the atria into the ventricles. A fourth heart sound may be caused by atrial contraction. These sounds are often produced because blood from the atria is flowing into a distended ventricle, e.g., in congestive heart failure. The third heart sound may be heard normally in individuals less than 30 years of age, but it is not present after that. The fourth heart sound is not commonly heard in persons with normal hearts. The presence of the third or fourth heart sound produces a "gallop" rhythm.

CARDIAC OUTPUT AND INDEX

Cardiac output is equivalent to *stroke volume* (i.e., amount of blood ejected with each beat) times *heart rate* (i.e., number of beats per minute).

Cardiac output = stroke volume × heart rate.

1. Stroke volume is approximately 70 ml. of blood ejected per heart beat.
2. Heart rate is normally 72 beats per minute.
3. Cardiac output is, thus, approximately 5040 ml. of blood per minute, i.e., 70 × 72. Cardiac output depends upon (a) venous return, (b) cardiac rate, and (c) strength of contraction. Cardiac output can increase four to five times when the healthy body is subjected to strenuous exercise.

The *cardiac index* may be computed from the cardiac output. To obtain the cardiac index, the cardiac output is divided by the body surface area. Therefore, the cardiac index describes the cardiac output in terms of liters/minute/square meter of body surface. The cardiac index gives a better indication of how well the tissues are being perfused than the cardiac output alone.

CARDIAC RESERVE

Cardiac reserve is the ability of the heart to adjust and to adapt to increased demands placed upon it from stresses such as exercise, excitement, fever, cold, acceleration, deceleration, or disease states. Normally the heart is able to greatly increase its output of energy to meet demands made upon it.

BLOOD PRESSURE

This is defined as the pressure exerted by the blood against the walls of the vessels — i.e., arteries, veins, capillaries.

The *difference* in blood pressure in arteries, capillaries, and veins, or *blood pressure gradient,* is the force that enables blood to flow throughout the body. The farther blood flows *from* the heart, the lower the pressure. Pressure is highest in arteries, drops significantly in capillaries, and is almost zero in great veins. There are *three types* of blood pressure; arterial, venous, and capillary.

Arterial Pressure. Arterial pressure is the pressure of blood against arteries' walls. (a) *Systolic pressure* is *maximum* pressure of the blood exerted against the artery walls when the heart *contracts* and is working; it is normally 115 to 120 mm. Hg. (b) *Diastolic pressure* is the force of blood exerted against the artery walls when the

*Refer to Chapter 15 for discussion of assessment of cardiac cycle (p. 345) and heart sounds (p. 347).

heart is *relaxing;* it is normally 75 to 80 mm. Hg. (c) *Pulse pressure* is the *difference* between systolic and diastolic pressures; it is normally 40 mm. Hg.

Circulatory factors influencing arterial pressure include:

a. *Cardiac output:* Increased output increases arterial pressure; decreased output decreases arterial pressure.

b. *Peripheral resistance:* Narrowed arterioles increase blood pressure; dilated arterioles decrease blood pressure.

c. *Arterial elasticity:* Elastic vessels accommodate to changes in blood flow, whereas rigid sclerotic vessels cause increases in systolic and pulse pressures.

d. *Blood volume:* Decreased blood volume (e.g., due to hemorrhage) results in decreased pressure.

e. *Blood viscosity:* Increased blood viscosity, due to overabundance of RBC's or plasma proteins, results in *high* pressure; decreased viscosity from anemia or lack of RBC's results in *lower* pressure.

Other factors influencing arterial pressure are:

a. *Age:* BP is lowest in newborn babies and highest in adults.

b. *Weight:* BP increases with excess weight.

c. *Emotions:* BP increases with release of epinephrine, caused by strong emotion.

d. *Exercise:* Extreme physical activity increases blood pressure. (Note: conditioned athletes often have lowered blood pressures at rest.)

Venous Pressure. Venous pressure is the blood pressure in the veins. In small veins there are no pulsations; the pressure is around 12 mm. Hg. In large veins leading to the heart, pulsations are reflected back from right atrial contractions; blood pressure is around 0 atmospheric pressure.

Capillary Pressure. Capillary pressure is the pressure exerted by the blood against the capillaries. It is 22 mm. Hg at the arterial end of the capillaries and 12 mm. Hg at the venous end. Capillary pressure is important in the formation of interstitial fluid. (Capillary blood pressure and filtration were discussed in Chapter 12.) When capillary pressure is *high,* capillary filtration increases and the fluid shifts from the vascular system into tissues (edema). When capillary pressure is *low,* capillary filtration decreases and fluid is drawn from the tissues into the circulatory system, which raises blood pressure.

FACTORS REGULATING CIRCULATION

The *nervous system* acts to regulate heart rate, degree of arteriolar constriction, and arterial blood pressure, in order to maintain homeostasis. Neural reflexes are controlled via the *vasomotor center* in the medulla oblongata. This comprises four centers controlling the heart and blood vessels:

1. *Vasoconstrictor* center, which *reduces* diameter of blood vessels.
2. *Vasodilator* center, which *increases* diameter of blood vessels.
3. *Cardioaccelerator* center, which *increases* heart rate.
4. *Cardioinhibitory* center, which decreases the heart rate.

The four centers are stimulated or inhibited by:

1. *Pressoreceptors,* or baroreceptors — specialized nerve endings affected by changes in pressure of blood in arteries.

a. *Arterial* pressoreceptors are located in the walls of the aortic arch and the carotid sinuses. When arterial pressure *increases,* arterial pressoreceptors are stimulated and impulses are carried to the medulla oblongata, where vasodilator and cardioinhibitory centers are stimulated. As a result, heart rate and arterial pressure *decrease.* When arterial pressure *decreases,* arterial pressoreceptors receive inadequate stimulation and fewer impulses are carried to the medulla oblongata. Thus, vasoconstrictor and cardioaccelerator centers are stimulated. As a result, heart rate and arterial pressure *increase.*

b. *Venous pressoreceptors* are located in terminal sections of the venae cavae and the right atrium. When blood pressure *increases* in venae cavae and the right atrium (e.g., from exercise), venous pressoreceptors and the cardioaccelerator center are stimulated. As a result, heart rate increases; blood is transferred rapidly into the arterial system; and systemic blood pressure rises *(Bainbridge reflex).* When pressure of blood *decreases* in venae cavae and the right atrium, the reverse occurs.

2. *Chemoreceptors:* receptors and organs located in the aortic arch and carotid bodies. Chemoreceptors are primarily sensitive to *oxygen* lack and secondarily to *increased blood carbon dioxide* and *decreased arterial pH.* When oxygen lack and carbon dioxide excess develop, chemoreceptors are stimulated, increased impulses are transmitted to the vasoconstrictor center, and arterioles constrict and blood pressure increases.

3. The *medullary ischemic reflex* produces vasoconstriction of small blood vessels in response to stimulation of the vasoconstrictor center by CO_2 excess and oxygen lack.

4. *Higher brain centers,* in the cerebral cortex and hypothalamus, transmit impulses to medullary centers when the individual experiences extreme emotion (e.g., fear, rage, embarrassment). Intense fear or anger causes vasoconstriction of arteries and cardioacceleration. Extreme embarrassment causes vasodilatation and blushing.

The *renal system* regulates circulation, blood volume, and blood pressure by controlling excretion or retention of water in urine (see also Chap. 12). When blood volume and BP *decrease* (due to hemorrhage, etc.), release of ADH and aldosterone is stimulated, glomerular filtration decreases, and urine production decreases. As a result, blood volume and blood pressure rise. The opposite set of events occurs with an *increase* in blood volume and blood pressure.

CHAPTER 32

ABNORMALITIES OF CARDIAC STRUCTURE AND FUNCTION: AN OVERVIEW

This chapter provides an overview of the following general concepts: (1) the causes of cardiovascular failure; (2) the effects of cardiovascular failure upon the body; and (3) methods by which cardiovascular failure can be reversed and its effects minimized.

THE CARDIOVASCULAR SYSTEM IN FAILURE

In the preceding chapter, we pointed out that it is the role of the cardiovascular system to deliver oxygen and nutrients to every cell and tissue of the body *without interruption,* and in amounts sufficient to meet the specific needs of each tissue and cell at any given moment. To meet the body's continuous metabolic demands, the cardiovascular system must fulfill the following requirements:

1. The heart must be able to adequately *pump blood* to all parts of the body. For effective pumping, the cardiac muscle and the cardiac conduction system must be in good working order.
2. The circulating *blood volume* must be sufficient to meet the body's needs.
3. *Peripheral vascular resistance* must be sufficient to maintain an adequate blood pressure.

When severe heart disease, hemorrhage, shock, or extreme hypotension, i.e., low blood pressure, develops, the heart and circulation will fail.

> Circulatory failure *is defined as the failure of the circulatory system to provide an adequate minute volume blood flow to keep pace with the metabolic needs of the body's tissues*

Circulatory failure can be either acute or chronic. *Acute* circulatory failure develops rapidly with severe symptoms; it is best exemplified by the clinical pictures of shock, cardiac arrest, syncope, and sudden death.

Shock and *cardiac arrest* are discussed in detail in Chapters 13 and 35, respectively. *Syncope* or fainting results from an intense, temporary, cerebral ischemia. Causes include emotional shock, extreme fear, various arrhythmias (disturbances of heart rate and rhythm), flying at high altitudes, and standing for long periods in one position. Syncope is characterized by a severe drop in blood pressure and a sudden loss of consciousness. Generally the individual who faints revives quickly when placed in a horizontal position, e.g., on a bed or on the floor, with the head level with the rest of the body.

Sudden death occurs when the heart swiftly and without warning stops pumping. The resultant intense cerebral anoxia brings life to a sudden end. Factors that may be responsible for the development of sudden death are (1) severe hemorrhage into the brain or pericardial sac; (2) massive pulmonary embolism resulting in obstruction of blood flow to the brain; (3) ventricular fibrillation; and (4) sudden brain injury due to trauma, toxins, metabolic factors, or vascular occlusion. Other precipitating factors are extreme fear or rage, heavy exercise in very hot or cold weather, straining while defecating, anesthesia, and withdrawal of fluid from the pleural or peritoneal cavities.

Chronic circulatory failure, on the other hand, develops gradually with more moderate symptoms; chronic failure is more specifically described by the term *"chronic congestive heart failure."*

Failure of the heart and circulation adversely affects all organs throughout the body, causing them to function poorly. In particular, the brain, kidneys, and liver are vulnerable to circulatory failure; striking symptoms characteristically develop from oxygen lack and the build-up of metabolic products in these organs.

CAUSATIVE FACTORS PRODUCING CARDIAC DYSFUNCTION

Table 32–1 lists factors associated with the development of cardiovascular diseases and their clinical manifestations. Although these factors are discussed throughout the unit, we shall briefly define them now and state their role in the causation of heart disease.

Disturbances of Blood Volume

A normal *inflow* of blood from the venous system is a basic requirement for adequate cardiac function and output. The volume of blood entering the heart must be neither too small nor too great. Too *small* a blood volume entering the heart will cause a *decrease* in cardiac output and circulatory collapse; too *great* a volume of blood entering the heart will overwork the heart and result in circulatory overload.

Fluid Loss. A *decreased* blood volume results from fluid loss, which may have developed as a result of dehydration, hemorrhage, or shock. *Dehydration,* you recall, results from severe fluid losses as a result of vomiting, diarrhea, profuse diaphoresis, draining wounds, etc. (Dehydration is discussed at length in Chapter 12.) These fluid losses, in turn, rapidly deplete the extracellular fluid, leading to an inadequate cardiac output with consequent shock and circulatory collapse.

Hemorrhage is a second important factor that lowers blood volume, decreasing the inflow of blood to the heart. Hemorrhage is defined as the escape of blood from the vessel in which it is normally confined. Factors causing hemorrhage are *trauma* that results in a vessel's rupture; *spontaneous* rupture of the vessel, e.g., a ruptured aortic aneurysm* or the rupture of a vessel in the brain of a hypertensive patient; *defects of the clotting mechanism* as a result of a deficiency of certain blood factors; and the effects of certain medications that interfere with the clotting mechanism, e.g., heparin, warfarin sodium (Coumadin).

Bleeding may be local or systemic. *Small* local hemorrhages are not dangerous unless they occur within the pericardial sac (where blood collection can cause cardiac tamponade) or in the brain.

On the other hand, *large systemic* hemorrhages are always dangerous because they adversely affect circulatory dynamics by drastically reducing blood volume, venous return to the heart, cardiac output, and the arterial blood pressure. To compensate for these dangerous changes, the cardiovascular system reflexively reacts in the following ways:

1. The *heart* beats more rapidly (tachycardia), in order to speed circulation to vital organs.
2. The *vessels* of the skin and abdominal viscera constrict. This increases arterial blood pressure and increases blood distribution to the vital organs, while reducing blood volume within the vessels of the skin and abdominal viscera.

*An aortic aneurysm is an abnormal dilatation and weakening of a localized area of the aorta.

TABLE 32–1. FACTORS ASSOCIATED WITH THE DEVELOPMENT OF CARDIOVASCULAR DISORDERS

Causative Factors	Cardiovascular Disorders
Disturbances of blood volume	Shock; hemorrhage; fluid overload
Obstructions of blood flow	Thrombosis; embolism; infarction
Ischemia of heart muscle	Angina pectoris; myocardial infarction; coronary insufficiency
Cardiac infectious processes	Rheumatic heart disease; subacute bacterial endocarditis; syphilitic heart disease
Cardiac structural abnormalities	Congenital defects; acquired pathologic changes in structure of valves and heart walls
Hypertension	Arterial hypertension; pulmonary hypertension
Cardiac tumors	Primary; secondary
Trauma to heart	Penetrating cardiac lesion; nonpenetrating cardiac lesion
Alterations in cardiac rate, rhythm, and conduction	Disturbances of impulse formation; failures of conduction
Additional noncardiac factors	Prolonged fevers; anemia; hyperthyroidism; severe anxiety; polycythemia

3. The *liver* and *spleen* discharge additional red blood cells, which are stored for emergencies.

4. The *colloidal osmotic pressure,* i.e., oncotic pressure, within the capillaries increases owing to the decreased filtration pressure within the capillaries. Increased colloid osmotic pressure causes tissue fluid to be sucked back into the blood vessels, thereby increasing blood volume and the arterial blood pressure. (Fluid transport between compartments is discussed in Chapter 12.)

5. The *kidneys* slow urine production, thereby conserving body fluid and blood volume.

When these mechanisms fail to bring the hemorrhage under control and bleeding continues without medical treatment, irreversible shock soon develops, followed by death.

Shock, a third factor resulting in decreased blood volume and cardiac output, results not only from hemorrhage, but also from other events such as burns, severe blows to the body, severe allergic reactions (anaphylactic shock), terrifying or upsetting emotional experiences, severe sepsis, and from heart failure or mechanical abnormalities that hinder cardiac function, i.e., cardiogenic shock.

Cardiogenic shock occurs when the heart fails as a pumping device and cardiac output is grossly inadequate to meet the body's needs. This form of shock results most frequently from damage to the heart muscle, severe arrhythmias, and compression of the heart as a result of cardiac tamponade. Cardiogenic shock is discussed further in Chapter 34 of this unit.

Fluid Overload. An abnormally *increased* blood volume results from a fluid overload. In Chapter 12, we discussed the problem of extracellular volume excess. You will recall that patients who are most prone to a circulatory overload are those who have received excessive IV fluids; patients with heart, kidney, liver, or brain disease; and patients receiving steroid therapy. When administering fluids to patients with heart disease, remember this rule:

Be extremely careful not to overload a patient with heart disease with rapidly administered infusions of IV solutions. Acute pulmonary edema may result because the damaged heart muscle will be unable to pump out and circulate the excess fluid.

Obstructions of the Blood Flow

For adequate circulation to take place, not only must the blood volume be adequate, but the blood must also be able to reach the heart so that it can circulate properly through the lungs and heart chambers and out into the arterial system. Blood flow to the heart can be disturbed or obstructed by thrombi, emboli, areas of infarction, and constrictive pericarditis.

Thrombosis. A *thrombus* (plural, thrombi) is a blood clot that has formed within a blood vessel or within the heart. Thrombus formation is dangerous because: (1) thrombi can occlude blood vessels, thereby obstructing blood flow to vital organs; and (2) thrombi can break free from their attachments to the vessel walls and travel in the blood stream to the heart, lungs, and brain, thus forming emboli.

Thrombi do not normally form within blood vessels because (1) the healthy blood vessel has an inner wall lined with endothelial tissue which is so *smooth* that fibrin and platelets cannot adhere to form the genesis of a clot; and (2) blood flow through the vessels is generally so *rapid* that there is little chance that formed elements within the blood will settle out to form clots. Instead, these formed elements are swept swiftly and smoothly along the circulatory route.

Consequently, factors which lead to the formation of blood clots are those which (1) decrease the smoothness of the endothelial lining of the vessel walls and the heart valves; (2) decrease the rate of blood flow; and (3) increase blood coagulability and the viscosity of the blood. Table 32–2 describes the physiologic disturbances that cause these factors.

A thrombus is formed when intact and ruptured platelets adhere together on a vessel wall. This tiny mass of platelets, which projects slightly into the vessel lumen or out from the heart lining, is called a *plaque.* The platelets that compose the plaque cause the precipitation of fibrin and the accumulation of formed blood elements, which form a blood clot. This fibrinous mass, which started as a small plaque, is now called a *mural* thrombus, i.e., a thrombus attached to the wall of a vessel or the heart. Once formed, a thrombus may (1) partially obstruct the lumen of a blood vessel; (2) completely obstruct the vessel's lumen (*occlusive* thrombus); (3) grow in size as a result of the addition of more platelets and formed blood elements (*progressive* or *propagating* thrombus); or (4) break free from the wall and travel in the blood stream (*embolus*).

Thrombosis may affect either the arterial or venous systems. Thrombi which occlude *arteries* usually result from extensive lesions of the arterial walls; because these thrombi obstruct the flow of blood to tissues, they may lead to ischemia or infarction of the dependent tissues.

Venous thrombosis is more common than arterial thrombosis since venous blood flow is slower than arterial, and also because the vein walls are thinner and more delicate than arterial walls and, thus, more susceptible to injury. Clots most

TABLE 32–2. CAUSATIVE FACTORS IN THROMBUS FORMATION

Major Factors	Contributing Factors
Damage to endothelial lining of blood vessels and heart	Hardening or sclerosis of vessels due to aging; injury to arterial walls; neoplasms affecting arteries; scarring and calcification of heart valves due to rheumatic heart disease and bacterial endocarditis
Decrease in rate of blood flow	Lack of muscular contraction in legs due to immobility and prolonged bedrest; spasm of arterial walls as in hypertension; narrowing of arterial walls as result of disease such as atherosclerosis; increased viscosity of blood due to polycythemia or dehydration; pooling of blood in atria due to atrial fibrillation
Increase in blood coagulability	Increase in platelet count or platelet stickiness (often seen following surgery or trauma); use of vitamin K

commonly form within the veins of the legs and pelvis. The major danger in venous thrombosis is that the clot will break loose from the vein wall and embolize to the lungs.

Embolism. An *embolus* is a mass of undissolved matter in a blood or lymphatic vessel, brought there by the blood or lymph flow. Emboli are composed of various types of materials: fat globules, bubbles of air, clumps of bacteria, tumor cells, foreign bodies (e.g., bullets), and clusters of parasites. The most common types of emboli, however, arise from preexisting thrombi in the veins and arteries which have become fragmented. In Table 32–3 we have listed the four most important types of emboli along with their causative factors and pathologic consequences.

Infarction. An *infarct* is a localized area of tissue, within an organ or part, which has become ischemic and necrotic due to the complete or total blockage of its blood supply. The occurrence of an infarct in the lung, usually as a result of a pulmonary embolus, is called a *pulmonary infarction.* An infarct in the myocardial tissue

TABLE 32–3. TYPES OF EMBOLI: SOURCES AND POSSIBLE PATHOLOGIC CONSEQUENCES

Classification	Sources of Emboli	Pathologic Consequences
Venous emboli	Fragmented thrombi within leg veins, most commonly deep calf muscles; fragmented thrombi within pelvic veins; thrombi on walls of heart's right side	May occlude a pulmonary vessel, coronary artery, or cerebral vessel; small emboli may cause small area of infarction; large emboli may cause death
Arterial emboli	Mural intracardiac thrombi; vegetative masses on heart valves as result of bacterial endocarditis; atherosclerotic plaques; aortic aneurysms; calcifications breaking loose from diseased heart valves	As above
Fat emboli (minute globules of fat which are carried in the blood)	Fractures of the long bones; severe burns; soft tissue injuries; fatty changes in the liver, iatrogenic causes; orthopedic procedures; IV injections of oily radiographic media	Globules usually remain in lungs; globules may travel to the brain, kidneys, and liver, producing severe damage and death; globules may pass to the brain, causing unconsciousness and severe neurologic damage
Air or gas emboli (bubbles of air or gas within the circulation)	Chest injuries (air may enter a large vein during inspiration); air may enter a large artery or vein which is pierced when needles are introduced into the chest during various procedures; cardiac surgery (air may enter the circulation as the patient is being removed from cardiopulmonary bypass)	Frothy masses may form which can occlude vessels, particularly in the lungs; large masses of gassy bubbles may become caught in right atria and ventricles and block pulmonary artery

owing to blockage of the coronary arteries is called a *myocardial infarction.*

The commonest causes of infarction are thrombosis and embolism. Other causes are twisting of an internal organ or its parts so that the organ's blood supply is impaired, e.g., twisting of a testis or bowel loop; and compression of arteries and veins, thereby cutting off circulation to the tissues they supply.

The development of an infarction can be extremely dangerous, and infarctions are common causes of critical illnesses and deaths. Exactly how damaging an infarct will be depends upon its size and location.

Whether an organ will become infarcted as a result of thrombosis or embolism depends upon the *organ's blood supply.* Some organs, e.g., spleen and kidney, receive their blood supply from a *single* vessel called an "end artery." While the end artery has branches, it does not have any blood vessels *between* the branches, i.e., anastomoses.* Thus, if an end artery becomes obstructed, there are no "detour channels" or anastomoses to carry the blood to the organ's tissues by bypassing the obstruction. In such a situation infarction is almost inevitable.

In structures with a *double* blood supply, one vessel can take over for the other in event of thrombosis or embolism. For example, the arms are supplied with blood from both the ulnar and radial arteries, while the legs receive blood from both the tibial and fibular arteries. Finally, structures, e.g., the bones, muscles, uterus, thyroid gland, and skin, are served by blood vessels with *many anastomoses,* consequently they do not often develop infarcts.

Unfortunately the coronary arteries that supply the myocardium contain very few anastomoses. However, numerous anastomoses exist between the heart's *small* vessels; these vascular connections can grow and provide the heart with sufficient *collateral circulation* if the artery occludes gradually over a period of time, or if the occlusion is only partial. But, if a *large* embolus *suddenly* blocks a coronary artery, infarction of the myocardium is inevitable because of the lack of anastomoses between the large arteries and the inability of the channels between the small vessels to swiftly provide collateral circulation under these circumstances.

Ischemia of the Heart Muscle

If the coronary arteries, which supply the myocardium, become blocked, the heart muscle will suffer from oxygen deprivation (i.e., *ischemia*). Insufficient blood supply to the myocardium results in such disorders as obliterative atherosclerotic heart disease, angina pectoris, coronary insufficiency, and myocardial infarction. These four serious disorders are grouped under the terms *coronary artery disease* (CAD) or ischemic heart disease and are discussed in detail in Chapter 36.

*An arterial anastomosis is a branch of an artery that is attached either to another artery or to itself at a more distant point. There are also arteriovenous anastomoses.

Infectious Processes Affecting the Heart

The structures of the heart, like any other body structures, are vulnerable to attacks by microorganisms and can be adversely altered by the resulting inflammatory and fibrous processes. The walls of the heart (epicardium, myocardium, and endocardium) can become dangerously infected and inflamed. As a result, valves may become narrowed, deformed, and sclerosed, and their function may become seriously impaired.

The infectious processes that most commonly affect the heart are:

Rheumatic Fever. A systemic inflammatory disorder affecting the body's connective tissue, which may involve the endocardium, myocardium, and pericardium

Rheumatic Heart Disease (RHD). A chronic cardiac condition which usually follows one or several episodes of rheumatic fever, characterized by valvular deformity and dysfunction.

Bacterial Endocarditis (BE). A serious bacterial infection of the endocardium and valves, caused by several types of organisms.

Myocarditis. Infection and inflammation of the myocardium resulting from many types of viral, bacterial, and parasitic disorders.

Pericarditis. Inflammation of the pericardium, which may follow rheumatic fever, myocardial infarction, pneumococcal infections, and tuberculosis.

Syphilitic Heart Disease. A condition which may adversely affect the heart valves and aorta and which may not become evident until 10 to 20 years following the initial syphilitic attack. (See Unit XXII for a discussion of syphilis.)

Among the most serious complications arising from infectious processes within the heart are *damaged valves.* The valves may either develop *stenosis* (narrowing of the valves due to scar tissue formation) or *insufficiency* (the valves are so eroded by infection and scarring that they cannot close properly). Both stenosis and insufficiency eventually lead to heart failure unless corrective measures are taken.

Structural Abnormalities due to Factors Other than Infection

Structural abnormalities may be either congenital or acquired. *Congenital* heart disease results from faulty development of the heart's structures in utero. *Acquired* structural defects occur as a result of various disease processes that develop following birth.

Congenital malformations are of several types:*

1. The *valves* may be stenosed, deformed, or absent.
2. The *arteries* (pulmonary and aortic) may be stenosed or malformed.
3. Abnormal *shunts* may be present. As their name implies, *left-to-right shunts* carry *oxygenated* blood from the left atrium or ventricle to the right atrium or ventricle; examples of conditions with left-to-right shunting are atrial septal defect and ventricular septal defect. These disorders *do not produce cyanosis* because the blood passes through the lungs before being shunted back to the heart's right side.

Right-to-left shunts carry *venous, nonoxygenated* blood from the right atrium or ventricle to the left atrium, left ventricle, or aorta. These conditions *produce cyanosis* since the pulmonary circulation is bypassed.

Acquired structural changes occur in the heart valves, the endocardium, myocardium, and pericardium. *Valvular* diseases are most commonly the result of infection or congenital abnormalities; they may also result from trauma. *Endocardial* disease may result from disseminated lupus erythematosus — an autoimmune disorder. Also, endocardial changes are sometimes seen in conjunction with rheumatoid arthritis.

The *myocardium* can be affected by diverse factors — tumors, metastases, toxins, chemicals, physical trauma (electric shock, radiation), immunologic responses, autoimmune diseases, and nutritional disorders. The conditions resulting from the effects of these factors on the heart are grouped into a single category called *cardiomyopathies.* Most cardiomyopathies are rare and of obscure etiology.

Pericardial disease usually occurs in conjunction with another disease that is affecting either the heart itself or surrounding structures, e.g., metastatic tumors.

Hypertension – Arterial and Pulmonary

Hypertensive heart disease resulting from *arterial hypertension* is one of the most common forms of heart disease. (See also Chapter 37.) It is also a significant causative factor in death from heart failure. The major characteristic of hypertensive heart disease is hypertrophy of the left ventricle, which eventually leads to congestive heart failure. Left ventricular hypertrophy results from the heart's increased workload as it attempts to pump blood into resistive narrowed vessels.

There are two major types of arterial hypertension:

1. *Essential* hypertension: A common form of hypertension, of unknown origin.
2. *Secondary* hypertension: A less common form of the disease, which develops secondary to renal disorders, toxemia of pregnancy, endocrine disorders, and so forth.

Pulmonary hypertension is the analogue of hypertensive heart disease. In pulmonary hypertension, the pulmonary pressure is elevated rather than the arterial pressure. This condition most commonly results from chronic lung diseases such as emphysema; however, it may also be caused by thrombosis or emboli within the pulmonary circulation. Pulmonary hypertension leads to a thickening of the right ventricle. Because of the excessive workload placed upon the right ventricle, the right side of the heart eventually fails as a pump. Right-sided heart failure due to diseases of the lung is referred to as *cor pulmonale*.

Pulmonary hypertension may also develop as the result of a congenital heart defect when blood from the left side of the heart is shunted through a defect to the right side, e.g., a ventricular septal defect. The high pressure from the left side of the heart is reflected to the right side via the shunt. Consequently, the pressure in the pulmonary vasculature increases. This high pressure in the lungs leads to thickening of the walls of the pulmonary vessels and pulmonary hypertension. If the congenital heart defect is not corrected or a palliative measure is not done to relieve the pulmonary hypertension, the condition becomes irreversible. The patient then suffers from severe respiratory problems, and the prognosis is poor.

Tumors and Trauma

Primary tumors of the heart are exceedingly rare and are generally benign. On the other hand, *secondary* tumors, resulting from metastases, are not uncommon and often develop from the spread of bronchogenic carcinomas arising in the mediastinal nodes.

Traumatic heart disease may occur as a result of (1) *penetrating* wounds of the chest wall, e.g., bullets, needles; (2) nonpenetrating lesions, e.g., a blow to the chest; or (3) excessive physical strain or exertion.

Disturbances of Rate, Rhythm, and Conduction

Disturbances of rate, rhythm, and conduction, or arrhythmias, occur in both normal and

*For further information on congenital malformations, consult a textbook on pediatrics.

diseased hearts. Arrhythmias develop when the heart is unable to properly elicit and transmit electrical impulses. Arrhythmias produce their effects on the body by altering circulatory dynamics. The arrhythmias will be discussed in Chapter 35.

Noncardiac Factors in Heart Disease

The heart can be adversely affected by disease processes in other parts of the body, nutritional factors, and emotional factors. Noncardiac problems damage the heart by increasing the heart's workload, decreasing its oxygen supply, disturbing its metabolic processes, and interfering with its nutrition.

Disease processes most likely to strain the heart and result in heart failure are systemic infections, fevers, autoimmune disorders, anemia, leukemia, hyperthyroidism, and electrolyte imbalances. Malnutrition can also produce heart disease, as exemplified by beriberi heart and cardiac disease associated with alcoholism. Finally, emotional stress and anxiety may produce transient adverse effects on cardiac rate, rhythm, output, and blood pressure.

CLASSIFICATION OF HEART DISEASE

From this overview of some of the diverse factors that play a role in heart disease, you can see that there are several possible ways to classify the various heart maladies. For instance, heart diseases can be divided into two basic groups: *congenital heart disease,* and *acquired heart disease.* Another way to group heart diseases is according to the specific *structure* within the heart that is affected, e.g., valvular heart disease, diseases of the myocardium, pericardium, endocardium, and diseases of the coronary arteries. Or cardiac dysfunctions can be classified according to a *specific etiology,* e.g., ischemic heart disease, traumatic heart disease, and infectious processes within the heart.

Heart conditions may also be grouped according to which *side* of the heart they affect or whether they affect the *heart as a whole.* For example, conditions that affect the *right* side of the heart are right ventricular failure, chronic cor pulmonale, pulmonary hypertension, and congenital shunts. The *left* side of the heart is involved in left heart failure, mitral and aortic stenosis and regurgitation, myocardial infarction, and arterial hypertension. The heart as a *whole* is disturbed by the arrhythmias.

A particularly helpful way to classify a heart disease is according to the major type of *physiologic disturbance* responsible for its development.

Note that the different conditions listed in Figure 32–1 have one characteristic in common; they all eventually lead to a *reduction* in *cardiac reserve.* In other words, *the ability of the heart to meet the body's metabolic needs, under both basal conditions and stress, is impaired by all cardiovascular diseases.* Grades of reduction in cardiac reserve are discussed more fully in Chapter 34.

OVERVIEW OF THERAPY IN CARDIOVASCULAR DISEASE

Broad Goals of Clinical Care

The overall goals of clinical care for patients with cardiovascular ailments may be listed thus:

1. Prevention and early recognition of cardiovascular disease.
2. Preservation of life in event of critical cardiovascular illness by means of (a) mobile and hospital-based critical care units, (b) precise monitoring equipment, and (c) new resuscitation techniques.
3. Rehabilitation of patients with cardiovascular disease.

Prevention of Heart Disease. *Heart disease is the leading cause of incapacitation and death in the United States and Europe today.* The prevalence of cardiovascular ailments in these countries is possibly due to the fact that people are living longer and are more sedentary. Statistically, cardiovascular disease seems to most commonly affect obese, middle-aged persons who lead physically inactive lives. Also, some authorities believe that the high incidence of heart disease is linked to the constant emotional stress and anxiety under which many persons must function in their jobs and at home.

Because heart disease is so prevalent and because it can bring suffering and death in its wake, it is vitally important for the nurse to help to *prevent* heart ailments and to refer persons with signs of heart disease to their doctors for early diagnosis and therapy. In your relations with others at work and at home, you can stress by word and example the importance of proper diet, weight control, exercise, physical and mental relaxation, and a yearly physical examination. Should you become aware that a friend, neighbor, or co-worker is suffering from symptoms of heart disease, e.g., dyspnea, edema, chest pain, or extreme fatigue, emphasize the importance of seeking medical care without delay. Early medical referral lessens the chances of the development of a serious, incapacitating heart ailment.

Preservation of Life. The critically ill patient with heart disease has a greater chance today of living and recovering than ever before in the history of medicine. The life of even the most threatened patient can often be preserved and sustained by means of the following developments: (1) the creation of coronary or cardiac care units (CCU); (2) the invention and use of precise monitoring equipment; (3) the development of sophisticated resuscitation techniques; and (4) the rendering of expert emergency care following a heart attack both at home and en route to the hospital.

The *coronary care unit* (CCU) is a highly equipped, fully staffed area of the hospital that is reserved specifically for care of patients suffering from acute myocardial infarction, dangerous arrhythmias, and severe heart failure. Within the CCU the patient critically ill with heart disease receives the constant care and supervision of skilled nurses who have advanced education and experience in the field of cardiology. In the event of any emergency, the necessary equipment, drugs, and personnel are on hand to immediately and skillfully treat the patient.

Monitoring equipment — which continuously records the patient's electrocardiographic tracings, blood pressure, heart rate, and venous pressures — is the second factor which helps to preserve patients' lives. The majority of monitoring mechanisms now contain an alarm system which responds when an emergency arises or if the patient's vital signs deviate significantly from the norm. The use of these electronic devices allows nurses and doctors to care for several critical patients at once without worry that one will undergo dangerous alterations in condition without their knowledge.

Sophisticated *emergency techniques* constitute the third factor that has enabled physicians and nurses to save the lives of critically ill patients. The three major methods of resuscitation employed are:

- *Closed Chest Cardiac Massage.* A procedure employed in a patient whose heart has arrested. The doctor or nurse rhythmically presses the lower part of the sternum downward against the vertebral column. This squeezes the heart and forces the blood out of its chambers into the circulatory system.

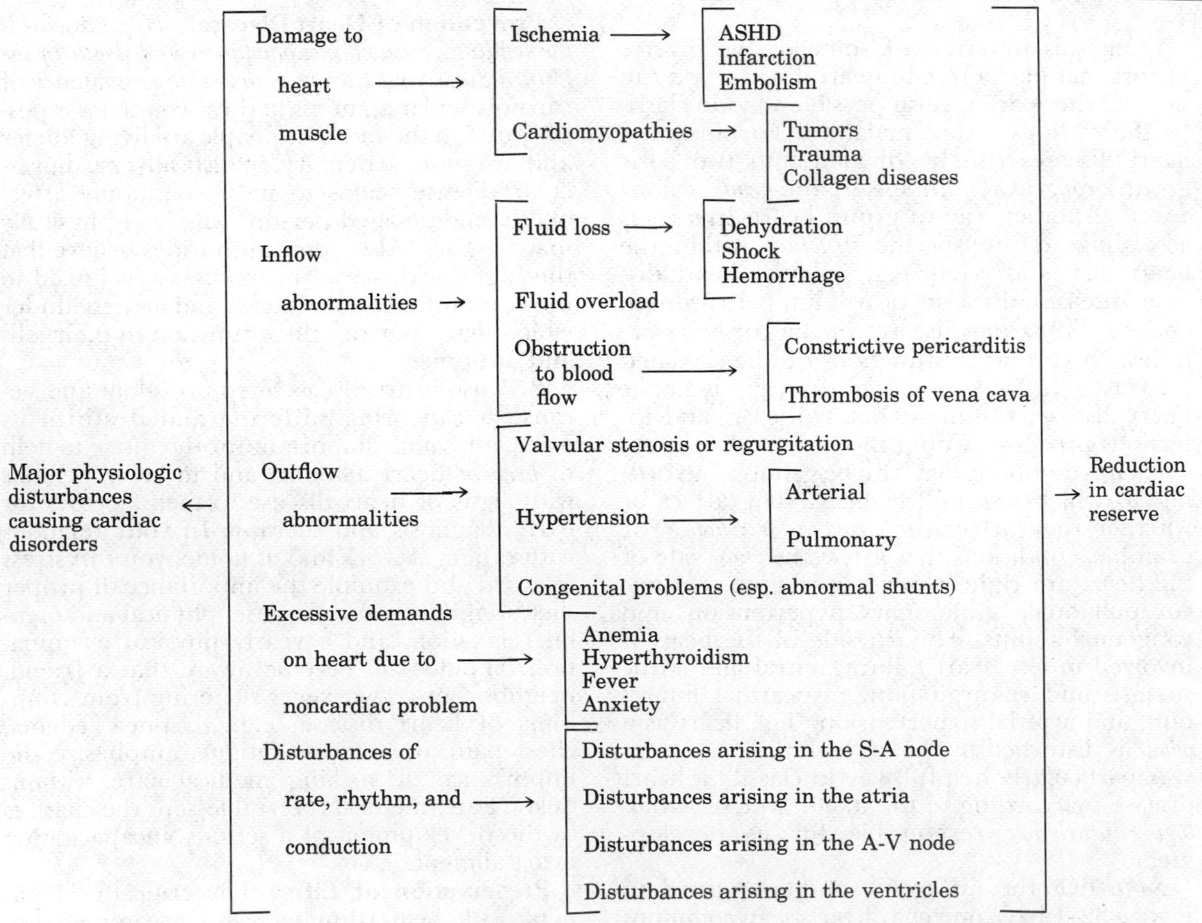

Figure 32–1. Classification of cardiac disorders according to the major type of physiologic disturbance.

- ▶ *Precordial Shock.* A procedure used to treat life-threatening arrhythmias, e.g., ventricular fibrillation. An electric shock of high intensity is delivered to the heart through the chest wall by a machine called an *external defibrillator.*

- ▶ *Cardiac Pacing.* A procedure used to restore the heart beat and circulation in patients with severe disorders in impulse formation and conduction, e.g., heart block. The artificial pacemaker is an electronic device that delivers short rhythmic discharges of low intensity via special pacing wires which are placed in the heart. These electrical discharges act to control the heart beat when the heart's natural pacemaker (the SA node) is defective or when there is a blockage at the AV junction which keeps the impulse from traveling to the ventricles and activating them.

These emergency techniques are considered in detail in Chapter 35.

Finally, many patients today receive expert emergency care at the *time* of their heart attack or *immediately afterwards,* which greatly increases their chances of survival. Modern firemen, policemen, and the lay public in most major cities are trained to render first aid to victims of acute myocardial infarctions. The techniques of cardiopulmonary resuscitation (CPR) are being taught in schools in many areas of the United States. Also, fully equipped mobile coronary care units give emergency care to a patient being transported to a hospital CCU. As a result, more patients with heart attacks *reach the hospital alive* today than ever before — patients who, only a few years ago, would have died either at home or on their way to the hospital.

Rehabilitation of Patients with Cardiovascular Disease*. In the recent past persons with damaged hearts frequently believed that heart disease would incapacitate them, making them "cripples" for life. Such patients often became despondent, even suicidal, because they felt that the joys and responsibilities of an active life would no longer be theirs. Today one of the prime goals of doctors and nurses is to teach the patient with heart disease to live as fully and as actively as possible with minimal strain on the heart. Thus, following serious illness a patient usually is instructed to increase his activities gradually until he is able to resume his former duties and recreations.

It is true that some patients with heart disease must make rather drastic changes in their life style. For example, heart patients who have worked at hard labor or those whose jobs are extremely stressful may have to change occupations; the homemaker with small children may have to hire help and rearrange the kitchen and house so that the workload is lighter; also, patients and their families may be forced to move from a two-story house to a one-story house to prevent overexertion from stair climbing.

However, the modern patient is not alone as he struggles to make these kinds of adjustments. The doctor, hospital nurse, public health nurse, occupational health nurse, physical therapist, occupational therapist, social worker, and the patient's employer and family can all assist him as he reestablishes his life following serious illness. In many cities, centers have been set up to help rehabilitate the cardiac patient. Also, patients who are compelled to make significant changes in their life style may obtain guidance from the Office of Vocational Rehabilitation and the American Heart Association.

*Because cardiovascular disorders currently more often affect men, we have deviated in this unit from our usual style and do use the masculine pronouns in a general way to refer to all persons.

Clinical Goals and Techniques

Specific therapeutic techniques and medications differ somewhat for each major cardiovascular problem. However, since the pathologic problems in all heart conditions tend to be somewhat similar, we can mention some important goals of care which generally apply to almost all dysfunctions of the cardiovascular system:

1. Improve cardiac output and increase cardiac reserve.
2. Correct arrhythmias and heart block.
3. Control sodium balance and edema.
4. Supply adequate fluid, nutrition, and oxygen to all tissues of the body.
5. Minimize the undesirable effects of therapy.

Drugs used in the treatment of cardiovascular disease are discussed later in this unit. The principal categories of drugs used include:

1. Cardiac glycosides (e.g., digitalis).
2. Antiarrhythmic agents (e.g., procainamide, quinidine).
3. Diuretics (e.g., thiazides, furosemide, mercurials).
4. Vasodilators (e.g., nitroglycerin).
5. Antihypertensive agents (e.g., phentolamine, hydralazine, ganglionic blocking agents).

CHAPTER 33

ASSESSING AND DIAGNOSING THE PERSON WITH HEART DISEASE

To diagnose heart disease the physician, assisted by the nurse:

1. Inquires about the patient's *present* symptoms and problems.
2. Determines the *etiology* of the heart ailment. The patient's past history, habits, and working schedule are explored; laboratory tests are ordered to verify the presence of infection, or any electrolyte abnormalities, abnormalities in the blood count, and so forth.
3. Determines, by physical examination and radiologic studies, what adverse *structural* changes have occurred within the heart, e.g., damaged valves.
4. Determines what *physiologic* problems and alterations have developed, e.g., a reduction in cardiac reserve.
5. Evaluates the extent of *cardiac reserve remaining,* and determines what *limitations* must be placed upon the patient to safely live within the limits of the heart's remaining functional capacity.

In this chapter we investigate the typical medical history of the patient with heart disease, the classic symptoms of heart disease, the typical physical examination, diagnostic procedures, and nursing evaluation of the patient.

THE PATIENT'S MEDICAL HISTORY

Asking a patient relevant questions about himself and his present and past life patterns is just as important diagnostically as taking an ECG reading or listening to the heartbeat.

What exactly do we want to know about the patient with suspected heart disease? First of all, the doctor explores the patient's *past medical history.* This reveals what type of person the patient is, his general health record throughout his life, and etiologic factors that may have contributed to the development of his present cardiovascular symptoms. Answers to the following questions are generally obtained:

1. What important childhood diseases did the patient have? Was there evidence of rheumatic fever? Does the patient remember having symptoms of rheumatic fever—sore throat, "growing pains," nosebleeds, nervousness?
2. Did the patient ever have tuberculosis or pneumonia? These diseases are sometimes associated with constrictive pericarditis.
3. Does the patient recall having had such viral infections as mumps, chickenpox, and influenza? These childhood disorders sometimes contribute to the later development of cardiac dysfunction.
4. What drugs has the patient taken — digitalis? quinidine? diuretics? tranquilizers?
5. Has the patient ever experienced a direct blow or heavy pressure upon the chest?
6. Has the patient ever had thrombophlebitis or any other clotting disorder? You will recall that thrombophlebitis can precede pulmonary embolism.
7. Does the patient have a history of gout or diabetes? Metabolic disorders tend to be linked with the development of atherosclerosis.
8. Has the patient's weight remained fairly stable since the age of 20, or has he tended to gain weight steadily over the past years? Obesity and lack of exercise appear to be important factors in the development of hypertension and coronary artery disease.
9. Has the patient ever had a venereal disease, particularly syphilis?
10. Has the patient suffered from any severe emotional problems in the past? How does he generally react to upsetting experiences?
11. What are the patient's living habits, e.g., alcohol, coffee, and tea consumption; number of cigarettes smoked per day, amount of daily physical exercise, hours of sleep per night, frequency and length of vacations? Cigarette smoking, lack of physical exercise, and lack of rest as a result of stress and overwork are linked to the development of cardiovascular disease.

Second, the doctor may ask about the patient's *family history.* Has any member of the patient's family had diabetes, tuberculosis, rheumatic fever, congenital heart disease, or have any relatives died prematurely as a result of hypertension or coronary disease?

The patient's *occupational* history, the third area of investigation, is of great importance in the diagnosis of heart disease. The doctor inquires into the physical and emotional demands of the patient's job, asking about what types of stresses the individual faces at work every day. The physician may also ask the patient about transportation to and from the job, since modern commuting is a definite source of stress. For example, does the patient commute a long distance? Does he drive his own car? Does he drive during peak hours of traffic?

Finally, the patient's *marital* history is investigated. Domestic problems are possibly even more significant than occupational stress in the development of heart disease. Thus, the physician inquires into the number of marriages, divorces, and separations and the number and ages of the patient's children; adequacy of sexual relations; and the physical and mental health of the patient's marriage partner.

SYMPTOMS OF HEART DISEASE

The six cardinal symptoms diagnostic of heart disease are chest pain, dyspnea, fatigue, palpitations, syncope, and edema.

Other important common symptoms are cyanosis, distended neck veins, murmurs, cough, and headache. When attempting to evaluate a patient's symptoms and their significance, answers are sought to the following questions:

1. *How long (days, weeks, months, years) has the patient been experiencing the symptom?*
2. *How much does the symptom bother the patient?*
3. *Does any particular type of incident or episode trigger the symptom?*

Chest Pain

Pain in the chest is a very common complaint, occurring in such cardiac diseases as angina pectoris, myocardial infarction, and pericarditis, and in such pulmonary diseases as pleurisy, pneumonia, and pulmonary embolism and infarction. Because chest pain can be caused by a number of different conditions, it is highly variable in its nature. To correctly evaluate chest pain and its causation, one must ask the patient about: (1) the *quality* of the pain (dull, sharp, crushing); (2) its *location;* (3) its *duration;* (4) points to which it *radiates* (arms, wrists, jaw, neck); (5) *factors that precipitate, aggravate.* or *relieve* the pain (exertion, emotion, movement, and deep breathing), and (6) the intensity of the pain, often graded on a scale of one to ten, with ten being the most severe pain one could imagine. It is essential to obtain an accurate description of a patient's chest pain whenever it occurs, because the doctor uses this information to help to decide whether the patient has a cardiac or a pulmonary condition.

Dyspnea

Dyspnea is defined as *labored* or *difficult breathing.* Like chest pain, this common symptom affects patients with cardiac diseases and also those with respiratory ailments. Dyspnea can also trouble patients experiencing anxiety, depression, and a psychosomatic condition called "cardiac neurosis."

Although dyspnea can develop in any form of heart disease, it almost always occurs in conjunction with cardiac enlargements and other pathologic structural and physiologic changes within the cardiovascular system. This symptom is most severe and incapacitating when the patient's lungs are congested and edematous and his heart is in failure.

There are several types of dyspnea or breathing patterns that are abnormal or difficult; e.g., exertional dyspnea, orthopnea, paroxysmal nocturnal dyspnea, cardiac asthma, and Cheyne-Stokes respirations.

Exertional dyspnea, the most common form of cardiac dyspnea, occurs when the patient exercises moderately and disappears when he rests. Such noncardiac conditions as poor physical health, old age, obesity, anemia, and obstructions of the nasal passages may also lead to dyspnea with mild exercise.

Orthopnea is difficult breathing that occurs when the patient is resting flat in bed and is relieved when the patient assumes an upright or semivertical position. Usually placing two or three pillows under the patient's head relieves orthopnea. This symptom is always indicative of advanced heart disease and is far more serious than is exertional dyspnea.

Paroxysmal nocturnal dyspnea is a form of difficult breathing that occurs in terrifying attacks during the night, thus the term "paroxysmal" (sudden attacks which occur periodically), "nocturnal" (night), "dyspnea" (difficult breathing). One author vividly describes the attacks:

> The patient is aroused from his sleep gasping for air, and must sit up or stand to catch his breath. He may sweat profusely. Sometimes he throws open a window widely to relieve the oppressive sensation of suffocation. The chest tends to become fixed in the position of forced inspiration. Both inspiratory and expiratory wheezes, often simulating typical asthma, are heard. . . . Occasionally these attacks may occur several times a night, necessitating sleeping upright in a chair.[146]

These attacks occur at night because, normally, when we lie down to sleep, body fluids are redistributed. A state of *hypervolemia* may then develop as blood which has pooled in the lower extremities while the patient is up and about now flows back toward the heart and lungs. The diseased heart, however, is unable to adequately pump the extra fluid out into the circulatory system. Thus, the lungs become congested, and this, in turn, leads to difficulty in breathing.

Paroxysmal nocturnal dyspnea is most common in those cardiovascular conditions that overwork the left ventricle; e.g., hypertension and aortic stenosis or insufficiency. Factors that can lead to attacks of paroxysmal nocturnal dyspnea in heart patients are coughing, nightmares, abdominal distention, full bladder, heavy evening meal, or frightening noises. These factors place an additional strain upon the heart, causing it to beat faster. Tachycardia, in conjunction with the hypervolemia, may tax the diseased left ventricle so much that it will be unable to pump all the blood which it is receiving out into the systemic circulation. Therefore, the blood will "back up" into the pulmonary circulation, and the blood pressure in the lungs will increase. This then leads to the development of lung congestion, and possibly pulmonary edema, as the increased pressure in the lungs forces fluid out of the pulmonary capillaries and into the alveoli.

Cardiac asthma is a term used to describe the *asthmatic wheezes* frequently heard in patients suffering from dyspnea in conjunction with pulmonary congestion and heart disease. The wheezes are caused by the following factors:

1. The lumens of the small bronchioles are reduced by the accumulation of edema fluids, which, in turn, increases resistance to airflow.
2. The walls of the bronchioles are thicker than normal because of the edema.
3. The small bronchioles are narrowed, and even collapsed, by the high intrathoracic pressure needed to overcome the obstruction to airflow within the bronchioles during expiration.*

The terms "cardiac asthma" and "paroxysmal nocturnal dyspnea" are sometimes used interchangeably, because cardiac asthma also occurs frequently at night when the patient is sleeping in a horizontal position.

Cheyne-Stokes respirations, or periodic breathing, is characterized by alternating periods of hyperpnea and apnea. In this form of dyspnea, the patient's breathing, at first shallow and slow, gradually becomes deeper and faster until it reaches a maximum point of depth. Next, the patient's breathing rate is slow and becomes more shallow until breathing stops all together, and a period of apnea lasting 10 to 20 seconds ensues. Following the apneic period, the breathing once again increases in depth and rate, and so on in a continuous cycle. This unusual breathing pattern characteristically appears in heart failure, certain neural disorders, in metabolic disorders, and following large doses of sedatives (Fig. 33–1).

Evidently the basic cause of Cheyne-Stokes respirations is an alteration in the sensitivity of the respiratory center in the brain to changes in the blood gases, particularly carbon dioxide.

Fatigue

Easy fatigability upon mild exertion, which is relieved by rest, is often the chief complaint of patients with heart disease. Fatigue due to heart ailments is a sign that the heart is unable to pump out sufficient blood and oxygen and to meet even a small increase in the metabolic demands of cells and tissues.

Palpitations

The term palpitation is derived from the Latin word *palpitare,* meaning "to throb." Palpitation is a common symptom in patients with organic heart disease as well as those patients whose cardiac symptoms have a neurotic basis. The individual with palpitations from whatever cause typically complains of the unpleasant sensation of being conscious of his heart's action. Thus, the patient may state that he can feel his heart "beating rapidly" or "forcefully" or "irregularly," i.e., he is overly aware of the beating of his heart to the exclusion of other sensations.

The major causes of palpitations are:

1. Nonfatal arrhythmias, e.g., premature beats and paroxysmal atrial tachycardia.
2. Noncardiac organic problems, e.g., anemia, hyperthyroidism, debility, infection.
3. Nonpathologic factors, e.g., excessive exercise, excitement, large meals, alcohol, tobacco, excessive intake of coffee or tea.
4. Nervous and emotional disorders in which there is undue worry over heart action and excessive fear of

*See the discussion of asthma in Unit XVI for further information.

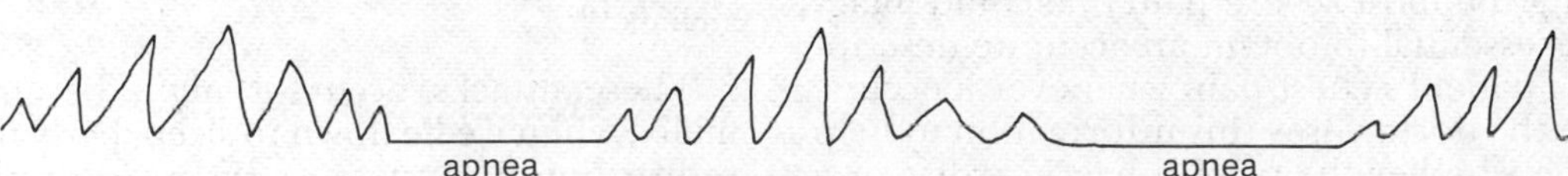

Figure 33–1. The pattern of Cheyne-Stokes respirations.

heart disease; e.g., palpitation is the chief symptom of cardiac neurosis.

Persons with cardiac neurosis are often so conscious of their heart's action that they may say they feel palpitations even when their heart rate and rhythm are absolutely normal. On the other hand, persons with organic heart disease may become so habituated to disturbances in cardiac rate and rhythm that the palpitations can occur without the patient's being consciously aware of the symptom.

The two most common types of palpitations are sinus tachycardia and premature ventricular systoles. *Sinus tachycardia* is a rapid forceful beating of the heart that may begin suddenly or slowly and subsides gradually. We have all experienced sinus tachycardia as it commonly occurs whenever we exert ourselves or become unduly excited. *Premature ventricular systoles* give one the unpleasant sense that the heart is "skipping a beat" or "doing flip-flops." The existence of these and other types of palpitations can be diagnostically confirmed by electrocardiography.

Syncope

Syncope or fainting, you recall, is the loss of consciousness as the result of a sudden decrease in blood flow to the brain. In patients with heart disease, syncope indicates that an adverse change in circulatory dynamics has suddenly and violently interfered with the individual's cardiac output and rhythm; e.g., there may have been the sudden development of heart block, cardiac arrest, or severe ventricular arrhythmias.

Edema*

Edema, a common sympton in many disorders, is defined as "accumulation of an abnormally large amount of fluid in the intracellular tissue spaces"; edematous fluid most commonly accumulates in the subcutaneous tissues. All edema fluid is drawn from the blood plasma and is similar in chemical composition to plasma. Edema may be localized to one specific organ or tissue, or it may be so severe that it affects the entire body (anasarca).

The major causes of edema in patients with heart disease and heart failure are (1) obstruction of the blood flow *into* the heart, which leads to venous congestion; (2) obstruction of the blood flow *from* the heart, which results in pulmonary edema; (3) fluid overload, which leads to circulatory overload; (4) abnormal renal retention of water and electrolytes in response to hormonal and neural regulatory mechanisms; (5) increased renal, arterial and venous pressure; (6) increased capillary permeability; (7) decreased colloid osmotic pressure due to loss or destruction of plasma proteins; and (8) disturbances in those factors that regulate the formation and flow of lymph.

When caring for patients with heart disease, watch carefully for the following signs indicative of edema:

- *Sudden weight gain which may precede the appearance of edema.*
- *Piffiness of ankles and hands in ambulatory patients.*
- *Swelling of tissues over the sacrum, buttocks, and posterior thighs in bedridden patients.*

Other Signs or Symptoms

Cyanosis. Cyanosis is a bluish discoloration of the skin that results from increased amounts of *reduced* hemoglobin within the blood. How *intense* the bluish skin hue is depends upon two factors: the *amount* of reduced hemoglobin present in the blood, and the extent to which one can *see the blood* within the superficial capillaries and venules of the skin. Visualization of blood within these vessels depends upon the patient's skin thickness, presence of edema, and pigmentation. In certain areas of the body, cyanotic discoloration may be intense, and in other areas it may be obscured entirely.

When examining patients for the presence of cyanosis:

- *Observe the color of ear lobes, lips, buccal mucosa, and fingernail beds.*
- *Observe the color of mucous membranes and retina of the eye in dark-skinned persons.*
- *Observe the patient in bright daylight if possible; fluorescent lighting distorts true color.*

Cyanosis may be either central or peripheral. *Central cyanosis* results from a low oxygen saturation of the arterial blood. Low arterial oxygen saturation may be caused by congenital right-to-left shunts (which cause the blood to bypass the lungs), or by pulmonary diseases, e.g., pneumonia. The central cyanosis appears on *warm* mucous membranes such as the conjunctiva and inside the lips and cheeks. The presence of central cyanosis is confirmed by testing the patient's

*Edema is discussed in detail in Chapter 12.

arterial blood for the level of arterial oxygen saturation. In some extreme cases, arterial oxygen saturation may be as low as 75 per cent or less, compared with the normal 94 to 100 per cent.

Peripheral cyanosis differs from central cyanosis in that the arterial oxygen saturation is normal; however, the oxygen saturation within the peripheral vascular bed is poor. Extensive lack of oxygen saturation within the peripheral bed results from slowed circulation within the capillaries and venules. Thus, peripheral cyanosis develops in conditions such as heart failure and shock (in which circulation time is prolonged), and in polycythemia (in which the blood is thick and sluggish in its flow), as well as in certain peripheral vascular diseases. In contrast to central cyanosis, peripheral cyanosis appears only on *cool* parts of the body such as the nose, cheeks, and ears.

Hypoxemia. Hypoxemia, or insufficient oxygenation of the blood, is common in patients with cardiac disease and also those with lung disease.

> *When caring for patients with serious cardiac ailments, watch carefully for the following signs of* hypoxemia:
>
> ▶ *An* increase *in* pulse rate; *the heart is trying to compensate for oxygen lack by pumping more blood more quickly.*
>
> ▶ *Signs of* cerebral anoxia; *e.g., irritability, restlessness, disorientation.*
>
> ▶ Asterixis *or* "liver flap"; *i.e., when the patient reaches for an object, his hands tend to flutter.*
>
> ▶ Cyanosis. *Cyanosis is a very* late *sign of oxygen lack. Do* not *wait for the appearance of cyanosis to notify the physician of suspected hypoxemia!*

Murmurs. *The identification of a murmur, or abnormal heart sound, is one of the most important diagnostic indications of valvular heart disease.* Normally blood flows through the heart valves and blood vessels in a smooth, quiet fashion, and no audible sounds are produced. However, when there is turbulence within the blood stream, abnormal sounds develop and are called murmurs. See Chapter 15 (p. 349) for a discussion of causes and classifications of heart murmurs.

Venous Engorgement of the Neck Veins

> *Distended neck veins are a common finding in congestive heart failure.*

Engorgement of the cervical veins indicates a high central venous pressure. In the section on diagnostic tests we shall discuss how to estimate venous pressure by examination of the neck veins.

Miscellaneous. Other symptoms of cardiac disorders that you may observe while giving patient care include:

Cough. Usually develops in patients suffering from heart failure and pulmonary edema.

Dizziness and headache. Commonly observed in patients with hypertension and cerebral arteriosclerosis.

Visual disturbances. An early sign of hypertension due to sclerosed vessels within the retina of the eye.

Abdominal pain. Usually occurs in persons with liver engorgement resulting from heart failure.

Nosebleed. Frequent nosebleeds in young persons may indicate rheumatic fever; in older persons, hypertensive heart disease.

THE PHYSICAL EXAMINATION OF THE HEART

The three main methods physicians and nurses use to examine the heart and its surrounding structures are percussion, palpation, auscultation. Refer also to Chapter 15 (pp. 350 and 351) for discussions of these techniques.

Percussion. When using percusson to examine the heart, the physician lightly but sharply taps the area of the chest overlying the heart. The pitch of the resulting sounds aids in determining the *position* and *size* of the heart. By the use of percussion, the doctor can often diagnose cardiac enlargement or displacement — signs indicative of congestive heart failure. This diagnostic method is not ordinarily used to examine obese persons, athletic persons with very muscular chest walls, or patients with emphysema.

Palpation. The precordium is that part of the anterior surface of the body that lies over the heart, the heart's great vessels, and the pulmonary structures that are located anterior to the heart. By palpating the precordium at the PMI (see Chapter 15), the physician is able to estimate *heart size;* it is also possible to detect certain *abnormal vibrations* originating in the heart that are difficult to hear through a stethoscope.

Auscultation. Auscultation, or listening to the patient's heart and chest with a stethoscope, is used to discover structural and functional abnormalities within the heart and lungs. Listening to the heart sounds is a particularly valuable diagnostic aid in thin individuals, because the sounds are far clearer than in obese persons. By careful auscultation with the stethoscope, the physician or specially trained nurse is able to:

1. Identify abnormal first or second heart sounds.
2. Note the appearance of abnormal heart sounds.

3. Analyze adventitious pulmonary sounds, e.g., rales and wheezes.
4. Note nonpathologic heart sounds.

The most important sounds to note are the first and second heart sounds. The *first* heart sound ("lubb"), which results from the closure of the mitral and tricuspid valves, indicates how well the left ventricle is contracting. If the sound is very loud, the left ventricle is probably contracting normally.

The second heart sound ("dubb"), which results from the closure of the aortic and pulmonic semilunar valves, gives information concerning the blood pressure within the vascular system — both arterial and pulmonary. Normally the second heart sound should be softer than the first sound at the apex of the heart. A very loud second heart sound may indicate either arterial or pulmonary hypertension.

Abnormal heart sounds can be differentiated from *normal* and *nonpathologic* sounds by means of auscultation. The normal heart sounds are usually of very brief duration, consisting only of a few vibrations, and are the result of a change in the velocity of the blood flow owing to closing of the valves. Examples of *nonpathologic* sounds are a "splitting" of the first sound (one semilunar valve closes before the other; this is due to respiratory influences), and an occasional added third heart sound. *Pathologic murmurs* are usually prolonged and have definite characteristics that are related to time, duration, intensity, location, and radiation.

Listening to the patient's *lungs* for abnormal sounds is an important method for diagnosing both heart and pulmonary abnormalities. *Moist rales,* which are fine crackling sounds like the crinkling of cellophane, are an important physical finding in patients with left ventricle failure. Rales may result from pulmonary infection, pulmonary edema, or aspiration of fluid; they generally indicate the presence of fluid within the patient's lungs.

Wheezes, a second type of abnormal chest sound, usually indicate narrowing of the bronchioles and the presence of bronchospasm. Wheezing is a common finding in acute pulmonary edema, asthma, and acute allergic reactions. See Chapter 15 for a more complete discussion of assessment of the heart and lungs.

DIAGNOSTIC PROCEDURES

The four most common types of diagnostic procedures used to diagnose cardiovascular disease are laboratory tests, measures of circulatory dynamics, radiology techniques, and graphic procedures.

Laboratory Tests

The major types of laboratory tests that physicians commonly order for patients with suspected heart ailments are (1) blood count, (2) erythrocyte sedimentation rate (ESR), (3) prothrombin time, (4) kidney function tests, (5) serum cholesterol, (6) blood smears and cultures, (7) blood serum protein, (8) serologic tests, (9) urinalysis, and (10) enzyme tests. Serum electrolytes, especially potassium, are also commonly ordered in selected patients such as those on potassium depleting diuretics and those receiving digitalis preparations. Let us briefly explore the purpose of each of these tests, the normal values, and the meaning of abnormal findings.

Blood Count.* A complete blood count is routinely ordered on all patients with suspected heart disease. The erythrocyte count is normally between 4 and 5.5 million/cu. mm. The erythrocyte count usually *decreases* in rheumatic fever and subacute bacterial endocarditis; it is usually *increased* in heart diseases in which inadequate oxygenation of tissues is a problem, e.g., right-to-left congenital shunts and heart conditions accompanied by pulmonary insufficiency.

The normal leukocyte count is from 5 to 10 thousand/cu. mm. The leukocyte count is *elevated* in infectious diseases of the heart (e.g., acute bacterial endocarditis), and following a myocardial infarction, because large numbers of white cells are necessary to dispose of the necrotic tissue resulting from the infarction.

Erythrocyte Sedimentation Rate. The sedimentation rate is a measure of the rapidity with which red blood cells settle out of the unclotted blood in one hour. The rate of settling is evidently influenced by changes in the levels of the blood proteins. The normal "sed" rate varies with the laboratory method used and with the sex of the patient. An approximately normal reading is between 6 and 20 mm. in 1 hour; the readings are generally higher for women than for men.

Examination of the blood sedimentation rate allows the physician to *roughly* follow the course of acute rheumatic fever, acute myocardial infarction, and infectious heart disease. However, the blood sedimentation rate is *not* a very accurate test, because it can be influenced by a number of physiologic factors other than disease. Although measuring the "sed" rate has been a helpful "old standby" in many hospitals, newer and more sophisticated tests are being developed which may eventually replace it.

Blood Coagulation Tests. As the name implies, blood coagulation tests examine the ability

*Leukocyte counts are discussed in Chapter 11; erythrocyte count is discussed in Unit XIV.

of a patient's blood to clot. Clotting is a complex physiologic phenomenon that depends upon the presence of blood clotting factors. (See Chapter 46.)

Prothrombin time determination, sometimes referred to as the "pro time," determines the activity of prothrombin, fibrinogen, and three other coagulation factors. This test is performed daily on the blood of patients receiving anticoagulant drugs that interfere with the synthesis of prothrombin in the liver, such as coumarin (Dicumarol) and warfarin sodium (Coumadin). The prothrombin time determination is also performed on patients suspected of having a tendency toward the formation of thrombi.

The *partial thromboplastin time* (PTT) measures all but three of the blood coagulation factors. The PTT is used in determining adequate levels of anticoagulation with heparin therapy and to aid in diagnosing clotting abnormalities.

Blood Urea Nitrogen (BUN). The BUN is a test of renal function. *Urea* is an important nonprotein nitrogenous substance that is formed in the liver and found in the blood, lymph, and urine. Urea is the final end product of protein metabolism and is the major nitrogenous factor within the urine. The BUN test measures the nitrogen faction of urea circulating in the blood.

The normal BUN is 8 to 28 mg./dl. of blood. BUN levels are elevated in kidney diseases and in heart ailments that adversely affect the renal circulation, e.g., congestive heart failure.

Serum Cholesterol. This laboratory test measures the level of cholesterol in the blood. Cholesterol is an alcohol released upon the breakdown of fats within the body. It is found in bile and blood and in the brain and spinal cord tissues. Cholesterol is most commonly ingested in egg yolk and in certain fats and oils.

The normal range for blood cholesterol is from 150 to 280 mg./dl. of blood. An increase in blood cholesterol is possibly associated with the development of atherosclerosis and coronary occlusion. We further consider the possible role of cholesterol in the etiology of coronary artery disease in Chapter 36.

For accurate results, patients should be *fasting* prior to the drawing of blood for the serum cholesterol test.

Serum Protein. You will recall from Chapter 12 that plasma proteins are large particles within the blood that exert a force called the *colloid osmotic pressure;* this pressure draws fluid from the interstitial fluid compartment into the vascular compartment or capillaries, thereby counterbalancing the force of hydrostatic blood pressure, which forces fluid out of the capillaries into the tissues. Thus, when the level of plasma proteins (especially serum albumin) drops below normal, the colloid osmotic pressure is diminished, and fluid escapes from the vascular compartment into the tissues. The result of diminished plasma proteins is *edema;* consequently the physician always checks the level of serum proteins in patients with edema.

The *normal* level of serum protein is 6 to 8 Gm./dl. of blood. A substantial decrease in the level of serum protein (below 5 Gm./dl.) results in edema. Hypoproteinemia (especially a reduction in serum albumin) is associated with long-standing cardiac failure as a result of malnutrition, decreased production of albumin by the liver in right-sided heart failure, and the loss of albumin in the urine and peritoneal effusions over a long period of time.

Blood Cultures. This form of laboratory study is ordered for patients with infectious diseases of the heart, e.g., bacterial endocarditis. The blood for the culture is obtained by venipuncture and is then inoculated into a culture medium. The bacterial colony that grows on the culture medium enables the doctor to identify the organism causing the infectious disease. Once the organism has been identified, the sensitivity of the organism to various antibiotics is tested to ascertain the proper course of therapy.

Serologic Tests. Because of the important role of syphilis in infections of the aorta and in the production of aortic aneurysms, the doctor frequently orders serologic examinations. The most common serologic tests for syphilis are (1) Venereal Disease Research Lab (VDRL) flocculation, used primarily as a screening test; (2) *Treponema pallidum* immobilization (TPI); (3) Fluorescent treponemal antibody absorbed (FTA-ABS); and (4) microhemagglutination treponemal antibody (MHA-TP), a simplification of the FTA-ABS. The FTA-ABS is the most sensitive. In patients in whom there is a strong suspicion of syphilis despite a negative VDRL or TPI, an FTA-ABS is usually indicated.

Urinalysis. Heart disease (in particular, congestive heart failure) can result in damage to the kidneys. Thus, in congestive heart failure, casts are usually present in the urine, albuminuria is common, and the urine's specific gravity is high.

You will recall from Chapter 12 that the specific gravity of urine (or the concentration of urine) is between 1.010 and 1.025. Patients suffering from congestive heart failure typically have a dark, concentrated urine with a *high* specific gravity of between 1.020 and 1.030; sodium content of the urine is very low. The urine is concentrated in these individuals because Na^+ and H_2O are being held in the tissues as edema fluid, cardiac output is reduced, and circulating blood volume is diminished. Diuresis and Na^+ restriction help to lower the specific gravity of the urine.

Albuminuria, as stated earlier, may also develop in patients suffering from congestive heart failure who have impaired renal function.

Enzyme Tests. Enzymes, which regulate metabolic activities within the cell, are released into the circulation when the cell membrane is damaged. The enzymes creatine phosphokinase (CPK) and lactic dehydrogenase (LDH) have isoenzymes which are found almost exclusively in cardiac muscle. Alpha-hydroxybutyrate dehydrogenase (HBD) is another enzyme found in the myocardium. Measurement of the serum levels of these enzymes in the patient suspected of having had a myocardial infarction or myocardial contusion will aid the physician in making a diagnosis and in following the progress of the myocardial damage. Normal values vary with different laboratories.

Measures of Circulatory Dynamics

Five important diagnostic procedures that measure how effectively the blood is circulating through the heart and vascular system are circulation time determination, measures of cardiac output, blood pressure readings, venous pressure measurements, and pulmonary artery and pulmonary artery wedge pressures.

CIRCULATION TIME DETERMINATION

The circulation time is the length of time it takes for a special solution (either sodium dehydrocholate or calcium chloride) injected intravenously to circulate from the patient's arm to his tongue, where it can be tasted. Sometimes this test is called a "circ time." This test is employed mainly to establish a diagnosis of congestive heart failure. or to follow the course of patients with this disease. The circulation time is *prolonged* in congestive heart failure because the patient's *blood volume* is *increased* (owing to fluid retention) and renal dysfunction, and because the *cardiac output* is reduced (owing to the heart's decreased pumping action).

The normal systemic circulation time (from arm to tongue) is *15 seconds.* Circulation time is *prolonged* in congestive heart failure, polycythemia vera, and myxedema; it is *reduced in* hyperthyroidism, anemia, pregnancy, fever, congenital heart disease with right-to-left shunts, and after eating and exercise. Because of the introduction of more reliable methods of evaluating cardiac status, the circulation time is rarely used at this time.

CARDIAC OUTPUT

You will recall from Chapter 31 that the cardiac output is the amount of blood pumped out of the left ventricle into the arterial system every minute; i.e., cardiac output is equal to the stroke volume (volume of blood pumped out with each beat) times the rate. Therefore, if the stroke volume of the left ventricle is between 50 and 90 ml., with an average of 70 ml., and the heart rate is 72 beats per minute, the normal cardiac output of the left ventricle is roughly between 4 and 7 L. The cardiac output of the right ventricle is considered equal to that of the left; this is because the right ventricle, while it is not so muscular as the left ventricle, pumps against lighter resistance.

There are two major methods for measuring cardiac output: application of the Fick principle, and indicator dilution methods.

Fick Principle. The Fick principle implies that the cardiac output per minute from the *right* ventricle (and consequently the *left* ventricle) can be determined by measuring the amount of blood that the right ventricle pumps into the lung capillaries within one minute. The amount of blood flowing through the capillaries of the lungs within 1 minute can be determined by (1) measuring the amount of *oxygen* that the blood has absorbed within 1 minute, which depends upon the patient's basal metabolic rate, and (2) measuring the difference between the oxygen content of the oxygen-poor venous blood entering the lungs and the oxygen-rich arterial blood that flows from the lungs into the left side of the heart and the arterial system.

To estimate the cardiac output by applying the Fick principle, three laboratory measurements are needed:

1. A measure of the patient's oxygen consumption in milliliters per minute when the patient is resting.
2. A measure of the oxygen content of arterial blood, which is obtained by direct arterial puncture.
3. A measure of the oxygen content of the mixed venous blood, which is customarily taken from the right ventricle or pulmonary artery during cardiac catheterization.

After obtaining the above measures, the physician next applies this formula to the data:

$$\frac{O_2 \text{ absorption ml./min.}}{\begin{array}{l}O_2 \text{ content of} \\ \text{arterial blood,} \\ \text{ml./L.}\end{array} - \begin{array}{l}O_2 \text{ content of} \\ \text{mixed venous} \\ \text{blood, ml./L.}\end{array}} = \text{cardiac output, L./min.}$$

As an example of the application of this formula, consider the following measurements for a typical patient.[67] (1) O_2 absorption per minute = 200 ml.; (2) oxygen concentration of arterial blood = 190 ml./L.; (3) oxygen content of the venous blood = 150 ml./L.

$$\frac{200 \text{ ml./min. } (O_2 \text{ absorption})}{\underset{(\text{arterial } O_2)}{190 \text{ ml./L.}} - \underset{(\text{venous } O_2)}{150 \text{ ml./L.}}} = \frac{200 \text{ ml./min.}}{40 \text{ ml./L.}} = 5 \text{ L. blood}$$

This is equal to (1) the cardiac ouput of the right ventricle, and (2) the amount of blood that has passed through the lungs in 1 minute. Because the outputs of both the right and left ventricles are approximately equal, 5 L. per minute is also the cardiac output of the left ventricle.

Indicator Dilution Methods. Indicator dilution methods provide a second means for obtaining a measure of cardiac output. In this procedure the patient receives a measured intravenous injection of dye. Next, blood samples are drawn from an artery, and the concentration of dye within the blood is calculated by means of precise measuring devices. Then this reading, which shows the amount of time required for the blood to absorb the measured amount of dye, is amplified; it appears as a curve on graph paper. The size of the curve indicates how much blood the heart has pumped out into the arterial system in a given amount of time, i.e., the cardiac output. Blood samples for the dye dilution method can be obtained during cardiac catheterization.

Thermodilution is another indicator dilution method which is frequently used for computing the cardiac output. This test can be easily carried out via a thermodilution catheter, a special catheter with one lumen opening into the right atrium and another opening into the pulmonary artery. In addition it has a lumen which contains a thermistor (temperature electrode) that allows for measurement of the temperature in the pulmonary artery.

Iced saline or 5 per cent dextrose in water of a known temperature is injected into the right atrium. Measuring the temperature changes in the pulmonary artery after injection of the cold fluid determines how much the blood has been diluted. From this information the cardiac output can be computed. The smaller the temperature change, the greater the cardiac output. The cardiac output of critically ill patients in intensive care units is usually determined by this method.

The *normal* cardiac output for the calm, resting patient (who has been NPO for 12 hours) spans a range of from 4 to 7 L. per minute, with an average of 5.3. Table 33–1 lists the conditions that elevate and depress cardiac output.

The *cardiac index,* as mentioned in Chapter 31, gives additional information about cardiac output by relating it to a person's size. A cardiac output adequate for a small person may be insufficient for someone who is large in stature.

TABLE 33–1. CONDITIONS THAT CAUSE A CHANGE IN CARDIAC OUTPUT

Conditions Decreasing Cardiac Output	Conditions Increasing Cardiac Output
1. Acute congestive heart failure	1. Hypoxia
2. Pericarditis with effusion	2. Hyperthyroidism
3. Old age	3. Excitement
4. Arterial hemorrhage	4. Exercise
5. Standing motionless, which decreases the venous return to the heart	5. Food intake
6. Myxedema	6. Oral and intravenous fluid intake
7. Atrial fibrillation	
8. Heart block	
9. Shock	
10. Valvular heart disease	

The normal cardiac index for a person at rest is 2.5 to 4 L./min./m².

ARTERIAL BLOOD PRESSURE

The most accurate blood pressure reading is obtained when the patient is truly resting, free of all physical and emotional stimuli that elevate blood pressure. Naturally this is an ideal state for which we strive but rarely, if ever, achieve.

In earlier courses you have probably studied the basic equipment needed and the method for taking a blood pressure reading.* In this section we shall briefly emphasize those factors that decrease or increase the chances of error. Because the blood pressure is a common diagnostic and evaluative measurement and because it is primarily a nursing procedure, we cannot emphasize enough the importance of an accurate reading and the elimination of error. Blood pressure readings are *most accurate* when you adhere to the following basic rules:

1. Instruct the patient to neither eat, drink, nor exert himself for at least one half hour prior to his blood pressure reading. Try to have the patient in a quiet room that has a comfortable temperature. If he is ambulatory, allow him to remain comfortably seated for at least 5 minutes before taking the reading.
2. Place the seated patient's arm on a table in such a way that it is at *heart* level; likewise, position the bed patient's arm at heart level, supporting it comfortably. If the patient's arm is *not* at heart level, both systolic and diastolic readings may be in error by as much as 10 mm. Hg.
3. Make certain that the blood pressure cuff is the *correct width.* A cuff that is too *narrow* for the arm will give a falsely high reading; a cuff too *wide* may result in a falsely low reading. Generally, a cuff 12 to 14 cm. (about 6 inches) wide is suitable for the average adult.
4. Make certain that you apply the cuff snugly and evenly and that the bag is *completley deflated* prior to the

*Refer to Sorensen and Luckman, *Basic Nursing: A Psychophysiologic Approach,* Chapter 29, for a complete discussion of measuring blood pressure.

first reading and between readings. Always center the cuff's bladder over the artery that you plan to occlude. Be sure that the stethoscope bell does not touch the tubes, cuff, or patient's clothing, as you may hear confusing extraneous sounds as a result.

5. Inflate the cuff as rapidly as possible (within 7 seconds or less) and deflate it at 2 to 3 mm. per heartbeat until you no longer hear Korotkoff's sounds.

6. When viewing the blood pressure gauges, remember these rules: (a) Observe the *aneroid* gauge from directly in front of it and from no farther than 3 feet away. (b) Observe the *mercury* gauge (which must be in a vertical position) with your eye at the level of the meniscus and from no farther than 3 feet away.

7. Take several blood pressure readings over a period of time; ask another nurse to take the patient's blood pressure so that you can compare readings.

8. Obtain orthostatic or postural blood pressures when appropriate.

9. When you record your findings: (a) Record the position of the patient during the reading. Blood pressure is usually higher in the standing position than in the lying position. Abbreviate lying (L) or standing (ST). (b) Record the arm used for the reading; right arm (RA) or left arm LA). (c) Record the *muffling* of Korotkoff's sounds as the diastolic reading. Also record the point at which Korotkoff's sounds disappear; e.g., 142/80/78; 142/76/76.*

What is a "normal" blood pressure reading? Insurance companies often place the normal blood pressure reading at around 120/80. However, it is essential to remember that blood pressure readings vary greatly among healthy individuals. For some persons a blood pressure of 120/80 would be abnormally high; for other persons it might be abnormally low. It is wise to consult the patient's former history or even the patient himself in regard to blood pressure readings taken in the past. What may appear to be an abnormal reading may actually be a normal reading for a particular individual.

Hypertension, a common problem, refers only to conditions in which the recorded pressure is *persistently* higher than normal. Generally a blood pressure that is persistently above 160 systolic or 100 diastolic is considered hypertensive.

VENOUS PRESSURE

The central venous pressure (CVP) is a measurement of the pressure within the superior vena cava. CVP reflects the pressure under which the blood is returned to the superior vena cava or the right atrium.

The normal CVP usually is between 5 and 10 cm. H_2O. In situations in which the blood volume is *reduced* (e.g., hemorrhage or fluid loss from other causes), the *CVP is lower than usual;* thus, values below 5 cm. H_2O may indicate a decreasing circulating volume.

In situations in which the circulatory system is *overloaded* (e.g., due to excessive administration of fluids or congestive heart failure) the *CVP will be higher than normal.* Thus, values above 10 cm H_2O may indicate overloading of the right heart.

Examination of the neck veins is an excellent means for estimating the venous pressure and "actually often exceeds in accuracy the measurement of venous pressure with a saline manometer in inexpert hands."[79]

To estimate the cervical or jugular venous pressure, the physician or nurse should follow this procedure:

1. Have the patient lie on a bed or table and raise the head of the bed so the patient is sitting at a 30- or 45-degree angle. Use a table or bed that breaks at the patient's hipline; otherwise, the patient's neck will be flexed, making it impossible to properly examine the neck veins.

2. Remove clothing that compresses the neck or upper thorax.

3. Use a pocket flashlight or place a gooseneck lamp in a position so that small shadows are cast on the patient's neck, thereby making the veins more apparent. Good lighting is important in this examination.

4. Locate the external jugular veins on each side of the neck and detect their pulsations.

5. Estimate the venous pressure by measuring the level to which the internal jugular veins are distended up the neck toward the head *above* the level of the manubrium (the upper bone of the sternum, which articulates with the clavicle) i.e., sternal angle; also estimate how high the venous pulsations extend. In a healthy individual seated at a 45-degree angle, the venous pulses should not ascend any higher than 1 or 2 cm. above the manubrium. In a patient with a high venous pressure of 25 cm. or more (e.g., in severe congestive heart failure), the cervical veins may be distended from the level of the manubrium up to the angle of the jaw (Figs. 33–2 and 33–3).

It is possible to roughly estimate the venous pressure by *examining the veins on the back of the patient's hand* as he raises and lowers his arm. As the patient raises his hand, watch for that point above the sternal notch at which the veins on the dorsum of his hand collapse. Normally collapse of the veins occurs when the back of the hand is a few centimeters above the sternal notch. When the venous pressure is elevated, the veins remain distended for several centimeters above the sternal notch.[4]

Finally, central venous pressure is measured by means of a *manometer* attached to an IV tubing and IV solution. This procedure is particu-

*For years there has been a lively debate between the "muffled sound" school of authorities and the "last sound" school concerning which level provides the more accurate index of the diastolic pressure. In 1967 the American Heart Association settled the dispute by recommending that clinicians record *both* muffling of sounds and the disappearance of sounds as the diastolic pressure.

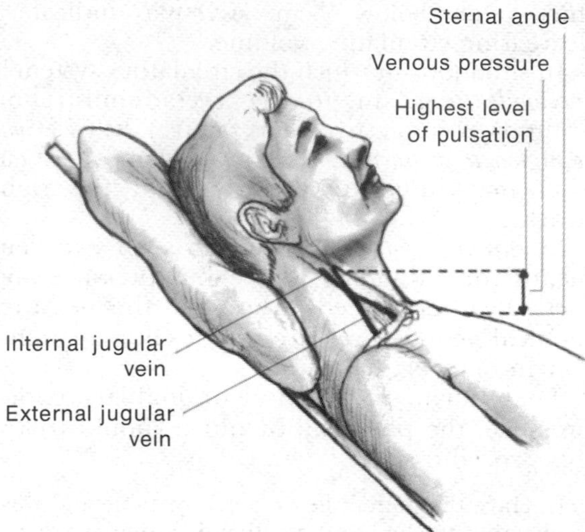

Figure 33–2. Estimation of jugular venous pressure. (1) Identify the external jugular veins. (2) Note the pulsations of the internal jugular vein; (3) Note the highest point at which it is possible to visualize the pulsations of the internal jugular vein. (4) Measure the vertical distance between this point and the sternal angle. (5) If the internal jugular pulsations cannot be visualized, locate the point above which the external jugular veins appear to be collapsed. (6) Record the vertical distance ascertained by either method in centimeters above the sternal angle together with the angle at which the patient is lying, i.e., at a 45-degree angle as in this figure. (From Bates, B.: *A Guide to Physical Examination.* Philadelphia: J. B. Lippincott, 1974, p. 142.)

larly helpful in assessing the status of critically ill patients because their CVP can be continuously monitored. A Teflon or polyethylene catheter is placed either in the right atrium or the superior vena cava. The catheter may be inserted through the median basilic or the cephalic vein in the antecubital space (known as a peripheral CVP line), or through a jugular or subclavian vein. Jugular or subclavian placement is often employed in emergency situations because the vessels are usually more accessible (especially in the patient in shock) and larger; the lines are shorter than peripheral CVP lines, thus allowing more rapid administration of fluid if necessary.

Once in place, the catheter is connected to IV fluid with a stopcock and manometer in-line. The CVP line may be used to administer fluids or may be used primarily for CVP measurements. When the line is used only for CVP measurements, a "flush bottle" of IV fluid, often containing heparin, is infused very slowly in order to maintain patency of the vein. A micro-dripper and/or IV drop-regulating pump may be added to the system. A chest x-ray is obtained as soon as possible to verify proper tube placement.

Remember that the fluid that the patient receives intravenously from the flush bottle could cause a circulatory overload unless it is carefully observed and adjusted to a slow rate of drip.

Kurihara and Moody offer the following information pertaining to establishing a baseline for the position of the monitor and measuring the pressure:

1. Establishing a Baseline for Manometer Position. The manometer is so positioned that the zero mark is at the level of the right atrium, using the left or right midchest (Fig. 33–4). The right atrium is located inferiorly to midsternum and halfway between the front to the back of the chest laterally. . . . If the patient has pulmonary emphysema, a lung disease, or a barrel chest, use the lower third of the lateral chest in locating the right atrium. This then establishes the reference position prior to each subsequent CVP measurement and reading. . . .

If the patient cannot tolerate a flat supine position because of orthopnea with left-sided heart failure, he may sit at a 45-degree angle with the zero point of the manometer adjusted to the level of the right atrium in

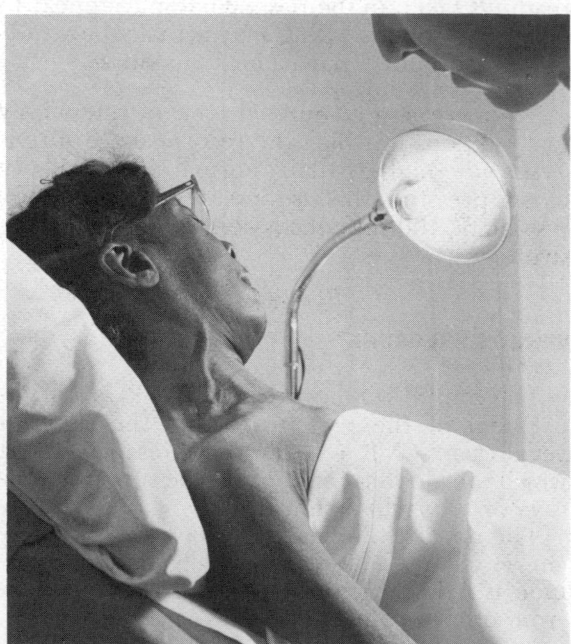

Figure 33–3. Close-up view of a patient, demonstrating greatly distended external jugular vein. The systemic venous pressure exceeded 30 cm. H_2O. (From Fowler, N. O.: *Examination of the Heart. Part 2: Inspection and Palpation of Venous and Arterial Pulses.* Prepared for the Committee on Medical Education of the American Heart Association. New York, American Heart Association, 1972.)

the sitting position. This then becomes the established reference position. Between measurements the patient may lie or sit in any position of comfort. Mark the baseline position of the manometer on the patient's chest so that all personnel will measure the CVP from the same point.

2. Measurement of Pressure

a. After the catheter has been properly positioned by the physician and the reference position is established, the nurse regulates the fluid from the flush bottle to run directly through the catheter into the vein ("solution arm" to "delivery arm" in diagram), in order to maintain the patency of the system.

b. By turning the stopcock from "solution arm" to "manometer arm," the manometer is then filled to a level of 20 to 25 cm.

c. The stopcock is then turned from the "manometer arm" position to "delivery arm" position for the actual pressure reading. With each respiration, the meniscus of the column of water in the "manometer arm" fluctuates. The reading is taken at the maximum level the meniscus reaches after it attains an average level in the column, indicating equal pressure in the manometer and the vena cava.

d. To keep the system open for subsequent readings, the stopcock is returned to its original position ("solution arm" to "delivery arm") and the flow is controlled by a microdrip method.

e. It is essential that the patient be relaxed at the time measurement is made, because straining, coughing, or any other activity that increases the intrathoracic pressure will cause spuriously high measurements. When CVP is measured while the patient is receiving mechanical ventilatory assistance, the ventilator must be temporarily disconnected to obtain a meaningful reading.[132A]

Frequently check the connections between the catheter and the attachments to be certain that they are secure; if they are not secure, the danger of *air embolism is present.* (See Chapters 13 and 95.) If the original reference position was established with the patient in a flat position, this same flat position must be resumed again at the time of repeated pressure readings. False readings can result from even a slight elevation of the head of the bed.

PULMONARY ARTERY AND PULMONARY ARTERY WEDGE PRESSURES

The CVP has not been a totally satisfactory means of measuring the status of left heart functioning, especially in critically ill patients, e.g., postoperative cardiac surgery patients or patients in cardiogenic shock. Significant changes

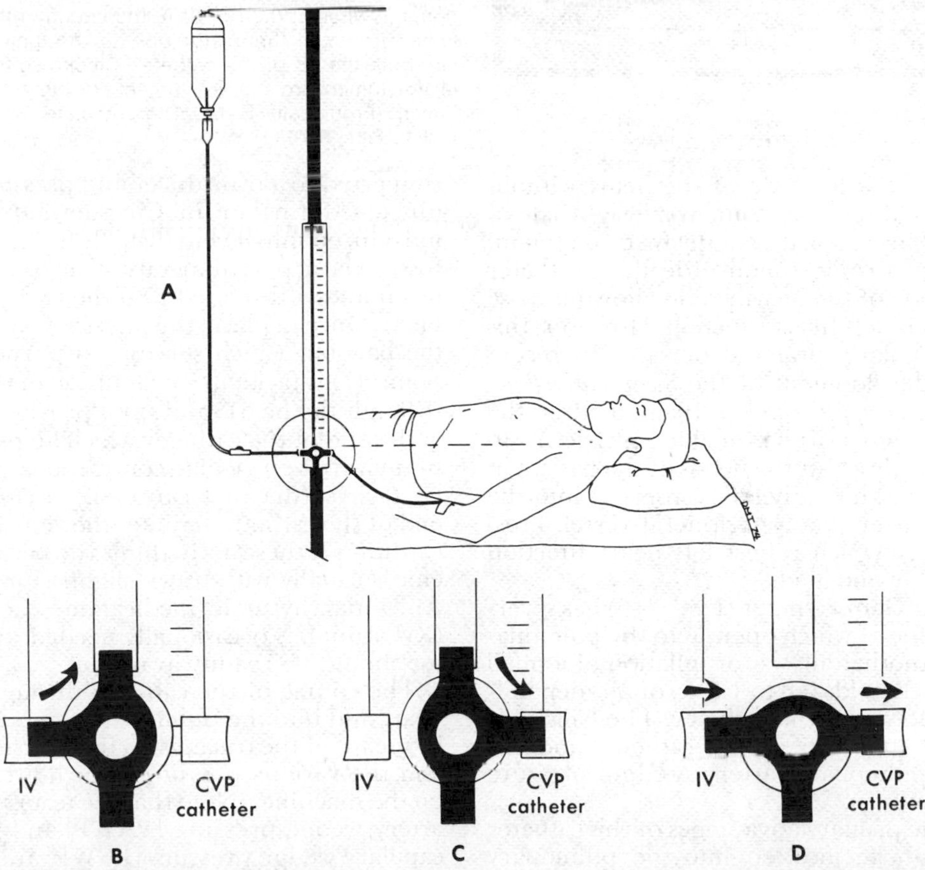

Figure 33–4. Procedure for measuring CVP with manometer. **A.** Manometer and IV tubing in place. **B.** Turn the stopcock so that the manometer fills with fluid above the level of the expected pressure. **C.** Turn the stopcock so that the IV is off and the fluid in the manometer flows to the patient. Obtain a reading after the fluid level stabilizes. **D.** Turn the stopcock to resume the IV flow to the patient. (From Schroeder, J. S., and E. K. Daily: *Techniques in Bedside Hemodynamic Monitoring.* St. Louis: C. V. Mosby Co., 1976, p. 70.)

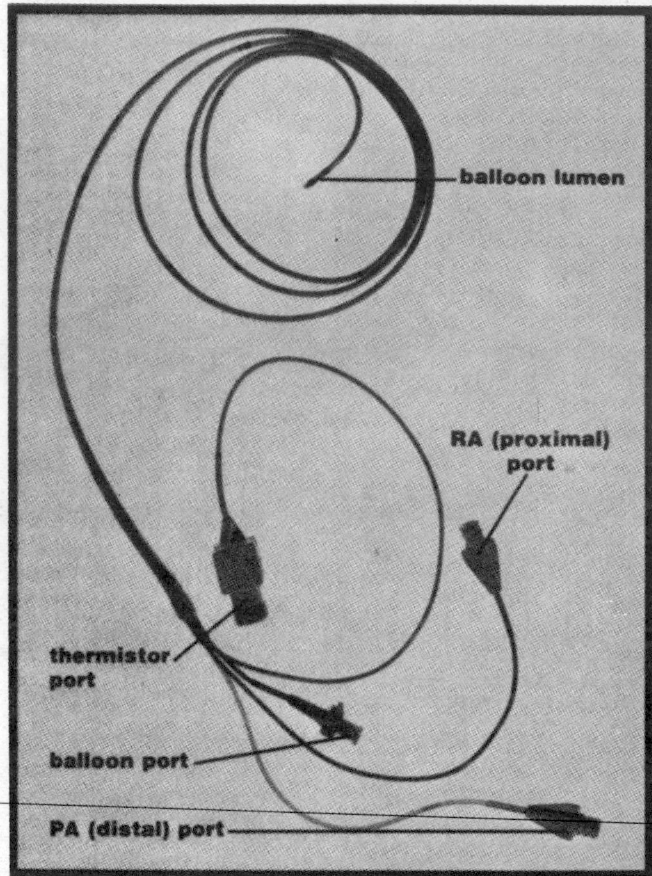

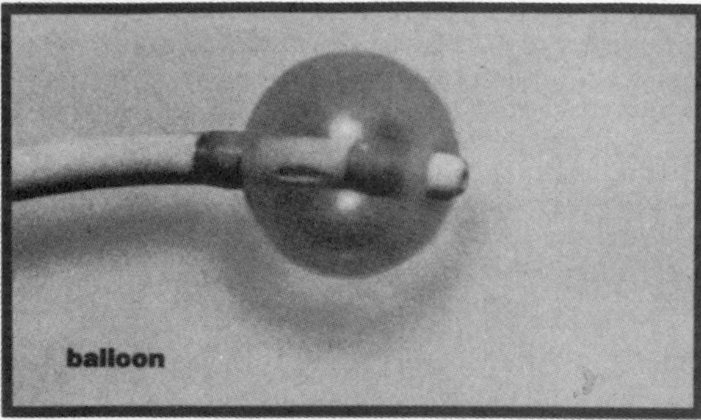

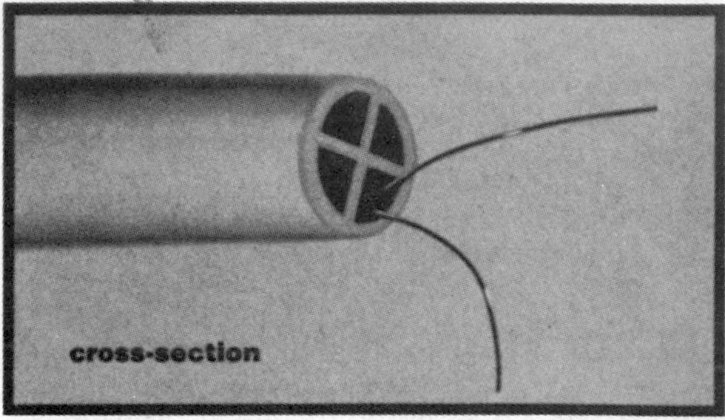

Figure 33–5. Three views of the Swan-Ganz catheter. The entire catheter with its four ports, a close-up of the inflated balloon, and a cross section of the four lumens and the thermistor wires inside the catheter. In the cross section, the wires at the right run the length of the thermistor lumen from the thermistor port to the lumen opening 4 cm. from the tip of the catheter. Clockwise from the thermistor lumen are the RA lumen, PA lumen, and balloon lumen. (From Lalli, S. M.: The complete Swan-Ganz. RN, 41:64, Sept. 1978.)

can occur in the left side of the heart without being reflected for some time in the right side of the heart. This can lead to a delay in treatment, or even improper treatment. Ideally, a catheter in the left side of the heart would allow for close observation of left heart function. However, this is not particularly practical or safe. In recent years, the development of the *Swan-Ganz flow-directed balloon-tipped catheter* (named after the men who designed it) has enabled physicians to more accurately assess the needs of the patient in heart failure. This catheter is inserted into the pulmonary artery via a peripheral vessel. Pressure readings which reflect left heart function can be readily obtained.

The Swan-Ganz catheter (Fig. 33–5) has several lumens, one of which opens into the pulmonary artery. Another allows for inflation of a small balloon which holds 0.8 to 1.5 cc. of air, depending upon the size of the catheter. The balloon is needed for insertion of the catheter and for obtaining pulmonary artery wedge pressure (PAWP) readings.

One of the primary advantages of this catheter is that it can be inserted into the pulmonary artery by the physician at the patient's bedside without the need for fluoroscopy (viewing the position of the catheter by means of a special x-ray machine). Before insertion, the catheter is connected to a transducer and pressure monitor (discussed further in Chapter 39). It is then introduced into a vein, usually in the antecubital fossa, via a percutaneous stick or venous cutdown and is threaded into the right side of the heart. Once in place, the physician injects air into the balloon, which serves two purposes at this point: (1) it facilitates propulsion of the catheter through the heart; and (2) it provides a cushion at the end of the catheter which helps to prevent premature ventricular contractions or ventricular tachycardia that can easily occur when the end of the catheter irritates the ventricular myocardium. If these arrhythmias do occur, the catheter is usually withdrawn slightly for a moment. An antiarrhythmic medication, e.g., lidocaine (Xylocaine), is occasionally needed. A defibrillator should be readily available.

The course of the catheter through the right heart and into the pulmonary artery is observed by means of the tracings on the pressure monitor and the various pressures which are registered on the machine. (Note that the terms pulmonary artery wedge pressure [PAWP] and pulmonary capillary wedge pressure [PCWP] are sometimes used interchangeably.) The values for normal pressures in the specific areas of the cardiovascular system are listed in Table 33–2.

Once it is in the pulmonary vasculature, the

TABLE 33–2. COMMONLY USED PRESSURES IN THE VARIOUS CARDIAC CHAMBERS AND MAJOR VESSELS (IN MILLIMETERS OF MERCURY)*

Right atrium	3	(0–5)
Right ventricle	24/4	(17–32/1–7)
Pulmonary artery	24/9	(17–32/4–13)
Left atrium	8	(2–12)
Left ventricle	130/9	(90–140/5–12)
Aorta	125/70	(90–140/60–90)

*Mean pressures are shown for the atria. In other chambers, the slash indicates systolic/diastolic pressures, figures in brackets show range of normal values.

(From Scher, A. M.: Electrocardiogram. *In* Ruch, T. C., and H. D. Patton (Eds.): *Physiology and Biophysics. II. Circulation, Respiration, and Fluid Balance,* 20th ed. Philadelphia: W. B. Saunders Co., 1974, p. 110.)

balloon finally reaches a point in the capillary where it becomes "wedged." The actual location of the catheter becomes evident on the oscilloscope of the monitor as the tracing changes from a pulmonary artery pressure tracing to an atrial pressure tracing (see Figure 33–6). When the Swan-Ganz catheter is wedged, it "looks" directly into the left side of the heart and is not influenced by pressure in the pulmonary artery. A direct relationship exists between the PAWP and the left ventricular end-diastolic pressure (LVEDP), therefore, the PAWP provides a reliable means of assessing difficulties which may be arising in the left side of the heart. (In patients with pulmonary hypertension the pulmonary artery pressures may be abnormally high, while the PAWP is normal.)

An elevated PAWP usually indicates that the strength of the myocardial contraction is not sufficient to empty the heart and provide an adequate cardiac output. The muscles are probably weakened because they are overstretched. Diuretic therapy will probably be the first method tried to decrease the PAWP.

If the decreased cardiac output is due to insufficient volume and pressure in the left ventricle just prior to systole, the PAWP will be low (Table 33–2). Therapy will then be directed at increasing the PAWP by administration of fluids. Higher pressures may be necessary, though, in a patient with a diseased heart who needs sufficient stretching of the myocardial muscle fibers to increase the strength of myocardial contraction. A PAWP of 16 to 18 mm. Hg may be necessary to accomplish this in some patients. Severe pulmonary congestion generally occurs when the PAWP is greater than 20 mm. Hg.

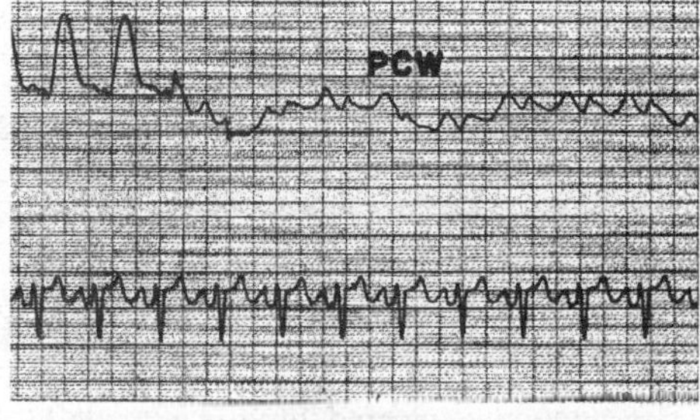

Figure 33–6. Characteristic pressure wave forms noted on the oscilloscope when the catheter is in the pulmonary artery (top left) and when it is "wedged" in a pulmonary arteriole. The pulmonary pressure wave flattens to a pulmonary capillary wedge (PCW) pattern as the balloon is inflated. The ECG (bottom) is recorded simultaneously. (From Woods, S. L.: Monitoring pulmonary artery pressures. *American Journal of Nursing,* 76:1765, Nov. 1976.)

The Swan-Ganz catheter also provides a means of readily obtaining samples of *mixed venous blood* from the pulmonary artery. (Mixed venous blood refers to blood from both the inferior and superior venae cavae.) The normal oxygen saturation of mixed venous blood is 75 per cent, whereas the oxygen saturation of arterial blood is 95 per cent. The difference between the arterial and venous oxygen saturation signifies the amount of oxygen extracted by the tissues of the body. In heart failure the oxygen saturation of mixed venous blood may fall considerably even though the arterial oxygen saturation may remain the same. This indicates that less blood is reaching the tissues owing to a decrease in the cardiac output, and more oxygen is therefore being extracted from the blood.

Pulmonary artery monitoring must be carried out in an ICU under the close scrutiny of an experienced nursing staff. Prior to insertion of the catheter, the nurse should explain to the patient that the procedure may be uncomfortable, but it should not be painful; a local anesthetic will be given at the catheter insertion site. The patient also should be aware that he will be covered with sterile drapes and that the physician doing the procedure will be in sterile attire. The nurse's support of the critically ill patient at this time is most essential.

Once the Swan-Ganz catheter is in place and PAWP readings have been obtained, the balloon is deflated. The *only* time the balloon should be inflated after it is in place is to obtain further PAWP readings. For the remainder of the time, the pulmonary artery pressure tracing should be visible on the oscilloscope. If a wedge tracing or a flat line appear on the scope when the balloon is not being inflated, the cause must be investigated. Simply irrigating the line to improve the patency may result in a normal pulmonary artery tracing. The catheter tip can float into a smaller portion of the pulmonary arteriole and become wedged without the balloon being inflated; this can also cause a flattened line on the monitor. If maneuvers to dislodge the catheter tip from this position (by having the patient cough or repositioning him) are not successful, it may be necessary for the physician to withdraw the catheter slightly. *Leaving the catheter in a "wedged" position can lead to infarction of the lung tissue being supplied by that vessel.*

When measuring pulmonary artery pressures and pulmonary artery wedge pressures, the patient should be lying flat, if possible. (Studies are currently under way to determine whether it is essential that the patient be positioned flat in order to obtain reliable pressure readings.) The transducer connected to the Swan-Ganz catheter should be at the level of the right atrium. If possible, remove the respirator from patients being mechanically ventilated while these pressures are being obtained.

Finally, the nurse caring for the critically ill patient whose left heart function is being monitored by the Swan-Ganz catheter should have a knowledge of what pressures are acceptable for each particular patient and the effects that the prescribed therapy is expected to have upon the patient's condition.

X-Ray Techniques

X-ray techniques are one of the major tools for diagnosing various types of heart disease. Some of the major purposes of x-ray techniques in making an evaluation of cardiac structure and function are:

1. To provide information about heart size and volume, the size of the individual chambers, the appearance of the vessels extending from the heart, and the presence and location of calcifications.
2. To reveal, by means of motion pictures (cineangiograms), any abnormal shunts or regurgitations within the heart.

The major types of x-ray techniques are fluoroscopy, angiocardiography, and cardiac catheterizaton.

Fluoroscopy. This simple, economical, and popular method of x-ray examination reveals the action of the heart at work. The patient stands in back of a fluorescent screen and in front of an x-ray tube. The examiner stands in front of the screen and is able to observe the continuous action of the heart.

This method of examination is used mainly to search for (1) abnormal tumors, structures, and calcifications within the heart; (2) signs of lung congestion; and (3) signs of pleural or pericardial effusion.

Fluoroscopy is a safe procedure with one exception — it is possible to overexpose the patient and examiner to ionizing radiation during the examination.

Angiocardiography. This procedure involves the intravenous injection of a radiopaque dye into the patient's heart during cardiac catheterization. Immediately after the dye is injected a series of x-ray films are taken which reveal the course of the dye as it circulates through the patient's heart, lungs, and great vessels. *Cineangiography* is the taking of moving pictures at this time; the cardiologist or cardiac surgeron can then carefully examine the heart in motion after the procedure. *Coronary arteriography* refers to the procedure when dye is injected directly into the coronary arteries during cardiac catheterization.

The purposes of angiocardiography are to:

1. Check the valves of the heart for competence.
2. Diagnose congenital septal defects.
3. Reveal calcifications or occlusions of the coronary arteries by means of selective coronary angiography.
4. Confirm diagnoses that cannot be confirmed by simpler means.
5. Study the structure and function of the heart in detail prior to cardiac surgery.

Angiocardiography is a complex and somewhat dangerous procedure and thus is performed only when absolutely necessary. Preparation of the patient is discussed under Cardiac Catheterization, next. The major types of angiocardiography are listed and defined in Table 33–3.

The *contrast medium* used for angiocardiography is usually an organic iodine medium such as diatrizoate sodium (Hypaque Sodium) or diatrizoate methylglucamine (Cardiografin). The physician calculates the dosage of contrast medium to be inserted into the patient's heart and vessels by determining the patient's weight in kilograms. Standard dosage for contrast media in angiography is 1 ml. per kg. of body weight.

Patients sometimes react allergically to iodine-base contrast media. In some cases the doctor may wish to skin test the patient for a possible

TABLE 33–3. MAJOR TYPES OF ANGIOCARDIOGRAPHY

Angiocardiography Procedure	Method Employed
Right-sided angiocardiography	Contrast medium is injected into the right heart chambers and pulmonary artery by means of a catheter threaded up a vein and into the heart during cardiac catheterization.
Left-sided angiocardiography	Contrast medium is injected into the left side of heart through a transvenous catheter passed through the atrial septum during cardiac catheterization or via a catheter passed retrograde through an artery into the left heart.
Selective coronary artery angiography	Contrast medium is injected directly into the ostium of each coronary artery via a catheter that is placed retrograde through an artery into the aorta.

allergic reaction on the day prior to the angiocardiography. Be on guard for such allergic symptoms as flushing, nausea and vomiting, tingling and numbness, weakness, and urticaria. Fortunately, anaphylactic shock is rare. Nevertheless, oxygen, antihistamine drugs, and epinephrine should be on hand whenever angiocardiography is performed.

Other complications that occasionally develop are *tissue slough* due to leakage of the contrast medium into the area surrounding the vein, and *venous thrombosis.*

Although fatalities rarely occur during angiocardiography, deaths can result from the rapid injection of large doses of contrast medium directly into the coronary arteries or cerebral vessels; the large bolus of medium evidently acts as a type of thrombus.

Nursing care of the patient following angiocardiography usually consists of checking the area of the incision for tenderness, swelling, infection, or thrombosis. If the area is excessively sore, warm compresses usually ease the pain.

Cardiac Catheterization. This complex procedure involves the insertion of a catheter into the heart and surrounding vessels to obtain detailed information about the structure and function of the heart, the valves, and the circulatory system. More specifically, cardiac catheterization is performed for the following reasons:

1. To confirm a diagnosis of heart disease and to determine the extent to which the disease has affected the structure and function of the heart.
2. To establish the existence of congenital abnormalities.
3. To obtain a clear picture of cardiac structure and function prior to heart surgery.
4. To obtain pressures within the heart chambers and the great vessels.
5. To inject contrast medium directly into the heart chambers and adjoining vessels in order to obtain x-ray films of the heart (i.e., angiocardiography).
6. To obtain estimates of cardiac output either by applying the Fick method or by indicator dilution studies.
7. To draw blood samples directly from the heart chambers and vessels in order to measure the O_2 content of the blood and the extent of oxygen saturation; this information indicates whether abnormal congenital shunts are present in the heart.
8. To enable the physician to perform specialized cardiac techniques, e.g., internal pacing of the heart.

Patients must be carefully prepared for this procedure, both physically and emotionally. Cardiac catheterization is important and frightening. Major steps in preparing the patient are:

1. Make certain that the patient has signed a *permit* for the procedure and that the doctor has explained the procedure — its purpose and its hazards — prior to the patient's signing the form.
2. Ask the patient whether he has ever suffered from allergies; the doctor may order a skin test with an iodine-containing solution on the day before the procedure.
3. Withhold solid foods for 8 hours and liquids for 3 hours prior to the procedure.
4. Drugs commonly ordered are penicillin injection on the day of the procedure to prevent possible infection if the patient has a history of rheumatic heart disease or congenital heart disease; and Nembutal, morphine, or diazepam (Valium), which may be administered 30 minutes prior to the procedure to relax and sedate the patient.
5. Be sure that the patient's height and weight are recorded in the chart. This is needed for calculating the amount of dye which will be given the patient.
6. Mark the patient's peripheral pulses with a pen prior to the catheterization and note the quality of the pulses in the chart. This will aid in locating the pulses after the procedure. They should be checked at this time in order to detect possible occlusion of the vessel where the catheterization was performed.

To prepare the patient psychologically for this procedure, it is helpful to include the following questions and information in your preparatory discussion.

1. Let the patient relate to you what the doctor has told him about cardiac catheterization. Ask the patient if he has any questions about the procedure. (Remember that many patients find it extremely difficult to express themselves freely to their doctor.)
2. Note the patient's general attitude toward the procedure. Does he seem extremely nervous, anxious, or apprehensive? If so, encourage him to express his fears openly. Patients may fear the cardiac catheterization procedure because they are frightened of being awake during the procedure and of having a foreign body passed into their heart. Worrying about what the results of the catherization will be and what treatment will be recommended (e.g., cardiac surgery) is another anxiety the patient may have before this procedure. If the patient continues to appear very anxious, report this to the doctor.
3. Tell the patient that he will experience little or no pain, as a local anesthetic is used to numb the catheter insertion site; however, he may feel fatigue because he will have to lie quietly for a period of 1.5 to 2 hours. Also, he may experience certain sensations; for example, he may at times have a fluttery sensation around his heart (this occurs if the catheter is being passed backward through an artery into the left side of the heart); his arm may feel like it is going to sleep; he may experience a flushed, warm feeling (this happens when contrast medium is injected for the angiocardiogram). He may also experience palpitations, if premature ventricular beats and short bursts of ventricular tachycardia occur owing to the tip of the catheter irritating the ventricles.
4. Explain to the patient that the procedure will be carried out in a special cardiac catheterization room that has the special x-ray equipment needed for this procedure. Explain that he will be on the x-ray table and that electrocardiogram leads will be attached to his extremities. Also inform the patient that the physi-

cians and nurses will be wearing scrub gowns and masks and that the room will be darkened at some point during the procedure to take x-ray films.

A cardiac catheterization is usually done on only one side of the heart, although sometimes it is necessary to insert the catheter into both sides of the heart. A *right*-sided cardiac catheterization is simpler and less dangerous than a left-sided procedure. For a right-sided cardiac catheterization, the physician first performs a cutdown on the antecubital vein and passes a sterile, radiopaque catheter 100 to 125 cm. long through the vein into the superior vena cava, then through the right atrium and ventricle into the pulmonary artery. The ECG is constantly monitored during the procedure. As mentioned earlier, premature ventricular contractions may occur as the catheter is being passed through the ventricles. If these become a problem, the catheter may need to be withdrawn temporarily or lidocaine (Xylocaine) may be administered. X-ray films are taken at some point during the proceedings. Pressures within the right atrium, ventricle, and pulmonary artery are measured, and blood samples are drawn. Dye may be injected into the right side of the heart, and films taken. A Swan-Ganz catheter may be inserted and advanced into the pulmonary artery so that a pulmonary artery wedge pressure reading can be obtained to assess left heart functioning.

Catheterization of the *left* heart can be performed in a number of ways:

1. The catheter can be passed retrograde from the brachial or femoral artery into the left ventricle.
2. During right heart catheterization, the atrial septum can be punctured with a special needle and the catheter passed *transseptally* from the right heart into the left heart.

Once the catheter is successfully maneuvered into position, the left side of the heart can be studied by means of pressure readings, blood studies, dye injection, or x-ray films. The coronary arteries can be studied during the left heart catheterization. The catheter is advanced to the base of the aorta and dye is injected into the opening of each coronary artery.

Pressures are valuable diagnostic tools in two ways: elevated pressures indicate stenosed valves, and an elevated left ventricular end-diastolic pressure is one of the first signs of left ventricular failure. (Average pressures are listed in Table 33–2.)

Whenever the doctor suspects the existence of congenital shunts or septal defects, samples of blood are drawn from the various chambers and arteries to determine oxygen content and the percentage of oxygen saturation. The oxygen content of the blood in the different chambers shows whether the blood is circulating in the proper sequence through the heart. For example, the doctor can confirm the existence of a left-to-right shunt by noting that the oxygen content of the blood is abnormally high in the right side of the heart and pulmonary artery. Normal oxygen saturation values are listed in Table 33–4.

TABLE 33–4. NORMAL OXYGEN SATURATION VALUES WITHIN THE CHAMBERS OF THE HEART AND GREAT VESSELS

Inferior vena cava Superior vena cava Right atrium Right ventricle Main pulmonary artery	65-80%	Wedged pulmonary capillary Left atrium Left ventricle	95-98%

From Stanton, A.: Cardiac Catheterization. *Nursing Times,* June 28, 1968, p. 860.

Remember that oxygen requirements of the tissues increase when an individual is excited or very restless; thus, the oxygen saturation values for patients who are frightened or restless may be quite inaccurate.

Care for patients following cardiac catheterization varies, depending upon the institution, but the following points are basic to good aftercare:

1. The extremity in which the catheter was inserted should be kept straight for several hours after the catheterization. If the catheter was inserted through the antecubital vein, the arm is immobilized on an arm board. If the catheter insertion site was in the groin, the patient must usually remain on bedrest for approximately 12 hours after the procedure. He may turn from side to side, but the head of the bed should not be elevated, in order to keep the leg straight at the groin.
2. Check the patient's pulse every 10 to 15 minutes during the first hour and then every 30 minutes for the next 3 hours or until stabilized. Observe for arrhythmias and blood pressure changes and report to a physician if these occur. Hypotension may develop after the cardiac catheterization if the patient voids a large amount; this is due to the diuretic effect of the dye.
3. Check the patient's temperature every 6 hours, as it may become slightly elevated.
4. Observe for nausea and vomiting.
5. Check the site of the cutdown or the percutaneous stick frequently for signs of swelling, infection, bleeding, or thrombosis. If the arm is painful, obtain an order for warm, moist compresses. If a hematoma develops, it may be necessary to apply pressure with a small sandbag.
6. Check the peripheral pulses in the extremity in which the catheter was inserted. Notify the physician of absent or weakening pulse — this could signify occlusion of the vessel.
7. Allow the anxious patient to discuss his experience with you if he wishes. Patients often recall the procedure vividly, particularly their sensations when the catheter was passed into the heart. "Talking out" feelings after a stressful experience often helps the patient to relax and to turn his mind to new experiences.

Complications are rare, but they can develop both during and following the cardiac catheterization procedure. During the catheterization, arrhythmias, including ventricular fibrillation, may develop as the catheter is passed into the ventricle; also *pneumothorax* and *hemopericardium* occasionally occur. Following the procedure there may be allergic reactions to the iodine-containing contrast medium (see Angiocardiography), thrombophlebitis of the vein used for the cutdown, or infection of the cutdown site.

Graphic Techniques

Graphic devices are used to record and graphically represent various aspects of cardiac function. Major graphic techniques are (1) the electrocardiogram (ECG), (2) the phonocardiogram, and (3) the echocardiogram.

Electrocardiogram. An electrocardiogram is a graphic record of the *electrical impulses* that are generated by depolarization and repolarization of the myocardium. These impulses are conducted to the external surface of the body where they are detected by electrodes and measured by a galvanometer.

The ECG is employed mainly to diagnose coronary heart disease and such abnormal cardiac rhythms as atrial fibrillation. However, as one authority warns:

> It is important to realize that the electrocardiogram (ECG) does not depict the actual physical state of the heart or its function. An ECG may be normal in the presence of heart disease unless the pathologic process disturbs the electrical forces.[163a]

You will recall from Chapter 31 that the SA node (pacemaker of the heart) initiates each heart beat by discharging an electrical impulse. These electrical impulses, which are normally discharged in a rhythmic manner 60 to 100 times per minute, spread throughout the atria and then the ventricles. As a result, atrial contraction is followed by ventricular contraction, and blood is propelled with each beat from the atria into the ventricles and from the ventricles into the aorta.

You will remember that each heart beat is equivalent to one cardiac cycle. Each cardiac cycle consists of (1) contraction or systole or *depolarization* of first the atria and then the ventricles, and (2) relaxation or diastole or *repolarization* of both atria and then both ventricles.

Through the action of the sodium pump, depolarization takes place as impulses move across cell membranes, and repolarization follows. Now let us apply this electrophysiologic process to cardiac muscle cells and to the myocardium as a whole. When the SA node elicits an electrical "spark" or impulse, the electrical spark stimulates the resting polarized myocardial cell. As a result, a wave of depolarization moves down the cell, causing the inside of the cell to become positively charged and the outside negatively charged. Soon a large group of myocardial cells is depolarized, which creates an electrical imbalance between the polarized section of the myocardium, which is *negative* in relationship to the depolarized section. The area of electrical imbalance produced is called an *electrical field.*

As the wave of depolarization spreads throughout the muscle cells of both atria and ventricles, first the atria and then the ventricles contract. When the depolarized cells become repolarized, the atria and then the ventricles relax. This process normally takes place with each beat of the heart — 60 to 100 times per minute.

The recording of the electrical activity of the heart generally takes place as follows:

1. The body, and in particular the body fluid, is an excellent *conductor* of electrical current.
2. When the depolarization process sweeps in a wave across the cells of the myocardium, the electrical current generated is conducted to the *body's surface* where it is detected by special *electrodes* placed on the patient's limbs and chest.
3. The electrodes are attached to *two* points on the body and are then connected to the ECG machine in order to complete the electrical circuit. Each pair of attachments is called a *lead.* The most commonly used leads (I, II, and III) are depicted in Figure 33–7.
4. The ECG machine graphically records the *differ-*

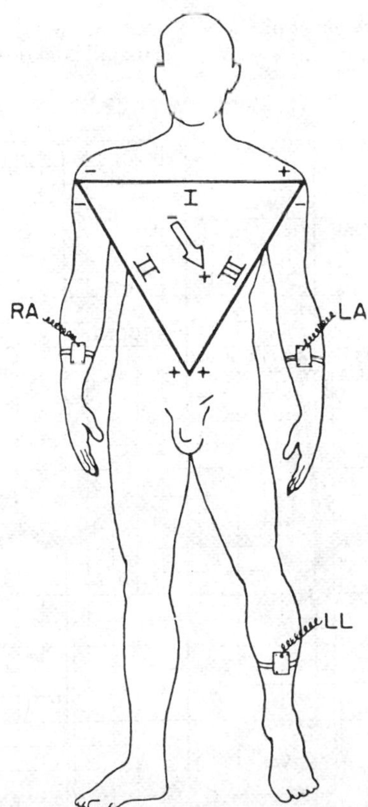

Figure 33–7. Points for obtaining ECG leads I, II, and III. The triangle formed is known as the Einthoven triangle. (From Berne, R. M., and M. N. Levy: *Cardiovascular Physiology,* 3rd ed. St. Louis, C. V. Mosby Co., 1977, p. 47.)

ence in voltage between these two points during cardiac depolarization and repolarization. For example, it records voltage differences between the right and left arm for lead I; between the right arm and left leg for lead II, and so on. The ebb and flow of the electrical impulses produced during each cardiac cycle are amplified and recorded by the ECG machine as deflections or waves.

The waves of excitation recorded by the ECG machine onto graph paper are arbitrarily designated by the following letters: P, Q, R, S, T. The QRS letters are generally referred to as the "QRS complex." The typical ECG pattern formed by these waves is illustrated in Figure 33–8. As you study Figure 33–8, note the following:

The P wave represents depolarization of the atria.

The PR interval represents the time it takes for the impulse to spread from the atria to the ventricles.

The QRS complex indicates ventricular contraction.

The T wave indicates repolarization of the ventricles.

The ST segment indicates that ventricular depolarization is completed and repolarization is about to begin.

The U wave (not shown) is a small wave that sometimes follows the T wave; it is usually diagnostic of K^+ depletion.

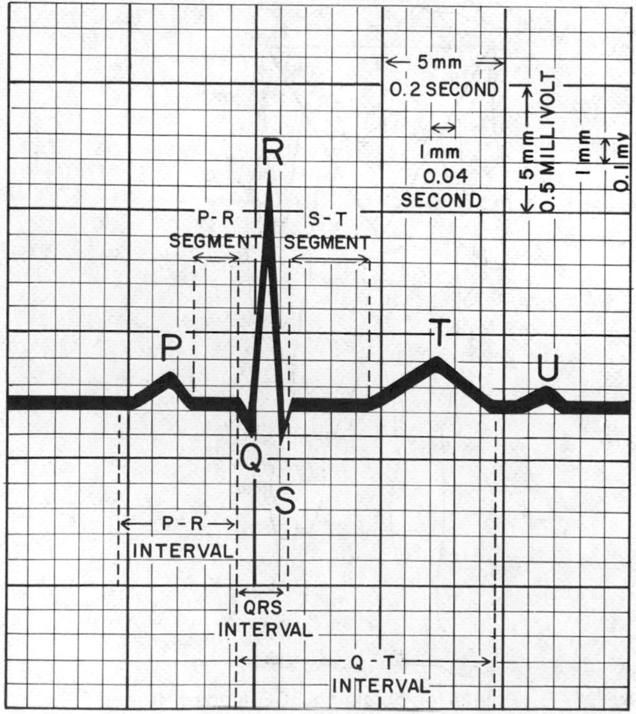

Figure 33–8. The normal ECG pattern. (From Sanderson, R. G.: *The Cardiac Patient.* Philadelphia: W. B. Saunders Co., 1972.)

An electrocardiogram tracing also shows the *voltage* of the waves and the *time duration* of both waves and intervals. As you can see in Figure 33–8, ECG graph paper is divided into horizontal lines and vertical lines, large squares and small squares. *Voltage* is represented by horizontal lines. Each small square is 1 mm. in height. Five small squares is equivalent to 5 mm. which, in turn, is equivalent to 0.5 mV. *Time* duration is measured by means of the vertical lines. Each *small* square signifies the passage of 0.04 second; and each *large* square, the passage of 0.20 second. Time durations for waves and intervals are as follows:

P wave — 0.08 second
PR interval — less than 0.20 second; average, 0.16 second
QRS complex — 0.08 second
ST segment — 0.12 second
T wave — 0.16 second

By studying the amplitude and time duration of the waves and intervals, doctors and nurses are able to diagnose disorders of both impulse formation and conduction.

When a serious arrhythmia or myocardial infarction is suspected, a standard 12-lead ECG is usually performed to comprehensively observe the electrical activity of the heart. The 12 leads are designated by Roman numerals and letters, e.g., I, II, III, V, aVR, aVL, aVF.

Classification of leads

- *Standard bipolar* limb leads* (three)
  - Lead I: Measures the difference in electrical potential between the left arm and right arm.
  - Lead II: Measures the difference in potential between the left leg and right arm.
  - Lead III: Measures the difference in potential between the left leg and left arm.
- *Precordial leads* (V_1 through V_6)
  - Electrodes placed at six different points on the chest wall overlying the heart.
- *Augmented unipolar limb leads* (modified standard limb leads — three)
  - aVR: Measures electrical potential between the center of the heart and the right arm (*a* stands for augmented, *V* for unipolar, *R* for right arm).
  - aVL: Measures electrical potential between the center of the heart and the left arm (*L* stands for left arm).
  - aVF: Measures electrical potential between the center of the heart and the left leg (*F* stands for left leg).

*Bipolar refers to leads where both the positive and negative electrodes are located on the body (e.g., in lead II the electrode on the right arm is negative and the electrode on the left leg is positive). The unipolar leads (i.e., the precordial leads and the augmented limb leads) have a positive electrode on the body and the negative electrode is considered to be infinity.

Augmented leads have wave deflections that are increased in amplitude by 50 per cent for easier reading.

Figure 33–9 illustrates the appearance of the normal cardiograph in each of the twelve leads. Generally a single lead ECG (employing lead II) is used for routine physical examinations, and for monitoring patients whose arrhythmias or cardiac disorders have already been diagnosed.

When an ECG is ordered, take a moment to reassure the patient that the procedure is absolutely safe and that he will *not* be electrocuted! Explain to the patient that an ECG simply records the electrical activity of his heart and that the procedure will help the physician to make a more accurate diagnosis if a cardiac problem is present.

An electrocardiographic tracing may be re-

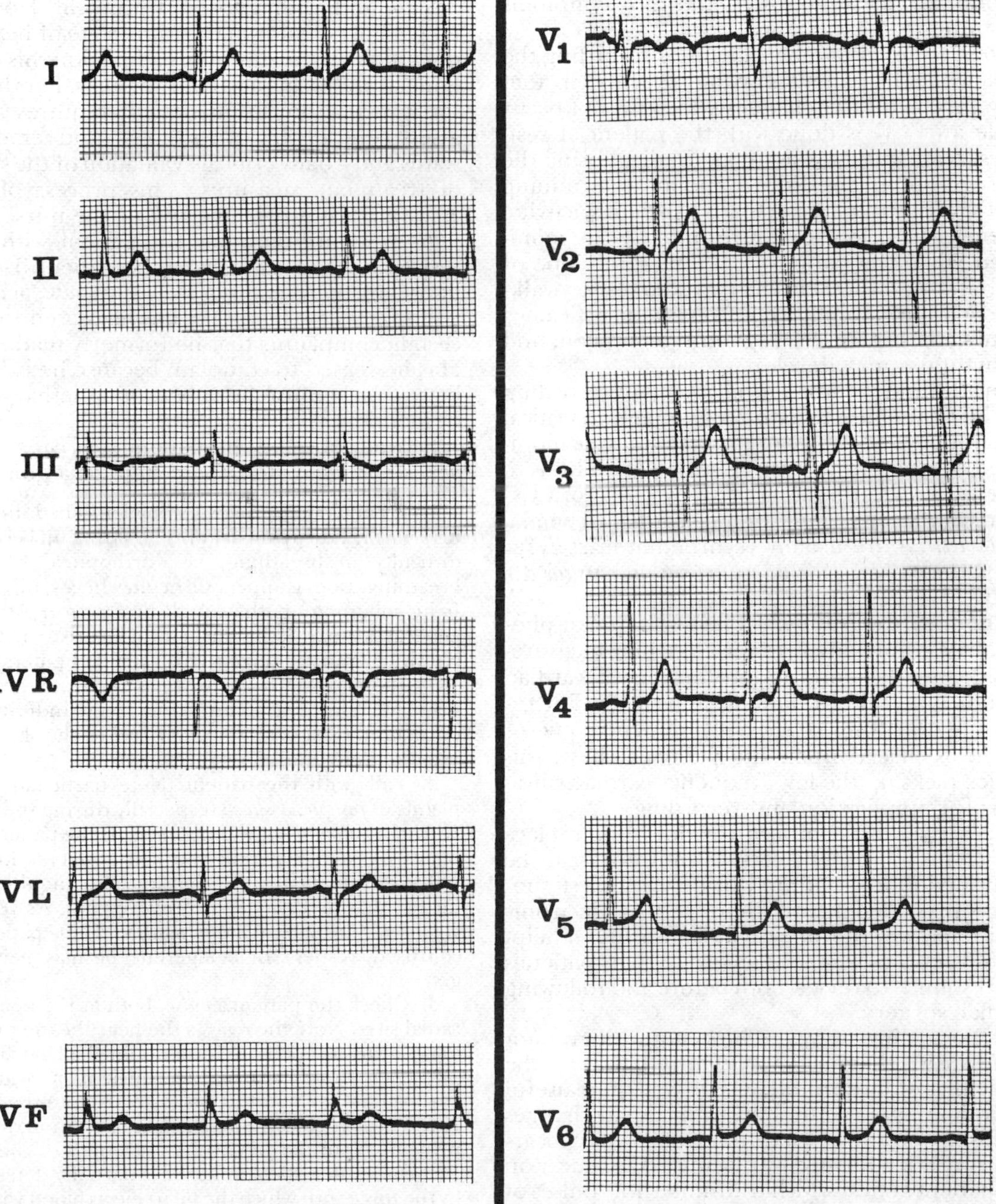

Figure 33–9. Standard 12-lead electrocardiogram with no significant abnormalities. (From Dubin, D.: *Rapid Interpretation of EKG's*; A Programmed Text, 3rd ed. Tampa, Fla., COVER Publishing Co., 1974, p. 280.)

corded continuously over a period of a day or more by having the patient wear a portable monitor called a *Holter monitor.* This is done to determine what arrhythmias may be causing specific symptoms in the patient which may not occur during the short period of time in which an electrocardiogram is taken. The patient goes about his daily activities and keeps a written account of these activities and any symptoms which he may experience.

Stress testing is another means of recording the ECG while the patient is engaging in activity that may produce ECG changes which do not occur while an ECG is done with the patient at rest. Stress testing is used as an aid in diagnosing the presence of heart disease and in determining how severely the disease limits a patient's activity. The patient's blood pressure and ECG are monitored while the patient performs some type of exercise, e.g., the Master's two-step test or walking on a treadmill. If coronary insufficiency occurs, chest pain, ST segment depression, and arrhythmias may develop.

In addition to these special means of recording the ECG, the heart rhythm of patients in critical care units, especially cardiac care units, is monitored continuously (usually in lead II). This is to observe for life-threatening arrhythmias or ECG changes that may indicate myocardial ischemia. *Rhythm strips* are usually recorded at least every 8 hours as a basis for comparison if changes do occur.

Phonocardiography. The technique of phonocardiography involves the electronic measurement, amplification, and recording of cardiac sounds onto special phonograph paper. For recording purposes a specially designed microphone is placed upon the patient's chest; this device picks up the low-frequency cardiac vibrations for amplication and recording.

This diagnostic procedure does not replace auscultation; indeed, certain murmurs can be identified more accurately by the use of a stethoscope in skilled hands than by this electronic device. However, some cardiologists find it helpful to keep a permanent record of their patient's heart sounds to review both before and following cardiac surgery.

Echocardiography. The echocardiogram, a noninvasive diagnostic procedure based on the principles of ultrasound, has proved quite useful in evaluating structural and functional changes in a wide variety of heart ailments. An echocardiogram is performed by placing a transducer on the patient's chest which transmits short pulses of high frequency sound through the heart. Wave pulses bounce off different heart structures and are reflected back to the transducer as a series of echoes. A graphic recording is made (see Fig. 33–10) from these echoes, and information regarding the heart is obtained from these recordings. Echocardiograms are helpful in such circumstances as diagnosing a pericardial effusion or determining the functioning of diseased valves or myocardial muscle.

NURSING ASSESSMENT OF THE CARDIAC PATIENT

It is generally the physician's task to thoroughly examine the newly admitted patient with heart disease and to diagnose his problem. However, no patient remains in the same state of health or disease as on the day of his admission; his condition naturally changes continuously. For this reason every seriously ill patient requires a *daily* assessment of his physiologic and emotional status and a daily critical evaluation of the success of treatment measures. This process of daily assessment is a primary task of the nurse.

As you care daily for the patient with heart disease, first of all *listen* to the patient. Does he have any new complaints, any new aches or pains, any new fears? Or has he ceased to make certain complaints that he formerly made daily? Has he ceased to complain because he is feeling better, or because he is becoming lethargic and despondent?

Second, observe the patient for *changes in his physiologic status.* Use these steps as a guide:

1. When you approach the patient's bed, first note his *position*. Is he lying flat or is he sitting up because of difficulty in breathing, i.e., orthopnea? Note his breathing. Does it appear difficult, wheezy, rapid, etc.? Is he coughing? Is the cough productive? Assess his general *coloring*. Is he flushed or feverish? Is there a bluish or cyanotic tinge to his skin? Is he perspiring? Take the patient's hand in yours and note the feel of his skin. A cold, clammy hand could indicate poor circulation or shock; a hot dry feel to the skin might indicate dehydration or fever.
2. Talk with the patient. Note particularly complaints of *fatigue, dyspnea* (especially during the night), *headache, palpitations,* and *chest pain.* If the patient complains of *pain*, learn all you can about its location, radiation, quality, and intensity; also inquire about factors that precipitate and relieve pain. As you converse with the patient, note his *affect.* If the patient acts confused, restless, or belligerent, he may need oxygen.
3. Check the patient's *pulse*, both at the apical and radial sites. Note the *rate.* Is the heart beating rapidly in order to compensate for a diminished cardiac output? Is it beating extremely slowly as a result of a blockage in the conduction system? Note the *rhythm.* Is the beat regular in its rhythm or is an arrhythmia present? Note the *amplitude* or strength of the pulse. Remember that the amplitude is partially determined by the force with which the heart ejects blood with each beat. A weak, fast pulse may signify shock and circulatory collapse.

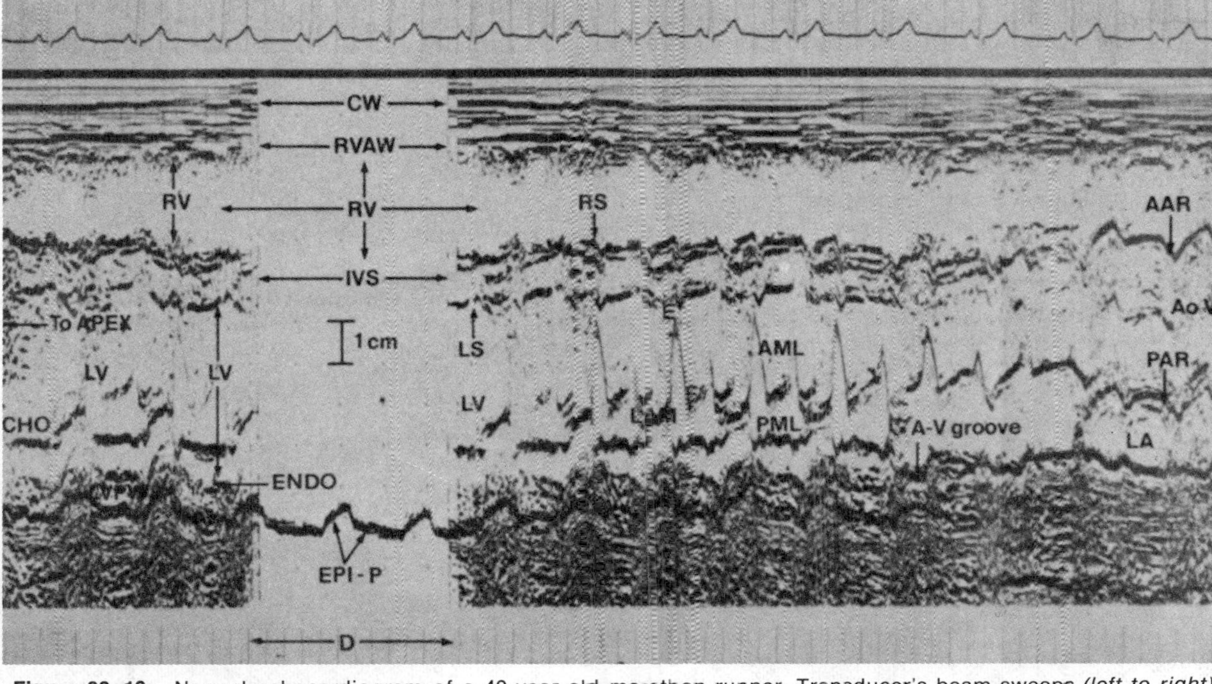

Figure 33–10. Normal echocardiogram of a 40-year-old marathon runner. Transducer's beam sweeps *(left to right)* from immediately above cardiac apex to base of heart. Damping permits only strongest echoes to be recorded. The ECG tracing *(top)* serves as a reference for diastole and systole. (From: Ultrasonography; Interpreting echoes from the heart. *Patient Care,* 13:135, Feb. 1979.) Abbreviations:

AAR, anterior aortic root
AML, anterior mitral leaflet
AoV, aortic valve fragments
A–V groove, atrioventricular groove
CHO, chordae tendineae of mitral valve
CW, chest wall
D, damped portion of echocardiogram
E, F, E-to-F slope of anterior mitral leaflet
ENDO, endocardium of left ventricular posterior wall
EPI-P, epipericardial echo
EPS, echo-poor space
IVS, interventricular septum
LA, left atrial chamber
LAM, normal linear anterior motion of mitral valve seen in systole
LS, left side of interventricular septum
LV, left ventricular chamber
LVPW, left ventricular posterior wall
MYX, cloud of echoes
NCC, non-coronary aortic cusp
PAR, posterior aortic root
PML, posterior mitral leaflet
RAC, right aortic cusp
RS, right side of interventricular septum
RV, right ventricular chamber
RVAW, right ventricular anterior wall
SB, systolic buckling

4. Take the blood pressure on *both* arms. Always know the patient's normal *baseline* for blood pressure. Remember that a blood pressure reading that is considered abnormal for the population at large may not be abnormal for this patient.

5. Check the patient's *neck veins*. Look for engorgement of the external jugular vein; this is an important sign of congestive heart failure.

6. Listen to the patient's *chest* with a stethoscope. Listen for the presence of rales and wheezes.

7. Note that patient's *intake* and *output* record and his daily *weight.* If daily intake exceeds daily output and if the patient has suddenly gained weight, he is probably retaining fluid.

8. Examine the patient's *back, buttocks,* and *ankles* for signs of pitting edema.

If pitting edema, dyspnea, chest pain, and distended neck veins are present at the same time, the patient probably has heart failure.

9. Carefully evaluate the patient's *response to treatment*. Are symptoms lessening, remaining the same, or becoming worse? Does the patient feel that his treatment is not helping him, or is he optimistic about his program of care? Are any untoward symptoms developing as a *result* of treatment?

Your findings from your daily examination and assessment of the patient need to be carefully charted and discussed in conference with the physician and other staff members. Your observations, if carefully done, will give the physician valuable clues as to the course of the disease and the type of therapy that should be instituted.

CHAPTER 34

CHRONIC CONGESTIVE HEART FAILURE

Heart failure is the result of undue stress upon the heart; essentially it represents failure of the cardiac muscle to pump sufficient blood to meet the body's metabolic needs. As stated in Chapter 32, cardiac failure may be either acute or chronic. *Acute* heart and circulatory failure develop swiftly when the heart muscle suddenly, and often totally, fails in its function as a pump; the dramatic results of sudden failure are shock, cardiac arrest, syncope, and sudden death. On the other hand, heart failure that develops slowly and has milder symptoms manifests itself in a clinical syndrome called *chronic congestive heart failure* (CHF). This syndrome, which eventually affects 50 to 60 per cent of all patients with organic heart disease, results from the inability of the heart to expel enough blood to meet the metabolic demands of the body. Basically, CHF is identified by the following characteristics:

1. The development of *compensatory mechanisms* which enable the weakened heart to continue to function. The three major mechanisms are tachycardia (rapid heart beat), ventricular dilatation, and hypertrophy of the heart.
2. A *low cardiac output* that is inadequate to meet the metabolic needs of the body's tissues.
3. The accumulation of *abnormal amounts of blood* in the systemic or pulmonary circulations, or both, with resultant *congestion* of these sytems.

CAUSATIVE FACTORS

A person's heart may gradually fail when one or more of the following conditions persists.

1. The *inflow* of blood to the heart is greatly *reduced* because of hemorrhage, dehydration, and so forth.
2. The *inflow* of blood to the heart is greatly increased as a result of excessive IV fluids, Na+ and water retention, and so on.
3. The *outflow* of blood from the heart is *obstructed* owing to damaged valves and narrowed arteries.
4. The *heart muscle* itself is *damaged* from either ischemia or inflammatory processes.
5. The *metabolic* needs of the body are increased as a result of fever, pregnancy, and so forth.

Clinical entities that most commonly result in congestive heart failure and that develop as a result of the above factors are arteriosclerotic heart disease, hypertensive cardiovascular disease, valvular heart disease, ischemic heart disease, rheumatic heart disease, constrictive pericarditis, the cardiomyopathies, circulatory overload, pulmonary diseases, and such noncardiac entities as hyperthyroidism, obesity, pregnancy, anemia, fever, and infection.

▶*Arteriosclerotic heart disease:* Arteriosclerosis, a condition characterized by a hardening and loss of elasticity in the walls of the arteries, increases the peripheral resistance against which the heart must pump. The resulting overwork forces the cardiac muscle to enlarge slowly. Sooner or later the muscle outgrows its blood supply and fails.

▶*Hypertensive cardiovascular disease:* Hypertension, if sustained for a long period of time, causes irreversible degenerative changes within the arterial walls. These changes, in turn, result in a permanent narrowing of the arteries, which overtaxes the heart, causing it to enlarge and finally fail.

▶*Valvular heart disease:* Narrowed or *stenosed* valves increase the work of the heart by forcing the heart to pump blood into the arterial system against considerable resistance. Dilated valves, which allow blood to regurgitate backward, also add to the work of the heart by increasing the amount of blood that it must try to pump forward with each stroke.

▶*Ischemic heart disease:* The myocardium may not receive sufficient oxygen and nourishment as a result of either (1) narrowing of the coronary arteries owing to atherosclerotic changes or thrombosis, or (2) enlargement of the heart muscle fibers to the extent that they outgrow the blood supply.

▶*Rheumatic heart disease:* Rheumatic fever usually damages the heart valves, causing them to become either narrowed or incompetent, which consequently puts strain on the heart.

▶*Constrictive pericarditis:* As a result of infection, the pericardium may become inflamed and later scarred and constricted. When the heart becomes encased by the dense fibers of the scarred pericardium, the inflow of blood to the heart is obstructed; also, constriction may prevent the heart from expanding and filling with blood between contractions. The result of decreased cardiac expansibility is a low cardiac output and increased venous pressure.

▶ *Cardiomyopathies:* This group of conditions can cause such extensive damage to the myocardium that it eventually fails.

▶ *Circulatory overload:* Too much fluid input to the heart, as a result of an overload of IV fluid, excessive Na+ retention, or renal shutdown, can overwhelm the heart's pumping capacity.

▶ *Pulmonary diseases:* Chronic emphysema, bronchiectasis, silicosis, and chronic tuberculosis all damage and constrict the arterioles of the lungs. Constriction of the pulmonary arterioles greatly augments the work of the *right* heart as it struggles to pump blood into the pulmonary circulation. As a result of these pulmonary diseases, the right ventricle enlarges and eventually fails, followed by failure of the left ventricle. The term cor pulmonale is used to describe right-sided heart failure associated with pulmonary disease.

▶ *Hyperthyroidism, obesity, pregnancy, anemia, fever,* and *infection:* These conditions increase the demands of the tissues for oxygen as well as the amount of metabolic waste materials that must be eliminated. If any of the above problems continue for too long or are too severe, the heart eventually fails from overwork. Additionally, in pregnancy the total body water and plasma volume increase greatly. "By term, plasma volume attains levels approximately 40 per cent above those of nonpregnant normal women."[166]

Factors that may *precipitate* CHF in *individuals with diseased hearts* are pregnancy and childbirth, severe tachycardia or bradycardia, severe overexertion and overwork, great mental strain, and a sudden elevation of the environmental temperature and humidity. These factors should be guarded against in individuals with known heart conditions.

CARDIAC RESERVE, COMPENSATION, AND DECOMPENSATION

The seriousness of a patient's cardiac disability is directly correlated with the extent to which the cardiac reserve is diminished. You will recall from Chapter 31 that cardiac reserve is the ability of the heart to adjust to increased demands placed upon it by exercise, excitement, fever, and so forth. When the heart loses its ability to adjust to various stresses by increasing its output, symptoms of heart disease develop.

> *The most typical first sign of reduced cardiac reserve is* a decreased tolerance to exercise.

While cardiac reserve is most often lost gradually it can also be lost *suddenly*, with resulting death.

In cases of gradual failure, how does the heart compensate for a loss in cardiac reserve? How does it augment its output in order to meet any increased demands placed upon it? The three major mechanisms by which the heart is sometimes able to increase its output are ventricular dilatation, ventricular hypertrophy, and tachycardia.

Ventricular dilatation refers to an increase in the length of the muscle fibers and is characterized by an increase in the *volume* of the heart chambers. With dilatation comes an increase in the systolic output because (according to Starling's law), a muscle when stretched contracts more forcefully. However, dilatation as a compensatory mechanism is limited. First, muscle fibers, if *stretched beyond a certain point*, cease to increase the contractile power of the heart. Second, a greatly dilated heart requires more oxygen to meet its metabolic needs. Thus, the dilated heart with a normal coronary blood flow can suffer from a serious lack of oxygen. Hypoxia of the heart muscle will, in turn, *decrease* the muscle's ability to contract.

Ventricular hypertrophy, on the other hand, refers to an increase in the *diameter* of the muscle fibers. It is characterized by a *thickening of the walls* of the chambers and a corresponding increase in the weight of the heart. Hypertrophy generally follows *persistent* dilatation, further increasing the contractile power of the muscle fibers.

However, hypertrophy, like dilatation, is limited as a compensatory mechanism. A hypertrophied heart does far greater work than a normal heart and, as a consequence, has greater demands for oxygen. Unfortunately, as the heart's muscle mass increases, the capillaries supplying the muscle fibers remain the same in number. Thus, in time, the hypertrophied heart, with its increased muscle mass, may simply *outgrow* its coronary blood supply and become hypoxic. Its contractile power then lessens.

Tachycardia, or an acceleration in heart rate, is the least effective compensatory mechanism. When the heart rate becomes too great, the ventricles are unable to fill adequately, with resultant hypotension and shock.

When these three mechanisms — tachycardia, dilatation, and hypertrophy — *succeed* in maintaining an adequate flow of blood to the tissues, *without symptoms* and in the presence of pathologic changes, the heart is in a state of *compensation*. *Cardiac decompensation* occurs when the heart, despite these mechanisms, is *unable* to cope with the work demands put upon it and must expend most of its reserve. At this point, symptoms develop upon activity, because the heart is unable to maintain adequate circulation.

FORMS OF CONGESTIVE HEART FAILURE

The heart is composed of two pumps — right and left — each of which bears its own stresses and has its own role in maintaining the circulation. For this reason, it is possible for one pump or side of the heart to fail independently of the other pump or side, which is termed *left-sided* or *right-sided* heart failure. Generally, however, because the circulatory system is a closed circuit and because the work of the heart depends upon the smooth functioning of *both* pumps, left- and right-sided heart failure occur almost together — one closely following the other.

Left-sided heart failure practically always results from damage to the left ventricular myocardium. Clinical entities which most frequently cause left ventricular damage are (1) hypertensive heart diseases; (2) ischemic heart disease; and (3) aortic valvular disease resulting from rheumatic heart disease, syphilis, and congenital anomalies. Occasionally, left-sided heart failure may begin in the left atrium as a result of mitral stenosis.

Thus, in left-sided heart failure, the basic fault lies in the heart muscle itself. The muscle may be diseased and unable to meet normal circulatory demands, or the heart muscle may be intrinsically normal but unable to meet increased circulatory needs. When failure first begins, the left ventricle fails to eject its full quota of blood. At this point the compensatory mechanisms of tachycardia, dilatation, and hypertrophy come into play. When these mechanisms fail, some residual blood remains in the dilated ventricle. This residuum, in turn, decreases the ventricle's capacity to receive blood from the left atrium. The left atrium, because it must now work harder to eject its blood, hypertrophies and dilates. As a result, it is unable to receive the full amount of incoming blood from the pulmonary veins. This leads to congestions of the *pulmonary system* and to symptoms that are *respiratory* in nature.

The *right* ventricle, because of the increased pressure in the pulmonary vascular system, must now dilate and hypertrophy in order to meet its increased workload. It eventually fails. Engorgement of the venous system then extends backward to produce congestion in the gastrointestinal tract, viscera, and kidneys, with *edema* as the main manifestation. This condition is referred to as *right heart failure.*

Right-sided heart failure almost always follows left-sided heart failure; it develops as a result of the stress placed upon the right ventricle as it attempts to pump blood against resistance into the patient's congested lungs. Occasionally, however, right-sided heart failure does develop *independently* of left-sided heart failure. Some causes are:

1. Infarction of the right ventricle (rare).
2. Pulmonary diseases, e.g., chronic emphysema and chronic tuberculosis, which force the right ventricle to pump blood against damaged and obliterated arterioles within the lungs.
3. Constrictive pericarditis, which obstructs the inflow of blood to the heart from the venous system.
4. Tricuspid stenosis and congenital pulmonic stenosis, causing undue exhaustion of the right ventricle.

Eventually the venous congestion created by right-sided heart failure causes the circulation of blood to slow, thereby lowering the output of the heart's left side.

At this point we must emphasize that only in the *early* stages of cardiac failure do left- and right-sided heart failure occur independently of each other. In the later stages of CHF *both* sides of the heart fail to function and both pulmonary and venous congestion are present.

Both right- and left-sided heart failure are sometimes referred to as *low output* failure because these two clinical entities are basically characterized by a reduction in cardiac output. *High output failure*, on the other hand, develops when the heart's output of blood is adequate or high but the metabolic demands of tissues are above normal. While low output failure results mainly from *primary* heart disease (i.e., the adverse alterations have developed within the heart itself), high output failure results from heart disease that develops secondary to other conditions. Hyperthyroidism, severe anemia, beriberi, arteriovenous fistula, and pregnancy often make such exorbitant demands upon the pumping action of the heart muscle that the heart, exhausted by its excessive efforts, finally fails.

MANIFESTATIONS OF CONGESTIVE HEART FAILURE

The symptoms of CHF result from a *decrease in cardiac output.* They involve congestion of either the pulmonary circulatory system, the venous system, or both. Almost all the manifestations of congestive heart failure affect tissues and organs that are located *away* from the heart, e.g., kidney, brain, liver and extremities.

In the following discussion, we have divided the symptoms of CHF into symptoms of left-sided heart failure and symptoms of right-sided failure. Again we wish to emphasize that in advanced CHF, *both* sides of the heart fail and all the symptoms discussed below are present.

Symptoms of Left-Sided Heart Failure

The following symptoms of left-sided heart failure develop as a result of congestion of the lungs with fluid owing to the back pressure of blood, and a decrease in cardiac output.

Dyspnea, Orthopnea, and Paroxysmal Nocturnal Dyspnea. These symptoms are caused by lung congestion and by the failure of the left side of the heart to maintain cardiac output. Dyspnea, you recall, means shortness of breath. It results from congestion of the patient's lungs owing to pulmonary engorgement. This congestion can eventually reduce the vital capacity to 1500 ml. or less.

The severity of dyspnea depends on the amount of pulmonary engorgement and resultant decrease in vital capacity, but also on the volume of air respired per minute. A patient with moderate pulmonary engorgement may not experience dyspnea at rest. However, when the same patient exercises, dyspnea may be experienced because a greater volume of air is required.

Because dyspnea is a *subjective* complaint it cannot always be closely correlated with the extent of CHF. Thus, an apprehensive person with moderate, pathologic changes may be more aware of dyspnea than a phlegmatic person with advanced disease.

Orthopnea, you recall, is a more advanced stage of dyspnea in which the patient cannot lie flat in bed because recumbency increases the difficulty in breathing. Blood pools in the lower body while the patient is sitting up. When the patient lies flat, the blood returns from the lower part of the body via the venous system to the lungs and heart, which are already congested. The result is orthopnea or increased dyspnea in the recumbent position.

Paroxysmal nocturnal dyspnea is often one of the first signs of left ventricular failure. This most frightening form of dyspnea awakens people from their sleep and forces them to get out of bed and catch their breath.

Cheyne-Stokes Respirations. We stated earlier that Cheyne-Stokes respirations are a cyclical type of breathing in which periods of apnea are replaced by periods of rapid deep breathing and then by apnea, and so forth. The exact reason why Cheyne-Stokes respirations develop in CHF is not known. They may occur as a result of the prolonged circulation time between the pulmonary circulation and the central nervous system, which, in turn, affects the respiratory center. This symptom may also be related to the respiratory alkalosis that so often develops in patients with congestive heart failure. (Respiratory alkalosis is discussed in Chapter 12.)

Pleural Effusion and Pulmonary Edema. These problems are the result of pulmonary congestion which is so severe that the distended capillaries leak fluid into the interstitial and alveolar spaces of the lungs. (Pulmonary edema is discussed on p. 810.)

Cough and Cardiac Asthma. Cough is a common symptom of left-sided heart failure. The cough is usually productive of large amounts of frothy, blood-tinged sputum. The patient coughs because a large amount of edema fluid is trapped within the pulmonary tree, irritating the delicate mucosa of the lungs. The expectoration of mucus is a result of severe pulmonary congestion and edema.

Wheezing or *cardiac asthma* is another sign of CHF; its exact etiology is as yet unknown.

Decreased Renal Function, Edema, and Weight Gain. Kidney function is adversely affected by the development of CHF, with the result that sodium and water are retained within the body. The probable sequence of events causing edema in left-sided heart failure is as follows: (1) Cardiac output is decreased because of heart failure; as a result, arterial pressure in the kidneys is diminished, reducing glomerular filtration and the output of sodium chloride and water. (2) Reduced effective circulating blood volume in some way triggers an increase in aldosterone secretion by the adrenal cortex; this then increases the rate of reabsorption of sodium by the renal tubules. (3) Because aldosterone causes sodium to be reabsorbed, the concentration of the extracellular fluid is increased. (4) The resulting increased osmotic pressure causes an increase in the release of antidiuretic hormone (ADH) from the neurosecretory cells of the hypothalamus, which results in the increased tubular reabsorption of water. The final result is edema.

See Chapter 12 for a detailed explanation of the role of hormones and the kidney in the development of edema.

Cerebral Anoxia. A decrease in the amount of oxygen carrying blood to the patient's brain causes irritability, restlessness, and a shortened attention span. Cerebral anoxia develops because of the decrease in cardiac output characteristic of left-sided heart failure. Impaired ventilation, with resultant hypercarbia, may also interfere with cerebral function.

Fatigue and Muscular Weakness. The profound exhaustion that patients with congestive heart failure experience is due to a decrease in cardiac output and prolonged circulation time. Decreased cardiac output diminishes oxygen to the tissues and decreases the speed with which metabolic wastes are swept up into the circulation for excretion.

Symptoms of Right-Sided Heart Failure

When the right side of the heart fails, the symptoms produced center on edema and venous congestion within the organs.

Liver Enlargement and Abdominal Pain. As the liver becomes congested with venous

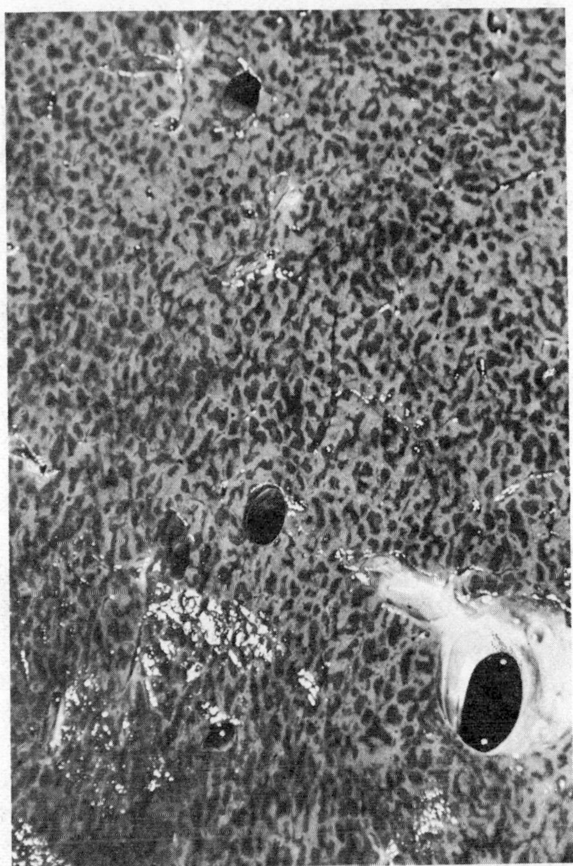

Figure 34–1. A close-up view of the transected surface of the liver with marked chronic passive congestion – the so-called nutmeg pattern associated with right-sided congestive heart failure. (From Robbins, S. L., and R. S. Cotran: *Pathologic Basis of Disease,* 2nd ed. Philadelphia: W. B. Saunders Co., 1979, p. 847.)

blood, it enlarges. If this occurs rapidly, stretching of the capsule surrounding the liver causes severe discomfort. The patient may either complain of a constant aching in the right upper quadrant or of sharp pain.

In severe congestive heart failure, lobules of the liver may become so congested with venous blood (see Fig. 34–1) that they become anoxic. Anoxia leads to necrosis of the lobules. In long-standing CHF, these necrotic areas may become fibrotic and then sclerotic. As a result, the patient develops a condition called *cardiac cirrhosis*, manifested by ascites and jaundice — symptoms of liver damage (Fig. 34–2).

Anorexia, Nausea, and Bloating. These symptoms develop secondary to venous congestion of the gastrointestinal tract. Anorexia and nausea may also result from digitalis toxicity — a common problem because digitalis is the drug of choice in treating congestive heart failure.

Dependent Edema. Among the early signs of right-sided heart failure are edema of the ankles and lower extremities (Fig. 34–3). Evidently edema results from venous congestion of the kidneys, producing compensatory vasoconstriction that, in turn, decreases renal blood

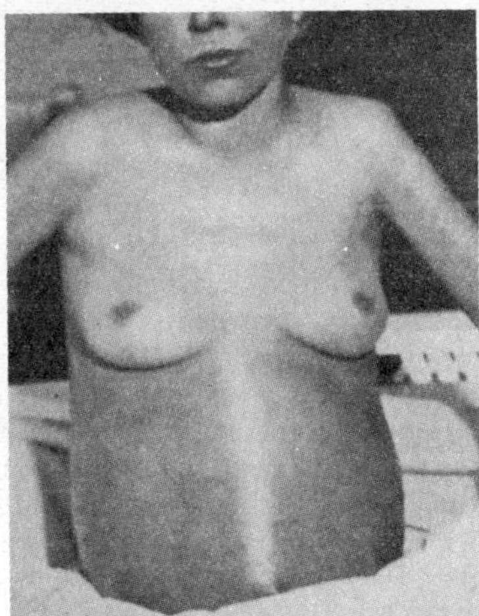

Figure 34–2. Ascites with cardiac failure. Note dark shade of the lips resulting from cyanosis. (From Delp, M. H., and R. T. Manning: *Major's Physical Diagnosis,* 8th ed. Philadelphia: W. B. Saunders Co., 1975, p. 554.)

flow. As a result, sodium excretion is impaired and edema fluid is retained.

Coolness of the Extremities. Venous congestion throughout the body reduces peripheral blood flow. As a result, the extremities are cool and the nail beds are often cyanotic.

Anxiety and Fear. Every lay person knows that the heart pumps blood through the body, and that without the vital work of the heart, life ends. For this reason, most individuals with a

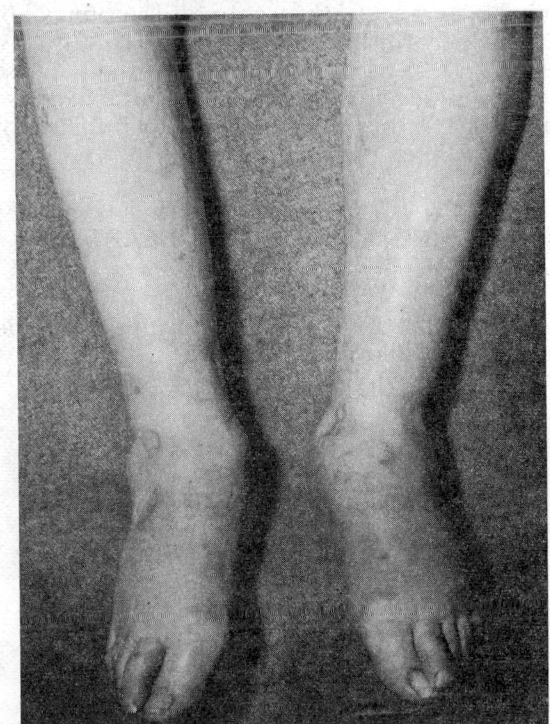

Figure 34–3. Dependent edema of the lower legs, illustrating "pitting" about the ankles. (From Robbins, S. L., and R. S. Cotran: *Pathologic Basis of Disease,* 2nd ed. Philadelphia: W. B. Saunders Co., 1979, p. 111.)

diagnosis of CHF feel anxious and depressed about their condition. As the course of the disease progresses and symptoms worsen, the fear of permanent disability and death may overwhelm even the most stoic patient. Patients express their fears in a number of ways; for example, they may have frequent nightmares, they may suffer from acute anxiety states or deep depressions, or they may withdraw completely from reality.

Symptoms of Advanced Congestive Heart Failure

Weight Loss and Cachexia. The individual with advanced congestive heart failure suffers from malnutrition of the tissues as a result of low cardiac output and venous congestion. Indeed, malnutrition may be as pronounced as it is in patients with advanced malignancies. However, because of the severe edema, patients with CHF look puffy and bloated and appear to be overweight. If diuresis is successful and edema is relieved, the patient's cachexic state becomes obvious.

Shock Syndrome. The typical clinical picture of shock usually appears during the terminal stages of CHF. Common symptoms are stupor, pallor, rapid thready pulse, cold sweats, restlessness, and profound hypotension. These symptoms develop because of a critical decrease in cardiac output due to almost total failure of the heart in its pumping action.

DIAGNOSING CONGESTIVE HEART FAILURE

Heart failure is generally diagnosed on the basis of the following:

- Presence of characteristic symptoms
- Muffled heart sounds
- Abnormal heart sounds
- Rales at the bases of the lungs
- X-ray film showing hazy lung fields, prominent distended pulmonary veins, and evidence of enlarged heart
- Elevated venous pressure
- Distended neck veins
- Prolonged circulation time
- Reduction in cardiac output.
- Presence of albuminuria
- Elevated BUN

Early recognition of these signs can forestall the development of advanced CHF and its complications.

*Functional and Therapeutic Classification of Heart Disease**

Functional Capacity (four classes)

- Class I: No limitation of physical activity. Ordinary physical activity does not cause undue fatigue, palpitation, dyspnea, or anginal pain.
- Class II: Slight limitation of physical activity. Comfortable at rest, but ordinary physical activity results in fatigue, palpitation, dyspnea or anginal pain.
- Class III: Marked limitation of physical activity. Comfortable at rest, but less than ordinary physical activity causes fatigue, palpitation, dyspnea, or anginal pain.
- Class IV: Unable to carry on any physical activity without discomfort. Symptoms of cardiac insufficiency, or of the anginal syndrome, may be present even at rest. If any physical activity is undertaken, discomfort is increased.

Therapeutic Classification (five classes)

- Class A: Physical activity need not be restricted.
- Class B: Ordinary physical activity need not be restricted, but unusually severe or competitive efforts should be avoided.
- Class C: Ordinary physical activity should be moderately restricted, and more strenuous efforts should be discontinued.
- Class D: Ordinary physical activity should be markedly restricted.
- Class E: Patient should be at complete rest, confined to bed or chair.

GOALS OF CARE

The overall goal of care for patients suffering from CHF is to reduce or eliminate those causative factors that lead to symptoms and complications.

Individual goals of care to reduce or alleviate the causative factors responsible for CHF are as follows:

1. Enlist the cooperation of the patient and significant others in pursuing a plan of care.
2. Diagnose and eliminate disease conditions and circumstances within the work and domestic environments that could contribute to the development of congestive heart failure.
3. Strengthen the heart and decrease its workload.
4. Reduce venous congestion in the lungs and body.
5. Supply oxygen and better nutrition to the heart muscle and to body tissues.
6. Decrease sodium and water retention.
7. Recognize, minimize, and alleviate the untoward effects of therapy: digitalis toxicity, thrombophlebitis, other complications of bed rest, low salt syndrome, and potassium deficiency resulting from mercurial diuretics.

*These classifications were delineated by the Criteria Committee, New York Heart Association.

Therapy in CHF

1. *Physical and mental rest*
2. *Digitalization*
3. *Adequate nutrition*
4. *Vasodilators; e.g., hydralazine and isosorbide dinitrate*
5. *Reduction of H_2O and Na^+ retention by means of:*
   a. *Low Na+ intake*
   b. *Diuretics*
   c. *Reduced fluid intake*
   d. *Reduction of anxiety*
6. *Oxygen therapy*
7. *Mechanical removal of pleural and peritoneal effusions*
8. *Education of the patient*

Rest

For patients suffering from CHF, bed rest is truly beneficial; some of its advantages for such patients are:

1. Reduction in heart's workload
2. Promotion of diuresis
3. Reduction in work respiratory muscles (decreases dyspnea)
4. Reduction in demands of tissues for oxygen (lessens circulatory demands)
5. Decrease in venous return (lessens pulmonary congestion and dyspnea)
6. Lowered blood pressure (diminishes arterial resistance against which heart must pump)
7. Lowered heart rate (prolongs the recovery period of cardiac muscle, thereby resulting in a more efficient cardiac contraction)

Whether a physician will prescribe complete bed rest or a program of modified bed rest depends upon the seriousness of the patient's condition. As a guide to the amount of activity that is safe for a patient, the doctor may refer to the functional and therapeutic classifications of heart disease and assign the patient to one of the classes.

The length of time patients are confined to bed and restricted in their activities varies. Patients are generally confined to bed for a long enough period to regain cardiac reserve but not so long that disability and other complications of bed rest are promoted. The optimum period of bed rest for patients with heart failure of varying degrees of severity is still under study.

The patient with heart disease who is confined to bed must *rest physically and mentally* to benefit from this program of care. To help the patient rest, the physician may order a mild sedative or small doses of barbiturates and tranquilizers to overcome problems of restlessness and insomnia. The following nursing actions are also helpful in promoting rest:

1. Place the patient in a cool, quiet room, not next to excessively noisy or talkative patients.
2. Keep the patient's toilet articles, books, radio, water, and so forth, close at hand so that the patient does not have to strain to reach them.
3. Allow the patient to use a bedside commode rather than a bedpan. Sitting on a bedpan is uncomfortable and does not promote proper elimination.
4. Make the patient as comfortable as possible. Give backrubs, prop the pillows, change the position as necessary.
5. Have a confident reassuring attitude with the patient; endeavor to reduce anxiety. Studies show that fear and anxiety can produce various transient cardiovascular responses; e.g., changes in heart rate, cardiac output, abnormalities in rhythm, change in blood pressure, peripheral resistance, blood viscosity, blood clotting time, and serum cholesterol level.

When a patient is placed on a program of prolonged complete bed rest, you will observe for, and attempt to prevent thrombophlebitis, pulmonary embolism, hypostatic pneumonia, renal calculi, and mental depression

The rate at which the patient is allowed to return to normal activities depends upon the severity of the condition. The patient who has been on prolonged complete bed rest usually resumes activities very gradually. At first a walk to the bathroom once a day may be allowed; later full bathroom privileges and sitting up for meals may be allowed. As the patient becomes more independent and active, it is important to observe for weight gain, edema, dyspnea, and distended neck veins; the appearance of such symptoms is a warning that a longer period of bed rest is necessary.

When the patient finally leaves the hospital and returns home, schedule adjustments will be needed to avoid overexhaustion. A nap in the afternoon, shorter working hours, early retirement at night, and frequent vacations may be necessary. As the patient's condition continues to improve, mild exercise may be undertaken gradually, e.g., walking short distances on level ground, playing a few holes of golf, and simple calisthenics. Such exercises, when performed sensibly, can strengthen the heart muscle and improve its performance.

Digitalization

The most important cardiac action of digitalis is a direct beneficial effect on myocardial contraction. Digitalis also increases the force of systolic contraction, the completeness of ventricular emptying, and the capacity of the heart for work. Digitalis preparations cause a sustained increase in the output of the failing heart.

Other effects of cardiac glycosides are reduction in the size of the dilated failing heart, depression of conduction through the bundle of

His, reduced refractoriness and increased myocardial instability, a facilitation of vagal effect on the sinoatrial node, and diuretic action leading to salt and water elimination.

There are a number of different digitalis preparations, and all have approximately the same effect upon the heart action. However, digitalis drugs differ significantly in their potency, speed of action, elimination from the body, and the extent of irritating action on the gastrointestinal tract. Table 34–1 lists commonly used digitalis preparations, along with their distinguishing characteristics.

The *rate* of digitalization and the *method of administration* depend upon the severity of the patient's condition. Oral digitalis preparations are generally employed in less serious cases and are given in divided doses. The patient may receive the total digitalizing dose of an oral digitalis drug within 24 to 72 hours. In emergency situations when the patient is critically ill, the doctor generally orders deslanoside (Cedilanid-D) or digoxin intravenously for rapid digitalization. Intravenous and intramuscular preparations are generally employed only in acute situations in which the patient's life is threatened; otherwise, digitalis drugs are almost always administered orally.

When administering digitalis, one must constantly be on guard for signs of *digitalis toxicity* or intoxication. Patients most prone to digitalis toxicity are the elderly and persons with advanced heart disease, severe arrhythmias or acute myocardial infarction. Also, individuals with cor pulmonale, hypothyroidism, hepatic disease, hypokalemia, or alkalosis readily develop signs of toxicity.

Major symptoms of digitalis toxicity are:

- *Gastrointestinal tract:* Anorexia, nausea, vomiting, diarrhea. These symptoms are common (in 50 per cent of patients with digitalis toxicity) and are often the first indication of toxicity.
- *Central nervous system:* Headache, fatigue, lethargy, depression, restlessness, irritability, drowsiness. CNS symptoms may be profound — convulsions, delusions, hallucinations, aphasia, memory loss, coma. Pain similar to trigeminal neuralgia may occur.
- *Cardiovascular system:* Arrhythmias, tachycardia or bradycardia with pulse rate *below 60,* heart block, cardiac failure.
- *Eyes:* Flickering flashes of light; "colored vision" — usually yellow, sometimes blue; photophobia; blurring, shimmering, scotomata, diplopia.
- *Endocrine:* Gynecomastia (excessive development of male mammary tissue), usually disappears when drug is stopped.
- *Allergic: Urticaria* and eosinophilia are *rare* manifestations.

If any of these manifestations are present, *do not* give the drug, report the symptoms at once to the physician. If digitalis toxicity is present the physician will probably order the following:

1. Discontinue the drug.
2. Administer potassium salts intravenously to aid in correcting arrhythmias if serum potassium level is low.
3. Administer *Dilantin, lidocaine,* or *procainamide* (Pronestyl) intravenously to correct premature ventricular contractions if present.
4. Administer *propranolol (Inderal)* intravenously to control tachyarrhythmia if present.

Because of the danger of digitalis toxicity, observing the following guidelines is important:

1. *Read the labels of all digitalis preparations with extreme care; these drugs have* similar names *(digitalis, digitoxin, digoxin) but* different strengths *and* dosages!
2. *Always take the patient's pulse for* one full minute *apically before giving a dose of digitalis.*
3. *Carefully note both the rate and rhythm of the pulse and chart them accurately.*
4. *If the heart beat is very rapid, below 60, or irregular (if normally regular), withhold the drug and notify the doctor.*
5. Observe *the patient carefully for all signs of digitalis toxicity; when severe symptoms are present, call the physician before giving the drug.*
6. *Insure that the patient and significant others*

TABLE 34–1. CARDIAC GLYCOSIDE PREPARATIONS

Agent	Onset of Action (IV)	Peak Action	Average Half-Life	Average Digitalizing Dose Oral	Average Digitalizing Dose IV	Usual Daily Oral Maintenance Dose
Ouabain	5–10 min.	0.5–2 hr.	21 hr.	–	0.3–0.5 mg.	–
Deslanoside	10–30 min.	1–2 hr.	36 hr.	–	0.8 mg.	–
Digoxin	10–30 min.	1.5–5 hr.	36 hr.	1.0–1.5 mg.	0.75–1.0 mg.	0.25–0.50 mg.
Digitoxin	25–125 min.	4–12 hr.	4–6 days	0.7–1.2 mg	1.0 mg.	0.1 mg.
Digitalis leaf	–	–	4–6 days	–	–	0.1 gram

are aware of the need to monitor the pulse rate daily when discharged home. The importance of taking potassium supplements, if ordered, or dietary means of potassium supplementation e.g., bananas, should also be reinforced.

Diet

Diet for the patient with CHF should be low calorie (unless the patient is underweight), bland, low residue, divided into small feedings, and low in Na^+ content.

The *low caloric diet,* supplemented with vitamins, benefits the patient with heart failure in several ways: weight loss is promoted, thereby reducing the workload of the heart; cardiac output, pulse rate, and blood pressure are decreased and basal metabolic rate is lowered, reducing the demands of tissues for nourishment and oxygen.

A *bland, low residue* diet is generally more palatable for patients with congestive heart failure. Raw fruits and vegetables are usually poorly tolerated because they cause gastric distention and heartburn. Also, patients should avoid foods belonging to the cabbage family, pastries, carbonated water, and fried foods because they tend to create flatulence and distention.

Small frequent feedings are preferable to three heavy meals a day. Large meals tend to create gastric distention, flatulence, and heartburn.

Reduction of Sodium and Water Retention

Methods employed to reduce edema are bed rest, digitalization, restriction of Na^+ in the diet, fluid restriction, diuretics, and reduction of anxiety.

Sodium-Restricted Diets. Healthy adults on a regular diet generally ingest from 3 to 12 Gm. of Na^+ daily, depending upon their individual tastes. The most common source of Na^+ in the diet is table salt added to food, during preparation or at the table. Other less common sources of Na^+ are medications containing Na^+, baking soda, baking powder, and sodium-containing toothpastes. Foods and drinks that are particularly high in Na^+ are smoked meats and fish, canned soups and vegetables, beer, cola drinks, meat extracts, potato chips, olives, pickles, catsup, salad dressings, most candy bars, spaghetti, macaroni, breads, and crackers.

Patients who must restrict their Na^+ intake are usually placed on one of the diets described in Table 34–2. The strictness of the diet prescribed depends upon the severity of the patient's heart condition.

Low Na^+ diets can be made more palatable by

TABLE 34–2. CLASSIFICATION OF LOW SODIUM DIETS

Diet	Amount Na^+ Allowed/Day	Indications	Food Substances and Beverages Restricted
Mild Na^+ restriction	2–3 Gm.	For patients with mild CHF	Do not add table salt; avoid obviously salty foods, e.g., salted nuts, potato chips, smoked meats, bouillon
Moderate Na^+ restriction	800–1200 mg.	For patients with serious CHF	Do not add salt to food at the table *or* during cooking; avoid salt-preserved foods and highly salted foods, condiments (e.g., catsup, soy sauce, chili sauce), cheese, peanut butter, canned vegetables and soups, frozen vegetables to which salt has been added, baking powder, prepared mixes, baking soda, and regular breads and rolls; use low Na^+ products
Strict low Na^+ diet	500 mg.	Patients with severe CHF	Observe all restrictions indicated for the moderate low Na^+ diet; avoid commercial salad dressings and mayonnaise, commercial candies, ice cream, ice milk, milk shakes, artichokes, beet greens, beets, carrots, celery, dandelion greens, mustard greens, spinach, Swiss chard, white turnips. Use no more than one pint skimmed milk a day (including milk used in coffee and on cereal).
Severe Na^+ restriction	250 mg.	Patients with very severe or intractable CHF	Observe all restrictions noted above; avoid regular milk (use low Na^+ milk only), no more than 2 to 4 oz. meat daily and no more than 3 eggs per week

adding salt substitutes to foods in place of table salt. Popular salt substitutes include Diasol, Adolph's salt substitute, Cosalt and Neocurtasal. (Many of the salt substitutes contain potassium; therefore, the patient's need for potassium supplements may warrant consideration.) Cooking with imagination and making food servings attractive can also help to make the low Na^+ diet more appetizing. Seasoning foods with onions, pepper, lemon and lime juice, vinegar, basil, bay leaves, chili powder, dill, mint, caraway seeds, paprika, garlic, mushrooms, tarragon, and wine greatly improves the flavor of low Na^+ foods which might otherwise taste flat.

Sodium restriction is generally tolerated fairly well by most patients. However, patients sometimes develop *low salt syndrome*. Manifestations of Na^+ deficit include weakness, nausea, and vomiting. Generally, increasing the patient's Na^+ intake corrects this problem.

Diuretics. Because diuretics are powerful, potentially dangerous drugs, they are usually ordered only when digitalization and Na^+ restriction have failed to correct Na^+ and water retention. When diuretics are used, both physician and nurse should carefully observe the laboratory reports for abnormalities in electrolytes, pH, and BUN. Both electrolyte balance and kidney function may be disturbed when diuretics are used for prolonged periods.

Table 34–3 lists agents for treating the degrees of heart failure. The most rapid-acting diuretics, furosemide (Lasix) and ethacrynic acid (Edecrin), used for severe and refractory heart failure, are described in Table 34–4.

All diuretics, when used in conjunction with a low Na^+ diet, may produce *dilutional hyponatremia* (water intoxication) unless the patient's water intake is curtailed. For the symptoms and treatment of dilutional hyponatremia, see Chapter 12.

Fluid Restriction. Generally fluid restriction is unnecessary, as Na^+ restriction and diuretics provide adequate diuresis. However, patients with severe refractory heart disease may need to restrict their fluid intake to less than 1000 ml. per day, and in extremely severe cases to 500 ml. per day.

Reduction of Anxiety. A reassuring attitude on the part of doctors and nurses is important in ensuring diuresis. A study by Barnes and Schottstaedt points out that a prolonged state of tension or depression can precipitate retention of sodium and water, whereas reassurance on the part of the physician or nurse can result in diuresis.[21]

TABLE 34–3. USE OF DIURETICS IN VARIOUS DEGREES OF HEART FAILURE

Degree of Heart Failure	Agent	Possible Supplemental Therapy	Side Effects
Mild (NYHA Class II)	Chlorothiazide *or* Hydrochlorothiazide *or* Chlorthalidone	KCl or dietary supplementation	Potassium depletion; arrhythmia with or without digitalis; precipitation of hepatic encephalopathy in cirrhotic patients; alkalosis; hyperglycemia; hyperuricemia
Moderate (NYHA Class III)	Chlorthalidone *or* Hydrochlorothiazide *or* Furosemide	KCl or dietary supplementation	See above
Severe (NYHA Class III or IV)	Furosemide *or* Ethacrynic acid	Hydrochlorothiazide *or* Chlorothiazide *or* Trichlormethiazide	See above; hypovolemia; hypotension
Cor pulmonale	Furosemide	KCl	"Contraction alkalosis" from vigorous diuretic therapy; increased HCO_3 reduces sensitivity of ventilatory controls, especially dangerous in patient with chronic CO_2 retention
Refractory heart failure or pulmonary edema	Furosemide plus Chlorothiazide if needed		

*Spironolactone is frequently of additional benefit because of the association of secondary hyperaldosteronism with severe heart failure.

(From Costrini, N. V., and W. M. Thomson (Eds.): *Manual of Medical Therapeutics,* 22nd ed. Boston, Little, Brown & Co., 1977, p. 90.)

TABLE 34–4. RAPID ACTING DIURETICS

Agent	Onset of Action	Peak Action	Duration of Action	Uses	Cautions
Furosemide (Lasix)	5 min. (IV) 30 min. (IM) 30 min. (PO)	30 min. 1–2 hr. 1–2 hr.	2 hr. 6–8 hr. 6–8 hr.	Acute pulmonary edema; severe CHF; hypertensive emergencies; CHF not responsive to less potent diuretics	Transient or permanent deafness possible when given rapidly IV; sudden death due to cardiac arrest possible after IM and IV administration; contraindicated in persons hypersensitive to sulfonamides, and in pregnant women and nursing mothers; K^+ depletion; alkalosis; volume depletion
Ethacrynic acid (Edecrin) (not given IM)	15 min. (IV) 30 min. (PO)	30 min. 2 hr.	2 hr. 6–8 hr.	Same as above Same as above	Extremely irritating to tissues, so dilute as recommended by manufacturer; may precipitate or aggravate gout, diabetes; severe Na^+, K^+, Cl^- depletion; agranulocytosis

Nursing Actions and Observations in Edema

1. Carefully record intake and output. Stress the importance of accurate records to all personnel caring for the patient.
2. Weigh the patient daily on the same scale, at the same time (usually in the morning before breakfast), and wearing the same amount of clothing.
3. Help the patient to rest as much as possible because recumbency favors diuresis in patients with heart failure.
4. Observe the patient for signs of dehydration from rapid diuresis. Observations of stability of blood pressure, fullness of the neck veins, hematocrit, urinary output, and skin turgor are helpful in determining the presence of dehydration.
5. Give the patient meticulous skin care, because edematous tissue is likely to break down. Check bony prominences at least daily. If possible, place the patient on an alternating pressure mattress, thereby lowering the possibility of decubitus development.

Criteria for evaluating the success of dietary and diuretic therapy in the patient with CHF are a decrease in pitting edema, weight loss, good urinary output, absence of neck vein distention, decrease in pulmonary congestion as evidenced on x-ray film, absence of rales and dyspnea, and a decrease in the circulation time and in the venous pressure.

Oxygen Therapy

Dyspnea is often greatly relieved by the administration of oxygen by means of nasal cannulas or masks. Oxygen therapy is particularly helpful in patients with CHF complicated by pulmonary disease or coronary thrombosis. Caution should be exercised, however, in the administration of oxygen to patients with chronic obstructive pulmonary disease (COPD). Unlike the normal individual whose respiratory drive is regulated by CO_2, the COPD patient, because of chronic elevations in CO_2 requires varying degrees of hypoxemia in order to stimulate the respiratory center. The use of high flow oxygen may cause respiratory arrest in these patients.

*Paracentesis and Thoracentesis**

Occasionally patients suffer from such severe peritoneal effusion that agonizing dyspnea and abdominal distention result. Today, with modern diuretic drugs, excess peritoneal effusion is relatively rare. However, when excess fluid does accumulate within the peritoneal cavity, the physician can mechanically remove the fluid by means of abdominal paracentesis.

Excess fluid can also collect in the chest, causing severe dyspnea. Rarely, when diuretic drugs and Na^+ restriction fail to relieve pleural effusion, thoracentesis is indicated. However, repeated thoracenteses are dangerous, because they may cause Na^+ depletion, hypotension and shock.

Education of the Patient and Significant Others

The treatment of CHF involves a long, often difficult period of adjustment for the patient and for significant others. Patterns of activity, eating, and drinking must often change radically; furthermore, some changes must be accepted as lifelong. Thus, without the patient's wholehearted cooperation, the treatment program may fail once the patient goes home from

*Abdominal paracentesis is discussed in Unit XVII; thoracentesis is discussed in Unit XVI.

the hospital. Four reasons why patients fail to adhere to their prescribed treatment plan are:

- *Lack of knowledge concerning the disease process.* Patients who understand the mechanisms causing their heart to fail and the methods by which heart failure can be reversed are usually much more cooperative.
- *Lack of motivation.* Some patients believe that their condition is hopeless and that there is little point in undergoing the rigors of a treatment program, particularly the Na^{+} restricted diet. It is difficult to change such attitudes. However, the constant encouragement and reassurance of physician and nurse are helpful.
- *Cultural and personal patterns.* Patients who are accustomed to spicy foods may find it extremely difficult to eat a diet that differs so radically from the natural diet of their friends and family. Energetic persons whose self-image involves being active and outgoing may be unable to restrict their activity without becoming severely depressed. In such patients the nurse and physician may have to tolerate occasional lapses from the program and settle for less than total cooperation from the patient.
- *Economic deprivation.* Some patients cannot afford expensive medications or special low Na^{+} foods. Also, elderly, debilitated individuals may be unable to prepare special diets for themselves. These individuals will lapse from their treatment program unless they receive financial assistance.

COMPLICATIONS OF CONGESTIVE HEART FAILURE

The major complications of CHF are the complications of bed rest, acute pulmonary edema, and refractory heart disease.

Acute Pulmonary Edema

Acute pulmonary edema is a medical emergency that usually results from left-sided heart failure. In patients with severe cardiac decompensation, the capillary pressure within the lungs may become so elevated that fluid pours from the circulating blood into the alveoli, bronchi, and bronchioles. The resulting pulmonary edema, if untreated, may cause death from suffocation. Patients literally drown in their own fluids (Fig. 34–4).

Symptoms of acute pulmonary edema are dramatic to view and terrifying for the patient. Typical manifestations include severe dyspnea, orthopnea, pallor, tachycardia, expectoration of large amounts of frothy, blood-tinged sputum, fear, wheezing, sweating, bubbling respiration, and cyanosis.

Treatment of acute pulmonary edema must be instituted immediately! Therapy includes the following steps:

1. *Positioning:* Place the patient in a semi-Fowler's position or in a chair in order to ease dyspnea.
2. *Sedation:* The physician generally orders morphine sulfate, 5 mg. IV slowly, to avoid hypotension; in less urgent cases, 10 to 15 mg. subcutaneously, to alleviate anxiety, decrease pulmonary reflexes, and reduce venous return.
3. *Oxygen:* Administer oxygen in high concentrations by mask, 40 to 60 per cent at 8 liters/minute, to relieve hypoxia and dyspnea and to lessen pulmonary capillary permeability. Intubation to facilitate removal of secretions and administration of intermittent positive pressure breathing (IPPB) also helps to improve ventilation. Alcohol may be added to the nebulizer to decrease secretions.
4. *Digitalization:* Rapid digitalization also promotes diuresis.
5. *Diuresis:* Rapid-acting diuretics usually help to promptly relieve fluid retention. The drug of choice in acute pulmonary edema is furosemide (Lasix), 40 to 120 mg. IV slowly. Patients taking Lasix at home may require much larger doses.
6. *Relief of bronchospasm:* Aminophylline, 250 to 500 mg. IV given slowly, helps to relieve severe bronchospasm and to increase cardiac ouput, renal flow, and urinary output of sodium and water.
7. *Reduction of blood volume:* Three methods for reducing blood volume are rotating tourniquets, phlebotomy, and the use of vasodilator drugs.

a. *Rotating tourniquets:* Soft rubber tourniquets or blood pressure cuffs are applied to three limbs with enough force to obstruct venous flow but not arterial flow, and are rotated every 15 minutes. Because approximately 700 ml. of blood are trapped in the patient's extremities, this procedure acts to retard venous return to the heart. Remember that rotating tourniquets is a potentially dangerous procedure.

Some hospitals use special electric automatic rotating tourniquet machines which have advantages over the manual application of tourniquets. First, timing

Precautions when rotating tourniquets

1. *Occlude the vessels of each limb for no more than 45 minutes at a time.*
2. *Prepare a diagram of the procedure so that each member of the hospital team will know at what time to move the tourniquets and in which direction (Fig. 34–5).*
3. *Observe the patient's skin carefully throughout the procedure for signs of beginning irritation.*
4. *When discontinuing, remove tourniquets* gradually, *or all the fluid trapped in the limbs will flood the heart at one time.*
5. *Use a wide BP cuff or tourniquet in order to minimize tissue damage and discomfort.*
6. *Modification of the procedure may be necessary if the patient has an IV in one extremity.*

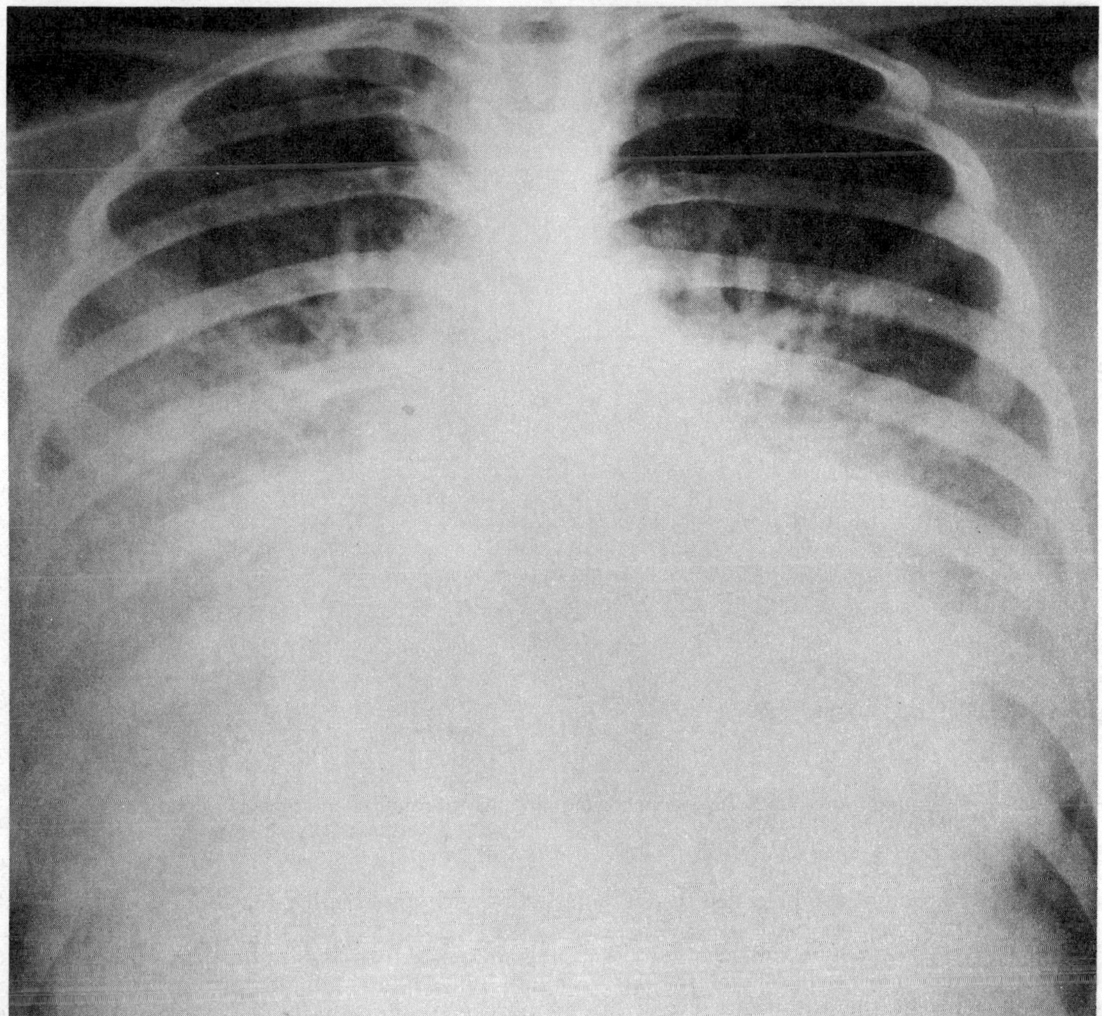

Figure 34–4. *Acute pulmonary edema secondary to left ventricular failure.* A posteroanterior roentgenogram reveals extensive consolidation of both lungs extending out to the visceral pleural surfaces. Much of the consolidation is homogeneous but individual acinar shadows can be identified in the upper lung zones. The heart is moderately enlarged. (From Fraser, R. G., and J. A. P. Paré: *Diagnosis of Diseases of the Chest,* 2nd ed. Vol. II. Philadelphia: W. B. Saunders Co., 1978, p. 1247.)

of the inflation and deflation of the cuffs is precise, every 11¼ minutes. One cuff automatically deflates while the other cuffs automatically inflate. A complete rotation of the tourniquets takes place every 45 minutes.

Second, the correct amount of pressure is automatically applied to the blood vessels so that venous flow to the extremities is properly obstructed, but arterial flow is not.

b. *Phlebotomy:* Removal of 300 to 700 ml. of blood can be performed when the rotation of tourniquets is unsuccessful in curtailing venous return to the heart. If circulatory collapse and shock have already developed, phlebotomy should not be performed, as it will aggravate the shock state.

c. *Vasodilator drugs: Venous dilators,* e.g., nitroglycerin and isosorbide dinitrate, dilate the venous capitance vessels and peripheral arterioles, thus reducing the amount of blood returned to the right side of the heart. *Arterial dilators* reduce impedance to ventricular ejection of blood to the body, thus decreasing the work load of the heart. Medications such as nitroprusside and trimethaphan are commonly used. Ideally the patient is in an intensive care unit with pulmonary artery and pulmonary artery wedge pressure monitoring when these agents are being administered.

8. *Controlled ventilation. Intubation* (orotracheal or nasotracheal) may be lifesaving when breathing is hindered by thick tracheobronchial secretions. Intubation makes possible aspiration of secretions and use of intermittent positive pressure breathing.

Refractory Heart Failure

Heart failure is termed "refractory" or "intractable" when recommended diet, drugs and treatments fail to alleviate symptoms and restore at least partial cardiac reserve, i.e., refractory heart disease is stubborn and difficult to manage.

To treat refractory heart disease, the physician usually reviews the patient's entire course and reassesses the medical treatment. Measures that the physician may then take include:

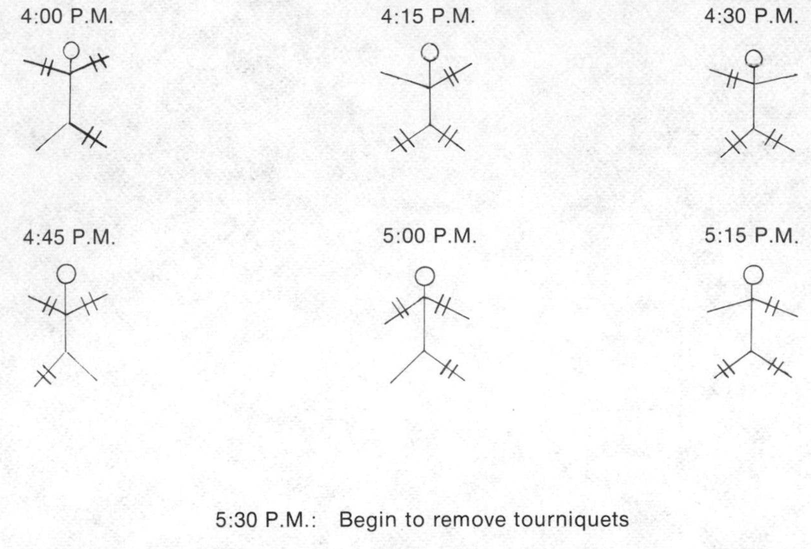

Figure 34–5. Rotating tourniquets: Diagram showing direction of rotation and time of rotation and removal.

1. A prolonged period of complete bed rest in the hospital.
2. Severe Na^+ restriction, e.g., 250 mg. Na^+ diet.
3. Fluids restricted to less than 500 ml. per day.
4. Combined diuretic therapy using several different types of diuretics.

PROGNOSIS

The prognosis for patients with CHF depends upon (1) the patient's age, (2) the degree of cardiac hypertrophy, (3) the amount of cardiac reserve, and (4) the presence of other heart or associated disorders. The prognosis can generally be predicted by observing the patient's response to therapeutic measures. If the patient responds slowly or inadequately to prescribed medications, special diets, bed rest, and so forth, the prognosis is poor. Also, the patient's life and health are endangered if any of the complications of bed rest, e.g., pneumonia, pulmonary embolism, develop.

CHAPTER 35

THE ARRHYTHMIAS

Arrhythmias (also called dysrhythmias) are disorders of the heart rate and rhythm that often lead to dramatic alterations in circulatory dynamics. For example, a *rapid* ventricular rate can precipitate angina pectoris, myocardial infarction, acute heart failure, pulmonary edema, syncope, and cerebral thrombosis. Conversely, abrupt *slowing* of the ventricular rate can lead to fainting and convulsions.

Arrhythmias affect both normal and diseased hearts. Persons with normal hearts may develop arrhythmias secondary to exercise, fever, hyperthyroidism, emotion, shock, and anemia. In other cases, arrhythmias arise as a direct result of coronary artery disease, rheumatic heart disease, and arteriosclerotic heart disease. Finally, many arrhythmias are caused by drug toxicities (e.g., digitalis toxicity) and electrolyte imbalances.

The most *frequently encountered* arrhythmias are sinus arrhythmia, sinus tachycardia, sinus bradycardia, atrial and ventricular premature beats, paroxysmal atrial tachycardia, and atrial fibrillation. Five arrhythmias that can produce *critical alterations in circulatory dynamics* are (1) ventricular fibrillation, (2) cardiac standstill, (3) ventricular tachycardia, (4) bradyarrhythmias, and (5) complete atrioventricular heart block.

> *The two potentially lethal arrhythmias are ventricular fibrillation and cardiac standstill; patients stricken by these arrhythmias must receive* immediate medical attention *or they will die within a few minutes or suffer irreversible brain damage.*

THE NORMAL AND ABNORMAL ECG

In Chapter 31 we discussed the normal electrophysiology of the heart. In Chapter 33 we considered the normal electrocardiogram which is, as you recall, a graphic tracing of the *electrical activity* (not mechanical activity) of the heart as it completes each cardiac cycle. In this chapter we shall consider abnormalities in the electrocardiogram resulting from disturbances in the heart's electrophysiology. In Table 35–1 we briefly compare the significance of the waves

TABLE 35–1. WAVES OF EXCITATION SEEN IN A TYPICAL ELECTROCARDIOGRAM

Wave	Meaning and Significance	Time Period	Abnormalities
P Wave	Signifies depolarization and contraction of the atria	0.08 sec.	Abnormal or absent P waves imply that another area of the heart muscle is acting as pacemaker in place of SA node
PR Interval	Section from beginning of P wave to beginning of QRS complex; signifies time it takes impulse to pass from atria to ventricles	Average time = 0.16 sec. Usually less than 0.20 sec.	Prolonged PR interval: Impulse being conducted more slowly than normal through AV node *Shortened PR interval:* impulse being conducted over a shortened abnormal route from atria to ventricles
QRS Complex	Depolarization and contraction of ventricles	0.06–0.12 sec.	Prolonged QRS complex signifies abnormal conduction or delay of conduction through the ventricles
ST Segment	Period following completion of depolarization of ventricles and preceding repolarization of ventricles	0.12 sec.	*Elevation* or *depression* of ST segment indicates ischemia or infarction of the heart muscle
T Wave	Repolarization of ventricles following contraction	0.16 sec.	*Inverted* T wave: implies ischemia or infarction of heart muscle

and intervals of the *normal* ECG with the significance of *abnormal* waves and intervals.

Remember when studying arrhythmias that the shapes of the P waves and QRS complexes remain normal in appearance as long as the wave of depolarization travels the normal route from atria to ventricles; i.e., from the SA node to the AV node, to the bundle of His, and down the right and left bundle branches into the specialized network of the Purkinje system. The P wave and QRS complex become *aberrant* in appearance when abnormalities arise either in impulse formation in the SA node, or along the pathway of impulse conduction. As one authority points out, *the key to the diagnosis of any arrhythmia is the presence and appearance of P waves, or atrial activation, and their relationship to QRS or ventricular complexes.*

DIAGNOSING AND ANALYZING ARRHYTHMIAS

Arrhythmias are diagnosed on the basis of the patient's medical history, the cardiovascular examination, and the ECG tracings. First, the patient may give a history of suddenly developing one or more of the following conditions: tachycardia, palpitations, anginal pain, extreme dyspnea, edema, and faintness.

Second, upon physical examination the doctor or nurse may discover the following evidence which points to the presence of a significant arrhythmia:

- A heart rate that is below 40 or above 140 beats/minute.
- An extremely irregular heart rhythm.
- A heart rate that does not increase with exercise or holding of the breath.
- A first heart sound which varies in intensity.
- The presence of the symptoms of congestive heart failure, shock, angina pectoris, syncope, or significant heart murmurs; these conditions may develop as a result of the effect of arrhythmias upon circulatory dynamics.

Finally, the physician will order a 12-lead electrocardiogram for the purpose of diagnosing the type of arrhythmia and the location of the cardiac disturbance. When examining an ECG tracing, one must carefully consider the following aspects:

Rate. The rate can be calculated by determining the distance between R waves (Fig. 35–1). Note: If there are two large squares between R waves, the rate is 150 beats per minute. Three large squares between R waves signifies a heart rate of 100 beats per minute, four large squares is equivalent to 75 beats per minute, and five large squares is equivalent to 60 beats per minute. Remember that the heart rate per minute is equal to the number of squares between R waves divided into 300; for example, if there are two squares between R waves, 300 divided by 2 equals 150 beats per minute.

Another way to calculate the rate, particularly when the rate is irregular, is to count the number of full complexes that occur within a 6 second period. The ECG paper is marked at three second intervals. To find the rate you simply multiply the number of full complexes in 6 seconds by ten. For example, if there are ten full complexes in a 6 second strip, the rate is 100.

Regularity of Rhythm. The ventricular rhythm is regular if the R waves occur at *regular* intervals; the rhythm is *irregular* if the succession of RR intervals fails to occur in a regular, normal time sequence. Some irregularities of rhythm occur regularly, whereas others occur spasmodically; the first group of arrhythmias are called *regular irregularities,* while the latter group are called *irregular irregularities.*

Appearance of the Waves or Deflections. *P waves,* when normal, are identical in contour and precede the QRS complexes. P waves remain *normal* in appearance in arrhythmias in which the SA node continues to act as pacemaker, e.g., sinus tachycardia. P waves become *abnormal* in contour, inverted, or buried in the QRS complex in arrhythmias characterized by *ectopic foci* (i.e., when the impulse arises in irritable tissue in either atria, AV junction, or ventricles). Ectopic foci disturb heart rate and rhythm by initiating impulses at a faster rate than the SA node, thereby taking over the role of pacemaker (e.g., atrial tachycardia).

The *QRS complexes* appear normal in arrhythmias in which the ventricles contract normally, e.g., all disturbances arising in the SA node, atria, and AV junction. QRS complexes, on the other hand, appear grotesque and bizarre in ventricular arrhythmias. In disturbances arising in the AV junction, QRS complexes often *precede* P waves owing to the abnormal upward spread of impulses from the AV junction.

The *T waves* may be inverted following ventricular muscle damage resulting from myocardial infarction.

Length of the ECG Intervals. *Prolonged* intervals indicate disturbances in the rate of conduction of impulses from atria to ventricles. *Shortened* intervals may indicate an *abnormal route* of conduction of impulses from atria to ventricles.

Elevation or Depression of the ST Segment. ST segment elevation or depression is measured in millimeters from the base-line or isoelectric line. Elevation or depression of the ST segment may indicate myocardial injury, electrolyte disturbances, or drug toxicities, especially digitalis toxicity.

CLASSIFICATION OF THE ARRHYTHMIAS

Arrhythmias may be classified in a number of ways, e.g., tachyarrhythmias (fast rhythm) or bradyarrhythmias (slow rhythm), regular or irregular, atrial or ventricular, paroxysmal or constant, due to disturbances in impulse formation or due to disturbances in conduction. In this discussion the arrhythmias are classified according to the part of the heart in which they originate, as follows:

A. Disorders arising in the sinoatrial node
   1. Sinus tachycardia
   2. Sinus bradycardia
   3. Sinus arrhythmia
   4. Sinus arrest
B. Disorders arising in the atria
   1. Premature atrial contractions (P.A.C.)
   2. Paroxysmal atrial tachycardia (P.A.T.)
   3. Paroxysmal atrial tachycardia with AV block
   4. Atrial flutter
   5. Atrial fibrillation
C. Disorders arising in the AV junction
   1. Disorders in which the AV junction takes over the role of pacemaker
      a. Junctional rhythm
      b. Premature junctional contractions (P.J.C.)
      c. Paroxysmal junctional tachycardia (P.J.T.)

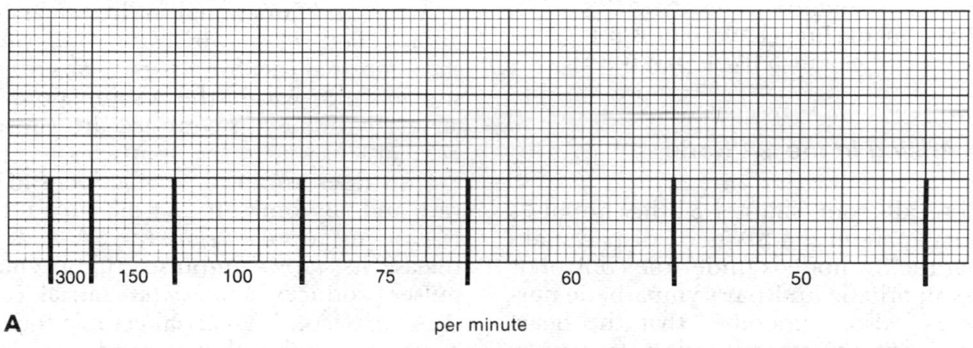

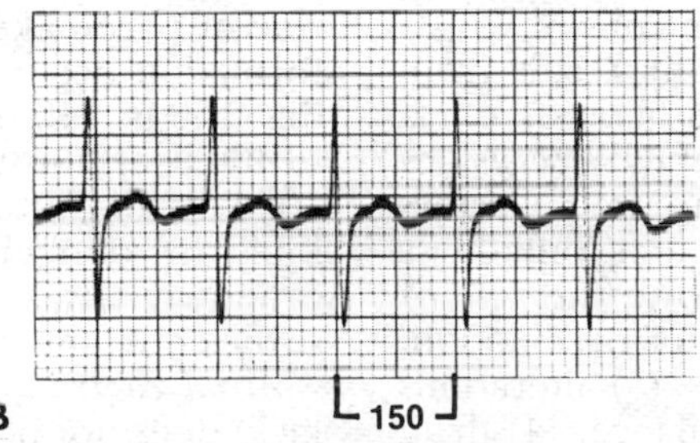

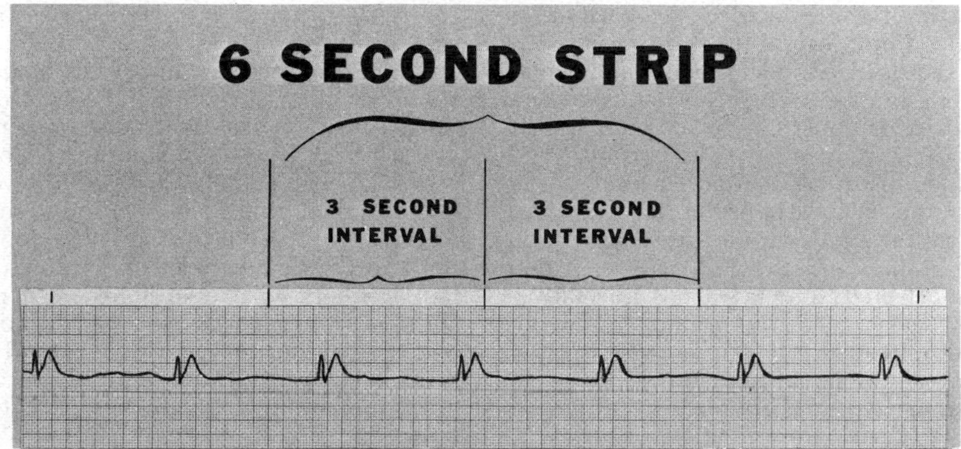

Figure 35–1. Ways of calculating heart rate. **A.** Calculating the rate by determining the distance between the R waves. If there are two large squares between the R waves, the rate is 150; if three large squares, the rate is 100, and so on. **B.** Since there are two large squares between the R waves, the rate is 150. **C.** Another method of calculating the rate is to count the number of QRS complexes occurring within 6 seconds and multiply by ten; the rate in this example is 30. (*B* from Phillips, R. E., and M. K. Feeney: *The Cardiac Rhythms.* Philadelphia: W. B. Saunders Co., 1973. *C* from Dubin, D.: *Rapid Interpretation of EKG's; A Programmed Text.* Tampa, Fla., Cover Publishing Co., 1974, p. 67.)

2. Disorders of conduction through the AV node
   a. First-degree heart block
   b. Second-degree heart block
   c. Third-degree heart block

D. Disorders arising in the ventricles
   1. Disorders caused by ventricular irritability
      a. Premature ventricular contractions (P.V.C.)
      b. Ventricular tachycardia
      c. Ventricular fibrillation
   2. Disorders of conduction
      a. Right bundle branch block (R.B.B.B.)
      b. Left bundle branch block (L.B.B.B.)

Disorders Arising in the SA Node

You will recall from Chapter 31 that impulses normally originate in the SA node of pacemaker, and that the SA node is under the control of both the sympathetic and parasympathetic nervous systems. Also, remember that the heart rate speeds when the sympathetic nervous system is in control and slows when the parasympathetic nervous system is in control.

SA node disturbances generally result from overactivity of either the sympathetic or parasympathetic nervous systems and only occasionally from disease of the SA node itself. Factors that affect the sympathetic and parasympathetic nervous systems and interfere with the role of the pacemaker are (1) excitement or emotion, (2) changes in the metabolic rate, (3) alterations in blood chemistry and fluid balance, (4) drug effects, (5) noncardiac diseases such as anemia and thyrotoxicosis, and (6) heart disease. As a result of any of these factors, the pacemaker may produce impulses too quickly (sinus tachycardia) or too slowly (sinus bradycardia); it may fail to initiate one or more beats (sinus arrest); or impulse formation may be affected by the individual's respirations (sinus arrhythmia).

In SA node disturbances the heart *rate* varies between 40 and 180 beats per minute, the *rhythm* is regular with the exception of sinus arrest and sinus arrhythmia, and the ECG configuration remains unaffected. The P wave is normal because impulses are originating (as they should) in the SA node; the QRS is normal because ventricular contraction is undisturbed.

The sinus arrhythmias are often of minor significance. However, prolongation of sinus tachycardia may place a strain on the heart muscle, and marked sinus bradycardia may lead to a severe decrease in cardiac output. Also, sinus tachycardia is an extremely dangerous arrhythmia in the postmyocardial infarction patient because the amount of work the heart is doing is greatly increased at a time when it needs to rest. Sinus bradycardia may be particularly harmful in persons with heart disease or in postoperative cardiac surgery patients; in these individuals the heart is often unable to increase the stroke volume and maintain an adequate cardiac output when the heart rate falls below 60.

Disorders Arising in the Atria

Atrial arrhythmias are caused by ectopic foci which develop in one of the atrial walls and which act to "take over" the role of the SA node or pacemaker.

Atrial and junctional arrhythmias are sometimes called *supraventricular arrhythmias* because the abnormal foci for ectopic beats originate at a site above or within the AV junction. Ventricular arrhythmias, in contrast, are caused by abnormal foci within the ventricles.

How does an atrial ectopic focus affect heart rate and rhythm? First of all, such a focus may release an impulse *before* the SA node is due to release its *normal* impulse; this premature impulse produces a *premature* atrial contraction (P.A.C). Second, an atrial ectopic focus may become so irritable that it produces impulses *extremely rapidly,* thereby totally taking over the role of pacemaker. Such rapid rates of impulse formation occur in paroxysmal atrial tachycardia (160 to 240 beats/minute), atrial flutter (250 to 400 beats/minute), and atrial fibrillation (over 400 beats/minute). These extremely rapid atrial rates are dangerous because the heart muscle cannot contract efficiently, nor can it recover sufficiently between contractions.

Atrial contraction (often referred to as atrial kick) does not occur at all in patients with atrial fibrillation. Normally, when the AV valves open, the blood flows rapidly from the atria into the ventricles. Just prior to the closure of the AV valves and ventricular contraction, the atria contract to expel an extra amount of blood into the ventricles. The blood which flows into the ventricles during atrial contraction often contributes significantly to the volume of blood in the ventricles just prior to systole (left ventricular end-diastolic volume — LVEDV). In patients with heart disease it is especially important that the LVEDV be adequate so that the myocardial muscle fibers will be stretched to a point that allows for maximum ventricular contractility and cardiac output (Starling's law). Ineffective ventricular contractions result in decreased coronary blood flow, which gives rise to anginal pain and congestive heart failure.

Atrial arrhythmias sometimes occur in conjunction with atrioventricular block. When atrial rates of impulse formation are very rapid (as in atrial tachycardia and flutter), the AV node is unable to respond to each beat; it may respond only to every *other* beat (2:1 block), every *third* beat (3:1 block) or every *fourth* beat (4:1 block). In these arrhythmias with block, the ventricular rate is *always slower* than the atrial rate. Thus, the pulse (which reflects ventricular rate) may be normal in persons with atrial flutter or tachycardia even though the atrial rate is very rapid.

When atrial flutter first appears, the ventricular rate is often very rapid. It may be one half the atrial rate, i.e., 125 to 200 beats per minute. In addition, the rhythm is usually regular at the onset of atrial flutter. But after therapy, the block at the AV node may increase, and only every third to fourth (sometimes only every sixth to seventh) impulse will be conducted to the ventricles. Generally the AV block varies (e.g., 4:1, 7:1, 3:1, and so on) with every beat leading to an irregularly irregular pulse.

In atrial fibrillation, conduction through the AV node occurs in a "hit or miss" fashion. The patient with atrial fibrillation also has a rapid heart rate at the onset of the arrhythmia and, as in atrial flutter, the ventricular rate decreases after therapy. The rhythm of atrial fibrillation, though, is always irregularly irregular.

Characteristics of atrial arrhythmias are *abnormally shaped P waves* due to abnormal foci in the atria which initiate impulses rather than the SA node, and normal QRS complexes because the conduction through the ventricles is usually unaffected by the atrial disturbances.

Treatment of atrial arrhythmias centers on: (1) stimulation of the vagus nerve, which normally acts to slow the heart (digitalis and mechnical measures such as carotid sinus massage); (2) depression of myocardial irritability (quinidine, propranolol, and procainamide are drugs of choice); and (3) rapid conversion to normal sinus rhythm with drugs (e.g., quinidine and digitalis) and precordial shock (see later in this chapter).

In Figure 35–2, ECG's of the chief atrial arrhythmias are shown.

*Disorders Arising in the AV Junction**

Two major types of arrhythmias arise in the AV junction: (1) disturbances in which the pacemaker role of the SA node is taken over by the AV junction; and (2) disturbances in which the AV junction blocks impulses journeying from the AV junction to the ventricles. These arrhythmias may occur because of ischemia or trauma in the area of the AV junction, e.g., after a myocardial infarction or cardiac surgery. Digitalis toxicity is also a cause of junctional arrhythmias.

The *first* group of disturbances is characterized by the *upward* spread of impulses from the AV junction to the atria rather than the normal downward transmission of impulses from the SA node to the AV junction. The abnormal upward direction of impulses is evident on the ECG; e.g., P waves are usually inverted as the impulse is traveling through the atria in a direction opposite to that found in normal sinus rhythm, and the PR interval is shortened. The impulses may spread through the atria at the same time that the ventricles are being activated. In this instance, the P wave may be buried in the QRS complex. Finally, the atria may contract after the ventricles, and the QRS complex will then precede the P wave. The QRS complex is normal because the ventricles are contracting normally.

The major junctional arrhythmias are junctional *escape rhythm* and junctional *tachycardias.*

The principal danger in untreated junctional arrhythmias is overwork of the heart and decreased output. In junctional rhythms, as with some atrial arrhythmias, the cardiac output may be decreased in patients with heart disease because atrial contraction may not always occur prior to ventricular contraction. Treatment of rapid junctional rhythms centers on drug therapy and precordial shock. A junctional escape rhythm is occasionally treated with a pacemaker. This may be required in patients who no longer have higher pacemakers in the SA node or atria initiating an impulse. The inherent rate of the AV junction is 40 to 60 beats per minute. This rate may not be rapid enough to maintain an adequate cardiac output in the patient with a diseased heart.

HEART BLOCK

In the second group of disturbances arising in the area of the AV junction, impulses passing from the atria to the ventricles are *blocked* at the AV node, so that the conduction of impulses from atria to ventricles slows or stops entirely.

Normally the impulse coming from the SA node is delayed at the AV junction for less than 0.20 seconds before traveling on to the bundle of His. However, when the AV junction has been damaged by ischemia, rheumatic fever, or drug toxicity, impulses are delayed at the AV

*Recent investigations have shown that previous conceptions of the atrioventricular node as an entity which possessed a high degree of automaticity, and hence could be regarded as a pacemaker, may be incorrect. Current terminology often refers to the AV "node" as the AV "junction," a term that embraces a somewhat larger area than was previously designated as the node. There is also some uncertainty as to the precise mechanisms by which the so-called nodal rhythms arise, and these arrhythmias are frequently referred to currently as "junctional arrhythmias."

junction for abnormally long periods of time, depending upon the degree of heart block.

In *first-degree heart block,* conduction in the AV node is slowed, so that the PR interval is longer than 0.20 second. This type of block is often associated with coronary artery disease, and may result from treatment with digitalis. The rate and rhythm are normal and regular. The P wave is normal, but there is a prolonged PR interval because of the prolonged AV conduction time (Fig. 35–3). The person with first-degree AV block is usually asymptomatic.

In *second-degree heart block,* every second, third, or fourth impulse from the atria is fully blocked; this creates a discrepancy between the atrial and ventricular rates, as mentioned in our

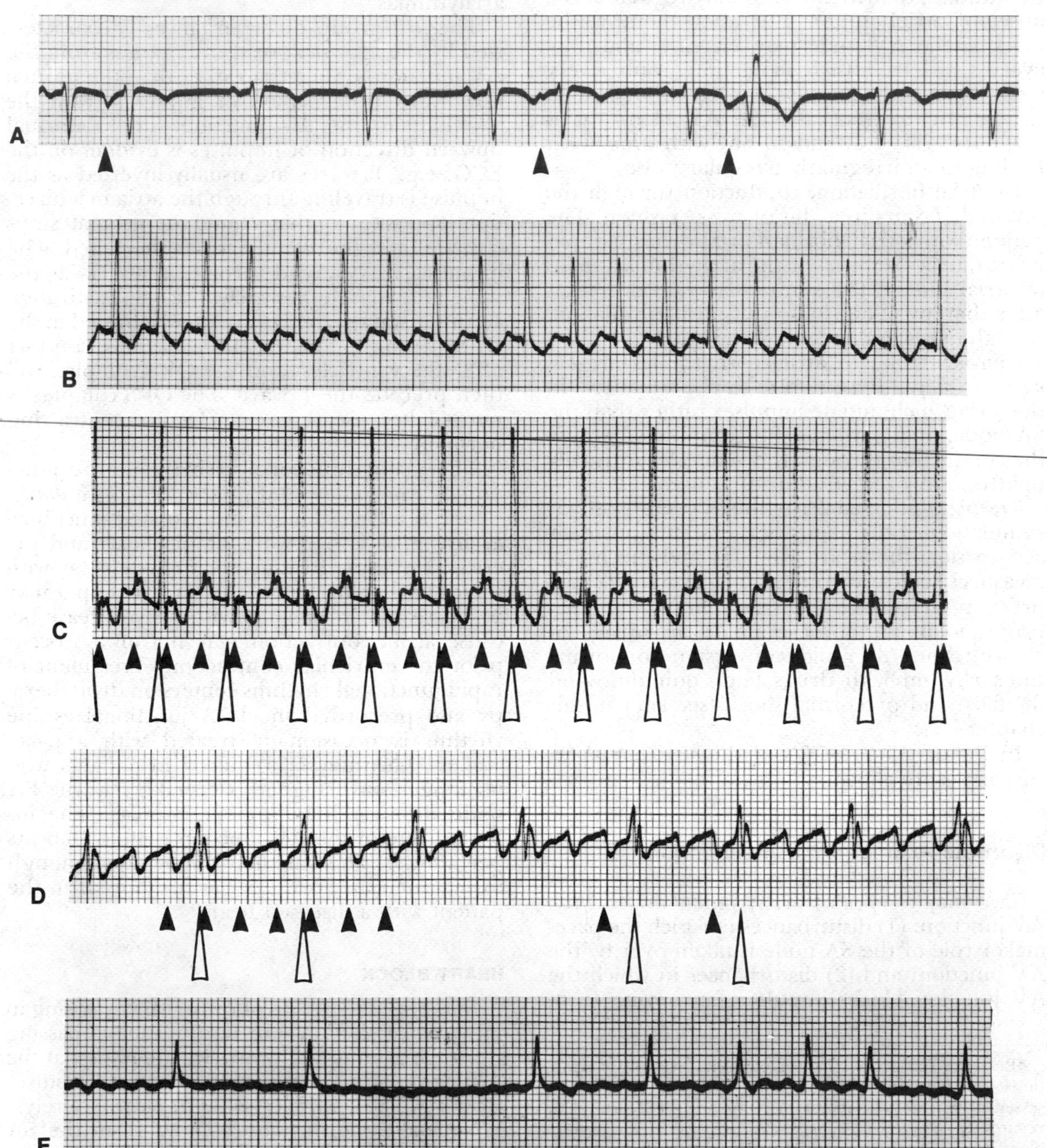

Figure 35–2. Common atrial arrhythmias. **A.** Sinus rhythm with premature atrial contractions (PAC's). **B.** Paroxysmal atrial tachycardia, also called supraventricular tachycardia. **C.** Atrial tachycardia with block (2:1 conduction). **D.** Atrial flutter. **E.** Atrial fibrillation. (Dark arrows indicate the P waves; white arrows indicate ventricular response.) (From Phillips, R. E., and M. K. Feeney: *The Cardiac Rhythms; A Systematic Approach to Interpretation.* Philadelphia: W. B. Saunders Co., 1973, pp. 91, 99, 103, 110, 119.)

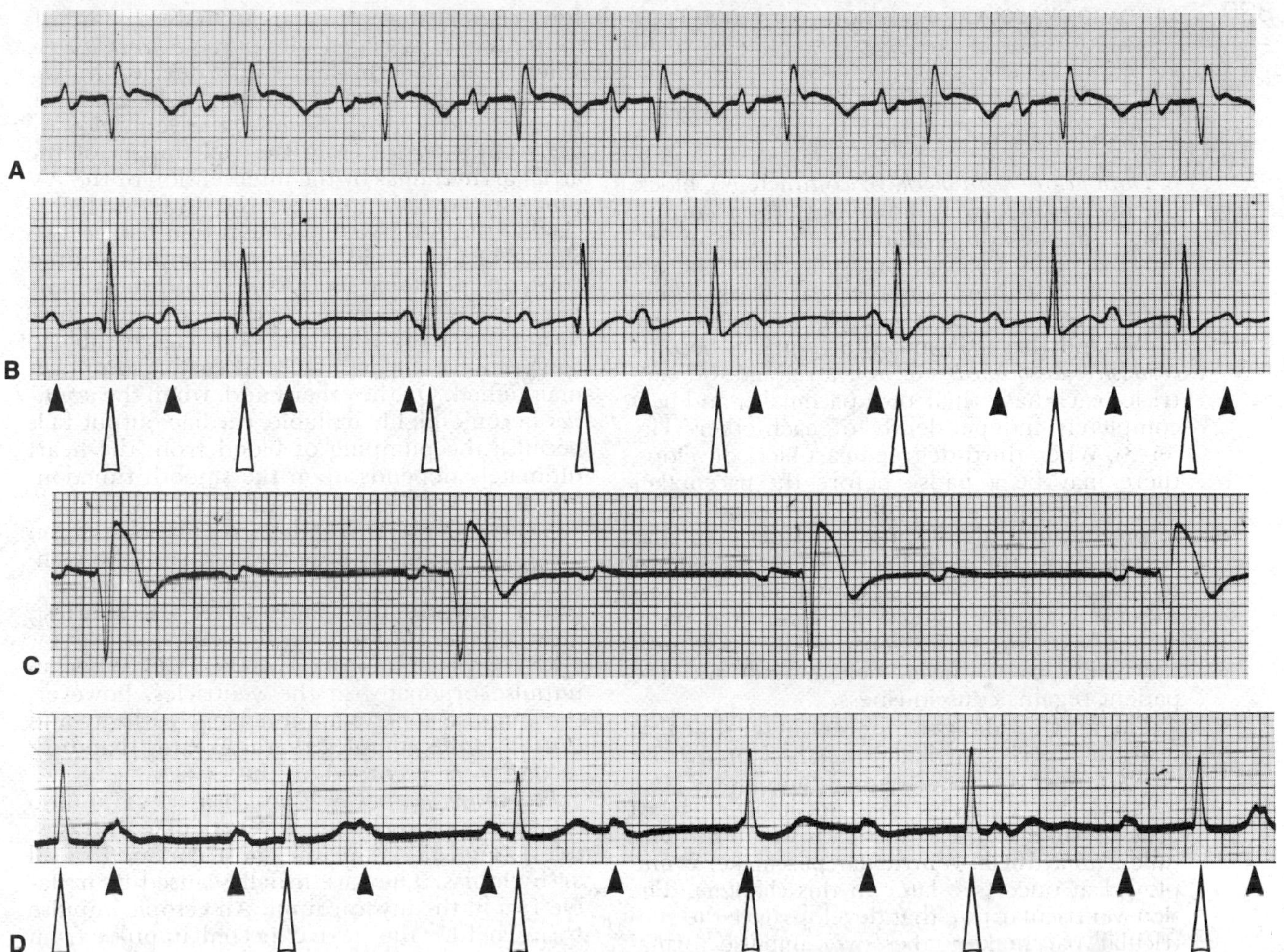

Figure 35–3. Heart blocks. **A.** First-degree heart block, characterized by prolongation of the PR interval. **B.** Second-degree Mobitz I (Wenckebach) heart block characterized by gradual prolongation of the PR interval until finally a P wave is not followed by a QRS complex. **C.** Second degree Mobitz II heart block, characterized by a normal PR interval when there are ventricular responses, but instances in which the P wave is not followed by a QRS complex. **D.** Complete or third degree-heart block, characterized by a variable PR interval and a lack of association of the P wave with the QRS complex, i.e., the atria and ventricles fill irrespective of each other. (From Phillips, R. E., and M. K. Feeney: *The Cardiac Rhythms; A Systematic Approach to Interpretation.* Philadelphia: W. B. Saunders Co., 1973, pp. 149, 161, 169, 178.)

discussion of atrial arrhythmias. If the ventricular rate becomes extremely slow in second-degree heart block, the patient may experience symptoms which are the result of a decreased cardiac output. This degree of block often occurs after an MI and with chronic lesions of the conduction system, and also sometimes results from digitalis or quinidine therapy. It may proceed to third-degree block.

There are two recognized subdivisions of second-degree block: (1) The Wenckebach phenomenon, or Mobitz Type I block, is composed of recurrent cycles in which the PR interval is progressively prolonged, until eventually no QRS complex follows the P wave. The cycle is then repeated (Fig. 35–3). (2) The Mobitz Type II block differs in that the PR interval is constant in length. The P waves are normal and are followed by normal QRS complexes at regular intervals, until suddenly a ventricular beat is dropped (Fig. 35–3).

Atropine and isoproterenol (which speed the rate of impulse conduction), pacemakers, and withholding drugs, e.g., digitalis, are some of the measures that may be used to treat second degree heart block. Mobitz II second-degree heart block is usually considered quite serious in the patient who has had an acute myocardial infarction, particularly when the infarction is an *anterior* one. The reason for concern is that complete AV block, which is characterized by complete AV dissociation, may *suddenly* occur in these patients. Third-degree heart block and the resultant decreased heart rate may have serious consequences after a myocardial infarction. For this reason, a temporary pacemaker is usually inserted prophylactically when Mobitz II heart block develops in this setting.

Third-degree heart block, or complete AV block, usually results from infections, from chronic lesions of the conduction system, after an MI, from digitalis toxicity, or from congenital abnormalities. In third-degree heart block, *all* impulses from the atria are blocked at the AV node, and the atria and the ventricles become *completely dissociated;* i.e., the atria and the ventricles each have their own pacemaker and beat completely independently of each other (Fig. 35–3). When third-degree heart block develops, there may be a pause before the pacemaker within the ventricles becomes active and begins to produce impulses. During this delay, cardiac output from the ventricles ceases and the patient faints or develops convulsions (Stokes-Adams syndrome). Once the ventricular pacemaker takes over, the ventricles begin to beat slowly (30 to 40 beats per minute) and the patient regains consciousness.

The greatest danger inherent in third-degree heart block is ventricular *standstill* or *asystole,* characterized by the Stokes-Adams attack. If a focus in the ventricles does not initiate a heart beat, asystole will lead to death within minutes unless an artificial ventricular pacemaker is employed at once (see later in this chapter). The slow ventricular rate that develops once the ventricular pacemaker takes over impulse formation may lead to *impaired cardiac output and circulatory function.* Isoproterenol, atropine, and artificial pacemakers are used to treat patients in third-degree heart block.

Disorders Arising in the Ventricles

Disorders of ventricular origin can be divided into the following two groups:

- Arrhythmias that result from irritability of the ventricles.
- Disturbances of impulse conduction through the ventricles as a result of injury of either the right or left bundle branches.

Arrhythmias That Result from Irritability of the Ventricles. The first group of ventricular arrhythmias is characterized by ectopic impulses which result from myocardial irritability and which arise *below* the level of the AV junction. Irritability of the ventricles progresses on a scale from slight (occasional premature ventricular contractions) to marked (ventricular tachycardia) to extreme (ventricular fibrillation).

Ventricular arrhythmias are generally more serious and life-threatening than are atrial or junctional arrhythmias. One reason for this difference is that ventricular arrhythmias are almost always associated with *intrinsic heart disease,* whereas atrial arrhythmias may develop in *normal* hearts that have been affected by emotion, fatigue, and so forth. Second, the ventricles are generally *protected* from the full impact of the atrial arrhythmias by the intervention of the AV junction. For example, in atrial flutter or tachycardia, the AV junction blocks one half to two thirds of the rapid, abnormal impulses fired from atrial ectopic foci. As a result, the abnormal impulses never reach the ventricles; thus, despite atrial disorders, the ventricles are able to contract at a normal rate and cardiac output is maintained. On the other hand, when the *ventricles* become highly irritable, cardiac output fails because the pumping of blood from the heart ultimately depends upon the smooth functioning of the ventricular muscles.

Ventricular arrhythmias are manifested on the ECG tracing by wide and bizarre QRS complexes. Normally the pathway by which impulses traverse the ventricles is the shortest, most efficient route; consequently, a narrow QRS complex is inscribed on the ECG. When an impulse originates in the ventricles, however, the impulse follows an abnormal pathway and causes a QRS complex that is greater than 0.12 second to be recorded on the ECG.

Premature ventricular contractions (PVC's) (also called ectopic beats and ventricular extrasystoles) (Fig. 35–4) are the most common of all arrhythmias. They are usually caused by irritable foci in the myocardium. An ectopic impulse forms before the next expected impulse from the SA node and takes the place of the normal beat. Therefore, no P wave appears ahead of the QRS in the ECG. PVC's are innocuous when they are infrequent or isolated and require no treatment. They are dangerous when they are (1) frequent (more than five per minute); (2) coupled with normal beats *(bigeminy);* (3) multifocal; (4) following a period of bradycardia; (5) occurring in pairs; (6) in a patient with an acute myocardial infarction; and (7) falling on the T wave.

This last occurrence is referred to as the *R on T phenomenon.* The downward slope of the T wave is considered the *vulnerable period of the cardiac cycle.* If the heart is stimulated at this time, it often cannot respond to the stimulus in an organized fashion because the muscle fibers are in various stages of repolarization. Therefore, PVC's occurring during this vulnerable period can precipitate the more life-threatening arrhythmias of ventricular tachycardia and ventricular fibrillation.

Ventricular tachycardia (Fig. 35–4) occurs when an irritable ectopic focus in the ventricles takes over the role of pacemaker. There are rapidly occurring series of PVC's with no normal beats in between. In the ECG the P waves are often buried in the QRS complex. The PR interval is

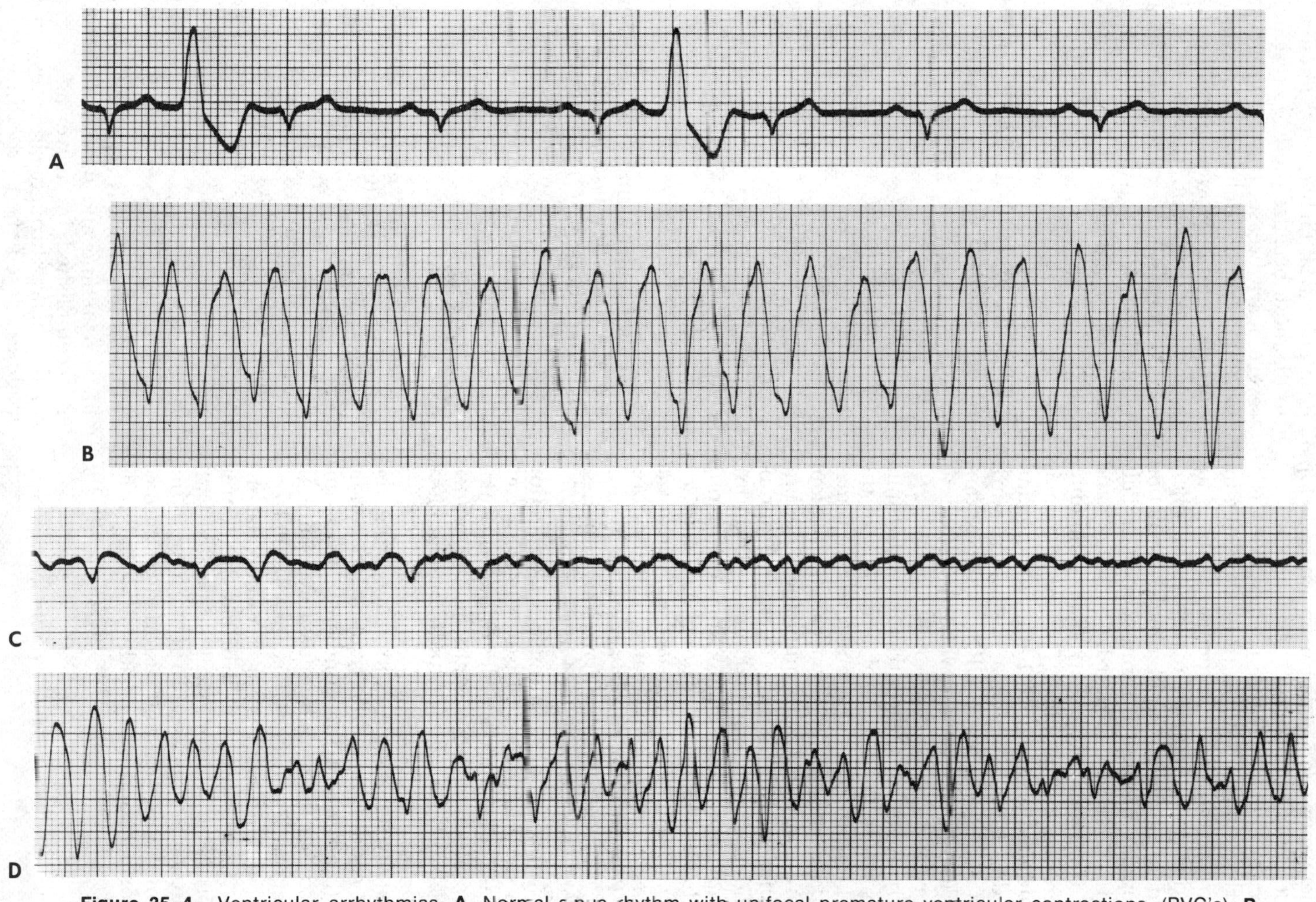

Figure 35–4. Ventricular arrhythmias. **A.** Normal sinus rhythm with unifocal premature ventricular contractions (PVC's). **B.** Ventricular tachycardia. **C.** Fine ventricular fibrillation. **D.** Coarse ventricular fibrillation. (From Phillips, R. E., and M. K. Feeney: *The Cardiac Rhythms; A Systematic Approach to Interpretation.* Philadelphia: W. B. Saunders Co., 1973, pp. 232, 250, 262.)

not measurable. The heart rate is 140 to 250/minute. Ventricular tachycardia is an *extremely dangerous* arrhythmia, producing a very low cardiac output which can quickly lead to myocardial infarction and cerebral ischemia. At any time ventricular tachycardia can develop into ventricular fibrillation.

Ventricular fibrillation (V.F.) (Fig. 35–4) is a *lethal* arrhythmia, and death results within minutes if treatment is not immediate. This is an advanced stage of ventricular tachycardia characterized by extremely rapid impulse formation and irregular impulse transmission. It usually results from severe myocardial damage, and may be the result of toxicity from quinidine, isoproterenol, or digitalis. The heart rate is rapid and chaotic, and no rhythm of any kind can be discerned. The ECG has bizarre wave patterns and P waves and QRS complexes cannot be identified. V.F. may be described as coarse or fine.

The treatment of the ventricular arrhythmia depends upon the degree of irritability of the myocardium. Infrequent premature ventricular contractions are usually not treated. Frequent PVC's are controlled with quinidine, lidocaine (Xylocaine), procainamide (Pronestyl), propranolol (Inderal), diphenylhydantoin (Dilantin), and disopyramide phosphate (Norpace), among others. *Ventricular tachycardia and fibrillation are emergencies that are swiftly treated with precordial shock and drug therapy* (lidocaine, Dilantin, bretylium, Pronestyl, inotropic agents, and vasopressors). The actual steps in dealing with these emergencies are summarized in Chapter 95.

Disturbances of Impulse Conduction through the Ventricles. Disturbances of conduction through the ventricles (intraventricular block) result in either a right bundle branch block (R.B.B.B.) or a left bundle branch block (L.B.B.B.).

The arrhythmia derives its name from the fact that conduction in the right or left bundle branch (branches of the bundle of His) is impaired, so that the impulse must travel through a different pathway. The defect may result from myocardial fibrosis or after a myocardial infarction. Of the two, L.B.B.B. has the poorer prognosis because it is usually associated with left ventricular disease. In both types, the QRS complex is wide and distorted because of the abnormal conduction pathway through the ventricles. There is no specific treatment for these arrhythmias.

WOLFF-PARKINSON-WHITE SYNDROME

This arrhythmia falls into the category of a pre-excitation syndrome, that is, the sinus impulse bypasses, partially or completely, the normal conduction pathway. The ventricular muscle thus is activated earlier than normal. The condition, also called the "accelerated conduction syndrome," is often referred to as the W-P-W syndrome. It is manifested by sudden attacks of supraventricular arrhythmias, especially atrial tachycardia. These are difficult to diagnose because the ECG resembles that of severe heart disease. It is thought that about 60 to 70 per cent of adults with this syndrome have normal hearts. However, if the tachycardia attacks are frequent, they may lead to myocardial fatigue and exhaustion. The attacks are treated by various drugs, chiefly digitalis, propranolol, quinidine, and procainamide.

GENERAL CLINICAL CARE IN THE ARRHYTHMIAS

The four major goals of care in the treatment of patients with arrhythmias are:

1. To convert an abnormal heart rhythm to a normal sinus rhythm.

2. To slow the ventricular rate when rapid.

3. To prevent further attacks of paroxysmal arrhythmias.

4. To decrease the degree of atrioventricular block if one exists.

Medical and nursing care generally revolves around the following therapeutic approaches: (1) drug therapy, (2) precordial shock (defibrillation and cardioversion), and (3) artificial cardiac pacing.

Drug Therapy

Drugs commonly used in the treatment of patients with arrhythmias are: quinidine, procainamide (Pronestyl), lidocaine (Xylocaine), propranolol (Inderal), isoproterenol (Isuprel), atropine, diphenylhydantoin (Dilantin), bretylium, digitalis, and a few others. Facts concerning these drugs are summarized in Table 35–2.

Precordial Shock[101]

Precordial shock is a procedure used to halt life-threatening and dangerous arrhythmias; it is accomplished by delivering electric current to the heart through either externally placed paddles (closed chest procedure) (Fig. 35–5) or paddles applied directly to the myocardium (open chest procedure). The two principal forms of precordial shock are defibrillation and cardioversion (sometimes called countershock).

How does precordial shock stop arrhythmias? When a high voltage electrical current is delivered to the heart for a brief period of time, the entire myocardium is completely depolarized at the moment of the shock. Total depolarization of the cells generally terminates myocardial fibrillation and other arrhythmias; as a result, the SA node can once again take over regulation of cardiac rate and rhythm.

DEFIBRILLATION

Defibrillation is an emergency procedure in which an electric current is delivered to the heart to terminate a *life-threatening* arrhythmia. Defibrillation is indicated in ventricular fibrillation. The patient with ventricular tachycardia who is not responding to lidocaine and who is losing consciousness is also defibrillated. Specially trained physicians and nurses may be called upon to perform the procedure in case of emergency.

Preliminary Measures. When a patient is being monitored and the monitor alarm sounds, or when a threat to life is noted in some other manner, the patient's condition is evaluated immediately. The ECG reading is checked, and the leads are checked for loose connections. The patient's pulses are checked. If the emergency is confirmed, the code alarm is given over the hospital intercom system to summon the emergency team (e.g., "Dr. Blue, Code 99," or whatever). In the meantime, resuscitation measures are started by the first person on the scene. These include cardiac massage and mouth-to-mouth resuscitation (see below). Critically ill patients may have an endotracheal or tracheostomy tube in place and be on a mechanical ventilator. Under these circumstances the patient should be disconnected from the ventilator and ventilated manually with a resuscitation bag. During this time the defibrillator is being set up, turned on, and allowed to warm up. The machine is set at 400 watt-seconds (joules) unless the patient is in digitalis toxicity or is small in stature, in which case a lower setting is used. The synchronizer switch on the machine is turned to "off" (synchronization is not possible during ventricular fibrillation).

Preparation of Patient. Unless an IV is already running, one is started immediately. Sodium bicarbonate is given to combat acidosis, and lidocaine to prevent development of arrhythmias during or following shock. No anesthesia is used.

Administration of Shock. The paddles are lubricated with electrode paste to prevent burning the skin. The paste should not extend beyond the paddles, and the paddles should lie flat against the body in order to avoid burns from sparks jumping across the skin. Moist saline pads may be used instead of paste. To save time, one paddle is usually placed over the *left sternal border*—the second intercostal space—and the other over the *apex of the heart.* The paddles can also be placed anteroposteriorly if convenient. All personnel, including the person administering the shock, *must stand back from the bed! Never touch bed or patient* when shock is being administered. (In some instances immediate defibrillation may be attempted before an IV has been inserted.)

Evaluation of Procedure. Immediately after defibrillation an ECG tracing is taken. Most of the newer cardiac monitors and ECG machines can withstand the shock when they are connected to a patient being defibrillated. Some may not record the ECG for several seconds after the patient has been shocked, though. Some defibrillators are equipped with paddles that are capable of monitoring the patient's ECG, even immediately after defibrillation. Therefore, if the paddles are left in place after the shock has been delivered, the pateint's response can be quickly evaluated.

A successful response is indicated by cessation of fibrillation, restoration of sinus rhythm, and normal contraction of heart muscle. A poor or dangerous response is indicated by failure of the arrhythmia to convert to normal rhythm or development of asystole.

If the patient remains in ventricular fibrillation after defibrillation, epinephrine may be administered directly into the heart before another shock is delivered. This helps to strengthen the heart muscle and may aid in converting the heart to a normal rhythm when the pateint is again defibrillated. If the ventricular fibrillation progresses to asystole, cardiac massage is instituted.

Aftercare. A special steroid cream is applied to the skin where the paddles had been applied. The patient is observed carefully, especially pulse, state of consciousness, and patency of airway. Ventricular fibrillation can recur!

CARDIOVERSION

This is an elective procedure in which electric current is delivered to the heart to terminate potentially dangerous or exhausting arrhythmias that have been refractory to drug therapy. The usual indications are tachycardias developing in patients who have had a myocardial infarction, e.g., atrial, nodal, or ventricular tachycardia. It is also used at times for atrial flutter or fibrillation. The procedure is performed *only* by specially trained physicians.

Preliminary Measures. ECG readings are taken to diagnose the type of arrhythmia present. The procedure is scheduled for a specified hour. It can be performed at the patient's bedside, but emergency equipment should be close at hand in case the patient develops a life-threatening arrhythmia when shocked. The patient is given a full explanation of the procedure.

Preparation of Patient. If the patient has been receiving digitalis, it is desirable to hold the drug the morning of the procedure, as digitalis may predis-

TABLE 35–2. DRUGS COMMONLY USED IN THE CARE OF PATIENTS WITH ARRHYTHMIAS

Drug	Action	Indications	Contraindications	Route of Administration	Side Effects
Quinidine	Depresses myocardial excitability; slows conduction time in atria and ventricles, prolongs PR and QRS intervals; prolongs refractory period; depresses myocardial contractility; reduces vagal tone.	Ventricular tachycardia; premature ventricular contractions; atrial flutter and fibrillation; ectopic beats (atrial or ventricular)	Sensitivity or allergy to drug; usually not given to persons with complete heart block, bundle branch block, thyrotoxicosis, acute rheumatic fever, or subacute bacterial endocarditis	Orally, as maintenance dose I.M. I.V., quinidine gluconate given in emergency situations	Hypersensitivity: fever, rash, hypotension; neurologic effects: tinnitus, diplopia, confusion, headache, delirium; gastric effects: anorexia, nausea, vomiting, diarrhea; myocardial effects: heart block, nodal rhythm, ventricular arrhythmias; emboli when the heart is converting to normal rhythm
Procainamide (Pronestyl)	Depresses ectopic pacemakers; action on heart similar to quinidine	Premature ventricular contractions; ventricular tachycardia; ventricular fibrillation when defibrillator not available; atrial tachycardia	Severe heart damage and shock because of hypotensive effect; complete heart block; allergy	Orally I.M. I.V. I.V. drip	Same as quinidine; severe hypotension with parenteral use; a lupus erythematosus–like syndrome may develop in some patients
Lidocaine (Xylocaine)	Rapid-acting local or topical anesthetic agent; depresses myocardium; decreases excitability, conduction, and force of contraction	Ventricular arrhythmias; sometimes used in open heart surgery as a direct topical anesthetic	Bradycardia; heart block; give with caution in liver disease, as drug is metabolized by liver	I.V. push I.V. drip	Neurologic signs: dizziness, blurred vision, sweating, progressing to coma, hypotension, and convulsions; cardiac signs: large doses occasionally cause decreased myocardial contractility
Propranolol (Inderal)	Beta adrenergic blocking agent; blocks the actions of the catecholamines upon the heart; decreases heart rate and contractility; decreases rates of SA node and ectopic pacemaker sites; decreases AV node conduction and ventricular irritability	Prolonged angina (see Chap. 36); premature ventricular contractions; atrial and ventricular tachycardias; tachycardia in Wolff-Parkinson-White syndrome; myocardial infarction.	Congestive heart failure and cardiogenic shock because patients in congestive heart failure or shock require catecholamine effects to stimulate force of myocardial contractions; AV or bundle branch block; bronchospasm, brittle diabetes	Orally I.V.	Bradycardia; hypotension; acute heart failure in persons with a damaged myocardium

Isoproterenol (Isuprel)	Increases heart rate, stroke volume, coronary blood flow; increases rate in AV block by acting on sinus node and AV node	Stokes-Adams syndrome; sinus bradycardia; sinus arrest; heart block, cardiac arrest	Use with caution in patients with hyperthyroidism, glaucoma, and limited cardiac reserve; myocardial infarction	I.C. (directly into heart) I.V. push I.V. drip	Tachycardia; palpitations; weakness; sweating; nausea; angina; headache
Atropine	Vagolytic drug; abolishes vagal reflexes during cardiac arrest or hypoxia	Bradyarrhthymias that the patient is not tolerating	Glaucoma; parotitis; tachycardia	I.V. I.M. Subcutaneously	Dry mouth with thirst; blurred vision from dilated pupils; disorientation; hallucinations; delirium; difficulty voiding; decreased respirations
Diphenylhydantoin (Dilantin)	Suppresses myocardial irritability	Most useful in the treatment of arrhthymias caused by digitalis toxicity	Drug allergy; hepatic disease because drug is inactivated in liver	I.V. Orally	Transient hypotension due to peripheral vasodilatation; respiratory or cardiac arrest; shock
Edrophonium hydrochloride (Tensilon)	Enhances action of vagus nerve; decreases heart rate	Paroxysmal supraventricular arrhythmias unresponsive to mechanical maneuvers to stimulate vagus nerve, e.g., carotid sinus massage	Hypotension	I.V. push	Nausea, salivation, bronchospasm, bradycardia, diaphoresis, hypotension (a very short-acting drug, so side effects last only minutes)
Bretylium tosylate (Bretylol)	Suppresses ventricular tachycardia and ventricular fibrillation; has a positive inotropic effect; does not decrease conduction across the AV junction significantly	Life-threatening ventricular arrhythmias *which have failed to respond to other types of therapy*	Digitalis toxicity	Various routes of administration, depending on needs of patient	Nausea and vomiting—less if administered slowly; hypotension
Disopyramide phosphate (Norpace)	Decreases myocardial excitability. Action on heart similar to quinidine	Premature ventricular contractions, ventricular tachycardia	Preexisting AV block; shock; glaucoma; urinary retention	Given daily orally, in divided doses	Heart block; CHF; urinary retention; dry mouth; blurred vision

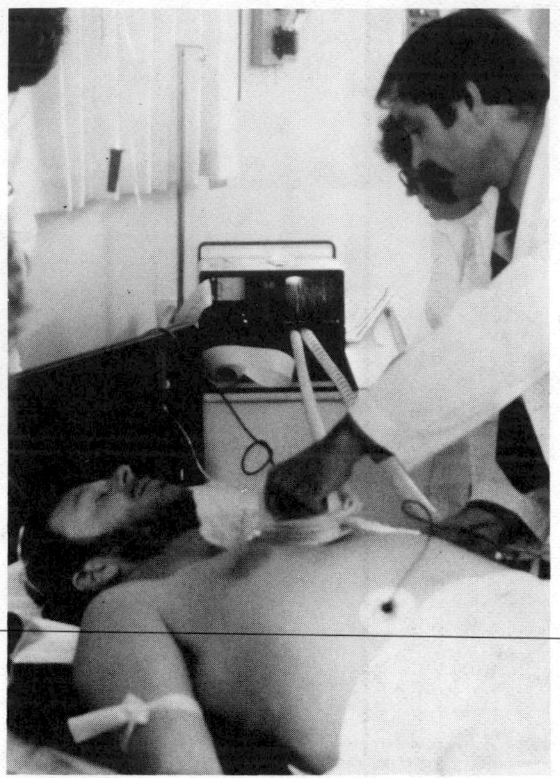

Figure 35–5. Position of defibrillator paddles during emergency administration of precordial shock. (Courtesy Physio-Control Corporation, Redmond, Washington.)

pose the patient to the development of ventricular arrhythmias during the procedure. A low serum potassium level also increases the patient's chance of developing life-threatening arrhythmias. Therefore, potassium salts should be administered if necessary.

Quinidine may be given for several days prior to cardioversion is an attempt to convert the arrhythmia. Quinidine will also make it easier to convert the arrhythmia to normal sinus rhythm if cardioversion is necessary, and prior administration of this drug will increase the patient's chance of remaining in sinus rhythm after countershock.

The patient is kept NPO for several hours before cardioversion. An IV is started. To reduce fear and pain, short-term anesthesia (diazepam [Valium]) is commonly used. Lidocaine should be readily available in the event the patient develops ventricular arrhythmias during the procedure.

Operation of the Machine and Administration of the Shock. The machine is set within a range of 50 to 400 watt-seconds. The synchronizer switch is turned to "on" in order to deliver the shock during the QRS complex and not on the downslope of the T wave. The paddles are lubricated with electrode paste. One paddle is placed on the patient's back, slightly medial to the tip of the left scapula, and the second is placed anteriorly over the base of the heart. The same precautions are observed during administration of the shock that were mentioned under defibrillation.

Evaluation of Procedure. An ECG tracing is obtained immediately after the procedure. In some cases ventricular fibrillation or tachycardia may occur. This indicates a poor response to the treatment; a successful response, of course, is indicated by the termination of the arrhythmia.

Aftercare. If the result is favorable, the patient is usually discharged the following day.

As noted, cardioversion may not always restore normal heart rhythm in patients with severe arrhythmias. If patients have long standing arrhythmias, e.g., atrial fibrillation or atrial flutter secondary to severe heart disease, the chances of cardioversion being successful are decreased. This procedure is most likely to permanently convert patients to normal sinus rhythm who have had the arrhythmia for a relatively short amount of time and who do not have chronic heart disease. *Hypoxia, acidosis,* and *drug toxicity* may also prevent the patient's heart from converting to a normal rhythm following precordial shock. The physician usually treats these disorders before precordial shock is attempted for the second time.

Artificial Cardiac Pacemakers

An artificial cardiac pacemaker is an electronic apparatus that is used to initiate the heart beat when the SA node is seriously damaged and unable to act as pacemaker or when impulses from the SA node and atria are not adequately transmitted through the AV junction to the ventricles. The artificial pacemaker controls the heart beat by means of electrical stimulation of the ventricles.

Artificial pacemakers are used to stimulate the heart beat in the following conditions:

1. Partial or complete AV block with Stokes-Adams attacks that do not respond to medical therapy.
2. Complete heart block.
3. Acute myocardial infarction with partial or complete heart block.
4. Acute myocarditis with heart block.
5. Heart block following cardiac surgery.
6. Intermittent sinus arrest.
7. Bradyarrhythmias with syncope (e.g., sinus bradycardia, atrial fibrillation, and junctional or ventricular escape rhythm or atrial flutter with a slow ventricular response).
8. To override ectopic foci which are causing tachyarrhythmias that are compromising cardiac output (e.g., paroxysmal supraventricular tachycardias, ventricular tachycardia). Pacemakers are used in

these instances when the arrhythmia has become refractory to medications.

TYPES OF PACEMAKERS

There are two major types of pacemakers: *temporary* and *permanent.* Temporary pacing may be initiated in an *emergency situation* to correct asystole which is not responding to other forms of therapy. Methods of artificially pacing the heart in emergency situations include the following:

1. *Percutaneous insertion* of electrodes through the chest wall directly into the myocardium. A large bore cardiac needle is inserted into the heart, and the pacing wire is then passed through the needle. (This is called *emergency transthoracic pacing.*)
2. *Insertion* of an insulated electrode wire *through a vein* in the arm to the right atrium, and then through the tricuspid valve into the right ventricle where it is wedged under the trabeculae; this method is called *emergency or temporary transvenous pacing.*

Short-term pacing, another form of temporary pacing, is useful in such disorders as myocardial infarction with temporary heart block, sinus arrest, and sinus bradycardia. The most popular method of short-term pacing is the insertion of a temporary transvenous pacing catheter as described above. Pacing wires may also be placed in the heart following cardiac surgery. They are usually sutured into the epicardium and are brought out through small puncture wounds in the chest wall or through the incision. Temporary pacing can be employed for several weeks if necessary.

The pacing catheter may be *bipolar,* meaning that both the negative and positive electrodes are located in the heart, or *unipolar.* With the unipolar catheter the negative electrode is in the heart and the positive electrode is located outside of the heart.

After the temporary pacing catheter has been inserted, it is connected to an *external* pacemaker box (see Fig. 35–6). The pacemaker is then turned on and the heart is stimulated with a low voltage electric shock which the patient generally does not feel.

When weaning the patient from a temporary pacemaker upon which the patient has relied for several weeks, the nurse and physician must frequently evaluate the patient's cardiac rate and rhythm; also they must give the patient encouragement and emotional support.

To discontinue use of the pacemaker, the physician turns the *external* pacemaker off, but leaves the temporary pacing catheter in the right ventricle as a safety precaution. If heart block continues or if the SA node is still unable to initiate its own beats, artificial pacing can be quickly resumed. It is important to reassure a nervous patient that the artificial pacemaker will be activated immediately in event of any heart problem during this weaning period.

In contrast to temporary pacemakers, *permanent* pacemakers can be used for months to years. The most important indication for permanent pacing is persistent *chronic heart block with Stokes-Adams attacks.*

There are two principal types of electrode placement for permanent pacing: endocardial and epicardial. The procedure for inserting an *endocardial,* or transvenous, pacemaker (the most common type) is similar to the insertion of a transvenous temporary pacemaker. Under fluoroscopic observation, a transvenous pacing catheter is passed through the *right external jugular vein* or through the *subclavian vein* beneath the clavicle (note that a superficial arm vein is *not* used as in temporary pacing) into the right atrium and then the right ventricle. The catheter is then attached to a battery-operated *pulse generator* (Fig. 35–7). The pulse generator is buried in a subcutaneous pocket, surgically placed beneath the clavicle or under the axilla (Fig. 35–8). A small stab wound is made in the "pocket," and a drainage catheter is inserted and attached to low suction; the pocket is usually drained for 24 hours to prevent the accumulation of drainage and the possibility of infection.

The major early complication of endocardial pacing is *displacement of the endocardial leads* within the right ventricle. When endocardial leads become dislodged, the myocardium is only stimulated spasmodically and sometimes receives no stimulation at all. Generally the malpositioned electrode can be manipulated back into position without serious consequences. The pacemaker can also pace the diaphragm when the pacing catheter is lying close to the apex of the heart. This is very uncomfortable for the patient as it causes continuous hiccoughing. Repositioning of the catheter may be needed to correct this situation.

Implantation of an *epicardial* pacemaker is a much more dangerous and complicated procedure than that described above and is infrequently used. It may be indicated, though, when transvenous pacing has not been successful in a particular patient. To institute epicardial pacing, the surgeon must perform a thoracotomy, expose the heart, and then sew electrodes onto the epicardium or heart's outer surface. Wires from these electrodes are then attached to a battery-operated pulse generator placed surgically in the anterior abdominal wall.

The major early complications of epicardial pacing are like those arising from any type of thoracic surgery. Patients (who are generally in

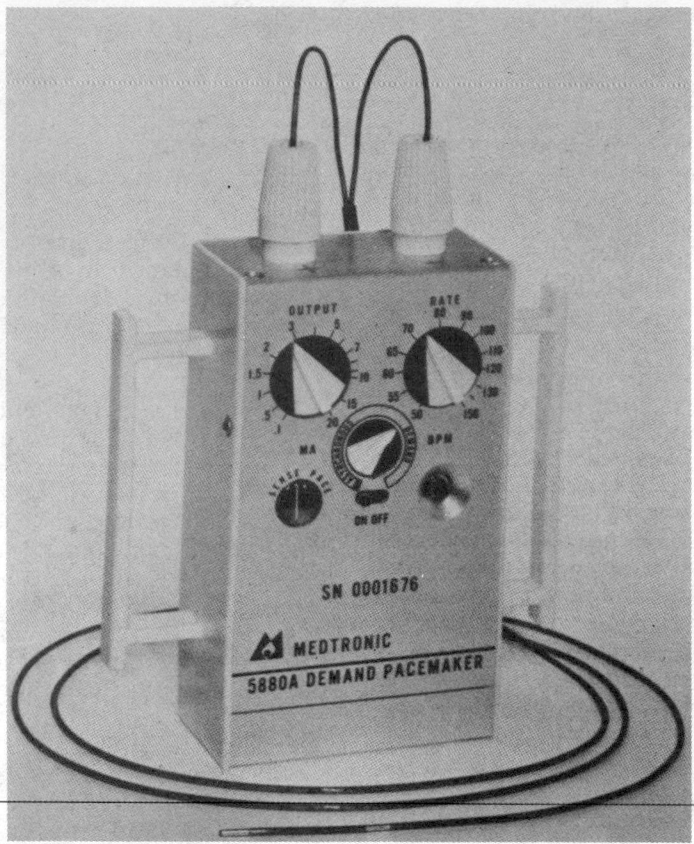

Figure 35–6. External pacemaker box. The Medtronic is a battery-powered pacemaker that operates in either the demand or fixed-rate mode. It incorporates filtering circuitry that blocks the AC leakage currents and built-in shielding to prevent most electrical interference. If interference is stronger than 100 mV, the pacemaker output is suppressed. (Photograph courtesy of Medtronic, Inc., Minneapolis, Minn.) (From Aspinall, J. J.: *Nursing the Open-Heart Surgery Patient.* New York, McGraw-Hill, Inc. 1973, p. 195.)

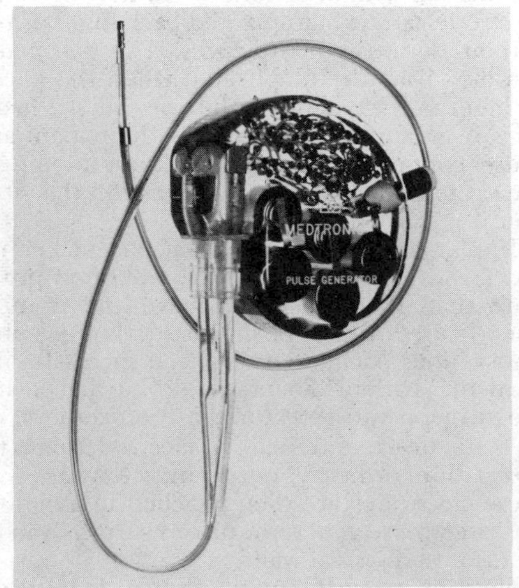

Figure 35–7. A pulse generator. A permanent transvenous (endocardial) pacemaker. (Courtesy of Medtronic, Inc.)

an older age group) may develop pulmonary infections, thrombophlebitis, decubitus, and all the other complications that accompany a prolonged immobilization period.

A *later* complication of epicardial pacing is the development of infected and inflamed areas around the electrodes which, in turn, necessitates increased power to stimulate the heart to contract. If infection is truly severe, epicardial pacing is discontinued in favor of endocardial pacing.

In sum, the major advantage of implanted pacemaker systems (endocardial and epicardial) is that they are entirely subcutaneous. As a result, the patient is free to move, turn, bathe, ambulate, and, in time, lead a normal life.

METHODS OF PACING

The three major methods of cardiac pacing are (1) fixed rate asynchronous pacing; (2) demand or standby pacing; and (3) atrial pacing.

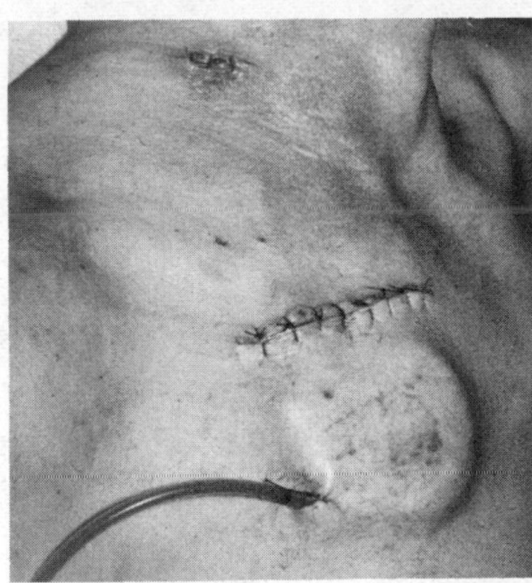

Figure 35–8. Pulse generator in subcutaneous pocket. (Courtesy of Medtronic, Inc.)

The *fixed rate continuous asynchronous pacemaker* was the first pacing device to appear on the market. It is called a "fixed rate" pacemaker because it stimulates the ventricles to contract at a fixed or preset rate regardless of the body's metabolic requirements at the time. The term "continuous asynchronous" means that the pacemaker is not synchronized to the patient's ECG pattern; thus it fires as set regardless of the ECG configuration.

The major advantage of the fixed rate pacemaker is its relative simplicity of operation. However, fixed rate pacemakers have three major disadvantages: First, the rate of firing does not increase with the patient's metabolic needs. Second, some patients, following insertion of a fixed rate pacemaker, convert back to a normal rhythm; as a result, impulses released by the SA node *compete* with impulses released by the artificial pacemaker. If the voltage is low, competition may not be a serious problem; an irregular pulse is generally the only sign. But, fixed-rate pacemakers can precipitate ventricular fibrillation if an artificial pacemaker impulse is released during the vulnerable period of ventricular repolarization following release of a normal impulse by the SA node. Certain drugs, electrolyte imbalances, and myocardial infarction are some circumstances which can increase the likelihood of ventricular fibrillation if the pacemaker fires during this vulnerable period.

Demand pacemakers fire on demand, or when needed to stimulate ventricular contraction. Therefore, if the SA node stimulates the appearance of a QRS wave, the demand pacemaker does not fire. On the other hand, when the SA node is unable to trigger the appearance of a normal QRS, the demand pacemaker goes into action and stimulates ventricular action. To function in this manner the demand pacemaker has a mechanism built into it that can *sense* when the patient has an independent heartbeat. If a certain amount of time has elapsed without an intrinsic heartbeat, the pacemaker stimulates the heart. Thus, the ECG readings of patients on demand pacemakers indicate the presence of an artificial pacemaker only when the natural QRS is not present. Figure 35–9 provides examples of ECG tracings of patients with artificial pacemakers.

Demand pacemakers are advantageous for patients who are frequently in normal sinus rhythm, but who nevertheless suffer periodically from attacks of severe bradycardia or syncope. In recent years, this type of pacing has supplanted the fixed rate type to a large degree.

Atrial pacing may be used in patients without AV conduction disturbances. This type of pacing may be used to help treat supraventricular arrhythmias (e.g., P.A.T. and atrial flutter) that are refractory to medical therapy. An advantage of atrial pacing is the benefits derived from atrial contraction. Atrial pacing wires are often sewn into the atrial epicardium during cardiac surgery to aid in the diagnosis and treatment of arrhythmias postoperatively. In other types of patients, a catheter may be introduced transvenously into the right atrium.

TECHNICAL PROBLEMS ASSOCIATED WITH CARDIAC PACING

Technical problems that interfere with pacemaker operation are decreasing as scientists continue to perfect pacemaker design. Still to be solved:

1. Dislodgement and migration of endocardial leads.
2. Infection of the site where the pulse generator is inserted.
3. Battery exhaustion. This problem usually becomes manifest by a gradual slowing of the heart rate below the rate at which the pacemaker has been set. Most batteries now last between 5 and 10 years. The implanted unit is replaced, when necessary, in the operating room under local anesthesia.

CLINICAL CARE OF PATIENTS WITH ARTIFICIAL PACEMAKERS

The nurse has many responsibilities when caring for patients with pacemakers. In Table 35–3 the care of patients with temporary and with permanent pacemakers is outlined and compared.

The patient who is to be discharged with a pacemaker permanently implanted needs to receive several special cautions and instructions. Some of these are:

1. Take pulse once daily for 1 full minute and note and report to the physician irregularities in rate and rhythm.
2. Take frequent rest periods at home and at work.
3. Prolonged hiccoughs should be reported to the doctor; rarely, the catheter tip might perforate the heart and migrate to the diaphragm, causing hic-

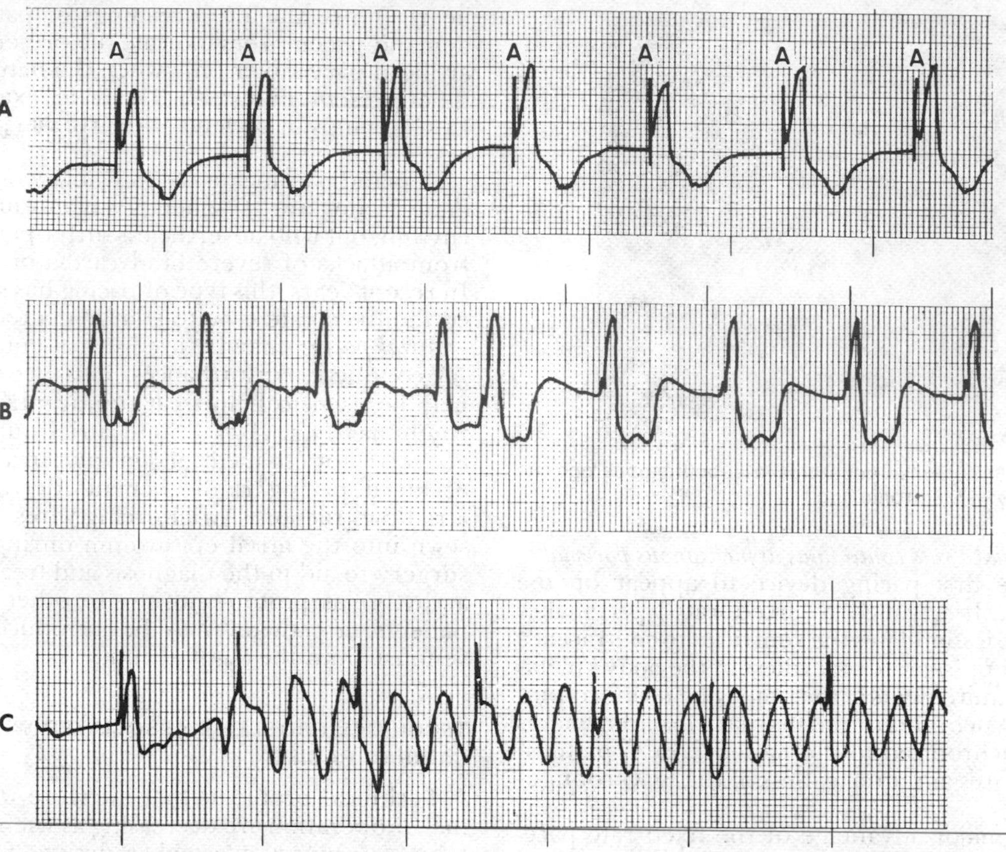

Figure 35–9. **A.** Continuous discharging ventricular pacemaker. The pacemaker stimulates each ventricular contraction in this tracing. Atrial activity is not readily apparent. Pacemaker artifacts are labeled *A.* **B.** Unlike the previous figure, spontaneous ventricular activity competes with the pacemaker for control of the cardiac rhythm. A poorly defined P wave precedes the first four QRS complexes, indicating spontaneous sinus rhythm. Pacemaker spikes "march through" these first four beats but remain completely uninfluenced by spontaneous activity. Finally, the ventricles are in a non-refractory state in time to be discharged by the fourth pacemaker spike. The last five QRS complexes are each initiated by a small spike and represent pacemaker-driven beats. Both conducted and pacemaker-induced QRS complexes have similar contours because the patient has intrinsic left bundle branch block which is mimicked by pacing the right ventricle. **C.** Continuously discharging ventricular pacemaker. The initial pacemaker-stimulated QRS complex is followed by a spontaneous premature ventricular contraction. The next pacemaker discharge occurs during the vulnerable period of this beat and precipitates ventricular tachycardia–fibrillation. (From Andreoli, K., et al.: *Comprehensive Cardiac Care—A Text for Nurses, Physicians, and Other Health Practitioners.* St. Louis, C. V. Mosby Co., 1976, p. 253.)

coughs. The catheter may also be lying in the right ventricle near the diaphragm and stimulate the diaphragm without actually perforating the myocardium.

4. Return to the clinic or private physician every 3 months.

CARDIAC ARREST AND CARDIOPULMONARY RESUSCITATION

Cardiopulmonary resuscitation (CPR) techniques are used to artificially maintain both circulation and ventilation in persons suffering from *cardiac arrest.* Cardiopulmonary resuscitation techniques involve: (1) external (closed chest) cardiac massage (manual heart compression), and (2) artificial ventilation by either mouth-to-mouth, mouth-to-nose, or mouth-to-airway techniques.

The term *cardiac arrest* is synonymous with the term *sudden death;* it means that the victim's heart beat, circulation of blood, and respirations have *suddenly* and *unexpectedly* stopped as a result of trauma, electrical shock, disturbed electrical activity within the heart, and so forth. Table 35–4 lists principal causes of cardiac arrest.

The terms *sudden* and *unexpected* are important in this definition because only the victims of *sudden* death are generally resuscitated. For example, a young healthy telephone company worker who suddenly receives a powerful jolt of electric current while working on telephone lines will undoubtedly suffer both cardiac and respiratory arrest; this person is a candidate for immediate resuscitation measures. On the other hand, an elderly person who dies from cancer does *not* experience a cardiac arrest in the strictest sense of the term. When this patient's heart ceases beating, death comes as a *natural* event for which the patient and the family are prepared. Therefore, this patient is *not* a candidate for resuscitation measures; indeed, such measures would only prolong suffering.

The Responsibilities of the Resuscitator

Cardiac arrest or sudden death can occur *anywhere* — in the home, on the street, in a general hospital ward, or in a highly specialized critical care setting, e.g., the CCU. For that reason both professional persons and trained laypeople are qualified to perform emergency cardiopulmonary resuscitation procedures. Within the hospital setting *nurses,* in particular, must be experts in resuscitation measures, because they are generally the first persons to discover a patient who has "arrested." It is typically nurses who must diagnose the problem, start cardiac massage, call for medical help, prepare emergency drugs, set up and sometimes even use the defibrillator. Because these tasks must be carried out *immediately,* every nurse needs accurate knowledge of resuscitation procedures of life-saving techniques.

Immediate Responsibilities of the Resuscitator:

> *1.* Recognize *the* signs *of cardiac arrest.*
> *2.* Protect *the patient's* brain *from* anoxia: *(a)* rapidly begin *artificial ventilation of the lungs; (b) immediately begin external cardiac massage in order to provide continuous artificial circulation to brain and vital organs.*
> *3.* Summon help — *either doctor, resuscitation team, or ambulance.*

Signs of Cardiac Arrest

> *Signs of cardiac arrest are as follows:*
> *1. Abrupt and complete unconsciousness.*
> *2. Apnea or gasping respirations.*
> *3. Absence of heartbeat and femoral, radial, and carotid pulsations.*
> *4. Dilation of the pupils.*

The outstanding sign of cardiac arrest is the absence of a carotid pulse. In some cases, however, the carotid, femoral, and radial pulses may be present but very feeble. In these instances it is still necessary to begin resuscitation measures at once, because cardiac output is undoubtedly poor, and the patient's brain, kidneys, and liver will suffer from inadequate oxygenation without artificial resuscitation.

If the resuscitator is unable to make a definite diagnosis of cardiac arrest based on the signs listed above, most authorities recommend that she or he begin resuscitation measures anyway, and leave the final decision to stop resuscitation for the judgment of the physician.

As mentioned, two groups of individuals should *not* be resuscitated: patients in the last stages of an incurable illness and persons whose heart beat and respirations have been absent for more than 6 minutes. There are, however, exceptions and it is generally safer to initiate resuscitative measures when in doubt. Resuscitation is often started in some cases of arrest associated with near drowning, hypothermia, and in children even after prolonged arrest. If a decision has been made in advance (with the significant others, staff, physician, and sometimes the patient), a written "no code" (i.e., do not attempt resuscitation) order may be included in the chart.

Protection of the Brain from Anoxia. An individual who has suffered a cardiac arrest is considered *clinically* dead; i.e., the heart has stopped beating. The patient, however, is still *biologically* alive, i.e., brain tissues and other organs still contain some oxygen and are therefore living. Indeed, the brain and other central nervous system tissues remain alive for a period of from 4 to 6 minutes, while other body tissues survive for even longer periods of time. Unfortunately, once this grace period of from 4 to 6 minutes following cardiac arrest passes, *biologic* death ensues and the patient's brain, now irreparably damaged, dies. Once biologic death occurs, resuscitation attempts are futile because the brain tissues are already severely damaged.

> Remember:
> *External cardiac massage and artificial ventilation* must *be started within* 4 to 6 minutes *following cardiac arrest or* irreversible brain damage *will develop as a result of oxygen deprivation and lack of circulation.*

Summon Help. It is extremely difficult for one person to carry out a successful cardiopulmonary resuscitation alone. It is almost mandatory that two persons assist the victim — one providing artificial ventilation, and the other providing cardiac compressions. Even when two persons are present, it is still absolutely essential to obtain expert medical help. The patient may need special drugs, countershock, intubation, and other emergency measures in order to reactivate the heart and respiratory system.

Within the hospital setting, special notification systems are generally used to quickly gather

TABLE 35–3. CLINICAL CARE OF PATIENTS WITH TEMPORARY AND PERMANENT PACEMAKERS

Therapeutic Measure	Temporary Pacemakers	Permanent Pacemakers
Activity	Immobilize extremity where transvenous catheter is inserted through a superficial vein; guard against *any* tension being placed on pacing catheter, in order to prevent displacement of catheter within ventricle	Moderately restrict patient's activities during first 24 hours following pacemaker insertion to observe pacemaker function under basal conditions; promote deep breathing, leg movements, and early ambulation following thoracotomy
Prevention of sepsis	Check temperature immediately following procedure and every 4 hours thereafter; report elevations of temperature at once; daily cleanse arm in which transvenous catheter is inserted, cover the area with an antibiotic ointment and sterile dressing; use sterile technique; oil the skin surrounding the catheter in the area outside the dressing where the wires of the external pacemaker may touch the skin; pad site under the catheter wires to prevent tissue injury	Same; antibiotics administered for 5 to 7 days following procedure; low suction to subcutaneous pouch following implantation of pulse generator in order to prevent accumulation of drainage
Postoperative care	Watch for signs of thrombophlebitis and infection at site of entry of transvenous catheter	Following pacemaker insertion: check vital signs q. ½ hour until stable; examine dressing for drainage; record I and O; give small amount of analgesic to relieve pain; ambulate day after surgery; regularly exercise arm on operated side to prevent frozen shoulder.
Promote environmental safety	Check all equipment in patient's room for *proper grounding* when externally powered pacemaker is used; improperly grounded equipment may allow the escape of small amounts of electrical current which could reach the heart through the pacing catheter and cause ventricular fibrillation; if the tips of the pacemaker wires are exposed when connected to the pacemaker box, cover them with a material that will prevent any electrical currents in the air from being conducted to the heart, e.g., part of a rubber glove; also make sure that the tips of the pacemaker wires are covered when they are not connected to the pacemaker box	Not applicable because entire pacemaker unit is subcutaneous
Monitor heart rate and rhythm	A paced beat is immediately preceded by a pacer spike or artifact on the ECG tracing; the QRS complex of the paced beat is wide and bizarre and resembles a premature ventricular contraction because the paced beat is initiated in the ventricles In fixed rate pacemakers, a pacemaker spike should precede every QRS complex on ECG; a pacer spike not followed by a QRS complex usually indicates that the pacemaker is not capturing the ventricles; This may be due to malposition of the pacer wires in the ventricles or insufficient voltage to stimulate the heart; the absence of a pacer spike may indicate a loose connection between the power source or a depleted battery in pacemaker box; also check for signs of competition between natural pacemaker and artificial pacemaker	Same; the permanent pacemaker does not just suddenly stop working, rather, it gradually slows over a period of time; if patient's heartbeat is dependent upon the pacemaker, he will notice his heart rate gradually decreasing; if he does not totally rely on the pacemaker, the integrity of the battery can be checked by means of a magnet: when magnet is held over pacemaker, the electrical field around the magnet interferes with pacemaker's ability to sense electrical activity from heart, consequently, the pacemaker should fire at the rate at which it has been set

TABLE 35–3. CLINICAL CARE OF PATIENTS WITH TEMPORARY AND PERMANENT PACEMAKERS (*Continued*)

Therapeutic Measure	Temporary Pacemakers	Permanent Pacemakers
Monitor heart rate and rhythm (*Continued*)	In demand pacemakers it is necessary to determine that the pacemaker is sensing when the patient has an adequate independent heart rate—this will be evident by the absence of pacer spikes; a pacer spike should not immediately follow the patient's own heartbeat, e.g., occur on or near the T wave; this indicates the pacemaker did not sense the heart's own activity and competition is occurring; the pacemaker must also sense when the patient has an insufficient heart rate—there should be evidence of a paced beat at this time; a long pause may indicate that the pacemaker is not firing in the absence of the patient's own heartbeat	
Provide emotional support	Give full explanation of function and use of pacemaker; explain that patient will not feel the electrical stimulation of the heart and will not be electrocuted; some patients with a pacemaker in place may think that the cardiac monitor is the pacemaker—they fear that when the leads are changed, their heart will stop beating; project a confident attitude when the patient is being weaned from the pacemaker	Encourage the patient throughout convalescent period; explain that battery failure is not a problem if patient reports to doctor or clinic for periodic checkups.
Discharge home	Patients usually discharged once they have been completely weaned from temporary pacemaker and cardiovascular function has stabilized	Patients usually in hospital for one week following implantation of pacemaker; this time interval gives staff sufficient time to evaluate pacemaker function and wound healing. See text for special patient cautions and instructions.

emergency resuscitation team members at the patient's bedside. Various codes are used; for example, "Alert — Room ____." "Doctor Blue — Room ____ stat." or "Code 99 — Room ____ stat." Once the team arrives, each person performs the specific task for which she or he is especially trained.

Treatment of Cardiac Arrest

Treatment of victims of cardiac arrest can be divided into three stages: emergency care, specific medical therapy, and postresuscitation care. Treatment must also take into consideration the possible complications and the psychologic support needed by the patient and significant others.

EMERGENCY CARE

Cardiopulmonary Resuscitation. Cardiopulmonary resuscitation (CPR) is the technique of manually compressing the heart and ventilating the lungs in the event of a cardiac arrest or inadequate heart rate. The technique is a psychomotor skill that requires practice on a teaching manikin in addition to formal classroom lecture presentations. All health care providers must be proficient in CPR, practice frequently, and be recertified yearly. New techniques are developed as more experience and research data are avail-

TABLE 35–4. CAUSES OF CARDIAC ARREST

Causes Associated with Surgery*	Causes Not Associated with Surgery
Hypotension	Acute myocardial infarction
CO_2 retention	Electrical shock
Reactions to anesthesia	Hypersensitivity or anaphylactic reactions
Depression from anesthesia	Hypothermia
Coronary occlusion	Suffocation, e.g., in plastic bag or abandoned refrigerator
Acute myocardial infarction	Airway obstruction, e.g., due to a foreign body
Inadequate ventilation of lungs	Digitalis poisoning
Anoxia due to airway obstruction	Cardiac catheterization
	Drowning
	Poisoning, e.g., carbon monoxide, cyanide, tricyclic antidepressants
	Pulmonary embolism

*Approximately one cardiac arrest occurs in every 1200 operations.

able; it is essential that the latest American Heart Association or American Red Cross standards be reviewed and the techniques mastered.

Even when CPR is performed perfectly, only about one third of the cardiac output is delivered. It is important, then, that CPR is performed with perfection. It is equally important that CPR not be interrupted for more than *5 seconds.* Exceptions to this rule are (1) when the patient is being moved; and (2) when endotracheal intubation is being carried out. The maximum amount of time allowed for these two procedures is *15 seconds.*

In addition to possessing skill in CPR, nurses must also take an active role in supporting CPR training for the public. Much of the success in decreasing mortality in out-of-hospital cardiac arrest in certain communities, e.g., Seattle, has been attributed to citizen-initiated CPR. Families/significant others of patients with cardiac problems should be asked if they know how to apply CPR, and referred to the appropriate agency if they lack this skill. It is important that this aspect be included in patient/family teaching. *Remember, CPR must be initiated within 3 to 4 minutes in order to prevent permanent brain damage.* Speed and precision are vital.

The Precordial Thump. The *precordial thump* is a blow which is delivered to the lower half of the patient's sternum *not more than one minute* after the person has suffered a cardiac arrest. The intent of this blow is to convert ventricular tachycardia or ventricular fibrillation of recent onset to a normal rhythm. *Therefore it is administered only when the arrest is witnessed and monitored.* If the heart has become anoxic, the precordial thump is not effective and it is important not to waste any time before beginning artificial ventilation and cardiac massage. The precordial thump is delivered by striking the middle of the sternum with the fleshy part of the fist from 8 to 12 inches above the patient's chest, as shown in Figure 35–11.

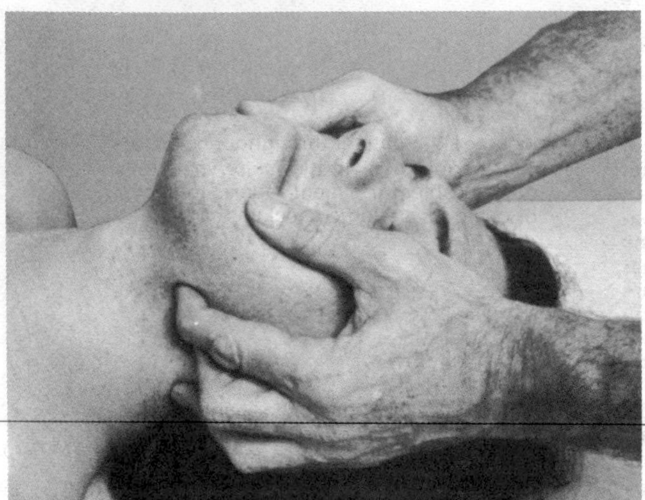

A

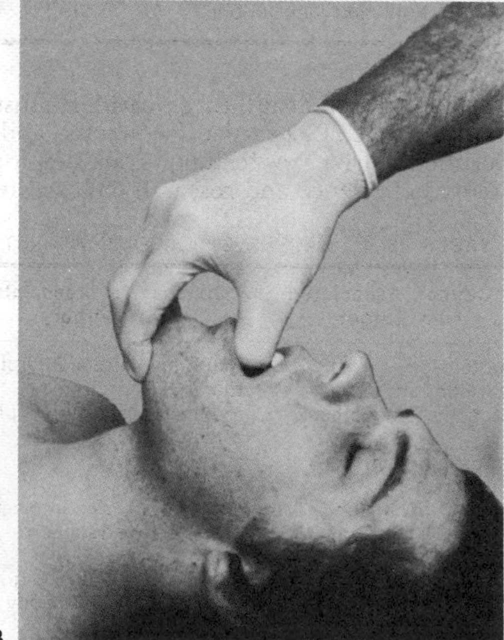

B

Figure 35–10. Positioning of the airway. **A.** Head tilt, with one hand placed on the patient's forehead, and the other placed under the patient's neck. Alternatively, the hand may be placed on the chin rather than under the neck; this is then called the chin lift–head tilt method. **B.** With the fingers at the angle of the jaw, the jaw is lifted upward and the neck hyperextended, opening the airway. (From Cosgriff, J. H.: *An Atlas of Diagnostic and Therapeutic Procedures for Emergency Personnel.* Philadelphia: J. B. Lippincott Co., 1978, pp. 96, 97.)

Technique

Step 1: Identify whether CPR is needed by the "*shake and shout*" method. Try to rouse the patient by shaking him and yelling in his ear, "Hey, are you all right?" If the patient was sleeping or somnolent due to alcohol, etc., he will usually respond. If no response, call for help and place the patient on a firm surface.

Step 2: Assess the airway. Open the airway, using either the chin lift–head tilt, jaw thrust, or neck lift techniques. (See Fig. 35–10.) Place your face over the patient's face with your head turned toward his chest. *Look, listen,* and *feel.* Look to see the chest rise and fall with breathing, listen for the sound of ventilations against your ear, feel for the exchange of air against your face. If the patient is not breathing, deliver four quick ventilations in rapid succession. Do not allow the patient to completely exhale between breaths. If the patient has not been breathing, the small airways are probably collapsed. The increasing volume in the lungs is needed to open up the airways.

In order to perform mouth-to-mouth ventilation, place one hand on the patient's forehead and pinch the nostrils with the thumb and index finger of the same hand. Place your other hand with the index and middle fingers under the chin at the angle of the jaw. Do not place all of your fingers on the patient's neck as you may occlude the airway. Alternatively, the hand may be placed under the neck to open the airway. With the hands in those positions, lift up on the jaw and tilt the head backward in order to open the airway. Dentures may be removed if they are loose-fitting; otherwise they are left in place to aid in maintaining a good seal.

Open your mouth widely and take a full breath, then blow the exhalation into the patient. Look at the chest to insure that the ventilation is being delivered. If you are unable to force air into the patient because of an obstruction, re-position the airway and repeat the attempt. If you are still unable to ventilate, there is a possibility that the patient has an airway obstruction such as food. Such an airway obstruction may be removed by delivering four quick blows to the back between the shoulder blades. If these are unsuccessful, it may be necessary to perform either the chest thrust or the abdominal thrust (Heimlich maneuver). These are discussed in Chapter 95.

When mouth-to-nose ventilation is done, the mouth is placed over the patient's nose and the patient's mouth is closed during ventilation. Open the mouth to allow exhalation.

Step 3: Once the airway is opened and ventilations have been delivered, the next step is to *assess the pulse* to determine whether cardiac compression is necessary. The carotid pulse is best assessed by palpating for it in the groove of the sternocleidomastoid muscle. (Remember that this muscle originates on the sternum and inserts on the mastoid process behind the ear.) *Do not palpate both carotid arteries at the same time as you may occlude the blood supply to the brain.* If there is no pulse, yell for help again and initiate closed cardiac massage.

Step 4: Expose the patient's chest. Using the middle finger of the hand that correlates with the side of the patient where you are positioned (e.g., use the left hand if you are positioned at the patient's left side), run the finger along the costal (rib) border toward the sternum. When your finger is in the groove between the rib and the sternum, place your index finger down on the chest. Keeping the index finger as a landmark, place the heel of the opposite hand next to the index finger on the sternum proximally (e.g., toward the head). It is important to avoid placing the hands on the xiphoid process because the xiphoid can lacerate the liver during chest compression. Additionally, improper hand placement often results in inadequate compression of the heart between the sternum and the vertebrae. The hand is placed with the heel of the hand on the middle of the sternum, and perpendicular to the sternum. The other hand, which was the original landmark, is then lifted off the chest and placed on top of that hand. Your body is positioned so that your shoulders are directly over the patient's chest, and your arms are straight with the elbows locked. (See Fig. 35–12.)

Step 5: Cardiac compression is accomplished by pressing straight downward on the chest, using the back and shoulders (rather than the wrists and elbows) for strength. The ratio of compressions to ventilations is 15:2 for one-person CPR, and 5:1 for two-person CPR. Whenever your hands leave the chest, e.g., to ventilate the patient, you must locate the proper hand position again, using the technique described. The chest is compressed 1.5 to 2 inches for an adult. For children, only one hand is used for compression and the depth is 0.75 to 1.5 inches. Compression in infants is done with the index and middle fingers of one hand at a depth of 0.5 to 0.75 of an inch.

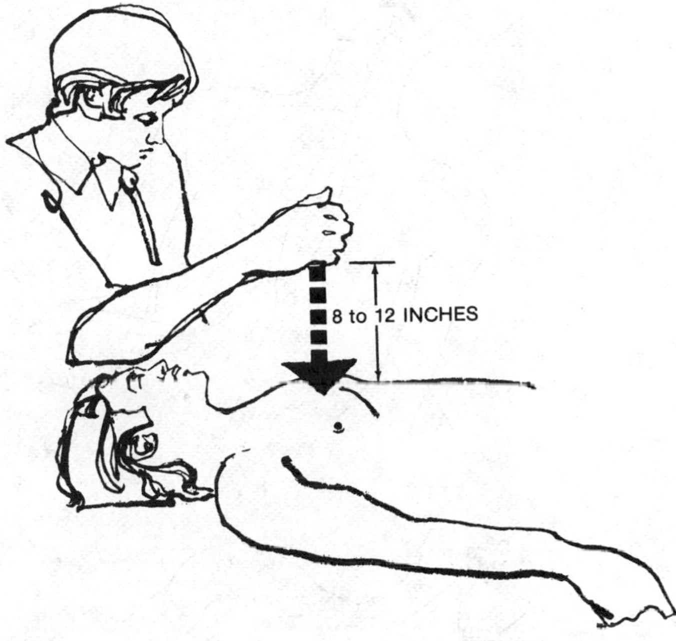

Figure 35–11. The precordial thump. (From Standards for cardiopulmonary resuscitation (CPR) and emergency cardiac care (ECC). Reprinted from the Supplement to Journal of the American Medical Association, February 18, 1974. © Copyright 1974, the American Medical Association. Reprinted with permission from the American Heart Association.

Step 6: The carotid pulse is assessed at frequent intervals to determine whether CPR is still required.

Step 7: CPR is carried out until one of the following occurs: (1) the patient regains a satisfactory pulse and no longer needs CPR; (2) the patient is pronounced dead by a physician; or (3) the rescuer is exhausted and unable to continue, and there is no one else available to take over performing CPR.

Signs of Effective Resuscitation. As resuscitation efforts continue, the resuscitator must decide whether the attempts to reestablish the patient's circulation are effective. For resuscitation efforts to be judged *effective,* at least *one* of the following signs must be present.

1. *Constriction of the pupils* — key sign *that the brain is sufficiently oxygenated.*
2. *Distinct carotid pulsations with each cardiac compression.*
3. *Blinking upon stimulation of the eyelid.*
4. *Breathing that begins spontaneously.*
5. *Movement and struggling.*
6. *Decreased cyanosis.*

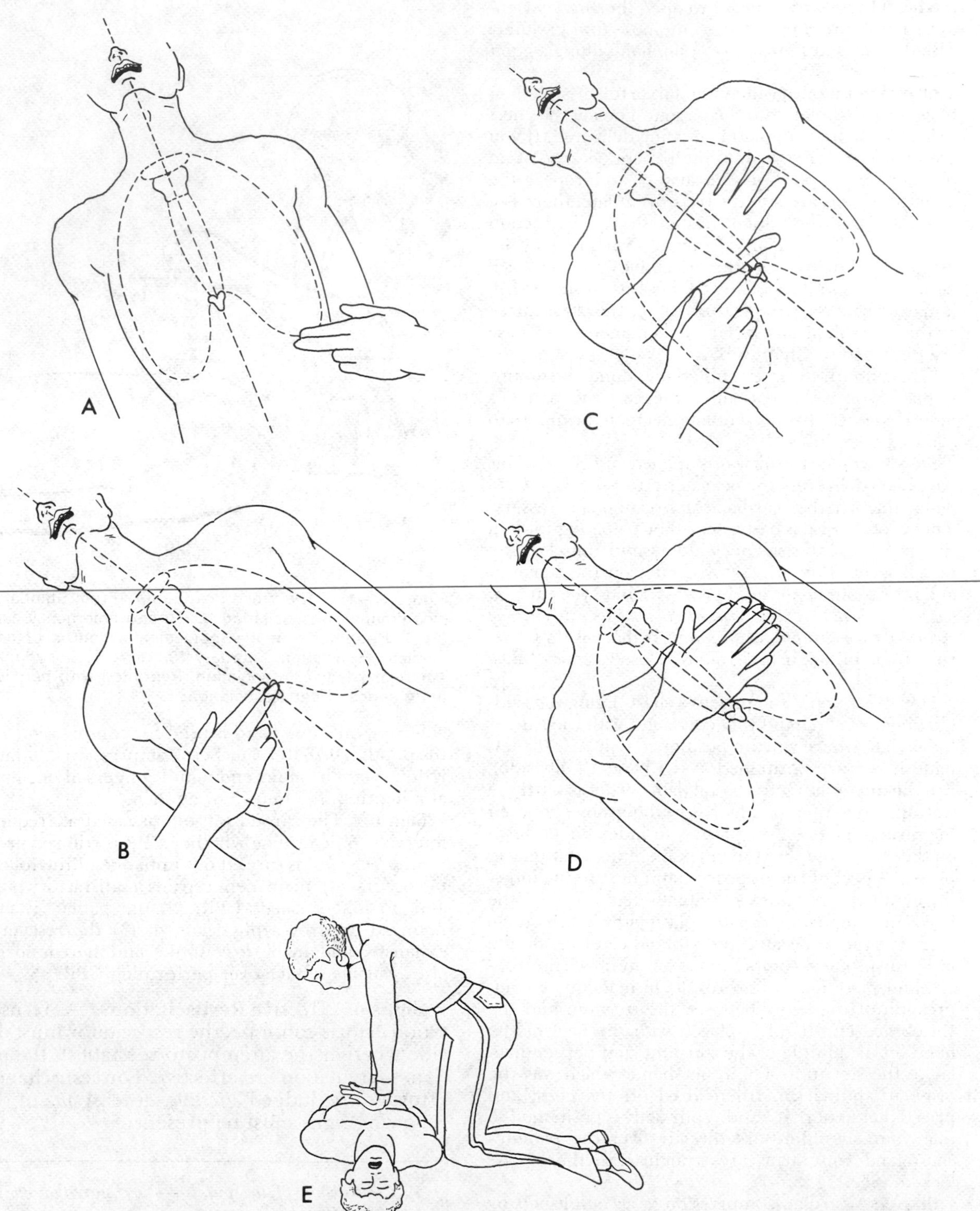

Figure 35–12. Proper hand position for cardiac compression. **A.** The index finger and middle finger of the rescuer's hand nearer the patient's feet are slid along the costal margin to the notch in the center of the chest, where the sternum and ribs join. **B.** The middle finger is placed high into the notch. The index finger is placed just above the middle finger, on the lower portion of the sternum. **C.** The heel of the second hand is placed on the lower portion of the sternum, touching the index finger of the first hand. **D.** The first hand is then removed from the notch and applied over and parallel to the hand on the patient's chest. **E.** Rescuer's shoulders are directly over the patient's mid chest. (From *Emergency Care and Transportation of the Sick and Injured,* 2nd ed. American Academy of Orthopaedic Surgeons, 430 North Michigan Ave., Chicago, 1977, pp. 96, 97.)

Ineffective Resuscitation. Unfortunately, resuscitation does not always succeed in reviving the patient. Factors responsible for *ineffective resuscitation* include the following:

1. Incorrect resuscitative techniques.
2. Heart is drained of its blood by hemorrhage or cardiac tamponade.
3. Blood supply to the heart is obstructed by presence of a pulmonary embolus.
4. Severe chronic lung disease has destroyed lung's capacity to oxygenate blood.
5. Lungs are filled with vomitus as a result of aspiration during cardiac massage.

Ineffective resuscitation is characterized by continuous coma, absence of compression pulsations, and persistence of dilated pupils. Even though resuscitation appears to be ineffective, authorities recommend that the resuscitation effort continue for at least one hour following the initiation of resuscitation procedures.

SPECIFIC MEDICAL THERAPY

Definitive medical therapy commences once the patient has either been admitted to the emergency room or a special resuscitation team has arrived to take over the patient's care. At this time, three considerations become paramount:[40] (1) What is the underlying cause of the cardiac arrest and can it be corrected? (2) What type of arrest has occurred? Is asystole or ventricular fibrillation present? (3) What treatment should be instituted?

Continued Resuscitation Efforts. While some resuscitation team members prepare drugs, IV infusions, the defibrillator, and so forth, two team members must continue to give the patient cardiac massage and respiratory assistance.

> *Cardiopulmonary resuscitation must* never *be interrupted to perform other procedures for more than 5 seconds at a time!*

Interruption of resuscitation procedures can result in a further loss of valuable oxygen to the brain.

Drug Therapy. The major drugs used during cardiopulmonary resuscitation are discussed in Table 35–5.

Electrocardiogram. The typical ECG reading during cardiac arrest is diagnostic of ventricular fibrillation; less commonly a reading will show asystole or a complete lack of wave configurations. However, an ECG may be normal in

TABLE 35–5. DRUGS USED IN CARDIAC RESUSCITATION

Drug*	Route of Administration	Uses in Cardiac Resuscitation
Epinephrine	Administered directly into myocardium with 3.5-inch 22-gauge needle (intracardiac) or IV push	Stimulates heart action; strengthens contractions of the heart; converts fine ventricular fibrillation to coarse ventricular fibrillation, thus allowing for easier defibrillation
Isoproterenol (Isuprel)	IV drip	Increases irritability and contractility of the myocardium; beneficial in treatment of complete asystole
10% Calcium chloride or Calcium gluconate	IV	Strengthens cardiac contractions
Sodium bicarbonate	IV	Corrects metabolic acidosis that develops due to tissue anoxia
Metaraminol (Aramine)	IV drip	Corrects severe hypotension, shock, and cardiovascular collapse
Lidocaine (Xylocaine) 1% solution	IV push	Used to treat ventricular arrhythmias
Lidocaine 4%	IV drip	Controls ventricular arrhythmias
Dopamine (Intropin)	IV drip	Increases BP by increasing strength of myocardial contraction; produces mild vasoconstriction in skeletal muscles; selectively dilates mesenteric and renal vessels
Bretylium tosylate (Bretylol)	IV push	For ventricular fibrillation that is not responsive to normal antiarrhythmic therapy
	IV drip	For ventricular tachycardia unresponsive to normal antiarrhythmic therapy

*Many of these emergency drugs are available in pre-filled syringes to facilitate their administration during cardiac resuscitation.

appearance although the heart is actually pumping very feebly with little cardiac output. Thus, ECG tracings cannot be used to rule out the possibility of cardiac arrest.

Remember that ECG tracings show only the electrical activity of the heart; they cannot serve as a guide to the heart's pumping efficiency.

Precordial Shock. When the patient's heart is in ventricular fibrillation, the doctor uses a direct current (D.C.) defibrillator to shock the heart, thereby halting the chaotic bizarre movement of the ventricles. The defibrillator is not used when the heart is in complete asystole, as defibrillation has no effect on cardiac standstill.

Oxygen. The patient is given 100 per cent oxygen by means of an endotracheal tube in order to fully oxygenate the brain and other vital organs.

Nasogastric Intubation. The patient with a full stomach is intubated at once to prevent vomiting and aspiration of vomitus. Even patients with an empty stomach often require intubation, because gastric dilatation may result from mouth-to-mouth and mouth-to-nose resuscitation.

POSTRESUSCITATION MEASURES

Skilled aftercare of the patient who has suffered cardiac arrest is crucial to survival. Typical orders and their rationale are given below:

1. If not already in the ICU or CCU the patient is admitted there because of the need for constant observation, monitoring equipment, defibrillators, and so forth.
2. Monitoring of the ECG, CVP, and blood pressure is instituted.
3. Temperature is taken every hour. A high temperature usually indicates cerebral damage or cerebral edema.
4. A hypothermia blanket is used if temperature is over 101°F. or 38.5°C. Hypothermia helps to lessen cerebral edema.
5. Blood gas and pH determinations are done to detect metabolic acidosis, which may have developed owing to poor tissue oxygenation during arrest. If the tissues are not properly oxygenated, anaerobic instead of aerobic oxidation takes place. Lactic acid is produced during anaerobic oxidation and this leads to a metabolic acidosis.
6. Amobarbital sodium is given intravenously in case of convulsions, which may occur because of brain damage or acidosis. Dilantin is given if convulsions continue.
7. A chest x-ray film is obtained using portable equipment. Ribs often are accidentally fractured during cardiac massage.
8. Insert endotracheal tube if not already in place. This maintains an open airway for the unconscious patient who cannot clear secretions by coughing.
9. Give oxygen continuously for 48 hours following resuscitation, by endotracheal tube or mask. This is required because respirations are depressed for some time after arrest.
10. Insert Foley catheter. Urine output is one measure of cardiovascular status. A very low urine output after cardiac arrest indicates cardiovascular collapse. Notify the physician if the urinary output is below 30 ml. per hour.

COMPLICATIONS

The patient may develop complications due to the cardiac arrest itself or as a result of the resuscitation measures used to save his life. Common complications are the following:

Pneumothorax as a result of ribs fractured during cardiac massage.

Hemorrhage from a ruptured liver or spleen due to faulty resuscitation techniques. Damage to liver and spleen can occur if the resuscitator applies pressure over the epigastrum rather than over the sternum.

Brain damage as a result of cerebral hypoxia.

Seizures due to either brain damage or metabolic acidosis.

PSYCHOLOGIC SUPPORT

Although it is easy to forget, the need for psychologic support for the patient and significant others during cardiac emergencies is extremely important. Talk as though the patient were completely awake and alert. Advise the patient in advance of the various procedures that will follow. Be specific, e.g., "You will feel a needle stick in your left arm." Many patients who have been resuscitated have a very clear recall of the events surrounding the resuscitation, including the verbal communication that occurred. Keep your voice well modulated and communicate in a calm, clear manner. Insure, too, that the spiritual needs of the patient and significant others have been met.

CHAPTER 36

CORONARY HEART DISEASE

For the heart muscle to contract properly, it must have an adequate blood supply. You will recall from Chapter 31 that the myocardium receives its blood supply from the coronary arteries. Should one or both of these arteries be blocked for any reason or should collateral circulation fail to develop, ischemia and infarction of the heart muscle are inevitable. The *major disorders* resulting from an insufficient blood supply to the myocardium are arteriosclerotic heart disease, angina pectoris, coronary insufficiency, and myocardial infarction; all these entities are grouped under the term *coronary heart disease* (CHD), also known as coronary artery disease (CAD) and ischemic heart disease (IHD).

Blockage of blood to the myocardium may be partial and temporary (e.g., angina pectoris) or complete and protracted (e.g., myocardial infarction).

OVERVIEW OF CORONARY HEART DISEASE

Incidence of CHD[56, 196, 241]

> *Coronary heart disease ranks* first *as a cause of death among persons in North America and Western Europe.*

Although between 1963 and 1973 coronary mortality rates declined 18.4 per cent among persons aged 35 to 74 years, over a million people continue to die every year of CHD and its complications. One of every five men in the United States develops CHD before the age of 60. Furthermore, researchers estimate that 3.1 million Americans over 18 years old definitely have CHD and 2.4 million probably do. For persons between 20 and 64 years old, CHD is the most common cause of death.

Death rates due to CHD are influenced by the age, sex, and race of patients and the social and economic environment in which they live.

- *Age.* Pathologic changes within the coronary arteries, which are severe enough to cause symptoms, appear predominantly in persons over age 40. However, individuals in their 30's and even 20's have been known to suffer anginal attacks or myocardial infarction.
- *Sex.* As a group, men are *four* times as likely to suffer from CHD as are women. However, this marked difference in susceptibility to CHD between the sexes decreases as age increases. For example, men below the age of 40 are much more likely to be stricken with CHD than are young women; however, by the age of 70, almost as many women as men are diagnosed with CHD. Also, women who take oral contraceptives are more likely to develop CHD, whereas women with an early menopause experience a three times greater risk of CHD than do women with a normal or late menopause.
- *Race.* White men die more frequently from CHD than do nonwhites. On the other hand, the rate of deaths among white women is generally a little lower than among nonwhite women. However, among elderly women death rates tend to be about the same for both whites and nonwhites.
- *Environment.* CHD is seven times more prevalent in North America, Australia, Europe, and New Zealand than in Japan, Africa, and South America. Also, incidence is higher among urban populations than among those in rural areas.

Causative and Precipitating Factors

The major cause of CHD is the development of *obliterative atherosclerotic* lesions within the coronary arteries, which act to narrow or obstruct these vital vessels.

> Atherosclerosis, *a disorder of lipid metabolism (characterized by deposits of fat-containing substances along the intima of blood vessels), is the commonest underlying cause of cardiovascular disease and death.*

In fact, 99 per cent of all cases are caused by narrowing of the coronary arteries due to atherosclerotic changes. Other, rare causes of CHD are (1) congenital abnormalities of the arteries; (2) luetic changes in the arteries due to earlier syphilitic infection; (3) vascular changes due to autoimmune disorders; and (4) coronary embolism.

Predisposing Factors. Robbins and Cotran explain the *pathogenesis* of coronary heart disease (ischemic heart disease) as follows: "The pathogenesis of all forms of IHD at the most fundamental level is an imbalance between myocardial oxygen supply and demand. Three factors are involved: (a) the adequacy of the coronary arterial flow, (b) the level of myocardial metabolic demands, and (c) the oxygen transport capacity of the blood. Among these the first is overwhelmingly the most important."[199]

Factors which apparently precipitate the onset of CHD include:

Personal Factors

1. *Genetic predisposition:* Frequently members of the patient's family have suffered from CHD at an early age.

2. Certain *personality traits:* Hard driving, competitive individuals who worry excessively about deadlines and who consistently overwork are *possibly* more prone to coronary disease. These persons are said to have Type A personalities and are described in Chapter 6.

3. *Professional stresses:* Doctors and executives seem to be more readily stricken with CHD than persons with occupations imposing less responsibility.

Disease Patterns

1. *Hypertension:* Sustained BP of over 160/95 mm. Hg. Compared to a person with a systolic blood pressure of 120 mm. Hg, an individual with a systolic blood pressure over 150 mm. Hg faces *double* the risk of suffering a heart attack.

2. *Obesity:* Weight 30 per cent or more above that considered standard for an individual of a certain height and build.

3. *Lipid abnormalities:* Serum cholesterol of over 200 mg. per 100 ml., or a fasting triglyceride of more than 250 mg. per 100 ml.

Currently it seems clear that elevated serum lipids (lipoproteins) are associated with an increased risk of atherosclerotic heart disease and peripheral vascular disease. An elevation of lipoproteins is called *hyperlipoproteinemia.* When only one of the classes of lipoproteins is elevated, the condition is called *hyperlipidemia.*[141]

Lipoproteins in the plasma are produced in the intestinal wall following the ingestion, digestion, and absorption of exogenous fat after eating, and in the liver. The five basic groups of lipoproteins classified according to lipid content are (a) *chylomicrons* which have the highest lipid content and the lowest density, (b) *very low–density lipoproteins* (VLDL) which have a large lipid content plus around 20 per cent cholesterol, (c) *low-density lipoproteins* (LDL) which carry at least two thirds of the plasma cholesterol, (d) *intermediate-density lipoprotein* (IDL), and (e) *high-density lipoproteins* (HDL) which carry more protein and less lipid.[249] The five types of hyperlipoproteinemia abnormalities and their clinical features are outlined in Table 36–1.

Recent investigations have documented the difference between high- and low-density lipoproteins (HDL and LDL) in predisposing persons to heart disease. Persons with high serum levels of HDL in proportion to LDL are less likely to develop CHD than persons with low HDL. It appears that HDL may even protect individuals against CHD and that the cholesterol carried in HDL does not become incorporated into atheroma (fatty plaques which form within the intima of blood vessels) as does LDL.[141, 253]

4. *Diabetes:* Fasting blood sugar of more than 120 mg./dl., or a routine blood sugar of 180 mg./dl.; evidence of sugar in the urine; decreased glucose tolerance.

TABLE 36–1. TYPES OF HYPERLIPOPROTEINEMIA

Type	Abnormality	Clinical Features	Differential Diagnosis
I	↑ Chylomicrons	Abdominal pain, pancreatitis, eruptive xanthomas, lipemia retinalis	Insulinopenic diabetes, dysglobulinemia, lupus erythematosus
II	IIa: ↑ LDL IIb: ↑ LDL + VLDL	Tendinous and tuberous xanthomas, xanthelasma, premature corneal arcus, premature vascular disease	Obstructive liver disease, hypothyroidism, nephrosis, porphyria, myxedema
III	↑ IDL	Glucose intolerance, unusual palmar deposits, tuberous xanthomas, premature vascular disease	Myxedema, dysgammaglobulinemia, possibly hypothyroidism
IV	↑ VLDL	Glucose intolerance, obesity, hyperuricemia, rare eruptive xanthomas	Diabetes, nephrosis, pregnancy, stress, glycogen storage disease, alcoholism
V	↑ VLDL + chylomicrons	Abdominal pain, pancreatitis, hepatosplenomegaly, eruptive xanthomas, sensory neuropathy, lipemia retinalis, obesity, glucose intolerance, hyperuricemia	Insulinopenic diabetes, nephrosis, alcoholism, myeloma

From Levy, R.I.: Hyperlipoproteinemia: From trial and error toward scientific precision. *Consultant,* 7:32, Oct. 1978, p. 32.

5. *Gout:* Uric acid level elevated over 7.5 mg./dl.; past history of gout.

6. *ECG abnormalities:* e.g., left ventricular hypertrophy, intraventricular block, unexplained atrial fibrillation, myocardial infarction. Persons with left ventricular hypertrophy have a four times higher mortality rate than do persons without this finding.

Adverse Environmental Problems

1. *Heavy cigarette smoking:* Evidently large amounts of nicotine absorbed into the blood stream may severely damage blood elements or the intima of arteries. Smoking two packs of cigarettes per day causes the incidence of CHD to increase four-fold.

2. *Sedentary occupation and life style:* Lack of exercise tends to promote mental depression and obesity.

3. *Stressful situations:* Emotional problems tend to indirectly promote compensatory overeating and excessive drinking and smoking. Also, nervous tension elevates blood pressure. However, to what extent emotional stress may *directly* cause CHD is still not known, and all theories are highly speculative.

4. *High-caloric, high-fat diet:* Overeating and consuming fatty rich foods promotes obesity, lipid abnormalities, and diabetes.

The major risk factors for CHD are shown in Figure 36–1. Hypertension and heavy smoking are two risks which have the greatest predictive value, "the presence of which results in a five-fold increase in incidence of atherosclerosis as compared to that in individuals with neither of these risk factors."[196]

Manifestations of CHD. As we stated earlier, the major cause of CHD is the development of obstructive atherosclerotic plaques in the coronary arteries (arteriosclerotic heart disease). Usually, symptoms of CHD do not appear until the lumen of the coronary artery is narrowed by 75 per cent.

> *Manifestations of CHD may take three basic forms: (1) angina pectoris, (2) acute myocardial infarction, and (3) sudden death.*

In addition, patients may develop heart failure, chronic arrhythmias, conduction disturbances, and a condition known as unstable angina or intermittent coronary syndrome which we describe later.

Myocardial infarction (i.e., heart attack) is the most common sign of CHD for which patients seek professional help. Each year over a million myocardial infarctions occur, with a survival rate of only 60 per cent. One quarter of myocardial infarctions do not produce symptoms (silent MI) and are diagnosed only by an ECG reading.

Angina pectoris which is characterized by transient attacks of substernal or precordial pain, is not nearly as common as myocardial infarction or sudden coronary death. Persons with newly diagnosed angina pectoris constitute only about

Nonmodifiable Risk Factors	Modifiable Risk Factors
	Major
1. Age	1. Elevated serum cholesterol and triglycerides
2. Sex	2. Habitual diet high in total calories, fats, cholesterol, carbohydrates, and salt
3. Familial history	3. Hypertension
	4. Cigarette smoking
	5. Carbohydrate intolerance
	Minor
	1. Obesity
	2. Sedentary living
	3. Personality type
	4. Psychosocial tensions

Figure 36–1. Risk factors for coronary heart disease. (Adapted from Hurst, J. W., et al.: *The Heart,* 3rd ed. McGraw Hill: New York, 1974.

one fourth of those who experience sudden death due to CHD.

Sudden death is the most typical manifestation of CHD when sudden death is defined as "death within the first 24 hours of the onset of symptoms, whether or not associated with myocardial infarction."[196] Approximately 65 per cent of persons who die suddenly and unexpectedly from CHD usually do so outside the hospital. For one fifth of these persons, sudden death is the first and only manifestation of CHD. In these cases, death usually results from ventricular fibrillation.

Diagnosis of CHD. The two major goals of diagnosis in CHD are to identify individuals with CHD, and to assess risk factors. Briefly outlined are the most important diagnostic techniques used:[13, 196]

Clinical history and careful assessment of life style.

Physical examination.

ECG, phonocardiography, apexcardiography.

Exercise stress testing.

Blood tests for lipoproteins and glucose.

Quantification of risk. The more risk factors a patient presents, the greater the chances of developing CHD. Recall that the risk factors most predictive of CHD are hypertension and heavy smoking, together.

Cardiac catheterization to assess the function of the left ventricle.

Coronary angiography to identify lesions in the coronary arteries.

These tests are discussed in Chapter 33 and mentioned again throughout the chapter.

Prevention and General Treatment of CHD

Concerning prevention, Kannel writes: "Preventive approaches to cardiovascular disease should include a public health approach to alter the ecology to one more favorable to cardiovascular health, hygienic measures initiated by an informed public on its own behalf, and preventive medicine for highly vulnerable persons. . . . If the appalling toll of cardiovascular disease is to be halted, more must be learned about the influences that promote the risk factors, and steps must be taken to prevent or correct these influences."[117]

A typical prevention and treatment program includes the following factors:

WEIGHT REDUCTION. This is achieved by means of a low-calorie diet. Instruct the patient to reduce *gradually*. Rapid weight loss can suddenly overload the blood with an excess of fatty substances which can, in turn, precipitate an anginal attack or a myocardial infarction. Patients with hypertension should be advised to restrict their salt as well as caloric intake.

MODIFIED LOW-CHOLESTEROL DIET. To reduce elevated serum lipid levels, patients generally restrict their intake of saturated fat, cholesterol, and simple sugars, and substitute *polyunsaturated* fats for saturated fat whenever possible. Recommended diets for the five types of hyperlipoproteinemia are summarized in Table 36–2. It is important to remember, however, that the role of diet in the pathogenesis of CHD is still controversial.

AVOID STRESS. Avoidance of situations that can precipitate anginal attacks is imperative. Patients should avoid large, heavy meals, intense emotional states, unusual strenuous exercise, and excessively hot or cold environments. Methods for reducing emotional stress are also outlined in Chapter 6.

CORRECTION OF PREEXISTING MEDICAL PROBLEMS. Treat problems that might contribute to the development of CHD (e.g., hypertension, anemia, hyperthyroidism, aortic valvular disease).

TABLE 36–2. DIETS FOR PRIMARY HYPERLIPOPROTEINEMIA

Factor	Type I	Type II	Type III	Type IV	Type V
Dietary prescription	Low fat (25 to 35 Gm.)	Low cholesterol, polyunsaturated fat increased	Low cholesterol; caloric distribution about 20% protein, 40% fat, 40% carbohydrate	Controlled carbohydrate (about 40% to 45% of calories), moderately restricted cholesterol	Restricted fat (30% of calories), controlled carbohydrate (50%), moderately restricted cholesterol
Calories	Not restricted	Not restricted except in type IIb, where weight reduction is often indicated	Achieve and maintain "ideal" weight; reducing diet if necessary	Achieve and maintain "ideal" weight; reducing diet if necessary	Achieve and maintain "ideal" weight; reducing diet if necessary
Protein	Total intake not limited	Total intake not limited	High intake	Not limited other than for weight control	High intake
Fat	Restricted to 25 to 35 Gm.; kind of fat not important	Intake of saturated fat limited; intake of polyunsaturated fat increased	Controlled to 40% to 45% of calories (polyunsaturated fat recommended in preference to saturated fat)	Not limited other than for weight control (polyunsaturated fat recommended in preference to saturated fat)	Restricted to 30% of calories (polyunsaturated fat recommended in preference to saturated fat)
Cholesterol	Not restricted	Less than 300 mg. or as low an intake as possible; only source is meat	Less than 300 mg.; only source is meat	Moderately restricted to 300 to 500 mg.	Moderately restricted to 300 to 500 mg.
Carbohydrate	Not restricted	Not restricted (may be controlled in type IIb)	Controlled; most concentrated sweets eliminated	Controlled; most concentrated sweets eliminated	Controlled; most concentrated sweets eliminated
Alcohol	Not recommended	May be used with discretion	Limited to two servings (substituted for carbohydrate)	Limited to two servings (substituted for carbohydrate)	Not recommended

From Levy, R.I.: Hyperlipoproteinemia: From trial and error toward scientific precision. *Consultant*, 7:32, Oct. 1978, p. 37.

Physical Examination. Yearly physical examinations and additional examinations are given as necessary; persons with recurrent indigestion, "heartburn," chest pain, and pain above the waistline that is associated with activity or emotional stress should see their physician.

Drug and Hormonal Therapy. *Anticoagulants* are used to treat and to prevent thrombosis. *Heparin* and *estrogens* have beneficial effects upon blood lipoproteins; however, these drugs have dangerous side effects. Heparin can cause bleeding, hematoma at the injection site, and dangerous allergic reactions. Estrogens can cause menorrhagia, breast soreness, and edema. *Nicotinic acid* given orally in large doses (3 to 6 Gm. daily in divided doses) substantially reduces serum cholesterol levels. Side effects are gastrointestinal irritation, nausea, vomiting, and diarrhea. *Thyroid* extract also lowers serum cholesterol but produces many undesirable side effects, e.g., nervousness, insomnia, palpitations.

Exercise. Regular exercise improves myocardial efficiency and reduces the many risk factors associated with the development of CHD. Payne states: "Indeed, a recent study has shown that lack of exercise may be the single risk factor that most clearly indicates a future manifestation of coronary heart disease."[188]

The ideal exercise for promoting myocardial efficiency and preventing CHD is *aerobic exercise.* Aerobic exercise is ". . . any activity that stimulates heart and lung activity sufficiently to increase oxygen uptake and delivery to body tissues, an adaptation which occurs over a period of weeks."[188]

For the prevention of heart disease, the following four characteristics of exercise must be considered:[56]

1. *Type of exercise:* Suitable exercises for stimulating cardiovascular and respiratory fitness include walking, jogging, swimming, cross-country skiing, rope jumping, bicycling, and so on. The relative merits of various exercises in inducing cardiovascular fitness are outlined in Table 36–3.
2. *Frequency:* A person should engage in at least three exercise sessions per week.
3. *Duration:* For cardiovascular training, 15 to 60 minutes of continuous exercise are required.
4. *Intensity:* Exercise should be sufficiently intensive to maintain the person's heart beat at 70 to 80 per cent of its maximum rate. However, it is important to instruct patients not to exceed this intensity level.

Any person starting a serious physical fitness program needs to be thoroughly instructed in how to exercise safely and efficiently. The following points are important:

- ▶ Each *exercise period* should consist of (a) 5 minutes of *warm-up exercises* (calisthenics, stretching); (b) 20 to 60 minutes of *aerobic exercises* at a heart rate of 70 to 80 per cent of maximum; and (c) 5 minutes of *cool-down exercises* (calisthenics, stretching exercises).
- ▶ An exercise program should begin *slowly;* beginners with heart disease must exercise at an intensity which does not produce dyspnea and at which they can still carry on a conversation.
- ▶ An exercise program should ideally be scheduled on a regular basis and at a definite time of the day. Spasmodic exercise sessions are not beneficial and may, in fact, be harmful.

Surgical Techniques. The goals of surgery in managing patients with CHD are to relieve pain, reduce the heart's workload, and supply the heart muscle with sufficient blood to carry on its tasks. Today surgeons seek to control CHD by increasing the bloodflow to the heart by means of a *coronary artery bypass graft.* As the disease usually involves the proximal one third to one half of the coronary artery, it is possible to enhance the circulation by using a graft from the saphenous vein to connect the aorta to the distal portion of the occluded vessel (see Figure 36–2).

Coronary bypass surgery has proved highly beneficial in relieving the symptoms of CHD. Indeed, in 90 per cent of patients, it relieves the pain of angina pectoris. Furthermore, there is increasing evidence that coronary bypass surgery prolongs life significantly in certain subgroups of coronary patients. For example, in a randomized study by the Veterans Administration, the lives of patients with left main artery occlusion were clearly prolonged in comparison to patients treated medically.[126] (See Figure 36–3). However, despite its benefits, this procedure does have its risks and is not universally accepted.

Forms of CHD

The major forms of CHD are (1) arteriosclerotic heart disease (ASHD), also known as obliterative atherosclerotic heart disease; (2) angina pectoris; (3) coronary insufficiency; and (4) myocardial infarction (MI).

Authorities disagree concerning the classification of these disorders. Some group angina pectoris, coronary insufficiency, and MI under ASHD. Others consider ASHD to be a specific type of CHD which differs in its manifestations from the other conditions listed. However, all authorities agree that there is much overlap between these disorders. Thus, some view ASHD, angina pectoris, coronary insufficiency, and MI as *stages* within a common, continuous disease process; this is the viewpoint we assume in this unit.

TABLE 36-3. RELATIVE MERITS OF VARIOUS EXERCISES IN INDUCING CARDIOVASCULAR FITNESS

Energy Range	Activity	Comment
1.5-2.0 Mets* or 2.0-2.5 Cals/min. or 120-150 Cals/hr.	Light housework such as polishing furniture or washing small clothes	Too low in energy level and too intermittent to promote endurance.
	Strolling 1.0 mile/hr.	Not sufficiently strenuous to promote endurance unless capacity is very low.
2.0-3.0 Mets or 2.5-4.0 Cals/min. or 150-250 Cals/hr.	Level walking at 2.0 miles/hr.	See "strolling".
	Golf, using power cart	Promotes skill and minimal strength in arm muscles but not sufficiently taxing to promote endurance. Also too intermittent.
3.0-4.0 Mets or 4-5 Cals/min. or 240-300 Cals/hr.	Cleaning windows, mopping floors, or vacuuming	Adequate condition exercise if carried out continuously for 20-30 minutes.
	Bowling	Too intermittent and not sufficiently taxing to promote endurance.
	Walking at 3.0 miles/hr.	Adequate dynamic exercise if low capacity.
	Cycling at 6 miles/hr.	As above.
	Golf—pulling cart	Useful for conditioning if reach target rate. May include isometrics depending on cart weight.
4.0-5.0 Mets or 5-6 Cals/min. or 300-360 Cals/hr.	Scrubbing floors	Adequate endurance exercise if carried out in at least 2 minutes stints.
	Walking 3.5 miles/hr.	Usually good dynamic aerobic exercise.
	Cycling 8 miles/hr.	As above.
	Table tennis, badminton and volleyball	Vigorous continuous play can have endurance benefits but intermittent, easy play only promotes skill.
	Golf—carrying clubs	Promotes endurance if reach and maintain target heart rate, otherwise merely aids strength and skill.
	Tennis—doubles	Not very beneficial unless there is continuous play maintaining target rate—which is unlikely. Will aid skill.
	Many calisthenics and ballet exercises	Will promote endurance if continuous, rhythmic and repetitive. Those requiring isometric effort such as push-ups and sit-ups are probably not beneficial for cardiovascular fitness.

*Met = multiple of the resting energy requirement; e.g. 2 Mets require twice the resting energy cost, 3 Mets triple, etc. (From Dedmon, R. E.: A prescription for fitness. *Consultant,* 18:44, November, 1978.)

ARTERIOSCLEROTIC HEART DISEASE (ASHD)

Arteriosclerotic heart disease (ASHD)* is a slowly progressive heart condition characterized by (1) internal thickening and plaque formation within the coronary arteries due to the deposition of fatty substances along the intima; (2) resultant fibrosis, calcification, and narrowing of the coronary arteries; and (3) a slow constriction of the blood supply to the myocardium, which can finally give rise to symptoms of angina.

Atherosclerotic changes within the coronary vessels as well as within the aorta and cerebral vessels generally occur in the following three stages:

Stage 1: Fatty Streak Formation. Fatty streaks, which

*ASHD is one type of obliterative atherosclerosis. Obliterative atherosclerosis occurs not only in the heart, but also affects the aorta and the larger arteries of the brain. In this unit, obliterative atherosclerosis is discussed only in relation to heart disease.

TABLE 36–3. RELATIVE MERITS OF VARIOUS EXERCISES IN INDUCING CARDIOVASCULAR FITNESS (*Continued*)

Energy Range	Activity	Comment
5.0-6.0 Mets or 6-7 Cals/min. or 360-420 Cals/hr.	Walking 4 miles/hr.	Dynamic, aerobic and of benefit.
	Cycling 10 miles/hr.	As above.
	Ice or roller skating	As above if done continuously.
6.0-7.0 Mets or 7-8 Cals/min. or 420-480 Cals/hr.	Walking 5 miles/hr.	Dynamic, aerobic and beneficial.
	Cycling 11 miles/hr.	Same.
	Singles tennis	Can provide benefit if played 30 minutes or more by skilled player with an attempt to keep moving.
	Water skiing	Total isometrics; very risky for cardiacs, pre-cardiacs (high risk) or deconditioned normals.
7.0-8.0 Mets or 8-10 Cals/min. or 480-600 Cals/hr.	Jogging 5 miles/hr.	Dynamic, aerobic, endurance building exercise.
	Cycling 12 miles/hr.	As above.
	Downhill skiing	Usually ski runs are too short to significantly promote endurance. Lift may be isometric. Benefits skill predominantly. Combined stress of altitude, cold and exercise may be too great for some cardiacs.
	Paddleball	Not sufficiently continuous but promotes skill. Competition and hot playing areas may be dangerous to cardiacs.
8.0-9.0 Mets or 10-11 Cals/min. or 600-660 Cals/hr.	Running 5.5 miles/hr.	Excellent conditioner.
	Cycling 13 miles/hr	As above.
	Squash or handball (practice session or warmup)	Usually too intermittent to provide endurance building effect. Promotes skill.
Above 10 Mets or 11 Cals/min. or 660 Cals/hr.	Running 6 miles/hr. = 10 Mets 7 miles/hr. = 11.5 8 miles/hr. = 13.5	Excellent conditioner.
	Competitive handball or squash	Competitive environment in a hot room is dangerous to anyone not in excellent physical condition. Same as singles tennis.

Note: Energy range will vary depending on skill of exerciser, pattern of rest pauses, environmental temperature, etc. Caloric values depend on body size (more for larger person). Table provides reasonable "relative stenuousness values" however.

Reprinted from *Beyond Diet . . . Exercise Your Way to Fitness and Heart Health,* by Lenore R. Zohman, M.D. Copyright CPC International, Inc., Englewood Cliffs, N.J.

are thin, slightly elevated, smooth, yellow lines or dots, first appear during childhood. In some cases, these streaks regress completely.

Stage 2: Fibrous Plaque Formation. The development of fibrous plaques reflects both a low-grade inflammatory reaction and a healing response. When this stage is reached, there is likelihood of further progression of the disease.

Stage 3: Stage of Complication. This stage involves necrosis, calcification, and vascularization of the plaque, with or without hemorrhage into the plaque. Such changes predispose to thrombosis.

The various types of atherosclerotic lesions which develop during these stages are illustrated in Figure 36–4.

ASHD is the *most common clinical form of CHD.* Predisposing factors leading to ASHD are the same as those related to CHD.

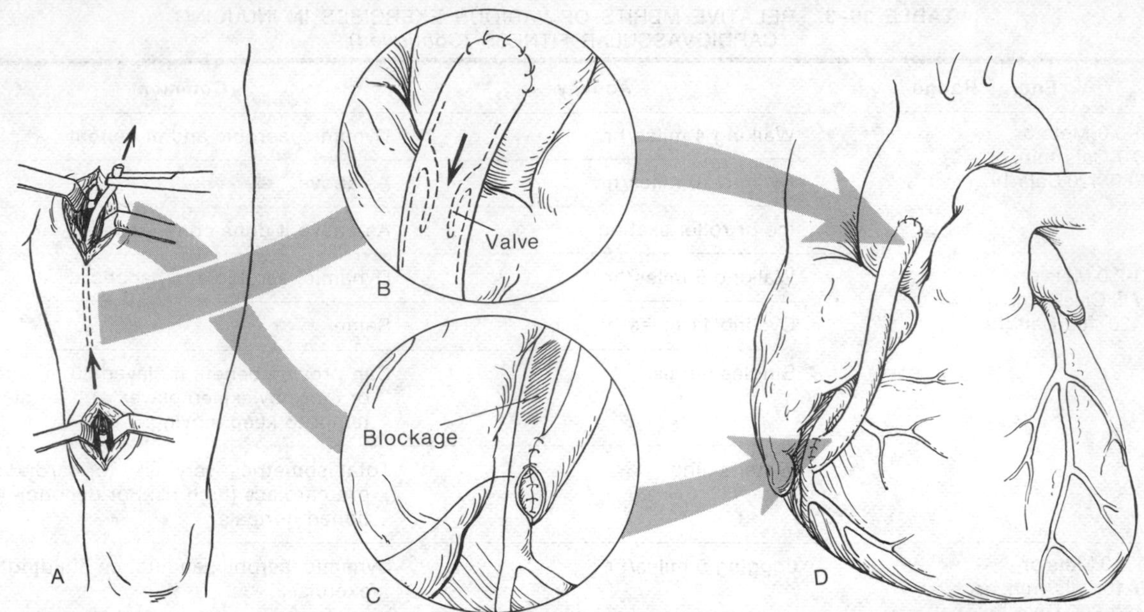

Figure 36–2. Saphenous vein revascularization surgery. **A.** A section of the saphenous vein is taken from the patient's leg; to prevent interference with blood flow, the valves are reversed. **B.** The distal end of the saphenous graft is sutured to the ascending aorta. **C.** The vein is next sutured to the coronary artery at a point below the blockage. **D.** Circulation is now reestablished.

Theories of Causation

Although it is a dangerous, crippling, and often deadly disease, the exact cause of atherosclerosis is unfortunately unknown. More questions have been posed than answers given, and conflicting etiologic theories are constantly argued. The most pertinent questions troubling medical researchers are these:

1. Is atherosclerosis an integral, uncontrollable part of the aging process? Or is atherosclerosis a pathologic condition resulting from disease-producing factors that are subject to human control?

2. Are the atherosclerotic changes within the major blood vessels the result of primary abnormalities of the vessels themselves? Or do the atherosclerotic changes in the vessel walls develop secondary to a primary metabolic abnormality that is present elsewhere in the body?

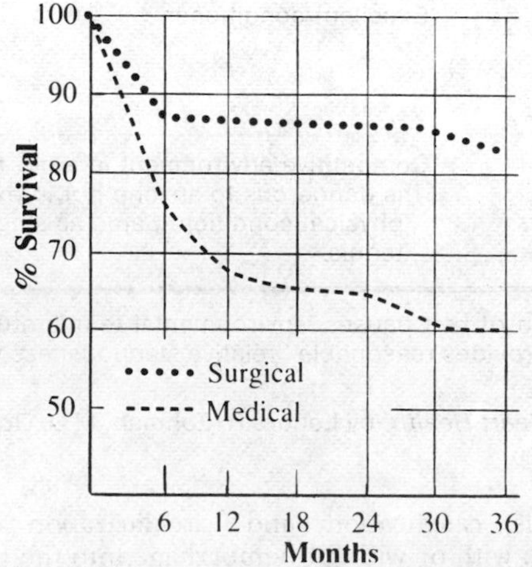

Figure 36–3. Results of the Veterans Administration randomized study, showing survival rates of patients with left main coronary artery disease treated surgically and medically. (From Takaro, T., H. N. Hulgren, M. J. Lipton, et al.: The VA Cooperative randomized study of surgery for coronary arterial occlusive disease. II. Subgroup with significant left main lesions. *Circulation*, 54(Suppl. III): III-107, 1976.)

In an attempt to answer these questions several theories have evolved — the aging theory, the metabolic theory, the stress theory, the hormonal theory, the viral or toxic agent theory, and the multifactoral theory.

According to the *aging theory*, the development of atherosclerotic changes within the arteries is a normal part of aging, which affects *all* persons to a greater or lesser degree. Some authorities believe that atherosclerotic changes begin even in the very young, and that these changes almost universally affect persons over age 20. Objections to the aging theory are based mainly on findings at autopsy; some elderly persons show no signs of atherosclerotic changes at autopsy, whereas young persons may show severe atherosclerotic changes.

Advocates of the *metabolic* theory state that atherosclerosis is the result of disturbances in *lipid metabolism* — in particular, cholesterol metabolism. Large numbers of research projects and studies have focused upon the role of cholesterol in the causation of atherosclerosis. Evidence for the metabolic theory:

1. Laboratory analysis of atherosclerotic lesions reveals the presence of large amounts of lipids, especially cholesterol esters and free cholesterol.

2. Numerous population studies conducted throughout the world show a correlation between *elevated serum cholesterol levels* and the development of CHD.* For example, advocates of the metabolic theory point out that serum cholesterol levels are as high as 200 to 250 mg./dl. In the United States where the disease is common, whereas serum cholesterol levels are as low as 100 to 150 mg./dl. in Japan and Korea where the disease is uncommon.

3. Other comparative population studies reveal a correlation between a *high intake of animal fats* and the development of atherosclerosis. For example, deaths from CHD were statistically lower during World War II when fatty foods were scarce than during postwar years. Figure 36–5 dramatically demonstrates the fall in deaths due to cardiovascular illness during World War II. With the postwar improvement in the economy, both the consumption of animal fat and the death rate from atherosclerosis rose. Another study comparing Japanese populations living in Japan, Hawaii, and Los Angeles revealed that CHD is relatively low among Japanese living in Japan, and moderately high among the Japanese in Hawaii; Japanese living in Los Angeles (Nisei) had rates comparable to those of the Caucasian population.

Other observers believe that the high incidence of atherosclerosis among persons in the United States, Denmark, and other highly technological countries is due to the economic and social *stresses* that are so abundant in Western civilization. Supporters of this theory point out that ASHD occurs far less frequently among less technological peoples. However, advocates of the "stress theory" cannot explain precisely how life stresses cause atherosclerotic changes within the major arteries. Anxiety and stress may well increase the needs of the heart for blood over and above the normal demands; however, it is not likely that stress could cause hemorrhage into an atheroma or rupture of a plaque.

Others point to *endocrine factors* — in particular, the *estrogens* — as a possible explanation for the onset and progress of atherosclerosis. The theory that sex hormones play an important role in the development of atherosclerosis rests upon the following evidence:

1. Atherosclerosis is prevalent among men, whereas women *prior* to the menopause are relatively immune to the process.

2. Young women (prior to the menopause) have a lower serum level of certain types of lipoprotein than do young men.

3. Serum levels of lipoprotein tend to equalize between the sexes during the years following the women's menopause; also, during the middle and late periods of life, atherosclerosis is equally prevalent among members of both sexes.

On the basis of these facts, some authorities conclude that the estrogenic hormones affect the release and distribution of plasma lipoproteins, which, in turn, influence the time of onset of atherosclerosis in each sex.

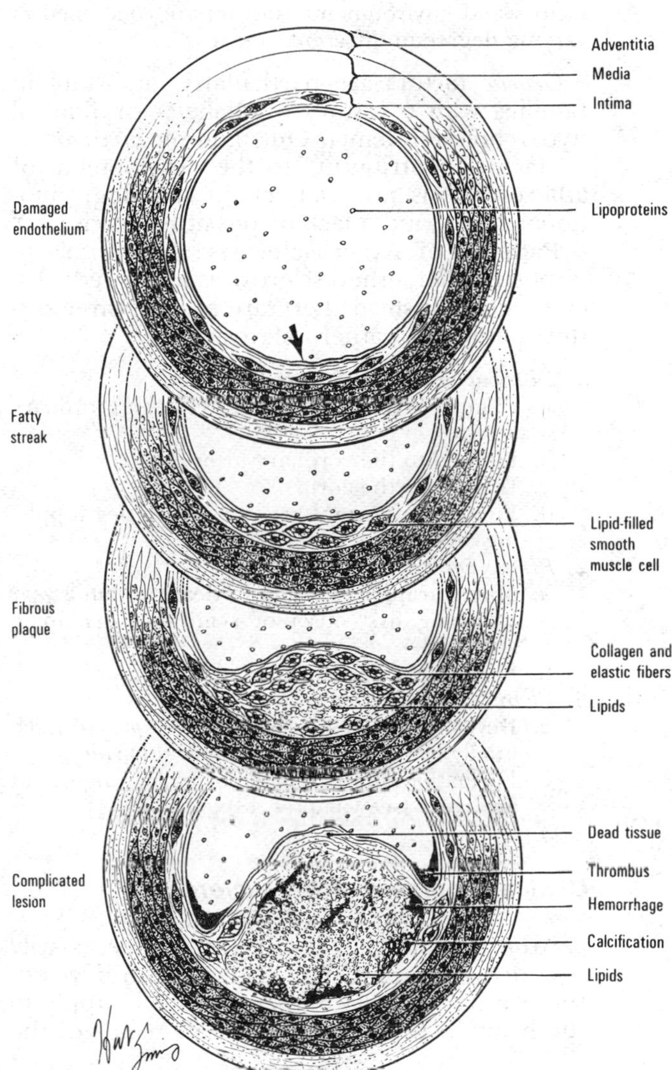

Figure 36–4. Types of atherosclerotic lesions. (From Debakey, M., and A. Grotto: *The Living Heart.* New York: Charter Books, 1977, p. 151.)

The *viral* or *toxic agent theory* has been proposed by Benditt and associates, who believe that an atherosclerotic lesion is derived from a single cell type. They have found in their work with laboratory rats that the number of cells in the arterial walls undergoing division is about ten times higher in rats with high blood pressure than in normotensive rats. They propose that viruses or toxic agents may initiate the transformation of a sensitive cell located in the arterial wall. As a result atherosclerotic lesions may later evolve. Benditt speculates that this pathologic process may be similar to the process by which cancer possibly develops.[55]

*In reviewing these and other population studies, it is important to remember that the statistical data upon which the research is based are often inconclusive or unreliable.

Finally, the *multifactoral theory* of atherosclerosis has many supporters. One authority states:

It is more probable that atherosclerosis is a disease of multifactoral etiology in which inborn or genetic factors and environmental factors are concerned in varying degree in different persons.[66]

Genetic factors are particularly important in families with a history of diabetes or familial hypercholesterolemia. Outstanding *environmental* factors contributing to the development of atherosclerosis are diet, chain smoking, emotional stress, and a lack of physical exercise.

Patterns of Atherosclerosis.[55] Contrary to popular belief, atherosclerosis is *not* a single disease entity. Instead there are at least three distinct patterns of atherosclerosis:

1. *Distribution of lesions*
   a. Limited to the peripheral arteries and coronary arteries
   b. Limited to the coronary arteries
   c. Limited to the aorta
   d. Limited to visceral arteries or arteries supplying kidneys
2. *Progression of lesions*
   a. May be rapid, resulting in death within a year following first onset of symptoms (galloping atherosclerosis)
   b. Very slow with long remissions
3. *Characteristics of lesions*
   a. Development of an atherosclerotic *plaque* which finally leads to the occlusion of an artery
   b. Formation of an *aneurysm* or ballooning-out of an artery (see Chapter 48)

Clinical Course of Atherosclerosis

Atherosclerosis, by itself, does not necessarily produce symptoms, For symptoms to develop, there must be *critical deficit* in blood supply to the heart in proportion to the demands of the myocardium for oxygen and nutrients. When atherosclerosis progresses slowly, the collateral circulation that develops can generally meet the heart's demands under normal conditions. Thus, whether or not symptoms of ASHD develop depends upon the *total* blood supply to the myocardium (by way of coronary arteries *and* collateral circulation) and not just upon the condition of the coronary arteries alone.

Because the extent of collateral circulation varies from person to person, the development and progress of atherosclerosis follow one of the following courses:

1. *Unrecognized ASHD:* The individual suffers no symptoms during his life time; atherosclerotic changes are found at autopsy.

2. *Asymptomatic ASHD:* The arteries undergo extensive pathologic changes, but the patient remains symptom free as a result of establishment of good collateral circulation.

3. *Clinical ASHD:* Signs of heart disease are present. Cardiac manifestations of obliterative atherosclerosis include episodes of chest pain, angina pectoris, myocardial infarction, congestive heart failure, arrhythmias, heart block and sudden death. The pathophysiology underlying these cardiac manifestations of obliterative atherosclerosis is outlined in Table 36–4.

Diagnosis

ASHD is diagnosed by the following methods:

1. A *history* of attacks of anginal pain.

2. *Coronary arteriography* helps to demonstrate the presence of calcification within the coronary arteries, and the degree to which the arteries are obstructed.

3. *ECG tracings* are examined for evidence of past myocardial infarction and the presence of T waves and Q waves.

4. *Laboratory tests* for total blood cholesterol. Hy-

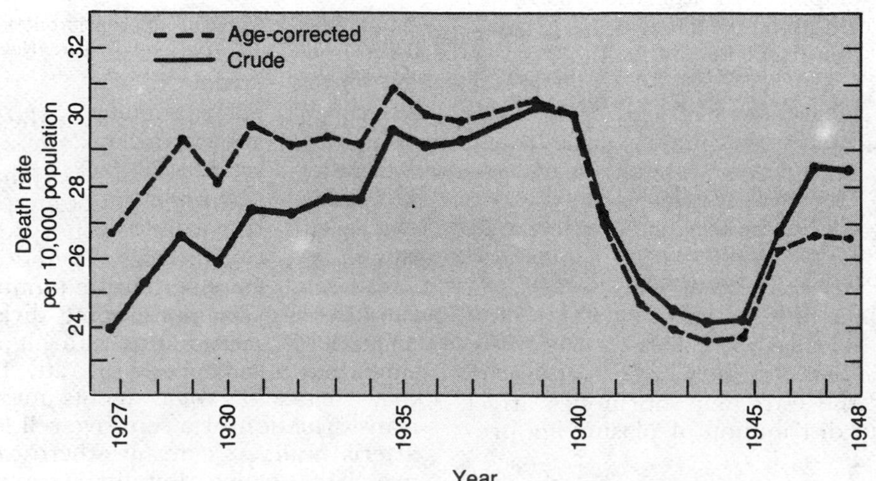

Figure 36–5. Mortality from circulatory disease in Norway from 1927 to 1948. (From Walker, W. J.: Success story: The program against major cardiovascular risk factors. *Geriatrics.* 31:97, Mar. 1976.)

percholesterolemia or a total blood cholesterol of more than 250 mg./dl. suggests the presence of atherosclerosis.

5. *Stress testing* on a treadmill or other exercise device helps in determining how much activity the patient can engage in before pain develops.

Clinical Care

Clinical care of the patient with ASHD generally centers on prevention and treatment of the specific manifestations of the particular disease process, e.g., angina pectoris, MI, CHF. General treatment and prevention of ASHD is the same as that for CHD. The specific treatment for angina pectoris and MI is discussed in the next sections.

ANGINA PECTORIS

Angina pectoris, which is also known as "cardiac pain of effort and emotion," is a clinical entity characterized by transient paroxysmal attacks of substernal or precordial pain that may radiate to the left shoulder and down the inner side of the left arm. (Other patterns of pain radiation also may occur with angina pectoris.)

The word "angina" is derived from a Greek word meaning "strangling," while the word "pectoris" refers to the breast or breast bone.

The pain of angina is precipitated by exertion, emotion, and exposure to cold, and is relieved by rest and the use of nitroglycerin tablets. *Unlike acute MI, the anginal pain is temporary, and myocardial tissues are not permanently damaged.*

Patterns of Angina Pectoris

Classic angina pectoris may be subdivided into the following basic patterns:[243]

▶ *Stable angina:* Paroxysmal chest pain or discomfort which is brought about by a predictable degree of exertion or emotion, characterized by a stable pattern of onset, duration, and intensity of symptoms.

▶ *Unstable angina* (preinfarction angina, crescendo angina, or intermittent coronary syndrome): Paroxysmal chest pain triggered by an unpredictable degree of exertion or emotion, which may occur at night, characterized by an increase in the number of attacks, the duration of attacks, and the intensity of the pain.[79]

In addition, anginal attacks may assume the following characteristics:

▶ *Nocturnal angina:* Occurs only during the night and is possibly associated with the REM sleep that accompanies dreaming.[9]

▶ *Angina decubitus:* Paroxysmal chest pain which occurs when the patient is reclining, and relieved by sitting or standing up.

▶ *Intractable angina:* Chronic incapacitating angina unresponsive to medical treatment.

TABLE 36–4. PATHOPHYSIOLOGY UNDERLYING CLINICAL MANIFESTATIONS OF ARTERIOSCLEROTIC HEART DISEASE

Clinical Expression	Mechanism
1. Angina pectoris	1. Transient, localized myocardial ischemia
2. Acute myocardial infarction	2. Arterial occlusion
3. Intermediate coronary syndrome (unstable angina)	3. Prolonged myocardial ischemia, with or without myocardial necrosis
4. Heart failure, acute and chronic arrhythmias, conduction disturbances, abnormal ECG	4. Gradual fibrosis of myocardium or conduction system; may result from (2) or (3) also
5. Sudden death	5. Any of the above, plus ventricular arrhythmia, or Stokes-Adams attacks

(From Krupp, M.A., and M.J. Chatton, (Eds.). *Current Medical Diagnosis and Therapy.* Los Altos, CA: Lange Medical Publications, 1978.)

Causative Factors and Underlying Pathology

Angina pectoris is a temporary state of myocardial hypoxia, the exact cause of which is still obscure. However, each of the variables listed below can result in myocardial ischemia and anginal pain.

1. *Decrease in myocardium's oxygen supply* (delivered by the coronary arteries)
   a. *Vessel factors:*
      (1) *Atherosclerosis,* narrowing of the lumen of coronary vessels, is the most common cause of anginal attacks.
      (2) *Arterial spasm* and *reflexive narrowing* of coronary vessels, resulting from cold, emotional stress, and smoking.
      (3) *Coronary arteritis,* or inflammation of the coronary arteries, due to infections, autoimmune disease, and so forth.
   b. *Circulatory factors:*
      (1) *Hypotension* due to spinal anesthesia, potent antihypertensive drugs, blood loss, and so forth, resulting in decreased blood return to the heart.
      (2) *Aortic stenosis* or *aortic insufficiency,* due to congenital anomalies or infectious process-

es, resulting in decreased filling pressure of the coronary arteries.

c. *Blood factors:*
   (1) *Anemia* and *hypoxemia,* resulting in decreased oxygen flow to myocardium.
   (2) *Polycythemia,* causing increased blood viscosity, which slows blood flow through the coronary arteries.

2. *Need for an increased cardiac output which may cause the heart to become overworked*
   a. *Physiologic factors:* Exercise, emotion, digestion of a large meal.
   b. *Pathologic factors:* Anemia, hyperthyroidism.
3. *Increased myocardial need for oxygen*
   a. *Damaged* myocardium unable to properly utilize oxygen.
   b. *Hypertrophied* myocardium that has "outgrown" its normal blood supply and requires added supplies of oxygen.
   c. *Aortic stenosis* or *insufficiency* and *diastolic hypertension,* causing heart to work harder.
   d. *Thyrotoxicosis,* increasing oxygen consumption.
   e. Strong *emotion* and heavy *exertion,* increasing heart's and body's need for oxygen.

Atherosclerosis is by far the most common cause of angina pectoris. As you recall, if atherosclerosis develops gradually, collateral circulation is usually established. However, while collateral circulation can supply the heart muscle with *just* enough blood to meet normal circulatory requirements, it is generally unable to oxygenate the myocardium when the body is undergoing excessive stress, e.g., heavy exercise, running up a flight of stairs, walking against the wind, great emotional excitement, and digestion of a heavy meal. It is at these critical moments that the pain of angina strikes, generally forcing the individual to stop his activities and rest.

Diagnosis of Angina Pectoris

Patient's History. The key to the proper diagnosis of angina is a complete, detailed history of the patient's attacks, which the patient is encouraged to describe in his own words. Typically the patient describes the attacks as usually following exertion, emotion, or a heavy meal.

The *pain* of angina, the most important aspect of the history, usually has the following characteristics:

Sensation. Squeezing, burning, pressing, choking, aching, bursting. The patient often says the pain feels like "gas" or "heartburn" or "indigestion." Pain is never described as sharp or knifelike.

Location. In 80 to 90 per cent of patients the pain is experienced as retrosternal or slightly to the left of the sternum.

Radiation. Usually the pain radiates to the left shoulder and upper arm; it may then travel down the inner aspect of the left arm to the elbow, wrist, and fourth and fifth fingers. The pain may also radiate to the right shoulder, neck, jaw, or epigastric region. On occasion the pain may be felt only in the area of radiation and not in the chest. The patient rarely experiences the pain as localized to any one single small area over the precordium.

Duration. Anginal attacks are usually of *short* duration, lasting less than 3 minutes. However, attacks precipitated by a heavy meal or extreme anger may last from 15 to 20 minutes.

Relief. Most anginal attacks quickly subside with the administration of nitroglycerin and with rest.

The typical "exertion — pain — rest — relief" symptom pattern is the major clue to the diagnosis of angina pectoris. Other symptoms accompanying the pain of angina are dyspnea, pallor, sweating, faintness, palpitations, dizziness, and digestive disturbances.

Physical Examination. Twenty-five to 40 per cent of patients with angina pectoris have no signs of cardiac pathology. Thus, the physical examination is rarely diagnostic.

ECG Findings and Angiocardiography. The electrocardiogram tracings are normal in 25 to 30 per cent of patients with angina pectoris. However, 70 per cent of patients with angina have ECG abnormalities following mild exercise. X-ray films of the coronary arteries may reveal atherosclerotic changes and evidence of CHD.

Nitroglycerin Test. The diagnosis of angina pectoris is fairly certain if glyceryl trinitrate (nitroglycerin), 0.4 mg. or 1/150 gr., invariably shortens an attack of anginal-type pain or increases tolerance to exercise.

Clinical Care

The care of patients with angina pectoris centers on two goals: relief of acute attacks, and prevention of further anginal attacks.

RELIEF OF ACUTE ATTACKS

To relieve the severe pain of angina, the patient is instructed to do the following:

1. Stop all activity and sit down or lie down as soon as the attack begins, remaining quiet until the pain subsides. Patients must be warned against trying to "heroically" continue on with their normal activities in spite of the pain.
2. Take glyceryl trinitrate (nitroglycerin) as soon as the pain begins.

Nitroglycerin has been the drug of choice against anginal attacks since 1867, and today is still the physician's major weapon against acute attacks. Administered sublingually, nitroglycerin acts to relieve the pain of angina within 1 or 2 minutes. Nitroglycerin acts by causing vasodilation and a decrease in the systemic blood pressure, which consequently decreases the amount of work the heart must do. The usual dose is 0.3 mg. (1/200 gr.). If this dosage proves ineffective, the physician may then increase the dosage to 0.4 to 0.6 mg. (1/150 to 1/100 gr.). Side effects of nitroglycerin include headache, hypotension, dizziness, and flushing. Patients taking nitroglycerin need the following special instructions to receive full benefit from the drug:

a. Carry nitroglycerin tablets at all times. Persons who live with the patient should know where the supply is kept.

b. Place one tablet under the tongue at the first indication of an attack and allow the tablet to dissolve completely. Retain saliva briefly before swallowing. If possible, lie down for a while after using the drug.

c. Always have "fresh" nitroglycerin tablets, as they lose their potency after 6 months. Nitroglycerin tablets should be stored in a dark bottle and in a dry place. The patient will experience a burning sensation on the tongue and a full, throbbing, sensation in the head if the tablets have full potency.

d. Repeat the drug dosage every 5 to 10 minutes until relief is obtained. If the pain is not subsiding or relieved after 3 to 5 tablets, the patient is generally instructed to call the physician or go to the nearest emergency room.

e. Warn the patient that effects, such as headache and flushing, will be felt, but that the discomfort from side effects tends to lessen as tolerance develops.

PREVENTION OF ATTACKS

Measures that may be helpful in the prevention of attacks:

Control of Precipitating Conditions and High Risk Factors

1. Anxious, nervous persons are often referred for psychiatric help. Also, they may be given mild, tranquilizing drugs.

2. Overweight patients are urged to reduce. All patients are encouraged to eat small meals, avoid high-calorie and high-cholesterol diets, abstain from gas-forming foods, and rest for short periods following meals. In addition, it appears that a high-fiber diet may not only reduce constipation and other intestinal tract ailments, but also lower the number and severity of anginal attacks. In one study, a high-fiber diet reduced intestinal transit time from 70 to 80 hours to 35 hours and also reduced cardiac output and intracolonic and intra-abdominal pressures.[10]

3. A regular program of daily exercise is planned for most patients in order to promote improved coronary circulation.

4. Patients who smoke must be instructed to quit smoking at once. Patients need to realize that smoking cigarettes raises carboxyhemoglobin in the blood, which then reduces the amount of oxygen available to the myocardium, which then can precipitate an anginal attack. In addition to stopping smoking, patients must avoid "passive smoking" (e.g., being in smoke-filled rooms) if they are to reduce the risk of anginal attacks. One study of passive smoking makes this point: "Being in the presence of a smoker, or in a room in which people have been smoking, is hazardous for the angina patient and should be avoided."[11]

5. The patient who leads an active, hectic life must learn to adjust activities to a level below that which precipitates anginal attacks. Brief rest periods throughout the working day, an early bedtime, and longer vacations are "musts."

6. The physician tries to protect the patient from further anginal attacks by correcting any coexisting medical or cardiovascular problems, e.g., hyperthyroidism, hypertension, congestive heart failure. The doctor may prescribe digitalis and diuretics to lessen the workload of the heart.

Drug Therapy

The two major types of drug therapy in the treatment of angina pectoris are *vasodilators* (e.g., nitroglycerin, isosorbide dinitrate and nitroglycerin ointment) and *beta-adrenergic blocking agents* (e.g., propranolol). The action of these two classes of drugs upon the heart and circulatory system is outlined in Figure 36–6.

1. *Nitroglycerin,* a vasodilator, may be used freely to prevent attacks. Patients must be taught to place a nitroglycerin tablet under their tongue *prior* to exercising, eating a large meal, engaging in emotionally stressful situations, or having sexual intercourse.

2. *Long-acting nitrates* act to maintain *coronary artery vasodilatation,* thereby promoting a greater flow of blood and oxygen to heart muscle. Isosorbide dinitrate (Isordil) and long-acting nitroglycerin preparations (e.g., nitroglycerin ointment) are the primary drugs used at the present time. These long-acting nitrates produce the same general side effects as nitroglycerin, i.e., severe headache, flushing of the skin, nausea and vomiting, hypotension, vertigo, and syncope. Route of administration and action are listed in Table 36–5.

Although long-acting nitrates are helpful in preventing anginal attacks, they are disappointing in that many patients develop tolerance to them within a few weeks. Once tolerance has developed, patients must resort again to the use of nitroglycerin sublingually. Regularly and carefully question all patients receiving long-acting nitrates concerning the degree of relief that they are receiving from the drug. Remember that tolerance develops rapidly.

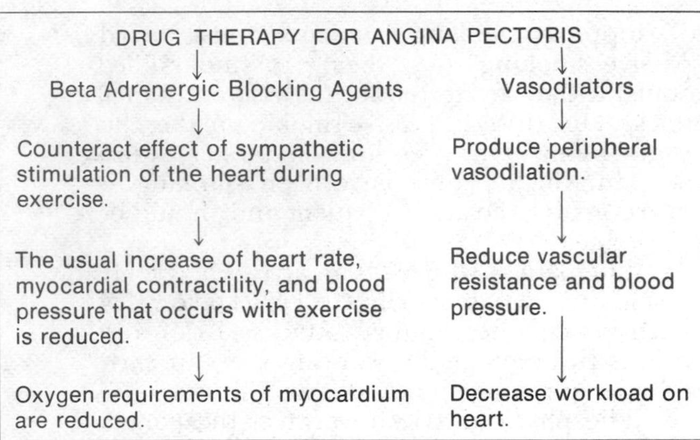

Figure 36–6. Rationale for drug therapy of angina pectoris.

3. *Propranolol (Inderal),* a beta adrenergic blocking agent, is given orally to decrease the number of anginal attacks and the consumption of nitroglycerin. Inderal acts by reducing the oxygen requirements of the myocardium. This, in turn, increases the exercise tolerance of patients with reduced coronary blood flow. However, because Inderal interferes with the pumping action of the heart, use extreme caution when administering this drug to persons with any degree of heart failure. Also, Inderal should not be administered to persons with a history of bronchial asthma, significant mitral or aortic valvular disease, allergic rhinitis during the pollen season, or brittle diabetes. It should never be given in conjunction with monoamine oxidase inhibitors.[79] Side effects of Inderal are usually transient and include nausea, vomiting, mental depression and mild diarrhea. Inderal given in combination with nitrates on an around the clock schedule appears to be superior to giving either type of drug alone.

4. *Sedatives, tranquilizers,* and *antidepressants* may lessen the frequency and severity of attacks. Commonly used tranquilizing drugs are phenobarbital, meprobamate (Equanil, Miltown), and diazepam (Valium). Drugs helpful against depression are nortriptyline (Aventyl) and amitriptyline (Elavil).

Surgical Techniques. Surgical procedures, discussed earlier, are sometimes employed in angina pectoris to increase coronary blood flow. Coronary angiography is used to more precisely locate lesions and points of narrowing within the coronary arteries preoperatively, which, in turn permits more precise corrective surgery. Nevertheless, at present, surgical methods only ease the patient's symptoms; surgery as yet cannot halt the process of atherosclerosis, although, as noted, life is prolonged in some cases.

In summary, there is to date no cure for the syndrome of angina pectoris. Nitroglycerin remains the drug of choice for alleviating the pain of angina and preventing further anginal attacks. Long-acting nitrates, propranolol, and surgery are all useful methods for reducing anginal attacks, but they remain controversial. Selective coronary angiography may enable more accurate diagnosis and treatment of angina pectoris.

Prognosis

The prognosis for angina pectoris depends upon the underlying disorder, the amount of collateral circulation, and the patient's ability to control those personal and environmental factors that precipitate attacks. The course of this disorder is generally prolonged. Attacks, which are typically interrupted by periods of remission, tend to become more severe and increasingly frequent. Patients usually survive from 5 to 10 years following the initial attack. One half of all sufferers from angina pectoris die suddenly; one third die following acute myocardial infarction.

ACUTE MYOCARDIAL INFARCTION (MI)

Acute myocardial infarction (MI), also known as coronary occlusion or just "a coronary," is a life-threatening condition characterized by the formation of localized *necrotic areas within the myocardium.* MI usually follows the sudden occlusion of a coronary artery and the abrupt cessation of blood and oxygen flow to the heart muscle.

Because heart muscle must function continuously, blockage of blood to the muscle and the

TABLE 36–5. LONG-ACTING NITRATES

Drug	Route of Administration	Action: *Onset*	Action: *Duration*	Comments
Isosorbide dinitrate (Isordil)	Oral Sublingual	30 min. 2–3 min.	3–4 hr. 1.5–4 hr.	Action may be hastened by chewing tablets
Nitroglycerin ointment (Nitrol and Nitro-Bid)	Applied to skin		3–4 hr.	May cause skin rash

development of necrotic areas within the myocardium represent a catastrophic blow to the body which may claim the patient's life. Indeed, even if the patient survives the initial attack, a host of deadly complications arise, and the dreaded but real possibility of suffering a second or third heart attack — attacks which may finally prove fatal.

Observation of a patient suffering from an acute MI leaves an unforgettable impression. The patient, sensing strongly that death is impending, is almost always frightened and in extreme pain. Even if he or she lives, fear and the remembrance of the pain remain long after recovery and the difficult struggle to reconstruct a life begins.

Incidence and Predisposing Factors

Myocardial infarction is the leading cause of death in North America, Australia, Europe, and New Zealand. In the United States, 15 to 20 per cent of Caucasians die from "coronaries;" the figure is somewhat lower among blacks.

Predisposing factors for myocardial infarction are the same as for all forms of CHD.

Etiologic and Pathologic Factors

The most common cause of myocardial infarction is complete or nearly complete occlusion of a coronary vessel by thrombus formation. Other less common causes are:

1. *Hemorrhage* of an atheromatous plaque, which initiates thrombosis or completes a partial thrombotic occlusion.
2. *Hypertrophy* of the heart muscle, causing the myocardium to outgrow its blood supply. Myocardial hypertrophy results from congestive heart failure and hypertension.
3. *Embolism* to a coronary artery.
4. *Gradual sclerotic occlusion* of a vessel without thrombosis.
5. Temporary *reduction in blood flow* to the coronary arteries resulting from postoperative or traumatic shock, gastrointestinal bleeding, severe dehydration, and hypotension from any cause.

> *When a coronary artery is suddenly blocked and blood and oxygen can no longer reach the heart muscle, the myocardial tissue supplied by that artery dies and becomes necrotic.*

Morphologic changes following an infarction include the following:

1. First 12 hours. Heart tissue appears normal upon gross examination.
2. 18–24 hours. Infarcted area looks anemic and gray-brown in contrast to normal red-brown color of myocardium.
3. 2nd to 4th day. Necrotic area becomes sharply defined.
4. 4th to 10th day. Necrotic area very apparent. Central tissue soft and may contain areas of hemorrhage.
5. 10th day. Necrotic tissue beginning to be replaced by ingrowth of gray, fibrous, vascularized scar tissue.
6. 10th day to 6th week. Scar tissue continues to advance and replace necrotic tissue.

The most common site for myocardial infarction is the *anterior wall of the left ventricle* near the apex. Infarction of the anterior left ventricles results from thrombosis of the descending branch of the left coronary artery. Other common sites for a myocardial infarction are the *posterior wall of the left ventricle* near the base and behind the posterior cusp of the mitral valve, and the inferior or diaphragmatic surface of the heart. Infarction of the posterior left ventricle results from occlusion of the right coronary artery or circumflex branch of the left coronary artery. An inferior infarction occurs when the right coronary artery is occluded.

The right ventricle and the atria are affected only 5 per cent of the time; the left ventricle is almost always affected because it carries a far heavier workload.

Symptoms

The major symptoms of an MI vary, depending upon whether pain, shock, or pulmonary edema dominates the clinical picture. Typical symptoms and their causation are listed in Table 36–6.

To understand more fully how an individual experiences pain and discomfort during an acute MI, pause to perform this brief experiment. Grasp firmly your lower left arm with your right hand. Tighten your grip to occlude circulation to your lower arm and hand and then pump your left hand. Continue this pumping action (while occluding the circulation) and you will feel an increasing sense of tension and painful discomfort. Magnify this feeling in your thoughts *many* times and imagine that it is occurring like a band around your chest and down your arm. These feelings are similar to those experienced during acute MI.

Diagnosis

The diagnosis of acute myocardial infarction is based upon the following findings:

1. Typical *pain* of infarction — an intense crushing, substernal, anterior chest pain of longer duration than anginal pain and not relieved by nitroglycerin.

2. Development of profound *hypotension* and *shock*.

3. The only reliable diagnostic *ECG* sign of myocardial infarction is QRS changes. ST-segment and T wave abnormalities may appear prior to the QRS abnormalities, but they are not truly diagnostic of acute MI.[31]

4. *Laboratory* findings include:* (a) *leukocytosis* of 10 to 20 thousand cells/cu. mm. appearing on the second day following MI and disappearing in one week, (b) *elevated sedimentation rate;* (c) *elevated SGOT* (serum levels rise within 4 to 6 hours following infarction, reach a peak in 24 to 36 hours, and decrease to normal in 4 to 7 days) and (d) *elevated LDH* (serum levels may remain elevated for from 8 to 9 days).

The serum level of *CPK MB* (an isoenzyme of CPK which is found only in cardiac muscle) is *increased* 4 to 6 hours after the onset of chest pain, reaches a peak in 12 to 18 hours, and returns to normal levels in 3 to 4 days; the serum levels of two *LDH isoenzymes* which are plentiful in heart muscle are *elevated* 12 hours after the onset of chest pain, peak in 24 to 48 hours, and usually remain increased for 10 days; the *HBD serum level rises* within the first 12 hours after a myocardial infarction, reaches a peak level in 2 to 3 days, and remains elevated for as long as 1 to 3 weeks.

*Laboratory findings and serum enzyme levels have been discussed in Chapter 33.

5. *Myocardial scintigraphy* is a new method for diagnosing myocardial infarction. A scintigram or scintiscan is a visual representation of the gamma rays emitted by a radioisotope; this visual "map" gives evidence about the concentration of the radioisotope in a particular tissue of the body, i.e., heart, kidney, and so on. Technetium-tagged pyrophosphate is used to label an infarcted myocardium and it appears on the scintigram as a "hot spot." However, because this test does not give positive results for 24 hours, it cannot be used to diagnose an acute MI during the early stages. Thallium-201, another radioisotope, produces a "cold spot" on an infarcted or ischemic area. Its diagnostic value is limited however, in that it cannot be used to differentiate between a new infarcted area and old scar from an earlier infarct.

Prognosis

Since the advent of coronary care units and devices which aid in promptly recognizing and treating life-threatening arrhythmias, 70 to 80 per cent of those suffering from an acute MI survive the initial attack. Chances for patient survival are greatly diminished by the presence of the following:

Old age
Evidence of other cardiovascular diseases, respiratory diseases, or uncontrolled diabetes mellitus

TABLE 36–6. PATHOPHYSIOLOGIC BASES OF SYMPTOMS IN MYOCARDIAL INFARCTION

Symptom	Bases of Symptoms
Pain: Crushing, severe, prolonged, unrelieved by rest or nitroglycerin, often radiating to one or both arms, the neck, and back.	Complete stoppage of blood supply to myocardium caused by thrombotic occlusion evidently causes accumulation of unoxidized metabolites within ischemic part of myocardium; this affects the nerve endings.
Shock: Systolic BP below 80 mm. Hg, gray facial color, lethargy, cold diaphoresis, peripheral cyanosis, tachycardia or bradycardia, weak pulse.	In some cases, shock caused primarily by the severe pain; in others, by a severe reduction in cardiac output and by inadequate tissue perfusion resulting in tissue hypoxia.
Oliguria: Urine flow of less than 20 ml./hr. as measured by indwelling Foley catheter.	Inadequate urine flow indicates renal hypoxia owing to inadequate tissue perfusion resulting from shock.
Low-grade fever: Temperature rises within 24 hours and lasts 3 to 7 days; usually 37.5 to 39.5°C. (100 to 103°F), accompanied by leukocytosis, elevated sedimentation rate, LDH, and SGOT.	Fever and elevated white counts result from destruction of myocardial tissue and the ensuing inflammatory process; fever drops when fibroblasts begin to replace leukocytes and scar tissue starts to form.
Apprehension, great fear of death, restlessness.	The severe pain of a heart attack is terrifying; also, most lay people are aware of the heart's importance and the significance of a heart attack; restlessness results from shock and pain.
"Indigestion," "gas pains around the heart," nausea and vomiting.	Patients may prefer to believe that their pain is caused by "gas" or "indigestion" rather than by heart disease; nausea and vomiting may result from severe pain or from vagovagal reflexes conducted from the area of damaged myocardium to the gastrointestinal tract.
Acute pulmonary edema: Sense of suffocation, dyspnea, orthopnea, gurgling; bubbling respirations.	In some cases, the left ventricle becomes severely crippled in pumping action owing to infarction; severe pulmonary congestion results, accompanied by low cardiac output and shock.

History of previous infarcts
Occlusion by a large thrombus
Sudden rapid occlusion

> *The danger of death from myocardial infarction is greatest during the first two weeks, but is particularly severe during the first 24 to 48 hours.*

Deaths generally result from the following complications:

Severe arrhythmias — in particular, ventricular fibrillation (which causes 40 to 50 per cent of deaths following acute MI)
Shock due to severe myocardial damage (9 per cent of deaths)
Congestive heart failure (40 per cent of deaths)
Rupture of the heart (5 to 10 per cent of deaths)
Recurrent myocardial infarction (5 per cent of deaths)

Patients fortunate enough to avoid the development of complications following MI still require a period of from 6 to 12 weeks for complete recovery. Unfortunately, however, 50 per cent of those individuals who do completely recover from their first coronary will die within 5 years; 75 per cent will die within 10 years from massive infarctions.

Clinical Care of the Patient with a Myocardial Infarction

The major *goals of care* for patients with acute MI are (1) successful treatment of the acute attack and prompt alleviation of symptoms; (2) prevention of complications and further attacks; and (3) rehabilitation and education of the patient and significant others.

TREATMENT OF ACUTE ATTACK

The patient who is suffering from an acute MI must be treated immediately! The severe pain must be alleviated, the ensuing shock reversed, and restlessness and fear eased. Complete rest, sedation, narcotics, oxygen, IV fluids, continuous monitoring, observation, and additional care are essential if the patient is to survive the first crucial 48 hours following the attack.

Typical therapeutic measures ordered for the newly admitted CCU patient with an MI are listed in Table 36–7, along with the rationale for each measure and the supportive nursing care.

PREVENTION OF COMPLICATIONS AND FURTHER ATTACKS

The possibility of death from complications always accompanies an acute MI. Thus, the prevention of life-threatening complications or at least their early recognition is one of the prime goals of clinical care. The major complications, their incidence, cause, prevention, and treatment are briefly outlined below.

Arrhythmias.* Specifically, ventricular premature beats, ventricular tachycardia and fibrillation, supraventricular tachycardia, heart block.

Significance. Forty to 50 per cent of deaths occur because of arrhythmias.

Causation. Ectopic rhythms arise in or near borders of intensely ischemic and damaged myocardial tissues. Damaged myocardium may also interfere with the conduction system, causing dissociation of the atria and ventricles (heart block). Supraventricular tachycardia may occur owing to heart failure.

Symptoms. Typical rate, rhythm, and ECG findings for specific arrhythmias; heart block with Stokes-Adams syndrome characterized by syncope.

Prevention. Continuous cardiac monitoring and PVC counts every 2 hours; report to physician if more than three PVC's per minute; prompt treatment of arrhythmias.

Treatment. *Frequent PVC's* — quinidine sulfate or lidocaine intravenously. *Ventricular tachycardial* — quinidine, Pronestyl, lidocaine, Dilantin, precordial shock. *Ventricular fibrillation* — immediate precordial shock. *Supraventricular fibrillation* — digitalis, quinidine, treatment of heart failure, precordial shock. *Heart block* — atropine, isoproterenol (with caution), use of temporary pacemaker.

Shock†

Significance. Shock is responsible for 9 per cent of the deaths from myocardial infarction; an estimated 80 per cent of patients who develop shock die from the complications.

Causation. Severe pain, decreased myocardial contraction and diminished cardiac output; undetected arrhythmias.

Symptoms. Systolic BP significantly decreased below patient's normal BP, diaphoresis, rapid pulse, restlessness, cold clammy skin, gray skin color.

Prevention. Rapid relief of pain and sufficient IV fluids to prevent circulatory collapse may help to prevent shock, rapid identification of arrhythmias is also important.

Treatment. Vasopressors such as levarterenol, dopamine, and Aramine to raise blood pressure by increasing peripheral resistance. In other cases vasodilators such as nitroprusside to promote better blood flow in the microcirculation. Positive isotropic agents such as dopamine sometimes used to increase cardiac contractility and cardiac output, and to improve tissue perfusion. Oxygen therapy; continuous interarterial and pulmonary artery monitoring; antiarrhythmic agents.

Congestive Heart Failure

Significance. Some authorities maintain that some degree of CHF and pulmonary edema is always present following acute MI.

Causation. Left or right ventricular failure.

Symptoms. CHF may be present at the onset of the infarction or it may develop weeks later. Typical

*See Chapter 35 for a complete discussion of arrhythmias, antiarrhythmic drugs, resuscitation measures, and precordial shock.

†Shock is discussed in detail in Chapter 13.

TABLE 36-7. TYPICAL THERAPEUTIC ORDERS EMPLOYED IN THE TREATMENT OF MYOCARDIAL INFARCTION: RATIONALE AND SUPPORTIVE NURSING CARE

Typical Order	Rationale	Supportive Nursing Care
Admit to CCU stat	CCU ensures constant supervision, monitoring, expert nursing care, and immediate attention in event of emergency	Relieve anxiety; reassure patient and family about CCU; explain in simple terms use of monitor; explain that skilled nurses and physicians are in constant attendance
Semi-Fowler's position	Position is comfortable; lowers diaphragm, thereby increasing lung expansion and promoting better ventilation; decreases venous return to heart, which prevents excessive pooling of blood within pulmonary vessels	If possible, have bed prepared prior to admission; support patient's shoulders and head adequately; reposition frequently (do not allow patient to slide down in bed); do not use Gatch bed (flexed knees promote thrombus formation)
Complete bed rest for 24 hours	Bed rest decreases stress and strain on damaged heart; if patient stable, sitting up in chair helps prevent venous stasis, promote bowel and bladder evacuation, and improve respiratory functioning	Place call light, water, bedside stand within easy reach of patient; if necessary, feed and turn patient; omit baths until critical stage has passed; give care in a calm, quiet, efficient manner; limit visitors; promote emotional and mental relaxation; give reassurance; allow patient to discuss problems; watch for and prevent complications of bed rest
Bedside commode for bowel movements; allow patient (if male) to stand with help by bedside to void (critically ill patients have Foley catheter)	Using a bedpan or urinal in bed is fatiguing; also, elimination is almost always incomplete; constipation, impaction, and urinary retention can result	Place call light within easy reach; assist patient out of bed; lift critically ill patient to commode with help of other nurses or an orderly; warn patient *not* to strain at stool; carefully chart bowel movements and voidings
Colace, orally, daily	Stool softness prevents constipation and straining	Give Colace (liquid) in fruit juice to mask bitter taste; if patient fails to have a bowel movement, notify doctor and obtain laxative order
Patient may feed and shave self (if mild attack)	Feeding and shaving self usually lessens emotional trauma and sense of helplessness; activity allowed depends upon severity of infarction, development of complications, presence of other illnesses, and patient's response to the activity	Arrange patient's tray or shaving equipment so that little exertion is required; watch patient carefully for signs of fatigue, and chart; consult doctor if patient appears to be overly tired from activities
Clear liquid diet for 48 hours, then 1200 calorie, soft, 2 gram Na^+ diet in 6 small feedings; very hot or cold beverages should be avoided	Clear liquids reduce hazard of vomiting and aspiration should resuscitation be necessary; small and soft, meals are easily digested; low Na^+ diet diminishes fluid retention, thereby decreasing work of heart; extremely hot or cold fluids may cause vagal stimulation and precipitate arrhythmias	Explain purpose of diet; serve food attractively; if diet unpalatable for patient, have dietitian consult with patient
Analgesia: morphine sulfate, 1–4 mg. IV, as needed for pain	Severe pain of infarction requires use of a powerful drug, e.g., morphine; pain persisting longer than 24 hours may indicate extension of the myocardial infarction or pericarditis	When patient complains of pain, evaluate situation immediately; carefully check BP, pulse, and respirations before and after giving drug (morphine causes hypoventilation and hypotension); *do not* give morphine if respirations less than 12 per minute; morphine and other narcotics may cause dizziness and fainting if patient stands; always put bedside rails up following injection of narcotics; encourage deep breathing to prevent pneumonia and atelectasis
Hypnotics: phenobarbital, orally, or chlordiazepoxide (Librium), diazepam (Valium), orally; chloral hydrate, orally, HS or flurazepam (Dalmane), orally, HS	Rest of the total patient (heart, body, and mind) is absolutely essential following trauma of acute MI; sedatives and hypnotics reduce fear and restlessness	Observe patient for effect of drugs; if restlessness continues, consult with physician; provide patient with as restful an atmosphere as possible; schedule "quiet periods" during the day when patient will not be disturbed

TABLE 36-7. TYPICAL THERAPEUTIC ORDERS EMPLOYED IN THE TREATMENT OF MYOCARDIAL INFARCTION: RATIONALE AND SUPPORTIVE NURSING CARE (*Continued*)

Typical Order	Rationale	Supportive Nursing Care
Oxygen, 3 liters per minute per nasal prongs	Arterial pO_2 may decrease following MI; oxygen helps to relieve dyspnea, chest pain, shock, cyanosis, and pulmonary edema	Check humidifier for H_2O level ("dry" oxygen can damage bronchial tubes); enforce safety precautions when O_2 being used, e.g., no smoking
BP, pulse, respiration q. 1–2 hours (vital signs may be continuously monitored by electronic means)	Vital signs give essential information; hypotension may foreshadow development of shock; rise in pulse rate may indicate shock; changes in pulse rhythm may precede life-threatening arrhythmia; very slow respirations may indicate morphine toxicity; gasping respirations (air hunger) may indicate oxygen lack; gurgling respirations indicate pulmonary edema	Explain to patient and family that frequent taking of vital signs is routine; report immediately BP above 170 or below 100, pulse above 110 or below 60, arrhythmias, respiration below 12 or above 24, and dyspnea and respiratory distress
Temperature q. 4 hours	Patient usually develops fever 24–48 hours after MI	Report temperature over 38.5,C. or 101°F. Report fever that persists after 6 or 7 days (pulmonary infection may be developing); observe for signs of dehydration; use measures to reduce temperature as necessary*
Twelve-lead ECG stat; continuous ECG monitoring, rhythm strip q. 2 hours; PVC count q. 2 hours for 48 hours	Twelve-lead ECG done soon after admission to evaluate cardiac status; rhythm strips used to observe changes in heart rhythm; frequent frequent PVC's (3 per min.) indicate ventricular irritation and may precede ventricular fibrillation	Reassure patient; explain use of ECG monitor; explain that ECG alarm going off is usually due to patient moving about in bed or lead coming off, not usually due to cardiac irregularities, explain that *static* on monitor indicates muscular movement; have emergency drugs and defibrillator on hand in event of life-threatening arrhythmia
Intake and output	Fluid *intake* should be just adequate (around 2000 ml. daily); too much may result in CHF, too little may cause dehydration—especially with elevated temperature	Inform all personnel that patient on I & O; label bed, Kardex, etc.
Foley catheter to measure urine output and specific gravity q. 1–2 hours. (this order for critically ill patient)	Oliquria indicates inadequate renal perfusion and shock; concentrated urine (high specific gravity) usually indicates dehydration	Report urine output below 30 ml. per hour and specific gravity of 1.020 or higher; maintain sterile technique when inserting and irrigating Foley catheter to prevent bladder infection
IV fluids: 5% dextrose in water; keep open with 10–20 cc. per hour	Vein should be kept open in case emergency IV drugs or a rapid phlebotomy is necessary	Watch IV infusions closely; if IV runs too rapidly, circulatory overload and pulmonary edema will result; maintain sterile technique in IV procedures
Twelve lead ECG and enzymes for 3 days	To aid in diagnosis	Explain reasons for test to patient
Special orders in event of complications include: anti-arrhymic agents, digitalis, diuretics, anticoagulants, K medications, vasopressors, or vasodilators	These orders discussed under Complications of MI	
Standing orders which the nurse may carry out in the event of life-threatening situations include: administration of anti-arrhythmic drugs; precordial shock; atropine, isoproterenol drip, lidocaine	These orders are carried out in life-threatening situations when a physician may not be readily available *Standing orders vary among institutions.*	Notify physician immediately of situation

*Controversy exists as to the safety of rectal temperatures following acute MI. Some studies have concluded that the insertion of a rectal thermometer stimulates the vagus nerve and causes a dangerous bradycardia. However, McNeal found in her study that taking a rectal temperature was a safe procedure and had no dangerous consequences.[155]

symptoms are dyspnea, orthopnea, weight gain, edema, enlarged tender liver, distended neck veins, basal rales.

Prevention. Low-sodium diet, restricted fluid intake, strict monitoring of IV fluids to prevent circulatory overload, bed rest.

Treatment. CHF — bed rest, digitalization, sodium-restricted diet, fluid restriction, diuretics. *Pulmonary edema* — morphine, ethacrynic acid or furosasemide intravenously, phlebotomy of 300 to 500 ml. or rotating tourniquets; intermittent positive pressure breathing.

Pulmonary Embolism. This may be secondary to phlebitis of the leg or pelvic veins.

Significance. Occurs in 10 to 20 per cent of patients at some point during either the acute attack or convalescent period.

Causation. Prolonged bed rest, increased blood viscosity, increased blood coagulability, use of the Gatch for flexing patient's knees.

Symptoms. *Venous thrombosis* — pain and swelling of the affected leg, pain in the calf upon dorsiflexion of the foot, fever. *Pulmonary embolism* — dyspnea, tachycardia, tachypnea, cough, pleuritic pain, pulmonary rales, cyanosis, fever, sometimes shock and cardiac arrest.

Prevention. Encourage patient to move legs and feet frequently; avoid placing pressure under patients' knees with pillows or bed Gatch; apply Ace bandages or elastic stockings to legs; administer sufficient fluids to prevent dehydration and increased blood viscosity; anticoagulant therapy.*

Treatment. Sedation, IV therapy, oxygen, heparin intravenously, oral anticoagulants, pulmonary artery embolectomy.

Recurrent Myocardial Infarction

Significance. Occurs in about 5 per cent of patients during the period of recovery from the first acute attack.

Causation. Possible overexertion, embolization, further thrombotic occlusion of a coronary artery by an atheroma.

Symptoms. Same as for first acute MI.

Prevention. Bed rest, oxygen, sedation, anticoagulants.

Treatment. Same as for the original acute attack.

Shoulder-Hand Syndrome

Significance. A rare disorder that is preventable.

Causation. Prolonged immobilization of the patient's arms and shoulders.

Symptoms. Affected shoulder becomes painful and tender; next, the hand becomes swollen, painful, and weak.

Prevention. Daily active or passive exercise of the arms and shoulders, physical therapy.

Treatment. Physical therapy.

Complications Due to Necrosis of Myocardium. These include ventricular aneurysm, rupture of the heart, ventricular septal defect (VSD); ruptured papillary muscle.

Significance. Infrequent but serious complications that usually occur 7 to 10 days after an MI.

Causation. Necrotic myocardial tissue is very weak and friable and therefore these complications may develop.

Symptoms. Signs and symptoms of congestive heart failure develop with ventricular aneurysm, rupture of the ventricular septum, and rupture of the papillary muscle. Symptoms of severe mitral insufficiency often develop when the papillary muscle of the left ventricle ruptures; ventricular arrhythmias, e.g., frequent PVC's and ventricular tachycardia, occur often in the presence of a ventricular aneurysm (the necrotic tissue is very irritable). Signs of cardiac tamponade develop with rupture of the heart.

Prevention. Measures to decrease the workload of the heart and increase the oxygen supply to the heart in an effort to keep area of infarction and necrotic tissue as small as possible.

Treatment. Usually surgery in 4 to 6 weeks: (1) excise ventricular aneurysm, (2) replace mitral valve if papillary muscle ruptured, or (3) repair VSD. Pericardiocentesis must be done immediately to relieve cardiac tamponade occurring after rupture of the heart.

Postmyocardial Infarction Syndrome (PMIS)[109]

Significance. A relatively rare complication which develops in 3 to 4 per cent of patients following myocardial infarction.

Causation. Possibly caused by a virus or an autoimmune reaction. Antiheart antibodies have been found in the sera of patients with PMIS and may have arisen in response to cardiac necrosis.

Symptoms. Chest pain, fever, dyspnea, pleuritis, pneumonitis, leukocytosis, pericarditis, pleural effusion. Cardiac tamponade most severe complication.

Prevention. Unknown.

Treatment. Watch for syndrome to appear up to several weeks following acute MI. Observe carefully for above symptoms. Reassure patient and encourage rest. Administer analgesics for pain.

REHABILITATION OF PATIENT

A successful rehabilitation program begins the moment a patient with a "coronary" enters the CCU for emergency care and continues for months and even years following discharge home from the hospital.

The overall goal of rehabilitation is to help the patient to live as full, vital, and productive a life as possible and yet remain within the limits of the heart's ability to respond to increases in activity and stress. In sum, the patient must avoid both invalidism and reckless overexertion.

Four important subgoals of rehabilitation are

*Anticoagulant therapy as a general preventive measure against thrombus formation and embolization following MI is highly controversial. In severe cases of myocardial infarction, however, most physicians do order intravenous administration of heparin upon the patient's admission, followed by an order for oral anticoagulants some days later. Anticoagulant therapy is discussed in detail in Unit XIV.

(1) to develop a program of progressive physical activity; (2) to educate the patient and the family concerning cause, prevention, and treatment of CHD; (3) to help the patient accept the limitations imposed by illness; and (4) to aid the patient in adjusting to changes in occupational goals.

Program of Physical Activity. Patients who have suffered a heart attack usually remain on bed rest for only 24 hours, unless complications such as congestive heart failure or arrhythmias develop. The typical program of activity for patients recuperating from an acute MI is:

First week postinfarction (*immediate* phase):

1. Admission to the coronary care unit. Room should be equipped with a calendar, clock, and window to help keep patient oriented.
2. Complete bed rest for first day or so with use of bedside commode for bowel movements.
3. Liquid diet for first 48 hours.
4. Shaving and feeding self, moving around in bed, and brushing teeth may be allowed once blood pressure and vital signs have stabilized; passive exercises should be started by coronary care nurse or physiotherapist.
5. As patient gains strength, sitting for brief periods on side of bed and dangling the feet is permitted.
6. Ambulation to a bedside chair for 15 to 20 minutes often permissible after first day.

Second and *third weeks* postinfarction (*intermediate* phase):

1. After fifth day, discharge from CCU to intermediate or regular unit if no complications have developed. Monitoring of vital signs by wireless telemetry may be continued. Bathroom privileges and shaving allowed from 7th day.
2. Self-care of majority of hygiene needs encouraged during second week. Brief supervised walks in hall allowable if no signs of complications.
3. Patient must avoid fatigue. Dyspnea, chest pain, tachycardia, and a sense of exhaustion are warning signals that patient is attempting to do too much.

Fourth week through *third month* postinfarction (*long-term* phase):

1. If no complications arise, patient is discharged home after third week. Essential to counsel family against treating patient as an invalid.

A recent trend is toward *early* discharge of persons with uncomplicated myocardial infarcts. A team at Duke Hospital has discharged post MI patients at the end of the first week. However, patients are allowed to go home early only if their households have adequate help and are conducive to rest. Also, such patients are followed carefully by trained nurse-clinicians who come to their homes and supervise thier medical status, exercise, diet, and so on, on an alternate-day basis. It is hoped that earlier discharge for MI patients will reduce patient depression as well as the expense of hospitalization.[14]

2. Sexual intercouse may be allowed four to eight weeks after an MI. Caution patient not to eat or drink alcoholic beverages immediately prior to intercourse.
3. Smoking must be completely discontinued.
4. Frequent walks are permissible, but strenuous activities such as shoveling snow must be avoided. The walking program aims toward a goal of 2 miles in less than 60 minutes.
5. Jogging may be undertaken during the eighth week, provided the patient tests out satisfactorily using a treadmill or other graded exercise testing device. A schedule for exercise at home for the 4th to 16th weeks postinfarction is presented in Table 36–8.
6. Some patients may be able to return to work at

TABLE 36–8. STARTING EXERCISE AT HOME* (FOUR WEEKS AFTER MYOCARDIAL INFARCTION)

Speed: 1.5 mph (1.8 Mets†)

Distance: 1/4 mile, 1315 ft., 2 long blocks, or 3 short blocks

Time: 11 minutes

Heart rate: increase 25; maximum 100; 60% age-adjusted maximum

Depending on symptoms and heart rate, change speed to 1.0 or 2.0 mph by adjusting time. After reaching 2.0 mph, increase distance to 1/2 mile, then speed to 2.5 mph, then distance to 1 mile, then speed to 3.0 mph.

Speed and Distances Walked After Myocardial Infarction

Weeks	*Speed (mph)*	*Distance (miles)*	*Time (minutes)*	*Mets*
4	1.5–2.0	0.25	8–11	1.8–2.2
6	2.0	0.5	15	2.2
8	2.0	1.0	30	2.2
10	2.5	1.0	24	2.8
12	3.0	1.0	20	3.1
14	3.5	1.0	17.5	3.6
16	4.0	1.0	15	4.0

**Colorado Heart Association.*

†For definition, see Table 36–3.

(From Mead, W. F.: Exercise rehabilitation after myocardial infarction. *American Family Physician,* 15:124, Mar. 1977.)

the end of 8 or 9 weeks if they remain asymptomatic. Persons with professional or white-collar jobs may be able to work full time, but manual laborers may have to work part time or find more sedentary work.

7. Between the 8th and 10th weeks, the patient should receive a complete physical examination, including ECG, excercise stress tests, lipid analysis, and chest x-ray film.

Education of Patient and Family. Following an acute MI, the patient and significant others must make many changes in their work patterns, life styles, diet, and so forth. Changes in life style are easier to make if a person understands the basic reasons for changes and the benefits to be obtained.

It is helpful to follow these steps when teaching the patient:

1. Consult with the physician as to when the patient will be ready for the instruction. Find out what information the doctor has already given the patient and significant others, and especially find out if there is any information that you are to withhold.
2. Select the proper time to begin instruction, make certain that the patient is calm, comfortable, rested, and receptive to learning.
3. Find out what the patient already knows or believes about CHD; correct any false notions or misconceptions.
4. Encourage the patient to ask questions about the condition. Give the patient paper and pencil for writing any questions that come to mind throughout the day; later these questions can be discussed with you or the doctor.
5. Do not overload the patient with information; allow learning at the patient's own pace. If the patient appears bored, tired, or preoccupied, continue your discussion at a later time.

The family and friends also need help and instruction, especially when the patient is discharged home. In particular, family members will need to know: (1) exactly how much activity the patient can tolerate at first; (2) medications the patient will be taking and their side effects; (3) details of a special diet if one is ordered; and (4) signs of complications (such as CHF) that they should report to the physician.

Emotional Support for Patient and Significant Others. As indicated, suffering an acute MI is one of the most terrifying events that a person can experience. Because the pain and fear are so devastating, most patients react to their heart attacks in distinct and dramatic ways. There are several coping devices that patients use to adjust to the realities (or to *obscure* the realities) of their illness. Common ways by which patients cope with the fact they have had a "coronary" are denial, euphoria, intellectualization, anger, hypochondriasis, regression, and depression.

Kucharski writes that patients who have suffereed an acute myocardial infarction fall into four basic groups: (1) patients who are able to master the situation although they may experience some anxiety and depression; (2) patients who experience extreme anxiety and depression but who are able to eventually master the situation; (3) patients who deny that the situation exists and who react with few emotional symptoms; and (4) patients who act dependent and who regress and decompensate throughout the entire rehabilitation period. These four types of emotional responses and some appropriate therapeutic methods for treating them are outlined in Table 36–9. Note that types 1 and 2 require (a) reassurance, (b) an opportunity to express their fears and feelings, (c) helpful information about their illness and how to cope with it, and (d) medication. Type 3 patients are best helped by positively stressing and utilizing their own strengths. Supervising Type 4 patients in a detailed and very specific treatment and rehabilitation program to prevent regression and invalidism is best.[132]

According to Hackett and Cassem, anxiety, depression and denial tend to emerge in the

TABLE 36–9. FOUR RESPONSES IN AND PRINCIPAL TREATMENT METHODS FOR POSTINFARCTION PATIENTS

	Type 1	*Type 2*	*Type 3*	*Type 4*
Response	Signal anxiety (fear) Reactive depression	Secondary anxiety Prolonged grief reaction	Denial (cognitive, major)	Denial Dependency Pathologic grief Regression Secondary gain
Treatment	Ventilation Clarification (medication)	Medication, e.g., haloperidol (Haldol), diazepam (Valium) Ventilation Clarification	Reinforce patient's time schedule and way of coping with stress	Limit-setting Structured treatment plans

(From Kucharski, A.: Psychologic stress in myocardial infarction. *American Family Physician,* 17:154, Mar. 1978.)

GUIDELINES FOR SEXUAL INTERCOURSE TO GIVE TO CARDIAC PATIENTS

These guidelines are presented to help you and your partner enjoy a satisfying sexual relationship while minimizing the work load on patients' hearts. Of course, your own feelings and beliefs will affect your choice of sexual expression.

1. Sexual intercourse should be resumed in the usual surroundings. Strange environment adds to heart stress.
2. A comfortable room temperature should be maintained during intercourse. Extreme room temperatures – and extremely hot or cold showers or baths – add to heart stress.
3. Foreplay is desirable. It will help prepare your heart gradually for the increased activity of intercourse.
4. Positions for intercourse should be comfortable, relaxing, and should permit unrestricted breathing. The following are appropriate:
   a. Side-lying rear entry
   b. Side-lying front entry
   c. Back-lying with the cardiac patient on the bottom
   d. With feet flat on the floor – the cardiac patient seated on a broad armless chair.
5. Oral-genital sex places no undue strain on the heart and may be a satisfactory means of sexual expression for you, depending on your and your partner's preferences.
6. Rest is beneficial before intercourse. Morning is an ideal time, but intercourse need not be restricted to this period.
7. Postpone intercourse for 3 hours after eating a heavy meal. Alcohol may be enjoyed in moderation, but again, wait 3 hours after drinking before having intercourse.
8. A relaxed atmosphere during intercourse will reduce stress on the heart. If you are tense or tired, you should postpone intercourse until after a good night's sleep.
9. Extramarital affairs may add increased stress to your heart and should be discussed with your doctor.
10. Clothing is sexually stimulating for some sex partners, but wear clothing that is loose-fitting.
11. Medications, such as nitroglycerin or isosorbide dinitrate (Isordil), may be taken before intercourse to prevent chest pain. Check this with your doctor.
12. Masturbation may require more energy than intercourse but usually does not. Therefore, masturbation should be discussed with your doctor or a nurse before resuming this type of sexual expression. You can sexually satisfy your partner without the stress of intercourse by manual manipulation.
13. Anal intercourse adds more stress to your heart and should be avoided until you discuss it with your doctor.

Figure 36–7. Guidelines for sexual intercourse to give cardiac patients. (From Moore, K., et al.: The joy of sex after a heart attack: Counseling the cardiac patient. *Nursing 77,* 7:54, June 1977.)

coronary care unit. Patients become most anxious on the second day, followed by vacillating denial. Depression typically strikes on the third day, then levels off by the sixth day and continues even after the patient goes home. Following discharge, the vast number of patients adjust well to their situation, especially after they are able to return to work and to normal sexual functioning.[98] However, all post-MI patients need continued encouragement and support. The pain may be gone but the fear of suffering another heart attack may continue indefinitely.

Remember also that close relatives to the patient may experience depression and anxiety and consequently need emotional support too. One study of the wives of MI patients indicated that they suffered considerable amounts of anxiety which took a variety of distressing forms: worries over possible problems, overeating, crying, headaches, constipation, and so on. The wives studied felt that the two areas of their conjugal lives most seriously affected by the MI were communications patterns with their husbands, and sexual relations. For example, there was a tendency for the wives to avoid direct confrontations with their husbands and to suppress anger; also, 30 per cent of the wives stated that they had sexual intercourse less frequently. They felt that they could be helped most by information and advice about their situation, and by someone who would listen to them.[135]

Return to Normal Sexual Relations. Patients and their sexual partners may become depressed if they feel that after an MI their sex life is "dead." Thus it is extremely important to educate patients and their loved ones that this is definitely not the case and that a normal sex life can be resumed — provided certain precautions are observed. Figure 36–7 provides important guidelines to patients and their sexual partners for safe sexual activities.

Moore and associates point out danger signs that signify that sexual intercourse is causing physiologic problems:[172]

Dyspnea or increased heart rate which persists for more than 15 minutes following intercourse
Extreme fatigue the day following intercourse
Chest pain during intercourse
Palpitations following intercourse, which last for 15 minutes or longer
Sleeplessness following intercourse

These symptoms of possible cardiac stress should be reported at once to the physician.

Return to Occupation. Approximately two thirds of patients who have suffered a first myocardial infarction are able to return to their former occupations. However, certain occupations, such as driving public vehicles or working in heavy construction, are too hazardous. For example, the patient might have a second MI while driving a bus and endanger the lives of others. In some cities, there are *cardiac work classification teams* composed of cardiologists, psychiatrists, social workers, and nurses who help patients who are bus drivers, heavy laborers, and so forth find more suitable work.

Self-employed and professional persons also need special guidance. The demands of the business and professional worlds are great, and competition is keen. The person with a heart condition who is a doctor, lawyer, or executive must learn to delegate duties to associates and to make time for recreation and rest.

Homemakers are another group of workers who need special counseling. They need to be instructed in how to simplify household chores and arrange working areas for maximum efficiency. In certain cases, additional household help may need to be employed.

Finally, some patients are forced to retire completely from work. These persons may become depressed and bored unless they find interesting and useful ways to spend their time. Hobbies, crafts, volunteering, television, movies, and cards and other games and sports are all helpful diversions.

CHAPTER 37

ARTERIAL HYPERTENSIVE CARDIOVASCULAR DISEASE

DEFINITION AND SIGNIFICANCE

Although hypertension is a common cardiovascular ailment, no single definition of the term is universally recognized. However, most definitions are similar to the following one accepted by the World Health Organization and many life insurance companies:

> *Hypertension is a persistent elevation of the systolic blood pressure above 140 mm. Hg and of the diastolic pressure above 90 mm. Hg.*

Many writers feel that the term "hypertension" does not necessarily denote a disease process, but is simply a physical finding that may or may not be medically significant. As Page explains:

"It should be remembered that blood pressure in itself is not a disease. Blood pressure provides the force to move the blood to perfuse the tissues. Since the need of tissues for blood changes from minute to minute, the demands on blood pressure vary. The enormous complexity of the problem of distributing the body's limited supply of blood to tissues with varying needs over time, a process which entails withdrawing blood from one area and shifting it to another, must be evident. It becomes clear why the body has so many ways of doing roughly the same thing, i.e., assessing the proper distribution of blood to meet the changing demands of life. If one regulator is destroyed, another can take over without much loss of flexibility in organ perfusion. The fact that so many regulatory mechanisms exist explains why there are so many ways to treat hypertension."[185]

Despite disagreement about the exact definition of hypertension, authorities do agree that a sustained elevation of blood pressure is of clinical significance because of its effects upon the heart, the vascular system, the kidneys, and the eyes. These effects are important medically because they can lead to such conditions as *hypertensive heart disease,* with resultant heart failure, myocardial infarction, cerebral vascular accidents, and kidney failure; *arteriolar nephrosclerosis,* with eventual renal failure; and *retinal abnormalities* terminating in blindness.

CLASSIFICATION

The three general ways of classifying hypertensive cardiovascular disease are:

Systolic and Diastolic Hypertension

Systolic hypertension is apparently related to loss of elastic tissue and to arteriosclerotic changes occurring in the aorta and other large blood vessels with advancing years; the systolic blood pressure is also influenced by emotional stress. Systolic hypertension is a serious condition because cardiac enlargement, heart failure, coronary artery disease, and strokes complicate an elevated systolic blood pressure more often than an elevated diastolic pressure.

Diastolic hypertension is a true disease phenomenon. It reflects the amount of pressure exerted on the arterial walls of the small arteries, exclusive of the pulse pressure (i.e., pressure caused by contraction of the left ventricle). It results from a decreased caliber of arterioles coupled with an increased blood viscosity, which leads to increased vascular resistance that ultimately causes an increased pressure within the arterioles.

Intermittent and Continuous Hypertension

Intermittent hypertension occurs when the blood pressure is variable, fluctuating between normal and moderately elevated. Caused by alternating constriction and then relaxation of the blood vessels, intermittent hypertension may continue for months and even years.

Continuous hypertension develops when the arterioles throughout the body are seriously damaged.

Primary and Secondary Hypertension

Primary hypertension, also known as *essential* or *idiopathic hypertension, constitutes 90 per cent of all cases of hypertension.* Its etiology is unknown. Types of primary hypertension are:

1. *Benign* hypertension. Characterized by a gradual onset and prolonged course.

2. *Malignant* hypertension. Characterized by abrupt onset and a short dramatic course which is rapidly fatal unless treated. Diastolic blood pressure is usually in excess of 150 mm. Hg and may rise above 180 mm. Hg. Pathologic changes in the kidney (petechial hemorrhages and medial necroses of the renal arterioles) characterize this potentially deadly form of hypertension. Severe and possibly fatal complications include hypertensive encephalopathy (neurologic abnormalities, convulsions), cardiac failure, renal failure, murmurs, left ventricular decompensation, and pulmonary edema.

Secondary hypertension develops as a result of other primary diseases of the cardiovascular system, renal system, adrenal glands, or neurologic system.

Low Renin, Medium Renin, and High Renin Hypertension[55, 97, 111, 244]

Hypertension may also be classified according to plasma renin activity. *Renin* is a peptide substance which is produced by the kidney and released under these conditions: a fall in blood pressure, a decrease in blood flow to the kidney, sodium depletion, stimulation to the sympathetic nervous system, secretion of catecholamines, adoption of the upright position, and the administration of drugs including diuretics and antihypertensives. Renin output is decreased by a rise in blood pressure and by the administration of beta-blockers and mineralocorticoids.

To understand renin activity and its effect on blood pressure, one must first consider the *renin-angiotensin-aldosterone* cybernetic blood pressure regulating system. As just noted, renin is released when blood pressure falls, and so on. Renin then passes through certain physiologic processes and is converted first to angiotensin I and then to angiotensin II, which is an active and powerful component of this system. Angiotensin II stimulates constriction of arterioles and also stimulates the adrenal cortex to release *aldosterone* — a hormone which causes the retention of sodium and the release of potassium, and consequently an increase in the volume of the blood. (See Chapter 12.) In sum, the vasoconstriction stimulated by angiotensin II and the increased blood volume generated by aldosterone causes the blood pressure to rise. Normally, if the blood pressure rises too high, negative feedback causes natriuresis (the excretion of abnormal amounts of sodium in the urine); in addition, the release of renin (the substance which started this cycle of physiologic events) ceases until blood pressure again drops too low. The renin-angiotensin-aldosterone system is diagrammed in Figure 37–1.

Using this physiologic cycle as a basis for classification and also treatment (see p. 874), patients with essential hypertension can be divided into the following groups:

1. *High renin essential hypertension* apparently affects 15 to 18 per cent of hypertensives. This form of the disease is primarily a disorder of *vasoconstriction* due to the excessive release of renin. Patients in this group are particularly at risk of heart disease, malignant hypertension, stroke, and kidney failure. These susceptible individuals need a carefully planned treatment program in order to reduce these cardiovascular-renal risks.

2. *Medium renin essential hypertension* is a "mixed" condition in which renin, mineralocorticoids and alpha-adrenergic agonists together cause the blood pressure to rise. It affects approximately 55 per cent of the hypertensive population.

3. *Low renin essential hypertension* is found in 30 per cent of the hypertensive population. It is essentially a disorder of *sodium retention* and is associated with abnormalities of mineralocorticoid release.

Secondary forms of hypertension for which the renin system of classification is sometimes employed are primary aldosteronism and renovascular hypertension. Patients with renal artery stenosis are usually found in the high plasma renin group. Patients with primary aldosteronism are typically classified as a low plasma renin group.[17]

Be aware that this method of classifying hypertensive patients according to renin activity is a new approach and, as such, represents a distinct departure from the traditional manner of classifying and treating hypertensive patients.

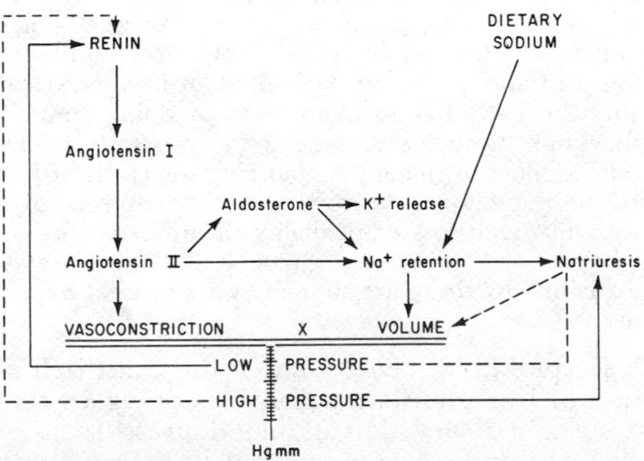

Figure 37–1. The renin-angiotensin-aldosterone system regulating vasoconstriction and volume components of blood pressure. Dotted lines indicate negative feedback. (From Weber, M. A., and J. H. Laragh: Hypertension. *In* Conn, H. F.: *Current Therapy 1978.* Philadelphia: W. B. Saunders Co., 1978, p. 210.)

BENIGN PRIMARY (ESSENTIAL) HYPERTENSION

Incidence and Predisposing Factors. Primary (essential) hypertension affects at least 1 person in every 10 in the United States or about 5 to 15 per cent of the adult population. Hypertensive heart disease, the result of a longstanding elevation of blood pressure, takes approximately 60,000 lives per year. In addition, hypertension is the principal risk factor for stroke and is one of the three major risk factors for coronary artery disease and myocardial infarctions. Strokes and heart attacks combined cause another 800,000 deaths in the United States per year. Even more alarming, at least half of the hypertensive population is undiagnosed and only a small number of those who have been diagnosed are receiving adequate treatment. Among those who are being treated, many cease to comply with their regimen; e.g., they skip doctors' appointments, eat a high-sodium diet, fail to take prescribed medications, and so forth. From these facts, it is apparent that essential hypertensive disease is currently a national problem of tremendous magnitude.[55, 119]

Essential hypertension most commonly develops in middle-aged and older persons, although it can strike youths and even infants. Women develop hypertension more frequently than men but are less dramatically affected by a sustained elevation of blood pressure. Blacks in the United States develop hypertension more readily than the white population; also, persons living in stressful urban environments and those frequently subjected to emotional trauma become hypertensive far more frequently than persons who live in rural or tropical environments and those living relaxed lives. Finally, studies show a link between obesity and hypertension and consistently demonstrate that a reduction in weight is usually accompanied by a reduction in blood pressure.

The malignant form of essential hypertension affects 1 to 5 per cent of those diagnosed as hypertensive. Men and black people are particularly prone to this deadly form of the disease.

Theories of Causation. The causative factors of primary (essential) hypertension are unknown. However, several theories of causation are being investigated. Briefly, these theories are (1) hypertension is caused by an excessive flow of vasoconstrictor nerve impulses from the vasomotor centers to the blood vessels; (2) hypertension results from kidney failure of unknown cause; (3) psychogenic factors such as continuous emotional disturbance can cause high blood pressure; (4) ischemia or irritated lesions of the brain cause hypertension; (5) hypertension is caused by a masked hormonal imbalance; (6) hypertension is a result of an inherited factor causing an increased thickness in the arterial walls; and (7) hypertension is the result of abnormal plasma renin activity.

Some investigators propose that hypertension results from many different factors interacting together. Page has advanced a multicausal theory of hypertension called the *mosaic theory*. He points out that because multiple factors regulate blood pressure, it follows that multiple factors are involved in the causation of high blood pressure. Factors which may together cause hypertension include (1) humoral factors, (2) neural factors, (3) hemodynamic factors, (4) endocrine factors, and (5) cardiovascular factors.[185]

Other researchers believe that hypertension develops as a result of the interaction of two chains of events. (See Figure 37–2.) One involves the genetic, personality, social, and emotional background of the individual and the interaction of these components with the body's neural, humoral, and vascular processes. The other chain is temporal and involves the gradual pathologic development of hypertension throughout the person's life, from prehypertension, to early and established hypertension, to complicated hypertension. A diagram of this theory and further explanation are included in Figure 37–2.[107]

Pathophysiology. From a pathologist's viewpoint, essential hypertension is a disorder in which the arterioles offer abnormal resistance to blood flow; also, there is usually a concurrent elevation of systolic blood pressure attributable to changes in the aorta's distensibility.

Early in the course of essential hypertension there may be no obvious pathologic changes in the blood vessels and organs, and few or no symptoms occur other than intermittent elevations of the blood pressure. However, as time passes widespread pathologic changes take place in both the large and small blood vessels and in the vital organs supplied with blood and oxygen by these vessels, namely, the heart, kidneys, and brain.

The *large* vessels such as the aorta, coronary arteries, basilar artery to the brain, and peripheral vessels in the limbs become sclerosed and tortuous; also, their lumens narrow, resulting in decreased blood flow to the heart, brain, and lower extremities. As the damage continues, large vessels may become completely occluded or hemorrhage may occur.

Small vessel damage is equally dangerous, causing additional adverse structural changes within the heart, kidney, and brain. The se-

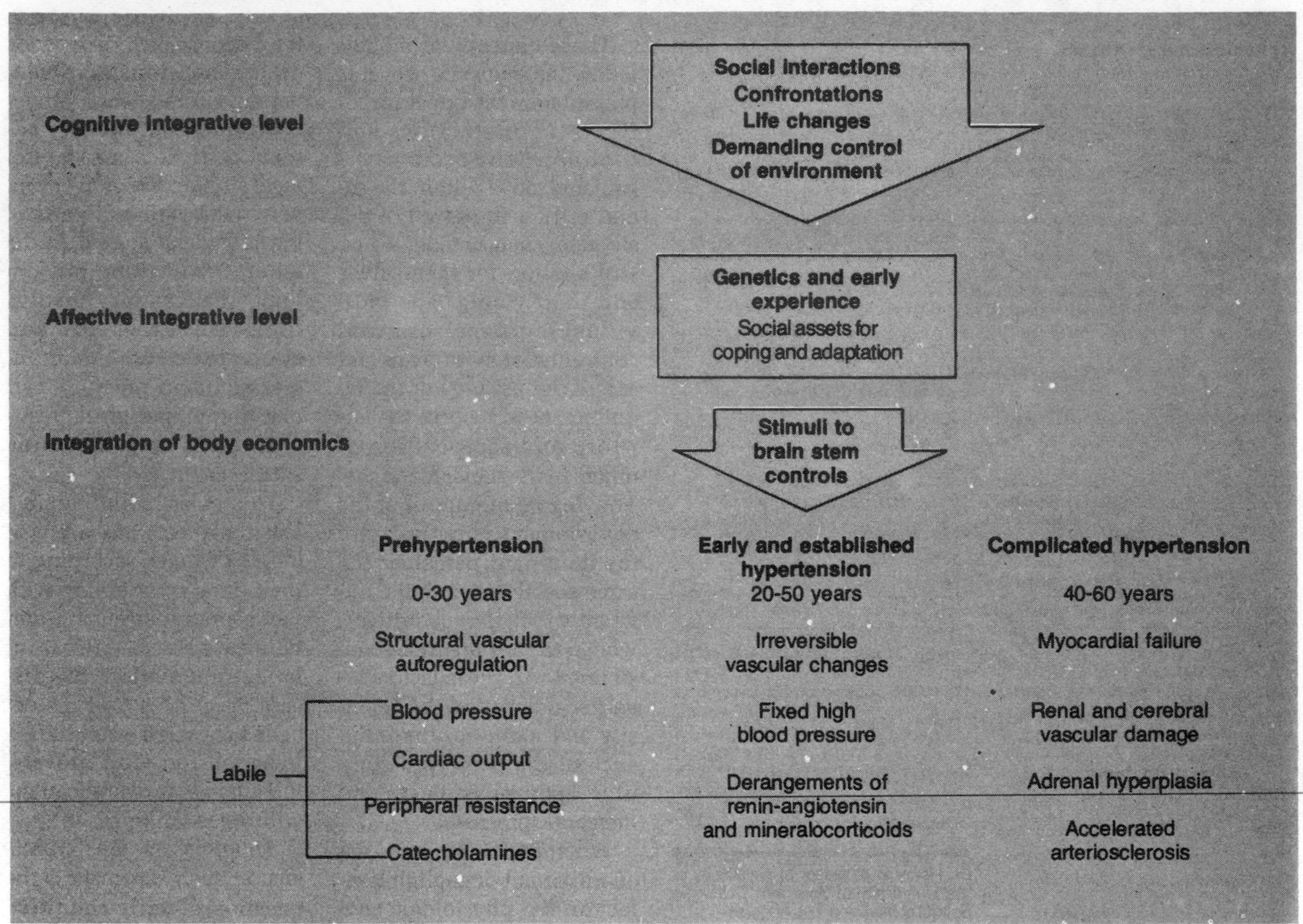

Figure 37–2. Essential hypertension develops as a result of the interaction of two chains of events. The first is shown in the upper part of the diagram by a large cognitive arrow representing the pressure of events as the individual searches for desiderata, deals with life changes, and attempts to control his environment. The affective "gain control" block below the arrow represents his genetic endowment, early experience, and social assets, which modify the stimuli to brain stem controls. The lower part of the diagram shows the role of time, as the induced changes progress from labile prehypertension with structural vascular autoregulation through fixed hypertension with cardiac hypertrophy to complicated hypertension with organ damage. (From Henry, J. P.: Understanding the early pathophysiology of essential hypertension. *Geriatrics,* 31:59, Jan. 1976.)

verely elevated diastolic blood pressure causes damage to the intima of the small vessels. Because of intimal damage, fibrin accumulates in the vessels, local edema develops, and intravascular clotting may occur. The final result of these adverse changes is a decreased blood supply to the tissues of the heart, brain, and kidneys and progressive functional insufficiency of these organs.

As stated earlier, one of the results of a long-sustained elevation of diastolic pressure is hypertensive heart disease, which may terminate in kidney failure. In the development of hypertensive cardiovascular disease, one sees the following vicious circle of pathologic changes in which each new manifestation of the disease further complicates all other manifestations of the disease: (1) the heart is meeting increased peripheral resistance because of constricted arterioles, but must continue to maintain normal cardiac output for the body to function without symptoms; (2) to accomplish this augmented work, the heart increases its *expenditure of energy* (this is accomplished by physiologic stretching of muscle fibers); (3) the stretching of muscle fibers leads to *hypertrophy* of the heart; (4) hypertrophy of the heart may lead to coronary insufficiency and *resultant myocardial infarction* because the enlarged heart muscle has outgrown its blood supply; (5) if the hypertrophied state of the heart is able to maintain proper cardiac output, a state of *compensation* exists but as left-sided cardiac failure progresses and; (6) the diastolic pressure rises in the failing left ventricle and atrium, the congestion extends back to involve the entire pulmonary tree, leading to a state of *pulmonary congestion,* which, in turn, leads to right-sided heart failure and blood backing up into the systemic circulation — this can then cause increased pressure in the *renal vasculature;* (7) the increased pressure of blood in the arteries coupled with the fact that arteriosclerosis weakens the blood vessels can cause blood ves-

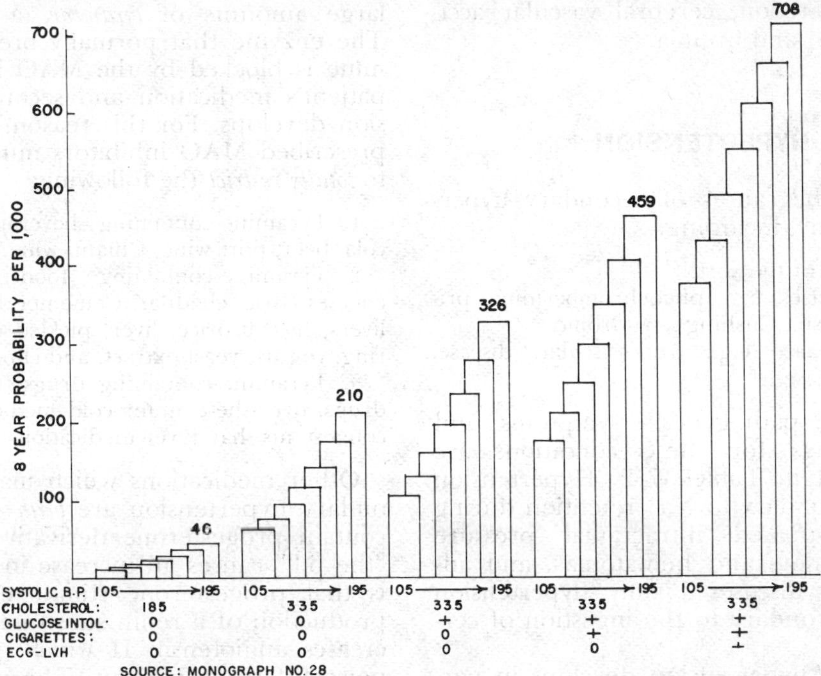

Figure 37–3. Risk of cardiovascular death according to systolic blood pressure. (From Beeson, P. B., W. McDermott, and J. B. Wyngaarden: *Cecil Textbook of Medicine,* 15th ed. Philadelphia: W. B. Saunders Co., 1979. With permission of Dr. W. B. Kannel.)

sels to rupture, producing *hemorrhage;* (8) when a blood vessel ruptures in the *kidney,* the latter becomes thrombosed. The area of the kidney supplied by the vessel becomes ischemic and dies, and this further aggravates the hypertension. Eventually, as this process occurs again and again, the kidney fails.

Death due to hypertensive cardiovascular disease results either from irreparable damage to the kidneys, brain, and myocardium as a result of small vessel damage, or from occlusion of a large vessel (e.g., acute MI) or hemorrhage from a large vessel (e.g., CVA). The risk of cardiovascular death is depicted in Figure 37–3.

Basis of Symptoms and Complications. As stated previously, the symptoms of prolonged, primary (essential) hypertension are due to pathologic changes in large and small vessels throughout the body. Typical symptoms and their causation are listed in Table 37–1.

Like the symptoms, the *complications* of hypertension also affect the heart, brain, eyes, and kidneys. Thus, patients with longstanding primary (essential) hypertension may eventually suffer from congestive heart failure, acute

TABLE 37–1. SYMPTOMS OF ESSENTIAL HYPERTENSION AND THEIR BASES

Symptoms	Base of Symptoms
BP persistently elevated above 140/90	Arterioles are constricted, causing abnormal resistance to blood flow
Anginal pain	Insufficient blood flow through coronary arteries to the myocardium
*Intermittent claudication**	Decrease in blood supply from peripheral vessels to the legs
Retinal hemorrhages and exudates	Damage to arterioles that supply the retina
Severe *occipital headaches* associated with nausea and vomiting, drowsiness, giddiness, anxiety, and mental impairment	Vessel damage within the brain
Polyuria; nocturia; diminished ability of kidneys to concentrate urine; protein and RBC's in urine	Arteriolar nephrosclerosis (hardening of arterioles within the kidney)
Dyspnea upon exertion	Left-sided heart failure
Edema of the extremities	Right-sided heart failure

*Intermittent claudication is a severe pain that develops in the calf muscles when a patient walks and subsides at rest; this is a symptom of peripheral vascular disease.

myocardial infarction, cerebral vascular accidents, blindness, and uremia.

SECONDARY HYPERTENSION

Etiology. The causes of secondary hypertension are many, including:

1. Coarctation of the aorta.
2. Adrenal causes, e.g., pheochromocytoma, primary aldosteronism, Cushing's syndrome.
3. Renal disease, e.g., renovascular disease, parenchymal disease.

The etiology, pathogenesis, symptoms, and physical findings for these conditions are briefly outlined in Table 37–2. Hypertension can also be secondary to Na^+ retention during pregnancy, increased intracranial pressure from brain tumors and hematomas, and advanced collagen diseases. Finally, hypertension can develop secondary to the ingestion of certain drugs.

For instance, hypertension develops in persons who are taking medications (usually antidepressants) which contain *monoamine oxidase* (MAO) *inhibitors* and who are (at the same time) ingesting food substances which contain large amounts of *tyramine,* a pressor agent. The enzyme that normally breaks down tyraminc is blocked by the MAO inhibitor in the patient's medication and secondary hypertension develops. For this reason, patients taking prescribed MAO inhibitors must be instructed to *totally restrict* the following:

1. Tyramine-containing beverages: coffee, tea, cola, beer, port wine, Chianti wine.
2. Tyramine-containing foods: broad beans, cheeses (Brie, cheddar, Camembert, Stilton) chicken livers, figs, licorice, liver, pickled or kippered herring, yogurt, yeast extract, and chocolate.
3. Tyramine-containing drugs: sympathomimetic drugs, over-the-counter cold medications, nasal decongestants, hay fever medications.[142]

Other medications which may result in secondary hypertension are *birth control pills* that contain progesterone derivatives. One reason "the pill" causes an increase in blood pressure is that progesterone stimulates an increased production of a renin substrate which then increases angiotensin II which, you recall, is a powerful pressor agent. The vast majority of women who take birth control pills experience a slight increase in blood pressure and approximately 2 per cent actually develop hypertension.[164]

TABLE 37–2. SECONDARY HYPERTENSION

Cause	Etiology	Symptoms	Physical Findings
Coarctation of aorta	Constriction of portion of aorta causes elevated blood pressure proximal to obstruction	Absence of femoral pulses; decreased BP in legs as compared to arms; weight loss	X-ray shows notching of ribs; intercostal bruits on auscultation
Pheochromocytoma	Adrenal medullary tumor causes excess secretion of catecholamines	Half of all patients have sudden attacks of severe headache with palpitation; hypermetabolic state; excessive sweating; meat intolerance; flushed, anxious appearance	Elevated BMR; elevated fasting blood sugar; excess excretion of catecholamines in urine
Primary aldosteronism	Functioning adenoma of adrenal cortex	Moderate elevation of blood pressure; muscular weakness; polyurea; nocturia; polydipsia; tetany; paresthesias; headache	Dilute alkaline urine; persistently low serum K^+ levels
Cushing's syndrome	Excess glucocorticosteroids excreted from adrenal cortex; cause may be an adrenocortical adenoma (or carcinoma) or adrenocortical hyperplasia	Mild hypertension; moon facies; "buffalo" hump on back; edema; hirsutism	Excretion of large amounts of 17-hydroxycorticoids and 17-ketosteroids in urine
Renovascular hypertension	Narrowing of renal artery due to atherosclerosis, fibrosis of wall of renal artery, or trauma to renal area	Hypertension; fluid retention with edema	Difference in length of kidneys; delayed appearance of dye from one kidney during intravenous pyelogram (IVP); decreased urine and Na^+ output
Parenchymal disease (acute and chronic glomerulonephritis)	Allergic response to infection in body (usually streptococcal), causing inflammatory changes in glomeruli	Hypertension; sodium and water retention; edema; oliguria; orthopnea; dyspnea; pulmonary edema; uremic odor	Cardiac enlargement; evidence of myocardial failure on ECG; elevated nonprotein nitrogen (NPN)

Diagnostic Approaches. The physician who examines a hypertensive patient carefully evaluates the following four areas:

1. The *form* of hypertension, i.e., essential or secondary. To make a diagnosis of essential hypertension, the doctor first rules out all secondary causes of hypertension by means of the history, physical examination, and laboratory studies.
2. Whether a *curable* form of hypertension is present. Hypertension caused by coarctation of the aorta, adrenal dysfunction, primary aldosteronism, renovascular disease, or brain tumors is potentially curable.
3. The *severity* of the hypertension is evaluated on the basis of the degree of adverse changes within the arterioles supplying the retina, the presence of ECG abnormalities, the extent of cardiac enlargement, and the degree of renal failure.
4. The *rate of progression* of cardiovascular damage. Cardiovascular pathology is evident if the patient complains of anginal pain or suffers from the symptoms of CHF.

The *diagnosis* of hypertension is confirmed by the patient's history, physical examination, and laboratory studies.

Questions to Include in History-taking:

1. At what age did the patient's blood pressure first become elevated?
2. Has anyone in the family suffered from high blood pressure?
3. Has the patient suffered at any point in life from renal or cardiovascular disease?
4. Has the patient recently experienced dyspnea, fatigue, weakness, anginal-type pain, swelling of the feet, or nocturia?
5. Has the patient suddenly lost weight (sign of pheochromocytoma) or suddenly gained weight (edema)?
6. Has the patient recently experienced severe headaches or drenching sweats (signs of pheochromocytoma)?

In talking with the patient, the doctor or nurse notes whether or not the hard driving personality usually associated with the hypertensive individual is present. Appearance is also observed. Does the patient have the moon facies and peculiar distribution of fat characteristic of Cushing's syndrome? If a woman, is hirsutism present? Does the patient have a flushed appearance and anxious expression, as characteristic of pheochromocytoma?

Points to Note in the Physical Examination:

Blood pressure readings taken on both arms in the supine and erect positions and on one leg. To obtain a truly reliable estimation of the patient's average blood pressure, serial readings should be taken every 1 to 2 hours over an 8 hour period for one to two days.

> Remember:
> *A single blood pressure reading is almost always inaccurate.*

Equally important is to be certain that the patient's forearm is kept at the *level of the heart* and is slightly flexed. If the arm is raised above the heart level, the reading will be a false low. If the arm is dropped below the heart, the reading will be a false high. (See Figure 37–4.)

Ophthalmoscopic examination for evidence of such vascular changes as arteriolar tortuosity, increased light reflex, narrowing, and irregularity of the arteries. Vascular damage within the retina has definitely occurred if hemorrhages, soft exudates, and papilledema are present.

Examination of the *heart* and *aorta* by means of auscultation, ECG readings, and aortography; radiology is also used to determine heart size.

Palpation of the arteries in the neck, wrists, femoral areas, and feet for evidence of coarctation of the aorta.

Neurologic examination for signs of cerebral thrombosis or hemorrhage. Signs of pathologic changes within the cerebrum range from a positive Babinski or Hoffman reflex to hemiplegia or paralysis of one side of the patient's body. (See Unit X for discussion of neurologic reflexes.)

Laboratory Studies:

1. General screening tests
   Urinalysis to determine the presence of protein, RBC's, pus cells, and casts — all evidence of possible renal disease
   Blood count and sedimentation rates
   Serum sodium, potassium, chloride, and carbon dioxide
2. More specific laboratory tests include:

Test for *renin-sodium profile:* Plasma renin activity is assayed and then plotted against mEq. of sodium excreted in the urine in a 24-hour urine sample. On the basis of this test, patients are classified as having low, medium, or high renin hypertension.

Test for *pheochromocytoma:** Analysis of urinary catecholamine metabolites, histamine test, and cold pressor test.

Tests for *primary aldosteronism:* Repeated electrolyte determinations of potassium, sodium, and carbon dioxide.

Tests for *Cushing's syndrome:* Urine 17-ketosteroids, blood corticoids.

Tests for *renal disease:* Intravenous pyelogram,

*Tests for pheochromocytoma, primary aldosteronism, and Cushing's syndrome are discussed in Unit XIX. Renal tests are discussed in Unit XIII.

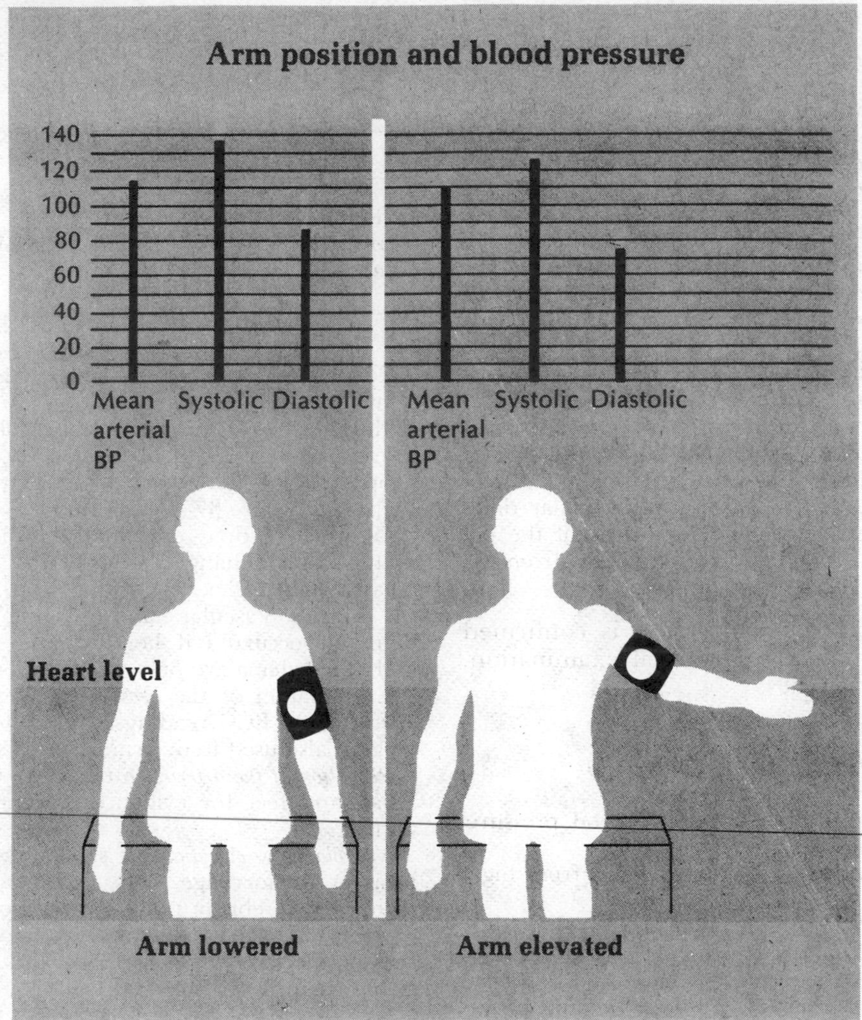

Figure 37–4. Importance of arm position during blood pressure monitoring. (From Finnerty, F. A.: Current Management: Part 1. Selecting and evaluating the patient. *Consultant*, 18:164, Jan. 1978.)

urine cultures, radioisotope renogram, renal arteriography, intravenous urograms.

If the clinical work-up produces no evidence of coarctation of the aorta, adrenal disease, or primary renal disease, the doctor then diagnoses the condition as *essential hypertension.*

Because the beginnings of adult hypertension often lie in childhood and adolescence, it is essential that *all children over the age of 3 years* receive yearly blood pressure determinations. Asymptomatic youngsters who on three separate occasions have an elevated blood pressure reading (in relationship to other children of their age) require a careful work-up and follow-up program. One system for identifying and evaluating asymptomatic children with elevated blood pressure is diagrammed in Figure 37–5. Note here that children at the 95th percentile are diagnosed as having high blood pressure rather than hypertension. This is because the term hypertension carries a connotation which could be psychologically damaging to some children and their parents.[231]

CLINICAL CARE OF THE PATIENT

Current treatment and nursing care of patients with hypertension is based upon the following five goals:

> *The goals of management are to:*
> *1. Control the blood pressure at the desired level, as close to normal as possible for each individual patient.*
> *2. Increase the patient's understanding of hypertension.*
> *3. Eliminate or reduce the adverse effects of therapy.*
> *4. Prevent the complications of hypertension.*
> *5. Maximize the ability of the patient and family to cope with the ramifications of a chronic health problem.*[7]

The following therapies are used to treat patients suffering from hypertension: general nonspecific therapeutic measures including supportive nursing care, drug therapy, surgical techniques, and specific therapies for hypertension of varying severity.

General Nonspecific Measures

1. Weight reduction if the patient is obese.
2. Moderate salt-restricted diet.
3. Planned program of regular physical exercise.
4. Changes in job or domestic setting for patients who work or live under considerable stress.
5. Mild tranquilizing drugs for patients who are nervous and apprehensive.
6. Short period of psychotherapy for individuals with serious emotional problems.
7. Daily periods of meditation and autohypnosis that may help the patient relax and induce a sense of well-being.

General *nursing care* of the patient with hypertension includes:

1. Provision of a restful, quiet hospital atmosphere.
2. Explanation of all procedures and diagnostic studies. Remember that some patients with hypertension are nervous, high-strung, compulsive individuals who may find it difficult to relax while undergoing renal function tests, ECG readings, and so forth.
3. Listening to the patient's fears and worries and offering reassurance when appropriate.
4. Explanation of diet restrictions (caloric and sodium restrictions). Patients suffering from CHD in addition to hypertension should also be instructed to reduce their consumption of animal fats.
5. Careful and accurate recording of the patient's blood pressure in both the standing and lying positions two or three times a day.
6. Administration of potentially dangerous hypotensive drugs with close observation of the patient for side effects.

Drug Therapy. The specific form of therapy today for the control of essential hypertension is chemotherapy. Important drugs for its control are summarized in Table 37–3. The three basic groups:

1. *Diuretics:* These drugs, particularly the thiazide diuretics, have proved effective in at least 50 per

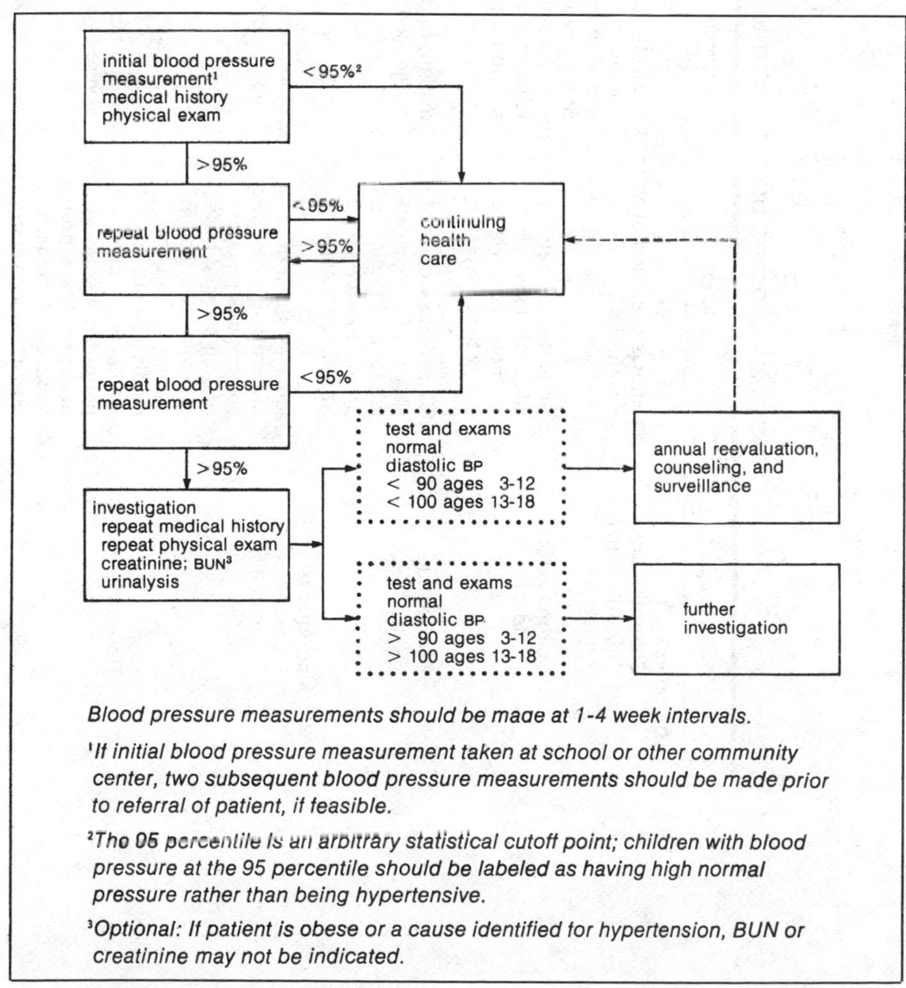

Figure 37–5. Identification and evaluation of asymptomatic children with elevated blood pressure. (From the beginnings of hypertension. *Emergency Medicine*, 9:97, July 1977.)

TABLE 37–3. DRUGS USED TO CONTROL HYPERTENSION

Drug	*Action*	*Indications For Use*	*Side Effects*
Diuretics			
Chlorothiazide (Diuril), other thiazides	Promotes excretion of Na^+ H_2O, and K^+	May be effective alone or in combination with reserpine in the treatment of mild hypertension	Hypokalemia; hyperuricemia; hyperglycemia
Spironolactone (Aldactone)	Inhibits Na^+-conserving effect of aldosterone; promotes renal Na^+ excretion without depleting K^+	Helps to combat hypokalemia produced by chlorothiazide	Breast stimulation (rare)
Furosemide (Lasix)	Inhibits reabsorption of Na^+ and Cl^- in ascending loop of Henle; promotes excretion of Na^+, Cl^-, K^+, and HCO_3^-	Excellent for treatment of reduced renal function	Severe electrolyte depletion, hypotension
Blocking Agents			
Propranolol (Inderal)	Decreases strength of myocardial contraction and inhibits response of an increased heart rate to usual stimuli, leading to reduced cardiac output	Moderately severe hypertension	Precipitation of congestive heart failure; bronchospasm
Reserpine	Depletes brain and peripheral tissues of norepinephrine; produces sedation; decreases peripheral vasoconstriction, heart rate, and standing blood pressure	Mild and moderately severe hypotension	Depression; nasal stuffiness; peptic ulceration; insomnia; Na^+ retention
Guanethidine (Ismelin)	Produces postganglionic sympathetic blockade, depletes tissue stores of norepinephrine	Severe, moderately severe, renal, and essential hypertension	Severe orthostatic hypotension; diarrhea; inability to ejaculate

Alpha-methyldopa (Aldomet)	Suppresses CNS sympathetic outflow; lowers supine and standing blood pressures; dilates peripheral arterioles; usually increases glomerular filtration and cardiac output	Severe and moderately severe hypertension	Initial drowsiness; skin eruptions; dryness of mouth; fluid retention; fever; occasionally liver damage
Clonidine (Catapres)	Suppresses CNS sympathetic outflow	Severe and moderately severe hypertension	Sedation, dry mouth, constipation, impotence; also, with abrupt cessation, withdrawal syndrome has occurred consisting of anxiety, headache, GI symptoms, severe hypertension
Trimethaphan (Arfonad)	Promotes pulmonary and peripheral vasodilation and emptying of the left ventricle	During surgery to control hypertension; also in hypertensive crises and in pulmonary edema resulting from hypertension	Urinary retention; orthostatic hypertension; anginal attacks in angina patients
Vasodilators			
Hydralazine (Apresoline)	Dilates peripheral blood vessels; antihypertensive effect is somewhat counteracted because vasodilation causes a reflex increase in cardiac output; renal blood flow is increased	Moderately severe hypertensive crisis	Tachycardia; angina pectoris; gastric irritation; palpitations; headache; arthritis; lupus erythematosus
Sodium nitroprusside (Nipride)	Decreases peripheral vascular resistance	Hypertensive crisis, to lower BP rapidly	Hypotension
Diazoxide (Hyperstat)	Promptly decreases peripheral vascular resistance and blood pressure	Injected IV in hospitalized patients in hypertensive crisis	Hypotension to shock levels; cerebral ischemia leading to convulsions and coma
Prazosin (Minipress)	New drug; specific action unknown; seems to act as smooth muscle relaxant	Mild to moderately severe hypertension	Severe postural hypotension may appear during first hours of treatment

cent of cases of hypertensive disease. They reduce blood pressure by reducing extracellular fluid volume. The most serious side effect of prolonged diuretic therapy is hypokalemia. (See Chapter 12.)

2. *Sympathetic nervous system blocking agents:* These drugs are employed in patients who are unresponsive to diuretics alone. Reserpine (an antiadrenergic agent) is the least potent of the group, followed by propranolol (a beta-adrenergic blocking agent); guanethidine (a ganglionic blocking agent) is the most potent. These medications lower blood pressure by interrupting the activity of the sympathetic nervous system and by lowering renin activity. (Remember that both the activation of the sympathetic nervous system and the release of renin result in vasoconstriction.) Blocking agents usually are given in conjunction with diuretics because the relative vasodilation they produce usually causes fluid retention.

3. *Vasodilators:* This group lowers blood pressure by dilating blood vessels. They are usually given with diuretics to prevent peripheral pooling of body fluids due to vasodilation.

Currently medications for control of hypertension are administered either on the basis of (a) the stepped-care drug treatment approach or (b) the patient's renin profile. The *stepped care-approach* "calls for the initiation of treatment with a small dosage of an antihypertensive drug, increasing the dosage of that drug, and then adding, in sequence, other drugs as needed."[72] The initial dosage of each drug is low and is increased only if the patient's blood pressure is not successfully responding to the medication. Of course, the dosage can be adjusted either up or down on the basis of the patient's periodic blood pressure readings. Administration of the lowest possible dosage needed for blood pressure control is always the goal of chemotherapy.

The four steps* of this chemotherapeutic regimen[202] are summarized here:

	Thiazides	Propranolol HCl	Methyldopa	Reserpine	Clonidine HCl†	Prazosin HCl†	Hydralazine HCl	Guanethidine sulfate
Step 1	●							
Step 2		●	●	●	●	●		
Step 3					●	●	●	
Step 4								●

*Chart adapted from Moser, M., J. R. Guyther, F. Finnerty, Jr., et al.: Report of the Joint National Committee on Detection, Evaluation, and Treatment of High Blood Pressure. *Journal of the American Medical Association,* 237:255, 1977.

†Experience is limited with clonidine HCl and prazosin HCl, newly approved, moderately potent antihypertensive agents that may be added or substituted for step 2 or step 3 drugs.

Because the *thiazide diuretics* are considered to be the cornerstone of antihypertensive therapy by the majority of physicians, they are the first drugs to be prescribed. Their beneficial effects usually become apparent after one to two weeks of diuretic therapy. However, if the patient's hypertension cannot be controlled by thiazides alone, moderately potent antihypertensive drugs (propranolol, methyldopa, reserpine) are added during Step 2 of the regimen. If the patient's blood pressure still remains elevated, then hydralazine, a more potent antihypertensive, is added in Step 3. If at this point the patient's blood pressure still fails to respond to the medications, the nurse and doctor must make an assessment. Is the patient complying with the program, and taking the medications? Is the diet high in sodium? Also, the patient may now need further diagnostic tests to confirm whether or not cardiovascular complications have developed. Finally, if there are no problems, Step 4 is taken and guanethidine is either added to the program or substituted for another drug. Unfortunately, guanethidine has some upsetting side effects; e.g., postural hypotension, diarrhea, and retrograde ejaculation.

This stepped-up drug regimen is also applied to children and adolescents.[231] Be aware that reserpine is not administered to children because of its side effects and propranolol has not received FDA approval for pediatric administration. Only those children who manifest persistent elevations of blood pressure are considered for chemotherapy, and then only after the child has attempted weight reduction as needed, salt restriction, and an exercise program.[231]

The second and newest chemotherapeutic approach to hypertension control is based upon the patient's *renin-sodium index.* Essentially, the rationale for choice of drugs utilizing this method is:[111, 244]

High renin hypertension: As explained earlier, high renin hypertension is a disease caused by vasoconstriction rather than by an excess of mineralocorticoid activity with resultant sodium retention. Thus the cornerstone of therapy for these patients is a *sympathetic nervous system blocking agent* which reduces renin activity (e.g., propranolol, methyldopa, and clonidine) rather than a diuretic.

Low renin hypertension: This is a problem involving sodium retention and thus responds best to *diuretics* (thiazides, chlorthalidone)

Medium renin hypertension: This form of hypertension responds reasonably well to both diuretic and sympatholytic drugs.

A treatment utilizing renin profiles is shown in Figure 37–6. Observe that drugs are added and subtracted as necessary until the patient's blood pressure is stabilized at the goal desired. For example, the patient with a high or normal renin profile is given propranolol; if this does not improve the hypertension, propranolol and a diuretic are then prescribed. Later, when the patient is stabilized on the two drugs, the physician may attempt to subtract the propranolol and see how the patient responds. If the response is good, the patient only need remain on diuretic therapy; if the response is unfavorable, the propranolol is resumed. On the other hand, if the diuretic and the propranolol together fail to control the hypertension, then other drugs are added or subtracted until just the right drug or drug combination is found.

Patients receiving antihypertensive drug therapy may develop acute hypotensive reactions, which are characterized by faintness, weakness, nausea, and vomiting. Patients on drug therapy must be taught how to prevent acute hypotensive reactions as well as what to do should a reaction occur. When discharge nears, you will alert the patient and significant others to these precautions:

1. Lie down immediately if faintness, weakness, nausea, and vomiting occur; put feet higher than head; flex thigh muscles and wiggle toes. This position promotes cerebral blood flow and lessens pooling of blood in limbs. Muscular activity decreases pooling of blood in lower extremities.
2. Avoid hot baths, excessive amounts of alcohol, and immobility following exercise which promote vasodilatation and may cause fainting.
3. Always rise *slowly* from a lying to a sitting position and from a sitting to a standing position, to allow the vascular system to adjust to positional changes.
4. Avoid standing motionless (e.g., at bus stops, in telephone booths, on subways, in supermarket lines, in the shower), especially within the first hour or two after receiving the medication. Standing causes vessels within the legs to relax, which allows blood to pool within the lower extremities; draining of blood from the brain and other vital organs can cause fainting.
5. Use caution in driving an automobile or operating machinery, especially within 2 hours after taking the drug. An accident could occur if acute hypotension develops suddenly.
6. Avoid cheese, beer, or wine when taking a monoamine oxidase inhibitor, (e.g., pargyline, Eutonyl). A severe reaction may occur, with the possibility of cerebral hemorrhage.
7. Avoid constipation; ask the doctor for a gentle laxative should bowels fail to move regularly. Exercise daily and take adequate fluids and roughage. Constipation may cause either an increased or irregular absorption of hypotensive drugs, which can result in critical hypotensive reactions.
8. Should hypotensive crises occur frequently, Ace bandages or elastic support stockings should be worn when ambulating. Ace bandages and elastic stockings promote venous return from the lower extremities and decrease pooling of blood within the legs.
9. When taking diuretics, watch for signs of hypokalemia (K^+ deficit) and notify doctor at once.

Surgical Techniques. Surgical techniques for the control of primary hypertension have decreased greatly in popularity with the advent of potent antihypertensive agents. Surgery, however, is still employed in the correction of secondary forms.

In *repair of coarctation of the aorta* the constriction is removed from the aorta and the upper and lower ends of the aorta are united, sometimes by means of a graft.

Adrenalectomy, or surgical excision of the ad-

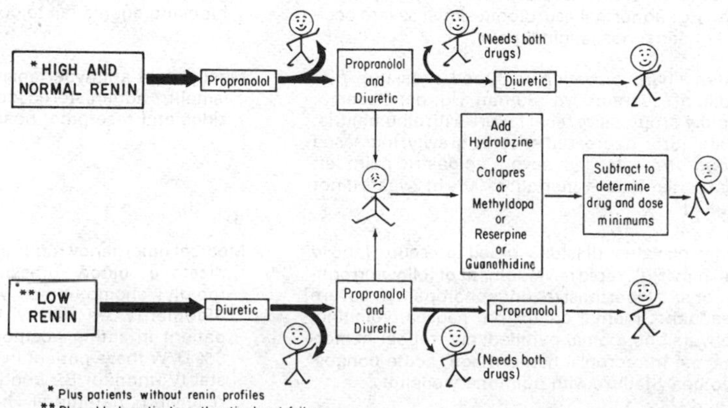

Figure 37–6. New hypertension treatment system: with or without baseline renin profiles. (From Weber, M. A., and J. H. Laragh: Hypertension. *In* Conn, H. F.: *Current Therapy 1978.* Philadelphia: W. B. Saunders Co., 1978, p. 216.)

renal tumor, is employed to correct pheochromocytoma, primary aldosteronism, and Cushing's syndrome.

Correction of renal artery stenosis may be done to alleviate hypertension caused by renal vascular disease.

Specific Therapies for Hypertension of Varying Severity. There are six different phases of hypertensive disease: the prehypertensive, mild benign, moderately severe benign, severe benign, malignant, and acute emergency (acute hypertensive crisis).

Each of these phases has certain characteristics and requires a specific type of therapy; this information is briefly summarized in Table 37–4.

REHABILITATIVE AND EDUCATIONAL APPROACHES

The nurse caring for the patient with hypertension usually has the responsibility for educating the patient in a program of lifelong blood pressure control as well as reinforcing the physician's instructions and explanations. As a general rule, physician and nurse must carefully tailor the rehabilitation program to the specific needs and personality of the patient. They must take into consideration the patient's habits, life style, and general outlook. Patients who are depressed or belligerent, who drink excessively, who are severely neurotic, or who have deteriorated mentally must be given special consideration in any teaching plan.

The most important point that the hypertensive individual and significant others must understand is that *essential hypertension is a chronic condition* that cannot be cured but can be *controlled.* When control fails, the reason must be determined. *The most common cause of treatment failure is a reluctance on the patient's part to comply with the program.* Poor compliance is most often due to inadequate instruction concerning hypertension and its care, uncomfortable side effects from the medications, mental depression, poor rapport with the doctor or nurse, and long waiting periods in the clinic or doctor's office for follow-up care. Other causes are an inadequate drug regimen and the presence of unsuspected forms of secondary hypertension (e.g., renal artery stenosis, pheochromocytoma.)

Nurses, in particular, can help prevent the main cause of treatment failure — patient noncompliance — by means of careful patient instruction. As you and the physician set up a teaching program for the patient about to be discharged home, make certain you include the following areas in your discussion:

Home Blood Pressure Recordings. The patient will need to learn how to wrap the blood pressure

TABLE 37–4. PHASES OF HYPERTENSION

Phase	Characteristics	Therapy
Prehypertensive	Blood pressure mildly elevated: systolic pressure below 200 mm. Hg, diastolic pressure below 100 mm. Hg; symptoms of anxiety may be present: headache, insomnia, irritability, forgetfulness	No specific therapy; occasionally tranquilizers or sleeping medication
Mild benign	Systolic pressure remains below 200 mm. Hg, diastolic pressure above 100 mm. Hg; vague symptoms of anxiety; headache, fatigue, palpitations	Weight reduction; Na^+-restricted diet; mild antihypertensive drugs; diuretics with K^+ replacements
Moderately severe benign	Systolic blood pressure above 200 mm. Hg, diastolic pressure above 110 mm. Hg; no evidence of vascular damage	Weight reduction; Na^+-restricted diet; more potent drugs: Aldomet, Apresoline
Severe benign	Systolic blood pressure up to 250 mm. Hg or higher, diastolic blood pressure persistently above 120 mm. Hg; abnormal neurologic signs: severe occipital headaches, anginal pain	Postganglionic blocking agents, e.g., Ismelin; ganglionic blocking agents if postganglionic blocking agents fail to control BP, e.g., Nipride
Malignant	Sudden sharp elevation in blood pressure: diastolic pressure above 130 mm. Hg; papilledema; rapidly progressive renal failure with albuminuria, proteinuria, decreased specific gravity, increased blood urea nitrogen; severe epigastric pain; left ventricular failure; mortality 100% in 2 years if not treated	Most potent antihypertensive drugs available, e.g., Ismelin, administered concomitantly with thiazides and reserpine; hospitalize promptly
Acute	Greatly elevated diastolic blood pressure (above 140 mm. Hg); rapid development of following conditions: Hypertensive encephalopathy, severe headache, mental confusion, nausea, vomiting, convulsions, coma, papilledema, retinal hemorrhages; intracranial hemorrhage; acute congestive heart failure with pulmonary edema	Medical emergency requiring immediate treatment; diastolic blood pressure must be reduced rapidly; chemotherapy with reserpine IM or IV, Aldomet IV, Arfonad IV diluted in 5% D/W (have patient in sitting position), Nipride IV diluted in 5% D/W (have patient in supine position), Hyperstat IV; monitor BP continuously while patient is receiving parenteral medications; when BP controlled, patient started on potent oral antihypertensives

TEACHING GUIDELINES for SODIUM RESTRICTED DIETS

Discuss salt, sodium chloride, and other sodium-containing compounds:

1. Sodium is a mineral essential for life. It is found in almost all foods and beverages, including water. It cannot be seen and often is not tasted.
2. Table salt is sodium chloride, and 40 percent of it is sodium.
3. Lite Salt contains about half the sodium per unit that regular table salt contains.
4. Sodium is present in flavored salts commonly used for seasoning. (garlic salt, celery salt, and onion salt)
5. Sodium is found in large amounts in such common commercial preparations as baking soda, baking powder, monosodium glutamate, meat tenderizer, and soy sauce.
6. Sodium is added to flavor or to preserve frozen, canned, and boxed foods.

Explain the relationship of sodium to high blood pressure and the rationale for eliminating sodium from the diet.

1. Normally, sodium exists in body fluids and tissues.
2. Extra sodium is removed from the body by the kidneys.
3. In some diseases, extra sodium may remain in the body and cause water retention and possibly more resistance in blood vessels.
4. Severely restricted dietary sodium (<3 Gm./day) and diuretics are equally effective in lowering arterial blood pressure.
5. Excessive amounts of retained sodium and water decrease the effectiveness of diuretic therapy and other antihypertensive medications.

Stress avoidance of foods and medications that contain multiple sodium compounds; stress importance of reading labels carefully.

1. Sodium is added to preserve or flavor commercially prepared foods. Labels can be read for such ingredients as salt and sodium compounds. (*Prepare by draining off the canned liquid and heating the food in tap water. *Eat recommended exchange amounts of canned foods. *Avoid all canned food.)
2. Fresh meat and fresh or plain frozen vegetables contain less sodium and are less expensive than those canned without salt.
3. All dietetic foods are not sodium free. Labels must be checked carefully.
4. Over-the-counter medications, such as Alka-Seltzer, antacids, cough medications, and laxatives, often contain large amounts of sodium and should not be taken without the doctor's permission.

Alter the diet while eliminating excessive sodium intake.

1. Eating three well-balanced meals a day with emphasis on foods naturally low in sodium is possible and can be appetizing. Snacks can be included without exceeding the sodium restriction. Many stores sell no-salt snack foods.
2. Limiting salt intake to the equivalent of one level teaspoon per day requires that
   - no salt be added at the table
   - no salt be used during food preparation
   - foods excessively high in sodium, including canned foods, be eliminated
3. Limiting salt intake to 5 Gm. per day requires that
   - no salt be added at the table
   - food be salted lightly during food preparation
   - canned, frozen, fresh foods be selected in measured amounts.
4. Calculation of sodium exchanges permits rationing of daily intake of sodium. This requires menu planning and allows for individual choices of foods moderate in sodium (100-250 mg./serving) and occasional limited intake of small amounts of foods high in sodium (300 mg./serving). (Preferred reference is Wilson. Additional calculations of sodium, protein, and potassium are available in hospital dietary manuals.)

Season food without using sodium-containing compounds.

1. Spices, herbs, fruits, and many other substances do not contain sodium. Lemon, particularly, enhances flavors of meat, chicken, fish, seafood, and snacks. Lists of acceptable flavors as substitutes and recipes using them should be given to patients
2. Fresh or powdered garlic and onion may be substituted for garlic or onion salt without difficulty.
3. Low-sodium cookbooks are available, but they are not necessary for patients with uncomplicated essential hypertension.

Consider salt substitutes.

1. Seek advice from patient's physician before suggesting them.
2. Most salt substitutes contain potassium as the flavor component. These may be useful in preventing potassium deficiency if the patient is taking a thiazide diuretic.
3. The potassium in salt substitutes may cause hyperkalemia in patients taking potassium-sparing diuretics or potassium supplements or in patients who have renal impairment.

Figure 37–7. Teaching guidelines for hypertensive patients using sodium restricted diets. An asterisk (*) indicates controversial material. Parentheses enclose directions for patients that are contraindicated by some authorities. (From Hill, M.: Helping the hypertensive patient control sodium intake. *American Journal of Nursing*, 79:906, May 1979.)

cuff, position the arm correctly, listen for systolic and diastolic sounds and record pressure accurately. Except perhaps in the extremely anxious patient, taking one's own blood pressure reading is often a great incentive for the patient to take medications as prescribed and to control weight and diet. The patient can see that blood pressure remains lower when the treatment program is followed, and that it rises when drugs and diet are ignored or the patient becomes unduly angry or excited.

Self-medication with Antihypertensive Drugs. As emphasized, antihypertensive drugs have dangerous side effects. Patients who are going to administer their own drugs need to be given the following precautions:

1. *Never take a larger dose of drug than prescribed without consulting the doctor.*
2. *Always take the drug on time; do not skip doses.*
3. *Never suddenly discontinue a drug without the doctor's permission, because severe hypertension may develop.*
4. *Always report untoward effects to the physician.*

Also, patients need to be cautioned about *acute hypotensive reactions;* they need specific rules for preventing and treating hypotension should it occur.

Dietary Restrictions. The doctor will probably want the patient to see a dietitian before discharge. You or the dietitian can give the patient printed information listing low-calorie, low-sodium foods. (Teaching guidelines for sodium restricted diets are listed in Figure 37–7.) Also, caution the patient to avoid eating large heavy meals, because the digestion of large amounts of food puts an unnecessary burden on the heart, and avoid drinking large amounts of fluid, because excess fluids increase the blood volume, which, in turn, increases blood pressure.

Exertion. Heavy, overly strenuous exercise is harmful for patients with hypertension; however, a planned, moderate exercise program is beneficial. Daily walks are an excellent means of exercise, although hills and stairsteps should be avoided. Gardening and golf are also enjoyable forms of exercise for many people.

Interpersonal Relations. The patient with hypertension recovers best in home and working environments that are relatively harmonious and peaceful. If the patient works under a supervisor who constantly harasses and pressures him, it may be necessary for the patient to find a more suitable employer.

An upsetting domestic atmosphere may not be so easily changed. However, you and the physician can counsel the patient's spouse, older children, or others living in the home concerning the importance of making the patient's home environment relaxed. Once the patient's family understands the correlation between high blood pressure and emotional tension, it is hoped they will ease the patient's home responsibilities and provide greater emotional support.

Hobbies. Encourage the patient to engage in hobbies that are stimulating and interesting but do not cause great anxiety or high emotion. Because people vary widely in their emotional responses to different activities, the selection of a hobby is a highly individual matter. For example, card playing for some persons is a pleasant social pastime, whereas for others it is competitive and nerve wracking. Likewise, spectator sports, political rallies, or horse races may have special significance for some people. As you discuss various activities with the patient, try to evaluate emotional responses. Guide the patient as much as possible into hobbies that are engrossing but not stressful.

PROGNOSIS

With the advent of effective antihypertensive chemotherapy, the outlook for patients suffering from hypertension is far brighter. Before, 70 per cent of patients with hypertension died of heart failure, 15 per cent of cerebral hemorrhage, and 10 per cent of uremia. Within the last decade, since the advent of effective antihypertensive agents, the mortality rate has decreased 40 per cent.[40] Today, most patients with hypertension die of complications of the basic atherosclerotic process, which affects the cerebral arteries, renal arteries, and coronary arteries, e.g., "stroke," renal failure, myocardial infarction. When hypertension arises as a secondary process, patients may die of the primary disease, e.g., polyarteritis, Cushing's disease, or nephritis.

Patients with malignant hypertension also have a far more favorable prognosis today. Before the advent of antihypertensive drugs, such patients rarely lived for more than two years following the onset of the disease. Today, 50 to 60 per cent of patients are still living five years following diagnosis.

CHAPTER 38

DISORDERS THAT AFFECT SPECIFIC STRUCTURES OF THE HEART

You recall from Chapter 31 that the major structures of the heart are the pericardium, the myocardium, and the endocardium. Many different factors are capable of adversely affecting these vital structures, e.g., viruses, bacteria, toxins, tumors, trauma, and various systemic diseases. In some cases these factors affect only one structure of the heart; in other cases, all structures of the heart undergo pathophysiologic changes.

PANCARDITIS: RHEUMATIC FEVER AND HEART DISEASE

Rheumatic fever is an acute or chronic systemic inflammatory process characterized by attacks of fever, polyarthritis, and carditis; the latter may eventually result in permanent valvular damage.

While CHD and hypertension mainly affect individuals over age 50, rheumatic fever is the most common cause of heart disease in persons under 50, and is rare in people over 50.[40] No one knows the exact incidence of rheumatic fever because it is not reportable. Authorities estimate that 2 to 3 per cent of persons who have suffered a beta-hemolytic streptococcal infection will develop rheumatic fever. Because most children and young people suffer at some time from a streptococcal infection, we can assume that the incidence of rheumatic fever is high. It is rapidly becoming less common as a result of prophylactic antibiotic therapy. Now physicians immediately administer antibiotics to patients with streptococcal infections, thereby preventing the later development of rheumatic fever.

Predisposing Factors. What are the major factors that *predispose* an individual to rheumatic fever and control *distribution* of the disease throughout the population?

First, *age* is a major consideration. Rheumatic fever primarily strikes children and teenagers. Children between the ages of 5 and 15 are particularly vulnerable; indeed, 90 per cent of first attacks of the disease affect this age group. Also, rheumatic fever is the principal cause of fatalities among youngsters between 5 and 19. While rheumatic fever mainly affects the young, it also attacks the aged, causing severe cardiac disability and death.

Second, rheumatic fever is influenced by *economic* factors; it strikes the slum dweller much more frequently than the suburbanite, the city dweller more frequently than the farmer. Evidently poor persons living in urban areas are more prone to rheumatic fever because of malnutrition, greater exposure to bacterial infections, and less money for medical and dental care.

Finally, rheumatic fever may possibly have a *genetic* basis. Some authorities suggest that persons can inherit a mendelian recessive trait for rheumatic fever. Other authorities point out that rheumatic fever may appear "to run in families" only because all family members are exposed to the highly infectious group A streptococcus when one family member has an infection.

ETIOLOGY

The exact cause of rheumatic fever is unknown. A few authorities believe that viruses are the major etiologic agents, whereas others feel that rheumatic fever develops as a hypersensitivity reaction to certain allergens. However, most evidence points to the *poststreptococcal hypersensitization* theory. Facts supporting this hypothesis are as follows: Rheumatic fever almost always develops following upper respiratory tract infection by the *beta-hemolytic group A streptococcus.* The *time* interval between the development of the streptococcal upper respiratory infection and the advent of rheumatic fever is almost always around five weeks; this is the approximate amount of time needed for the patient to become sensitized to the organism and to undergo an immune reaction.* However,

*See Chapter 11 for a discussion of the immune reaction.

since only 2 to 3 per cent develop rheumatic fever following streptococcal infections, researchers hypothesize that these susceptible persons have a greater immunologic response to streptococci.

PATHOPHYSIOLOGY

Rheumatic fever is classified by most authorities as a hypersensitivity "collagen" disorder; thus, it is characterized by an inflammatory process that affects connective tissue in organs throughout the body, i.e., the heart, joints, nervous system, respiratory system, and so forth.

While the effects of rheumatic fever upon the joints, tendons, skin, respiratory system, and serosal membranes are temporary and fairly benign, it often produces permanent damage of the heart. As one author states:

> The heart bears the brunt of the attack, suffers the most disabling injuries, and damage to it is the reason for the importance of rheumatic fever as a cause of disability and death.[142]

Rheumatic carditis is the most important consequence of rheumatic fever; this condition develops in approximately 75 per cent of patients. Carditis generally appears during the first or second week following the development of rheumatic fever, and it involves one or all three layers of the heart (myocardium, endocardium, and pericardium). When all three layers are affected simultaneously, the condition is called *pancarditis.*

Table 38–1 summarizes the pathophysiologic effects of rheumatic fever upon the myocardium, endocardium, and pericardium.

Rheumatic fever can lead to permanent heart damage if the endocardium and valves become involved in the inflammatory process. Damage is permanent because the valve leaflets encrusted with vegetations become shriveled and shortened, producing valvular dysfunction and poor cardiac activity. First, the damaged valve may become narrowed or *stenosed,* greatly increasing the heart's labors as it struggles to propel blood forward through its chambers and into the aorta. Second, the valve leaflets may become so shortened that they cannot close securely. As a result, blood *regurgitates* or leaks backward through the damaged valve into the chamber from which it was ejected. The final consequence of both valvular stenosis and regurgitation is heart failure owing to strain and overwork.

Noncardiac changes that result from the widespread inflammatory process are (1) red, swollen, tender joints; (2) tissue edema; (3) large subcutaneous nodules under the skin; (4) thickened, red, granular synovial membranes; and (5) occasionally, pneumonitis.

ONSET AND SYMPTOMS

As we stated earlier, rheumatic fever almost always follows a streptococcal infection. There are typically three phases in its onset.

Phase 1: The patient suffers from an acute streptococcal infection, e.g., scarlet fever, streptococcal sore throat, or streptococcal tonsillitis. During this period the patient experiences chills, fever, swollen lymph nodes, and sore throat.

Phase 2: Patient recovers from the acute infection and appears symptom-free. This latent period of sensitization lasts from one to five weeks.

TABLE 38–1. EFFECTS OF RHEUMATIC FEVER UPON THE MYOCARDIUM, ENDOCARDIUM, AND PERICARDIUM

Condition	Characteristic Lesion	Factors in Causation of Lesion	Significance of Pathophysiologic Involvement
Rheumatic myocarditis	Aschoff bodies, minute nodules, usually found in connective tissue around small arteries in myocardium	Formed by leukocytes that mass in inflamed tissues	Nodules may eventually become fibrotic; damage from fibrosis may eventually damage arteries in myocardium; myocarditis may cause a temporary loss in contractile power of the heart; permanent damage rarely results
Rheumatic endocarditis	Tiny *vegetations* resembling little beads form along line of closure of valve flaps	Probably result from inflammation, ulceration, and erosion of valve flaps	Inflammatory damage of valves results in *permanent* severe heart disease
Pericarditis	Nonspecific lesions	Result from a diffuse, nonspecific fibrinous or serofibrinous inflammatory reaction	May cause pericardial friction rub; usually no serious sequelae

Phase 3: Symptoms of rheumatic fever develop and the patient is once again acutely ill.

While symptoms of the acute streptococcal infection result from the direct invasion of tissues by bacteria, the manifestations of rheumatic fever evidently result from a *hypersensitivity reaction* to those streptococci that invaded weeks earlier and were vanquished by the body's defense mechanisms. (See Chapter 10.) Thus, the symptoms result mainly from inflammation of connective tissues. The symptoms are many and varied:

Arthralgia or joint pain is the most prominent manifestation of rheumatic fever. Joints affected are the ankles, knees, shoulders, elbows, and wrists. Arthralgia usually has a rapid onset and subsides after a period of several hours to several days. During this time young patients may complain of "growing pains."

Carditis is the second most common manifestation of rheumatic fever; it is by far the most dangerous and destructive consequence of this disease (Table 38–1).

Fever of 38°C. (100.4°F.) or higher temperature elevations alternate with periods when temperature is normal (relapsing fever).

Subcutaneous nodules are small nodules that adhere loosely to the patient's tendon sheaths; they usually occur in children and are evident only during the first week or so following the onset of the disease.

Erythema marginatum is a migratory rash that usually appears on warm areas of the body. The lesions are crescent-shaped and have clear centers.

Abdominal pain is a common symptom that varies in site and severity; the pain may be related to engorgement of the liver.

Sydenham's chorea, also called St. Vitus dance, is a nervous disorder characterized by grimacing and constant jerky purposeless movements. It is common in children, especially young girls; characteristically, chorea does not appear until the late stages of the disease.

Malaise, asthenia, weight loss, and anorexia probably develop as a result of fever, pain, and the general debilitation that is characteristically linked with any serious illness.

DIAGNOSTIC MEASURES

Laboratory Studies. No specific laboratory studies diagnose rheumatic fever. At best, laboratory findings only serve to confirm the presence of acute infection. Thus, one finds an elevated sedimentation rate and an elevated leukocyte count of from 15,000 to 30,000. One helpful, nonspecific laboratory finding that occurs in 85 to 90 per cent of these patients is an elevation of *antistreptolysin serum titers.* A positive finding indicates that the patient's body has formed antibodies against one or more streptococcal antigens. Also, 50 per cent of patients with active rheumatic fever have a throat culture positive for *beta-hemolytic group A streptococci.*

ECG Findings. The presence of rheumatic carditis is best established by serial ECG tracings. A prolonged PR interval, irregular rhythm, and signs of atrial fibrillation are the major evidence of myocardial damage.

Physical Examination. The final diagnosis of rheumatic fever rests upon the following physical findings: (a) the presence of two or more of the following symptoms — carditis, Sydenham's chorea, subcutaneous nodules, erythema marginatum, and polyarthritis, (b) evidence of a recent beta-hemolytic streptococcal infection; and (c) prompt relief of fever and joint pain by salicylate administration.

Evidence of rheumatic *carditis* is based on typical ECG findings; presence of mitral or aortic diastolic murmurs; and signs of fibrous or pleuritic type pericarditis and/or CHF.

CLINICAL CARE

The major goals of care in the treatment of patients with rheumatic fever are:

1. To control and alleviate the infecting streptococci.
2. To protect the heart against the highly damaging effects of carditis.
3. To relieve joint pain, fever, and other symptoms.

Typical measures used in the care of patients with rheumatic fever are bed rest, proper diet, and chemotherapy with penicillin, salicylates, and steroids.

Bed Rest. A patient with rheumatic fever must rest for two reasons: to reduce strain on the heart, and to minimize metabolic needs during the acute, febrile stage of the disease.

When on bed rest the patient may be allowed to perform certain self-care activities, e.g., turning, oral hygiene, feeding, grooming. Nonstrenuous diversional activities such as watching television, reading and listening to the radio may be permitted. Short vistis from relatives and friends are usually permitted, provided the visitors are free from colds, flus, and sore throats.

The patient must generally remain on bed rest for a period of several weeks or longer. Ambulation and self care are not permitted until the following criteria are met: *temperature* remains normal without the use of salicylates; *resting pulse* (in adults) remains under 100; *ECG* tracings show no signs of myocardial damage; and *sedimentation rate* returns to normal.

Once up and about, the patient must still be cautioned not to overdo. How long activities must be restricted depends upon whether carditis develops and the extent of permanent heart damage resulting from such carditis.

Restrictions may extend for many months; in severe cases of rheumatic carditis, patients may even be forced to undergo restrictions on a permanent basis; e.g., they may have to change occupations if their job is strenuous, move from a two-story house to a one-story house, and so forth. When significant changes in life style are necessary, patients can obtain guidance from the Crippled Children's Division of the Federal Children's Bureau and from the American Heart Association.

Diet Therapy. The patient with rheumatic fever needs a bland, high-protein, high-carbohydrate diet to maintain adequate nutrition in the face of fever and infection. The doctor may also order supplements of vitamins and minerals. The intake of oral fluids is encouraged to prevent dehydration due to fever. If the patient shows signs of severe carditis or CHF, a low-sodium diet is necessary; fluids may also be restricted.

Encourage the patient (who is often anorexic) to eat all meals. Nursing personnel may have to feed the patient if activity has been severely curtailed because of cardiac involvement.

Drug Therapy. The three major groups of drugs used to treat rheumatic fever are antibiotics, salicylates, and steroids. The antibiotics employed are *penicillin* and the *sulfonamides.* These drugs are given for 10 days following the onset of rheumatic fever in order to destroy any streptococci remaining alive in the upper respiratory tract. Following this period, prophylactic doses of these drugs are given to prevent fresh attacks of streptococcal infection.

The *salicylates* are given to control fever and to relieve joint pain. *Sodium salicylate* is the most commonly used drug in the salicylate group. The maximum adult dose of this drug is 1 to 2 Gm. (15 to 30 gr.) every 2 hours orally. For patients with heart failure, aspirin is ordered in place of sodium salicylate. Observe patients taking salicylates carefully for early signs of toxicity.

Early signs of salicylism include tinnitus, nausea, and vomiting.

To reduce gastric irritation, salicylates are usually given with an antacid, or enteric-coated tablets are used.

Steroids are frequently given to patients with severe rheumatic fever to relieve symptoms. Fever, joint pain, and swelling are often dramatically reduced within 24 to 48 hours. However, steroid therapy probably neither prevents nor minimizes rheumatic carditis and its damaging after effects.

PROPHYLAXIS

First attacks of rheumatic fever are entirely preventable today, provided patients with streptococcal infections receive prompt antibiotic therapy. Also, patients who have recovered from an attack of rheumatic fever may prevent *subsequent* attacks by taking prophylactic doses of antibiotics and observing good health practices. Patients should be told that it is important that they avoid subsequent attacks of rheumatic fever, since repeated attacks may lead to serious heart disease, which can result in permanent cardiac disability and failure.

Penicillin is the prophylactic drug most frequently given, although the sulfonamides may be ordered if the patient is sensitive to penicillin. Two typical orders are penicillin, 200 to 250 thousand units orally before breakfast, or benzathine penicillin (Bicillin), 1 million units monthly. Additional doses of prophylactic penicillin must be taken before and after undergoing surgical procedures and dental manipulations of any kind. Prophylactic drugs are usually given for a period of five years following the initial attack; after five years, recurrences are uncommon.

The patient must also take good care of teeth and gums and receive prompt dental care for cavities and gingivitis. Persons who have upper respiratory infections or who have had a streptococcal infection within the last three months should be avoided. Finally, the physician should be called immediately if any of the symptoms of streptococcal sore throat (pharyngitis) develop; it is extremely important that antibiotic therapy be received promptly for any infection.

The symptoms of streptococcal sore throat are an elevated temperature of 38.9° to 40° C. (102 to 104° F.), chills, sore throat, and enlarged painful lymph nodes. Patients must take excellent care of themselves and guard against infections for the *rest of their lives* to avoid the possible development of heart disease.

PROGNOSIS AND COMPLICATIONS

Since the advent of antibiotic therapy, the prognosis for patients with rheumatic fever is generally good. Today, only 1 to 2 per cent of patients die during the initial attack; in these cases, death usually results from acute myocarditis. Most patients recover rapidly; laboratory and clinical signs generally completely subside within one to two months following therapy. However, some patients have residual heart damage, which may lead to either valvular stenosis or regurgitation. Should these patients have recurrent attacks of rheumatic fever, residual heart damage may eventually terminate in congestive heart failure. Fortunately, in some cases valvular disease can be successfully corrected by surgery before failure ensues.

Serious complications of rheumatic fever that may disable or kill the patient are CHF (the major cause of death); infarctions of the brain or kidneys due to embolization of valvular vegetations or mural thrombi within the heart; bacterial endocarditis; and pulmonary congestion due to left-sided heart failure, which may result in deadly pulmonary infections.

DISEASES THAT AFFECT THE ENDOCARDIUM

You will recall from Chapter 31 that the endocardium is a layer of endothelial tissue that lines the heart's cavities and aids in the formation of the valves. Diseases that may affect the endocardium are bacterial endocarditis (acute and chronic), chronic valvular heart disease, and rheumatic endocarditis.

Bacterial Endocarditis

DEFINITION AND CHARACTERISTICS

Bacterial endocarditis is a severe bacterial infection of the endocardium. It is characterized by the formation of friable vegetations on the heart valves, and by the metastatic spread of bacteria from the valves via the blood stream to organs and tissues all over the body. Bacterial endocarditis is usually fatal unless the patient receives antibiotic therapy.

There are two classic forms of bacterial endocarditis: acute bacterial endocarditis (ABE) and subacute bacterial endocarditis (SBE).

Acute bacterial endocarditis is a severe infection of fulminating onset characterized by high fever, heart murmurs, embolic phenomena, and splenomegaly. It is usually caused by highly pathogenic organisms capable of producing widespread damage, such as *Staphylococcus aureus,* pneumococci, beta-hemolytic streptococci, and gonococci. The infection follows a rapid course, and the endocardium may be severely damaged early in the disease. It is responsive to antibiotic therapy.

Subacute bacterial endocarditis is a smoldering infection manifested by a continuous fever, weight loss, fatigue, joint pains, and splenomegaly. The causative organisms are indigenous to the body and cause relatively little destruction; they include *Streptococcus viridans, S. faecalis,* and *Staphylococcus aureus.* The onset is insidious and the course prolonged, but with adequate antibiotic therapy, there is little or no damage to the endocardium.

The incidence of bacterial endocarditis is much lower today than in the past because of the development of antibiotics. It is estimated that it currently represents less than 1 per cent of all cardiac disorders. Persons between the ages of 20 and 40 are most susceptible to this disorder; however, bacterial endocarditis is currently striking older persons far more often than formerly.

PREDISPOSING FACTORS

How do bacteria enter the body, overcome the body's natural barriers against invasion, and reach the heart valves? Specifically, what factors predispose an individual to bacterial invasions of the heart valves? By what portals of entry do the organisms enter into the valves?

One factor that *predisposes* the patient's heart valves to bacterial invasion is *preexisting disease or injury* of the heart valves as a result of rheumatic, syphilitic, or arteriosclerotic heart disease or congenital anomalies. Also, patients with artificial heart valves are more prone to develop bacterial endocarditis. A second factor to consider is the *virulence* of the attacking bacteria. Bacteria of low virulence attack only damaged valves, but bacteria of high virulence can attack and destroy normal valves in patients with no preexisting heart disease.

Bacterial endocarditis usually follows *acute infection* of the tonsils, kidneys, gums, teeth, or lungs. However, bacteria can also enter the circulation following such simple maneuvers as vigorous brushing of the teeth or chewing hard foods or candies. It may also follow *heart surgery.* Bacterial endocarditis following cardiac surgery is often very severe, with the mortality rate (with aggressive antibiotic therapy) approximating 59 per cent. Patients may develop endocarditis shortly after surgery, or several years later. Regardless of the time frame, the symptoms may be subtle. An elevated temperature is the most common finding in these patients. Finally, bacteria can be introduced into the body by contaminated needles and careless technique in the parenteral administration of drugs. For this reason, drug addicts are often victims of bacterial endocarditis.

CAUSATIVE ORGANISMS

In recent years, antibiotic therapy has brought about a substantial change in the organisms responsible for bacterial endocarditis. The incidence of infections caused by staphylococci has at least doubled in the last 30 years while frequency of infections due to *Streptococcus viridans* has been cut almost in half. The increased incidence of the staphylococci and *S. faecalis* as causative factors is evidently due to the development of antibiotic-resistant strains of these organisms. Other antibiotic-resistant organisms that are causing increased numbers of infections are fungi and gram-negative bacilli. On the other hand, pneumonococci, gonococci, and meningococci have been virtually eliminated as causative agents because these organisms are so highly sensitive to penicillin and other antibiotics.

PATHOPHYSIOLOGY

As in rheumatic endocarditis, the lesion characteristic of bacterial endocarditis is a *friable vegetation* (Fig. 38–1) that forms on the valve leaflets. Such vegetations can severely damage not only the heart valves but other organs located throughout the body. The amount of damage caused depends on the type and virulence of organisms causing the infection; e.g., staphylococci are far more virulent organisms than is *Steptococcus viridans* and thus they cause larger vegetations more rapidly. Common complications resulting from the growth of vegetations on the valves are perforation of the valve leaflets; extension of the bacteria to the aorta or to the pericardium; metastatic spread of the infecting organism from the valves through the blood stream, causing abscess formation within the myocardium, spleen, kidneys, and brain; and infarction of the spleen, brain, gastrointestinal tract, and other sites as a result of shedding of vegetations into the blood stream as *emboli.*

SYMPTOMS AND COMPLICATIONS

Bacterial endocarditis signs can be categorized into three major groups: infection, cardiac involvement, and emboli.

The signs of *infection* comprise the most outstanding manifestations of bacterial endocarditis. The most reliable sign of infection is *fever,* a manifestation of bacterial endocarditis present in all patients. Typically the fever is *remittent* in nature, with afebrile periods lasting from days to weeks. Other signs of infection are chills, night sweats, fatigue, anorexia, weight loss, "aches and pains," cough, and loss of libido.

Signs of *cardiac involvement* are usually related to the presence of either rheumatic heart disease or congenital heart disease. Typical manifestations include tachycardia, splenomegaly, petechiae of the skin and mucous membranes, clubbing of the fingers and toes in longstanding cases of heart disease, pallor, joint swelling and pain, arthritis, and painful nodes of the finger

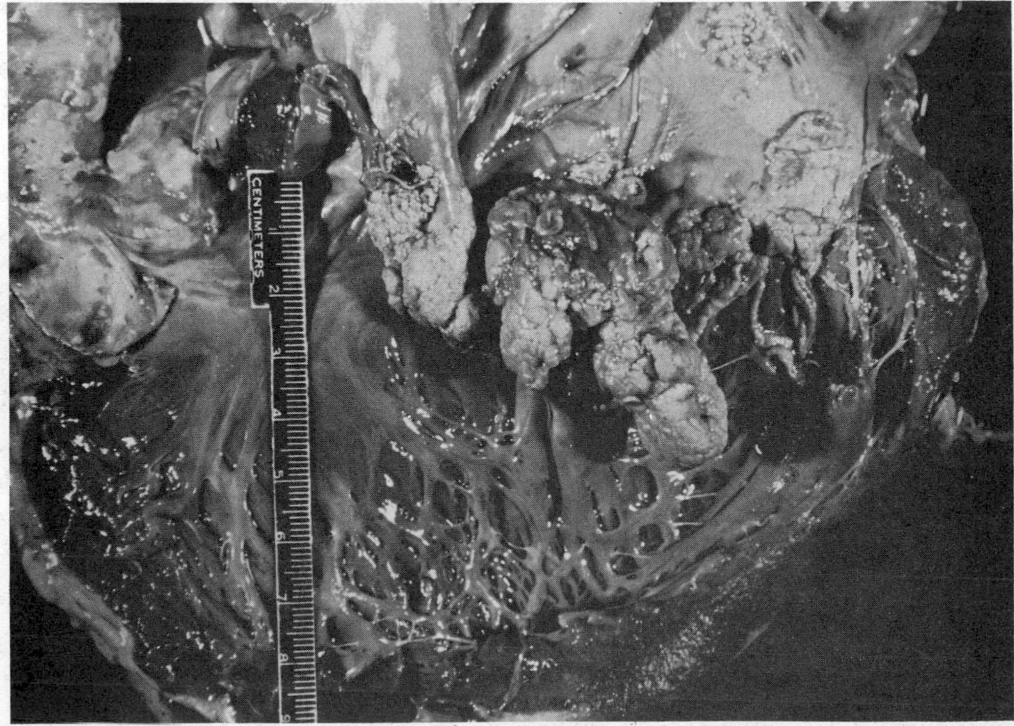

Figure 38–1. Infective bacterial endocarditis of the mitral valve with massive friable masses and extension of the vegetations to the atrial endocardium. (From Robbins, S. L., and R. S. Cotran: *Pathologic Basis of Disease,* 2nd ed. Philadelphia: W. B. Saunders Co., 1979, p. 684.)

and toe pads which occasionally result from endothelial swelling.

The most important cardiac sign is a *cardiac murmur,* which varies in character from day to day. These variations represent the growth and fragmentation of the valvular vegetations.

Finally, *embolic phenomena* disrupt organ functions all over the body, causing widely divergent symptoms. When the left side of the heart is involved, vegetation fragments are swept into the arterial circulation, which carries them to the spleen, kidneys, gastrointestinal tract, brain, and extremities where they then create large and small areas of infarction. When the right heart is involved, emboli pass into the pulmonary circulation; these fragments may then clog the arterioles of the lungs, causing pulmonary infarction.

The *spleen* is the organ most commonly affected by emboli, followed next by the kidney. Signs of splenic infarction are tenderness and enlargement of the spleen, and pain in the upper abdomen. Key signs of *renal* involvement are flank pain and hematuria. When the arterioles of the *brain* are obstructed by emboli, the patient typically experiences sudden visual problems, an inability to speak, and paralysis of one side of the body. When emboli lodge in the arterioles of the *extremities,* gangrene of the toes or fingertips may result. Finally, *pulmonary* embolism is characterized by severe dyspnea, hemoptysis, cough, and pleuritic pain.

The symptoms of ABE and SBE were mentioned previously. Patients afflicted with ABE suffer higher fevers than those with SBE. Also they experience severe chilling, and rapid weight loss. The vegetations produced on the valve leaflets are larger, and embolic phenomena are far more severe than in the subacute form of the disease. Patients with SBE appear to be chronically rather than acutely ill, they look thin and drawn, are tired, and are ashen in color.

The *complications* of bacterial endocarditis are many; the most dangerous are congestive heart failure, which often results directly from endocarditis; perforation or destruction of the aortic valve; infarction of the spleen, kidney, and so forth; embolism; anemia; and metastatic abscess formation.

DIAGNOSIS

Correctly diagnosing bacterial endocarditis is a challenging task even for the most experienced physician. The reason the disease is so difficult to diagnose is because the majority of its symptoms are vague and nonspecific and could easily be attributed to several different infections and cardiac ailments. Even though embolic phenomena produce dramatic specific symptoms, the organs involved are generally far removed from the heart; consequently, many physicians fail to connect splenic or renal infarction with infectious heart disease.

The major method of diagnosis is examination of *blood cultures.* Typically, three to five blood specimens are drawn over a 36- to 48-hour period. In 85 to 90 per cent of patients blood cultures are positive by the third day. Other helpful but nonspecific laboratory findings in bacterial endocarditis are elevated sedimentation rate, anemia, leukocytosis, and microscopic hematuria, proteinuria, and casts.

CLINICAL CARE

The five major aims of clinical care for patients with bacterial endocarditis are:

1. To identify the infectious organism.
2. To destroy the infectious organism, thereby halting the growth of vegetations on the heart valves.
3. To protect the heart from permanent damage and valvular destruction.
4. To prevent relapses and recurrent fevers.
5. To surgically correct reparable valvular deformities, congenital defects, and so forth.

These goals are met by means of general therapeutic measures, antibiotic therapy, and surgical techniques.

General Therapeutic Measures. Patients are generally hospitalized for from two to six weeks. Complete bed rest is generally not enforced unless fever or signs of heart damage are evident. Fever, when present, is relieved by means of rest, cooling measures, forced fluids, and the administration of aspirin. As in most infectious processes, the patient should be encouraged to eat a nutritious diet, to drink sufficient fluids, and to rest mentally and physically.

Antibiotic Therapy. The mainstay of treatment in bacterial endocarditis is the administration of antibiotics. Before the advent of antibiotics almost all persons afflicted with bacterial endocarditis died; patients still die when antibiotic therapy is not adequate.

The major principles of antibiotic therapy in the treatment of bacterial endocarditis are:

By means of blood cultures, the physician must discover to which antibiotic the infecting organism is *sensitive.*

The antibiotic used must be *bactericidal* rather than bacteriostatic.

The antibiotic must be ordered in *sufficiently large doses;* the serum level of the drug should be at least five to 10 times that needed to destroy the organism.

Drug therapy needs to be continued for at least *four to six weeks* or the patient may suffer a severe relapse once the drug is discontinued.

Antibiotics must be administered *exactly at the specified time intervals* or the blood levels of the antibiotic will fall, which, in turn, leads to the further multiplication and growth of organisms.

For most cases of bacterial endocarditis the ideal antibiotic is *penicillin;* this drug is particularly useful in the control of *Streptococcus viridans* infections. The dosage prescribed depends upon how sensitive the organism is to penicillin. Dosages range from 2.4 million units per day (for sensitive organisms) up to 100 million units per day (for penicillin-resistant organisms). In some cases streptomycin is given concurrently with penicillin. The combination of streptomycin and penicillin is particularly effective against *S. faecalis.*

Penicillin is usually given IV piggyback for a six-week period. Because of the long term IV therapy, it is important to prevent complications from inactivity. Encourage the patient to turn, move, and deep breathe. If the IV catheter is securely in the vein and the IV tubing is sufficiently long, movement should not disrupt the infusion. Once the patient begins to ambulate, obtain a movable IV stand so that the patient can push the stand and IV bottle along. Emphasize to patients that they should not remain immobile simply because they have an IV running.

Some patients are allergic to penicillin. In these cases the doctor may attempt to control the allergy with antihistamines and steroids. If severe allergies persist, the doctor then discontinues penicillin altogether and orders another antibiotic such as tetracycline, erythromycin, or chloromycetin. Unfortunately these drugs are not so effective as penicillin, and the patient will almost always suffer a relapse following therapy.

Criteria indicating control of the infection are the following:

- Fever, sweats, fatigue, tachycardia, and anorexia should gradually disappear within three to five days following the beginning of therapy.
- Weight gain and improvement in the blood picture should occur during the second week.
- Urinary function should steadily improve over the four- to six-week period of therapy.

Two major *complications* that can arise during the treatment period or soon afterward are embolic episodes and relapses. *Emboli* are fairly common during the first three months following the initial administration of antibiotics. Evidently emboli result from the shrinking and shedding of vegetations as the endocardium undergoes healing and repair. Fragmentation of vegetation with resultant embolism sometimes continues for as long as one to two years following the beginning of therapy.

Relapses usually occur within one to two weeks following cessation of therapy, although patients sometimes relapse months after treatment. Some reasons for relapses are ineffective antibiotic therapy, too short a period of treatment, drug reaction, embolism, metastatic abscess formation resulting from seeding of the blood with bacteria, thrombophlebitis, superinfection with other organisms, or the presence of an underlying disease such as rheumatic fever. Relapses are diagnosed on the basis of symptoms (a rise in fever, nodules, anorexia) and positive blood cultures. The physician generally treats the patient with a higher dosage of antibiotic given over a longer period of time or with a different antibiotic.

Surgical Techniques. Although surgery is sometimes a factor in causing bacterial endocarditis, it also plays a significant role in its cure. Some of the current uses of surgery in treating bacterial endocarditis and its sequelae are removal of infected valves, drainage of abscesses in the heart and elsewhere, removal of congenital shunts, repair of injured valves and chordae tendineae, and splenectomy for splenic abscess or infarction.

PROGNOSIS

Only 10 per cent of patients with bacterial endocarditis die of the primary disease; deaths are due to antibiotic-resistant infections or occur during relapse. Another 20 per cent die from complications: *cardiac failure* as a result of valvular damage, *embolization* due to fragmentation of vegetations, or *renal insufficiency* caused by renal infarction. Renal failure from pyelonephritis may also occur. Of the 70 per cent of patients remaining, some will recover almost totally, whereas others may be burdened with a permanently damaged heart and possibly renal insufficiency.

Factors that determine the prognosis of bacterial endocarditis are (1) the presence of preexisting heart damage; (2) the development of distorted valves and/or cardiac failure during the course of the disease; (3) the severity of embolic episodes; (4) the nature of the infecting organism (virulent or nonvirulent); (5) the duration of time between onset of the disease and therapy; (6) response of the organism to the antibiotic (antibiotic-sensitive or -resistant); (7) degree of kidney damage; and (8) the valve affected (aortic valve involvement is more serious than mitral valve involvement). The outlook is excellent for patients who are properly treated early in the course of the disease and who do not develop serious cardiac or renal lesions.

Chronic Valvular Heart Disease

The heart valves, when healthy, keep blood flowing through the heart and lungs in the proper direction. Diseased valves may *impede* the flow of blood from one chamber to the next (valvular *stenosis*) or they may allow blood to leak or regurgitate back into the chamber from which the blood is being propelled (valvular *insufficiency* or *regurgitation*). Either problem places great stress upon the heart. For a time the heart may be able to compensate for the additional strain by myocardial hypertrophy. However, if valvular damage worsens and the patient is not treated, CHF will eventually develop.

While any valve can be damaged, the mitral valve is the most commonly affected, followed in incidence by the aortic valve and the tricuspid valve. It is rare for the pulmonary valve to be involved. Below is listed the incidence of various forms of valvular disease.

Mitral valvular disease — 50 to 60 per cent of all cases.

Combined mitral and aortic valvular disease — 20 per cent.

Aortic valvular disease — 10 per cent.

Pulmonic valvular disease — very rare.

The *diagnosis* of valvular heart disease is based upon: the patient's past history of heart disease (e.g., evidence of rheumatic fever or bacterial endocarditis); the presence of a significant murmur; and the detection of valvular lesions on x-ray fluoroscopy, angiography, or ECG studies, or during cardiac catheterization.

Valvular heart disease is almost always treated *surgically*. The damaged valve may be repaired or it may be removed and a prosthetic valve sutured into its place.

One commonly used prosthetic valve is the *tilting disc* type, which is sewn into the valvular opening when the diseased valve is removed (Fig. 38–2). The valve is made of a special material upon which endothelial cells will grow rapidly.

Complications resulting from the insertion of artificial heart valves are: (1) displacement of the valve due to broken sutures, (2) heart block, (3) leakage within the artificial system, resulting in regurgitation, (4) infection of the prosthesis, (5) destruction of red blood cells by the prosthetic valve, and (6) formation of emboli around the prosthesis.

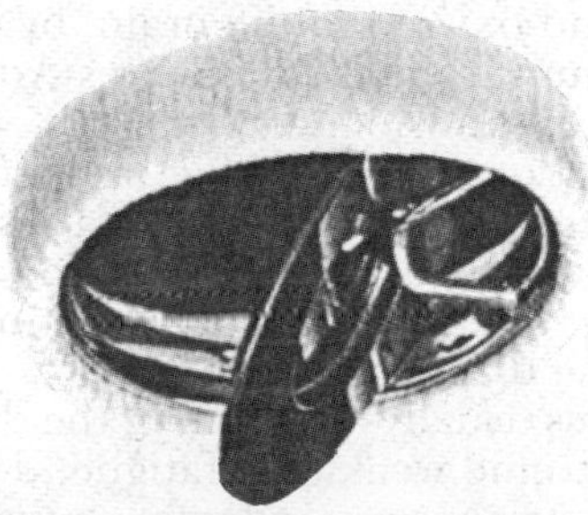

Figure 38–2. The Björk-Shiley cardiac valve prosthesis (tilting disc type). (Courtesy of Shiley Laboratories, Inc., 17600 Gillette Ave., Irvine, Cal.)

MITRAL VALVULAR DISEASE

The mitral or bicuspid valve lies between the *left* atrium and ventricle. It is the primary task of the mitral valve to promote blood flow *forward* from the left atrium to the left ventricle and to prevent the *backward* leakage of blood from the ventricle to the atrium. Lesions of the mitral valve tend either to obstruct the flow of blood from atrium to ventricle (stenosis) or to allow blood to leak back from ventricle to atrium (regurgitation). In either case, the left atrium is overworked. As a result, left atrial hypertrophy develops, followed by pulmonary congestion, overwork of the right ventricle, and right heart failure. Without treatment, patients with either mitral stenosis or regurgitation will die in CHF.

Mitral Stenosis. Mitral stenosis is the commonest lesion of the mitral valve. About three fourths of the patients are women under the age of 45. As acute rheumatic endocarditis heals, the valve leaflets retract, the chordae tendineae contract and shorten, and the mitral commissures fuse. As the valves become calcified and immobile the valvular orifice narrows, preventing normal passage of blood from left atrium to left ventricle. The left atrium hypertrophies to compensate for the strain of pushing blood through the narrowed orifice. The overload of blood trapped in the atrium causes pulmonary hypertension and congestion; the congestion, in turn, overworks the right ventricle and causes right ventricular failure. The inadequate filling of the left ventricle leads to reduced cardiac output and fatigue. In longstanding cases the left ventricle may shrink and even atrophy.

The symptoms of mitral lesions may appear gradually or quite suddenly. The first symptom is usually excessive fatigue, but this may be accompanied by shortness of breath, cough, bronchitis, orthopnea, paroxysmal nocturnal dyspnea, cyanosis, and pulmonary edema. Failure of the right heart may cause enlargement of the liver, edema, increased venous pressure, and abdominal discomfort.

On auscultation there is a rumbling, low-pitched presystolic murmur and a snapping, loud, first heart sound. Atrial fibrillation develops in 50 to 80 per cent of patients and may precipitate acute dyspnea and pulmonary congestion. During episodes of atrial fibrillation the pulse is irregular and faint; the blood pressure may be low.

Thrombi may form in the left atrium due to stagnation of blood when there is no effective atrial contraction during fibrillation. Emboli may then be released into the systemic circulation, and travel to the kidneys, spleen, extremities, and brain, causing tissue infarction.

Hemoptysis is common and results from longstanding pulmonary venous hypertension; it may be mild or severe.

Mitral stenosis may be diagnosed by angiography, cineangiography, catheterization of the left heart, ECG to determine signs of right ventricular hypertrophy, or ultrasound techniques to determine mobility of the mitral valve.

Treatment is surgical and consists of commissurotomy or prosthetic valve replacement. (See Chapter 39.)

Mitral Regurgitation. Mitral regurgitation is a less common phenomenon than mitral stenosis. The majority of patients are men. Although rheumatic fever is the principal cause, it may be a congenital anomaly or develop secondary to bacterial endocarditis or aortic valvular disease.

When the mitral valves atrophy, the left atrium dilates and hypertrophies to compensate for the increased load of blood leaking back from the left ventricle through the valve. This also causes pulmonary congestion and resulting right heart failure and its sequelae.

Many patients never develop cardiac symptoms, but most feel great fatigue, followed by dyspnea on exertion, and cough. The pulmonary symptoms are less severe than in mitral stenosis, but when the right heart is affected, the symptoms are the same.

On auscultation there is a blowing, high-pitched systolic murmur, and a third heart sound is present. Atrial fibrillation may occur, but does not precipitate acute pulmonary congestion.

The pulse is usually normal and adequate in volume, but will become irregular if fibrillation occurs. The blood pressure is normal or low.

Although emboli and hemoptysis do occur, their appearance is far less frequent than in mitral stenosis. Fatigue is quite pronounced because of the left ventricular failure.

Diagnosis is made by fluoroscopy and by injection of indicator dye into the left ventricle; prompt appearance of the dye in the left atrium gives a positive diagnosis.

Treatment is surgical and may be either valvuloplasty or valve replacement.

AORTIC VALVULAR DISEASE

The aortic valve lies between the aorta and left ventricle. During systole it opens so that blood can flow from the ventricle into the aorta; during diastole it closes to prevent leakage of blood from the aorta back into the left ventricle.

Aortic valvular disease is far less common than is mitral valvular disease, although it often occurs in conjunction with mitral disease. Lesions of the aortic valve act to obstruct the flow of blood forward from the left ventricle into the aorta and systemic circulation (stenosis) or they allow blood to leak back from the aorta into the left ventricle (regurgitation or insufficiency). Both aortic stenosis and regurgitation overwork the left ventricle. Left ventricular hypertrophy develops as a compensatory measure and, in turn, is followed by atrial hypertrophy, pulmonary congestion, and right ventricular failure. Thus, aortic valvular disease, like mitral valvular disease, ends in CHF.

Atrial fibrillation and embolic phenomena are characteristic of mitral valvular disease, whereas angina pectoris and syncope result from aortic valvular disease.

Aortic Stenosis. Aortic stenosis accounts for one fourth of the patients suffering from chronic valvular disease; 80 per cent are male. It may be either congenital or acquired. Acquired disease may result from rheumatic endocarditis or, among the elderly, atherosclerosis.

In stenosis the aortic valve opening narrows, and the valve flaps fuse as a result of inflammation or growth of atherosclerotic plaques. The left ventricle hypertrophies without dilating to compensate for the stress of pumping blood through the narrowed opening. The cardiac output is low. The left atrium cannot empty normally, and pulmonary circulation becomes congested, placing the right ventricle under such stress that it will fail if treatment is not received.

Patients may remain asymptomatic until they are 30 or 40 years old. The first symptom is usually fatigue, followed by angina pectoris and dyspnea on exertion. The dyspnea is caused by the elevation of the left ventricular end-diastolic pressure, which also increases left atrial and capillary pressures. Late in the disease orthopnea, paroxysmal nocturnal dyspnea, and pulmonary edema may occur. The anginal pain develops because of the decreased blood flow to the heart through the stenotic valve.

Syncope often occurs on exertion or change in position and may be caused by insufficient cardiac output which produces inadequate flow of blood and oxygen to the brain, by overactive carotid sinus reflex, by Stokes-Adams syndrome, or by transient arryhthmias.

A harsh, rough midsystolic murmur may be heard on auscultation, as well as a systolic thrill over the aortic area. The pulse is slow and small in volume. The systolic blood pressure is normal, but the diastolic is high.

Symptoms usually arise late in the disease and include extreme weakness, fatigue, debilitation, venous hypertension, edema, hepatomegaly, and ascites.

Diagnosis is made by left heart catheterization; aortic, coronary, and left ventricular angiograms; and ECG.

Surgery is the treatment of choice but is performed only when lesions are severe, because of the high risk. Either valvulotomy or valve replacement by a prosthesis may be done.

Idiopathic Hypertrophic Subaortic Stenosis (IHSS). IHSS is a congenital heart defect in which the outflow tract of the left ventricle is constricted just below the aortic valve by a hypertrophied fibrinous ring. This can greatly impede the outward flow of blood through the aortic valve during systole. The symptoms are very similar to those of aortic stenosis. A left heart catheterization aids in the diagnosis of IHSS. This defect can be treated medically with drugs to relax the left ventricle, e.g., propranolol, or surgically by excising the fibrinous ring during open heart surgery.

Aortic Regurgitation. Aortic regurgitation occurs one half as frequently as aortic stenosis, and once again the majority of patients are male (75 per cent). It, too, may be congenital or acquired. Rheumatic endocarditis is the principal cause; syphilis may be an occasional etiologic factor.

The opening of the aortic valve widens, and valve flaps, deformed by infectious processes, fail to close properly during diastole, allowing blood to regurgitate from the aorta back into the left ventricle. The left ventricle dilates and hypertrophies to compensate for the greater load of blood. Unless treated, left ventricular failure will be followed by right heart failure.

The first symptom is usually sinus tachycardia or premature systoles, and is followed by dyspnea on exertion and angina pectoris. These symptoms may not appear until the patient is aged 30 or 40. The exertional dyspnea, as well as orthopnea and paroxysmal nocturnal dyspnea, develops as a result of pulmonary congestion. Late in the disease the patient may experience dyspnea at rest. Anginal pain develops for the same reasons as in aortic stenosis. Late in the disease the symptoms are similar to those experienced by patients with aortic stenosis.

On auscultation there is a soft, blowing aortic diastolic murmur and a forceful apical impulse. The systolic blood pressure is normal or slightly elevated, but the diastolic is low.

Diagnosis is made by angiocardiograms, ECG, and indicator dilution studies with opaque dye.

Treatment by surgery is undertaken only when disease is severe, and consists of the removal of the damaged leaflet and the suturing of the two normal cusps together to form a bicuspid valve, or replacement of the cusp or valve by a prosthesis.

Women of child-bearing age with mitral or aortic valve disease should carefully discuss the risks of pregnancy with their cardiologists and obstetricians. Depending upon the severity of the disease, pregnancy may be contraindicated because of the excessive strain it places upon the heart.

TRICUSPID VALVULAR DISEASE

The tricuspid valve guards the opening between the right atrium and right ventricle. Pure lesions of the tricuspid valve are relatively uncommon. Usually tricuspid stenosis or regurgitation develops in combination with other structural disorders of the heart.

Lesions of the tricuspid valve place great stress on the right side of the heart. As a result, these disorders inevitably produce *right heart failure.* Treatment involves correction of the valvular deformity and alleviation of the heart failure.

Tricuspid Stenosis. Tricuspid stenosis occurs predominantly in women. It is a relatively rare phenomenon and usually occurs in combination with mitral and/or aortic valvular disease. It may be congenital. It is most commonly a sequela of rheumatic fever.

The valve opening narrows and the valve flaps fuse as a result of endocardial inflammation. Blood is blocked on its return to the heart and lungs, with resulting venous engorgement and right heart failure. Failure of the right heart produces hepatomegaly, dependent edema, ascites, extreme fatigue, and cardiac cirrhosis. The resulting jaundice and cyanosis give the patient a slate-colored complexion.

Auscultation shows a rumbling diastolic murmur. There is a presystolic pulsation in the liver.

Chest x-ray films show an enlarged right atrium. The diagnosis is confirmed by angiogram.

Treatment may be medical (low-sodium diet, diuretics, and digitalis) or surgical (valve repair or prosthetic replacement).

Tricuspid Regurgitation. Tricuspid regurgitation is relatively rare; it is found more frequently in children than in adults. It may be congenital, but more frequently follows rheumatic fever, bacterial endocarditis, or trauma.

As a result of inflammation the tricuspid valve widens and the valve flaps are unable to close securely. Blood leaks back into the right atrium as well as being pushed forward into the pulmonary circulation, causing venous engorgement and right heart failure.

Symptoms are the same as in tricuspid stenosis and the slate-colored complexion is sometimes seen.

A blowing, holosystolic murmur is heard on auscultation. Atrial fibrillation is usually present.

An angiogram is diagnostic. Chest x-ray films show an enlarged right atrium and ventricle.

Treatment is the same as for tricuspid stenosis.

PULMONIC VALVULAR DISEASE

Lesions of the pulmonic valve are extremely rare and are not discussed in this text.

DISEASES THAT AFFECT THE MYOCARDIUM: MYOCARDITIS

Acute myocarditis is an inflammatory condition of the myocardium. It develops either during or following diseases of viral, bacterial, rickettsial, spirochetal, fungal, or parasitic origin. Frequently acute myocarditis develops secondary to acute endocarditis or pericarditis.

The major cause of acute myocarditis is *rheumatic fever;* diphtheria, subacute bacterial endocarditis, trichomoniasis, and influenza are also associated with the development of this condition.

The symptoms are generally vague and nonspecific. In mild cases of myocarditis, symptoms are absent and diagnosis is made only on the basis of serial ECG readings, which typically reveal T wave abnormalities. In more severe cases the manifestations of myocarditis are generally obscured by the manifestations of the primary disorder, e.g., rheumatic fever, SBE, diphtheria. Thus, the patient may experience a variety of symptoms: fever, leukocytosis, fatigue, nausea and vomiting, anorexia, tachycardia, and chest pain. Shock and death may occur in young adults affected with severe myocarditis.

Myocarditis is diagnosed on the basis of ventricular enlargement and heart failure that develops suddenly and without apparent cause; i.e., there is no evidence of valvular heart disease or any other heart condition that can cause failure.

Patients with acute myocarditis are treated with digitalis and placed on complete bed rest until symptoms of infection and inflammation lessen and disappear. Overexertion and stress during the critical symptomatic period of myocarditis can result in sudden death.

DISEASES OF THE PERICARDIUM: ACUTE AND CHRONIC PERICARDITIS

Pericarditis is an inflammation of the visceral or parietal pericardium, or both, often resulting in compression of the heart, critical decrease in ventricular filling and emptying, and cardiac failure. This inflammatory process may develop either as a primary condition or secondary to a number of different diseases and circumstances, e.g., rheumatic fever, uremia, tuberculosis, collagen diseases, various infections (bacterial, viral, fungal), cancer, myocardial infarction, toxic overdose, and trauma.

Pericarditis is classified as either acute or chronic. Acute pericarditis, in turn, is classified as *dry* (fibrinous) or *exudative* (pericarditis with effusion). The exudate may be serous, purulent, or hemorrhagic. When fluid accumulates very rapidly or accumulations are large, *cardiac tamponade* develops and the heart is unable to expand and fill with blood; decreased filling, in turn, leads to drastically reduced cardiac output, shock, and death.

Chronic pericarditis is usually called *chronic constrictive* or *adhesive* pericarditis. A constrictive, sometimes calcified membrane around the heart prevents filling and emptying of the ventricles, eventually resulting in cardiac failure.

Acute Pericarditis

As stated previously, acute pericarditis is an acute inflammation of the pericardium that may be either dry or exudative.

Acute Fibrinous Pericarditis. This may result from virus infections, myocardial infarction, tuberculosis, bacteremia or septicemia of the pericardium, or spread from a contiguous organ. Delicate, "violin string" adhesions form and may completely obliterate the pericardial sac, but they rarely spread to the thoracic wall, diaphragm, or lungs, and cardiac action is infrequently hampered.

On auscultation there is a to-and-fro friction rub over the precordium that is synchronous with the systole and diastole. The sound, which usually persists for 7 to 10 days, may be soft and scratchy, loud and leathery, or low and grating.

Dyspnea is often present. Chest pain varies from mild to severe over the precordial or substernal area. It radiates to the shoulder and neck and down the left arm; it is aggravated by swallowing, coughing, and lying supine. Typically, the pain is relieved by leaning forward. The temperature may be elevated to 37.8 to 39.4° C. (100-103° F.), depending on the underlying infection. Fever also increases the pulse rate. Tachycardia is usually present. The patient is pale, anxious, and restless, and appears acutely ill.

Blood tests show a leukocytosis of 10,000 to 20,000. Chest x-ray film will usually reveal cardiac dilatation. ST-T changes on the ECG are probably related to the myocarditis that so frequently accompanies pericarditis.

Treatment includes bed rest, analgesics (acetylsalicylic acid for mild pain, morphine sulfate for severe), and appropriate antibiotics.

The pathologic effects of acute pericarditis upon the heart are illustrated in Figure 38-3.

Acute Pericarditis with Effusion. Acute pericarditis with effusion may follow acute fibrinous or acute purulent pericarditis or be caused by tuberculosis, malignant disease, myxedema, nephrosis, or advanced congestive heart failure.

Fluid accumulates within the pericardial sac, compressing the heart and reducing ventricular filling and arterial pressure. Cardiac action is severely hampered, leading to heart failure. Dyspnea and orthopnea are always present.

The friction rub heard in acute fibrinous pericarditis usually disappears when effusion develops but may occasionally be heard.

Pain may or may not be present; when present it may resemble that caused by acute fibrinous pericarditis or be dull, diffuse, and oppressive. The distended pericardium compresses the bronchi and lungs, causing a cough and making it necessary for the patient to sit up and lean forward to breathe.

The temperature may be elevated. The pulse is paradoxic; it fluctuates with respiration and is lowest at the end of each full inspiration. Neck veins are distended as a result of the reduced ventricular filling. The patient is acutely ill.

Leukocyte counts are elevated to 10,000 to 20,000. Pericardial fluid is aspirated for culture, for cytologic examination, and for determination of specific gravity and protein content. With large effusions the normal contours of the heart may not be discernible on chest x-ray films. Fluoroscopy will reveal a decrease in the pulsations of the heart. Cardiac catheterization and angiocardiography are also useful diagnostic aids.

Bed rest, analgesics, and antibiotics are ordered. The physician may tap the pericardial sac, aspirating the collected fluid and instilling antibiotics directly into the sac. Drainage may require incision of the chest wall.

Complications of Acute Pericarditis. The only important complication of acute fibrinous pericarditis is *pericardial effusion.* The major complication of pericarditis with effusion is *cardiac tamponade.*

Cardiac tamponade signifies an acute compression of the heart due to an accumulation of fluid within the pericardial sac. This critical condition develops when either the amount of fluid within the pericardial sac is very large or fluid has accumulated rapidly; e.g., sudden hemorrhage into the pericardial sac. Large or rapidly accumulating effusions raise the intrapericardial pressure to a point at which venous blood is unable to flow into the heart, which, in turn, decreases ventricular filling. As a result, venous pressure rises and cardiac output and arterial blood pressure fall; a narrowing pulse pressure is a sign of cardiac tamponade. The heart attempts to compensate in this emergency by beating rapidly (tachycardia). However, tachycardia can sustain the patient's cardiac output for only a short period of time; without immediate treatment, the patient is doomed to die in shock. The pathophysiology of pericardial tamponade is illustrated in Figure 38–4.

The symptoms of cardiac tamponade are the same as the manifestations of shock, pericarditis with effusion, and venous congestion. In shock the patient experiences hypotension, tachycardia, cyanosis of lips and nails, restlessness, pal-

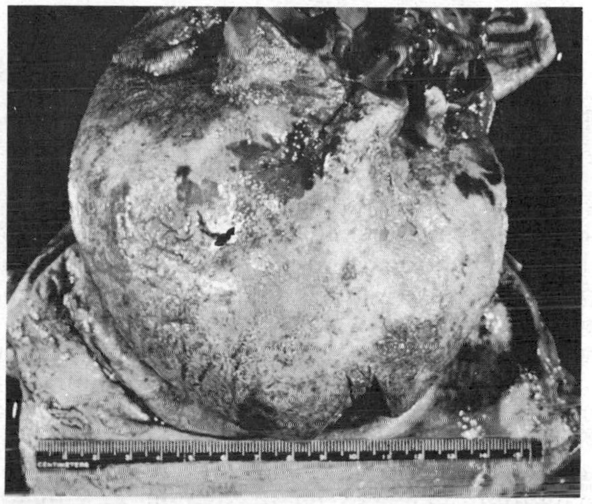

A. Pericarditis is almost always secondary to another disorder. Inflammations extend to the pericardium by continuity, blood vessels, or lymphatics.

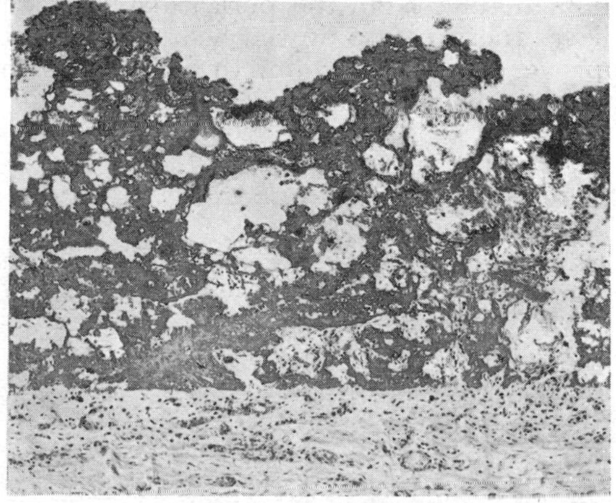

B. With severe inflammation, there is an outpouring of large amounts of plasma protein, including fibrinogen, and serous fluid into the pericardial sac.

Figure 38–3. A. Acute pericarditis, a gross view of the heart. **B.** The microscopic appearance of the fibrinous exudate in pericardial effusion. (From Robbins, S. L., and R. S. Cotran: *The Pathologic Basis of Disease,* 2nd ed., Philadelphia: W. B. Saunders Co., 1979, p. 81.)

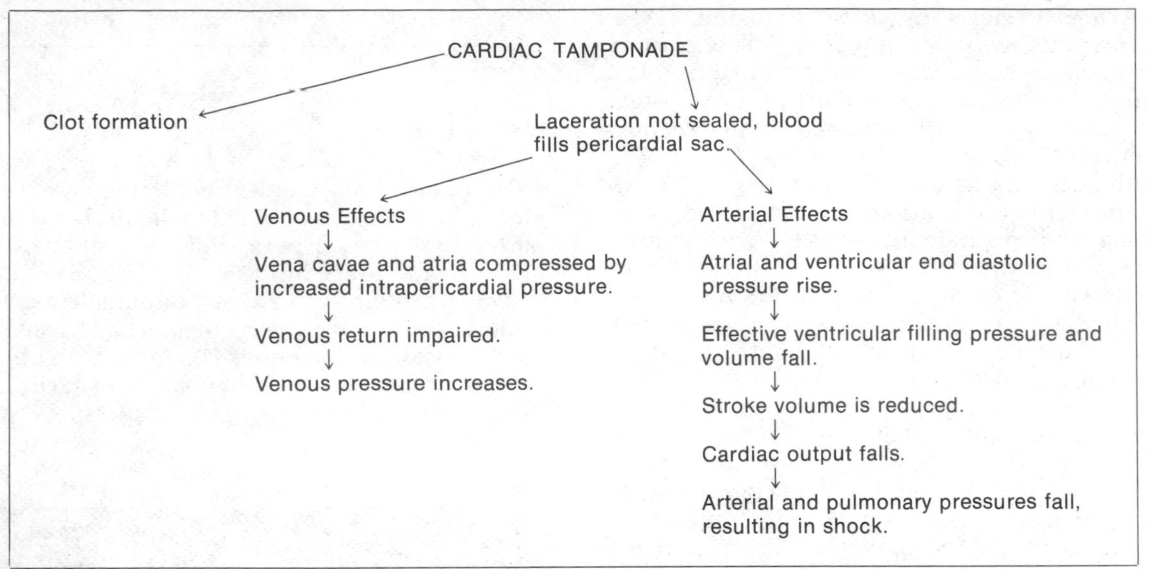

Figure 38-4. Summary of the pathophysiology of pericardial tamponade. (Adapted from Shoemaker, W. C.: Early diagnosis and management of pericardial tamponade. *Hospital Medicine,* 14:7, Nov. 1978.)

lor, and diaphoresis. A paradoxical pulse, muffled heart sounds, and dyspnea result from the pericardial effusion. When the veins become congested those in the neck are distended, there is increased venous pressure, liver enlargement, ascites, and edema of the legs. The combination of distended neck veins (indicating an elevated venous pressure), distant heart sounds, and arterial hypotension is called *Beck's triad.* All three symptoms may not be present in all patients with pericardial tamponade.

The patient with cardiac tamponade needs immediate treatment! The emergency treatment of choice is a pericardiocentesis (i.e., aspiration of fluid from the pericardial sac). This relieves the pressure on the heart and thereby improves cardiac function. In many cases this procedure is lifesaving.

Chronic Constrictive Pericarditis

Chronic constrictive pericarditis is a chronic inflammatory condition in which the pericardium changes into a thick, fibrous, sometimes calcified band of unyielding tissue that encircles, encases, and compresses the heart, thereby preventing proper ventricular filling and emptying. The eventual result of this slow, unrelenting compression is cardiac failure.

Frequently a sequel to tuberculosis, chronic constrictive pericarditis is characterized by symptoms of right heart failure and inadequate cardiac output; e.g., fatigue on exertion, dyspnea, leg edema, ascites, low pulse pressure, distended neck veins, and prolonged circulation time. However, this condition is occasionally asymptomatic.

Chronic constrictive pericarditis is treated both medically and surgically. The patient is treated to relieve symptoms of congestive heart failure, with the doctor ordering digitalis, diuretics, and a low sodium diet. Surgical treatment involves excision of the damaged, constricting pericardium (i.e., pericardectomy). Surgery offers hope of cure to approximately 60 per cent of persons disabled by constrictive pericarditis.

CHAPTER 39

CARE OF PATIENTS UNDERGOING HEART SURGERY

In 1925 Sir Henry Soutlar of London performed the first heart surgery — a closed repair of a stenosed mitral valve. Since that time heart surgery has been revolutionized by the development of open heart techniques that allow surgeons to directly visualize the heart while they explore, cut, repair, and suture. Such optimal operating conditions have enabled modern surgeons to replace diseased valves with prosthetic valves, to repair severe congenital lesions, and to perform heart transplants.

TYPES OF HEART SURGERY

There are two major types of cardiac surgery: closed and open. *Closed heart* surgery is performed without the benefit or hazards of *extracorporeal circulation* (ECC; cardiopulmonary bypass). ECC is a procedure in which a machine (the *pump oxygenator* or *heart-lung machine*) completely controls cardiopulmonary function, thereby enabling surgeons to operate for lengthy periods without the patient's becoming anoxic. Examples of closed heart procedures are closed mitral commissurotomy to correct mitral stenosis (Chapter 38) and procedures that correct some congenital defects.

Conversely, *open heart procedures,* because of their lengthiness and complexity, must be performed with the aid of ECC. Examples of major open heart procedures are total replacement of a diseased valve with a prosthetic valve (Chapter 38) and heart transplants.

Heart Transplants

Since the 1960's heart transplants have been widely publicized and discussed throughout the world. The first successful human heart transplant was performed in South Africa by the then obscure surgeon, Christiaan Barnard. By the end of 1970, 166 more heart transplants had been performed, but only 23 patients were living; i.e., the heart transplant procedure had had a discouraging 85 per cent mortality rate.[233A]

The greatest single problem in performing heart transplants is not the surgical procedure itself but the *rejection* process by which the patient's body rejects the donor's heart. (Allograft rejection is discussed in Chapter 11.) This process is poorly understood; however, physiologists do know that following implantation of the donor heart, plasma cells attack the donor cells and destroy them by upsetting their metabolic processes. Also, the patient forms antibodies against the foreign heart tissue, which leads to an antigen-antibody reaction. As a result, the heart's lining hemorrhages, the heart walls thicken, and the myocardium assumes a mottled appearance; finally, the new heart fails to function altogether and circulatory collapse ensues.

Nonetheless, at the present time a few medical centers in the United States perform heart transplants on a routine basis. In these centers, patients rarely die due to the rejection process during the first year, and the survival rate after one year is approximately 50 per cent.

Open Heart Surgery: Benefits and Problems

The greatest advantage of open heart surgery is that it allows the surgeon to directly visualize the heart during the operation. However, before open heart procedures could be developed, surgeons had to discover how to either (1) slow or halt the patient's circulation for a period of time without causing brain anoxia (hypothermia), or (2) detour the blood that would normally enter the heart and lungs through an artificial heart-lung machine (ECC).

Hypothermia was the first technique to make open heart surgery possible. One purpose of hypothermia is to *decrease* the patient's *metabolic needs,* thereby automatically lowering the rate at which the body uses oxygen. Another purpose is to provide the surgeon with a *bloodless field* in which to operate. The patient's reduced need for oxygen allows the surgeon to clamp off the venae cavae and azygos veins, thereby halting circulation through the heart for a period of time.

How long circulation can be stopped depends upon the *depth* of hypothermia. At normal body temperature the circulation can be stopped for only 2 to 3 minutes without tissue damage from anoxia. However at 28° C. (moderate hypothermia), circulation can be stopped for a period of

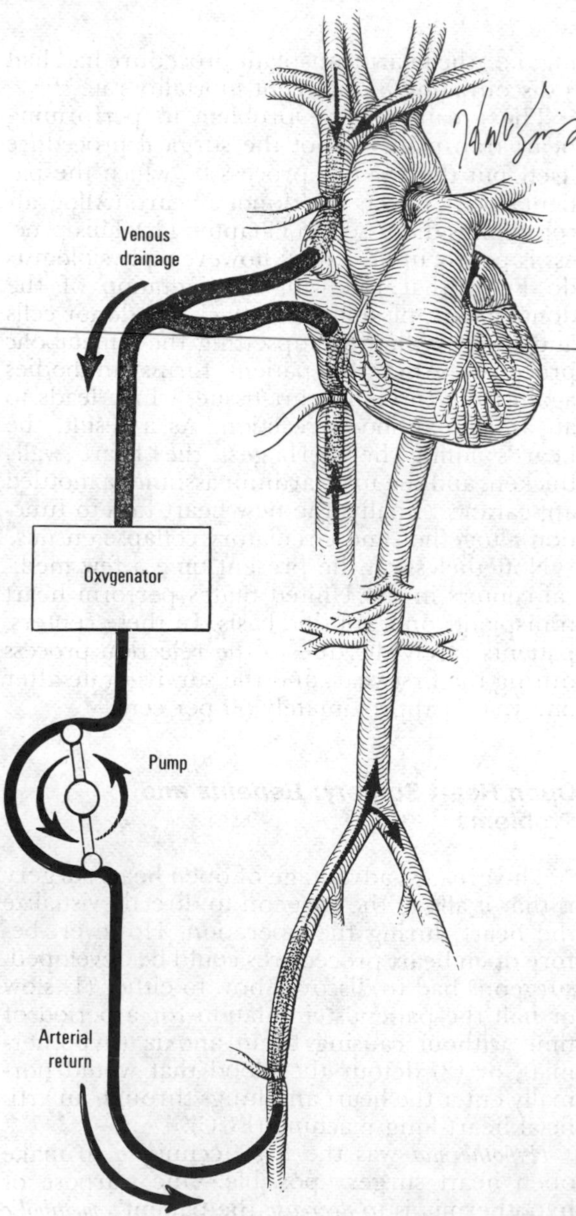

Figure 39–1. The heart-lung machine. (From DeBakey, M., and A. Gotto: *The Living Heart.* New York: Charter Books, 1977.)

15 to 20 minutes — adequate time to complete certain simple procedures. At 10° C. (profound hypothermia) circulation can be halted for about 1 hour, during which time the blood is pumped through a heat exchanger; however, surgery must be completed within the hour or the patient may die unless rewarmed.

To induce hypothermia, the patient is anesthetized. Next, the body is cooled in a hypothermia blanket that maintains body temperature at the desired level. (Use of the hypothermia blanket is discussed in Chapter 26.)

The major danger of hypothermia is *ventricular fibrillation,* which occurs when the temperature drops to around 26° C. Other complications are cardiac arrest and cardiac failure.

Today, hypothermia is being almost universally replaced by total cardiopulmonary bypass (ECC). However, some surgeons continue to use moderate or profound hypothermia in combination with ECC.

While hypothermia is suitable for surgery of short duration, only ECC can be used for extremely complex surgical procedures such as valve replacement or heart transplants. Thus, the heart-lung machine, more than any other apparatus, has made sophisticated open heart surgery possible.

The first pump-oxygenator was used with a human patient in 1951 in an unsuccessful attempt at ECC. Two years later the machine was used again in the successful repair of an atrial septal defect; the patient lived for 30 minutes while on cardiopulmonary bypass. Since 1955 improved versions of the machine have been built, and ECC is now routinely used throughout the world for open heart surgery.

The purposes of the heart-lung machine are four: (1) to divert the circulation from the heart and lungs which, in turn, provides the surgeon with a bloodless field in which to operate; (2) to perform all gas exchange functions for the body while the patient's heart and pulmonary systems are at rest (i.e., O_2-CO_2 exchange); (3) to filter, rewarm, or cool the blood; and (4) to circulate the oxygenated, filtered blood back into the patient's arterial system.

Briefly, the procedure for ECC is:

First, the machine is primed (filled) with 3 or 4 liters of either heparinized blood or a blood substitute such as low molecular weight dextran (Rheomacrodex) or Ringer's lactate solution. When the patient's chest is opened the surgeon inserts two large-bore cannulas through the right atrium into the superior and inferior venae cavae. The venous blood is next aspirated from the venae cavae by a vacuum pump into the heart-lung machine (Fig. 39–1). An oxygenator removes CO_2 from the blood and adds oxygen. The oxygenated blood is then pumped to a heat exchanger where it is rewarmed (or cooled if the surgeon desires hypothermia). Next the blood passes through a filter that removes air bubbles and other emboli. Finally, the blood is returned to the body via either the aorta or femoral artery.

Despite its beneficial effects, the use of the heart-lung machine is not without its dangers. For example, the pump can crush and destroy blood cells; also, sludging of cells sometimes occurs, leading to thrombus formation. Finally, air emboli can form as a result of excess oxygen absorption.

Other specific complications which are apparently related to ECC are: low cardiac output syndrome (shock), hemolysis and hemorrhage, lung damage, and kidney damage. These complications will be discussed under postoperative care.

PREOPERATIVE CARE

In Unit VIII we discussed in detail the preparation of a patient for general surgery. All the information given in Unit VIII is applicable to patients about to undergo heart surgery. However, because heart surgery is a particularly stressful experience, special preparation and instruction in certain areas are needed.

Patient's History. The patient you admit for heart surgery has probably suffered from cardiac and pulmonary symptoms for months or years. The extent of the disability will naturally affect the outcome of surgery as well as the type of care required during the postoperative period. Facts you need to know about the patient's physical status are:

- The heart condition for which the patient is being surgically treated and its duration.
- The purpose of the surgery and the risk involved.
- Past cardiopulmonary illnesses that may predispose the patient to postoperative complications, e.g., bacterial endocarditis, pulmonary embolus, allergy, abnormal bleeding.
- The degree of cardiac impairment that the patient suffers; i.e., are there symptoms or is the patient asymptomatic? Does the patient have symptoms when at rest or only during exertion?
- The types of medications and therapeutic measures that the patient has received or is currently receiving, e.g., digitalis, quinidine, IPPB, oxygen.

Psychologic Preparation. All patients facing surgery, of whatever nature, are somewhat apprehensive. Those facing *heart* surgery often develop feelings of fear, depression, and despair that are overwhelming. Because fear can adversely affect the patient's *physiologic* response to surgery, it is important to allow the patient to ask questions and freely express emotions about the coming operation. A preoperative program of instruction designed to reduce anxiety concerning heart surgery and the recovery period should include these areas:

General Information. Information should be given concerning hospital rules and regulations; visiting hours in the ICU; the priest, rabbi, or minister who will be on duty and the visitation hours; and the house doctors, clinical nurse specialist, or nursing supervisor whom the patient's family can contact for information on the day of surgery and throughout the postoperative period.

Most patients benefit from a tour of the recovery room and intensive care unit. It is helpful to introduce patients to the staff who will be caring for them. Familiarize the patient with the equipment that will be used in the ICU, e.g., chest drainage tubes, oxygen apparatus, cardiac monitors, and IV setups.

Verbal Instruction. Instruct the patient concerning the contemplated surgery, preoperative care, and convalescence. However, before giving instruction in these areas, always ask the doctor what information has already been given the patient; also find out if the doctor wants any information withheld. Let the patient tell you in his or her own words the understanding held about the heart problem. Correct any misconceptions the patient may have about the disease and the surgery. Simple graphic charts and a model of the heart and its valves will help the patient to learn and to remember more easily.

Preparing for surgery is an area of concern for many patients. One study indicates that patients want to learn about the following aspects of preoperative care: diagnostic tests (electrocardiograms, electroencephalograms, and pulmonary function tests); blood replacement therapy; the surgical prep; and anesthesia (sleeping medications, anesthesiologist's visit on the eve of surgery, and state of consciousness immediately prior to the operation).

Patients tend to ask the greatest number of questions about the *recovery room* and *ICU;* therefore, it is wise to discuss these two areas thoroughly. If the patient has not toured the facilities, a description of the areas will be of benefit. Patients feel far more confident once they learn that highly skilled nurses will care for them in a well-equipped, heavily staffed, special area of the hospital.

Prepare patients for what to expect as they regain consciousness in the recovery room. For example, mention that the patient will awaken with a chest tube, which drains blood and air from the chest so the lungs can reexpand. Also discuss the tube through the mouth or nose into the trachea that will be attached to a machine that will breathe for the patient the first 18 to 24 hours postoperatively. Explain that an IV or blood transfusion will be running into an arm, and that the patient will be attached to various equipment to continuously monitor vital signs and heart rhythm. Emphasize that although the patient will experience pain, the pain will be relieved by medication and comfort measures.

Finally, explain that the patient will be awakened frequently in the ICU to receive vital nursing care. Give examples of the types of scheduled activities: vital signs every 15 minutes; temperature every 2 hours; frequent turning; coughing, deep breathing every hour; blood drawn for tests every morning, and so forth.

Patients also need information concerning discharge from the ICU and hospital. Of interest are the average length of stay in the ICU, the room to which the patient will return from the ICU, the average length of stay in the hospital, and the diet and activities permitted on return home. Be very general in your discussion of these points; remember that many unforeseen events can arise in surgery and in the ICU that can greatly alter the patient's postoperative course.

DEMONSTRATIONS AND PRACTICE SESSIONS. Demonstrate deep breathing and coughing, range of motion, and use of the IPPB machine. Allow the patient to practice these activities under your supervision. Emphasize the vital importance of proper breathing, coughing, and movement.

Postoperative patients have expressed conflicting views about what they felt patients should be told beforehand concerning pain, hallucinations, and so forth. It is evident that patients differ significantly in the types of information they find helpful. Some wish to know everything and others nothing. Thus, the instruction of patients prior to heart surgery *must be highly individualized.*

Physiologic Preparation. It is important for patients to be in the best physical condition possible before undergoing the stresses of heart surgery. Thus, patients are generally admitted to the hospital a few days prior to the surgery for a thorough medical evaluation. During the preoperative period the goals of care are (1) to conduct diagnostic and laboratory studies, (2) to correct any metabolic imbalances, infections, and arrhythmias, and (3) to establish baselines for vital signs, weight, ECG, and so forth —signs that can be used for comparison during the postoperative period.

Preoperative *laboratory tests* include urine tests and blood electrolyte, enzyme, and coagulation studies. Important *diagnostic studies* that give valuable information about cardiac status are the ECG, phonocardiogram, vectorcardiogram, chest x-ray films, and cardiac catheterization.

Existing imbalances and *cardiac and pulmonary ailments* are corrected by means of rest, diet, and drugs. For example, CHF is treated with digitalis, low-sodium diet, rest, and diuretics. Arrhythmias are corrected with quinidine or cardioversion. Latent or residual infection is corrected by antibiotic therapy. K^+ imbalance is controlled by potassium supplements.

Finally, to establish *baselines* for postoperative comparisons, weigh preoperative patients daily and take their vital signs (including apical-radial pulse) every 4 hours.

Immediate Preoperative Care. The preparation of patients on the evening before and the day of heart surgery is essentially the same as the preparation of patients for chest surgery.* The patient's skin is prepped for a thoracotomy; if a coronary artery bypass graft is to be done, the legs are also shaved and prepped.

POSTOPERATIVE CARE

General Observations and Orders

Following heart surgery the patient is admitted to the recovery room or intensive care unit. For the first 48 hours the patient needs constant professional observation and care, for it is during this period that the most serious complications arise. Figure 39–2 exemplifies a postoperative cardiac surgery patient in an intensive care unit.

Typical observations and orders for patients immediately following general surgery have been discussed in Unit VIII. In addition to these general duties, you will also perform special tasks when caring for patients following heart surgery.

Monitor blood pressure and heart rate continuously; record every 15 to 30 minutes till patient stabilizes, then every hour; report systolic BP below 90 mm. Hg.

Check all pulses (apical, radial, and pedal).

Note level of consciousness; report to surgeon if patient does not awaken within 1 hour after surgery.

Check pupils for size, equality, and reaction to light. Report to physician if pupils are unequal in size, are dilated, or fail to react to light.

Central venous and pulmonary artery pressures should be continuously monitored and values recorded with the vital signs; changes should be reported to the physician as specified in the postoperative orders.

If the patient's BP is adequate, elevate head of bed to semi-Fowler's position to facilitate chest drainage and lung reexpansion.

Continuously monitor ECG. Note and report frequent premature contractions (atrial, nodal, or ventricular). These arrhythmias foreshadow more serious arrhythmias.

---

*Review immediate preoperative care for patients undergoing general surgery, Unit VIII, particularly Chapter 19.

Most patients have an endotracheal tube in place after surgery and are ventilated by means of a mechanical ventilator for 18 to 24 hours; this is to ensure adequate ventilation in the immediate postoperative period. If stable the morning after surgery, the patient is usually weaned from the ventilator, the tube is removed, and oxygen given by means of a high humidity face mask; the endotracheal tube should be taped securely in place, and the ventilator tubing should be secured so that undue strain is not placed on the tube (see Chapter 54 for care of the patient on a ventilator).

Milk chest tubes hourly to dislodge clots; prevent kinking of tubing; record amount and color of drainage hourly.

Measure urine volume hourly. Report to surgeon if urine output is below 30 ml. an hour for 2 consecutive hours. Note color of urine and record specific gravity. Keep a cumulative hourly intake and output record.

Begin range of motion exercises as soon as patient stabilizes.

Measure temperature hourly; report elevation of over 101° F. or 38.5° C.

Administer IV infusions and blood transfusions per cutdown according to physician's orders.

Schedule chest x-ray film and ECG daily per doctor's order.

Schedule daily bloodwork as ordered, e.g., serum electrolytes, coagulation studies, CBC, arterial blood gases.

Goals of Care for Patients Following Cardiac Surgery

Goal 1: Promote cardiovascular function, tissue perfusion, and stabilization of vital signs.

Goal 2: Promote respiratory function by promoting chest drainage and adequate ventilation of the lungs.

Goal 3: Promote fluid, electrolyte, and nutritional balance.

Goal 4: Promote renal function.

Goal 5: Promote rest, comfort, and relief from pain.

Goal 6: Promote neurologic function.

Goal 7: Promote psychologic adjustment to postoperative period.

Goal 8: Promote early movement and ambulation.

Goal 9: Prevent postoperative complications.

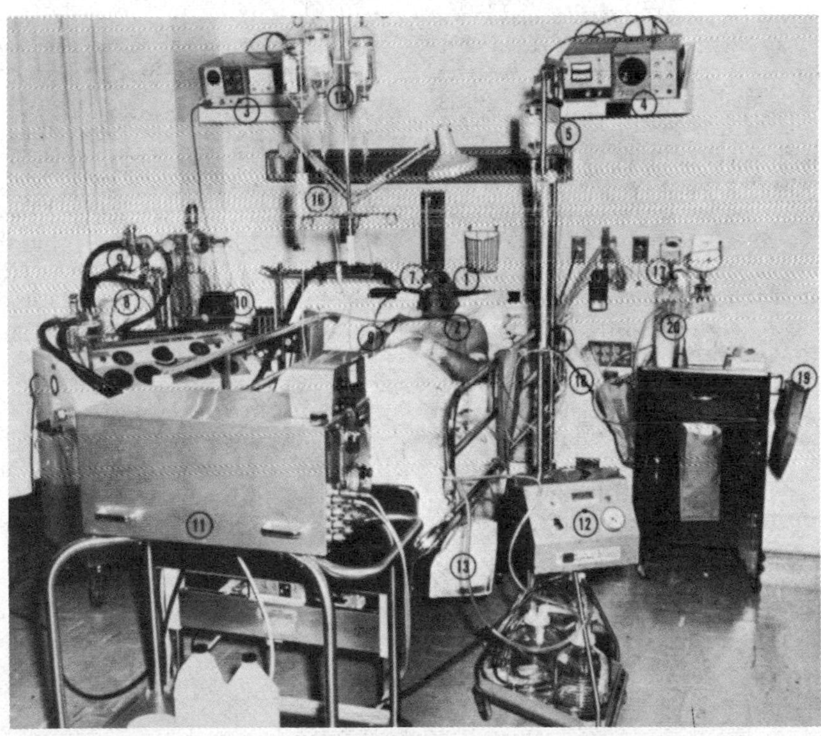

Figure 39–2. The environment of the intensive care unit with its many machines can be a source of stress. Depicted are: (1) patient 24 hr after aortic valve replacement; (2) ECG monitoring leads on chest; (3) ECG oscilloscope and heart rate meter; (4) central arterial pressure wave form and read out meters; (5) arterial pressure Infusor bag with transfer pack containing heparinized solution for maintaining patency of the arterial line; (6) sphygmomanometer with blood pressure cuff for comparison measurement; (7) endotracheal tube with tubing from Engstrom respirator connected; (8) spirometer on Engstrom respirator for measuring expired minute volume; (9) airway pressure gauge, which shows pressure that is required to deliver volume of air and oxygen; (10) Ambu bag for manual sighing or for use in power failure; (11) hypothermia machine with reserve supply of alcohol solution; (12) Emerson suction for chest tube drainage; (13) Cystoflow bag for urinary drainage; (14) CVP manometer; (15) IV fluid administration system; (16) buretrol for addition of antibiotics to IV line; (17) suction for endotracheal suctioning; (18) sterile catheters for endotracheal suctioning; (19) bag for soiled suction catheters; and (20) sterile saline and cups for suctioning use. (From Aspinall, J. J.: *Nursing the Open-Heart Surgery Patient.* New York: McGraw-Hill, Inc., 1973, p. 160.)

Goal 1: Promote Cardiovascular Function, Tissue Perfusion and Stabilization of Vital Signs

The most reliable measures of cardiovascular function and tissue perfusion are the vital signs. Stabilization of vital signs following heart surgery usually indicates adequate cardiovascular function, whereas severe deviations indicate complications such as hemorrhage, shock, cardiac tamponade, or infection. The normal ranges for each vital sign following cardiac surgery and the meaning of deviations are as follows:

Arterial Blood Pressure

1. To obtain an accurate BP postoperatively, an 18 or 20 gauge Teflon catheter is placed *intra-arterially,* usually in the radial artery. This catheter is then attached to a *transducer* (sometimes called a *strain gauge*) via stiff connecting tubing called *pressure transmission tubing.* Regular IV tubing should not be used; it can cause inaccurate pressure readings. The transducer, which converts the mechanical energy of the patient's blood pressure to electrical energy, is connected to an electronic *pressure monitor.* The electrical energy then produces a continuous tracing of the patient's arterial pressure wave form on the *oscilloscope* of the pressure monitor, as shown in Figure 39–3. A numerical value for the systolic, diastolic, and mean blood pressure can also be obtained from the pressure monitor. The arterial line is irrigated continuously or at intervals with heparinized water or saline. The arterial line may be used as a route for obtaining blood for all types of blood work which the patient may require except coagulation studies.

The Swan-Ganz catheter is also attached to the pressure monitor in the same manner. Most pressure monitors are able to monitor the pulmonary artery and arterial pressures simultaneously. The ECG tracing is also usually displayed on the same oscilloscope as the pressure tracings. This is helpful in determining the effect that various arrhythmias, e.g., PVC's, atrial fibrillation, junctional rhythms, may have on the cardiac output. (Refer to Chapter 13, particularly Figure 13–17, for further details on the equipment used in pressure monitoring.)

2. Maintain BP between 20 mm. Hg above and 20 mm. Hg below normal baseline BP taken preoperatively. Following mitral and aortic valve surgery, patients may tolerate a low systolic blood pressure of 90 mm. Hg without difficulty. Following surgery on coronary arteries, patients cannot tolerate systolic BP drops of more than 10 mm. Hg below preoperative baseline because the myocardium will be inadequately perfused. Maintaining a sufficient diastolic BP is also very important as the myocardium receives 70 per cent of its blood supply during this phase of the cardiac cycle; blood flows more easily through the coronary arteries while the ventricles are relaxed. In addition, hypertension is also dangerous in the patient who has had a coronary artery bypass graft as the high BP may cause the new grafts to break loose.

With the pressure monitoring equipment available today, the *mean arterial pressure (MAP)* can also be monitored on the postoperative cardiac surgery patient. The MAP is significant because it is the average blood pressure in the systemic circulation. Since diastole is longer than systole, the mean pressure is nearer in value to the diastolic BP. The mean arterial blood pressure is normally 70 to 90 mm. Hg.

3. Causes of decreased blood pressure following heart surgery are pain, inadequate movement, cardiac tamponade, fear, low cardiac output syndrome, thrombosis blocking site of graft or anastomosis, metabolic acidosis, hemorrhage, overmedication with narcotics, arrhythmias, and hypovolemia.

4. Complications resulting from persistent hypotension are cerebral ischemia, renal shutdown, and myocardial infarction.

Pulses (Radial, Apical, Temporal, Posterior Tibial, and Dorsalis Pedis)

1. Check *radial pulse* for rate, rhythm, and volume. *Rapid* radial pulse may indicate ar-

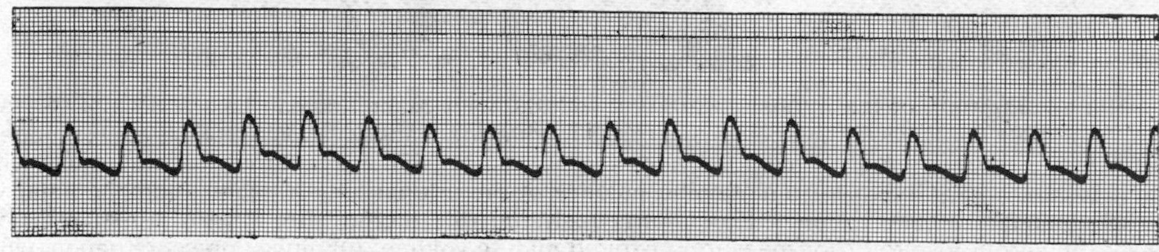

Figure 39–3. An arterial pulse wave obtained from an intra-arterial catheter. The normal pulse wave is characterized by an initial rather rapid anacrotic rise to a rounded peak or "anacrotic" shoulder. After the peak pressure is reached, the pressure falls gradually, making the descending limb of the pressure pulse wave less steep than the ascending limb. The descent is interrupted by the closure of the aortic valve (predicrotic notch), which results in a small rise in the pulse wave (dicrotic wave), followed by a gradual descent until the next ejection of blood from the ventricle. (From Aspinall, J. J.: *Nursing the Open-Heart Surgery Patient.* New York: McGraw-Hill, Inc., 1973, p. 108.)

rhythmias, shock, fear, fever, hypoxia, CHF, or hemorrhage. *Slow* radial pulse may indicate heart block or severe anoxia.

2. Check *apical-radial pulse* for a difference in number of beats per minute. *Pulse deficit* may indicate atrial fibrillation—a frequent complication of mitral stenosis.

3. Check for presence of *pedal pulses* (over posterior tibial artery and dorsalis pedis artery). Absence of pedal pulses may indicate presence of peripheral emboli blocking blood vessel in extremity, report immediately to surgeon. If pulses are absent, check skin of lower extremities for coldness and cyanotic appearance.

Venous Pressure and Left Heart Filling Pressures

1. The central venous pressure and pulmonary artery pressures are usually monitored postoperatively. A pressure higher than normal is often acceptable in the postoperative open heart surgery patient. This is because a heart which has not only been diseased but also subjected to the trauma of surgery is weakened and needs the higher filling pressure to aid in strengthening the force of myocardial contraction and maintaining an adequate cardiac output. Therefore, the surgeon will usually specify parameters for venous and pulmonary artery pressures which are acceptable for a particular patient, taking this into consideration.

2. Some patients may also have a left atrial catheter in place as another means of monitoring the status of left heart functioning in the early postoperative period. Again, acceptable values for the left atrial pressure vary with each patient. Left atrial catheters must be handled with *extreme care* to prevent clots or air from being injected into the left atrium and on into the systemic circulation.

3. Causes of abnormally *elevated* CVP and left heart filling pressures are hypervolemia, and ineffective myocardial contractions.

4. Abnormally *decreased* CVP and left heart filling pressures result from hypovolemia.

Temperature

1. Normally the temperature rises 2 or 3 degrees above normal during the first or second day postoperatively and remains elevated for 3 to 4 days. Treat with aspirin or Tylenol suppositories (on doctor's orders) and minimal bed covering; for persistent elevations, icebags or a hypothermia blanket may be ordered.

2. Reportable abnormal findings are elevation to 38.5°C. (101°F.) or higher, or an elevation that persists for more than 4 or 5 days. Abnormal temperature elevation may be caused by infection, dehydration, hemolysis due to transfusion reaction, or atelectasis. The untoward effects of the elevated temperature are increased metabolic demands, which augment work of the heart, and dehydration and hypovolemia.

Abnormally low temperatures range from 34.4° C. (94° F) to 36° C. (96.8° F.) and may be caused by shock or cardiac decompensation. The physician may order an electric blanket to increase temperature.

Electrocardiogram. Electrical activity of patient's heart is monitored continuously for at least 3 or 4 days following surgery. Observe carefully for abnormal ECG tracings; heart block, ventricular tachycardia, and atrial fibrillation are common complications of open heart surgery.

Goal 2: Promote Respiratory Function and Sufficient Oxygenation by Promoting Chest Drainage and Adequate Ventilation of the Lungs

Adequate respiratory function depends upon the maintenance of a clear and open airway, removal of excess pulmonary secretions, proper aeration of lungs and oxygenation of blood, and the maintenance of chest tube patency and drainage. Observations of respiratory function and care of respiratory problems and complications include the following:

Observe Respirations

1. *Rate:* The ventilator is usually set at a rate which will provide adequate ventilation of the patient along with the appropriate tidal volume and oxygen percentage. An awake patient may initiate respirations in addition to those delivered by the artificial ventilator. Note whether or not the patient is assisting the ventilator (usually the assist light will come on when the patient is assisting the ventilator). In some cases the rate may need to be increased to assure adequate ventilation of the lungs and oxygenation of the blood. This can be determined by arterial blood gas analysis.

2. *Depth:* Shallowness of patient's own respirations may be due to pain. Give a narcotic if vital signs are stable.

3. *Dyspnea:* The patient may *"fight"* the ventilator. In other words, breathe *against,* instead of *with,* the machine. This can lead to inadequate ventilation. The patient may feel a sufficient amount of air is not forthcoming. Airway obstruction (possibly due to excessive secretions), pain, fear, anoxia, acidosis, hemorrhage, and improper placement of the tube may cause the patient to have difficulty in breathing and should be investigated immediately. Arterial blood gas studies and a chest film are usually obtained. The ventilator settings may need ad-

justment; sedation of the patient may be necessary.

> *While the patient is on the artificial ventilator, make sure the ventilator alarms are functioning.*

4. *Wheezing* results from pulmonary edema, bronchospasm, or airway obstruction.
5. *Postextubation:* It is vital that the patient be observed closely for indications of respiratory distress. The rate, depth, and character of respirations should be checked frequently. The patient's color and vital signs should also be noted as changes may indicate inadequate ventilation and the need for reintubation. Arterial blood gases will also be drawn to determine whether the patient is breathing adequately after extubation.

Prevent Retention of Pulmonary Secretions

1. Avoid *complications* of retained secretions, e.g., atelectasis, pneumonia, and subsequent inadequate oxygenation of the tissues, by frequently turning patient; suctioning intubated patient or helping the extubated patient take deep breaths and cough every 1 to 2 hours; nasotracheal suction of extubated patient if temperature becomes greater than 101° F. (38.5° C.) and patient is coughing ineffectively. In addition, the patient should wear a high-humidity oxygen mask after the endotracheal tube is removed to help loosen the secretions. IPPB and chest physiotherapy are other measures used to rid the lungs of secretions. In rare cases, bronchoscopy may be indicated for removal of secretions.
2. Observe *amount* of pulmonary secretions: copious or scant.
3. Observe *color:* white or pale yellow secretions are normal; green and brown secretions may indicate pulmonary infection; large amounts of frothy secretions usually indicate pulmonary edema.
4. Observe for *accompanying signs* of retained secretions: apprehension, perspiration, rapid pulse, dyspnea, cyanosis, gurgling respirations.

Observe Skin. Observe patient's skin coloring for duskiness, mottling, or frank cyanosis. If duskiness appears, oxygen is usually given at 5 liters/min. per nasal cannula.

Chest Drainage. Check chest drainage from chest tubes.* Chest tubes are inserted to drain air and fluid from the pleural cavity, thereby allowing the lungs to reexpand following surgery. They are also used for drainage of the pericardial sac (these tubes are referred to as mediastinal tubes).

Measure and observe chest drainage by collecting drainage in a calibrated cylinder. Measure findings and record hourly. In *normal findings* the amount of drainage varies with the nature of the surgery and the patient's general condition. Up to 100 ml. of drainage may be lost during the first hour postoperatively as a result of reexpansion of the lungs, which forces drainage through chest tube. There will be approximately 500 ml. of drainage over the first 24 hours, with an average of 20 to 30 ml. lost per hour. Large gushes of drainage are sometimes expelled when the patient turns or coughs. Drainage is usually dark red during the early postoperative period; it gradually becomes more serous as time passes.

Abnormal findings, which are reportable, include amounts of drainage in excess of 5 ml./kg. of body weight/hour; a sustained hemorrhage that lasts for more than 1 minute; and sudden cessation of chest drainage accompanied by increase in venous pressure, dyspnea, and oliguria, which may indicate intrathoracic bleeding with accumulation (i.e., cardiac tamponade). The patient may need to return to the operating room for control of excessive bleeding or relief of cardiac tamponade.

Blood is replaced by transfusion. The chest drainage is usually replaced milliliter for milliliter with intravenous blood. In some cases, blood transfusions continue until the CVP is normal.

Chest tubes are milked every hour to express clots, which could block drainage, and checked for kinks or bending. If clots cannot be removed by milking the tube, the physician may need to declot the tube using a long catheter with an inflatable balloon on the end. Chest wound infection is prevented by prophylactic administration of antibiotics. Portable chest films are taken daily until lungs have reexpanded.

Goal 3: Promote Fluid, Electrolyte, and Nutritional Balance

Following heart surgery, the patient typically receives parenteral fluids, blood transfusions, water within 12 hours after surgery, clear liquids, solid foods, and then a full diet, which is usually low in sodium.

Parenteral Fluids. IV fluids are administered judiciously for the first 3 days postoperatively to avoid overload of the circulatory system, which can result in overwork of the heart. Typically administer 500 to 700 ml. per square meter body surface per 24 hours (including oral intake).

The parenteral fluid most commonly used is

*Care of patient with chest tubes is discussed in Unit XVI.

dextrose in water. Sodium-containing fluids are rarely used, as they may lead to circulatory overload (hypervolemia) and heart failure.

Blood Transfusions. These are administered to replace blood lost in chest drainage.

Oral Liquids and Solids. Water is allowed 12 hours postoperatively if the patient is fully responsive and not nauseated; clear liquids are allowed next, followed by solid foods. Watch for signs of abdominal distention and paralytic ileus (see Unit VIII); if either of these conditions develops, stop oral fluids at once and notify the physician.

Electrolyte Balance. Daily electrolyte studies are ordered to determine blood levels of Na^+, K^+, and Cl^-; electrolytes are replaced parenterally if deficient. Hematocrit, hemoglobin, and prothrombin time are ordered daily to determine extent of blood loss or hemorrhage. Blood gases are drawn to determine the pH, pCO_2, and pO_2 of arterial blood (see Chapter 12).

Nursing Duties. Careful measurement and recording of intake and output; daily weighing to determine whether patient is retaining fluids within tissues or losing excessive fluid rapidly: significant fluctuations in weight act as a guide to fluid replacement.

Goal 4: Promote Renal Function

To estimate the adequacy of the patient's renal function, carefully note and record volume, color, and specific gravity of urine; also check patient for signs of suprapubic distention.

Volume. Measure hourly for first 8 to 12 hours following surgery; patient almost always has a Foley catheter. *Normal* is an output of 20 to 30 ml. per hour. Reportable *abnormal* findings: Urine output less than 30 ml. per hour.

Causes of oliguria or anuria are hypovolemia; hemolysis of erythrocytes during cardiopulmonary bypass, which causes sludging of blood in renal tubules; hypotension; and low output failure. *Treatment* of oliguria involves increase in fluid intake if dehydration is present; correction of shock or low output failure; furosemide intravenously, if indicated; and use of peritoneal dialysis or the artificial kidney in patients with renal shutdown.

Color. Urine color may be bloody as a result of hemolysis of erythrocytes during ECC.

Specific Gravity. Normal finding: 1.015 to 1.020. Specific gravity may be *elevated* because of oliguria or presence of RBC's. *Lowered* specific gravity results from overhydration and inability of kidney tubules to filter waste products.

Nursing Observations. Note intake and output; observe patient carefully for signs of bladder distention; weigh patient daily.

Goal 5: Promote Rest, Comfort, and Relief from Pain

If the patient is to rest and sleep comfortably, pain must be relieved. (Causes of pain and restlessness and their treatment are discussed in Unit VIII.)

Pain Medication. Administer Demerol or morphine sulfate for pain postoperatively; administer judiciously, because large doses of narcotics suppress cough reflex. Avoid overmedicating a patient who is still recovering from hypothermia. The body at this time is unable to metabolize the narcotic as quickly as normal, and the drug may accumulate in the patient's system.

Attempt to relieve patient's pain and restlessness with comfort measures prior to administering narcotic; e.g., change patient's position, splint incision during coughing, properly place pillows for support.

Splint Incision. Splint patient's incision firmly during coughing and deep breathing exercises. Use small pillow or hands to splint a sternotomy. Use towel or hands to splint a lateral thoracic incision.

Goal 6: Promote Neurologic Function

Following heart surgery, you must carefully observe the patient's level of consciousness, pupil size and reaction, orientation, and ability to move extremities.

Level of Consciousness. Patient should awaken within 1 to 2 hours following surgery. Failure to awaken may result from embolization of air, calcium, fat, or thrombotic particles to the brain. *Slow* return of consciousness (over 2 to 4 days) may result from a diffuse neurologic deficit owing to poor cerebral capillary perfusion during ECC.

Eyes. Check pupils hourly during early postoperative period for size, equality in size, and reaction to light. Pupils dilate when blood contains excess carbon dioxide.

Orientation. Disorientation and restlessness may indicate anoxia or embolization to the brain. Mental confusion may also result from great fatigue or fear.

Ability to Move Limbs. Hemiplegia, inability to move an extremity, or extreme weakness of an extremity may indicate embolization to the motor area of the brain. Check pedal pulses; absence of pulses may indicate presence of peripheral emboli blocking blood vessel to extremity.

Goal 7: Promote Psychologic Adjustment to the Postoperative Period

Following cardiac surgery, patients may become disoriented, delusional, and frankly psychotic; the majority of patients experience auditory or visual hallucinations. Also, severe depressions are not uncommon.

Causes of Confusion, Hallucinations, and Psychotic Behavior. Isolation within ICU, sensory deprivation; lack of rest and sleep over an extended period of time; fear and anxiety; depersonalization of the patient because of staff's preoccupation with monitors and machines; absence of normal day and night patterns (ICU's are active and well lighted 24 hours a day).

Causes of Postoperative Depression. Extreme fatigue and debility following surgery; prospect of future responsibilities to be faced as patient grows strong and well.

Prevention of Mental Confusion, Undue Fear, Anxiety and Tension

1. Always address the patient by name and introduce yourself by name.
2. Place a calendar and clock at the bedside to orient the patient to the date and time of day.
3. Take an active interest in the patients; do not ignore *them* as you work with monitors, IPPB apparatus, and so forth.
4. Position cardiac monitor so that it is out of the patient's view. Many patients are made unduly nervous by witnessing their own heart action.
5. Schedule the patient's day so that periods of nursing care alternate with periods of rest and relaxation.
6. Encourage patients to freely discuss their fears and anxieties.
7. Prepare patient's significant others for changes in patient's sensorium following surgery. Before the visiting hour, warn family members if the patient is hallucinating or is severely depressed so that they are not unduly shocked.

Goal 8: Promote Early Movement and Ambulation

Prolonged periods of bed rest following heart surgery (or any surgery) may cause weakness, pooling of respiratory secretions, atelectasis, thrombophlebitis, osteoporosis, urinary retention, renal calculi, and a negative nitrogen balance. *Planned activity* is the most important single factor in preventing the complications of bed rest. The type and amount of activity that each patient is allowed will depend upon the type of surgery and the patient's general postoperative condition.

Position in Bed. Patient usually remains flat in bed until systolic blood pressure is over 100 mm. Hg; then patient may be placed in a semi-Fowler's position. Check BP again 5 minutes after patient assumes new position. *Never elevate the patient's knees,* because this position exerts pressure against the vessels of the lower extremities and may cause thrombosis.

Turning and Exercising. If stable, patient may be turned from side to side at intervals for back care. Passive exercises and leg flexion every 2 hours to prevent thrombosis of lower extremities.

Typical Ambulation Schedule. Day after surgery, patient usually dangles for short period. On evening of first postoperative day or on second postpostoperative day, patient is generally allowed to sit in chair for a brief period of time. Fifth to seventh day postoperatively, patient begins to ambulate in room and down hallway. By twelfth to fourteenth day patient is usually fully ambulatory.

Eight to 10 weeks is the normal length of time usually needed for patients to fully regain strength following surgery. Upon discharge home, the patient gradually increases activity until achieving moderate walks and climbing stairs without undue fatigue. The patient usually returns to work 2 to 3 months following surgery.

Goal 9: Prevent Postoperative Complications

Observe the patient constantly for the following postoperative complications.*

1. Postoperative hemorrhage.
2. Shock due to hemorrhage, pain, or trauma.
3. Cardiac tamponade.
4. Renal insufficiency and renal shutdown due to shock, hemolysis, and afferent arteriolar vasoconstriction during ECC procedure.
5. Cardiac arrhythmias caused by K^+ imbalance, cardiovascular drugs, trauma caused by operating on the heart, hypoxia, and acidosis. As mentioned before, temporary pacemaker wires are usually inserted at the time of surgery in case a pacemaker should be required to treat certain arrhythmias in the postoperative period.
6. Low cardiac output syndrome resulting from heart failure and metabolic acidosis. Decreased arterial blood pressure and low cardiac output which is due to weakening of the left

*Postoperative complications are also discussed in Unit VIII.

ventricular muscle are usually accompanied by increased CVP or pulmonary artery wedge pressure. These changes indicate that the heart is receiving an adequate amount of blood but is not able to pump the blood out into the systemic circulation. Consequently, the blood accumulates in the pulmonary vessels and the right side of the heart. Treatment for decreased blood pressure due to a failing heart muscle often is administration of inotropic agents, e.g., dopamine, isoproterenol, or epinephrine, which make the heart beat stronger. Much care must be taken when inotropic agents are administered, though, as they also increase the work of the heart and the need for oxygen.

7. Hypovolemia may become evident as the patient's body temperature begins to increase in the first few hours postoperatively. The hypothermia of the patient in the operating room causes an increase in peripheral vascular resistance. As the body warms after surgery, vessels dilate and blood pressure often falls if the blood volume is inadequate due to postoperative bleeding. The CVP and pulmonary artery wedge pressure are decreased in hypovolemia. These two parameters must be carefully monitored as the blood is replaced.

8. Hypervolemia from fluid overload. The patient may need diuresis while the pulmonary artery wedge pressure is closely monitored.

9. Electrolyte imbalances.

10. Respiratory insufficiency caused by inadequate exchange of respiratory gases during ECC or inadequate postoperative ventilation.

11. Pneumothorax (inadequate lung expansion) resulting from blockage of chest tubes by kinks, blood clots, and so forth.

12. Wound infection, usually resulting from staphylococcal invasion.

13. Convulsions, hemiplegia, or limb weakness owing to embolization.

14. "Stress" ulcer resulting from reaction of body to prolonged physiologic stresses imposed by extensive surgery. (See Unit XVII.)

DISCHARGE PLANNING

As discharge time approaches, encourage the patient to express any fears about the future, e.g., having to assume more responsibility upon recovery. If patient remains debilitated after surgery, anxieties about being a burden to the family, inability to go to work, and so on, may arise.

Depending upon the type of surgery and possible postoperative complications, the patient may need to take various medications or follow a special diet or activity regime upon return home and will need instruction regarding the therapy. Coumadin, an oral anticoagulant medication, may be prescribed for patients with prosthetic valves to prevent embolic formation around the prosthesis. Some patients require a permanent pacemaker postoperatively. Digitalis, diuretics, and a low-sodium and high-potassium diet are other types of therapy that may be prescribed upon discharge.

BIBLIOGRAPHY (Unit XII)

1. Aagaard, G. N.: Treatment of hypertension. *American Journal of Nursing,* 73:621, Apr. 1973.
2. Agarwala, B., et al.: Why does a child with a normal heart undergo cardiac catheterization? *American Family Physician,* 17:117, June 1978.
3. Alderman, E. L.: Propranolol and heart disease. *Consultant,* 17:24, July 1977.
4. Alexy, B. J.: Monitoring cardiovascular status with non-invasive techniques. *Nursing Clinics of North America,* 13:423, Sept. 1978.
5. A look at high blood pressure — part 1. *The Harvard Medical School Health Letter,* IV:1, June 1979.
6. A look at high blood pressure — part II. *The Harvard Medical School Health Letter,* IV:1, July 1979.
7. Altman, G. B.: Management of the hypertensive patient. *Nurse Practitioner,* 1:98, Jan.-Feb. 1976.
8. Andreoli, K., et al.: *Comprehensive Cardiac Care — A Text for Nurses, Physicians, and Other Health Practitioners.* St. Louis: C. V. Mosby Co., 1976.
9. Angina after bedtime. *Emergency Medicine,* 10:52, Jan. 1978.
10. Angina, other geriatric ills improved by high fiber diet. *RN,* 41:116, Oct. 1978.
11. Angina patients are at risk in smoke-filled rooms. *RN,* 41:107, Dec. 1978.
12. Angina pectoris: Rationale of drug therapy. *Hospital Medicine,* 15:65, Jan. 1979.
13. Antman, E., and P. F. Cohn: Coronary artery disease: Correlation between clinical and angiographic findings. *Hospital Medicine,* 15:8, Mar. 1979.
14. A quick return from MI. *Emergency Medicine,* 10:169, Oct. 1978.
15. Arbeit, S., et al.: Recognizing digitalis toxicity. *American Journal of Nursing,* 77:1936, Dec. 1977.
16. Aspinall, M. J.: *Nursing the Open-Heart Surgery Patient.* New York: McGraw-Hill, Inc., 1973.
17. Ayers, C. R.: Hypertension: Checklist for management. *Hospital Medicine,* 12:6, Nov. 1976.
18. Badeer, H. S.: Axioms on athelete's heart syndrome. *Hospital Medicine,* 13:70, Apr. 1977.
19. Baden, C. A.: Teaching the coronary patient and his family. *Nursing Clinics of North America,* 7:563, Sept. 1972.
20. Bailey, R.: Diuretics in the elderly. *British Medical Journal,* 1:1618, June 1978.
21. Barnes, R., and W. W. Schottstaedt: The relation of emotional state to renal excretion of water and electrolytes in patients with congestive heart failure. *American Journal of Medicine,* 29:227, Aug. 1960.
22. Beeson, P. B.: Infective endocarditis. *In* Beeson, P. B., and W. McDermott (Eds.): *Cecil Loeb Textbook of Medicine,* 14th ed. Philadelphia: W. B. Saunders Co., 1975.
23. Bergersen, B. S., and E. E. Krug: *Pharmacology in Nursing,* 13th ed. St. Louis: C. V. Mosby Co., 1976.
24. Berne, R. M., and M. N. Levy: *Cardiovascular Physiology,* 3rd ed. St. Louis: C. V. Mosby Co., 1977.

25. Bragg, T. L.: Psychological response to myocardial infarction. *Nursing Forum,* XIV:383, 1975.
26. Brest, A. N.: Antiarrhythmic therapy: How to select the right method. *Consultant,* 19:23, Jan. 1979.
27. Bretylal: A unique new antiarrhythmic, clinical aid. McGaw Park, Ill., *Arnar-Stone Laboratories, Inc.,* July 1978.
28. Bruckheim, A. H.: Practice patterns in the management of hypertension. *American Family Physician,* 17:209, Mar. 1978.
30. Burch, G. E.: Axioms on myocardial infarction. *Hospital Medicine,* 14:8, Sept. 1978.
31. Burch, G. E.: The special problems of heart disease in old people. *Geriatrics,* 32:51, Feb. 1977.
32. Butler, H. H.: Atrioventricular block. *Consultant,* 16:206, Nov. 1976.
33. Calcium in cardiac resuscitation. *Consultant,* 19:60, March 1979.
34. Caldwell, J. R.: Practical approach to hypertension: 1. Diagnostic evaluation. *Postgraduate Medicine,* 65:66, May 1979.
35. Caldwell, J. R.: Practical approach to hypertension: 2. Treatment. *Postgraduate Medicine,* 65:81, May 1979.
36. Campbell, W. B.: Axioms on malignant hypertension. *Hospital Medicine,* 12:6, July 1976.
37. Carlson, R. W., and H. G. Becker: Preventing or managing cardiopulmonary arrest. *Consultant,* 19:58, June 1979.
38. Carnes, G. D.: Understanding the cardiac patient's behavior. *American Journal of Nursing,* 71:1187, June 1971.
39. *Chardack-Greatbatch Implantable Cardiac Pacemakers: Endocardiac and Myocardial Systems.* Technical information distributed by Corvek Medical Equipment Company, Portland, Oregon, for Medtronic, Inc.
40. Chatton, M. J., et al.: *Handbook of Medical Treatment,* 15th ed. Los Altos, Cal.: Lange Medical Publications, 1977.
41. CHF diagnosis and treatment today. *Emergency Medicine,* 11:109, Aug. 1979.
42. Ciuca, R.: Cor pulmonale. *Nursing '78,* 8:46, Dec. 1978.
43. Clark, D. A., et al.: Cardiac transplantation in man. *American Journal of Medicine,* 54:563, May 1973.
44. Cogen, R.: Cardiac catheterization: Preparing the adult. (Pictorial.) *American Journal of Nursing,* 73:77, Jan. 1973.
45. Cogen, R.: Preventing complications during cardiac catheterization. *American Journal of Nursing,* 76:401, Mar. 1976.
46. Conn, H. F.: *Current Therapy 1979.* Philadelphia: W. B. Saunders Co., 1979.
47. Conner, T. P.: A little about patent ductus arteriosus. *Consultant,* 16:83, Nov. 1976.
48. Conover, M. H., and E. G. Zalis: *Understanding Electrocardiography — Physiological and Interpretative Concepts.* St. Louis: C. V. Mosby Co., 1976.
49. Correcting common errors in blood pressure measurement. (Programmed instruction.) *American Journal of Nursing,* 65:133, Oct. 1965.
50. Costrini, N. V., and W. M. Thomson: *Manual of Medical Therapeutics.* Boston: Little, Brown and Co., 1977.
51. Cromwell, R. L., et al.: *Acute Myocardial Infarction: Reaction and Recovery,* St. Louis: C. V. Mosby Co., 1977.
52. Dack, S.: Acute pulmonary edema. *Hospital Medicine,* 14:112, Mar. 1978.
53. Davis, M. Z.: Socioemotional component of coronary care. *American Journal of Nursing,* 72:1426, Aug. 1972.
54. Davis, R., et al.: Treatment of chronic congestive heart failure with Captopril, an oral inhibitor of angiotensin converting enzyme. *New England Journal of Medicine,* 301:117, July 1979.
55. DeBakey, M., and A. Gotto: *The Living Heart.* New York: Charter Books, 1977.
56. Dedmon, R. E.: A prescription for fitness. *Consultant,* 18:44, Nov. 1978.
57. Derrick, H. F.: How open heart surgery feels. *American Journal of Nursing,* 79:227. Feb. 1979.
58. Dines, D. E.: The dyspneic patient. *Hospital Medicine,* 12:6, Jan. 1976.
59. DiPalma, J. R.: Drug-induced changes in vital signs and blood pressure. *RN,* 42:46, June 1977.
60. Diuretics: Adverse reactions and precautions. *Nurses' Drug Alert,* Nov. 1978.
61. Dolgin, M.: Bundle-branch block: When to consider cardiac pacing. *Consultant,* 18:71, Sept. 1970.
62. Dowdall, S. A.: Breathing techniques that help reduce hypertension. *RN,* 40:73, Oct. 1977.
63. Dracup, K. A.: Unraveling the mysteries of cardiomyopathy. *Nursing '79,* 9:84, May 1979.
64. Dunphy, J. E., and L. W. Way: *Current Surgical Diagnosis and Treatment,* 3rd ed. Los Altos, Cal.: Lange Medical Publications, 1977.
65. Durbin, D.: *Rapid Interpretation of EKG's,* 3rd ed. Tampa Fla.: Cover Publishing Co., 1974.
66. Early signals of a heart attack. Information sheet. Metropolitan Life Insurance Co., 1977.
67. Ebert, P. A.: Ventricular aneurysm. *Hospital Medicine,* 14:36, Feb. 1978.
68. Effler, D. B.: Myocardial revascularization 1978. *Postgraduate Medicine,* 63:98, Jan. 1978.
69. Eliot, R. S., and E. A. Salhany: Sudden death and acute myocardial infarction. *Postgraduate Medicine,* 64:52, Oct. 1978.
70. Endocarditis goes to the head. *Emergency Medicine,* 10:208, Nov. 1978.
71. Ferrer, M. I.: Axioms on heart block. *Hospital Medicine,* 13:25, July 1977.
72. Finnerty, F. A., Jr.: Hypertension: Current management. Part 1. Selecting and evaluating the patient. *Consultant,* 18:163, Jan. 1978.
73. Finnerty, F. A., Jr.: Hypertension: Current management. Part 2. Therapy — the stepped-care approach. *Consultant,* 19:126, Feb. 1978.
74. Finnerty, F. A., Jr.: Hypertension: Current management. Part 3. Drug and patient resistance. *Consultant,* 19:53, Mar. 1978.
75. Finnerty, F. A.: Hypertension in the elderly. *Postgraduate Medicine,* 65:119, May 1979.
76. Fowler, N. O.: *Examination of the Heart: Part 2: Inspection and Palpation of Venous and Arterial Pulses.* Prepared for the Committee on Medical Education of the American Heart Association. New York: American Heart Association, 1972.
77. Fowler, N. O.: Sinus tachycardia — how to identify common causes. *Consultant,* 12:47, Mar. 1972.
78. *Framingham Heart Study: Detection of Factors Increasing Risk of Coronary Disease.* Bethesda, Md.: The National Heart Institute, 1964.
79. Frank, M. J.: What to do for the patient with unstable angina. *Consultant,* 19:117, Jan. 1979.
80. Frank, M. J., and C. Alvarez-Mena: *Cardiovascular Physical Diagnosis.* Chicago: Year Book Medical Publishers, Inc., 1973.
81. Franklin, S. S.: Guide to Prognosis in Hypertension. *Hospital Medicine,* 13:49, Mar. 1977.

82. Frantz, A., and M. Galdys: Keeping up with automatic rotating tourniquets. *Nursing '78,* 8:31, Apr. 1978.
83. Friedman, H. H. (Ed.): *Problem-Oriented Medical Diagnosis.* Boston: Little, Brown and Co., 1975.
84. Frohlich, E. D.: Hypertensive crisis. *Hospital Medicine,* 13:32, Jan. 1977.
85. Futral, J. E.: Postoperative management and complications of coronary artery bypass surgery. *Heart and Lung,* 6:477, May-June 1977.
86. Gazes, P. E.: Guiding MI patients to recovery. *Consultant,* 19:34, Mar. 1979.
87. Goldberger, E.: *Treatment of Cardiac Emergencies,* 2nd ed. St. Louis: C. V. Mosby Co., 1977.
88. Goldring, D., et al.: Cardiovascular emergencies in infants and children. *Hospital Medicine,* 12:20, Mar. 1976.
89. Gordon, F. S.: Geriatrics medications: Tailoring cardiovascular therapy to the patient. *RN,* 41:56, Mar. 1978.
90. Gould, L.: Guide to recognition of digitalis toxicity. *Hospital Medicine,* 13:93, July 1977.
91. Gould, L., et al.: Pericardial effusion as an early complication of acute myocardial infarction. *American Family Physician,* 19:107, Apr. 1979.
92. Green light for oral nitrates. *Emergency Medicine,* 10:173, Sept. 1978.
93. Greenwald, J. G.: Echocardiography in the cardiac work-up. *American Family Physician,* 18:137, Sept. 1978.
94. Grollman, A.: How drugs work: Diuretics. *Consultant,* 12:53, July 1972.
95. Gronim, S. S.: Helping the client with unstable angina. *American Journal of Nursing,* 78:1677, Oct. 1978.
96. Gross, P.: Drugs to start the heart. *Emergency Medicine,* 10:127, Feb. 1978.
97. Guyton, A. C.: *Textbook of Medical Physiology,* 5th ed. Philadelphia: W. B. Saunders Co., 1976.
98. Hackett, T. P., and N. H. Cassem: Coronary Care: *Patient Psychology.* Booklet prepared by the American Heart Association, 1975.
99. Hammond, C. E.: Protecting patients with temporary transvenous pacemakers. *Nursing '78,* 8:82, Nov. 1978.
100. Hammond, J. J., and W. M. Kirkendall: Antihypertensive drugs for the aging. *Geriatrics,* 34:27, June 1979.
101. Harris, R.: The aging heart: insight into biologic changes and their clinical significance. *Geriatrics,* 32:41, Feb. 1977.
102. Hart, R.: A review of CPR for adults. *Nursing '79,* 9:54, Feb. 1979.
103. Hart, R.: Giving artifical ventilation. *Nursing '78,* 8:48, June 1978.
104. Hatcher, C. R., Jr.,: Surgical management of unstable angina pectoris. *Medical Times,* 107:75, Mar. 1979.
105. Hathaway, R.: The Swan-Ganz catheter, a review. *Nursing Clinics of North America,* 13:389, Sept. 1978.
106. Heger, J. J., and C. Fisch: Axioms on cardiac arrhythmias. *Hospital Medicine,* 15:20, Jan. 1979.
107. Henry, J. P.: Understanding the early pathophysiology of essential hypertension. *Geriatrics,* 31:59, Jan. 1976.
108. Hill, M.: Helping the hypertensive patient control sodium intake. *American Journal of Nursing,* 79:906, May 1979.
109. Hirsch, A. T.: Postmyocardial infarction syndrome. *American Journal of Nursing,* 79:1240, July 1979.
110 Hollander, G., and E. Lichstein: Guide to evaluation of ischemic heart disease. *Hospital Medicine,* 16:46, July 1979.
111. Hollifield, J. W.: Essential hypertension: Renin levels as guides for therapy. *Consultant,* 18:147, Sept. 1978.
112. Home one week after MI. *American Journal of Nursing,* 78:1553, Sept. 1978.
113. Hurst, J. W. (Ed.): *The Heart, Arteries and Veins.* New York: McGraw-Hill Book Co., 1978.
114. In cardiac arrest, resuscitate with care. *Emergency Medicine,* 10:219, Nov. 1978.
115. Important nonrheumatic causes of mitral regurgitation. *Hospital Medicine,* 14:55, Nov. 1978.
116. Jokl, E.: Exercise and the heart. *Consultant,* 12:46, July 1972.
117. Kannel, W. B.: Office evaluation of coronary candidates. *Hospital Medicine,* 15:38, Feb. 1979.
118. Kapoor, A. S., and N. S. Dang: Reliance on physicial signs in acute myocardial infarction and its complications. *Heart and Lung,* 7:1020, Nov.-Dec. 1978.
119. Katz, F. H.: Primary hypertension. *Hospital Medicine,* 13:26, Apr. 1977.
120. Kennedy, J.: Myocardial infarction in coronary artery disease. *Cardiovascular Nursing,* 12:23, Nov.-Dec. 1976.
121. Kent, S.: Does exercise prevent heart attacks? *Geriatrics,* 33:95, Nov. 1978.
122. Kent, S.: Hormones and heart disease. *Geriatrics,* 34:97, June 1979.
123. Kent, S.: Vitamin C therapy: Colds, cancer, and cardiovascular disease. *Geriatrics,* 33:91, Oct. 1978.
124. King, G., and G. M. Folger: The nurse in the cardiac catheterization laboratory. *Supervisor Nurse,* 9:37, Oct. 1978.
125. King, S. B., III.: Classification of patients with coronary atherosclerotic heart disease. *Medical Times:* 107:38, Mar. 1979.
126. King, S. B., III,: Indications for bypass in atherosclerotic heart disease. *Medical Times,* 107:51, Mar. 1979.
127. King, S. B., III,: To what extent does bypass relieve pain and prolong life? *Medical Times,* 107:87, Mar. 1979.
128. Kirkendall, W. M., et al.: *Recommendations for Human Blood Pressure Determinations by Sphygmomanometers.* Authorized by the Central Committee for Medical and Community Programs of the American Heart Association on May 5, 1967. New York: American Heart Association, 1967.
129. Kleiger, R. E.: Chest pain in patients seen in emergency clinics. *Journal of the American Medical Association,* 236:595, Aug. 1976.
130. Kloth, H. H.: Axioms on rheumatic heart disease. *Hospital Medicine,* 13:8, Mar. 1977.
131. Krupp, M. A., and M. J. Chatton: *Current Medical Diagnosis and Treatment.* Los Altos, Cal.: Lange Medical Publications, 1978.
132. Kucharski, A.: Psychologic stress in myocardial infarction. *American Family Physician,* 17:154, Mar. 1978.
132a. Kurihara, M., and Moody, F. G.: The complications of general surgery. *In* Meltzer, L. E., et al.: *Concepts and Practices of Intensive Care for Nurse Specialists.* Philadelphia: Charles Press Publishers, Inc., 1969.
133. Lalli, S. M.: The complete Swan-Ganz. *RN,* 41:65, Sept. 1978.
134. Lancour, J.: How to avoid pitfalls in measuring blood pressure. *American Journal of Nursing,* 76:773, May 1976.
135. Larter, M. H.: M.I. wives need you. *RN,* 39:44, Aug. 1976.

136. Lavin, M. A.: Bed exercises for acute cardiac patients. *American Journal of Nursing,* 73:1226, July 1973.
137. Learn the ABC of life support. Information sheet. Metropolitan Life Insurance Co., 1977.
138. Lehmann, J.: Auscultation of heart sounds. *American Journal of Nursing,* 72:1242, July 1972.
139. Lemberg, L., and S. Hamer: Arrhythmias complicating acute myocardial infarction: A self-teaching program. *Heart and Lung,* 5:576, July-Aug. 1976.
140. Leon, A. S., and H. Blackburn: Exercise rehabilitation of the coronary heart disease patient. *Geriatrics,* 32:66, Dec. 1977.
141. Levy, R. I.: Hyperlipidemia: From trial and error toward scientific precision. *Consultant,* 7:32, Oct. 1978.
142. Loebl, S., et al.: *The Nurse's Drug Handbook.* New York: John Wiley & Sons, 1977.
143. Loggie, J. M. H.: Identification and management of juvenile hypertension. *Postgraduate Medicine,* 65:103, May 1979.
144. London, S. B., and R. E. London: Critique of indirect diastolic end-point — "muffling" vs. "last" sound. *Archives of Internal Medicine,* 119:34, Jan. 1967.
145. Long, M., et al.: Hypertension. What patients need to know. *American Journal of Nursing,* 76:765, May 1976.
146. Lukas, P. S.: Dyspnea. *In* MacBryde, C. M., and R. S. Blacklow (Eds.): *Signs and Symptoms: Applied Pathologic Physiology and Clinical Interpretation,* 5th ed. Philadelphia: J. B. Lippincott Co., 1970.
147. MacBryde, C. M., and R. S. Blacklow (Eds.): *Signs and Symptoms: Applied Pathologic Physiology and Clinical Interpretation,* 5th ed. Philadelphia: J. B. Lippincott Co., 1970.
148. Maloney, R.: Helping your hypertensive patients live longer. *Nursing '78,* 8:26, Oct. 1978.
149. Manwaring, M.: What patients need to know about pacemakers. *American Journal of Nursing,* 77:825, May 1977.
150. Manzi, C. C.: Cardiac emergency! How to use drugs and c.p.r. to save lives. *Nursing '78,* 8:30, Mar. 1978.
151. Manzi, C. C.: Edema — how to tell if it's a danger signal. *Nursing '77,* 7:66, Apr. 1977.
152. Materson, B. J.: Beta-adrenergic blocking agents in hypertension: Pro and con. *Consultant,* 18:98, Oct. 1978.
153. Mayer, G. G., et al.: Arrhythmias and cardiac output. *American Journal of Nursing,* 72:1597, Sept. 1972.
154. Mayer, G. G., and C. W. Peterson: Theoretical framework for coronary care nursing education. *American Journal of Nursing,* 78:1209, July 1978.
155. McNeal, G. J.: Rectal temperatures in the patient with an acute myocardial infarction. *Image,* 10:18, Feb. 1978.
156. McNeal, G. J.: Tracing arrhythmias. *American Journal of Nursing,* 79:98, Jan. 1979.
157. McNeer, J. F., et al.: Hospital discharge one week after acute myocardial infarction. *New England Journal of Medicine,* 298:229, Feb. 1978.
158. Mead, W. F.: Exercise rehabilitation after myocardial infarction. *American Family Physician,* 17:121, Mar. 1977.
159. Mead, W. F.: The aging heart. *American Family Physician,* 18:73, Aug. 1978.
160. Mechner, F.: Patient assessment: auscultation of the heart — part II. *American Journal of Nursing,* 77:1, Feb. 1977.
161. Mechanisms of edema in myocardial failure. *Hospital Medicine,* 12:79, Aug. 1976.
162. Mehlman, D. J., and M. F. Arnsdorf: Antiarrhythmic therapy for the elderly: A two-edged sword. *Geriatrics,* 34:29, May 1979.
163. Meltzer, L. E., et al.: *Concepts and Practices of Intensive Care for Nurse Specialists,* 2nd ed. Bowie, Md.: Charles Press Publishers, Inc., 1976.
163a. Meltzer, L. E., et al.: *Intensive Coronary Care.* Philadelphia: Charles Press Publishers, Inc., 1970.
164. Merrill, J. P.: Curable hypertension. *Hospital Medicine,* 12:6, Apr. 1976.
165. Meserko, U.: Preoperative classes for cardiac patients. *American Journal of Nursing,* 73:665, Apr. 1973.
166. Metcalfe, J.: The heart in pregnancy: Guide to practical considerations. *Hospital Medicine,* 14:95, Sept. 1978.
167. Metheny, M. M., and W. D. Snively: *Nurse's Handbook of Fluid Balance,* 2nd ed. Philadelphia: J. B. Lippincott Co., 1974.
168. Meyer, R. M. S., and D. T. Morris: Alcoholic cardiomyopathy: A nursing approach. *Nursing Research,* 26:422, Nov.-Dec. 1977.
169. Missri, J.: Hematologic toxicity of drugs used in cardiovascular disease. *Postgraduate Medicine,* 65:165, Jan. 1979.
170. M. I. update. *Emergency Medicine,* 10:110, May 1978.
171. Money savers; An inexpensive source of potassium replacement. *Nurses' Drug Alert,* II:22, Mar. 1978.
172. Moore, K., et al.: The joy of sex after a heart attack: counseling the cardiac patient. *Nursing '77,* 7:53, June 1977.
173. Moore, M. A.: Hypertension in the ambulatory patient. *American Family Physician,* 16:188, Nov. 1977.
174. Moore, S. J.: Pericarditis after acute myocardial infarction: manifestations and nursing implications. *Heart and Lung,* 8:551, May-June 1979.
175. Morris, D. C.: Valve disease. *Medical Times,* 107:47, Jan. 1979.
176. Moss, A. J., et al.: The early posthospital phase of myocardial infarction: Prognostic stratification. *Circulation,* 54:58, 1976.
177. Mundth, E. D.: Surgical considerations in management of angina pectoris. *Postgraduate Medicine,* 61:130, Mar. 1977.
178. New guidelines for endocarditis. *Emergency Medicine,* 9:35, Aug. 1977.
179. Niven, R. G.: Psychologic adjustment to coronary artery disease. *Postgraduate Medicine,* 60:152, Nov. 1976.
180. Noble, J.: An approach to refractory heart failure. *American Family Physician,* 15:138, Apr. 1977.
181. Notter, D., E. R. Giblet, and C. A. Finch: *General Medicine.* Seattle: University of Washington Medical School, 1970.
182. Nutter, D. O.: Cardiomyopathies. *Medical Times,* 107:57, Jan. 1979.
183. Okoniewski, G. A.: Sexual activity following myocardial infarction. *Cardio-Vascular Nursing,* 15:1, Jan. 1979.
184. Pacemaker protocol. *Emergency Medicine,* 10:50, June 1978.
185. Page, I. H.: Hypertension — the fledgling of modern medical practice. *Postgraduate Medicine,* 61:203, Jan. 1977.
186. Parker, B. M.: Mitral valve prolapse: What "popping, click and crescendo murmur" mean. *Consultant,* 19:78, Feb. 1979.
187. Parmley, W. W.: Axioms on congestive heart failure. *Hospital Medicine,* 13:44, Oct. 1977.

188. Payne, F. E.: A practical approach to effective exercise. *American Family Physician,* 19:76, June 1979.
189. Phillips, R. E., and M. K. Feeney: *The Cardiac Rhythms: A Systematic Approach to Interpretation.* Philadelphia: W. B. Saunders Co., 1973.
190. Preston, T., et al.: Three therapeutic approaches in tachycardia. *Geriatrics,* 28:110, Mar. 1973.
191. Peart, W. S.: Arterial hypertension. *In* Beeson, P. B., and J. W. McDermott (Eds.): *Cecil-Loeb Textbook of Medicine,* 14th ed. Philadelphia: W. B. Saunders Co., 1975.
192. Price, S. A., and L. M. Wilson: *Pathophysiology: Clinical Concepts of Disease Processes.* New York: McGraw Hill Book Co., 1978.
193. Rackley, C. E., et al.: Glucose-insulin-potassium infusion in acute myocardial infarction. *Postgraduate Medicine,* 65:93, Feb. 1979.
194. Remington, R. D.: Blood pressure: The population burden. *Geriatrics,* 31:48, Jan. 1976.
195. Reno, D. J.: Swan-Ganz. *RN,* 41:5, Dec. 1978.
196. Ratts, T. E.: Axioms on coronary artery disease. *Hospital Medicine,* 14:36, Mar. 1978.
197. Robinson, A.: Detection and control of hypertension: Challenge to all nurses. *American Journal of Nursing,* 76:778, May 1976.
198. Robinson, P. H.: Pericarditis. *Medical Times,* 107:73, Jan. 1979.
199. Robbins, S. L., and R. S. Cotran: *Pathologic Basis of Disease,* 2nd ed. Philadelphia: W. B. Saunders Co., 1979.
200. Russell, R. O., Jr., et al.: Acute myocardial infarction: Diagnosis, pitfalls, management. *Hospital Medicine,* 14:6, Dec. 1978.
201. Russell, R. O., and C. E. Rackley: *Hemodynamic Monitoring.* Mt. Kisco, N.Y.: Futura Publishing Co., 1974.
202. Ryan, C.: Guidelines for evaluating and treating hypertension. *Geriatrics,* 34:43, July 1979.
203. Sacksteder, S., et al.: Common congenital cardiac defects. *American Journal of Nursing,* 78:264, Feb. 1978.
204. Segal, B. L., et al.: IHSS: Echocardiography can uncover the diagnosis. *Consultant,* 19:191, Mar. 1979.
205. Selzer, A.: *Principles of Clinical Cardiology.* Philadelphia: W. B. Saunders Co., 1975.
206. Scalzi, C. C.: Behavioral responses following an acute myocardial infarction. *Heart and Lung,* 2:69, Jan.-Feb. 1973.
207. Schroeder, J. S., and E. K. Daily: *Techniques in Bedside Hemodynamic Monitoring.* St. Louis: C. V. Mosby Co., 1976.
208. Sher, P. P.: Cardiac isoenzymes: Better tests for diagnosing myocardial infarction. *Consultant,* 18:166, Oct. 1978.
209. Shoemaker, W. C.: Early diagnosis and management of pericardial tamponade. *Hospital Medicine,* 14:7, Nov. 1978.
210. Simon, A. B.: Axioms on sudden coronary death. *Hospital Medicine,* 14:54, May 1978.
211. Skydell, B., and A. S. Crowder: *Diagnostic Procedures: A Reference for Health Practitioners and a Guide for Patient Counseling.* Boston: Little, Brown, and Co., 1975.
212. Slessor, G.: Auscultation of the chest — a clinical nursing skill. *Canadian Nurse,* 69:40, Apr. 1973.
213. Smith, C. A.: Body image changes after myocardial infarction. *Nursing Clinics of North America,* 7:663, Dec. 1972.
214. Smith, J. W., et al.: Post-MI: To stress or not to stress. *Geriatrics,* 33:25, Oct. 1978.
215. Sochocky, S.: Axioms on chronic cor pulmonale. *Hospital Medicine,* 12:7, Sept. 1976.
216. Sochocky, S.: Ventricular septal defect due to myocardial infarction. *American Family Physician,* 18:153, Oct. 1978.
217. Sodeman, W. A., and W. A. Sodeman, Jr.: *Pathologic Physiology,* 5th ed. Philadelphia: W. B. Saunders Co., 1974.
218. Sokolow, M., and M. B. McIlroy: *Clinical Cardiology.* Los Altos, Cal.: Lange Medical Publications, 1977.
219. Sopko, J., and R. Freeman: Salt substitutes as a source of potassium. *Journal of the American Medical Association,* 238:608, Aug. 1977.
220. Spodick, D. H.: Acute pericarditis and pericardial effusion: Guide to diagnosis and management. *Hospital Medicine,* 15:72, May 1979.
221. Standards for cardiopulmonary resuscitation (CPR) and emergency cardiac care (ECC). *Journal of the American Medical Association,* 227(Suppl.):837, Feb. 1974.
222. Steelman, R. B.: About arteriosclerotic heart disease. *Consultant,* 18:143, June 1978.
223. Storlie, F.: *Patient Teaching in Critical Care.* New York: Appleton-Century-Crofts, 1975.
224. Strong, A. B.: Caring for cardiac catheterization patients. *Nursing '77,* 7:60, Nov. 1977.
225. Surawicz, B.: Pitfalls in interpretation of ECG stress tests. *Postgraduate Medicine,* 65:54, Feb. 1979.
226. Sweetwood, H.: Patients with pacemakers. *Nursing '77,* 7:44, Mar. 1977.
227. Symptoms in cardiac tamponade. *Hospital Medicine,* 15:79, June 1979.
228. Tarazi, R. C.: Should you treat systolic hypertension in elderly patients? *Geriatrics,* 33:25, Nov. 1978.
229. Tegtmeyer, C. J.: Complications of cardiac pacemakers. *American Family Physician,* 14:66, July 1976.
230. Thadepalli, H.: Infective endocarditis: How to recognize its new look. *Consultant,* 18:190, Nov. 1978.
231. The beginnings of hypertension. *Emergency Medicine,* 9:97, July 1977.
232. The not-so-mild-mannered MI. *Emergency Medicine,* 10:206, Jan. 1978.
233. Thomas, J.: Care and rehabilitation after myocardial infarction. *In* Conn, H. F. (Ed.): *Current Therapy 1975.* Philadelphia: W. B. Saunders Co., 1975.
233A. Thompson, T.: The year they changed hearts. *Life,* 71:56, Sept. 1971.
234. Thorpe, C. J.: A nursing care plan — the adult cardiac surgery patient. *Heart and Lung,* 8:690, July-Aug. 1979.
235. Tucker, R. M.: Renovascular hypertension: Current status. *Hospital Medicine,* 15:57, May 1979.
236. Tyzenhouse, P. S.: Myocardial infarction: Its effect on the family. *American Journal of Nursing,* 73:1012, June 1973.
237. Upping the dosage for cardiomyopathy. *Emergency Medicine,* 11:89, Apr. 1979.
238. Van Meter, M., and P. G. Lavine (Eds.): *How to Read an EKG Correctly.* Jenkintown, Pa.: InterMed Communications, 1975.
239. Vinsant, M. O., et al.: *A Commonsense Approach to Coronary Care — A Program,* 2nd ed. St. Louis: C. V. Mosby Co., 1975.
240. Walinsky, P.: Acute hemodynamic monitoring. *Heart and Lung,* 6:838, Sept.-Oct. 1977.
241. Walker, W. J.: Success story: The program against major cardiovascular risk factors. *Geriatrics,* 31:97, Mar. 1976.
242. Waller, J. L., and J. A. Kaplan: Advances in monitoring during coronary bypass. *Medical Times,* 107:63, Mar. 1979.

243. Walton, C., and B. Hammond: Angina — teaching your patient how to prevent current attacks. *Nursing '78,* 8:33, Feb. 1978.
244. Weber, M. A., and J. H. Laragh: Hypertension. *In* Conn, H. F. (ed.): *Current Therapy 1978.* Philadelphia, W. B. Saunders Co., 1978.
245. Weldon, C. S.: What's new in surgery: Cardiothoracic surgery. *Emergency Medicine,* 11:131, June 1979.
246. Weinberg, S. L.: Prognosis after acute myocardial infarction. *Consultant,* 18:139, Dec. 1978.
247. Weinberg, S. L.: 'Quinidine syncope' without quinidine. *Heart and Lung,* 7:779, Sept.-Oct. 1978.
248. When hyper- is normotension. *Emergency Medicine,* 9:57, Dec. 1977.
249. Williams, S.: *Nutrition and Diet Therapy,* 3rd ed. St. Louis: C. V. Mosby Co., 1977.
250. Wiggers, C. J.: The heart. *Scientific American,* May 1957.
251. Winslow, E. H.: Visual inspection of the patient with cardiopulmonary disease. *Nursing Digest,* p. 20, Winter 1976.
252. Winsor, T.: How much exercise for the cardiac patient? *Consultant,* 18:43, June 1978.
253. Witztum, J. J.: Diagnosis and treatment of hyperlipidemia. *Hospital Medicine,* 14:60, June 1978.
254. Woods, S. L.: Monitoring pulmonary artery pressures. *American Journal of Nursing,* 79:1765, Nov. 1979.
255. Wunsch, C. M.: Rehabilitating the patient who has had a heart attack. *Consultant,* 17:74, Dec. 1977.
256. Yalof, I.: The multidisciplinary team: An effective approach to management of the cardiac surgery patient. *Heart and Lung,* 8:699, July-Aug. 1979.
257. Yokes, J. A., and W. A. Reed: Heart surgery. *In* Meltzer, L. E., et al. (Eds.): *Concepts and Practices of Intensive Care,* 2nd ed. Philadelphia: Charles Press, Inc., 1976.

UNIT XIII

NURSING PEOPLE EXPERIENCING DYSFUNCTION OF THE KIDNEY AND THE URINARY TRACT

by Barbara Innes, R.N., B.S.N., M.S.

INTRODUCTION AND STUDY GUIDE

The nursing of patients experiencing dysfunction of the kidneys and urinary tract encompasses all aspects of nursing from the care of patients with short-term, easily cured difficulties to long-term maintenance care or care of the dying. Both physical and psychologic components are equally important. Particularly with the long-term problems, both the patient and people who live with the patient are integral parts of the problems and their solutions. Continuity of care between the hospital, out-patient department, and home must be considered. It is important to use all resources on the health care team.

Urology and *nephrology* are terms often used to distinguish disease entities. Urology refers to the study of disorders of the urinary tract — that is, ureters, bladder, and urethra — while nephrology refers to the study of disorders of the kidney itself. This is often an inadequate division, as disorders of the lower urinary tract soon affect the kidney and vice versa. These terms, *urology* and *nephrology*, are also used to designate specialties in medicine: the urologist is a surgeon most concerned with anatomic disorders, and the nephrologist is an internist concerned with physiologic disorders.

It is important to realize that the nurse's role in the care of patients with urinary dysfunction is changing, especially with patients being treated for end-stage renal disease. The number of patients undergoing dialysis and renal transplantation is growing. While much of the care required remains within the realm of the specially trained clinician, nurses in general practice or specialties other than nephrology will come into contact with renal patients much more frequently also. More patients who have had or will be having dialysis or transplant will be seen in general hospitals or out-patient settings for other disorders. More patients contemplating such treatment will be looking for information and advice. And more families and friends of renal patients will be asking questions and seeking support. Thus, it is necessary for all nurses to understand what is involved in these treatments and the kind of care and support patients and significant others will need.

This unit provides you with enough information to accurately identify the needs of patients with urinary tract disorders and to effectively provide the care required to meet these needs. The following guidelines will help you achieve maximum learning from this unit:

1. Prior to studying this unit, you should have a good understanding of fluid and electrolyte balances and imbalances. See Chapter 12.
2. Since so many urinary tract disorders are long-term, you should be familiar with the concept of adaptation to chronic illness.
3. This unit assumes that you are familiar with specific procedures, such as catheterization, catheter care, and bladder irrigation. If you need to review these techniques, consult an appropriate source.
4. As you study this unit, familiarize yourself with the following terms:

renal
urethra
ureter
micturition
nephron
tubules
glomerulus
parenchyma
renal pelvis
calices
blood urea nitrogen
creatinine
reflux
sphincter
strictures
incontinence
nocturia
hematuria
pyuria
voiding
fluid balance
catheter
catheterization
meatus
retention
specific gravity
creatinine clearance
urinalysis
concentration
pyelography
cystoscopy
urethrography
angiography
retrograde
pyelonephritis
perinephric
ureteritis
cystitis
urethritis
nephritis
hydronephrosis
calculi
lithiasis
polycystic
glomerulonephritis
nephrotic
dialysis
diffusion
hemodialysis
peritoneal dialysis
dialysate
semipermeable membrane
homograft
immunosuppression
autoimmune
renal transplantation
cannula
arteriovenous shunt
internal arteriovenous fistula

Upon completion of this unit, you should be able to

- Describe the normal anatomy and physiology of the urinary tract.
- Describe in detail a plan for complete assessment of a patient's urinary status.
- Interpret results of specified diagnostic tests in relation to their impact on nursing care.
- Describe the role of the nurse in caring for the patient undergoing selected diagnostic tests.
- Utilize assessment data to accurately identify needs of the patient with specific disorders of the kidney and lower urinary tract.
- Design effective care plans based on identified needs for patients with specified disorders of the kidney and lower urinary tract.
- State rationale for decisions made in the care of patients with specified disorders of the kidney and lower urinary tract.
- Demonstrate consideration for continuity of care in all situations in which the patient needs care.
- Include those who live with the patient in all aspects of the care process.

CHAPTER 40

NORMAL ANATOMY AND PHYSIOLOGY OF THE URINARY TRACT

The main functions of the urinary system are (a) to remove waste products from the body and (b) to regulate the fluids, electrolytes, and acid-base balances and osmotic pressures within the body. Thus, the urinary tract plays a major role in the maintenance of homeostasis. These functions are accomplished through the formation of urine, a complex task involving the processes of filtration, reabsorption, and secretion. The formed urine is then excreted from the body.

The kidneys also have several nonexcretory metabolic and endocrine functions. Their role in blood pressure regulation, red blood cell production, insulin degradation, prostaglandin synthesis, and regulation of other substances in the body will be discussed below.

ANATOMY OF THE URINARY TRACT

The urinary tract is composed of four organs: kidneys, ureters, bladder, and urethra. Figure 40–1 illustrates the position of these structures within the body. Supporting musculature, blood supply, and nervous innervation complement the system.

In males, the reproductive system is anatomically connected to the urinary tract; both of them share the same outlet from the body — the urethra. The prostate gland, although not a direct part of the urinary system, can have a major impact on the functioning of the urinary tract. This gland is located below the bladder neck and completely surrounds the urethra. Normally, this relationship causes no problem, but if the gland enlarges, it constricts the urethra and obstructs the outflow of urine. Further discussion of the male reproductive system is found in Chapter 82.

Kidneys

The two kidneys are located retroperitoneally in the posterior aspect of the abdomen on either side of the vertebral column. They lie between the twelfth thoracic and the third lumbar vertebrae, with the left kidney usually positioned slightly higher than the right. Adult kidneys average approximately 11 cm. in length, 5 to 7.5 cm. in width, and are 2.5 cm. thick. They are loosely supported in place by a mass of perirenal fat and connective tissue called renal fascia.

Each organ is shaped like a kidney bean, with the distal edge being convex and the medial boundary being concave. In the innermost part of the concave section is the hilus, through which pass the renal artery, renal vein, lymphatics, nerves, and the renal pelvis, which is the natural upper extension of the ureter. A firm, tough, fibrous capsule surrounds and adheres to the renal parenchyma. Inside this capsule, each kidney is divided into three major areas: cortex, medulla, and pelvis. Figure 40–2 demonstrates the gross anatomy of the kidney. The *cortex* lies just under the renal capsule and portions of it extend down into the medullary layer to form the renal columns. The *medulla* is divided into 8 to 18 cone-shaped masses called renal pyramids. Their bases are positioned on the corticomedullary boundary and the apices extend toward the renal pelvis, forming papillae. The papillae have 10 to 25 openings on the surface of each through which the urine empties into the renal pelvis. The inner area, or *renal pelvis*, is a sinus lined with transitional epithelium. The wall opposite the hilus of the kidney forms two or three outpouchings called major calices which extend outward from the hilus. Each major calyx is divided into minor calices which extend toward the papillae. The combined volume of the pelvis and calices is approximately 8 ml. The renal pelvis narrows as it reaches the hilus and becomes the proximal end of the ureter.

The functioning unit of the kidney is the *nephron*, and each kidney contains more than one million of these units. A nephron is a microscopic structure consisting of a glomerular capsule and tubular system which empties into the renal pelvis. Figure 40–3 illustrates a functioning nephron. Located in the cortical layer of the kidney, the proximal end of the nephron is a double-walled cup, called the *glomerular* or *Bowman's capsule*, which is lined with a simple squamous epithelium to allow easy filtration from the blood. Inside the capsule is the *glomerulus*, which is a tuft of nonanastomosing capillaries fed by an afferent arteriole and drained by an efferent arteriole. The *proximal tubule* is a convoluted portion about 15 cm. long with innumerable microvilli lining its lumen forming a brush border and vastly increasing its membrane surface area. As it nears the medullary layer, the tubule abruptly narrows and forms the descending *loop of Henle*. This then turns back on itself as the ascending limb of the loop of Henle, which is larger in diameter than the descending limb. The loop of Henle, as it moves back into the cortex of the kidney, becomes the *distal convoluted tubule*, which joins a *collecting duct*. Each collecting duct receives the terminal end of several nephrons as it courses through the cortex and medulla of the kidney. As the collecting ducts within a renal pyramid get closer to the apex of the pyramid, several coalesce to form a larger *duct of Bellini*, which opens into a minor calyx of the renal pelvis.

The *macula densa* lies between the afferent arteriole and the distal convoluted tubule, where it passes close to the arteriole. The *juxtaglomerular cells* are found between the macula densa and the afferent arteriole just before it enters the glomerular capsule. Together these two cellular structures form the *juxtaglomerular apparatus*, which is felt to play a major role in the renin-angiotensin system.

Renal Circulation. The kidneys receive 20 to 25 per cent of the cardiac output under resting conditions, which averages more than one liter per minute. The *renal arteries* branch from the abdominal aorta at the level of the second lumbar vertebra. Passing laterally to the hilus of the kidney, each artery usually divides into an anterior and posterior branch, which supply the anterior and posterior portions of the kidney, respectively. Further subdivisions of the primary branches of the renal artery are called *lobar arteries*; these vessels supply the papillae. These arteries divide into *interlobar arteries* which run between the renal pyramids until they reach the corticomedullary zone where they form incomplete arches, *arcuate arteries*, around the bases of the pyramids. Branching from the arcuate arteries are the *interlobular arteries* which supply the cortical substance and renal capsule. The interlobular arteries also give rise to the afferent arterioles which become the *glomerulus*.

The *efferent arterioles* carry blood from the glomerulus. They then divide into a network of *peritubular capillaries* which supply the tubules and re-

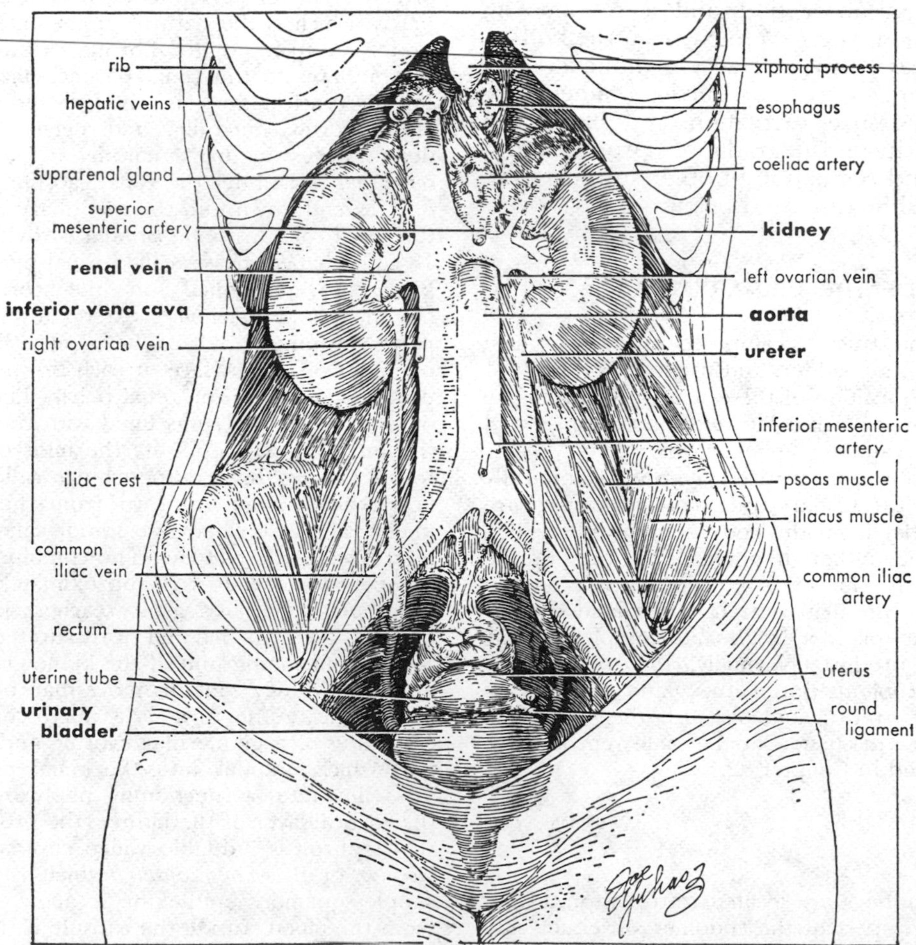

Figure 40–1. Anterior view of the posterior abdominal wall with peritoneum removed showing kidneys, ureters, bladder, and related structures. (From Crouch, J.: *Functional Human Anatomy.* Philadelphia: Lea and Febiger, 1972.)

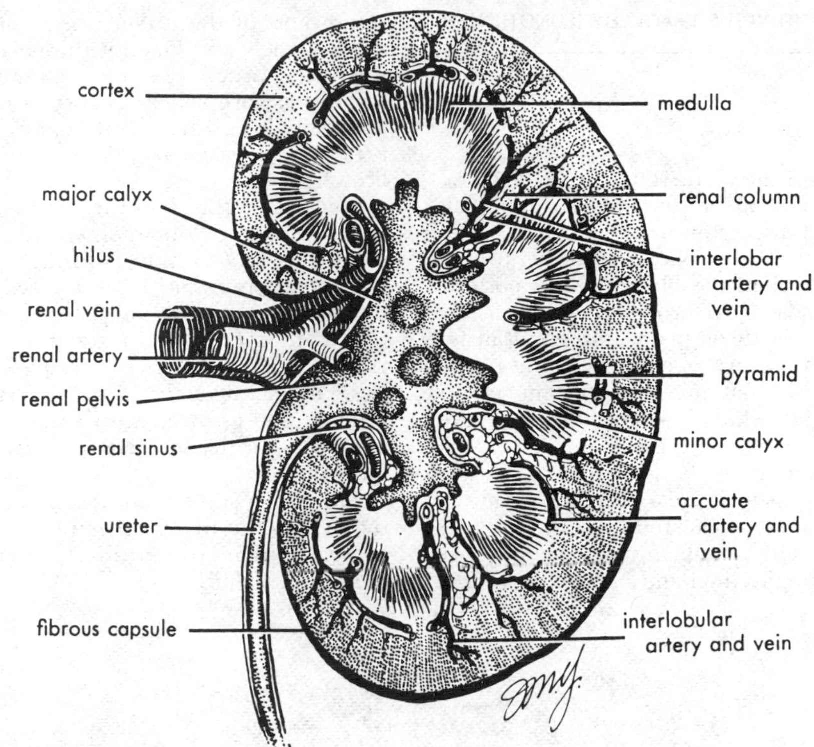

Figure 40–2. Sagittal view of the kidney. (From Crouch, H.: *Functional Human Anatomy.* Philadelphia: Lea and Febiger, 1972.)

ceive the materials reabsorbed by the tubular structures. This segment of renal circulation, where capillaries empty into other arterioles which proceed to a second set of capillaries, is a unique arrangement that allows a high filtration pressure in the glomerulus. Some of the efferent arterioles from juxtamedullary glomeruli do not form a peritubular capillary network, but instead drain into a network of vessels forming hairpin loops called the *vasa recta*; these loops dip into the medulla for variable distances and play a role in the renal concentrating mechanism. The blood then leaves the kidney in a venous system closely corresponding to the arterial system: *interlobular veins* to *arcuate veins* to *interlobar veins* to *lobar veins* to the *renal vein.* The renal circulation then empties into the inferior vena cava.

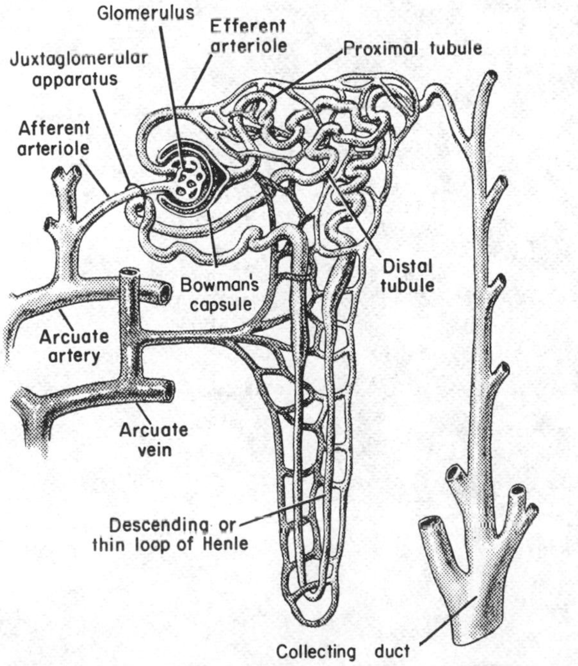

Figure 40–3. Diagram of a functioning nephron. (From Guyton, A.: *Textbook of Medical Physiology.* Philadelphia: W. B. Saunders Co., 1976.)

Innervation. The kidney receives both sympathetic and parasympathetic innervation. The renal nerves course along the renal blood vessels as they enter the hilus of the kidney. The sympathetic nerve supply comes from the twelfth thoracic to the second lumbar nerves via the splanchnic nerves and the celiac plexus. Parasympathetic nerves branch from the vagus nerve and also travel through the celiac plexus. There are also contributions from the superficial hypogastric plexus and intermesenteric, upper splanchnic, and thoracic nerves. The nerves terminate primarily on the walls of the blood vessels rather than in the tubules and are believed to have a vasomotor function. Adrenergic fibers also end in close proximity to the juxtaglomerular cells and renal tubules. It is important to note that a completely denervated kidney will continue to form urine.

Ureters

The ureters form from the medial tapering of the renal pelvis at the hilus of the kidney and are

25 to 35 cm. long in the adult. They lie in the extraperitoneal connective tissue and descend vertically along the psoas muscle toward the pelvic cavity. After dipping into the pelvic cavity, the ureters course anteriorly to join the bladder in its posterolateral aspect. At each ureterovesical junction, the ureter runs obliquely through the bladder wall for about 1.5 to 2 cm. before opening into the lumen of the bladder. This anatomic arrangement usually functions as a valve which prevents the backward flow, or reflux, of urine into the kidney.

Each ureter has definite elastic characteristics and is made of three tissue layers — an inner mucosa lining the lumen, a muscular middle layer, and a fibrous outer layer. The musculature is generally designated as inner longitudinal and outer circular, but along most of the ureter, the muscle fibers actually run obliquely and blend with one another to form a meshlike tissue. The muscle arrangement allows urine to be propelled down the ureter by peristaltic action. This peristalsis is thought to be regulated by a myogenic pacemaker located near the renal calices.[208]

Blood is supplied to the ureters by one or more vessels that run longitudinally along the tube. Because the ureters travel through several anatomic areas, these ureteral vessels are fed by several of the following arteries: renal artery (frequently), testicular or ovarian artery, aorta and common iliac arteries, internal iliac artery (frequently), vesical arteries, umbilical artery, and uterine artery. The number and assortment of contributing arteries anastomosing with the ureteric vessels varies with each individual.

The ureter's innervation comes from the eleventh thoracic to the first lumbar nerves. The network of nerves becomes progressively more dense toward the terminal end.

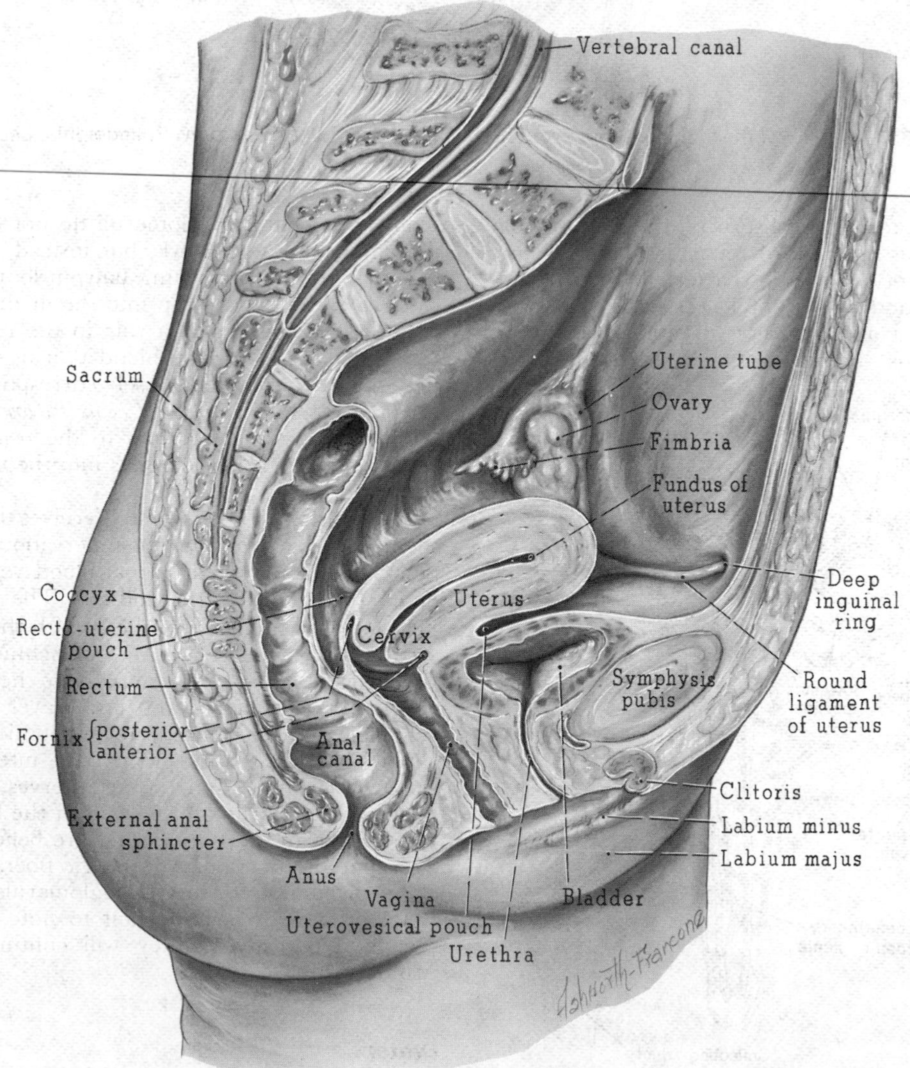

Figure 40–4. Mid-sagittal section of the female pelvis. (From Jacob, J., C. Francone, and W. J. Lossow: *Structure and Function in Man*, 4th ed. Philadelphia: W. B. Saunders Co., 1978.)

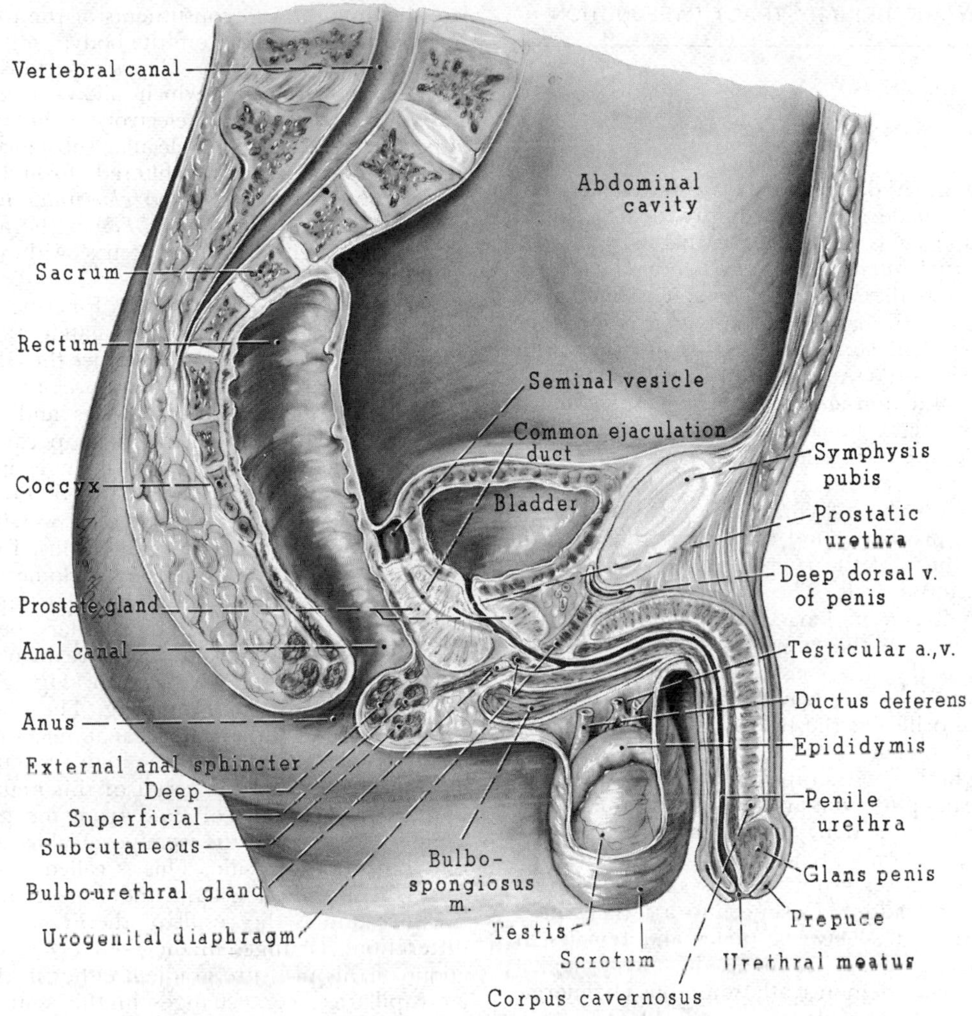

Figure 40–5. Mid-sagittal view of the male pelvis and external genitalia. (From Jacob, J., C. Francone, and W. J. Lossow: *Structure and Function in Man*, 4th ed. Philadelphia: W. B. Saunders Co., 1978.)

Bladder

The urinary bladder is a hollow organ located in the anterior half of the pelvis behind the symphysis pubis. Figures 40–4 and 40–5 illustrate the position in the female and male, respectively, of the bladder and urethra in relation to the other anatomic structures of the pelvis. The space between the bladder and the symphysis pubis is filled with a loose connective tissue which allows the bladder to rise cranially as it fills. The peritoneum covers the top border of the bladder, while the base is held loosely in place by the true ligaments. The bladder is also enveloped by a loose fascia.

The bladder wall has several tissue layers. The internal lining of the vesical is transitional epithelium with some mucus-secreting glands. Then there are three muscle layers. Although the direction of the muscle fibers in each layer is not as distinct as previously thought,[175] the inner and outer layers tend to have fibers running longitudinally, while those of the middle layer are circular. The meshlike arrangement of the layers makes up the *detrusor muscle*. This allows the bladder wall to be very elastic, while also maintaining strength. Bundles of these smooth muscle layers come together at the base of the bladder to form the internal spincter or opening into the urethra. The *trigone* describes the triangular area cornered by the ureterovesical junctions and the internal sphincter.

The superior and lateral aspects of the bladder are served by the superior vesical artery, which branches from the umbilical artery and internal iliac artery. The inferior vesical artery, which supplies the underside of the bladder, may arise independently or in common with the middle rectal artery.

Innervation for the bladder comes from the hypogastric sympathetic, pelvic parasympathetic, and pudendal somatic nerves. Ganglia are most commonly found in the bladder base and around the ureteral orifices. Neurologically these areas tend to act in continuity with each other and their functions seem to be coordinated by both the sympathetic and parasympathetic nervous systems.

Urethra

The urethra is a tube that starts at the base of the bladder and extends to the surface of the body.

There is a great difference between females and males. The female urethra is approximately 4 cm. in length and curves slightly forward as it reaches for its external opening or *meatus* located between the clitoris and the vaginal orifice. It is lined with epithelium, which has in it some mucus-secreting glands. The circular muscle layer is continuous with that of the bladder. As the urethra passes through the urogenital diaphragm, the circular muscle fibers form the external sphincter.

The male urethra is about 20 cm. long and is divided into three main sections. The *prostatic* urethra extends about 3 cm. below the bladder neck through the prostate gland to the pelvic floor. The ejaculatory ducts of the reproductive system empty into its posterior wall. The *membranous* urethra is about 1 to 2 cm. in length and ends where the muscle layer forms the external sphincter. The distal portion is the *cavernous* urethra. It is approximately 15 cm. long and travels through the penis to the urethral orifice at the tip of the penis. It is also lined with epithelial cells.

The urethral blood supply is provided primarily by the internal pudendal artery and urethral artery. This is supplemented by those vessels feeding the surrounding anatomic structures.

Innervation arises from sources similar to those supplying the bladder. Gosling and associates have found a difference between males and females in distribution of nerve terminals in the proximal urethra. Females demonstrate numerous cholinergic nerves, but only rare adrenergic ones. However, in males, the area is richly supplied by adrenergic nerves, indicating direct sympathetic control.[109]

PHYSIOLOGY OF THE URINARY SYSTEM

The main function of the urinary system is the formation of urine. This is the role of the kidneys and, in this process, several constituents of the body can be regulated. The other organs of the urinary tract work to transport the urine from the kidneys out of the body.

Kidneys

Urine is formed in the nephrons by three processes: filtration, reabsorption, and secretion. *Filtration* is the passage of a liquid through a filtering membrane as the result of a pressure differential. In the kidney this takes place in the glomerulus. The tubular portion of the nephron is the site for *reabsorption*, the taking back of fluids and other substances through body tissues, and *secretion* which involves the active transport of certain chemicals from the blood stream into the tubules. Figure 40–6 shows how each of these processes is utilized in different anatomic portions of the nephron to regulate the amount and constituents of the urine being formed and excreted from the body.

Glomerular Filtration. The glomerulus is a semipermeable membrane which allows free passage across it of water and electrolytes but is usually impermeable to larger molecular substances such as protein. The fluid that is filtered through this glomerular membrane is called *glomerular filtrate* and the *glomerular filtration rate (GFR)* is the amount of glomerular filtration that occurs within a given period of time.

The glomerular filtration rate for a normal adult male of average size is approximately 125 ml. per minute. Several factors can influence the GFR. These include hydrostatic and oncotic pressure gradients between the glomerular capillaries and Bowman's capsule, rate of renal blood flow, permeability of the glomerular membrane, and changes in the total area of the glomerular capillary bed. Probably the most important is the amount and pressure of the blood supply reaching the glomerulus, for without any blood flow there would be no glomerular filtration. Pressure within the glomerular capillaries is usually higher than in other capillary beds in the body. Whereas hydrostatic pressure in other capillaries is normally 15 to 20 mm. Hg, glomerular capillary pressure is 70 mm. Hg. The higher pressure is caused by the unique anatomic structure of the afferent arterioles and the high resistance in the efferent arterioles. The result of this high pressure is the "pushing out" of fluid from the glomerular capillaries through the semipermeable membrane into Bowman's capsule. This is called *ultrafiltration*, since the filtration occurs under exceedingly high pressure and is the result of the *hydrostatic pressure* differential. Changes in the GFR occur with alterations of this pressure gradient either in the glomular capillaries, e.g., changes in the systemic blood pressure, or in Bowman's capsule, e.g., renal edema or ureteral obstruction. The kidney does have some resistance to changes in systemic blood pressure through the process of *autoregulation*. This capability allows the kidney through intrinsic regulation of renal circulation to maintain a relatively constant renal blood flow and thus GFR over a range of arterial blood pressure from 70 to 200 mm. Hg. Outside of these limits, the pressure of the blood flow and GFR varies with the systemic blood pressure. It is important to note that certain medications may modify the kidney's autoregulatory ability.

The *oncotic pressure* is the pulling pressure exerted by the plasma proteins within the capillaries (see Chapter 12). This force works in opposition to the capillary hydrostatic pressure so that the GFR is the result of the hydrostatic pressure minus the oncotic pressure. Changes in the concentration of the plasma proteins, e.g., fluid depletion and hypoproteinemia alter the influence of this force.

Closely allied with the pressures affecting GFR is the amount of *renal blood flow* reaching the glomerulus. Anything enhancing or interfering with renal circulation will alter the GFR. Such things as direct trauma to or obstruction of any of the blood vessels interrupts this flow. Medications may alter renal blood flow. For instance, dopamine and glucagon

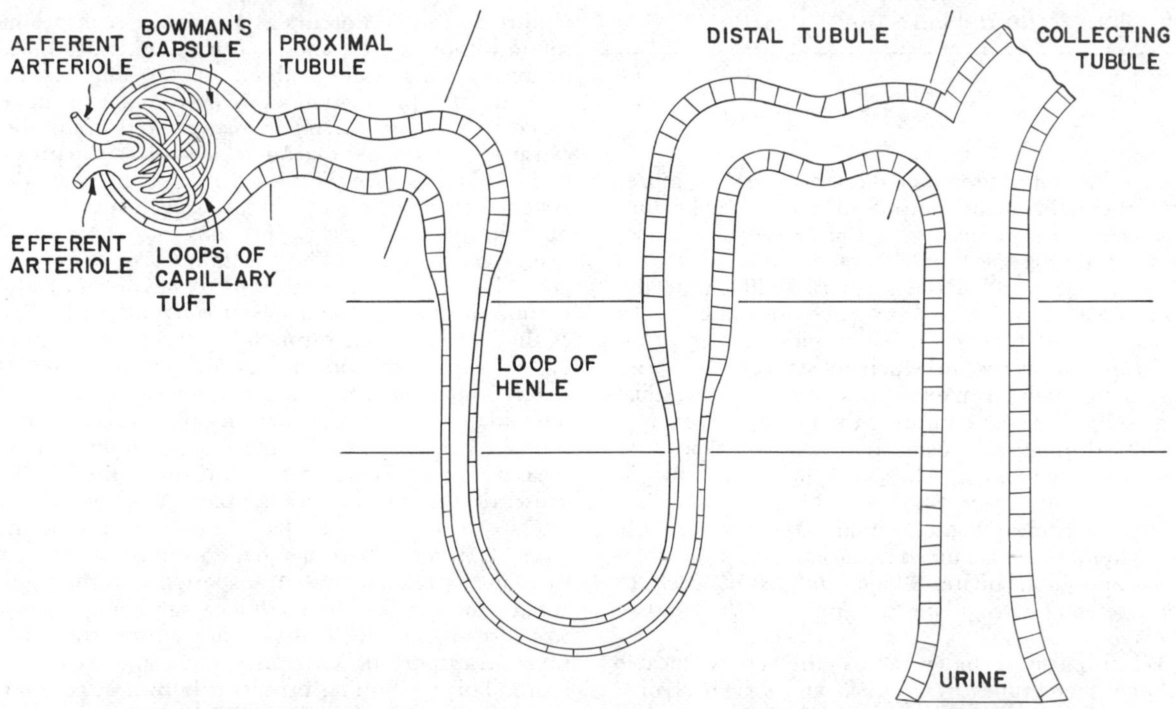

Glomerulus	Proximal tubule	Henle's loop	Distal tubule	Collecting duct
Filtration	65 percent Na^+ and water reabsorbed ADH not required All glucose, K^+, urate reabsorbed HCO_3^- reabsorbed H^+ secreted Fluid leaves isotonic	Na^+ transport from ascending limb Countercurrent establishes hypertonic interstitium Fluid leaves hypotonic	Na^+ reabsorbed ADH required for H_2O reabsorption K^+ and urate secreted HCO_3^- reabsorbed H^+ secreted NH_3^+ secreted Leaves hypotonic or isotonic	Water reabsorbed in final concentrating operation ADH required

Figure 40–6. The major functions of each portion of the nephron. (Adapted from Koushanpour, E.: *Renal Physiology: Principles and Functions.* Philadelphia: W. B. Saunders Co., 1976, and Papper, S.: The effects of age in reducing renal function. *Geriatrics,* May 1973.)

produce direct renal vasodilatation without apparent effect on the systemic blood pressure. Some diuretics cause vasoconstriction, while others lead to increases in renal blood flow. Activation of the adrenergic nervous system may decrease blood flow either through release of norepinephrine from the renal sympathetic nerves or by epinephrine from the adrenal medulla.[205] Bacterial pyrogens prompt vasodilation. It has been found that a high-protein diet increases renal blood flow, although the mechanism for this is as yet unknown.[100] As demonstrated, the list of influential factors is long.

As mentioned above, normal *capillary permeability* interferes with the passage of plasma proteins into the filtrate. Any pathology that changes this relationship interferes with the normal oncotic pressure gradient.

Changes in the *total area* of the *capillary glomerular bed* modify the structure available to filter the blood. These usually involve a reduction in the functioning area and result from glomeruli-destroying diseases or partial nephrectomy.

The results of the filtration process represent the first stage in the formation of urine. The composition of this ultrafiltrate is approximately 94 per cent water and 6 per cent solutes. The list of normal solutes includes sodium, potassium, calcium, magnesium, chloride, bicarbonate, phosphate, sulfate, and organic acids.

Tubular Reabsorption. Although the kidneys

initially filter 180 liters per day, this does not represent the daily urine output of the normal adult. The main reason for this is the reabsorptive function of the renal tubular system, which returns about 99 per cent of the glomerular filtrate to the body. Reabsorption takes place through active transport and passive diffusion and osmosis. *Active transport* is a process in which substances are moved across the tubular membranes into the interstitial space by the expenditure of metabolic energy, usually through adenosine triphosphate. Once into the interstitial tissues, these substances are picked up by the capillaries. Substances reabsorbed in this manner include glucose, amino acids, protein, uric acid, sodium, potassium, magnesium, calcium, chloride, and bicarbonate. Blood and tissue levels of these elements regulate the rate of their active transport.

Water passively moves across the semipermeable tubular membranes by *diffusion* and *osmosis* according to the concentration gradient. As solutes are transported into the interstitial spaces, the concentration of solutes outside the tubule rises, causing water to shift out of the tubular system. This process occurs without the aid of antidiuretic hormone (ADH) in the proximal tubule, but, as illustrated in Figure 40–6, ADH is required in the distal tubule and collecting ducts. This hormone increases the permeability of these membranes, allowing the water to move more freely along its concentration gradient. Current evidence indicates that the ADH binds to the peritubular surface of the cells and initiates reactions leading to the permeability changes.[138]

Some substances are poorly reabsorbed through the tubular membranes. These include urea, phosphate, sulfate, uric acid, nitrate, and phenols, which are waste products that need to be excreted from the body. As water is reabsorbed by osmosis, the concentration of these substances inside the tubule rises, causing some of the molecules to pass through to the interstitial spaces. However, this process is very inefficient, and this inefficiency allows the body to rid itself of metabolic wastes.

Tubular Secretion. Tubular cells are also capable of secretion, which is a chemical activity allowing transport of substances from the blood into the tubules. The two physiologic elements most involved in this process are potassium and hydrogen.

Regulation of Fluids and Electrolytes. The regulation of fluids and electrolytes in the body occurs primarily because of feedback systems between the nephrons and the body fluids and tissues. These systems alter the processes described above — filtration, reabsorption, and secretion — to determine the amount and composition of the urine excreted from the body.

Assuming renal blood flow to be adequate, the fluid volumes are maintained principally through the diluting and concentrating mechanisms of the nephrons. Dilution occurs as a result of reabsorbing solute without water, and concentration is produced by reabsorbing water without solute. The process allowing the production of hyperosmolar urine is called the *"counter-current" mechanism* and occurs because of the anatomic arrangement of the nephron and capillaries (see Fig. 40–3). A counter-current system occurs when the inflow travels parallel to, opposite to, and in close proximity to the outflow over some distance. There continues to be debate about how this mechanism works, but the end result is concentration of the urine. It is hypothesized that as the filtrate travels through the ascending loop of Henle where the membrane is impermeable to water, sodium and chloride are moved out into the intersitial space by active transport. This reduces the salt concentration in the distal tubule and increases the concentration in the interstitium. Because of the concentration gradient, some of the interstitial salt diffuses back into the descending loop of Henle, where it moves around the hairpin turn and is again actively transported into the interstitial tissues. Since the medullary salt concentration was already slightly higher than before, the additional transport of salt raises the osmolarity even more. This continuing process is known as counter-current multiplication.[199] Figure 40–7 illustrates the effect of this mechanism on the osmolarity, and thus concentration, of the filtrate as it travels through the tubules. The resulting hypertonicity of the interstitial fluid is maintained because the vasa recta, which follow the course of the loop of Henle, operate as counter-current exchangers. Solutes move out of the blood vessels going toward the cortex and into vessels descending into the pyramids. At the same time, water diffuses out of the descending vessels and into the ascending vessels. This recirculation preserves the solute concentration in the interstitium.

If this process were to continue unmediated, the urine produced would be very dilute, since the membranes of the distal tubule and collecting ducts are relatively impermeable to water without the activity of ADH. In the presence of ADH, these membranes become permeable to ADH and allow water reabsorption to take place freely. Thus, the hyperosmolar fluid delivered to the distal tubule becomes iso-osmolar with the interstitial spaces by the time it reaches the papillae. The fluid reabsorbed in this manner diffuses into the vasa recta and is returned to the general circulation through the renal circulation. Because of the influence of ADH on the concentrating and diluting abilities of the nephrons, anything that affects the release of ADH affects the amount of urine produced.

Urea works to augment the concentration of urine. As water is reabsorbed from the tubule, the concentration of urea increases. The inner medullary portion of the collecting duct is permeable to urea, and it is reabsorbed freely along the concentration gradient into the interstitium. This helps maintain the high osmolarity of the interstitial space so that more water is reabsorbed in the presence of ADH.

The regulation of electrolyte excretion by the kidney is influenced by a variety of factors, including hydrostatic and oncotic pressures and the circulating effect of aldosterone and other adrenocortical hormones. The movement of sodium also affects the regulation of several other electrolytes. For instance, the active reabsorption of sodium causes passive reabsorption of chloride and bicarbonate. The reabsorption of potassium has some reverse correlation to the reabsorption of sodium, although this is not a rigid process; however, if body levels of potassium are too high, excess potassium is secreted into the tubules.

Chapter 12 further discusses the role of the kidney in water and electrolyte regulation.

Regulation of Acid-Base Balance. Regulation of pH within the body is done primarily by the kidney. Metabolic acids, e.g., phosphoric, keto, uric, and sulfuric acids, are normally excreted as they are formed. Then, in the presence of acid-base imbalances, the kidneys excrete either hydrogen or bicarbonate ions as appropraite to restore balance.

Normally the cells of the renal tubules secrete equivalent amounts of hydrogen and bicarbonate. Hydrogen ions are secreted into the proximal and distal tubules and the collecting ducts through the hydration of carbon dioxide in the presence of carbonic anhydrase. The carbonic acid goes on to split into carbon dioxide and water. The carbon dioxide is reabsorbed from the tubules and excreted by the lungs, while the water is excreted in the urine.

In the case of acidosis, excess hydrogen ions are secreted into the proximal and distal tubules and collecting ducts and excreted in the urine. There is a limit to the hydrogen gradient and, without buffers to tie up the free hydrogen in the urine, this limit would be reached quite rapidly. As mentioned above, the hydrogen reacts with bicarbonate to form carbon dioxide and water. It also reacts with dibasic phosphate to form monobasic phosphate and with ammonia to form ammonium ion. The formation of these compounds allows the secretion of more hydrogen. The excess acid is excreted in the urine, lowering its pH.

With alkalosis, the excretion of hydrogen ions ceases. At higher levels of bicarbonate concentrations in the body, bicarbonate may actually be excreted in the urine, resulting in increased systemic pH levels.

Further discussion of the kidney's contribution in acidbase regulation is included in Chapter 12.

Regulation of Blood Pressure. Recall from Chapter 37 that in the event of blood volume depletion, the renin-angiotensin-aldosterone system works to maintain the blood pressure. As arterial blood pressure drops, there is reflex vasoconstriction in the splanchnic circulation which effectively reduces renal blood flow and thus glomerular filtration rate. This stimulates the release of *renin* from the juxtaglomerular cells. The mechanisms regulating the release of renin may be classified as (a) intrarenal, including baroreceptors in the afferent arterioles and natrioreceptors in the macula densa which are sensitive to changes in sodium concentration; (b) sympathetic, including renal nerves as well as the action of catecholamines; and (c) humoral, including the effects of sodium, potassium, vasopressin, and angiotensin II.[344] The renin is released into the blood stream where it acts on angiotensin I, which is produced in the liver and has a very weak vasconstrictive effect on peripheral vessels. As this substance passes through the lungs, it is converted

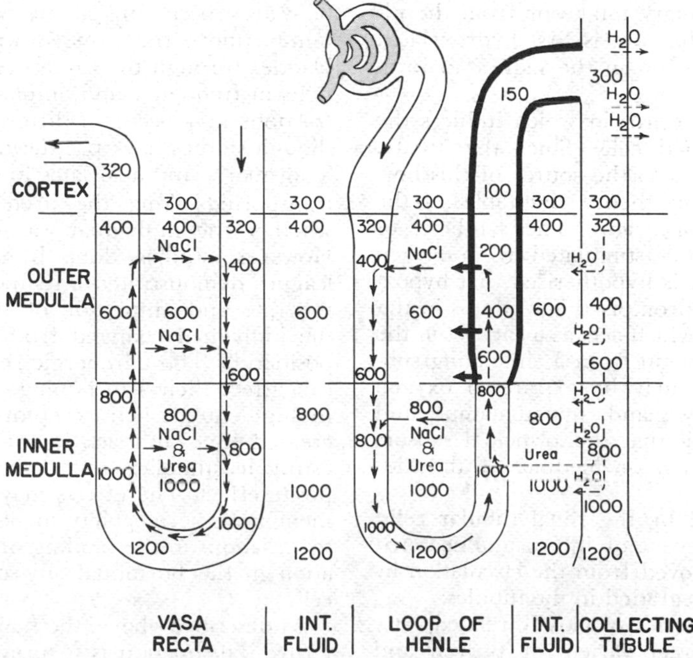

Figure 40–7. The "counter-current" mechanisms for concentrating the urine. (Values are in milliosmols.) (From Guyton, A.: *Textbook of Medical Physiology.* Philadelphia: W. B. Saunders Co., 1976.)

to angiotensin II, which is a powerful vasoconstrictor and exerts its effects on the smooth muscle of the arteriolar walls. This increases the peripheral resistance and, thus, the blood pressure, causing a drop in renin secretion in the kidney. Aldosterone production may be stimulated by angiotensin I, and it also helps raise the blood pressure by facilitating the reabsorption of sodium and water from the distal tubule, resulting in increased blood volume.[81]

There has been an enzyme found in urine called *kallikrein* which catalyzes the formation of vasodilator hormones. It appears that this urinary kallikrein may be derived in the kidney and thus it is different from plasma kallikrein. There is still much controversy regarding its correlation to blood pressure regulation. Levy and associates, in studying normotensive and hypertensive black and white males, found that while all groups had increased urinary kallikrein activity when put on a low sodium diet, black males with hypertension had the smallest gain. They also found a direct correlation between urinary kallikrein activity and renal blood flow. This seems not only to indicate a definite role in blood pressure regulation, but may also account for some of the racial differences in the resistance of the renal vasculature.[181]

Other Metabolic and Endocrine Functions. In addition to the production of renin, the kidney has several other metabolic and endocrine functions. These include the synthesis of 1,25-dihydroxycholecalciferol, biogenesis of erythropoietin, degradation of insulin, synthesis of prostaglandins, and the provision of energy required to perform its own functions.

1,25-dihydroxycholecalciferol (DHCC) is a hormone derived from vitamin D which helps to stimulate absorption of calcium from the intestine and which works with parathyroid hormone to encourage osteoclastic bone resorption. This helps maintain calcium homeostasis in the body. Cholecalciferol, which is obtained through dietary intake or from the ultraviolet radiation of the sun, is first hydroxylated in the liver and then again in the kidney to form DHCC.

Erythropoietin is a glycoprotein which induces the production of red blood cells. Since the 1950's, there has been debate as to the source of this hormone; however, current theory re-establishes the kidney as the point of origin. The synthesis of erythropoietin seems to be stimulated by an oxygen deficit in the kidney. It is hypothesized that hypoxia, whatever its cause, prompts the synthesis in the enzyme, erythrogenin, which acts as a catalyst in the formation of erythropoietin from a circulating substrate. Although there may be extrarenal oxygen sensors in the pituitary gland, hypothalamus, and carotid bodies, it is felt that the principal sensors are located in the cortex or medulla of the kidney.[80, 199]

Insulin is deactivated by the renal tubular cells. Approximately 20 per cent of the insulin secreted by the pancreas is removed from the circulation by the kidneys and then degraded in the tubules.

Prostaglandins are a series of closely related fatty acids which have a great variety of proven and hypothesized physiologic actions. They are formed in most, if not all, organs of the body. Further discussion of prostaglandins and their actions is found in Unit XXII. In the kidney, they are synthesized in the collecting tubules and medullary interstitial cells. They are then removed from the kidney by the renal vein and in the urine. They may play a role in the autoregulation mechanism in the kidney and may function as antihypertensive hormones. However, there is still much work to be done in the identification of specific functions of prostaglandins in the kidney.

The active transport system of the kidney requires the generation of significant amounts of energy with which to carry out this function. The *provision of this energy* is probably the major metabolic activity of the kidney. Because of the primary usage of energy being the active transport of sodium, there is a close correlation among the sodium reabsorption rate, renal blood flow, and gomerular filtration rate, and the rate of renal oxygen consumption. The kidneys extract relatively little oxygen from the renal blood flow, and this rate remains stable even in states of low blood flow.[199]

Movement of Urine Through the Kidney. As the above functions are carried out, the forming urine moves through each nephron. It travels through the collecting ducts toward the apex of the pyramids, where it flows through the openings in the papillae into the renal pelvis. As the urine enters and distends the pelvis, the muscle wall contracts, propelling the urine across the ureteropelvic junction into the ureter. This movement of urine into the ureter is a relatively constant process, since the maximum safe capacity of the adult renal pelvis is 3 to 5 ml. Amounts above this level cause renal tissue damage due to pressure.

Ureter

The chief purpose of the ureter is to transport urine from the renal pelvis to the bladder. Peristaltic waves occurring about one to five times per minute move the urine down the ureter into the bladder through the ureterovesical junctions. Variations in frequency and amplitude of peristaltic contractions may occur in different body positions, although studies have produced contradictory results. Thornberry and associates found that the urine was transported along the ureters at the same rate whether the individual was inverted or supine.[308] However, studies done by MacKinnon and colleagues demonstrated a temporary increase in both the rate and amplitude of peristaltic waves when the individual changed from the supine to prone position.[190] The adrenergic receptors in the ureters can affect their functioning. Progesterone appears to augment the beta receptors, which produces decreased tone and activity of the ureters, whereas estrogens stimulate alpha receptors, causing the opposite effect. The effects may be due to changes in membrane permeability to potassium and chloride, to variations in the binding of calcium, and to alteration in the hormonal environment of the muscle cells.[43]

As described above, the main function of the ureterovesical junction is to prevent backflow of urine to the kidney during voiding or when the bladder becomes overdistended. Intactness of this valve is essential to prevent pressure damage to the renal tissue. In addition to its anatomic placement, the valve works because of the lack of smooth muscle in its wall just proximal to its entry into the bladder. Thus, the usual intravesical pressure tends to keep it collapsed except when urine is spurting through it. During the act of micturition, the ureter passing though the muscle layers is squeezed shut.

Bladder

The bladder acts as a storage vessel for the urine received from the ureters until such time as it is to be passed from the body. The urine enters in propulsive waves filling the bladder. There is a slight increase in the intravesical pressure for approximately the first 25 ml. accumulation. Then the pressure stays relatively stable until about 400 to 500 ml. have collected. The accommodation occurs because of the slow stretching of the detrusor muscle. The pressure curve rises markedly as the bladder fills with more than 500 ml. and soars as the act of micturition is initiated. Electromyographic tracings demonstrate that electric activity of the detrusor muscle increases during the filling process. In controlled studies, when filling of the bladder was stopped before distention, the electrical impulses slowed; this provides evidence of detrusor accommodation. Upon full distention of the bladder, electrical activity remains high and increases further when voiding is initiated. After micturition, the electrical impulses decrease rapidly.[171]

Micturition, also called *urination* and *voiding*, is the act of emptying the bladder. As the bladder fills and the muscle fibers expand, stretch receptors in the bladder wall are stimulated. The first urge to void is felt at about 150 ml. and a marked feeling of fullness usually occurs around 400 ml., although this level can be increased or decreased through habit patterns. Impulses are sent to the sacral portion of the spinal cord where the micturition reflex is initiated, causing the bladder to contract and the urethral sphincters to open. As the bladder musculature contracts, the pressure is transmitted to the urine, forcing it out through the urethra. The bladder muscle fibers extend longitudinally down the urethra and, as they contract, they shorten the urethra and pull the bladder down toward a point of fixation at the distal portion of the pubis. Unless the reflex is mediated at this point, urination will occur immediately.

However, the impulses initiating the micturition reflex are also sent to the cerebral cortex. After a period of successful toilet training in early childhood, the external sphincter is usually under voluntary control. If the person feels that environmental conditions are not right for urination, the external sphincter countracts, stopping the flow of urine. The micturition reflex can also be intiated by the cerebral cortex when necessary.

One side effect of urination, affecting primarily healthy young to middle-aged men, is *micturition syncope*. Although it occurs very infrequently, its results are dangerous for the individual. After arising from bed in the early morning or evening to void, the person becomes light-headed and faints during or immediately after urination. Recovery is usually rapid and complete. Although the etiology of this episode is unclear, it is thought to be the result of vagal stimulation during bladder contraction. This alters cardiac output. Other theories include nocturnally increased vagal tone, bladder neck obstruction, postural hypotension, Valsalva's maneuver, autonomic imbalance, and a form of epilepsy.[271]

Urethra and Meatus

The urethra is the only normal passageway for the urine to leave the body. It has been demonstrated that detrusor contraction during micturition is preceded by about 5 seconds by a significant fall of pressure within the urethra. This facilitates movement of urine from the bladder with its higher pressure into the urethra. The contraction phase of voiding is the result of interruption of the sympathetic effect.

As mentioned above, the urethra ends at the urethral meatus, which is usually under voluntary control in the adult. When voiding is not appropriate, the meatus contracts, holding back the flow of urine until the reflex stimulation ceases.

Following the act of micturition, the female urethra empties by gravity. The male urethra is emptied of remaining urine through drainage by several contractions of the bulbocavernous muscle.

Supplementary Muscle Action During Micturition. In addition to contraction of the detrusor muscle and relaxation of the sphincters, voluntary contraction of the abdominal muscles facilitates micturition by increasing pressure on the bladder wall. During urination, the perineal muscles must be relaxed. Conversely, contraction of the perineal muscles assists the external sphincter to resist the outflow of urine.

EFFECTS OF AGING ON URINARY FUNCTION

As part of the natural aging process, the kidney becomes smaller. The cause of this loss of tissue, which occurs especially in the renal cortex, is uncertain; it may be focal as the result of scarring or diffuse due to renal blood vessel changes.[114]

Partly because of this loss of functioning nephrons and partly because of generalized circulatory changes, renal function decreases with advancing age. Affected are the glomerular filtration rate, tubular reabsorption, and ability to concentrate the urine. All normal regulatory and metabolic functions of the kidney become less efficient, and there is little or no reserve with which to respond to periods of increased stress.[233, 234]

The aging process also affects the act of micturition. The bladder becomes funnel-shaped due to alterations in the supporting connective tissue and weakening of pelvic floor muscles. Irritability of the bladder wall increases, causing more urgency to the normal desire to void. Finally, impairment of the detrusor's ability to elongate results in decreased bladder capacity. Because of these changes, the elderly person has problems with incontinence, frequency, retention, and dysuria.[242]

CHAPTER 41

ASSESSMENT OF URINARY SYSTEM FUNCTION

Adequate assessment is essential to accurate diagnosis of urinary system problems. The sources of information for this data base include history and physical examination and a variety of specific studies using the laboratory, x-ray, radioisotopes, ultrasound, pressure profiles, endoscopy, and biopsy. The extent of testing needed is determined by information previously obtained.

For most people in the American culture, urinary elimination is a private thing. The embarrassment caused by having to discuss the topic with others has a great impact on the assessment process. Many people are so reluctant to discuss problems involving the urinary tract that they may delay seeking medical assistance until the disorder is quite advanced. When they do come for help, their feelings of humiliation may continue to interfere with the gathering of important information.

While not everyone is uncomfortable talking about their urinary system, several of the tests involved in the assessment process can be rather distressing. Providing a urine specimen may be quite embarrassing, especially if the patient has to handle it, such as when carrying the container down the hall or bringing it from home. Some of the studies even require that the patient urinate in front of a camera or with people watching. What this all means is that the nurse and other health professionals involved in the data collection process must be very empathetic with the patient. Realizing the patient's discomfort, they should take measures to provide as much privacy as possible. Well-developed communication skills will be necessary to obtain complete and accurate information from the patient. Allowing the patient to express anxiety and reassuring the patient that you will do whatever is possible to ease any embarrassment will help communicate to the patient your understanding and caring. But, above all, you must be very alert to what the patient is communicating, both verbally and nonverbally, because subtle clues may be crucial to the final decision about the patient's problem.

HISTORY

As with other systems, the history-taking is probably the most important part of the assessment process. Most problems are usually discovered during this process. Using carefully organized questions and clarifying answers given by the patient, the nurse will be able to learn the following pieces of information needed to make an accurate diagnosis and plan the appropriate intervention.

Physical Factors

Usual patterns of micturition. Frequency? Times of day and night? Behaviors used to stimulate urination?

Change in usual pattern resulting from current illness or stress.

Presence of *artificial orifice.* If present, what kind? For how long? Why was it done? How is it usually managed? Is it now or has it ever caused problems?

Difficulty starting and maintaining stream.

Does patient feel like the bladder is being emptied?

Feeling of *urgency.*

Anything *unusual* noticed about the *urine.*

Incontinence. Amount? Frequency? Constant dribbling? Occurs with what kind of stress? Is patient aware of having been incontinent? Duration of the problem? Is it getting worse? What does patient normally do about it?

Pain associated with the urinary tract. Location? Kind? Severity? Duration? Is it getting better or worse? What seems to bring it on? What relieves it? Painful urination (dysuria)? If dysuria present, when during act of micturition does it occur? (See description of pain below.)

History of any *disease process, surgical procedure, or trauma* affecting the urinary tract. When did it occur? What was its effect? How was it treated? What was the result of the treatment?

Relevant medications, e.g., diuretics, antibiotics, narcotics, cholinergics, nephrotoxins, phenazopyridine, rifampin.

Allergies.

Activity level. Amount and kind of activity? What assistance with mobility does patient need? Does patient use toilet, commode, or bedpan?

Fluid status. Amount and kind of fluid intake? Times during day? Unusual losses, e.g., diarrhea, heavy perspiration? Weight gain/loss pattern?
Bleeding tendencies.
Pruritus.
Numbness or tingling of extremities.
Gastrointestinal symptoms. Anorexia? Nausea or vomiting? Diarrhea?

Much of the information sought is primarily related to the urinary tract, but it is also necessary to involve other systems when they have direct impact on or are affected by urinary function. For instance, data about the patient's level of activity will provide a gross estimate of the tone of the musculature needed to achieve or inhibit micturition. It will also help you approximately plan the facilities needed for meeting the patient's elimination needs. Although they are not definitive in and of themselves, gastrointestinal symptoms, bleeding, itching, tingling, and numbness may be part of the picture of renal disease. Knowledge about the patient's allergies can be an important factor in decisions about diagnostic tests ordered and medications used to treat identified disorders.

Pain. Careful description of the patient's pain may help pinpoint the source of the problem. *Kidney* pain, which is usually caused by sudden distention of the renal capsule, is felt as a dull, constant ache in the *costovertebral angle* just lateral to the sacrospinalis muscle below the twelfth rib; this pain often spreads along the subcostal area to the umbilicus. Radiculitis often mimics renal pain, so it is important to differentiate between the two. Radicular pain is a hyperesthesia of the skin area supplied by the irritated peripheral nerve which can be stimulated by pinching both the skin and fat of the abdominal and flank regions. Exerting pressure over the costovertebral angle with the thumb may elicit local tenderness of the involved peripheral nerve at its point of emergence, while a gentle pounding over the angle may be necessary to elicit renal pain, indicating a deeper, more visceral sensation. Figure 41–1 illustrates percussion over the costovertebral angle (Murphy's percussion). *Ureteral* pain is manifested as back pain resulting from capsular distention and a colicky pain, produced by spasm of the renal pelvis and ureteral muscle, which radiates from the costovertebral angle down across the abdomen to the genital area. In males, pain originating in the upper ureter is usually felt in the ipsilateral (same side) testicle, while lower ureteral pain is referred to the scrotal wall. Females describe ureteral pain in the ipsilateral labium. The most common *bladder* discomfort arises from overdistention and is felt in the suprapubic area. Bladder infection causes a burning pain in the distal urethra for females or prostatic urethra in males during micturition.[286] *Urethral* pain is usually felt along the course of the urethra or at the meatus.

Determining precisely when, during the act of micturition, burning occurs will help differentiate between bladder and urethral origins. Burning at the beginning of urination, as the bladder contracts the inflamed tissue, indicates urethritis. A bladder infection is suspected when the burning occurs during and after the voiding process.

Renointestinal Reflexes. Renointestinal reflexes may cause gastrointestinal and renal symptoms to occur simultanteously. Afferent stimuli originating in the renal capsule or pelvic musculature may cause pylorospasm or other changes of the smooth muscle of the enteric tract and adnexa. In addition, anatomic proximity of the kidneys with the gastrointestinal structures may mean that renal disorders are mimicked by intestinal disturbances. The right kidney lies close to the hepatic flexure of the colon, duodenum, head of the pancreas, common bile duct, liver, and gallbladder, while the left kidney is bordered by the splenic flexure of the colon, stomach, pancreas, and spleen. This partially explains why patients experience nausea and vomiting, anorexia, diarrhea, and abdominal discomfort concomitantly with their urinary tract symptoms. Renal inflammation may also produce signs of peritoneal irritation.[286]

*Psychosocial Factors**

Psychologic. During the history-taking process described above, and continuing

*See also Chapter 14.

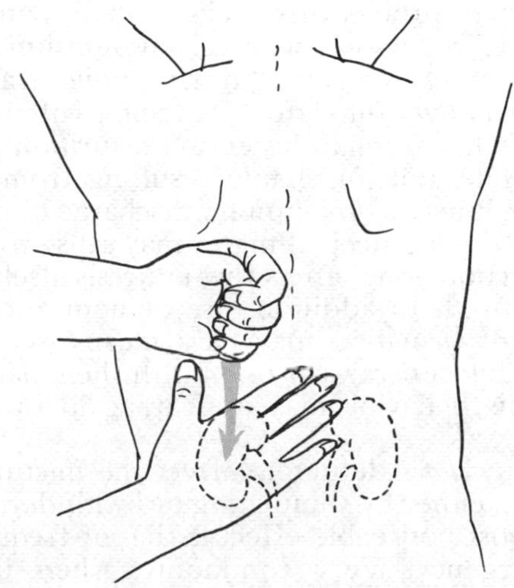

Figure 41–1. Percussion over the costovertebral angle (CVA) is done to evaluate renal pain.

through the rest of the examination, it is also important to be assessing the psychologic elements of the patient. The psyche can have great influence on the functioning of the urinary system, as well as being markedly affected by performance of the system. One of these influences is the *power of suggestion.* The micturition control center is connected to the various sensory portions of the brain, allowing micturition to be initiated by any number of auditory, visual, or somesthetic stimuli. The nurse frequently uses this factor to help patients who are having difficulty voiding, e.g., running water in the sink. In doing this, the nurse must be careful, because the activity may have unexpected results, since anyone within hearing distance may be likewise stimulated. Just the mere act of thinking about voiding may be enough to stimulate the reflex, which can be helpful or bothersome depending on where you are—in your sailboat in the middle of a lake, on a bus caught on the freeway, or lying on an x-ray table waiting for the films to be developed.

Past experiences produce varying effects on the process of voiding. As mentioned before, the cultural teachings of most people have led them to consider the act of micturition as a private thing. American society supports this by providing locks on bathroom doors, separate public restrooms for men and women, etc. This frame of reference may cause inhibition of the micturition reflex if the person is in an environment where the element of privacy is missing. Common situations include a moderately busy restroom (a problem almost exclusively for women), on a commode behind the curtain in a multi-bed room, or in the bathroom with the nurse standing just outside the door waiting. Experiences linked with toilet-training during childhood can have long-lasting effects. A person's negative or positive attitudes toward bladder elimination can sometimes be traced back to this developmental period. Rewards or reinforcement for positive behavior tend to result in continued problem-free elimination patterns. However, a person who received punishment as the primary motivator during toilet-training may carry over into adult life feelings of guilt or anxiety that are manifested in micturition problems. The guilt or shame resulting from prolonged enuresis (involuntary discharge of urine, usually during sleep at night) may cause voiding dysfunction long after the enuresis itself has been cured. In addition, use or nonuse of the toilet for urination may be a means by which some children reward or punish their parents, and this behavior may appear again in adult life.

Anxiety states definitely affect the micturition pattern, either by stimulating or by hindering it. The most noticeable effect is that of frequency and urgency. Very commonly, when facing stressful situations, people have a strong urge to void, even though they may have urinated just moments before. Conversely, anxiety characterized by general muscle tension can interfere with urination, since relaxation of the perineal muscles is essential to completing the act of micturition. Anxiety may also intensify the signs and symptoms of urinary tract disorders; fear of the unknown and wondering what the outcome will be, for instance, make the pain seem worse, and health professionals believe that such things as bleeding, degenerative processes, and healing can be greatly affected by the patient's emotional state. In terms of the fear of pain, it is certainly true that once a person has moderate to severe burning pain on urination, he or she will be most reluctant to repeat that experience again, thus inhibiting the act of micturition.

Incontinence (involuntary loss of urine from the bladder) may be the result of severe depression or "giving up." The person no longer feels that it is worth the energy needed to maintain continence. It is postulated that this is a common cause of incontinence in the elderly. The progression of incontinence also seems to be a vicious cycle: the patient does not care any more and so is incontinent; the nursing staff and those who live with the patient "accept" the condition by protecting the patient's clothing and bed linen and just passively cleaning up when the patient becomes wet, thus communicating, "I do not really care either." The patient thinks, "I must be even more worthless than I thought, since no one cares" and is incontinent even more, and on and on.

On the other hand, the *functioning, or malfunctioning, of the urinary system often has tremendous consequences for the patient's psyche.* The entire gamut of emotions and defense mechanisms may be seen. Occurrence of the very common emotion of embarrassment was described above. Feelings of joy and happiness may occur when a suspected diagnosis is ruled out or when an existing problem is corrected, allowing the patient to return to the desired life style. Conversely, developing problems which interfere with a person's life style may result in anxiety, depression, and/or anger. Many urinary disorders necessitate a change in body image, ranging from a feeling that "my body is not as strong and invincible as I though it was" to extreme anatomic changes by which the urine leaves the body through an opening "abnormally" created in the abdominal wall or in which no urine is produced at all and a machine must perform this vital cleansing function. The adaptation process following the serious disruption of body image leads the patient and significant others through denial, anger, depression, and hopefully to acceptance and internalization of a new self-concept. During this time, the patient and significant others will experience conflicts involving dependence/independence and changes in life-role responsibilities and in interpersonal relationships. The patient may regress to previous coping behaviors, which further frustrate others.

Although closely allied with body image, the fear of death is a real concern of patients with urinary tract problems. It is well-known that a functioning renal system is essential to the continuation of life. Whether the problem is large or small, there is always the reality that it could progress to a terminal stage. Some patients may be able to discuss this fear openly, while others may not even be able to admit such a possibility. Many times this fear is suggested by behaviors such as "acting out," denial, and social withdrawal.

The nurse can learn much information about the state of the patient's psyche by carefully listening to the patient's conversation and observing the patient's behavior pattern. Cues may be given indirectly through the way the patient answers questions and initiates conversation, subtlely through camouflaged statements, or directly — he or she may come right out and say "I'm afraid of dying." Depending on the amount of trust developed in the relationship, the nurse may also successfully employ the direct route; the patient may be asked outrightly, "Are you afraid your husband might not love you any more?" or "How will you feel if this transplant does not work?" Whatever communication techniques are used, it is crucial that the nurse consciously assess the patient's emotional state, since no one else on the health team may be assisting the patient and significant others in this realm.

Social. As mentioned above, urinary problems may cause a change in life style. In order to predict the kind and extent of changes that may or should occur, it is necessary to know the patient's current status. Information that will complete this section of the data base includes:

Living conditions. House or apartment, etc.? Location? Proximity to supporting services, e.g., groceries, transportation, medical facilities? Adequacy of environment for patient's needs?

Support system. Spouse? Children? Parents? Siblings? Friends? Interrelationships? Their willingness and ability to help if needed? Appropriate community agencies?

Financial status. Adequate income or resources to meet patient's need? Medical insurance?

Work. Kind of work? Place of work? Hours of work? What happens if patient is away from job?

Other life responsibilities, e.g., scout troop leader, volunteer firefighter, chairperson for upcoming social event.

Hobbies.

Mental. Finally, the nurse needs to assess the patient's mental status in order to plan appropriately for safety and learning needs. Relevant information encompasses:

State of orientation.

Level of *knowledge* about urinary function and problems involved.

Ability to *learn.* Memory? Attention span? Communication skills? Expressed interest?

Ability to follow directions

PHYSICAL EXAMINATION

The physical examination is guided by the information obtained during the history-taking process. Most of the data needed comes directly from examination of the organs of the urinary system; however, to complete this portion of the data base, it is also necessary to consider portions of other systems.

Urinary Tract Organs

Kidneys. Inspect for masses in the upper abdomen and flank areas. Because of the location of the kidneys, normally only the lower pole of the right kidney can be felt on deep palpation. With the patient lying supine on a hard surface, deep palpation is accomplished in the following manner: For the right kidney, stand on the right side of the patient, place your right hand on the abdomen between the rib cage and the iliac crest, and position your left hand posteriorly in the costovertebral angle. Support the area from below with the left hand and have the patient take a deep breath. As the patient inhales, the right hand should compress the tissues in deep palpation. Instruct the patient to exhale and then hold the breath. Slowly release the pressure with the right hand; the pole may be felt at this time. Instruct the patient to breathe normally, and remove your hands. The left kidney may be palpated in the same manner. If you stand at the patient's left side while examining the left kidney, reverse your hand positions so that the right hand is placed posteriorly and the left anteriorly. Because this kidney is located higher up in the rib cage, it is not normally felt.

Depending on the size of the patient and the skill of the examiner, it may be possible to outline the kidneys both anteriorly and posteriorly by percussion. This technique is particularly helpful when pain and muscle spasm prevent proper palpation. Costovertebral angle tenderness may be assessed by placing the left hand over the area and striking it with the fist. Ordinarily this percussion would produce a dull sound and no discomfort.

Auscultation should be done in the costovertebral angle and upper abdominal quadrants. A systolic bruit is often associated with stenosis or aneurysm of the renal artery.[286]

Bladder. As the bladder distends, it rises out of the pelvic cavity above the symphysis pubis. In a very thin person or one with a very distended bladder, it may be visible on inspection. It may also be palpable. The adult bladder can be percussed if it has at least 150 ml. of fluid in it. After the initial assessment, have the patient empty the bladder and then palpate and percuss it again to distinguish the bladder from a possible mass.

Urethra. Primarily, examination of the urethra involves inspecting the external meatus and the perineal area for signs of discharge, abnormal tissue growth, cleanliness, and anatomic integrity. Aberrant location of the meatus should be noted. The penis may be palpated for masses along the distal portion of the male urethra and the perineal area can be palpated for tenderness.

The size and patency of the meatus and the urethra may be evaluated by passing instruments of varying diameters through the urethra. Different sizes of rubber or plastic catheters may be used or special urologic implements may be preferred. A *bougie* is a rod with an olive-shaped tip on one end and an acorn-shaped tip on the other. These rods range in size from 8 to 32 Fr.; and the acorn tip is particularly useful in locating strictures, since the flared part of the acorn gets hooked on the constriction as the bougie is pulled out. A *sound* is a smooth, cylindrical rod with a rounded tip. Its size range includes the even sizes from 8 to 32 Fr. Figure 41–2 illustrates examples of bougies and sounds. These instruments, which may also be used to dilate the meatus and urethra, are passed under aseptic conditions beginning with a small size and increasing the diameter until the largest caliber that can be easily inserted is found. Strictures, which will be discussed in Chapter 42, may cause the insertion process to be more difficult.

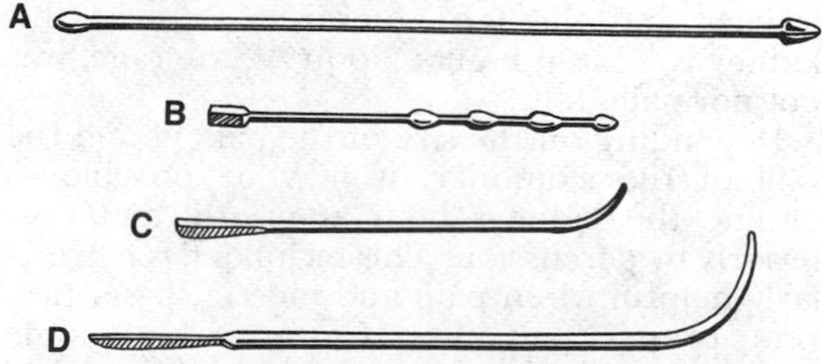

Figure 41–2. Bougie and sounds used to calibrate urethral diameter: *A* and *B*, bougies. *C*, female sound; *D*, male sound. (Adapted from Winter, C., and A. Morel: *Nursing Care of Patients With Urologic Diseases.* St. Louis: C. V. Mosby Co., 1977.)

Alternative Urinary Outlets. If the patient has had a urinary diversion procedure, such as an ileal conduit, he or she will have an opening created in the abdominal wall. This stoma should be inspected and its location, size, shape, color, intactness, and odor noted. The quality and quantity of drainage should be observed. In addition, the condition of the peristomal skin should be evaluated for color, cleanliness, intactness, and absence of lesions, such as maceration and irritation. Observation of the cleanliness and appropriateness of the urine collection system will provide clues to possible patient-teaching needs. Finally, patients' responses during this part of the examination may also indicate their stage of acceptance of the stoma and their altered urinary function.

The patient may have catheters that are responsible for the partial or complete removal of urine from the body. These drainage catheters may be inserted into the bladder, ureters, or kidneys and may come out of the body through either the urethra or the abdominal or flank wall. In the presence of these catheters, the examiner should inspect them for patency, location, and cleanliness. The tubing can be palpated for crystallization by rolling it between the fingers, feeling for a "gravelly" sensation. The tissues around the catheter as it enters the body should be observed for cleanliness and the absence of lesions such as inflammation and ulceration.

Related Body Systems

Selected information from other body systems is crucial to the correct identification of urinary tract problems and the ensuing plan of intervention. As described before, the urinary system, with its excretory and regulatory functions, is closely allied with these other systems, both anatomically and physiologically. For each of these systems, a more complete assessment is described in the appropriate unit in this book.

Fluid Status. An accurate *intake and output measurement* is important to determine the balance in the patient's fluid status; disproportionate amounts of either one may lead to volume excess or depletion. When interpreting these figures, consideration must be given to other gains and losses, such as an unusual intake of highly liquid foods, diarrhea, fever, and humid climate. Keeping track of the patient's intake and output helps identify the presence of important signs of abnormal kidney function: oliguria, anuria, and polyuria. The normal adult on a regular diet and taking in about 1200 ml. of measurable fluids in a day is expected to excrete

1200 to 1500 ml. of urine in a 24-hour period. *Oliguria* is a urine volume significantly below this amount, usually less than 400 ml. per 24 hours, while *anuria* means the absence of urine production. These two conditions may indicate shock, poisoning, or any other process that would interfere with urine formation in the kidney. Anuria would, of course, be a normal finding in patients who had had bilateral nephrectomies (removal of the kidneys). *Polyuria* implies significantly larger than normal amounts of urine output and could be caused by chronic renal failure, diabetes mellitus, diabetes insipidus, diuretic administration, etc. In the presence of polyuria, it is important to discriminate between water diuresis and solute diuresis; this is done on the basis of urinary specific gravity, urinary osmolarity, and serum sodium values, which are discussed below. *Water diuresis* is designated by a low urinary specific gravity, low urinary osmolarity, and a normal or elevated serum sodium and indicates either a lack of ADH, such as after trauma to the posterior pituitary gland, or unresponsiveness of the renal tubules, such as may occur with hypokalemia or hydronephrosis. *Solute diuresis* is the result of impaired tubular absorption of a particular solute, as may accompany diabetes mellitus or relief of an acute bladder obstruction. It is recognized by a high urinary specific gravity, elevated urinary osmolarity, and a normal or low serum sodium level.[22]

Body *weight* is a good indicator of fluid gains and losses when it is carefully measured on a daily basis and compared to previous findings. Dry *mucous membranes* may signal volume depletion, while the presence of *edema* may be a sign of volume excess. In assessing edema, it is important to determine its progression or recession; measuring the girth of the edematous parts on a daily basis provides an accurate, objective means to record and communicate this information. Discussion of a complete fluid status assessment is found in Chapter 12.

Neurologic Status. Renal dysfunction may interfere with normal activity within the nervous system, as when a build-up of calcium causes tetany or as the toxins accumulate in chronic renal failure. Conversely, the urinary tract depends on an intact nervous system in order to carry out its main function of waste removal. Any abnormality in nervous stimulation to the urinary organs or their surrounding tissue interferes with the propulsion and expulsion of urine. In addition to assessment of gross nervous function, e.g., the ability to walk and maintain balance, the examiner may test the intactness of innervation specific to urinary tract function. Since the anal and urinary sphincters are supplied by branches of the same nerve, intactness of one may indicate a similar level of functioning of the other. Sensation of the perianal skin can be tested by stroking it. Anal sphincter tone can initially be evaluated by inserting a gloved, lubricated finger into it, noticing the amount of resistance felt. While the finger remains in the rectum, the bulbocavernous reflex can be tested; squeezing the glans penis or clitoris or jerking on an indwelling bladder catheter causes contraction of the external anal sphincter and bulbocavernous muscle when this reflex is intact, indicating an unimpaired sacral 2 to 4 arc. Other tests evaluating relevant neurologic activity are described later in this chapter.

Integumentary Status. The *color* of the skin can be very indicative of renal dysfunction. For instance, pallor may result from erythropoietin-deficiency anemia, or deposits of a carotene-like substance, caused by failure of renal excretion, may give the skin a yellow-gray cast. *Dry skin* may be a sign of chronic renal failure and may also indicate volume depletion. *Bruises* or *petechiae* may represent bleeding tendencies. *Crystal deposits* on the skin (found primarily in areas of concentrated perspiraton) is a secondary sign of severe, prolonged renal failure.

Musculoskeletal Status. General body tone can be demonstrated by observing the patient walk and otherwise move around during the examination. Ability to do this will provide a gross impression of the patient's muscle tone and will enable the examiner to come to some conclusion about the patient's physical ability to handle urinary elimination needs. Specific muscle groups involved in the act of micturition are the perineal and abdominal muscles. The strength of these can be assessed by having the patient consciously contract or tighten the perineal and abdominal muscles. The changes in tautness can be seen and palpated. The ability of the patient to purposely interrupt the flow of urine midstream also indicates adequate perineal musculature.

Cardiovascular Status. Monitoring of the cardiovascular system can identify signs of fluid and electrolyte imbalances. Most specific to the urinary tract is *blood pressure* measurement. Hypertension is a finding in many renal diseases and may be the result of fluid volume overload or of disturbance of the renin-angiotensin system. Increasing hypotension will eventually lead to renal shutdown, a condition which can become irreversible. Both of these findings call for medical intervention and, while serial readings are most helpful, single readings at the far ends of the gauge may indicate the need for immediate action.

Respiratory Status. The quality of respirations can be indicative of the patient's fluid and acid-base balances. Further discussion of respiratory assessment can be found in Chapter

52. In addition, during renal failure, the breath may have an odor of urine resulting from the build-up of toxins in the blood stream.

Other Systems. A vaginal and rectal examination is routinely done in the assessment of urinary problems. Inspection and palpation of these two orifices will help to identify fistulas, masses, prolapses, and diverticula.

DIAGNOSTIC TESTS

There is a large scope of diagnostic tests available to evaluate the status of the urinary system. These include laboratory tests, x-ray, ultrasound, radioisotopes, pressure profiles, endoscopy, and surgical exploration. The decision about which procedures to employ is made on the basis of the history and physical examination and the results of previous studies.

The nurse's role during this testing phase is several-fold: Preparation of the patient — both physically and psychologically — requires that the nurses be knowledgeable about the purpose of the test, what it entails, and what will be expected of the patient. Patient teaching can then include these items. The patient should also be given the opportunity to express concerns and questions. The nurse may be directly involved in the collection and testing of specimens, and assistance during the procedure may be needed by the examiner and the patient. Specific studies require particular post-test care, such as watching for hemorrhage after a kidney biopsy. Finally, the nurse must understand the test results so that this information can be explained to the patient and so that the findings can be appropriately utilized in the patient's care plan.

Laboratory Tests

Collection of Specimens. The accurate outcome of any laboratory test depends on the collection of the right kind of specimen in the proper manner in the right container at the right time. Once the specimen has been collected, it must be stored properly until the correct testing procedure is done on it and the findings are accurately interpreted. The nurse and other people — patient, people in the patient's household, laboratory personnel — will share this responsibility.

The types of urine specimens include random, clean-catch (midstream), catheter, 24-hour, and double-voided. A *random* specimen is one that can be collected at any time, although an early morning specimen gives more definitive results for some values. Usually no special preparation of the patient is needed, although the female patient may be asked to wash the perineal area to clean away any collected debris. The specimen is then collected in any clean container. This type of specimen cannot be used for culture and sensitivity, since the lack of specific cleaning and the use of an unsterile container contaminate the specimen.

A *clean-catch,* or *midstream,* specimen is collected if the urine is to be cultured. The goal of this procedure is to reduce as much as possible the contamination of the specimen by external organisms. Meticulous cleansing of the penis or perineal area is done with either soap and water, benzalkonium chloride, or iodine preparations, but studies have shown that iodine is the most effective agent.[50, 218] It is important that the agent be completely removed after cleansing, since contamination of the specimen with the agent may sterilize the urine, possibly resulting in a false negative. After the cleansing process, the patient begins to void into the bedpan, commode, or toilet (to wash out the distal urethra), stops the stream of urine while a sterile container is appropriately positioned, and then continues voiding into the container until enough urine has been obtained. The container is then removed and the patient finishes voiding into the original receptacle.

A *catheterized* specimen may be used for culture, although the procedure is not commonly used because of the risk of introducing organisms during the catheterizing procedure. A straight or indwelling catheter is inserted under aseptic conditions and the urine is allowed to flow directly from the end of the catheter into a sterile specimen container.

A specimen may also be collected from an indwelling catheter already in place. Urine can be obtained from the collection bag for tests that would use a random sample. However, this procedure is controversial. It cannot be used for culture or sensitivity or when testing for the presence of glucose and ketones when insulin administration will result from the findings. Most prefer to get a fresh specimen from the catheter itself. Because of the high risk of introducing pathogens whenever the urinary drainage system is opened, it is best to obtain the specimen from the catheter with a needle and syringe. Using aseptic technique, a small gauge (21 to 25) needle is inserted into the catheter distal to the sleeve leading to the balloon. The puncture of the catheter should be done at an angle to allow resealing by the catheter after the needle is withdrawn. Also, slant the needle toward the drainage tubing to avoid entering the balloon lumen.

A special procedure must be used when obtaining a urine for culture from a person with an *ileal conduit,* a type of urinary diversion created from segments of the ileum or sigmoid colon. It is virtually impossible to insert a catheter directly into the conduit without contaminating it with organisms from the stoma or the first few centimeters of the ileum. After cleansing the stomal area with soap and water and antiseptic and rinsing it with sterile water, change sterile gloves and cut a No. 18 Fr. rubber whistle-tip catheter to about 10 cm. length. Then cut a pediatric feeding tube to approximately 30 cm. from the connector end. Lubricate the rubber catheter and insert it into the stoma about 5 cm., gently rotating it if resistance is felt. Holding the outer catheter in place, thread the feeding tube through it for about 7.5 cm. Put the connector end of the inner tube into a test tube or specimen container and allow the urine to flow by gravity. If there is no urine flow within several minutes, have the patient move around or apply gentle suction on the catheter with a 5 cc. syringe. When the specimen has been collected, remove both catheters and replace the collection bag.[338]

A *24-hour* specimen is usually collected in one large container. Some of the specimens may need to have a chemical preservative in the container and/or be refrigerated during the collection period. When the specimen collection is begun, the patient voids and this specimen is discarded. All urine voided in the next 24 hours is placed in the container. Twenty-four hours from the time of the first voiding, the patient is instructed to void and this urine is added to the specimen.

One of the major needs during this collection process is careful communication among all persons involved; if any single urine specimen is inadvertently discarded, the entire procedure must be begun again.

A *double-voided* specimen is usually needed when the urine is being tested for glucose and ketones. This is necessary to assure that the urine being tested reflects the current status of these two substances being filtered from the blood. The first voided specimen may or may not be tested. In some agencies, this urine is tested and, if found to be negative, no further specimen is obtained; in other agencies, it is tested in case a second specimen cannot be obtained. If a second specimen is needed, the patient is instructed to urinate again 20 to 30 minutes after the first voiding.

Examination of the Urine. The urine can be examined by direct visualization, microscopically, and by performing a variety of tests on it in order to determine the presence of substances in the urine. The results of these examinations may indicate pathology in the urinary tract as well as in other parts of the body.

A *routine urinalysis* is usually done on a single, random specimen, although a midstream or catheterized specimen may be used. Table 41–1 summarizes the usual observations made during this testing procedure and the normal values.

The *color* of the urine normally ranges from pale yellow to deep amber, depending on its concentration. Some color changes occur because of medications or food ingested, while other colors indicate pathology. Foods often causing red urine include blackberries, rhubarb, beets, and red dyes. Ingestion of large amounts of carotene causes a bright yellow urine. Common medications producing urinary color changes include the following:

anthraquinone laxatives	reddish brown in acid urine; red in alkaline urine
chloroquine	rusty yellow
chlorzoxazone	orange or purple-red
methylene blue	green
phenazopyridine	orange-brown, orange-red or red
phenolphthalein	pink-red in alkaline urine
rifampin	bright orange-red

It has been shown that aniline, a substance contained in some hair dyes, is absorbed through the scalp and excreted by the kidneys and may make the urine dark.[198]

The most common significant color change indicating pathology results from *bleeding in the urinary tract.* Bleeding in the upper tract produces dark red or smoky-grey urine, while bleeding in the lower tract is seen as red urine. Other color changes resulting from pathologic conditions include red-brown or "tea-colored," from the release of myoglobin from severely damaged muscle tissue, dark yellow indicating

TABLE 41–1. NORMAL FINDINGS IN A ROUTINE URINALYSIS

Component	Normal Values
Color	Pale yellow to deep amber
Opacity	Clear
Specific gravity	1.002–1.035
pH	4.5–8
Glucose	Negative
Ketones	Negative
Protein	Negative
Bilirubin	Negative
Red blood cells	None to 3
White blood cells	None to 4
Bacteria	None
Casts	None
Crystals	None

the presence of urobilin or bilirubin, and green produced by *Pseudomonas* organisms.

Freshly voided urine is normally transparent. It becomes cloudy on standing, but this can be reversed with the additon of a few drops of acid. Increases in the *opacity* denoting pathology usually result from the presence of bacteria, crystals, or other foreign material in the urine.

Specific gravity indicates the concentration of the urine and can be used to estimate the patient's general fluid status. Since one of the major functions of the kidney is to maintain fluid balance, usually the more concentrated the urine, the more fluid-depleted the patient. In terms of renal function, this measurement is used primarily to indicate the patient's concentrating and diluting ability. When the kidneys have lost these abilities, the urine no longer reflects physiologic stimuli and the specific gravity becomes fixed at a level equal to that of the plasma, usually 1.010. This occurs with tubular disease or endocrine disease involving ADH insufficiency. Contrast media used during x-ray procedures can produce readings above 1.040. Other substances in the urine, e.g., molecules of glucose and protein, can also cause high values.

Urinary *pH* is usually reflective of the plasma pH, with alkalinization or additional acidification occurring in order to maintain the body's acid-base balance. Alkaline urine is found with metabolic alkalosis, low protein diets that are high in vegetables and citrus fruits; alkalinizing medications such as soda bicarbonate and acetazolamide; and in the presence of ammonia-splitting bacteria. It also indicates renal tubular acidosis in which tubular absorption is impaired. Strongly acid urine results from metabolic acidosis, metabolic alkalosis in potassium deficiency, a high-protein diet, uncontrolled diabetes, and some medications, such as ammonium chloride and mandelic acid.

The appearance of *glucosuria* depends on the plasma glucose level and the renal threshold, which indicates the point of blood sugar level at which the kidney begins to excrete glucose. Glucosuria may normally result from eating a heavy meal or from emotional stress. Intravenous solutions containing glucose may also raise the serum glucose level above the renal threshold. Abnormal findings of glucose in the urine are found with uncontrolled diabetes and other pancreatic disorders and impaired proximal tubular reabsorption.

Urine glucose testing is frequently done in the home, clinic, or hospital unit. Diabetic patients and others in their households routinely perform this test. The most important factor in successful performance of the variety of tests available to determine the presence of glucosuria—copper reduction, e.g., Clinitest, or enzyme glucose oxidase, e.g., Testape, Clinistix, Ketodiastix— is meticulous following of accompanying directions, including use of reference charts with bright colors for comparison. Williams observed 122 nursing personnel at all levels; she found no relation between the accuracy of findings and the educational level of the person performing the test. The major source of errors resulted from failure to follow steps of the procedure and a tendency to be influenced by previous findings.[58] Correct instructions can be found in any fundamental nursing text* and on the package insert included with the testing equipment. In evaluating results of these tests, it is also important to remember that many outside factors can cause false negatives and positives. A partial list of these include ascorbic acid, cancer metabolites, cephalosporins, chloramphenicol, ethanol, levadopa, metaxalone, methyldopa, nalidixic acid, paraldehyde, phenazopyridine, probenecid, salicylates, fulfonamides, and tetracyclines; pregnant women have lactose in their urine during the third trimester, necessitating use of the enzyme testing method.[189, 274]

Ketones are found in the urine when the body's fat stores are being metabolized for energy, producing an excess of metabolic end products. This occurs with uncontrolled diabetes, fasting, pregnancy and lactation, and severe infections accompanied by vomiting and diarrhea.

The *protein* usually measured during a routine urinalysis is albumin. Albuminuria often denotes abnormal glomerular permeability due to blood pressure changes as in renal vein abnormality, pre-eclampsia, and hypertension, or intrinsic glomerular disease. Massive proteinuria is indicative of a nephrotic syndrome due to such disease processes as systemic lupus erythematosus and amyloidosis. Fever can produce increased urinary protein excretion, possibly because of immunologic injury to the glomerular and/or tubular basement membrane during infection.[141] There is also documentation that a small percentage of healthy individuals, usually males, have a postural proteinuria with protein leakage occurring only in the upright position. Mahurkar and associates studied 120 normal males and found that protein excretion increased on standing in 20 per cent of the men, although the rate of excretion generally remained within normal limits;[192] most studies report the incidence rate of orthostatic proteinuria as approximately 5 per cent.[328] Exercise proteinuria is considered to be the result of

*See Sorensen and Luckmann, *Basic Nursing: A Psychophysiologic Approach,* Chapter 30.

partial failure of tubular reabsorption of filtered proteins. Any finding of proteinuria should be further evaluated as described below.

Bilirubinuria is usually indicative of extrehepatic biliary tract obstruction. Other causes include hepatitis, portal inflammation, and hepatocellular damage. When a urine specimen containing bilirubin is shaken, a yellow foam is produced.

Hematuria may or may not be accompanied by other symptoms. Asymptomatic hematuria often presents a challenging diagnostic problem and requires very meticulous evaluation. It has recently been found that the occurrence of hematuria, sometimes with clots, is rather common among long-distance runners. This condition usually reverses itself after the run and is thought to be the result of mild, benign lower urinary tract lesions.[305] Red blood cells in the urine often indicate pathology, although it is not unusual to never find the etiology of this phenomenon. Poliak and associates did renal biopsies on 402 patients with asymptomatic hematuria with the following results: normal kidneys or minimal unclassifiable lesions — 21 per cent; focal proliferative glomerulonephritis — 54 per cent; diffuse proliferative glomerulonephritis — 20 per cent; chronic glomerulonephritis — 3 per cent; pyelonephritis — 1 per cent; and other — 1 per cent.[245] Hematuria may also be found in such disease states as tuberculosis, renal pelvis calculi, sickle cell anemia or the trait, tumors, IgA–IgG nephropathy, systemic lupus erythematosus, and polyarteritis nodosa. Anticoagulation and excessive use of analgesics leading to papillary necrosis can also produce red blood cells in the urine. It is important when collecting urine from a woman to note whether she is menstruating, since contamination of the specimen with menstrual blood will give a false positive. It is also necessary to observe whether the bleeding occurs at the beginning or end of the voiding, since this information can help differentiate the source.

The presence of *white blood cells* designates an infectious process somewhere in the urinary tract. When accompanied by casts, renal epithelial cells, a few red blood cells, and bacteria, the leukocytosis is usually the result of a kidney infection. Bladder infections give rise to leukocytosis with red blood cells and bladder epithelial cells, but no casts. Noninfectious inflammatory diseases of the urinary tract may also produce white blood cells in the urine.

Since the urine is normally sterile, *bacteriuria* represents infection within the urinary tract. Presence of bacteria in the urine, whether or not it is accompanied by physical signs and symptoms of urinary tract infection, needs further evaluation with urine cultures.

Casts are formed elements organized in the nephrons by the agglutination of protein. They are most likely to be formed in the distal tubules and the collecting ducts and are excreted in the urine. Their presence indicates tubular or glomerular disease. There are several varieties of casts, and the identification of the specific type helps pinpoint the contributing problem. A few *hyaline casts* can be found normally, especially after strenuous exercise, although some hypothesize that their presence in people at rest may indicate future renal or cardiovascular disease; these clear, colorless cylinders are also found in acute glomerulonephritis, acute pyelonephritis, malignant hypertension, chronic renal disease, congestive heart failure, and diabetic nephropathy. *Red cell casts* may be yellow or clear and denote bleeding within the nephron as the result of glomerulonephritis, acute renal allograft rejection, and acute tubular necrosis and may be the only manifestation of renal involvement in such pathologic conditions as systemic lupus erythematosus, subacute bacterial endocarditis, arteritis, and diabetic nephropathy. *White cell casts,* or *leukocyte casts,* which indicate bacterial infection and noninfective inflammatory disease, are often hard to distinguish from *epithelial casts,* which denote sloughing of renal tubular epithelium due to eclampsia, poisoning with heavy metals, amyloidosis, acute renal allograft rejection, etc.; these two types of casts are frequently intermixed. *Granular casts* come from two sources: gradual breakdown of cellular material or the aggregation of serum proteins and other elements; their presence indicates such things as renal parenchymal disease, acute renal rejection, pyelonephritis, chronic lead poisoning, and viral disease. The final stages of tubular inflammation and degeneration produce *waxy casts;* chronic renal failure and chronic and acute renal allograft rejection cause the formation and excretion of this type of cast. Casts formed in the tubules are usually of a narrow caliber, while those shaped in the collecting ducts are wider. Normal urine flow is generally too swift to allow the formation of these wide-bore casts, so their presence in the urine indicates substantial slowing of the urinary stream and malfunctioning of the renal system. In general, the wider the casts, the poorer the patient's prognosis.[275, 309, 328]

Crystalluria may or may not indicate pathology. Common findings are calcium oxalate, uric acid, and urate in acid urine and phosphate and carbonate crystals and amorphous phosphates in alkaline urine. The presence of crystals in the urine is an important predisposing factor in calculus formation.

Although not generally included in the routine urinalysis, the determination of osmolality, proteins other than albumin, and porphobilinogen in a single specimen may be done to further delineate renal pathology. *Urine osmolality* is considered by some to be a more precise measurement of urine concentration than specific gravity, since osmolality reflects only the number of solute particles and is not influenced by the size or composition of those particles. The range of urine osmolality is 50 to 1400 mOsm./kg. and, as a comparison, a specific gravity of 1.022 corresponds to an osmolality of 800 mOsm./kg.[328]

One of the classic proteinurias not attributed to albumin is Bence-Jones protein, which is found in multiple myeloma. Bence-Jones protein is a low molecular weight polypeptide which is detected either by heating the specimen or by electrophoresis. Other protein components may be found in macroglobulinemia and various tubular defects.

Porphobilinogen is a hemoglobin precursor. Porphyrins excreted in the urine occur because of hereditary metabolic diseases, impaired hematopoiesis, decreased liver function, carbon tetrachloride or benzene toxicity, heavy metal poisoning, Hodgkin's disease, and some kinds of anemia. In the presence of porphyrins, standing urine turns wine-colored. The urine can be further evaluated by the addition of various chemicals or by screening the specimen with ultra-violet light looking for an orange to red fluorescent color.

Twenty-four hour urine specimens are utilized to determine the excretion rate of a number of elements. Frequently used tests measure urinary levels of sodium, potassium, calcium, chloride, phosphorus, uric acid, and quantitative determination of proteins.

Clearance Studies. While direct examination of the urine gives a gross estimate of renal function, more definitive measures are needed to determine the adequacy of kidney activity. One type of renal function test to determine the glomerular filtration rate and tubular excretory ability involves measuring clearance rates of creatinine, urea, inulin, para-aminohippuric acid, phenolsulfonphthalein, and radioactive isotopes. The concept of *clearance* is defined as the amount of plasma totally cleared of a given substance in one minute. Quantitative renal excretory function is the difference between the rate of filtration of any given substance across the glomerular wall and the rate at which this substance is excreted in the urine.

In looking for a substance with which to measure glomerular filtration rate, it is necessary to find one that is freely filtered in the glomerulus, but is unable to pass through the tubular epithelium in any direction. *Inulin* is a fructose polysaccharide with these characteristics. A loading dose of inulin is administered intravenously and a constant infusion is maintained to produce a steady plasma concentration. At given points during the process, timed urine and plasma levels of inulin must be obtained. Accurate timing of these specimen collections is crucial to the outcome of the tests; bladder catheterization may be necessary to accomplish this. Normal values for this test are 124 plus or minus 15 ml. plasma/min./1.73/m.^{2} of body surface for men and 110 plus or minus 15 ml./min./1.73 m.^{2} for women. Values decrease slightly with aging.

Because the measurement of plasma and urine levels of inulin must be done so frequently and so accurately, this test is not widely used in general practice. Creatinine and urea clearance tests are more widely employed. Both of these substances are endogenous, which eliminates the need to establish and maintain a plasma level. *Creatinine* is filtered in the glomerulus, but is also secreted by the tubule, so that the final value provides only an estimate of glomerular filtration rate. This factor becomes more problematic as renal function is increasingly impaired, since these patients often have high serum creatinine levels which then enhance the secretion of creatinine. Thus it is recommended that serial determinations be done to illustrate the developing situation. Urine is collected over a 24-hour period, preferably beginning and ending in the early morning. At the end of this period, a fasting blood sample is collected. An adult female normally excretes 0.8 to 1.7 gm./24 hours and a male 1 to 1.9 gm./24 hours. Care must be taken in applying these values in the elderly. Longitudinal studies demonstrate declining creatinine clearance rates after the age of 34 years, with the rate of decline increasing after the age of 65 years. This is probably due to reduction in muscle mass and reduced renal blood flow.[263]

Urea clearance is sometimes used but, because the rate of tubular secretion varies with the rate of urine flow, its findings are not as useful as creatinine clearance. When employing this procedure, it is essential to assure a urine flow of at least 2 ml./min. Before the test is begun, the patient fasts for several hours. The patient empties the bladder and then drinks two or more glasses of water. Exactly one hour later, the patient voids and a blood sample for a blood urea nitrogen (BUN) is taken. At this point, the patient drinks another two or more glasses of water, and in exactly one hour, voids again. At each voiding, the entire specimen is kept, carefully labelled as to the time, and sent to the laboratory. If necessary, the bladder is catheterized in order to get an accurate specimen. The normal level of clearance is 75 ml./min. or more and 54 ml./min. if the flow was below 2 ml./min. Reference values for the test range from 75 to 125 per cent of normal. In addition to urine flow rate, the amount of protein intake and protein catabolism within the body can also affect the clearance rate.

Tubular transport is partially measured through the excretion rate of para-aminohippuric acid (PAH) or phenolsulfonphthalein (PSP). PAH is almost completely removed from the plasma through filtration and secretion. The findings are compared with the values of glomerular filtration rate procured through inulin clearance determination. The difference between PAH and inulin values represents tubular functioning capacity. Like inulin clearance testing, the determination of PAH excretion involves the need for a high degree of technical accuracy and thus is not as widely used as the PSP test.

Phenolsulfonphthalein is secreted by the proximal tubule at a rate proportionate to the renal blood flow. Ninety-four per cent of this red dye is secreted in the tubules and the remaining 6 per cent is filtered in the glomerulus. After the patient empties the bladder, 6 mg. of PSP is injected intravenously and urine specimens are collected at specified intervals. Various laboratories have different time intervals, but all require that the patient void 15 minutes after the injection of PSP; this is the most crucial specimen. In order to assure that the patient will be able to void when necessary, fluids may be encouraged before and during the test. Patients should also be warned that the dye may turn the urine red, so they will not think that they are bleeding.

In the laboratory, the urine is compared to a standardized color chart or a colorimeter to determine the amount of dye being excreted. Since the dye is not visible in acid, an alkaline solution may be added to the specimen. The dye begins to appear in the bladder 3 to 6 minutes after its administration, and 20 to 30 per cent of it is excreted in 15 minutes. Sixty-five to 75 per cent of the initial dose is normally excreted within an hour. Chlorothiazide, penicillin G, and hypoproteinemia may cause false findings.

Other methods of measuring renal function are being developed. One of these is the use of *radioisotopes* to determine clearance rates. This procedure is called a *renogram* and involves the intravenous injection of a minute amount of a radioactive compound such as iodohippurate sodium (Hippuran). The patient is placed in a sitting or supine position with radiation counters positioned on the skin over the kidneys. A third counter may be placed over the chest to monitor disappearance of the isotopes from the blood. The rate of radioactive emission is counted over a period of 15 to 20 minutes by a recording meter. The test measures renal blood flow, active tubular transport, and excretion, and each kidney can be compared with the other. The test requires no special preparation of the patient and no special precautions are required with the patient or the urine, since the dose of radioactivity is so low. The primary restriction in the widespread use of the renogram is its limited availability.

Other techniques using radioisotopes to measure renal function utilize blood determinations to calculate clearance rates. For example, ^{99m}Tc-Sn-DPTA, a radiopharmaceutical, is injected, and plasma samples are drawn at given intervals to determine the amount of remaining isotope.[160] The clearance of ^{51}Cr-EDTA requires only a single, very accurately timed blood sample.[220]

Concentration and Dilution. The loss of the kidney's ability to concentrate and dilute urine indicates significant renal tubular damage. Normally, as the body becomes fluid-depleted through decreased intake or increased losses through the gastrointestinal tract, respiratory tract, or perspiration, larger volumes of water are reabsorbed, resulting in more concentrated urine. Conversely, with increased fluid intake, more water is excreted, causing more dilute urine. One of the first kidney functions to be lost is this ability to concentrate and dilute. In severe renal damage, the specific gravity may become fixed at a level of 1.008 to 1.012, regardless of the amount of fluid intake.

There are several tests that can be performed to evaluate this aspect of renal function. Two frequently used procedures measuring concentration ability are the Fishberg and Addis tests. The *Fishberg concentration test* involves denying the patient any food or fluid intake after the evening meal. Early-morning specimens are collected and their specific gravity determined. A reading of less than 1.024 suggests renal function impairment. In this instance, the period of fluid depletion may be extended for up to a total of 22 hours, with periodic urine specimens evaluated for their specific gravity. The *Addis concentration test* calls for severe restriction of fluid intake for 24 hours; the amount of fluid allowed to the patient differs with each laboratory. A 12-hour specimen is collected during the last half of the fluid-restricted period. This sample is analyzed for the quantitative presence of protein, white blood cells, red blood cells, and casts. Factors that can interfere with the normal concentrating ability of the kidney include decreased sodium intake, low protein diet, and glucosuria.

During *dilution tests,* the patient empties the bladder and then drinks 1200 ml. of water or fruit juice within 30 minutes. Physical activity should be kept to a minimum during the test to prevent fluid losses through other routes. Urine specimens are collected at specified intervals — usually every 30 minutes — for 3 hours. The volume is measured and the specific gravity determined for each specimen. With normal renal function, the entire 1200 ml. should be voided, and the specific gravity will be about 1.002.

The patient's cooperation in following the procedures of these tests is essential for accurate findings, particularly with concentration tests in which the patient must resist the temptation to drink any fluids for many hours. It is very important that the patient fully understand the procedure and why fluids are not allowed. The nurse may also need to intervene to help the patient cope with thirst.

Blood Chemistry. Measuring selected components in the blood aids in the evaluation of renal function. Probably the most frequently used determination is the *blood urea nitrogen (BUN)*. Urea is the end product of the metabolism of protein and is normally excreted from the body through the kidneys. Therefore, any impairment of renal function causes an increase in the plasma level of urea. The BUN starts to rise when the glomerular filtration rate falls below 50 ml./min.[309] Unfortunately, the BUN can also be elevated by such nonrenal factors as high protein intake or protein catabolism within the body. This single value must be evaluated very cautiously.

The *serum creatinine* level is usually measured along with the BUN. Creatinine is also excreted through the kidney, so increased serum levels indicate decreased renal function. It is also felt by many to be a more accurate indicator of renal function than the BUN.

The ratio of BUN to creatinine is helpful in identifying the etiology of kidney malfunction. The normal ratio is 10 to 15:1. Elevations of BUN in relation to serum creatinine denote renal impairment due to prerenal causes such as blood loss, severe diarrhea, heart failure, and liver disease.

Hematology. The inspection of a random blood sample provides some data about renal function as well as the progress of disease processes within the urinary tract. Decreased red blood cells, hemoglobin, and/or hematocrit may indicate bleeding from the urinary tract or may signal reduced erythropoietic function by the kidney. An increased white blood cell count with increased neutrophils may denote an infectious process, while return of these values to normal represents recovery from the infection.

Bacteriologic Studies. Since the kidneys, ureters, and bladder are normally sterile, the urine formed and transported in them is also sterile. The distal portion of the urethra is usually colonized with organisms, but these bacteria ordinarily do not reach further up the urinary tract. Therefore, the presence of organisms in the urine is an abnormal finding. Any signs and symptoms of urinary tract infection reported by the patient and/or the presence of bacteriuria or urinary leukocytosis indicates the need to further examine the urine so that specific treatment can be instituted.

The existence of pathogens in the urine is usually determined by *culture*. The urine specimens for this testing are collected by catheterizing the bladder or by obtaining a midstream, or clean-catch, voided specimen as described above. The main goal is to provide the laboratory with a specimen that has not been contaminated with organisms outside the urinary tract. Many authorities suggest that this specimen should be obtained in the early morning to allow adequate accumulation of organisms within the urine being cultured. Once the specimen has been obtained, it should be transported to the laboratory immediately. If the urine will not be examined right away, it should be refrigerated, since the bacteria will continue multiplying at room temperature.

Frequently the first screening test done is a Gram stain on the uncentrifuged urine. The treated urine is then examined under a microscope and an initial report of the type and gross amount of organisms may be given. Whether or not a Gram stain is done, the identification of specific pathogens must be done by culturing the urine. The urine is swabbed onto media plates which are placed into an environment appropriate for growth for 24 to 72 hours. Any colonies present are further studied to specifically name and quantify the organisms present. The mere finding of organisms does not signify clinical infection. Each colony seen represents 1000 organisms per ml. and levels below 10,000 organisms per ml. usually represent contamination of the specimen. It is generally agreed that concentrations of 10^5 organisms per ml. constitute significant infection.

Once the causative organisms have been identified, sensitivities should be done to designate the antibiotics to be used to combat their growth. This is becoming even more important as the number of resistant organisms is increasing, owing in part to the misuse of antibiotics. Treatment with the wrong antibiotics is costly to the patient in terms of both money and time lost. Sensitivity tests are usually done on agar plates which have on them small paper disks impregnated with the drugs to be tested. The growth of organisms sensitive to any given antibiotic is inhibited in the area around the disk.

Nurses must be aware of sensitivity reports, since occasionally these are overlooked and treatment with the wrong medication will continue much longer than necessary.

As an alternative to the more common culturing technique, there are several other screening devices used to detect significant bacteriuria. These depend on chemical reactions mediated by the metabolic effect of bacteria on the indicator substance used. Dip sticks with chemically treated pads are typically used for this type of testing. This technique has the advantage of being simple to perform and relatively inexpensive, and it allows patients to more conveniently test their morning specimens. However, there is controversy regarding the accuracy of these devices. While some authorities claim a high correlation between the results of dip sticks and the conventional laboratory culture, others assert that too many false negatives are reported.[184, 333]

Cytologic Examination. The examination of urine for malignant cells can provide early evidence of urinary tract cancer. It frequently demonstrates the presence of tumors before they are visible endoscopically.

Radiologic Studies

In most diagnostic protocols, x-ray examination of the urinary tract is the next step in identifying actual or potential malfunction. These studies may be done with or without the injection of contrast material and may involve static and/or dynamic films. Since these examinations are done in the x-ray department, the nurse's main responsibility is to have patients adequately prepared for the procedure so that the results will be as accurate as possible. And, as with any procedure, the nurse must be sure that patients fully understand the process and their role in it.

Kidneys, Ureters, Bladder. An x-ray of the *kidneys, ureters, and bladder (KUB)* is a simple film of the lower abdomen. It involves no contrast medium and thus no risk to the patient and can be done without consideration of the amount of remaining kidney function. The outline of these organs demonstrates their size, shape, and location. This helps to identify soft tissue masses, malformations, and radiopaque calculi.

Excretory Urogram. The *excretory urogram (EUG)*, also called *intravenous pyelogram (IVP)*, involves intravenous injection of a radiopaque dye that is filtered by the kidney and excreted through the urinary tract. Through this examination, it is possible to identify the absence or presence, location, size, and configuration of the kidneys, ureters, and bladder. Filling of the renal calices and pelvis can be determined, and post-voiding films showing abnormal retention of dye can indicate bladder neck obstruction.

Physical preparation of the patient normally involves restricting fluids and cleaning out the bowel. Food and fluids are withheld from at least midnight prior to the examination. This relative fluid depletion allows the radiopaque dye to be more concentrated when it enters the kidney, thus providing clearer films. If the patient is receiving intravenous fluids, the rate of infusion may be slowed for several hours prior to the study. Fluid depletion is contraindicated in patients with multiple myeloma, severe diabetes, or uric acid nephropathy; these conditions make the kidney sensitive to the contrast medium and this sensitivity, combined with reduced renal perfusion due to decreased renal blood flow, predisposes the patient to the development of acute renal failure. If these patients must have an EUG, it must be performed with the patient in a well-hydrated state.

Because the kidneys are located retroperitoneally, the bowel must be cleared of gas and fecal material that may cause partial or total obscuring of the kidneys. Cathartics are usually administered the evening before the examination. However, this part of the preparation may be omitted in patients with suspected or known inflammatory bowel disease or when vigorous colonic activity is otherwise contraindicated. If cathartics were not effective or not given for any reason, enemas or a rectal suppository may be administered early in the morning before the x-ray.

The combination of fasting and catharsis may cause weakness, especially in patients already debilitated by age and illness. Thus the nurse must take precautions to assure the comfort and safety of the patient. Bedtime sedation should be omitted, and the call bell should be kept handy. The patient should be instructed to call for assistance with ambulation, and the side rails should be kept up if necessary. The staff should be alerted to the need to answer the patient's call light with special promptness.

The patient is placed in a supine position on the x-ray table. Initially, a KUB film is taken as a scout film. This helps to assure that the bowel is clear enough to continue with the rest of the procedure. It also screens for calculi in the renal collecting system; since the contrast medium in the collecting ducts is the same density as any calcification in this area, stones can easily be missed during the EUG.

The radiopaque dye is injected intravenously, usually as a bolus, although an infusion drip may be used if the patient's vein cannot tolerate a rapid injection or if there are poorly functioning kidneys. The dyes currently used are di- and tri-iodinated derivatives of benzine and pyridine. Two commonly used substances are diatrizoate sodium (Hypaque) and meglumine diatrizoate (Renografin). The compounds normally cause flushing of the face, a feeling of warmth, and a salty taste in the mouth. These effects are transitory and do not mean that the study should be stopped. However, the *iodine* in the substances may cause *severe allergic reactions* in hypersensitive people. In a collection of 32,964 patients undergoing EUG, 5.1 per cent had minor reactions; 1.72 per cent, acute; and 0.09 per cent, severe. The incidence of allergic reactions was 2.5 times higher in patients with a positive allergy history.[336]

> *Before the examination is begun, the patient should be carefully questioned about any allergy history. A known sensitivity to iodinated contrast media is an absolute contraindication to continuation of the procedure.*

A positive allergy history other than to iodine requires skin testing prior to intravenous injection, and this procedure is recommended for all patients, since sensitivity to the material is inconsistent from examination to examination. *However, a negative skin test is no assurance that there will be no reaction.* Any signs of allergic response, such as itching, hives, wheezing, or other respiratory distress call for immediate discontinuation of the injection. Antihistamine, epinephrine, vasopressors, oxygen, and resuscitation equipment must be available to definitively treat the anaphylactic response.

In addition to the possibility of anaphylactic reactions due to the contrast medium, there have also been documented cases of *acute renal failure* following injection of the dye. Although the incidence rate is low, this side effect should be kept in mind. Out of 7800 patients receiving intravascular contrast media, 8 developed acute renal failure. Predisposing factors include vascular disease, diabetes, and pre-existing renal insufficiency. Diatrizoate sodium itself reduces the renal blood flow and enhances blood viscosity through its induced changes in erythrocyte level. These factors, added to the fluid depletion state, increase the patient's risk markedly.[8] Treatment of acute renal failure is discussed in Chapter 43.

Films are usually taken 2, 5, 10, 15, 20, 30, and 60 minutes after the dye is injected; the later films may also be post-voiding. The patient is normally kept in the supine position throughout this time, although upright, oblique, and lateral films may also be obtained. Ureteric compression is frequently done to enhance distention of the collecting system and upper ureters. A compression band with inflatable balloons is applied across the patient's lower abdomen after the 5-minute film and left in place until the 10-minute films are obtained. Sometimes, with delayed renal functioning, additional x-rays may be needed one to two hours later; if the patient is to remain on the x-ray table during this time, care must be taken to insure comfort as much as possible.

In the case of advanced renal failure or with a unilateral, non-visualized kidney, a large bolus of undiluted dye may be used to produce better visualization of the urinary system; this technique is called *high-bolus urography*.[195] In preparing the patient for this examination, it is usually unnecessary to have a period of fluid restriction. There is some increased risk with this technique. Potentially serious *electrocardiographic abnormalities* have occurred in older patients with evidence of previous heart disease. Identified risk factors include abnormal electrocardiogram, coronary artery disease, and congestive heart failure.[293] However, the occurrence rate of cardiac arrhythmias during the procedure is very low, and the beneficial effects seem to show that the technique is worthwhile. There is some controversy as to whether the bolus or drip procedure is more useful, although this depends somewhat on the intended progress of the rest of the study, e.g., the drip technique delivers dye over a longer period of time.

When the patient is returned to the floor following completion of the examination, observation for reactions to the dye must be continued. Food, and especially fluids, should be given to the patient to counteract fast and fluid depletion.

Retrograde Pyelogram. A *retrograde pyelogram* involves the passage of small caliber catheters through a cystoscope into the ureters to the level of the renal pelvis. (The procedure for cystoscopy is described below.) Small amounts of contrast media are injected into the kidney through the catheters and x-ray films are taken to delineate the collecting system. The patient may feel some discomfort in the kidney region when the dye is injected, but there is no actual pain unless the renal pelvis has been overdistended. As the catheters are withdrawn, more dye is injected and films are taken to record the outline of the ureters. Preparation and care of the patient during and after the procedure is the same as that needed for a patient undergoing cystoscopy.

The performance of retrograde pyelography is indicated when there has been unsatisfactory visualization of the renal collecting system or ureters during an EUG. It is also helpful in the assessment of the degree of ureteral obstruction. It can be used in patients who are hypersensitive to intravenous radiopaque dye, although this procedure does not provide any information about the status of blood flow to the kidney or about nephron function.

There are no particular contraindications to

this procedure, although it does carry some risk for the patient. Entering the urinary tract occasionally causes primary urinary tract infection or stirs up pre-existing infections. Manipulation of the ureters may cause edema resulting in temporary obstruction to the flow of urine.

Cystourethrography. X-ray examination of the bladder and urethra can be done separately or in combination. During *cystography* contrast medium or air is injected into the bladder through a catheter. When the bladder is full, films are taken to profile the size and shape of the bladder and to detect the presence of vesicoureteral reflux. The patient is then frequently asked to void and a follow-up x-ray is done. This final film measures the amount of residual urine.

Urethrography is done to outline the inner size and shape of the urethra and to check for extravasation. In male patients, x-rays are taken after a very thick, jelly-like radiopaque substance is injected through a wide-mouthed syringe into the urethral meatus. This material usually reaches only as far as the urogenital diaphragm. The procedure in females requires a less viscous contrast agent and a special catheter.

The combination of these two procedures, called *voiding cystourethrography*, provides visualization of urethral lesions, vesicoureteric reflux, and bladder or urethral obstructions. The radiopaque material is instilled into the bladder through a urethral catheter as for a cystogram. The catheter is then removed and the patient asked to void. Films are taken during the voiding process to observe the flow of the contrast medium. The micturition process may be recorded on movie film in order to better visualize the movement of the contrast medium. Being required to void in the presence of other people can be very embarrassing to the patient and may even interfere with the ability to void. Emotional support and the judicious placement of screens may help put the patient more at ease.

Renal Angiography. *Renal angiography* is done to visualize renal vasculature. It is helpful in diagnosing renal artery stenosis or renal vein thrombosis, studying renovascular hypertension, demonstrating vascular damage after trauma, investigating causes of acute renal failure, and differentiating highly vascular tumors from avascular cysts when space-occupying renal lesions have been identified.

Renal arteriography involves the injection of a radiopaque dye into the renal vascular tree and the taking of serial x-ray films to outline blood vessels. Access to the circulation is usually achieved through the femoral artery. A guide wire is threaded into the artery through an arterial needle. The needle is then removed, leaving the guide wire in place, and a radiopaque flexible catheter is passed over the guide wire. Using fluoroscopy to help in the guidance, the catheter and wire are advanced through the femoral and iliac arteries into the aorta. The guide wire may be removed and dye injected when the catheter is in position at the level of the renal arteries, or the wire and catheter may be guided into the renal artery itself before the dye is injected; this is called *selective renal arteriography*. Once the dye has been injected, films are taken at the rate of 2 to 3 per second for several seconds to show filling and emptying of the renal artery tree. Delayed films are usually done to visualize function of the renal veins.

There are alternate sites for vascular access. A *translumbar aortogram* involves direct puncture of the aorta at the level of the renal arteries with a long needle. Puncture of the axillary artery or antecubital vein may also be done.

In addition to anaphylactic reactions and possible renal damage due to the radiopaque dye used, there are several other serious potential complications resulting from this procedure. Hemorrhage along the route of the vessel puncture may be either external or, especially with a translumbar aortogram, internal. Vascular injury may occur at the puncture site or anywhere along the path of the guide wire and catheter. Thrombosis or embolism may occur as a result of dislodgement of plaque from vessel walls during the procedure.

Pre-examination preparation of the patient is the same as for EUG, including testing the patient for hypersensitivity to the dye being used. The procedure is usually done under a local anesthesia, although the patient frequently receives pre-procedure sedation. One of the chief potential side effects of this examination is post-vessel puncture hemorrhage. Pressure dressings are applied over the puncture site immediately after the catheter is removed. The area is observed frequently for several hours for signs of fresh bleeding. The patient is usually placed on bedrest for several hours to allow complete sealing of the puncture site. If a femoral puncture has been done, pedal pulses are also checked frequently to detect any reduced circulation to the feet which may occur as a result of vascular injury. Especially after a translumbar aortogram, vital signs should be monitored frequently to disclose the presence of hemorrhage.

Another method by which to study the venous system of the kidneys is *renal phlebography*. Because of the small caliber of the renal artery and the copious blood flow in the renal veins, renal arteriography is often inadequate for satisfactory visualization of these vessels, necessitating an alternate procedure. During renal phlebography, the femoral vein is punctured and a catheter is threaded through the inferior vena cava and into the renal veins. The rest of the procedure, as well as the care of the patient, is the same as for renal arteriography.[36]

Computerized Axial Tomography. The use of *computerized axial tomography*, also called CAT scan, CT scan, or EMI scan, can be beneficial in the determination of kidney pathology. CAT scanning involves an x-ray beam which sweeps around the body allowing measurement of various tissue densities. This ability permits evaluation of a nonfunctioning kidney and presence of subcapsular and perirenal bleeding as well as the presence of other abnormal tissue formations.[166, 268]

Intravenous administration of contrast media may be used for image enhancement. As with the use of dyes for other kidney radiograms, this implies some risk for the patient. *Acute renal failure* has been documented in patients with long-standing hypertension, diabetes, or elevated serum nitrogenous levels. Adequate hydration of the patient before the examination may reduce the incidence of this complication.[121]

Ultrasonography

Ultrasound projects high-frequency waves into the abdomen. These waves are reflected back from the surfaces of retroperitoneal structures and converted into electrical energy to be shown on an oscilloscope. Instant-developing time-lapse pictures are taken of the oscilloscope image to record the outline of the structures.

Ultrasonography of the kidneys has many uses. Probably the prime value is in the differentiation between fluid-filled cysts and solid masses. Other applications include localization and mapping out of the kidney before biopsy by percutaneous aspiration, evaluation of transplanted kidneys, determination of hydronephrosis in nonfunctioning kidneys, identification of renal calculi, and estimation of residual urine.[95, 236, 286] Additional uses are continually being discovered.

The procedure has been found to be entirely safe and to have a high accuracy rate. It is noninvasive, involves no contrast media, and has produced no ill effects in any patients or the offspring of pregnant women. Studies have documented accuracy rates of 92 to 98 per cent for cysts and 60 per cent for carcinomas.[279, 287]

Radioisotope Studies

In addition to the renal function tests done with radioisotopes that were described above, radioactive compounds can also be used to delineate the kidneys. As with the clearance studies, the radioisotope is injected intravenously and a gamma scintillation camera or probe and/or computer is used to record the size and shape of the kidneys. The isotope compounds used, however, are ones that are retained in the kidneys for several hours or days rather than being cleared immediately. Lesions in the kidney, such as tumors or infarcts, do not absorb the radioactivity and thus appear as "cold" or "blank" spots on the scanner; in this situation, further study is needed to determine the actual cause of the cold spot.

Cystometrography and Urethral Pressure Profile

A cystometric examination is a procedure which evaluates the motor and sensory functioning of the bladder and the efficiency of micturition. It is used primarily in the work-up of patients having voiding problems and/or difficulty with incontinence. Through a series of measurements, diagnostic information can be obtained about bladder capacity, pressure profiles before and during micturition, and the dynamics of the urinary stream.

No pre-procedure preparation of the patient is necessary. At the beginning of the examination, the patient is asked to void while the examiner notes the time and effort needed to initiate micturition; size, force, and continuity of the stream; and dribbling after voiding ceases. A retention catheter is then passed through the urethra and the balloon is inflated. Any residual urine is removed and measured. In order to test the sensory function of the bladder, a specific amount of cold water may be instilled through the catheter followed by warm water. The distal end of the catheter is attached to the apparatus which will be used to deliver the fluid or air to the bladder and to measure the intravesicular pressures. Figure 41–3 illustrates the set-up of this equipment. Either air or saline may be used to distend the bladder; the latter is utilized most frequently, but many examiners feel that carbon dioxide insufflation permits better visualization than water. The saline is instilled through the catheter at a constant rate of about 1 ml./min. or in periodic amounts of 50 ml. The intravesicular pressure is recorded continuously and the patient is asked to inform the examiner when the urge to void is first felt and again when the bladder feels quite full. These points are accurately noted on the intravesicular pressure record. Figure 41–4 shows normal intravesical pressures during a cystometrogram. The urethral catheter is removed and the patient is asked to cough so that stress incontinence may be identified. The patient empties the bladder while the examiner makes the same observa-

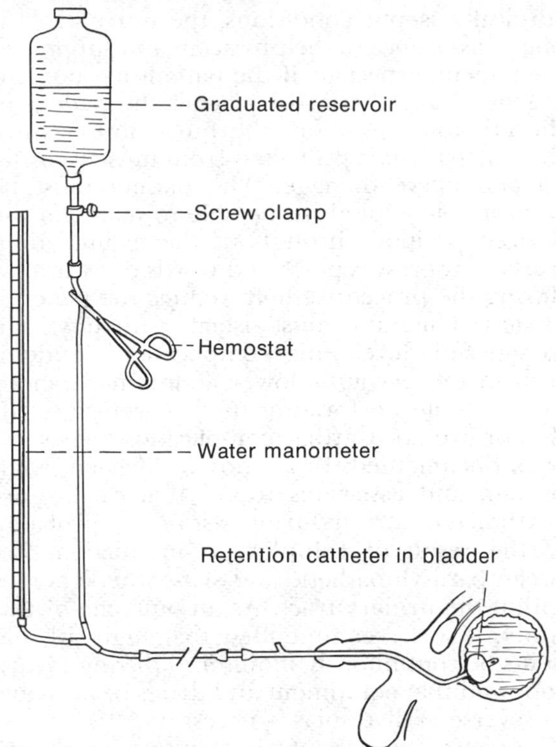

Figure 41-3. Equipment used for cystometrography.

tions as during the initial voiding; the amount of residual urine is again determined. The entire procedure may be repeated several times and bethanechol may be administered to further differentiate any neurologic impairment of bladder function. In order to measure bladder pressures during micturition, a tiny urethral catheter may be inserted and left in place during voiding; intraabdominal pressure can be measured with a small rectal catheter.

Although not always done as part of a cystometrogram, *urethral pressure profiles* may also be evaluated, particularly to decide the urethra's role in incontinence. The main factors measured are the intraluminal urethral closing forces and effective urethral length. Using a double-lumen catheter, urethral pressures must be determined at several levels of bladder fullness, including maximum capacity.

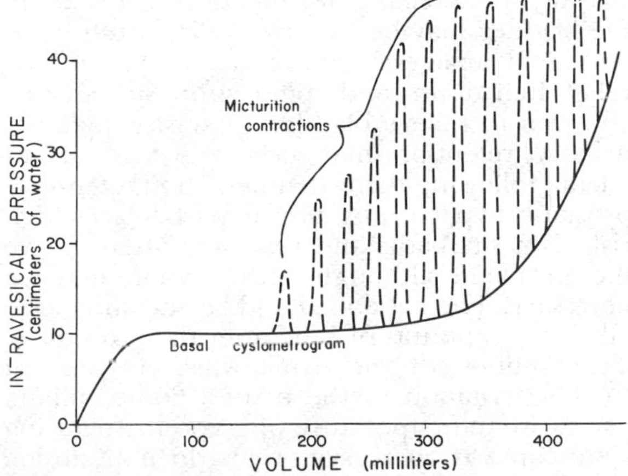

Figure 41-4. A normal cystometrogram. (From Guyton, A.: *Textbook of Medical Physiology*. Philadelphia: W. B. Saunders Co., 1976.)

Direct Visualization of the Urinary Tract

The oldest method of direct visualization of the urinary tract is *cystoscopy*, which involves insertion of a cystoscope into the bladder via the urethra. This procedure may be useful for both diagnostic and therapeutic purposes. Its diagnostic uses include (1) direct inspection of the bladder, making it possible to see tumors, calculi, ulcers, or other defects; (2) collection of urine directly from the kidney pelvis and from each kidney separately; (3) x-ray visualization through the retrograde pyelogram as described above; (4) measurement of bladder capacity and evidence of vesicoureteral reflux; and (5) biopsy of the bladder and urethra. Treatment uses of the cystoscope include (a) resection of tumors or diverticula, (b) removal of stones and foreign bodies, (c) fulguration of bleeding areas, (d) dilatation of the ureters, (e) emptying of the renal pelvis, and (f) implantation of radium seeds.

The first recorded attempt to examine internal body cavities was in 1806 in Vienna when Bozzini used candles and reflecting mirrors. The first practical cystoscope was developed in Berlin in 1879 by Leiter, Nitze, and Heyman.[322] Today's cystoscope consists primarily of a sheath, obturator, and optical lens system. The sheath is a solid metal tube which, with the obturator in place, can be passed through the urethra into the bladder without trauma. Once the cystoscope is in position, the obturator is removed from inside the sheath and the lighted lens system is introduced. Figure 41-5 shows a cystoscope in place. Several attachments can be used with the cystoscope to accomplish various functions. Forceps may be passed through the sheath to obtain tissue samples for biopsy or to remove foreign bodies. A guide can be used to help direct small catheters into and up the ureters to the level of the renal pelvis so that specimens can be obtained from each kidney separately. Scissors, needles, and electrodes may also be introduced into the bladder or urethra as needed.

Cystoscopy may be done either in the hospital or in the physician's office. It may also be performed under either local or general anes-

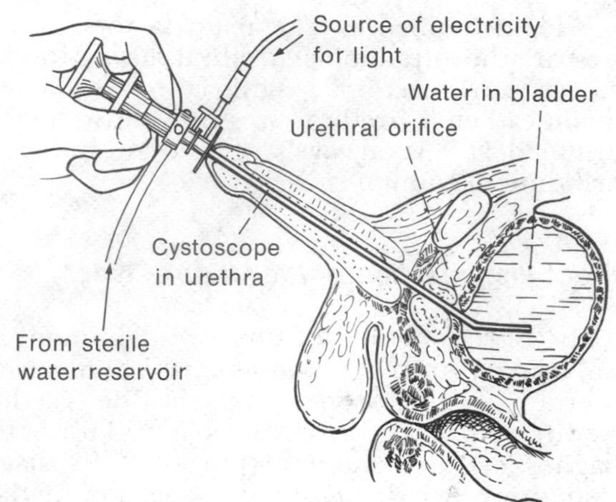

Figure 41–5. A cystoscope in place inside the bladder.

thesia. It is crucial that the patient remain very still during the examination to avoid trauma to the urinary tract; thus the decision about the type of anesthesia to be used may depend on the patient's reliability to maintain the necessary position without moving.

Preparation of the patient involves both physiologic and psychologic realms. Patients are usually given enemas before the procedure to clear the bowel. Some patients, especially those receiving a general anesthesia, may be required to fast for several hours prior to the examination. Patients having a local anesthesia may be instructed to maintain an adequate fluid intake to ensure an adequate flow of urine for the collection of specimens and for retrograde pyelography if it is to be performed; fasting patients may receive intravenous fluids. Usually a sedative or narcotic, and sometimes an anticholinergic, is administered before the procedure.

As with any procedure, effective patient teaching is important in the alleviation of anxiety and assurance of optimum cooperation by the patient. This is particularly important if the cystoscopy is done under local anesthesia. Since the procedure is usually done with the patient in the lithotomy position, the patient should be informed that this position can be very tiring and uncomfortable, but that it is very important to remain still throughout the examination. You can help the patient with deep breathing and general relaxation exercises to decrease discomfort as the cystoscope is introduced. The desire to void will be pronounced as the cystoscope passes the neck of the bladder and also when bladder capacity is measured by filling it with water.

During the procedure, which is done under surgically aseptic conditions, the nurse's role is one of assistance to the physician and support to the patient, especially if the patient has not had a general anesthesia. In placing the patient in the lithotomy position, the nurse must assure that the patient is protected from musculoskeletal and nerve damage. The patient must be comfortable enough to be able to maintain the desired position throughout the examination. Verbal progress reports and words of assurance during the procedure help reduce the patient's anxiety. The nurse must also alert the physician to signs of developing complications. Sudden pain in the pelvic or lower abdominal regions may indicate perforation of the urethra, bladder, or ureters. Cardiac complications have also been documented. In a study of 69 men, Kimbrough and associates found that cardiac arrhythmias occurred during cystoscopy, probably as the result of complicated interactions between parasympathetic and sympathetic nerves within the urinary tract. As an outcome of this study, it was recommended that high-risk patients be continuously monitored during cystoscopy and that equipment and drugs be available to reverse arrhythmias if necessary.[154]

Care for the patient after cystoscopy should include bed rest for a short time. If the patient has had a general anesthesia, this will include the expected recovery period during which time the usual post-anesthesia recovery monitoring of the patient should be done. Even if the procedure is done on an ambulatory basis under local anesthesia, patients should not stand immediately after removal of their legs from the stirrups, as this sudden circulatory change may cause dizziness and syncope; this is especially true for elderly patients.

Pink-tinged urine is quite common following cystoscopy, but any bright red bleeding or clots in the urine should be reported to the physician. If dyes have been used in the procedure, the patient should be warned that the urine may have an unusual color. Pain in the back, bladder spasms, and a feeling of fullness and burning in the bladder may be expected. Warm tub baths and mild analgesics are usually sufficient for relief. Belladonna and opium suppositories may be given to relieve bladder spasms. Sometimes urinary retention may occur as a result of edema following the instrumentation; men with prostatic hypertrophy are at particularly high risk. Hot sitz baths and relaxants often relieve the problem, although catherization may be necessary. The patient should be encouraged to take large amounts of fluid after the procedure. This dilution of the urine will help prevent further irritation to the tissues. Some chilling and a rise in temperature often occur following cystoscopy. If these symptoms do not subside readily as a result of providing extra warmth and offering frequent fluids, further investigation should be done. Cystoscopy may spread infection in the urinary tract and can cause a bacteremia. Although quite controversial, prophylactic use of antibiotics following urinary tract instrumentation is recommended by some authorities because of the high risk of infection. If the patient complains of abdominal pain following the procedure, the physician should be notified immediately, as accidental perforation of the urinary tract organs might be the cause.

Patients are often discharged within a couple of hours after cystoscopy. Written as well as verbal instruction should be given, as the patient may not be able to remember instructions given immediately following this stressful procedure.

One of the major problems with the standard cystoscope is that it is rigid, and thus the examiner may be unable to visualize parts of the bladder. The evolution of flexible endoscopic instruments has helped to solve this problem. Continued development of these instruments increases their contributions to the diagnostic process.

Instrumentation advances also allow for direct visualization of the kidney. Done under strict aseptic technique, *nephroscopy* allows the examiner to observe the renal pelvis, calices, fundus, and collecting system. It can be done to locate and remove calculi; diagnose etiology of hematuria; and biopsy, fulgurate, and resect tumors. It is a safe procedure with no significant complications reported. Care of the patient before and after the procedure is similar to that needed by a patient having a renal biopsy, as discussed below.

Renal Biopsy

Obtaining a specimen of renal tissue for biopsy may be done using either open or closed techniques. *Open* biopsy requires the surgical procedure, nephrostomy, involving an incision through the flank. This procedure allows direct visualization of the kidney, and the tissue obtained is adequate 100 per cent of the time. However, the procedure also has a prolonged recuperation period for the patient and is costly to the patient in terms of direct costs and indirectly through work time lost. Care of the patient having this procedure is discussed in Chapter 43.

One method of *closed* biopsy is the *retrograde renal and ureteral brush* procedure. This technique is used to collect tissue specimens from the renal pelvis and ureters. The initial part of the procedure is done as a cystoscopy with the patient under general anesthesia. A whistle-tip ureteral catheter is introduced and its proper positioning guided by fluoroscopy or multiple x-rays. A biopsy brush is then passed through the catheter and the lesion is brushed over several times. The brush is removed and any tissue adhering to the bristles is sent to the laboratory. If no tissue is found on the brush, 20- to 48-hour urine specimens may be collected to catch any cells that may have been dislodged by the bristles. Postoperatively, the patient may be given intravenous fluids at a rapid rate to reduce the possibility of clot formation at the biopsy site and to facilitate specimen collection. Some oozing of blood may be expected for 24 to 48 hours. Some patients experience severe renal colic, which is usually relieved by narcotics and fluids.[106]

Probably the most frequently used procedure is the *percutaneous renal biopsy*. During this procedure, a specially designed needle is inserted, piercing the skin and entering the kidney to obtain a small sample of tissue. When it was first demonstrated in 1934, it was not widely accepted because adequate tissue yield was only 40 to 67 per cent. However, since the development and use of fluoroscopy and ultrasound techniques to allow more precise localization of the biopsy needle, adequate results are achieved approximately 95 per cent of the time.[83] It is now considered a very important diagnostic tool, especially in any disease process that is evenly distributed through all parts of the kidney; it is helpful both as a one-time examination and when done serially to monitor the progress of a disease. Contraindications to the performance of percutaneous biopsy include a single functioning kidney, infection, tumors (because of the danger of dissemination), hydronephrosis, severe hypertension, coagulation disorders, and an uncooperative patient. Severe renal failure has previously been regarded as a contraindication; however better procedures for localization of the kidney have reduced the dangers associated with the technique. Pregnancy is usually considered a contraindication because of the high doses of radiation that may be necessary during localization of the needle; the use of ultrasound eliminates this risk.

Before the biopsy is done, a battery of x-ray and laboratory studies is done. These usually include excretory urogram, urine culture, hematocrit and blood urea nitrogen determinations, and bleeding and coagulation studies. Renal arteriography is mandatory if an aneurysm is suspected to avoid puncture of this vascular defect. Blood for replacement may be ordered as stand-by.

The procedure is usually done under local anesthesia with little or no premedication. The patient is placed in a prone position with a firm pillow or sandbag under the abdomen to straighten the natural lordosis of the spine. The kidney to be biopsied is located with ultrasound and/or fluoroscopy with dye injected intravenously. After careful skin preparation, the skin is infiltrated with the anesthetic agent. The patient is instructed to take in as deep a breath as possible and hold it. The probe needle is then inserted through the skin and positioned inside the renal capsule slightly lateral to the midline of the kidney. After the correct position of the distal end of the needle is confirmed, the probe needle is removed and the biopsy needle is inserted. The patient may now be allowed to breathe normally, but must be in full respiratory inspiration each time a tissue specimen is taken. When enough tissue has been obtained, the needle is removed and firm pressure is immediately applied to the site; after several minutes, a pressure dressing is applied.

The reported incidence of complications ranges from 0.75 per cent for major complications to 10 per cent for minor ones, which include microscopic hematuria, pain, fever, and extravasation of the contrast medium.[174] The mortality rate is 0.2 per cent.[48] Because of this, biopsy is usually not performed unless the knowledge gained would be likely to affect the treatment regimen for the patient. The most common major complication is *hemorrhage*. This may be suggested by gross or microscopic hematuria, flank or abdominal pain, hypotension, and a decreasing hematocrit. It must be noted, however, that low hematocrit or hypotension alone cannot be used as good indicators of hemorrhage, since some patients develop these conditions without significant bleeding; it is hypothesized that this may occur because of hemodilution or as a result of massive sympathetic stimulation caused by penetration of the needle.[33] Continued bleeding or the resultant hematoma may require surgical exploration and may further lead to removal of the involved kidney. Intrarenal arteriovenous fistulae may occur, causing an audible bruit over the kidneys, and may lead to hypertension. Because of the chances of a pneumothorax, especially when the upper pole of the kidney is biopsied, some authorities recommend a routine expiratory chest x-ray after the procedure; this is especially important for elderly patients with an already compromised cardiopulmonary reserve. Other complications include infection, traumatic urinoma, and laceration or perforation of the kidney or adjacent structures.

The patient should remain prone for approximately 30 minutes after completion of the procedure, with the vital signs and puncture site being monitored every 5 to 10 minutes. He or she may then be transferred to bed and should remain on bed rest and avoid straining for at least 24 hours. Vital signs and the puncture site are checked regularly during this time. A sample of each voiding is kept and placed consecutively in order to facilitate comparison and evaluate bleeding. Dip sticks may be used to determine the presence of hematuria, and specimens may be sent to the laboratory to more precisely determine the amount of bleeding. The patient should be encouraged to drink large amounts of fluid to avoid clot formation and retention which could obstruct urine flow. The period of bed rest will likely be extended in the presence of continued hemorrhage. A hematocrit and hemoglobin study is usually done within 8 to 10 hours to test for anemia. The patient may also need emotional support during this time of waiting for the diagnosis and its implications.

Upon discharge, advise the patient to avoid strenuous activity for approximately 2 weeks. Also instruct the patient about the signs of hemorrhage and what to do if these occur, since delayed bleeding may occur several days after the biopsy.[83]

CHAPTER 42

DISORDERS OF THE URETERS, BLADDER, AND URETHRA

The principal function of the ureters, bladder, and urethra — sometimes called the lower urinary tract — is to transport urine from the kidney out of the body. Anything that obstructs the flow or interferes with the neuromuscular ability to move and expel urine when desired reduces the ability of these organs to fulfill this role. Disorders can be expected to cause both physical and psychological problems, while at the same time both these components can influence the severity and progress of the disorder. The nurse must consider both realms in identifying patient problems and planning and implementing solutions to these problems.

CONGENITAL ANOMALIES

As with any congenital anomalies, some may produce signs early in life, while others may go undetected until adulthood. Some require intervention to prevent further damage; other disorders need no treatment.

Ureter

An *abnormal course* or *distal opening* of the ureter is the most common ureteral congenital anomaly. A retrocaval ureter, usually the right one, hooks around behind the vena cava before it returns to the proper side of the pelvis and enters the bladder appropriately. This is more significant in males, since the deviation probably represents a normal variation in most females. Other deviations may also be found. Rather than opening normally into the bladder, the ureters may open directly into the urethra or vagina. Openings into the bladder itself may be into abnormal portions of the wall, which often results in a backflow of urine during micturition. Treatment of these problems may involve reimplantation of the distal ends of the ureters or replacement of the ureters; these procedures are described below.

Duplicate ureters are found, each arising from a renal pelvis. There are several variations to this anomaly: (a) the ureters on one side may unite at some point along the way; (b) both may open in the normal portion on the trigone; or (c) one or both may open into the urethra or vagina.

Abnormal dilatation of the ureter is another type of congenital defect. A *ureterocele* is dilatation and pouching of the ureteric wall just adjacent to the vesicoureteral junction. This condition may also be called *mega-ureter* and causes problems because of its refluxing and/or obstructive effects. While it may be asymptomatic, the defect may result in loin pain due to backflow pressure on the kidney. These patients frequently have recurrent urinary tract infections.

Congenital pelvic ureteric obstruction occurs at the junction of the renal pelvis and the ureter. This occurs bilaterally about 10 per cent of the time and causes hydronephrosis from the backup of urine.

Bladder

Exstrophy of the bladder is a condition resulting from a lack of closure of the symphysis pubis. There is no abdominal wall and the open bladder protrudes through the surface. Since the bladder is not closed, urine leaks continuously, keeping the child wet and damaging the surrounding tissue. Treatment alternatives include dressing and diapering the area, functional closure, and urinary diversion following surgical removal of the bladder. Techniques for urinary diversion are discussed below. Whatever treatment is selected, both the child and the family require much skilled nursing care to help them cope with the difficult situation.

Two conditions, occurring more often in females, that cause recurrent urinary tract infections are *bladder-neck contractures* and *megalocystis.* Tightening of the lumen of the bladder can be caused by a fibrous ring at the point of insertion of the urethra at the base of the bladder. Megalocystis is a large-capacity bladder lacking in muscle tone.

Fistulas, or abnormal openings into the bowel or vagina, sometimes occur, as well as *separated bladder compartments* and *diverticula*. Fistulas and diverticula will be discussed below.

Urethra

Urethral anomalies are rare in females. Those that do occur include absence or atresia of the urethra, misplacement of the meatus, urethral stricture, and fistulas.

Congenital defects of the male urethra are not common. In addition to strictures, fistulas, atresia and megalourethra, misplacement of the meatus can occur. In *hypospadias,* the meatus is located along the under surface of the penis or, occasionally, in the scrotum or perineum. *Epispadias* is much less common and almost always accompanies exstrophy of the bladder. In this condition, the dorsal urethra is not closed or is absent. Both conditions require surgical-repair, usually done in several stages.

URINARY REFLUX

Probably the most common consequence of the congenital anomalies described above is *urinary reflux* or the backward flow of urine within the urinary tract. This problem usually occurs at the vesicoureteral junction so that urine backflows into the ureter and frequently into the renal pelvis. However, there can also be reflux at the urethrovesical junction when the urethra is improperly connected to the bladder. In addition to congenital malformations, reflux can also be caused by infectious processes in which edema and fixation of the intramural ureter or urethra interfere with the normal valve action. Neuromuscular malfunctions can contribute to reflux, as can bladder neck obstruction which causes increasing intravesical pressure to a point where it finally overrides the resistance of the ureteral sphincters.

The main result of urethrovesical reflux is an ever-present residual urine which is an important factor in the incidence of urinary tract infection. The continual presence of urine can also lead to changes in detrusor tone, increasing the bladder's capacity and raising the threshold at which the micturition reflex is initiated.

Infection and *renal damage* are the two primary problems resulting from vesicoureteral reflux. The kidneys are usually protected from ascending infections by the vesicoureteral sphincters; however, with reflux, any pathogens in the bladder are carried up the ureters to the kidney. Since the capacity of the renal pelvis is only 5 ml., any larger amounts of urine, whether they result from ureteral obstruction or from reflux, cause renal parenchymal changes. The increased hydrostatic pressure leads to renal cortical atrophy and calicectasis. The destruction of kidney tissue, often asymptomatic and undetected, can proceed to end-stage renal disease.

Treatment of urinary reflux includes conservative methods as well as surgical approaches. The decision about which to use depends on the age of the patient and the degree of kidney damage that has occurred or is expected to occur. Conservative treatment may be prescribed for children until puberty, at which time there will be increased bladder tonicity and elongation of the intramural portion of the ureter. The nonsurgical techniques include good perineal hygiene, early identification and treatment of urinary tract infections, and frequent bladder emptying. In a study of 102 patients with vesicoureteral reflux, 42 per cent had a spontaneous cessation after conservative treatment.[179]

The presence of renal damage usually dictates the need for surgical intervention. This group of patients includes almost all adults with urinary reflux. Other indicators for surgery include obstruction at the ureteropelvic junction, intractable infection, and lack of desired response to the maturation process. Since the most common causes of reflux are defects along the ureter, the most frequent surgical procedures used involve the ureter, e.g., reimplantation of the ureter(s).

Preoperative preparation of the patient having ureteral surgery is similar to that required by any patient. See Chapter 17.

Postoperatively, there will be a urethral or suprapubic catheter in place to keep the bladder empty in order to reduce tension on the suture line. A *ureteral catheter* will also be inserted into each ureter involved in the surgical procedure. This tiny catheter is made of a semirigid plastic material which contains a radiopaque strip so that its position can be determined by x-ray. It is inserted into the ureter with its tip frequently being placed in the renal pelvis; the distal end extends through the bladder and out through the urethra or through an abdominal incision. The placement of a ureteral catheter serves three purposes: to splint the ureter to facilitate healing, to prevent obstruction from edema following surgery or other trauma in the area, and to drain urine.

> *Since the renal pelvis holds only 5 ml. before tissue damage due to pressure begins, it is absolutely essential that ureteral catheters be kept patent. They are never clamped for any reason.*

The catheters are easily plugged with mucous shreds, blood clots, and chemical sediment. The doctor should be questioned before irrigation is done. If catheter irrigation is ordered, aseptic techniques must be used. A maximum of 5 ml. of irrigating solution, usually normal saline, should be allowed to flow in by gravity. If patency cannot be established, the doctor should be notified immediately.

If the catheter is not sutured in place, it should be secured to the patient's skin to avoid accidental removal. Each catheter — ureteral and urethral — should drain into its own collection bag so that reduced flow from any source will be immediately noticeable. Output from each of the catheters should be measured and recorded every hour for the first 24 hours and then every 4 to 8 hours until they are removed. It is expected that most of the urine will drain from the ureteral catheters for the first 48 to 72 hours postoperatively; then as the inflammation recedes, urine will flow around the ureteral catheters and be drained by the urethral or suprapubic catheter. It is also expected that as the patient recovers from the surgery, the color of the urine will progress from bright red to clear yellow over a matter of days. Fluid intake must be adequate to assure a good flow of urine.[136, 239]

URINARY RETENTION

Urinary retention means that the urine is retained in the bladder. Urine production continues, but accumulated urine is not released. One of the most common causes is obstruction at or below the bladder outlet. Prostatic hypertrophy occurs in 30 to 50 per cent of males after the age of 50 years. As the prostate gland enlarges, it constricts the urethra. Urethral valves, which are now considered to be congenital diaphragms in the urethra; urethral strictures; meatal stenosis; calculi; fibrosis; and tumors also obstruct the outflow of urine from the bladder. The pathologic effects of this obstruction include hypertrophy of the detrusor muscle; formation of bladder trabeculae, or development of connective tissue in the bladder wall; and diverticula of urinary organs proceeding to hydroureteronephrosis if the retention and increased intravesical pressure is not relieved.

Retention may also be the result of decreased sensory input to and from the bladder, muscle tension, and emotional anxiety. Surgery has traditionally been considered a contributory factor. In a study of 840 postoperative patients, it was found that 13.3 per cent needed catheterization before normal voiding could be re-established. One of the most significant variables was the administration of a spinal anesthesia either alone or in combination with general or regional anesthesia; 23.3 per cent of these patients required catheter drainage.[136] Medications, such as opiates, sedatives, antihistamines, antispasmodics, and psychotropic drugs can interfere with the normal neurologic function of the micturition reflex. Anorectal problems, such as hemorrhoids or fecal impaction, contribute to urinary retention, probably owing to either obstructive properties or to secondary spasm of the perineal musculature hampering the ability to relax. Poor fluid intake reduces glomerular filtration rate, and very slow urine production fills the bladder just as slowly. This may allow the detrusor muscle to accommodate to the increased volume in such a manner that the stretch receptors are never fully activated. Once the detrusor muscle fibers are stretched beyond a certain point, they become incapable of contracting at all, so micturition never occurs.

The cardinal sign of urinary retention is the absence of voided urine. However, it is necessary to differentiate between retention and oliguria or anuria. A distended bladder is the most important finding. As the bladder fills, it rises above the level of the symphysis pubis, sometimes being displaced to either side of midline. Percussion over the bladder produces a "kettledrum" sound. The patient may complain of increasing discomfort and the need to urinate and may become increasingly restless and diaphoretic. Intake and output measurements help predict the expected amount of urine production.

Frequent (more often than once an hour) voiding of 25 to 50 ml. of urine at a time may indicate *retention with overflow.* As the bladder continues filling, the intravesical pressure rises. At some point, this pressure overcomes the restraining ability of the sphincter. Enough urine flows out of the bladder to reduce the intravesical pressure to the level at which the external sphincter can again control the flow of urine. The patient may complain that the bladder does not feel really empty. The bladder starts filling again, and the cycle is repeated over and over. Specific gravity determinations of the voided urine aid in the differentiation of retention with overflow from oliguria.

The initial treatment of retention involves the use of independent nursing actions. Providing the patient with privacy, warming the bedpan before offering it to the patient, and placing the patient in a sitting position to enlist the aid of gravity and increased intra-abdominal pressure may also help to relieve the problem. Making use of the power of suggestion advocates running water within hearing of the patient or flushing the toilet. The use of an audio tape recording of aquatic sounds has been effective, although it is highly recommended that the patient use earphones for the "protection" of others. Pouring warm water over the perineum or sitting in a warm bath not only appeals to the power of suggestion, but also promotes muscle relaxation. Dabbling the hands in water sometimes works. Applying ice to or stroking the inner thigh with light pressure may stimulate trigger points which activate the micturition reflex. If the person is very tense and anxious, any measure that will help relaxation may aid in relieving the situation.

If the above measures are unsuccessful, then more definitive methods must be used to relieve the problem. Cholinergic medications may be used to stimulate bladder contraction, although they must never be used if mechanical obstruction is present. In this instance, intravesical pressure is increased against an obstructed outlet, which could result in vesicoureteral reflux or a ruptured bladder. Neostigmine and bethanechol are often administered. Bethanechol increases detrusor tone, but also increases bladder outlet and urethral resistance. To counteract this effect, it has been suggested that this medication be given with phenoxybenzamine, which is a potent alpha-adrenergic blocker. There is some indication that this drug combination may reduce the incidence of surgical intervention now used to increase intravesical pressure and decrease outlet and urethral resistance.[152]

Catheterization

If all other measures fail to effect urination, the bladder needs to be catheterized. Two routes of catheterization may be used: suprapubic or urethral.

The *suprapubic catheter* is inserted by the physician, often under a local anesthesia and frequently in the patient's room. A general anesthesia may be used if another surgical procedure is being performed too. The patient must have a distended bladder. The suprapubic skin is prepped. Using sterile technique, the catheter may be inserted through a small surgical incision or a trocar/cannula is passed through the skin into the bladder. Once the trocar/cannula is in place, the trocar is removed and the catheter is threaded through the cannula. Figure 42–1 shows the suprapubic catheter in position. The catheter is then attached to a closed drainage system as with the urethral catheter. The catheter may be sutured in place and/or secured with a commercially made retention body seal. Care of the patient with a suprapubic catheter is similar to that of a patient with a urethral catheter, although there may be no routine daily insertion site care. The most frequent problem is poor drainage due to mechanical obstruction, obstruction of the catheter tip by the bladder wall, or obstruction by sediment or clots. Disconnection of the catheter from the drainage tubing can disrupt the siphon drainage. When the catheter is removed, the muscle layers of the bladder immediately contract over the puncture site and the surface wound is small, negating the need for closing sutures.

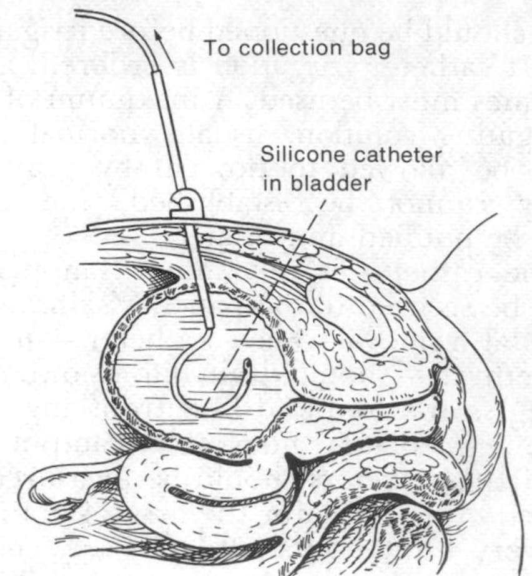

Figure 42–1. Suprapubic catheter in place within the bladder. (Adapted from Greena, W., et al.: Nonoperative suprapubic urinary drainage. *American Family Physician*, 16:136, Oct., 1977.)

A lower rate of urinary tract infections, ease in evaluating the patient's ability to void normally, and increased comfort for the patient are cited as advantages of the suprapubic catheter over the urethral catheter. However, the procedure is not without its risks. Potential complications include dislodgement of the catheter; hematuria, especially after the use of large-bore catheters; and bowel perforation during trocar insertion.

The *urethral catheter* is by far the most common one used. With appropriate orders from the physician, either a straight or retention catheter is inserted through the external meatus into the urethra beyond the internal sphincter into the bladder. A straight catheter is used when the catheter will be removed as soon as the urine is drained from the bladder. The retention or indwelling catheter is retained for an undetermined period, being kept in place with an inflated balloon near the tip of the catheter.

Regardless of the type of catheter being used, it is inserted using strict aseptic technique; the exception to this is the use of clean technique for out-patients on an intermittent catheter program. (See further discussion under neurogenic bladder.) The retention catheter is attached to either a bedside drainage bag or a leg bag. A *leg bag* is frequently used with long-term catheter draining, especially if the patient is going home with an indwelling catheter; this device allows the patient more mobility and eliminates the embarrassment of having to carry a drainage bag with its long tubing around for everyone to see. Figure 42–2 shows a leg bag in position on the calf. Because of the bag's small capacity, it must be emptied frequently. At night, a conventional drainage system is usually used so that the patient can sleep through the night without emptying the leg bag. This frequent opening of the system increases the chance of infection. The rubber straps holding the bag to the leg can cause skin irritation, thrombophlebitis, and ulcer formation if they are attached too tightly. Even if the straps are applied loosely, they tend to tighten as the bag fills. Meticulous skin care and periodic removal of the bag help prevent these problems. Cleanliness and odor control are managed by washing the apparatus with soap and water and soaking it in a 1 per cent acetic acid (vinegar) solution overnight.

The use of indwelling catheters is accompanied by several physical hazards, including urinary tract infection and tissue trauma. The incidence of urinary tract infection as a result of catheterization has been cited as ranging from 35 to 95 per cent, and a direct relationship between the development of bacteriuria and the length of time the catheter is left in place has been well documented.[40, 49, 276] Andriole reports that bacteriuria occurred in 50 per cent of the catheterized patients after 24 hours and increased to 98 to 100 per cent after 4 days.[100] The most common causative organisms are *Escherichia coli, Proteus, Klebsiella, Aerobacter, Pseudomonas aeruginosa, Streptococcus,* and *Staphylococcus.* These organisms may enter the urinary tract via the inside of the system when it is opened for any reason or up the exterior of the catheter in the thin layer of fluid and exudate that forms around the catheter. Further discussion of the development and treatment of urinary tract infection after the introduction of the organisms is included below.

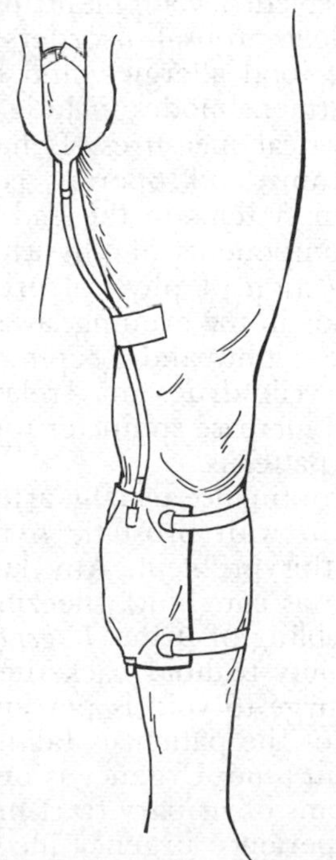

Figure 42–2. Condom drainage and leg bag. Leg bag may be attached to calf of leg, as shown, or to thigh.

Tissue trauma may occur during the catheterization procedure. Tissue necrosis may also be the result of use of an oversized catheter or of continuous pressure, as when not enough slack is left between the meatus and the site of taping on the leg or abdomen. An indwelling catheter continually moves in and out of the distal urethra. This constant friction can cause tissue breakdown, and the process is further enhanced if encrustation on the outside of the catheter is allowed to occur.

Assuring proper operation of the drainage system and preventing complications are primarily functions of nursing intervention. Patency must be maintained. Actions used to prevent infection include meticulous perineal care, maintaining a closed drainage system, avoiding backflow of urine, adequate fluid intake, urine acidification, and the prophylactic use of antimicrobial medications.

If the urinary retention is being caused by obstruction, removal of the occlusion is necessary for long-term relief. Dilatation of the urethra may be done with a rubber, indwelling catheter, inserting a larger diameter catheter each day. The urethra may be dilated more quickly with size-graduated sounds, filiforms and followers, or other dilating instruments; this is usually done under general or local anesthesia. Surgical intervention is sometimes necessary. If the bladder neck has become rigid due to inflammation, a cystoplasty may be done to insert an elastic wedge into the area. Removal of urethral strictures can be done with plastic repair of the urethra to return it to its proper functioning.

URINARY INCONTINENCE

Urinary *incontinence* is the inability of the urinary sphincters to control passage of urine from the body. There may be totally uncontrolled emptying of the bladder or a constant dribbling of urine. Whatever its form, this condition is highly embarrassing to patients, destroys their self-esteem, and can become the overwhelming force controlling their lives. Lack of control of voiding is associated with an infantile state and may lead to feelings of helpless-

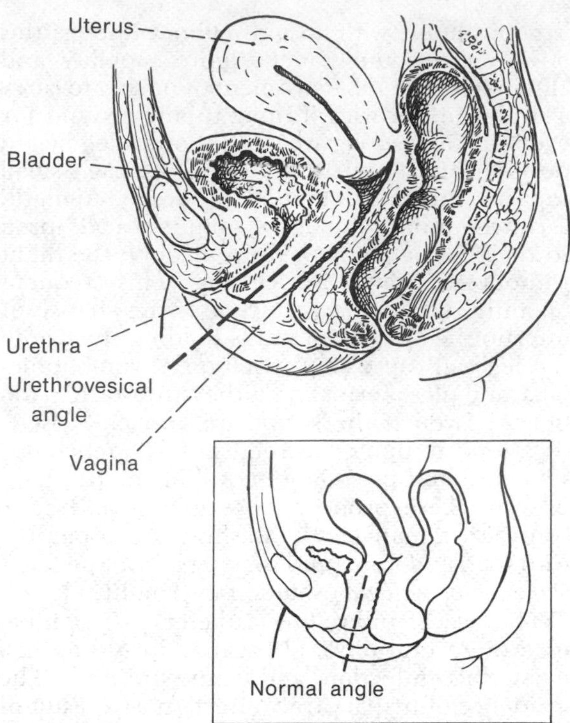

Figure 42–3. Alteration in the urethrovesical angle contributes to the occurrence of incontinence in the female. (Drawn from Butts, P.: Assessing urinary incontinence in women. *American Journal of Nursing*, 79:72, Mar., 1979.)

ness, hopelessness, and frustration. See Chapter 41 for further discussion of the psychosocial impact.

Incontinence can be caused by anything that interferes with sphincter control. This includes both psychologic and physiologic factors. Psychologic mechanisms that are important in the etiology of incontinence include regression, dependence on the part of the "mother" and/or the "child," rebellion, insecurity, manipulative attention-seeking, sensory deprivation, and a disturbance of conditioned reflexes which may result in the patient's failing to void on the toilet or bedpan but urinating when coming into contact with clean clothes or sheets.[331] Anatomic causes of incontinence result from sphincter weakness or damage, detrusor muscle instability, and weak abdominal perineal musculature. Common causes of sphincter damage are obstetrical trauma, postoperative weakness, and congenital weakness. The potential origin of detrusor instability includes local bladder lesions, e.g., infection, neoplasm, and senile "trigonitis"; lower motor neuron lesions, e.g., tumor, prolapsed disk, complication of pelvic surgery, and osteoarthritis of the lumbosacral spine; upper motor neuron lesions, e.g., cerebral vascular accident, multiple sclerosis, and transection of the spinal cord; and large bowel disease, e.g., spastic colon and diverticular disease. Recurrent urinary tract infections, previous gynecologic surgery, obstetric trauma, and senile vulvitis can lead to urethral narrowing.[217] Figure 42–3 shows how alteration of the urethrovesical angle in the female reduces the competency of the internal sphincter. It has also been found that women with stress incontinence have shorter urethras, which tend to telescope when the women stand; longer urethras are inclined to be more continent. Other factors that contribute to the development and maintenance of incontinence are medications, e.g., narcotics, sedatives, antihistamines, atropine-like substances, and ganglionic-blocking drugs; alcohol; fecal impaction; and scarring of the bladder and urethra with adhesion formation. Incontinence may be a sign of "giving up" or may be a matter of no one's answering the patient's call light.

TYPES OF INCONTINENCE

There are five main types of incontinence: enuresis, stress, urgency, paradoxical, and continuous. *Enuresis* is usually a problem of childhood, but does extend into adulthood in 1 to 3 per cent of the cases.[53] It involves incontinence of urine, especially at night. *Primary* enuresis means that there has never been a dry period; *secondary* enuresis is a resumption of night incontinence after a successful period of dryness. Theories regarding the etiology of this problem include delayed development, parental failure, genetics, sleep arousal disorders, toilet-training difficulties, food allergies, and behavior problems. Treatment modes include psychotherapy and/or physical measures. Behavior modification programs and operant conditioning by using alarm systems in the bed have met with success. Components of physical programs include correction of physical problems, restriction of fluids in the evening, awakening to void during the night, and keeping the bedroom warm. Tricyclic drugs may relax the detrusor muscle and increase sphincter tone or they may alter sleep patterns.

Stress incontinence usually affects women, although men with prostatic hypertrophy may also have this problem. Any kind of physical stress, such as coughing, sneezing, or laughing causes dribbling of urine. *Urgency* incontinence is the inability to hold back the flow of urine when the urge to void is perceived. The chief complaint of the patient is failure to reach the bathroom in time. Urgency is one of the cardinal symptoms of urinary tract infections. Some women experience urgency incontinence for a few days prior to the beginning of their menstrual period. *Paradoxical,* or overflow, incontinence is retention with overflow when the passing of small amounts of urine is not voluntary. *Continuous* incontinence is similar to that of the toddler before toilet-training. The act of urination is uninhibited and occurs whenever the micturition reflex is stimulated. The patient may or may not be aware of this kind of incontinence. The patient suffering with incontinence will have one or a combination of these forms.

MANAGEMENT OF INCONTINENCE

Management of incontinence, regardless of its form, requires first a complete diagnostic evaluation to identify causative factors that can either medically or surgically be alleviated. Urinary tract infection must be eliminated to reduce its continued irritation of the detrusor muscle. Measures should be taken to suppress any chronic cough. Some drugs can contribute to the problem, e.g., antihistamines, atropine-like and ganglionic-blocking agents, and should be stopped. Other medications can be used to decrease detrusor irritability, e.g., emepronium bromide, flavoxate hydrochloride, amobarbital, and propantheline bromide alone or in combination with thiopropazate hydrochloride. Although their use is controversial, topical or systemic estrogens are sometimes given to post-menopausal women to treat atrophic vaginitis and urethritis.

Weight reduction, if necessary, and pelvic exercises not only help in regaining of bladder control, but may also prevent occurrence of the problem. *Kegel exercises* are used specifically for resolution of stress incontinence. With the patient sitting in a chair with the feet planted on the floor and the knees spread, she is instructed to contract the perineal muscles as though stopping the expulsion of urine. This exercise should be repeated 10 times at four periods during the day. She should also try to start and stop the stream of urine whenever she voids.

A successful *bladder training program* requires patience of both the nurse and the patient and significant others. The first step in instituting the program is to discuss the procedure and expected outcome with the patient. Overall, the patient must be given hope that something, indeed, can be done about the incontinence problem.

A bladder training program revolves around an adequate fluid intake, a muscle-strengthening exercise program (as described above), and carefully scheduled voiding times. A specialized modification, called intermittent catheterization, is discussed below. During the program, although the patient's bed and clothing may be padded to protect them from becoming wet, actual diapering of the patient should be avoided. Diapering further demeans the patient and gives "permission" to be incontinent.

Many patients suffering from incontinence reduce their fluid intake, thinking this will result in no urine to be expelled and thus better control. Actually, adequate urine production is necessary to stimulate the micturition reflex. Therefore, unless contraindicated by the patient's physical status, daily fluid intake should be maintained at 2000 to 2500 ml. These fluids are carefully spaced through the day and are limited at bedtime to allow the patient to sleep for longer periods.

In the meantime, the patient is placed on the commode or toilet every 30 minutes to 2 hours and aided to void. The intervening time span is determined by the frequency of bladder emptying. As the program progresses, the patient is encouraged to hold the urine longer and the intervals are lengthened.

Electrical inhibition of the micturition reflex has been successful for many patients. These devices which deliver a barely perceptible electrical stimulation, may either suppress uninhibited detrusor contractions or increase outflow resistance by lengthening the urethra, increasing the tension of the urethral wall, decreasing the radius of the urethral lumen, and increasing the vesicourethral angle. The electrodes may be implanted surgically within the pelvic muscles for indirect stimulation, or direct stimulation may be achieved by using either intravaginal or anal devices. Figure 42–4 shows the three main types of electrical stimulators. The intravaginal or anal plugs can be removed and reinserted as necessary; the anal plug must be removed for defecation and needs to be cleaned frequently. Whatever apparatus is used is attached to a control box. The patient can activate the system as desired to alleviate the occurrence of incontinence.

Mechanical pressure is sometimes used to interfere with the outflow of urine. A *pessary* is inserted into the vagina where it exerts pressure on the bladder neck area. Some of these devices have inflatable balloons which can periodically be released to permit voiding. The use of pessaries had been linked with complications, including discomfort, leukorrhea, ulceration, fistulas, and malignancy. A *penile clamp*, as illustrated in Figure 42–5, can be used to compress the urethra in the male. The use of this appliance is controversial. If it is utilized, it must be removed and repositioned frequently to prevent pressure sore development on the penis.

Sometimes none of the conservative measures described above are effective. The nursing intervention must be aimed at protecting the patient's skin, clothing, bed linen, etc. If the skin

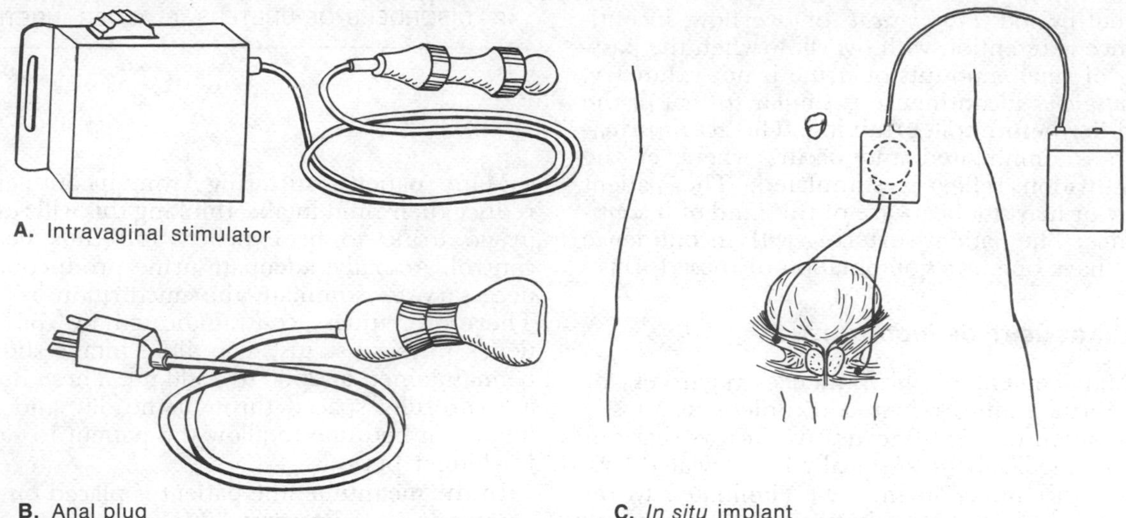

Figure 42–4. Devices used for electrical stimulation of the micturition reflex. The varieties include (*A*) an intravaginal stimulator, (*B*) an anal plug, and (*C*) an *in situ* implant with the electrodes placed within the muscle tissue and the aerial wires taped to the skin. (Adapted from Willington, F.: *Incontinence in the Elderly.* London: Academic Press, 1976.)

does become wet, it must be meticulously cleaned and dried to prevent the severe rashes and skin breakdown which result from maceration and ammonia production. However, the best way to accomplish this goal is to drain the urine away before it touches any of these surfaces. Indwelling catheters should be used only as a last resort because of their frequent contribution to bacteriuria. External drainage systems have been developed for men, but no successful device, except waterproof pants, has been created for women. *External condom drainage* involves a thin rubber or plastic sheath which is put over the penis and is connected to either a leg bag or a bedside drainage bag. Thus, when the urine is released from the bladder, it runs down the tube into the collecting device. The main problems with this system are leakage with or without detachment of the condom, twisting of the condom, and stasis of urine, which can cause maceration of the penis. Attachment of the condom sheath so that it stays in place and yet does not compromise circulation to the distal penis can sometimes be a challenge. It may be necessary to shave off the pubic hair before prepping the skin. The penis should be washed with soap and water and allowed to dry thoroughly; the penis is wiped with alcohol to remove skin oils and, if it is to be used, an adhesive is applied. When rolling the condom sheath up over the penis, care must be taken to allow at least 1.5 cm. between the distal end of the penis and the internal end of the sheath in order to reduce skin irritation (see Fig. 42–6). Only elastic tape should be used to allow for expansion during erections. A suggested method for applying the tape is to place two strips longitudinally and then another piece in a spiral fashion. Patency of the system should be checked frequently, and the condom should be removed periodically to allow the skin to be cleansed and to dry.

Another drainage system involves a *pubic pressure urinal*, as shown in Figure 42–7. This device is considered especially helpful for the patient with a small or receding penis. The flange is placed over the penis and attached to the waist belt, the thigh straps are fastened to the belt; then the cone-shaped top is fit over the penis and stretched to fit on the flange. If the patient is ambulatory, the penis cover is positioned diagonally, but otherwise, it is placed vertically, which prevents kinking.[17]

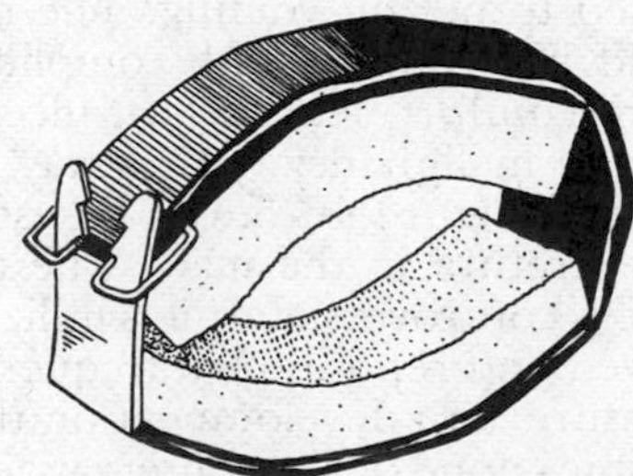

Figure 42–5. A penile clamp can be used to compress the urethra to prevent incontinence. (Drawn from Winter, C., and A. Morel: *Nursing Care of Patients with Urologic Diseases.* St. Louis: C. V. Mosby Co., 1977.)

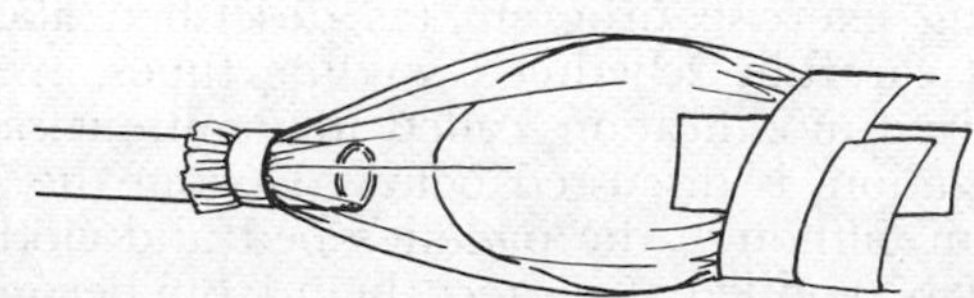

Figure 42–6. External condom drainage for the male patient. (Drawn from Winter, C., and A. Morel: *Nursing Care of Patients with Urologic Diseases.* St. Louis: C. V. Mosby Co., 1977.)

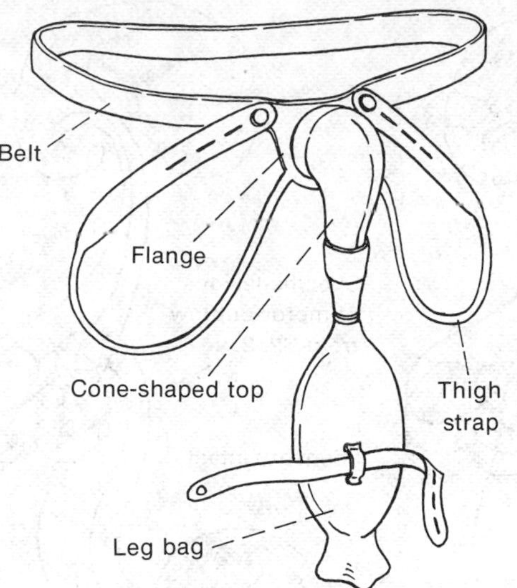

Figure 42–7. A pubic pressure urinal. (Drawn from Baum, M.: I want to be dry! *Nursing 78,* 8:75, Feb., 1978.)

SURGICAL INTERVENTION FOR INCONTINENCE

Surgical intervention may be utilized to correct or compensate for anatomic defects that are contributing to the incontinence. The most common surgical procedures are those intended to restore the normal urethrovesical angle. Frequently this involves elevation and suspension of the bladder using either tissue or inorganic materials for support. Marshall-Marchetti-Krantz and Pereyra are two commonly used techniques. Suspension procedures are also done on the urethra. Postoperatively, these patients frequently have suprapubic catheters for approximately eight days, during which time they are maintained on a high fluid intake to prevent occurrence of infection. During this time, constant patency of the drainage system must be preserved, since the pressure of a filling bladder may hinder the healing process. A *clamp and release program* is then initiated to help the detrusor muscle regain its tone. The catheter is clamped off for ever-lengthening intervals while urine collects in the bladder during the period of catheter occlusion. The catheter is opened periodically to let the bladder empty. The patient may void at any time that the desire to void is felt. After voiding, the amount of residual urine is measured to determine the effectiveness of bladder emptying; the amount of residual urine helps determine when the catheter can be removed.

Other surgical procedures used are aimed at providing an intact, patent route for the transport of urine. Removal is necessary for any scar tissue that may be interfering with the normal function of the bladder neck. If urethral or sphincter narrowing is contributing to the problem of incontinence, these must be dilated or the obstruction removed.

NEUROGENIC BLADDER DYSFUNCTION

Neurogenic bladder refers to a collection of bladder dysfunctions all of which are caused by lesions of the central or peripheral nervous systems. The signs and symptoms demonstrated by the patients depend on the site of the lesion.

There are five main types of neurogenic bladder dysfunction (Fig. 42–8):

- The *uninhibited neurogenic bladder* produces an "infant-like" voiding; as soon as the first urge to void is felt, urine is excreted. This type is caused primarily by lesions in the corticoregulatory tracts, e.g., cerebrovascular accident, multiple sclerosis, myelomeningocele.
- The *sensory paralytic bladder* is the result of interruption in the lateral spinal tracts, e.g., tabes dorsalis and diabetic neuropathy. Because of the sensory loss, the patient cannot perceive bladder filling; this leads to chronic retention with overflow incontinence.
- A *motor paralytic bladder* is the most uncommon type and is caused by defects in the motor outflow from sacral vertebrae 2, 3, and 4. Disease processes that can cause this dysfunction include poliomyelitis, tumor, trauma, and infection. Although the patient has full sensation of bladder filling, even to the point of pain, he or she is unable to initiate micturition.
- The patient with an *autonomous neurogenic bladder* can neither perceive bladder fullness nor initiate or maintain urination without employing some means of assistance, such as applying external pressure on the abdomen; stress incontinence is a common complaint. It occurs following destruction of all nerve connections between the bladder and the central nervous system, e.g., trauma, inflammatory processes, and malignancy.
- Finally, transection of the spinal cord above the sacral segments causes a *reflex neurogenic bladder*. There is no sensation and the bladder contracts reflexly, but does not completely empty. The patient's neurogenic bladder may be one of the above types alone or a combination of more than one.

Neurogenic bladder dysfunctions may also be classified according to the level of the lesion within the central nervous system. *Upper motor neuron* causes occur above the sacral segments of the spinal cord, while lesions in or below the sacral vertebrae produce a *lower motor neuron* bladder.

"Cord" bladder results from acute injury to or disease of the spinal cord. In the acute stage, the bladder is atonic or flaccid. This period is called the *spinal shock phase* and may last from weeks to months. In the *recovery stage,* the motor and sensory functions of the bladder begin to return and the patient is started on an active rehabilitation program.

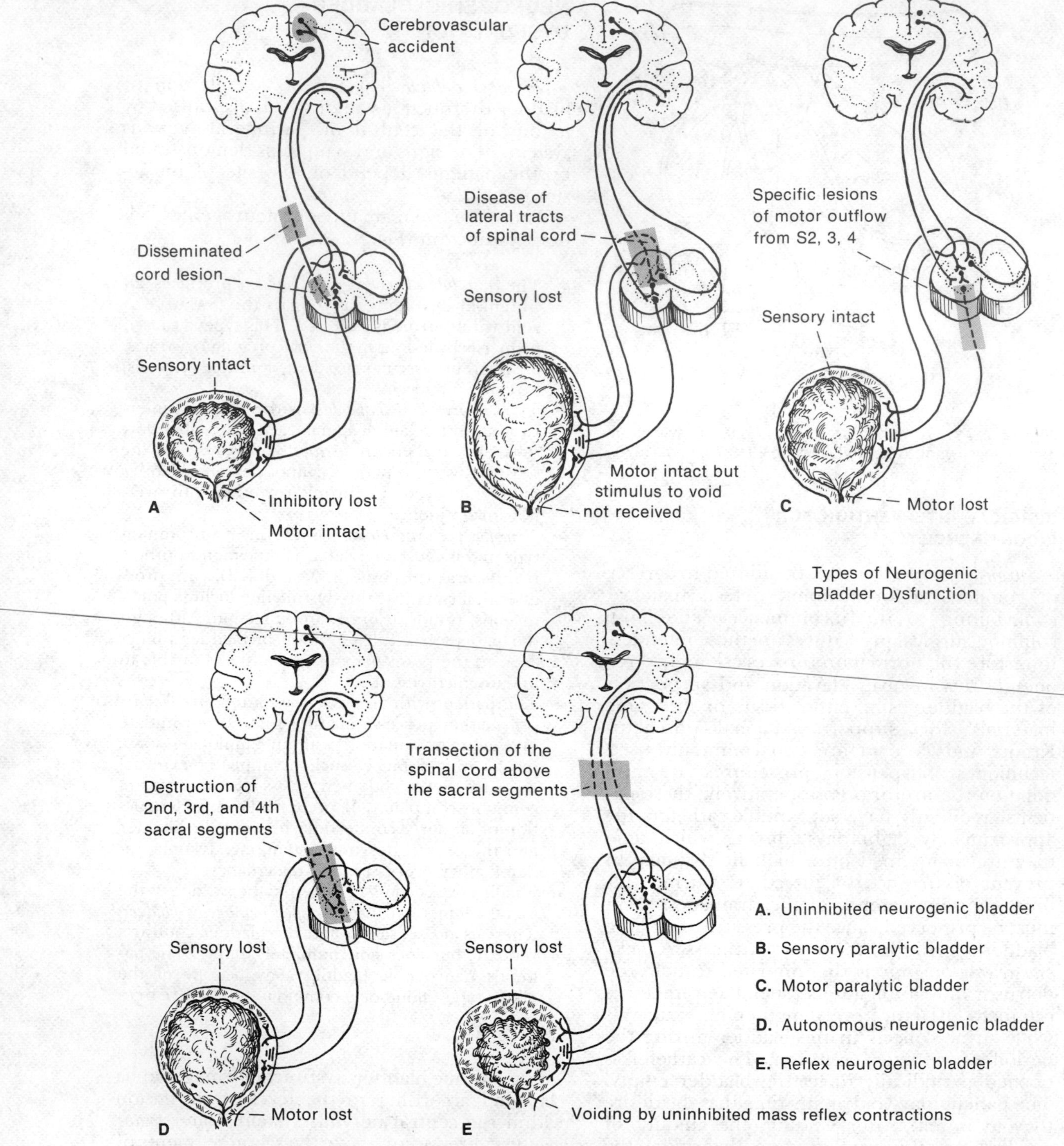

Figure 42–8. Types of neurogenic bladder dysfunction.

Rehabilitation of the patient with a neurogenic bladder includes a bladder training program with or without the use of intermittent catheterization, chemotherapy, and sometimes surgical intervention. A bladder training program, with its suggestions for fluid intake, scheduled bladder emptying, and exercises was described above. Because patients with a neurogenic bladder may have difficulty initiating and maintaining urination, they may need to be taught ways to help stimulate the reflex. Providing external pressure on the abdomen augments the force of the contracting detrusor muscle. This may be accomplished by simply leaning forward, bending at the waist, and/or pushing on the abdomen with the hand or arm. Taking a deep breath pushes the diaphragm down. The patient may be instructed to wear a corset or girdle as a source of external pressure. The *Credé maneuver* involves placing the fingers over the bladder and pressing down slowly; the pressure is exerted downward toward the symphysis pubis as though "milking" the urine out of the urinary system. This technique, which can be done by either the nurse or the patient, must be used with care. If used in patients with upper motor neuron lesions, the maneuver can cause urethral dyssynergia, and any obstruction to outflow from the bladder could result in ureteral reflux.

The patient can utilize several methods to initiate and maintain micturition. Trigger points on the body, e.g., lower abdomen, inner thighs, and pubic area, are located and stimulated by stroking, pinching, or applying ice. Because they are both innervated by the pudendal nerve, stretching of the anal sphincter also causes reflex relaxation of the external urethral sphincter. The patient leans forward while sitting on the toilet and inserts two gloved fingers into the anus. The fingers are then either stretched apart or pulled posteriorly. The male must be careful to avoid touching the glans penis, which stimulates the bulbocavernous reflex resulting in contraction of the external sphincter.

Autonomic hyperreflexia, also called *autonomic dysreflexia*, is a serious, potentially life-threatening complication that occurs to spinal cord–injured patients during a bladder training program (or if their urinary drainage system becomes obstructed). This condition is the result of an excessive autonomic response to normal stimuli and affects primarily patients with upper motor neuron lesions. Although it can be triggered by any visceral distention or stimulation of pain receptors on the skin, bladder distention is the most frequent cause. The most common symptoms are excessively increased blood pressure, bradycardia, throbbing headache, flushing, diaphoresis below the level of the lesion, blurred vision, nasal congestion, nausea, and pilomotor spasm. If left untreated, the hypertension can lead to seizures and/or stroke. The patients must be taught to recognize the symptoms so they can summon help immediately when manifestations first appear.

> *Autonomic hyperreflexia is considered a medical emergency. The initial treatment is to remove the triggering stimuli, e.g., re-establishing the urine flow and removing a fecal impaction if necessary – but only after inserting a topical anesthetic into the rectum to offset further stimulation.*

Catheterization may be necessary or, if a catheter is already in place, patency of the system must be restored. Vital signs should be monitored every five minutes and the head of the bed should be placed in a semi-Fowler's position. Medications, such as diazoxide, phenoxybenzamine, guanethidine sulfate, propantheline bromide, and mecamylamine hydrochloride may be used to relieve the acute symptoms and chronic occurrence of the episodes. Intrathecal instillation of tetracaine hydrochloride may be used to block nerve conduction. Surgical intervention may finally be needed to prevent recurrence.[84, 148]

INTERMITTENT CATHETERIZATION PROGRAMS

For treatment of long- or short-term bladder atony, an *intermittent catheterization* program may be instituted as an alternative to long-term indwelling catheterization. The program consists of inserting a straight urethral catheter into the bladder at specified time intervals, draining the urine, and removing the catheter. The catheterization procedure may be done by the patient (self-catheterization) or by anyone in the environment who has been properly trained. Patients are encouraged to learn self-catheterization as soon as possible, since it greatly increases their independence and allows for expansion of their environment.

Clean technique rather than a sterile one is usually recommended for the catheterization procedure, especially for patients outside the hospital with its high risk of nosocomial infections. Studies have shown that clean technique produces no increase in the rate of urinary tract infections as compared with sterile technique. The main procedural differences between these two methods are that, in clean catheterization, gloves are not worn, so good handwashing or the use of treated towelettes is essential; a clean rather than a sterile catheter is used; and, because of the natural lubrication of the female urethra, females use no lubricant on the catheter. Males do use a water-soluble lubricant because of the length of the urethra; they are more susceptible to traumatic urethritis. Most authorities advocate washing the catheter with soap and water after the procedure, rinsing and drying, and then storing the catheter in a plastic sandwich bag or other clean container. The catheter may be periodically sterilized by boiling.

The patient's position during self-catheterization may be either sitting or standing. When the female utilizes a standing posture, she usually has one foot on the floor and places the other on a chair or the toilet seat to allow better identification of the meatus. A mirror may be used at first by the female as she is learning to locate the meatus, but she should not be allowed to become dependent upon it, since she may frequently find herself in situations without a mirror.

Timing is the key factor in the success of intermittent catheterization programs. Catheterizations must be carried out at specified time intervals throughout the 24-hour period. A patient who is incapable of adhering to this schedule is not an appropriate candidate for the program. The time interval between catheterizations is set for each individual according to the degree of continence. The initial time interval for adults is every four hours. This interval is gradually lengthened as the patient progresses.

There is much variety in the amount of fluids allowed. Some programs allow the patient to have fluids as desired, while others restrict fluid intake to varying degrees. This particular aspect of the program needs systematic investigation.

Although not 100 per cent effective with all people, intermittent catheterization programs seem to be a viable alternative. Success is measured by two main parameters: catheter-free bladder and absence of bacteriuria. Studies report sterile urine in 39 to 77 per cent of the patients and achievement of a catheter-free bladder in 72 to 91 per cent of the program participants.[232, 238, 346] Other advantages include increased independence, better hygiene, and ease of sexual relations.

Intermittent catheterization is not, however, a panacea. The literature documents cases in which the program was not successful for a variety of reasons. The program does require a lot of responsibility on the part of the patient. Also, some patients have developed a silent hydronephrosis secondary to obstruction, infection, or reflux due to abnormally high resting bladder pressures. This condition is discovered only by means of an excretory urogram and monitoring of renal function, both of which should be done frequently. The problem can be reversed by insertion of an indwelling catheter.[137]

MEDICAL AND SURGICAL INTERVENTION

Medications can be used to treat neurogenic bladder dysfunction. Antispasmodics and anticholinergics, e.g., dicyclomine, propantheline, and flavoxate, may be given to relieve uninhibited or reflex bladder contractions. Phenoxybenzamine and other alpha-adrenergic blocking agents may be utilized. Bethanechol chloride is frequently administered to stimulate an atonic bladder.

If the above conservative measures are ineffective, surgical intervention may be necessary. External sphincterotomy or repair of the bladder neck may restore normal bladder function. An uninhibited bladder may be helped by interrupting innervation to the bladder reflex. Injection of alcohol into the subarachnoid space or rhizotomy (cutting) of the sacral nerves is done to increase bladder capacity by inhibiting reflex bladder contractions without interfering with normal sphincter function. Sometimes, temporary sacral nerve blocks are done before permanent surgical interruption to help evaluate potential candidates. In another procedure, electrodes may be implanted in the thoracic or cervical levels of the spinal epidural space and then attached to a percutaneous stimulator. As soon as the patient gets the intensity of the electrical stimulation properly regulated, the device can be used to interfere with reflex bladder contractions. Finally, if all else fails, urinary diversion (see discussion below) may be done to give the patient a more manageable urinary system.

URINARY TRACT INFECTION

Urinary tract infection is a very prevalent problem. Primarily because of the anatomy of the female urethra and perineum, women are more often affected than men, and sexually active or pregnant women are most vulnerable. The most common causative organisms are *Escherichia coli, Klebsiella, Aerobacter, Proteus,* and *Pseudomonas,* and the source of most of these organisms is the patient's own colon. In the past, *Serratia marcescens* was considered to be a nonpathogen but has recently become identified more and more with serious infections.

Several pathophysiologic mechanisms are implicated in the development of urinary tract infections. The principal factor is the overcoming of the host's resistance by invading organisms. Normally the bladder is inherently resistant to infection. Even though numerous pathogens reach the bladder, sterility of the urine is usually quickly re-established. This resistance to infection is probably due to antibacterial properties of the bladder mucosa, and maybe of the urine, and to phagocytosis. The mechanical action of voiding also removes organisms from the lower urinary tract. Anything that breaks down these defenses opens the way for an infectious process. Loss of the integrity of the mucosal lining may be caused by an indwelling catheter, calculus, or parasites. Lapides has postulated that many urinary tract infections are the result of bladder distention. As the bladder wall overdistends, blood flow decreases. The ischemic tissue is now more vulnerable to organism invasion. Common causes of overdistention include urethral obstruction and suppression of voiding. Infection can also occur from the patient's own gut via the hematogenous or lymphogenous route.[175]

Female anatomy makes women more susceptible to urinary tract infection. The short urethra mechanically reduces the distance between the bladder and the external environment. The location of the external meatus makes it very vulnerable to contamination. Studies have identified colonization of the vaginal introitus with enterobacteria as a significant variable characteristic of women who suffer recurrent urinary tract infections; this increases the bacterial environment of the perineum.[92]

There are a number of other predisposing factors. Sexual intercourse increases the susceptibility of women because of the resultant inflammation of the urethra; this can further lead to strictures which result in urinary stasis and pooling of a good growth medium. Hormonal changes in the aging woman cause alteration of the vaginal pH and thus vaginal flora. Previous urinary tract infection makes the patient more vulnerable to recurrent infections. The convalescent bladder is less resistant to bacterial invasion, and studies show that this period of susceptibility increases in length with each successive infection.[172] The presence of an indwelling bladder catheter greatly increases the risk of urinary tract infection for the patient. Undergarments made of synthetic fibers have been implicated. Studies are also being done to determine the relationship of stress to the development of infection.

Ureteritis

Ureteritis is associated with pyelonephritis, which is discussed in Chapter 43. Curing the kidney infection cures the ureteral inflammation, except when chronic infection causes the ureter to become fibrotic and strictures occur.

Cystitis

Cystitis is an inflammation of the bladder wall. It is the most frequent site of infection within the urinary tract, and infection in the ureter and kidney are frequently caused by ascending bacteria.

The symptoms are usually localized to the urinary tract: burning on urination, frequency, and urgency. Low back pain is commonly present. Other symptoms include hematuria, cloudy urine, abdominal pain, malaise, chills, fever, nausea and vomiting, and flank pain. It must be remembered that approximately 10 per cent of the patients with bacteriuria are asymptomatic so that accompanying signs and symptoms are not necessarily the best way to diagnose the presence of urinary tract infection. The final diagnosis is based on the results of urine cultures.

Treatment is multifaceted and may be different for a patient suffering an initial acute infection than for a patient with recurrent infections. The principal component is an antibiotic specific to the causative organisms. Commonly used *pharmacologic agents* include trimethoprim-sulfamethoxazole, nitrofurantoin, ampicillin, gentamycin, sulfasoxazole, methenamine mandelate, phenazopyridine, and the cephalosporins. Medications containing azo dyes are thought to have an anesthetic effect on the urinary tract mucosa and may be used to treat the burning. The antibiotic therapy usually must be continued for some time after the symptoms subside to ensure elimination of the organisms; however, some studies are being done to determine the effectiveness of single-dose therapy. Patients with recurrent urinary tract infections may be on antibiotics for months. There is controversy concerning the prophylactic use of antibiotics with high-risk patients, such as those that have an indwelling catheter. While some feel that this practice delays or prevents the onset of urinary tract infection, others propose that, partially because of the large number of potential causative organisms, choosing the appropriate drug would be very difficult. There is also documented evidence of a growing number of resistant organisms in the urinary tract. One of the most frequent uses of prophylactic antibiotics is with women whose recurrent infections seem to be related to sexual intercourse. These patients may be instructed to take a single dose of medication post-intercourse; the most widely used drugs include nitrofurantoin, nalidixic acid, and the cephalosporins.[319]

Other than *surgical correction* of strictures or other anatomic abnormalities, further treatment of cystitis can be done through independent nursing intervention. *Increased fluid intake* keeps the urine osmolarity low and facilitates frequent voiding to rid the bladder of infected urine. It has been documented that *acidifying the urine* decreases the rate of bacterial multiplication. The most common method of doing this is to have the patient drink cranberry juice. Cranberries contain rather large amounts of quinic acid which is excreted in the urine as hippuric acid. This is unlike other fruits which actually have an alkaline metabolic end reaction. Other sources advocate the use of therapeutic doses of vitamin C, or ascorbic acid. The literature is somewhat contradictory regarding both the long- and short-term therapeutic effects of either of these measures and indicates the need for further investigation.[201, 224] An acid-ash diet is an effective means of acidifying the urine. Foods encouraged in this diet are meats, eggs, cheese, prunes, cranberries, plums, and whole grains. Forbidden foods include carbonated beverages, anything made with baking powder or soda, fruits other than those mentioned above, most vegetables, olives, pickles, and nuts other than peanuts. The nurse can help the patient select an appropriate diet.

Many nursing measures are aimed also at preventing recurrences. Patients are encouraged to void at least every 2 to 3 hours during the day and one or two times at night to prevent bladder distention. They may be instructed to empty their bladder and drink two glasses of water immediately after sexual intercourse. Good perineal hygiene is important, and female patients must be taught to wipe from front to back. Patients must be taught to avoid all predisposing factors discussed above.

Urethritis

Urethritis is an inflammation of the urethra. It can occur as a sudden, acute infection, or it may be found in a chronic state. Causes include bacterial invasion, bubble bath, perfumed soaps, feminine hygiene sprays, and spermicidal jellies. Urethritis is frequently a component of venereal disease. (See Chapter 85 for further discussion of this entity.)

Symptoms, as with cystitis, include burning on urination, frequency, and nocturia. There may be pain in the urethra with movement. There is redness and irritation of the lining of the urethra, and the lips of the meatus may be swollen. There is frequently a discharge in the male, but not usually in the female.

Treatment includes removal of the cause of the urethritis and administration of systemic and/or topical antibiotics if it is caused by an infection. Sitz baths and forcing fluids may be helpful. Sexual intercourse should usually be avoided until the symptoms subside and then different positions and the use of lubrication should be discussed with the patient. Contributory factors should be avoided to prevent recurrence.

URINARY BLADDER CALCULI

Urinary *calculi*, or stones, are formed primarily in the kidney, with some originating in the bladder. This section will discuss only bladder stones — their causes, signs and symptoms, and treatment. Renal stones and their movement into the ureter as well as a full discussion of the etiology and types of, treatment for, and measures used to prevent recurrence of urinary calculi in general is included in Chapter 43.

Formation of bladder calculi may be induced by infection, presence of any foreign body, failure to empty the bladder normally, and obstruction. Stones originally formed in the kidney may continue to grow while in the bladder. As long as these stones remain in the bladder, they frequently cause no symptoms at all, although many patients complain of cystitis symptoms. A very large stone may produce a heavy feeling in the suprapubic region and a decreased bladder capacity and may cause an intermittent urinary stream if it lodges against the bladder neck during micturition. The stone may cause partial or total obstruction and/or mucosal trauma if it enters the urethra.

If it is suspected that the patient has urinary stones, the nurse may need to strain all urine voided through at least four layers of gauze pads. After straining, the nurse inspects the pads carefully for any stones filtered from the urine. During this time, the nurse may also need to encourage the patient to drink 3000 to 4000 ml. of fluid per day unless otherwise contraindicated. This helps wash stones out of the bladder and hinders the continued formation by keeping the urine dilute.

It is hoped that just waiting will allow the stones to be passed from the bladder naturally. However, if this does not happen, or if cystograms show that the calculus is too large to pass through the urethra safely, surgical intervention will be necessary. One of two approaches is used: suprapubic or transurethral. A suprapubic incision may be made into the bladder and the stones removed. The procedure is called a *cystolithotomy.* Postoperative care of the patient is similar to that required by a patient having a suprapubic prostatectomy (see Chapter 82). Transurethrally, removal of small stones may be done with a cystoscope. Large stones may be broken up with an instrument called a lithotrite (stone crusher). This process is called *lithotripsy.* Another method, *litholapaxy*, involves crushing the stone and then irrigating the bladder to wash out the pieces. Postoperatively, the nurse must monitor the patient for signs of hemorrhage, urinary retention, infection, and stone recurrence.

NEOPLASMS

Cancer of the urinary tract accounts for 9 per cent of all cancers among men and 4 per cent among women. Approximately 38,000 people die each year from cancer arising in the urinary system and male genital tract.[93] See Unit IX for a general discussion of patients with neoplastic disorders.

Ureter Neoplasms

Tumors arising primarily in the ureter are rare. Usually these are an extension of renal or bladder neoplasms or of tumors originating in the bowel, uterus, or ovary. Those primary neoplasms that do occur are usually a papillary transitional-cell or squamous-cell carcinoma and are most frequently found in the lower third of the ureter. Ureteral cancer occurs predominantly in males in the sixth and seventh decades of life.

One protocol for *staging ureteral cancer* is as follows: Stage A — submucosal infiltration; Stage B — muscular invasion; Stage C — periureteral fat involvement; Stage D — extension outside the ureter to adjacent structures, regional lymph nodes, or distant metastases.[16] Common sites for metastasis include the lungs and liver.

Usually the first sign of ureteral malignancy is gross hematuria. Development of the tumor is normally painless until obstruction has occurred, when the patient may complain of flank pain. Confirmation of the diagnosis is made through urine cytology, excretory urogram, and cystoscopy.

Treatment of ureteral cancer almost exclusively involves surgical intervention, although radiation may be used in advanced cases with local extension. Customarily, the surgical procedure used is removal of the kidney, ureter, and attached segment of the bladder on the involved side. Some investigation is being done on long term results of local excision of the tumor. If removal of all or part of the ureter is to be done, consideration must be given to replacement of the ureter in order to retain an intact urinary system. The material used must be chemically inert, flexible yet able to keep its inner shape and remain free of urinary stasis, capable of maintaining water-tight anastomosis lines, resistant to urinary salt deposits, resistant to reflux, and able to last the patient's lifetime. Substances that have met these criteria include silicone rubber, Teflon, and bovine carotid heterografts.[3, 11] Pre- and postoperative care of the patient is similar to that suggested for patients having nephrectomy, ureteral reimplantation, and/or segmental resection of the bladder, depending on the procedure performed.

If the decision is made not to do any of the above procedures, some palliative measure may be needed to prevent or alleviate obstruction of the ureter by the malignancy. Urinary diversion, as described below, may be done, or a ureteral stent catheter may be placed into the ureter to maintain its patency. This catheter has wings on it to prevent its dislodgement by ureteral peristaltic waves or by gravity and a flange to prevent its migration up the ureter.[104] It is placed during cystoscopy.

Bladder Cancer

Bladder cancer is the most frequent neoplasm of the urinary tract and accounts for approximately 3 per cent of the deaths due to cancer. It occurs most frequently in the fifth to seventh decades and affects men 2.3 times as often as women.[93]

Etiology of this disease process may come from several sources. Industrial exposure to certain substances may cause bladder cancer. Exposure to aniline dye used in rubber and cable manufacture may be linked to tumors occurring up to 20 years later. Workers in the textile and leather industries also seem to be at greater risk. Although reports are somewhat contradictory, there seems to be a link between smoking and bladder malignancies, thought to be the result of carcinogenic metabolites produced by abnormal tryptophan metabolism.[96] Pelvic radiation and the use of cyclophosphamide and azothioprine therapy increase the patient's risk. For several years, the artificial sweeteners saccharin and cyclamate have been under suspicion as causative factors. Cyclamates were banned by the United States government in 1969.

Investigation continues regarding saccharin. Studies in which rats were fed massive doses of saccharin demonstrated an increased incidence of bladder tumors; however, human studies have failed to show this. Kessler compared the saccharin intake of 209 patients with recently diagnosed bladder cancer and 209 similar patients without bladder disease and found no difference.[151] Studies on diabetic patients with relatively high intakes have not demonstrated an increased number of bladder tumors. Cohen states that for the overweight person, the ingestion of one diet soft drink carries with it a risk equal to the risk of taking in one additional kilocalorie.[57] Chronic cystitis, bladder calculous disease, schistosomiasis, or a large phenacetin intake may also predispose the patient to bladder cancer.

Most bladder cancers are papillomatous growths within the bladder lumen, although these may also infiltrate the bladder wall. Nodular tumors are less frequent and have a tendency to invade the bladder wall. Cellular proliferation is chiefly of the transitional epithelium, although squamous cell or adenocarcinoma may occur. Rhabdomyosarcoma is a tumor with a very poor prognosis, occurring primarily in infancy.

Bladder tumors are frequently graded as a way to communicate their cell-type. *Grade I tumors* are called atypical transitional-cell papillomas or transitional-cell carcinomas because they resemble benign papillomas. *Grade II growths* are transitional-cell papillary carcinomas that are larger and have a more extensive attachment to the bladder wall. *Grades III and IV* are poorly differentiated and usually nodular.

Staging of the tumor indicates the depth of its penetration into the bladder wall and its degree of metastasis. This determination is crucial in the decision about treatment mode. Clinical staging requires the results of at least an excretory urogram, cystoscopy, biopsy, and bimanual examination under anesthesia. Figure 42–9 demonstrates the usual staging schema used. Stage 0 is limited to the mucosa, while Stage A indicates invasion no further than the submucosa. A Stage B_1 tumor extends not more than halfway through the muscle layer, and Stage B_2 is more deeply into the muscle layer but not into the fat. A Stage C neoplasm has infiltrated beyond the muscle layer but is not metastatic or invading adjacent structures. Stage D tumors are metastatic with D_1 to the pelvic lymph nodes and/or adjacent organs and D_2 beyond the pelvis.[78] Common sites for metastasis include the liver, bones, and lungs. The "prognostic dividing line" seems to be between Stages B_1 and B_2 with tumors staged higher on the scale having a much poorer outlook.

Painless hematuria is the most frequent first sign, occurring in up to 75 per cent of patients. Unfortunately, this bleeding is usually intermittent in the early stages, which accounts for frequent delays on the part of the patient in seeking medical advice and on the part of the physician in further evaluation. As the disease progresses, the patient may complain of bladder irritability with frequency and dysuria. Symptoms of obstruction or the development of a fistula may cause the patient to seek help.

In addition to the diagnostic tests used for staging the tumor, other measures may be used to detect the presence of bladder tumors. Biologic markers may be a valuable aid. A 90 per cent accuracy has been found in correlating cytology results and the presence of urinary fibrinogen degradation products with the disease activity.[321] Measuring the concentration of epithelial cells in the urine may be helpful. Since tetracycline is held in necrotic tissue for a prolonged time and fluoresces under ultraviolet light, this drug may be administered prior to cystoscopy. The detection of leukoplakia, or grayish-white lesions within the bladder indicate a high potentiality for malignancy.

CHEMOTHERAPY AND RADIATION THERAPY IN BLADDER CANCER

In the treatment of bladder cancer, several *chemotherapeutic agents* are being used. Work is continuing in the search for an effective standard protocol. Cyclophosphamide and adriamycin have had some success, although results seem to be better when they are used in combination. In preliminary studies, a compound of cis-platinum diamine dichloride, cyclophosphamide, and doxorubicin hydrochloride (CISCA) has shown a good response.[296] Instillation of alkylating agents, such as thiotepa or mitomycin-C, into the bladder has had some success with superficial tumors. Local application of formalin may be used to control bladder hemorrhage which may result from the cancer itself or from radiation or cyclophosphamide trauma. Under anesthesia, necrotic tissue and clots are removed and the bleeding points treated with fulguration. The formalin is instilled, allowed to remain in the bladder for a time, and then drained. Care must be taken to prevent vesicoureteral reflux of the chemical. 5-Fluorouracil can be used systemically or may be infused directly into the hypogastric artery for advanced disease. The use of *immunotherapy*, e.g., bacille Calmette-Guerin (BCG) vaccine, is

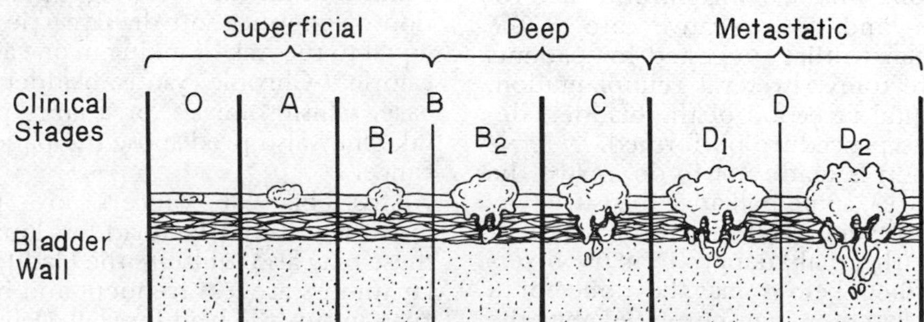

Figure 42–9. Jewett-Marshall clinical staging of bladder cancer. (Adapted from Whitmore, W.: Bladder Cancer. *Ca—A Cancer Journal for Clinicians*, 28:170, May–June, 1978.)

being investigated for its treatment value resulting from stimulation of the immune system or from direct alteration of the tumor's genetic material (see Chapter 23).

Radiation therapy is an accepted treatment mode, primarily for more advanced disease, although its value in early stage disease is gaining recognition. *Intracavitary* radiation is achieved by inserting an indwelling catheter with its balloon filled with isotopes or, infrequently, by implanting radium, tantalum, or gold seeds or wires around the base of the bladder. Radium may also be implanted in the uterus or vagina. This type of therapy is used to treat superficial tumors. The urine from these patients may need to be saved and sent to the radioisotope department for monitoring, and the patient may be isolated from others. *External supervoltage* radiation has not been very successful when used alone, but has been effective when used in combination with surgery or chemotherapy. It may be used preoperatively for advanced malignancies, although frequently surgery is done to determine the stage of the tumor, and temporary diversion procedure is done before radiation is begun. In a study of 724 patients, Miller found that those having preoperative radiation followed by cystectomy had significantly fewer local failure rates and more 10-year survivals than those having only radioisotope treatment or postoperative radiation; there were, however, more major complications.[212] *Megavoltage* techniques, which allow a more precise aiming of the rays, have improved the possibilities of using radiation for superficial tumors. Palliative radiation may be used to relieve pain, bowel obstruction, and leg edema secondary to venous or lymphatic obstruction, or to control bladder hemorrhage.

The patient receiving radiation therapy has a significant risk for developing complications. The most frequently occurring ones include severe cystitis and proctitis, causing dysuria, frequency, urgency, nocturia, and diarrhea. Treatment includes antispasmodics, increased fluid intake, and urinary tract antiseptics for the cystitis and a low residue diet and agents which decrease intestinal motility for the proctitis. Delayed effects, such as ileitis and colitis, persistent cystitis, and bladder ulceration and hemorrhage may occur as late as 6 to 12 months after the radiation.

SURGICAL TREATMENT OF BLADDER CANCER

Surgical treatment ranges from local resection and fulguration of the tumor to total cystectomy, which necessitates diversion of the normal urinary flow. *Transurethral resection* of the tumor and *fulguration* (destruction of tissue by electric current through electrodes placed in direct contact with the growth) are usually used for some superficial malignancies. Hematuria is expected postoperatively and the patient will usually have an indwelling catheter until the bleeding ceases. Sometimes, the catheter will be attached to a continuous or intermittent closed bladder irrigation system to prevent clots from obstructing the catheter. Care of the patient is similar to that needed after a cystoscopy or transurethral prostatectomy (see Chapter 82). This includes an adequate fluid intake and analgesics and antispasmodics as necessary.

A *segmental resection*, or *partial cystectomy*, is used for tumors located in the mobile parts of the bladder which can be sacrificed, such as the dome and those involving the ureteral orifice. In this procedure, up to half the bladder may be removed. During the initial postoperative period, the bladder capacity will be markedly reduced; the postoperative bladder may be able to hold no more than 60 ml. However, over a period of several months, the bladder tissue will regenerate, increasing the volume capability to 200 to 400 ml.

In addition to the usual postoperative care for patients having had a segmental resection of the bladder, *it is absolutely crucial that the bladder be continuously drained.* Because of its small capacity, it is very easy for the bladder to become overdistended, thereby putting too much stress on the suture line. So the patient usually returns with two catheters in place — a suprapubic and a urethral catheter — so as to obviate the possibility of drainage interruption. Low, continuous suction may be attached to either or both catheters to further avoid the potentiality of obstruction. Early ambulation is encouraged and care must be taken to avoid tangling and kinking of the drainage tubings. The amount of urine draining from each catheter should be observed frequently so as to avoid prolonged occlusion of any catheter. The presence of the two catheters frequently causes severe bladder spasms and antispasmodics may be necessary. The suprapubic catheter is usually removed one to two weeks postoperatively and the urethral catheter is left in place until the cystotomy incision is well-healed; if the healing time is prolonged, the patient may be discharged home with the catheter remaining in place. If the latter occurs, the patient must be carefully taught how to properly care for the bladder and catheter at home.

When both catheters have been removed, the patient will become acutely aware of the reduced bladder capacity. It is customary to need to void as often as every 20 minutes. The patient needs to be well-informed of this before the catheter is removed and then will need repeated reassurance during this time that the bladder capacity will increase. In the meantime, it is very important that the patient maintain a fluid intake of at least 2000 ml. per day. The nurse can help the patient avoid becoming a "prisoner of the bathroom" by advising him or her to drink large quantities of fluid at a time when a bathroom is conveniently near. When the patient wants to go out fluid intake can be restricted for several hours; fluids should also be restricted in the evening to allow for minimal sleep disruption during the night. It must be remembered that, although bladder capacity will increase, it is unlikely that it will ever reach preoperative volume. Thus, return to presurgical voiding habits may not be complete, and the patient may need to be counseled in adjusting to this change in life style.

Total cystectomy entails removal of the bladder and urethra in females and the bladder, urethra, prostate, and seminal vesicles in the male. Radical cystectomy also involves dissection of the pelvic lymph nodes. This procedure is indicated when the tumor is invasive, involves the trigone, or whenever the malignancy cannot be adequately treated by less radical methods. In choosing this treatment, the patient's potential life expectancy should be considered, since the postoperative period requires a great deal of emotional and physical adjustment by the patient and significant others.

Since the bladder and urethra are removed, permanent urinary diversion is necessary. Several alternatives for this are possible and will be discussed below more fully. The surgical procedure may be done in one step, with urinary diversion and cystectomy performed at the same operative time; or the surgery may be done in two stages, with urinary diversion done during the first operation and cystectomy performed several weeks later. Radiation therapy may be given between these two stages. The literature presents contradicting views regarding which technique is most desirable, and the surgeon's final choice is made after discussing with the patient such things as therapeutic benefit, length of hospital stay, costs, and expected absence from work and family responsibilities.

Urinary diversion is essential after total cystectomy and may also be done to establish adequate urinary drainage in patients with meningomyelocele or other congenital anomaly, neurogenic bladder, mechanical obstruction to the outflow of urine, severe interstitial cystitis, or trauma to the lower urinary tract interfering with its normal function. The ureters may be implanted into the colon so that the urine exits through the rectum, or the ureters may empty through an opening in the skin; openings into the kidney may be established to allow urine to drain directly from the renal pelvis into an external collection system. Figure 42–10 illustrates the variety of urinary diversion methods used.

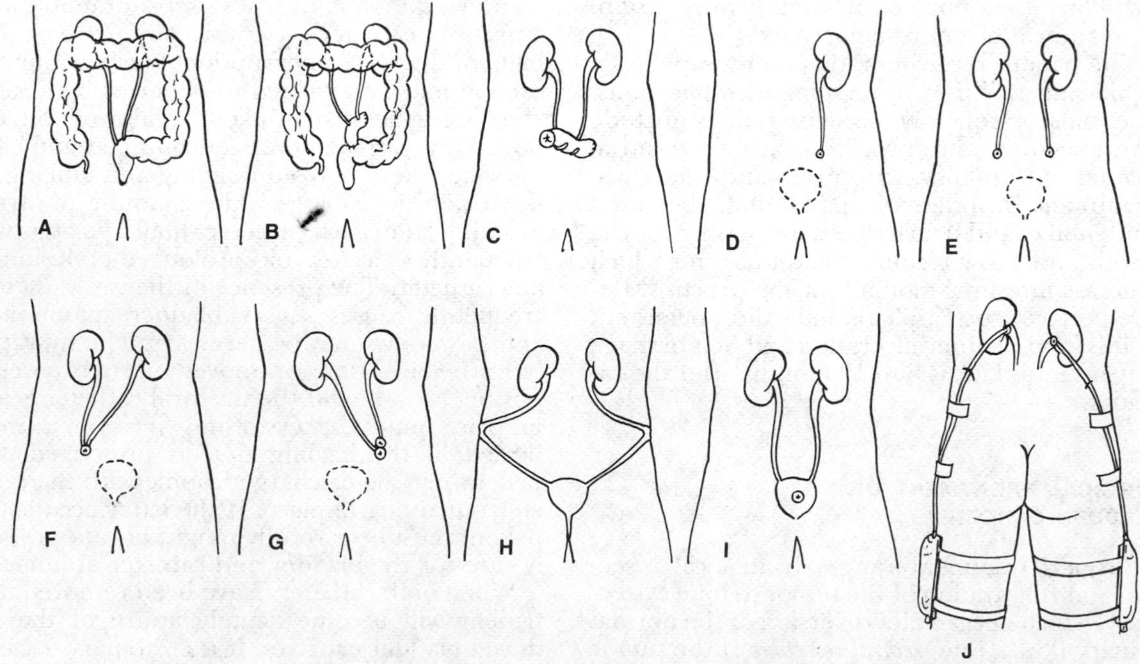

Figure 42–10. Alternative methods used for urinary diversion: *A,* Ureterosigmoidostomy. *B,* Ureteroileosigmoidostomy. *C,* Ileal conduit. *D,* Single ureterostomy. *E,* Bilateral ureterostomy. *F,* Transureteroureterostomy. *G,* Double-barrel ureterostomy. *H,* Loop ureterostomy. *I,* Vesicostomy. *J,* Nephrostomy.

Whatever diversion alternative is selected, it can be assumed that the patient and the patient's friends and relatives are going to need a great deal of emotional support. Changing the normal route of urine flow and eliminating the patient's usual micturition pattern necessitates a change in body image. It is expected that alterations in the patient's normal emotional, psychological, and perceptual reactions will occur. In preoperative teaching, be sure to include the expected anatomic and physiologic alterations, how these will affect the patient's life style, and how the patient's current life style can be maintained. Hope is an important need! Community resources, such as ostomy clubs and the American Cancer Society, may be of tremendous help to the nurse in anticipating and meeting the patient's needs. Postoperatively, the patient must be helped to look at the stoma, if there is one, and to accept it as a part of the total self. He or she must be carefully guided in learning how to care for this new drainage system and to integrate it into the usual daily activities. The people in the patient's household also need this support from the nurse.

Two diversionary methods result in urine being excreted through the rectum. These are *ureterosigmoidostomy* and *ureteroileosigmoidostomy.* In the former procedure, which is the more common of the two, the ureters are implanted into the sigmoid colon. There are two major complications: chronic pyelonephritis and hyperchloremic acidosis. Intrarectal pressure that is higher than normal intravesical pressure facilitates reflux of fecal material into the ureters and even into the renal pelvis. The colonization by intestinal organisms initiates and maintains chronic infection. Persistent inflammation may cause strictures or obstructing fibrosis in the ureters, which can contribute to the development of hydronephrosis as the fluid volume within the kidney increases. Normally, excess chlorides are excreted from the body in urine. Ureterosigmoidostomy creates hyperchloremic acidosis in both ways. Chronic infection and hydronephrosis interfere with normal tubular function and thus the excretion of enough chloride load in the urine. In addition, because of its absorptive properties, the sigmoid colon itself may absorb chlorides that are present in the urine. In ureteroileosigmoidostomy, a segment of the ileum is isolated and anastomosed to the sigmoid colon; the ureters are implanted into the ileal segment. This procedure is purported to reduce the incidence of pyelonephritis and hyperchloremic acidosis, but these complications can still occur. In both methods, the urine mixes with the fecal material, causing very liquid stools. The result is frequent trips to the bathroom. This inconvenience is heightened by the frequent complaint of anal leakage and "stress incontinence." Flatus will be a permanent problem for the patient, who must be taught to expel gas only in the toilet. Gas-forming foods must be avoided.

Another procedure using a segment of the intestine as a conduit constructs the system so that it empties through an opening in the skin. An *ileal conduit,* also called *ureteroïleostomy, ileal bladder,* or *Bricker's procedure,* is the most common urinary diversion alternative used. Usually, a portion of the terminal ileum, which has the least reabsorptive power, is isolated, and the continuity of the intestine is reestablished with an end-to-end anastomosis. Portions of the sigmoid colon and jejunum may also be used for this procedure, but the ileum is most commonly utilized. The proximal end of the segment is closed and the distal end is brought out through a hole created in the abdominal wall and is sutured to the skin to form a stoma. The ureters are then implanted into the ileal segment. The urine flows into the conduit and is continually propelled out through the stoma by peristalsis. Since the ileal segment does not act as a reservoir, minimal absorption of electrolytes occurs, thus avoiding the imbalances that occur when the rectum serves as a reservoir. This procedure requires that the patient permanently wear a collection appliance. The most common complication of this drainage system is the late development of obstruction at the ureteroileal anastomosis. Other complications include urinary tract infection, leakage at the anastomosis site, stenosis anywhere along the system, hydronephrosis, calculi, peristomal hernia, uremia, skin irritation and ulceration, and stomal defects.

Cutaneous ureterostomy brings the ureter(s) to the surface of the abdomen where the urine drains directly into a drainage appliance without the use of an intermediary conduit. There are several variations of this procedure. A *single* or *bilateral ureterostomy* brings the distal end of the ureter directly out through the abdominal wall, creating one or two stomas as appropriate. A *transureteroureterostomy* produces only one stoma as one ureter is brought over and implanted into the other ureter. A *double ureterostomy* forms two stomas in very close proximity as both ureters are brought to the surface together. A *loop ureterostomy* is usually a temporary diversion, with mid-sections being brought to the skin surface for drainage; the rest of the urinary tract is left intact, allowing normal urinary functioning to be reestablished later. Infection and obstruction to urinary flow are constant potential problems. A *vesicostomy* creates a hole in the abdomen directly over the bladder. After the bladder is sutured to the abdominal wall, a stoma is formed from the bladder wall and the bladder empties directly out through this stoma.

Nephrostomy is insertion of drainage catheters into the renal pelves through a surgical incision. This procedure may be permanent, such as when the ureters have also been removed as part of a cystectomy, or temporary so as to divert urine flow when plastic repair has been done on the ureters. Balloon- or mushroom-tipped catheters are inserted into the kidneys and connected to an external drainage system. Because of the high risk of infection and calculus formation, this procedure is a last resort and is usually considered only a palliative measure. Other complications include erosion of the collecting system by the catheter, hemorrhage, mucosal edema, and perforation of the calyx during catheter insertion.

Preoperative Preparation

Preoperative preparation of the patient having diversionary surgery includes listening to and teaching the patient about urinary diversion as described above. In addition to the general physical preparation of the patient, the bowel may need special preparation: a nonresidue diet for several days, sterilization of the bowel with neomycin, and/or cleansing of the bowel with cathartics and enemas. If a stoma is to be created, the site should be selected during the preoperative period. The main criterion for stomal placement is that it allows the faceplate of the drainage appliance to bond securely to the abdominal surface. This means that the umbilicus, rib margins, pubis, and iliac crests must be avoided. Placement directly on the patient's waistline will cause excessive pressure on the stoma by the patient's clothing. The patient is observed in the supine, standing, and sitting positions during the selection process. Usually the stoma is created in the right or left lower quadrant of the abdomen.

Postoperative Care and Complications

Postoperative care of the patient includes routine monitoring of vital signs and incision integrity. Normal supportive measures as described in Chapter 19 are provided for the patient. The patient will frequently have a nasogastric tube in place, since postoperative ileus is a common occurrence. If nephrostomy tubes are present, they will be connected to a bedside drainage system; the tubing must be kept patent to prevent obstruction to the free flow of urine and the drainage system must be maintained as a closed system as much as possible to prevent pyelonephritis. If the patient has had a stoma created, there will be a temporary clear plastic pouch over the stoma which is usually connected to a gravity drainage system allowing continual drainage and measurement of the urine flow. There may also be ureteral catheters in place to splint the ureters during the healing process. These catheters, which are usually removed before the patient is discharged, may extend out through the stoma, but are ordinarily visible just inside the stomal opening. Measure urine output every hour for the first 24 hours and then at least every eight hours. Check the ostomy bag frequently for leaks and the skin under it for irritation. It is also important to frequently observe the stoma itself. Inspect the stoma as soon as the patient returns from surgery so you will have a baseline from which variations can be quickly detected. Note its size, shape, and color. An edematous stoma is expected in the immediate postoperative period. However, other changes may indicate the onset of complications, necessitating notification of the physician.

> *A dusky or cyanotic color of the stoma may denote an embarrassed blood supply and the onset of necrosis. This is an emergency!*

The reduced blood supply may be the direct result of the surgical technique or may be caused by a too small or improperly centered appliance faceplate or poorly applied peristomal protective materials. Other stomal complications include prolapse, or protrusion from the skin, or retraction into the abdomen below the level of the skin. Leakage at the site of the anastomoses or ureteral separation from the conduit may cause signs of peritonitis as urine seeps into the peritoneal cavity. Although bleeding from the stoma may indicate a surgical defect, it is very common for the intestinal mucosa, which is very fragile, to bleed during an appliance change or with a poorly fitted or placed collection bag.

Long-Term Nursing Care and Self-Care

Long-term care of the patient is geared toward maintenance of a functional urinary system and prevention of any complications that may interfere with this. It is also important to help the patient and significant others adjust to the patient's changed body. Even though there may have been excellent counseling during the preoperative period, actual reality of the diversion will probably stimulate further expression of the grief process. Anger and/or depression are to be expected. In dealing with a stoma, the patient may first have to be helped to just look at and talk about it. Then, as soon as possible, the patient must begin to help care for it, gradually assuming more responsibility, until independence in the care of the stoma, peristomal skin, and drainage system is achieved.

Skin irritation or breakdown is a constant threat. The main preventive measure is to keep urine from contact with the skin, primarily by means of a well-fitted and properly applied appliance. The opening in the adhesive backing of the temporary pouch or faceplate of the permanent appliance should be approximately 3 mm. larger than the stoma. The faceplate opening will have to be remeasured after the edema in the stoma recedes. Each time the bag is changed, the skin around the stoma is cleaned with soap and water and thoroughly dried. Any adhesive material adhering to the skin must be removed with adhesive remover, if necessary. If crystals are present on the skin, washing with a dilute vinegar solution may help remove them. During and after the cleansing process, a gauze or tissue roll should be placed over the stoma to prevent urine from flowing out over the skin; this roll is removed just as the appliance is being reapplied. It is also suggested that appliance changes be done in the early morning whenever possible, since urine production is slowest at this time.

Since urine is not as corrosive to the skin as feces, a skin barrier is not always used. However, many authorities do suggest that a *skin barrier* be applied prophylactically. If a barrier is to be used, its stoma opening is cut just large enough to fit over the stoma and is applied next to the skin before the pouch or faceplate is put on. A skin bond cement or adhesive disc may be used to help the faceplate stick to the skin more securely. A non–water-soluble adhesive spray is available which allows the patient to go swimming.

Once the skin has been properly prepared, application of the appliance can be completed. With a *temporary pouch*, the paper is removed from the adhesive backing and the opening cut in the back is placed over the stoma. The adhesive portion is pressed firmly to the skin with creases or wrinkles carefully avoided. With a *permanent appliance*, the pouch is stretched onto and adhered to the faceplate so that it lies smoothly. Then the faceplate is carefully centered over the stoma and adhered to the skin. Nonallergic adhesive tape strips may be placed around the edges of the temporary pouch or the faceplate for additional security. A belt can be used to hold the faceplate in place, especially if the patient will be engaging in strenuous activities; patients may also feel more secure if this belt is worn continuously. If a belt is used, the patient must be cautioned against excessive tightness, which may lead to formation of pressure sores under the faceplate. Whatever type of pouch is being used, the opening at the bottom should be toward the patient's feet to assure adequate drainage. As mentioned above, the temporary pouch may be attached to a continuous, closed drainage system. A permanent pouch usually has a valve-type opening in the bottom which can be closed, allowing urine to collect in the pouch, or open so that the pouch can be emptied or attached to gravity drainage, using either a bedside collection bag (especially at night) or a leg bag. Being able to have a self-contained pouch drainage system allows the patient to resume most, if not all former activities with very little, if any, change needed in style of dress. However, the patient must be cautioned to empty the pouch frequently, since the weight of accumulating urine may pull the faceplate away from the skin and cause leakage. The seal should also be checked more frequently whenever the patient is perspiring.

If *skin irritation* occurs, treatment must begin immediately. The pH of the urine should be checked, since strongly alkaline urine is irritating to the skin. Urine cultures may identify a urinary tract infection which must be treated. The appliance should be checked carefully to find any leakage and to determine if the skin is sensitive to anything used in the process of application. Skin irritation may also result from too frequent changing of the pouch; because of this, it is usually recommended that the bag be left in place for several days at a time as long as it is not leaking. The skin should be left open to the air as much as possible using absorbent pads to catch the urine. A heat lamp may be used to facilitate healing. When the appliance is used, dust the skin with karaya powder followed by the application of a karaya seal pouch, one especially designed for urinary stomas. Antibiotic creams or nystatin may be necessary if the irritation is being caused by bacteria or Monilia.

Odor control is another common problem with urinary stomas. Noxious odor often results from poor hygiene, alkaline urine, infection, and the ingestion of certain foods like asparagus. Control of this odor can be achieved. Reusable appliances should be washed thoroughly with soap and lukewarm water; hot water may cause excessive brittleness of the plastic pouch. If this does not remove the odor, the bag can be soaked in a dilute white vinegar solution or a commercial deodorant product for at least 20 to 30 minutes. The bag is then rinsed and allowed to dry. There are deodorant tablets available which can be placed in the pouch while it is being used. Ingestion of methionine can alleviate the smell of ammonia. As described in the discussion of cystitis, some authorities recommend cranberry juice, ascorbic acid, and/or an acid-ash diet as a means of acidifying the urine.

Dilute urine is usually less odiferous than concentrated urine, so an adequate fluid intake is helpful in preventing embarrassing odor.

During and after the acute postoperative period, the patient must be monitored for development of complications in addition to those described above. *Urinary tract infection* is a constant threat because of the open nature of the urinary tract. *Obstruction* anywhere along the course interferes with normal urine flow. One example of this is stenosis of the stoma, which may occur as the result of scarring during stomal maturation. If the opening on the faceplate is too large, epithelial hyperplasia, or thickening of the peristomal skin, may occur causing contracture of the stoma. Patients with urinary diversion are also prone to uric acid and calcium stone disease, with some studies reporting incidence rates as high as 30 per cent. The onset of urinary stone development usually occurs at least two years postoperatively and sometimes as much as 5 to 10 years later.[115]

Helping these patients regain their independence greatly helps them accept their new body image. This requires a well-thought-out management plan. As mentioned before, patients should begin taking an active role in their care as soon as possible. Creating an environment as close as possible to that in the patient's home, the nurse should help the patient organize the equipment and procedure necessary for caring for the stoma. Most patients prefer to have two permanent appliances so that one can be soaking and drying while the other is being worn. Patients must be able to remove and reapply the appliance, care for the appliance, empty the pouch and attach it to the night drainage system if necessary, and care for the stoma and peristomal skin with a high degree of confidence. They need to be able to make adaptations while traveling or visiting. They may need help in selecting clothing that will not obstruct the drainage system. They must know the importance of maintaining a daily fluid intake of at least 2000 ml. and be able to select the correct food and fluids. Furthermore, patients must know when to contact their physician, e.g., changes in urine color or quantity of urine output, cloudy or foul-smelling urine, or stomal color changes. A well-planned teaching-learning program, including both the patient and significant others, is essential and it is very helpful to arrange for follow-up home visits after the patient is discharged from the hospital.

Surgical Procedures That Maintain Continence

Some surgeons are employing a procedure which eliminates the need to wear an external appliance, since urine does not flow continuously from the reservoir. The *continent vesicostomy* requires that the bladder be left in place. In this procedure, the urethral neck is closed and a vesicostomy is performed, with a nipple valve being fashioned from the bladder wall (see Fig. 42–11). As the bladder fills, the pressure of the urine causes the nipple to intussuscept, preventing urine flow from the bladder. In order to drain the bladder, the patient catheterizes the stoma using clean technique. The patient having this procedure returns from surgery with a suprapubic catheter and an indwelling catheter placed in the bladder through the stoma. These catheters are usually sutured in place and remain for up to six weeks postoperatively. The catheters and surrounding skin are meticulously cleaned every day using sterile technique, and catheter irrigations may be ordered. The main problem reported by patients is severe bladder spasms. This is treated by maintaining a good fluid intake and using belladonna and opium suppositories as necessary. The patient usually goes home with these catheters and must be able to continue the required care. Following the healing process, the catheters are removed and the patient is taught intermittent catheterization technique. He or she should wear a gauze pad over the stoma for protection and is advised to wear some type of medical identification to alert others to the presence of the vesicostomy in case of an emergency.[15]

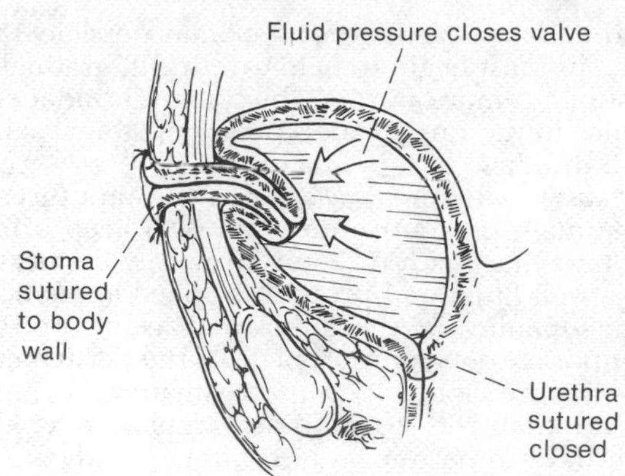

Figure 42–11. A continent vesicostomy. (Drawn from Barrett, N.: Continent vesicostomy: The dry urinary diversion. *American Journal of Nursing,* 79:462, Mar., 1979.)

Another diversion procedure used to maintain continence is the *continent cecoileal conduit.* In this technique, a part of the cecum acts as the reservoir. Figure 42–12 shows how the terminal ileum intussuscepts into the cecum to form a nipple while the other end is brought to the abdominal wall to form a stoma. As above, the reservoir is drained by catheterization. Postoperatively, the patient is usually denied oral food and fluid for approximately a week. Intravenous fluids help maintain a high urine output. Ureteral catheters help splint the ureters during the healing process. Because of the normal volume capacity of the cecum, the conduit is initially catheterized every two hours and, as this capacity increases, the interval between catheterizations is also lengthened. The need for emptying is usually signalled by a full sensation in the abdomen.[345]

Some patients who have had urinary diversion without cystectomy or urethrectomy may face at some time in their lives a possibility of *undiversion.* Because of some change in their condition, they may be able to have the normal continuity of their urinary tract re-established. Careful evaluation of the patient must be done before the decision is made, with high priority given to near normal renal function and the ability of the bladder to regain its normal function. The procedure carries a significant failure risk and it must be decided that the chances for success are very high. The reconstruction procedure selected is usually one of three alternatives: direct ureterovesical anastomosis, autotransplantation of the kidneys to the iliac fossa followed by ureterovesical anastomosis, or the use of a bowel segment to replace ureteral length. The main problem with the last technique is the continuous formation of mucus and the electrolyte reabsorption that occurs.[155]

OTHER TREATMENTS FOR BLADDER CANCER

Other treatment modalities for cancer of the bladder include hydrostatic pressure and heat. When treating the bladder with *hydrostatic pressure,* a rubber balloon is inserted into the bladder and inflated by gravity flow, or normal saline is instilled directly into the bladder. This distention puts pressure on the bladder wall, causing tissue anoxia. It is hypothesized that the normal mucosa can withstand the ischemic periods while the tumor cells are particularly vulnerable and become necrotic. There is also evidence that tumor cells are more susceptible to *heat* than normal cells. Based on this data, some physicians are instilling heated saline solutions into the bladder in the treatment of superficial transitional-cell carcinomas.

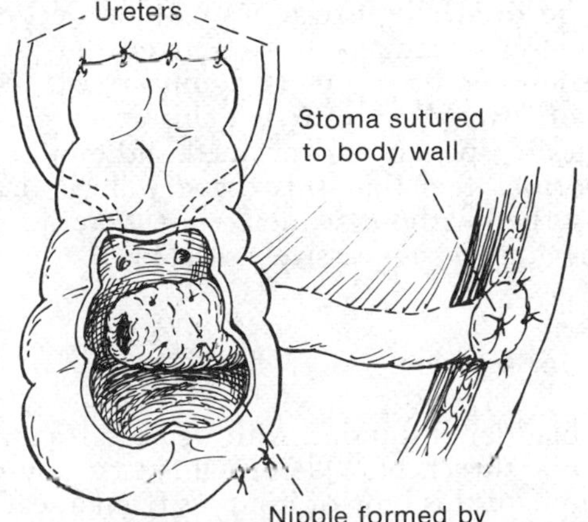

Figure 42–12. A continent cecoileal conduit. (Drawn from Zingg, E., and R. Tscholl: Continent cecoileal conduit: Preliminary report. *Journal of Urology,* 118:725, Nov., 1977.)

Patients with treated bladder cancer have a high rate of recurrence. In a study of 114 patients, the interval between the original treatment and the recurrence of tumor ranged from three months to 27 years. In 19 per cent of the patients, the new tumor was of a higher grade and 22 per cent of the recurrences were of a higher stage.[14] Thus, the patient must be strongly encouraged to continue the follow-up program suggested by the physician.

Urethral Neoplasms

The most commonly occurring benign urethral tumors are condylomas in the male and caruncles in women. Caruncles are common in women ages 40 to 65 and are considered to be the result of chronic irritation. Malignant neoplasms are uncommon in either sex, occurring more frequently in women than in men. Histologically, the tumors found most often in men are squamous-cell and transitional-cell carcinomas, while neoplasms in the female are usually adenocarcinomas or squamous-cell carcinomas. Because of the anatomy of the urethral wall and the degree of lymph drainage, localized metastasis is fairly common, primarily to the inguinal and iliac lymph nodes. In women, the infiltration may involve the vulva and vagina. Further metastasis usually involves the lung, liver, bone, and brain.

Whether the tumor is benign or malignant, the symptoms are similar. These include bleeding, urinary obstruction, dysuria, palpable urethral mass, urethral discharge, perineal pain, and urinary incontinence. Diagnosis is confirmed by endoscopic examination and biopsy. If a malignant tumor is found, it is important that the lymph nodes be examined meticulously to determine whether or not there has been metastasis.

Treatment of benign tumors is usually done by transurethral fulguration or excision, although total or subtotal urethrectomy may be necessary for larger lesions. Other treatment modes that have had some success include podophyllum cream, thiotepa or colchicine instillations, and BCG injections. Recurrence is common.

As with any cancer, the recommended treatment of malignant urethral tumors depends on the degree of invasion by the tumor. Surgery and/or irradiation are the acceptable choices. If surgery is done, radical procedures are usually performed. Partial or total urethrectomy may be done, requiring permanent urinary diversion, although some work is being done on replacing urethras with silicone rubber tubing. In addition, men may face partial or total penectomy, while women may need anterior pelvic exenteration and vulvectomy. Radical excision of the pelvic lymph nodes may be done as part of, or in addition to, the above surgical procedures. Besides providing the demanding physical postoperative care required by these patients, the nurse must also be ready to recognize and intervene with tremendous psychologic problems. Destruction of the external genitalia deals a crushing blow to a person's body image and empathetic counselling will be needed by the patient and relatives and friends. Elimination of urine from the body will be accomplished by one of the methods of urinary diversion described above if a cystectomy has been done; otherwise, the external sphincter may be salvaged and a perineal orifice created. Five- to 10-year survival rates for patients with urethral cancer average 32 per cent.[34]

DIVERTICULA

A *diverticulum* is a pouch or sac resulting from the herniation of the mucous membrane lining through a defect in the muscular wall of an organ. These may be either congenital or the result of high pressures in the urinary tract from obstructive pathology. Ureteral diverticula are very rare, while vesical and urethral diverticula are much more common. The main problems caused by urinary diverticula are recurrent urinary tract infections due to stasis of the urine and malignancies probably due to chronic irritation from the persistent infection. Treatment usually involves removal of contributing factors, such as obstruction and urinary tract infection followed by surgical excision of the pouch and reestablishment of normal patency of the urinary tract. Postoperatively, the patient will have catheter drainage of the urine to allow complete tissue healing. Since these patients have usually had long-term infections, medication therapy will likely be continued for some time following the surgical procedure.

TRAUMA TO THE LOWER URINARY TRACT

Anything that interrupts the integrity of the urinary tract can be considered trauma, including planned surgical procedures. However, this section will discuss only those interruptions that occur as the result of unplanned injury.

Ureteral Injuries

Most accidental injury to the ureters occurs during surgery. Perforation or tearing may occur during the manipulation of intraureteric catheters or other instruments. The ureters may be occluded by ligating sutures or a misplaced hemostat or may be transected during pelvic surgery. To prevent the latter, many surgeons insert ureteral catheters before pelvic procedures to facilitate easy identification of the ureters. Gunshot or stab wounds may also traumatize the ureters and, although not very common, blunt trauma or rapid deceleration has been known to cause tearing of these structures.

Visualization of the injury may be the first indication of its presence, especially if it has occurred as a complication of surgery. However, frequently the trauma is not discovered until signs and symptoms have occurred. Hematuria may be present, but the most common indications are anuria and kidney pain and/or symptoms of extravasation of urine. As urine seeps out into the tissues, pain may develop in the lower abdomen and flank. As the extravasation continues, there may be signs of sepsis, paralytic ileus, palpable intraperitoneal mass, and appearance of urine in the external wound. An excretory urogram and cystoscopy are the most definitive means by which to diagnose the problem.

Treatment primarily involves surgical repair of the defect. An end-to-end anastomosis is most desired. However, it may be necessary to do more radical procedures, such as cutaneous ureterostomy, transureteroureterostomy, and reimplantation. Prosthetic ureteral implants may be used. Nephrectomy may be needed if severe renal damage has occurred due to obstruction and/or sepsis. If significant extravasation of urine has occurred, this space may be surgically opened and drained, although some authorities feel that this urine will be readily reabsorbed without sequelae if it is sterile. Any sepsis must be aggressively treated.

Bladder Injuries

A bladder distended with urine can rupture when a direct blow is sustained; a common example of this type of injury is from a seat belt during an automobile accident. The bladder may also be punctured by bullets, knives, bony splinters from a fractured pelvis, or from internal instruments such as catheters, sounds, and cystoscopes.

When the bladder ruptures, whatever the cause, urine spills out into the peritoneal cavity and continues to leak out as long as the bladder is not intact. Pain low in the abdomen and hematuria, in addition to a history of injury or blow to the abdomen, should always arouse suspicion of bladder injury. Specific signs and symptoms of a ruptured bladder depend on the location and extent of the tear. Pelvic cellulitis or peritonitis may occur. The patient may also demonstrate urination difficulties, e.g., voiding small amounts of bloody urine or inability to urinate at all.

Treatment involves establishment of urinary drainage through either a suprapubic or a urethral catheter and surgical repair of the bladder wall. Postoperatively, urinary drainage is maintained to prevent tension on the suture line.

Urethral Injuries

The urethra, as well as the bladder, may be injured in pelvic fractures. Falling astride an object with force or a blow to the groin may also cause urethral contusion and laceration. Instrumentation injuries may occur during medical or surgical treatments or may be self inflicted. Penetrating wounds may also cause urethral damage.

The main indication of urethral damage is the partial or total inability to pass urine through the urethra. Even if some urine does get through, urinary extravasation occurs during voiding, causing increasing swelling in the scrotal or inguinal areas; this may produce sepsis and necrosis. Bleeding may be present at the external meatus; blood may also extravasate into the surrounding tissues, giving the area an ecchymotic appearance. Localized pain may also be experienced. The most common complications of urethral trauma are the development of urethral strictures and the incidence of impotence in men. Impotence, which occurs because of damage to the cavernous tissue of the penis or the blood vessels or nerves supplying this area, has been reported in as many as 40 per cent of the cases.[58]

Treatment of urethral injuries is controversial. It is generally agreed that urinary drainage must first be established with either a urethral or a suprapubic catheter. Some authorities then suggest an immediate primary surgical repair of the urethra, while others prefer to wait for two to three weeks to see if the urethra will heal itself before surgically intervening. The patient must be carefully monitored for signs of developing sepsis.

FISTULAS IN THE URINARY TRACT

Fistulas are abnormal passages between two organs or between an organ and the skin which allow intercommunication of secretions and other substances. They may be congenital or may result from trauma, inflammation, or malignant invasion. Long-term urethral catheterization has been identified as a cause of fistula formation in men because of the constant pressure on the penile-scrotal junction. Common fistulas found in the urinary tract include ureterovaginal, vesicovaginal, and colovesical (particularly in men).

The presence of a urinary tract fistula is suspected when urine leaves the body from an unnatural site or when abnormal constituents appear in the urine, such as air or fecal material. Urinary tract infection is a common finding. Diagnosis may be confirmed by excretory urogram, cystoscopy, and sigmoidoscopy. To further delineate the path of the fistula, a dye, such as congo-red or indigocarmine, is instilled into the urinary tract and the outlet is then identified.

Before surgical repair of the fistula is undertaken, the continuous flow of urine from the kidney must be guaranteed through temporary urinary diversion, either externally as described above or with catheters. The specific surgical procedure to be used depends on the preference of the surgeon; some repairs may be done in one stage, some in as many as three. The primary outcome is excision of the fistula and re-establishment of tissue integrity. Postoperatively, the patient will usually continue with urinary diversion until the surgical site is well-healed. If catheters are in place, irrigations should be done only after consultation with the physician.

CHAPTER 43

DISORDERS OF THE KIDNEY

As described in Chapter 40, the kidneys carry out a number of dynamic functions that help the body maintain homeostasis. In addition to producing urine and thus regulating the body's fluid, electrolyte, and acid-base balances, the kidneys have a number of other functions, e.g., erythropoietin and prostaglandin production, insulin degradation, and a role in the renin-angiotensin-aldosterone system. These latter activities have become extremely important in medical decisions about the prognosis and treatment of patients with renal disorders. For instance, although it is known that complete loss of renal function is incompatible with life, medical advances have made dialysis and transplant much more readily available. Thus, albeit very serious and requiring significant life-style changes for the patient, the loss of the kidneys and/or their functions has recently been considered less of a risk to the patient than 20 years ago. Treatment of some renal diseases and injuries has reflected this philosophy. However, as more is learned about the full scope of kidney function, it is being recognized that dialysis cannot entirely substitute for the normal kidney. Therefore, surgical removal of the kidney, or nephrectomy, may not be done as readily.

Because of the close alliance between the kidneys and other body processes, any alteration in the kidney will eventually have some effect on other organ systems and physiologic activities. Likewise, changes in other parts of the body will often affect kidney function and sometimes renal tissue itself. This chapter will discuss the common disease processes and injuries that interfere with normal renal function. Although there will be a brief description of the effects of extrarenal influences on the kidneys, the primary purpose of this chapter is to discuss specific renal pathology: etiology, clinical course, and the medical and nursing care required by it. Because of the potential seriousness of any renal problem, the patient and significant others will have both physical and psychological needs, and the nurse must be knowledgeable about both aspects and be constantly alert to patients' needs.

EFFECT OF CHEMICALS AND EXTRARENAL DISEASE PROCESSES

As mentioned above, many disease processes with primary foci in other parts of the body produce effects within the kidney. Examples of these include diabetes mellitus, cardiovascular pathology, and sepsis. Description of the renal implications of these pathologies will be brief; the reader is referred to the appropriate units in this book for a more complete discussion.

Extrarenal Disease Processes

One of the most common extrarenal diseases affecting the kidney is *diabetes mellitus.* Diabetic nephropathy is a progressive process frequently leading to renal failure. It is estimated that as many as half the patients with diabetes mellitus have renal lesions at the time of death, and renal failure is the cause of death in approximately 6 per cent of adult-onset diabetics and 50 per cent of those with juvenile-onset diabetes.[108, 199] The most frequent pathologic change is a characteristic intercapillary *glomerulosclerosis.* These lesions can be diffuse or nodular and are produced by a progressive enhancement of the basement membrane in the mesangial matrix and, to some extent, the glomerular capillary walls. The mean mass of glomeruli in a diabetic patient has been found to be 2.5 times larger than that of a nondiabetic.[41] There is also progressive microangiopathy of the arterioles servicing the glomeruli. Initially, the sclerotic, or hardening, process increases the renal vascular resistance, contributing to systemic hypertension, but does not cause renal insufficiency; in fact, the glomerular filtration rate may be increased during the early period. However, as more nephrons are destroyed, available functioning renal tissue decreases and the patient begins to demonstrate proteinuria, hypertension, edema, and signs and symptoms of renal failure. The progression of this process is significantly related to the age of the patient at onset of the disease and to the success in controlling the disease and the patient's weight, but not to the actual duration of the diabetic process.[302]

Other lesions found in diabetic nephropathy include recurrent pyelonephritis and renal papillary necrosis. Glycogen deposition in the renal tubules is not considered to be significant.

Since the kidneys receive such a large share of the cardiac output, renal function can both affect and be affected by alterations within the cardiovascular system. *Hypertension* is a prototype of a condition that can be both a cause and an effect of renal disease. Renovascular hypertension occurs as a result of renal artery stenosis or renal infarction, which activates the renin-angiotensin-aldosterone system, producing increased systemic blood pressure. Renal hypertension arising from parenchymal renal disease usually results from the kidneys' decreasing ability to excrete salt and water. Other causes, although not as common, include increased renin release due to decreased glomerular perfusion and developing inadequacy of renal vasodilator substances such as occurs with analgesic nephropathy. Renovascular and renal hypertension together cause an estimated 6 to 8 per cent of the cases of systemic hypertension.[221] On the other hand, sustained systemic high blood pressure adversely affects the kidneys. It has been estimated that in patients having uncontrolled hypertension lasting more than 5 years, microscopically evident nephrosclerosis is present even though all other renal diagnostic tests may be normal. This kidney damage is the direct result of degenerative changes in the arterioles and interlobular arteries caused by increased blood pressure. There is direct correlation between the duration and degree of elevated blood pressure and the severity of the renal vascular disease, and progression of the disease can frequently be halted or slowed by bringing the hypertension under control.

Cardiovascular *shock,* or *hypotension*, also affects renal function. Renal vasoconstriction reduces the renal blood flow. However, because of the autoregulatory capabilities of the kidneys, as described in Chapter 40, glomerular filtration rate is maintained at a functional level until advanced stages of systemic shock, at which time acute renal failure ensues. Restoration of the systemic blood pressure usually reverses the renal vasoconstriction and kidney function returns. There may be a period of polyuria following correction of hypovolemic episodes; the mechanism for this is unclear. Then, before renal function returns to normal, there may be another oliguric period followed by a "mobilization phase" during which there is a massive movement of sequestered fluid into the intravascular space. This may cause some hypertension until the kidneys can remove the extra fluid. Careful fluid management of the patient is crucial during these recovery phases.

Cardiac disease influences kidney function primarily through its effect on cardiac output and circulating blood volume. The hemodynamic and hormonal changes may lead to decreased ability of the kidneys to excrete sodium and water. This causes increased intravascular congestion and edema and establishes a pathologic cycle.

Peripheral vascular disease is an important factor. *Atherosclerosis* was discussed with diabetic nephropathy. *Thromboembolic disease* can affect the renal circulation and cause infarction of the tissue supplied by the affected blood vessel. The interstitial hypertonicity and low oxygen pressure found in the renal medulla seem to favor the sickling of red blood cells in the juxtamedullary region of the kidney in patients with *sickle-cell disease*. These cell masses cause gross hematuria as venules are ruptured, papillary necrosis, renal infarction, concentrating disturbances due to interference with the "counter-current mechanism," nephrotic syndrome, pyelonephritis, and finally renal failure. The kidney is the most affected organ in *disseminated intravascular coagulation*, in which inactivation of clotting mechanisms causes hemorrhage from affected areas.

Extrarenal *sepsis* may affect kidney function either through its effect on the systemic circulation or through its stimulation of the immune system. Renal reactions to septic shock would be similar to those described above, while immunologic injury leading to glomerulonephritis is described below. It is also possible for pathogens to break away from extrarenal foci of infection and travel to the kidney, where additional sites can be established.

Although not a disease, *pregnancy* has definite influence over kidney function. Dilation of the collecting system and kidney enlargement begins during the first trimester and may persist 9 to 12 weeks postpartum. Renal blood flow and glomerular filtration rate increase by 30 to 50 per cent, which contributes to increased creatinine clearance and decreased uric acid excretion. These normal changes must be taken into account when interpreting laboratory findings in pregnant women. Also expected in pregnancy are increased proteinuria, including orthostatic proteinuria; increased glycosuria, which is usually transient; and polyuria and nocturia due partially to external compression of the bladder but also possibly due to alterations in antidiuretic hormone metabolism.[122]

Many other extrarenal disease processes influence kidney function. These include neoplastic disease, connective tissue disorders, and metabolic disturbances.

Nephrotoxins

Many chemicals, including drugs, can affect renal function in a positive and/or negative way. This discussion will be limited to those substances which have adverse effects on the kidney. *Nephrotoxins* are substances which have specific destructive effect on renal cells.

These toxic agents can cause five types of renal injury: acute tubular necrosis, defects in the tubular transport system, interstitial nephritis, vasculitis, and nephrotic syndrome.

Nephrotoxic substances found in the environment include heavy metals, such as mercurial compounds, lead, cadmium, bismuth, arsenic, copper, and phosphorus; carbon tetrachloride; ethylene glycol; trichloroethylene; carbon monoxide; and chlorinated hydrocarbons. Exposure to many of these occurs in industrial locations. Snake venom and certain mushrooms also fall into this category. The most frequent renal result of these substances is acute tubular necrosis, with some also causing tubular transport defects and nephrotic syndrome.

Nephrotoxic reactions from drugs cover the gamut of all five types of kidney damage. The two most common drug classifications causing renal damage are antibiotics and certain analgesics. Since the kidneys are the major route of excretion of many antibiotics, renal tissue is directly exposed to the compounds. The longer the duration of exposure, the higher the risk of renal damage. Factors such as preexisting renal disease, changes in renal blood flow, electrolyte imbalances, and concurrent use of other nephrotoxic drugs enhance the effect of any given medication. Antibiotics that place the patient at high risk include penicillins, cephalosporins, sulfonamides, gentamicin, kanamycin, neomycin, polymixins, amphotericin B, and streptomycin. Besides using these drugs for as short a time as possible, maintaining a high fluid intake may be the main preventive intervention against the nephrotoxic effects. A high urine output keeps the medication dilute within the kidney and helps prevent any crystallization of the compound.

The risk of renal damage from overuse of certain analgesics has received more attention in recent years. Most suspect are the salicylates and phenacetin, which are frequently used in combination. The process of injury, which is enhanced by fluid depletion, begins in the renal medulla where the medication is concentrated. It is probable that local damage to the endothelium of the vasa recta causes anoxia, resulting in papillary necrosis. The necrotic tissue sloughs and blocks the collecting tubules.[320] Patients receving long-term therapeutic doses of salicylates should have periodic monitoring of their renal function, since early renal changes can frequently be reversed by decreasing or eliminating the dosage.

Anesthesia itself reduces the kidney's vasoconstrictive ability, by which it helps protect itself against drops in systemic blood pressure, thus making the kidney more vulnerable to the effects of shock. In addition, certain anesthetic agents, particularly methoxyflurane, have a direct nephrotoxic effect. Administration of this general anesthetic can cause acute tubular necrosis and has been associated with fatal acute renal failure. Halothane may also have adverse effects on renal function. Sodium thiopental has been shown to be present in higher serum concentrations in patients with renal disease than in subjects with normal kidney function receiving the same dose.

Other commonly used medications which can have nephrotoxic effects include furosemide, thiazides, probenecid, phenytoin, intravenous amphetamines, low molecular weight dextran, phenylbutazone, rifampin, phenindione, and gold therapy. Radioiodinated contrast agents used in x-ray studies have been associated with acute tubular necrosis. While receiving these agents, the patient should receive an adequate fluid intake, and renal function should be observed before and after administration.

CONGENITAL AND HEREDITARY ANOMALIES OF THE KIDNEY

Renal congenital anomalies usually occur in regard to the number, position, form or size, and structure. There may be an abnormal blood supply, although malformations that significantly affect renal function are rare. Anomalies of the ureteropelvic junction usually cause obstruction at that point and resultant hydronephrosis. This situation is usually discovered and treated during childhood.

Renal agenesis indicates the absence of one or both kidneys. A single kidney presents no difficulty if its functional status is adequate, and it is frequently discovered for the first time during an excretory urogram being done for some unrelated reason. A person can live normally with one well-functioning kidney, as aptly demonstrated by people who donate a kidney to a relative needing a kidney transplant. Bilateral agenesis, on the other hand, is incompatible with life. It has also been found that in unilateral agenesis, the functioning kidney is at high risk for additional anomalies.

Supernumerary kidneys may occur, although their incidence is rare. This condition is usually asymptomatic and the presence of additional kidneys, as with unilateral renal agenesis, is found during excretory urogram. The extra ureter enters either the ipsilateral ureter or the bladder.

Ectopic, or malpositioned, kidneys are usually found in the pelvis, although thoracic kidneys have been documented. Problems associated with this anomaly include respiratory difficulties, pain from pressure on nerves or surrounding structures, and management of labor during the birthing process. One kidney may also be found across the midline so that both are on the same side. This condition is usually undiscovered until infection or obstruction necessitates x-ray examination.

Anomalies of form or size include aplasia, hypoplasia, dysplasia, and horseshoe kidney. *Aplastic* kidneys contain no functioning renal tissue; the kidney is small and contracted. *Renal hypoplasia* produces miniature kidneys with some functioning tissue. Clinically this condition may be completely asymptomatic; however, it may be the origin of hypertension and recurrent urinary tract infection. *Dysplastic* kidneys are essentially hypoplastic with abnormal tissue. They may contain such things as cysts, cartilage, striated muscle, and primitive glomeruli. This anomaly is rare and usually found during an excretory urogram. *Horseshoe kidney* occurs in 1:500 to 1:8000 births[61] and involves the joining of the two kidneys so that they form one organ somewhat resembling a horseshoe (Fig. 43–1). The kidneys are connected, usually at the lower poles, by an isthmus of tissue. Since the developmental error interferes with the normal ascent and medial rotation, the kidney is usually located in the lower lumbar region with its pelvis facing anteriorly. Although this condition may be asymptomatic, there is predisposition to hydronephrosis and infection secondary to ureteropelvic junction obstruction and calculus formation.

Congenitally abnormal structure of the kidney usually denotes the presence and progression of cysts within the renal tissue. This plight ranges from a simple, solitary cyst through almost complete replacement of the functioning renal structures by cystic tissue. A *simple renal cyst* commonly originates superficially within the renal parenchyma. It is slow-growing and usually produces no symptoms until the patient has reached adulthood, when it may cause a heaviness and pain in the abdomen and may become a palpable mass. When discovered, it presents a diagnostic challenge, as differentiation must be made between a cyst and a malignant tumor. As long as the cyst remains asymptomatic, no treatment is usually undertaken. If necessary, the cyst may be aspirated with a needle or a partial nephrectomy may be done to surgically remove the cyst. Injection of the cyst with iophendylate has been successful, although there is a risk of chronic inflammatory changes within the kidney. Iophendylate is an iodized fatty acid compound usually used as a contrast medium during x-ray procedures. It apparently causes a proliferative inflammatory reaction within the cyst wall leading to a reduction in size.

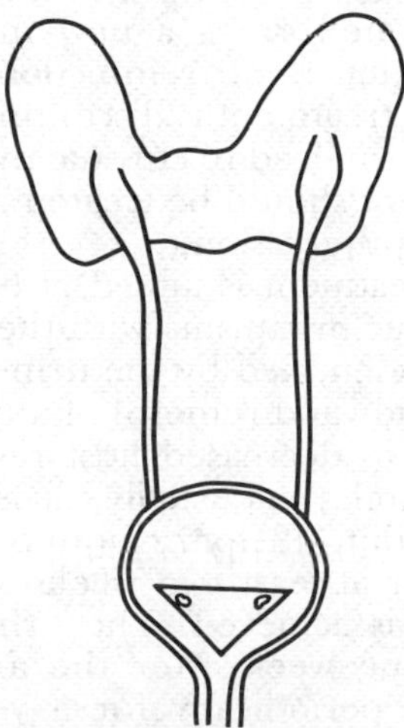

Figure 43–1. Horseshoe kidney (From Lapides, J.: *Fundamentals of Urology*. Philadelphia: W. B. Saunders Co., 1976.)

Multicystic disease is usually found in conjunction with dysplastic kidneys, although it may occur in otherwise normal kidneys. If the condition is bilateral, the child usually dies in infancy. However, if the disease is unilateral and the contralateral kidney is normal, prognosis for the patient is excellent.

Polycystic disease of the kidney is a hereditary disorder in which grapelike cysts replace normal tissue of the kidney. It may be of an infantile or adult type, depending primarily on the age of onset of signs and symptoms. The prognosis for infantile polycystic disease is poor, although renal transplantation may improve the outlook. Adult polycystic disease has an incidence rate of 1:250 to 1:5000 and accounts for about 5 per cent of the patients receiving hemodialysis.[51, 61] It is inherited as an autosomal dominant trait. It is usually bilateral and affects males and females equally. Symptoms usually appear in middle age, although they may begin as early as age 20 or as late as 80.

Symptoms of adult polycystic disease are varied. The most common presenting symptoms are dull, aching lumbar or lateral abdomen pain which may be colicky in nature, and hematuria. Other common urinary tract findings are proteinuria, palpable kidneys, pyuria, calculi, and renal insufficiency. Hypertension with resulting cardiac enlargement and heart failure occur in approximately 50 per cent of the patients. The kidney can become so enlarged as to cause severe pressure on other organs, producing additional extrarenal symptoms. The ultimate result of this disease is renal failure. As the disease slowly progresses, renal nephrons are destroyed, renal function deteriorates, and uremia ultimately results. The mean duration of the disease from the onset of symptoms to the development of uremia is approximately 16 years.[51]

There is no known way to arrest the progress of the destructive cysts, so conservative treatment is directed toward preservation of kidney function. Urinary tract infection is the most common complication because of the distorted renal architecture. Therefore, prevention and/or treatment of infection is important. Hypertension is aggressively controlled. Unlike patients with increasing creatinine clearance rates caused by other kidney diseases, patients with polycystic kidney disease seem to waste rather than retain sodium. Thus, these patients need to have an increased sodium intake. Principles of nursing care of the patient once the renal failure is evident are the same regardless of the cause of the failure. These principles will be discussed later in this chapter.

Treatment methods available to patients with renal failure are also used with patients with polycystic kidney disease. Surgical nephrectomy may sometimes be done if conservative therapy has been ineffective with severe recurrent pyelonephritis or in the event of intractable hemorrhage. Hemodialysis and renal transplantation are being done with increasing frequency and success.

Because of the hereditary nature of the disease, genetic counseling should be done, particularly if the disease is diagnosed during the childbearing years. Prospective parents who are at risk for development of the disease need to be monitored throughout this period. Progress is being made on tests that can be done before age 30 with confidence in the results. These include ultrasound, renal scan, and maximal concentrating ability of the kidney, which tends to be decreased in polycystic kidney disease.[51]

Adult-onset medullary cystic disease, sometimes called uremic sponge kidney or medullary polycystic disease, is also an autosomal dominant disorder. It is similar to polycystic disease in all apsects except that its progress to uremia occurs very rapidly after its onset in the second or third decade of life. Prognosis is poor.

Medullary sponge kidney is a cystic disorder that produces spaces at the apex of the renal pyramids. Onset peaks during adolescence or in the third to fourth decade. Infection, calculi, pain, and hematuria are potential complications, but renal function usually does not deteriorate unless the infection or calculi are uncontrolled.

There are several other hereditary renal disorders including chronic nephritis, congenital nephrotic syndrome, distal renal tubular acidosis, idiopathic hypercalciuria, and nephrotic diabetes insipidus. Many of these are fatal during childhood, but some persist into adulthood and will be discussed in the appropriate units of this text.

RENAL INFECTIOUS PROCESSES

Pyelonephritis

Pyelonephritis is an inflammation of the kidney caused by a bacterial infection. Sometimes an infection may be a primary disease. This is facilitated by the presence of a calculus, malignancy, hydronephrosis, or trauma that has reduced host resistance. However, most kidney infections appear to be extensions of infectious processes located elsewhere, with the bladder being the most common site. The etiology and pathogenesis of infections in the lower urinary tract are discussed in Chapter 42. The bacteria spread to the kidney primarily by traveling up (ascending) the ureter to the kidney; blood and lymphatic circulation also provide channels for the organisms. Ureteral reflux, which allows infected urine back into the ureter, and obstruction, which causes stagnation of urine allowing multiplication of the organisms, are the most common causes of ascending urinary tract infections.

There are two main types of pyelonephritis — acute and chronic. They differ particularly in their clinical picture and long-term effects.

Acute Pyelonephritis

Acute pyelonephritis may cause minimal symptoms and may even be asymptomatic. Typically, though, the patient presents in acute distress and appears quite toxic. He or she may report a one to two day history of dysuria, frequency, urgency, and other signs of cystitis. Fever, chills, nausea, and flank pain on the involved side are frequent findings. Percussion or deep palpation over the costovertebral angle elicits marked tenderness. The urine may be cloudy or bloody and foul-smelling and may contain many bacteria, red blood cells, and pus cells. The white blood count is usually elevated. Urine cultures will document the presence of bacteriuria and identify the invading pathogens.

The course of this acute infection is usually short, and it may even subside without treatment. However, recurrence is very frequent, either as a relapse of a previous infection not totally eradicated or as a new infection. The greatest incidence of reinfection is at four months after treatment is discontinued. Repeated infections can lead to chronic pyelonephritis, and the patient should be treated adequately to prevent this progression.

Medical treatment is aimed at eradication of the pathogenic organisms with the appropriate antibiotic as identified by the urine culture and sensitivity study and removal of any component contributing to decreased host resistance. The correct antibiotics will usually cause the urine to be sterile within 48 to 72 hours. The drug is continued for at least two weeks after the first sterile urine is achieved. The urine should be recultured one week after the antibiotics are stopped and periodically for a year after the infection. Surgery and/or additional medication therapy may be needed to correct any predisposing factor, such as obstruction or calculus.

Nursing care during the acute attack of pyelonephritis is directed toward symptomatic relief. *Forcing fluids* will offer the quickest relief for the burning on urination and will help to control the fever. The increased urine flow will also help to wash bacteria out of the urinary tract. Fluids should not be overforced, however, to avoid dilution of the antimicrobial. Appropriate measures should be taken to relieve the discomfort caused by the fever, nausea, and pain.

When the acute infection has subsided, the patient should be instructed in the importance of continuing follow-up care to prevent further infection, which can lead to chronic pyelonephritis and kidney failure. Patients must understand the importance of continuing the antibiotic even though they may feel fine. They should also be instructed in ways to prevent further infections anywhere in the urinary tract. See Chapter 42 for more discussion of prevention.

Chronic Pyelonephritis

Chronic pyelonephritis is a slowly progressive disease usually asssociated with recurrent acute attacks, although there may be no previous history of acute pyelonephritis. The kidney becomes contracted and the number of functioning nephrons decreases as they are replaced by scar tissue. The tubules become occluded and then dilated proximal to the point of obstruction. The end point of this disease process, unless halted, is renal failure.

Since it has no specific symptoms of its own, chronic pyelonephritis is frequently recognized on the basis of abnormal laboratory findings when the patient is being evaluated for hypertension and its complications, which are the most frequent manifestations of the disease. The laboratory studies may show azotemia (elevated nitrogenous substances in the blood), pyuria, anemia, acidosis, and/or proteinuria. They also demonstrate a poor concentrating ability.

Medical and nursing treatment are aimed at preventing further renal damage. If bacteria are found, appropriate antibiotics are given as in acute pyelonephritis. Hypertension must be controlled. Additional treatment depends on the degree of renal failure that has already occurred.

Another, less common, type of pyelonephritis is *emphysematous* pyelonephritis. It is found almost exclusively in patients with diabetes mellitus. The disease, which is usually caused by *Escherichia coli*, is ordinarily unilateral and is associated with renal parenchymal necrosis and spontaneous gas formation within the kidney. Possibly because of the high glucose levels in the renal tissue, the organisms produce carbon dioxide through fermentation of the sugar. The treatment for this condition is surgical removal of the involved kidney.[46]

Renal Carbuncle

A *renal carbuncle*, or *kidney abscess*, is a localized infection contained wtihin the cortex of the kidney. It is usually formed by the coalescence of smaller infectious foci or microabscesses in the renal parenchyma. The most common causative organism has been *Staphylococcus aureus*, but gram-negative organisms are quickly becoming the more prevalent cause. As with other kidney infections, the organisms may have spread along the hematogenous route from extrarenal sites or may have ascended from the lower urinary tract. However, most authorities feel that the hematogenous spread is more common, with organisms coming particularly from the skin or respiratory tract. Very frequently the patient will give a history of recent cutaneous furuncles.

The most common presenting symptoms are high fever and moderate to severe pain. The pain is usually constant in nature and is felt either in the upper quadrant of the abdomen or in the costovertebral area; it sometimes resembles renal colic. Unlike pyelonephritis, the urine is usually sterile, since the carbuncle does not communicate with the urinary collecting system. Other symptoms of infectious process are usually demonstrated by the patient: weakness, anorexia, diaphoresis, and leukocytosis.

Medical and nursing care is similar to that needed for acute pyelonephritis. Aggressive antibiotic treatment is usually successful. A needle aspiration of the carbuncle may be done in order to do a culture and sensitivity study on the contents; this helps pinpoint the appropriate antimicrobial to be used. It is sometimes necessary to do a surgical incision and drainage of the abscess. If this is done, nursing care expands to include care of the incision postoperatively. A drain will likely be left in place for some time.

Perinephric Abscess

A *perinephric abscess* involves the fatty tissue surrounding the kidney. It may be an extension of a renal infectious process (most common) or may have been spread hematogenously from an extrarenal infection. As with renal carbuncle, gram-negative organisms are rapidly emerging as the most common cause, replacing staphylococci. The abscess may spread in several directions and the patient may present with a draining flank abscess or a subphrenic abscess.

Signs and symptoms are the same as with a kidney abscess — fever, tenderness, flank or loin pain, and other signs of sepsis — with the addition of possible swelling over the site.

Medical and nursing care are also almost identical to that required for renal carbuncle. Appropriate antibiotics are administered and symptomatic interventions are undertaken. Because of the nature of a perinephric abscess, incision and drainage are needed more frequently than with renal carbuncle. When this surgical procedure has been done, there may be profuse drainage from the wound requiring frequent dressing changes.

Renal Tuberculosis

Tuberculosis of the kidney, which affects men more frequently than women, occurs when the causative agent, *Mycobacterium tuberculosis*, is brought to the kidney via the blood stream from another source in the body, usually the lungs. Once the organisms have reached the kidney, they may become dormant for many years. By the time they again become active, the original infection is often well healed. Frequently, the primary tubercular site was asymptomatic, making it difficult to identify the renal tuberculosis on the basis of history.

Pathologically, the clinical course of renal tuberculosis is generally very slow, and clinical signs and symptoms often do not become evident until the later stages of the disease. Early disease involves the renal cortex or medulla. Tissue destruction extends in all directions, eventually eroding into a calyx at the tip of a papilla, and then progresses to rupture into the renal pelvis. Once the infection reaches the pelvis, it spreads along the mucosa; this allows the organisms full access to the rest of the kidney and also permits them to move down the urinary tract where they can infect any of the other urinary organs. If untreated, the destructive process continues to form large, caseating masses which coalesce to destroy kidney tissue. X-ray examination at this time shows the kidneys to have a "moth-eaten" appearance and, as these lesions calcify later in the disease, their characteristic appearance becomes known as "putty kidney." Organisms reaching the lower urinary tract cause infection of these organs, with the most problematic results being fibrosis and stricture formation and destruction of the ureterovesical valve. If these processes stenose the ureter, reducing the exit for pus and urine from the infected kidney, renal destruction is accelerated. Descending tubercle bacilli may also lodge in the male reproductive organs, causing reduced function.

When the renal tuberculosis does become clinically evident, the signs and symptoms are often nonspecific. Renal symptoms may be preceded by general malaise, weight loss, low grade fever, and night sweats, but these are not as frequent as with pulmonary tuberculosis. Symptoms of cystitis, as described in Chapter 42, are often the presenting indications. Flank pain may be present, and hematuria and pyuria are common. Males frequently have signs and symptoms of epididymitis. Definitive confirmation of the diagnosis is made on the basis of culture of *Mycobacterium tuberculosis* from the urine. The specimens for culture are collected on at least three successive *mornings.* Because tubercle bacilli are shed intermittently, three to twelve negative cultures are needed to absolutely exclude the diagnosis of active renal tuberculosis.

When collecting the urine specimen, the nurse must remember that the urine from patients with renal tuberculosis is infectious. Special precautions are necessary when handling this urine.

Chemotherapy with antituberculosis drugs has reduced the need for surgical intervention. Multiple drug therapy is used, usually combining at least three of the following medications: streptomycin, rifampin, ethambutol, isoniazid, cycloserine, pyridoxine, and sodium para-aminosalicylate. Because of the slow division time of tubercle bacilli and to make it easier for the patient, the medications are usually given in a single daily dose, although, if patients are having difficulty with side effects, the day's quota may be given in divided doses. Chemotherapy is usually continued for a minimum of 2 years, though some physicians are studying the long-term effect of drug courses lasting a total of 6 to 9 months.

Surgical intervention includes total or partial nephrectomy or cutaneous ureterostomy. Permanent urinary diversion may be necessary if severe strictures or bladder damage is irreparable. Indications for surgery include persistent infection which has not responded to chemotherapy, intractable pain, hemorrhage, uncontrollable hypertension, suspicion of renal malignancy, and progressive strictures. The issue of whether to do partial or total nephrectomy is very controversial.

When planning nursing care for the patient with renal tuberculosis, the nurse must keep in mind that the patient has a prolonged illness and will require long-term care and support. During the initial stages, while the patient is hospitalized, the nurse assists with the diagnostic tests and helps get the patient regulated on medications. If surgery is necessary, pre- and postoperative care is similar to that for any patient having renal surgery. Measures must be instituted to improve the patient's general health: good nutrition, adequate rest, good hygiene. Tuberculosis is a disease that arouses a great deal of fear and feeling of social isolation. The nurse should help the patient discuss and work through such feelings. Especially for patients who are to be hospitalized for a prolonged period of time, help may be needed in making arrangements regarding home and job. Some may have to change occupations temporarily or permanently. The nurse may use other resources on the health team, such as social services, to help meet these needs.

Once the patient has been discharged from the hospital, one of the biggest problems is continued compliance with the prescribed medical and nursing regimens, especially when the patient begins to feel better. The nurse should help the patient understand the need for the prescribed long course of continuous drug therapy and the necessity for continuing follow-up examinations. During this time, the patient should be given positive feedback for adhering to the regimens if this is appropriate. And, if not, the patient and nurse should utilize problem-solving techniques in helping to reestablish compliance.

INTERSTITIAL NEPHRITIS

The characteristic finding in *interstitial nephritis* is an inflammatory reaction within the interstitium of the kidney. Although other diseases, such as radiation nephritis, and acute tubular necrosis, have a similar reaction as part of their morphology, the term interstitial nephritis usually refers to two specific situations: during a septic illness and as an allergic reaction. These two specifications give rise to the classifications of infectious and noninfectious. *Infectious* interstitial nephritis is also known as pyelonephritis and occurs as the result of pathogens in the renal parenchyma. See the full discussion of pyelonephritis above. The *noninfectious* form is associated with nephrotoxic agents, many of which are common medications. These agents may cause immunologic injury at the tubular level; immune complexes have been found. (See the section on nephrotoxic agents for more discussion of this pathology.) Interstitial nephritis is also found in some chronic, slowly progressive diseases, e.g., sarcoidosis and Sjögren's syndrome. Work is being done to identify more definitive boundaries for this disease.

Another, more commonly used, classification for this disease process is acute and chronic. *Acute interstitial nephritis* includes both septic and allergic etiologies. Its onset is usually rapid and its signs and symptoms are the result of tubular cell injury. Progress of the disease process can take one of three courses: complete recovery, rapid progression to renal failure and death, or movement to chronic interstitial fibrosis. Clinical diagnosis is established on the basis of such findings as glycosuria, high urine sodium concentration, and acute renal failure in a patient who is septic or is being exposed to nephrotoxic agents known to cause intrarenal allergic reactions. Eosinophilia and skin rash may also be found in the latter patients. Elimination of the infection in the septic patient and/or discontinuing offending medications will usually bring about recovery. Although corticosteroids are frequently used, there is no clear evidence of their worth. Nursing care is based on the patient's symptoms and, depending on the patient's condition, may need to encompass the care needed by a patient with acute renal failure.

In *chronic interstitial nephritis* there is progressive interstitial fibrosis and chronic inflammatory cell infiltration with tubular atrophy. Common stimuli include analgesic abuse, lead poisoning, and radiation. People from certain areas of Bulgaria and Yugoslavia are prone to a variation called *Balkan nephritis.* In the terminal stages, the altered renal vasculature and renal structure make the disease indistinguishable from chronic pyelonephritis. Therefore, the care of the patient is similar to that of the patient with either chronic pyelonephritis or chronic glomerulonephritis.

GLOMERULONEPHRITIS

Glomerulonephritis is a term that encompasses a variety of disease entities, most of which are caused by immunologic reaction resulting in proliferative and inflammatory changes within the glomerular structure. Since the primary function of the glomerulus is to filter blood, 80 per cent of the cases of glomerulonephritis are the result of trapping of antigen-antibody complexes within the glomerulus. Approximately 5 per cent are caused by circulating antibodies to the glomerular basement membrane.[175] The different pathologies are classified in various ways, but this unit will discuss the following types: acute, subacute, latent, membranoproliferative, rapidly progressive, chronic, and minimal change.

Acute Glomerulonephritis

Although another organism may be responsible, the stimulus for *acute glomerulonephritis* is usually a beta-hemolytic streptococcal infection elsewhere in the body. The disease characteristically occurs 10 days to 3 weeks after the primary infection. It appears that upon being exposed to the streptococcal antigens, the body produces antibodies. The complexes being deposited in the glomerulus cause a proliferative and inflammatory reaction. The mechanism for this injury is not clearly understood. The kidney becomes swollen, fatty, and congested. A bloody exudate seeps from the capillaries, infiltrating the renal parenchyma and causing decreased renal function.

This disease process is most often seen in children and young adults. Some authorities feel that its occurrence in older people is actually an exacerbation of earlier subclinical disease. It is customarily a self-limiting disease with full recovery, especially in children, but does progress to subacute or chronic glomerulonephritis in 25 to 40 per cent of the adults. A fatality report of 1.3 per cent has been given.[265]

Onset of the disease may be sudden or insidious. With sudden onset, the patient may experience fever, chilling, weakness, pallor, anorexia, nausea and vomiting, and dizziness. Generalized edema, particularly facial and periorbital swelling, is a typical finding. Accompanying the edema, physical examination may reveal ascites, pleural effusion, and signs of congestive heart failure with pulmonary edema. The patient frequently has headache and moderate to severe hypertension. Visual acuity may be reduced owing to retinal edema. There may be abdominal or flank pain, probably caused by kidney edema and distention of the capsule. Oliguria, and even anuria, may be present for several days; the longer this persists, the more irreversible kidney damage occurs. On the other hand, the disease may be so mild that the patient reports vague weakness, anorexia, and lethargy. The disease may even be initially discovered on the basis of a routine urinalysis.

Examination of the urine provides the data necessary for definitive diagnosis of acute glomerulonephritis. Gross hematuria and proteinuria are the cardinal findings. The urine, which may be scanty in amount, is typically smoky, red, or brown in color and has a low pH and a specific gravity in the mid- to high-normal range. It might be expected that the low urine production would result in a higher specific gravity, but the kidneys have decreased ability to concentrate. There are many red blood cells, white blood cells, and granular and hyaline casts. Mirroring reduced renal function, serum urea nitrogen and creatinine levels will be elevated and clearance rates will be down. C-reactive proteins and antistreptolysin titer are usually elevated.

Acute glomerulonephritis can become a fulminant process proceeding quickly to uremia or may become chronic glomerulonephritis. However, most patients start to evidence recovery within 10 to 14 days. Most clinical signs return to normal within several weeks, although the hematuria and proteinuria may persist for several months. Increased activity during the convalescent period may contribute to increased hematuria and proteinuria. If complete recovery has not occurred within 2 years, it is not likely that it will come. Some use the term *subacute glomerulonephritis* to designate disease which lasts more than 6 to 8 weeks. While most of the signs and symptoms of acute disease may have disappeared, the patient is still very susceptible to recurrent streptococcal infections, which will readily cause exacerbations of the glomerulonephritis. *Latent glomerulonephritis* sometimes refers to a situation in which the patient is asymptomatic but still has significant levels of albumin and casts in the urine more than a year after the acute onset; these elements indicate continued slow parenchymal changes.

Since nothing will heal the glomerular lesions already present, treatment is aimed at preventing further renal damage and improving kidney function. Medically, drug therapy is used to eliminate antigens, alter the immune balance of the patient, and inhibit or alleviate the inflammatory process. Initially, the patient is evaluated for other sites of streptococcal infection and, if found, appropriate antibiotics, e.g., penicillin, are used. Corticosteroids, immunosuppressives, alkylating agents, purine antagonists, and folic acid antagonists may be used to achieve the latter two goals. Dosages may be administered in one of several ways: "pulse" method, in which high doses are given once a day on alternate days; daily; or by interrupted regimens. It appears that side effects are less evident on "pulse" and intermittent dosing. Continued research is being done attempting to find more effective medications with which to treat this disease. In the meantime, other drugs may be used to symptomatically treat the patient, such as anticonvulsants and antihypertensives.

Nursing Care in Glomerulonephritis

Much of the care needed by the patient is in the realm of nursing. In line with the overall goals of therapy, the nursing care plan should contain planned interventions for avoidance of additional concurrent infections, diet, fluid balance, activity, skin care, and monitoring for complications. Because the patient will be immobilized for a period of time, all aspects of the body's response to immobility must be considered. The disease itself markedly diminishes the patient's natural defenses to infection, particularly streptococcal organisms. Treatment with immunosuppressives and corticosteroids even further reduces patient resistance. While isolation is not necessary, precautions should be taken to protect the patient from people with obvious infectious processes. General supportive measures help to boost the patient's defense mechanisms. He or she must be taught to avoid infections.

The diet ordered by the physician is generally a high-carbohydrate, low-protein one. This allows the patient to receive adequate calories to avoid protein catabolism while allowing the kidney to rest as it handles fewer protein molecules and metabolites. The degree of protein restriction depends on the amount being lost in the urine and the individual requirements of the patient. Sodium will also be restricted depending on the amount of edema present. In addition, anorexia, nausea, and vomiting caused by the disease may interfere with the taking in of enough calories. A dietician can help plan the patient's diet around these restrictions.

Fluid balance is important. Careful monitoring of daily weights and intake and output help determine the progress of the edema and thus provide an estimate of renal function. Daily measurement of edematous parts, e.g., legs and abdomen, also provides helpful objective data. The patient's allowable fluid intake will be based on the results of the above measurements. Most likely, fluid intake will be restricted. Thirst may be reduced by allowing the patient to suck on hard candies or by taking small amounts of water to sip. Meticulous oral hygiene will help alleviate thirst as well as prevent parotitis, which may be a complication of the reduced fluid intake.

Rest is essential — both physical and emotional. As mentioned above, there is a direct correlation between activity and the amount of hematuria and proteinuria. Exercise also increases catabolic activity. The amount of activity allowed to the patient depends on the results of serial urinalyses. The period of bedrest followed by a period of very limited activity may be prolonged for several weeks to months. Therefore the patient may need assistance in making arrangements concerning family, home, job, finances, community responsibilities, etc. He or she must be encouraged to talk about fears and concerns and must be helped to deal with the emotional reactions expected during a long-term illness with a questionable prognosis. Only after these problems are dealt with will the patient be able to have emotional rest. Appropriate diversionary activities must be found to help the patient deal with the prolonged physical immobilization.

Edema interferes with cellular nutrition, making the patient more susceptible to skin breakdown. Therefore, measures must be taken to prevent this complication. These include good hygiene, massage, and position changes as well as the use of other prophylactic equipment, such as eggshell mattress and sheepskin.

Early recognition of complications facilitates prompt medical attention. Common complications are pulmonary edema, cardiac failure, and increased intracranial pressure. Progression to renal failure is also a possibility. Appropriate monitoring must be done.

Membranoproliferative Glomerulonephritis

Membranoproliferative glomerulonephritis is a process that was recognized only a few years ago and is gaining importance. It is differentiated from acute glomerulonephritis by the facts that it affects the mesangial cells of the kidney rather than the endothelium and that it characteristically follows a progressive course to renal failure over a period of a few years. The chances for recovery are very poor.

As with acute glomerulonephritis, this disease is most common in children and young adults. Although it might be preceded by a streptococcal infection, much more frequently there is no apparent predisposing condition. Gross hematuria and persistent proteinuria are often the initial signals. If the nephrotic syndrome (see below) is not present at the outset of the disease, it will almost certainly evolve later. Medical and nursing care is a combination of that required for acute and chronic glomerulonephritis.

Rapidly Progressive Glomerulonephritis

Rapidly progressive glomerulonephritis is a fulminant variation of the disease. Its stimulus may be a streptococcus, pneumococcus, staphylococcus, or virus, or a collagen disease—or something thus far unknown. It is a disease primarily of young adults which usually begins undramatically and slowly and then relentlessly progresses to renal failure and uremia within a period of weeks to months. Morphologically, it is a diffuse proliferative inflammation of the glomerulus with its hallmark being epithelial crescents, this proliferation encircles the glomerulus, encroaching on Bowman's capsule and apparently compressing the glomerular tufts. The diagnosis is made on the basis of large numbers of these crescents being found on renal biopsy.

Early in the disease process, it is usually very difficult to distinguish between this disease and acute glomerulonephritis, unless a biopsy is done. However, as the disease progresses, oliguria and eventually anuria ensue. Edema and proteinuria become massive, and other signs and symptoms of uremia become paramount. Some patients have survived with immunosuppressives and corticosteroids being used to halt the progression of the disease. Dypyridamole, an anticoagulant, has also been used. However, these medications are not very successful and death usually occurs. On the basis that abnormalities of local coagulation play a role in the disease progression, some physicians have been trying low-dose heparin with some success in arresting and partially reversing the renal failure.[99] Dialysis may also be able to prolong the patient's life. Nursing care includes that needed for the other forms of glomerulonephritis plus the need for dealing with the issue of death and dying because of the rapid progression of the disease.

Chronic Glomerulonephritis

Chronic glomerulonephritis is also considered to be an immunologic disease, although it seems to represent a much milder antigen-antibody reaction. The immunologic injury apparently occurs at a continuous rate, as demonstrated by the fact that when presumably healthy kidneys are transplanted into patients with a history of glomerulonephritis, there is a recurrence of disease in the transplanted kidney. As glomeruli and their tubules are destroyed, the kidneys shrink in size and become contracted. Functioning renal tissue is replaced by fibrous and scar tissue. Sclerosis of renal blood vessels also occurs. The rate of destruction is variable.

This disease process has a very insidious onset. The patient may remain clinically asymptomatic, showing intermittent or persistent hematuria and proteinuria for several years. It may frequently be found when the patient is being evaluated for the cause of hypertension and its complications. Common presenting symptoms include malaise, weight loss, edema, increasing irritability, polyuria and nocturia due to the kidney's inability to concentrate urine, headache, dizziness, and digestive disturbances. Visual disturbances are caused by papilledema and retinal hemorrhages and include seeing black spots and flashes of light, dimming of vision, and transitory blindness. As the disease progresses, these symptoms intensify and the patient begins to experience respiratory difficulty and angina.

Examination of the patient demonstrates characteristic findings. Hypertension is probably the cardinal finding. Its complications are frequent. It is not uncommon for the patient to have nosebleed, signs of arteriosclerosis, cardiomegaly, and hemorrhage into the kidneys, lungs, retina, or cerebrum. Edema increases as heart failure becomes more severe and the serum albumin decreases. Examination of the eyegrounds shows vascular changes and edema of the discs. Urinalysis shows a fixed specific gravity, small amounts of proteinuria except during acute exacerbations, casts, white blood cells, renal tubular cells, and consistent hematuria. Anemia tends to be severe.

Chronic glomerulonephritis progresses over a period of several to as many as 30 years. The late stage of the disease is called the nephrotic stage. The most disturbing finding at this point is the massive anasarca, or generalized edema. The patient is essentially water-logged. The eyes are swollen almost shut and the patient suffers from ascites, hydrothorax and orthopnea, increased intracranial pressure, and sometimes pericardial effusion. Although a few patients survive this stage and enter a phase of remission, most die within 1 to 2 years.

Treatment — both medical and nursing — is mainly symptomatic and aimed at avoiding acceleration of the renal damage. Chemotherapy regimens that have been tried have included anti-inflammatory agents and anticoagulants, such as indomethacin and cyproheptadine. Because of the length of the disease, the patient is usually ambulatory, and restrictions being imposed on the patient must strike a balance with his or her life-style. This will facilitate long-term compliance. Hypertension must be treated and kept under control. Intercurrent infections at any site must be identified and aggressively treated. Diet and fluid intake may be regulated to control the edema and hypertension. Protein and sodium may be restricted. However, if the nonprotein nitrogen blood level is not elevated, the prescribed protein intake may be increased to over 80 grams per day. It is hypothesized that this replaces protein being lost in the urine and avoids hypoproteinemia, which contributes to edema. Anemia may require blood transfusions. Constipation must be avoided. The patient's activity level must be carefully adjusted depending on such things as energy reserve and cardiac status. Dialysis may be used to treat the uremia. It is important for women to avoid pregnancy, since they are highly susceptible to toxemia and spontaneous abortion. Because of the long course of this illness, with all its accompanying physical, emotional, and social problems, all possible resources should be mobilized to help the patient cope.

Other Forms of Glomerulonephritis

Minimal change glomerulonephritis, also called lipoid nephrosis, and idiopathic membranous glomerulonephritis are two additional forms. They both have many similarities to the types described above as well as some differences. Both appear to be related to immunologic injury, but do not have the proliferative or inflammatory characteristics of the other forms. Both disease processes are associated with the nephrotic syndrome (see below for description).

Minimal change glomerulonephritis is much more frequently found in children than in adults, and most patients report an incident representing an immunologic challenge, e.g., bacterial infection, bee sting, and poison ivy. As the disease progresses, electron microscopy shows thickening of the basement membrane and mesangial cells. Onset is usually abrupt, often with massive edema which appears out of proportion to the amount of proteinuria. The protein lost is primarily albumin. Hypertension, microscopic hematuria, and azotemia are infrequent. The characteristic features of this disease are its good prognosis, especially with the administration of steroids, its tendency for spontaneous remission, and the tendency for exacerbations. Spontaneous remissions have occurred in 30 to 50 per cent of the patients without using steroids. With the administration of high-dose steroids, the recovery rate comes up to 75 per cent.[335] Most patients have at least one, and usually more, exacerbations, usually within a year of the initial onset or of each other. The longer a patient has been in remission, the less likely he will have another relapse, with a 3 year span being the most indicative. Exacerbations seem to have no deleterious effects on the kidneys. Approximately 80 per cent of the children with minimal change glomerulonephritis achieve complete recovery,[108] but this rate decreases as the age of the patient increases. It is known that dramatic remissions are sometimes triggered by a viral infection, especially measles; it is thought that this may be the result of adrenal cortical stimulation.

Idiopathic membranous glomerulonephritis is primarily a disorder of adults. The singularly most characteristic morphologic change is thickening of the glomerular capillary wall and the development of spike-like projections in the basement membrane. The report of immunologic challenge is not as frequent as with other types of glomerulonephritis, although the onset is usually very insidious, and the antigen source may not be recognized or remembered. Hypertension and hematuria may be found in some patients and the proteinuria consists of both albumin and globulins. Spontaneous remission is infrequent, and many patients progress slowly to renal failure in a few years. Steroids and immunosuppressives may help the remission rate, although evidence of this is not definite. Exacerbations are frequent, and progressive glomerular scarring occurs during these episodes. Later stages of the disease become indistinguishable from chronic glomerulonephritis.

NEPHROTIC SYNDROME (NEPHROSIS)

Nephrosis is a term referring to any disease of the kidney characterized almost exclusively by degenerative lesions of the renal tubular epithelium and is marked by the *nephrotic syndrome,* which is a constellation of symptoms: massive proteinuria, hypoalbuminemia, and edema. Although some people use the terms interchangeably, nephrosis itself is primarily a disease of young children. The reader should consult a standard pediatrics textbook for more information.

The nephrotic syndrome results from diffuse glomerular damage. Its causes are numerous, with the most common being glomerulonephritis or some other systemic disorder, such as diabetes mellitus or lupus erythematosus. Other predisposing factors include allergic reactions, renal vein thrombosis, secondary syphilis, malaria, lymphoma, and preeclampsia.

The pathophysiology of this disorder finds the glomerular basement membrane becoming abnormally permeable to protein molecules, particularly albumin. There is some evidence of a decreased ability of the tubules to reabsorb filtered protein, although this theory is not yet universally accepted. The resultant hypoalbuminemia alters the oncotic pressure within the vascular tree, which starts the development of edema. This stimulates decreased elimination of sodium and water by the kidney and augmentation of aldosterone production. So the cycle goes.

Based on this physiology, the clinical picture of the nephrotic patient includes, as mentioned above, proteinuria, hypoalbuminemia, and edema. Edema is usually the patient's chief complaint. Although its onset may be insidious, it becomes massive and complications of the swelling may be seen. The skin frequently has a characteristic waxy pallor due to the edema rather than the anemia. Other symptoms include anorexia, malaise, irritability, and amenorrhea or abnormal menses. The amount of proteinuria may range from daily losses of 4 to 30 grams. Serum albumin concentrations may be as low as 1 to 2.5 grams per 100 ml. There may be hyperlipidemia, currently thought to be increased hepatic lipoprotein synthesis in response to the decreased serum albumin. A mild normocytic anemia is common. The urine typically contains granular and epithelial cell casts and fat bodies. There may be some hematuria.

The primary aim of medical therapy is to heal the leaking glomerular basement membrane and stop the massive loss of protein in the urine. The cycle of edema would then be broken. *Steroids* are used successfully with some patients, depending on the cause of their disease. Studies are being done on the effect of long-term steroid administration with favorable results, although it is known that patients can become steroid-dependent. Chlorambucil and cyclophosphamide, which are both nitrogen mustard derivatives, may be used as an alternative to prednisone; their mechanism of action is unclear, but they have been successful in reducing proteinuria.[225] Indomethacin has also been effective in some patients, probably through its inhibiting action on prostaglandin synthesis.[9]

Much of the treatment regimen is directed toward decreasing the patient's edema. A *high protein diet* is prescribed to replace body proteins and thus restore normal oncotic pressure. Because of the massive urinary losses, an intake of 120 to 150 grams daily for an adult is recommended in order to achieve a positive protein balance. A *high calorie intake* is also necessary for the body to utilize the additional protein. Since the kidneys have a reduced capacity to excrete sodium, a *salt restriction* is usually imposed. There is some controversy as to how much restriction there should be and for how long. Because it is so vital that the patient take in the necessary protein and calories, it is important that the diet be as palatable as possible. The amount of edema is used as the main criterion for this decision, and many times the restriction will be lifted during convalescence or when the edema is minimal.

Unless the patient is hyponatremic, fluids are not usually restricted. The patient's fluid balance should, however, be carefully monitored via daily weights, girth measurements, and intake and output determinations.

Supplementary to the diet control of the edema, medications may be used. *Diuretics* are frequent parts of the regimen. Spironolactone is often the primary agent because of its blocking action on aldosterone. Other commonly used diuretics include furosemide, ethacrynic acid, thiazides, and carbonic anhydrase inhibitors (see Chapter 37). In adjunct to the diuretics, plasma volume expanders, e.g., salt-poor albumin, plasma, and dextran, may be administered to raise the oncotic pressure within the vascular tree. This pulls fluid from the extracellular spaces and makes it available for filtration in the kidneys. Diuresis must be handled with particular caution with elderly patients because of their reduced capability to tolerate sudden shifts in intravascular volume.

There is a high incidence of renal vein thrombosis among patients with the nephrotic syndrome. Because of this, some patients may be placed on *long-term anticoagulation.* The nurse must teach the patient how to monitor for possible hemorrhage; the patient should also carry some identification describing medications being taken.

In addition to supporting the parts of the treatment regimen described above, the nurse helps the patient achieve and maintain maximal health. The amount of exercise allowed the patient is based on the severity of the edema. Bedrest is imposed only during severe edema and, as the fluid balance moves toward normal, the patient is allowed more activity. Hospitalization is usually not prolonged. Skin care is important because of the high potentiality of breakdown due to the interference with cellular nutrition by the edema. During acute stages, the patient and significant others may need much assistance in dealing with the accompanying malaise, anorexia, and depression.

HYDRONEPHROSIS

Hydronephrosis is the distention of the renal pelvis and calices by an obstruction to normal urine flow. Urine production continues and the urine is trapped proximal to the obstruction. The occlusion itself may be caused by several things, including calculus, tumor, scar tissue, inflammation, or a kink in the ureter. Whatever the cause, the damming up of the urine exerts pressure on the renal pelvic wall. Over time, sustained or intermittent high pressure will cause irreversible destruction of nephrons. However, at moderate to low pressure levels, the kidney may just continue to dilate with no observable loss of function. There is always a great risk of pyelonephritis because of the urinary stasis and reflux.

Treatment is aimed at preventing infection and permanently relieving the obstruction. Care must be taken in the management of the patient just after relief of the obstruction to prevent the untoward effects of a syndrome called *postobstructive diuresis.* Removal of the obstruction causes a sudden release of the pressure on the renal parenchyma which was being caused by the trapped urine. This leads to a reflexive diuresis which normally ceases as the kidneys readjust, but can lead to fluid depletion if it continues. There are three types of diuresis. In ascending order of frequency, these are (1) water diuresis due to a lack of response by the distal nephrons to anitdiuretic hormone; (2) urea diuresis; and (3) salt diuresis which is caused by either improper fluid management or a defect in tubular reabsorption. Salt diuresis may cause failure of the "counter-current mechanism" (see Chapter 40).

Because of the dangers involved in this condition, it is crucial to closely monitor the patient after an obstruction is released. Frequent observations that should be made include hourly urine output; weight; vital signs every 30 minutes for the first 24 hours and then every two hours; urine for specific gravity, albumin, and sugar; and presence of edema. Periodic serum electrolyte and glucose determinations should be made. Nursing care of the patient must take into account the expected presence of severe fatigue caused by urinary losses and the need for frequent observations. *Fluid management during this period is crucial.* It is usually recommended that hourly fluid replacement be based on the previous hour's urinary output.[318]

RENAL CALCULI

Although renal stones can be formed anywhere in the urinary tract, the most frequent site is the kidney. These stones may travel down the urinary tract with or without resultant damage, may lodge anywhere along the tract, or may stay within the kidney. It has been estimated that in the United States, over 200,000 people per year are admitted to hospitals because of renal calculus disease. This figure grossly underestimates the total number of people who are developing stones, since many urinary calculi are passed through the urethra without knowledge of the patient and many other patients are treated in outpatient visits to emergency rooms and clinics.

The formation of urinary stones follows some general principles regardless of the specific type of calculus. The process of stone formation is one of crystallization. Crystal growth occurs in the following manner: nucleation, in which crystallites are formed from supersaturated urine, is the initiating step, with growth proceeding by aggregation to form larger particles. This process may continue as is or a particle may travel down the urinary tract until it is trapped at some narrow point, at which it may become the nidus for formation of a stone. There is also evidence that a fibrous matrix made of proteins may be formed in the kidney or bladder into which the crystallites are deposited and trapped; this then becomes the nucleus of the stone. The excessive production of this mucoprotein may account in part for the frequent finding of family history of renal stones.

There are a number of *etiologic factors* that influence the formation of renal stones. The *presence of precipitators* in the urine includes the protein matrix as described above and bacteria or inflammatory elements. Increased *solute concentration* occurs because of fluid depletion and/or an increased solute load; this increased concentration predisposes precipitation of crystals, such as calcium, uric acid, and phosphate. Urinary pH influences the solubility of certain crystals with some crystal types precipitating readily in acid urine and some in alkaline urine. *Abnormal pH* levels are seen in renal tubular acidosis, administration of carbonic anhydrase inhibitors, presence of urea-splitting organisms, and severe chronic diarrhea. Normal urine contains substances that inhibit the aggregation of certain crystals. Therefore, *deficiency of* these "*solubilizers*" facilitates some formation. These substances include pyrophosphates, citrate, magnesium, and sodium. There may be "*antisolubilizers*" in the urine, such as aluminum, ferric iron, and silicone. Drinking water and magnesium trisilicate are common sources of silicone. Certain *medications* may induce stone formation through various modes. Commonly used drugs with this potential side effect include acetazolamide; absorbable alkali, such as calcium carbonate and sodium bicarbonate; aluminum hydroxide (prolonged use); oral orthophosphate; and allopurinol. Massive doses of vitamin C increase urinary oxalate concentration.[175] Anything that results in *urinary stasis* predisposes the patient to stone formation, since the crystals in unmoving urine precipitate more readily. Common conditions causing this problem include urinary tract obstruction and immobilization. It is probable that the development of urinary lithiasis (calculi) is not the result of one of the above factors, but of multiple phenomena. One of the biggest questions still not completely answered regarding renal calculi is why some people form stones and some do not. This problem is particularly important when working with recurrent "stone-formers."

TYPES OF STONES

There are a variety of types of renal calculi formed. Stones may be of one type solely or may be a combination. Approximately 75 per cent of all urinary tract stones contain calcium, usually as calcium phosphate or calcium oxalate. Calcium stones may range in size from very small particles, which are often called *sand* or *gravel*, to giant *staghorn* calculi which may fill the entire renal pelvis. They have a peak onset in the third decade and afflict primarily men. Hypercalciuria, or an increased solute load of calcium in the urine, is caused by three main components: (a) high rate of bone resorption which frees up calcium (hyperparathyroidism; immobilization; Paget's disease; osteolysis caused by malignant tumors of the breast, lung, and prostate; Cushing's disease); (b) absorption from the gut of abnormally large amounts of calcium (milk-alkali syndrome, sarcoidosis, excessive intake of vitamin D); and (c) impaired renal tubular absorption of filtered calcium (renal tubular acidosis). About 35 per cent of all calcium stone formers do not have high serum levels of calcium and have no apparent cause for their hypercalciuria. This condition is called *idiopathic hypercalciuria.* It is thought that the excess calcium excretion comes from either interstitial overabsorption of calcium or defective renal tubular reabsorption ("calcium wasters").

The second most frequent crystal to cause stones is *oxalate*, which is relatively insoluble in urine. Its solubility is only slightly affected by changes in the urinary pH. The mechanism for oxalate availability is unclear. It is felt by many to be at least closely related to diet and nutrition. The disease is most common in areas where cereals are a major component in the diet and least common in dairy farming regions. Some conditions in which the incidence of oxalate stones increases may be related to hyperabsorption of oxalate, e.g., inflammatory bowel disease, post–ileal resection or small bowel bypass, overdosage of ascorbic acid, and methoxyflurane anesthetic. There is also some thought that a concurrent fat malabsorption causes the binding of calcium, which frees oxalate for absorption. Recent research has identified a possible congenital metabolic defect in which decreased activity of the glycolytic enzyme aldolase leads to an accumulation of oxaloacetate and oxalic acid.[124] There findings add to the knowledge base about the congenital condition of *primary hyperoxaluria* and *oxalosis* in which there is excessive tissue deposition and urinary excretion of oxalate.

Struvite stones, also called *triple phosphate*, are caused by certain bacteria, usually *Proteus*, which contain the enzyme urease. This enzyme splits urea into two ammonia molecules which raise the pH of the urine. Phosphate precipitates in alkaline urine. This action has caused the label "urea-splitters" to be given to these organisms. The stones formed in this manner are *staghorn* calculi which grow to fill the renal pelvis and caliceal system. These stones are particularly hard to eradicate because the hard stone forms around a nucleus of bacteria, protecting them from any antibiotic therapy. Any small fragment left after surgical removal of the stone begins the cycle again.

Uric acid stones are caused by increased excretion of urate, fluid depletion, and a low urinary pH. Hyperuricuria is the result of either increased uric acid production or the administration of uricosuric agents. Approximately 25 per cent of the patients with primary gout and 50 per cent of those with secondary gout develop uric acid stones. There may also be a link between hyperuricuria and calcium stone formation in that uric acid crystals seem to absorb some of the crystal formation inhibitors normally found in the urine.

Cystinuria is the result of a congenital metabolic error inherited as an autosomal recessive disorder. Acid urine helps precipitation of the crystal to form *cystine* stones. Appearance of these stones usually occurs during childhood and adolescence with development after that very rare.

Xanthine stones also occur as the result of a rare hereditary condition in which there is a deficiency of the enzyme xanthine oxidase. It also precipitates readily in acidic urine.

SIGNS AND SYMPTOMS

Despite the type of stone that has been formed, the potential damage is essentially the same: pain, obstruction, and tissue trauma with secondary hemorrhage and infection. Thus, there tends to be one general clinical picture of signs and symptoms for all stone types. The rest of this discussion will deal primarily with stones affecting the kidneys and ureters. For further information about bladder and urethral stones, see Chapter 42.

The most characteristic symptoms of renal or ureteral calculi is a sharp, severe pain with a sudden onset. Depending on the site of the stone, this pain may be called either renal colic or ureteral colic. *Renal colic* originates deep in the lumbar region and radiates around the side and down toward the testicle in the male and the bladder in the female. It is caused by distention of the renal pelvis and proximal ureter by an increase in hydrostatic pressure. *Ureteral colic* radiates toward the genitalia and thigh and is the result of ureteral distention. When the pain is severe, the patient appears to be in acute distress and will usually exhibit nausea and vomiting, pallor, and diaphoresis, and be quite anxious. Diarrhea and abdominal discomfort may be present due to activated renointestinal reflexes. There may be frequency, although little urine may be voided. The pain may last for minutes to days and may be somewhat resistant to narcotic interference. It may be intermittent, which usually means that the stone has moved. It is hypothesized that the ureter dilates just proximal to the calculus, which allows urine to pass through, relieving the ureteral distention. Then, as the stone moves and sets up a new site of obstruction, the pain returns. The pain subsides when the stone has reached the bladder.

Pain caused by renal stones is not always severe and colicky in nature. It may be a dull, aching, or heavy feeling. This is particularly true during the early stages of developing hydronephrosis. Sometimes there may be no sensation and the first clue the patient may have is when a "clink" against the toilet bowl is heard when the stone is passed.

As with any disease process, the history given

by the patient is very important in identifying the problem. Full information about the onset of symptoms and the pattern of pain is vital. Family history of calculi is suggestive. Recent dietary habits should be evaluated. For instance, a large intake of purines may be significant, and drinking large amounts of fruit juices and tea facilitates precipitation of oxalates. The patient should be asked about recent medications and the presence of any contributing factors, such as urinary tract infection or gout.

Physical findings are primarily centered on two things: the urine and x-ray studies. It is important to strain *all* urine being voided through several layers of gauze. This may be done by the patient or nurse. All debris in the bedpan or urinal is carefully examined. Any stone material must be saved, partially so the composition of the stone can be analyzed as a basis of treatment and partially to show how much has passed through the urinary tract. The urine should also be monitored for hematuria. A routine urinalysis gives important information about the pH, the specific gravity, and the presence of red blood cells, white blood cells, crystals, and casts. Twenty-four–hour urine specimens may be collected to determine the daily output of possible causative crystals. A urine culture will help to identify urinary tract infection, whether it be a primary or a secondary problem. Blood levels of constituent elements, such as calcium, phosphorus, and uric acid may be determined. Stones containing calcium and cystine are radiopaque and will show up on a kidney, ureter, bladder (KUB) x-ray. Excretory urogram and retrograde pyelography will usually also be done.

TREATMENT OF RENAL STONES

The primary aim of treatment is to preserve renal function. *Medical and nursing management* is concerned with three main phases of patient need: (1) care of the patient during the acute phase; (2) elimination of any stones; and (3) long-term prevention of recurrence. During the *acute phase* when the patient is very ill with renal or ureteral colic, care is mainly symptomatic. Narcotics and antispasmodics are used for control of the pain and antiemetics for the nausea and vomiting. Warm baths and moist heat to the flank may provide relief. The patient should remain on bedrest, although he or she may be too uncomfortable to do so during the most severe period. Fluid intake should be at least 3000 ml. per day. Intravenous fluids may be needed until the nausea and vomiting are controlled.

Methods for *elimination of the stone* range from simply waiting through removal of the kidney. A small renal calculus entrapped in the calyx which is asymptomatic and apparently causing no complications will probably be left entirely alone, although the patient will be instructed in a preventive program. Even if the stone is causing severe discomfort, the medical intervention may be a matter of waiting, since almost 90 per cent of all renal calculi pass through the urinary tract spontaneously. During this time, fluid intake is kept high and the patient is kept as comfortable as possible with medication if necessary. The urine is meticulously strained and the patient is continually monitored for hematuria and urinary tract infection. Any infection found is treated aggressively with the appropriate antibiotic. Measures may be instituted to prevent formation of additional stones. Oral methylene blue has been used to help dissolve stones, with contradictory results.

If it is decided that the stone will not be passed before undesirable complications occur, *mechanical intervention* will be used. Depending on the position of the calculus, a cystoscopy may be done and one or two ureteral catheters inserted past the stone. From this point, several different treatment modes may be tried. The catheters may be left in place for 24 hours. Their presence drains the urine trapped proximal to the stone and dilates the ureter, which may facilitate spontaneous movement of the calculus, or the catheters may mechanically guide the stone downward as they are removed. A continuous renicidin irrigation may be established in an effort to dissolve the stone. Sometimes when an irrigation system is established, a nephrostomy tube is placed in the kidney as a safety valve in case the ureteral drainage is occluded. Care of this tube is like that of a wound and drain, with strict aseptic technique required. Finally, an attempt may be made to manipulate or dislodge the stone. A variety of special catheters with loops and expanding baskets may be inserted through the cystoscope and may be used to snare the stone. The postoperative care of these patients is the same as that following cystoscopy (see Chapter 41). Chapter 42 describes the care of a patient with indwelling ureteral catheters.

If the above techniques are unsuccessful in removing the stone, *surgical removal* will be necessary. A stone lodged in the ureter will require a *ureterolithotomy*, which involves an incision into the affected ureter. The approach may be through a lower abdominal or flank incision. The stone is removed, any strictures are repaired, and the incision is closed. One technique that may be used for recurrent urolithiasis is the placement of an ileal segment between the renal collecting system and the bladder. This segment provides an additional large-caliber channel for urine flow which helps avoid recurring ureteral obstruction by stones.[215]

Postoperative care needed by the patient will depend, to a large extent, on the location of the incision and the type of drainage tubes present. With a flank incision, the care will be that needed after kidney surgery as described below, while the patient with an abdominal incision is cared for as any patient having major abdominal surgery. The nurse will need to know that the incision may be expected to drain large amounts of urine for days to weeks after the surgery; the ureter is frequently not sutured with a water-tight seal in order to prevent further hydronephrosis from ureteral occlusion. Frequent dressing changes will be needed or a colostomy bag may be applied around the drain or incision to catch the drainage and reduce the frequency of dressing changes. A ureteral catheter or T-tube may be left in place to splint the ureter during the healing process.

Removal of a stone from the renal pelvis is done by a *pyelolithotomy* and from the renal parenchyma by a *nephrolithotomy*. In the case of extensive staghorn calculi, the kidney may need to be split end-to-end in order to facilitate complete removal. There is a very high recurrence of struvite stones unless all fragments are removed. This patient has a greatly increased risk of postoperative hemorrhage. An irrigation system with a stone-dissolving solution, e.g., hemiacidrin, may be established. If kidney damage has been too severe, it may be necessary to do a *nephrectomy,* partial or total removal of the kidney. Care of the patient having surgery on the kidney is described below.

PREVENTION OF RECURRENCE OF RENAL STONES

The third aspect of patient management is *prevention of further stones.* Although most persons who have a urinary tract stone will never have another, approximately 25 per cent of the patients develop recurrent lithiasis. And the ability to predict who will and who will not is still not very reliable. Recurrence of a stone usually happens within a 2- to 3-year period, but may occur as much as 20 years later. As the number of recurrences increases, the interval between stones tends to become shorter.[55] Prevention involves a lifelong program.

The three main components of a preventive regimen are fluids, diet, and medications. The patient's *fluid intake* should be at least 3000 to 4000 ml. per day. This amount may need to be increased as insensible losses increase, e.g., hot climate, fever, diarrhea. The increased urine volume resulting from this high fluid intake decreases the concentration of solutes and alleviates urinary stasis. The kind of fluids the patient drinks depends upon what dietary restrictions are necessary. It is important that the fluid intake be as consistent as possible throughout the 24-hour period. Patients are usually advised to drink 1 glass every hour during the day and 2 large glasses just before going to bed. This will usually mean that patients will need to void about mid-way through the night, at which time they should drink another glass. The patients will likely need help in adjusting their life-styles to accommodate the frequent need for bathroom breaks.

In order to plan necessary *dietary restrictions,* it is essential to have the results of a stone analysis. Several stone constituents require specific diet adjustments to avoid stone formation. Hypercalciuria may be reduced by decreasing the intake of calcium. This is usually accomplished by restricting all dairy products. This precaution should be taken with immobilized patients even if they do not have a history of calculus formation, since immobility itself causes freeing of calcium from the bones. Excessive intake of vitamin D and vitamin D–enriched food should be avoided in order to prevent stimulation of parathyroid hormone production. Patients with oxalate stones need to avoid high oxalate foods, e.g., tea, cocoa, instant coffee, cola drinks, beer, rhubarb, beans, spinach, and certain fruits (citrus, apple, grape, and cranberry). An acid-ash diet is recommended for patients with triple phosphate or struvite stones and an alkaline-ash diet for propensity toward uric acid calculi. An acid-ash diet encourages eggs, meat, poultry, fish, cereals, and specific fruits and vegetables, including cranberries, prunes, grapes, asparagus, pumpkin, tomatoes, and corn. Foods allowed on an alkaline-ash diet are milk; fruits, except cranberries, plums, and prunes; rhubarb; vegetables, especially legumes and green vegetables; and small amounts of ham, beef, halibut, trout, and salmon. It may be necessary to markedly restrict protein intake in order to decrease dietary methionine in patients with cystine stones; however, this is quite rare. The reader should consult a therapeutic diet guide for specific details about these diets.

Medications may also be used to reduce the incidence of recurrent calculi. Drugs frequently used to control calcium stone formation include cellulose phosphate, a calcium-binding resin which decreases intestinal absorption of calcium, and hydrochlorothiazide, which increases renal tubular reabsorption of calcium. The use of cellulose phosphate typically causes mild, transient diarrhea. Methylene blue may decrease calcium oxalate crystal formation. These patients should avoid calcium-containing antacids. Cholestyramine is commonly used with oxalate stone-forming patients. It is an anion-exchange resin which adsorbs oxalate. Its important potential side effect is a severe vitamin K depletion. Orthophosphate may increase the urinary concentration of oxalate solubilizer, although the mechanism of action is not totally clear. Pyridoxine is given to patients with oxalate stones on the basis that its deficiency interferes with the metabolism of gloxylic acid and therefore increases excretion of the crystal. Magnesium oxide also decreases oxalate excretion, and isocarboxazid apparently also blocks the metabolism of oxalate. One of the most frequent components of the medication regimen for triple phosphate or stuvite stones is long-term antibiotics as an attempt to control the infection. Methylene blue and phosphate binders may be used. The patient may need a phosphorus supplement. A specific urease inhibitor, e.g., acetohydroxamine acid, may be of value. The primary medication used for uric acid stones is allopurinol, which is a xanthine oxidase inhibitor. Uricosuric drugs should be avoided whenever possible, since they increase uric acid excretion in the urine, thus increasing the solute concentration. Cystine stone-formers are treated with D-penicillamine or mercaptopropionylglycine, which transforms L-cystine into a water-soluble disulfide derivative. Patients treated with these drugs usually need supplemental vitamin B_6.

It is frequently helpful to adjust the urinary pH as a means to control precipitation of crystals. An acidic urine, with a pH below 6, is used to prevent possible calcium and triple phosphate or struvite stones. Chapter 42 describes methods used for acidifying the urine. In addition, methionine or ammonium salts may be used. Uric acid and xanthine stones require alkaline urine, which is usually accomplished with sodium bicarbonate or citrate.

Two other objectives need to be achieved as part of the preventive program. Any underlying contributing problem must be corrected, e.g., metabolic and anatomic. Infection must be avoided and/or aggressively treated for all stone types, since its incidence places additional stress on the kidneys.

RENAL NEOPLASM

Benign tumors of the kidney are rare. Classifications include lymphangioma, lipoma, medullary fibroma, adenoma, and leiomyoma. When large ones occur, it is relatively impossible to distinguish them from malignant tumors by x-ray. If other diagnostic tests are also inconclusive, nephrectomy is frequently done.

About 85 per cent of all renal tumors are malignant. There are approximately 7300 deaths per year due to adult kidney cancer, representing 1 to 3 per cent of all malignancies.[93, 267] The tumors are most frequently discovered in the fifth and sixth decades. *Adenocarcinoma,* or *renal cell carcinoma* or *hypernephroma*, is the most frequent type of tumor, accounting for 80 per cent of all kidney neoplasms. Tumor growth begins in the renal cortex and usually goes on for some time before it produces symptoms. It can grow very large and tends to compress adjacent renal parenchyma rather than infiltrate it. The tumor, which is usually hypervascular, tends to surround blood vessels and stenose them. The lungs and mediastinum are the most frequent site of metastasis for this tumor, with liver, bone, skin, spleen, renal vein, and brain being other common sites.

Other types of renal cancers include nephroblastoma, sarcoma, and epithelial tumors within the renal pelvis. *Nephroblastoma,* or *Wilms' tumor,* is primarily a disease of children, although it has occasionally been found in adults. For further discussion of this type of cancer, refer to a pediatric text. *Sarcoma* is found infrequently and is considered to arise in the renal capsule. Most tumors of the renal pelvis are primarily *urothelial* in origin and include three different tissue types: transitional cell, squamous cell, and adenocarcinoma. These neoplasms represent about 15 per cent of total renal cancers.

SIGNS AND SYMPTOMS OF RENAL CANCER

Symptomatology for renal malignancies is varied and, as mentioned above, tumor growth may be quite advanced by the time the disease is discovered. Frequently, suspicion is first aroused when a palpable abdominal mass is found during a routine physical examination. It has been established that the average time delay between the onset of hematuria and diagnosis is 23 months, and 14 months between the initial pain and diagnosis.[93] Many times, extrarenal manifestations are found before renal cancer itself is confirmed. It has been established that as many as 35 per cent of the patients have metastasis when the final diagnosis is made.

The common triad of presenting symptoms includes *hematuria, flank pain, and a palpable abdominal or flank mass.* The hematuria is usually gross and intermittent, which helps explain the patient's delay in seeking medical advice. The clinical picture also contains a combination of the following frequent signs and symptoms: fever, weight loss and cachexia, fatigue, hypertension, amyloidosis, thrombophlebitis, anemia, erythrocytosis, and an elevated sedimentation rate. Less frequent findings include peripheral neuropathy, inferior vena cava obstruction, priapism, and varicocele. Hydronephrosis may occur if the tumor obstructs the ureteropelvic junction. The incidence of pulmonary embolus as a presenting manifestation may be more frequent than previously thought owing to the high rate of vena cava and renal vein involvement. Plasma erythropoietin, renin, and chorionic gonadotropin levels are elevated and prostaglandin production increases in renal cell carcinoma. Diagnosis is confirmed on the basis of several diagnostic tests, including excretory urogram, nephrotomography, ultrasound, CAT scan, selective arteriography, and biopsy after ureteral brushing or needle aspiration.

Staging

Staging of the tumor helps delineate the appropriate treatment mode to be used. One classification is as follows: Stage I — confined to the kidney; Stage II — involves perirenal fat, but is confined to Gerota's fascia; Stage III — vascular or lymphatic involvement; and Stage IV — distant metastasis.[64]

TREATMENT OF RENAL CANCER

The conventional and principal *treatment* for renal cancer is *nephrectomy*. Radiation and/or chemotherapy may be part of the medical regimen but are adjunctive to surgical removal of the kidney. For renal cell adenocarcinoma, the surgical procedure of choice is radical nephrectomy, including lymph node dissection. When the tumor is located in the renal pelvis, a nephroureterectomy is usually done because of the tendency of transitional cell cancer to "seed" down the ureter into the bladder; with this procedure, a cuff of the adjacent bladder is removed. Even in advanced cases, when the prognosis is poor, nephrectomy may be done as palliation for pain and hematuria. If the nephrotic disease is bilateral, partial nephrectomy may be done on at least one kidney, depending on the extensiveness of the tumor. Partial nephrectomy may also be done if the cancer is in the only functioning kidney. If partial nephrectomy is not possible in these cases, the entire kidney(s) will be removed and the patient placed on long-term dialysis. These patients are candidates for transplant in the future, but they are usually maintained on dialysis for at least a year to observe for recurrence of the disease.

Preoperative treatment may help shrink the tumor and make it easier to resect during surgery. Irradiation has been shown to reduce the size of the tumor. Renal artery embolization of the affected kidney may be done to infarct the tumor and reduce its vascularity. This is usually done by placing one of several things into the renal artery to occlude it: absorbable gelatin sponge, barium, autologous skeletal muscle, or a Swan-Ganz catheter. This procedure may also be done to control hemorrhage in an inoperable kidney.

As a treatment method, irradiation seems to be most useful in preoperative preparation of the tumor. It is sometimes used postoperatively to destroy any residual or recurrent tumor cells. Radiation of the kidney may also be used in patients whose tumor has been deemed inoperable.

Clinical investigation continues to seach for an effective chemotherapeutic regimen. Medroxyprogesterone and testosterone have been used as hormonal therapy. Cyclophosphamide and 5-fluorouracil, both antineoplastic drugs, have been used. Stimulants to the immune system, e.g., BCG, have shown some positive results. Transfer factor, which is a polypeptide that can restore or initiate cellular immunity, is being studied with a positive outlook.[216] Ribonucleic acid also mediates immune reaction and has had some success in patients with pulmonary metastasis.[248] Other drugs are being studied.

It must be noted that there have been numerous reports of spontaneous regression of renal adenocarcinoma. Authorities consider these episodes as more evidence that the disease has a definite immunologic or hormonal link.

NURSING CARE IN RENAL CANCER

Nursing management of the patient with renal cancer must consider the general aspects of care needed by any patient with neoplastic disease (see Chapter 23). Most specific to the patient with a kidney malignancy is the care required for a patient having a nephrectomy or nephroureterectomy. The pre- and postoperative care for nephrectomy is the prototype for any kind of renal surgery; the care required for other procedures can be variations of this model.

Preoperative preparation of the patient having renal surgery includes general guidelines as described in Chapter 17. Fluid intake may be increased to assure adequate excretion of waste products before surgery. In addition to the usual anxiety associated with having surgery, the patient may be very concerned about his urinary function postoperatively. If there will be a remaining kidney with good function, the patient can be assured that this kidney will be able to take over to fully meet the body's elimination needs. (See the discussion about renal transplantation for more information about this.)

The position of the patient during the surgical procedure depends on the incision to be used. For a flank incision, the patient will be placed in a hyperextended side-lying position. Some surgeons use a combination of a thoracoabdominal and subcostal abdominal incision. For this approach, the patient is placed in an oblique position with rolled towels situated to elevate the flank. This incision extends from the posterior axillary line to the lateral border of the rectus abdominis muscle in the midline abdomen.

Postoperative care is similar to that for a laparotomy. One of the biggest challenges is the *prevention of atelectasis and pneumonia*. Deep breathing and coughing are very difficult for the patient because the incision is so close to the diaphragm. So the patient will want to splint the chest protectively. In addition, if a thoracoabdominal approach was used, there will be chest tubes in place. Judicious use of narcotics to relieve the pain and mechanical external support to the chest with the hands will help the patient do his deep breathing and coughing exercises more effectively. Intermittent positive-pressure breathing apparatus may also be used to aid in respiratory exchange and the expectoration of secretions. Surgically induced or spontaneous pneumothorax does occur occasionally after nephrectomy, so the nurse should be prepared for this possibility.

Careful monitoring of renal function is essential. Urine output is measured hourly in order to identify renal failure as early as possible. Other serial observations about fluid balance to make frequently include intake and output and weight.

Because of the patient's position during the operation, *muscular pain* may occur. This may be relieved by massage, moist heat, and analgesics.

Paralytic ileus is a fairly common postoperative occurrence. The nurse should evaluate the patient's gastrointestinal status carefully before starting oral food and fluids. Treatment of an ileus includes nothing by mouth, nasogastric and/or rectal tubes, exercise as possible, and sometimes medications to stimulate intestinal peristalsis.

Wound care is routine and depends on the condition of the incision. With nephrectomy, there frequently is no drain inserted. There may be clamps in place with the handles extending out through the incision. These may be necessary when it is impossible to ligate the renal vessels. If present, these instruments should not, under any circumstances, be dislodged, and the patient should not be allowed to lie on the affected side.

Other components of nursing care needed include exercise, nutrition, elimination, and the prevention of complications.

RENAL TRAUMA

Serious injury to the kidney is relatively rare because of the protection afforded by the rib cage and the heavy muscles of the back. Traffic accidents and falls in which the person lands on the abdomen, flank, or back are the most common cause of injury. This type of situation usually causes blunt trauma. Although protected, the kidney is able to move a distance of one to three vertebral levels on its pedicle and to be bounced against the ribs. Kidney lacerations are also associated with fractures of the spine and ribs as well as with penetrating injuries from bullets and knives.

Figure 43–2 illustrates the five levels of traumatic injury that can occur to the kidney: contusion with intrarenal hemorrhage, rupture with subcapsular hemorrhage, rupture into the renal pelvis, shattered rupture, and pedicle injury. A contusion involves the development of a hematoma which remains confined within the renal parenchyma. Rupture of the kidney may cause hemorrhage between the capsular wall with or without bleeding also into the renal pelvis. A shattered or "fractured" kidney results in hemorrhage throughout the renal tissue. The pedicle holds the renal artery and other vital circulatory and nervous system connections for the kidney; injury to this may well jeopardize the life of the kidney. A pedicle injury may occur with or without intrarenal hemorrhage.

In addition to the immediate problems of hemorrhage and loss of functioning renal tissue, kidney trauma makes the patient highly susceptible to a number of other problems. Even in closed injuries, there is a high risk for sepsis leading to the development of kidney and perinephric abscesses. Secondary hemorrhage is not uncommon. Other complications include hypertension due to fibrosis and ischemic kidney, renal artery thrombosis, arteriovenous aneurysms, fistula formation due to the extravasation of urine, and the development of urinomas and pseudocysts.

The first key to identifying renal trauma is suspicion because of the type of injury the patient suffered. There are frequently multiple injuries, and the renal trauma may well get lost in the shuffle. *Hematuria* (gross or microscopic) is a cardinal sign, being found in approximately 80 per cent of the patients. However, it must be remembered that serious renal injury can occur without hemorrhage, so a clear urine should not negate the possible diagnosis. Other findings include shock, flank pain, and the development of a palpable mass in the affected flank area. Loss of intestinal peristalsis may also occur.

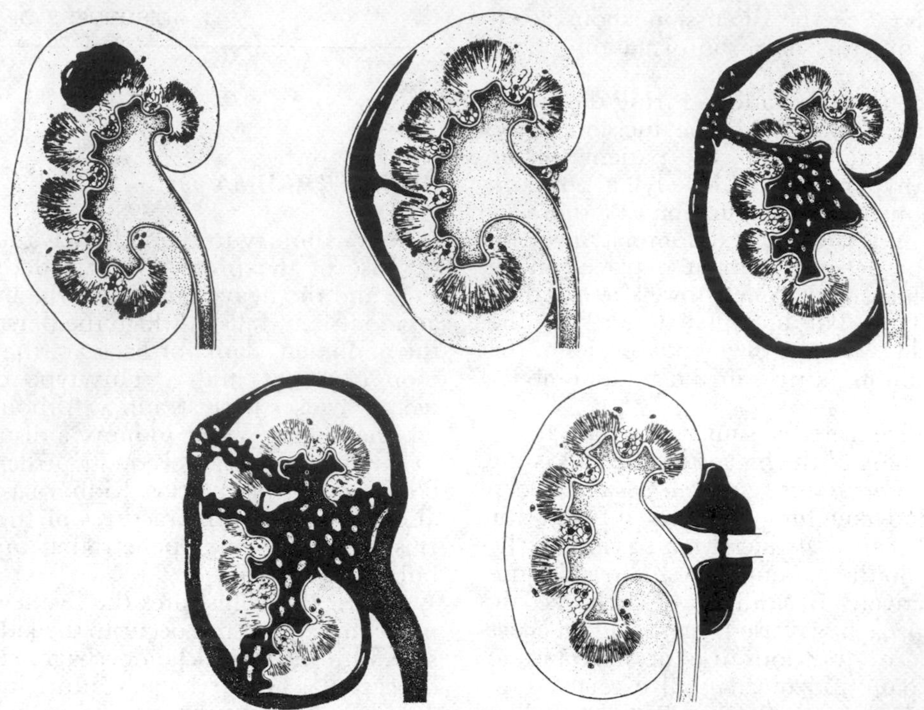

Figure 43–2. Levels of traumatic injury to the kidney. (From Derrick, F., and R. Kretkowski: Trauma to the kidney, ureter, bladder, and urethra. *Postgraduate Medicine,* 55:183, Jan., 1974.)

Excretory urogram, retrograde pyelography, renal scan, and renal arteriography help confirm the kind and amount of injury to the kidney.

The *treatment* of renal trauma is greatly controversial, with the decision necessary being whether to pursue a conservative or surgical pathway. It is generally accepted that kidney contusion calls for conservative treatment and that penetrating injuries require surgical exploration to determine the extent of the injuries and to repair damage to the tissues along the line of penetration. However, there is diversity of opinion on how to handle the renal damage found in this instance and on how to approach the ruptured kidney. Some recommend free use of nephrectomy as a treatment mode in order to avoid later sequelae, while others feel that the goal should be to salvage maximum renal function. The latter group advocates giving the conservative approach, sometimes called expectant management, a fair trial and, if surgery is necessary, to attempt to repair the kidney before removing it. In one retrospective study, 84 patients with renal damage, excluding pedicle injury, were treated by expectant management. The data seemed to show that the final rate of nephrectomy was much lower and that kidneys will often heal themselves without further intervention.[307]

Conservative treatment is possible because the retroperitoneal space allows for tamponade and primarily involves waiting and watching. In the absence of other injuries, a patient with microscopic hematuria and a normal excretory urogram may not even be hospitalized but followed on an outpatient basis. If there is gross hematuria, the patient is placed on bedrest until the urine clears. Serial observations of the urine, hematocrit, and vital signs are made to watch the progress of the hemorrhage. Rotating urine specimens may be collected in order to compare current and previous urine color and turbidity. Even if replacement fluids are not needed, a prophylactic intravenous line may be established and a type and cross-match for blood may be done. If a hematoma is present or the excretory urogram demonstrates extravasation of urine, antibiotics may be given to prevent sepsis. Blood transfusions may be given if the hematocrit indicates the need for replacement. After the urine has totally or almost cleared, the patient will be allowed to increase his activity. After discharge from the hospital, it is important for the patient to follow through on the recommended blood pressure checks and follow-up excretory urograms. These are necessary to rule out the development of secondary hypertension and anatomic derangement of the kidney.

Renal hemorrhage may be controlled by injection of an autologous clot into the secondary arteries supplying the bleeding site. Blood is drawn from the patient and allowed to clot. The clot is then injected angiographically. Normal endothelium has a strong clot-lysing effect, so the clot disappears after a period of several hours from the normal adjacent vasculature and affects only the damaged portion.

Possible indicators for surgical exploration

include continued moderate to severe hemorrhage and continued extravasation of urine. Extravasation itself is not definite grounds for surgery, since sterile urine usually resolves or encapsulates spontaneously. However, sometimes it produces severe tissue reaction and causes the formation of fistulas. The pocket of extrarenal urine may also become obstructive.

If repair of the kidney is to be tried rather than nephrectomy, the surgical procedure aims to debride devitalized tissue, achieve hemostasis, establish a water-tight seal of the collecting system, approximate the renal parenchymal edges, and drain the renal fossa. Two surgical techniques have increased the successful outcome of repair attempts. *Extracorporeal* or *bench surgery* allows the kidney to be removed from the body so that better visualization and manipulation is possible during the repair process; the kidney is then returned to the body by autotransplantation. During the time outside the body, the kidney is maintained either by hypothermia or by a perfusate mechanically pulsed through it. The *slush technique*, involving immersion of the kidney in iced saline slush, decreases the metabolism and oxygen requirement of the renal tissue, allowing longer intraoperative ischemic times. This does cause some systemic hypothermia, but not a significant amount. Pedicle vascular injury may also be repaired. If these goals cannot be attained, nephrectomy is necessary. Postoperative care of these patients is as described above.

RENAL VASCULAR ABNORMALITIES

The kidneys depend on adequate blood circulation to nourish the tissues and to provide blood for filtration so they can perform their intended functions. Anything that interferes with the normal circulatory flow significantly reduces the renal capabilities.

Renal Artery Disease

Two progressive disease processes that can lead to stenosis or thrombosis of the renal artery are atherosclerosis and fibrous dysplasia. Acute *obstruction* can be caused by embolism or thrombosis. Trauma, as described above, can also interrupt normal blood flow. The renal artery may be purposely occluded in order to produce a "*medical nephrectomy*" or total renal infarction; this may be done preoperatively in the case of renal adenocarcinoma or to control proteinuria or hypertension. Shredded Gelfoam may be used, or a liquid substance which polymerizes instantly when it contacts blood may be injected into the renal artery. Renal circulation may also be interrupted by a dissecting *aneurysm* in the renal artery. Corrective surgery may be indicated in the possibility of pregnancy or when functional disease can be attributed to the aneurysm. The end result of any of these conditions, if severe enough, is reduced renal blood flow, which causes renal parenchymal ischemia and finally renal tissue atrophy.

The symptoms of acute renal artery obstruction include sudden flank pain over the affected kidney and fever. The urinalysis may be normal, and blood chemistries may show an elevated serum glutamic oxaloacetic transaminase and lactic dehydrogenase. An excretory urogram will demonstrate a nonfunctioning kidney, and a renal scan will show no arterial blood flow. Progressive occlusion may cause the same symptoms, although compensatory mechanisms may obviate some of the acute reactions. Hypertension and increased erythropoietin production are results of long-term stenosis.

The *ischemic kidney* is a major consideration in the treatment and prognosis of renal artery occlusion. Collateral circulation does develop in response to the reduced renal circulation. Intrarenal vessels have been found to arise from several different sources. This process helps preserve the kidney if there has been sufficient growth time prior to the total obstruction. In this instance, ischemic periods may be tolerated for up to several weeks. This is because a lack of filtration is accompanied by a marked reduction in renal work and oxygen requirement so that collateral circulation can handle the needs. However, there is always a question of relationship between the duration of the ischemia and the possibility of restoring adequate renal function.

Treatment of the ischemic kidney, unless the ischemia was therapeutically caused, involves surgical revascularization of the kidney. An adequate blood supply must be reestablished. Procedures commonly used are aortorenal and splenorenal bypasses. This anastomosis establishes communication between the kidney and another major artery.

Renal Vein Disease

The primary process involving the renal vein is *thrombosis*. Obstruction in venous drainage increases interstitial pressure, which reduces renal function. Signs and symptoms of this condition include severe lumbar pain, renal enlargement, proteinuria, and hematuria. If the obstruction is bilateral, there will be oliguria and azotemia. Frequently found underlying diseases include diabetic nephropathy, chronic glomerulonephritis, renal amyloidosis, collagen vascular disease, hypercoagulable states, pregnancy, use of oral contraceptives, and nephrotic syndrome.

Survival of the kidney depends, in large part, on the degree of collateral circulation development before the vessel was totally occluded. Embolectomy or ligation of the renal veins may be done. Anticoagulants may also be administered. Dextran-70 may be given for its antithrombotic effects in order to dissolve the clot. If enough renal damage has occurred, nephrectomy may be necessary.

RENAL FAILURE

The Uremic Syndrome

Uremia literally means "urine in the blood." This term and the term *uremic syndrome* are used to describe a set of symptoms that result from loss of renal function. This loss may be sudden or may develop over a long period; it may be self-limiting or irreversible. Sudden loss of kidney function, such as occurs in damage from trauma, shock, toxins, or acute glomerulonephritis, brings on uremia rapidly and usually causes a severe deterioration of the patient's condition. Gradual loss of kidney function over an extended period may occur with glomerulonephritis, hypertension, chronic pyelonephritis, and other diseases. When the loss of renal function is a gradual process, the patient may be able to function quite well for a long time in spite of uremia.

As might be expected from the wide variation of functions performed by the kidneys, the effects of uremia are found not only within the kidneys themselves, but also within all other organ systems in the body. Because of the time component, chronic renal failure produces more degenerative changes in the body systems than does acute uremia. However, both types have many of the same consequences and the ultimate result, unless the process can be halted, is coma, convulsions, and death.

A more complete discussion of acute and chronic uremia, or renal failure, follows.

Acute Renal Failure

Acute renal failure refers to the abrupt loss of kidney function. Over a period of hours to a few days, the glomerular filtration rate falls, accompanied by a concomitant rise in serum creatinine and urea nitrogen. A healthy adult eating a normal diet needs a minimum daily urine output of approximately 400 ml. in order to excrete the body's waste products through the kidneys. Less than this amount indicates a decreased glomerular filtration rate. Oliguria usually refers to daily urine outputs between 50 and 400 ml., and anuria refers to outputs below 50 ml.

The *pathogenesis* of acute renal failure is not totally clear. One hypothesis is that the damaged tubules cannot conserve sodium normally, which leads to activation of the renin-angiotensin-aldosterone system. This redistributes the renal vascular supply by increasing the glomerular arteriolar resistance and reducing the renal blood flow. The result is decreased glomerular pressure, glomerular filtration rate, tubular flow, and thus oliguria.[94, 156] There is also a theory that cellular and protein debris within the tubule obstruct the lumen, which raises the intratubular pressure; this increasing pressure opposes filtration pressure until glomerular filtration stops. Other possible pathogenic mechanisms include leakage of filtered urine through the damaged tubules back into the peritubular capillaries and chemical and/or morphologic changes in the basement membrane of the glomerular capillary, which decrease nephron filtration.[63, 178]

CAUSES OF ACUTE RENAL FAILURE

The numerous *causes* of acute renal failure can be categorized into three major areas: prerenal, renal, and postrenal. *Prerenal* causes interfere with renal perfusion. The kidneys depend on an adequate delivery of blood to be filtered by the glomeruli. Therefore, a reduced renal blood flow obviously decreases the glomerular filtration rate. Conditions that contribute to decreased renal blood flow include volume depletion, such as vomiting, diarrhea, hemorrhage, excessive use of diuretics, burns, renal salt-wasting conditions, and glycosuria; volume shifts, e.g., "third space" sequestration of fluid, vasodilating drugs, and gram-negative sepsis; and volume expansion, such as in cardiac pump failure, hepatorenal syndrome, and severe nephrotic syndrome. *Renal* causes refer to parenchymal changes from disease or nephrotoxic substances. Acute tubular necrosis, or lower nephron necrosis, is the most frequent renal cause of acute oliguria, accounting for as many as 90 per cent of the cases. This destruction of the tubular epithelial cells is the result of impaired renal perfusion and/or direct damage from nephrotoxins. The former cause — ischemia – is similar to prerenal hypoperfusion except that in the case of prerenal failure, correction of the underlying problem usually leads to immediate return of renal function, while in renal hypoperfusion, correction of the causative factor may be followed by continued oliguria for as long as 30 days. In addition to the nephrotoxins described above, other causes of acute tubular necrosis include the presence of heme pigments, such as myoglobin and hemoglobin, which are liberated from damaged muscle tissue, and the toxins produced in gram-negative septicemia. Additional renal causes of acute renal failure include glomerulonephritis; microvascular and large vascular occlusion as in hemolytic-uremic syndrome; thrombosis; vasculitis; scleroderma; trauma; atherosclerosis; tumor invasion; and cortical necrosis which is caused by prolonged vasospasm of the cortical blood vessels. Finally, acute renal failure due to *postrenal* causes occurs because of obstruction in the urinary tract anywhere from the tubules to the urethral meatus. Common sources of obstruction include prostatic hypertrophy, calculi, invading tumors, surgical accidents, and retroperitoneal fibrosis. This particular cause is frequently difficult to identify unless the obstruction is bilateral. This is because the unobstructed kidney continues to function normally and, if the affected kidney is only partially obstructed, it may even become polyuric as it loses its ability to concentrate. In managing the patient with acute renal failure, it is important to determine from which of the above categories the disease arises before treatment is started.

Although each of the following causative factors can be classified in one of the above categories, it is important to be aware of the incidence of iatrogenically induced acute renal failure. McMurray and associates found that in one group of 278 patients with acute oliguria, 91 cases were provoked by health care personnel in the course of therapy for other conditions. These factors included administration of potentially toxic agents, such as antibiotics, anesthetics, and radiographic contrast media; failure to adjust the dosage of drugs whose primary site for excretion is the kidneys; failure to use prophylactic preventive measures, such as adequate hydration and diuresis; surgical complications; and delay in recognizing and responding to the primary disease.[203]

SIGNS AND SYMPTOMS OF ACUTE RENAL FAILURE

> *The most common overall sign of acute failure is alteration in the expected urine output.*

Usually there is a marked diminution of the 24-hour output, although not always. There are two varieties of acute renal failure: oliguric and nonoliguric. *Oliguric* acute renal failure is the much more common of the two and its specifics dominate this discussion of acute renal failure. There is some controversy as to whether the *nonoliguric* or *high-output* variety is an entity in and of itself or just a phase of oliguric acute renal failure. It does not occur very frequently but is associated with less morbidity and mortality than the oliguric type, probably because of the lesser degree and shorter duration of azotemia. The urine produced in the nonoliguric variety is dilute and nearly isomolar, indicating that not all nephrons have stopped filtering. The urine in oliguric acute renal failure is reduced to less than 400 ml. per day.

As mentioned above, it is important to determine the cause of acute renal failure before deciding on the treatment mode. It is necessary to recognize the *symptomatology* in order to do this. The signs and symptoms of prerenal failure are quite diverse, depending on the causative condition. The patient will frequently have a history of increased fluid loss, such as diarrhea or hemorrhage, and/or will demonstrate signs of imbalanced fluid status. The urine has a high specific gravity and osmolality and there is little or no proteinuria. Urine sediment is usually normal, although it may contain a few hyaline and granular casts. There is very little urinary sodium excretion. Intrinsic renal failure symptomatology also depends on the contributing condition. Systemic signs may include edema, weight gain, hemoptysis from elevated left ventricular end-diastolic pressure, weakness from anemia, and hypertension. The urine has a fixed specific gravity, a high sodium concentration, and definite proteinuria. In the case of glomerulonephritis, there will be hematuria and red blood cell and hemoglobin casts. Acute tubular necrosis will cause "muddy brown" granular casts. If there has been significant tissue damage, elevated levels of serum creatine phosphokinase and potassium can be expected. Urine produced in postrenal failure may have fixed specific gravity and elevated sodium concentration with little or no proteinuria. Urine sediment is generally normal. The most definitive signs are those indicating obstruction as described with calculi and neoplasms.

COURSE AND EFFECTS OF ACUTE RENAL FAILURE

The course of acute renal failure is marked by several *phases*. The *onset* covers the period from the precipitating event to the development of oliguria. In the *oliguric-anuric* phase, the urine output falls to below 400 ml. per day (except in nonoliguric acute renal failure). The duration of this aspect is from one day to 8 weeks, with 8 to 15 days being the average time. The longer the persistence, the poorer the prognosis. A gradual or abrupt return of glomerular filtration and leveling of the blood urea nitrogen signal the *diuretic* phase. Some break this up into two periods: *early*, marked by halting of the blood urea nitrogen rise, and *late*, or *recovery*, signified by a falling blood urea nitrogen. The *convalescent* stage begins when the blood urea nitrogen becomes stable and ends when the patient has returned to his normal activity. This phase may take several months.[39]

The *effects* of acute renal failure are widespread. The major consequences include (1) fluid and electrolyte imbalances — fluid overload, hyperkalemia, hyponatremia, hypocalcemia, and hypermagnesemia; (2) acidosis; (3) increased susceptibility to secondary infections; (4) anemia; (5) platelet dysfunction; (6) gastrointestinal complications — anorexia, nausea and vomiting, diarrhea or constipation, and stomatitis; (7) increased incidence of pericarditis; and (8) uremic encephalopathy characterized by apathy, defective recent memory, episodic obtundation, dysarthria, tremors, convulsions, and coma.[180] Wound healing is impaired. Other symptoms are usually a result of these sequelae.

TREATMENT OF ACUTE RENAL FAILURE

Medical and nursing management of the oliguric patient is largely based on preventing and treating the above effects. As with any disease process, prevention is the primary treatment. Attaining and maintaining adequate hydration and diuresis in high-risk patients is crucial, as is the prevention of contributing factors. Once acute renal failure has developed, quick action facilitates full restoration of normal renal function. In the case of prerenal causes, correction of the underlying condition may be all that is necessary. Postrenal causes must be rectified. In the meantime, development of the sequelae of acute renal failure requires specific interventions.

Treatment of acute renal failure is an intensive care type of situation. Much of the care revolves around physiologic monitoring and intervention. However, it must be remembered that the patient, as well as significant others, will be very anxious and frightened. Frequent, careful explanations should be given. The nurse must be constantly alert to the emotional and psychologic needs of the patient and significant others and be ready to intervene.

Fluid and Electrolyte Balance

Restoration of fluid balance requires careful monitoring of the intake and output, daily weight, orthostatic changes in the blood pressure, pulse rate, respiratory rate, skin turgor, and mucous membranes. Serial central venous pressure values may be measured. Urine specific gravity, usually an indication of fluid balance, may be negated by intrinsic renal disease. Heart sounds, breath sounds, and the patient's mental status may indicate the presence of fluid imbalance. Fluid replacement must be done very carefully to avoid fluid overload. Replacement is often calculated on the basis of urine output plus the 600 to 800 ml. of insensible water loss that usually occurs in 24 hours. Some physicians use a daily weight loss of 0.2 to 0.5 kg. per day as a measure of the success of their fluid replacement program. It is felt that this represents usual daily weight loss from protein catabolism.

Electrolyte balance must be maintained. Probably the most dangerous imbalance is *hyperkalemia* because of its contribution to cardiac arrest. In addition to the kidney's inability to excrete potassium, this electrolyte is released in greater quantities from the body cells when acidosis is present and is further increased by rapid tissue catabolism as in fever, severe infection, and trauma. Electrocardiogram monitors are frequently used. Cation exchange resins may be administered orally or rectally to facilitate the excretion of potassium. Sorbitol is also given to prevent impaction and to eliminate the sodium released by the exchange resins. Potassium-containing foods and medications should be avoided. The administration of 50 per cent glucose and regular insulin, with sodium bicarbonate, if necessary, or calcium gluconate intravenously can temporarily prevent cardiac arrest in an emergency. Hyponatremia is usually an effect of hemodilution rather than true lack of sodium. Therefore, treatment is actually a factor of proper fluid replacement. Hypocalcemia may require intravenous administration of calcium gluconate. Hypophosphatemia is treated with decreased dietary intake and phosphate binders. Antacids containing magnesium should be avoided. Physostigmine may be used for hypermagnesemia and intravenous magnesium sulfate for hypomagnesemia.

Metabolic acidosis usually results from the accumulation of acid waste products. Correction of this state must be done slowly with sodium bicarbonate. In the meantime, oxygenation is supported and attempts are made to reduce protein catabolism.

Nutrition

Proper nutrition is crucial. A diet high in calories and low in protein is usually prescribed. It may also be a low sodium, low potassium diet. The protein needs to be of high biologic value, containing the essential amino acids in order to reduce nitrogenous waste products. Adequate carbohydrate intake reverses the process of gluconeogenesis. If tolerated, butter balls, made with butter and powdered sugar, may be used to provide enough calories. Because of the frequent anorexia, nausea, and stomatitis accompanying renal failure and the general unpalatability of the diet, adequate nutrition often presents a major challenge for the nurse. If oral intake is not sufficient to meet requirements, tube feedings or total parenteral nutrition may be instituted. The use of hyperalimentation has caused two problems for patients with acute renal failure. Intolerance to the high carbohydrate content, which can lead to *nonketotic, hyperosmolar, hyperglycemic coma*, seems to be the result of catecholamine action on carbohydrate metabolism. *Secondary hyperchloremic acidosis*, the second problem, is treated with sodium bicarbonate or by adding acetate to the solution. Intralipids are administered intravenously. Androgens have been used by some to reduce protein catabolism.

Other Aspects of Care

Secondary infections are the causative factors in as many as 50 to 90 per cent of the deaths from acute renal failure.[180] The patient should be monitored carefully for the incidence of infectious processes and, if they occur, they should be treated aggressively. Use of urethral catheters should be avoided because of their great potential for inducing infection. Nursing care must be designed to prevent infection in the usual high-risk sites, e.g., respiratory tract, wounds, and the mouth.

Pericarditis occurs in as many as 18 per cent of the patients. Be aware of its signs and symptoms: pleuritic pain that may be relieved by an upright position, pericardial friction rub, tachycardia, and fever. Treatment is usually begun with steroids, but pericardiocentesis and pericardiectomy may be necessary if cardiac function is compromised.

Other treatments are used for symptomatic relief. Convulsions may be relieved by intravenous phenytoin or diazepam or by phenobarbital. Anemia is treated with transfusions only when necessary. Bleeding tendencies may be helped by correcting vitamin K deficiencies. The use of mannitol, loop diuretics, furosemide, and ethacrynic acid to stimulate renal output is controversial.

It may become necessary to use dialysis to treat the patient. Duration of the condition and/or the failure of the above measures to correct fluid and electrolyte imbalances may require the use of peritoneal dialysis or hemodialysis. The care of patients having these treatments is described below.

Chronic Renal Failure

Chronic, or *irreversible*, renal failure is a progressive reduction of functioning renal tissue so that the remaining kidney mass can no longer maintain the body's internal environment. It can develop insidiously over a period of many years or can occur as a result of a bout of acute renal failure from which the patient fails to recover. Because of the wide diversity of contributing elements and disease processes, the early stages of renal failure are quite varied. However, as the destruction of nephrons progresses to its end-stage, the manifestations become very similar and are classified as the uremic syndrome. The end result for the patient with renal failure is uremia and death, or treatment by dialysis and/or transplant. Conservative treatment does not cure the disease but retards its progress so that the patient may never actually reach the need for more radical treatment during his lifetime. Even the successful use of dialysis and transplant will require continued extraordinary emphasis for the rest of the patient's life. Some patients have described the position of the patient with chronic renal failure as the "marginal man"—one who is neither dying nor returned to society "healed" but is still in limbo.[173] It is definite, then, that a diagnosis of chronic renal failure implies a lifelong process for the patient and significant others.

CAUSES AND COURSE OF CHRONIC RENAL FAILURE

The *causes* of chronic renal failure are numerous. Throughout Chapters 42 and 43, discussions of various injuries and disease processes have cited renal failure as an end result. Chronic glomerulonephritis, polycystic kidney disease, obstruction, repeated bouts of pyelonephritis, and nephrotoxins are examples. (See acute renal failure for a complete discussion of prerenal, renal, and postrenal causes of failure.) Systemic diseases, such as diabetes, hypertension, lupus erythematosus, polyarteritis, sickle cell disease, and amyloid disease, may also produce renal failure.

The *pathogenesis* of chronic renal failure portrays slow deterioration and destruction of renal nephrons with progressive loss of their normal function. As the total glomerular filtration rate falls and clearance is reduced, the serum urea nitrogen and creatinine levels rise. Remaining functioning nephrons hypertrophy as they are required to filter a larger load of solutes. One of the consequences of this is that the kidneys lose their ability to concentrate urine adequately. In an attempt to continue excreting the solutes, a large volume of dilute urine is passed, making the patient susceptible to fluid depletion. The tubules gradually lose their ability to reabsorb electrolytes. This can result in "salt-wasting," in which the urine contains very large amounts of sodium, which leads to more polyuria. As renal damage advances and the number of functioning nephrons decline, the total glomerular filtration rate decreases further and the body becomes unable to get rid of water, salt, and other waste products through the kidneys. When the glomerular filtration rate is below 10 ml. per minute, clinical uremia is evident. The body becomes increasingly toxic until its status is no longer compatible with life.

The projected *course* of irreversible renal disease is as follows:

- Normal functioning.
- In reduced renal reserve, the blood urea nitrogen may be high normal, but there are no clinical symptoms. Normal function is evident as long as the patient is not exposed to unusual physiologic or psychologic stress.
- Renal insufficiency demonstrates more advanced pathology by a mild azotemia when the patient is on a general diet, impaired urine concentration with nocturia is commonly found, as is mild anemia. Renal function is easily impaired by stress.
- Renal failure causes severe azotemia, acidosis, impaired urine dilution, severe anemia, and a number of electrolyte imbalances, such as hypernatremia, hyperkalemia, hypocalcemia, and hyperphosphatemia.
- Finally, end-stage renal disease (ESRD) is characterized by two groups of clinical symptoms: deranged excretory and regulatory mechanisms and a distinctive grouping of gastrointestinal, cardiovascular, and neuromuscular symptoms.[228]

MANIFESTATIONS OF CHRONIC RENAL FAILURE

The *manifestations* of chronic renal failure, with its retention of nitrogenous waste products and changes in fluid and electrolyte and acid-base balances, are present in every body system. *Renal* alterations were described above and include the kidney's inability to concentrate urine and regulate electrolyte excretion. Polyuria progressing to anuria develops, and the patient loses normal diurnal patterns of voiding.

Electrolyte balances are upset by impaired excretion and utilization. The salt-wasting properties of the failing kidneys, vomiting, and diarrhea cause hyponatremia. Most patients are very susceptible to salt loss accompanied by fluid depletion, so that sodium must be continually replaced. Later in the disease, and earlier with some patients, salt and water retention may contribute to hypertension and congestive heart failure. However, there is also some evidence that salt-wasting may reverse itself late in the disease as an adaptation process. Therefore, sodium levels are very individualized. The kidneys are very efficient potassium excretors so that potassium imbalances usually do not occur until late in the disease. In oliguric renal failure, hyperkalemia is common and can become suddenly dangerous. The potassium excess is contributed to by catabolism, potassium-containing drugs, trauma, blood transfusions, and acidosis. Hypokalemia occurs in nonoliguric renal failure, since the kidneys cannot conserve potassium. Hypocalcemia is the usual finding. As described below in the pathophysiology of renal osteodystrophy, early retention of phosphorus causes a fall in serum calcium; however, in later stages of the disease, more phosphorus accumulates, causing hyperphosphatemia. Elevated serum magnesium levels are found early, but these do not usually reach a dangerous level unless the patient is receiving magnesium-containing laxatives or antacids.

One of the main *metabolic* signs of advancing renal failure is a rising blood urea nitrogen and serum creatinine caused by the accumulation in the blood of waste products of protein metabolism. The proteinuria accompanying renal disease often causes hypoproteinemia within the body, which has a direct effect on the intravascular oncotic pressure. Carbohydrate intolerance is the result of impaired insulin production and metabolism. Four mechanisms are responsible: peripheral insulin antagonism, impaired secretion, prolonged half-life directly related to kidney malfunction, and abnormalities in circulating insulin. This characteristic means that special care is needed when adjusting insulin dosages for diabetic patients with renal failure. Results of glucose tolerance tests must be carefully interpreted, however, since the values can be affected by malnutrition, medications, and infection. The high incidence of hyperlipidemia is thought to be caused by increased production of lipids by the liver in response to the elevated blood sugar and insulin levels. At the same time, there seems to be reduced assimilation of the lipids in the peripheral tissues, possibly owing to the blockage of lipoprotein lipase activity. Metabolic acidosis occurs because of the kidneys' inability to excrete hydrogen ions due to decreased reabsorption of sodium bicarbonate and decreased formation of dihydrogen phosphate and ammonia.

The most frequent manifestation within the *cardiovascular* system is *hypertension*. This is produced through the mechanisms of volume overload and stimulation of the renin-angiotensin system. Any of the many systemic complications of prolonged high blood pressure may be found. The effects of volume overload on the heart are seen, including left ventricular hypertrophy and congestive heart failure. Pericarditis is recognized with increasing frequency. Symptoms include pericardial pain, tachycardia, and fever. The condition may progress to pericardial effusion and cardiac tamponade. Arrhythmias may be the result of hyperkalemia, acidosis, hypermagnesemia, and decreased coronary perfusion. Atherosclerosis is accelerated, probably owing to the hypertension and hyperlipidemia. Arterial calcifications have been identified, with the ankles being the most common early location. Other sites include the abdominal aorta, feet, pelvis, hands, and wrists. Peripheral sites are usually asymptomatic, but gangrene may develop.[207]

The primary *hematologic* effect of renal failure is *anemia*. Frequently, it is the fatigue, weakness, and cold intolerance accompanying the anemia that originates the evaluation leading to the diagnosis of renal disease. The proposed contributors to this condition are numerous: reduced red blood cell production due to a deficiency of erythropoietin; reduced red blood cell life span; iron and folate deficiencies; and increased losses due to hemolysis and bleeding. Occasionally, polycystic disease or renal adenocarcinoma may cause a markedly elevated hematocrit. Bleeding tendencies are the result of impaired platelet aggregation and a lack of platelet Factor III or Factor VIII.

The entire *gastrointestinal* system is affected. Transient anorexia, nausea, and vomiting are almost universal. Patients often experience a constant, bitter, metallic taste, and their breath commonly smells fetid, fishy, or ammoniacal. Stomatitis, parotitis, and gingivitis are common problems due to poor oral hygiene and the formation of ammonia from salivary urea. Accumulations of gastrin due to the decreased degradation by the diseased kidneys may be the main factor in the development of ulcer disease. Esophagitis, gastritis, colitis, gastrointestinal bleeding, and diarrhea are found. Acute pancreatitis has been reported.

Some of the *respiratory* effects can be attributed to *fluid overload*, such as pulmonary edema. A characteristic condition, called uremic lung, is a kind of pneumonitis that responds very well to fluid removal. Acidosis causes a compensatory increase in respiratory rate as the lungs try to eliminate excess hydrogen ions.

The *musculoskeletal* system is affected fairly early in the disease and *bony reabsorption* found on x-ray may be the first sign of renal failure in some patients. The most prevalent problem, affecting up to 90 per cent of the patients with chronic renal failure, is *renal osteodystrophy*, which takes several forms: osteomalacia, osteitis fibrosis, and/or osteosclerosis. The development of this manifestation results from interrelationships between the kidney-bone-parathyroid and calcium-phosphorus-vitamin D connections. As the glomerular filtration rate decreases, phosphorus excretion decreases and calcium elimination increases. The decreased serum calcium stimulates the release of parathyroid hormone, which mobilizes calcium from the bones and facilitates phosphorus excretion. This returns the serum levels of both elements to normal, a situation which is maintained through hyperparathyroidism until the glomerular filtration rate is below 25 to 30 ml. per minute. At that point, the kidneys no longer convert vitamin D, which is absorbed from the intestine and synthesized in the skin to its active form, 1,25-dihydroxycholecalciferol. The lack of this substance interferes with calcium absorption from the intestine and paradoxically facilitates phosphate retention and, thus, mineralization of the bone with calcium and phosphate is impaired.[284] Demineralization of the bone frees more calcium and phosphorus into the blood. This process may also account for calcifications that occur in other body parts, such as soft tissues, joints, heart, eyes, and arteries. Patients with this complication may have diffuse bone pain and bone deformities, but the outstanding symptom is weakness, particularly of the proximal muscles. They frequently have much difficulty getting out of a chair. X-ray is the definitive diagnostic tool, and the alkaline phosphatase level is usually elevated.

Dermatologic problems are particularly uncomfortable for the patient. The skin is usually dry owing to atrophy of the sweat glands. Pruritus often leads to excoriated skin because of the continued scratching. The pruritus may be caused by peripheral nerve damage, high plasma concentrations of parathyroid hormone, and the presence of uremic frost. *Uremic frost* occurs late in the uremic syndrome and consists of white or yellowish crystals of urate that are secreted through the skin in a highly inefficient attempt by the body to rid itself of accumulated waste products. The etiology of the retained urochrome pigments, making the skin orange-green or gray in color, is not clear. Pallor of anemia is evident. The bleeding tendencies produce ecchymosis and purpura. Hair is brittle and tends to fall out and nails are thin and brittle. Bower and associates have observed a nail pattern, called a "half and half" nail, in which the proximal half is normally white and the distal portion is brownish.[98]

Neurologic signs are present from early in the disease. *Peripheral neuropathy* causes many symptoms, such as burning feet, inability to find a comfortable position for the legs and feet (restless leg syndrome), gait changes, foot drop, and paraplegia. These symptoms move up the extremities and may extend to include the upper extremities. Nerve conduction becomes slower. *Central nervous system* changes include increased nervous irritability, nystagmus, twitching, seizures, central nervous system depression, and coma. Involvement of the cranial nerves may alter any of the senses. Hearing threshold levels show a definite high-frequency deficit early in the disease, and hearing progressively deteriorates. Uremic amaurosis is a very sudden onset of bilateral blindness which seems to reverse itself in hours to days. Eyes often contain a deposit of calcium salts which give them an irritative red appearance. It is usually assumed that mental function is impaired, as evidenced by decreased attention span, ability to concentrate, memory, reasoning, and judgment. The nurse must be careful not to label the patient permanently, however, since some studies have shown that this state is reversible with treatment of the renal failure.

Reproductive system changes can be very alarming to the patient. The female often experiences menstrual irregularities, particularly amenorrhea and infertility. Completing a pregnancy is rare. Males can expect impotence, testicular atrophy, oligospermia, and reduced sperm motility. Both sexes report decreased libido.

Psychologic changes occur, probably as the result of both the physiologic alterations and the extreme stress placed on the pateint by the presence of a life-threatening disease. Behavior changes are remarkable and are greatly influenced by the patient's underlying personality structure. Expected alterations include marked personality changes, labile emotions, increased demands on others, withdrawal, depression, agitation, delusions, and psychosis.

Impairment of the *immunologic* system makes the patient very *susceptible to infection.* This is in addition to the many factors that otherwise reduce resistance. Several factors are involved, including depression of humoral antibody formation, suppression of delayed hypersensitivity, and decreased chemotactic function of the leukocytes.

Finally, renal failure has a serious effect on *drug metabolism.* The uremic patient is at very high risk for *drug toxicity* owing to the effect of renal changes on the metabolism and excretion of otherwise therapeutic medications. There are three main causes of this toxicity: (a) a high plasma level of the drug due to either impaired renal excretion or impaired hepatic metabolism of the drug, (b) increased sensitivity to the drug due to uremia-induced changes in the target organ or in the protein-binding of the drug, and (c), a metabolic load because of administration of the medication. There are a variety of tables and formulas that help guide dosage decisions. The nurse must remember that drug dosages often must be altered and that the usual dosage ranges stated in the drug literature may not be safe for the patient with chronic renal failure. Familiarity with and alertness in observing for toxic reactions are crucial.

MANAGEMENT OF CHRONIC RENAL FAILURE

After correction of any contributing factors, fluid and dietary adjustments are the mainstays of *conservative management* of the patient with chronic renal failure. The goals of medical and nursing care are to preserve renal function and to delay the need for dialysis or transplant as long as feasible, improve body chemistries and alleviate extrarenal manifestations as much as possible, and provide for a maximum quality of life for the patient and significant others.

Stringent regulation of the patient's *fluid intake* is usually not necessary until later in the disease process, although this may become necessary any time the patient develops significant overload or depletion. Progress of the fluid status is monitored by observing daily weight, orthostatic blood pressure, skin turgor and mucous membrane moisture, and by intake and output comparison if the patient is hospitalized. When patients are being cared for on an outpatient basis, the nurse should teach them how to weigh themselves and how to interpret the relationship of daily weight loss or gain to their need for sodium and water. Patients should learn to take their blood pressure as an additional indication. Early in the disease, there is usually no fluid restriction, and diuretics may be used to stimulate excretion of water by the kidneys. Forcing fluids should be avoided, however, since this facilitates excessive urinary excretion of salt. Later in the disease progression, there may be a restriction of free water.

As the kidneys lose their concentrating ability, care must be taken to avoid fluid depletion.

> *Dehydration can quickly precipitate a crisis, causing the patient to become uremic.*

The patient must understand that vomiting or diarrhea or working or playing in a hot environment can cause uncompensated fluid loss and must be prevented or controlled. The appearance of edema indicates fluid overload, but some physicians prefer the patient to have a little end-of-the-day edema so that it is more evident that fluid depletion is not a danger. Thirst is not a reliable indicator of fluid needs; if used as a guide, fluid overload would be inevitable. As the failure progresses, it usually becomes necessary to restrict fluid intake. Although authorities differ in their exact figures, daily fluid allowances may be 400 ml. plus measured output. Diuretics that interfere with electrolyte reabsorption or that antagonize aldosterone may be used to get rid of extra fluid, but this practice is controversial.

Dietary adjustment is dictated by many components of chronic renal failure, including accumulation of nitrogenous waste products, impaired excretion of electrolytes, vitamin deficiencies, and continued catabolism. The *wasting syndrome* is a major problem. The renal failure patient constantly loses body weight, muscle mass, and adipose tissue. Many of the manifestations of irreversible renal failure plus emotional depression induce anorexia which, when complemented by a frequently unpalatable diet, constitutes a major nursing challenge — getting the patient to take in adequate nutrition while minimizing uremic toxicity. Measures to relieve nausea and vomiting, stomatitis, and other gastrointestinal manifestations must be taken in an attempt to stimulate the patient's appetite. Diet counseling is essential for compliance, and the nurse needs to arrange for dietary consultation if possible. The patient needs to know how to translate the dietary regimen into a palatable, understandable food program. You can help the patient learn to select and prepare foods and learn where to obtain special foods.

Specific adjustments of dietary elements depend on the results of blood chemistries. There is some debate as to whether and how *protein intake* should be *restricted*. Early in the disease, it is generally well accepted that no restriction is necessary, although the patient should be advised to avoid high-protein fad diets. However, once the disease has advanced to the point where gastrointestinal symptoms of uremia become evident, restraint of protein intake is usually needed. The main problem is determining the proper level that will allow the ideal amount of protein to maintain internal nitrogen equilibrium without causing an extensive protein load. The blood urea nitrogen and serum creatinine may be used to monitor this. The allowable number of grams per day differs from no restriction to 20 to 40 grams daily. The more protein included, the more palatable the diet. Sometimes, more important than the actual number of grams of protein is their quality. Giordano and Giovanetti determined that proteins of high biologic value with their higher percentage of essential amino acids can be used more efficiently with less nitrogenous waste than other proteins. They developed a special diet based on this rationale, and many physicians are using a modification of this. In order to increase the intake of amino acids, patients' diets are sometimes supplemented with mixtures of these elements presented in different forms. Research on the use of keto acid analogue diets has indicated that this source of nitrogen may produce less urea than the use of amino acids, although it is costly and difficult to obtain the necessary components. It is crucial that the patient receive adequate calories to avoid catabolism of body proteins. One recommendation is that at least 35 kcal. per kg. per day be taken in order to prevent the wasting syndrome. Since protein intake may be restricted, it may be necessary to rely on carbohydrate and fat for the needed calories. Breads, cookies, and pasta made from a low-protein wheat-starch–based flour; cane sugar; oils, butter, and cream are among the foods that can be encouraged. There are also commercial preparations of electrolyte-free, nonsweet substances and emulsions of oil in water available to use as supplements. Because of the high incidence of hyperlipoproteinemia, the intake of triglycerides may be restricted; if this happens, receiving adequate calories becomes even more difficult. Vitamin supplements of water-soluble folic acid, pyridoxine hydrochloride, and ascorbic acid are usually given, since low protein diets are typically deficient in them. If the patient is unable to take in the above diet through normal food, or for more control over the components of a patient's food intake, liquid elemental diets or hyperalimentation may be used instead of or in addition to regular foodstuffs.

Dietary *electrolytes* may be encouraged or restricted. The kidneys cannot adjust to excesses of sodium at either end of the continuum and the regulation of this element is a delicate matter. At times the kidneys are salt-wasters and sodium must be encouraged to replace that which is lost; at other times, the kidneys retain sodium and dietary intake must be restricted. There is much debate as to how *sodium intake* should be managed. Some feel that there should be a moderate restriction with careful monitoring of urinary sodium excretion as a guideline. Many different regimens are used. Serial monitoring of data indicating fluid status also gives important information about sodium needs. *Potassium* is frequently not restricted as long as the urine output is above one liter per day. Serum potassium levels provide the primary necessary information. Patients must be reminded not to use salt substitutes since they contain potassium chloride. When hyperkalemia becomes evident, restriction of potassium in food and fluids is instituted. In an emergency situation, when the serum potassium is above 7.0, intravenous glucose, insulin, and calcium gluconate or oral or rectal sodium polystyrene sulfonate, a cation-resin exchange, may be given. Dissolving the resin in ginger ale helps to prevent its sticking to the teeth and to mask its gritty taste. Sorbital is usually given with the resin to avoid constipation and counteract the sodium retention that can occur. A high *calcium* intake is started early and encouraged throughout the disease. Dietary sources may be supplemented with calcium carbonate, calcium lactate, or calcium gluconate. *Phosphorus* is restricted in a step-wise pattern in direct correlation to the decreasing glomerular filtration rate. Phosphate-binding antacids, such as aluminum hydroxide and aluminum carbonate gels, may be used to further reduce phosphorus levels.

Sorbents are chemicals which adsorb gases, liquids, or dissolved substances. These compounds are currently being used in dialysis equipment. Research is being done on the administration of these agents orally to remove uremia toxins through the gut. Activated charcoal and oxidized starch are now being used, and work is being done to develop others. Their use is not universally accepted.

Acidosis contributes to many of the undesirable effects of chronic renal failure. Sodium bicarbonate is often used to correct this imbalance. Another agent is Shohl's solution, which is a combination of sodium citrate and citric acid; the use of this substance may promote stomatitis.

Iron sulfate and folic acid may be used to treat the *anemia* of irreversible renal failure with uncertain results. Parenteral iron is frequently given. Oral or parenteral androgens are thought by some to stimulate erythropoiesis. Histidine and pyridoxine supplements are under investigation. Measures should be taken to avoid iatrogenic blood loss, such as avoiding the use of aspirin. Transfusions are avoided unless absolutely necessary because of the risk of sensitization of histocompatibility antigens, hepatitis, and the further suppression of erythropoiesis. Patients with chronic renal failure have usually adapted so that they can tolerate very low hemoglobins quite well.

Much of the treatment for *renal osteodystrophy* involves dietary and medication regulation of calcium, phosphorus, and acidosis as described above. The parathyroidism must also be brought under control. Vitamin D in its active form is frequently used, although it must be administered with care because of its severe side effects from metastatic calcifications. Calcifediol may be used to promote bone mineralization by increasing the intestinal absorption of calcium and decreasing circulating parathyroid hormone and alkaline phosphatase.[303] Some advocate subtotal parathyroidectomy as a means of reducing parathyroidism.

Fluid and sodium regulation are major ways of treating congestive heart failure. Other *cardiovascular* manifestations are managed much the same as in a patient without chronic renal failure. *Hypertension* must be controlled. Diuretics may be used, although precautions must be taken to avoid fluid depletion. Some consider alpha-methyldopa, guanethidine, hydralazine, and propanolol to be the medications of choice, since they do not interfere with renal blood flow. Pericarditis calls for pericardial aspiration and/or pericardiectomy.

Pruritus is very aggravating, both to the patient and to the health care worker trying to help the patient. Moisturizing oils put into the bath or applied directly help correct the dry skin. Phototherapy has been used successfully. Other treatments that have met with varied success include cholestyramine, oral trimeprazine, antihistamines, heparin, and intravenous lidocaine. Subtotal parathyroidectomy has provided some patients with immediate relief, although there are also reports of reoccurrence.

Neurologic manifestations require safety measures to protect the patient from injury. Anticonvulsants and sedatives may be used. Phenothiazines are potentiated by uremia and should be avoided. Reduction in mental function requires more patience in explaining and reexplaining things to the patient.

Rest is important to the patient, whose body is under a great deal of stress. Encourage frequent naps. Exercise is also important, but discourage strenuous exercise, which increases catabolism.

Patient teaching is a crucial part of the management plan. Most of the time the patient will be treated as an outpatient, responsible for his or her own care and progress. Patients and significant others must know about normal renal function and how their disease has altered it, the details of their medical and nursing care and how they can best comply with them, and a number of self-observation skills as described above. A careful teaching plan must be worked out with patients and their families and friends. Patient learning must be continually evaluated throughout implementation of the plan.

Dialysis

There are two major types of dialysis: *peritoneal dialysis and hemodialysis.* Each may be used to relieve symptoms of renal failure temporarily until the patient regains kidney function; both are also used to sustain life in the person with irreversible kidney disease. In the latter case, the dialysis must continue intermittently for the rest of the person's life. Dialysis is also used to overcome uremia and physically prepare the patient to receive a transplanted kidney. Dialysis is frequently necessary to keep the patient alive until a suitable donor kidney is found. If the transplanted kidney does not function adequately immediately, dialysis may be used to prevent uremia until the kidney functions sufficiently.

Dialysis, or diffusion, refers to the passage of particles (ions) from an area of high concentration to an area of low concentration across a semipermeable membrane, one with pores large enough to allow certain particles to pass through but too small to allow the passage of larger particles. When the two solutions are separated by a semipermeable membrane, solute particles will move toward the solution with lesser concentration. Simultaneously water will move, by the process of osmosis, toward the solution in which the solute concentration is greater.

When dialysis is used as a substitute for kidney function, the semipermeable membrane used is either the peritoneal membrane (for peritoneal dialysis) or an artificial membrane (for hemodialysis). This membrane must have pores large enough to allow the passage of electrolytes, urea, and creatinine, but too small to allow passage of blood cell and other protein molecules. The two solutions used on opposite sides of the membrane are (1) the blood and (2) a specially prepared electrolyte solution called dialysate.

There are four basic *goals of dialysis therapy:*

- Removal of the end products of protein metabolism, such as urea and creatinine, from the blood.
- Maintenance of a safe concentration of the serum electrolytes.
- Correction of acidosis and replenishment of the blood's bicarbonate buffer system.
- Removal of excess fluid from the blood.

It must be remembered that solute particles and water can move freely across the membrane in either direction between the blood and the dialysate. With this in mind, note that if the patient's blood has a higher concentration of urea, creatinine, and certain electrolytes other than the prepared dialysate solution, these particles will move into the dialysate solution, thus lowering the level in the blood. Likewise, if the blood is deficient in a substance, such as bicarbonate, a higher concentration of this substance in the dialysate will cause it to move into the blood, raising the blood level. Excess fluid can be removed from the blood by increasing the particle concentration of the dialysate with a solution such as dextrose. This increased particle concentration will cause water to move into the dialysate while, at the same time, the dextrose moves into the blood. The tendency is always toward an equalization of concentration of the two solutions.

PERITONEAL DIALYSIS

Peritoneal dialysis involves the instillation of dialysate into the peritoneal cavity, allowing time for substance exchange and then removal of the dialysate. This cycle is repeated several times during a dialysis period. The procedure is useful for both acute and chronic renal failure and for fluid and electrolyte imbalances. It has been used for overdoses of drugs and toxins, but, because its clearance is much slower than hemodialysis, it may not be satisfactory for this purpose. Peritoneal dialysis is used for patients with severe cardiovascular disease or with bleeding tendencies, for those with poor vascular access which makes them inappropriate for hemodialysis for any reason. Some people prefer to use this technique with small children and the elderly.

Although there may be no absolute contraindications, some conditions may be considered as deterrents to this procedure, such as acute renal failure complicated by hypercatabolism or heat stress, peritonitis, recent abdominal or chest surgery or trauma, ileus and bowel distention, diffuse intra-abdominal adhesions, and respiratory insufficiency. One of the primary advantages of this technique is its relative ease, which allows it to be used in community hospitals without all the sophisticated equipment needed for hemodialysis. One of the major drawbacks in using peritoneal dialysis, as compared with hemodialysis, is the time factor involved. Chronic intermittent peritoneal dialysis usually lasts 10 to 12 hours and must be done three to five times a week, depending on the patient's condition; hemodialysis is much less time-consuming.

Technique of Peritoneal Dialysis

The *technique* for peritoneal dialysis involves inserting the catheter, instilling the dialysate, monitoring the patient, and removing the dialysate. Prior to the catheterization, the patient must be fully prepared. Usually there will have been some time to discuss with the patient the renal disease and the proposed treatment. The patient must know exactly what will happen and what to do during the dialysis process, and what kind of results can be expected from the treatment. Informed consent must be obtained.

Baseline weight, vital signs, and blood chemistries provide important data for later comparison. A central venous pressure line may be inserted and a cardiac monitor attached for continuous observation. Mild sedation may be provided. The bladder and bowel should be emptied. The abdomen is shaved and prepped. The equipment is entirely ready with the dialysate warmed to 38° C. and all tubings flushed to prevent air from entering the cavity.

The catheter insertion may be done in the operating room or at the bedside under local or general anesthesia. The preferred site for insertion is about 3 to 5 cm. below the umbilicus, an area which is relatively avascular and has less fascial resistance. Using strict aseptic technique, the skin is cut and a trocar is inserted through the abdominal tissue layers into the peritoneal cavity. The catheter is then inserted and the tip is usually positioned so that it lies deeply within the pelvic gutter; the correct position will often give the patient the urge to defecate. A small amount of dialysate may be allowed to run through the catheter to facilitate insertion. The catheter is generally sutured in place to avoid accidental dislodgement. Figure 43–3 shows the different appliances which may be used in chronic intermittent dialysis. The subcutaneous and Deane prostheses are inserted and left in place to provide permanent fistula tracts for insertion of the dialysis catheter each time the procedure is done. The skin is closed over the top of the apparatus which remains movable under the skin. Each time the catheter is needed, the skin is pierced with a stylet and the catheter inserted. The Tenckhoff catheter has two Dacron-felt cuffs bonded to the catheter. The catheter is inserted and left in place. Over a period of one to two weeks, there is an ingrowth of fibroblasts and blood vessels into the cuffs, which fix the catheter in place and provide an effective barrier against dialysate leakage and bacterial invasion. The life-span of the Tenckhoff catheter has been reported to range from 2 weeks to 27 months (average: 13 months), with outlet obstruction being the most common reason for removal. Heparin may be added to the catheter to prevent plugging between dialyses.

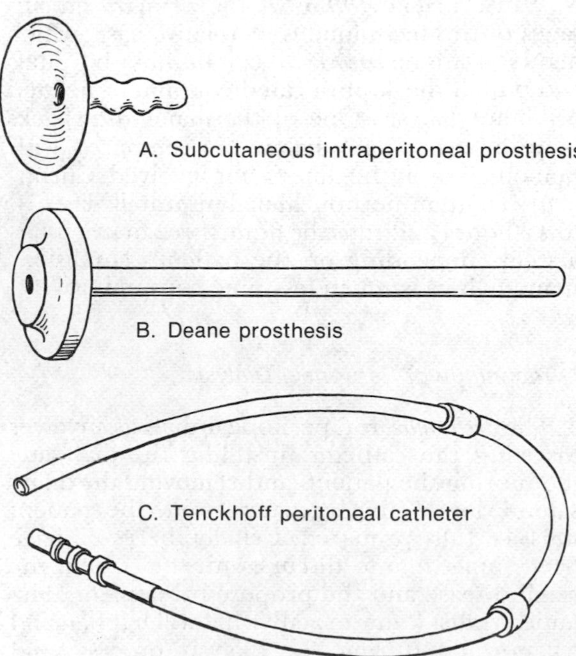

Figure 43–3. Types of permanent abdominal appliances used in peritoneal dialysis.

The dialysate is usually allowed to run into the peritoneal cavity by gravity flow, although an electronic drip regulator may be used. The dialysate is warmed to prevent chilling the patient and to dilate the peritoneal blood vessels, thus facilitating substance exchange. Two liters is usually instilled in adults, although smaller amounts may be needed at first until the patient adjusts. Care must be taken to prevent air entering the peritoneal cavity throughout the entire procedure. "Dwell time" is the period during which the dialysate is left in the cavity. Equilibrium between the dialysate and the body fluids usually occurs within 15 to 30 minutes, with the maximum change happening within the first five minutes. Therefore, the solution is typically left in place 30 to 45 minutes and then allowed to flow out through the catheter by gravity and siphon flow. Machines are available to automatically handle the entire cycle.

The number of dialysis cycles depends on the normalization of body fluids and blood chemistries, as indicated by laboratory studies. A dialysis period may take from 10 to 36 hours. Peritoneal clearance is influenced by several factors, including size of the membrane area, blood flow to the peritoneum, and alterations in the permeability of the peritoneal membrane.

Complications of Peritoneal Dialysis

Although considered a safe procedure, there are a number of *complications* that can be attributed to peritoneal dialysis. *Catheter problems* include displacement and plugging. Obstruction may be due to malposition, adherence of the catheter tip to the tissue wall, or infection. *Constipation* can reduce the catheter flow, although the mechanism for this is unclear. Leakage usually indicates improper catheter function or poor abdominal muscle support. *Bowel perforation* is most likely to occur in cachectic patients or where there are abdominal adhesions. Signs of this complication include return of fecal material in the dialysate, and/or massive diarrhea after instillation of the dialysate. *Blad-*

der perforation may also occur if it has not been emptied prior to catheter insertion. *Peritonitis* is signaled by cloudy returns and signs of peritoneal irritation. Antibiotics may be given systemically or with the dialysate. *Pain* during dialysis may be the result of rapid instillation, incorrect dialysate pH, or excessive suction during outflow. Any air introduced usually collects along the diaphragm and causes shoulder pain. *Hernia* formation may occur. Systemic *cardiovascular and neurologic effects* are usually the result of fluid and electrolyte imbalances. *Hyperglycemia* may occur in diabetic patients as a result of absorption of glucose from the dialysate and electrolyte changes. *Respiratory* difficulties may occur during dwell time because of pressure on the diaphragm.

Nursing Responsibilities in Peritoneal Dialysis

With the exception of insertion and removal of the peritoneal catheter, peritoneal dialysis is primarily a nursing procedure. Throughout the process, careful monitoring of the patient's temperature, pulse, respiratory rate, blood pressure, weight, and intake and output is necessary. Urine fractionals may be done to check for glycosuria. It is important to watch for the development of hypovolemia and the retention of dialysate. Outflow each time should be approximately 100 to 200 ml. more than the inflow except for the first and possibly the last couple of cycles. If there is retention, have the patient move around to bring the fluid to the catheter tip where it can be picked up. The system should be checked for kinks or other obstruction. Fluid accumulations of over 300 ml. should be reported to the physician.

> *Since peritonitis is the main complication of peritoneal dialysis, it is crucial that aseptic technique be used throughout the procedure.*

Dressings over the insertion site should be changed at least daily using an iodine solution as the cleansing agent. Some authorities recommend use of topical antibiotic ointment. The dressing should be kept dry and should be arranged so that the catheter does not lie in direct contact with the skin.

Relief of discomfort may be achieved in several ways, including slowing the rate of flow, elevating the head of the bed, massaging the abdomen, or having the patient move around. Analgesics may be given. If eating makes the patient uncomfortable, small meals may be served frequently. It is also helpful to coordinate the meals with drainage periods.

Food and fluid restrictions are frequently liberalized during treatment. Approximately 10 to 20 grams of protein are lost with each dialysis process; this must be replaced in the diet.

Because of the immobilization and the intermittent pressure on the diaphragm reducing its full excursion, the patient is at high risk for respiratory complications. Encourage the patient to cough and deep breathe regularly. Positive-pressure breathing exercises may be instituted prophylactically.

Unless the dialysis can be completed during the patient's sleep time, diversionary activities will be necessary. Also, if the patient will be having long-term intermittent dialysis, the nurse, patient, and significant others will be having a prolonged relationship and the nurse should be constantly working to establish and maintain a supportive, therapeutic rapport with them. See hemodialysis for a more complete discussion of the psychologic aspects of dialysis.

Peritoneal Dialysis Outside the Hospital

The development of permanent catheters and automated machines to control dialysis has made home peritoneal dialysis a viable option for many patients. The ease of hooking the patient up to the system makes it especially useful for people who live alone. The patient has both hands free to make the one necessary tube connection. Patients going onto a home program need a complete training program so that they can independently handle the entire dialysis process at home.

Another development, which allows the patient more mobility and independence, is the technique of *continuous ambulatory peritoneal dialysis.* With this procedure, the dialysate is drained from the peritoneal cavity approximately 5 times a day and replaced with fresh solution. The permanent catheter is capped and the patient can resume his daily activities. This change of solution can be done anywhere. In one study, 9 patients have been maintained in this manner for 136 weeks and report increased appetite, energy, and sense of well-being. There is a continuing problem of recurrent peritonitis which responds well to antibiotics, but the procedure seems to be able to clear the toxins from the body adequately.[246]

HEMODIALYSIS

Hemodialysis is used for patients with acute or irreversible renal failure. It can be used for the same purposes as peritoneal dialysis, although it is usually the treatment of choice when toxic agents, such as barbiturate overdose, need to be removed from the body quickly.

The first development of an "artificial kidney" was in 1943 in the Netherlands. In 1960, Scribner reported the first successful treatment of patients with chronic renal failure. In the early years, although the technology was available, the exorbitant cost and the lack of equipment required that a stringent selection process be done in the choosing of patients who would be allowed to have hemodialysis. Patients were screened as to their motivation, intelligence, emotional stability, and rehabilitative potential; in essence, it had to be decided who among the many potential candidates would best be able to cope with the program and who would make the biggest contribution to society.

In 1972, an amendment to the Social Security Act assured that any patient with chronic renal failure would be able to have any life-saving treatment needed. In 1973, Medicare took over the financial responsibility for many patients on hemodialysis. Thus, the availability of this treatment mode for patients with irreversible renal failure has become much more prevalent. The selection criteria can be applied more freely and the patient population receiving hemodialysis now represents a wider cross-section in terms of age, rehabilitative potential, and socioeconomic status. However, the question of suitability for long-term hemodialysis continually undergoes revision. For instance, previously, elderly patients with chronic renal failure were not considered acceptable candidates for hemodialysis. However, a study by Rathaus and Bernheim of 26 elderly patients showed that these people actually complied with the diet and self-limitation required by hemodialysis better than younger patients and that their life-style and outlook on life led to a higher rate of success with the hemodialysis program.[251] Although there continues to be controversy regarding the long-term effects of underlying cardiovascular disease, their results and those of others indicate that age alone should not be considered a contraindication for hemodialysis.

Procedure for Hemodialysis

The *procedure* for hemodialysis involves allowing blood to flow from the patient's body into a membrane package and then returning the dialyzed blood to the patient. Strict asepsis must be maintained throughout the procedure. While the blood is within the external membrane compartment, the dialysate solution is delivered by a mechanical pump to flow on the outside of the membrane. Diffusion takes place between the blood and dialysate solution. Typical hemodialysis systems consist of a means of (a) *blood access*—dialyzer; dialysate; tubing; blood pump; heparin pump; and (b) *devices to monitor* conductivity, temperature, flow rates, and pressures of blood and dialysate, and to *detect* blood leaks and presence of air in the venous line.

One of the vital aspects of hemodialysis is the *establishment and maintenance of adequate blood access.* Without it, hemodialysis cannot be done. The major routes of access are external arteriovenous shunts and internal arteriovenous fistulas. The *external arteriovenous shunt* requires the surgical placement of two tubes, or cannulas, into the patient's forearm, upper arm, or leg. The radial artery and cephalic vein are the most common vessels used. Figure 43–4 illustrates how one cannula is inserted into an artery and the other into a vein. The two Silastic tubes are brought out to the surface of the skin and connected together with a U-shaped segment called a shunt. Blood flows from the patient's artery through the shunt into the patient's vein. When he is to be attached to the hemodialyzer, a tube leading to the membrane compartment is connected to the arterial cannula. Blood then fills the membrane compartment and flows back into the patient by way of a tube connected to his venous cannula. When the dialysis is completed, the arterial cannula is clamped. When the blood in the membrane compartment has been returned to the body, the venous cannula is clamped and the U-shaped shunt reapplied to connect the artery and vein. This access can be created quickly and so is particularly suited to situations in which dialysis must be started right away. *Infection* at the site of insertion and *clotting* are frequent complications and often require moving the cannula sites. Other problems that occur with shunts are accidental dislodgement, hemorrhage, and skin erosion.

Creation of an *internal arteriovenous fistula* is also a surgical procedure in which an artery in the arm is anastomosed to a vein in a sideways or end-to-end fashion (Fig. 43–5). This creates an opening or fistula between a large artery and a large vein. The leaking of arterial blood into the venous system causes the veins to become engorged. This process takes at least 1 to 2 weeks and sometimes as long as 12 weeks to develop enough for the site to be used, making this approach inappropriate for immediate use. Peritoneal dialysis and external areteriovenous shunts may be used while the fistula is forming. Once the fistula is developed, the large veins may be punctured, using 14- or 16-gauge needles. When the patient is to go on dialysis, a needle is placed in the prominent vein. Another needle is placed in a different vein or in the opposite direction to the first needle in the same vein. By the use of a blood pump of the tubing

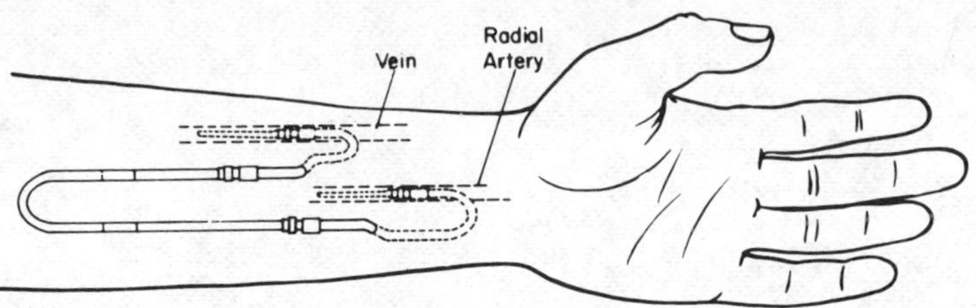

Figure 43–4. External arteriovenous shunt for hemodialysis blood access. (From Harrington, J., and E. Brenner: *Patient Care in Renal Disease.* Philadelphia: W. B. Saunders Co., 1973.)

leading to the hemodialyzer, arterial blood is pulled out of the vein by way of the fistula. Blood returns to the patient by a tube connected to the other needle. Another method of accessing the fistula is with *single needle dialysis.* Figure 43–6 shows the needle apparatus used to puncture the fistula; this device means that only one puncture is required each time, but there may be significant recirculation of dialyzed blood, meaning that clearance rates are decreased. Internal arteriovenous fistulas have been documented to cause severe hand swelling or ischemia ("steal syndrome"), hemorrhage, thrombosis, and aneurysm. Infection is less frequent than with external shunts.

If direct arteriovenous anastomosis is inappropriate for a patient, a *graft* may be used between the artery and vein. This technique is often necessary when there are no suitable peripheral vessels owing to such things as multiple external shunts and intravenous drug abuse. Autogenous grafts usually use the saphenous vein. However, this procedure has not been highly successful on a long-term basis owing to stenosis, aneurysm, and dilatation. Bovine carotid artery grafts have been widely used and have been shown to have long-range effectiveness. Synthetic materials used for grafting include polytetrafluoroethylene, Dacron velour, and Sparks mandril.

There are several types of dialyzers available. These include coil, parallel flow, and hollow fiber. Choice of a particular system is mostly a matter of preference. The dialysate solution can be altered to fit the patient's need.

Hemodialysis as a treatment for irreversible renal failure must be continued intermittently for as long as the patient lives. A typical schedule would be 6 to 10 hours of treatment three days each week. This schedule will vary with the size of the patient, the type of dialyzer used, the rate of blood flow, the personal preference of the patient, and several other factors. Work is being done on different schedules which better fit the patient's life-style while also producing better physiologic effects. Preliminary results have shown that a schedule of two hours of dialysis time every day produced significant improvement in all physical parameters, and patients on this schedule report increased energy and feeling of well-being.

The purpose of hemodialysis used in chronic renal failure is to clear the waste products from the body; restore fluid, electrolytes, and acid-base balances; and reverse some of the untoward manifestations of irreversible renal failure. Success is varied. Excess fluid, potassium, urea nitrogen, and acid ions are removed, but only temporarily; between dialyses these elements will build up again. Nutritionally, carbohydrate intolerance is alleviated. Amino acids, protein, glucose, and water-soluble vitamins are lost. The anemia is generally enhanced. The predialysis causative factors are still present and additional losses occur during dialysis owing to blood sampling, residual blood left in the dialyzer, and bleeding secondary to anticoagulation during dialysis. Serum iron stores are also further depleted. Hyperlipidemia seems to increase and is associated with accelerated atherosclerosis. Renal osteodystrophy usually improves; this can be further facilitated by adding calcium to the dialysate. Pruritus may occur for reasons not yet under-

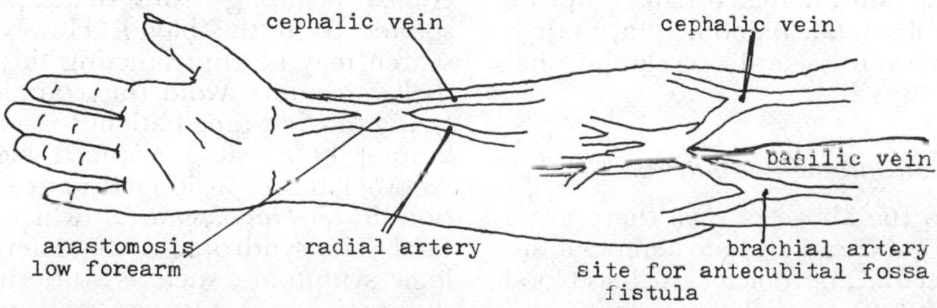

Figure 43–5. Internal arteriovenous fistula for hemodialysis blood access. (From McNamara, R.: The bioinstrumentation of hemodialysis. *Nursing Clinics of North America,* 13:611, Dec., 1978.)

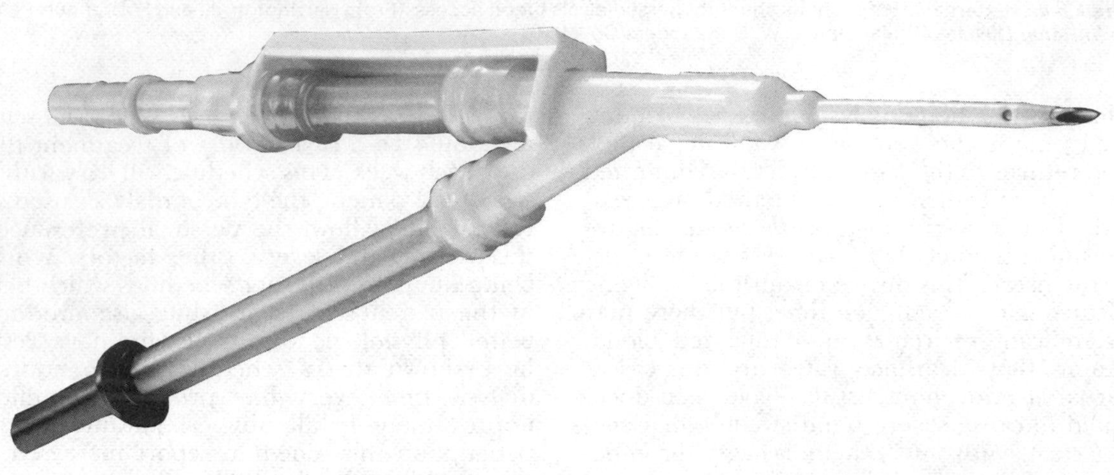

Figure 43–6. Unipuncture catheter for single needle dialysis. (From McNamara, R.: The bioinstrumentation of hemodialysis. *Nursing Clinics of North America*, 13:611, Dec., 1978.)

stood. Men on maintenance hemodialysis often develop gynecomastia, which is usually transient; this occurs because of low testosterone levels. However, many of the other sexual manifestations of uremia are reversed after a period of adaptation.

The usual effect of hemodialysis on serum concentration of medications is increased clearance of the drug. This is therapeutic in the case of drug overdose. Otherwise, it is frequently necessary to supplement medication dosages. Examples of drugs requiring higher doses include aminoglycosides, cephalosporins, penicillins, ethambutol, sulfonamide, trimethoprim, salicylates, phenobarbital, aminophyllin, methyldopa, methotrexate, and cyclophosphamide.[191]

Complications of Chronic Hemodialysis

In addition to the above effects. there are a number of *complications* of chronic hemodialysis. These include technical problems, such as blood leaks, overheating of the dialysate solution, insufficient blood loss, improper concentration of salts in the dialysate, and clotting; hypotension or hypertension; cardiac arrhythmias from potassium imbalance; air embolus; hemorrhage from heparinization; and pyrogenic reactions. Gastrointestinal ulcer disease is often complicated by hemorrhage. Muscle cramps often occur as a result of hyponatremia or hyposmolality. *Dialysis disequilibrium syndrome* is a complication that can occur particularly during the patient's first dialysis episode. It is characterized by mental confusion and deterioration of level of consciousness and may last for several days. Its etiology is unclear. Previous theories attributed this problem to the development of cerebral edema resulting from the rapid removal of solutes from the blood. However, recent research may be contradicting this theory. Many dialysis centers avoid this complication by dialyzing the first-time patient for a short period of 2 to 4 hours at a reduced blood flow rate. Another more prolonged neurologic complication is *cerebral dyspraxia,* which is frequently fatal. The syndrome is characterized by neurologic symptoms, such as stuttering, dysarthria, dyspraxia, and seizures and psychiatric disorders, such as paranoia, anxiety, depression, and progressive dementia.

Cardiac disorders, cerebrovascular disease, and infections are the most common causes of death. However, the long-term survival rate of patients receiving maintenance dialysis is encouraging. An overall 3-year survival rate of 66 per cent has been reported, with the ratio increasing with younger patients — 60 per cent for patients over 60 years of age and 72 per cent for those 20 to 29 years old. The presence of diabetes in the patient markedly lowers these figures, as does cardiovascular disease.[119]

Nursing Care in Hemodialysis

Most of the care required by the patient during and after hemodialysis falls within the realm of nursing. Providing this care requires specialized training.

Continuous monitoring during dialysis provides vital information about the progress of the treatment and allows early diagnosis of potential complications. There should be a well-organized plan for observing and recording vital signs, dialysate composition and temperature, functioning of the entire dialysis system, blood flow, and clotting times. The nurse should also be alert to early signs of potential complications as listed above.

Care of the shunt site is designed to prevent clotting and infection. The shunt is usually filled with undiluted heparin. The skin at the puncture site is cleaned daily with an antiseptic solution. An antimicrobial ointment may be applied followed by a dressing. A waterproof covering is necessary when the patient plans to bathe or swim. The site must be protected from trauma. Blood pressure readings should not be taken on or blood specimens drawn from the arm with the cannula. Between dialysis periods, the skin over an internal arteriovenous fistula requires only routine care with soap and water.

Providing adequate nutrition is often easier during dialysis and for a time afterwards. Dialysis usually relieves many of the gastrointestinal problems that frequently interfere with adequate intake. Food and fluid restrictions are usually liberalized during actual dialysis and then reimposed after the treatment. However, dietary noncompliance remains a major problem during maintenance hemodialysis, as it does with all patients with chronic renal failure. In a study of 192 patients exhibiting life-threatening behavior, 117 died because of noncompliance with the treatment regimen. One of the main factors was consuming forbidden food and fluids.[29] Research is needed to find motivation techniques to help these patients.

Psychosocial Aspects of Hemodialysis

Much of the care required by patients and significant others revolves around the psychosocial aspects of dialysis. Patients on maintenance dialysis often have ambivalent feelings. On one hand, they realize that hemodialysis is their tie with life. Yet, the many restrictions and life-style changes imposed on patients and significant others make continuation of the program extremely difficult. Patients frequently report that they feel in limbo between the worlds of life and death.

It is not uncommon for patients to feel quite grateful and optimistic at the start of their treatments. Usually they have felt poorly for some time and they view the treatment as a route to survival and a hope for feeling well again. It takes a few days or weeks for the full realization of the permanence of the treatment in their lives to occur. Depression during this period is expected. The suicide rate among dialysis patients has been estimated at 100 times that of the general population.

Three of the most frequent psychologic problems are *change in body image, dependency-independency conflict,* and *daily facing potential death.* The patient's own feelings of weakness and illness plus the presence of the arteriovenous shunt and hemodialysis equipment are constant reminders to the patient that he or she is no longer a "whole" person. Relationships with relatives and friends, job, and community roles and responsibilities will likely be altered. Changes in sexuality emphasize the problem even further. The patient's normal need for independence is continually threatened by dependence on the dialysis machinery and the staff in charge of care. This is especially true of adolescents and young adults. Other emotional problems that have been identified include the need for identity, safety and control of the environment, love, esteem, and communication. The stress on marital and family relationships and friendships is extreme.

Assistance for the patient and significant others must begin before dialysis is started. They need to fully understand the treatment and its implications. They should be encouraged to discuss their feelings. It is often difficult for them to voice concerns about continuing the treatment because of its significance to the patient's life. These feelings are often, albeit subconsciously, supported by the staff; it is very difficult for the personnel to accept a patient's decision to stop treatment and choose ultimate death instead. The staff, who often become a kind of "family" to the patient, must provide a continued unified, supportive approach and be ready to accept the whole gamut of reactions to dialysis by the patient and significant others. It is helpful to know the patient's usual patterns of response to stress. If patients have sound psychologic coping mechanisms and help from those around them, they usually accommodate themselves to this situation and plan their lives realistically. Patients who handle stress poorly or who have little support from others sometimes never make an adequate adjustment. Active participation by patients in their care is a valuable tool in helping to meet several of the needs identified above.

Cost of Hemodialysis

The monetary cost of hemodialysis is high. In 1977, the United States government paid $901 million for the treatment of patients with end-stage renal disease.[119] One means for reducing this cost is the use of *self-dialysis* with appropriate patients. The dialysis procedure is carried out by a trained patient either at home or in an outpatient dialysis facility. In addition to reducing the number of personnel needed during dialysis, this program is one means of allowing patients to actively participate in their care. Another advantage to the patient is less disruption of close relationships due to a more flexible schedule. However, success in the program requires that the patient have a strong internal motivation and continuous support from significant others and the staff. The training program to prepare the patient and others involved should cover normal anatomy and physiology of the kidney, principles of osmosis, construction and care of the access route, venipuncture, how to monitor and record specific parameters of the patient and machine, sterilization and aseptic technique, how to begin and terminate dialysis, how the equipment works and how to trouble-shoot problems with it, medications to be used, and medical complications of dialysis and how to avoid them.[82]

Home Dialysis

Home dialysis is self-dialysis done in the patient's home. Usually this program improves the patient's quality of life because is is less disruptive to the patient and others in the household than having to go to the dialysis center for treatment. Home dialysis offers the patient more access to significant others and greater feelings of independence and control. However, this treatment mode also produces definite stresses and personal relationships. Spouses have voiced concerns about their lack of free time, decreased mobility, and increased responsibility. In group therapy session, they have often talked about depression, anger, guilt, fear of making a mistake, and feelings of being burdened forever. Patients for this program must be carefully selected. Criteria might include stability of relationships, psychologic stability, financial support, and lack of severe physical complications. Elderly patients without contraindicating physical conditions have been found to be particularly suited to home dialysis, probably because of their maturity and social status. A successful program requires a staff who are advocates of home dialysis, a good training program as described above, and the provision of good support services, e.g., medical, nursing, and social services; provision of supplies; equipment maintenance; dietary counseling; psychiatric counseling; home visits; and retraining as necessary.[31]

Two developments that have offered added mobility for the patient are the "kidney in a suitcase" and the wearable artificial kidney. Both are small, portable machines that allow the patient to dialyze almost anywhere and also may be viable alternatives for rural community hospitals. Neither is widely used yet.

Renal Transplantation

Renal transplantation, or *renal homograft,* is the surgical transfer of a human kidney from one individual to another. This procedure is usually done as a treatment for irreversible renal failure, but may also be done whenever bilateral nephrectomy or removal of a solitary functioning kidney is necessary. This may occur in the case of trauma or renal malignancy.

The first successful kidney transplant was performed in the early 1950's and has been accepted as a viable alternative for the treatment of end-stage renal disease. A successful transplant prolongs patients' lives and markedly improves the quality of their lives. They are freed from the restrictions of dialysis and from the reversible manifestations of uremia. However, the procedure is certainly not without its risks. In addition to those risks attending the surgical procedure itself, the patient will have to live the rest of his or her life with the possibility of *graft rejection* and the hazards of immunosuppression. Over the years, patient survival rates have greatly improved, although there has not necessarily been parallel progress in the duration of grafts. Survival rates differ between patients receiving HLA-antigen-identical kidneys and those receiving grafts without this compatibility. One source cites patient survival rates of 90 per cent with antigen-identical kidneys and 70 per cent with nonidentical grafts; 3-year survival rates of HLA-antigen–identical kidneys are 65 per cent from a living relative and 40 per cent with a cadaver. Nonantigen-identical grafts have had a 50 per cent survival rate.[119] Another source reports overall graft survival rates of 94 per cent at 1 year, 81 per cent at 3 years, and 72 per cent at 4 to 5 years.[74] The presence of diabetes markedly reduces these figures.

The primary limiting factor in the number of transplants done is the availability of kidneys.

Many states have instituted a Uniform Anatomical Gift Act, which allows people to give permission before their own death for the use of their organs after death for transplant. This alleviates some of the problem of obtaining cadaver kidneys. However, the loss of potentially useable kidneys is still very high, owing to lack of awareness and acceptance by health care professionals, relatives, and the community as a whole. Solution of this problem requires professional and public education and work for enabling legislation. Medical and nursing personnel in rural communities must be trained in the technical aspects of removing, preserving, and transporting kidneys to metropolitan centers for transplant. Regional networks are being organized for referral and to facilitate distribution of kidneys.

Selection of a transplant *recipient* is based on careful evaluation of the patient's medical, immunologic, psychologic, and social statuses. The decision is usually made by an interdisciplinary team. Important psychosocial concerns include the patient's (a) feelings about transplant, (b) understanding and acceptance of the risks and chances of graft survival, and (c) family and social obligations. Although there are few absolute contraindications to transplantation, the presence of some physical conditions markedly increases the risk for the patient, primarily because of the long-term immunosuppressive administration that is necessary to avoid graft rejection. Acute infection and malignancy that cannot be controlled, oxalosis, and the presence of chronic obstructive pulmonary disease are definite contraindications. Patients with liver disease, psychologic disorders, diabetes, and advanced atherosclerosis need particularly careful consideration.

OBTAINING KIDNEYS FOR TRANSPLANTATION

As suggested by the survival rates cited above, the most desirable *source* of kidneys for transplant is living, related donors with histocompatibility. Willing family members are screened for ABO blood group and human leukocyte antigen (HLA) suitability. These grafts have the highest chance for survival. However, the location of enough suitable living, related donors for patients needing transplants is essentially impossible. Therefore, most kidneys for transplantation are cadaver organs. Potential kidney grafts can be obtained from recently deceased patients who had no systemic disease, such as infection, cancer, and advanced cardiovascular disease, no urinary tract disorders, and no prolonged hypoxia or hypotension prior to death. As with other organs, the harvesting of cadaver kidneys has raised a number of ethical problems, such as determining the point of death of the patient. Many times there is a conflict of interest between trying to prolong a dying patient's life and the need for a kidney for transplant. Many hospitals have a team that makes the decision about when the kidney may be taken and then works with the family of the dying patient to obtain permission to remove the kidneys.

Once permission has been obtained to harvest a suitable cadaver kidney for transplant, the major problem becomes one of preserving the kidney during transportation to the recipient so that maximal renal function is maintained. Preservation methods also allow adequate time for tissue typing, for full investigation of the donor for underlying disease, and to prepare the recipient for surgery. Commonly used methods for preservation include simple cold storage, in which the kidney is flushed with chilled electrolyte solution and placed in a sterile electrolyte slush, and hypothermic pulsatile perfusion. A variety of perfusates have been used and preservation times of 6 to 12 to 72 hours have been reported. Graft survival times may also be increased by pretreatment of the donor to prevent acute tubular necrosis before removing the kidney from the body. Once brain death has been determined, the patient should be well hydrated with Ringer's lactate to improve renal perfusion. Mannitol or furosemide may be used to achieve diuresis. Diabetes insipidus frequently occurs in cadavers between the time of death and the harvesting of the kidney. It may be prevented by the administration of Pitressin. Other medications given may include heparin, phenoxybenzamine to prevent renal vasospasm, methylprednisolone, and cyclophosphamide. Allopurinol may partially protect the kidney from ischemic cellular damage.

If the potential donor is a living relative, careful physical and psychologic evaluation is necessary. After histocompatibility has been established, probably the main physical criterion is that the donor have two well-functioning kidneys, since continued life after the unilateral nephrectomy depends on adequate renal function in the remaining kidney. Full evaluation of the entire urinary tract is done. The patient also receives a complete examination to rule out any systemic disease that may render the donor unsuitable. Psychologically, potential family donors must be evaluated as to their real desire to donate a kidney and their ability to make a lifelong adjustment to voluntarily losing a kidney. Frequently, evaluation of the donor is done by a team different from that caring for the recipient in order to avoid ambivalence and conflict of interest. Discussions with the donor should be held in strictest confidence and, if the person decides not to donate, the medical team frequently cites a physical contraindication to help assure continued acceptance of the potential donor by the family.

Personal and family relationships are very important factors in the decision to accept a potential donor. A variety of motivations have been reported including strong altruistic drives, hopes to restore previously destroyed family ties, and religious beliefs. It is usually easier to find a donor for a child than for an adult family member.

There frequently is tremendous pressure brought to bear on the potential donor by the recipient and the rest of the family.

The donor and family must also be prepared for postsurgical psychologic reactions. Strong emotional ties often develop between the donor and recipient during the evaluation period, and the donor frequently feels very responsible for the success or failure of the graft postoperatively. Graft rejection is usually devastating to these people. Also the need to protect the remaining kidney may give rise to later feelings of anger. Postoperative traumatic reactions by the donor are less likely in patients who have good inner resources, flexible defense mechanisms, and good mental health. Another source of postoperative stress for the donor is the fact that families tend to pay more attention to the recipient because of the continued possibility of graft rejection. The donor often feels abandoned. However, strong, long-lasting, positive effects are usually reported. These include identification of a source of inner strength, a more positive self-image, and a general "sense of feeling good" about saving someone's life.

If the potential donor is a minor, special legal precautions must be taken during the evaluation period. To neutralize conflict of interest, the court usually assigns guardians ad litem for the child. The final decision is made by these people and the court. The use of small children is controversial, with strong opinions found on both sides of the issue.

The donor may be assured that the remaining kidney will assume adequate total renal functioning for his body. The renal blood flow and glomerular filtration rate of the remaining kidney have been reported to increase to 70 to 80 per cent of the preoperative levels of both kidneys together. Within 2 to 6 years, the 24-hour creatinine clearance levels often recover 85 to 87 per cent. It is hypothesized that this increased function is facilitated by tubular hypertrophy and hyperplasia. Men tend to do slightly better than women, possibly because of the effect of testosterone.[68]

PREOPERATIVE PREPARATION AND TRANSPLANTATION PROCEDURE

Preoperative preparation of both the donor and the recipient include all aspects of general preoperative care as outlined in Chapter 17. In addition, there are several concerns unique to the recipient. The patient must be in as optimal condition as possible. This means that adequate conservative management and dialysis should have placed the patient in as close to a non-toxic state as is feasible. All infections must be eradicated. Gastrointestinal ulcers must be treated. Any lower urinary tract malfunctions must be corrected. Sometimes, when the bladder will be unacceptable to receive urine from the transplanted kidney, a urinary diversion procedure, such as an ileal conduit, may be done prior to the transplant itself. The patient's low hematocrit level increases his surgical risk, but there is much debate as to whether or not the patient should be transfused before surgery. The controversy is based on the question of whether transfusions actually stimulate an antigen presensitization. Many who utilize transfusions preoperatively recommend leukocyte-poor packed red blood cells. Immunosuppressive therapy may be started at least 24 hours before surgery.

Prior to the actual transplant procedure, some surgeons may choose to do one or more pretransplant procedures in an attempt to improve the chances of graft survival. There is a great deal of debate about the efficacy of performing bilateral nephrectomy. Definite indications for nephrectomy include uncontrollable hypertension, renal infection, and vesicoureteral reflux. Some also consider polycystic kidneys to require nephrectomy. Reasons given for this procedure include prevention of recurrent glomerulonephritis, removal of sources of infection, facilitation of blood pressure control, avoidance of recurrence of some renal diseases, elimination of massive proteinuria, and facilitation of postoperative monitoring of urine output from the transplanted kidney. However, opponents of this procedure cite irreplaceable endocrine and metabolic kidney functions, such as erythropoiesis and vitamin D metabolism, as rationale for leaving uninfected kidneys in place. Pretransplant nephrectomy also requires rigid fluid restriction postoperatively and increases the need for transfusion. Long-term effects of not doing nephrectomy are still being studied. One study of 74 patients, 27 with pretransplant nephrectomy and 47 without, demonstrated that the latter group had better survival and fewer graft rejections; the incidence of postoperative hypertension was similar in both groups.[19] Pretransplant splenectomy may be done in some centers, but the benefits of this procedure are controversial.

The transplantation operative procedure consists of placing the donor kidney in the recipient's body. Although the kidney is occasionally placed into the thigh, it is usually positioned in the iliac fossa and the renal vessels are anastomosed to the recipient's iliac vessels (Fig. 43–7). The surgical procedure is done swiftly to decrease the time the donor kidney is without a blood supply. Periods of ischemia longer than 30 minutes can damage the function of the newly transplanted kidney.

Usually the kidney begins to function immediately. There is usually a period of diuresis for the first 8 to 24 hours owing to a defect in the proximal tubular transport of sodium and glucose. This syndrome and its treatment are similar to postobstructive diuresis described above. Sometimes adequate functioning is delayed a few days. Hemodialysis may be performed intermittently until good function is established.

COMPLICATIONS OF KIDNEY TRANSPLANTATION

Except in the case of identical twin donor and recipient, the major postoperative complication is *homograft rejection reaction.* This is an immunologic attack against the foreign donor organ in an attempt to get rid of it. The reaction is stimulated by *foreign histocompatibility antigens.* There are four main types of clinical rejection: hyperacute, accelerated, acute, and chronic. *Hyperacute* rejection occurs any time from the moment of vascularization of the kidney to 48 hours postoperatively. It appears to be the result of circulating cytotoxic antibodies in a presensitized patient which quickly destroy the graft. The kidney and frequently the patient become toxic. Treatment is immediate removal of the transplanted kidney. *Accelerated* rejection occurs abruptly after an apparently adequate onset of kidney function. The reaction occurs within the first week, sometimes within 12 to 24 hours of kidney transplantation. It is thought to be caused by undetectably low levels of antibodies against the donor's antigens. Although antirejection therapy may solve the problem, transplant nephrectomy is usually needed. *Acute* rejection usually occurs within the first six weeks post-transplant, with two weeks being the most common time; it can be stimulated years later by a change in medication or unusual immunologic stress. It is a cell-mediated process which produces interstitial edema and vasculitis within the

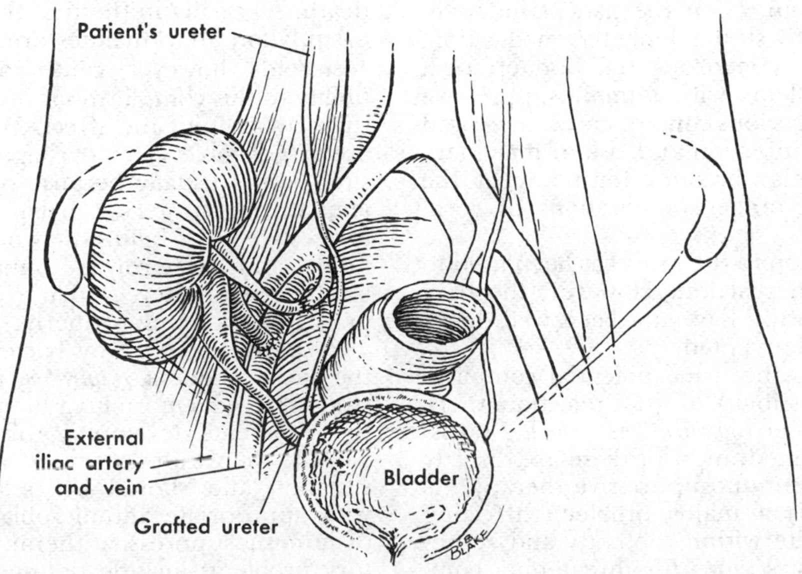

Figure 43–7. Transplanted kidney in place. (From Brundage, D.: *Nursing Management of Renal Problems.* St. Louis: C. V. Mosby Co., 1976.)

kidney. Clinical signs of this reaction include fever, an elevated white blood cell count, acute hypertension, and signs of deteriorating renal function. It is usually treatable with steroids and radiation. *Chronic* rejection occurs slowly over a period of months to years. It mimics chronic renal failure and is resistant to therapy.

When signs of transplant rejection occur, it is necessary to differentiate between this diagnosis and others with symptoms similar to those of rejection. Examples include acute renal failure, renal thrombosis, obstruction, and leakage. It is essential to pinpoint the cause before treatment is begun. Urography, renal scan, and ultrasound are among the diagnostic tools used.

Antirejection therapy revolves around the use of immunosuppressive drugs, which block the body's normal immune responses. Without these agents, almost all transplants would be lost. Azathioprine and prednisone or methylprednisolone are the most frequently used drugs. Steroids may be given in high-dose "bolus" or "pulse" therapy. Cyclophosphamide is sometimes used in place of azathioprine. The injection of antilymphocyte globulin (ALG) or antilymphocyte serum (ALS) causes a decreased response to specific antigens, although their long-range therapeutic effect in humans is still under investigation. In the case of documented and sometimes suspected graft rejection, usual daily doses of the immunosuppressive drugs are significantly boosted. The administration of these agents continues indefinitely, usually for the patient's lifetime. Sudden discontinuance, such as may occur when the patient independently decides to stop taking the medication, usually triggers a vigorous rejection episode. The main problems with immunosuppressive therapy are two serious consequences: increased susceptibility to infection and risk of malignancy. These sequelae account for many of the short- and long-range complications of renal transplant.

Local irradiation to the graft has been used to reverse rejection reaction. However, the benefits of this therapy have not been well documented nor well accepted.

In addition to the usual potential complications and the possibility of graft rejection, there are a host of other *complications* of renal transplant. As mentioned, most of these are directly attributable to immunosuppressive therapy. As cited, *infection* is a major problem, affecting every possible site within the body and representing the most serious life-threatening complication. Gram-negative bacteria are the most common causative organisms. There is also a high incidence of viral infections, particularly cytomegalovirus. Adding to the problem is the fact that immunosuppressive agents mask early signs of sepsis so that by the time infections are recognized, they are fairly well advanced. Sometimes, immunosuppressive therapy is reduced for a short time while the infection is brought under control.

The most frequent renal complication is *rejection.* Spontaneous rupture of the kidney usually occurs within 14 days of the transplant. It is thought to be caused by rejection or ischemic damage or by some intrinsic renal disease and produces intense pain and swelling over the transplant site and signs of systemic shock. There may be hemorrhage from the operative site. Attempts may be made to surgically repair the laceration, but the usual result is loss of the kidney. Calculi are usually calcium stones secondary to hyperparathyroidism. Fistula formation includes caliceal-cutaneous, ureteral, and vesical. Long-term uremia and anemia and steroid therapy may be predisposing factors. Surgical repair may be undertaken, as well as tapered alternate-day steroid treatment. Other urinary tract complications include ureteral, bladder, or pelvic leaks; obstruction; reflux, lymphocele; and malignancy. Urethral catheter drainage is used until spontaneous voiding occurs to prevent overdistention of the bladder.

Cardiovascular complications may be local or systemic. Renal artery stenosis is a frequent cause of systemic hypertension. Treatment may call for resection of the stenosed segment and reanastomosis. The use of dipyridamole may inhibit platelet aggregation and may significantly protect against stenosis. Renal (iliac) vein thrombosis has been documented. Thromboembolism may be the second leading cause of death, especially in the first three weeks before coagulation abnormalities are corrected. Corticosteroids, however, cause continuing susceptibility to this complication, probably because of their hyperlipidemic effect. Mycotic aneurysms are predictable. Hemorrhage at anastomoses sites occurs usually because of technical problems during surgery. Cardiac arrhythmias and congestive heart failure may occur as a result of fluid and electrolyte imbalances. Plasma erythropoietin titers return to normal when the graft is functioning properly.

Pneumonia, caused by bacteria and fungi, is the most frequent *respiratory complication.* One study showed a mortality rate of 51.5 per cent in those patients developing this problem.[134] Obviously, then, respiratory infections are a crisis situation and should be treated immediately with appropriate antimicrobials and reduction of immunosuppressive therapy. Other respiratory problems include pulmonary edema, pulmonary emboli, and reactivated tuberculosis. "Transplant" lung is a syndrome characterized by an alveolar-capillary block, splotchy lung on x-ray, and few other signs. Antirejection therapy seems to clear the disease, giving credence to the idea that it is an immunologic problem.[39]

Infections, especially oral and esophageal, are common *gastrointestinal sequelae.* Heparin and cirrhosis occur and may be associated with the use of hepatotoxic drugs, such as azathioprine. Peptic ulcer disease is a particularly problematic consequence. Impaired gastrin metabolism and increased secretion due to stress-induced epinephrine release enhance the development of ulcers. Elevated histamine levels, hyperparathyroidism, and hypercalcemia may also contribute. Antacid therapy should be continued prophylactically for at least six months post-transplant. Uremia, ischemic colon, immunosuppressives, overgrowth of pathogens, and radiation all advance the development of colitis. Pancreatitis also occurs, although its pathogenesis is not entirely clear.

Skin carcinomas are particularly common. Other dermatologic sequelae include infection, purpura, acne, and alopecia. Wound healing is markedly slowed, directly attributable to the use of steroids.

Other systems are also affected by post-transplant complications. *Musculoskeletal sequelae* include hyperparathyroidism, osteoporosis, and myopathy. Aseptic bone necrosis is probably due to corticosteroid therapy, although the pathogenesis is controversial. The *reproductive problems* described in chronic renal failure frequently disappear after transplantation. However, hydrocele and testicular atrophy are common. The incidence of gynecologic malignancies is significantly higher than in the general population, with cervical cancer dominating. Successful pregnancies have been completed after transplant. Steroid-induced cataract glaucoma and retinitis secondary to cytomegalovirus are common *ocular consequences.*

NURSING CARE IN TRANSPLANTATION PROCEDURES

Much of the *nursing care* is aimed at prevention, early recognition, and treatment of these complications plus measures to facilitate maximum renal function and help the patient attain an optimal quality of life. Immediate postoperative care of both the donor and recipient encompasses the care required by any patient having surgery, as described in Chapter 19. Care of the donor resembles that of any patient having a nephrectomy. The additional care required by the recipient is partially suggested by the potential complications. The nurse must be constantly aware of the signs and symptoms of these sequelae.

Reverse, or protective, isolation may be used because of the patient's susceptibility. However, precautions are usually not this strict, and measures are taken to protect the patient from potential sources of infection within the environment. For instance, when patients go to x-ray, they may be dressed in gown and mask and visitors are usually restricted.

Monitoring of renal function and fluid balance is crucial during the postoperative period. Vital signs, central venous pressure, weight, hourly or half-hourly urine output, and intake are measured frequently. Serial laboratory determinations of hemoglobin, hematocrit, blood urea nitrogen creatinine, and electrolytes will be followed closely. All urine should be saved and its specific gravity measured. Intravenous replacement of fluids must be managed carefully and is frequently based on the previous hour's urine output. A high urine output is usually desired. Care must be taken to avoid obstruction of any ureteral or urethral catheters.

Because of the high incidence and seriousness of pneumonia to the renal transplant patient, preventive respiratory treatment is essential. Coughing and deep breathing exercises are begun immediately. This is painful for the patient, and the nurse can use analgesics judiciously and put external pressure over the incision to help the patient do this more effectively. Positive pressure breathing apparatus may also be employed.

Wound care must be done using the strictest aseptic technique, since the patient does not have much resistance to bacterial invasion. Delayed wound healing makes the patient susceptible to dehiscence longer than usual. If the patient has a shunt for hemodialysis, it will be left intact in case dialysis is needed postoperatively. Measures must be taken to preserve the shunt.

Oral hygiene is important because of the high incidence of stomatitis, bacterial and fungal infections, and the fact that the patient is usually on nothing by mouth postoperatively. Antifungal mouthwashes may also be used.

Because of the common occurrence of paralytic ileus, the patient will usually have a nasogastric tube for at least 24 hours. As bowel peristalsis returns, the diet is advanced. Unless the patient is demonstrating rejection or hypertension, there may be no dietary restrictions, although some physicians prescribe alterations in protein, sodium, and carbohydrate intake. As soon as the patient is taking oral food and fluids, antacid therapy is begun.

Early ambulation is necessary to prevent cardiovascular and pulmonary complications and to stimualte gastrointestinal function. In addition, since sodium excretion is increased in the recumbent position, it is important for the patient to be kept in an upright position.

Psychologic Support

Psychologically, the patient must be helped to incorporate a new kidney into his or her body image. Four stages of a healthy adjustment process have been identified:[222]

- *Foreign body stage,* during which the patient feels he or she is carrying around something that is very fragile and needs to be carefully protected
- *Stage of partial internalization,* which indicates gradual acceptance and decreased interest in the graft
- *Complete internalization,* in which the patient is usually not aware of the transplant unless it is specifically mentioned by someone else
- *Regression to the foreign body stage,* which can occur during any routine evaluation procedure

However, not all patients proceed normally through these steps. Many experience depression as they realize their continued vulnerability to rejection. Overdependency and excessive drinking are examples of behaviors caused by the depression. If the graft fails, expected reactions include anger, hostility, guilt, and a helplessness-hopelessness syndrome. Relatives and friends may mirror these feelings.

Long-term care usually covers the rest of the patient's lifetime. Continued physical and psychologic support is needed. The importance of complying with recommended medical regimens and follow-up evaluation schedules must be emphasized and periodically reinforced. The patient will need to arrange activities and lifestyle so as to avoid infections and highly stressful situations. In essence, the patient and family will need assistance in adjusting to a lifelong chronic condition.

BIBLIOGRAPHY (Unit XIII)

1. Adler, S.: Managing chronic renal failure. *Consultant,* 16:41, Dec., 1976.
2. Agus, Z.: What to do for the patient with kidney stones. *Consultant,* 17:21, Aug., 1977.
3. Albert, P., et al.: Carotid heterograft for segmental ureteral substitution. *American Journal of Surgery,* 131:556, May, 1976.
4. Altshuler, A., et al.: Even children can learn to do self-catheterization. *American Journal of Nursing,* 77:97, Jan., 1977.
5. Anderson, E.: Woman and cystitis. *Nursing '77,* 7:50, Apr., 1977.
6. Andriole, V.: Hospital acquired urinary infections and the indwelling catheter. *Urologic Clinics of North America,* 2:451, Oct., 1975.
7. Appel, G., and H. Neu: The nephrotoxicity of antimicrobial agents. *New England Journal of Medicine,* 296:663, Mar. 24, 1977.
8. Appel, R., et al.: Reversible renal failure following intravascular contrast radiography. *Journal of the American Medical Association,* 238:1947, Oct. 31, 1977.
9. Arisz, L., et al.: The effect of indomethacin on proteinuria and kidney function in the nephrotic syndrome. *Acta Medica Scandinavia,* 199:121, 1976.
10. Arnold, S., and A. Ginsburg: Understanding and managing enuresis in children. *Postgraduate Medicine,* 58:73, Nov., 1975.
11. Auvert, J.: Trends in Alloplastic Replacement of Segments of the Urinary Tract. *Urological Research,* 4:143, Dec., 1976.
12. Awad, S., et al.: The treatment of the uninhibited bladder with dicyclomine. *Journal of Urology,* 117:161, Feb., 1977.
13. Banowsky, L.: The role of adjuvant operations in renal transplantation. *Urologic Clinics of North America,* 3:527, Oct., 1976.
14. Barnes, R., et al.: Changes in grade and stage of recurrent bladder tumors. *Journal of Urology,* 118:177, July, 1977.
15. Barrett, N.: Continent vesicostomy: The dry urinary diversion. *American Journal of Nursing,* 79:462, Mar., 1979.
16. Batata, M., and H. Grabstald: Upper urinary tract urothelial tumors. *Urologic Clinics of North America,* 3:79, Feb., 1976.
17. Baum, M.: "I want to be dry!" *Nursing '78,* 8:75, Feb., 1978.
18. Beard, M.: The impact of hemodialysis and transplantation on the family. *Critical Care Quarterly,* 1:87, Sept., 1978.
19. Bennett, W.: Cost-benefit ratio of pretransplant bilateral nephrectomy. *Journal of the American Medical Association,* 235:1703, Apr. 19, 1976.
20. Bennett, W., et al.: Drug-related syndromes in clinical nephrology. *Annals of Internal Medicine,* 87:582, Nov., 1977.
21. Bergreen, P., et al.: Therapeutic renal infarction. *Journal of Urology,* 118:372, Sept., 1977.
22. Berman, L.: An abundance of urine. *Journal of the American Medical Association,* 229:203, July 8, 1974.
23. Berman, L.: Sickle cell nephropathy. *Journal of the American Medical Association,* 228:1279, June 3, 1974.
24. Berman, L.: Urine isn't everything. *Journal of the American Medical Association,* 231:978, March 3, 1975.
25. Berman, L.: When the urine is red. *Journal of the American Medical Association,* 237:2753, June 20, 1977.
26. Biller, D.: Patient's point of view: Diet in chronic renal failure. *Journal of the American Dietetic Association,* 71:633, Dec., 1977.
27. Bissada, N., et al.: Medical management of urolithiasis. *American Family Physician,* 13:89, May, 1976.
28. Bissada, N., et al.: Renal carcinoma: Diagnostic and therapeutic aspects. *American Family Physician,* 16:100, Aug., 1977.
29. Blackburn, S.: Dietary compliance of chronic hemodialysis patients. *Journal of the American Dietetic Association,* 70:31, Jan., 1977.
30. Bladder Cancer and Saccharin. *Lancet,* 2:592, Sept. 17, 1977.
31. Blagg, C.: Home dialysis. *Dialysis and Transplant,* 6:14, Oct., 1977.
32. Bloodless cure for a kidney. *Emergency Medicine,* 9:91, Apr., 1977.
33. Bolton, W.: Nonhemorrhagic decrements in hemato-

crit values after percutaneous renal biopsy. *Journal of the American Medical Association,* 238:1266, Sept. 19, 1977.

34. Bracken, R., et al.: Primary carcinoma of the female urethra. *Journal of Urology,* 116:188, Aug., 1976.
35. Bradley, W., et al.: Neurology of micturition. *Journal of Urology,* 115:481, May, 1976.
36. Braedel, H., et al.: Renal phlebography: An aid in the diagnosis of the absent or non-functioning kidney. *Journal of Urology,* 116:703, Dec., 1976.
37. Brenner, B., and Rector, F.: *The Kidney.* Volumes I and II. Philadelphia: W. B. Saunders Co., 1976.
38. Brenner, B., et al.: Mechanics of glomerular ultrafiltration. *New England Journal of Medicine,* 297:148, July 21, 1977.
39. Brundage, D.: *Nursing Management of Renal Problems.* St. Louis: C. V. Mosby Co., 1976.
40. Bultitude, M., and Eykyn, S.: The relationship between the urethral flora and urinary infection in the catheterized male. *British Journal of Urology,* 45:678, Dec., 1973.
41. Butcher, D., et al.: Size and weight of glomeruli isolated from human diabetic and nondiabetic kidneys. *Journal of Laboratory and Clinical Medicine,* 89:544, Mar., 1977.
42. Butts, P.: Assessing urinary incontinence in women. *Nursing '79,* 9:72, Mar., 1979.
43. Caine, M., et al.: Some clinical implications of adrenergic receptors in the urinary tract. *Archives of Surgery,* 110:247, Mar., 1975.
44. Caldwell, W.: Radiotherapy: Definitive, integrated and palliative therapy. *Urologic Clinics of North America,* 3:129, Feb., 1976.
45. Can this kidney be saved? *Emergency Medicine,* 9:51, Dec., 1977.
46. Carris, C., et al.: Emphysematous pyelonephritis. *Journal of Urology,* 118:457, Sept., 1977.
47. Champion, V.: Clean technique for intermittent self-catheterization. *Nursing Research,* 25:13, Jan./Feb., 1976.
48. Chan, J.: Kidney biopsy: Analysis of patient data and indications for kidney biopsies. *Journal of Urology,* 118:641, Oct., 1977.
49. Chavigny, K.: The use of polymixin B as a urethral lubricant to reduce the post-instrumental incidence of bacteriuria in females. An exploratory study. *International Journal of Nursing Studies,* 12:33, Mar., 1975.
50. Chavigny, K., and Nunnally, D.: A comparison of methods for collecting clean-catch urine specimens in a clinic population of obstetric patients. *American Journal of Obstetrics and Gynecology,* 122:34, May 1, 1975.
51. Chester, A., et al.: Polycystic kidney disease. *American Family Physician,* 16:94, Dec., 1977.
52. Chezem, J.: Urinary diversion: Select aspects of nursing management. *Nursing Clinics of North America,* 11:445, Sept., 1976.
53. Cline, F.: Enuresis: A frequent problem with multiple causation and generally manageable. *Nurse Practitioner,* 1:36, July/Aug., 1976.
54. Coe, F.: Treatment and prevention of renal stones. *Consultant,* 18:47, Oct., 1978.
55. Coe, F., et al.: The natural history of calcium urolithiasis. *Journal of the American Medical Association,* 238:1519, Oct. 3, 1977.
56. Coffield, K., et al.: Experience with management of posterior urethral injury associated with pelvic fracture. *Journal of Urology,* 117:722, June, 1977.
57. Cohen, B.: Relative risks of saccharin and calorie ingestion. *Science,* 199:983, Mar. 3, 1978.
58. Colapinto, V.: Urethral trauma. *Canadian Medical Association Journal,* 117:791, Oct. 8, 1977.
59. Confer, D., et al.: Dramatic palliation for painful, fixed bladder squamous cell carcinoma with 5-fluorouracil infusion. *Journal of Urology,* 118:483, Sept., 1977.
60. Cook, J., et al.: Ultrasonic demonstration of intrarenal anatomy. *American Journal of Roentgenology,* 129:831, Nov., 1977.
61. Correa, J., et al.: Polycystic horseshoe kidney. *Journal of Urology,* 116:802, Dec., 1976.
62. Crabtree, M.: How to assess a patient's urologic complaint. *RN,* 38:79, Nov., 1975.
63. Cronin, R., et al.: Acute renal failure: Diagnosis, pathogenesis and management. *Hospital Medicine,* 12:26, Aug., 1976.
64. Cronin, R., et al.: Renal cell carcinoma: Unusual systemic manifestations. *Medicine,* 55:291, July, 1976.
65. Cross, P.: Ureteral reimplantation: Nursing care of the child. *American Journal of Nursing,* 76:1800, Nov., 1976.
66. Crowe, L., et al.: Evaluating renal function: Current status of clinical tests. *Postgraduate Medicine,* 62:58, July, 1977.
67. D'Afflitti, J., et al.: Group sessions for the wives of home-hemodialysis patients. *American Journal of Nursing,* 75:633, Apr., 1975.
68. Davison, J., et al.: Renal function studies after nephrectomy in renal donors. *British Medical Journal,* 1:1050, May 1, 1976.
69. Debenedictus, T., et al.: Intraurethral condylomas acuminata: Management and review of the literature. *Journal of Urology,* 18:767, Nov., 1977.
70. Decenzo, J., and G. Leadbetter: The interaction of host immunocompetence and tumor aggressiveness in superficial bladder carcinoma. *Journal of Urology,* 115:262, May, 1976.
71. DeGroot, J.: Catheter-induced UTI's. How can we prevent them? *Nursing '76,* 6:34, Aug., 1976.
72. Devine, H., et al.: The permanent Tenckhoff catheter for chronic peritoneal dialysis. *Canadian Medical Association Journal,* 113:219, Aug. 9, 1975.
73. Dhar, S., and E. Smith: Renal transplantation. *Heart and Lung,* 4:894, Nov./Dec., 1975.
74. Diethelm, A., et al.: Retrospective analysis of 100 conservative patients undergoing related living donor renal transplantation. *Annals of Surgery,* 183:502, May, 1976.
75. DiPalma, J.: Drugs that induce changes in urine color. *RN,* 40:34, Jan., 1977.
76. Donadio, J.: Glomerulonephritis: Approach to diagnosis and treatment. *Hospital Medicine,* 14:36, Apr., 1978.
77. Dowd, J.: Methods of urinary diversion. *American Operating Room Nurses Journal,* 23:37, Jan., 1976.
78. Dretter, S., et al.: Managing carcinoma of the bladder. *Geriatrics,* 29:75, Sept., 1974.
79. Eknoyan, G.: Axioms on acute oliguria. *Hospital Medicine,* 13:32, Dec., 1977.
80. Erslev, A.: Renal biogenesis of erythropoietin. *American Journal of Medicine,* 58:25, Jan., 1975.
81. Federspiel, B.: Renin and blood pressure. *American Journal of Nursing,* 75:1462, Sept., 1975.
82. Feegle, J.: Teaching self-dialysis to adults in a hospital. *American Journal of Nursing,* 77:270, Feb., 1977.
83. Fennell, S.: Percutaneous renal biopsy. *American Journal of Nursing,* 75:1292, Aug., 1975.
84. Feustel, D.: Autonomic hyperreflexia. *American Journal of Nursing,* 76:228, Feb., 1976.
85. Fiberoptics in the urinary tract. *Emergency Medicine,* 10:82, Oct., 1978.

86. Firlit, C.: Urethral abnormalities. *Urologic Clinics of North America,* 5:31, Feb., 1978.
87. Flanagan, M.: Acute urinary retention. *Hospital Medicine,* 12:60, Sept., 1976.
88. Fleisch, H., et al.: *Urolithiasis Research.* New York: Plenum Press, 1976.
89. Ford, L.: A question of balance: The effects of chronic renal failure and long-term dialysis. *Canadian Nurse,* 73:19, Mar., 1977.
90. Fost, N.: Children as renal donors. *New England Journal of Medicine,* 296:363, Feb. 17, 1977.
91. Foster, J.: Dialysis: A treatment modality in renal failure. *Critical Care Quarterly,* 1:25, Sept., 1978.
92. Fowler, J., and T. Stamey: Studies of introital colonization in women with recurrent urinary infections: The role of bacterial adherence. *Journal of Urology,* 117:472, Apr., 1977.
93. Frank, I., et al.: Urologic and male genital cancers. *In* Rubin, P. (Ed.): *Clinical Oncology for Medical Students and Physicians: A Multidisciplinary Approach.* New York: American Cancer Society, 1978.
94. Freedman, P., and E. Smith: Acute renal failure. *Heart and Lung,* 4:873, Nov./Dec., 1975.
95. Freimanis, A., and M. Absher: Ultrasonic diagnosis in and about the kidney. *Journal of the American Medical Association,* 234:1263, Dec. 22, 1975.
96. Freni, S., et al.: Erythrocyturia, smoking and occupation. *Journal of Clinical Pathology,* 30:341, Apr., 1977.
97. Friedman, E.: Sorbents in the management of uremia. *American Journal of Medicine,* 60:614, May 10, 1976.
98. Friedman, E.: *Strategy in Renal Failure.* New York: John Wiley and Sons, 1978.
99. Fye, K., et al.: Low-dosage heparin in rapidly progressive glomerulonephritis. *Archives of Internal Medicine,* 136:995, Sept., 1976.
100. Ganong, W.: *Review of Medical Physiology.* Los Altos: Lange Medical Publications, 1977.
101. Gault, P.: How to break the kidney stone cycle. *Nursing '78,* 8:24, Dec., 1978.
102. George, C., and Farrell, P.: A preliminary assessment of daily dialysis. *Dialysis and Transplant,* 6:10, Mar., 1977.
103. Ghoneim, M., and Pandya, H.: Plasma protein binding of thiopental in patients with impaired renal or hepatic function. *Anesthesia,* 42:545, May, 1975.
104. Gibbons, R., et al.: Experience with indwelling ureteral stent catheters. *Journal of Urology,* 115:22, Jan., 1976.
105. Gittes, R.: Operative nephroscopy. *Journal of Urology,* 116:148, Aug., 1976.
106. Gittes, R.: Retrograde renal and ureteral brush biopsy. *American Journal of Nursing,* 78:410, Mar., 1978.
107. Gleason, D., et al.: Urodynamics. *Journal of Urology,* 115:356, Apr., 1976.
108. Golden, A., and Maher, J.: *The Kidney.* Baltimore: The Williams and Wilkins Company, 1977.
109. Gosling, J., et al.: The autonomic innervation of the human male and female bladder neck and proximal urethra. *Journal of Urology,* 118:302, Aug., 1977.
110. Gottlieb, M., et al.: Immunologic test for rejection. *Urologic Clinics of North America,* 3:553, Oct., 1976.
111. Gow, J.: Genitourinary tuberculosis: A study of short course regimens. *Journal of Urology,* 115:707, June, 1976.
112. Greem, T.: Urinary stress incontinence: Differential diagnosis, pathophysiology, and management. *American Journal of Obstetrics and Gynecology,* 122:368, June 1, 1975.
113. Greene, W., et al.: Nonoperative suprapubic urinary drainage. *American Family Physician,* 16:136, Oct., 1977.
114. Griffiths, G., et al.: Loss of renal tissue in the elderly. *British Journal of Radiology,* 49:111, Feb., 1976.
115. Grimes, J.: Stone disease in urinary diversion. *Southern Medical Journal,* 68:494, Dec., 1975.
116. Gross, J., and Kokko, J.: The influence of increased tubular hydrostatic pressure on renal function. *Journal of Urology,* 115:427, Apr., 1976.
117. Grossman, R.: A pratical approach to managing acute oliguria. *Consultant,* 19:42, Jan., 1979.
118. Gutman, R.: Manipulation of allograft immunogenicity by pretreatment of cadaver donors. *Urologic Clinics of North America,* 3:475, Oct., 1976.
119. Gutman, R., and Amara, A.: Outcome of therapy for end-stage uremia: An informed prediction of survival rate and degree of rehabilitation. *Postgraduate Medicine,* 64:183, Nov., 1978.
120. Guyton, A.: *Textbook of Medical Physiology.* Philadelphia: W. B. Saunders Co., 1976.
121. Hanaway, J., et al.: Renal failure following contrast injection for computerized tomography. *Journal of the American Medical Association,* 239:205, Nov. 7, 1977.
122. Harris, J., et al.: The kidney and pregnancy. *American Family Physician,* 18:97, Oct., 1978.
123. Harvey-Smith, W.: Renal cell carcinoma. *Nurse Practitioner,* 4:39, Jan./Feb., 1979.
124. Hautman, R., and Lutzeyer, W.: Calcium oxalate stone disease: Congenital defect of metabolism? *Journal of Urology,* 116:687, Dec., 1976.
125. Heenrich, M., and Slevin, S.: Patients' attitude toward hemodialysis frequency: A pilot study. *Dialysis and Transplant,* 6:12, May, 1977.
126. Henrich, W., and Anderson, R.: Drug use in renal failure. *Postgraduate Medicine,* 64:153, Nov., 1978.
127. Henrich, W., et al.: Therapeutic renal arterial occlusion for elimination of proteinuria: Medical nephrectomy. *Archives of Internal Medicine,* 136:840, July, 1976.
128. Hepinstall, R.: Interstitial nephritis: A brief review. *American Journal of Pathology,* 83:213, Apr., 1976.
129. Herr, H.: Intermittent catheterization in neurogenic bladder dysfunction. *Journal of Urology,* 113:477, Apr., 1975.
130. Hill, G., et al.: Perfusion-related injury in renal transplantation. *Surgery,* 79:440, Apr., 1976.
131. Hirvas, J., et al.: Psychological and social problems encountered in active treatment of chronic uraemia: The living donor. *Acta Medica Scandinavia,* 200:17, 1976.
132. Hollenberg, N., and Adams, D.: The renal blood supply in oliguria states: When is a kidney ischemic? *American Heart Journal,* 91:255, Feb., 1976.
133. Hosking, D.: Disease of the urinary system: Renal osteodystrophy. *British Medical Journal,* 2:110, July, 1977.
134. Huertas, V., et al.: Pneumonia in recipients of renal allografts. *Achives of Surgery,* 111:162, Feb., 1976.
135. Ihels, L., et al.: Aseptic necrosis of bone following renal transplantation: Experience in 194 transplant recipients and review of the literature. *Medicine,* 57:25, Jan., 1978.
136. Innes, B., and Bruya, M.: Postoperative voiding patterns and related contributing factors. *Washington State Journal of Nursing,* 49:13, Summer/Fall, 1977.
137. Intermittent catheterization: A small warning. *Emergency Medicine,* 6:274, Apr., 1974.
138. Jamison, R., et al.: The urinary concentrating mechanism. *New England Journal of Medicine,* 295:1059, Nov. 4, 1976.

139. Jeffs, R.: Extrophy and cloacal exstrophy. *Urologic Clinics of North America,* 5:127, Feb., 1978.
140. Jenkins, P., et al.: Self-hemodialysis: The optimal mode of dialytic therapy. *Archives of Internal Medicine,* 136:357, Mar., 1976.
141. Jensen, H., et al.: Proteinuria in non-renal infectious diseases. *Acta Medica Scandinavia,* 196:75, July/Aug., 1974.
142. Jensen, V.: Better techniques for bagging stomas: Urinary ostomies. *Nursing '74,* 4:60, July, 1974.
143. Juliani, L.: Assessing renal function. *Nursing '78,* 8:34, Jan., 1978.
144. Juliani, L., and Reamer, B.: Kidney transplant: Your role in aftercare. *Nursing '77,* 7:46, Oct., 1977.
145. Kafkas, M.: The diagnosis of bladder tumors by concentration of epithelial cells in the urine and by the help of the fluorescence property of tetracycline. *Journal of Urology,* 117:581, May, 1977.
146. Karow, A.: Solutions to the organ acquisition problem. *Dialysis and Transplant,* 5:48, Feb./Mar., 1976.
147. Kasprak, M.: Spinal stimulation: Pre- and postoperative care. *American Operating Room Nurses Journal,* 23:1221, June, 1976.
148. Kavchak-Keyes, M.: Autonomic hyperreflexia. *American Rehabilitation Nursing Journal,* 2:17, Sept./Oct., 1977.
149. Kennedy, G., et al.: Subacute toxicity studies with sodium saccharin and two hydrolytic derivatives. *Toxicology,* 6:133, Aug./Sept., 1976.
150. Kent, S.: Urinary tract problems in women are linked to sexual activity. *Geriatrics,* 30:145, July, 1975.
151. Kessler, I.: Non-nutritive sweeteners and human bladder cancer: Preliminary findings. *Journal of Urology,* 115:143, Feb., 1976.
152. Khanna, O.: A new pharmacologic approach to the non-emptying bladder. *American Family Physician,* 17:162, May, 1978.
153. Kimble, M.: Diabetes. *Nursing Digest,* 2:113, Nov./Dec., 1974.
154. Kimbrough, H., et al.: Cardiac rhythm in men during cystoscopy. *Journal of Urology,* 113:846, June, 1975.
155. King, L.: Undiversion: When and how? *Journal of Urology,* 115:296, Mar., 1976.
156. Kintzel, K.: *Advanced Concepts in Clinical Nursing.* Philadelphia: J. B. Lippincott Co., 1977.
157. Kiviat, M., et al.: Sphincter stretch: A new technique resulting in continence and complete voiding in paraplegics. *Journal of Urology,* 114:895, Dec., 1975.
158. Kjellstrand, C., et al.: Kidney transplants in patients over 50. *Geriatrics,* 31:65, Sept., 1976.
159. Klein, K., and Karokawa, K.: Metabolic and endocrine alterations in end-stage renal failure. *Postgraduate Medicine,* 64:99, Nov., 1978.
160. Klopper, J., et al.: Measurement of glomerular filtration rate. *New England Journal of Medicine,* 296:284, Feb. 3, 1977.
161. Kokko, J.: The role of the renal concentrating mechanisms in the regulation of serum sodium concentration. *American Journal of Medicine,* 62:165, Feb., 1977.
162. Kollins, S., et al.: Roentgenographic findings in urinary tract tuberculosis: A 10-year review. *American Journal of Roentgenology Radium Therapeutic Nuclear Medicine,* 121:487, July, 1974.
163. Kopple, J.: Nutritional management of chronic renal failure. *Postgraduate Medicine,* 64:135, Nov., 1978.
164. Koushanpour, E.: *Renal Physiology: Principles and Functions.* Philadelphia: W. B. Saunders Co., 1976.
165. Krassnitzky, O.: The use of frozen blood. *Dialysis and Transplant,* 6:18, Aug., 1977.
166. Kreel, L.: Computerized transverse axial tomography. *Nursing Times,* 72:17, June 24, 1976.
167. Kress, H.: Adaptation to chronic dialysis: A two-way street. *Nursing Digest,* 5:26, Spring, 1977.
168. Kroes, R., et al.: Long-term toxicity and reproductive study (including a teratogenicity study) with cyclamate, saccharin, and cyclohuylamine. *Toxicology,* 8:285, Dec., 1977.
169. Kumar, S., et al.: Intravesical formalin for the control of intractable bladder hemorrhage secondary to cystitis or cancer. *Journal of Urology,* 114:540, Oct., 1975.
170. Kussman, M., et al.: The clinical course of diabetic nephropathy. *Journal of the American Medical Association,* 236:1861, Oct. 18, 1976.
171. LaJoie, W., et al.: Electromyographic evaluation of human detrusor muscle activity in relation to abdominal muscle activity. *Archives of Physical Medicine and Rehabilitation,* 57:382, Aug., 1976.
172. Landes, R.: Urinary tract infection — More than a one-time thing. *Consultant* 15:32, Feb., 1975.
173. Landsman, M.: The patient with chronic renal failure: A marginal man. *Annals of Internal Medicine,* 82:268, Feb., 1975.
174. Lang, E.: Renal cyst puncture and aspiration: A survey of complications. *American Journal of Roentgenology,* 128:723, Apr., 1977.
175. Ladides, J.: *Fundamentals of Urology.* Philadelphia: W. B. Saunders Co., 1976.
176. Laver, M.: Acute urinary tract infections in women. *Consultant,* 16:230, Nov., 1976.
177. Lawson, S., and Cook, J.: Condom urinals. *Nursing Mirror,* 145:19, Dec. 1, 1977.
178. Leman, J.: Acute renal failure. *American Family Physician,* 18:146, Sept., 1978.
179. Lenaghan, D., et al.: The natural history of reflux and long-term effects of reflux on the kidney. *Journal of Urology,* 15:728, June, 1976.
180. Leste, G.: Nondialytic treatment of established acute renal failure. *Critical Care Quarterly,* 1:11, Sept., 1978.
181. Levy, S., et al.: Urinary kallikrein and plasma renin activity as determinants of renal blood flow: The influence of race and dietary sodium intake. *Journal of Clinical Investigation,* 60:129, July, 1977.
182. Lindeman, R.: Drug treatment of the chronic idiopathic glomerulopathies. *Postgraduate Medicine,* 62:135, Sept., 1977.
183. Linton, A.: Diagnosis and treatment of infections of the urinary tract. *Heart and Lung,* 5:607, July/Aug., 1976.
184. Litvak, A., et al.: A clinical evaluation of a screening device (Microstix) for urinary tract infections. *Southern Medical Journal,* 69:1418, Nov., 1976.
185. Llach, F.: Current status of amino acid and keto-acid diets in chronic renal failure. *Dialysis and Transplant,* 6:24, May, 1977.
186. Logan, D.: The female urethral syndrome. *Consultant,* 17:78, May, 1977.
187. Low, J.: Urethral behavior during the involuntary detrusor contraction. *American Journal of Obstetrics and Gynecology,* 128:32, May 1, 1977.
188. Lucas, C.: The renal response to acute injury and sepsis. *Surgical Clinics of North America,* 56:953, Aug., 1976.
189. Lundin, D.: Reporting urine test results: Switch from + to %. *American Journal of Nursing,* 78:878, May, 1978.

190. MacKinnon, K., et al.: The influence of position on urine transport. *Journal of Urology,* 109:631, Apr., 1973.
191. Mahar, J.: Principles of dialysis and dialysis of drugs. *American Journal of Medicine,* 62:475, Apr., 1977.
192. Mahurkar, S., et al.: Relationship of posture and age to urinary protein excretion. *British Medical Journal,* 1:712, Mar. 29, 1975.
193. Magnusson, M., and Stowe, N.: Controversy in organ preservation. *Urologic Clinics of North America,* 3:491, Oct., 1976.
194. Malgieri, J., et al.: The changing clinicopathological pattern of abscesses in or adjacent to the kidney. *Journal of Urology,* 118:230, Aug., 1977.
195. Mamdani, B., et al.: High-bolus urography: A superior technique in advanced renal failure. *Journal of the American Medical Association,* 234:1054, Dec. 8, 1975.
196. Maney, J.: A behavioral therapy approach to bladder training. *Nursing Clinics of North America,* 11:179, Mar., 1976.
197. Marchant, D.: Urinary incontinence in the female. *Hospital Medicine,* 13:60, Mar., 1977.
198. Marshall, S., et al.: Dark urine after hair coloring. *Journal of the American Medical Association,* 226:1010, Nov. 19, 1973.
199. Maude, D.: *Kidney Physiology and Kidney Disease: An Introduction to Nephrology.* Philadelphia: J. B. Lippincott Co., 1977.
200. May, H.: *Enterostomal Therapy.* New York: Raven Press, 1977.
201. McLeod, D., and Nahata, M.: Inefficacy of ascorbic acid as a urinary acidifier. *New England Journal of Medicine,* 296:1413, June 16, 1977.
202. McMillan, D.: Deterioration of the microcirculation in diabetes. *Diabetes,* 24:944, Oct., 1975.
203. McMurray, S., et al.: Iatrogenic factors in acute renal failure. *Postgraduate Medicine,* 63:85, May, 1978.
204. McNamara, R.: The bioinstrumentation of hemodialysis. *Nursing Clinics of North America,* 13:611, Dec., 1978.
205. McNay, J.: Pharmacology of the renal circulation. *American Journal of Medicine,* 62:507, Apr., 1977.
206. McPherson, B., et al.: Nursing in slush surgery. *American Operating Room Nurses Journal,* 25:227, Feb., 1977.
207. Meema, H., et al.: Arterial calcifications in severe chronic renal disease and their relationship to dialysis treatment, renal transplant and parathyroidectomy. *Radiology,* 121:315, Nov., 1976.
208. Melchior, H.: Urodynamics. *Urological Research,* 3:51, Aug., 1975.
209. Mendez, R.: Renal trauma. *Journal of Urology,* 118:698, Nov., 1977.
210. Menon, M., and Jeffs, R.: Structural incontinence. *Urologic Clinics of North America,* 5:175, Feb., 1978.
211. Merrill, R.: Review of vascular access. *Dialysis and Transplant,* 6:22, Dec., 1977.
212. Mieler, L.: Bladder cancer: Superiority of preoperative irradiation and cystectomy in clinical stages B2 and C. *Cancer,* 39:973, Feb., 1977.
213. Mitchell, J.: Axioms on uremia. *Hospital Medicine,* 14:6, July, 1978.
214. Mitchell, M., et al.: Ileal loop stenosis: A late complication of urinary diversion. *Journal of Urology,* 118:957, Dec., 1977.
215. Monnig, J., et al.: The ileal ureter in recurrent urolithiasis. *Journal of Urology,* 116:699, Dec., 1976.
216. Montie, J., et al.: Immunotherapy of disseminated renal cell carcinoma with transfer factor. *Journal of Urology,* 117:553, May, 1977.
217. Moolgaoker, A.: Management of stress incontinence in women. *Geriatrics,* 31:60, June, 1976.
218. Moore, D., and Bauer, C.: Effect of Prepodyne[R] as a perineal cleansing agent for clean catch specimens. *Nursing Research,* 25:259, July/Aug., 1976.
219. Moore, G.: Psychiatric aspects of chronic renal disease. *Postgraduate Medicine,* 60:140, Nov., 1976.
220. Moore, W., et al.: Estimation of glomerular filtration rate. *British Medical Journal,* 3:704, Sept. 20, 1975.
221. Moser, M.: Diagnosis and treatment of renal and renovascular hypertension. *Hospital Medicine,* 13:81, Nov., 1977.
222. Nelson, B.: A nursing approach to patients with long-term renal transplants: A practical application of nursing theory. *Nursing Clinics of North America,* 13:157, Mar., 1978.
223. Nemer, F., et al.: How to manage colovesical fistula. *Geriatrics,* 33:86, Oct., 1978.
224. Nickey, K.: An investigation of the urine pH of selected subjects on prescribed regimens of cranberry juice and ascorbic acid. Unpublished Masters Thesis, University of Washington, Seattle, Washington, 1973.
225. Nortman, D., and Coburn, J.: Renal osteodystrophy in end-stage renal failure. *Postgraduate Medicine,* 64:123, Nov., 1978.
226. Novak, D.: Selective renal occlusion phlebography with a balloon catheter. *British Journal of Radiology,* 49:589, July, 1976.
227. O'Brien, K., et al.: Long-term hemodialysis for patients over 50. *Geriatrics,* 31:55, Sept., 1976.
228. Oestreich, S.: Rational nursing care in chronic renal failure. *American Journal of Nursing,* 79:1096, June, 1979.
229. Olsson, C., and Krane, R.: Extracorporeal surgery: New route to greater kidney salvage. *RN,* 37:1, June, 1974.
230. O'Neill, M. (Ed.): Symposium on care of the patient with renal disease. *Nursing Clinics of North America,* 10:411, Sept., 1975.
231. Opelz, G., and Terasakis, P.: Blood transfusions in hemodialysis units: Yes or No? *Dialysis and Transplant,* 6:46, Nov., 1977.
232. Orikasa, S., et al.: Experience with non-sterile intermittent self-catheterization. *Journal of Urology,* 115:141, Feb., 1976.
233. Papper, S.: The effects of age in reducing renal function. *Geriatrics,* 28:83, May, 1973.
234. Parsons, V.: What decreasing renal function means to aging patient. *Geriatrics,* 32:93, Jan., 1977.
235. Pattison, A.: Treatment of bladder carcinoma using hydrostatic pressure therapy. *Nursing Times,* 72:249, Feb. 19, 1976.
236. Pedersen, J., et al.: Residual urine determination by ultrasonic scanning. *American Journal of Roentgenology Radium Therapeutic Nuclear Medicine,* 125:474, Oct., 1975.
237. Peirce, S., et al.: Slush technique in renal surgery. *American Operating Room Nurses Journal,* 25:223, Feb., 1977.
238. Perkash, I.: An attempt to understand and to treat voiding dysfunction during rehabilitation of the bladder in spinal cord injury patients. *Journal of Urology,* 115:36, Jan., 1976.
239. Perry, S.: Ureteral reimplantation for uretero-vesical

reflux in a pediatric patient. *Heart and Lung,* 6:297, Mar./Apr., 1977.

240. Persijin, G.: Effect of blood transfusions in renal transplantation. *Dialysis and Transplant,* 6:44, Dec., 1977.

241. Peters, P., and Bright, T.: Blunt renal injuries. *Urologic Clinics of North America,* 4:17, Feb., 1977.

242. Pinell, C.: Disorders of micturition in the elderly. *Nursing Times,* 71:2019, Dec. 18, 1975.

243. Platt, M.: Genetic aspects of renal disease: A survey of the various recognized forms. *Clinical Pediatrics,* 15:1024, Nov. 1976.

244. Plourde, M.: Reflections on urinary diversion. *American Operating Room Nurses Journal,* 23:45, Jan., 1976.

245. Poliak, V., et al.: Asymptomatic hematuria: Diagnostic approach. *Postgraduate Medicine,* 62:115, Sept., 1977.

246. Popovich, R., et al.: Continuous ambulatory peritoneal dialysis. *Annals of Internal Medicine,* 88:449, Apr., 1978.

247. Raff, M., et al.: Infectious diseases complicating renal transplantation: A survey and recommendations for prevention, recognition and management. *Southern Medical Journal,* 69:1603, Dec., 1976.

248. Ramming, K., et al.: Immune RNA therapy for renal cell carcinoma: Survival and immunologic monitoring. *Annals of Surgery,* 186:459, Oct., 1977.

249. Rao, M., et al.: Infusion pyelography in anuric patients. *Journal of Urology,* 116:297, Sept., 1976.

250. Raskin, M., et al.: Effect of intracystic pantopaque on renal cysts. *Journal of Urology,* 114:678, Nov., 1975.

251. Rathaus, M., and Bernheim, J.: Are your elderly patients good candidates for dialysis? *Geriatrics,* 33:56, Sept., 1978.

252. Ray, J., et al.: Surgical treatment of colovesical fistula: The value of a one-stage procedure. *Southern Medical Journal,* 69:40, Jan., 1976.

253. Reece, R., and Koontz, W.: Leukoplakia of the urinary tract: A review. *Journal of Urology,* 114:165, Aug., 1975.

254. Reed, R., et al.: Acute renal vein thrombosis with dextran treatment. *Journal of Urology,* 118:851, Nov., 1977.

255. Relief for frequent relapsers. *Emergency Medicine,* 10:167, Sept., 1978.

256. Renkin, E., and Robinson, R.: Glomerular filtration. *New England Journal of Medicine,* 290:785, Apr. 4, 1974.

257. Richard, C.: Nursing implications in prevention of complications in peritoneal dialysis. *Heart and Lung,* 4:890, Nov./Dec., 1975.

258. Richie, J., and Sacks, S.: Complications of urinary undiversion. *Journal of Urology,* 117:362, Mar., 1977.

259. Roberts, A.: Systems of life, ureters and bladder. *Nursing Times,* 72: center pages, Dec. 2, 1976.

260. Rodman, M., and Smith, D.: *Clinical Pharmacology in Nursing.* Philadelphia: J. B. Lippincott Co., 1979.

261. Ronald, A., et al.: Bacteriuria localization and response to single-dose therapy in women. *Journal of the American Medical Association,* 235:1854, Apr. 26, 1976.

262. Rosenberg, I.: Renal hemodynamic effects of sepsis. *Heart and Lung,* 5:777, Sept./Oct., 1976.

263. Rowe, J., et al.: The effect of age on creatinine clearance in men: A cross-sectional and longitudinal study. *Journal of Gerontology,* 31:155, Mar., 1976.

264. Rowlands, D., et al.: The pathology of renal homograft rejection: A review. *American Journal of Pathology,* 85:773, Dec., 1976.

265. Sanjad, S., et al.: Acute glomerulonephritis in children: A review of 153 cases. *Southern Medical Journal,* 70:1202, Oct., 1977.

266. Santopietro, M.: Meeting the emotional needs of hemodialysis patients and their spouses. *American Journal of Nursing,* 75:629, Apr., 1975.

267. Say, C., and Hori, J.: Malignant tumors of the kidney. *Hospital Medicine,* 13:46, Aug., 1977.

268. Schaner, E., et al.: Computed tomography in the diagnosis of subcapsular and perirenal hematoma. *American Journal of Roentgenology,* 129:83, July, 1977.

269. Scharf, J., et al.: Carcinoma of the bladder with azothioprine therapy. *Journal of the American Medical Association,* 237:152, Jan. 10, 1977.

270. Schlegel, J., and Hamway, S.: Individual renal plasma flow determination in 2 minutes. *Journal of Urology,* 116:282, Sept., 1976.

271. Schoenberg, B., et al.: Micturition syncope — Not a single entity. *Journal of the American Medical Association,* 229:1631, Sept. 16, 1974.

272. Schulman, C., et al.: New concepts of ureterovesical innervation. *Journal of Urology,* 109:381, Mar., 1973.

273. Schumann, D.: The renal donor. *American Journal of Nursing,* 74:105, Jan., 1974.

274. Schumann, D.: Tips for improving urine testing techniques. *Nursing '76,* 6:23, Feb., 1976.

275. Schumann, G., et al.: An improved technic for examining urinary casts and a review of their significance. *American Journal of Clinical Pathology,* 69:18, Jan., 1978.

276. Shapiro, S., et al.: Catheter-associated UTIs: Incidence and a new approach to prevention. *Journal of Urology,* 112:659, Nov., 1974.

277. Shapiro, S., et al.: Fate of 90 children with ileal conduit urinary diversion a decade later: Analysis of complications, pyelography, renal function and bacteriology. *Journal of Urology,* 114:289, Aug., 1975.

278. Sherwood, T.: Radiology now: Dynamic bladder studies. *British Journal of Radiology,* 49:977, Dec., 1976.

279. Sherwood, T.: Renal masses and ultrasound. *British Medical Journal,* 4:682, Dec. 20, 1975.

280. Shinaberger, J., and Blumenkrantz, M.: Dialysis therapy and transplantation in uremia: Which to use when. *Postgraduate Medicine,* 64:169, Nov., 1978.

281. Shipley, S., and Wrye, S.: Myoglobinuria. *Heart and Lung,* 5:950, Nov./Dec., 1976.

282. Silber, S.: Renal trauma: Treatment by angiographic injection of autologous clot. *Archives of Surgery,* 110:206, Feb., 1975.

283. Simon, H., et al.: Genitourinary tuberculosis: Clinical features in a general hospital population. *American Journal of Medicine,* 63:410, Sept., 1977.

284. Simon, N., et al.: Chronic renal failure: Pathophysiology and medical management. *Cardiovascular Nurse,* 12:7, Mar./Apr., 1976.

285. Simonds, J.: Enuresis: A brief survey of current thinking with respect to pathogenesis and management. *Clinical Pediatrics,* 16:79, Jan., 1977.

286. Smith, D.: *General Urology.* Los Altos: Lange Medical Publications, 1975.

287. Smith, E., and Bennett, A.: The usefulness of ultrasound in the evaluation of renal masses in adults. *Journal of Urology,* 113:525, Apr., 1975.

288. Smith, E., and Freedman, P.: Dialysis: Current status and future. *Heart and Lung,* 4:879, Nov./Dec., 1975.

289. Smith, L., et al.: Nutrition and urolithiasis. *New England Journal of Medicine,* 298:87, Jan. 12, 1978.

290. Smith, R., and Ehrlich, R.: The surgical complications of renal transplantation. *Urologic Clinics of North America,* 3:621, Oct., 1976.

291. Smith, S.: Concepts in renal transplantation. *Critical Care Quarterly,* 1:53, Sept., 1978.

292. Sperling, K.: Intermittent catheterization to obtain catheter-free bladder function in spinal cord injury. *Archives of Physical Medicine and Rehabilitation,* 59:4, Jan., 1978.

293. Stadalnik, R., et al.: Electrocardiographic response to intravenous urography: Prospective evaluation of

275 patients. *American Journal of Roentgenology,* 129:825, Nov., 1977.

294. Stamm, W.: Guidelines for prevention of catheter-associated UTIs. *Annals of Internal Medicine,* 82:386, Mar., 1975.
295. Steele, B., et al.: Interpretation of renal function tests. *Geriatrics,* 29:63, Jan., 1974.
296. Sternberg, J., et al.: Combination chemotherapy (CISCA) for advanced urinary tract carcinoma: A preliminary report. *Journal of the American Medical Association,* 238:2282, Nov. 21, 1977.
297. Stone, W.: Vitamin supplementation of hemodialyzed patients. *Dialysis and Transplant,* 6:51, June, 1977.
298. Streltzer, J., et al.: The spouse's role in home dialysis. *Archives of General Psychiatry,* 33:55, Jan., 1976.
299. Sturdy, D.: *Essentials of Urology.* Bristol: John Wright and Sons, Limited, 1974.
300. Swendseld, M.: Nutritional needs of patients with renal disease. *Journal of the American Dietetic Association,* 70:488, May, 1977.
301. Szwed, J.: Pathophysiology of acute renal failure: Rationale for signs and symptoms. *Critical Care Quarterly,* 1:1, Sept., 1978.
302. Takazakura, E., et al.: Onset and progression of diabetic glomerulosclerosis: A prospective study based on serial renal biopsies. *Diabetes,* 24:1, Jan., 1975.
303. Teitlbaum, S., et al.: Calcifediol in chronic renal insufficiency: Skeletal response. *Journal of the American Medical Association,* 235:164, Jan. 12, 1976.
304. Tenckhoff, H.: *Chronic Peritoneal Dialysis.* Seattle: University of Washington, 1974.
305. The hematuria of the long-distance runner. *Emergency Medicine* 10:84, May, 1978.
306. Thomas, W.: *Renal Calculi: A Guide to Management.* Springfield, Ill.: Charles C Thomas, Publisher, 1976.
307. Thompson, I.: Expectant management of blunt renal trauma. *Urologic Clinics of North America,* 4:29, Feb., 1977.
308. Thornbury, J., et al.: Effect of gravity on ureteral peristalsis in normal human adults in the inverted position. *Journal of Urology,* 3:465, Apr., 1974.
309. Tilkian, S., and Conover, M.: *Clinical Implications of Laboratory Tests.* St. Louis: C. V. Mosby Co., 1975.
310. Torrens, M., and Griffith, H.: Management of the uninhibited bladder by selective sacral neurectomy. *Journal of Neurosurgery,* 44:176, Feb., 1976.
311. Trew, P., et al.: Renal vein thrombosis in membranous glomerulonephropathy: Incidence and association. *Medicine,* 57:69, Jan., 1978.
312. Truesdale, B., et al.: Perinephric abscess: A review of 26 cases. *Journal of Urology,* 118:910, Dec., 1977.
313. Turcotte, J., et al.: Adjuvant immunosuppression in renal transplantation. *Urologic Clinics of North America,* 3:597, Oct., 1976.
314. Types of neurogenic bladder dysfunction. *Hospital Medicine,* 13:86, July, 1977.
315. Vaamonde, C.: Peritoneal dialysis: Current status. *Postgraduate Medicine,* 62:148, Sept., 1977.
316. Venkateswara, K., et al.: Thromboembolic disease in renal allograft recipients: What is its clinical significance? *Archives of Surgery,* 111:1086, Oct., 1976.
317. Visel, J.: Clinical aspects of renal biopsy. *Heart and Lung,* 4:900, Nov./Dec., 1975.
318. Vogel, C.: Keeping patients alive in spite of postoperative obstructive diuresis. *Nursing '79,* 9:50, Mar., 1979.
319. Vosti, K.: Recurrent urinary tract infections: Prevention by prophylactic antibiotics after sexual intercourse. *Journal of the American Medical Association,* 231:934, Mar. 3, 1975.
320. Wagoner, R.: Analgesic nephropathy — A continuing problem. *Postgraduate Medicine,* 60:50, Dec., 1976.
321. Wajsman, Z., et al.: Evaluation of biological markers in bladder cancer. *Journal of Urology,* 114:879, Dec., 1975.
322. Wallace, D.: The evolution of the cystoscope. *Nursing Mirror,* 141:60, July 17, 1975.
323. Walser, D.: Behavioral effects of dialysis. *Canadian Nurse,* 70:23, May, 1974.
324. Wear, J.: Solving selected problems of the aging urinary tract. *Postgraduate Medicine,* 58:179, Nov., 1975.
325. Wheldon, D., and Slack, M.: Multiplication of contaminant bacteria in urine and interpretation of delayed culture. *Journal of Clinical Pathology,* 30:615, July, 1977.
326. Whitmore, W.: Bladder cancer. *CA* — A Cancer Journal for Clinicians, 28:170, May/June, 1978.
327. Whyte, J., and Thistle, N.: Male incontinence: The inside story of external collection. *Nursing '76,* 6:66, Sept., 1976.
328. Widmann, F.: *Clinical Interpretation of Laboratory Tests.* Philadelphia: F. A. Davis Co., 1973.
329. Williams, D., and Chisholm, G.: *Scientific Foundations of Urology.* Volumes I and II, Chicago: Wm. Heinemann Medical Books, Limited, 1976.
330. Williams, S.: Diabetic urine testing by hospital nursing personnel. *Nursing Research,* 20:444, Sept./Oct., 1971.
331. Willington, F.: *Incontinence in the Elderly.* London: Academic Press, 1976.
332. Wilson, M.: Bladder training for the chronically ill. *RN,* 38:36, June, 1975.
333. Winter, C.: Rapid miniaturized tests for bacteriuria: Microstix and Bactercult urine tests. *Journal of Urology,* 114:755, Nov., 1975.
334. Winter, C., and Morel, A.: *Nursing Care of Patients with Urologic Diseases.* St. Louis: C. V. Mosby Co., 1977.
335. Wintrobe, M. (Ed.): *Principles of Internal Medicine.* New York: McGraw-Hill Company, 1974.
336. Witten, D., et al.: Acute reactions to urographic contrast medium: Incidence, clinical characteristics and relationship to history of hypersensitivity states. *American Journal of Roentgenology Radium Therapeutic Nuclear Medicine,* 119:832, Dec., 1973.
337. Wollam, G., et al.: The kidney as a target organ in hypertension. *Geriatrics,* 31:71, Aug., 1976.
338. Wood, R.: Catheterizing the patient with an ileal conduit stoma. *American Journal of Nursing,* 76:1592, Oct., 1976.
339. Woodrow, M., et al., Suprapubic catheters — A direct line to better drainage. *Nursing '76,* 6:40, Oct., 1976.
340. Wynder, E., et al.: The epidemiology of bladder cancer: A second look. *Cancer,* 40:1246, Sept., 1977.
341. X-rays in focus: The IVP in renal disease. *Nursing Times,* 73:17, May 19, 1977.
342. Yagoda, A., et al.: Adriamycin in advanced urinary tract cancer: Experience in 42 patients and review of the literature. *Cancer,* 39:279, Jan., 1977.
343. Yu, T.: Nephrolithiasis in patients with gout. *Postgraduate Medicine,* 63:164, May, 1978.
344. Zanchetti, A.: Neural regulation of renin release: Experimental evidence and clinical implications in arterial hypertension. *Circulation,* 56:691, Nov., 1977.
345. Zingg, E., and Tscholl, R.: Continent cecoileal conduit: Preliminary report. *Journal of Urology,* 118:724, Nov., 1977.
346. Zrubecky, G.: Intermittent catheterization with unsterile instruments. *Paraplegia,* 11:179, Aug., 1973.

UNIT XIV*

NURSING PEOPLE EXPERIENCING DISTURBANCES OF THE BLOOD AND BLOOD-FORMING ORGANS

INTRODUCTION AND STUDY GUIDE

Blood is part of the inner sea of body fluid that bathes, nourishes, and oxygenates every one of our cells and tissues. In addition, the blood carries cells and other substances that both protect the body from invading microorganisms and stop bleeding by inducing coagulation of the blood upon injury to a vessel. It is not surprising, then, that blood disorders affect any or all organs of the body and that the three problems basic to blood disease are *tissue hypoxia, susceptibility to infection,* and *hemorrhage.*

Because the manifestations of blood diseases are widespread and the causes are multiple, the nursing of patients with hematologic disorders is demanding and complex. The nurse must be knowledgeable in many diverse areas in order to give competent care.

1. A knowledge of the *anatomy* and *physiology* of the hematologic system is needed to understand the numerous laboratory studies presented in this unit, the symptoms of different blood dyscrasias (a special term often used for blood disorders), and many of the therapies.

2. A review of *immune* and *autoimmune responses* (see Chapter 11) is necessary, because certain blood conditions are the result of antigen-antibody reactions.

3. Because some blood disorders are caused by deficiency states, principles of *nutrition* should be reviewed, including the roles of vitamins and iron in blood production.

4. A precise understanding of *drug action* is needed, because many blood disorders are caused by drug toxicity. For instance, myelotoxins (drugs that damage bone marrow) cause the pancytopenia of bone marrow failure; administration of oxidizing agents to persons with certain enzyme deficiencies causes hemolytic anemia; and other drugs can precipitate antigen-antibody reactions. It is important to learn which drugs fall into these three categories and to be aware of early clinical and laboratory indications of drug toxicity.

5. Hematologic nursing includes *cancer* nursing. Many diseases discussed in this unit are caused by malignant changes within the blood-forming organs, e.g., the leukemias, Hodgkin's disease, multiple myeloma, and possibly polycythemia vera. Consequently, a careful review of Unit IX is important (especially the sections on the psychologic impact of cancer, cancer chemotherapy, irradiation of tumor masses, radioisotope therapy, and general nursing care).

6. The theories and practices underlying blood transfusions are not

*Phyllis Coindreau Patterson, R.N., M.S., critically reviewed and acted as a consultant for this unit.

presented in this unit. Consequently, it is necessary for the student to review the chapter on administration of blood transfusions in Sorensen and Luckmann, *Basic Nursing: A Psychophysiologic Approach,* or in a similar source.

7. Some knowledge of *genetics* is necessary to educate and counsel patients with genetically transmitted blood disorders, e.g., sickle cell anemia, the thalassemias, and hemophilia.

8. It is necessary to be aware that patients with blood dyscrasias often have *psychologic problems* related to their disease because of prolonged pain and other discomforts. Most hematologic disorders are chronic in nature and some (particularly those that are malignant) are ultimately fatal. To help patients deal with the acute and chronic stresses that accompany many hematologic disorders, reconsider carefully Chapter 6 — Responses to Stress-Producing Factors — and apply principles of stress reduction when planning patient care.

Upon completion of this unit, you should be able to apply the knowledge obtained to patient care in the following ways:

- ▶ Assess, evaluate, and report the general signs and symptoms of blood disorders.
- ▶ Assist in the safe administration of blood transfusions and blood component therapy.
- ▶ Develop a teaching program (with the aid of the dietician) that will educate persons who are particularly susceptible to the development of anemia in the principles of good nutrition.
- ▶ Be aware of the susceptibility of patients with certain blood dyscrasias (e.g., aplastic anemia, leukemia) to the development of life-threatening infections and take appropriate precautions.
- ▶ Guard all patients with bleeding disorders from trauma; observe for signs of bleeding and hemorrhage and take appropriate action.
- ▶ Assist patients in overcoming the anxiety and depression that accompany many of the more serious and chronic blood disorders.

Study Guide

1. As you read this unit, familiarize yourself with the following terms and concepts:

blood
plasma
hematocrit
differential blood count
blood dyscrasia
blood component therapy
tissue typing
splenomegaly
blood film
bone marrow transplant
petechiae
ecchymosis
occult bleeding
erythrocyte
erythropoiesis
hematopoiesis
hemoglobin
anemia
polycythemia
iron combining capacity
positive iron balance
extrinsic factor
intrinisic factor
leukocyte
leukopenia
agranulocytosis
leukocytosis
thrombocyte
thrombocytopenia
pancytopenia
myelotoxin
enzymopathy
hemolysis
hemolytic crisis
plumbism
hapten
dominant and recessive traits
heterozygous
homozygous
hemostatic mechanism
fibrinolysis
hematoma
hemarthrosis

2. Acquaint yourself with the actions and untoward effects of the following drug groups: oral and parenteral iron preparations, vitamin B_{12} and folic acid preparations, vitamin K preparations, chelating agents, myelosuppressant agents, alkylating agents, corticosteroids, MOPP combination chemotherapy, and anticoagulants.

3. Be aware of the nurse's responsibilities to the patient prior to and during the following special procedures: bone marrow aspiration and biopsy, fecal and urinary urobilinogen tests, Schilling test (see pernicious anemia), blood administration, reverse isolation, venesection (see polycythemia vera), sodium cyanate therapy (see sickle cell anemia), splenectomy, x-ray therapy, radioisotope therapy, platelet transfusions (see leukemia), and cancer immunotherapy (see Chapter 23).

CHAPTER 44

INTRODUCTORY CONCEPTS

REVIEW OF THE ANATOMY AND PHYSIOLOGY OF THE HEMATOPOIETIC SYSTEM

Blood: Definition, Functions, Characteristics, and Formation

Chapter 12 stated that the total body water (TBW) is divided into intracellular fluid and extracellular fluid. The extracellular fluid (ECF), in turn, is divided into *interstitial fluid* and *plasma.* Interstitial fluid occupies the intercellular spaces, whereas plasma occupies the vascular space. *Blood* is a mixture of cells (red blood cells, white blood cells, platelets) and plasma.

Blood circulates continuously through the heart and vascular system. As the blood is propelled through the body by the heart's pumping action, it performs many vital functions: It transports oxygen to the cells and carries carbon dioxide from the cells to the lungs for removal from the body. The blood also carries absorbed food products from the gastrointestinal tract to the tissues; at the same time, it removes metabolic wastes from tissues and carries them to the kidney, skin, and lungs for excretion. In addition, various hormones are carried by the blood from the endocrine glands (where they originate) to other parts of the body. Also, the blood protects the body from dangerous microorganisms by carrying leukocytes and antibodies to the site of infection, injury, or inflammation. Finally, the blood is instrumental in regulating body temperature by transferring heat from within the body to the small vessels supplying the skin, from which it can be released into the surrounding atmosphere.

Major characteristics of blood are as follows:

- *Color: Arterial* blood is bright red, owing to the mixture of oxygen with hemoglobin within the red blood cells. *Venous* blood is dark red because of loss of oxygen from the reduced hemoglobin.
- *Viscosity:* Blood is three to four times more viscous than water.
- *Reaction:* Blood has a slightly salty taste and a slightly alkaline reaction of pH 7.35 to 7.45.
- *Volume:* An adult has approximately 70 to 75 ml. of blood per kg. of body weight; thus, the average adult body contains around 5 to 6 liters of blood.

The organs involved in the formation of blood and its constituent cellular elements are the bone marrow, spleen, liver, and lymph nodes. Cells produced by these organs include erythrocytes, leukocytes, thrombocytes, plasma cells, and reticuloendothelial cells.

Blood Composition. Blood is composed of plasma, which makes up 55 per cent of the blood; and solid suspended particles (blood cells and thrombocytes), which comprise the other 45 per cent of the blood. The *hematocrit* (Hct) is the term used to describe the percentage of blood that is cellular.

Plasma, the liquid portion of the blood, is a straw-colored watery substance composed of:

- 92 per cent water.
- 7 per cent proteins, which include (1) serum albumin, $alpha_1$ globulin, $alpha_2$ globulin, beta globulin, and gamma globulin — all necessary for exerting colloidal osmotic pressure. (See Chapter 12.) The gamma globulin fraction also contains the immunoglobulins (antibodies) IgM, IgG, IgA, IgD, and IgE, which are essential in the body's defense against microorganisms. (See Chapter 11.) (2) Fibrinogen and prothrombin, which are essential for blood coagulation.
- Less than 1 per cent antibodies, nutrients, metabolic wastes, respiratory gases, enzymes, hormones, other clotting factors, and inorganic salts.

The major *function* of plasma is the maintenance of blood volume within the vascular compartment.

Blood cells are thought to be derived from "one pluripotential 'stem' cell, which goes through a series of divisions and maturation changes to result in the mature cells found in the circulating blood."[108] This entire mechanism is not well understood. Figure 44–1 is a representation of the stem cell divisions resulting in the development of mature cells.

The *particles* that travel suspended in the plasma include erythrocytes (red blood cells), leukocytes (white blood cells), and thrombocytes (platelets). Erythrocytes are principally involved in oxygen transport; leukocytes, in the defense of the body against microorganisms; and thrombocytes, in hemostasis.

In the adult the *bone marrow stem cell* gives rise to all the cellular elements in blood; that is, to erythrocytes, leukocytes (granulocytes, monocytes, and lymphocytes), plasma cells, and megakaryocytes which evolve into platelets. Recall from Chapter 11 that further differentiation of lymphocytes occurs in the thymus, where they become *T-lymphocytes* responsible for *cellular* immunity. The *B-lymphocyte* is differentiated, at a site unknown, to a plasma cell which produces *humoral immunity.* The plasma cell produces the circulating antibodies IgM, IgA, IgG, IgE, and IgD. B-lymphocytes and T-lymphocytes are found in the lymphoid tissue of the body, the spleen, the liver, and the bone marrow. These organs also contain fixed and migratory macrophages, which act as the reticuloendothelial system to phagocytize foreign invaders and red blood cells. (See Chapter 10.) The spleen is particularly active in the destruction of red blood cells. Each of the cellular elements of the blood is discussed in more detail throughout this unit.

OVERVIEW OF ABNORMALITIES OF THE BLOOD AND BLOOD-FORMING ORGANS

Disorders of the blood and blood-forming organs are usually divided into diseases primarily involving: (1) erythrocytes, (2) leukocytes, (3) platelets, (4) reticuloendothelial cells, and (5) clotting mechanisms.

The four basic physiologic disturbances characterizing hematopoietic disorders are as follows:

Decrease in Number of Cells (Cytopenia). When erythrocytes decrease, the result is *anemia,* a condition characterized by a reduction in the oxygen-carrying capacity of the blood. A *decrease* in leukocytes is termed *leukopenia,* while a reduction in granulocytes (one category of leukocyte) is called *granulocytopenia.* Patients with leukopenia have a greatly increased vulnerability to *infection.* Finally, a decrease in the *thrombocyte* or platelet count is called *thrombocytopenia.* Hallmarks of thrombocytopenia are: easy bruising, petechiae, and a tendency to bleed readily from the gums, perirectal area, and gastrointestinal tract.

Overproduction of Either Normal or Defective Cells. An abnormal increase in erythrocyte production is called *polycythemia;* an increase in the manufacture of abnormal, immature *leukocytes* is termed *leukemia;* the abnormal malignant proliferation of plasma cells results in a condition called *plasma cell myeloma* or *multiple myeloma.* These conditions (polycythemia, myelogenous and monocytic leukemia, and plasma cell myeloma) are usually classified as *myeloproliferative diseases* because the malignant overproduction of cells takes place within the *bone marrow.*

When cellular overproduction occurs within the *lymphatic tissues,* the resulting conditions are classified as *lymphoproliferative disorders.* Examples include: (1) Hodgkin's disease (the malignant proliferation of one form of reticuloendothelial cell within the lymph nodes); (2) lymphocytic leukemia (overproduction of lymphocytes within the lymph nodes which are released into the blood; and (3) lymphosarcoma (the abnormal proliferation of lymphocytes or lymphoblasts within the lymph nodes).

Defects in Coagulation Mechanism. This is caused by *depletion* or *absence* of one or more *clotting* factors. This group of disorders, which is characterized by persistent bleeding and hemorrhage, includes the hemophilias, hypoprothrombinemia, and disseminated intravascular coagulation.

Disorders of the Spleen. These include *enlargement of the spleen* (splenomegaly), which occurs in association with numerous blood dyscrasias. Another disorder of the spleen is a clinical syndrome termed "hypersplenism." This syndrome arises from "the overactivity or exaggeration of one or more of the spleen's functions."[73] It is characterized by peripheral blood cytopenia and may involve erythrocytes, granulocytes, thrombocytes, or any combination of the three.

General *causative factors that can result in disorders of the hematopoietic system* include: hemorrhage, dietary deficiencies, malabsorptive disorders, infection, toxicity of drugs, malignant overproduction of cells, increased destruction of cells by an overactive spleen, genetic predisposition to faulty blood cell production, immunologic defects, and metabolic disturbances. In

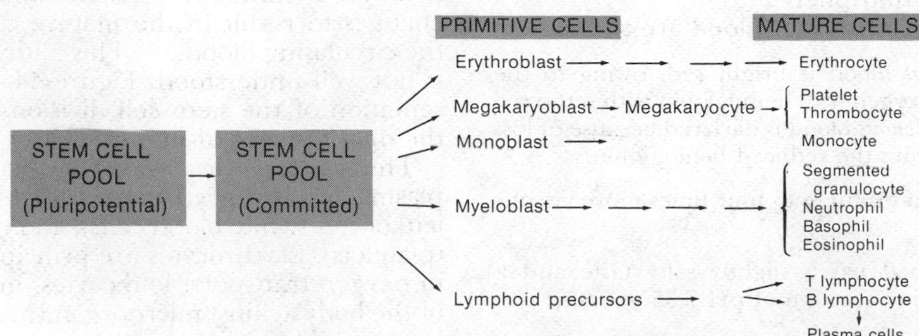

Figure 44–1. Theory of formation of blood cells: ⟶ indicates that maturation steps are occurring. (From Schumann, D., and P. C. Patterson: The adult with acute leukemia. *Nursing Clinics of North America,* 7(4):743, Dec. 1972.)

addition, a large number of blood disorders result from unknown (idiopathic) causes.

GENERAL PROBLEMS AFFECTING PATIENTS WITH HEMATOPOIETIC DISORDERS

As we have said, any disorder of the blood or blood-forming organs may adversely affect all organs and tissues; as a result, the major manifestations of blood disease are diffuse. Signs and symptoms that characterize the majority of blood dyscrasias and their underlying bases are shown in Table 44–1.

OVERVIEW OF DIAGNOSTIC TESTS AND THERAPEUTIC MEASURES

Blood disorders are primarily diagnosed in the laboratory. Although dozens of specific laboratory tests are used to diagnose individual disorders, the three major tests that are performed in all cases are: (1) complete blood count and differential to determine the number of erythrocytes and leukocytes as well as the percentage of the different types of leukocytes; (2) bone marrow biopsy; and (3) the blood film, i.e., a study of the morphology of blood cells within a peripheral blood smear.

Specific *clinical care* for patients with blood dyscrasias may involve either specific curative measures or palliative measures that relieve symptoms and prolong life. There are several general medical and nursing care measures that are used to treat the majority of patients with blood disorders. *Bed rest* is usually prescribed for persons suffering from severe anemias, hemorrhage, or bleeding diseases. Rest counteracts the fatigue and weakness caused by the blood's decreased oxygen-carrying capacity. To help *maintain muscle tone,* the patient who is confined to bed should be encouraged and assisted with passive, isotonic exercises. The *diet* in blood dyscrasias should be high in protein, iron, and vitamins. *Drug* administration is one of the nurse's responsibilities. Iron salts and vitamins B_{12} and K are given to correct deficiency states. Cancer chemotherapeutic agents are used to suppress the malignant proliferation of blood cells and reticuloendothelial cells. *Irradiation* and *radioisotope* therapy also play a vital role in the control of both myeloproliferative and lymphoproliferative disorders. *Reverse isolation* is a commonly employed procedure for patients with leukemia or with leukopenia from any cause. Isolation is needed to protect the patient with few mature, functioning leukocytes and a compromised immune system from being over-

TABLE 44–1. SIGNS AND SYMPTOMS CHARACTERISTIC OF BLOOD DYSCRASIAS

Signs and Symptoms	Bases
Chronic fatigue and dyspnea	Decrease in erythrocytes (anemias, leukemias, and hemorrhagic disorders) causes a reduction in the oxygen-carrying capacity of the blood.
Increased susceptibility to infection	Decrease in mature circulating leukocytes (leukemia, leukopenia, and lymphoma) decreases the number of cells available to combat invading microorganisms and produce antibodies.
Gastrointestinal symptoms (anorexia, weight loss, indigestion, sore mouth and tongue)	Decrease in gastric secretions (as seen in pernicious anemia); abnormal changes in mucous membrane cells; and the effects of certain drugs and extreme fatigue all contribute to the lack of desire or inability to eat.
Hemorrhage and bleeding into tissues and joints (hemarthrosis) and from mucous membranes	Hemorrhage results either from a decrease in the platelet count (as a result of drugs, infections, or autoimmune causes) or from absence of one or more clotting factors.
Bone pain and deformity	Hyperactivity of bone marrow (seen in myeloproliferative disorders) and pathological fractures (seen in multiple myeloma) both produce bone pain and deformity.
Jaundice (yellow discoloring of the skin and sclerae)	Rupture and hemolysis of abnormal erythrocytes (characteristic of hemolytic anemias and pernicious anemia) cause release of large amounts of bilirubin into the circulation, resulting in yellowing of the skin.
Enlarged liver and spleen and hyperplasia of bone marrow	Caused by either: (1) congestion from overproduction of cells (e.g., polycythemia, leukemia, etc.) or (2) excessive demands upon these organs to destroy defective cells (e.g., hemolytic anemias).
Mental depression	Chronic depression results from the chronicity of most blood diseases and the fatigue and discomfort characteristic of these disorders.

whelmed by infection. *Special mouth care* is needed for patients with blood dyscrasias because bleeding from the teeth and gums is extremely common. Special care for the perirectal area is important because of susceptibility to breakdown, bleeding, and infection: proper, early care could prevent an abscess or fistula.

Operations performed upon patients with hematopoietic diseases include: (1) *staging laparotomy,* as deemed necessary for the lymphoma population; (2) *surgical excision of tumor masses* (performed in lymphosarcoma); and (3) *splenectomies* for hypersplenism, hemolytic and hemorrhagic disorders, and to relieve symptoms in chronic lymphocytic leukemia and Hodgkin's disease.

Infections are treated with conventional therapy. Gamma globulin and granulocytes may be used as necessary.

Blood component therapy is used to replace specific deficient elements in the blood. For example, patients with hemophilias need cryoprecipitate or concentrates of factor VIII or IX. Disseminated intravascular coagulation may require fresh plasma, platelets, or both. The different cytopenias need replacement of only the depleted cell: erythrocytes, granulocytes, or thrombocytes (platelets).

Obviously, *blood transfusions* are a vital part of the therapy for many of the blood dyscrasias. As we stated in the study guide, the principles, techniques, and complications associated with blood transfusions are presented in detail in Sorensen and Luckmann, *Basic Nursing: A Psychophysiologic Approach.* We advise the student to carefully consider the questions concerning blood transfusions in the study guide and to review an appropriate basic nursing text.

CHAPTER 45

NURSING PERSONS WITH DISORDERS PRIMARILY AFFECTING THE ERYTHROCYTES

THE NORMAL ERYTHROCYTE

Review of Anatomy and Physiology

The word *erythrocyte* is taken from the Greek terms *erythros* (red) and *kykos* (cell). Other terms used interchangeably with erythrocyte are "red blood cell" (RBC) and "red blood corpuscle," a phrase which means "little red body."

Red blood corpuscles are composed of two principal parts: (1) the supporting stroma and encircling membrane, which are responsible for approximately 2 to 5 per cent of the red cell's weight; and (2) the conjugated protein called *hemoglobin,* which is responsible for approximately 95 per cent of the red cell's mass.

Erythrocytes, along with leukocytes and thrombocytes, travel throughout the body as suspended particles in a river of plasma. As you recall, erythrocytes greatly outnumber both leukocytes and thrombocytes; thus, in a cubic millimeter of blood there are approximately 5 million erythrocytes, 250 thousand thrombocytes, and only 8 thousand leukocytes. In an adult human body, the total number of circulating erythrocytes approaches the fantastic sum of 35 trillion cells. Erythrocytes have a diameter that ranges between 6 and 9 μ, with 7.7 μ as an average. One micron is equivalent to one thousandth of a millimeter or 1/25,000 of an inch.

The *functions* of erythrocytes are threefold: the transport of oxygen from the lungs to the tissues and carbon dioxide from the tissues to the lungs, the promotion of normal hydrogen ion balance, and the maintenance of blood viscosity.

The *structure* of a red blood cell is admirably designed to enable it to carry out its most important function — oxygen and carbon dioxide transport. Normal erythrocytes, microscopic in size, are shaped like biconcave discs with rather thin centers and thicker outer edges. Such a shape gives the red cell two advantages: First, its biconcave shape provides a relatively *large surface area* for the efficient, rapid absorption and release of oxygen and carbon dioxide. Second, the biconcave discs have great *flexibility* and *elasticity,* which enable them to adapt their shapes to the diameter of the various blood vessels through which they circulate.

As discussed later, it is disastrous when disease causes erythrocytes to lose this biconcave shape and become spherical, elongated, or crescent-shaped. Abnormally shaped erythrocytes cannot carry the blood gases efficiently. Furthermore, these cellular anomalies are easily broken and fragmented as they travel through the smaller vessels; eventually these fragments jam together within the capillaries, thus blocking circulation to the tissues.

STRUCTURE AND FUNCTION OF HEMOGLOBIN

Hemoglobin, the major constituent of the red blood cell, is composed of a simple protein called *globin* and a red-colored compound called *heme.* Heme is a complex molecule containing iron and the red pigment porphyrin, which gives blood its color. There are approximately 200 to 300 million molecules of hemoglobin within each erythrocyte.

The most important characteristic of hemoglobin is its ability to *combine chemically* with oxygen in a loose and easily reversed connection. The compound that results from the union of oxygen and hemoglobin is called *oxyhemoglobin.*

Oxyhemoglobin, which causes arterial blood to be bright red, is formed as the red blood corpuscles pass through the alveoli of the lungs. As the blood leaves the capillaries of the lungs and passes into the arteries, oxyhemoglobin releases its oxygen, which diffuses out of the blood vessels into the tissue fluid where it satisfies the oxygen requirements of cells and tissues.

Once hemoglobin loses its oxygen, it is called *reduced hemoglobin.* Because venous blood contains reduced hemoglobin, it is dark red in color.

In addition to combining with oxygen, hemoglobin also combines with *carbon dioxide.* As carbon dioxide is released from the body's cells, it diffuses into the tissue fluid and then into the blood where it is picked up and carried by hemoglobin to the lung capillaries. In the lungs, carbon dioxide separates from hemoglobin and diffuses into the alveoli; from there it is exhaled into the atmosphere.

The third gas with which hemoglobin readily combines is *carbon monoxide.* When hemoglobin is combined with carbon monoxide, it is no longer able to transport oxygen to cells and tissues. Consequently the major pathologic alteration occurring in carbon monoxide poisoning is *tissue hypoxia.* The most common cause of carbon monoxide poisoning is inhalation within a closed area of fumes from auto exhaust systems, sewers, and gas or oil heaters. The victim of carbon monoxide poisoning may die from asphyxiation; if the person lives, permanent brain damage may remain.

The numerous forms of hemoglobin, and the disorders affecting hemoglobin production, are discussed later in this chapter.

ERYTHROCYTE PRODUCTION AND STORAGE

During infancy *erythropoiesis* (i.e., red blood cell production) takes place within the marrow of both the long and short bones of the body. However, as the young child develops into an adult, the marrow of the long bones is replaced by fatty tissue. Consequently, in adulthood, erythropoiesis occurs only in the proximal ends of the femora and humeri and in the bones that form the ribs, sternum, skull, vertebrae, hands, and feet.

The bone marrow produces approximately 200 billion erythrocytes daily. Normal red blood cell production depends basically upon three factors: (1) the presence of normal genetic precursors for erythrocyte formation; (2) a healthy bone marrow which has not been damaged by drugs, toxins, and so forth; and (3) a proper diet that includes an adequate intake of iron, vitamin B_{12}, folic acid, protein, pyridoxine, and traces of copper. If any of these factors is missing or faulty, production of erythrocytes will be insufficient; the erythrocytes produced may be misshapen, overly fragile, excessively small or abnormally large; and hemoglobin production may be inadequate or defective.

The red blood cell has an average life span of approximately 120 days. Erythrocytes originally arise from primitive stem cells, called *hemocytoblasts,* located within the bone marrow; hemocytoblasts can evolve into either erythrocytes, leukocytes, or platelets. The differentiation of a hemocytoblast into an erythrocyte is stimulated by *erythropoietin* — a factor within the plasma which regulates red blood cell production. The evolving red blood cell finally loses its nucleus, leaves the bone marrow by a venous route, and enters the general circulation; it is now called a *reticulocyte.* Within the blood stream the young reticulocytes circulate for another 4 days; during this time they mature into adult erythrocytes.

The majority of erythrocytes are actively involved in the transport of oxygen and carbon dioxide; however, some erythrocytes are held in storage by the *spleen* — the body's blood reservoir. These "reserve corps" of erythrocytes are released by the spleen whenever the circulating red blood cell count begins to drop significantly below normal levels, e.g., during periods of great physical or emotional stress, during pregnancy, and during emergencies such as hemorrhage, shock, or carbon monoxide poisoning.

As the adult erythrocyte carries out its tasks, it is subjected to considerable stress as it squeezes and twists its way through the blood vessels. In time, the aging cell becomes worn and fragile and eventually ruptures. At this point, hemoglobin leaves the cell and the withered remaining membrane is called a "ghost cell." Both the ghost cell and the hemoglobin it once contained are quickly phagocytized by macrophages within the liver, spleen, and red bone marrow. (See Chapter 10.) Hemoglobin, when phagocytized, breaks down into its globin and heme fractions. The *iron* of the heme fraction returns to the liver where it is reused in making fresh hemoglobin. The *porphyrin* molecules from the heme fraction are converted by the liver into *bilirubin,* an orange bile pigment. Bilirubin is excreted from the liver into the bile; it is finally excreted from the body in the feces and urine. During periods of severe red blood cell destruction (for example, in hemolytic anemia), large amounts of bilirubin are formed as a result of the massive breakdown of hemoglobin.

Under normal conditions, the approximately 180 million aged erythrocytes that are destroyed every minute are replaced that same minute by approximately 180 million young erythrocytes. As a result, the population of red blood cells within the healthy body remains fairly constant. What happens, however, if the erythrocyte loss or destruction begins to *exceed* erythrocyte production? When the erythrocyte count becomes abnormally low, an inadequate amount of hemoglobin is available to carry oxygen to the tissues and, as a result, *hypoxia* develops. Hypoxia stimulates the release of erythropoietin, which then stimulates the bone marrow to produce more red blood cells (Fig. 45–1). Because the healthy bone marrow is capable of producing six to eight times the amount of red blood cells that it normally produces, the red blood

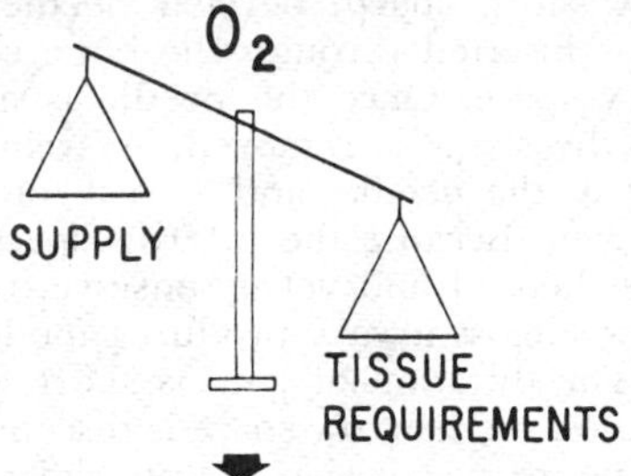

Increased Humoral Erythropoietic Activity

Increased Marrow Erythropoietic Activity

Increased Oxygen-Carrying Capacity of the Peripheral Blood

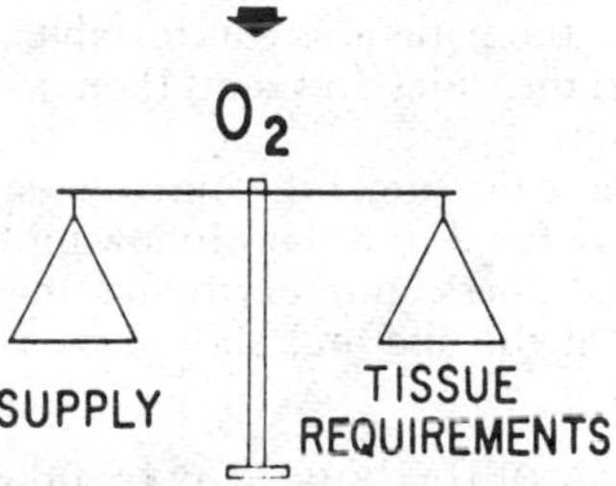

Figure 45–1. Erythropoietic stimulation via the humoral regulatory mechanism. (From Linaman, J. W.: Hematology. New York: Macmillan Co., Inc., 1975.)

cell count increases so that erythrocyte production keeps pace with erythrocyte destruction. As a result of this homeostatic mechanism, erythrocyte concentration within the circulation remains remarkably constant.

ABNORMALITIES OF ERYTHROCYTE STRUCTURE, PRODUCTION, AND LIFE SPAN

Causes of Abnormalities

There are numerous diseases involving red blood cells. However, only two basic pathophysiologic developments underlie all erythrocyte disorders:

1. A *decrease* in the hemoglobin concentration, the number of red blood cells, and the volume of packed red cells per hundred milliliters of blood. Levels below the physiologically normal or normal for the individual are due to one or all of the following: (a) insufficient erythrocyte production because of abnormal production by the bone marrow, (b) defective erythrocyte synthesis because of the absence of an essential factor, (c) increased erythrocyte destruction caused by hereditary factors or an acquired condition, or (d) increased erythrocyte loss caused by acute or chronic blood loss.

2. An *increased* number of circulating red blood cells *(polycythemia)* due to either: (a) a disorder of unknown etiology, which is apparently similar to cancer, or (b) a compensatory mechanism that develops in response to tissue hypoxia (secondary polycythemia).

Detecting Abnormalities of Erythrocytes

A number of laboratory tests are used to detect abnormalities of erythrocyte production, structure, function, and life span and to diagnose various erythrocyte disorders. The most commonly employed tests are discussed here.

The *red blood cell count* (RBC count) measures the concentration of erythrocytes per cu. mm. of blood. Normal values are 4.7 to 6.1 million erythrocytes per cu. mm. for *men* , and 4.2 to 5.2 million erythrocytes per cu. mm. for *women.* The erythrocyte count is *increased* in polycythemia vera and in those cardiac and pulmonary disorders characterized by cyanosis; it is *decreased* in the anemias.

The *hemoglobin (Hgb* or *Hb) determination* evaluates the hemoglobin content of the erythrocytes. More specifically, it measures the number of grams of hemoglobin per 100 ml. of blood. Normal values for *men* are 14.5 to 16.0 Gm./100 ml. blood, and for *women* 13.0 to 15.5 Gm./100 ml. blood. The hemoglobin content of the blood *increases* in polycythemia vera and in dehydration; it *decreases* in hemodilution of the blood as a result of fluid overload and in certain anemias, e.g., iron deficiency, and pernicious, hemolytic, or hemorrhagic anemia.

The *hematocrit* (Hct) test, also known as the "packed red cell volume test," is sometimes used in place of the RBC count. To obtain a hematocrit reading, a sample of whole blood, usually 4 ml., is centrifuged until the erythrocytes separate from the plasma; the volume of red blood cells is then determined and expressed as either cubic milliliters of packed cells per 100 ml. blood or in volumes/100 ml. Normal values are 42–53 volumes/100 ml. of blood for *men,* and 38–46 volumes/100 ml. blood for *women.* The hematocrit is *increased* in polycythemia vera and in hemoconcentration resulting from fluid loss and dehydration; it is *decreased* in the anemias.

The *reticulocyte count* determines the effectiveness and speed of red blood cell production and the responsiveness of the bone marrow to a diminished number of circulating red blood cells. Specifically, this test measures the number of reticulocytes released from the bone marrow into the blood. The normal value is 25,000 to

75,000 reticulocytes per cu. mm. of blood, or 1 to 2 per cent of the total erythrocyte count, providing the erythrocyte count is within a normal range. An *increase* in the reticulocyte count indicates an abnormal increase in erythrocyte production, which is probably due to excessive red blood cell destruction (e.g., hemolytic anemia), or loss (e.g., hemorrhage). A *decrease* in the reticulocyte count may indicate bone marrow failure or pernicious anemia. This test is used routinely to check the efficiency of erythropoiesis in persons working with radioactive materials and to evaluate the effectiveness of treatment in cases of pernicious anemia and bone marrow failure.

BONE MARROW ASPIRATION EXAMINATION

This is an extremely important diagnostic procedure employed in the diagnosis of most blood dyscrasias (including aplastic anemia, the leukemias, pernicious anemia, and thrombocytopenia). Examination of the bone marrow reveals the number, size, and shape of red cells, white cells, and platelets as they evolve through their various developmental stages. Hematologists study the marrow cells for various maturational abnormalities. Bone marrow samples are most commonly taken from the posterior iliac crests. Other possible sites for sampling include the sternum and the anterior iliac crests. The procedure may be performed by a specially trained physician, nurse, or laboratory technician. Equipment for the procedure and the method of handling the sample vary widely from institution to institution.

Preparation of the patient for a bone marrow aspiration involves the following steps:

1. Explain to the patient the purpose of the procedure: state that a small sample of bone marrow will be taken and sent to the laboratory for examination.
2. Ask the patient to sign a special permit prior to the aspiration.
3. Obtain an order for sedation if the patient appears to be extremely apprehensive.
4. Position the patient properly according to the site to be used. The site and proper positioning will vary from institution to institution.
5. Ensure that the aspiration site is meticulously cleaned and that the area is draped with sterile towels.

The *procedure* for aspirating the bone marrow is as follows:

1. The skin and subcutaneous tissue down to the periosteum are usually anesthetized with a local anesthetic.
2. A short, sharp, beveled needle containing a stylus is inserted through the bone cortex into the marrow space. Once the needle is in the marrow space, the stylus is removed. A syringe is then attached to the needle, and 1 to 2 ml. of marrow is withdrawn. Because the marrow space itself cannot be anesthetized and yet is sensitive, removal of the marrow almost always produces moderate to acute pain. The duration of pain is short; it stops as the suction on the marrow space is discontinued.
3. The marrow is ejected onto slides.

Care following the procedure is outlined below:

1. Some bleeding following the aspiration usually occurs. Firm pressure should be applied directly to the site for as long as needed. Ice packs, combined with pressure, can help control prolonged bleeding. Failure to stop the bleeding promptly can result in a hematoma, which may cause the patient discomfort for many days.
2. Make the patient as comfortable as possible.
3. Label the slides and send them to the laboratory immediately.
4. Observe the site of the marrow aspiration at least twice a day for 2 to 3 days following the procedure. Local tenderness and erythema may be signs of infection at the site and should be reported to the physician.

A biopsy of the bone may be taken at the time of marrow aspiration. This bone specimen is ejected into a jar containing a preservative and is sent to the laboratory along with the marrow.

OTHER TESTS

Blood Film. A blood film is an examination of the blood to determine variations and abnormalities in erythrocyte size, shape, and hemoglobin content. Cells that are *normal* in size and shape are termed *normocytes;* cells that are *normal* in *hemoglobin content* are called *normochromic* (meaning normal color). Abnormalities of erythrocyte size, shape, and color are numerous; usually they indicate some form of anemia (Table 45–1).

Erythrocyte Indices. Erythrocyte indices are measurements of erythrocyte size and hemoglobin content. These values are derived from the erythrocyte count, hemoglobin, and hematocrit and are obtained by laboratory study of a peripheral blood film. The three erythrocyte indices, mean corpuscular volume (MCV), mean corpuscular hemoglobin (MCH), and mean corpuscular hemoglobin concentration (MCHC), are described in Table 45–2. The indices are extremely helpful in the diagnosis of various anemias.

Erythrocyte Fragility Test. The erythrocyte fragility test measures the rate at which erythrocytes become increasingly fragile and finally burst when suspended in a graded series of hypotonic saline solutions. The solutions range

TABLE 45–1. ABNORMALITIES OF THE ERYTHROCYTE

Cellular Abnormality	Characteristics of Abnormal Cell	Conditions Characterized by Abnormality
Anisocytosis	Erythrocytes vary in size from normal	Any of the anemias
Poikilocytosis	Erythrocyte abnormally shaped, e.g., tear-shaped, club-shaped	Any of the anemias; most bizarre shapes seen in the most severe anemias
Microcyte	Erythrocyte abnormally small ($<6\mu$)	Microcytic anemias, e.g., iron deficiency anemia, thalassemia major
Macrocyte	Erythrocyte abnormally large ($>9\mu$)	Macrocytic anemias, e.g., pernicious anemia, folic acid deficiency anemia
Hypochromic cell	Erythrocyte appears pale because of abnormally low hemoglobin content	Any of the anemias
Spherocyte	Erythrocyte relatively small and round rather than biconcave in shape	Thalassemia major; hemoglobin C disease
Schistocyte	Fragmented erythrocytes with extremely bizarre shapes, e.g., triangles, spirals	Hemolytic anemia
Sickle cell	Erythrocyte crescent- or sickle-shaped owing to presence of abnormal hemoglobin (hemoglobin S)	Sickle cell anemia
Target cell	Erythrocyte thin, with small amount of hemoglobin in center	Thalassemia major
Metarubricyte	Nucleated erythrocyte	Severe anemia

from 0.85 per cent saline solution (0.9 per cent is normal or physiological saline) to 0.30 per cent solution. Normal values are:

- Hemolysis starts at 0.45 to 0.39 per cent saline solution.
- Hemolysis is completed at 0.33 to 0.30 per cent saline solution.

Fragility *increases* (that is, cells burst at a higher than normal saline concentration) in congenital hemolytic anemia and in hereditary spherocytosis. Fragility is *normal* in acquired hemolytic anemias and is *decreased* in obstructive jaundice, that is, cells do not burst until a lower than normal concentration is reached.

Erythrocyte Life Span Determination. The erythrocyte life span determination estimates the rate at which erythrocytes that are tagged with chromium-51 disappear from the circulation over a period of days or weeks; i.e., it measures the life span or survival rate of circulating red blood cells.* This test is primarily

*See Unit IX for discussion of radioisotopes and their use in diagnosis.

TABLE 45–2. THE ERYTHROCYTE INDICES

Mean Corpuscular Volume (MCV)	Mean Corpuscular Hemoglobin (MCH)	Mean Corpuscular Hemoglobin Concentration (MCHC)
Measures average size or volume of individual erythrocyte	Measures hemoglobin content within erythrocyte of average size	Measures average hemoglobin concentration within 100 ml. of packed red cells
Formula for: $\frac{HCT}{RBC}$	Formula for: $\frac{HGB}{RBC}$	Formula for: $\frac{HGB}{HCT}$
Normal value: 87 ± 5 cu.μ	Normal value: 29 ± 2 $\mu\mu$g.	Normal value: 30–36 Gm./100 ml. packed red cells
MCV < 80 means abnormally small, i.e., *microcytic,* cells	MCH < 27 indicates hemoglobin deficiency (*hypochromic* cells)	MCHC < 32 indicates hemoglobin deficiency
MCV > 94 means abnormally large, i.e., *macrocytic,* cells	MCH > 32 indicates *macrocytic* cells with abnormally large volume of hemoglobin	MCHC remains normal when MCH > 32 because cells are oversized, i.e., fewer cells can be packed together within 100 ml.

employed in the differential diagnosis of the anemias.

The test varies among institutions but involves basically the following procedures:

1. A blood sample (25 ml.) is drawn from the patient into a heparinized syringe and is then mixed with chromium-51. The sample is incubated for approximately 30 minutes, during which time the red blood cells become "tagged" with the chromium-51.

2. The blood sample is then reinjected into the patient. Twenty-four hours later a 10 ml. blood sample is drawn. (The 24-hour interval assures that the tagged blood cells have been adequately circulated.) The radioactivity and hematocrit are determined for the sample, which then becomes the baseline for further comparison.

3. Every 2 to 3 days for approximately 2 weeks, 10 ml. samples are drawn to determine the amount of radioactive red blood cells remaining. These samples are then compared with the initial baseline values.

The rapidity with which the chromium-51 tagged cells disappear is indicative of the severity of the hemolytic disease process.

Coombs' Test. The Coombs' test is used to: (1) detect certain antigen-antibody reactions between serum antibodies and red cell antigens; (2) differentiate between various forms of hemolytic anemia; (3) determine unusual or minor blood types; and (4) test for the possible development of erythroblastosis fetalis. The *direct Coombs' test* is used to examine erythrocytes for the presence of antibodies (agglutinins) that damage erythrocytes but will not cause clumping or hemolysis. It is employed to cross match blood for blood transfusions, to test umbilical cord blood for the possible presence of erythroblastosis fetalis, and to diagnose acquired hemolytic anemia. The *indirect Coombs' test* is used to identify antibodies to erythrocyte antigens in the serum of patients with a greater than normal chance of developing transfusion reactions. Both tests are agglutination procedures performed using a suspension of the patient's red blood cells.

Urobilinogen Test. The fecal and urinary urobilinogen test determines the amount of urobilinogen excreted in the urine and feces. Urobilinogen is a compound that results when bilirubin is broken down by intestinal tract bacteria (you recall that bilirubin results from the breakdown of hemoglobin following destruction of red blood cells). Normally, 99 per cent of the urobilinogen formed is excreted in the feces and only 1 per cent is excreted in the urine. Normal values are:

Urinary urobilinogen: 1 to 4 mg. in 24 hours.
Fecal urobilinogen: 50 to 300 mg. in 24 hours.

Both urinary and fecal urobilinogen are increased in hemolytic anemia, owing to the excessive destruction of cells and resultant breakdown of large amounts of hemoglobin.

There is no special preparation for this test, and the procedure is very simple. The patient's urine is collected in a container either for a 24-hour period or for a 2-hour period during the afternoon. Afternoon specimens are used because urinary excretion of urobilinogen reaches its peak during the time span from midafternoon to early evening.

Nursing responsibilities are: (1) to note the exact times at which the urine collection is started and ended; and (2) to transport the *total* urine collected to the laboratory as soon as possible in order to prevent bacteria within the urine from converting urobilinogen to urobilin by oxidative processes.

THE ANEMIAS

Definition and Incidence

Anemia is usually defined as "a reduction below the normal level in the number of red blood cells, the quantity of hemoglobin, and the volume of packed red cells per hundred milliliters of blood."[108] As you can see from this definition, anemia is *not* a disease in itself, but a *laboratory diagnosis* which takes many different forms; e.g., the cells may be microcytic, macrocytic, hypochromic, and so forth.

However, although anemia is not a specific disease, it is the *principal manifestation* of a number of abnormal conditions such as: (1) deficiency states caused by a dietary lack of iron, vitamin B_{12}, folic acid, and so forth; (2) hereditary disorders of the erythrocyte; (3) disorders involving the hematopoietic tissues (bone marrow damage or a hyperactive spleen); and (4) bleeding from the gastrointestinal tract because of cancer, or hemorrhage from any organ as a result of trauma.

The *incidence* of anemia is extremely high. This is particularly true in underdeveloped countries where nutrition is poor, and in tropical regions where the hookworm (which sucks blood from the intestinal wall of its host) is endemic. Some epidemiologists calculate that at least one half of the world's population suffer from anemia at some time in their lives.

General Causes and Effects of Anemia

Major Causes of Anemia

1. *Excessive blood loss.*
2. *Deficiencies and abnormalities of erythrocyte production.*
3. *Excessive destruction of erythrocytes.*

In turn, the three factors listed above may result from the following problems: bleeding due to trauma or cancer; dietary deficiencies; the ingestion or absorption of poisons or drugs that suppress the bone marrow; chronic infections; and genetic abnormalities that result in faulty erythrocyte genesis and/or structure.

We stated earlier that the major role of the erythrocyte is to transport oxygen to the tissues. Consequently, the major physiologic *effect* of anemia is to *reduce the capacity of the patient's blood to carry oxygen* to the tissues. This results in tissue hypoxia. *Tissue hypoxia* is the *basic underlying cause of all symptoms accompanying anemia.*

Symptoms accompanying anemia differ, depending upon the severity and chronicity of the anemia, the age of the patient, and whether the patient is afflicted with another malady. Patients with *mild* anemia (hemoglobin, 10 to 14 Gm.) are almost always asymptomatic unless they suffer, at the same time, from another disorder. If symptoms occur, they typically follow strenuous exertion. For example, following exercise, the patient may notice palpitations, dyspnea, and excessive diaphoresis, owing to the additional effort required by the heart and lungs to provide the body tissues with sufficient oxygen.

Patients with *moderate* anemia usually suffer from increased dyspnea, palpitations, and diaphoresis upon exertion as well as chronic fatigue, which occurs whether the patient is at rest or active.

When anemia is *severe,* patients appear pale and exhausted all the time; also, they complain of severe palpitations, sensitivity to cold, loss of appetite, profound weakness, dizziness, and headache. The severely anemic person (particularly the elderly person) can eventually develop serious cardiac complications. Congestive heart failure (CHF) may arise as a result of increased demands upon the heart to beat faster and harder in order to transport more oxygen to the tissues. Angina pectoris may also develop, either alone or in conjunction with CHF. In severe anemia, angina pectoris results from insufficient oxygenation of the myocardium.

Diagnosis of Anemia

Anemia is diagnosed on the basis of the various blood tests just described, the physical examination, and the patient's history. The three basic laboratory tests confirming the presence of anemia are the total erythrocyte count, the hemoglobin determination, and the hematocrit. To determine the *specific type* of anemia present, the hematologist (a specialist in the study of blood) examines both the patient's bone marrow specimen and the blood film. Also, the erythrocyte indices and, in some cases, the rate of erythrocyte destruction are calculated. In addition to ordering laboratory tests the physician also conducts a complete physical examination to determine the general state of the patient's health. Moreover, a careful medical and social history is helpful in determining the cause and the severity of the anemia.

Both doctor and nurse need to question the patient about the following:

- Symptoms (presence of fatigue, dizziness, headache, sensations of "pins and needles" in the fingers and toes, premature graying of hair, stomatitis, and others)
- The color of urine and stools over the past weeks or months (tarry stools and/or brown, hazy, or smoky urine indicate internal bleeding)
- The adequacy of the person's diet
- The person's tolerance for exercise
- Medications being taken or taken in the recent past
- Whether the person has been exposed recently to insecticides or any other poisonous substances
- Whether the person has been treated for chronic infections, cancer, renal disease, liver disease, bleeding ulcers, or hemorrhoids

A family history is also useful. Some blood disorders are hereditary (e.g., hereditary spherocytosis); others are linked with race (e.g., sickle cell anemia) and place of birth (e.g., thalassemia major).

Clinical Care of the Patient With Anemia

The goals of care for patients with anemia are to: (1) alleviate or control the causative factors; (2) relieve symptoms; (3) prevent complications; and (4) develop, for patients with chronic anemia, a realistic, practical, lifelong plan of care.

Therapy for the anemias ranges from specific treatment to purely symptomatic care. Therapy also varies in intensity and duration; some anemias can be cured within a few weeks or months, whereas others require lifelong treatment.

The anemias that respond best to *specific* treatment are those caused by deficiency states. For example, iron deficiency anemia is cured with iron preparations and diet, while pernicious anemia is controlled with injections of vitamin B_{12}. Other anemias (e.g., aplastic anemia due to bone marrow failure and some of the acquired hemolytic anemias) can often be successfully treated by discontinuance of a damaging drug or chemical agent. Anemia due to blood loss is usually corrected by investigation of the cause of the bleeding, medical and surgical control of the bleeding, and use of transfusions. Symptomatic care for *all* patients with anemias includes the following measures:

Rest. Rest is essential for lowering the patient's oxygen requirements and for reducing strain on the heart and lungs. Patients with *mild* anemia are rarely hospitalized and are usually fully ambulatory. However, these individuals should be encouraged to rest or nap frequently throughout the day, to shorten their working hours whenever possible, and to retire early. If the ambulatory patient experiences dizziness or lightheadedness while at work or at home, tell her or him to lie flat on a bed, couch, or floor for a few minutes. Lying down without a pillow helps to relieve dizziness by increasing the circulation of blood and oxygen to the brain.

Patients with *severe* anemia are usually hospitalized and placed on bed rest until their blood picture improves. An extremely weak patient needs help in bathing, turning, eating, and caring for teeth or dentures. Also, to ensure sufficient rest, protect the severely anemic patient from frequent visitors, continuous telephone interruptions and excessive noise. Planned rest periods are advisable.

Skin Care. *Frequent turning* is essential for patients with severe anemia if skin breakdown is to be prevented. Because of the reduction in circulating red blood cells, the tissues of the anemic patient do not receive adequate amounts of oxygen. Without preventive measures, the resultant tissue hypoxia can quickly lead to decubitus formation. (See Sorensen and Luckmann, *Basic Nursing: A Psychophysiologic Approach,* for a discussion of ways to prevent skin breakdown in bedridden and debilitated patients.)

Diet. The diet in anemia should be high in protein, iron, and vitamins. These substances are essential for normal erythrocyte formation. Unfortunately, patients with anemia may have little appetite for the nourishing foods that they need so badly. Anorexia often results from weakness and profound fatigue. Also, patients with pernicious anemia or iron deficiency anemia often have difficulty eating because of a sore mouth, tongue, or esophagus. The following measures are helpful in combating anorexia: (1) serve six small, easily digested meals a day instead of three large meals; (2) avoid hot spicy foods if the patient suffers from a sore mouth or throat; (3) give oral hygiene before and after the patient eats; and (4) feed the patient who is too exhausted to do it.

Anemic patients and the persons who live with them need practical instruction on how to plan and prepare a nourishing diet at home. To teach patients about the dietary prevention and treatment of anemia, you can: (1) arrange for private consultation between the dietitian, the patient, and significant others; (2) provide booklets on nutrition and meal planning and discuss the information with the patient; (3) provide for the patient appetizing recipes for foods high in iron, vitamin B_{12}, and other vitamins; (4) ask the dietitian to help the patient prepare several weeks of sample menus containing nutritious foods that the patient enjoys, can afford, and knows how to prepare; and (5) arrange for a public health nurse to visit the patient at home for continued dietary supervision.*

Mouth Care. Special mouth care is a necessity for all patients with severe anemia because they often suffer from a sore mouth or tongue. Special oral hygiene measures include: (1) cleansing the teeth before and after meals with a soft-bristled toothbrush or applicators; (2) allowing the patient to rinse his or her mouth every 2 hours with mouthwashes that are cool and slightly alkaline; and (3) lubricating the lips frequently with mineral oil or petrolatum to prevent dryness or cracking.

Transfusions. Blood transfusions are not administered routinely to all patients with anemia because they can result in dangerous reactions and complications. However, blood transfusions are valuable in the treatment of patients with anemia due to *acute* blood loss. The administration of several pints of blood is often lifesaving for the individual with a hemoglobin of less than 10 Gm. as a result of hemorrhage.

Blood transfusions may be used to treat patients with *severe chronic anemia* (hemoglobin less than 6 Gm.) who have responded poorly to other forms of therapy. However, in spite of its benefits, giving whole blood to persons with severe chronic anemia is extremely hazardous because they need the RBC's and not the other components of the blood.†

> *Patients who have a heart condition in addition to anemia are particularly vulnerable to circulatory and pulmonary complications.*

To help alleviate the dangers of circulatory overload in the patient with cardiac complications, the doctor may order the administration of a small volume of *packed red cells* in place of whole blood. Additionally, the physician may

*Usually books on nutrition and sample menus and recipes can be obtained from the dietitian in your hospital or from the local public health department.

†Other potential complications caused by blood tranfusions can be found in Sorensen and Luckmann, *Basic Nursing: A Psychophysiologic Approach,* Chapter 39.

attempt to reduce the patient's plasma volume *before* the transfusion by: (1) administering diuretics to promote the elimination of large amounts of water or (2) by withdrawing an amount of plasma from the patient which equals in volume the amount of blood ordered for the transfusion.

As you administer blood to the patient with chronic anemia and heart disease, take the following precautions: (1) administer the blood *very slowly* to prevent overloading the heart and lungs; (2) check the patient's *pulse* every 15 minutes for tachycardia — an indication that the heart is overworking as a pump; (3) examine the patient's *neck veins* for fullness and monitor the *central venous pressure* (elevation of the central venous pressure over 10 cm. H_2O indicates a circulatory overload); (4) observe the patient for symptoms of *respiratory distress* and listen for the sound of *rales* in the patient's basilar lung regions; and (5) stop the transfusion at once and notify the physician if the patient's pulse becomes rapid (over 120 beats per minute), if the central venous pressure is elevated, or if the patient develops symptoms of pulmonary edema.

Oxygen Therapy. This is rarely ordered for patients with mild anemia. However, patients with *severe* anemia need oxygen because their blood is so greatly reduced in its capacity to carry this life-sustaining gas. In these cases, the administration of oxygen helps to prevent tissue hypoxia and also lessens the work of the heart as it struggles to compensate for the deficiency of oxygen-carrying hemoglobin.

Protection of Patient. Protection of the patient from *chilling* and *burns* is an important nursing function. Because of poor circulation, patients with anemia typically say they feel cold and chilled. Warm clothing and blankets help anemic patients to feel more comfortable and, consequently, to rest and sleep better.

Avoid applying heating pads or hot water bottles to patients with anemia, because their skin (which is poorly supplied with blood and oxygen) burns easily. Also, patients may not be aware of any burning sensation.

The patient with pernicious anemia, in particular, suffers from a decreased sensitivity to heat. A severe burn may result from a heating device before the patient or nursing staff becomes aware of the condition.

Isolation. Isolation of the patient from possible *sources of infection* is one therapeutic technique. Severely anemic patients are typically exhausted and debilitated and, consequently, develop infections easily. Do not care for patients with anemia if you have a cold or sore throat; also, do not permit infected visitors, patients, or other personnel to come into close contact with the patient. *Reverse isolation techniques* may be used to protect patients with aplastic anemia; these individuals suffer from leukopenia (a reduced leukocyte count) as well as anemia and are therefore particularly vulnerable to infection. Many of the infections this patient population acquires may be self-originating rather than coming from external contaminants.

Classification of the Anemias

Anemias are generally classified according to either the morphologic characteristics of the erythrocytes (i.e., normocytic, microcytic, etc.) or the etiology of the condition (i.e., hemolytic hemorrhagic, etc.). In many instances the etiologic method of classification is inappropriate since anemia is merely a symptom of an underlying pathophysiologic process whose nature and etiology may be obscure. Nurses should therefore be familiar with morphologic classification, which is in common usage because it is objective, descriptive, and independent of etiologic factors.[112]

Although our discussion of the individual anemias will consider them from an etiologic standpoint, a brief review of the more common morphologic categories usually employed is given. You will recall that in earlier portions of this chapter, particularly in Tables 45–1 and 45–2, the terms macrocytic and microcytic have already been introduced and the standards for applying these terms to cells, based on the mean

MORPHOLOGIC CLASSIFICATION OF ANEMIAS

Type of Anemia	Criteria	Clinical Examples
Normocytic (normochromic)	MCV 80–94 c.μ MCHC >30%	Anemia of sudden blood loss, anemia of pregnancy, anemia of chronic disease, e.g., cancer, some hemolytic anemias
Macrocytic (normochromic)	MCV >94 c.μ MCHC >30%	Pernicious anemia, anemia in myxedema, folic acid deficiency, some hemolytic anemias
Microcytic (normochromic)	MCV <80 c.μ MCHC >30%	Anemia of chronic disease
Hypochromic microcytic	MCV <80 c.μ MCHC <30%	Iron deficiency anemia

corpuscular volume (MCV), were indicated. The mean corpuscular hemoglobin (MCH) and the mean corpuscular hemoglobin concentration (MCHC) are the foundation by which the designations of normochromia, hypochromia, or hyperchromia are predicated.[113]

The etiologic classification given below, which we follow in this text, is used here because it is easier to relate patient care and teaching to the etiology of an anemia than to its cellular characteristics.

*Anemias: Etiologic Classification**

I. Anemias resulting from excessive blood loss
  A. Acute posthemorrhagic anemia
  B. Anemia due to chronic blood loss
II. Anemias resulting from reduced erythrocyte production
  A. Anemias due to a deficiency of factors necessary for red cell production
    1. Iron deficiency anemia
    2. Anemias due to deficiencies of vitamin B_{12} and folic acid (megaloblastic anemias)
      a. Pernicious anemia
      b. Other anemias due to vitamin B_{12} deficiency
      c. Anemia due to folic acid deficiency
  B. Anemias of bone marrow failure
III. Anemias resulting from excessive erythrocyte destruction (hemolytic anemias)
  A. Hemolytic anemias resulting from intrinsic erythrocyte defects
    1. Glucose-6-phosphate dehydrogenase (G6PD) deficiency
    2. Hereditary spherocytosis
  B. Hemolytic anemias mainly resulting from extra-erythrocyte factors (acquired hemolytic anemias)
    1. Hemolysis due to trauma
    2. Hemolysis due to chemical agents and drugs (toxic hemolytic anemia)
    3. Hemolysis due to infectious agents
    4. Hemolytic disease secondary to systemic disease (secondary hemolytic anemia)
    5. Hemolysis due to isoimmune hemolytic reactions
    6. Hemolysis due to autoimmune disorders
    7. The paroxysmal hemoglobinopathies
IV. Anemias resulting both from disturbances of erythrocyte production and from increased erythrocyte destruction
  A. Anemias due to defective hemoglobin synthesis
    1. Hemoglobinopathies (e.g., sickle cell anemia)
    2. Thalassemias
  B. Secondary anemias (also called anemias of relative bone marrow failure or simple chronic anemias)

*Classification adapted from Berkow, R., and Talbott, J. H. (Eds.): *Merck Manual of Diagnosis and Therapy.* 13th ed. Rahway, N.J.: Merck, Sharp & Dohme Research Laboratories, 1977.

Anemias Resulting from Excessive Blood Loss

ACUTE POSTHEMORRHAGIC ANEMIA

Definition, Etiology, and Symptoms. Acute posthemorrhagic anemia is a normocytic, normochromic anemia that develops following the rapid loss of large numbers of erythrocytes during a massive hemorrhage.

Common *causes* of acute bleeding are:

- Severed blood vessels due to trauma
- Spontaneous rupture of an aneurysm
- Hemorrhagic disorders
- Erosion of an artery by a cancerous growth or ulcerative lesion

The adverse *effects* of acute hemorrhage are due to the rapid decrease in blood volume and the reduced oxygen-carrying capacity of the blood that results from the loss of erythrocytes. The severity of the patient's symptoms and the prognosis depend upon: (1) the *rate* of bleeding; (2) the *site* of the hemorrhage; and (3) the *volume* of blood lost. A gradual loss of a large amount of blood is less threatening than the rapid loss of a smaller volume of blood.

The clinical manifestations of acute hemorrhage include: restlessness; dizziness; syncope; thirst; pallor; diaphoresis; rapid thready pulse; hypotension; rapid deep respirations, which later become shallow; severe headache; and disorientation. Disorientation indicates cerebral anoxia. In addition to these symptoms, internal hemorrhage into body organs and tissues causes fever, pain in the area of bleeding due to distention of tissues, and symptoms of organ displacement (e.g., hemothorax can result in a mediastinal shift). If internal or external hemorrhage remains uncontrolled, the blood pressure continues to drop and shock develops. Untreated, the shock becomes irreversible and death swiftly ensues.

Laboratory Findings. Following acute hemorrhage, the patient's blood picture is in a state of flux for several weeks. The erythrocyte count, hemoglobin, and hematocrit findings are completely unreliable for the first 24 to 48 hours following hemorrhage because *vasoconstriction* (a compensatory mechanism which occurs during shock) and *loss of plasma volume* mask the actual degree of erythrocyte and hemoglobin loss. In other words, the erythrocytes that remain following hemorrhage are concentrated within a smaller space and a smaller volume of plasma than normal. Consequently, the erythrocyte, hemoglobin, and hematocrit appear deceptively high when, in fact, they may be dangerously low. However, after 1 to 2 days, extracellular fluid from the tissues and prescribed intravenous fluids enter the patient's vascular compartment and dilute the red blood cell concentration. As a result, the remaining (greatly diminished) erythrocytes circulate in a more normal amount of plasma. Consequently, the erythrocyte count, hemoglobin, and hematocrit reflect more accurately the degree of anemia present.

If there is no further bleeding, blood restoration begins within 4 to 5 days. The erythrocyte count and hemoglobin usually return to normal within a month to six weeks. During this period, large numbers of reticulocytes appear in the blood, sometimes accompanied by a few normocytes if the anemia is severe.

Clinical Care. Emergency treatment of patients with acute hemorrhage centers on controlling and stopping the hemorrhage, treating shock, and restoring the blood volume as rapidly as possible.

> *Blood transfusion is the treatment of choice if the patient's blood loss is greater than 20 per cent of the total blood volume.*

The patient is generally treated with intravenous infusions of plasma while blood is being typed and crossmatched. Other supportive measures for the hemorrhaging patient are sedation, rest, and oral fluids if the patient can tolerate them and if she or he is not going to surgery.

Once the patient's blood volume has been restored and shock has abated, the next goal of care is to *replenish the iron stores* that were lost during hemorrhage. A nutritious diet helps the patient to overcome an iron deficiency. Encourage the patient to eat foods high in protein, iron, and vitamins. If diet therapy proves inadequate, the doctor may order the administration of iron supplements.

ANEMIA DUE TO CHRONIC BLOOD LOSS

The major *causes* of chronic blood loss are bleeding peptic ulcers, prolonged or excessive menses, bleeding hemorrhoids, and cancerous lesions within the gastrointestinal tract. The *results* of chronic bleeding are: (1) continuous loss of small numbers of erythrocytes, which are usually adequately replaced by the bone marrow, and (2) continuous loss of iron, which may result in a total depletion of the patient's iron stores. Because of the severe iron losses, the anemia of chronic bleeding is identical in symptoms and laboratory findings to *iron deficiency anemia* (see discussion in following section). To treat anemia due to chronic blood loss, the physician must locate the site of bleeding, control the cause of bleeding, and correct the patient's iron deficiency with proper diet and iron supplements.

Anemias Resulting from Reduced Erythrocyte Production

ANEMIAS DUE TO DEFICIENCIES OF FACTORS NECESSARY FOR RED CELL PRODUCTION

We stated earlier that effective erythropoiesis depends upon the adequate intake and proper assimilation of iron, vitamin B_{12}, folic acid, protein, pyridoxine, and traces of copper. Inadequate intake, defective assimilation, or excessive loss of any one of these factors will result in a deficiency of that nutrient, followed by the development of anemia. The *most common* deficiency state is iron deficiency. Deficiencies of vitamin B_{12} and folic acid are also prevalent. Protein deficiency, also frequently encountered, is discussed in Chapter 12. Pyridoxine deficiency occurs infrequently in humans; copper deficiency is extremely rare.

Iron Deficiency Anemia

DEFINITION AND INCIDENCE. Iron deficiency anemia is a chronic, microcytic, hypochromic anemia caused by either inadequate absorption or excessive loss of iron.

The *incidence* of iron deficiency anemia throughout the world is extremely high. It is the most prevalent of the anemias and it affects at least twice as many persons as all the other anemia put together.

The *distribution* of this condition is related to geographic location, economic class, age groupings, and sex. Viewed on a worldwide basis, iron deficiency anemia most commonly strikes persons in underdeveloped countries such as India where nutrition is extremely poor. This problem is also prevalent in tropical zones and in Southern United States, Mexico, and Puerto Rico, where blood-sucking parasites such as the hookworm are endemic.

The poor of all nations suffer far more frequently from iron deficiency than do the middle and upper classes. Also, women between the ages of 15 and 45 and young children are extremely vulnerable to iron deficiency. On the other hand, adult males and postmenopausal females are rarely troubled by this problem unless they suffer, at the same time, from conditions causing chronic blood loss. Population studies reveal that 10 to 30 per cent of all women suffer from iron deficiency, 10 to 60 per cent of pregnant women and young infants have this condition, while only 3 per cent of men have symptoms of iron lack.[14]

IRON BALANCE. The adult human body contains approximately 50 mg. of iron per 100 ml. of blood. Total body iron ranges between 2 to 6 Gm., depending upon the size of the individual and the amount of hemoglobin the person's cells contain. Approximately two thirds of this iron is contained in hemoglobin ("essential iron"); the other third is stored in the bone marrow, spleen, liver, and muscle. If an individual develops an iron deficiency, the iron stores are depleted first, followed later by a reduction in hemoglobin formation.

We obtain iron from food, important sources being liver (the richest source), oysters, lean meats, kidney beans, whole wheat bread, kale, spinach, egg yolk, turnip tops, beet greens, carrots, apricots, and raisins.

An adequate diet supplies the body with approximately 12 to 15 mg. of iron per day, of which only 5 to 10 per cent (0.6 to 1.5 mg.) is absorbed. The amount of iron normally absorbed daily is *just sufficient* to meet the needs of healthy men and older women past the childbearing age, but is *not* sufficient to supply the greater needs of menstruating and pregnant women, adolescents, infants, and children. Note in Table 45–3 that these five groups of individuals must have a higher daily intake of iron if iron deficiency is to be prevented. Fortunately, if iron intake is inadequate during childhood or pregnancy or if bleeding develops, the gastrointestinal tract is capable of increasing the absorption of iron to around 20 to 30 per cent of the total daily intake or iron instead of only 10 per cent. In this way the body often compensates for diminishing iron stores due to inadequate iron intake or excessive iron loss.

Iron is *excreted* in urine, sweat, bile, and feces and from the skin as desquamated cells. Daily iron excretion is normally less than 1 mg. The normal monthly menses causes women of child-bearing age to lose another 0.4 to 1.0 mg of iron daily, or 12 to 30 mg. monthly. The only *abnormal* source of iron loss is *hemorrhage* or *chronic bleeding*. A chronic blood loss of as little as 2 to 4 ml. per day can result in iron deficiency anemia because 1 mg. of iron is lost in every 2 ml. of blood. To compensate for abnormal iron losses or an insufficient iron intake, the body excretes less than 0.5 mg. of iron daily rather than the 1 mg. normally excreted.

In sum, the maintenance of a positive iron balance depends upon an intake of iron sufficient to meet the needs of the individual during the various phases of his or her life and to compensate for any abnormal iron losses. Iron balance is regulated first by controlled absorption of iron and secondly by controlled excretion of iron. In this way, the body compensates for mild degrees of iron deficiency. If iron deficiency is severe, pharmacologic iron supplements are necessary to restore positive iron balance.

ETIOLOGY OF IRON DEFICIENCY ANEMIA. Acute or chronic bleeding is the principal cause of iron deficiency anemia in adults. The major causes of excessive blood loss are *trauma, excessive menses* (more than 12 pads used per period), and *gastrointestinal tract bleeding*. Gastrointestinal tract bleeding may result from peptic ulcers, hiatus hernia, gastritis, cancer, hemorrhoids, diverticula, ulcerative colitis, or salicylate poisoning. Bleeding from the gastrointestinal tract is usually chronic in nature and occult (i.e., obscure or not readily apparent).

Blood donation, a form of blood loss, is also a source of iron depletion. Each time a blood donor gives a pint of blood, a certain percentage

TABLE 45–3. ESTIMATED DIETARY IRON REQUIREMENTS*

	Absorbed Iron Requirement (mg./day)	Daily Food Iron Requirement† (mg./day)
Normal men and nonmenstruating women	0.5–1.0	5–10
Menstruating women	0.7–2.0	7–20
Pregnant women	2.0–4.8	20–48‡
Adolescents	1.0–2.0	10–20
Children	0.4–1.0	4–10
Infants	0.5–1.5	1.5 mg./per kg.§

*Brown, E. B.: Hypochromic anemias. *In* Beeson, P. B., W. McDermott, and J. B. Wyngaarden (Eds.): *Cecil Textbook of Medicine.* 15th ed., 1979.

†Assuming 10 per cent absorption.

‡This amount of iron cannot be derived from diet and should be met by iron supplementation in the latter half of pregnancy.

§To a maximum of 15 mg.

of iron is lost, depending upon the person's hemoglobin level prior to donation. To make up for this iron loss, the blood donor should increase daily intake of iron for a full year following the blood donation.

A second cause of iron deficiency anemia is an *inadequate intake* of foods high in iron, as we have just disussed. Finally, iron deficiency anemia results when adequate iron is ingested but is *not absorbed* properly. Causes of defective assimilation of iron are:

- Chronic diarrhea
- Malabsorption syndromes (e.g., celiac disease, tropical and nontropical sprue, cystic fibrosis)
- A high intake of cereal products coupled with a low intake of animal protein
- Partial or complete gastrectomy, which causes a decrease in both the assimilation and absorption of food iron
- Clay-eating (pica), a common practice of women and children in socioeconomically disadvantaged areas, which causes iron to precipitate as an insoluble substance within the intestinal tract

Symptoms. In mild cases of iron deficiency anemia, the patient is generally asymptomatic. However, in more severe cases all the general symptoms of anemia discussed earlier appear, e.g., palpitations, dizziness, and sensitivity to cold. Later in the course of the disease, patients usually develop brittleness of hair and nails. In severe cases, patients may experience dysphagia (difficulty in swallowing), stomatitis (inflammation of the mucosa of the mouth), and atrophic glossitis (tongue is inflamed and also smooth due to atrophy of papillae). This triad of symptoms is called the *Plummer-Vinson syndrome.* Despite the weakness and discomfort associated with iron deficiency anemia, patients rarely die from this condition unless severe cardiac complications develop.

Diagnostic Tests. The diagnosis of iron deficiency anemia is based upon examination of the patient's blood and bone marrow. The *morphology* of the erythrocytes in this anemia is highly characteristic. The individual red blood cells are small (microcytic) and pale (hypochromic) because they are deficient in hemoglobin. The blood *hemoglobin* level is markedly reduced and may fall as low as 3.6 Gm./100 ml. However, the *total erythrocyte count* is usually only moderately reduced, rarely dropping below 3,000,000 cells per 100 ml. The MCV, MCH, and MCHC are all reduced. The *serum iron level* (normally between 50 and 150 μg. per 100 ml. of blood) may decrease to 10 μg. Total iron-combining capacity is elevated to 350 to 500 μg. per 100 ml. (normal is 250 to 350 μg. per 100 ml.).[68] *Hemosiderin* (an insoluble form of storage iron) is completely absent from the bone marrow. Finally, there is a newly available commercial test that involves an immunoradiometric assay of the serum for ferritin. In patients with iron deficiency anemia, levels are below normal.

Once the diagnosis of iron deficiency anemia is confirmed, studies are conducted to find the *cause* of the anemia. If gastrointestinal tract bleeding is suspected, the doctor orders a battery of tests to determine the approximate amount of blood lost daily, locate the site of bleeding, and pinpoint the lesion responsible for the blood loss. Diagnostic tests commonly employed in the study of gastrointestinal tract bleeding are x-rays of the gastrointestinal tract (GI series), stool examinations for occult blood, esophagoscopy, gastroscopy, and sigmoidoscopy. (See Unit XVII for discussion of these procedures.)

Clinical Care. Therapeutic goals for patients with iron deficiency anemia are: (1) to diagnose and correct the underlying cause of the anemia, and (2) to correct the iron deficit by means of medicinal iron preparations and a diet high in food iron.

Medicinal iron can be administered orally or parenterally; however, it is administered orally whenever possible. The drugs of choice for *oral* administration are ferrous sulfate or ferrous gluconate.

It is important to administer oral iron preparations correctly. First of all, because iron salts are *gastric irritants,* they *should always be given following meals or a snack.* Iron preparations taken on an empty stomach cause dyspepsia, abdominal discomfort, and diarrhea. Second, undiluted liquid preparations of iron salts cause staining of the teeth; consequently, liquid iron preparations should be diluted well and administered through a straw. Third, whenever possible, give ferrous salts with *orange juice* because ascorbic acid promotes better iron absorption. Finally, warn the patient that iron preparations will change the color of stools because iron is excreted in the bowel movements; emphasize that the tarry appearance of the feces is a harmless side effect.

Parenteral iron therapy is administered to patients: (1) who have an intolerance to oral iron preparations, (2) who habitually forget to take their medications, or (3) who are continuing to suffer from blood losses. Iron-dextran is the parenteral drug of choice.

Iron-dextran causes darkening and discoloration of the skin around the injection site unless administered properly. When giving iron-dextran IM, remember these points:

1. Use one needle to withdraw iron-dextran and another needle to administer it. Failure to change needles will result in staining of the patient's tissues.

2. When drawing up the medication, leave 0.5 ml. of air in the syringe.
3. Give the injection with a 2- or 3-inch, 19- or 20-gauge needle, *deep* into the upper outer quadrant of the buttock; never use the patient's arm or any other exposed area.
4. Use the "Z" tract injection technique (i.e., form the outline of a "Z" by pulling the subcutaneous tissue to one side) when giving the injection; this method prevents the medication from leaking into the tissues.
5. Make certain that the needle is not in a vein; then give the injection followed by the 0.5 ml. of air. The air removes iron-dextran from inside the needle's shaft, thereby preventing leakage of the drug as the needle is removed from the tissues.
6. Never massage the site of injection.
7. Encourage the patient to ambulate, because walking hastens drug absorption. However, caution the patient not to exercise vigorously or wear constricting garments or a girdle.
8. Throughout the course of injection therapy, observe for pain at the site of injection, the development of sterile abscesses, lymphadenitis, fever, headache, urticaria, hypotension, or anaphylactic shock. Fortunately, anaphylaxis is rare.

A favorable response to iron therapy typically occurs within 48 hours; the patient usually feels more energetic and less irritable and has a better appetite. "In the peripheral blood, the reticulocyte count begins to increase in a few days, usually reaching a maximum at about 7 to 12 days, and thereafter decreases."[126] Under optimum conditions, the patient's hemoglobin is restored at a daily rate of around 0.3 Gm./100 ml. of blood. However, because iron stores are replenished at a slower rate than hemoglobin, patients must continue to take iron preparations for 2 or 3 months following return of their hemoglobin to normal.

PROGNOSIS. In the majority of cases, iron therapy is successful in reversing the symptoms of iron deficiency anemia. However, approximately one third of women and one fourth of men have a recurrence. In these cases the anemia itself was evidently cured but not the underlying cause, e.g., severe bleeding or prolonged menses.

Anemias Due to Deficiencies of Vitamin B_{12} and Folic Acid (Megaloblastic Anemias). *Vitamin B_{12}*, which contains cobalt, has two major functions: it is essential for normal red blood cell maturation, and it is necessary for normal nervous system function. Dietary sources of vitamin B_{12} are animal products such as liver, milk, and eggs; it is not contained in vegetables. Vitamin B_{12} is also produced by bacteria within the intestines of humans and animals. Other names for vitamin B_{12} are cyanocobalamin, antianemic factor, and extrinsic factor, which means a factor of external origin. The *extrinsic factor* (i.e., vitamin B_{12} obtained from foods) cannot be absorbed by the small intestine unless a substance called the *intrinsic factor* (i.e., a factor of internal origin) is present. A condition called *pernicious anemia* develops when the intrinsic factor is missing.

Like vitamin B_{12}, *folic acid* (a B-group vitamin) is necessary for red blood cell formation and maturation. However, folic acid does not play a role in nervous system function. The major dietary sources of folic acid are green vegetables and liver.

Anemias due to deficiencies of vitamin B_{12} and folic acid are called *megaloblastic anemias* because they are characterized by the appearance of megaloblasts (large primitive erythrocytes) in the blood and bone marrow. Other common features of the megaloblastic anemias are: (1) the development of leukopenia and thrombocytopenia in addition to anemia; (2) oral, gastrointestinal, and neurologic symptoms; and (3) a favorable response to injections of either vitamin B_{12} or folic acid.

The underlying defect in the megaloblastic anemias is *disturbed synthesis of deoxyribonucleic acid (DNA)*, the basic substance composing chromosomes. Deficiencies of either vitamin B_{12} or folic acid evidently impede the formation of essential DNA precursors. As a result, maturation of erythrocytes, leukocytes, and platelets is defective.

The same basic *etiologic factors* — dietary inadequacies, impaired absorption, and metabolic disturbances — underlie both vitamin B_{12} deficiency and folic acid deficiency. In vitamin B_{12} deficiency, the diet is deficient in meat and dairy products, and in folic acid deficiency vegetables are lacking in the diet.

As mentioned, the principal cause of impaired absorption of vitamin B_{12} is deficiency of the intrinsic factor. Folic acid absorption and utilization may be impeded by the administration of compounds known as folic acid antagonists, by the use of anticonvulsants, or by liver disease. Intestinal malabsorption of both vitamins can be due to any of a group of conditions such as sprue, celiac disease, steatorrhea, or surgical resection of the small intestine. Such additional conditions as tapeworm, excessive accumulation of intestinal bacteria, or intestinal diverticuli may also cause impaired absorption of vitamin B_{12}.

Metabolic disturbances such as hyperthyroidism, pregnancy, or cancer may lead to additional requirements for both these vitamins, thus producing deficiency states.

Because pernicious anemia is the most prevalent form of vitamin B_{12} deficiency in the United States and Canada, we discuss this formerly fatal condition in some detail. Other vitamin B_{12}

deficiency anemias and folic acid deficiency anemia are considered briefly.

Pernicious Anemia

DEFINITION AND INCIDENCE. Pernicious anemia is a chronic progressive, macrocytic anemia of adults, caused by a *deficiency* of the *intrinsic factor.* Major characteristics of pernicious anemia are: (1) abnormally large erythrocytes (macrocytic), (2) hypochlorhydria (deficiency of hydrochloric acid in the gastric juice), (3) neurologic and gastrointestinal symptoms, and (4) a fatal outcome without lifelong injections of vitamin B_{12}.

Although pernicious anemia is the most common of the megaloblastic anemias, it is not a common disease. Only 0.1 per cent of the population have this ailment.

Pernicious anemia mainly strikes men and women over 50. It most commonly affects blue-eyed persons of Scandinavian origin. However, pernicious anemia is occasionally seen in people under 35 and in blacks.

ETIOLOGY. Lack of the intrinsic factor (the basic defect in pernicious anemia) is caused by atrophy of the glandular mucosa of the gastric fundus. The exact factor or factors causing this mucosal atrophy and the associated hypochlorhydria remain unknown. However, the following theories of causation are gaining widespread acceptance. First, a *hereditary* basis for the disease seems likely but is currently unproved. Pernicious anemia does tend to "run in families" and is probably inherited as a single, dominant, autosomal factor. Prolonged *iron deficiency,* which can cause gastric atrophy, is a second possible predisposing factor. However, the most promising etiologic theory to date is that pernicious anemia is an *autoimmune disorder.* Ninety per cent of patients with pernicious anemia have autoantibodies that react specifically against parietal gastric cells, while 40 per cent of patients have a 7S gamma autoantibody that acts against the intrinsic factor.

Unless controlled with vitamin B_{12}, pernicious anemia always develops following *total gastrectomy;* also, 15 per cent of patients develop pernicious anemia following partial gastrectomy or gastrojejunostomy for peptic ulcer.

BASES OF SYMPTOMS. As stated earlier, vitamin B_{12} deficiency diminishes DNA synthesis; reduced DNA synthesis, in turn, results in defective maturation of cells. The cells most disturbed by defects in DNA synthesis are the more rapidly dividing body cells, i.e., cells of the bone marrow and gastrointestinal tract. Thus, consequences of vitamin B_{12} deficiency are *macrocytic anemia* and *gastrointestinal disorders.* Both these problems can be reversed with injections of vitamin B_{12}. Second, lack of vitamin B_{12} can alter the structure and disrupt the function of the peripheral nerves, spinal cord, and the brain. Thus, the third major consequence of this disorder is *disturbed nervous system function* and, in extreme cases, *permanent neurologic damage* occurs which cannot be reversed by treatment with parenteral vitamin B_{12}. Central nervous system symptoms develop in three quarters of patients.

More specifically, the signs and symptoms of pernicious anemia and their bases are shown in Table 45–4.

Patients with pernicious anemia have a high incidence of *benign gastric polyps* and *gastric carcinoma.* For this reason, persons undergoing treatment for pernicious anemia should be routinely examined for signs of gastric bleeding or obstruction due to tumor growth.

Untreated pernicious anemia terminates in death; *delayed* treatment results in *permanent disabilities.* In addition to the nervous system damage already mentioned, severe macrocytic anemia of long duration can trigger the development of congestive heart failure and angina pectoris in the elderly.

TABLE 45–4. SIGNS AND SYMPTOMS OF PERNICIOUS ANEMIA

Signs and Symptoms	Bases
Anemia: weakness; pallor; dyspnea; palpitations; fatigue	Reduced erythrocyte count (less than 3 million RBC/cu mm blood) impairs oxygen-carrying capacity of blood.
Gastrointestinal symptoms: sore mouth; smooth, beefy red tongue; weight loss; indigestion; constipation or diarrhea	Gastric lesion involves atrophy of gastric mucosa and causes reduced secretion of *hydrochloric acid* as well as intrinsic factor; HCl plays important role in chemical digestion of food.
Neurologic symptoms: tingling, numbness of hands and feet; paralysis; irritability; depression; psychotic behavior	Lack of vitamin B_{12} causes degeneration of dorsal and lateral columns of spinal cord, peripheral nerve degeneration and even brain damage.
Jaundice: pale yellow tinge to the skin	Rupture and hemolysis of abnormally large erythrocytes as they pass through capillaries.

DIAGNOSTIC TESTS. Pernicious anemia is diagnosed on the basis of: (1) the presence of the triad of symptoms described above (anemia, gastrointestinal symptoms, neurologic disorders); (2) laboratory blood and bone marrow tests; (3) the absence of hydrochloric acid in the gastric juice, and (4) a favorable response to a "therapeutic trial" with vitamin B_{12}.

Laboratory findings that confirm a diagnosis of pernicious anemia include the following:

- *Erythrocyte count:* Erythrocytes are usually reduced to below 3 million RBC/100 ml.
- *Blood film:* Erythrocytes are oval and macrocytic and contain an amount of hemoglobin which is proportionate to their size.
- *Bone marrow examinaton:* Bone marrow contains high numbers of megaloblasts (an abnormal form of erythrocyte maturation) but few normoblasts and normally maturing erythrocytes. The bone marrow also shows defects in the maturation of leukocytes.
- *Bilirubin:* Unconjugated bilirubin (a product of hemoglobin breakdown) is usually elevated, owing to hemolysis of defective erythrocytes.
- *Serum LDH* (lactate dehydrogenase) activity is extremely high.
- *Schilling test:* This measures the absorption of radioactive vitamin B_{12} (tagged with cobalt-60) both before and after parenteral administration of the instrinsic factor. This procedure is the *definitive test for pernicious anemia;* it is used to detect lack of the intrinsic factor, the basic defect in this disease.

  The test is performed in two, and sometimes three, stages. If after the first stage, during which only vitamin B_{12} has been given, the patient's urinary excretion of the vitamin is in the normal range, pernicious anemia probably is not present and the test is terminated. If the excretion is abnormal, a second stage is performed in which intrinsic factor is given with the vitamin B_{12}. If the results of this are equivocal, a third stage is sometimes used to determine whether an alteration in intestinal bacteria is causing the malabsorption of the vitamin.
- *Gastric juice analysis* for the presence of free hydrochloric acid is another important test. Almost all individuals with pernicious anemia secrete gastric juice that has: (1) an abnormally low volume, (2) an abnormally high pH, and (3) no free hydrochloric acid. Furthermore, in pernicious anemia, gastric secretions remain scanty and the pH elevated even *after* the patient is given an injection of *histamine*—a substance which normally stimulates the flow of gastric juice.
- *Therapeutic trial with parenteral vitamin B_{12}.* For this test the patient is given IM injections of vitamin B_{12} for 10 days. The patient who has pernicious anemia responds quickly and favorably to the medication, e.g., an increased sense of well-being results and the blood picture improves. The diagnosis of pernicious anemia is confirmed if large numbers of reticulocytes appear in the blood 4 to 5 days following the vitamin B_{12} injection.

CLINICAL CARE. Patients with pernicious anemia need both immediate care and lifelong therapy with maintenance vitamin B_{12}.

During the *acute* phase of illness, the patient may be treated with injections of vitamin B_{12}.

Generally the patient responds quickly and dramatically to vitamin B_{12} injections. Within 24 to 48 hours the person usually begins to feel less weak, irritable, and depressed, and appetite begins to return. Within 72 hours, reticulocytes begin to increase, and by the end of the first week following initiation of therapy, the patient's total erythrocyte count is significantly higher. With improvement of the blood picture, patients with cardiovascular involvement usually experience a gradual lessening of cardiac symptoms. Although the function of the peripheral nerves may improve with treatment, any spinal cord or brain damage is almost always permanent.

Ferrous sulfate or ferrous gluconate may be given orally following meals, if hemoglobin level fails to rise in proportion to increases in the total erythrocyte count.

As stated earlier, iron deficiency may play a role in the etiology of pernicious anemia; consequently an iron deficit, if present, must be corrected. Also, iron deficiency anemia can develop in the *course* of treating pernicious anemia. Injections of vitamin B_{12} can cause such a rapid regeneration of erythrocytes that the patient's iron stores become depleted. As a result of iron depletion, the hemoglobin level remains low even though the total erythrocyte count rises.

Folic acid is sometimes given, in conjunction with vitamin B_{12}, to patients with a history of poor nutrition. However, folic acid can be a potentially dangerous drug when used to treat pernicious anemia, because it reverses the anemia and the gastrointestinal tract disorders, but it does *not* reverse the neurologic manifestations and may even intensify them.

Some physicians state that folic acid is *contraindicated* in the treatment of pernicious anemia; others point out that folic acid can probably be used safely if given in small doses but vitamin B_{12} should always be given simultaneously.

In addition to medicinal therapy, a number of *supportive measures* may help to sustain the patient through the acute phase of his illness.

- *Blood transfusions.* Generally blood transfusions are not necessary, because patients with pernicious anemia respond quickly and favorably to vitamin B_{12} injections. Occasionally, however, anemia may be so severe that the patient is in danger of developing circulatory collapse and shock. In these extreme cases, blood tranfusions may be life-saving.

► *Nutritious diet.* Encourage patients with pernicious anemia to eat foods high in iron, protein, and vitamins, e.g., fish, meat, milk, and eggs. Instruct the patient who has dyspepsia or a sore mouth to avoid foods which are either coarse, highly seasoned, or difficult to digest. If the patient's appetite is poor because of severe glossitis, administer oral hygiene both before and after meals to clean the mouth and ease discomfort.

► *Bed rest.* A patient with severe anemia is usually kept on bed rest until the acute phase of illness is over and the blood picture improves. If progress is satisfactory, the patient usually begins to ambulate within 2 to 3 weeks following the beginning of vitamin B_{12} therapy.

The patient on bed rest needs special care because of the neurologic and mental disturbances associated with the illness. The individual who is confused or disoriented will need *side rails* on the bed to prevent falls; if the patient is extremely restless or delusional, *restraints* may be necessary. To prevent contractures, joint stiffness, muscle atrophy, and other complications of bed rest, do complete *range of motion exercises* with the patient at least three times daily. Footdrop can be prevented by using a *bed cradle* or *footboard* to lift the weight of bedclothes off the patient's feet. *Physical therapy* is usually ordered for persons with severe neurologic damage to prevent flaccid and spastic paralysis.

Once the patient begins to ambulate, protection from falls is needed, especially at night. Patients with pernicious anemia often have great difficulty walking in the dark; instruct the hospitalized patient to ring for help should he or she need to get up at night.

► *Protection from burns.* When applying hot compresses, hot water bottles, or heating pads, watch the patient carefully for reddening of the skin. Remember that persons with pernicious anemia have reduced sensitivity to sensations of heat and pain.

MAINTENANCE THERAPY. Once the acute stage of the illness is past, the patient with pernicious anemia must enter a *lifelong program of maintenance therapy* with vitamin B_{12}. The nurse plays a vital role in educating patients with this disorder concerning the importance of continuous care.

In addition to lifelong drug therapy, patients with permanent neurologic disabilities need an intensive program of physical therapy and rehabilitation. All patients should be encouraged to see their doctors at least twice a year for a complete physical examination.

PROGNOSIS. If therapy is adequate and uninterrupted, the patient can expect to feel free of the symptoms of anemia for the rest of his or her life; also the person can be assured that the neuropathy will not progress further. However, should the patient fail to take vitamin B_{12} as ordered, symptoms of anemia will return and the neuropathy will worsen within 2 months to 3 years following interruption of therapy.

Other Anemias Due to Vitamin B_{12} Deficiency

While pernicious anemia arises from lack of the intrinsic factor, another group of anemias results from *lack* of the *extrinsic factor* (vitamin B_{12}). Deficiency of the extrinsic factor may be caused by: faulty diet, defective absorption due to intestinal disease, or metabolic disturbances. Although the megaloblastic anemia that develops in these conditions is the same as that seen in pernicious anemia, hypochlorhydria and degenerative neurologic changes *do not occur.* Treatment of vitamin B_{12} deficiency depends upon the specific cause.

An *inadequate dietary intake* of vitamin B_{12} can be corrected by the oral administration of 25 μg. of the vitamin daily, in conjunction with a more balanced diet. Diets deficient in vitamin B_{12} are rarely seen in the United States except among the very poor who cannot afford meat and among strict vegetarians; however, they are common in India and other countries with large poor populations.

Poor absorption of vitamin B_{12} results from: (1) an overgrowth of bacteria within the intestinal tract due to intestinal stasis, (2) infestation with the fish tapeworm, or (3) one of the malabsorption syndromes. Bacteria that proliferate within intestinal blind loops and diverticula (small blind pouches that form in the walls of the colon) cause anemia by competing with the host for available vitamin B_{12}. This problem can be corrected by surgical removal of the pouches or blind loops and by administration of broad-spectrum antibiotics to control infection. The fish tapeworm, which is ingested in raw fish, also competes with its host for vitamin B_{12}. Treatment involves removal of the tapeworm and the temporary administration of vitamin B_{12} until the anemia is corrected.

To treat the anemia caused by malabsorption syndromes (e.g., sprue and celiac disease), the patient is given 100 μg. of vitamin B_{12} IM daily for 10 days, followed by 100 μg. of vitamin B_{12} monthly until the absorption dysfunction is corrected.

Supplemental vitamin B_{12} is given orally to individuals who have an increased need for the vitamin due to metabolic disturbances or changes, e.g., in pregnancy or hyperthyroidism.

Anemia Due to Folic Acid Deficiency

Etiology. Anemia associated with folic acid deficiency is very common. This condition has many causes, the majority of which are identical to the causes of vitamin B_{12} deficiency. Usually folic acid deficiency results from a *poor diet* lacking in such foods as green leafy vegetables, liver, citrus fruits, and yeast. *Chronic alcoholics,* because of their typically inadequate diets, are particularly susceptible to this problem; also, high levels of alcohol in the blood partially block the response of the bone marrow to folic acid, thereby interfering with erythropoiesis.

Second, folic acid deficiency, like vitamin B_{12} deficiency, can develop in conjunction with *malabsorption syndromes* (e.g., sprue, celiac disease, steatorrhea, etc.). Also, certain drugs can impede folic acid absorption and utilization. For example, a serious anemia may develop in conjunction with the long-term use of anticonvulsant drugs (e.g., primidone, diphenylhydantoin, and phenobarbital); the administration of antimetabolites (e.g., folic acid antagonists, purine analogs, and pyrimidine analogs) to patients with cancer and leukemia; and the administration of certain oral contraceptives.

Finally, folic acid deficiency is extremely common in women during the *third trimester of pregnancy.* At this time, expectant mothers have a six times greater than normal need for folic acid.

Bases of Symptoms. Folic acid, like vitamin B_{12}, is necessary for the synthesis of DNA. Both vitamin B_{12} and folic acid deficiencies cause symptoms of megaloblastic anemia (fatigue, cardiac symptoms, slight jaundice) and gastrointestinal tract disturbances (e.g., dyspepsia, smooth beefy tongue); however, *unlike* pernicious anemia, a lack of folic acid does *not* cause neurologic manifestations.

Anemia due to folic acid deficiency has a slow and insidious onset. The patient usually appears quite ill and is often thin and emaciated. Because of the patient's malnourished and debilitated state, symptoms of folic acid deficiency (fatigue, weakness, dyspnea, etc.) are often obscured by other disorders. For example, the patient may suffer from deficiencies of iron, protein, minerals, and all the vitamins and also may be suffering from electrolyte imbalances. Some individuals additionally have neurologic symptoms owing to thiamine, calcium, or magnesium deficiencies; these problems are frequently linked with alcoholism. Cirrhosis of the liver and bleeding varices may further complicate the anemia.

Diagnostic Tests. The megaloblastic anemia caused by folic acid deficiency is identical to that seen in pernicious anemia. It is diagnosed on the basis of blood film and bone marrow examination. Once the presence of a macrocytic anemia is confirmed, the physician must next decide whether the anemia is the result of folic acid or vitamin B_{12} deficiency. If folic acid deficiency is the cause: (1) the serum folate level is less than 4 nanograms (normal is 7 to 20 nanograms); (2) the Schilling test is normal; (3) hydrochloric acid is probably present in the gastric juice; (4) neurologic symptoms are absent; and (5) the patient responds favorably to a therapeutic trial of 50 to 100 μg. of folic acid IM daily for 10 days.

Clinical Care. To treat anemia due to folate deficiency the patient is given oral doses of folic acid (0.1 to 5 mg.) daily until the blood picture improves or until the cause of intestinal malabsorption is corrected. Patients with malabsorption syndromes may need parenteral folic acid initially, followed by maintenance therapy with oral doses.

Folic acid is administered parenterally in the form of folinic acid (Leucovorin Calcium injection).

Vitamin C is sometimes prescribed in addition to folic acid because it augments the role of folic acid in promoting erythropoiesis.

ANEMIA OF BONE MARROW FAILURE

General Considerations. The anemia of bone marrow failure has several names, each of which is descriptive of some aspect of the disease, i.e., aplastic, hypoplastic, aregenerative, or primary refractory anemia. *Aplastic anemia* is the term most commonly used. The word "aplastic" means "having deficient or arrested development." Thus, aplastic anemia is a deficiency of circulating erythrocytes owing to the arrested development of red cells within the bone marrow.

Although aplastic anemia sometimes occurs alone (pure RBC aplasia), it is usually accompanied by *agranulocytosis* (a reduction in leukocytes, particularly granulocytes), and *thrombocytopenia* (reduction in thrombocyte or platelets). These three problems occur together because the bone marrow produces not only erythrocytes but leukocytes and thrombocytes as well. Consequently, if the bone marrow is abnormal for any reason or if it has suffered exposure to a myelotoxin (any substance that is toxic and damaging to bone marrow), production of erythrocytes, leukocytes, and thrombocytes slows greatly, and a deficiency of all three types of cells develops; this condition is called *pancytopenia* (i.e., depression of all cellular blood elements). Pancytopenia affects people of all ages; both sexes are equally susceptible. The incidence of aplastic anemia is approximately four cases per million population.

Etiology. In approximately one half of patients, the etiology of aplastic anemia is *unknown;* the cause may possibly be asociated with chromosomal aberrations or tumors of the thymus gland (thymomas). Exposure to a specific myelotoxin is thought to be the causative agent in many other patients presenting with aplastic anemia or pancytopenia.

There are three groups of myelotoxins:

1. Agents that *always* cause marrow damage when given in sufficiently large doses; e.g., radiant energy (x-rays, radium, radioactive isotopes of gold, phosphorus, etc.); benzene and benzene derivatives; and the alkylating agents and antimetabolites used to treat malignant tumors.
2. Agents that are *occasionally* responsible for marrow failure; chloromycetin (the drug most commonly linked with aplastic anemia), sulfonamides, quinacrine, phenylbutazone, the anticonvulsants diphenylhydantoin and mephenytoin, and the gold compounds.
3. Suspicious agents that have been linked with aplastic anemia in *only a few cases,* e.g., streptomycin, tripelennamine, DDT, meprobamate, hair and aniline dyes, and carbon tetrachloride.

Why do the above agents cause the bone marrow to stop producing blood cells? Radiant energy inhibits mitosis or cell division. The antimetabolites employed in cancer chemotherapy block the synthesis of purines or nucleic acids. However, in the majority of cases, the exact mechanism by which the above agents cause marrow failure is unknown. Also, it is not known why certain drugs and chemicals cause a pancytopenia in some persons and not in others. To date, the most plausible reason is that some individuals are hypersensitive to certain drugs; consequently, the development of marrow failure in these cases is an *idiosyncratic reaction.*

Symptoms and Laboratory Picture. The onset of aplastic anemia may be insidious or rapid. In idiopathic or hereditary cases, the onset is usually gradual. However, when bone marrow failure is the result of a myelotoxin, the onset may be explosive and the patient may quickly develop distressing symptoms.

The manifestations of pancytopenia are particularly severe because not only is the erythrocyte count reduced, but the leukocyte and platelet counts are lowered as well. Consequently the patient develops the following three conditions:

1. *Normocytic anemia.* The *erythrocyte count* is usually below 1 million/cu. mm., and the *reticulocyte count* is also low. The patient reports progressive fatigue, lassitude, and dyspnea.
2. *Granulocytopenia.* The leukocyte count may be less than 2000/cu. mm. (normal is 6000 to 9000/cu. mm.). The patient suffers from an increased susceptibility to infection because, without leukocytes, the body cannot adequately battle bacteria and other invading organisms. (See Chapter 10.) If the leukocyte count drops below 1000 cells per cu. mm. the patient becomes vulnerable to severe fulminating bacterial infections.
3. *Thrombocytopenia.* The platelet count may fall to less than 30,000/cu. mm. (normal is 200,000 to 350,000/cu. mm.). Reduced thrombocyte levels usually cause bleeding into the skin and mucous membranes; if thrombocytes are severely reduced, the patient will hemorrhage.

The diagnosis of aplastic anemia and pancytopenia is based on graphic representation of the differential blood count, the patient's symptoms, a history of exposure to a myelotoxin, and a bone marrow examination. In pancytopenia, the bone marrow is fatty and contains very few developing blood cells.

Clinical Care. The patient with pancytopenia is often critically ill; prompt medical attention and skillful nursing care are necessary. The first step in halting the process of aplastic anemia is *immediate withdrawal of the offending agent or drug.* Any patient who is either undergoing radiotherapy or who is receiving a drug that is a suspected myelotoxin must be protected from marrow failure by frequent hemograms. The signal for withdrawal of the drug in question is a significant drop in the erythrocyte, leukocyte, or platelet count. Usually, prompt termination of a suspicious agent is followed by a rise in the blood count. Unfortunately, in the case of the antibiotic chloramphemicol (Chloromycetin), marrow failure may progress despite discontinuation of the drug.

If aplastic anemia does develop, *blood transfusions* are the mainstay of therapy. However, transfusions are discontinued as soon as the bone marrow begins to produce blood cells. Repeated transfusions can result in hemosiderosis (an increase in tissue iron stores) and an enlarged spleen. Extensive trials have been performed with chelating agents, especially desferrioxamine.[126] They are used as a substitute method for iron removal in patients whose anemia is severe enough to preclude a phlebotomy.[126] *Corticosteroids* and *androgens* are sometimes prescribed on a trial basis to help to stimulate bone marrow function. Unfortunately, in a large number of cases, these drugs fail to restore bone marrow activity.

Splenectomy is considered when the patient has an enlarged spleen which is either destroying normal cells or suppressing the development of blood cells within the bone marrow. However, for patients with decreased leukocyte and platelet counts, splenectomy is a dangerous operation because of the risk of infection and hemorrhage.

Bone marrow transplantation can be performed in specialized centers for those patients who have a matched sibling. Tissue typing techniques determine the presence of a "match." Patients who survive bone marrow transplantation for aplastic anemias are capable of living totally normal, healthy lives.

The prevention and treatment of *complications* resulting from pancytopenia is the final important aspect of care. The two major complications of this condition are *infections* (respiratory, urinary, etc.) and *bleeding*.

> *The prevention of infection is largely a nursing responsibility.*

Patients must be isolated from other patients and from personnel with infections of any type. If the patient's white count drops below 1000 per cu. mm., strict reverse isolation is necessary.* To build resistance against infection, encourage the patient to eat foods high in vitamins and protein. If the patient has a sore mouth, administer oral hygiene before and after meals. Observe the patient carefully for signs that an infectious process is beginning, e.g., a rise in temperature, the "sniffles," a sore throat, severe anorexia, the appearance of ulcerations on mucous membranes, pain and burning upon urination. When an infection develops, the physician determines the causative organism and orders a specific antibiotic. Antibiotics are rarely administered prophylactically to patients with pancytopenia because such a practice encourages the development of drug-resistant organisms.

To control *bleeding* (which results from thrombocytopenia) corticosteroids are occasionally given to increase capillary resistance; also, the physician may order the administration of platelet-rich transfusions. In order to reduce platelet antibody formation, patients should receive, when possible, platelets from HL-A compatible donors. Depending upon the severity of their disease, women of childbearing age may be considered for a prophylactic amenorrhea program to prevent blood loss. These programs vary among institutions but usually involve administration of an estrogen or possibly progesterone compound. Such intervention diminishes the actual blood loss during menstruation.

*Reverse isolation procedures are considered in the discussion of leukemia. (See Chapter 46.)

Nursing measures and precaution that help to prevent episodes of bleeding are as follows:

- Caution the patient not to pick at the nose; advise use of a *soft* toothbrush and use of an *electric* razor, to prevent injuries.
- Obtain orders for the *oral* administration of medications whenever possible; if you must administer a medication by injection, use a dry sponge to exert mild pressure over the injection site until bleeding has *stopped completely*.
- Carefully record the patient's bowel movements and at the first sign of constipation obtain an order for a stool softener or laxative if necessary. Hard stools can damage the rectal mucosa and straining at stool can increase intra-abdominal pressure and thereby cause internal bleeding.

Prognosis. Over 50 per cent of patients with severe pancytopenia die, usually either from hemorrhage or from overwhelming infection. Death usually occurs within a few months following the onset of the anemia. Of the 40 to 50 per cent who survive, approximately 25 per cent die by the end of the third year following development of the condition; the other 25 per cent of patients either recover completely or remain semi-invalids for years. The prognosis for this condition is best when the myelotoxic agent is identified and discontinued *early* in the course of the disease.

Anemias Resulting from Excessive Erythrocyte Destruction (Hemolytic Anemias)

General Considerations. Aged, dead, and defective cells are removed from the circulation by reticuloendothelial cells (located mainly within the liver, spleen, and bone marrow). Normally, erythrocytes survive in the circulation for approximately 120 days before removal. However, in hemolytic anemia, the rate of erythrocyte destruction is greatly accelerated. Thus, the three major hallmarks of hemolytic anemia are:

1. A shortening of the erythrocyte life span
2. An abnormal increase in the numbers of erythrocytes destroyed by reticuloendothelial elements
3. Failure of the bone marrow to produce sufficient erythrocytes to compensate for the vast numbers of red cells lost

What are the causes of hemolytic anemia? Hemolysis of erythrocytes is the result of either: (1) an *intracorpuscular defect* within the erythrocyte itself, which is sometimes triggered by an extracellular factor (e.g, drugs, plasma components, or splenic hyperactivity), or (2) an *extracorpuscular factor* (a factor or mechanism *external* to the erythrocyte, e.g., infections and chemical or physical agents).

Symptoms and Laboratory Findings. Hemolytic anemia may be acute or chronic. There are also chronic forms of hemolytic anemia punctuated by severe acute episodes of hemolysis called *hemolytic crises.*

The patient with hemolytic anemia suffers from all the general manifestations of *anemia* discussed earlier, i.e., lassitude, fatigue, and so forth. The specific signs and symptoms that characterize hemolytic anemia are listed and explained in Table 45–5. In addition, some patients experience hemolytic crises. These are, in some cases, precipitated by the development of an acute infection. The major symptoms of hemolytic crisis are malaise, chills, fever, aches and pains in the abdomen or back, and red or black urine. The major complication of an acute hemolytic crisis is *acute renal failure* resulting from ischemic necrosis of renal tubules.

Laboratory findings diagnostic of hemolytic anemia usually include: normocytic anemia, reticulocytosis due to increased efforts of the bone marrow to compensate for excessive erythrocyte destruction, increased red cell fragility, shortened erythrocyte life span, hyperbilirubinemia, increased fecal and urinary urobilinogen, and hemoglobinemia in cases of massive intravascular hemolysis.

Clinical Care. The *treatment* of hemolytic anemia includes the following basic clinical steps:

- Pinpoint and *eliminate,* whenever possible, *causative factors* that precipitate episodes of hemolysis, e.g., infections, exposure to certain chemicals.
- Maintain *fluid and electrolyte balance.* Administer intravenous infusions as ordered, carefully check and record patient's intake and output.
- Maintain *renal function.* In cases of severe hemolysis, infusions of either sodium bicarbonate or sodium lactate are administered to alkalize the urine.
- *Combat anemia* and *shock* with the cautious administration of blood transfusions. Caution is necessary because the transfused cells will be rapidly destroyed if the patient has an autoimmune hemolytic disease. If an autoimmune mechanism is responsible for hemolysis of cells, the patient is treated with steroids. When corticosteroids fail to halt hemolytic reactions in autoimmune disorders, splenectomy is usually the treatment of choice.

HEMOLYTIC ANEMIAS DUE MAINLY TO INTRINSIC ERYTHROCYTE DEFECTS

Glucose-6-Phosphate Dehydrogenase (G6PD) Deficiency. G6PD is an important red cell enzyme; consequently G6PD deficiency can be defined as an *enzymopathy,* a *genetic defect* that involves the partial or complete deficiency of certain essential enzymes. The specific detrimental effect of G6PD deficiency upon erythrocytes is to make them more susceptible to hemolysis following ingestion of those drugs and foods classified as *chemical oxidants.*

An inherited sex-linked disorder, G6PD deficiency is a common problem, affecting at least 100 million persons in the world. Among Americans, G6PD deficiency affects 10 to 15 per cent of American blacks and about 1 to 2 per cent of American whites. It is also fairly common among people who live close to the Mediterranean, e.g., Greeks, Italians, Arabs. Individuals with this enzymopathy may remain completely asymptomatic throughout their lives, since, typically, symptoms develop only following exposure to certain agents. Occasionally, however, Caucasian persons develop spontaneous attacks of hemolytic anemia that have not been precipitated by a known external factor.

G6PD deficiency causes hemolysis of red cells because erythrocytes require glucose for energy; the enzyme G6PD is responsible for approximately 10 per cent of the glucose metabolized by erythrocytes. When red cells are exposed to oxidative drugs and foods, the amount of glucose that the red cell must metabolize is greatly increased above normal. If a G6PD deficiency exists, the red cells are unable to adequately metabolize glucose, and, consequently, they can-

TABLE 45–5. SIGNS AND SYMPTOMS OF HEMOLYTIC ANEMIA

Signs and Symptoms	Bases
Jaundice (yellowness of the skin and eyes)	Abnormally large amounts of bilirubin accumulate within the blood, owing to excessive destruction of erythrocytes.
Splenomegaly, hepatomegaly, and hyperplasia of bone marrow	Reticuloendothelial elements within the spleen, liver, and bone marrow become hyperactive because of the increased demands upon them to phagocytize defective erythrocytes.
Cholelithiasis (pigment gallstones)	Excessive accumulation of bilirubin due to destruction of erythrocytes leads to development of pigment stones within the gallbladder.

not cope with the oxidative effects of certain substances. As a result, hemolysis occurs. Because young, newly released erythrocytes contain a substantial amount of G6PD, only aging erythrocytes are destroyed upon exposure to causative agents.

More than 40 oxidative drugs and foods produce hemolytic anemia in persons with G6PD deficiency, e.g., primaquine, quinine, aspirin, sulfonamides, phenacetin, vitamin K derivatives, chloramphenicol (Chloromycetin), the thiazide diuretics, and the fava bean.

Following exposure to any of the above agents, the individual with G6PD deficiency develops *acute intravascular hemolysis* lasting about 7 to 12 days. During this acute phase, the patient suffers from anemia and jaundice. Laboratory findings include moderate hemoglobinemia and hemoglobinuria, an elevated serum bilirubin, reticulocytosis, and the appearance of Heinz bodies (small particles of oxidized hemoglobin) within the red cell. Following the acute hemolytic stage, the patient's blood picture *automatically* begins to improve, whether or not the offending drug is discontinued. The hemolytic reaction of persons with G6PD deficiency is self-limiting because, as mentioned, only *older* erythrocytes are destroyed when in contact with a chemical oxidant. However, if drug exposure continues for long, the patient will develop chronic hyperhemolysis until contact with the offending agent is ended.

Treatment of this condition involves the identification and total removal of the drug or food precipitating the hemolytic reaction. Care of the patient during the week of acute hemolysis is purely symptomatic, i.e., rest, fluids, nutritious diet, and so forth.

Because drugs that precipitate hemolytic reactions in G6PD deficiency are common (e.g., aspirin, phenacetin), and because G6PD has a high worldwide incidence, screening tests for this enzymopathy should be a part of every public health program. Careful screening is particularly important for the black population. Tests must be performed when the patient is well, or the results are unreliable. One of the most striking laboratory signs of this condition is the appearance of "bite" cells in the peripheral blood. "Bite" cells are erythrocytes that look as if they have had "bites" taken from their peripheries, possibly because Heinz bodies have been removed from the cells by the spleen.[9] It is important that persons be screened for G6PD deficiency before donating blood, because the administration of cells deficient in G6PD can be hazardous for the recipient.

Hereditary Spherocytosis (Congenital Hemolytic Jaundice, Congenital Spherocytic Anemia)

General Considerations. Hereditary spherocytosis is a common form of chronic hemolytic anemia found in all races and all ages. This condition is *inherited* as a simple mendelian dominant trait. Because the trait is *dominant*, a child can inherit hereditary spherocytosis if only one parent carries the abnormal gene.

The two most distinctive characteristics of hereditary spherocytosis are the appearance of large numbers of *spherical-shaped erythrocytes* ("spherocytosis"), and an *enlarged spleen*. *Spherocytosis* develops because the erythrocytes have a defective cellular membrane, extremely permeable to the influx of sodium ions. In order to curtail the flow of sodium ions through its defective membrane, the erythrocyte must increase its metabolic work and, consequently, its expenditure of glucose. Eventually, glucose and cellular energy become depleted and sodium ions flow through the cellular membrane without resistance. Thus, the red cell interior becomes *hypertonic*. Intracellular hypertonicity, in turn, draws water to the cell, causing the erythrocyte to swell and become spherical in shape. Because spherocytes are thick and relatively inflexible, they are easily trapped within the splenic venous sinusoids, where they are devoured by phagocytes. As a result, the *spleen* becomes greatly enlarged owing to overwork, and the patient suffers from *anemia* and *jaundice* as a result of the massive hemolysis of red cells within the spleen.

Symptoms and Laboratory Findings. The symptoms of hereditary spherocytosis are the same as the general symptoms of hemolytic anemia discussed earlier, e.g., malaise, anemia, jaundice, gallstones, and splenomegaly. Splenomegaly is more pronounced in this condition than in any other form of hemolytic anemia. Because of the massive size of the spleen, patients with hereditary spherocytosis experience left upper quadrant fullness and abdominal pain. Occasionally *acute* abdominal pain develops as a result of splenic infarction. Persons with this disorder suffer from severe hemolytic crises, which are sometimes fatal.

Laboratory findings are distinctive and include: (1) spherocytes in the blood smear, (2) reticulocytosis, (3) lowered red cell count and hemoglobin values, and (4) increased osmotic fragility. Osmotic fragility is increased because the spherocyte has a smaller surface area than the normal biconcave erythrocyte and a larger cell content than normal because of the excessive inflow of water and sodium into the cell. As a result of these two factors, spherocytes rupture quickly when placed in hypotonic saline solutions, because they cannot tolerate a further influx of water.

Clinical Care. Although the administration of blood transfusions may benefit the patient in hemolytic crisis, the only treatment indicated in all cases of hereditary spherocytosis is splenectomy. Ninety per cent of patients who undergo splenectomy experience complete reversal of symptoms. Although spherocytes continue to circulate, these misshaped cells usually have a more normal life span once the spleen is removed. Nonetheless, this condition cannot be completely cured.

HEMOLYTIC ANEMIAS DUE MAINLY TO EXTRA-ERYTHROCYTE FACTORS (ACQUIRED HEMOLYTIC ANEMIAS)

The major extracorpuscular factors that can result in hemolytic anemia include: trauma, chemical agents and drugs, infectious agents, systemic diseases, isoimmune reactions, and autoimmune disorders.

Hemolysis Due to Trauma. Hemolytic anemia may develop swiftly following severe *burns.* Clinical findings include a large drop in the erythrocyte count, hemoglobinemia, and hemoglobinuria. Also, hemolysis of red cells sometimes occurs following replacement of defective heart valves with prosthetic valves or the repair of cardiac septal defects. Trauma to erythrocytes caused by either burns or surgery causes the cells to fragment. Fragmented erythrocytes (schistocytes) are quickly destroyed by phagocytes.

Hemolysis Due to Chemical Agents and Drugs (Toxic Hemolytic Anemia). Many drugs and chemicals can cause hemolysis of red cells. Chemical and drug reactions are generally due to one of the following factors: the *oxidant effects* of the drug or chemical, or an *immune reaction* precipitated by the drug.

Chemical oxidants vary greatly in their potency and consequently in their ability to destroy erythrocytes. Some chemical oxidants are relatively mild and cause hemolytic reactions in only a small segment of the world population (for example, persons with G6PD deficiency). Other chemical oxidants are so toxic that they cause hemolytic reactions in every person exposed to a sufficient dose of the substance, e.g., benzene, phenylhydrazine, nitrites, potassium chlorate, arsenic, colloidal silver, and lead. These powerful compounds are capable of damaging the red cell membrane. As a result, the cell becomes more fragile and is quickly destroyed.

One of the most common examples of hemolysis due to contact with a chemical agent is *lead poisoning (plumbism).* Lead poisoning causes characteristic changes in the brain, nervous system, spinal cord, and digestive tract. Industrial workers who are daily exposed to lead vapors, mist, or dust may become victims of plumbism. Also, small children can develop lead poisoning when allowed to chew on furniture or windowsills covered with lead-based paint or to eat chips of flaking lead-based paint, found in older, deteriorating buildings. The symptoms of plumbism are illustrated in Figure 45–2. Treatment of this condition involves administering mild saline cathartics in order to promote the elimination of lead salts from the intestinal tract, followed by the giving of a chelating agent such as calcium disodium edetate.

An *immune* response, the second major cause of toxic hemolysis, is the result of an antigen-antibody reaction. (See Chapter 11.) Drugs that can precipitate antigen-antibody reactions in susceptible individuals are quinine, quinidine, methyldopa, sulfonamides, phenacetin, and penicillin. The most common example of an immune response to a drug is the "penicillin reaction." Penicillin is a potentially dangerous drug because it is a hapten. As you recall from Chapter 11, a *hapten* is a substance that is normally nonantigenic but which has the capacity to combine with a body protein. When this combination takes place, the body protein is modified in such a way that it can act as a foreign antigen. As a result, the body builds antibodies that react with the altered body protein in an antigen-antibody reaction.

Finally, certain snake and spider venoms as well as some vegetable poisons (e.g., some mushrooms) cause hemolytic reactions that are frequently fatal.

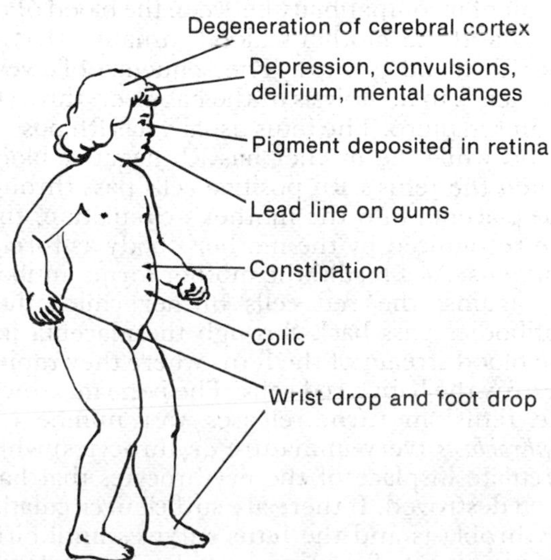

Figure 45–2. Effects of lead poisoning.

Hemolysis Due to Infectious Agents. Hemolytic anemia may develop as a complication of several different conditions caused by microorganisms, e.g., bacterial endocarditis, malaria, miliary tuberculosis, infectious hepatis, infectious mononucleosis, and meningococcemia.

Infectious organisms can cause hemolytic anemia in three ways: by releasing toxins that act as hemolyzers, by entering the red cell and destroying it, and by promoting antigen-antibody reactions. For example, the organism may attach itself to the surface of the cell; as a result, the cell surface becomes so altered that it acts as a foreign antigen. In response to the altered red cell, antibodies form and an immune reaction takes place.

Hemolytic Anemia Secondary to Systemic Diseases. Hemolytic anemia sometimes complicates the following systemic conditions: Hodgkin's disease, leukemias, renal cortical necrosis, lymphomas, and systemic lupus erythematosus.

Hemolysis Due to Isoimmune Hemolytic Reactions. An isoimmune hemolytic reaction is an antigen-antibody reaction in which erythrocytes are destroyed by antibodies that have developed in response to antigens from another individual of the same species. One example of an isoimmune hemolytic reaction is the *transfusion reaction.* The most severe transfusion reactions involve the hemolysis of the *donor* red cells by antibodies within the blood of the recipient.

Erythroblastosis fetalis, a disorder seen in the newborn, provides a second example of a hemolytic isoimmune reaction. This condition is the result of incompatibility between the blood of the fetus and the mother's blood, usually affecting the Rh blood groups. The sequence of events that leads to hemolysis of the baby's erythrocytes begins in utero. The fetus usually has Rh positive blood while the mother has Rh negative blood. When the fetus's Rh positive cells pass through the placenta into the mother's circulation, they are recognized by the mother's body as foreign antigens. As a result, the mother forms antibodies against the red cells of her child; these antibodies pass back through the placenta into the blood stream of the fetus where they rapidly destroy the baby's red cells. The bone marrow of the fetus, in turn, releases vast numbers of *erythroblasts* (very immature erythrocytes) which circulate in place of the erythrocytes that have been destroyed. If there are sufficient circulating erythroblasts and the fetus survives until birth, the treatment of choice is an *exchange* transfusion in which the fetus's Rh positive blood is replaced by Rh negative blood, thereby halting the hemolytic process.*

Hemolysis Due to Autoimmune Disorders. Autoantibodies, like isoantibodies, are capable of destroying red blood cells. Unlike isoantibodies, autoantibodies do not develop against an antigen from *another* individual of the same species; instead they arise in response to autoantigens that have developed within the body of the *individual.* (See Chapter 11.)

Autoimmune hemolytic anemia is a disorder of the immune mechanism in which the patient's immune system produces antibodies that agglutinate his or her *own red cells* in an antigen-antibody reaction. As a result, the agglutinated cells clump together and are phagocytized within the spleen.

This condition arises in two ways: First, it may develop *secondary* to other autoimmune disorders or following the administration of certain drugs. Autoimmune conditions sometimes complicated by hemolytic anemia include systemic lupus erythematosus and the lymphoproliferative diseases (leukemia, lymphosarcoma). Drugs that sometimes precipitate autoimmune hemolytic anemia include penicillin (which acts as a hapten), quinidine, quinine, and methyldopa. Second, this disease can develop spontaneously and without a history of prior autoimmune disease; this is known as *idiopathic autoimmune hemolytic anemia.* This condition is characterized by a mild to moderate hemolysis. The red blood cells become coated with IgG antibodies that arise spontaneously or following ingestion of one of the above drugs.

The symptoms of autoimmune hemolytic anemia differ little from those of other hemolytic anemias. Profound, sometimes fatal, sporadic *hemolytic crises* are common. Other complications include gallstones and thrombocytopenic purpura.

Autoimmune hemolytic anemia is mainly diagnosed on the basis of a positive Coombs' test. As you recall, the Coombs' test is a method for detecting whether the patient's red cells are coated with antibodies.

The *treatment* of secondary autoimmune hemolytic anemia includes treatment of the underlying autoimmune condition and termination of the use of any suspicious drugs.

The idiopathic form of the disease is treated with steroids, transfusions, and splenectomy when indicated. The *steroid* of choice is prednisolone.

Transfusions may give temporary relief from symptoms. However, they do not adequately restore the patient's erythrocyte level, because

*More sophisticated techniques are being developed for the treatment of erythroblastosis fetalis. For information, consult a textbook of pediatrics.

the donor cells are often rapidly destroyed by the patient's antibodies.

Splenectomy is the treatment of choice if steroids fail to produce a remission or if the side effects of steroid therapy are too severe. Once the spleen is removed, recurrences of hemolytic anemia may develop, but they are far less severe than the hemolytic crises prior to surgery. Such minor hemolytic episodes are usually controlled by steroid therapy.

The Paroxysmal Hemoglobinurias. A "paroxysm" is an episode or occurrence of abrupt onset and termination. *Hemoglobinuria* means that hemoglobin is present in the urine. In sum, the term "paroxysmal hemoglobinuria" describes a rare and serious condition in which the patient suffers from acute episodes of intravascular hemolysis which result in the passage of hemoglobin into the urine.

Attacks of paroxysmal hemoglobinuria can be precipitated by: (1) *sleep* (paroxysmal nocturnal hemoglobinuria); (2) exposure to *cold* temperatures (paroxysmal cold hemoglobinuria); and (3) extreme *exertions,* as in marching for long distances (march hemoglobinuria). Because paroxysmal nocturnal hemoglobinuria is the most common of these three conditions, it is discussed in more detail.

PAROXYSMAL NOCTURNAL HEMOGLOBINURIA (PNH). This condition is a rare, severely incapacitating blood dyscrasia which most commonly strikes young men in their twenties. The exact cause of this disease remains a mystery. However, PNH evidently results from an unknown defect within the erythrocyte itself that makes the red cell vulnerable to hemolysis when in contact with components normally found in plasma (e.g., magnesium, properdin, and complement). Extrinsic factors that can precipitate hemolytic episodes include infection, menstruation, and the administration of iron or vaccines.

The anemia produced by PNH is both normocytic and normochromic. Symptoms are similar to those of other hemolytic anemias, e.g., jaundice, chronic fatigue, scleral icterus, splenomegaly. In addition to these manifestations, the patient's urine, following sleep, is often dark brown or the color of port wine because of acute hemolytic episodes. When hemoglobinuria continues for days or weeks, substantial losses of iron eventually result in the development of *iron deficiency anemia.* In severe cases of PNH, *complications* include leukopenia, thrombocytopenia, and thrombosis. Thrombi may develop following a severe hemolytic episode and commonly cause death.

Because PNH cannot as yet be cured, *treatment* is directed toward alleviation of symptoms. The treatment of choice is the administration of red blood cells that have been washed in saline. Whole blood transfusions are usually *not* given, because factors within the donor plasma may precipitate further hemolysis of the patient's erythrocytes. Also, iron salts are given to patients with iron deficiency anemia. Androgens are occasionally administered to promote erythropoiesis.

Although an individual with this condition may live a normal number of years, the disease is *chronic,* and debilitating attacks of hemolytic anemia may occur throughout life. However, in many cases the patient is able to lead an active normal life between attacks.

Anemias Resulting from Both Disturbances of Erythrocyte Production and Increased Erythrocyte Destruction

IMPAIRED HEMOGLOBIN SYNTHESIS

The Hemoglobinopathies. As mentioned earlier, each molecule of hemoglobin is composed of four molecules of an iron-porphyrin complex called *heme* and one molecule of a simple protein called *globin.* It is the *globin* portion of hemoglobin that is defective or deficient when hemoglobin synthesis is abnormal. In order to understand anemias due to defective hemoglobin synthesis, we must first review the basic structure of a globin molecule.

Each globin molecule is composed of two pairs of polypeptide chains; one pair of chains is called the "alpha" chain, the other pair, the "beta" chain (Fig. 45–3). Each alpha chain contains 141 amino acid residues, while each beta chain contains 146 amino acid residues, making 574 amino acid residues in all. The number and sequence of amino acids on the alpha chain is regulated by one gene called a "structural" or "regulatory" gene; another gene controls the amino acid sequence on the beta chain. The

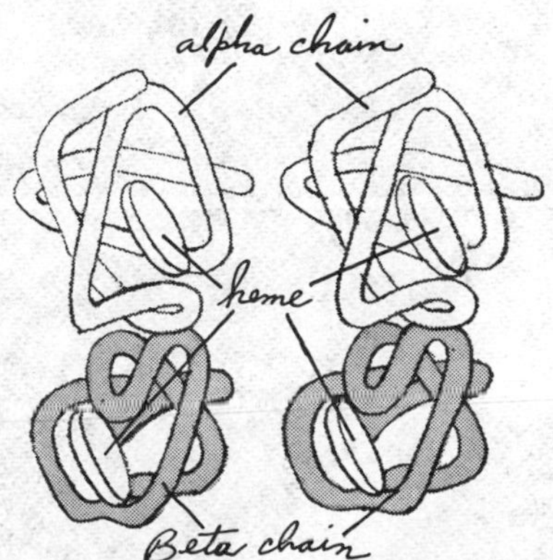

Figure 45–3. Structure of the hemoglobin molecule. (From Foster, S.: *American Journal of Nursing, 71*:1952, October, 1971.)

arrangement of amino acids on each pair of chains does not normally vary from person to person. *Any deviation* in the precise number or sequence of amino acid residues results in a disorder of hemoglobin synthesis.

Hemoglobinopathies are a group of conditions characterized by the formation of abnormal hemoglobin. Specifically, they are due to abnormalities of the polypeptide chains forming the globin molecule. In the majority of cases, the beta chains are defective. The abnormalities of alpha or beta chains, resulting in defective hemoglobin, are generally caused by *minute variations* in the sequence of the amino acid residues composing the chains. As one author writes of sickle cell anemia (the most important hemoglobinopathy): "Of the 574 amino acid residues which compose the globin of a hemoglobin molecule, the substitution of only two [amino acid residues] causes 50 per cent of homozygous Hb S (sickle cell hemoglobin) carriers to expire before age 20 and is lethal to most of the remaining sufferers by middle age."[102a] Thus, while the difference between normal hemoglobin and abnormal hemoglobin is minute, it is extremely important.

The three major forms of normal hemoglobin are hemoglobin A, hemoglobin A_2, and fetal hemoglobin (hemoglobin F); 97 per cent of the hemoglobin of a normal person is composed of hemoglobin A and 2 to 3 per cent is hemoglobins A_2 and F. *Variants* of hemoglobin A number over 100. They include hemoglobins C, D, E, G, H, I, J, K, L, M, N, O, P, Q, and S. Fortunately the majority of these abnormal hemoglobins are not detrimental to health and do not cause anemia or symptoms of any kind. In the United States, the only abnormal hemoglobins that are of consequence are hemoglobin S (sickle cell hemoglobin), hemoglobin C, and hemoglobin D. These forms of abnormal hemoglobins produce a relatively mild disorder in persons who are heterozygous carriers of the trait (those who inherit the gene from only one parent), and profound sometimes fatal anemia in homozygous carriers (those who inherit the gene from both parents).

SICKLE CELL ANEMIA AND SICKLE CELL TRAIT. Sickle cell anemia (Hb SS disease) is a chronic hereditary hemolytic disorder, primarily affecting the black population of the world. It is characterized by the presence, in the patient's red blood cells, of an abnormal type of hemoglobin: hemoglobin S (Hb S) instead of hemoglobin A (Hb A). These cells assume a sickle or crescent shape when oxygen in the blood decreases (Fig. 45–4). Once they "sickle," these abnormal cells are easily destroyed by the thousands as they attempt to circulate through the body's smaller vessels.

Sickle cell trait is generally a relatively mild condition that may produce few or no symptoms. It is present in persons who are *heterozygous* for sickle cell hemoglobin.

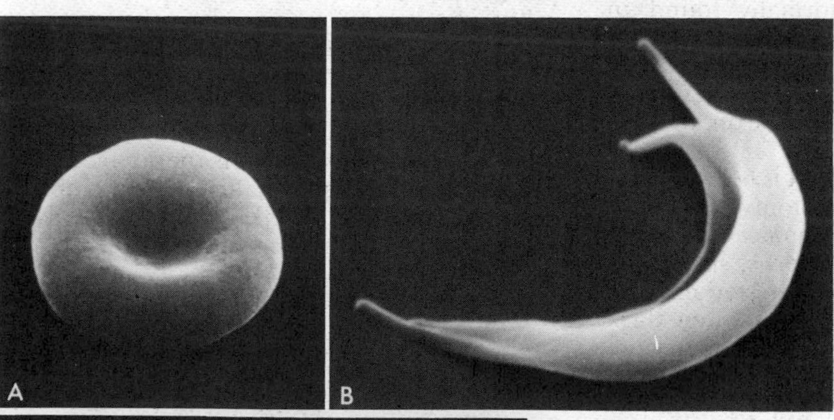

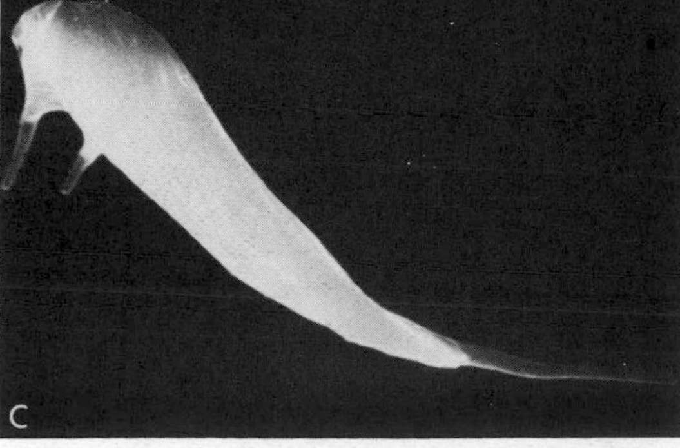

Figure 45–4. Scanning electron micrograph of erythrocytes. Comparison of a normal cell (*A*) and deoxygenated sickled cells (*B* and *C*). (Courtesy of Dr. James White, from Bunn, H. F., et al.: *Human Hemoglobins.* Philadelphia: W. B. Saunders Co., 1977.)

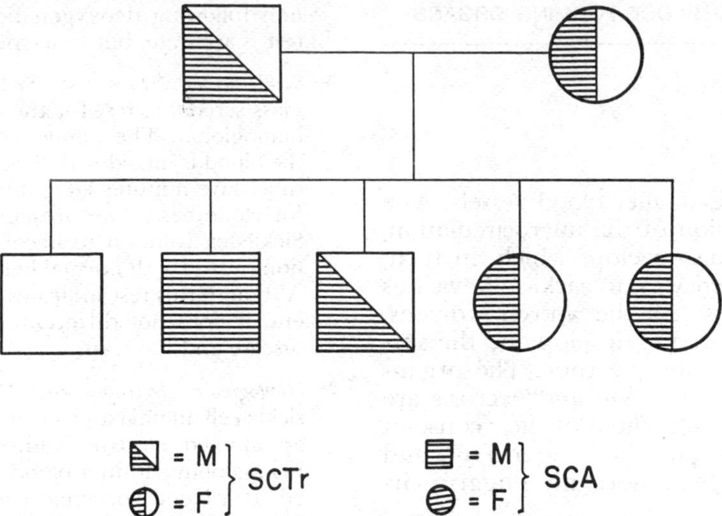

Figure 45–5. Possible inheritance pattern of sickle cell anemia with parents heterozygous for hemoglobin S. SCTr = sickle cell trait and SCA = sickle cell anemia (homozygous sickle cell disease). (From Leavell, B. S., and O. S. Thorup: *Fundamentals of Clinical Hematology.* Philadelphia: W. B. Saunders Co., 1976.)

Incidence and Pathogenesis. As shown in Figure 45–5, whether a person will have sickle cell anemia, sickle cell trait, or neither, depends upon the genes for hemoglobin that the person has inherited from each parent. Persons who are homozygous for Hb S are estimated to have erythrocytes that contain 80 to 100 per cent abnormal Hb S and only up to 20 per cent normal Hb A. The erythrocytes of persons with sickle cell trait contain approximately 25 to 40 per cent Hb S and 60 to 75 per cent Hb A.

Both sickle cell anemia and sickle cell trait are found predominantly among black people. Within the United States alone, "two million black Americans, or 1 in every 10, carry a gene for sickle hemoglobin and have sickle cell trait. One in every 500 black newborn infants in the country has sickle cell anemia and at present about 27,000 to 36,000 people are affected. Each person with sickle cell anemia has only a fifty per cent chance of reaching his twentieth birthday."[50]

Sickle cell anemia develops as a result of a genetic mutation that is transmitted from parent to child. The sickle hemoglobin is an inherited variant of adult hemoglobin. As mentioned earlier, the presence of Hb S in the hemoglobin molecule causes deformation of the red blood cell's round shape into a sickle or crescent. This occurs when the oxygen in the blood decreases.

The underlying problem that causes the occurrence of the sickle cell hemoglobin at the molecular level is the substitution of valine* on each beta chain where a glutanic acid should occur. (See earlier explanation of the hemoglobin molecule.) This valine substitution causes an abnormal reaction between hemoglobin S molecules when the oxygen in the blood decreases. During the abnormal reaction, the alpha and beta chains in the sickle hemoglobin line up in a pathologic chain and a deformed, elongated, ('sickle') red blood cell results.

The exact mechanisms that precipitate sickling crises or "attacks," which take varying forms in different persons, remain somewhat unclear. However, two major factors are definitely linked with the sickling of cells; these are *hypoxia,* owing to low oxygen tensions, and an *elevated blood viscosity,* owing to an increased concentration of sickled cells.

Hypoxia develops in persons with Hb S whenever they are exposed to low oxygen tensions as a result of climbing to high altitudes, flying in nonpressurized planes, exercising strenuously, or undergoing anesthesia without receiving adequate oxygenation. Although both Hb S and Hb A have the same solubility when oxygenated, *deoxygenation* of the blood drastically affects Hb S. Thus, when normal hemoglobin is deoxygenated, it becomes only half as soluble as when oxygenated, whereas sickle cell hemoglobin becomes 50 times less soluble. According to various investigators, the decreased solubility of Hb S causes it to become more viscous and to crystallize, thereby deforming the shape of the cell, through the process previously described. The heavy concentration of misshapen cells during a sickling crisis makes the blood abnormally viscous; as a result, the circulation becomes extremely sluggish. If dehydration due to vomiting, diarrhea, excessive sweating, or the ingestion of diuretics is also present, the blood becomes even thicker and the pathologic situation is compounded. Because of the viscous blood, the sickle cells tend to pack together or

*Valine is an amino acid that tends to form strong hydrophobic bonds (strong nonpolar bonds that prevent a molecule from reacting with molecules of water).

"log jam" within the smaller blood vessels. As a result of this occlusion of the microcirculation, more severe hypoxia develops which, in turn, causes more erythrocytes to sickle. A vicious circle thus develops. As the anoxia worsens, thrombosis and infarction develop and the surrounding tissues become necrotic. The organs most vulnerable to infarction and necrosis are the brain and kidneys, because of their constant demand for oxygen, and the bone marrow and spleen, because of their normally sluggish circulation.

Bases of Symptoms. Sickle cell anemia usually manifests itself during childhood, but occasionally symptoms do not appear until the patient has reached adulthood. Young children who develop the disease fail to grow properly. They typically have spindly legs, a short trunk, and a tower-shaped skull because of hyperactivity of the bone marrow.

Symptoms, whenever they occur, are due to the following three underlying factors: hemolytic anemia resulting from the destruction of sickle cells; thrombosis and infarction owing to occlusion of the microcirculation by the sickled cells; and an elevated bilirubin owing to the release of hemoglobin, which results in gallstone formation (cholelithiasis). These three problems profoundly affect all the organs and tissues of the body with severe, often fatal, consequences. Organs such as the spleen, liver, and penis are affected by the collection of sickled erythrocytes and undergo enlargement and, later, dysfunction. The interference with the circulation affects the brain, the kidneys, the heart, the lungs, and the skin. Leg ulcers are found in about 75 per cent of older children or adults with the disease. The proliferation of the bone marrow leads to osteoporosis and, later, osteosclerosis. These are only a few of the forms that symptoms may take in sickle cell anemia.

Cerebral hemorrhage or shock claims the lives of many patients during childhood. However, some individuals manage to survive until they are 50 years of age or older. Death, when it comes, is usually the result of *uremia,* caused by progressive renal damage.

Diagnosing Sickle Cell Anemia and Trait. There are currently four laboratory procedures that are used to diagnose the presence of sickle cell hemoglobin in either homozygous or heterozygous carriers:

- *Stained blood smear.* Examination of a stained blood smear for the presence of sickle cells.
- *Sickle cell slide preparation* (sickle prep). Observation of a specimen of blood for the sickling phenomenon following deoxygenation of the blood. This test is accurate, but time-consuming to perform.
- *Sickle-turbidity tube test* (Sickledex). An excellent mass screening test for the detection of sickle cell hemoglobin. The patient's finger is pricked and the blood is mixed with Sickledex solution in a test tube. Five minutes later the specimen is observed for cloudiness. The presence of Hb S causes the Sickledex solution to become turbid, while solutions mixed with normal hemoglobin remain clear. Although this test indicates whether Hb S is present, it does not differentiate between sickle cell disease and the trait.
- *Hemoglobin electrophoresis.* Differentiates between sickle cell anemia and sickle cell trait. By means of an applied electric field, the various types of hemoglobin within a blood specimen are separated. If a blood specimen contains both Hb S and Hb A, the person has sickle cell trait; if only Hb S is present, the person has sickle cell anemia.

Clinical Care. The treatment of sickle cell anemia consists chiefly of supportive care, e.g., rest, oxygen, I.V. administration of fluids and electrolytes, sedation, and the prescription of analgesics. In some cases the slow administration of packed red cells or partial exchange transfusions help to relieve severe anemic symptoms. Anticoagulants, steroids, and cobalt treatments have all been tried in the past without success in reversing the sickling process.

One newer experimental approach in the treatment of sickle cell anemia is the use of *sodium cyanate.* When this drug is used over a long period of time, it apparently modifies the hemoglobin molecule so that the tendency to sickle lessens. Unfortunately, cyanate causes neurotoxic side effects. To avoid these effects, cyanate must be given in dosages that may be too low to improve the anemia. Further therapeutic trials are needed to confirm the usefulness of this treatment approach.

In addition to treating sickle cell crises, one must also treat the complications of sickle cell anemia. *Leg ulcers* are cleansed with warm saline soaks and an enzyme debridement agent (Biozyme, Elase, Panofil, or Travase) and are then covered with a sterile dressing. The patient is placed on bed rest, and the legs are elevated. A bed cradle is usually ordered to alleviate pressure on the legs. In cases of severe ulceration, skin grafts may be needed to close the wound. *Cholelithiasis* and/or *pathologic fracture* may require surgery. *Cardiac arrhythmias* can be treated by routine methods. Patients with eye disorders are referred to an ophthalmologist.

Educational Aspects. Many blacks are totally unaware that they carry the sickle cell trait and that they can transmit this trait to their offspring. For this reason, mass screening tests for the detection of Hb S are being perfected for use among the black population. Persons having only the sickle cell trait may never be detected unless they are exposed to extremely low tensions (e.g., in mountain climbing or flying in a nonpressurized plane), which may cause sickling to occur. However, extremely hard work or exercise, or such stress as pregnancy, may cause the trait to be evidenced through collapse or other effects.

When counseling people about sickle cell anemia or sickle cell trait, it is important to include the following points in your discussion:

- Explain the nature of the disease to the involved persons and give them a chance to vent their feelings and ask questions.
- Encourage black parents to have not only themselves but their children tested for the presence of Hb S.
- If a person does have sickle cell disease or trait, provide information on how to prevent crises.

Warn the patient to avoid high altitudes or flying in unpressurized planes, because oxygen tension is lowered under these conditions. Encourage the patient to have routine medical exams that include a red blood cell count. Also, caution the patient to guard against becoming dehydrated. Advise the person to call a physician should vomiting, diarrhea, a high fever, or any other cause of water loss develop.

- Encourage young black people who are carriers of Hb S to ask their physician for genetic counseling before marrying or having children.
- Warn young women with sickle cell anemia that pregnancy carries a very high risk for them; they may develop pulmonary and/or renal complications.

Other Variant Abnormal Hemoglobins. As stated earlier, the only abnormal hemoglobins that produce anemias of consequence within the United States are hemoglobins S, C, and D.

Homozygous hemoglobin C disease (Hb CC disease) is found in one out of every 6000 blacks; 2 to 3 per cent of American blacks carry the hemoglobin C trait. Individuals with Hb CC disease suffer from a fairly severe anemia that is accompanied by manifestations similar to those of sickle cell anemia, with the exception that their erythrocytes do not assume the sickle shape. Persons who carry the trait (i.e., they have A-C hemoglobin) usually remain asymptomatic. Treatment of the disease centers around the alleviation of symptoms; occasionally blood transfusions are required.

S-C hemoglobin disease is more common than Hb CC disease because so many blacks are heterozygous carriers of the sickle cell trait. Manifestations of this condition include sicklemia, anemia, or splenomegaly. Hematuria, retinal hemorrhages, and aseptic necrosis of the femoral head may also be present.

Hb S-D disease is uncommon; apparently it affects both blacks and nonblacks. Symptoms are similar to those of sickle cell anemia, but less severe.

The Thalassemias. The thalassemias are a group of inherited chronic hemolytic anemias that predominantly affect persons with Mediterranean or Southern Chinese ancestry and are characterized by the production of extremely thin, fragile erythrocytes called *target cells.* Because the thalassemias were first discovered among people living around the Mediterranean, this group of conditions was named for the sea (*thalassos* meaning "sea"). The group has also been called Mediterranean anemia or Cooley's anemia. The thalassemias also affect American blacks and people from Central Africa and Southern Asia.

The severity of the anemia produced by the thalassemias depends upon whether the afflicted individual is homozygous or heterozygous for the thalassemia trait. *Thalassemia major* and *intermedia,* characterized by a *profound* anemia, appear in homozygotes. *Thalassemia minor* is characterized by a relatively *mild* anemia and develops in heterozygotes.

Etiology. You recall that hemoglobin is composed of two pairs of polypeptide chains called alpha chains and beta chains. Unlike sickle cell anemia, the polypeptide chains in the thalassemias are completely normal in structure. This group of disorders, instead, is characterized by an *insufficient amount* of polypeptide chains as a result of a genetic defect. Either alpha or beta chains can be affected by diminished synthesis. In *alpha thalassemia,* alpha chain synthesis is slowed; in *beta thalassemia,* beta chain synthesis is retarded.

Beta thalassemia is by far the most common form of the disease. For this reason, beta thalassemia is simply referred to as "thalassemia" or "classic thalassemia."

Manifestations. The symptoms of thalassemia major are generally the same as those of other hemolytic anemias, e.g., jaundice, cholelithiasis, leg ulcers, enlarged spleen. However, one distinctive characteristic of thalassemia is a *pronounced bone hyperactivity* that results in thickening of the cranial bones. As a result of cranial bone hyperplasia, persons with this disorder have a *mongoloid* appearance or facies.

Laboratory findings in thalassemia (beta form) include the following:

- *Target cells* (abnormally thin fragile cells) and other bizarrely shaped erythrocytes appear in the circulation.
- The *serum bilirubin* and *fecal* and *urinary urobilin-*

ogen are greatly elevated because of the severe hemolysis of abnormal cells.

- *Fetal* hemoglobin (Hb F) is greatly elevated; in some cases it rises to as high as 90 per cent.
- *Hb* A_2 (a normal variant of Hb A) is also elevated and may rise to as high as 6 per cent instead of the normal 1.5 to 3.0 per cent.

The high percentages of Hb F and Hb A_2 are evidently a result of the decrease in beta chains characteristic of this anemia, which forces the bone marrow to produce abnormally large numbers of *alpha chains, gamma chains* (which are normally made only during fetal life), and *delta chains.* The compensatory increase in fetal hemoglobin results from the combination of alpha and gamma chains, while the increase in Hb A_2 results from the combination of alpha and delta chains.

Thalassemia minor is usually asymptomatic, with the exception of a mild anemia. Also, the blood smear of patients with this condition contains small, defective erythrocytes.

Clinical Care. Transfusion therapy is the only treatment available today. Patients with thalassemia major are treated with transfusions of packed red cells, which may be administered: (1) on a monthly or bimontly basis (regular transfusion regimen); (2) whenever the patient's hemoglobin falls below 3–4 Gm./100 ml. (nonsystematic transfusion); or (3) every 15 days in order to maintain the patient's hemoglobin at 12–15 Gm./100 ml. (hypertransfusion regimen). When it becomes evident that transfused cells are being rapidly destroyed by the spleen (causing a severe hemolytic anemia), *splenectomy* is necessary.

Because patients with thalassemia must receive so many transfusions, they are in danger of developing an *iron overload,* which may eventually lead to myocardial hemosiderosis and resulting cardiac arrhythmias. Excessive iron can be removed from the blood to some extent by *chelating agents* such as desferrioxamine.

Thalassemia minor is generally so mild that patients do not require treatment. However, all persons who carry the thalassemia trait need genetic counseling.

Prognosis. The outlook for patients with thalassemia major is usually poor. Children are retarded in their growth and development and many fail to live past puberty. Thalassemia minor, on the other hand, does not affect life expectancy.

SECONDARY ANEMIAS

The secondary anemias, as the name implies, arise in association with other conditions such as chronic systemic diseases, (e.g., rheumatoid arthritis, malnutrition, leukemia, the lymphomas, multiple myeloma); chronic infections (lung abscess, empyema, pelvic inflammatory disease); acute and chronic renal disease complicated by uremia; cirrhosis of the liver; endocrine disorders (myxedema); and cancer.

The anemia accompanying cancer results from one of the following three factors: chronic blood loss, hemolysis of cells, or the development of space-occupying lesions within the bone marrow (myelophthisic anemia).

While the etiology of the secondary anemias varies with the underlying condition, all these anemias have two factors in common: the erythrocytes have a shortened life span, and the bone marrow, although functioning normally, is unable to produce enough red cells to compensate for erythrocyte losses. For this reason, the secondary anemias are also called "the anemias of *relative bone marrow failure.*"

The anemia which develops in these conditions may be moderate to severe, depending upon the underlying cause. *Treatment* involves correction of the underlying condition. Blood transfusions are sometimes given to patients with hemoglobin levels below 8–9 Gm./100 ml.

THE POLYCYTHEMIAS

Polycythemia is defined as an increase in both the *number* of circulating *erythrocytes* and the *concentration of hemoglobin* within the blood. In this condition, red blood cells may number as high as 8 to 12 million per cu. mm., and the hemoglobin concentration may rise to 8 to 25 Gm/100 ml. The three forms of polycythemia (polycythemia vera, secondary polycythemia, and relative polycythemia) are considered below.

Polycythemia Vera. Polycythemia vera is classified as a *myeloproliferative disorder* (meaning "overgrowth of bone marrow"). It usually develops in middle age and is particularly common among Jewish men.

Although the precise etiology of this disease remains unknown, it is believed to be a form of malignancy analogous to leukemia. The three major hallmarks of this condition are: (1) the relentless, unrestrained production of massive numbers of erythrocytes; (2) the production of excessive myelocytes (leukocytes within the bone marrow); and (3) an overproduction of thrombocytes. The overproduction of all three of these cell lines results in the following three pathologic consequences: an increase in the *viscosity* of the blood; an increase in the total *volume* of blood, which may be twice or even three times greater than normal; and severe *congestion* of all tissues and organs with blood. Because of these three problems, the patient suffers from numerous symptoms. The most important signs and symptoms of polycythemia vera and their causation are listed in Table 45–6.

Thrombotic complications claim the lives of around 30 per cent of patients, another 10 to 15

TABLE 45–6. SIGNS AND SYMPTOMS OF POLYCYTHEMIA VERA

Signs and Symptoms	Bases
Ruddy complexion and dusky redness of mucosa	Great volume of blood causes congestion of capillaries supplying skin and mucous membranes.
Hypertension accompanied by dizziness, headache, and a sense of fullness in the head	Increased volume and viscosity of blood causes increased blood pressure.
Congestive heart failure (shortness of breath, orthopnea, etc.)	Increased blood volume and viscosity increase work of the heart, leading to failure.
Thrombus formation, particularly within vessels supplying the brain, heart, lungs, and lower extremities; cerebral vascular accidents, myocardial infarction, and gangrene of the feet can result	Increased viscosity of blood causes the circulation to slow, promoting thrombus formation; also, increased platelet count causes blood to clot more easily.
Bleeding and hemorrhage in the gastrointestinal tract, oropharynx and brain, especially following minor accidents or surgery	Congestion and distention of capillaries, venules and arterioles causes rupture of the vessels, resulting in hemorrhage.
Enlarged liver and spleen	Large numbers of erythrocytes collect within the liver and spleen; increased volume of blood within the portal circulation also causes organ congestion.
Peptic ulcer (See Unit XVII)	Gastric secretions are increased in polycythemia.
Gout (painful swollen joints—usually of the big toe)	Increased cell production results in increased cell destruction; this leads to increased released nucleoprotein; one product of nucleoprotein breakdown is uric acid, and increased uric acid levels in blood cause gout.

per cent die from *hemorrhage.* Finally, for obscure reasons, approximately 15 per cent of patients die from either *myelogenous leukemia* or *myelofibrosis* accompanied by pancytopenia.

The goals of treatment in polycythemia vera are: (1) reduction of blood volume and viscosity; and (2) reduction of bone marrow activity. Methods of treatment are as follows:

▶ *Venesection* (phlebotomy regimen). Emergency treatment of the patient involves removal of 500 to 2000 ml. of blood until the hematocrit is 45 per cent. Once the hematocrit has been reduced, the doctor usually removes 500 ml. of blood from the patient every 2 to 3 months. Caution patients undergoing venesection to avoid foods high in iron (clams, oysters, liver, legumes) because a high iron intake somewhat counteracts the therapeutic effects of venesection.

▶ *Myelosuppressive agents.* The administration of radioactive phosphorus (^{32}P) sometimes produces remissions that last for 6 months to 2 years. (See also Chapter 23.) Other drugs useful for combating polycythemia are nitrogen mustard, busulfan (Myeleran), Chlorambucil, and cyclophosphamide.

▶ *Activity.* In order to prevent the development of thrombi as a result of circulatory stasis, encourage patients with polycythemia vera to ambulate if possible. Patients who are bedridden require frequent turning and passive exercise of their extremities.

▶ *Fluid balance.* To reduce the viscosity of the patient's blood, force fluids and carefully record intake and output.

Secondary Polycythemia. You recall that the major function of erythrocytes is to carry oxygen to the body tissues. Consequently, when the body's demand for oxygen increases for any reason, the bone marrow is forced to produce more erythrocytes to prevent tissue hypoxia. Whenever red cells must increase excessively as a compensatory response to *tissue hypoxia,* the condition is called *secondary polycythemia.*

Hypoxia that is sufficiently prolonged to cause polycythemia results from chronic lung disease (particularly emphysema), congenital heart disease, and prolonged exposure to altitudes of 10,000 feet or more. It is interesting that people who live in the Andes and other mountainous areas for prolonged periods are usually without symptoms of hypoxia because their blood has literally "thickened." These mountain dwellers produce high numbers of red blood cells, which increases the oxygen-carrying capacity of their blood and enables them to live and work at an altitude that would incapacitate a newcomer.

The *symptoms* and laboratory findings for persons with secondary polycythemia are the same as for those with polycythemia vera, except that the leukocyte and thrombocyte counts are normal and splenic enlargement does not occur.

To *treat* secondary polycythemia, the physician must treat the underlying disease or condition causing hypoxia.

Relative Polycythemia. Whenever the body loses plasma without losing red blood cells, the concentration of erythrocytes increases *relative* to the amount of plasma contained within the vascular system. The *causes* of relative polycythemia are fluid loss and dehydration as a result of insufficient fluid intake, diarrhea, vomiting, burns, excessive administration of diuretics, and so forth. *Treatment* of this condition simply involves the re-establishment of fluid and electrolyte balance.

CHAPTER 46

NURSING PERSONS WITH OTHER MAJOR DISTURBANCES OF THE BLOOD AND BLOOD-FORMING ORGANS

NURSING PATIENTS WITH DISORDERS PRIMARILY AFFECTING LEUKOCYTES AND PLASMA CELLS

The leukocytes or white blood cells* are one of the body's major defenses against infectious and parasitic organisms. Normally leukocytes number between 5000 and 10,000/cu. mm. A rise in the white cell count over 10,000/cu. mm. is called *leukocytosis;* white cell usually increase in response to the entry of infectious organisms into the body. Conversely, a *decrease* in the white cell count below 5000/cu. mm. is called *leukopenia;* leukocytes may decrease as a result of viral infections and exposure to drugs or myelotoxic agents.

Plasma cells, or plasmocytes, are mononuclear cells that are probably the primary producers of *gamma globulin;* they are formed within the bone marrow and lymph nodes. Pathologic conditions involving plasma cells are called *plasma cell dyscrasias.*

Agranulocytosis

Agranulocytosis (granulocytopenia, malignant neutropenia) is an acute, potentially fatal blood dyscrasia characterized by profound neutropenia. *Neutropenia* is a reduction in the number of circulating polymorphonuclear neutrophils (granulocytes).

The most common cause of agranulocytosis is *drug toxicity* or *hypersensitivity.* There are two major groups of drugs that are capable of suppressing granulocyte production:

1. Agents that *always* produce neutropenia when given in sufficiently large doses over a period of time, e.g., nitrogen mustard and other cancer chemotherapeutic agents and therapies (radiation, radioisotopes) and benzene.
2. Agents that produce neutropenia only in persons who are *particularly sensitive* to the drug, e.g., certain tranquilizers (Thorazine), antithyroid agents (propylthiouracil), anticonvulsants (diphenylhydantoin), and antibiotics (chloramphenicol).

Agranulocytosis can occur in patients who have anemias related to diminished erythropoiesis (aplastic anemia, megaloblastic anemia), and it may also develop during the course of certain diseases, e.g., tuberculosis, overwhelming infection, typhoid fever, malaria, and uremia.

Agranulocytosis occurs throughout the world — particularly in areas where the drugs listed above are in common use. For as yet undiscovered reasons, women are much more susceptible to this condition than are men. However, even among females, agranulocytosis is relatively rare.

The *symptoms* of agranulocytosis arise as a result of its characteristic severe neutropenia. You recall that neutrophils, which constitute 50 to 70 per cent of all circulating leukocytes, are one of the body's swiftest and most powerful lines of defense against invading microorganisms. Consequently, any decrease in neutrophils results in a severe increase in the body's susceptibility to bacterial invasion, particularly of the highly vulnerable mucous membranes of the throat and mouth.

Typically the onset of this acute disease is rapid. For the first 2 or 3 days the person complains of severe fatigue and weakness. Next the person develops a sore throat, ulcerative lesions of the pharyngeal and buccal mucosae, dysphagia, prostration, high fever, weak rapid pulse, and severe chills. Without prompt treatment with antibiotics, the disorder is usually fatal within less than a week.

*The classification and function of both leukocytes and plasma cells are discussed more thoroughly in Chapter 10.

Diagnosis of agranulocytosis is based upon the following findings:

▶ *Leukopenia* (500 to 3000 WBC/cu. mm.) with an extreme reduction in polymorphonuclear cells (0 to 2 per cent).

▶ Bone marrow examination, revealing an *absence of polymorphonuclear leukocytes,* or, in some cases, a maturational arrest of young developing cells.

▶ Cultures of the urine, blood, and ulcerative lesions within the throat and mouth that are *positive for bacteria* (usually gram-positive cocci).

▶ A *history* of exposure to an offending drug, plus all the above findings. Because many people medicate themselves with potentially dangerous drugs, it is important to investigate all drugs the patient takes.

The *clinical care* of patients with agranulocytosis involves the following steps:

▶ *Halt bone marrow arrest early.* Observe patients who are receiving potentially toxic drugs or anticancer therapy for extreme fatigue, the development of a sore throat or mouth, and fever. Check the patient's hemogram daily for a drop in the white blood cell count; immediately notify the physician should even a mild leukopenia develop.

▶ *Eradicate the infection.* The doctor will order cultures of urine, blood, throat secretions, any open lesions, and stool as possible sources of infection. Antibiotic sensitivity testing is also done. Antibiotics of choice are carbenicillin and cephalothin. Both are given IV.

▶ *Guard* the patient from *further infection* during treatment. Bed rest and a high-protein, high-vitamin, high-caloric diet will prevent excessive weakness and debilitation. The patient may be placed in *reverse isolation* in order to reduce exposure to infectious organisms.

▶ Give *meticulous mouth care* and assess the mouth daily. To remove necrotic exudate from the oral and pharyngeal mucosa, irrigate the patient's mouth and throat with warm saline solution every 1 or 2 hours. An ice collar, anesthetic lozenges, and prescribed analgesics help to relieve the severe pain. Request soft bland foods and protein concentrates for the patient until throat condition and dysphagia improve. The patient may also require sedation for sleep.

▶ *Relieve fever* with cooling measures (alcohol rub, tepid baths) and antipyretic drugs. Force fluids to 2500 ml. per day to prevent dehydration as a result of diaphoresis.

▶ *Prevent constipation.* Hard stools damage the intestinal and rectal mucosa and thus increase the risk of infection. Gentle enemas may be ordered, but enemas are usually avoided because of potential damage to rectal mucosa, with resultant infection and abscess formation. Stool softeners are usually ordered routinely.

▶ *Educate patients* to avoid medicating themselves without their doctor's direction. Explain the dangers of taking antibiotics or tranquilizers that have been prescribed for a friend or relative. Inform the patient that one person may be hypersensitive to a drug that is safe for another individual.

With antibiotic therapy, many patients recover from agranulocytosis within 2 to 3 weeks. However, without antibiotics, the mortality rate from this condition is approximately 80 per cent.

The Leukemias

Leukemia (which literally means "white blood") is a fatal neoplastic disease that involves the blood-forming tissues of the bone marrow, spleen, and lymph nodes. Its outstanding characteristic is the abnormal, uncontrolled, and destructive proliferation of one type of white cell (i.e., granulocyte, lymphocyte, or monocyte) and its precursors. Victims of leukemia and the lymphomas account for 6 per cent of all individuals suffering from cancer. Although leukemia strikes people of all ages, it is the leading cause of death among *children* between the ages of 4 and 14 years (with the possible exception of congenital anomalies). The cause of leukemia remains essentially unknown. Some experts believe a virus is responsible; others believe that these may be a hereditary predisposition. Still others feel that it is caused by increased and excessive radiation exposure.

CLASSIFICATION OF THE LEUKEMIAS

There are several forms of leukemia, each of which affects a different age group. Leukemias are classified according to the following criteria:

Course and Duration of Disease. *Acute* leukemia has a *rapid onset* and typically progresses to a fatal termination within days to months if untreated. The massive numbers of leukocytes produced are very immature and they accumulate rapidly within the blood-forming organs, causing organ malfunction. The *chronic* leukemias have a *gradual onset* and a slower, more protracted course than the acute leukemias; in some cases the patient lives for 5 or more years. The white cells produced are more mature and consequently better able to carry out their task of defending the body against invading microorganisms. Acute leukemia is more common among children and young adults, whereas chronic leukemias tend to strike people between the ages of 25 and 60.

Type of Cell and Tissue Involved. Abnormal proliferation of one type of white cell (lymphocyte, myelocyte, or monocyte) occurs in both acute and chronic leukemias. Thus, there are six major types of leukemia: (1) acute lymphocytic leukemia, (2) acute myelocytic leukemia, (3) acute monocytic leukemia, (4) chronic lymphocytic leukemia, (5) chronic myelocytic leukemia, and (6) chronic monocytic leukemia (rare). Variations of this classification are often employed. For example, the acute leukemias are sometimes classified as lymphoblastic, myeloblastic, or monoblastic because of the preponderance of immature cell forms in these categories of disease.

Lymphocytic leukemia is characterized by hyperplasia of lymphoid tissues, whereas myelocytic leukemia is characterized by hyperplasia of the bone marrow and spleen. Lymphocytic leukemias are much more common in children, whereas myelocytic leukemias are mostly found in adults.

Number of Leukocytes in Blood and Bone Marrow. Occasionally, patients with acute leukemia have a normal or even *lower* than normal leukocyte count. In these instances, the condition is called *aleukemic leukemia* or *subleukemic leukemia.*

ETIOLOGY, PATHOGENESIS, AND SYMPTOMS

As with other cancers, the exact etiology of leukemia is unknown. There is a great amount of evidence indicating that no single factor is responsible for the disease process. "In most instances, leukemia appears to result from concatenation of host susceptibility factors, chemical or physical injury to chromosomes, and clearly in animals and presumably in humans as well, the incorporation of genetic information of viral origin into susceptible stem cells."[125]

While the exact cause of leukemia remains elusive, the widespread and devastating effects of this malignant disease upon the body have been studied for years. The three major effects of leukemia are: (1) the *proliferation* of *high numbers of abnormal, immature leukocytes,* (2) the *accumulation* of these cells within the lymph nodes, (3) the eventual *infiltration* of these cells into tissues all over the body. These three developments, in turn, lead to other pathologic changes and many symptoms. Abnormal bleeding combined with an infection is the most common clinical sign of leukemia. Table 46–1 lists some major signs and symptoms accompanying all forms of leukemia.

There is not an organ that is not eventually involved in the leukemic process. Hemorrhages into the retina may cause blindness, while hemorrhages into the brain tissue may cause a cerebral vascular accident. The lungs, mouth, throat, skin, and kidneys are all vulnerable to infection. Anorexia, nausea, and vomiting cause malnutrition. As you will see, the reactions to therapeutic measures cause further symptoms. It becomes evident then why the victim of leukemia needs constant and meticulous nursing care and observation.

DIAGNOSIS AND CLINICAL CARE

Leukemia, during its early stages, may be discovered by accident during a routine physical examination that includes blood work. An elevated leukocyte count with a "shift to the left" (a term indicating the presence of large numbers of immature leukocytes) usually alerts the physician to the possible presence of leukemia. Tests

TABLE 46–1. SIGNS AND SYMPTOMS IN LEUKEMIA

Signs and Symptoms	Bases
Severe infections, e.g., ulcerations of the mouth and throat, pneumonia, septicemia	Although leukocyte count is high (15,000–500,000/cu. mm. or higher), leukocytes are immature or abnormal and consequently unable to fight and destroy microorganisms
Anemia accompanied by fatigue, lethargy, hypoxia, etc., and hemorrhage (gum bleeding, ecchymoses, petechiae, retinal hemorrhages) due to thrombocytopenia	Rapidly proliferating leukocytes evidently "crowd out" the developing erythrocytes and thrombocytes
Enlarged organs cause pressure on adjacent structures (e.g., splenomegaly, hepatomegaly, lymphadenopathy, bone marrow hypercellularity)	High numbers of white cells accumulate within the liver, spleen, lymph nodes, and bone marrow, causing distention of the tissues
Increased metabolic rate accompanied by weakness, pallor, and weight loss	Increased production of leukocytes requires large amounts of amino acids and vitamins. Increased destruction of cells leads to increased release of metabolic wastes which must be disposed of by the body
Hyperuricemia (excess of uric acid in the blood), causing renal pain, obstruction from stone formation, and infection	Large amounts of uric acid are released as a result of the destruction of mass numbers of leukocytes in part by antileukemic drugs
Renal insufficiency with uremia (a late development)	Abnormal leukocytes infiltrate into the kidneys
Central nervous system symptoms, e.g., headache, disorientation	Abnormal white cells infiltrate into the central nervous system

and symptoms that later confirm a diagnosis of leukemia include: (1) a differential leukocyte count in which one type of white cell is overwhelmingly predominant; (2) a bone marrow specimen that contains massive numbers of abnormal leukocytes (this being the most definitive test); (3) a blood film that reveals many "blast" cells; and (4) the presence of anemia, bleeding tendencies, sternal tenderness, and organ enlargement.

The *treatment* of leukemia varies with each form of the disease. However, the *goal of care* in all forms of leukemia is the same: to halt the destructive proliferation and infiltration of abnormal and immature leukocytes and to obtain a *remission* (i.e., lessening or cessation of symptoms) for as long a period as possible.

To date there is no cure for leukemia. However, a number of measures are used to temporarily halt the malignant process, alleviate symptoms, and prevent complications, e.g., radiation therapy; radioisotope therapy; chemotherapy; corticosteroid therapy; blood platelet and granulocyte transfusions; antibiotics; bone marrow transplants; immunotherapy; reverse isolation techniques; and supportive nursing care. When these measures are successful, patients may experience remissions that last for as long as 15 years.

Table 46-2 lists the various drugs used against different types of leukemia and also in Hodgkin's disease and other lymphomas (discussed in later sections).

TABLE 46–2. CHEMOTHERAPEUTIC AGENTS USED IN THE LEUKEMIAS AND LYMPHOMAS*

Acute Lymphoblastic Leukemia
- Adriamycin
- Carmustine (BCNU)
- Cyclophosphamide (Cytoxan)
- Cytarabine (Cytosar, Ara-C)
- Daunorubicin (Daunomycin)
- Hydroxyurea (Hydrea)
- Immunotherapy: BCG, Levamisole
- L-Asparaginase
- Mercaptopurine (Purinethol)
- Methotrexate (formerly Amethopterin)
- Prednisone (Deltasone, Merticorten, et al.)
- Thioguanine
- Vincristine (Oncovin)

Chronic Lymphocytic Leukemia
- Chlorambucil (Leukeran)
- Cyclophosphamide (Cytoxan)
- Prednisone (Deltasone, Merticorten, et al.)
- Triethylenemelamine (TEM)

Chronic Myelocytic (Granulocytic) Leukemia
- Busulfan (Myleran)
- Chlorambucil (Leukeran)
- Cyclophosphamide (Cytoxan)
- Cytarabine (Ara-C, Cytosar)
- Hydroxyurea (Hydrea)
- Mercaptopurine (Purinethol)
- Triethylenemelamine (TEM)
- Vincristine (Oncovin)

Acute Myeloblastic (Granulocytic) Leukemia
- 5-Azacytidine
- Carmustine (BCNU)
- Cyclophosphamide (Cytoxan)
- Cytarabine (Cytosar)
- Daunorubicin (Daunomycin)
- Mercaptopurine (Purinethol)
- Methotrexate (formerly Amethopterin)
- Methyl-Gag
- Rubidazone
- Thioguanine

Hodgkin's Disease and Other Lymphomas
- Bleomycin
- Carmustine (BCNU)
- CCNU (Lomustine)
- Cyclophosphamide (Cytoxan)
- Doxorubicin (Adriamycin)
- DTIC (Imidazole carboxamide)
- Mechlorethamine (Mustargen; nitrogen mustard)
- Methyl CCNU (Semustine)
- Prednisone (Deltasone, Meticorten, et al.)
- Procarbazine (Matulane)
- Streptozotocin
- Thiotepa (triethylenethiophosphoramide)
- Triethylenemelamine (TEM)
- Vinblastine (Velban)
- Vincristine (Oncovin)

*Some of these drugs are still experimental.

VARIETIES OF LEUKEMIA: CLINICAL COURSE AND CLINICAL CARE

Acute Leukemia. Acute leukemia is a disease primarily of the young; its peak incidence occurs in children between the ages of 1 and 5 years. As mentioned earlier, acute lymphocytic anemia is most commonly found in children.

The onset and manifestations of all forms of acute leukemia are somewhat similar. Typically there is a prodromal period during which the child experiences fatigue, headache, sore throat, night sweats, and shortness of breath. Following this, the patient develops acute symptoms of severe tonsillitis, ulcerations and sometimes gangrenous lesions within the mouth, bleeding from the gums and rectum, bleeding into the skin, and severe joint and bone pain. The lymph nodes, liver, and spleen enlarge; and severe anemia, accompanied by debilitation and exhaustion, develops. Without therapy, the patient's life terminates in either overwhelming infection or severe hemorrhage within a few days to a few months. However, with therapy (such as combined chemotherapeutic agent usage, supportive therapy, transplantation, and immunotherapy) some patients obtain a remission that may last for many years.

Examination of the blood of a patient with acute leukemia usually shows an elevated white count; sometimes, however, leukopenia is present. A bone marrow examination and blood film are needed to differentiate acute leukemia from a severe infection, thrombocytopenia, or rheumatic fever (the latter disorder too is characterized by joint and bone pain).

The clinical care of persons with acute leukemia is structured to allow the patient to continue to pursue as full a life as possible for as long as possible. When feasible, the patient should live at home, continue going to school or work, and engage in an active social life. To sustain the patient during this illness, the patient's family, teachers, and employers need information concerning the nature of leukemia — it symptoms, treatment, and prognosis.

The mainstay of therapy for acute leukemia is *chemotherapy* and the investigational use of immunotherapy. (See Table 46–2.) In addition, patients also receive *blood transfusions* to correct anemia; *platelet transfusions* to prevent hemorrhage as a result of thrombocytopenia (granulocyte transfusions are used in the neutropenic patient); specific *antibiotics* to combat infection; and a drug called *allopurinol* (Zyloprim), to inhibit the formation of uric acid crystals within the renal tubules. When allopurinol is given, the patient should drink up to 1500 ml. of water per day to promote an adequate urine output. Bone marrow transplants are also being investigated for use in the leukemic patient population.

Chronic Myelocytic or Granulocytic Leukemia (CML). This form of leukemia usually strikes individuals between the ages of 25 and 60 years. It is characterized by the abnormal proliferation of granulocytes (mostly mature, but some are less mature), which flood the peripheral circulation, accumulate densely within the bone marrow, and infiltrate the liver, spleen, and other tissues.

The symptoms of CML are generally the same as those general symptoms discussed earlier (e.g., anemia, bleeding, and so forth). However, the outstanding characteristic of this particular form of leukemia is a *massive spleen,* which may grow so large that it fills the abdomen and part of the pelvis. The liver may also be greatly enlarged. In contrast to chronic lymphocytic leukemia, the lymph nodes tend to swell very little. Also, patients with CML suffer from severe pain in the long bones; this results from the engorgement of the marrow with abnormal leukocytes.

The most serious problem facing a patient with CML is *extreme vulnerability to infection.* The invasion of microorganisms poses a severe threat because the neutrophils, which constitute the majority of the body's leukocytes, are extremely immature. Moreover, the drugs used to treat CML tend to injure or kill the few normal circulating neutrophils, which further increases the patient's susceptibility to infection.

The onset of CML is usually insidious. For many months or even years the patient may complain of weakness and weight loss. The first specific sign may be a heavy sensation in the abdomen (due to the enlarged spleen) and a sense of extreme abdominal distention after meals. The patient may also suffer from sternal tenderness and mild lymph node enlargement. Bleeding problems due to thrombocytopenia do not usually develop for many years.

The *treatment* of CML includes the following measures:

- *X-ray therapy.* X-rays are either administered to the entire body or focused on the spleen or liver.
- *Radioisotope therapy.* Radioactive phosphorus (^{32}P) may be given in place of x-ray therapy; it yields results similar to total body irradiation. The advantage of radioisotope therapy is that ^{32}P produces almost no radiation sickness.
- *Chemotherapy.* A drug used in the treatment of CML is busulfan (Myleran), an alkylating agent. Once the WBC count lowers to around 10,000, the drug is stopped or given periodically. The major toxic effect resulting from prolonged treatment with busulfan is *irreversible thrombocytopenia.*
- Investigative treatment procedures include splenectomy and immunotherapy.

Platelet counts should be performed daily on patients receiving busulfan. Steadily decreasing platelet counts may be an indication for stopping administration of the drug.

Other useful drugs are also listed in Table 46–2.

Patients may live for 3 to 5 years following the onset of the disease, whether or not they have received treatment. Death usually follows infection or an episode of either acute bleeding or thromboembolism.

Chronic Lymphocytic Leukemia (CLL). This form of leukemia is characterized by the uncontrolled proliferation of *lymphocytes,* which accumulate in the lymph nodes and lymphoidal tissues and eventually infiltrate the bone marrow, liver, and spleen. Although the cause of CLL is unknown, this neoplastic disorder appears related to the lymphomas, discussed later.

CLL principally affects older persons between 50 and 70 years of age. For unknown reasons, it is three times more common in men than in women.

The onset of CLL is insidious. Many patients are asymptomatic for years. Indeed, 25 per cent of cases are diagnosed from a routine blood examination that reveals an elevated WBC (up to 600,000/cu. mm.), in which 80 to 98 per cent of the leukocytes are small, mature-looking lymphocytes (Fig. 46–1).

Early symptoms of CLL are chronic exhaustion, anorexia, and swollen lymph nodes all over the patient's body. In some cases, the patient may also have a slightly enlarged liver and

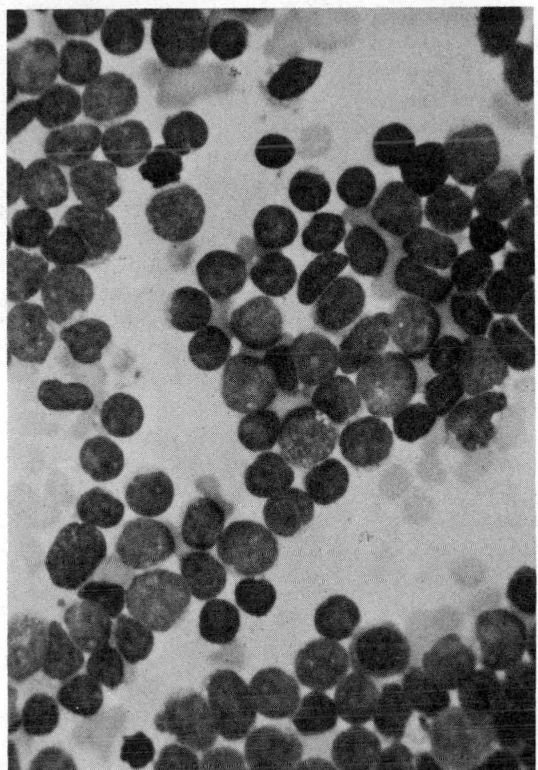

Figure 46–1. A peripheral blood smear in a patient with chronic lymphocytic leukemia, crowded with mature and slightly immature lymphocytes. (WBC 120,000–92% lymphocytes.) (From Robbins, S. L., and R. S. Cotran: *Pathologic Basis of Disease,* 2nd ed. Philadelphia: W. B. Saunders Co., 1979, p. 780.)

spleen. Later, as the disease progresses, anemia, fever, susceptibility to infections, cachexia, and mild hemorrhagic tendencies develop. Leukemic infiltrations into the retina of the eye and the skin cause visual disturbances and skin lesions. Pressure of the enlarged lymph nodes upon various nerves causes pain and even paralysis. In approximately one third of all patients with CLL, mediastinal lymph node enlargement results in respiratory symptoms. Finally, during the last stages of this disorder, the patient's immune system may become involved in the disease process. Thus, two late complications of CLL are: (1) hemolytic anemia due to an autoimmune disorder and (2) hypogammaglobulinemia — a condition that further increases the patient's susceptibility to infection.

The *treatment* of CLL centers around x-ray therapy and chemotherapy. Commonly used drugs include these *alkylating agents:* chlorambucil (Leukeran), triethylenemelamine (TEM), and cyclophosphamide (Cytoxan). In addition, the patient is also given small daily doses of *corticosteroids.*

The complications of CLL also require treatment. Anemia usually responds to transfusion therapy and to doses of corticosteroids. Severe hemolytic anemia must sometimes be controlled by splenectomy. Antibiotics, which are always ordered on the basis of culture and sensitivity tests, are given to control infections. Patients with *recurring* infections due to low gamma globulin levels are treated with prophylactic doses of gamma globulin.

In most patients, drug therapy does promote long periods of remission. With repeated remissions, some patients live for 15 years or longer following the inception of chemotherapy.

GENERAL NURSING CARE FOR PATIENTS WITH LEUKEMIA

The preceding discussions demonstrate that patients with leukemia suffer from multiple problems and from numerous symptoms involving every organ of the body.

Some of the most critical problems facing patients with leukemia are:

1. Suppression of normal bone marrow function, owing to uncontrolled proliferative disease and/or antileukemia therapy (i.e., the use of chemotherapeutic agents), which in turn results in the following:
   a. Extreme susceptibility to infections, owing to the predominance of immature and abnormal white blood cells.
   b. A drop in platelet count to less than 50,000 per cu. mm. or a progressively falling platelet count, which can cause bleeding, bruising, and even hemorrhage.
   c. A drop in red blood cell count, which leads to the manifestations of anemia, i.e., fatigue, dyspnea, and other problems.
2. Extreme discomfort and iatrogenic problems that arise from antileukemia therapy; e.g., radiation therapy can cause radiation sickness, and the various antileukemic drugs may cause bone marrow depression, alopecia, and uric acid accumulation.
3. Pain due to distention of tissues, caused by the accumulation of huge numbers of white cells within the liver, spleen, lymph nodes, and bone marrow.
4. Depression, anxiety, and realistic fears of death and dying.
5. Long-term care and its attendant problems — incurred expenses, family and social problems, and employment difficulties.

Supportive nursing measures that alleviate some of the pain and depression accompanying leukemia and that also help to prevent complications include:

1. Prevent, control, and treat infection
2. Assess and control bleeding
3. Provide adequate rest

4. Control pain
5. Provide adequate food and fluid intake
6. Mimimize the discomfort and side effects of antileukemic therapy
7. Provide psychologic support

Prevent, Control and Treat Infection. When caring for patients with leukemia, take time to review normal values for peripheral white blood cell counts; also, frequently review your patient's white cell count. Granulocyte counts below 55 per cu. mm. signal the possibility of the patient developing an infection. Check the patient's vital signs at least every 4 hours. Increases in temperature, pulse, and respiration may indicate systemic infection and should be reported to the patient's physician. Progressive hypothermia is seen in some types of infection.

If the patient's vital signs indicate that an infection may indeed be "brewing," it is imperative that blood, throat, urine, stool, and wound cultures (when applicable) be obtained and sent to the laboratory quickly. Local infections in the granulocytopenic patient often appear as tender, erythematous areas. Such areas are often without pus, as the patient does not have sufficient white cells to produce pus. Culture any drainage from such an area. Also, pain or burning upon urination is a signal to obtain a clean-catch midstream urine for culture.

The *mouth* is a choice site for infection and bleeding in the leukemic patient with impaired granulocyte function and decreased platelet levels. The mouth problem is characterized by swollen, easily bruised or abraded mucous membranes. Crater-type ulcerations of bacterial, fungal, or viral origin may be present. The mouth problem is often acute enough to prevent oral intake of nourishment. It may produce constant pain, requiring systemic analgesics. It often prevents normal verbal communication. When the leukemic patient achieves a remission, the mouth lesions resolve rapidly.

Methods for preventing mouth lesions are, as yet, undetermined. Methods of palliating the problem are, at best, only marginally effective. It is an area of nursing care in desperate need of meaningful research.

Currently, attempts to care for the mouth involve the following:

- Conscientious and careful cleansing of the mouth as often as every 2 hours, with soft, cotton tip applicators. Lubricate lips afterwards.
- Frequent examination of the mouth for new lesions. Frequent culturing of the mouth for the presence of organisms that can be treated locally.
- Avoiding trauma to the mouth, especially by rough textured foods.
- Possible prophylactic antimicrobial agents.

Remember that a *high fever* may accompany the infections that strike patients with leukemia. Ice packs, hypothermia units, cool body sponging and nonaspirin oral antipyretics are used to control fever. Application of extra blankets and warming of the patient's room air may help in relieving discomfort due to hypotension. Unfortunately, these measures only *control* body temperature; they do not have an effect on the *source* of the abnormal temperature.

When systemic *antibiotics* are ordered to combat infection, administer them immediately. Take great care to administer them on schedule, so that blood levels of the antibiotic are maintained.

> Remember:
> *The leukemic patient with a low granulocyte count is in an extremely vulnerable position and may die of overwhelming infection if not given treatment promptly and on schedule!*

Granulocyte transfusions are also used in the leukemic patient who has suppressed bone marrow caused by chemotherapy or the underlying disease process and who, therefore, has an increased susceptibility to infection.

Patients who appear to be developing an infection or who have developed any degree of hematopoietic depression may be placed in *reverse isolation.* Move the patient to a single room and allow only persons who are in good health to visit or give nursing care. At this time, explain to the patient that isolation is a necessary protective measure.

Unfortunately, traditional reverse isolation procedures to protect patients from exposure to infectious organisms are of questionable value for the patient with severely compromised granulocyte production. Even small numbers of bacteria may produce a lethal infection. Also, many patients are thought to become infected with organisms from *within their own GI tracts.* An isolation package offering greater protection is the Laminar Air Flow environment or a similar system, which uses sterilized air flow, sterile equipment, and special procedures designed to protect the patient from her or his own native flora. Such procedures involve the administration of oral nonabsorbable antibiotics to sterilize the gut and the use of local antibiotic ointments, powders, and sprays to decontaminate body areas normally high in organisms. The goal is to make the environment *totally sterile,* not just to reduce the numbers of organisms (Fig. 46–2).

Even when sterile environments are being used effectively, the constant monitoring of the agranulocytic patient for signs of infection is a crucial part of the nursing effort. In addition, it is important to teach patients and the people close to them to participate in the constant observation for infection. Patients and their significant others may be very helpful in this regard during the patient's hospitalization. Also, knowledge of the signs of infection may help patients to care for themselves better when discharged home.

Assess and Control Bleeding and Anemia. Peripheral platelet counts of less than 50,000 per cu. mm. or progressively falling platelet counts should alert the nurse to increase surveillance of the patient for signs of bleeding. Inspect the patient's *urine* and *stool* routinely, both grossly and microscopically, for signs of blood. Check the patient's *skin* thoroughly for petechiae and bruising. Examine the patient's *mouth* for palatal petechiae, bleeding, and bruising. Interruptions in the integrity of the *skin* (as for injections, venipunctures, IV therapy) should receive special local care to prevent bruising at the site. Teach the patient about the significance of the *platelet count.* Advise the patient to avoid trauma and bruising, to use a soft toothbrush, and to avoid eating mechanically abrasive foods. Also, warn patients to report headaches and changes in vision. *Constipation* must be prevented because it can cause bleeding of the rectal mucosa.

Some patients can tolerate platelet counts as low as 5000 to 10,000 per cu. mm. without showing signs of bleeding. Other patients will show signs of bleeding with a platelet count at 50,000 per cu. mm. Because of this wide variation in tolerance, it is most important to do everything you can to identify the onset of signs of bleeding. Platelet transfusions are often given on the basis of your information. Platelet transfusions are given to prevent life-threatening bleeding.

Platelet transfusions are generally obtained from blood banks. They are usually administered according to blood type. Because few red cells are transfused with platelets, cross matching is not necessary. Platelets should be administered as soon as they are received and given as rapidly as the patient can tolerate. The physician may request a platelet count 1 hour after the infusion, to determine the effectiveness of the transfusion in increasing the patient's peripheral count. Patients with active bleeding may show a *change* in that bleeding during or following the transfusion. That information is

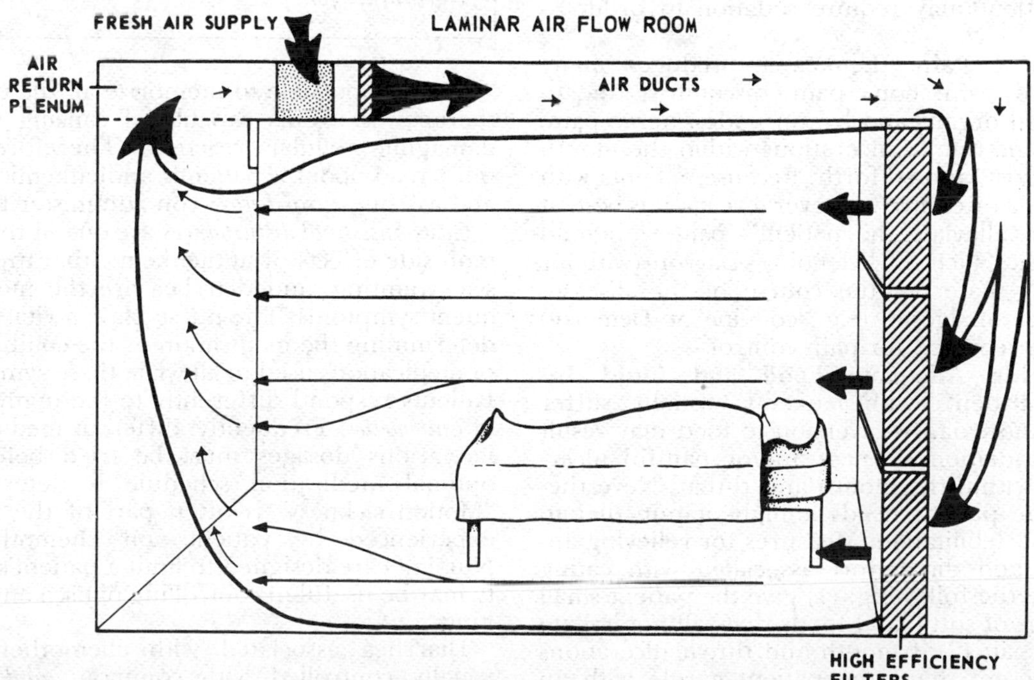

Figure 46–2. Diagram of air circulation in a laminar air flow room. By combining high-efficiency air filtration with air flowing in a horizontal pattern at 90 feet per minute (to prevent particles from settling), a sterile environment can be achieved. Outside air is caught in the laminar flow and filtered before it reaches the patient. Ninety per cent of air samples from a laminar air flow room are sterile.[2a] (From Brodey, G. P.: Infection in patients with cancer. In Holland, J. F., and E. Frei, III: *Cancer Medicine.* Philadelphia: Lea & Febiger, 1973.)

an important observation, usually made by the nurse.

Patients may have *reactions* to platelet transfusions. Most commonly the reactions are allergic in nature and are treated with Benadryl. Chills and fever occur uncommonly. Intravenous Demerol usually aborts the chills. The patient should receive a fever work-up, including cultures of his or her blood and the transfused platelets. Patients with a history of frequent allergic reactions to platelet transfusions may receive Benadryl before the transfusion.

Patients with marrow suppression also experience *anemias,* because erythrocytes are crowded out by the wildly proliferating white cells. This condition is treated with red cell transfusions or transfusions of whole blood.

Provide Adequate Rest. Encourage the ambulatory patient to sleep at least 8 hours every night and to take naps during the day as needed. As you recall, patients with leukemia experience an increased metabolic rate because of the massive overproduction of leukocytes; they also suffer from hypoxia due to anemia. Consequently, these individuals need additional rest because they are chronically fatigued and exhausted (a state that increases susceptibility to infection). In far advanced cases of leukemia, the patient may require sedation in order to sleep.

Control Pain. Leukemia produces many types of pain: bone pain, discomfort due to enlarged organs and lymph nodes, nerve pain, dysphagia due to ulcerations within the mouth and throat, and so forth. Because patients with leukemia often live for several years, it is best, at first, to alleviate the patient's pain with mild analgesics such as Tylenol or Darvon (without aspirin). Later in the course of the disease, stronger analgesics (e.g., codeine or Demerol) may be required for pain control.

Provide Adequate Food and Fluid Intake. Patients with leukemia usually suffer from anorexia. An aversion to food may result from radiation sickness and/or painful ulcerations within the mouth and throat. Nevertheless, the patient needs a high-vitamin diet to prevent debilitation. Measures for relieving anorexia and discomfort associated with eating include the following: (1) give the patient small servings of soft bland foods that will not irritate the throat; (2) if mouth and throat ulcerations are present, have the patient gargle with an anesthetic solution immediately prior to eating; (3) when throat discomfort is severe, order nutritious cold or frozen foods such as ice cream, fruit sherbet, malted milk shakes, chilled fruit and vegetable juices, concentrated diet drinks that are high in protein, and so forth; (4) contact the dietitian if the patient continues to be dissatisfied with the diet; (5) if nausea and vomiting persist, obtain an order for intravenous infusion therapy.

In addition to eating an adequate diet, the patient with leukemia must also drink at least *3000 to 4000 ml. of fluid every day.* Fluids are needed to prevent dehydration resulting from fever and diaphoresis, and to dilute the high levels of uric acid that result from destruction of abnormal leukocytes by the chemotherapeutic agents. The nurse must keep an accurate record of fluid lost through emesis or diarrhea. Proper management of fluid and electrolyte balance is impossible without this information. Weighing the patient daily can provide additional information useful in managing the patient's fluid balance.

Minimize the Discomforts and Side Effects of Antileukemic Therapy. Antileukemic therapy is often difficult to administer, and it has many unpleasant side effects. The single most important nursing aspect of administering chemotherapy is related to the intravenous route of administration. *Remember that the veins are the lifeline sustaining leukemic patients!*

> *Meticulous care in administering chemotherapy greatly prolongs the life of veins. A* single episode of infiltration *of a chemotherapeutic agent can damage many veins, in addition to causing the patient considerable discomfort.*

It is not possible to memorize all the chemotherapeutic agents capable of causing such a damaging cellular reaction. Therefore, you must read about a patient's antileukemic drugs and ask questions *before* you administer them.

Gastrointestinal disturbances are one of the common side effects of antileukemic therapy. Nausea, vomiting, and diarrhea are the most frequent symptoms. The nurse plays a vital role in determining the medication or the combination of medications used to alleviate these symptoms. Patients respond differently to the many kinds of *antiemetics.* Frequently, different medications in various dosages must be tried before an optimal medication schedule is determined. "Motion sickness" is often part of the nausea experienced by patients on chemotherapy. Nursing care designed to limit a patient's activity may be useful in controlling nausea and vomiting.

Diarrhea associated with chemotherapy is usually controlled with common *antidiarrheal agents.* Severe cases may be treated with *IV morphine.* Systemic analgesics known to slow the motility of the gut may be an analgesic of choice for the patient with diarrhea. Patients receiving *antacids* should receive those that tend to produce constipation. The patient with diarrhea has an increased risk of perianal irritation and infection. Meticulous cleaning of the area after each stool will reduce that risk. Prophylactic sitz baths are often effective.

Provide Psychologic Support. Whether or not patients should be told that they have leukemia is a vital question. (See Unit IX.) Patients with this disease often suffer from depression. Patients who know they have leukemia often need psychologic support throughout the difficult weeks, months, or years following diagnosis. Fortunately, most patients and the persons close to them are encouraged once they realize that the patient can lead an almost normal life during the period of remission obtained by chemotherapy and radiotherapy.

Before patients are discharged, arrange for them to visit the social worker if there is a financial problem. The social worker and community agency representative (American Cancer Society) can be contacted for information concerning home nursing; housekeeping and cooking services; and purchase of wheelchairs, bandages, hospital beds, drugs, and so forth. Patients suffering from *severe* depression or other psychologic problems may benefit from a psychiatric referral. It is the nurse's responsibility to assess such symptoms as withdrawal, constant weeping, inability to concentrate, total loss of appetite, insomnia, and threats of suicide and take appropriate action (i.e., develop a plan of nursing care; refer patient to a psychiatrist, social worker, or religious advisor; suggest prescription of antidepressant drugs, or suggest occupational therapy).

Leukemic patients who feel depression associated with relapse and acute illness can get over that depression when their clinical state improves. They should be reassured that the depression will pass, just as many of the other discomforts associated with relapse eventually pass.

If the leukemic patient's nurse is well informed about leukemia and openly teaches that knowledge, and if the nurse is conscientious and intelligent in appraising and treating clinical problems, the patient will experience a true sense of psychologic support. Likewise, the nurse who is willing to work within a close and productive relationship with the patient and physician will observe that the relationship has a profound effect upon the patient's feelings of well-being, trust, and confidence.

When working with a patient with a life-threatening illness, remember that the person is living. The whole emphasis of care of the person should not be on dying.

Multiple Myeloma (Plasma Cell Myeloma)

Multiple myeloma is a neoplastic condition characterized by: (1) the abnormal malignant proliferation of plasma cells; (2) the development within the bone marrow of either single or multiple tumors composed of abnormal plasma cells; and (3) bone destruction throughout the body, followed later by dissemination of the disease into the lymph nodes, liver, spleen, and kidneys.

This condition most commonly occurs in people over 40 years of age; it affects twice as many men as women. Although multiple myeloma was once considered a relatively rare disease, its incidence has increased in recent years and now approaches that of Hodgkin's disease.

The onset of multiple myeloma is usually gradual and insidious. Most patients pass through a long *presymptomatic period* that lasts from five to 20 years. During this phase of the disease, some individuals suffer from recurrent bacterial infections, particularly pneumonia. Increased susceptibility to infection is evidently linked to disturbances of antibody formation resulting from abnormalities of plasma cells.

Once symptoms finally appear, they typically involve the skeletal system, particularly the pelvis, spine, and ribs. Some patients have backache or bone pain that worsens upon movement. Other suddenly suffer a pathologic fracture accompanied by severe pain. As time goes on, skeletal destruction increases and the patient may develop deformities of the sternum and rib cage. Some patients shrink 5 inches or more in stature as a result of shortening of the spine. Diffuse osteoporosis is also usually present, accompanied by a negative calcium balance. The skull shows multiple osteolytic lesions (Fig. 46–3). Drainage of calcium and phosphorus from the damaged bones eventually leads to the development of renal stones, particularly if the patient is immobilized.

In addition to bone destruction, multiple myeloma is characterized by disruption of erythrocyte, leukocyte, and thrombocyte production as a result of replacement of the bone marrow with plasma cells. Impaired production of these three cell forms causes: anemia, hemorrhagic tendencies as a result of thrombocytopenia, and increased vulnerability to infection owing to granulocytopenia.

Complications of multiple myeloma include hypercalcemia and renal and neurologic disorders. The major neurologic complications are compression of the spinal cord by tumors, later

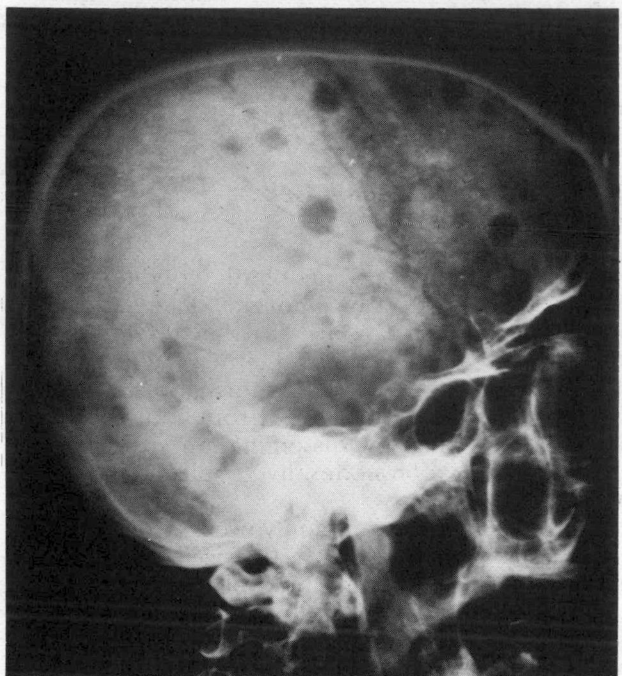

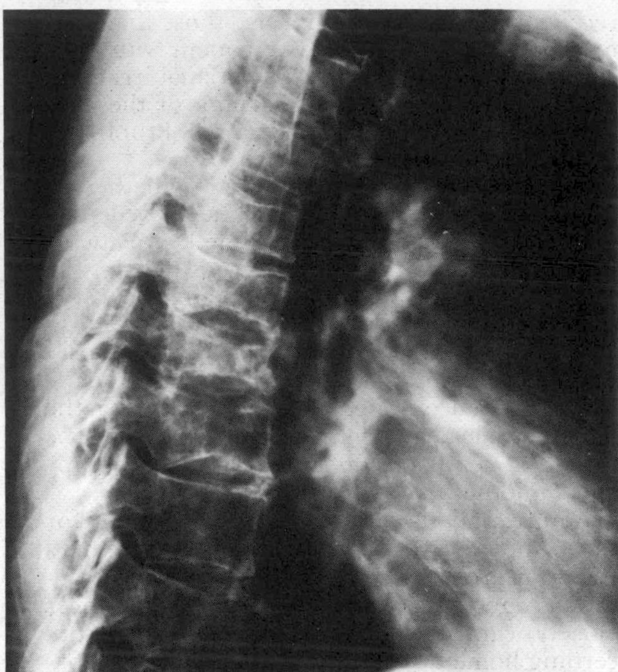

Figure 46–3. Characteristic x-ray abnormalities in multiple myeloma. Skull shows multiple osteolytic ("punched out") lesions. Thoracic spine shows extensive osteoporosis and partial collapse of several vertebral bodies. (From Osserman, E. F.: Plasma cell dyscrasias. *In* Beeson, P. B., W. McDermott, and J. B. Wyngaarden: *Cecil Textbook of Medicine*. Philadelphia: W. B. Saunders Co., 1979, p. 1859.)

followed by the development of paraplegia. Renal disease results from blockage of the convoluted tubules by particles of coagulated protein.

Diagnosis of multiple myeloma rests upon x-ray studies, a bone marrow aspiration and biopsy, and laboratory examinaton of blood and urine. X-ray studies reveal diffuse lesions in the bone, widespread demineralization, and osteoporosis. The bone marrow contains large numbers of immature plasma cells. Normally, plasma cells constitute only 5 per cent of the marrow cellular population, but in multiple myeloma, plasma cells make up between 30 and 95 per cent of the cell population. Because of the abnormal proliferation of plasma cells, blood studies generally reveal a high concentration of serum globulins. Another diagnostic sign of multiple myeloma is the appearance of an abnormal globulin in the urine that is called *Bence Jones protein.**

GOALS OF CARE

Once multiple myeloma is diagnosed, the treatment is purely symptomatic. The four major goals of care for persons with this fatal condition are as follows:

Reduce Tumor Mass. Radiotherapy and chemotherapy are currently used to reduce bone tumor size and growth. Tumors composed of plasma cells are usually radiosensitive; consequently only small doses of radiation are necessary to control symptoms and tumor size. The two alkylating agents used to treat multiple myeloma are melphalan (Alkeran) and cyclophosphamide (Cytoxan). Alkeran has been the most successful drug to date in the treatment of multiple myeloma. The major toxic effect of Alkeran is *pancytopenia.* For this reason, observe the patient's hemogram daily for signs of bone marrow depression. Cytoxan, while helpful, is not as consistently effective as Alkeran. Side effects of Cytoxan include leukopenia, nausea, alopecia and hemorrhagic cystitis.

Control Pain. Patients with multiple myeloma suffer from severe bone pain and sometimes from spontaneous fractures. However, relief from pain can often be obtained by the administration of analgesics.

Promote Adequate Ambulation and Hydration. You recall that multiple myeloma is characterized by osteoporosis and the resultant loss of calcium from the bones into the blood and urine. Calcium loss leads to hypercalcemia, hypercalciuria, renal stones, and potentially fatal renal damage. Osteoporosis and calcium loss always worsen if the patient is immobilized. To prevent complications, it is essential to move or to ambulate the patient frequently and to force fluids.

Ambulating patients with multiple myeloma is a major nursing challenge. Many patients, because of pain or fear of falling, prefer to remain immobilized in their beds. Analgesics and orthopedic supports and braces can be used to reduce the patient's pain and sense of insecurity. Because persons with multiple myeloma are particularly vulnerable to pathologic

*In 1848 Henry Bence Jones identified a protein substance that is usually excreted in the urine of persons with multiple myeloma and other bone tumors.

fractures, always accompany the patient who is walking, in order to prevent accidents and falls.

The administration of fluids is another important nursing responsibility. Patients with multiple myeloma require between 3000 and 4000 ml. of fluid per day. If fluid intake is adequate, patients have a 24-hour urine output of approximately 1500 ml. Sufficient fluid is needed not only to counteract the calcium overload but also to prevent protein from precipitating in the renal tubules.

The necessity to ambulate and hydrate the patient with multiple myeloma cannot be stressed enough! As Osserman explains:

> *"Unless mobilization and hydration are accomplished by these measures, it is usually impossible to maintain a patient for the time required to accomplish a remission with chemotherapy."*[89]

Treat Complications. Anemia is treated with transfusion therapy. Infections are managed with antibiotics. To prevent recurrent infection, the doctor may order the administration of gamma globulin, 10 ml. IM every 2 weeks. Corticosteroids and Mithramycin are prescribed for severe hypercalcemia accompanied by nausea and vomiting. Patients suffering from spinal cord compression must sometimes undergo a laminectomy.

Drug and x-ray therapy together with excellent nursing care can extend the life of some patients with multiple myeloma for many years. However, patients usually die within 1½ to 2 years following diagnosis of the disease.

NURSING PATIENTS WITH DISORDERS PRIMARILY AFFECTING THE LYMPH NODES AND SPLEEN

The Lymphoproliferative Disorders (Malignant Lymphomas)

The lymphomas are a group of neoplastic tumors that chiefly affect lymphatic structures and are composed of either lymphocytes or reticulum cells. Lymphomas may be classified as follows: (1) Hodgkin's disease and (2) non-Hodgkin's lymphomas, such as (a) lymphosarcoma, (b) reticulum cell sarcoma, and (c) Burkitt's lymphoma (a disease primarily affecting children who live in Central Africa).

HODGKIN'S DISEASE

Definition and Incidence. Hodgkin's disease is a chronic, progressive, neoplastic disorder. It is initially characterized by enlargement of the lymph glands, spleen, and liver, followed later by the pathologic involvement of tissues and organs throughout the body. The cause of Hodgkin's disease is unknown.

A disorder of young adults, Hodgkin's disease principally occurs between the ages of 20 and 40. Among adults, men affected outnumber women by a ratio of 2:1; among children, boys are striken five times more often than are girls.

Over the past 20 years there has been a significant improvement in the survival rate of patients stricken with Hodgkin's disease. Some researchers state that "with early diagnosis and aggressive treatment 90% of patients with localized Hodgkin's disease can now be cured — that is, have a 10 year survival without recurrence. This compares with 35% only ten years ago."[66]

Pathogenesis. You will recall that each neoplastic blood disorder is characterized by the abnormal proliferation of one particular type of blood cell. In Hodgkin's disease the proliferating cells are abnormal histiocytes (one category of reticuloendothelial cells) called *Reed-Sternberg* cells. As these atypical giant cells multiply, they eventually replace the normal cellular elements within the lymph nodes. In time, the structure of the lymph nodes is damaged and areas of necrosis and fibrosis develop.

Typically, Hodgkin's disease initially affects one lymph node and then travels to other lymph nodes throughout the body via lymphatic channels. In some cases, the neoplastic process may extend to other organs and structures. For example, nodules of varying size may appear in the liver and spleen; the vertebrae may be affected, resulting in vertebral collapse; and organs such as the ureters and bronchi may be invaded because of their close proximity to involved lymphatic structures.

Hodgkin's disease is often divided into categories or stages, classified according to the microscopic appearance of the involved lymph nodes, the extent and severity of the disorder, and the prognosis. One method of staging is shown in Table 46–3.

Bases of Symptoms. The first symptom of Hodgkin's disease is the painless enlargement of the lymph nodes, caused by the massive proliferation of Reed-Sternberg cells. Later, as the disease disseminates throughout the reticuloendothelial system (a process which may be slow or swift), numerous and varied manifestations appear. The major signs and symptoms of Hodgkin's disease are outlined in Table 46–4.

During the late stages of the disease, the patient becomes severely anemic and cachexic. Also, as lymphatic obstruction worsens, large amounts of fluid accumulate in the patient's chest and abdomen. Eventually the patient dies in a state of shock and debilitation.

TABLE 46–3. ANN ARBOR CLINICAL STAGING

Stage	Description
I	Involvement of a single lymph node region (I) or of a single extralymphatic organ or site (IE).
II	Involvement of two or more lymph node regions on the same side of the diaphragm (II), or localized involvement of extralymphatic organ or site and of one or more lymph node regions on the same side of the diaphragm (IIE).
III	Involvement of lymph node regions on both sides of the diaphragm (III), which may also be accompanied by localized involvement of extralymphatic organ or site (IIIE) or by involvement of the spleen (IIIS), or both (IIISE).
IV	Diffuse or disseminated involvement of one or more extralymphatic organs or tissues with or without associated lymph node enlargement.
A	No general symptoms.
B	Presence of one or more general symptoms: (1) unexplained weight loss of more than 10% of the body weight in the 6 months before admission; (2) unexplained fever with temperatures above 38°C; (3) night sweats.

Notes: 1. The lymphatic structures are defined as the lymph nodes (N), spleen (S), thymus, Waldeyer's ring, appendix, and Peyer's patches.

2. The reason for classifying the patient as Stage IV is defined further by defining sites by symbols:

H–liver	L–lung
M–marrow	O–bone
P–pleura	D–skin

3. Liver involvement is always considered Stage IV disease, as is bone marrow involvement away from a site of an involved lymph node.

From Le Blanc, D. H.: People with Hodgkin disease: The nursing challenge. *Nursing Clinics of North America,* 13(2):281, June 1978. (As reprinted from Carbone, P. P., et al.: Report of the committee on Hodgkin's disease staging classification. *Cancer Research,* 31:1860, 1971.)

Diagnosis. *Lymph node biopsy* is the definitive examination for diagnosing Hodgkin's disease. When peripheral lymph node enlargement is present, one entire lymph node is removed and examined for the presence of Reed-Sternberg cells. However, some patients do not have enlarged peripheral lymph nodes but may simply notice pruritus, intermittent fever, and weakness. In these cases, Hodgkin's disease can often be diagnosed by x-raying the patient's chest for evidence of mediastinal or hilar adenopathy.

Blood studies typically reveal a normocytic normochromic anemia. Also, because of disturbances of the immune mechanism, patients with Hodgkin's disease are usually unable to react normally to skin tests for tuberculosis.

Clinical Care. Patients in stages I or II of Hodgkin's disease can sometimes be cured with wide-field megavoltage radiation. Doses of 3500 to 4500 roentgens (r) given over a 4- to 6-week period can possibly eradicate the disease for life, provided the neoplastic process has not spread beyond the lymph node chains, spleen, and nasopharynx. If sites other than the three listed above require irradiation therapy, the radiologist protects the vital organs (i.e., the heart, lungs, liver, bone marrow, kidneys) with tailor-made leaded shields in order to prevent permanent organ damage.

Unfortunately, patients with stage III or IV disease cannot be cured by radiation therapy. However, they usually experience symptomatic relief when treated with radiotherapy and chemotherapy combined. See Table 46–2 for the drugs currently used for chemotherapy. Many institutions use a combination of chemotherapeutic drugs. The doses and drug schedules vary with the institution and the individual patient, but a "basic pattern is to give the drugs in six courses: each course being a 28-day period in which the patient receives drugs for 14 days, then 'rests' for 14 days to permit bone marrow recovery."[66] (See Table 46–5.)

Despite the symptomatic relief that the chemotherapeutic drugs bring, many patients are unable to tolerate them. The most distressing and immediate side effect of the chemotherapeutic drugs is severe *nausea and vomiting,* which may last for hours. To reduce nausea: (1) give the medication in the evening following a light lunch and no dinner; (2) request an order for sedation and an antiemetic drug; and (3) keep the patient's room cool and quiet following administration of the agent. A second and more dreaded toxic effect of chemotherapy is *pancytopenia,* which may develop within 10 to 14 days following the IV injection. If the patient's hemogram reveals any degree of leukopenia, anemia, or thrombocytopenia, chemotherapy must be discontinued.

Surgery, a third form of therapy, is sometimes employed to remove tumors that are placing undue pressure upon an organ or nerve; e.g., surgical excision of a tumor that is pressing on the spinal cord will relieve pain and paralysis.

In addition to reducing the size of tumor masses, therapy is also directed toward the relief of symptoms. *Fever* is reduced with acetylsalicylic acid, given every 4 hours, and the administration of cooling measures; *anemia* is controlled with transfusions; *pruritus* (an often intractable problem) is sometimes relieved by the administration of either colchicine or chlorpromazine (Thorazine); *infections* may be guarded against by reverse isolation techniques.

Prognosis. There is a 95 per cent cure rate for patients who are diagnosed in stage I or II of the disease and who are treated with intensive radiotherapy. Patients who are diagnosed stage III or IV now have an arrest rate greater than 70 per cent with the use of combined conventional and experimental chemotherapy. When untreated, patients with Hodgkin's disease have a life expectancy of 5 years.

TABLE 46-4. SIGNS AND SYMPTOMS OF HODGKIN'S DISEASE

Signs and Symptoms	Bases
Severe pruritus is an early sign	Cause unknown.
Irregular fever usually present; typically, temperature is elevated for a few days and then drops to normal or subnormal for several days or weeks; continuous high fever may indicate impending death	Temperature elevation is apparently related to neoplastic involvement of the internal nodes or viscera.
Splenomegaly and hepatomegaly	Dissemination of the disorder from the lymph nodes to other organs of the reticuloendothelial system.
Jaundice	Obstruction of the bile ducts as a result of liver damage causes the pigment bilirubin to accumulate in the blood and discolor the skin.
Edema and cyanosis of the face and neck	Enlarged lymph nodes may place pressure on the superior vena cava and cause edema of the areas which it drains.
Pulmonary symptoms including cough, stridor, dyspnea, chest pain, cyanosis, and pleural effusion	Mediastinal lymph node enlargement, involvement of the lung parenchyma, and invasion of the pleura occurs in more than one half of patients.
Progressive anemia accompanied by fatigue, malaise, anorexia, etc.	Erythrocyte life span is shortened, and erythropoiesis is unable to keep pace with erythrocyte destruction.
Bone manifestations include pain, vertebral compression and, infrequently, fracture	Dissemination of the disease from the lymph nodes to the bones.
Nerve pain	Compression of the nerve roots of the brachial, lumbar, or sacral plexuses.
Paraplegia	Compression of the spinal cord resulting from extradural involvement.
Increased susceptibility to infection	Impairment of immune mechanisms from unknown causes.
Alcohol-induced pain: bone pain or pain around the mediastinum occurs immediately after drinking alcohol and lasts for 30 to 60 minutes	Cause unknown.

TABLE 46-5. MOPP COMBINATION CHEMOTHERAPY REGIMEN FOR HODGKIN DISEASE*

Drug	Abbreviation	Schedule
Nitrogen mustard (Mustargen)	M	Given IV on day 1 and day 8.
Vincristine (Oncovin)	O	Given IV on day 1 and day 8.
Procarbazine	Pr	Given orally, day 1 through day 14.
Prednisone	P	Given orally day 1 through day 14, in 1st and 4th cycle only.

*Minimum of six 2-week cycles with 2-week rest between cycles. Doses of M, O, and Pr are reduced as WBC falls below 4000/cu. mm. and platelets fall below 100,000/cu. mm., or if neurotoxicity develops.

Dose is stopped if WBC reaches 1000/cu. mm. and platelets, 50,000/cu. mm. Hemorrhage is possible at counts below 20,000/cu. mm.

Modified from Le Blanc, D. H.: People with Hodgkin disease: The nursing challenge. *Nursing Clinics of North America*, 13(2): 281, June 1978, p. 282.

NON-HODGKIN'S LYMPHOMAS

Lymphosarcoma and Reticulum Cell Sarcoma. Lymphosarcoma and reticulum cell sarcoma are considered together because they have much in common. Their symptoms, physical abnormalities, laboratory findings, and treatment modalities are very similar. Like Hodgkin's disease, they are malignant conditions of unknown etiology that primarily involve lymphatic tissues. Lymphosarcoma and reticulum cell sarcoma are neither common nor rare, developing in persons of all ages; however, they principally strike middle-aged persons.

The earliest sign of lymphosarcoma or reticulum cell sarcoma is *painless lymphadenopathy,* which is usually unilateral.

The first lymph nodes to enlarge are usually in the neck, although axillary or inguinal lymph nodes may sometimes enlarge initially. As the disease progresses, the neoplastic process spreads along lymphatic channels to other lymph nodes. Eventually lymphosarcoma and

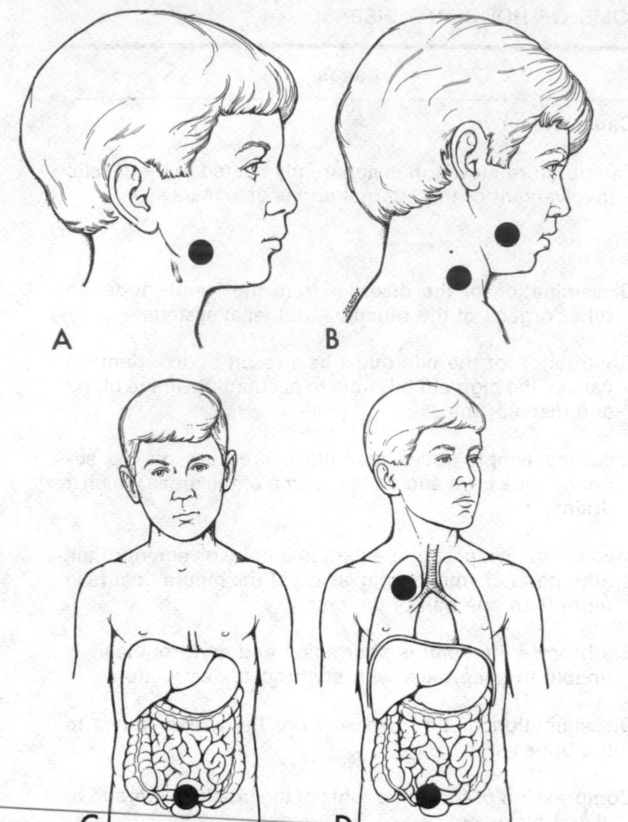

Figure 46–4. Tumor staging for Burkitt's lymphoma is an indicator of the person's prognosis. Stage A is a tumor localized to a single extra-abdominal site; Stage B, tumor involves two or more extra-abdominal sites; Stage C, intra-abdominal tumor with or without facial involvement; Stage D, intra-abdominal tumor with involvement of anatomic sites other than facial. The later the stage, the less likely the cure. (From Wackenhut, J. S., and R. A. Barnwell: Burkitt's lymphoma. *American Journal of Nursing,* 79(10):1766, Oct. 1979.)

reticulum cell sarcoma invade the *bone marrow;* this is one of the outstanding features of these diseases. Other organs that may be involved include the liver, spleen, skin, gastrointestinal tract, and nervous system. Pressure on these organs and organ obstruction, in turn, produce symptoms; e.g., abdominal pain, nerve pain or paralysis, and so forth. Other general problems that accompany lymphosarcoma and reticulum cell sarcoma include anemia, malaise, fever, weight loss, sweating and pruritus.

The *diagnosis* of lymphosarcoma or reticulum cell sarcoma is based on *lymph node biopsy.* When either disease is present, destruction of lymph node architecture is evident, and normal cellular elements are replaced by huge numbers of lymphocytes or lymphoblasts. Once the diagnosis is confirmed, the patient is further evaluated in order to discern the stage of the disease. Staging for lymphosarcoma and reticular cell sarcoma is the same as for Hodgkin's disease.

Like Hodgkin's disease, lymphosarcoma and reticulum cell sarcoma are treated with irradiation, chemotherapy and, occasionally, surgery. However, for patients with lymphosarcoma or reticulum cell sarcoma irradiation is only a palliative rather than a curative measure, as it is in stage I and II of Hodgkin's disease. Irradiation is less successful in lymphosarcoma and reticulum cell sarcoma because: (1) lymphosarcoma and reticulum cell sarcoma tend initially to strike several sites at once, whereas Hodgkin's disease tends to limit itself to one site for a period of time; and (2) the dosage of radiation must be lower in lymphosarcoma and reticulum cell sarcoma than in Hodgkin's disease because the bone marrow, which is involved in lymphosarcoma and reticulum cell sarcoma, is easily injured by radiotherapy.

The drugs used to treat lymphosarcoma and reticulum cell sarcoma are the same as those used for Hodgkin's disease, e.g., cyclophosphamide (Cytoxan), vincristine (Oncovin), and prednisone.

On rare occasions, surgical excision of an involved lymph node is performed and is curative. For a successful operation, the disease must be discovered in its early stages and be limited to a single lymph node.

The prognosis for patients with lymphosarcoma or reticulum cell sarcoma is poor. Adults generally survive for about 2 years following the onset of the disease, while children under 16 usually die within less than 1 year.

Burkitt's Lymphoma. This malignant lymphoma was first discovered in 1957 by Burkitt among children in Central Africa. This condition is most common in tropical Africa, although a similar tumor occurs in the United Sates and accounts for 5 per cent of all childhood malignancies. Characteristically, Burkitt's lymphoma:

- ▶ Affects children (2 to 14 years of age)
- ▶ Develops in extranodal sites (usually jaw, abdomen, and CNS)
- ▶ Responds remarkably well to chemotherapy. Approximately one third of all patients achieve a complete remission that lasts for 2 years.

Staging of the tumor is determined by site, as seen in Figure 46–4.

Burkitt's lymphoma responds rapidly to cancer chemotherapeutic agents (the treatment of choice). The tumor cells proliferate at a doubling time of 24 hours; this accounts for the sensitivity to the drugs. Other modalities of treatment include surgery for removal of rapidly enlarging tumors, radiation for CNS involvement and treatment of medical emergencies resulting from obstruction by the tumor mass.

Nursing care revolves around (1) the effects of the diagnosis of cancer on the patient and significant others, (2) the effects of the lysing cells (i.e., hyperkalemia, hyperphosphatemia, hypocalcemia, hyperuricemia), and (3) the effects of toxic chemotherapeutic agents.

Infectious Mononucleosis

Infectious mononucleosis (also known as "glandular disease" and the "kissing disease") is a benign self-limiting condition characterized by painful enlargement of the lymph nodes, lymphocytosis, and fever. The cause of infectious mononucleosis is a herpes-like virus called the Epstein-Barr virus (EBV). Although it is possibile that the disease is transmitted by direct contact such as kissing, the exact mode of transmission remains unknown.

Primarily a disease of the young, infectious mononucleosis usually strikes children between the ages of 3 and 5 and young persons between the ages of 15 and 25. It has its greatest incidence among college students, medical students, and nurses. Although infectious mononucleosis usually occurs sporadically, it also sweeps in epidemic form through colleges and children's homes.

Although infectious mononucleosis is a relatively mild disorder, its effects upon the body are widespread. The lymph nodes enlarge; the blood picture reveals a lymphocytosis; the spleen may swell two to three times its normal size; liver function is sometimes impaired; and both the peripheral and central nervous systems may be involved in the disease process.

The onset of infectious mononucleosis follows an incubation period of uncertain length that is believed to extend from a few days to several weeks. The patient complains of fever, chills, malaise, severe headache, sore throat, and painful, swollen lymph nodes that are located mainly in the posterior, cervical, axillary, and groin regions. Ten to 15 per cent of patients develop a macular rash that closely resembles the rash seen in rubella. Splenic enlargement causes left upper quadrant pain. Nervous system involvement causes the severe headache. In rare cases, liver involvement may result in the development of a hepatitis-like syndrome. When infectious mononucleosis is severe, the patient risks developing the following complications:

- Splenic rupture as a result of the infiltration of the spleen by massive numbers of lymphocytes.
- Streptococcal pharyngitis or Vincent's angina owing to secondary bacterial invasion of the throat.

The diagnosis of infectious mononucleosis is based upon the following three criteria: (1) the clinical picture (i.e., fever, lymphadenopathy, sore throat, splenomegaly); (2) the blood picture, which includes a white count of 12,000 to 18,000 leukocytes per cu. mm., of which 60 per cent are large, atypical lymphocytes (known as Downey cells); and (3) a positive Paul-Bunnell heterophil test. The term *heterophil* means "having an affinity for more than one group or species."[44] In 1932 Paul and Bunnell discovered that the blood of patients with infectious mononucleosis contained antibodies that would clump or agglutinate the red blood cells of sheep. Normally human beings do not produce agglutinins against sheep erythrocytes; consequently, a positive heterophil test helps to confirm the diagnosis of infectious mononucleosis, though positive tests sometimes occur in other conditions.

There is no specific medical therapy for patients with this condition that will either alleviate or hasten the disease process. Infectious mononucleosis must simply run its course. However, it is possible to relieve the patient's symptoms and to provide comfort. Thus, the patient is confined to bed until fever, malaise, fatigue, and headache lessen. Salicylates, cool sponge baths, and a large fluid intake are important measures for controlling fever. Warm saline throat irrigations are occasionally administered to very ill patients with beneficial results. Although steroids do not in any way alter or accelerate the course of the disease, these drugs tend to increase the patient's sense of well-being.

In addition to providing symptomatic relief, a second goal of care is to prevent and to treat complications. When caring for patients with infectious mononucleosis, remember the following points:

1. Caution the patient against engaging in excessive activity; this may result in splenic rupture or a lowered resistance to infection.

2. Watch the patient closely for the two signs of splenic rupture: abdominal pain, and shock. Report these signs at once and prepare the patient for emergency surgery.

3. Isolate the patient from possible sources of bacterial contamination. If throat pain worsens, report this immediately so that appropriate antibiotic therapy can be started.

Although complications sometimes develop, the prognosis for patients with infectious mononucleosis is generally excellent. The febrile phase of this disorder, which generally lasts from 2 to 4 weeks, is followed by a long convalescent period during which time the patient slowly regains strength and energy.

The Spleen and Its Disorders

The spleen, a glandlike organ that is located in the upper part of the abdominal cavity on the left side of the body, has long been an enigma. The ancients called the spleen "a dark organ . . . full of mystery." The spleen was once believed to harbor a person's irritations, melancholy, and anger; thus, we still say that a man who expresses rage is "venting his spleen." Today, while we no longer regard the spleen as the site of negative emotion, we still fail to fully understand its physiologic role. As part of the reticuloendothelial system, the spleen apparently performs a vital but not essential function in purifying the blood and protecting the body from various stresses. Known functions of the spleen include the following:

- Acts as a blood reservoir in animals and to a lesser extent in human beings. When the body is subjected to excessive stress (e.g., extreme exertion, bleeding, carbon monoxide poisoning), the spleen contracts and expels its store of erythrocytes into the circulation.

- Purifies blood and captures circulating antigens.
- Acts as a primary source of antibodies in infants and small children; produces lymphocytes, plasma cells, and antibodies in adults.
- Performs extramedullary hematopoiesis (production of erythrocytes outside the bone marrow). The spleen normally produces red cells in the fetus. In adults, however, extramedullary hematopoiesis is *abnormal;* it occurs only in individuals with bone marrow depression and a resultant pancytopenia. If prolonged, extramedullary hematopoiesis leads to splenomegaly.
- Destroys red blood cells when they reach the end of their 120-day life span.
- Traps and destroys fragile or defective red blood cells (spherocytes).
- Is responsible in part for iron metabolism.
- Pitting ("removes particulate inclusions from red cells without destroying the cell itself"[125]).

Splenectomy. *Despite the important functions listed above, the spleen can be removed (splenectomy) without harm to the adult patient.* (You will recall that *all* surgeries carry the risk of postoperative complications. See Chapter 20.) The role of the spleen can be completely taken over by other reticuloendothelial organs (e.g., the liver, lymph nodes, and bone marrow). However, because the spleen is a major source of antibody formation in children, pediatricians do not recommend splenectomy during the early years of a child's life. If splenectomy is absolutely necessary, the child must receive prophylactic antibiotics following surgery in order to prevent infection.

The most frequent indication for splenectomy is *rupture of the spleen* complicated by severe hemorrhage. Causes of splenic rupture include the following: (1) trauma, which can result from automobile accidents, penetration with a bullet or knife, a severe blow to the spleen, and so forth; (2) accidental tearing of the splenic capsule during surgery on neighboring organs; and (3) diseases of the spleen that cause softening or damage (e.g., infectious mononucleosis and malaria).

Hypersplenism is a second important indication for splenectomy. The term hypersplenism implies that the spleen is destroying, in excessive numbers, one of the cellular elements of the blood (i.e., erythrocytes, leukocytes, or platelets). Signs of hypersplenism include splenomegaly, anemia or leukopenia, and a compensatory increase in the production of the sequestered blood cells by the bone marrow. Overactivity of the spleen develops either as a primary condition of unknown origin or secondary to another disease. *Primary* hypersplenism occurs in idiopathic thrombocytopenic purpura and congenital spherocytosis. *Secondary* hypersplenism occurs in association with leukemia, the lymphomas, Hodgkin's disease, tuberculosis, and portal hypertension resulting from liver disease. Primary hypersplenism can be alleviated by splenectomy. However, splenectomy is simply a palliative measure for patients suffering from secondary hypersplenism, since the surgery has little or no effect on the course of the primary illness.

Once the indication for splenectomy is certain, the surgery itself is relatively simple unless the spleen is greatly enlarged or surrounded by adhesions. The pre- and postoperative care of patients is generally the same as that discussed in Unit VIII. However, there are a few specific observations to remember when caring for patients following splenectomy.

1. Observe the patient carefully *for hemorrhage* and *shock.* Patients with thrombocytopenic purpura suffer from bleeding tendencies as a result of their decreased platelet levels. Transfusions of platelets at the time of surgery may help to diminish the threat of hemorrhage but will not alleviate it. Also, accident victims may have suffered other serious injuries in addition to splenic rupture that may lead to shock and bleeding, e.g., fractured ribs, a head injury, broken limbs.
2. Observe the patient for an *elevated temperature.* For unknown reasons, patients usually run a fever as high as 38.3° C. (101° F.) for 10 days or more following splenectomy. Usually this temperature elevation is *not* the result of infection, and consequently the patient does not benefit from antibiotic therapy. Occasionally, however, the fever is associated with complications such as pneumonia, wound infections, and so forth. For this reason, carefully observe the patient for *all* the symptoms of the various postoperative complications and do not simply rely upon temperature elevation as the major symptom heralding infection.
3. Observe the patient for *abdominal distention* and *discomfort.* Removal of an enlarged spleen may cause the stomach and intestines to expand in order to fill the void. Abdominal distention can be relieved by application of a tight abdominal binder and the parenteral administration of neostigmine (Prostigmin).

Any infection in a young child who has had a debilitating hematologic disease and has had a splenectomy should be considered a life-threatening situation, because of the child's compromised defense system. Many experts feel these patients should "be given prophylactic antibodies for a few years after splenectomy."[125]

NURSING PATIENTS WITH DISORDERS PRIMARILY AFFECTING PLATELETS AND CLOTTING FACTORS

Hemostasis

Hemostasis is defined as the "arrest of the escape of blood by either natural (clot formation or vessel spasm) or artificial (compression or ligation) means."[82] The promotion and control of hemostasis depend upon the hemostatic mechanism, the fibrinolytic inhibitor mechanism, and natural anticoagulants circulating in the blood.

The Hemostatic Mechanism. The three components of the hemostatic mechanism are the blood vessels, platelets or thrombocytes, and coagulation factors.

Blood Vessels. Whenever there is bleeding as a result of injury or disease, the blood vessels supplying the damaged site *constrict;* vasoconstriction, in turn, slows the flow of blood to the injured area, thereby decreasing blood loss. Vasoconstriction is the result of reflex nervous system and muscular tissue reactions. *Serotonin* (a powerful local vasoconstrictor secreted by cells in the small intestine and absorbed by released platelets) also promotes blood vessel constriction upon injury.

Platelets or Thrombocytes. The precise meaning of the word thrombocyte is "clot cell"; however, platelets are not cells in the true sense of the word. They are tiny disc-shaped fragments derived from giant cells called *megakaryocytes* that are located in the bone marrow. Platelets perform four vital hemostatic functions: (1) they form a temporary clot by adhering to each other (aggregation) and to the vessel wall (adhesion); (2) they release incomplete thromboplastin which, along with other substances, aids in the formation of a permanent clot; (3) they release a contractile protein that causes the soft permanent clot to contract, shrink, and grow firm; and (4) they contribute to vascular integrity. Hemostasis is largely controlled by platelets, unless large blood vessels have suffered damage and bleeding is severe. In the case of hemorrhage, the coagulation factors must join with the platelets in the formation of a permanent clot. Normally the platelet count is 200,000 to 350,000/cu. mm. A decrease in platelets is called *thrombocytopenia,* while an increase is called *thrombocytosis.*

Coagulation Factors. The 13 coagulation factors are listed in Table 46–6 along with their sources, characteristics, and functions. Note that the factors are designated by Roman numerals in accordance with the standard international nomenclature.

The exact manner in which the different components of the hemostatic mechanism work together to form a clot is not totally understood. However, physiologists recognize that blood coagulation (which involves an intricate and complex cascade of events) occurs upon activation of the intrinsic and extrinsic pathways, which are diagrammed in Figure 46–5. Note that the extrinsic pathway begins with trauma to tissues that lie outside vessels. The intrinsic pathway involves the blood itself and damage to the blood vessels, i.e., endothelial damage or the release of platelet factors.

The end result of the clotting cascade is the conversion of prothrombin to thrombin and soluble fibrinogen to a fibrin clot. An insoluble protein, fibrin is composed of dense interlacing threads that entrap erythrocytes and platelets. At this stage of the clot formation process, the platelets, by releasing a contractile protein, perform their final hemostatic function — shrinkage and retraction of the clot into a firm insoluble fibrin mass. In the process of retraction, a clear yellow substance called *serum* is squeezed from the clot; serum differs from plasma in that it does not contain clotting substances.

In some cases hemostasis is complete at the earlier stage and the formation of a permanent fibrin clot is not necessary; in other cases such clot formation is not sufficient to stop hemorrhage. For example, bleeding from a small pinprick can normally be terminated by a platelet plug, whereas more serious cuts require the interaction of the various coagulation factors. When an artery is severely traumatized or severed, surgical intervention with tourniquets, ligation, or cautery is needed to halt hemorrhage.

Fibrinolysis (Clot Dissolution). Once the tough fibrin clot has served its purpose (i.e., halting hemorrhage), it must be dissolved by the fibrinolytic or clot-lysis mechanism in order to prevent permanent thrombosis and occlusion of the injured blood vessel. The fibrinolytic mechanism is active in less than a day following the formation of a clot. The two substances involved in the lysis of a clot are *plasminogen* and *plasmin,* the active substance in fibrinolysis. Plasmin is a proteolytic enzyme capable of digesting such protein materials as fibrin, fibrinogen, and factors V and VIII. *Plasminogen,* a serum globulin, is the inactive precursor of plasmin. Plasminogen can be activated by a number of natural activators found in blood, urine, and so forth. In clinical practice the doctor may activate plasminogen and induce fibrinolysis in patients with pulmonary emboli by administering either streptokinase or urokinase intravenously.

Normally the fibrinolytic mechanism remains localized to the site of clot formation. Occasionally, however, the mechanism may become overactive (resulting in hemorrhage) or underactive (resulting in excessive thrombosis of blood vessels).

Control of Hemostasis. By what means is the coagulation system controlled so that it functions effectively when needed, but *only* when needed? First, as you recall, the normal epithelium does not attract platelets, nor does the normal blood contain activators of coagulation. Second, the blood contains natural anticoagulants that act continuously to inhibit coagulation, e.g., heparin, antithrombin, and antithromboplastin. Finally, the blood contains the proteolytic enzyme plasmin, which, upon activation, performs fibrinolysis and thereby clears the vessels of clots.

Hemorrhagic Disorders

Causes and Classification. Normal clot formation and lysis depend upon the presence of the following: (1) strong healthy blood vessels, (2) normal numbers of circulating platelets, (3) the 13 clotting factors, and (4) a well-controlled fibrinolytic system. Conversely the four basic problems underlying hemorrhagic (bleeding) disorders are: (1) weak, damaged vessels that rupture easily or spontaneously; (2) platelet deficiency (thrombocytopenia) due to either hypoproliferation, excessive pooling of platelets in the spleen, or excessive platelet destruction; (3) deficiency or total lack of one of the clotting factors; or (4) excessive or insufficient fibrinolysis.

The major bleeding disorders can be classified as follows:

I. *Purpura* (extravasation of blood into the tissues and mucous membranes)
   A. Vascular purpuras

TABLE 46–6. COAGULATION FACTORS

Factor	Name or Substance	Source, Characteristics, Function
I	Fibrinogen	Produced in the liver; protein present in plasma at an average level of 300 mg. %; when acted upon by thrombin, forms fibrin
II	Prothrombin	Produced in the liver, with vitamin K an essential part; glucoprotein present in plasma and measured according to its activity; when acted upon by thromboplastin, forms thrombin
III	Thromboplastin	Tissues and platelets (incomplete); plasma (complete); incomplete forms require factors V, VII, X; complete form is a product of interaction between factors VIII, IX, XI and platelets; acts upon prothrombin to form thrombin
IV	Calcium	Obtained from diet; present in serum levels of 4.8–5.2 mEq./l.; is an inorganic ion required in all stages of coagulation as an activator of enzyme activity
V	Labile factor	Derived from plasma globulin; found in normal plasma; used up in the clotting process; deteriorates rapidly at room temperature; accelerates conversion of prothrombin to thrombin
VI	Unassigned	In early studies, was thought to be the active form of factor V
VII	Stable factor	Produced in the liver; not consumed in clotting, therefore present in normal serum; stable to heat and storage; accelerates the conversion of prothrombin to thrombin
VIII	Antihemophilic globulin	Derived from plasma globulin; completely consumed in clotting; unstable at room temperature; essential to the formation of thromboplastin and conversion of prothrombin to thrombin
IX	Plasma thromboplastin component (Christmas factor)	Produced in the liver; not consumed during clotting; influences amount of thromboplastin generated
X	Stuart-Prower factor	Probably produced in the liver, with vitamin K essential; present in normal plasma and serum; stable at room temperature; similar to factor VII; essential to generation of thromboplastin and activity of prothrombin
XI	Plasma thromboplastin antecedent	Site of synthesis unknown; present in normal plasma and serum; stable; essential to formation of plasma thromboplastin
XII	Hageman factor	Site of synthesis unknown; relatively stable; activated on contact with glass; physiologic role not completely known
XIII	Fibrin stabilizing factor	Site of synthesis not known; high levels in plasma; deficiency associated with mild bleeding tendency, poor wound healing; maintains firm clot after formation.

Modified from French, R. M.: *Nurses' Guide to Diagnostic Procedures*, 4th ed. New York: McGraw-Hill Book Co., Inc., 1975.

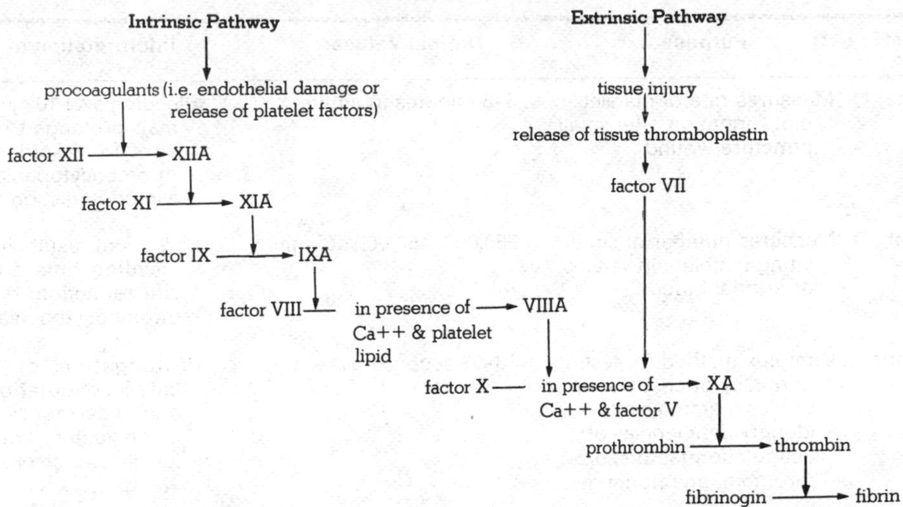

Figure 46–5. The clotting cascade. (From O'Brian, B. S., and S. Woods: The Paradox of DIC. *American Journal of Nursing*, 78(11):1879, Nov. 1978.)

B. Purpura due to platelet disorders
   1. Idiopathic thrombocytopenic purpura
   2. Secondary thrombocytopenias

II. Coagulation disorders
   A. Hemophilia
   B. Hypoprothrombinemia
   C. Defibrination syndrome
   D. DIC (Disseminated intravascular coagulation)

Diagnosis and Laboratory Studies. The diagnosis of hemorrhagic disorders rests upon the patient's medical and familial history, the physical examination, and a battery of specific laboratory tests for platelet and clotting defects. The patient's *history* usually offers numerous clues to the type of bleeding problem present and its cause. Questions typically included in the history-taking procedure are:

- How long has the patient had a bleeding problem? Was it present in childhood or has it appeared only recently?
- Do any members of the patient's family have a history of bleeding episodes?
- Is bleeding linked with any specific event or procedure? For example, does severe bleeding occur following minor trauma? a tooth extraction? minor surgery? participation in contact sports? during shaving? during the menses in female patients?
- Does the patient have frequent nosebleeds? Is there a history of bleeding into joints or cavities? Does the patient bruise easily? Is there evidence of petechiae or epitaxis?
- Does the patient have a history of hepatic, splenic, or renal disease? (These three conditions are often characterized by hemorrhagic manifestations.)
- How severe are the individual bleeding episodes and what is their duration? More precisely, is there prolonged oozing of blood from a site or sudden massive hemorrhage? (Sudden hemorrhage is a far less common manifestation of bleeding disorders than is oozing of long duration.)
- Has the patient recently taken either anticoagulant drugs or drugs that tend to suppress bone marrow function (e.g., chloramphenicol, antineoplastic drugs)? or drugs that interfere with platelet function (e.g., ASA)?

If the patient's history points to the presence of a bleeding disorder, the physician next examines the individual for the overt signs of bleeding. *Petechiae* (tiny hemorrhagic spots caused by intradermal or submucosal bleeding) are usually present in the vascular and thrombocytopenic purpuras. The presence of *ecchymoses* (large blotchy subcutaneous hemorrhagic areas), *hematomas* (blood tumors), and *hemarthrosis* (blood within the joints) is diagnostic of hemophilia. However, ecchymoses may be present in any hemorrhagic disorder. Patients who hemorrhage severely from several areas during a major surgical procedure or during childbirth may have a fibrinogen deficiency. In addition to examining the patient for evidence of bleeding, the physician also searches for evidence of cirrhosis of the liver (hepatomegaly, jaundice, and so forth) and splenomegaly.

The most crucial evidence for pinpointing the type and cause of a bleeding disorder is obtained from laboratory studies. Initially the physician usually orders the following four basic laboratory tests in order to determine if the bleeding problem is due to a vascular, a coagulation, or a platelet defect: bleeding time, prothrombin time (one stage), platelet count, and partial thromboplastin time (PTT). Ninety-five per cent of all bleeding disorders are diagnosed by the PTT and prothrombin time. Once

TABLE 46–7. LABORATORY TESTS USED IN THE DIAGNOSIS OF HEMORRHAGIC DISORDERS

Name of Test	Purpose	Normal Values	Interpretation of Findings
Bleeding time (Bl time)	Measures rate of platelet clot formation after small puncture wound	3–8 minutes in adults	Bleeding over 10 minutes abnormal; prolonged bleeding occurs in vascular maladies, thrombocytopenia, and after aspirin ingestion
Platelet count	Measures number of circulating platelets in venous or arterial blood	250,000–450,000/cu. mm.	Low count results in prolonged bleeding time and impaired clot retraction; diagnostic of thrombocytopenia
Partial thromboplastin time (PTT)	Complex method for testing normalcy of coagulation process; employed to identify deficiencies of coagulation factors, prothrombin, and fibrinogen	39–53 seconds	Prolongation of time indicates coagulation disorder due to deficiency of a coagulation factor; not diagnostic for platelet disorders
Prothrombin time (Pro time)	Determines activity and interaction of factors V, VII, X, prothrombin, and fibrinogen; used to determine dosages of anticoagulant drugs	12–15 seconds (one-stage method)	Prolongation of time indicates: patient receiving anticoagulants; abnormally low fibrinogen concentration; deficiencies of factors II, VII, V, and X; presence of circulating anticoagulants as seen in lupus erythematosus; impaired prothrombin activity
Coagulation (clotting time)	Crude measure of coagulation process in venous blood; used to control heparin therapy	9–12 minutes (Lee-White method)	Prolonged time occurs in: severe coagulation problems; therapeutic administration of heparin
Thrombin time	Measures functional fibrinogen available, as shown by time needed to form fibrin clot	10–13 seconds	Prolonged time indicates: hypofibrinogenemia; presence in blood of excess heparin or other anticoagulants
Thromboplastin generation test (TGT)	Measures generation of thromboplastin; if result abnormal, second stage is done to identify missing coagulation factor	12 seconds or less (100%)	Abnormal values found in hemophilia
Fibrinogen level	Measures level of fibrinogen in plasma	200–400 mg./100 ml.	Abnormally low values may indicate liver disease, congenital afibrinogenemia, or acquired afibrinogenemia
Clot retraction	Indicates function and number of platelets; measures time needed for contraction of an undisturbed clot	Clot retraction begins within 2 hours and is finished within 24 hours	Clot retraction retarded in thrombocytopenia; clot is small and soft in thrombasthenia (functional disturbance of platelets)
Tourniquet test (Rumple-Leeds test; capillary fragility test)	Crude test of vascular resistance and platelet number and function; done by placing blood pressure cuff on arm for 5 minutes and then counting petechiae	No petechiae	Petechiae appear in thrombocytopenia and vascular purpura

primary laboratory screening has been performed, the doctor may decide to order other more sophisticated tests of hemostatic function (Table 46–7).

General Clinical Care. Specific medical measures for treating the various hemorrhagic diseases differ. However, there are a number of general observations, precautions, and nursing actions that apply to all patients suffering from bleeding disorders. Important points to remember are:

1. Instruct the patient and significant others about the signs and symptoms of bleeding and about the importance of reporting them promptly.
2. *Observe* the patient continuously for *signs of bleeding.* Examine the skin and the interior of the mouth for petechiae and ecchymosis. Observe stools for bright red blood as well as for the tarry appearance that indicates the passage of old blood. Observe urine for the smoky color that signals hematuria. Report and chart the development of nosebleeds, their severity and duration. Remember to observe for the subtle signs of *internal* hemorrhage, e.g., faintness, tachycardia, hypotension, confusion, disorientation, and air hunger.
3. *Guard the patient from trauma.* If the patient is bedridden, turn gently but frequently (every 1 to 2 hours). Assist weak or elderly ambulatory patients to the bathroom, particularly at night, in order to prevent bumps and falls. Caution both male and female patients to use electric razors rather than blades for shaving, to avoid cuts. Also, to prevent bleeding of gums, instruct the patient to use a soft toothbrush soaked in warm water for cleaning the teeth.
4. *Prevent constipation.* Hard stools, straining at stool, and fecal impactions all traumatize the rectal and anal mucosa, causing bleeding as well as increased intra-abdominal pressure and increased intracranial pressure. If constipation does develop, notify the physician. A gentle laxative, stool softener, or enema may be necessary.
5. *Administer intramuscular injections with special care.* Remember to: (1) use a small needle, (2) apply pressure to the site of the injection for several minutes following administration of the medication, and (3) examine the injection site for continued bleeding for several hours following the injection.
6. *Instruct the patient to carry an identification card* at all times, stating: (1) the patient's blood disorder, (2) the name of the patient's doctor or clinic, and (3) the patient's blood type.
7. Observe the laboratory data to correlate clinical signs of bleeding and to anticipate critical times of possible bleeding.
8. Instruct the patient not to take any medication without first consulting the nurse or physician.

Purpura

Purpura is defined as the extravasation of small amounts of blood into the tissues and mucous membranes. As you recall, the smallest hemorrhages are called *petechiae,* while larger hemorrhagic lesions are called *ecchymoses.* These two forms of bleeding may result from either vessel damage or rupture (vascular purpura) or a platelet deficiency (thrombocytopenic purpura).

VASCULAR PURPURA

The major characteristic of vascular purpura is easy rupture of the smaller blood vessels upon any undue pressure, with resultant bleeding into the tissues. The causes of vascular purpura are many, e.g., heredity, allergy, exposure to drugs and poisons, poor nutrition, infection, and hypertension. Major forms of vascular purpura include the following:

Familial Hemorrhagic Telangiectasia. This hereditary condition is characterized by episodes of nosebleed or gastrointestinal bleeding and telangiectatic lesions (small red lesions of the skin and mucous membranes resulting from dilated capillaries, arterioles, or venules). There is no cure for this condition. Severe gastrointestinal tract hemorrhage is treated with iron therapy and transfusions. Because this condition is hereditary, genetic counseling is appropriate.

Anaphylactoid Purpura (Allergic Purpura). This form of vascular purpura evidently arises from an *allergic reaction* that damages the vascular epithelium. Its major characteristic is acute or chronic inflammation of blood vessels supplying the skin, joints, gastrointestinal tract, and kidneys. Symptoms include arthritic pains, abdominal pain, hematuria, gastrointestinal hemorrhage, fever, and malaise. Treatment is symptomatic. Steroids are often used to relieve distress. Typically, attacks of the disease automatically subside within 1 to 6 weeks; however, episodes of bleeding tend to recur over the years.

Toxic Purpura. This condition is characterized by damage to blood vessels following exposure to certain medications and poisons (e.g., snake venom). Treatment involves identification and cessation of the offending drug.

Symptomatic or Secondary Purpuras. These disorders arise secondary to other diseases and are not caused by intrinsic or inherited disorders of the vasculature. Conditions that can result in secondary purpura include: (1) serious tissue trauma arising from a blow or a burn; (2) arterial hypertension resulting in increased capillary pressure; (3) blood stream infections that damage the vascular epithelium (e.g., subacute bacterial endocarditis); (4) scurvy (the result of vitamin C deficiency), which causes increased capillary fragility; and (5) uremia and cachexia, which, for unknown reasons, result in vessel weakness. The alleviation of the secondary purpuras is based upon treatment of the primary disorders.

PURPURAS DUE TO THROMBOCYTOPENIA

The term "thrombocytopenia" means a *reduction in platelets below 200,000 per cu. mm.* The two major problems that follow a serious reduction in the platelet count are: (1) spontaneous bleeding into the skin, mucous membranes, and internal cavities and organs; and (2) oozing of long duration from tiny lacerations and needle pricks. The two principal types of thrombocytopenia are: idiopathic thrombocytopenic purpura (ITP), and secondary thrombocytopenia.

Idiopathic Thrombocytopenic Purpura (ITP). The major characteristic of this bleeding disorder is the *premature destruction of platelets.* Normally platelets survive within the circulation for 8 to 10 days; however, platelet survival in ITP is as brief as 1 to 3 days or less. Although the exact etiology of ITP is unknown, the majority of authorities currently support the *autoimmune theory* of causation. For unidentified reasons *autoantibodies develop* which either interrupt megakaryocyte development (which then results in reduced platelet production) or sensitize platelets, so that they become more vulnerable to destruction by the spleen.

Acute ITP is primarily a disease of children; 85 per cent of patients are under 8 years of age. Chronic ITP is primarily a disease of adults. Women are affected three times as frequently as men.

The onset of this disorder is often sudden and acute, but in most cases, ITP is characterized by remissions and exacerbations which, in untreated cases, may occur for years. Symptoms include petechiae, ecchymosis, epistaxis, bleeding from the gums, and easy bruising. Women may have extremely heavy menses or bleeding between periods. *Complications* of ITP include:

- Cerebral hemorrhage, which proves fatal in 1 to 5 per cent of patients.
- Severe hemorrhages from the nose, gastrointestinal tract, and urinary system.
- Bleeding into the diaphragm, which can result in pulmonary complications.
- Nerve pain, anesthesia of extremities, and/or paralysis as a result of the pressure of a hematoma upon nerves or brain tissues.

Laboratory findings which confirm the presence of ITP include: (1) a platelet count below 100,000 per cu. mm.; (2) prolonged bleeding time *but* normal coagulation time (all coagulation factors are present and normal); and (3) increased capillary fragility as demonstrated by the tourniquet test.

The two basic treatments for ITP are steroid therapy and splenectomy. *Steroids* are given to patients suffering from severe bleeding of short duration; they are also administered preoperatively prior to splenectomy. The purpose of steroid therapy in ITP is to reduce the bleeding tendency and to elevate the platelet count; however, steroids are rarely able to produce a permanent cure. A commonly used steroid is prednisone.

The treatment of choice for patients with ITP is *splenectomy.* In 60 to 80 per cent of patients, removal of the spleen results in a complete and permanent remission. No one knows exactly why splenectomy is so successful. If the autoimmune hypothesis is correct, removal of the spleen probably halts the premature destruction of sensitized platelets. Since young children often recover spontaneously from ITP, pediatricians do not usually recommend splenectomy until the child is at least 6 years of age.

Nursing care for patients with ITP is directed toward observing for and preventing internal hemorrhage, particularly *cerebral hemorrhage.* Patients with severe ITP are usually placed on *bed rest* in order to prevent excessive activity and consequent exhaustion. It is extremely important to observe for and to prevent: *constipation,* which is accompanied by straining at stool, and *upper respiratory infections,* which lead to coughing and sneezing.

> Remember:
> *Both straining at stool and coughing cause an increase in intracranial pressure, which can result in cerebral hemorrhage.*

The *prognosis* for patients with ITP is good. Eighty per cent of children and 10 to 20 per cent of adults with this disorder recover spontaneously without any treatment.

Secondary Thrombocytopenic Purpuras. Unlike idiopathic (primary) thrombocytopenic purpura, the secondary thrombocytopenias have identifiable causes. For example, these purpuras may arise secondary to viral infections, bone marrow failure, the defibrination syndrome, disseminated lupus erythematosus, lymphoproliferative disorders, and infectious mononucleosis. Drug hypersensitivity is another important cause of thrombocytopenia. Common offending drugs include quinidine, quinine, the sulfonamides, phenylbutazone, and chlorothiazide derivatives. Symptoms and laboratory findings are the same as those found in ITP.

TREATMENT

Treatment of these conditions centers around the total removal or at least partial alleviation of the underlying cause as well as the control of bleeding. All potentially toxic drugs must be identified and discontinued. Usually the platelet count begins to rise in a few days and is normal within a week following removal of toxic agents. To control bleeding the physician may order the administration of *corticosteroids.*

Platelet transfusions are given either prophylactically, when the platelet count falls below 20,000 to 30,000 per cu. mm., or as a treatment for hemorrhage. Patients can be supported with platelet transfusions for periods of time ranging from weeks to years. Transfused platelets do not have a normal life span but may function effectively for as long as 5 to 6 days. Long-term platelet support is usually complicated by the patient's ability to develop antibodies to the transfused platelets. Platelet counts obtained 1 hour after transfusion that show no resultant rise in the patient's peripheral platelet count, or which even show a decrease in the count, indicate the presence of platelet antibodies. Platelet support at that point can be continued only by obtaining specially matched donors. Perfectly matched donors can provide platelet support for years.

Coagulation Disorders

The coagulation disorders are characterized by a *defect in the clotting mechanism* resulting from the depletion or absence of one or more of the clotting factors. The three important coagulation disorders discussed here are the hemophilias, hypoprothrombinemia, and disseminated intravascular coagulation (the defibrination syndrome.)

THE HEMOPHILIAS

The hemophilias are relatively common disorders characterized by prolonged bleeding, particularly following accidental, surgical, or dental trauma. There are three major types of hemophilia: hemophilia A (classic hemophilia), hemophilia B (Christmas disease), and von Willebrand's disease. The major characteristics of these three disorders are compared in Table 46–8. Because *classic hemophilia* is by far the most common of the hemophilias (includes 80 per cent of all hemophilia cases), our discussion of symptoms and treatment refers only to this type.

Hemophilia A is classified as a childhood disorder; however, because of new developments in treatment that prolong life, this disease now extends into the patient's adult years. Manifestations of hemophilia A include the following:

- *Slow, prolonged, persistent bleeding* from cuts, scratches, and other minor traumas, which may finally result in massive, deadly hemorrhage unless medically controlled.
- *Delayed hemorrhage* following trivial injuries. Bleeding may not start from a site until hours or even days have passed following the moment of trauma.
- Severe *hemorrhaging* from the gums following dental extraction or even brushing the teeth with a hard toothbrush.
- Severe, sometimes fatal, *epistaxis* following injury to the nose, e.g., a blow or "punch" on the nose.
- Overwhelming *gastric hemorrhage,* which may be linked with gastric disorders such as ulcers.
- Recurrent *hematomas,* which may form in the deep subcutaneous tissue, intramuscular tissues, and around the peripheral nerves. If nerves are compressed by the hematomas, the patient suffers severe pain, anesthesia of the innervated part, and sometimes permanent nerve damage, paralysis, and muscular atrophy.
- Recurrent *hemarthrosis* (bleeding into the joints) is common in untreated cases and may result in serious joint deformity and permanent crippling. Hemarthrosis affects the knees, ankles, elbows, wrists, fingers, hips, and shoulders, in that order.

TABLE 46–8. A COMPARISON OF THE THREE FORMS OF HEMOPHILIA

Form of Hemophilia	Etiology	Transmission	Major Laboratory Findings
Hemophilia A (classic hemophilia)	Inherited Factor VIII (antihemophilic globulin) deficiency	Transmitted as a sex-linked *recessive* trait; transmitted by females; occurs in males and, rarely, homozygous females	Coagulation time prolonged but bleeding time normal; factor VIII missing from plasma
Hemophilia B (Christmas disease)	Inherited Factor IX (plasma thromboplastin component) deficiency	Transmitted as a sex-linked *recessive* trait; transmitted by females; occurs in males and, rarely, homozygous females	Laboratory findings and symptoms same as in hemophilia A.
Von Willebrand's disease	Inherited Factor VIII deficiency and defective platelet dysfunction	Transmitted as an autosomal *dominant* trait to both sexes; occurs in both males and females	Both coagulation time *and* bleeding time prolonged; low factor VIII levels; platelet adhesiveness decreased

The five goals of treatment for patients with hemophilia are: (1) to stop topical bleeding as quickly as possible; (2) to raise the level of antihemophilic factor (AHF) in the patient's plasma, thereby temporarily supplying the missing factor causing hemorrhage; (3) to prevent crippling deformities from hemarthrosis; (4) to prevent unnecessary trauma; and (5) to educate the patient.

Topical bleeding can usually be temporarily controlled by applying pressure to the injured site, packing the area with Gelfoam or fibrin foam, and applying topical hemostatics such as thrombin. However, to permanently halt the bleeding episode, fresh plasma, fresh frozen plasma, cryoprecipitate, commercial concentrates, or fresh whole blood must be administered to the patient in order to supply vitally needed AHF.

Because AHF deteriorates quickly, the blood product must be given to the patient within 6 hours following withdrawal from the donor.

In addition to fresh whole blood and fresh plasma, AHF levels may also be raised by the administration of commercial AHF concentrates, e.g., cryoprecipitate, Hemophil, AHF, and Fibro-AHG. Concentrates are also available for supplying factors VII, IX, X, and prothrombin. Commercial concentrates rich in the missing factors are also administered *prophylactically* to patients prior to dental extractions and surgical procedures.

There is one major *complication* linked with repeated transfusion and AHF therapy: about 5 per cent of hemophiliacs become sensitized to AHF and develop *autoimmune anticoagulants* (*Anti-AHF factor*). There are various experimental methods being used to combat this problem. One such method is the use of immunosuppressive therapy.

Hemarthrosis is usually treated with AHF or fresh whole blood administration, resting the joint (sometimes in a protective cast), and packing ice around the joint. Analgesics and corticosteroids are often given to reduce joint pain and swelling. If pain is severe, the doctor may be forced to aspirate blood from the joint. Once bleeding stops and the swelling is reduced, the patient is encouraged to move the joint. However, the patient should be cautioned not to put weight on an affected lower extremity until swelling completely subsides and muscle strength is normal.

Prevention of injury is dependent upon certain precautionary nursing measures as well as a willingness on the part of the patient to live sensibly with his disorder. Points to remember when caring for persons with hemophilia are as follows:

- ▶ Teach young patients to avoid all unnecessary sources of trauma, e.g., elective surgery, contact sports.
- ▶ Instruct patients to always inform doctors, dentists, teachers, and employers that they have hemophilia. Of course, the patient must also carry an identifying card.
- ▶ Should surgery or tooth extraction be necessary, request the patient to ask friends and family to donate blood so that a sufficient amount of blood is on hand.
- ▶ When administering intramuscular injections, always check the injection site every hour for *several days* following the injection.

Remember:
In hemophilia, bleeding and hemorrhage are often delayed for substantial periods of time following trauma.

The *prognosis* for patients with hemophilia has greatly improved since the discovery of AHF. Formerly, 50 per cent of patients with this disorder died before they reached their fifth birthday. Today, death rarely occurs as a result of bleeding from minor trauma. Some centers are training patients to infuse themselves after recognizing the symptoms of bleeding. This treatment plan involves strict guidelines but has resulted in less time lost from work or school and in a decreased number of emergency room visits. Fatalities mainly follow the development of autoimmune anticoagulants (anti-AHF factors) and bleeding into the retroperitoneal space following internal hemorrhage.

HYPOPROTHROMBINEMIA

The term "hypoprothrombinemia" means that the amount of prothrombin circulating in the blood is deficient. *Prothrombin* is a complex globulin protein produced in the liver and normally found in the blood. For prothrombin synthesis to take place, *vitamin K* (a fat-soluble vitamin) must be present in the liver to act as a catalyst.

Hypoprothrombinemia develops as a result either of vitamin K deficiency or of overdosage with Dicumarol.

Vitamin K deficiency. This fat-soluble vitamin is normally obtained in a balanced diet; also (in all but the newborn) vitamin K is synthesized by certain intestinal tract bacteria. Once ingested or manufactured internally, vitamin K, because it is fat-soluble, is dependent upon the presence of *bile* for absorption. When absorbed, vitamin K is ready to catalyze prothrombin synthesis within the liver cells. Vitamin K *deficiency,* then, is the result of: (1) improper diet; (2) gastrointestinal tract disorders which interfere with the absorption of vitamin K (e.g., malabsorption syndrome and obstructive jaundice due to bile duct obstruction); (3) liver damage that is so extensive that the liver cells cannot produce bile or synthesize prothrombin; or (4) prolonged sulfonamide or antibiotic administration which sterilizes the bowel, thereby halting the manufacture of vitamin K by intestinal tract bacteria.

Overdosage with Dicumarol. Bishydroxycoumarin (Dicumarol) is an effective anticoagulant used to reduce the danger of clot formation in persons with heart disease and peripheral vascular disorders. Dicumarol acts by interfering with the conversion of vitamin K to prothrombin within the liver cells. If dosage is excessive, the patient's prothrombin time is prolonged (usually below 40 or 50 per cent). If the prothrombin time drops below 10 to 15 per cent, the patient is in danger of bleeding or hemorrhaging spontaneously.

The major manifestations of hypoprothrombinemia are: ecchymosis following minimal trauma, epistaxis, postoperative hemorrhage from the incision, hematuria, gastrointestinal tract bleeding, and prolonged bleeding from a venipuncture. The outstanding laboratory finding is a *prolonged prothrombin time.*

Treatment of hypoprothrombinemia is directed at the underlying cause. For example, vitamin K deficiency as a result of malabsorption is corrected by the administration of a parenteral preparation of vitamin K. The two drugs of choice are: menadione sodium bisulfite (Hykinone), IM; and menadiol (Synkayvite), IM. If Dicumarol overdose is the underlying problem, anticoagulant therapy is stopped. In order to normalize the prothrombin time, the patient is given phytonadione (fat-soluble vitamin K; Mephyton) orally for minor bleeding problems or Aqua-Mephyton IV for hemorrhage. Finally, if the prothrombin deficiency is the result of liver disease, prothrombin can temporarily be replaced directly by transfusion therapy; or concentrates of prothrombin and factors VII, IX, and X may be given.

DISSEMINATED INTRAVASCULAR COAGULATION (DIC)

The term "disseminated intravascular coagulation" means diffuse or widespread coagulation within arterioles and capillaries all over the body. DIC is a complex and important coagulation disorder characterized by two apparently conflicting sets of manifestations: (1) *diffuse fibrin deposition* within arterioles and capillaries all over the body with resultant *widespread clotting;* and (2) *hemorrhage* from the kidneys, brain, adrenals, heart, and other organs. The disorder is sometimes called the "defibrination syndrome."

"The patients who develop DIC are usually critically ill with obstetrical, surgical, hemolytic, or neoplastic disease."[61] Table 46–9 lists conditions that may precipitate DIC. In caring for a patient with one of these conditions, the nurse must be alert for the signs of DIC. Although the cause of DIC is unknown, possibly its onset is linked with the entry into the blood of thromboplastic substances (e.g., in metastatic cancer, obstetric complications, shock, sepsis, tissue damage from burns or trauma, and snake bites).

The pathologic chain of events characterizing DIC apparently is as follows: (1) certain disease states (toxemia of pregnancy, cancer, etc.) cause the release of thromboplastic substances which evidently promote the deposition of fibrin throughout the microcirculation; (2) as a result, microthrombi form in the brain, kidneys, heart, and other organs, causing microinfarcts and tissue necrosis; (3) red cells become trapped in the fibrin strands and are destroyed (hemolysis); (4) platelets, prothrombin, and other clotting factors are consumed in the process, which then leads to bleeding; (5) the excessive clotting activates the fibrinolytic mechanism, which causes

TABLE 46–9. COMMON CONDITIONS THAT MAY PRECIPITATE DIC

I. Conditions that may cause the release of thromboplastin from the tissues:
   1. *Obstetrical conditions* such as abruptio placentae, retained dead fetus, and amniotic fluid embolism.
   2. *Neoplastic growths* such as prostatic cancer, acute leukemias, giant cavernous hemangioma, and bronchogenic cancer.

II. Conditions that may cause the release of platelet factor III.
   1. *Hemolytic processes* such as transfusions of mismatched blood and acute hemolysis from infection or immunologic disorders.
   2. *Tissue damage* from extensive burns and trauma, transplant rejections, heat stroke, or surgery—particularly following extracorporeal circulation.
   3. *Fat emboli.*
   4. *Snake bite.*

III. Conditions that *may* cause DIC, although the mechanisms are not understood.
   1. *Acute bacterial and viral infections.*
   2. *Glomerulonephritis.*
   3. *Purpura fulminans.*
   4. *Thrombotic thrombocytopenic purpura.*
   5. *Cirrhosis.*
   6. *Acute fulminant hepatitis.*
   7. *Shock.*

Modified from Jennings, B. M.: Improving your management of DIC. *Nursing 79,* 9:60, May 1979.

the production of fibrin split products; these end products act to inhibit platelet clotting functions, which causes further bleeding.

The onset of DIC is usually acute; chronic cases of DIC characteristically develop in persons with cancer or in mothers who are carrying a dead fetus. Manifestations may be either mild or extremely severe. Symptoms include the following:

- Petechiae and ecchymoses on the skin, mucous membranes, heart lining, lungs, etc.
- Prolonged bleeding from a venipuncture
- Severe, uncontrollable hemorrhage during surgery or childbirth
- Oliguria and acute renal failure
- Convulsions and coma, which may terminate in death

Laboratory findings, in severe cases of DIC, indicate that the hemostatic mechanism has failed totally. A prolonged prothrombin time, very low platelet count, and incoagulable blood are typical findings. Table 46–10 lists the laboratory tests used in diagnosis of DIC.

The clinical care of a patient with DIC involves: (1) treatment of the basic problem (e.g., shock, delivery of a fetus, surgery for or irradiation of cancer); (2) the reversal of pathologic clotting; and (3) the control of bleeding and shock. To reverse clotting, the physician usually orders heparin IV, every 4 to 6 hours.

Blood transfusions are administered to replace blood and lessen shock. Finally, human fibrinogen is sometimes given in cases of severe fibrinolysis; however, human fibrinogen is a dangerous medication because it can cause *hepatitis.* The patient is also given platelets, cryoprecipitate, fresh plasma to replace consumed platelets, and coagulation factors.

The prognosis for patients with DIC varies. The condition may be self-limiting, or the patient may die from hemorrhage and organ damage within a few days.

The survival of a patient with DIC may depend upon good nursing care. Care of the patient should be centered around these five goals:

1. To detect occult bleeding.
2. To prevent further bleeding.
3. To measure blood loss.
4. To administer blood products and medications skillfully.
5. To support the patient's other needs.[60]

TABLE 46–10. LABORATORY TESTS USED IN DIAGNOSIS OF DIC

Test	Results in DIC Patient
Screening tests to assess depletion of clotting factors and platelets	
Prothrombin time (PT)	Prolonged in DIC. Also prolonged in patients with liver disease or vitamin K deficiency and in patients receiving coumarin treatment.
Partial thromboplastin time (PTT)	Usually prolonged in DIC, but not always. Also prolonged in patients with hemophilia and in patients receiving heparin treatment.
Thrombin time	Usually prolonged in DIC and in liver disease.
Fibrinogen level	Usually depressed in DIC and in liver disease.
Platelet count	Usually depressed in DIC.
Tests frequently used to measure effect of DIC on specific blood components	
Fibrin split products (FSP)	Elevated in DIC and in liver disease.
Protamine sulfate test	Strongly positive in DIC (weakly positive in liver disease, thrombosis, or after surgery).
Factor assays	Several tests are used; each measures the level of a different coagulation factor in the plasma. Assays for II, V, and VII are commonly done for DIC. These levels will be reduced.

Adapted from Jennings, B. M.: Improving your management of DIC. *Nursing 79*, 9:60, May 1979.

BIBLIOGRAPHY (Unit XIV)

1. Adamson, J. W., et al.: Polycythemia vera: Stem-cell and probable clonal origin of the disease. *New England Journal of Medicine,* 275:913, Oct. 1976.
2. Alderman, D. B.: Therapy for essential cutaneous telangiectasia. *Postgraduate Medicine*, 61:91, Jan. 1977.

2a. Altman, A. J., and A. D. Schwartz: *Malignant Diseases of Infancy, Childhood, and Adolescence.* Philadelphia: W. B. Saunders Co., 1978.

3. Amaral, B. W.: Immune thrombocytopenia purpura: An overview. *Postgraduate Medicine*, 61:197, Apr. 1977.
4. Asperheim, M. K., and R. A. Eisenhauer: *The Pharmacologic Basis of Patient Care*, 3rd ed. Philadelphia: W. B. Saunders Co., 1977.
5. Barnes, A., Jr.: Infections mononucleosis. *Nursing Digest,* 4:51, Jan–Feb. 1976.
6. Beck, W. S.: New outpost on the trail of polycythemia vera. *New England Journal of Medicine*, 295:951, Oct. 1976.
7. Beeson, P. B., W. McDermott and J. B. Wyngaarden (Eds.): *Cecil Textbook of Medicine*, 15th ed. Philadelphia: W. B. Saunders Co., 1979.
8. Bell, W. R., and W. L. Cook: What to do when the patient bleeds too much. *Consultant*, 17:94, Aug. 1977.
9. Berkow, R., and J. H. Talbott (Eds.): *The Merck Manual of Diagnosis and Therapy*, 13th ed. Rahway, N.J.: Merck Sharp and Dohme Research Laboratories, 1977.
10. Beutler, E.: Sickle cell anemia: How to detect and combat it. *Consultant*, 12:21, Apr. 1972.
11. Bissell, D. M.: Porphyria. *In* Conn, H. F. (Ed.): *Current Therapy 1979*. Philadelphia: W. B. Saunders Co., 1979.
12. Blackburn, E. K.: Acute leukemia. *Nursing Times*, 67:509, Apr. 1971.
13. Bonnett, J. D.: Normocytic normochromic anemia. *Postgraduate Medicine*, 61:139, June 1977.

14. Bouchard, R., and N. F. Owens: *Nursing Care of the Cancer Patient*, 2nd ed. St. Louis: C. V. Mosby Co., 1972.
15. Brown, E. B.: Hypochromic anemias. *In* Beeson, P. B., W. McDermott and J. B. Wyngaarden (Eds.): *Cecil Textbook of Medicine*. 15th ed. Philadelphia: W. B. Saunders Co., 1979.
16. Buickus, B. A.: Administering blood components. *American Journal of Nursing*, 79:937, May 1979.
17. Burrow, J. P., and J. K. Luce: Platelet changes in women taking oral contraceptives. *Postgraduate Medicine*, 62:52, Aug. 1977.
18. Byrne, J.: A review of the CBC: Stained red cell examination. *Nursing 76*, 6:15, Dec. 1976.
19. Byrne, J.: Coagulation studies: Part I. Tests of vascular and platelet function. *Nursing 77*, 7:8, May 1977.
20. Byrne, J.: Coagulation studies: Part II. Tests of plasma-clotting factors. *Nursing 77*, 7:24, June 1977.
21. Byrne, J.: Hematology studies: Part IV. Tips for interpreting the sedimentation rate and reticulocyte count. *Nursing 77*, 7:9, Jan. 1977.
22. Byrne, J.: Hematology studies: Part V. How to evaluate the shape of red blood cells. *Nursing 77*, 7:17, Feb. 1977.
23. Byrne, J.: Hematology studies: Part VI. A review of mean corpuscular values and red cell indices. *Nursing 77*, 7:10, Mar. 1977.
24. Byrne, J.: Hematology studies: Part VII. A review of less common blood tests. *Nursing 77*, 7:20, Apr. 77.
25. Byrne, J.: Review of the CBC: The differential white cell count. *Nursing 76*, 6:15, Nov. 1976.
26. Carmel, R.: Iron-related anemias: Look for more than deficiency. *Consultant*, 19:135, Mar. 1979.
27. Castle, W. B.: Megaloblastic anemia. *Postgraduate Medicine*, *64*:117, Oct. 1978.
28. Chaplin, H.: Transfusion reactions. *In* Beeson, P. B., W. McDermott, and J. B. Wyngaarden (Eds.): *Cecil Textbook of Medicine*, 15th ed. Philadelphia: W. B. Saunders Co., 1979.
29. Conley, C. L.: Hemoglobin, the hemoglobinopathies, and the thalassemias. *In* Beeson, P. B., W. McDermott and J. B. Wyngaarden (Eds.): *Cecil Textbook of Medicine*, 15th ed. Philadelphia: W. B. Saunders Co., 1979.
30. Conn, H. F. (Ed.): *Current Therapy 1979*. Philadelphia: W. B. Saunders Co., 1979.
31. Cross-match. Avoiding the cross-match mismatch. *Emergency Medicine*, 9:101, Jan. 1977.
32. Cullins, L. C.: Blood therapy: Preventing and treating transfusion reactions. *American Journal of Nursing*, 79:935, May 1979.
33. Desotell, S.: A brighter future for leukemia patients. *Nursing 77*, 7:19, Jan. 1977.
34. Diggs, L. W.: Screening tests for sickle cell anemia. *Postgraduate Medicine*, 51:267, Feb. 1972.
35. Doswell, W. M.: Sickle cell anemia: You *can* do something to help. *Nursing 78*, 8:65, Apr. 1978.
36. Eichner, E. R.: Anemia due to iron deficiency. *In* Conn, H. F. (Ed.): Current Therapy 1979, Philadelphia: W. B. Saunders Co., 1979.
37. Eosinophils.: Too many eosinophils. *Emergency Medicine*, 10:89, Nov. 1978.
38. Eyster, M. E.: Hemophilia: A guide for the primary care physician. *Postgraduate Medicine*, 64:75, Nov. 1978.
39. Factor VIII.: Extra mileage from factor VIII. *Emergency Medicine*, 10:105, June 1978.
40. Finch, C. A.: Anemia of chronic disease. *Postgraduate Medicine*, 64:107, Oct. 1978.
41. Flynn, K. T.: Iron deficiency among the elderly. *Nurse Practitioner*, 3:20, Nov.–Dec. 1978.
42. Foley, G., and A. M. McCarthy: The child with acute leukemia: The disease and its treatment. *American Journal of Nursing*, 76:1108, July 1976.
43. Foster, S.: Sickle cell anemia: Closing the gap between theory and therapy. *American Journal of Nursing*, 71:1952, Oct. 1971.
44. French, R. M.: *Nurse's Guide to Diagnostic Procedures*, 4th ed. New York: McGraw-Hill Book Co., Inc., 1975.
45. Getting blood from a baby. *Emergency Medicine*, 10:192, 1978.
46. Graenicke, H. R.: Intravascular coagulation: 1. Differential diagnosis and conditioning mechanisms. *Postgraduate Medicine*, 62:68, Nov. 1977.
47. Green, J. B.: Macrocytic anemias. *Postgraduate Medicine*, 61:155, June 1977.
48. Hauer, B. A., et al.: A time for autotransfusion. *Emergency Medicine*, 9:125, Apr. 1977.
49. Hayhurst, M., et al.: Asthmatics may react adversely to I.V. hydrocortisone. *South African Medical Journal*, 53:259, Feb. 1978.
50. Herbert, J. T., et al.: False-positive epidemic infectious mononucleosis. *American Family Physician*, 15:119, Feb. 1977.
51. Hillman, R. S.: Blood loss anemia. *Postgraduate Medicine*, 64:88, Oct. 1978.
53. Holcroft, J. W.: The loss of blood. *Emergency Medicine*, 11:179, May 1979.
54. Horowitz, C. A.: Practical approach to diagnosis of infectious mononucleosis. *Postgraduate Medicine*, 65:179, June 1979.
55. Infection: Delaying infection in leukemics. *Emergency Medicine*, 11:82, Jan. 1979.
56. ITP under the knife. *Emergency Medicine*, 10:120, Oct. 1978.
57. Jacob, H. S.: Severe bone marrow failure: Possible pathophysiologic mechanisms. *Postgraduate Medicine*, 64:97, Oct. 1978.
58. Jacobs, P.: Tumours of bone. *Nursing Times*, 68:1572, Dec. 1972.
59. Jarowski, C. I., and M. Coleman: Multiple myeloma. *Hospital Medicine*, 14:58, Mar. 1978.
60. Jennings, B. M.: Improving your management of DIC. *Nursing 79*, 9:60, May 1979.
61. Jennings, J. C.: Hemoglobinopathies in pregnancy. *American Family Physician*, 15:104, Jan. 1977.
62. Kardinal, C. G.: Chronic melocytic leukemia. *Hospital Medicine*, 13:97, Sept. 1977.
63. Kass, L.: The spectrum of chronic lymphocytic leukemia. *Postgraduate Medicine*, 60:95, Oct. 1976.
64. Kazak, A.: Blood therapy: Processing blood for transfusion. *American Journal of Nursing*, 79:931, May 1979.
65. Keating, M. J., et al.: Acute leukemia. *CA: A Cancer Journal for Clinicians*, 27:2, Feb. 1977.
66. Keaveny, M. E.: Hodgkin's disease: The curable cancer. *Nursing 75*, 5:48, Mar. 1975.
67. Krishnamurthy, M., et al.: Bland cholestasis: Unusual hepatic sequela in sickle cell anemia. *Postgraduate Medicine*, 64:215, Sept. 1975.
68. Krupp, M. A., and M. J. Chatton: *Current Medical Diagnosis and Treatment*. Los Altos, Calif.: Lange Medical Publications, 1978.
69. Lamon, J. M., and D. P. Tschudy: The porphyrias. *In* Conn, H. F. (Ed.): *1978 Current Therapy*. Philadelphia: W. B. Saunders Co., 1978.
70. Le Blanc, D. H.: People with Hodgkin's disease: The nursing challenge. *Nursing Clinics of North America*, 13:281, June 1978.
71. Leventhal, B. G., and S. Hersh: Modern treatment of childhood leukemia: The patient and his family. *Nursing Digest*, 3:12, July–Aug. 1975.
72. Lewis, S. M.: The blood and spleen. *In* Conn, H. F. (Ed.): *Current Therapy 1978*. Philadelphia: W. B. Saunders Co., 1978.
73. Linman, J. W.: *Hematology*. New York: Macmillan Co., Inc., 1975.
74. MacBryde, C. M., and R. S. Blacklow (Eds.): *Signs and*

Symptoms: Applied Pathologic Physiology and Clinical Interpretation, 5th ed. Philadelphia: J. B. Lippincott Co., 1972.
75. Mann, F. D.: Platelets, thrombosis, coagulation, and atherosclerosis. *Postgraduate Medicine*, 62:15, Aug. 1977.
76. Marengo-Rowe, A. J., and J. E. Leveson: Evaluation of the bleeding patient. *Postgraduate Medicine*, 62:171, July 1977.
77. Mason, C. C.: The physician's office laboratory: How does yours measure up? *Postgraduate Medicine*, 63:65, Apr. 1978.
78. McCredie, K. B.: Current concepts in acute leukemia. *Postgraduate Medicine*, 61:221, Jan. 1977.
79. McCurdy, P. R.: Microcytic hypochromic anemias. *Postgraduate Medicine*, 61:147, June 1977.
80. McFarlane, J. M.: The child with sickle cell anemia: What his parents need to know. *Nursing 75*, 5:29, May 1975.
81. Metz, J.: Pernicious anemia and other forms of vitamin B_{12} deficiency. *In* Conn, H. F. (Ed.): *Current Therapy 1979*. Philadelphia: W. B. Saunders Co., 1979.
82. Miller, B. F., and C. B. B. Keane.: *Encyclopedia and Dictionary of Medicine and Nursing*, 2nd ed. Philadelphia: W. B. Saunders Co., 1978.
83. Moore, K.: How patient education can reduce the risks of anticoagulation. *Nursing 77*, 7:24, Sept. 1977.
84. Nachman, R. L.: Hematologic and hematopoietic diseases: Introduction. *In* Beeson, P. B., W. McDermott, and J. B. Wyngaarden (Eds.): *Cecil Textbook of Medicine*, 15th ed. Philadelphia: W. B. Saunders Co., 1979.
85. Nathan, D. G.: Regulation of erythropoiesis. *New England Journal of Medicine*, 296:685, Mar. 1977.
86. Newton, P. A.: Multiple myeloma: Uncommon or uncommonly diagnosed? *Postgraduate Medicine*, 61:107, May 1977.
86a. Niederman, J. C.: Infections mononucleosis. *In* Beeson, P. B., W. McDermott, and J. B. Wyngaarden (Eds.): *Cecil Textbook of Medicine*, 15th ed. Philadelphia: W. B. Saunders Co., 1979.
87. Nolan, J. W.: Infectious mononucleosis. *Nurse Practitioner*, 4:12, Apr. 1979.
88. O'Brian, B. S., and S. Woods: The paradox of DIC. *American Journal of Nursing*, 78:1878, Nov. 1978.
89. Osserman, E. F.: Plasma cell dyscrasias. *In* Beeson, P. B., W. McDermott, and J. B. Wyngaarden (Eds.): *Cecil Textbook of Medicine*, 15th ed. Philadelphia: W. B. Saunders Co., 1979.
90. Palmer, R. L.: Intravascular coagulation and fibrinolysis. *Postgraduate Medicine*, 62:181, 1978.
91. Parker, A. L.: Blood therapy: Massive transfusions. *American Journal of Nursing*, 79:944, May 1979.
92. Pisciotta, A. V.: The anemic patient. *American Family Physician*, 18:144, Nov. 1978.
93. Pochedly, C.: Acute lymphoid leukemia in children. *American Journal of Nursing*, 78:1714, Oct. 1978.
94. Rapp, C. E., Jr.: Infectious mononucleosis: The "holiday" disease. *Consultant*, 18:21, Nov. 1978.
95. Ratnoff, O. D.: Heritable disorders of blood coagulation. *In* Beeson, P. B., W. McDermott, and J. B. Wyngaarden (Eds.): *Cecil Textbook of Medicine*, 15th ed. Philadelphia: W. B. Saunders Co., 1979.
96. Robbins, S. L., and R. S. Cotran: *The Pathologic Basis of Disease*, 2nd ed. Philadelphia: W. B. Saunders Co., 1979.
97. Rodgers, J. M.: Hodgkin's disease: Hope is the key to nursing care. *Nursing 75*, 5:55, Mar. 1975.
98. Rodman, M. J.: Anticancer chemotherapy against the leukemias and lymphomas. Part 3. *RN*, 35:49, Apr. 1972.
99. Rossman, M., et al.: Pheresis therapy: Patient care. *American Journal of Nursing*, 77:135, July 1977.
100. Rutman, R., et al.: Blood therapy: Screening donors and the phlebotomy procedure. *American Journal of Nursing*, 79:926, May 1979.
101. Schumann, D., and P. Patterson: Multiple myeloma. *American Journal of Nursing*, 75:78, Jan. 1975.
102. Shanbrom, E.: A systematic approach to the diagnosis of the anemias. *Medical Counterpoint*, pp. 30–3, Dec. 1971.
102a. Sherman, L. A.: Disseminated intravascular coagulation (DIC). *In* Conn, H. F. (Ed.): *Current Therapy 1979*. Philadelphia: W. B. Saunders Co., 1979.
103. Sickle Cell Anemia. *Medical World News*, Dec. 3, 1971, p. 37.
104. Sickle cells: Unplugging sickle cells. *Emergency Medicine*, 11:145, July 1979.
105. Silberman, S.: Less waste — and fewer complications in blood component therapy. *Consultant*, 18:97, Mar. 1978.
106. Smith, S. E.: Drug therapy 1972: Drugs and the blood. Part 5. *Nursing Times*, 63:383, Mar. 1972.
107. Snively, W. D., and D. R. Beshear: *Textbook of Pathophysiology*. Philadelphia: J. B. Lippincott Co., 1972.
108. Stefanini, M.: Diffuse intravascular coagulation versus fibrinolysis. *Postgraduate Medicine*, 51:215, Apr. 1972.
109. Stoutenborough, K. A.: Hematological disorders. *In* Price, S. A., and L. C. Wilson: *Pathophysiology: Clinical Concepts of Disease Processes*. New York: McGraw-Hill Book Co., Inc., 1978.
110. Three tests can tell why babies bleed. *Emergency Medicine*, 9:181, Mar. 1977.
111. Transfusion Committee: Guidelines for granulocyte transfusion therapy. Medical Staff, University Hospital, Seattle, Washington, Dec. 1978, pp. 1–3.
112. Trowbridge, A. A.: Neutropenia: When and when not to treat. *Postgraduate Medicine*, 61:208, Apr. 1977.
113. Vaz, D. D. S.: The common anemias: Nursing approaches. *Nursing Clinics of North America*, 7:711, Dec. 1972.
114. Walker, P.: Bone marrow transplant: A second chance for life. *Nursing 77*, 7:24, Jan. 1977.
115. Wallerstein, R. O.: Polycythemia vera — who needs therapy? *Consultant*, 17:148, Apr. 1977.
116. Ward, P. C. J.: Investigation of macrocytic anemia. *Postgraduate Medicine*, 65:203, Feb. 1979.
117. Ward, P. C. J.: Investigation of microcytic anemia. *Postgraduate Medicine*, 65:235, Jan. 1979.
118. Ward, P. C. J.: Investigation of poikilocytic normochromic normocytic anemia. Part 2: Spiculated forms. *Postgraduate Medicine*, 65:229, Apr. 1979.
119. Ward, P. C. J.: Red cell indices revised: Review with test cases. *Postgraduate Medicine*, 65:282, May 1979.
120. Waters, W. E.: Anaemia in women. *Nursing Mirror*, 134:20, Apr. 1972.
121. Weiss, R. B., and S. Shah: When "lymphoma" is not lymphoma: Diagnosing immunoblastic lymphadenopathy. *Postgraduate Medicine*, 63:101, May 1978.
122. Whitehead, J. A., and M. M. Chohan: Paraphrenia and pernicious anemia. *Geriatrics*, 27:148, May 1972.
123. Whitehouse, J. M. A.: The leukaemias: Acute leukaemia. Part 1. *Nursing Times*, 68:703, June 1972.
124. Whitehouse, J. M. A.: Chronic leukaemias. Part 2. *Nursing Times*, 68:737, June 1972.
125. Williams, W. J., et al.: *Hematology*, 2nd ed. New York: McGraw Hill Book Co. Inc., 1977.
126. Wilson, P.: Iron-deficiency anemia. *American Journal of Nursing*, 72:502, Mar. 1972.

UNIT XV

NURSING PEOPLE EXPERIENCING DISTURBANCES OF PERIPHERAL VASCULAR FUNCTION

by Rosemary Pittman, R.N., B.S.N., M.S., Marie Cowan, R.N., B.S.N., M.S., and Joan Luckmann, R.N., B.S., M.A.

INTRODUCTION AND STUDY GUIDE

The study of peripheral vascular disease focuses upon disorders of the arteries, veins, and the lymphatics, as well as upon the tissue trauma that develops when the vascular system is damaged. More specifically, this unit covers diseases of the aorta, functional and organic diseases of the arteries and veins, and the anatomy and physiology relative to these disorders. Since the lymphatic system is closely related to the circulatory system, common lymphatic disorders are also discussed. Also, lower limb amputations are considered in this section because amputation may be necessary when peripheral vascular damage results in gangrene.

Although we discuss disorders of the aorta as well as conditions affecting the hands (e.g., Raynaud's disease and Raynaud's phenomenon), the primary emphasis in this unit is upon disease of the lower extremities. Also heavily stressed is the role of *atherosclerosis* in vascular disease. In Unit XII we pointed out that atherosclerosis is a disorder of unknown etiology, which is characterized by deposits of fat-containing substances along the intima of blood vessels. Peripheral arterial disease must be looked at in relationship to atherosclerosis because the majority of arterial disorders are due to this important disease process. Atherosclerosis is a lifelong process and is not a single lesion or syndrome. The disease begins in infancy and progresses in episodic fashion over the individual's entire life.

Peripheral vascular diseases are an important group of disorders because they are so common. Few members of our population will escape some degree of vascular degeneration as they pass through the aging process. The majority of patients afflicted with vascular problems are middle-aged or older. They often suffer from other diseases that affect their vessels, e.g., diabetes, heart disease. Also, these patients often become depressed, and with good reason. Vascular diseases are usually chronic, painful, incapacitating and debilitating. Moreover, long-term medical care is costly, causing a severe strain on family finances. Patients with vascular disturbances need psychologic support as well as physical care.

The role of the nurse in caring for patients with peripheral vascular disease focuses heavily on patient education. Vascular conditions usually cannot be cured; however, extensive tissue damage can often be prevented by teaching the patient some simple measures for increasing his or her circulation. To reverse or at least to control the advance of vascular disease, nurse, doctor, and patient must all work closely together in developing a total plan of care that the patient will carry on at home and throughout life.

While reading this unit, the student should become thoroughly familiar with the following terms:

- ischemia
- arterial ischemic leg ulcer
- venous stasis ulcer
- Buerger-Allen routine
- aortography
- reaction-to-injury hypothesis
- angiography
- treadmill exercise
- lumbar sympathetic block
- oscillometry
- Doppler ultrasound flow detector
- plethysmography
- arterial thrombosis
- Trendelenburg's test
- venography
- arterial embolism
- pulmonary embolism
- intermittent claudication
- rest pain
- rubor
- trophic changes
- gangrene
- aneurysm
- acute arterial occlusion
- thromboangiitis obliterans
- functional vascular disease
- Raynaud's phenomenon
- Raynaud's disease
- bypass graft
- varicosities
- venous insufficiency
- thrombophlebitis
- phlebothrombosis
- vein ligation
- embolectomy
- lymphadenopathy
- lymphedema
- lymphangitis
- Symes amputation
- below-knee amputation
- above-knee amputation
- temporary prosthesis
- cosmetic prosthesis
- delayed prosthesis fitting
- immediate prosthesis fitting
- rigid dressing
- phantom limb sensation
- replantation

By the end of this unit, the student should be able to achieve the following objectives:

a. Detect deviation from normal in the peripheral vascular system.

b. Recognize the importance of taking the pulse in the posterior tibia and dorsalis pedis arteries and of comparing the limbs for symmetry; discover the patient's sensitivity to cold, nutritional damage as shown by lack of hair, tissue atrophy, and nail changes, and symptoms of numbness and pain on exercise or rest.

c. Help the patient understand the pathologic changes that are occurring, understand the diagnostic tests being performed, and understand the rationale and procedures of planned treatment.

d. Assist the patient in establishing a meticulous care plan for the affected limbs, as well as a plan for changing those life patterns that contribute to the exacerbation of the disease.

e. Assist in establishment of the overall care plan for the patient.

f. Understand the pathophysiology of the peripheral arterial, venous, and lymphatic systems.

g. Understand the symptoms, diagnosis, and treatment of disease processes affecting these systems.

CHAPTER 47

INTRODUCTORY CONCEPTS

ANATOMY AND PHYSIOLOGY OF THE PERIPHERAL VASCULAR SYSTEM

THE STRUCTURE OF THE VASCULAR SYSTEM

Blood flow is essential to life. It is dependent upon the efficiency of the heart as a pump and the patency of the blood vessels. Circulation is influenced by viscosity, hydration, mechanisms affecting coagulation and fibrinolysis, local changes in the size of the vessels, as well as iatrogenic, inflammatory, and neurogenic processes.

Vessels are grouped into six categories:

1. The *aorta* and large *arteries,* which constitute a distribution system
2. The *arterioles,* sometimes called the resistance vessels, which act as a regulating system
3. The *microcirculation,* in which metabolites pass to and from the tissues across the endothelium of capillaries
4. A collecting system of *veins* carrying blood to the heart
5. The *larger veins* acting as a storage system
6. *Lymphatic vessels,* which collect lymph from the tissues and return it to the blood at the junction of the internal jugular and subclavian veins.

The *anatomic pattern* of the blood vessels of the upper and lower extremities is similar. A large main artery (axillary, external iliac) enters the limbs and runs the length of the proximal segment (brachial, femoral). In the lower limb there is an additional major source of supply to the buttocks through the obturator and gluteal branches of the internal iliac artery. At the elbow or knee the main artery divides into two branches (radial and anterior and posterior tibial), which supply the forearm or leg and finally anastomose to form the plantar or palmar arch. From these arteries the digital arteries run to the fingers or toes. In sum, main arterial trunks give off branches, and each branch gives off further branches of arteries of smaller caliber until, from the smallest arteries, the blood passes into the arterioles and then into capillaries, where it nourishes the tissues.

Arterioles are small thick-walled vessels with an overall diameter of about 0.2 cm. and are important regulators of the peripheral circulation.

Capillaries are thin-walled vessels from 5 to 10 μ in diameter. Red blood cells must alter their shape to pass through the smallest of these vessels. From the capillaries, the blood flows into the venules and then into the veins. The main venous drainage of the upper and lower limbs is similar and is through a superficial and deep set of veins.

Arteriovenous anastomoses are special structures present only in certain sites. They are generally believed to regulate both local and general temperature.

Except for capillaries, all blood vessels are similar in *structure.* They consist of an outer layer of connective tissue (the *adventitia*), a middle coat (the *media*), and an endothelial lining called the *intima.* Between the media and intima there is a well-defined layer of elastic tissue named the internal elastic lamina. *Veins* have a thinner medial coat than the arteries, a greater proportion of white fibrous tissue, and less muscle and elastic tissue. Also, veins contain valves that direct the blood proximally. Finally, the walls of *capillaries* consist of two components: endothelial cells and a basement membrane surrounded by a pericapillary sheath of connective tissue.

Major arteries and major veins of the body are illustrated in Figures 47–1 and 47–2.

FACTORS REGULATING THE PERIPHERAL VASCULAR SYSTEM

All arteries are contractile in that they can decrease (vasoconstriction) or increase (vasodilatation) their caliber in response to appropriate stimuli. The mechanism regulating vasomotor activity is complex, consisting of central nervous influences, chemical substances in the blood stream, and the autonomous action of the arterial wall itself.

Vascular Nerves. There is evidence that the *hypothalamus* is the chief regulating center for peripheral vasomotor activity, but the cerebral center also exerts some influence.

Arteries have a relatively rich nerve supply from the sympathetic nervous system. Stimulation of the sympathetic nerves causes vasoconstriction and sympathectomy causes vasodilatation. Evidence for the presence of sympathetic vasodilator nerves to the blood vessels of the skin is unsatisfactory, but there is good evidence

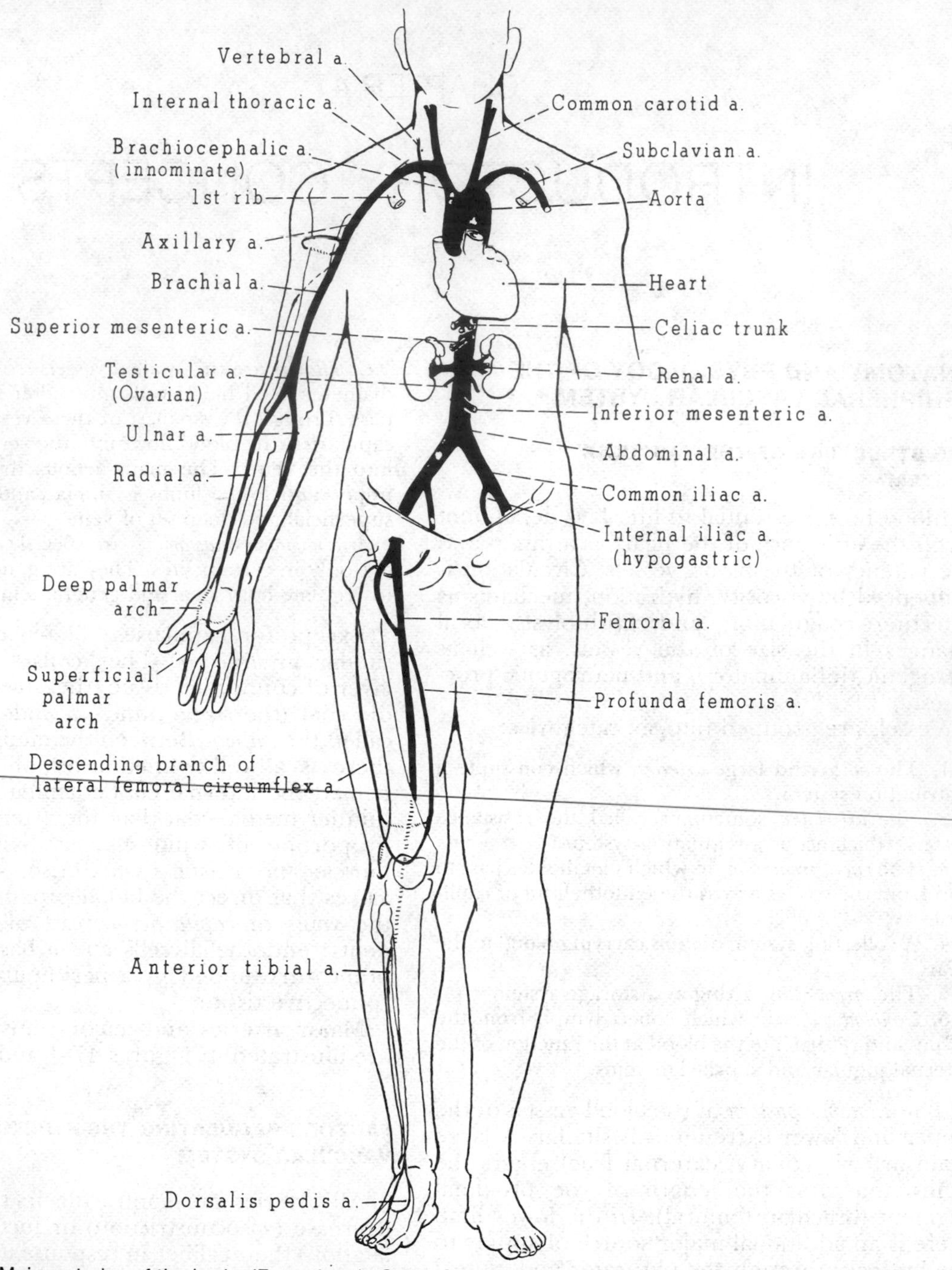

Figure 47–1. Major arteries of the body. (From Jacob, S. W., C. A. Francone and W. J. Lossow: *Structure and Function in Man,* 4th ed. Philadelphia: W. B. Saunders Co., 1978.)

that both constrictor and dilator nerves supply the muscles.

Hormonal and Chemical Control. There are three powerful substances within the blood that help to control the caliber of blood vessels; they are epinephrine, norepinephrine, and angiotensin II.* *Epinephrine* constricts superficial blood vessels, but in small doses dilates vessels supplying the muscles, brain, and heart. *Norepinephrine* constricts all blood vessels; it particularly affects the peripheral vessels. *Angiotensin* is a substance formed by the interaction of renin and a serum globulin fraction; it constricts arteries.

Local Regulatory Mechanisms. The following substances act locally on blood vessels, although they circulate in the systemic circulation:

▶*Histamine* is a potent vasodilator of small blood vessels, although it may also constrict the large arteries.

*Epinephrine and norepinephrine are discussed in Unit XIX and in Chapter 6.

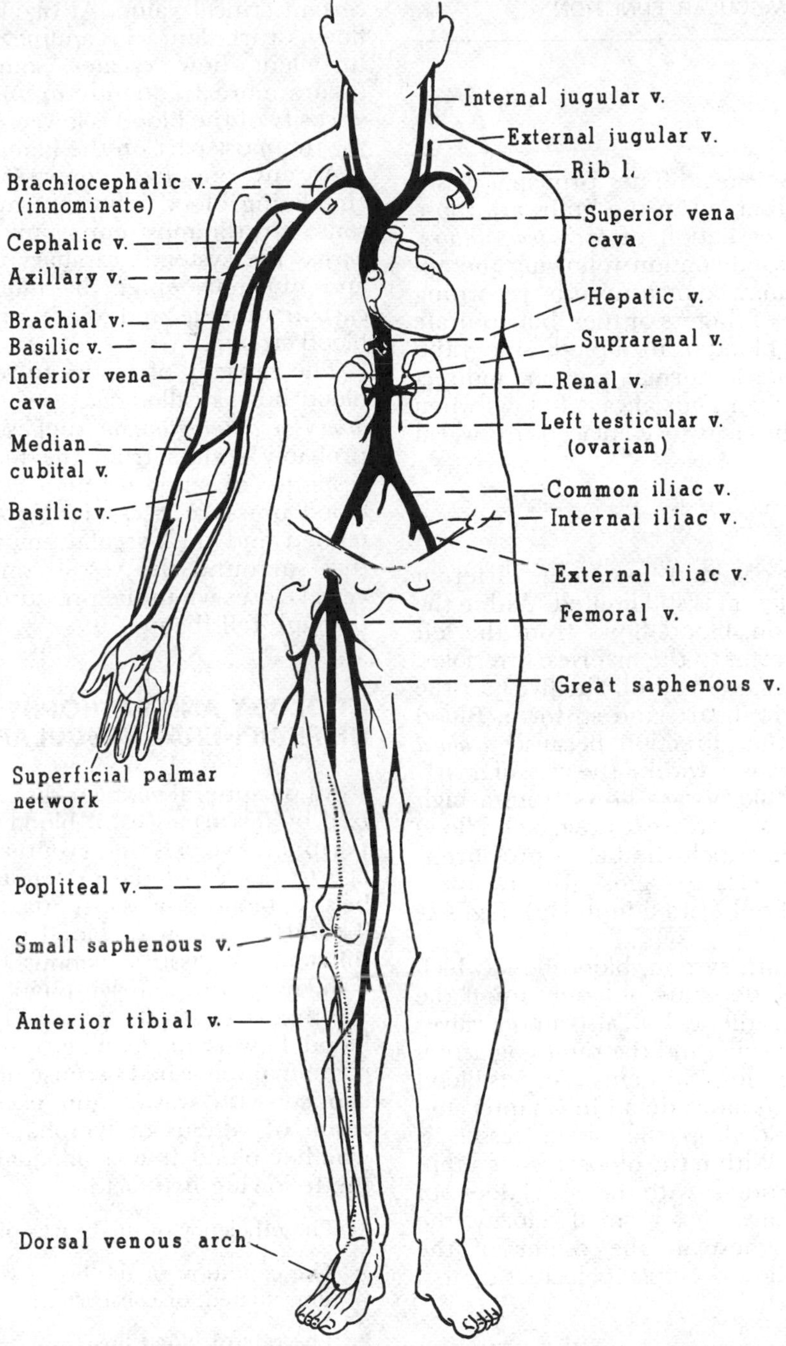

Figure 47–2. Major veins of the body. (From Jacob, S. W., C. A. Francone and W. J. Lossow: *Structure and Function in Man*, 4th ed. Philadelphia: W. B. Saunders Co., 1978.)

▶ *Bradykinin* is one of a group of vasoactive peptides and is a powerful vasodilator, especially of cutaneous vessels.

▶ *Muscle metabolites* have a strong vasodilator action.

▶ *Acetylcholine* is another vasodilator substance, but its action is transient and is more apparent in the face and upper limbs than in the lower limbs.

▶ *Serotonin* is liberated from platelets that stick to the vessel wall in the injured area. It is a powerful constrictor of cutaneous arterioles but dilates capillaries.

▶ *Vasopressin,* often called the antidiuretic hormone (ADH), is secreted by the posterior pituitary and released into the blood stream by impulses in the nerves from the hypothalamus. In large doses, vasopressin elevates arterial blood pressure by action of the smooth muscles of the arterioles. Vasopressin is probably not secreted in amounts sufficient to produce appreciable vasoconstriction.

In addition, trauma to an artery causes it to constrict. Also, moderate *heat* dilates the arteries; *cold* constricts isolated segments of the artery, but after 10 to 15 minutes the cooled artery relaxes.

Vasomotor Reflexes. The principal vasomotor reflexes observed in the limbs are those concerned with regulation of *body temperature.* The degree of vasodilatation following the application of heat may be measured by recording skin temperature of fingers or toes, but accurate measurements of blood using a plethysmograph are preferable. In a normal person, indirect vasodilatation in the hands always follows when the trunk or the legs are placed in warm water.

BLOOD FLOW

Understanding of blood flow to the different parts of the circulation is still limited. Within the systemic circulation, blood flows from the left ventricle to the aorta, to the arteries, arterioles, capillaries, venules, veins and, finally, into the right atrium of the heart, and so forth. Blood always flows in this direction because a *blood pressure gradient* exists within the vascular system. Because a fluid always flows from a high pressure area to a low pressure area, blood flows from the aorta (in which the blood pressure is around 100 mm. Hg) to veins (which have a blood pressure of only 1 to 6 mm. Hg) (Fig. 47–3).

Within the venous system, blood flow (which is against gravity) depends not only upon the blood pressure gradient, but also upon valves located within the veins and the pumping action of muscles surrounding the veins. Venous blood flow is described in more detail in Chapter 49.

The flow of blood in the blood vessels is normally *laminar.* Within the blood vessels a thin layer of blood in contact with the vessel does not move. The next layer has a small velocity, the velocity being highest in the center of the stream. Laminar flow occurs at velocities up to a

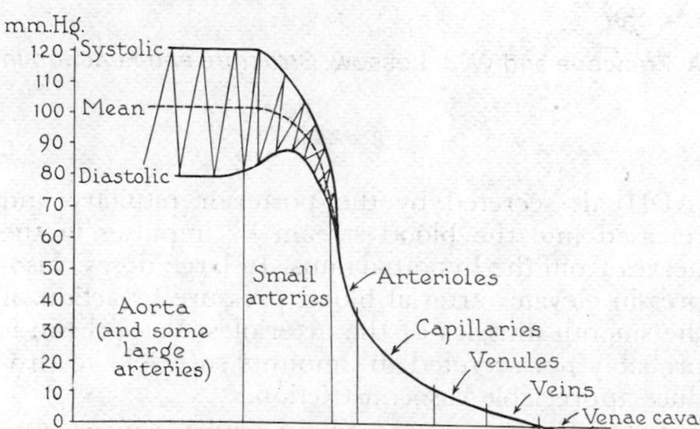

Figure 47–3. Diagram showing pressure gradients in different divisions of the circulatory system. (From King, B. G., and M. J. Showers: *Human Anatomy and Physiology,* 6th ed. Philadelphia: W. B. Saunders Co.)

certain critical value. At or above this velocity, flow is turbulent. Streamline flow is silent, but turbulent flow creates sounds. Turbulence occurs more frequently in anemia because the viscosity of the blood is lower. Viscosity depends for the most part on the hematocrit.

At any one time, only 5 per cent of the circulating blood is in the capillaries; but in a sense it is the most important part, because it is across the systemic capillary walls that oxygen and nutrients enter the interstitial fluid and carbon dioxide and waste products enter the blood stream.

The capacity of tissues to regulate their own blood flow is called *autoregulation.* The *myogenic theory of autoregulation* suggests that regulation probably results from the intrinsic contractile response of smooth muscle to stretch. As the blood pressure rises, the blood vessels are distended and the vascular smooth muscle fibers that surround the vessel contract. The blood vessel closes when the pressure of blood flowing through falls below 70.

ETIOLOGY AND PATHOPHYSIOLOGY OF PERIPHERAL VASCULAR DISEASE

All peripheral vascular diseases are characterized by disturbances of blood flow through the peripheral vessels that eventually result in damage to tissues of the extremities. As we stated before, blood flow is essential to life and health. The arterial flow of blood carries oxygen and nutrients to tissues; venous flow carries away cellular wastes; and lymphatic flow conveys tissue fluid back to the general circulation. When blood flow is inadequate, cells and tissues become malnourished because of oxygen lack and choked with wastes and excessive fluid as a result of venous or lymphatic stasis. Basically, whether blood flow is adequate depends upon the following five factors:

- The efficiency of the heart's pumping action
- The condition of the blood vessels (whether patent, dilated, or constricted)
- The rate of blood flow
- The needs of the tissues for oxygen and nutrients as well as for removal of waste products
- Nervous system activity

THE ROLE OF THE HEART

We stressed in Unit XII that blood flow ultimately depends upon the continuous and efficient pumping of the blood by the heart to all parts of the body. When, for any reason, the heart begins to fail as a pump, blood flow becomes abnormal. Recall that in left-sided failure, blood backs up into the lungs, causing congestion coupled with a decrease in cardiac output. These factors, in turn, reduce blood flow to the more peripheral vessels. When the right side of the heart fails, the patient suffers from severe venous congestion within the liver, gastrointestinal tract, and kidneys as well as edema of the ankles and lower extremities. Eventually, with failure of both the right and left pumps, the patient suffers severe malnutrition of tissues as a result of venous congestion and low cardiac output. In the end, the patient usually dies in severe shock and circulatory collapse.

THE ROLE OF THE BLOOD VESSELS

Arteries. To carry the blood adequately, arteries must be patent and must be capable of dilating and constricting normally in response to thermal, hormonal, neural, and chemical stimulation. When arteries become obstructed or damaged, there is a decreased flow of oxygen and nutrients to the tissues, which leads to *ischemia* (a temporary and localized deficiency of blood to tissues), malnutrition of tissues, and, ultimately, tissue necrosis and gangrene. Causes of arterial narrowing and obstruction include the following: atherosclerosis and arteriosclerosis,* arterial thrombosis and emboli; damage due to chemical or physical agents; infectious processes; vasospastic disorders (also called functional disorders) which cause constriction of blood vessels, e.g., Raynaud's disease; and congenital malformation.

Whether the patient with arterial occlusion will develop tissue necrosis and gangrene depends upon the *extensiveness* of the block as well as upon the *speed* at which arterial obstruction develops. For example, total or near total occlusion of an artery by a thrombus or embolus is far more critical than is the partial narrowing of an artery as a result of arteriosclerotic changes. Likewise, the patient with an arterial obstruction that develops swiftly has a much poorer prognosis than does the patient with arteries that have gradually narrowed over the years. The gradual development of arterial disease is less dangerous because *collateral circulation* (the growth of new vessels to replace many of the damaged ones) has had an opportunity to develop.

Veins. The efficiency of veins in returning blood to the heart depends upon patency of the veins, competent valves within the veins, and adequate pumping action of the muscles surrounding the veins. Blood flow through the veins can be slowed by the following:

- *Defective valves,* which usually result either from *stretching* of the veins as a result of prolonged venous pressure or from *inflammation* of the veins. Defective valves eventually result in *varicose veins* (which are dilated, tortuous superficial veins) and in *venous insufficiency.* (See Chapter 49.)
- *Thrombus formation* within the veins, which may be caused by either stasis of blood flow, hypercoagulability of the blood, or damage to the endothelial lining of the veins.* Venous thrombi may or may not be accompanied by inflammation. The greatest danger when thrombophlebitis (thrombus formation with inflammation) or phlebothrombosis (venous thrombosis without inflammation) occurs is that the clot will break free of the vessel wall and travel as a deadly embolus to the heart, lungs, or brain.

Blockage of blood through the veins (whether caused by venous insufficiency, inflammation, or a blood clot) results in *increased venous pressure.* Increased venous pressure, in turn, causes the hydrostatic pressure to rise within the capillaries, which decreases the amount of fluid that the capillaries can reabsorb from the tissues. *Edema* results. Edematous congested tissues cannot receive the oxygen and metabolites which they need; also waste products, which cannot be transported back into the circulation, build up within the swollen tissues. The consequence of severe venous stasis is *malnutrition* of tissue. Malnourished tissue is highly susceptible to bacterial infection; consequently, patients with venous insufficiency are susceptible to *leg ulcers* and *cellulitis.*

Lymphatics. The lymphatic system drains intracellular fluid from the interstitial spaces and routes it back to the circulation. *Obstruction* of lymphatic flow can result from infection of lymphatic structures, trauma to lymphatic vessels, and blockage of the lymphatics by tumors. The most outstanding manifestation of lymphatic obstruction is *edema,* which is often massive in nature. Important disorders of the lymphatic system include localized lymphadenopathy, generalized lymphadenopathy, lymphedema, and tuberculosis of the lymphatic system.

RATE OF BLOOD FLOW

The rate of blood flow controls the amount of oxygen and nutrients that the tissues receive. When the blood flow through the vessels is seriously decreased, the tissues which those vessels supply become ischemic and malnourished. Major causes of a decrease in the *rate* of blood flow include: (1) increased viscosity of blood as a result of polycythemia or dehydration; (2) atherosclerotic narrowing of the arteries; (3) spasm of the arterial walls as in hypertension; and (4)

*Atherosclerosis and arteriosclerosis are described at length in Chapter 36 and Chapter 48.

*Thrombus formation is discussed in Chapters 32, 36, 48, and 49.

decreased pumping action of muscles surrounding the veins, which can result from immobility.

METABOLIC NEEDS OF TISSUES

The needs of the tissues for blood and oxygen are *constantly changing*, depending upon the individual's activity level, thermal environment, and state of health. When the metabolic needs of the body *increase*, more blood flow to tissues is needed and the arteries normally *dilate*. When the metabolic needs of the tissues *decrease*, the needs of the tissues for blood also decrease and the vessels *constrict*.

Body tissues demand a *greater* than normal blood flow under the following conditions:

- *Increased physical activity* or strenuous exercise, which raises the needs of tissues for oxygen and the demands of the tissues for blood.
- The direct application of *heat* to a part of the body (e.g., by a hot water bottle or heating pad), which results in arterial dilatation; an increased blood flow to the tissues exposed to the source of heat; and the consequent dissipation of excess heat.
- *Infection*, which leads to dilatation of the vessels supplying the involved tissues, resulting in more protective antibodies and leukocytes being conveyed to the infected site.

On the other hand, tissues require a *smaller* than normal blood flow under these circumstances:

- *Decreased physical activity* or rest, which lowers the tissue's needs for oxygen.
- *Chilling* of the body or direct application of cold (e.g., an ice pack) to a body part, which results in vasoconstriction, decreased blood flow to the chilled part, and the conservation of body heat.

Normally, blood vessels, by dilating and constricting, are able to vary the amount of blood that the tissues of the extremities receive. However, sclerosed, obstructed, damaged, inelastic blood vessels are unable to dilate and constrict normally. Consequently, these vessels fail to supply tissues with the additional blood that they require when physical exercise increases, heat is applied, or infection develops. For this reason, patients with peripheral vascular disease experience pain in their legs upon walking, tissue damage when heat is applied directly to an extremity, and leg ulcers and cellulitis when infection develops.

NERVOUS SYSTEM ACTIVITY

Blood flow also depends upon *sympathetic nervous system stimulation*. Stimulation of the sympathetic nervous system results in *vasoconstriction* and decreased blood flow to the tissues of the extremities. *Removal* of sympathetic nervous system stimulation by adrenergic blocking agents or by lumbar sympathectomy (an operation that interrupts sympathetic nerves) causes vasodilatation and increased blood flow to the extremities.

In sum, any factor that narrows, obstructs, or damages the blood vessels impedes blood flow. When blood flow slows, tissue nutrition decreases, cellular waste products increase, ischemia develops, and the danger of thrombus and embolus formation escalates. Without treatment, tissue damage may advance to the point of cellulitis, leg ulceration, or gangrene. Eventually, the limb may have to be amputated.

BASES OF SYMPTOMS

Patients with peripheral vascular disease all experience *ischemia*. Consequently, despite the wide variety of specific peripheral vascular disorders, patients with vascular problems suffer from many of the same symptoms. The most common nonspecific manifestations of peripheral vascular disease and their bases are listed in Table 47–1.

Nurses in ambulatory care facilities should be alert to the *early* manifestations of peripheral vascular disease, e.g., nail changes, skin color changes, pallor or redness of extremities, tissue changes, atrophy, edema, lack of hair, the presence or absence of pedal pulses, hyperesthesias, and paresthesias. Also it is important to note whether the changes are unilateral or bilateral. Some patients are reluctant to bring up minor complaints, and careful questioning and observation by the nurse may elicit important information about early signs and symptoms of this insidious condition.

CLINICAL CARE OF PATIENTS WITH PERIPHERAL VASCULAR DISEASE: OVERVIEW

As a general rule, patients with peripheral vascular disease suffer from one or more of the following problems: (1) decreased arterial blood flow to peripheral tissues, (2) venous stasis, (3) prolonged vasoconstriction, (4) vascular obstruction, (5) ischemic pain, and (6) tissue damage (either ulcerations, infections, or gangrene). Consequently, the five major goals of care are as follows:

1. *Increase arterial blood flow to the extremities and increase venous return to the heart*
2. *Promote vasodilatation*
3. *Prevent and treat vascular obstruction*
4. *Relieve ischemic pain*
5. *Prevent tissue damage and infection and promote healing of ulcerated areas*

Goal 1: Increase Arterial Blood Flow and Venous Return

The principal methods for augmenting the patient's circulation are proper positioning, prescribed exercise, and patient education.

Positioning. To safely position a patient with peripheral vascular disease, you must first learn whether the disorder is arterial or venous in nature. Patients with *arterial* blood disorders suffer from a deficit of oxygenated blood to their extremities. Because blood flows to *dependent* parts of the body (i.e., parts lower than the heart), position individuals with arterial disease so that blood flows toward their legs and feet. In serious cases of arterial insufficiency, the doctor may order the *head* of the patient's bed to be elevated on six-inch blocks so that blood from the heart flows more easily to the extremities whenever the patient is asleep or resting. In milder cases, patients can benefit from simply sitting for periods of time with their feet flat on the floor. Remind all patients with arterial insufficiency to avoid raising their feet above heart level unless this is specifically prescribed by their physician as an exercise measure. (See Buerger-Allen exercises below.)

In contrast to arterial disease, patients with *venous insufficiency* suffer from a pooling of deoxygenated blood in their extremities and poor venous return to the heart. To overcome the pull of gravity which further impedes venous return, instruct the patient with venous stasis to elevate his or her legs above heart level frequently and to avoid prolonged standing or sitting. Also, these individuals should sleep with the *foot* of the bed elevated on six-inch blocks.

Teach patients with either arterial or venous insufficiency to avoid standing in any one position for more than a few minutes, because prolonged standing interferes with circulation.

TABLE 47–1. SIGNS AND SYMPTOMS OF PERIPHERAL VASCULAR DISEASE

Signs and Symptoms	Bases
Intermittent claudication (severe pain in the calf muscles, which occurs upon walking or exercise of the limbs and which is relieved by rest)	Exercise increases the metabolic needs of tissues; damaged arteries are unable to dilate and supply the tissues with oxygen; evidently ischemia coupled with a build-up of metabolites creates a painful muscle spasm that forces the patient to stop walking or exercising.
Rest pain (pain in the extremities, which occurs when the patient is resting)	Blockage of a vessel by a thrombus or embolus or severe arterial disease may so reduce the blood supply to the tissues of the extremities that the patient experiences ischemic pain even at rest. The pain is possibly due to the release of a metabolic factor that is related to tissue anoxia.
Coldness and pallor of the extremities	An adequate blood supply gives the tissues a rosy hue; also, the warmth of the blood warms the extremities. When blood flow is deficient, the extremities feel cold and look pale. When a patient with peripheral vascular disease raises the legs above heart level, the extremities appear even whiter (blanching) because arterial blood flow is more critically reduced.
Rubor (tissues of the extremities are reddish blue in color)	Rubor indicates peripheral vessel damage that is so severe that the vessels are no longer able to constrict, but remain *permanently dilated.* Rubor typically develops after prolonged anoxia or exposure to severe cold.
Cyanosis or blueness of the tissues	When the blood contains too little oxygen, the tissues turn a bluish color, indicating the presence of abnormal amounts of deoxygenated hemoglobin.
Trophic changes (adverse changes in the skin and nails of the extremities, e.g., dryness, scaling of the skin, brittle toenails)	The word *trophic* pertains to nutrition; thus, trophic changes in peripheral vascular disease result from prolonged ischemia and malnutrition of tissues.
Leg ulcers and cellulitis	*Arterial ischemic leg ulcers* are caused by chronic occlusion of small arteries and arterioles. *Venous stasis ulcers* are a consequence of venous insufficiency; stagnant blood pooling in the tissues of the extremities provides an excellent medium for bacterial growth and resultant infection and ulcerations.
Gangrenous changes (death and decay of tissues of the extremities)	Severe and prolonged ischemia due to complete or almost total stoppage of blood flow to a part results in gangrene.

Exercise. A moderate prescribed program of exercise and rest is a most helpful method for increasing the circulation. For example, the patient often benefits from taking short walks followed by periods of rest. Instruct the patient to walk as much as possible every day. The exercise program should begin judiciously and progress gradually until the patient has substantially lengthened his or her walking distance. Tell the patient to let pain be the guide to the amount of activity to undertake. Pain in the extremities signals the patient that the muscles and tissues of the legs are not receiving enough oxygen. If severe discomfort in the calf is experienced after walking a block, the person should stop and rest before walking further.

A popular form of exercise for patients with vascular disorders is the *Buerger-Allen routine.*

These exercises are divided into three parts.

1. The patient lies on a bed or couch and elevates both feet on a special board for from a half minute to 3 minutes. A straight-backed chair may be used instead of the board, with the top of the chair back and the front of the seat resting on the bed or couch. The chair back or board should be padded with a pillow or other soft material.

2. The patient then sits on the edge of the bed or couch with legs spread out and relaxed and the heels resting on the floor. The feet are bent up and down as far as possible, and then turned inward and outward. After this, the person bends the toes up and spreads them, then down to close them. Each set of movements should be continued about 3 minutes. The feet should become entirely pink. If they should become blue or painful, the patient should lie down and elevate the feet until rested.

3. After the first two parts, the patient lies down with the legs horizontal and covered to keep them warm. The person remains in this position for about 5 minutes.

The three steps involved in Buerger-Allen exercises are illustrated in Figure 47–4.

Patients who cannot perform active postural exercises such as the Buerger-Allen routine or who have severe circulatory involvement of the lower extremities may benefit from using an *oscillating bed.* This electrically operated bed (also called the "rocking bed") rocks up and down in smooth continuous cycles of approximately 3 minutes each. The motion of the bed is such that the patient's feet are first raised about 6 inches above the horizontal position, and then lowered about 12 to 15 inches, then raised, then lowered, and so forth. This steady rocking motion provides the patient with continuous passive postural exercise.

If the doctor orders an oscillating bed for your patient, give the following instructions and care:

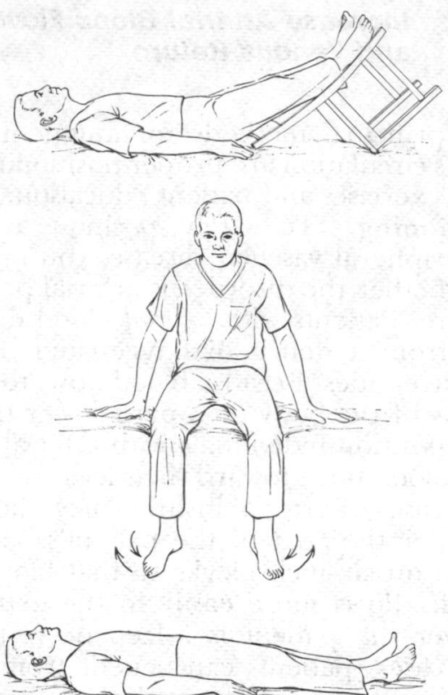

Figure 47–4. Buerger's exercises. (From Barker, W. F.: *Peripheral Arterial Disease,* 2nd ed., W. B. Saunders Co., 1975.)

- Explain the purpose of the oscillating bed to the patient, give reassurance that circulation will improve with the use of the bed and that pain and discomfort in the legs will lessen.
- Show the patient how to operate the switch that rocks the bed. Give instructions to stop the bed for a short time should dizziness or nausea develop — symptoms which are sometimes experienced when the bed is first used.
- Encourage patients to operate the bed as much as they can tolerate, both day and night.
- Place a padded footboard at the foot of the bed to support the patient's feet.

Although exercise may help the majority of patients with vascular disorders, there are some patients for whom exercise is absolutely contraindicated. Patients who must not exercise are those with *leg ulcers, cellulitis,* or *gangrene.* As you recall, exercise and activity increase the metabolic needs of tissues and, consequently, tissue requirements for oxygenated blood. For this reason, patients with tissue breakdown or necrosis are placed on bed rest; even minimal activity raises the oxygen requirements of their tissues above that which their damaged arteries can provide.

Bed rest is also ordered for patients with *arterial or venous thrombosis.* Activity is dangerous because a thrombus could become detached and travel as an embolus to the heart, lungs, or brain.

Patient Education. Patients with peripheral

vascular disease need special instruction in how to increase circulation to their extremities and prevent venous stasis. Four rules you should emphasize to all patients with vascular problems are as follows:

> 1. *Avoid obesity; extra pounds exhaust the heart, decrease circulation, and increase venous congestion. A low lipid diet seems to be particularly helpful in controlling atherosclerosis (See Chapter 36).*
> 2. *Avoid standing in any position for an extended period of time; prolonged standing promotes venous stasis.*
> 3. *Never wear constricting clothes: e.g., garters, girdles, tight belts, tight shoelaces.*
> 4. *Never cross the legs at the knee because this constricts the popliteal vessels.*

Goal 2: Promote Vasodilatation

Dilated arteries have a greater capacity for carrying blood to the extremities. Measures which promote vasodilatation are discussed below.

Warmth. Warmth can be both a blessing and a curse for patients with vascular disease. Warmth is beneficial for the patient only when it acts as insulation against cold and chilling. For example, encourage the individual with vascular disease to set the thermostat at home at around 70 to 72°F. If possible, keep the hospital room comfortably warm. Remind the patient to wear gloves, scarves, and socks when going outside on a chilly day. If chilling occurs, tell the patient to have a warm drink or take a warm bath. It is also safe to apply a hot water bottle to the abdomen; this procedure causes reflex dilatation of arteries in the extremities, thereby increasing blood flow without untoward effects.

On the other hand, applying any source of heat *directly to the extremities* is especially dangerous.

> *The use of hot water bottles, heating pads, and hot foot soaks is strictly contraindicated unless specifically ordered by the physician.*

As stated earlier, heat increases tissue metabolism. If the arteries are unable to dilate normally, blood flow to the extremities will be inadequate, and the tissues will become ischemic.

Prevention of Vasoconstriction. Factors that cause vasoconstriction are nicotine (which causes vasospasm), high emotion (which stimulates the sympathetic nervous system), and chilling. You can help patients to avoid the damaging effects of prolonged vasoconstriction in the following ways:

- ► Explain the dangers of smoking to the patient who uses tobacco. Encourage the person to stop smoking completely. The patient who realizes that smoking literally threatens life and limbs may develop sufficient motivation to abstain permanently. The severe vasoconstricting effect of nicotine on the circulation is dramatically displayed in Figure 47–5.
- ► Protect the patient, whenever possible, from upsetting, emotionally charged situations. Encourage the patient to try and relax, both mentally and physically. Counseling services may be indicated for very nervous, high-strung individuals.
- ► Prevent the patient from becoming chilled, using the methods described above.

Vasodilators. Drugs that dilate the peripheral vessels either act *directly* on the smooth muscles of the arteries or by *blocking* the constricting effects of epinephrine and norepinephrine upon the nerve endings supplying arteries (adrenergic blocking agents). Vasodilators currently used include cyclandelate, ethaverine hydrochloride, nicotinyl alcohol, and nylidrin hydrochloride. Alcohol, in moderation, is also an excellent vasodilator.

However, for vasodilators to work, arteries must still be capable of dilating. For this reason, vasodilators of any kind are of little benefit to patients with severely sclerosed and damaged vessels. Also, they are of no value in the care of the elderly.

Lipid-Reducing Drugs. Because hyperlipidemia plays a role in the development of atherosclerosis, lipid-reducing drugs such as clofibrate may be prescribed.

Sympathectomy. Sympathectomy is a surgical procedure in which sympathetic nerve fibers supplying the peripheral vessels are severed, causing relaxation of the arterioles and better blood flow. As is the case with vasodilators, sympathectomy is successful only in those patients in whom the vessels are still elastic enough to dilate. To determine how successful a sympathectomy might be, a doctor sometimes injects the vertebral sympathetic ganglia with alcohol, thereby temporarily interrupting sympathetic impulses to the extremities.

Goal 3: Prevent and Treat Vascular Obstruction

Any form of vascular obstruction hinders circulation — sometimes dramatically. Arteries can become clogged with accumulations of lipids, calcium deposits, complex carbohydrates, and fibrous tissue. Both arteries and veins can be obstructed by thrombi and emboli. How can vascular obstruction be prevented? As you recall from Unit XII the prevention of atherosclerosis and arteriosclerosis is still an enigma, because the precise cause of these conditions remains unknown. Researchers have suggested low cholesterol diets, exercise, control of obesity, avoidance of tobacco, and the development of a calm, rational frame of mind as possible preventive measures.

In contrast, methods for preventing venous thrombosis are more clear-cut. (See also Chapter 49.) Thrombus formation is usually caused by venous stasis, hypercoagulability of the blood, injury to the venous wall, or combinations of these. Preventive measures designed to counteract the above factors include: avoidance of *prolonged* bed rest; ample fluids to prevent dehydration and resultant hypercoagulability; range-of-motion exercises for the bedfast; proper positioning in bed (e.g., avoidance of use of the knee gatch and lateral recumbent position); and the use of anticoagulant therapy.

Unfortunately, vascular obstruction may develop despite attempts to prevent it. When a vessel becomes partially or totally occluded, how is the condition treated? Severely sclerosed, obstructed arteries can be replaced with synthetic vessels; this procedure, called a *bypass graft,* is frequently used for femoropopliteal disease. (See Chapter 48.) Also, an *endarterectomy* may be performed to open clogged arteries and "ream out" obstructing atheromatous material. In cases of *acute arterial occlusion* owing to an embolus or thrombus, *embolectomy* (surgical removal of the embolus) is the treatment of choice.

Venous thrombosis, in contrast to acute arterial thrombosis, usually responds to more conservative treatment. Facets of care include bed rest, elevation of the legs above heart level, elastic

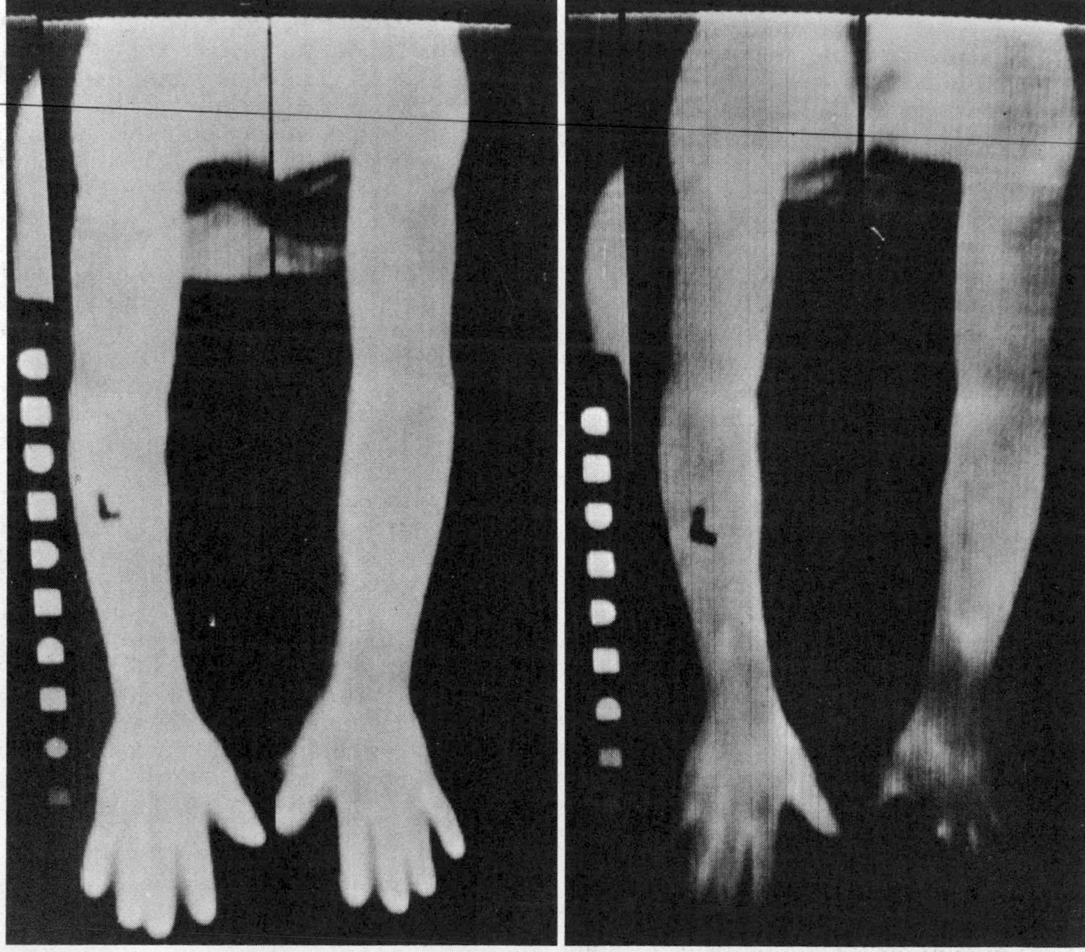

Figure 47–5. Effect of nicotine on the circulation is seen in thermograms of a man's arms before he smoked (*left*) and 15 minutes after he smoked a cigarette (*right*). Nicotine has constricted blood vessels, reducing the amount of blood in the arms and lowering their temperature. (By permission: J. Gershon-Cohen, M.D. Previously published Scientific American, February 1967). (From Jacob, S. W., C. A. Francone, and W. J. Lossow: *Structure and Function in Man,* 4th ed. Philadelphia: W. B. Saunders Co., 1978.)

support hose, continuous warm moist packs, anticoagulant therapy and fibrinolytic drugs (drugs which dissolve thrombi), and dextran 70, which helps to prevent further thrombus formation. Thrombi can also be removed surgically from large veins (thrombectomy).

Goal 4: Relieve Ischemic Pain

The pain of ischemia is usually chronic and continuous in nature. For this reason, patients with peripheral vascular disease are often depressed and irritable. Pain limits their activities, disturbs their sleep, saps their energy, and demoralizes their spirits. Thus, pain must be relieved if the patient is to rest and to improve.

Any measure that increases circulation to the extremities will help to alleviate ischemic pain; e.g., warmth, proper positioning, the oscillating bed, vasodilators, avoidance of tobacco, and so forth. Also, pain can be subdued by the use of analgesics, although therapies that augment circulation are preferable.

Goal 5: Prevent Tissue Damage and Infection and Promote Healing of Existing Lesions

Because of their poor circulation, patients with peripheral vascular disease are highly susceptible to infections, ulcerations, and gangrene of the extremities. Moreover, once a lesion develops, it tends to heal poorly or not at all. Without normal vessels and adequate blood flow, the damaged tissues fail to receive needed oxygen, nutrients, antibodies, and protective leukocytes, and the process of tissue damage continues. Eventually it may become necessary to amputate the limb. Consequently, the prevention of circulatory complications cannot be stressed enough.

Patients must be taught to avoid injury to their extremities. For example, remind patients to check bath water with a bath thermometer instead of with their toes, in order to prevent burns; to wear shoes to avoid injury to the feet; to avoid creating open lesions by scratching flea or mosquito bites on the legs; to use mild soaps; and to rub soothing lotions or lanolin on hands, feet, legs, and arms to discourage dryness. Also teach patients to observe for trophic changes, e.g., dryness and cracking of the skin on the feet, thickening of the nails, and so forth. Such changes should be reported to the patient's doctor promptly.

FOOT CARE

Foot care is particularly important to any person who has a problem with peripheral circulation, and preventive measures are easier to initiate than corrective ones.* Health care personnel should ascertain whether the patient is wearing adequate footwear and hosiery, and whether nails and skin on the feet are cared for properly. Minor foot problems in peripheral vascular disease can easily become serious.

Corns and Calluses. A *corn* is a traumatic keratosis caused by friction and pressure of a shoe when a step is taken. Corns most commonly occur on the fourth or fifth toe, generally over a joint or bony prominence. The typical corn is conical, with its base on top and its apex reaching to deeper structures. The keratosis is removed with a scalpel or other instrument, with care taken not to cut too deeply. After the cornified layer is removed, regrowth may be inhibited by placing a U-shaped pad of felt directly behind the corn to eliminate or disperse the pressure.

A *callus* is a flat, ill-defined mass of keratotic material, usually found on the bottom of the foot under a bony protuberance. Pressure of a shoe and uneven walking are usual causes. Pressure can be alleviated with padding and protective devices and various types of inlays in the shoe. The overall care of the skin is very important. Lanolized cream keeps the skin soft and prevents cracks in dry, hyperkeratotic skin.

Ingrown Toenail. An ingrown toenail can be a serious problem in a person with impaired circulation. As many as 46 causative factors have been cited by various authors. Three basic types of lateral nail problems are described: (1) incurvated nail, (2) ingrown nail, and (3) hypertrophic ungual labium. The patient may have one or more of these conditions.

The symptoms of a *simple incurvated nail* are tenderness, pain on walking, and pain on digital pressure. Prophylactic care consists in trimming the nail properly by cutting it straight across. Stockings and shoes should be long enough to allow for lengthening of the foot during weight-bearing.

Active treatment consists of removing the cellular debris and callus tissue from the margin of the nail gently with a probe. The nail groove should be packed so the nail plate grows forward and the soft tissue of the nail lip will not be impinged upon. The first packing should be done with cotton or lamb's wool, after lubrication of the groove with an emollient ointment containing a topical anesthetic. Elderly persons should not undertake this procedure for themselves; they should be under supervision of a

*The principles of foot care are described in Unit XIX, Chapter 72. Please refer to this section for basic information.

podiatrist, nurse, or doctor for the 3 or 4 months it takes the nail to grow the length of the toe plate.

The *ingrown toenail* or *onychocryptosis* is not so common but has more harmful results. If the lateral border of the nail is mutilated by improper trimming, a pointed sliver frequently remains attached. As the nail plate grows forward, pressure compresses the soft labium against the sharp point, which penetrates the skin. Treatment consists first of removing the sliver. After removal, warm boric acid soaks for 20 to 30 minutes every 4 hours may be instituted. A dry sterile dressing should be applied and a broad-spectrum antibiotic prescribed. Rest in bed or hospitalization is advised. After the infection has cleared, the same treatment is used as described for the incurvated nail.

Hypertrophic ungual labium is a condition in which the nail lip is massively enlarged, frequently overriding a good portion of the nail plate. This is caused by irritation of the epithelium of the nail groove by the lateral nail margin as a result of repeated improper nail trimming. Confining footwear presses the lip against the nail border, producing irritation and chronic inflammation and leading to eventual permanent hypertrophy. Both ingrown toenail and incurvated nail lead to a hypertrophied lip if care is inadequate or lacking. Surgical intervention may be indicated if the condition is chronic and infection returns repeatedly.

Although the feet are most frequently the focus of trauma in vascular disease, the *legs* are also subject to tissue breakdown. Indeed, leg ulcers are a common complication of peripheral arterial occlusive disease and of varicose veins. *Arterial ischemic leg ulcers* are treated with topical corticosteroid and antibiotics. The ulcers are kept clean, dry, and pressure-free. Often skin grafting is necessary. *Varicose ulcers* are treated with bed rest, elevation of the feet above heart level, continuous warm moist compresses, antibiotics, special bandages, proteolytic enzymes such as streptokinase (Varidase) and trypsin (Tryptar), and skin grafting. As with all the complications of vascular disease, leg ulcers are far more easily prevented than cured.

BIBLIOGRAPHY

References for Chapter 47 are included in the bibliographies for Chapters 48, 49, and 50.

CHAPTER 48

DISEASES OF THE AORTA AND ARTERIES

DISORDERS OF THE AORTA

STRUCTURE OF THE AORTA

The aorta is the main artery of the body. It is divided into the ascending aorta, the arch of the aorta, and the descending aorta. The aorta is an elastic artery, composed chiefly of plates of elastic tissue remarkably able to withstand the systolic blood pressure and provide elastic recoil, although elasticity diminishes with age. The walls of the aorta contain pressor receptors which, when stimulated by a rise in blood pressure, lead reflexly to a fall in blood pressure and heart rate. The ascending aorta is about 3 cm. in diameter and has a course of about 5 cm. The root is dilated because of the three bulges in its wall, i.e., the sinuses of the aorta, each named for a cusp of the aortic valve.

The branches of the ascending aorta are the right and left coronary arteries. The ascending aorta continues into the arch, the branches of the arch of the aorta being the brachiocephalic trunk, the left common carotid artery, and the left subclavian artery. The thoracic aorta descends from the arch through the aortic opening in the diaphragm and becomes the abdominal aorta. The branches of the thoracic aorta may be classified as parietal and visceral. The parietal arteries supply the diaphragm and intercostal area; and the visceral, the bronchial, esophageal, pericardial, and mediastinal areas. The abdominal aorta divides into the right and left common iliac arteries. The aorta is under greater stress than the rest of the arterial system because of its large diameter and the pressure of each systolic ejection of blood. Major diseases affecting the aorta are aortitis, aneurysms, and arteriosclerotic occlusive disease.

AORTITIS

Aortitis is inflammation of the aorta; primarily it damages the arch of the aorta. Causes include arteriosclerosis and syphilis.

By far the most common site of cardiovascular syphilis is the ascending portion of the aorta. In most cases, involvement of the aorta produces only moderate dilatation of the ascending aorta (uncomplicated aortitis). However, it may lead to such complications as aortic insufficiency, aortic aneurysm, or narrowing or obstruction of the coronary ostia. These complications occur in 35 to 40 per cent of patients with syphilitic aortitis. The main finding is roentgenographic indication of dilatation and occasional calcification of the ascending aorta. This may also be produced by atherosclerosis in persons over 50 years of age. If a patient under 45 has roentgenographic findings in the absence of other heart disease and has a history of syphilis or a positive serologic test, syphilitic aortitis should be suspected.

Serologic tests are positive in 75 to 95 per cent of patients with untreated syphilitic aortitis. The prognosis of treated uncomplicated aortitis is relatively favorable, since complications are prevented by treatment. Penicillin is the most effective agent.

Aortic insufficiency is the most frequent complication of syphilitic aortitis, occurring in approximately one third of the patients. Generally it becomes manifest 10 to 25 years after the primary infection, although in 7 per cent it may occur within the first 5 years. The prognosis is poor, as only 35 to 45 per cent survive 10 years after the diagnosis is made. If the patient is symptomatic, the chances for survival are much better.[9]

AORTIC ANEURYSMS

An aneurysm is a sac formed by the dilatation of an artery as a result of localized weakness and stretching of the arterial wall. While aneurysms occur most commonly in the aorta, they may develop in any artery or vein in the body. Aortic aneurysms are very dangerous because they can *rupture*, causing death due to internal hemorrhage and shock.

Robbins and Cotran classify aneurysms according to the following:[40]

1. *Location:* Aneurysms are designated as either venous or arterial; they are also described according to the specific vessel in which they develop (e.g., aorta, splenic artery, femoral vein) and, more precisely, according to the exact

area of the vessel that they affect, e.g., descending thoracic aorta, lower abdominal aorta.

2. *Etiology:* In broadest terms, any vascular disease (under certain conditions) can give rise to an aneurysm. However, the most common cause of aneurysms is *atherosclerosis,* followed by syphilis and cystic medionecrosis — a degenerative condition that affects the musculoelastic media of the aorta and predisposes it to dissecting aneurysm (see discussion below). Other causes of aneurysms include congenital defects of the arterial wall, trauma, and infections that result in weakness of the vessel walls.

3. *Gross appearance:*[33] This classification lists aneurysms according to their shape, anatomic features, and the size of the aneurysmal dilatation. Accordingly, the following types of aneurysms are recognized: (1) *true aneurysm,* in which one or all three layers of the arterial wall (adventitia, media, intima) are involved; (a) *fusiform aneurysm,* a uniform, spindle-shaped dilatation of a segment of an artery; (b) *saccular aneurysm,* an outpouching from an artery caused by localized thinning and stretching of the medial coat; (c) *dissecting aneurysm,* a cavity formed by blood that has been forced between the layers of the arterial wall; and (2) *false aneurysm,* one resulting from a complete rupture or wounding of all coats of the artery, the blood then being retained by the surrounding tissues. The types of aneurysms, as classified by their anatomic features, are diagrammed in Figure 48–1.

Arteriosclerotic aneurysms usually develop at a site in the artery that is not surrounded by skeletal muscle or where the artery is subject to frequent bending during physical activity. Fusiform arteriosclerotic aneurysms occur most often in the aorta, especially the abdominal aorta, and in the iliac arteries. Saccular arteriosclerotic aneurysms are most often seen in the abdominal aorta and the popliteal arteries; they may also occur in the femoral artery. As noted below, aneurysms of the thoracic aorta presently are usually caused by arteriosclerosis rather than syphilis, and are usually fusiform rather than saccular. Aneurysms of arteriosclerotic type usually develop after the age of 60 years and are about 10 times as frequent in men as in women.

> *"The common factor in all pathologic processes responsible for aneurysm is the damaged media which cannot withstand the systolic blood pressure and leads to progressive dilatation."*[33]

Thoracic Aortic Aneurysms. One sixth of aortic aneurysms are thoracic. Syphilis was formerly the commonest cause of thoracic aortic aneurysms but is now second to atherosclerosis. Indeed, because antibiotics have significantly reduced the incidence of syphilitic aneurysms, the majority of thoracic aneurysms are caused by atherosclerosis. The symptoms are variable and depend on the rapidity with which the aneurysm dilates and the effect of the pulsating mass on the surrounding structures. Most are asymptomatic unless large.

The thoracic aorta is the most common site of a *dissecting* aneurysm, with other arteries usually

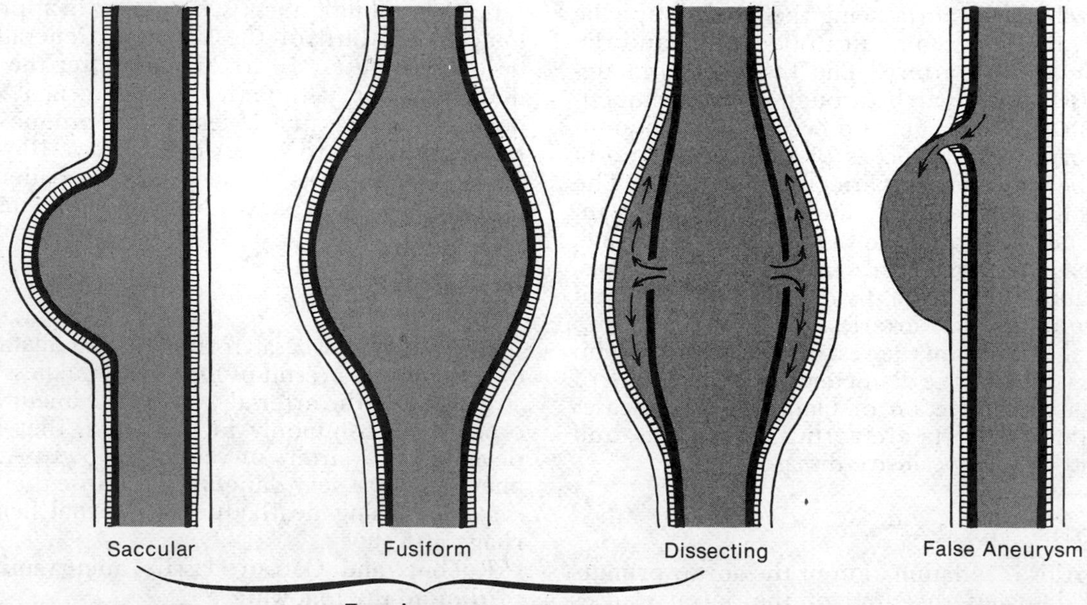

Figure 48–1. Aneurysms classified according to gross appearance and anatomic features. In *true aneurysms,* one layer or all three of the layers of the vessel wall may be involved. In *false aneurysm,* the vessel wall has ruptured and the blood clot is being retained in an outpouching of tissue from the vessel wall. The three types of true aneurysms are: the *saccular aneurysm,* characterized by a bulbous outpouching of one side of the vessel; the *fusiform aneurysm,* characterized by a uniform spindle-shaped dilatation of a segment of the artery; and the *dissecting aneurysm,* in which the layers of the vessel wall split, creating a cavity.

involved by extension of the dissection. Dissecting aneurysms were once considered rare but "are now considered to be the most common catastrophic illness involving the aorta. . . ."[40] Within the United States alone, 2000 new cases of dissecting aneurysm are diagnosed each year. However, because most cases remain undiagnosed, some authorities estimate that up to 60,000 persons per year may develop this potentially deadly condition! Dissecting aneurysms are extremely dangerous, resulting in death, if untreated, within 15 minutes for 35 per cent of cases and within 1 week for 75 per cent of cases.[40] Fortunately, more persons with dissecting aneurysms are now being more swiftly diagnosed and treated, with a substantial saving of human life.

The cause of dissecting aneurysm of the thoracic aorta is not known, but a genetic predisposition is suggested. Hypertension is the most commonly associated clinical condition, being diagnosed in 94 per cent of cases.[40] Arteriosclerosis does not appear to be causally related, and syphilis appears to be a deterrent because it produces fusion of the layers of the aorta. Dissection usually begins in the medial layer and frequently extends partially around the aorta and occasionally completely around it. The most frequent cause of death in a dissecting aneurysm of the aorta is external rupture of the hematoma.

The clinical picture of dissecting aneurysm of the aorta is extremely variable. The symptoms arise from three sources: (1) the dissection itself, (2) the pathology that resulted in the development of the aneurysm, and (3) the pressure of the aneurysm upon nearby structures — the trachea (dyspnea, stridor, brassy cough), the esophagus (dysphagia), the left recurrent laryngeal nerve (hoarseness), or the superior vena cava (edema of neck and arms, distended neck veins).

Generally, men affected outnumber women; and, although the condition can occur at any time, it usually affects persons between 40 and 70 years of age. The onset is usually sudden; there is severe and persistent pain, described as "tearing" or "ripping." The pain usually begins in the anterior thorax but may be between or below the scapulae. It may begin high in the epigastrium or in some unusual site such as face or neck. If sudden collapse or syncope occurs, the pain can be absent.

The early symptoms in the patient are often pallor, sweatiness, and mild shock, with moderately or even markedly elevated blood pressure. Hypertension or a history of it has been found in about 94 per cent of patients. Blood pressure may be markedly different in both arms, and there may be lowered arterial pulsations and varying degrees of ischemia in one or more of the extremities. The heart rate may be moderately increased and there may or may not be murmurs. Abdominal tenderness may also be present. Because of the variable clinical picture, early diagnosis is not accurate in about 40 to 50 per cent of patients. The condition may be mistaken for acute myocardial infarction, cerebrovascular accident, acute abdomen, and acute peripheral arterial occlusion. The aneurysm may also be mistaken for a neoplasm or a cyst. Electrocardiograms, roentgenograms, and angiography may help in diagnosis and in localizing the dissection. The prognosis is poor in untreated patients and is unfavorably influenced by age, location of primary tear (ascending or arch portion of the aorta), hypertension, and other cardiovascular disease.[15] Aortography may be used to determine the size of the aneurysm in some cases. Ultrasound is also used as a diagnostic technique. Continuous ultrasonic B scanning will give information concerning the size of the aneurysm, thickness of the walls, and the size of the intraluminal clot; and it can be used serially to determine progress. Size and presence of other arteriosclerotic vascular diseases affects the prognosis. Aneurysms larger than 6 cm. have a 45 to 50 per cent chance of rupture.[11] Five-year survival of unoperated patients without clinically associated coronary disease was 50 per cent and with ischemic heart disease, 20 per cent.[11]

Pain is the predominant symptom of *nondissecting* aneurysms of the thoracic aorta; it usually develops in the anterior chest and is frequently substernal, but sometimes it occurs in the back or shoulders. It is usually described as a steady ache and may be felt only when the patient is in the supine position. Obstruction of the superior vena cava or subclavian vein may occur; dysphagia, dyspnea, and stridor may be present, as may hoarseness and cough because of pressure on the recurrent pharyngeal nerve. Sometimes no physical signs develop. The electrocardiogram is not of value in making the diagnosis. The most helpful procedure is roentgenoscopy, and often the aneurysm is discovered only by x-ray. In arteriosclerotic aneurysms, deposits of calcium are frequently seen near the edges of the outline of the aneurysm.

Treatment of thoracic aortic aneurysms depends upon the type of aneurysm present (Fig. 48–2). Evidence indicates that medical management is effective in 80 to 85 per cent of patients with Type III (descending aorta acute dissecting aneurysms), whereas surgery is the treatment of choice for Types I and II (involving ascending dissecting aortic aneurysms).[52]

Once a diagnosis of acute dissecting aneurysm has been made, patients are placed into an intensive care unit, and an intensive medical and surgical monitoring program is immediately started. In a *medically* oriented program, the goals of therapy are to lower systolic blood pressure to 100 to 120 mm. Hg and to reduce the pulsatile aortic flow by means of potent medications. Methyldopa (Aldomet) and propranolol (Inderal) are given to decrease blood pressure and myocardial contractibility and to lessen the pulsatile nature of the blood flow through the aorta. Other medications that can be administered are reserpine (Serpasil) and guanethidine (Ismelin). (These medications are discussed in Chapter 37.)[52] To monitor the effects of these medications upon the patient's condition, the patient's electrocardiogram is continuously recorded. An intra-arterial needle is placed for accurate monitoring of the arterial pressure; a Swan-Ganz catheter is inserted for measuring left-sided and right-sided heart pressures, and a Foley catheter is inserted into the patient's bladder to monitor urinary output. Pain is controlled with medication. The physician usually orders daily chest x-rays, and an aortogram is typically obtained shortly after admission. If the patient's condition stabilizes, he or she can then be transferred from the intensive care unit to the ward. Food by mouth is usually permitted after 3 days and ambulation within 2 weeks.

On the other hand, if the medical program fails to control the symptoms of the aneurysm, and if impending rupture or leakage of the aneurysm seems possible, *cardiovascular surgery* is indicated. The objectives of *surgical treatment* of dissecting aortic aneurysm are: (1) preventing further dissection, (2) eliminating the possibility of external rupture, (3) correcting aortic valve damage if present, and (4) restoring the patency of occluded vessels. Surgical mortality is high during acute dissection. In some treatment centers the acute stage is managed with drug therapy, followed in 2 to 3 weeks by corrective surgery.

The prognosis for persons with thoracic aortic aneurysms is not so poor as that for those with an abdominal aortic aneurysm. In a Mayo Clinic series, 68 per cent of patients survived 3 years; 50 per cent, 5 years; and 30 per cent, 10 years. Age greater than 50 years, a large aneurysm, and diastolic hypertension all affected the prognosis unfavorably.[15] Death is often caused by rupture of the aneurysms. Rupture occurs in about a third of patients.

Abdominal Aortic Aneurysms. The common cause of aneurysm of the abdominal aorta

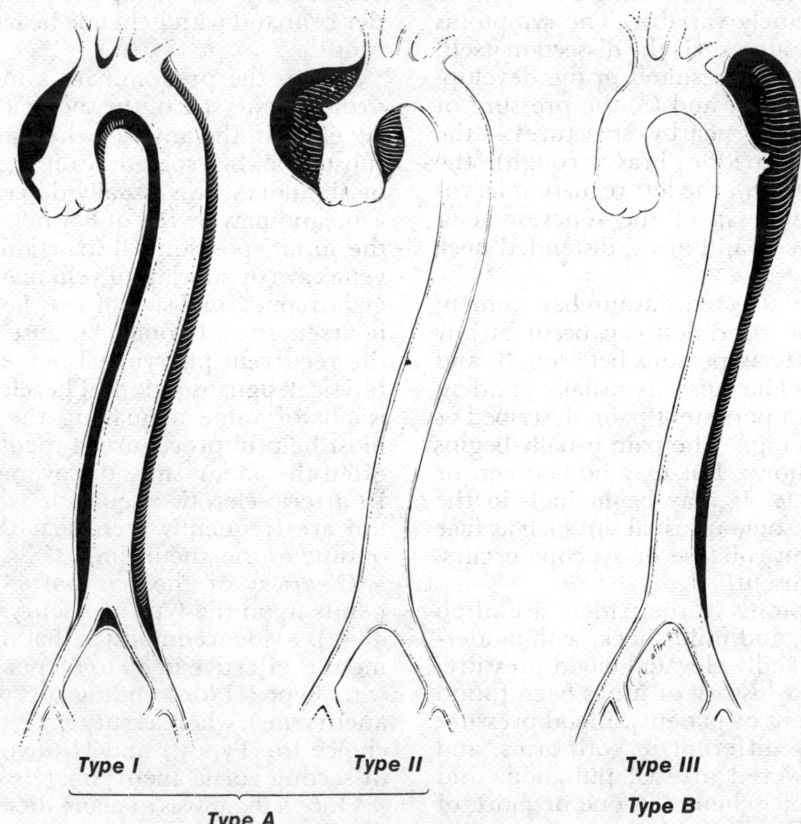

Figure 48–2. DeBakey classification of dissecting aneurysms. (From Robbins, S. L., and R. S. Cotran: *Pathologic Basis of Disease,* 2nd ed. Philadelphia: W. B. Saunders Co., 1979, p. 625.)

is arteriosclerosis. Figure 48–3 presents a photograph of an atherosclerotic aneurysm of the abdominal aorta. Syphilis is present in from 5 to 10 per cent of the patients, but arteriosclerosis is usually also present. The aorta and iliac arteries are the most frequently involved abdominal vessels. Approximately 40 per cent of patients with abdominal aortic aneurysms have symptoms, abdominal pain being the most common. It may be persistent or intermittent and is most frequently felt in the middle or lower part of the abdomen at the left of the midline. Another frequent complaint is back pain, usually low in the back; this is frequently caused by rupture of the aneurysm. Less commonly an abdominal mass appears or abdominal throbbing occurs.

A pulsating abdominal mass is the most frequent and important physical sign. Determination of blood pressure in the arm and thigh of a patient in a supine position is of value in differential diagnosis. Normally the blood pressure in the thigh is higher than that in the arm by 15 mm. or more of mercury. However, in most patients with abdominal aortic aneurysm the systolic pressure in the thigh is abnormally low compared with that of the arm. However, normal comparative blood pressures in the arm and thigh do not rule out aneurysm. A systolic bruit can often be heard over the aneurysm. However, the best means of confirming the diagnosis is x-ray examination of the lumbar spine in the anteroposterior and lateral positions.

Rupture is the most deadly complication of abdominal aortic aneurysm, and it thus must be diagnosed quickly and accurately. The symptoms compose a triad of (1) pulsating abdominal pain combined with intense back pain, (2) a pulsating abdominal mass, and (3) shock. In addition, the red blood cell count falls and the white blood cell count rises. Note in Figure 48–4 that an abdominal aneurysm may rupture in several different directions. The rupture may be: (a) into the peritoneum — with almost universally fatal results; (b) intramesenteric; (c) retroperitoneal, which is the most common type of rupture and has the best prognosis; or (d) into the inferior vena cava, which results in shock and heart failure due to the creation of a massive arteriovenous fistula. Finally, the aneurysm may rupture into the duodenum or rectum and cause severe gastrointestinal hemorrhage.[32]

The diagnosis of ruptured abdominal aneurysm is frequently missed. Consequently, physicians and nurses must be aware of this critical possibility when caring for middle-aged persons reporting of acute abdominal pain or severe low back pain.[32]

Because of the danger of rupture, *surgical intervention* is definitely the treatment of choice for patients with abdominal aortic aneurysm. Newer surgical and grafting techniques now permit resection of abdominal aortic aneurysms and their replacement by grafts. Replacement of an abdominal aortic aneurysm with a synthetic bifurcation graft is diagrammed in Figure 48–5. A surgical mortality of approximately 5 per cent for elective resection and graft of abdominal aortic aneurysms has been reported, with the mortality higher (30 to 50 per cent) in surgical treatment of ruptured aneurysms. However, without immediate surgery following rupture, mortality is almost 100 per cent. For all persons suffering from abdominal aortic aneurysms, survival rates are nearly twice as good for patients who have surgical treatment as for those who are not operated on.

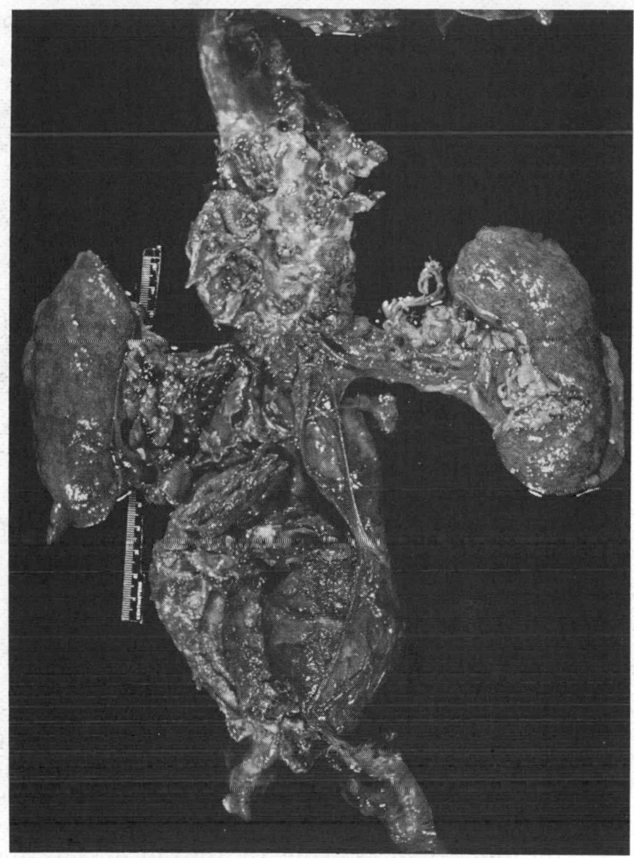

Figure 48–3. Atherosclerotic aneurysm of the abdominal aorta. (From Robbins, S. L., and R. S. Cotran: *Pathologic Basis of Disease*, 2nd ed. Philadelphia: W. B. Saunders Co., 1979, p. 622.)

Other Sites of Aneurysms. Aneurysms are found less commonly in the upper extremities than in the lower extremities. The most common sites in the lower extremities are the popliteal space and Scarpa's triangle.

Popliteal aneurysms are important causes of ischemic symptoms in the lower limbs. Although the patient may be aware of a swelling behind the knee, he or she seldom complains unless symptoms such as rest pain, coldness, or numbness develop. A peripheral aneurysm is dif-

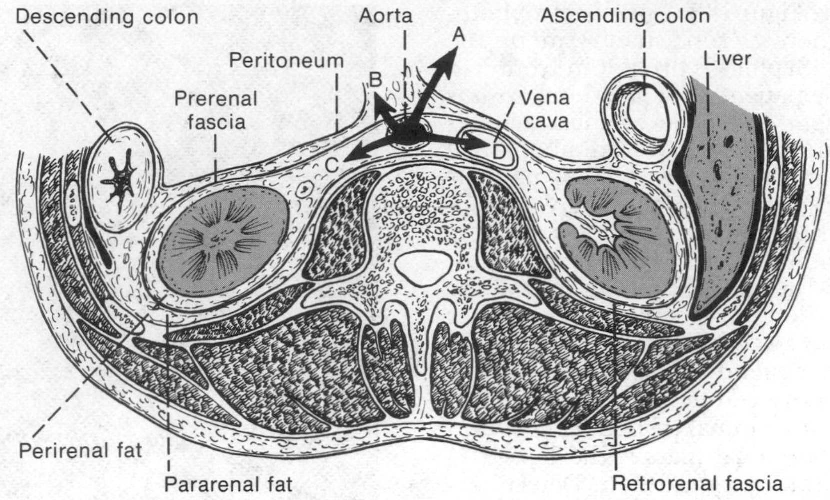

Figure 48–4. Abdominal aortic aneurysms can rupture in these directions: *A,* Intraperitoneal; *B,* Intramesenteric; *C,* Retroperitoneal; *D,* Into the inferior vena cava. Also rupture may develop in the duodenum or rectum.

ferentiated from other swellings by the presence of expansile pulsation. Complications of popliteal aneurysms frequently occur and may lead to loss of an extremity or to death. The most dangerous complications are embolus distal to the aneurysm, leaking of the aneurysm, and pressure from the aneurysm on a neighboring vein or nerve. Thrombosis may occur, resulting in severe ischemia with development of gangrene and loss of the limbs. Surgical treatment is the only satisfactory method of dealing with aneurysms of the popliteal artery and should be done before complications occur.

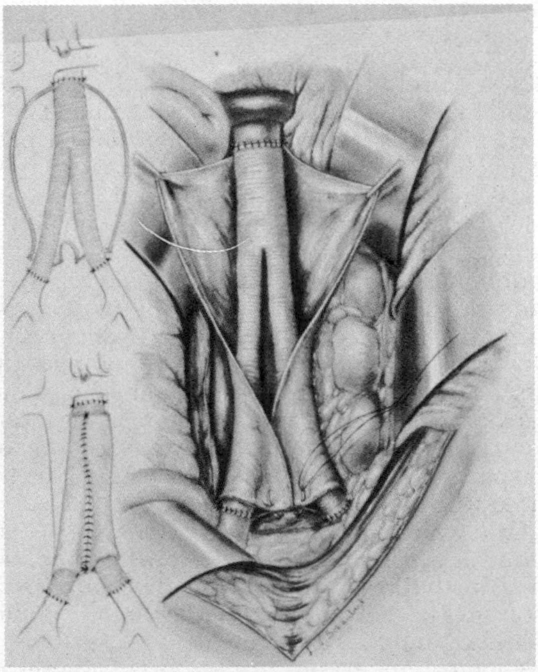

Figure 48–5. Replacement of an aortic aneurysm with a synthetic bifurcation graft. The laminated clot within the aneurysm has been removed and the outer wall is closed over the graft. (From Wylie, E. J., et al.: Arteries. *In* Dunphy, J. E., and W. W. Lawrence: *Current Surgical Diagnosis and Treatment,* 3rd ed. Los Altos, Calif.: Lange Medical Publications, 1977, p. 712.)

Surgical Treatment of Aneurysms. Aortography is advised in patients suspected of having an aneurysm of the *ascending* aorta to establish the diagnosis and to assess the condition of the aortic valve, which may require graft replacement. Surgery usually involves resection of the aneurysm and replacement of the excised segment with a graft. Extracorporeal circulation with a pump oxygenator is sometimes employed. When the aneurysm has been opened, a coronary cannula is inserted. A woven Dacron graft is sutured to the proximal and distal aortic segments, and the remaining wall of the aneurysm is approximated over the graft. Hospital mortality for resections of the ascending aorta, even when valve replacement is also required, is about 10 per cent.[15]

Aneurysms of the *transverse aortic arch* are rare, with the decreasing incidence of untreated syphilis in the population. Because of the high surgical mortality, operation is advised only in those patients who experience symptoms and in whom the aneurysm is enlarging.

Aneurysms of the *descending* portion of the thoracic aorta usually occur just distal to the origin of the left subclavian artery. The cause is most often atherosclerosis, although this is also a common site for traumatic aneurysms. Since the aorta must be interrupted for the insertion of a graft, it is necessary to provide flow in the distal aorta to allow circulation to continue. Some form of bypass is instituted, using either the left atrial femoral artery or the femoral vein and femoral artery. After bypass is instituted, the aneurysm is incised and a woven Dacron graft is inserted and covered with the trimmed wall of the aneurysm. The current hospital mortality rate is about 10 to 12 per cent.[15]

Aneurysms involving the descending thoracic aorta plus the upper abdominal aorta are difficult to correct surgically because it is often necessary to reconstruct the celiac, mesenteric, and renal arteries. The operative mortality is high, but the risk may be justified because of the poor prognosis of patients with aneurysms in this area. A graft is attached to the side of the thoracic aorta proximal to the aneurysm and attached distally at the aortic bifurcation. Side branches are constructed from the main graft to the visceral arteries and the aneurysm is excised.

The *terminal aorta* distal to the origin of the renal arteries is a common site for aneurysm formation. Surgery is indicated for such an aneurysm if the patient is capable of withstanding an abdominal operation.

The excision of *popliteal* aneurysms is done preferably before the aneurysm becomes symptomatic or complicated. The results of operation are excellent in uncomplicated cases. The long-term effectiveness of the graft is determined by the extent of occlusion in the distal vessels. Patients with popliteal aneurysms have a high incidence of disease in the abdominal aorta and the iliac and femoral arteries.

Resection is generally indicated for aneurysms of the iliac and femoral arteries, with use of a prosthetic graft or an autogenous saphenous vein graft.[15]

PERIPHERAL ARTERIAL DISEASES

Peripheral arterial diseases can be divided into two groups: (1) conditions characterized by organic changes and (2) conditions in which no organic changes develop. Organic changes are *present* in atherosclerosis and arteriosclerosis, thromboangiitis obliterans (Buerger's disease), acute arterial occlusion, and arterial embolism. Organic changes are *absent* in Raynaud's disease.

Atherosclerosis and Arteriosclerosis

Definitions. The commonest form of arterial disease is atherosclerosis, atheroma, or arteriosclerosis. Some authors differentiate between arteriosclerosis and atherosclerosis by considering the latter to indicate focal changes, and using arteriosclerosis to refer broadly to "hardening of the arteries." Atherosclerosis rarely occurs in the absence of arteriosclerosis. Major sites of peripheral arteriosclerotic occlusive disease are diagrammed in Figure 48–6.

Atherosclerosis has been defined by the World Health Organization as a complex of changes in the intima of arteries consisting of "the focal accumulation of lipids, complex carbohydrates, blood products, fibrous tissue and calcium deposits and associated with medial changes." Atherosclerosis is a *generalized* arterial disease, and when it is present in the limbs, it is usually present elsewhere in the body. It chiefly affects the main arteries, often in a patchy manner (Fig. 48–7). The branch arteries are unaffected except at their point of departure from the main artery, and the small arteries are also unaffected. The two most common loca-

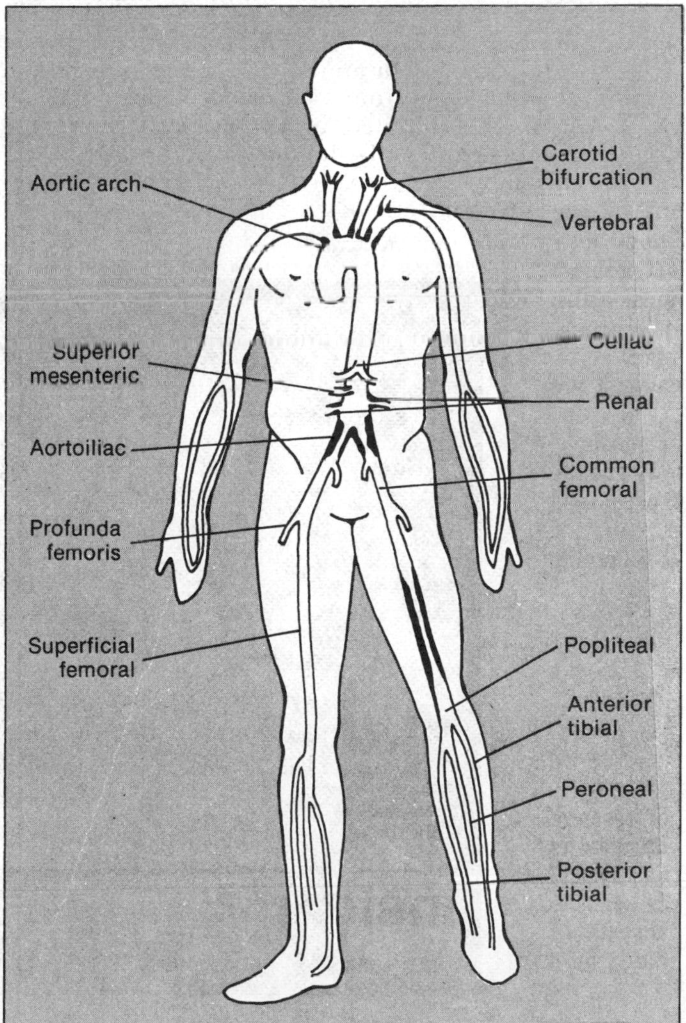

Figure 48–6. Major sites of peripheral arteriosclerotic occlusive disease. (From Hoyster, T. S., et al.: Peripheral arterial disease. *Postgraduate Medicine,* 62:154, Nov., 1977.)

tions for the stenosis due to atherosclerosis that occurs in cerebrovascular insufficiency are the carotid bifurcation and the origin of the vertebral artery. Symptoms indicating stenosis or small emboli from plaques in the carotid bifurcation are mental confusion, transient weakness of an extremity, and monocular blindness. Occasionally there is a loss of consciousness. When the vertebral artery is impaired, there is likely to be dizziness and motor instability.[44] Atherosclerosis is more common in the lower than the upper limbs, although it may be an important cause of vascular disturbance in the hands. The lesions cause narrowing of the arterial lumen and critically reduce blood flow, and thrombosis or aneurysm may result.

Etiology. The etiology of atherosclerosis, remains a mystery. The condition is present to some degree in almost all adults and many develop to an advanced degree without ischemic complications, or an individual may have severe complications from a localized plaque.

As we indicated in Chapter 36, there are many theories of why and how atherosclerosis develops. Yet another modern hypothesis concerning the etiology of atherosclerosis is the *reaction-to-injury* or the *response-to-injury hypothesis.*[40] This theory is summarized in Figure 48–8. According to this viewpoint, atherosclerotic lesions begin to develop as a response to some form of injury to the arterial endothelium. The injury itself may be: (a) either small or significant in nature and (b) either a one-time-only event or a repeated and chronic problem. Further, the *response* to injury may be (a) short and self-limiting, followed by regeneration of the endothelium, or (b) pathologic, resulting in the development of an atheromatous plaque. The latter especially occurs when injury is repeated or becomes chronic in nature.

While this theory is, in the words of Robbins and Contran "the neatest theory" of atherosclerosis, it is by no means conclusive. As we emphasized in Chapter 36, the notion that there may be one single cause of atherosclerosis appears highly unlikely. Robbins sums up the mystery surrounding this enormous problem in this way:

> It may well be that there is no one cause of atherosclerosis, no single initiating event, and no exclusive pathogenic mechanism. *Clinically significant atherosclerosis appears to be a disease of multiple origins.*[40]

Risk Factors. Various risk factors have been reputed to be associated with the condition; e.g., no population on a regular low-fat diet has been shown to have a high prevalence of the coronary heart disease. It is on this basis that cholesterol

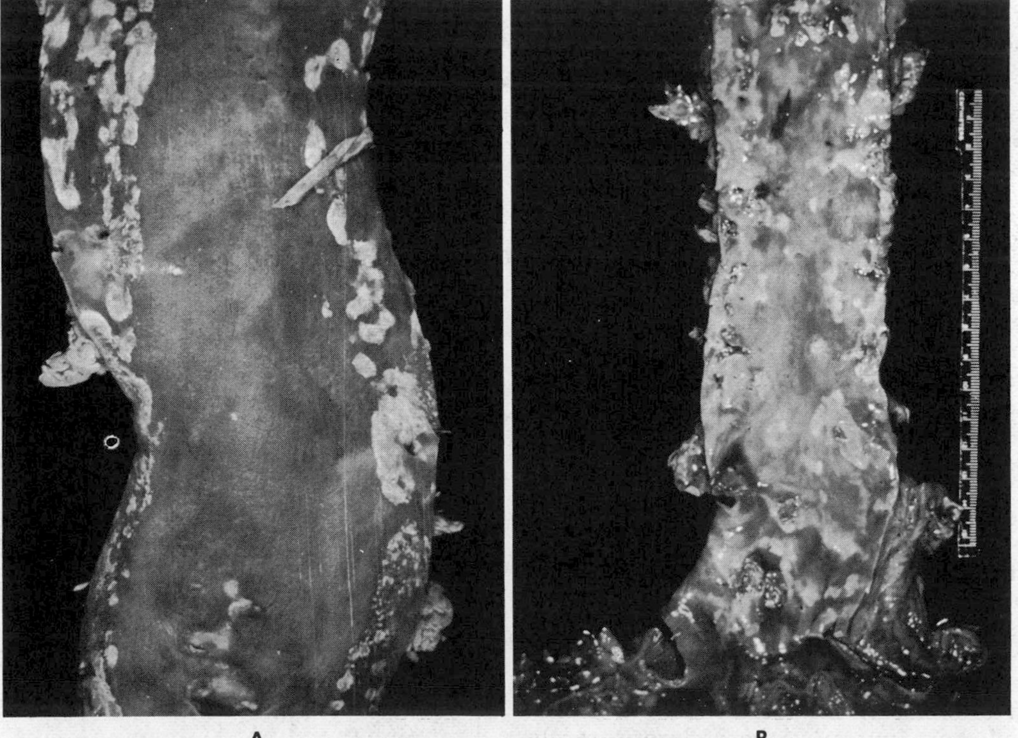

A B

Figure 48–7. **A.** Atherosclerosis. An early stage with widely scattered, barely elevated intimal plaques. **B.** More extensive lesions. (From Robbins, S. L., and R. S. Cotran: *Pathologic Basis of Disease,* 2nd ed. Philadelphia: W. B. Saunders Co., 1979, p. 602.)

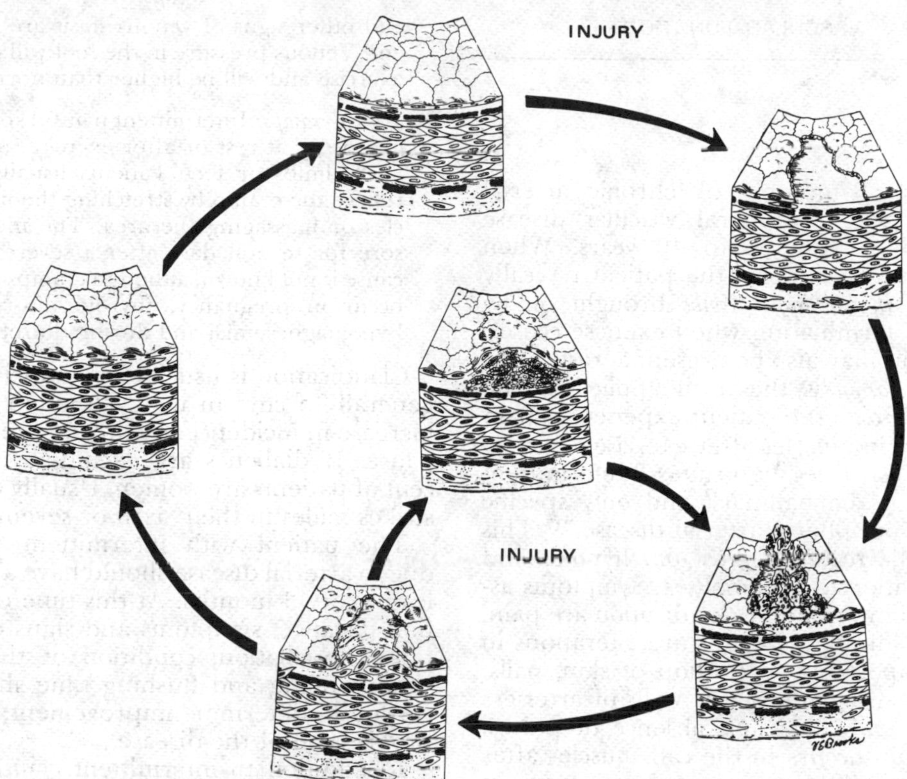

Figure 48–8. Two possible different cycles of events in the response-to-injury hypothesis. The larger cycle represents limited endothelial injury. Endothelial injury may lead to desquamation, platelet adherence, aggregation, and release, followed by smooth muscle proliferation and connective tissue formation. If the injury is a single event, the lesions may go on to heal and regress, leaving a slightly thickened intima. The smaller, inner cycle demonstrates the possible consequences of repeated or chronic injury to the endothelium in which lipid deposition may occur and smooth muscle proliferation may continue, leading to a complicated lesion containing newly formed connective tissue and lipids, which may eventually calcify. (From Ross, R., and J. A. Glomset. The pathogenesis of atherosclerosis. *New England Journal of Medicine*. 295:420, 1976.)

has been implicated as a causative factor, but this is not yet proved. Associated diseases such as diabetes and hypertension appear to accelerate atherosclerosis.

Cigarette smoking is implicated by autopsy studies that show an increasing degree of coronary atherosclerosis with increasing age and the number of cigarettes smoked during life. *Effects of tobacco* have not been documented as etiologic factors in peripheral vascular disease. However, since tobacco smoking does decrease cutaneous blood flow, patients with diseases that limit extremity blood flow should be advised to stop smoking. Of patients with arteriosclerosis obliterans who continued to smoke, 11.4 per cent required amputation during a 5-year period, whereas none who stopped smoking needed an amputation.[23]

Hormones, particularly estrogen, have a potent effect on atherogenesis. Obesity, physical inactivity, and emotional stress are all implicated as factors. Genetic factors seem to be important in combination with environmental factors. For further discussion of the etiology of atherosclerosis, see Chapter 36.

> *"Among the killers in the Western world, atherosclerosis is overwhelmingly in first place."*[40]

Incidence. Atherosclerosis is the most common disease in the elderly. It is the most frequent reason for death in persons over 65, and in the sixth and seventh decades kills ten times as many people as cancer. Over half of all persons between the ages of 60 and 70 will die of some manifestation of atherosclerosis. Because the major target organs of atherosclerosis are coronary and cerebral vessels, atherosclerosis usually clinically appears in the form of a myocardial infarction (heart attack) or a cerebral vascular accident (stroke). About 50 per cent of patients with peripheral arterial insufficiency have other clinical signs of atherosclerosis.

Today, there is evidence that the incidence of atherosclerosis is increasing in the younger age group. As a group, it contains a greater number of cigarette smokers than the general population.

Symptoms. Symptoms of chronic arterial occlusion due to peripheral vascular disease may not appear for 20 to 40 years. When manifestations do appear, the patient typically reports *pain in the lower limbs* brought on by exercise and terminating when exercise ceases, although pain may also be present at rest. *Intermittent claudication* is the term applied to the symptom in which the patient experiences pain or discomfort in muscles after exercise, which is relieved by rest. Friedman states: "Intermittent claudication is the hallmark and only specific symptom of peripheral arterial disease."[17] This problem is the result of muscular hypoxia and the accumulation of metabolites. Symptoms associated with intermittent claudication are pain, coldness, or numbness. Signs are alterations in color or temperature; condition of skin, nails, tissue, and hair; condition of walls of arteries; auscultation or bruits; and absence of pulses. Typically, pain occurs in the calf muscles after walking and disappears on rest. It can occur in muscles other than the calf but is frequently not recognized.

One classic characteristic of intermittent claudication is that it is *reproducible*; i.e., the same situation produces the same response every time almost without exception. As Hertzer explains: "The individual who cannot negotiate the width of a parking lot because of leg pain on one day, but is able to walk indefinitely the next, does not have intermittent claudication."[20]

Intermittent claudication, while it is the outstanding manifestation of arterial disease, may also appear in a number of other disorders that are unrelated to arterial disease. Other conditions that cause intermittent claudication or a similar type of leg pain include the following:

- *Arthritis:* Patients who have arthritis of the knees may have calf pain on walking, but it is also present at rest. The pain connected with arthritis of the hip is generally more severe when the patient starts to walk and lessens as the patient continues to walk.

- *Lumbar disk disease:* The patient's pain usually occurs at rest but may be aggravated by walking. Presence of normal pulses and the distribution of pain laterally in the hip or thigh help rule out arterial disease.

- *Neurogenic claudication:* This is secondary to compression or intermittent ischemia of the lower cord. This diagnosis is confirmed by myelography.

- *Venous claudication:* Patients with iliofemoral venous obstruction may have symptoms of venous obstruction much like arterial disease. Swelling and other signs of venous stasis are usually present. Venous pressure in the foot will increase with exercise and will be higher than normal.

- *Muscle cramps:* Intermittent painful spasms of muscles occur at rest or after exercise, usually in the lower limbs or feet. Patients usually attempt to relieve the cramp by stretching the involved muscles or massaging the area. The muscle may be sore for several days after a severe cramp. The cause is not known, although cramps are known to occur in pregnancy, thyroid disorder, uremia, hypomagnesemia, and during diuretic therapy.

Claudication is usually insidious in onset and generally occurs in men, although there is an increase in incidence in females after the menopause. If diabetics are excluded, only 10 per cent of patients are women. Usually claudication strikes males in their sixth or seventh decade.

The patient with intermittent claudication due to arterial disease should have a check-up at least every 3 months. At this time the claudication distance, symptoms and signs of ischemia, pulses, oscillation, condition of the feet, and venous filling and flushing time should be recorded to determine improvement, stability, or progression of the disease.

In addition to intermittent claudication, patients with arterial insufficiency of the lower limbs may develop *ischemic rest pain.* "By definition, ischemic rest pain is a persistent form of dull or aching pain that occurs initially in the distal tissues of the foot, such as the digits, the region of the metatarsophalangeal joint, the dorsum of the foot or the heel area."[4] As with intermittent claudication, the cause of rest pain is unknown; however, authorities believe that it results from the release of a metabolic factor that is related to tissue anoxia. Pain at rest signifies that the blood flow to the extremity is too limited to maintain even very small tissue requirements. Patients often have a dependent reddish blue discoloration of the toes, which then become white when the legs are elevated. The toes are cold to the touch; also hypertrophied toenails, tissue atrophy, ulcers, or gangrene may be present. Occlusion of the deep femoral artery or of the large three calf arteries is usually present in patients with ischemia at rest. Both intermittent claudication and ischemic rest pain can be completely relieved by successful arterial reconstructive surgery in the ischemic limb.

Diagnosis and Assessment. The physician bases the diagnosis on the patient's symptoms (e.g., complaints of intermittent claudication, numbness of the legs), observable changes in the appearance of the limbs, palpation of the peripheral pulses, and a variety of diagnostic tests.

Signs observed by the doctor are alterations in color or temperature of the affected extremity. Nutrition of the limb may be inadequate, resulting in thickened and opaque nails, shiny and

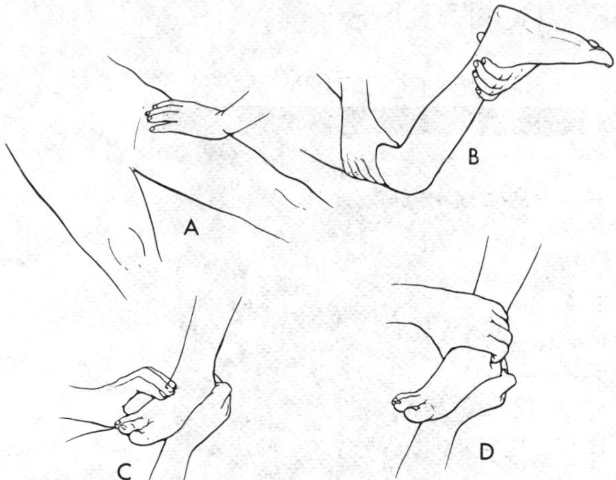

Figure 48–9. The method of palpation for pulsations in the peripheral arteries. *A*, Femoral artery. *B*, Popliteal artery. *C*, Dorsalis pedis artery. *D*, Posterior tibial artery. (From: Fairbairn, J. F., II, J. L. Jurgens, and J. A. Spittell, Jr.: *Peripheral Vascular Diseases*, 4th ed. 1972.)

atrophic skin, decreased hair growth, dry or fissured heels, and loss of subcutaneous tissue in the digits.

The most important part of the examination is palpation of the peripheral pulses. Absence of a normally palpable pulse is the most reliable sign of occlusive arterial disease, since in the lower limb the femoral pulse in the groin and the posterior tibial pulse behind the medial malleolus are easily felt (Figs. 48–9 and 48–10). Comparison of pulses in both extremities is helpful. The popliteal pulse is often difficult to feel in obese or muscular patients. The position of the dorsalis pedis artery in the foot is variable. It is absent on one side in about 15 per cent of normal subjects, so that absence of the dorsalis pedis pulse is not a very reliable sign of arterial disease. When pulses are being palpated, it should also be ascertained whether the arterial wall is palpable, tortuous, or calcified. Auscultation over the main arteries is useful, as a systolic bruit usually indicates an atheromatous plaque.

There are a number of tests that can be performed as a part of the clinical examination of the patient. Seven commonly used tests include: Oscillometry, skin temperature studies, angiography, exercise tests for intermittent claudication, lumbar sympathetic block, use of the Doppler ultrasound velocity detector, and plethysmography.

Oscillometry. Alterations in the pulse volume are measured by placing a pneumatic cuff around the extremity at different levels, attached to an oscillometer (an aneroid system). The arterial pressure with each pulsation is transmitted via a sensitive diaphragm to a needle attached to a dial. The reading is recorded in units called the *oscillometric index.* Abnormal findings help to pinpoint the level of arterial occlusion, but the results may vary in different patients and the information is not always conclusive. Figure 48–11 illustrates an oscillographic tracing of wave patterns produced by arterial flow velocity signals in normal and obstructed vessels.

Skin Temperature Studies. These are done in various ways: (1) palpating and comparing skin warmth or coolness in opposing limbs; (2) the use of direct-reading skin temperature thermometers; (3) immersing one extremity in warm water, and observing for *rise* in skin temperature in other extremity, which should follow normally owing to reflex vasodilatation; (4) placing a hot water bottle on the patient's abdomen and observing extremities for reflex rise in skin temperature. Coldness of one or both extremities under normal room temperature implies poor circulation; the failure of the arteries in an extremity to dilate as described in (3) and (4) indicates arterial damage. However, these tests can be unreliable if the patient is anxious and, in general, are only of limited value in diagnosis.

Angiography (Arteriography). Contrast dye is injected into the arteries and x-ray films are made of the vascular tree. The films may indicate abnormalities of blood flow due to arterial obstruction or narrowing. Disadvantages are the possibility of allergic reactions to the radiopaque dye, and the fact that the inspection site may become irritated or thrombosed.

Exercise Tests for Intermittent Claudication. The patient walks or performs some other

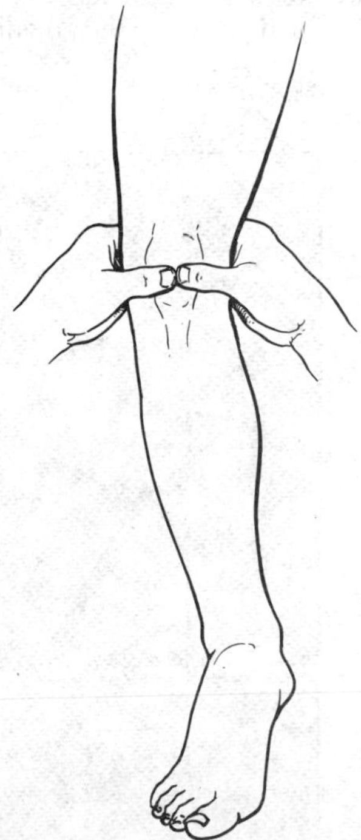

Figure 48–10. An alternative method for palpating pulsations in the popliteal artery. (From: Fairbairn, J. F., II, J. L. Juergens, and J. A. Spittell, Jr.: *Peripheral Vascular Diseases*, 4th ed. 1972.)

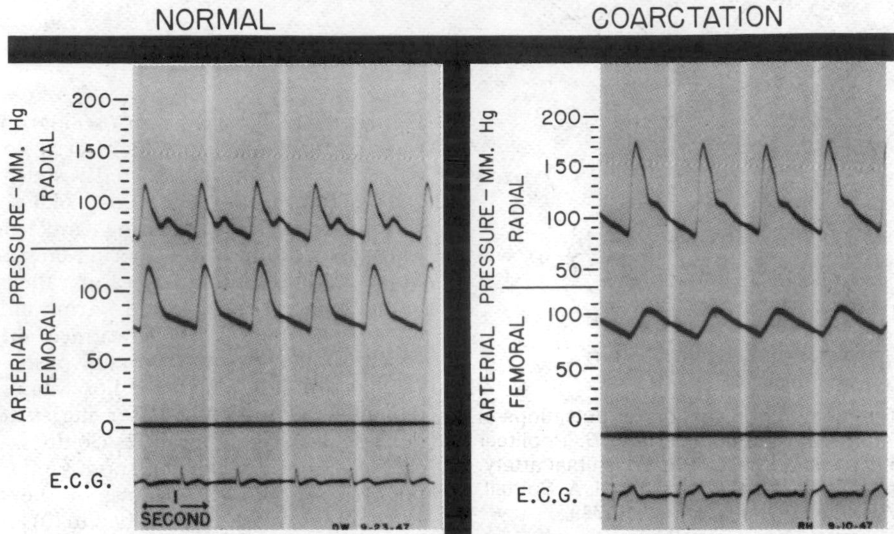

Figure 48–11. Arterial pulse contours. Simultaneous recordings of pulse waves in radial and femoral arteries of a normal young adult and a young patient with coarctation of the thoracic aorta. (From Fairbairn, J. F., II, J. L. Juergens, and J. A. Spittell, Jr.: *Peripheral Vascular Diseases,* 4th ed. 1972.)

form of exercise until pain occurs; the length of time required for onset of calf pain following start of exercise is recorded. Claudication on exercise indicates the failure of damaged arteries to adjust the blood flow to the increased tissue requirements for oxygen. *Treadmill exercise* is most useful in evaluating patients with peripheral vascular disease. In this simple test, the patient lies down for 5 to 10 minutes, while ankle pressures are recorded with the Doppler flow meter. The patient walks the treadmill until the pain of claudication appears. Then the patient lies down again. Normally arm and ankle pressures rise during exercise; in patients with claudication, ankle pressures fall.[27] (See Figure 48–12.)

Lumbar Sympathetic Block. Local anesthetic is injected into the sympathetic ganglia, thereby temporarily blocking the sympathetic vasomotor nerve fibers supplying an ischemic limb. A decrease in limb pain and increase in skin temperature indicates that sympathetectomy could improve circulation to the

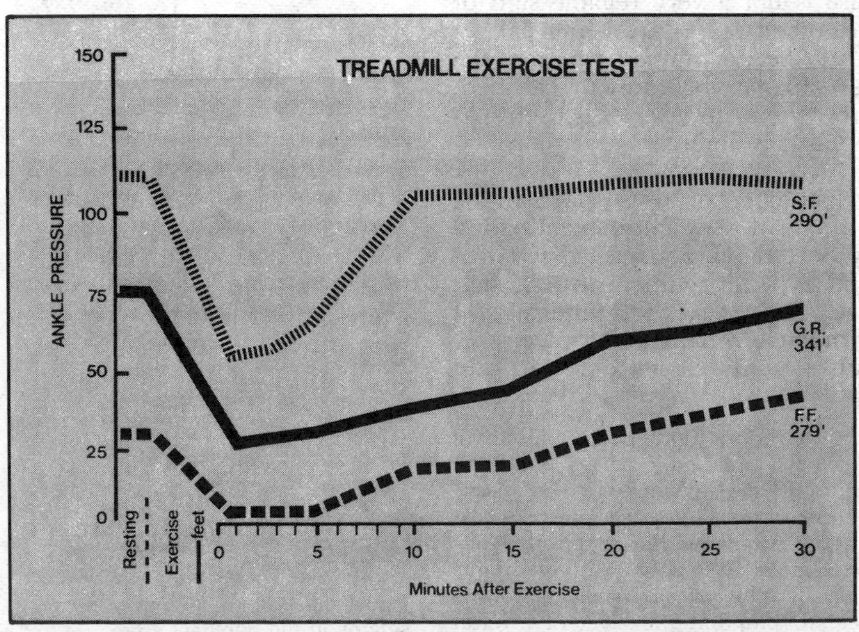

Figure 48–12. Ankle pressure tends to fall appreciably during exercise in a patient with claudication. (From Lennihan, R., and M. Mackereth: Proper evaluation of intermittent claudication. *Consultant,* 16:201, Oct. 1977.)

extremities. A possible adverse reaction may be *shock* as a result of movement of the blood from the vital organs into the peripheral vessels.

The Doppler Ultrasound Flow Detector. This electronic stethoscope is most helpful in obtaining qualitative and quantitative information about blood flow and for evaluating intermittent claudication. With the Doppler, it is possible to listen to blood flow through the femoral, dorsalis pedis, popliteal, and posterior tibial arteries even when the arteries are not palpable. Normally, *healthy* arteries produce an explosive swish as the blood is propelled through them with each beat of the heart. Blood flow distal to *obstructed* arteries sounds low and slurred. In addition, the Doppler can be attached to a blood pressure cuff to obtain thigh, calf, and ankle pressures as indicated above. The Doppler is discussed further in Chapter 49.

Plethysmography. This diagnostic device monitors and graphically records pulse changes and changes in the size of the legs with each heart beat. Plethysmography is considered further in Chapter 49.

In addition, all patients with signs of peripheral vascular diseases should undergo diagnostic studies for diabetes and for lipoprotein abnormalities. These studies usually include a 3- to 5-hour glucose tolerance test and lipoprotein electrophoresis. (See Chapter 72 for discussion of diabetes and Chapter 36 for lipid abnormalities.)

Examination generally places the patient in one of three groups, depending on the area of the principal occlusion:

1. About 80 per cent of the patients with occlusive arterial disease of the lower limbs have disease in the femoropopliteal segments. The adductor region is the most common, followed by the popliteal artery just above the knee joint and the popliteal bifurcation.
2. The patients with aorto-iliac lesions make up about 15 per cent; here there is an occlusion in the common iliac artery or at the aortic bifurcation.
3. Patients with femoropopliteal lesions may also have one or more occlusions in the arteries of the leg, and the incidence of these combined lesions increases as the patient ages.

Prognosis. The significance of peripheral arterial occlusion is that it indicates the presence of atherosclerosis. Atherosclerosis of the coronary or cerebral arteries is more likely to cause death or disability than is intermittent claudication or other peripheral effects. Of patients with claudication, more than half die from myocardial infarction.

Moreover, existence of symptomatic aorto-ilio femoral occlusive disease results in approximately a 10-year decrease in life expectancy compared to the normal population. However, a significant proportion of the cumulative mortality appears to be due to coronary artery disease and diabetes. Neither the presence nor the anatomical location of occlusive disease distal to the common femoral bifurcation by itself decreases life expectancy. A low operative mortality rate, excellent long-term patency, and potentially normal life expectancy has increased the desirability of vascular surgery for patients who have symptoms of peripheral vascular disease but who are free of diabetes mellitus and coronary artery disease.[30]

Treatment. It is important to reassure the patient that the limbs are in no immediate danger and to give some general information about necessary changes in living habits.

General Care Measures. The patient should be encouraged to walk, and a program of graduated walking should be planned, with the patient's participation.

Several studies have shown that patients generally *feel* better on an exercise program and may improve their walking distance. Some believe these benefits are due to increased collateral circulation, whereas others believe that muscle strength in general may be improved. Overweight patients should be encouraged to reduce and to improve those dietary habits that contribute to overweight. There is no evidence that a special diet will alter the course of atherosclerosis once clinical evidence of it has appeared. Cigarette smoking may influence vascular disability. Patients who stop smoking and start exercising may improve their walking capacity. Some patients are not aware of chest pain, shortness of breath, and simple fatigue because their attention is focused on their leg discomfort. They should be questioned carefully about these symptoms, as medical or surgical treatment may improve their walking ability if they have coronary artery disease or chronic pulmonary insufficiency.

Meticulous care of the feet should be advised, using warm water, drying gently and thoroughly, using lubricants to keep the skin soft, and wearing clean cotton or wool socks daily. Shoes and slippers should be well fitted. Patients should never go barefooted. The patient should not wear constricting garters, foundation garments, or hosiery. Bed socks should be worn to bed, and the bed warmed by an electric blanket rather than hot water bottles or heating pads.

Drug Therapy. Various *drugs* may be used in treatment of peripheral arterial disease. Drugs given are usually vasodilators, anticoagulants, and/or drugs that lower the serum cholesterol.

Drugs that cause dilatation of the peripheral blood vessels act as *adrenergic blocking agents* (such drugs as pentolamine and phenoxybenzamine); they interfere with the actions of epinephrine and norepinephrine when these substances are released at the nerve endings in the blood vessels, or they act directly on the smooth muscles in the walls of the blood vessels. There is question about their effect when there is generalized atherosclerotic disease. Although the drugs are not toxic, there are unpleasant side effects such as facial flushing, tachycardia and palpations, nervousness and excitability, dizziness, shivering, nausea, and weakness. Since most patients do better when they are receiving treatment, even placebos, there may be merit in prescribing drugs that act directly on the blood vessels rather than adrenergic blocking agents, which dilate mainly the cutaneous blood vessels and divert blood away from the muscles. *Alcohol* is a very good vasodilator and for occasional use is as good as any of the adrenergic blocking agents. *Vitamin E* has been used, and some patients seem to improve but probably no more than with a placebo. However, it is harmless.

Cyclospasmol (Cyclandelate) is an oral peripheral vasodilator. It relaxes the vascular smooth muscles and has no significant adrenergic stimulating or blocking action.[38] It should be used with caution in patients with severe obliterative coronary artery, cerebral vascular disease, or glaucoma. In a double blind cross-over study, Reich found that during treatment with 1600 mg. of cyclospasmol, measurements of circulatory efficiency improved daily. Patients found relief from the leg pain that had occurred after walking short distances and relief from symptoms of ischemic cerebral vascular disease, e.g., memory loss, dizziness, loss of personal neatness.

Although *anticoagulants* can be used effectively in patients with venous thrombosis, there is little evidence that they can reduce or prevent arterial thromboses, and they are generally not used unless there is some additional indication.

Finally, drugs *that lower serum cholesterol are sometimes ordered*. Although there is an association of atherosclerosis with a high concentration of cholesterol and lipid substances in the blood, there is no clear evidence that by the use of special diets and drugs the course of atherosclerosis will be modified. The safest method is to reduce the total fat intake in the diet and to replace saturated fat with oils rich in polyunsaturated fatty acids. A drug that has been found to lower serum cholesterol is clofibrate (Atromid-S). When given in appropriate doses, this drug reduces serum cholesterol 20 to 25 per cent in the majority of patients. Side effects are mild gastrointestinal upsets, drowsiness, and occasional skin rashes.

SURGICAL TREATMENT. Patients should not be referred for surgical treatment unless the claudication is sufficiently severe as to interfere with life or with ordinary day-to-day activities. The number of patients who can be helped by endarterectomy or a bypass graft is small, probably about 10 per cent. Lumbar sympathectomy has also been employed to improve the collateral circulation and may have a limited place in some patients with intermittent claudication.

THE CHRONIC ISCHEMIC LIMB AND ITS CARE. Patients with a chronic ischemic limb have a disability that is usually of rather long duration. Such patients commonly have intermittent claudication, but their main complaint is either pain in the foot or areas of necrosis.

As mentioned previously, the care of the chronically ischemic limb should be meticulous, with careful attention to cleanliness and keeping the foot dry. Socks should be soft, preferably woolen, and well-fitted footwear should be worn. The feet should not be allowed to become cold. Localized areas of gangrene should be kept dry and should not be treated unless there is an infection. It is probably best for the patient to be up and about.

Individuals with chronic ischemic limb are prone to the development of ischemic *leg ulcers*. Arterial ischemic ulcers are caused by small vessel disease. They are typically very painful, while the leg itself is cool to the touch, has a loss of hair, and lacks a palpable pulse. The goal of treatment for leg ulcers is to eliminate infection, reduce inflammation, and encourage granulation of new tissue. General care includes keeping the area of ulceration clean, dry, and free from pressure. Sometimes topical corticosteriods and topical antibiotics are applied. Bedrest is helpful because it reduces the oxygen needs of the impaired tissues. Often, skin grafts are needed to cover the site once the ulcerated area is free from infection and granulation tissue is evident.[10,42]

The pain of severe ischemia is difficult to relieve. When strong analgesics such as morphine are necessary, the patient should be prepared to accept amputation.

Sympathectomy may be done to relieve the circulation in the chronic ischemic foot. Arterial surgery is sometimes done to improve circulation when the patient has an aorto-iliac block or a femoropopliteal occlusion. The arteries in the leg must be healthy enough to carry sufficient blood to the foot once the block has been removed or bypassed.

Acute Arterial Occlusion

Acute occlusion of the main artery of a limb may be caused by trauma, embolism, or thrombosis and may occur in a healthy or diseased artery. About 90 per cent of the clinically recognized cases are in the lower limbs.

It is important to differentiate between arterial thrombosis and arterial embolism. *Acute arterial thrombosis* is usually due to arterial obstruction by a blood clot that forms in an artery damaged (usually) by atherosclerosis. Arterial thrombosis may also develop in an arterial aneurysm, especially aneurysms that form in the popliteal artery.

In *arterial embolism* the wall of the artery is often healthy and the obstruction in the artery comes most frequently from a thrombus within the heart. Sometimes portions of a blood clot, such as platelet emboli, may form at points of turbulence and lodge at a bifurcation and may initiate a thrombus, or atheromatous emboli may block small arteries. In the lower extremity, over half of the emboli will lodge in either the superficial femoral or the popliteal artery. Nurses should be alert to symptoms of emboli in patients with rheumatic valve disease or myocardial infarction and in patients with artificial heart valves. Atrial fibrillation is a very common cause of arterial emboli.

Because arterial thrombosis is usually superimposed upon atherosclerosis, and consequently develops in a damaged vessel, more extensive surgery is required to correct thrombosis than to correct arterial embolism. Surgery for arterial thrombosis usually involves an arterial reconstructive procedure for revascularization of the leg. Arterial emboli can be fairly easily removed by a simple embolectomy.

Signs and Symptoms. Occlusion usually has a dramatic onset but may pass unnoticed if the patient is seriously ill and confined to bed. Burning or aching pain in the tissues distal to the site of the occlusion is usually the first symptom, which rapidly increases in intensity and subsides slowly over a period of hours. Active or passive movement of the limb aggravates the pain. Occasionally the occlusion is painless and attention may be called to it by the appearance of the limb, or by numbness or paresthesias. In addition, weight bearing may suddenly become difficult and the person may even experience paralysis of the limb. The early symptoms are followed by a sense of coldness, numbness in the extremity, and muscle weakness. Arterial pulsation is absent or weakened distal to the site of the occlusion.

The circulatory changes that follow arterial occlusion, and that predict outcome, are complex and depend on varied factors. Acute occlusion produces a fall in the mean and pulse pressures in the distal arteries and a decrease in tissue pO_2. In a normal artery, normal blood flow is restored by collateral channels, but patients with acute arterial occlusion may have a weakened heart, and other factors such as immobility, anemia, or dehydration may be present.

Treatment. The first decision is whether an operation should be performed to remove the occluding embolus or thrombus. Any surgery should be performed as quickly as possible. Patients can have a successful embolectomy performed under local anesthesia. If the patient is not seen until some hours have elapsed since the occlusion, the viability of the limb will determine if the operation can be performed.

While decisions concerning surgery are being made, the patient should be put to bed in a comfortable warm room. To ease the pain of vasospasm, a small dose of papaverine hydrochloride is sometimes given. If this medication is ordered, administer it very slowly and make certain that the patient has not received morphine earlier. Also, an alcoholic beverage acts as a potent vasodilator, but one cannot be given if the patient is going to surgery and must remain NPO.

The limb should be protected from pressure and other trauma and kept at room temperature, neither warm nor chilled. The best position for the limb is level or slightly dependent. The affected leg should be gently covered by an occlusive dressing to protect it from trauma.

If the decision is for medical treatment or there is a delay in procuring a surgeon, anticoagulants are generally started immediately. Heparin, 10,000 to 15,000 units as the initial dose followed by 10,000 units at 8-hour intervals, is recommended. If the patient has a cardiac condition, the heparin should be given by a single intravenous injection rather than as a continuous drip, to prevent overloading the circulation. Heparin should be continued for a minimum of 48 hours to 7 days, after which a change to an oral anticoagulant may be made. It is the prevailing practice to treat all patients who have a definite source of embolism and who have made a satisfactory recovery from an acute episode of occlusion with long-term anticoagulant therapy for an indefinite period.

Aside from surgery, fibrinolytic agents may be used for removal of an occluding thrombus or embolus. At present two substances are available for use, streptokinase and urokinase. The drugs are expensive, difficult to monitor, and require some hours to clear the arterial lumen.

Prognosis. Because most patients have either a cardiac lesion or arterial disease, their ultimate prognosis is uncertain and there is insufficient evidence to suggest significant improvement with long term anticoagulant therapy.

Thromboangiitis Obliterans (Buerger's Disease)

In 1908 Buerger proposed the name thromboangiitis obliterans for an arterial disease which he felt was distinct from atherosclerosis in that acute inflammatory lesions and occlusive thrombosis of the arteries and veins were characteristic findings. The condition is sometimes called *Buerger's disease*.

The criteria accepted as favoring this diagnosis rather than atherosclerosis are the following.:[39]

- The patient is a male of less than 40 years at the onset of the symptoms.
- The patient is a heavy cigarette smoker.
- Superficial thrombophlebitis may be present.
- Involvement of arteries of upper limbs or viscera is common.
- Arteriography reveals occlusive peripheral arterial disease.

Pain is the outstanding symptom. Intermittent claudication is a common complaint and occurs in almost all patients at some stage of the disease. It is frequently the first symptom noted by the patient and occurs most commonly in the arch of the foot. It is somewhat less common in the calf of the leg but may be noted in both sites. Rest pain with signs of persistent ischemia of one or more digits may be one of the first clinical indications. Coldness or sensitivity to cold may be an early symptom. Various types of paresthesias may occur. Pulsations in any or all the posterior tibial and dorsalis pedis arteries may be impaired or absent. In advanced cases the extremities may be abnormally red or cyanotic, particularly when dependent. The color changes are more significant if they involve only one extremity or only certain digits or portions of digits. Sometimes certain digits are colder than others on the same extremity.

Ulceration and gangrene are frequent complications and may occur early in the course of the disease. These lesions may appear spontaneously but often follow trauma. Gangrene usually occurs in one extremity at a time. Edema of the legs is fairly common in advanced cases. Changes in the nails and skin appear, and segmental thrombophlebitis affects the smaller veins in about 40 per cent of patients.

Diagnostic studies include leg arteriography, skin temperature determination, oscillometry, blood studies, and x-ray examinations. The clinical course of the disease is greatly influenced by whether the patient smokes, and if so, stops smoking. In the majority of patients who continue to smoke, the course of the disease is slowly and episodically progressive, with the development of first minor and later more extensive ulcerative gangrenous lesions after a period of months or years.

The *prognosis* as to survival of digits or limbs and the necessity for amputation depend on the stage of the disease when treatment is initiated, whether the patient continues to smoke, and whether he avoids major or minor trauma to the ischemic tissues. In a 10-year period, in one study, 6 per cent of the patients required amputations of fingers, 6 per cent amputation of toes, and 13 per cent amputation of a leg.[15] Patients in the study had a practically normal survival rate.

Treatment is generally the same as for atherosclerotic peripheral vascular disease. In essence, care is pointed toward (1) arresting progress of the disease, (2) producing vasodilatation, (3) relieving pain, and (4) treating ulcers and gangrene. All patients are advised to abstain completely and permanently from use of tobacco in any form. The use of whisky or brandy may be of some value during periods of exacerbation. Exposure to cold should be avoided. Patients should be carefully instructed to prevent mechanical, chemical, and thermal injuries to the feet. Regional sympathetic ganglionectomy produces vasodilatation and may be of some value.

Amputation should be deferred until conservative treatment has been given a reasonable trial. It is almost always unwise to delay amputation of the leg when the gangrene extends well into the foot, and it should not be delayed if pain is severe and cannot be controlled or if severe infection or toxicity occurs. It is seldom necessary in these patients to carry an amputation above the knee.

Functional Vascular Disease

Raynaud's Disease. A confusion of terminology has existed in connection with this condition since its first description by Raynaud in 1862. The terms "Raynaud's disease" and "Raynaud's phenomenon" have both been used over the years, sometimes to describe the same set of findings. At present the consensus is that "Raynaud's phenomenon" should be used to refer to intermittent episodes of constriction of small arteries or arterioles of the extremities, causing changes in the color and temperature of the skin of the extremities. These local changes are not necessarily related to the status of the peripheral vascular system as a whole. Unlike Raynaud's disease (which is a bilateral affliction), Raynaud's phenomenon is generally unilateral and may affect only one or two digits. Raynaud's phenomenon may occur after trauma; for instance, after the use of high-speed vibrating tools under conditions of cold. It may also be related to various neurogenic lesions, certain occlusive arterial diseases, and various other miscellaneous conditions. Irrespective of the causes, Raynaud's phenomenon is due to reduction of blood flow to the upper extremity secondary to an arterial lesion.

Raynaud's disease, in contrast to Raynaud's phenomenon, is of unknown etiology, although immunologic abnormalities seem to be present in many patients.

The criteria for making the diagnosis of *Raynaud's disease* are:

- Intermittent attacks of pallor or cyanosis of the digits by exposure to cold or from emotional stimuli.
- Bilateral or symmetrical involvement.
- No evidence of occlusive disease in the digital arteries or any primary systemic disease to which the changes might be secondary.
- Gangrene which, when it occurs, is limited in large part to the skin of the tips of the digits.
- A history of symptoms for at least 2 years.

There are a large number of diseases associated with cold sensitivity of the Raynaud type categorized into intravascular disorders, e.g., cold agglutinins, diseases of the vessel walls such as thromboangiitis obliterans, occupational trauma and vascular injury, collagen disorders, and extravascular disorders. One of the first problems is establishing the diagnostic category for a patient with cold sensitivity.

Raynaud's disease is most likely to have an early age of onset, often commencing in the teens. The process will initially involve only the distal portion of one or more digits, although as the disease becomes more severe all the digits are involved. The feet are rarely as symptomatically involved as the hands. A careful history should be taken to elicit the possibility of other disease. On physical examination, normal-appearing fingers without ulceration suggest Raynaud's disease. Radial and ulnar pulses should be present and normal. Eighty per cent of patients with Raynaud's disease are women.

Reassurance of the patient that the condition is not likely to lead to a serious disability is desirable. Keeping the extremities warm and avoiding smoking are important. Vasodilator drugs may be prescribed. Reserpine drugs, which decrease the store of norepinephrine in the peripheral arteries, have been tried and found to have few side effects. Although sympathectomy has been used in treatment, its effectiveness is very limited in advanced cases. However, it appears to be beneficial at an earlier stage of the disease. Symptoms may disappear entirely and should they recur, they seem to be milder and less frequent.

Acrocyanosis. In acrocyanosis, the extremities tend to be blue and cold even when the environmental temperature is normal. Generally both hands and feet are affected, and the changes are often found with increased sweating. The condition occurs most often in women.

Chilblains and Frostbite. Chilblains is a common vascular disorder due to cold, in which the skin becomes discolored and there is pain, swelling, and itching. Acute chilblains occur mainly on the fingers and toes and consist of subcutaneous nodules over which the cyanosed skin is thinned and may break down into an indolent and painful ulcer. *Frostbite* occurs when tissues are frozen hard. This happens when they are exposed suddenly to temperatures of −4°C. or lower.

Vasospasm of Disuse. The most common causes of long-term disuse of the limbs are anterior poliomyelitis, traumatic denervation, cerebrovascular accidents, and reflex sympathetic dystrophy.

At an early stage the arterioles of a limb with vasospasm from disuse will dilate fully when the subject becomes warm, but with long continued disuse and exposure to cold, atrophic changes proportional to the extent and duration of the disuse gradually occur. Natural wrinkles over the knuckles tend to smooth, fingers taper, the pulp atrophies, and the nails curve and thicken. Breaks in the skin due to minor trauma become painful and heal with difficulty. Over the limb as a whole, the venules of the skin lose tone and become telangiectatic. Lymphatic drainage slows, and the legs in particular develop edema readily. Sympathectomy may effect an improvement in circulation in some patients, but it is simpler and more effective to keep the skin warm at all times.

Surgical Restoration of Primary Circulation

Arteries may be operated on when there is the possibility of removing the obstruction and restoring the patient to gainful employment or more enjoyment of living. Physician and patient may decide to attempt salvage rather than amputation.

Endarterectomy. Angiography is used to identify the exact nature and extent of disease. Endarterectomy is intended to open orifices of collateral arterial branches as well as segments of the main channel. Patches of autologous vein or Dacron may be necessary after removal of the atheroma. The surgery is generally fitted to the specific needs of the patient, and a combination of bypass and thromboendarterectomy may be required.

Bypass Graft for Femoropopliteal Disease. The repair of lesions in the femoropopliteal area is one of the principal concerns in vascular surgery today. This is one of the commonest arterial lesions of the lower extremity, especially in patients over 70 years of age. Of the 73,000 reconstructions of major arteries in the United States every year, more than 20,000 (27 per cent) involve the femoral popliteal segment.[30] The preferred surgical method is an autogenous saphenous vein bypass graft. Three specific bypass procedures are pictured in Figure 48–13. Plastic prostheses have been used less because they have often failed to remain open. Knitted Dacron bypass grafts are used when it is difficult to obtain autologous tissues. Bovine heterografts may also be used.

The method of selecting patients with femoropopliteal disease for grafting will affect the results, but one group reports overall long patency rates of 70 to 90 per cent with this method.[15] Elderly patients are now considered for arterial reconstruction. In recent years, with the use of noninvasive methods to evaluate vascular status (e.g., the use of the Doppler flowmeter), the once prevalent negative attitude toward bypass grafts for older patients has changed to greater acceptance. The operative risk is only about 1 per cent if the surgeon is a well-trained specialist; more attempts at surgical repair of this type of occlusion probably should be attempted.

Pre- and Postoperative Care. Adequate circulating blood volume must be maintained to permit good perfusion throughout the period of arterial repair. Careful preoperative attention to the total body potassium stores is important, to prevent cardiac arrhythmias. Also, it is important to screen elective cases for focus of infection or an infectious process *before* surgery is undertaken. Tooth abscesses, active urinary tract infections, or respiratory infections must be treated preoperatively.

Postoperatively, central venous pressure is monitored, and observation of kidney function is important. Every effort should be made to prevent thrombosis. The patient's legs should be elevated above the level of the heart. Anti-

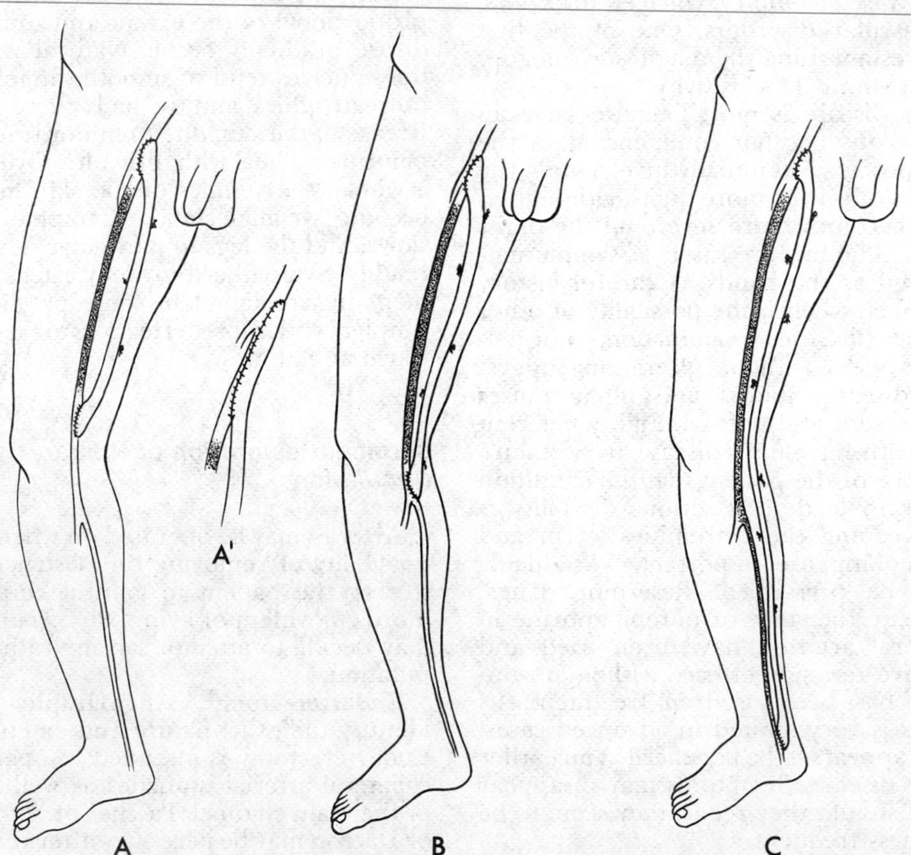

Figure 48–13. *A,* Femoropopliteal bypass from common femoral artery to proximal popliteal; *B,* bypass to tibioperoneal trunk; *C,* long bypass to ankle. (From Nora, P. F.: *Operative Surgery: Principles and Techniques.* Philadelphia: Lea & Febiger, 1972, p. 785.)

coagulants are used during the operation and postoperatively if the patient's condition warrants.

Infection is one of the commonly dreaded outcomes of vascular prosthetic repair. The most common presentation of infection is purulent wound drainage and graft exposure. There may or may not be hemorrhage, low grade fever, sinus tracts, graft occlusion, local hemorrhage, false aneurysms, upper GI bleeding or emboli. *Staphylococcus aureus* is the most frequently cultured organism and infections are most often in the groin. 80% of infections are noted within 5 weeks of the date of the operation. Dacron and Teflon prostheses function well unless they become infected.[28]

Nursing Considerations

Preoperative Care. If vascular surgery is not an emergency, the nurse may be able to assist the patient and significant others by explaining the various procedures involved, and by offering the patient and concerned others psychologic support. The nurse will be assessing the patient's readiness and desire to learn about the surgery and the postoperative care involved. The nurse obtains baseline data on the patient's vital signs and the character of the peripheral pulses. Prior to going to the operating room, the patient may have an IV and a Foley catheter inserted, and is weighed. Just before surgery, an arterial line and a central venous pressure line will generally be inserted. It is usual practice to give the patient broad-spectrum antibiotics for 48 hours preoperatively.

Postoperative Care. The nurse is responsible for monitoring the patient to determine the adequacy of blood flow and other complications following surgery. It is helpful if the distal pulses are marked on the skin with ink, since they are sometimes difficult to localize. Pulse, blood pressure, and renal output are important measures of patient status. Bleeding and emboli are the main complications following aortic repair. Homan's sign (pain on dorsiflexion of the foot) might indicate a blood clot in the calf. The patient should not have pillows under the knees or have the knee gatch raised, as pressure may increase the possibility of clotting. The patient may wear thromboembolic stockings.

The nurse should be alert for such signs of hemorrhage as increase in pulse rate, decreasing blood pressure, anxiety, restlessness, pallor, cyanosis and thirst. Oliguria, clammy skin, and venous collapse occur later. The patient's alertness and consciousness must be checked regularly. In surgery on the ascending aorta, a thrombolic occlusion of a major artery feeding the brain is an emergency. Occlusion of a cerebral vessel for a few minutes may cause irreparable damage to the brain!

Coronary occlusion may cause chest pain, increased central venous pressure, shortness of breath, pallor, and apprehension. In surgery of the thoracic aorta, interruption of the blood flow to the lumbosacral area of the spinal cord may result in weakness or paralysis of the lower extremities, which may appear as long as 72 hours after surgery. If spinal shock occurs, there may be a very low diastolic blood pressure, paralytic ileus, mesenteric emboli, and atony of the bladder. Cardiac and respiratory failure may follow. Distention of the neck veins and a rising central venous pressure may indicate left heart failure.

In abdominal aorta surgery, the nurse should observe for abdominal distention, bowel sounds, and rigidity. Vital signs need to be continually checked for signs of hemorrhage and shock. Urinary output must be monitored. There may be injury to adjacent veins, bleeding from the graft, injury to the ureters, ileus, and necrosis of the sigmoid colon.[6]

The patient must be helped to take deep breaths, must be turned, and must be encouraged to cough vigorously every hour if there is a long thoracotomy incision. Suctioning may be used if coughing is not successful. It is important to instruct patients about the necessity and method of coughing prior to surgery.

Home Care After Peripheral Vascular Surgery. Most patients with aneurysm repair will not require home visits, but individuals who have healing incisions from arterial reconstruction and ulcers on the heel or lower leg because of poor circulation will need home visits. The nurse may instruct the patient in wound and ulcer care, early identification of complications, safety, ambulation, diet, and continuity of care. Providing the family with a readily available source of consultation by telephone may identify and resolve concerns.[43] Home care leaflets are published by the American Heart Association that give helpful guides for home care following vascular surgery.

BIBLIOGRAPHY (Chapter 48)

1. Atchison, J. S., and J. Murray: Post-vascular surgery — When happiness can be a warm foot. *Nursing 78*, 8:36, Dec. 1978.
2. Barnes, R. W.: Axioms on acute arterial occlusion of an extremity. *Hospital Medicine*, 14:34, June 1978.
3. Barnes, R. W.: Diagnosing vascular disease with noninvasive tests. *Consultant*, 17:56, Dec. 1978.
4. Baron, H. C.: Chronic arterial insufficiency of the lower limbs. *Hospital Medicine*, 14:33, Sept. 1978.
5. Blowup in the arteries. *Time*, p. 85, July 1978.

6. Bordicks, K. J.: Nursing implications. *Nursing Digest*, p. 8, Sept.–Oct., 1973.
7. Bouhout, J., et al.: Unilateral Raynaud's phenomenon in the hand. *Surgery*, 82:547, Nov. 1977.
8. Cobey, J., and J. H. Cobey: Chronic leg ulcers. *American Journal of Nursing*, 74:258, Feb. 1974.
9. Conn, H. L., Jr., and O. Horowitz: *Cardiac and Vascular Disease*. Vol. II. Philadelphia: Lea and Febiger, 1971.
10. Connors, P.: Treating leg ulcers. *Nursing 77*, 7:66, May 1977.
11. Dallen, J. E.: Diseases of the aorta. *In* Thorne, G. W., et al. (Eds.): *Harrison's Principles of Internal Medicine,* 8th ed. New York: McGraw-Hill Co., Inc., 1977.
12. Deykin, D.: Antithrombotic therapy. *Postgraduate Medicine*, 65:135, Jan. 1979.
13. Dunphy, J. E., and L. W. Way: *Current Surgical Diagnosis and Treatment*, 3rd ed. Los Altos, Calif.: Lange Medical Publications, 1977.
14. Fagan-Dubin, L.: Atherosclerosis: A major cause of peripheral vascular disease. *Nursing Clinics of North America*, 12:101, Mar. 1977.
15. Fairbairn, J. F., II; *Peripheral Vascular Diseases*, 4th ed. Philadelphia: W. B. Saunders Co., 1972.
16. Fenn, J. E.: Reconstructive arterial surgery for ischemic lower extremities. *Nursing Clinics of North America*, 12:129, Mar. 1977.
17. Friedman, S. A.: Guide to diagnosis of peripheral arterial disease. *Hospital Medicine*, 15:87, Jan. 1979.
18. Garrett, W. V., and R. W. Barnes: Degenerative arterial disease. *In* Conn, H. F. (Ed.): *Current Therapy 1978*, Philadelphia: W. B. Saunders Co., 1978.
19. Hazzard, W. R.: A pathophysiologic approach to managing hyperlipemia. *American Family Physician*, 14:78, Aug. 1976.
20. Hertzer, N. R.: Abdominal aortic aneurysm: Guide to diagnosis and management. *Hospital Medicine*, 15:65, Mar. 1979.
21. Hertzer, N. R.: Surgical management of intermittent claudication. *American Family Physician*, 16:108, Sept. 1977.
22. Jackson, D. R.: How to treat peripheral artery disease. *Consultant*, 17:105, Sept. 1977.
23. Jurgens, J. L., et al.: Arteriosclerosis obliterans. *Circulation*, 21:188, 1960.
24. Karmody, A. M.: Three lifelines for a broken lifeline. *Emergency Medicine*, 9:210, Oct. 1977.
25. Kessro, B.: Peripheral arterial insufficiency — Postoperative nursing care. *Nursing Clinics of North America*, 12:143, Mar. 1977.
26. Lang, G. D.: Managing the patient with abdominal aortic aneurysm. *Nursing 78*, 8:24, Aug. 1978.
27. Lennihan, R., and M. Mackereth: Proper evaluation of intermittent claudication. *Consultant*, 17:193, Oct. 1977.
28. Lukweg, W. C. Jr., and L. J. Grandfield: Vascular prosthetic infections: Collected experience and results of treatment. *Surgery*, 82:335, Mar. 1977.
29. Margolis, I. B., and D. Hayes: Managing peripheral vascular disease secondary to arteriosclerosis. *Geriatrics*, 32:75, June 1977.
30. Malone, J. M., et al.: Life expectancy following aortofemoral arterial grafting. *Surgery*, 82:551, May 1977.
30a. Mannick, J. A., and J. D. Coffman: *Ischemic Limbs; Surgical Approach and Physiological Principles*. New York: Grune and Stratton, 1973.
31. Miller, K. M.: Assessing peripheral perfusion. *American Journal of Nursing*, 8:1673, Oct. 1978.
32. Mullen, D. C.: Abdominal aortic aneurysm. *Hospital Medicine*, 12:60, Aug. 1976.
33. Nemir, P. Jr., and R. C. Vrachnos: The surgical management of abdominal aneurysms. *Hospital Medicine*, 12:40, Jan. 1976.
34. On blue toes. *Emergency Medicine*, 9:113, Mar. 1977.
35. Peripheral vascular disease — A diagnostic guide. *Emergency Medicine*, 9:127, Jan. 1977.
36. Pierce, P. F.: Gains and losses of vascular surgery patients. *Nursing Clinics of North America*, 12:119, Mar. 1977.
37. Ream, I.: Counseling patients with leg pain; a review of peripheral vascular disease. *Nursing 77*, 7:54, Oct. 1977.
38. Reich, R.: Cyclandelate: Effect on circulatory measurement and exercise tolerance in chronic arterial insufficiency of the lower limbs. *Journal of the American Geriatric Society*, 25:202, 1977.
39. Richards, R. L.: *Peripheral Arterial Disease*. Baltimore: Williams and Wilkins Co., 1970.
40. Robbins, S. L., and R. S. Cotran: *Pathologic Basis of Disease*, 2nd ed. Philadelphia: W. B. Saunders Co., 1979.
41. Rodman, M. J.: Thromboembolic disorders: Part 2. Arterial thrombosis and embolism. *RN*, 39:61, July 1976.
42. Roenigk, H. H., Jr.: Leg ulcers in the elderly. *Geriatrics*, 34:21, July 1979.
43. Rose, M. A.: Home care after peripheral vascular surgery. *American Journal of Nursing*, 74:260, Feb. 1974.
44. Royster, T. S., et al.: Peripheral arterial disease. *Postgraduate Medicine*, 62:153, Nov. 1977.
45. Ryzewski, J.: Factors in the rehabilitation of patients with peripheral vascular disease. *Nursing Clinics of North America*, 12:161, Mar. 1977.
46. Seminar on vascular disorders. *The Practitioner*, May 1977.
47. Sexton, D. L.: The patient with peripheral arterial occlusive disease. *Nursing Clinics of North America*, 12:89, Mar. 1977.
48. Sounding the popliteals. *Emergency Medicine*, 9:67, Dec. 1977.
49. Taggart, E.: The physical assessment of the patient with arterial disease. *Nursing Clinics of North America*, 12:109, Mar. 1977.
50. Thorne, G. W., et al. (Eds.): *Harrison's Principles of Internal Medicine,* 8th ed. New York: McGraw-Hill Book Co., Inc., 1977.
51. Witkowski, J. A., and L. C. Parish: Leg ulcer: Treat the cause, too. *Consultant,* 16:83, Aug. 1976.
52. Wheat, M. W.: Acute dissecting aneurysms. *Emergency Medicine,* 9:137, June 1977.

CHAPTER 49

DISEASES OF THE VEINS AND LYMPHATICS

This chapter provides an overview of the following general concepts: (1) the physiology of the veins pertinent to understanding their dysfunction, (2) the main causes of venous dysfunction, (3) the effects of venous dysfunction on the body, and (4) nursing interventions by which venous dysfunction can be eliminated or minimized.

PHYSIOLOGY OF THE VEINS

The veins function as channels to transport blood from the capillaries to the right side of the heart. The veins are low pressure, high volume reservoirs. The venous pressure in the recumbent person is approximately 13 mm. Hg in the foot and approximately 3 mm. Hg in the right atrium. The veins contain 70 to 80 per cent of the total blood volume. The veins are very distensible because of their thin, elastic walls sparsely covered with vascular smooth muscle. Therefore, for small changes in pressure, there is a large change in volume. For example, a rise of 1 mm. Hg may increase the capacity of a vein three times; a rise of 10 mm. Hg increases the volume six times. Beyond this pressure level, the venous wall becomes progressively stiffer and does not expand as much with further increases in pressure.

What is regulated in the venous system and how is it regulated? The relationship between pressure and volume or compliance ($\Delta V/\Delta P$) is regulated in one of two ways — actively or passively. *Active* regulation is by neurogenic venoconstriction caused by the alpha adrenergic nerves. "Alpha receptors" in veins vary from region to region. The skin and splanchnic veins are the most densely innervated. However, the muscle veins have little or no active regulation by sympathetic venoconstriction. *Passive* regulation of venous volume takes place by a reduced distending pressure in the vein. As the distending pressure falls below the level necessary to hold the vein in a rounded shape, the vein collapses from elastic recoil of the wall, causing a major fraction of volume to be passively dispelled.

Valves of the Veins. Veins that carry blood against the force of gravity are usually equipped with valves. Valves are most common in the veins of the lower extremities. The venae cavae and the portal, cerebral, intra-abdominal, and pulmonary veins do not have valves. Functioning valves permit venous flow only toward the heart and from the superficial to the deep veins. Valves break the hydrostatic column of blood and reduce the hydrodynamic load in the propulsion of blood toward the heart. A valve consists of two frail cusps composed of endothelial folds. The competence and function of the valves depend on the normal integrity of the vein wall.

Effects of Posture on Venous Pressure and Volume. In the recumbent position, the pressure gradient between the peripheral venous circulation (approximately 10 to 15 mm. Hg) and right atrium (approximately 3 mm. Hg) is the major driving force for propulsion of the blood. The valves will restrict blood flow to one direction. Inspiration facilitates the flow of blood into the right atrium; expiration decreases the inflow. The most negative intrathoracic pressures occur during inspiration. This negative pressure tends to increase the transmural pressure of the thoracic vena cava. The elevated transmural pressure distends the lumen facilitating influx of blood into the thorax and right atrium. If intrathoracic pressure is increased by contraction of the thoracic muscles, as in forced expiration, lifting a heavy weight, or the Valsalva maneuver, the intrathoracic pressure will rise enough to compress the vena cava. Initially this will increase the blood flow to the right atrium and later prevent inflow of blood into the thorax.

In the upright position, the venous return of blood from the lower limb to the heart depends almost entirely on the contraction of the calf muscles. When the muscle of a leg is contracted, the muscle presses against the veins of the leg so that the veins are compressed. Blood tends to flow away from the areas of compression toward the heart. This pumping action is called the "muscle pump." When a person is standing still, the "muscle pump" does not work and the venous pressures in the lower part of the leg rise.

Why do distal venous pressures increase in the upright position? When a person stands up, a continuous hydrostatic column develops from the heart level to the foot. The venous valves remain open because the flow is essentially unidirectional. Therefore, the pressure in the veins of the foot will be equal to the weight of the hydrostatic column of blood between the foot and the level of the atria. This is defined by the equation $P=\rho gh$, where P=pressure; ρ=rho, a constant for density of blood; g=force of gravity; and h=height of the column. The venous pressure in the foot would therefore be approximately 80 mm. Hg in the upright position. This increase in venous capillary pressure results in decreased reabsorption of fluid from the tissues into the capillaries, and edema tends to develop (see Chapter 12). The increased volume of blood trapped in the distal veins can be mobilized by skeletal muscular activity, either exercise or isometric contraction of the leg muscles. After taking only 7 to 10 steps, the venous pressure at the ankle level can return to normal levels of 10 to 15 mm. Hg because the continuous hydrostatic column has been broken by the muscular contraction and the closure of the valves.

In summary, muscular pumping action, as occurs in walking or isometric exercise, has two important functions: (1) it lowers the venous and capillary hydrostatic pressures, thereby preventing edema, and (2) it reduces the volume of blood contained within the veins of the legs and facilitates the return of blood to the right heart. This is ultimately reflected in maintaining left cardiac output and arterial blood pressure. In the upright position the force of gravity opposes the return of blood to the heart. If the feet are elevated above the heart in the supine position, blood flow to the heart is facilitated by the force of gravity.

VENOUS INSUFFICIENCY

Venous insufficiency is caused by *incompetency of the valves* of the leg veins. Varicose veins are due to incompetent valves in the *superficial* veins. Leg ulcers or stasis ulcers are due to incompetent valves in the *perforating* veins. Valvular incompetence of the deep veins is more serious because it can lead to the postphlebitic syndrome.

Pathophysiology. Frequently the valves of the venous system are defective. This incompetency occurs when the veins have been overstretched by an excess of venous pressure for a prolonged period of time, as occurs in pregnancy, obesity, or an occupation that requires standing for long periods. The vein walls are weaker than those of the arteries. After prolonged periods of pressure they distend, preventing the leaflets of the valves from closing tightly and thus making them incompetent. Therefore, the valves will not block reverse flow in the dilated veins. Owing to this valvular incompetency there is venous stasis and increased venous pressure. The "venous pump," or the compression of the deep veins by skeletal muscle, cannot pump blood effectively to reduce the elevated venous pressure that results from the standing position. The high venous pressure results in increased hydrostatic pressure in the capillary, preventing reabsorption of fluid into the capillary from the tissues and promoting edema.

VENOUS LEG ULCERS

Venous leg ulcers or stasis ulcers are due to incompetence of valves in the perforating veins. The perforating veins connect the deep veins to the superficial veins. During exercise in the upright position, the high pressure produced by the contraction of muscle in the deep veins is transmitted to the superficial veins. In the presence of incompetent perforating vein valves over a period of many years, the high pressure causes rupture of the small skin veins and venules, resulting in stasis ulcers. Extravasation of red blood cells occurs into the surrounding subcutaneous tissues. The red blood cells disintegrate, leaving a deposit of hemosiderin that stains the tissues a characteristic brownish color. This pigmentation is usually noted on the distal third of the lower extremity and the malleolar areas. Thus, the subcutaneous hemorrhage leads to pigmentation, subcutaneous fibrosis, cutaneous atrophy, and lymphatic obstruction. All these chronic changes contribute to the development of stasis ulcers, characteristically located in the malleolar area. Figures 49–1 and 49–2 show examples of pigmentation and stasis dermatitis (in varicose veins) resulting from chronic venous insufficiency. Once the skin is broken, infection occurs, usually due to either staphylococcus or streptococcus.

VARICOSE VEINS

Varicose veins are abnormally lengthened, dilated, tortuous, superficial veins whose *valves are incompetent*. The greater and lesser saphenous veins are most commonly involved. The pathophysiology of varicose veins is related to the disturbances in hemodynamics that result from the incompetency of the valves of the

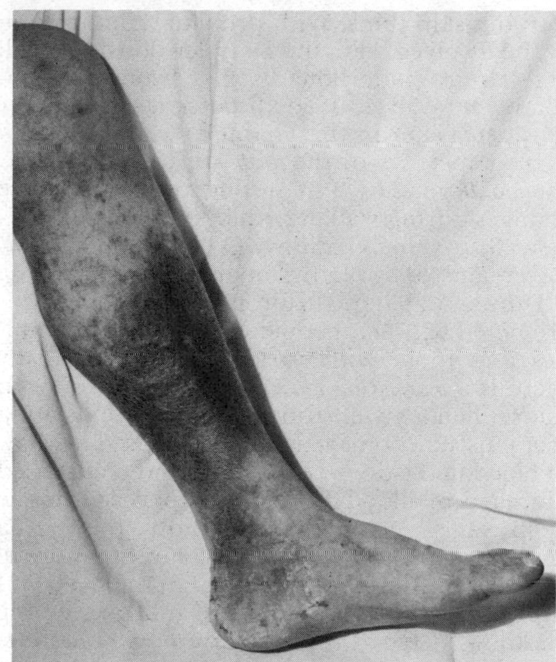

Figure 49–1. Pigmentation of leg resulting from chronic venous insufficiency of long standing. (From Fairbairn, J. F., II, J. L. Juergens, and J. A. Spittell, Jr.: *Allen-Barker-Hines Peripheral Vascular Diseases,* 4th ed. Philadelphia: W. B. Saunders Co., 1972.)

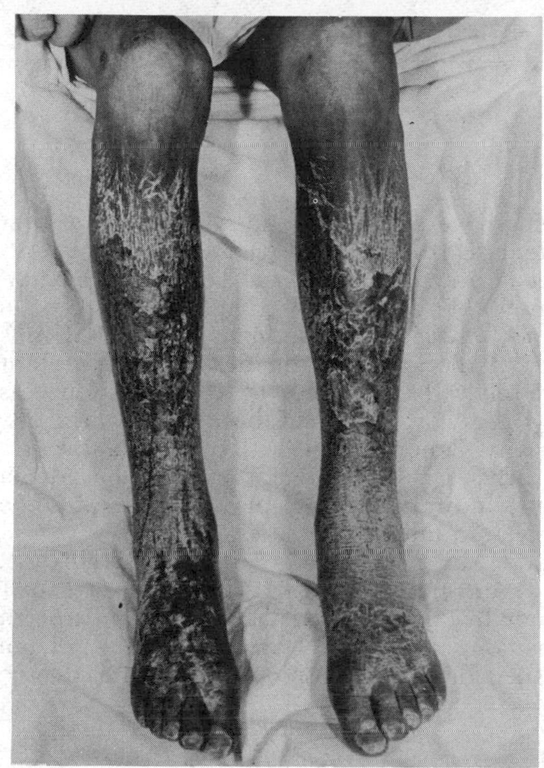

Figure 49–2. Stasis dermatitis in varicose veins of the lower extremity. (From Robbins, S. L., and R. S. Cotran: *Pathologic Basis of Disease,* 2nd ed. Philadelphia: W. B. Saunders Co., 1979.)

major superficial veins. A comparison of a normally functioning venous system and an incompetent venous system complicated by varicosities is given in Figure 49–3.

Varicose veins are a fairly common problem in our society, affecting an estimated 10 per cent of the adult population. Furthermore, 40 to 50 per cent of adults may have minor varicosities of the lower limbs that do not produce symptoms but are unsightly. Persons in occupations that require long periods of standing (e.g., police, operating room nurses, cooks, dentists) are particularly affected by varicosities.

The pathogenesis of varicose veins is unknown. Genetic factors are important but are poorly understood. Possibly there may be a primary weakness in the walls of the veins or a congenital lack of valves. External factors such as prolonged standing, obesity, pregnancy, and extreme height aggravate the condition.

Varicose veins may be either primary or secondary. *Primary* varicose veins occur in the absence of deep venous insufficiency and usually are uncomplicated except for a cosmetic deformity. *Secondary* varicosities occur because of obstruction and valvular incompetence of the deep veins. Secondary varicosities are usually due to thrombophlebitis (postphlebitic syndrome) but can also be secondary to acquired or congenital arteriovenous fistulas and extrinsic pressure, such as from a tumor, on the inferior vena cava or iliofemoral veins.

Assessment of Patient with Varicose Veins. Many persons with dilated, tortuous skin

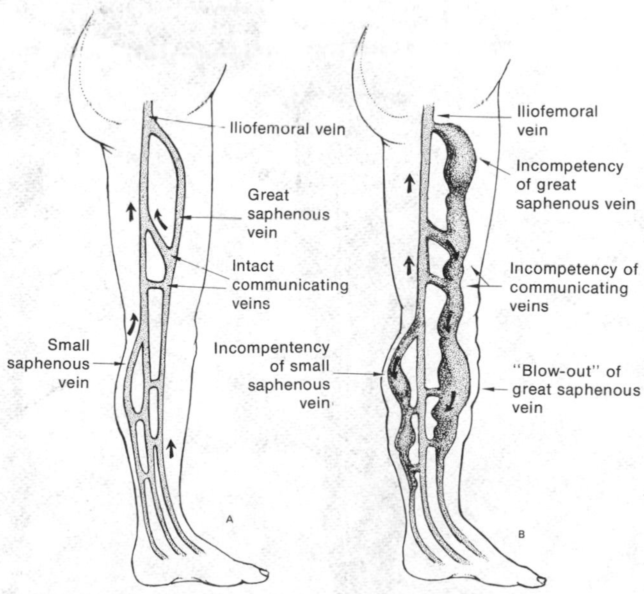

Figure 49–3. **A.** Diagram of the venous circulation of the healthy lower limb. Note that the blood ascends in both the superficial and deep systems and in health the blood passes into the deep veins via the communicating veins. **B.** Varicosities produced in the superficial venous system as a result of incompetency of the valves in the communicating veins. In both drawings the arrows indicate the flow of blood in the superficial and deep systems and in the communicating veins. (Adapted from Abramson, D. I.: *Vascular Disorders of the Extremities,* 2nd ed. New York: Harper & Row, 1974, p. 514.)

veins have minimal or no symptoms, not even edema of the leg. The venous pump may not fail if only the superficial veins are incompetent. Other people may complain of diffuse dull aches, muscle cramps, and fatigability of muscles of the lower extremities. These symptoms are relieved by elevation of the leg, thus increasing the flow of blood back to the heart by gravity. Other patients with concomitant venous insufficiency of the deep veins exhibit edematous, indurated, scaly, pigmented, and sometimes ulcerated extremities.

The diagnosis of *primary* varicose veins (i.e., only incompetent superficial veins) is usually made by (a) inspection of the legs in the upright position, and (b) the Doppler flowmeter. Upon inspection the varicosities will appear as dilated, tortuous skin veins. With proximal compression of the involved vein, the Doppler flowmeter will detect retrograde flow distally through the incompetent valves. (See discussion of Doppler flowmeter later in this chapter.)

Incompetency of the *deep* and *superficial veins* can be *diagnosed* (1) by noting venous pressure changes during walking, (2) by Trendelenburg's test, (3) by phlebography, (4) by Doppler flowmeter, and (5) by plethysmography.

During walking, different venous pressures are noted between people with normal extremities and those with varicose veins. Normally there is a *marked decrease* in venous pressure in the saphenous vein during walking, indicating that muscular contraction has increased the flow of blood in the deep veins and allowed increased drainage of blood from the superficial to the deep veins. When exercise stops there is a *gradual return* of venous pressure to normal levels, indicating that the valves in the deep and superficial veins are closing and preventing backflow of blood. *Extremities with varicose veins have less of a decrease in venous pressure during*

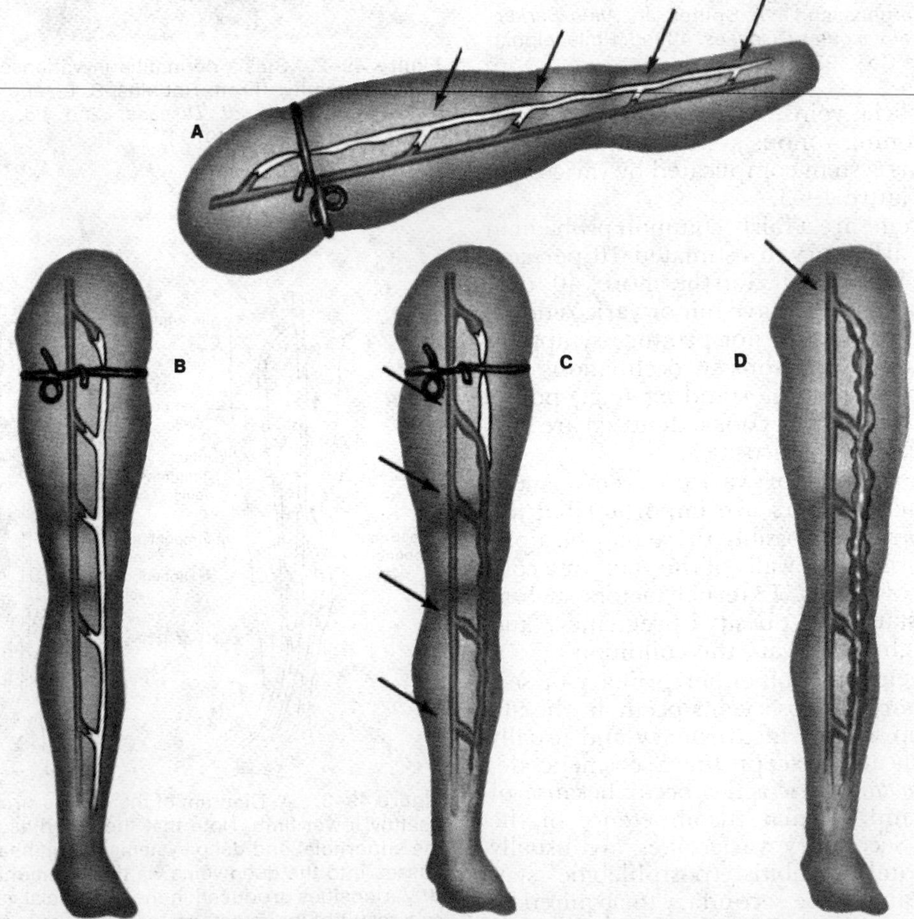

Figure 49–4. Trendelenburg test. **A.** With the leg elevated, the superficial veins empty by gravity and then a tourniquet is applied at the groin. **B.** Normal patient is standing upright with superficial venous system remaining empty; valves of the communicating veins are intact. **C.** Varicosities fill within 30 seconds, owing to incompetence of the communicating veins. **D.** Upon release of the tourniquet, veins become further distended, indicating incompetence at the saphenous-femoral junction. (From Weintraub, A. M., and M. N. Gomes: Varicose veins. *American Family Physician,* 13:110, Mar. 1976.)

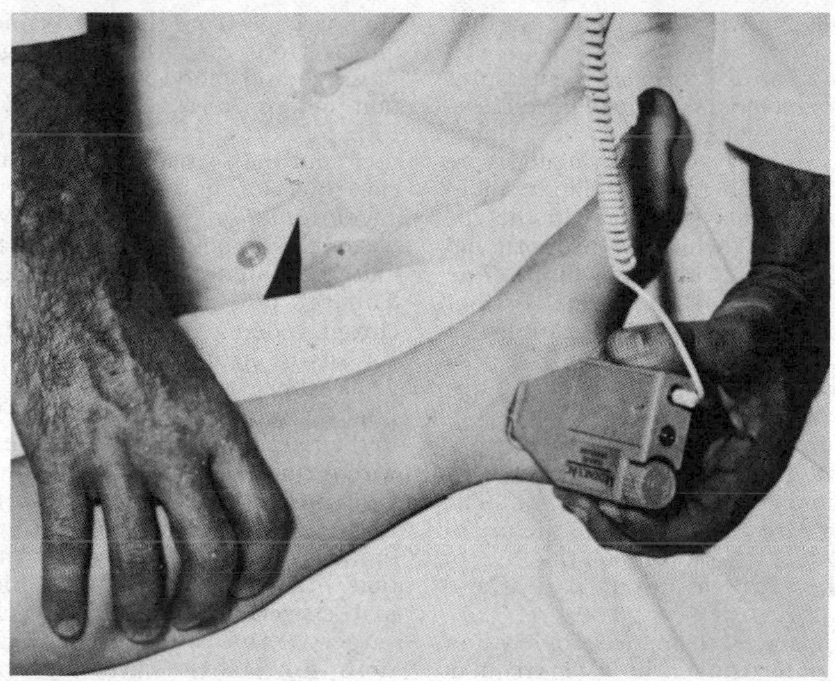

Figure 49–5. Doppler ultrasound transducer being used in screening for major deep vein thrombosis. Some of the newer Doppler instruments are even smaller than the one shown here, being no larger or thicker than a pen. (From Barnes, R. W.: Diagnosing vascular disease with noninvasive tests. *Consultant*, 18:57, Dec. 1978.)

walking and, upon cessation of walking, have a more rapid return to normal pressure. Because of incompetent valves between the saphenous and deep veins, there is incomplete emptying of the saphenous veins during muscle contraction, and when walking ceases, the superficial veins, because of their incompetent valves, fill very rapidly.

Backward flow of blood through incompetent valves into the saphenous vein can be shown with Trendelenburg's test, also called the *retrograde filling test*. The person being tested is put in the recumbent position with the affected leg raised above the heart, thus emptying the veins (Fig. 49–4). Then a tourniquet is applied around the leg to occlude the superficial veins. The person then stands and the tourniquet is taken off. If the valves of the superficial veins are incompetent, the varicose veins distend *very quickly* with the backflow of blood held by the tourniquet. To assess the deep vein system the tourniquet is placed on the thigh while the person is standing, thus filling the veins. He or she is told to lie down with the legs elevated. The emptying of blood from the superficial veins indicates that the deep venous system is patent.

In phlebography, 50 ml. of angiographic contrast material is injected into the deep and/or superficial veins. Overhead radiographs are then taken while the person performs various leg movements and exercises. Both normal and abnormal veins as well as the cusps of the valves can be visualized.

The Doppler ultrasound probe or flowmeter is a noninvasive method to determine blood flow in the larger blood vessels as well as the patency of vessels. The Doppler probe is a small instrument that contains a piezoelectric crystal to transmit sound and another crystal to receive backscattered sound signals. (See Figure 49–5 for a picture of a Doppler transducer.) The Doppler probe determines blood flow in this way: (1) it emits a beam of ultrasound into the patient's tissues, (2) the sound wave is reflected from moving erythrocytes, (3) the *difference* in the frequency of the transmitted sound and the reflected sound is called the *Doppler shift or effect,* which depends upon red blood cell velocity and is proportional to blood flow, (4) the reflected ultrasound is amplified by the Doppler as an audible signal or a recorded analogue wave. If the Doppler flowmeter is placed over the femoral, popliteal, or saphenous vein and the calf or thigh is compressed, a large surge of venous blood will be evident if the peripheral venous system is patent and the valves are competent. A diagnosis of valvular incompetence in the femoral, saphenous, or popliteal veins is based on the demonstration of retrograde flow following calf or thigh compression. No blood flow will be heard after calf or thigh compression because the blood will flow back through incompetent valves.[2] In the vertical position, the demonstration of a reverse flow occurring during expiration, enhanced by the Valsalva maneuver, is diagnostic of valvular incompetence.

The *plethysmographic technique* measures changes in venous blood volume. The plethysmograph apparatus consists of a thin rubber tube filled with mercury or an insulated wire that is wrapped around the limb. Plethysmography graphically displays changes in the circumference of the legs, which are proportional to changes of volume within the limbs. The difficulty with these measurements is that slight movements from the patient can distort the record and given false readings. These methods are discussed further later in this chapter.

Nursing Intervention and Treatment. Patients with venous insufficiency cannot be cured but can be maintained in optimal health. The goals of nursing care are to promote the use of antigravity measures, to promote the use of elastic support hose, to reassure the patient, and to prevent leg ulcers.

Antigravity measures to increase blood flow from the veins to the heart include: (1) frequent elevation of the legs above the heart level, (2) avoiding prolonged standing or sitting, crossed legs, beds gatched at the knee, chairs that are too high for the patient's feet to touch the floor or that are too deep, placing pressure on the popliteal area, and (3) avoiding sources that would increase pressure above the legs, such as tight girdles and round garters. Note that blood flows from a higher to lower pressure, and if the intra-abdominal pressure is greater than the pressure in the extremities, there will be an impediment of venous flow and dilatation of leg veins. The patient should sleep with the foot of the bed elevated 6 inches by placement of blocks under the leg of the bed. At least one third of every 24 hours should be spent with the feet and legs elevated.

Increased venous pressure on the surface of the leg can be counteracted by the compression of elastic support hose. Ideally this support should just balance the increased pressure. Thus, since in the standing position there is more pressure at the ankle than just below the knee, the stocking should be fitted individually to the patient's legs. Measurements are usually taken of the circumference at the ankle and calf, and from 1 inch below the knee or 1 inch below the groin to the bottom of the foot. Measurements are taken after the patient has been recumbent to reduce edema. Stockings that extend above the knee often bind the popliteal space and act as a tourniquet, especially when the knee is bent; knee-length elastic stockings are preferable.

Many patients fear rupture of varicose veins with massive hemorrhage. This is an uncommon complication. Should it occur, the patient should be reassured that there is time to get to the hospital before bleeding to death is likely. Hemorrhage from the veins is not so threatening as from the arteries owing to the lower pressure and blood flow in the veins. In addition, hemostasis is achieved by vascular spasm, formation of a platelet "plug," blood coagulation, and the formation of fibrous tissue in the clot, thus closing the rupture in the vein.

Vein Ligation. When surgery of the superficial veins is being considered, the deep veins must be patent, as demonstrated by Trendelenburg's test; otherwise, the patient will have chronic edema and discomfort. The surgery consists of ligating the saphenous vein at the groin where it joins the femoral vein and stripping the saphenous vein system from the groin to the ankle. An incision is made in the ankle; a wire is threaded through the lumen of the vein from groin to ankle; then the wire together with the vein is pulled from the groin incision. The branches of the vein break off near their junction with the saphenous vein. Bleeding is minimal, especially if the legs are elevated during surgery. Some surgeons make additional incisions to remove varicosities of the smaller branches of veins.

Following surgery, the legs are wrapped with a pressure bandage evenly from foot to thigh. This bandage is left untouched until the seventh day, when the stitches are removed. The three most important postoperative objectives for the first week are (1) maintenance of firm elastic pressure over the whole limb, (2) promotion of regular movement and exercise of the legs, and (3) elevation of the foot of the bed 6 to 9 inches so that the legs are above the heart level when the patient is in bed. The patient gets up for short periods of active walking starting 24 to 48 hours after surgery. Before walking, the calf and knee are wrapped in extra firm elastic bandages put on over the original bandage to counteract the high venous pressure. The patient is told not to stand still or to sit. After walking he or she gets back into bed with feet up. On the seventh day, the stitches are removed and the patient usually goes home. Elastic bandages and active walking exercises are usually necessary for 3 weeks after leaving the hospital. In cases of ankle perforating vein exploration, support for an additional 2 weeks may be necessary. Elderly persons need support for a longer time. The beneficial effect of surgery upon severe varicosities is dramatically illustrated in Figure 49–6.

Complications following varicose vein surgery are hemorrhage, infection, nerve damage, and deep vein thrombosis.

The most common site for *bleeding* is the *wound in the groin* following high ligature and stripping. It is retrograde bleeding from the stripped canal. Usually, careful wrapping of the leg from foot to groin and compression applied especially to the upper thigh and groin will decrease the risk of serious bleeding. Some discoloration and bruising along the stripper track are normal. One week after stripping, the patient's leg looks "black and blue." It is important to warn the patient about this to avoid alarm.

Nerve damage involving the *saphenous nerve* may develop following venous surgery. In the distal third of the leg, the saphenous nerve has a very close relation to the saphenous vein. If the distal third of the saphenous vein is stripped by a bulky stripper head, some temporary or permanent nerve damage occurs. A feeling of "pins and needles" with hypersensitivity to touch occurs in the area. If the damage is temporary,

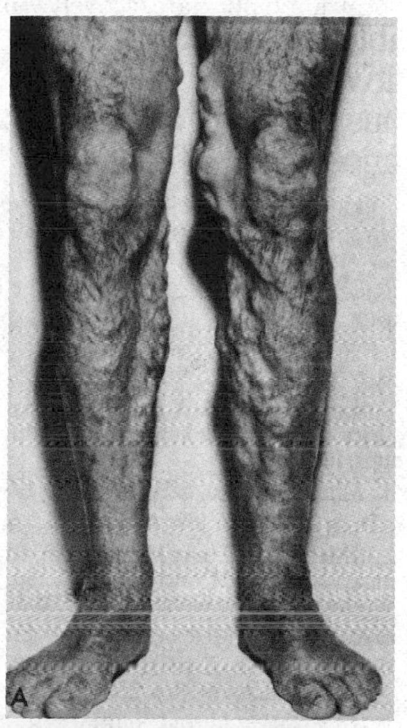

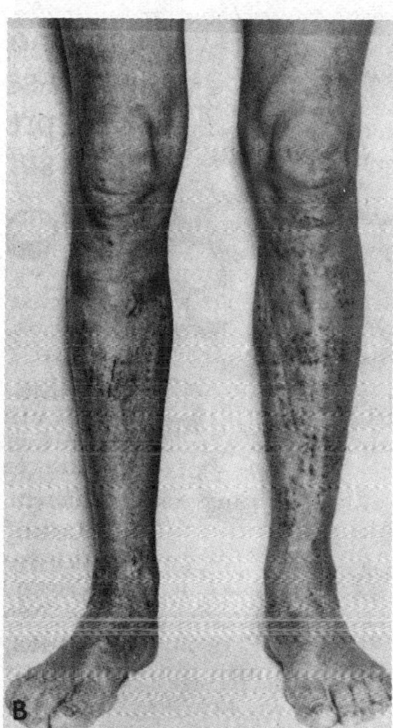

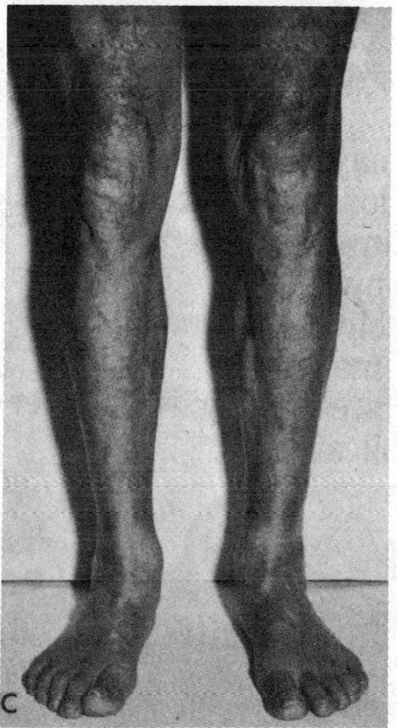

Figure 49–6. Extensive varicosities (incompetency of greater saphenous systems). **A.** Appearance preoperatively. **B.** Two weeks postoperatively. **C.** Fifteen years postoperatively. (*A* and *B* from Lofgren K. A.: Varicose veins. *In* Haimovici, H. (Ed.): *Vascular Surgery: Principles and Techniques*. New York, McGraw-Hill Book Co., 1976. Used by permission of publisher. *C* from Lofgren, K. A.: Varicose veins: Their symptoms, complications and management. *Postgraduate Medicine,* 65:131, June 1979.)

the symptoms last 2 to 3 weeks and normal sensation returns. If there is permanent damage, the symptoms change to a central area of anesthesia with a peripheral zone of hypersensitivity. This is loosely called "saphenous neuritis."

Deep vein thrombosis and embolism are no more frequent after these operations than they are after surgery in general. Indeed, if all the postoperative precautions (bandaging, movement, exercise) are taken, thrombosis should be less frequent. *Infection* is rare following venous stripping.

Sclerosant Injection. Sclerosing solutions such as 5 per cent sodium morrhuate or 1 to 3 per cent sodium tetradecyl sulfate (Sodium Sotradecol) or ethanolamine oleate are injected into the vein, producing a localized phlebitis and thrombosis of the veins. Sclerotherapy is palliative, not curative. It can successfully close unsightly tortuous skin veins (spider bursts) for the cosmetic gratification of the patient (see Fig. 49–7). One of the best applications of sclerotherapy is to close off annoying residual superficial veins *after* vein ligation. The slcerosing agent is contraindicated during vein surgery owing to risk of deep vein thrombosis. Within minutes after injection, elastic compression and active walking should be promoted. Elastic bandages are worn for about 6 weeks.

Treatment of Varicose Ulcers. The main principles in controlling varicose ulcers are (1) to control the abnormal venous hypertension caused by the incompetent perforating veins, and (2) to clear and control infection.

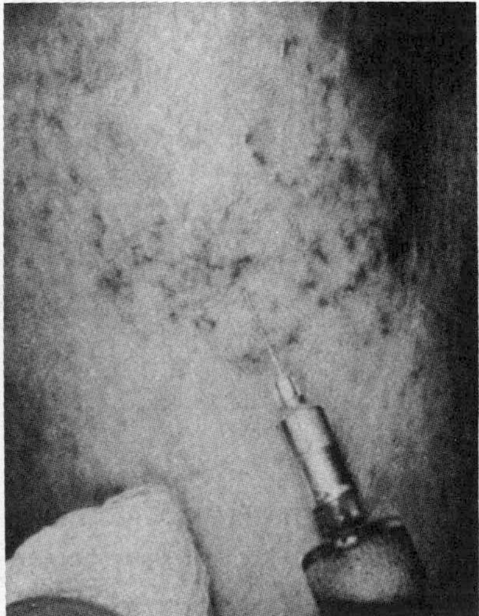

Figure 49–7. Spider burst being injected with foamy sclerosing solution. (From Lofgren, K. A.: Varicose veins: Their symptoms, complications and management. *Postgraduate Medicine,* 65:131, June 1979.)

Controlling venous hypertension can be achieved by elastic compression bandaging and by bed rest with the feet elevated above the level of the heart. When elastic bandaging is used to control ulcers, the bandage must be strong enough to counteract the very high venous pressure (80 to 100 mm. Hg) efficiently. A light elastic stocking will not do; only a heavy webbing elastic bandage will achieve this.

Almost all ointments, creams, powders, and local antibiotics are actively *harmful* to ulcers. They contribute to skin sensitivity problems, which complicates healing of the ulcer. Therefore, sepsis is treated not with local antibiotics but with oral antibiotics. Antibiotics specific for the offending organism are started after cultures have been taken from the ulcer. Clean the ulcer with sterile normal saline or boric acid. Then place a piece of nonadherent gauze (such as Terylene) followed by four layers of dry gauze over the ulcer. The elastic bandage is then put on from the toes to just below the knee. During the night or when the patient is in bed, the ulcer can be exposed to air.

Three big don'ts need to be emphasized in the care of leg ulcer:

- ▶ *Don't* use dressings that exclude air. These dressings stop evaporation, thus making the skin moist and soggy — a condition that is an ideal culture medium for bacterial growth.
- ▶ *Don't* use antibiotic creams or paraffin gauze impregnated with sulfa drugs. They increase the risk of skin allergies that are difficult to control.
- ▶ *Don't* use steroid ointments. They are anti-inflammatory and prevent healing.

In some instances an *Elastoplast boot* can be applied so the patient can be ambulatory. Other types of bandaging are Unna's paste boot and the zinc gelatin bandage. After 1 or 2 days of bed rest in order to decrease the edema, the boot is applied from the distal metatarsal level to the knee. At first it may be necessary to change the boot every 3 to 4 days because of edema and in order to cleanse the ulcer. But as the edema decreases and the ulcer heals, the boot can be changed every week.

Healing can be hastened by applying skin grafts after the ulcer has become clean and granulation has started. If the arterial blood supply is not obstructed, healing usually occurs quickly.

Occurrence of leg ulcers should be prevented by the wearing of elastic support hose, elevation of the feet and legs a certain portion of each day, the avoidance of extremes of heat and cold and of too tight shoes and stockings, and the wearing of a foam rubber pad around the ulcer-bearing region, around and above the malleolus. This area tends to be very sensitive to trauma because the underlying venous insufficiency is still present.

THROMBOPHLEBITIS AND PHLEBOTHROMBOSIS

Thrombophlebitis is inflammation of a venous wall with clot formation. Phlebothrombosis is clot formation in the vein without or followed secondarily by inflammation. It is difficult to tell in some patients which condition came first; after several days, inflammation and thrombus are coexistent. Throughout this discussion, we shall use the term "thrombophlebitis" to designate this group of conditions.

Pathophysiology. When a thrombus develops, the process begins locally by platelets coming into contact with a damaged vessel wall and adhering to the endothelium. Where the platelets adhere to the collagen, adenosine diphosphate (ADP) is released. ADP is also released from the damaged tissues and disrupted platelets. The ADP produces an aggregation of platelets which make up a "platelet plug." The platelets undergo "viscous metamorphosis" or structural degeneration. Thrombin is necessary for this viscous metamorphosis. Thrombin can come from extrinsic or intrinsic sources (note Fig. 49–8). Once viscous metamorphosis begins, the platelets release phospholipid platelet factor 3, which forms an intrinsic thromboplastin that acts on prothrombin to form thrombin. These thrombi build up by the coagulation of plasma. Thus, there will be erythrocytes, leukocytes, and platelets with fibrin strands throughout. Deep vein thrombi vary from 1 to 2 mm. in diameter to long tubular masses filling main veins. Small thrombi are found commonly in the pockets of the valves of the deep veins.

The newly formed venous thrombus has a "tail" that may become detached and give rise to a pulmonary embolism. Probably 24 to 48 hours after thrombus formation, the "tail" will undergo lysis or become organized, and adhere to the vessel wall. Thus, the risk of embolization is eliminated. As the thrombus becomes larger in diameter and length, it obstructs the veins. The inflammatory process can destroy the valves of the veins, thus initiating venous insufficiency.

If a thrombus occludes a major vein (e.g., femoral, iliac, inferior or superior vena cava, axillary, subclavian), the venous pressure rises in the distal limb, leading to engorgement of the veins with blood. Initially the edema is nonpitting because it is due to increased intravascular volume and venous pressure in the capillaries, which prevents resorption of fluid from the tissues into the capillaries. Eventually the increased venous and capillary pressures lead to increased transudation of fluid into the tissues, with the formation of pitting edema.

Usually there is little functional disturbance as a result of thrombophlebitis of the superficial veins (saphenous) and the deep small veins (femoral, tibial, and popliteal). Abundant collateral venous channels usually evolve to relieve the increased venous pressure and volume.

The pathogenesis of thrombus formation is usually attributed to venous stasis, hypercoagulability, and/or injury to the venous wall (Virchow's triad). It is thought that at least two of the three conditions must be present for thrombi to form.

Conditions that may cause *venous stasis* are varicose veins, obesity, surgery, pregnancy, *prolonged bed rest*, and congestive heart failure.

Conditions that may cause hypercoagulability are malignant neoplasms (especially visceral and ovarian tumors); blood dyscrasias that raise the platelet count, decrease fibrinolysis, increase the clotting factors or increase the viscosity of the blood; and oral contraceptive (anovulatory) drugs.

In light of recent research on hypercoagulability in the development of intravascular coagulation in patients who suffer from thromboembolism, there may be an alteration in the factors of the coagulation system (Fig. 49–8) or the fibrinolytic system (Fig. 49–9). Thus, a malfunc-

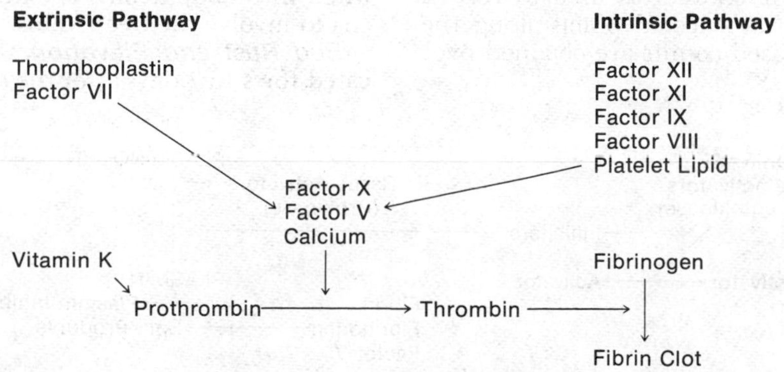

Figure 49–8. The factors of coagulation.

tion of one or both systems that would produce hypercoagulability and/or hypofibrinolysis could hypothetically produce widespread thrombosis.

Conditions that may cause *endothelial injury* are IV injections, thromboangiitis obliterans (Buerger's disease), fractures and dislocations, and chemical injury from slcerosing agents, opaque media for x-ray, and certain antibiotics such as chlortetracycline.

The divisions just mentioned are not strict. For example, postoperative venous thrombosis is probably due to slow venous flow during bed rest as well as vein wall injury due to tight strapping during surgery and to the activation of clotting factors in the postoperative period.

Assessment of the Patient with Thrombophlebitis. Table 49–1 gives a summary of the causative factors and signs and symptoms of thrombophlebitis of the superficial and deep veins.

Tests helpful in making the *diagnosis* of thrombophlebitis are phlebography, venous pressure measurements, isotope studies, ultrasonic flow detection and plethysmography.

Phlebography or venography was mentioned earlier in this chapter. Thrombi are identified as areas of radiolucency in opaque filled veins; lack of filling of a vein is indicative of venous occlusion due to a thrombus. Venography is the single most useful diagnostic device for confirming the presence of venous thrombosis.

Venous pressures can be taken easily in the saphenous veins. When there is venous occlusion in one leg, the venous pressure will be higher than in the unaffected leg. This test is significant only in the early course of thrombophlebitis before collateral veins have developed.

Isotope studies are helpful only in diagnosing the early formation of thrombi.[39] Fibrinogen labeled with radioactive iodine molecules makes up a clot along with naturally occurring fibrinogen. A scintillator counter is used to record radioactive counts at selected points along the extremities. Increased counts are obtained over thrombi.[32]

The ultrasonic Doppler flow detector transmits high frequency sounds through the skin, utilizing the principle known as the Doppler effect. As mentioned, ultrasonic waves are reflected from the red blood cells in a large vein and are shifted in frequency by an amount proportional to the velocity of flow of blood. In normal persons velocity of flow of blood is increased during inspiration and decreased during expiration. If a deep vein such as the iliac vein is fully obstructed with a thrombus, then the ultrasonic detector transmits a continuous blood flow with no respiratory modulations. If the vein is partially obstructed, the instrument detects only poor respiratory modulations.[72] The instrument is used to study blood flow in the major arteries and veins.

As mentioned previously in this chapter, calf blood volume can be measured with an *electrical impedance plethysmograph*. The test is based on the fact that sustained deep inspiration decreases venous return from the legs by increasing intra-abdominal and intrathoracic pressures and partially compressing the inferior vena cava. Blood is trapped in the calf and thus volume increases. With expiration, venous return to the heart resumes and consequently blood volume in the limb decreases. Figure 49–10 illustrates the normal respiratory waves that are found when the venous system is unobstructed between the calf and diaphragm. Figure 49–11 shows the greatly diminished respiratory waves that indicate venous thrombosis. Plethysmography often produces false negative results because the patient (1) cannot sustain deep inspiration long enough to cause pooling of the blood in the deep veins; (2) is unable to lie flat; (3) is in congestive heart failure; or (4) has peripheral arterial occlusion.

Nursing Intervention and Treatment. The primary goals of clinical care are to prevent thrombi already formed from becoming emboli, and to prevent new thrombi from forming. Care measures include (1) improving blood flow by physical means such as bed rest, elevation, elastic support hose, (2) applying warm moist packs, and (3) preventing hypercoagulability by drug therapy: anticoagulants, fibrinolytic drugs, and dextran. Superficial venous thrombosis usually requires anticoagulant therapy only when thrombophlebitis is extensive and threatens to involve the deep veins.

Bed Rest and Elevation. Bed rest is indicated for 4 to 7 days after the onset of thrombus

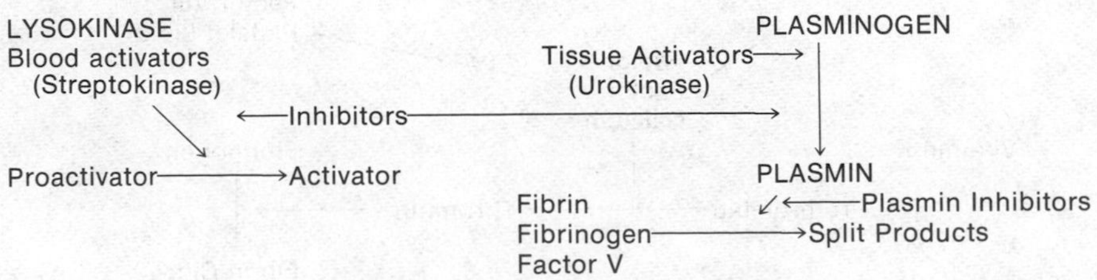

Figure 49–9. The fibrinolytic system.

TABLE 49–1. CLINICAL APPRAISAL OF THROMBOPHLEBITIS

Veins	Causative Factors	Signs and Symptoms	Edema	Pulmonary Embolism	Venous Insufficiency
Superficial Veins: saphenous, median cephalic, median basilic	Varicose veins, IV injections, Buerger's disease, blood dyscrasias, cancer	Tender, indurated, red, visible palpable cord along vein; ovoid nodules in skin	Rare	Rare	Rare
Deep Small Veins: femoral, tibial, popliteal, pelvic	Post operative, post partum, prolonged bed rest, congest ve heart failure, blood dyscrasias, cancer, oral contraceptives, fractures and dislocations	Increased muscle turgor over tenderness on affected vein; pressure; minimal or no venous distention; deep muscle tenderness; limb may be warmer than opposite limb; dorsifluxion of foot may cause calf pain (Homans' sign); occasionally fever—rarely exceeds 101°F.	Occasional edema may be masked and revealed by measuring circumference of extremities	Always a possibility	Rare
Major Deep Veins: femoral, iliac, axillary, subclavian, superior and inferior vena cava		No superficial signs of inflammation; cyanosis of extremity; venous distention of limbs	Usually	Always a possibility	Frequent

formation in order to allow the "tail" to become firmly adherent to the vessel wall, thus decreasing the possibility of emboli. Bed rest also prevents fluctuations in pressure in the venous system that occur with walking.

Elevation of the legs above the level of the heart facilitates blood flow by the force of gravity. The increase of blood flow prevents venous stasis and the formation of new thrombi. Elevation of the legs also decreases venous pressure, thus relieving edema and pain. Elevation is best accomplished by raising the foot of the bed 6 to 8 inches on blocks. Use of pillows or gatching the bed too frequently results in elevation of the knee above the foot and interferes with proper flow.

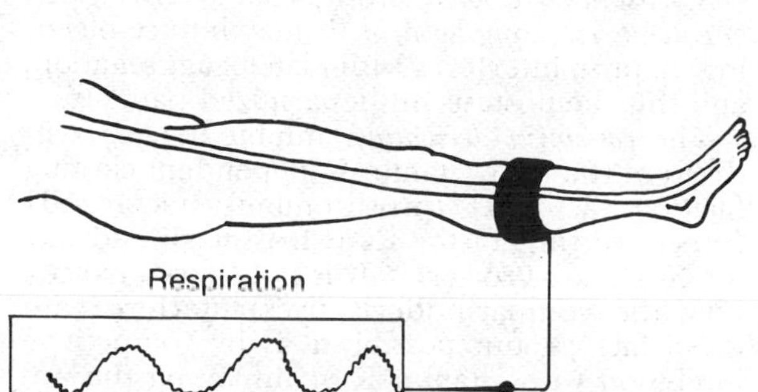

Figure 49–10. Normal respiratory waves measured with plethysmography. (From Berkowitz, H. D.: Two easier ways to diagnose deep vein thrombosis. *Consultant,* 19:100, May 1979.)

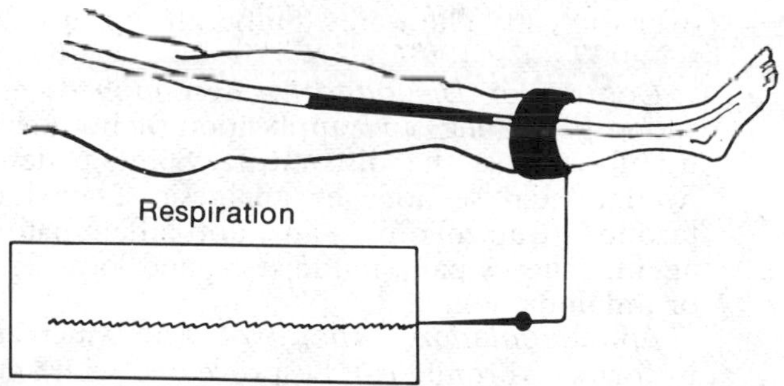

Figure 49–11. Abnormal respiratory waves in deep vein thrombosis. (From Berkowitz, H. D.: Two easier ways to diagnose deep vein thrombosis. *Consultant,* 19:100, May 1979.)

Elastic Support Hose and Exercise. Elastic support is not required with adequate elevation of the lower extremities. When the patient walks, elastic support hose or bandages must be used. The elastic support compresses the superficial veins and, with walking, blood flow in the veins is increased and venous pressure kept to a minimum. *Standing and sitting are not allowed,* since they increase the hydrostatic pressure in the capillaries, promoting edema. Once the threat of embolization is over, walking and exercises in bed should be encouraged to decrease venous pressure and to promote blood flow by the contraction of muscles compressing the veins. A recommended exercise in bed is dorsiflexion of the feet against a footboard.

Sometimes pneumonic vascular compression (PVC) leggings will be ordered to aid blood flow.[35] These leggings or boots are attached by polyethylene tubing to an electric pump. Air is pumped into each legging alternately for 1 minute at a pressure of 40 to 45 mm. Hg. Use of these leggings is usually discontinued when the patient starts walking.

After thrombosis of a deep calf vein, the patient should wear elastic support for 6 to 8 weeks.

Continuous Warm Moist Packs. Warm packs around the involved area should be given initially for 20 hours of every 24, decreasing the time as the condition improves. The purpose of the heat is to relieve venospasm, produce analgesia, and hasten resolution of inflammation.

A convenient method of applying heat is to use a plastic pad through which hot water circulates from a thermostatically controlled reservoir. This device maintains heat without frequent changing. A light dressing, not necessarily damp, is placed around the limb under the plastic pad and then a dry wrapping is applied over the pad. The water temperature is usually set at 37.8°C. (100°F.).

Control of Discomfort. Rest in bed, elevation of the leg, and application of hot packs usually relieve the discomfort. Some patients need a mild sedative or analgesic. Phenylbutazone (Butazolidin), an anti-inflammatory agent, relieves pain, tenderness, and local signs of inflammation.

Anticoagulation Therapy. Any increase in formed thrombi can be prevented with anticoagulants such as heparin or one of the coumarin derivatives. There is no evidence that heparin has any action on emboli already formed except to prevent propagation and platelet adhesiveness on the surface of thrombi.[12] Vascular occlusion that is resolved during heparin treatment is due primarily to the body's own mechanisms: thrombolysis, recanalization of the vein, and development of collateral vessels.

Heparin is thought to act by preventing the activation of clotting factor IX and inhibiting the action of thrombin in conjunction with a plasma cofactor.[12] Its effect can be determined by measuring the Lee-White clotting time, the activated partial thromboplastin time, and the partial thromboplastin time. The normal mean values are (1) Lee-White clotting time is 7 minutes, rising to 15 minutes 4 hours after heparin injections; (2) activated partial thromboplastin time is 40 seconds, rising to 47 seconds 2 hours after heparin injection.[59] A clotting time value may be determined before heparin injections in order to adjust the dosage. Propagation of emboli can be prevented if the clotting time is at least twice normal.

Heparin is *contraindicated* in the following conditions: severe hypertension, cerebrovascular hemorrhage, active ulceration, and overt bleeding from the gastrointestinal, genitourinary, or respiratory tract.

There are different opinions about the dosage and frequency of heparin administration for thrombophlebitis. Some authorities recommend 5000 units IV every 4 hours; others recommend 10,000 to 15,000 units IV every 4 hours for 48 hours, then reduced to lower levels (usually 5000 units); still others recommend 15,000 to 20,000 units subcutaneously every 12 hours. Heparin therapy is advised for varying lengths of time, from 1 day to 7 days, based on the time when the thrombi present have become firmly adherent to the vein wall. Anticoagulation therapy is usually started with heparin and continued with coumarin.

Complications of heparin treatment are bleeding and arterial emboli. Bleeding is usually first observed in fresh surgical incisions, injection sites, or the urine. As mentioned, arterial thrombi are formed from the aggregation of platelets, and since the primary hemostatic defense in heparinized patients is platelet aggregation, these patients are susceptible to arterial emboli.

> *While patients are receiving heparin, it is vital to avoid intramuscular injections, invasive procedures, and minor types of trauma – all of which could lead to minor bleeding or even hemorrhage.*

The specific antidote to heparin is protamine sulfate, 50 to 100 mg. IV or 1 mg./100 units of the last injected dose of heparin. Unfortunately, excess of protamine may prolong clotting.

Acetylsalicylic acid (aspirin) should never be given to patients receiving heparin. It may induce bleeding. Aspirin interferes with platelet aggregation, and thus hemostasis, in heparinized patients.

The *coumarin derivatives* inhibit hepatic synthesis of the four vitamin K–dependent clotting factors: factor II (prothrombin); factor VII (proconvertin); factor IX (Christmas); and factor X (Stuart-Prower).[34] It is not known exactly how the coumarin derivatives interfere with these factors, but possibly it is by competitive inhibition with vitamin K or inhibiting the uptake of vitamin K at its site of action.[47]

The coumarins include acenocoumarol (Sintrom), bishydroxycoumarin (Dicumarol), ethyl biscoumacetate (Tromexan), phenprocoumon (Liquamar), and warfarin sodium (Coumadin).

The effect of the coumarin derivatives can be determined by measuring the prothrombin time, which is measured every day before coumarin is given. An effort is made to keep the prothrombin time at one and one half to two times the normal time (normal reading are 12 or 13 seconds by the Quick method and 13 to 17 seconds by the Link-Shapiro method). (See Unit XIV.) The most serious complication from these drugs is bleeding: purpura, ecchymosis, hematuria, bleeding from the gums. The antidote for the coumarin derivatives is vitamin K (Mephyton, menadione, Hykinone, Synkayvite). If bleeding does occur, the drug is discontinued for a period of time.

The coumarin derivatives require a period of time (24 to 48 hours) before becoming effective. Therefore heparin, which is fast-acting, is used initially with a coumarin and then discontinued when the desired effect is achieved. Then therapy is continued with oral coumarin derivatives. Anticoagulation is usually continued approximately 4 weeks after an acute venous thrombosis and 3 to 6 months after pulmonary embolism (discussed later in this chapter).

The following drugs should not be given with coumarin derivatives: (1) drugs that *inhibit* coumarin action (increased tendency to clot), i.e., the following hypnotics — the barbiturates, glutethimide (Doriden), and ethclorvynol (Placidyl); (2) drugs that *potentiate* coumarin action (increased tendency to bleed), i.e., the anabolic steroids, chloral hydrate, chloramphenicol, glucagon, neomycin, phenylbutazone (Butazolidin), quinidine, and aspirin.[13, 34, 47, 70]

Fibrinolytic Drugs. Fibrinolytic drugs *dissolve thrombi*. Streptokinase and urokinase are fibrinolytics; Arvin is not, but it removes plasma fibrinogen and renders the blood incoagulable. These drugs have been experimental; most of the clinical studies have been done on streptokinase.

Streptokinase is an enzyme derived from cultures of beta hemolytic streptococci. Its effect depends on the activation of plasminogen, which breaks down fibrin (Fig. 49–9). Complications involve bleeding and allergic reactions. The antidote for streptokinase is Epsikapron (aminocaproic acid).

Because streptokinase is highly antigenic, it must be given carefully, observing for symptoms of an allergic reaction and anaphylactic shock (hypotension, tachycardia, fever, chills, and rash). A typical dosage would be 600,000 units of streptokinase in 500 ml. of 5 per cent dextrose intravenously at a rate of 80 ml. per hour.[16] Other regimens have been reported using streptokinase initially, then heparin, followed by maintenance with warfarin sodium.[6]

Dextran 70. Low molecular weight dextran (1) decreases blood viscosity, thus reducing hypercoagulability, (2) coats the vascular endothelium and blood elements, thus reducing contact factors that trigger coagulation, (3) reduces aggregation of blood cells, and (4) improves blood flow. Best results are obtained when treatment is started 4 to 8 hours after onset of symptoms of deep vein thrombosis or pulmonary embolism. The usual dose is 500 ml. of a 10 per cent solution every 6 hours intravenously. Because dextran also is antigenic and produces sensitive reactions, it is not widely used in treating venous thromboses.

Surgical Measures. Surgery is indicated if (1) anticoagulant therapy is not advised, (2) anticoagulant therapy is not effective (unusual), or (3) there is extreme thrombosis with impending gangrene. Thrombi can be successfully removed (thrombectomy) from major veins such as the subclavian, iliac, or femoral.

Embolus rarely complicates thrombectomy, but despite the use of heparin, thrombosis occasionally occurs, probably secondary to injury of the vein wall. There are two methods employed to disrupt the flow of blood and thus prevent pulmonary embolism: (1) Vein ligation traps the thrombus in the vein distal to the operative ligature. This procedure is usually done in massive iliofemoral thrombosis. (2) Plication of the inferior vena cava is done to partially interrupt blood flow, thus allowing normal flow by trapping emboli. This procedure is done by suturing parts of the vena cava or by insertion of a grid or umbrella-like prosthesis into the lumen of the vena cava. A frequent complication is the formation of new thrombi at the surgical site. Figure 49–12 shows various techniques and devices for attempting to prevent fatal embolism without interrupting vena caval flow.

Complications. The three major complications of thrombophlebitis are venous insufficiency, postphlebitic syndrome, pulmonary embolism, and postphlebitic neurosis.

Postphlebitic neurosis usually occurs in anxious, apprehensive people who have the misconception that their veins harbor clots that are going to break loose and move to the heart, causing sudden death. They refuse to bear weight on their extremities or walk, so that disuse atrophy prolongs the disability. Often the nurse or doctor enhances the patient's fantasies by careless remarks. For example, the use of the word "clot" in the presence of the patient tends to be more threatening than "thrombus" or "inflammation."

Prophylaxis. The prevention of thrombophlebitis and pulmonary embolism entails two problems: methods to prevent the formation of thrombi in the deep veins, and methods to prevent embolization after thrombi have formed. Prophylaxis, like treatment, is geared toward prevention of stasis of blood flow, injury to the endothelial wall, and hypercoagulability.

Some preventive measures that can be taken or taught to the patient are:

Prevention of stasis

Passive dorsiflexion of the foot and then active exercises in bed postoperatively, post partum, and for patients on prolonged bed rest.

Tilting the surgery table head down by 15 degrees if the surgery warrants it.

Electrical stimulation of the calf muscles and/or intermittent compression of the calf by pneumonic leggings during surgery.

Early ambulation post surgery and post partum.

Elastic support hose during and after surgery.

Deep breathing exercises postoperatively to promote thoracic pumping action.

Avoidance of tight garters and girdles.

Prevention of hypercoagulability

Dextran 70 on day of surgery and 1 or 2 days postoperatively.

Prophylactic preoperative low-dose heparin therapy for elderly patients with hip fractures, obese patients undergoing gynecologic surgery, or patients with severe varicosities, or, actually, all patients undergoing major surgery.[32]

Avoidance of taking the "pill" as a contraceptive.

Avoidance of dehydration after surgery or prolonged bed rest.

Prevention of injury to the vein wall

Avoidance of infiltration during intravenous therapy.

Heel cushions during surgery to elevate the calves and avoid damage to the intima of the vein.

Avoidance of gatch position in bed or putting pillows under calves postoperatively to avoid damage to endothelium of veins.

PULMONARY EMBOLISM

Pulmonary embolism means that a foreign object, usually a "tail" of a thrombus, has been deposited in some branch of the pulmonary artery with or without damage to the lung tissues. If necrosis has occurred in the lung tissue, the term "pulmonary infarction" is used.

Pathophysiology. Pulmonary emboli can be caused by air, fat, amniotic fluid, neoplasms, or thrombi. Thrombus is the most common cause of embolus. Pulmonary embolism has been reported in varying ranges of 4 to 60 per cent occurrence after deep vein thrombosis.

The "tail" of the thrombus breaks loose and travels through the veins to the right side of the heart and into the pulmonary artery. Most frequently the embolus is broken into multiple small particles by the churning and pumping action of the heart. The pulmonary pathophysi-

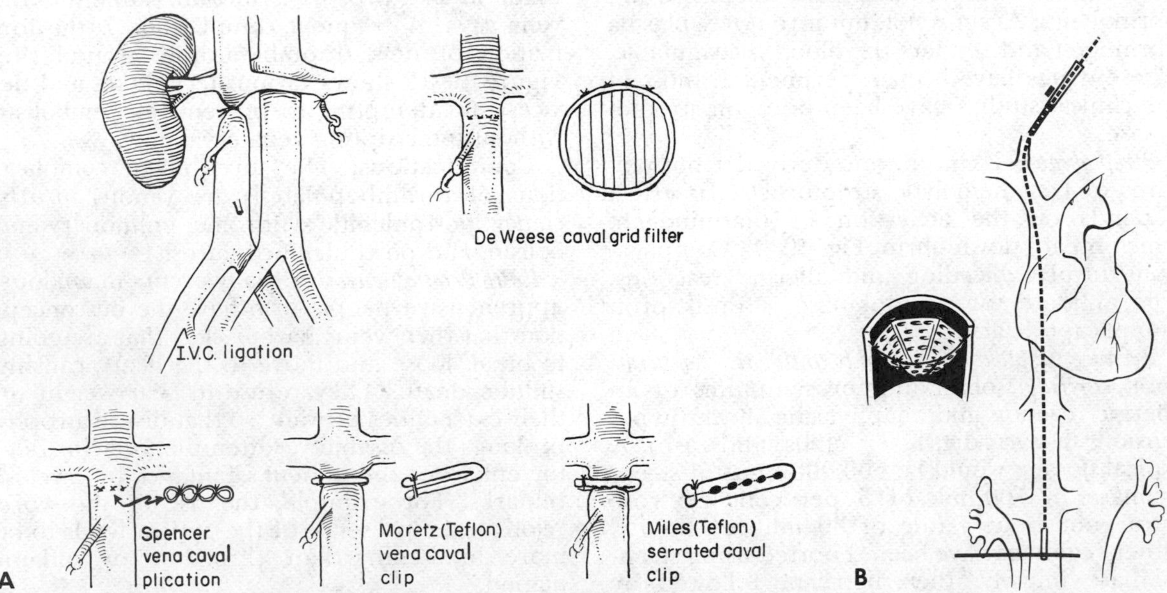

Figure 49–12. **A.** Drawings illustrating various surgical techniques available for preventing embolism from pelvic and lower extremity veins. Spermatic or ovarian vein ligation provides additional protection and is accomplished at time of vena caval procedure. **B.** Transvenous method of vena caval interruption using a caval prosthesis of umbrella design (Mobin-Uddin). Insert illustrates the opened umbrella. Both sieve-like and nonfenestrated prostheses have been used. (From Fairbairn, J. F., II, J. L. Juergens, and J. A. Spittell, Jr., *Allen-Barker-Hines, Peripheral Vascular Diseases,* 4th ed. Philadelphia, W. B. Saunders Co., 1972.)

ology occurs as a result of obstruction of blood flow with increasing venous pressure in the pulmonary artery, and perhaps the presence of reflex vasoconstriction as a result of thromboembolism. Serotonin, a vasoconstrictor, may be released from platelets, causing pulmonary hypertension.

Pulmonary embolism occurs abruptly. It may be severe to minor, depending on the size and number of the emboli. The right lower lobe is the most frequently involved; the left lower lobe is the second most important site of predilection. Of the patients who die, approximately one half die within a half hour of the onset, two thirds within 1 hour, and three fourths within 2 hours. The mortality rate is approximately 38 per cent.[29]

The significant hemodynamic consequences of pulmonary embolism are related principally to the strain placed on the right side of the heart by elevation of the pulmonary arterial pressure. It is estimated that approximately 65 per cent of the pulmonary circulation must be obstructed in order to produce significant strain on the right heart and that approximately 79 per cent must be obstructed in order to produce persistent pulmonary hypertension.[43]

Complete obstruction of a major pulmonary artery causes immediate death secondary to right ventricular failure, decreased stroke volume, poor diffusion of carbon dioxide and oxygen, and finally shock. Reduction of 50 to 60 per cent of the cross-sectional area of pulmonary arteries will cause respiratory and circulatory changes.[43] The obstruction due to the emboli causes increased pressure in the pulmonary artery. The "backward effects" are decreased emptying of the right ventricle, increased volume and pressure in the right ventricle, and increased volume and pressure in the great veins. The "forward effects" are decreased volume in the left atrium, decreased stroke volume, and stimulation of the baroreceptor reflex, thus maintaining arterial blood pressure and increasing contractility of the left ventricle for a period of time. Then shock ensues.

There has been considerable interest in the arterial oxygen tension following pulmonary embolism. Szucs and associates found the arterial pO_2 to be decreased in each of the 36 patients with angiographically documented pulmonary embolism; as a rule there was a decrease of arterial pCO_2 and elevated pH with respiratory alkalosis.[61] Perhaps as many as 10 per cent of patients with pulmonary emboli will have normal oxygen tensions.

If there is a partial obstruction, the lung probably survives, and fibrinolysis resolves the emboli; resolution is slow (approximately 2 weeks, provided there is no cardiac or pulmonary disease).

Poor circulation to the lung tissue can lead to necrosis and infarction. *Lung infarction* occurs in the presence of pulmonary emboli when there is also systemic hypotension. Infarction occurs when there is permanent occlusion of blood to a tissue. The lung has two arterial systems: the pulmonary arterial system and the bronchial arterial system. If some part of the pulmonary arterial system is occluded by emboli and there is minimal or no perfusion through the bronchial arterial system because of low cardiac output, then a lung infarction will occur. This has been reported to occur 2½ to 79 hours following obstruction of a pulmonary artery by embolus. Pulmonary infarction disables but does not in itself cause death.[1]

Assessment of the Patient with Pulmonary Embolism. Pulmonary embolism may be silent, varied in symptomatology, and recurrent. It can be manifested by dyspnea, substernal oppressive chest pain, tachycardia, hemoptysis, cough, cerebral ischemia (restlessness, anxiety, syncope, convulsions), electrocardiographic changes, shock, right-sided failure, fever with elevated leukocyte count and erythrocyte sedimentation rate, and/or sudden death.[49]

The pain is described as a crushing substernal pain if a large embolus is lodged in a major pulmonary artery. Other descriptions are sharp, localized, stabbing, occurring with breathing, and "pleuritis" pain.

Signs that infarction has occurred are hemoptysis, cough, fever, and friction rub. The patient may cough up small or massive amounts of blood. The fever is characteristically 101 to 102° F. A friction rub may be heard transiently over the infarcted area. Both pain and friction rub may disappear with the development of pleural effusion.

Shock (hypotension, tachycardia, cold, clammy extremities) and low arterial pCO_2 and pO_2 are ominous signs of massive emboli.

Pulmonary embolism can be *diagnosed* by chest x-rays, electrocardiogram, blood enzyme levels, pulmonary angiograms, measurement of arterial blood gases, and radioisotope lung scan.

Chest x-rays show a wedge-shaped opacity if infarction is present. Other signs of pulmonary embolism are elevation of the diaphragm, decreased vascularity, and dilated pulmonary arteries.

ECG patterns, if present, that are highly suggestive of the diagnosis of pulmonary emboli are inverted T on leads V_1 to V_4, transient right bundle branch block, right axis deviation, right ventricular hypertrophy, and tall P waves in leads II, III, and aVF.[28]

Blood enzymes show an elevation in the blood lactic dehydrogenase (LDH) level. There is usually no rise of serum glutamic oxaloacetic transaminase (SGOT). The serum bilirubin level rises in cases of increased pressure and blood volume in the great veins owing to right ventricular strain.

Pulmonary angiograms are the most effective means of diagnosing pulmonary emboli. This procedure is done by injecting radiopaque dye into the right atrium and pulmonary artery via a catheter threaded through a peripheral vein. Visualization of any filling defects of the heart and right pulmonary artery is done by taking sequential x-rays.

Arterial blood gases indicate an arterial hypoxemia (low pO_2) and hypocapnia (low pCO_2) in massive pulmonary embolism. There may be a severe respiratory alkalosis.[61]

Radioisotope lung scan is done by injecting intravenously particles of human serum albumin that have been labeled with radioactive iodine (^{131}I) or technetium (^{99m}Tc). These macroaggregated particles are trapped in the pulmonary microvasculature and are distributed according to pulmonary flow. Both lungs are scanned with a scintillation counter and the amount of radioactivity counted gives an indication of obstruction to flow.

Nursing Intervention and Treatment. The general goals of the care of the patient with pulmonary embolism are (1) anticoagulant and fibrinolytic therapy (refer to previous section); (2) prevention of formation of additional thrombi (refer to previous section); (3) treatment for shock, if warranted, giving vasoconstrictors such as levarterenol (Levophed) or metaraminol (Aramine) (see Chapter 13); (4) treatment of respiratory distress by continuous oxygen by nasal catheter or oxygen mask, positioning patient with the head of bed elevated at least 30 degrees to ease breathing or use of a respirator (see also Unit XVI); and (5) allaying fear and apprehension.

The patient's fear is associated with the sudden onset of severe chest pain and the inability to breathe. The patient becomes anxious, restless, and apprehensive. Many times such patients will not reveal their innermost fears to others. Since sudden death can ensue from pulmonary embolism, the doctor may discuss the potential seriousness of the disease with the patient. The nurse's firm emotional support can be a stabilizing factor at this time. This support can effectively be shown by staying with the patient and giving honest assurances of the advances that have been made in the treatment of pulmonary embolism. In addition, the nurse should give intensive care efficiently and unhurriedly and not display the emotional strain of caring for a seriously ill or dying patient.

There are three *surgical treatments* for pulmonary embolus: venous interruption by vein ligation to prevent the embolus from traveling to the heart (see previous section); vena cava plication to allow blood flow but to trap emboli (see previous section); and embolectomy.

An *embolectomy* is the surgical removal of emboli from the pulmonary arteries. Before the advent of the cardiopulmonary bypass, the procedure had an extremely high mortality rate. Even now embolectomy concurrently with anticoagulant therapy still carries a high risk,[48] partly because of possible misdiagnosis and partly because of the problems involved in operating on patients in profound shock.

DISORDERS OF THE LYMPHATIC SYSTEM

*Review of Anatomy and Physiology of the Lymphatic System**

Structure of the Lymphatic System. The lymphatic system comprises (1) plexuses of small, thin, vein-like vessels (lymphatics) that empty lymph (a fluid similar to plasma and tissue fluid except for an absence of proteins of high molecular weight) into the left and right brachiocephalic veins; (2) lymph nodes, which are small, oval bodies situated so that lymph flows through them on its way to the veins; (3) collections of lymphoid tissue situated in the walls of the intestinal tract and in the spleen and thymus; and (4) the circulating lymphocytes. The lymphatic system and drainage are illustrated in Figure 10–1.

The lymphatic vessels tend to lie near the veins. The peripheral lymphatics join larger lymphatics and pass through regional lymph nodes before entering the blood stream. Ultimately all lymphatics converge into two main trunks, the thoracic duct, and the right lymphatic duct, which empty into the junctions of the subclavian and internal jugular veins on the left and right sides, respectively. The *thoracic duct* drains most of the lymph vessels of the body: lower extremities, pelvis, abdominal cavity, left thorax, and left head, neck, and upper extremity. The *right lymphatic duct* is the common trunk for the lymph flow from the right side of the head, neck, thorax, and upper arm.

There are active and passive mechanisms to transport the lymph along the lymph vessels. Smooth muscles within the wall of the lymphatic vessels contract synchronously along segments between valves. This serves to actively propel

*The lymphatic system (lymphatics, lymph nodes, spleen, lymphocytes) is discussed in Chapter 10. For more detailed information consult an anatomy and physiology text.

the lymph from one segment to the next. The valves restrict movement toward the thoracic duct. Passive transport can occur by compression from skeletal muscle and other surrounding tissues. The larger lymph vessels are innervated, and stimulation of these nerves may alter lymph flow — although this has not as yet been conclusively proved.

Functions of the Lymphatic System. The three fundamental functions of the lymphatic system are (1) the development and maintenance of the immune system, (2) the transport of fluids and proteins (and other colloid substances) from the interstitial spaces back to the veins, and (3) the reabsorption of fats from the small intestine. Let us briefly consider each function.

Recall from Chapter 11 that the *immune response* involves two separate but interdependent mechanisms. One mechanism involves antigen-sensitive lymphocytes and is known as *cell-mediated* or *delayed type immunity.* Circulating antibody is not involved in this reaction. This form of immunity is responsible for rejection of foreign cells, tumors, and resistance to many viral and fungal infections. Cell-mediated immunity is controlled by T-lymphocytes. In the cell-mediated immune response, lymphocytes attack the antigenic agent. The second mechanism is known as *humoral* or *immediate type immunity.* It involves the synthesis of antibodies by plasma cells in response to some antigen. B-lymphocytes, whose progeny produce antibodies, participate in the humoral response. The cells themselves do not interact with the antigen but produce antibodies that do. In addition, *macrophages* within the lymph nodes play an important role in the immune response by trapping antigen so that it can be presented to reactive lymphocytes. These immunologically competent cells respond by generating clones of specificially reactive (sometimes called "killer") lymphocytes. Phagocytosis of antigen by macrophages or reticuloendothelial cells in the lymph nodes can also occur.

Second, the lymphatics are an important element in the fluid exchange and protein transport between blood and tissue. The lymphatic capillaries permit free entry of fluid, small and large molecules, and cellular elements from the interstitial space. In infections, bacteria and leukocytes with phagocytized bacteria are generally transported into the lymphatics. Unfortunately, neoplastic cells are also transported into the lymphatics to invade lymph nodes and other distant organs.

The mechanisms of transport of fluid and other substances between the lymphatics and the interstitial spaces are explained by the *Starling-Landis hypothesis of the capillary.* Hydrostatic pressure in the lymphatic capillaries (1 to 2 mm. Hg) measures about the same as the hydrostatic pressure in the interstitial space.[71] The wall of a lymphatic capillary is similar to a blood capillary except that it has larger "pores." That is, there are large spaces between the endothelial cells through which large molecules can pass (see Fig. 49–13). This wall structure coupled with the same pressure in the interstitial spaces and the lymph capillaries suggests that there is relatively free communication between the interstitial spaces and the lymph capillaries. Thus, any increase in the interstitial pressure will increase lymph flow. Any agent or procedure that increases the rate of filtration from the blood capillaries will increase lymph flow. Interstitial pressures and lymph flow can be increased by raising venous pressure or reducing plasma oncotic pressure or by inflammation. A general increase in systemic arterial pressure does not significantly increase lymph flow, but hypotension decreases or stops lymph flow. Ordinarily, the volume of lymph represents the difference between capillary filtration and reabsorption, which is approximately 2 to 4 liters daily.

Finally, the third function of the lymphatic system is the *absorption of digested fat.* This function is performed by the lymph capillaries of the intestine which are called *lacteals.* Lymph that is laden with fat is called *chyle.*

Examination of the Lymphatic System

Although over 60 groups of lymph nodes are listed by anatomists, only three regional groups are usually examined: the cervicofacial and supraclavicular, the axillary and epitrochlear, and the inguinal and femoral. The standard examination of the lymph nodes involves inspection and palpation. Usually lymph nodes cannot be felt in the adult, but enlarged nodes, perhaps as

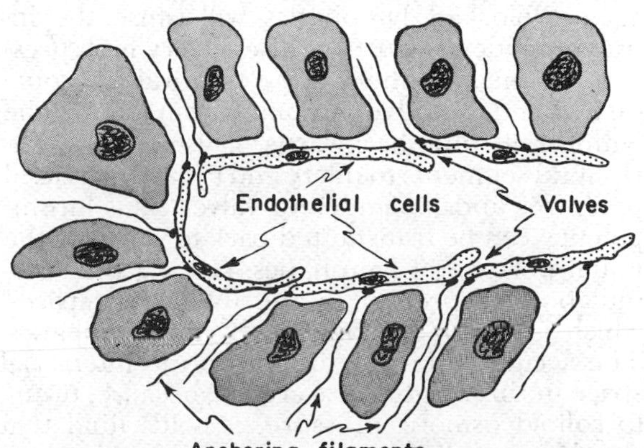

Figure 49–13. Special structure of the lymphatic capillaries that permits passage of substances of high molecular weight back into the circulation. (From Guyton, A. C.: *Textbook of Medical Physiology,* 5th ed. Philadelphia: W. B. Saunders Co., 1976.)

a result of some previous inflammation, are frequently palpable. Cervical nodes up to 1 cm. in diameter can always be felt in children up to 12 years of age. Palpable nodes are most common in the occipital, axillary, and inguinal regions. Femoral lymph node enlargement more often indicates a pathologic state. Any node, whether palpable or not, may show microscopic changes indicative of neoplasm.

Localized lymphadenopathy (lymph node enlargement) is usually due to either inflammation or neoplasm. Acute inflammation (lymphadenitis) causes enlarged, tender, rather soft nodes, sometimes associated with red streaks, indicating lymphangitis. Adenopathy due to neoplastic metastasis is usually hard, nontender, and somewhat fixed to the underlying structures.

Since the lymphatic system plays an important role in various diseases, its study by the injection of radiopaque material and roentgenographic visualization *(lymphography)* has become an important diagnostic tool. One purpose for which this method is especially valuable is the investigation of swelling in the lower extremities, which is often difficult to diagnose by other means.

Lymphedema

Pathophysiology. Lymphedema means *edematous tissues* with high concentrations of *protein* in some part of the body due to *insufficiency of lymph drainage.* It is produced by (1) the relative absence of lymphatics, (2) partially or completely blocked lymphatics, or (3) the inadequate or faulty transport of lymph.

Lymphedema arises in the following way. Contractions of the collecting lymphatic vessels against blocked lymphatics will cause the intralymphatic pressures to rise to very high pressure in the periphery. The thin walls become dilated and the valves become incompetent. The lymph will flow backwards, causing more peripheral segments to dilate and to have increased pressures and incompetent valves. This incompetency can be transmitted back to valves of the initial peripheral lymphatics, causing the accumulation of protein in the interstitial spaces, which is normally removed by the lymphatics. The accumulation of protein in the interstitial space in this condition is crucial, because, owing to colloid osmotic pressure, it holds fluid that should normally be reabsorbed by the blood capillaries.

The consequence of chronic lymph congestion is *fibrosis.* After a period of lymph stasis, there is a proliferation of fibroblasts, resulting in the formation of dense connective tissue in the subcutaneous tissue. The mechanism for this is unknown.

Primary Lymphedema. Lymphedemas are best classified into primary and secondary lymphedemas. Other names for primary lymphedema are "lymphedema of unknown origin" or 'idiopathic lymphedema." The primary lymphedemas may be classified according to age of onset: congenital (present at birth), praecox (early in life), tarda (late in life). Primary lymphedemas can also be classified according to radiologic findings: aplasia (no lymph vessels), hypoplasia (where they are smaller or fewer than normal), or hyperplasia (where they are larger or more numerous). Congenital and familial lymphedema is also called Milroy's disease. It is inherited as an autosomal dominant trait.

Of the primary forms, *lymphedema praecox* is the largest group, with a peak in the second decade. It is more common in females than in males. The edema usually appears spontaneously and without known cause. A dull, heavy sensation is present but actual pain is absent. Elevation of the limb and rest in bed cause a reduction but not its disappearance. Smooth skin becomes roughened and the edema is nonpitting. Acute lymphangitis and cellulitis are infrequent. Ulceration of the skin does not occur. However, the limb may become greatly enlarged, uncomfortable and unsightly (see Fig. 49–14).

Secondary Lymphedema. Secondary lymphedema occurs because of some damage or obstruction to the lymph system by another disease process or procedure: surgical excision or trauma, neoplasms (primary or metastatic), filariasis, inflammation, or high doses of irradiation.

Postsurgical lymphedema is usually seen following surgical excision of axillary, inguinal, or iliac nodes, usually as a prophylactic or therapeutic measure for metastatic tumor. For example, lymphedema of the upper arm is encountered after radical amputation of the breast (see Chapter 81). Figure 49–15 illustrates the stages in development of post surgical lymphedema.

The irregular interval at which lymphedema occurs after lymphadenectomy is remarkable. There may be an initial edema after surgery, but weeks, months, or years may pass before the extremity becomes edematous.

Filariasis, caused by the nematode *Wuchereria bancrofti,* is the prevalent endemic disease in Western Samoa. It is one of the most common diseases of the world. It is transmitted by mosquitoes from human to human. The living embryos (microfilariae) of the adult female worm are found in the blood stream. The larvae migrate to the lymphatics, where they mature into adult worms. Lodgment of the adult worms in the lymph nodes and vessels leads to lymph flow obstruction, lymphedema, and elephantiasis. Most patients have intermittent attacks of high fever, chills, malaise, fatigue, tender regional lymphadenopathy, severe muscle pain, and areas of erythema with increased edema. They are classicially referred to as "mumu attacks." Present public health measures include the mass distribution of diethylcarbamazine (Hetrazan), a microfilaricidal drug to lower the risks of becoming infected. However, for the individual with advanced disease, there is little that can be offered in terms of cure.

Lymphedema secondary to neoplasms in the lymph nodes is common. The malignant disease may be primary, such as lymphomas or Hodgkin's disease, or metastatic from some other site (see Chapter 46).

Chronic lymphedema secondary to inflammation is relatively uncommon, probably as a result of early control with antibiotics. The chronic lymphedema is due to recurrent lymphangitis and cellulitis caused usually by bacterial organisms.

Radiation in moderate amounts does not appear to damage the lymph vessels. However, heavy radiation for a particularly resistant tumor usually leads to lymphatic obstruction.

Treatment of Lymphedema. There are three current general modes of treatment of lymphedema: physical therapy, coumarin therapy, and surgery.

Physical therapy, in the treatment of arm or leg lymphedema, is a mechanical or manual forced squeezing of the soft tissue in order to press the stagnant lymphatic fluid to the proximal part of the limb. This is followed by specific active and passive exercises to transport the lymph further into the lymphatic system and finally into the blood stream. A number of pneumatic pumping devices for intermittent compression are available. The pressure is defined as 30 mm. Hg for the deeper and 20 mm. Hg for the more peripherally situated lymphatic vessels. Evaluation of the intervention is done by measuring the perimeters of both extremities before and after treatment.

Coumarin and related compounds are valuable drugs in the treatment of lymphedema. Their basic action is to remove the protein in the interstitial spaces. Then the fluid will reenter the blood capillaries in the absence of the proteins' colloidal osmotic pressure, which held the fluid in the tissue. Piller and Casley-Smith injected radioprotein (^{51}Cr) and a nonmetabolizable tracer (^{125}I-labeled polyvinylpyrolidine, PVP) into the legs of rats with lymphedema.[51] The addition of coumarin caused the ratio of protein to PVP to fall significantly. This shows that coumarin causes protein to leave the injection site more rapidly than PVP. These experiments did not trace the fat of the protein — whether it entered blood capillaries or lymph capillaries or underwent endocytosis (i.e., increased uptake of protein by lysosomes in the tissue) or proteolysis. There is some experimental evidence that supports the argument that coumarin removes protein by proteolysis.[9]

There are two basic types of *surgical procedure* for lymphedema: the excisional type, in which the markedly edematous subcutaneous tissue is removed, and the transfer of superficial lymphatics into the deep lymphatic system by a buried shaved subcutaneous skin flap.[63, 64] The latter procedure is designed to improve lymphatic drainage over a 10-year period in cases of

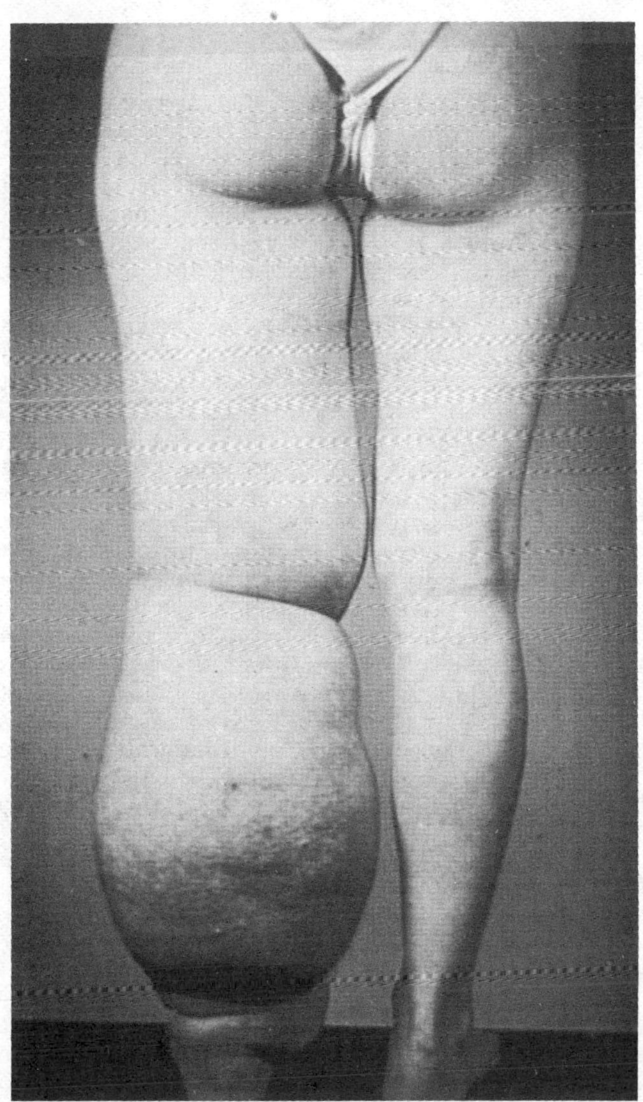

Figure 49–14. Lymphedema praecox of the leg in 20-year-old woman. (From Young, J.: The swollen leg. *Am. Fam. Physician,* 15:163, Jan. 1977.)

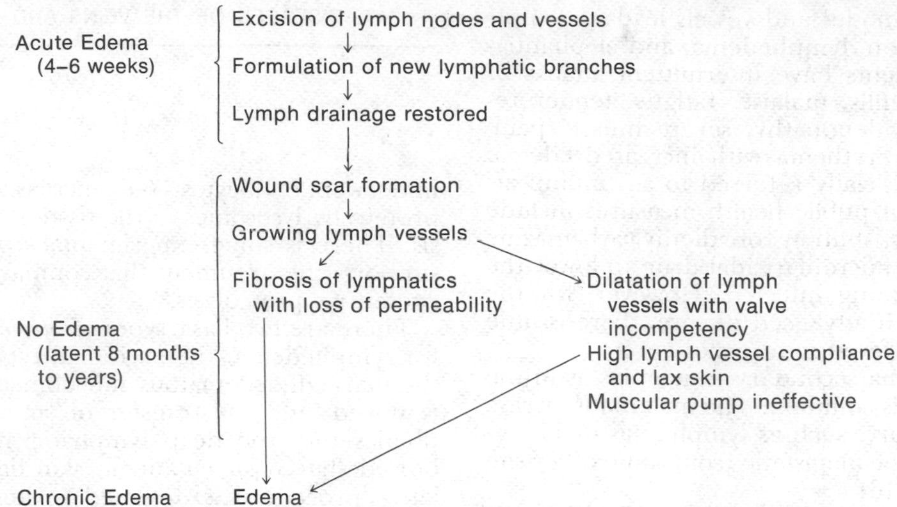

Figure 49–15. Sequence of development of postsurgical lymphedema. (From Olszewski, W.: On the pathomechanism of development of postsurgical lymphedema. *Lymphology,* 6:35, 1973.)

chronic lymphedema of the extremities.[63] The results were satisfactory in 92 per cent of patients with primary lymphedema and 100 per cent of patients with secondary lymphedema. Depending on the condition of the overlying skin, grafts may have to be obtained from other healthy areas (Charles procedure). The chief indications for surgery are (1) to reduce the weight of the bulky part, (2) to make it possible for patients with elephantiasis to wear normal clothes and footwear, (3) to reduce the incidence of inflammatory attacks, (4) to control skin changes, such as thickening, induration, hyperkeratosis, and dermatitis, and (5) to improve the cosmetic appearance of the limb.

The objectives of *postoperative nursing care* are (1) provide constant postoperative elevation of the extremity even during ambulation; (2) provide extensive suction drainage underneath the flap to prevent hematoma formation for approximately 7 days postoperatively; (3) administer prophylactic antibiotics for 5 to 7 days postoperatively; (4) careful sterile dressing changes; and (5) observation for complications — flap necrosis, abscess formation, hematoma, ulceration, cellulitis, joint stiffness, and epithelial cysts.[12, 33]

Palliative treatment of lymphedema includes oral diuretics (thiazides), elevation of the affected extremity and elastic or Ace bandage support. Use of *diuretics* is controversial in lymphedema. Diuretics do not remove the excess protein. They shift the Starling equilibrium towards resorption, but the resulting dehydration leads to secretion of aldosterone and antidiuretic hormone. This stimulates retention of water and sodium. Once fibrosis occurs, the less efficient the above-mentioned methods become.

Lymphadenitis

Lymph nodes act as defensive barriers and are secondarily involved in virtually all systemic infections and in many neoplastic disorders arising elsewhere in the body. Generalized lymphadenopathy (enlargement of two or three regionally separated lymph node groups) is usually due to inflammation, neoplasm, or immunologic reactions. Lymphomas and Hodgkin's disease are discussed in Chapter 46. Disorders of the immune system, such as hypersensitivity, are discussed in Chapter 11.

The infections that lead to lymphadenitis are so numerous and varied that a detailed description would involve a list of all systemic microbiologic diseases. The specific node or nodes affected in infectious diseases depend upon location of the infection, nature of the invading organism, and severity of the disease. Lymphadenitis can be classified nonspecifically as acute or chronic.

Acute Lymphadenitis. Acute lymphadenitis is usually one of two pathologic patterns: (1) suppuration in lymph nodes that drain infections caused by pyogenic organisms, or (2) reticuloendothelial hyperplasia, edema, and leukocyte infiltration of the nodes caused by nonpyogenic organisms, such as spirochetes, rickettsiae, and viruses. Acutely inflamed lymph nodes are most commonly seen locally in the cervical region in association with infections of the teeth or tonsils or in the axillary or inguinal regions secondary to infections of the extremities. Generalized lymphadenopathy is characteristic of the secondary stage of syphilis, viral infections, and bacteremia. Clinically, in acute lymphadenitis, the lymph nodes are enlarged, tender, warm, and reddened.

Chronic Lymphadenitis. In the long-standing course of infection, the lymph nodes frequently become extensively scarred, with fibrous connective tissue replacement. Clinically, these nodes are enlarged, firm to palpation and not tender or warm.

The nursing care of lymphadenitis depends upon administration of the appropriate antibiotic and treatment of the primary infection.

BIBLIOGRAPHY (Chapter 49)

1. Alpert, J. S., et al.: Experimental pulmonary embolism: effect on pulmonary blood volume and vascular compliance. *Circulation,* 49:152, 1974.
2. Barnes, R. W.: Diagnosing vascular disease with noninvasive tests. *Consultant,* 18:56, Dec. 1978.
3. Baron, H. C.: Valvular incompetence and varicose veins. *Hosp. Med.,* 12:24, April 1976.
4. Berkowitz, H. D.: Two easier ways to diagnose deep vein thrombosis. *Consultant,* 19:100, May 1979.
5. Breslau, R. C.: Intensive care following vascular surgery. *Amer. J. Nurs.,* 68:1670, 1968.
6. Brown, G. Streptokinase therapy for pulmonary embolism. *Postgrad. Med.* 49:262, 1971.
7. Brown, N. L. Prophylaxis of pulmonary embolism. *Br. Med. J.,* 2:780, 1970.
8. Brown, N. L., et al.: Prevention of recurrent pulmonary embolism. *Br. Med. J.,* 3:382, 1969.
9. Casley-Smith, J. R., and N. B. Piller: The mode of action of coumarin and related compounds in the treatment of edema. *In* Clodius, L. (Ed.): *Lymphedema.* Stuttgart: Georg Thieme Publishers, 1977.
10. Chappell, M. B.: Pulmonary embolism. *Nurs. Mirror,* 132:26, 1971.
11. Clarke, M. B., et al.: Use of labelled fibrinogen in the detection and management of deep vein thrombosis. *Br. J. Radiol.,* 43:829, 1970.
12. Clodius, L.: *Lymphedema.* Stuttgart: Geog Thieme Publishers, 1977.
13. Coon, W. W.: Anticoagulant therapy for venous thromboembolism. *Postgrad. Med.,* 63:157, April 1978.
14. Couch, N. P.: Axioms on venous thrombosis. *Hosp. Med.,* 13:68, June 1977.
15. Craddock, C. G.: Lymphocytes and the immune response. *N. Engl. J. Med.,* 285:324, 1971.
16. Davies, M.: Streptokinase therapy for deep vein thrombosis. *Nurs. Times,* 69:211, 1973.
17. Dee, R.: New interest in sclerotherapy for varicose veins. *Consultant,* 17:123, June 1977.
18. Deykin, D.: The use of heparin. *N. Engl. J. Med.,* 280:937, 1969.
19. Deykin, D.: Warfarin therapy I. *N. Engl. J. Med.,* 283: 691, Sept. 24, 1970.
20. Deykin, D.: Warfarin therapy II. *N. Engl. J. Med.,* 283: 801, Oct. 8, 1970.
21. Dodd, H., and F. B. Cockett: *The Pathology and Surgery of the Veins of the Lower Limbs.* New York: Churchill Livingstone, 1976.
22. Fairbairn, J. F., et al.: *Peripheral Vascular Diseases,* 4th ed. Philadelphia: W. B. Saunders Co., 1972.
23. Foley, W. T., and I. S. Wright: *Color Atlas and Management of Vascular Disease.* New York: Appleton-Century-Crofts, 1959.
24. Goldstone, J.: Veins and lymphatics. *In* Dunphy, J. E., and L. W. Way (Eds.): *Current Surgical Diagnosis and Treatment,* 3rd ed. Los Altos, Cal.: Lange Medical Publications, 1977.
25. Guyton, A. C.: *Textbook of Medical Physiology,* 5th ed. Philadelphia: W. B. Saunders Co., 1976.
26. Hills, N. H., and S. S. Calnan: Deep vein thrombosis after surgery. *Nurs. Mirror,* 135:29, 1972.
27. Hume, M.: Massive thrombophlebitis of the lower extremities. *In* Conn, H. F. (Ed.) *Current Therapy 1978.* Philadelphia: W. B. Saunders Co., 1978.
28. Humphries, J., et al.: Criteria for the recognition of pulmonary emboli. *J.A.M.A.,* 235:2011, 1976.
29. Hurst, J. W., and R. B. Logue: *The Heart, Arteries and Veins,* 2nd ed. New York: McGraw-Hill Book Company, 1970.
30. Johnson, B. J.: The hazards of immobilization: effects on cardiovascular function. *Amer. J. Nurs.,* 67:781, 1967.
31. Juergens, J. L.: Venous thromboembolism. *Cardiov. Clin.,* 3:234, 1971.
32. Kakkar, V. V.: Deep vein thrombosis. *Circulation,* 51:8, 1975.
33. Kinmouth, J. B., et al.: Comments on operations for lower limb lymphedema. *Lymphology,* 8:56, 1975.
34. Koch-Weser, J., and E. M. Sellers: Drug interactions with coumarin anticoagulants. *N. Engl. J. Med.,* 285:547, 1971.
35. Lee, B. Y.: Noninvasive prevention of deep vein thrombosis. *Am. Fam. Physician,* 14:128, Nov. 1976.
36. Lofgren, K. A.: Primary varicose veins. *In* Conn, H. F. (ed.): *Current Therapy 1978.* Philadelphia: W. B. Saunders Co., 1978.
37. Lofgren, K. A.: Varicose veins: their symptoms, complications, and management. *Postgrad. Med.,* 65:131, June 1979.
38. Maki, D. G.: Septic thrombophlebitis (Part 2). *Hosp. Med.,* 13:6, Jan. 1977.
39. Mayor, G. E., et al.: Peripheral venous scanning with ^{125}I-tagged fibrinogen. *Lancet,* 1:661, 1972.
40. Miller, G. A. H.: Massive pulmonary embolism — medical management. *Br. J. Med.,* 2:777, 1970.
41. Miller, J. F.: Cellular basis of the immunological defects in thymectomized mice. *Nature,* 214:992, 1967.
42. Monks, B. E.: Venous thrombosis. *Nurs. Mirror,* 132:40, 1971.
43. Nelson, J. R., and J. R. Smith: The pathologic physiology of pulmonary embolism: a physiologic discussion of the vascular reactions following pulmonary arterial obstruction by emboli of varying size. *Am. Heart J.,* 58:916, 1959.
44. Oakley, C. M.: Diagnosis of pulmonary embolism. *Br. Med. J.,* 2:773, 1970.
45. O'Brien, J. R., and V. V. Kakkar: Peripheral venous scanning with ^{125}I-tagged fibrinogen. *Lancet,* 1:909, 1972.
46. Olszewski, W.: On the pathomechanism of development of postsurgical lymphedema. *Lymphology,* 6:35, 1973.
47. O'Reilly, R. A., and P. M. Aggeler: Determinants of the response to oral anticoagulant drugs in man. *Pharmacol. Rev.,* 22:35, 1970.
48. Paneth, M.: Surgical management of massive pulmonary embolism. *Br. Med. J.,* 2:778, 1970.
49. Parker, B. M., and J. R. Smith: Pulmonary embolism and infarction. *Am. J. Med.,* 24:402, 1958.
50. Paulose, K. P., et al.: Diagnosis of pulmonary embolism, a correlative study of the clinical, scan and angiographic findings. *Br. Med. J.,* 3:67, 1970.
51. Piller, N. B., and J. R. Casley-Smith: The effect of coumarin on protein and PVP clearance from rat legs with various high protein edemas. *Br. J. Exp. Pathol.,* 56:439, 1975.
52. Price, S. A., and L. M. Wilson: *Pathophysiology: Clinical*

Concepts of Disease Processes. New York: McGraw-Hill Book Co., 1978.

53. Robbins, S. L., and R. S. Cotran: *Pathologic Basis of Disease,* 2nd ed. Philadelphia: W. B. Saunders Co., 1979.
54. Roenigk, H. H.: Leg ulcers in the elderly. *Geriatrics,* 34:21, July 1979.
55. Rushmer, R. F.: *Cardiovascular Dynamics,* 4th ed. Philadelphia: W. B. Saunders Co., 1976.
56. Sasahara, A. A., and V. L. Foster: Pulmonary embolism: recognition and treatment. *Amer. J. Nurs.,* 67:1634, 1967.
57. Schatz, I. J., et al.: Disability after real or alleged venous thrombosis. *Postgrad. Med. J.,* 31:358, 1962.
58. Sexton, D. L.: Symposium on patients with peripheral vascular disease. *Nurs. Clin. North Am.,* 12:87, Mar. 1977.
59. Silverglade, A.: Biological equivalence of beef lung and hog mucosal heparins. *Curr. Ther. Res.,* 18:91, 1975.
60. Statham, L.: Pulmonary embolism. *Nurs. Times,* 68:284, 1972.
61. Szucs, M., et al.: Diagnostic sensitivity of laboratory findings in acute pulmonary embolism. *Ann. Intern. Med.,* 74:161, 1971.
62. Tikoff, G., and S. M. Prescott: Axioms on thrombophlebitis and phlebothrombosis. *Hosp. Med.,* 15:36, April 1979.
63. Thompson, N.: Buried dermal flap operation for chronic lymphedema of the extremities. *Plast. Reconstr. Surg.,* 45:541, 1970.
64. Thompson, N.: The surgical treatment of advanced postmastectomy lymphedema of the upper limb. *Scand. J. Plast. Surg.,* 3:54 1969.
65. Turpie, A. G. G., and J. Hirsh: When and how to use heparin prophylaxis and treatment. *Geriatrics,* 34:59, June 1979.
66. Vermeulen, W. J.: Experience with the Thompson procedure as treatment for filarial elephantiasis of the extremities. *In* Clodius, R. (Ed.): *Lymphedema.* Stuttgart: Georg Thieme Publishers, 1977.
67. Wadsworth, T. G.: Postoperative deep vein thrombosis. *Nurs. Mirror,* 134:28, 1972.
68. Wallach, R.: Dextran therapy for pregnancy-associated deep thrombophlebitis. *Am. J. Obstet. Gynecol.,* 112:613, 1972.
69. Weintraub, A. M., and M. N. Gomes: Varicose veins. *Am. Fam. Physician,* 13:107, Mar. 1976.
70. Wessler, S., and S. N. Gitel: Heparin and warfarin therapy: recommendations concerning efficacy and safety. *Postgr. Med.,* 65:103, Feb. 1979.
71. Wiederhielm, C. A.: The capillaries, veins and lymphatics. *In* Ruch, T. C., and H. D. Patton (Eds.): *Physiology and Biophysics,* 12th ed. Philadelphia: W. B. Saunders Co., 1974.
72. Yao, S. T., et al.: Detection of proximal vein thrombosis by Doppler ultrasound flow-detection method. *Lancet,* 1:1, 1972.
73. Young, J. R.: Axioms on thrombophlebitis and phlebothrombosis. *Hosp. Med.,* 12:6, Oct. 1976.
74. Young, J. R.: The swollen leg. *Am. Fam. Physician,* 15:163, Jan. 1977.

CHAPTER 50*

NURSING THE PERSON UNDERGOING AN AMPUTATION

Amputation is the surgical removal of all or part of an extremity. The most frequent indication for amputation of the *lower extremities* is *peripheral vascular disease.* Indeed, according to McCollough, "Recent major surveys of lower limb amputations have revealed that up to 85 per cent of civilian amputations performed today are for complications of peripheral vascular disease."[48] Because peripheral vascular disease is associated with the aging process and is also one of the several complications of diabetes mellitus, the seemingly concurrent increased life span and increase of diabetic patients possibly may account for this high incidence.

In contrast, the most common indication for amputations of the *upper extremities* is *severe trauma* due to electrical, chemical, and thermal burns; frostbite; armed conflict; war injuries; or explosions. Only rarely are upper limb amputations performed to control peripheral vascular disorders.

Children most frequently require amputations because of trauma, congenital malformation, or limb deficiency.

Other reasons for amputating either upper or lower extremities, in order of most frequent occurrence: acute or chronic infections, e.g., chronic osteomyelitis, fulminating gas gangrene, trophic ulcers, and septic wounds; severe crushing wounds; malignant tumors and frostbite; congenital deformities.

A recent study by Kay and Newmann[36] revealed that men undergo more amputations than women, especially of the upper extremities. In addition, amputations in men were more frequently due to trauma than disease; the reverse was true for women. In comparing their findings with a similar study done in 1964, a definite trend in the reduction of trauma-related amputations and an increase in disease-related amputations was observable.[29] The decreasing number of trauma-related amputations may indicate stricter safety control factors in industry. The industrial nurse has a definite role in developing safety programs that will alert both employer and employee to risk factors and preventive solutions.

Faced with increasing numbers of amputees, the health professions have striven in recent years to improve the care of these patients. At one time, major goals of care were limited to removal of the injured or diseased limb and avoidance of infection and contractures. Today the goals have greatly expanded to include the *total rehabilitation* of the amputee, thereby insuring return to full function and a normal active life. In Friedmann's words, attainment of full function includes "reconstructive amputation without procrastination, prompt healing of the stump, fast patient preparation to use a good artificial limb provided promptly, and training.[28]

Despite tremendous improvements in the care of amputees, the individual undergoing amputation still faces a severe — sometimes catastrophic — trauma that strikes not only the body but the mind and emotions as well. We live in a highly mobile society. Also, our society admires "the doer," the independent achiever, the individual who "gets around," and who "gets things done." Moreover physical attractiveness is presented in all media as being almost essential for survival in a competitive world. The youthful, beautiful, intact body is upheld as the ideal to the United States public night and day on billboards, in magazines, and on television. For these reasons amputation signifies much more to the average person than simply the loss of a limb; it symbolizes the end of the mobility that was previously enjoyed and the loss forever of a whole, intact body and a satisfying self-image. These losses, in turn, cause the patient to fear further losses on the job market and in family and social relationships.

To help the amputee to overcome these fears and anxieties and to return to full function is

*Henrietta P. Gaines, R.N., B.A., critically reviewed and assisted with the revision of this chapter.

the major task of the nurse and the rehabilitation team: physician, nurse, physical therapist, occupational therapist, prosthetist, social worker, and psychologist. If the amputee is to reach these goals, the health team must design a total plan of care in keeping with the individual patients' personality and needs. Friedmann summarizes the "ideal" care plan when he states:

> Evaluating the patient's needs is central to good care, and should determine the total plan for that individual, which he understands, and in which he concurs. It includes the decision to operate, the type and timing of surgery, the postoperative care, fitting and training — physical, psychological, and vocational. This is what is necessary in treating the person rather than the diseased limb.[28]

SURGICAL EVALUATION OF THE PATIENT

When surgeons evaluate a patient for possible amputation, they must decide upon (1) whether to amputate; (2) the type of amputation (i.e., open or closed); (3) the level of amputation required; (4) the patient's rehabilitation potential; and (5) the type of postoperative prosthetic fitting and rehabilitative program desired. Let us briefly explore each of these problems.

The Decision to Amputate. The surgeon's decision about whether to amputate depends primarily upon the patient's condition, results of tests of peripheral vascular function, and the general attitude of the surgeon and the patient toward amputation. First of all, an amputation is in order if the patient's life is in danger (e.g., in severe toxicity resulting from gangrene) or if the patient suffers from intractable limb pain. Also, the surgeon may amputate if the patient's ability to function is hopelessly impaired by a damaged extremity. Limb impairment may result from either severe injury, congenital deformity, or chronic ischemia resulting from extensive peripheral vascular disease.

Secondly, when peripheral vascular disease is the major indication for amputation, the surgeon orders diagnostic tests before making a final decision. Studies of peripheral function include oscillometry, tests for intermittent claudication, angiography, skin temperature studies, and palpation of the popliteal arteries. These tests were discussed in Chapter 48.

Through the consideration of these test results, the physician must also determine if revascularization procedures are indicated and the prognosis for circulatory return after vascular reconstruction. Once gangrene is present in an extremity, no amount of revascularization will reverse the situation, nor can circulatory impairment owing to small vessel disease be restored by vascular reconstruction.[15]

In addition, the decision to amputate is determined, in part, by the surgeon's attitude toward the procedure. Friedmann implies that amputation is equated in the minds of some doctors with failure, and that these surgeons may strive to save the patient's extremity "at all costs." On the other hand, Friedmann states, "When the surgeon views the problem as attempting to improve the overall function of his patient, he appreciates that proper amputation, and postoperative care, can restore the patient to a level of function only slightly different from the preamputation state.[28]

Like some surgeons, some patients may resist amputation even though it would greatly improve their function. For example, one of the authors (JL) once cared for a young woman whose hand had been horribly crushed and mangled in a wringer accident. Even though her hand was deformed, painful and useless, this patient refused to consider amputation; unfortunately, she regarded amputation as a further form of multilation. Finally, after many months and great effort, her doctors convinced the young woman that a well-fitted, functioning, prosthetic device would be superior to a hand that was useless and unsightly. The patient underwent surgery and prosthesis training and eventually learned to accept her artificial hand as a functioning part of herself.

However, the elderly who suffer considerably from the pain of ischemia may often desire to have the source of the pain removed without such intense fear of loss of body image or function. In providing support for the patient facing an inevitable amputation, the nurse should consider those values relative to the *patient's age* and *maturity level.*

Type of Amputation. There are two types of amputation procedures: the open or guillotine amputation and the closed or "flap" amputation. The major indication for *guillotine amputation* is *infection.* The fact that the stump is not closed over with a skin flap allows the free drainage of purulent or infectious material. Patients undergoing an open amputation require antibiotic therapy and the use of strict aseptic technique whenever the incision is cleansed, the dressing is changed, and so forth. Once the infection is completely eradicated, the patient then undergoes *stump revision* closure.

The *closed* or *flap* amputation is one in which the stump is closed or covered by a flap of skin sutured over the bone end of the stump. This type of amputation, illustrated in Figures 50–2 and 50–3, is performed when there is *no evidence of infection* and consequently no need for extensive open drainage. However, to prevent accu-

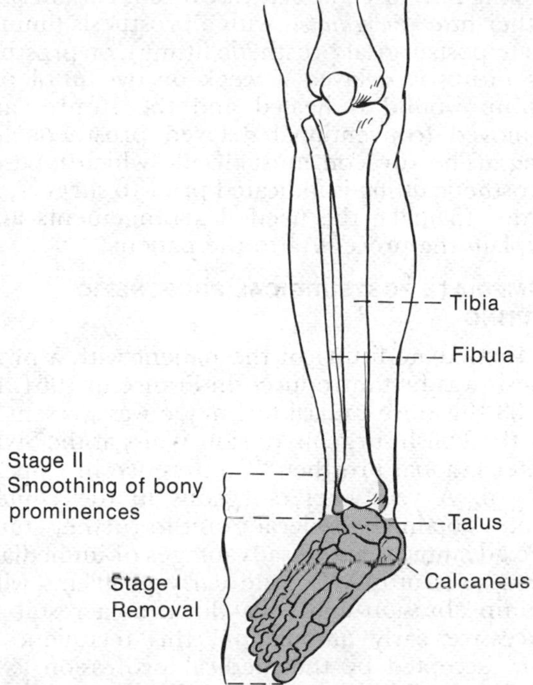

Figure 50–1. Syme's amputation. Note that there is no invasion of bone during Stage I.

mulations of blood and serous fluids, some surgeons elect to insert small drains into the incision site to allow drainage of these fluids. Nursing care of these drains entails: (a) prevention of inadvertently dislodging the tubing during positioning of the patient, (b) assuring patency by avoiding external pressure or "pinching" of the tubing, and (c) frequent emptying of accumulated drainage from the drainage bag. If the tube becomes dislodged, the nurse *should not* attempt to reinsert it as this will introduce contamination into the surgical wound. If a rigid dressing is applied during surgery, drains are not necessary because the dressing compresses the stump and alleviates swelling. (See discussion of the rigid dressing below.)

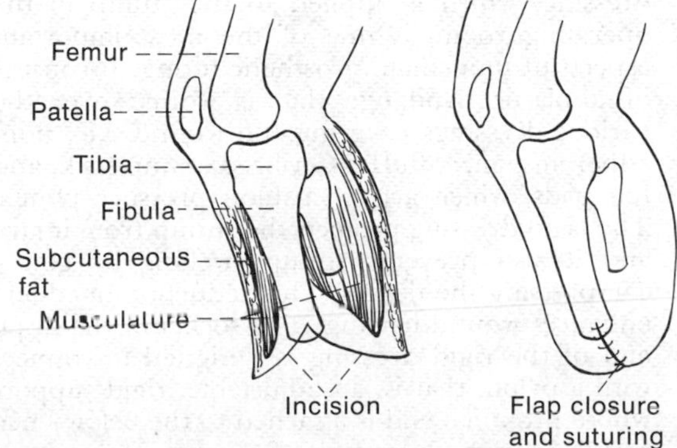

Figure 50–2. Below-knee amputation. Note contouring of muscle tissue and skin flap to accommodate flap closure.

Level of Amputation. Specific amputation levels for the *lower extremities* are as follows:

- Amputation in the foot.
- Amputation at the ankle level (Syme's operation) (Fig. 50–1).
- Below the knee (B/K) amputation (Fig. 50–2).
- Knee disarticulation (bones separated at the knee).
- Above the knee amputation (Fig. 50–3).
- Hip disarticulation (amputation through the hip or pelvis, which is performed for malignant tumors, massive injuries, and extensive gangrene).

Specific amputation levels of the *upper extremities* are:

- Wrist disarticulation
- Below-elbow amputation
- Elbow disarticulation
- Above-elbow amputation

The level of amputation for either lower or upper extremities should never be higher than absolutely necessary. In the case of lower extremity amputations, the percentage of *energy expenditure* by the patient increases with each higher level of amputation as follows:[28]

- Unilateral B/K amputation: 10 per cent higher than in the nonamputee
- Bilateral B/K amputation: 20 per cent higher than in nonamputee
- Unilateral A/K amputation: 60 per cent higher than in nonamputee

The surgeon tentatively decides upon the level of amputation prior to surgery. Circulation

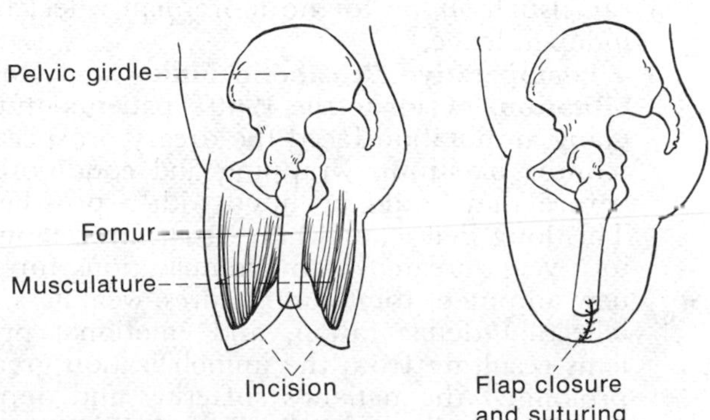

Figure 50–3. Above-knee amputation. Note contouring, as in Figure 50–2.

to the skin of the extremities must be adequate for the stump to heal satisfactorily. To evaluate circulatory status, the surgeon examines the patient's extremity for warmth, sensation, and hair growth; also arteriography, oscillometry, and other procedures discussed earlier may be ordered. There also must be consideration of the age of the patient relative to the rehabilitation goals. Assurance of ambulation is greater for the elderly if the knee joint is saved.[30]

However, it is not until the patient is in the operating room that the surgeon makes a final decision concerning stump length. The selection of amputation level at that time is based upon the extent of bleeding from the incised skin edges. If skin bleeding is normal, then the amputation is performed at the level selected preoperatively. If skin bleeding is scant, then the surgeon is forced to operate at a higher level to ensure adequate postoperative healing.

Evaluation of Rehabilitative Potential. Ideally, patients should attain independent function with the use of a prosthesis. However, prosthetic rehabilitation requires patient cooperation, good coordination, and a tremendous expenditure of energy. Unfortunately some patients, because of age or disease, are unable to undertake prosthesis training. Conditions that prohibit prosthesis fitting and ambulation include the following:

- Severe neurologic disease
- Disorientation, senility, psychosis, or severe mental retardation
- Chronic heart failure accompanied by greatly reduced cardiac reserve
- Chronic obstructive pulmonary disease
- Progressive, severe complications of diabetes, e.g., nephropathy, neuropathy

Individuals burdened with these problems can usually hope for no more than wheelchair independence.

Postoperative Prosthetic Fitting and Rehabilitation. Prior to the 1960's, patients undergoing amputation faced the dreary prospect of months of stump wrapping and conditioning before they could be fitted with a prosthesis. This long delay (anywhere from three months to a year) created many complications for the new amputee. Joint contractures, weakness, intellectual deterioration, and emotional problems resulting from the immobilization greatly prolonged the patient's suffering and dependency as well as hospitalization. Today, old-fashioned methods of protracted stump conditioning have been largely discarded. Patients are either fitted *immediately* with a prosthesis (immediate postsurgical prosthetic fitting), or prosthesis fitting is delayed a week or two until the stump wound is healed and the sutures are removed (conventional delayed prosthetic fitting). The surgeon must decide which type of prosthetic fitting is indicated prior to surgery, in order to make the needed arrangements and explain the procedure to the patient.

IMMEDIATE POSTSURGICAL PROSTHETIC FITTING

Immediate fitting of the patient with a prosthesis was first introduced in France in 1961. In 1963 this once radical technique was presented by the Polish surgeon Marion Weiss at the Sixth International Prosthetic Conference in Copenhagen. A year later, surgeons in the United States obtained a federal grant to further study the advantages and disadvantages of immediate prosthetic fitting. Despite early problems with stump abrasion and breakdown as a result of excessive early ambulation, this technique is now accepted by the medical profession as a highly useful procedure, and it is currently employed in medical centers throughout the world.

The program for immediate postsurgical prosthetic fitting typically involves the following aspects:[1, 28]

- *Myoplastic surgery.* Myoplasty is the plastic repair of muscles whereby severed muscles are reattached to one another and to the bone. It is employed during closed amputation in order to restore normal muscle tension, and to restore muscle and tendon sensory feedback loops which, in turn, make the stump sensitive and responsive to stimuli. A stump which acts as a sensory-motor end-organ enables the amputee to use a prosthesis more effectively, learn a more graceful gait, and regain the sense of balance. However, some authorities believe that the use of myoplastic techniques is unnecessary and even unwise in some amputations, and that they should be used only in young patients with adequate circulation.
- *Application of a total contact rigid dressing.* The rigid dressing, which is applied to the stump in the operating room, is one of the most important aspects of immediate prosthetic fitting. It consists of a plastic bandange that is wound over the various dressings covering the wound, i.e., nonadherent gauze, fluffs, sterilized stump sock, and felt pads, which act to cushion pressure points. The rigid dressing protects the stump from injury and it also prevents stump swelling by gently compressing the tissues. This reduction in edema enhances wound healing. The socket of the distal end of the rigid dressing is designed to connect with a pylon, that is, an adjustable, rigid support whose proximal end is attached to the below-knee socket or to the knee unit of an above-knee prosthesis. The distal end is connected to a foot-ankle assembly (Fig. 50–4). The rigid dressing is usually

changed three to four times before a permanent prosthesis is applied. Cast changes are necessary because, as the stump heals, it tends to shrink and is consequently no longer compressed by the original cast. In fact, through the cast changes, stump shrinkage can be easily monitored.

- *Early ambulation.* The real purpose of early ambulation with an immediate postsurgical prosthesis is to condition and prepare the patient's stump for later gait traning. A desirable secondary effect is in the reduction of postoperative complications and a quicker fitting for the permanent prosthesis. The patient usually begins to ambulate the first postoperative day. Ambulation time is brief (3 minutes once or twice that day) and weight-bearing is strictly limited (see below).

- *Controlled progressive ambulation.* The patient ambulates a little more each day, depending upon the specific rehabilitation program and the patient's tolerance of increased activity. At first, simply standing at the bedside with help takes place; next, learning to walk between parallel bars; gradually progression to crutches and then a cane is accomplished. Finally the amputee is able to walk without assistance of any kind. This gait training period usually extends for approximately three months. During these exercise periods, the before and after standing pulse and blood pressure are monitored by the physical therapist or nurse, who is also alert to any complaints of pain under the cast. In patients who have been on prolonged bedrest, a "tilt table" for slowly adjusting the patient to an upright stance is used.

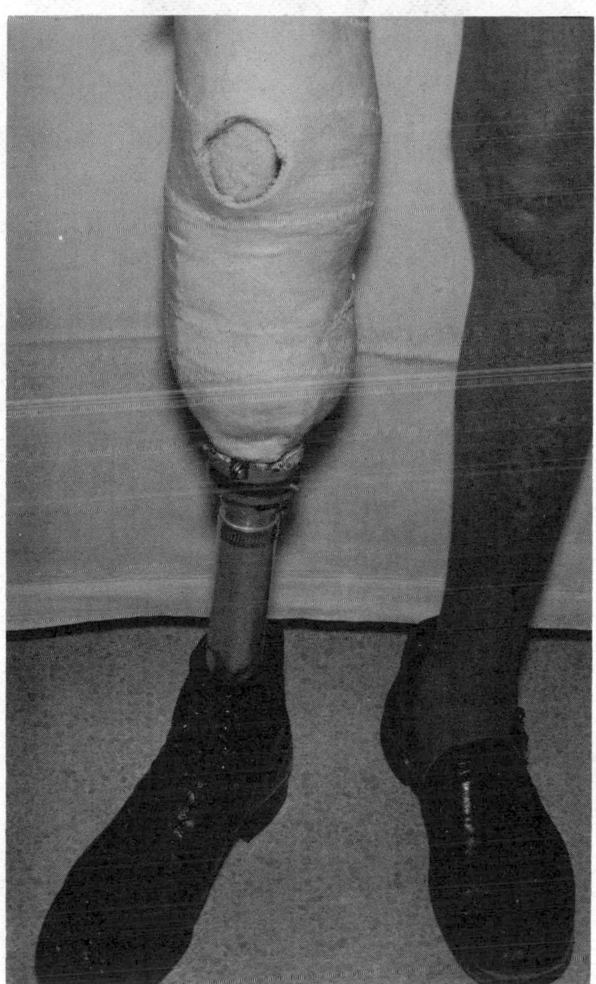

Figure 50–4. Immediate postsurgical prosthesis in place after below-knee amputation for occlusive arterial disease. Note rigid dressing, pylon, and foot-ankle assembly. (From Fairbairn, J. F., II, J. L. Juergens, and J. A. Spittell, Jr.: *Peripheral Vascular Diseases,* 4th ed. Philadelphia: W. B. Saunders Co., 1972.)

- *Limited weight-bearing.* Weight-bearing must be strictly limited during the first weeks of ambulation, because the wound is still healing. To learn to control weight-bearing, new amputees are placed on paired scales and told to note the amount of weight that they are placing on their prosthesis as compared with the unamputated limb. During the first two weeks following amputation, patients are instructed to *never place more than 20 to 25 pounds of weight* on the prosthetic limb.[1] As healing increases, weight-bearing increases. Because it is difficult for most patients to remember the "feel" of the proper weight, one hospital is now using a "beeper," which is placed between the prosthetic foot and the rigid dressing. The "beeper" is sensitive to pressure and it "beeps" to warn the patient whenever the assigned weight-bearing capacity is exceeded.[7]

- *Patient cooperation.* The patient is truly a prime member of the rehabilitation team. If immediate postsurgical prosthetic fitting is to be successful, the patient must be willing to limit weight-bearing, learn and apply the principles of stump and prosthesis care, and wholeheartedly enter into a program of progressive ambulation and gait training.

Benefits. Immediate prosthetic fitting offers the amputee many advantages. First of all, emotional adjustment to the amputation is better if the patient awakens from surgery with a substitute limb already attached to the stump. In addition, the rigid dressing acts as a compression bandage, molding and shrinking the stump. This continuous sustained compression reduces stump edema, pain, phantom sensations, and contractures. Also, by alleviating the need for months of stump wrapping and preprosthetic conditioning, the rigid dressing shortens the patient's rehabilitation period and speeds return to social and economic independence. Finally, the program of early progressive ambulation alleviates the complications of immobility, stimulates the circulation, and fosters a sense of hope and optimism in the patient and significant others.

Indications and Contraindications. Immediate postoperative prosthetic fitting is almost always indicated for children and juveniles. It is also highly beneficial for individuals with below-knee and below-elbow amputations.

On the other hand, immediate fitting is contraindicated for the following patients:

- Above-knee amputees, because these patients are usually severely debilitated from the condition which resulted in amputation; e.g., diabetes, gangrene, osteomyelitis.
- Above-elbow amputees, because these individuals have usually suffered extensive trauma and are in poor or critical condition.
- Patients with incapacitating medical disorders; e.g., neurologic disease, severe heart disease, extensive vascular pathology, anemia, and hypoproteinemia.
- Patients who are unable or unwilling to control weight-bearing during the early postoperative period; e.g., confused senile persons, patients who do not understand the language in which instructions are given, the psychotic, and mentally retarded.
- Patients who have undergone vascular reconstruction or who have an infected stump.

In addition, immediate fitting should not be attempted in small hospitals with inadequate prosthetic facilities.

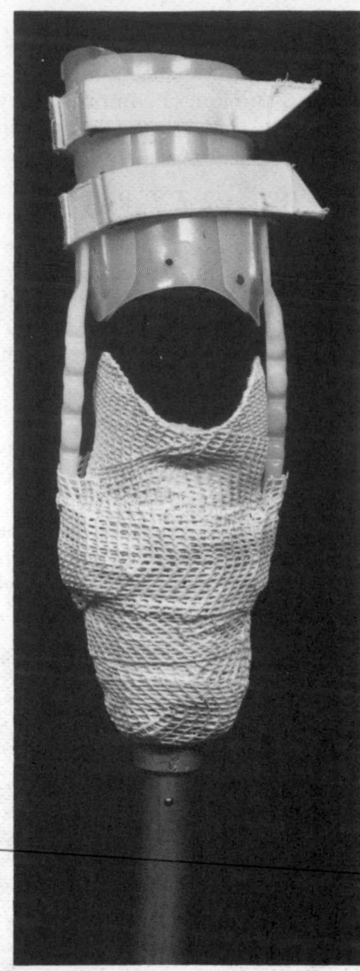

Figure 50–5. Temporary prosthesis for a below-knee amputation, frequently referred to as "light-weight intermediate prosthesis." It provides construction that is capable of full weight bearing. Note the plastic thigh cuff with Velcro straps. The plastic, flexible knee joints facilitate more normal joint activity. Decreased weight plus ease in putting on are both important features. (Courtesy of Rancho Los Amigos Hospital, Downey, Cal.)

CONVENTIONAL DELAYED PROSTHESIS FITTING

Immediate prosthetic fitting is not always possible; however, authorities agree that every amputee capable of eventually ambulating should receive a temporary prosthesis *as soon as possible* following surgery. Early prosthesis fitting and training benefits the patient psychologically. Also early ambulation prevents the complications associated with immobility; moreover, the pumping action afforded by walking reduces stump edema more effectively than does stump bandaging.

The timetable for patients undergoing delayed prosthesis fitting is approximately as follows:

- The patient returns from surgery with the stump dressed and covered with either Ace bandages or stump socks; note that the rigid dressing is generally not used for conventional delayed fittings.
- During the following one to two postoperative weeks, the patient's stump is wrapped in the manner shown in Figures 50–6 and 50–7; note the differences in technique from wrapping an above-knee stump and a below-knee stump.
- During the second or third postoperative week, the sutures are removed. If the stump has healed satisfactorily and no complications are present, the patient is then fitted with a provisional temporary prosthesis made of plaster of Paris or plastic, as shown in Figure 50–5. At this time the patient begins to ambulate; however, only partial weight bearing is allowed.
- By the sixth week, the patient is allowed to put full weight on the prosthesis.
- By the tenth to twelfth week the patient is fitted with a permanent prosthesis, provided progress has been satisfactory.

Which prosthetic fitting technique is generally more successful — the immediate or the delayed? Choice of technique depends upon the patient's needs and upon the surgeon's personal preference. On the one hand, the immediate technique is usually selected for young patients and for those who need the psychologic "lift" provided by immediate replacement of the amputated limb. Also, the use of the rigid dressing offers many advantages. On the other hand, delayed fitting may be preferred by some surgeons because it is generally safer. Wound disruption rarely occurs with delayed fitting because the wound must be almost completely healed before the patient can begin to ambulate. Further, the amount of rehabilitation time saved by using the more risky immediate fitting is only one to two weeks at most.[28] Finally, the use of immediate fitting techniques is limited to large medical centers where prosthetic experts are available.

THE COSMETIC PROSTHESIS

Those patients who are not prosthetic candidates for whatever reasons but who, for cultural or personal reasons, cannot accept reentry into society minus a limb may be referred for a cosmetic prosthesis. Its functional use is for enhancing the patient's self-esteem. Because its construction does not allow the patient to bear weight, the patient should be cautioned to not attempt any kind of transfer or ambulation activities using it.

CARE OF THE PATIENT UNDERGOING AMPUTATION OF THE LOWER EXTREMITIES

PREOPERATIVE CARE

Psychologic Preparation. As we emphasized earlier, it is extremely difficult for the average person to accept amputation of one or more extremities even though it is absolutely necessary.

Amputation is dreaded because it destroys the patient's idealized body image, imposes both physical and social limitations, and temporarily (and sometimes permanently) disrupts one's life style. In sum, amputation signifies a painful venture into a frightening unknown.

We know that fears and anxieties that remain unchallenged and unresolved during the preoperative period can adversely affect the patient's progress during the postoperative period. To help the potential amputee feel less fearful of the coming surgery, put into practice the following six suggestions:

- *Establish open, honest communication.* Allow the patient to freely express fears and negative feelings over the coming loss of the limb. Try to analyze how the patient perceives the amputation procedure. Report to the physician if you note the presence of extreme depression, great fear and anxiety, or suicidal tendencies. Utilize also the services of the social worker or psychologist or both.

- *Give and reinforce information.* Most patients feel less anxious when they know what to expect upon awakening after surgery. Ask the surgeon what the patient has been told about the coming amputation. Typically the surgeon reassures the patient

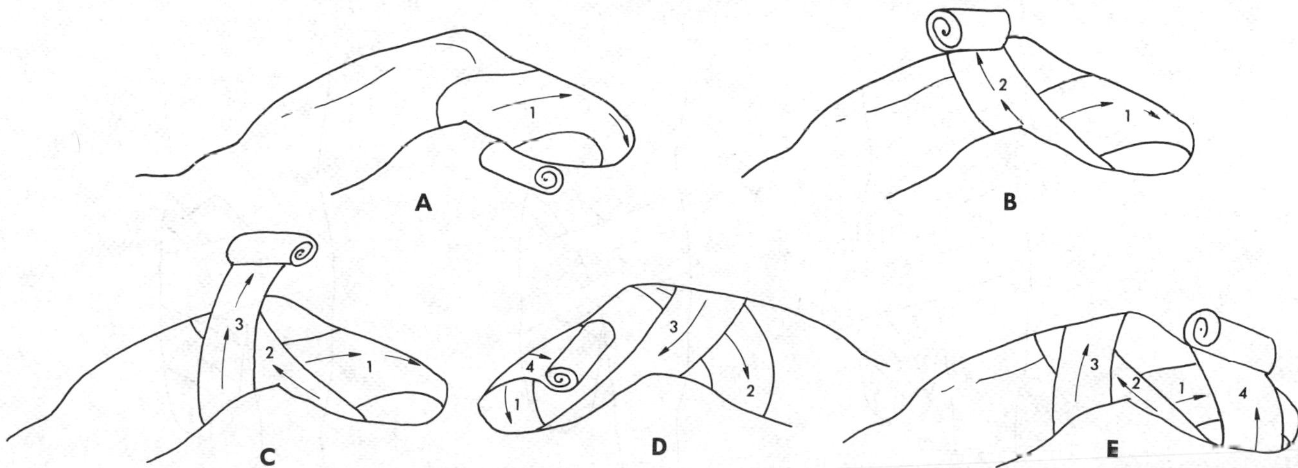

Figure 50–6. Bandaging a below-knee amputation stump. If a second bandage is needed, it should be started over the medial condyle, reversing the procedure shown. Anterolateral aspect: **A,** Start 4″ elastic bandage above lateral condyle. Enclose medial, distal end of stump. Apply pressure via bandage at distal end. Use diagonal, not circular, turns. Hold roll so it is upward for ease in unwinding. **B,** Bring roll around posterior aspect of calf, enclosing beginning of roll. Make turn around thigh above patella. Be sure there is *less* tension on bandage above knee than on end of stump. **C,** Turn No. 3 goes diagonally above knee and down to include medial condyle. Anteromedial aspect: **D,** Turns 3 and 4 continue to posterior aspect of calf. **E,** Turns 3 and 4 enclose lateral, distal end of stump. Continue to above knee as shown with turns 2 and 3. Finish enclosing end of stump using diagonal and figure-of-8 turns. Be sure greatest pressure is on end of stump. (Courtesy of Physical Therapy Department, Harborview Medical Center, Seattle.)

that as much of the extremity as possible will be saved. The doctor also discusses the type of prosthetic fitting that the patient will undergo (immediate or delayed) and the approximate amount of time that will lapse before the patient receives the final prosthesis and is at least 90 per cent independent. The surgeon may also describe the immediate postoperative period and the discomforts, problems, and possible complications that may accompany it. Once you know what the surgeon has said, you can then safely discuss any points that worry or confuse the patient. Be certain that what you say is well thought out, accurate and considerate of the person's psychologic needs.

- *Prepare for phantom limb sensation*, By informing patients that these sensations occur and are normal, the nurse may avert misunderstandings. Patients who have these sensations may indeed feel they are "verging on insanity," but they may also refuse to tell anyone for fear that their suspicions will be confirmed. Unable to talk about their feelings, these patients may become withdrawn or they may act out behaviors that further compound the problem.
- *Establish expectations.* Not only do patients want to know what to expect after surgery, they need to know what the staff *will expect of them.* Emphasize that the patient is the most important member of the rehabilitation team. If patients want to achieve independence, then they will have to exercise several times a day, strictly limited weight-bearing (if they are losing part of a leg) until instructed otherwise, learn all the intricacies of stump and prosthesis care, and master the use of the protheses.
- *Build confidence.* The patient will feel more confident of successful rehabilitation if he or she meets the rehabilitation team prior to surgery. If at all possible, arrange to introduce the patient to the physical and occupational therapy staffs, the prosthetist, and the vocational counselor; in some institutions the team also includes a social worker and psychologist.

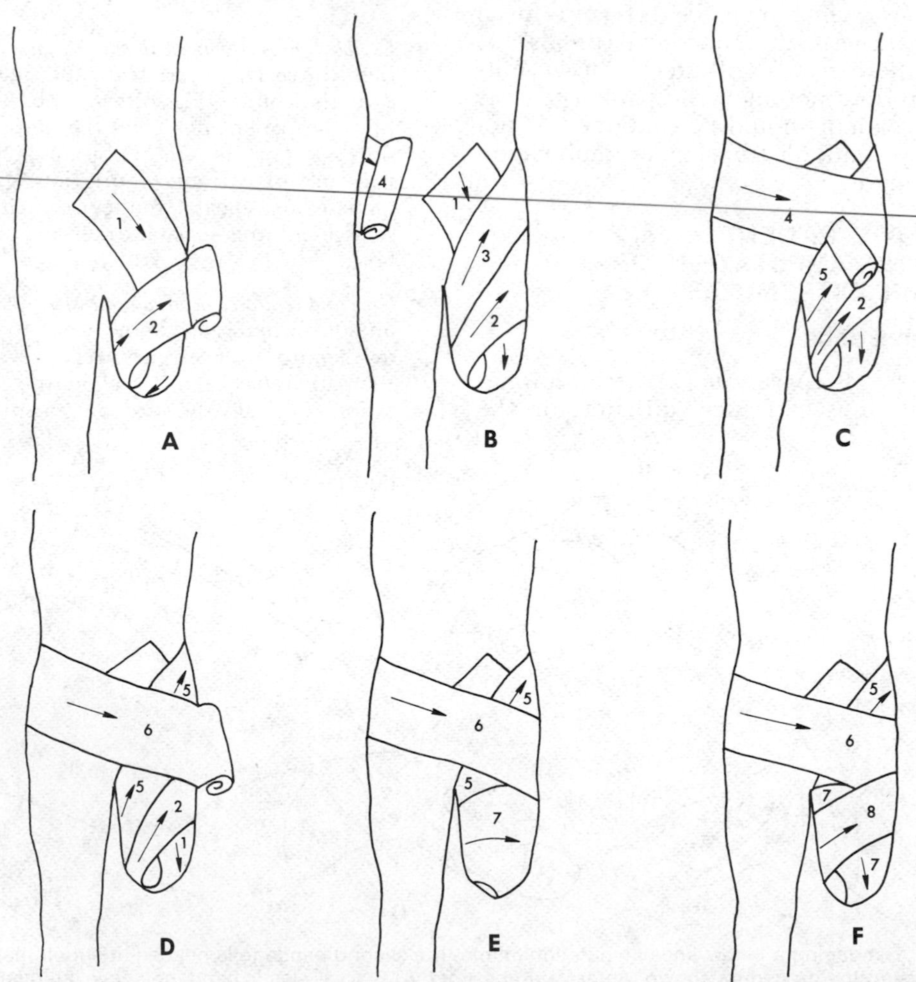

Figure 50–7. Bandaging an above-knee amputation stump. **A,** Use 6″ elastic bandage. Enclose medial, distal end of stump. Apply pressure via bandage to end of stump. Use diagonal, not circular, turns. **B,** Turn No. 3 must be high in groin and then turn made around waist to hold No. 3 in place. Do not pull hip into flexion. (A second 6″ roll may be needed.) **C,** Turn No. 5 must be high in groin and a loop made around waist again. **D,** See diagram. **E,** Enclose lateral, distal end of stump. (A 4″ roll may be needed.) Continue diagonal and figure-of-8 turns around stump. **F,** Continue turns to shape end of stump. (Courtesy of University of Washington Department of Prosthetics, from booklet *Prosthetics-Orthotics.*)

- *Sustain hope and optimism.* Like the patient who faces mastectomy, laryngectomy, or permanent colostomy, the future amputee often feels that social, vocational, and love lives virtually end with surgery. To counteract this hopeless outlook, it is extremely helpful to introduce the patient to other amputees who are mastering their prostheses and achieving independence. The support, encouragement, and understanding of other amputees often provides the hope and courage that many future amputees so desperately need.

Physical Preparation. Physical preparation of patients for amputation focuses upon controlling or alleviating underlying illnesses and infections, correcting nutritional and fluid imbalances, and preparing patients for postoperative ambulation by increasing their strength and endurance.

Diabetics are considered a surgical "risk" group and have special considerations in preoperative preparation.[45] Persons with ulcerated legs or osteomyelitis may be treated with antibiotics and bed rest. Debilitated persons are nourished with foods high in protein; they may also be given supplements of vitamins and minerals. The severely anemic are treated with iron preparations and blood transfusions, and dehydrated patients receive intravenous fluids to correct their fluid imbalances.

Finally, if time and the patient's condition permit, the patient is started on a somewhat strenuous program of exercise and mobility training that will be beneficial during the postoperative period. With guidance from the physical therapist and nurse, the patient performs a number of exercises at least once or twice a day. Recommended exercises include active hip extension, abduction, straight leg raising, and quadriceps setting for below-the-knee amputations; hip extension, abduction, and adduction for above-the-knee amputations. Also the patient learns how to transfer from bed to a wheelchair to the toilet and then back again. In addition, the patient ideally is taught to ambulate in a walker and on crutches and also how to control and modify weight-bearing on the affected side. Upper extremity weakness hinders the use of ambulatory aids, i.e., crutches, walker, cane. Occupational therapists will prescribe and begin a strengthening program to promote rehabilitation potential. If patients can master these essential exercises and skills during the preoperative period, they are almost assured of a smoother postoperative course.

POSTOPERATIVE CARE

Goals and Basic Principles of Care. According to Friedmann, the goals of postoperative care for all new amputees are as follows:

(1) The preservation and improvement of the patient's general health, with particular attention to the cardiovascular respiratory system and the vascular state of the remaining leg; (2) the creation of the kind of stump which can most effectively utilize the modern total contact prosthesis with redevelopment of proprioception and sensory feedback from floor reaction forces as a means of communication for the optimal development of skillful, automatic gait; (3) diminishing the adverse consequences of the amputation in the functional, psychic, social, economic and vocational spheres. All of the above must be consistent with the individual patient's abilities and problems, and the conditions under which he must live and function.[28]

Basic postoperative goals are the same, but the actual postoperative care of amputees varies, according to whether the patient: (1) has been immediately fitted with a prosthesis while in surgery, (2) will be fitted at a later time, (3) is ineligible for prosthesis fitting for reasons cited earlier, or (4) has undergone a guillotine type of amputation because of infection. Let us begin by considering the first two groups.

In Table 50–1 we have compared and contrasted postoperative care for patients undergoing immediate prosthesis fitting and those undergoing conventional delay prosthesis fitting.

The third group of patients, which includes the elderly, senile, and debilitated, need continuous and conscientious nursing care throughout the postoperative period if their condition is not to worsen. These individuals may be seriously dehydrated and may consequently need intravenous fluids. Elderly and senile patients and those with neurologic conditions may be incontinent of both urine and feces. To prevent gross contamination of the stump wound, place a plastic material (such as Saran Wrap) around the outside bandage and secure it with adhesive tape. Do not apply adhesive tape directly to the skin of a patient with circulatory impairment.

In addition, the elderly and debilitated are usually unable to perform active exercises; passively exercise these patients' limbs several times a day until strength increases. Take care to turn debilitated amputees every one to two hours and have them cough and deep breathe frequently. Remember that patients in this group are highly susceptible to all the complications of immobilization The main cause of death postoperatively among the elderly is bronchopneumonia. Observe these patients continuously for signs of hypostatic pneumonia, contractures, and bladder and kidney problems. Also, the new amputee who is old, ill, weak, and exhausted usually suffers from severe depression, which results in further immobilization.

Finally, there are the patients who undergo a *guillotine* amputation. As you recall, the indica-

TABLE 50–1. POSTOPERATIVE CARE: COMPARISON OF AMPUTEES UNDERGOING DELAYED AND IMMEDIATE PROSTHESIS FITTING

Type of Care	Delayed Prosthesis Fitting	Immediate Prosthesis Fitting
Stump care	Stump covered with dressings and Ace bandage or stump socks; note if Penrose drains were inserted during surgery to remove blood and serous fluid; check tubes for patency.	Stump covered with dressings and rigid plastic dressing; Penrose drains usually not inserted because rigid dressing helps to prevent bleeding by compressing the stump.
	Observe dressings for signs of excessive bleeding; *always have large tourniquet on hand* to apply around stump in event of hemorrhage.	Observe rigid dressing for signs of oozing; if oozing occurs, mark blood stain with a pen and observe stain every 10 minutes for increase in size; report excessive oozing at once.
	Reinforce or change dressings as ordered; wrap stump with Ace bandages as shown in Figures 50–6 and 50–7, or cover dressings with stump socks; *check bandages frequently*—they can slip and form a tourniquet around stump, occluding blood supply.	Provide *cast care* as discussed in Unit XX and outlined in Table 50–2. *Guard against cast slipping off stump* because edema and wound disruption rapidly develop; if slippage occurs, compress stump at once with tightly wrapped plastic bandage; observe for loosened cast that "turns" on stump; *notify surgeon.*
	Sutures removed in 10 to 14 days if wound healing well; temporary prosthesis fitted at that time.	Sutures usually removed in 10 to 14 days during first cast change; cast changed one to two more times thereafter, to compensate for stump shrinkage.
Pain relief	Narcotics (Demerol and codeine) may be needed to control severe incisional and phantom pain (Unit XI).	Darvon usually sufficient for pain control because rigid cast greatly reduces pain and phantom sensation.
Positioning	Elevate stump on pillow for 24 to 48 hours to hasten venous return, prevent edema, and promote patient comfort; *do not* elevate for more than 48 hours or hip contracture may result.	Elevation of stump for 24 hours usually sufficient; rigid cast acts to control swelling. Provide padding between casted and other extremity to avoid skin abrasion.
Turning	Turn patient to prone position for short time first postoperative day and then 2 to 3 times daily to prevent hip contracture; have patient roll from side to side.	Same; rigid cast, however, acts to prevent both hip and joint contractures and turning is not so essential.
Exercises	Exercises to prevent contractures started as soon as possible (1st or 2nd day postoperative), including: active range of motion, especially of remaining leg; strengthening exercises for upper extremities; hyperextension of stump.	Exercises not so essential because rigid dressing prevents contractures; also, early ambulation prevents all immobilization disabilities.
Ambulation	Transfer to wheelchair and back within 1st or 2nd postoperative day. Crutch walking is started as soon as patient feels sufficiently strong (Unit XX).	Ambulate patient in walker for short period first day. Ambulate longer time each day; in physical therapy, patient uses parallel bars, then crutches, then cane.
Psychologic support	Observe carefully for signs of depression or despondency; remind depressed patients that they will receive prosthesis when wound heals.	Observe for depression; patients usually less depressed if they awaken with prosthesis attached.

tion for this type of amputation is *infection.* The stump is left open and unsutured to permit free drainage. To prevent retraction of the skin, traction is applied, either Buck's extension traction or a Thomas splint may be used. (See Unit XX.)

Infection is treated with bedrest and antibiotics. The choice of antibiotic is initially determined through culture and sensitivities taken from the infected wound prior to surgery. When sensitivities are not available, initial antibiotic treatment may be started with a broad-spectrum antibiotic, e.g., cephalosporins, and given IV piggyback as the method of choice for administration. This preoperative treatment reduces the inflammatory process, thus reducing edema. The reduction of both bacteria and edema give the surgeon a more favorable "tissue environment" on which to perform surgery. Intraoperative cultures may be taken from deep within the infected tissue. These will invariably be more accurate and consequently provide the physician with the choice of the most appropriate postoperative antibiotic. Once the infection is controlled, the patient returns to surgery for closure of the stump.

Postoperative Complications. These vary with the type of prosthetic fitting the patient receives. Persons who are scheduled for *delayed* prosthesis fitting are subject to the following preprosthetic complications:

- *Hemorrhage.* Some oozing and drainage is normal following amputation. However, excessive bleeding should be reported at once to the surgeon. Also, always keep a large tourniquet at the bedside in event of massive hemorrhage.

▶ *Hematoma.* A hematoma is a tumor-like mass of coagulated blood that has escaped into the tissues or into a cavity. The surgeon can usually prevent stump hematoma by carefully clamping off vessels in surgery and by inserting drains into the wound. Hematoma is a dangerous postoperative complication because it delays wound healing and also provides culture media for infection-causing bacteria. To treat hematoma, the surgeon aspirates the blood from the tissues and firmly bandages the stump.

▶ *Stump edema.* A certain amount of stump edema is *inevitable* in patients who are not fitted with a rigid dressing in the operating room. However firm, correct stump bandaging may lessen not only the degree of stump edema, but also the problem of asymmetric edema ("dumbbell" edema). Figure 50–8 shows detrimental and inadequate stump wrapping. In contrast, note the firm, smooth, proper stump wrapping shown in Figure 50–9.

▶ *Skin complications.* The major skin problems following amputation include delayed healing of the surgical wound and necrosis of the incisional skin edges. Treatment of these problems may involve a return to surgery for stump revision.

▶ *Joint contracture.* Without the rigid dressing, the postamputation patient may develop various joint contractures, including hip joint flexion contracture, stump adduction contracture, knee flexion contracture, and footdrop. Contractures can be prevented by instituting the following nursing measures: (1) do not elevate the patient's stump on a pillow for more than 24 to 48 hours following surgery; (2) avoid positioning the stump in an externally rotated, abducted position; (3) prevent abduction contracture by adducting the stump on a scheduled basis; (4) put the patient through range-of-motion exercises (passive or active) at least three times a day; (5) position the patient in a prone position for several hours each day; (6) place a footboard on the end of the bed to prevent footdrop of the remaining limb; and (7) observe for and provide promptly the prescribed analgesic for associated surgical pain. When pain is experienced, the involved limb will be "drawn up" or flexed as a response to the pain. Without pain relief, the patient will be unable to relax and extend the limb as required to prevent contractures.[31]

▶ *Phantom limb sensation.* As mentioned, the majority of new amputees experience the peculiar sensation that their amputated limb is still present. This sensation may or may not be painful; it may disappear within hours following amputation or it may continue for years. There is no cure or treatment for phantom limb sensation because the causation is not fully understood. However, it is helpful to warn patients about phantom limb sensation prior to amputation and to reassure them that these sensations are "normal."

▶ *Phantom pain.* Between 1 and 10 per cent of all amputees develop painful phantom limb sensation. However, children undergoing amputation of congenitally deformed limbs experience no phantom limb pain. With amputations of previously normal and intact limbs, children under 5 years of age seldom experience phantom limb pain while those over 10 or 12 years of age experience pain with the same frequency as adults though not to the same degree.[41] The causation and treatment of phantom pain are discussed in Unit XI.

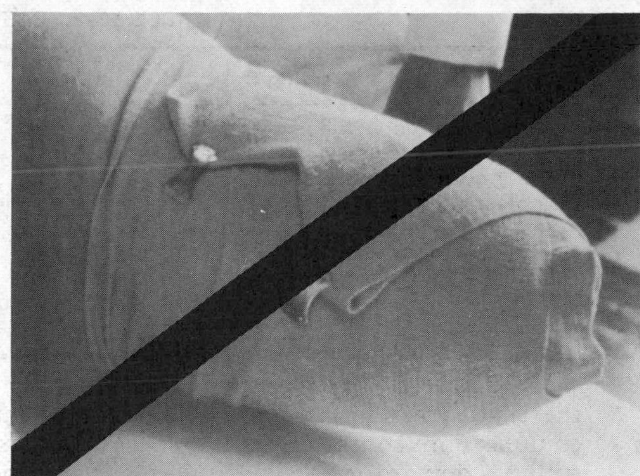

Figure 50–8. Inadequate stump wrapping. (From Thompson, R. G.: *Orthopedic Clinics of North America, 3*:323, July 1972.)

Patients who undergo *immediate* prosthesis fitting and receive conscientious nursing care do *not* experience many of the complications listed above (See Table 50–2 for care of the amputee in a rigid dressing or cast.) Also, incisional pain and phantom limb pain are often greatly lessened by the rigid dressing. However, serious complications may develop *because* of the rigid dressing and early ambulation program. First of all, the opaque rigid dressing makes it impossible for the surgeon and nursing staff to inspect the stump for beginning signs of skin breakdown, wound disruption, and so forth. Second,

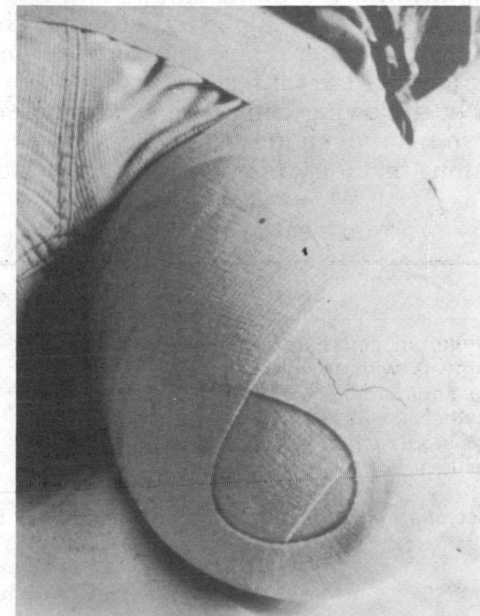

Figure 50–9. Proper stump wrapping. (From Thompson, R. G.: *Orthopedic Clinics of North America, 3*:329, July 1972.)

TABLE 50–2. CAST CARE FOR THE AMPUTEE

Nursing Care	Purpose
Allow plaster to dry 24 hours prior to weight bearing.	To prevent cracking or abnormal molding
Do not position so supports or pressure occurs over or under bony prominences.	To prevent abnormal molding
Do not encase plaster with plastic nor place plastic under cast.	To permit rapid and complete drying of plaster
Support cast with palm of hands during positioning.	To prevent abnormal molding
Check cast for looseness (easily slides up and down).	To prevent skin abrasion
Check cast for tightness (inability to insert finger between cast and skin).	To prevent constriction of nerves and circulation

the rigid dressing can fall off the stump; this complication constitutes an *emergency* because stump edema forms in minutes and wound disruption may occur within half an hour following slippage of the cast. With elective removal of the cast to view a wound, stump swelling also immediately begins. Too prolonged an interval between cast removal and cast replacement may create a slippage problem (Table 50–1) as the edema reduction mechanism of the replaced cast resumes. To prevent this likelihood, apply a firm Ace bandage immediately around the stump after cast removal and keep the stump elevated until cast replacement. Finally, too much weightbearing during the first days of ambulation before the wound is healed may result in wound disruption and skin breakdown. Because of this grave danger, some doctors prefer delayed prosthesis fitting to the immediate technique. See also Ch. 76.

The possibility of an *operative wound infection* is present for any type of amputation procedure; therefore, the nurse must remain alert to any "signs and symptoms" of infection: temperature spikes, fever associated with chills and diaphoresis, an increasing sedimentation rate, and an above normal white blood cell count. These symptoms are general and may indicate pneumonia, urinary tract infection, or wound infection. The following clinical signs and observations in conjunction with the above are indications that *wound infection* may be present:

- Increased complaints of pain at the operative site,
- Areas of extreme tenderness with or without erythema along the surgical incision,
- Increased stump edema,
- Necrosis along the suture line,
- Purulent drainage from *the wound.*

REHABILITATION AND PROSTHESIS TRAINING

The purpose of postamputation rehabilitation is to help the new amputee attain the highest possible level of independence. For elderly debilitated patients who cannot receive a prosthesis, the highest level of independence obtainable may be simply wheelchair independence. Table 50–3 defines levels of ambulatory status in regard to anticipated functional abilities within the home. The discharge plans of an amputee returning home should be made with consideration of the ambulatory level and what chores the patient may need assistance with. For the majority of new amputees the goal of rehabilitation is to achieve at least 90 per cent independence with the use of a prosthesis.

Amputation of a limb displaces the center of gravity which is normally located just below the umbilicus. In any movement, whether ambulatory or positional, an individual must keep this

TABLE 50–3. LEVELS OF AMBULATORY STATUS (IN HOUSEHOLD MANAGEMENT)

Level	Functional Abilities
I. *Community ambulator.* Can walk 2000 feet with prothesis, with or without aids.	Essentially independent in all activities. Able to shop, do own household chores, and attend social outings.
II. *Household ambulator.* Can walk 100 feet with prosthesis, with or without aids.	Able to do most household chores. Requires assistance in shopping and long trips.
III. *Physiologic ambulator.* Can walk 10 feet with prosthesis, with or without aids.	Unable to do some heavy household chores. May need assistance with cooking. Unable to ambulate in community. Requires someone to do shopping.
IV. *Wheelchair independent.* Uses wheelchair at all times.	Unable to do most heavy household chores. May need assistance with cooking. Requires someone to do shopping.
V. *Wheelchair assisted.* Needs assistance with transfer.	Requires assistance with household chores, all shopping, large meal preparation, and personal hygiene.
VI. *Wheelchair dependent.* Uable to do transfers. May not be able to operate wheelchair.	This patient cannot live alone without assistance in all areas of maintaining self and home.

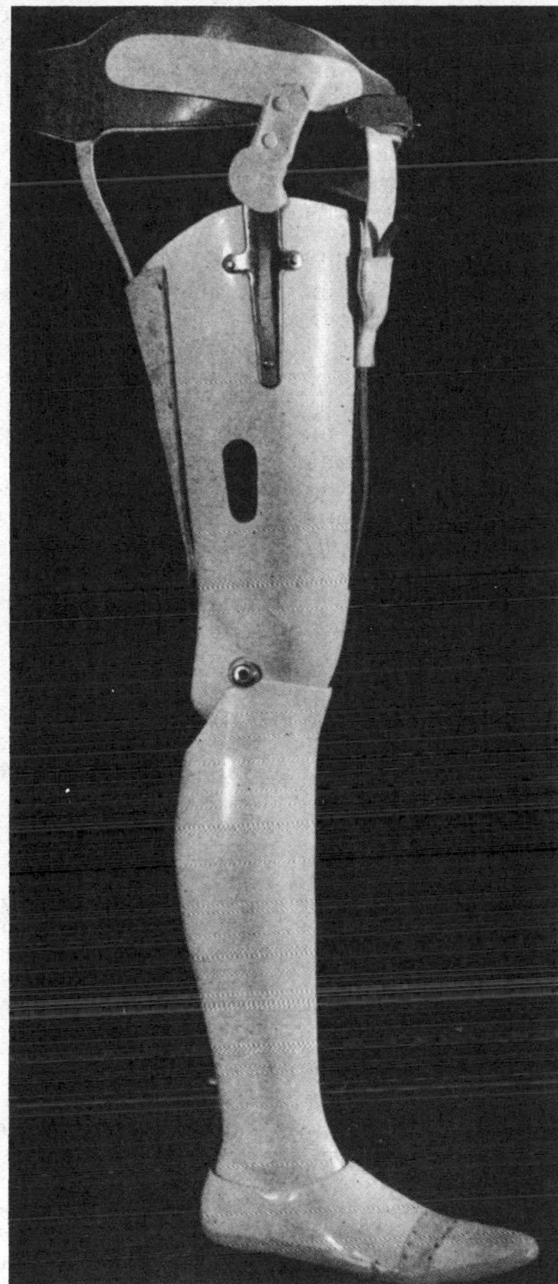

Figure 50–10. Conventional above-knee wood socket with hip joint and pelvic band; single axis knee and ankle. (Institute of Rehabilitation Medicine, New York University Medical Center, New York, N.Y.)

center of gravity in balance, otherwise, one falls. We learn this automatically from birth; therefore, we rarely consider it on a conscious level. An amputee must relearn this because the prosthesis, however similar, will not be an exact replica in weight and movement as the lost limb.

When the prosthesis is not being worn, as during the night, turning will also require a readaptation in body balance. Because of this, the immediate postoperative patient who was prior to surgery totally independent in position changing may require the nurse's assistance until adjustment is made to this new center of gravity.

The Prosthesis Prescription. Prostheses are prescribed by physicians and constructed by prosthetists who, ideally, have been examined and certified by the American Board for Certification of Prosthetists. Basically, lower limb prostheses are composed of the following four components: the socket, joints (hip and knee), suspension (suction system, pelvic band, waist belt, or leather thigh corset), and foot and ankle (Figs. 50–10 and 50–11). However, each of these four components can be modified in numerous ways to meet the needs of the patient. Describing the complicated task of prescribing a prosthesis, Friedmann explains as follows:

> To send a patient to a prosthetist with a "prescription" for an "above-knee prosthesis" is equivalent to sending a patient to a pharmacist with a prescription

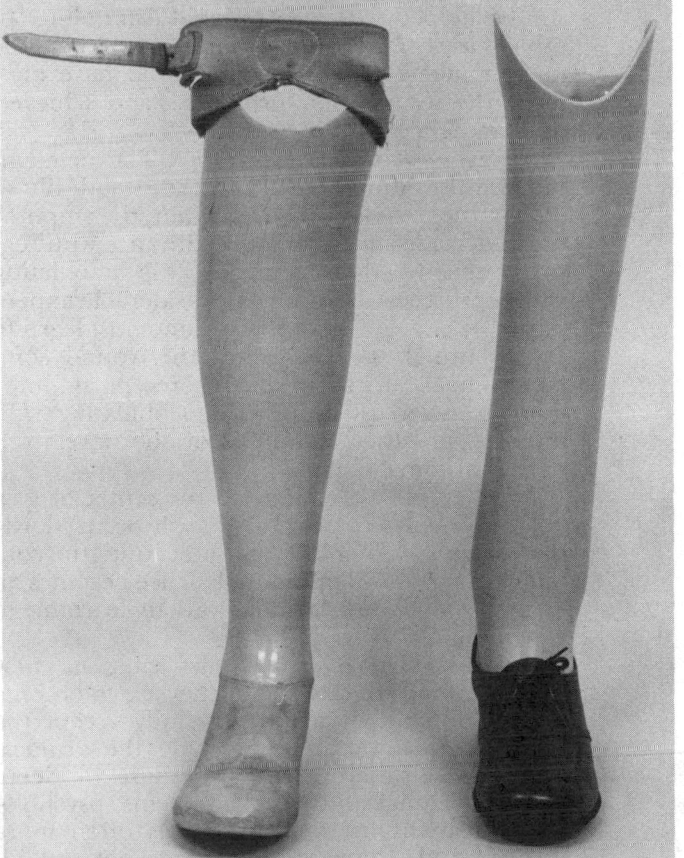

Figure 50–11. *Left,* Prosthesis for a below-knee amputation. Strap is worn above the knee for support of prosthesis. *Right,* Prosthesis for a Syme's amputation. A strap is not necessary. Note the larger ankle diameter to allow for insertion of bulbous stump. (Courtesy of Rancho Los Amigos Hospital, Downey, Cal.)

for "heart medicine." To illustrate the complexity of above-knee prosthetic prescription, there are at least fifteen varieties of feet and ankles. There are five types of friction, six of brake and six extension aids for prosthetic knees. There are eight types of socket designs and the same number of suspensions.... Prosthetically we fit not the stump but the individual.[28]

To tailor a prosthesis prescription to the individual, physicians must evaluate many factors. They must first consider the length and condition of the stump. They must also assess the patient's age, weight, agility, endurance, general state of health, finances, occupational goals, social and family situation, mental health, intelligence, and motivation to become independent. Irons et al. discuss further physiologic criteria for anticipation of successful prosthesis use: "The residual limb" (stump) "must also have adequate strength. . . . in order to control the prosthesis. . . The sound limb must have adequate strength and tolerance for weight bearing."[34] In addition, motivation is one of the most important factors to be considered, because without sufficient motivation the patient will be unwilling to undertake the hard work and training that mastering a prosthesis requires. Sometimes the poorly motivated person can be helped with professional counseling. In other cases, motivation is increased when the patient meets other amputees who have mastered the use of their prostheses and achieved independence.

Adjustment to a Prosthesis. The new amputee must adjust to the prosthesis both physically and psychologically. *Physically*, the amputee must increase strength and endurance with regularly scheduled exercise, because ambulating with a prosthesis requires a considerable expenditure of energy. Also, the patient must learn to control weight-bearing until the wound completely heals. In addition, the recent amputee must conscientiously practice ambulating with the new prosthesis until he or she develops a skillful automatic gait.

Adaptation to a change in the center of gravity, as discussed previously, will occur slowly but progressively in the amputee, until the conscious effort of maintaining balance becomes an unconscious control, analogous to learning to ride a bicycle.

Psychologically, patients must integrate new prosthesis into themselves if they are to become truly independent again. To fully accept the prosthesis, patient must include the artificial limb in their body image. Because of deep-seated personal and social problems, psychologic adjustment to a prosthesis is often more difficult and may take longer than physical adjustment.

Postprosthetic Complications. Once the patient starts using a prosthesis he or she may develop skin complications and/or stump and generalized weakness. *Skin breakdown* on the stump is extremely serious because it interrupts prosthesis training and prolongs hospitalization. Specific skin complications include breakdown of the previously healed scar and blistering or ulceration of the stump. Diabetics are particularly susceptible to skin complications as peripheral neuropathy may obliterate the diabetic's awareness of stump pain.

The stump should be inspected hourly when the patient first begins to ambulate on the prosthesis. If skin irritation and abrasion develop, prosthesis use must be temporarily discontinued and the stump must be firmly wrapped in bandages until the skin irritation is alleviated. If ulcerations appear on the stump or the stump fails to heal, the patient may have to undergo surgical stump revision before being able to resume prosthesis training.

Stump weakness and generalized weakness are problems that particularly plague elderly amputees and discourage them during prosthesis training. A carefully designed program of exercise will help strengthen weak muscles and also increase the patient's general endurance level.

Stump and Prosthesis Care. Teaching the patient the stump and prosthesis care in the hospital and at home is an important part of the total rehabilitation program. When discussing *stump care* with the patient, emphasize the following points:

- The stump should be *inspected daily* for redness, blistering, or abrasions. A mirror can be used to examine all sides and aspects of the stump. Caution the patient against ever putting a Band-Aid on the stump; Band-Aids may irritate the skin and may cause sores and infection when they are pulled off.
- *Daily stump hygiene* is essential. The stump should be washed with a mild soap and then carefully rinsed and dried. Both soap left on the skin and dampness are very irritating and can eventually cause skin breakdown and infection. Also, nothing should be applied to the stump after it is bathed. Emphasize that alcohol dries and cracks the skin while oils and creams soften the skin too much for safe prosthesis use.
- *Woolen stump socks*, which are worn over the stump for cleanliness and comfort, must be washed in cool water and mild soap to prevent shrinkage. To prevent stretching, socks should be washed gently. Stump socks should be dried lying flat on a towel. If the socks tear, they must be replaced; the wrinkling caused by mending the socks is highly irritating to the skin.
- *Stump swelling* can be prevented by instructing the patient to put on the prosthesis immediately upon arising and keeping it on all day once the wound has healed completely. Emphasize that the more the patient wears the prosthesis, the more the stump will shrink.

The patient must also learn how to *care for the*

prosthesis. Important points to stress are listed below:

- Sweat and dirt should be removed from the prosthesis socket daily. Tell the patient to wipe out the inside of the socket with a damp soapy cloth. To remove the soap, use a clean damp cloth; never pour water into the socket because the water may ruin the leather parts of the prosthesis and also rust the prosthetic joints. Remind the patient to dry the prosthesis socket thoroughly; a damp socket can irritate the skin and cause stump breakdown and infection.
- The patient should never attempt to adjust or mechanically alter the prosthesis. If problems develop, tell the patient to immediately consult the prosthetist for professional help.
- The prosthesis should be examined by the prosthetist for mechanical defects on a regular yearly basis.

CARE OF THE PATIENT UNDERGOING AMPUTATION OF THE UPPER EXTREMITY

Amputations of the upper extremities occur with far less frequency than amputations of the lower limbs; indeed the ratio is currently approximately 1 upper extremity amputation to every 11 lower extremity amputations.[36] As we stated earlier, the major indication for upper extremity amputation in the adult is severe trauma; vascular disease is a rare causative factor.

Because of the trauma and shock that is suffered, the patient who is undergoing upper extremity amputation requires extensive *preoperative care prior to surgery*. Blood transfusions, intravenous infusions, and antibiotics may all be necessary.

In addition, upper extremity strengthening exercises should begin preoperatively as the patient can tolerate. Maintaining shoulder joint movement through passive range of motion done by the nurse or occupational therapist will prevent contractures. Begin to accustom the patient to the use of one hand so that following surgery he or she will be able to be more independent in such activities as feeding and grooming.

Psychologic preparation also is an extremely important aspect of care. Loss of a lower extremity is traumatic, but loss of an arm may be truly catastrophic. The functions of the arm and hand are highly specialized, and the loss of these functions threatens the patient in every aspect of life. To obtain a slight sense of how incapaci-

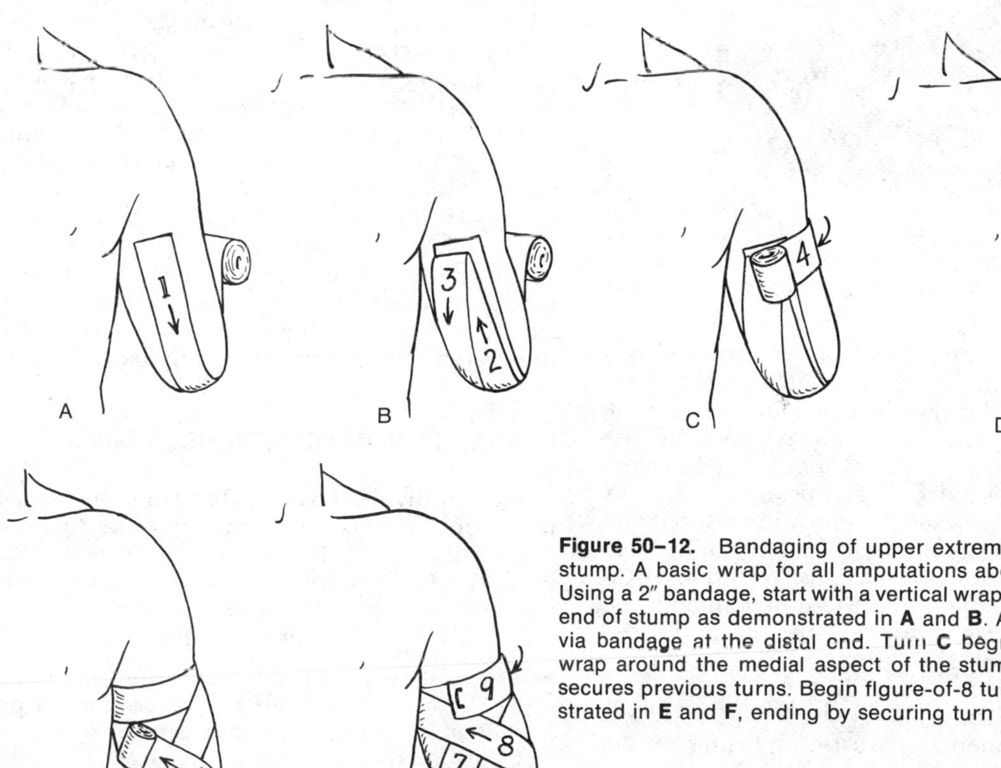

Figure 50–12. Bandaging of upper extremity amputation stump. A basic wrap for all amputations above the elbow. Using a 2″ bandage, start with a vertical wrap over the distal end of stump as demonstrated in **A** and **B**. Apply pressure via bandage at the distal end. Turn **C** begins a diagonal wrap around the medial aspect of the stump, and turn **D** secures previous turns. Begin figure-of-8 turns as demonstrated in **E** and **F**, ending by securing turn 9 with tape.

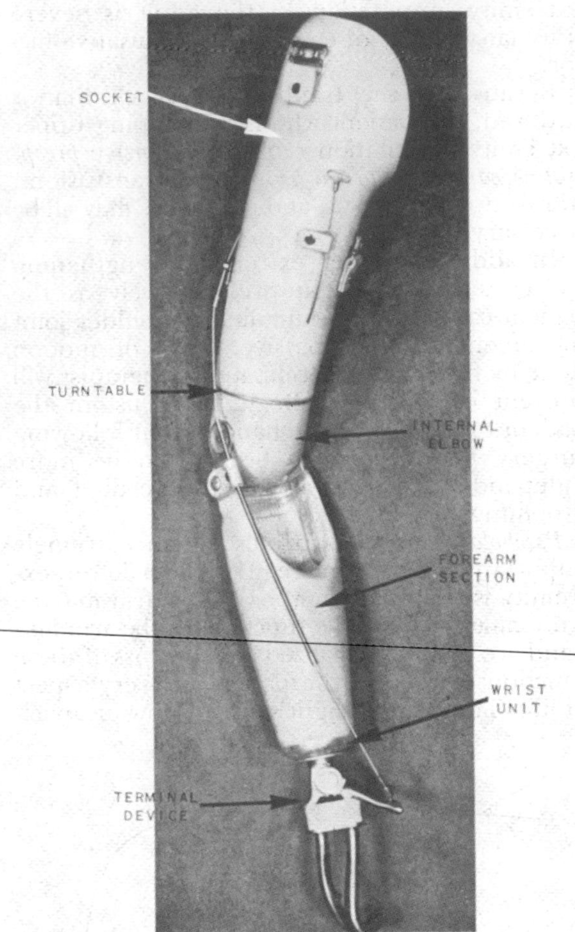

Figure 50–13. Standard above-elbow prosthesis. (From Stoner, E. K.: *In* Krusen, F. H., F. J. Kottke, and P. M. Ellwood, Jr.: *Handbook of Physical Medicine and Rehabilitation,* 2nd ed. Philadelphia: W. B. Saunders Co., 1971.)

tating the loss of an arm is, place your dominant hand and arm in a sling for a full day. Note how frustrated you become when you cannot write with customary ease, carry a heavy package, use a can-opener, use a zipper, and so forth. Imagine how you would feel if you knew that your arm was to be *permanently* removed and that you would have to spend months relearning arm and hand functions with the use of a hook. It is not surprising, then, that these patients may be deeply depressed prior to surgery and need constant psychologic support.

The *postoperative course* for upper extremity amputees depends upon whether the patient undergoes immediate prosthesis fitting or delayed fitting. As with lower limb amputations, there are several pros and cons for each type of prosthetic fitting procedure. Sarmiento points out that immediate fitting is useful for *below*-elbow amputees, but offers few benefits for those with above-elbow amputations.[64] Also, immediate prosthesis fitting may or may not offer psychologic benefits. Some patients may be relieved when they awaken from surgery with a prosthetic hook in place, whereas other patients may be frightened or repulsed by the hook. In addition, the immediate fitting may be dangerous for the amputee who has suffered extensive injuries, because the opaque rigid cast prevents the physician and nursing staff from examining the stump.

If the patient does receive an *immediate* prosthesis, the patient returns from surgery with a rigid plaster of Paris dressing and a temporary prosthesis in place. The prosthesis socket is changed within 7 to 10 days after surgery. Two to three weeks postoperatively, the surgeon removes the sutures from the stump and changes the socket again. The patient receives a definitive prosthesis within four to eight weeks following surgery.

When delayed prosthesis fitting is chosen over immediate, the patient returns from surgery with the stump covered with soft dressings and an elastic bandage. Unlike the care of lower extremity stumps, an upper extremity stump is bandaged, as illustrated in Figure 50–12, quite *gently* because compression of the traumatized area is to be avoided until healing takes place. The patient usually begins exercises the day following surgery. Within 10 to 14 days postoperatively, the patient's sutures are removed and a temporary prosthesis is provided.

The prescription for an upper extremity prosthesis is just as complicated as is a lower limb prosthetic prescription. A standard type of upper arm prosthesis is illustrated in Figure 50–13. Also note the cosmetic hands illustrated in Figure 50–14.

As with lower limb amputees, the individual who has lost an upper extremity must be highly motivated to master the prosthesis and achieve independence. Also, if rehabilitation is to be successful, the prosthetic arm and hand must be integrated into the patient's total body image.

REPLANTATION OF SEVERED LIMBS

Every individual who suffers traumatic amputation of a limb is not a candidate for replantation of the severed limb, but the procedure is entirely feasible for some individuals under certain conditions. Whether a limb can be reattached successfully depends upon:

- the physical and mental condition of the patient. The best candidates for this procedure are persons who are young, in good general health, and highly motivated to master a reattached limb.
- the condition of the stump. Immediate first aid must be given to the stump at the scene of the accident to prevent hemorrhage.

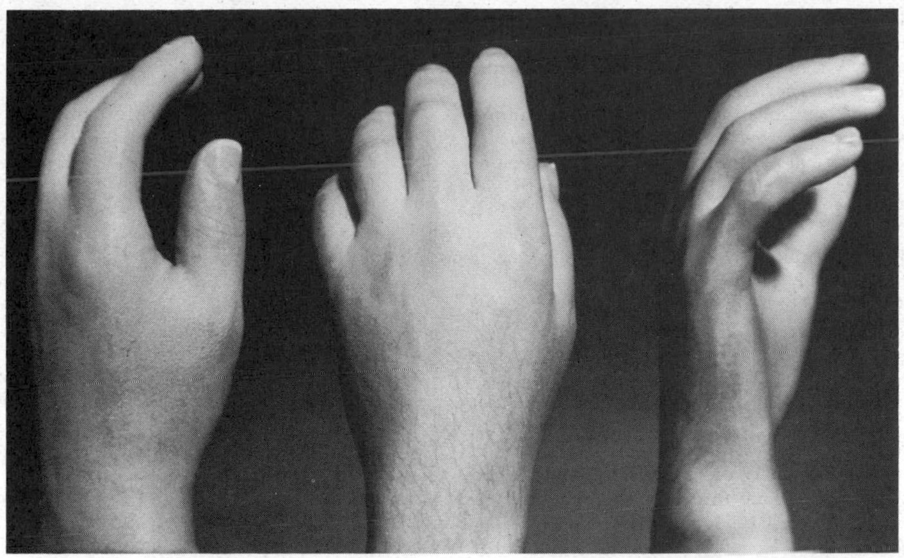

Figure 50–14. Cosmetic (nonprehensile) hand. (From Peizer, E., and T. Pirrello: *Orthopedic Clinics of North America, 3*:397, July 1972.)

- the condition of the severed limb. It is vital that the detached limb be wrapped in a sterile drape, put into a plastic bag, and refrigerated until surgery.
- the availability of a properly equipped operating room and an operating team experienced in microvascular surgery.

Since 1962, hundreds of severed fingers, hands, and arms have been replanted with considerable success. Unfortunately, because the sciatic nerve (the largest nerve in the body) must be rejoined if the leg is to have normal sensation and function, reattachment of severed lower limbs has been much more difficult for surgeons to master. Recently, a few cases of reattached lower limbs have been reported in the news and medical literature. (See also Chapter 95.)

BIBLIOGRAPHY (Chapter 50)

1. Alexander, A. G.: Immediate postsurgical prosthetic fitting. The role of the physical therapist. *Journal of the American Physical Therapy Association*, 51:152, Feb. 1971.
2. Alves, R., and T. A. Martin: An overview of orthotics and prosthetics. *ONA Journal*, 4:231, Sept. 1977.
3. An alternative to amputation. *Emergency Medicine*, 11:42, Aug. 1979.
4. Baker, J. L.: Nursing care study: Traumatic sub-total amputation of the right hand. *Nursing Times*, 74:323, Feb. 1978.
5. Baker, W. H. et al.: The healing of below knee amputations; A comparison of soft and plaster dressing. *American Journal of Surgery*, 133:716, June 1977.
6. Batzdorff, J.: A non-standard above-elbow prosthesis for a multiple handicapped patient. *Orthotics and Prosthetics*, 30:37, Setp. 1976.
7. Beeper keeps amputee on toes. *Journal of the American Medical Association*, 209:634, Aug. 1969.
8. Biedermann, W. G.: Management of short above-knee amputees. *Orthotics and Prosthetics*, 4:21, Dec. 1976.
9. Borrell, R. M., and D. G. Simons: Heart rate as an indicator of exercise stress response in lower extremity amputees. *American Corrective Therapy Journal*, 25:173, Nov.–Dec. 1971.
10. Brogden, R. N., et al.: Streptokinase: A review of its clinical pharmacology, mechanism of action and therapeutic uses. *Drugs*, 5:357, 1973.
11. Buck, B., and A. D. Lee: Amputation: Two views. *Nursing Clinics of North America*, 11:641, Dec. 1976.
12. Burgess, E. M.: Disarticulation of the knee. *Archives of Surgery*, 112:1250, Oct. 1977.
13. Burgess, E. M.: Immediate postsurgical prosthetic fitting: A system of amputee management. *Physical Therapy*, 51:139, Feb. 1971.
14. Burgess, E. M.: Wound healing. *Bulletin of Prosthetic Research*, p. 109, Fall 1974.
15. Burgess, E. M., and F. W. Marsden: Major lower extremity amputations following arterial reconstruction. *Archives of Surgery*, 108:655, May 1974.
16. Burkhalter, W. E., et al.: The upper extremity amputee. Early and immediate postsurgical prosthetic fitting. *American Journal of Bone and Joint Surgery*, 58:46, Jan. 1976.
17. Buttrup, E., and E. E. May: The child amputee and his parents. *Rehabilitative Literature*, 33:139, May 1972.
18. Cheney, R.: Immediate postsurgical prosthetics in the management of below-knee amputees. *ONA Journal*, 4:260, Oct. 1977.
19. Clark, M., with D. Shapiro: Life and limb. *Newsweek*, Jan. 15, 1979.
20. Cooper, S. B., et al.: Individualized nursing care for a patient with bilateral A-K amputations. *ONA Journal* 3:253, Aug. 1976.
21. Copley, I. J.: No matter what you call it, it's still pain to the patient. *RN*, 41:64, Feb. 1978.
22. Cummings, V.: Amputees and sexual dysfunction. *Archives of Physical Medicine and Rehabilitation*, 56:12, Jan. 1975.
23. Effeney, D. J., et al.: Transmetatarsal amputation. *Archives of Surgery*, 112:1366, Nov. 1977.
24. Engstrand, J. L.: Rehabilitation of a patient with a lower extremity amputation. *Nursing Clinics of North America*, 11:659, Dec. 1976.
25. Fairbairn, J. F., II, et al.: *Peripheral Vascular Diseases*, 4th ed. Philadelphia: W. B. Saunders Co., 1972.
26. Foort, J.: Amputee management procedures. *Orthotics and Prosthetics*, 28:3, Mar. 1974.

27. Foort, J.: How amputees feel about amputation. *Orthotics and Prosthetics*, 28:21, Mar. 1974.
28. Friedmann, L. W.: The prosthesis — immediate or delayed fitting. *Angiology*, 23:518, Oct. 1972.
29. Glattly, H. W.: A statistical study of 12,000 new amputees. *Southern Medical Journal*, 57:1373, Nov. 1964.
30. Gonzales, E. G., et al.: Energy expenditure in below-knee amputees; correlation with stump length. *Archives of Physical Medicine and Rehabilitation*, 55:111, Mar. 1974.
31. Harding, J. M.: Amputation of the lower limb. *Nursing Times*, 70:1025, July 1974.
32. Harris, P. L., et al.: The fate of elderly amputees. *British Journal of Surgery*, 61:665, Aug. 1974.
33. Humm, W.: Care of the lower limb amputee. *Nursing Times*, 70:1935, Dec. 1974.
34. Irons, G., et al.: A light-weight above-knee prosthesis with an adjustable socket. *Orthotics and Prosthetics*, 31:3, Mar. 1977.
35. Kahn, O., et al.: Mortality of diabetic patients treated surgically for lower limb infection and/or gangrene. *Diabetes*, 23:287, April 1974.
36. Kay, H. W., and J. D. Newman: Relative incidences of new amputations: Statistical comparisons of 6,000 new amputees. *Orthotics and Prosthetics*, 2:3, June 1975.
37. Kegel, B., et al.: Functional capabilities of lower extremity amputees. *Archives of Physical Medicine and Rehabilitation*, 59:109, Mar. 1978.
38. Kerstein, M. D., et al.: Associated diagnoses complicating rehabilitation after major lower extremity amputation. *Angiology*, 25:536, Sept. 1974.
39. Kerstein, M. D., et al.: Successful rehabilitation following amputation of dominant versus nondominant extremities. *American Journal of Occupational Therapy*, 31:313, May–June 1977.
40. Laforest, N. T., and L. W. Regon: The physical therapy program after an immediate semirigid dressing and temporary below-knee prosthesis. *Physical Therapy*, 53:497, May 1973.
41. Lambert, C. N.: Amputation surgery in the child. *Orthopedic Clinics of North America*, 3:473, July 1972.
42. Lane, H. J.: Working with problems of assault to self-image and lifestyle. *Social Work in Health Care*, 1:191, Winter 1975–1976.
43. Little, J. M., et al.: Vascular amputees: A study in disappointment. *Lancet*, 1:793, April 1974.
44. MacInnes, M. S.: Bilateral amputation of the legs — patient care and rehabilitation. *Nursing Times*, 73:1033, July 1977.
45. *Managing Diabetics Properly*. Nursing '77 Books. Horsham, Pa.: Intermed Communications, 1977, p. 187.
46. Marsden, F. W.: Limb loss and limb replacement: A new confidence. *Medical Journal of Australia*, 1:132, Jan. 1973.
47. McClinton, V. S.: Nursing of the upper extremity amputee and preparation for prosthetic training. *Nursing Clinics of North America*, 11:671, Dec. 1976.
48. McCollough, N. C.: The dysvascular amputee. *Orthopedic Clinics of North America*, 3:303, July 1972.
49. McVittie, C. K.: Nursing care study. Traumatic amputation of the right arm. *Nursing Mirror*, 141:47, Aug. 1975.
50. Meador, R.: Learning to live with a new leg. *Amer. Journal of Nursing*, 79:1339, Aug. 1979.
51. Miller, M. B.: Advanced occlusive arterial disease (gangrene) in the aged, and decision-making for amputation. *Journal of the American Geriatric Society*, 22:321, July 1974.
52. Mooney, V., and F. W. Wagner, Jr.: Neurocirculatory disorders of the foot. *Clinical Orthopaedics and Related Research*, 122:53, Jan.–Feb. 1977.
53. Moore, W. S., et al.: Below the knee amputation for ischemic gangrene. Comparative results of conventional operation and immediate postoperative fitting technique. *American Journal of Surgery*, 124:127, Aug. 1972.
54. Pasnau, R. O., and B. Pfefferbaum.: Psychologic aspects of post-amputation pain. *Nursing Clinics of North America*, 11:679, Dec. 1976.
55. Peizer, E., and T. Pirrello: Principles and practice in upper extremity prostheses. *Orthopedic Clinics of North America*, 3:397, July 1972.
56. Pfefferbaum, B., and R. O. Pasnau: Post-amputation grief. *Nursing Clinics of North America*, 11:687, Dec. 1976.
57. Rehabilitation of a left below-knee amputee. *Nursing Mirror*, 142:60, Feb. 1976.
58. Reyburn, T. V.: A method of early prosthetics training for upper extremity amputees. *Artificial Limbs*, 15:1, Autumn 1971.
59. Reyes, R. L., and E. B. Leahey, Jr.: Elderly patients with lower extremity amputations: Three-year study in a rehabilitation setting. *Archives of Physical Medicine and Rehabilitation*, 58:116, Mar. 1977.
60. Roach, L. B.: Traumatic amputation. *Nursing '72*, 2:40, Nov. 1972.
61. Roon, A. J., et al.: Below-knee amputation: A modern approach. *American Journal of Surgery*, 134:153, July 1977.
62. Rozier, C. K.: Three-dimensional work space of the amputee. *Human Factors*, 19:525, Dec. 1977.
63. Sarmiento, A.: Recent trends in lower extremity amputation. *Nursing Clinics of North America*, 2:399, Sept. 1967.
64. Sarmiento, A.: Postoperative management. *Orthopedic Clinics of North America*, 3:435, July 1972.
65. Saving severed limbs. *American Journal of Nursing*, 75:2072, Nov. 1975.
66. Stern, P. H., and P. A. Skudder: Amputee rehabilitation. I. Lower limb amputations. *New York State Journal of Medicine*, 77:1436, Aug. 1977.
67. Stoner, E. K.: Care of the Amputee. *In* Krusen, F. H., et al. (Eds.): *Handbook of Physical Medicine and Rehabilitation*, 2nd ed. Philadelphia: W. B. Saunders Co. 1971.
68. Stubbins, J.: *Social and Psychological Aspects of Disability: A Handbook for Practitioners*. Baltimore: University Park Press, 1977.
69. Taggart, M.: Body image: Looking beyond the mirror. *Journal of Practical Nursing*, 27:25, Aug. 1977.
70. Tooms, R. E.: Amputation surgery in the upper extremity. *Orthopedic Clinics of North America*, 3:383, July 1972.
71. Wagner, F. W., Jr.: Amputations of the foot and ankle. Current status. *Clinical Orthopedics and Related Research*, 122:62, Jan.–Feb. 1977.
72. Wagner, F. W., Jr.: The diabetic foot and amputations of the foot. *In* Mann, R. A. (Ed.): *Duvries' Surgery of the Foot*, 4th ed. St. Louis, C. V. Mosby Co., 1979.
73. Waters, R. L., et al.: Energy cost of walking of amputees: The influence of level amputation. *American Journal of Bone and Joint Surgery*, 58:42, Jan. 1976.
74. Whitehead, A. S.: Nursing care study: Neglect of diabetes leading to bilateral amputation. *Nursing Times*, 74:1490, Sept. 1978.
75. Williams, J. W., et al.: Pulmonary embolism after amputation of the lower extremity. *Surgery in Gynecology and Obstetrics*, 140:246, Feb. 1975.
76. Wilson, A. B., Jr.: *Limb Prosthetics*. Huntington, N.Y.: Robert E. Krieger Publishing Co., 1972.
77. Yao, S. T., and Dean, R. H.: Hemodynamic measurements in peripheral vascular disease. *Current Problems in Surgery*, 13:5, Aug. 1976.
78. Zalewski, N., et al.: Hemipelvectomy: The triumph of Ms. A. *American Journal of Nursing*, 73:2073, Dec. 1973.

UNIT XVI*

NURSING PEOPLE EXPERIENCING DISTURBANCES OF RESPIRATORY FUNCTION

INTRODUCTION AND STUDY GUIDE

Breathing is a physiologic function almost synonymous with being alive. "Life" and "breath" are intertwined in the minds of all of us. To have difficulty breathing, then, is to have difficulty staying alive. People with respiratory disorders are often very frightened — frightened that they cannot breathe and sometimes frightened that they may die — perhaps very uncomfortably. Whether such fears are reasonable is irrelevant. The fears may still be experienced.

Nurses participate in the care and rehabilitation of patients with both acute (short-term) and chronic (long-term) respiratory illnesses. These illnesses are common causes of disability. Respiratory illnesses are the most common type of acute disorder. For example, acute respiratory infections, e.g., "flu" and "colds," seem to affect almost everyone at some time. Respiratory allergies distress many persons throughout the year. Chronic respiratory illnesses cause millions of people to lose work time, retire early, and lose years of productive life. The incidences of chronic respiratory illnesses and lung cancer are increasing at alarming rates. Chronic lung diseases are second only to heart disease as a cause of death in the United States.

> *Many respiratory disorders could be prevented, e.g., chronic bronchitis, chronic obstructive pulmonary emphysema, lung cancer, tuberculosis, pneumonia, and lung abscess. Nurses participate both directly and indirectly in the prevention of respiratory disorders.*

Nurses' direct actions include (1) encouraging periodic deep breathing, coughing, and turning among patients likely to develop atelectasis or pneumonia (e.g., postoperative patients, patients confined to bed rest); (2) preventing aspiration (e.g., in obtunded or paralyzed patients); (3) safely administering respiratory therapy and chest physical therapy (e.g., postural drainage) when indicated; (4) performing suctioning to maintain a patent airway; (5) encouraging passive activities; (6) encouraging active goal-oriented exercise; (7) coordinating activities of daily living with breathing retraining; (8) aiding patients and their significant others to cope with a

*Rosemary Jo Craig, B.S., R.N., C.R.T.T., R.R.T., critically reviewed and assisted in the revision of this unit.

chronic illness; (9) assessing and monitoring lung function and status; and (10) providing nursing care for persons requiring critical respiratory care.

Indirectly, nurses may help to prevent numerous respiratory disorders through education. Topics on which nurses may give information include: (1) hazards associated with pulmonary irritants, e.g., cigarette smoke, air pollutants; (2) dangers of foreign body aspiration, e.g., in children; (3) emergency care following airway obstruction or chest injuries; (4) methods of preventing spread of air-borne infections; (5) use of influenza vaccines; and (6) importance of early investigation and treatment of respiratory symptoms, e.g., cough, sputum production, shortness of breath. A nurse is often instrumental in urging persons with respiratory conditions to seek and to accept treatment. Early treatment of *acute* respiratory problems and an adequate period of convalescence afterwards are important in preventing *chronic* disorders.

Respiratory care is important not only for persons with intrinsic respiratory disorders but also for people with other primary problems. For example, the first priority of emergency care in *any* situation is to maintain function of the lungs and heart; e.g., the airway is cleared and cardiopulmonary resuscitation is performed as indicated. During *any* surgery performed under general anesthesia, the anesthesiologist maintains adequate respiration. Following surgery the nurse maintains a patent airway and prevents postoperative pulmonary complications, e.g., atelectasis, pneumonia. *All* patients in intensive care units or confined to bed, regardless of their basic illnesses, are continuously cared for to prevent the development of respiratory complications associated with inactivity. An important part of *many* rehabilitative programs is to help patients improve lung function. Prevention of respiratory complications is imperative, since these disorders can be fatal.

Increasingly, intensive respiratory care units are being established to provide skilled care for patients with serious respiratory conditions. Nurse clinicians, with advanced training and skills in respiratory care, are functioning effectively in these settings. The quality of nursing care given to seriously ill patients with respiratory disorders strongly influences the success or failure of treatment programs. Successful respiratory care requires the effective participation of a treatment team that basically consists of physicians, nurses, respiratory therapists (formerly called inhalation therapists), and physical therapists.

Pulmonary surgery has advanced tremendously in recent years. However, in spite of both medical and surgical advances, many patients suffer with and succumb to pulmonary conditions that cannot yet be successfully reversed or treated. In the future, lung transplantation or insertion of artificial lungs may restore health to persons whose own lungs are irreparably damaged.

Occupational and community health nurses have important roles in the prevention and treatment of respiratory disorders. For example, occupational health nurses are active in helping employers find ways to protect workers from industrial substances that can cause respiratory disease, e.g., dusts, gases, fumes, sprays, liquids, bacteria, fungi. Community health nurses participate in home care and community education.

Disorders of the upper respiratory tract, i.e., nose, throat, pharynx, and larynx, are presented in Unit XXIV. Included in that unit are discussions of endotracheal intubation and tracheostomy. Acute pulmonary edema is discussed in Unit XII; discussion of pulmonary embolism is in Unit XV. This unit focuses on disorders of the pleurae, pleural spaces, tracheobronchial tree, and lungs. Included in Chapter 51 is a brief overview of the anatomy and physiology of the respiratory system. Chapter 52 discusses diagnostic and evaluative procedures for assessment of the patient with a respiratory disorder. In Chapter 53, common nonspecific manifestations of respiratory disorders are considered, e.g., abnormal patterns of breathing, abnormal secretions, cough, hypoxia, respiratory failure. Common respiratory therapeutic measures are reviewed in Chapter 54, e.g., factors of general importance as well as medications, chest physiotherapy, and other forms of respiratory therapy. Chapter 55 considers in depth specific disorders of the pleurae, pleural spaces, tracheobronchial tree, and lungs, e.g., pleurisy, pneumothorax, atelectasis, pulmonary tumors, pneumonias, tuberculosis, and chronic obstructive pulmonary disease. In Chapter 56 tracheobronchial, diaphragmatic, and chest injuries are discussed. The unit's final chapter, Chapter 57, presents information about closed chest drainage and chest surgery.

Overview: Basic Types of Respiratory Disorders

The respiratory system is subject to a wide variety of disorders. Examples of some of these problems are briefly summarized here. In some conditions more than one causative factor is operative, e.g., infection and irritation are often coexistent.

TYPICAL EXAMPLES OF RESPIRATORY DISORDERS

Causative Factor	Examples of Disorders
Airway obstruction; aspiration	Chronic obstructive pulmonary disease (COPD); atelectasis; bronchiectasis; lung abscess; aspiration pneumonia
Allergic reactions	Bronchial asthma
Breakdown of alveolar walls	Pulmonary emphysema
Bronchopulmonary irritation	Pulmonary emphysema; lung cancer; chronic bronchitis; COPD; pneumoconioses ("dust diseases")
Bronchospasm	Extrinsic vs. intrinsic asthma; psychogenic asthma; COPD; chronic bronchitis; pulmonary emphysema
Infection	Influenza; pneumonia; pulmonary emphysema; pulmonary tuberculosis; pleurisy; thoracic empyema; bronchopleural fistula; lung abscess; bronchiectasis; atelectasis; bronchitis; tracheobronchitis; fungus infections; pulmonary infections caused by bacterial, viral, and atypical organisms
Trauma	Penetrating chest injuries; nonpenetrating chest injuries (e.g., blunt or crushing injuries); pulmonary laceration; hemothorax; pneumothorax; flail chest; fractured ribs; tracheobronchial injuries; diaphragmatic injuries
Tumors	Benign pulmonary tumors; metastatic pulmonary tumors; primary malignant tumors (bronchogenic carcinomas)
Ventilation-perfusion abnormalities	May accompany various disorders; in some instances pulmonary capillaries are inadequately perfused with blood although alveoli are adequately ventilated, e.g., pulmonary emboli (ventilation without perfusion); in other cases alveolar ventilation is impaired although blood flow is normal, e.g., atelectasis (perfusion without ventilation)
Alveolar-capillary membrane permeability abnormalities	May develop with interstitial fibrosis and progressive granulomatous diseases; total area of the alveolar-capillary membranes may be reduced in disorders such as pulmonary emphysema, pneumoconiosis, and far advanced pulmonary tuberculosis; antineoplastic drugs; O_2 toxicity
Arteriovenous (AV) shunting	Hypoxia results from venous dilution of the arterial blood stream, or if large groups of alveoli are nonfunctioning and blood passes through pulmonary capillaries without gaseous exchange occurring
Restrictive pulmonary disorders	Expansion of the chest cage, diaphragm, or lungs may be limited by paralysis of the muscles of respiration, phrenic nerve paralysis, pulmonary fibrosis, kyphoscoliosis, pleural thickening, scarring, third trimester pregnancy, obesity
Obstructive lung disorders	Emphysema, chronic bronchitis, asthma (COPD)
Extrapulmonary	Hiatal hernia; neuromuscular disorders

Objectives and Study Guide

After carefully studying the information presented in this unit and applying it during your clinical experience, you can expect to be able to:

- Demonstrate an accurate and clear understanding of the normal anatomy and physiology of the respiratory system.
- Prepare patients and their significant others physically and psychologically for the procedures and emotions they may experience during diagnosis and evaluation of a respiratory disorder.
- Understand and recognize common manifestations experienced by people with respiratory disorders.
- Skillfully observe patients for signs and symptoms of respiratory problems and interpret such observations accurately and appropriately.
- Perform emergency measures safely and responsibly during a respiratory crisis.
- Offer appropriate psychosocial support to patients and their significant others during respiratory problems.
- Skillfully carry out nursing and delegated medical responsibilities related to therapeutic measures for respiratory disorders.
- Know the usual clinical care and surgical procedures of respiratory pathologic conditions and be able to understand the principles involved when such care varies from usual.
- Communicate relevant and accurate information concerning respiratory anatomy, physiology, pathology, diagnostic procedures, treatment regimens and rehabilitative processes to patients and their significant others.
- Be able to effectively teach accurate and realistic measures that may prevent the occurrence of respiratory disease.
- Plan competent, personalized nursing care with people experiencing respiratory problems on a short- and long-term basis.

In preparation for studying this unit, review in appropriate textbooks: (1) normal *anatomy* and *physiology* of the tracheobronchial tree, lungs, muscles of respiration, and pleural space; (2) *pharmacologic agents* useful in treating respiratory disorders (e.g., antihistamines, antimicrobials, bronchodilators, cough medications, gases, narcotic antagonists, vasoconstrictors, and decongestants); and (3) *microbiology* of microorganisms which may produce diseases of the respiratory tract (e.g., *Mycobacterium tuberculosis, Hemophilus influenzae,* pneumococcus, staphylococcus, streptococcus, fungi, atypical organisms resembling tuberculosis).

As you study this unit, refer back to other sections of this text as necessary for review. Possible review areas include: *fluid-electrolyte imbalances,* especially respiratory acidosis and respiratory alkalosis (Chap. 12); mechanisms of *hypersensitivity* to more completely understand bronchial asthma (Chap. 11); the body's response to *injury* and *infection* (Chap. 10); *physiologic shock* (Chap. 13); nursing patients experiencing *surgery* (Unit VIII) and *pain* (Unit XI) in association with chest injury, chest surgery, and painful conditions involving the respiratory system; *disturbances of cellular function* as a review when studying lung cancer (Unit IX); and *cardiopulmonary resuscitation* (Unit XII).

The scope of this text does not allow for specific information and instruction in the use of the equipment and medications utilized to treat respiratory impairments. You are referred to texts and journals that deal directly with respiratory therapy concepts, equipment, pharmacology, practical aspects of intensive respiratory care, adaptations, and practical aspects of care of persons with chronic obstructive pulmonary disease. Suitable references may be found in the bibliography at the end of the unit.

As you proceed through the unit, carry out the following:

1. Summarize the principles and aspects of care for patients undergoing bronchoscopy, thoracentesis, collection of sputum specimens, arterial blood gas analysis, and pulmonary function studies.
2. State in your own words the value of blood gas analyses and auscultation, inspection, percussion, and palpation of the chest.
3. List some observations of importance in assessing patients with respiratory disorders.
4. Summarize care of (a) a dyspneic patient; (b) a patient experiencing hemoptysis; and (c) a patient in acute respiratory insufficiency or failure.
5. Identify ways in which nonproductive coughing can be minimized and productive coughing stimulated and made more effective.
6. State the indications of a person having hypoxemia and hypercapnea.
7. Summarize nursing activities useful in promoting maintenance of a clear airway and removal of respiratory secretions.
8. List physical clues indicative of chronic lung disease.
9. List some pulmonary irritants which should be avoided by persons with respiratory problems.
10. Practice abdominal breathing so you will be able to effectively teach this exercise to patients.
11. Observe a patient receiving pulmonary physiotherapy (e.g., breathing exercises, postural drainage, clapping, vibrating). Review the patient's condition and identify specifically how pulmonary physiotherapy is therapeutic.
12. Visit the respiratory therapy department or observe patients being treated with aerosolization, humidification, oxygen, and positive pressure ventilation. Review these procedures with a qualified person. Identify hazards associated with oxygen therapy and positive pressure respirators. If medications are being given by IPPB, familiarize yourself with the medications and how they are prepared for administration.
13. State why a patient with chronic respiratory insufficiency and CO_2 retention should *not* be given high concentrations of O_2 even though the PaO_2 is low, i.e., why is the goal of treatment *not* one of attempting to rapidly raise the PaO_2 to "normal" by giving high concentrations of O_2?
14. Identify some hazards of deep tracheal suctioning and ways in which potential dangers may be avoided.
15. Summarize key points in the prevention of the following disorders and identify major patient-teaching points of importance in working with patients who have these disorders: atelectasis, lung abscess, bronchiectasis, pulmonary tuberculosis, lung cancer, pneumonia, influenza, chronic obstructive pulmonary disease, bronchial asthma, chronic bronchitis, chronic pulmonary emphysema, and pneumoconiosis.
16. Familiarize yourself with research reports which document the harmful effects of cigarette smoking and air pollution.
17. Describe the "atypical" organisms that produce pulmonary diseases similar to tuberculosis.
18. Name some fungus infections of the lungs, i.e., pulmonary mycoses, and review the etiology of these infections.
19. Identify some of the economic, social, and emotional pressures patients and their significant others must learn to cope with and experience in the following disorders: lung cancer, pulmonary tuberculosis, and COPD (asthma, bronchiectasis, chronic bronchitis, emphysema).
20. Describe how an open chest wound or chest surgery disrupts normal intrapleural pressure. What therapeutic procedures are used to restore normal intrapleural pressure?

21. Describe paradoxical motion, mediastinal shift, and mediastinal flutter. How can these complications occur in chest injuries? What treatment is indicated?

22. Summarize factors of importance in pre- and postoperative care following chest surgery.

23. Make a drawing of three-bottle, closed chest drainage and state the purpose of each bottle. What is meant by closed chest drainage? What is meant by a water seal? Identify potential problems that can occur with closed chest drainage (e.g., the chest catheter is accidentally pulled out of the chest) and appropriate immediate care.

24. Describe the difference between a pressure limited (controlled) ventilator and a volume limited (controlled) ventilator.

25. List the basic aspects of care for a patient receiving continuous mechanical ventilation.

26. List the criteria and methods of weaning a patient from continuous mechanical ventilation.

27. Briefly discuss the difference between PEEP and C-PAP; list beneficial and adverse effects.

28. List normal values for arterial blood gases. Why are venous samples not used? Observe an arterial puncture.

29. Oxygen is a drug. List other drugs administered to a patient via the respiratory tract and describe their actions, uses, and side effects.

30. List alternate methods of aerosolization of medications into the respiratory tract other than IPPB. Observe these methods of administration during your clinical experience. What are three basic elements essential for deposition of aerosol medications in the airway?

31. List four methods of providing hydration to the respiratory tract.

32. Become familiar with aspects of breathing retraining such as control of breathing using dyspnea positions, use of pursed lip breathing, diaphragmatic breathing, and effective coughing techniques.

33. Define the principle utilized with incentive respiratory devices; be able to demonstrate the correct procedure to a patient.

34. List three causes of restrictive lung disease. Relate the patient's pulmonary impairment to potential problems you may encounter in both the medical and surgical care of these patients. Do the same for obstructive diseases.

35. State the route and method of infection the *Mycobacterium tuberculosis* takes. List some important methods of control of this disease. Consider the following question: Who is more hazardous, the identified patient who is on drug therapy or a neighbor with unknown tuberculosis?

36. List five causes of adult respiratory distress syndrome (ARDS) and the general course of therapy for such patients.

37. List four indications for hyperbaric oxygen therapy and side effects and contraindications to this form of respiratory therapy.

CHAPTER 51

OVERVIEW OF ANATOMY AND PHYSIOLOGY OF RESPIRATORY SYSTEM

The lungs are vital organs, that is, they are necessary to sustain life. Without the lungs, life-giving and life-sustaining oxygen would not be supplied to the body tissues. The cardiovascular (heart and blood vessels) system's function is to supply oxygen (O_2) to all body tissues via the circulating blood. Blood circulated by the cardiovascular system also removes carbon dioxide (CO_2) produced by metabolism in the body tissues. This waste product is carried in the blood to the lungs. There the CO_2 is exchanged for O_2. The volume of blood which has circulated to the lungs from the body is called *unoxygenated* or *desaturated blood.* The blood that exchanges CO_2 for oxygen and then circulates from the lungs to the tissues is called *oxygenated* or *arterialized blood.* The removal of CO_2 from the blood by the lungs and the addition of fresh O_2 into the blood by the lungs is referred to as an *exchange of gases.*

THE RESPIRATORY SYSTEM

Figure 51–1 shows the anatomy of the respiratory system.

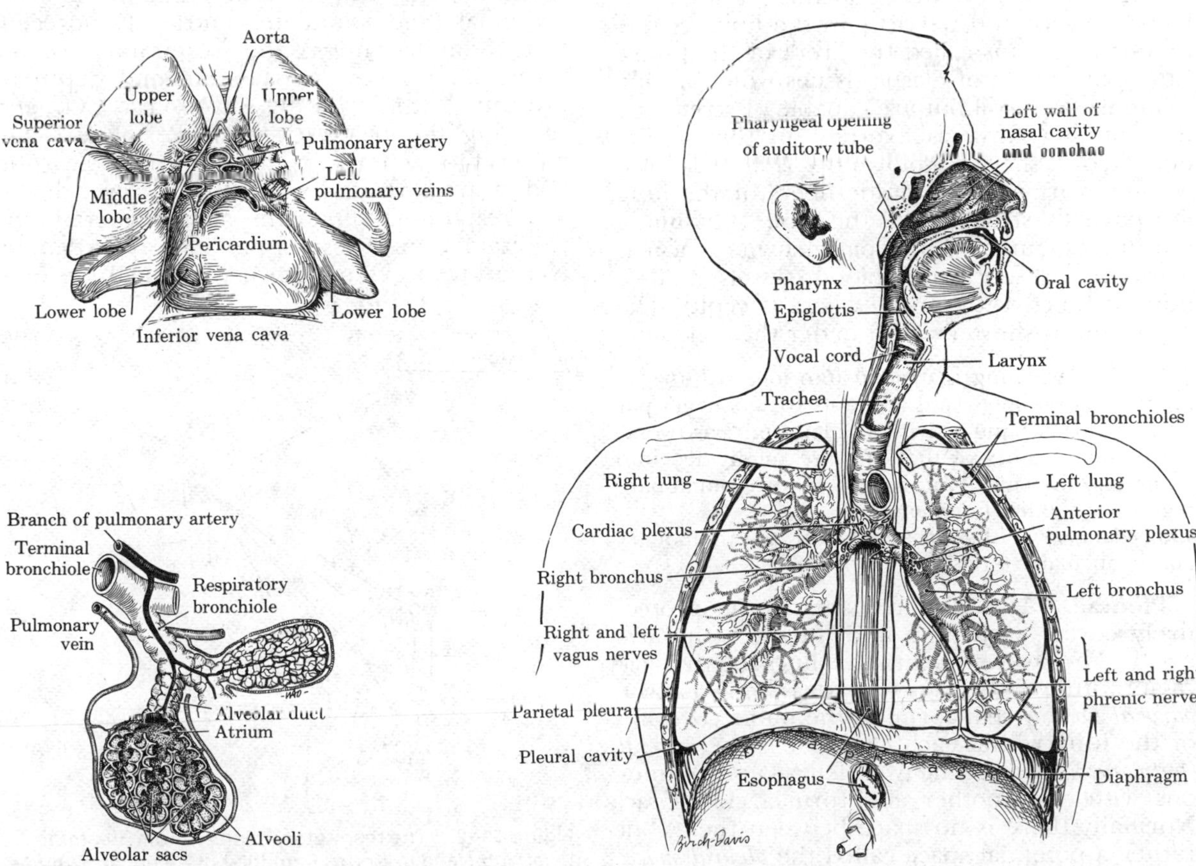

Figure 51–1. Organs of the respiratory system. (From *Dorland's Illustrated Medical Dictionary,* 25th ed. Philadelphia: W. B. Saunders Co., 1974.)

Gross Anatomy

Thoracic Cavity. The thoracic cavity has four subdivisions: (1) *right pulmonary space,* which contains the right lung surrounded by visceral and parietal pleura; (2) *left pulmonary space,* which contains the left lung surrounded by visceral and parietal pleura; (3) *pericardial space,* which contains heart and pericardial sac; and (4) *mediastinal space,* the center of the thoracic cavity, located between pulmonary spaces; this contains the esophagus, trachea, and great blood vessels and heart.

Lungs (Right and Left). These main organs of respiration are located within the thoracic cavity on either side of the heart. Light, spongy, porous, elastic, cone-shaped organs, they inflate with inspiration of air and deflate (but do not completely collapse) with expiration. They extend from the diaphragm to just above the clavicles; i.e., the *base* of lung rests on diaphragm while the *apex* (top) extends above the first rib. The *hilus* or *hilum* is the notch or depression in the medial surface of the lung at which the mainstem bronchus, pulmonary blood vessels, and nerves join the lung. Sometimes the hilus is called the "root of the lung." Lungs are made of elastic tissues which have a tendency to recoil but are capable of stretching if a pulling force is exerted on them from outside or if they are "blown up" (inflated) from within. Normally the elastic fibers of the lung are partially stretched all the time, thus filling the lung chamber. Lung parenchyma is a network of air tubes and blood vessels, and is honeycombed with air-filled sacs (alveoli). The right lung is shorter and broader than the left.

Lobes. Each lung is divided into lobes: the right lung has three lobes and accounts for about 55 per cent of normal lung activity; the left lung has two.

Segments. Lobes of the lung are subdivided into segments: the right lung has 10 bronchopulmonary segments; the left lung, eight.

Blood Supply. Blood is supplied by the pulmonary and bronchial arteries.

Pleurae. A two-layered membrane protectively covers each lung and lines the thoracic cavity. The layer of pleura that lines the thoracic cavity within each lung chamber is known as the *parietal pleura;* that forming the outer covering of the lung within each chamber is the *visceral (pulmonary) pleura.* The two pleurae are continuous with one another and form a closed sac. Normally there is no space between them, but rather a potential space called the *pleural space.* A thin film of serous fluid, i.e., *pleural fluid* (only a few ml.), is present between the two pleurae in the pleural space. This film acts as a lubricant and also causes the moist pleural membranes to adhere somewhat, the cohesion producing a tensile strength or pulling force that helps to hold the lungs in an expanded position. Normally, pressure within the pleural space is always negative (i.e., subatmospheric). Resting intrapleural pressure is usually about 755 mm. Hg, but prior to inspiration it decreases to about 751 mm. Hg. A constant negative intrapleural pressure is essential for normal respirations. This pressure is another factor that prevents the lungs from recoiling and holds them expanded. Negative pressure exerts a sucking or pulling force.

Diaphragm. A muscular partition separating the thoracic and abdominal cavities, the diaphragm is innervated on either side by a phrenic nerve.

Respiratory Center. Located in the stem portion of the brain, i.e., medulla, immediately above spinal cord (Fig. 51–2), this center controls breathing. Normally, the respiratory center is stimulated by the increased concentration of CO_2, and to a lesser degree by the decreased amounts of O_2 in arterial blood. This mechanism is mediated by sensitive chemoreceptors located in the medulla and in the walls of the arch of the aorta and carotid arteries. Centrally, CO_2 and hydrogen ions in the cerebrospinal fluid stimulate central chemoreceptors. Stimulation of the respiratory center causes an increase in the rate and depth of breathing, thus blowing off excess CO_2 and reducing the blood's acidity. Peripheral chemoreceptor reflexes from the aortic and carotid bodies are activated when the O_2 level drops. The respiratory center dispatches orders to the respiratory muscles, stimulating contraction. Nerve fibers extend down the spinal cord. In

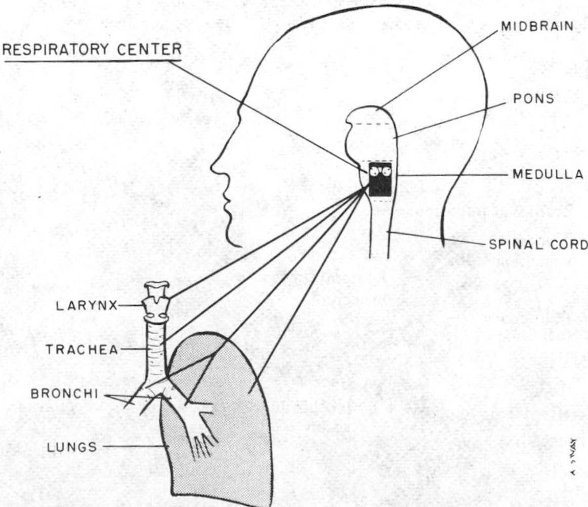

Figure 51–2. The respiratory center. (From *Breathing . . . What You Need to Know.* Pamphlet of American Lung Association, 1968.)

the cervical (neck) region of the cord these fibers continue via the *phrenic nerves* to innervate either side of the *diaphragm*. If one phrenic nerve is damaged, the diaphragm on the affected side is paralyzed in an elevated position.

Conducting System

Following is a brief review of the conducting pathways of the respiratory system. The conducting system is a network of airways that provides the pathway for the transport and exchange of oxygen and carbon dioxide. The pulmonary conducting system is typically divided into the upper airway and the lower airway.

Upper Airway. The upper airway is a combination of the nose, pharynx, larynx, and epiglottis. Major functions of the upper airway are (1) conduction of air to lower airway; (2) protection of the lower airway from foreign matter; and (3) warming, filtering, and humidification of the inspired air.

Lower Airway. The lower airway (also called the tracheobronchial tree) is composed of the (a) trachea, (b) right and left main stem bronchus, (c) segmental bronchi, (d) subsegmental bronchi, and (e) terminal bronchioles. The *carina* is an anatomic landmark important for the placement of endotracheal tubes. It is located at the base of the trachea where the trachea divides into the right and left main stem bronchi.

The major functions of the lower airway are (1) *conduction of air* through many branches of airways to the alveolar level. Diameters of the airways diminish as the airways branch. This increases the total cross-sectional area of the lungs. Many nerves, lymphatics, and bronchial arteries surround the bronchi. (2) *Mucociliary clearance* and (3) *production of pulmonary surfactant* are discussed later.

Trachea. Smooth, flexible, muscular, tube-like air passage about 1 inch wide and 4 to 5 inches long, reinforced on sides and in front by 15 to 20 C-shaped rings of cartilage. Opening of the "C" faces posteriorly. Cartilage rings protect trachea and keep it open by preventing its collapse. The trachea extends from larynx to mainstem bronchi; it serves as passage to and from lungs. The inner surface is lined with ciliated epithelium.

Mainstem Bronchi (Right and Left). These are also called *primary* or *main bronchi.* Two subdivisions of the trachea branch off from the tracheal bifurcation, and one mainstem bronchus enters each lung. These tubular passages conduct air between trachea and pulmonary bronchi. Walls contain cartilaginous rings and ciliated mucous lining. The right mainstem bronchus is shorter and wider, and extends downward more vertically than the left. (Aspiration thus more frequently occurs into the right main bronchus.)

Secondary Bronchi. These are also referred to as *bronchial tubes, air tubes,* and the *bronchial tree.* Subdivisions of main bronchi spread in an inverted tree-like formation, branching through each lung field. These tubular passages convey air within the lung between the mainstem bronchi and bronchioles. There are lobar and segmental bronchi.

Bronchioles. These are the smallest subdivisions of bronchi; they conduct air from secondary bronchi into alveoli (air sacs). Segmental bronchi divide into smaller bronchioles within the bronchopulmonary segments. The final branches of bronchioles, i.e., terminal respiratory bronchioles, communicate directly with clusters of alveoli. The smooth muscle of bronchioles is supplied by both divisions of the autonomic nervous system: the sympathetic promotes relaxation, the parasympathetic promotes constriction.

Lung Parenchyma. The lung is metabolically very active. Approximately 10 per cent of oxygen consumption is accounted for by the lung. The lung parenchyma is the working area of lung tissue. It consists of millions of alveolar units. Alveoli, small air sacs located at the end of the terminal bronchioles, are the structures that allow the exchanges of gases (oxygen and carbon dioxide). The entire alveolar unit is made of repiratory bronchioles, alveolar ducts, and alveolar sacs. Gas exchange actually begins in the respiratory bronchioles. By the age of 8 years, the number of alveoli has grown from 24 million to 300 million. The total working alveolar surface area is approximately 70 to 80 square meters. The large number of alveoli and the large surface area are necessary to meet both resting and exercise oxygen requirements. Each alveolar unit is supplied with 9 to 11 prepulmonary and pulmonary capillaries. The blood supply for these capillaries comes from the right ventricle of the heart. The major function of the lung parenchyma is the passage and exchange of molecular oxygen and carbon dioxide from the pulmonary capillaries and the alveoli.

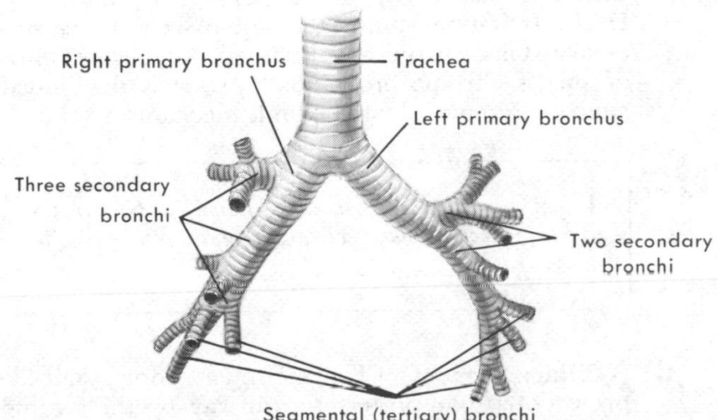

Figure 51–3. Branches of the bronchial tree. (From Dienhart, C. M.: *Basic Human Anatomy and Physiology,* 3rd ed. Philadelphia: W. B. Saunders Co., 1979.)

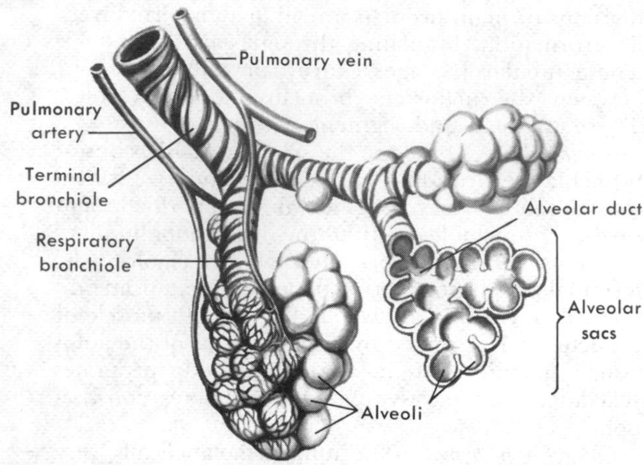

Figure 51–4. Functional lung lobule. (From Dienhart, C. M.: *Basic Human Anatomy and Physiology*, 3rd ed. Philadelphia: W. B. Saunders Co., 1979.)

Normal Protective Mechanisms of the Respiratory System

Five mechanisms protect the integrity of the respiratory system: (1) the mucus blanket, (2) ciliary action, (3) macrophages, (4) surfactant, and (5) cough. Respiratory dysfunction may affect these protective mechanisms, or external forces may alter these mechanisms, thereby causing respiratory dysfunction.

Mucus Blanket. *Mucus* is secreted by special cells called "goblet cells." They are located in the lining of the tracheobronchial tree. The function of the mucus is to entrap debris that has entered the tracheobronchial tree. The debris and mucus is then carried by the cilia upward toward the mouth where it is expectorated or swallowed. The normal production of mucus is about 100 ml. per day. Mucus is composed of water (95%); lipds (1%); glycoprotein (2%); carbohydrates (1%); and a very small amount of DNA. Irritation causes the goblet cells to become enlarged and chronically inflamed. A typical example of this is chronic bronchitis. *Sputum* is that mucus which is removed by the cough mechanism.

> *When mucus is retained and allowed to pool in the lungs, infection may occur. Oxygenation may also be impaired.*

Ciliary Action. Cilia are microscopic, hair-like projections that protect the airway by their rapid, coordinated, unidirectional beating. The movement of the cilia propels a sheet of mucus ("mucus blanket") upward toward the oropharynx. The mucus carries entrapped cells, inhaled particles, and agents of infection toward the mouth where they may be expectorated by a cough, or swallowed into the stomach and rendered harmless by gastric secretions. The action of the cilia is impaired by hypoxia (lack of oxygen), hyperoxia (too much oxygen), dehydration and drying, and pollutants such as smoke. Ciliary function is enhanced with hydration and with the administration of bronchodilators.

Macrophages. Macrophages are located in the alveoli. These phagocytic scavengers of the respiratory system ingest both exogenous and endogenous debris. They move with pseudopodial motion.

Surfactant. Surfactant is one of the most important secretions of the alveoli. Surfactant is a detergent-like phospholipid compound. It reduces the surface tension of the fluid lining of alveoli. Without surfactant, the surface tension in the lung would be so great that it would collapse. When the production of surfactant is impaired, the lung becomes stiff and the alveoli collapse. Reexpansion of these collapsed alveoli requires high inflating pressures.

Many conditions can interfere with the production of surfactant and its balance in the alveoli. Some of them are hypoxia, hyperoxia, pulmonary edema, atelectasis and pneumonia, drowning, and aspiration of foreign material.

PHYSIOLOGY

Movement of Gases

The lungs and circulation act together to convey respiratory gases between the atmospheric air and body tissues. The lungs perform their function by *ventilation* and by *exchange of gases.*

Ventilation. Movement of air into and out of the lungs along bronchial airways is a cyclic process of inspiration and expiration, bringing freshly oxygenated air into the lungs and removing "stale" air and CO_2. The amount of ventilation that occurs is affected and regulated by (1) respiratory centers in the brain and in the periphery, (2) chemicals in the cerebral spinal fluid, (3) the partial pressure* of carbon dioxide (pCO_2), (4) the partial pressure of oxygen (pO_2), (5) the pH, and (6) other factors such as pain, temperature, emotions, physical activity.

Effective ventilation requires patent airways; elastic, expansile lungs and tracheobronchial tree; efficient, adequate musculoskeletal apparatus of the chest wall and related structures; and normal relation between amounts of air inspired per breath and amounts within lungs. The effectiveness of ventilation can be meas-

*Partial pressure, abbreviated "pp," is the pressure of a gas which is a portion of the total pressure exerted by a gas mixture. For example, ambient air pressure (atmospheric) is 760 mm. Hg at sea level. The partial pressure of oxygen is 159 mm. Hg. This is calculated by multiplying the per cent of oxygen by 760 mm. Hg. That is, 760 × 21 per cent = 159 mm. Hg.

ured by a laboratory test called *arterial blood gas analysis.*

Exchange of Gases. Exchange of gases between the air and blood in the terminal alveolar capillary system is part of the process of *respiration* (Fig. 51–5). Specifically, respiration refers to the exchange of O_2 and CO_2 in the body within the lungs, between the cells and their environments, and in intracellular metabolism. The exchange of CO_2 and O_2 at the alveolar-capillary level is termed *external respiration.* The exchange of O_2 and CO_2 at the tissue-cellular level is termed *internal respiration.* (CO_2-O_2 transport is discussed in Chap. 12.) During respiration body tissues are supplied with O_2 for metabolism and CO_2 is released from the tissues.

Normal Body Respiration. This requires:

1. Adequate O_2 concentration in the alveoli.
2. Adequate amount of hemoglobin capable of combining with this O_2.
3. Diffusion of O_2 from the alveoli in concentrations sufficient to saturate the blood adequately before it leaves the lung.
4. Transportation of the oxyhemoglobin to the tissues at a rate commensurate with tissue needs.
5. Availability of the body cells to use the O_2 supplied to them.

Gas Exchange. This occurs at two places within the body: the lungs (in pulmonary alveoli), and the tissues. Pulmonary gas exchange is effected by: *ventilation; perfusion* (i.e., supplying of the lungs with blood from the right side of the heart); and *diffusion* (i.e., the movement of O_2 and CO_2 between the gas phase (in alveolar air) and the blood phase (in capillaries).

Gas exchange is also affected by the availability of an adequate concentration of O_2 in the inspired air. Gas exchange will be affected by changes in the partial pressure of O_2 due to changes in altitude.

Hydrogen Ion Imbalances. The lungs perform important functions in governing the body's hydrogen ion balance. This important homeostatic function is discussed in Chapter 12. Respiratory malfunctioning can cause serious hydrogen imbalances, e.g., respiratory acidosis and respiratory alkalosis. *Respiratory acidosis* is a serious result of *hypercapnia,* i.e., the retention of excessive amounts of CO_2. *Respiratory alkalosis* is a manifestation of *hypocapnia,* i.e., the excessive blowing off (loss) of CO_2.

The major stimulus to ventilation is a mild elevation of the pCO_2. Normally, if the pCO_2 rises, ventilation is stimulated by this increase and the level of ventilation increases to correct the mild elevation of the pCO_2.

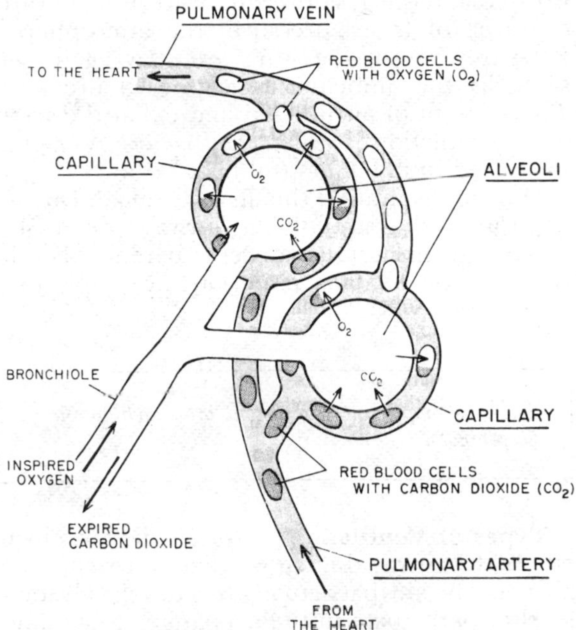

Figure 51–5. Action of the alveoli in the circulatory system. (From *Breathing . . . What You Need to Know.* American Lung Association, 1968.)

The Mechanism of Ventilation: "Anatomy of a Breath"

The process of ventilation occurs in two phases. The movement of air into the lungs is termed *inspiration* or *inhalation.* This is an *active* process involving movement of muscles and the thorax. The movement of air out of the lungs is termed *expiration* or *exhalation* and is normally a *passive* process.

Thousands of times each day the "message" to breathe is transmitted through the body in the form of a chemical stimulus. This chemical stimulus originates in the cerebral spinal fluid and is transmitted to the brain's medulla. The message is then directed down through the *vagus nerve* to the other central and peripheral mechanisms.

As the message to inhale is recognized by the receptors in the chest, the chest cavity enlarges. This enlargement occurs as the major muscle of respiration, the *diaphragm,* contracts, flattens, and descends into the abdomen. Increasing the capacity of the thorax in this way provides space for lung expansion.

As mentioned earlier, the outer surface of the lungs and the inner surface of the chest wall are covered with membranes called *pleurae.* Pressure changes in the intrapleural space (intrapleural pressure) and pressure changes within the lung (intrapulmonic pressure) combine to pull the lungs open. This produces a pressure gradient (that is, a pressure difference) that causes air to flow into the lungs from the atmosphere. Atmospheric air is also called *ambient air.* Inspiration continues until the pressure gradient between the atmospheric air and the air in the lungs is equal. Air flow then ceases and expiration commences.

Normally, exhalation is quiet and passive. This means that air is expelled as the thorax recoils to its resting position. As the lung volume decreases, the air within the airways is compressed and the gas flows out of the lung toward the area of lesser pressure (the atmosphere). Pressures within the lung are now again the same as the ambient (atmospheric) pressure. The amount of air inhaled and exhaled during quiet ventilation is called *tidal volume* (V_T). It is measured in milliliters (ml.).

During inspiration the airways dilate. During expiration the size of the airways decreases. This is an important concept to remember in the care of patients experiencing respiratory dysfunction.

The most important and potent bronchodilator is a deep breath.

Types of Ventilation. Not all the air which enters the airway during ventilation reaches the alveoli. The air that actually reaches the alveolar level to participate in the exchange of CO_2 and O_2 is called *alveolar ventilation* (V_A). The efficiency of ventilation is determined by the alveolar ventilation. The only means of assessing the effectiveness of the alveolar ventilation is by arterial blood gas analysis. Specifically, the pCO_2 is the portion of the arterial blood gas that demonstrates the adequacy of ventilation.

The air that does not reach the alveolar level but only enters the conducting airway is called *anatomic dead space* ($V_D$anat). Anatomic dead space is approximately equivalent in volume to the body weight of the individual. For example, a 150-pound person would have 150 ml. of anatomic dead space. The term dead space universally refers to movement of air without an exchange of gases.

Another term relating to ventilation is *minute ventilation.* This is the total amount of air moved in and out of the lungs in 1 minute. Minute ventilation ($\dot{V}$) is measured in liters per minute (LPM). Normal adult minute ventilation is in the 5 to 12 LPM range.

Alveolar minute ventilation ($\dot{V}_A$) is the volume of air that reaches the alveoli in a minute and participates in gas exchange. If ventilation is inadequate, and the pCO_2 is elevated, this is termed *hypoventilation.* If ventilation is excessive and the pCO_2 is below normal, *hyperventilation* ensues.

CHAPTER 52

DIAGNOSIS AND EVALUATION OF PERSONS WITH RESPIRATORY DISORDERS

Nurses are usually responsible for preparing patients for respiratory diagnostic tests. This involves discussing the preparation, actual procedure, and postprocedure activities with patients and their significant others as well as carrying out any physical preparation for the procedure or as ordered by the physician. Because anxiety influences respirations, it is especially important for the patient to be psychologically well prepared for diagnostic procedures and to be as relaxed as possible during them. Because pulmonary diagnosis may involve numerous diagnostic tests (some of which are acutely uncomfortable), the patient may become discouraged and irritable. Patients who are dyspneic tire easily and often require planned rest periods during the diagnostic process. When nurses are present during tests they not only assist the physician but also help patients by calming them, eliciting their cooperation and confidence, informing them of progress during the procedure, instructing them what to do (or not do) during the procedure, and appropriately offering praise and encouragement. (Review a basic nursing text for details concerning anxiety reduction.)

CHEST ROENTGENOGRAPHY

Common Chest Film Procedures

Chest x-ray films are often made for *screening* purposes, i. e., to detect pulmonary lesions such as tuberculosis, in large selected population groups, and they are frequently a part of the routine admission data base collection. The films are read by experts, and persons with suspicious findings usually have further chest films and other diagnostic tests. Chest x-ray screening programs not only help to detect pulmonary tuberculosis, but they also frequently call attention to other pulmonary problems and disorders involving the heart and other mediastinal structures, e.g., tumors, pulmonary bullae, cardiac disease, structural abnormalities. Some respiratory disease screening programs also include simple breathing tests (helpful in detecting such disorders as pulmonary emphysema).

Routine chest films are an important part of any complete physical examination. These routine films may demonstrate lesions in the chest which are asymptomatic and thus would otherwise go undetected in time for early treatment. When a lesion is detected, a chest film helps provide information about the lesion's size, location, and nature. Chest films not only furnish information about disorders involving lung tissue but can also detect problems involving numerous related structures. For example, they may reveal: (1) disorders of the soft tissues and bones of the chest wall; (2) abnormal diaphragmatic contours; (3) limited ranges of diaphragmatic excursions on respiration; (4) abnormalities in heart position, size, contour, and other abnormal mediastinal configurations; (5) tracheobronchial abnormalities; (6) pleural thickening; (7) fluid in the pleural space; and (8) grossly abnormal changes in the caliber or distribution of pulmonary arteries and veins.

Before chest films are taken patients are briefly told about the procedure and what they will be required to do. Clothing and metal objects are removed down to the waist and patients are given a protective drape or gown. (Metal objects show up on the developed film and thus obscure the body structures in the area they cover.)

Chest films may be made at the patient's bedside or in the radiology department, depending on the patient's state of health. The films may be taken with the patient standing, sitting erect, or lying down. Most chest films are taken with the patient sitting or standing up. The patient is positioned correctly and is then usually instructed to take a deep breath and hold it for a few seconds while the x-ray film is being taken. The maximal inspiration of air fills the lungs, thereby enabling a clearer view of pulmonary structures.

Although a variety of x-ray techniques may be employed in evaluating pulmonary disorders, the most common views are a *posteroanterior* (PA or "flat plate") with the x-ray beam passing from the body's posterior to anterior surface; *lateral* views taken through the right or left side of the chest; and various *oblique* views which are slanting or inclined at specified angles (Fig. 52–1). Additionally, a *lordotic* film may be taken to more clearly view the apices, i.e., the rounded upper portions of each lung which extend upward as high as the first thoracic vertebra. Of the oblique views the most common are the right and left anterior obliques; these permit views of structures obscured in the PA position and of the mediastinal contents. The recumbent lateral position (also called "decubitus") helps to localize fluid in the pleural space, i.e., pleural effusions.

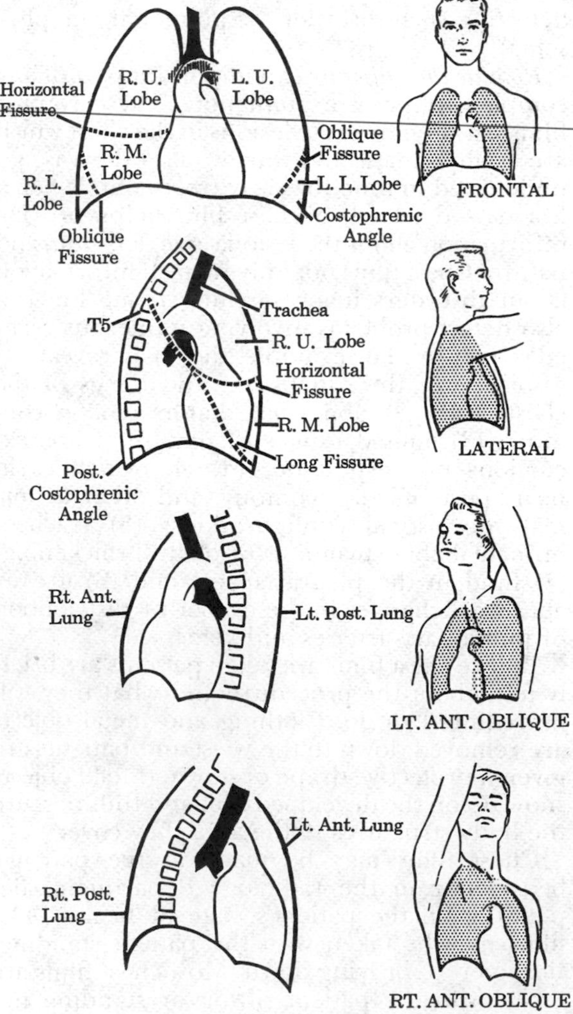

Figure 52–1. Pulmonary projections and relationships. (From *Merck Manual,* 12th ed. Rahway, N.J.: Merck Sharp & Dohme, 1972.)

Body Section Roentgenography; Stereoscopic Roentgenography

In addition to the x-ray views discussed above, special techniques of *body section roentgenography* may also be employed in pulmonary diagnosis. These techniques show detailed images of structures lying in a predetermined plane of tissue, while blurring the images of structures in other planes. It is thus possible to study areas normally concealed by overlying structures. These x-ray films of structures at selected layers of the body are obtained by various methods known by such names as *laminagraphy, planigraphy, stratigraphy,* and *tomography.* In performing body section roentgenography, numerous films are taken at differing planes of the chest until the area being studied is in clear focus. This technique is especially helpful in evaluating pulmonary densities, cavities, and tumors. *Stereoscopic roentgenography* (three-dimensional views) enables more accurate spatial localization of questionable areas than do the usual two-dimensional films.

Bronchography

A *bronchogram* is an x-ray film of the tracheobronchial tree and lung taken after an opaque medium (a radiopaque oil or water-soluble dye) is instilled into a bronchus (via a tube passed nasally into the trachea or via a bronchoscope). Bronchoscopes and bronchoscopy are discussed below. The opaque material coats and outlines the bronchial tree, thereby enabling visualization of this structure when the x-ray film is taken. (See Figure 52–2.)

Because regurgitation and aspiration are potential dangers associated with bronchography, it is important that patients receive special pre- and postprocedure care.

Prior to bronchography the following nursing activities are typically of importance:

- Instruct the patient to perform thorough oral hygiene the evening before and the morning of the procedure.
- Withhold oral intake for 6 to 12 hours (to prevent possible regurgitation and aspiration).
- Assist the patient with postural drainage as ordered the morning of the procedure (clearing the bronchi of secretions enables the radiopaque material to enter these areas and produce a more informative film.

- Ask the patient about any loose teeth, capped teeth, dental bridges, or oral inflammations and chart their presence (loose teeth or dental prostheses can be broken off or dislodged and aspirated during the procedure).

- Remove and safely store removable dental structures.

- Report oral inflammations to the physician (it may be necessary for you to inspect the patient's mouth).

- Have the patient sign a consent permit if required by hospital policy.

- Administer preprocedure medications as ordered. Inform the patient that the medications will promote relaxation by reducing awareness of the surroundings. Atropine may be ordered to minimize secretions and a short-acting barbiturate to sedate the patient and reduce the stimulating effects of anesthetic agents.

Although local anesthesia (cocaine, lidocaine, or tetracaine) prevents coughing and gagging when the tube is being passed (during bronchography or bronchoscopy), it can also cause serious (sometimes fatal) toxic reactions. Symptoms of *cocaine toxicity* include palpitations, excitation, rapid and bounding pulse, euphoria, elevated blood pressure, and rapid, deep respirations. These are symptoms of stimulation of the nervous system from above downward. Overstimulation is followed by depression of the nervous system in this same descending order. Unless symptoms of overactivity are promptly observed, reported, and treated, *fatal respiratory failure may occur.* Treatment may include continuous mechanical ventilation (CMV) via an artificial airway, controlled oxygen administration, and the intramuscular or intravenous administration of a rapid-acting barbiturate, e.g., secobarbital sodium (Seconal).

Preparation of the patient for bronchography (or bronchoscopy) also involves giving appropriate *patient education* concerning the procedure itself, what is expected of the patient during the procedure, and any pre- or postprocedure restrictions (and the reasons for these restrictions).

Relaxation is important during intubation since a relaxed person experiences less discomfort and the procedure can also be performed more rapidly and more successfully. Reassure patients that they will be able to breathe at all times since the tubes passed into the trachea are hollow. It is desirable, however, if patients can learn before the procedure to more consciously govern their breathing. For example, have them practice breathing through the mouth only, with the mouth open; then have them practice breathing through the nose only, with the mouth open.

Inform patients that their throat will be anesthetized during the procedure to increase comfort and prevent gagging. The local anesthesia sprayed into the throat tastes bitter. Instruct the patient not to swallow this medication, but rather to spit it out into facial tissues or an emesis basin which will be provided.

Finally, tell the patient that nothing should be taken by mouth following the procedure until the gag reflex returns, and demonstrate how the gag reflex will be tested.

Once the physician has properly positioned the bronchoscope or catheter in the trachea the radiopaque material is introduced. The patient is tilted into various positions, which causes the liquid material to run along the walls of the tracheobronchial tree, into the bronchi and bronchioles (Fig. 52–2). After a series of x-ray films, postural drainage is used to help the dye to flow back out of the tracheobronchial tree so it can be expectorated. Postural drainage sessions should be supervised by the nurse while the patient is hospitalized. (Postural drainage is discussed on p. 1233). It is desirable for as much dye as possible to be removed after bronchography. Some dyes are absorbed by the body within 12 to 24 hours; others may remain in the tracheobronchial tree for several months. Follow-up films are commonly taken. Surgery may be postponed for several months following bronchography if the physician believes that dye remaining in the tracheobronchial tree may jeopardize the patient's recovery. Oxygenation may be impaired if the dye is not removed. This precaution is particularly necessary if the dye used had an oil base.

Following bronchography the patient is not allowed oral intake until it is certain that the local anesthesia has worn off and the patient's gag reflex has been restored. (See Unit X.) The gag reflex may return as soon as 2 hours following the procedure or it may not return for 6 to 8 hours. *Post a sign on the patient's bed clearly stating intake restrictions.* Tracheal intubation may cause the patient's throat to feel irritated and sore following the procedure. Observe the patient closely for indications of cocaine or other topical anesthetic toxicity and for symptoms of laryngospasm or laryngeal edema (resulting from laryngeal trauma during intubation). Impaired respirations may occur, necessitating immediate lifesaving treatment. To help remove the radiopaque substance from the lungs the physician may order the use of a large volume nebulizer for hydration and mobilization of the dye and secretions, followed by postural drainage. Effective coughing and deep breathing exercises may also be carried out.

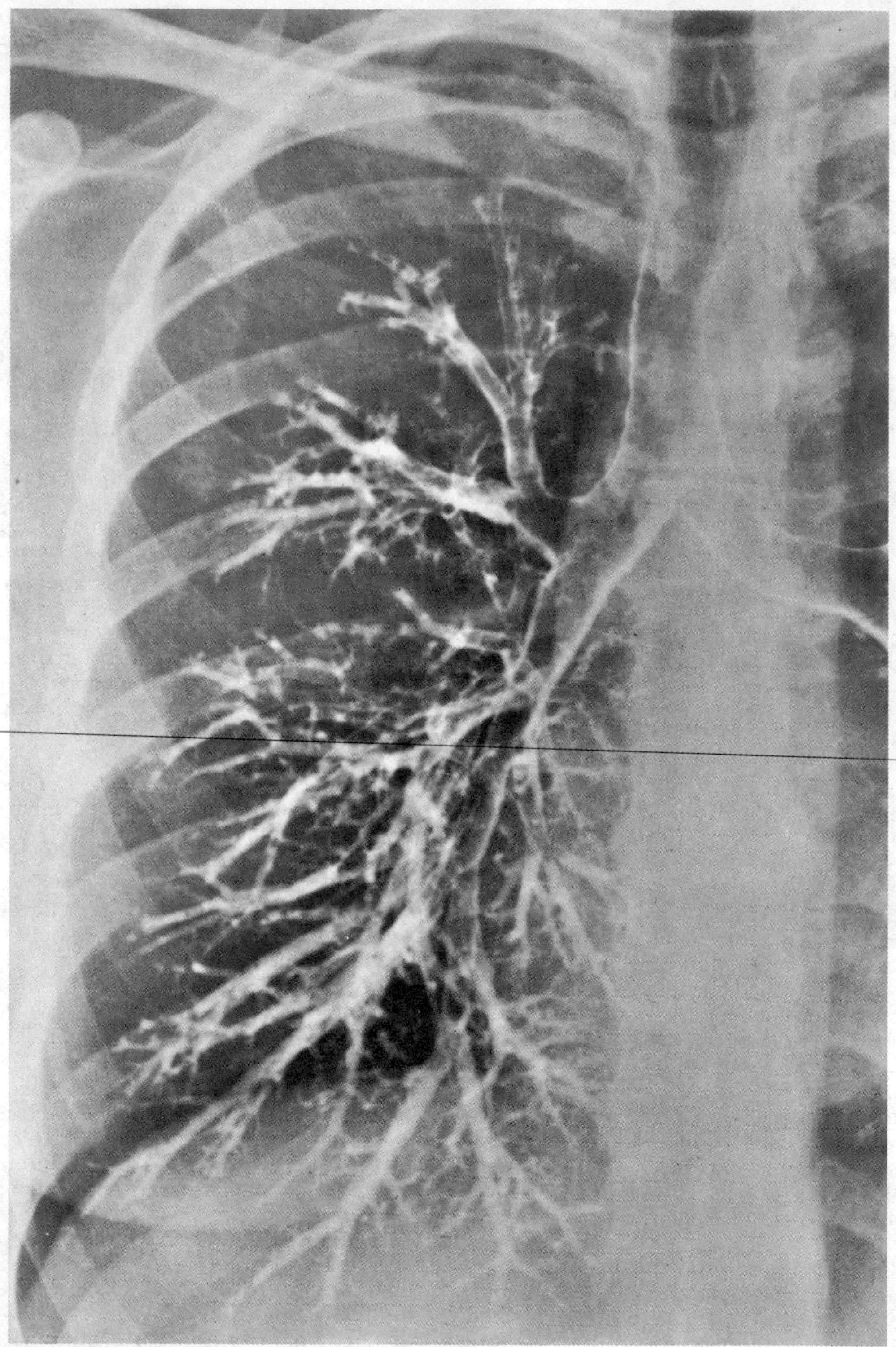

Figure 52–2. Right bronchial tree (frontal projection). Normal bronchogram of a 39 year old woman. (From Fraser, R. G., and Paré, J. A. P.: *Organ Physiology: Structure and Function of the Lung.* Philadelphia: W. B. Saunders Co., 1977.)

Pulmonary Angiography

Angiography (i.e., the roentgenographic visualization of blood vessels following injection of a contrast medium) is useful in evaluating pulmonary disorders as well as disorders of the brain, heart, and other body systems. Pulmonary angiography is helpful in diagnosing such conditions as pulmonary embolism, lung tumors, aneurysms, vascular changes associated with emphysema, congenital defects, blebs, or bullae. Indeed, any space-occupying lesion within the thorax may be an indication for pulmonary angiographic investigation.

Angiography may demonstrate various pulmonary mechanical abnormalities, e.g., displacement of vessels from their normal positions (possibly due to bullae), or reduced blood flow to an area (perhaps caused by congenital defects, emboli, or tumorous obstruction).

Although numerous *techniques* for performing pulmonary angiography have been developed, in essence the procedure involves passing a catheter from a vein in the arm, into the heart (through the right atrium and right ventricle), and up into the pulmonary artery. Local anesthesia is used for the procedure. As the catheter is being progressively inserted pressures can be measured (e.g., in the right atrium, right ventricle, and pulmonary artery) and blood samples can be removed from various regions of the pulmonary circulatory system. Once the catheter is properly positioned a radiopaque substance is rapidly injected with a pressure injector and pulmonary x-rays are immediately taken and recorded on film or video tape. Manual injection of the dye into a peripheral vein may produce satisfactory blood vessel visualization and is less hazardous than catheterization, but it is not routinely used because the pictures obtainable are limited in number and may be of poorer quality, and also a larger volume of contrast substance is necessary.

Complications associated with pulmonary angiography include: (1) mechanical problems associated with use of a catheter (e.g., local vascular problems, myocardial perforation with the catheter, or rupture, fragmentation, or perforation of the catheter itself); (2) pharmacologic problems (e.g., untoward allergic or toxic reactions to the contrast material or reactions to local anesthesia); and (3) cardiac complications (e.g., myocardial irritability caused by the catheter's presence in the heart's chambers). During the procedure the patient is closely monitored by continuous electrocardiography for cardiac arrhythmias. (See Unit XII.)

The patient is told before the contrast medium is injected into the lung that the injection may cause a temporary flushed, warm feeling. It is not uncommon for the injection to also provoke cough.

CHEST FLUOROSCOPY

Examination of the chest with fluoroscopic equipment enables the physician to view both lungs at the same time during the breathing process. Thus it is possible to actually view the dynamic activity of such cardiopulmonary mechanisms as cardiac action, diaphragmatic action, and lung expansion and contraction. By observing the movements of the thoracic wall and diaphragm during breathing, considerable information can be obtained about ventilation. Formerly it was not possible to have a permanent record of a fluoroscopic examination. Now, if desired, *spot films,* i.e., localized instantaneous x-rays, may be taken of questionable areas for later study. Modern special *image intensifier equipment* projects the fluoroscopic examination onto a *television screen* and may also record the entire examination on *film* for future study.

Sometimes mass roentgenographic surveys use techniques of *photofluorography* instead of routine chest x-ray survey films. This is the photographic recording of fluoroscopic images on small films with the use of a fast lens.

The room may need to be darkened for *fluoroscopy.* The patient sits or stands in front of the fluoroscope. The procedure is painless. The physician gives the patient directions while looking into the fluoroscope, e.g., "take a deep breath and hold it for a few seconds." Physicians and nurses attending the patient during fluoroscopy wear lead-lined aprons and gloves for protection against unnecessary exposure to radiation. Properly maintained modern equipment minimizes radiation exposure.

LUNG SCINTIGRAPHY

Lung scintigraphy produces a graphic record of particles in the lung (as registered by a scintiscanner) following administration of a radioisotope. A scintiscanner is an apparatus used to record the concentration of a gamma ray emitting isotope in a tissue or organ. Lung scintigraphy may also be accomplished by using a scintillation camera. Lung scintiscanning may be carried out in different ways, e.g., radioaerosol inhalation, xenon-133 gas inhalation, and perfusion lung scan studies. (See also p. 1191.)

Perfusion studies evaluate the perfusion of the lung with blood. Perfusion lung scanning procedures are performed by intravenous injection of macroaggregated albumin labeled with radioactive isotopes (e.g., ^{131}I or ^{51}Cr) and counting of the emissions of the radioactive isotopes with a scintiscanner. This determines the distribution of radioactivity in the pulmonary vascular structures. The results are recorded on a diagram of the lungs, which then clearly shows which areas are well perfused with blood (indicated by a high uptake of radioactive substances) and which areas are poorly perfused (indicated by only small amounts of radioactive uptake). Areas of poor perfusion may result from emboli, tumors, or other disorders.

ENDOSCOPIC EXAMINATION OF THE TRACHEOBRONCHIAL TREE (BRONCHOSCOPY)

Bronchoscopy refers to the examination of the tracheobronchial tree and many of its bronchopulmonary segments. Formerly, visualization of the tracheobronchial tree was limited by the large straight metal bronchoscope, and only the larger airways were visible. Within the past decade endoscopic examination of the tracheobronchial tree has been facilitated by the advent of long, pliable, flexible scopes that utilize fiber light bundles. (See Fig 52–3.) These light bundles transmit a true picture of the airway. The flexible fiberoptic bronchoscopes are small enough in diameter to allow easy passage through the transoral or transnasal route with or without the passage of an endotracheal tube. If an endotracheal tube is used to facilitate the passage of the scope, the endotracheal tube must be of a large enough inner diameter (8.5 mm. or greater) to provide for maintenance of the patient's ventilation around the bronchoscope during the procedure.

Both rigid and flexible bronchoscopes may be used to obtain samples of pulmonary tissues and cells for cytologic examination. Bronchial washings may also be obtained by flushing the airway with a saline solution. These samples may be examined for abnormal cellular structure or bacteriologic examination. Special attachments designed to facilitate the biopsy of specimens, bronchial washings, brushings, suction, and instillation of anesthetic agents are part of the accessories used with the flexible fiberoptic bronchoscope (Fig. 52–3).

The procedure may be performed in surgery, in an endoscopic procedure room, at the bedside, or under fluoroscopy. Many procedures for diagnostic purposes are done on an outpatient basis. The patient arrives at the hospital or clinic "fasting" and may have preprocedure arterial blood gas and ventilatory screening tests performed, especially if subsequent surgery is a possibility. Following the procedure, nursing observations and interventions are the same as for the postbronchogram patient. If biopsies were taken the patient must be cautioned to observe sputum for blood. The nurse must always note the presence of blood. Sudden dyspnea following the procedure may indicate a pneumothorax, especially if peripheral lung tissue was biopsied.

Therapeutic bronchoscopies are often carried out in the critical care units caring for ventilator-dependent patients with thick inspissated sputum or possible airway obstructions. The bronchoscope may also be passed through a tracheostomy tube to facilitate removal of secretions. The flexible fiberoptic bronchoscope may be passed through a specially designed adapter so that continuous mechanical ventilation (CMV) and bronchoscopy may be carried out simultaneously.

The rigid bronchoscope is still required to remove foreign objects, to obtain specimens for biopsy of large vascular tumors which may hemorrhage, and to suction large volumes of blood or mucus too excessive for the channel in the flexible fiberoptic bronchoscope.

Preparation of the patient for bronchoscopy is similar to that for bronchography, except for the following: (1) the procedure will be performed in a darkened room (often an operating room) so the doctor can more clearly see the structures lighted by the scope, (2) 30 to 60 minutes prior to the procedure morphine sulfate, meperidine, or a similar sedative may be ordered; and (3) a general anesthetic (e.g., intravenous anesthesia) may or may not be used.

For more detailed discussion of fiberoptic bronchoscopy see the article by Landa[97] and another by Marici.[104] *During bronchoscopy* the pa-

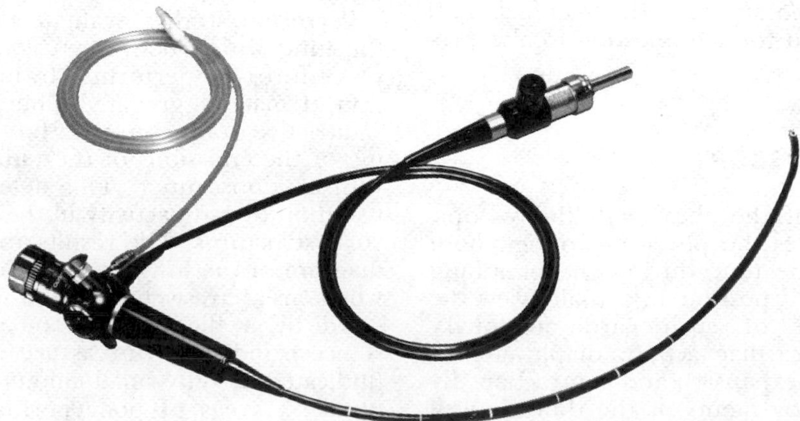

Figure 52–3. A flexible fiberoptic bronchoscope. (Courtesy of The Olympus Corporation, New Hyde Park, N.Y.)

tient lies on the back with neck hyperextended so the bronchoscope can more easily be inserted. Hyperextension is obtained by placing a small pillow under the patient's shoulders in such a manner that the head drops back over the edge of the pillow. Hyperextension elevates the pharynx so it is in a straight line with the trachea. During the procedure the conscious patient is reminded to keep arms to the sides, breathe through the nose, relax, and not clench fists.

After bronchoscopy the patient is closely observed for possible serious complications. The following aspects of clinical care are of special importance:

- Position the patient as ordered and as indicated. For example, the conscious patient may be ordered to be kept flat or in semi-Fowler's position, lying on either side. If a general anesthetic was used and the patient is not fully conscious, he or she is positioned flat, with head and body turned to one side to prevent aspiration.
- Instruct the conscious patient with impaired swallowing to let saliva run from the side of the mouth (while lying on the side with a basin or tissues under the mouth) rather than attempt to swallow.
- Save all sputum expectorated for laboratory studies (cytology and culture). Copious amounts of sputum may be produced as a result of the trauma caused by passing the scope.
- Observe the patient closely for indications of impaired respiration. Laryngospasm or laryngeal edema (see Unit XXIV) may occur owing to laryngeal trauma. Notify the physician immediately of such symptoms as laryngeal stridor, dyspnea, and shortness of breath. Have emergency resuscitation equipment available (including tracheostomy tray). Provide emergency resuscitation as necessary. Set up and administer warm mist treatments if prescribed (to prevent laryngeal edema).
- Give the patient nothing by mouth until the gag reflex returns. Once the gag reflex is present (2 to 8 hours following the procedure) give small amounts of fluids unless nausea or vomiting occurs. Because of sore throat and difficulty in swallowing after bronchoscopy, warm or soothing liquids may be more easily taken. A soft diet may be tolerated 8 hours after the procedure; after 24 hours a regular diet may be prescribed.
- Observe the patient's sputum closely for indications of hemorrhage (frank blood) if biopsy was performed. Sputum is expected to be slightly bloodstreaked for several hours, or perhaps for one or two days; however, excessive bleeding is reported immediately.
- Observe the patient for subcutaneous emphysema (around the face and neck) and dyspnea. If present, immediately report these symptoms, for they indicate the serious (and fortunately rare) complication of perforation of the trachea or bronchus. (Subcutaneous emphysema is discussed in Chapter 57.)
- Observe the patient closely for symptoms of toxicity caused by local anesthetic agents, e.g., cocaine, as described on pp. 1172–1173.
- Provide appropriate treatment if the patient has a sore throat. An ice collar may be used to minimize edema and soreness. Once the patient is able to swallow, lozenges or soothing liquids to gargle may be given.
- If diazepam was administered during the procedure, observe the patient closely for irrational behavior. A transient (24 hours) episode may occur. Patients must not be allowed to operate motor vehicles or leave the hospital unattended if bronchoscopy was performed on an outpatient basis.

THORACENTESIS

Thoracentesis, also called thoracocentesis, refers to needle puncture through the chest wall into the pleural space for the purpose of removing pleural fluid (and/or possibly air). Thoracentesis may be performed for diagnostic or therapeutic reasons.

Therapeutically, pleural fluid accumulations may be drained off to relieve lung compression and respiratory distress, or to remove excessive pleural fluid which could become infected and cause empyema. Thoracentesis may be therapeutically useful in treating such pulmonary disorders as pleurisy with effusion, empyema, hydrothorax, and hemothorax (see below).

Diagnostically, pleural fluid obtained by thoracentesis is subjected to careful study of its chemical, bacteriologic, and cellular composition. In the clinical laboratory the specimen's consistency, color, and the presence or absence of blood are noted. Evaluations are also made of glucose and protein content, specific gravity, white and differential blood counts, and the presence of bacteria and cells. Cellular composition may reveal the presence of neoplastic cells. Effusions characterized by lymphocytosis occur most often in patients with tuberculosis, lymphoma, or carcinoma. (See Table 52–1.)

Before thoracentesis the nurse prepares the patient psychologically, assembles necessary equipment, and properly positions the patient. Patient education includes briefly explaining the procedure, telling the patients that they help by not moving during the procedure, and informing them that after the procedure they should have only minimal discomfort at the puncture site. If patients move suddenly during the procedure they can force the needle through the pleural space and injure the visceral (pulmonary) pleura or lung.

Equipment for thoracentesis includes: 5-ml. syringe and needle for local anesthesia, local anesthetic drug, 50-ml. syringe, 17-gauge aspirating needle, three-way stopcock, sterile

TABLE 52–1. DIFFERENTIAL DIAGNOSIS OF PLEURAL EFFUSION

I. Transudative pleural effusions
- Congestive heart failure
- Cirrhosis
- Nephrotic syndrome
- Acute glomerulonephritis
- Myxedema
- Peritoneal dialysis
- Hypoproteinemia
- Meigs' syndrome
- Sarcoidosis

II. Exudative pleural effusions
- Infectious diseases
  - Tuberculosis
  - Bacterial infections
  - Viral infections
  - Fungal infections
  - Parasitic infections
- Neoplastic diseases
  - Mesotheliomas
  - Metastatic disease
- Collagen vascular diseases
  - Systemic lupus erythematosus
  - Rheumatoid pleuritis
- Pulmonary infarction
- Gastrointestinal diseases
  - Pancreatitis
  - Esophageal rupture
  - Subphrenic abscess
  - Hepatic abscess
  - Whipple's disease
  - Diaphragmatic hernia
- Injury
  - Hemothorax
  - Chylothorax
- Drug hypersensitivity
  - Nitrofurantoin
  - Methysergide
- Miscellaneous diseases
  - Asbestos exposure
  - Pulmonary and lymph node myomatosis
  - Uremia
  - Postmyocardial infarction syndrome
  - Trapped lung
  - Congenital abnormalities of the lymphatics

From Light, R. N.: Pleural fluid analysis: How to interpret the tests. *Consultant,* 18:97, May 1978.

tubing, hemostats, sterile specimen tube and collecting vial, sterile towels, materials for skin preparation, collodion, and small sterile dressing. A biopsy needle should also be on hand. (See p. 1180.)

It is important that the needle and syringe used for thoracentesis fit tightly to prevent atmospheric air from entering the pleural space. Since pleural exudates tend to coagulate easily, specimens are usually collected in tubes containing either sodium citrate or potassium oxalate.

Positioning is important. Thoracentesis is most effectively performed with the patient sitting upright (pleural fluid can then accumulate for removal at the base of the chest) with neck and dorsal spine flexed and arms and shoulders raised (this elevates and separates the ribs, thus ensuring less traumatic needle insertion). Have the patient sit on the edge of the bed with feet supported on a chair. Then roll an overbed table in front of the patient, place a pillow or folded bath blanket on this table, and have the patient raise arms and shoulders and lean over the padded surface, resting the head on the padding. Remain by the patient's side. Physically support the patient especially if he or she is very nervous or weak. Two nurses may well be required — one to assist the patient and one to assist the doctor.

If the patient cannot sit up for thoracentesis, turn the person on to the unaffected side and place the arm on that side up over the head.

Throughout the thoracentesis observe the patient's condition, reassure and advise, assist the physician, and take the patient's pulse and respiratory rates several times. Tell the patient what is happening, e.g., when an injection will be made, to avoid the patient being startled into sudden movement. Observe the patient closely for shock chills, pain, nausea, coughing, pallor, dyspnea, cyanosis, weakness, increased respiratory rate, or diaphoresis. Call the physician's attention to these symptoms.

Thoracentesis is performed aseptically with local anesthesia. The site of needle insertion for fluid removal is most often just below the angle of the scapula at the seventh intercostal space. At times the physician uses a chest x-ray film for purposes of measuring the level at which the

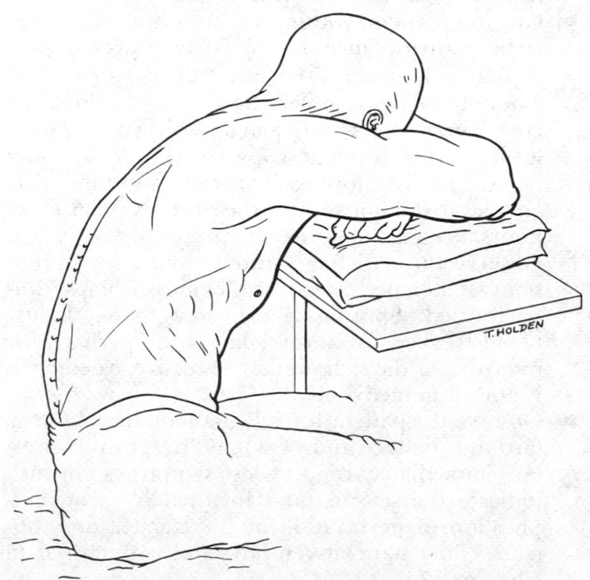

Most effective position for thoracentesis. (From Zimmerman, C. E.: *Techniques of Patient Care,* 2nd ed. Boston: Little, Brown and Co., 1976.)

aspiration should be performed. The lower tip of the scapula is used as a landmark and then the distance of the fluid below this landmark is measured. With the patient positioned as for the x-ray film, the physician then carries out the same measurements on the patient's back and performs the aspiration. If thoracentesis is performed too low, the liver or spleen may be punctured, causing serious aftereffects.

A small gauge needle and a 5-ml. syringe are used to locate the pleural space and to inject the anesthetic agent. Then a larger needle (17-gauge) is used for the fluid removal. This needle is attached to a three-way stopcock (to prevent air from entering the pleural space) and a 50-ml. syringe. Hemostats (or artery clamps) may be used to hold the needle in place after insertion or to mark the desired depth of insertion.

As the needle passes through the parietal pleura (lining the walls of the parietal cavity), the patient may feel pressure or pain even though a local anesthetic has been injected.

Fluid in the pleural space is slowly and gently aspirated. Not more than 1200 ml. are removed at one time in order to reduce the dangers of circulatory collapse or acute pulmonary edema. Rapid removal does not provide sufficient time for the lung to reexpand and the patient may become short of breath, may cough, and may have chest pain. These symptoms indicate possible mediastinal shift toward the side of the thoracentesis. (See Chapter 56.) Precautions are taken to avoid tearing the lung and thus causing a pneumothorax during thoracentesis; for the same purpose, care is taken to maintain negative pressure. Excessive traction on the syringe plunger during fluid removal can cause lung puncture by drawing the lung forcefully against the needle point.

Occasionally the physician may wish to visualize the pleural space by inserting the flexible fiberoptic bronchoscope into this space.

After the needle is removed, pressure is applied over the puncture site. The site is usually sealed with collodion and covered with a small sterile dressing. Specimens are sent immediately to the clinical laboratory. The patient may be positioned recumbent for an hour with punctured chest side up. This position minimizes possible fluid seepage by gravity into the pleural space and allows the pleural puncture site to seal over. The nurse charts the procedure, including comments about the amount and character of fluid removed, and the patient's tolerance of the procedure, e.g., pulse, color, appearance, how patients say they feel. Any relief that the patient may have obtained from the procedure, e.g., breathing more comfortably, is noted and charted.

Following thoracentesis the nurse observes the patient for indications of *complications* or fluid reaccumulation in the pleural space. Specific observations include the following:

- ► Observe for symptoms of *shock,* e.g., faintness, falling blood pressure, weak rapid pulse, rapid respirations. Shock is a rare complication, but can result from fluid shifting into the pleural space from the vascular space. This shift decreases the circulating blood volume, thereby causing shock.
- ► Check the *puncture site* for indications of leakage.
- ► Observe for the following symptoms, of possible *lung damage* (e.g., *pneumothorax,* p. 1267, or *tension pneumothorax,* p. 1342) or possible *reaccumulation of fluid:* (1) blood-tinged sputum or hemoptysis, (2) excessive, uncontrollable coughing or persistent cough, (3) indications of respiratory distress (e.g., dyspnea, cyanosis, tightness in the chest); and (4) subcutaneous emphysema.
- ► Ausculate the entire chest. Compare breath sounds and listen for abnormal breath sounds.
- ► Watch for indications of *mediastinal shift* if large amounts of fluid were removed. Symptoms include those of cardiac distress or pulmonary edema (indicated by blood-tinged frothy sputum). These symptoms are caused by sudden shift of the mediastinal contents toward the side from which the fluid was removed.
- ► Observe for indications of *pyogenic infection* (due to contamination).

Frequently serum electrolyte blood studies are ordered after thoracentesis to guide planning for intravenous electrolyte replacement therapy. Replacement therapy is necessary if large amounts of fluid are removed since pleural fluid is isotonic. (See Chapter 12.)

A chest film may also be ordered following thoracentesis to determine the effects of the procedure. The physician reading the x-ray film notes whether pleural fluid remains, air was accidentally introduced during the procedure, or mediastinal shift occurred, and if the lung is reexpanding satisfactorily to fill the space previously occupied by the fluid accumulation.

Patients who develop pleural effusions as a sympathetic response to tumors may have tetracycline, Cytoxan, or other agents injected into the pleural space to cause the formation of an inflammatory process. These sclerosing agents will aid in the prevention of further fluid formation.

PULMONARY ECHOGRAMS

Reflected ultrasound, using the echo-ranging technique, can be useful in detecting and localizing pleural effusion. Not only is the ultrasound technique useful diagnostically (in detecting pleural effusion which may not show up on chest x-rays or by thoracentesis), but it may also be of value in selecting sites for therapeutic pleural aspiration.

BIOPSY

Biopsy may be taken of various tissues during the process of investigating respiratory disorders. We have previously mentioned that biopsy may be taken of *tracheobronchial* structures at the time of bronchoscopy. Biopsies of *scalene* and *mediastinal nodes* may be performed (under local anesthesia) to obtain tissue for pathogenic analysis by culture, animal inoculation, or microscopic inspection.

Pleural biopsy was initially performed surgically through a small thoracotomy (open biopsy). Today pleural biopsy is most commonly performed with a special biopsy needle. Needle biopsy is a safe, simple, very useful diagnostic procedure of value in determining the etiology of many pleural effusions. The needle removes a small fragment of parietal pleura which is used for microscopic examination and culture. If bacteriologic studies are to be performed the biopsy specimen is obtained before chemotherapy is started. Pleural biopsy can easily be performed at the time of routine thoracentesis; thus, a biopsy needle, e.g., a Cope needle, should be available whenever pleural fluid is removed by thoracentesis.

In performing biopsy it may be necessary for the physician to make multiple needle insertions at different sites. Both the skin and pleura are injected with a local anesthetic. Then a small skin incision is made with a scalpel blade to facilitate insertion of the biopsy needle.

The specific diagnoses most frequently established from pleural needle biopsy specimens are tuberculosis, other granulomatous diseases, and tumors (primary or metastatic to the pleura). Disease processes that occur in the periphery of a lung often involve the parietal pleura and commonly are associated with pleural effusion. Thus, pleural biopsy is considered whenever there is radiologic evidence of fluid in the pleural space.

The preparation and positioning of a patient for pleural biopsy is similar to that for thoracentesis. Rare complications include temporary pain resulting from intercostal nerve injury, pneumothorax, and hemothorax. Following the biopsy the patient is therefore observed closely for indications of these conditions, e.g., dyspnea. The danger of pneumothorax associated with needle pleural biopsy can be reduced by using special needles designed to obtain the specimen while the needle is being withdrawn, rather than upon insertion. Follow-up chest x-ray films may be taken a few hours after the procedure. Possible hemothorax is indicated by a substantial increase in fluid in the pleural space. This finding indicates the need for immediate thoracentesis.

As with pleural biopsy, *lung biopsy* may be accomplished either by surgical exposure of the lung or by use of a needle. Tissue removed is examined microscopically and bacteriologically. Lung biopsies are most often performed to identify pulmonary tumors.

Needle puncture aspiration biopsy of chest lesions is performed under fluoroscopic monitoring. After the lesion is found on a chest film and localized under fluoroscopy, topical anesthesia is administered and a needle is inserted through the chest wall into the lesion. A small sample of cells is then aspirated for microscopic study and the needle is withdrawn. Aspiration biopsy may enable the definitive diagnosis of malignant neoplasms, granulomas, or other nonmalignant growths. Possible complications of needle aspiration biopsy of the lung are hemoptysis and pneumothorax. After the procedure the nurse examines the patient's sputum closely for evidence of blood and observes the patient for respiratory distress associated with possible pneumothorax.

Indications of complications following any biopsy are reported immediately to the physician.

ASSESSMENT OF RESPIRATORY FUNCTION AND DYSFUNCTION

The assessment of respiratory dysfunction calls for the participation of many departments

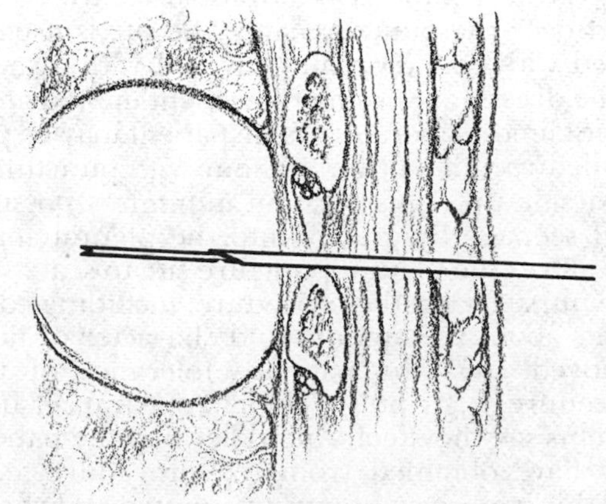

Lung tumor biopsy. The carrier needle is advanced over the forked needle and removed. The tissue is in the groove of the forked needle. (From Nealon, T. J.: *Fundamental Skills in Surgery*, 3rd ed. Philadelphia, W. B. Saunders Co., 1979.)

within the hospital. The efforts of the clinical laboratory, pulmonary function laboratory, respiratory therapy department, and radiology department all combine to provide information to assist the physician and health care workers treat and assess respiratory function and dysfunction.

Bacteriologic Examination of Sputum

To determine the cause of an infection, fresh sputum specimens are obtained either by deep effective coughing or by suctioning the patient's tracheobronchial tree. The sputum that is collected is then *cultured* in the laboratory. This means that the sample is streaked onto a special plate with a coating of nutrients. This is called a *culture and sensitivity* (C and S) determination. If bacteria are present, they will grow and form colonies. The bacteria then can be further identified. Subcultures can be made, if desired. When the bacteria are identified, specific antibiotic therapy may be instituted.

Some microorganisms are very slow growing. For example, it may take 3 to 12 weeks to obtain a positive culture of tubercle bacilli. Bacteria which cause disease are pathogenic. Both pathogenic and nonpathogenic bacteria may be found in sputum cultures with some lung diseases. Thus, after all findings have been correlated, the physician decides on their significance.

Specimens obtained for culture (bacteriologic examination) are always collected before the patient receives any bactericidal medications (antibiotics, sulfonamides), unless the culture is being taken to evaluate the effectiveness of medications already given. If bactericidal medications are given prior to the initial bacteriologic examination, it is impossible to obtain accurate antimicrobial drug sensitivity test results.

Antimicrobial drug sensitivity tests may be ordered to identify to which specific medications a patient's bacteria are sensitive, i.e., which antibiotics will be therapeutically effective. The collection procedure for a specimen for these tests is the same as that for any sputum culture, i.e., the specimen is protected so it is uncontaminated and so the organisms in the specimen remain viable.

Another sputum examination may be ordered when tuberculosis is suspected. The organism causing tuberculosis is *Mycobacterium tuberculosis.* For this test, the specimens are collected early in the morning for 3 or more successive days. The tuberculosis organism is an acid-fast organism and the test for tuberculosis in the sputum is called an *AFB* (acid-fast bacillus).

Respiratory tract cytology is another type of sputum examination in which the sputum is examined for abnormal, cancerous cells. Sputum contains epithelial cells because of the constant exfoliating of old and diseased cells into the airways. Respiratory tract cytology can be used in the diagnosis and typing of malignant lesions and in identifying benign respiratory conditions, e.g., granulomas and inflammations. While not conclusive, cytology can lend support to the diagnosis of bacterial, granulomatous, viral, or fungal diseases. Sputum specimens for cytologic examinations are usually collected in the early morning and often more than one specimen is required.

Sputum Specimen Collection. Before obtaining a sputum specimen give patients the necessary instructions. Tell them to be sure that they furnish as a specimen only those secretions coming from below the larynx ("Adam's apple"). Next, help patients to rinse out the mouth with *water* to remove food particles. Do not brush the teeth or use an antiseptic mouthwash. Antiseptic solutions affect the viability of microorganisms in the sputum specimen. Specimens are obtained by asking patients to cough deeply, not just clear the throat. Instruct patients to fill the lungs with a "pillar of air" behind the mucus, expectorate the sputum with short blasts, and to cough deeply. A deep, vigorous cough brings up a specimen from deep within the tracheobronchial tree. (See discussion of coughing in Chapter 57.)

It is desirable to collect sputum specimens when the patient first awakens in the morning. Secretions tend to pool and collect in the lungs during sleep and, thus, early morning coughing is likely to be more productive of sputum; also, a higher concentration of organisms tends to occur in secretions that accumulate at night. Give the patient the specimen jar the evening before the specimen is to be collected so that mucus brought up in the *first* cough upon awakening in the morning can be expectorated. At least one teaspoonful of sputum is necessary for laboratory examination.

Patients who have difficulty "raising" sputum may need to have a specimen collected with the help of a *heated aerosol.* In this procedure the patient inhales 10 per cent saline in distilled water from a heated nebulizer. This solution has a drawing effect on airway secretions and is irritating enough to precipitate a cough. The nebulizer is powered by compressed oxygen or air; thus, a fine mist of saline is produced. The production of secretions is also stimulated by vapor condensation within the tracheobronchial tree; the patient can then more easily cough up these secretions. This procedure must be used with caution as bronchospasm due to the irritating effects may occur. Auscultate the chest prior to, during, and after the procedure.

Prior to the first heated aerosol sputum collection patients are told that they will inhale a fine mist of warm saline and that this will help them to cough effectively so they can raise sputum. The patient is then shown how to: (1) place the mouthpiece into or the mask over the airway; (2) deeply inhale the mist vapor until coughing begins; and (3) cough effectively. (Aerosol treatments are discussed further in Chapter 54.)

Sputum specimens are collected in covered wide-mouthed jars or waterproof, disposable sputum cups or boxes. If a culture is to be performed the container's opening and inside must be sterile. Instruct the patient to expectorate directly into the center of the container without touching the container with the mouth. Also tell the patient to be careful that sputum does not contaminate the outside of the container.

Always keep sputum containers covered. This not only is esthetically desirable (because the odor and sight of sputum are offensive), but also prevents spread of air-borne microorganisms from the sputum and prevents air contamination of the specimen. Cover the outside of glass containers with a paper towel held on with a rubber band. Sputum specimen containers should never become completely full. Provide extra containers as necessary.

Provide tissues so the patient may cover the mouth when coughing up sputum and wipe his or her mouth after expectorating the sputum specimen. Keep used tissues picked up and discarded. When the patient is coughing be certain you keep your head turned away from the direction of the cough to protect yourself from air-borne infections. Always wash your hands thoroughly after handling used tissues or sputum specimen containers. If a patient has suspected or known tuberculosis and has not been on chemotherapy, it may be desirable to wear a mask if you need to be present during the time the patient is coughing up the specimen. (See Chapter 55.)

If sputum is being obtained for laboratory study, the specimen should be promptly delivered to the laboratory bacteriology refrigerator and not remain at the bedside. If it is not possible to *immediately* send the specimen to the laboratory after collection, refrigerate it on the ward, making sure it is clearly marked for identification. If a patient is in isolation, the container's outside is considered to be contaminated and must be appropriately handled to prevent spread of infection.

Blood Tests

White Blood Cell (Leukocyte) Counts. A *total white blood cell count* (normally 6000 to 9000/mm.^{3}) and a *differential count* may help to diagnose respiratory inflammations, allergies, and infections. These tests may also help to distinguish between acute and chronic infections. The necessary blood sample is obtained from a venipuncture or a finger prick. White blood cells are discussed in detail in Chapter 10. Here we summarize only a few relevant points.

White blood cell counts usually increase with infections. Although *acute infections* usually produce a radical increase in circulating WBC's (i.e., leukocytosis), *chronic infections* may increase the total number of leukocytes only slightly. In fact, occasionally a marked decrease (i.e., leukopenia) occurs with tuberculosis or severe debilitation.

With acute infections, increases occur mostly in the *polymorphonuclear leukocytes,* i.e., the neutrophils, eosinophils (acidophils), and basophils. Most bacterial infections elevate *neutrophils.* These phagocytic cells normally form 50 to 70 per cent of the total WBC's; i.e., they are normally 3000 to 7000/mm.^{3} of blood. Allergic disorders, such as allergic asthma, elevate *eosinophils* (normally 50 to 400/mm.^{3} or 0 to 1 per cent of WBC's). *Basophils* (normally 0 to 50/mm.^{3} or 0 to 1 per cent of WBC's) may prevent coagulation in inflammatory conditions.

Chronic infections may increase the number of *mononuclear leukocytes,* i.e., lymphocytes and monocytes. *Lymphocytes* (normally 1500 to 3000/mm.^{3} or 25 to 33 per cent of WBC's) increase with some bacterial infections. *Monocytes* (normally 285 to 500/mm.^{3} or 4 to 6 per cent of WBC's) are typically increased in tuberculosis and chronic inflammatory conditions. These phagocytes are also increased during recovery phases of infections.

Red Blood Cell (Erythrocyte) Evaluations. Evaluations of red blood cells used in diagnosing and treating respiratory disorders include red blood cell count, hemoglobin concentration, hematocrit test, and erythrocyte sedimentation rate.

The hemoglobin in erythrocytes transports oxygen from the lungs throughout the body. Hemoglobin not only gives up oxygen to the cells but also carries carbon dioxide from the tissues back to the lungs. It is clinically important to determine not only a patient's *red blood cell count* (total number of RBC's) but also the amount of hemoglobin in the RBC's. Normal RBC counts for men are 4.8 to 5.5 million/mm.^{3} of blood, and 4.4 to 5.0 million/mm.^{3} for women. *Hemoglobin concentration* for men is normally 14.5 to 16.0 Gm./dl. of blood, and 13.0 to 15.5 Gm./dl. of blood for women. Inadequate cellular respiration can occur if a patient's RBC count or hemoglobin concentration is deficient.

Additional information about the number, capacity, and size of RBC's can be obtained by combining information about hemoglobin concentration with that obtained from a *hematocrit* test. This test determines the volume percentage of erythrocytes in whole blood. Normally

RBC's comprise 45 to 50 per cent (expressed as volume per cent) of the volume of whole blood in men, and 40 to 45 volume per cent for women.

An *erythrocyte sedimentation rate* measures the rate of speed with which RBC's settle to the bottom of a volume of drawn blood. This test provides a rough measurement of abnormal concentrations of fibrinogen and serum globulins that accompany certain inflammatory or infectious disorders which destroy cells, e.g., tuberculosis and cancer. The normal values for this test vary with the method used to perform the test, e.g., Cutler, Westergren, Wintrobe. (RBC functions and laboratory evaluations are discussed more completely in Unit XIV.)

Arterial Blood Gas Analysis. The effectiveness of respiratory function and the degree of respiratory dysfunction may be determined by analysis of a sample of arterialized (oxygenated) blood. The arterial blood gas (ABG) analysis is the only method of assessing the efficiency of ventilation. Blood gas analyses are essential in the evaluation and management of critically ill and acutely ill patients, in caring for patients being mechanically ventilated (i.e., on respirators), in evaluating acute and chronic pulmonary disorders (e.g., chronic obstructive pulmonary diseases), and as part of total electrolyte evaluations.

Blood gas measurements evaluate such factors as rate of cellular metabolism and oxygen status, ventilation efficiency, the ability of hemoglobin to transport oxygen and carbon dioxide, the level of arterial oxygen status. They also reflect the state of buffer systems. Since the lungs are the principal regulators of acid-base balance, blood gas studies are important determinants of the state of pulmonary function.

Key Terms*

pO_2 *Partial pressure of oxygen in the air. This is measured in millimeters of mercury. Atmospheric pressure (760 mm. Hg) is the sum of the pressure of all gases in the air, and the pressure of any one is referred to as* partial pressure.

PaO_2 *Partial pressure of arterial oxygen. When speaking of venous blood, a small v is substituted for the a.*

SaO_2 *Arterial oxygen saturation. This is the oxygen carried bound to hemoglobin (hemoglobin-oxygen saturation).*

CaO_2 *Total oxygen content of arterial blood.*

The arterial blood sample is obtained by puncturing one of the more accessible arteries of the limbs. The radial, brachial, and femoral arteries are the sites generally used. (See Figure 52–4). To obtain accurate test results, specimens for blood gas analyses must be correctly collected and handled as *anaerobic* samples. Unclotted blood is necessary, and specimens may be collected in a glass syringe flushed with heparin. Small amounts of heparin will not significantly dilute the specimen; larger amounts would affect pH and a more acidotic reading will be obtained. In obtaining the specimen care is

*From Waldron, M. W.: Oxygen transport. *American Journal of Nursing,* 79:272, Feb. 1979.

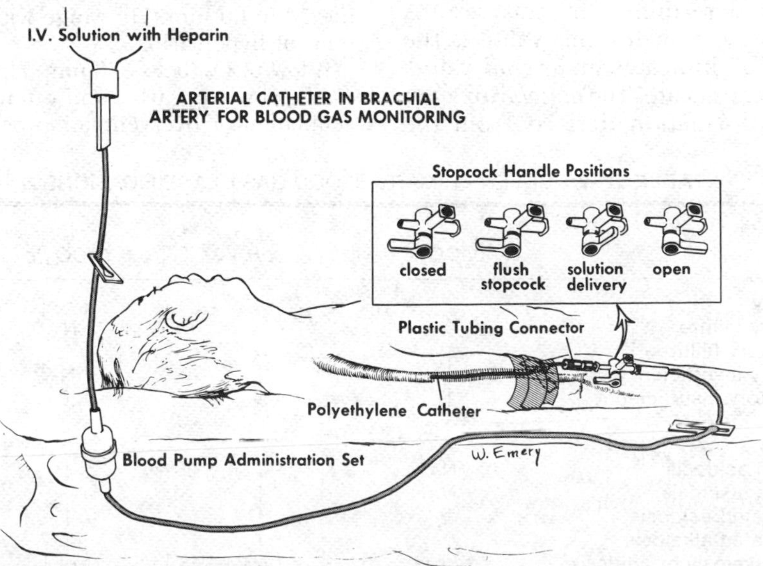

Figure 52–4. Catheter in place in brachial artery for blood gas monitoring. (From Kurihara, M.: *Nursing Clinics of North America,* 3:65, Mar. 1968.)

taken to avoid getting any air bubbles into the sample, since the air would affect the blood gas measurements. Air (ambient) in the syringe will give erroneous pCO_2 (too low) and pO_2 (higher than actual) results. A blood specimen of 2.5 ml. is adequate for most blood gas measurements; 0.5 ml. is sufficient for some gas analyzers. Placing the sample in a container of ice reduces the rate of metabolic activity in the syringe so that the pO_2 will remain stable, as will the pH and pCO_2.

The puncture site must be observed following the puncture for leaking of blood into the tissues. To prevent the complications of leaking and hemorrhage, firm pressure is maintained over the puncture site for 5 to 10 minutes with a sterile gauze dressing. Patients receiving anticoagulant drug therapy must have firm pressure applied to the site for 10 to 15 minutes or longer. Carefully observe the site for leaking through the puncture site.

The basic information obtained by the arterial blood gas includes: (1) *the pH* — a means of determining the acidity or alkalinity (acid-base balance) of the blood and the degree to which the body has adjusted to dysfunctions through its buffering mechanisms; (2) *the* pCO_2 (carbon dioxide tension) — the key to effective ventilation. An above normal measurement is hypoventilation. The pCO_2 of a patient with chronic respiratory disease may be chronically elevated, termed *chronic* CO_2 *retention.* A below normal pCO_2 is *hyperventilation* or *overventilation;* (3) the pO_2 (oxygen tension) — the adequacy of oxygenation may be determined by this test. A more specific abbreviation for this value is the p_aO_2. The small "a" indicates an *arterial* value. (A large "A," p_AO_2, indicates the *alveolar* oxygen tension.) Other information derived from the arterial blood sample includes the *level of bicarbonate* (HCO_3) in the plasma, which represents the metabolic component of the acid-base status of the patient, and the per cent of oxygen saturating the hemoglobin (S_aO_2).

Normal Arterial Blood Gas Values

pH 7.38–7.42 pCO_2 35–45 mm. Hg

pO_2 above 80 mm. Hg (80–100 mm. Hg)
Except: Newborn = 40–60 mm. Hg
Over 60 years of age: subtract 1 mm. Hg for each year over 60 years

HCO_3 22–26 mEq./L. O_2 saturation = 97%

Table 52–2 is an aid to determine the classification of arterial blood gas values.

Blood pH. This measurement gives important information on a patient's metabolic state and the effectiveness of respirations. Blood pH levels depend on the amount of CO_2 in the blood. The pH is thus important in evaluating the blood's acid-base balance.

Carbon Dioxide Tension (pCO_2)*.* This reflects the effectiveness of ventilation. An elevated pCO_2 indicates *respiratory acidosis* or hypercarbia, i.e., excessive carbonic acid. An elevated pCO_2 may occur with hypoventilation because the CO_2 is not being effectively "blown off" by the lungs and, thus, the CO_2 builds up in the blood. Such hypoventilation may result from "splinting" the chest (breathing shallowly) because of pain upon breathing, e.g., pleuritic pain, incisional pain, pain from injured ribs, excess sedation.

Patients with chronic obstructive pulmonary diseases are often able to tolerate elevated pCO_2 levels in the 50 to 60 mm. Hg range without showing symptoms of hypercarbia.

A low pCO_2 (below 38 mm. Hg) indicates *respiratory alkalosis* or hypocarbia and often results from hyperventilation or overventilation, which causes the CO_2

TABLE 52–2. SEVEN PRIMARY BLOOD GAS CLASSIFICATIONS

	$paCO_2$	*pH*	*(HCO_3^-)p*	*Base Excess*
Primary ventilatory				
1. Acute ventilatory failure	↑	↓	N	N
2. Chronic ventilatory failure	↑	N	↑	↑
3. Acute ventilatory insufficiency	↓	↑	N	N
4. Chronic ventilatory insufficiency	↓	N	↓	↓
Primary acid-base				
1. Uncompensated acidosis	N	↓	↓	↓
Uncompensated alkalosis	N	↑	↑	↑
2. Partly compensated acidosis	↓	↓	↓	↓
Partly compensated alkalosis	↑	↑	↑	↑
3. Compensated alkalosis or acidosis	↑ or ↓	N	↑ or ↓	↑ or ↓

Arrows indicate depressed or elevated values. N = normal.
From Shapiro, B. A.: *Clinical Interpretation of Blood Gases.* Chicago, Yearbook Medical Publishers, Inc., 1973.

to be blown off excessively. The pCO_2 decreases because the blood's CO_2 content is low. Hysteria and salicylate overdose are examples of conditions that can cause hypocarbia. Hypocarbia may be a serious manifestation, as it leads to decreased cerebral blood flow, paresthesias, and seizures. Pharmacologically, carbon dioxide is a vasoconstrictor.

Oxygen Tension (pO_2). The pO_2 measures the effectiveness of the lungs in oxygenating the blood, i.e., the ability of the lungs to diffuse inspired oxygen across the alveolar membrane into the circulating blood. Patients with chronic obstructive pulmonary diseases may be able to tolerate an arterial pO_2 as low as 55 to 60 mm. Hg without showing symptoms of distress and hypoxemia. An awareness of this tolerance is highly important, since it is unnecessary (in fact, it can be fatal) to try to raise the pO_2 in these patients to within laboratory normal levels; the *patient's individual known normal* pO_2 becomes the guide for oxygen therapy in these patients.

Arterial pO_2 may be elevated by administering oxygen and by changing the patient's position. Position change can improve pulmonary ventilation and reduce the return of unoxygenated blood to the left atrium of the heart.

Because the pO_2 reflects the amount of oxygen passing from pulmonary alveoli into the blood, it is directly influenced by the amount of oxygen being inspired. When pO_2 measurements are being made to evaluate a patient's "normal" ventilatory effectiveness, the blood sample is taken before supplemental oxygen therapy is started. The pO_2 may also be determined once a patient is receiving oxygen therapy to evaluate the effectiveness of the therapy so necessary adjustments can be made. Oxygen administration does not *cure* hypoxemia; it relieves the symptoms.

As expected, the venous pO_2 is normally quite a bit lower than the arterial pO_2, since much of the blood's oxygen has been given up to the cells. Factors affecting venous pO_2 are tissue perfusion adequacy, blood volume (a low blood volume will be apparent from a low central venous pressure), the effectiveness of gaseous exchange, and cardiac output. Venous blood pH is about 7.36 and venous pCO_2 is between 40 and 41 mm. Hg.

For further discussions of the clinical significance of blood gas measurements and treatment of hydrogen ion imbalances (metabolic acidosis, metabolic alkalosis, respiratory acidosis, and respiratory alkalosis) see Chapter 12 and bibliography entries 18 and 143.

Serum Electrolyte Analyses. Serum electrolyte analyses are frequently of importance in monitoring the fluid-electrolyte status of patients with respiratory disorders. Examples of two electrolyte imbalances that may be related to respiratory function are hyperpotassemia (potassium elevation) caused by chronic hypoventilation, and hyperchloremia (chloride elevation) caused by hyperventilation. (For further discussion of serum electrolytes and fluid-electrolyte imbalances see Chapter 12.)

C-Reactive Protein Test (CRP). A positive reaction (precipitate formation) occurs in the presence of tissue inflammation or destruction, such as that caused by widespread cancer or active tuberculosis. Normally C-reactive protein is not present in venous blood.

Lactic Dehydrogenase Level (LDH). Lactic dehydrogenase (LDH) is an intracellular enzyme that affects the speed of intracellular metabolic processes. Blood serum LDH is normally 165 to 300 units. Five isoenzymes, or variants, of LDH have been identified. The isoenzyme that occurs in the lungs is LDH-3. Cellular injury or destruction of cells containing LDH causes the release of the enzyme into the blood stream. Elevated plasma concentrations of LDH thus may aid in diagnosing conditions causing cellular injury or destruction. Pulmonary infarction increases serum LDH-3. (LDH has also been discussed in Unit XII.)

Pulmonary Function Tests

Evaluation of pulmonary function involves two groups of measurements. The first group of tests evaluates the physical activities necessary for assessment of ventilation and pulmonary mechanics. These tests are sometimes said to be evaluations of the bellows actions of the lungs, i.e., the abilities of the chest wall, diaphragm, and lungs to move air in and out, and to *distribute* it to pulmonary alveoli. This first group of measurements are called "ventilatory function tests" and are discussed in this section. They assist the physician in further classification of pulmonary function by differentiating between *obstructive* and *restrictive* pathology.

The second group of pulmonary function tests measure the effectiveness of *gaseous distribution and diffusion* across the alveolar capillary membrane and the effectiveness of *vascular perfusion* of the lungs by capillaries. Blood gas measurements assist in evaluating gaseous diffusion; these tests were discussed in the previous section. At the end of this section we shall briefly discuss the carbon monoxide diffusing test and some measurements of pulmonary vascular perfusion.

Pulmonary function testing is highly valuable in objectively:

- ▶ detecting impaired pulmonary function,
- ▶ characterizing or generally classifying the impairment,
- ▶ estimating severity of the impairment,
- ▶ following the course of pulmonary disease and evaluating treatment responses, and
- ▶ providing information helpful in planning care and in caring for patients having thoracic surgery.

Certain tests may aid in the identification of patients who may have reduced motivation and thus an increased incidence of postoperative problems result-

TABLE 52–3. PULMONARY FUNCTION ABBREVIATIONS

Abbreviation	Meaning	Abbreviation	Meaning
CC	Closing capacity	MVV	Maximal voluntary ventilation
C_{dyn}	Dynamic lung compliance	$paCO_2$	Arterial partial pressure of CO_2 (mm. Hg)
C_{STAT}	Static lung compliance	paO_2	Arterial partial pressure of O_2 (mm. Hg)
CV	Closing volume (L.)		
DL_{CO}	Diffusing capacity for carbon monoxide (ml./min./mm. Hg)	PEF	Peak expiratory flow (L./sec.)
ERV	Expiratory reserve volume	P_{TP}	Transpulmonary pressure (mm. Hg)
FEV_1	Forced expiratory volume in 1 sec. (L.)	$\dot{Q}$	Perfusion (L./min.)
FEV_3	Forced expiratory volume in 3 sec. (L.)	R_{AW}	Airway resistance
		RV	Residual volume
FVC	Forced vital capacity	TLC	Total lung capacity
FRC	Functional residual capacity	V	Lung volume (L.)
$[H^+]$	Concentration of hydrogen ions (nanomoles/L.)	VC	Vital capacity
		$\dot{V}$	Ventilation (L./min.)
IRV	Inspiratory reserve volume	$\dot{V}_A$	Alveolar ventilation (L./min.)
$MEF_{50\ per\ cent\ VC}$	Mid-expiratory flow at 50% vital capacity (L./sec.)	$\dot{V}_{CO_2}$	CO_2 production (L./min.)
$MIF_{50\ per\ cent\ VC}$	Mid-inspiratory flow at 50% vital capacity (L./sec.)	$\dot{V}_{O_2}$	O_2 consumption (L./min.)
MMEF	Mean maximal expiratory flow (L./sec.)		

ing from poor coughing and deep breathing effort. Respiratory function tests are especially helpful in evaluating the respiratory status of patients with reduced lung capacities and chronic obstructive pulmonary disease. Pulmonary function may be seriously compromised by generalized pulmonary disorders, e.g., obstructive pulmonary disease, pulmonary fibrosis, pneumoconiosis. Some of the simpler pulmonary function tests are often employed for various screening purposes, e.g., periodic physical examinations, pre-employment health examinations, evaluating insurance and disability claims. Others may be performed in an attempt to predict or estimate the per cent of impairment in ventilation following a lobectomy or pneumonectomy.

Some *limitations* of pulmonary function tests are:[58] (1) an etiologic or anatomic diagnosis is not directly given; (2) lesions are not precisely located; (3) a fairly large deviation from the predicted normal findings is necessary before the tests have meaning; (4) the gross ventilatory tests lack the sensitivity necessary to identify early localized changes; and (5) misleading or useless test results can occur unless both the patient and the person performing the test give maximum cooperation and exertion.

The nurse participates in pulmonary function tests by helping to explain to the patient the general value of the tests, basically how the tests are performed, and what is expected of the patient during the tests. Patients with breathing difficulties are often apprehensive about having "breathing tests" performed. Many fear their air supply will be inadequate during the testing or that they will become too exhausted; others dread any anxiety-provoking situation, since anxiety usually increases their breathing difficulties. Pulmonary function tests may indeed be very tiring. Because various tests must be repeated two to three times to insure reproducible results, many patients need planned rest periods during and after testing. The patient must be cautioned to not smoke or take bronchodilator medications for 4 to 6 hours prior to the test.

The nurse carries out any orders for physically preparing a patient for pulmonary function tests. Spirography (discussed below) generally requires no special preparation of the patient. During the test the patient is given necessary instructions, e.g., "take a deep breath," "exhale and try to push all the air out of your lungs," and so forth. Pulmonary function tests are usually performed in a laboratory setting by a technician or physician.

The following information is of basic importance in understanding respiratory function:

Respiratory rate: Rate of respirations during a normal resting state; normally 12 to 20 respirations per minute; exercise and emotions influence this rate.

Oxygen consumption: Normally about 110 to 150 ml./min. during rest, while *carbon dioxide elimination* is about 88 to 120 ml./min.

Respiratory quotient: Normally 0.8; obtained by dividing the value of carbon dioxide elimination by the oxygen consumption.

VENTILATORY FUNCTION TESTS

As their name implies, ventilatory function tests are performed to evaluate how well the lung is ventilating. The tests most commonly performed are made with a *spirometer* and a recording device. A spirometer contains a floating drum which moves up and down with changes in pressure. The excursions of the drum are recorded on a rotating chart. From this graphic record it is possible to calculate the quantity of gas moved during each excursion of the drum. This type is classified as a *water seal* spirometer. The other categories are dry-rolling seal, wedge (or bellows), and the Wright spirometer (see Fig. 52–5).

Ventilation studies are performed with the patient breathing only through the mouth. To ensure mouth breathing a *nose clip* is often applied, and the patient is given time to adjust to the clip. A mouthpiece and connecting tube connect the patient's respiratory system and the spirometer.

No single factor adequately expresses pulmonary ventilation; rather a composite of values is necessary to give the full picture. The values most commonly measured in ventilatory function testing will be discussed below. Naturally the volumes of air inhaled and exhaled vary, depending upon such factors as weight, height, sex, age, activity, and the body's demands. Predicted normals for the various ventilation function tests are calculated for a given patient on the basis of the preceding factors. The examples of "normal" in the following discussions are average for a normal young adult man (Fig. 52–6). Averages for the normal young adult woman are often 20 to 25 per cent less.

Tidal Volume (*V_T or TV*). Amount of air inspired or expired with each breath during quiet, normal breathing. This measurement is called tidal volume

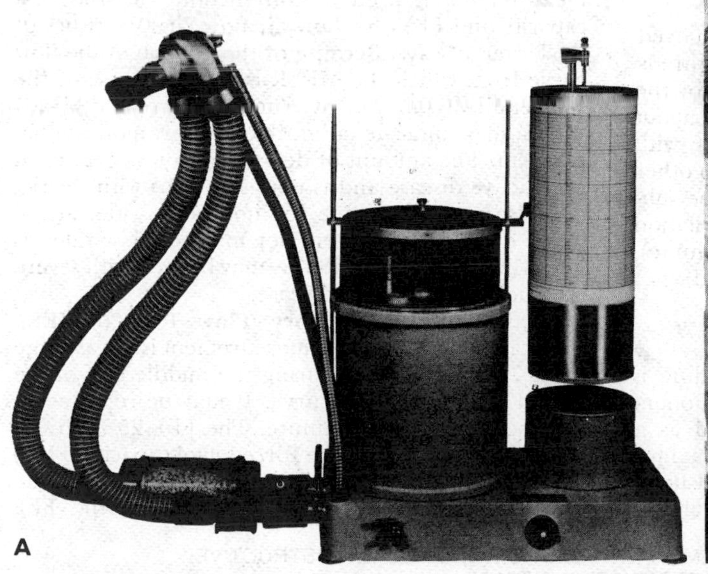

A

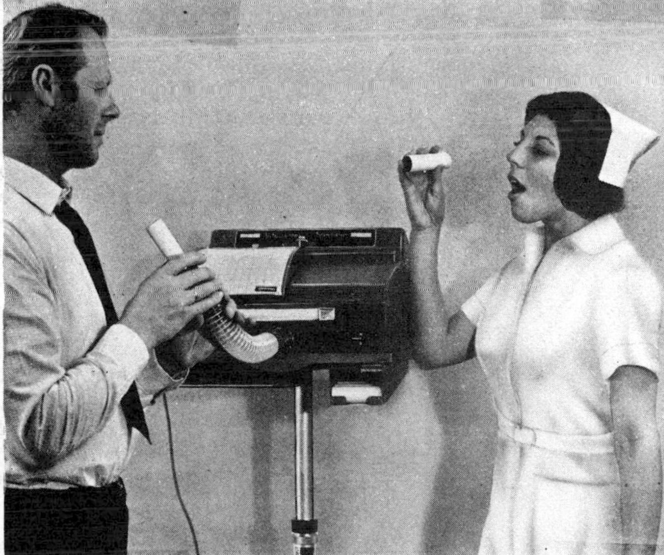

B

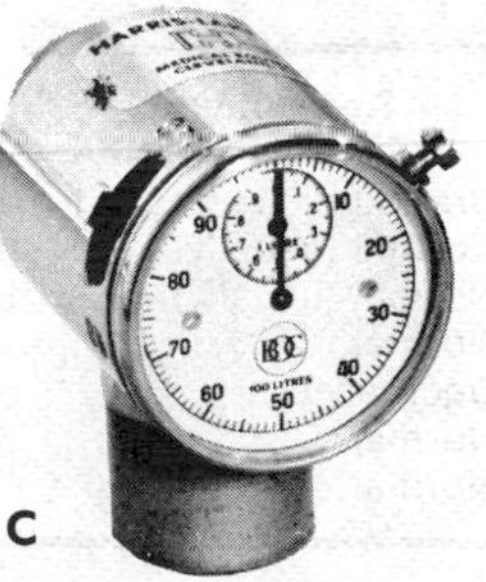

C

Figure 52–5. Types of spirometers. **A.** A water seal spirometer. **B.** A wedge or bellows type. This is useful for bedside procedures. **C.** Wright spirometer, used to measure exhaled tidal volume and minute ventilation. (*A*, courtesy of Warren E. Collins Co., Braintree, Mass.; *B*, courtesy of Vitalograph, Ltd., Kansas City, Mo.; *C*, courtesy of Harris-Lake, Inc., Cleveland, Ohio.)

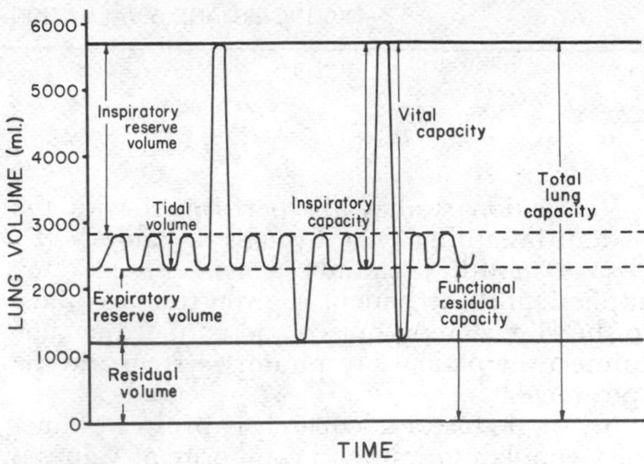

Figure 52–6. A spirogram, showing the divisions of the respiratory air. (From Guyton, A. C.: *Function of the Human Body,* 4th ed. Philadelphia: W. B. Saunders Co., 1974.)

because it measures the flow of air coming in and out like the tides, during one respiratory cycle. Sometimes V_T is measured during exercise to evaluate dyspnea. (Exercise tests are discussed later.)

V_T is normally about 500 ml. Of this, anatomic dead space gas (V_D) equals about 150 ml. or 1 ml. per pound of body weight. *Dead space air* refers to that air in the conducting airways from the nose and mouth down to the bronchioles. Air in the dead space does not exchange gases with the blood since it does not reach alveolar membranes. A dead space volume greater than one third of tidal volume indicates the need for an increase in total ventilation to prevent hypercarbia (alveolar hypoventilation).

Minute Respiratory Volume ($V_{min.}$). *Also called "minute ventilation,"* this is the total volume of air moved in or out of the lungs during 1 minute. The figure is obtained by multiplying the tidal volume (V_T) by the respiratory rate per minute (f). Normal $V_{min.}$ = about 6000 to 7500 ml. A normal $V_{min.}$ may occur with emphysema, but a reduced $V_{min.}$ can occur with other pulmonary disorders. Minute ventilation can be subdivided into two divisions: (1) alveolar ventilation (about two thirds of the total air taken in 1 minute), and (2) dead space ventilation (about one third).

EXPIRATORY MEASUREMENTS

Vital Capacity (VC). A vital capacity reading is one of the most important portions of the pulmonary function spirogram. Vital capacity is defined as a maximal amount of air exhaled after a maximal inspiration. The normal vital capacity is based upon predicted values. This normal or predicted value is determined by sex, age, and height. Men have greater predicted vital capacities than women. For example, a man 24 years old and 6 feet tall would have a greater predicted vital capacity than a man aged 60 who is 5 feet, 7 inches tall.

The vital capacity maneuver provides much information and is the basis for many of the pulmonary function measurements. The patient must be well instructed and familiar with the breathing pattern. Encouragement during the procedure is important. The test is usually repeated at least three times to assure the patient's best effort and validity.

The total forced vital capacity is measured in liters per minute.

Forced Expiratory Volume (FEV). The graph is measured in timed intervals, usually 1, 2, and 3 seconds. This measurement is termed the forced expiratory volume timed (FEV_t). During a normal vital capacity maneuver the FEV_1 sec. (first second) should be 83 per cent of the total vital capacity; the FEV_2 sec., 93 per cent of the total vital capacity; and the FEV_3 sec., 97 per cent of the total vital capacity. The patient should be able to exhale the total vital capacity in 4 seconds. A prolonged expiratory time and decreased forced expiratory volumes are associated with obstructive lung diseases (see Table 52–4).

The FEV_t is often expressed as a ratio of the forced vital capacity (FEV_t/FVC). Other measurements associated with the flow curve of the vital capacity are shown in Table 52–4.

Maximal Expiratory Flow Rate (MEFR). This measurement, also called the FEF 200–1200, measures the flow rate of the first 1000 ml. exhaled. This measurement is used in conjunction with the vital capacity and FEV_t to show air flow characteristics of the larger airways. Because of the portion of the flow curve from which the MEFR is taken, disease of the smaller airways may be overlooked. Decreased MEFR values may indicate a mechanical or motivational problem. The amount of decreased flow is greater in obstructive disease and is not as obvious with restrictive diseases. The range for normal is wide, in the range of 250 to 450 liters per minute. Flow rates as low as 60 L./minute, or lower, may be seen with severe obstructive pulmonary disease.

Maximal Mid-Expiratory Flow Rate (MMEF). Also called the FEF. This measurement is the average 25 to 75 per cent flow during the middle half of the forced expiratory flow curve. It may be reported in liters/second, or liters/minute. The FEF 25%–75% is based on a segment of the forced vital capacity (FVC) that includes more than the initial portion of the exhaled breath. The normal values for the FEF

TABLE 52–4. EXPECTED PULMONARY FUNCTION FINDINGS IN OBSTRUCTIVE AND RESTRICTIVE DISEASE

	Obstructive	Restrictive
Vital capacity	Decreased	Normal or Decreased
FEV	Decreased	Normal (usually)
$FEF_{25-75 \text{ per cent}}$	Decreased	Normal (usually)
MVV	Decreased	Normal
RV	Increased	Decreased
Expiratory time	Prolonged	Normal
FRC	Increased	Normal

25%–75% are smaller than those for the FEF 200–1200. The values for healthy young men may average 282 L./min. The FEF 25%–75% is more reliable in indicating smaller airway disease. It is also less effort-dependent than the MEFR.

Maximal Voluntary Ventilation (MVV). This test was formerly called the maximal breathing capacity (MBC). It is a test of air flow, muscular strength, and coordination compliance of the lung and thorax, and the resistance offered by the airways and tissues and patient effort. It is measured by having the patient voluntarily breathe as deep and fast as possible for 10, 12, or 15 seconds. The total volume of air moved is extrapolated through a mathematical calculation and reported in liters/minute. Normal values vary ve-tween 20 and 30 per cent. The MVV for an average (1.7 m.^{2}) adult man is 170 L./min. Values are lower in women and with increasing age. The patient with moderate to severe obstructive disease will have an obvious decrease in the MVV. The patient with restrictive disease may have a normal or decreased MVV.

Expiratory Reserve Volume (ERV). This measurement is defined as the volume of air which can be exhaled after a normal exhalation. It is usually about 1000 ml.

Peak Flow Rate (PFR). This is the maximal flow rate attainable at any time during the forced expiratory volume. It may be recorded in either liters/second or liters/minute. It is an effort-dependent measurement. A decreased peak flow rate indicates a mechanical problem, largely of a nonspecific nature. Normal young men may be able to generate peak flow rates of up to 600 liters/minute.

Expiratory Force (EF). This measurement is made with a manometer. It is an indication of the expiratory force generated by a patient and may demonstrate a lack of sufficient expiratory force to successfully expel mucus and foreign debris. It is often used when an artificial airway is considered, i.e., removal or insertion of an endotracheal tube. The minimal acceptable value is +60 cm. H_2O.

INSPIRATORY MEASUREMENTS

Inspiratory Capacity (IC). This is the maximal amount of air which may be inhaled from the resting expiratory level. It is recorded in liters or milliliters. A normal adult man (1.7 m.^{2}) may have an inspiratory capacity of 3600 ml.

Forced Inspiratory Volume (FIV). This is the same maneuver as an FVC but is performed by beginning at maximal expiration and inspiring as forcefully as possible.

Forced Inspiration Flow (FIF). The measurement of the FIF may clarify the nature of the decreased flow rates, as to whether the cause is due to upper or lower airway disorders. This test may be designated FIF 200–1200 or MIFR. The validity of this test depends upon cooperation and effort from the patient. Healthy young men may be able to attain inspiratory flow rates of 300 L./min.

Inspiratory Force (IF). This is the amount of negative force a patient can generate on inspiration and often gives an indication of the ability to maintain the integrity of the airway with an effective cough, to deep breathe, and to maintain ventilation. The minimal acceptable value is −25 cm. H_2O. This measurement is performed with a manometer and should be a standard measurement in the assessment of the patient who may require mechanically assisted ventilation.

OTHER PULMONARY TESTS

Total Lung Capacity (TLC). The total lung capacity is the amount of gas contained in the lungs at the end of a maximal inspiration. It is measured in liters or milliliters. It may be a calculated value obtained by adding the FRC and the IC or by addition of the VC and the RV.

If available, a body plethysmograph may be used. This air-tight chamber in which the patient sits is also called a "body box." Through a special fluorescent device (pneumotach) and a shutter valve, the patient in the body plethysmograph may breathe comfortably and thoracic gas volumes, airway resistance, and alveolar pressures may be measured.

The TLC is decreased in edema, atelectasis, neoplasms, restrictive lesions, pulmonary congestion, pneumothorax, and thoracic restriction. TLC may be normal or increased in bronchiolar obstruction with hyperinflation and emphysema. Even if TLC is increased or normal, ventilation and the surface area for gas diffusion may not be normal.

TLC may be expressed in milliliters or liters. A normal adult male TLC is 6000 ml.

Functional Residual Capacity (FRC). Residual Volume (RV). The FRC is the volume of gas remaining in the lungs at the resting end-expiratory level. It is usually measured with the residual volume (RV). The residual volume is that volume of gas remaining in the lungs at the end of a full, complete, maximal expiration. The lungs cannot be completely emptied of air as long as the chest remains closed. The FRC = ERV + RV. The method of determining the RV and the FRC is indirect. For example, the patient inhales a known percentage of a gas such as helium. Its point of equilibrium with the gas in the patient's lung is then measured. The remaining concentration of helium is then recorded. The value of helium in the spirometer can then be calculated. Once the initial volume of helium is known, the FRC and RV may be calculated.

An elevated FRC indicates a pathologic condition, e.g., hyperinflation of the lung which is seen with emphysematous changes or asthmatic or fibrotic obstruction; compensatory overinflation of lung tissue to fill a space created by surgical removal of a portion of the lung; or deformity of the thorax. An increase in the FRC leads to muscular and mechanical inefficiency. If the FRC is greatly enlarged, the inspiratory capacity is reduced so the ability of a patient to increase ventilation on demand is limited.

The significance of an increased RV indicates that certain changes have occurred in the thorax, respiratory muscles, or pulmonary tissues. Except in young people with asthma, these changes are not reversible.

RV may be decreased in diffuse pulmonary restrictive disease and in diseases in which alveoli are occluded in many areas of the lung.

Closing Volume (CV) and Closing Capacity (CC). These tests are more sophisticated and require more extensive and expensive equipment. Patient coordination and effort are essential. The value of the test is not universally accepted for the margin of error is great.

Tests showing an increased CV and CC are significant, indicating early small airway disease. A patient with a normal spirogram (VC, FEV_t, and so on) may have an abnormal CV and CC. However, evaluation and early diagnosis of small airway disease is not one of the routine pulmonary function tests done in most hospital settings at this time.

Flow Volume Loop (FVO). A flow volume loop shows the relationship between flow and volume. This is measured during a forced expiratory volume maneuver, followed in the same cycle by a forced inspiratory volume maneuver. This is plotted against the volume expired. The flow is reported in liters per second and the volume in liters.

The advantage of this test is that significant decreases in flow, volume, or both are available in a single graphic display.

The shape of the loop aids in diagnosing the respiratory problem. The FVO is mainly sensitive to changes in the lower airways and only slightly sensitive to changes in the upper airway.

Radioactive Gas Function Tests. Significant advances in the study of regional pulmonary function have been made possible by the use of radioactive isotopes, multiple fixed or moving detectors, and scintillation cameras. For example, various aspects of pulmonary function can be evaluated by having a subject inhale a small amount of a relatively insoluble radioactive gas, e.g., xenon (Xe)-133. Radiation counters positioned over various portions of the chest can evaluate specific locations of uneven pulmonary ventilation; a high level of radioactivity occurs in well-ventilated regions of the lung, while poorly ventilated regions are identified by a low level of radioactivity.

These are sensitive indicators of airway obstruction which can help to distinguish emphysematous, bronchitic, and mixed types of obstructive airway disease. These inhalation scans are useful counterparts to perfusion scans (discussed below) and also can help to evaluate response to treatment.[80]

Use of a scintillation camera and xenon-133 permits visualization of slowly ventilated spaces. The photographs (called *scintiphotographs*) are examined for irregularities in distribution and clearance of radioactivity. (See also earlier discussion of lung scintigraphy.)

Exercise Tests. Some ventilation tests are done with the patient exercising as directed. During exercise, arterial blood specimens are taken for analysis of blood gases, and pulmonary function tests are performed. *Exercise tolerance tests* evaluate the amount of exercise a subject can experience before becoming dyspneic. Patients with very low respiratory reserves may become dyspneic after walking only a few steps; some are dyspneic even at rest (see Table 52–5). Exercise tolerance may be tested by simply having the subject walk down a hallway and up and down a flight of stairs. It may more accurately be measured by having the patient pedal a stationary bicycle, walk a treadmill, or step up and down on a single stair step in the laboratory.

Bronchospirometry. This method of lung examination was formerly used to assess the ventilatory function of either the right or left

TABLE 52–5. CLASSIFICATION OF DYSPNEA

Grade I	Can keep pace walking on the level with a normal person of similar age and body build, but not on hills or stairs.
Grade II	Can walk a mile at own pace without dyspnea, but cannot keep pace with a normal person.
Grade III	Becomes breathless after walking about 100 yards, or for a few minutes on level.
Grade IV	Becomes breathless while dressing or talking.

Modified from Committee on Diagnostic Standards, American Thoracic Society, 1962.

lung or the individual bronchopulmonary segments. This procedure is rarely performed today, having been replaced with sophisticated scanning tests (discussed below).

INTERPRETATION OF VENTILATORY TESTS

When ventilatory tests are interpreted by the pulmonary physician, the reported values (those measurements of the patient) are compared with the predicted values. The physician is thus able to categorize generally the patient's lung function. Diagnosis of specific disease processes is not possible with only the information provided by the tests of ventilatory function. Two broad categories of pulmonary disorders can be determined: obstructive diseases and restrictive diseases. (See Table 52–6). To see how various deviations from normal values aid in categorization, refer again to Table 52–3.

Data from pulmonary function tests must be correlated with data obtained from arterial blood gas analysis, occupational and environmental history, medical history, social history (including history of smoking), physical assessment, and pulmonary history.

Pulmonary function spirometry is termed *within normal limits* if the actual values produced by the patient are within 15 to 20 per cent of the predicted normal values.

REVERSIBILITY AND BRONCHODILATOR RESPONSE

Ventilatory tests such as the vital capacity, FEV_t, MVV, and FEF 25%–75% are frequently performed before and after the administration of an inhaled or aerosolized bronchodilator such as a solution of Bronkosol. The results of the test before and after are calculated and noted. The patient is said to have "significant reversibility" if the improvement following administration of the aerosol bronchodilator is 15% or more.

Chronic lung disease cannot be cured. Only subjective and symptomatic relief can be given a patient. The importance of "reversibility" or temporary improvement in lung function is obvious. Not all chronic lung diseases respond or improve with bronchodilator administration.

Tests of Pulmonary Circulation

Radioactive Gas Perfusion Tests. The use of radioactive gases has made possible evaluation of not only regional pulmonary function but also the regional distribution of blood flow, i.e., regional pulmonary perfusion. Capillary blood flow in the lungs can be measured by giving a radioactive tracer, e.g., xenon-133, intravenously. The xenon comes out of solution as it courses through the pulmonary capillaries, and it enters the alveolar gas. Radiation detectors then demonstrate a high concentration of xenon in areas well perfused with blood (i.e., those with good capillary blood flow); low concentrations of xenon occur in poorly perfused areas of the lung.

A *lung scan* may be useful in evaluating pulmonary perfusion when space-occupying disorders or pulmonary infarction are suspected (these conditions reduce perfusion). A lung scan is performed by intravenously injecting iodinated (^{131}I) serum albumin aggregated or techne-

TABLE 52–6. OBSTRUCTIVE AND RESTRICTIVE DISEASE

Obstructive	Restrictive
Disorders or diseases affecting the patency and/or elasticity of the airways, leading to an increase in airway resistance. Expiration primarily affected.	Those diseases and disorders causing an interference or change in the chest wall or lung parenchyma; space-occupying lesions which result in decreased distensibility of the chest wall. Inspiration primarily affected.
Emphysema	Kyphoscoliosis
Mucosal edema of airways	Ankylosing spondylitis
Bronchitis	Scleroderma
Asthma	Abdominal distention
Inhalation of noxious gas; smoke	Obesity
Bronchiectasis	Third trimester of pregnancy
Airway inflammation in response to irritants, viral or bacterial infections	Pulmonary fibrosis
Allergic response	Paralysis of ventilating muscles
	Neuromuscular diseases
	Chest wall trauma
	Inflammatory changes of the lung tissue and pleura
	Tumors
	Pulmonary edema

tium (^{99m}Tc) serum albumin aggregated. These aggregates lodge in the pulmonary capillaries when injected, and scanning of the lung then permits detection and mapping of areas of impaired perfusion. The clumps of albumin collect in regions of the lung which have good blood flow and these areas thus show a high level of radioactivity. The clumps are not able to enter vessels obstructed by disease processes; thus, poorly perfused areas have a low level of radioactivity.

Pulmonary scintigraphy may be performed to evaluate both the ventilation and perfusion of the lung of a patient. This dual function testing offers both qualitative and quantitative comparisons of ventilation and perfusion.

Uneven distribution of ventilation with air trapping in the lung can be readily demonstrated by the inhalation of xenon-131. Pulmonary arterial obstruction (e.g., due to a pulmonary embolus or a mass such as a tumor) can be detected by the perfusion scan. The V/Q scan is perhaps most frequently used in the diagnosis of a pulmonary embolism.

V/Q scans may also be used in preoperative evaluation of the patient scheduled for thoracic surgery. Predictions of expected postoperative pulmonary function may be made for the patient who may require a lobectomy or pneumonectomy. If the preoperative study determines a certain percentage of lung function arising from the affected section of lung, then postsurgical lung function may be estimated. With this information, the surgeon may treat the patient with a nonsurgical method of therapy and thus avoid severe pulmonary incapacitation for the patient.

Cardiac Catheterization. Cardiac catheterization is another important means of studying pulmonary circulation. During catheterization the pulmonary blood flow, pulmonary arterial pressure, and pulmonary end-capillary pressure may be determined. Evaluation may be made of changes that occur during exercise. Blood gas analyses may also be made of blood samples obtained during catheterization. (Cardiac catheterization is discussed in Unit XII.)

Other Evaluations of Cardiopulmonary Circulation. Developing cardiopulmonary complications in critically ill patients may be detected by evaluating the *central venous pressure* (CVP) and by *pulmonary artery catheterization.* The CVP provides information about the filling pressure of the right ventricle and is useful in diagnosing right ventricular failure. (CVP is discussed in Unit XII.) Pulmonary artery catheterization measures left-sided heart pressure and is valuable in diagnosing left ventricular failure, pulmonary edema, and pulmonary hypertension, all of which may develop without right ventricular failure.

The *Swan-Ganz catheter* is a flow-directed balloon-tipped catheter which is floated into the heart via the right side of the heart. (See also Unit XII.) The catheter is directed into the pulmonary artery. The pressure within the pulmonary artery and in the pulmonary capillary may be measured. Other possible measurements include cardiac output and mixed venous oxygen tension ($P_{\bar{v}}O_2$) and content ($C_{\bar{v}}O_2$). These two parameters are valuable in the assessment of tissue oxygen utilization and the ability of tissues to extract O_2. Venous blood will vary in O_2 tension and O_2 content owing to the varying O_2 consumption rates in different parts of the body.

The thermodilution method of cardiac output determination is now the popular choice in the intensive care setting. A 5 to 10 ml. sample of saline or dextrose is injected into the pulmonary artery. A heat-sensitive thermistor is located in the pulmonary artery. It registers the drop in temperature resulting from injecting a cool (room temperature to ice cold) solution. A thermal dilution curve is recorded and a cardiac output may be determined.

For details about pulmonary artery catheterization and significant findings consult Gernert and Schwartz's article, "Pulmonary Artery Catheterization,"[68] and Kurpershoek and Pierce, "Bedside Cardiopulmonary Techniques.[95]

Carbon Monoxide Diffusion Tests. Three methods may be used to evaluate the diffusing capacity of the lungs (DL), i.e., the rate of gas exchange across the alveolar membrane. These three methods are the single-breath method, the rebreathing technique, and the steady-state technique. All three methods use carbon monoxide (CO) to measure the DL, because the blood's hemoglobin has a special affinity for CO such that CO combines with the hemoglobin more rapidly than does oxygen, and CO can be easily measured.

The *single-breath* CO test is performed by: (1) having the patient inhale a very low concentration of CO; (2) having the patient hold his or her breath for 10 seconds before exhaling; and (3) calculating the CO rate of diffusion by determining the difference between the CO concentration in the inspired air and that in the expired air. Normally the CO rate of diffusion is 25 ml./min./mm. Hg. Normally the rate at which CO disappears from the alveolar gas is directly proportional to its rate of diffusion.

The *rebreathing* CO test is performed by having the patient *rapidly* rebreathe for about 90 seconds from a bag containing a low concentration of CO and air. The diffusing capacity is then calculated.

The *steady-state* CO test is performed by having the patient breathe (at a normal rate) about 12 to 14 breaths of a mixture of air and a low concentration of CO. An arterial blood sample is then taken and a pCO_2 is obtained. From this the mean alveolar pCO is calculated. Normally the CO rate of diffusion with this test is 17 ml./min./mm. Hg.

Slow diffusion rates may result from the presence of abnormal fluids or thick, fibrosed alveolar membranes.

Skin Tests

Skin tests performed in diagnosing and evaluating respiratory disorders include: tests to determine sources of hypersensitive (allergic) reactions, the Schick test to determine susceptibility to diphtheria, tuberculin tests to identify tuberculosis infection, and tests with other antigens to help in the differential diagnosis of fungus or nontuberculous mycobacterial infections.

Skin Tests for Allergies. Inhalant allergens (e.g., plant pollens and dusts) may cause seasonal hay fever, seasonal asthma, and allergic rhinitis. Skin tests may be performed to identify a patient's specific allergens. The patient may then be slowly hypersensitized against that particular allergen. (See Chapter 11.)

Schick Test. The Schick test is a measure of immunity to diphtheria. The test is performed by intracutaneously injecting a quantity of diphtheria toxin diluted in salt solution equal to one fiftieth of the minimal lethal dose. One thirtieth of a unit of antitoxin per cubic centimeter of blood is adequate to neutralize the toxin. If the subject receives less than this amount of antitoxin, the toxin is not neutralized and an area of inflammation appears at the site of the skin injection. Thus, lack of immunity to diphtheria is indicated by redness and edema at the injection site five to seven days following the injection.

Tuberculin Skin Tests. Tuberculin skin tests are used for diagnosis and case-finding for tuberculosis. (Tuberculosis is discussed in Chapter 55.) These skin tests identify persons who require further diagnostic investigation, i.e., positive tuberculin reactors who show sensitivity to tuberculin. Tuberculin skin tests are based on the fact that infection with *Mycobacterium tuberculosis* produces a specific sensitivity to certain chemical products of the organisms which are contained in culture extracts. These extracts are called *tuberculins.*

A *tuberculin reaction* is a delayed, acute, local, specific inflammation resulting from the injection of specified amounts of tuberculin. The intradermal injection of tuberculin in sensitized persons produces an area of *induration* (i.e., an abnormally hard place) 48 to 72 hours later which varies in size and intensity according to the individual's sensitivity and the amount of tuberculin injected. The degree of sensitivity is then determined by measuring the reaction. Let us emphasize that erythema (i.e., redness) may or may not surround the area of induration. Erythema without induration is without significance. (Reading or interpreting the tests is discussed later.)

A positive tuberculin reaction indicates that the individual being tested has, at some time, been infected somewhere in the body by tubercle bacilli. The infection may have been minor and may no longer be active. A positive reaction does *not* provide definite proof of an infection and does *not* indicate whether the individual's infection is currently active or inactive. Further diagnostic tests are necessary to obtain this information. Note that a positive tuberculin skin test does *not* mean the subject was merely exposed to someone with active tuberculosis; it means that somewhere within the body the subject has a healed or active site of tuberculous infection.

Tuberculin tests are routinely given to children, young adults, persons known to have been exposed to tuberculosis, persons with radiographic findings suggestive of tuberculosis (especially if sputum examinations are negative), and hospital personnel in direct contact with persons having active tuberculosis. The value of the tuberculin test as a screening procedure is increasing as the prevalence of tuberculosis in the population decreases; it is particularly valuable in identifying persons who require chemoprophylaxis.

Tuberculin converters are tuberculin reactors who are known to have been nonreactors within the previous 12 months (Chap. 55); those persons who do not have clinically detectable progressive disease are often given isoniazid prophylactically. Persons with positive tuberculin reactions who are proved to have clinically active tuberculosis by further diagnostic studies are given appropriate treatment.

With few exceptions, once acquired, definite sensitivity to tuberculin persists throughout life. The sensitivity may vary in intensity and temporarily may decrease or disappear in the course of certain severe illnesses. It may also decrease or disappear if chemoprophylactic treatment is given in the earliest stages of infection. Also, the skin reaction to tuberculosis is frequently abolished or reduced in intensity during the administration of corticosteroid drugs. A very small number of persons occasionally fail to react to tuberculin even after a natural infection or after administration of vaccine prepared from living or dead tubercle bacilli. Tuberculin sensitivity may also decrease in old age.

Although no direct or proportional relationship exists between the level of hypersensitivity to tuberculin and the extent or severity of the tuberculosis infection, the intensity of the tuberculin reaction is at times significant. For example, it appears that the greater the size of the tuberculin reaction, the greater the possibility that active disease exists or will appear in the subject and close contacts. Generally, relatively high levels of sensitivity are found in persons with recently acquired infection, in those with caseous, nonpulmonary tuberculosis, and in persons in continuous contact with individuals with active tuberculosis but who are not themselves infected.

Test Procedures. Two kinds of tuberculin are currently widely used for tuberculin skin testing; *old tuberculin* (OT), which is obtained from heat-sterilized cultures of tubercle bacilli; and *purified protein derivative* (PPD), which consists of the protein of dead tubercle bacilli obtained from filtrates of autoclaved cultures of tubercle bacilli that have been grown on synthetic medium. *PPD is the preferred tuberculin preparation* because its strength is standardized and tests with the same dose are comparable. PPD and OT dilutions (in buffered diluents) can retain their potency for as long as six months if protected from contamination and kept refrigerated. Dilutions in physiologic saline should not be used after one week.

Contraindications to tuberculin testing include any rash, allergic dermatitis, scabies, or current reactions to smallpox vaccinations. The nurse checks for these contraindications prior to administering a tuberculin skin test.

Before discussing specific techniques of tuberculin testing, consider the following points of importance in any skin testing procedure.

Before giving the test, briefly explain the test procedure and its significance to the patient. Explain that a positive reaction does not mean active tuberculosis. Your explanation before the test may reduce a patient's anxiety if a positive reaction develops.

Keep tuberculin testing equipment separate from that used for any other injection. Tuberculin and other antigens (e.g., blastomycin, coccidioidin, and histoplasmin) are difficult to remove from glassware and other materials. Thus, bottles, syringes, needles, jet guns, and other equipment used for one antigen should not subsequently be used for another.

Record any tuberculin test given. State the date the test was given; the type of test used; the type and dose of tuberculin administered; the date the test was read; and factual comments about any reactions to the test, e.g., millimeters of induration.

A *variety of techniques* are available for administering the tuberculin test. These include: the intracutaneous or intradermal (Mantoux) test, jet gun injection, multiple-puncture tests (e.g., Heaf, Sterneedle, Mono-Vacc, or tine), von Pirquet scratch test, and Vollmer patch test. Of all these techniques, *the method of choice for administering tuberculin is the Mantoux test* because it introduces a measured amount of tuberculin into the skin and produces the most consistent and reliable results. Jet injection and multiple-puncture techniques may be used for survey and screening purposes. Often a Mantoux test is subsequently performed on persons who have reactions to these screening tests. The von Pirquet and Vollmer tests are not recommended because of relative unreliability.

Intradermal (Mantoux) Tuberculin Test. This test is routinely performed for differential diagnosis and survey by the intradermal injection of 5 tuberculin units (TU) of intermediate strength PPD (0.001 mg.). The injection is given into the upper third of the inner surface of the left forearm after the skin is cleansed with an alcohol sponge. When possible a disposable tuberculin syringe with an attached 26-gauge, ½-inch beveled needle is used. If a nondisposable tuberculin syringe is used, a very sharply beveled steel or platinum (25- or 26-gauge) needle is used. The needle bevel is held upward and the needle tip is inserted between the layers of the skin.

When the 0.1 ml. of PPD is properly injected into the skin a discrete, pale elevation of the skin resembling a mosquito bite is produced (Fig. 52–7). If this wheal is less than 6 mm. in diameter the injection is repeated, with another syringe, about an inch diagonally below the first. Skillful administration is necessary, so that the test material is injected intradermally rather than subcutaneously or outside the skin. A dressing is not applied over the injection site.

The Mantoux test is read 48 to 72 hours after the injection. The reading is made in good light, with the subject's forearm slightly flexed. The injection site is inspected visually and palpated. The site is observed from the side against the light as well as by direct

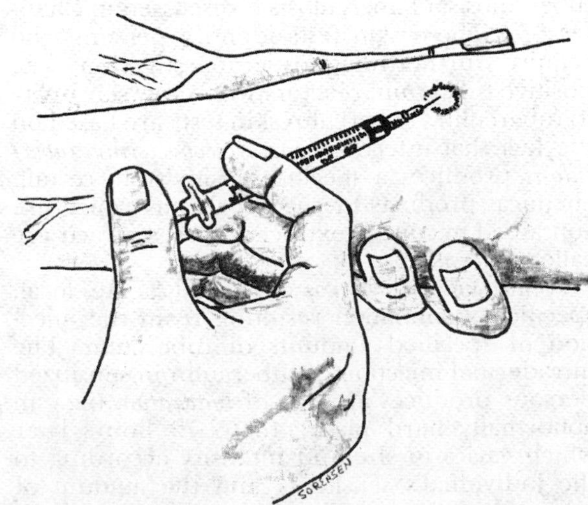

Figure 52–7. Mantoux tuberculin skin test. Note: skin is tightly stretched for the injection.

light. Palpation is performed by gently stroking the area with the fingers. *A Mantoux skin test can be properly read only if the area is palpated;* merely looking at the puncture site is not sufficient. The diameter of the area of induration is measured transversely to the long axis of the forearm and is precisely recorded in millimeters. Erythema is also measured if present; however, as mentioned earlier, erythema without induration is insignificant. In some severe reactions necrosis may occur at the injection site; its presence is recorded.

An area of induration of 10 mm. or more is considered a *positive reaction.* Induration from 5 to 9 mm. in diameter is classified as a *doubtful reaction.* (Sometimes such a reaction indicates infection with unclassified atypical mycobacteria rather than the true tubercle bacilli.) Persons with doubtful reactions are routinely given further diagnostic tests. Induration of 4 mm. or less is considered to be a *negative* reaction.

Jet Injection Tuberculin Test. A jet gun delivers 5 TU of PPD intradermally under high pressure. As with the Mantoux test, the wheal produced should be 6 to 10 mm. in diameter. If it is less than 6 mm. the injection is repeated at another site. This test is read, recorded, and interpreted in the same manner as that discussed above for the Mantoux.

Multiple-puncture Tuberculin Tests. There are several different types of applicators for multiple puncture tests. All such tests are less accurate than the Mantoux because unknown amounts of tuberculin are administered and the reactions are less precisely defined and more difficult to measure. The tests are most often used for testing large groups of subjects. Multiple-puncture tuberculin tests puncture the skin either by pressing into the skin an applicator which has points on which tuberculin is dried (e.g., the tine test) or by puncturing the skin through a film of liquid tuberculin (e.g., the Sterneedle test). These techniques may introduce more than 5 TU of tuberculin because they all use concentrated tuberculin.

The time intervals between injection and reading vary with multiple-puncture tests according to the type of test given. Manufacturer's instructions must be followed carefully. Less skill is necessary to administer multiple-puncture tuberculin tests than to administer the Mantoux test; however, the subject's skin must be prepared and the test given and interpreted strictly.

Reactions to multiple-puncture tests may be in the form of discrete, separate papules at various puncture points, or coalescent reactions may occur in which several papules fuse together to form one larger reaction. The diameter of the largest single papule or the largest single coalescent reaction is measured as described for the Mantoux test.

Details of administering and reading multiple-puncture tuberculin tests can be obtained from the manufacturers of these products or from the American Lung Association. (Contact your local branch or write A.L.A., 1740 Broadway, New York, N.Y. 10019.)

Skin Tests with Other Antigens. Respiratory disorders caused by certain pathogenic fungi are sometimes diagnosed by skin tests. Three *fungal antigens* are currently commercially available for skin testing: coccidioidin, histoplasmin, and blastomycin. Reactions to these fungal antigens do not prove active disease, but rather suggest a possible diagnosis. Cross-reactions occur between fungal antigens.

Animal Inoculation

Sometimes animal inoculation is necessary to differentiate between pathogenic and nonpathogenic organisms. The guinea pig, for example, is highly sensitive to tuberculosis. Specimens which may be used for guinea pig inoculation include: sputum, urine, ground-up or homogenized material from resected lung lesions, pleural fluid, or cerebrospinal fluid. At least two animals are used. Multiple subcutaneous inoculations of specimen material are made in the inguinal and axillary regions. Six to nine weeks after inoculation the animals are examined at autopsy for evidence of infection.

Gastric Content Analysis (Gastric Washings)

Some patients are unable to raise sputum for specimens, e.g., they are not producing enough sputum to raise or they are unable to cooperate enough to raise a specimen (unconscious, aged, young children, severely debilitated). In these patients pulmonary disease may be diagnosed or evaluated by examining gastric contents when the patient is in a fasting state. Gastric contents are aspirated for study through a nasogastric tube or a tube passed orally to the stomach. An analysis of gastric contents may reveal pathogenic organisms causing pulmonary infections, because these organisms are often swallowed.

Gastric aspiration is rarely necessary nowadays, as deep tracheal suction and mobilization maneuvers are usually effective in obtaining the desired specimens.

See Unit XVII for further discussion of nasogastric intubation.

HISTORICAL ASSESSMENT

The following information presented in brief outline form is important in determining the type and level of respiratory dysfunction. You may wish to consult texts which deal with the topic of historical assessment in more detail. The format used here may aid nurses in obtaining valuable information and knowledge about patients. (See also Chapter 15.)

1. *General state of health*
   a. Family health history; e.g., is asthma, emphysema, tuberculosis, or lung cancer present in the family?
   b. Medications. Is the patient taking bronchodilators, diuretics, antibiotics, heart medications, or any other drugs for a chronic or acute medical condition?
2. *Specific respiratory history*
   a. *Chest pain.* Is it associated with breathing, exercise, etc.?
   b. *Shortness of breath.* When does it occur, is it painful, what causes it to improve?
   c. *Cough.* When does it occur, is sputum produced, is it associated with pain; how often does it occur, is blood observed in the sputum?
   d. *Sputum production.* How much; what color; what time of day is the most productive, does position affect the amount of production; is there any odor to the sputum?
   e. *Hemoptysis* (blood in the sputum). How often, when does it occur, is pain associated with the raising of blood?
3. *Exercise tolerance.* How much activity can the patient usually perform, what limits the degree of activity; when did a change in the amount of exercise tolerated start?
4. *Wheezing.* What causes the wheeze (exercise, emotions, exposure to allergens or other external factors)?
5. *Allergies* that produce respiratory distress, e.g., pollens, molds, etc. When did the allergic symptoms begin? When were they diagnosed?
6. *Occupational history.* Length of time exposed to occupational irritants, e.g., welding, coal mining, sandblasting, etc.
7. *Personal pollution history*—this includes smoking history. Smoking history is reported in number of "pack years." To determine this figure, multiply the number of years cigarettes have been smoked by the average number of packs of cigarettes smoked per day. Two packs per day × 40 years of smoking = 80 pack years.

PHYSICAL ASSESSMENT*

A brief description of the general observations and clues which may indicate the presence of existing lung disease may be found in Table 52–7. See also Figure 52–8 for a picture of classic manifestations of chronic respiratory dysfunction. It is important to observe the patient for physical clues of chronic respiratory dysfunction, as the presence of chronic lung disease may determine the type and expected outcome of therapy.

Assessment of Dyspnea. Dyspnea is a subjective symptom. It may be caused by numerous factors, as noted in the preceding discussion. Patients will perceive shortness of breath in varying manners. (See Table 52–5). It is important to pay complete attention to this complaint. The patient with dyspnea has experienced a significant change in the work of breathing. These changes lead to metabolic oxygen demands which act as a stimulus to increase ventilation. The physiologic need to increase ventilation to meet these demands leads to an increased level of dyspnea. As you can see, dyspnea is part of a vicious cycle. Assessment of the cause of dyspnea must be followed by intervention. Assessment includes:

- Observation of the patient's appearance, including the breathing pattern;
- Determination of activities and mental and emotional states prior to and during episodes of shortness of breath;
- Physiologic data such as chest x-ray film, arterial blood gases, pulse, blood pressure, breath sounds, vital capacity, and tidal volume;
- Familiarity with the patient's medical therapy, including drugs the patient is receiving which may have adverse effects that lead to feeling short of breath; and
- Other predisposing factors.

Intervention must be aimed at the factors causing dyspnea, decreasing dyspnea, increasing the patient's ability to tolerate dyspnea, and assisting the patient to deal with dyspnea-provoking situations. Evaluation of the effects of your intervention must be noted in the patient care plan. This information is valuable to the continuity of care.

TABLE 52–7. PHYSICAL CLUES TO CHRONIC RESPIRATORY DYSFUNCTION

1. Overdeveloped "strap" muscles (sternomastoid muscles)
2. Elevated sternum
3. Increased anteroposterior diameter of chest
4. A flaring, barrel-shaped chest
5. Classic breathing patterns using pursed-lip breathing or a prolonged expiratory phase
6. Characteristic posture that elevates the ribs and increases the size of the thorax (shoulders usually elevated)
7. Clubbing of the fingers and toes (see Chapter 53, Fig. 53–3, p. 1216)
8. Signs of heart failure, e.g., swelling of the feet and ankles; noisy respirations
9. Cough and noisy respirations
10. Nicotine stains on fingers
11. Retraction of the spaces between the ribs during inspiration

Skin Color Changes

Evaluation of skin color changes requires practical observation and experience. Accurate observation requires adequate illumination. Diffuse over-bed lighting and the glow of a flashlight are inadequate. A lamp with a 60-watt bulb

*See also Chapter 15.

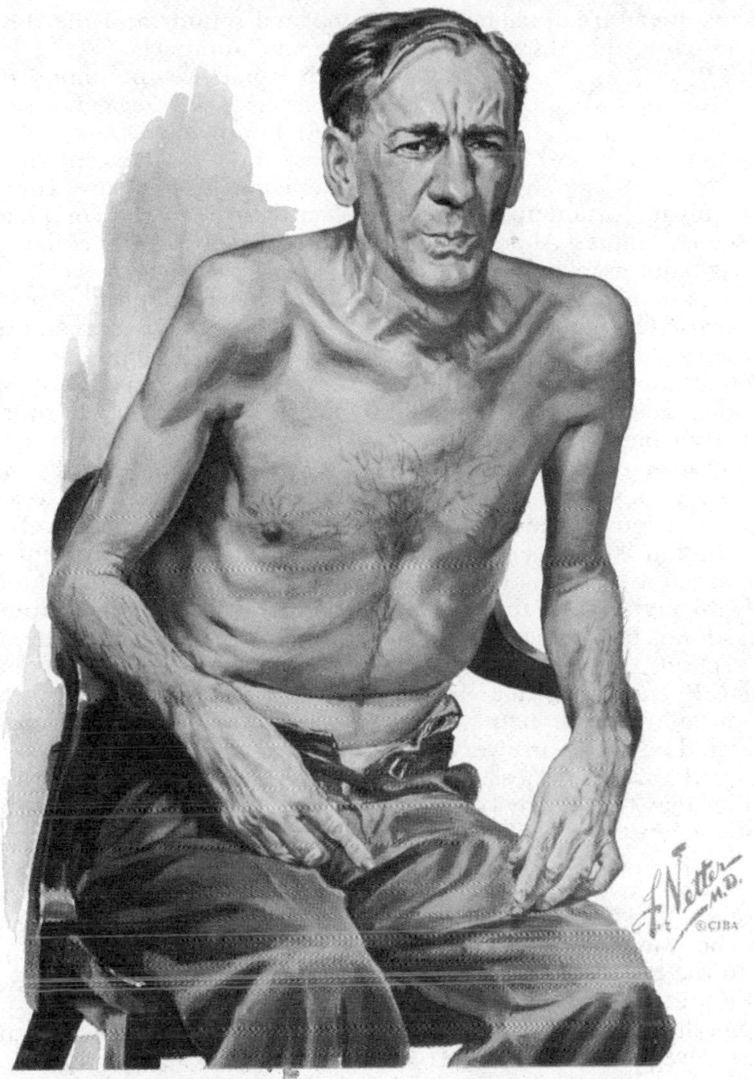

Figure 52–8. Typical posture of a patient with chronic lung disease. (From CIBA Clinical Symposia, 20:No. 2, Apr.-June 1968.)

which may be moved close to the patient in minimally acceptable nonglare daylight offers the best illumination. Examination of a limb should be made at heart level with the patient in a low, semi-Fowler's position. Ambient temperature and the emotional status of the patient may either mask or alter the actual skin color. When examining the color of the nail beds, it is important to determine the length of time since the patient smoked a cigarette. One of the effects of cigarette smoking is peripheral vasoconstriction.

For best observation, the skin ideally should be clean and dry. Bathing should not immediately precede inspection, however, as friction, warm water, or harsh soaps may alter the skin.

Edema reduces the intensity of skin color changes by increasing the distance between the skin's surface and the pigmented and vascular layers.

The identification of *cyanosis* in some persons of Mediterranean background and those of full-blooded black origin is difficult. A bluish tinge to the lips and gums is often part of the normal pigmentation of the mucous membranes of persons of these origins. The sclera of the eye may also be pigmented with melanin. Many blacks have freckle-like pigmentation of the gums, mouth, tongue, and nail beds. Color changes are best observed where pigmentation is least: the sclera, conjunctiva, nail beds, lips, oral cavity, tongue, palms, and soles of the feet. When cyanosis is questionable, apply light pressure to create pallor. If cyanosis has developed, the color will reappear from the outer edge and spread to the center. Color should return in one second.

For accurate evaluation of color changes in dark-skinned persons, observe the patient frequently. Know and compare your observations of color and behavior. Be aware of the behavior changes that accompany the disorders that cause color change.[130]

Auscultation

Auscultation is highly important in evaluating a patient's pulmonary status. Although the stethoscope was originally used only by physicians to listen to a patient's heart and lungs, today it is also widely used by nurses. By carefully auscultating patients' lungs, nurses may detect evidence of pneumonitis, congestive heart failure, or secretion accumulations. When a stethoscope is not available, abnormal respiratory sounds may be detected by listening with the ear against the patient's chest and placing the hand on various portions of the chest.

Pulmonary auscultation is best performed if the patient is encouraged to open the mouth and breathe deeply through it while the examiner listens to breath sounds by placing the stethoscope on various sections of the patient's back (Fig. 52–9). Normal and abnormal breath sounds are most often relatively high pitched and easily auscultated. A few are very low pitched, however, and can be felt easier than heard. The examiner may thus gently place the palms of the hands against the patient's chest wall in an attempt to pick up the vibrations of these low-pitched sounds.

Breath sounds reveal important data useful in the evaluation of the patient's condition. The nurse must listen to the breath sounds of many patients, as practice and supervision are essential to the development of expertise. The technique of auscultation requires a knowledge of normal sounds and the development of a systematic approach.

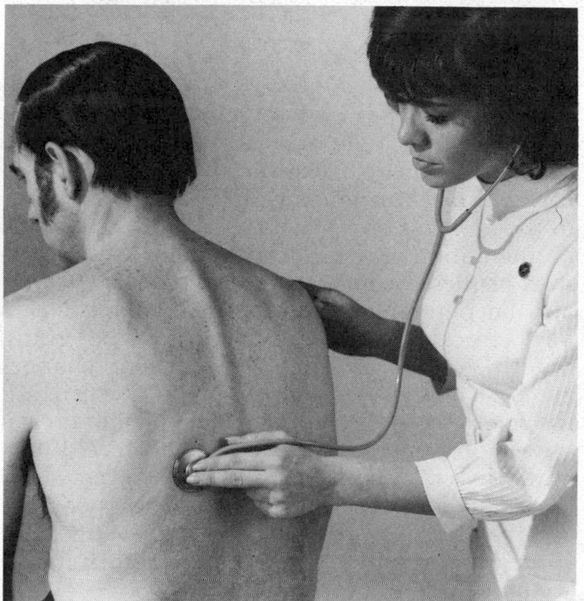

Figure 52–9. Auscultation. (From Littmann, D.: *American Journal of Nursing*, *72*:1238, July 1972.)

Normal breath sounds have four classifications. *Vesicular sounds* are soft, whisper-like, and low pitched, and are usually heard over most of the chest except the major large airways. Vesicular sounds are composed of a sound heard through the complete inspiratory phase and partially during exhalation.

Tracheal and *bronchial breath sounds* are loud, harsh, and tubular sounding, normally heard over the trachea and the large conducting airways. Inspiration is often not as loud as expiration and is slightly shorter in duration than expiration. These sounds are abnormal if heard over other regions of the thorax.

Bronchovesicular breath sounds are a combination of bronchial and vesicular sounds. They are heard best over the central airway (e.g., the sternum or the intrascapular area). This sound is often heard over the anterior and apical lung segments of the right upper lobe. It is more muffled than bronchial breath sounds. Inspiration and expiration are equal in length and intensity.

Abnormal or pathologic breath sounds are termed *adventitious* sounds. Included in this category are (1) absent breath sounds; (2) rhonchi and wheezing, (3) stridor, (4) rales, and (5) pleural friction rubs.

Absent, or *diminished,* breath sounds may be noted with apnea, improper use of the stethoscope, pneumothorax, severe emphysema, severe obesity, severe asthma, and/or severe pleural thickening. Diminished sounds are diagnostic of emphysema. A silent chest in a patient with obvious apparent distress is an emergency situation. Prompt attention to the ventilatory status of the patient is crucial to the viability of the patient.

Rhonchi and *wheezing* are easily recognized. Rhonchi are usually expiratory; wheezing may be either inspiratory or expiratory. Both generally involve the integrity or patency of the airway and indicate that an accumulation of fluid, airway mucosal edema, or smooth muscle spasm (bronchospasm) is present. Rhonchi are usually lower pitched. Wheezes are often described as having a musical quality. Wheezing is generally associated with asthma but may be present in many other diseases and conditions. Rhonchi often can be eliminated by clearing the airway of accumulated secretions.

Stridor is characterized by a crowing or snoring sound on inspiration. This sign is associated with upper airway obstruction found in croup (laryngotracheobronchitis) and foreign body aspiration. Stridor is usually accompanied with sternal retractions and an obvious increase in the work of breathing.

Rales are adventitious sounds related to the sound of air entering fluid in the alveoli and small airways. The sound is similar to the crinkling of cellophane or the sound heard by wetting the thumb and forefinger and opening and closing them near the ear. Rales are inspiratory phase sounds indicative of congestive failure, pulmonary edema, or pneumonia.

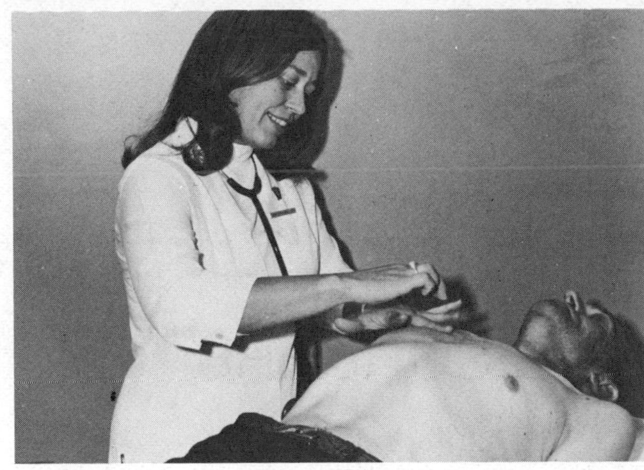

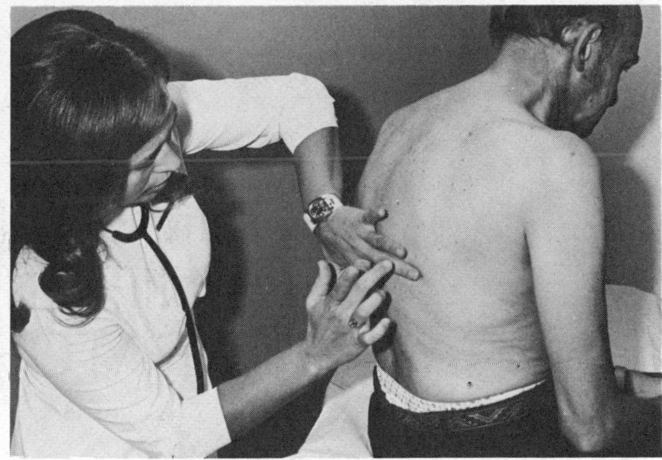

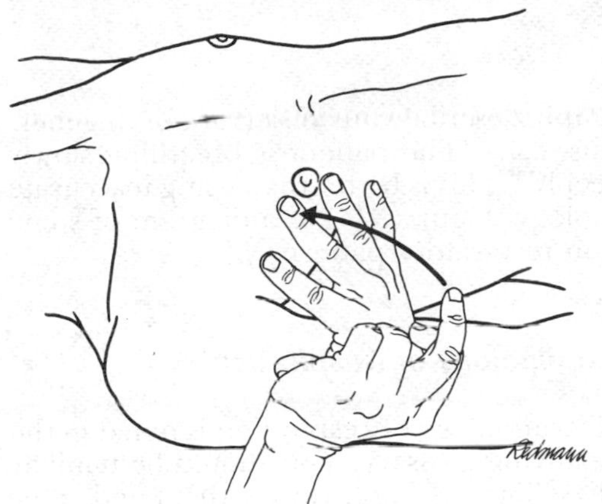

Figure 52–10. Percussion of the lungs. (From Traver, G. A.: *American Journal of Nursing*, *73*:466, Mar. 1973.)

A *pleural friction rub* is a loud, creaking, leather-like sound heard over parts of the thorax where the two pleural layers are rubbing together owing to inflammation. The patient may describe discomfort directly over this part of the thorax. This sign is diagnostic of pleurisy. (See discussion of pleurisy, p. 1263.)

Inspection, Percussion, and Palpation

In addition to auscultation, the chest may also be examined by inspection, percussion, and palpation. *Inspection* of the chest may reveal changes in its contour or mobility, e.g., both sides of the chest may not rise and fall evenly during inspiration and expiration. Intercostal ballooning or retraction in the intercostal spaces occurs when a patient has tremendous difficulty in ventilating the lungs and must exert extreme effort when trying to move air in and out of the lungs. Reduced chest wall movement on the affected side occurs with pneumothorax, atelectasis, and extensive parenchymal obstruction. Obviously if the nurse is going to properly inspect chest movements, the patient's clothing must be lowered so that a comparison of both sides of the chest can be made. In addition to the preceding observations, the rate and rhythm of ventilation are evaluated by inspection.

Percussion (striking an area with short, sharp blows as an aid to diagnosing the condition of the parts beneath the blow by the sound obtained) may demonstrate significant changes in density in the lungs (Fig. 52–10). Percussion over "normal" lung tissue produces resonance, i.e., intensification and prolongation of sound caused by the transmission of the sound vibrations to a cavity. When the density of lung tissue is increased, e.g., by the presence of fluid, percussion elicits dullness.

Palpation is the least useful method of physical examination of the chest. Palpation may detect *changes in muscle tone* and *fremitus,* i.e., a vibration or thrill perceptible upon palpation. A rhonchal (or bronchial) fremitus is produced by air moving through a large, mucus-filled bronchus. A friction fremitus occurs when two dry surfaces rub together. Pleural fremitus is specifically a vibration of the thoracic wall felt when the pleural surfaces rub together, causing friction. Palpation may also be used to delineate areas of thoracic pain or masses.

Respiratory disorders may produce a variety of changes from normal functioning which may be detected by auscultation, inspection, percussion, and palpation. Many of these alterations are discussed throughout the unit. (See also article by Traver.[170])

CHAPTER 53

COMMON NONSPECIFIC MANIFESTATIONS OF RESPIRATORY DISORDERS

To properly assess a patient and give appropriate care, nurses need to be familiar with some of the more common nonspecific indications of respiratory disorders. In Chapter 52 we discussed tests and activities used in the detection and evaluation of certain manifestations of respiratory disorders. We shall now consider a number of additional indications of respiratory disorders.

CONSTITUTIONAL SYMPTOMS

Among a variety of constitutional symptoms that respiratory disorders may produce are those indicative of

- *general debilitation,* e.g., anorexia, weight loss, fatigue, weakness, apathy, irritability;
- *infection,* e.g., increased pulse rate, elevated temperature; and
- *trauma,* e.g., symptoms of shock such as weak rapid pulse, drop in blood pressure.

ABNORMAL PATTERNS OF BREATHING

Breathing, or respiration, is difficult to evaluate because it can be voluntarily altered and is subject to emotional influences. In spite of this fact, much can be learned about the body's internal environment and respiratory disorders by assessing the nature of a patient's breathing.

It is a nursing responsibility to accurately observe, describe, and report abnormalities of breathing. This can be difficult since medical terminology is often inconsistent and many terms are not defined precisely or are used carelessly. Greater attempts must be made by all health care professionals to standardize definitions and to carefully describe the distinguishing characteristics of various patterns of breathing. If you are uncertain about which terms to use, simply describe your observations in general terms, e.g., "The patient is breathing slowly and deeply." This is better than using inaccurate terminology. Figure 53–1 is a diagram of some common respiratory patterns.

The Terminology of Respiration

The terminology of respiration is noted in the accompanying glossary. You should be familiar with these terms; if not, review them and refer to a basic nursing text (e.g., Chapter 36 of Sorensen and Luckmann: *Basic Nursing: A Psychophysiologic Approach*) as needed.

Abdominal respirations. Breathing accomplished mostly by the abdominal muscles and diaphragm. Abdominal breathing can be highly effective. Often patients are taught abdominal breathing to increase the effectiveness of the ventilatory process, e.g., patients with diffuse obstructive lung disorders or following chest surgery.

Apnea. Temporary or permanent cessation of breathing.

Biot's respirations. A type of periodic breathing in which periods of tachypnea, and usually hypopnea, alternate abruptly with apnea. The irregular periods of apnea alternate with periods in which four or five breaths of uniform depth are taken. The duration of the periods is more variable than that in Cheyne-Stokes breathing, and Biot's breathing is viewed as an "irregular irregularity." It may occur with increased intracranial pressure, head injury, meningitis, encephalitis, brain abscess, and heat stroke.

Bradypnea. Slow breathing (less than 10 cycles/min.) with no significant changes in depth. Frequently occurs with increased intracranial pressure and following administration of depressing amounts of narcotics and sedatives.

Cheyne-Stokes respirations. The best known type of periodic breathing, characterized by rhythmic waxing and waning of the depth of respirations, with regularly recurring episodes of apnea or marked hypoventilation. The periodicity of this type of breathing is fairly regular. A series of ventilations gradually increase in tidal volume and rate, then gradually decrease until they lapse into another apneic period. Cheyne-Stokes breathing occurs typically in severe heart failure, uremia, and coma caused by neurologic disorders.

Diaphragmatic respirations. Performed mainly by the diaphragm. Also called *abdominal* or *belly breathing.*

Dyspnea. Difficult, labored, or painful breathing. While dyspnea may be "normal" at times (e.g., as a result of extreme physical exertion), it may also be symptomatic of numerous disorders, that interfere with adequate ventilation or perfusion of the blood with oxygen. The dyspneic patient is subjectively aware of difficulty with breathing and experiences such feelings as being smothered or unable to breathe.

Eupnea. "Normal," easy, quiet breathing. The normal adult respiratory rate is between 10 and 24 cycles/min.

Gasping. Rhythmic or irregular spasmodic inspiratory effort which is typically brief and maximal and terminates abruptly.

Hyperpnea. Abnormally deep breathing, i.e., an increase in tidal volume. Although rate may be increased to some degree, increased depth of breathing is the main abnormality. Occurs, for example, in well-conditioned athletes following strenuous exercise.

Hyperventilation. Increased minute ventilation. Abnormally rapid, deep, and prolonged breathing, e.g., caused by central nervous system disorders, drugs which increase sensitivity of respiratory centers, or acute anxiety. Often produces respiratory alkalosis; increased amounts of air enter the lungs, causing a reduction in CO_2 tension. Some experts prefer using "hyperventilation" to refer to increased minute ventilation (regardless of whether due to increased rate or to tidal volume) and "polypnea" when a striking increase occurs in both rate and depth of breathing. (Hyperventilation is discussed further below.)

Hypopnea. Greatly reduced depth of breathing with less striking reduction in rate. For example, may occur during sleep or following administration of narcotics or sedatives. Also, may result from poor posture or the partial paralysis of respiratory muscles.

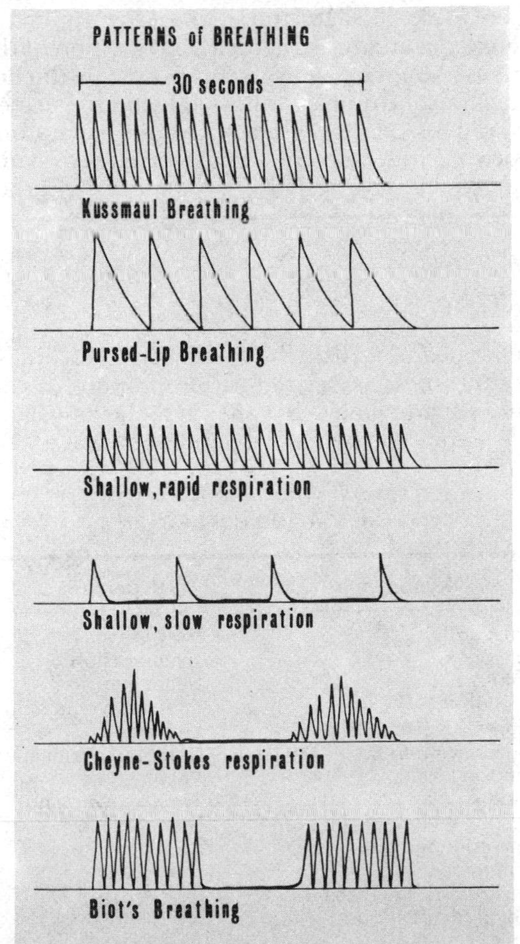

Figure 53–1. Respiratory patterns suggesting specific etiologic problems. (From Hodgkin, J. E.: Respiration as a vital sign. *Respiratory Therapy, 7*:35, Sept.-Oct. 1977.)

Hypoventilation. Reduced minute ventilation. Abnormally low amounts of air enter the lungs. Causes an elevation of CO_2 tension. Some experts prefer using "hypoventilation" to refer to reduced minute ventilation (regardless of whether due to reduced rate or to tidal volume) and using "oligopnea" for states in which both rate and depth are reduced significantly. (Hypoventilation is discussed below.)

Interrupted respirations (cogwheel or wavy respirations). Jerky breathing pattern, the inspiratory and expiratory sounds are clearly split into two or more sounds rather than occurring as a normal continuous sound.

Kussmaul's respirations (air hunger). Paroxysmal dyspnea. Often precedes diabetic coma. While Kussmaul's breathing is sometimes an example of hyperventilation, it is more often truly dyspneic.

Oligopnea. See hypoventilation.

Orthopnea. Inability to breathe except when the trunk is in an upright position. Dyspnea may or may not be present with the erect posture. Seldom occurs with primary pulmonary disorders; frequently accompanies heart failure. The erect posture reduces venous pressure and pulmonary congestion and thereby reduces resistance to breathing. Commonly the degree of orthopnea is described in terms of the number of pillows the patient needs to elevate the head so he or she can breathe, e.g., "two-pillow orthopnea" or "three-pillow orthopnea."

Paradoxical respirations. Breathing pattern in which a lung (or portion of lung) inflates during inspiration, i.e., acts opposite to normal. (Discussed further in Chapters 56 and 57.)

Periodic breathing. Respiratory arrhythmias in which the rate, depth, or tidal volume changes markedly from one interval to the next and the pattern of change is periodically reproduced, e.g., Cheyne-Stokes breathing, Biot's breathing.

Polypnea. See hyperventilation.

Rales. Gurgling, bubbling sounds, synchronized with breathing, which occur when the moving air passes through fluids in the small airways and alveoli as in pulmonary edema.

Shortness of breath (SOB). Quick respiration which is not necessarily dyspneic, i.e., difficult or painful. At times SOB is a result of emotions, exercise, metabolic activity, e.g., fever.

Stridor. Noisy respirations characterized by harsh crowing sounds caused by the forcing of air through a partially obstructed larynx or trachea in spasm.

Tachypnea. Rapid breathing (rate more than 24 cycles/min.) which does not significantly change in depth; occurs during emotional states, e.g., periods of passion and states of fear.

Thoracic respirations. Breathing accomplished by the thoracic muscles, e.g., intercostal muscles and others.

Hyperventilation

It is important to determine the causative factors of *hyperventilation,* among which are

- Acute or chronic anxiety;

- Neurocirculatory asthenia;
- Central nervous system lesions including meningitis, encephalitis, cerebral hemorrhage or trauma, and tumors;
- Hormones and drugs such as epinephrine, progesterone, large doses of analeptic drugs, and massive doses of salicylates;
- Increased metabolism from hyperthyroidism and fever;
- Hypoxia leading to a compensatory attempt to correct the decrease in arterial oxygenation;
- Acidosis caused by metabolic imbalance stimulating an increase in alveolar ventilation in an attempt to compensate through the respiratory system;
- Pulmonary reflexes when alveoli collapse, when deflation receptors are irritated, when pulmonary hypertension occurs, and when certain receptors in the respiratory tract are irritated;
- Hypotension causing stimulation of chemo- and pressure receptors;
- Mechanical overventilation from any form of positive pressure ventilation; and
- Somatic pain.

Blood gases will show a decreased pCO_2 ,an increased pO_2 and an elevated pH (above 7.45). The elevation of the pH and the reduction of the pCO_2 result in an erroneous pO_2 value. The blood gas study may report an arterial oxygen tension that is within "normal limits." Unfortunately, due to the relationship between hemoglobin and oxygen in the presence of hypocapnia, the oxygen is more closely bound to the hemoglobin and is not as readily supplied to the tissues.

Symptoms of alveolar overventilation (hypocapnia) include numbness and tingling in extremities and face, anxiety, cerebral vasoconstriction leading to dizziness, tremors and twitching, transient paralysis of extremities, and convulsions.

Hypoventilation

Hypoventilation results when alveolar ventilation is insufficient to meet metabolic demands. It is a symptom, not a disease. Causes of hypoventilation are:

- Depression of respiratory centers from general anesthesia, excessive doses of narcotics and sedatives, cerebral trauma, increased intracranial pressure, prolonged cerebral anoxia or ischemia, high concentration of inhaled CO_2;
- Interference with nerve impulse conduction and/or neuromuscular transmission to respiratory muscles by neuromuscular blocking agents such as curare or pancuronium bromide, polio, spinal cord lesions, peripheral nerve block by nerve gas, myasthenia gravis;
- Disease affecting use of respiratory muscles;
- Thoracic movement impairment by arthritis, emphysema, thoracic deformities;
- Limited chest excursion from pleural effusion or pneumothorax; and
- Pulmonary diseases such as pneumonia, atelectasis, tumors, obstructive and restrictive lesions in the upper or lower respiratory tract.

The arterial blood gases produced by hypoventilation include an elevated pCO_2, a decreased pH (below 7.35) and a decreased pO_2 if the patient is breathing room air. If the patient is receiving supplemental oxygen, the pO_2 may be satisfactory but CO_2 retention will continue. CO_2 retention can be corrected only by adequate alveolar ventilation.

See Table 53–1 for the signs and symptoms of hypoxemia and hypercapnia. Recognition of the signs of abnormal oxygen and carbon dioxide status must be quickly followed by both objective (arterial blood gas) and subjective (symptoms improved) assessment. Progression of symptoms could have lethal consequences. (Carbon dioxide narcosis is discussed in Chapter 54.)

Dyspnea

Dyspnea is a disturbing subjective feeling of breathlessness associated with sensations of ventilatory inadequacy. Dyspnea may be associated with hypo- or hyperventilation. Much of the

TABLE 53–1. SIGNS AND SYMPTOMS OF HYPOXEMIA AND HYPERCAPNIA

Hypoxemia	Hypercapnia
Tachycardia	Restlessness
Tachypnea	Hypertension
Confusion	Headache
Agitation	Impaired ventilation
Progressive irritability	Lethargy
Progressive muscle weakness	Cerebral vasodilation
Cyanosis	Papilledema
Diplopia	Tremor, twitching
Difficulty with coordination	Somnolence
Impaired judgment	Coma
Somnolence	
Loss of consciousness	
Bradycardia; cardiac arrhythmias	
Bradypnea, hypoventilation	
Coma	
Apnea	

sensation of dyspnea probably results from the sustained work of breathing (especially breathing against obstruction) necessary to try to maintain adequate gas exchange. Patients with moderate to severe difficulty in breathing typically become fatigued and mentally distressed from the increased physical and mental effort required. Dyspnea is a common clinical problem which requires skilled nursing intervention and sensitive care.

Numerous *respiratory problems* produce dyspnea, e.g., damaged lung parenchyma, airway obstruction, chest pain, reduced lung compliance, impaired alveolar-capillary gas exchange, overworked or weakened respiratory muscles. Specific respiratory disorders which may produce dyspnea include pleurisy, aspirated foreign bodies, and parenchymal as well as tracheobronchial lesions that cause inflammation and obstruction. Other examples are mentioned throughout this discussion. In addition to being caused by respiratory disorders, dyspnea may be *psychogenic* in origin or may result from *cardiac disorders* (e.g., cardiac insufficiency) or *anemia.* Changes in the blood's components may make the blood unable to effectively transport the respiratory gases.

Types of Dyspnea. There are various types of dyspnea (see discussion of the Assessment of Dyspnea in Chapter 52). *Exertional dyspnea* is induced by physical exertion or effort. This is the most common type and may occur with any condition that impairs ventilation, e.g., obstructive or restrictive pulmonary disorders, with diffusion defects, or from inefficient mechanics of breathing. Dyspnea is seldom produced by early pulmonary disease but is more common with chronic disorders, e.g., diffuse obstructive lung disease. (See Table 52–5 in Chapter 52 for the ATS Classification of Dyspnea.)

Cardiac dyspnea refers to dyspnea caused by heart disease. Left ventricular failure from aortic insufficiency or mitral stenosis may cause *paroxysmal dyspnea.* Paroxysmal dyspnea occurs in attacks, usually while the patient is sleeping at night but also during the daytime. Paroxysmal dyspnea may be relieved by having the patient sit upright for 30 to 60 minutes and breathe deeply several times.

Some patients are dyspneic even when resting, i.e., *dyspnea at rest.* Dyspnea at rest does occur with chronic pulmonary disease but it is more typical of congestive heart failure. It may occur with diffuse pulmonary diseases causing alveolar-capillary block and in conditions in which secondary factors are superimposed on a reduced pulmonary reserve, e.g., in patients with both bronchitis and pulmonary emphysema. Marked dyspnea at rest also is produced by some acute pulmonary disorders, e.g., bronchial asthma, pneumonia, massive atelectasis, pneumothorax.

Clinical Care During Acute or Severe Dyspnea. Severe or acute dyspnea, e.g., during an asthmatic attack, is frightening for both patient and nurse. The patient struggles to breathe and is acutely uncomfortable. A person experiencing dyspnea is often overwhelmed by feelings of panic, extreme anxiety, and fears of suffocation and death. The gasping patient may plead with the nurse, "Help me breathe! I can't get air!"

In order to work effectively with a dyspneic patient the nurse must have in mind a plan of care, be sensitive to his or her own reactions to extreme respiratory distress, and efficiently perform clinical actions directed at giving the patient relief. The nurse who panics when a patient develops acute dyspnea conveys anxiety to the patient, thereby adding to already devastating problems. Also, the anxious nurse's judgment may be impaired, increasing chances of error. For example, a nurse, overwhelmed with a desire to terminate the dyspneic attack and calm the patient, may administer excessive sedation or excessive oxygen. Both of these actions may have serious, possibly fatal consequences.

Activities important in caring for a dyspneic patient are summarized below:

▶ Maintain a clear airway, promote and assist effective ventilation and respiration, promote bronchodilation. Encourage the patient to practice controlled diaphragmatic breathing.

▶ Stay with the patient, maintain a positive, calm approach, allay the patient's stresses, anxieties, and fears; act in an efficient, quiet, and reassuring manner.

▶ Place the patient in the position that allows the most comfortable breathing.

▶ Conserve the patient's energy for the work of breathing, anticipate needs, promote rest, relaxation, and relief of tension. Do not excessively or unnecessarily increase fatigue. Do not require the patient to talk or to move more than is minimally necessary. Do not excessively sedate or tranquilize the dyspneic patient.

▶ Interpret and carry out orders, e.g., for O_2, sedatives, tranquilizers, bronchodilators. If in doubt about whether to use a PRN order, consult with the physician.

▶ Remove the cause of the dyspnea when possible. Carry out treatments directed at the underlying disorder responsible for the dyspneic attacks.

▶ Conduct procedures in such a way that they do not increase dyspnea, e.g., take rectal rather than oral temperatures, avoid use of heavy bedding over the patient's chest.

▶ Maintain a quiet environment that is relatively cool and moist.

▶ Protect the severely dyspneic patient from injury, e.g., by side rails. The patient's judgment may be poor because of a dire psychophysiologic state.

- Prevent fluid-electrolyte imbalances. Intravenous infusions may be necessary during severe attacks of dyspnea because the patient cannot take adequate food and fluids orally. Record intake and output.
- Make observations and evaluations of the dyspneic episode; report and use these observations and evaluations to plan and give clinical care directed at reducing the severity of the present dyspneic episode and preventing future periods of dyspnea if possible.
- Assess the presence of hypoxemia and/or hypercapnia by drawing an arterial blood gas sample.

If the airway seems obstructed encourage the patient to cough productively; minimize ineffective coughing. Suction as necessary but not excessively. Suction removes air and oxygen as well as secretions and thus can increase the severity of breathlessness.

Oxygen, nebulized bronchodilators, nebulized medications to thin thick secretions, and other forms of respiratory therapy must be administered correctly. The effectiveness of all forms of therapy should be noted — both beneficial and adverse reactions. Oxygen is the most common drug administered to the patient exhibiting dyspnea. Its need is governed by an arterial blood gas determination. The dose of oxygen may be ordered in liters per minute or in a percentage. The effects of therapy should be assessed; for instance, did the oxygen improve the pre-therapy hypoxemia without causing CO_2 retention? Dyspneic patients receiving oxygen by mask may become anxious since this method of O_2 administration increases the sense of suffocation. Dyspneic patients typically are most comfortable with O_2 administered per nasal cannula.

Do not leave the patient alone during an acute dyspneic attack. Often the mere presence of the nurse helps the patient to relax somewhat. Talk to the patient; give instructions; explain what you are doing. Listening helps to distract, relax, and rest the patient. Calmly reassure the patient and help her or him to control breathing and to exhale more slowly so as to slow the rate of breathing. This causes ventilation to be more efficient also.

Assist the patient to a position which facilitates ventilation. Often, but not always, the preferred position is one with the head of the bed elevated. Respect the patient's preferences for positioning. Patients usually know how they can breathe most comfortably, e.g., sitting upright, bending forward over a table, lying semi-upright. (See Fig. 53–2.) After you have helped the patient to assume the position of choice, place pillows, supports, padding, and so forth, so the person can maintain that position without fatigue or discomfort. Leaning forward facilitates use of the accessory muscles of respiration, e.g., abdominal, cervical, dorsal, and pectoral muscles. These muscles are used during conscious expiration, e.g., to expel trapped air.

During attacks of dyspnea remind the patient to practice controlled breathing. As stated, dyspnea usually causes the affected person to expend increased amounts of energy to breathe, and the person often breathes more rapidly. Unfortunately these reactions only worsen the patient's condition by reducing the effectiveness of ventilation and by increasing O_2 requirements and airway obstruction. To prevent these detrimental effects, persons subject to dyspnea should be taught controlled breathing methods (e.g., diaphragmatic breathing) that reduce the effort necessary to breathe and improve the effectiveness of ventilation. Pursed-lip breathing is one of the most important techniques in the control of breathing. A detailed discussion of breathing exercises in provided later in this unit.

Observations important to make when a patient experiences dyspnea include:

- Notation of events which preceded the attack and what the patient was doing when the attack began
- Patient's reaction to the attack and any accompanying symptoms, e.g., diaphoresis, emotional state, sputum, cough, color, pulse, rate and character of respirations
- Severity of the attack and how long it lasted
- Responses to treatment

If episodes of dyspnea appear to be regularly recurrent, this observation should also be noted.

Following an acute attack of dyspnea ensure that the patient rests to relieve exhaustion from the effort of breathing and the anxiety accompanying the attack. Also, the dyspnea may have caused loss of sleep.

Because the dyspneic patient is commonly frightened, frustrated, fatigued, and uncomfortable, the patient may be short-tempered. The nurse must be able to overlook abusive behavior and recognize and respond to the cause of the patient's behavior. Be certain that a dyspneic patient always has a call bell within easy reach. Respond rapidly to the patient's summons so the person is reassured that help is nearby when needed. Periodically "drop in" to visit the patient without being summoned. These actions reinforce the feeling of being "looked after" in an anxious person.

Care in Chronic Dyspnea. The individual with chronic dyspnea, e.g., with emphysema or chronic obstructive lung disease, must be taught how to live with breathlessness. For example, teach the patient about the following factors which will facilitate ease in breathing: dietary modifications, diaphragmatic breathing, improved breathing habits, pursed-lip breathing, control of breathing, proper posture, graded

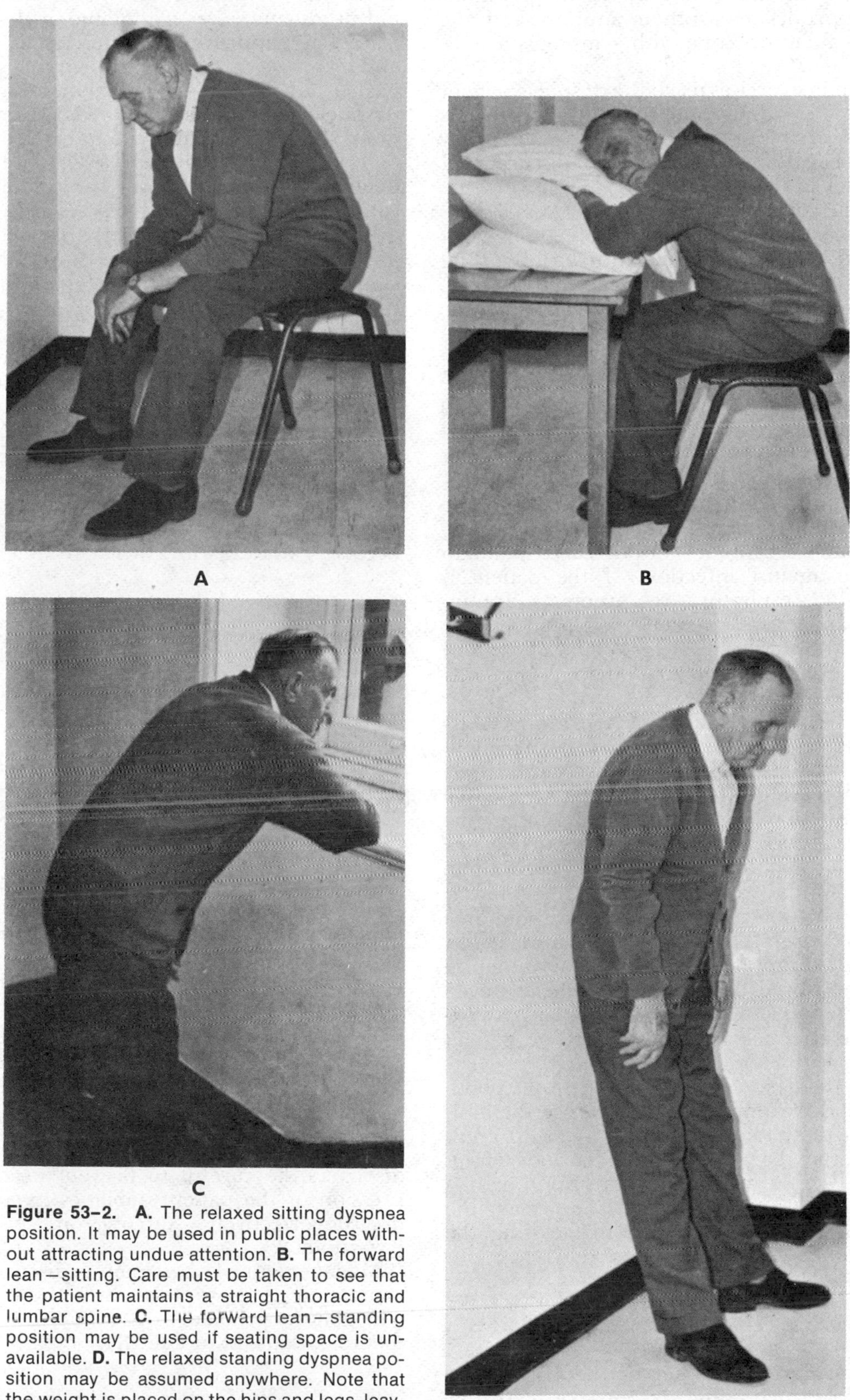

Figure 53–2. **A.** The relaxed sitting dyspnea position. It may be used in public places without attracting undue attention. **B.** The forward lean – sitting. Care must be taken to see that the patient maintains a straight thoracic and lumbar spine. **C.** The forward lean – standing position may be used if seating space is unavailable. **D.** The relaxed standing dyspnea position may be assumed anywhere. Note that the weight is placed on the hips and legs, leaving the diaphragm and thorax relaxed. (From Gaskell, D. V., and B. A. Webber: *The Brompton Hospital Guide to Chest Physiotherapy,* 2nd ed. Oxford: Blackwell Scientific Publications, 1974.)

goal-oriented exercise, and room ventilation. Include significant others in teaching sessions when appropriate, as their support and the patient's ability to cope with symptoms are directly related.

Breathing exercises teach the dyspneic patient controlled breathing and breathing techniques that promote more efficient and easy lung ventilation. Breathing exercises are discussed in detail later in this unit.

General comfort measures can greatly help the dyspneic patient to relax and feel somewhat refreshed. Keep the patient in dry clothes and bed linens, and at a comfortable temperature. Minimize feelings of suffocation by keeping the patient's environment open to circulating air. Frequent oral hygiene is of importance, especially if the patient is mouthbreathing. Massage of the upper back, neck, and shoulders helps to relieve physical tension resulting from labored breathing.

Adequate nutrition is required by the dyspneic patient. This is important because of the large amount of energy such a person is expending and because it is important to maintain resistance against infection. If the patient is overweight, respiratory requirements are increased and excessive work is placed on the heart. If the patient is underweight, expiration may be impaired because the diaphragm tends to flatten.

Small, frequent feedings of nourishing foods and liquids are better than larger, less frequent intake. If the stomach is excessively full it distends, increasing pressure on the abdominal muscles and diaphragm; this impairs abdominal breathing. Advise the patient subject to dyspnea to avoid liquids and foods that are gas-forming, e.g., ice water, cabbage, onions, cauliflower, radishes, cucumbers, turnips, melons, and lima and navy beans. The administration of airway clearance therapy before meals may minimize fatigue produced by eating. Nonetheless, even the minimal exertion necessary to eat may exhaust the dyspneic patient. Offer the patient assistance with eating as required.

Permit the dyspneic patient to help plan both activity and treatment schedules since the individual's activity tolerance may vary at different times of the day. Two typical periods of increased dyspnea and fatigue are upon arising for the day and following meals, especially the last meal of the day. When first arising the patient's lungs are often congested by secretions that have pooled during the period of relative inactivity in bed. At the end of the day the patient is usually exhausted from the day's exertions.

The nurse closely observes the patient for evidence of increasing dyspnea or excessive fatigue upon exertion. Unnecessary invalidism is undesirable, but at times it is necessary to conserve the patient's energy by minimizing the number of self-help activities. Because of the beneficial effects of ambulation, it is encouraged as long as the patient can tolerate activity without producing excessive fatigue or dyspnea.

Exercise improves the muscles in the body and increases the ability of the muscles to utilize oxygen, and must not be eliminated from the dyspneic patient's activities. An exercise program should be instituted and carried out on a daily basis. The reasons for exercise must be explained to the patient, who should be encouraged to keep progress records. Because achievement is important, progressively graded. goal-oriented exercise is used. Walking is the simplest and best form of exercise, a distance that the patient is able to accomplish should be chosen. If increased dyspnea occurs during exercise, patients must be encouraged not to panic but to remember they can control their breathing. Patients set the pace and should take their time. When an objective is attained, goals should be expanded. Successfully achieving goals will help people have feelings of self-worth, which are essential to the establishment and maintenance of the coping mechanisms necessary to deal with chronic dyspnea.

CHEST PAIN

Pulmonary disorders may produce pain in the chest wall (including its bony and cartilaginous structures), parietal pleura (the visceral pleura is insensitive to pain), bronchi, and trachea. The pain associated with pleural inflammation is often quite incapacitating if untreated and is worsened by changes in intrathoracic pressure, e.g., sneezing, coughing. (Pleurisy and pleural pain are discussed in Chapter 55.) Chest pain also commonly occurs with bronchogenic carcinoma, pneumonia, and tracheobronchial inflammations. The latter condition produces pain of a burning nature which patients frequently describe as a raw feeling in the lining of the throat and windpipe. Coughing aggravates this pain, but respirations do not worsen it. Chest injuries and chest surgery often produce moderate to severe pain. (See Chapters 56 and 57.) When administering pain-relieving drugs for any chest pain associated with respiratory disorders, be careful to prevent excessive depression of the patient's abilities to cough and breathe effectively. Narcotics are particularly hazardous.

Management of chest pain is discussed more completely as appropriate throughout this unit. The general problem of pain and pain management is discussed in Unit XI.

BRONCHOSPASM

Bronchospasm (wheezing) is the spasmodic contraction of the walls of the bronchi, with mucosal edema, increased mucus secretion, and narrowing of the airway, resulting in reduced expiratory flow. Bronchospasm is a component of numerous respiratory disorders, e.g., asthma, chronic bronchitis, chronic pulmonary emphysema, foreign body aspiration. Other causes are aspiration of gastric contents, inhalation of toxic substances, exercise, viral infections, heart failure, and many other asthma-like and nonasthma conditions. Reduction of the size of the bronchial lumina predisposes the patient to retention of secretions and infection, in addition to making ventilation of the lung more difficult. The airway resistance as well as the work of breathing is increased. Severe bronchospasm is a life-threatening condition.

The specific treatment of bronchospasm is the administration of bronchodilators to open the airways by relaxing contracted muscles. Bronchospasm may also be reduced by preventing unnecessary irritation of the tracheobronchial tree, e.g., avoidance of irritating smokes, gases, and other air pollutants, avoidance of cold air, and prevention of unnecessary nonproductive coughing. Treatment of bronchospasm is discussed in greater detail elsewhere throughout this unit.

NURSING ACTIONS TO AID IN PREVENTION OF RESPIRATORY DYSFUNCTION

A nurse has many opportunities to teach both hospitalized persons and those in the community. A nurse is often thought of as the most accessible member of the health care team and thus often has more opportunities to practice prevention of diseases than a physician. The death rate from chronic lung disease has increased significantly over the past 15 years, therefore recognition of hazards to respiration and action to reduce or correct them can aid in combating this trend. Some of the information that may be included in *patient-family teaching sessions* includes:

▶ *Avoidance of irritants.* Noxious chemicals, environments which contain fumes, dust, and other irritants to the respiratory system may cause pulmonary diseases. Diseases and conditions that cause respiratory dysfunction as a result of occupational exposure to irritants are called *pneumoconioses.* Aerosol sprays such as for cleaning and grooming may also irritate the respiratory system. Inhalation of these irritating sprays may induce bronchospasm.

▶ *Reduction of personal pollution.* Various occupations pollute the air we breathe. Worse, in a way, is air pollution caused by the "personal pollution" of cigarette smoking, and "second-hand" smoke (cigarette smoke breathed by nonsmokers). The hazardous effects of cigarette smoking are well known. Nonetheless, many people choose to ignore these facts. Not only are smokers increasing the risks to themselves by continuing to smoke, but they also cause lung problems and damage to persons around them who breathe in the second-hand smoke.

Persons with diagnosed respiratory disorders should not continue to smoke. Cessation of smoking may not reverse the effects caused by smoking, but it will decrease the progression of irritation to the airway and contribute to a reduction or improvement of respiratory dysfunction symptoms.

Your local Lung Association can provide you with facts about smoking which you may find helpful in your personal and professional life.

▶ *Adequate fluid intake.* The importance of hydration is discussed elsewhere in this chapter. Adequate hydration is of great importance in treating both acute and chronic respiratory dysfunction. Patients with chronic lung disease should be encouraged to drink 2 to 3 quarts of water per day. A nurse can help patients more comfortably meet this intake requirement by making fresh water available.

▶ *Specific actions for the patient with chronic respiratory disease.*

Avoid crowds—especially during seasons when colds and flu are prevalent. This reduces the risk of exposure to respiratory disorders. Avoid situations where cigarette smoke or other respiratory irritants will be encountered.

Avoid temperature extremes—a sudden change from a warm to a cold environment can cause increased shortness of breath. Many persons with chronic lung disease feel they should move to a dry climate. This may not benefit everybody. Before making a permanent move, patients should be encouraged to discuss the decision with a respiratory medical specialist, and to consider all the factors involved.

ABNORMAL SECRETIONS

A typical adult produces about 100 ml. of mucus daily. This mucus is produced by mucous cells and goblet cells lining the tracheobronchial tree. Mucus acts to entrap inspired particles and to moisten tracheobronchial membranes. Mucus is carried upward in the tracheobronchial tree by cilia lining the walls of the airway. Coughing and clearing the throat are other actions that move secretions into the pharynx.

Irritations or inflammation of the nasal mucosa or sinuses may cause *rhinorrhea,* i.e., copious mucus discharge from the nose. (Disorders of the nose and sinuses are discussed in Unit XXIV.) Tracheobronchial or pulmonary irritations or infections often cause an increase in mucus production, and sputum frequently changes in consistency and/or color. *Sputum* is composed of mucus (from the tracheobronchial tree), leukocytes, epithelial cells, dirt, bacteria, and nasopharyngeal secretions. Saliva is not sputum. Certain pulmonary disorders produce sputum with specific characteristics:

Abscess — foul odor (anaerobic infection); large quantities
Asthma — mucoid
Bronchiectasis — periodic large quantities; separates into three layers upon standing
Bronchitis (chronic) or emphysema — very tenacious; thick
Carcinoma (bronchogenic) or tuberculosis (advanced) — contains frank blood
Edema — frothy; large quantities; pink
Pneumonia (pneumococcus) — sticky, small amounts, rusty or pink
Suppuration — purulent; large quantities; yellow or green (bacterial infection)
Tracheobronchitis — mucoid

The defense mechanisms of the lung, including mucociliary clearance of collected debris in the airway, may be impaired if certain conditions exist. Retardation of mucociliary activity is caused by alcoholism, dehydration, airway trauma, hyperoxia (too much oxygen), hypoxia, cold ambient temperature, infection, drugs such as atropine, noxious gases such as sulfur dioxide and nitrous dioxide, and cigarette smoking. Mucociliary clearance may be enhanced by hydration, ambient temperatures in the 28 to 33° C. range, certain drugs, and chemicals such as iodine, epinephrine, xanthines, and acetylcholine.

Secretions may accumulate in the lower tracheobronchial tree as a result of an increase in secretion production, depression or failure of the normal tracheobronchial cleansing mechanisms, or both. Some possible detrimental effects of these accumulated secretions are (1) airway obstruction, (2) prevention of normal alveolar gas exchange, (3) hypoxia (due to inadequate oxygenation of the blood), (4) respiratory acidosis (due to inadequate CO_2 elimination), and (5) pulmonary disorders such as atelectasis, tracheobronchitis, and bronchopneumonia. Hypoxia is particularly serious in patients with head injuries since hypoxia increases cerebral edema and thus elevates intracranial pressure. If secretions are retained in the lungs and tracheobronchial tree they easily become sites of infection since they provide an excellent medium for the growth of pathogens in a dark moist place. Retained secretions also may form mucous plugs which can obstruct airways, impair ventilation and respiration, and produce atelectasis, i.e., collapse of a portion of the lung. Atelectatic lung easily becomes infected.

The average diameter of the smaller bronchial tubes is less than that of a broom straw, thus they can easily be obstructed. Airways normally lengthen and widen during inspiration and shorten and narrow during expiration. If the airways are partially obstructed, air cannot bypass obstructions during expiration.

Various factors may prevent a patient with a respiratory disorder from being able to move secretions effectively. For example, the patient may not be able to cough effectively because of postoperative pain, sedation, weakness, tracheostomy, or endotracheal intubation. Tracheostomies and endotracheal tubes not only reduce a patient's ability to cough but also increase secretion formation. The combination of these two factors is obviously dangerous and the tracheostomized or intubated patient must be closely observed to ensure maintenance of a patent airway. The cough reflex is weak in elderly persons, and respirations tend to be shallow.

A patient with thick, voluminous bronchopulmonary secretions may experience suffocation-like sensations and so panic when unable to cough up secretions. Feelings of fear, anxiety, and panic further increase the patient's respiratory difficulties. Calmly the nurse attempts to reassure the patient and to enlist cooperation in nursing activities that help to clear these distressing, sometimes life-threatening, secretions.

Care of the Patient with Sputum Abnormalities

Activities important in helping to mobilize and to remove tracheobronchial secretions include:

Coughing effectively and productively; breathing exercises.
Suctioning.
Humidifying inspired air.
Maintaining body hydration, e.g., forcing fluids.
Changing positions frequently. Causes secretions to move within the tracheobronchial tree and lungs; prevents pooling of secretions and stimulates coughing.
Postural drainage.
Chest percussion, clapping, tapping, vibrating. Increases force of expiration and moves secretions.
Administering prescribed medications, e.g., bronchodilators, expectorants, proteolytic enzymes, mucolytic agents, heated aerosols.
IPPB treatments. Increase inspired volume and increase diameter of bronchioles for more effective coughing.
Artificial airway. When there are profuse secretions

and cough is ineffective it is often desirable to place an artificial airway (endotracheal tube) so that proper tracheobronchial hygiene can be performed. Tracheostomy may sometimes be preferable to endotracheal intubation because secretions are usually more difficult to remove through endotracheal tubes.

Therapeutic bronchoscopy.

Some patients find it helps to loosen mucus if they take a hot drink upon arising, inhaling the steamy vapor, sipping the drink, and holding the liquid momentarily in the mouth before swallowing.

Often secretion removal poses serious problems in giving clinical care. For example, a patient's secretions may be thick and tenacious and the patient may be unable to raise them, or secretions may be so copious that the person becomes fatigued by constantly trying to clear the tracheobronchial tree. A more forceful cough is necessary to dislodge dry, thick, or tenacious secretions (low in water content and high in viscosity) than thinner secretions. Secretions must be fluid enough that they can be moved up the tracheobronchial tree by effective coughing. Once in the pharynx, sputum may either be swallowed or expectorated.

Patients producing large amounts of sputum or having infected sputum, e.g., in tuberculosis, should be instructed to expectorate sputum into a sputum collection cup rather than swallowing it. The expectorated sputum is then available for observation and laboratory evaluation or it can be disposed of safely. Large amounts of swallowed sputum may reduce a patient's appetite. If a patient who is producing sputum cannot adequately protect you from contamination (e.g., by covering the mouth and nose when coughing) it may be advisable to mask the patient or to wear a gown and mask yourself. (See Chapter 54.)

Provide the patient who has a productive cough with ample tissues, a sputum collection cup, a paper bag (fastened to the bedside or a chair) for tissue disposal, and disposable hand wipes. Instruct the patient to protect others and to prevent contamination of the environment by covering the nose and mouth with several tissues when coughing or sneezing. Tell the patient to fold used tissues over before disposing of them in the toilet or tissue bag. The patient should wash frequently or use disposable hand wipes after handling contaminated tissues. (See Chapter 54.) Always provide equipment so the patient may wash before eating.

Impress upon the patient the importance of raising secretions from the lungs and tracheobronchial tree. Teach proper methods of productive coughing. When caring for a patient who is producing abnormal secretions (rhinorrhea or sputum), periodically observe and chart the color, character, and amount of secretions and the patient's response to treatments. Be certain to mention if the secretions have a foul odor.

Keep the patient as clean and comfortable as possible and maintain an orderly, pleasant environment. Used tissues not only are unsightly and often malodorous, but also are sources of contamination and should be removed from the bedside and properly disposed of. When a tissue collection bag becomes half full, remove, close securely, and dispose of it; then replace the bag. Always wash thoroughly after handling sputum-contaminated articles (e.g., tissues, tissue bags, sputum cups, soiled linens) and after giving mouth or nose care. Provide good room ventilation. Sputum produced with some pulmonary disorders is quite foul smelling.

Frequent mouth and nose care helps to minimize mouth and breath odors and the collection of thickened secretions in these areas. This care is especially important when a patient is mouth-breathing and/or producing large quantities of sputum. Even though cleansing a patient's nose and mouth and cleaning up expectorations are activities that are often unpleasant to perform, they are an important part of total patient care (particularly when the patient has a respiratory disorder). Nurses must take care not to communicate to the patient any distasteful or repulsive feelings they may have while performing these activities. Periodically examine the patient's oral and nasal mucous membranes for indications of lesions, inflammation, or other disorders. These inspections can easily be made while giving nose and oral care.

The unpleasant taste and odor of sputum often causes patients to have a poor appetite. Provision for frequent oral hygiene helps to refresh the mouth and may improve appetite. Chewing gum or sucking on hard candy between meals may also freshen the mouth. It is desirable to provide oral hygiene before as well as after meals. The sight of contaminated tissues and sputum collection cups may adversely affect appetite. Before serving trays be certain the bedside environment is picked up and sputum containers are out of sight.

Medications that may be prescribed for patients producing excessive or abnormal bronchopulmonary secretions include *expectorants* and *mucolytic enzymes.* Mucolytic and enzyme preparations may be given by aerosol. Water (either oral or parenteral) is the best expectorant. Aerosol administration of saline, water or of 0.45 per cent normal saline, may also be used to hydrate the patient to promote mucus expectoration. Sedatives and analgesics should be used judiciously to prevent oversedation and depression of the cough reflex.

Pulmonary congestion (or inflammation) causes the respirations to become more rapid and shallow. Respirations of this nature may indicate to the nurse that the patient needs to be encouraged or assisted to cough productively, or that suctioning is necessary if the person is unable to cough effectively. Noisy, moist respirations also indicate that secretions are accumulating in the lungs. Auscultate the patient's chest and observe respirations before and after encouraging coughing or performing suctioning. Be certain to chart your observations. Contact the physician for necessary orders if a patient is having excessive difficulty in coughing up secretions or if you are unable to clear the airway.

> An obstructed airway is an emergency! *The nurse must be familiar with the following cardinal indications of laryngeal and/or tracheal obstruction: gurgling and rattling respirations, stridor, cyanosis, rib retraction, the use of accessory muscles of respiration. Occasionally oral fluids are regurgitated through the nose.* The airway must immediately be cleared.

Retained secretions lead to ineffective oxygenation and carbon dioxide retention. The patient with excessive secretions should have an arterial blood gas sample drawn to assess the efficiency of oxygenation and ventilation.

Hemoptysis

Hemoptysis is the expectoration of blood or blood-tinged sputum; it may vary in degree from slight amounts of blood in the sputum to large quantities of frank blood. Massive hemoptysis obstructs the airway. Death due to severe hypoxemia occurs more commonly than death from exsanguination. Although hemoptysis can be fatal, it most typically is a nonfatal, self-limited disorder.

Conditions that most typically produce hemoptysis are those that cause inflammation of the tracheobronchial tree, or erosion and necrosis of blood vessels and lung parenchyma. Hemoptysis may thus result from pneumonia or other acute respiratory infections (e.g., due to trauma of the tracheobronchial tree produced by repeated or severe coughing or other irritations) or from such other serious respiratory disorders as pulmonary infarction, aspirated foreign body, benign bronchial adenoma, crushing or penetrating chest injuries, bronchogenic carcinoma, tuberculosis, pulmonary abscess, or bronchiectasis. Nonrespiratory disorders that may produce hemoptysis include aortic aneurysm (in which the vessel has eroded into and ruptured into a bronchus), mitral stenosis (in which a blood vessel has ruptured within the congested pulmonary circulation), and congestive heart failure due to mitral stenosis. Sometimes disorders that cause a bleeding tendency or failure of the clotting mechanism produce hemoptysis.

Whatever the extent of hemoptysis, it is essential that the patient receive a thorough medical evaluation to determine the cause of the bleeding so appropriate treatment can be given. This investigative process may include history, general physical examination, chest films, tomograms, bronchograms, bronchoscopy, and fluoroscopy.

Important points to consider when taking a history are:[2]

- ▶ Previous episodes of hemoptysis
- ▶ History of chest disease
- ▶ Exercise tolerance
- ▶ Medication history
- ▶ Bleeding tendencies
- ▶ Careful investigation of current episode (duration, quantity, and rate of bleeding)

The physical examination should include:

- ▶ State of consciousness
- ▶ Changes in pulse and blood pressure
- ▶ Evidence of chest trauma
- ▶ Splinting of chest wall
- ▶ Breath sounds (may help localize area of bleeding)
- ▶ Clubbing, adenopathy, wasting in cancer patients, increased AP diameter and low diaphragm in severe emphysema are all signs which may suggest the underlying process

When blood is expectorated, nursing observations of the expectorated material can be helpful in ascertaining the point of origin of the bleeding in the body and determining whether the blood is venous or arterial. Often it is desirable to save the specimen for the physician or laboratory to examine. Bloody secretions expectorated from the mouth can originate from such body areas as esophagus (e.g., bleeding esophageal varices), nose (e.g., epistaxis), nasopharynx, mouth, tongue, gums, lungs or tracheobronchial tree (hemoptysis), or stomach (hematemesis). Bleeding originating in the nose or nasopharynx often causes bloody discharge to appear in the nares, and sniffling usually precedes or accompanies the expectoration of blood. (See Unit XXIV.)

Several points, as shown in Table 53–2, help to differentiate hemoptysis from hematemesis and therefore should be considered when charting observations of expectorated bloody secretions.

Other symptoms of hemoptysis may include

apprehension, salty taste in mouth, burning or bubbling feeling in chest, feelings of being smothered or drowning, and tickling sensation in throat. (See Table 53–2.)

Hemoptysis, especially if moderate to severe, is frightening for both patient and nurse. The nurse attempts to quiet and reassure the patient by staying with the person and giving appropriate instructions. Tell the patient not to try to talk, to breathe slowly and deeply, and to expectorate (not swallow) the blood and secretions. The fearful patient tends to hyperventilate; this not only causes the lungs to be excessively active but also interferes with effective respiration.

One goal of clinical care is to provide rest for the affected lung tissue without unduly suppressing the protective cough reflex necessary to clear the airway. The patient with hemoptysis should immediately be placed on complete bed rest, kept warm, and positioned so that the drainage of blood from the bronchi is encouraged. A receptacle for expectoration is provided. When possible, codeine and sedatives are avoided in order to preserve those reflexes necessary to maintain a patent airway. However, if the patient is quite anxious, a sedative such as phenobarbital may be ordered. If violent coughing occurs, codeine may be prescribed in amounts which suppress but do not abolish the cough reflex. Morphine is contraindicated.

IPPB is contraindicated until the cause of hemoptysis is determined, but oxygen may be prescribed to relieve dyspnea, cyanosis, and hypoxemia. Suctioning is performed only as necessary to clear the airway. A laryngoscope and bronchoscope should be available for the physician to perform deep suctioning and endotracheal intubation if required. Hemoptysis can cause atelectasis and pneumonia if bronchi are obstructed by blood.

Observe the patient's vital signs. Severe hemoptysis may produce shock as a result of blood loss. (See Chapter 13.) If shock appears to be developing, a blood transfusion and other measures may be employed. Formerly, in treating severe hemoptysis, an artificial pneumothorax was sometimes performed on selected patients in an attempt to rest lung tissue by temporarily collapsing the lung. Currently emergency surgery is occasionally performed in an attempt to save a patient's life, e.g., if prolonged severe hemoptysis occurs in a patient with cavernous tuberculosis. Emergency surgery for resection offers the best chances for survival. Thoracoplasty may be indicated. When hemoptysis is believed to have resulted from defective blood coagulation, vitamin K_1, calcium gluconate, and blood transfusions may be ordered. Usually in treating hemoptysis infusions are administered slowly to prevent a rapid increase in blood

TABLE 53–2. DIFFERENTIAL FEATURES OF HEMOPTYSIS AND HEMATEMESIS

Hemoptysis	Hematemesis
Blood is coughed up, not vomited. Retching and nausea may come from pharyngeal irritation from blood.	Blood is vomited.
A portion of the blood should be frothy.	Blood is never frothy.
Blood is usually, but not always, bright red in color.	Blood is dark red in color.
Blood is alkaline in reaction.	Blood is acid in reaction.
Hemoptysis is preceded by a gurgling noise or a sensation stimulating a cough reflex. This may be absent in massive hemoptysis.	Hematemesis is preceded by nausea and vomiting.
There is sometimes a history of past cough.	There may be a history of alcoholism and/or gastric disturbances, plus clinical findings of liver disease.
There is continued blood-tinged sputum, which lasts for several days.	Blood-tinged sputum is usually absent.
Blood is mixed with pus, organisms or macrophages; some of the macrophages may contain hemosiderin particles.	Vomited blood may contain food particles.
Anemia may or may not be present.	There are often clinical and laboratory findings of blood loss before the actual hematemesis.

From Lyons, H. A.: *Basics of RD.* New York: American Thoracic Society, 1976.

volume and consequently an increase in bleeding.

Provide the patient with fresh linens as indicated, i.e., remove any blood-stained linen. Oral hygiene helps to freshen the patient's mouth. Following hemoptysis the patient may have nothing by mouth for a while. If oral intake is permitted, cool liquids may be refreshing. Instruct the patient to avoid physical exertion until the physician approves. Give only gentle back care to a patient who has recently had hemoptysis to prevent possibly reactivating bleeding.

COUGH

A cough is the sudden, noisy expulsion of alveolar air from the lungs, the air being under very high pressure. Coughing is usually a normal protective act that cleans the tracheobronchial tree (acting in cooperation with airway cilia) in an attempt to prevent aspiration or to remove irritants. Coughing may be a symptom of numerous thoracic and laryngeal disorders (acute, chronic, inflammatory, neoplastic). *Cough appears to be the most common symptom of respiratory disease.* Cough is a protective mechanism in health, but it can become a disturbing phenomenon during disease. A nonproductive cough is both useless and damaging.

Generally coughing is an involuntary reflex act; however, it can be produced voluntarily. Although coughing can often be consciously inhibited, this voluntary control is limited. Reflex coughing results from the chemical or mechanical stimulation of receptors in the pharynx, larynx, or tracheobronchial tree or stimulation along the vagus nerve. Mechanical factors that commonly induce coughing include cooling, drying, irritation or inflammation of the tracheobronchial mucosa and/or lung parenchyma; foreign body or foreign particle aspiration; and accumulations of secretions within the tracheobronchial tree. The "cough center" is composed of a group of neurons in the brain's medulla. Impulses reach this center by way of the glossopharyngeal or vagus nerve.

A *chronic cough* is any cough that persists for a month or longer, even though the cough occurs only when getting up for the day or when lying down at the end of the day. Inhaled cigarette smoke is the commonest cause of chronic cough. All persons with chronic coughs should be medically evaluated, because this symptom may indicate a serious pulmonary or cardiac disorder that should be treated. Respiratory diseases that may produce chronic cough include tuberculosis, lung cancer, bronchiectasis, and bronchitis. Often people tend to overlook, minimize, or self-treat chronic coughs. These persons should be helped to realize that coughing is not itself a disease, but rather is symptomatic of other disorders. *"Short-term"* coughs should always be investigated if they are accompanied by pain, shortness of breath, or production of blood-tinged sputum. Nonpulmonary disorders that may produce cough include otitis media, subdiaphragmatic irritation, congestive heart failure, and mitral valve disease.

In addition to the fatigue and loss of appetite that cough may cause in most persons, in some patients (e.g., with increased intracranial pressure or cardiac disorders) coughing causes dangerous muscular exertion or hazardous elevations in intrathoracic, intracranial, and blood pressures. These alterations may, in turn, precipitate such life-threatening problems as heart failure or aneurysm rupture. Severe episodes of coughing not only produce muscular soreness and pain, but have been known to fracture ribs.

Nursing observations concerning a patient's cough may be helpful in establishing diagnosis and treatment. Important observations to make and chart include:

- ▶ Factors that induce the coughing episode and measures that relieve coughing.
- ▶ Character of the cough, e.g., frequency, episodic, paroxysmal, productive or nonproductive, sound and depth (deep, shallow, whooping, rattling, dry, hacking, hard, croupy, racking).
- ▶ Time at which coughing episodes typically occur, e.g., "Patient coughed violently and productively upon awakening in the early A.M.."
- ▶ Events apparently associated with or resulting from the coughing, e.g., nausea, vomiting, decreased appetite, interrupted sleep, fatigue, pain, changes in vital signs, dyspnea, anxiety.

Effective Coughing. An effective cough is one in which the patient has been taught to use the diaphragm, posture, slow deep stacked breaths and short expulsive blasts of air to mobilize and expectorate the secretions.

Six steps are involved in creating an effective cough:

1. A slow deep inspiration to open the trachea and adequately inflate the lungs with air.
2. A quick tight closure of the glottis. This builds up pressure in the thorax. This is called a *Valsalva maneuver*. It increases intrathoracic and intra-abdominal pressure, necessary to insure the production of a force great enough to expel the bolus of mucus and debris.
3. Contraction of both the intercostal and abdominal muscles, causing compression of the thoracic and abdominal cavities.
4. At peak intrathoracic pressure, the glottis is opened.
5. The open glottis creates a pressure difference between the abdomen (higher) and the thorax (lower). The diaphragm is pushed upwards.
6. The motion of the diaphragm produces a violent and explosive current of air. This air flow is often called a "pillar of air."

The preceding steps are necessary to assure that the muscular energy expended by the patient is not wasted.

The nurse must teach the patient the proper method of coughing. To aid the patient in understanding what is required, phrases like "get air behind the mucus," "cough from your boots," and "pillar of air" often help illustrate your instructions.

Forced coughing may cause adverse effects in patients with severe chronic lung disease. The forced cough may collapse airways, resulting in air trapping, or it may cause a rupture of thin-walled alveoli (blebs). A pneumothorax could be produced. Patients with unstable cardiac and cerebral function must also be cautioned against forced coughing.

Measures to facilitate effective coughing include:

- *Changing positions*. Roll the patient from side to side to promote drainage of secretions into the large airways.
- *Increase the patient's level of activity*. Place the patient in a chair; ambulate the patient. Encourage deep breathing and slow exhalation during ambulation.
- *Prolongation of exhalation*. Breathing in through the nose and exhaling through pursed lips. Exhalation should continue until secretions are moved to one of the tracheobronchial cough reflex centers and a cough is elicited.
- *Vibrations/End-expiratory assist*. The nurse's hands are placed around the lower ribs. As the patient exhales or coughs, firm, upward vibrating pressure is applied. This method often supports the thorax enough to assist the patient to achieve an expulsive cough and expel secretions.
- *Sips of water*. A few sips of water may stimulate a cough.
- *Discuss alternatives to coughing*. The alternatives include suctioning.
- *Manual stimulated cough*. The patient is given a deep inflation with a manual self-inflating resuscitation bag. This often loosens secretions and promotes a cough in the patient with an artificial airway.
- *Splinting*. Place a pillow over the patient's abdomen. During exhalation have the patient press firmly against the pillow and cough. At the same time, the nurse may support either the abdomen or thorax to assist the expulsive cough.

Caring for a Patient with a Cough

Effective clinical care of a patient with a cough is based on consideration of the patient's condition and the cause and character of the cough. When possible, cough is relieved by treating the underlying disorder. A patient who is coughing and expectorating is potentially infectious; therefore, personnel must take appropriate precautions when giving patient care. These precautions include: (1) instructing the patient to cover the mouth and nose with a tissue when coughing and to properly discard the tissue afterward, (2) teaching the patient how to correctly use sputum containers, (3) practicing appropriate self-protective measures, e.g., maintaining one's own level of health, wearing mask and/or gown if indicated, staying out of the direct line of a patient's cough, properly handling and disposing of contaminated sputum containers and tissues, and practicing thorough handwashing before and after caring for the patient. (See Chapter 55.)

Factors important in caring for patients with chronic coughs include: (1) minimizing respiratory irritants in the air (e.g., avoiding use of aerosol products, prohibiting smoking and use of powders); (2) providing uninterrupted rest periods; (3) administering appropriate medications (e.g., mucolytic enzymes, bronchodilators, expectorants); (4) relieving mucous membrane inflammation (e.g., by humidification of inspired air); (5) providing well-balanced meals; (6) increasing fluids to help to liquefy secretions; and (7) preventing respiratory infections.

Sometimes medication is prescribed to mildly depress a nonproductive cough. Note: *cough depressants are typically inadvisable if a patient has a productive cough or retained secretions*. Medications that depress the cough reflex act on the cough center in the medulla and are called *antitussive* medications. Prior to giving cough medications check the patient's respirations to see if they are "noisy." If rhonchi or other adventitious sounds are present encourage the patient to cough productively and clear the airway prior to administration of the medication. Also, instruct the patient not to take a drink soon after taking the medication, because the liquid swallowed will remove the soothing coating of cough mixture from the throat.

Often it is the nurse's responsibility to teach patients to breath deeply and cough effectively. Periodic effective coughing and deep breathing not only help to prevent secretion accumulation within the tracheobronchial tree, but also provide the lung expansion necessary for efficient breathing. Patients who should receive coughing–deep breathing instructions include all patients who have respiratory disorders that increase secretion production, have retained bronchopulmonary secretions, have chest injuries, are going to have or have had thoracic or high abdominal surgery, or have restricted activity and are therefore subject to the complications of immobility. Effective, periodic coughing and deep breathing can often prevent complications which might otherwise develop from retained secretions and poor pulmonary aeration. Details of instructing the surgical patient in coughing are given in Chapter 57 of this unit.

Coughing and deep breathing sessions must be performed as needed to maintain a patent airway. The patient should be told that coughing removes secretions from the lungs and that deep breathing reexpands the lungs and dilates the bronchi.

A deep breath is the most potent bronchodilator.

During the time patients are actually coughing and deep breathing, position them with the head and chest upright if possible. This position facilitates maximal chest expansion. During coughing–deep breathing exercises observe the patient's condition carefully, provide rest periods, and give appropriate emotional support. Auscultate the patient's chest before and after coughing and deep breaths so you can evaluate the effectiveness of the procedure.

A patient whose coughing produces pain (e.g., a patient with pleurisy or chest injury, or who has had chest surgery) usually tends to try to suppress coughing because it is painful. This may permit secretions to accumulate within the lungs and tracheobronchial tree. Such a patient benefits from mechanical support or "splinting" of the chest during vigorous coughing. Splinting is discussed in Chapter 57.

HYPOXIA AND ANOXIA

In its broadest sense *hypoxia* refers to a deficiency of oxygen in body tissues. This condition has numerous internal and external causes (discussed further below) and may be acute or chronic. When the tissues are virtually without oxygen, the condition is correctly termed *anoxia*. In common practice, however, precise distinctions are not made between a deficiency and a total lack of O_2 and, therefore, the terms hypoxia and anoxia are frequently used interchangeably. *Hypoxemia* means a deficiency in the O_2 content of the blood (arterial blood usually). If correctly used, *anoxemia* would mean the complete lack of O_2 in the blood.

Effects of Anoxia. Anoxia produces irreversible tissue damage and, ultimately, tissue death. The length of time that passes before these changes occur varies, depending upon the affected tissue's metabolic rate. For example, brain damage occurs rapidly if the brain is anoxic for longer than 4 to 5 minutes. The heart and retina are also highly sensitive to O_2 deprivation.

Classifications. Hypoxia (or anoxia) may be classified as follows:[78]

Hypoxic (anoxic or arterial) hypoxia: oxygenation of the arterial blood is deficient, even though the blood has a normal O_2-carrying capacity.

Anemic hypoxia: Reduction in the blood's O_2-transporting capacity, i.e., hemoglobin deficiency. (See discussion of the anemias in Unit XIV.)

Stagnant (circulatory) hypoxia: Reduced capillary blood flow prevents adequate oxygenation of the body tissues, even though the blood's O_2 content and O_2-transporting capacity are normal.

Histotoxic (metabolic) hypoxia: Impaired oxidative–enzyme cellular mechanisms prevent the cells from utilizing O_2. Even though the arterial blood may have a normal O_2 concentration, the cells may be hypoxic, e.g., if the cellular demand for O_2 is excessively high. Cyanide poisoning is an example of histotoxic hypoxia.

Clinical Manifestations. Clinical manifestations of hypoxia (anoxia) depend upon such factors as the severity and type of hypoxia, whether it is acute or chronic, and the prehypoxic physiologic adequacy of the involved tissues. Earliest indications of hypoxia include hyperventilation, tachycardia, and hypertension. Hypertension occurs because hypoxia induces increased sympathetic nervous system activity which causes tissue vasoconstriction and increased peripheral resistance. Other early symptoms of hypoxia are restlessness and possibly headache and slight confusion. Because of their relatively mild nature, the early symptoms of hypoxia may be overlooked except by the most careful of observers. (See Table 53–1.)

Cyanosis, a classic sign of hypoxia, is an unreliable indicator since it often does not appear until the hypoxia is far advanced, and, at times, may occur in the absence of arterial hypoxia. Oxygen saturations above cyanotic levels may exist in spite of severe tissue hypoxia. (Cyanosis is discussed below.) When hypoxia occurs in debilitated elderly patients or when it is of an advanced degree, the blood pressure falls to a hypotensive level and the heart rate markedly decreases (indications of failure of the sympathetic response).

The symptoms of *local hypoxia* depend upon the affected region of the body. For example, varicose veins may produce discoloration and ulceration of hypoxic tissues. Hypoxia of the lower extremities causes intermittent claudication. Angina pectoris results from myocardial hypoxia; hypoxia of the brain may result in attacks of syncope.

When hypoxia develops slowly and is *chronic*, the body usually adapts physiologically by increasing the respiratory rate and increasing the blood's oxygen-transporting capacities. Bone marrow (which is sensitive to hypoxia) increases its production of RBC's. The blood's oxygen-carrying power can be evaluated by the hematocrit and the hemoglobin level. Both may be elevated in chronic hypoxemia not caused by anemia. (See discussions of polycythemia below and in Unit XIV.)

Clinical Care. Clinical care of the hypoxic (anoxic) patient is directed at relieving the underlying disorder, increasing O_2 supply, and maintaining effective ventilation of the lungs. The patient is kept at rest to minimize oxygen needs. The effectiveness of O_2 therapy and the amount of O_2 indicated vary from patient to patient. (Oxygen therapy is discussed in Chapter 54.) Rest and the administration of relatively low concentrations of O_2 relieve many hypoxic individuals. However, O_2 therapy alone may be only slightly helpful in treating anemic, stagnant, or histotoxic hypoxia. Persons with these disorders require additional specific treatments. High O_2 concentrations may be indicated to correct hypoxia and maintain the oxygen requirements of the tissues. O_2 administration and need must be assessed and documented with an arterial blood gas determination.

In the presence of impaired alveolar ventilation (indicated by an increased $PaCO_2$), treatment is directed at maintaining a patent airway and mechanically assisting ventilation. (Respirators are discussed in Chapter 54.)

It is important that the nurse develop skill in recognizing *early* indications of mild hypoxia so treatment can be started well before there is danger of tissue damage. Severe dyspnea and cyanosis usually indicate that serious hypoxia has developed. Hypoxia is particularly serious in patients with head injuries, since it increases cerebral edema and thus elevates intracranial pressure.

Because morphine and sedatives depress respiration they are contraindicated in the presence of significant hypoxia. If these medications must be administered (e.g., to combat physiologic shock) it is important to be certain that equipment is at the bedside to assist ventilation if necessary and to observe the patient closely for indications of ventilatory impairment.

HYPERCAPNIA (CARBON DIOXIDE RETENTION)

The retention of CO_2, with pH below 7.35, produces respiratory acidosis. (See Chapter 12.) Pulmonary disorders may produce hypercapnia as a result of severe airway obstruction, e.g., secretions blocking large portions of the tracheobronchial tree or severe bronchospasm. If the arterial pCO_2 ($PaCO_2$) rises suddenly and markedly, the following symptoms may occur: tremor, altered mentation, headache, somnolence, or asterixis. With extremely high acute $PaCO_2$ levels (above 65 mm. Hg) the patient may need constant stimulation to breathe. Unless respiratory acidosis is corrected early, continuous mechanical ventilation is necessary. Patients with chronic lung disease may tolerate higher $PaCO_2$ levels as the CO_2 retention occurred progressively over a period of time, allowing the regulatory mechanisms of respiration to be reset.

Severe hypercapnia narcotizes the respiratory center in the medulla. When this happens the respiratory drive then originates from the peripheral chemoreceptors, i.e., carotid and aortic bodies. These chemoreceptors are sensitive to the low PaO_2. High concentrations of oxygen must be avoided in treatment, or else this hypoxic respiratory drive will be suppressed. Controlled-flow oxygen therapy is given according to the patient's requirements, as indicated by blood gases.

CYANOSIS

Cyanosis is a bluish discoloration of the skin, mucous membranes, and nail beds which occurs with changes in the circulating blood (rather than from pigmentary changes in the skin). Cyanotic discolorations may be gray, pale violet, blue, purple, or almost black. Although anoxemia is the most common cause of cyanosis, this discoloration may also result from other pulmonary or extrapulmonary factors, occurring singly or in combination. Pulmonary abnormalities that may produce cyanosis include insufficient alveolar ventilation, impaired diffusion from alveoli to capillaries, and abnormal perfusion-ventilation relationships. Pulmonary and extrapulmonary disorders that produce severe cyanosis include advanced chronic pulmonary disease, polycythemia, congestive heart failure, and some congenital cardiovascular defects.

As mentioned previously, *cyanosis is not a reliable indication of hypoxia*. In cyanosis resulting from a lack of O_2 in the blood the presence and depth of the cyanotic discoloration results from the amount of reduced hemoglobin (Hgb) present in the blood. Cyanosis does not appear until an excess of reduced Hgb is present, i.e., 5 Gm. or more of reduced Hgb/100 ml. of blood. A marked and even dangerous reduction of arterial O_2 tension (PaO_2) can occur before observable cyanosis appears. Cyanosis usually develops when the blood is about 85 per cent saturated with O_2 (PaO_2 about 50 mm. Hg). In patients with anemic or histotoxic hypoxia, severe hypoxemia may occur without cyanosis. In contrast to this situation, only slight hypoxemia may produce cyanosis in a patient with polycythemia. See the discussion of assessment of color changes in dark-skinned patients in Chapter 52.

POLYCYTHEMIA

Disorders causing chronic pulmonary insufficiency (e.g., chronic obstructive pulmonary diseases) produce chronic hypoxemia (anoxemia). In turn, chronic hypoxemia often causes an impressive increase in the total erythrocyte mass, i.e., polycythemia. The polycythemia develops as a compensatory response to hypoxemia and represents the body's attempt to increase the blood's oxygen-transporting capacity by increasing the number of RBC's. This compensatory response is not without its problems, however, because the increase in the number of RBC's also thickens the blood, thereby increasing the likelihood of embolism and thrombosis and making it difficult for the heart to pump the thickened blood. Usually the disadvantages of the increased blood viscosity outweigh the advantage of increased O_2 capacity. Polycythemia is particularly dangerous in the patient who has cor pulmonale. (Polycythemia is discussed in Unit XIV.)

PULMONARY OSTEOARTHROPATHY

Pulmonary osteoarthropathy is also called *secondary hypertrophic osteoarthropathy*, or sometimes is loosely referred to as simply *clubbing of the fingers and toes*. Although such clubbing is one manifestation of pulmonary osteoarthropathy (Fig. 53–3), there are others, e.g., arthralgia and subperiosteal proliferation in the long bones. These changes in bones and soft tissues of the extremities occur in chronic pulmonary as well as nonpulmonary disorders (e.g., congenital heart disease, hepatic cirrhosis) and may also occur as a congenital trait. Pulmonary conditions that may produce osteoarthropathy include bronchial carcinoma, pulmonary abscess, and bronchiectasis. Although the pathogenesis of pulmonary osteoarthropathy is not well understood, it is believed to result from increased vascularity developing in response to chronic hypoxia.

COR PULMONALE

Cor pulmonale (CP) refers to the chronic or acute enlargement of the heart's right ventricle, secondary to a disorder of respiration (e.g., neuromuscular disorders of the muscles of respiration) or disease of the lungs or pulmonary vasculature. Most commonly CP is chronic and results from chronic obstructive pulmonary diseases, e.g., pulmonary emphysema, chronic bronchitis. A massive pulmonary embolism may produce acute cor pulmonale. Heart failure may or may not accompany the condition. Acute pulmonary infections or other conditions that acutely increase arterial hypoxemia may produce acute, reversible episodes of CP in patients with chronic pulmonary disorders.

Factors in the development of CP and right-sided heart failure may include: (1) reduction in the size of the pulmonary vascular bed as a

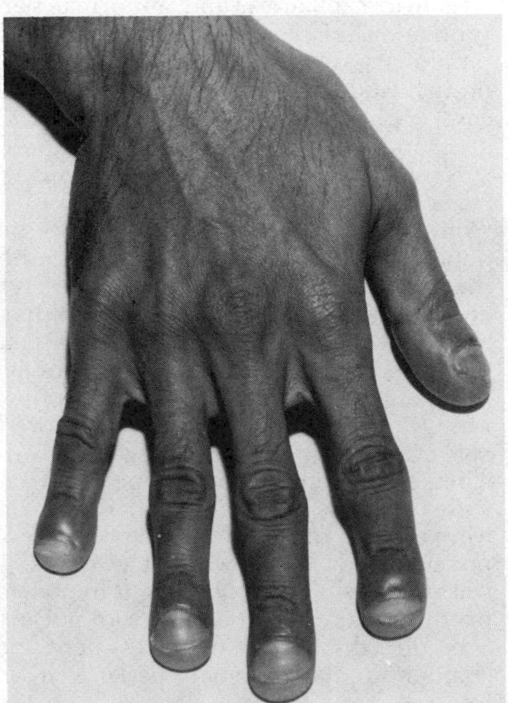

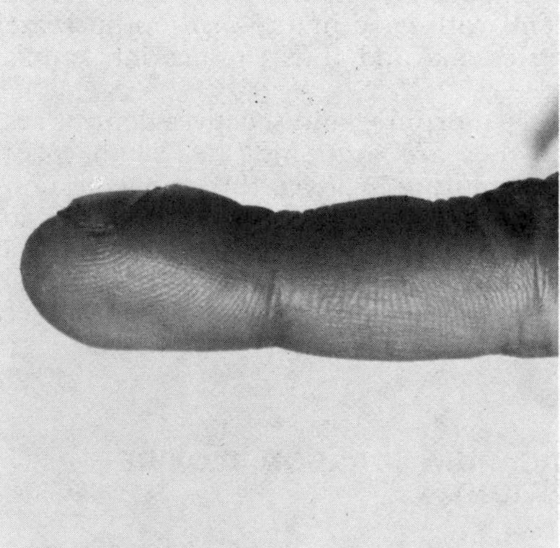

Figure 53–3. Top view of the right hand and side view of the index finger of a patient with advanced clubbing of the digits secondary to diffuse interstitial lung disease. (From Hinshaw, H. C., and J. F. Murray: *Diseases of the Chest,* 4th ed. Philadelphia: W. B. Saunders Co., 1979, p. 21.)

result of destruction of pulmonary capillaries or loss of large amounts of lung tissue; (2) increased resistance in the pulmonary vascular bed; (3) shunting of unaerated blood; and (4) the effect of reduced blood O_2 in causing pulmonary vasoconstriction and elevation of pressure in the pulmonary artery. The most common direct cause of CP is pulmonary arterial hypertension.

The hypertensive effect of arterial hypoxemia is increased by the respiratory acidosis that occurs with advanced chronic obstructive pulmonary disease. Arterial hypoxemia can induce an increase in cardiac output and produce a secondary polycythemia (which increases blood viscosity and volume). The hypoxemia thus exacerbates the effect of pulmonary hypertension.

Clinical indications of CP may include dyspnea, cyanosis, cough, substernal pain, syncopal attacks upon exertion, a loud pulmonic second sound (P_2), and a precordial systolic lift. In the presence of heart failure the patient develops orthopnea, peripheral edema, and distended jugular veins. With CP the chest films demonstrate the enlarged pulmonary artery and right ventricle. In advanced CP there is evidence on the electrocardiogram of right ventricular hypertrophy.

Pulmonary hypertension may initially occur only when pulmonary blood flow is increased (e.g., with exercise or fever), but eventually it becomes continuous. Hypertrophy and dilation of the muscle of the right ventricle of the heart then develop and eventually heart failure occurs. Right-sided heart failure increases the work of the right ventricle and reduces cardiac output. Many patients with chronic obstructive pulmonary disease eventually die from heart failure when the overloaded heart reaches its limit of muscular compensation.

The *treatment* of congestive heart failure due to CP is complex and may include O_2 therapy, sodium restriction, rest, diuretics and digitalis. Digitalis toxicity must be closely watched for because it commonly occurs in patients with CP. (Heart failure and its management are discussed in Unit XII.)

RESPIRATORY INSUFFICIENCY AND RESPIRATORY FAILURE

Respiratory insufficiency and failure are common clinical disorders. In simple terms, *respiratory insufficiency* means that respiratory function is inadequate to meet the body's needs *during exertion*. Exertional dyspnea is a common symptom of respiratory insufficiency and is caused by inability of the lungs to exchange gases efficiently during physical effort. *Respiratory failure* means that *even while resting*, respiratory function is inadequate; the lungs fail to maintain normal arterial blood gases because of thoracopulmonary or neuromuscular disorders that affect respiration. Focusing on abnormal blood gas levels as evidence of "respiratory failure" is analogous to identifying abnormalities of the blood urea as evidence of "renal failure." Most commonly respiratory failure develops as a continuation of unrecognized or inadequately treated respiratory insufficiency.

In spite of the fact that respiratory insufficiency and failure have rather precise definitions, it is not unusual to find the terms used interchangeably. For example, instead of saying that a patient is in "respiratory failure," some physicians indicate the patient is in a "severe or extreme state of respiratory insufficiency." Possibly the two states can most easily be envisioned as existing on a continuum progressing from mild respiratory insufficiency to severe respiratory failure and death (if unrelieved by treatment).

> *Early recognition and treatment of respiratory insufficiency is imperative to prevent development of respiratory failure.*

Etiology. Respiratory insufficiency and failure may develop from a wide variety of conditions. Basically these conditions can be divided into three major groups: impaired ventilation, impaired diffusion and gas exchange, and ventilation-perfusion abnormalities and venous admixture.

The development of respiratory insufficiency is illustrated in Figure 53–4. Frequent causes are listed in Table 53–3.

In *acute respiratory failure* (ARF), the lung is unable to maintain adequate arterial oxygenation with or without the impairment of CO_2 elimination. To determine the degree of impairment an arterial blood gas determination must be obtained. It is generally accepted that a PaO_2 of 50 mm. Hg or less and a $PaCO_2$ of 50 mm. Hg or greater are conclusive of the diagnosis. (Some use the term *ventilatory failure* if the pCO_2 is elevated.) Even verification of arterial oxygenation does not insure that minimal tissue oxygen needs are being met. Arterial pO_2's of 30 mm. Hg may be tolerated only for a few minutes. Other body systems will sustain often irreparable damage if their oxygen needs are not satisfied. The brain, kidney, and heart are first affected.

Persons with chronic lung disease who are clinically stable may tolerate pO_2's in the 50 mm. Hg range and elevated pCO_2's. These patients are designated as having *chronic respiratory failure.* Development of a pulmonary infection, heart failure, bronchospasm, and prolonged surgical procedures may undermine their stability and precipitate acute respiratory failure.

Acute respiratory failure may also occur with pulmonary embolism, pulmonary edema, neurologic conditions, chest trauma, surgery, and drug overdose (accidental or intentional).

Respiratory insufficiency often develops in two phases.

- A period of adequate compensation occurs in which the patient compensates for abnormal gas exchange by increasing perfusion and/or ventilation. Increasing the cardiac and pulmonary work in this way enables the maintenance of nearly normal blood gases.

- The patient enters a phase of inadequate compensation in which alveolar hypoventilation develops as a result of increased resistance to breathing. This phase is characterized by severe hypoxia and CO_2 retention. Also, secondary polycythemia, cor pulmonale, and tissue edema frequently develop.

The patient in chronic pulmonary insufficiency or failure may be able to compensate for a high $PaCO_2$ level for a while. However, this delicate balance can easily be upset if the patient experiences added stress. For example, the patient with chronic obstructive pulmonary disease (COPD) may be able to manage fairly well from day to day even though blood gas levels are not "normal." But if a respiratory infection develops (i.e., an added stress) acute respiratory failure may develop rapidly in which $PaCO_2$ levels continue to spiral upward while pH levels decline.

Clinical Manifestations. Because respiratory insufficiency and respiratory failure both result from impaired alveolar gas exchange, the predominant clinical findings in these disorders are abnormal arterial blood gas values. The abnormalities that may be present are *hypoxemia*, indicated by a fall in the arterial oxygen pressure (PaO_2), and *hypercapnia* or hypercarbia, indicated by an elevated arterial CO_2 pressure ($PaCO_2$). For practical purposes it is possible to identify two clinical patterns distinguishable by the presence or absence of hypercapnia: (1) hypercapnia develops only when hypoventilation and/or ventilation-perfusion disorders are present; (2) hypoxemia without hypercapnia may occur when the pulmonary capillary bed is reduced or the alveolar-capillary membrane is thickened. Symptoms of hypoxia and hypercapnia are summarized in Table 53–4.

Symptoms vary, depending upon the underlying disorder and the severity and acuteness or chronicity of the pulmonary insufficiency or failure.

The *early* cerebral manifestations of acute respiratory failure are anxiety, restlessness, dyspnea, and headache; *late* cerebral manifestations are somnolence, mental confusion, increased spinal fluid pressure, papilledema, and coma.

The following symptoms and signs indicate impending or actual *inadequacy of the muscles of respiration:*

- Gradual increase in blood pressure and pulse rates.
- Restlessness and irritability.

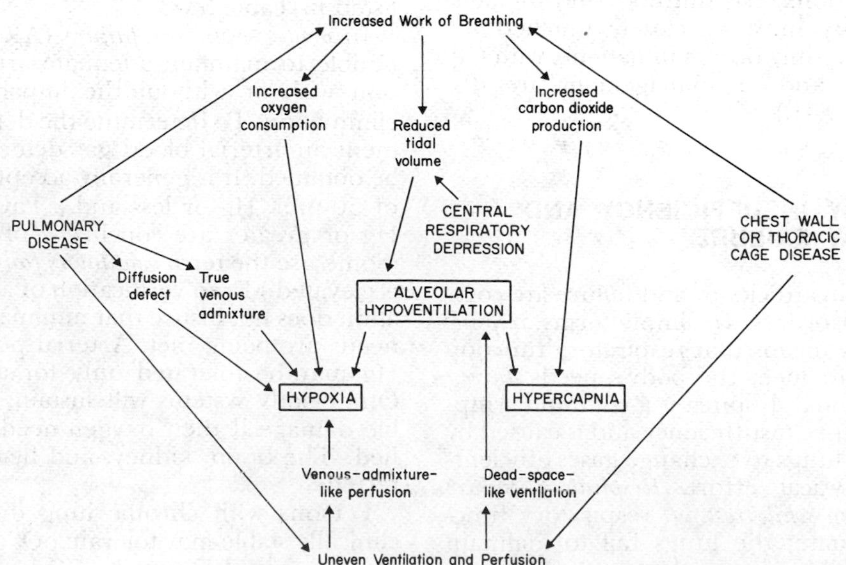

Figure 53–4. The mechanism of development of respiratory insufficiency. (From Cherniack, R. M., L. Cherniack, and A. Naimark: *Respiration in Health and Disease,* 2nd ed. Philadelphia: W. B. Saunders Co., 1972.)

- ▶ Shallow, rapid respirations with flaring of the alae nasi, i.e., the cartilaginous expansions that form the outer, curving side of each nostril.
- ▶ Inability to repeat three or four numbers without pausing for breath.
- ▶ Use of the accessory muscles of respiration or purely diaphragmatic breathing.
- ▶ Absence of normal retraction of the lower intercostal spaces during inspiration.
- ▶ Asymmetry of movement of the thorax, particularly with deep respirations.
- ▶ Inability to sniff (an activity related to the diaphragm).*

The nurse has an important role in observing for and promptly reporting symptoms of acute respiratory insufficiency or failure. *Early detection* of these disorders improves chances of providing effective treatment.

Diagnosis. In reaching a diagnosis the physician correlates clinical observations with knowledge of the patient's blood gases, pulmonary function tests, and the basic clinical disorder. Ultimately accurate diagnosis of respiratory insufficiency or failure requires demonstration of abnormal blood gas levels and pH values, since there are no specific physical symptoms upon which a purely clinical diagnosis can be made. The suggested figures for a diagnosis of pulmonary failure are a $PaCO_2$ of 50 mm. Hg or more, and a PaO_2 of less than 50 mm. Hg.

Laboratory tests are essential. Arterial blood is drawn as soon as possible for blood gas (PaO_2 and $PaCO_2$) determinations. This procedure is repeated with each change in oxygen administration or ventilation and each change in the patient's status, e.g., increased agitation or lethargy, until the patient's condition is stabilized. These laboratory evaluations monitor changes in alveolar ventilation and are the only methods for accurately identifying dangerously abnormal levels. On the basis of laboratory findings therapy is planned to correct respiratory acidosis and to ensure adequate oxygenation of body tissues.

Simple spirometric measurements may be performed at the bedside. Usually a chest film, electrocardiogram, sputum culture and sensitivity, blood count, and determination of blood electrolytes are also ordered while emergency care is being given. The hematocrit is useful in detecting a reduced O_2-carrying capacity (anemia) or an excessive increase in the number of RBC's (polycythemia). Although polycythemia may result from increased bone marrow activity in response to chronic hypoxemia, it may also be due to hemoconcentration resulting from dehydration.

TABLE 53–3. FREQUENT CAUSES OF ACUTE RESPIRATORY INSUFFICIENCY

Airway obstruction
Foreign body: aspiration, vomitus, trauma
Inflammation: epiglottitis, laryngitis, asthma, "croup"
Airway burns: heat or chemicals
Chronic obstructive lung disease
Fibrocystic disease
Pulmonary edema
Drowning or near-drowning
Restriction of thoracic cage or damage to pleura
Flail chest
Multiple rib fractures
Penetrating wounds of chest
Ruptured diaphragm
Spontaneous or traumatic pneumothorax
Abdominal surgery
Ascites
Peritonitis
Severe obesity
Kyphoscoliosis
Spinal arthritis
Neuromuscular inadequacy
CNS depression: drugs, trauma, CVA, uncontrolled O_2 therapy
Coma: diabetic, uremic, etc.
Diseases: Guillain-Barré syndrome, polio, multiple sclerosis, myasthenia gravis
Myoneural junction involvement
Toxins: botulism, tetanus
Organophosphates (insecticides)
Parenchymal disease
Traumatic: pulmonary contusion, "shock lung"
Tumors: benign or malignant
Disturbances of pulmonary perfusion
Emboli, fat emboli
Pulmonary hypertension

From Sweetwood, H.: Acute respiratory insufficiency: How to recognize this emergency . . . how to treat it. *Nursing 77,* 7:24, Dec. 1977.

TABLE 53–4. CLINICAL MANIFESTATIONS OF RESPIRATORY FAILURE

Hypoxia	Hypercapnia
Restlessness: impaired motor function and judgment	Headache
Confusion, delirium	Dizziness
Unconsciousness	Confusion
Hypotension	Unconsciousness
Tachycardia	Twitching
Central cyanosis	Miosis, engorged fundal veins, papilledema
Warm extremities (vasodilatation) ?	Hypertension
	Sweating

*From Bigelow, D. B., et al.: *Medical Clinics of North America, 51*:323, March, 1967.

Clinical Care. Treatment of *chronic pulmonary insufficiency* is basically symptomatic and supportive. Clinical care focuses on the administration of oxygen to relieve hypoxemia, ventilatory assistance to control the $PaCO_2$, treatment of the underlying disorder, maintenance of effective tracheobronchial hygiene, prevention of infection, avoidance of bronchial irritation, and limitation of activity.

Correction of hypoxemia does not always correlate with the adequacy of tissue oxygenation. If cellular oxygen requirements are not met, hypoxia exists. The nurse must continue to assess the patient for signs of the adequacy of the cardiac output. If the cardiac output is adequate and no other conditions exist which would impair oxygen uptake by body tissues, the respiratory, cardiac, renal and neurologic systems will react normally. Some parameters that the nurse should monitor include cardiac output determinations, urinary output, pulse, blood pressure, ECG for arrhythmias, tidal volume (7 to 10 ml./kg. body weight), vital capacity maneuver (double or triple the V_T), arterial blood pH, and absence of or improvement in the clinical signs of hypoxemia and hypercapnia. (These aspects of care are discussed more completely in the section on chronic obstructive pulmonary diseases, Chapter 55.) Endotracheal intubation is indicated in acute exacerbation of respiratory failure superimposed on chronic obstructive pulmonary insufficiency.

Episodes of acute respiratory failure often may be prevented by the early detection and treatment of mild respiratory insufficiency. When acute respiratory failure does develop, the patient is best cared for in an intensive care setting staffed by personnel who are: skilled in observation and the performance of clinical care, which often involves the use of complex mechanical devices; experienced in dealing with respiratory emergencies, and aware of the pathophysiology of the disorder being treated. The intensive care unit should be equipped with the necessary therapeutic aids and monitoring equipment. The patient in respiratory failure is highly susceptible to infection and may therefore be cared for in an isolation setting at times.

> *Acute respiratory failure is a medical emergency which, without proper treatment, rapidly progresses to irreversible cardiorespiratory failure and death.*

The chances of successfully managing a patient in acute respiratory failure have improved in recent years as a result of increased understanding of the physiologic changes characteristic of pulmonary failure, perfected methods of clinical care, and the development of precise laboratory techniques for measuring blood gases. With the provision of excellent care, many situations may be reversed which initially appear hopeless.

Because untreated respiratory failure is a terminal event, questions often arise about the advisability of heroic treatment. If the physician knows the patient and realizes that heroic treatment will at best only restore a miserable existence, the physician may decide to treat the patient in a conservative, routine manner, e.g., insertion of an oral or nasal endotracheal tube to facilitate removal of secretions but no mechanical ventilation or other heroic measures. Factors that influence the physician's decision in this matter include the expressed wishes of the patient and/or significant others and the patient's history prior to the episode of failure.

Clinical care of patients with acute respiratory failure is directed basically at relieving hypoxia, hypercapnia, hypotension, and dyspnea by maintaining respiration and supporting circulation as necessary. Essential aspects of the management of acute failure are summarized in Table 53–5.

In providing *intensive nursing care* for the patient in acute respiratory failure, do not leave the patient unattended. Observe carefully for indications of significant changes, e.g., worsening of hypoxia and/or hypercapnia. Frequently assess the patient's status, i.e., vital signs, level of consciousness, effectiveness of coughing, as well as the V_T, respiratory rate and pattern, and the inspiratory force and vital capacity. If these values deteriorate along with the $PaCO_2$, continuous mechanical ventilation must be instituted. Chart and report appropriate observations.

Calm and reassure the patient while giving care. Hyperactivity increases O_2 requirements; relieve the patient's anxieties and fears as much as possible by acting in an efficient, reassuring manner and providing supportive mental care. If the patient experiences confidence in your ability to help he or she may be able to relax somewhat and to breathe more comfortably and effectively.

MAINTENANCE OF VENTILATION AND OXYGENATION. Position the conscious patient sitting upright in a supported, forward-leaning position. Instruct the patient how to breathe most effectively. Meticulously maintain a patent airway. Suction as necessary. Caution must be employed when suctioning a hypoxemic patient. The vacuum removes oxygen as well as mucus and may cause microatelectasis. Suctioning also stimulates the vagus nerve. Vagal stimulation and hypoxemia may lead to lethal cardiac arrhythmias. Check for upper airway obstruction and relieve it if present. Prevent aspiration. If the patient is stuporous or unconscious insert an oropharyngeal airway to prevent airway obstruction and to facilitate secretion removal (until endotracheal intubation can be performed). Perform emergency resuscitation if indicated.

Assist with bedside bronchoscopy, tracheostomy, or endotracheal intubation when these procedures are indicated. Bedside bronchoscopy may be required to remove mucus plugs or foreign objects from the tracheobronchial tree. At the time of bronchoscopy, specimens may be obtained and sterile saline may be instilled (to liquefy secretions).

Prevent depression of the respiratory and cough centers by medications or excessive O_2. Sedatives and narcotics that depress these centers are typically contraindicated in the presence of acute respiratory insufficiency or failure. However, if they are ordered, use these medications cautiously and be prepared to mechanically support ventilation, to artificially stimulate coughing, or to remove secretions via suctioning.

Oxygen therapy is started immediately to correct hypoxemia; however, precautions must be observed to prevent depression of the respiratory centers and further retention of CO_2. The danger of administering high concentrations of O_2 to hypercapnic patients has been discussed previously. Controlled concentrations of O_2 may be administered via a Venturi mask. (see also p. 1238). Nasal cannulas do not provide predictable O_2 concentrations.

Ventilation must be improved immediately. Be prepared to help initiate and supervise mechanical ventilation, e.g., with a volume ventilator. (See discussion of ventilators in Chapter 54.) Some patients do not require total ventilatory support but do benefit from IPPB treatments, low-flow O_2, and aerosolized medications and hydration solutions. Those in extreme respiratory failure require continuous mechanical ventilation via endotracheal tube.

A variety of therapeutic measures may be used to mobilize, liquefy, and remove secretions. (See Care of the Patient with Sputum Abnormalities, p. 1208.)

Treatment of Fluid-Electrolyte Imbalances. Excessive administration of parenteral fluids must be avoided; however, dehydration needs to be relieved by replacement of lost fluids. Maintaining body hydration helps to thin secretions. Activities useful in guiding fluid replacement therapy include evaluation of serum sodium and hematocrit levels, measurements of fluid intake and output, notation of skin turgor, and recording of daily body weight.

Serious acid-base imbalances develop when an episode of acute respiratory failure occurs in a patient who has chronic respiratory failure. Respiratory acidosis usually develops, and metabolic acidosis may also occur if there is severe hypoxemia.

The clinical features of acute respiratory acidosis are[92a]:

- Disturbances of consciousness, headache, restlessness
- Papilledema and asterixis (flapping tremor) (likely

TABLE 53–5. MANAGEMENT OF ACUTE RESPIRATORY FAILURE

1. Improve ventilation and oxygenation
   a. Insure clear airway by tracheal suction, oral or nasal endotracheal intubation, tracheostomy, mucolytic agents; combat bronchospasm by intravenous aminophylline, hydrocortisone, and nebulized bronchodilator
   b. Give oxygen for hypoxemia
   c. Humidification of O_2 or air, especially with tracheostomy or endotracheal tube
   d. Assist ventilation with IPPB device (cuffed tracheostomy tube when indicated); control ventilation with automatic cycling with or without muscle paralyzing agents
2. Treat cardiac and circulatory status
   Obtain history of recent medications, particularly digitalis, steroids; obtain ECG; treat congestive heart failure, arrhythmias, venesection if necessary for hematocrit of 60 or over
3. Combat bronchopulmonary infection
   Obtain sputum smear, culture and sensitivity tests; start antibiotic therapy; take chest x-ray film, by portable equipment if necessary, and compare with previous films
4. Monitor laboratory values
   a. Arterial pH, pCO_2, pO_2, SaO_2
   b. Serum bicarbonate, sodium, potassium, chloride
   c. Hematocrit
5. Attend to fluid and electrolyte balance
   Chart fluid intake and output; intravenous fluids, usually glucose in water; supplement potassium intake if indicated; intravenous sodium bicarbonate if needed for refractory respiratory acidosis

Avoid use of opiates, barbiturates and excessive digitalis.

Modified from *Chronic Obstructive Pulmonary Disease: A Manual for Physicians.* Portland, Ore.: Oregon Thoracic Society, 1965.

to be associated with hypercapnia, even when hypoxemia is controlled)

- Apnea or coma with gasping respirations
- Hypertension (in very severe instances hypotension may result from generalized sweating and vasodilation)
- Tachycardia and bounding pulse
- Cyanosis (especially likely to be found around nose, lips and nail beds)

Severe acidosis (pH below 7.15) is a life-threatening condition, sodium bicarbonate is immediately administered intravenously. After 15 minutes the pH is again checked and treatment is re-evaluated. It is not uncommon for alkalosis to develop *during the treatment* of respiratory failure. This may occur because bicarbonate levels are often elevated and bicarbonate excretion by the kidneys is slower than the excretion of CO_2 by the lungs (if the lungs are being mechanically ventilated).

The evaluation and treatment of electrolyte imbalances may be complicated by the effects of steroid and diuretic therapy and the presence of compensated respiratory acidosis and/or congestive heart failure. With compensated respiratory acidosis the patient may have a serum chloride level that is low in relation to bicarbonate and a low body potassium in spite of a normal serum potassium and, hence, a heightened sensitivity to digitalis. If congestive heart failure develops, the levels of sodium and potassium are commonly reduced because of dilution due to an increased blood volume.

Often potassium depletion is present in patients with chronic respiratory failure. If these persons develop acute respiratory failure the potassium depletion is seriously worsened and must be replaced. Potassium is usually not given early in the course of mechanical ventilation. When respiratory acidosis increases in severity rapidly, the pH falls, potassium leaves the cells, and total body potassium depletion may occur even though serum potassium is normal. These processes are reversed and the serum potassium may be low, once the respiratory acidosis is corrected. When normal ventilation is achieved, potassium may be replaced in the form of oral potassium chloride, because chloride depletion may also have occurred. (For complete discussion of fluid-electrolyte balance and imbalances see Chapter 12.)

TREATMENT OF COMPLICATIONS. Prevent the complications of inactivity.* Remember to give *total* patient care and not focus your attention exclusively on the patient's respiratory system. Prevent the infections that can be introduced if unclean respiratory therapy equipment or unsterile suction catheters are used.

If infection is present, e.g., tracheobronchial or pulmonary infection, administer antibiotics as ordered. In some instances antibiotics are ordered prophylactically, before culture and sensitivity reports are returned, to prevent superinfection. In treating patients who are critically ill, penicillin (or cephalothin) and kanamycin may be started; in less critical situations ampicillin or tetracyclines may be used. Often in chronic obstructive pulmonary disease, infection is the precipitating cause of the episode of respiratory failure.

Relieve bronchospasm if present by administering prescribed bronchodilators. Beta-adrenergic drugs (terbutaline, isoetharine, isoproterenol, metaproterenol, and others) and the methylxanthines (aminophylline) may be used in combination for optimal bronchodilation. Drugs are administered by the best route. In an acute state, the most rapid absorption is through the systemic and pulmonary routes. Some of these drugs are for aerosol administration only. Adrenocortical steroids are usually given for bronchospastic or inflammatory pulmonary disorders, via the IV, oral, and aerosol routes.

Correcting hypoxemia and acidosis, improving ventilation, and reversing the basic causes of the acute episode of respiratory failure are typically the most effective methods of treating right heart failure, if present. Other therapeutic procedures are to digitalize the patient and administer diuretics as indicated once ventilation is established. Digitalis must be used cautiously because, as mentioned earlier, the patient may have a heightened sensitivity to it.

Intestinal and gastric decompression may be necessary to relieve abdominal distention, which impairs ventilation by elevating the diaphragm.

Hydration is essential to facilitate airway patency and reduction of airway resistance.

---

*See Sorensen and Luckmann: *Basic Nursing: A Psychophysiologic Approach* for complete discussion of the dangers of immobility.

CHAPTER 54

COMMON RESPIRATORY THERAPEUTIC MEASURES

GENERAL MEASURES*

Posture; Positioning. People experiencing respiratory disorders can usually breathe most comfortably if positioned with head and chest elevated. Severely dyspneic people often need to sit completely upright; people with less severe respiratory distress may find a semi-upright position suitable. Elevation of the chest and head makes ventilation of the lungs easier by permitting the lungs and respiratory muscles to function without being cramped. Sitting with the shoulders slightly pulled back enables unrestricted movement of the diaphragm and, hence, facilitates diaphragmatic breathing. To position the patient correctly, place a pillow lengthwise behind the back and head. Do not flex the head forward with another pillow.

The person who is weak or severely dyspneic (e.g., during an asthmatic attack) commonly finds it more comfortable if positioned upright, using a padded overbed table to lean on. Place a pillow on the overbed table and encourage the person to rest head and arms upon the pillow while leaning slightly forward. Raise siderails if indicated and be certain the patient has call bell, sputum cup, and tissues within easy reach.

A person with a chronic respiratory disorder can breathe more effectively by maintaining correct posture while standing, sitting, or lying down. Encourage the patient to observe his or her posture in a mirror and to maintain a straight posture with shoulders pulled back.

Room Environment. Patients with respiratory disorders are generally most comfortable in a cool environment. Individual preferences concerning room temperature should be respected. Air-conditioning may facilitate respirations by keeping the air cool and fresh. Maintain an environment that is free of unnecessary air pollution, e.g., smoke, aerosolized room deodorant sprays. Adequate humidification of air is important to prevent drying of secretions.

Activity; Rest. Some respiratory disorders force the patient to modify normal daily activity patterns. With many acute disorders, e.g., influenza, the patient may need to rest in bed for several days but may return to the usual level of activity upon recovering. Chronic respiratory disorders may make it necessary for the patient to gradually curtail or modify daily activities. The patient may be advised to change to more sedentary work or to retire. Unless prohibited by the physician, ambulation and other activities are encouraged within the limits of a patient's abilities. Remaining as active as possible not only helps a patient's general morale but also prevents the complications that result from inactivity. (See discussion of activity in section on dyspnea in Chapter 53.)

Adequate rest is also necessary. Often it is difficult to obtain sufficient rest because of disruptive symptoms, e.g., dyspnea, cough. The nurse attempts to identify and to correct conditions that are inhibiting rest, e.g., positioning a dyspneic patient in such a way that breathing is facilitated and insuring adequate room humidification if a hacking cough is present. When prescribed, cough depressant medications given prior to the night's rest help to ensure a quiet night. Often planned periods of uninterrupted rest during the day are helpful, since respiratory disorders can be especially fatiguing.

Oral Hygiene. Frequent oral hygiene is important when a patient has a respiratory disorder, because cleansing of the mouth temporarily removes the unpleasant taste and odor of sputum. Oral hygiene is refreshing and makes the patient pleasant for others. Also, it may improve the patient's appetite and general feeling of well-being. When antiseptic mouthwashes are used, the number of pathogens in the mouth is reduced, thereby also reducing the possibilities of pulmonary infec-

*Many of these points of general importance are discussed as appropriate in greater detail elsewhere in this unit. Others of a basic nursing nature are discussed in detail in Sorensen and Luckmann, *Basic Nursing: A Psychophysiologic Approach.*

tion. Oral hygiene is essential following administrations of aerosolized mucolytics, steroids, antibiotics, and enzymes.

Nutrition; Appetite; Hydration. As noted, the patient with a respiratory ailment may have a poor appetite because of the unpleasantness of sputum production. Appetite may also be impaired because of dyspnea, fatigue, nausea, or other unpleasant symptoms. To enhance the patient's appetite, maintain a pleasant environment (e.g., place sputum bottles out of sight, replace soiled linens) and offer oral hygiene and handwashing before and after meals. Smaller, more frequent servings of food are generally tolerated better than three large meals. Gas-forming foods are undesirable, since they may restrict ventilation by producing abdominal distention. A variety of foods and liquids that do not form gas should be offered, so that the patient can have a choice.

Optimal hydration helps to liquefy bronchopulmonary secretions so they can be more easily removed (thick, tenacious secretions are difficult to cough up and expectorate), and to prevent constipation and fluid imbalances. The patient with tenacious secretions is encouraged to have a high fluid intake (3000 to 4000 ml. daily) and to be sure that a large amount of fluid intake is water. Milk products may cause thick sputum although this has not been proved scientifically.

Frequently it is desirable to maintain an intake-output record. When appropriate the patient may participate in keeping this record. If the patient's activities are restricted, make certain that ample fresh fluids are within easy reach at the bedside. Emphasize the importance of maintaining hydration and instruct the patient to develop a regular routine for taking fluids to ensure that daily intake reaches the prescribed amount. For the patient with chronically retained secretions, fluid intake may be assessed by observing the color of the urine. If fluid intake is adequate, the urine should be pale yellow. Fluid intake may need to be restricted in the presence of renal or circulatory insufficiency.

Infection Prevention and Control. Instruct the patient with a respiratory disorder to remember the following points of importance in preventing the development of new respiratory infections:

- Wear warm, dry, protective clothing if it is necessary to be outside in cold or damp weather.
- Avoid excessive exertion in very cold or humid environments.
- Maintain a balanced pattern of work, rest, and recreation.
- Avoid crowds during periods when respiratory infections are prevalent and where there is heavy smoke.
- Do not smoke.
- Follow the doctor's advice concerning influenza shots and antibiotics.
- Observe the sputum for indications of infection (e.g., increased amounts of sputum, change in color of sputum).
- Consult the doctor if a new infection seems to be developing.

The patient with a chronic respiratory problem should seek early treatment of any new, acute infection. Even those infections that appear "minor" must be treated vigorously to prevent the development of a progressive, serious superinfection.

The nurse has many opportunities while giving patient care to prevent the development of new infections or to control existing infections. Patients especially susceptible to the development of pulmonary infections include those who are bedridden or otherwise immobilized, e.g., in traction, paralyzed; in respiratory failure; tracheostomized; or being treated with respiratory therapy equipment, antibiotics, antimetabolites, or corticosteroids.

Opportunistic infections are of increasing importance. These may be hospital-acquired (nosocomial) or drug-induced, e.g., superinfections may develop during the administration of antibiotics, or infection may develop in patients receiving antimetabolites or corticosteroids. Nosocomial infections include those a patient may acquire from the use of contaminated equipment such as suction or urethral catheters or aerosol generators, room humidifiers, and other forms of respiratory equipment. The development of nosocomial infections from contaminated equipment indicates a serious error in technique.

To effectively control infections or prevent their development, the nurse observes prophylactic measures such as:

- Observing isolation, gown, mask, and handwashing techniques as necessary to prevent cross-contamination.
- Turning and repositioning patients frequently while they are in bed; encouraging activity, coughing, deep-breathing to mobilize secretions.
- Maintaining a clear airway and preventing atelectasis. When suctioning is indicated it should be gently performed and carried out as a sterile procedure. All care given to a patient's airway must be performed aseptically.
- Sterilizing respiratory therapy equipment frequently, e.g., IPPB valves, tubes, humidifiers.

Restricting the number of visitors or staff members who have contact with a patient who is susceptible to infections or who has a communicable infection.

▶ Protecting patients from persons with upper respiratory or other infections, i.e., from staff members, visitors, other patients.

▶ Locating patients within a ward in such a way that spread of infection is not promoted; overcrowding should be avoided and patients with communicable infections should be segregated from noninfected patients.

▶ Maintaining an optimal level of personal resistance and of resistance in patients, e.g., ensure adequate rest, nutrition, hydration.

▶ Teaching patients methods of preventing the spread of air-borne infections. For example, teach the patient to cover nose and mouth with disposable tissues when sneezing or coughing.

▶ Observing closely for indications of infections in patients receiving antimetabolites or corticosteroids and the development of superinfections in patients receiving antibiotics.

▶ Administering antibiotics as prescribed. Specific antibiotic therapy is based on bacteriologic culture and sensitivity reports. At times broad-spectrum antibiotics are prescribed before culture sensitivity reports are available.

Avoidance of Pulmonary Irritants. Chronic pulmonary diseases, such as chronic bronchitis and pulmonary emphysema, represent a major health hazard that has become of increasing significance in the past few decades. The incidence of lung cancer has also increased markedly during the 20th century. *Cigarette smoking* is related to the increase in deaths from these diseases and is the major cause of chronic bronchitis and lung cancer in the United States (Fig. 54–1). *Air pollution* may be an additional factor in the increased incidence of these devastating pulmonary disorders.

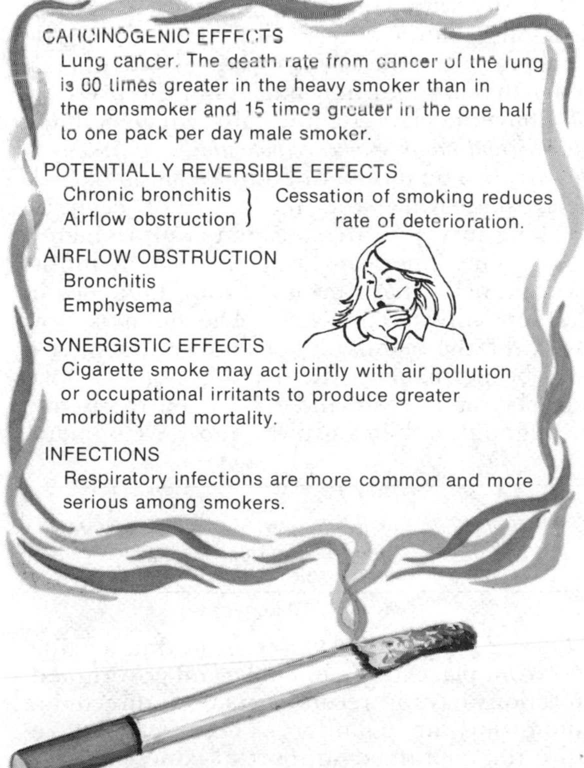

Figure 54–1. Hazards of cigarette smoking.

> *The one most important cause of respiratory irritation is cigarette smoking.*

Experimental studies indicate that certain gases in cigarette smoke and polluted air may damage bronchopulmonary function in the following ways: (1) cilia are destroyed, thus impairing the removal of mucus via action of the cilia; (2) mucous cells enlarge (hypertrophy) and secrete excessive mucus; (3) bronchial walls thicken and lose their elasticity; (4) alveolar-capillary membranes (through which O_2 and CO_2 exchange occurs) thicken; and (5) alveolar walls may rupture, producing large cavities in the lung parenchyma. These events cause numerous pulmonary problems. For example, reduced mucus flow, increased mucus production, and narrowing of the airways all contribute to *retention of secretions.* Retained secretions are an ideal site for the development of *infection.* Secretion retention and tracheobronchial irritation produce *coughing.* Narrowing and loss of elasticity of the bronchi produce *difficulties in moving air in and out of the lungs.* Expiration is usually abnormally prolonged and may be accompanied by wheezing sounds. Impaired lung capacity causes the patient to experience *dyspnea upon exertion.* Thickening of the alveolar membranes and breaking down of alveolar walls causes *impaired gas exchange.* Thickened membranes impede the transfer of gases across the membranes; normally alveolar membranes are extremely thin, delicate structures. Destruction of the alveolar walls not only reduces the amount of alveolar membrane surface available for gas exchange, but also reduces the blood supply coursing through the lungs because destruction of alveolar walls destroys the capillaries within the walls.

Cigarette smoking and air pollution are preventable situations; however, their prevention is not easily achieved. Habitual cigarette smoking is a practice that involves complex psychosocial-economic factors. The manufacturing and sale of cigarettes is financially a profitable business. Legislators are reluctant to prohibit by law behavior such as smoking.

Smoking is clearly contraindicated in the presence of bronchopulmonary and numerous other disorders involving the heart, blood vessels, stomach, trachea, and larynx. However, habitual smokers with such disorders often find it extremely difficult, perhaps impossible, to stop smoking. Nurses participate actively, but not judgmentally, in trying to help patients to stop smoking by providing encouragement and education. Educational materials designed for patient use may be obtained from agencies such as the American Heart Association, American Cancer Society, the American Lung Association, and equivalent organizations in other countries. Numerous opportunities arise for nurses to present factual information about cigarette smoking to patients as well as community members. Of course, nurses who refrain from smoking encourage others to make a similar individual decision. It is especially important for young people to be convinced that they should never begin to smoke.

For example, a man with a pulmonary disorder who smokes may believe that his condition will not improve if he discontinues cigarette smoking. He should be told that if he stops smoking he may prevent or at least slow down further deterioration of lung function, his cough should decrease, and his sputum production will decrease in amount. He should understand that if he cannot completely stop smoking it is certainly desirable to reduce the number of cigarettes smoked and to stop inhaling. However, smoking even one cigarette can worsen the symptoms of pulmonary disorders by causing bronchospasm and irritation of the mucosa of the tracheobronchial tree.

Smoking threatens health not only because of its relationship to lung cancer but also because it is a factor in other serious disorders. For example, smoking is known to be a factor in cardiac and circulatory disorders. Also, the mortality ratio of cigarette smokers compared with nonsmokers is high in other disorders such as oral cancer, peptic ulcer, and cancer of the larynx and esophagus.

> *"The life expectancy of an average 30-yr-old who smokes 15 cigarettes/day is shortened by more than 5 yr. The incidence of cigarette smoking in the USA declined somewhat after 1964 when the health risks associated with smoking were first widely stressed, but it is again on the increase and poses one of the greatest public health problems in the Western World."*[16]

During the process of breaking the habit of smoking the ex-smoker may be quite irritable and nervous. The physician may prescribe a tranquilizer as a means of helping the patient through this difficult time. A person trying to stop smoking should be assisted to find ways of relieving anxieties and tensions other than by smoking. For example, physical activities such as exercising or performing small repetitive motor movements (chewing gum, or handling a pen or pencil) may be helpful. Or the patient may obtain some relief by periodically inhaling deeply, as if inhaling from a cigarette. Assistance, encouragement, and understanding given the patient by others during the withdrawal period can be very helpful. Even if the patient occasionally "slips" and "lights up," the overall progress made in cutting down on smoking should be praised. People who are trying to stop smoking should not be treated like children (e.g., "scolded") if they smoke. They are in the process of making a serious adult decision upon which their lives may depend.

As mentioned, some people cannot stop smoking. Psychosocial reasons that are difficult to identify, and that may be more important to the involved individuals than health and life, compel them to continue smoking. These people may become highly defensive about their smoking, even though they may inwardly be deeply distressed about being unable to control their own behavioral patterns. Feelings of guilt, depression, and loss of self-esteem often occur when such persons develop illnesses that they view as self-inflicted as a result of habitual smoking, e.g., lung cancer, chronic bronchitis.

Smoking can be viewed as both a private and a public concern, since cigarette smoke not only "pollutes" the body of the smoker but also contributes to general air pollution around the smoker and thus affects other persons. Increasing attempts are being made to permit nonsmokers to be segregated from smokers if they so wish.

Persons who smoke increase their risk of developing lung cancer 14-fold. Not only do smokers suffer the harmful side effects of cigarette smoking, but nonsmokers in the presence of a burning cigarette must also inhale polluted air. *Second-hand smoke is potentially hazardous to the airway.* The number of adult male smokers is decreasing while the incidence of cigarette smoking in young persons and adult women is rising. The American Lung Association and its local branches have been a strong influence in the new anti-smoking laws. The public is now aware of the rights of nonsmokers. If success is to be permanent, the decision not to smoke must be made early and reinforced frequently throughout a child's growth and development.

> *"Cigarette smoking would seem to be a deep-seated death wish, a true twentieth century plague."*[9a]

General air pollution varies from time to time and from place to place. Public and governmental actions have in recent years been directed at minimizing air pollution. These activities require the continued support of concerned citizens. It has been clearly demonstrated that

LUNGS
AT WORK
NO SMOKING
YOUR LUNG ASSOCIATION
The "Christmas Seal" People

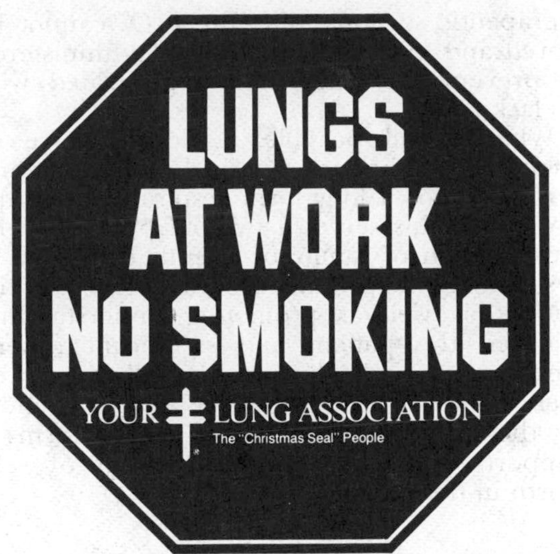

Figure 54–2. Local Lung Associations distribute this and other antismoking materials without charge.

acute episodes of air pollution, e.g., in heavily industrialized communities, are associated with increased death and illness rates. These rates are particularly high among persons with chronic cardiac and pulmonary disorders. Persons with such disturbances who live or work in environments that have a high level of air pollution may be advised by their physicians to move or to change occupations.

Other pulmonary irritants that should be avoided by persons with pulmonary disorders are airborne allergens, excessively cold or dry air, and all aerosolized products, e.g., spray deodorants, hair sprays. (See discussions elsewhere in this unit.)

Nurse-Patient Relationships. Chronic pulmonary disorders and cancer of the lung are examples of some respiratory conditions that may be especially difficult for patients to accept. As previously mentioned, patients with these disorders who have smoked heavily for a number of years often have feelings of guilt and anger about the possible association of their smoking habits with their illnesses. The nurse is *not* being helpful in situations of this kind by adopting a vituperative "you should have known better" attitude. Both nurse and patient must have realistic attitudes about the patient's condition and set realistic goals. For example, lungs that have been severely damaged cannot be permanently or markedly improved in function. However, some improved function may be possible, and that degree of improvement may be enough to make the patient feel better and increase activity. An attitude of hopelessness on the part of nurse or patient is defeating. With encouragement and a sense of confidence, much can be accomplished, and symptomatic relief may be obtained even though the prognosis is guarded. Patients must feel that the nurse not only *gives* care, but also cares about them as individuals.

Some symptoms caused by respiratory disorders may be disturbing for both patient and nurse. For example, the patient who is producing large amounts of foul-smelling sputum may feel unclean and be embarrassed. The nurse may have feelings of repulsion when handling contaminated articles or when the patient expectorates. Some respiratory conditions produce life-threatening feelings of suffocation or choking, causing the patient to panic and fight for air. Events such as acute respiratory failure, crushing chest injuries, or chest surgery are often highly anxiety-provoking and may evoke concerns about dying. The nurse's attitude can help to calm the fearful, struggling patient while administering necessary care. The patient must be relieved of disturbing anxieties whenever possible since these feelings worsen such bronchopulmonary symptoms as dyspnea and bronchospasm.

The patient's behavior may be influenced not only by psycho-emotional disturbances but also by physical factors. For example, metabolic imbalances such as abnormal blood gas levels may affect behavior. Fatigue, caused perhaps by the effort of breathing or lack of sleep, may cause the patient to be irritable and depressed. The nurse helps staff members and the patient's significant others to try to understand what the patient may be experiencing and to learn effective ways of being helpful.

Numerous serious problems must often be dealt with by a patient with a chronic pulmonary disorder, such as socioeconomic concerns. Prolonged illness is expensive; the patient may need to pay for hospitalizations, physicians, and medications. Special equipment may need to be bought or rented, e.g., oxygen, IPPB machine. Illness may not only force the patient to leave work but also make participation in enjoyable social activities difficult or impossible. Infectious conditions such as tuberculosis may cause patients to feel that a stigma has been placed on their lives. Chronic respiratory disorders like emphysema impair normal sexual activity and thus remove the patient even further from a normal life pattern and the pre-illness self-image.

The patient with chronic pulmonary disease must learn to adapt to limitations imposed by the illness. The goal of care is to *preserve* existing lung function and make the most out of what lung function still exists. This is sometimes hard for the patient to accept. In this learning-adjustment process patients can be helped by others, and must also help themselves. When an effective, therapeutic nurse-patient relationship exists, the nurse provides services both directly and indirectly beneficial to the patient. In addition to providing help within the boundaries of the nursing role, the nurse participates in making referrals to qualified persons who are of assistance in other ways, e.g., social workers, respiratory therapists.

Like many other illnesses, chronic respiratory disorders, lung cancer, or other pulmonary disorders may be denied by the affected persons until symptoms eventually force recognition of the illness. Once they do seek medical care, some patients hesitate to participate in the recommended therapy programs. These reluctant patients must be assisted to understand ways in which therapy will actually be of benefit. Emphasize that therapy is helpful even though improvement may not be rapidly apparent. Patient participation in many aspects of pulmonary therapy programs is essential. Each patient has special problems with activities of daily living. These problems must be solved before self-care activities may be successfully taught. For example, hair grooming may be extremely difficult. Instruction in control of breathing and modifications in breathing patterns may be necessary before postural drainage and exercise can be taught.

Self-care activities may include performing postural drainage and breathing exercises, forcing fluids, taking medications, and administering respiratory therapy. Praise patients who faithfully follow their recommended therapy regimens and encourage those who feel discouraged.

Respect for a patient's preferred activity schedule is especially important when caring for a patient with a pulmonary disorder. The dyspneic patient may require frequent rest periods and usually knows when he or she can most comfortably be active during the day. The patient who is producing large amounts of sputum may require pulmonary therapy techniques, e.g., postural drainage, before getting out of bed in the morning. Nett and Petty observe that patients with emphysema may develop ritualistic, compulsive tendencies concerning their bronchial hygiene and physical therapy programs.[118] These tendencies should not be interfered with but rather should be viewed as useful and necessary for the patient.

Hypoxemia decreases visual acuity. It also impairs mentation and cognitive functions. Patients who are hypoxemic must be provided with supplemental oxygen. The oxygen must be administered during any instructive and therapeutic sessions. (Of course O_2 cannot be stored and must be continuously administered to prevent the complications associated with O_2 lack.)

When at all possible, a close relative or friend should be included in the planning and instruction of a long-term respiratory therapy program. This serves a twofold purpose. The participation of family or friends can serve as a source of help and encouragement for the patient as well as promoting understanding between the patient and significant others. The person with chronic lung disease often feels a burden to others. The encouragement by the nurse and significant others forms a support system to promote feelings of self-worth in the patient.

PHARMACOLOGIC AGENTS

A variety of pharmacologic agents may be used to treat patients with pulmonary disorders. Some of the more common of these drugs are presented briefly in the following overview. Medications are discussed further throughout the unit in relation to specific conditions. Space does not permit detailed discussions of individual medications, consult a textbook of pharmacology for necessary details.

Antihistamines. Antihistamines are used to treat disorders caused by allergic reactions, e.g., bronchial asthma. Examples of antihistamines include brompheniramine maleate (Dimetane), chlorpheniramine maleate (Chlor-Trimeton), diphenhydramine hydrochloride (Benadryl), and tripelennamine citrate (Pyribenzamine). Drug hypersensitivity is discussed in Chapter 11.

Antimicrobials. Examples of antimicrobials used to combat pulmonary infections are tetracyclines, penicillin, cephalosporin antibiotics (cephalothin, Keflin), streptomycin, sulfonamides, and erythromycin. At times antibiotics are administered via aerosol to treat tracheobronchial infections, so that the particles of the drug may reach the air passages.

Antibiotics most commonly administered via aerosol are Polymixin B, Kanamycin, and Colistin. They have the same side effects by aerosol as they do if administered by more traditional routes. Oral hygiene is very important following aerosolization of antimicrobials.

Bronchodilators. Bronchodilating agents are administered via several different routes: IV, subcutaneously, rectally, orally, or by inhalation (by hand nebulizer, in a premeasured pressurized hand cartridge, or in an IPPB device, or other form of aerosol generator).

Bronchodilators act *directly* on bronchial smooth muscle to relieve bronchospasm. They are commonly divided into two groups: sympathomimetic medications, e.g., epinephrine hydrochloride (Adrenalin), isoproterenol hydrochloride (Isuprel), and ephedrine sulfate; and theophylline preparations, e.g., aminophylline. In recent years this category has increased to include bronchodilators with a more selective action on bronchial mucosa and muscle and a minimum of undesired side effects. They are called *beta-2 agonists.* Currently included in this list are terbutaline, isoetharine, and metaproterenol. Atropine sulfate is at times used as a bronchodilator. However, its action differs from that of the beta-active drugs.

Other medications *indirectly* improve bronchial function; antibiotics and adrenocorticosteroids are good examples. Antibiotics combat infections that tend to increase mucus production and thus block bronchi, and adrenocorticosteroids such as prednisone reduce inflammation, which causes bronchial walls to thicken and thereby reduces the size of bronchial lumina.

Cough Medications. *Antitussive agents* inhibit the cough reflex in the cough center. Examples are benzonatate (Tessalon), codeine phosphate (methylmorphine), dextromethorphan hydrobromide (Romilar), and hydrocodone bitartrate (Dicodid, Hycodan).

Expectorants aid in the expectoration of secretions. *Water is the best expectorant.* Acetylcysteine (Mucomyst) may be aerosolized or instilled into the trachea to reduce the viscosity of secretions; glyceryl guaiacolate (incorporated in Robitussin) increases flow of secretions and reduces viscosity of inflammatory exudate in the tracheobronchial tree; terpin hydrate is used to reduce abundant sputum.

Many cough medications are prepared in syrup form. By reducing local irritation these soothing syrups may reduce afferent nerve impulses which arise in the respiratory tract. Cough syrups may be made by adding various medications to demulcents or emollients that coat and protect the mucous membranes. Instruct the patient *not* to take water for a while after swallowing a cough medication. Swallowing water (or other liquids, foods, or medications) washes the medication off the pharyngeal mucosa, thus circumventing the desired local soothing effect.

Enzymes. Enzymes are rarely used to liquefy secretions as they are extremely irritative to tracheobronchial mucosa. Some institutions may use pancreatic dornase (Dornavac) to help to liquefy thick purulent sputum by digestion or to debride the lesions of empyema.

Gases. Examples of gases that may be used therapeutically are carbon dioxide (CO_2), a respiratory stimulant (generally contraindicated in the presence of respiratory failure, cardiac decompensation, or pulmonary edema); oxygen (O_2), used to correct hypoxemia (in some situations high concentrations of O_2 can produce the serious problems of CO_2 narcosis, see p. 1238); and helium, an inert gas used as a vehicle for the administration of other gases, e.g., with O_2 or general anesthetics. Carbon dioxide (in 5, 7, or 10 per cent mixtures with oxygen) may be used to treat hiccoughs. Oxygen therapy is discussed later in this chapter. Light, inert helium (in an 80 per cent mix with oxygen) may be used to replace the nitrogen content of air; it is believed this provides a gas mixture that can be transported with less effort in the airways.

Narcotic Antagonists. Narcotic antagonists are used to overcome respiratory depression caused by narcotic drugs. Respiratory depression can be a serious side effect of narcotic analgesics, barbiturates, and numerous tranquilizers and nonbarbiturate sedatives. In some situations (e.g., chest injury, pulmonary failure) respiratory depression is a life-threatening complication. Examples of narcotic antagonists are nalorphine hydrochloride (Nalline), levallorphan tartrate (Lorfan), and naloxone (Narcan).

Respiratory Stimulants. Central nervous stimulants that increase the activity of respiratory centers include doxapram hydrochloride (Dopram) and ethamivan (Emivan). Stimulants are rarely used unless the cause of respiration can be rapidly reversed. Stimulation may only cause an increased oxygen need by the tissues.

Vasoconstrictors and Decongestants. Medications in this classification may be used to treat allergic reactions and are given by diverse routes, e.g., topically (as nosedrops, sprays, and aerosols), parenterally, and orally. Examples are cyclopentamide hydrochloride (Clopane), ephedrine sulfate, and phenylephrine hydrochloride (Neo-Synephrine).

PULMONARY PHYSIOTHERAPY

Activities that are part of a pulmonary physiotherapy program include breathing exercises, productive coughing techniques, and postural drainage with vibration and cupping. Emphasis is placed on teaching patients the above techniques so they can effectively participate in their own care and continue it as long as necessary on an outpatient basis. Significant others who will assist the patient with pulmonary physiotherapy at home are often included in teaching sessions. In many large hospitals and clinics, pulmonary physiotherapy is performed by respiratory and/or physical therapists. However, in other settings not staffed with these specially trained persons, it is often the nurse's responsibility to perform and teach techniques of pulmonary therapy. Even when physiotherapists and respiratory therapists are available, the nurse often becomes involved in the program by providing continued patient teaching, supervision and support.

Pulmonary physiotherapy is useful in the treatment of numerous respiratory disorders, e.g., bronchiectasis, chronic obstructive pulmonary disease, pulmonary emphysema, chronic bronchitis, bronchial asthma, and following chest surgery and chest injury. The patient with a chronic pulmonary problem should be told that it may take several weeks before the physical therapy program produces noticeable improvement. For example, it may take several weeks of practicing breathing exercises before a patient feels able to breathe more comfortably and with less effort. If the patients expect rapid improvement, they may become discouraged and not participate in the therapy schedule. *For pulmonary physiotherapy activities to be effective they must be performed routinely and diligently.*

For example, as a woman with a severe respiratory disorder learns the techniques of pulmonary physiotherapy she gradually realizes that *she can* relax and control her breathing; *she can* breathe more effectively during dyspneic periods (if she practices slow controlled breathing rather than breathing rapidly and forcefully); and *she can* feel generally better and improve her lung function by faithfully following the prescribed schedule of exercises and postural drainage.

Space does not permit detailed discussion of the techniques of pulmonary physiotherapy; breathing exercises and postural drainage will be discussed briefly. For additional detail, consult specialized references in the bibliography.

Breathing Retraining*

Acute or chronic respiratory dysfunction often predisposes a patient to poor breathing habits. *Breathing retraining* involves a number of methods designed to promote improvement in a patient's breathing patterns to assure maximal use of respiratory function. Breathing retraining allows patients to "get the most out of what they have," i.e., to improve the quality of life and breath. Breathing retraining teaches the patient how to *control* breathing.

Unlike other forms of therapy, breathing retraining must be learned and then performed on a constant basis. It must, therefore, become part of the person's way of life. Breathing retraining is not effective if practiced only periodically, e.g., 10 minutes four times a day.

The major muscles of respiration are the diaphragm and the intercostals. The diaphragm is a potentially strong, dome-shaped muscle, separating the thorax and the abdomen. During inspiration the diaphragm descends and enlarges the thorax (air rushes into the lungs); during exhalation the diaphragm relaxes, recoils, and moves upward toward the lungs (forcing air out). By learning to use the diaphragm properly, a person may learn to breathe more effectively. Patients with chronic and acute respiratory dysfunction can greatly benefit by learning *diaphragmatic breathing* as a means to control breathing. (See Fig. 54–3.) They thus obtain maximal beneficial effects from breathing. In order for breathing exercises to be most helpful the patient needs also to maintain the general muscle tone of the body by following a recommended program of regular exercises.

Prior to beginning breathing exercises the patient should attempt to clear the respiratory tract of secretions. The nurse helps as necessary, e.g., by suctioning or stimulating productive coughing. Aerosol treatments may be given immediately before the breathing exercises are

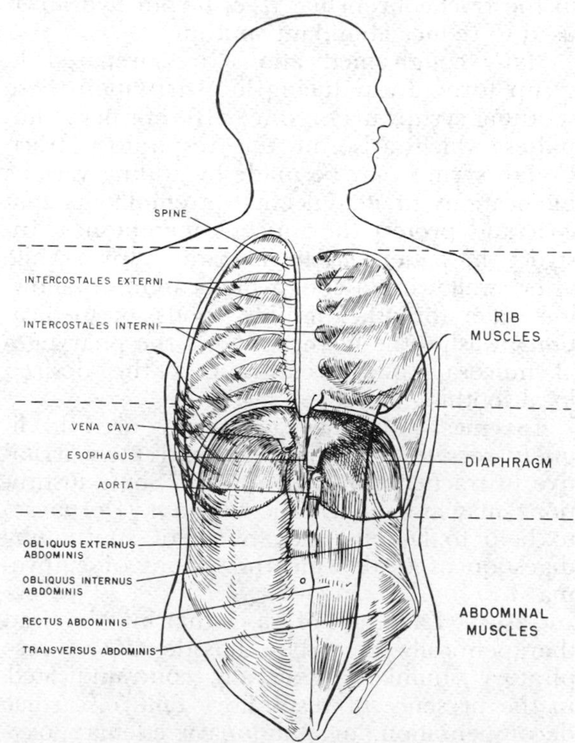

Figure 54–3. The most important of the breathing muscles. (From *Breathing . . . What You Need to Know.* American Lung Association, 1968.)

*See also discussion of a coughing–deep breathing regimen in Chapter 57.

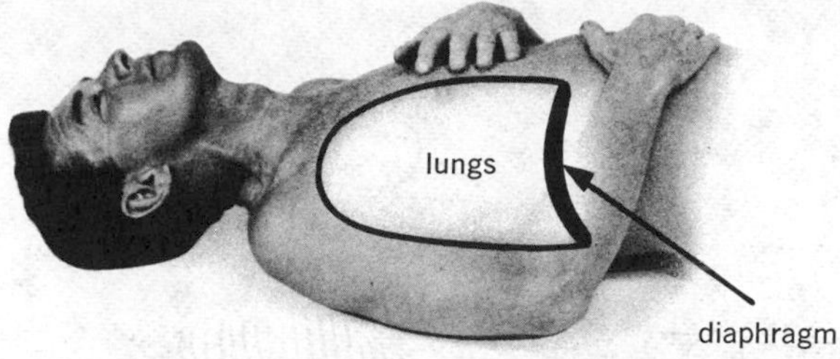

Figure 54–4. Basic position of hands during breathing exercises. The chest should move as little as possible. Note that the abdomen enlarges during inspiration and lowers during expiration. (From *Living with Asthma, Chronic Bronchitis, and Emphysema.* Northridge, Cal.: Riker Laboratories, 1969.)

started to relax and open the air passages and to loosen tenacious mucus. Following aerosol treatments the patient is encouraged to cough effectively. Postural drainage may be employed to help remove secretions. The nasal passages should also be cleared. If blowing the nose does not relieve nasal congestion, prescribed medications may be used to open nasal passages and shrink the nasal lining.

Many breathing retraining procedures are performed with the patient lying flat (no pillow) on a firm surface or in a position in which breathing is optimal. Breathing retraining must be adapted to the individual patient's needs. It must not cause undue stress or increase dyspnea. *The goal of retraining is to enhance breathing patterns.*

Abdominal ("Belly" or Diaphragmatic) Breathing. During abdominal breathing the abdomen visibly rises during deep inhalation and contracts during exhalation. With expiration the patient should feel the abdominal muscles tighten. Tightening the abdominal muscles helps the diaphragm to squeeze air out of the lungs. By placing one hand on the abdomen and the other on the chest, the patient can feel if he or she is breathing correctly while sitting up or reclining. The basic position of the hands during breathing exercises is illustrated in Figure 54–4.

How to Teach Diaphragmatic Breathing

To instruct a patient in the effective use of the diaphragm, follow the step-by-step guidelines outlined here.

- Place the patient in a comfortable and relaxed semi-Fowler's position.
- Place your thumbs in the patient's epigastric notch, i.e., just below the xiphoid process.
- Spread your hands around the patient's lower ribs with your fingers comfortably spread.
- Instruct the patient to *inhale through the nose* while relaxing the abdomen and while the patient *pushes your thumbs "out"* with her or his abdominal wall. By so doing, the diaphragm is being used.
- Instruct the patient to pause naturally and briefly at the end of inspiration. This effects a smooth pattern of ventilation and an even distribution of air into and out of the lungs.
- Gently press inward and upward on the epigastric notch with your thumbs as you instruct the patient to contract the *abdominal muscles during exhalation.* Instruct the patient to "purse" the lips during exhalation (discussed further below).
- Ideally, the length of exhalation should be two to three times longer than the time to inhale. This is especially important for patients with chronic lung disease as they have difficulty breathing out effectively.
- Do not excessively emphasize the amount of exhalation time. If undue effort is placed on counting, the patient generally becomes anxious. This leads to dyspnea and defeats the goal of breathing retraining.
- After the patient has mastered this exercise in a semi-Fowler's position, it is practiced and performed in lying, standing, and sitting positions and then during exercise. A weighted object (such as a 5 to 10 pound sandbag) or a hand placed on the upper abdomen will remind the patient to use the diaphragm.

Gradually the patient learns to adjust this controlled breathing pattern to the rhythm of body movements, e.g., walking. The person develops a rhythm to ventilation in which it takes at least twice as long to exhale as it does to breathe in. Some patients use a metronome to help them to establish this rhythm.

Various breathing exercises are directed at *forced exhalation,* forcing "trapped" air out of the lungs while using an abdominal breathing pattern. A method of forcing air from the lungs is to push on the chest with the flattened palms of the hands. Another exercise is to pull a band of material snugly around the chest while exhaling and relaxing the band during inhalation. Even tension should be applied during this exercise; the band of cloth should be a piece of tightly woven fabric (e.g., drapery pleating tape) that is at least 3 inches wide.

Pursed-Lip Breathing. One of the best techniques for controlling breathing is the use of pursed-lip breathing during exhalation.

In chronic lung disorders, the airways lose their elasticity and may collapse during exhalation — especially during forced or labored exhalation. When airways collapse, air is trapped beyond (distal) to the point of collapse. The patient is then unable to efficiently exhale and experiences a feeling of shortness of breath

(SOB). This may lead to anxiety which will, in turn, lead to further dyspnea.

The nurse may easily *teach pursed-lip breathing* to anyone who requires the ability to control their breathing. Instruction is conducted as follows:

- Encourage the patient to relax.
- Instruct the patient to breathe in through the nose.
- Then instruct the patient to slowly exhale through pursed lips, so that a "blowing" effect occurs during exhalation. "Blow out as if you are slowly blowing on the flame of a candle."
- Encourage the patient to breathe out through pursed lips slowly and completely for a comfortable length of time.

Pursing of the lips slows or retards the flow rate of exhaled air. This also creates a back pressure in the airway, maintaining "flabby" airways in an "open" position. This helps the patient to more completely empty the lungs, while preventing the collapse of the airway (see Figure 54–5). Pursed-lip breathing can be practiced during any activity.

Coaching is very important when teaching a patient breathing retraining techniques. Coaching involves instruction, demonstration, discussion and practice with the patient. When coaching a patient in breathing retraining techniques, discuss with the patient ways in which the technique will help, e.g., being able to be more active without experiencing the fear of being short of breath. Demonstrate *how to do it,* then have the person practice while you supervise. Maintain a soft, calm voice while repeating the steps of the exercise. Such a tone of voice helps relax the patient. Your genuine encouragement and praise can help obtain the patient's interest.

The main objective in teaching control of breathing is to allow the patient with respiratory dysfunction to obtain or maintain a sense of normality without creating undue respiratory distress. *As patients learn to control breathing, they gain the ability to reduce and control anxiety-produced dyspnea while preventing disease from controlling their lives.* The techniques learned by the patient must be applied in all situations, not just "practiced" on a scheduled basis. Pursed-lip and diaphragmatic breathing must be used while performing all levels of activity and activities of daily living. In order to fully achieve control of breathing and maintenance of effective patterns of ventilation, the patient must first learn to relax.

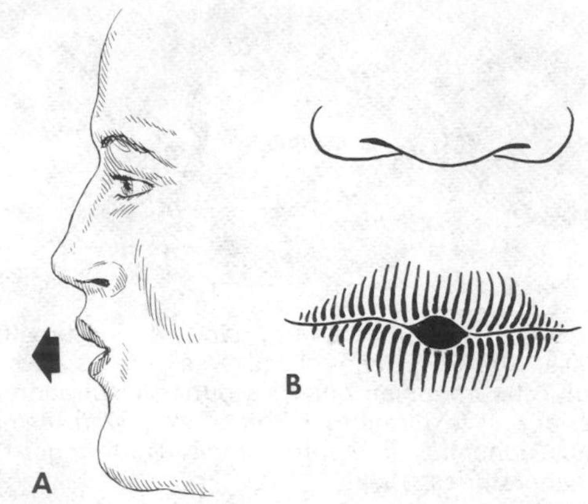

Figure 54–5. Pursing the lips has two advantages. Aside from increasing the pressure within the bronchus, it also prolongs the expiratory phase of breathing and converts the inefficient rapid panting into a slower respiratory rate which facilitates emptying the lung. This technique may be likened to gently blowing on a candle flame, so that it flickers but does not go out. (*A* from Dirschel, K. M.: *Nursing Clinics of North America,* *8*:617, Dec. 1973. *B* from American Lung Association: What You Can Do About Your Breathing, p. 29.)

Relaxation. Patient relaxation can be encouraged if staff members maintain an unhurried and calm approach to the patient. Tight restrictive clothing worn by the patient should be loosened or removed. The patient then assumes a position favorable to muscular relaxation and comfort. The recommended *dyspnea positions* (Chapter 53) are designed to facilitate breathing and the use of the diaphragm without requiring the work of other muscles. Patients should be shown these positions and then instructed to assume an appropriate position should they become dyspneic. Such positions will assist them in regaining control of breathing. Diaphragmatic breathing and slow, relaxed, pursed-lip exhalation are used by patients while in a dyspnea position.

If the patient requires additional assistance in relaxation, the following *relaxation exercises* may be tried. (See also Unit III.)

- Slow *head rolling* to the left and right in a circular pattern. Coordinate with breathing: inhale as the head goes from left to right; exhale on the head swing from right to left.
- *Shoulder rolling* (backward and forward) coordinated with breathing. Inhaling while the shoulder is rolling backward; exhaling while the shoulder is brought forward.
- *Arm swinging* (backward and forward) coordinated with breathing. Inhaling while the arm swings upward and forward; exhaling on the downward, backward swing.
- *Tightening all muscle groups* — from head to toe while inhaling. Relaxing all muscle groups while exhaling.

During these exercises, inhalation should be

through the nose and exhalation through pursed lips. The pattern of ventilation must be relaxed and unhurried and must feel comfortable. Exhalation should be longer than inhalation to allow for adequate time to empty the lungs of air.

Teach the patient to make a conscious effort to exhale slowly and as completely as possible. The patient may practice taking a deep breath, leaning forward from the waist and exhaling as completely as possible. Bending forward while walking also helps to make forced expirations possible.

Postural Drainage/Chest Physiotherapy

Postural drainage and chest physiotherapy (chest percussion and vibration) are effective therapies which have been in use for many years. These therapies are often used in combination with other forms of respiratory therapy to promote optimal respiratory function.

Proper *postural drainage* consists of positioning the patient to *effectively* drain particular segments of the lung requiring drainage to remove retained secretions. (See Fig. 54–6.) Postural drainage uses *gravity* to move the secretions from the affected segments of the lung. The segment of the lung which is *uppermost* (with its bronchus in the vertical position) is the section that will drain retained secretions into the larger conducting airways. There the secretions may be removed either by an expulsive cough or by suctioning. The various positions for postural drainage differ, depending upon the anatomic position of the segment(s) to be drained. Positions may need to be modified according to patient condition and tolerance. One example of a postural drainage exercise is shown in Figure 54–7.

Once properly positioned, the patient holds the position for 5 minutes or more in each position. Patients may require close supervision during postural drainage.

Stop or change positions during postural drainage when the patient cannot tolerate that position any longer; when no more secretions are heard, felt, or drained; when the patient's cough becomes nonproductive; or when the patient becomes tired, dyspneic or cyanotic.

Chest physiotherapy consists of chest percussion

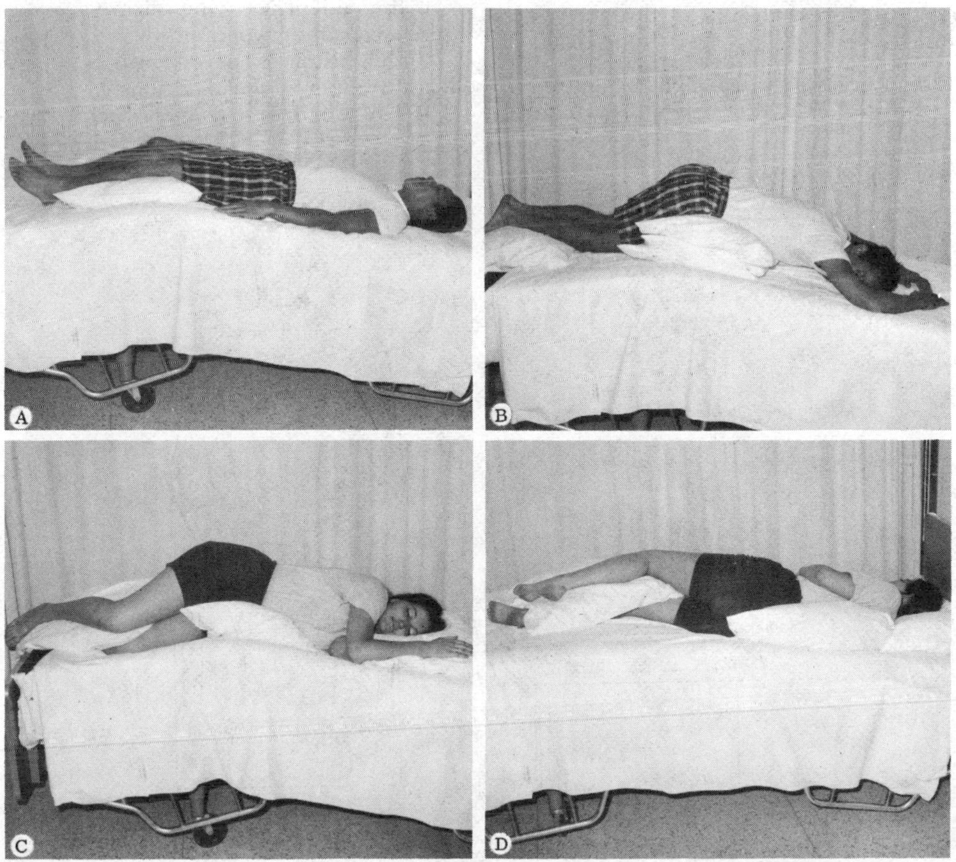

Figure 54–6. Some postural drainage positions. (From Krusen, F. H., F. J. Kottke, and P. M. Ellwood, Jr.: *Handbook of Physical Medicine and Rehabilitation,* 2nd ed. Philadelphia: W. B. Saunders Co., 1971.)

and vibration. *Percussion* is done by hitting the thorax with a cupped hand over the affected area. The cupped hand "captures" a pocket of air (see Figure 54–8) as it strikes the chest. The percussion loosens those secretions in the affected areas of the lung. The percussion must be performed directly over the affected area and should be performed with both hands in a rhythmical pattern. *The hands must not slap the chest wall.* A hollow, deep sound is produced when this is done correctly. The effective performance of chest percussion requires practice and direct supervision. It must not be attempted without adequate preparation and practice. *Vibration* is another method of using energy waves from the hand to move secretions from the affected portion of the lung. It is more difficult and requires demonstration and practice.

Indications for postural drainage and chest physiotherapy are:

- Preoperative patients with excessive secretions from any cause (chronic bronchitis, smoking, and so on).
- Postoperative patients with excessive secretions due to an ineffective cough (from pain, splinting, sedation, or obtunded mentation).
- Bronchial or lobar pneumonia which is productive of secretions.
- Lung abscess (if abscess does *not* involve the vascular system).
- Any disease process in which abnormal sputum may be produced and the patient is prone to recurrent infection (cystic fibrosis, bronchiectasis, chronic bronchitis).
- When bronchospasm or extreme tenacity of the sputum makes effective raising of secretions either difficult or exhausting (asthma, bronchiectasis).
- When musculoskeletal abnormalities interfere with the effective expulsive cough mechanism (scoliosis, quadriplegia, "barrel chest").
- When the patient is unable to initiate a voluntary cough (infancy, unconsciousness).
- When the patient is obese or otherwise a very inactive person.

Contraindications for postural drainage are:

When cyanosis or exhaustion are increased by its use.

If suction equipment is unavailable and the patient is unable to manage his or her own airway.

A patient with unstable vital signs, including increased intracranial pressure; any pre-emergent situation—medical or surgical in nature.

Contraindications for percussion and vibration are:

Over an area of known or suspected carcinoma or metastatic disease.
When bronchospasm is increased by its use.
When there is the likelihood of hemorrhage.
If the patient is having seizure activity.
When pain is experienced.
With a history of predisposition to pathologic fractures (use percussion judiciously).
If the patient is extremely obese (the energy wave

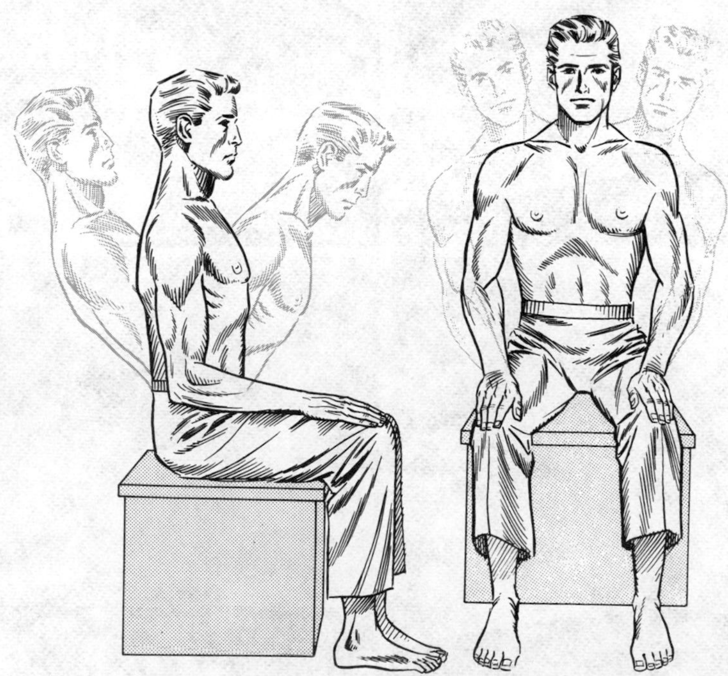

Figure 54–7. Postural drainage exercise to drain upper lobes. (From Secor, J.: *Patient Care in Respiratory Problems.* Philadelphia: W. B. Saunders Co., 1969.)

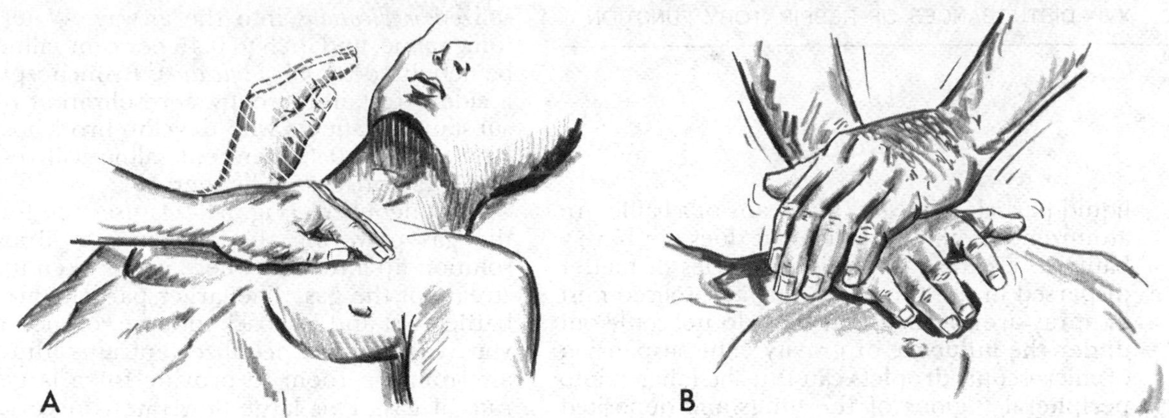

Figure 54–8. Positions of the hands for percussion (*A*) and vibration (*B*). (After Kurihara, M.: Postural drainage, clapping and vibrating. *American Journal of Nursing, 65*:76, Nov. 1965.)

will not sufficiently penetrate through the fat tissue).

How to determine the correct position for drainage:

X-ray — check the x-ray reports and position the patient in the drainage position for that section of the lung.

Auscultation — listen with a stethoscope to all areas of the chest. Low-pitched and rumbling noises can be cleared with drainage.

Hands — place the flat of your hand on various parts of the chest wall. You may feel the secretions vibrating through your hand when the patient breathes or speaks.

Trial and error

History — you may know by experience and medical history that a particular area of the lung is involved.

IMPORTANT HINTS

- ▶ Do not attempt chest physiotherapy and drainage following a meal. The session must be two hours after a meal or immediately preceding the next meal.
- ▶ Never percuss or vibrate over areas of soft tissue, the spine, or areas of increased pain.
- ▶ If many areas are being drained, schedule apical section drainage positions (sitting) in the middle of the series.
- ▶ If one position produces discomfort or dyspnea, change positions rather than totally stop the session.
- ▶ For maximal effect, the secretions must be loosened, the airways opened, and the cough effective and expulsive.

Patients cannot effectively perform percussion or vibration procedures on themselves but they can help to move secretions by making *tapping* movements on the chest. These movements, made with the fingertips of both hands, cause vibrations in the chest that help to dislodge secretions. Significant others can also perform tapping.

For a good summary of a bronchial hygiene program using physiotherapeutic techniques, see the article by Foss.[60]

RESPIRATORY THERAPY

Techniques of respiratory therapy are of vital importance in the clinical care of patients with pulmonary disorders and in the prevention of pulmonary complications in other groups of patients. Respiratory therapy, formerly known as inhalation therapy, is a relatively recent area of clinical specialization. The scope of this field is rapidly enlarging owing to increasing knowledge and improved therapeutic techniques. Activities of importance in respiratory therapy include maintaining a clear airway, e.g., via endotracheal intubation or tracheostomy suctioning; providing humidification of inspired air or gases; administering aerosolized medications via nebulizers; administering oxygen or other gases; and assisting or completely controlling ventilation via respirators, as well as performing various tests to assess patients' lung function.

Respiratory therapy procedures should be performed by trained therapists or by nurses who have received advanced instruction in the techniques. Space does not permit detailed discussions in this text of the specialized procedures of respiratory therapy, but this section provides general descriptions of some of the more common procedures. For additional information consult with respiratory therapists and refer to textbooks and manufacturers' instruction materials prepared for use with specific types of equipment. Endotracheal intubation and tracheostomy are discussed in Unit XXIV.

Nebulization (Aerosolization)

A nebulizer is a mechanical device that produces an aerosol, i.e., a suspension of solid or liquid particles in a gas, by means of a baffle. An atomizer is a similar device but does not have a baffle to create a fine mist. Particles of matter dispersed in the form of a fine aerosolized mist or spray are so small that they do not settle out under the influence of gravity. The suspension of microscopic droplets can thus be inhaled into peripheral regions of the lungs and deposited directly onto the tracheobronchial mucosa.

Nebulizers are used for airway *hydration* (discussed in the next section) and to deliver aerosolized *medications* into the airway. Water, isotonic saline, and 0.25 to 0.45 per cent saline may be nebulized for *humidification.* Bronchospasm is a side effect induced by aerosolization of any substance. Patients who develop bronchospasm from 0.25 to 0.45 per cent saline will respond better to antispasmodic therapy.

A jet nebulizer (Fig. 54–9*A*) uses the force of the gas powering the nebulizer to draw the solution up a tube to where it is broken up by a stream of the gas. The larger particles are then baffled out and fall back into the solution reservoir. Usually, the nebulizer entrains (draws in) air from the room to provide for a large flow rate of gas. This large flow rate is necessary in order to exceed a patient's minute ventilation to reduce the work of breathing and to insure stable concentration of oxygen. They are pow-

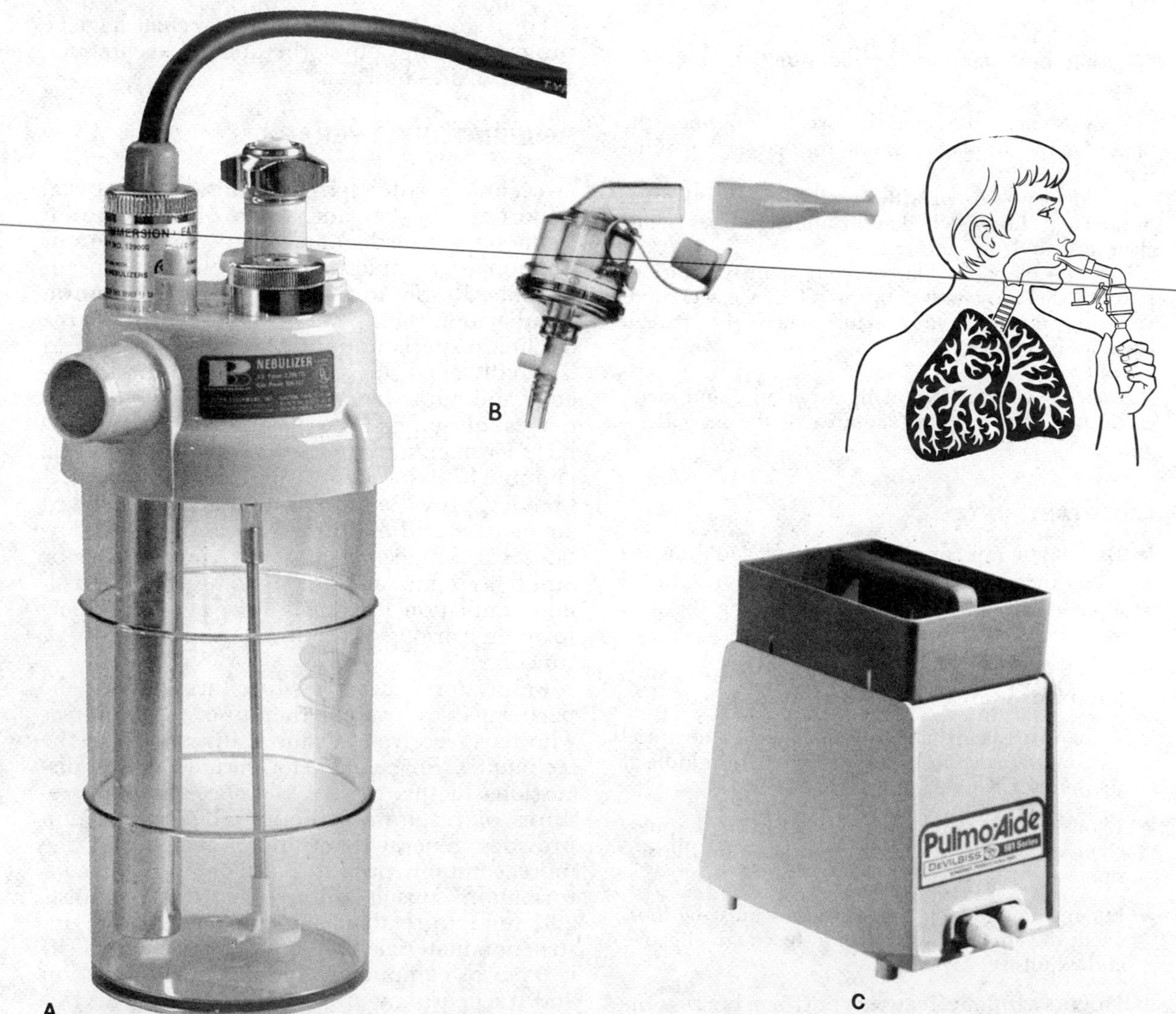

Figure 54–9. **A.** A jet nebulizer used to deliver large-volume hydration therapy. **B.** The hand-held nebulizer is the simplest form of small-volume nebulization therapy. Its major hazard is overuse by the patient. Since it is used to specifically deliver medications, adverse reactions or fastness to the drug may result. **C.** Medicated aerosols may be nebulized via compressors. (*A,* courtesy of Puritan-Bennett Corp., Kansas City, Mo.; *B* and *C,* courtesy of The DeVilbiss Co., Somerset, Pa.)

ered in various ways; the simplest is manual compression of the rubber bulb of an atomizer (Fig. 54–9*B*). The pocket-sized metered-dose cartridge nebulizer is popular. Other methods are compressors (Fig. 54–9*C*), compressed gas, or an intermittent positive-pressure breathing machine.

Those used for hydration are called *large-volume nebulizers* (Fig. 54–9*A*). *Small-volume nebulizers* deliver medications to the respiratory system and are often referred to as "dry" aerosols. Medications administered via small-volume nebulizers include bronchodilators, mucolytics, antibiotics, and steroids.

Ultrasonic nebulization produces particles of such extremely small size that they may reach the pulmonary alveoli. These minute particles are produced when high-frequency sound waves vibrate through water or isotonic saline. Ultrasonic mists can be fanned as a "cold fog" into tents, i.e., high humidity tent therapy, or fog nebulizers can be attached to oxygen masks or face tents.

Mist therapy is sometimes ordered prior to IPPB treatments or postural drainage. Some patients tolerate mist therapy better than others. The high water content of the air used for mist treatments may contribute to a patient's feelings of shortness of breath due to bronchospasm. Relief is usually obtained when the patient is able to clear airways of water-laden secretions or a bronchodilator is administered. It is important for a patient to be adequately prepared psychologically for mist treatments. Also, the patient should be closely supervised during these treatments until he or she becomes familiar with the procedure and experiences the benefits of mist therapy. Instruct the patient to cough effectively during and following the mist treatment. Charting should include a description of the patient's tolerance of the procedure (emotionally and physically) and the effectiveness of the treatment (e.g., amount of sputum produced). Complete charting helps the physician to determine the type and amount of mist that are of greatest benefit to the patient.

Nebulization therapy may be ordered as a continuous or intermittent procedure. Specific instructions are given by the physician relative to the amount of medication to be inhaled and the frequency of the nebulization therapy. If hand-powered nebulizers are used, a specific number of inhalations are ordered. If other types of aerosol generators are used, the treatment may take 10 to 20 minutes. The nurse or therapist must be alert for the development of adverse reactions to the nebulized medications. It is essential that the person administering the therapy also assess its effectiveness. For instance, if bronchospasm was evident before therapy, did the administration of the bronchodilator improve the quality of the breath sounds? Were adverse effects avoided? The evaluation of therapy is important and must be charted along with the therapy given.

It is the responsibility of all personnel caring for the patient receiving nebulization therapy to insure that the solution nebulized is sterile and that the tubings, nebulizer, and patient connections are changed and sterilized at least every 24 hours. The water reservoir and the moist tubing provide an excellent breeding ground for bacterial colonization and infection.

Following aerosol treatments, postural drainage, chest percussion, and expulsive coughing may be employed. Nasal and oral hygiene should be performed.

Humidification

Humidifiers are devices that add water vapor (humidity) to the inspired gas. Oxygen and other compressed gases are dry. The addition of water vapor decreases the drying effects of these gases and makes the patient more comfortable.

- ▶ Moist air prevents drying and irritation of the mucous membranes within the respiratory system.
- ▶ Moist air prevents drying and thickening of respiratory tract secretions and loosens these secretions so they can more easily be removed. By keeping secretions thin and liquid in nature, moist air makes them easier to raise. Dry thick secretions can form plugs and crusts within the tracheobronchial tree that can be life-threatening if they obstruct airways.

Extra moisture can be added to room air by relatively simple methods, e.g., placing a vaporizer or kettle of boiling water in a patient's room. Other methods of providing humidification include use of nebulizers (e.g., with IPPB machines), heated aerosols, high humidity tracheostomy collars, high humidity oxygen tents, and ultrasonic mist units of various sorts (e.g., to humidify room air or for use with tents, hoods, or masks). Bedside nebulizers and room humidifiers are more effective in treating disorders of the upper airways than those deeper within the bronchopulmonary system. These devices produce an aerosol output that is typically restricted to larger particle size; hence, the particles do not penetrate deeply within the lungs.

Oxygen may be humidified by bubbling it through water. The water may be at room temperature or heated to body temperature. Heating increases the efficiency of humidification because a gas will carry more humidity if the water is heated.

Vaporizers are especially helpful to patients with irritation of the nose, throat, or bronchi. Large electric vaporizers (which use a gallon size water jar) may be used in hospitals; smaller electric vaporizers (with pint or quart size jars) are available from drug stores for home use. A vaporizer produces steam by heating water placed in the water jar. The steam is then either directed toward the patient or is permitted to flow generally into the room.

When directing steam toward a patient be certain the vaporizer and flow of steam are far enough away from the patient to prevent accidental burns.

If humidification is being obtained by simply boiling water on a hot plate in a pan or teakettle, be certain to place the apparatus at a safe distance from the patient and keep the water container more than half full.

Adequate humidification is necessary during continuous mechanical *ventilation.* Humidifying devices can cause problems in ventilatory therapy: for example, condensed water can partially obstruct the inspiratory tube of a respirator and thereby markedly reduce effective ventilation; and a bolus of water may be projected into the patient's tracheobronchial tree with the inspiratory phase of ventilation if water condenses in the tubes leading from the nebulizer to the patient.

Humidification and warming of inspired air or air-oxygen mixtures is important following *tracheostomy (or endotracheal intubation)* whether or not the patient is using a respirator. Tracheostomy creates an artificial air passage that bypasses the upper airway (see Unit XXIV); thus, the "new airway" is exposed to atmospheric air that is not warmed, moistened and filtered by upper respiratory mucosa. To compensate for loss of the normal functions of the upper airway, it is desirable to use heated nebulization immediately after tracheostomy is established. The object of heated humidity is to project into the tracheostomy tube air-oxygen mixtures at body temperature that are saturated with water vapor. A relative humidity of over 100 per cent at about 37° C is desirable. If the temperature is in doubt, it should be monitored to prevent possible hyperthermia. High humidity tracheostomy collars are available that permit easy access for suctioning.

High humidity tracheostomy masks (Fig. 54–10*A*) may be used if humidification and not oxygenation is the therapeutic objective. For patients who require specific inspired oxygen concentrations, a high volume variable O_2 concentration volume nebulizer is used (Fig. 54–10*B*). The large bore tubing is attached to a Briggs adapter (also called an aerosol T-piece) (Fig. 54–10*C*). The maintenance of a stable O_2 concentration requires an additional 6 inch length of large-bore aerosol tubing which provides a reservoir of oxygenated gas, because as the patient inhales oxygenated gas is inhaled from both sides of the aerosol T-piece. The shorter length of aerosol hose is often referred to as an "after burner."

OXYGEN THERAPY

Oxygen is used to treat the effects of hypoxemia. Oxygen administration does not cure the disease or the condition. O_2 is used to alleviate the harmful and possible lethal effects of hypoxemia. O_2 need must be assessed by arterial blood gases and the monitoring of the patient for the signs and symptoms of hypoxemia. O_2 may be used in both acute and chronic conditions. For example, airway obstruction, pulmonary edema, acute respiratory failure, chronic respiratory insufficiency, cardiac disorders, metabolic disorders, shock, and many other pulmonary and nonpulmonary disorders may cause hypoxemia and the need for supplemental oxygen.

Oxygen must never be withheld from the hypoxemic patient. The effects of oxygen administration must be monitored by objective and subjective measures.

When hypoxia is accompanied by apnea or dyspnea it may be necessary to ventilate the patient manually or mechanically while administering O_2. Oxygen may then be administered by adding supplemental O_2 to an IPPB system driven by compressed air. Methods of administration of O_2 are discussed further below.

Like a drug, O_2 should be given in amounts that are safe for the individual patient. In some instances high concentrations of O_2 can be fatal, while low concentrations can be lifesaving. Thus, it is *not* always true that if a little O_2 helps, a lot of O_2 will be even more helpful. Oxygen therapy prescriptions should be governed by blood gas levels, just as insulin prescriptions are governed by blood sugar levels. Knowledge of arterial blood gas values is mandatory. Recently, with the development of techniques that enable delivery of high O_2 tensions to patients, O_2 toxicity has become a major problem. This and other hazards of O_2 therapy are discussed further below.

Administration of Oxygen. Oxygen therapy is administered in many modes. In many cases a nasal cannula at low flow rates may be sufficient to relieve hypoxemia. If ventilation is inadequate, oxygen administration is performed in conjunction with mechanical ventilation.

The optimal dose of O_2 is the concentration that reverses potentially lethal hypoxemia without causing undesired and harmful side effects.

Oxygen is supplied for administration either from a portable tank (cylinder) or from a wall outlet (which leads via pipes to a large stored O_2 supply). Oxygen can be administered by masks, nasal cannula, face tent, ventilator, or nebulizer. Much of the equipment used for O_2 administration is disposable.

Some patients with chronic respiratory diseases need to have supplementary O_2 accessible in their homes; various types of O_2 equipment are available. Lightweight portable units with liquid oxygen can easily be carried with the patient while ambulatory or exercising. Ambulatory oxygen therapy is particularly useful in treating patients who have marked respiratory disability as a result of chronic obstructive pulmonary disease.[122]

The nurse must be familiar with the different methods of administering O_2, be able to supervise O_2 therapy, and be able to detect malfunction of the apparatus in use. The percentages of O_2 delivered by most equipment are only approximate. The gas delivered to the patient should therefore be periodically monitored with an oxygen meter when the O_2 concentration must be closely governed. A nurse responsible for oxygen therapy also must be familiar with the hazards of O_2 therapy and clinical indications of hypoxia, respiratory acidosis, CO_2 narcosis, respiratory alkalosis, and O_2 toxicity.

General clinical care measures of importance during O_2 administration include maintenance of a patent airway by correct positioning, suctioning, and productive coughing; mouth and nose care every 3 to 4 hours; periodic repositioning; skin care; changes of equipment as necessary (e.g., tanks should be changed before

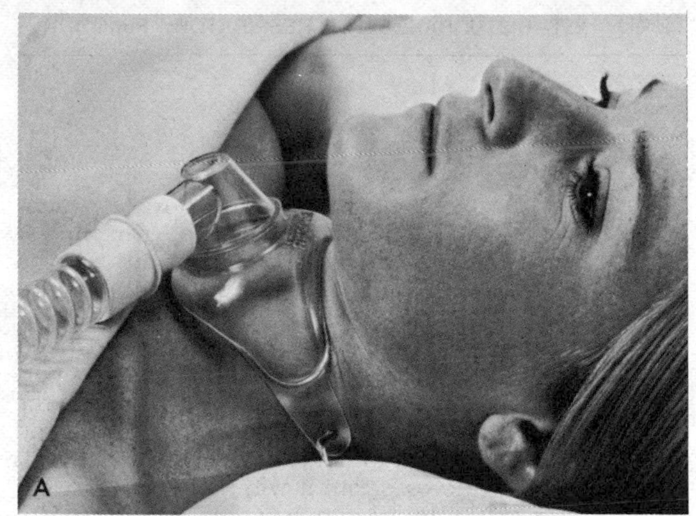

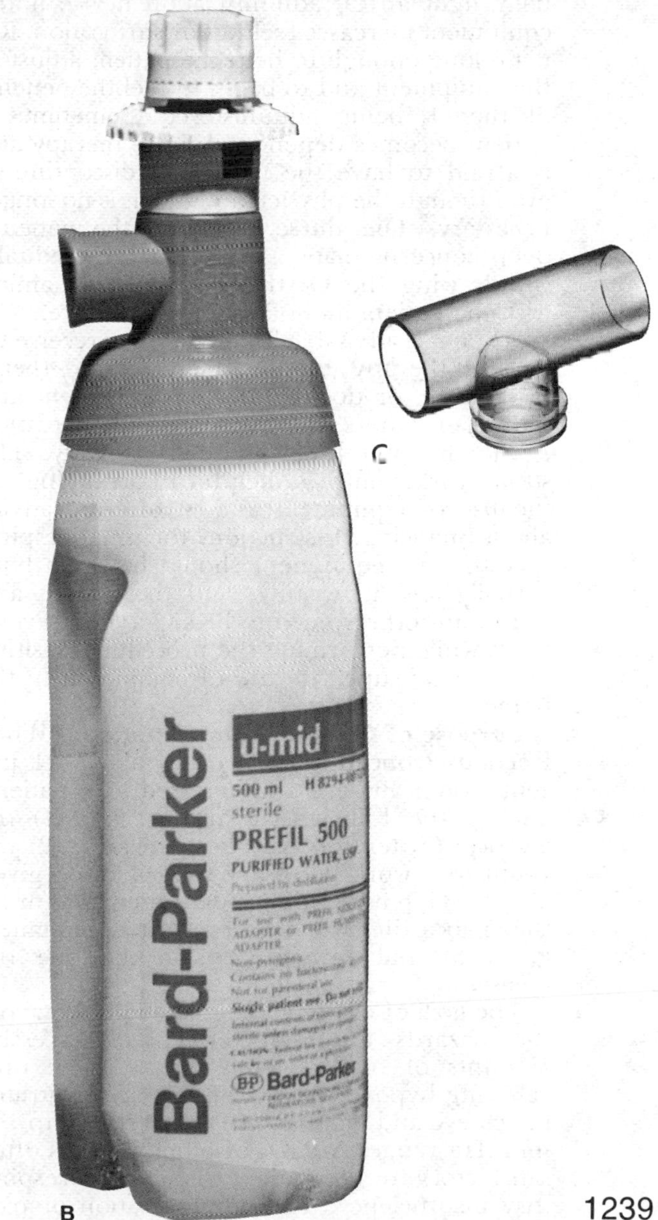

Figure 54–10. **A.** A tracheostomy mask, to administer supplemental humidity to a patient when the normal warming and humidification mechanisms have been bypassed. **B.** One type of variable FIO_2 nebulizer. By rotating the collar, varied amounts of air are entrained and specific oxygen concentrations obtained. **C.** A Briggs adapter for administering oxygen and supplemental hydration to the patient with an artificial airway—either a tracheostomy or endotracheal tube. (*A* and *C*, courtesy of Hudson Oxygen Sales Co., Temecula, Cal.; *B*, courtesy of Bard Parker, Lincoln Park, N.J.).

they become empty), and appropriate patient teaching and reassurance. Once oxygen administration is begun, the O_2 source must not be removed or the PaO_2 may be reduced more severely than it was before therapy.

The first time O_2 is to be given to a patient, explain the procedure and familiarize the person with the equipment to be used. Discuss the benefits of oxygen therapy. Some patients (and their significant others) are frightened by O_2 therapy and associate it with being near death. These attitudes need to be explored and realistically discussed. The dyspneic patient may initially fight an O_2 administration device if the equipment increases feelings of suffocation. Remain long enough to help the patient adjust to the equipment and to begin to feel the benefits of the O_2 being administered. Sometimes a patient becomes dependent on O_2 therapy and is afraid to have the treatment discontinued, even though the physician knows it is no longer necessary. The nurse, realizing the patient's deep concern, plans a program for gradually withdrawing the O_2 therapy while remaining with the patient and offering reassurance.

When it is advisable for a patient to receive O_2 or IPPB therapy at home, the respiratory therapist, nurse, or doctor informs the patient and significant others where to obtain the necessary equipment and how to use it correctly. The social worker may be helpful in arranging for the use of equipment and in offering advice about financing. Instructions for using respiratory therapy equipment should be given both verbally and in writing, and the patient and significant others need to be supervised several times while performing the procedure. Visiting nurses may supervise use of equipment in the home.

Purpose of Oxygen Administration. When fractions (concentrations) of O_2 above 21 per cent (room air) are administered to a patient, one of the following results occurs: (1) the alveolar O_2 tension may be increased; (2) the ventilatory work necessary to maintain a given alveolar O_2 tension may be decreased; and/or (3) the myocardial work necessary to maintain a given arterial oxygen tension may be decreased.

The goal of oxygen administration is to avoid the hazards and side effects of excessive amounts of oxygen while at the same time relieving hypoxemia. Oxygen dosage is titrated to achieve and maintain a PaO_2 in the 70 to 100 mm. Hg range. A PaO_2 of 60 mm. Hg is often satisfactory for the patient with chronic respiratory insufficiency. The administration of oxygen must never proceed without monitoring the effectiveness of therapy. Arterial blood gases must be determined and documented, along with nursing observations.

Hazards of Oxygen Administration. *Infection.* The use of contaminated equipment can infect the patient. Infecting organisms may be present in such places as suction catheters, tracheostomy or endotracheal tubes, connecting tubing, humidifier water, and masks. A few organisms, e.g., *Pseudomonas aeruginosa,* can even grow in some chemical disinfectants. The resultant infections are difficult to treat. To prevent infections of this nature, equipment must be properly sterilized and each person giving patient care must practice appropriate aseptic technique. Positive pressure oxygen equipment is particularly subject to contamination. These items should be changed daily when equipment is in use on a given patient.

Combustion. Oxygen itself does not burn but it supports combustion. Hence, fire is a potential hazard when O_2 is being administered. Flatter comments: "The greater the amount of oxygen present, the more easily fires start and the more rapidly they burn. . . . With the oxygen concentration increased above that of normal air, ignition becomes much easier, the rate of combustion is much faster, and extinguishment of such a fire may be extremely difficult."[57a] The following *factors are of importance in preventing fires during O_2 administration:*

- Properly ground all electrical plugs and electrical equipment.
- Do not permit use of electric razors on the patient.
- Enforce no smoking rules; post no smoking signs. Remove the patient's cigarettes, pipe, cigars, and matches from the room.
- Do not permit open flames, frayed electrical wires, or extension cords within the patient's environment.
- Do not use oils (e.g., oily hair dressings, mineral oil as a lip lubricant), greases, or flammable solutions (e.g., alcohols, ether, antiseptic tinctures) on the patient. If lubricants are necessary use a product with a water base such as K-Y jelly.
- Never use oil on O_2 equipment. In pure O_2, fuels can ignite without a spark.
- Prevent static electricity. Electrical sparks can easily ignite fires in an O_2-enriched environment. Sparks from static electricity are also hazardous. Woolen blankets and other items that may produce static electricity should not be used during O_2 administration.

Drying of Respiratory Tract Mucosa. As discussed previously, O_2 is a very drying gas when delivered into the respiratory system under pressure. To prevent hazardous drying and irritation of the respiratory mucosa, impaired ciliary action, and thickening of secretions within the respiratory tract, O_2 must *always* be humidified when administered. When O_2 is administered through a tracheostomy tube, special humidification is necessary so the gas mixture that enters the trachea is nearly saturated at body temperature. Oxygen can be passed through water or solutions (saline or medicated solutions) to humidify the gas before it is inhaled. Little O_2 is lost in the humidifying liquid because O_2 is only slightly soluble in water.

Oxygen Toxicity. The development of oxygen toxicity is *time*- and *dose*-related. That is, the development of pathophysiologic changes that occur within the lung is progressive, taking between 24 to 48 hours to become evident. Pulmonary oxygen toxicity has not developed when the fraction of inspired oxygen (FIO_2) has been under 60 per cent. Table 54–1 shows that the most common method of oxygen administration, the nasal cannula, provides a maximal FIO_2 of 40 per cent. Patients receiving *low flow* oxygen therapy (discussed later) do not develop pulmonary oxygen toxicity.

Pulmonary oxygen toxicity is included among the diseases and conditions classified under the heading of adult respiratory distress syndrome (ARDS). (See Chapter 13.) The symptoms of oxygen toxicity initially include those of a mild tracheobronchitis beginning as a tracheal irritation and a cough. The cough may become more severe, the substernal irritation may increase in severity, and dyspnea may become apparent. As symptoms progress, there is a marked reduction in vital capacity. Because many patients requiring high dose oxygen therapy may be receiving continuous mechanical ventilation, they may be unable to communicate the onset of symptoms. The nurse must provide for communication with the patient if at all possible. The most definitive symptom is apparent when serial arterial blood gas reports are reviewed. As the course of therapy progresses, the arterial blood gas values will reflect a decreasing PaO_2 as the FIO_2 is increased. At the same time, an increase in the inspiratory airway pressure needed to deliver a tidal volume will be noted on the manometer. This indicates a change in the lung compliance. *Compliance is the ability of the lung to accept a given volume of air.* A decreased compliance is an indication that oxygen toxicity is developing. The nurse must be alert for any of these insidious signs.

The pathophysiologic changes that occur with O_2 toxicity, as discussed here, can be classified as *acute.* The prolonged exposure to a high O_2 environment causes structural damage to the pulmonary tissues. Interstitial edema, thickened alveolar-capillary membranes, intra-alveolar hemorrhage, alveolar edema, and atelectasis develop. Oxygen transport is impaired. As damage continues, exudates of protein and fibrin and cellular debris coalesce to form hyaline membranes in the alveoli. The exact mechanisms for the development of oxygen toxicity are not known.

The findings at the end-stage of oxygen toxicity include progressive atelectasis and consolidation along with fibrosis of the lung. Chest films show progressive opacification of the lungs. As the progression continues, oxygenation is further impaired and the patient becomes more difficult to ventilate due to decreasing compliance. On auscultation breath sounds may be diminished and rales may be audible.

Treatment and management are aimed at the maintenance of adequate oxygenation and treatment of the underlying, precipitating disease. Early recognition of the signs of toxicity is essential. Maintenance of adequate oxygenation may require both ventilatory assistance with a volume ventilator as well as end-expiratory pressure. (See the discussion of C-PAP and PEEP later in this chapter.) The use of corticosteroids in the treatment of O_2 toxicity has been found to be of no benefit.

The nursing assessment of and intervention for people with O_2 toxicity include:

- emotional support to the patient and significant others;
- evaluation of fluid and electrolyte status;
- monitoring and documenting arterial blood gas response to any change in therapy;
- analyzing and documenting the inspired O_2 concentration following any change in the FIO_2;
- aseptic airway care (due to the damage within the lung, infection is an even greater hazard);
- prevention of any further damage or complications.

Atelectasis. Collapsed alveoli develop as a result of increased oxygen concentrations in the inspired air. The mechanism for this O_2-induced side effect is the elimination of nitrogen (N_2) from the lung due to displacement of N_2 by O_2, and the effect of oxygen on pulmonary surfactant. Hyperoxia retards the production of surfactant. Loss of surfactant also causes the forces of surface tension to collapse the affected alveolar units.

Atelectasis may result from many other situations, e.g., hypoventilation, impingement of a portion of the lung by space-occupying lesions, mucus plugs, the effects of anesthesia, the postoperative period, and so on.

The resultant collapsed, airless alveoli will continue to be perfused with blood. However, they cannot function to provide O_2. This condition is termed *intrapulmonic shunting*. The result is hypoxemia.

It is important to observe patients receiving high doses of O_2 for signs of hypoxemia: vague discomfort, anxiety, tachypnea, fever, cough, tachycardia, shortness of breath, sternal retractions. The symptoms vary depending on the degree of atelectasis. Arterial blood gases reports must be obtained. The chest film should be assessed during the course of high dose O_2 administration and performed serially if atelectasis develops. On auscultation, the affected areas will have diminished or absent breath sounds. The degree of impairment may also be assessed by serial parameter checks of vital capacity, inspiratory force, and tidal volume.

Nursing actions appropriate for patients with atelectasis include deep breathing with an inspiratory hold, adequate fluid intake and output, and proper positioning. The patient should not be positioned with the affected area in the dependent position as the degree of hypoxemia may be thus increased owing to the gravitational effects on blood flow.

Retrolental Fibroplasia (RLF). The hazards of oxygen therapy may affect the eye. RLF was noted in premature infants who required an oxygen-enriched environment. However, the damage was not immediately noted as the assessment of visual acuity is not routine. We now know that infants exposed to oxygen concentrations which cause an O_2 tension of 200 mm. Hg or more in the blood will develop fibrotic changes behind the lens which impairs light penetration to the retina.

The eye of the adult may also be damaged by oxygen. Tearing, edema, and visual impairment result from the toxic effects on the cornea and lens of the adult.

Oxygen-induced Apnea. The patient with chronic CO_2 retention has already been discussed. The stimulus for respiration in such a patient is no longer the central receptor site in the medulla and pons, but rather the peripheral pressoreceptors located in the arch of the aorta and the carotid arteries. These receptors are sensitive to oxygen lack. Administration of supplemental oxygen may dampen this secondary stimulus to respiration, leading to hypoventilation and respiratory failure.

It is the nurse's responsibility to observe the patient for the physical signs and clues of chronic lung disease. Administration of O_2 must be carried out only following assessment of arterial blood gas status. The arterial blood gas response to the O_2 must be documented, especially the response of the pCO_2. Unmonitored O_2 administration to the patient with a hypoxic respiratory drive may result in hypoventilation or apnea.

Nevertheless, oxygen therapy is often indicated in treating chronic respiratory insufficiency. When a patient with chronic respiratory insufficiency or CO_2 retention requires O_2 therapy, the O_2 is administered cautiously in *low concentrations* (25 to 35 per cent) at a low flow rate (1 to 2 liters per minute) to prevent CO_2 narcosis.

Oxygen Flow Rates

The terms low flow and high flow refer to the rates of oxygen delivered to the patient by the equipment. Systems that deliver to the patient flow rates of oxygen less than the inspiratory flow rate requirements are termed low flow systems. Those that provide the total inspiratory flow rate needs are called high flow systems.

Low Flow Systems. These deliver O_2 concentrations in a wide range — from 21 to 90 per cent. The variables that control the fraction of inspired oxygen (FIO_2) include (1) the capacity of the anatomic reservoir (the nasopharynx, oropharynx, and nose); (2) the amount of the oxygen reservoir; (3) flow rate of oxygen (liters per minute); and (4) the patient's pattern of ventilation. Low flow systems are the most familiar and allow ease of administration with a minimum of interference in the patient's care. However, the variables involved in the determination of the oxygen concentrations do not allow either accuracy or dependability. Nasal cannulas, masks, and masks with reservoir bags are the most common types of low flow systems.

Table 54–1 shows the concentrations of O_2 available at various liter flows with the three standard low flow systems. The per cent of oxygen as it comes out of the wall is 100. It is the amount of air entrained by patients to meet their inspiratory flow needs and the dilution of the oxygen with 21 per cent room air that determines the inspired O_2 concentration. Table 54–1 assumes that the pattern of ventilation is regular. Shapiro, Trout, and Harrison caution that the FIO_2 in a low flow system varies tremendously with changes in tidal volume and ventilatory pattern. In a low flow system, the larger the tidal volume, the lower the FIO_2; or the smaller the tidal volume, the higher the FIO_2.

A *nasal cannula* (also called nasal prongs) requires patent nasal passages (see Figure 54–11*A*). Mouth breathing does not affect the FIO_2 as the oxygen in the nose is drawn into the trachea by the air in the oral cavity. Flow rates of O_2 administered by nasal cannula are in the range of 1 to 6 LPM. Liter flow above 6 LPM has no effect on administering higher FIO_2 as the anatomic reservoir's capacity is about 6 liters.

TABLE 54–1. GUIDELINES FOR ESTIMATING THE PERCENTAGE OF OXYGEN DELIVERED BY LOW FLOW SYSTEMS

	FIO_2 (%)*
Nasal Cannula	
1 L.	24
2 L.	28
3 L.	32
4 L.	36
5 L.	40
6 L.	44
Standard O_2 Mask	
5–6 L.	40
6–7 L.	50
7–8 L.	60
Mask with Reservoir	
6 L.	60
7 L.	70
8 L.	80
9 L.	90
10–15 L.	99+

*The FIO_2 assumes a normal pattern of ventilation.
(From Shapiro, B. A., R. Harrison, and C. A. Trout: *Clinical Application of Respiratory Care.* Chicago: Year Book Medical Publishers, Inc., 1975.)

Masks (see Figure 54–11*B*) may be used to increase the anatomic reservoir and thereby administer oxygen concentrations above those produced by the nasal cannula. (See Table 54–1.) A danger exists of exhaled air accumulating in the mask's reservoir, which could result in a patient rebreathing exhaled air. This is avoided by the practice of never administering O_2 by low flow mask at rates less than 5 to 6 LPM.

A *mask* (see Figure 54–11*C*) with a *reservoir bag* must be used if percentages above 60 per cent are desired with a low flow system (see Table 54–1). If there is a one-way valve between the bag and the mask, the system is a nonrebreathing mask. The patient will breathe all the inspired air from the reservoir. If there is no one-way valve between the bag and mask, the system is called a partial rebreathing mask. This

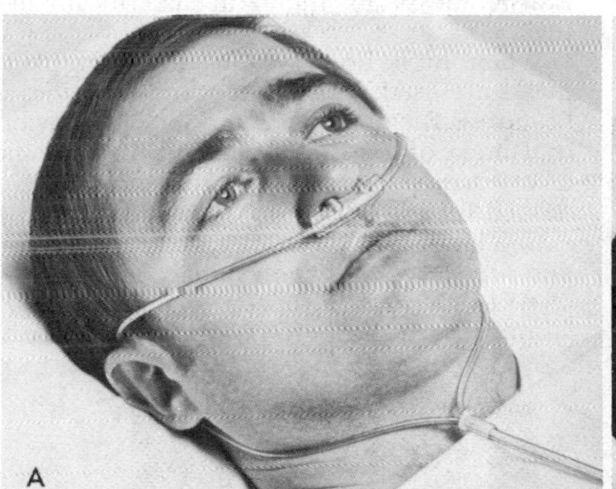

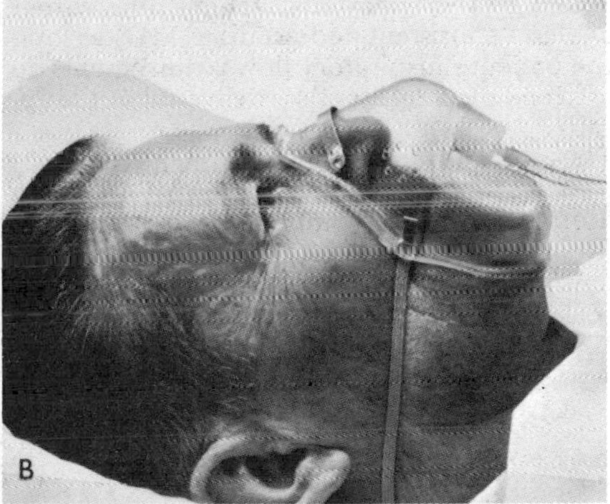

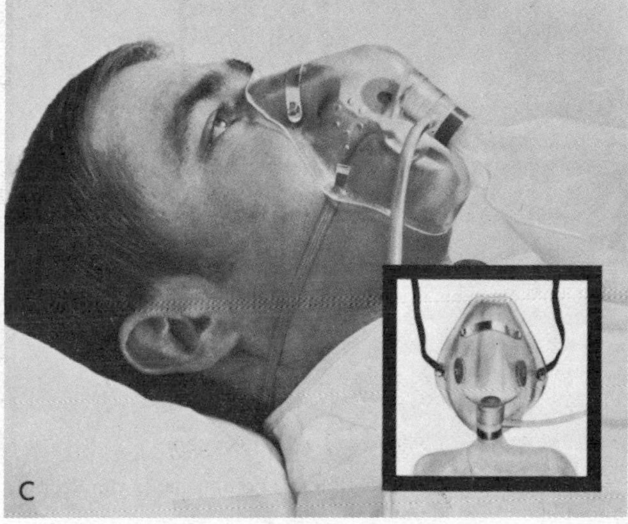

Figure 54–11. **A.** A nasal cannula (nasal prongs) is the most common mode of low flow oxygen delivery. **B.** The standard oxygen mask. **C.** Reservoir bag attached to the mask. (Courtesy of Hudson Oxygen Sales Co., Temecula, Cal.)

bag is an *oxygen reservoir,* not a carbon dioxide rebreathing bag. Whenever a reservoir bag is used, the nurse must observe the bag during inhalation. The bag must never collapse more than half per breath. Flow rates used are 6 to 12 LPM. Oxygen concentrations will be in the 60 to 90+ per cent range, depending on the pattern, depth, and rate of ventilation. Masks must fit securely.

Because the O_2 must be given with precision therapy is guided by frequent blood gas monitoring. The goals of O_2 administration with such a patient are to preserve a hypoxic state (low PaO_2 level) and thus preserve the source of the respiratory drive, while also preventing an additional $PaCO_2$ buildup and increasing the transportation of O_2 in the blood to obtain adequate tissue respiration.

High Flow Systems. These provide a flow rate and reservoir capacity adequate to supply the total inspired air needs. The patient using a high flow system breathes only the gas being supplied by the apparatus. A high flow system provides a consistent and accurate FIO_2 as long as the patient's inspiratory flow requirements do not exceed the total liter flow delivered by the apparatus.

The capability of high flow systems includes the ability to deliver either high or low oxygen concentrations. The combination of providing accuracy and inspiratory flow demands is usually accomplished by the use of a *Venturi* device, which utilizes a principle of fluid physics called the *Bernoulli principle.* This mechanism entrains a specific proportional amount of room air for each specific liter flow of oxygen. This air/O_2 entrainment ratio provides a specific O_2 percentage and large total flow rates of air and oxygen. For instance, if a Venturi system set for 40 per cent O_2 is used, it has an air-to-oxygen entrainment ratio of 3:1. If the flowmeter is set at 10 LPM, and for each liter of O_2, three liters of air are entrained, total liter flow will be 40 LPM. Each FIO_2 has its own air/O_2 entrainment ratio, thus each FIO_2 has a different total liter flow. The higher the FIO_2, the lower the total liter flow.

High flow systems can provide O_2 concentrations of from 24 to 100 per cent. Venturi-type masks (see Figure 54–12) provide 24 to 55 per cent O_2. Nebulizers utilizing the Venturi principle provide 30 to 100 per cent O_2 concentrations. Volume ventilators are also considered high flow systems. They will be discussed later in this chapter.

High flow systems have three major advantages: (1) consistent FIO_2; (2) control of the entire inspired atmosphere, including temperature and humidity; and (3) ease of analyzing the FIO_2 with an oxygen analyzer (see Figure 54–13). This is a significant advantage in the critically ill patient.

When high flow systems like Venturi-type masks are used, some patient care activities may be more difficult to perform. The most obvious is oral intake of food and fluids. An alternate short-term form of oxygen therapy should be prescribed for the patient to use while eating.

Good judgment, caution, and careful observation are necessary when initially administering O_2 to a patient whose history is unknown. Supervision is particularly important during the first

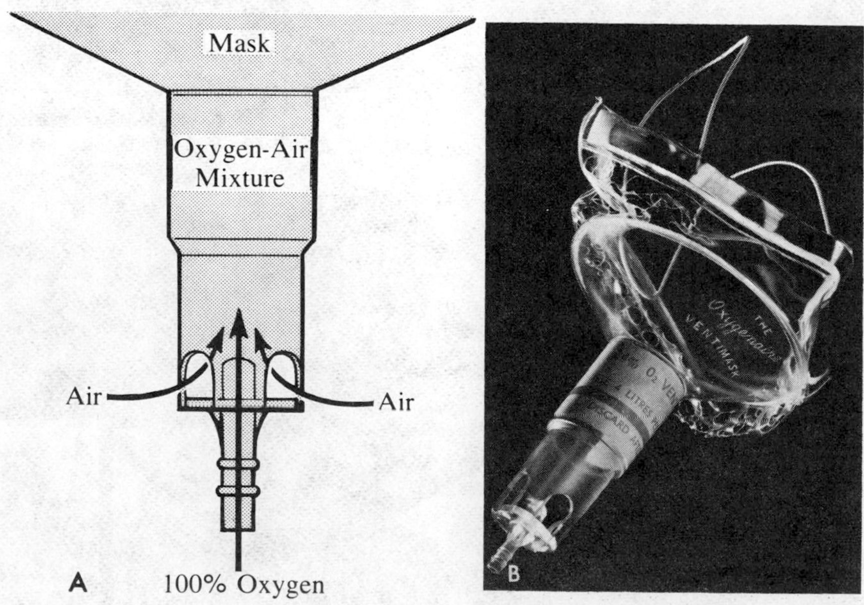

Figure 54–12. *A*, Venturi principle. *B*, Ventimask. (From Secor, J.: *Patient Care in Respiratory Problems.* Philadelphia, W. B. Saunders Co., 1969.)

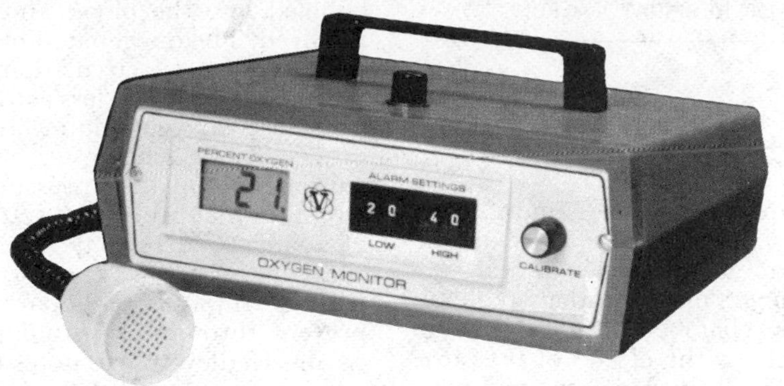

Figure 54–13. An oxygen analyzer is essential to the accurate determination of inspired O_2 concentrations. This model may be placed in line in the delivery system of many high flow oxygen systems. (Courtesy Hudson Oxygen Sales Co., Temecula, Calif.)

30 to 60 minutes because apnea can occur, e.g., if the administration of O_2 abruptly removes the hypoxic respiratory stimulus. If this occurs the patient may "pink up and die." This phrase summarizes the following sequence of events: the patient's color may improve (as blood PaO_2 level rises), but the person hypoventilates, becomes increasingly stuporous and then comatose, loses the cough reflex, becomes apneic and dies. Correction of the hypoxemia "pinks up" the patient but proves to be fatal by removing the respiratory drive, and death occurs. Close observation and prompt treatment may break this fatal chain of events. Indications of the development of respiratory depression (e.g., reduced rate or depth of breathing, reduced levels of consciousness) or increasing hypercapnia signal the need to immediately lower the O_2 concentration, contact the physician, and prepare to manually ventilate the patient.

Oxygen administration must never be interrupted. It must be carried out during all activities, including eating, transport to other departments, bathing, and ambulation.

Withdrawal of the oxygen source may result in a reflex hypoxemia, with resulting pO_2's at levels lower than pretherapy levels. It is the responsibility of all personnel caring for the patient to realize the importance of the maintenance of continuous oxygen administration.

The safest method of administering O_2 in the presence of CO_2 retention is by careful observation for the signs and symptoms of an increasing $PaCO_2$ and by serial blood gas determinations.

Hyperbaric Oxygen Therapy (OHP)

This term is used to describe the administration of oxygen, usually of 100 per cent concentration, in an environment of increased atmospheric pressures. The abbreviation OHP, signifying *oxygen under high pressure,* may be used.

Research continues to find new uses and applications other than decompression sickness (bends). Among the most frequent are treatment of patients with anaerobic infections, degenerative bone diseases, burns, cyanide poisoning, carbon monoxide poisoning, air emboli caused by decompression sickness, and emboli caused by nondiving incidents such as hemodialysis, arteriograms, and open heart surgery. The use of OHP is controversial in the treatment of radionecrosis due to the effects of OHP on some carcinomas. Hyperbaric oxygenation is infrequently used in cardiovascular diseases owing to the vasoconstrictive effects of hyperoxia. The use of OHP during sickle cell crisis is still in the research phase.

Normal barometric atmospheric pressure is 760 mm. Hg at sea level. Sea level atmospheric pressure is considered to be "1 atmosphere." The percentage or fraction of O_2 in the atmosphere at any elevation is .21. At 760 mm. Hg oxygen exerts a partial pressure of 159 mm. Hg (760 mm. Hg × .21 = 159 mm. Hg). The alveolar pO_2 will be approximately 100 mm. Hg. If 100 per cent oxygen is administered at 1 atmosphere, the partial pressure of oxygen in the alveolus will be approximately 673 mm. Hg. The arterial pO_2 may be either within this range or significantly lower, depending on the patient's pre-existing pulmonary status, such as alveolar or circulatory impairments, which would affect oxygen transport. At an FIO_2 of 1.0 (100 per cent) the hemoglobin is maximally saturated. To increase the available oxygen supply, oxygen must be administered at pressures above 1 atmosphere. In this way the oxygen is carried in the plasma compartment of the circulating blood. The administration of 100 per cent O_2 at 3 atmospheres provides an alveolar pO_2 of 2193 mm. Hg. The arterial pO_2 usually falls in the range of 1600 to 1800 mm. Hg. This large alveolar-arterial (A-a) difference is probably due to the vasoconstrictive effect of hyperoxia and microatelectasis induced by hyperoxia. Oxygen under pressure is most often administered at 2 to 3 atmospheres. The length of time of the treatment varies.

Hyperbaric chambers may be either single or multiple occupancy chambers. Patient care is complicated not only by the effects of pressure on equipment but also by lack of accessibility to patients, especially those treated in the single occupant chamber. The pressure changes make mechanical valves "sticky," affect air-filled balloons such as those in artificial airways, and create volume changes in IV drip. The pressure changes during both compression and decompression also may cause discomfort and damage to the paranasal sinuses and the middle ear. Patients must be taught to clear their ears by swallowing and yawning. During treatment at the prescribed pressure, the patient must be observed for respiratory rate, pattern of ventilation, and general overall tolerance of the procedure. Claustrophobic reactions are not uncommon, especially in single occupant chambers. *Convulsions* may occur when O_2 is breathed at greater than normal atmospheric pressures.

OHP is contraindicated for metastatic carcinoma, viral infections, pneumothorax, uncontrolled high fevers, CO_2 narcosis, bronchospasm, and patients with excessive feelings of claustrophobia.

Extracorporeal Membrane Oxygenation (ECMO)

The use of prolonged extracorporeal oxygenation is still in the investigative stage. The expensive equipment is available only in large institutions. Protocols and criteria for this mode of oxygen therapy are currently being determined and evaluated in a national program in the United States.

Patients selected for this mode of therapy are those who are not responding to the conventional critical respiratory care procedures used to treat severe hypoxemia. A dilemma is to select patients who have potentially reversible disease soon enough in the course of disease. ECMO must be instituted before pulmonary damage from high ventilator inflation pressures and toxic levels of oxygen have caused irreversible pulmonary damage. ECMO is contraindicated in patients who are actively bleeding, have terminal illnesses, and have acute respiratory failure superimposed on chronic obstructive pulmonary disease.

The procedure involves circulation of venous blood through a membrane where oxygen is bubbled into the blood and carbon dioxide is removed. The oxygenated blood is then infused into the arterial circulation. In this way the pulmonary system is less active and may recover while tissue oxygenation is insured. If mechanical ventilation is being utilized inspired oxygen tensions and inflation pressures may be reduced to nontrauma-producing settings. Other aspects of ventilator care may be continued, such as chest physiotherapy and tracheal suctioning.

Large amounts of heparin must be used to prevent thrombosis within the extracorporeal circuit. Hedley-Whyte notes that this presents a great risk as serious hemorrhage occurs in approximately 20 per cent of patients on prolonged extracorporeal oxygenation. Bleeding problems also result owing to a fall in the platelet count of patients receiving ECMO.[75]

Nursing care includes maintenance of aseptic conditions, as sepsis is also a major complication, and attention to all data obtained from parameters monitoring vascular, pulmonary, and circulatory status.[75]

MECHANICAL RESPIRATORY AIDS

Indications and Types of Equipment

Some patients are unable to ventilate their lungs effectively. We have discussed previously the wide variety of disorders that may result in respiratory insufficiency or failure. These patients require immediate assistance, which includes either establishment of an artificial airway (e.g., by endotracheal intubation or tracheostomy) and mechanical ventilation of the lungs with a positive pressure ventilator. (See Table 54–2.)

Positive pressure ventilators may be broadly categorized as those for short-term therapeutic use, such as those used to administer *intermittent positive pressure breathing* (IPPB), and those capable of maintaining all aspects of ventilation and oxygen administration, or *continuous mechanical ventilators* (CMV). The CMV category may be further divided into pressure-limited and volume-limited ventilators, which will be discussed later in this chapter.

Negative pressure ventilators, such as the Drinker, at one time were extremely important in saving the lives of persons with polio. They were large and cumbersome, and provided no means for specific oxygen concentrations or tidal volumes. They were of use primarily in neuromuscular disorders that caused respiratory failure. A compact negative pressure device, called a *chest cuirass*, has had some acceptance. Again, this form of ventilation is for the patient with no need for oxygen enrichment and other essential aspects of modern mechanical ventilators.

Physiologic Effects of Positive Pressure

A decrease in cardiac output is the most common physiologic effect of concern to nurses caring for patients receiving either intermittent or continuous mechanical ventilation. As the positive pressure inflates the lungs, the pressure in the thorax also affects the flow of blood in the vena cava. Blood flow to the right side of the heart is retarded. The heart is accustomed to functioning with subatmospheric pressures. The normal action of the thorax as a pump assists in the return of blood to the heart and also in maintenance of an adequate cardiac output. Normal, unassisted respiration begins with a subatmospheric pressure that continues to negatively increase during inhalation and decreases during exhalation but never exceeds atmospheric pressure except under conditions of stress. Positive pressure applied to the airway has the opposite effect.

During an assisted breath, the positive pressure inflates the lung during inhalation. As the lung expands, the intrapulmonary pressure increases. The increase in the intrapulmonary pressure is transmitted through the lung into the pleural space, which elevates the intrathoracic pressure during inhalation. Exhalation is passive and pressures return to their normal resting subatmospheric level as the patient exhales into the ambient atmosphere. Positive pressure impairs venous return to the right heart, right heart arterial filling, and pulmonary blood flow. The positive pressure also affects the left side of the heart by increasing left heart filling and output. This effect only occurs for a short time.

When a patient is inhaling under positive pressure, the nurse must monitor both pulse and blood pressure. In critical patients, measurement of the pulmonary vascular pressures is necessary.

Other body systems are affected by the application of positive pressure. As the diaphragm descends into the abdomen during the inspiratory phase, blood flow to the splanchnic area is decreased. Portal vein pressure is increased by the increased intra-abdominal pressure. Oxygen transport to the mesenteric bed and the liver is also decreased.

Positive pressure also causes a decrease in urine flow and an increase in vasopressin. The action of elevated vasopressin levels leads to the reabsorption of free water in the renal tubular cell. Salt and water retention occur as ADH secretion is increased. Lymphatic flow is also decreased due to the effects of positive pressure.

Positive pressure breathing may also cause neurophysiologic changes. When blood gas changes improve in the patient in acute, uncompensated respiratory failure, improved cerebral oxygenation status results. The patient with compensated respiratory acidosis may be adversely affected due to the "blowing-off" of CO_2. The resulting acute alkalosis causes faintness, dizziness, light-headedness, anxiety, and, if the pCO_2 is reduced moderately, paresthesia. If the pCO_2 is severely reduced, convulsions and cardiac arrhythmias result. Ziment notes that patients on continuous mechanical ventilation may develop a degree of cerebral edema. The cerebral edema may actually contribute to ICU psychosis syndrome.[195]

It is important to avoid rapid changes in the blood gases. In this way the physiologic manifestations of rapid changes in $PaCO_2$ and pH may be avoided. A general rule of practice:

TABLE 54–2. INDICATIONS OF NEED FOR AN ARTIFICIAL AIRWAY

Parameter	Normal Value	Consider Intubation
Respiratory Rate (f)	12–20/min.	>35/min.
Tidal Volume (V_T)	10–15 ml./kg. body weight	<5 ml./kg.
Vital Capacity (VC)	65–75 ml./kg. body weight	<10 ml./kg.
Inspiratory Force (IF)	75–100 cm. H_2O	<−25 cm. H_2O
PaO_2	75–100 mm. Hg (room air)	<70 mm. Hg on 50% O_2
$PaCO_2$	35 45 mm. Hg	>55 mm. Hg
A-a DO_2	25–65 mm. Hg	<450 mm. Hg after 10 min. on 100% O_2
V_D/V_T	0.25–0.40	>0.60

The above parameters may be used as criteria for intubation. Reversal of the lower limits leading to intubation may be used as criteria for weaning/extubation.

Changes in $PaCO_2$ must not be more than 10 mm. Hg per hour. Changes in arterial pH must not be more than 0.1 pH unit per hour.

Principles of Nursing Care

Nurses caring for patients with inadequate ventilation must be familiar with clinical indications of respiratory distress (restlessness, apprehension, irritability, wakefulness, use of accessory muscles of respiration, pallor, increasing pulse rate, and increasing laborious respirations) and must have advanced training in the various types of mechanical respiratory aids that may be used to improve ventilation. Whenever possible patients are given respiratory assistance well before a crisis develops. This anticipatory care requires close observation and availability of necessary equipment.

Assisted ventilation is often initially alarming to conscious patients and their significant others. The appearance of the machine may be frightening. Also, since respiration is vital, the patient may have fears that the machine will fail. Psychologic preparation of a patient for use of a ventilator helps to ensure successful treatment. The patient who is inadequately prepared may panic and defeat the purpose of the ventilator by "fighting" the cycle of the machine and breathing ineffectively. As time permits, the patient is told how the apparatus will help, what he or she will feel while on the machine, how to cooperate, and the basic mechanics of the respirator. Because patients with respiratory difficulties are usually tense and apprehensive, the transition to the mechanical respiratory equipment needs to be carried out as smoothly and as calmly as possible. Patients who require continuous mechanical ventilation must never be left unattended. Only experienced nursing and respiratory therapy personnel should care for such patients.

Respirators in use should be checked frequently to ensure their proper operation. The plug should be taped in place to the wall outlet and should be checked periodically to be certain the connection is maintained. Also, cords should be placed so they are not underfoot, so that they will not cause accidents or be accidentally pulled loose. A self-inflating (Ambu) bag with a nonrebreathing exhalation valve should always be kept at the bedside of a patient being mechanically ventilated. Then emergency manual resuscitation (maintain a respiratory rate of 15/min.) can be given if the respirator fails to operate properly or if power failure occurs. Manual ventilation is also used at other times, e.g., if it is necessary to temporarily disconnect the respirator for tests or treatments or to change apparatus on the machine and during suctioning of the tracheobronchial tree.

Modern mechanical ventilation is almost entirely automatic, but it is accompanied by various nursing problems, such as maintaining prescribed inspired O_2 concentrations, supplying adequate humidification, preventing trauma and infection, preventing mechanical problems such as loose connections and kinks in tubing that may interrupt proper functioning of the equipment, and maintaining patency of endotracheal and tracheostomy tubes. (Endotracheal intubation and tracheostomy are discussed in Unit XXIV.)

At times when patients are surrounded by a lot of machines it becomes easy to overlook "the person" being treated and instead focus attention on "the machines." This is indeed unfortunate. Patients dependent on ventilators require complete care, which requires comprehensive planning and meticulous attention to detail. It is especially important to establish a satisfactory way of communicating with the patient as he or she will be unable to talk. A "magic slate" may be useful.

Indications for Continuous Mechanical Ventilation (CMV)

Many causes alter a patient's ability to maintain effective alveolar ventilation. These factors may or may not initially include hypoxemia. Table 54–2 shows the criteria for placement of an artificial airway. These parameters have been adopted by many hospitals as protocols for intubation.[125A]

Artificial airways are established in the following situations:

- Any patient who is unable to maintain a patent airway due to impaired cough and airway clearance mechanisms
- Acute respiratory failure with or without pneumonia, pulmonary embolism, status asthmaticus, heart failure, COPD
- Postoperative respiratory insufficiency
- Post-traumatic respiratory insufficiency
- The comatose patient unable to maintain a patent airway and adequate ventilation
- Upper airway embarrassment such as laryngeal edema
- Neuromuscular diseases causing respiratory failure, adult respiratory distress syndrome (ARDS), drug and chemical intoxication causing respiratory depression

BASIC ASPECTS OF CARE FOR A PATIENT ON CMV

Regardless of the type of ventilator used to deliver continuous mechanical ventilation, the nurse must determine, provide, and monitor certain aspects of care to assure the optimal safe environment for patients:

▶ Maintain the correct level of oxygenation — use of an accurately calibrated O_2 analyzer to check the FIO_2. Never remove the oxygen source.
▶ Maintain optimal arterial blood gases by efficiently reporting the results of arterial blood gas reports to the physician; notify respiratory therapy personnel regarding ventilator setting changes; rigorous attention to the correct functioning of the ventilator.
▶ Provide a means of communication for the patient — an alphabet chart, magic slate, pencil and paper.
▶ Provide round-the-clock nursing care. *Never leave the patient unattended.*
▶ Maintain a patent airway using strict aseptic technique, hyperinflation, and hyperoxygenation.
▶ Provide optimal humidification of all inspired gas.
▶ Protect the patient's airway from nosocomial infection with good handwashing technique, sterile solutions for humidification, frequent changes and sterilization of the ventilator circuit and all the equipment that comes in contact with the patient's airway.
▶ Be familiar with the ventilator; know the signs of malfunction.
▶ Be prepared to manually ventilate the patient with a self-inflating or anesthesia bag in the event of a ventilator malfunction or a power failure.
▶ Check vital signs, inspiratory pressures, breath sounds, and ventilatory parameters every hour. Document, report trends or abnormal findings.
▶ Provide for the maintenance of muscle tone by performing ROM exercises. Dangling, sitting in a chair, and ambulation may also be included in the activity program as the patient's status improves.
▶ Provide for nutritional needs through parenteral administration. Oral intake may be given if the patient has a tracheostomy tube and does not have a tracheoesophageal fistula and is able to swallow.
▶ Keep accurate intake and output records.
▶ Stabilize the artificial airway. Mark nasal and oral endotracheal tubes with a marking pen just before they enter the mouth or nose. The position of the tube may then be determined. If an oral tube is used, stabilize with an oral airway. Move the airway and tube to the opposite side of the mouth every shift to avoid necrosis.
▶ Monitor the respiratory status with blood gases, chest film, auscultation, and tracheal aspirate cultures.
▶ Turn the patient every two hours. If possible, always keep the affected lung uppermost.
▶ Hematest stools. The stress incurred from critical care situations frequently precipitates the development of stress ulcers.
▶ Administer prophylactic antacids hourly.
▶ Maintain a calm, reassuring atmosphere.
▶ Provide for the sleep needs of the patient. Plan activities and periods of nonactivity.
▶ Administer oral care every 2 to 4 hours.
▶ Make certain the disconnect (low inspiratory line pressure) and other ventilator alarm systems are working.

WEANING THE PATIENT FROM CMV

The decision to begin weaning the patient from continuous mechanical ventilation is made by the physician. The observations and documentation of the patient's medical and respiratory status by the nurse and respiratory therapist are of great importance. The task of weaning a patient from mechanically supported respiration may cause both psychologic and physiologic changes. The length of time required to successfully wean the patient from the ventilator is generally related to the underlying disease process and to the state of health prior to commitment to the ventilator. A young person who has had an overdose of drugs generally weans rapidly. The patient with COPD who develops an acute respiratory failure and has little or no pulmonary reserve, however, often requires much patience and skill from all members of the team.

Weaning the patient from mechanical ventilatory support is not synonymous with the removal of the artificial airway. The assessment of the need for the airway must be made after the patient demonstrates successful spontaneous ventilation for 12 to 48 hours and that the respiratory mechanics are capable of maintaining a patent airway.

Criteria for a weaning trial are:

Reversal of the indications for intubation and ventilation.
Correction and stabilization of the causes for ventilation.
Improvement in the active disease process.
Nutritional and fluid status sufficient to maintain increased metabolic needs and demands of spontaneous respiration.
Physical strength and mental alertness present.
Afebrile — infections controlled.
Stable cardiovascular, renal, and cerebral status.
Arterial blood gases, electrolytes, hemoglobin, and other laboratory tests at optimal levels.
Physiologic parameters listed in Table 54–3.

Weaning should not be begun late in the day, or when the patient is tired. All conditions must be optimal.

METHODS OF WEANING

Selection of the appropriate technique generally depends upon the initial causative factors

TABLE 54–3. PARAMETERS FOR WEANING FROM CONTINUOUS MECHANICAL VENTILATION

Mechanical Considerations	
1. Inspiratory force (IF)	>25 cm. H_2O
2. Tidal volume (V_T)	>5 ml./kg.
3. Vital capacity (VC)	>10–15 ml./kg.
4. Expiratory force (EF)	>+60 cm. H_2O
5. Resting minute ventilation (can be doubled with MVV maneuver)	>10 L./min.
Ventilation/Oxygenation	
1. $PaCO_2$	within normal range
2. PaO_2	minimally 70–80 mm. Hg on 0.5 FIO_2
3. Dead space to tidal volume (V_D/V_T)	0.55–0.60
4. PaO_2 on 100% O_2	>300 mm. Hg
5. Shunt fraction	<15%

leading to continuous ventilation. The three most often used methods are (1) intermittent mandatory ventilation (IMV), (2) T-piece trial with periodic return to the ventilator, and (3) T-piece with continuous positive airway pressure (C-PAP).

IMV is a method originally used to wean patients from CMV who had required long-term ventilation or who for other reasons were difficult to wean. There are many ways to set up a ventilator to deliver IMV. However, the basic concept is the same. Patients remain connected to a ventilator; between the ventilator and the patient in the inspiratory line a system of valves and humidified O_2 is inserted. The ventilator is placed on control mode; a tidal volume and rate are selected. The beginning rate is usually one half the patient's spontaneous respiratory rate. On IMV patients set their own respiratory rate and tidal volume. The ventilator gives the patient the preset volume and rate. The rate is gradually reduced until patients are totally supporting their own ventilation.

Positive end-expiratory pressure (PEEP) or continuous positive airway pressure (C-PAP) may be used in conjunction with IMV. This modality is discussed in more detail later.

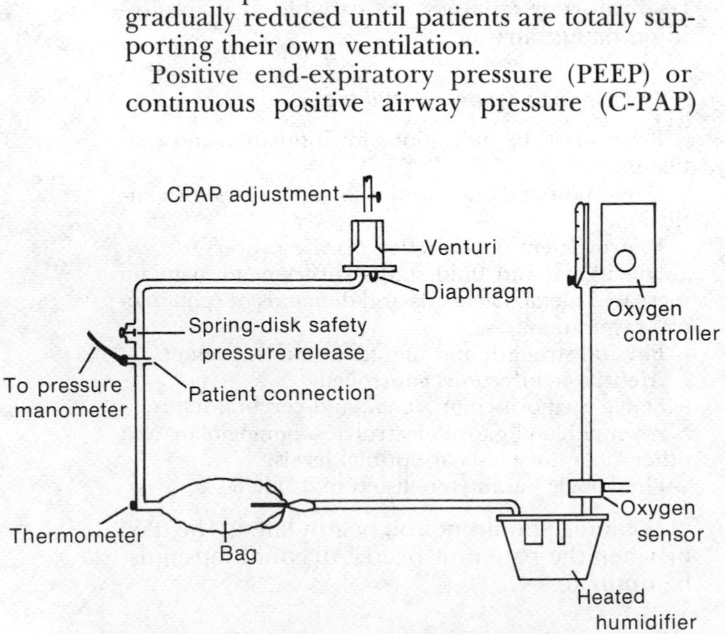

The *T-piece* (also called a Briggs adapter) (Fig. 54–10*C*) has been discussed earlier. It is attached to a heated nebulizer. Specific oxygen concentrations are then delivered via large-bore aerosol hose to the Briggs adapter. All respiratory and anesthesia fittings are either 15 or 22 mm. in size. The standard fitting on the end of the tracheostomy or endotracheal tube is 15 mm. The connecting portion of the Briggs adapter fits onto the 15 mm. portion of the artificial airway. The remaining open end of the T-piece is fitted with a short tube that functions as a reservoir to maintain a constant FIO_2. The flow rate of the humidified oxygen-air mixture is fast enough to flush exhaled gas from the circuit to prevent rebreathing of exhaled air.

T-piece with C-PAP refers to the application of continuous positive airway pressure. (See Figure 54–14.) This pressure is maintained in the patient circuit during both the inspiratory and the expiratory phases of ventilation. An aerosol generator (nebulizer) provides both humidification and precise inspired oxygen concentrations. The generator may be powered by an oxygen blender to insure that the total liter flow delivered on the inspiratory side of the system is three times greater than the patient's minute ventilation. The expiratory circuit may be placed into a column of water or a special valve may be placed in the expiratory line that exerts the required amount of airway pressure. One-way valves may be used to insure unidirectional flow patterns. A manometer is also incorporated into the system so that the amount of pressure applied to the airway may be measured.

C-PAP has the same uses, effects, hazards, and contraindications as does PEEP (positive end-expiratory pressure). The difference between C-PAP and PEEP lies in the patient's ventilatory status. C-PAP is applied to a spontaneously breathing patient and PEEP refers to positive airway pressure while on a mechanical ventilator. (The application of positive airway pressure will be discussed later in this chapter.)

If the patient is being weaned successfully,

Figure 54–14. A C-PAP system is used to maintain the oxygen status of a patient who is unable to maintain a PaO_2 but who is able to maintain an adequate $PaCO_2$. A Boehringer valve provides the positive airway pressure. (From McPherson, S.: *Respiratory Therapy Equipment.* St. Louis: C. V. Mosby Co., 1977.)

certain physiologic changes may occur. Among these changes is an increase in the vital capacity, tidal volume, and inspiratory force. The $PaCO_2$ will probably increase slightly as CMV tends to tip the patient into the hypocapneic side of carbon dioxide tensions. An increase in the alveolar-arterial oxygen difference will usually occur. If it remains within the 55 to 100 mm. Hg range (on 100 per cent O_2) the patient will probably be successful. The reason for an increased A-a gradient is probably the development of rapid alveolar collapse. The cardiac output may or may not rise following discontinuance of mechanical ventilation. A fall in cardiac output may indicate a return to CMV.

Oxygen consumption during weaning is directly related to the rise or fall of the cardiac output. It is increased if the CO_2 increases, and vice versa. Blood pressure and pulse may increase during weaning owing to an increased sympathoadrenal response occurrence.

The first attempt at weaning may not be successful. Failure is generally attributed to (1) decreased muscular strength due to poor nutritional status or certain disease processes, or the discoordination of respiratory muscles due to prolonged disuse because of prolonged CMV, (2) increased work of breathing due to an increase in airway resistance, abdominal distention, a small-diameter artificial airway, upper airway obstruction, and unresolved acute lung diseases, and (3) increased ventilation requirements.

If the first attempt is not successful, it is important to determine the reason(s) and try to eliminate these deterrents in subsequent attempts. Table 54–4 lists factors that indicate unsuccessful weaning. In this event, the patient must be returned to the continuous mechanical ventilator. The nurse and respiratory therapist must continue to closely monitor the patient's status. They must monitor, measure, and document spontaneous tidal volume; vital capacity; maximal voluntary ventilation; inspiratory effort; breath sounds; cardiovascular, renal and cerebral status; and arterial blood gases.

C-PAP and PEEP

C-PAP or PEEP may be used in the adult respiratory distress syndrome (ARDS). ARDS is composed of a wide variety of situations that cause adverse pulmonary effects due to alveolar collapse and loss of compliance.

Normal respiration returns the intrathoracic pressures to ambient atmospheric pressure. Application of positive airway pressure during *expiration* prevents the return of the intrathoracic pressures to atmospheric pressure. Instead, a new *above*-atmospheric expiratory-inspiratory baseline is established. (See Figure 54–15.) As noted, C-PAP is positive airway pressure applied during expiration on a spontaneously breathing patient, and PEEP refers to the application of positive pressure on patients being mechanically ventilated.

Physiologic Effects of PEEP/C-PAP. The FRC is that volume of air remaining in the lung after a normal expiration. If end-expiratory alveolar volumes remain above their critical closing point, the alveoli will remain open and functioning. However, if they close, the alveoli collapse. If alveolar collapse occurs, the volume of the FRC also decreases. When the alveoli collapse, hypoxemia results and the airway becomes "stiffer" or less compliant. (See Figure 54–16.)

Alveolar volume may be affected by (1) an alteration in the amount of surfactant. The less surfactant in the alveolus, the greater the forces of surface tension and thus the greater potential for alveolar collapse. (2) The volume of air actually present in the alveolus at end-expiration is important. The relationships of alveolar volume, volume of nitrogen in the alveolus, and inspired oxygen concentrations are important considerations in maintenance of alveolar integrity. The alveolar filler gas is nitrogen. A decreased concentration may cause alveolar collapse. Nitrogen is rapidly replaced by high concentrations of inspired oxygen. This depletion causes quick collapse. (3) The closing volume is greater than the patient's FRC. Bronchiolar closure during expiration may reduce alveolar ventilation.

When alveoli collapse, pulmonary blood flow continues. Although perfusion (blood flow) con-

TABLE 54–4. FACTORS INDICATING AN UNSUCCESSFUL WEANING ATTEMPT WITH MANDATORY RETURN OF THE PATIENT TO CONTINUOUS MECHANICAL VENTILATION

1. Change in blood pressure: a rise or fall of 20 mm. Hg systolic and/or 10 mm. Hg diastolic.
2. Pulse rate: increase of 20 beats/minute or pulse greater than 110.
3. Respiratory rate: an increase of 10/minute or a rate of more than 30 to 35/minute.
4. Tidal volume: less than 250 to 300 ml. (adult).
5. Significant ECG changes.

6. PaO_2	60 mm. Hg	Acceptable values in patients with COPD may be lower PaO_2 and pH and higher $PaCO_2$.
7. $PaCO_2$	55 mm. Hg	
8. pH	7.35	

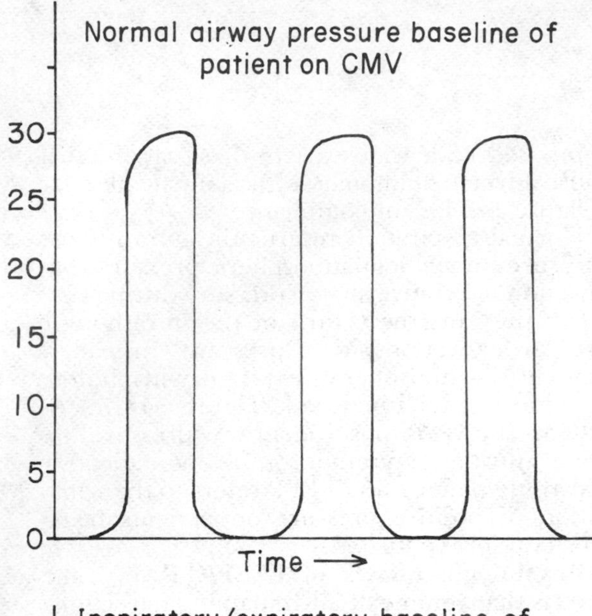

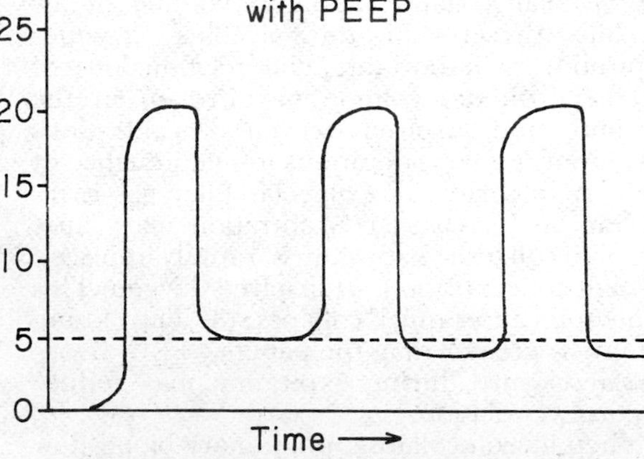

Figure 54–15. The reset resting inspiratory/expiratory levels for patients on CMV, PEEP, and C-PAP. Zero represents ambient pressure.

tinues, oxygenation of the blood flow to that alveolus does not occur. As alveoli collapse, the residual volume is decreased. A decreased RV also causes a reduced FRC. This results in a true intrapulmonary shunt. (A shunt refers to perfusion without oxygenation.) Lung compliance is also affected. Once alveolar collapse occurs, reinflation requires very high opening pressures. The generation of these high opening pressures significantly increases the work of breathing. The resulting hypoxemia from alveolar collapse and the increased oxygen consumption caused by the increased work of breathing may severely compromise the patient.

C-PAP and PEEP are used to maintain the alveolus in an open state. Thus oxygen status is improved. The major advantage of positive end-expiratory pressure is that oxygenation is improved and, generally, this may be accomplished by lower FIO_2's. In this way, the body's metabolic oxygen requirements may be met without the toxic effects of higher doses of oxygen.

Hazards of PEEP and C-PAP. The physiologic effects of positive airway pressure on inspiration-expiration are basically the same as those effects discussed in the section on IPPB and CMV. There are a few added risks such as rupture of the lung from increased intrathoracic and intra-airway pressures (barotrauma). Patients may develop pneumothorax, subcutaneous emphysema, and pneumomediastinum. Cardiovascular embarrassment may also occur. If the cardiac output cannot be improved with vasopressors or expansion of the blood volume,

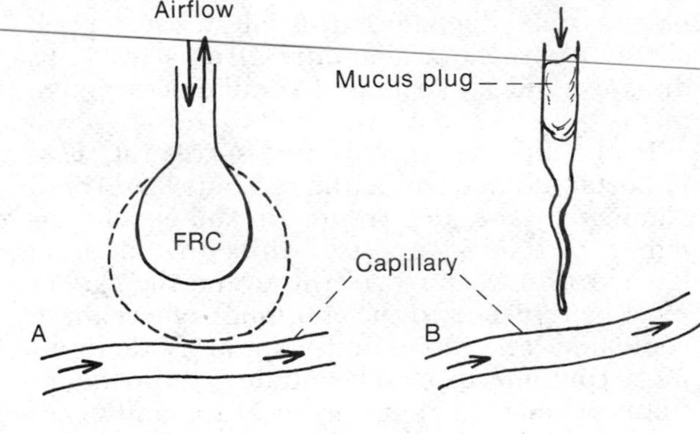

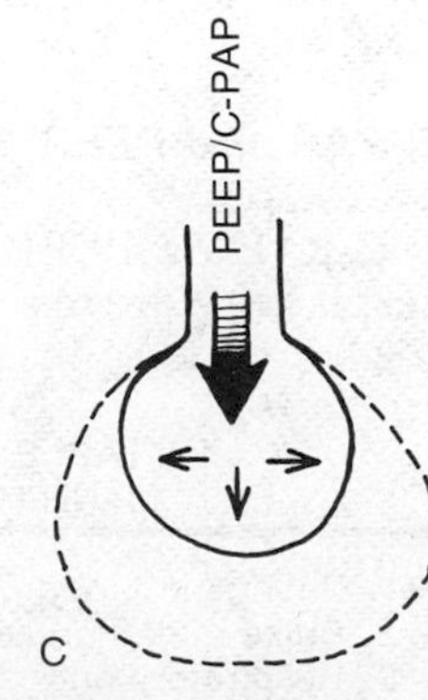

Figure 54–16. Effects of positive airway pressure on the alveolus. **A,** Normal alveolus. Dotted line represents expansion during inspiration. **B,** Collapsed alveolus. Perfusion continued. **C,** Alveolus opened by positive pressure. Dotted line indicates alveolus during inspiration and solid line indicates end-expiratory alveolar volume.

hepatic and renal function will be compromised. C-PAP or PEEP must be discontinued. The development of free air in the thorax also constitutes a potential emergency. The pressure must be relieved or cardiac tamponade may occur. C-PAP and PEEP also increase the intracranial pressure. In neurologic patients this is an added medical problem.

The nurse must observe the patient for untoward signs and symptoms. The basic parameters to be monitored are:

- blood pressure and heart rate;
- breath sounds;
- urinary output;
- signs of increased heart failure;
- chest film (before and following the institution of positive airway pressure);
- presence of free air in subcutaneous tissue (always feel both the posterior as well as the anterior subcutaneous tissue); and
- the arterial blood gas response.

The aim of C-PAP or PEEP is to find the amount of pressure that produces the best PaO_2 and reduces the amount of shunt without producing adverse effects such as hypotension. The search for this value is called *Best PEEP*. Positive airway pressure may be applied in adult levels of +5 to +20 cm. H_2O. Pressures greater than +20 cm. H_2O are often referred to as *Super PEEP*.

IPPB

Today the use and effectiveness of, and alternatives to, IPPB are being discussed and evaluated. At one time IPPB was the "miracle therapy," a panacea, and because much of the equipment required a degree of operational skill, it appeared that "everything was being done for the patient." The past few years have seen much soul searching and research into the actual benefits and uses of IPPB. The pendulum of pro versus con in respect to the value of IPPB seems to have finally settled into an in-between, realistic position.

IPPB does have its place in respiratory therapy but, like any form of therapy, it must be used with a therapeutic goal in mind, and must be evaluated frequently as to its efficacy. IPPB must be administered only for the correction of specific abnormalities. IPPB is not the only therapeutic modality employed in respiratory care; if IPPB is the *best therapy* for a specific abnormality then it must be administered therapeutically. The physician, nurse, and respiratory therapist must ascertain the effects of therapy.

The *indications* for IPPB include inability or unwillingness to deep breathe; impaired or ineffective cough mechanism; relief of acute shortness of breath, as in severe asthma and pulmonary edema; for delivery of aerosolized medications into the respiratory tree in patients unable or unwilling to deep breathe; to reverse acute hypoventilation and avoid intubation if frequent IPPB is successful in reduction of an acutely elevated $paCO_2$; as one method of weaning a patient from CMV; and subjective claims by patients that IPPB makes them feel better, after objective assessment. In patients with chronic CO_2 retention, IPPB may actually be harmful.

Contraindications for IPPB: uncorrected pneumothorax (this includes the optimal function of the chest tube and associated equipment); tracheoesophageal fistula that may cause gastric insufflation, vomiting, and aspiration; undiagnosed hemoptysis; bullous emphysema and other conditions with evidence of airtrapping; exacerbation of undesired cardiovascular effects and other adverse physiologic effects; inability of patient to correctly use this mode of therapy; and inadequate equipment and facilities as well as personnel untrained and unskilled in the proper techniques of IPPB administration.

IPPB may only be given if ordered by a physician. Therefore it is the physician who determines whether IPPB is the appropriate therapy, or whether therapeutic objectives could be attained by simpler, less expensive methods. The responsibility lies with the physician, but it is the nurse and therapist who administer and monitor therapy and who generally suggest alterations in therapy that will assist the patient in achieving the therapeutic goal.

Types of Positive Pressure Ventilators. There are two general types of mechanical ventilators: pressure-cycled and volume-cycled. Most of these machines can provide either controlled or assisted ventilation, intermittently or continuously. Pressure-cycled ventilators are most commonly used for elective intermittent therapy. Volume-cycled ventilators are used when continuous mechanical ventilation is indicated.

Pressure-cycled ventilators (see Fig. 54–17) are commonly powered by wall or tank oxygen. Usually this is for the sake of convenience and not therapeutic effectiveness. Because most pneumatically powered ventilators internally incorporate a Venturi device to entrain additional room air to meet the inspired ventilation needs of the patient, the FIO_2 delivered to the patient is variable. The FIO_2 at the beginning of in-

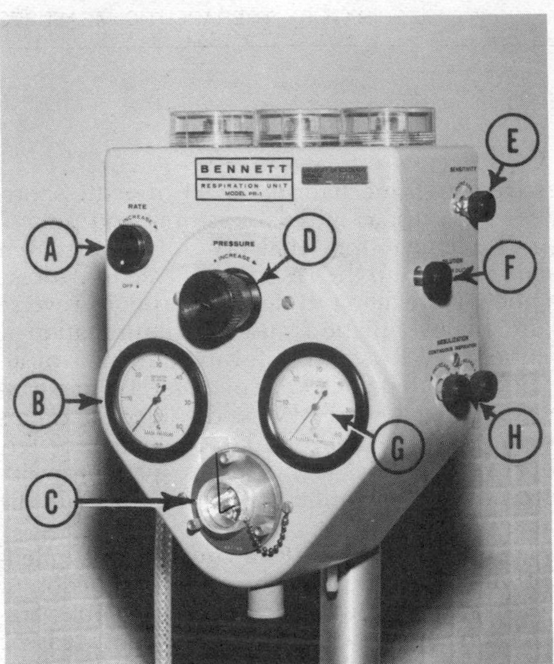

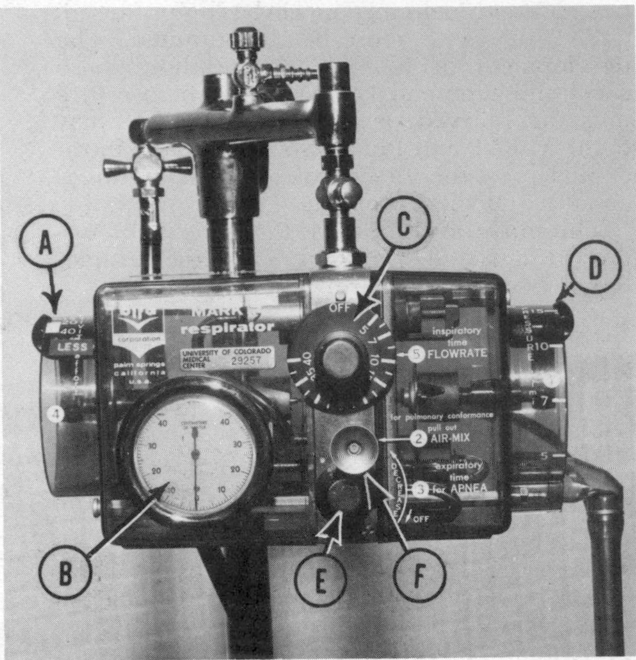

Figure 54–17. The Bennett PR-1 (left) has the following features: A = rate control; B = airway pressure indicator; C = flow-sensitive valve; D = pressure control; E = sensitivity control; F = oxygen diluter; G = machine pressure indicator; H = humidifier controls. The Bird Mark 7 (right) has: A = sensitivity control; B = airway pressure indicator; C = flow control; D = pressure control; E = rate control; F = oxygen diluter. (From Nett, L.: *Nursing Clinics of North America,* 9:128, Mar. 1974.)

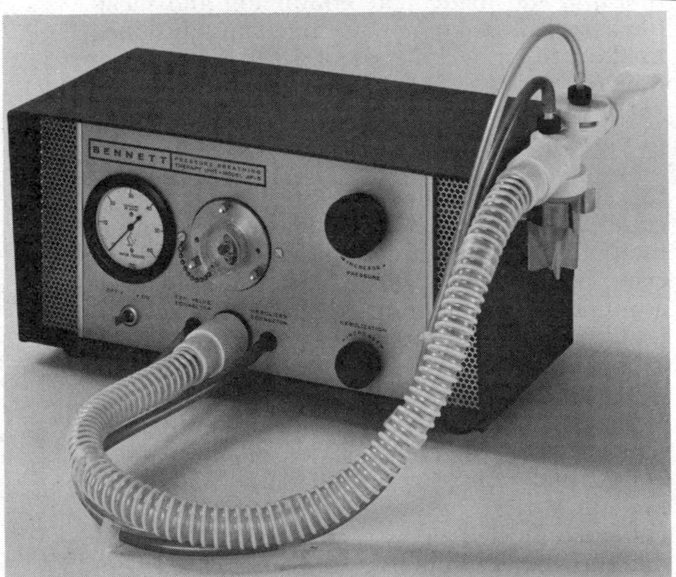

Figure 54–18. A portable pressure breathing therapy unit for home and hospital use. (Courtesy of Puritan-Bennett Corp., Kansas City, Mo.)

spiration may be 40 per cent, but during the final one third of the inspiratory phase, the FIO_2 is 100 per cent. Oxygen-driven IPPB ventilators must not be used on patients with chronic CO_2 retention, hypoxic-drive ventilatory stimulus, and those whose conditions would be compromised by varied, nonspecific oxygen tensions. If IPPB is indicated for these patients, compressed breathing air (21 per cent O_2) may be used to power the ventilator. If available, electrically powered, compressor-driven IPPB ventilators should be used. (See Figure 54–18.)

Pressure-cycled Ventilators. Also called "pressure-controlled" or "pressure-limited" ventilators, these include machines such as the Bird Mark 7 and Bennett (PR series) (Fig. 54–17). These ventilators are set by the nurse or respiratory therapist to deliver a specified amount of positive pressure (e.g., 10 to 30 cm. H_2O). Gas is delivered into the airway during inspiration until the proximal airway pressure equals the predetermined amount of pressure. When the preset pressure is reached in the airway, the machine is triggered into expiration and the patient exhales without assistance. With each inspiration the same pressure is reached. In the presence of increased pulmonary resistance and according to the therapeutic goal, it may be necessary to increase the pressure required to deliver the gas. The amount of resistance with the system (including the lungs) governs to some extent the volume of gas delivered.

When pressure-sensitive ventilators are being used, the total volume being expired is periodically measured by a *Wright respirometer* to ensure an adequate tidal volume. The machine is then adjusted as necessary, since the volume of gas that the patient receives is not always maintained at a constant level.

All models of pressure-cycled respirators have as primary controls: a *pressure control* with a pressure gauge that governs the tidal volume delivered (commonly the control is initially set at 15 to 20 cm. H_2O), and a *sensitivity control* that determines how much negative pressure the patient's inspiratory effort must have to cycle the respirator. Other controls that pressure-cycled machines may have include: (1) a *respirations control* or automatic cycling device (this must never be used for intermittent therapy purposes) (2) *inspiratory flow-rate control,* which determines the length of the inspiration cycle (i.e., the rate of speed at which the amount of inspiratory pressure set on the pressure-control dial will be delivered).

Volume-cycled Ventilators. These are also called "volume-controlled" or "volume-limited" ventilators. (See Figure 54–19.) These ventilators are used after the *volume* of inspired air to be delivered is preset. Within physiologic limits a pre-determined total volume is delivered regardless of airway pressure. The patient receives air at whatever amount of pressure is required to deliver it within safe limits. As stated, volume-controlled ventilators may be used for continuous mechanical ventilation.

A mouthpiece or mask can be used with pressure-cycled ventilators during IPPB, but an artificial airway is necessary for use of volume-cycled ventilators. (Pressure-cycled ventilators may also be used on intubated patients.)

Specific information regarding various brands of volume- and pressure-cycled ventilators will not be discussed in this text. The student is encouraged to refer to manufacturers' materials and respiratory therapy textbooks dealing with ventilators. It is essential that only persons fully educated and skilled in management of ventilators be allowed to administer and care for the patient on either pressure-limited or volume-cycled ventilators.

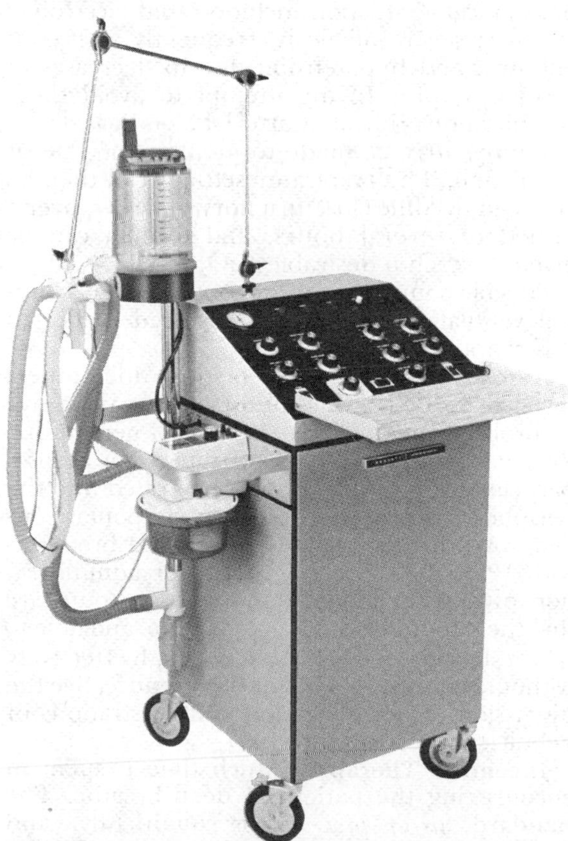

Figure 54–19. A Volume ventilator used either to assist or control a patient's respirations. (Courtesy of Puritan-Bennett Corp., Kansas City, Mo.)

Assisted (Patient-cycled) and Controlled (Machine-cycled) Ventilation. With *assisted* ventilation the patient's own inspiratory effort turns on ("trips") the respirator, thus initiating the mechanical inspiratory phase. The force of inspiration is then accelerated by the machine. Because some patients can make only weak inspiratory efforts, the respirator may be adjusted to respond to the individual patient's respiratory abilities. Thus, even a slight inspiratory effort may activate the positive pressure phase, causing the lungs to be rapidly inflated. When the flow of gas stops, the patient exhales without assistance from the machine. Some machines can be set to automatically trigger another inspiration if, after a period of delay, the patient does not spontaneously trigger the respirator. Setting the automatic cycling control thus safely assures ventilation if a patient's inspiratory efforts cease or become too weak to regularly trigger the machine.

Although the patient's own inspiratory efforts typically govern assisted ventilation, with *controlled* ventilation the patient's rate of ventilation is automatically cycled by the respirator at the predetermined number of cycles per minute. The respiratory cycle should allow for an expiratory time conducive to return of blood flow to the right heart.

An artificial airway (e.g., nasal or oral endotracheal tube, tracheostomy tube) is required for controlled ventilation. Cuffed tubes are used in the airway to insure adequate tidal volume. (Cuffed endotracheal and tracheostomy tubes are discussed in Unit XXIV.) Humidification of inspired air and gases is imperative in treating the intubated patient. Also, a patent airway must be maintained by suctioning the patient as necessary, using sterile technique.

Some patients who have spontaneous respirations "fight" the respirator during controlled ventilation because they cannot synchronize their respirations with the machine's cycle. Ungoverned respiratory efforts that are out of phase with the respirator exhaust the patient and cause ineffective alveolar ventilation. If the nurse is unable to help the patient to relax and to breathe in cycle with the machine, the physician should be contacted. When a patient is breathing out of cycle with the respirator, it is not advisable to overventilate the person in an effort to reduce spontaneous respiratory attempts. It is helpful to adjust the frequency of the automatic cycling to the patient's respiratory cycle when placing the patient on the respirator and then gradually change the machine's automatic cycling to the desired frequency and stroke volume.

When an artificial airway is in place, a patient who is fighting the respirator may safely be sedated or narcotized to reduce ventilatory efforts and successfully maintain automatic ventilatory control. Medications that may be given for this purpose are morphine, diazepam (Valium) and meperidine (Demerol). Some physicians administer small intravenous doses of D-tubocurarine (curare) to depress spontaneous ventilation, although it is not the paralyzing agent of choice if bronchospasm and increased airway resistance are evident or potential problems. Curare causes the release of a bronchoconstrictive agent, histamine. Bronchoconstriction and possibly hypotension may result. One of the newer nondepolarizing muscle relaxants is pancuronium bromide (Pavulon). It is five times as potent as d-tubocurare. Its actions resemble those of curare but with minimal histamine release. It is essential that the mechanical ventilators and disconnect alarms be in optimal functioning condition as these patients are unable to ventilate themselves due to myoneural blocking effects of the paralyzing agents. Nursing care must be at its best. Personnel caring for the paralyzed, continuously ventilated patient must realize that sensorium is *not* impaired by these agents. Nursing and respiratory care personnel must not act as if the patient were comatose or deaf; careful reassurance and explanation must also be incorporated into the patient's care.

The usual IV dose of curare is 9 to 30 mg. for 30 to 60 minutes of paralysis. It may be administered in divided doses to maintain relaxation effects. Optimal action of the drug is obtained when the diaphragm is paralyzed. The average effective dose of Pavulon is 4 to 6 mg. for 30 to 60 minutes of paralysis. Reversal of these effects is by drugs that inhibit acetylcholinesterase and allow an excess of acetylcholine to accumulate at the myoneural junction. Neostigmine (Prostigmine) and edrophonium (Tensilon) are the drugs administered to reverse the paralysis. However, serial doses may need to be administered if overcurarization occurred, as recurrence of paralysis is possible.[105]

Muscle-paralyzing agents may also be administered in continuous IV drip with the rate of infusion titrated to control the prolonged paralytic effects.

Controlled respiration is frequently used if the patient has muscle spasms, is bucking the ventilator, or is confused or tachypneic, or if respiratory efforts are out of phase with the mechanical ventilator. Paralyzing agents may also be used to insure effective mechanical ventilation in the management of patients who have sustained head injury, flail chest, seizure disorders, or tetanus.

Once a patient begins to ventilate spontaneously continuous ventilation is stopped and the person is given assisted ventilation.

A patient receiving continuous, controlled, positive-pressure ventilation is totally dependent and therefore requires constant supervision by skilled personnel.

When patients are initially placed on a ventilator they must be closely observed to evaluate effectiveness of the therapy and to prevent complications. Blood gases may be monitored and critical adjustments made on the mechanical apparatus. The most common serious complications that arise during the initial period of mechanical ventilation include rapid electrolyte changes; severe alkalosis, frequently with convulsions; and hypotension due to decreases in cardiac output. In an attempt to avoid these complications repeated arterial blood gas determinations may be made to monitor the rate of ventilation. The respirator settings can then be adjusted to come close to a normal $PaCO_2$ over a period of several hours, and oxygen can be given to reach a desirable PaO_2 level.

Possible complications of continuous mechanical ventilation have been discussed earlier in this chapter.

Aerosol Therapy. Patients who do not meet the criteria for IPPB administration may receive aerosolized medications via aerosol generators. Recent studies have demonstrated that aerosol particles are more uniformly deposited into the peripheral airway if carried by a spontaneous deep breath rather than by a forced breath as with IPPB. The major criteria for administration of aerosol medications via this route are that the patient be alert, cooperative, and able to take a slow, deep breath and to cough effectively without requiring mechanical assistance. See the discussion of aerosolization and illustrations of nebulizers on pp. 1235–1237.

Incentive Therapy. Much time is spent in encouraging the patient to deep breathe. The standard *stir-up procedure* is cough, turn, and deep breathe. Studies have shown that, if properly done, deep breathing plays a key role in the prevention of atelectasis. A deep breath is also the most potent bronchodilator. A deep breath is also *essential* for production of an effective cough. A number of patients may have impairments that seriously affect their ability to cough and deep breathe. These patients will require a combination of respiratory therapy modalities to effectively maintain the patency of the airway and prevent serious pulmonary complications. However, a great many patients, especially postoperative patients, may have no serious pulmonary impairments. These people still need to cough and deep breathe to prevent secretion retention but are able to cooperate and perform these modalities with a minimum of mechanical assistance.

A slow, spontaneous deep breath, with an inspiratory hold for 3 to 5 seconds, has been shown to significantly reduce the incidence of pulmonary complications. Spontaneous deep breaths are effective, but the effects are better if an *incentive device* is used. (See Figure 54–20.) These devices offer visual reward as well as a means of assessment of the inspired volume. Incentive breathing devices affect the inspiratory capacity (IC) and work on the principle of *sustained voluntary maximal inflation.* This is a form of *goal-directed therapy.*

For the best effect, the use of these devices must be taught preoperatively and not when the patient is heavily sedated or in pain. Patients with pneumonia, neuromuscular weakness, and medical conditions that may predispose to fluid collection also benefit from incentive devices. They are always left at the bedside. The patient is instructed to perform the sustained voluntary maximal inflation maneuver 10 to 20 times an hour. The patient should be supervised and goals increased frequently.

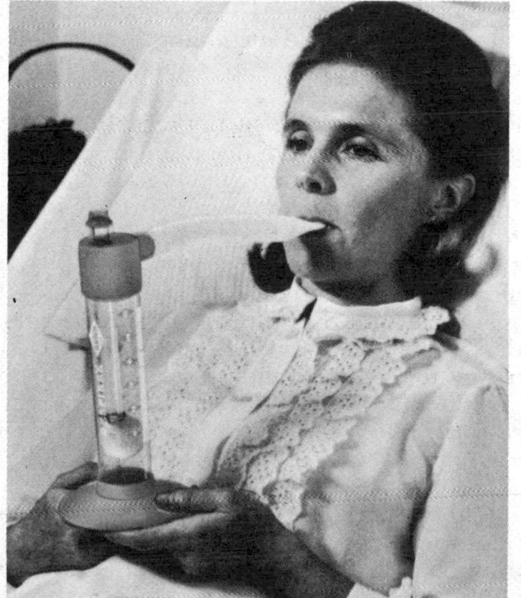

Figure 54–20. A type of incentive device used to promote effective deep breathing. (Courtesy of John Bunn Co., Buffalo, N.Y.)

Incentive exercise procedure:

1. The goal is set for the patient.
2. The patient is instructed to exhale slowly and completely, then told:
3. Place the mouthpiece between the teeth and close lips around mouthpiece.
4. Using the mouth *only,* take a slow, deep breath until the preset goal is reached.
5. Sustain the inflation pressure in the chest for 3 to 5 seconds.
6. Exhale slowly.
7. Repeat steps 1 through 6.

Patients may be overzealous and require verbal caution not to rush. The effects of overventilation have been mentioned: dizziness, lightheadedness, and so on. It must be remembered that incentive therapy is not effective in patients unable to take a deep breath due to lack of cooperation, pain, discoordination of respiration, lack of motivation, weakness, obtundation, or senility.

Other forms of respiratory therapy may be incorporated into the incentive therapy program: (1) hydration; (2) aerosolization of medications; (3) mobilization maneuvers such as turning, position changes, and ambulation; (4) breathing retraining; (5) postural drainage and chest physiotherapy; and (6) assistance and instruction in effective coughing techniques. As with all forms of respiratory therapy, it is essential that the effectiveness of therapy be frequently evaluated.

SUCTIONING*

Suctioning (aspiration of secretions) is a common nursing activity employed to remove secretions from the nose, mouth, or tracheobronchial tree and to stimulate productive coughing. Suctioning of the nose and mouth is a relatively simple, safe procedure, details for which can be found in textbooks of nursing fundamentals. This discussion focuses on tracheal suctioning.

Tracheal Suctioning

Tracheal suctioning is also called "deep" suctioning. Suctioning of the trachea and proximal portions of each mainstem bronchus may be performed by passing a sterile catheter through the mouth ("orotracheal"), through the nose

*For a more complete discussion of suctioning, refer to Sorensen and Luckmann, *Basic Nursing: A Psychophysiologic Approach.*

("nasotracheal"), or through an endotracheal or tracheostomy tube. Nurses most commonly perform tracheal suctioning through the nose or via an artificial airway. Suctioning through a tracheostomy is discussed in Unit XXIV.

When properly performed, tracheal suctioning can be helpful and relatively painless and will promote the comfort (indeed, perhaps, save the life) of a patient in respiratory distress. If improperly performed, this procedure can be detrimental, painful, and possibly even fatal.

The various complications of tracheal suctioning are infection, hypoxemia, hypoxia, mechanical trauma to the airway, alveolar collapse, vagal stimulation, bradycardia, rupture of a bronchial suture line, and cardiac arrhythmias and death.

Preoxygenation and hyperinflation of the patient before, during, and following the suction process help to prevent complications. *Lobar collapse* occurs when air cannot enter a portion of the lung. Suctioning may produce lobar collapse if a catheter is too large in diameter for the size of the airway being suctioned. It is important to carefully select a catheter of appropriate size for suctioning and not to force or wedge the catheter into a bronchus. (The diameter of the bronchus becomes smaller as it extends away from the trachea.) Caution is necessary when performing deep tracheal suctioning following pulmonary surgery because a suture line may be traumatized by the catheter, i.e., the catheter may be *accidentally pushed through a sutured bronchus.*

Continuous suctioning for 15 to 30 seconds can produce *sudden death.* Possible causes include prolonged suctioning, which causes anoxia and then *severe cardiac arrhythmias;* respiratory tract reflexes, which stimulate *bradycardia* and *bronchospasm;* and *distention of the heart with blood* from the superior vena cava and pulmonary artery. Critically ill patients should never be suctioned longer than 15 seconds, and it is safe to suction for that long *only* if the patient has been preoxygenated and is carefully monitored for indications of complications. It is generally safest to apply suction intermittently for no longer than 5 to 8 seconds.

Because it is a potentially hazardous procedure, deep tracheal aspiration should not be performed without advanced training in the procedure. In some settings the physician's permission is necessary for this procedure. *Techniques to mechanically stimulate coughing should be used before resorting to suctioning.* These techniques (e.g., direct external mechanical stimulation of the trachea and internal mechanical stimulation of the trachea produced by prolonged exhalation of the patient) are discussed on p. 1213. Coughing is frequently stimulated by passage of a catheter through the nose or mouth.

Ungvarski comments as follows about the need for endotracheal suctioning:[173a]

> It should be kept in mind that most patients, unless they are extremely debilitated, are quite capable, physiologically, of coughing up sputum into the pharynx and then expectorating or swallowing it. Therefore, the primary purpose of introducing a catheter into the trachea is not vigorous suctioning but, simply, tracheal stimulation with a catheter.
>
> Actual endotracheal suctioning need only be used for patients with tenacious secretions (which must be physically removed by suction) or impaired pulmonary function (which may interfere with the cough reflex), or for those who are extremely debilitated and too weak to bring up secretions even after vigorous coughing.

The goals of all suctioning procedures are to remove secretions and stimulate productive coughing without causing prolonged airway obstruction, infection, damage to delicate mucous membranes, or other complications.

Factors of General Importance. *Observe the patient closely for indications of the need to be suctioned,* such as noisy respirations, restlessness, and increased pulse and respiratory rates. Cyanosis is a late sign of upper airway obstruction and hypoxemia. The conscious patient is usually aware of the need to be suctioned and can inform the nurse. Obtunded patients must be carefully observed and suctioned promptly when indicated. Keep operable suctioning equipment and ample suctioning supplies at the bedside of any patient who is unable to clear the tracheobronchial tree.

Patients who require suctioning often benefit from humidification of inspired air, since this tends to liquefy secretions and make them easier to remove by suction. Prior to suctioning, attempt to move secretions up into higher levels in the tracheobronchial tree by using postural drainage with percussion and vibration. To loosen tenacious, thick mucus the physician may order the nurse to instill a few milliliters of sterile water, normal saline, or sodium bicarbonate solution (5 per cent) into the trachea immediately prior to aspiration. Additionally, liquefying agents may be instilled through the catheter. The instillation of small amounts of sterile normal saline (1 to 2 ml.) may reduce the tendency of plastic catheters to stick to the walls of plastic intratracheal or tracheostomy tubes. The solution is inserted in this instance while the suction catheter is being passed.

As mentioned, infection is one hazard of

suctioning. Nasal or oral suctioning is a clean procedure; wash your hands before suctioning. *Tracheal suctioning is a sterile procedure;** wear sterile gloves and use sterile solutions and catheters. *Storage of suction catheters in an antiseptic solution is not acceptable practice.* Studies have revealed that this practice only encourages the growth of bacteria, especially gram-negative bacteria. Additional harm may be done if droplets of the solution are deposited on the mucous membrane of the airway. Disposable gloves and catheters reduce the possibility of introducing infection into the lungs. Infection is risked each time a catheter is introduced into the tracheobronchial tree, since normally this is a sterile structure. *Always use separate equipment to suction the nose or mouth;* i.e., never suction the trachea with a catheter used previously for nasal or oral suctioning. Frequently exchange suction equipment kept at the bedside to prevent possible use of contaminated equipment.

Select an Appropriate Suction Catheter. Never use a closed-tip catheter, such as a urinary catheter. A straight whistle-tip catheter is most frequently used and 90 per cent of the time will only cannulate the right mainstem bronchus. Cannulation and suctioning of the left mainstem bronchus is facilitated by use of a coudé-tip catheter. Soft plastic catheters are now available, and a transparent catheter is useful because suctioned material can be observed.

Catheter sizes used for suctioning vary, depending on the diameter of the orifice to be intubated, e.g., nostrils, endotracheal or tracheostomy tube lumen, and so forth. Frequently No. 14 or 16 (Fr.) catheters are used for tracheal suctioning in an adult. The catheter should be one half to two thirds the diameter of the tube to be intubated. If the catheter's diameter is too small it may be impossible to remove thick secretions or mucus plugs. On the other hand, too large a catheter occludes the orifice's opening and causes excessive negative pressure, which may predispose to atelectasis or lobar collapse. It is most desirable to have available several sizes (Fr. Nos. 12, 14, and 16) of sterile suction catheters for adult suctioning.

Prior to suctioning be certain the patient is well oxygenated. Some sources[148A] recommend administering 100 per cent O_2 for 5 minutes to increase the patient's PaO_2 before suctioning. Because tracheal suctioning removes O_2, it lowers the PaO_2 and can trigger cardiac arrhythmias.

Evaluate a patient's pulse (for bradycardia) and heart action (for indications of heart block) on a cardiac monitor if possible when preparing to suction and while suctioning. Monitor the patient throughout the suctioning procedure, observing for the following sequence of events, which may occur as a result of excessive suctioning, or in patients with a low PaO_2 or marginal cardiopulmonary reserve before suctioning: initial tachycardia, followed by cardiac irritability and downward shifting of the natural pacemaker, i.e., premature contractions; nodal rhythm, resulting from myocardial hypoxia and acidosis; bradycardia; and, finally, asystole. If tachycardia occurs during tracheal suctioning, evaluate the severity of the symptom and proceed only if it is mild. *Discontinue suctioning immediately if bradycardia develops and ventilate the patient with high O_2 concentrations.* Report untoward effects of suctioning at once.

Perform the suction procedure gently; lubricate the catheter, insert it carefully, avoid excessive suction pressures, and do not move the catheter up and down within the trachea with poking or jabbing motions. Respiratory tract mucosa is easily damaged and is subject to edema, bleeding, ulceration, and infection. Rough or prolonged suctioning and excessive pressures traumatize tracheobronchial mucosa and may produce tracheobronchitis and perhaps its feared complications of tracheal or bronchial stenosis. Even with gentle suction technique the trachea's walls are irritated and traumatized slightly each time suction is performed. *Suction a patient as frequently as indicated but no oftener.* Excessive suctioning not only is traumatic but also stimulates production of increased secretions. Never insert a dry catheter into the trachea. Before insertion lubricate the catheter's distal end with sterile water, sterile normal saline, or a fine coating of a nonreactive, water-soluble lubricant, e.g., K-Y jelly. Release suction if you feel the catheter "grab" against mucous membranes; otherwise, the mucosa will avulse into the catheter openings.

Keep suction periods brief. Do not apply suction while inserting the catheter (Fig. 54–21). Application of suction during insertion causes suction on tracheal mucosa (thus irritating and traumatizing the mucosa) and removes more oxygen while creating microatelectasis; remember that suction removes air as well as secretions. As mentioned, it is recommended that suctioning periods *never* exceed 15 seconds. *Prolonged suctioning may worsen respiratory insufficiency and produce hypoxia, asphyxia, and cardiac arrest.* Hypoxia may result from use of too large a catheter, use of suction that is too high, or not allowing the patient time to adequately hyperoxygenate and hyperinflate between periods of suctioning[173a] (Fig. 54–21). Overstimulation or prolonged irritation at the bifurcation of the trachea during

*In some instances "clean technique" is used in caring for patients with permanent tracheostomies, e.g., the hands are thoroughly washed before suctioning.

deep endotracheal suctioning may produce multiple premature ventricular contractions, leading to cardiac arrest.

Avoid excessive suction pressure. Adjust the suction to correspond with the nature of the secretions being removed. Use the lowest level of negative pressure that will be effective. Withdraw the catheter slowly while applying suction. During removal rotate the catheter around your forefinger. This exposes the catheter's openings to a greater tracheal surface area, enabling more effective removal of secretion and less localized mucosal trauma.

If it is necessary to continue the suctioning procedure, *allow the patient to rest,* and administer O_2 if indicated for about 3 minutes before the next insertion. If the patient is on a respirator, ventilate the patient for a while and *administer O_2 before suctioning again.* At the termination of tracheal suctioning, again raise the patient's PaO_2 to presuctioning levels by administering high O_2 concentrations.

Beware of patients for whom tracheal suctioning is particularly dangerous. Suction these patients only if absolutely necessary. Jacquette[82] identifies the following high-risk situations: (1) PaO_2 below 70 mm. Hg (suctioning would further reduce the arterial O_2 tension); (2) large alveolar-arterial gradient* (indicates very low cardiopulmonary reserve); and (3) generally poor condition, e.g., inadequate oxygenation, hypotension, arrhythmias, acid-base imbalances.

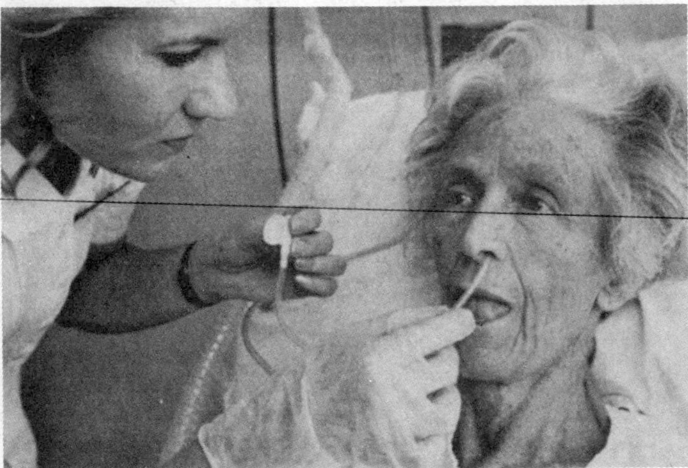

A

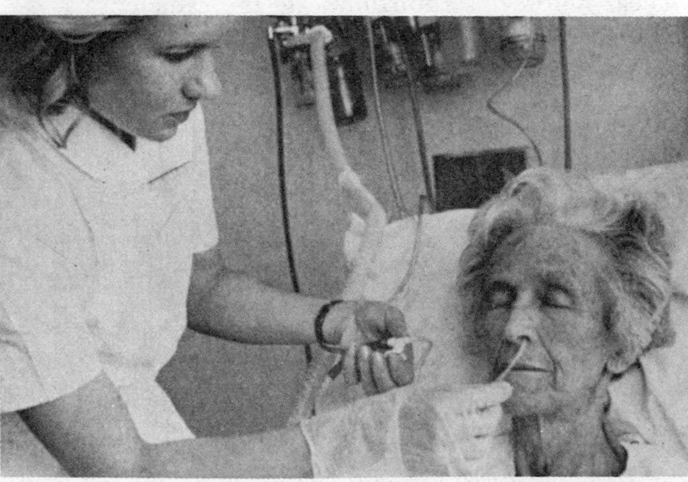

B

Figure 54–21. Precautions important with tracheal suctioning. *A,* Catheter is not attached to suction while it is being passed, but oxygen and suction tubing, placed across the pillow, are readily accessible for connection. *B,* Between suction attempts, the catheter is connected to oxygen and the patient rests. (From Jacquette, G.: *American Journal of Nursing, 71*:2362, Dec. 1971.)

Nasotracheal Suctioning Procedures

Nasotracheal suctioning is performed using sterile (preferably disposable) gloves, catheter, lubricant, and irrigating solutions. A catheter is inserted past the posterior oropharynx, around the epiglottis, through the vocal cords, and finally down into the trachea. The vocal cords open with inspiration. If passage of the catheter through the vocal cords is difficult, instruct the patient to "take a deep breath" as you insert and pass the catheter. This opens the cords wider to allow easier passage of the catheter.

Various problems can make it difficult to gain access to the trachea with a catheter; among these are presence of obstructing material in the nostrils, of swollen mucous membranes, and of nasal polyps or deviated nasal septum. Additionally, nasal passages are extremely tender; thus, pain is easily produced. Another problem that can occur is that the catheter may go into the esophagus if the patient swallows when the catheter reaches the epiglottis, or the catheter may coil in the nasopharynx instead of passing through the epiglottis.

The trachea bifurcates into the right and left mainstem bronchi. The right mainstem bronchus typically has a 15 degree angle to the vertical, while the left mainstem bronchus is angled at about 25 to 35 degrees. The more acute angulation of the left bronchus makes it more difficult to intubate than the right. Nonetheless, it is possible to intubate either mainstem bronchus during tracheal suctioning by angulation of the head and neck toward the side

*The alveolar-arterial gradient is normally a difference of about 50 to 55 mm. Hg. It represents the difference between the O_2 tension of alveolar air and of the arterial blood once respiration has occurred. Large alveolar-arterial gradients signify poor ventilation/perfusion ratio, poor ventilation of segments of the lung with air, and poor perfusion of pulmonary segments with blood.

opposite the bronchus to be entered, using a suction catheter with a slightly curved tip, and rotating the catheter's tip so it points toward the bronchus to be entered. To enter the right mainstem bronchus, position the patient partially on the right side, turn the head to the left, and point the chin up. Reverse these positions to enter the left mainstem bronchus.

Effective tracheal suctioning is a gentle yet swift procedure in which timing is important. The person performing the procedure works with deliberate, controlled actions. Deep suctioning is best accomplished through an artificial airway, especially a tracheostomy. The need to remove secretions from this patient will be evident due to loud, wet respirations and visible mucous bubbling into the tubing; by auscultation and the recognition of rhonchi; and through an increase in the peak airway pressure visible on the manometer if the patient is on CMV. The suctioning procedure must be particularly well coordinated when a patient is attached to a respirator. If the patient has a cuffed endotracheal or tracheostomy tube, suctioning is performed, when possible, when the cuff is deflated and the patient's position is changed, or when other treatments are given to facilitate gravitation of the secretions in the airway. By planning nursing care activities so they coincide it is possible to provide the patient with more periods of undisturbed rest.

When performing tracheal suctioning on a patient with chest tubes, the tubes are temporarily clamped. This is done because violent coughing may be stimulated, and clamping the tubes limits dissipation of the effort and force of coughing. If the tubes are not clamped, a significant reduction occurs in the peak negative and positive pressures, and energy is used during inspiration to draw water up the tubing (from the underwater seal) and to expel the air in the pleural space during expiration.

Endotracheal suctioning is an uncomfortable, often frightening procedure for a patient. Once the catheter passes between the vocal cords the patient cannot talk because the cords cannot approximate. The catheter's presence in the trachea may make the patient highly anxious and acutely restless. The patient benefits from directions about what to do to help during the procedure and from frequent reassurance. Often during tracheal suctioning the patient instinctively wants to pull at the catheter, especially when the cough reflex is stimulated. Cooperative patients can be asked to try to control this instinct.

Some patients tolerate tracheal suctioning better if they are given an analgesic half an hour before the procedure. Occasionally it is necessary to spray the nasopharynx and hypopharynx with a topical anesthetic in patients with extremely active gag reflexes. However, the use of an anesthetic is generally to be avoided because it depresses the cough reflex and increases the risk of aspiration if the patient vomits.

In preparation for nasotracheal suctioning, place an emesis basin and tissues within easy reach for use when the patient expectorates. Have the patient blow the nose to clear the nasal passageways. With a flashlight inspect the patient's nostrils for possible obstructions (e.g., deviated nasal septum) before inserting the suction catheter. Select the least obstructed nostril for suctioning. If both nostrils appear free of obstruction, use them alternately for the different suctioning sessions so you do not excessively irritate one nostril. (Remember to chart which nostril was used.)

Nasotracheal suctioning may be facilitated if a *nasal airway* (Fig. 54–22*A*) is inserted into one of the external nares. This device facilitates proper entry into the trachea. Available in both millimeter and French sizes, the correct size airway may be lubricated with water-soluble or anesthetic jelly and left in place for a few days. It prevents repeated mechanical irritation and trauma. It is especially helpful in the nonintubated patient who requires frequent nasotracheal suctioning.

An *oropharyngeal airway* (Fig. 54–22*B*) is useful not only in keeping the tongue out of the posterior oropharynx, but also as a guide for the suction catheter as it is introduced into the posterior oropharynx. It may be left in place in the obtunded patient. Patients who are alert rarely allow one to be left in place.

Procedure. Nasotracheal suctioning may be accomplished as follows (see Fig. 54–23).

Position the patient sitting up, leaning slightly forward, with back supported. The patient's face should look straight ahead, with the head extended and neck slightly flexed. An assistant (if present) should stand behind the patient.

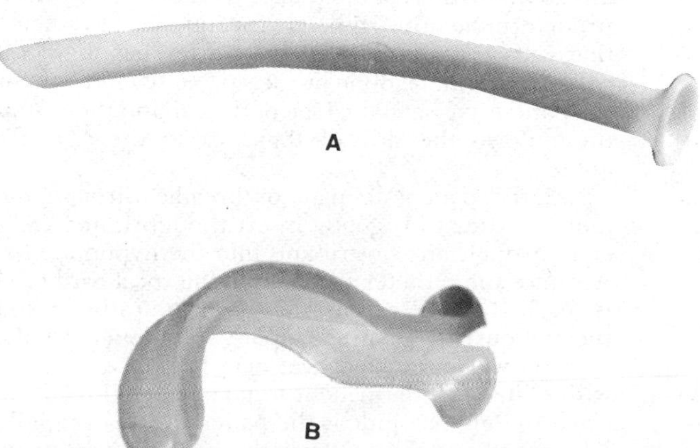

Figure 54–22. **A.** The placement of a nasal airway may facilitate effective and less traumatic nasal tracheal suction. **B.** An oropharyngeal airway may be used in the obtunded patient. This is a Berman-style airway. (Courtesy of Portex Co., Inc., Wilmington, Me.)

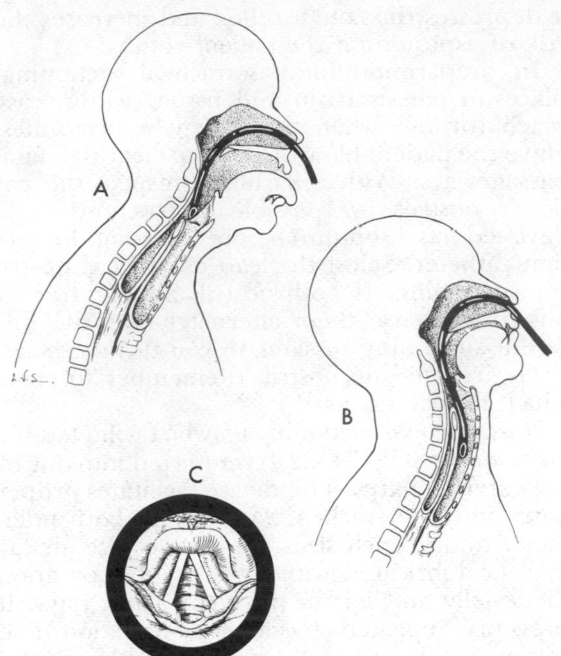

Figure 54–23. Technique of nasotracheal suctioning. *A,* Optimal position of head in order to direct catheter tip anteriorly into the trachea. *B,* After the catheter has been advanced into the trachea, the tongue is released and the patient's head may be more comfortably positioned. *C,* View of the vocal cords from above. The cords are most widely separated during inspiration. (From Sanderson, R. G. (Ed.): *The Cardiac Patient.* Philadelphia, W. B. Saunders Co., 1972.)

Have the patient extend the jaw, open the mouth widely and stick out the tongue. The assistant grasps the tongue with a dry 4 × 4 gauze. Pulling the tongue forward displaces the epiglottis forward and helps to prevent deflection of the catheter into the esophagus. (Once the catheter reaches the trachea the tongue is released and the patient can position the head more comfortably.)

Note the position of the curved catheter tip in relation to the Y connector, so you will know in which direction the tip is pointed once it is out of sight. Also, predetermine approximately the amount of catheter that will be inserted when the tip reaches the vocal cords. This can be done by measuring from the tip of the patient's nose to the lobe of the ear and then from there down the side of the neck to the "Adam's apple."

Ask the patient to pant or breathe through the mouth. After this, gently insert the lubricated catheter through one nostril and into the hypopharynx. Advance the catheter slowly until the vocal cord level is reached. Make certain the tip of the catheter and the patient's head are properly positioned so the catheter will enter whichever mainstem bronchus you wish. Then ask the patient to take a deep breath (to open the glottis) and, as the patient does so, rapidly advance the catheter through the larynx into the trachea, unless resistance is met. To stabilize the position of the catheter and thus prevent its accidental withdrawal, hold the catheter near the patient's nose. Up to this time tracheal suction should not be applied.

Apply suction by *intermittent* occlusion of the Y connector orifice or vent with the thumb for 5 to 8 seconds after any possible wedging of the catheter tip is corrected by withdrawing the catheter for 1 or 2 cm. Suction is applied only while the catheter is being withdrawn. During suctioning, listen for air-sucking sounds at the level of the catheter tip. (If these sounds cease, or if the catheter tip feels as if it were stuck against the tracheal wall and is not easily withdrawn, stop suctioning.) While intermittently applying suction, progressively withdraw the catheter a short distance until the entire length of the trachea is suctioned.

Allow the patient sufficient rest periods as you advance down each mainstem bronchus and as you suction that bronchus during withdrawal of the catheter. During rest periods the catheter may be left in place, but suction is not applied. If the patient appears anoxic, administer O_2 temporarily by mask or through the catheter. If indicated, instill 5 ml. of sterile water or sterile saline into each mainstem bronchus and repeat the suctioning.

If the catheter cannot be inserted to the expected depth, a mucus plug may be obstructing the lumen of the trachea. Instillation of a small amount of sterile water or normal saline is useful in such a situation to liquefy the mucus sufficiently for the suction catheter to withdraw the mucus, and the catheter can then be inserted to the desired depth. Injection of a mixture of acetylcysteine (Mucomyst) in normal saline may be ordered through the catheter to help loosen and liquefy secretions.

Following tracheal suctioning, auscultate the chest to determine the effectiveness of the procedure. Repeat suctioning as indicated after letting the patient rest for at least 3 minutes and administering O_2. Chart the effectiveness of the procedure, the character and amounts of secretions removed, and the patient's tolerance of the procedure. Aspiration of blood-tinged mucus may indicate that suction has been too forceful and has damaged the mucous membranes.

EMERGENCY CARDIOPULMONARY RESUSCITATION

If a patient's respirations cease, immediately begin ventilation through the nose or mouth. Feel the carotid pulse after inflating the lungs a few times. If the pulse is not detectable, begin external cardiac compression in an attempt to restore circulation. Then continue both respiratory and circulatory resuscitation. If obstruction prevents artificial ventilation or if the airway cannot be cleared, emergency establishment of an airway is indicated to bypass the obstruction, i.e., tracheal intubation is indicated. (Cardiopulmonary resuscitation is discussed in detail in Unit XII. Mouth-to-neck resuscitation is discussed in Unit XXIV.)

CHAPTER 55

DISORDERS OF THE PLEURAE, PLEURAL SPACES, TRACHEOBRONCHIAL TREE, AND LUNGS

DISORDERS OF THE PLEURAE OR PLEURAL SPACES

Pleurisy (Pleuritis)

Inflammation of the pleura may be *fibrinous* (dry) or *serofibrinous* (wet). A *wet pleurisy* is accompanied by pleural effusion as a result of an abnormal increase of nonpurulent pleural fluid. In *dry pleurisy* the amount of pleural fluid does not increase.

DRY PLEURISY

This condition frequently accompanies pneumonia and other inflammatory pulmonary diseases, and may complicate such disorders as chest trauma, cancer, pulmonary infarction, chest wall infections, mediastinitis, and pericarditis. The size of the area affected may range from a small portion to most of the pleural surface.

Dry pleurisy typically develops suddenly and is easily diagnosed by characteristic pleuritic pain and a friction rub, which can be detected by auscultation.

Pleuritic pain associated with dry pleurisy results from the rubbing together of the two inflamed pleural surfaces during breathing. The pain is caused only by inflammation of the parietal pleura, since the visceral pleura contains no pain receptors. Some patients with dry pleurisy have vague discomfort or pain only when coughing or breathing deeply, whereas others have severe, sharp stabbing pains. Often pleuritic pain is (a) more severe during inspiration (which stretches the inflamed pleura) and (b) localized to one side of the chest.

The characteristic *pleural friction rub* results from the rubbing together of the congested, inflamed pleurae. If effusion develops and fluid separates the pleurae, the friction rub ceases. A pleural friction rub most commonly is heard 24 to 48 hours after the beginning of pleuritic pain. The sounds of a pleural friction rub vary in intensity and are heard during both inspiration and expiration.

The patient with a dry pleurisy may have fever and malaise. Often pain causes the person to breathe shallowly and rapidly. The breathing motions of the affected side may be observed to be limited since the patient may use accessory muscles to help breathing rather than fully expanding the lower chest. In an attempt to limit respiratory movements the patient may press the affected side of the chest with the palm of the hand while breathing or coughing, or may lie on the affected side.

Treatment of dry pleurisy involves identifying and treating the underlying disease, placing the patient at rest, and providing symptomatic treatment directed at pain relief. In order to help minimize the patient's pain, position the patient on the affected side to splint the chest. Also, manually splint the patient's chest during coughing (if the person is unable to do this alone effectively). The correct method of splinting a patient's chest during coughing is discussed on p. 1365. The patient on bed rest must be frequently turned and periodically encouraged to cough and deep breathe to prevent complications of inactivity. Since the patient's natural tendencies are to avoid coughing and to breathe shallowly, the lungs may be poorly aerated. Thus, periodic expansion of lung tissue (by turning and deep breathing) and clearing of the tracheobronchial tree (by coughing and turning) are essential. Formerly a routine treatment of pleurisy was to strap the patient's chest with strips of adhesive tape or bind it with a chest binder in an effort to minimize the pain associated with breathing. These methods of treatment are currently seldom used because it is realized that they may detrimentally interfere with adequate aeration and respiration and foster the development of atelectasis and pneumonia.

Obtaining pain relief may require an antitussive medication (if a hacking, nonproductive cough is present) and analgesics. Some patients obtain relief from aspirin, but others require stronger analgesics, e.g., codeine, morphine, or meperidine (Demerol). Narcotics are administered cautiously to prevent further reduction of coughing and ventilation (by depressing the cough and breathing centers of the brain). Applications of heat over the painful area may provide comfort.

Some physicians treat mild pleuritic pain by spraying ethyl chloride over the area of greatest pain for about 1 minute, and then spraying along the body's long axis through the entire area of pain in such a way that a line of frost about one inch wide is produced. This procedure often gives relief for 1 to 10 hours. Severe pleuritic pain may be treated with a series of subcutaneous injections of procaine hydrochloride solution in the area of greatest pain. Occasionally to relieve pleuritic pain it is necessary to block the intercostal nerves by the paravertebral infiltration of an anesthetic agent. (See Chapter 30.)

WET PLEURISY

As stated, *wet pleurisy* is accompanied by an abnormal increase in the pleural fluid. The fluid is nonpurulent. (If it is purulent, the disorder is called "empyema." See p. 1265.) A wet pleurisy is also called *pleurisy with effusion* or *serofibrinous pleurisy*. As many as 5 liters of fluid may collect in the pleural cavity.

Etiology. Pleural effusion is actually a symptom (not a specific disorder) that may be produced by numerous conditions, e.g., bronchial carcinoma, leukemias, lymphomas, breast cancer, trauma, acute pneumonia, pulmonary edema, pulmonary infarction, subdiaphragmatic abscess, cirrhosis of the liver, systemic infections, cardiac and renal diseases (e.g., congestive heart failure, nephrosis), and some of the collagen diseases (e.g., disseminated lupus erythematosus, periarteritis nodosa).

When there is a history of malignancy, pleural metastasis is a likely cause of effusion. Other important features in the history are:[155]

- Fever and purulent sputum
- Chest trauma
- Arthralgia
- Pleuritic chest pain
- Congestive heart failure
- Medication history, especially use of anticoagulants
- Occupational exposure to asbestos

The abnormal quantity of fluid in the pleural space (with pleural effusion) may be either an exudate or a transudate. *Exudates* are substances that have escaped from blood vessels; *transudates* are substances that have passed through a membrane or tissue surface.

Symptoms. The onset of pleurisy with effusion depends on the underlying disorder and may be dramatically sudden or insidious. Symptoms may include dyspnea (possibly developing rapidly), pallor, fatigue, weight loss, prostration, high fever, pleural pain, and possibly a dry cough. Inspection of the side of the chest that has pleural effusion typically reveals distention and absence of movement during breathing. The area is commonly flat when percussed if more than 350 ml. of fluid are present. On auscultation breath sounds are very decreased or absent. Large collections of fluid in the pleural space collapse the lung on the affected side. This reduces pulmonary volume and vital capacity, produces dyspnea and impaired pulmonary ventilation, and may cause embarrassment of the heart and mediastinal shift as a result of pressure. (Refer to discussion of mediastinal shift on p. 1342.)

Diagnosis. Procedures used to diagnose pleurisy with effusion include history, physical examination, pleural biopsy, x-ray studies, reflected ultrasound, and exploratory thoracentesis. Etiology can be definitely established only by aspirating some pleural fluid for laboratory investigation.

In the clinical laboratory a specimen of pleural fluid may be given a cytologic examination to detect cancer cells, and a bacteriologic examination in which Gram and acid-fast smears are done and cultures are made on appropriate media. Additional laboratory investigations include counts of erythrocytes and leukocytes, measurement of specific gravity and protein content, determination of glucose level, and examination for cholesterol crystals.

Bloody pleural fluid commonly occurs with carcinomatous effusions and may also occur following pulmonary infarction or with tuberculous effusions.

Small amounts of pleural effusion can be difficult to identify by x-ray films. Generally 300 to 500 ml. of free pleural fluid must be present in the pleural space before this fluid is detected by a routine posteroanterior chest film. A film taken with the patient in the lateral recumbent position is most useful in detecting small pleural effusions. Lateral decubitus films may help determine whether fluid or a thickened pleura is present. Recently, reflected ultrasound has proved useful in detecting and localizing even small amounts of pleural fluid.

Treatment. Treatment of pleurisy with effusion is directed at the underlying disorder. Thoracentesis is performed to establish diagnosis and relieve any respiratory distress resulting from the presence of the space-occupying fluid. Pleural effusion caused by metastasized cancer often recurs, requiring repeated thoracentesis. When large quantities of fluid accumulate after a thoracentesis, the physician may insert a small chest catheter (14 or 16 Fr.) and connect it to closed chest drainage without suction. The catheter may be left in place for three days. Catheter drainage enables easier pleural space drainage and aids repositioning of the visceral and parietal pleurae.

Nonpyogenic (sterile) pleural effusions tend to absorb spontaneously if the patient remains on bed rest. Those effusions related to pyogenic infections are treated as an empyema (see below). Pleuritic pain, if present, is managed as outlined in the discussion of dry pleurisy.

> *Observe persons with pleural effusion closely for indications of respiratory embarrassment.*

Report such findings at once so the physician can immediately perform thoracentesis and remove fluid that has reaccumulated and is compressing the lung on the affected side. Keep a thoracentesis tray available for emergency thoracentesis.

When a pleural effusion is neoplastic in origin the patient may be treated with x-ray therapy to the pleural space and by instillation of chemotherapeutic agents into the pleural space (after as much fluid is removed as possible). Agents that may be used include nitrogen mustard, mechlorethamine hydrochloride, quinacrine hydrochloride, or radioactive gold. When chemotherapy is used in this manner, the patient's position is changed every 15 minutes so the entire pleural space may have contact with the drug. (See also Chapter 23.)

Thoracic Empyema (Pyothorax, Suppurative Pleurisy)

Although the term *empyema* is frequently used to refer to the accumulation of pus in the *chest* it actually means the collection of pus in *any* body cavity. Hence, this section is correctly titled *thoracic empyema.* For the sake of expediency, however, the term "empyema" is used in the remainder of this discussion to refer to thoracic empyema.

Etiology. The accumulation of purulent exudate in the pleural cavity may occur in several ways. For example, empyema may be directly introduced (by penetrating chest wounds, chest surgery, or other penetrating therapeutic procedures) or it may result from the spread of infection from neighboring structures (e.g., lungs, mediastinum, chest wall). Also, empyema may complicate such disorders as pneumonia (especially staphylococcal pneumonia), tuberculosis, pulmonary abscess, or bronchiectasis.

Empyema is a serious disorder that fortunately occurs less often since the use of carefully selected antibiotic therapy. When it does develop, and is treated *early* with appropriate antibiotics, empyema can usually be effectively controlled.

The size of the area affected by an empyema varies from only a small area of inflammation to involvement of the whole pleural cavity. The *exudate* present varies in consistency from thin to thick pus. The appearance of the pleura may be essentially normal or, with long-term infections, may be grossly distorted and thickened.

The natural history of a pleural space infection falls into three stages.[12a]

- Exudative stage (thin pleural fluid and low leukocyte count)
- Fibropurulent stage (increase in leukocyte count, appearance of fibrin, frank pus may be aspirated and adhesions occur)
- Organization stage (thick exudative membrane and fixation of lung)

When a *chronic empyema* develops it is usually a recurrent infection of the pleural space that results from the incomplete treatment of an acute empyema. Chronic empyema may be caused by such disorders as foreign body in the pleural space, bronchopleural fistula, tuberculosis, or osteomyelitis of a rib. Chronic empyema may be difficult to treat effectively, since the pleura often becomes extremely thick, and a tough exudate or fibrous tissue binds the lung to the chest wall. Enclosed in such an inelastic covering, the compressed lung cannot easily expand and contract to ventilate effectively. Pleural fibrosis with shrinkage may cause the involved side of the chest to appear shrunken. Scoliosis may develop along with the displacement of mediastinal structures as they are pulled toward the affected side. Multiloculated cavities filled with pus may be present between the chest wall and lung. Clubbing of the fingers often occurs with chronic empyema.

Diagnosis. Empyema may be difficult to diagnose, since it may be obscured by symptoms of the primary disorder. All patients with pulmonary infection or chest injuries are closely observed for indications of empyema. Empyema is strongly suspected in patients with pulmonary infection who do not respond to treatment.

Physical indications of empyema are the same as those of pleural effusion, e.g., dullness to percussion over the involved area. Severity of symptoms is variable, but typically a spiking fever is present. Pleural pain may occur. Some persons with empyema are chronically ill, with weight loss, malaise, and fever. Others are acutely ill, with a high fever and prostration.

In the process of establishing diagnosis special projection chest x-rays are usually taken in an attempt to identify the location(s) of accumulations of pus. After the physical examination and x-rays are completed, the physician selects a site for *thoracentesis.* Thick pus is difficult to aspirate, and a large bore needle must be used. Diagnosis is confirmed by examining the pleural exudate removed by thoracentesis. In addition to evaluating the specimen's color, specific gravity, and cell count, Gram stains and aerobic and anaerobic cultures are performed. By means of culture the causative organisms are identified and their specific sensitivity to antibiotics is determined.

Treatment. Treatment of empyema focuses on complete drainage of the localized collection of pus and obliteration of the pleural space, and administration of antibiotics to clear the infection and prevent its spread. Antibiotics may be given systemically, or may be instilled directly into the pleural space. Fibrinolytic enzymes (e.g., trypsin, streptokinase, streptodornase) may help decrease the viscosity of the pus and dissolve fibrin clots. Intrapleural aspirations and instillations may be performed daily via thoracentesis or thoracotomy tube.

Some patients cannot be effectively treated with enzymatic debridement, intermittent aspirations, and instillations of antibiotics. For example, these treatment methods are ineffective if a multiloculated empyema is present. Such empyemas are treated with open or closed chest drainage through a large-diameter chest tube.

Closed chest drainage may be used if the visceral pleura remains flexible (so the lung can reexpand and the pleural space will be obliterated once the pus-filled cavity is drained), and if the pus is relatively thin. The chest catheter may be inserted in a treatment room or at the bedside. (See p. 1368.)

Open drainage of thoracic empyema is possible only if there is no danger of collapse of the lung when atmospheric pressure enters the pleural space (i.e., through the incision in the chest wall and the drainage tube which is placed through that incision and left open to atmospheric pressure to drain). Open chest drainage may be used if an empyema is localized within strong "walls" (boundaries) which bind the lung to the chest wall or which otherwise prevent lung collapse. It is often necessary to remove portions of one or two ribs to place a chest drainage tube. With open drainage the tube is left in place and covered with a large absorbent dressing. Dressing changes are carefully performed to prevent introducing new infection and to prevent infection of the person changing the dressing (from the contaminated material on the dressing). The physician changes the tube periodically.

Patients with uncomplicated empyema are usually kept on bed rest while febrile. Care given during this period is directed at preventing the complications of inactivity and helping the patient to overcome infection. The patient with a chest drainage tube is helped to be ambulant as soon as the physician gives approval. Improvement is indicated by a reduction in pus production, general symptomatic improvement, and a fall in temperature and WBC count.

In addition to medications and drainage of the pus-filled cavity, treatment also includes the performance of *breathing exercises* to help ensure adequate lung expansion and pulmonary function. Breathing exercises are started as soon as possible. The patient is instructed to breathe deeply (perhaps every hour while awake). See Chapter 54 for discussion of Incentive Devices. Breathing exercises help prevent the contraction and binding down of lung tissue in an unyielding fibrous encasement of thickened pleural tissue. If compression of lung tissue is severe, arterial blood gases must be assessed, and O_2 administered if hypoxemia is present.

Persons with empyema should be observed for indications of pneumothorax (see below). Occasionally an untreated empyema drains spontaneously through the chest wall. *Complications* of empyema may also include brain abscess, meningitis, pericarditis, or endocarditis.

Persons with open chest drainage can often be discharged home and treatment continued on an outpatient basis. Provision must be made for dressing changes at home. The patient and a significant other are taught how to properly change dressings and dispose of contaminated items. A visiting nurse may periodically provide assistance as indicated and inspect the wound.

Unfortunately, but characteristically, *empyema tends to drain and heal slowly.* Thus, drainage is usually necessary for a prolonged period of time. Sometimes the physician instills a radiopaque substance into the cavity to evaluate progress in the healing process. At times the cavity is irrigated periodically with a sterile solution. The visiting nurse may perform these irrigations at home. As the cavity heals the physician may slowly withdraw the drainage tube. The cavity must close before the drainage system can be discontinued. After the drainage tube is removed the chest wound is covered with appropriate dressings.

Some patients cannot be effectively treated even with tube drainage, e.g., if they have thick pus or extensive pleural damage. These persons require *thoracotomy* to resect the empyema cavity and surgically remove the binding fibrinous peel that tends to form in chronic infections. Stripping off the thickened membrane is called *decortication.* It permits reexpansion of the lung. (See Chapter 57.)

Hemothorax

Hemothorax is a collection of blood (e.g., from severed or torn vessels) in the pleural space. The bleeding may occur following injury (e.g., pulmonary laceration, puncture by fractured rib) or chest surgery.

Symptoms. Symptoms may include chest pain, cyanosis, decreasing blood pressure, increased pulse and respiratory rates, dyspnea, decreased or absent breath sounds, and dullness over the affected side of the chest. Mediastinal shift may occur, i.e., displacement of mediastinal contents toward the unaffected side of the chest.

> *Closely observe patients with hemothorax for indications of shock and/or respiratory distress.*

Diagnosis. Diagnosis of hemothorax is confirmed by chest film and/or finding blood in the pleural space upon performing thoracentesis. *Treatment* is directed at evacuating the pleural space and completely reexpanding the lung. It consists of needle aspiration (thoracentesis) or closed chest drainage via thoracotomy tube if thoracentesis is ineffective. If these measures are unsuccessful, surgery is indicated to control bleeding and evacuate blood and clots. Blood replacement may be indicated. A minor hemo thorax may resolve without specific treatment. *Often pneumothorax and hemothorax occur together, i.e., hemopneumothorax.* Both reexpansion exercises and O_2 (if indicated) must be instituted. (For additional discussion of hermothorax see Chapter 56.)

Pneumothorax

A *pneumothorax* is a collection of air or gas in the pleural cavity. It may result from (1) *thoracentesis* (if the needle "nicks" the lung); (2) *thoracic surgery* (in which the pleural cavity is entered); (3) *accidental injury* (e.g., from a torn lung, fractured bronchus, or penetration of the chest wall; (4) barotrauma from positive pressure ventilation. These causes of pneumothorax are discussed in appropriate sections of this unit.

- An *open pneumothorax* exists when communication is present between the outside of the body and the pleural space, e.g., through an opening in the chest wall.
- With a *closed pneumothorax* there is no communication between the outside of the body and the pleural space. Air enters the pleural space internally from ruptured alveoli or a bronchus. Closed pneumothorax is most common. (See also Chapter 56.)
- *Spontaneous pneumothorax* may develop from air leaking from pulmonary alveoli or erosion of a disease process through the pulmonary pleura. For example, a large emphysematous bulla may rupture or a tubercular lesion may erode into the pleural space (see Fig. 56–1*A* in Chapter 56 for illustration of pneumothorax). Spontaneous pneumothorax is a form of closed pneumothorax.

A *spontaneous pneumothorax* is most commonly the result of a rupture of a small bleb close to the pleura, but may also occur as a complication of a wide variety of intrapulmonary or mediastinal disease processes. Subpleural bleb rupture occurs 85 per cent of the time. The remaining 15 per cent result from congenital causes, scarring from inflammatory diseases such as tuberculosis, and other diseases such as asthma, bronchiectasis, emphysema, and pneumoconioses. At one time physical exertion was thought to play a role in the development of the spontaneous pneumothorax. This theory has been discarded, since the majority of patients were at rest when the pneumothorax occurred. Any process that disrupts pulmonary architecture can lead to bleb formation.

Spontaneous pneumothorax occurs most commonly in young men between 15 and 35 years of age. The right side appears to be more involved than the left. Frequently these persons have no previous history of respiratory disease.

Symptoms. *Indications of pneumothorax* include sudden, sharp chest pain; cough; sudden shortness of breath with violent but futile respiratory effort; fall in BP; weak, rapid pulse; hyperresonance over the affected thoracic space; apprehension; anxiety; restlessness; diaphoresis; pallor or cyanosis; faintness; feeling of tightness in the chest; decreased or absent breath sounds over the collapsed lung; and cessation of normal chest movements on the affected side.

Diagnosis; Treatment. Respiratory insufficiency and other complications of a large pneumothorax may be rapidly fatal if not recognized and promptly treated. Untreated pneumothorax is a serious condition because it collapses lung tissue and may cause mediastinal shift. Immediately report indications of pneumothorax. *Diagnosis* is definitely established by chest x-ray film.

The following aspects of *clinical care* are important if a patient develops symptoms of a pneumothorax:

- Remain with and keep the patient as calm and quiet as possible. Place the person in a sitting position and encourage him or her to try to control coughing and gasping.
- Without communicating undue alarm to the patient, have another nurse immediately notify the physician and bring thoracentesis equipment to the bedside so the physician can aspirate air quickly if indicated.
- Obtain arterial blood gases.
- Administer O_2 to relieve dyspnea if necessary. (Note: Administer O_2 cautiously in presence of chronic obstructive pulmonary disease or chronic respiratory insufficiency from other causes to prevent CO_2 narcosis).
- Evaluate pulse and respiratory rates for indications of shock, increasing respiratory distress, and mediastinal shift.

A small pneumothorax may require no specific treatment except restricted activity, mild cough suppression, and O_2. The air in the pleural space is gradually reabsorbed by the body. A larger pneumothorax may be treated by: (1) needle aspiration of the air with needle and syringe (thoracentesis); (2) insertion of a small polyethylene catheter through a needle and removal of air by a suction machine or with a syringe connected to a three-way stopcock; or (3) closed chest drainage, with or without suction, via an intercostal catheter (inserted under local anesthesia through a trocar). Closed chest drainage aspirates air and promotes lung reexpansion. Occasionally thoracotomy is necessary to treat pneumothorax adequately.

Following pneumothorax the patient is advised to avoid physical exertion until the physician recommends resumption of normal activities. Observe the patient for indications of a persistent air leak or recurrent pneumothorax. With a spontaneous pneumothorax the air leaks occur most often in persons with chronic obstructive pulmonary disease (COPD) because of their overinflated lung tissue, chronic cough, and heightened expiratory effort. During recovery from pneumothorax the physician periodically checks for subcutaneous emphysema, and reexpansion of the lung with x-ray films and possibly fluoroscopy.

Bronchopleural Fistula

A *bronchopleural fistula* is a persistent communication between the pleural cavity and the bronchial tree. Bronchopleural fistula is typically seen today in patients with "old" healed tuberculosis. Prior to use of antimicrobial medications bronchopleural fistula also occurred commonly with other pulmonary disorders such as bacterial pneumonia, bronchiectasis, lung abscess, pulmonary infarction, and postpneumonic empyema.

Presently this complication is less common and more amenable to treatment. *Surgical procedures* are necessary to correct bronchopleural fistula, and may be employed to fill the pleural space, e.g., decortication, staged thoracoplasty. (See Chapter 57.)

DISORDERS OF THE TRACHEOBRONCHIAL TREE AND LUNGS

Atelectasis

Pathophysiology. *Atelectasis* is an area of lung tissue (or at times even a complete lung) that is collapsed, airless, and shrunken. An atelectasis may be *complete* or *incomplete* (partial) and may be an *acute* or *chronic* disorder.

Atelectasis occurs frequently in association with various pulmonary disorders, e.g., infections, pleural effusions, tumors; as a postoperative complication, e.g., following thoracic surgery or high abdominal surgery; and as a complication of immobility.

> *Atelectasis can often be prevented by efficient nursing care.*

The main *cause* of atelectasis is bronchial obstruction by secretions, tumors, bronchospasm, or foreign bodies. Within a few hours after a bronchus is obstructed the air is absorbed from the blocked lung tissue and the affected lung tissue collapses or shrinks. Trapped alveolar air is absorbed by the circulating blood. Frequently infection (e.g., pneumonia) and impaired regional circulation complicate atelectasis. If untreated, the airless, poorly perfused atelectatic area deteriorates into an infected, retracted, fibrotic portion of lung with bronchiectatic changes. (Bronchiectasis is discussed later.) If prompt treatment is given and the obstruction is removed before these destructive changes occur, air reenters the distal lung tissue and expands it, inflammation and infection subside, and effective circulation is restored.

Atelectasis can result not only from the *internal* obstruction of a bronchus but also from pressure applied to the *outside* wall of a bronchus, as by an enlarged lymph node or tumor, or to the outside of a lung, e.g., by an elevated diaphragm or accumulations of air or fluids in the pleural space or pericardial sac.

Symptoms. *Symptoms* of atelectasis are basically determined by the rapidity with which bronchial obstruction develops, by the degree of alveolar collapse, and by the presence or absence of secondary infection. Increased hypoxemia, dyspnea, and weakness are almost the only symptoms of a slowly developing atelectasis. A massive, rapidly developing collapse with infection typically causes sudden severe dyspnea, cyanosis, decreased blood pressure, tachycardia, shock, anxiety, and temperature elevation. Additionally, pain occurs on the affected side, and breath sounds and ventilatory excursions of the chest are reduced or absent. Ventilatory movements on the unaffected side may appear exaggerated as the patient struggles to breathe.

Percussion over the collapsed lung demonstrates dullness to flatness. X-ray examination reveals a solid lack of radiance of the airless area of the lung and diminished lung size. In the presence of large atelectatic areas the diaphragm is elevated on the affected side, the rib spaces are narrowed, and the heart, mediastinum, and trachea deviate *toward* the atelectatic area. (*Note*: Massive pleural effusion and spontaneous pneumothorax cause similar clinical symptoms, but with these disorders x-ray films show the mediastinal structures pushed *away* from the affected side.) Bronchoscopy may or may not reveal bronchial obstruction.

Prevention. *Preventive measures* include:

- Prevention of aspiration and maintenance of a clear airway by correct positioning and removal of bronchopulmonary secretions. Indications of bronchial obstruction include wheezing or a sharp, forced expiration. (See discussion of prevention of pneumonia, p. 1281).
- Maintenance of effective aeration of the lung, e.g., by frequent deep breathing–coughing sessions.
- Use of IPPB (with air, not O_2) to improve ventilation and bronchial drainage.
- Turning and repositioning every hour while the patient is obtunded or bedridden.
- Avoidance of large doses of sedatives and opiates, which depress cough reflex and respirations.
- Avoidance of tight dressings and restraints.
- Prevention of abdominal distention.
- Encouragement of mobility.
- Reduction of bronchospasm, e.g., by administering nebulized bronchodilators.
- Promotion of liquefaction of secretions by administration of aerosols of saline and water, humidifying inspired air, and maintaining body hydration.
- Avoidance of anesthetic agents with a long post-anesthetic narcosis; avoidance of very high O_2 concentrations with too little nitrogen during anesthesia; and leaving the lung filled with air (not O_2) at the termination of operative anesthesia.

Clinical Care. When *acute atelectasis* develops it is treated when possible by removal of the underlying cause. Treatment is rapidly instituted to prevent destructive changes and other complications. Thoracentesis may be performed to remove accumulations of air or fluid from the pleural space if they are causing atelectasis. To remove bronchial obstruction, treatment may include: (1) stimulation of productive coughing; (2) suctioning; (3) positioning the patient with the involved side elevated (so drainage of the affected area can occur); (4) stimulation of deep breathing; (5) administration of aerosols with a nebulizer; (6) bronchoscopy (to remove obstructions directly when they can be visualized in the tracheobronchial tree; (7) oxygen; and (8) CMV and/or continuous positive airway pressure. Antibiotics are administered to treat or to prevent pulmonary infection. Once the obstruction is removed the patient is helped to regain normal lung function by IPPB, incentive devices, turning, coughing, and ambulation. *Chronic atelectasis* may be successfully treated by surgically removing the affected area — segment or lobe — and treating secondary infection.

Influenza ("Flu," Grippe, Catarrhal Fever)

Epidemiology and Immunology. This acute, highly contagious respiratory disease is viral in origin. The influenza virus can be observed only with an electron microscope, since it is smaller than a bacterium.

Influenza may occur sporadically or in epidemics. Occasionally pandemics (i.e., epidemics spreading to all parts of the world) develop, characterized by a rapidly fatal pulmonary infection. In such fulminant fatal cases, dyspnea, cyanosis, hemoptysis, pulmonary edema, and death may result as soon as two days after onset of the illness.

An example of an influenza pandemic was that of 1918, which took the lives of more than 21 million persons. As a medical catastrophe this pandemic was second only to the Black Death in the 14th century. More recent examples of influenza pandemics are the 1957–58 ("Asian flu") infections, caused by a new mutant strain of Type A influenza virus, and the 1968–69 ("Hong Kong flu") illness.

Three types of influenza virus are recognized; A, B, and C. *Type A* is further classified into different serotypes which are numbered, N_0N_1, H_1N_1, H_2N_2, and H_3N_2. (H_3N_2, the most recent serotype, is the only one that causes epidemics of a type A variety.) Older strains disappear as new strains emerge. *Type B* does have strain-specific variations but as there are a lot of cross-relationships between the strains they are not numbered. *Type C* is not prevalent and serotypes are not defined.[26A]

Influenza is most commonly caused by type A virus producing sporadic respiratory illness every year. Acute epidemics occur about every three years — usually in the autumn and winter. Acute major pandemics occur about once a decade when a change occurs in the prevalent type of influenza A virus. Influenza B virus is hardly ever associated with pandemics but produces epidemics about every five years. Influenza C is an endemic virus which causes mild sporadic respiratory disease.[26A]

The influenza virus has a selective affinity for the respiratory tract's epithelial lining and causes inflammation of the airways, with patches of necrotic, sloughing epithelium. Influenza is basically an airborne infection, most commonly spread by droplet nuclei containing the virus. These infected droplet nuclei are spread by coughing, sneezing, kissing, and the use of towels, drinking glasses, and similar objects that have been freshly contaminated.

Symptoms. Following the incubation period of about 48 hours, the nonimmune infected person suddenly becomes acutely ill. Symptoms include prostration, fever 37.7 to 40°C. (100 to 104° F.), severe headache with photophobia and retrobulbar aching, chills, weakness, generalized muscular aches and pains (most severe in the legs and back), anorexia, sore throat, anxiety, dry cough, coryza, sneezing, mild substernal distress, flushed face, and the formation of herpetic lesions on the mouth and lips. Temperature elevates rapidly and may remain high for two or three days in mild cases or four to five days in severe cases. Possible complications include secondary bacterial pneumonia, cardiovascular disease, cervical lymphadenitis, sinusitus, tracheobronchitis, and otitis media. Vasomotor collapse can occur with severe influenza.

Persons with chronic lung disease and minimal pulmonary reserve may develop acute respiratory failure if they get the flu. Some pulmonary physicians feel that persons with COPD should be vaccinated against flu in the early fall before flu season.

Once the fever abates after two to three days (occasionally up to five days), the other acute symptoms rapidly disappear. However, fatigue, cough, weakness, and sweating may persist for several more days or, perhaps, weeks.

Treatment. Treatment is symptomatic and consists of measures such as bed rest (until 24 to 48 hours after fever abates), antipyretics and analgesics, light diet, increased fluid intake, mild codeine cough mixture, warm isotonic saline gargles, cool vapor or steam inhalations, humidification of inspired air, nasal instillations of phenylephrine in sodium chloride solution, and prevention of chilling and fatigue. General comfort measures, such as back rubs, oral hygiene, and sponges, can greatly reduce aggravating discomforts. Laxatives may be ordered. Observe the patient closely for indications of complications and report these immediately. The patient is gradually ambulated as improvement occurs. Full activity out of bed is not permitted until easy fatigue, weakness, and dizziness have subsided. A convalescent period following recovery from acute symptoms is advisable to prevent relapse or secondary infection.

Persons with uncomplicated influenza usually recover without residual impairment. However, fatalities may occur, e.g., among pregnant women, the aged, diabetics, and persons with chronic lung disease or chronic cardiac disease. Most fatalities result from bacterial complications.

Control; Prophylaxis. Infected persons should be isolated and given instruction about measures they can take to minimize the spread of their airborne disease. (Methods of preventing the spread of droplet-nuclei infections are discussed on pp. 1209, 1213, 1224.)

While most city dwellers cannot avoid some influenza infections, the severity of these infections may be minimized by the maintenance of an optimum level of general health, avoiding crowds during periods when the "flu" is prevalent, and attempting to stay out of the path of coughing, sneezing persons.

Polyvalent vaccines are now available against the prevalent types of influenza. They reduce influenza infection for about one to two years after vaccination. These influenza immunizations are recommended annually for persons most likely to succumb to influenza infections, e.g., debilitated, aged persons with chronic diseases. When epidemics are predicted, vaccination is recommended for other groups, e.g., pregnant women, persons performing vital public services.

It is recommended that the primary vaccination and annual booster doses be given in the early fall. The primary immunization usually consists of one vaccine — subcutaneous or intramuscular (never intradermal). When new strains arise, two or three doses containing the new strains are given at monthly intervals.[26A] Before administering the vaccine, inquire if the person has a sensitivity to eggs, since the vaccine is made of virus propagated in chick embryos. Epinephrine should be kept available in case of a severe immediate reaction. (See Chapter 11.) Severe reactions are rare, but local or constitutional reactions are not uncommon. These can be minimized by giving the vaccine in divided doses at one- to two-day intervals. It takes about two weeks following vaccination for immunity to develop. New vaccines are always being studied. One presently under development is an attenuated live virus vaccine that when administered intranasally will elicit secretory antibodies where the virus enters the body.[26A]

Acute Bronchitis; Acute Tracheobronchitis

Pathophysiology. *Bronchitis,* i.e., bronchial inflammation or infection, may be either an *acute* or *chronic* disorder. (*Chronic bronchitis* is discussed on p. 1325). Bronchitis may occur as a primary disorder or in company with numerous other pulmonary disorders, e.g, bronchiectasis, tuberculosis, chronic obstructive pulmonary disease, pulmonary emphysema. Bronchitis may be diffuse or localized and may be caused by infections or by physical or chemical agents, e.g, dust, fumes, smoke.

Acute tracheobronchitis is an acute inflammation of the mucous membranes of the tracheobronchial tree; usually the disorder is self-limited and does not permanently impair structure or function. If only the bronchi appear involved the condition is called "bronchitis"; if the trachea is also involved the condition is accurately called "tracheobronchitis." Tracheobronchitis is the more common disorder.

When tracheobronchitis results from an infection the condition is usually an extension into the trachea and bronchi of a general acute upper respiratory infection (URI). Temporary impairment of the self-cleaning mechanisms of the bronchi (e.g., cilia) permits bacterial invasion. Once bacteria invade the normally sterile bronchi, mucopurulent exudate and cellular debris accumulate. These accumulations must be expectorated.

Acute tracheobronchitis occurs most often during winter months. This disorder is only a mild illness for most persons, but it can be life-threatening in infants and small children (because their bronchi are easily obstructed) and in persons who have chronic pulmonary or heart disease or who are otherwise debilitated. *Prompt, thorough treatment of upper respiratory infection is important in the prevention of acute tracheobronchitis,* especially in the above described population. Acute tracheobronchitis may also occur with generalized infections such as chickenpox, measles, whooping cough, and influenza.

Symptoms. Acute tracheobronchitis is characterized by *early* symptoms of an acute URI (substernal tightness, chills, coryza, sore throat, muscle and back pain, and slight fever); *later* onset of cough, which is initially dry, irritating, and nonproductive and then progresses to become productive of mucopurulent to purulent sputum; and no x-ray film densities and only a few pulmonary signs, e.g., musical rhonchi, wheezes. Persistent localized pulmonary signs may indicate serious complications. In uncomplicated cases, sputum cultures produce the common mouth organisms. At other times specific pathogens are demonstrated, e.g., pneumococci, beta-hemolytic streptococci. A temperature elevation (38.5 to 39° C., or 101 to 102° F.) may last three to five days in some of the more severe uncomplicated illnesses. Usually acute symptoms subside within two to five days; however, a cough may be present for as long as 14 to 21 days. Bronchospasm (which results from bronchial irritation) may cause the patient to be dyspneic, and sometimes may produce hypoxemia and hypoventilation. Secondary infections may include sinusitis and/or laryngitis.

Clinical Care. Clinical care is basically symptomatic and is similar to that given with any acute URI. Factors of importance include:

- ▶ Bed rest; aerosolized hydration; expectorants; increased fluid intake (3000 to 4000 ml./day); moist heat applications to the chest wall; hot drinks (to stimulate productive coughing and relieve congestion), light or soft nourishing diet; antipyretic analgesic medications (to reduce fever and relieve malaise).
- ▶ Prevention of relapse or secondary infection. Protect patient from fatigue and chilling. Take precautions to prevent pneumonia. (See discussion on p. 1281.) Encourage productive coughing and periodic deep breathing. Administer antibiotics if ordered.
- ▶ Relief of bronchospasm if present. Ephedrine, aminophylline, isoproterenol (Isuprel), and isoetharine are bronchodilators that may be prescribed. (See discussion of bronchodilators below.)
- ▶ Prevention of spread of tracheobronchitis to others during period of communicability.

Antibiotics are not indicated initially if the causative organism is a virus. However, in the presence of bacterial infection antibiotics may be ordered if the patient is not rapidly improving or is more than mildly ill. A broad-spectrum antibiotic, e.g., tetracycline, may be ordered until sputum culture reports are available to guide specific antibiotic therapy. Antibiotics may be given in an attempt to prevent secondary infection in patients for whom severe acute infections could be fatal.

Cough depressants are not usually given, since it is important that the lungs be cleared of accumulated secretions. However, sometimes the physician mildly suppresses cough (e.g., with a codeine or another cough mixture) if the cough is unproductive and excessively fatiguing.

As can be seen, treatment of tracheobronchitis is generally conservative and is directed at preventing extension of the infection and the development of complications. Persons for whom tracheobronchitis can be serious are observed especially closely for indications of worsening of their conditions. It is advisable for the patient to observe a period of convalescence with reduced activity to ensure complete recovery.

Bronchiectasis

Bronchiectasis is a disorder of the medium-sized bronchi, characterized by *chronic dilatation* of these air passages and the destruction of bronchial elastic and muscular structures.

Pathophysiology. Bronchiectasis may affect the bronchial tube(s) uniformly *(cylindric bronchiectasis),* may produce irregular pockets *(sacculated bronchiectasis),* or may produce terminal bulbous enlargements at the end of the dilated tube *(fusiform* or *spindle-shaped bronchiectasis).* Cylindrical bronchiectasis is of doubtful clinical significance. The characteristic bronchial dilatations become apparent when a diagnostic bronchogram is performed. The lower and middle lobes of the lungs are most often affected. Involvement varies, and may be bilateral or extensive.

Microscopic inspection of sections of bronchi affected with bronchiectasis reveals that the wall of the bronchus in the dilated sections has been replaced with scar tissue. The dilated bronchial sections may be surrounded by areas of pneumonia.

Etiology. Causes of bronchiectasis are *obstruction* and *infection.* Obstructions, e.g., mucus, pus, or foreign bodies, block the bronchi and eventually cause them to dilate. If the dilated bronchial walls become infected and damaged from the infection, the dilatation becomes irreversible. Bronchiectasis can also occur distal to an obstruction when infection develops beyond the point of obstruction.

Bronchiectasis may be present at birth, but most often begins in early childhood as an acquired disorder resulting from a pulmonary infection which complicates influenza, measles, or whooping cough, or is the result of foreign body aspiration. Bronchial obstructions leading to bronchiectasis also may occur as a result of such disorders as bronchial tumor, pulmonary tuberculosis, and cystic fibrosis (mucoviscidosis). Because children have bronchi that are small and soft, bronchial obstruction and damage can more easily occur at younger ages. However, since infection and bronchial obstruction do not routinely produce bronchiectasis, unknown intrinsic factors are believed to be important in its etiology.

Permanently damaged bronchial walls cannot move effectively and ciliary action is absent as a result of destroyed or damaged mucous membranes. *Ectatic* (i.e., distended) *bronchi* may collapse when intrapleural pressure is rapidly increased during cough. Because secretions cannot be adequately removed, infection subsequently occurs. Infected secretions then collect constantly in the bronchial dilatations. Changes in body position cause these secretions to flow into regions of healthy bronchial tissue. The infected secretions are raised from here as a result of ciliary action, bronchial wall movements, and coughing. Bronchial damage is more serious when it occurs in the lower regions of the lungs, since gravity cannot help to drain the affected bronchi, as would occur from the upper lung fields.

Symptoms. Bronchiectasis is basically characterized by:

- Chronic profuse discharge of thick sputum containing pus
- Fetid breath
- Hemoptysis (This occurs in about half the patients.)
- Chronic, severe, frequent paroxysms of coughing

Other common symptoms include fatigue, weight loss, shortness of breath upon exertion, and moist rales and rhonchi over the lower lobes. Sinusitis is frequently present. Persons with advanced bronchiectasis often appear weak, emaciated, and cyanotic, and have clubbing of the fingertips. Typically persons with bronchiectasis have a history of developing winter colds which usually progress to pneumonia.

Diagnosis. Characteristic history and symptoms are indicative of bronchiectasis. Bronchograms confirm the diagnosis. Bronchoscopy may be helpful in demonstrating bronchial obstruction and in identifying involved pulmonary segments. Persons with advanced bronchiectasis may show decreased ventilation when lung function studies are performed. Characteristic laboratory findings do not occur with bronchiectasis. The characteristic appearance of the sputum is often of diagnostic value in bronchiectasis. When allowed to stand, the sputum has a typical three-layered appearance. Frequently a highly mixed bacterial content is revealed when sputum is microscopically examined.

Clinical Care. Treatment of bronchiectasis may involve both medical and surgical procedures. *Surgical resection* of involved portions of the lung (e.g., segment, lobe) is the only way by which bronchiectasis can be eliminated. However, not all patients are candidates for surgery. Pulmonary resection may be performed on young patients with recurring symptoms or persons up to age 60 who have severe symptoms, such as recurrent hemoptysis, caused by unilateral localized bronchiectasis. Segmental resections or lobectomies are most often performed, but sometimes pneumonectomies or bilateral procedures are carried out. (Care of the patient having chest surgery is discussed in Chapter 57.)

The *medical management* and *general clinical care* of a patient with bronchiectasis focus on the following activities:

- ▶ Periodic postural drainage, e.g., the first drainage upon awakening, the last at bedtime. Some patients with mild involvement require postural drainage only when they develop a cold. Others with severe involvement require postural drainage several times a day. Patients with severe bronchiectasis may be positioned for several hours in a tipped-up position on a special bed. Some patients with severe disease are advised to permanently elevate the foot of the bed 4 to 6 inches.
- ▶ Treatment of complications with respiratory therapy is indicated for chronic respiratory insufficiency. Chronic sinus infections are treated appropriately. (See Unit XXIV.)
- ▶ Liquefaction of sputum by keeping the patient hydrated systemically, and administering aerosol hydration and mucolytic agents. Bronchodilators are also indicated.
- ▶ Bronchoscopic removal of bronchial obstruction and/or dilation of a stenosed bronchus.
- ▶ Avoidance of upper respiratory infections and air-polluted environments. The patient is advised not to smoke and to avoid dusty, smoky, or otherwise polluted atmospheres. The physician may advise the patient to live in a warm, dry climate. Tell the patient to avoid contact with persons who have influenza or respiratory infections and to contact a physician early if symptoms of superimposed infection develop.
- ▶ Promotion of rest. Bed rest is often advised for persons with severe bronchiectasis and those with acute respiratory infections. The bronchiectatic person should avoid fatigue and chilling.
- ▶ Improvement of resistance to acute respiratory infections by encouraging a well-balanced diet and a program of balanced exercise and rest that is individualized for the patient's condition.
- ▶ Promotion of effective cough and deep breathing exercises. Instruct the patient how to cough productively. Deep breathing exercises improve alveolar ventilation and help to move secretions out of the inflated lungs.
- ▶ Frequent oral hygiene, because of the copious sputum production. Always provide oral hygiene prior to meals.
- ▶ Administration of antimicrobial medications suppresses bacteria in the pockets of infection; reduces cough, sputum, and other symptoms; and treats the areas of pneumonia that occur around the bronchial dilatations.
- ▶ Awareness of the "normal" color, volume, and characteristics of the sputum. A sudden increase, or decrease, or change may be a signal of impending medical problems.

Patient-family education is of importance in the care of a patient with bronchiectasis. The nurse participates actively in this instruction in a variety of settings, e.g., office, clinic, hospital, and home. Whereas persons with severe bronchiectasis require year-round medical supervision, those with only mild involvement may need care only during and after acute respiratory infections.

Complications. Possible *complications* of bronchiectasis include chronic pulmonary suppuration, progressive pulmonary insufficiency, hemoptysis, amyloidosis, and chronic cor pulmonale. Cardiac complications develop because of the extra burden placed upon the heart.

Prevention

The cause of chronic cough should always be investigated. Severe childhood respiratory infections should be prevented when possible.

When severe respiratory infections occur they should be promptly and completely treated. Aspirated foreign bodies must be promptly removed via bronchoscopy. Parents require instruction from health personnel to seek *early* treatment for children with persistent coughs or evidence of bronchial obstruction, before disease can become established.

Preventive measures are helping to reduce the incidence of bronchiectasis. Formerly a common disorder, today bronchiectasis occurs far less often because of the use of immunizations and antibiotics.

Pulmonary Abscess (Lung Abscess)

A *pulmonary abscess* is a localized collection of pus within a cavity that has been formed by the necrosis of surrounding inflammatory tissue and lung tissue. The areas of the lungs most often affected by abscess formation are the superior segment of the lower lobe or the lower part of the upper lobe. The right lung develops abscesses more often than the left. Multiple abscesses occur occasionally.

Etiology. Lung abscesses usually develop *secondary to localized bronchial obstruction*, which may occur from a neoplasm (e.g., bronchogenic carcinoma), from pneumonia (or other infections such as tuberculosis, fungus infection, and extension of amebic abscess of liver), or following aspiration of secretions or foreign objects.

Pathology. Abscess formation represents an attempt by the body to wall off infection and inflammation and to keep it localized and encapsulated so it does not spread to adjacent structures. Early in the course of development of a pulmonary abscess, an area of consolidation (lobar or segmental) occurs. Gradually this consolidation assumes a round shape as a pus-filled cavity forms. For a while the abscess may remain somewhat isolated and not communicate with a bronchus. Eventually, however, most pulmonary abscesses erode and rupture into a bronchus.

When this has occurred, the patient begins to expectorate the contents of the pus-filled cavity as *foul sputum*. Satisfactory, rapid healing can occur if the abscess is able to drain freely and completely through its bronchial opening. If all the contents of the cavity are removed by drainage through the tracheobronchial tree, the cavity becomes air-filled and the walls of the abscess collapse and contract, eventually obliterating the cavity. However, if the cavity drainage is incomplete and prolonged, a chronic condition develops and healing is prevented by the retention of pus and the development of firm, fibrotic, epithelium-lined abscess walls.

Infrequently a pulmonary abscess perforates into the pleural space, rapidly producing an empyema and perhaps also shock and a bronchopleural fistula. Occasionally pulmonary abscesses erode into blood vessels, resulting in hemorrhage and possibly the transmission of infected emboli to the brain. These emboli develop into brain abscesses secondary to the pulmonary abscess.

Symptoms. The person with a pulmonary abscess may be subacutely (but chronically) ill, or acutely ill, e.g., toxic, prostrate, febrile. Symptoms of pneumonia are often the first to appear, that is, sweats, chills, malaise, anorexia, fever (39.5°C. [103°F.] or higher), cough, dyspnea (if a large area is involved), and perhaps chest pain (if there is pleural involvement). Moist rales may be heard. Sputum is characteristically purulent (often dark brown) unless the abscess is totally walled off and does not have access to a bronchus for drainage. Hemoptysis may occur with a communicating lung abscess. A person with a *chronic* pulmonary abscess develops anemia, weight loss, and clubbing of the fingers.

Diagnosis. Before a lung abscess perforates a bronchus (and begins to drain) it may be difficult to detect. Once bronchial drainage is established, the patient begins to expectorate large quantities of purulent sputum. Sputum may be streaked with blood, may contain pieces of gangrenous lung tissue, and may have a foul odor. This excessive sputum production may last only for several hours or may continue for several days. As the fluid drains out of the abscess, a cavity with a fluid level in it can be observed on the patient's chest film. To establish diagnosis and obtain information necessary for proper treatment the physician usually: (1) performs a physical examination; (2) performs bronchoscopy to rule out tumor or foreign body and to obtain a specimen; (3) orders serial x-rays and tomography; and (4) orders sputum and bronchoscopy specimens for bacteriologic and cytologic evaluation. Sometimes it is necessary to perform a needle aspiration of the abscess to obtain a specimen for laboratory examination. Lung abscesses are commonly caused by anaerobic, staphylococcal, and aerobic gram-negative organisms.

Clinical Care. Treatment is aimed at maintaining effective drainage of a lung abscess and eliminating infection. *Early treatment is important to prevent the development of a chronic condition*. Most patients can be treated without surgical procedures.

Drainage of the abscess is encouraged by the use of postural drainage. Often the daily volume of sputum is measured and recorded. Decreasing amounts of sputum usually indicate effective treatment. The patient is also given instruction about how to cough effectively so that the purulent sputum collecting in the lungs will be raised and expectorated. Suctioning may help to keep the airway patent. Medications may be ordered to help the patient raise sputum. If a patient is unable to cough effectively (e.g., if paralyzed or weakened) a tracheostomy may be necessary so sputum can be suctioned from the lung. Occasionally the physician uses a bronchoscope to aspirate thick, tenacious drainage. Hydration and oxygenation are also indicated.

Chemotherapy of a pulmonary abscess is started as soon as a specimen of the abscess contents has been sent to the laboratory for sensitivity tests and culture. The most effective antibiotic is generally penicillin. As a rule, large doses are administered to make certain effective tissue levels of the antibiotic are maintained in the abscess walls. Kanamycin or gentamicin may also be administered if a gram-negative organism is believed to be present. Generally a combination of medications is necessary, because various organisms are usually present. Typically, chemotherapy is continued for 6 to 8 weeks.

After a course of appropriate antibiotics, symptoms resulting from suppuration of lung tissue are usually relieved. The patient is then reevaluated because the disappearance of symptoms does not always mean that cure has been accomplished. Every attempt is made to prevent the abscess from developing into a chronic condition.

Bronchograms, and perhaps *planigrams,* are routinely performed several weeks after the ordinary chest film has cleared. The results of these procedures are carefully evaluated to determine whether adequate healing has occurred or whether a persistent cavity or bronchiectatic changes are present.

Surgery is necessary if causative organisms are resistant to chemotherapy or if residual cystic cavities or bronchiectasis occurs. Resectional pulmonary surgery, e.g., lobectomy, pneumonectomy, is the procedure of choice. (See Chapter 57.)

Pulmonary (Lung) Tumors

Pulmonary tumors may be *benign* or *malignant* and *primary* or *secondary*.

> *The most common pulmonary tumors are primary bronchogenic carcinomas. This means that* most *pulmonary tumors first arise within pulmonary structures rather than metastasizing to the lungs (i.e., most are not secondary tumors), arise specifically within the bronchial epithelium, and are malignant.*

BENIGN AND METASTATIC PULMONARY TUMORS

Very few nonmalignant pulmonary tumors occur. When they do, benign and metastatic (i.e., secondary) pulmonary tumors are generally asymptomatic. However, they sometimes cause symptoms as a result of local pressure. One exception is a benign bronchial adenoma, which typically bleeds and produces recurrent hemoptyses. Whenever possible, benign pulmonary tumors are surgically excised. When viewed by x-ray, these tumors often have clearly defined margins and smooth outlines. Benign pulmonary tumors may become malignant.

> *The lungs are the most common site of tumors that have metastasized from other organs.*

Metastatic tumors in pulmonary structures most often come from malignant tumors in the breast, stomach, prostate, kidney, thyroid, testis, or bone.[100] Secondary bronchial carcinoma is difficult to differentiate from primary bronchial carcinoma because it produces similar x-ray densities, symptoms, and cytologic findings. The cytologic identification of malignant cells in sputum (or bronchial aspirate) only indicates malignant disease in the lung. It does not clarify whether the cells are from primary or secondary disease.

Persons suspected of having *primary lung cancers* need to be thoroughly evaluated to rule out the presence of an extrathoracic carcinoma. The most definitive diagnostic procedure for confirming diagnosis of metastatic bronchial carcinoma is careful histologic examination of specimens of bronchial tissue obtained by biopsy or surgical resection. Diagnosis is clearly established by finding cells that are characteristic of extrathoracic carcinomas. For example, colloid-containing cells typify thyroid cancers, whereas clear and opaque cells typify renal cancers. When possible, a patient may benefit from the removal of a metastatic pulmonary lesion if it is a solitary lesion.

PRIMARY MALIGNANT PULMONARY TUMORS (BRONCHOGENIC CARCINOMAS)

Primary pulmonary tumors have an extremely high rate of malignancy. Of those that are malignant, the vast majority arise from the bronchial epithelium (hence are called *bronchogenic carcinomas*). The right lung is affected more often than the left. Centrally located pulmonary tumors occur more often than tumors in the peripheries of the lungs. The central location is, unfortunately, more frequently inoperable because of the tumor's proximity to the mediastinum. If untreated, bronchogenic carcinoma is usually fatal within 9 months. Patients who survive the longest usually have well-circumscribed, slowly growing, peripheral tumors which can be surgically treated by lobectomy.

Pathology. More than 90 per cent of all lung cancers develop from the bronchial tree's epithelium. While the pathogenesis of lung cancer is not clearly understood, it is speculated that the following sequence occurs:[27]

- "Nonspecific inflammatory reaction with hypersecretion, followed by desquamation down to, but not including, the basal cells.
- Nonspecific reactive hyperplasia of the basal cell and metaplasia, especially at the site of bifurcations of the bronchial tree.

TABLE 55–1. WORLD HEALTH ORGANIZATION CLASSIFICATION OF LUNG TUMORS (CATEGORIES I TO IV)

	Incidence (Per Cent)
I. Epidermoid carcinoma	42
II. Small-cell anaplastic carcinoma	15–37
1. Fusiform	
2. Polygonal	
3. Lymphocyte-like	
4. Others	
III. Adenocarcinoma	10
1. Bronchogenic	
a. Acinar	
b. Papillary	
2. Bronchioloalveolar	
IV. Large-cell carcinoma	20
1. Solid tumor with mucin	
2. Solid tumor without mucin	
3. Giant cell	
4. Clear cell	

- Increasing atypia of the metaplastic cells. These findings were present in 93 per cent of active smokers, 6 per cent of ex-smokers 5 to 15 years after they stopped smoking, and 1 per cent of nonsmokers.
- Carcinoma in situ.
- Invasive carcinoma."

The four major histologic types of invasive lung cancer are *epidermoid (squamous), adenocarcinoma, large cell anaplastic*, and *small cell anaplastic*.

Table 55–1 presents the World Health Organization classification of lung tumors and includes the incidence of the four main types of invasive lung cancer.

The most common type of primary pulmonary neoplasm is *squamous cell (epidermoid) carcinoma*. Squamous cell carcinomas develop in the main bronchi or larger bronchial branches. Generally they spread by direct extension and lymph node metastasis and metastasize more slowly than other types. They occur most often in males and are almost always associated with cigarette smoking. Well-differentiated squamous cell carcinomas offer a better prognosis than less clearly differentiated types.

Women tend to live longer than men following surgery for lung cancer. This sex difference in survival rates is partially related to the type of tumors women more commonly have, the extent of the disease, and the amount of surgery performed.

Primary lung tumors may cause malignant invasion of the brain, adrenal glands, liver, bones, and opposite lung. Mediastinal and cervical lymph nodes are often involved in spread of the tumor. The diaphragm and pleural cavity may also be affected by neoplastic extension. As mentioned, squamous cell carcinomas usually spread by direct extension and lymph node metastasis. The other major types tend to spread via the bloodstream.

Incidence and Etiology. Lung cancer is the leading cause of male cancer deaths. The mortality rate for men has increased more than 15-fold in 40 years. The rate for women has also increased steadily. (See Figure 55–1).

> *The incidence of primary cancer of the lung is increasing and it is the most common fatal cancer.*[16] Lung cancer is the only form of cancer that is showing a rapid, almost epidemic increase.

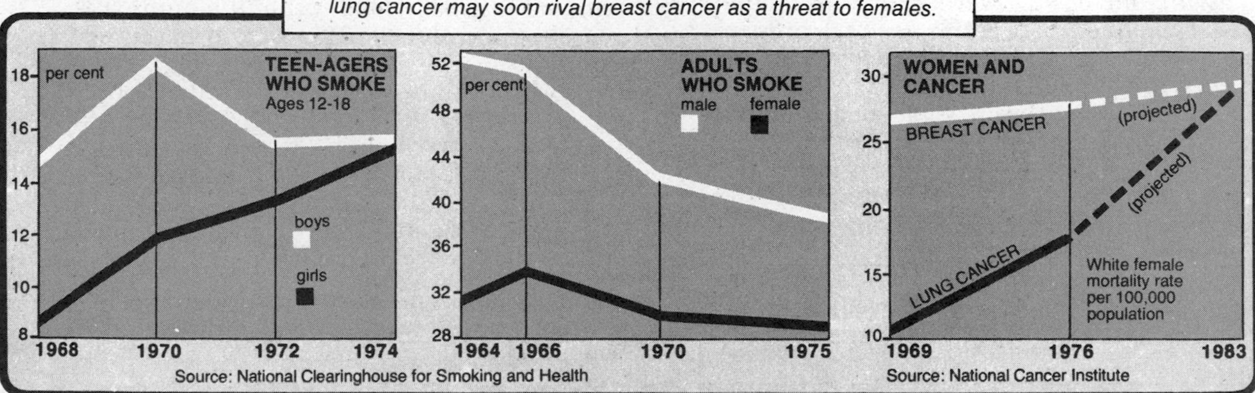

Figure 55–1. "In women, lung cancer increased 30 per cent between 1973 and 1976 in 11 areas across the United States and most victims died within three years, the National Cancer Insitute reported." (*Seattle Post-Intelligence.* October 20, 1978.) (Graph, courtesy of *Newsweek Magazine,* 43:83, Jan. 22, 1977.)

The mortality rate is high because early diagnosis (the time when cure is most possible) of pulmonary cancer is difficult. However, cancer of the lung (like other types of cancer) may be cured if detected *early* enough. Primary lung cancer most often occurs between ages 40 and 70.

Cancer of the lung is a particularly tragic condition because it is largely a self-imposed, preventable disease caused most frequently by cigarette smoking. Bronchogenic carcinoma occurs far more often among heavy smokers than among nonsmokers. The bronchogenic cancer rate for women has quadrupled in the past 40 years; this is thought to be a direct result of cigarette smoking.

Cigarette smoke contains numerous chemical carcinogens (i.e., agents that assist the action of cancer-producing chemicals). The risk of developing lung cancer increases in proportion to the number of cigarettes smoked, length of time an individual has smoked, how deeply the smoker inhales, and the age at which the smoking habit began.

Cigarette smoking causes progressive cellular changes of the kind that precede cancer. These cellular changes increase in degree as more cigarettes are smoked, and they diminish if the smoker stops smoking before invasive lung cancer develops. Additionally, it is statistically clear that a decrease in lung cancer death rates occurs among persons who stop smoking. This decrease is roughly proportional to the time elapsed since smoking was stopped.

Other irritating inhalants also appear to be significant in the development of lung cancer. The incidence of lung cancer is increased among persons working with: uranium ore, asbestos, chromates, nickel dust, or bischloromethyl ether. Suggestive evidence indicates that prolonged exposure to air pollution promotes pulmonary neoplasms.[16] (See Table 55–2.) It is therefore important that air pollution be minimized or alleviated and that industrial workers exposed to irritants be given appropriate health supervision and protection in order to reduce the incidence of lung cancer.

The prevention of lung cancer also requires education concerning the importance of annual physical examinations that include chest x-ray films and of seeking medical evaluation promptly if any symptoms of lung cancer or any of "Cancer's Seven Warning Signals" appear. (See also Unit IX.)

TABLE 55–2. RISK FACTORS FOR BRONCHOGENIC CANCER

Cigarette smoking
Uranium mining
Asbestos exposure
Working with chromate
Working with arsenic
Chlormethyl-methyl ether exposure
Previous upper respiratory tract cancer
High inducibility of aryl hydrocarbon hydroxylase (not yet substantiated)

From Anderson, H. A.: Preoperative evaluation of bronchogenic cancer. *Consultant,* 18:196, Sept. 1978.

The *nurse's role* in the prevention and early detection of pulmonary cancer includes:

- encouraging persons with chronic cough or with a change in the character of a cough to seek medical evaluation;
- encouraging persons who are habitual heavy smokers to have a chest x-ray film every six months;
- recommending medical evaluation to persons with recurring or chronic respiratory infections;
- participating in community and other educational programs that present the facts about the harmful effects of smoking and other sources of air pollution;
- informing persons in the community about local cancer detection clinics, symptoms that may indicate pulmonary cancer, and diagnostic tests used when pulmonary cancer is suspected; and
- emphasizing the need for the early detection and treatment of all malignant lesions.

Symptoms. Pulmonary cancer is a "silent disease" in its earliest stages, giving no indication of its presence and often being undetectable by physical examination. Asymptomatic tumors developing in "silent areas" of the lung are detected only by chest film. By the time symptoms begin to appear the cancer may have progressed beyond the point of cure. When symptoms of lung cancer do occur they may include blood in the sputum, chest pain, symptoms of a lingering pulmonary infection, and persistent cough. *All coughs or other evidences of respiratory infection which last longer than two to three weeks should be medically investigated*, particularly in heavy cigarette smokers.

The symptoms produced by pulmonary cancers vary, depending upon the location and size of the tumor. If the cancer begins in a bronchus, as it grows it tends to irritate and partially obstruct the bronchus. *The most common symptom of bronchogenic carcinoma is the development of a cough or a change in the severity or nature of a cough* (if chronic cough has been present). Tumors that block off a bronchus may cause numerous problems in the area distal to the stenosis or obstruction, e.g., atelectasis, dilating of bronchi beyond the block, abscess formation, bronchiectasis or pneumonitis. Retained secretions may cause recurring episodes of pneumonia or bronchitis. These symptoms may also result from tumors compressing bronchi. The symptoms resulting from infection associated with bronchial obstruction or stenosis may be the symptoms, e.g., dyspnea, chills, fever, that initially prompt a person with pulmonary cancer to seek medical attention.

Pulmonary tumors located near the pleura may produce pleuritic pain and bloody pleural effusion. Tumors located near the bottom of the lung may irritate the diaphragm and involve the phrenic nerve, producing referred pain along the top of the shoulder, as well as breathing difficulties. As tumors located at the top of the lung enlarge they may involve the ribs, the sympathetic nerve chain (producing pupil changes), or the brachial plexus (causing arm pain). Invasion of the mediastinal structures, e.g., esophagus, by tumor may produce ulceration, bleeding, and difficulty in swallowing. Obstruction of the superior vena cava or invasion of a portion of the heart may occur as a tumor extends within the thorax. Tumors which enlarge in such a direction that they press against the trachea produce tracheal symptoms. The recurrent laryngeal nerve may be involved, producing hoarseness and vocal cord paralysis.

Weakness, weight loss, anemia, and anorexia often occur with advanced lung cancer. These nonspecific systemic effects of malignancy are discussed more completely in Unit IX.

Various *systemic syndromes* often occur in association with lung cancer. Among these are *nonmetastatic* neuromuscular syndromes (occurring in patients with bronchogenic carcinoma), arthralgias and clubbing of the fingers and toes, and metabolic disorders such as hypercalcemia, polycythemia, inappropriate ADH secretion, Cushing's syndrome, and (in males) bilateral mammary gland hypertrophy. The destruction or removal of the primary cancer or performance of a bilateral adrenalectomy may correct adrenocortical hyperplasia caused by production of ACTH by the tumor.

Diagnosis. Procedures that may be used to diagnose lung cancer include x-ray examinations; sputum cytology; mediastinoscopy; biopsy of scalene nodes or enlarged cervical or axillary lymph nodes (when mediastinal or hilar involvement is believed to be present); thoracentesis with evaluation of pleural fluid (if pleural effusion is present); bronchoscopy (with biopsy of the tumor and/or examination of bronchial washings); needle biopsy of the tumor (directly through the chest wall); lung scanning; pleural biopsy; and possibly thoracotomy and biopsy. (Diagnostic procedures are discussed in detail in Chapter 52.)

During the diagnostic investigation the physician not only establishes the location and type of tumor, but also evaluates the operability of the tumor and the extent of its spread. The *ideal* means of detecting lung cancer early in persons who continue to smoke habitually (and have smoked for 15 to 20 years or longer) would be to periodically examine sputum specimens and perform bronchoscopy and to perform a yearly complete physical examination, with chest films made every 3 to 4 months even though the individual is asymptomatic.

The best *routine* means of detecting lung cancer *early* is to encourage people to have a large chest x-ray film annually (preferably more often in persons who have smoked heavily for a number of years). As mentioned earlier, in asymptomatic persons who are harboring a lung cancer an abnormal chest film is often the only change found during a routine physical evaluation. Such an x-ray may reveal such findings as: thick-walled cavities, pleural effusion, small peripheral nodules, masses in the hilar region, lung infiltrations, atelectasis, pleural thickening, indications of pulmonary infection, bone erosion, or emphysematous dilatation of alveoli.

Pulmonary angiography is useful in diagnosing bronchogenic carcinoma. To determine the hilar and mediastinal extent of the cancer, contrast visualization of the vena cava and pulmonary artery and veins is performed in both frontal and lateral projections. Pulmonary veins can be evaluated only by cineradiography, i.e., a motion picture record of successive images appearing on a fluoroscopic screen. Persons with lung tumors involving major pulmonary vessels have a poor prognosis following surgical resection. Therefore, the angiographic demonstration of such involvement may contraindicate attempts at surgical treatment.[29A]

Table 55–3 summarizes characteristics of main types of lung cancer.

Treatment. Persons with resectable lung cancers are treated by *surgery*. It is possible, under favorable circumstances, for pulmonary cancer to be cured by complete surgical excision of affected tissue. The amount of lung tissue resected depends upon the extent of the disease. Although a lobectomy may suffice if a tumor is well localized, pneumonectomy is often required. Involved contiguous structures may also be removed. It appears that careful block removal of mediastinal lymph nodes draining the involved lobe or lung increases chances of survival. This procedure is employed when pulmonary nodes contain metastasis but mediastinal nodes are free of metastasis. Some physicians believe that administering *high voltage radiation* to the tumor site and the adjacent pulmonary hilum prior to surgical resection minimizes the risk of metastasis. Sometimes irradiation shrinks previously inoperable tumors in such a way that surgery is then possible.

As with many other malignant tumors, the five-year survival rate increases if surgery is performed while the tumor is localized; the rate decreases if the tumor has spread to regional lymphatics and other structures.

TABLE 55–3. CHARACTERISTICS OF MAIN TYPES OF LUNG CANCER

Cell Type	Epidemiology	Radiographic Presentation	Primary Symptoms, Signs and Pathogenesis	Metastatic Potential	Therapeutic Response Factors: Growth Rate	Resectability	Response to Drugs	Response to Radiation
Epidermoid	High correlation to cigarette smoking, exposure to uranium ores Environmental	40–60% present with hilar or perihilar mass or infiltrate 25–30% with single peripheral nodule from 4–8 cm. in diameter 8–10% show central necrosis and cavitation of mass with thick walled cavities	Secondary to local growth: cough, hemoptysis, stridor Secondary to bronchial obstruction: atelectasis, pneumonitis, dyspnea Secondary to extension to pleura: pleural effusion, chest pain, restrictive dyspnea Secondary to extension to chest wall: chest pain, increasing dyspnea, involvement of the first thoracic and eighth cervical nerve resulting in severe shoulder pain radiating down the ulnar distribution of the arm (the superior sulcus or Pancoast's syndrome)	Uncommon, but may occur in this order: (a) lymph nodes, (b) adrenals. (c) liver	Slow	Good, 8% cure	Limited	Poor Controls local disease Palliative
Small cell	High correlation to cigarette smoking, exposure to uranium ores Environmental	69–75% present with hilar or perihilar mass Infrequently peripheral mass less than 4 cm. in diameter Hemidiaphragm elevation (results from paralysis of phrenic nerve)	Secondary to local and regional lymphatic spread–cough, hemoptysis, stridor Hoarseness from paralysis of recurrent laryngeal nerve Dyspnea from phrenic nerve involvement Dysphagia from extrinsic compression of esophagus Pleural effusion from obstruction of mediastinal lymphatics Venous distention of face, neck, chest, back from obstruction of superior vena cava Involvement of pericardium/heart causes pericardial effusion, tamponade, arrhythmia	Highly metastatic; 80% have metastasis with symptoms of 3 months' duration 45% have bone marrow involvement, 8% brain 50% liver, adrenals and kidney may be involved	Rapid	Poor, not advised because of high rate of metastasis	Dramatic, but disease recurs	Dramatic, but response ineffective due to wide metastasis
Adenocarcinoma	Unknown; may occur in nonsmokers, most frequently in women	60–70% located in periphery, usually less than 4 cm. in diameter	Pleural involvement by direct extension –pleural effusion, chest pain, restrictive dyspnea Frequently, no symptoms at time of discovery on chest x-ray Involvement of first thoracic and eighth cervical nerve	Intermediate	Slow		Better than epidermoid Poorer than small cell	Most radio resistant
Large cell anaplastic	Cigarette smoking	Peripheral lung mass, alone or combined with other lesions Cavitation may occur, leaving thick-walled cavity with or without air-fluid level	Principal symptoms same as for epidermoid	Intermediate metastasis in this order: (a) kidney, (b) liver, (c) adrenals	Relatively slow	Intermediate–between small cell and epidermoid	Poor	Intermediate–between epidermoid and adenocarcinoma

From Boyer, M. W.: Treating invasive lung cancer. *American Journal of Nursing*, 77:1918, Dec. 1977.

Depending on the source of the figures, the percentage of patients with lung cancer having resectable tumors ranges from 25 to 50 per cent. Lung tumors sometimes prove to be inoperable at the time of surgical exploration. Some patients are unable to tolerate chest surgery because of severe cardiac or pulmonary conditions. Other *contraindications to surgery* include evidence that the cancer has metastasized either distantly (e.g., to the central nervous system or bone) or locally (e.g, as evidenced by pleural effusion, hilar lymph node metastases, obstruction of the superior vena cava, or laryngeal nerve involvement). Surgery may be performed on some persons with pericardial invasion or chest wall invasion if the involved area is technically resectable.

Some patients benefit temporarily from pulmonary surgery even though the total lung cancer cannot be resected. For example, such *palliative resection* may be performed if a patient has developed a lung abscess distal to an obstructed or stenotic bronchus.

Postoperative radiation therapy is usually given following pulmonary resection when metastases to adjacent structures are suspected. During radiation therapy unrecognized hypercalcemia (e.g., caused by parathormone production by the tumor) may be exaggerated or hyperuricemia may occur. When detected, these conditions are treated medically.

Palliative irradiation often helps to make people with inoperable lung cancer more comfortable for a while. The objective of palliative therapy is to minimize or eliminate the acutely distressing aspects of the disease (e.g., pain, cough, shortness of breath) by producing a temporary regression of tumor size. Thus, the patient is more comfortable even though the lesion continues to progress. Palliative radiation may also somewhat prolong life; however, this is not the primary goal of the therapy. Severe blockage of the superior vena cava or innominate veins is an acutely distressing, potentially fatal complication of pulmonary cancer which causes respiratory embarrassment, distention of neck veins, cyanosis of the head and neck, and edema of the face and orbits of the eyes. Temporary relief may be given by irradiation of the involved mediastinal region.

Palliative therapy for nonresectable pulmonary cancer may be provided by a course of *supervoltage radiation* carefully directed at the primary site and the mediastinal area of lymph node drainage. Another means of palliative therapy is the *implantation of an isotope* at the primary site, e.g., gold-filtered radon seeds or ^{125}I permanent implants. (See also Unit IX.)

Following pulmonary resection some physicians administer prophylactic long-range low-dose *chemotherapy*. Medications may be given singly or in combination. (See Table 55–4.) Sometimes chemotherapeutic agents are instilled locally through a bronchial arterial catheter. This method provides intensive local treatment, since the bronchial arterial system may be the major arterial supply to pulmonary neoplasms.

Palliative chemotherapy may alleviate some distressing symptoms and provide a general improvement of a transient nature in some persons with extensive inoperable bronchogenic carcinoma. However, medical treatment of relapses is usually less effective than the first course of therapy, and remissions are usually of brief duration. (Chemotherapy of cancer is discussed in Unit IX.)

Most recently *immunotherapy* has been used as a means of stimulating the body to produce antibodies to suppress the cancer cells. The success of this form of therapy will not be completely known for a few years.

Prognosis of pulmonary cancer is very poor if cancer cells are found in a pleural effusion. This means the cancer cells have spread into the lymphatics. When pleural effusion is detected, thoracentesis is performed. Once all the fluid is removed from the pleural space a *sclerosing agent* is instilled to stop this component of the cancer activity and to produce a pleural seal. Preparations that may be used for this purpose include radioactive gold, radioactive phosphorus, or a freshly prepared mixture of water and nitrogen mustard. Following the injection of one of these substances into the pleural cavity, the patient is turned in various positions to facilitate spread of the medication. Occasionally it is necessary to use closed chest drainage with high suction (e.g, 30 to 60 cm. of water) to accomplish complete drainage of the pleural effusion prior to instillation of the medication.

Any person with primary pulmonary cancer, whether or not surgical resection has been performed, is carefully followed for evidence of metastases, e.g., to the brain, bones, contralateral lung. Routinely examinations are scheduled each month for the first year and at longer intervals thereafter. Before discharge the patient is told to contact a physician if additional symptoms develop, e.g., chest pain, dyspnea, hoarseness, dysphagia, or pain upon swallowing. These symptoms may indicate metastasis.

Nursing care of patients with cancer is discussed in Unit IX.

Pneumonias

A *pneumonia* is an acute inflammation of the alveolar spaces of the lung that causes consolidation of lung tissue as alveoli fill with exudate. There are a variety of types of pneumonias, with different causative agents. Most pneumonias are caused by infection. However, some result from *chemical irritants such as noxious gases*. Generally pneumonias are referred to as *bacteri-*

al or *nonbacterial*, or they may be more precisely identified according to the specific etiologic agent, e.g., pneumococcal, Friedländer's, staphylococcal, rickettsial, fungal, mycoplasmal, or viral pneumonia. This classification, based on the etiologic organism, is the most commonly used. Pathogenic bacteria range in length from 0.5 micron (pneumococci) to 3.0 microns (enteric bacteria). Particles of mucus in this size range may carry bacteria into the alveoli where they are retained.

At times pneumonias are designated in terms of their *structural distribution*. For example, bronchopneumonia involves only those alveoli in contact with bronchi. Bronchopneumonias usually consist of diffuse patches of pneumonia scattered throughout both lungs. Another name for bronchopneumonia is lobular pneumonia, i.e., pneumonia involving only a portion of a lobe. A pneumonia that involves an entire lobe is termed lobar pneumonia (Fig. 55–2).

With any pneumonia it is essential that the etiologic agent be accurately identified so appropriate antimicrobial medications can be given. Sometimes mixed infections occur in which more than one type of organism is present. Reductions in the morbidity and mortality from pneumonias have occurred as a result of specific antimicrobial therapy; nonetheless, patients continue to die from pneumonia. Early diagnosis and vigorous therapy are therefore essential.

The clinical courses of various pneumonias and their specific chemotherapeutic management may vary, but the general supportive care given is basically the same regardless of the etiologic agent.

> *The recovery of patients seriously ill with pneumonia often depends on skilled nursing care.*

Predisposing Factors. Numerous conditions and factors *predispose* an individual to pneumonia. Among these are chronic illness and debility, cancer, thoracic surgery, atelectasis, common cold and other viral respiratory infections, chronic respiratory infections and disorders, influenza, smoking, fibrocystic disease, malnutrition, cardiac failure, tracheostomy, exposure to noxious gases, exposure to cold, treatment with immunosuppressive agents, hypoventilation, hypostasis, impaired ciliary action in the tracheobronchial tree, impaired alveolar phagocyte function, depression of cerebral function, and aspiration.

The previous state of health of the person is the major deciding factor in the course of bacterial pneumonia. Preexisting pulmonary disorders — both chronic and recent —predispose the airways to bronchopneumonia.

Aspiration of secretions, liquids, foods, vomitus, pills, and so forth, can result from disorders that depress cerebral function, impair swallowing, and obliterate or depress the cough or epiglottal reflex. Examples of patients in danger of aspirating include persons who have had application of a local anesthetic to the throat or have been under a general anesthetic, comatose or stuporous patients, and persons with central nervous system conditions that impair swallowing, e.g., bulbar paralysis. Comatose and stuporous patients hypoventilate and generally are inactive; these conditions promote retention of secretions in the lungs — an ideal medium for infection. Chronic ethanol abuse often leads to pneumonia owing to both aspiration and malnourishment.

Pneumonia commonly develops among aged and debilitated persons. It most often occurs during those times of the year when upper respiratory infections are prevalent.

Prevention. Prophylactic administration of antibiotics is not effective in preventing pneumonia in predisposed individuals. Immunization against influenza is useful in preventing pneumonia that can complicate influenza.

Efforts directed at preventing pneumonia are most often those that maintain optimal respiratory function, prevent aspiration, and vigorously treat underlying diseases. Clinical states and medications that tend to suppress local bronchopulmonary defense mechanisms (e.g., ciliary action and pulmonary macrophages) are avoided when possible. Among these are hypoxemia, acidosis, narcotics, sedatives, and adrenocorticosteroids.

> *Skilled nursing care can help prevent some pneumonias, e.g., those related to aspiration, hypoventilation, immobility.*

Many *nursing activities* focus on preventing pneumonia. Some of the more important of these are summarized below:

- Correctly position unconscious and semiconscious patients to prevent aspiration, e.g., postoperatively, or following strokes.
- Never administer food, fluids, or medications by mouth to comatose or stuporous patients or to patients who lack a gag reflex, e.g., those who have not recovered from a local throat anesthetic.
- Frequently turn and reposition patients who are immobilized.

TABLE 55-4. CHEMOTHERAPEUTIC AGENTS USED IN LUNG CANCER

Agent and Route of Administration	Excreted by	Nadir	Side Effects	Nursing Actions
methotrexate MTX Amethopterin PO IV	kidneys	6 days (WBC) 9 days (platelets)	GI: stomatitis, nausea and vomiting, gingivitis, sore throat, GI bleed, diarrhea liver toxicity: 20% develop cirrhosis, acute liver atrophy kidney toxicity with renal failure endocrine: menstrual problems, reduced sperm adult-onset diabetes CNS complications: headache, drowsiness, blurred vision aplastic anemia (rare) bone marrow depression	give antiemetic before treatment medicate to numb mouth and throat areas small, frequent feedings I & O; guaiac stools be supportive, especially to younger patients who may develop sexual problems closely observe for infection, bleeding
cyclophosphamide Cytoxan Endoxan CTX IV PO	kidneys body tissue and fluids	10–14 days	nausea and vomiting alopecia, up to 90% interferes with wound healing hemorrhagic cystitis, colitis GI: oral, mucositis, stomatitis endocrine: amenorrhea, male—loss of virility bone marrow depression nonspecific dermatitis, fingernails and skin darker	give antiemetic before treatment offer support for change in body image, alopecia, sexual changes IV hydration or force fluids to keep patient hydrated I & O, observe urine for hematuria closely observe for infection/bleeding
CCNU **cyclohexyl chloroethyl nitrosourea** PO	body tissue and fluids	4–6 weeks 4 weeks (platelets) 5 weeks (WBC)	thrombocytopenia and leukopenia nausea and vomiting anorexia	prevent infections; check temperature frequently antiemetics helpful; small frequent feedings; bland diet give CCNU with fluids on an empty stomach closely observe for infection and bleeding
MeCCNU **methyl CCNU** PO	body tissue and fluids	29–43 days	nausea, vomiting, anorexia reduced platelet count leukopenia bone marrow depression	helpful to give antiemetic before treatment, give on an empty stomach 4 hours PC watch for infection/bleeding
BCNU IV	body tissue and fluids		nausea, vomiting, anorexia reduced platelet count leukopenia bone marrow depression	helpful to give antiemetic before treatment, give on empty stomach, small, frequent feedings watch for infection/bleeding
doxorubicin HCl Adriamycin IV	liver	7–10 days	nausea, vomiting stomatitis, mouth ulcerations alopecia bone marrow depression cardiac toxicity: premature ventricular contractions, congestive heart failure (CHF) thrombophlebitis at injection site	helpful to give antiemetic before treatment, good oral hygiene inject into tubing of running IV, check for infiltration check apical pulse for irregularity, assess for possibility of CHF watch for infection/bleeding

TABLE 55–4. CHEMOTHERAPEUTIC AGENTS USED IN LUNG CANCER *(Continued)*

Agent and Route of Administration	Excreted by	Nadir	Side Effects	Nursing Actions
bleomycin sulfate Blenoxane IV	not known	usually not myelosuppressant	anaphylaxis nausea, vomiting, anorexia chills, fever mucositis alopecia pulmonary fibrosis in about 5% of patients dermatologic changes—tightening and hardening of palmar and plantar skin, with discoloration	observe frequently for change in B P or pulse give antiemetic before treatment; provide extra blankets, frequent temperature observations use antipyretics, soft bland diet strict oral hygiene
hexamethylmelamine PO	urine	14 days	thrombocytopenia, leukopenia nausea, vomiting, diarrhea neurologic: paresthesias, hyporeflexia, motor weakness, decreased position sense, vibratory sense, and touch mental: depression, somnolence, dysphasia, insomnia, hallucinations weight loss, slight anemia	watch for infection/bleeding give antiemetics and antidiarrheals assist as needed observe frequently soft, bland diet
vincristine sulfate Oncovin IV	liver	mild myelosuppressant	nausea, vomiting neurotoxicity: paresthesias, neurotic pain, loss of deep tendon reflexes, muscular weakness, hoarseness alopecia, up to 50% of patients constipation	give antiemetics adequate hydration stool softeners or laxatives observe for weakened grip, foot drop, muscle weakness, paresthesias (first observed in fingertips) assist with dressing and buttoning if necessary
hydroxyurea Hydrea PO	urine	24–48 hrs.	bone marrow depression occasional GI and oral ulceration, nausea and vomiting may occur maculopapular rash (rare)	soft diet capsule can be opened and dissolved in warm tea or orange juice watch for infection/bleeding
mechlorethamine HCl nitrogen mustard HN 2 Mustargen HCl IV	body fluids	7–10 days	nausea, vomiting leukopenia, thrombocytopenia alopecia may occur, temporary amenorrhea, impaired spermatogenesis, maculopapular skin eruptions diarrhea, anorexia	premedicate with antiemetic and/or sedative avoid contact with skin, eyes wear gloves when reconstituting, use immediately watch for infection/bleeding sodium thiosulfate–antidote for skin contact or infiltrated IV
ifosfamide IV	kidney	7–10 days	leukopenia nausea, vomiting occasionally alopecia (with high doses) hemorrhagic cystitis transient mental confusion	watch for infection/bleeding, medicate for nausea p.r.n. closely observe urinary output, microscopic exam daily for hematuria IV hydration, push PO fluids
epipodophyllotoxin derivative VP-16 IV	probably liver	10–14 days	hypotension nausea leukopenia	check BP 2–3 times during infusion run solution in over 1 hour watch for infection

Table continued on the following page.

TABLE 55–4. CHEMOTHERAPEUTIC AGENTS USED IN LUNG CANCER (*Continued*)

Agent and Route of Administration	Excreted by	Nadir	Side Effects	Nursing Actions
streptozotocin IV	probably kidney	rarely myelosuppressant	nausea, vomiting proteinurea renal toxicity mild hepatotoxicity diabetes (reversible) abdominal cramps	premedicate with antiemetic check urine for protein, glucose hydrate with IV fluids, push fluids by mouth good oral hygiene bland diet, soft foods
procarbazine Matalene PO	kidney and body fluids	14 days	nausea, vomiting, anorexia bone marrow depression mental depression, restlessness some alopecia orthostatic hypotension	give antiemetics but not phenothiazines, give h.s. to reduce nausea and vomiting avoid alcoholic beverages, narcotics, sedatives, ripe cheeses, bananas instruct on way to stand up to avoid dizziness watch for infection/bleeding
5-FU, fluorouracil IV	kidney	9–14 days	stomatitis bone marrow depression nausea, vomiting diarrhea dermatitis	strict oral hygiene watch for infection/bleeding give antiemetics

Modified from Boyer, M. W.: Treating invasive lung cancer. *American Journal of Nursing,* 77:1920, Dec. 1977.

- Encourage periodic coughing and deep breathing in patients who are recovering from surgery, are immobilized, or have retained pulmonary secretions.
- Maintain a patent tracheobronchial tree, e.g., by suctioning, hydration, deep breathing, coughing.
- Prevent overmedication with sedatives, narcotics, and cough-suppressive medications. Oversedation and respiratory depression predispose to secretion accumulation in the lungs.
- Observe for early indications of possible pneumonia; call symptoms to the physician's attention so early treatment can be instituted if necessary.
- Encourage prompt treatment of colds and "flu," especially in persons susceptible to pneumonia.
- Prevent spread of communicable respiratory infections by using appropriate medical asepsis and isolation. Keep the very young and very old away from close contact with a person who has pneumonia. Encourage good room ventilation and minimize crowding. Properly clean respiratory therapy equipment to prevent spread of infection.
- Give frequent oral hygiene to dependent persons in your care.
- Observe necessary precautions that minimize the likelihood of aspiration when giving food or liquids to patients who are likely to aspirate. Make certain nasogastric tubes are correctly positioned in the stomach before administering a tube feeding or medication.

CONSOLIDATION OF ONE LOBE

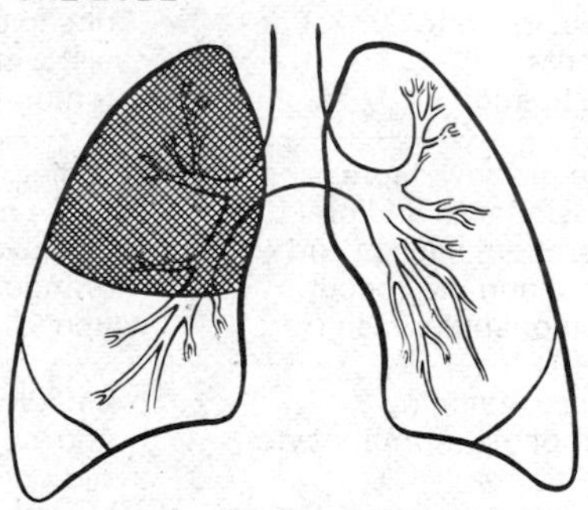

PATCHY CONSOLIDATION

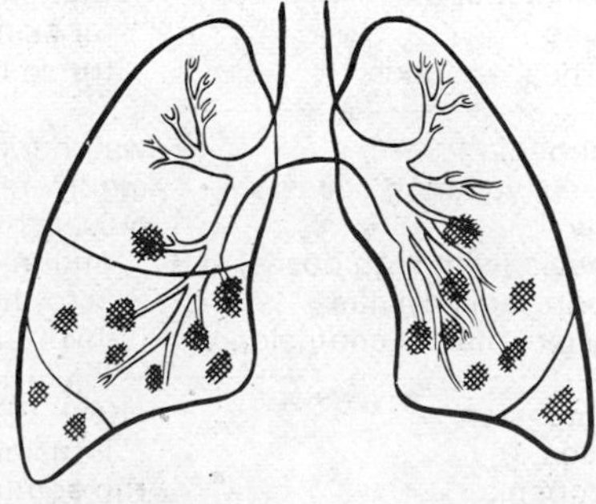

AREA OF CONSOLIDATION

Figure 55–2. Two types of pneumonia: consolidation of one lobe (lobar) and patchy consolidation (lobular or bronchopneumonia). (Modified from *Introduction to Respiratory Diseases,* 4th ed. Copyright American Lung Association.)

BACTERIAL PNEUMONIAS

Most bacterial pneumonias are caused by *Diplococcus pneumoniae,* i.e., the pneumococcus. Other microorganisms that may cause bacterial pneumonias include *Staphylococcus aureus,* group A hemolytic streptoccocci, *Escherichia coli, Hemophilus influenzae,* Klebsiella-Enterobacter-Serratia group, *Francisella tularensis,* Proteus species, or Pseudomonas. Commonly aspiration pneumonias, hypostatic pneumonias, and "terminal" pneumonias are mixed infections. Often healthy carriers are responsible for infecting others. Pathogenic organisms that cause bacterial pneumonias are frequently present among the normal flora of the respiratory tract.

Because pneumococcal pneumonia is the most common type of bacterial pneumonia and because it generally typifies pneumonias caused by all etiologic agents, this discussion focuses in detail on pneumococcal pneumonia.

Bacterial Invasion. Bacteria may enter the lungs through the airways or the blood. Sterility of the lower airway depends upon steady transport of mucus by ciliary motion that removes most particles greater than 5 microns. The integrity of the lower airway depends upon optimal conditions. This process is disturbed by adverse factors such as hypoventilation, hyperoxia, hypoxia, chemical irritants, and acute viral infections.

PNEUMOCOCCAL PNEUMONIA

Pathology. Pneumonia caused by pneumococci usually involves one or more lobes of the lung. Pneumococci are not the only organisms that cause lobar pneumonias. However, whatever the etiologic organism(s) may be, lobar pneumonias classically have the following four histologic stages: congestion, red hepatization, gray hepatization, and resolution. (Consult a textbook of pathology for details.)

Pneumococci initially reach the alveoli via the respiratory passages. During the course of the infection the sputum becomes rusty-colored because of the red blood cells which escape from the blood vessels and pass through the alveolar membrane. As alveolar fluids spill into the bronchioles they are eventually coughed up through the tracheobronchial tree. Inflammation of the mucous membranes of the bronchi, trachea, pharynx, and nose occurs. Thus, the entire respiratory system is involved. During the periods of consolidation (when the alveoli are filled with thick exudate), adequate gas exchange cannot occur in involved areas of the lungs; pulmonary ventilation and diffusion are impaired, and the blood oxygen tension is subnormal.

Symptoms. Pneumococcal pneumonia, usually has a sudden onset, with shaking chills, high fever, cough, blood-flecked or pinkish (progressing to rust-colored) sputum, and "stabbing" chest pains (worsened by respiratory movements and, in some instances, referred to the shoulder, abdomen, or flank). Chest pain is caused by pleuritic involvement. Occasionally gastrointestinal symptoms such as nausea, vomiting, diarrhea, and jaundice occur. Often herpes simplex is present and the cheeks are flushed. Frequently history reveals that the patient has had a recent respiratory illness, e.g., an upper respiratory infection was present for several days before the infection worsened and moved rapidly into the lower respiratory tract. The patient may experience a chill followed by fever at the beginning of pneumonia. Body temperature may rise within a few hours to 40 or 40.1°C. (104 to 106°F.).

Typically the patient with pneumonia appears severely ill and may be found lying on the affected side in an attempt to splint her or his painful chest. Toxic delirium often occurs with severe pneumonia, particularly in alcoholic patients. If conscious and alert, the patient with pneumonia usually experiences aching pains, weakness, headache, and general malaise. Dyspnea and hypoxemia are common and cyanosis may develop. Respirations are shallow. The nares may flare with inspiration and the patient grunts with expiration. Flaring nares and an expiratory grunt are manifestations of respiratory distress. An expiratory grunt is a physiologic attempt at maintaining alveolar patency. (It is also frequently observed in neonates with idiopathic respiratory distress syndrome.) Marked tachypnea (30 to 45 respirations per minute) occurs. The pulse rate is also frequently increased, e.g., tachycardia may be present with 100 to 130 heart beats per minute. Abdominal distention and a pleural friction rub may also be present. Profuse perspiration is common.

Initially the cough tends to be dry, short, painful, and hacking. Later in the illness the cough becomes productive and pain decreases. Early in the course of pneumonia chest excursion on the affected side is diminished. Respiratory rales may be heard; breath sounds may be suppressed. Sputum is rusty during the earlier stages of the disease; it becomes yellow and mucopurulent during resolution. Sputum may be tenacious and difficult to expectorate.

Course of Illness. Patients with pneumococcal pneumonia who are treated early, vigorously, and appropriately usually respond well. Without treatment the mortality rate increases. The higher mortality rates occur in patients over age 50 and those with complications or other diseases, e.g., heart failure. Untreated persons whose illness is uncomplicated usually experience resolution by *crisis* about 7 to 10 days after onset of the pneumonia. The crisis period, in untreated cases, is the period when the patient's temperature "breaks" and declines rapidly. Typically the temperature remains elevated until the crisis occurs.

Diagnosis. The presence of rusty sputum is practically diagnostic of bacterial pneumonia. In addition to the previously described symptom pattern, other key factors in the diagnosis of pneumococcal pneumonia include lung infiltration visible on x-ray film, leukocytosis (20 to 35 thousand/mm.^{3}), and pneumocci present in the sputum and frequently also in the blood.

Sputum smears (Gram's stain) and cultures determine the bacterial etiology; blood cultures are also performed in bacteremic cases and are positive in about one fourth of the patients. Special laboratory procedures, e.g., the capsular swelling technique, may be used to type pneumococci. Types I to VIII most commonly occur in adults. Sputum from persons with pneumonia typically contains numerous pneumococci and red and white blood cells. The WBC count is usually elevated but it is sometimes normal or low; a low WBC indicates a poorer prognosis.

Sputum specimens for smear and culture and a blood culture should always be collected prior to giving the patient any antimicrobial medications.

It may be impossible to culture out, and hence identify, the infecting organism if antibiotics are started before the specimen is collected. When a good sputum specimen cannot be obtained, tracheal aspiration may be performed to obtain a specimen. (Be certain to collect sputum specimens in sterile containers). Sputum cultures require at least 24 to 48 hours to grow.

X-ray findings with bacterial pneumonias vary, depending on the stage of the disease. For example, initially vague haziness appears in the involved area. Later, well defined areas of consolidation appear and pleural fluid may blunt the costophrenic angles. An electrocardiogram may be necessary to help the physician to evaluate the patient's cardiac status. Blood specimens may be collected for blood gas and electrolyte evaluations. Urinalysis is routinely ordered.

A *pneumococcal vaccine* is now available. It is a bivalent type of vaccine made up of the eight most common types of pneumococcal organisms which cause eighty per cent of all pneumococcal infections. The indications for immunization of a person are much the same as the criteria used for influenza inoculations: persons who are chronically ill, debilitated, with little or no pulmonary reserve, with abnormal or depressed abilities to form antibodies. Examples of conditions in which inability to form specific antibodies occurs are hypogammaglobulinemia (congenital or acquired) and multiple myeloma.

Clinical Care. Clinical care of any patient with pneumonia is to provide chemotherapy that will be effective against the specific etiologic agent, provide symptomatic or supportive care to relieve symptoms associated with the pneumonia, and prevent complications of pneumonia. Essential activities include:

- Observe and evaluate response to care.
- Observe for and treat complications.
- Carry out and/or assist with diagnostic procedures.
- Ensure adequate physical and mental rest.
- Prevent chilling and exposure to drafts.
- Prevent spread of infection.
- Give frequent oral hygiene and lip and nose care.
- Provide fluid-electrolyte replacements and treat imbalances.
- Provide appropriate diet and fluid intake.
- Promote good tracheobronchial hygiene to help the patient breathe more comfortably and effectively, using appropriate respiratory care maneuvers applicable to the patient's level of illness.
- Administer specific chemotherapy and observe for side-effects or toxicity.
- Instruct the patient concerning convalescence and prevention of future respiratory infections.

Observations. When caring for a patient with pneumonia the nurse observes for indications of hypoxemia, respiratory insufficiency, or failure, shock, pulmonary edema, hyperthermia, spread of infection, atelectasis, pleurisy, abdominal distention, paralytic ileus, herpes simplex, fluid-electrolyte imbalances, and mental aberrations. Pneumonia may precipitate congestive heart failure in elderly patients or patients with preexisting heart disease. Observe closely for *early* indications of complications and report pertinent symptoms *immediately.*

Shock and pulmonary edema are the most frequent causes of death in pneumonia.

Space does not permit a detailed summary of all reportable symptoms. However, some are production of copious amounts of frothy sputum; increasingly labored respirations; temperatures below 37°C (98.6°F.) or above 39.4°C (103°F.); marked alterations in pulse rate and/or blood pressure (abnormal increases or decreases); indications of increasing hypoxemia (e.g., marked restlessness, disorientation, cyanosis, and increasing pulse rate); and toxic delirium. The nurse also reports any situations for which orders are required, e.g., abdominal distention, pleuritic pain.

Evaluate restlessness carefully and attempt to identify and relieve its cause when possible. The restless patient may require oxygen, suctioning, position change, dry linens, assistance to use the urinal or bedpan, relief from abdominal distention or pleuritic pain, encouragement to cough and deep breathe, or mild sedation. Also, evaluate hypotension carefully. It may indicate shock, bacteremia or hypoxia.

Observe also the patient's general response to therapy. One measure of a patient's condition and response is the temperature curve. The effect of antipyretics must be considered when evaluating a temperature curve.

Other measures a nurse uses to evaluate a patient with pneumonia include periodic measurements of vital signs, intake and output; observations of the patient's respiratory movements, including inspection of the movements of both sides of the chest; inspection and palpation of the skin and abdomen; inspection and measurement of sputum; evaluation of cough, pain and sensorium; inspection of lips and mucous membranes; and evaluation of laboratory findings such as arterial blood gases and WBC count.

During the acute stages of pneumonia, vital signs are taken and recorded at least every four hours. If complications appear to be developing or if a patient's condition is otherwise changing rapidly, vital signs are taken more often. Because the patient with pneumonia is dyspneic and coughs frequently, rectal temperatures are taken to obtain more accurate readings.

Rest. Ensure adequate rest, both physical and mental. Exertion and activity fatigue the patient and increase the need for oxygen. The patient usually remains on bed rest and avoids unnecessary activity until the infection begins to respond to therapy. During the acute phase, complete bed rest is imperative except for the mildest of infections. Patients who respond rapidly to treatment may be allowed out of bed after having a normal temperature for two or three days. Longer periods of bed rest are necessary with more severe or complicated illnesses. Check activity orders. Some patients are allowed to use a commode rather than bedpan while on bed rest. With improvement, activity is gradually increased but is interspersed with rest periods.

During the acute period of illness, soporifics, e.g., chloral hydrate or short-acting barbiturates, may be prescribed to help the patient to sleep.

Talking is fatiguing to a person who is acutely ill and dyspneic. The nurse therefore minimizes "social" conversation and expresses interest in the patient in other ways. Visitors may be restricted during the acute period of illness; those permitted are instructed to avoid excessive talking.

Keep the patient's environment pleasant and restful and provide planned, uninterrupted rest periods. Assist with personal hygiene as indicated by the patient's condition. During the period of bed rest turn the patient frequently and exercise the lower limbs. Place items needed by the patient, such as tissues, sputum cup, water, hand wipes, paper bag, call bell, within easy reach to minimize exertion. Smoking is not permitted.

A diagnosis of pneumonia is feared by some patients, especially older persons. Also, with severe infections various aspects of the illness itself may be highly anxiety-provoking, e.g., dyspnea, pain, bloody sputum. Help reduce fears and apprehension by maintaining a calm, efficient manner and giving appropriate reassurance and explanations. Anxiety is carefully evaluated because it may indicate hypoxemia.

Maintaining Warmth and Dryness. Protect from chilling and exposure to drafts and keep comfortably warm, unless the person is hyperthermic and cooling measures are being used. To prevent possible chilling and unnecessary fatigue, omit a total bed bath while the patient is acutely ill. However, be certain to provide necessary skin care without chilling the patient. Frequently check an acutely ill patient to determine whether bed linens or gown is damp from perspiration. Damp linens must be changed immediately.

Prevention of Spread of Infection

> *Because bacterial and viral pneumonias are communicable as long as the patient is febrile, appropriate precautions must be employed to prevent the spread of infection to others.*

The patient's room should be well ventilated to minimize air contamination. Instruct the patient to turn the head away from persons nearby and to cover the nose and mouth with disposable tissues when sneezing or coughing. This helps to prevent infected droplets from becoming airborne. After use, tissues should immediately be placed in a paper bag so they can later be burned. Provide disposable, covered sputum cups if sputum is copious or specimens are necessary. Change the paper bags used to hold contaminated tissues and sputum cups at least three times daily, as they become half full. Before disposing of sputum make certain it is not necessary to save a specimen. Always cover sputum containers before properly disposing of them.

Frequent handwashing is also important in preventing infection transmission. Always wash after contact with the patient or with articles that could be contaminated. Nurses also always wash prior to giving care, to protect the patient from secondary infection. Persons with respiratory infections should not care for or visit the patient who has pneumonia.

To ensure medical asepsis it is often desirable for nurses to cover their uniforms with gowns when caring for patients who are acutely ill with pneumonia and who may be unable to properly protect the nurse.

Pneumococcal pneumonia is not highly communicable. However, the causative agent can be carried from one patient to another by a healthy person. Staphylococcal pneumonia can also be spread by human carriers. In addition, it can apparently be spread by the dust from dry sweeping or from bedding. The nurse should take care not to unnecessarily "flourish" or shake bed linens while giving care. Dust-laying sweeping compounds should be used and bedding should be treated with germicidal compounds as a preventive measure. Ultraviolet lights may be placed in strategic locations to decontaminate the air.

Specific isolation precautions are usually not necessary with most pneumonias. However, agency policies vary. Some hospitals practice isolation during the acute phase of certain pneumonias, e.g., staphylococcal pneumonia, which has a tendency to cause periodic outbreaks in hospitals. It is always advisable during the acute phase to keep a patient with pneumonia away from other patients predisposed to pneumonia, e.g., persons seriously ill, elderly, debilitated, postsurgical, or those with chronic obstructive pulmonary disease. Single rooms are best during the acute period of illness.

Inform visitors of necessary precautions if they visit an infectious patient.

Oral Hygiene; Lip and Nose Care. Give frequent oral hygiene and lip and nose care. These nursing activities can make patients more comfortable and are particularly important if they are febrile and dehydrated, have herpes simplex lesions, are mouth breathing, or producing foul sputum. Oral hygiene may prevent spread of the infection to the ears, and is necessary to prevent stomatitis, i.e., inflammation of the oral mucosa. Lung abscess formation also may be prevented by frequent oral hygiene, since the most common cause of lung abscess is aspiration of anaerobic mouth flora. When giving oral hygiene be certain to clean the patient's tongue well and to lubricate the lips.

Dryness and crusting of the nares can be a minor but distressing problem. Soothing water-soluble creams or ointments may be applied around the nares. Crusts may be gently removed with swabs moistened in water or hydrogen peroxide.

Maintaining Fluid-Electrolyte Balance. Fluid-electrolyte replacement must be provided. Maintain and evaluate the patient's intake and output record carefully for indications of imbalances and look for clinical symptoms of imbalances. (See Chapter 12.)

Fluid replacement is tailored to the individual patient's needs. Persons with pneumococcal pneumonia lose a great deal of fluid and salt because they usually perspire heavily. As mentioned, vomiting and diarrhea sometimes occur. Also, patients with bacterial pneumonias often require increased hydration because of elevations in insensible fluid loss caused by fever and hyperventilation, and because pulmonary secretions are increased. Maintaining adequate hydration is important not only to prevent fluid imbalances but also to facilitate expectoration of bronchopulmonary secretions.

Frequently it is necessary to supplement hydration by mouth with intravenous fluids (75 to 150 ml. per hour). It is advisable to monitor the central venous pressure when replacing fluids in some patients (e.g., those with impending congestive heart failure) to prevent the development of pulmonary edema. (See Unit XII.)

Diet. Intravenous fluids are sometimes ordered to provide nutrition as well as fluid intake for anorexic, nauseated, or vomiting patients. Or, anorexic, dyspneic persons may best tolerate a liquid diet during the acute period of pneumonia. With improvement they progress to a soft-solid and then general diet. Persons with complications whose illness is prolonged may be given a high-protein, high-caloric diet with vitamin supplements. Increased metabolism and the loss of plasma and cells in the pneumonic exudate make it desirable for the caloric intake to be a minimum of 1200 to 1500 calories daily. Caloric intake can be increased by adding food concentrates to fluids, e.g., adding lactose to milk. Dyspneic, congested people often have difficulty taking fluids and may find it fatiguing to drink.

Some physicians prescribe a diet of solid food early because they believe such a diet may prevent the possible complication of paralytic ileus. It is recommended that gas-forming foods be avoided to minimize the occurrence of abdominal distention or paralytic ileus.

Respiratory Care. Respiratory therapy is frequently necessary in the presence of pneumonia because effective ventilation and gas exchange may be impaired by the presence of inflammatory exudate in the alveoli, atelectasis, increased bronchopulmonary secretions, and secondary bronchospasm. Respiratory care is individualized. Elderly people often have a diminished cough reflex and require intensive respiratory care to help them to remove secretions. Seriously ill patients and those with underlying pulmonary disease may develop severe hypoxemia and respiratory failure. The nurse participates actively in promoting good tracheobronchial hygiene and helping the dyspneic patient to breathe more comfortably and effectively.

Oxygen administration may be required to help the patient breathe and rest more easily. Oxygen therapy may help relieve restlessness and cough, prevent pulmonary edema, and also prevent or relieve abdominal distention. Indications for oxygen therapy include cyanosis, dyspnea, weakness, delirium, circulation disturbances, painful or lowered respirations, and a pO_2 of 70 mm. Hg or lower. The most appropriate route to produce adequate oxygen status to the tissues is used. The efficacy of oxygen therapy needs to be monitored periodically by determining blood gas levels. This is of special importance in patients with underlying chronic pulmonary or ventilatory disease in order to prevent suppression of respiration. (See previous chapters in this unit.) Arterial pO_2, pCO_2, and pH values are determined several times a day in seriously ill patients.

Some patients may require controlled mechanical ventilation to maintain effective respiration. In the presence of obvious *bronchospasm* the physician may order aminophylline (given intravenously over a period of several hours) and/or dyphylline (Lufyllin), and beta-adrenergic drugs. Because an adequate airway must be maintained it may be necessary to use *nasotracheal suction* (by sterile technique) and to *endotracheally intubate* the patient.

Effective coughing is necessary to remove secretions from the tracheobronchial tree. The patient is instructed how to cough effectively; if coughing is painful it may be helpful to splint the patient's chest. (See Chapter 57.) Ineffective coughing is discouraged since it tires the patient. Emphasize to the patient the importance of coughing up and expectorating rather than swallowing sputum. Observe expectorated sputum and record your observations.

Respiratory physiotherapy, e.g., *percussion, clapping*, may be necessary to help move tenacious secretions so they can be expectorated or removed by suction. Often supervised postural drainage (for 5 to 30 minutes three or four times daily) is necessary. *Intermittent positive pressure breathing* (IPPB) may be ordered two to four times daily. Various substances (e.g., acetylcysteine, isotonic saline solution, bicarbonate 4.2 per cent, or a bronchodilator such as isoproterenol or other more selective beta-agonists like isoetharine, terbutaline) may be nebulized, depending upon the patient's needs.

Supervise planned coughing and *deep breathing sessions* and provide assistance as required. Plan these sessions to coincide with periods when the patient is awakened for other care, e.g., medications. During such sessions, protect yourself by having the patient cover the nose and mouth with tissues and by keeping your face away from the path of expiration. The frequency of planned coughing and deep breathing sessions depends upon a patient's condition. Deep breathing exercises help prevent reductions in vital capacity and pulmonary compliance.

When hacking cough interferes with a patient's rest and is debilitating, medications may be used to partially suppress (but not abolish) the cough.

Excessive depression of the cough reflex dangerously encourages the retention of bronchopulmonary secretions and the development of atelectasis.

Although *cough suppressant medications* may be ordered early in the acute phase of illness (while the cough is typically painful and nonproductive), during the latter phase of pneumonia expectorants may be prescribed. *Expectorants* help to clear the lungs and tracheobronchial tree of secretions and exudate. Topical nebulization may be used to help liquefy secretions as well as humidify inspired air.

Antimicrobial Medications. *Before* antimicrobial therapy is started, sputum and blood are collected for culture. Antibiotics to which the organism(s) is known to be sensitive are prescribed after its identification. Generally antibiotics are selected that have as narrow a spectrum as possible, since the use of broad-spectrum antibiotics may lead to complicating superinfections.

Often it is necessary to begin antibiotic administration before the specific infecting organism can be identified by culture. The physician makes a presumptive diagnosis (based tentatively on the patient's history and physical examination and interpretation of a Gram stain of sputum and a capsular swelling test) and begins initial chemotherapy. Once laboratory results are available from blood and sputum cultures and the offending organism is precisely identified, the antibiotic therapy is changed if indicated. Except in mild infections, antibiotics are typically administered parenterally when treating pneumonia.

Pneumococcal pneumonia is generally best treated

with crystalline penicillin G. This medication may be given intravenously in the presence of shock. Potassium penicillin V may be given orally to patients who are not severely ill and who do not have gastrointestinal symptoms. It may also be used when conditions preclude parenteral therapy or make it difficult. The cephalosporins, tetracyclines, lincomycin, and erythromycin are also useful.

Before the first dose of penicillin or other antibiotic is given the patient's history is carefully reviewed for evidence of possible hypersensitivity to the drug prescribed. An intravenous sensitivity test is advisable with a small amount of penicillin prior to giving the first dose. If a patient is hypersensitive to penicillin, or is suspected of being hypersensitive, another antibiotic such as erythromycin or cephalosporins may be used.

Administer antibiotics at the time ordered to maintain the desired blood level of medication. Observe the patient closely for indications of side effects or toxicity of the antibiotics, e.g., diarrhea, vomiting, nausea, soft tissue reactions, pruritus, skin rash, or indications of anaphylactic shock. *Report indications of allergy or cross-allergy immediately.*

Persons with pneumococcal pneumonia who receive adequate chemotherapy early in the course of their illness have about a 5 to 10 per cent mortality rate. Fatalities usually occur in patients younger than 3 years of age and older than 50. Prognosis is less favorable and convalescence longer in the presence of the following conditions: involvement of two or more lobes; a positive blood culture; WBC below 5000; BUN higher than 70 mg./dl.; endocarditis; meningitis; or underlying chronic disease.

If appropriate antibiotic therapy is started early enough, symptoms usually begin to subside rapidly during the first two to three days of treatment. If this response does not occur, the patient is reassessed for the presence of complications, possible drug fever, other disease, or superinfection.

Chemotherapy is continued in uncomplicated cases until bacteriologic evidence of infection has disappeared and an obvious improvement occurs clinically. Prolonged chemotherapy is advisable in some destructive pneumonias (e.g., staphylococcal pneumonia) in an attempt to prevent relapse.

Complications of Pneumonia. Effective diagnostic and treatment methods have reduced the incidence of complications of pneumonia, but problems still occur. Some are life-threatening; therefore, the nurse observes closely for indications of delayed resolution of disease or the development of complications in persons acutely ill with pneumonia and reports these observations promptly. Complications most frequently occur in aged patients, patients suffering from chronic illnesses, and patients who did not receive early, appropriate treatment. Both pulmonary and nonpulmonary complications may occur.

Pulmonary Complications. Pulmonary complications that may be associated with pneumonia include: pulmonary edema, pulmonary abscess, atelectasis, respiratory failure, and superinfection with other bacteria as a consequence of therapy. Some patients infected with drug-resistant or highly virulent organisms experience a spread of the pneumonic activity or delayed resolution of the infection. These problems can usually be effectively managed by changing prescribed medications to include agents to which the infecting organisms are sensitive.

Nonpulmonary Complications. Nonpulmonary complications include: dry pleurisy, pleurisy with effusion, empyema, and various other infections, particularly septicemia, acute otitis media, acute sinusitis, septic shock, disseminated intravascular coagulation, herpes simplex, abdominal distention, paralytic ileus, mental aberrations, and hyperthermia.

- *Dry pleurisy* fairly often accompanies pneumonia and may progress to *pleurisy with effusion. Empyema* necessitates total removal of the exudate by repeated thoracentesis or tube or open surgical drainage. At times antibiotics are instilled locally. Sterile pleural effusions usually require no treatment. All aspirated pleural fluid is examined by smear and culture, so that early treatment can be started if empyema is present.

- *Other extrapulmonary infections* may accompany bacterial pneumonias. Among these are nephritis, peritonitis, pericarditis, endocarditis, meningitis, and purulent arthritis. These infections result from *septicemia*, i.e., invasion of the blood stream by bacterial toxins that are carried to other tissues or organs. Extrapulmonary infections require prolonged therapy with increased doses of specific antibiotics.

- Acute *otitis media* and *acute sinusitis* may occur if the bacterial infection extends into the middle ear and sinuses.

- *Septic shock* may develop in pneumonias: (1) with delayed or inadequate treatment; (2) those complicated by the presence of other debilitating illnesses; or (3) those caused by highly virulent or drug-resistant organisms. Early symptoms of peripheral vascular collapse occurring with septic shock include reductions in blood pressure, temperature, and level of consciousness; weak, rapid pulse; and cool, clammy skin. (Septic shock is discussed in Chapter 13.)

- Patients with pneumonia who have underlying heart disease may experience *cardiovascular failure* associated with congestive heart failure. In such cases the physician evaluates the patient's heart size, peripheral edema, and CVP and prescribes appropriate treatment, e.g., digitalis, diuretics, or both. (See Unit XII.)

- *Disseminated intravascular coagulation* may complicate some severe pneumonias. Full doses of heparin may be administered once the condition is identified. (See Unit XIV.)
- *Herpes simplex* (fever sores or cold sores) is a minor complication which frequently occurs, particularly with bacterial pneumonias. Palliative treatment of these lesions in the vesicular stage may include applications of tincture of benzoin or spirits of camphor. Ointments may be prescribed once the lesions are encrusted.
- *Abdominal distention* frequently complicates severe pneumonia and usually results from air swallowing by a severely dyspneic patient. It may also result from decreased peristalsis, which allows fluids and gas to collect in the intestinal tract. Abdominal distention is uncomfortable and, more seriously, may interfere with pulmonary expansion and further compromise respirations. It elevates the diaphragm and restricts diaphragmatic excursions, compressing the lower regions of the lungs. (See Unit XVII.)
- *Paralytic ileus*, i.e., absence of intestinal peristaltic action, may occur with severe pneumonia. To prevent this a nurse should: (1) record all bowel movements and report constipation; (2) observe the abdomen for tenderness, rigidity, or abdominal distention and report the occurrence of these symptoms; (3) report vomiting (with ileus the vomitus may contain fecal matter); and (4) periodically listen to the abdomen for bowel tones (in the absence of peristalsis no bowel tones can be heard). Enemas are usually not given in the absence of peristalsis because the fluid will be retained and will further increase abdominal distention unless the fluid is siphoned back. Treatment is basically decompression of the abdomen accomplished by insertion of a Miller-Abbott tube. (See Unit XVII.)
- *Mental aberrations* of various kinds may occur with pneumonia. Toxicity, hyperthermia, and hypoxemia each contribute to such abnormal mental states as confusion or disorientation, toxic delirium, or acute anxiety states. The nurse therefore periodically evaluates the patient's mental status and observes closely for indications of these complications. (Refer to Unit X.)

  Report mental aberrations to the physician and help significant others to understand the patient's behavior. It is especially important that the patient not be restrained. A restrained patient may panic, become combative, and struggle against restraints. Such exertion and anxiety can critically worsen the condition of a toxic dyspneic patient. Abnormal behavior is carefully assessed in a patient acutely ill with pneumonia to be certain the symptoms are not caused by pneumococcal meningitis. If meningitis is suspected, a diagnostic lumbar puncture is performed.

  When you give patients sedatives or tranquilizers, remember to check the sensorium periodically and chart your observations. Avoid oversedation since it depresses the cough reflex and respiratory center. Short-acting sedatives may be used if absolutely necessary.

- *Hyperthermia* may also complicate pneumonia. Temperature elevations greater than 39.4°C. (103°F.) should be lowered by cooling measures or antipyretic medications. Antipyretics may help to relieve muscular aches and malaise in addition to reducing fever. Patients with extremely high temperature elevations may require hypothermia. (See Unit X.)

Convalescence. Pneumonia is a physically taxing illness. Therefore, the patient may feel weakened and may fatigue easily for some time after acute symptoms have been relieved. Instructions during the period of convalescence should be followed carefully. A fairly long period of convalescence is necessary for aged or chronically ill persons. Rest periods are usually advisable even after only brief acute pneumonias. A physician decides when a patient can return to work. Prior to hospital discharge, caution persons with pneumonia against overexertion and encourage them to keep follow-up medical appointments. During the period of convalescence chest x-ray films are taken to evaluate clearing of the lung. Typically a patient is advised to continue deep breathing exercises for six to eight weeks after discharge.

Pneumonia tends to make the affected person susceptible to recurring respiratory infections. Therefore, advise the patient how such infections can possibly be prevented and emphasize the need for early medical evaluation of any symptoms. Influenza vaccination may be recommended, since secondary bacterial pneumonias can occur with influenza.

OTHER BACTERIAL PNEUMONIAS

Space does not permit detailed discussion of the various bacterial pneumonias. As stated earlier, the clinical courses and supportive treatments are generally similar to those of pneumococcal pneumonia. However, specific antibiotic therapy varies, depending on the infecting organism and its drug sensitivities. Summarized below are comments about the more common of these.

- *Streptococcal pneumonia* (most frequently caused by hemolytic organisms of Lancefield's Group A) is usually a complication of influenza or measles, but may follow scarlet fever or streptococcal sore throat. A large pleural effusion, often bloody, may occur early. Empyema may develop. Streptococcal pneumonia usually appears suddenly and is severe with marked toxemia.

- *Staphylococcal pneumonia* (usually caused by coagulase-positive *Staphylococcus aureus*) may occur as a primary infection in the very young or aged, but otherwise most commonly develops as a complication of influenza. Also it may develop in hospitalized patients as a superinfection or as a complication of tracheostomy, immunosuppressive therapy, surgery, debility, or diseases affecting host defenses against infection. Staphylococcal pneumonia is a serious infection with a high mortality rate. Tracheostomy may be required because of copious respiratory secretions.

- *Pneumonia caused by Hemophilus influenzae* (most commonly by Types A and B) may occur in adults as a lobar pneumonia, bronchopneumonia, or bronchiolitis. Recovery is typical. Sputum is characteristically tenacious and "apple-green" colored.

- *Friedländer's bacillus (Klebsiella pneumoniae) and other enterobacterial pneumonias.* Although any of the types of Friedländer's bacillus may cause pneumonia, the most common invaders are Types 1 and 2. Other organisms that can cause similar pneumonias include *Escherichia coli,* Proteus species, Salmonella species, *Pseudomonas aeruginosa, Pseudomonas pseudomallei,* and anaerobic Bacteroides species. Prompt treatment of pneumonias caused by these organisms is imperative. The mortality rate is particularly high if treatment is delayed beyond the second day of illness. These pneumonias cause critical illness. Cavitation may develop and pleural involvement is typical.

- *Legionnaires disease* is a pneumonia-like condition (caused by a rod-shaped, gram-negative, nonacid-fact bacterium). It was brought dramatically to public attention in 1976 when it affected more than 180 people attending an American Legion convention in Philadelphia. Twenty-nine of those affected died.

Incidence and Epidemiology. The causative bacteria thrive in stagnant water and have been found in small streams. Air-conditioning and other cooling systems using water are therefore good mediums for their growth. The disease thus usually occurs among people in buildings where water-operating air-conditioning systems have been used, or on excavation and construction sites. There is a tendency for Legionnaires disease to be severe and epidemic during summer, most commonly in middle-aged and elderly people. It typically occurs in people who have attended the same event or worked in the same building. However, Legionnaires disease also has been identified in young people and children and has occurred throughout the year. Mild, sporadic cases (Pontiac disease) also have been reported.

Symptoms. A person with Legionnaires disease may experience many symptoms including severe chest pain, dyspnea, a nonproductive cough or a cough with some mucoid or blood-stained sputum, extreme weakness, malaise, myalgia, rapid rise in temperature (38.8 to 41.1°C. [102 to 106°F.]), bradycardia, diarrhea, abdominal pain, vomiting, increased muscle tone, and unsteady gait. Sometimes the person may become confused and delirious and consciousness may be impaired. Renal and respiratory failure may occur.

Diagnosis. Legionnaires disease should be suspected in persons with the above symptoms and erythromycin treatment commenced. Definitive diagnosis, by culture of lung tissue or pleural fluid, takes 7 to 10 days. Treatment cannot wait that long. (Autopsy confirmation may be made in a few hours.)

Other laboratory findings include slightly elevated leukocyte count, marked elevation of erythrocyte sedimentation rate (ESR), mildly abnormal liver function findings, moderate proteinuria, microscopic hematuria, hypoxemia, and hypocapnia. Lung x-ray films show progression from patchy infiltrate with interstitial or consolidated appearance to unilateral or even bilateral nodular consolidation.

Antibiotic treatment. Erythromycin is the most effective antibiotic for Legionnaires disease. It is administered intravenously when the person is acutely ill and orally once the person has begun responding to treatment. Tetracycline and chloramphenicol may also be used.

General Management. Care is similar to that appropriate for people experiencing other kinds of pneumonia. A person with Legionnaires disease is likely to be not only acutely ill but also very frightened by having a mysterious, highly publicized disease. *Excellent symptom-related care and genuine emotional support are imperative.*

The person may be cared for in an intensive care unit during the acute stage. Careful observation may be necessary. If status becomes further and emotional status, vital signs, signs of impaired consciousness, respiratory status (including arterial blood gases), and intake and output measurements (as determined with indwelling Foley catheter and daily weights).

Generally, oxygen therapy is instituted. If respiratory failure occurs, endotracheal intubation may be necessary. If status becomes further impaired, continuous mechanical ventilation must be instituted. IV fluids may be administered. Temperature control may require the use of a hypothermia blanket.

Other than thorough handwashing precautions, isolation procedures are not necessary since the disease is not transmitted from person to person.

Although pneumococcal pneumonia seldom causes any permanent damage to the lung, residual defects may result from other infections. Organisms such as staphylococcus, Friedländer's bacillus, and tubercle bacillus, which cause tissue death in the center of the involved area, may leave abscess cavities and scarring of the lung. Also, empyema development may cause permanent pleural thickening.

PRIMARY ATYPICAL PNEUMONIAS

Primary atypical pneumonia (PAP) is a respiratory syndrome that may be caused by various agents (e.g., *Mycoplasma pneumoniae* or certain viruses) and usually differs from the "typical" bacterial pneumonias by having a more insidious, gradual onset and with constitutional symptoms (e.g., headache, fatigue, fever) that may prevail over respiratory tract symptoms. Other common findings with PAP include x-ray evidence of infiltration but very few physical signs upon examination of the chest, WBC count that is normal or low (leukopenia), and gradually increasing cough with scanty sputum production and fever. Sputum is usually mucopurulent but occasionally may be blood-tinged.

Mycoplasma pneumoniae is also called the *"Eaton agent." Mycoplasmal pneumonias* occur year round and may have peak incidence in the summer. Often mycoplasmal infection causes severe frontal headaches. This type of pneumonia typically occurs in children and young adults. Death is rare, but sometimes the illness extends for several weeks. Cold agglutinins (autohemagglutinins for human type O erythrocytes) occur in about half of mycoplasmal infections and can be identified by a simple serologic test. *Mycoplasma pneumoniae* can be cultured from respiratory secretions.

Mild cases of mycoplasmal pneumonia usually do not require antimicrobial medications. Severe cases may be treated with erythromycin or tetracycline. General symptomatic care is similar to that for pneumococcal pneumonia.

VIRAL PNEUMONIAS

Viral pneumonias can be severe, even fatal illnesses (particularly with the virus of influenza A), but usually these infections are mild, and may be undetected. Among the numerous agents that may cause viral pneumonias are influenza and parainfluenza viruses, adenoviruses, rhinoviruses, respiratory syncytial virus, herpes simplex, cytomegalovirus, and coxsackie-, echo-, and rheoviruses.

> *About 75 per cent of all acute pulmonary infections are viral pneumonias.*[16]

Viral infections are indicated by the *absence* of respiratory pathogens when sputum is cultured. Commonly the diagnosis is made on the basis of clinical findings and serologic tests, since many agencies are not equipped to isolate viruses. Symptoms range from those of a common cold to respiratory insufficiency, which may progress rapidly. Prognosis is variable. *Antibiotics are not indicated in the treatment of viral pneumonia*. If the infection is an influenza A_2 viral infection, the patient may be given amantadine (Symmetrel) early in the course of the infection. Experimentally, cytomegalovirus and varicella pneumonias have been treated with inhibitors of normal DNA synthesis given parenterally, e.g., idoxuridine or cytosine arabinoside, and rhinoviral infections have been treated with the intranasal administration of interferon inducers, e.g., polyinosinic-polycytidylic acid (poly I:C). However, treatment of viral pneumonias is presently essentially symptomatic and is similar to that given for pneumococcal pneumonia.

Prophylactic vaccination with influenza A and B is available. This may be used for high-risk persons, e.g., pregnant women, persons over age 50, persons with chronic heart or lung disease.

Work is under way to develop effective *vaccines* against respiratory viruses, but these are difficult to prepare because of the numerous distinct antigenic serotypes. Possibly in the future vaccines will be available that can be administered via the respiratory route. This would be desirable, since such vaccines would induce the formation of local antibodies that would control respiratory infections more effectively than circulating antibodies.

Pulmonary Tuberculosis

Definition and Etiology. *Tuberculosis* is a reportable, communicable, infectious, inflammatory, acute or chronic disease that may occur in almost any part of the body. Pulmonary infection is the most common; however, tuberculosis can spread to any other organ through the blood stream and lymphatics. Because the lungs are most frequently infected, this discussion is chiefly limited to *pulmonary tuberculosis*. Tuberculosis located in areas other than the lungs is called *"extrapulmonary."*

Tuberculosis is caused by *Mycobacterium tuberculosis,* the true "tubercle bacillus." Various atypical mycobacteria have recently been identified that resemble the true tubercle bacillus and produce diseases similar to true tuberculosis. (See discussion of atypical mycobacteria on p. 1305.)

Mycobacterium bovis (bovine tubercle bacillus) formerly caused numerous cases of tuberculosis in human beings as a result of the human ingestion of raw milk from infected cattle. Currently bovine tuberculosis has been practically eliminated in the United States because of the pasteurization of milk and tuberculin skin testing programs for cattle. (Infected cattle are destroyed.) Bovine tuberculosis continues to be a problem in other countries where similar public health programs are lacking and tuberculosis commonly occurs in cattle.

Unless otherwise stated, the discussion in this section is limited to the most common human form of tuberculosis, i.e., pulmonary tuberculosis resulting from infection by *Mycobacterium tuberculosis*.

Characteristics of the Tubercle Bacillus. Tubercle bacilli are *rod-shaped, aerobic* (i.e., require oxygen to live), *nonmotile* (i.e., do not move), *gram-positive, acid-fast* microorganisms that *reproduce very slowly* within the human body (they divide approximately every 18 to 24 hours) and cannot reproduce outside the body (except under laboratory conditions). Tubercle bacilli have a high lipid content that contributes to their acid-fast staining characteristics.

The tubercle bacillus can be destroyed by heat, e.g., burning, boiling for 5 minutes, autoclaving, pasteurization of milk; exposure to direct noonday sunlight for varying lengths of time, depending upon the strength of the sun's rays; contact with certain germicides (ordinary disinfectants are ineffective, coal tar preparations are most penetrating); and ultraviolet radiation (very effective).

Routes of Infection. Tuberculosis infections can occur by inhalation (*most common*); ingestion (relatively uncommon since reduction of bovine infections); or direct infection, e.g., through a cut in the skin or mucous membranes (extremely rare).

Tubercle bacilli are present in the air as a result of coughing, sneezing, and expectorating by infected persons. Infected minute droplet nuclei may then be inhaled into pulmonary peripheral alveoli or, transported by air currents, may remain suspended in the air for long periods of time. Large droplets are not inhaled into the alveoli because they tend to drop to the ground or be filtered out by the lung's protective mechanisms if inhaled. *Tuberculosis is*, thus, *essentially an airborne infection* transferred from person to person via inhalation of infected droplet nuclei.

Pathology. If inhaled and implanted in healthy lung tissue bacillus-laden droplet nuclei can become a focus of infection. Infection is established if the bacilli survive and begin to multiply in the susceptible lung tissue. When tubercle bacilli infect the lung, the body's defensive mechanisms attempt to isolate and destroy the bacilli. Phagocytosis and lymphocytosis occur, and epithelioid cells and fibrous tissue attempt to wall off the infected area, with tubercles.

Tuberculosis infections are characterized by the formation of *tubercles*. Tubercles are gray translucent masses composed of small spherical cells that contain giant cells and are surrounded by a layer of epithelial connective tissue cells. The central portions of tubercles typically undergo a process of caseous degeneration (i.e., caseation), liquefaction, and cavitation.

Caseation is a necrotic process that is unique to tuberculosis. During the process of caseation the tissue changes into an amorphous cheeselike mass that consists of tubercle bacilli, dead white blood cells, and necrotic lung tissue. Large portions of caseous material may become encapsulated and form nodules that may be detected by x-ray. Caseous material is semisolid and gray-white in appearance.

At the peripheries of *caseous nodules* the tubercle bacilli and the body's white blood cells continue to battle in a zone of inflammatory reaction which consists of exudate, lymphocytes, multiplying connective tissue cells, and dilated capillaries. The center of the caseous nodule is avascular; thus, thrombosis formation occurs. Avascular, necrotic lung tissue that is sealed off in the lung and cannot be evacuated through the tracheobronchial tree provides an excellent medium for the bacilli. Tubercle bacilli located in caseous nodules live in an environment that is difficult to penetrate therapeutically, e.g., via the blood stream or tracheobronchial tree.

Eventually the caseous material in the nodule's center tends to soften and liquefy. If erosion into a bronchus occurs, this liquefied material spills out into the tracheobronchial tree and is coughed up as *sputum*. Sputum may be highly infectious. Some of this infected material may spread throughout the lung or into the opposite lung via the tracheobronchial tree. As the liquefied material drains out of the nodule, an air-filled sac remains, i.e., a *cavity*. (See Fig. 55–3.)

Not all lesions progress to cavitation. Sometimes active inflammation subsides and some of the inflammatory products are removed by resolution, i.e., absorption of the inflammation. Some healing by resolution occurs, but most tuberculous lesions heal by scarring or fibrosis. Fibrous organization and healing occur, and the caseous lesions become encapsulated and gradually are infiltrated with deposits of calcium; *calcified lesions* are often visible on x-ray film.

Primary (First) Infection. The first time one is infected with tuberculosis the individual is said to have a *primary infection*. Generally primary infections are located in the lower part of the upper lobe of the lung or near the pleura in the lower lobe. Although a primary infection may be only microscopic in size (and hence never even appear on x-ray film), the following sequence of events typically occurs.

A small area of tuberculous pneumonic exudation develops in the lung parenchyma (*Ghon tubercle*); the center of this area quickly becomes caseous. Wandering white blood cells engulf the infecting mycobacteria and carry some of them to regional lymph nodes. Thus, the infection (although minute) is rapidly spread to the regional bronchopulmonary (hilar) lymph nodes, and the area of caseous pneumonia in the lung is referred to as a *primary complex* (Fig. 55–3).

Primary infections cause the body to develop a state of sensitivity that is manifest by a positive reaction to tuberculin skin tests. This development of tuberculin sensitivity in all body cells occurs 3 to 10 weeks after the primary infection and is maintained as long as living bacilli remain in the body (perhaps for life). This allergic reaction to tubercle bacilli or their proteins (tuberculins) is believed to be related to the continued presence of tubercle bacilli within caseous lesions (even though these lesions may be only microscopic in size).

The term *tuberculin converter* is used to refer to persons who do not show roentgenographic or bacteriologic evidence of pulmonary tuberculosis, but in whom the tuberculin skin test converts from a known negative reaction to a known positive reaction, i.e., from less than 5 mm. of induration with a Mantoux skin test to 10 mm. or more.

Primary tuberculous infections often are never recognized because they usually are relatively asymptomatic. In most cases body defenses are adequate to arrest primary infections, and they heal by fibrosis and calcification. Occasionally, however, a primary infection is not

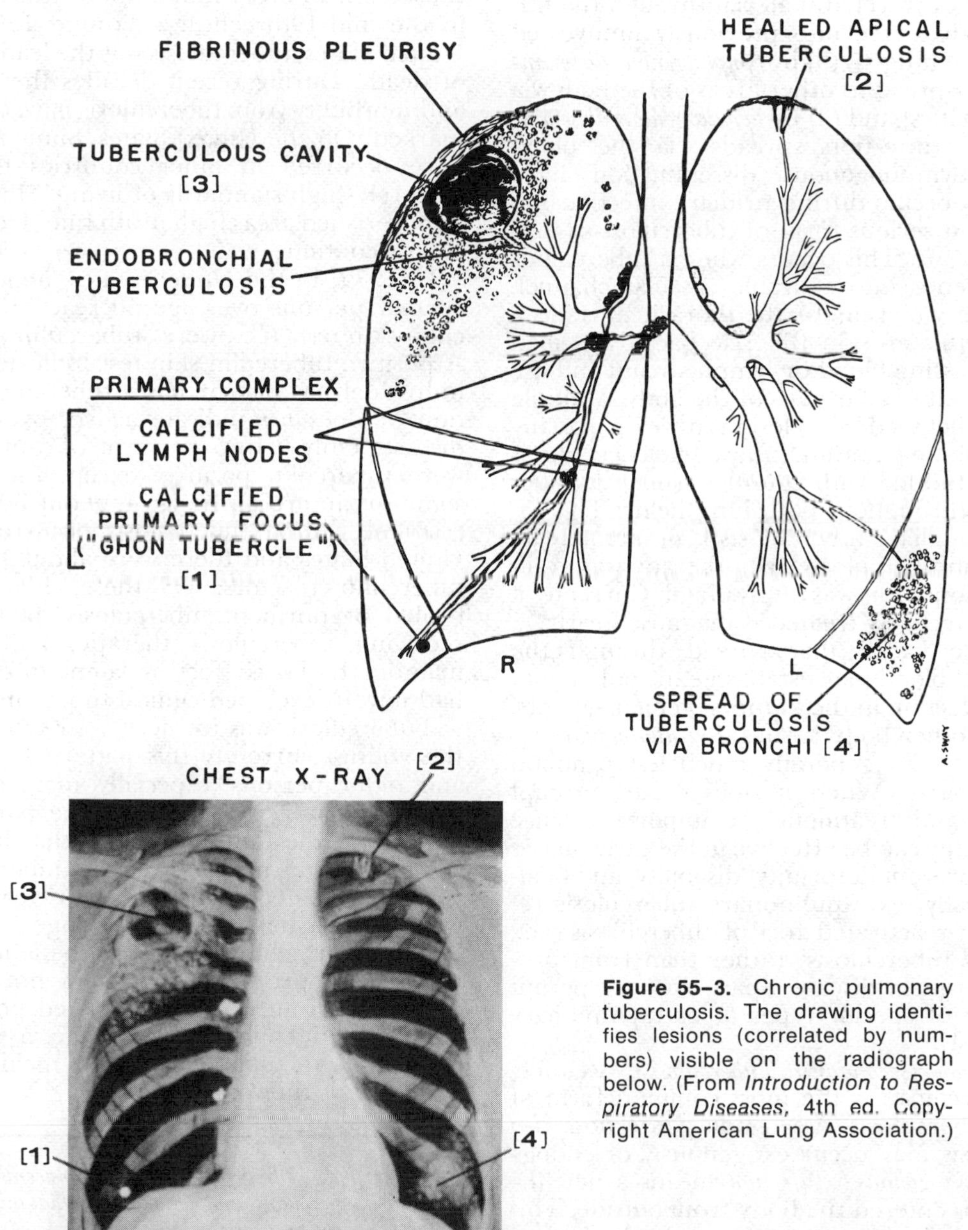

Figure 55–3. Chronic pulmonary tuberculosis. The drawing identifies lesions (correlated by numbers) visible on the radiograph below. (From *Introduction to Respiratory Diseases*, 4th ed. Copyright American Lung Association.)

controlled, and *progressive primary tuberculosis* develops. In this situation the primary complex sites progress and worsen, possibly causing cavitation and spread of active infection.

Progression of Tuberculous Lesions. Basically tuberculosis lesions can progress or extend in four ways: (1) by *local progression*, e.g., the local enlargement of a lesion by erosion through its capsule; (2) by *bronchogenic dissemination*, e.g., aspiration of infected material through the tracheobronchial tree into previously uninvolved areas of the lung(s); (3) by *lymphogenous dissemination*, e.g., spread to other areas of the body via the lymphatics; and (4) by *hematogenous dissemination*, e.g., infection spreads via the blood stream. Lymphogenous dissemination most commonly occurs during primary infections.

The most serious form of tuberculosis is *miliary tuberculosis*. This occurs when a tuberculous lesion extends into a sizable vascular channel, either artery or vein, or the thoracic duct. As a result of this erosion tubercle bacilli are shed into the passing blood or lymph stream and are disseminated to all organs of the body. Multiple small ("millet seed" size) lesions develop in many body tissues, e.g., brain, lungs. The chest film is typically studded with countless small densities scattered throughout both lung fields. The patient with miliary tuberculosis is desperately ill. Before antituberculosis drug therapy was available this condition was always fatal. Currently it may be effectively treated if diagnosed early.

Tubercle bacilli that spread through the lymph and blood may establish extrapulmonary sites of infection in the kidneys, genitalia, joints, brain, or other body tissues. *Extrapulmonary tuberculosis* is now generally much less common than formerly. When it does occur, prompt diagnosis and treatment are important, since drug therapy can be effective in the early phases and may prevent deformity, disability, and fatality. Typically, extrapulmonary tuberculosis results from reactivated foci of tuberculosis, i.e., secondary tuberculosis, rather than from progressive primary disease. Space does not permit discussion of specific types of extrapulmonary tuberculosis.

Reinfection (secondary) Tuberculosis. Reinfection tuberculosis is the most common form of clinical tuberculosis. A secondary infection with tuberculosis may occur exogenously or endogenously. *Exogenous reinfection* means a new infection has entered the body from outside. This type of reinfection rarely occurs in the United States, but may occur in countries where tuberculosis is prevalent. In the United States most tuberculosis reinfection results from the post-primary progression of the first infection, *i.e., endogenous reinfection.* This represents *reactivation* of a previously dormant focus of tuberculosis. It typically occurs in the lungs' apical (upper) regions (Simon foci).

Primary sites containing tubercle bacilli may remain latent (alive but dormant) for years and then reactivate if the person's resistance becomes lowered. Because reinfection is possible (infection does not provide total immunity) and because dormant lesions may reactivate, *it is extremely important for persons who have had a tuberculosis infection to be reevaluated periodically for evidence of active disease.*

Incidence. Tuberculosis is believed to have caused one of every four adult deaths in Europe in the mid-19th century. Around 1900 in the United States, tuberculosis was the leading cause of death. During recent decades the mortality and morbidity from tuberculosis have decreased markedly in the United States. Similar declines have occurred in other countries that have relatively high standards of living. However, in impoverished areas high death rates from tuberculosis continue.

In 1972, in the United States, about 25 per cent of persons over age 50 reacted to tuberculin skin tests (i.e., were "tuberculin positive"). A positive tuberculin skin test indicates that an individual has had or has a tuberculosis infection; it does *not* indicate active, overt clinical disease. Only 2 to 5 per cent of young adults were tuberculin positive (except for those in some urban areas). In 1974, about 30,000 new cases of clinical tuberculosis occurred in the United States and there were about 15 million tuberculin reactors. Of these, 500,000 had healed or dormant tuberculosis; 60,000 were receiving tuberculosis therapy, and the remainder harbored foci of latent infection but had never developed clinical tuberculosis.[162]

Tuberculosis was formerly a disease affecting the young, currently this pattern has shifted, and older persons, especially men, are more commonly infected. This may be partially explained by the fact that lesions that have been controlled and inactive for a number of adult years reactivate during the later years of life when health may decline. Younger people of the present generation have benefited from health care programs that were not available during the youth of the now aged population. Infants and children below age 5 are quite susceptible to tuberculosis. The incidence also increases during puberty.

> *Many persons have adopted a complacent attitude toward tuberculosis and do not realize that this disease continues to be a serious public health problem in the United States and other countries, and is especially serious in overpopulated, poor countries.*

Predisposing Factors

- Overcrowded, poor living conditions. Increasingly, tuberculosis is becoming more common among city dwellers, particularly those who are in the lower socioeconomic groups, are poorly nourished, and live in crowded, poorly ventilated quarters. Tuberculosis commonly affects men about twice as often as women. Blacks and North American Indians are highly susceptible. Tuberculosis thrives in catastrophic situations (e.g., war, large-scale disasters). Mental and physical stress, exhaustion, and poor nutritional status may modify the course of tuberculosis.
- The virulence of the organisms to which an individual is exposed and the length of exposure. Some organisms are more virulent than others. Infection with tuberculosis most often occurs from prolonged close associations with an individual who has active tuberculosis, but it is also true that many persons do not develop tuberculosis in spite of such associations.
- Tuberculosis infections are not inherited, but it is possible that some hereditary factor(s) causes some individuals to be more or less susceptible to infections than others.

Reactivation of tuberculosis in previously infected individuals tends to occur most often among persons at the low end of the socioeconomic scale, persons who live alone, and alcoholics. Other factors include inadequate drug therapy of previous tuberculosis infections, and the presence of such conditions as diseases of the lymph system, diabetes mellitus, peptic ulcer, and silicosis. Reinfection may also occur (1) following gastric resection; (2) among persons receiving oncolytic or immunosuppressive agents; (3) among persons who have converted to a positive P.P.D. within the past year; and (4) among long-term steroid dependent individuals.

- Persons who are going to receive prolonged adrenocorticoid therapy, e.g., for arthritis, should be carefully evaluated prior to the administration of these medications to be certain no active tuberculosis infection is present. Also, during the course of steroid therapy the patient should be periodically evaluated for indications of active tuberculosis, since steroid preparations depress inflammation and antibody and lymphocyte production and thus may predispose to tuberculosis.

Symptoms. Because of its typically insidious onset, tuberculosis infection may be actively present and progressing even though the patient is relatively asymptomatic. When symptoms do appear they may be both local and systemic.

- *Local symptoms* commonly include cough and sputum production. Cough usually occurs with cavitary disease in which material drains into the bronchi, and it is therefore not typically an early symptom. Sputum tends to be yellowish and mucoid. Less common symptoms are dyspnea, hemoptysis, and pleuritic pain (with pleural involvement). Rales may be heard over the affected lung. Sometimes tuberculosis is marked by symptoms indicative of influenza, a lingering cold, or cigarette cough.
- *Constitutional symptoms* tend to be nonspecific, e.g., fatigue, night sweats, irritability, lassitude, rapid pulse rate, malaise, late afternoon low-grade fever, weight loss, anorexia, indigestion, pallor, irregularity or suppression of menses, vomiting.

Often persons with active tuberculosis appear amazingly well in spite of the fact that they may have far advanced disease with large cavities in their lungs and other extensive lung damage.

> *Individuals with active tuberculosis must be identified and properly treated not only for their own welfare but also to prevent transmission of the disease to others.*

Diagnosis. Diagnostic procedures used to establish a diagnosis of tuberculosis *routinely* include complete medical and social history, complete physical examination, chest x-ray films, tuberculin testing, and the bacteriologic examination of sputum or other specimens. Other diagnostic procedures may be performed, including photofluorography, bronchography, bronchoscopy, pleural biopsy, lung biopsy, and mediastinal and scalene node biopsies.

Routine laboratory tests include acid-fast smears and the planting of cultures to identify the specific organism(s) present. Drug-sensitivity cultures are also performed. Occasionally guinea-pig inoculations are made with urine. Several sputum specimens (each a minimum of 5 to 10 ml.) are taken *before* drug treatment of any kind is started. Heated aerosol treatments with hypertonic saline may help to induce sputum for specimen purposes in persons who have difficulty raising sputum. Aspiration of fasting gastric contents may be done in patients who are unable to cough and raise sputum, who are in a comatose state, and very young children. The aspirate may be examined for acid-fast bacilli, as with aerosol-induced sputum specimens. (Diagnostic procedures are discussed in detail in Chapter 52.)

The following findings typically confirm a suspected diagnosis of pulmonary tuberculosis: (1) a positive tuberculin skin test; (2) appearance of areas of infection visible on chest films; and (3) the specific identification of *M. tuberculosis* from cultured specimens. Because tubercle bacilli reproduce slowly, a minimum of three weeks is necessary to obtain a positive culture report and at least eight weeks for a negative report.

A positive reaction to a tuberculin skin test indicates that the individual has been infected with tuberculosis, but such a reaction does not indicate whether the infection is currently active or inactive. A positive tuberculin reaction merely indicates tissue sensitivity or allergy to tuberculin.

Positive tuberculin tests are usually followed by chest x-ray films for evidence of active pulmonary tuberculosis. Usually even very small lesions can be seen. Films may be taken from several different positions. Calcified primary lesions or other healed lesions may be detected on the film, as well as evidence of active disease, e.g., pulmonary infiltration, nodules, cavities, or other abnormalities such as pleural effusion.

A negative bacteriologic report does not routinely mean absence of active tuberculosis. Numerous sputum specimens may need to be examined before a positive specimen is located. Typically three or more specimens are examined to confirm diagnosis. Some patients have a positive smear but a negative culture after they have taken antituberculosis medications for a while. This situation occurs because the organisms are still present in the patient's sputum (or whatever specimen is being observed) and thus can be identified on a smear, but they are too weak to reproduce and grow out on a culture. Often it is possible to identify disease caused by unclassified or anonymous mycobacteria only by culturing the organisms.

Because the tubercle bacillus may affect any body tissue, the symptoms of tuberculosis are highly variable, and depend upon the site of infection. A differential diagnosis is made with care.

The erythrocyte sedimentation rate (ESR) is accelerated in active tuberculosis, paralleling the severity of the disease.

CLINICAL MANAGEMENT

Trends in Treatment. "Open air" treatments and "rest cures" were advocated in the first half of this century. Patients were hospitalized for months, even years. The discovery of effective drug therapy for treating tuberculosis about 1944 revolutionized the treatment of this disease. Since that time the number of patients hospitalized for treatment of tuberculosis has dramatically decreased. Persons are now admitted to general hospitals for a period of time. The length of hospitalization is far shorter, and outpatient services have become extremely important.

The treatment and management of tuberculosis depends on four basic factors: (1) drug therapy; (2) education of the patient and significant others; (3) exposure to ultraviolet light; and (4) adequate ventilation of the room in which the patient is staying.

Drug Therapy: The only effective manner of eliminating active tuberculosis is by the administration of drugs. *Failure to take the drugs for the prescribed length of time may result in reactivation of the disease at a later date.* The importance of drug therapy must be continually stressed. Patients must be made aware that although they may feel well and be asymptomatic, they must not fail to take medicine. Antituberculosis medications are typically taken for 1 to 2 years.

Education: Proper education concerning the nature of the disease and the course and purposes of the treatment regimen. Prevention of the spread of infection by careful coughing, tissue disposal, and handwashing is important. Perhaps the most important aspect of education is teaching the patient to cough into tissues, thereby preventing the aerosolization of the droplet nuclei.

Ultraviolet light: Rooms set up to deal with persons with active tuberculosis ideally have an ultraviolet light installed. Ultraviolet light is lethal to the tubercle bacillus. The light must be installed above direct eye contact level to prevent damage to the eyes of both the patient and the other health care workers.

Ventilation: Ventilation of the room is important to clear the ambient air of the droplet nuclei. Health regulations in each community specify the minimal amount of air exchange per hour in a room housing a person diagnosed as having active disease.

Hospitalization. The initial hospitalization of new cases may be helpful for the following reasons: (1) complete clinical evaluation can be made; (2) early indications of drug toxicity can be detected; (3) a regimen for administration of medications can be accomplished; and (4) infectious patients, who might spread the disease if unhospitalized, can be isolated until chemotherapy renders them noninfectious. Weg comments: "The primary reason for hospitalization is to establish diagnosis rapidly and efficiently. . . . The least important reason for hospitalization today is isolation of the patient."[181A]

During hospitalization the extent of the patient's disease is determined, reaction to chemotherapy is evaluated, and laboratory reports are obtained. As with any hospitalized patient, care is not complete unless education is given during this period of time about the nature of the illness and its treatment.

Chronic illnesses of any kind cause numerous problems for patients and their significant others. Persons with communicable chronic diseases who must be confined to hospitals often suffer additionally because of their isolation. Time passes slowly and with difficulty for persons who prefer being at home and actively participating in their "normal," pre-illness life styles. During the time of hospitalization, occupational therapists and nurses can often help patients to participate in projects that are individually meaningful and help to make time pass more pleasantly.

Criteria upon which the decision to discharge a patient is based include:[181A] (1) the patient's clinical well-being; (2) roentgenographic evidence that disease has stabilized or improved; (3) bacteriologic evidence that the number of acid-fast bacilli being excreted has been reduced; and (4) most important, the physician's judgment that the patient, home situation, and local outpatient care system will assure completion of the prescribed chemotherapy.

Typically, discharge is permitted when organisms can no longer be detected by a sputum smear, provided the patient understands the nature of the illness and the need for prolonged medication. Once discharged, the patient is followed closely as an outpatient. Initially smears and cultures are usually taken weekly. After the patient has three *consecutive* negative sputum cultures (i.e., cultures in which no tubercle bacilli appear), permission is typically given to return to work. The intervals between outpatient visits are then gradually lengthened.

Home Care. Most people with tuberculosis can accept responsibility for their own care and most (perhaps all) of their treatment is carried out at home. Home care, rather than hospital care, is possible largely because antituberculosis medications effectively control transmission of tuberculosis. Hence, the presence of the patient in the home is not hazardous. Public health nurses usually make frequent home visits to patients undergoing outpatient treatment for tuberculosis.

Patient Education. Frequently nurses are responsible for providing patient education. Make certain your educational materials and comments are realistic and not outdated. Provide factual, current information about tuberculosis. Patient teaching materials of various kinds are available from local branches of lung associations and health departments. Educational materials should not merely be handed to patients, but should be reviewed with them. The patient should be encouraged to ask questions and to discuss any concerns.

> *Tuberculosis tends to be a relapsing disease that may lie quiescent for years and then reactivate. It is not possible with present methods of treatment to totally "cure" a patient of tuberculosis. Instead the patient's disease is considered to be "controlled."*

Patients need help to understand that for the rest of their lives they may carry in their bodies tubercle bacilli that are capable of causing reinfection, if resistance is lowered. Often a patient can be helped to understand tuberculosis better if it is compared with diabetes, in the sense that the condition may be controlled but lifetime medical care and supervision are required.

The person with active disease may require instruction in the following areas: drug therapy, diet, protective precautions, complications, chest surgery (if appropriate), and follow-up care. (Chest surgery is discussed in Chapter 57.)

Patient-family teaching can often be conducted effectively in group sessions (in the hospital, clinic, or at home) with the patient and significant others assembled together.

Specific details important in patient education are presented throughout this discussion of tuberculosis.

Prevention of Disease Transmission.* People with active (communicable) tuberculosis require information about how tuberculosis is spread and ways in which *they* can prevent the spread of their disease to others. Instead of expecting others to protect themselves, the patient must take the initiative and accept the responsibility for carrying out protective measures.

Major ways in which *patients* with communicable tuberculosis can prevent spreading their tuberculosis to others include:

Take antituberculosis medications regularly as instructed. "Chemical isolation" is achieved on antituberculosis medications. Effective drug therapy rapidly causes patients to become noninfectious even before alterations in smears or cultures occur, i.e., even though sputum remains positive. Patients taking antituberculosis medications are unlikely to transmit tuberculosis even though resistant organisms may still be present.

Cover the nose and mouth with several layers of disposable tissues when coughing, sneezing, or laughing.

Expectorate sputum into a disposable sputum container or tissues.

Avoid close contact with others until a physician advises such contact is safe. The physician decides whether a patient on home care should occupy a room alone. The patient receiving home care should understand that it is necessary to adequately protect infants and children below age 5 from infection.

Ensure adequate air ventilation.

*Isolation techniques are discussed in detail in Sorensen and Luckmann: *Basic Nursing: A Psychophysiologic Approach.*

Precautions are individualized and based on knowledge of whether a patient's tuberculosis is communicable. For example, how long has the patient been receiving antituberculosis medications and is sputum positive?

In the hospital setting, measures to prevent air contamination by tubercle bacilli and the cleansing or decontamination of infected air are the main means of protecting personnel from infection when caring for a person with communicable tuberculosis. Because tuberculosis is an airborne infection, *adequate room ventilation* is essential. Decontamination of the air can be achieved by the use of nonrecirculating air conditioning or *ultraviolet lighting*. Recirculated air is decontaminated by using ultraviolet lights in air ducts.

Ultraviolet light destroys the tubercle bacilli. These lights may be strategically placed in hospital areas in which newly admitted infectious patients are cared for and in areas where undiagnosed patients are treated, e.g., emergency rooms and admitting rooms. Irradiation of upper room air with ultraviolet light is the most effective method for decontaminating the immediate environment. This procedure can rapidly make room air noninfectious. Good ventilation is important, but it is usually much slower than ultraviolet light in reducing the concentration of airborne organisms.

In the recent past it was common practice for persons caring for patients with tuberculosis to attempt to protect themselves from infection by wearing masks, gowns, and hair coverings. It is now realized that these practices are generally unnecessary and may be psychologically damaging to the patient. Occasionally a patient who is unable to protect persons giving care (e.g., by covering the nose and mouth when sneezing and coughing) may be *masked* during periods of close contact while direct, face-to-face, patient care is being given. Only certain types of masks are effective, e.g., the Ultra-Filter mask.

At times *face masks* must be worn by personnel, e.g., when having intimate contact with patients who are just beginning chemotherapy and who are unable (or unwilling) to take actions necessary to protect the nurse by wearing a mask, covering their noses or mouths when coughing, or properly disposing of sputum.

- *Gowns* are no longer considered necessary in caring for patients with tuberculosis. However, gowns may be worn to keep one's uniform clean when caring for patients who are unable or unwilling to protect the nurse, e.g., by properly disposing of sputum, feces, emesis, and so forth.
- Because tuberculosis is not transmitted by fomites (i.e., inanimate objects which can harbor pathogenic microorganisms and transmit them to others), special care is not necessary for personal belongings, linens, or eating utensils.
- *Handwashing* is an effective means of removing those organisms that might possibly be picked up from direct contact with infectious body discharges or from fomites. It is *always* advisable for a nurse to keep fingernails short and clean and to avoid habits like nail chewing or habitually having hands close to the face or hair. Hygienic measures routinely followed in caring for any patients are adequate when caring for patients with tuberculosis who have negative sputum.

> *Many misconceptions exist about the communicability of tuberculosis. These misconceptions unfortunately occur among some nurses.*

It is the obligation of nursing personnel to participate whenever possible in spreading correct information. This important educative process can greatly help to reduce unnecessary isolation and fears associated with tuberculosis. The fears and concerns which surround a diagnosis of tuberculosis are deeply rooted in past associations and practices.

General Aspects of Clinical Care. Tuberculosis is a diagnosis that is difficult to accept. Often people with tuberculosis sense a social stigma attached to their illness. Feelings of guilt commonly occur if a patient believes he or she has infected others. The nurse can be of help during the difficult period in which a patient and significant others must adjust to this diagnosis.

A nurse's ability to be helpful to persons with tuberculosis is directly related to his or her own attitude toward tuberculosis. Fortunately knowledge of the origins of diseases like tuberculosis have brought rational acceptance of it as an illness like all others.

Helping a patient to adjust to the diagnosis is an important aspect of the care of patients with tuberculosis, but other activities are also of clinical importance. These activities include:

- Preparing the patient for assisting with diagnostic and investigatory procedures.
- Measuring the patient's vital signs and weight periodically. Evaluating sputum production.
- Evaluating the patient's apparent general state of health, appetite, and mental-emotional status.
- Administering antituberculosis medications as prescribed and observing for toxic effects from these medications. (Sometimes drug therapy for tuberculosis is called chemotherapy.)
- Managing cough and other related symptoms. As with other pulmonary disorders, sedatives and narcotics are used with great caution to prevent

excessive depression of cough and respirations. Because of the chronicity of tuberculosis, special caution is required to prevent drug dependency.

- Performing cooling measures if the patient has a high body temperature, and providing dry linens if perspiring heavily.
- Observing for and treating complications such as pleurisy, hemoptysis, atelectasis, bronchopleural fistula, spontaneous pneumothorax, and airway disorders. Pulmonary impairment associated with obstructive airway disease is a common complication of advanced tuberculosis.
- Participating in designing and implementing a program of treatment and rehabilitation for the individual patient.
- Giving appropriate pre- and postoperative care if the patient is treated surgically.

It has been established that once an effective program of drug therapy has begun, a special diet, climate control, and prolonged bed rest are of no value in treating tuberculosis.[181A] Rest is valuable as long as the patient is symptomatic, but with adequate drug therapy prolonged rest appears to be unnecessary. A well-balanced diet is important for adequate healing and recovery from tuberculosis, but a special diet is unnecessary. Addington comments, "Adequate chemotherapeutic regimens produce uniformly excellent results. Prognosis is not determined by factors other than chemotherapy; for example, rest, the amount of fresh air or sunshine, diet, smoking habits, length of hospitalization, and alcohol use or abuse by themselves do not influence outcome. All that matters is that the patient receive the medication!"[1]

Drug Therapy of Active Tuberculosis. Tuberculosis may be particularly difficult to treat medically because of the kinds of pathologic changes associated with this disease. For example, tissue tends to become ischemic and necrotic because blood vessels do not effectively perfuse involved tissue, and bronchioles and small bronchi become stenosed. Drug therapy is also difficult because (1) the bacilli may develop drug resistance and (2) there is currently no medication that can be given in amounts large enough to completely destroy all the bacilli in the body. Some medications used to treat tuberculosis are bacteriostatic, others are bactericidal. Antituberculosis medications act by hampering reproduction of the tuberculous organisms in various ways.

Persons receiving antituberculosis drug therapy rapidly become noninfectious.

When prolonged effective drug therapy can be administered to persons with newly discovered disease, the outlook for recovery is favorable. Prognosis is not so favorable for far advanced disease.

Drug therapy of active tuberculosis requires uninterrupted, intensive, prolonged administration of medications to which the patient's specific organisms are sensitive.

In order for the drug therapy of tuberculosis to be effective certain *basic principles of therapy* must be applied. Some of the more important principles are:

- *Prior to starting drug therapy, adequate sputum specimens should be obtained* for bacteriologic and biochemical studies. Results of drug-sensitivity and other tests form a baseline for continued therapy.
- *Multiple drug therapy (combination drug therapy) is always used in treating active tuberculosis.* Single drugs are never administered because this fosters the development of organisms that are resistant to the medication being administered.
- *New medications are always introduced in combination* if a drug treatment regimen appears to be ineffective. Single medications are never added to a failing treatment program for the above stated reasons.
- *Drug therapy for tuberculosis is continued long after all radiographic, bacteriologic, and clinical evidence of active disease has vanished.* Typically drug therapy is given for 18–24 months or longer in treating active tuberculosis. Tuberculosis heals very slowly and the disease process is likely to reactivate if drugs are stopped prematurely. Some patients continue medication for the remainder of their lives.
- *Antituberculosis medications are most effective when administered in a single daily dose* rather than in divided doses throughout the day. The full dose of oral medications is usually taken on an empty stomach shortly after arising. Injectables are administered about one hour after oral medications so the peak concentrations of both the parenteral and oral medications will occur simultaneously.
- *Antituberculosis medications are commonly divided into "first-line" and "second-line" drugs.* (See Table 55–5.) The first-line drugs (or primary medications) are those most effective and most commonly used. Second-line (secondary) antituberculosis drugs are used only if a patient's organisms are resistant to the first-line medications or to replace first-line drugs in people for whom they are contraindicated.
- Factors assessed in deciding upon a specific patient's tuberculosis drug therapy may include:

TABLE 55–5. TREATMENT OF MYCOBACTERIAL DISEASE

	Most Common Side Effects	*Tests for Side Effects*	*Remarks*
		First-Line Drugs	
Isoniazid	Peripheral neuritis, hepatitis, hypersensitivity	SGOT/SGPT (not as a routine)	Bactericidal; pyridoxine, 10 mg. as prophylaxis for neuritis; 50–100 mg. as treatment
Ethambutol	Optic neuritis (reversible with discontinuation of drug; very rare at 15 mg./kg.), skin rash	Red-green color discrimination and visual acuity	Use with caution with renal disease or when eye testing is not feasible
Rifampin	Hepatitis, febrile reaction, purpura (rare)	SGOT/SGPT (not as a routine)	Bactericidal; orange urine color; negates effect of birth control pills
Streptomycin	Eighth nerve damage, nephrotoxicity	Vestibular function audiograms; BUN and creatinine	Use with caution in older patients or those with renal disease
		Second-Line Drugs	
Viomycin	Auditory toxicity, nephrotoxicity, vestibular toxicity (rare)	Vestibular function audiograms; BUN and creatinine	Used with caution in older patients; rarely used with renal disease
Capreomycin	Eighth nerve damage, nephrotoxicity	Vestibular function audiograms; BUN and creatinine	Used with caution in older patients; rarely used with renal disease
Kanamycin	Auditory toxicity, nephrotoxicity, vestibular toxicity (rare)	Vestibular function audiograms; BUN and creatinine	Used with caution in older patients; rarely used with renal disease
Ethionamide	Gastrointestinal disturbance, hepatotoxicity, hypersensitivity	SGOT/SGPT	Divided dose may help gastrointestinal side effects
Pyrazinamide	Hyperuricemia, hepatotoxicity	Uric acid, SGOT/SGPT	Combination with an aminoglycoside is bactericidal
Para-aminosalicylic acid (aminosalicylic acid)	Gastrointestinal disturbance, hypersensitivity, hepatotoxicity, sodium load	SGOT/SGPT	Gastrointestinal side effects very frequent, making cooperation difficult
Cycloserine	Psychosis, personality changes, convulsions, rash	Psychologic testing	Very difficult drug to use; side effects may be blocked by pyridoxine, ataractic agents, or anticonvulsant drugs

From Addington, W. W.: Tuberculosis and other mycobacterial diseases. *In* Conn, H. F. (Ed.): *Current Drug Therapy 1978.* Philadelphia: W. B. Saunders Co., 1978, p. 148.

category of disease, previous treatment, patient acceptance, drug toxicity, and cost.

► When *corticosteroids* are employed in treating tuberculosis they must *always* be given in combination with antituberculosis chemotherapy. Corticosteroids may be used in tuberculosis when a patient is in an overwhelming or life-threatening situation, e.g., tuberculous pneumonia or tuberculous meningitis. In these situations the anti-inflammatory and detoxifying effects of corticosteroids and corticotropin are helpful. Also, corticosteroids may be given in less serious situations to promptly produce symptomatic recovery (e.g., fever, anorexia) and to repair the anemia of infection.

Frequently any symptoms of tuberculosis that a patient with active disease may have tend to disappear or abate after a few days of chemotherapy. It must be emphasized to the patient to continue taking antituberculosis medications long after symptoms disappear. Since most people with tuberculosis are treated on an outpatient basis, the responsibility for staying on the necessary medication regimen rests with the patient. *Patient education is a highly important aspect of tuberculosis drug therapy.* Medications must be taken regularly, exactly as prescribed for as long as prescribed. The patient is advised to see the doctor if medication is upsetting in any way, and is told not to stop taking medication or to cut back on the number of pills taken.

Teach patients the names, doses, time of administration and reportable side effects of their antituberculosis medications. Drug therapy of outpatients may be supervised by clinic or public health nurses. Because therapy for tuberculosis is prolonged (and patients must continue to receive medical supervision for the remainder of their lives) long-term support and guidance are important aspects of care.

When the medical treatment of tuberculosis fails, the failure can generally be attributed to errors in drug choice or dosage; initial improper use of multipe drugs; failure of the patient to take medications as prescribed; or cessation of chemotherapy prior to complete healing. Although it is relatively rare, a few persons are initially infected with drug-resistant organisms.

Surgical Treatment of Pulmonary Tuberculosis. Drug therapy is the major method of treatment of tuberculosis. However, surgery may, on *rare* occasions, be performed. Patients with tuberculosis are carefully selected for surgical treatment. Some cannot tolerate surgery even though it might be helpful. Surgery is never performed on patients with tuberculosis without providing preoperative multidrug antituberculosis drug therapy to prevent spread of the disease at the time of surgery. (Chest surgery is discussed in Chapter 57.)

TUBERCULIN CONVERTERS

Persons who are exposed to active tuberculosis must be skin tested to determine whether they have been infected with the organism. A positive skin test (usually a P.P.D.) does not mean that active disease is present. It means that the process of *cellular immunity* has developed. Persons who develop positive skin tests are said to be *converters.* That is, they have "converted" their tuberculin skin test from a negative to a positive reaction. These persons are at high risk to develop active tuberculosis should the conditions be right.

Once conversion has occurred, a P.P.D. is typically not repeated, as it usually remains positive. Tuberculosis screens and re-evaluation for persons who may be re-exposed or become symptomatic consist of a chest x-ray film and, occasionally, bacteriologic evaluation of the sputum for the presence of acid-fast organisms. Converters are usually given a prophylactic course of isoniazid (INH) for one year. INH is useful because of its low cost, efficacy, and ease of administration.

Persons who may benefit from the chemoprophylactic administration of antituberculosis medications include:

Tuberculin converters who do not show evidence of clinically active disease, i.e., no x-ray evidence of tuberculosis and no positive laboratory tests that identify the presence of the tubercle bacillus in body secretions or tissues. Any child with a positive tuberculin test who is less than five years of age is considered to be a converter and is treated chemoprophylactically. Additionally, the preschool friends or sibling of any child with a positive tuberculin test are given INH prophylactically (even though the tuberculin test has not converted).

Persons who have been in close contact with individuals proved to have active tuberculosis.

Individuals receiving long-term corticosteroid therapy.

Persons with silicosis.

Medical supervision and follow-up are necessary with any chemoprophylactic program. Periodic chest films and tuberculin tests are important in the follow-up program. It is particularly important that children at high risk or children who are converters be under close medical supervision to detect active disease early if it develops. Occasionally chemoprophylaxis is given to tuberculin-negative persons in an attempt to prevent infections in high-risk situations, e.g., in households with recalcitrant infectious patients.

TUBERCULOSIS CONTROL PROGRAMS

Tuberculosis is a disease that could be eliminated through intensified public health control programs. Physicians, public health nurses, and clinic nurses are often active in providing health services necessary for tuberculosis case-detection and follow-up care. Groups active in tuberculosis control programs in the United States include local health departments, the United States Public Health Service (USPHS), and local organizations of the American Lung Association. Activities of importance in these control programs are summarized below:

- Intensified case finding directed at identifying every infected individual, e.g., conducting tuberculin test surveys and mass chest film programs among high-risk groups.
- Long-range medical follow-up of individuals who have been treated for active tuberculosis and of persons suspected of having a tuberculosis infection. "Suspects" are persons with positive skin tests and x-ray indications of tuberculosis but who do not yet have provable active tuberculosis.
- Identification, evaluation, and follow-up of contacts of persons with active disease. Contacts are given skin tests and chest x-ray films are taken. Medical follow-up is particularly important for the first year following exposure to active tuber-

culosis. Nurses frequently participate in identifying and following up persons who were in contact with a patient before active tuberculosis was diagnosed.

- Dissemination of facts about tuberculosis.
- Provision of necessary diagnostic and long-term treatment facilities for all persons with active disease and provision of prophylactic treatment for converters and high-risk individuals.

As the preceding discussion demonstrates, persons who are carefully followed in tuberculosis control programs include (1) persons with active tuberculosis, (2) those with inactive tuberculosis, i.e., those previously treated for active tuberculosis, persons with positive skin tests, converters, and (3) those considered to be at high risk of developing active infection. *Persons with positive skin tests considered to be at high risk* include those who are debilitated, are on immunosuppressive drugs, have diseases of the lymph system, are postgastrectomy, are diabetic, are long-term steroid users, are recent converters (within the past year), are young, are alcoholic, or have sarcoidosis or silicosis.

Case finding by means of *chest x-ray* screening is most successful among high-incidence groups in the population, e.g., close associates or contacts of active cases, low economic groups, and general hospital admissions. However, in order to avoid unnecessary exposure to radiation it is recommended that the *tuberculin test* (rather than the chest film) be used as a preliminary screening tool. This is particularly important in screening children and young adults. Tuberculin tests are recommended as part of annual physical examinations. Persons who are at high risk of infecting children, e.g., school employees, should receive routine tuberculin tests followed by x-ray films of positive tuberculin reactors.

Routine tuberculosis screening programs are usually conducted among foodhandlers, armed service personnel, and persons in large institutions. Routine admission chest x-ray films are taken in many general hospitals, clinics, lodging houses, and jails, and among welfare clients and migrant farm workers. These are of value in detecting not only tuberculosis but also other chest disorders, e.g., lung cancer.

Some persons with active tuberculosis refuse to accept treatment or to take the precautions necessary to prevent transmission of their disease to others. Unreliable persons of this nature seriously impede attempts to control and eventually eradicate tuberculosis. Occasionally legal action is necessary to commit these persons to hospital care.

Alcoholics under treatment for tuberculosis as outpatients often do not take their antituberculosis medications regularly, and if they are transient and move about from city to city they often do not keep or make the necessary follow-up appointments for medical supervision. These circumstances favor the development of drug-resistant organisms. Ideally, when patients who are alcoholic are hospitalized for the treatment of tuberculosis, they should simultaneously receive treatment directed at the concomitant problem of alcoholism. (Alcoholism is discussed in Chapter 94.)

GUIDELINES FOR HOSPITALS

The trend to close tuberculosis sanatoria and to care for persons with active disease in general hospitals and as outpatients is possible because of the development of drug therapy and increased knowledge about the disease and its transmission and control.

In the United States, the Communicable Disease Center, Atlanta, publishes guidelines for the care of hospitalized active tuberculosis patients. These are used by each state to develop its own policies and procedures. State health departments are responsible for establishing and monitoring these policies and programs in their states. Information regarding the handling of in- and outpatients with tuberculosis may be obtained from local health departments.

Hospitals caring for persons with active tuberculosis are required by law to have an ongoing tuberculosis screening program for those personnel who care for these persons. Physicians, nurses, and respiratory therapy personnel are usually evaluated every six or twelve months.

BCG (BACILLE CALMETTE-GUÉRIN)

BCG is a vaccine given in an attempt to produce increased resistance to clinical tuberculosis. BCG contains live, attenuated bovine tubercle bacilli incapable of producing active disease. Although BCG offers some protection from tuberculosis, it is not completely prophylactic.

Considerable difference of opinion exists concerning the best method of administration. One method is to administer the vaccine intradermally (with a multiple puncture disc) to assure the administration of a controlled dose. Successful vaccination may be confirmed by demonstrating a positive tuberculin reaction six to ten weeks after vaccination. BCG is typically administered to young children and then may be repeated 12 to 15 years later. BCG can be given *only* to persons with a negative tuberculin skin test. It should *never* be given in the presence of active tuberculosis or skin disorders.

The advisability of using BCG is debatable, and practices vary from country to country. In the United States, BCG vaccination is seldom used, but quite successful BCG vaccination programs have been carried out in the United Kingdom and some European countries. BCG programs have also been used in developing countries.

Because BCG changes the tuberculin skin test from a negative to a positive reaction for varying lengths of time, it interferes with the usefulness of tuberculin testing case-finding programs and the goal of eventually having all persons in the United States be tuberculin-negative. Attainment of this goal is highly important since endogenous reinfection is believed to cause most clinical tuberculosis in countries such as the United States.

The United States has effective methods of case finding, controlling, preventing, and treating tuberculosis. The battle against tuberculosis in this country is directed mainly at tuberculin reactors by providing them with chemoprophylaxis (especially if the reactors are persons who have a high risk of developing tuberculosis). It is therefore important to maintain the skin test as a means of case finding.

Most physicians in the United States believe that the risk of tuberculosis among nonreactors is too low to justify using BCG vaccination in that group, and that the vaccine possibly gives only a low level of protection.

Several large studies have shown that (a) persons vaccinated with an effective strain of BCG who do develop tuberculosis develop less progressive forms of illness; and (b) a significant reduction in the incidence of clinical tuberculosis results from BCG vaccination.

Possible complications following the administration of BCG include local ulcers and (less commonly) lymph node abscess formation or suppuration.

During screening programs it is advisable to ask patients: (1) have you ever been skin tested for tuberculosis before; (2) what were the results (positive or negative); (3) have you ever lived in another country; and (4) have you ever received BCG?

Pulmonary Disease Produced by Atypical Organisms

Persons with atypical tuberculosis are not infectious. Atypical tuberculosis is caused by saprophytic acid-fast organisms picked up from the environment. The disease process differs from that of *Mycobacterium tuberculosis.* The atypical acid-fast organisms usually grow on diseased lung tissue.

It is debatable whether all these varied mycobacterial diseases should be called "tuberculosis" or "mycobacteriosis." Currently the practice is to reserve the term tuberculosis for those infections caused by the *M. tuberculosis* or *M. bovis* (the so-called mammalian tubercle bacilli), or *M. avium.* Diseases caused by atypical mycobacteria, collectively termed the atypical mycobacterioses, are sometimes referred to by naming the particular species or group, e.g., "disease of the lung due to Battey bacillus." Although these diseases resemble tuberculosis they have different therapeutic and public health implications.

It is impossible to differentiate between typical and atypical acid-fast bacilli by means of *smears* performed in the clinical laboratory. However, the atypical organisms differ in cultural characteristics from "typical" forms of *M. tuberculosis.* Therefore, laboratory *cultures* are necessary for precise diagnosis. These culture results often are not available for two to three months after a patient has been started on antituberculosis drug therapy. Once a physician realizes that a patient does not have tuberculosis appropriate changes are made in drug therapy according to the specific causative organism. Atypical organisms are frequently resistant to medications currently available, e.g., isoniazid, streptomycin, and para-aminosalicylic acid. When a patient is discovered to have atypical organisms, drug susceptibility tests are usually made with both primary and secondary drugs (see preceding discussion of antituberculosis medications) to identify the most effective drug combination.

Infections with atypical organisms are common; however, only a few actually produce disease. Persons with atypical microorganisms are treated in open wards and are not considered to be infectious. Atypical organisms are widely distributed in nature, e.g., in water, vegetable matter, soil, and raw milk. Also, they may be recovered from the gastric contents and sputum of healthy persons.

It is believed that a weak reactivity to tuberculin skin testing frequently indicates a subclinical dormant infection with atypical mycobacteria. When clinical infection with these organisms occurs, it tends to be more apparent in persons who have some other chronic lung damage, e.g., silicosis, chronic bronchitis, emphysema.[162]

Some facts about the four groups of atypical mycobacteria:

- Group I: *M. kansasii* and *M. marinum (balnei).* Also called photochromogens. Yellow pigment develops rapidly only after exposure to light during growth phase. Most reported cases in the U.S. are from Texas, Kansas, and Illinois. These infections respond to antituberculosis medications less well than *M. tuberculosis* infections, but they do show some susceptibility to the usual antituberculosis drugs in higher doses.
- Group II: *M. scrofulaceum* and *M. aquae.* Also called scotochromogens. Yellow to orange pigmentation appears without exposure to light. Occurs in soil in most areas of the U.S; also commonly found in water. Seldom produces pulmonary disease in humans. Often found as harmless saprophytes in sputum. May produce scrofula

in children. Drug treatment may give enough inhibition to permit surgical excision of the nodes if they are fluctuant or draining.

- Group III: *M. intracellularis* (Battey bacillus), *M. avium,* and *M. xenopei*. Also called nonchromogens. White or ivory appearance; no pigment produced when exposed to light. Found in soil and in tissues of certain domestic animals, e.g., cattle, swine. Battey infections are more common in the southeastern U.S., especially Florida and Georgia. Typically these infections are difficult to treat because the organisms usually are highly resistant to the usual concentrations of all anti-tuberculosis medications. Some patients respond to a five-drug program of prolonged treatment but must be closely observed for the numerous side effects that can occur. If the disease cannot be controlled it produces widespread pulmonary disease which slowly progresses until death occurs from cor pulmonale and pulmonary insufficiency. Some patients with localized disease may have surgical resection (e.g., lobectomy) performed if they have adequate pulmonary function. (Group III organisms which do not produce disease in humans include *M. terrae* ["radish" bacillus] *M. gastri,* and *M. trivale* ["V" subgroup]).
- Group IV: *M. fortuitum.* Organisms in this group are also called "rapid growers." The only pathogen in the group is *M. fortuitum.* Only rarely causes pulmonary disease.

Pulmonary Mycoses (Fungus Infections)

It is not uncommon for the respiratory tract to be infected with fungi (molds). Some fungus infections are increasing in incidence. The mode of infection, immunologic status, and best means of prevention have not been identified for most fungus infections of the lungs. However, specific drug treatments are available and have improved the prognosis of many fungus infections. Without drug therapy some fungus infections, e.g., blastomycosis, may be progressive and fatal.

The fungicidal antibiotic *amphotericin B* has been especially valuable in reversing the prognosis of many fungus infections which were previously critical. The patient is hospitalized for the administration of this medication because cautious administration and close observation for toxic effects are necessary. Be certain to follow the manufacturer's directions carefully when preparing infusion solutions of amphotericin B, and consult a textbook of pharmacology for discussions of the procedure for administering this medication, dosage, toxic effects, and so forth. Saline solutions should not be used, since saline precipitates this medication.

Because of the specificity of treatment for pulmonary mycoses, it is essential that an accurate *diagnosis* be made so the proper chemotherapy can be given. Precise diagnosis may be difficult because mycotic diseases involving the lungs commonly produce clinical symptoms and radiologic findings indistinguishable from those produced by bacteria (e.g., tuberculosis), viruses, or carcinoma. The diagnosis of a mycosis depends upon either actually isolating the organism from sputum, gastric washings, spinal fluids, blood, urine, bone marrow, joint fluid, skin and mucous membrane lesions, prostatic secretion, bronchial aspirates, or biopsy specimens or demonstrating specific measurable immunologic changes in host response.

Skin tests with commercially available antigens are possible only for coccidioidomycosis and blastomycosis at this time. *Before* skin tests are applied to a patient suspected of having a systemic mycosis, 15 to 20 ml. of venous blood is drawn for serum separation. If skin tests have been applied before the blood serology sample is drawn, be certain this information and the date and result of the test are sent with the serum specimens.

Often it takes two to eight weeks for some fungi to be isolated and specifically identified from clinical materials. When cultures have not been performed or are negative, the physician may make a diagnosis based on correlating the morphology of the organism with skin tests, serologic reactions, and residential and occupational data. In contrast to viral and bacterial diseases, it is possible to diagnose fungus diseases with a high degree of reliability by examining specially stained tissue sections. Although the tissue reaction to the fungus is not diagnostic, the distinctive morphology of the fungus may permit a skilled histopathologist to make a specific etiologic identification.

Two relatively common pulmonary fungus infections are histoplasmosis and coccidioidomycosis. Both these disorders are fairly clearly localized geographically.

Histoplasmosis. *Histoplasmosis* is also called "histo," cave fever, or cytomycosis. This chronic granulomatous disease of the reticuloendothelial system principally affects the lungs and occasionally spreads by hematogenous dissemination. The causative fungus is *Histoplasma capsulatum.* This disorder occurs most commonly in the East and Midwest, particularly in the Ohio and Mississippi river valleys. Millions of Americans are believed to have been infected, but few fatalities occur. Histoplasmosis does not appear to be transmitted from person to person but rather the fungus spores grow in moist, dark protected soil such as that found in old chicken houses, pigeon lofts, belfries, and bat-infested caves. The fungus is lightweight enough to float when infected dust is stirred up and is small enough to be inhaled.

In the lungs the fungus causes *pathologic changes* which closely resemble those of tuberculosis, e.g., tubercle formation, central caseation, scarring, cavity formation, and calcification. Symptoms vary (from flu-like to more serious symptoms), depending upon the degree of exposure. Treatment of the more severe infections may include administration of amphotericin B and/or surgical removal of sections of lung imbedded with spores.

Public health nurses in rural areas are active in the prevention of histoplasmosis by urging farmers to keep farm buildings clean and dry and reminding them to wet down the floor before sweeping out farm buildings (to prevent dust from rising). Chicken droppings should always be wetted down before chicken houses are cleaned out. Storm cellars should be kept clean and dry. Of course, it is desirable to avoid bat-infested belfries and caves. Persons raising pigeons should be advised how to properly care for these birds and clean their lofts.

Coccidioidomycosis. Other terms for coccidioidomycosis are "the bumps," San Joaquin valley fever, and desert fever. This granulomatous disease, caused by the fungus *Coccidioides immitis*, produces acute and chronic pulmonary lesions. In the United States coccidioidomycosis occurs almost exclusively in the Southwest. The primary form of this disorder is typically a benign, acute, self-limited respiratory disease. The progressive form is a chronic (possibly fatal) infection involving not only the lungs but other structures such as skin or bone. Disease is produced in humans by inhalation of dust contaminated with spores. An animal reservoir may occur in some rodents. The only effective medication is amphotericin B.

Other Pulmonary Mycoses. Four other generalized fungus infections involving the lungs, which are relatively less common and less well localized geographically, are:

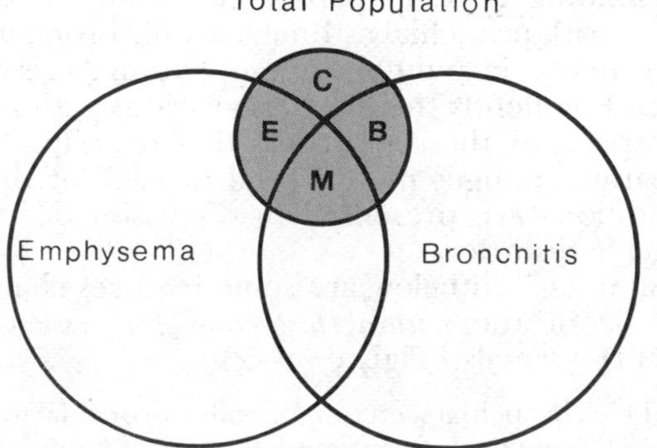

Figure 55–4. Relationship of emphysema, bronchitis, and chronic obstructive pulmonary disease (COPD). The small circle denotes patients with COPD. E, emphysematous disease; B, bronchial disease; C, COPD without bronchitis or anatomic emphysema; M, mixed-type disease. (After *Chronic Bronchitis and Emphysema*, Das Medizinische Prisma, No. 4, p. 4, 1971. Copyright 1971 by C. H. Boehringer Sohn.)

- *Blastomycosis:* A chronic granulomatous infection caused by *Blastomyces dermatitidis,* which has a predilection for the skin and lungs.
- *Cryptococcosis* (torulosis): A generalized granulomatous infection caused by *Cryptococcus histolyticus,* with a predilection for the meninges and lungs.
- *Actinomycosis* ("lumpy jaw"): A chronic granulomatous infection caused by *Actinomyces bovis,* which is characterized by abscess formation with numerous draining sinus tracts, e.g., through the chest wall.
- *Nocardiosis* (streptothricosis): A chronic granulomatous disease caused by *Nocardia asteroides*, which produces numerous abscesses and sometimes sinus tracts.

CHRONIC OBSTRUCTIVE PULMONARY DISEASE (COPD)

Chronic obstructive pulmonary disease (COPD) is a term applied to respiratory disorders that involve persistent obstruction of bronchial air flow. COPD is a* functional *category (rather than a specific disease). This means the patient has* persistent *airway obstruction that is a chronic problem and tends to slowly and progressively worsen.*

Various diseases may be associated with COPD, e.g., pulmonary tuberculosis, bronchiectasis, silicosis, pulmonary fibrosis. However, *the conditions that most frequently give rise to COPD are bronchial asthma, chronic bronchitis, and anatomic pulmonary emphysema.*

Numerous diseases of the respiratory tract, including those referred to as COPD, produce similar physiologic alterations and symptoms. These similarities may make an accurate diagnosis difficult. Figure 55–4 illustrates the relationship of emphysema, bronchitis, and COPD. Each disorder can occur alone or in combination with another; each may or may not be associated with COPD. *Bronchitis and emphysema coexist most frequently.*

In England the terms "chronic bronchitis" and "emphysema" are used synonymously. However, in England chronic bronchitis is the

*Other terms to refer to this group of conditions include: diffuse obstructive pulmonary syndrome (DOPS); diffuse obstructive lung disease (DOLD); chronic airway obstruction (CAO); chronic obstructive lung disease (COLD); chronic obstructive pulmonary emphysema (COPE); obstructive airway disease (OAD); obstructive ventilatory disease (OVD); OVD of the lungs; and chronic obstructive airway disease (COAD).

diagnosis most commonly used when a patient has combined chronic bronchitis and emphysema (and possibly also bronchial asthma). In the United States it has been more usual for emphysema to be diagnosed as the more important component of such combined disease, and the presence of bronchitis has tended to be ignored. Currently, attempts are being made to focus on the common problem of COPD rather than emphasizing one predominant diagnosis, since a more definitive diagnosis is not necessary for treatment.

Incidence

Chronic obstructive pulmonary diseases are on the increase at alarming rates.

Statistics are difficult to obtain for the overall incidence of COPD because of confusion and varying interpretations of pertinent definitions. However, COPD is clearly a major cause of disability and death. COPD ranks second only to heart disease as a cause of disability in the United States. Mortality rates for COPD are reported to be *doubling* about every *five years*! It is believed that the actual mortality from COPD exceeds that from lung cancer. The incidence in women appears to be increasing. However, at present men are affected eight to ten times more often than women with symptomatic COPD. Probably this is because men have smoked more heavily, more often, and for a more prolonged time than women.[16] In addition to suffering and death, COPD causes serious socioeconomic problems.

Other factors of importance in the increasing incidence of COPD include (1) increasing survival rates of patients because of improved treatment procedures, (2) increasing age of the population, and (3) the increasing ability to recognize COPD and identify it as a cause of morbidity and mortality.

Etiology. The exact cause(s) of COPD has not been identified. However, the following etiologic factors are considered to be of importance as possibly causing, aggravating, or exacerbating COPD: smoking, recurrent or chronic bronchopulmonary infection, air pollution, pneumoconiosis (and other occupational exposures, e.g., to molds, fungi, coal dust, cotton fibers, asbestos, irritating gases), allergic factors, genetic factors, aging of the lung, and vascular changes. *Currently the factor that appears to be of greatest etiologic importance is smoking.*

Prevention. Public education about the hazards of pulmonary irritants (smoking, air pollution) and the value of having respiratory disorders promptly investigated and treated is important, since the early detection of COPD is difficult, and affected persons are unable to recognize the development and progression of this disorder. By the time a person seeks medical help, structural lung damage is often very advanced and the person does not have the cardiopulmonary reserve needed to meet physiologic needs. *Persistent coughs* (including those referred to as "smoker's cough" or "morning cough") should always be evaluated *early* and treated. Periodic physical examinations (e.g., annually) are important in the prevention or early detection of COPD.

Symptoms. Early symptoms of COPD develop insidiously and progress slowly; *a common triad that occurs with COPD is dyspnea (especially upon exertion), intermittent cough, and fatigue following exertion.* These symptoms may begin as only a slight shortness of breath, a mild morning cough, and a bit of fatigue, e.g., from walking upstairs. Because of the mild nature of the symptoms, the affected person commonly does not seek medical evaluation. Gradually, however, symptoms worsen and the patient develops COPD which, even in its mild to moderate forms, is a distressing chronic illness.

In its more severe forms, COPD is a crippling condition which increasingly causes the victim to struggle for air. COPD typically causes a *forced exhalation* which is always noticeable with chronic anatomic pulmonary emphysema, occurs in some patients with chronic bronchitis, and is present during an attack of bronchial asthma. Wheezing, weight loss, general debilitation, and abnormal blood gas levels are other common symptoms of COPD. Pulmonary function tests demonstrate retardation of expiratory flow, which, if progressive, causes dyspnea, hypoxemia, and hypercapnia.

Pathology. The pathologic changes that occur with bronchial asthma, chronic bronchitis, and anatomic pulmonary emphysema are distinct. Frequently there are also various pathologic aspects of these disorders that overlap. The separate changes most typical of each of these conditions are presented in discussions of the specific disorders.

Summarized below are some features characteristic of the *natural history of progression* of COPD. (See also Figure 55–5.)

- Thick bronchial secretions, swollen bronchial walls, and unequal alveolar ventilation result from infectious or allergic processes.
- Some alveoli may become hyperinflated; others become atelectatic.
- Thoracic excursion is reduced by chronic bronchial obstruction, air trapping, and thoracic overdistention.

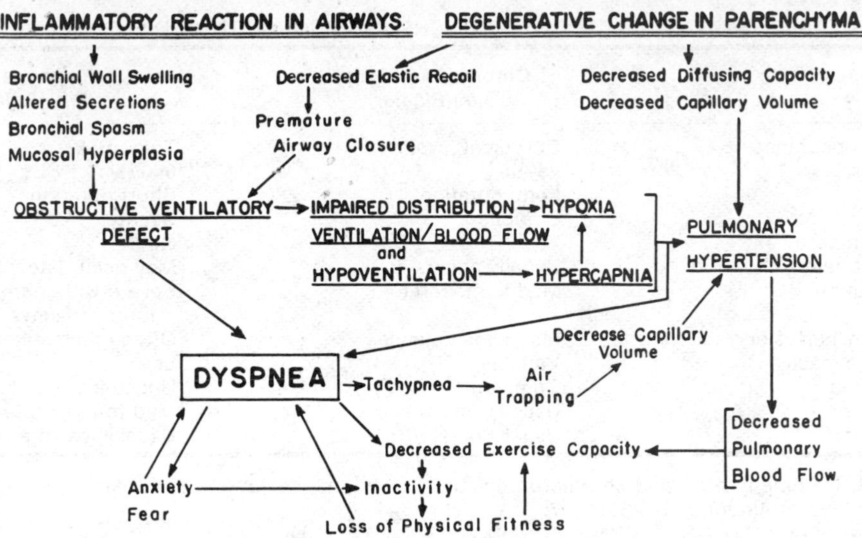

Figure 55–5. The nature of chronic obstructive lung disease. (From Miller, W. F.: *Medical Clinics of North America, 51*: 349, Mar. 1967.)

- Gradual destruction of lung parenchyma and loss of the lung's elastic contractility (ability to recoil) occurs. These factors cause an increased (less negative) intrapleural pressure, which contributes to the collapse of bronchioles and poorly supported bronchi.
- The weight of the abdominal viscera lowers the diaphragm because of the lung's weakened elastic recoil.
- Tidal volume, vital capacity, and the inspiratory reserve necessary for effective coughing are diminished by the reduced thoracic excursion.
- Increased work of breathing occurs, fatiguing the patient and perhaps causing confinement to chair or bed. In order to breathe, the patient involuntarily employs the accessory muscles of respiration, uses the shoulder girdle and abdominal muscle groups, and purses the lips to keep the airways open to allow exhalation.
- Eventually the patient develops permanently reduced alveolar ventilation, carbon dioxide retention, hypoxia, and chronic respiratory acidosis owing to the syndrome of bronchial obstruction, alveolar air trapping, patchy atelectasis, and chronic muscle fatigue.
- As the patient's condition worsens, hypoxemia leads to further debilitation by weakening the myocardium, interfering with renal function, increasing capillary permeability, and causing polycythemia, anorexia, and weight loss.
- Increasingly body buffers are consumed by attempts to compensate for chronic respiratory acidosis.
- The patient's ability to meet life's stresses is reduced. Recurrent episodes of pulmonary infections (e.g., acute bronchitis, pneumonia) may eventually cause cor pulmonale, respiratory failure, coma, and death.

Many patients with COPD who are persistently hypoxic have an increase in hematocrit beyond the normal range. (See "Polycythemia," Unit XIV.) *The association of hypoxemia, polycythemia, and cor pulmonale occurs most often in those persons with COPD who have severe chronic bronchitis.* Because of their appearance, these individuals have been described as *"blue bloaters"* (abbreviated as "BB"). Persons with dyspnea caused by severe emphysema, who do not have accompanying cyanosis or indications of congestive heart failure, have been described as *"pink puffers"* ("PP"). (See Table 55–6.) These two contrasting types of chronic airway obstruction are distinguishable by clinical criteria alone. This classification is therefore useful in the early identification of COPD, before laboratory measurements of physiologic function are made.

Detection of COPD. Because many patients in a nurse's care may have COPD (and therefore require special care to make them more comfortable while preventing possible complications), *nurses must be able to assess patients in such a manner that COPD can be detected.* One cannot rely on the Kardex or the patient's chart for the identification of COPD, because often only the primary diagnosis or impression may be available. In emergency situations no chart or Kardex information may be available. Nurses must, therefore, be capable of rapidly making their own assessments. Essential changes produced by COPD are summarized in Table 55–7. Many of these key observations are discussed further in this text.

Awareness that a patient has COPD is especially important to prevent CO_2 narcosis when giving O_2 therapy.

TABLE 55–6. CHARACTERISTICS OF CHRONIC BRONCHITIS AND EMPHYSEMA

	Chronic Bronchitis *(Blue Bloater)*	**Emphysema** *(Pink Puffer)*
General appearance	Corpulent, cyanotic	Thin, pink
Age, years	45–65	65–75
Cough	Long duration	Short duration
Sputum	Copious	Scanty
Cardiac enlargement	Yes	No
Cor pulmonale with failure	Usually occurs early	May occur late
Hyperinflation	Mild to moderate	Severe with increase in total lung capacity
Ventilation/perfusion ratio	Marked imbalance	Often minimal imbalance
Diffusing capacity	Variable	Low
Hypercapnia	Common	Unusual until late
Hypoxemia	Usually severe	Mild to moderate
Hematocrit	Usually greater than 60%	Usually less than 65%

From Filley, G. F.: Emphysema and chronic bronchitis: Clinical manifestations and their psychologic significance. *Medical Clinics of North America,* 51:283, 1967.

Complications. Complications of COPD include carbon dioxide narcosis, acute respiratory failure, metabolic alkalosis, uncompensated respiratory acidosis, bronchopulmonary infections, cor pulmonale (observe for digitalis toxicity when digitalis is prescribed to treat cardiac failure), spontaneous pneumothorax (due to ruptured pulmonary bleb or bullae), arteriosclerotic and hypertensive heart disease (because many patients with COPD are middle-aged or

TABLE 55–7. DETECTION OF CHRONIC OBSTRUCTIVE LUNG DISEASE

Primary Changes	**Secondary Changes**
Chest	*Blood Pressure*
Increased A-P diameter ("barrel chest"); chest fixed in inspiratory position; expanded lower rib margin; due to air trapping and enlargement of lungs with loss of ability to recoil	Pulsus paradoxus (reduction of arterial pulse during inspiration); due to effect on cardiac filling from accentuated respiratory effort; during inspiration increased negative intrathoracic pressure occurs
Enlarged accessory muscles of respiration; use of these muscles and abdominal muscles during ventilation to help force air out of lungs	*Red Blood Cells*
Prolonged expiratory time; due to air trapping and collapse of airways upon expiration	Polycythemia develops in response to hypoxia
Expiratory wheezing (high-pitched, whistling sound); due to bronchospasm	*Heart*
Rhonchi (loud snoring sounds or low-pitched rattling sounds at end of expiration); due to mucus in airways	Right ventricular strain and enlargement (cor pulmonale); due to pulmonary hypertension which results from hypoxia and acidosis; liver engorgement, peripheral edema also occur; evidence of cor pulmonale; apical sound in epigastric area; right ventricular lift or thrust; loud P_2; tall, pointed P waves; and right axis deviation
Decreased breath sounds; due to reduced air flow, pleural effusion, or lung parenchyma destruction	
Fingernails and Hands	*Blood Vessels*
Clubbing; vertical fingernail ridging	Venous engorgement (which elevates venous pressure); results from impeded venous return to heart (due to elevated pressures in right side of heart and altered intrathoracic pressure); indications of venous engorgement; jugular venous distention; hepatojugular reflux; peripheral edema; pleural effusion (typically right-sided); or ascites
Hyperemia; due to excess blood supply as CO_2 build-up causes arteries to dilate	
Fine twitching of extremities; asterixis ("metabolic flap"); due to hypoxemia, hypercapnia	
Neurologic	*Electrolytes*
Restlessness, agitation, lethargy, coma, headaches (during night or upon arising), nightmares, difficulty sleeping; due to alterations in O_2, CO_2, and hydrogen levels; brain sensitive to changes	Low serum chloride and elevated serum CO_2; resulting from retention of bicarbonate ions (in an attempt to buffer additional carbonic acid formed by excess CO_2) and excretion of chloride ions in their place

Modified from Sedlock, S. A.: *American Journal of Nursing,* 72:1407, Aug. 1972.

elderly), pulmonary thromboembolic disease (especially if significant polycythemia is present), and peptic ulcer.

Because almost one of four persons with COPD is estimated to have a *peptic ulcer* at some time, the nurse observes closely for indications of this complication (especially if a patient is receiving steroid or anticoagulant therapy). Symptoms of peptic ulcer include abdominal soreness, hematemesis, and epigastric pain. Abdominal pain may diminish the patient's appetite and contribute to weight loss. Among the factors that may predispose to the development of peptic ulcer are increased gastric secretion, psychosomatic influences, CO_2 retention, and reduced arterial oxygen saturation.

Clinical Care of Patients with COPD. Providing appropriate, comprehensive clinical care for the patient with COPD is highly challenging and may tax a nurse's knowledge, ingenuity, and patience. Meticulous attention to detail is essential. The nurse's expertise is necessary in making clinical judgments and in skillfully performing nursing procedures. Additionally, the nurse must provide the emotional care required by a chronically ill, dyspneic patient.

Clinical care attempts to maintain existing lung function, prevent additional irreversible lung damage and loss of pulmonary function, promote symptomatic relief (with bronchodilators, antibiotics, tranquilizers, IPPB therapy), and provide a vigorous program of total rehabilita-

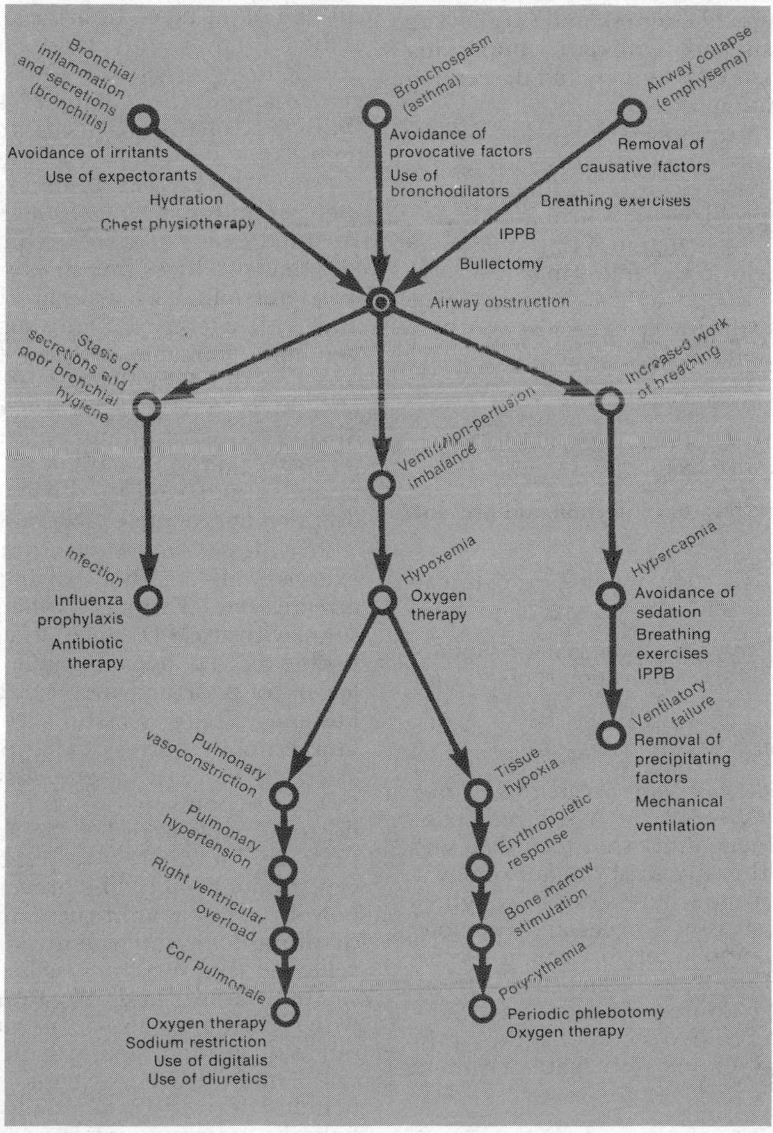

Figure 55–6. Overview of physiologic approach to therapy of COPD. (From Golish, J. A., and M. Ahmad: Management of COPD *Postgraduate Medicine*, 62:132, July 1977.)

tion (through patient education, postural drainage, breathing retraining exercises with supplemental oxygen therapy, and vocational training or retraining).

Basically the treatment of obstructive pulmonary disease is directed at making the most of remaining lung function and maintaining patency of the peripheral bronchial tree. This means that therapeutic procedures are employed to (1) remove viscid and inspissated secretions from occluded bronchioles; (2) improve ventilation, enlarge air passages, and reduce resistance to the flow of gases into and out of the alveoli (by reducing in thickness the walls of bronchioles that are swollen by cellular infiltration and submucosal edema); and (3) alleviate respiratory acidosis and hypoxia by improving alveolar exchange of CO_2 and O_2 and decreasing the work of breathing.

Summarized and discussed below are factors important in the care of all patients with COPD regardless of the basic disorder. Clinical care is directed at the problem of chronic, diffuse, irreversible airway obstruction.* Care measures to be discussed include the following:

- Cleanse and dilate the tracheobronchial tree. Promote bronchial drainage.
- Assist ventilation and respiration.
- Remove, avoid and/or minimize bronchial irritants and other provocative factors.
- Control chronic respiratory infection and prevent acute infections.
- Observe for and treat complications, e.g., prevent heart failure.
- Provide patient-family education, general supportive and emotional care, stimulation routines, and total rehabilitation.
- Provide long-term supervision and care.

Cleansing and Dilating Tracheobronchial Tree; Promoting Bronchial Drainage. Assist with postural (gravity) drainage and other techniques of pulmonary physiotherapy to stimulate removal of retained secretions to where it can be coughed up, or removed by suction if necessary. Promote effective coughing and deep breathing. Some patients with COPD cannot cough effectively, so cough stimulation routines are necessary. Suction as indicated to remove secretions. Promptly remove liquefied secretions, if the patient cannot do so alone, to prevent suffocation. Maintain hydration to thin secretions and encourage appropriate physical activity (e.g., ambulation) to move secretions. Force fluids as indicated. Maintain humidification of inspired air, e.g., with heated aerosol generator or ultrasonic nebulizer. Administer medications ordered to cleanse and dilate the tracheobronchial tree, e. g., bronchodilator aerosols, mucolytic (mucus-dissolving) aerosols, wetting agents, detergents, expectorants, systemic bronchodilators, antibiotics, steroids.

Bronchospasm commonly occurs with COPD. Normally bronchi have a tremendous ability to change the size of their lumina; damaged bronchi may require bronchodilator medications to relax the smooth muscle surrounding the bronchi.

Assisting Ventilation and Respiration. Administer respiratory therapy (IPPB, oxygen) as required by the patient's condition. Oxygen (O_2) may be required if the arterial oxyhemoglobin is reduced significantly. *When giving O_2 to a patient with COPD, give low concentrations to prevent carbon dioxide narcosis.* (See Chapter 54.) Management of fluid-electrolyte imbalances is discussed in Chapter 12.

Oxygen therapy is administered in the treatment of most moderate to severe cases of COPD. In some cases, it is only required during exercise that produces breathlessness or hypoxemia (as determined by arterial blood gases at rest and with exercise). Lightweight, portable oxygen equipment may be used during ambulation or when the patient is out of bed. At times it is necessary to give *total ventilatory support.* (See discussion of respiratory insufficiency and respiratory failure, Chapter 53.) Provide appropriate supportive care during periods of severe dyspnea and acute exacerbations.

Provide *patient education* concerning breathing exercises and methods of improving breathing effectiveness. Fatigue is a major enemy of persons with COPD since it adds to breathing problems. To avoid fatigue the patient must learn to plan activities carefully and thereby budget energy. Restful sleep is also important. Emotional stress and unpleasantness impair sleep and increase fatigue. Advise the patient not to take sleeping pills or tranquilizers without a doctor's explicit order, because these medications tend to depress respirations during sleep. Constipation should be prevented, since the full bowel pushes against the diaphragm, impeding diaphragmatic movement. Measures helpful in relieving dyspnea are discussed in Chapter 53.

Ambulation and Breathing. The person with COPD must also be instructed in the importance of graded, goal-oriented, *progressive exercise.* The improved psychologic and physiologic benefits derived from a daily exercise program help the patient maintain a feeling of self-worth. Physiologically, exercise stimulates the mitochondria in muscle tissue to better utilize the

*Detailed discussions of various procedures, e.g., suctioning, postural drainage, IPPB, breathing exercises, oxygen therapy, and so forth, have been presented in Chapter 54.

available oxygen for tissue metabolism. In this way the patient's exercise tolerance is improved.

Exercise must also be accompanied by instruction in breathing retraining exercises. Techniques for walking, stair climbing, and other forms of exercise must be demonstrated by the nurse or respiratory therapist and practiced by the patient until they feel natural.

It is important that an exercise program be realistic for the patient. The home environment must be considered. If the patient is a city dweller who lives in an apartment on the top of a hill, walking outside may not be possible or even advisable. Stationary bicycles offer an alternative. The goal of the exercise is to develop and condition the large muscle groups. (See Chapter 54 on breathing retraining.)

Before exercise is taught, the patient must be comfortable with *pursed lip breathing (PLB), diaphragmatic breathing (DB)* and *dyspnea positions.* These techniques are also utilized by the patient as they exercise. (See Chapter 54.)

Inspiration and expiration are easily synchronized with ambulation. The patient should be instructed to exhale using PLB. Exhalation should take longer than inhalation. Going up and down stairs is also included. Instruct the patient to inhale while standing still and then to climb or descend the stairs on exhalation. Prior to opening a door or lifting an object, the patient with COPD is instructed to inhale and then perform the activity on exhalation. Teach the patient to not hurry.

Frequent, positive reinforcement and encouragement is necessary, as the patient with COPD often becomes easily discouraged. Goals set for the level of exercise must be realistic. As they are achieved, they may be increased.

Removing, Avoiding and/or Minimizing Bronchial Irritants. Smoking is clearly contraindicated in the presence of COPD, but often it is difficult to give up this habit. Smoke-filled rooms and activities that send dust into the air should be avoided. Dust-producing articles (e.g., feather-filled bedding) and strong cooking odors (e.g., smoke from frying, barbequeing) can also irritate the respiratory tract.

Instruct the patient with COPD to avoid inhaling excessively cold air (cover the mouth and nose with a scarf when outside in very cold weather.) Inhalation of extremely cold air may precipitate bronchospasm. Excessive heat should also be avoided since it increases oxygen requirements. Sudden temperature changes (hot or cold) are undesirable. The avoidance of specific allergens (foods, pollens, animal danders) to which a patient is known to be sensitive is particularly important in extrinsic bronchial asthma. (See discussion of bronchial asthma, p. 1315.)

Advise the patient to avoid using powders and aerosolized commercial products (e.g., spray deodorants, hair sprays), and to stay away from air-polluted environments, since air pollutants may cause bronchospasm. The physician may advise occupational changes if the patient works in a polluted environment. Some patients benefit from the use of a home air conditioning unit equipped with an effective filter system. Maintenance of a high relative humidity in the home (40 to 50 per cent) is also helpful, particularly during the winter.

In some cases the physician advises the patient to move to a climate that has minimal shifts in humidity and temperature. Very warm, dry climates are as undesirable as those that are very cold or very humid. High altitudes are also undesirable; they worsen hypoxia. Commonly persons with COPD can live more comfortably at altitudes between 300 and 600 feet. However, some people prefer altitudes up to 3000 feet. Flying in pressurized aircraft at high altitudes should not give the patient added respiratory distress.

Nosedrops should be used only if prescribed, since some over-the-counter products contain oils that may damage the lungs.

Excessive, forceful coughing irritates the tracheobronchial tree. Although productive coughing is essential to clear the tracheobronchial tree of secretions, nonproductive coughing should be controlled. The patient should try to avoid situations that may produce a coughing spell.

Infection Control and Prevention. Control *chronic* respiratory infections and prevent *acute* respiratory infections in the patient with COPD, since infections cause further lung damage and deterioration of lung function. In addition to possibly structurally damaging the lung, infections increase mucus production and further restrict ventilation. Also, drug-resistant infections can become a problem. An acute respiratory infection can be fatal to the patient with COPD.

Acute pulmonary infections constantly threaten the patient with COPD because of the patient's lowered resistance. In an attempt to minimize the severity of acute infections some physicians prescribe daily prophylactic doses of antibiotics during cold damp months or if the patient has been exposed to an acute respiratory infection. Upper respiratory infections often precipitate attacks of asthma and chronic bronchitis.

The lung in COPD is always chronically infected. The goal of therapy in such a situation becomes one of suppressing the bacteria rather than eliminating them. This may be accomplished by giving the patient intermittent doses of antibiotics, e.g., on any two consecutive days of the week. Encourage the patient to stay on the prescribed routine.

Instruct the patient concerning the following actions, which are of importance in *preventing infections:* (1) avoid close contact with persons who have respiratory infections or "flu"; (2) avoid crowds during times of the year when respiratory infections most commonly occur; (3) maintain a high resistance (e.g., by getting adequate rest and relaxation, eating a nourishing diet high in vitamin C, and avoiding stressful situations and exposure to temperature extremes, dampness, and drafts); and (4) practice frequent thorough oral hygiene.

Influenza vaccines are usually advised prophylactically as a precaution against the development of severe acute infections. Chronically infected tonsils and obstructive adenoids may be removed and sinus infections treated.

Teach the patient to observe sputum for indications of infection, e.g., increased sputum production or changes in color (from clear or white to gray, yellow, or brown). Other symptoms of acute infection include excessive drowsiness, chest pain, chills, increased dyspnea, cyanosis, leukocytosis, and increased tightness in the chest. Instruct the patient to seek medical care promptly if an acute infection appears to be developing.

During periods of acute infection continuous daily antibiotic treatment is usually indicated. Before the results of sputum culture and sensitivity tests are available, broad-spectrum antibiotics may be prescribed.

Excessive, unproductive coughing is usually mildly suppressed in the patient with COPD because it traumatizes the respiratory system and thus increases the susceptibility of this system to infections.

Complications. Observe for indications of worsening of the patient's condition such as: increased sputum production, cough, dyspnea, or wheezing, cyanosis, edema, and mental confusion. In order to evaluate a patient's condition, daily charting should include notation of: sputum (amount, character); coughing (amount, productivity); skin, mucous membrane and nail bed color; amount of dyspnea and/or wheezing; appetite; and mental state. Weigh the patient as requested by the physician or as indicated. Right-sided heart failure (cor pulmonale) is a chronic problem with COPD. Heart failure is controlled by rest, salt restriction, diuretics, and heart muscle strengthening medications. (See Unit XII.)

Patient-Family Education; General Supportive and Emotional Care; Rehabilitation. Include the patient's significant others at appropriate times during patient teaching sessions. Carefully evaluate and meet learning needs. Areas that may need to be covered include: explanation of the basic respiratory disorder; preventative measures; activity adaptations; and such treatment procedures as medications (actions, side effects, methods and times of administration), dietary restrictions, pulmonary physiology (postural drainage, breathing exercises, exercise retraining programs, effective coughing techniques) and respiratory therapy techniques (oxygen administration, aerosol, and IPPB administration).

Establish individualized programs to help each patient to achieve and attempt to maintain an optimal level of activity. Assist the patient to accept realistic long-term goals and to be as comfortable and independent as his or her condition permits. Help the person to adapt daily activities to the respiratory limitations without encouraging unnecessary passivity or invalidism. The more active a patient can be (without excessively increasing dyspnea), the better and stronger the person will feel. Activity also minimizes complications that tend to accompany inactivity. Physical activity tolerance varies from patient to patient, and a given patient's tolerance may vary from day to day or even within the same day.

Rehabilitation of persons with COPD can be as successful as that of persons with neuromuscular and skeletal disabilities. Rehabilitative procedures will not reverse the permanent structural pulmonary damage caused by COPD, but they can teach the patient ways to live with limited cardiorespiratory reserve, and they can prepare the person for employment or self-care attuned to his or her mental and physical capacities. Successful rehabilitation programs involve participation by the patient, significant others, physician, nurses and other paramedical personnel. A multidisciplinary approach is desirable.

It is estimated that with proper rehabilitation techniques about half of the people who are already disabled by respiratory disease can be restored and improved enough that they can return to work or at least to self-care. Most people with chronic respiratory diseases are able to pursue some form of regular employment. Vocational retraining may be necessary to enable the patient to perform work that is compatible with respiratory limitations. Some communities have COPD rehabilitation programs sponsored by hospitals, clinics, or local agencies, e.g., of lung associations. Social workers and employees of state rehabilitation services may be helpful if change of employment is advised to avoid bronchial irritants or to reduce physical exertion. Social workers may also make appropriate referrals to: obtain equipment necessary for home care, to relieve socioeconomic problems, or to obtain total care if indicated. Over a period of years costs of equipment, oxygen, medications, and hospitalizations are considerable.

A variety of informative materials are available through health or lung associations.

Long-Term Supervision and Care. A person with COPD requires long-term follow-up care which may involve community nurses as well as personnel in outpatient departments. The visiting nurse is helpful in (1) assessing the home situation; (2) giving or supervising home care; (3) helping the patient to adapt treatment procedures (e.g., dietary restrictions, humidification, postural drainage, oxygen administration) to the home environment; (4) suggesting ways in which the home environment can be modified to minimize energy expenditure; (5) making needed referrals; and (6) counseling, teaching, and emotionally supporting the patient and significant others. The support, encouragement and participation of significant others in the care of a person with COPD can greatly help the patient to improve. Significant others often require assistance in increasing their acceptance and tolerance of the problem.

Because of the distressing nature of COPD it is not uncommon for a person with this disorder to become discouraged and depressed. COPD may force the affected person to make numerous changes in life style and to abandon pleasurable activities. Emotional support must be realistic, sensitive, flexible, and freely given.

It is essential that the patient not neglect any aspects of the treatment regimen. In general, the patient can most thoroughly follow the prescribed treatment program by establishing and adhering to a scheduled routine. The nurse can help the patient construct a timetable that lists in order the various recommended treatment activities and when they should be performed.

People with COPD commonly experience their greatest difficulty upon arising. It may take an hour or longer before the routine activities of the day can be started, e.g., grooming, eating, dressing. The patient may need to get up earlier or arrange to start work later than formerly to allow time for necessary morning treatments, e.g., aerosolized bronchodilator, IPPB, oxygen, steam inhalation, postural drainage, breathing exercises.

Factors adversely affecting prognosis *with COPD include: (1) cor pulmonale, particularly if one or more episodes of congestive heart failure have occurred; (2) polycythemia; (3) impaired gas exchange (low diffusing capacity); and (4) severe ventilatory impairment with hypoxemia and hypercapnia.*

Bronchial Asthma

Definition. Although chronic bronchitis and pulmonary emphysema both produce continuous airway obstruction, bronchial asthma produces obstruction of an intermittent nature (unless complicated with COPD). The word "asthma" comes from the Greek word for "panting" and refers to *attacks* of shortness of breath (dyspnea). The asthmatic patient experiences recurrent *paroxysms* of dyspnea that characteristically are of a wheezing type, produced by obstruction of air flow in the bronchioles and smaller bronchi. Asthma is characterized by bronchospasm, mucosal edema, and excessive mucus.

Bronchial asthma is typically an intermittent *or* reversible *type of obstructive lung disease in which the widespread narrowing of bronchial lumina (bronchospasm) changes in severity over brief periods of time either spontaneously or as a result of treatment. Bronchial asthma is also characterized by an increased responsiveness of the tracheobronchial smooth muscle and mucous glands to various stimuli.*

Some people have mild, uncomplicated asthma that produces symptoms only occasionally, whereas others have chronic, severe asthma. *Persons who have had asthma for years commonly develop anatomic pulmonary emphysema and cor pulmonale; bronchitis and bronchiectasis are other possible complications.*

Asthmatics classified as having COPD have some degree of *persistent* airway obstruction. Persons who have both asthma and bronchitis, in addition to persistent (although variable) airway obstruction, are said to have "chronic asthmatic bronchitis" and are classified as having COPD.

Bronchial asthma is not due to cardiovascular disease. The condition called *cardiac asthma* (due to left ventricular failure) also produces wheezing respirations. The clinical management of this condition is entirely different from that of bronchial asthma and is not discussed here.

Etiology. Bronchial asthma has basically two forms, extrinsic or intrinsic. (See Table 55–8.)

- *Extrinsic (atopic) asthma* is caused by external agents such as dust, lint, insecticides, mold spores, pollens, food items, synthetic drugs (e.g., aspirin), animal danders, and feathers. This form is best understood and is a reaction to specific allergens. (See Chapter 10.) In many cases the history of hypersensitivity to external agents can be confirmed by skin testing. Most commonly extrinsic asthma develops in children or young adults. While attacks are acute, they are often self-limiting. Often this condition is outgrown; however, it may become chronic.

TABLE 55-8. CLINICAL CHARACTERISTICS OF EXTRINSIC (ATOPIC) AND INTRINSIC (NONATOPIC) ASTHMA

	Extrinsic, Atopic (Allergic)	Intrinsic, Nonatopic (Infective/Idiopathic)
Onset of symptoms	Usually during childhood	Usually in adults over age 35
Family history of atopy	Positive	Usually negative
History of infantile eczema	Positive	Negative
Identifiable allergy to inhaled and ingested substances	Positive	Negative
Passive transfer of IgE (skin-sensitizing) antibody	Positive	Negative
Reactions to skin test with inhalant allergens	Positive	Negative
Association with Type I, IgE reaction	Positive	Negative
Eosinophilia	Positive	Positive
In vitro release of histamine from washed leukocytes	Positive	Negative
Hyposensitization therapy	Favorable response	Equivocal
Typical attack	Acute and usually self-limiting	Often fulminant and severe
Relationship of acute attack to infection	May be present	Often present
Symptoms and physical findings	Identical for both types of asthma	
Aspirin sensitivity	Negative	Positive
Prognosis	Generally favorable	Less favorable
Death during acute attack	Rare	May occur

From Weiss, E. B.: Bronchial asthma. *Clinical Symposia,* 27:39, 1975.

The prognosis is generally favorable and death rare.

Extrinsic asthma results from the sensitization of an atopic person to specific allergens, so that exposure to even minute amounts of those allergens precipitates an acute asthmatic attack. The main component of the attack is the production of histamine in the cells of the bronchial mucosa. Allergic disorders of the respiratory tract are most commonly caused by such inhalant allergies as pollens (particularly the ragweed family), household dusts, and animal danders. Patients with extrinsic asthma commonly smoke cigarettes and have chronic bronchitis (with or without pulmonary emphysema). Any of these conditions may produce dyspnea, wheezing, hypersecretion of mucus, and severe, paroxysmal episodes of coughing.

► *Intrinsic (nonatopic) asthma* is also called "infectious" or "infective asthma" — an unsuitable phrase which incorrectly implies that asthma can be communicable. Intrinsic asthma, in which the specific cause frequently cannot be identified, is difficult to understand. Often the precipitating cause is predominantly infection in the upper (nose, sinuses) or lower (bronchi, lungs) respiratory tract. Enlarged adenoids, nasal polyps or spurs, or sinus infections may be present. Intrinsic asthma may begin at any age, but most commonly develops after age 35. Attacks tend to be more fulminant and severe. Prognosis is poorer. It develops into a lifelong chronic condition in which attacks gradually increase in frequency and severity. The condition often merges into asthmatic bronchitis; at times emphysema coexists. Death may occur.

With intrinsic asthma the respiratory tract reacts to infections, but it is usually not possible to prove the presence of sensitivity to specific infecting organisms by skin tests. Also, a correlation does not exist between the development of reinfections and attacks of asthma. A theory of etiology which focuses on probable hypersensitivity to bacteria has been proposed to explain why intrinsic asthma occurs; however, evidence for this theory is not convincing. It is not uncommon for patients who have had extrinsic asthma to later develop intrinsic asthma.

The basic cause of bronchial asthma is an inherited tendency (called *atopy*) to develop a hypersensitivity reaction of the antigen-antibody type. The reaction is manifested physically by bronchospasm and skin wheals. Usually persons with asthma (extrinsic or intrinsic) give a family medical history which includes hypersensitivity (e.g., asthma, rhinitis, eczema) as well as a personal medical history of allergic disorders such as eczema, urticaria, dermatitis, or hay fever. When both parents have allergies, about 75 per cent of their children will also be allergic.

Secondary factors may perpetuate asthmatic attacks and may profoundly influence the severity and frequency of these attacks. Examples of these factors are emotional stress, fatigue, endocrine changes (menopause, pregnancy, puberty, menstruation), environmental changes (in humidity and temperature), and exposure to noxious fumes (paints, chemicals, smoke). These factors precipitate symptoms by upsetting the delicate balance maintained between the patient and his allergic environment.

> *"Asthmatic" attacks occurring in persons with chronic bronchitis and/or emphysema may indicate that the patient is experiencing an acute exacerbation of established chronic airway obstruction. Such a condition can progress rapidly to hypoxia, hypercapnia, and respiratory acidosis.*

Pathology. Pathologically a bronchial asthma attack is characterized by: (1) bronchi plugged with thick, tenacious, slightly cloudy mucus; (2) bronchial walls contracted (owing to spasm or increased bronchial smooth muscle tone) and thickened (as a result of acute inflammation and edema); (3) hyperactive mucous glands; and (4) hyperinflation of alveoli, alveolar ducts, and respiratory bronchioles. Note that breakdown of the alveolar walls is *not* characteristic of asthma, as it is with anatomic pulmonary emphysema, and that mucous glands are *not* increased in number (as with chronic bronchitis).

General pathophysiologic considerations in asthma are:[158]

- Control of bronchi by autonomic nervous system.
- Bronchoconstriction may be produced by vagal cholinergic stimulation and with beta-adrenergic blockers.
- Histamine may also produce bronchoconstriction.
- Most of the sympathetic influence on the lung is humoral.

The following pathophysiologic events typically occur *during an asthmatic attack*: airway resistance is increased; residual volume of the lung is increased; abnormal intrapulmonary gas-mixing occurs; CO_2 is retained; and arterial O_2 saturation is decreased. Respiratory alkalosis (arterial pH ↑ 7.45) may occur early if there is hyperventilation, or respiratory acidosis (arterial pH ↓ 7.35) may develop as a result of airway obstruction. Respiratory function tests are often normal between asthmatic attacks. However, ventilatory impairment remains with some patients, especially persons who have had asthma for a number of years.

During an acute asthmatic attack, air movement is impaired during expiration because of constricted edematous bronchial lumina, which are filled with excess secretions. Characteristically a wheeze occurs and expiration is prolonged. The wheeze is produced as air is forced through the constricted bronchi. The lungs appear hyperextended and voluminous. The alveoli are greatly distended. As the attack worsens, a temporary emphysema-like situation occurs with air trapping and ballooning. Air trapping occurs after air enters the alveoli because the bronchial lumina narrow during the expiratory effort. Air trapping not only distends alveolar walls but also weakens them.

In allergic forms of asthma the local bronchial reaction is due to antigen-antibody combination. In addition to the tissue changes already mentioned, increased capillary permeability occurs and increased numbers of eosinophils appear in the tissues, peripheral blood, and secretions.

Symptoms. As stated, asthmatic attacks are paroxysmal and vary in frequency, intensity, and duration. Most commonly the attacks are of short duration. Between attacks the patient may be asymptomatic, or some symptoms may persist, especially upon exertion or during extremes in emotion.

Attacks frequently begin suddenly, without warning, even when the patient is at rest. Typically the patient suddenly becomes short of breath and feels as if suffocating or drowning. In an attempt to obtain relief the person sits up or stands up and leans forward. Devoting enormous amounts of energy to breathing, the patient struggles to try to breathe slowly and deeply. Expiration is prolonged. Wheezing is most pronounced during expiration and can often be heard at some distance from the patient. Respirations are difficult, but the rate is frequently normal. Most often the patient is pale rather than cyanotic. However, cyanosis may occur with severe attacks.

Cough and sputum production commonly occur. Rales are easily auscultated. Initially the cough is dry and minimal, but as the attack increases in severity the cough becomes more pronounced and productive of large amounts of sputum. If infection is present the sputum is mucopurulent. Often termination of the attack is indicated by severe coughing and the expectoration of thick, tenacious sputum followed by a feeling of relief and clearing of the airways.

During severe attacks the chest is markedly distended and the neck veins bulge, owing to increased intrathoracic pressure caused by air trapping in the lungs. The increase in negative intrapleural pressure is also indicated by marked retraction of the intercostal, supraclavicular, and suprasternal spaces. The chest appears fixed in the inspiratory position, and accessory muscles of respiration are used in an attempt to increase the effectiveness of ventilatory efforts. Profuse perspiration often occurs as a result of increased sympathetic innervation, indicating the stress to which the patient is being subjected and the effort being expended. After a severe attack the patient's chest may be quite sore.

Symptoms may subside in less than an hour, may persist for several hours, or may last for several days if status asthmaticus develops. *Status asthmaticus* is an acute, critical, distressing episode of bronchospasm that is not relieved by conventional bronchodilator therapy. This is an exhausting condition of sustained shortness of breath that is intractable to ordinary treatment methods and produces respiratory insufficiency and hypoxia. These attacks may last for days without relief and may terminate in death. (Treatment is discussed later in this section.)

Other types of acute asthmatic attacks are seldom fatal. They are, however, serious, frightening, and exhausting experiences. Acute asthmatic attacks may be dangerous in persons with cardiac disorders and in elderly persons. *During asthmatic attacks sudden death from respiratory exhaustion may occur, especially if sedatives are administered unwisely and too freely.*

Diagnosis. The differential diagnosis of bronchial asthma is usually made easily from : (1) a history of recurrent, paroxysmal attacks of dyspnea, cough, wheezing and production of mucoid sputum; (2) a family or personal history of allergy; (3) prolonged expiration with wheezing noises and musical rales; and (4) eosinophils in the sputum or blood.

Asthma does not produce characteristic chest x-ray findings. Pulmonary function studies are unnecessary for diagnosis. However, if performed, they may indicate that between attacks some air trapping continues (producing an increased volume of residual air). Often persons with extrinsic asthma have *elevated serum levels* of immune globulin E (IgE). Arterial hypoxemia (low PaO_2 may be present during severe attacks in which acute bronchospasm develops.

"All that wheezes is not asthma" is a phrase to remember during the process of establishing a differential diagnosis. Other conditions that produce symptoms similar to asthmatic attacks include heart failure (cardiac asthma), pulmonary embolism, endobronchial tuberculosis, obstructive pulmonary emphysema, bronchogenic carcinoma, and bronchial obstruction due to a foreign body.

Although it is relatively easy to make a differential diagnosis of bronchial asthma, it is more difficult to diagnose the specific etiology of the asthmatic attacks. When possible, a careful search is made to identify the causative agent. A thorough *history* is taken and includes exploration of familial susceptibility, environmental exposure, and secondary modifying factors such as psychogenic stimuli. Often nurses can compile such a history. *Skin testing* is employed to attempt to identify specific extrinsic allergens. (See Chapter 11.) The patient is also investigated for evidence of respiratory infections. Persons with asthma are investigated for both *sensitization* and *infection,* because they are often affected by both external allergens and infective factors.

Prevention of Asthmatic Attacks. Clinical care of persons with asthma is directed at providing immediate relief from acute attacks, reducing chronic symptoms (wheezing, coughing, shortness of breath), relief of hypoxemia, and minimizing the frequency of attacks. A calm reassuring manner aids in the control of the breathing pattern to produce more complete exhalation. Often the nurse participates in teaching ways in which to try to prevent asthmatic attacks. Long-term care, directed at controlling the causes of attacks, may include treatment of infection, emotional disorders, and allergies.

When *specific allergens* are identified as precipitating extrinsic asthmatic attacks, the patient is instructed about possible ways to avoid these allergens. Specific hyposensitization is also commonly performed by the physician. Food extracts are not used for hyposensitization. Foods to which the patient may be sensitive include milk, eggs, chocolate, wheat, and shellfish. Examples of medications to which the asthmatic may be sensitive include acetylsalicylic acid (aspirin), antibiotics, horse serum, and iodine preparations. (See also Chapter 11.)

When disorders such as chronic sinusitis, nasal polyps, and tonsillitis are present and are believed to contribute to asthmatic attacks, these conditions are treated appropriately. Currently tonsils and adenoids are less often removed than formerly because of their recognized importance in the immune response.

If *infection* is believed to contribute to asthmatic attacks, care is directed at preventing recurrent respiratory infections and instructing the patient to see a doctor promptly if infection appears to be developing.

Commonly *vaccines* are beneficial in chronic intrinsic asthma. Stock catarrhal vaccines are used cautiously because asthmatics may be highly sensitive to them. Autogenous vaccines may be prepared (from nasopharyngeal cultures or sputum cultures) and injected weekly. Some physicians give combinations of equal part of stock and autogenous vaccine to protect the patient against bacteria commonly acquired with respiratory infections as well as those bacteria that the patient is known to harbor.

The patient with asthma must also learn to avoid or to minimize *secondary factors* that can precipitate attacks of asthma, e.g., fatigue, emotional stress. Psychotherapy may be useful in helping some patients maintain an optimal state of mental well-being. Sometimes small amounts of tranquilizers or sedatives are prescribed to promote calmness, relaxation, and rest. Observations concerning a patient's activities immediately prior to an attack may be helpful in identifying factors that precipitate an attack. Such observations should be charted, they may help to prevent future attacks.

Persons with asthma should be informed of the importance of maintaining adequate *hydration.* Some asthmatic attacks are precipitated by dehydration of the mucous membranes. A person with asthma should drink 3000 to 4000 ml. of fluids per day, unless contraindicated by cardiac or renal disease.

Changes of climate (e.g., moves to warmer, drier climate) are sometimes recommended for a person with severe asthma that is refractory to usual medical treatment. The benefits to be derived from climatic changes vary, depending upon the specific etiology of a patient's asthma. Permanent

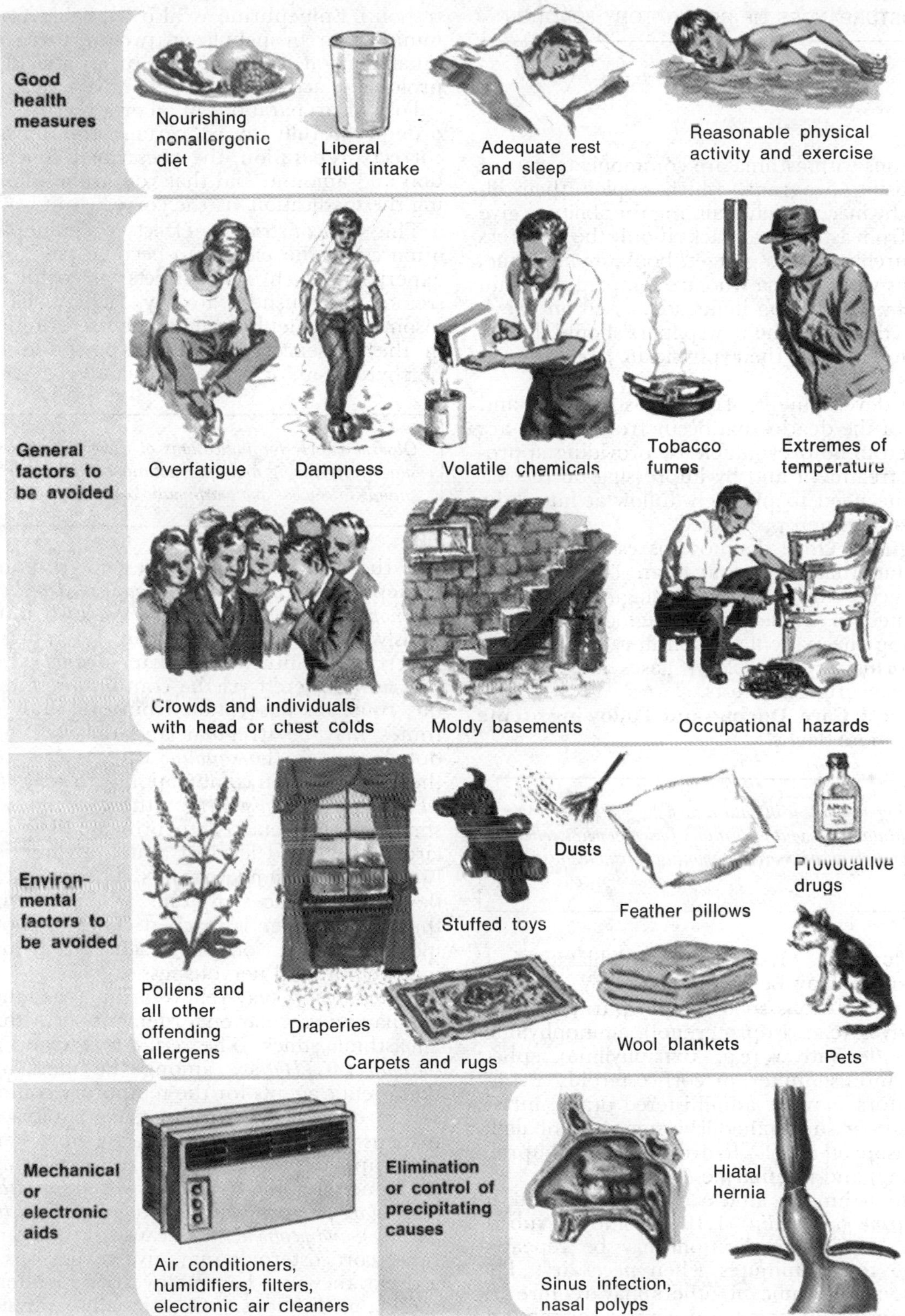

Figure 55–7. General management principles for the asthmatic patient. (© Copyright 1975 CIBA Pharmaceutical Company, Division of CIBA-Geigy Corporation. Reproduced, with permission, from *Clinical Symposia,* illustrated by Frank H. Netter, M.D. All rights reserved.)

moves should not be made until the patient has had a trial residence to determine the beneficial effects of such a change. It may be desirable for the patient to avoid fog, smog, and extremely cold weather.

Some patients benefit from the use of air conditioners equipped with special devices to filter out pollens. Keeping environmental air humidified may also be helpful. Some types of "air purifiers" are ineffective.

Persons with asthma are commonly targets of advertising programs which exploit their illnesses by inaccurately claiming the ability to give relief from asthmatic attacks if only the sufferers will purchase some gadget, book, or medicine. Persons with asthma who are tempted to obtain relief by purchasing items advertised on television, radio, or in the newspapers should discuss such items with their physician *prior* to purchase.

The development of status asthmaticus and many of the deaths that occur from asthma are believed to be preventable by providing appropriate treatment and by impressing on the patient the need to precisely follow at home the medical regimen prescribed.

Staging. Once diagnosis is established it is important that the severity of an acute asthmatic be staged. One method of staging asthma is presented in Table 55–9. Staging is done by assessing the patient's respiratory distress and monitoring arterial blood gases and bedside pulmonary function tests.

Clinical Care During and Following Acute Asthmatic Attacks.*

> *During an acute asthmatic attack the goals of care are to maintain efficient respiratory function while relieving bronchial spasm and promoting the expulsion of secretions.*

Medications. Relaxation and dilatation of the bronchi may be accomplished by administering medications such as epinephrine and its derivatives (e.g., isoproterenol), aminophylline and its derivatives (e.g., oxtriphylline), ephedrine, antihistamines, or corticosteroids. Bronchodilators may be administered orally, intravenously, or subcutaneously; some are inhaled, e.g., isoproterenol hydrochloride (Isuprel, Aludrine) and isoetharine (Bronkosol).

Most asthmatic attacks initially respond to *epinephrine (adrenalin)* 1:1000 solution, subcutaneously. The medication may be repeated after 5 to 15 minutes when necessary. The patient and significant others may require instructions about how to administer the medication by the subcutaneous route. In acutely ill patients, epinephrine 1:1000 may be administered intravenously — *cautiously* and *very slowly* because of vasoconstricting effects. (Monitor pulse rate and blood pressure during administration.) Epinephrine is also available for administration by nebulizer (two or three deep inhalations at the beginning of an attack). For prolonged activity it may be given intramuscularly in preparations in oil or glycerin. Check orders carefully to be certain you have the correct preparation, the prescribed concentration and amount, and that you are administering the medication via the correct route.

The vasoconstricting effects of epinephrine often cause the patient to become pale and to experience such side effects as palpitation, tremor, nervousness, anxiety, tachycardia, and insomnia. Epinephrine must be used cautiously in the presence of severe hypertension, hyperthyroidism, or heart disease.

> *Observe closely for indications of drug toxicity and side effects during and after administration of medications to combat acute asthmatic attacks.*

If the asthmatic attack does not respond to epinephrine, then *theophylline ethylenediamine (aminophylline)* may be given very slowly intravenously in saline (taking about 10 minutes to inject) or by intravenous drip. *Aminophylline* is best administered via the continuous intravenous route, as absorption from oral and rectal routes may be irregular and delayed. Aminophylline is in the *xanthine* category of drugs; these work well in combination with *sympathomimetic* or *beta-agonist drugs* (those drugs which stimulate the beta cell to bronchodilate). The circulating blood level of aminophylline is between 15 and 20 micrograms. The patient may develop systemic symptoms when the upper therapeutic range is reached. These symptoms include nausea, vomiting, tachycardia, insomnia, tremor, and nervousness.

Antihistamines may relieve asthma, as mucosal edema and vascular engorgement occur during an asthma attack. The *corticosteroids* and *corticotropin (ACTH)* are among the most useful therapeutic agents for the temporary control of severe or intractable asthma, e.g., status asthmaticus. It is not known exactly how steroids interrupt an asthmatic attack. Corticosteroids are generally used. *Corticosteroids are contraindicated in the presence of diabetes, tuberculosis (active or inactive), and peptic ulcer.* Because of the dramatic relief corticosteroids may give to persons with asthma, they may become overly dependent on these medications. Occasionally physicians maintain some patients on long-term therapy with prednisone or a similar corticosteroid. Sometimes, the use of an inhaler, e.g., Beclomethasone, provides the beneficial effects of corticosteroids with a minimum of side effects. In order to use the inhaler properly the patient is told that this inhaler must be used *regularly*, as prescribed, rather than for immediate relief.

*Emergency management is discussed in Chapter 95.

TABLE 55–9. STAGING OF THE SEVERITY OF AN ACUTE ASTHMA ATTACK

Stage	Symptoms and Signs	FEV_1 or FVC	pH	PaO_2	$PaCO_2$
I (mild)	Mild dyspnea; diffuse wheezes; adequate air exchange	50–80% of normal	N* or ↑	occasionally N or most often ↓	N or ↓
II (moderate)	Respiratory distress at rest; hyperpnea; marked wheezes; air exchange N or ↓	50% of normal	generally ↑	↓	generally ↓
III (severe)	Marked respiratory distress; marked wheezes or absent breath sounds; check for pulsus paradoxus >10 mm.; sternocleidomastoid retraction	25% of normal	N or ↓	↓	N or ↑
IV (respiratory failure)	Severe respiratory distress; lethargic; confused; prominent pulsus paradoxus; sternocleidomastoid retraction	10% of normal	↓ ↓	↓	↑ ↑

*N = normal. (Reproduced from The Merck Manual, 13th ed. Copyright under the Universal Copyright Convention and the International Copyright Convention 1977 by Merck & Co., Inc., Rahway, N.J., U.S.A.)

Numerous combination preparations are available for treating asthmatics, e.g., ephedrine hydrochloride or sulfate, aminophylline, and a sedative such as phenobarbital. The actions of *ephedrine* are similar to those of epinephrine but are milder. Since ephedrine taken by itself often evokes anxiety and tachycardia, it is desirable to give it in combination with medications that minimize these stimulatory effects. Ephedrine, epinephrine, and isoproterenol all reduce bronchospasm by relaxing the smooth muscle that lines the larger bronchioles and bronchi. Isoproterenol may cause adverse cardiac side effects. The trend now is toward *beta-selective adrenergic sympathomimetics.*

Sedatives are contraindicated in the treatment of severe asthma. Nervousness in persons with severe asthma is frequently caused by hypoxemia; the respiratory depression produced by sedation aggravates this. In addition, sedatives may depress the cough reflex. However, sedation is used at times in treating mild cases to counteract the overstimulation that bronchodilator medications sometimes produce. In a situation of this kind, phenobarbital or diazepam (Valium) may be administered orally. *Narcotics* are generally contraindicated because they depress respirations. However, at times they are used cautiously provided respirators are available if needed to mechanically support respiration. Morphine not only depresses respiration but also causes bronchoconstriction.

Persons with asthma may be given *mildly sedative cough mixtures* such as antihistamine mixtures with codeine or elixir of terpin hydrate with codeine to relieve excessive, nonproductive cough. *Expectorants,* (ammonium chloride or potassium iodide) may loosen thick, tenacious bronchial secretions.

Oxygen is usually administered during an acute asthmatic attack due to the hypoxemia associated with bronchospasm and excess mucus production. Prior to the administration of oxygen arterial blood gases must be drawn. The typical blood gas during the acute phase is one in which the pH and pCO_2 are alkalotic. The pO_2 will usually be reduced.

TABLE 55–10. ASTHMA THERAPY

Acute asthma
Mild to moderate
Ephedrine (oral)
Terbutaline (oral)
Metaproterenol (oral)
Aminophylline (oral)
Epinephrine (SC)
Terbutaline (SC)
Severe (status asthmaticus)
Oxygen by nasal cannula
Intravenous fluids
Aminophylline (I.V.)
Epinephrine (SC) or Terbutaline (SC)
Hydrocortisone (IV)
Chronic asthma
Ephedrine (oral)
Terbutaline (oral)
Metaproterenol (oral)
Aminophylline (oral)
Cromolyn sodium (inhalation)
Beclomethasone (inhalation)

Adapted from Sokol, W. N., and G. N. Beall: Asthma. *Hospital Medicine,* 13:10, May 1977.

TABLE 55–11. SIDE EFFECTS OF SOME COMMONLY USED ANTIASTHMATIC DRUGS

Drug	Side Effects
Sympathomimetic drugs (beta-stimulators)	
Epinephrine Ephedrine Isoproterenol Isoetharine Metaproterenol	Restlessness, anxiety, tremor, headaches, dizziness, palpitations, tachycardia, hypertension, cardiac arrhythmias, weakness, hyperglycemia, and urinary retention
Terbutaline	Same as above, plus muscle tremors
Aminophylline (theophylline)	Nausea, vomiting, epigastric pain, headaches, tachycardia, arrhythmias, nervousness, irritability, excitement, convulsions, diuresis, and vertigo
Cromolyn sodium	Cough, hoarseness, rash, hypersensitivity pneumonitis, and, rarely, anaphylaxis and vasculitis
Steroids	
Oral or parenteral	Fluid retention, hypertension, acne, weight gain, adrenal suppression, cataracts, gastritis, gastric ulcers, cushingoid state, hypokalemia, and psychosis
Inhaled (beclomethasone)	Cough, minor wheezing, hoarseness, and candidiasis of mouth and pharynx

From Ahmed, M., and C. Lindquist: Bronchial asthma: Some aspects of pathogenesis and therapy. *Postgraduate Medicine,* 62:111, July 1977.

An asthmatic patient with a normal pH and pCO_2 is in impending respiratory failure. Arterial blood gases must be frequently performed. Intubation equipment and a mechanical ventilator must be readily at hand. If the pH and pCO_2 should become acidotic, an artificial airway and ventilation must be instituted.

Infections that may be present are treated specifically when possible with *antibiotics* and *sulfonamides* to which the infecting organisms are known to be sensitive. Recurrent infections are common. Tetracyclines may be given before laboratory culture and sensitivity results are available. Although penicillin is a useful antibiotic for gram-positive infections, it (like horse serum) often tends to produce serious and sometimes fatal allergic reactions in asthmatics. Moreover, cross-allergenicity exists between the penicillins and the newer semisynthetic derivatives, e.g., ampicillin and oxacillin. A *sensitivity test* is performed prior to administering the first dose of penicillin when penicillin is ordered.

Penicillin and other related medications, e.g., ampicillin and oxacillin, must be used cautiously in asthmatic patients because of possible serious allergic reactions.

Once an acute asthmatic attack has passed, the patient may be started on *disodium cromoglycate* (sodium cromolyn, Aarane, Intal), a long-term maintenance drug. The action of this drug is to prevent the release of histamine, serotonin, and SRS-A by the mast cell in an antigen-antibody reaction causing bronchospasm. This drug, in powder form, is inhaled by the patient on a routine daily basis. The powdered medication is administered via a capsule placed in a device called a Spinhaler. The nurse must stress the importance of taking this drug on a *routine basis.* It must be used when the airway is at its most patent, that is, following the administration of bronchodilators and other therapy to open the airways. The patient must also be warned that this is a prophylactic medication and not one for treatment of an acute asthmatic attack. Disodium cromoglycate is primarily of value in the prevention of bronchospasm from extrinsic mechanisms. However, there has been success with this drug in the prevention of exercise-induced bronchospasm, especially running and swimming. Because it is not a stimulant, this drug may be legally used during competitive sports events.

Persons with asthma are given medications for *home use* during attacks. Because asthmatic attacks tend to vary in their severity and their response to chemotherapy, medications given the patient for home use may include (in the order to be used if necessary): (1) an adrenergic aerosol; (2) an oral preparation of ephedrine and/or theophylline; (3) aerosol steroid; and (4) sodium cromolyn if indicated.

Care Measures. Summarized below are activities of importance in the clinical care of a person *during* an acute asthmatic attack:

- Administer medications (bronchodilators, steroids, and oxygen) promptly to provide relief as soon as possible after the onset of attack.
- Observe for toxic affects of medications as well as therapeutic effects.
- Position the patient to breathe more comfortably

(Fig. 55–8); manually assist ventilation if indicated.

- Maintain clear airway; suction if indicated.
- Offer appropriate reassurance; provide constant care (do not leave patient alone during acute attack).
- Maintain quiet, restful environment; restrict visitors; minimize environmental irritants (e.g., remove feather pillows, prohibit smoking and flowers, maintain effective air conditioning); maintain emotional atmosphere in which patient feels comfortable expressing anxieties. Some patients are admitted to the hospital temporarily during an acute attack and are placed in an area where environmental control of allergies can be maintained.
- Minimize patient's exertion and fatigue by anticipating needs and providing assistance, e.g., with eating, drinking, as necessary. Discourage unnecessary talking.
- Evaluate frequently: rate and character of respirations; pulse; color of nail beds, mucous membranes and skin (observe for cyanosis); amount of perspiration; frequency and character of cough; amount and character of sputum (color, viscosity); emotional state; activity (e.g., restlessness); and physical stamina (fatigue, exhaustion). Monitor vital signs every four hours, or more frequently if indicated. Observe for indications of untoward side effects of therapy, e.g., arrhythmia, tachycardia, nausea and vomiting.
- Evaluate patient frequently for indications of need for respiratory therapy (e.g., indications of hypoxia, respiratory insufficiency). Provide oxygen therapy as indicated and ordered.
- Provide humidification of inspired air (steam, cool vapor).
- Prepare for and assist with emergency care, e.g., bronchoscopy, intubation, and continuous mechanical ventilation.

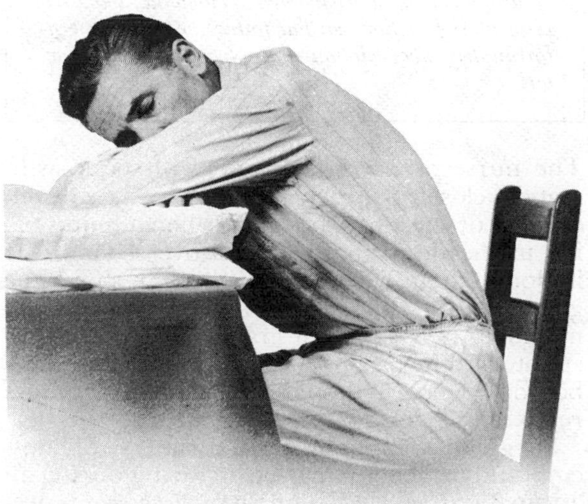

Figure 55–8. A comfortable position during an asthma attack. (From *Living with Asthma, Chronic Bronchitis, and Emphysema.* Riker Laboratories.)

- Observe for and report indications of infection, congestive heart failure, or other complications.
- Control excessive, unproductive cough without depressing respiratory reflexes.
- Use sedatives cautiously if ordered and indicated.
- Observe for indications of fluid-electrolyte and acid-base imbalances; provide appropriate care to prevent or correct. Maintain hydration and nutrition. Record intake and output. If indicated, force fluids to thin secretions.
- Protect against chilling; keep patient dry if diaphoretic; prevent drafts.

See Chapter 54 for the discussion on criteria for the institution of mechanical ventilation.

IPPB is contraindicated in some patients with asthma because it decreases the pulmonary capillary blood volume and thus decreases perfusion and arterial pO_2. During an asthmatic attack the patient may obtain some relief by practicing *breathing exercises* that enable control of breathing pattern and breathing efficiency.

The administration of topical bronchodilators and steroids may be accomplished by small-volume nebulizer or by IPPB. Deposition of particles is best accomplished when carried on a spontaneous deep breath. If the patient is too fatigued or uncooperative, positive pressure may be used.

It has long been recognized that patients with chronic bronchial asthma are unusually sensitive to *emotional factors.* Some patients appear to improve significantly when given reassurance, attention and optimistic treatment. Realizing that a patient may be frightened of another attack, the nurse stops in frequently and keeps the patient's call bell within easy reach. If the patient signals, the summons is answered quickly. At night it is reassuring to some patients to keep the room dimly lighted. Attempt to maintain an atmosphere that promotes relaxation. The nurse and the patient's significant others should realize that asthmatic attacks that may be precipitated by emotional factors *cannot* be controlled or stopped "if only the patient makes up his or her mind to do so." Because of the stressful nature of severe asthmatic attacks some patients are reluctant to leave the security of the hospital environment.

Following an acute asthmatic attack:

Attempt to identify and report any conditions you observed that may have *precipitated* the attack.

Ensure a period of undisturbed *rest* because the patient is usually exhausted. *Expectorants* may be given to help to remove tenacious secretions. *Postural drainage* with clapping and vibrating may be ordered to help to clear the tracheobronchial tree. Ample *fluid intake* is important following an attack to prevent dehydration.

Provide appropriate *patient-family teaching* based on identified needs. Areas emphasized may include: (1) describing the nature of asthma; (2) clarifying diagnostic tests, e.g., skin tests, and desensitization procedures; (3) preventive measures, e.g., prevention of respiratory infections, environmental control to avoid irritants, minimizing emotional strain, dietary restrictions, fluid intake; (4) care during an attack, e.g., medications used (their names, purposes, dosages, frequency of administration, undesirable side-effects, routes of administration) and how to administer them (e.g., injections, suppository insertion, aerosols); (5) pulmonary physiotherapy (e.g., breathing exercises, effective coughing, postural drainage); (6) any necessary activity restrictions; and (7) need for long-term medical supervision, follow-up care, long-term planning, rehabilitation procedures, and maintenance therapy. Advise the patient not to buy advertised medications or quack remedies, and that no medication should be taken without a doctor's permission. If the patient has known drug allergies, encourage wearing of a bracelet or tag that states the allergy.

Treatment of Status Asthmaticus. Status asthmaticus is a *medical emergency*. It is frequently caused by respiratory infection but may also occur as a result of a medication (e.g., acetylsalicylic acid), severe stress (worry, fatigue), persistent exposure to an allergen, withdrawal of previous corticosteroid medication, dyspnea (e.g., due to exposure to air pollutants, the presence of emphysema, or the occurrence of complications such as myocardial failure).

The use of antimicrobial and corticosteroid medications has improved the treatment of patients with status asthmaticus. The patient is always admitted to a hospital for environmental control, rest, close supervision, and intensive diagnostic and treatment procedures.

Once a patient is hospitalized for the treatment of status asthmaticus the *initial orders* typically include the following:

- Bed rest in orthopneic position. This promotes rest and relieves dyspnea.
- Cover pillows with allergen-proof covers; eliminate pollen contact, dust factors, and other irritating inhalants (e.g., smoke); give no acetylsalicylic acid, penicillin, or opiates. This prevents exposure to allergens and medications to which patient may be sensitive. Avoid overuse of medications such as sedatives and narcotics, *which cause respiratory depression.*
- Soft (5 Gm. salt) diet; force fluids; monitor intake and output. Maintain hydration and nutrition. Food allergens to which the patient is known to be sensitive are eliminated from the diet. IV's may be given slowly to maintain adequate hydration until sufficient oral intake is possible. During prolonged IV administration, serum electrolytes are monitored and adjusted.
- Sputum for culture and drug-sensitivity tests and eosinophil count (guide to future specific treatment). Specimen is taken prior to giving first dose of antimicrobial drugs.
- Tetracycline. *(Immediate antimicrobial treatment* is started before sputum culture reports are returned because respiratory infection often precipitates status asthmaticus).
- Corticosteroids. *(Corticosteroids are very effective* in treating status asthmaticus. Infusions of hydrocortisone are given separately from other infusions.)
- Bronchodilators, e.g., aminophylline. IV, stat; IV drip. Methylxanthines and $beta_2$-adrenergic drugs work well in combination and are the drugs of choice.
- Chloral hydrate, if necessary for sleep. *(Use minimal effective dose to ensure rest without depressing respiratory reflexes.)*
- Chest roentgenogram, stat (necessary to make differential diagnosis). Roentgenogram of nasal sinuses (to locate foci of infection).
- Electrocardiogram, stat. If present, heart failure is appropriately treated.
- Complete blood count and urinalysis.
- Blood for urea nitrogen, CO_2, sodium, potassium, chloride, sugar, sedimentation rate. Arterial blood gases are always followed carefully. Arterial blood gas values are determined as soon as possible and are repeated every 30 to 60 minutes until the patient is clearly improved. A normal or rising $PaCO_2$ is serious. The patient will require an artificial airway and CMV.

At times patients in status asthmaticus die. The causes of death are most commonly pneumonia, impaired respiratory function, cardiac failure, or acidosis. Unfortunately, oversedation is also too frequently a factor.

The nurse observes the patient in status asthmaticus closely for early indications of the development of these *complications.* When administering medications guard against oversedation. If in doubt about whether a medication should be given, check with the attending physician. Remember, it is more desirable to preserve respiratory reflexes, even though the patient may be somewhat restless, than to depress these reflexes by oversedating the patient.

Surgical Treatment of Asthma. Bronchoscopy and intubation may be lifesaving during an asthmatic attack. Occasionally *bronchoscopy* is necessary to aspirate secretions trapped in the tracheobronchial tree or to irrigate the airways. Secretions blocking the airways may seriously impair alveolar oxygen and carbon dioxide exchange and may produce atelectasis and respiratory insufficiency. Endotracheal *intubation* facilitates repeated secretion aspiration, irrigation of the airways, humidification, and ventilation when indicated.

Numerous *surgical procedures* have been suggested to treat patients with chronic bronchial asthma; however, these procedures are unsuccessful. Various functional types of surgery have attempted to relieve bronchospasm by inhibiting nervous influences traveling via the sympathetic or parasympathetic (vagal) system, or both.

Chronic Bronchitis

Definition and Incidence. *Chronic bronchitis is a chronic inflammation of the tracheobronchial tree with recurrent cough and sputum production.* Chronic bronchitis is more precisely defined as a *clinical* disorder characterized by the hypersecretion of bronchial mucus, and accompanied by a chronic or recurrent productive cough. The symptoms must occur for a minimum of three months a year for at least two consecutive years before the condition can be accurately diagnosed as chronic bronchitis. Also, other possible causes of the symptoms must be excluded.

> *Chronic bronchitis is almost always associated with heavy cigarette smoking. Heavy smokers have a* very high *incidence of chronic bronchitis.*

Chronic bronchitis occurs principally among middle-aged or elderly men, particularly in city dwellers.

The prevalence and activity of chronic bronchitis increase during periods of fog and cold, wet weather. It is thus not surprising that there is an extremely high incidence of chronic bronchitis in England — a foggy, highly industrialized country. Also, in the United States *chronic bronchitis is a leading cause of disability, and its incidence continues to increase.*

As stated in the discussion of COPD, both chronic bronchitis and pulmonary emphysema are present in the vast majority of patients with COPD. These conditions present similar clinical features, appear to have a common etiologic basis, and are treated by essentially the same procedures. Chronic bronchitis commonly precedes and complicates pulmonary emphysema. Nonetheless, some patients with chronic bronchitis, at autopsy, have almost no structural pulmonary emphysema, and some patients with terminal destructive pulmonary emphysema have almost no bronchitis.

Etiology. Chronic bronchitis develops in response to repeated irritation, e.g., from cigarette smoke, air pollution (toxic industrial gases, irritating dusts, smokes, chemicals), and infections (low-grade chronic pulmonary infections, pneumonia, influenza). Possibly heredity is important. Other factors that promote the progression of chronic bronchitis include inadequate bronchial drainage; narrow compressed or constricted bronchi; inadequate circulation; pulmonary fibrosis; and mechanical distortions. In addition to commonly occurring with pulmonary emphysema, chronic bronchitis also frequently accompanies pulmonary tuberculosis, chronic bronchial asthma, pulmonary fibrosis, chronic sinusitis, bronchiectasis, and kyphoscoliosis.

Onset. Chronic bronchitis is a serious, progressive, potentially fatal illness of insidious onset. Some persons with chronic bronchitis never experience more than a chronic or recurrent cough productive of mucoid sputum (cough may persist for years without causing respiratory distress), whereas others suffer progressive breathlessness, repeated pulmonary infections, and eventually succumb to respiratory failure. Commonly chronic bronchitis progresses over a period of years and is punctuated with periodic acute exacerbations. Bronchopneumonia is a frequent complication of acute periods.

Many people neglect chronic bronchitis until it is advanced. The bronchitic individual's *medical history* typically includes habitual cigarette smoking, a habitual morning cough (commonly ascribed to smoking), and an increasing tendency to expectorate for progressively longer periods after every cold. Gradually the duration of cough and the amount of sputum increase over the years until these symptoms are steadily present. Because these symptoms develop gradually, the patient may not notice their worsening.

This pattern of insidious development is indeed unfortunate because if the patient followed relatively simple precautions and received vigorous treatment when the bronchitis was of a mild degree, permanent lung damage might be limited.

> *Unhappily, chronic bronchitis often becomes increasingly severe and eventually becomes merely a part of progressively fatal disorders, e.g., cor pulmonale, pulmonary emphysema.*

Prevention. Like lung cancer, pulmonary emphysema, and some other respiratory disorders, *chronic bronchitis can often be prevented* by relatively simple precautions. Since chronic bronchitis seldom occurs among nonsmokers, the *prevention* of this disorder is possible to a large extent by the elimination of cigarette smoking. It is also important to prevent or alleviate air pollution and occupational exposure to fumes and dust. Nurses play an important role in the prevention of chronic bronchitis by providing instruction about the hazards of cigarette smoking and air pollution, and by encouraging persons with symptoms of respiratory disorders to seek *early* evaluation and treatment.

Pathology. Pathologically chronic bronchitis is characterized by chronic inflammation of the bronchial wall, mucosal edema, and hypertrophy, hypersecretion, and hyperplasia of bronchial mucous glands and epithelial mucous goblet cells. The increase in the size and number of mucous glands and cells is noticeable clinically by the increased production of sputum. Additionally, there is usually some emphysema (enlargement of the air spaces caused by breakdown of the alveolar walls).

Chronic bronchitis causes the bronchi to appear thick and inelastic. The bronchial surface may be dry or covered with mucus and pus, and is dark red in color. Cilia are absent. The epithelium, mucous glands, and muscular layers are deformed. Diverticula ("pockets") in the bronchi result from the openings of enlarged mucous glands. Bronchiectasis is frequently present in the form of cylindrical bronchial dilations.

Because of degenerative changes in the bronchi (e.g., destruction of cilia), the patient's normal mechanisms for removing sputum, bacteria, and so forth, from the lungs are ineffective and it is necessary to cough increasingly in order to try to clear the lungs. Ineffective bronchial drainage promotes the retention of pus and mucus and the obstruction of air passages. Hence, repeated pulmonary infections occur frequently, and the mucous membranes are usually chronically inflamed and infected. Bronchospasm may aggravate the various dysfunctions associated with chronic bronchitis. Narrowing of the smaller airways produces dyspnea, wheezing, and impaired gas exchange.

It is not unusual for chronic bronchitis to progress with structural destruction of the alveolar walls and alveolar capillary bed. These irreversible lung changes may cause *serious obstructive problems.* Chronic bronchitis with obstruction may produce the following lung function findings: *increased* residual lung volume, and *reduced* vital capacity, maximum breathing capacity, and timed vital capacity (slow retarded expiration). Increased resistance to airflow is the first change in pulmonary function caused by chronic bronchitis. This produces some degree of alveolar hypoventilation; i.e., even though the tidal volume may be normal, the O_2 and CO_2 exchange is insufficient. Obstructed expiratory air flow may result from bronchial scarring, bronchial spasm, mucus obstructing the bronchi, and thickening of bronchial walls (from edema and inflammation). All these factors reduce the size of the lumina of the bronchi. Air trapping in the alveoli and bronchioles results from obstruction of air flowing during expiration.

As chronic bronchitis progresses, *hypoventilation* is indicated by an increased arterial pCO_2 and reduced pO_2. Pulmonary hypertension, cor pulmonale (right ventricular hypertrophy), right heart failure, and respiratory failure often develop.

Symptoms. Commonly the symptoms of chronic bronchitis worsen during cold, damp weather. *Persistent cough* and *sputum production* are principal symptoms. Often more than one ounce of odorless sputum is produced daily; it may be white (mucoid), gray, mucopurulent, or purulent. Microscopic examination of sputum reveals many kinds of bacteria. Organisms most commonly isolated include the influenza bacillus, pneumococci, staphylococci, streptococci, and Friedländer's bacillus. Occasionally sputum is blood-tinged following severe coughing. Usually sputum is tenacious. The cough may be loose, rattling, and constant or paroxysmal, with severe spasms lasting several minutes. Commonly the cough is worse in the morning and the evening. Chest expansion is usually reduced. Bronchial exudate may produce rales that are sonorous and moist, squeaking or wheezing. The patient may experience a sensation of heaviness in the chest.

Acute episodes of febrile infection tend to occur several times each winter. Between these episodes the patient with chronic bronchitis is characteristically afebrile, with no change in WBC or ESR. Attacks of bronchopneumonia may cause a sudden worsening in the patient's condition.

During periods of acute exacerbations the patient may suddenly develop severe, potentially fatal hypoxia, hypercapnia, acidosis, and cor pulmonale. These abnormalities may not be present between periods of exacerbation. However, gradually, with disease progression, chronic hypoxia, hypercapnia, and cor pulmonale may develop.

With progression and worsening of chronic bronchitis the patient develops: obstructive symptoms (e.g., uses accessory muscles for ventilation and purses the lips during prolonged expiration); symptoms of hypoxia and hypercapnia; increasing dyspnea of an asthmatic nature; wheezing respirations; and incapacitating paroxysms of coughing. The patient's color is usually dusky or cyanotic. Emphysema may gradually be superimposed and obstructive symptoms predominate. Exertional dyspnea gradually curtails the patient's physical activity. Dyspnea does not usually occur in early chronic bronchitis, but appears with COPD. Death may result from irreversible respiratory failure or may occur during an acute, possibly reversible, exacerbation.

Diagnosis. Chronic bronchitis is easily *diagnosed* from a history of a chronic, productive cough. Ventilatory function and respiratory gas exchange tests are performed to evaluate the severity of the condition. Also, the patient's respiratory system is carefully examined to establish a differential diagnosis and to detect other serious pulmonary disorders. The volume of sputum raised per day may be measured to evaluate severity of the disorder.

An ordinary chest film does not demonstrate characteristic abnormalities in the presence of chronic bronchitis, but bronchograms will show the following characteristic changes: diverticula, cylindrical dilations, "accordion-like" irregularities, and small round terminal expansions of the bronchial tree. Routine bacteriologic sputum examination seldom provides information of value. Cytologic examination of sputum, however, may be useful. For example, some "purulence" may be caused by eosinophils. This indicates the need to investigate and treat allergic aspects of the disorder.

Clinical Care. Clinical care of persons with chronic bronchitis (and pulmonary emphysema) is basically the same as that previously discussed for people with COPD. *Care focuses on* reducing or controlling symptoms, e.g., improving ventilation and respiration, relieving bronchospasm; minimizing progression of disease by reducing bronchial irritation; preventing additional tissue damage by preventing or controlling complications. Success of therapy rests largely upon the nurse's ability to skillfully give and coordinate the necessary clinical care and the patient's ability to thoroughly perform aspects of self-care that are essential for functioning at an optimal level.

Discussed below are some factors of particular importance in the *clinical care of patients with chronic bronchitis (and pulmonary emphysema).*

► *Minimize bronchial irritation,* e.g., by removing or reducing chemical irritants and by avoiding acute respiratory infections. Reduce exposure to general air pollution and occupational atmospheric hazards. It is imperative that smoking be stopped. Job changes may be necessary. The patient may be advised by the physician to live in a mild climate. A home air-conditioning unit with an effective filtration system may help to minimize bronchial irritation. A relatively high humidity should be maintained in the home, especially during cold months, Nasal breathing (rather than mouth breathing) is

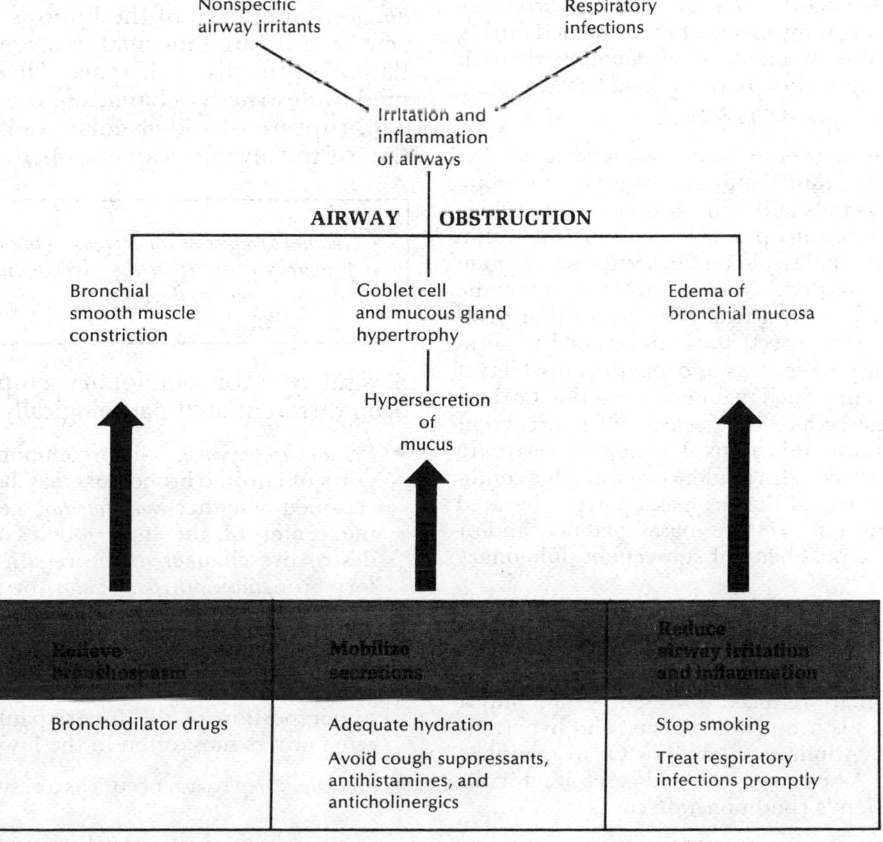

Figure 55-9. Causes and treatment of chronic bronchitis. (From Speir, W. A., Jr.: How to improve management of chronic obstructive lung disease. *Consultant*, 17:168, May 1977.)

encouraged, so inspired air can be normally warmed, filtered, and humidified in the nasal passages. Known allergens should be avoided. (See discussion of allergens in previous section on bronchial asthma). Cold drinks may precipitate coughing. Also, coughing may be precipitated by rhinitis and postnasal drip. Antihistamines may be given to control these nasal and postnasal problems. Codeine phosphate or a comparable antitussive may be used to mildly suppress nonproductive, irritating cough.

- *Control chronic respiratory infections and promptly treat intercurrent acute infections,* e.g., with antibiotics, expectorants, bronchodilators. The patient should seek medical care at the *beginning of any* respiratory infection or "flu." If sputum becomes purulent, antibiotics may be indicated.
- *Relieve bronchospasm and combat air trapping.* Bronchospasm may be relieved with ephedrine sulfate or related drugs, or isoetharine in solution by nebulization. Aminophylline may also be used to relieve bronchospasm. Antihistamines may help to relieve bronchial inflammation. Persistent bronchospasm that cannot be relieved with simple bronchodilators and physiotherapy may be treated with a course of corticosteroids to reduce bronchial inflammation. Many bronchitics are helped during winter months by taking small amounts daily of prednisone and they have no problem stopping the drug once winter passes.
- *Prevent or minimize acute intercurrent respiratory infections* by having annual influenza injection, avoiding exposure to colds and "flu" at home or in public, and maintaining an optimal level of general health. Undue emotional strain and excessive weight gain should be avoided. During winter months the patient may prophylactically be given either penicillin or a broad-spectrum antimicrobial medication to reduce the severity and length of disability if infection occurs. Such maintenance antibiotic therapy does not reduce the *frequency* of intercurrent acute respiratory infections. The upper airways are carefully inspected for evidence of treatable conditions (e.g., infected sinuses, nasal polyps, deviated nasal septum) to restore nasal patency and/or minimize the possibility of subsequent pulmonary infections.
- *Minimize dyspnea* by breathing retraining and control of breathing. An electrocardiogram is performed for diagnostic purposes, and obesity and hypertension are reduced if present. Commonly a triad of chronic bronchitis, obesity, and hypertension occurs. Administer low flow O_2 to minimize hypoxemia. Assess arterial blood gases at intervals and if a patient's condition worsens.
- *Facilitate raising of sputum and clearing of air passages; support ventilation and respiration.* Frequently a physiotherapist can best support these activities, following them with postural and breathing exercises. The patient is taught how to cough effectively, perform breathing exercises, and perform postural drainage. It is necessary to *meticulously* follow a pattern of thorough tracheobronchial and oral hygiene and to force fluids to prevent dehydration and drying of secretions. Steam, mist, or other inhalants may help the patient to clear air passages. Nebulization with warm normal saline may be employed to moisten the respiratory mucosa. Postural drainage is especially important if bronchiectasis is also present.

IPPB using air, combined with bronchodilator aerosols, may be useful if marked bronchial obstruction is present and ventilatory capacity is reduced. These treatments may be given for 10 to 20 minutes several times per day. If oxygen therapy is necessary it is given cautiously to prevent CO_2 narcosis.

Pulmonary Emphysema

Definitions and Types. The word "emphysema" comes from the Greek word *emphysan,* meaning to "puff up with air." Emphysema is actually a *pathologic diagnosis* only, not a clinical diagnosis. In the United States the term "emphysema" has been overused and misused as a clinical diagnosis. "Emphysema" means that destruction of lung tissue has occurred and an *anatomic* alteration of the lungs is present, characterized by an abnormal enlargement (overinflation) of the distal air spaces (alveoli) accompanied by destructive changes of the alveolar walls, e.g., rupture of the alveolar walls and destruction of the alveolar capillary bed.

> *Pulmonary emphysema is not a single entity but rather is primarily a defect in the alveolar walls that may result from various diseases.*

Several *types* of pulmonary emphysema have been differentiated pathologically.

- *Primary emphysema,* which commonly occurs after years of chronic bronchitis, may be pathologically classified as either *centrilobular,* i.e., beginning in the center of the lung lobules and producing destructive changes in the region of the respiratory bronchiole; or *panlobular* (or panacinar), i.e., occurring throughout the lung and characterized by the generalized dilatation of air spaces of secondary lobules.* The centrilobular type is the most common and has a predilection for the upper portion of the lungs; panlobular emphysema occurs most often in the lower lungs.
- *Secondary emphysema* occurs as a result of any condi-

*Secondary lobules consist of three to five terminal bronchioles and their associated respiratory tissue.

tion that causes scarring or fibrosis in the lung. This type of pulmonary emphysema is pathologically classified as the *paracicatricial* (or traction) type and is characterized by alveolar wall destruction and alveolar overdistention adjacent to fibrotic pulmonary lesions. The focal air cysts produced are generally called "blebs," "bullae," or "pneumatoceles." Usually the smaller lesions are referred to as "blebs," whereas the larger air cysts (over 1 inch in diameter) are called "bullae."

Paracicatricial emphysema and the lobular types of emphysema, e.g., centrilobular or panlobular, may occur within the same lung. When large, thin-walled air spaces (bullae) are created by the destruction of numerous alveoli and interlobular septa, a bronchial communication is commonly present which acts like a check valve and causes air trapping.

The type of pulmonary emphysema under discussion in this section is chronic destructive pulmonary emphysema associated with obstructive lung disease. This discussion does *not* pertain to (1) *senile or atrophic emphysema,* a decreased state of pulmonary elasticity which normally occurs with aging and is accompanied by only minimal impairment of function; (2) *compensatory emphysema,* the simple and nonobstructive overinflation of lung which occurs as lung tissue expands to fill a space produced by the contraction or surgical removal of another pulmonary segment or lobe; (3) *nondestructive overinflation of alveoli* secondary to a check-valve, air-trapping type of bronchial obstruction (produced by tumors, secretions, or foreign bodies obstructing a bronchial lumen or occurring during acute bronchial asthmatic attacks); (4) *skeletal emphysema,* associated with distortion and immobility of the thorax due to kyphosis; or (5) *subcutaneous, mediastinal, or interstitial emphysemas,* which are not pulmonary disorders but result from injuries that cause air leakage into other body tissues or spaces.

Incidence

> *Emphysema is by far the most common chronic lung condition and is the major cause of pulmonary disability. Emphysema occurs more often than tuberculosis and lung cancer combined.*

It is believed that more than 10 million persons in the United States have frank emphysema, and more than 20 million others have some form of COPD (e.g., bronchitis, asthma) bordering on emphysema. Chronic bronchitis and emphysema most often occur in cold, damp climates among white males who are middle-aged or older (50 to 70). The incidence of these disorders is increasing among females, however, presumably owing to increasing habitual cigarette smoking among women.

Most persons over age 40 who have asthma and chronic bronchitis also have pulmonary emphysema. *Chronic bronchitis and emphysema are the fastest rising causes of death in the United States. Only heart disease surpasses emphysema as a major cause of disability.*

Etiology. We have previously discussed factors of *etiologic* significance in the development

TABLE 55-12. DIFFERENTIATING BETWEEN CHRONIC BRONCHITIS AND EMPHYSEMA

	Chronic Bronchitis	Emphysema
Exposure to airway irritants	Almost invariably a history of cigarette smoking	Usually a history of cigarette smoking
Presenting symptom	Persistent cough and sputum production	Gradually progressive exertional dyspnea
Dyspnea	Variable	Persistent
Respiratory infections	Frequent episodes of wheezing, dyspnea, and purulent sputum	Infrequent respiratory infections
Physical examination	Tendency to overweight Expiratory wheezes	Tendency to thinness Expiratory wheezes may not be prominent Diminished basilar breath sounds that do not increase in intensity with deep breathing
Chest film	May be normal "Dirty chest" with increased bronchovascular markings	Overinflation Flattened hemidiaphragms Increased retrosternal air space Increased lucency of lower third of lung fields
Pulmonary function tests	Reduction in FEF (forced expiratory flow) 25% to 75% (early) Reduction in FEV_1 (later) Normal diffusing capacity	Reduction in FEF 25% to 75% Reduction in FEV_1 Reduction in diffusing capacity

From Speir, W. A., Jr.: How to improve management of chronic obstructive lung disease. *Consultant,* 17:168, 1977, p. 172.

of COPD and chronic bronchitis. These factors are of importance also in the development of emphysema. Emphysema is frequently believed to be a late result of chronic bronchial irritation or infection.

> *It is estimated that more than 90 per cent of persons with pulmonary emphysema smoke heavily; however, emphysema can also occur among nonsmokers.*

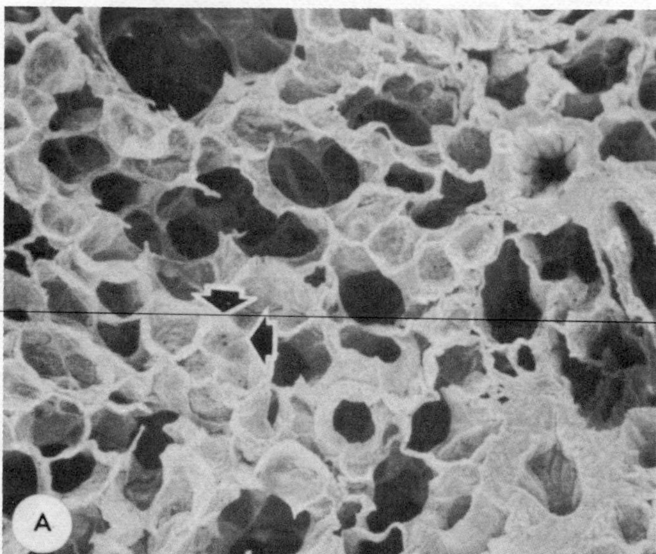

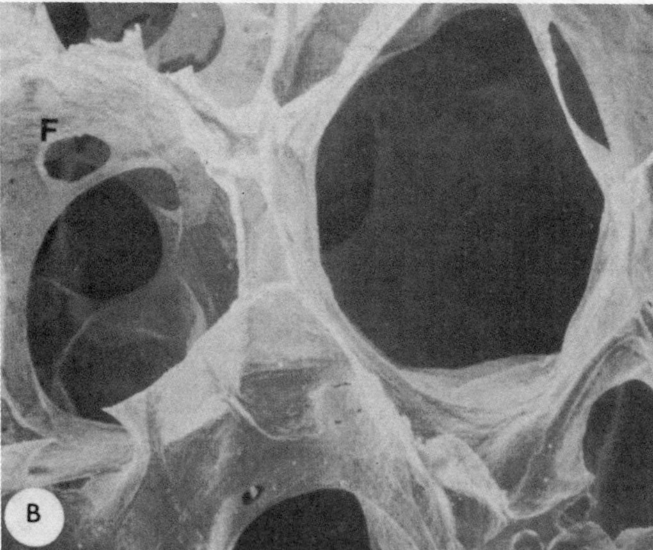

Figure 55–10. A. Scanning electron micrograph of normal lung. Arrows indicate pores of Kohn. (×50.) **B.** Scanning electron micrograph of emphysematous lung with destructive air-space enlargement and fenestrations (F). (×50). (From Benjamin, S. P., and L. J. McCormack: Structural abnormalities in COPD. *Postgraduate Medicine,* 62:103, July 1977.)

Persons with emphysema often live where air pollution is a constant problem. Possibly a genetic factor is also important in the etiology of emphysema.

Prevention. Measures of importance in the prevention of pulmonary emphysema are the same as those discussed previously pertaining to the prevention of COPD and chronic bronchitis. Because preventive measures may be unsuccessful, efforts are directed also at the early detection of emphysema and related pulmonary disorders.

Pathology. Chronic pulmonary anatomic emphysema is characterized by breakdown of the alveolar walls, alveolar ducts, and respiratory bronchioles. This results in a reduction in the total number of alveoli and the formation of enlarged air spaces in the lung as several alveoli coalesce and form one larger space. (See Figure 55–10.)

At the time of autopsy or surgery the lungs do not collapse when the chest is opened (normal lungs collapse when atmospheric pressure enters the chest). Grossly, emphysematous lungs appear enlarged, dry, relatively bloodless, and pale. Commonly they contain numerous superficial blebs (air blisters) of different sizes along the margins of the lungs. When cut, the lung surface contains numerous large air spaces which are so enlarged they are visible with the naked eye. Microscopically it can be seen that the alveolar walls are thin, stretched out and, frequently, broken down. The alveoli appear ragged, disrupted, and distended and have lost their elasticity. Instead of multiple minute alveoli honeycombing the lung parenchyma, large air cysts haphazardly occur.

Commonly the bronchi show evidence of chronic bronchitis or atrophy. With atrophy the bronchial walls become thin and dilated and collapse easily. Other pathologic changes typical of *chronic bronchitis* are frequently also present.

With emphysema a vicious circle of events becomes established that increases the patient's susceptibility to respiratory irritation, infection, and allergic reactions. Some events that perpetuate the circle of repeated pulmonary infection include: (1) increased mucus formation; (2) collapse of bronchi during expiration (trapping air, mucus, and germs); (3) ineffective coughing (due to impaired forceful expiration); (4) narrowed bronchial lumina; (5) destruction of cilia (loss of a normal mechanism for cleaning the tracheobronchial tree); (6) mouth breathing (which dries out pulmonary secretions, making them more difficult to expel); and (7) mucus retention (retained mucus serves as a medium for bacterial growth). *Infections increase tissue damage in the already damaged lung, thus setting the stage for reinfection.*

Destruction of alveolar walls results in the destruction of portions of the pulmonary capillary bed located in the alveolar walls. Thus, the total alveolar surface area of the lungs, where gas exchange occurs, is reduced. Air trapping and the reduction in the number of alveoli (with the subsequent reduction in the blood supply available for gas exchange) produce ventilation and perfusion imbalances that are typically indicated by an elevated $PaCO_2$ and a reduced PaO_2.

The resultant *hypoxia* causes numerous responses throughout the body. For example, hypoxia produces vasoconstriction and thus further decreases pulmonary blood flow. (Refer back to Chapter 53 for a discussion of the effects of hypoxia.)

Pulmonary hypertension develops because of the reduction in space that has occurred in the pulmonary vascular bed. Eventually the patient develops *cor pulmonale* and *right-sided heart failure.*

Symptoms. Pulmonary emphysema (like chronic bronchitis) has an insidious onset and the illness is often denied until the condition is far advanced. In the earlier stages patients with emphysema commonly attempt to treat themselves with home remedies or over-the-counter patent medicines. Eventually symptom progression forces the patient to seek medical help. Commonly emphysema becomes disabling when the patient is between 45 and 55 years of age.

The major symptom of pulmonary emphysema is shortness of breath, resulting from collapse of the airways upon expiration. Exertional dyspnea is an early symptom, but eventually the patient may become dyspneic even when at rest, especially during episodes of acute bronchial disease. Persistent dyspnea forces the patient to work increasingly harder to move air in and out of the lungs. *The greatest difficulty is experienced in exhaling.* Although expiration is normally an involuntary action, it becomes an active muscular effort for the emphysematous person. Expiration is prolonged and deflation of the lungs becomes increasingly difficult. The patient must actually "squeeze" the air out of the lungs by producing a positive pressure in the chest. This pressure may collapse the air passages during expiration. Commonly during expiration the neck veins increase in prominence and the patient breathes through the mouth, pursing the lips (to help to keep the air passages open). Wheezing may be audible during expiration. Inspiration is usually short and rapid.

Wheezing and rales occur in proportion to the amount of bronchitis present. When percussed the lungs give an exceptionally resonant note. Breath sounds are faint. Respirations tend to be shallow and rapid. The patient may breathe as frequently as 25 to 30 times per minute and still not get enough oxygen. People with established emphysema have clubbing of the fingertips. The face may be pale or may be ruddy to ruddy-cyanotic. Persons with emphysema are sometimes characterized as "pink puffers." (Refer back to Table 55–6.)

Gradually changes occur in the shape and size of the chest as a result of pulmonary overdistention and air trapping. Eventually the patient develops a characteristic "barrel-shaped" chest in which the chest appears hyperinflated, i.e., rounded chest and back (dorsal kyphosis), ribs in a more horizontal position, and enlarged anteroposterior diameter of the chest (Fig. 55–11). The chest is then rigid and fixed in an inspiratory position and the lungs are chronically hyperexpanded. A reduction occurs in the normal rise and fall of the chest during ventilation; the entire thorax tends to move vertically as a unit. The ribs become fixed at their joints, and the work of breathing increases greatly. The patient experiences a feeling of tightness in the chest. Diaphragmatic movement is absent or severely impaired and the diaphgram becomes flattened. The flattened diaphragm depresses the liver.

The rigid chest cage forces the patient to overuse the abdominal and upper intercostal muscles and also to use the accessory muscles of respiration (sternocleidomastoids, scaleni, pectorals) to ventilate the lungs. The muscles in the chest and upper neck are held taut to help with ventilation. Even during quiet ventilation the

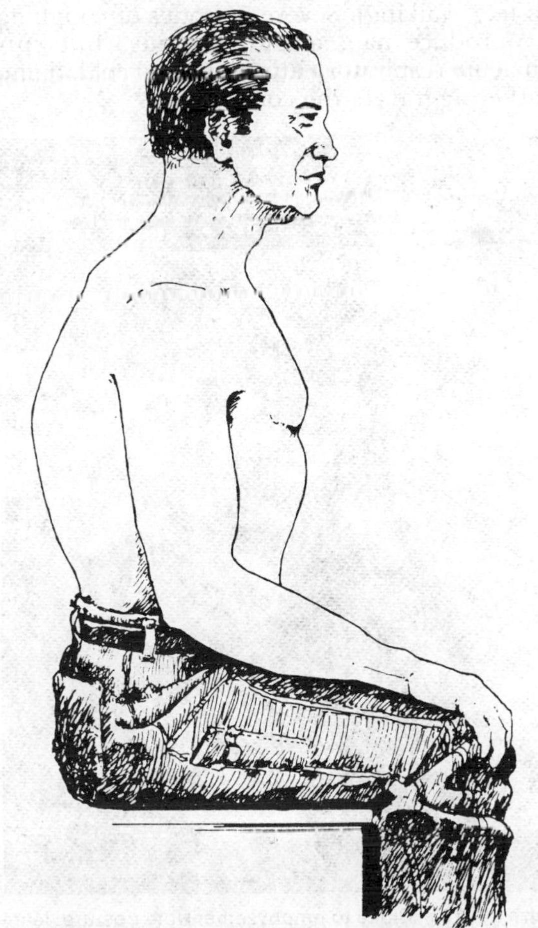

Figure 55–11. "Barrel chest" typical of pulmonary emphysema. (From Block, E. R.: Pitfalls in diagnosing and managing pulmonary diseases. *Geriatrics,* 34:70, Feb. 1979.)

neck muscles are used. The neck appears to be shortened because the neck muscles are tense and contracted. Typically the patient sits leaning forward, hands on knees and shoulders elevated (Fig. 55–12). This position helps to elevate the diaphragm. During expiration the patient sometimes manually presses on the diaphragm. The patient with emphysema speaks in short jerky sentences and usually appears anxious and gaunt. Even minor physical exertion may produce extreme respiratory distress and fatigue.

In addition to dyspnea, a chronic productive cough is another frequent symptom of emphysema. Even though the cough is productive, it is usually inefficient. Thus, only small amounts of sputum are raised. Morning paroxysms of coughing commonly occur that produce thick, viscous sputum. Cough is typically spasmodic, fatiguing, hard, and initiated by even minimal exertion (e.g., talking). Severe episodes of coughing may produce nausea and vomiting. Intercurrent acute respiratory infections and cold, damp weather aggravate the cough.

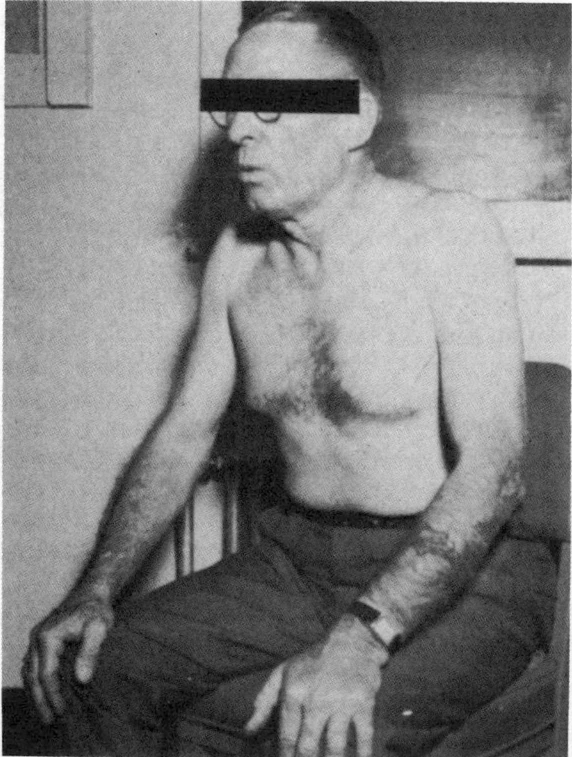

Figure 55–12. Clues to emphysema. Note posture: leaning forward, arms on knees, to elevate the diaphragm. Pursed lips help keep air passages open while exhaling. Muscles in neck, upper chest are taut as they help in work of breathing. (From Whatley, J. L.: Battle for breath. *Today's Health,* Feb. 1967.)

Symptoms of right-sided heart failure (e.g., peripheral edema, venous distention) may be present with advanced emphysema. Prior to the development of heart failure, dyspnea may be relieved by lying down flat. However, once heart failure develops, dyspnea becomes continuous and is not relieved by reclining. Persons with advanced emphysema have a rapid heart rate.

Hypoxia, respiratory acidosis, and the increased muscular effort necessary for ventilation produce lethargy, anorexia, weakness, and weight loss. Respiratory function is severely impaired in advanced emphysema. Deficient oxygenation of the brain and high CO_2 levels in the blood may produce mental changes, e.g., impaired memory, poor judgment, confusion, lethargy, possibly coma. With severe ventilatory insufficiency the patient may experience impairments of sensorium and headache; papilledema, miosis and asterixis (flapping tremor) are observable.

In persons with pulmonary emphysema death most usually results from heart failure (caused by cor pulmonale), an acute bronchopulmonary infection, or respiratory failure. Other complications that can be fatal include spontaneous pneumothorax, pulmonary thromboembolism, or peptic ulcer.

Diagnosis. *History and physical examination* demonstrate many of the characteristic symptoms discussed above, e.g., exertional dyspnea with an insidious onset, wheezing, prolonged, expiration, chronic productive cough, barrel chest, use of accessory muscles of respiration. Medical history frequently includes heavy smoking for a number of years and repeated pulmonary infections which have increasingly left the patient short of breath upon exertion.

- Chest x-ray films may appear normal until emphysema is in its advanced stages. With advanced emphysema x-ray findings may include: (1) overaeration of the lungs (i.e., on x-ray film lung parenchyma does not appear normally darkened); (2) increased vascularity at lung peripheries; (3) abnormal heart size and position; (4) increased anteroposterior chest diameter; (5) enlarged lungs; (6) low flat diaphragm images; (7) widening of the rib spaces; and (8) large cysts that appear as ring-like or annular translucencies. The latter changes are referred to as "vanishing lung."
- *Fluoroscopy* may reveal difficulty with expiration, low, flat diaphgrams that move poorly during ventilation, and limited rib motion during inspiration.
- *Scintillation scanning* and *pulmonary angiography* help to evaluate non-affected areas of the lungs (especially helpful if pulmonary surgery is being considered). Radioactive gas studies of ventilation-perfusion relationships show that people with pulmonary emphysema have abnormalities of both perfusion and ventilation. Bronchograms usually demonstrate a characteristic "tree in winter" effect, in which the smaller "branches" and "foliage"

are not outlined. Also, bronchograms show changes in the bronchi typical of chronic bronchitis.

- *Pulmonary function tests* are useful in confirming a diagnosis of pulmonary emphysema and evaluating the condition. Characteristic findings are reduced maximal breathing capacity, reduced forced expiratory volume, slow maximal midexpiratory flow, increased residual volume, and reduced expiratory reserve volume. The timed vital capacity is commonly reduced, as are the FEV_1 and MMEF. Exercise tolerance tests may produce severe, frightening respiratory distress.

- If equipment is not available to measure pulmonary function it is possible to *roughly evaluate lung function* in the following ways: First, see if the patient can blow out a lighted match that is held 6 inches from the open mouth. The match must be blown out by exhaling air forcefully through the open mouth, i.e., without pursing the lips. If this "*match test*" cannot be performed, severe ventilatory obstruction is generally present. The second test consists of timing (with an ordinary watch that has a second hand, or with a stop watch) the rate at which the total vital capacity can be exhaled with maximum effort. Normal emptying time is 3 seconds; moderate obstructive disease is present if emptying time is 5 to 6 seconds. Severe obstructive disease is present if emptying time is greater than 7 seconds.

- Measurements are made of *blood gases* and blood pH (acid-alkali balance). Arterial oxyhemoglobin saturation is reduced. Ventilatory insufficiency results in alveolar hypoxia and, hence, the blood's PaO_2 is reduced. Also, because the lungs cannot effectively blow off CO_2, the $PaCO_2$ increases (hypercapnia). Although this developing *respiratory acidosis* can be compensated for at first by the retention of bicarbonate by the kidneys, eventually this compensatory mechanism fails (indicated by falling of blood pH) and the respiratory acidosis worsens progressively. Blood pH may remain normal, even in the presence of respiratory acidosis, until failure of the compensatory mechanisms occurs. To buffer increased amounts of carbonic acid the serum bicarbonates are elevated.

- As a result of *secondary polycythemia,* the red blood cell count and packed cell volume (sedimentation rate) may be increased. The white blood cell count is normal with emphysema; however, it is elevated in the presence of acute infections.

- An electrocardiogram may be performed to evaluate the patient's cardiac status.

Clinical Care. Clinical care for patients with pulmonary emphysema is basically similar to that previously discussed for COPD, chronic bronchial asthma, and chronic bronchitis. Similarities in care occur because bronchospasm is a problem common in all these disorders. (Refer back to previous sections as necessary. Specific procedures, e.g., oxygen therapy, postural drainage, are discussed more completely in Chapter 54.)

> *Treatment of emphysema is basically palliative and focuses on helping the patient to maintain tidal respiration (without excessive effort) during the greatest possible range of exercise.*

To accomplish this goal, efforts are directed at preventing or minimizing pulmonary infections, improving pulmonary circulation and ventilation, and reducing bronchial spasm and edema and hypersecretion of mucus. Techniques of pulmonary physiotherapy are employed to make the maximum use of the respiratory muscles. Aerosol therapy is frequently used to deliver medications to decrease airway obstruction. The patient must work hard to maintain an optimal level of activity in spite of increasing rigidity of the chest wall in a position of expansion. Because pulmonary emphysema forces the affected individual to make numerous life changes, emotional care is highly important.

Plan nursing care of a person with emphysema in such a manner that the patient's breathlessness will not be excessively worsened. Provide frequent rest periods. In writing about his own experiences as a victim of emphysema W. R. Jones comments:

> Anyone working with this breathless part of the population should have some physical realization of how these people must live and breathe. Take a *full* deep breath, then let out only *one third* of it, and continue to breathe out while retaining that *two thirds* of the original breath for the better part of a day. Each breath will be only partial; the retained portion becomes essentially toxic, and every tissue of your body takes the rap. If you do this conscientiously, you will be breathing somewhat in the manner of a patient with emphysema — except that he will do this about 20,000 times a day and over 7,000,000 times a year.

Assisting Ventilation. Some patients with pulmonary emphysema subjectively feel better following the administration of IPPB. Depending upon the severity of impaired inspiratory flow, bronchodilators, mucolytics, or both may be delivered by small volume nebulizer or IPPB. IPPB administered to a patient with any form of COPD should be powered by compressed air. Because most of these patients are stimulated to breathe owing to hypoxemia, oxygen-powered IPPB machines may depress the patient's ventilatory drive. If low flow O_2 is concurrently administered, it must *not* be removed. O_2 is a drug; it cannot be stored and must be continuously administered to maintain tissue oxygenation.

Oxygen is used with great caution at low flow rates, 2 to 3 liters per minute nasally. The patient is observed frequently for indications of *CO_2 narcosis.* (See Chapters 12 and 53.) When oxygen therapy is started the PaO_2, $PaCO_2$ and arterial blood pH are monitored.

> *Patients who give their own IPPB or oxygen treatments at home must be warned that the excessive use of O_2 can be dangerous and may actually suppress breathing rather than making breathing easier. By emphasizing that oxygen is a drug that must be used only as prescribed, you can help the patient realize that excesses can be dangerous.*

It is essential that a person with emphysema be well hydrated (to prevent dehydration and to thin secretions) and that optimum tracheobronchial hygiene be maintained by postural drainage, expectorants, aerosols, and humidification of inspired air. Suctioning is performed as necessary.

Controlling Cough. Mild cough depressants are indicated if cough is very fatiguing or nonproductive; sedatives and narcotics are contraindicated since they depress respirations. Ineffective coughing is discouraged since it worsens the patient's disorder by enlarging emphysematous cystic spaces, slowing down even further the escape of air from the alveoli, and compressing normal lung tissue. Coughing produces a sudden increase in intrabronchial pressure, which is not evenly distributed throughout the emphysematous lung. This pressure increase, associated with unequal airway resistance in the bronchi, may increase alveolar damage.

Breathing Exercises. Breathing exercises and exercises that strengthen abdominal muscles and facilitate more complete exhalation are taught to persons with emphysema. The patient learns to become aware of the diaphragm, how to use it more effectively during ventilation (by developing a slow, relaxed pattern of abdominal breathing), and how to maintain its optimal mechanical efficiency. During exercise the patient may benefit from long-term oxygen therapy administered from lightweight portable containers of liquid oxygen. Breathing exercises, improved posture, and mild physical exercise help combat respiratory insufficiency as a result of reduced lung compliance and restricted pulmonary excursion.

Other Measures. Allergic responses increase bronchospasm and must therefore be prevented or controlled by desensitization to known allergens. (Refer back to discussion of bronchial asthma.) Bronchodilators are administered to relieve bronchospasm and increase airway patency. Adrenal corticosteroids, e.g., prednisone, may be required if other measures fail to relieve bronchospasm.

Complications. Observe the patient closely for the development of possible *complications of emphysema,* e.g., spontaneous pneumothorax (as a result of rupture of a bleb or bulla), acute respiratory infections, peptic ulcer, anemia, cor pulmonale, respiratory failure. *Early* treatment of these conditions is imperative and may be started as a result of a nurse's alert observations. Because acute respiratory infections can be fatal in the presence of emphysema, make every attempt to prevent or minimize them, e.g., by annual influenza immunizations. Patients should know the danger signals of infection and see a doctor if they begin to develop. Antibiotics are given to control chronic infections and to treat acute infections. Some patients require prolonged antimicrobial therapy. When specific bacterial sensitivity cannot be determined, tetracycline may be given.

> *Cor pulmonale and respiratory failure are late complications. Emphysema is the most common cause of chronic cor pulmonale and chronic pulmonary insufficiency.*

(Treatment of patients with respiratory insufficiency or respiratory failure was discussed earlier in this unit.)

Rehabilitation and Emotional Care. The nurse focuses rehabilitation on helping persons with emphysema (and their significant others) to learn ways of controlling symptoms and minimizing their effects. Self-care is encouraged for as many activities as possible, for as long as possible. Patients must learn to live within their limitations and to routinely follow recommendations made by physicians and other health services personnel. Patient teaching may be difficult if a patient is severely hypoxic, because mental acuity may be reduced.

Chronic destructive pulmonary diseases, such as COPD and pulmonary emphysema, create numerous *emotional* and *socioeconomic problems* for patients and their significant others. Progressive invalidism is both emotionally and financially burdensome, requiring changes in life patterns and withdrawal from many normal activities of daily life. Often people with these disorders pass through periods of denial of their illnesses, before their obvious loss of health forces them to seek help. Even then many are unable to stop smoking or to comply with other recommendations, even when told that the prohibited activities worsen their physical disorders.

Obviously, crushing psychologic problems occur with diseases that are as devastating as pulmonary emphysema and COPD.

Effective patient care must include recognition of psychopathologic reactions in addition to awareness of pathophysiology. Suicide occurs fairly commonly in men with emphysema.[118]

Surgical Treatment. Some persons with pulmonary emphysema benefit from the *surgical resection* of large, solitary bullae (confined to one area of the lung) or the removal of nonfunctioning pulmonary tissue. Bullae may compress the normal lung tissue next to them. Breathing efficiency is improved by the removal of nonfunctioning lung tissue in some persons. Only selected patients with emphysema are candidates for surgical therapy. Surgical procedures that attempt to improve pulmonary blood circulation or cut nerves to make breathing easier (i.e., carotid body surgery or glomectomy) have not been successful.

Adult Respiratory Distress Syndrome (ARDS)

Adult respiratory distress syndrome (ARDS) refers to a group of diseases, insults, and conditions that result in acute lung injury. Synonyms to describe this syndrome include *wet lung syndrome, shock lung, oxygen toxicity, congestive lung syndrome, stiff lung,* and many other similar terms.

The ARDS syndrome was first recognized during World War II. During the Vietnam conflict it was described and studied owing largely to traumatic circumstances such as large volume blood loss, massive trauma, rapid evacuation from battle areas, rapid treatment and recovery from the shock and injury, followed by subsequent development of respiratory failure 12 to 48 hours later. Parallels to wartime respiratory problems were recognized in civilian practice.

Etiology. No specific etiology describes ARDS. The injury to the lung may be from *direct* or *indirect causes.* (See Table 55–13.) Among the many *factors contributing* to ARDS syndrome are smoke inhalation, aspiration, ingestion and inhalation of toxic chemicals, drug overdose, fat or air emboli, drowning, viral pneumonia, prolonged cardiopulmonary bypass, severe hypotension, thoracic trauma and contusions, D.I.C., neurogenic pulmonary edema, sepsis, oxygen toxicity, renal failure, pancreatitis, or radiation injury to lung.

Clinical Findings. Classic symptoms of ARDS are dyspnea, tachypnea, and sometimes intercostal retractions. Cyanosis in spite of oxygen therapy may also be observed. The lung compliance is greatly compromised. If the patient is on a ventilator, peak inspiratory pressures will be high in order to achieve the re-

TABLE 55–13. DISORDERS ASSOCIATED WITH ARDS

Shock of any cause	Inhaled toxins
	Oxygen
Infection	Smoke
Gram-negative sepsis	Corrosive chemicals
Pneumonia	Nitrous oxide, chlorine, ammonia, phosgene, cadmium
Viral	
Bacterial	
Fungal (rare)	
Pneumocystis carinii (rare)	Hematologic disorders
	Intravascular coagulation
Trauma	Massive blood transfusion
Fat emboli	Postcardiopulmonary bypass (?)
Lung contusion	
Nonthoracic trauma	
Head injury	Metabolic and toxic disorders
	Pancreatitis
Liquid aspiration	Uremia
Gastric juice	Paraquat ingestion
Fresh or salt water	
Hydrocarbon fluids	
	Miscellaneous
Drug overdose	Lymphangitic carcinomatosis
Heroin	Increased intracranial pressure
Methadone	Eclampsia
Propoxyphene (Darvon)	Postcardioversion
Barbiturates	Radiation pneumonitis

From Brown, M., and J. L. Andrews, Jr.: How to manage adult respiratory distress syndrome. *Geriatrics,* 34:39, April 1979, p. 41.

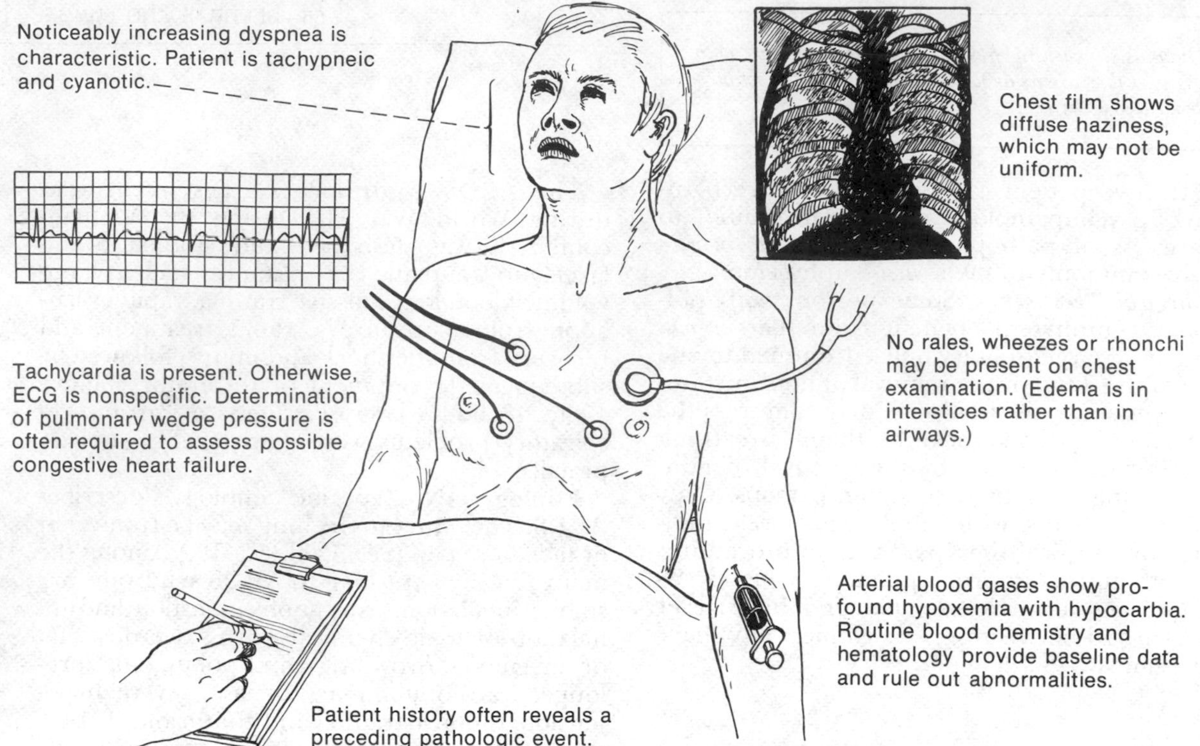

Figure 55–13. Clinical features of ARDS. Determination of pulmonary wedge pressure often necessary to assess possible congestive heart failure.

quired tidal volume. The lungs are edematous with fluid. The most remarkable laboratory sign is the PaO_2. Even at remarkably high FIO_2's the resulting PaO_2 is low. Carbon dioxide transport is rarely impaired and the $PaCO_2$ may be low or normal. The chest film usually will show a progressive bilateral parenchymal infiltration with air bronchograms and a ground glass appearance. On auscultation breath sounds may be somewhat diminished and inspiratory rales may be heard (Fig. 55–13).

Pathophysiology. Early in the course of the disease process interstitial edema is present. As the disease progresses, the lungs get wetter and become heavy and "liver-like." Alveolar collapse and filling with edema fluid occurs and oxygen transport and pulmonary compliance are impaired, i.e., the lungs get "stiffer." Congestion, hyaline membrane formation, and hemorrhage develop. Pulmonary compliance and oxygen transport become more compromised (Table 55–14). (For further discussion, see p. 243.)

Treatment. Patients with ARDS must receive aggressive, prompt, and intensive clinical care. The *treatment objective* is to maintain adequate alveolar ventilation and tissue oxygenation. Treatment must include prevention or correction of the underlying disorder and maintenance of adequate systemic blood pressure — the longer the hypotensive episode, the graver the consequences of the disease. Arterial blood gas levels are absolutely essential. Improved oxygenation may be obtained if C-PAP or PEEP is included in the therapy. Corticosteroids are sometimes used, depending upon the causative factors. Antibiotics are indicated in some instances. Fluid and electrolyte management is also of great importance. (See Table 55–14.)

The *nurse's role* includes a full understanding of the precipitating cause and appropriate treatment; ventilator and airway management; monitoring of hemodynamic and arterial blood gas levels, intake and output, breath sounds, and vital signs and all laboratory data; and assessment of pulmonary performance to include inspiratory pressure, inspiratory force, tidal volume, FIO_2, and level of end-expiratory pressure.

Management of ARDS involves maintaining the arterial oxygen tension at 50 to 60 mm Hg while administering an inspired oxygen tension below 50 per cent. It may be necessary to employ positive airway pressure (see Chapter 54: PEEP and C-PAP and Care of a Patient on a Ventilator). Fever, chills, restlessness, and other factors increasing oxygen demands by the body must be appropriately managed.

Continuous airway pressure is usually begun at +5 cm. H_2O. The level of expiratory pressure is increased or decreased as deemed necessary by arterial blood gas levels.

Patients who require blood transfusions may develop metabolic acidosis if stored blood depleted of 2,3-diphosphoglycerate (2,3-DPG) is administered. The depletion of 2,3-DPG prevents the release of O_2 by the hemoglobin to the tissues of the body.

Nurses caring for patients with ARDS work closely with physicians and respiratory therapists.

TABLE 55–14. ADULT RESPIRATORY DISTRESS SYNDROME

Stages of ARDS

Stage 1
- Interstitial pulmonary edema
  - Pulmonary capillary congestion
  - Electron microscopy findings: widening of junction of endothelial cells and swelling of endothelial cells

Stage 2
- Intra-alveolar pulmonary edema
  - Eosinophilic proteinaceous fluid in alveoli

Stage 3
- Cellular response
  - Hyaline membrane formation
  - Type II pneumocyte hyperplasia
  - Capillary endothelial regeneration
  - Fibrogenesis, then fibrosis

Therapeutic Modalities

Oxygen (controlled dose)
Mechanical ventilation with positive end-expiratory pressure (PEEP)
Fluid restriction
Diuretics
Cardiotonic/vasopressor agents
Hypothermia
Antibiotics
Steroids (?)
Heparin (?)
Extracorporeal membrane oxygenation (?)

Adapted from Brown, M., and J. L. Andrews, Jr.: How to manage adult respiratory distress syndrome. *Geriatrics,* 34:39, April 1979.

Pulmonary Embolism and Pulmonary Infarction

Refer to Unit XV for discussion of these topics.

Pulmonary Hypertension

Pulmonary hypertension is almost always directly caused by heart and lung disease. As lung tissue is destroyed by disease, the mean pulmonary artery pressure increases. The increases may be transient and largely reversible, or relatively permanent and resistant to therapy (as in emphysema or widespread thromboembolism). The destruction of tissue by disease obliterates the pulmonary vascular reserve. Normally, this reserve prevents dyspnea on exertion because the vascular bed enlarges three or four times normal resting level.

Pulmonary hypertension is generally *diagnosed* through electrocardiogram and radiologic findings. The most common *symptoms* that occur as a result of pulmonary hypertension are dyspnea and weakness. The pulmonary reserve is unable to compensate for the oxygen needs demanded by increased exercise. The compression and obliteration of pulmonary vasculature reduce the effective capillary bed for perfusion. This in turn raises the pulmonary vascular resistance. The administration of low flow oxygen for 16 to 20 hours has been shown to reduce the hypertension. If the patient's PaO_2 is satisfactory, oxygen may be administered for this period of time. This is the only instance in which noncontinuous O_2 administration is acceptable. Often, however, oxygen is administered on a continuous low flow basis.

Primary pulmonary hypertension is not associated with either cardiac or pulmonary disease. This condition occurs in people between the ages of 20 and 40, more often in women than men. The exact mechanisms are not known, but pulmonary emboli are thought to play a significant role. The symptoms are palpitations, substernal and left-sided chest pain (usually on exertion), exertional dyspnea, and syncopal attacks. Death may occur suddenly from a rapidly developing right heart failure. This disorder is quite rare.

Pneumoconioses (Dust Diseases)

The word *pneumoconiosis* is a very general term which simply means that dust is retained in the lungs. Disease-producing dusts typically cause a fibrous tissue reaction in the lungs and produce symptoms such as shortness of breath, chronic cough, and mucus production. Disease-producing dusts tend to be those associated with certain occupations. The familiar dusts of smoke-filled cities, gravel or dirt roads, and household dusts do not produce pneumoconioses.

Silicosis is the best known of the pneumoconioses because it is the most common and most crippling. Silicosis was formerly called silicotuberculosis; other common names for silicosis include *"stonecutter's disease," "miner's phthisis," "potter's asthma,"* and *"grinder's rot."* Silicosis results from the occupational inhalation of dust containing free silica. This disorder may occur in mining, granite cutting and polishing, foundries, sandblasting, pottery manufacturing, and concrete breaking. Silicosis produces fibrous pulmonary nodules or diffuse pulmonary fibrosis, which may increasingly impair lung function. Silicosis develops in direct proportion to the percentage and concentration of silica and the duration of exposure.

Symptoms of advanced silicosis may include shortness of breath upon exertion, cough, wheezing, expectoration of dark gray to black sputum with pulmonary infections, and chest pains. Chronic bronchitis and pulmonary emphysema often occur with advanced silicosis. *The main complication of silicosis is pulmonary tuberculo-*

sis. Multiplication of tubercle bacilli appears to be stimulated by the cellular toxicity of silica. Silicosis causes irreversible lung damage. *Treatment* of advanced cases is similar to that previously described for COPD, e.g., IPPB, bronchodilators, and the antimicrobial treatment of intercurrent infections. Treatment of chronic bronchitis and pulmonary emphysema has also been discussed.

Examples of other pneumoconioses include:

Anthracosilicosis, caused by inhalation of a combination of coal dust and silica.

Asbestosis, caused by inhalation of asbestos fibers.

Bagassosis, caused by inhalation of dust from pressed sugar cane stalks.

Baritosis, caused by inhalation of dust from barium sulfate.

Berylliosis, caused by inhalation of beryllium dust (a metal that is inert except in sensitized individuals).

Byssinosis, caused by inhalation of cotton dust.

Farmer's lung, caused by inhalation of dust from moldy hay.

Siderosis, caused by inhalation of dust of iron oxide.

Stannosis, caused by inhalation of dust of tin oxide.

Of the above pneumoconioses, the following are benign, i.e., they do not cause pulmonary fibrosis, impaired lung function, or increased susceptibility to tuberculosis: bagassosis, baritosis, byssinosis, farmer's lung, siderosis, and stannosis.

Because pneumoconioses result from occupational exposures to certain dusts, the *prevention* of these disorders is often possible. Most pneumoconioses can be prevented by the implementation of safety practices designed to reduce hazardous dust levels. Nurses in public health and occupational health positions are active in the prevention and early detection of pneumoconioses.

CHAPTER 56

INJURIES TO THE CHEST

"The thorax presents a fairly large exposed portion of the body that is particularly vulnerable to impact forces. Grave thoracic injuries are becoming more frequent; injuries to the thorax and vital structures contained in the thoracic cavity cause more severe and fatal injuries than do head and facial injuries. Chest injury is a major killing injury, necessitating urgency of treatment."[138A] Injuries to the chest are also discussed in Chapter 95.

CAUSES AND TYPES OF INJURIES

Accident prevention is the key to reducing the number of chest injuries, since these injuries often result from falls, the use of machines, and the use of potentially lethal weapons, e.g., knives, guns. Many chest injuries result from automobile accidents in which the driver is thrown against the steering wheel and the occupants are thrown against the dashboard or front seat. Nurses can contribute to accident prevention by participating in safety education programs and encouraging safety precautions, e.g., slip-proof mats in bathtubs and showers, the use of seat belts in automobiles. Some chest injuries result from seemingly innocuous activities. For example, the ribs may be fractured from the strain of severe coughing or sneezing.

Normal respiratory function requires integrity of the tracheobronchial tree, lungs, diaphragm, pleurae, and thoracic wall. Additionally, the heart and cardiovascular system must be intact. All of these structures may be damaged by chest injuries. The major dangers associated with chest injuries are punctured organs deep within the body (e.g., heart, lungs) and internal bleeding. As with other injuries, chest injuries range from relatively minor bumps and scrapes to severe crushing or penetrating injuries that are rapidly fatal because of cardiopulmonary damage.

Chest injuries may be of a penetrating or nonpenetrating (blunt) nature. Blast injuries, e.g., caused by explosions, may rupture pulmonary alveoli and vessels. Hemorrhage and asphyxiation then often cause death. Crushing chest injuries may fracture ribs and seriously compress and damage the lungs and heart. Penetrating chest wounds (e.g., from bullets, knives, flying shrapnel, or splinters) may cause an open chest wound that permits atmospheric air to enter the pleural space and disrupt the normal mechanisms of ventilation. Additionally, penetrating chest wounds may seriously damage the lungs, heart, and other thoracic structures.

Head injuries frequently coexist with chest injuries and may modify the treatment of the chest injury. Patients with concomitant head injuries must be protected from hypoxia, which may result from inadequately treated chest injuries. Therefore an artificial airway may need to be established even though it may not be necessary for treatment of the chest injury.

GENERAL MANAGEMENT OF THE CHEST-INJURED PATIENT

After receiving emergency care, the person who has chest injuries is examined more thoroughly and a chest film is taken to identify and evaluate injuries. An electrocardiogram is also performed to ascertain possible cardiac injury. A complete history may help the physician to rapidly evaluate the extent of the injury.

Nurses may help obtain information concerning the accident from the patient or witnesses. It is beneficial to know[67A] the identity, velocity, and pathway of the wounding agent; the type and speed of the vehicle; and, if the patient was in a car, whether seat belts were being worn or whether the patient was thrown by the impact. Information of this nature helps the physician to assess injury to regional as well as distant anatomic structures.

A thorough physical examination of the chest (front and back) with the patient completely undressed is performed to look for indications of injury. Subtle changes or physical findings can be highly important in evaluating the chest-injured patient.

Geiger summarizes some of the important basic techniques used for the physical diagnosis of chest injuries.[67A]

► *Inspection and observation:* (1) Determine the level of consciousness, emotional state, or degree of apprehension; (2) note the color of mucosa, nail beds, and the presence and degree of cyanosis or pallor; (3) evaluate the respiratory pattern and rate, and the use of accessory muscles of respiration; (4) note the status of cervical pulses and veins; (5) determine whether injury is closed or contused and search for wounds of entrance and exit; (6) note character and amount of sputum or tracheal secretions.

- *Palpation and percussion:* (1) Determine equality and amplitude of pulses; (2) determine cardiac size and location of apical impulse; (3) evaluate chest expansion and check for areas of hyperresonance or dullness; (4) determine areas of tenderness or pain, abnormal mobility of ribs or sternum, tracheal shift, or crepitation.
- *Auscultation:* (1) Evaluate breath sounds; (2) assess cardiac sounds; (3) determine blood pressure in both arms and legs, when indicated.

Treatment of chest injuries may include closed chest drainage and/or thoracotomy. (Both topics are discussed in Chapter 57.) Thoracotomy is necessary for only about 1 out of 10 chest-injured patients. Whether or not chest surgery is necessary, much of the clinical care given the chest-injured patient is similar to that given postoperatively following chest surgery. (Refer to Chapter 57 as necessary.) Some general activities of importance in caring for any chest-injured patient are discussed briefly below.

Maintain Patent Airway. This can be done by correctly positioning the patient to prevent aspiration, suctioning as necessary, turning, "coughing," and "deep breathing" the patient at least hourly. The airway may be obstructed by mucus, bone fragments, broken teeth or dentures, blood and/or vomitus. An artificial airway (endotracheal tube) may be inserted to facilitate airway patency.

Ensure Adequate Ventilation. Some patients require oxygen, endotracheal intubation, tracheostomy, or mechanical ventilation. Carefully evaluate blood gas reports and the patient's general respiratory status, e.g., rate of respiration, chest movements, dyspnea, spontaneous tidal volume. Administer oxygen and titrate dosage according to subsequent arterial blood gases. The head-elevated position makes breathing easier and is usually the most comfortable position for the conscious chest-injured patient. (Positioning and care of unconscious patients is discussed in Unit X. Tracheostomy and endotracheal intubation are discussed in Unit XXIV.)

If a patient does not ventilate normally after the upper airway is established, or if the condition continues to deteriorate without an obvious cause, undetected injuries may be present, e.g., hemothorax, pneumothorax, flail chest, ruptured bronchus, cardiac tamponade, ruptured thoracic aorta. Immediately notify the physician of the patient's condition so further evaluation can be made. (Treatment of complications is discussed below.)

Assist with Diagnostic and Therapeutic Procedures as Indicated. Thoracentesis, bronchoscopic aspiration, chest drainage tube insertion, or endotracheal intubation may need to be done. *Maintain effective functioning of equipment* such as that used for respiratory therapy and closed chest drainage.

Replace Blood Loss and Prevent or Treat Shock. Shock often accompanies chest injuries and should be closely observed for and treated early. (See Chapter 13.) Upon admission of the patient a blood sample is taken for typing and cross-matching, so that blood loss can be replaced. Until these laboratory results are available the patient is given a blood substitute, such as plasma or dextran. Examine the patient carefully for external bleeding and estimate blood loss. Observe also for symptoms of internal bleeding: pallor, restlessness, cold clammy skin, low blood pressure, empty veins, and rapid thready pulse. Internal bleeding may result from injuries to the thoracic or abdominal viscera, torn muscles, or fractures. Bleeding into the pleural space may be of a large amount (e.g., 2 or more liters) but can usually be rapidly detected. Hemorrhage into areas such as the chest wall, as from torn intercostal muscles, is more difficult to detect. A liter of blood can accumulate between the chest wall muscles within the chest wall planes without producing much swelling.

Immediately call to the physician's attention any indications of hemorrhage. The volume of blood replacement is determined by the physician after evaluation of clinical findings, laboratory reports (e.g., hemoglobin, packed cell volume), and central venous pressure. Rapid blood replacement is essential in the management of thoracic injuries. Additional blood loss on top of hypoxemia will even further compromise the patient's oxygen status.

Prevent, Observe for, and Treat Other Complications. Observe the patient closely for symptoms of cardiopulmonary dysfunction. Report immediately symptoms indicative of complications, e.g., dyspnea, sudden sharp chest pain, blood-streaked sputum, agitation. Because indications of complications may not appear immediately, continued close observation is essential for the newly injured patient. Observe for symptoms of previously undetected injuries, e.g., fractures, abdominal injuries.

Promote effective tracheobronchial secretion movement and removal. Supervise and encourage periodic coughing, deep breathing, turning, and exercise. Instruct the patient to make a conscious effort to breathe normally. The patient will tend to breathe shallowly to minimize pain. Encourage productive coughing and airway clearance because it removes sputum and other tracheobronchial secretions and prevents them from pooling and becoming potential sources of infection and obstruction. It is helpful to assist the cough effort by supporting the affected chest area with your hands and/or pillows. Administer antibiotics as prescribed to combat pulmonary infection, caused by trauma and infected secretions.

Control Pain Without Causing Excessive Depression of Respirations or Cough. Cautiously administer analgesics as indicated. Analgesics help by making the patient more comfortable in taking deep breaths and coughing, by minimizing pain, and by permitting periods of rest and relaxation. Pain associated with coughing may be minimized by "splinting" the patient's chest during coughing. (See Chapter 57.) Atropine, morphine, and barbiturates are contraindicated because they cause respiratory depression. Mild sedation and frequent small doses of meperidine (Demerol) may control pain. Nerve blocks may also be helpful.

Maintain Fluid-Electrolyte Balance and Nourishment. When administering IV's to the chest-injured patient remember the possible danger of pulmonary edema and watch for symptoms of this complication. Pulmonary edema can occur if impaired pulmonary circulation is overloaded with fluid. Maintain an accurate intake and output record to guide fluid replacement. IV feedings are given until it is safe for food to enter the stomach. Oral intake may be temporarily contraindicated because of abdominal injury, nausea, surgery, or impaired consciousness. Once it is no longer necessary to keep the stomach empty, unconscious patients are given nasogastric tube feedings and conscious patients are started on a light diet.

Attempt to Calm and Gain the Cooperation of the Patient. The chest-injured patient may be in extreme cardiopulmonary distress and therefore highly fearful and anxious. Efficient, skillful actions on the part of calm, reassuring attending personnel can help the patient relax somewhat and breathe more effectively. Intensive nursing care is essential for the severely injured patient.

COMPLICATIONS OF CHEST INJURIES

Severe trauma to the chest may produce numerous complications. Among these are:

- Hemothorax, pneumothorax (open or closed), hemopneumothorax, pneumomediastinum
- Mediastinal flutter, mediastinal shift
- Lung compression, lung laceration, lung contusion
- Fractured ribs, flail chest, paradoxical motion
- Subcutaneous or mediastinal emphysema
- Injuries to the diaphragm and/or mediastinal contents, cardiac tamponade
- ARDS
- Shock, severe pain, dyspnea, hypoxemia
- Tracheal and/or bronchial tears

Hemothorax; Pneumothorax; Hemopneumothorax

Chest injuries frequently cause *hemothorax* (blood in the pleural space), *pneumothorax* (air in the pleural space), or *hemopneumothorax* (both blood and air in the chest cavity). These conditions were briefly discussed in Chapter 55. Blood in the chest cavity results from pulmonary lacerations, torn intercostal blood vessels from fractured ribs, and a ruptured intrathoracic aneurysm. Air may enter the pleural space directly through a hole in the chest wall ("open" pneumothorax) or diaphragm, or it may escape into the pleural space from a puncture or tear in one of the internal respiratory structures, e.g., bronchus, bronchioles, alveoli. The latter form of pneumothorax is called a "closed" or "spontaneous" pneumothorax.

Never pull a penetrating object, e.g., a piece of steel or wood, out of the chest when giving first aid following chest injury. To do so could precipitate serious internal hemorrhage or pneumothorax (the presence of the object in the wound may be preventing air from entering). Leave the object in place for a physician to remove when appropriate.

Indications of pneumothorax include hyperresonance on percussion, diminished breath sounds, and pain. Pneumothorax must be considered if the patient becomes restless, reports sudden chest pain, or shows increasing pulse and respiratory rates. Chest films may reveal a slight shift of the trachea away from the affected side and retraction of the lung back from the parietal pleura. If a pneumothorax is suspected (but the patient's respiratory distress is so severe that there is not enough time for x-ray confirmation), the physician may insert an 18-gauge needle into the second interspace in the midclavicular line. Aspiration will then demonstrate whether free air is present.

Accumulations of blood, fluids, and air in the

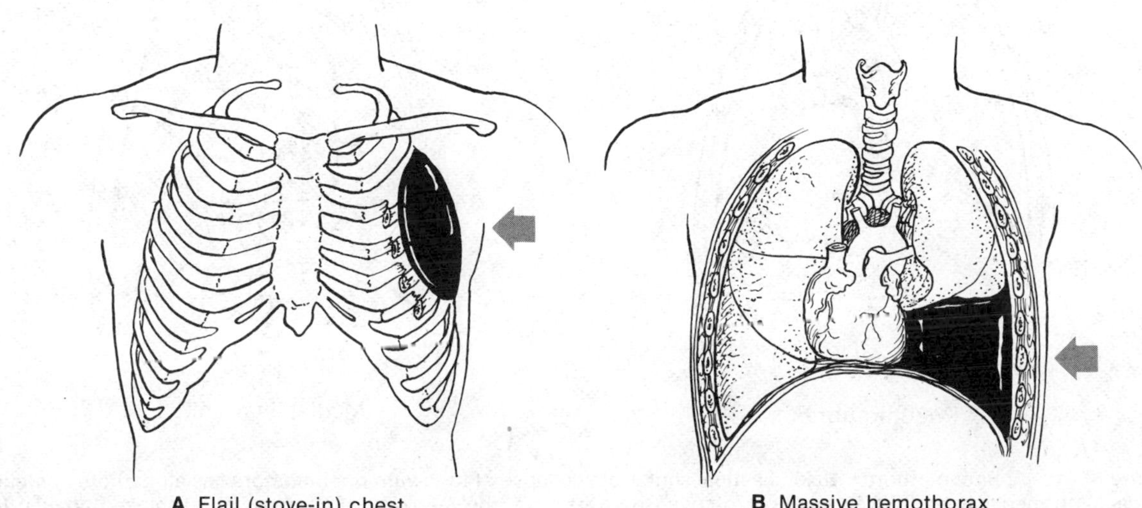

A Flail (stove-in) chest

B Massive hemothorax

pleural space cause positive pressure to build up in that area. (Remember: negative pressure normally exists in the pleural space.) As the pressure build-up increases, it begins to collapse the lung and impair respiratory exchange; the patient becomes dyspneic and frequently goes into shock (Figure 56–1*A*).

Immediately after chest injury, *emergency thoracentesis* may be performed to remove accumulations of air, blood, or secretions. These emergency needle aspirations may prevent death from cardiopulmonary failure. Next, a catheter may be placed in the pleural space and connected to *closed-chest drainage*. The catheter permits the continuous escape of air, secretions, and blood and helps the lung to reexpand by reestablishing the subatmospheric pressure (i.e., negative pressure in the pleural space) necessary for normal pulmonary ventilation. Sometimes a *thoracotomy* is necessary to explore the chest and surgically repair the site of origin of the pneumo- or hemothorax.

Tension Pneumothorax; Mediastinal Shift. A tension pneumothorax is a serious valvular type of pneumothorax in which air enters the pleural space with each inspiration, becomes *trapped* there, and is not expelled during expiration. The trapped air continues to build up pressure in the chest as the amount of air accumulating in the pleural space increases with every inspiration.

If untreated, as the intrapleural pressure or tension increases it *collapses the lung* on the affected side and then may cause a *mediastinal shift* (Fig. 56–1*B*). A mediastinal shift means that the contents of the mediastinum (heart, trachea, esophagus, great vessels) are pushed or "shifted" toward the unaffected side of the chest. Mediastinal shift may cause compression of the lung in the direction of the shift (i.e., the lung opposite the pneumothorax) and compression, traction, torsion, or kinking of the great vessels (e.g., vena cava), thus dangerously impairing blood return to the heart.

Tension pneumothorax produces serious circulatory and pulmonary impairment that can rapidly be fatal. Tension pneumothorax is a high priority surgical emergency that must be promptly diagnosed and treated.

Symptoms of tension pneumothorax include: marked dyspnea; subcutaneous emphysema (trapped air escapes into the subcutaneous tissue of the chest wall causing the tissue to swell up and feel spongy); cyanosis; acute chest pain; shift of the trachea to the opposite side; tympany on percussion, hyperresonance, and reduced or absent breath sounds on the affected side; increased pulse and respiratory rates; feeling of pressure within the chest; and decreased movement of the affected side of the chest on inspiration.

Indications of *mediastinal shift* include cyanosis, severe dyspnea, deviation of the larynx and trachea from their normal midline position in the neck toward the side of the chest opposite the pneumothorax, and a change either medially or laterally in the heart beat's position of maximum impulse (normally near the midclavicular line in the fifth interspace). Some symptoms of mediastinal shift are similar to those produced by congestive heart failure, e.g., displacement of the trachea to one side, distended neck veins, dyspnea, and increased pulse and respiratory rates. Because no blood is available

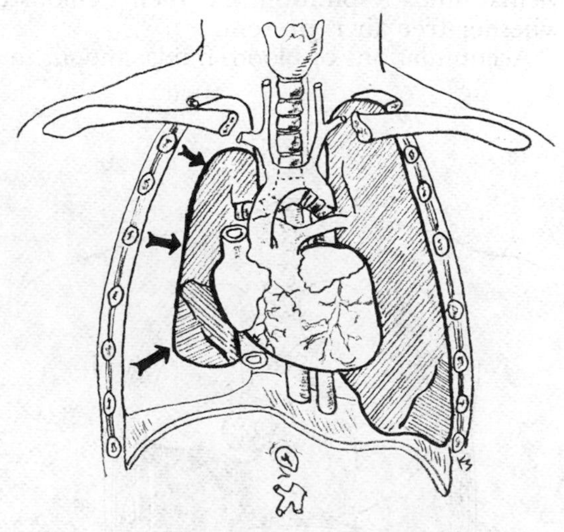

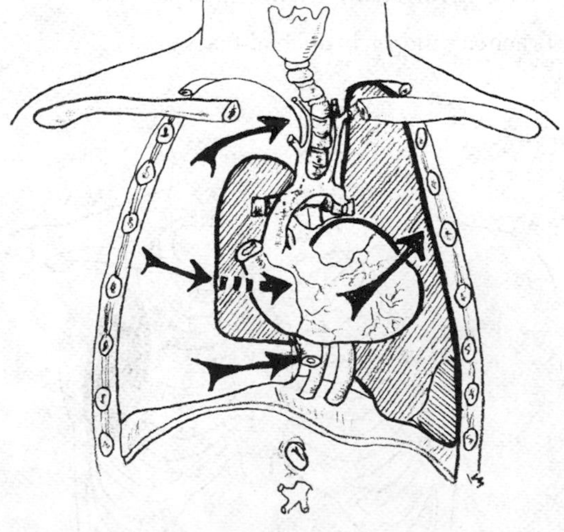

Figure 56–1. **A.** Pneumothorax. **B.** Mediastinal shift. Note collapse of lung with pneumothorax as air gathers in pleural space. With mediastinal shift, in addition to collapse of the lung, the mediastinal contents are displaced against the unaffected side of chest.

for cardiac output, the patient's blood pressure cannot be obtained in the presence of severe mediastinal shift. A suspected mediastinal shift may be confirmed by x-ray film or by directly measuring intrapleural pressure with an open-end "U" manometer. Laryngeal and tracheal deviation can be detected by gentle palpation as well as by x-ray film.

The *immediate treatment* of a tension pneumothorax is to convert the tension pneumothorax into an open pneumothorax (a less serious disorder) by providing an escape route for the air or fluid in the pleural space on the affected side. This can be accomplished most easily and rapidly by simply inserting a needle into the pleural space. If thoracentesis equipment is available (instead of merely a needle), lifesaving treatment may be prompt thoracentesis, using a three-way stopcock in the anterior 2nd intercostal space at the midclavicular line. As the trapped air rushes out, tension is relieved and the lung reexpands. Once the lung has been expanded, closed chest drainage (often with suction) is instituted. This permits air and fluid to leave the pleural space, but will prevent them from reentering.

Antibiotics are usually given because of the danger of empyema resulting from leakage of pulmonary secretions into the pleural space.

Iatrogenic Pneumothorax. *Iatrogenic pneumothorax* is the most common form of pneumothorax. The term iatrogenic indicates that the condition is a result of medical treatment. Iatrogenic pneumothorax may be intentional, as in diagnostic procedures, or unavoidable and unintentional, as those occurring following a needle biopsy.

Open Pneumothorax; Mediastinal Flutter. An open pneumothorax occurs with *"sucking" chest wounds.* In this type of wound the traumatic opening in the chest wall is large enough that air moves freely *in and back out* of the chest cavity during ventilating movements (Fig. 56–2). This abnormal movement of air through the chest wound produces a "slurping" or "sucking" noise that *is audible if the environment is quiet.*

To prevent possibly fatal complications from open pneumothorax, the opening in the chest wall must immediately be covered, thus preventing the abnormal passage of air.

Open sucking chest wounds may result not only from accidental injuries but also from surgical trauma. For example, if a chest drainage tube is accidentally pulled out of the chest, the remaining puncture incision in the chest wall may become a sucking wound.

When an open sucking chest wound is detected the emergency treatment is to securely cover the wound immediately with anything present. An airtight covering usually prevents a tension pneumothorax from developing and preserves ventilation of the opposite lung. Time is not wasted to obtain a sterile gauze petrolatum dressing (the ideal covering for such a wound) if such a dressing is not immediately available. Instead, at the scene of an accident the wound may be temporarily covered with a folded scarf or handkerchief, or possibly the heel of the examiner's hand.

In a hospital or clinic setting if you discover a sucking chest wound, immediately cover it with whatever is at hand, e.g., a towel, until someone else can bring a petrolatum dressing. *Never leave the patient unattended while you go off to find the proper dressing.* Administer appropriate first aid treatment, stay with and reassure the patient, and continue to apply pressure over the chest opening while you summon help. When your summons is answered, ask that the physician be notified and that a proper dressing or other needed equipment be brought to you. When possible, fix the temporary dressing firmly in place with several strips of wide tape.

If conscious and cooperative, the patient with

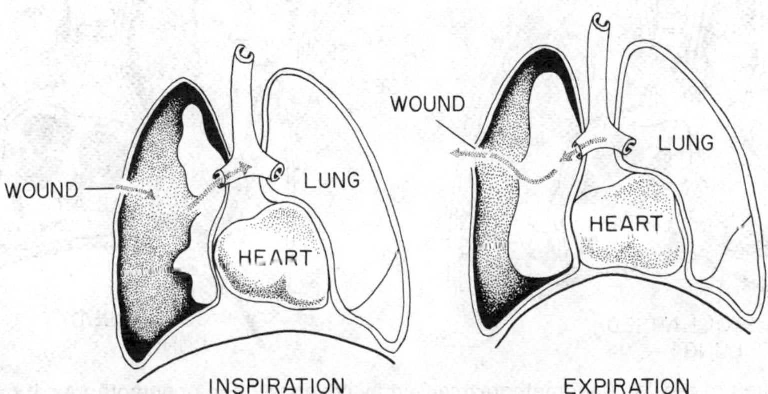

Figure 56–2. Open pneumothorax, i.e., "sucking" chest wound. (From Grant, H., and R. Murray: *Emergency Care.* Robert J. Brady Co., 1971.)

an open pneumothorax can help you. Instruct the person to take a very deep breath and then to try to blow it out while keeping the mouth and nose closed. This pushing effort against a closed glottis helps to push air out through the chest wound and helps to reexpand the lung. When the patient does this, apply the dressing before the patient can again inhale.

After a sucking chest wound on a chest-injured patient has been covered with an emergency air-tight dressing, remain with the patient and observe closely for indications of tension pneumothorax and mediastinal shift until the physician is present. It would be possible for these complications to occur if the patient had an air leak from the lung or a bronchus that was permitting the escape of air into the pleural space. In such a situation, closing the chest wall wound with an airtight dressing would prevent the outflow of the escaping air (from the lungs or bronchus), and thus a previously open pneumothorax would be converted into a tension pneumothorax. Although it is dangerous to have air moving in and out of the pleural space with each respiration (open pneumothorax), it is far more dangerous to have a situation in which air moves only into the pleural space and cannot move back out (tension pneumothorax). If the patient appears to be developing tension pneumothorax after sealing of the wound, immediately unplug the seal (Fig. 56–3).

The physician usually orders chest films to determine the amount of air in the pleural space and displacement of thoracic structures. Closed chest drainage may be necessary to remove the air and allow the lung to reexpand if it is collapsed. A closed chest drainage system permits air to move out of the pleural space but not into it. If the patient is in severe respiratory distress, the physician may need to perform emergency procedures, e.g., thoracentesis. Be certain that equipment that may be needed is available at the bedside when the physician arrives.

In addition to *dyspnea* and *collapse of the lung* on the affected side, the patient with an open pneumothorax may experience *mediastinal flutter.* This complication results from the rush of air in and out of the thoracic cavity on the affected side. With inspiration, the mediastinal structures and collapsed lung are pushed toward the injured side. Then, with expiration, these structures move back toward the unaffected side. These fluttering back and forth movements of the vital structures produce severe cardiopulmonary embarrassment which is fatal if not treated promptly.

Because infection can complicate an open pneumothorax, antibiotics are usually prescribed.

Hemothorax. To confirm a diagnosis of hemothorax the physician may aspirate blood by inserting a needle into the 8th interspace. To drain intrathoracic accumulations of blood the physician inserts two large-caliber chest tubes — one anteriorly, the other posteriorly. The tubes may then be connected to a single water-sealed drainage bottle to maintain closed chest drainage. Thoracotomy is indicated if bleeding continues for an abnormally long period of time or if the patient is losing large quantities of blood.

Fractured Ribs

Chest injuries frequently fracture one or more ribs. Indications of rib fractures include pain and tenderness over the fracture area, bruising at the injury site, protruding bone

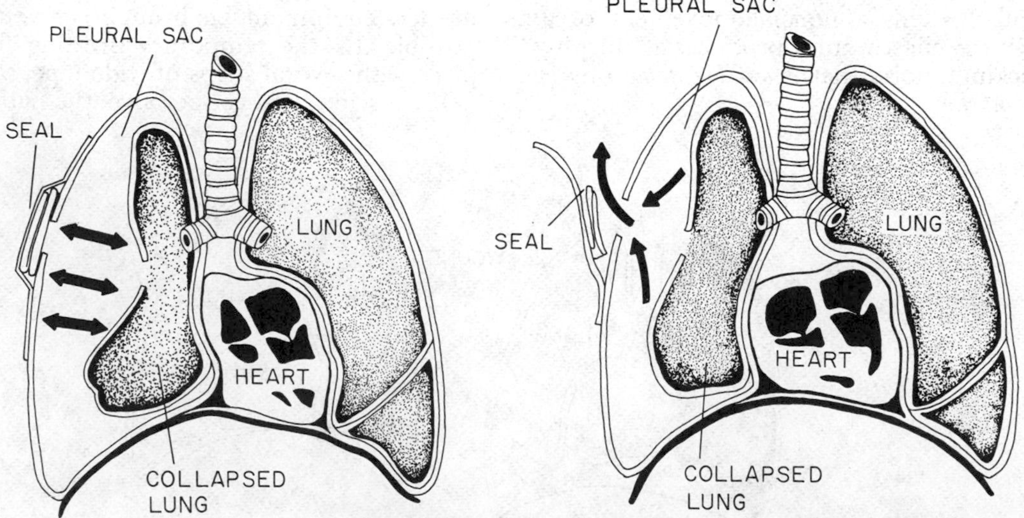

Figure 56–3. Correction of tension pneumothorax caused by covering open pneumothorax. If patient's condition declines after puncture wound is sealed, unplug the seal immediately. (From Grant, H., and Murray, R.: *Emergency Care.* Robert J. Brady Co., 1971.)

splinters if the fracture is compound, shallow respirations, and the tendency of the patient to splint the chest, i.e., to hold the chest or breathe shallowly to minimize chest movements.

The ribs most frequently fractured are numbers 4 through 8. Rib fractures can interfere with respiratory function by producing pain as the rib cage expands or contracts during breathing, or by puncturing or injuring the pleura and lung (and thus causing pneumo- and/or hemothorax) if splinters or fragments of bone penetrate inward. Fractured ribs predispose the patient to atelectasis and pneumonia because pain causes the patient to breathe shallowly and prevents effective coughing. Secretions therefore accumulate, obstructing bronchi and becoming a focus of infection. Shallow breathing also reduces lung compliance, i.e., causes "stiff" lungs. All these problems can be combated by frequent coughing, deep breathing, and position changes. Adequate pain coverage and splinting the chest during coughing and deep breathing help the patient to carry out these painful but vital activities more comfortably.

Care in Rib Fractures. Pulmonary function may be inhibited if more than two ribs are fractured. Severe crushing injuries to the rib cage seriously interfere with the mechanics of respiration. The pain from multiple rib fractures may cause the newly injured patient to go into shock. In an attempt to prevent shock, nerve blocks may be performed (e.g., by injecting procaine) in the intercostal nerves above and below the fractured ribs or by continuous segmental thoracic extradural nerve blocks. Pain relief obtained in this way makes it possible for the patient to breathe deeply, cough, and move about. Pain caused from simple fractures of only one or two ribs may be relieved by injecting a local anesthetic at the fracture site itself. Analgesics may be ordered for pain relief.

Analgesics are administered cautiously to the chest-injured patient. Narcotics may worsen respiratory depression and may depress the cough reflex (particularly in older persons).

Pain must be managed cautiously, e.g., with mild sedatives and small frequent doses of meperidine (Demerol).

In the past the affected side of the chest was immobilized if a patient had fractured ribs and no visceral damage was present. Immobilization was accomplished by "strapping" the ribs with strips of adhesive tape, an Ace bandage, or chest binder. This was done to try to reduce pain upon ventilation. Today strapping is condemned since it is realized that by restricting deep breathing strapping can cause complications such as hypoxia, hypoventilation, hypercapnia, pneumonia, or atelectasis.

Bone splinters from fractured ribs may cause pneumothorax or hemothorax by puncturing the lung and pleura. Chest x-ray films are carefully reviewed for indications of these complications. The nurse watches for symptoms of pneumothorax or hemothorax and reports them promptly if they appear. Bright red sputum may be coughed up by the patient if the lung has been penetrated.

Fractured ribs are generally treated conservatively unless the lung or pleura has been penetrated.

Crushed Chest; Flail Chest; Paradoxical Motion

Severe chest injuries that compress the rib cage often produce a crushed chest (sometimes called "stove-in chest"), in which the ribs are pushed in on the lung, and a "flail chest," which disrupts the normal bellows action of the thorax by causing paradoxical motion. (Note: Paradoxical motion may also result from surgical removal of several ribs, as in thoracoplasty, or from diaphragmatic paralysis, which impairs the action of the thoracic bellows.) (See figure on p. 1341.)

With crushed chest it is common for a fractured rib end to tear the pleura and lung surface, thereby producing hemopneumothorax. Both sides of the chest may be involved. Also, with a crushed chest it is common for several *adjacent ribs to be fractured in two or more places.* These double-line fractures produce a flail slab of the chest wall (i.e., flail chest) which no longer has bony or cartilaginous connections with the rest of the rib cage. Lacking attachment to the thoracic skeleton, the section of chest wall between the fractures "floats" and moves independently during ventilation.

In flail chest the detached portion and its underlying lung tissue move *paradoxically* in opposition to the remainder of the chest cage and lungs. Paradoxical respirations permit little movement of gases during inspiration and expiration. During *paradoxical motion* the flail portion of the chest and its underlying portion of lung are "sucked in" upon inspiration (instead of expanding normally outward) and they are ballooned out ("blown out") upon expiration (instead of collapsing normally inward) (Fig. 56–4). Severe cardiovascular disturbances and respiratory insufficiency progressing to hypoxia and carbon dioxide retention can result from these maverick actions unless rapid treatment is instituted.

Flail chest is one of the most critical of all chest injuries. The majority of patients who die from thoracic trauma in traffic accidents die from the effects of flail chest.

Loss of rigidity of the thoracic cage makes it impossible for the lungs to expand fully. Paradoxical motions neutralize the normal respiratory excursions of the chest wall and not only move air up and down in the trachea but also shunt stale air back and forth from one lung to the other. During inspiration some already used air ("pendulum air") may move from the affected to the non-affected lung and thus further reduce effective ventilation. Upon inspiration some air is sucked from the flail portion of the lung into the expanding regions of both lungs. During expiration some expiratory air is pushed into the flail portion of lung which is blowing out. These exchanges of stale air further reduce the effectiveness of respiration.

Paradoxical motion not only severely impairs normal breathing but also makes effective coughing impossible; therefore, secretions collect in the lung and hypoventilation and hypoxemia result. This may lead to acute respiratory failure. Secretions tend to be copious and thick and often are blood-tinged. Additionally, the mediastinal structures tend to swing back and forth during ventilatory movements. With a large area of paradoxical motion, these "swings" may seriously affect circulatory dynamics, producing elevated venous pressure, impaired filling of the right side of the heart, and decreased atrial blood pressure.

Severe cardiac or pulmonary failure causes a high mortality rate in persons with crushing chest injuries. Pulmonary edema, pneumonitis, and atelectasis often develop rapidly when the chest is crushed because fluids tend to increase and collect at the injured site.

In sum, paradoxical motion causes ineffective respiration (hypoxemia and hypercapnia), accumulation of pulmonary secretions, and impaired filling of the right side of the heart as a result of a lowering of the intrapleural negative pressure, which eventually progresses to right-sided heart failure and death.

Symptoms and Diagnosis. The patient with untreated flail chest suffers extreme distress while desperately trying to ventilate in spite of the excruciating pain. Hypoxia is worsened as the effort necessary to try to breathe further depletes the diminished available oxygen supply. The patient is usually cyanotic and severely dyspneic; respirations are typically rapid, shallow, and grunty. Large amounts of tracheobronchial secretions are produced. Shock commonly occurs and the patient may be hemorrhaging from the lungs or major vessels. Symptoms of paradoxical respirations include breathlessness or dyspnea with tachycardia as well as obvious paradoxical chest movements.

The patient who has sustained blunt trauma to the thorax and abdomen should be disrobed for emergency evaluation to observe for flail chest. Flail chest and paradoxical motion may result from sternal and rib fractures or from costochondral separations which cannot be detected by x-ray film. Commonly the 3rd to the 9th ribs are fractured at the necks posteriorly and also in the midaxilla. Paradoxical motion is frequently present soon after injury; however, sometimes it does not develop for several hours.

When multiple rib fractures are present, observe the patient's chest movements closely for paradoxical motion. Report this complication immediately.

Clinical Care. Clinical management of flail chest may include:

- Intensive nursing and respiratory care.
- Suction to maintain airway. When tracheal aspiration fails to maintain a clear airway the physician must perform bronchoscopy.
- IPPB and O_2 for a small degree of flail chest may suffice until the chest wall stabilizes.

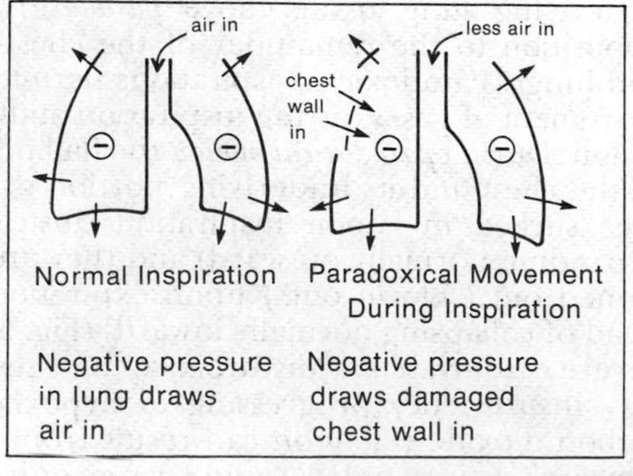

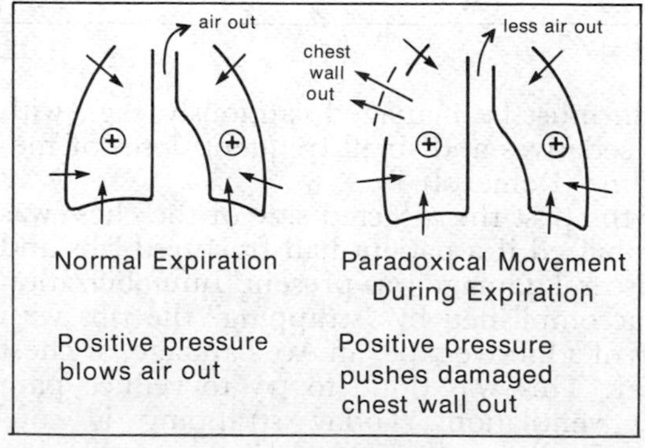

Figure 56–4. Paradoxical motion. (Drawn by K. C. Sorensen.)

- ▶ Internal stabilization with continuous mechanical ventilation via an artificial airway and controlled oxygen administration.
- ▶ Control of shock, hemorrhage, and pain. Control of hemorrhage helps to treat shock and hypoxia. Pain may be managed by nerve blocks and meperidine. Carefully evaluate agitation and restlessness to determine whether they are caused by pain or hypoxia.
- ▶ Prevention and treatment of infection. Administer antibiotics. Turn, cough, and deep breathe the patient to prevent pneumonia. Prevent aspiration.
- ▶ Relief of abdominal distention.
- ▶ Promotion of pulmonary reexpansion.
- ▶ Stabilization of flail portion of chest wall (internally) to eliminate paradoxical motion. (See emergency management.)

Rapid, effective treatment of flail chest and continued close supervision and nursing care are mandatory. As an emergency measure, e.g., at the scene of an accident, while waiting for help to arrive, apply pressure with a firm pad or the palm of the hand over the flail portion of the chest wall. Even though the underlying lung is compressed, the patient's respiratory distress will be somewhat relieved by stopping the paradoxical motion. Another means of applying pressure is to simply turn the patient onto the affected side.

In the hospital various treatments may be used to internally stabilize a portion of flail chest and thus prevent paradoxical motions during ventilation. *External* stabilization using towel clips and weights is rarely used today.

The patient with a flail chest has lost the mechanical ability to maintain adequate ventilation (owing to lack of maximal negative pressure in the pleural space). The treatment of choice is to place an artificial cuffed airway in the trachea and institute positive pressure ventilation. These actions immediately expand the lungs, reduce hypoxia and hypercapnia, restore adequate ventilation, decrease paradoxical motion, remove pendulum air, relieve pain by decreasing movement of the fractured ribs, provide an avenue for suctioning and cough stimulation, and combat the development of atelectasis, pneumonia, and pulmonary edema. Also, the use of a mechanical respirator provides fixation of the chest wall by *internal pneumatic stabilization.* This stabilizes the chest in the inflation position and keeps the fractured ribs properly aligned for healing.

The patient is commonly managed with an endotracheal tube. Internal stabilization with a continuous mechanical volume ventilator may require 10 to 14 days. Intravenous muscle relaxant medication may be administered. Some physicians may ventilate the patient in the *Control* mode to establish a controlled respiratory pattern. In this way the patient will not initiate respirations and there is less risk of separating healing costochondral junctions. Muscular skeletal paralyzing agents such as pancuronium bromide and D-tubocurare are administered to the patient who requires control of ventilation.

Frequent evaluations of blood gases and electrolytes are necessary to maintain effective respiration and combat possible fluid-electrolyte imbalances. A variety of factors may produce metabolic and respiratory acidosis in chest-injured patients (Fig. 56–5). Frequent roentgenograms are also necessary to evaluate the chest.

If a thoracotomy (chest wall incision) is necessary for other problems, e.g., diaphragmatic rupture, persistent bleeding, the surgeon may fixate the fractures internally when the chest is open. *Operative fixation* of a flail chest may be achieved by applying various devices to stabilize the flail portion of the chest wall, by passing sutures through the intercostal muscles, or by passing wires through holes drilled in the ribs if the intercostals are too damaged to hold stitches. Operative fixation of the flail chest segment is necessary when an air leak is present, e.g., from lacerated lung, or positive pressure ventilation may cause a tension pneumothorax in spite of the use of closed chest drainage.

Subcutaneous Emphysema

Frequently fractured ribs and other chest injuries cause air to escape into the subcutaneous tissues. This may also occur after thoracic surgery. The escaped air may then travel through the tissue for some distances under the skin; the presence of air causes the affected areas to puff out. (The word "emphysema" means a swelling or inflation caused by the presence of air.) If the skin is gently palpated over the air-expanded areas a crackling sensation which sounds similar to crackling cellophane may be noted (crepitus).

Although various areas of the body may be affected, some of the regions that may appear most grossly distorted by subcutaneous emphysema are the face, neck, and scrotum. Because of the bloated look of the face and neck, the patient's appearance may be alarming and visitors should be forewarned and given a simple explanation of the condition. Usually subcutaneous emphysema is not serious; however, the patient should be closely observed for respiratory distress if the neck is quite swollen.

Subcutaneous emphysema may occur with

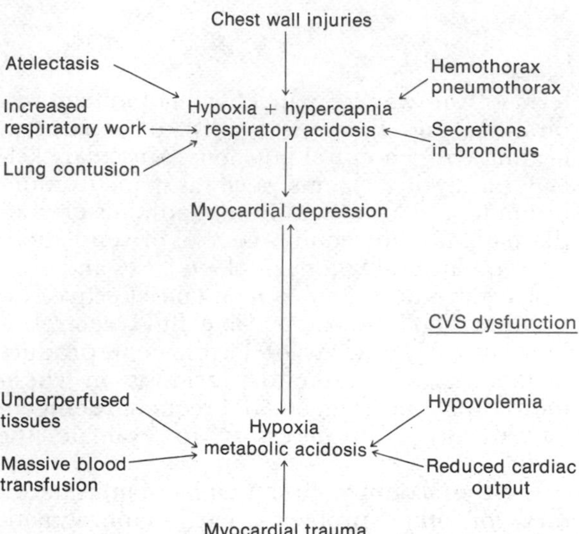

Figure 56–5. Factors producing metabolic and respiratory acidosis in chest injuries. (Modified from Reid and Baird, 1965.)

ventilator therapy, C-PAP, and PEEP. Its presence should be noted at once, a chest film made, and its progression followed. Subcutaneous emphysema may frequently reabsorb spontaneously in the body or may require treatment.

Pneumomediastinum; Pneumopericardium

Pneumomediastinum and pneumopericardium are serious medical problems. The air pressure exerted on these structures may compress the great vessels and prevent cardiac filling and emptying. This occurrence is not uncommon in pediatric ventilator care and also occurs in adults on a ventilator following a pneumothorax resulting from iatrogenic or other causes.

Cardiac Tamponade

Cardiac tamponade is acute compression of the heart resulting from the collection of blood or fluid in the pericardial sac. This may occur following either blunt or penetrating chest or upper abdomen trauma. It may also occur as a complication following vigorous cardiopulmonary resuscitation (CPR) and if the auricular appendage or right ventricle is accidentally perforated during cardiac catheterization or insertion of pacing wires, central venous pressure (CVP) lines, or Seldinger wires. Bleeding into the pericardium may be caused by rupture of the heart or coronary vessel. Even a small quantity of blood in the pericardial cavity will embarrass cardiac action and lead to cardiac arrest unless treatment is given promptly.

Rapid pericardiocentesis can be lifesaving. The removal of as little as 10 to 20 ml. of blood may relieve symptoms, and the patient's vital signs may immediately improve. As long as the patient continues to improve the physician withdraws as much blood as can be easily obtained. An 18-gauge needle is inserted through the xiphocostal angle to aspirate the pericardial sac. The patient is closely observed for repeated episodes of tamponade and several pericardiocenteses may be necessary. Usually thoracotomy is performed after tamponade has been relieved so the cardiac wound can be repaired surgically.

Cardiac tamponade is suspected when an injured patient is received in the emergency room in shock without evidence of blood loss. In some instances tamponade does not appear until one or two hours later. The nurse must therefore closely observe the chest-injured patient for symptoms of cardiac tamponade. These symptoms include high central venous pressure, narrowed pulse pressure (with or without cyanosis), paradoxical pulse, distant and muffled heart sounds, declining blood pressure, decreased pulse pressure, dyspnea, and reduced consciousness owing to impaired cerebral circulation. Electrocardiographic monitoring is advisable, and an aspirating needle and syringe should be readily available to prevent myocardial injury. Once the pressure of the accumulated fluids in the pericardial sac is relieved, the heart can again attempt to function normally.

ARDS (Wet-Lung Syndrome)

The wet-lung syndrome is a complication of chest injuries. This topic is discussed in detail in Chapter 55.

Shock

The chest-injured patient may require large quantities of blood to treat hypovolemic shock. When possible, surgery is delayed until the blood volume is restored. Although shock is frequently the result of hypovolemia, in the chest-injured patient it may also be caused by pericardial tamponade, flail chest, respiratory obstruction, or tension pneumothorax. Central venous pressure readings are carefully interpreted, since cardiac tamponade can be hidden by hypovolemia with a normal venous pressure; i.e., in the presence of hypovolemia the CVP may be normal even though cardiac tamponade is present. Once the physician correctly identifies the etiology of a patient's shock, treatment is rapidly administered. (Shock is discussed in Chapter 13.)

CHAPTER 57

CHEST SURGERY

Specific thoracic conditions that may be treated surgically were discussed in Chapters 55 and 56. Successful thoracic surgery depends not only on skills of the operating team, but also on quality nursing care during the pre- and postoperative periods. Nurses caring for persons following chest surgery must be familiar enough with the chest's anatomy and physiology that they can recognize alterations from normal that have resulted (a) from the patient's underlying disorder and (b) from the operative procedure performed. Also nurses must be able to recognize changes from the chest's normal structure and function that occur if postoperative complications develop. Such basic knowledge forms the framework upon which a nurse plans and administers personalized patient care directed at an uncomplicated recovery from the operative procedure.

Emphasis in this chapter is primarily on pulmonary surgery. Surgical procedures performed on the heart are discussed in Unit XII. Refer to Unit VIII for a general discussion of nursing care given patients undergoing surgery.

> *Much of the clinical care given chest surgery patients is* preventive care *directed at averting the numerous complications that can develop following thoracic surgery.*

PREOPERATIVE CLINICAL CARE

As with any surgery, prior to thoracic surgery a patient is prepared both physically and psychologically. Additionally, thorough evaluation is made of the patient's cardiopulmonary and general physical status. A great deal of time is spent during the preoperative period in teaching the patient ways to effectively participate in care during the postoperative period.

Preoperative Physical Evaluation and Preparation

Evaluation is made during the preoperative period of a patient's vital signs, general health, state of nutrition and hydration, general cardiac status, and specific pulmonary function (including arterial blood gas) status. When possible, attempts are made *prior* to surgery to improve the patient's hydration and nutritional status to optimal levels. For example, fluids may be forced to help thin bronchopulmonary secretions, and a high-calorie, high protein, increased vitamin diet may be given. Additionally, problems detected during the preoperative work-up, e.g., cardiac disorders, are evaluated and treated. When conditions are observed that contraindicate surgery (e.g., acute respiratory infection or skin lesions), they are called to the surgeon's attention.

> *Smoking causes bronchopulmonary irritation, increases tracheobronchial secretions, decreases oxygen saturation, and increases carboxyhemoglobin in the blood.*

Because oxygen saturation and minimal secretion production are important during and following thoracic surgery, *the patient is advised not to smoke* during the pre- and postoperative period. This advice is often extremely difficult for patients to follow if they are habitual smokers. Anxiety over the surgery may increase the desire to smoke.

During the preoperative period the appearance of the oral cavity is noted. This is of importance prior to thoracic surgery because the mouth is a major entrance to the lower respiratory tract. If during administration of oral hygiene a nurse notes infected teeth or lesions in the mouth, these findings are reported to the surgeon and the anesthesiologist.

If a patient has a known pulmonary infection, broad-spectrum antibiotics are usually ordered prior to surgery to minimize the number of pathogens. Postural drainage may also be prescribed (e.g., if an abscess, bronchiectasis, or retained secretions are present) to promote drainage from the lung of infected matter. (Postural drainage was discussed in Chapter 54.) Usually the patient is placed on a sputum observation routine preoperatively and sputum is observed, measured, and recorded every 8 or 24 hours. Sputum specimens are sent to the laboratory as ordered. Patients with impaired pulmonary function may be treated preoperatively with antibiotic and bronchodilating medications and intermittent positive pressure breathing equipment. Supervised breathing exercises help to improve respiratory efficiency prior to thoracic surgery.

PREOPERATIVE TESTS

Special tests may be ordered prior to thoracic surgery and include sputum examination, pulmonary function tests, bronchospirometry, chest x-ray films (including tomograms), bronchoscopy, bronchogram, electrocardiogram, and possibly cardiac catheterization. Prior to a pneumonectomy or left lobectomy it is especially important to study distribution of pulmonary function between the two lungs to determine whether the patient can tolerate the proposed loss of lung tissue without becoming a "pulmonary cripple." (Pulmonary diagnostic tests and procedures are discussed in Chapter 52.) *Routine preoperative tests* are also ordered.

IMMEDIATE PREOPERATIVE PHYSICAL PREPARATION

Immediate physical preparation of a person for chest surgery, beginning the day before surgery, may or may not include an enema and postural drainage. Thorough oral hygiene is routinely performed the morning of surgery. When atropine is ordered preoperatively (to minimize secretion formation), it should not be given until postural drainage has been completed (if ordered for the morning of surgery). Because it is important to minimize secretions in the tracheobronchial tree during thoracic surgery, patients about to undergo thoracic surgery may be ordered to receive larger preoperative doses of atropine than patients scheduled for surgical procedures involving other areas of the body. (See Unit VIII for discussion of other aspects of the immediate preparation of a patient for major surgery.)

Preoperative Teaching and Psychologic Preparation

During the preoperative period a person about to undergo thoracic surgery is helped, emotionally and intellectually, to prepare for the experience. The physician discusses with the patient and significant others reasons why the proposed surgery will be helpful. Often patients and their significant others are reluctant to ask physicians questions or to express their emotional concerns about surgical procedures. Frequently nurses are helpful in these areas, answering questions when possible, facilitating expression of concerns, and making plans and referrals as appropriate.

People are naturally apprehensive about having surgery performed on vital organs like the lungs. Preoperative emotional support is therefore of major importance. Because pulmonary surgery involves surgery on the "breathing apparatus" it is not uncommon for patients to express concern about being unable to breathe effectively following surgery.

> *Give patients control when possible. Teaching patients preoperatively how to effectively help themselves during the postoperative period is especially important before chest surgery.*

Discuss with a patient what will be happening during the early postoperative period, and talk specifically about how the patient will participate during recovery. These aspects of patient education are carefully *planned* by the nurse and are carried out in detail. Notes are made in the patient's chart of teaching sessions, e.g., what was generally discussed, whether the patient appeared to understand the discussion, what procedures were demonstrated, whether the patient correctly redemonstrated exercises, and so forth.

All forms of respiratory therapy that will be used by a patient in the postoperative period should be taught preoperatively and performed by the supervised patient. Patients who have chronic impaired respiratory function may require ventilatory assistance in the immediate postoperative period. An explanation and visual acquaintance with the continuous mechanical ventilator should be included in teaching plans.

Unless it is explained to patients *before* surgery that they will be surrounded by a lot of equipment (e.g., chest drainage, oxygen, ventilator) when they awaken from the anesthetic, they will tend to think that the equipment is present because their condition is poor. It must, therefore, be emphasized preoperatively that it is *routine* procedure to use various types of equipment following surgery to help the patient recover more rapidly. Significant others should also be prepared for what will be happening to the patient following surgery, so they are not unnecessarily frightened by the equipment, procedures, and the patient's appearance.

Tell the patient preoperatively that long periods of rest will not be possible for several days following surgery. For example, for the first 24 postoperative hours the patient will be awakened hourly to deep breathe, cough, and change position. On subsequent days he or she may be awakened every four hours, day and night, to ambulate, exercise, cough, and deep breathe.

Incentive respiratory exercises are best performed following surgery if they are taught to patients *before* surgery. Preoperatively teach the patient how to effectively turn, deep breathe, cough, and carry out exercises that are important postoperatively. Teach leg exercises to prevent thrombi from forming in the calves of the legs. Teach arm and shoulder exercises on the operative side to maintain normal range-of-motion and correct posture. Breathing exercises are also important for effective pulmonary function. When available, a physical or respiratory therapist may do the preliminary teaching for these activities. The nurse, however, is often responsible for supervising activity sessions. Be certain to familiarize yourself with the physician's preference for the patient's activity program. Some physicians order specific exercises.

Tell the patient that turning, coughing, and deep breathing are important following chest surgery not only because these activities help to move secretions out of the lung, but also because they help to reexpand the lung (which is temporarily collapsed when the thoracic cavity is opened during surgery), and they help to force air and drainage out of the chest cavity when drainage tubes are used. (Note: Of course, if an entire lung is going to be removed [pneumonectomy], there will be no lung tissue to reexpand postoperatively on the operated side. Nonetheless, coughing and deep breathing are highly important to prevent complications in the remaining lung.) Practice sessions (for turning, coughing, deep breathing, exercising) are important during the preoperative period. Supervise patients during these practice sessions until they can correctly perform these activities. *Remember to give encouragement and praise!*

Discuss with the patient the frequency with which various postoperative activities need to be performed. Inform the patient that medications and personal assistance will be given to promote comfort while performing these activities. Emphasize, however, that not all discomfort can be removed postoperatively with medications and that the patient is expected to be active (deep breathe, cough, exercise, turn, sit up, ambulate) in spite of moderately severe pain.

Other areas important to include during preoperative patient teaching sessions include:

- Evaluating the patient's understanding of the anatomy of the thorax and of the anticipated surgical procedure. Provide appropriate instruction as indicated.
- Telling the patient that vital signs may be monitored or taken frequently during the postoperative period. It is desirable to show the patient monitoring equipment that may be used and to explain briefly the function of the equipment. If the patient's vital capacity will be measured by the nurse following surgery the patient should be familiarized with this procedure.
- Informing patients that various equipment will be used following surgery to help them breathe more comfortably and effectively. For example, oxygen will probably be given nasally, and other respiratory therapy equipment such as a nebulizer or respirator may be used. Appropriate teaching is given concerning all equipment to be used. If it is known preoperatively that an endotracheal tube will be inserted, the patient is prepared for this procedure. (Artificial airways are discussed in Unit XXIV.)
- Informing patients of the reasons for suctioning and closed chest drainage (if chest drainage tubes will be used). Basically a patient is told that suctioning helps to remove secretions from the lungs, and that because chest surgery normally causes fluids to accumulate inside the chest postoperatively, chest tubes will help to drain off this fluid and air from the chest cavity.
- Preparing patients for the fact that they will probably be receiving intravenous feedings and may have a central venous pressure line or an indwelling arterial line as part of routine care. A cut-down may be performed on a leg vein during surgery (to ensure a route for intravenous therapy if shock occurs).
- Discussing with patients the fact that they will have moderately severe pain postoperatively and encouraging them to discuss pain and discomforts with the nurse. State that pain-relieving medications will be available.

COMMON THORACIC SURGICAL PROCEDURES

During thoracic surgery endotracheal anesthesia is usually administered. In fact, thoracic surgery became routinely possible only after the endotracheal method of anesthesia was perfected. This form of anesthesia makes it possible for an anesthetist to maintain effective functioning of the unoperated lung during the operative procedure. Once the pleural space is entered, the lung on the operative side collapses due to the entrance of air under atmospheric pressure. (Anesthesia is discussed in Unit VIII.)

Exploratory Thoracotomy

As its name indicates, *exploratory thoracotomy* "explores" the thorax to locate sources of injury or bleeding, or to inspect and take a biopsy specimen of suspected carcinoma. The biopsy may be of a lymph node or a section of the lung or may be a wedge resection (to be discussed). Exploratory thoracotomy may be accomplished through either a posterolateral parascapular incision or an anterior incision through an intercostal space. With either approach, the incision is of major size, the pleura is opened, and the ribs are spread to clearly expose the entire lung and hemithorax. Usually closed chest drainage is necessary postoperatively.

Resectional Pulmonary Surgery

Resectional pulmonary surgery is a surgical procedure in which a lung or portion of lung is removed. The various types of resection procedures differ in the amount of lung tissue removed. Closed chest drainage is not routinely used following pneumonectomy (removal of an entire right or left lung), but it is always used following other pulmonary resections.

Pulmonary resections are performed either via a posterolateral parascapular approach (through the 4th, 5th, 6th, or 7th intercostal space) or via an anterior approach (through the 3rd, 4th, or 5th intercostal space). Typically the anterior approach causes less disability and pain. Pulmonary resections are used to treat numerous conditions, e.g., chronic localized infections, cysts, bronchiectasis, pulmonary tuberculosis (unhealed by chemotherapy), bronchial adenoma, bronchogenic carcinoma.

Resectional operative procedures commonly performed on the lung are briefly discussed below:

- *Pneumonectomy:* Removal of an entire lung, e.g., in the presence of bronchogenic cancer, extensive (unilateral) tuberculosis, bronchiectasis, or lung abscess. In order to remove a lung the surgeon severs and sutures the mainstem bronchus at its bifurcation and the large pulmonary artery and veins. A pleural flap is sutured over the bronchial stump as an added precaution against postoperative air leakage through the stump. Once the lung is removed the thoracic cavity is an empty space. To help to reduce the size of this cavity the surgeon severs or crushes the phrenic nerve on the affected side; this paralyzes the diaphragm in an elevated position.

  Closed chest drainage is generally not used after pneumonectomy because it is desirable for fluids to accumulate in the empty thoracic space. Eventually the thoracic space fills in with serous exudate which consolidates, preventing extensive mediastinal shift of the heart and remaining lung. Sometimes a surgeon places a chest tube and *leaves it clamped* upon completing pneumonectomy. The surgeon may use this tube during the postoperative period as an avenue for inspecting for frank bleeding and measuring and regulating pressure in the thoracic space. (It is desirable to leave a slightly negative pressure in the closed thoracic space.) Some physicians use a pneumothorax apparatus to measure intrathoracic pressure and to add or remove air in order to maintain the pressure at the desired level. Pneumonectomies are most often performed to remove lung cancer.

- *Lobectomy:* Removal of a lobe of the lung, e.g., when disease (bronchiectasis, abscess, tumor, fungal infection, tuberculosis, cyst, or bleb) or injury is confined to one lobe. Any lobes of the lungs can be removed. (*Remember:* The right lung has three lobes; the left lung, two.) The bronchus leading into the removed lobe is sutured. Following pulmonary resection some compensatory, nonpathologic emphysema occurs as the remaining lung tissue overexpands to fill in the portion of the thoracic space previously occupied by the resected tissue. Closed chest drainage is used postoperatively.

- *Segmental resection (segmentectomy):* Removal of one or more lung segments when the disorder is limited to only the segment(s) resected, e.g., bronchiectasis, tuberculosis. (*Remember:* The lobes of the lungs are divided into parts called "segments." The right lung contains 10 segments and the left has eight). By delicate dissection the surgeon identifies and ligates the appropriate segmental bronchus, pulmonary artery, and vein. The remaining lung tissue then overexpands to fill the space occupied by the removed segment. Closed chest drainage is used postoperatively.

- *Wedge resection:* Removal of a small, localized area of disease (e.g., tuberculosis) near the surface of the lung. The portion removed is triangular (wedge-shaped) and is only part of a segment. Because the area resected is so small, pulmonary structure remains relatively unchanged after healing. The area to be removed is isolated by clamps and then resected. Sutures and chest drainage tubes are then placed.

When performing pulmonary resectional surgery, a surgeon is careful to remove no more lung tissue than necessary and thus save as much functional tissue as possible.

Decortication

Decortication is the removal or "stripping off" of a thick fibrous membrane or "peel" that sometimes develops over the visceral pleura. Such a membrane interferes with the lung's normal ventilatory movements; it may develop as a result of empyema or the prolonged presence of blood or fluid in the pleural space. The lung may become constricted and "trapped" by an infection or organized clot.

During the blunt dissection necessary to remove this membrane, numerous lung leaks are inevitably created. Postoperatively it is necessary to have at least two chest catheters present to accomplish closed chest drainage. If the surgery is to be successful, it is necessary for the decorticated lung to be rapidly and completely reexpanded. Closed chest drainage with suction is used to help the lung to reexpand rapidly and fill the pleural space. If the fibrinous membrane has restricted the lung for some time, the lung may not effectively reexpand even after the peel is removed. In such instances, once the surgeon is convinced that the lung cannot expand sufficiently (even though "freed" from its restrictive cover), a thoracoplasty may be performed.

Thoracoplasty

A *thoracoplasty* is a plastic operation on the thorax in which ribs or portions of ribs are removed to reduce the size of the thoracic space. Removal of ribs weakens the chest wall and permits atmospheric pressure (pushing against the outside of the chest) to collapse the weakened portion. When thoracoplasty is performed, the periosteum is stripped from the ribs before the ribs are removed. The periosteum is left in place in the chest wall and eventually a bony substance re-forms which holds the chest wall in that area in a collapsed position. Although the surgeon attempts to remove the desired ribs while remaining *outside* the pleural space, the pleura is sometimes inadvertently entered. When this occurs, closed chest drainage or aspiration is necessary postoperatively to reexpand the lung.

Before it became possible to resect the lung or portions of it, thoracoplasty was frequently used as an extrapleural form of collapse therapy to treat cavitary pulmonary tuberculosis. Currently it is seldom used for this purpose, but may be used to close a chronic empyema space, or to help to reduce the thoracic space before or after resectional surgery. (*Note:* This procedure is not routinely performed with resectional surgery, but only when clearly indicated.) Prior to pneumonectomy, for example, a thoracoplasty (called a *"preresection"* or *"tailoring" thoracoplasty*) may be performed to minimize chances of a postresectional mediastinal shift. This procedure may also be performed prior to other resectional surgeries if a surgeon believes the remaining portions of lung will not be able to expand enough following the resection to fill the pleural space or that they may overstretch and become pathologically emphysematous. Following some resections a *"postresection" thoracoplasty* is necessary if the remaining portions of lung fail to adapt themselves to the pleural cavity.

Some of the earlier thoracoplasties were quite disfiguring because the surgical procedures interfered with the shoulder girdle in such a way that the shoulder on the operated side drooped noticeably below the "normal" shoulder, the scapula sank medially against the mediastinum, and the chest on the operated side appeared markedly "caved in." Newer surgical procedures have greatly reduced these problems, since the shoulder girdle is not disrupted and the number of ribs removed is fewer; generally no more than three ribs are removed.

> *The removal of many ribs at one time is incompatible with continued life, because the soft, unstable chest wall that results goes into paradoxical motion. Paradoxical motion seldom occurs following modern thoracoplasty.*

POSTOPERATIVE CLINICAL CARE

Chest surgery is traumatic; many of the aftereffects and complications are therefore similar to those that follow chest injuries (Chapter 56). MacVicar and Mendelsohn observe that following chest surgery (or chest injuries) patients may develop "important and dangerous physiological and biochemical alterations" that basically result from "inadequate pulmonary ventilation and/or inadequate pulmonary or systemic blood circulation."[102A] During the postoperative period the basic aim of care is, therefore "to obtain and maintain respiratory and circulatory efficiency and to prevent physiological and biochemical alterations that may result from inadequate pulmonary ventilation and tissue perfusion."[102A]

In general, following thoracic surgery the patient is kept on a "mobilization" and "stir-up" regimen for several days — coughing, deep breathing, sitting up, ambulating, turning, exercising. The necessary care typically demands that the patient be active during the early postoperative period. Well-meaning but inexperienced nurses sometimes hesitate to insist that patients be active during this critical time. For example, such "sympathetic" nurses may permit patients to sleep through periods when they should be awakened to cough or deep breathe; or they may tell patients that exercises can be "skipped this time." These attitudes of misplaced sympathy are a grave disservice to patients.

Sensitivity to a patient's postoperative anxieties and discomforts is also necessary during the stressful postoperative period. The skillful nurse discusses a patient's concerns and distresses and offers appropriate reassurance, encouragement and relief. The nurse also inspires confidence in patients by performing skillfully and self-confidently while giving postoperative care. These attitudes come, in part, with familiarization with routines and equipment used postoperatively.

Complications Following Thoracic Surgery

Numerous complications can occur following thoracic surgery. Among these are: respiratory insufficiency, hypoxia, function loss; hyperventilation, CO_2 retention, hypercapnia; mediastinal shift; paradoxical motion; pneumothorax; hemorrhage, hemothorax; shock, hypotension; cardiac arrhythmias, myocardial infarction; respiratory arrest, cardiac arrest; pulmonary embolism, thrombophlebitis; residual pleural space; bronchopleural fistula; atelectasis, pneumonia; infections, e.g., wound infection, empyema; adrenal exhaustion; gastric dilatation, abdominal distention, paralytic ileus; subcutaneous emphysema; and acute pulmonary edema. Many of these complications result from inadequate ventilation or inadequate circulation.

Following thoracic surgery *inadequate ventilation* (causing alveolar hypoventilation) may occur because of: (1) airway obstruction (caused by retained bronchopulmonary secretions); (2) atelectasis; (3) incisional pain and discomfort from chest tubes (causes the patient to breathe shallowly and ineffectively); (4) depression of the central nervous system (e.g., caused by narcotics, sedatives, anesthetic agents, and muscle relaxants); (5) preexisting disease of lung parenchyma; (6) compression of lung tissue (caused by pneumothorax, hemothorax, abdominal distention, or phrenic nerve injury); (7) reduction of the amount of lung tissue available for aeration; (8) paradoxical respirations; or (9) bronchiolar narrowing or spasm. Alveolar hypoventilation produces hypoxia and hypercapnia and lowers the ventilation-perfusion ratio.

Circulatory insufficiency (indicated by hypotension) following thoracic surgery may result from: hypovolemia caused by blood loss or fluid depletion (when hypovolemia causes low cardiac output the shock syndrome develops); cardiogenic disorders (e.g., underlying myocardial disease causing arrhythmias, hypotension, myocardial infarction); and neurogenic causes (e.g., pain-induced hypotension).[102A] Circulatory insufficiency produces hypoxia, acidosis, and ischemia of the vital organs.

Physical indications of possible complications include low systolic blood pressure (below 90), temperature elevation (above 37.2° C or 99° F.), indications of hemorrhage through the incision, bloody chest drainage, pallor, dyspnea, cyanosis, increased pulse rate, increased respiratory rate, and acute chest pain. Specific symptoms associated with some of the more common specific complications are discussed more completely.

RESPIRATORY INSUFFICIENCY; HYPOXIA; HYPOXEMIA; HYPERCAPNIA

These disorders, discussed in Chapter 53, can all develop following thoracic surgery. The nurse giving postoperative care must be particularly alert to *early* indications of the development of these complications so appropriate treatment can be given promptly. Some postoperative factors leading to hypoxemia are illustrated in Figure 57–1.

TENSION PNEUMOTHORAX; MEDIASTINAL SHIFT; PARADOXICAL MOTION

These complications have also been previously discussed in detail (Chapter 56). Tension pneumothorax can result from postoperative air leakage through pleural incision lines if closed chest drainage fails to function properly. A large pneumothorax (or hemothorax) causes mediastinal shift. Also, mediastinal shift can easily occur following pneumonectomy if the patient is incorrectly positioned. If three or more ribs have been removed, paradoxical motion may occur with respirations.

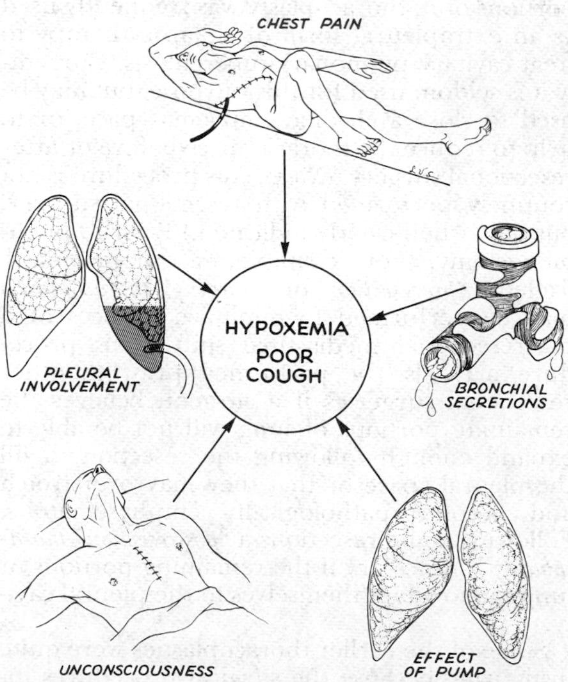

Figure 57–1. Postoperative factors leading to hypoxemia. (From Thomas, A. N.: *In* Sanderson, R. G., *The Cardiac Patient: A Comprehensive Approach.* Philadelphia: W. B. Saunders Co., 1972.)

HEMORRHAGE; HEMOTHORAX; HYPOVOLEMIC SHOCK

Blood loss during major thoracic surgical procedures may be greater than blood loss during most general surgical procedures because (a) blood vessels dissected within the thorax are of large caliber (a technical accident can produce considerable blood loss rapidly); (b) the incision is quite large and tends to have considerable capillary oozing; and (c) adhesions and tissue planes within the thorax are generally quite extensive and vascular.

Periodically check dressings or the incisional area (if a dressing is not present) for evidence of *bleeding* or *drainage.* Record findings, noting if the dressing is dry or the type and amount of drainage. Examine drainage in the closed chest drainage system for evidence of bleeding, and periodically evaluate the patient's pulse and blood pressure for indications of hypovolemic *shock,* i.e., an increasing pulse rate or a drop in blood pressure (lower than the preoperative blood pressure).

> *Manifestations of hemorrhage into the pleural space include bloody chest drainage, unstable blood pressure, increased pulse, dyspnea, and other symptoms of pulmonary collapse.*

Since progressive oliguria or anuria is another late symptom of shock, evaluate the patient's urinary output carefully each hour during the immediate postoperative period. Also observe for changes in sensorium that may indicate shock. Laboratory tests that may be employed to detect hypovolemia include a hematocrit and a determination of blood volume by means of radioactive albumin or dye-dilution techniques.

When a patient shows indications of hemorrhaging, have intravenous solutions, blood replacements, and plasma expanders readily available. The rate of fluid replacement can best be governed by continuously monitoring the CVP and arterial pressure. In the management of postoperative shock in a patient who has undergone thoracic surgery the Trendelenburg position is generally contraindicated since it causes the diaphragm and abdominal contents to elevate and, thus, restrict ventilation. *Hemothorax* may be treated with needle aspiration or closed chest drainage. Occasionally surgery is necessary. (Hemothorax was discussed in Chapter 56.)

As previously mentioned, not all hypotensive patients are in hypovolemic shock; shock may also develop as a result of cardiogenic or neurogenic causes. (Chapter 13 discusses shock in detail.)

CARDIAC ARRHYTHMIAS; MYOCARDIAL INFARCTION

A high percentage of persons requiring thoracic surgery have underlying cardiac disease. Thus, the cardiovascular system is carefully evaluated prior to surgery so patients can be managed safely during and following surgery. High-risk patients with underlying cardiac disease may have continuous electrocardiographic (ECG) monitoring during the postoperative period. Cardiac effectiveness can be severely limited by arrhythmias or myocardial infarction postoperatively. These disorders must be promptly treated since they may be life-threatening. (See Unit XII.)

> *Cardiac arrhythmias occur fairly often following thoracic surgery. The arrhythmia that occurs most often is atrial fibrillation; however, any of the arrhythmias may occur.*

RESPIRATORY ARREST; CARDIAC ARRREST

These grave complications and their clinical management are discussed in detail in Unit XII. Following thoracic surgery the nurse must be prepared to give appropriate *emergency cardiopulmonary resuscitation.*

PULMONARY EMBOLISM

Pulmonary embolism (producing obstruction of the pulmonary artery) is a serious potential complication following pulmonary surgery and is a significant cause of postoperative hypoxemia. Observe the patient closely for indications of this infarction of lung tissue. *Symptoms* of pulmonary embolism and infarction are variable, depending upon the location and degree of infarction. Small emboli may produce no pain, whereas large emboli may be associated with intense pain, suggestive of an MI. Other symptoms may include dyspnea, fever, hemoptysis, symptoms of right heart failure, hypoxia (producing metabolic acidosis), engorgement of neck veins (especially on inspiration), rapid and deep or shallow respirations, and symptoms associated with circulatory collapse, e.g., tachycardia, hypotension, pallor, apprehension, sense of impending doom, nausea, sweating, weakness, and breathlessness. Upon auscultation, localized wheezing may be noted over a specific portion of lung. The bronchospasm may be transient. (Pulmonary embolism is discussed in Unit XV.)

RESIDUAL PLEURAL SPACE

If a *persistent pleural space* develops from inadequate reexpansion of lung tissue, additional surgery such as a thoracoplasty may be required.

BRONCHOPLEURAL FISTULA

Bronchopleural fistula can result postoperatively from: (1) inadequate closure of the bronchus at the time of pulmonary resection; (2) inadequate blood supply to the bronchial stump, with resultant necrosis and "blow out" of the stump; (3) infection at the point of the bronchial amputation, with resultant "blow out" of the suture line; and (4) alveolar or bronchiolar tears on the surface of the remaining lung. When a bronchopleural fistula occurs, *air escapes into the pleural space* and is forced into the subcutaneous tissues around the incision, producing *subcutaneous emphysema* (see p. 1357), and/or *infection* occurs in the pleural space as a result of tracheobronchial secretions draining into the pleural space. Additional surgery may be necessary to correct bronchopleural fistula.

ATELECTASIS; PNEUMONIA

> *Maintenance of a patent airway is a primary goal of clinical care following thoracic surgery.*

If airway obstruction is allowed to develop, *atelectasis* typically results. Atelectasis, in turn, causes two major complications of thoracic surgery — *hypoxia* and *hypercapnia.* Also, once atelectasis occurs, *pneumonitis* may soon develop. Airway obstruction is indicated by restlessness, inadequate chest expansion, stridor, cyanosis, dyspnea, and noisy respirations. Indications of massive atelectasis include increased rate of respirations, rapid pulse, elevated temperature, profuse perspiration, and cyanosis.

If atelectasis is suspected, the physician orders arterial blood gas determinations and oxygen administration. Numerous *therapies* are employed in the treatment of pneumonia, e.g., antibiotics, IPPB, aerosol administration of both high-volume hydration aerosols and medicated aerosols, mucolytic agents, chest physiotherapy, and incentive breathing exercises. In some cases, intratracheal suctioning and irrigation, bronchoscopy, and insertion of an artificial airway may be needed. *Generally the development of postoperative atelectasis indicates that the patient's nursing care was inadequate and that all the necessary measures were not performed to maintain airway patency.* (Atelectasis and pneumonia are discussed in Chapter 55, see also Fig. 52–2.)

INFECTIONS

Prior to the use of more thorough preoperative preparation of the patient and before the advent of definitive antibiotic therapy, *pulmonary and pleural infections* commonly occurred following thoracic surgery. Currently routine prophylactic antibiotic coverage is *not* used with thoracic surgery. Antibiotics are administered if infected areas were surgically entered or if an infection is known to exist in the wound, pleurae, or tracheobronchial tree. Whenever possible, antibiotics are selected after sensitivity studies have identified the specific medication to which a patient's organisms are sensitive. If empyema occurs, additional surgery may be needed.

> *Postoperative infection may be prevented by aseptic suctioning technique, aseptic technique when caring for the closed chest drainage system (e.g., when emptying the fluid collection bottle), administration of antibiotics as ordered, hygienic nose, mouth and skin care, and maintenance of a patent airway.*

ADRENAL EXHAUSTION

Patients who have had long debilitating illnesses prior to surgery may experience *adrenal exhaustion* postoperatively because of the stress of surgery. Watch for early indications of hypoadrenalism. (See Unit XIX.) Treatment includes administration of adrenocortical steroids.

GASTRIC DISTENTION

Gastric distention may result from air swallowing as well as depression of gastric motility as a result of anesthesia. Additionally, insufflation of anesthetic gases into the stomach may occur during surgery. Observe for gastric distention by inspecting and percussing the patient's abdomen. *Abdominal distention is not only uncomfortable but is also potentially dangerous following thoracic surgery because the enlarged abdomen elevates the diaphragm and, thus, impairs the patient's ventilatory movements, which may already be precariously limited.* Gastric dilatation most commonly occurs following surgical procedures on the left hemithorax, and occurs early in the postoperative period. An upright chest x-ray establishes the diagnosis.

When gastric dilatation occurs, the physician

may order nasogastric suction to accomplish gastric decompression. The tube is left in place until gastrointestinal motility returns and the patient is taking adequate oral intake. Neostigmine (Prostigmin) may be prescribed to stimulate peristalsis and facilitate flatus expulsion. Ambulation and exercising also help the patient to expel flatus.

SUBCUTANEOUS EMPHYSEMA

Observe the patient for *subcutaneous emphysema* around the incision and in the chest and neck. To evaluate the rate of progression of the emphysema, periodically mark the patient's chest with a skin-marking pencil at the outer periphery of the emphysematous tissue. If subcutaneous emphysema reaches the level of the patient's neck, make periodic measurements of the neck's circumference.

Subcutaneous emphysema commonly occurs following thoracic surgery and usually is not dangerous (except in infants). However, a *progressive increase* in the amount of subcutaneous emphysema occurs if a patient's chest drainage tubes are not functioning effectively. Progressive emphysema is particularly serious following pneumonectomy, because it may signify air leakage through the bronchial stump. If the rate of increase is rapid, notify the surgeon. *Treatments* may include: (1) insertion of a new thoracotomy tube, (2) addition of suction to a closed chest drainage system (or increasing the amount of suction currently in use); or (3) aspiration of the mediastinum. Occasionally it is necessary to return a patient to surgery to repair a bronchial stump. Severe subcutaneous emphysema in the neck may require tracheostomy. Areas of subcutaneous emphysema may be tender and therefore should be handled gently and palpated no oftener than necessary. Severe subcutaneous emphysema may be quite uncomfortable.

ACUTE PULMONARY EDEMA

Circulatory overload resulting in *acute pulmonary edema* is a potential threat following any resectional procedure because operated lung does not immediately reexpand following surgery, and pulmonary tissue was removed during surgery. Both factors cause a reduction in size of the pulmonary vascular bed.

Fortunately acute pulmonary edema does not often occur following thoracic surgery. However, when failure of the left ventricle does occur as a result of surgery, it most typically develops following pneumonectomy or in patients who had congestive heart failure preoperatively. Acute pulmonary edema may occur rapidly following removal of one lung, not only because of the drastic reduction in the pulmonary circulatory system, but also because of the increased permeability of capillaries caused by hypoxia. *Acute pulmonary edema is a life-threatening compli*

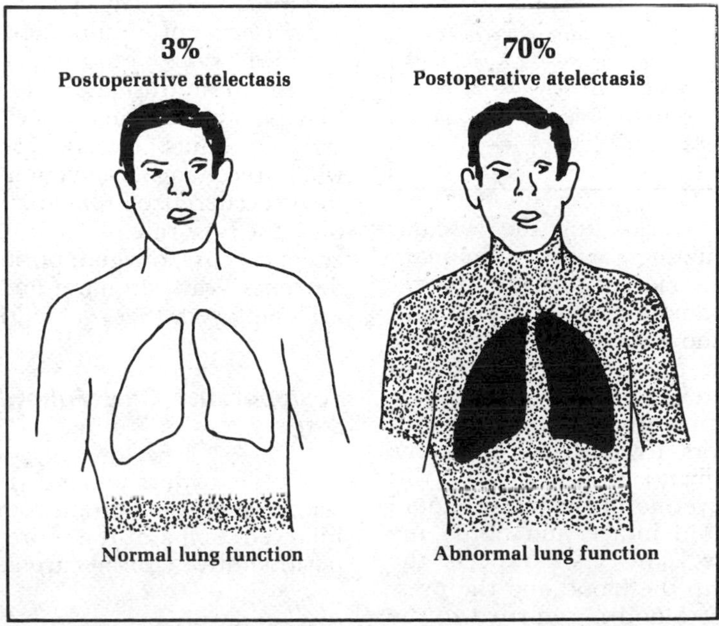

Figure 57–2. Postoperative atelectasis tends to occur in about 3 per cent of patients with normal lung function and in about 70 per cent of patients with abnormal lung function. (From Shafer, N.: Preparing the asthmatic patient for surgery. *Consultant,* 17:84, May 1977.)

TABLE 57–1. MANAGING A PATIENT WITH PULMONARY EDEMA

Stages of Pulmonary Edema	Symptoms	Nursing Responsibilities
Initial stage	Persistent cough—patient feels "like a cold coming on" Slight dyspnea/orthopnea Exercise intolerance Restlessness Anxiety Crepitant rales may be heard over the dependent portion of the lungs Diastolic gallop	Check color and amount of expectoration. Position patient for comfort. Auscultate chest for rales and third heart sound. Medicate as ordered. Monitor apical and radial pulses for rate and rhythm. Assist patient with all needs to conserve strength. Provide emotional support (through all stages) for patient and family.
Advanced stage	Acute shortness of breath Respirations—rapid noisy (audible wheeze, rales) Cough more intense and productive of frothy, blood-tinged sputum Cyanosis Diaphoresis—skin cold and clammy Tachycardia—arrhythmias Hypotension	Institute emergency measures: 1. Give oxygen—preferably by high concentration mask or IPPB. 2. Insert IV if not already done. 3. Aspirate nasopharynx p.r.n. 4. Apply rotating tourniquets. 5. Give digitalis and morphine as ordered. 6. Give potent diuretics (e.g., furosemide [Lasix] or ethacrynic acid [Edecrin]) as ordered. 7. Insert Foley catheter. 8. Calculate intake and output exactly. 9. Draw ABG's. 10. Attach cardiac monitor leads and observe ECG. 11. Prepare for phlebotomy, if necessary. 12. Have resuscitation equipment available.
Acute stage	Decreased level of consciousness Ventricular arrhythmias Shock Diminished breath sounds	Give emotional support to patient and family. Be prepared for cardioversion of tachyarrhythmias. Assist with intubation and mechanical ventilation. Resuscitate if necessary.

From Isacson, L. M.: Treating pulmonary edema. *Nursing 78,* 8:42, Feb. 1978, p. 44.

cation. Therefore, during the postoperative period the nurse directs efforts at *preventing* this complication. *Remember:*

> *Following thoracic surgery never administer intravenous fluids at a rate exceeding 84–125 ml./hr. (unless specifically ordered otherwise) because of the possibility of precipitating circulatory overload and causing pulmonary edema.*

The possibility of overloading the vascular system and precipitating acute pulmonary edema following thoracic surgery can be reduced by carefully evaluating intake and output and by monitoring the patient's hemodynamic status. Regulation of the rate of flow of intravenous fluids is determined by evaluating the CVP or pulmonary pressures determined with flow-directed catheters (Swan-Ganz catheter). (See Unit XII.) Usually it is specified that if this pressure reaches a given level the nurse should limit the patient's fluid intake and notify the surgeon immediately. The CVP reflects the heart's ability to pump the blood and the pressure under which the blood is returned to the superior vena cava or the heart's right atrium. Venous return to the right atrium is influenced by respiratory movements and intrathoracic pressure alterations. Resistance to the outflow of blood from the right side of the heart (causing elevation of the CVP) may result from reduction in the pulmonary vascular compartment following resectional surgery (see also below).

Symptoms of pulmonary edema include dyspnea, rales, gurgling respirations, frothy sputum, cyanosis and other signs and symptoms of hypoxemia. (See Chapter 54.) Observe patients closely for these symptoms while receiving intravenous infusions, report their occurrence immediately, and reduce at once the flow rate of the infusion. If pulmonary edema occurs, oxygen, positive airway pressure, diuretics, cardiotonics, and vasoactive drugs are employed. (See Table 57–1.)

Postoperative Care Following Thoracic Surgery

Specific orders are individualized after thoracic surgery, but certain routines are frequently followed. Some of the more common aspects of postoperative clinical care are discussed.

IMMEDIATE CARE

Upon receiving a patient in the recovery room or intensive care unit following chest surgery the nurse: (1) institutes oxygen therapy and suction as indicated; (2) positions the patient according to his/her condition; (3) evaluates and records vital signs (pulse, blood pressure, CVP and arterial pressure, temperature, and respirations), (4) makes certain thoracotomy tubes are correctly attached to the prescribed type of closed chest drainage apparatus (with or without suction, as ordered); (5) examines dressing or incision area (a dressing may not be present) for bleeding and/or drainage; (6) looks for evidence of subcutaneous emphysema; (7) checks flow rate of intravenous blood or fluid replacements; (8) evaluates patient's sensorium; (9) observes and auscultates patient's chest for indications of complications (e.g., retraction of the rib cage during ventilatory movements, paradoxical respirations, ease or difficulty of ventilation, presence of stridor or rales); and (10) evaluates other factors indicative of the patient's general condition (skin, nail bed, and mucous membrane color; skin texture; respiratory pattern; body position; movement or lack of movement of facial muscles and extremities). Observations are made as frequently as a patient's condition warrants.

EQUIPMENT

Equipment that *must* be available and in good working condition during the immediate postoperative period following thoracic surgery typically includes apparatus for suctioning, oxygen administration, closed chest drainage, arterial pressure monitoring, thoracentesis, respiratory therapy equipment including endotracheal intubation equipment and a volume ventilator, and intravenous therapy. The nurse should have a stethoscope.

Equipment for *emergency care* that should be readily available includes Ambu-type bag, respirator, tracheostomy set, laryngoscope, bronchoscope, endotracheal tubes, needles, syringes, vasoconstrictors, heart stimulants, and intravenous solutions.

VITAL SIGNS

Typically, for the first two or three postoperative hours, vital signs are taken every 15 minutes. Thereafter, if the pulse rate and blood pressure have started to stabilize at the preoperative level, vital signs are taken every 30 minutes for several hours and then hourly throughout the operative night. Blood pressure is closely evaluated for 24 to 36 hours postoperatively because it may fluctuate. A patient with a persistently low blood pressure is closely observed because this finding may be caused by cardiac disorders, hemorrhage, pain, hypoxia, or an inadequate circulating fluid volume. During the postoperative period patients are also closely observed for respiratory distress.

CENTRAL VENOUS PRESSURE (CVP) READINGS

As previously mentioned, the CVP is important following thoracotomy and may be measured continuously or at least frequently. The nurse observes the CVP for sudden increases or decreases. Since the CVP measures the heart's ability to adequately accept and put out the circulating blood volume, an elevated CVP signals impaired venous return to the heart. (See also Unit XII.)

When indicated, the CVP catheter may be used for such additional activities as drawing blood for laboratory tests, intravenous infusions, drug administration, and performing phlebotomy.

ARTERIAL PRESSURE MONITORING

Flow-directed catheters floated into the pulmonary artery are now commonly used to determine a patient's hemodynamic status. The *Swan-Ganz catheter* has replaced the CVP line in many intensive care settings. The Swan-Ganz catheter offers a more reliable means of monitoring patients with potentially severe cardiopulmonary decompensation. This method allows measurement of both the *pulmonary arterial (PA)* and *pulmonary capillary wedge pressure (PCW)*.

The PCW reflects the function of the left heart more than the CVP or PA pressure measurement. Other measurements to assess a patient's cardiopulmonary and circulatory status may be made through the pulmonary artery catheter. These include approximation of the activity of the left heart, collection of blood samples to assess arteriovenous O_2 difference, and performance of cardiac-output measurements.

FLUIDS AND NUTRITION

During or immediately following chest surgery the patient is given a blood transfusion followed by whatever intravenous fluids the surgeon orders. As discussed, *intravenous feedings and blood transfusions must be run slowly (unless specifically otherwise ordered) to prevent overloading of the vascular system, with resultant pulmonary edema.* Once the patient is fully conscious, is not nauseated, and is generally doing well, clear fluids are usually permitted. Diet then progresses to a soft and then a general diet as tolerated. Fluid intake is increased, also as tolerated, and is encouraged during the postoperative period, since fluid intake helps to liquefy tracheobronchial secretions so they can be more easily expectorated. Record intake and output and evaluate for imbalances.

PAIN MANAGEMENT

Following thoracic surgery knowledgeable pain management is imperative. Unless the patient is adequately medicated the extreme pain and discomfort of the first few postoperative days may indirectly result in complications. On the other hand, if a patient is overly medicated with narcotics the cough reflex and respirations will be depressed, again setting the stage for the development of complications.

Following chest surgery pain may cause the patient to experience neurogenic hypotension, as pointed out earlier. Also, the patient who is not given adequate pain relief may be unable to perform the essential postoperative activities of coughing, deep breathing, turning, exercising, sitting up, and ambulating. The patient in severe pain breathes shallowly and rapidly (in other words, ineffectively), and tries to avoid chest movements. Also, he or she resists other movements. As a result of this inactivity secretions are retained and the lung does not properly reexpand. Atelectasis and pneumonia rapidly ensue. These complications may be fatal. When possible, medicate the patient prior to deep-breathing, coughing, and exercise sessions so patient participation can be more effective.

In addition to the physical consequences of inadequate pain coverage the patient also suffers emotional anguish and is fearful. Obviously the nurse contributes greatly to a patient's total well-being by skillfully helping to relieve postoperative pain. Medications are, of course, not the only means of reducing pain. For example, correctly positioning and turning the patient are comfort measures that also provide relief (see below). (See also discussion of pain in Unit XI.)

During the first few days of postoperative care the patient may require frequent medication for pain relief. Commonly morphine or meperidine hydrochloride (Demerol) is prescribed. Some physicians do not prescribe morphine following thoracic surgery because of its depressing effects on the respiratory and cough centers; therefore, the medication of choice is meperidine. In addition to giving pain relief, meperidine also appears to dilate the bronchi. The opiates tend to have the opposite, detrimental effect of producing bronchospasm and thickening secretions.

If narcotics are ordered following chest surgery, they are used sparingly. Sometimes dosages smaller than usual are ordered so the medication can be administered more frequently without depressing the respiratory centers in the brain. Medications that have analgesic-potentiating properties, such as hydroxyzine (Atarax, Vistaril) may be prescribed to be given in combination with small doses of narcotics. Following the adminstration of narcotics, closely observe the patient's respiratory rate and quality for indications of depression.

Following thoracic surgery the patient's chest is often extremely painful not only because of the trauma of the surgery, but also because of the presence of large chest drainage tubes. Sometimes severance of intercostal nerves at the time of surgery produces postoperative sensations of pain, numbness, or heaviness in the operative region.

Usually these sensations are temporary. At the time of surgery some surgeons inject the intercostal nerves with a local anesthetic, e.g., procaine, to minimize pain during the immediate postoperative period. Occasionally an intercostal nerve block is necessary postoperatively for pain relief.

POSITIONING; TURNING

Following chest surgery a supine position is often the position of choice while the patient is unconscious. *Generally the Trendelenburg position is contraindicated* because it causes the abdominal organs to push against the diaphragm (and hence restrict lung excursions), and also because it creates pressure on the mediastinal contents. Such pressure decreases venous return and cardiac output. In some patients postoperative hypotension results from venous pooling of blood in the legs. This hypotension may be alleviated by applying elastic bandages to the legs or elevating the legs without elevating the hips.

Typically following thoracic surgery the patient remains flat until vital signs have stablized and consciousness is regained. Then repositioning occurs in a semi-Fowler position (head of the bed elevated 30 to 45 degrees). This position is desirable because it causes the diaphragm to drop down in a normal position (thus enhancing lung expansion); it makes possible ventilation with the least effort by the patient; and it facilitates chest catheter drainage. When moving a patient from a supine to a semi-Fowler position, elevate the head gradually.

Check positioning orders carefully for each patient. If these orders are unclear, clarify them before positioning the patient. Be certain you know if a patient is permitted to be on the operated side or if the preferred position is on the unoperated side or back. *Correct positioning is especially impor-*

tant following pulmonary resection. Following lobectomy it is generally permissible to use full lateral turning on both sides. This permits expansion of lung tissue on both the operated and unoperated sides. Occasionally a surgeon specifies that a patient is not to lie on the operated side. Lying on the operated side may also be forbidden *following segmentectomy or wedge resections* because it is desirable to foster expansion of remaining pulmonary tissue. *If the patient has a sternum-spliting incision,* positioning on either side or the back may be allowed (the back position is most comfortable).

Following pneumonectomy extreme lateral turning is avoided because the mediastinum is not held in place by lung tissue on both sides; typically the patient is permitted to turn only one quarter of the full lateral position to prevent mediastinal shift and compression of the remaining lung. Generally the patient is allowed to lie on the operated side for brief periods, e.g., to permit back care. Then, if the pulse and blood pressure remain stable while turned, permission may be given to turn onto either side 24 hours following surgery. Some surgeons permit the patient to be positioned only on the back or on the operated side. The patient is turned hourly from one position to the other.

When helping a patient to move about following chest surgery, e.g., to slide up in bed or to sit up, support the back of the head and assist from the unoperated side, e.g., do not tug or pull on the arm on the operated side. In many hospitals a piece of muslin or a rope (with a handle) long enough for the patient to grasp is tied securely to the foot of the bed. The patient is instructed to grasp this "*pull rope*" when pulling up to the sitting position or lowering to lie flat, during later convalescence. Also, *be careful not to exert traction on the chest tubes.* While in bed the patient may find it comfortable to have a pillow under the neck and head; a pillow under the back may be uncomfortable.

Turn the patient every one or two hours to mobilize and promote drainage of secretions within the tracheobronchial tree and the drainage of air and fluids from the pleural space (if closed chest drainage is employed). *Allowing the patient to remain in one position for too long predisposes to thrombus formation (because it slows blood flow) and may cause inadequate aeration of part of the lungs.* Turning improves circulation generally since it causes muscles to squeeze on blood vessels. Position changes also have favorable effects on the patient's general comfort. When changing the patient's position, reposition to maintain good posture and body alignment, and so thoracic movements are unrestricted. If the thorax cannot move freely to ventilate and expand the lungs, alveolar hypoventilation and its serious consequences occur. Also, when positioning the patient, *be certain chest and drainage tubes are correctly placed and are not kinked or compressed.*

Patients usually have very sore, aching chests after chest surgery. If ribs have been resected, the patient's rib cage may remain sore for weeks. The large rib-spreading retractors used during surgery also make the chest cage very sore. Gentleness in handling the patient is essential.

AMBULATION

As with other types of surgery, early ambulation following thoracic surgery helps to reduce postoperative complications since it improves ventilation, circulation, and patient morale. Even though the patient may be reluctant, ambulation is usually encouraged as soon as vital signs are stable postoperatively. It is thus not unusual for patients to ambulate on the evening of surgery or the morning of the first postoperative day. Closed chest drainage does not prevent a patient from getting out of bed, sitting up in a chair, or walking about. Some physicians order ambulation every four hours, around the clock, to prevent vascular stasis and its related complications. Patients with limited cardiovascular reserve or heart disorders may not be able to ambulate as soon as other patients with a stronger general state of health.

If oxygen is being administered to a patient, it must be administered *during all activities.* When large portions of lung tissue have been removed and pulmonary status has been surgically compromised, the flow rate of O_2 during ambulation may vary from the resting oxygen flow rate. Small portable tanks and portable liquid oxygen systems make oxygen administration easy. O_2 humidifiers are not necessary for short-term O_2 administration such as during ambulation.

EXERCISES

Exercising is another important aspect of postoperative care following thoracic surgery. As stated previously, exercises to be performed postoperatively are taught to the patient during the preoperative period whenever possible so the patient can become familiar with them and practice them at a time when not in acute discomfort. Postoperatively the exercises ordered by the surgeon are reviewed with the patient and are performed with assistance or under the supervision of the nurse or physical therapist. Nonvigorous exercises of the arms, trunk, and lower extremities begin soon after surgery.

Goals. Postoperative exercise following thoracic surgery are directed at:

- Preventing collapse of lung tissue, atelectasis, and impaired ventilation. Breathing exercises and abdominal breathing (see Chapter 54) are performed to reexpand the lung, improve ventilation, obtain maximal pulmonary function, and help the patient to cough more effectively. Abdominal breathing helps to minimize pain associated with ventilation.
- Preventing musculoskeletal and circulatory disorders. Complete range-of-motion (ROM) exercises are performed while the patient is confined to bed to prevent the complications of bed rest and to preserve body postural symmetry.
- Preventing ankylosis of the shoulder and stiffness and contractures of the arm on the operated side. Exercising the arm and shoulder on the operated side is directed at maintaining normal joint range-of-motion, reeducating injured or unused muscles, and minimizing postoperative discomfort (see below).
- Preventing a generally depressed mental state. Exercising improves the patient's general feeling of well-being.

Following thoracoplasty and pneumonectomy it is particulary important to maintain correct body alignment when positioning the patient and to have the patient practice maintaining good posture. The prevention of postoperative scoliosis is especially important following pneumonectomy.

Preparation. Prior to exercise sessions, encourage the patient to cough productively to clear the tracheobronchial tree. This ensures more effective oxygenation during the exercise activities. Provision of adequate pain coverage prior to exercise sessions has previously been discussed. Adequate hydration also enhances cough performance.

Tolerance. During periods of exercise, the patient is closely observed for indications of dyspnea, shortness of breath, or fatigue. A patient's ability to tolerate the exercise program is evaluated and recorded so the exercise program can be increased or modified according to the abilities. Care is taken to not fatigue the patient and to not perform exercises beyond the point of pain. Exercising is restricted if a patient has persisting dyspnea or shortness of breath, and the surgeon is notified of the patient's condition. It takes time for a patient's exercise tolerance to increase, because the body must gradually adjust to its reduced respiratory capacity following resectional surgery. The greater the amount of lung resected, the longer the period of adjustment.

Exercises are introduced in an orderly sequence and are increased in number as the patient's tolerance improves. Exercises are first performed with the patient lying in bed, later while sitting up and, finally, while standing. Planned rest periods are important during exercise periods. The activity tolerance that a patient has two to three months after discharge is about the maximal level that will be attained. Some patients find this level is below their presurgery exercise capacity level.

ARM AND SHOULDER POSTOPERATIVE EXERCISES.

Following thoracic surgery the arm and shoulder on the operative side are actively or passively taken through a full range of motion several times daily to prevent a "frozen" shoulder. *Passive exercises* on the operated arm and shoulder are usually initiated four hours following recovery from anesthesia. Exercises may be performed twice every four to six hours through the first 24 postoperative hours. Some surgeons believe that in order to prevent the dysfunction syndrome the arm and shoulder on the operated side should be exercised through a full range of motion approximately 20 times every two hours. Remember to support the patient's arm when performing passive exercises.

Active exercising is encouraged as soon as the patient's condition permits and the surgeon gives approval. Often on the first or second postoperative day the patient begins actively exercising the arm and shoulder. Supervise to be sure the exercises are performed correctly. Preoperatively a physical therapist measures the patient's joint range of motion; postoperatively the goal of physical therapy is to return the patient to this preoperative level of function.

Postoperative arm and shoulder exercises help prevent formation of adhesions between the muscles incised during surgery. During thoracotomy an incision is made across two separate layers of muscle. Normally these layers glide smoothly over one another. However, after each layer has been cut across and then sutured, the two layers tend to adhere at the suture lines postoperatively. Adhesions joining the two layers of muscle quickly form unless the muscles are repeatedly exercised.

Muscles typically transected by thoracotomy incisions include the trapezius, latissimus dorsi, rhomboideus major, and serratus anterior. These muscle groups form the shoulder girdle and maintain the trunk's posture. Unless these injured muscles are restored to efficient functioning, postural deformities result from overdevelopment of similar muscle groups on the other side of the body. Postoperatively some exercises are directed at hyperextending the arms with resistance (to strengthen the latissimus dorsi), adducting and flexing forward the upper extremities (to maintain shoulder girdle motion), and adducting the scapula (to strengthen the trapezius).

If you are unfamiliar with a surgeon's preferences for an exercise program following thoracotomy, obtain the necessary details. Some specific arm and shoulder exercises commonly prescribed following thoracic surgery are:

- ▶ Elevate the shoulders (thus elevating the clavicle and scapula). Hunch the shoulders forward and then pull them back as far as possible.
- ▶ Raise the elbow upward, keeping the elbow as close to the ear as possible and then extend the arm straight out at the level of the shoulder.
- ▶ Extend the arm up and back, then out to the side and back, and finally down at the side and back. This exercise extends and abducts the arm.
- ▶ Sit erect in an armchair and grip the arms of the chair in such a manner that pressing down on the palms of the hands will raise the body straight up in the chair. Next, while slowly inhaling, press down on the palms of the hands, pull in the abdomen and stretch up from the waist until the elbows are completely extended. After briefly holding this position, slowly exhale while slowly lowering the body back into the chair. This exercise depresses the shoulder in addition to exercising the lungs.
- ▶ Place the hands on the small of the back and attempt to push the elbows and shoulder blades toward one another. This exercise adducts and elevates the scapula.
- ▶ Reach over the head and push the arm in an upward and outward manner. This exercise rotates the scapula, fixing it against the rib cage.
- ▶ Place the arm bent at the elbow so the hand lies on the stomach (Fig. 57–3*A*). Then grasp the arm at the wrist (the patient can do this by using the "good" arm and hand) and raise the arm in an arc up off the abdomen and up directly over the top of the head. Return to the beginning position. This exercise flexes the operative arm. (This exercise can be performed while the patient lies flat in bed, as well as while sitting or standing erect.) Instruct the patient to inhale while raising the arm and to exhale while lowering it. This adds a breathing exercise to the arm exercise.
- ▶ Place the arm at the side, palm up, and raise the arm in an arc sideward up to the top of the head (Fig. 57–3*B*). Return to the starting position. (These exercises can be performed while the patient is in bed by sliding the arm on the mattress.) Again, have the patient inhale while raising the arm and exhale while lowering it. This exercise abducts and adducts the shoulder.
- ▶ Place the arm to the side at shoulder level with the elbow bent at a right angle. Then rotate the shoulder by moving the arm in an arc so it goes back (to touch the bed with the back of the hand), and then forward (to touch the bed with the palm) (Fig. 57–3*C*). This exercise rotates the shoulder outward and inward.

Throughout the postoperative period the patient is encouraged to further exercise the arm on the operated side by making a conscious effort to use that arm in the daily activities of eating, reaching for things, grooming, etc. Placing the bedside stand on the *operated side* encourages the patient to reach with the affected arm. Also, it is desirable for patients to pull themselves up to a sitting position by using the arm on the *operated side* to grasp the pull rope.

Patients are reluctant to carry out postoperative exercises after surgery because of pain and other discomforts. However, the patient must realize that if the arm and shoulder are not exercised, they will become stiff, and painful contractures will develop. Thus, some pain and discomfort must be tolerated during the postoperative period in order to avoid future disability and discomfort.

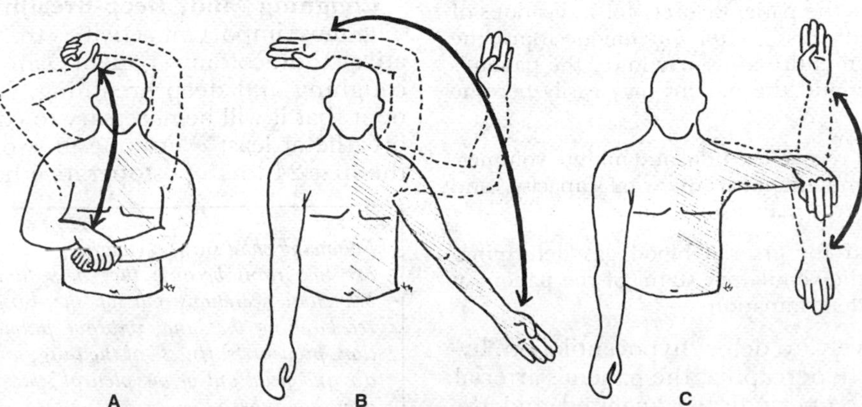

Figure 57–3. Some arm and shoulder exercises commonly prescribed following thoracic surgery. See text for discussion. (Drawn by K. C. Sorensen.)

RESPIRATORY THERAPY

Routinely following chest surgery the patient receives supportive oxygen therapy, follows a deep-breathing, coughing regimen (with chest "splinted" by the nurse), and is suctioned as indicated. Postural drainage may or may not be ordered. When ordered, postural drainage should be continued as scheduled until the cough is nonproductive and the patient is ambulatory. Techniques of chest percussion and vibrating are used in the early postoperative period cautiously owing to the presence of the wound.

Various other techniques of respiratory therapy may be ordered to mobilize tracheobronchial secretions following thoracic surgery. These include heated or cool aerosols for hydration and mucociliary clearance, coughing, deep breathing and the use of intermittent positive pressure breathing (IPPB), medicated aerosols, or incentive devices to cause pulmonary expansion and improve ventilation. IPPB treatments may be prescribed with bronchodilators or mucolytics. Consult Chapter 54 for discussion of most of these procedures.

Evaluation. Following thoracic surgery the patient's respiratory status is carefully evaluated, since temporary or permanent changes from normal respiratory function may result from thoracotomy. Usually the changes in ventilation and respiration that result from surgery are basically unilateral.

Assessment of the effectiveness of ventilation and respiration in a patient following chest surgery includes the following actions:

- Expose the patient's chest periodically to observe the rise and fall of both sides of the chest during ventilatory movements. (Following pneumonectomy the chest wall on the operated side is obviously not expected to move since the entire lung has been resected.) Decreased movement on one side of the chest during inspiration is one indication of possible pneumothorax.
- Auscultate the chest and carefully evaluate the quality of respiration; e.g., rales indicate congestion. Observe the patient closely for indications of respiratory distress. After pneumonectomy the removal of an entire lung may lower the patient's vital capacity and the patient may easily become dyspneic.
- Measure and record the tidal and minute volumes. Serial determinations of the vital capacity, and inspiratory force may also be done.
- Obtain blood for arterial blood gas determinations. Note the ventilatory status of the patient at the time of determination.

Postoperatively, to detect hypoventilation, hypoxemia, and hypercapnia, the patient's arterial blood gases are periodically analyzed and the ventilatory efficiency is evaluated by measuring tidal ventilation. The latter measurement is made with a spirometer, which may be attached to an artificial airway or may be used with a nose clip and mouthpiece or face mask. The nurse may be asked to measure the patient's ventilatory capacity. Additionally, the patient's pulse and respiratory rates and blood pressure are carefully evaluated and close observations are made for indications of respiratory insufficiency such as cerebral indications of hypoxia and hypercapnia, e.g., irritability, restlessness, disorientation, or (more seriously) stupor and coma; decreased respiratory excursion; retraction of the rib cage; and dyspnea, stridor, rales, or rhonchi. (See discussion of respiratory insufficiency and failure, Chapter 59. See also the discussion on intubation and extubation, Chapter 54.) A patient with respiratory insufficiency requires oxygen therapy, and mechanical ventilation via an artifical airway.

Oxygen Therapy. Oxygen administration during the immediate postoperative period ensures adequate oxygenation during the time that the patient's ventilation may be reduced from anesthetic depression, lethargy, and pain. Also, it is during the immediate postoperative period that the lung is the most fully collapsed. Collapse of the lung and resection of pulmonary tissue reduces the alveolar-capillary surface, where exchange of respiratory gases occur. This situation corrects itself as remaining lung tissue reinflates, or, following pneumonectomy, as the body adjusts to the loss of one lung.

Nasal oxygen is routinely administered by cannula or Venturi mask until the patient recovers from anesthesia, or longer if respiratory insufficiency is present. Oxygen must be administered continously until the oxygen status is stable and normal, as determined by the arterial blood gas.

If a patient requires O_2, it must be administered during *all* phases of postoperative care. Deteriorating arterial blood gases and ventilatory mechanics parameters require placement of an artificial airway and continuous mechanical ventilation (CMV).

Coughing and Deep-Breathing Regimen. The most important activities that the postoperative thoracotomy patient can perform are coughing and deep breathing. Inform the patient that it will be necessary to cough and deep breathe at least every one to two hours during the first 24 to 48 postoperative hours.

Following chest surgery coughing and deep breathing are important because they help to move tracheobronchial secretions out of the lung, assist with reexpanding the lung, improve pulmonary circulation, prevent "stiffness" of the lung, and help to force air and fluid out of the pleural space through chest drainage tubes.

Coughing is a protective mechanism by which foreign material is expelled from the air passages. Coughing loosens secretions and forces them into the upper respiratory tract, from which they may be expectorated or suctioned. Adequate ventilation cannot be obtained unless the airway is clear of secretions. *Deep breathing* dilates the airways, stimulates surfactant production, and expands the lung tissue surface, thereby increasing the area for respiratory gas exchange (O_2 and CO_2). Deep breathing also improves pulmonary circulation, because lung expansion decreases intrapleural pressure and this, in turn, stimulates blood flow to the lungs. If the lungs are not periodically stretched by deep breathing, they tend to become progressively stiffer and more difficult to inflate. Alveolar collapse, "shunt," and hypoxemia result.

These activities are especially important following thoracic surgery. If the lung is not promptly reexpanded, adhesions may form in the pleural space and keep the lung compressed. Infections may develop if secretions accumulate in the pleural space, collapsed lung, or tracheobronchial tree. Accumulations of secretions in the tracheobronchial tree also may cause obstruction, atelectasis, and ventilatory insufficiency.

Coughing and deep-breathing routines are started once the patient regains consciousness and are usually continued every hour (or oftener) for the first 24 postoperative hours. Turn the patient, take vital signs, administer medications, and perform other necessary nursing care when awakening hourly to cough and deep breathe; then it is not necessary to reawaken the patient later for these activities. In addition to coughing, the patient is instructed to take 10 to 20 deep breaths hourly. After the first 24 hours it is usually sufficient if the patient coughs and deep breaths every two hours. The routine varies, however, according to the patient's condition.

Effective coughing cannot occur if a patient's body alignment is poor, e.g., if slumped down or curled up in bed. The most effective coughing is achieved with the patient sitting erectly upright. Thus, as soon as the patient's blood pressure is stable provide assistance to sit up in bed and cough.

Often patients are afraid to deep breathe and cough following thoracic surgery because they fear they may "split open" their incisions or damage their lungs. These fears can be abated by patiently yet firmly reassuring the patient that the coughing and deep-breathing regimens are actually helpful. The patient is also reassured by having the nurse manually splint the incision. (Splinting is discussed later.)

Pain, fatigue, and fear may cause the patient to merely clear the throat rather than cough effectively. Also, the patient may tend to breathe shallowly rather than deeply. The nurse tactfully reminds the patient to deep breathe and to cough in the manner practiced preoperatively, e.g., to inhale deeply enough that the chest expands and the "voice box is shut off," then to let pressure build up in the chest, and finally to suddenly let the air out by coughing with the mouth and throat open. Keeping the glottis tight increases the intrapulmonary pressure. Before coughing it is helpful if the patient takes several deep breaths.

Additional details important in the proper coughing and deep-breathing routine are as follow: (1) give the patient two tissues to cover the mouth and nose when exhaling or coughing; (2) tell the patient to expand the chest by breathing in deeply enough so that the chest wall will move your hands as they rest lightly on the rib cage; (3) instruct the patient to relax the abdomen while breathing in, so the abdomen will expand while the chest expands; and (4) once the expansion is complete, have the patient forcibly cough while consciously tightening the abdomen and squeezing down the rib cage.

Because pain coverage is best 20 to 30 minutes after pain medication is given, schedule coughing and deep-breathing sessions at those times when possible. Remember that the less pain the patient experiences the more effectively it is possible to cough and deep breathe; remember also the hazards of overmedicating the patient.

After a patient coughs several times, listen to the chest with a stethoscope. If the breath sounds are still "wet," let the patient briefly rest and then assist with coughing again. Sips of warm water sometimes help a patient to cough more effectively. Encourage coughing until the patient's chest sounds clear of secretions.

Occasionally a patient momentarily loses consciousness (syncope) during the deep-breathing and coughing regimen. This may occur because: (1) cerebral ischemia develops because of the fact that the activities increase intrathoracic pressure and thus impede venous return to the heart and reduce cardiac output; and/or the blood's carbon dioxide content is suddenly reduced because hyperventilation "blows off" large quantities of CO_2 from the lungs.[102A] Usually the patient recovers within a few minutes, since syncope is typically a self-limited disorder.

See the discussion of coughing techniques in Chapter 53.

Splinting the Chest. The nurse splints a thoracic incision (or a painful chest) by placing the hands anteriorly and posteriorly around the incised area* (Fig. 57–4). (Be certain you wash prior to and after handling the patient.) When splinting a chest, keep the palms of your hands flat and your fingers spread (be very careful not to cause uncomfortable uneven pressure or squeezing). Apply firm even pressure over the incision without restricting chest expansion. Next, instruct the patient to cover nose and mouth with tissues and to take a deep breath and cough.

Note in Figure 57–4 that the nurse has positioned herself on the side of the patient opposite to his incision and she is standing so her head is behind the patient's chest. This protects her by keeping her out of the path of the patient's cough, and it also permits her to listen to the chest during the coughing. Because she has her hands on the patient's chest the nurse can feel if the patient expands his chest as he should while taking a deep breath.

Good body mechanics are important when you splint a patient's chest, so that neither you nor the patient experiences fatigue from the position assumed and so the patient feels securely supported but not painfully squeezed. Proper splinting does not depress the sternum and does not restrict the normal excursions of the diaphragm (by holding the lower part of the rib cage, i.e., the last five pairs of ribs). The diaphragm contributes over half to the ventilatory process and thus must be free to move. During inspiration the diaphragm flattens out and the sternum elevates. While properly splinting the chest incision the nurse helps to depress the rib cage during the expiratory phase of ventilation. This application of pressure during the expiratory phase helps the patient to expel secretions.

Correctly splinting a patient's chest, as described, promotes a sense of security in addition to reducing discomfort when coughing and deep breathing. Splinting decreases stretching of a chest incision and thus minimizes pain during the forceful ventilatory movements of deep breathing and coughing. For the first few postoperative days the chest is splinted by the nurse during deep-breathing and coughing sessions. However, the patient is soon able to be more independent and splint the operated side with one hand and to cover the mouth with the other while coughing and deep breathing.

*Splinting may also be performed by supporting beneath the incision with one hand and exerting downward pressure on the shoulder of the affected side with the other hand.

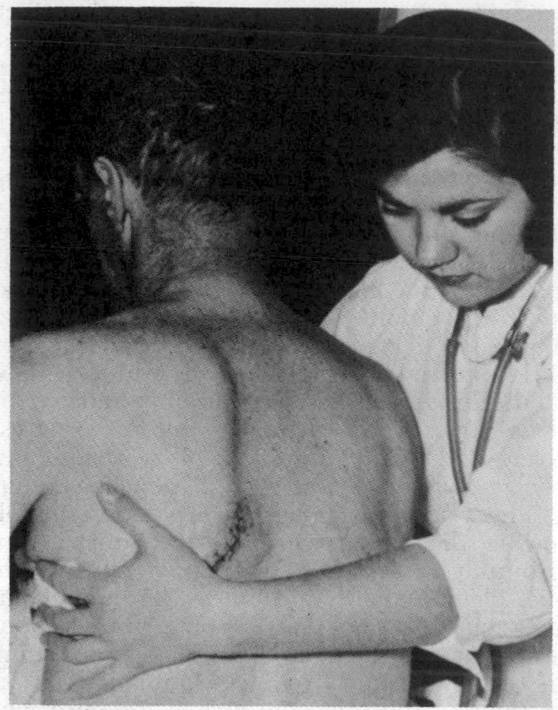

Figure 57–4. Correct position for "splinting" a patient's chest. See text. (From MacVicar, J. and H. J. Mendelsohn: *In* Meltzer, L. E., F. Abdellah, and J. R. Kitchell (Eds.): *Concepts and Practices of Intensive Care for Nurse Specialists.* Philadelphia, The Charles Press, 1969.)

Suctioning. The nurse caring for patients who have had thoracic surgery needs to become familiar enough with chest auscultation to determine when a patient should be suctioned. Suctioning is performed when lungs are congested and the person is unable to cough effectively enough to remove the secretions. Pharyngeal suctioning helps to remove secretions from the pharynx and also stimulates coughing. Endotracheal suctioning removes secretions from the tracheobronchial tree and also stimulates an excellent cough reflex. Suctioning is discussed in Chapter 54.

During the immediate postoperative period orders may be written for the patient to be suctioned at least every two hours and then p.r.n. Sometimes a tracheostomy is necessary to facilitate maintenance of a clear airway.

> *Following pulmonary resectional surgery there is the potential danger of accidentally traumatizing or actually pushing the suction catheter through a bronchial suture line while performing deep tracheal suctioning.*

In some settings deep tracheal suctioning is performed only by physicians. Certainly it should never be performed by a nurse who is unskilled in the procedure. The possibility of breaking through the bronchial suture line is greatest when pneumonectomy has been performed, because the suture line is at the tracheal bifurcation. With other resectional procedures, e.g., lobectomy, it is usually considerably more difficult to break the suture line since the suction catheter would have to make two turns before reaching the bronchial stump.

Improper tracheal suctioning will produce unwanted and hazardous side effects. Maintenance of oxygenation followed by hyperinflation to reexpand the lung is an essential part of the suctioning procedure. Adequate hydration will facilitate removal of secretions. Hydration may be performed either parenterally or topically. Thick, tenacious secretions may be more easily removed following the aerosolization of mucolytic agents such as Mucomyst or sodium bicarbonate.

Frequent nasotracheal suctioning may be less traumatically and more effectively performed if a nasal airway is inserted into one of the nares.

A mucous plug blocking one of the bronchi may cause a patient to become confused and cyanotic and to develop a rapid respiratory rate and tachycardia. Suctioning is necessary. In some instances the physician can remove the mucous plug only by suctioning through a bronchoscope.

The airway of the unconscious patient is carefully maintained with suctioning, correct positioning, and other appropriate measures to maintain its patency. (See Units VIII and X.)

Postural Drainage. Postural drainage in the Trendelenburg position may or may not be ordered to be routinely performed during the postoperative period. Do not carry out this procedure unless you have a specific order from the surgeon to do so. Some surgeons do not want patients placed in a head-low position following thoracic surgery because they believe it is too difficult for the patient to breathe while in that position. *If you do perform postural drainage following chest surgery, be certain to observe the patient closely for respiratory distress during the procedure,* and be certain to use only those positions authorized by the surgeon for a given patient. Do not leave the patient unattended during postural drainage sessions. (Postural drainage is discussed in Chapter 54.)

CHEST X-RAY FILMS

Chest films are often taken daily for several days following thoracic surgery so the surgeon can evaluate the patient's progress. The surgeon looks at the chest film for indications of pulmonary expansion or collapse; infection in the pleural space, lung parenchyma, or tracheobronchial tree; atelectasis; or air fluid collections in the pleural space. Treatment is then planned in accordance with the needs of the patient.

Closed Chest Drainage

As mentioned, during chest surgery atmospheric air enters the pleural space through the thoracotomy. This causes the lung to collapse on the operated side. Following thoracotomy it is thus generally necessary to use closed chest drainage to foster and permit the drainage of air and/or fluid from the pleural space and to prevent their reflux (i.e., backward or return flow); to help to reexpand remaining lung tissue by reestablishing negative pressure; and to prevent shifting of the mediastinum and collapse of lung tissue by equalizing pressure.

The nurse has numerous responsibilities associated with the use of closed chest drainage, e.g., to maintain proper functioning of the apparatus and to periodically observe the chest drainage.

Closed chest drainage means simply that the drainage system used is closed to atmospheric pressure. As explained in the following pages, various types of apparatus may be used. The classic form of closed chest drainage is a water-seal bottle (a one- or two-bottle set-up may be used). Controlled mechanical suction may or may not be applied to a water-seal set-up. When suction is used, two or three bottles are attached together and connected to a suction source such as a wall suction outlet or a portable suction motor.

In some settings bottle drainage systems have been replaced with newer equipment of simpler design and maintenance, e.g., Pleur-Evac units (discussed later). However, the nurse must still understand the water-seal forms of bottle chest drainage as these may still be used. Additionally, an understanding of the principles of bottle chest drainage is basic to understanding any type of closed chest drainage equipment.

When caring for a person with closed chest drainage it is important to:

- understand the principles and purposes of chest drainage;
- understand the specific apparatus being used so you can tell when it is functioning correctly, when it is malfunctioning, and, if possible, how to correct malfunctions;
- understand necessary precautions of importance;
- detect early symptoms of impending complications in the patient, e.g., tension pneumothorax.

It is necessary to be prepared for emergencies by keeping available a thoracentesis tray and an extra set of bottles, connectors, tubing, and so forth.

Before caring for a patient on closed chest drainage

be certain to familiarize yourself with the apparatus being used. Literature describing some closed chest drainage systems and their functions is available from the distributors of commercial equipment. Hospital procedure books are another source of information. Explain the basic purposes of closed chest drainage to the patient and significant others. Also, inform them of necessary precautions they should know. Show the patient how to be careful of the drainage tubes and other apparatus when moving about so the tubing is not kinked or pulled. Place a sign on the patient's bed which clearly cautions visitors and others not to handle the chest suction equipment and to be careful not to accidentally displace any of it. (See Table 57–2.)

USES AND OBJECTIVES

Closed chest drainage is used in the treatment of empyema and pneumothorax (e.g., following chest injuries or spontaneous pneumothorax), and postoperatively after thoracic or thoracicoabdominal surgery. Although it appears somewhat formidable initially, the apparatus for closed chest drainage is actually quite simple. Regardless of the type of apparatus used, all have the same objectives: to remove fluid and/or air from the pleural space; to reduce the size of the pleural space; to reestablish normal negative pressure in the pleural space; to promote reexpansion of the lung with apposition and cohesion of the parietal and pulmonary pleurae (so normal ventilation is restored); and to prevent reflux (i.e., backward or return flow) of air and/or fluid back into the pleural space from the drainage apparatus.

TABLE 57–2. DEFINITION OF TERMS RELATED TO CHEST DRAINAGE AND SUCTION

Movement of Gases: All gases, including air, will move from an area of higher pressure to an area of lower pressure. This is the basic principle involved in both respiration and chest suction.

Intrapulmonic: Pertaining to, or affecting, the spaces *within* the lungs.

Intrathoracic (intrapleural): Pertaining to, or affecting, the potential space between the parietal and visceral pleura.

Pneumothorax: The presence of air in the intrathoracic space which results in the collapse of the lung.

Atmospheric pressure: The sum total of the pressures exerted within the atmosphere. Standard (at sea level) pressure is 760 mm. Hg. Also called ambient pressure.

Positive pressure: A pressure *greater than* ambient or standard pressure of 760 mm. Hg pressure. Positive pressure is related to inflation of objects.

Negative pressure: A pressure *less than* 760 mm. Hg which exerts a suctioning or vacuum force.

Adapted from Rexilius, B. G.: *Chest Drainage and Suction.* Philadelphia: F. A. Davis Co., 1977.

INSERTION OF CHEST CATHETERS

Usually chest catheters are inserted in an operating room at the time of chest surgery. However, in some emergencies and in treating such disorders as empyema, a chest catheter may be inserted in a treatment room or at the bedside. (Chest catheters are sometimes also called "chest drains," "thoracotomy tubes," or "chest tubes.")

In the course of pulmonary surgery, the parietal pleura is incised and the pleural space entered. Atmospheric air then rushes into the pleural space. As a result, the lung recoils to its unexpanded size and remains compressed, and the cohesion of the parietal and pulmonary pleurae is disrupted. Chest surgery thus causes the patient to have a pneumothorax on the operated side.

During chest surgery the anesthetist carefully manages pulmonary function for the patient. As the surgeon prepares to close, the anesthetist mechanically expands the operated lung. The surgeon positions chest drainage catheters within the chest and then closes the chest wall while the anesthetist inflates the lung.

When the chest wall is closed, pressure within the pleural space is initially atmospheric. Additional air may continue to escape into the pleural space for a while through openings in the pulmonary pleural incision. Although the pleura is sutured it takes time for it to heal. The trauma of surgery causes serosanguineous fluid to collect in the patient's chest until healing occurs. Unfortunately this fluid is a good culture medium and may thus predispose to infection. Also, the fluid may cause pleural thickening, which reduces pulmonary compliance and reduces the lung's ventilatory and diffusion capacities by "stiffening" the lung. Closed chest drainage (via the chest catheters) is therefore used postoperatively to remove air and serosanguineous fluid from the pleural space.

Following resectional surgery (except pneumonectomy) two catheters are usually placed in the chest. One of these (the "upper" or "anterior" tube) is placed anteriorly through the second intercostal space to permit the escape of air rising in the pleural space. The other catheter (the "lower" or "posterior" tube) is placed posteriorly through the 8th or 9th intercostal space in the midaxillary line to drain off serosanguineous fluid accumulating in the lower portion of the pleural space. The lower tube may have a larger diameter than the upper to enhance free drainage. Chest catheters may be brought out of the chest wall through stab

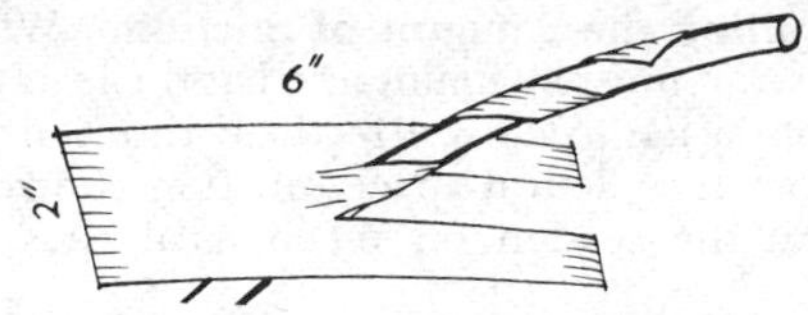

Figure 57–5. Tape attached to chest catheter to provide additional support on outside of chest dressing. (From Sutton, A. L., *Bedside Nursing Techniques in Medicine and Surgery,* 2nd ed. Philadelphia: W. B. Saunders Co., 1969.)

wounds or through the incisional line. Although the catheters are secured to the patient's skin with suture, the tubes also may be taped to the outside of the dressing, as shown in Figure 57–5 to provide security against displacement.

The two chest catheters may be joined to each other with a plastic or glass Y-junction (and then attached to one water-seal drainage set), but it is preferable to leave the two catheters separate and to attach them to two separate water-seal drainage systems. This makes it possible to monitor the air and fluid drainage from each tube and then to remove the nondraining tube without disrupting the rest of the system. Flexible drainage tubing connects the chest catheter with the drainage apparatus. Usually the catheters are connected to the drainage apparatus before the patient leaves surgery.

FACTORS AFFECTING CHEST DRAINAGE

Various factors may affect the removal of air and fluid through the chest drainage system.

Location of Chest Drainage Apparatus. The apparatus for closed chest drainage must always be located at a level *lower than the patient's chest* (unless for some reason the catheters are clamped). Drainage by gravity is thus maintained, and air and fluid are not forced back into the pleural space. The drainage apparatus may be located in a box or special rack (fastened to the patient's bed or on wheels at the bedside) or taped securely to the floor so it will not accidentally be knocked over. The preferred arrangement is the rack attached to the bed, because the danger of breaking, elevating, or upsetting the bottles is reduced. If drainage bottles are on the floor, be careful not to lower a high-low bed or side rails onto the bottles. Keep the drainage bottles about two to three feet below the patient's chest.

When moving the patient from surgery to the recovery room the tubing may be *double clamped* and the drainage apparatus may then be placed on top of the patient's bed during transportation. After the patient is situated in the recovery room the apparatus is lowered below the level of the patient's chest and then the clamps are opened. *Never open clamps on the drainage tubing if the apparatus is above the level of the patient's chest or the fluid in the drainage bottle will run down or be siphoned into the patient's pleural cavity.*

Position of the Patient. Positioning following chest surgery has been discussed. Positioning orders must be followed carefully. Frequently a semi-Fowler position is used. If the patient can be positioned on the side that has the chest catheters coming out of it, position in such a way that the person is not lying on (and compressing or kinking) the catheters or tubing, since this not only impairs drainage and causes retrograde pressure (which forces drainage back into the pleural cavity) but also greatly increases the patient's discomfort. When the patient is in a lateral position place a small sandbag or folded towel on either side of the tubing to prevent the patient's body weight from compressing the tubing.

Placement and Length of Drainage Tubing. Drainage tubing (connecting the chest catheters with the drainage apparatus) should be neither too short nor too long. Attach the tubing to the edge of the patient's mattress bedding in such a way that it falls in a straight line to the drainage apparatus with no dependent loops. Dependent loops of tubing that contain fluid obstruct flow and create back pressure, thus impairing drainage of air or fluid. Drainage tubing may be secured to the bedding in various ways. For example, place a rubber band or strip of adhesive tape around the tubing and then pin the other end of the rubber band or tape to the mattress. Or, make a trough in the drawsheet around the drainage tube, then pull the two sides of the trough up on either side of the tube and pin them together. Do not pin the tubing so tightly in the trough that it is constricted or cannot be moved. Sandbags, small pillows, or folded abdominal pads can also be positioned around the tube to make a trough.

From the mattress to the patient the tubing length should be adequate for the patient to turn and sit up without pulling on the chest catheters. Coil excess tubing flat on the bed. Excessive tubing length adds to problems with tangling and kinking of the tube. Each time the patient is turned or otherwise moved, check chest catheters to be certain they are not displaced, and check drainage tubing to be certain it is properly positioned.

Maintaining Patency of Drainage Tubing. Frequently check the patency of the drainage tubing and chest catheters. Make certain the patient is not lying on the tubing and that it is not otherwise kinked or compressed. Also, make sure the tube is not internally plugged, e.g., with blood clots. The flow of drainage fluids can easily be observed through clear plastic tubing. A glass adapter in rubber tubing makes observation of drainage possible. Also, observe the fluid collecting in the drainage bottles. *If the tubing is not patent, drainage of air and fluid from the pleural space is impossible.*

Sometimes when there is a great deal of bloody drainage from the chest, e.g., in the early postoperative period following chest surgery, drainage tubes are "milked" every 30 to 60 minutes. *"Milking" a drainage tube* means the tubing is gently compressed in the direction of the drainage apparatus (away from the patient) to remove air, fluid or blood clots. The tubing is gently clasped in the nurse's hand and then (with the other hand stabilizing the tube so it will not have traction on it and be displaced) the hand is slid over the tubing in a direction *away from* the chest and *toward* the drainage system. (Alcohol sponges held in the hand make it possible to slide more easily down the length of the tubing). ("Milking" is also called "stripping.") Another way to milk a chest tube is to clasp one hand around the tube as close to the chest as possible and squeeze the tube against the palm of the hand, and then proceed similarly downward, hand over hand toward the drainage apparatus. Some plastic chest tubes have a built-in bulb device for milking. Because milking the tubing changes intrapleural pressure and can be painful if performed too vigorously, the nurse is as gentle as possible during the procedure.

Taping the portion of the drainage tubing that enters the drainage bottle to a piece of tongue blade prevents kinking of the tube in this area, and is another way of maintaining tube patency.

The accumulation of blood, fluid, or air in the pleural space may eventually compress the lung, with the possibility of tension pneumothorax or mediastinal shift occurring. Therefore, if malfunction of the drainage apparatus occurs, the nurse tries to immediately correct the problem and to observe the patient closely for *early* symptoms indicative of complications. The *early* detection of tension pneumothorax, for example, can prevent mediastinal shift if appropriate treatment is given promptly.

The physician must be notified immediately if these complications are suspected. While waiting for the physician to come, the nurse attempts to locate and correct the cause of any problems within the chest drainage system. Perhaps a relatively simple action corrects the malfunctioning system, e.g., straightening a kinked tube or setting upright a water-seal bottle that has been knocked over accidentally. Sometimes milking the tube will dislodge a blood clot that is obstructing the tube. Occasionally it is necessary for the physician to irrigate the chest catheters to remove obstructions.

Maintaining an Airtight Drainage System. Closed chest drainage systems must be kept airtight (closed to atmospheric air). To accomplish this, *bottles in the drainage apparatus are sealed with tight-fitting stoppers and all connections are taped.* If air leaks into the drainage tubing it enters the pleural space and thus not only defeats the purposes of the drainage system, but can possibly cause complications such as tension pneumothorax. When the drainage system is not airtight it is impossible to reestablish negative pressure in the pleural space because atmospheric air continues to enter the pleural space through the air leak. Obviously if tubes in the drainage system are accidentally disconnected or if bottles in the apparatus are broken, the drainage system is no longer airtight.

Controlling the Amount of Suction. When suction is used it must be maintained at the level ordered by the physician to most effectively drain off air and fluid from the pleural space. Suction control is discussed in the section on mechanical chest suction below.

INFECTION PREVENTION WITH CHEST DRAINAGE

When properly used, closed chest drainage helps to prevent infections in the pleural space by removing serosanguineous fluids. However, unless careful aseptic technique is used in caring for chest catheters and the drainage system, infection may be introduced into the pleural space. *Observe strict asepsis whenever you are changing the apparatus or any of its connections.* If you disconnect the tubes, maintain a sterile field. Be certain to protect the tubes' open ends with sterile dressings. Always wash your hands thoroughly before and after caring for chest tubes. Because an infection can occur along the tube tract, chest catheters are usually not used for more than five to seven days.

ACTIVITY WITH CHEST DRAINAGE

The patient with water-seal chest drainage can sit up in bed, get in and out of bed, and ambulate without clamping the chest catheters as long as: (1) the water-seal bottle is kept upright (so the long glass tube in the bottle is kept below the fluid level in the bottle); (2) the bottle is kept lower than the chest; and (3) all connections remain intact. Be careful not to exert traction on the tubings. Various arrangements are used for keeping the chest bottles with a patient while moving around. If suction is to be maintained during ambulation the patient can walk only the few steps permitted by the length of the tubing.

Sometimes the physician orders a patient's chest catheters to be double clamped and disconnected during ambulation. However, *if air drainage has been occurring the tubes are never clamped because of the danger of tension pneumothorax.* With the tubes clamped, the air would continue to accumulate in the pleural space, thus exerting increasing pressure since there would be no means of escape.

Encourage the patient on closed chest drainage to *frequently cough and deep breathe.* In addition to clearing the bronchi of secretions these activities promote lung expansion and the expulsion of air and/or fluid from the pleural space (by increasing intrapulmonic and intrapleural pressures).

CLAMPING CHEST DRAINAGE TUBING

Rubber-shod clamps are routinely kept at the bedside of any patient on closed chest drainage. The clamps are 6- to 8-inch, strong hemostats with protective rubber placed over their tips. Two clamps are kept available for each chest catheter so each catheter can be *double clamped* (for extra safety) if clamping is necessary. When not in use, clamps should be stored in an easily visible place where they are readily available. They can be kept clamped to the bottom sheet at the head of the bed when the patient is in bed. When the patient is out of bed the clamps are usually kept clamped to the patient's bathrobe. Do not tape the clamps to the bed or they will be too difficult to release for emergency use. Also, do not leave the clamps merely lying on the bedside stand or in a drawer; if you do it is likely that they will not be there when you need them or they will be hidden by other articles. When clamps are attached to linens, be careful they are not accidentally sent to the laundry.

There are times when clamping a patient's chest tubes is definitely contraindicated. Clamps are currently not used on chest tubes as frequently as they formerly were.

> *Except for those emergencies in which clamping is clearly indicated, do not clamp chest drainage tubes without an order to do so.*

Occasionally it is necessary to *briefly* clamp a chest tube to locate a source of malfunction in the apparatus. Sometimes an order is given to clamp a patient's chest tubes for a few minutes during transportation to another area of the hospital, e.g., radiology. However, usually the tubes are not clamped when the patient is moved, but rather care is taken to keep the drainage system below the level of the patient's chest and the drainage system is transported too.

The best time to apply clamps to a chest catheter is following an expiration. The clamps should be removed again as soon as possible. Never cover the clamps with bedding while they are in use. If they are left clamped on the chest tube and are covered up they are easily forgotten and may not be released when they should be.

ONE-BOTTLE WATER-SEAL APPARATUS

Basic Set-up. This, the most simple apparatus for establishing closed chest drainage, consists of: (1) a sterile bottle that contains about 100 ml. of sterile normal saline or sterile water; (2) a tight-fitting rubber stopper with two holes in it (the stopper is placed in the opening of the bottle and is taped securely in place); and (3) two hollow tubes (inserted through the holes in the stopper and taped into place once they are positioned). One tube is short and acts as an *air vent;* the other tube is longer and acts as a *water-seal* (Fig. 57–6).

> *Water-seal drainage acts as a one-way valve, permitting the unidirectional flow of air and fluid out of the pleural space, but permitting none to enter from the drainage system.*

The longer tube in the water-seal apparatus is placed so it extends into the solution in the bottle and terminates about 3 to 5 cm. below the fluid level. The other end of the long tube (i.e., the end outside the bottle) is attached to the patient's chest drainage tubing. Once attached to the patient's drainage tubing *the end of the long tube in the bottle must always be kept below the fluid level in the bottle.* If this end of the tube is above the fluid level, atmospheric air passes through the bottle's air vent (short tube), into the open end of the long tube, through the drainage tubing, and in to the pleural space.

A "water-seal" means simply that the water in the bottle seals off the atmospheric air, preventing atmospheric pressure from entering the chest drainage tube and thus from entering the pleural space. Atmospheric air enters the air vent in the water-seal bottle, but it cannot penetrate the surface of the water and enter the end of the long tube under the water. Similarly, air and fluid can escape from the pleural space by passing through the long tube in the bottle and into the fluid in the bottle. Air escaping from the chest then bubbles up through the fluid in the bottle (because air is lighter than water), and escapes out of the bottle by passing through the air vent. The fluid in the

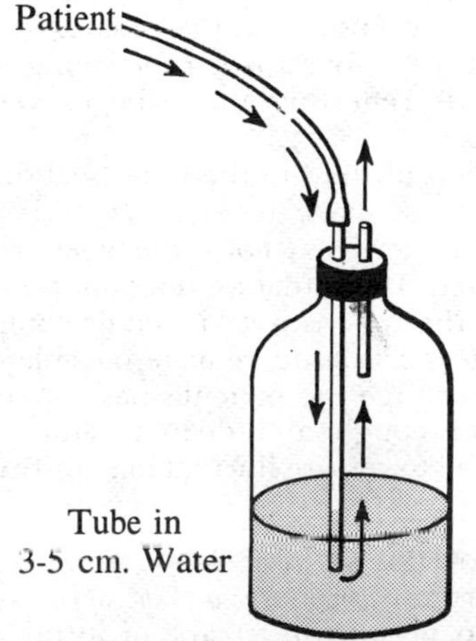

Figure 57–6. One-bottle system for closed chest drainage. (From Secor, J.: *Patient Care in Respiratory Problems.* Philadelphia: W. B. Saunders Co., 1969.)

water-seal bottle is not drawn up into the chest tube because the fluid is heavier than air and is thus held down in the bottle by gravity. Thus, water-seal drainage creates a *closed drainage system* that permits air and fluid to escape out of the pleural space but also prevents outside air or fluid from entering the pleural space. (Of course if the bottle is accidentally raised higher than the level of the patient's chest, the force of gravity will cause the fluid to run down the tube into the chest).

The one-bottle water-seal chest drainage apparatus does not produce suction, but rather operates by gravity. This system may be used following pneumonectomy (where suction is not necessary to expand the remaining lung tissue since the lung was removed) and in treating empyema. It may also be used following resectional surgery or open chest wounds if the physician does not think mechanical suction is necessary.

How to Tell if the Drainage Apparatus Is Functioning Properly. It is the nurse's responsibility to make certain the water-seal apparatus is functioning properly. The observations necessary to evaluate the functioning of a water-seal apparatus are discussed below.

- Observation of the water-seal tube. As previously discussed, pressure changes occur during respiration. During inspiration, fluid is sucked up into the tube a few centimeters because of the decreased intrapleural pressure. Conversely, during expiration the heightened intrapleural pressure forces the fluid back down the tube. When you observe this *fluctuating or oscillating movement of fluid* up and down in the long tube in the water-seal bottle, you know that the drainage tubes are patent and the apparatus is functioning properly because it is reflecting the patient's ventilatory movements.

  Fluctuation of fluid in the water-seal tube stops when the lungs have reexpanded (this point is discussed further below) or if the tubes are kinked or obstructed. If fluctuation does not occur check to be sure the tube is not kinked or compressed; try milking the tube to remove possible obstructions; and change the patient's position and have him or her cough and deep breathe. If these measures fail to restore fluctuation, notify the physician.

- Observation of the air-vent tube. Make certain that the short *air-vent tube is kept open* to the atmosphere to permit the escape of intrapleural air from the bottle. If this tube is stopped up, any intrapleural air being expelled into the bottle is trapped in the collection bottle and thus increases pressure within the bottle. If this pressure becomes great enough it prevents drainage of air and fluid from the pleural space and can produce tension pneumothorax and mediastinal shift.

- Observation of the fluid in the water-seal bottle. Watch for bubbling in the water-seal bottle. The bubbling is caused by air passing out of the pleural space and up through the liquid in the bottle. *Intermittent bubbling* is not abnormal; in fact, it indicates that the water-seal drainage is accomplishing one of its purposes, i.e., the removal of air from the pleural space. Intermittent bubbling may occur with the patient's normal expirations, since expiration increases intrapleural pressure and forces air through the tube.

  Continuous bubbling during both inspiration and expiration may indicate that air is leaking into the drainage system. Obviously this situation must be corrected, since air entering the system is also entering the pleural space. Attempt to locate the source of the *air leak* and repair it if you can. Begin by inspecting the chest wall where the catheters are inserted. If a chest catheter appears to be loose, gently squeeze the skin up around the catheter or apply sterile petrolatum gauze around the area of insertion and see if this stops the continuous bubbling in the bottle. If this does not stop the leak, check the tubing inch by inch and all connections. You may find a break in the tubing or a loose connection that can be sealed with tape. If you still cannot locate the leak it may be necessary to replace the drainage bottle with another sterile water-seal bottle.

  Rapid bubbling (in the absence of an air leak) indicates that considerable loss of air is occurring, e.g., from an incision or tear in the pulmonary pleura. The physician should be notified immediately so appropriate steps can be taken to prevent collapse of the lung or mediastinal shift. Thoracentesis may be necessary.

  When assigned to care for a patient on water-seal drainage, it is important to know if the patient is a "bubbling" patient, i.e., a patient who has air in the pleural space which has been bubbling up in the water-seal bottle. Knowing this enables you to observe for significant changes in the drainage pattern. For example, you can note if intermittent bubbling changes to constant bubbling, or if a patient who has not been bubbling begins to bubble. Also, knowledge about a patient's "bubbling status" prepares you to give appropriate emergency care if anything goes wrong with the drainage apparatus.

  Notify the physician of any accidents involving closed chest drainage.

What to Do if the Water-seal Bottle Is Broken. If the bottle is broken, you know that atmospheric air will enter the pleural space through the drainage tubing. This can be prevented by immediately clamping the chest catheter. It must be realized, however, that clamping the catheter also prevents air (or fluid) from leaving the pleural space; thus, clamping a chest catheter is not always the procedure of choice.[114A]

If a water-seal bottle is broken and the patient is known to have been bubbling (i.e., it is known that air has been coming out of the pleural space), the chest tube is not clamped but is left open until it can be attached to a new water-seal bottle. (A second water-seal bottle should always be kept available.) Even though an open pneumothorax will occur, this is far less serious than a closed tension pneumothorax, which will compress the lungs and progress to a mediastinal shift. If the bottle breaks and it is known that the patient has not been bubbling, the nurse immediately clamps the chest catheter; then wipes the exposed ends of the cateter with an antiseptic solution and reconnects them to another sterile water-seal bottle.

It can be seen that in such an emergency an evaluation is rapidly made of the extent to which exposure of the pleural space to atmospheric air would disrupt therapy, and of the pros and cons of shutting off airflow into and out of the chest cavity with clamps. The nurse must be prepared to make such a decision and immediately take appropriate action. Obviously it is necessary to know whether the patient has been bubbling air *before* the bottle is broken, since there is no way to observe this once the bottle is broken.

Once a patient's chest tubes are clamped, observe closely for symptoms of tension pneumothorax and mediastinal shift.

If you have applied clamps to a chest tube after a water-seal has been broken (or for some other reason) and you notice the patient is beginning to experience respiratory distress before being reconnected to a water-seal apparatus (e.g., the patient is breathing rapidly and shallowly, is apprehensive, and is becoming cyanotic), tension pneumothorax is probably occurring, possibly with mediastinal shift. Immediately release the clamps on the chest catheter and call for the physician. It is best to open the clamps and thus create an open pneumothorax, since at least with an open pneumothorax air can move both in and out and is not trapped in the pleural space, building up pressure.

What to Do if the Chest Tubing Accidentally Is Disconnected. A tube that is accidentally disconnected should simply be reconnected and the system observed to be certain it is functioning. Taping the tubing at the site of the disconnection should prevent another similar accident.

What to Do if the Water-seal Bottle Is Accidentally Kicked Over. If this happens, the water-seal breaks and atmospheric air begins to enter the pleural space. To correct this situation simply return the bottle to the upright position, thereby reestablishing the water-seal. Once the water-seal is again functioning, instruct the patient to take one or two deep breaths to force out of the pleural cavity any air that may have entered while the water-seal was broken.

What to Do if the Water-seal Bottle Is Accidentally Elevated to the Level of the Patient's Chest. Elevation of the bottle to this level causes any fluid in the tubing to flow back into the pleural space. Immediately lower the bottle to reestablish the drainage system.

What to Do if the Water-seal Bottle Is Accidentally Elevated above the Level of the Patient's Chest. This is serious, since fluid in the bottle will be siphoned or flow by gravity into the pleural space. If much fluid enters the pleural space from the drainage bottle, the patient's lung may be collapsed on the affected side and a mediastinal shift may occur. Lower the bottle at once and contact the physician immediately.

MEASURING AND OBSERVING CHEST DRAINAGE

The air being removed from the pleural space escapes through the water-seal bottle's air vent, but the fluid is simply evacuated into the collection bottle and stays there. Expiration causes intrapleural pressure to rise higher than the pressure exerted by the water on the end of the water-seal tube, and fluid (and air) is forced from the pleural space into the bottle. As drainage collects in the water-seal bottle of a one-bottle set-up, more pressure is required to force the fluid down in the submersed water-seal tube upon expiration in order to permit the escape of fluid and air from the pleural space. *The depth to which the water-seal tube is immersed below the fluid in the bottle determines the pressure exerted by the water.*

To reduce the amount of pressure that the drainage must overcome, the long water-seal tube may be periodically pulled up in the bottle as fluid accumulates. Thus, less of the tube is under the fluid in the bottle. (Remember never to pull the end of the tube above the fluid level line.) Of course, it may be necessary to change the drainage bottle as it fills. Be certain it is never allowed to become so full that it covers the opening of the air vent.

Because it is important to know the amount of drainage coming from the pleural space and its rate of accumulation, a piece of tape is placed on the bottle so levels can be noted. This record helps the physician to determine the amount of blood loss and the rate of flow of drainage from the pleural space. These facts are important in planning blood replacement therapy and in evaluating the patient's status. Patients with excessive drainage may need to be returned to surgery for exploration to determine the cause.

The *marking tape* is applied when the apparatus is first set up. As mentioned, usually 100 ml. of sterile saline or sterile water is initially placed in the water-seal bottle. A mark is then made on the tape indicating this fluid level. Above the initial fluid level mark, the tape is marked at intervals representing additional 50-ml. accumulations. The times at which these various marks are reached by the draining fluids are marked on the tape opposite the drainage level mark.

Carefully measure and record chest drainage. It is not unusual for as much as 500 to 1000 ml. of drainage to occur in the first 24-hour period following chest surgery. Between 100 and 300 ml. of drainage may accumulate during the first two hours; following this, the amount of drainage should lessen.

Chest drainage is normally grossly bloody immediately following surgery, but it should not continue to be so for more than several hours. If the drainage remains frankly bloody for an abnormal period of time or if bleeding recurs after it has obviously stopped, contact the surgeon. Blood loss is evaluated by observing the rising level in the fluid collection bottle. If the patient's blood pressure drops and the pulse is rapid, *hemorrhage* is suspected. The drainage collection bottles are checked for a rise in the fluid level. If the level has not risen, the tubes are checked for patency. The physician is always immediately notified since the patient may be bleeding rapidly within the chest.

Replacement of a One-bottle Chest Drainage Apparatus. Periodically the drainage collection bottle must be replaced with another sterile set-up. Usually water-seal bottles are changed only if the physician orders them to be or if they are broken or malfunctioning. The person changing the bottles must be qualified to do so.

A physician or nurse may change a one-bottle water-seal apparatus in the following manner.

- ▶ First assemble the necessary equipment: two clamps and a sterile water-seal bottle set up as the original bottle was with 100 ml. of sterile normal saline or sterile water, a labeled measurement tape on the side of the bottle, and a snug stopper with two tubes (one short, one long) properly positioned.
- ▶ Double clamp the chest catheters close to the patient's chest to prevent air from entering the pleural space through the disconnected tubing.
- ▶ Disconnect the bottle to be replaced and attach the new set, making certain the connections are airtight and that the end of the long tube in the bottle is below the fluid level.
- ▶ Be certain the bottle is located lower than the patient's chest.
- ▶ Unclamp the patient's chest catheter (be sure you remove *both* clamps) and make certain the system is functioning properly before leaving the patient. Do not clamp the chest catheters until you have everything ready to complete the replacement. Keeping the catheters clamped for too long may permit air and fluid to accumulate to dangerous levels in the pleural space.

TWO-BOTTLE WATER-SEAL DRAINAGE

Basic Set-Up. With a two-bottle water-seal apparatus one bottle collects drainage and the other bottle is the water-seal bottle. In this set-up the *empty drainage bottle* is between the patient and the *water-seal bottle* (Fig. 57–7). The empty drainage bottle: (1) has a strip of tape applied to the side of the bottle to record the rate and quantity of drainage; (2) is sealed off at

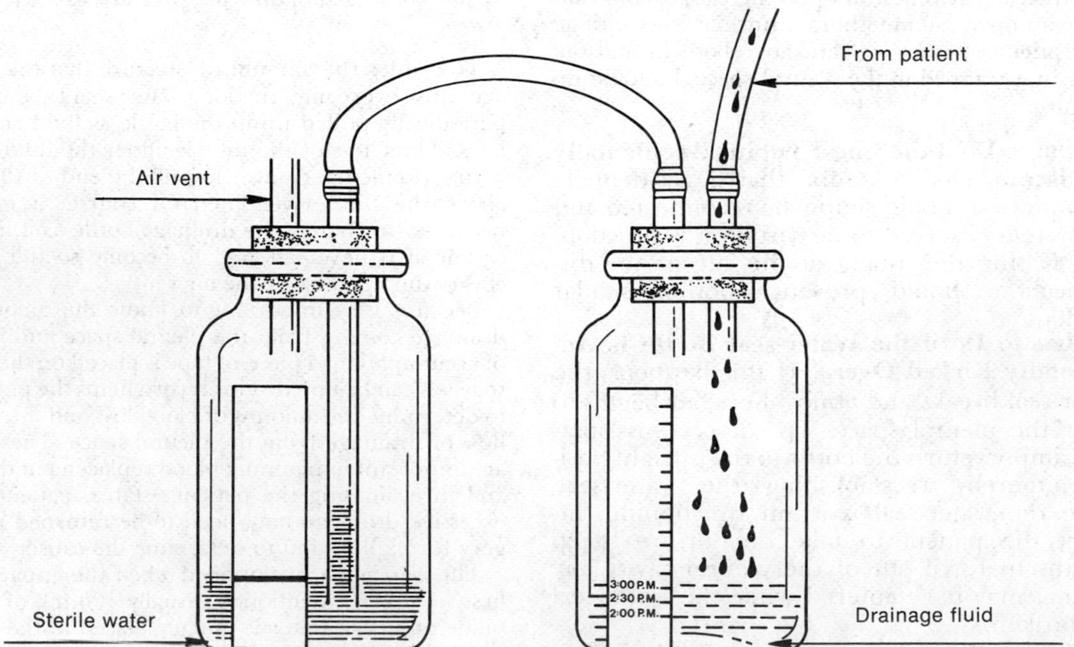

Figure 57–7. Two-bottle water-seal drainage. (After *Closed Drainage of the Chest*, U.S. Public Health Service Publication No. 1337, May, 1965.)

the top with a snug-fitting rubber stopper; and (3) has two short tubes that pass through holes in the stopper. Each tube extends into the bottle for about one inch. One of these short tubes is attached to the drainage tubing coming from the patient; the other is attached (with a small section of tubing) to the underwater tube of the water-seal bottle. Because drainage does not pass into the water-seal bottle in this set-up, the strip of tape on the outside of the water-seal bottle is marked only to indicate the initial level of the sterile saline or sterile water. As with the one-bottle water-seal apparatus, the air vent of the water-seal bottle must be left open to atmospheric air.

A two-bottle water-seal apparatus makes it easier to observe the amount and character of drainage from the patient's chest (since the drainage does not mix with the water or saline in the water-seal bottle). Also, the two-bottle set-up makes it easier to control the pressure within the system, and thus makes it easier for fluid and air to leave the pleural space. As mentioned earlier, when a one-bottle drainage apparatus begins to fill up with drainage fluid, the level of fluid in the underwater tube rises unless the tube is gradually pulled up as the fluid level increases. The higher the level of fluid in the tube, the more pressure is required to push the column of fluid down. Thus, air or fluid attempting to leave the pleural space must exert more pressure. This problem is solved by having a separate bottle for drainage collection.

Except for the differences just discussed, the one- and two-bottle water-seal systems perform similar functions in similar ways. The fluid in the underwater tube fluctuates with inspiration and expiration when the system functions properly, and air escapes from the air vent in the water-seal bottle.

HOW TO TELL WHEN WATER-SEAL DRAINAGE IS NO LONGER NECESSARY

The physician determines when to remove water-seal drainage. As mentioned, one indication that evacuation of intrapleural air and fluid is completed and the lung has reexpanded is the cessation of fluid fluctuation in the long tube of the water-seal bottle. The reexpanded lung blocks the catheters' openings in the pleural space, and thus the fluctuations of intrapleural pressure during inspiration and expiration are no longer transmitted to the water-seal apparatus. When the lung is completely reexpanded, no air or fluid passes through the chest catheters.

Usually the lung is fully reexpanded after two or three days of chest drainage postoperatively. Generally chest catheters are left in place for 24 hours after all air drainage and significant fluid drainage has stopped. Chest catheters may not be removed if the chest is draining more than 50 to 75 ml. of fluid daily. The sooner the tubes can be removed, the better, since their presence often contributes to the patient's postoperative pain and inactivity. Also, the longer the tubes are in place the greater the risk of infection. In treating empyema, chest drainage tubes may be used for longer periods of time than following chest surgery.

To confirm an impression that the lung has reexpanded the physician auscultates and percusses the patient's chest and orders a chest x-ray film. If the physician is convinced that it is safe to remove the chest catheter the physician then proceeds to do so. Although both chest tubes may be removed at the same time, it is more common for the upper chest tube to be left in place for a while longer than the lower. (Removal of chest catheters is discussed later.)

MECHANICAL SUCTION CLOSED CHEST DRAINAGE

Mechanical suction can be applied to the chest in various ways. For example, a special apparatus may be used with a built-in suction motor and a built-in device to control the amount of suction (negative pressure) exerted by the system. (See discussion of Thoracic Thermotic Pump, below). Or suction may be applied to the pleural space by attaching an electric suction pump or wall suction outlet to special two- or three-bottle water-seal set-ups* (Fig. 57–8). (Note: Often a small empty "trap bottle" is attached with tubing between the suction source and the suction control bottle. This trap bottle [not shown in the illustrations in Figure 57–8] prevents the suction motor from getting water in it if overflow of water should accidentally occur from the suction control bottle.)

Uses. Generally the normal ventilatory movements of the chest (during inspiration and expiration), coughing, and deep breathing adequately pump air and fluid from the pleural space and reexpand the lung, along with simple water-seal drainage. However, when these activities and gravity drainage are not adequate to promote reexpansion of the lung and emptying of the contents of the pleural space, a suction

*Space does not permit discussion of the two-bottle set-up for use with mechanical suction. However, this system can be easily grasped once the reader understands the discussions of the other set-ups we have presented, i.e., the one- and two-bottle water-seal apparatus and the three-bottle water set-up for use with mechanical suction. A two-bottle set-up for use with mechanical suction is illustrated in Figure 57–8.

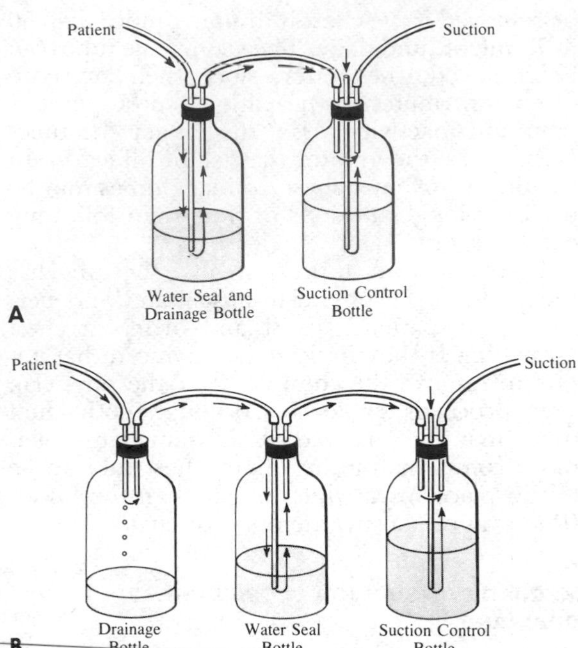

Figure 57–8. **A.** Two-bottle system for closed chest drainage with suction. **B.** Three-bottle system. (From Secor, J.: *Patient Care in Respiratory Problems.* Philadelphia: W. B. Saunders Co., 1969.)

apparatus of some type is necessary. Continuous gentle suction may be used when a patient's cough and respirations are too weak to force air and fluid out of the pleural space through the chest catheters. Suction may also be applied to closed chest drainage in the treatment of empyema. Additionally, suction may be used if air is leaking into the pleural space faster than it can be removed by a water-seal apparatus (e.g., if there is considerable air leakage through the pulmonary pleura) and/or to speed up the removal of air or fluid from the pleural space.

There are two ways to provide chest suction. Occasionally the physician attaches a chest catheter to a needle and then inserts the needle into a *vacuum blood donor bottle* (500 ml. capacity). This set-up provides very mild suction. More often, a *mechanical suction pump* is used, e.g., a Moe, Emerson, or Stedman pump or suction from a wall outlet.

The suction motor establishes and maintains suction (negative pressure) throughout the closed drainage apparatus and within the pleural space because the motor continually removes air from within the system (including air drawn into the system from the pleural space). As air is removed, the system's capacity increases and the pressure within it falls. The negative pressure thus created actively pulls or sucks air and fluid from the pleural space. The evacuated fluid collects in a bottle (in some set-ups this is the water-seal bottle, as will be discussed); the air drawn out of the pleural space is forced out of the system, with air from the system itself, through the motor's exhaust apparatus.

Because most suction motors create amounts of suction potentially damaging to the pulmonary pleura, the *degree of suction in the system* (and thus in the pleural space) *must be controlled.* To control the amount of pressure exerted by a wall suction outlet, a valve and meter may be inserted between the wall outlet and the water-seal bottle. When portable suction machines are used, a suction-control bottle (to be discussed) governs the amount of negative pressure permitted to build up within the system.

Suction may be applied to both chest catheters, but is more commonly applied to the upper tube (to remove intrapleural air). Because physicians vary in their use of suction with closed chest drainage, and because the type and amount of suction ordered varies from patient to patient, the nurse carefully reads the physician's orders. Suction is used immediately following decortication, but in other surgical procedures it may not be used for 24 hours postoperatively. Some surgeons believe the early use of suction enlarges the size of air leaks.

Three-bottle Water-seal Apparatus for Use with Mechanical Suction. The three-bottle suction set-up consists of: (1) a drainage collection bottle (the bottle closest to the patient); (2) a water-seal bottle (the middle bottle); and (3) a suction control bottle (connected to a suction source). (Refer back to Figure 57–8.) The set-up is the same as the two-bottle water-seal apparatus previously discussed, except that attached to the water-seal bottle's former air vent opening is the third bottle. The drainage and water-seal bottles are connected to each other as previously described.

Suction Control Bottle ("Breaker Bottle"). In a three-bottle water-seal apparatus for use with mechanical suction the purpose of the third bottle is to control the amount of pressure in the system. The suction control bottle contains water and a tight-fitting stopper with *three openings* in it. The stopper is taped to the bottle; all connections are also taped to prevent air leaks. Two short tubes are passed through two of the openings in the stopper. These tubes extend into the bottle about 1 inch. One tube is joined with flexible tubing to the former air vent of the water-seal bottle; the other short tube is connected with flexible tubing to the suction motor. Passing through the third opening in the stopper is a third tube much longer than the other two. One end of this is open to the atmosphere; the end in the bottle extends below the water level. This tube is the *suction control tube.*

The depth to which the suction control tube is inserted below the fluid level in the bottle controls the amount of pressure within the system. The physician orders how far the control tube is to be kept below the fluid level. For example, if the physician wants to limit the suction on the pleural space to 10 cm. of water* (approximately the normal intrapleural pressure during inspiration), it may be ordered that the tube be kept submerged 10 cm. below the fluid level in the suction control bottle. Then, regardless of the amount of negative pressure from the suction machine, the amount of negative pressure in the three-bottle system (and hence in the pleural space) will not exceed 10 cm. of water.

The level of water in the open tube of the suction control bottle sinks in proportion to the amount of negative pressure in the apparatus when the suction source is turned on. For example, if there are 10 ml. of water between the tip of the tube under the water and the water level, 10 cm. of water is the amount of negative pressure in the system. The water in the control tube would thus sink to the bottom of the tube when the suction source is turned on in order to reach this amount of negative pressure. If the amount of negative pressure in the system begins to increase (i.e., the pressure in the system falls below that for which the suction control tube is set), air is drawn into the system through the control tube and the suction breaks at the 10 cm. of water level. Excessive degrees of negative pressure are thus not permitted to build up in the system. As much air is pulled in as is needed to raise the pressure back up to the set level. It is important that the upper end of the suction control tube be kept open to atmospheric air for the apparatus to function properly.

The initial water level in the suction control bottle should be marked on a piece of tape placed on the side of the bottle. (Marking tapes needed for the drainage and water-seal bottles have been discussed.) It is the nurse's responsibility to periodically check the suction control tube to be certain it is submerged the prescribed distance beneath the fluid level in the bottle.

How to Tell if the Apparatus is Functioning Properly. Proper functioning of the suction control bottle is indicated by the periodic emptying of the fluid in the control tube, and by bubbling through the water of the air being drawn into this tube. In order to govern pressure within the system, the water in the suction control bottle bubbles almost constantly as outside air is drawn into the system.

> *Absence of bubbling in the suction control bottle means the system is not properly functioning and the correct suction level is not being maintained.*

Possible reasons for malfunctioning of a mechanical suction apparatus include air leaking into the pleural space or into the drainage apparatus, and mechanical problems in the pump. The most serious problem would be air leaking into the pleural space. Therefore, check for this problem first by briefly clamping off the chest drainage tube and then observing the suction control bottle. If you see the bottle bubbling, you know that nothing is wrong with either the drainage apparatus or the pump; the problem is therefore an air leak into the pleural space around the chest tubes. If you cannot effectively seal off this air leak, e.g., with petrolatum gauze, notify the physician immediately. If the suction control bottle fails to begin to bubble when the chest catheter is clamped, you know the problem is in the drainage connections or the pump. Check the system carefully, looking for loose connections, air leaks around bottle tops, or air leaks in the tubing, e.g., split tubing. Also, make certain the tubing is not kinked and that it is correctly positioned and there are no dependent loops. Because the chest catheter remains clamped during this inspection, observe the patient closely for indications of tension pneumothorax. As soon as you have corrected the problem with the system, the suction control bottle's fluid will begin to bubble. Then immediately remove the clamps on the chest catheter. If the suction motor appears to be causing the problem, i.e., the suction control bottle does not function properly after you have checked all the tubing and all connections, obtain another pump at once.

When the water in the suction control bottle fails to bubble and the nurse cannot identify and correct the source of difficulty, the physician is contacted. It may be that the amount of suction in the system needs to be increased if air is rapidly leaking from the pleura. If this is the cause of the system's malfunctioning, the physician will order the amount of suction to be increased so the escaping air can be more rapidly removed from the pleural space. To increase the amount of suction, water is added to the suction control bottle. Thus, the distance is increased between the tip of the tube and the water level in the bottle and the suction is proportionally increased.

In a mechanical suction arrangement (unlike the simpler water-seal set-ups discussed earlier) the fluid level in the long water-seal tube *does not* fluctuate with the ventilatory movements of the patient's chest because the suction holds the fluid level in the tube at a fixed level. Thus, you do not have the fluctuating of this fluid column to indicate proper functioning of the system or, conversely, the absence of fluctuation to indicate malfunction. However, as with the simpler water-seal arrangements discussed previously, *continuous bubbling in the water-seal bottle does indicate an air leak in the system.*

To detect an *air leak* in a closed-chest mechanical suction apparatus, first look for observable defects in the mechanical suction system and make certain all connections are taped. If the system continues to malfunction begin to look for a leak by clamping the tubing briefly. Start at the chest catheter end of the tubing and work your way toward the apparatus. If you place a clamp between the leak and the water-seal bottle, and the continuous bubbling in the water-seal bottle stops, you know the leak is located between the end of the catheter and the water-seal bottle. Thus,

*In some settings the usual suction applied postoperatively is 20 to 30 cm. of water. At times the suction has been increased as necessary up to 90 cm. of water without proving harmful.[102A]

when you have been able to place a clamp at a point between the air leak and the water-seal bottle you will be able to identify the area of the leak because the continuous bubbling in the water-seal bottle will stop.

Periodically, to see if the system is operating properly (e.g., to make certain the tubing is not obstructed), the mechanical chest suction apparatus may be modified so it becomes a simple water-seal system for a few moments. (Note: It is also modified in this way when the physician wants to check to see if the lung has reexpanded and the chest suction can be discontinued). Once the system has been converted to a simple water-seal system, the underwater tube in the water-seal bottle is observed. (Remember that fluctuation of the fluid in this tube indicates normal functioning, whereas cessation of this fluctuation occurs when the tubes are clogged or the lung has reexpanded.)

To modify the mechanical apparatus so it becomes a simple water-seal apparatus, the suction motor is turned off and the section of tubing running to the motor is disconnected and left open to atmospheric air. (If you prefer, disconnect the tube between the water-seal bottle and the suction control bottle.) Leaving this tubing open provides an air vent so any intrapleural air can escape from the system. If the tubing is not disconnected when the motor is off, the intrapleural air may build up in the system and cause a tension pneumothorax. (As stated earlier, when the motor is running and the tubing is connected, the intrapleural air escapes through the motor's exhaust system.) While the suction is briefly interrupted, the fluid level in the water-seal tube is observed for fluctuations.

REMOVAL OF CHEST CATHETERS

When chest catheters are to be removed, premedication for pain is usually given about one half hour before the procedure, since removal of the catheters is moderately painful. After premedicating the patient, the nurse assembles equipment for the physician, e.g., sterile scissors, a knife or suture set to cut the suture; sterile petrolatum gauze and a 4 × 4 gauze square to cover the wound; and three 2-inch wide strips of tape about 6 inches long.

The patient is positioned sitting on the edge of the bed or lying on the unoperated side. After clipping the stitches the physician quickly removes the catheters. Removal is accomplished either during expiration or at the end of a full inspiration to prevent air from being sucked back into the pleural space while the drain is being pulled out. Following removal of the chest catheter the wound may be closed with skin clips or covered with petrolatum gauze. A dressing is then firmly applied over the wound and is secured with wide strips of tape. The wound heals in a few days. Usually a chest x-ray film is ordered following removal of chest tubes.

Be certain to check the areas of the catheter skin incisions for air leakage for the first few hours after the catheter has been removed. Observe for subcutaneous emphysema of surrounding tissues. *Also, closely observe the patient during this time for indications of respiratory distress that could be caused by loss of negative intrapleural pressure or tension pneumothorax.* Notify the physician immediately who will reinstitute closed chest drainage if indicated.

ALTERNATE EQUIPMENT FOR CHEST DRAINAGE

Some newer species of equipment for chest drainage and suction will be mentioned briefly here.

Flutter Valve. A flutter valve can be used to replace underwater drainage bottles in closed chest drainage apparatuses (Fig. 57–9). The B-P Heimlich Chest Drainage Valve is presterilized, disposable, and about 7 inches long. When inserted between a chest catheter and a drainage collecting apparatus the valve permits the unidirectional flow of air and fluids from the pleural space into the collection apparatus, but it does not permit the reflux of air or fluid back into the chest.

The flutter valve itself is actually a single piece of wide, thin rubber tubing which is open at the end of the valve attached to the chest catheter and then is compressed at its other end so its flattened sides remain in contact with each other. Fluids draining from the intrapleural space thus can enter the open end of the tubing and pass out through the flattened ends of the valve, but they cannot reenter the flattened sides of the tubing because the two sides remain

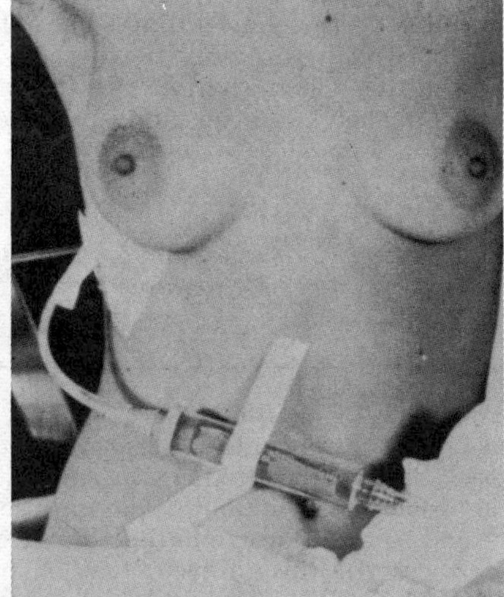

Figure 57–9. With catheter and Heimlich flutter valve secured in place, this patient with a spontaneous pneumothorax can go about her business while the leak is healing and the lung is reexpanding. (From: Something new in pneumothorax. *Emergency Medicine,* 9:231, April 1977.)

in contact with each other. The valve offers minimal resistance to the passage of air or fluids leaving the intrapleural space. The piece of rubber tubing is enclosed in a clear plastic case, which makes it easy to observe the passage of fluids, blood, and so forth, through the valve. Also, the expansion and contraction of the valve leaflets (caused by changes in the intrapleural pressure associated with ventilatory chest movements) can be observed. The flutter valve functions in any position; thus, the patient may assume any position.

Water-seal systems that use bottles are not only cumbersome but also tend to restrict the patient's mobility and are frequently the cause of accidents and a great deal of anxiety for both patient and staff. The plastic flutter valve is safer for the patient and easier for the nurse. It enables greater freedom of movement for the patient, a factor of importance in the postoperative course of chest surgery patients, who tend generally to want to be less active than is desirable. With the valve the patient can be comfortably ambulatory if the drainage tubing is connected to a portable plastic bag. Since it functions in the same manner as a water-seal bottle, the flutter valve can be attached to chest suction if necessary.

Pleur-Evac. The Pleur-Evac is a presterilized, disposable plastic apparatus that duplicates in principle the three-bottle closed chest drainage system (Fig. 57–10). Within the one apparatus there are three separate chambers which:

- collect drainage (the chest catheter attaches to this chamber which has a self-sealing diaphragm at the bottom for sterile removal of specimens);
- provide a water-seal (1 to 2 cm. of water are added to this chamber to form the water-seal);
- provide suction control (this chamber is filled with water to the desired height, e.g., 10 to 25 cm.).

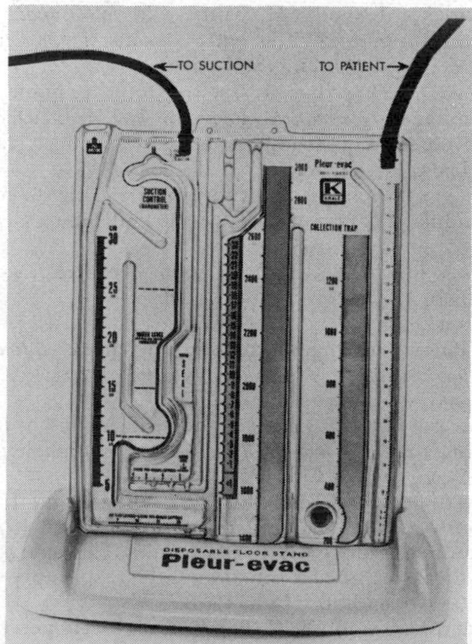

Figure 57–10. Pleur-Evac. (Courtesy of Deknatel, Inc., Queens Village, N.Y.)

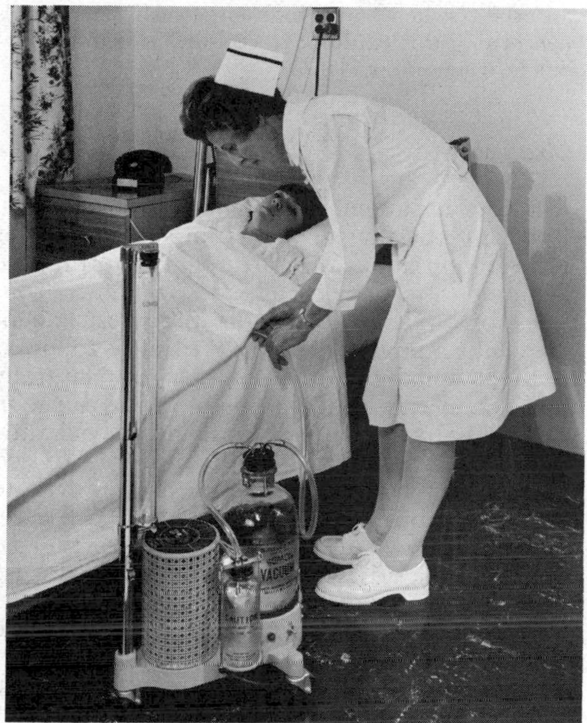

Figure 57–11. Gomco Thoracic Thermotic Pump for closed chest drainage. (Courtesy of Gomco Surgical Manufacturing Corp., Buffalo, N.Y.)

Tubing is attached from the suction chamber to the suction source. The Pleur-Evac may be placed in a floor stand or attached to the bedside. (For additional details consult the manufacturer's information sheet.)

Some of the newer equipment designed for closed chest drainage simplifies the nurse's responsibilities in caring for the equipment. However, the same high level of patient care and observation is necessary and the nurse must understand the basic principles of closed chest drainage.

Thoracic Thermotic Pump. This pump, manufactured by Gomco, is especially designed to create a controlled amount of suction for the purpose of removing air and fluid from the pleural space (Fig. 57–11). The apparatus contains a manometer (bubble type), with a long manometer tube which functions similarly to a suction-control bottle tube in a water-seal bottle set-up modified for use with suction. Either water or mercury may be used in the manometer. Mercury is used if suction greater than 25 cm. of water is desired. (Mercury is 13.6 times as dense as water. For example, 10 cm. of water equals 0.74 cm. Hg or 7.4 mm. Hg). If even greater suction is required, two pumps can be attached to the chest catheter with a Y connector. A water-seal can be set up as part of the drainage apparatus. The pump has an off-on switch and a high-low switch. (For details concerning this equipment, consult the manufacturer's instruction booklet.)

Discharge

Before a patient is discharged from hospital following chest surgery it is important to offer information about the care regimen to practice at home. Such advice includes continued routines of oral hygiene, nutrition, rest, deep-breathing, coughing, and exercising as followed in the hospital just prior to discharge. Naturally these activities are modified by the surgeon according to the patient's individual needs during recovery. Additionally, the patient is advised to avoid activities or environments that irritate the tracheobronchial tree and could cause severe coughing episodes. For example, the patient may be advised not to smoke, not to use aerosol products (e.g., spray deodorants), to avoid dusty areas, and to avoid exposure to persons who have upper respiratory infections. The patient should be told to contact the physician if symptoms of an upper respiratory infection or other ailments develop.

Plans for returning to work activities are individualized. Some persons are able to return to work within a few weeks after thoracic surgery, whereas others need occupational counseling because a change of occupation is necessary; still other patients are unable to work.

BIBLIOGRAPHY

1. Acinapura, A. J.: Check beneath the broken ribs. *Emergency Medicine,* 9:79, Nov. 1977.
2. Adams, F. V.: Respiratory tract hemorrhage: Guide to emergency management. *Hospital Medicine,* 14:66, Oct. 1978.
3. Adams, N. R.: The nurse's role in systematic weaning from a ventilator. *Nursing '79,* 9:35, Aug. 1979.
4. Addington, W. W.: Tuberculosis and other mycobacterial diseases. *In* Conn, H. F. (Ed.): *Current Therapy 1978.* Philadelphia, W. B. Saunders Co., 1978.
5. Ahmad, M., and C. Lindquist: Bronchial asthma: Some aspects of pathogenesis and therapy. *Postgraduate Medicine,* 62:111, July 1977.
6. American Cancer Society: *1973 Cancer Facts and Figures* (Pamphlet). New York: American Cancer Society, Inc., 1972.
7. American Cancer Society: *Answering the Most Often Asked Questions About. . .Cigarette Smoking and Lung Cancer* (Pamphlet). New York: American Cancer Society, Inc., 1965.
8. American Thoracic Society: *Basics of Respiratory Disease,* Vols. 1, 2, 3. New York: American Lung Association, 1975.
9. Andersen, H. A.: Preoperative evaluation of bronchogenic cancer. *Consultant,* 18:196, Sept. 1978.

9A. Ayres, S. M., et al.: Respiratory management of the critically ill patient. *New York State Journal of Medicine,* 68:2871, Nov. 1968.

10. Ayvazian, L. F.: Extrapulmonary manifestations of tumors of the lung. *Postgraduate Medicine,* 63:93, Feb. 1978.
11. Baker, P. J.: Postoperative atelectasis. *Nursing Digest,* 4:42, Spring 1977.
12. Bakow, E. D.: Sustained maximal inspiration — a rationale for its use. *Respiratory Care,* 22:379, April 1977.

12A. Bartlett, J. G.: Empyema. *Hospital Medicine,* 12:77, Feb. 1976.

13. Baum, G. L. (Ed.): *Textbook of Pulmonary Disorders,* 2nd Ed. Boston: Little, Brown and Company, 1974.
14. Benjamin, S. P., and L. J. McCormack: Structural abnormalities in COPD. *Postgraduate Medicine,* 62:101, July 1977.
15. Bergner, R. K., and A. Bergner: Outpatient management of asthma. *American Family Physician,* 15:141, May 1977.
16. Berkow, R., et al. (Eds.): *The Merck Manual of Diagnosis and Therapy,* 13th ed. Rahway, N.J.: Merck Sharp & Dohme Research Laboratories, 1977.
17. Bernstein, N. D., and A. R. Schwartz: Influenza vaccines — Fall 1978. *American Family Physician,* 18:156, Nov. 1978.
18. Betson, C.: Blood gases. *American Journal of Nursing,* 68:1010, May 1968.
19. Biddle, T. L.: Acute pulmonary edema. *Hospital Medicine,* 13:56, Dec. 1977.
20. Billops, D.: Would you recognize a plague victim in time? *RN,* 40:62, July 1977.
21. Blakey, D. L.: Drug resistant tuberculosis. *CDC-MNWR,* 51:417, Dec. 1977.
22. Block, E. R.: Pitfalls in diagnosing and managing pulmonary diseases. *Geriatrics,* 34:70, Feb. 1979.
23. Bobowitz, I. D.: Choosing the correct combinations against tuberculosis. *Consultant,* 17:217, Jan. 1977.
24. Bode, F. R.: Axioms on smoking and the respiratory tract. *Hospital Medicine,* 14:35, Nov. 1978.
25. Boldeker, E., and J. H. Dauber (Eds.): *Manual of Medical Therapeutics,* 21st ed. St. Louis: Department of Medicine, Washington University, 1974.
26. Boyd, A. D.: When to operate for carcinoma of the lung. *Postgraduate Medicine,* 63:127, Feb. 1978.
27. Boyer, M. W.: Treating invasive lung cancer. *American Journal of Nursing,* 77:1916, Dec. 1977.
28. Brown, M., and J. L. Andrews, Jr.: How to manage adult respiratory distress syndrome. *Geriatrics,* 34:39, April 1979.
29. Buck, M.: Why can't this patient breathe? *RN,* 42:73, Feb. 1979.

29A. Buckingham, W. B., D. W. Cugell, and L. J. Kettel: Pulmonary angiography in lung diseases. *Journal of the American Medical Association,* 200:122, June 1967.

30. Burton, G. G., G. E. Gee, and J. E. Hodgkin: *Respiratory Care, A Guide to Clinical Practice.* Philadelphia: J. B. Lippincott Co., 1977.
31. Byrd, R. B.: Current concepts in diagnosing the cause of pleural effusion. *Geriatrics,* 32:44, Oct. 1977.
32. Campbell, E. J., and S. S. Lefrak: How aging affects the structure and function of the respiratory system. *Geriatrics,* 33:68, June 1978.
33. Carr, D. T., and E. C. Rosenow: Bronchogenic Carcinoma. *Basics of RD,* Vol. 5. American Thoracic Soci-

ety. New York: American Lung Association, May 1977.

34. Ciuca, R.: Cor pulmonale. *Nursing 78,* 8:46, Dec. 1978.
35. Clarke, J. T.: Planning antibiotic therapy of pneumonia. *Geriatrics,* 32:51, Nov. 1977.
36. Codish, S. D., J. S. Tobias, and A. P. Monaco: Systemic mycotic infections. (Parts 1 and 2.) *Hospital Medicine,* 14:6 and 30, June and July 1978.
37. Comer, T. P., and A. A. Roscher: Which tests — and when — to diagnose lung cancer. *Consultant,* 17:95, June 1977.
38. Conn, H. F. (Ed.): *Current Therapy* 1979. Philadelphia: W. B. Saunders Co., 1979.
39. Cordasco, E. M., and H. S. VanOrdstrand: Air pollution and COPD. *Postgraduate Medicine,* 62:124, July 1977.
40. Costello, J. F.: Asthma: Diagnosis can be difficult. *Consultant,* 17:35, Dec. 1977.
41. Coyle, N., and E. Arbit: How to protect your patients against aspiration pneumonia. *Nursing '78,* 8:50, Oct. 1978.
42. Cugell, D. W.: Guide to modern lung function tests. *Hospital Medicine,* 14:57, Jan. 1978.
43. Dack, S.: Acute pulmonary edema. *Hospital Medicine,* 14:112, Mar. 1978.
44. D'Agostino, J. S., and P. L. Welch: The phrenic pacemaker. *Nursing '79,* 9:41, May 1979.
45. Davies, R. J., and J. E. Salvaggio: Occupational asthma: How to recognize, treat — and prevent it. *Consultant,* 18:201, Oct. 1978.
46. Del Bueno, D. J.: A quick review on using blood-gas determinations. *RN,* 41:68, Mar. 1978.
47. Dembert, M. L.: Physical examination of scuba divers. *American Family Physician,* 20:91, Aug. 1979.
48. Dolin, R.: Amantadine and influenza A. *American Family Physician,* 19:127, Jan. 1979.
49. Eisenberg, M., C. Furukawa, et al.: *A Manual of Antimicrobial Therapy and Communicable Disease.* Olympia: State of Washington Department of Social and Health Services, 1976.
50. Ennis, S., and T. R. Harris: Positioning infants with hyaline membrane disease. *American Journal of Nursing,* 78:398, Mar. 1978.
51. Falotico, J. B.: Pulmonary embolism: Don't overlook these subtle warnings. *RN,*42:47, Feb. 1979.
52. Farina, A. T., S. J. Alderman, and R. J. Carella: Radiotherapy for bronchogenic carcinoma. *Postgraduate Medicine,* 63:117, Feb. 1978.
53. Favorito, J., J. M. O. Pernice, and P. Ruggiero: . . .Beyond the hospital. Apnea monitoring to prevent SIDS. *American Journal of Nursing,* 79:101, Jan. 1979.
54. Fazzini, E. P.: Lung cancer: The pathologist's role in management. *Postgraduate Medicine,* 63:103, Feb. 1978.
55. Fergus, L. C., and E. M. Cordasco: Pulmonary rehabilitation of the patient with COPD. *Postgraduate Medicine,* 62:141, July 1977.
55A. Filley, G. F.: Emphysema and chronic bronchitis: Clinical manifestations and their physiologic significance. *Medical Clinics of North America* 51:283, March 1967.
56. Fink, J. N.: The asthmatic. *American Family Physician,* 18:124, Dec. 1978.
57. Fisher, M. L.: Helping acutely ill patients put out the fire. *American Journal of Nursing,* 79:1104, June 1979.
57A. Flatter, P. A.: Hazards of oxygen therapy. *American Journal of Nursing, 68*:80, Jan. 1968.
58. Foley, M. F.: Pulmonary function testing. *American Journal of Nursing,* 71:1134, June 1971.
59. Foley, M., J. Tomashefski, and E. Underwood, Jr.: Pulmonary function screening tests in industry. *American Journal of Nursing,* 77:1480, Sept. 1977.
60. Foss, G.: Postural drainage. *American Journal of Nursing,* 73:666, April 1973.
61. Francis, P. B.: Spirometry in office practice. *Postgraduate Medicine,* 63:72, Jan. 1978.
62. Frank, S. T.: 10 questions physicians most often ask — about treating pulmonary diseases. *Consultant,* 17:23, Oct. 1977.
63. Freiman, D. B., and W. T. Miller: Sarcoidosis: A multisystem disease. *American Family Physician,* 15:78, Jan. 1977.
64. Fuhs, M.: Patient teaching aid: Breathing and abdominal muscle-strengthening exercises. *Nursing '78,* 8:61, Sept. 1978.
65. Garfield, J. W.: Present-day diagnosis of lung cancer. *Postgraduate Medicine,* 63:82, Feb. 1978.
66. Gaskell, D. V., and B. A. Webber: *The Brompton Hospital Guide to Chest Physiotherapy,* 2nd ed. Oxford: Blackwell Scientific Publications, 1974.
67. Geelhoed, G. W.: Prevention of thromboembolism. *American Family Physician,* 19:147, Mar. 1979.
67A. Geiger, J. P.: Diagnosis of chest injuries. *Hospital Medicine,* 7:109, Oct. 1971.
68. Gernert, C. F., and Schwartz, S.: Pulmonary artery catheterization. *American Journal of Nursing,* 73:1182, July 1973.
69. Golbey, R. B.: Chemotherapy for lung cancer. *Postgraduate Medicine,* 63:137, Feb. 1978.
70. Golish, J. A., and Ahmad, M.: Management of COPD: A physiologic approach. *Postgraduate Medicine,* 62:131, July 1977.
71. Gong, H., Jr.: Fat embolism syndrome. *Postgraduate Medicine,* 62:40, Dec. 1977.
72. Greenberg, M. I., and J. Walter: Axioms on smoke inhalation. *Hospital Medicine,* 14:100, April 1978.
73. Guyton, A. C.: *Function of the Human Body,* 4th ed. Philadelphia: W. B. Saunders Co., 1974.
74. Hand, J.: Keeping anticoagulants under control. *RN,* 42:25, April 1979.
75. Hedley-Whyte, J., et al.: *Applied Physiology of Respiratory Care.* Boston: Little, Brown and Company, 1976.
76. Hildebrand, W. L., et al.: Use and abuse of oxygen in the newborn. *American Family Physician,* 18:125, Sept. 1978.
77. Hinshaw, H. C.: Management of tuberculosis. *Postgraduate Medicine,* 61:52, April 1977.
78. Holvey, D. N., et al. (Eds.): *The Merck Manual,* 12th ed. Rahway, N.J.: Merck Sharp and Dohme Research Laboratories, 1972.
79. Hutchinson, R.: The common cold primer. *Nursing '79,* 9:57, Mar. 1979.
79A. Isacson, L. M., and K. Schultz: Treating pulmonary edema. *Nursing '78,* 8:42, Feb. 1978.
80. Isawa, T., K. Wasserman, and G. V. Taplin: Lung scintigraphy and pulmonary function studies in obstructive airway disease. *American Review of Respiratory Diseases,* 102:161, Aug. 1970.
81. Isler, C.: What if Legionnaires' disease turns up in your hospital? *RN,* 41:23, Nov. 1978.
82. Jacquette, G.: To reduce hazards of tracheal suctioning. *American Journal of Nursing,* 71:2362, Dec. 1971.
83. Johnston, R. F., and Audet, P. R.: Antituberculosis chemotherapy. *American Family Physician,* 17:136, June 1978.

83A. Jones, W. R.: Living with emphysema. *Nursing Outlook,* 15:53, Sept. 1967.
84. Kanto, W. P., Jr.: Dealing with respiratory distress. *Emergency Medicine,* 9:67, Oct. 1977.
85. Kanto, W. P., Jr.: Resuscitation comes first. *Emergency Medicine,* 9:31, Oct. 1977.
86. Kanto, W. P., Jr., and L. J. Calvert: Neonatal resuscitation. *American Family Physician,* 16:76, Dec. 1977.
87. Kasik, J. E., and S. Schuldt: Why tuberculosis is still a health problem in the aged. *Geriatrics,* 32:63, Mar. 1977.
88. Kaspar, R. L.: Six effective ways to prevent Pseudomonas pneumonia. *Consultant,* 17:197, Jan. 1977.
89. Katz, S.: What is the air quality index? *American Family Physician,* 18:121, Oct. 1978.
90. Kavet, J.: A perspective on the significance of pandemic influenza. *American Journal of Public Health,* 67:1063, Nov. 1977.
91. Kent, S.: The aging lung. Part 1. Loss of elasticity. *Geriatrics,* 33:124, Feb. 1978.
92. Kent, S.: Vitamin C therapy: Colds, cancer, and cardiovascular disease. *Geriatrics,* 33:91, Oct. 1978.
92A. Kettel, L. J.: Acute respiratory acidosis. *Hospital Medicine,* 12:31, Feb. 1976.
93. Keys, T. F.: How to cope with infectious pneumonia in the immunologically compromised patient. *Geriatrics,* 33:68, Feb. 1978.
94. Kudla, M. S.: Emergency care of the patient with respiratory distress. *Critical Care Update,* 12:5, Dec. 1977.
95. Kurpershoek, C. J., and T. Pierce: Bedside cardiopulmonary techniques. *Critical Care Update,* 8:5, Aug. 1977.
96. Lance, E., and H. Sweetwood: Chest trauma when minutes count. *Nursing 78,* 8:28, Jan. 1978.
97. Landa, J. F.: Bronchofiberoscopy perspective, 1977. *Respiratory Therapy,* 5:59, Sept.-Oct. 1977.
98. Lemon, S. M., and J. S. Pagano: Fulminant pneumonia. *Hospital Medicine,* 13:79, Jan. 1977.
99. Light, R. W.: Pleural fluid analysis: How to interpret the tests. *Consultant,* 18:97, May 1978.
100. Lynne-Davies, P.: Influence of age on the respiratory system. *Geriatrics,* 32:57, Aug. 1977.
101. Lyons, H. A.: Differential diagnosis of hemoptysis and its treatment. *Basics of RD,* Vol. 5. American Thoracic Society. New York: American Lung Association, Nov. 1976.
102. MacDonnell, K. F., and M. S. Segal: *Current Respiratory Care.* Boston: Little, Brown and Co., 1977.
102A. MacVickar, J., and H. J. Mendelsohn: Chest surgery. *In* Meltzer, L. E., F. Abdellah, and J. Kitchell (Eds.): *Concepts and Practices of Intensive Care for Nurse Specialists.* Philadelphia: The Charles Press, 1969.
103. Marcott, M.: There's more to post-op extubation than just pulling out a tube. *RN,* 40:43, Sept. 1977.
104. Marici, F. N.: The flexible fiberoptic bronchoscope. *American Journal of Nursing,* 73:1776, Oct. 1973.
105. Mathewson, H. S.: *Pharmacology for Respiratory Therapists.* St. Louis: C. V. Mosby Co., 1977.
106. McCarthy, D. S.: Chronic obstructive lung disease: Guide to diagnosis and management. *Hospital Medicine,* 14:40, Dec. 1978.
107. McKaig, C., S. Steele, and M. P. Sullivan: Respiratory and cardiac conditions in children: A test of your nursing skill. *Nursing '79,* 9:94, May 1979.
108. McPherson, S. P.: *Respiratory Therapy Equipment.* St. Louis: C. V. Mosby Co., 1977.
109. Meador, B.: Pneumothorax: Providing emergency and long-term care. *Nursing '78,* 8:43, Nov. 1978.
110. Medicine: Slow-motion suicide. *Newsweek,* 93:83, Jan. 22, 1979.
111. Millen, D. L.: Aspiration: Foiling a silent killer. *RN,* 41:34, Aug. 1978.
112. Mitchell, R. S. (Ed.): *Synopsis of Clinical Pulmonary Disease.* St. Louis: C. V. Mosby Co., 1974.
113. Molyneux-Luick, M.: Water-sports injuries: The old and the new. *Nursing '78,* 8:50, Aug. 1978.
114. Moody, L. E.: Primer for pulmonary hygiene. *American Journal of Nursing,* 77:104, Jan. 1977.
114A. Morgan, C. V., Jr., and T. W. Orcutt: The care and feeding of chest tubes. *American Journal of Nursing,* 72:305, Feb. 1972.
115. Moses, R. M., and S. Steinberg: Does the MA-1 respirator make you nervous? *RN,* 42:35, April 1979.
116. Murray, J. F.: *The Normal Lung.* Philadelphia: W. B. Saunders Co., 1976.
117. Neff, T. A.: Meeting the challenge of pulmonary embolism. *Consultant,* 17:50, April 1977.
118. Nett, L. M., and T. L. Petty: Why emphysema patients are the way they are. *American Journal of Nursing,* 70:1251, June 1970.
119. O'Malley, P., and M. A. Zankofski: Disposable suction catheters: Nursing '79 Product Survey. *Nursing '79,* 9:70, May 1979.
120. Oslick, T.: Aerosol sympathomimetic amines. *American Family Physician,* 15:146, June 1977.
121. Peterson, L. D., and J. H. Green: Nurse-managed tuberculosis clinic. *American Journal of Nursing,* 77:433, Mar. 1977.
122. Petty, T. L.: Pulmonary rehabilitation. *Basics of RD,* Vol. 4. American Thoracic Society. New York: American Lung Association, Sept. 1975.
123. Petty, T. L.: *Intensive and Rehabilitative Respiratory Care,* 2nd ed. Philadelphia: Lea and Febiger, 1974.
124. Plummer, A. L.: Choosing a drug regimen for obstructive pulmonary disease. 1. Agents to achieve bronchodilatation. 2. Agents other than bronchodilators. *Postgraduate Medicine,* 63:36 and 113, April and May 1978.
125. Pons, V. G., and R. Dolin: Influenza. *Hospital Medicine,* 14:78, Oct. 1978.
125A. Pontoppidan, H.: Indications of respiratory failure. *New England Journal of Medicine,* 287:690, 1972.
126. Questions patients ask about smoking and health. *Consultant,* 17:163, Sept. 1977.
127. Rau, J., and M. Rau: To breathe or be breathed: Understanding IPPB. *American Journal of Nursing,* 77:613, April 1977.
128. Rexilius, B. G.: *Chest Drainage and Suction.* Philadelphia, F. A. Davis Co., 1977.
129. Rhodes, M. L.: How to manage respiratory failure. *Consultant,* 17:48, Nov. 1977.
130. Roach, L. B.: Assessment: Color changes in dark skin. *Nursing '77,* 1:48, Jan. 1977.
131. Rogers, R. M.: Respiratory failure: Base treatment on the patient's needs. *Consultant,* 18:83, June 1978.
132. Rothfeld, A. F., and P. A. Bromberg: Pneumothorax: Diagnosis and management. *Hospital Medicine,* 14:66, July 1978.
133. Rowlett, D. B., and D. L. Dudley: COPD: Psychosocial and psychophysiological issues. *Psychosomatics,* 19:273, May 1978.
134. Ruppel, G.: *Manual of Pulmonary Function Testing.* St. Louis: C. V. Mosby Co., 1975.
135. Sabiston, D. C., Jr.: *Davis-Christopher: Textbook of Surgery,* 11th ed. Philadelphia, W. B. Saunders Co., 1977.

136. Sackner, M. A.: The best of the old and the new in diagnosing pulmonary disease. *Consultant,* 17:158, May 1977.
137. Sandham, G., and B. Reid: Some Q's and A's about suctioning. *Nursing '77,* 7:60, Oct. 1977.
138. Schumann, G. G., and V. F. Colon: Sputum cytology. *American Family Physician,* 19:81, April 1979.
138A. Secor, J.: *Patient Care in Respiratory Problems.* Philadelphia: W. B. Saunders Co., 1969.
139. Seinfeld, E. D., and O. J. Balchum: Unsuspected pulmonary emboli in well persons: The incomplete pulmonary infarction syndrome. *American Family Physician,* 15:140, Feb. 1977.
140. Shafer, N.: Preparing the asthmatic patient for surgery. *Consultant,* 17:84, May 1977.
141. Shafer, N.: Travel alert: High altitude pulmonary edema. *Consultant,* 17:36, July 1977.
142. Shank, J. C., and R. F. Latshaw: Pleural effusion. *American Family Physician,* 18:143, Mar. 1978.
143. Shapiro, B. A.: *Clinical Application of Blood Gases.* Chicago: Year Book Medical Publishers, Inc., 1973.
144. Shapiro, B. A., R. Harrison, and C. A. Trout: *Clinical Application of Respiratory Care.* Chicago: Year Book Medical Publishers, Inc., 1975.
145. Sharma, O. P.: Diagnosing cryptogenic fibrosing alveolitis. *Consultant,* 17:127, Jan. 1977.
146. Sharma, O. P.: Finding the cause of PIE. *Consultant,* 17:54, Dec. 1977.
147. Sharma, O. P.: Sarcoidosis: Unusual pulmonary manifestations. *Postgraduate Medicine,* 61:67, Mar. 1977.
148. Sherry, S.: Prophylaxis for pulmonary embolism. *Consultant,* 17:59, Sept. 1977.
148A. Shim, C., et al.: Cardiac arrhythmias resulting from tracheal suctioning. *Annals of Internal Medicine,* 71:1149, Dec. 1969.
149. Shoemaker, W. C.: Early diagnosis and management of pericardial tamponade. *Hospital Medicine,* 14:7, Nov. 1978.
150. Simpson, C. M.: I saw the MA-1 through a patient's eyes my own. *RN,* 42:44, April 1979.
151. Sitzman, J.: Nursing assessment of the acutely ill respiratory patient. *Critical Care Update,* 9:20, Sept. 1977.
152. Sladen, A.: Maintenance of a patent airway. *Hospital Medicine,* 13:56, Aug. 1977.
153. Smith, B. J.: Safeguarding your patient after anesthesia. *Nursing '78,* 8:53, Oct. 1978.
154. Sokol, W. N., and G. N. Beall: Asthma. *Hospital Medicine,* 13:10, May 1977.
155. Sopko, J. A.: Pleural effusions: Guide to diagnosis. *Hospital Medicine,* 15:75, Feb. 1979.
156. Spector, S. L.: Asthma: Current pathophysiologic and therapeutic aspects. *Hospital Medicine,* 15:80, April 1979.
157. Speir, W. A., Jr.: How to improve management of chronic obstructive lung disease. *Consultant,* 17:168, May 1977.
158. Spragg, R. G.: Adult respiratory distress syndrome. *Hospital Medicine,* 15:31, Mar. 1979.
159. Stambaugh, D., and C. Wallace: What every nurse needs to know about massive chest damage. *RN,* 40:40, July 1977.
160. Stanley, L.: The near drowning victim: CPR is not enough. *RN,* 41:41, June 1978.
161. Stanley, L.: You really can teach COPD patients to breathe better. *RN,* 41:43, April 1978.
162. Stead, W. W., and J. Bates: Mycobacterial diseases. *In* Thorn, G. W., et al. (Eds.): *Harrison's Principles of Internal Medicine,* 8th ed. New York: McGraw-Hill Book Co., 1977.
163. Stone, D. J.: Bullous emphysema. *Hospital Medicine,* 13:72, Jan. 1977.
164. Sullivan, H. J.: Technical data: Tuberculosis. *Integral Asepsis Forum* of Aiken Laboratories, 1975.
165. Sweetwood, H.: Acute respiratory insufficiency: How to recognize this emergency . . . how to treat it. *Nursing '77,* 7:24, Dec. 1977.
166. Tecklin, J. S.: Positioning, percussing, and vibrating patients for effective bronchial drainage. *Nursing '79,* 9:64, Mar. 1979.
167. Thurlbeck, W. F.: *Chronic Airflow Obstruction in Lung Disease.* Philadelphia: W. B. Saunders Co., 1976.
168. Tiffany, P.: A look at incentive spirometry. *Respiratory Therapy,* 5:15, Sept.-Oct. 1977.
169. Tomashefski, J. F.: Definition, differentiation, and classification of COPD. *Postgraduate Medicine,* 62:88, July 1977.
170. Traver, G. A. (Ed.): Symposium on care in respiratory disease. *Nursing Clinics of North America,* 9:97, Mar. 1974.
171. Tsou, E., and S. Katz: Sickle cell lung disease. *American Family Practitioner,* 16:128, Oct. 1977.
172. Tucker, S. M., et al.: *Patient Care Standards.* St. Louis: C. V. Mosby Co., 1977.
173. Turndorf, H.: Beyond the opening of the airway. *Emergency Medicine,* 9:26, Nov. 1977.
173A. Ungvarski, P.: Mechanical stimulation of coughing. *American Journal of Nursing,* 71:2358, Dec. 1971.
174. UpJohn Laboratories: *The Asthmatic Patient in Trouble* (Pamphlet). 1976.
175. Up-to-date survey of tracheal tubes. *Nursing '76,* 6:66, Nov. 1976.
176. Varkey, B., and U. N. Kumar: Asbestos-related diseases of lung and pleura. *Postgraduate Medicine,* 63:48, June 1978.
177. Vogel, J. H. K.: Pulmonary hypertension: Evaluation and treatment. *Hospital Medicine,* 13:69, Sept. 1977.
178. Waldron, M. W.: Oxygen transport. *American Journal of Nursing,* 79:272, Feb. 1979.
179. Ward, J.: Cromolyn sodium: A new approach to treatment of asthma. *Heart and Lung,* 3:415, May-June 1975.
180. Webb-Johnson, D. C., and J. L. Andrews, Jr.: 10 questions physicians most often ask . . . about bronchodilator therapy. *Consultant,* 18:23, Sept. 1978.
181. Webster, J., and R. Davison: Aspiration pneumonitis: A serious problem. *Geriatrics,* 32:42, Dec. 1977.
181A. Weg, J. G.: *Treatment and Control of Tuberculosis* (Pamphlet). New York: American Lung Association, 1972.
182. Weiss, R. B.: Small cell carcinoma: The "different" type of lung cancer. *Geriatrics,* 32:75, April 1977.
183. West, D. W., et al.: Five year follow-up of a smoking withdrawal clinic population. *American Journal of Public Health,* 67:536, June 1977.
184. When to look to the Legionnaires. *Emergency Medicine,* 10:177, Oct. 1976.
185. White, S. J.: Respiratory drugs: When to give them . . . what to watch for. *RN,* 41:46, June 1978.
186. Wieczorek, R. R., and B. Horner Rosner: The asthmatic child: Preventing and controlling attacks. *American Journal of Nursing,* 79:258, Feb. 1979.
187. Wilson, R. F. (Ed.): A Self Study Text adapted from *Principles and Techniques of Critical Care.* UpJohn Laboratories, December,
188. Wilson, R. F.: Acute respiratory failure and how to manage it. *Consultant,* 18:25, May 1978.

189. Wolf, A. F.: Occupational lung disease. Part 2: Conditions caused by inorganic dusts. *Consultant,* 17:161, Jan. 1977.
190. Wylie, C. M., and M. R. Bear: Should we discourage cigarette smoking in elderly patients? *Geriatrics,* 33:95, Sept. 1978.
191. Zavala, D. C.: The threat of aspiration pneumonia in the aged. *Geriatrics,* 32:46, Mar. 1977.
192. Zelechowski, G. P.: Physiological and psychological implications of dyspnea. *Respiratory Therapy,* 7:18, Nov./Dec. 1977.
193. Zelis, R., et al.: The pulmonary edema symptom. *Nursing Digest,* 5:45, Spring 1977.
194. Ziment, I.: What to expect from expectorants. *Journal of the American Medical Association,* 2:193, July 1976.
195. Ziment, I.: *Respiratory Pharmacology and Therapeutics.* Philadelphia: W. B. Saunders Co., 1978.

UNIT XVII

NURSING PEOPLE EXPERIENCING DISTURBANCES OF DIGESTIVE FUNCTION

by Shirley Harlow, R.N., B.S., B.A., M.A.

INTRODUCTION AND STUDY GUIDE

The book of Proverbs in the Bible states, "A dry crust eaten in peace is better than steak every day along with argument and strife."[189] This ancient bit of wisdom is true today. One of the purposes of this unit is to make the student aware of the influence of the emotions of the functioning of the gastrointestinal tract.

A second purpose is to make the student cognizant of the types of disease entities that occur within the digestive system — abnormalities in structure, secretion and motility, tumors, infections, perforations, injuries, and vascular abnormalities — along with recognition of the effect that each of these may have.

A third purpose of this unit is to enable the student to understand the various tests and devices that are used in the diagnosis of disorders of the gastrointestinal tract and to know the nurse's responsibilities to the patient and to the physician prior to, during, and following these examinations.

The student should also know the various abnormalities in function that are created by the surgeon in attempting to help the patient. The nurse not only must understand the alteration in function that has occurred and its effect upon the patient's physiology, but also must understand the effect it has upon the individual's life.

The fifth purpose of this unit is to familiarize the student with the common manifestations of abnormal function (symptoms) which occur in the gastrointestinal tract, their cause, and the rationale for the treatments used to correct them.

Study Guide

1. Before you begin your reading ask yourself the following questions:

What would I do if I had a severe stomach ache?
What do I do when I am constipated or have diarrhea?
What would I recommend to a friend if she complained of abdominal pain, rectal bleeding, excessive gaseousness, vomiting, or diarrhea?
What would I say to a friend who said he had a stomach ulcer?

2. Familiarize yourself with the following prefixes: entero-, gastro-, oro-, ano-, colo-, ileo-, endo-, herni-.

3. Familiarize yourself with the following suffixes: -otomy, -ostomy, -orrhaphy, -itis, -oscopy.

4. Practice putting the prefixes in No. 2 with the suffixes in No. 3 to make words.

5. Familiarize yourself with these words: friable, diverticulum, polyp, herniation, prolapse, obstruction, adhesion, perforation, peritoneum, gland, enzyme, hormone, digestion, absorption.

6. Learn the meaning of these symptoms and their possible significance: tenesmus, heartburn, melena, hematemesis, anorexia, malaise.

7. Following your reading try to answer the following questions:

a. What is hunger? What causes satiety?

b. What is the specific digestive function of each of the organs of the digestive system?

c. What is the relationship of structure to function for each organ, including the protective mechanisms and physiologic processes taking place at each level?

d. What kinds of symptoms might be expected with disorders at various levels of the gastrointestinal system?

e. How do the various disorders of the gastrointestinal system affect the nutritional status of the individual?

f. How is the gastrointestinal system, and each of its component parts, controlled?

g. What are the common surgical procedures that are performed at each level of the tract? What problems does the patient face in adjusting to the changes in function created by each of these procedures?

h. What lay workers are very helpful, if not essential, in meeting the needs of the patient with an "ostomy"? Where would you find such a worker in your local community? Where would you refer a patient? Where can patients in your community secure equipment to use with an "ostomy"?

i. What diagnostic tests are used for gastrointestinal disorders? What are the nursing responsibilities for each? What preparation does the patient need for each? What follow-up care?

j. What are the various dietary modifications that are ordered for patients with diseases of the gastrointestinal tract? What is the rationale for each? What are the modifications for a patient with an "ostomy"? Why?

k. What is an "acute abdomen"? What observations should a nurse make of this patient? Why?

l. When is hyperalimentation a useful treatment? What are the major nursing responsibilities in relation to this treatment?

8. By the time you have completed this unit, you should be able to do the following:

a. Assess your patient's emotional status as it affects gastrointestinal functioning and attempt to create an environment conducive to ingestion, digestion and/or elimination.

b. Show your understanding of the nursing needs of patients with disorders in various portions of the digestive tract and of the different disease processes which occur in the gut. Show an understanding of both of these variables in your nursing care planning:

(1) Describe the affect disease has on digestive function in each portion of the tract and what nursing measures are appropriate.

(2) Explain the differences and similarities in care required by a person who has a congenital malformation of the tract, an infectious process, an ulcer or perforation, or a malignant lesion at various locations in the gut.

c. Prepare a patient mentally (including teaching) and physically for a diagnostic test to be done on the digestive system (such as endoscopy, x-ray barium studies, and aspiration of secretions) and care for him or her afterwards.

d. Give supportive physical care and make observations of the patient who is undergoing gastrointestinal decompression therapy.

e. Diagram the various surgical interventions commonly performed on various portions of the digestive tract and state the nursing implications for each and the rationale underlying the surgical approach.

f. Recognize symptoms caused by abnormal functioning of the gut and be able to instigate appropriate nursing measures for patient comfort.

g. Be able to care for a patient with a colostomy or ileostomy, understand the method of elimination control being employed, and state what the nurse can do to aid the patient in adjustment to the "ostomy."

h. Teach patients concerning normal and altered physiology of digestion and implications these have for body nutrition and fluid and electrolyte balance and the effects these can have on other body systems.

CHAPTER 58

REVIEW OF THE ANATOMY AND PHYSIOLOGY OF THE DIGESTIVE SYSTEM

The digestive tract, sometimes also called the alimentary canal, is a hollow muscular tube that extends from the mouth to the anus and has as its principal function the provision of the body with fluids, nutrients, and electrolytes. It is lined with secreting cells and glands and has accessory organs, all of which contribute to this function of providing the body with the materials it needs to function. Normally the digestive tract is the only source of intake for the body. Raw materials, taken in through the mouth, after proper chemical conversions are used by the body in all its functions. See Figure 58–1 for the structural arrangement of the tract and the names of the parts. The portion of the tract from the stomach to the anus is the gastrointestinal tract, where the major digestive activity takes place, but this term is often loosely applied to indicate the entire digestive apparatus.

A secondary function of the tract is to dispose of the waste residues from this digestive process. Only wastes from this tract are eliminated from it; wastes from body metabolism are excreted by other routes such as the lungs, kidneys, and skin.

ACTIVITIES OF THE TRACT

The activities of the tract are (1) the secretion of electrolytes, hormones, and enzymes to be used in the breakdown of the materials ingested and (2) the movement of ingested products through at the proper rate to ensure (3) complete digestion of the food and (4) absorption of the end products into the blood stream.

Motility. There are two types of movements in the gastrointestinal tract: mixing and propulsive. These are produced by rhythmic contractions of the smooth muscle fibers which lie in the stomach and gut. These fibers vary somewhat from one segment to another because of their different functions, but they usually consist of an outer longitudinal layer, an inner circular layer, and a thin layer in the deeper portion of the mucosa. See Figure 58–2 for a typical cross-section of the gut. The mixing movements, sometimes called segmentation contractions, consist of rhythmic contractions between individual segments, alternating with contractions occurring at the mid-point of each segment. A propulsive movement, called *peristalsis,* consists of a wave of contraction which moves forward, forcing the contents of the tube ahead of it. This type of movement occurs in all smooth muscle tubes of the body and can go in either direction from the point of stimulation; however, in the bowel the waves usually move toward the anus.

Innervation. Distention of a local segment of the bowel is the usual stimulus for the initiation of a peristaltic wave, but one can also be stimulated by any irritation of the mucosa or by the presence of a specific chemical substance. Nervous stimulation occurs by means of the intramural nerve plexuses, which lie within the layers of the bowel wall beginning at the esophagus. These are known as the myenteric plexus (Auerbach's) in the outer layer and the submucosal plexus (Meissner's) in the inner layer. (See Figure 58–2.) These nerves maintain the continuous tone of the bowel and also stimulate movements.

These plexuses are stimulated by the parasympathetic nervous system, and in general, cause an increase in the tone of the gut, a decrease in the tone of the sphincters, and an increase in the frequency, volume, and velocity of contractions. The cranial division of the parasympathetic nervous system mediates impulses via the vagus nerve to the area from the esophagus to the proximal colon, while the distance from the mid-colon to the anus is controlled by the sacral division. Sympathetic innervation comes via nerve fibers that leave the spinal cord between T–8 and L–3. The nerve impulses then pass through ganglia such as the celiac and mesenteric and spread to all parts of the gut. In general, they reduce peristaltic activity and increase the tone of

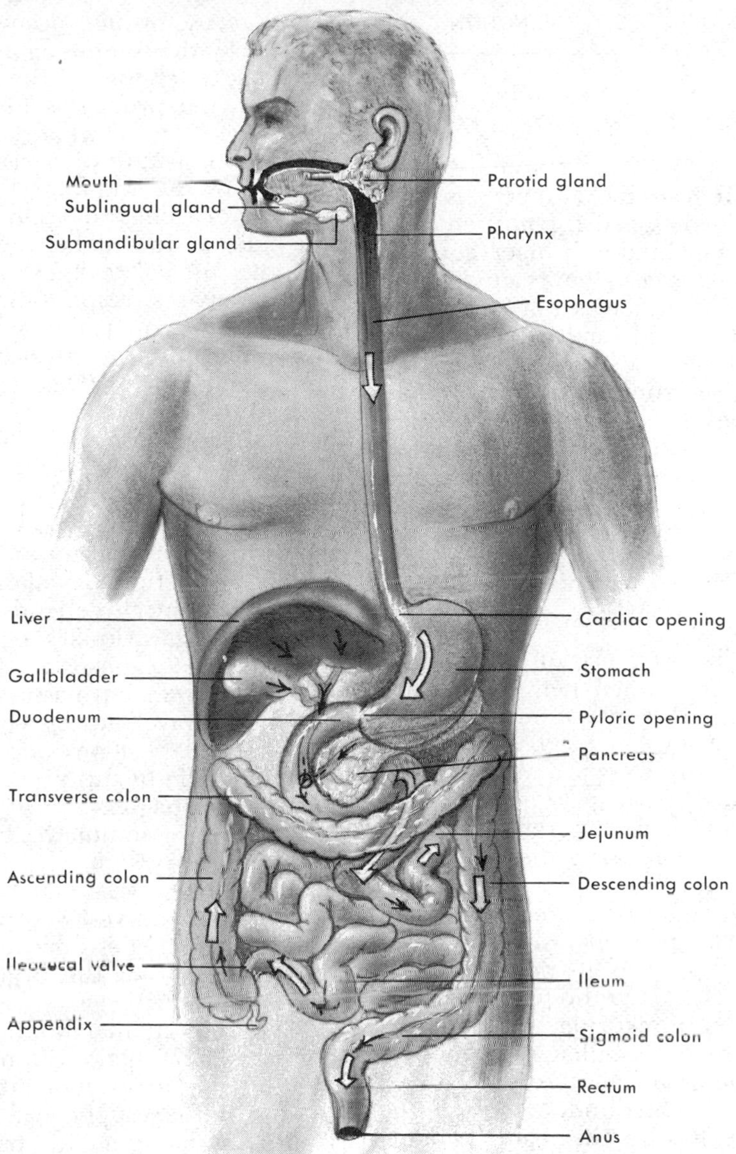

Figure 58–1. The digestive system. (From Dienhart, C. M.: *Basic Human Anatomy and Physiology,* 3rd ed. Philadelphia: W. B. Saunders Co., 1979, p. 184.)

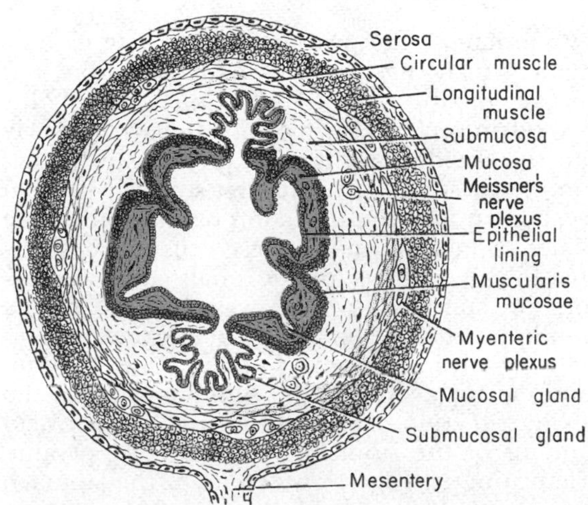

Figure 58–2. Typical cross-section of the gut. (From Guyton, A. C.: *Physiology of the Human Body,* 5th ed. Philadelphia: W. B. Saunders Co., 1979, p. 382.)

sphincters. Sympathetic effects on the bowel are minimal, as denervation has only short-term effects.

Secretions. There are two general types of secretions in the digestive tract: mucous secretions, which are produced from the mouth to the anus, and digestive secretions composed of enzymes and electrolytes, which are produced from the mouth to the end of the ileum. Mucus is produced to protect and to lubricate the walls of the tract and to ease the passage of food and partially digested products. Digestive juices are secreted to break down the various foods for absorption.

Digestion and Absorption. The digestive process is the breaking of food by digestive juices into compounds which are small enough in size and in the right chemical form for absorption. They are absorbed into the blood stream by diffusion and by active transport.

Controls on Ingestion. Hunger is the body's expression of its need for nutrients. In animals and in small infants hunger controls ingestion, but humans also have an appetite which is learned and which is not necessarily related to the body's need for food and fluids. Frequently we eat because we enjoy the taste sensations we derive from eating rather than because our bodies have a hunger for that particular nutrient. Satiety is the feeling we have when our hunger and/or appetite has been satisfied.

THE MOUTH, PHARYNX, AND ESOPHAGUS

The Mouth. The first act of digestion is chewing. This occurs immediately upon entry of food into the mouth and not only prepares the food for swallowing but meets a psychologic need. The teeth, tongue, walls of the cheeks, and palate all participate in this activity, which is controlled by reflex activity through the fifth cranial nerve and is stimulated by the presence of food in the mouth. The functions of chewing are to break the food products into smaller portions; to break down the fibrous coverings so as to provide access for the digestive enzymes to the food particles; and to prevent traumatizing the mucous membrane lining of the esophagus by making the food to be swallowed smoother.

Saliva acts to lubricate and to soften the food mass and to dissolve the readily soluble components of the food, thus stimulating the taste buds and increasing the enjoyment of the food. It contains the enzyme ptyalin (amylase), which acts to hydrolyze starches by splitting off maltase. If allowed to function long enough, amylase will break starches down to maltose.

Maintenance of dental health is important, since pressures ranging from 25 to 275 pounds are exerted during the chewing process, depending upon the nature of the food and the teeth involved. Artificial dentures are not as efficient in chewing as are natural teeth and can contribute to malnutrition, because poorly chewed foods are not so readily utilized in the digestive process.

Swallowing (Deglutition). After a mouthful of food, which is now called a bolus, has been sufficiently chewed, it is swallowed. The quantity in each bolus is approximately 5 ml. and consists of particles 2 mm. in size. The act of deglutition, which consists of three phases, is extremely complex. The first phase, called the *voluntary,* or *oral,* occurs when the food is pressed by the tongue against the palate, forcing it backward toward the pharynx. From this point on the process is involuntary. The second stage of swallowing, called the *pharyngeal,* begins with a wave of peristalsis, which was initiated by the voluntary act and causes a number of things to occur simultaneously. As the bolus is forced between the tonsillar pillars, the soft palate draws upward to close the posterior nares, respirations cease momentarily, the vocal cords approximate, and the larynx pulls upward, covering the vocal cords and stretching the opening of the esophagus. This causes the relaxation of the upper esophageal (hypopharyngeal) sphincter and begins the third (*esophageal*) stage, in which the peristaltic wave forces the bolus down the esophagus by the force of muscle contraction, by the momentum produced, and by the force of gravity. The time it takes for the bolus to reach the stomach depends upon its consistency and the individual's body position. Fluids tend to arrive ahead of the peristaltic wave, and the more solid masses may arrive after it. The bolus travels faster when the individual is in a vertical position. See Figure 58–3 for a representation of this process.

The Esophagus. Peristaltic waves in the esophagus are stimulated by primary and secondary means. Primarily, the act of swallowing activates the waves reflexly through the glossopharyngeal nerves. Secondary stimulation of esophageal peristalsis occurs from dilatation of the lower half of the organ and is probably reflex in origin.

All glands in the esophagus are mucus secreting. The function of mucus is lubrication of the bolus to promote its passage and protection of the esophageal mucous membrane from trauma due to passage of partially chewed food products.

THE STOMACH

Functions. The stomach is a muscular organ which has as its main function the storage, mixing, and liquefaction of the bolus of food into chyme, which it discharges slowly into the duodenum. The main digestive function of the stomach is the first stage of protein breakdown and the digestion of the connective tissues of meat to make these cells more accessible to the enzymes of the small bowel. Digestion of starches, which was begun in the mouth by the action of ptyalin, continues in the stomach in the center of the bolus and can continue for as long as 30 minutes or until the mixing function of the stomach allows the acid contents of the stomach to contact the ptyalin, inactivating it. Digestion of fats in the stomach is minimal and probably limited to butterfats. Other than alcohol, there is very little absorption in the stomach. (See Figure 58–4.)

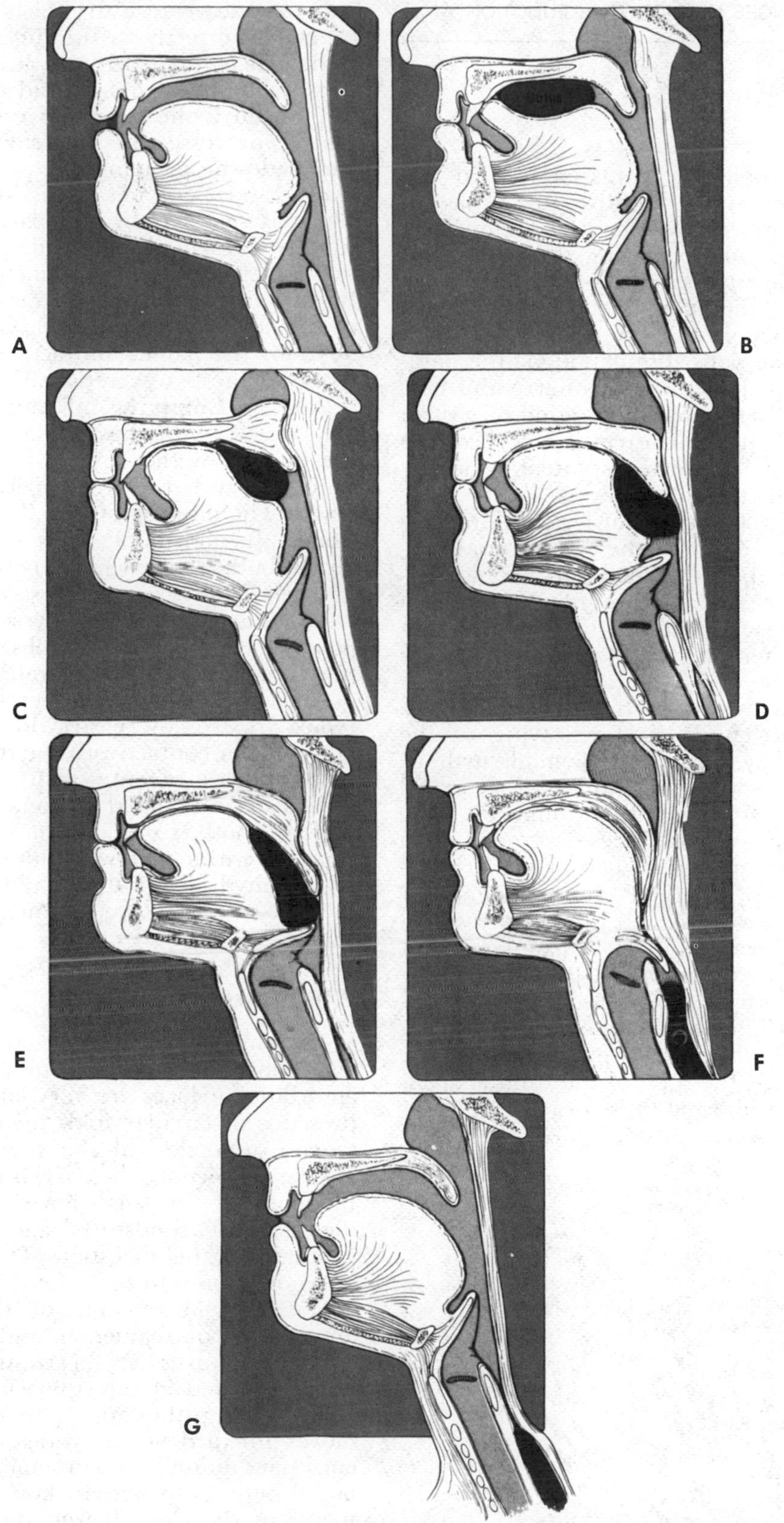

Figure 58–3. The mechanism of swallowing. **A.** Mouth and pharynx at rest. **B.** Early oral phase. **C.** Late oral phase. **D.** Early pharyngeal phase. **E.** Middle pharyngeal phase. **F.** Late pharyngeal phase. **G.** Esophageal phase. (From Dobie, R. A.: Rehabilitation of swallowing disorders. *American Family Physician*, 17:86, May 1978.)

Activity. When the bolus arrives in the stomach, secretion of digestive juices has already begun in response to the stimulus of smelling, tasting, and chewing the food. This is known as the *cephalic* stage of digestion. The *gastric* stage of digestion is stimulated by the presence of food in the stomach and is regulated both by nervous stimulation via the parasympathetic fibers of the vagus nerve and hormonal stimulation through secretion of gastrin by the gastric mucosa. Gastrin is absorbed into the blood stream and then stimulates motility and secretion by the stomach.

The stomach empties slowly, accommodating itself to the ability of the duodenum to receive and act upon the materials. Tonic contraction of the musculature of the stomach causes the pressure within it to remain almost constant whether it is empty or full. This is accomplished by expansion and contraction of the fundus as the stomach fills and empties. Mixing of the chyme and emptying of the stomach occur by means of slow mild rhythmic peristaltic waves which begin about every 20 seconds at the fundus and continue over the antrum to the pylorus. These waves gain in strength as they progress, becoming very vigorous at the pylorus. A few milliliters of chyme are forced through the pylorus with each peristaltic wave and the remainder is propelled back into the stomach, further mixing the mass. The rugae of the walls of the stomach also contribute to the mixing by digging deeply into the chyme with each wave. As the stomach empties, the tone of the fundus maintains a constant internal pressure.

Secretions. About 3000 ml. of gastric juices are secreted every 24 hours. Those that contribute directly to the digestive process include mucus, hydrochloric acid (HCl), pepsin, small amounts of lipase, and the intrinsic factor. Pepsin is the most active factor in the digestive processes of the stomach, acting to break down proteins to polypeptides, proteoses, and peptones. The hydrochloric acid which is secreted by the parietal cells in the fundus is essential to provide the acid medium that is necessary for the function of pepsin. It is secreted in response to vagal impulses, gastrin, and histamine. (See Tables 58–1 and 58–2 for the names and actions of the various types of digestive secretions.)

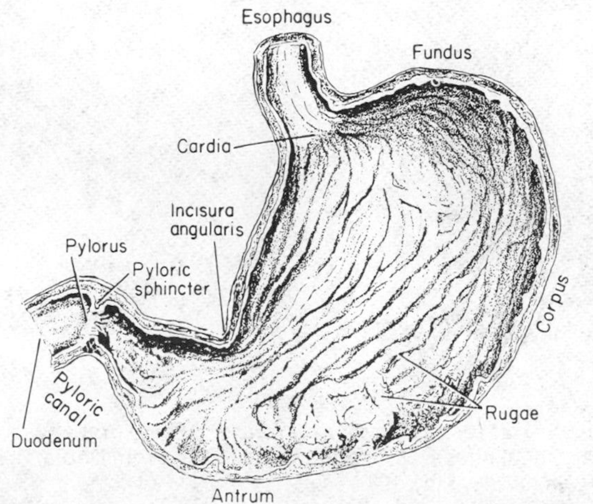

Figure 58–4. Physiologic anatomy of the stomach. (From Guyton, A. C.: *Physiology of the Human Body,* 5th ed. 1979, p. 384.)

Rate of Emptying. Factors that influence the rate of emptying of the stomach include: the fluidity of the chyme, the amount in the stomach, and the receptivity of the small bowel. The enterogastric reflex and enterogastrone, the hormone secreted by the small bowel, both act to inhibit the empyting of the stomach. Practically any stimulation of the duodenum — distention, presence of acid, hypotonic or hypertonic substances, and the presence of any carbohydrate, fat, or protein product — will cause the enterogastric vagus reflex arc to slow gastric motility and secretions. Fat in contact with the duodenal mucosa causes release of enterogastrone, which is absorbed into the blood stream and causes inhibition of both secretions and motility of the stomach within a few minutes. The presence of carbohydrates in the small bowel also causes the release of enterogastrone, but to a lesser extent.

THE SMALL BOWEL

The small bowel is only about 10 feet long and 1 inch in diameter, but the secreting and absorbing surfaces are very large owing to the presence of circular folds involving the mucosa and a portion of the submucosa and fingerlike projections called villi (Fig. 58–5). The functions of the small bowel are to complete digestion of foodstuffs and to absorb the products of this digestion. The waste residues are moved on into the colon.

Motility. Movements of the small bowel are mixing, or segmental, and peristaltic. The peristaltic waves are a continuation of the waves initiated in the stomach and propel the chyme along the gut. The chyme normally moves forward at an average rate of about 1 cm. per minute and remains in the small bowel between 3 and 10 hours. Mixing movements of the small bowel consist of the alternate contraction of circular muscle fibers. These mixing movements, in addition to mixing the chyme, also bring it into closer contact with the glands and juices for better digestion and into closer contact with the villi for absorption.

TABLE 58–1. DIGESTIVE HORMONES

Hormone	Source	Inhibition Factors	Stimulating Factors	Action
Gastrin	G cells of gastric antrum; duodenal mucosa	Acid in stomach	Distention of stomach by food; presence of products of protein digestion; vagal stimulation; elevated blood levels of calcium and epinephrine.	Stimulates secretion of HCl and pepsin; growth of gastric mucosa; relaxes ileocecal sphincter.
Enterogastrone	Intestinal mucosa		Fats, sugar and acid in small intestine.	Inhibits gastric acid secretion and mobility.
Secretin	Duodenal mucosa	Lack of stimulation	Acid gastric contents entering duodenum.	Stimulates secretion of watery alkaline pancreatic fluid. Augments CCK. Decreases gastric acid secretion. Stimulates secretion of pancreatic digestive enzymes.
Cholecystokinin (CCK)	Duodenal mucosa	Lack of stimulation	Products of protein and fat digestion in duodenum.	Augments secretin in stimulating secretion of alkaline pancreatic juice and digestive enzymes. Stimulates gall bladder contraction. Inhibits gastric emptying. Stimulates pepsin secretion. May weakly and selectively stimulate gastric acid secretion. Stimulates motility of small bowel.
GIP (Gastric inhibitory peptide)	Duodenal and jejunal mucosa		Presence of glucose and fat in duodenum. Not affected by acid.	Inhibits gastric acid secretion and motility. Stimulates secretion of intestinal juice and insulin.
VIP (Vasoactive intestinal peptide)	Intestinal mucosa		None reported as yet.	Stimulates insulin release. Intestinal secretion of electrolytes and water. Inhibits gastric acid secretion. Dilates peripheral blood vessels and lowers blood pressure.
Motilin	Duodenal mucosa			Diminishes speed of gastric emptying and stimulates gastric acid secretion and pepsin.
Substance P	Neurons of brain; gastrointestinal tract			Increases motility of small bowel.
Bombesin	Gastrointestinal tract(?)			Increases gastrin secretion and motility of small bowel.
Somatosin	Hypothalamus Gastrointestinal tract(?)			Inhibits secretion of gastrin, VIP, GIP, secretin, and motilin.

A *peristaltic rush* is a powerful peristaltic wave which begins in the duodenum and passes to the ileocecal valve in a few minutes. Its purpose is to relieve the intestine of an irritating substance. It can be caused by any intense chemical or mechanical irritation or by extreme distention.

Digestive Activity. Digestive secretions of

TABLE 58–2. DIGESTIVE ENZYMES

Enzyme	Source	Action and Products
		Carbohydrates
Ptyalin (salivary amylase)	Parotid and submaxillary glands	Breaks starch into maltose, maltotriose , limit dextrins (Polysaccharides into disaccharides)
Pancreatic amylase (more potent than ptyalin)	Pancreas	
Maltase*	Intestinal mucosa	Breaks maltose and maltoriose into glucose
Dextrinase	Intestinal mucosa	Breaks alpha limit dextrins into glucose
Lactase*	Intestinal mucosa	Breaks lactose into galactose and glucose
Sucrase*	Intestinal mucosa	Breaks sucrose into glucose and fructose
		Proteins
Pepsin I, II, III	Chief cells of gastric mucosa	Breaks dietary proteins into polypeptides of various sizes
Enterokinase	Duodenal mucosa	Activates trypsin
Trypsin	Pancreas	Splits polypeptide chains
Peptidases* (several)	Intestinal glands	Splits polypeptides into amino acids
		Fats
Gastric lipase (tributyrase)	Gastric mucosa	Digests butterfat
Pancreatic lipase	Pancreas	Splits emulsified fats into monoglycerides
Intestinal lipase*	Intestines	Splits neutral fats into glycerol and fatty acids

*Secreted mainly in the brush border of the epithelial cells; digest the food substances on the outside surfaces of the microvilli before or during absorption through the epithelium.

the small bowel are numerous and each has a specific function (Table 58–1). The small bowel also secretes several hormones that enter the blood stream and stimulate the pancreas to release its digestive secretions (Table 58–2). When the digestive functions are completed and the end products are ready for absorption, the following transformations have occurred:

Carbohydrates changed to: monosaccharides, disaccharides (few)

Proteins changed to: amino acids, dipeptides (minute quantity)

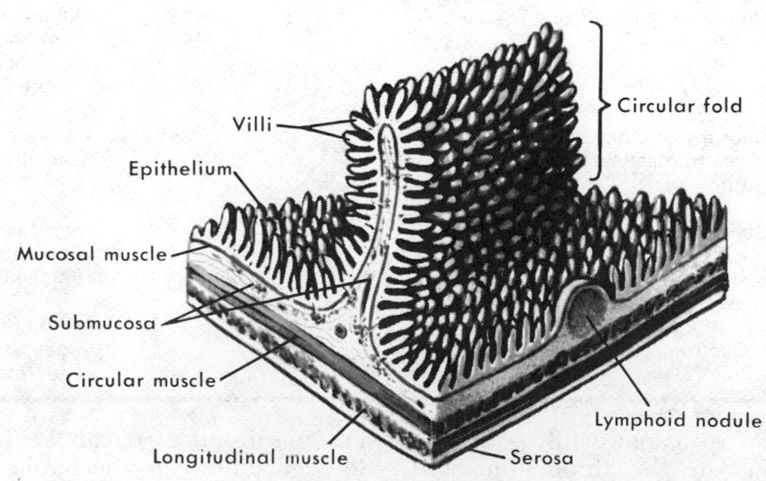

Figure 58–5. Section of wall of small intestine. (From Dienhart, C. M.: *Basic Human Anatomy and Physiology,* 3rd ed. 1979, p. 192.)

Fats changed to: fatty acids, monoglycerides, diglycerides, and triglycerides (few)

These products are absorbed along with water and electrolytes by diffusion and by active transport. Carbohydrates and proteins are absorbed by active transport along with sodium in a mutually dependent relationship in which neither material is transported without the other. The active transport of carbohydrates and amino acids is called a secondary type of active transport. Fatty acids are absorbed by diffusion, whereas most of the electrolytes are absorbed actively. Water diffuses by osmosis as a result of these other transport systems.

Digestion and absorption from the small bowel is very efficient. The chyme obtained from the terminal ileum contains no digestible carbohydrates, very few lipids, and only 15 to 17 per cent nitrogen-containing substances, most of which are bacterial or desquamated epithelial cells and the remains of digestive secretions.[172]

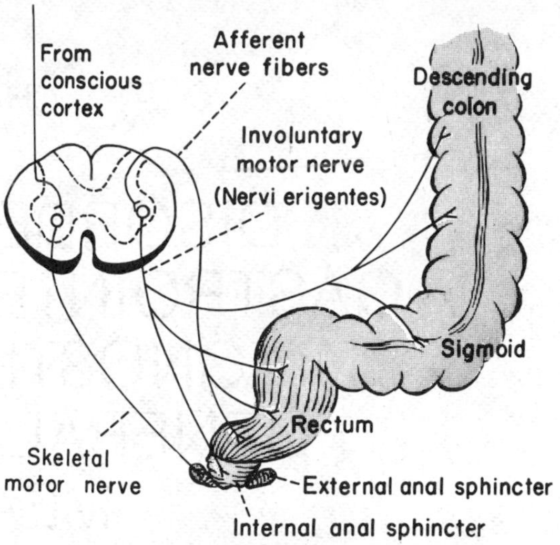

Figure 58–6. The afferent and efferent pathways of the parasympathetic mechanism for the defecation reflex. (From Guyton, A. C.: *Physiology of the Human Body,* 5th ed. 1979, p. 387.)

THE COLON, RECTUM, AND ANUS

The major function of the colon is absorption of water and electrolytes in the proximal half and storage of the feces in the distal half until defecation occurs. Anatomically the colon is larger in diameter than the small bowel and does not contain villi. The only significant secretion is mucus, and the cells are columnar absorbing cells and goblet cells.

Motility. The movements are, as in the small bowel, mixing and propulsive. The mixing movements, sometimes called haustral contractions, facilitate absorption by exposing all the fecal matter to the mucosal surfaces. The propulsive movements or mass movements occur three or four times a day and are initiated by distention of the colon walls and by the gastrocolic or duodenocolic reflex. These reflexes are strongest after the first meal of the day.

Secretion. The mucous secretion of the large intestine can be stimulated by the parasympathetic nerves but occurs mainly through tactile stimulation. It protects the bowel wall against excoriation from the fecal mass and from bacterial activity, and its alkalinity helps to counteract the effects of acid formation from this bacterial action. This is also aided by small amounts of actively secreted bicarbonate. The mucus has adherent qualities which aid in the production of a formed fecal mass.

Absorption. Absorption of sodium, chloride, and water occurs in the large bowel and reduces the volume of chyme from 500 ml. in the cecum to 100 ml. of fluid in the feces. The colon is capable of absorbing 90 per cent of the sodium and water presented to it.

Bacterial Action. Bacterial action in the large bowel causes the formation of gases, which provide bulk and help to propel the feces. These organisms also synthesize some important nutritional factors such as vitamin K, thiamin, riboflavin, vitamin B_{12}, folic acid, biotin, and nicotinic acid. Until recently it was thought that these were absorbed, but experiments have shown that only folic acid is absorbed in significant amounts.[74]

Defecation. Feces are three fourths water and one fourth solid matter. The organic constituents include undigested food residues, digestive secretions and enzymes, dead cells, bile pigments, and mucus. Thirty per cent of the mass consists of bacteria and another 30 per cent is fat. The nature of the diet does not change the contents of the stool except for the amount of cellulose present.

The defecation reflex is stimulated by distention of the rectum. (See Figure 58–6 for the neurological pathways of this reflex.) This occurs when feces and gas are propelled into the rectum from the descending colon during a mass peristaltic movement. This distention sets the defecation reflex in motion as the pressure within the rectum rises and the internal and external sphincters are relaxed. The individual may voluntarily suppress this defecation urge by contracting the striated muscles of the pelvic floor and the external sphincter. This slows the motility of the bowel. If the individual elects to defecate when the reflex is set in motion, he or she augments pressure within the colon by increasing the intra-abdominal pressure. This is done by lowering the diaphragm and contracting the abdominal muscles. The diaphragm is lowered by contracting the chest muscles on an inflated lung while the glottis is closed.

CHAPTER 59

DISORDERS OF THE GASTROINTESTINAL TRACT: DIAGNOSTIC TESTS AND GENERAL TREATMENT MEASURES

The major function of the gastrointestinal tract is the digestion and absorption of nutrients needed by the body for proper functioning. To accomplish this, the tract carries these nutrients along at a rate consistent with proper digestion and absorption. The mucous membrane lining, the glands which lie within it, and the accessory organs secrete digestive juices and enzymes which act chemically upon the foods and liquids to digest them. After this has taken place, the end products are absorbed into the blood stream and taken to the liver and other portions of the body for storage and use.

Abnormalities and disease conditions that occur in this tract manifest themselves through interference with one or more of these functions. The disease conditions may interrupt the continuity of the muscular or mucous layers, harm the tissues of the tract by damage to the blood or nerve supply, interfere with the flow of chyme through the tract, or hamper digestion of the material while it is in the gut. Abnormalities can be of mechanical, infectious, traumatic, neoplastic, vascular, nervous, or emotional origin.

COMMON CAUSES OF DYSFUNCTION OF THE GASTROINTESTINAL TRACT

Obstruction to Flow of Chyme

Motility of the gut can be stopped, slowed, or increased by an abnormality of the nervous system regulatory mechanism, and it can be interrupted by interference with the blood supply to the gut. Nervous system abnormalities usually result from some general toxic or traumatic condition. Interruption of the central nervous system, as by transection of the spinal cord, does not interfere with peristalsis, since that is mainly regulated by the intramural plexuses (Auerbach's and Meissner's).

Blood supply is necessary to a viable tissue and is essential to the health of the organ. Any local interruption of blood supply is an emergency.

Tumors. Neoplasms may be either intra- or extraluminal. Since the chyme is liquid except at the terminal end of the colon, a tumor must be relatively large to interfere with its flow through the tract. Total obstruction of gastrointestinal flow is a late symptom of tumor growth. Both benign and malignant tumors can cause such an interruption. Malignant tumors also cause other problems, since they invade the tissues and metastasize.

Loss of Structural Integrity. There are both developmental and acquired conditions that interfere with the structure of the bowel enough to impede flow through the tract. *Strictures* occur in the esophagus as a result of trauma, especially from drinking extremely hot foods or caustic substances. Strictures also occur in the lower tract, but here they are more often the result of healing of scars from ulcerations or surgical procedures. Bands of *adhesions* (scar tissue) from surgical operations sometimes cause constriction of the lumen when they encircle a loop of bowel. This is a common cause of bowel obstruction.

A *herniation* (protrusion through an abnormal opening) can occur in many portions of the tract. As the gut squeezes out through the internal or external opening, there is apt to be interference with the flow within it or with the blood supply to the herniated segment. The more common types of hernias are hiatus, inguinal, femoral, umbilical, and incisional. They are named by the location of the herniated portion.

The gastrointestinal tract has two structural deformities that occur within its wall; one is an outpouching, and the other an invagination (Fig. 59–1). The outpouching, called a *diverticulum,* may involve all layers of the bowel wall but usually occurs through a weakness in the muscular layer. These occur more commonly as the individual ages, since the muscle fibers gradually lose their tone. A *polyp,* or inward growth, involves the inner mucosal layers of the bowel wall. These may be large or small, single or multiple. Polyps are particularly dangerous in the bowel, as they tend to become malignant. A large polyp can obstruct the lumen of the bowel by occupying space; it can also become twisted on its pedicle and strangulate.

Trauma. Any type of trauma may occur — from blunt blows or knife and stab wounds to gunshot perforations. Trauma is apt to cause bleeding or contusions and may open the bowel lumen. Since bowel secretions contain digestive enzymes, they are very irritating to the peritoneal cavity. The bowel also contains bacteria, so whenever the lumen of the bowel is opened to the peritoneal cavity, there is danger of infection. A physical insult, the presence of chemical or infectious agents, or their sequelae, are apt to cause cessation of bowel motility.

Infections. Bacteria are normally present in the lumen of the bowel, and since all food is potentially contaminated, foreign organisms can be ingested. Most of these organisms are destroyed in the highly acid medium of the stomach, but some may survive and, if pathogenic, cause disease. Worms of many kinds, amoeba, and other parasites are commonly acquired when tourists visit certain tropical countries.

Toxins released from some bacteria, such as those which cause staphylococcal food poisoning, are very irritating to the lower tract. This type of condition usually causes diarrhea and vomiting in the body's effort to remove the offending substance. The major problem in these conditions is electrolyte balance, since digestive juices are not resorbed completely because of the increased rate of passage.

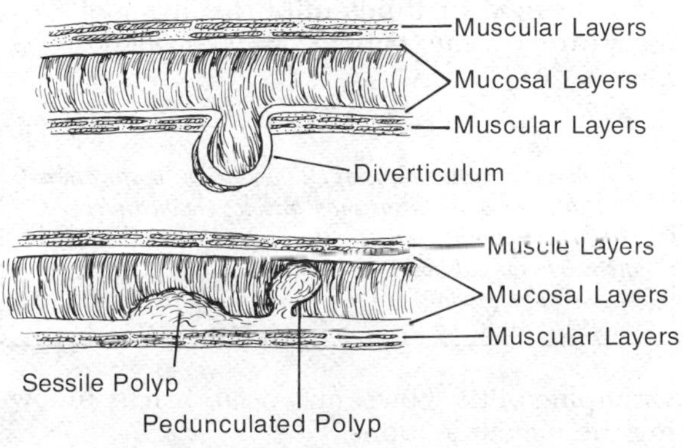

Figure 59–1. Diverticulum vs. polyp.

Interference with Digestive Function

Mechanical. Whenever the forward progress of chyme through the bowel is stopped, a chain of events is set in motion. Peristalsis usually increases in intensity and rate in an effort to overcome the obstruction. Pressure within the lumen of the bowel increases as gases and fluids begin to accumulate. Increased pressure within the lumen of the bowel causes the secretory function of the small bowel to increase without an increase in the absorptive process; thus, the problem is rapidly compounded. The patient can go into shock as a result of these fluid shifts.

Secretory Dysfunction. Inadequate or excessive amounts of some of the digestive juices will cause interruption in the digestive function, especially if the pH level is altered, since the acidity of the environment must be within very narrow limits for most of these enzymes to function. Diagnosis of the cause of these problems can be quite difficult. Tests are made of the levels of various substances in varied portions of the bowel and symptoms are considered.

An increase in the acidity of the stomach and duodenum is probably the main reason for the development of peptic ulcers. Excessive amounts of digestive juices can digest the mucosa because they overpower the normal protective mucous layer.

DIAGNOSTIC MEASURES

Since disease can occur any place in the gastrointestinal tract, diagnostic measures attempt to locate the level of the problem and identify the nature of the abnormality. The general methods of diagnosis are x-ray studies, endoscopy (viewing the inside through a lighted tube), analysis of the secretions from various parts of the tract, biopsies, cytologic studies, and radionuclide uptake tests.

X-rays

Since x-rays show shadows of the relative densities of the structures photographed, the inside of the gastrointestinal contract (GI) tract cannot be visualized unless a contrast medium is ingested or instilled into it. A flate plate (x-ray taken without contrast media) will show only general shadows, fluid levels, and gas. The usual terms given for x-ray studies of the gastrointestinal tract are: upper GI or barium meal, and lower

GI or barium enema. The two together are known as a GI series.

Upper GI. In an upper GI study, the patient drinks barium sulfate, which is a white chalky, radiopaque substance. It is frequently flavored to make it more palatable. As the patient swallows the substance, the swallowing mechanism is studied by fluoroscope to detect the presence of abnormalities. Pictures are taken as the barium passes through the esophagus to show structural and/or functional problems. In the stomach the barium outlines the walls and shows the presence of ulcer craters and filling defects that could be caused by tumors. The emptying time of the stomach is observed. Barium is usually followed through the small bowel with x-rays to determine its rate of passage and to look for structural abnormalities.

Lower GI. The large colon is studied with barium given per rectum. Sufficient barium is given to distend the bowel and show any abnormality in structure or a space-occupying tumor mass. Follow-up pictures are taken after the patient eliminates the barium to determine the efficiency of emptying the colon.

Preparation of the Patient. Preparation of patients for a gastrointestinal x-ray study includes explaining the procedure to them so they will understand what is happening and what the physician hopes to learn from the test. The upper GI or barium meal must be done on an empty stomach, so food and fluids are withheld for several hours. Since barium becomes solid when moisture is absorbed from it, a laxative is given following the test to empty the large bowel before a barium impaction can form. The normal diet is resumed after the x-ray study if there are no contraindications to it.

Enemas must be given before a lower GI study to empty the bowel of all feces. Any retained fecal matter will cause a filling defect to show on the x-ray and confuse the diagnosis. Since fecal matter is constantly entering the right colon from the cecum, the small bowel is emptied too, usually by means of a purgative such as castor oil, which is given the night before the test. Sometimes the patient is given only liquids the day or night before the test. Unless the bowel has been completely emptied by giving the individual no solid food for 24 hours, breakfast can usually be eaten the morning of the x-ray because the procedure will be completed before the food reaches the large bowel. Following the procedure, a cleansing enema is given if the follow-up x-ray shows retained barium.

Endoscopy

Endoscopy is the visualization of the inside of a body cavity by means of a lighted tube. The most common endoscopic examination of the digestive tract is done with a 25 cm. long, lighted, rigid tube — a sigmoidoscope — which is inserted through the anus to visually inspect the sigmoid colon. Today most examinations of the upper tract and the more extensive ones of the lower tract are performed with a flexible scope. Flexibility is achieved in these scopes by utilizing glass fibers in the lens systems. The esophagus, the stomach, and sometimes the duodenum are visualized by means of a tube inserted through the mouth, whereas a tube inserted through the anus can be maneuvered past the sigmoid colon into the left, transverse, and frequently even into the right colon. The scopes are equipped in various ways. Some are equipped with a camera to enable the physician to obtain color photographs which can be studied after the examination. Others have equipment for performing a biopsy (Fig. 75–2), removing a polyp, or securing cells for cytologic examination. Many single polyps of the bowel are removed during colonoscopy, thus avoiding a surgical approach.

Nursing Responsibilities. Better visualization of these cavities is possible when they are empty. Because of this and because of the danger of aspiration, the patient who has a gastroscopy usually fasts several hours before the examination. When the entire large bowel is examined, a clear liquid diet is given 24 hours before the test, followed by either a cathartic given orally the night before or a cleansing enema given the morning of the test, or both. Since the rectosigmoid is empty immediately after defecation, a suppository may be ordered prior to sigmoidoscopy to stimulate defecation.

Many patients find the intrusive entry of the gastrointestinal system by a lighted tube a traumatic experience. The musculature of the tract tends to react with spasms, causing the patient crampy pain; it is uncomfortable to swallow a tube and embarrasing to have the rectum entered. Thus, the patient who is undergoing these examinations needs understanding support from the nurse and clear explanations of what to expect and why the test is being performed.

The patient who has had a gastroscopy usually receives a local anesthetic to the posterior pharynx to ease discomfort from the introduction of the tube; following the examination, offer no food or fluids until this has warn off. (See care of the patient after bronchoscopy, Unit XVI.)

> *The major complications of endoscopy are perforation and hemorrhage. Signs may develop immediately or over a period of hours after the examination; therefore the nurse should observe the patient carefully for any hemorrhage, abdominal distention, or pain.*

Cramping of the bowel may occur briefly following these examinations.

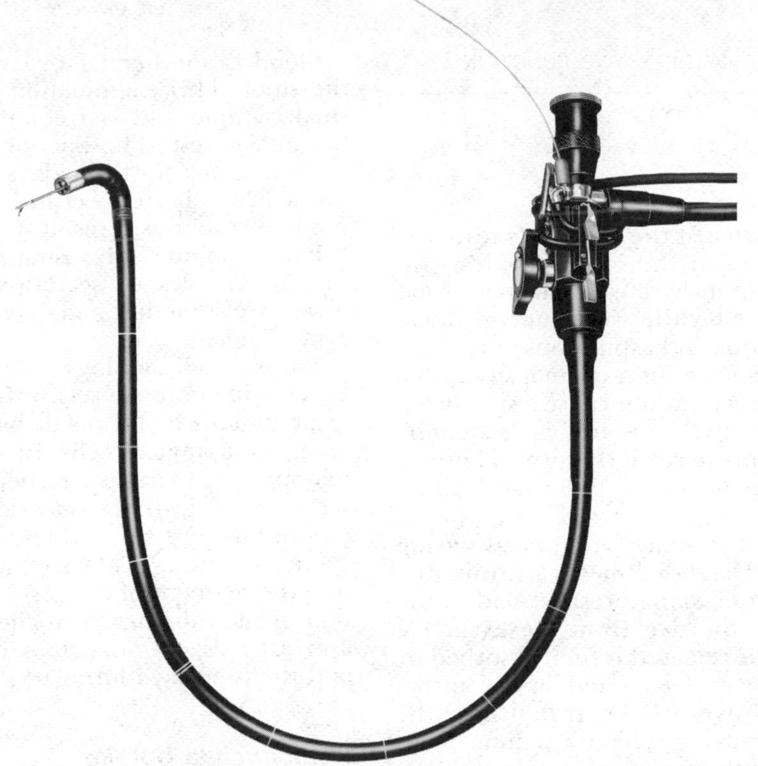

Figure 59–2. Fiberscope for gastric examination. (Courtesy of American Cystoscope Makers, Inc.)

Analysis of Secretions

Analysis can be made of the contents of the gastrointestinal tract for the presence or absence of digestive juices, bacteria, or parasites. Secretions can be secured at the time of endoscopy examination or, as is more common, by the insertion of a tube into the stomach or small bowel. Stool specimens and rectal aspirations are also used for analysis.

Gastric Analysis. The contents of the fasting stomach are aspirated and analyzed for free and total acid. If none is found, some means of stimulating the stomach may be used, such as a meal of crackers or bread (Ewald meal), ingestion of alcohol or caffeine, or the injection of histamine. Aspirations are made through a stomach tube at intervals after the injection of the stimulus. Gastric acidity is typically high in the presence of duodenal ulcers and low when the patient has pernicious anemia.

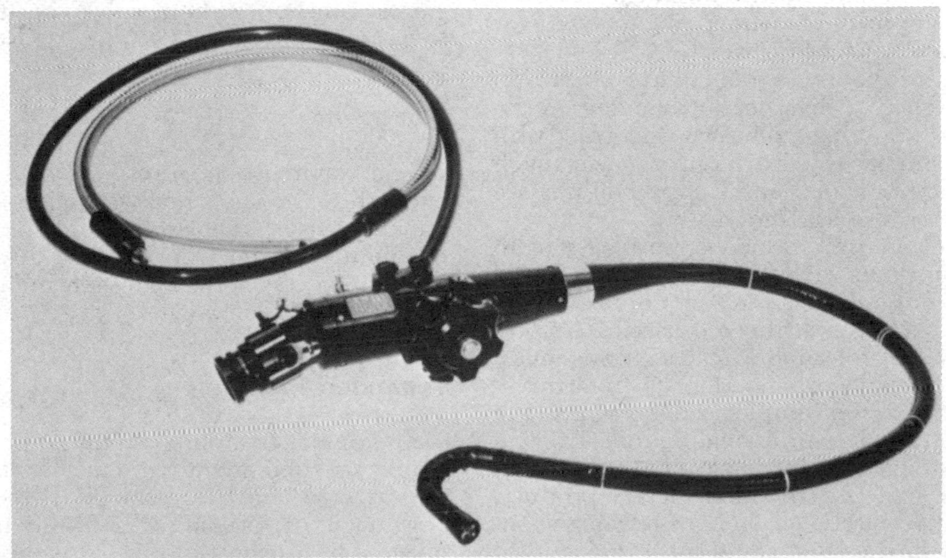

Figure 59–3. Sixty-five centimeter flexible fiberoptic pansigmoidoscope. (From Holt, R. W., and D. C. Wherry: Why flexible fiberoptic sigmoidoscopy is important in the geriatric patient. *Geriatrics*, 34:85, May 1979.)

Insulin is given to test the stomach's response to vagal stimulation in the Hollander test. Insulin given intravenously causes a drop in blood sugar which stimulates the vagus nerve. Blood sugar determinations and aspirations of the gastric secretions are done. In a normal stomach a drop in blood sugar does not cause a significant rise in gastric acidity. This test is frequently done after vagotomy to see if the surgical procedure was successful in reducing the vagal stimulation of gastric acidity.

The tubeless gastric analysis is done by having the patient ingest Diagnex Blue or azuresin (the dye azure A in an exchange resin). Acid in the stomach displaces the dye from the exchange resin. The dye thus released is then absorbed by the bowel mucosa and excreted in the urine. The amount of dye excreted indicates the amount of acid available. The test is done on an empty stomach and consists of having the patient empty the bladder and ingest an agent that stimulates gastric acid and the dye. At the end of the test, the bladder is emptied again and the urine tested for the dye. The total quantity of dye excreted in this time period is analyzed and an estimation made of the amount of acid in the stomach.

Tubercle bacilli may be present in the stomach of a person with active pulmonary tuberculosis because mucous secretions from the lungs are normally carried by ciliary action to the pharynx where they are propelled to the stomach. Therefore, gastric washings are sometimes taken of patients who do not raise sputum and in whom a diagnosis of pulmonary tuberculosis is difficult to obtain. Gastric washings are taken the first thing in the morning and analyzed for the presence of acid-fast bacilli.

Analysis of Stools. Stool cultures are taken in the presence of diarrhea or dysentery. Various parasites ranging from the microscopic protozoa and amebae to fairly large organisms such as worms are possible causes. Stool cultures are also done for bacteria and viruses.

The stool culture specimen must be sent to the laboratory for examination while it is still warm. Since these organisms are not necessarily passed in every stool, three consecutive stools are usually sent for analysis. Stools for chemical analysis are usually examined for the total quantity expelled, so the complete stool is sent to the laboratory rather than a small sample from it. Analysis for fat content is frequently made, as well as for some of the other dietary products and digestive secretions. An unusually high content of fat in the stool could mean inadequate absorption from the small bowel.

Blood is another factor commonly sought in the stool. This examination is done on a very small sample and is frequently performed by the guaiac test. The patient is sometimes on a meat-free diet for three days before these specimens are collected because of potential false positive results as a result of meat ingestion.

Examination of Small Bowel Secretions. Samples of secretions from the small bowel are sometimes analyzed for digestive enzymes and for bile.

Biopsy and Cytology. Specimens for cellular examination are secured during endoscopy examinations by means of biopsy forceps or by taking scrapings of cells. In addition, by means of a special apparatus attached to rubber or plastic nasogastric tubes, gastric and small bowel biopsies may be secured and washings done for cytologic studies. A nasogastric tube is passed into the segment of interest and, when the location of the tube has been checked by x-ray, the apparatus is operated to secure the specimen and the tube is withdrawn.

Radionuclide Uptake

The uptake of substances such as vitamin B_{12} (Schiller test), fat, and several protein molecules is sometimes studied by tagging the substances with a radioactive isotope (radionuclide) to assess the degree of absorption of these factors.

The radioisotope $^{99}Tc^{m}$, which has a half-life of 6 hours and emits gamma rays, has recently been used as a noninvasive method to estimate the acid secretory ability of the stomach. The amount of $C1^{-}$ secreted by the stomach is a good indicator of the acid or H^{+} secretory ability. Since the stomach handles $^{99}Tc^{m}$ in the same manner as $C1^{-}$, the administration of this tagged substance can give a good indication of gastric function without subjecting the patient to gastric aspiration.

Ultrasound

The major use of ultrasound as a diagnostic aid in the gastrointestinal system is to outline the pancreas, liver, gallbladder, and spleen. It also distinguishes fluid from adipose tissue and will show an abscess of the abdomen and the volume of fluid present in ascites.

Computed Tomography

Abdominal Computed Tomography (ACT) is mainly useful in identifying masses such as neoplasms, cysts, and abscesses. ACT does have the advantage of providing a three-dimensional image, but for most disorders of the gut, other diagnostic procedures are more helpful.

Blood Examinations

Analysis of the blood through hematologic studies and electrolyte determinations gives information concerning the general status of the patient.

Nursing Responsibilities for Specimen Collection

The nurse must know what specimen is to be collected and in what manner. You must know whether the whole specimen or only part of it is to be sent to the laboratory and whether it must be sent immediately (as a warm stool) or if it should be kept in the refrigerator. You should know the purpose for any specimen sent to the laboratory and collect it accordingly. You should also make sure that the patient understands what is being collected, how, when, and why, so he or she can cooperate with the test. The nursing assistants must also understand how the specimen is to be collected and when. A specimen that is inadvertently discarded or improperly collected usually makes it necessary for the patient to undergo the entire test a second time, necessitating extended hospitalization, increased cost and delay in starting treatment.

TREATMENT MEASURES

Decompression

Decompression is the removal of fluid and air from the gastrointestinal tract via a nasogastric tube attached to suction. Since any obstruction to the flow of chyme through the bowel causes many problems in homeostasis, patients with potential problems are frequently intubated, as well as those who have already developed symptoms of obstruction. Decompression may be used preoperatively and is almost universally used in the postoperative patient who has had surgery on the gastrointestinal tract.

Purpose. The purpose of decompression is to relieve the pressure caused by intestinal contents and gases that remain in the bowel because of some obstruction; it can also be used in diagnosis. Postoperatively, it is used to remove secretions that cannot pass because of swelling and edema in the area of surgery.

Types of Tubes. There are two types of tubes used to achieve decompression. Short tubes are used for the stomach and duodenum and long tubes for the remainder of the tract. Short tubes are the Levin and the Rehfuss, both rubber, and the newer plastic nasogastric tubes. These tubes are long enough to extend into the stomach but not into the bowel. The Rehfuss tube is sometimes threaded just through the pylorus to aspirate duodenal contents.

The long tubes are intended to extend the length or a portion of the length of the small bowel, so are between 6 and 10 ft. long. The more common ones are the Miller-Abbott, Cantor, and Harris (Table 59–1 and Figure 59–4). These tubes all have one thing in common, namely, some means of attaching a heavy substance, usually mercury, to allow peristalsis of the bowel to propel the tube through the tract. The tube is threaded from the nose into the stomach and then through the pylorus, where peristaltic activity of the bowel carries it to the desired area.

Sometimes it is quite difficult to get the tube to pass through the pylorus. The patient is instructed to lie on his or her right side. The physician may guide the tube through the pylorus under fluoroscopic visualization. Once the tube has passed into the duodenum, it is advanced an additional 2 to 4 inches every hour or half hour (as ordered by the physician) to give it slack so peristalsis can carry it along. When it has reached the desired location, it is taped securely into place to prevent further advancement.

Suction. Only low pressure suction is used, because excessive negative pressure within the stomach or bowel might cause the mucosa to be sucked into the openings on the tube, impairing the effectiveness of the suction. Intermittent electrical suction is commonly used. Since mucus tends to plug the openings of these

TABLE 59–1. GASTRIC AND INTESTINAL TUBES

	Length	Size (French)	Lumen	Other Characteristics
Short Tubes				
Levin type (plastic or rubber)	125 cm. (50″)	12, 16, 18	Single	
Rehfuss	120 cm (48″)	12, 14	Single	Metal tip
Salem sump	120 cm. (48″)	12, 14, 16, 18	Double	Sump type suction
	90 cm. (36″)	10		
Long Tubes				
Cantor	300 cm. (10′)	16	Single	Mercury-weighted
Harris	180 cm. (6′)	14, 16	Single	Mercury-weighted
Miller-Abbott	300 cm. (10′)	12, 14, 16, 18	Double	Mercury-weighted

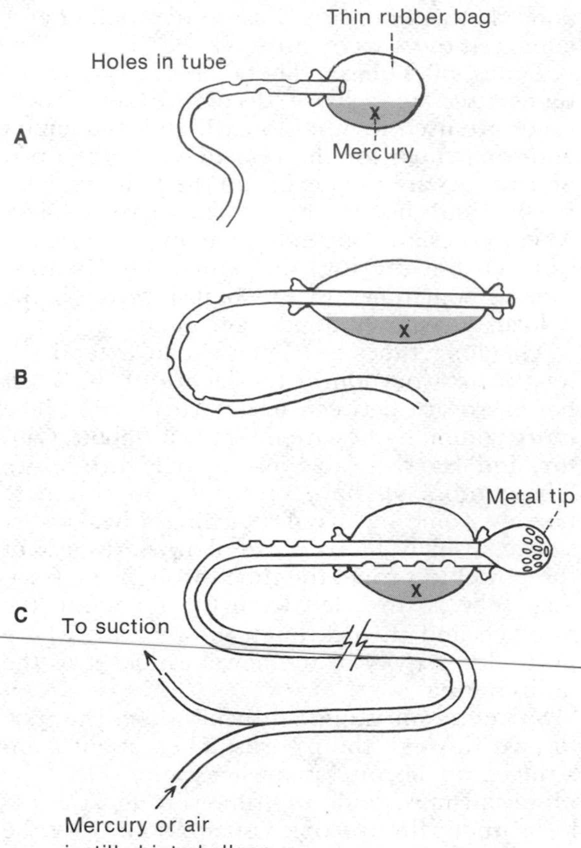

Figure 59–4. Three types of long intestinal decompression tubes. **A.** The Cantor tube. A single-lumen tube, mercury is instilled before insertion of tube. Suction is along both sides. **B.** The Harris tube. A single-lumen tube, mercury is instilled before insertion. Suction is at the end and along both sides. **C.** The Miller-Abbott tube. A double-lumen tube, mercury is instilled after insertion through the second lumen. Suction is at end, (through metal tip) and along one side.

tubes, it is often necessary to irrigate them to maintain or check their patency. The plastic Salem sump has a second lumen which is open to air, preventing the development of excessive negative pressure because the extra lumen brings air into the cavity continuously. This tube will not function effectively if attached to intermittent suction because the second lumen must be kept free of secretions by constantly aspirating air.

Insertion of Tubes. Nasogastric tubes are inserted through the nose or mouth into the stomach. The insertion of these tubes is frequently very frightening to the patient. The nurse must be understanding, gentle, and helpful to the patient in both explanations and manner. The explanation of what will be done should be adapted to the patient's need. Some wish to know all the details, whereas some prefer only brief instructions, as too much information increases their anxiety.

The tube is gently inserted through the nares into the posterior nasal pharynx and allowed to bend downward into the oral pharynx. It is well to have the patient swallow once the tube has rounded this curve, because the sphincter at the proximal end of the esophagus remains closed except during swallowing to prevent the introduction of air into the stomach during respiration. During swallowing the larynx rises, stretching the cricopharyngeus muscle and causing it to relax. Resistance might be felt at this sphincter when the tube is first inserted, but the sphincter will relax as the patient swallows. Swallowing also encourages the tube to enter the esophagus rather than the trachea. Swallowing water, if it is allowed, lubricates the tube, making it easier to pass. After passing the sphincter, the tube is advanced fairly rapidly until it is in the stomach. Its presence in the stomach can be verified by several means: by aspiration of gastric contents, by listening with a stethoscope to hear air pass into the stomach as it is rapidly instilled into the tube with a syringe, or by holding the end of the tube under water to see if air comes out (as it will if the tube is in the lungs).

Nursing Management of the Patient with Nasogastric Tube in Place. Maintaining comfort while the tube is in place is of utmost importance to the patient. The external nares may become sore from crusted secretions around the tube or from pressure. The tube should be gently cleaned to remove crystals that form from dried mucus. Water-soluble lubricants can be used on the tube and the external nares. The tube should be taped in such a manner as to prevent pressure. The patient's mouth is usually dry because of the absence of chewing, which is the normal stimulus to salivary secretions, and because of mouth breathing, which results from the presence of the tube. Frequent oral hygiene will increase the patient's comfort by removing debris and stimulating salivation. The teeth should be brushed even though the patient is not eating because bacterial action continues in the mouth and gingival stimulation is still needed.

> Remember:
> *Patients with a nasogastric tube in place need frequent oral hygiene for comfort and for maintenance of a healthy oral cavity.*

Sometimes the patient is allowed to chew gum or suck on sour candies or ice chips to aid in stimulating salivation.

Patients frequently complain of a sore throat from the presence of the tube. Anesthetic lozenges or gargles may be ordered for this. Sometimes the patient needs only the reassurance that this is a common feeling from the presence of the tube.

The material aspirated via the tube should be observed frequently for color, odor, and quantity, and any changes should be reported to the physician. Contents of the suction bottles must be measured to maintain an accurate count of fluid intake and output. It is important to record what area of the digestive tract the measured contents came from, because the electrolyte content of the small bowel is entirely different from that of the stomach. Sometimes samples of these secretions are sent to the laboratory for analysis. After the volume of the total specimen has been measured and thoroughly mixed, a small portion is sent for analysis.

It must be remembered that any irrigating solution that is instilled into a nasogastric tube is counted as intake for the patient. An accurate record must be kept of how much is instilled and how much aspirated from the tube during irrigations.

Solution that does not return during an irrigation will be returned in the suctioned fluids later, so it must be included as intake. Normal saline is frequently the irrigating solution of choice because water, a hypotonic solution, can increase the loss of electrolytes through osmotic action if too much of it is instilled. If the tube is irrigated often, this can be a significant factor.

Surgical Intervention

Surgical intervention is intended to restore the ability of the gut to propel the digestive materials through. Thus, many procedures involve repairing a structural abnormality, for example, reducing a herniation, releasing adhesions, or patching a perforation. Removal of a neoplastic growth or other pathologic condition such as an ulcer or polyp is also common. The removal of lesions frequently involves making changes in the route by which the chyme flows. Sometimes large segments are bypassed or a short circuit is created as segments are removed. After resections are done, the lumina of the various portions are sutured together by side-to-side, side-to-end, or end-to-end anastomoses.

In some instances it is necessary to divert the fecal stream to the surface of the abdomen, either to temporarily rest the portion distal to it or because the diseased portion extends to the anus and it is not possible or desirable to make an anastomosis there. In these instances a colostomy (opening of the colon onto the abdomen) or an ileostomy (opening of the ileum to the surface of the abdomen) is done. (See sections on colostomy and ileostomy below.)

Cecostomy. Following surgical procedures on the large bowel, there is swelling and impaired function for a few days. During this time the vast quantities of digestive juices (7 to 10 liters) continue to be secreted and, if they are not diverted, the patient may become very distended. A nasogastric tube is sometimes inserted into the stomach, but since most of this fluid is secreted in the small bowel, a tube is frequently inserted surgically into the cecum (cecostomy) to decompress this portion of the bowel. The tube is attached to a drainage bottle and drained by gravity. Irrigations are usually necessary, as this tube tends to become plugged with fecal material.

General Nursing Problems

Nursing care of patients with disease of the gastrointestinal tract is aimed at keeping the intestinal contents flowing freely through the gut, keeping tubes open, and maintaining the patient's electrolyte and nutritional balance. Since nutrition, eating, and elimination have deep emotional implications for many people, malfunction in these areas can cause deep distress to the patient. Cancer is a frequent diagnosis, and this disease in itself causes great emotional distress. Patients need support and understanding from the nurse, who must remember that people frequently express their concerns indirectly by their behavior rather than by words.

Eating is a social activity and when a person is unable to do this normally or must follow a severely restricted diet, some other means of meeting this need is necessary. The nurse can help by letting patients express their frustration and feelings about restrictions without making any judgmental comments and by making sure they understand the condition and the reasons for the restrictions.

Elimination is viewed as a very important function by many people, and many feel that a bowel movement every day is essential to good health. For this reason, patients tend to become quite upset when they have a disturbance of elimination. Patients who do not understand what normal elimination is and how it is achieved need even more instruction to understand the alterations that occur.

Many people feel that elimination is a shameful subject and are embarrased to be in the hospital for such a problem. You can help these people by your manner of acceptance of their condition and by making sure they understand what is happening to them. Avoid doing or saying anything in front of a visitor that might embarrass the patient.

Some special procedures for feeding patients and providing for their elimination processes when disease has interfered with normal functioning are discussed next.

Gavage. Feedings instilled into the stomach through a tube are called gavage feedings. They are given when the patient is unable to take foods normally owing either to an obstruction in the esophagus or to the inability to swallow. They are sometimes used temporarily after esophageal surgery. Tubes used include the nasogastric tube, gastrostomy tube, and jejunostomy tube. The first two lead into the stomach and the other, as the name implies, is in the jejunum.

Feedings given by the tube should be balanced nutritionally and not cause the patient gastrointestinal distress. Liquid feedings frequently cause diarrhea, either from the presence of concentrated ingredients or from improper storage, which allows organisms to grow or toxins to form. Liquid feedings can also cause constipation because of their lack of bulk.

Commercially prepared feedings are available in a number of different formulas that contain the basic nutrients in varying proportions and chemical states. Jejunal feedings must have nutrients in a form which can be absorbed in that area, because the gastric and duodenal digestive processes have been bypassed. If the patient's problems stem from too rapid transit through the tract, a higher rate of absorption can be accomplished by providing the nutrients in a form ready for absorption, so that little or no chemical transformation is needed, and the short time the chyme is in the small bowel is used to better advantage.

For convenience to the patient and also for ease of preparation, the regular diet of the hospital or the family at home can be liquefied in a blender, diluted to proper consistency, and given by tube. This is done only when the patient does not have special dietary needs. When chewing is important to the patient's mental state or when the digestive tract needs stimulation, allow the patient to chew the food and spit it out. It can then be placed in the feeding or discarded.

Several methods are used to administer tube feedings. They can run through a syringe or funnel which is attached to the tube or by drip from a bottle or bag (Murphy drip). Feedings can also be pumped through the tube at a set rate. Pumps are frequently used when the feeding is given continuously during the day and night.

For the patient in the home, feedings given at intervals through an Asepto syringe are common. When feedings are given in this way they should be allowed to run in by gravity and the bulb or plunger used only to start the flow when necessary; discomfort and nausea result from too rapid filling. The feeding should be at, or slightly below, body temperature. Heat will coagulate a feeding made from milk and eggs, and hot liquids could burn or irritate the gastric mucosa. Cold starts unfavorable gastric reactions by causing vasoconstriction, which reduces the flow of gastric digestive juices.

The patient should receive 2500 to 3000 ml. of fluid through the tube daily. Water is given prior to the feeding to make certain the tube is patent and to help to start the flow of the feeding solution. Following the feeding, the tube is cleansed by instilling 50 to 100 ml. of water. Air can be prevented from entering the tube during the feeding by not allowing the syringe to empty completely before adding more fluid or by pinching the tube while more fluid is added. Fluids can be instilled between meals as indicated.

Most patients are sensitive about taking food in this manner, and would prefer privacy while receiving feedings. Other patients in a ward usually do not like to watch this type of feeding while they eat their own food. Some patients enjoy joining others at the dinner table to participate in the social exchanges even though they cannot eat. Others cannot tolerate watching other people eat normally. Thus, arrangements as to timing and location for eating and tube feedings, both in the hospital and in the home, should be made to the satisfaction of everyone involved.

*Total Parenteral Alimentation (Hyperalimentation)**

Many patients with disorders of the gastrointestinal system are unable to ingest or digest sufficient nutrients to maintain themselves in a state of positive nitrogen balance or anabolism. These patients include those who have debilitating diseases such as malabsorption of the bowel, inflammatory diseases of the bowel or who for some reason are unable to eat adequate amounts, infants with major congenital abnormalities in the digestive tract, and patients who have excessive metabolic needs because they are losing vast quantities of protein-laden body fluids daily as a result of extensive burns or draining wounds. These patients are all candi-

*This procedure is also discussed in Chapter 12, p. 218.

dates for total parenteral alimentation or hyperalimentation, which is the intravenous administration of hypertonic solutions of glucose plus nitrogen (amino acids and polypeptides) and other nutrients sufficient to achieve tissue synthesis and anabolism in patients with normal or excessive nutritional needs. The composition of standard hyperalimentation solutions for adults are shown in Table 59–2.

Supplying the total nutritional needs of the body by intravenous infusion must be done by a special technique, because the amount of nutrients needed to achieve anabolism, dissolved in the volume of fluid that the body can tolerate daily, produces a solution which is so hypertonic it causes phlebitis, clotting, and local swelling of the blood vessel used for the infusion. For instance, intravenous fluid of 2500 ml. per day of 5 per cent glucose supply about 500 calories and no amino acids; this same volume of 10 per cent glucose would supply only 1000 calories, which is still below the basal caloric requirements of the resting adult and would contain no protein. A solution containing sufficient calories and protein, when diluted enough for toleration by the body, would be from 12 to 15 liters.

This problem has been circumvented two ways. The most common is by the insertion of a catheter into the superior vena cava via the right or left subclavian vein (Fig. 59–5). The hypertonic solution is rapidly diluted by the large amount of blood flowing through this vein. Among the complications that can occur during or following insertion of the catheter are those

TABLE 59–2. COMPOSITION OF STANDARD HYPERALIMENTATION SOLUTIONS FOR ADULTS

	Bulk Method	Stock Solution Method	Kit Method
	165 gm anhydrous dextrose USP plus 860 ml 5% protein hydrolysate in 5% dextrose	350 ml 50% dextrose plus 750 ml 5% protein hydrolysate in 5% dextrose	500 ml 8.5% Freamine II plus 500 ml 50% dextrose
	Sterilization by passage through 0.22 micron membrane filter under laminar-flow filtered-air hood	Aseptic mixing technique under laminar-flow filtered-air hood	Aseptic mixing with transfer apparatus
Volume	1000 ml	1100 ml	1000 ml
Calories	1000 kcal	1000 kcal	1000 kcal
Dextrose	208 gm	212 gm	250 gm
Hydrolysate	43 gm	37 gm	
Amino acids			42.5 gm
Nitrogen	6.0 gm	5.25 gm	6.25 gm
Sodium	8 mEq	7 mEq	5 mEq
Potassium	14 mEq	13 mEq	
Phosphate			10 mEq

Additions to each unit of base solution (average adult):

Sodium (chloride and/or acetate, lactate, bicarbonate)	40 to 50 mEq
Potassium (acetate, lactate, chloride, acid phosphate)	20 to 40 mEq
Magnesium (sulfate)	8 to 15 mEq
Phosphate (potassium acid salt)	12 to 18 mMol

Additions to only one unit daily:

Vitamin A	5000 to 10000 USP units
Vitamin D	500 to 1000 USP units
Vitamin E	2.5 to 5.0 IU
Vitamin C	250 to 500 mg
Thiamine	25 to 50 mg
Riboflavin	5 to 10 mg
Pyridoxine	7.5 to 15 mg
Niacin	50 to 100 mg
Pantothenic acid	12.5 to 25 mg
Calcium (gluconate)	4.8 to 9.6 mEq

Optional additions to daily nutrient regimen:

Vitamin K	5 to 10 mg	
Vitamin B_{12}	10 to 30 μg	Alternatively may be given I.M. in appropriate daily or weekly dosages
Folic acid	0.5 to 1.0 mg	
Iron	0.2 to 3.0 mg	

Micronutrients such as cobalt, copper, iodine, manganese, and zinc are present as contaminants in hydrolysate solutions, but may be given in plasma transfusion (10 mg/kg) once or twice weekly if desired.

From Dudrick, S. J.: A patient on I.V. therapy need not starve! *Consultant,* 18:142, Feb. 1978, p. 146.

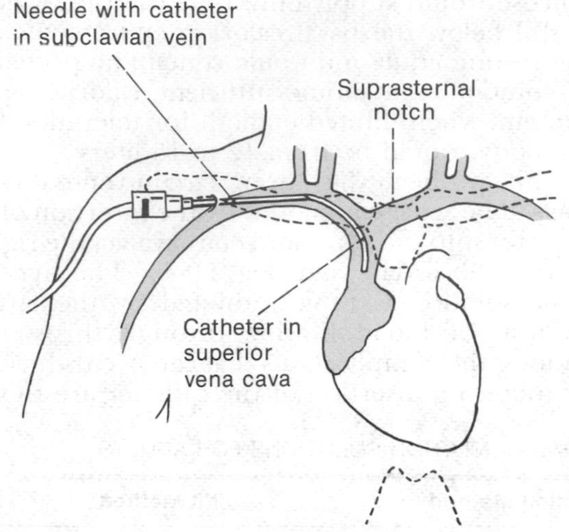

Figure 59–5. Insertion of catheter into superior vena cava via right subclavian vein.

due to accidental perforation of the pleura, injury to the brachial plexus or the artery, air embolism, or subclavian venous thrombosis.

The other approach is to make an external arteriovenous fistula, as is done in renal dialysis. (See Unit XIII.) The solution is infused into the plastic fistulous tract and is mixed and diluted there before it comes into contact with the patient's vein. Both methods have proved successful in large numbers of patients.

Complications. The major complications of total parenteral nutrition (TPN) therapy include:

Infection. Patients receiving TPN are very susceptible to infection, especially Candida septicemia. Concentrated glucose solutions provide a good medium for bacterial growth. Contamination of either the catheter, solution, insertion site, tubing, or filters can lead to the development of infection. Stringent asepsis must be exercised by the pharmacy when preparing TPN solutions. In order to reduce the possibility of infection developing from the solutions, they are mixed under rigid aseptic control in a closed location to minimize contact with airborne particles. Furthermore, no more than a 24-hour supply of solution should be prepared in advance. A filter is commonly used in the intravenous tubing to trap bacteria and particles. In addition, the dressing and administration equipment must be changed every 24 to 48 hours, using meticulous aseptic technique. Betadine or an antibiotic ointment are often applied to the catheter insertion site with each dressing change.

Hyperglycemia. When the rate of glucose infusion is faster than the rate of glucose metabolism by the body, hyperglycemia results. If hyperglycemia is allowed to persist, the renal threshold for glucose reabsorption is exceeded and osmotic diuresis with subsequent dehydration and electrolyte depletion occurs. To avoid this complication, TPN infusions should be administered at a constant rate and checked every 30 minutes. A mechanical infusion pump will provide greater accuracy in administration of solutions and help prevent wide fluctuations in rate.

Hypoglycemia. One of the body's major responses to high blood glucose levels, such as those found in patients receiving TPN, is increased insulin output from the pancreas. When a hypertonic glucose infusion is abruptly interrupted, insulin levels remain high while glucose levels decline, resulting in a rebound hypoglycemia. Kinking of the tubing or catheter by position changes, infiltration of the IV, failure of the mechanical pump, or allowing the infusion bottle to run dry can cause cessation of solution flow and subsequent hypoglycemia.

Nausea, headache, or lassitude. These untoward reactions may result from too rapid infusion of fluids.

Infiltration of the infusion catheter. When the catheter dislodges from the vein, the patient may complain of shoulder pain or burning at the insertion site. Edema of the neck and face may also be evident.

Nursing Responsibilities. Expert nursing care of the patient is essential to the successful outcome of this treatment. The nurse is an essential member of the team that manages a patient on hyperalimentation.

As mentioned, strict aseptic technique during the insertion of the catheter, during dressing changes, and during changes in the bottles, filters, and intravenous tubing is essential. Most hospitals that use the therapy have developed rigid procedures for accomplishing these duties, and some allow only specially trained nurses to do them.

Procedures vary in detail, but most hospitals change the tubing and filters routinely every 24 to 48 hours and the dressings around the catheter insertion site every 2 to 3 days. The skin is cleaned with a substance such as acetone or ether to remove oils, since they harbor bacteria; this also breaks down the cellular walls of the bacteria. The skin is then cleaned with an antiseptic solution such as iodine, and an antibiotic ointment is applied to the insertion site. After cleansing and application of a sterile dressing, tape is used to form an occlusive dressing that will be impervious to air and small amounts of moisture. A mask should be worn by all those near the wound to prevent the introduction of organisms from the nasal pharynx.[40]

Since too rapid a flow of a solution will cause hyperglycemia and too slow a flow will fail to instill the needed nutrients, it is vital that close attention be given to regulation. It is important that the flow rate not be increased in speed though it is behind schedule. Most institutions use a pump to regulate the flow and to eliminate the changes in rate of flow that occur with alterations in the patient's activity and position.

The flow rate of a hyperalimentation infusion must be maintained at its ordered rate – never speeded up!

It is essential that no air enter the system. This can easily occur when the catheter is in the vena cava since changes in thoracic volume, as from taking a deep breath, cause changes in the pressure within this vein. If this occurs while the catheter is open during a tubing change or during insertion, air could be sucked into the system, causing an air embolus that might be fatal. This possibility is avoided by having the patient in slight Trendelenburg (head down) position when the tube is being manipulated or by having the patient perform the Valsalva maneuver of increasing intrathoracic pressure by bearing down during the brief periods during which the tube is open.

Nursing observations are concerned with the patient's electrolyte balance, the presence of infection, untoward reactions to the hyperosmolar infusion, weight gain, and tissue repair. Accurate records of intake and output, including all the abnormal routes that are employed, are absolutely essential. The physician will monitor the patient's blood electrolytes, but an accurate count of what was taken and what was excreted is still essential. Blood pressure measurements and daily weights are frequently ordered to monitor the patient's progress. The presence or absence of sugar in the urine is usually tested every 6 hours to make certain the infusion is not running too rapidly for the body to metabolize the glucose.

Other observations of nausea, vomiting, lassitude, fever, and any other abnormal response should be reported, as they might indicate the presence of a complication.

Some essential nursing observations and routines which help safeguard patients receiving TPN are summarized in Table 59–3.

Home Therapy. In several medical centers patients who must remain on TPN for a prolonged period are successfully managed at home. Most receive the infusion during sleep, which presents a potential problem in maintaining the proper rate of infusion. A pump regulator can be used, but many individuals use only the gravity drip. Patients can either buy their solutions premixed or, as is less expensive, purchase the chemicals and mix their own. Several medical centers report patients being maintained successfully at home.[174, 92, 6]

Colostomy*

A colostomy, which is the opening of some portion of the colon onto the abdominal surface, is performed when it is impossible for the feces to progress through the colon and out the anus because of some pathologic condition, or when it is more desirable or manageable to divert the fecal stream, as for a paraplegic. Temporary colostomies are done to divert the fecal flow away from an area of inflammation or around an operative area. A permanent colostomy is created as a means of elimination when the rectum or anus are nonfunctional as a result of disease, birth defect, or a traumatic condition.

When only one loop of bowel is open on the abdominal surface, the patient has a single-barreled or end colostomy because there is only one stoma. A double-barreled colostomy is one in which both loops, the distal and proximal, are open on the abdominal wall (Fig. 59–6). A single-barreled colostomy is permanent if the bowel distal to it has been resected, while a double-barreled colostomy may be permanent or it may be closed at a later time, depending upon the disease present. A temporary colostomy is done most commonly at the midpoint of the left colon or the transverse colon, whereas a

*The author is indebted to Pat Starkovich, R.N., Enterostomal Therapist, who served as consultant for the sections on colostomy and ileostomy.

TABLE 59–3. DAILY CHECKLIST FOR MEMBERS OF TOTAL PARENTERAL NUTRITION (TPN) THERAPY TEAM

Examine label on TPN bottle to confirm that it contains correct formulation
Check TPN flow rate
Observe patient's appearance, color, mood, and orientation
Check record of vital signs on bedside chart
Check record of fluid intake and output and body weight
Check results of fractional urine tests for glucose and acetone
Check results of biochemical blood tests, especially determinations of glucose, inorganic phosphorus, and electrolyte levels
Examine dressing covering site of infusion
Read progress notes to maintain familiarity with patient's course, results of studies, and proposed plan
Make appropriate notes in chart to keep nursing and medical staff informed about nutritional progress

From Hodges, R. E.: Total parenteral nutrition. *Postgraduate Medicine,* 65:171, Mar. 1979, p. 174.

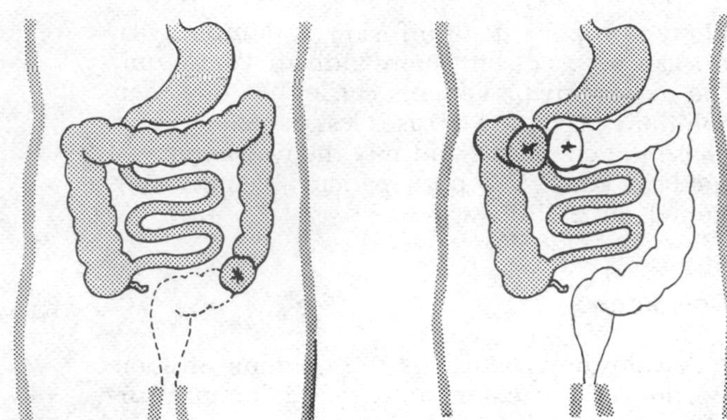

Figure 59–6. The location of colostomy stomas. Left, single-barreled colostomy. Right, double-barreled colostomy. (From *Colostomies: A Guide,* published by the United Ostomy Association, Los Angeles.)

permanent colostomy is usually at the sigmoid colon but may be anywhere. Since the main function of the large bowel is absorption of water, the stool is more formed and the colostomy is easier to manage when it is nearer the terminal (left) colon than in the transverse or right colon.

Management. The immediate postoperative care is the same as for any abdominal surgery patient, with the addition of watching for spillage through the colostomy if it is open and checking the color of the stoma. If it is dark — blue-black or magenta — the surgeon must be notified immediately. Fecal contents are highly contaminated with bacteria, so care should be taken to keep these secretions away from the surgical incision. When creating a temporary colostomy, the surgeon frequently brings a loop of bowel out through a wound which is separate from the surgical incision and keeps it from slipping back by placing a rod beneath it (Fig. 59–7). Two or three days postoperatively the bowel will be opened, usually with a cautery. Since there are no sensory nerve endings in the bowel wall, this procedure is painless to the patient, except for some cramping pain, which may occur if the trauma stimulates contractions.

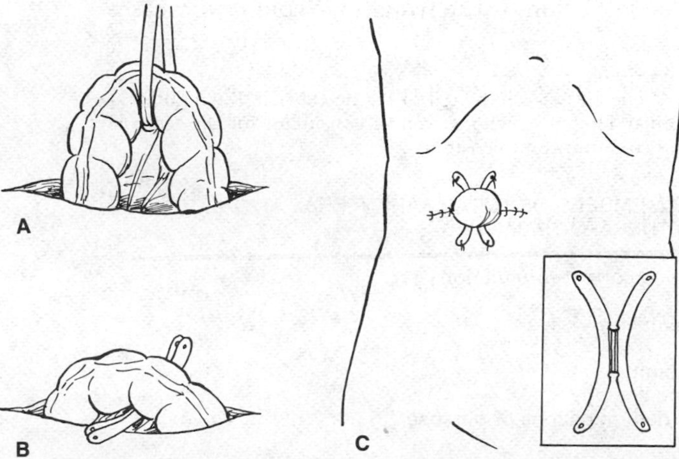

Figure 59–7. Formation of a loop colostomy. **A.** Loop of bowel brought out through incision. **B.** Plastic rod inserted under loop. **C.** Rod opened (unfolded) and lying flat against abdomen. Holes in each end may be sutured to the skin if desired. Insert shows detail of rod (bridge) unfolded.

The surgeon will usually indicate which loop is the proximal and which the distal. This is not always immediately obvious until feces begin to flow, since the loop is sometimes reversed as it is brought through the abdominal wall.

Emotional Response by Patient. The patient who has a colostomy usually has some difficulty adjusting to it. Feces are associated in most people's minds with "dirt" and shame, and bowel movements become a private function quite early in life. Depending upon the individual's attitude toward excretory functions, knowledge about colostomies prior to surgery, and general ability to adjust to stressful situations, the patient's reactions may range from apparently easy acceptance to a total withdrawal from social contacts. Some individuals refuse to look at the stoma and have a great deal of difficulty accepting its presence, while others "take it in stride" and immediately begin to participate in stoma care. The nurse's reaction and manner towards the patient and the care the patient requires can affect the person's adjustment. The patient's acceptance of any "ostomy" is also somewhat dependent upon the medical condition that necessitated its creation. For some, it represents a "cure," for others it is a temporary condition and for others it is merely a palliation, as with the patient who has extensive cancer.

The nurse must make a careful assessment of the patient and the patient's mental acceptance before attempting to teach ostomy self-care. Discussion with significant others to find out the patient's general reactions to life's stresses will give much needed information. The type of relationship between a husband and wife or any intimate partners is important to understand also. Is one a dominant figure? Is one person dependent on the other?

Watson has compared the phases of adjustment to an "ostomy" to the psychologic phases experienced by a person in any crisis. The stages are: (1) *shock,* (2) *defensive retreat,* (3) *acknowledgment,* and (4) *adaptation.** She points out that during the first two stages patients need much support, a realistic appraisal of their situation and encouragement to participate in their own care. Clients must reach the acknowledgment phase before they are able to

*See Chapter 26, p. 522.

achieve any real rehabilitative gains. However, as they begin to achieve the ability to care for the stoma, then they are able to reach the final or adaptive level.[196]

Teaching must be paced to the patient's level of acceptance of the colostomy as well as ability to perform the tasks of management. If physically able to do so, an adult usually prefers to care for the colostomy without involving significant others more than absolutely necessary. However, a husband or wife should be knowledgeable about the colostomy and the care required. He or she must also learn to accept this mode of elimination as a way of life for the mate; lack of acceptance by the spouse makes the patient's adjustment harder.

Control of Elimination. Elimination can be handled in two ways: Natural elimination patterns of the body can be utilized, with the patient wearing a bag to collect the feces whenever they come, or an attempt can be made at control by irrigations. If the colostomy is in the transverse or right colon, wearing a bag will be necessary, as the feces are still quite liquid in these areas. When irrigations are not used, then the attempt at control is made by adjusting the diet so as to obtain a stool of the desired consistency. Some people prefer to have rigid dietary regulation and not be bothered with irrigations, and some people are not physically or emotionally able to cope with the irrigation procedure. Some people are able to regulate a colostomy well enough by diet alone to avoid wearing a bag over the stoma.

When regulation by irrigation is attempted, irrigation is usually done daily. In this way the patient hopes to empty the colon and have no passage of stool until the next irrigation. This method also necessitates control of the patient's diet to avoid laxative foods that might cause an unexpected evacuation.

A colostomy irrigation, which is very similar to an enema, can be done at any time of day that is convenient for the patient but should be done at the same time each day and should always be done with the patient sitting on the stool. The purpose of the irrigation is to distend the bowel sufficiently to stimulate peristalsis, which will cause the evacuation to occur. Most patients can stimulate evacuation of the bowel with a relatively small amount of fluid (300 to 500 ml.). But, since there is no sphincter on a colostomy and the fluid tends to return as it is instilled, some individuals may need to use up to 1000 ml. to achieve complete evacuation. This problem is partially overcome on some commercial irrigating sets through the provision of cones or dams. Note in Figure 59–10 that the irrigating catheter has been passed through a cone which will help hold the fluid within the bowel during the irrigation.

The soft rectal tube or catheter that is used to instill the fluid is lubricated with a water soluble lubricant and inserted about 3 inches. Care should be used in inserting it to avoid perforation of the bowel; if any resistance is encountered, some solution should be instilled to distend the bowel ahead of the tube and thus ease its insertion. Frequently the bowel makes a turn shortly below the abdominal wall, and there may be a constriction owing to an attachment made during surgery, so the patient must become familiar with the contour of his bowel and learn to insert the tube without undue poking, which might damage the delicate mucous membrane. The temperature of the solution should be at or very slightly below body temperature, since warmer solutions tend to cause the bowel to relax. Every colostomy is different, and some people may need to use more solution than this or to insert the tube farther to avoid backflow. Each patient must learn the best method to manage his or her own bowel. See Figs. 59–8 and 59–9 for sample instruction sheets given to patients.

Many hospitals and some home health agencies employ an *Enterostomal Therapist* who is a registered nurse with postgraduate training in the management of "ostomies." This health worker (a) assists patients in finding equipment to meet their needs and (b) usually conducts teaching sessions with patients and with other nurses concerning proper management of ostomies.

There is a large assortment of commercial equipment available for irrigating a colostomy. Most physicians have a set purchased while the patient is hospitalized, for the patient to take home. The cost of these sets varies widely, and the type of apparatus used is largely a matter of personal preference. Fig. 59–10 shows a sample commercially made irrigation set. The patient should be referred to a convenient surgical supply house to see the variety of sets available and make a selection. Uusually, before investing in a new apparatus, the patient should use the "starter set" until familiar with the colostomy, its problems, and the problems of irrigating it.

In an emergency, a temporary irrigation set can be made from a plastic bread wrapper and a rubber canning ring (Fig. 59–11). Many people already own an enema bag, and with the addition of a connector, an irrigating catheter can be attached. The rigid rectal tube that comes with these sets should not be used on a colostomy because of the danger of trauma to the bowel wall.

Stoma bags are not necessary after the colostomy is regulated, but for a few hours after irrigations or when dealing with a bout of diarrhea, most people prefer to wear a bag to protect their clothing. In either case, they should always carry a pouch with them. Surveys have shown that a high percentage of patients with colostomies wear a bag at least part of the time. Bags are attached to the abdominal wall by an adhesive substance. Some bags are made with a karaya gum ring which adheres to the abdomen when held with a belt (Fig. 59–12).

COLOSTOMY IRRIGATION TECHNIQUE

Purpose: To establish control of fecal discharge.

1. Remove pouch.
2. Put sleeve faceplate over stoma and snap on belt.
3. Fill bag with 5 cups lukewarm water.
4. Let a little water run through catheter.
5. Lubricate catheter tip with water soluble lubricant such as K-Y or Lubrafax.
6. Push shield down to 2 inches from end of catheter.
7. With water running, insert catheter and press shield firmly against stoma.
8. When water is all in, remove catheter, fold down top of sleeve and clamp.
9. Let drain for 15 minutes.
10. Refill bag (or use pitcher) and rinse out sleeve.
11. Wear sleeve another 45 minutes approximately. Wipe off bottom of sleeve and fold in half, put top and bottom ends together and clamp.
12. Do what you wish for 45 minutes.
13. Remove sleeve, wash skin and stoma and put on new pouch.
14. To take care of equipment:
    A. Wash sleeve with warm water and mild detergent. Rinse well and hang up to dry.
    B. Hang up irrigating set to dry.

Note: Sleeves do wear out. It is recommended that you keep extra sleeves on hand.

Do not ever force catheter into stoma.
Do not insert catheter more than 4 inches maximum.
Do not use more than 1 quart water (1000 ml.).
Do not irrigate more than once a day.
Do not use Vaseline for lubrication, as it hardens catheter tip.
Do not irrigate if you develop diarrhea.

Figure 59–8. Typical irrigation technique instruction sheet given to patients. (Courtesy Group Health Cooperative of Puget Sound, Seattle, Washington.)

Mucous secretions from the bowel make some protection over the stoma necessary when the patient does not wear a bag. A piece of tissue or a thin gauze square with a piece of plastic over it to retain the moisture is usually sufficient. Commercial pads with a moisture-proof backing are available.

Diet. Diet is of utmost importance in the management of a colostomy, because the consistency of the stool and presence of gas depend on the type of foods ingested. Each individual is different: each person must discover by trial and error what can and cannot be eaten. In general, the foods that bothered a person before the

INFORMATION FOR PATIENT WITH COLOSTOMY

To Gain Control

1. Irrigate daily until you can go one week without spillage.
2. Begin adding one food at 3-day intervals. If you lose control, this may be a laxative food for you and should be avoided. During this period, continue daily with irrigations.
3. After you have tolerated all foods you want to include in your diet, you may try irrigating every other day. If after one week you have no spillage between irrigations, continue with every other day. Wear gauze pad lightly covered with water-soluble jelly over stoma between irrigations.
4. If you do have spillage with every other day irrigation, you will need to irrigate daily in order to gain control.

Problems You May Encounter

Diarrhea (frequent, loose stools)	*Cramping*
A. Frequent causes 1. Foods you cannot tolerate 2. Constipation 3. Certain medications 4. Illness	A. Frequent causes 1. Water flow too fast or 2. Amount of water too much
B. What to do: 1. Omit irrigation and call	B. What to do: 1. Slow the flow 2. Lower irrigation bag to shoulder height—have good hand control of on and off valve. 3. May use less water

Note: During cleaning, stoma may bleed as spotting on tissue or washcloth. This no cause for alarm.

Figure 59–9. Typical information sheet given to patients with a colostomy. (Courtesy Group Health Cooperative of Puget Sound, Seattle, Washington.)

surgery will be troublesome. Roughage, fresh fruits, and prunes and other laxative or bulk-forming foods will need to be eaten judiciously or diarrhea may develop. On the other hand, with a totally constipating diet, a person will have problems with hard stools. Thus patients must find out for themselves what balance of food creates the best consistency of stool with the least amount of gas.

Special Problems. *Diarrhea* is a serious problem for colostomy patients and can create havoc in the best managed life style. The person should contact the physician for instruction concerning medications that can be taken to slow the motility of the bowel. Many people keep such medications on hand and use them at the first indication of trouble.

Two further problems can result from diarrhea: *excoriation of the skin* from the digestive juices that have not been resorbed, and *electrolyte imbalance* when the condition persists. The individual should be encouraged to continue taking water and possibly plain tea when diarrhea begins, but it is usually best to take no food until bowel motility has returned to normal.

When *hard stools* are present, it is difficult to evacuate the bowel and may be difficult to get water into the colostomy for irrigation. Fecal impactions can also occur. Oil instilled directly into the stoma at bedtime or several hours before irrigation will usually help this situation. Only a small amount is needed; the individual might try 5 to 10 ml. first and await the results before trying more. Too much oil will cause the colostomy to leak oil after irrigation. Sometimes the physician has the patient take the stool softener dioctyl sodium sulfosuccinate to hold more fluid in the feces.

Gas is an embarrassing problem since the individual has no control over its passage and has no sensations to indicate when it is about to pass. The noise of the passage of gas and the resultant odor can cause the person to avoid social situations. Charcoal and bismuth subcarbonate are thought by some to help and can be taken orally with the physician's approval. Odorproof pouches and those with charcoal filter disks are available, but the most satisfactory method of control is dietary. Since each individual is different, the person will have to find out by trial and error which foods cause him problems. In general, nuts, cabbage, sauerkraut, broccoli, corn, cauliflower and legumes are gas-forming foods. Swallowing air by eating too rapidly, chewing gum, or drinking carbonated beverages can also be causes for intestinal gas.

Strictures of the stoma occur following some surgical techniques because the rectus muscles of the abdominal wall tend to close over the artificial opening made through them. Some physicians routinely teach their patients to dilate the stoma with a gloved finger before each irrigation. Other physicians feel that the passage of a formed stool is sufficient dilatation.

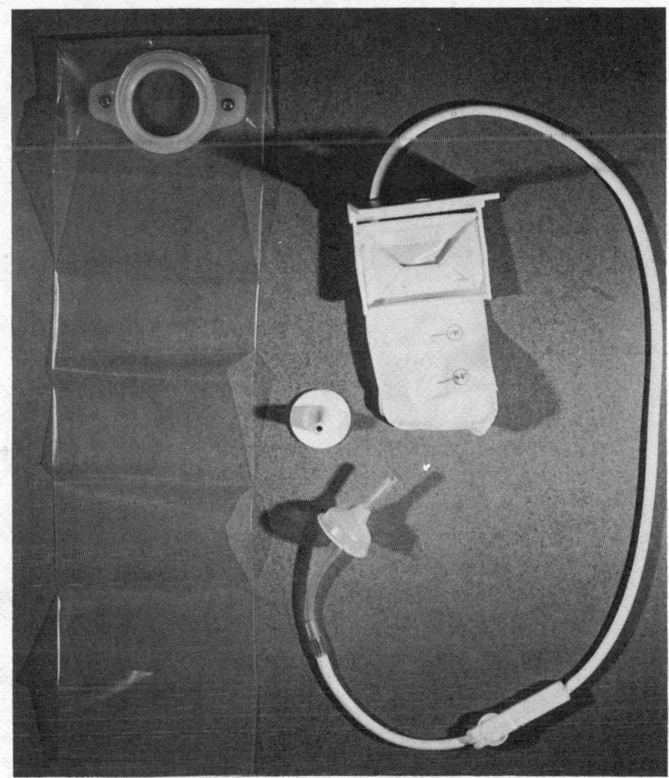

Figure 59–10. Commercially made irrigation set. On the right, a bag with irrigating tubing and tip. It can be hung from a hook on wall or from a standard. Note the cone close to the tip of the tubing. Another type of cone is adjacent in picture. Sleeve to direct returning solution into stool is on left. Patient wears the sleeve with the faceplate over the stoma, held in place with a belt.

Regular cleansing of the skin around the stoma is necessary to prevent irritation. Excoriation due to the constant presence of moisture can usually be prevented or healed with a light dusting of karaya powder, but too much powder will prevent the pouch from sticking.

Patient Adjustment. The person who has a colostomy can lead a completely normal life. He or she can engage in all the sports and social activities enjoyed before surgery. Travel is not a serious problem, but the patient must allow extra time in the itinerary for stoma care in unfamiliar situations. Many people do these things without difficulty. There are no restrictions in dress except that a change of undergarments should be carried in case of accidental soiling.

There is no physical reason why the person cannot enjoy normal sexual relationships, except for some men who become impotent after a radical perineal dissection. Psychologic barriers because of the supposedly "dirty" opening on the abdomen of one partner may cause some problems, but with love, patience, and understanding, and with good hygienic practices on the part of the person with the colostomy, there need be no problem. However, it may take several months after surgery before a couple manages to reestablish a satisfactory relationship.

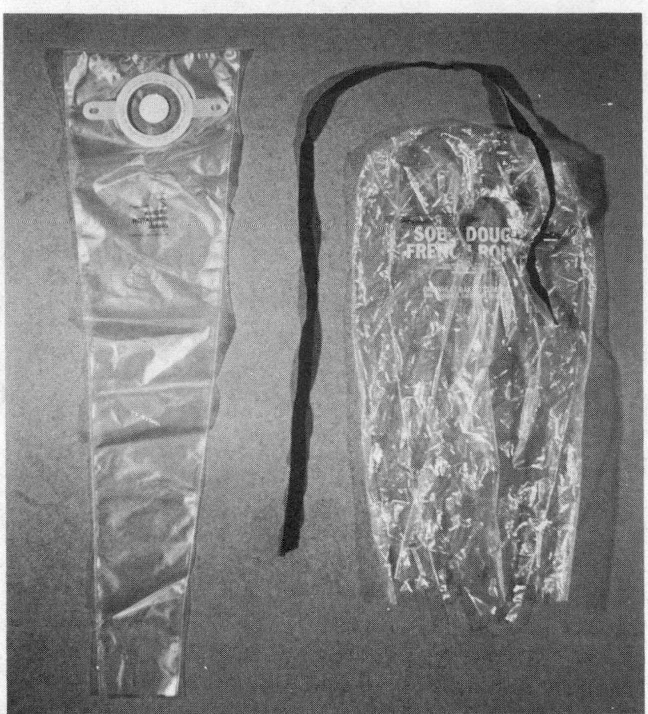

Figure 59–11. Disposable colostomy irrigation equipment. The bag on the left is commercially made. Note the wedged circle through which the irrigating catheter is inserted. The home-made irrigator (right) is made by creating a hole near the closed end of a plastic bread bag and wrapping the plastic around a rubber canning ring to form a snug bond. A belt to hold the apparatus close to the abdomen can be threaded through safety pins that pierce the rubber ring. A small hole can be made for insertion of the irrigation catheter. The bag is discarded after use. As with most other irrigating equipment, the patient uses these bags while sitting on the stool, with the open end of the bag held between the legs to direct the returning flow into the toilet.

The preceding discussion may make adjustment of the colostomy patient sound easy, but the average person has many problems in achieving this level of rehabilitation. Depression is common and "management" of anything as unpredictable as the human intestine is very difficult, if not impossible, without a sphincter. After the person has been provided with a pouch that not only does not leak, but produces neither odor nor skin problems, the resolution of difficulties is the patient's problem. Patients need much support and knowledgeable advice as they learn to live with the situation. Some cities have established "ostomy" rehabilitation clinics to help these patients with their problems. When an enterostomal therapist (ET) is available, this worker will assist the patient in learning to manage and accept the ostomy and will help the patient achieve a smooth transition from the hospital to the home and to the rehabilitated life.

In most large communities there is an "ostomy" club. These clubs are beneficial, as people share their concerns with others who understand and exchange "solutions" to their common problems. Information concerning the local club can be acquired from a local hospital, the local cancer society office, or from the United Ostomy Association, Incorporated, 1111 Wilshire Boulevard, Los Angeles, California 90017.

Ileostomy

An ileostomy is the opening of the ileum onto the abdominal surface. The colon may or may not be resected. The most frequent reason for doing an ileostomy is the treatment of ulcerative colitis, but the operation is also done as a treatment for regional enteritis (Crohn's disease), multiple polyposis, cancer of the bowel, and sometimes as a temporary diversion of the fecal stream. The vast majority of ileostomies are permanent.

The major difference between an ileostomy and a colostomy is the consistency of the fecal stream. The feces are liquid in the terminal ileum and contain digestive enzymes which can digest the skin. There is no way to regulate the fecal flow, so the traditional method of control is for the individual to wear a collection bag over the stoma.

A newer method of collecting fecal matter from the ileum is by the formation of a continent ileostomy (or ileal pouch). It consists of a reservoir that is created by the formation of a pouch from a portion of the terminal ileum. The open end of this pouch is threaded between the rectus muscles to form a valve seal and then opens onto the abdomen. Fecal material retained within this pouch is irrigated or drained out three to four times a day as the patient threads a small irrigating catheter through the valve. The main problem resulting from this procedure has been caused by incompetent valves that leak, making it necessary for the patient to wear a pouch.

After a traditional ileostomy, the patient returns from surgery wearing a temporary bag which adheres to the skin. It is very important to make sure that secretions do not leak from this bag, as they will cause a skin burn which keeps the bag from sticking and causes further leakage and further burning. Prevention of leakage is especially important while the surgical incision is healing. The patient must know how to apply and manage the appliance before leaving the hospital. The patient should practice this in a situation as closely resembling his or her own bathroom as possible. There are a number of appliances on the market, but none is perfect. The patient should seek help until one is found that fits well, does not leak, and that can be worn at least one day (preferably 3 to 5 days) without changing. It may be several months after surgery before the stoma achieves its final size, so the patient should not be in a hurry to purchase this expensive equipment. The patient should be provided with the names and locations of local surgical supply companies from which this equipment can be purchased and where help in procuring a properly fitting appliance can be obtained. An enterostomal therapist is a great help to these patients in finding the proper appliance.

Since no control over the fecal flow is possible, there is little reason for dietary control. These patients may find that some foods cause them to have excessive problems with gas and with odor and may have to make some minor dietary adjustments. The major difficulty patients have is with skin care, so their biggest problem is in achieving a good fit between the appliance bag and the skin.

If diarrhea develops from any source, the patient must seek medical care immediately, because a state of acute electrolyte imbalance can develop rapidly, owing to the excessively rapid loss of digestive juices. Since the potassium loss is especially serious, these patients should keep a high-potassium dietary supplement on hand at all times. Family and friends as well as the patient must be aware of this ever-present danger.

As mentioned, the most common reason for doing this surgery is an inflammatory condition of the bowel. The average patient has usually had the bowel disorder for a number of years before deciding to have surgery and is in a poor state of nutrition. The person frequently has many emotional problems as a result of the condition and has decided upon surgery as the lesser of two evils. The surgical procedure in which the colon is resected is a great physiologic shock to an already malnourished body, and the ileostomy is an equally great shock to a patient in a depressed emotional state. When the patient awakens after surgery and realizes what has been done, depression often sets in. A research study found that even though the nature of the surgery was discussed with patients preoperatively, they "were shocked and horrified after surgery when they realized what the operation entailed."[130]

In caring for this patient the nurse must remember that he or she has had an emotionally draining disease and that the decision to have this type of surgery was not made lightly. This person needs patient understanding and reassurance that the ileostomy will be "manageable" and that a normal life is still possible. Many of these patients are irascible, and consequently many nurses find them difficult to care for.

Members of ostomy clubs visit these patients in many communities. Patients in the previously mentioned study reported that a preoperative visit by one of the members was helpful in reassuring the patient that a person still looked normal after undergoing this surgery. Visits are made only on the invitation of the physician, so in many instances the person is not seen preoperatively. However, a visit from an ileostomy patient is helpful after surgery too, because the patient can identify with another person who has the condition better than with the doctors and nurses

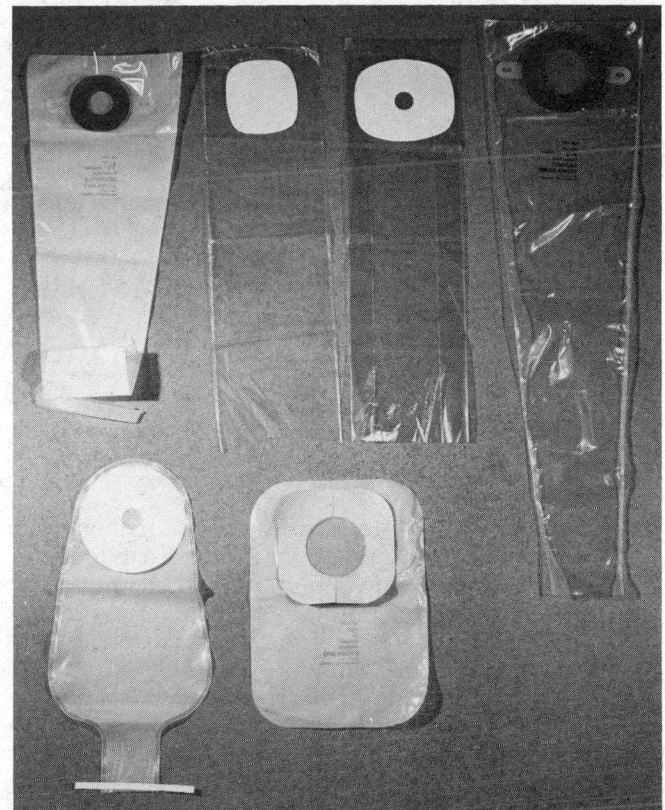

Figure 59–12. Commercially made colostomy and ileostomy pouches. Note that all but one are open at the bottom for emptying. Upper left and upper right have karaya gum seals; the others have a protective paper over an adhesive substance. The paper is peeled off before the bag is applied. Note the clamp closures on the two bags on the left.

who have had no personal experience with the problems involved.

The family of the ileostomy patient has as much of an adjustment to make as the patient does, and at the same time they must understand what the patient is going through and accept what may be unpredictable and trying behavior. Nurses can do much in the way of helping the family by listening to their reactions and interpreting the patient's problems to them. The family and intimate relationship problems are very similar to those of a colostomy patient.

It should be assumed from the beginning that patients will learn to manage the stoma and bag as soon as physically able to do so; this is as necessary to the ileostomy patient as learning to use a prosthesis is to the amputation patient. The patient, to achieve a satisfactory adjustment, should have an appliance which fits snugly, does not leak or cause odor or skin irritation, and stays in place for several days. Also, the patient should be able to (a) change the bag without undue problems or undue expenditure of time, (b) eat a balanced diet and, (c) live a normal life—socially, vocationally, recreationally, and sexually. These are the goals of nursing care.

CHAPTER 60

ABNORMALITIES OF THE MOUTH AND OROPHARYNX

DENTAL DISORDERS

Since dental care and dental hygiene are provided by workers in these disciplines, we shall discuss only conditions that the nurse needs to understand when caring for the sick person and when functioning as a health teacher and case finder.

One aim of dentistry is to preserve the natural teeth in good health as long as possible, because the natural teeth are almost always more functional in masticating food than a dental prosthesis. Efficient digestion of food depends on proper mastication, which in turn depends on functional dentures. So healthy teeth are important to gastrointestinal function.

Decay and periodontal disease are the major causes of tooth loss. Plaque has been cited as the major cause of both caries (decay) and periodontal disease and is also the initial stage in the formation of calculus.

Dental plaque is a soft mass of proliferating bacteria with a scattering of leukocytes, macrophages and epithelial cells in a sticky polysaccharide-protein matrix that adheres to the teeth, from which it can only be detached by mechanical cleansing. It is transparent and colorless and escapes detection unless it absorbs pigment from within the oral cavity or is stained in the dental office by disclosing solutions or wafers available for that purpose.[78]

Food affects plaque because bacterial enzymes liquefy food debris after a meal and utilize some of the carbohydrates along with saliva in plaque formation. The polysaccharide *dextran* is the major component of the intercellular matrix that envelops the plaque bacteria and attaches them to each other and to the tooth surface. The sticky organic film begins to form and mats of bacteria begin to collect within 2 hours of cleaning. All carbohydrates contribute to plaque formation because they supply energy used in biosynthesis of the macromolecules and the proliferation of bacteria.

Caries. Dental decay is a common condition. Its etiology is multifaceted and involves the resistance of the tooth enamel, the nature of the plaque, including its bacteria, and the diet ingested by the individual. Of these factors, the dental plaque is probably the most important. The most commonly accepted theory today is that acids produced by bacteria in the plaque begin to decalcify the inorganic tooth enamel when the pH goes as low as 5.5. However, plaque and saliva also offer some protection, since it has buffering qualities. Acid-producing cariogenic bacteria and carbohydrates must both be present in order for decay to develop. Any carbohydrate in the mouth stimulates acid production by bacteria, but sucrose seems to be the most effective form. The longer carbohydrate remains in the mouth after ingestion, the longer it takes for the pH to return to normal levels; therefore, increased frequency of ingestion and ingestion of sticky substances such as caramels or honey cause the acid level in the mouth to be elevated for longer periods of time with an increase in cavity production. The only treatment for caries is prevention.

Periodontal Disease. The early form of periodontal disease is gingivitis, inflammation of the gingiva. The late form of the disease is periodontitis or pyorrhea. In *periodontitis* the inflammation extends from the gums into the periodontal pockets, resulting in loosening of the teeth as their supporting structures are destroyed (Fig. 60–1).

Gingivitis is manifested by bleeding of the gums from minor trauma. There is usually some alteration in color of the gingiva and there may be swelling, but pain is not a prominent symptom. It is characterized by inflamed gingiva, with the formation of pockets that gradually deepen and eventually cause destruction of the underlying tissues and separation of the gingiva from the tooth.

Preventive Measures and Oral Hygiene. The only method of control of periodontal disease and caries is prevention. Caries can be prevented by either increasing the resistance of the enamel or decreasing the hazards which surround the tooth. The former is accomplished with the use of flourides while the latter, a multifaceted problem, is aided by thorough cleansing to remove plaque, decreasing the frequency of eating, and reducing the ingestion of between-meal sweets, especially sticky, adherent ones. Removal of plaque is the best defense against gingivitis and thus periodontal disease. Since plaque cannot be removed without friction, rinsing the mouth is ineffective alone. Toothbrushing, the use of dental floss, interdental cleansers, and water irrigation under pressure are the most important means of oral hygiene. The friction measures dislodge the plaque and debris and rinsing removes it.

Research has shown that reducing the carbohydrate content of the diet reduces the amount of decay that occurs. Since this is difficult to accomplish in the average person, other approaches have been to incorporate agents in the dentifrice that will either neutralize the acid or destroy the bacteria. This approach has not shown very promising results. The use of mouthwashes is of dubious value because their effect wears off in from one half to three hours, depending upon the strength of the solution; also, microorganisms tend to develop resistance to the solutions. To be most effective they should be used at least twice a day, and the brand should be changed routinely to prevent bacteria from building up resistance.[154]

Work is in progress to provide a means of *immunization against caries*. Saliva contains IgA plus an additional component, and it has been shown to contain antibodies against several strains of decay-producing bacteria. On this basis, immunizations have been given into the mucous membrane in the vicinity of the salivary glands in an effort to increase their antibody formation. These animal experiments indicate that it may be possible to develop a vaccine against caries, but it is too soon to predict the end result of this reserach. In addition to this possible antibacterial action, saliva also

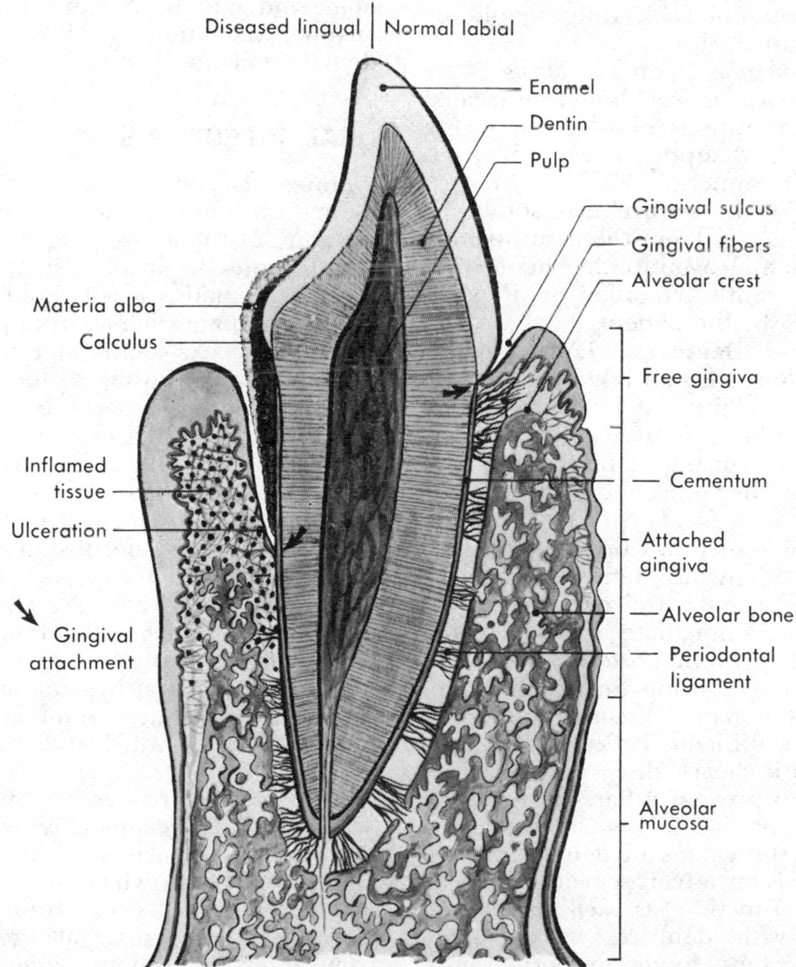

Figure 60–1. Periodontal disease. Diagramatic representation of a tooth. The right side illustrates normal healthy tissues. Note, on the left side, the destruction of alveolar bone and periodontal fibers which hold the tooth in place. (Courtesy Department of Dental Hygiene, University of Washington School of Dentistry.)

has an important role in caries protection due to its cleansing action to remove food debris mechanically and its buffering effect.

Dental Emergencies. A patient sustaining an injury that *fractures a tooth* must be seen by a dentist, as entry of bacteria into the pulp canal of the tooth can cause infection.

Postextraction hemorrhage can be either primary, occurring within an hour or two of the extraction and usually caused by dislodging of the clot, or secondary, probably caused by infection in the socket or a loose clot. Both types of hemorrhage can be treated in an emergency situation with the application of local pressure. A sterile gauze pad, applied over the extraction site with the patient biting upon it, frequently brings about hemostasis. Sometimes biting on a moistened tea bag is a successful home remedy since pressure is achieved and the tannic acid in the tea helps to promote hemostasis. Any continued bleeding should be treated by a dentist.

Emergencies such as deep *lacerations of the gums* and *fractures of the jaw* should be treated by a surgeon. Lacerations bleed freely owing to the excellent blood supply. Local pressure is the best first aid treatment.

In any wound of this nature, care should be taken to remove debris from the mouth gently to prevent accidental aspiration. This can be accomplished by gentle irrigation or, if possible, gentle rinsing by the patient.

Extractions and Dentures. Local application of ice for alternate half-hour periods will help to prevent swelling after a tooth extraction. Patients should eat only bland soft foods and avoid vigorous rinsing of the mouth. Frequent gentle oral hygiene will make the patient feel better.

Extractions are sometimes done in the hospital when the patient has complicating medical conditions or when a full denture extraction is to be done. Immediate insertion of the denture helps to prevent postoperative swelling and provides a covering for the open operative area, but makes subsequent fitting of the denture more difficult. Patients with a history of rheumatic heart disease are usually given penicillin to prevent a flare-up from the transient bacteremia that follows an extraction.

Regardless of the claims of dental adhesive products in television advertisements, artificial dentures never function as well as natural teeth. Patients with dentures usually need added time to chew foods properly. Since many individuals have dentures at the age when the gastrointestinal tract is less able to cope with improperly masticated food, this has an important influence on the total nutrition of the individual. Many people have poorly fitting dentures that are uncomfortable. Tissues of the mouth and jaw change during the lifetime, especially after the removal of teeth, so dentures may need to be modified to achieve proper fit and efficiency. Only 6 per cent of persons with dentures visit a dentist regularly for proper maintenance of the prosthesis. The extent of this problem is evident when one considers that there are an estimated 4 million denture wearers who have worn their dentures more than 23 years and another 15 million who have worn theirs more than 13 years.[135] Nurses should encourage patients to seek dental aid to achieve better mastication.

Persons who wear dentures should massage the gums twice daily when dentures are out of the mouth for cleansing. This stimulates circulation of the underlying tissues.

Since many individuals are sensitive about wearing dentures, partially because the dentures change their appearance, and partially because they equate dentures with aging, the nurse must be tactful in mentioning them. Some individuals do not wish to be seen by anyone, including their spouse, unless the dental appliance is in place.

ORAL INFECTIONS

Stomatitis. Stomatitis is an inflammation of the mouth; inflammation of the tongue is glossitis; and of the gums, gingivitis. These may be of infectious origin or a symptom of systemic disease. Stomatitis is commonly caused by mechanical trauma such as from jagged teeth, biting the cheeks, and mouth breathing; by chemical trauma owing to foods and drinks or sensitization to contactants such as mouthwashes and dentifrices; or by infection with organisms such as viruses, streptococci, borrelia, yeasts, and molds. Patients who are receiving chemotherapy for cancer frequently develop a severe, very painful stomatitis.

A person who has a sore mouth has little interest in eating, has excessive salivation, and may have a foul breath. Treatment, in addition to removal of the cause, consists of frequent soothing oral hygiene and topical medications, which are sometimes applied in mouthwashes. A soft bland diet is usually necessary.

Aphthous Stomatitis (Canker Sore). There is no agreement as to the etiology of these lesions, which are ulcers of the mouth and lips. Factors which have been suggested include emotional stress, trauma, vitamin deficiency, food and drug allergy, endocrine imbalance, viral infections; some consider them a manifestation of herpes. There is much evidence that they occur as a result of hypersensitivity. They heal spontaneously in from one to two weeks. Topical or systemic steroids shorten the healing time, and the routine administration of steroids has suppressed their recurrence in susceptible individuals.

Herpes Simplex. By the age of 5 years, 90 per cent of the population have had an infection, usually asymptomatic, of primary herpes simplex. The majority of the cases of recurrent herpes simplex take the form of herpes labialis (fever blister, cold sore). The lesions occur as clear vesicles, which are most frequently located at the mucocutaneous junction of the lips and face. They heal without scarring in about a week. People differ greatly in their susceptibility to the blisters. Some develop them following very short exposure to sunlight or heat or after a very short period of fever. Given sufficient stimulus, almost every adult will develop one.[15]

Unless the ulcer is secondarily infected, antimicrobial treatment does not affect the progress of the ulcer. The only treatment is symptomatic; local ointments and anesthetics may soothe the lesions. Some think that repeated vaccinations prevent the occurrence of these lesions, but reserach studies have not validated this.

Vincent's Angina. Formerly thought to be very contagious and frequently called "trench mouth," this infection is a gingivitis that is manifested by ulcers that are covered with a pseudomembrane. It is caused by fusiform bacteria and spirochetes that are resident in most people's mouths. It is now thought to be brought on by poor oral hygiene, nutritional deficiencies, local tissue damage, and debilitating disease. There are acute, subacute, and chronic forms, depending upon the severity of the symptoms. The acute form manifests itself by the sudden onset of a sore mouth, spontaneous bleeding of the gums, the presence of a membrane, and a foul odor. Treatment is the removal of the devitalized tissues and correction of the underlying cause by such measures as rest, bland diet, and vitamins. Pain medications and peroxide mouthwashes are also used to promote patient comfort.

ORAL TUMORS

Leukoplakia. Leukoplakia is an area of hyperkeratinization which is yellow-white or gray-white in color, occurs in any region of the mouth, is of varying sizes and shapes, is usually elevated with a roughened or leathery surface, and has clearly defined borders. This lesion is caused by chronic irritation of the mucosa by physical, thermal, or chemical means, and is sometimes related to systemic factors such as poor nutrition or syphilis. These lesions are frequently precancerous and sometimes cover an already malignant lesion. They should be watched carefully, and a biopsy should be taken if there is any question about the lesion or if it changes in character. Any irritating cause should be eliminated. Since these lesions can be readily seen in the mouth, the nurse should be alert for their presence and report them.

Cancer. The death rate for cancer of the mouth is much greater than it should be considering the incidence of this disorder and the availability of the oral cavity for inspection and case finding. The majority (90 per cent) of the malignant lesions in the mouth are squamous cell carcinomas, of which 70 per cent occur on the lips, lateral border of the tongue, and floor of the mouth. They are more than twice as common in men as in women.

Cancer of the tongue has the poorest prognosis because of the extensive vascular and lymphatic supplies to this organ and probably also because its vulnerable position exposes it to all manner of trauma inflicted from within the mouth. Cancer of the lip — with a cure rate of 80 to 90 per cent — has the best prognosis, probably due to early diagnosis.

The lesions ulcerate early, tend to be fixed and hard, and typically are not painful. Any lesion in the mouth which does not heal in 2 weeks should be examined by a competent physician, especially in persons over 55 who have a history of smoking and the use of alcohol. Previously it was thought that leukoplakia was the most common precursor to cancer in the mouth, but recent research has found that "red, velvety, erythroplastic lesions with white speckling" are most frequently the initial sign.[151] This same study identified the floor of the mouth, sides and underside of the tongue, and the soft palate complex as the most frequent sites.

Etiologic factors seem to be poor oral hygiene with bacterial irritation, physical trauma as from jagged teeth or improperly fitting dentures, or chemical and thermal trauma from tobacco, alcohol, and hot or spicy foods. Malnutrition, syphillis, and cirrhosis have also been found to be present in a large number of patients with this condition.

The cancer spreads primarily by local extension and to regional lymph nodes, but rarely invades the venous system to form distant metastases. The condition is diagnosed positively only by biopsy. Cytologic study has been shown to be of significant value in screening, but unfortunately is not used widely enough to have reduced the mortality rate. Cytologic examination, when used as a diagnostic aid, is performed on any suspicious appearing mucosa and is followed by biopsy when the reports show questionable cells. Cancer of the mouth, even when completely cured, tends to recur in another primary lesion. Studies have shown significant increases in the incidence of recurrence in patients who continue to use alcohol or tobacco after the first lesion is treated.[113, 149]

Treatment is primarily by surgical excision or by radiation, depending upon the location and type of cell.

Benign Tumors. The most common benign tumors of the mouth are fibromas, lipomas, neurofibromas, and hemangiomas. As with benign tumors in other parts of the body, they cause problems for the patient mainly by occupying space and by pressure. They can usually be excised when they cause the patient functional or cosmetic problems.

DISORDERS OF THE SALIVARY GLANDS

Inflammation. The most common inflammation of the salivary glands is parotitis, that is, inflammation of the parotid glands, or surgical mumps. However, any of the salivary glands can become inflamed. This is probably usually the result of inactivity of the gland caused by certain medications and lack of oral feeding. As secretions of the salivary glands diminish, oral bacteria have an opportunity to invade and multiply. Good oral hygiene to keep the bacterial count of the mouth as low as possible is probably the best preventive measure in addition to keeping the patient well hydrated and stimulating secretions of the glands by various means such as sucking on hard candies or chewing.

Calculus. Stones, or calculi, usually form in the salivary glands as a result of inacitivity of the gland combined with a metabolic condition favoring precipitation of salts. As with stones in other locations, a focus or nidus is necessary for stimulating the precipitation of the salt. Irritation from the stone causes local inflammation, swelling, and pain when the gland is called upon to secrete, as during chewing. Treatment is local excision. Stones occur most commonly in the submaxillary glands, probably because this duct is longer and the secretions are more viscous and alkaline than those from other glands.

Tumors. Most tumors occurring in the salivary glands are benign. The most frequent malignant tumor is adenocarcinoma; cancer occurs more often in the submaxillary glands than in the parotids. Enlargement is the main symptom of both types of tumors, with the malignant ones growing more rapidly than the benign. Pain occurs when expansion within the capsule of the gland creates pressure on sensory nerves.

Some of the malignant tumors spread predominantly by means of the lymphatics and some by means of the veins. Some are radiosensitive. The decision as to type of treatment will be made on the basis of the type of cell and the extent of growth or spread.

Ludwig's Angina. This is a fairly rare condition in which infection from the mouth, usually from an infected tooth, spreads into the soft tissues below the chin and around the submaxillary glands. The patient has a fever, local swelling, and tenderness. The treatment is by antibiotics and local heat. If the infection is not checked, the patient can suffer acute respiratory distress as a result of pressure on the adjacent trachea and pharynx. The nurse should observe the patient for respiratory problems (see Unit XVI) and notify the physician before the condition becomes acute.

ORAL SURGERY

In addition to procedures involving the teeth and gums, surgery done in the oral cavity includes the repair of injuries and the removal of tumors. Any portion of the oral cavity, including the sinuses and nasal structures, can be affected. (See Unit XXIV for nasal and sinus conditions.) Removal of malignant tumors frequently involves a fairly wide local excision of tissue along with removal of associated lymph nodes. Since removal of these structures can interfere with talking, chewing, and swallowing and frequently results in a cosmetic defect, the rehabilitation of these patients following surgery can be quite a challenge. Various types of trauma also frequently result in a cosmetic defect and may cause problems in eating and speaking. Prosthetic devices are available to replace some of the hard tissue structures such as the hard palate and to seal off openings into the sinuses. These improve the appearance and aid in chewing and swallowing with varying levels of effectiveness.

Glossectomy. The removal of the tongue has vast implications for the patient, since the tongue is the major organ of taste and speech and is active in chewing and swallowing. The most common reason for removal of this organ is carcinoma. Because the tongue is a very vascular organ and has excellent lymphatic drainage, the prognosis is poor even following removal early in the disease process. Following surgery the patient's speech is difficult to understand. See section on emotional reactions below.

Mandibulectomy. Cancer occurring on the floor of the mouth or near the lower jaw sometimes requires removal of a portion of the mandible to achieve adequate excision. This results in a very noticeable cosmetic defect and also presents a problem in achieving adequate mastication. As with oral surgery for cancer, it is usually done in conjunction with a radical neck dissection.

Radical Neck Dissection. Since death from cancer of the oral cavity most frequently comes from pressure on the trachea, esophagus, blood vessels, and nerves in the neck as a result of spread of the tumor into the cervical lymph nodes, a radical neck dissection is frequently done on patients with this condition. (See Unit XXIV.)

Mandibular Fractures. Trauma to the face or jaws sometimes results in fractures. As with fractures elsewhere, the segments must be immobilized in order to maintain alignment while healing takes place. Immobilization is accomplished by internal fixation with screws and plates or by wiring the teeth together. Wires are placed between the teeth and the two jaws are held together by means of rubber bands stretched between the upper and lower jaws. These can easily be removed in case the patient experiences difficulty such as choking or vomiting. The patient will be unable to chew while these wires are in place, so will be fed a liquid diet. Oral hygiene is important and, with the exception of the exterior surfaces of the teeth, can be done only by frequent rinsing or irrigation of the mouth. The diet is monotonous in consistency, and the patient tends to experience constipation because of a lack of bulk, but since these fractures heal fairly rapidly, the jaw immobilization usually lasts only from 4 to 5 weeks.

Nursing Management in Oral Surgery

The nursing care needed by this patient is determined by the extent of the procedure, the location of the incisions, whether a tracheostomy has been done, and whether the patient is able to talk and swallow. Catheters are frequently used under the skin flaps to eliminate the need for large bulky dressings. These will be attached to some source of suction. Dressings vary from none at all to large bulky ones. There may be packing present in the mouth, nose, or sinus cavities.

Airway. Maintenance of an airway is the most critical need for these patients. If the surgical procedure has been extensive, most of them will have a tracheostomy to prevent respiratory difficulty as a result of edema and swelling of the oral and pharyngeal structures. Patients are positioned in a sitting posture after surgery to promote venous and lymphatic drainage. They may have a dusky appearance about the face resulting from venous congestion rather than from poor aeration. Checking the color of the fingers and toes will show whether proper oxygenation is being achieved. Restlessness and apprehension in this patient may be symptoms of air hunger rather than pain. (See Unit XVI for nursing care of the tracheostomy patient.)

Nutrition. Normal eating may be difficult because of swelling, the location of suture lines, or because swallowing is impossible. A nasogastric tube, which is placed during surgery, is frequently used to provide nourishment. If it is accidentally dislodged, it should not be replaced without checking with the physician because of potential damage to the suture lines. Sometimes a gastrostomy is done for feeding purposes; occasionally the patient is able to drink a liquid diet.

Pain. Pain is not as much of a problem for these patients as their appearance would indicate. Frequently mild analgesics are all that is needed to keep them comfortable. Swelling is the cause of most of the discomfort.

Oral Hygiene. Mouth care gently and frequently given is mandatory for these patients. Some centers use a gentle spray to cleanse the tissues instead of irrigations or cotton-tipped applicators. Solutions frequently used are physiological saline, weak hydrogen peroxide, and weak sodium bicarbonate. Antibiotic solutions or dilute mouthwashes may also be ordered. Suction tips used to aspirate the irrigating solutions from the mouth should be handled with care to prevent trauma to the exposed sutures. Gentle care given frequently is essential to patient comfort and infection-free healing.

Saliva. When the patient is unable to swallow, the management of saliva becomes a problem. A wick placed in the mouth with the other end in an emesis basin is one way of collecting it when the patient is in bed. The basin should be emptied frequently, as the pan is apt to spill in the bed and because of the odor that results from decomposing saliva.

Complications

Hemorrhage. This can occur in the first few hours after surgery or several days postoperatively and can be massive because of the large vessels that supply this area. Local pressure is the best method of meeting this emergency until the physician can be reached. Usually the repair will have to be done in the operating room.

INFECTION. When this occurs there may be severe pain. Frequent oral hygiene is a preventive measure. Local medications may be used to treat a wound infection from anaerobic organisms, and systemic antimicrobial therapy may be employed.

Emotional Reactions of the Patient

Patients who undergo radical oral surgery and, to a lesser extent, those who have minor procedures done have a number of adjustments to make. We are all influenced by our physical appearance, and when this is altered, especially when the contours of the face and jaws become abnormal, the patient feels conspicuous and different. The head and neck are publicly visible, so deformities are evident to others. In addition to disfigurement, these patients also have normal fears about surgery and about having cancer, and they frequently experience difficulty in breathing and communication.

Fear, anger, and grief are normal reactions to this situation. Consider Mr. M.'s difficult adjustment to oral surgery. He probably has generalized fears of the future, the outcome of his condition, and his ability to live normally, as well as specific fears of rejection by others, of being alone, of being unable to communicate his needs, and of the occurrence of sudden complications. Anger at the general situation, his loss, and his helplessness to control it are part of the grieving process. It is necessary for him to go through this as he learns to accept his situation and reconstructs his life style.

The nurse must recognize these problems and give support to Mr. M. as well as to his family and friends as they attempt to work through the situation. The family may need explanations concerning the necessity for the patient to grieve and the normality of his reactions to the situation. They will probably also experience the same emotions.

When Mr. M. is unable to communicate, the problem is to help him express his needs and feelings adequately. The nurse can provide paper for him to write down his thoughts and his needs and should check on him frequently so he will know that he is not alone. A call bell should always be placed conveniently and should be answered promptly. Much communication can be accomplished by sign language and a few written words. The sensitive nurse can communicate compassion and concern to the patient and find out from writing and from nonverbal replies to verbal questions what his specific needs and problems are. The nurse's manner should communicate acceptance as he is to the patient. It is a temptation to treat persons who cannot talk as though they also cannot hear or understand. The nurse must be alert to any tendency on the part of staff or visitors to treat these individuals as though they are mentally incompetent.

Mr. M.'s inability to eat normally is another factor for him to accept and may be the one he feels safe in complaining about. Remember that his complaints are probably directed at his general situation rather than at the nurse as a person.

An attempt should be made to help this patient begin to meet others by walking about the hospital corridors. This type of patient is usually up and about quite soon after surgery, and social encounters and physical activity are both good for him.

CHAPTER 61

ABNORMALITIES OF SWALLOWING AND OF THE ESOPHAGUS

REVIEW OF ANATOMY AND PHYSIOLOGY

The esophagus is a hollow muscular tube that is collapsed in its resting state. It is composed of striated muscle in the upper portion and smooth muscle in the lower. There is a sphincter mechanism at both ends of this tube, and there are areas of natural narrowing where the aorta and left mainstem bronchus pass it. These four narrowed areas are also the points at which disease processes most frequently occur (Fig. 61–1).

The esophagus is innervated by the 10th and 11th cranial nerves and also has sympathetic nervous fibers from the cervical and thoracic areas. Its intrinsic nervous control comes from the intramural plexus (Auerbach's) in the mucosal layer. Although pressure within the esophagus is lower than pressure within the stomach, stomach contents do not normally regurgitate into the esophagus because of pressure at the cardiac sphincter (lower esophageal sphincter). The act of swallowing initiates a wave of peristalsis, or contraction, which moves down the esophagus to the stomach. This contraction is preceded by a wave of relaxation. Food from the esophagus is propelled into the stomach by this peristaltic wave, by gravity, and by the opening of the cardiac sphincter during the wave of relaxation.

Symptoms of Disorders. *Dysphagia*, or difficulty in swallowing, is the most prominent symptom of any disorder of the esophagus. This may be difficulty in initiating the act, pain in relation to the act, or a feeling that the food is meeting resistance and sticking or pausing as it passes a particular portion of the esophagus. Food and fluids may be aspirated or regurgitated through the nose when the difficulty is in the pharyngeal phase of swallowing. (See Fig. 58–3.)

Heartburn or *pyrosis* is another common symptom of esophageal disease. The term is frequently used by patients to describe very different sensations, so it is important to find out what this term means to the patient who uses it. It usually means substernal midline burning, which tends to radiate, generally in waves, upward to the neck. It is important to find out if the symptom is amplified when the patient lies down or bends over.

Esophageal regurgitation is the bringing of gastric contents up into the mouth without eructation and without the propulsive wave of reverse peristalsis present in vomiting. This tends to occur when stomach contents have refluxed into the esophagus or when the esophagus does not empty into the stomach.

Causes of Swallowing Problems. Swallowing is a highly complex act and causes of difficulty are numerous. Most problems are due either to some mechanical obstruction or to neuromotor malfunction. (See Chapter 58, especially Fig. 58–3.)

Constriction of the passageway by congenital defects or such acquired conditions as tumors, inflammation, strictures, or hiatus hernia will cause difficulty in passing food masses that are larger than the constricted area. The patient usually first experiences difficulty in swallowing solids and then liquids when the problem is mechanical.

Motor dysfunction can be caused by a problem in the reflex coordination of the act, by brain damage as from trauma or a CVA, or by a muscular disorder. Brain damage in the area of the medulla, which controls swallowing, or in the area of cranial nerves that coordinate the act (5th, 7th, 9th, 10th, and 12th) are common reasons for swallowing problems. In neuromotor disorders it is usually equally difficult to swallow solids and liquids. Neuromuscular disorders that can upset this delicately balanced act of swallowing include scleroderma, polymyositis, and diabetes mellitus. Myasthenia gravis can reduce the force of the propulsive wave.

Dysphagia may also result from cardiovascular abnormalities — particularly in the elderly. Specific conditions causing vascular dysphagia

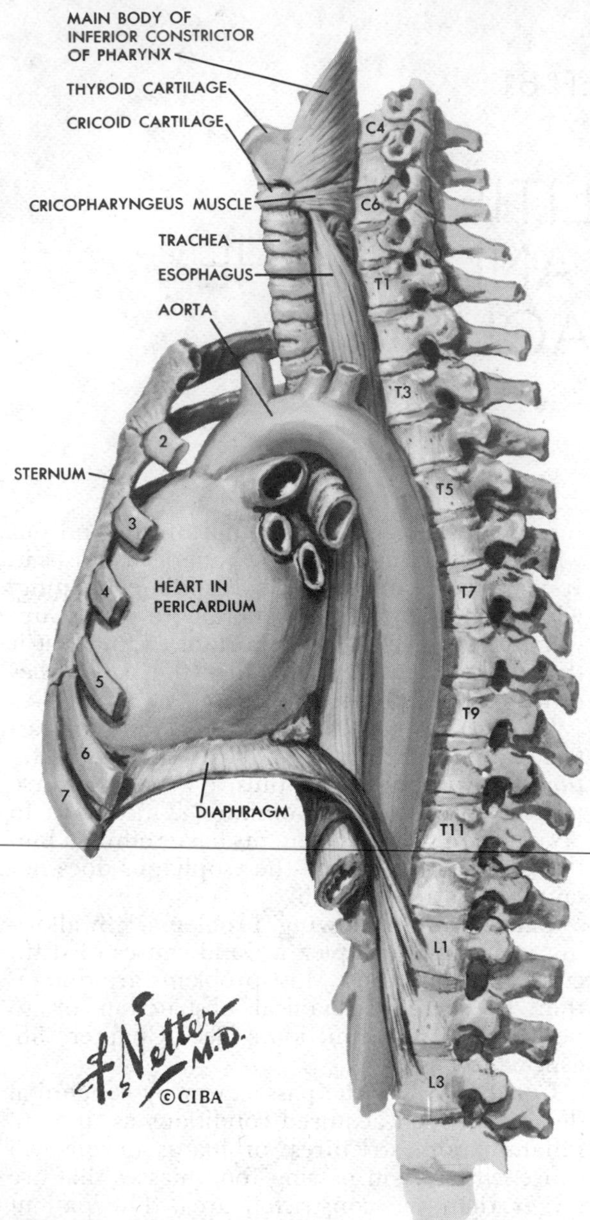

Figure 61–1. Relationship of esophagus to adjacent structures. © Copyright 1959 CIBA Pharmaceutical Company, Division of CIBA-GEIGY Corporation. Reproduced, with permission, from THE CIBA COLLECTION OF MEDICAL ILLUSTRATIONS by Frank H. Netter, M.D. All rights reserved.

include: an enlarged heart, aneurysm of the aorta, and calcification of the descending aorta. The relationship of the heart and great arteries to the esophagus is clearly shown in Figure 61–1.[93]

DISORDERS OF THE ESOPHAGUS

Structural

Congenital Anomalies. Several anomalies can occur during the embryonic development of the esophagus in its separation from the trachea. The two principal types of anomalies are atresia and fistula, which occur in several different forms. These become evident shortly after birth, since the infant is unable to swallow without either regurgitating the fluid or aspirating it into the lungs. The most common types of anomalies are pictured in Figure 61–2. All of these require prompt surgical repair if the infant is to survive. Consult a pediatrics nursing text for the details of diagnosis, treatment, and nursing care.

Diverticula. A diverticulum is a pouch opening out from a hollow viscus. They occur in the esophagus at the pharyngoesophageal sphincter, in the midesophagus at the level of the bifurcation of the bronchus, and in the region near the diaphragm. The second two are called traction diverticula, are relatively rare, and frequently cause no symptoms.

A pulsion diverticulum, also called Zenker's diverticulum, is seen most often in males over 50 years of age. It occurs on the posterior wall of the pharynx above the upper border of the cricopharyngeus muscle and results from excessive pressure during swallowing, usually the result of the pharynx contracting before the sphincter relaxes. The sac gradually enlarges and descends into the superior mediastinum. The major symptom is the sensation of a foreign body in the throat and dysphagia for both solids and liquids (Fig. 61–3).

As the diverticulum enlarges, it gradually alters the alignment of the esophagus and pharynx so that the most direct route from the pharynx is into the diverticulum rather than down the esophagus, causing an increasing volume of food to enter the diverticulum. Complications are malnourishment from inadequate intake and tracheal aspiration as a result of regurgitation from the sac when the person lies down. Perforation of the sac results in contamination of the mediastinum, with potentially grave sequelae. This could occur during the passage of a nasogastric tube or esophagoscope.

Strictures. Strictures may be of inflammatory, traumatic, or congenital origin. Esophagitis, radiation, and corrosive burns are the most frequent causes. Treatment includes removing the cause, if possible, and performing dilatations. Surgical excision may be necessary.

Achalasia. This condition is sometimes called cardiospasm or aperistalsis. It is caused by failure of swallowed food to enter the stomach and results in esophageal dilatation. It is probably due to the lack of a normal peristaltic wave, so that no stimulus for opening the cardiac sphincter occurs. A distended esophagus can cause pressure on the trachea, producing dyspnea and cough, and on the great vessels and heart, resulting in cardiac problems. Tracheal aspiration of foods retained in the esophagus occurs when the patient lies down.

The most probable cause of the condition is degeneration of innervation, either from the vagal motor nuclei or the myenteric plexus (Auerbach's). The interruption varies from mild to complete. Since innervation is destroyed, the only treatment is to dilate or cut the sphincter. This must be done extensively enough to allow the food to pass through but not so much as to allow the gastric contents to reflux back into the esophagus and cause esophagitis. In addition to dilatation, nonsurgical treatment includes helping the patient to learn to relax and to live with the condition.

Hiatus Hernia. This is a diaphragmatic hernia in which a portion of the stomach is herniated through the esophageal hiatus of the diaphragm. It can occur from sudden penetrating or compressive trauma or it can develop through congenital or acquired weaknesses in the diaphragm. In both the congenital and acquired weaknesses, intra-abdominal pressure, as from obesity, pregnancy, ascites, and physical exertion, can cause the abdominal contents to herniate upward through the defect (Fig. 61–4).

Symptoms of the disorder, which vary from none at all to acutely severe, come mostly from esophageal reflux of gastric contents. The extent of symptoms is determined by the size of the hernia and the amount of compression placed on the herniated portion of the stomach. The resulting venous congestion and increasing pressure cause interference with passage of food into the stomach. Traumatically induced herniation can cause shock, hemorrhage, and pneumothorax.

Surgical treatment reduces the hernia through an abdominal or thoracic approach, depending upon the size of the hernia and the nature of the defect. Medical management aims to control the symptoms by avoiding overdistention of the stomach, reducing acidity of the stomach, and reducing the intra-abdominal pressure. The patient is instructed to (a) eat frequent, small, bland meals, (b) take antacids, and (c) take no anticholinergic drugs because they delay emptying of the stomach. The patient should also avoid coughing and activities that involve bending forward. The patient usually has the head of the bed elevated to help to prevent esophageal reflux during sleep.

Neoplasms

Benign. There are very few benign lesions of the esophagus, and most of these are asymptomatic. Leiomyoma accounts for more than half of those that do occur.

Malignant. Cancer of the esophagus occurs predominantly in men over 50 and accounts for only 2 per cent of cancer deaths. The mortality rate for carcinoma of the esophagus in white males in this country has remained constant since 1930, while the incidence among nonwhite males has risen from 1.3 to 10.2 per 100,000 male population between 1934 and 1966. Nonwhite males acquire this disease at an average age of 55.2 as opposed to 62.3 for white males. The reason for these differences is not clear. The worldwide incidence of the disease varies from country to country and from one area of a country to another. The ratio of incidence between males and females also varies from location to location. The etiology is unknown, but study is being made of the environmental differences between the locations with a low and high incidence. It is generally agreed that smok-

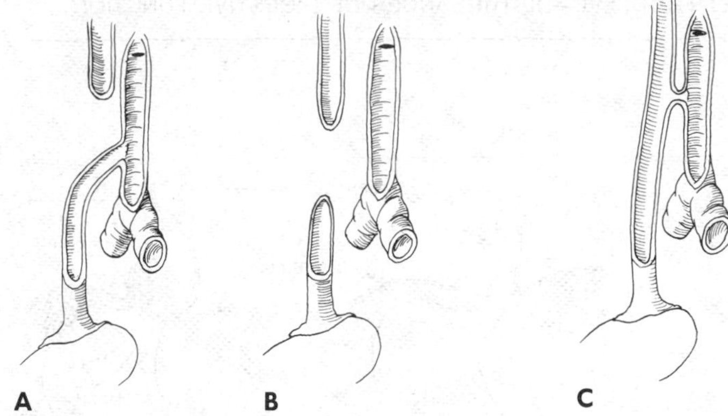

Figure 61–2. The most common forms of tracheoesophageal fistula and esophageal atresia. **A.** Atresia of the upper portion of the esophagus with a fistula connecting the lower portion of the esophagus to the trachea. **B.** Esophageal atresia without tracheal involvement. **C.** Fistulous connection of a normal trachea and esophagus (H-type fistula). (From Davis, L. A.: *Nursing Clinics of North America*, 8:443, Sept. 1973.)

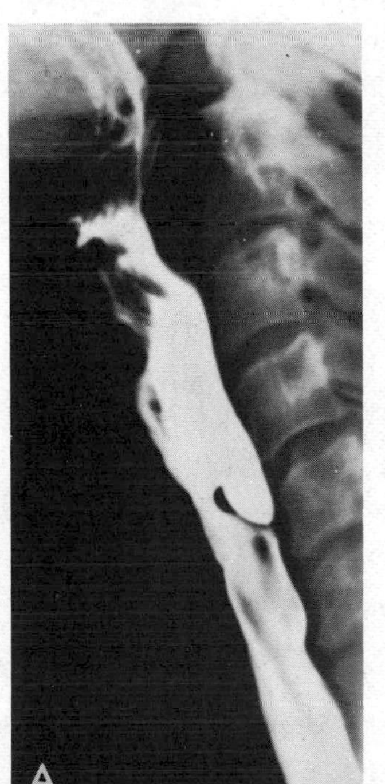

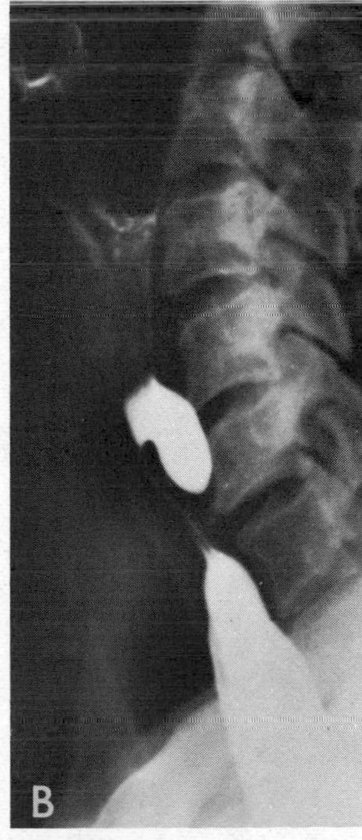

Figure 61–3. Zenker's diverticulum. **A.** Bolus filling diverticulum as it passes down the esophagus. **B.** Filled diverticulum with remainder of bolus in lower esophagus. (From Valdes-Dapena, A. M., and G. N. Stein: *Morphologic Pathology of the Alimentary Canal.* Philadelphia: W. B. Saunders Co., 1970, p. 61.)

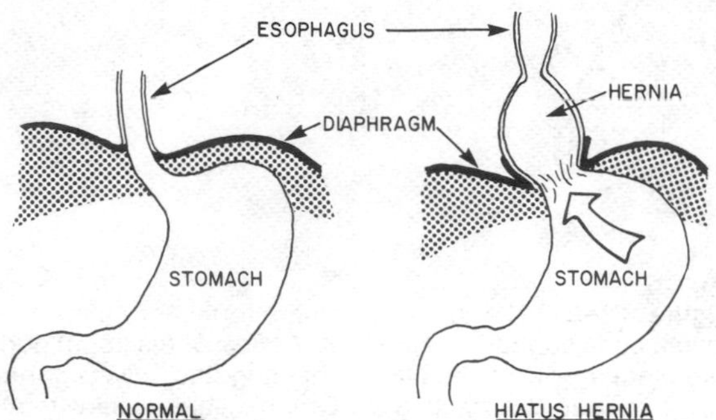

Figure 61–4. Diaphragmatic hernia. The normal esophagus and the mechanism of a hiatus hernia are shown. The diaphragm muscle stretches across the midpoint of the abdomen and the chest cavity. The hernia occurs at the juncture of the stomach and the esophagus as a result of weakness or relaxation of the opening in the diaphragm. (From Howard, R. B., and N. H. Herbold: *Nutrition in Clinical Care.* New York: McGraw-Hill Book Company, 1978, p. 351.)

ing and the ingestion of alcohol and hot foods and drinks are related to the development of this disease. Research data at present suggest that dietary deficiencies may increase susceptibility to the disease.

The prognosis of cancer of the esophagus is very poor, with a 3 year survival rate of 5 per cent. The reasons for this are the early lymphatic spread and late development of symptoms. The tumor growth causes a reduced amount of flexibility in the normally very distensible esophagus, causing most of the symptoms. The first symptom is typically dysphagia, but this usually does not occur until the tumor involves the whole circumference of the esophagus. By the time this symptom is reported to the physician, the tumor has frequently invaded the deeper layers of the esophagus and sometimes even adjacent structures such as the bronchus.

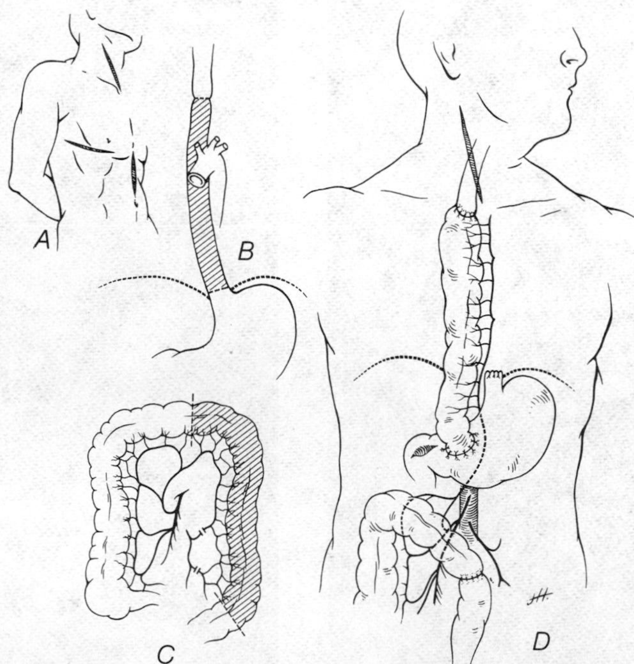

Figure 61–5. Esophagectomy with interposition of left colon. **A.** Incision. **B.** Shading indicates portion of esophagus to be resected. **C.** Mobilized portion of colon. **D.** Completed operation. (From Schwartz, S. I., et al.: *Principles of Surgery,* 2nd ed. New York: McGraw-Hill Book Co., 1974, p. 1036.)

Tumors occur in any part of the esophagus, but the majority are in the lower two thirds. Diagnosis is made by barium swallow, esophagoscopy, cytologic examination, and direct biopsy.

Treatment is mainly surgical, with the major objective being to enable the patient to continue eating. Even when the tumor is small enough to be resected, a cure is not achieved. Cobalt radiation produces palliation by reducing tumor size and slowing growth, but it tends to cause fistulas to develop. Dilatations can be done to maintain the size of the lumen. Chemotherapy using methotrexate has given symptomatic relief, and 5-FU and cyclophosphamide injected directly into the lesion have given relief from dysphagia.

Various approaches have been used to maintain continuity of the esophagus and to allow the patient to eat normally after resection of the tumor: the stomach may be brought up into the mediastinum after the esophagus is shortened by a resection; a segment of the colon may be implanted to replace the resected portion (Fig. 61–5); an artificial prosthesis may be inserted in the lumen; or a channel may be made to the exterior above and below the resected portion and an exterior tube used to connect them. None of these approaches is very satisfactory, but they have all achieved the purpose of allowing the patient to continue to eat normally for a longer period of time. When these approaches are impossible, a gastrostomy is usually done to maintain the patient's nutrition.

Trauma

The major traumatic conditions that affect the esophagus are chemical burns, foreign bodies, and injuries from external forces or from examination with an esophagoscope. Chemical burns occur from the ingestion of acids or alkalies and sometimes from the ingestion of highly spiced foods. Thermal burns can result from drinking extremely hot liquids. Foreign bodies are most apt to lodge in the natural narrow spots of the esophagus. Possible results of trauma are perforation with a resultant contamination of the mediastinum and stricture formation as healing occurs.

Treatment for strictures is by dilatation or

surgical excision of the diseased portion and re-anastomosis or interposition of a tube from the stomach or colon.

Vascular Disorders

Esophageal varices are the major disorder of vascular origin. Since these are the result of pressure in the portal system, they are discussed with liver conditions in Unit XVIII.

Inflammatory Disorders

Esophagitis is an inflammation of the mucosa and submucosa that is usually caused by the reflux of gastric juices into the lower esophagus. The most prominent symptoms are heartburn; intolerance of spices, alcohol, and caffeine; and regurgitation, sometimes with vomiting. The patient may also experience dysphagia. Esophagitis is usually associated with hiatus hernia, but it can also occur independently. It is due to failure of the cardiac sphincter of the stomach to maintain enough pressure to prevent gastric contents from entering the esophagus.

Treatment is aimed at preventing the gastric juices from damaging the esophageal mucosa by the use of oral antacids, a bland diet, avoiding eating before lying down, and sleeping with the head of the bed elevated. Surgical approaches are intended to reduce the acidity of the stomach, as by a vagotomy, or to reduce reflux by tightening the sphincter muscle.

NURSING CARE OF THE PATIENT WITH A DISORDER OF THE ESOPHAGUS

Even though conditions that affect the esophagus differ widely in etiology, the symptoms are similar, varying mostly in intensity and time of occurrence. Difficulty in swallowing and discomfort due to regurgitation of gastric contents are the major symptoms presented by these patients. Nursing care needs, which are determined in large measure by the symptoms, are related to maintaining nutrition because of the swallowing difficulties, preventing complications resulting from malnutrition, and minimizing discomfort, since regurgitation and inability to eat cause both physical and psychologic pain. Nursing care will be discussed on the basis of the symptoms that may be presented by the patient.

Dysphagia. This symptom varies from a mild feeling that food is sticking in the throat or esophagus to the total inability to consume foods or fluids. The patient who is admitted to a health care facility because of difficulty in swallowing should be closely observed by the nurse, since diagnosing the cause is one of the major aims of care. The nurse should record what kinds of foods are tolerated best — solids or liquids, hot or cold food – and whether the patient swallows better when alone or when in a social group, and whether the time of day makes a difference in swallowing ability. These observations will aid the physician in determining the cause, which might be psychogenic, neurologic, muscular, or a space-occupying lesion.

The patient who has a tumor within the lumen of the esophagus will experience increasing difficulty in taking food. More complete chewing and a diet that is thinner in consistency will aid in swallowing for a while. Encourage such patients to take only small bites and to chew the food thoroughly before attempting to swallow. Help them to relax during meals by making them physically comfortable and by minimizing sources of emotional stress.

Patients with acute dysphagia are frequently malnourished and may have problems as a result of altered electrolyte and metabolic balances. Thus, they are candidates for the complications of debilitating disease such as decubitus ulcers and pneumonia. They are particularly prone to developing respiratory complications from aspirated materials.

Aphagia. Many problems ensue when the patient is unable to swallow anything, even liquids, because of a tumor or stricture in the upper esophagus. Since saliva and other nasopharyngeal mucous secretions must go somewhere, the patient can easily choke and must spit frequently or else drool. Constant wiping of saliva from the lips can cause irritation, with cracking of the skin and open lesions. Since it is impractical to collect this quantity of secretions in tissues, the patient should carry a receptacle to receive them. As most people find the sight of a jar of expectorated saliva repugnant, it is helpful if the jar is covered or made of opaque material and has a screw lid. This jar should be emptied often, because of the odors which result from the presence of decomposing bacteria, pus, blood, and saliva. An exudate may be present, resulting from bacterial growth and necrosis of the devitalized tissues in the tumor mass.

When the tumor mass or stricture is in the lower two thirds of the esophagus, the patient's symptoms will come from distention of the esophagus and regurgitation.

Patients should have frequent oral care to maintain a tolerable taste in their mouths. A pleasant tasting mouthwash, a mild bicarbonate solution, or a physiological saline solution can be used. Diluted hydrogen peroxide is effective against anaerobic organisms and is sometimes mixed half and half with a mouthwash. The mouth should be rinsed often, and care taken to keep it in as healthy a condition as possible. Some patients chew food and expectorate it, to help maintain the health of the oral tissues. This also stimulates the secretion of digestive juices and is helpful when done just before a tube feeding.

GASTROSTOMY. When surgical methods of providing a route from the mouth to the stomach fail, a gastrostomy is frequently done. Occasionally a nasogastric feeding tube is left in place. In either method, the patient must be provided nutrition through a tube, which means that the pleasure of eating and chewing is lost and that all food ingested must be in liquid form. (See Chapter 59 for gavage techniques.)

A gastrostomy is made by suturing the anterior wall of the stomach to the abdominal surface and tightly suturing either a valve prosthesis or a tube (frequently a Foley catheter) into the opening. The tube prevents leakage of the acid gastric juices onto the abdominal wall, and the attachment between the wall of the stomach and the abdomen prevents the leakage of gastric contents into the abdominal cavity.

The skin about the opening should be washed with a gentle soap and thoroughly dried twice daily, or whenever secretions leak. Protective ointments such as zinc oxide can be applied to the skin for lubrication and for protection from secretions.

Intake of nutrients and fluids through the gastrostomy is essential to this patient's continued life. Significant others should also know how to manage the feedings. Frequently these patients remain at home, and nursing supervision will aid the family in coping with problems that arise. In addition to routine health supervision, the nurse should check facets of care related to the gastrostomy, such as urinary and bowel elimination. An inadequate urine output might mean that the patient is getting insufficient fluids via the gastrostomy tube or that the kidneys are overloaded with nitrogenous products. Constipation could indicate an inadequate fluid intake, or it could result from the liquid feedings. Diarrhea can be caused by improper storage of the feedings, or it could be due to the formula used in the feedings.

The nurse should check for evidence that the tube is patent and that the patient is using proper technique in caring for it and also is consuming a well balanced diet.

Since a gastrostomy, if done for cancer, is a palliative measure, the patient and significant others will need support from the nurse, as for any dying patient.

Discomfort. Heartburn is the usual symptom of regurgitation of stomach contents into the esophagus. Its origin is not certain, but is thought to be due to irritation of the esophageal mucosa by the acid secretions of the stomach. Antacids help by neutralizing the acid secretions. Emptying of the esophageal contents into the stomach is sometimes facilitated by having the patient maintain an upright position (never slumped) for several hours after meals and by promoting relaxation. Help the patient to relax. Of course, the cause of the retention of food in the esophagus may alter the approach to treatment.

When the esophagus is occluded and swallowed food is retained, discomfort comes mainly from the distention and the shortness of breath caused by pressure on the lungs. Little can be done except helping the patient to relax and encouraging ingestion of smaller amounts at one time. Dilatations of the stricture and sometimes surgery are the treatments of choice.

Observations to be Made on Patients with Esophageal Problems

In addition to the observations of the patient's ability to swallow, the nurse should also observe and report the patient's general *nutritional status, state of hydration* and *weight.* Some patients are able to obtain sufficient foods and fluids even with great difficulty in swallowing. Other patients may need supplementary fluids and nourishment.

Pain — its type, duration, location, and the time of its onset — is a significant factor, as is the presence of gaseousness as evidenced by eructations, abdominal distention with tympanites, and flatulence. Does the patient retain the food eaten? Is it regurgitated, or is it vomited? If the food is vomited from the stomach with propulsive waves, is this accompanied by nausea?

The patient's *acceptance of the condition* and *general mental state* are important in evaluating probable acceptance of some of the potential treatment measures. Significant others and their helpfulness to the patient as well as their emotional stability are also important factors to assess.

NURSING CARE OF THE ESOPHAGEAL SURGERY PATIENT

In addition to the usual factors involved in nursing care of the surgical patient, there are some specific things to consider when a patient has esophageal surgery, but they depend upon where in the esophagus the problem is located and the patient's nutritional status. A gastrostomy may be done to enable the patient to take a high-protein, high-caloric diet preoperatively, since a poorly nourished patient is not a good surgical risk. In most surgical procedures the patient should be prepared for a chest incision and be taught about chest tubes and coughing, as are other thoracic surgical patients. (See Chapter 57 for care of the thoracic surgical patient.)

Depending upon the procedure to be done, the patient's prognosis will vary from excellent to very poor. The surgical procedure may offer a hope of cure, as in a pulsion diverticulum or benign stricture, or it may offer only palliation, as in surgery for cancer of the esophagus. Procedures that are done for incompetency and overcompetency of the cardiac sphincter are only partially successful. The nurse should find out from the surgeon what the probable survival results will be before discussing anticipated surgery with the patient. Patients should not receive, even indirectly, an expectation of results that are impossible to achieve.

After surgery the patient will probably have both chest and gastric suction and an incision that extends from the thoracic region to the abdomen. A tracheostomy may be present. A nasogastric tube is usually placed in the stomach during surgery and attached to suction to remove fluids and drainage from the surgical site and to divert food and fluids away from the surgical anastomosis until healing has taken place. It should not be removed or adjusted, because the suture line might be damaged by trauma from the tube. It will remain in place postoperatively until enough healing has occurred to allow food and fluids to pass without danger of the formation of a fistula into the mediastinum.

In the immediate postoperative period, maintenance of patency of the chest, tracheostomy, and gastric tubes is the most important nursing responsibility.

The major goal of care in the convalescent surgical period is to aid in the healing of the esophageal suture lines by keeping the gastric suction open and functioning. This prevents tension from distention and keeps the tubes free from secretions, fluids, and food which might leak into the mediastinum, creating a fistulous tract and causing infection. The patient may be kept flat in bed immediately after surgery to prevent pulling and tension on the suture line when an anastomosis has been created in the esophagus.

In addition to the usual observations made on a postoperative patient, this patient should be observed especially for respiratory complications and for the occurrence of a fistula and/or infection. Mouth care is important in the prevention of both of these complications. Routine postoperative measures such as leg and arm and breathing exercises are also extremely important.

Patients who are not allowed to eat for 10 days to 2 weeks after surgery may have a gastrostomy for feeding purposes, or if a nasogastric tube is left in place, a diet may be instilled through it.

After an oral diet has been resumed, the patient who has had his or her stomach brought up into the thoracic cavity may experience discomfort because of the presence of a full stomach within the chest. Procedures in which the cardiac sphincter has been eliminated or made incompetent may leave the patient with heartburn from esophageal reflux of gastric acid. Ingestion of small meals, remaining upright after meals, sleeping with the head of the bed elevated, and taking antacids will help to control these symptoms.

When the patient is ready, oral feeding resumes with clear water and gradually progresses to soft foods as the ability to swallow develops. A high esophageal anastomosis may create difficulties for the patient in relearning to swallow.

CHAPTER 62

ABNORMALITIES OF THE STOMACH AND PROXIMAL DUODENUM

ANATOMY AND PHYSIOLOGY

Digestion, which has started in the mouth, continues in the stomach by the action of saliva in the center of the bolus. Gastric secretions begin the next phase of digestion by breaking down connective tissues and beginning the digestion of proteins, as described earlier in this unit. There is very little absorption within the stomach. Alcohol and acetylsalicylic acid are the two most important chemicals absorbed there. The chief functions of the stomach are to mix the chyme and to regulate the flow of gastric contents into the upper intestine. The rate of emptying depends upon the volume ingested, the thoroughness with which it has been chewed, and the nature of the ingested foods. Fats and foods that have been poorly chewed are retained longer.

SYMPTOMS OF DYSFUNCTION

Symptoms of dysfunction are caused by excessive gastric secretions (which feed upon the stomach mucosa), by excessive motility, or by retention of gastric contents. The most prominent symptoms are pain, acid eructations and belching, nausea, vomiting, hemorrhage, and diarrhea.

Pain, the most characteristic symptom, is caused mostly by acid in contact with eroded stomach mucosa resulting in chemical irritation of nerve endings. It is also caused by stretching and sudden contractions of the stomach, which results in a stretching of the nerve terminals. This can be caused by increased motility and increased smooth muscle tension, as found in an obstruction.

Anorexia, loss of appetite occurs in various diseases such as hepatitis and is also present in mental depression. Hunger is caused by a number of stimuli, including contraction of the empty stomach. When the stomach empties slowly, one normal stimulus of the hunger sensation is missing and anorexia can result.

Nausea is produced by any condition, such as unpleasant stimuli or distention, that increases tension on the walls of the stomach, duodenum, or lower end of the esophagus.

Vomiting can follow nausea or occur without it. Vomiting is caused by stimulation of the emetic center, which is in the medulla near the sensory nucleus of the vagus. It is influenced by the chemoreceptor trigger zone as well as by nerve impulses and can be excited by (1) direct mechanical stimuli, as in increased intracranial pressure; (2) chemical stimuli from bloodborne metabolites or toxic substances; and (3) sympathetic and parasympathetic afferent nerve impulses through the vagus, glossopharyngeal, vestibular, and the splanchnic nerves. In most people higher center impulses such as those caused by unpleasant odors, subjects, and sights can also stimulate vomiting. Drugs of the phenothiazine derivative group, such as chlorpromazine (Thorazine), promazine (Sparine) and prochlorperazine (Compazine), depress vomiting caused by chemoreceptor stimulation.

Bleeding results from local trauma or irritations that cause erosion or ulceration of the mucosa. Possible sources of upper gastrointestinal bleeding include:[183]

Esophagitis
Neoplasm in the esophagus
Varices
Esophageal ulcer
Hiatus hernia
Neoplasm in the stomach
Gastric ulcer
Gastritis
Anastomotic (marginal) ulcer
Duodenal ulcer
Duodenitis

While bleeding may arise from numerous causes, up to three quarters of all cases of upper gastrointestinal bleeding are caused by (a) esophagogastric varices, (b) hemorrhagic gastritis, or (c) peptic ulcer.

Diarrhea can be caused by increased peristalsis resulting from an increased gastrocolic reflex or from the effort of the stomach and intestines to eliminate a local irritant.

Belching and *flatulence* are caused predominantly by swallowed air. Frequently the individual attempts to belch to relieve a vague feeling of distress in the stomach. When attempting to belch with the mouth closed, the person sometimes adds more air to the stomach than he removes. Air is swallowed easily during eating and drinking, especially by nervous persons who ingest food rapidly.

FUNCTIONAL DISORDERS

Gastric functions are mediated through both the autonomic and central nervous system activities. The central nervous system is strongly influenced by social, environmental, and psychologic stimuli; these factors also affect the individual's gastric response. *The stomach mirrors the emotions.*

Indigestion (Dyspepsia)

Since the factors influencing digestion are so numerous, dyspepsia can be due to emotional problems, to disease of the gastrointestinal system, to disease processes elsewhere in the body, or to such things as eating too rapidly, chewing inadequately, eating during a period of emotional upset, poorly cooked foods, or ingestion of certain foods that tend to form gas. Food allergy may be responsible. Symptoms usually occur from altered gastric secretion or motor activity. They include a feeling of fullness, nausea, belching or eructations, heartburn, and flatulence. Table 62-1 lists causes of altered motility and secretion.

Anorexia Nervosa

This condition was first described over one hundred years ago; since that time many researchers have attempted to determine the cause and thus the treatment. It is a condition, predominantly of teenage females, in which they feel "too fat," find food very distasteful, and adamantly refuse to eat. Weight losses of 25 to 50 per cent of body weight result. Symptoms include periods of hyperactivity, compulsive overeating followed by vomiting (frequently self-induced), and a hysterical or obsessive personality. Other symptoms, probably due to the state of starvation, include amenorrhea, constipation, fine hair over the body, bradycardia, and hypotension. (See Figure 7-4.)

Although the etiology is unknown, most authorities feel it has a psychoneurotic basis; recently, however, an abnormality of hypothalamic function has been proposed to explain both the metabolic and psychologic malfunctions. Most authorities still attribute these abnormalities of thyroid, androgen, and cortisol metabolism to the state of starvation.

The first aim of treatment is to improve the state of nutrition so that therapy can be undertaken to overcome the underlying problem. Gentle persuasion to encourage the patient to eat is the preferred method of achieving weight gain, but this is difficult to accomplish and sometimes tube feedings are used. Psychotherapy and behavior modification are frequently used together in the total therapeutic approach. These patients are usually hospitalized to control the environment, provide a consistent approach, reduce physical activity, and monitor intake. Drugs of the phenothiazine group and tricyclic antidepressants are sometimes given to enhance the other means of therapy.

Obesity

The presence of an excess of adipose tissue in the body is termed obesity. It is caused by a caloric intake that exceeds the energy expenditure. Although it can be the result of a metabolic dysfunction, it is usually due simply to overeating. A number of metabolic abnormalities are present in obese persons, but they are probably the result of the obesity rather than the cause.

Recent studies have shown that individuals who are overweight in childhood, especially before the age of 2 years and immediately prior to puberty, develop an increased number of fat cells, which remain throughout life. After weight loss, the size of the cells become smaller, but the *number* of cells does not diminish. One

TABLE 62-1. CAUSES OF ALTERED GASTRIC MOTILITY AND SECRETION

Increased Motility	Decreased Motility
Hunger Prospect of appetizing food Pleasant sensory stimuli Moderate distention Alcohol Coffee Hostility Anxiety Resentment	Marked distention (overeating) Ingestion of fats Smoking Physical fatigue Unpleasant sensory stimuli Pain Fear Shock Depression Sadness
Increased Secretion	**Decreased Secretion**
Sight, smell, and taste of food Prolonged anxiety, guilt, conflict, hostility, or resentment Presence of food in stomach Removal of large part of intestines	Depression Release of enterogastrone Fear Gastric pH of 1.5 or less Fats, carbohydrates and acids in duodenum

theory states that these cells continue to stimulate overeating because the increased number of fat cells apparently release more hormonal or other appetite stimuli than would be released from a normal number of fat cells.[81] However, recent studies of fat babies have not shown a significant number to be obese in later childhood.[159, 185]

The average person balances food intake with metabolic needs so that weight remains fairly constant throughout adult life. A weight gain sometimes accompanies aging because the individual does not adjust food intake to a lowered metabolism and diminished activity.

Obesity tends to run in families, but this is probably the result of eating habits learned in the home rather than an inherited dysfunction. Some people eat to satisfy their emotional needs. This is encouraged when parents feed children to reward or comfort them. These individuals upon becoming adults, may reward or console themselves with food in any situation of joy, adversity, or sorrow. Food can become the individual's major source of gratification and solace.

Diet. The basic treatment for obesity is dietary. A number of diets are advocated but, at the present time, there is no basis for recommending one over another, except that a weight loss diet must provide fewer calories than the person's energy expenditure while — over the long term — supplying the nutrients necessary for health.

Fasting, or complete abstinence from food, can be tolerated for repeated periods of 10 to 15 days if fluids and vitamins are provided; it results in an average weight loss of one pound per day. Complications include postural hypotension, anemia, cardiac irregularities, and a decreased uric acid excretion with a hyperuricemia, which is reversed when the fast is halted and may then result in uric acid neuropathy and retention of sodium and water. It is best that the individual be hospitalized when this method of therapy is used.

Drugs. Appetite depressant drugs from the amphetamine group are sometimes used at the beginning of a diet. They are effective for only a few weeks and may cause problems because of their stimulating effects. More importantly, it is sometimes difficult to withdraw the person from their use because they are addictive.

Exercise. As a method of weight loss this is not of practical value because of the amount of exercise needed to lose one pound; however, any added activity increases the energy output and increases the caloric deficit of a patient who is following a weight loss diet. In some sedentary patients a little increase activity without any alteration in dietary habits can make the difference between maintaining weight and achieving a small weight loss. Any obese patient who is on a calorie-restricted program should have a planned, gradually increasing program of energy output to aid in weight loss and to tone muscles.

Support Groups. Most obese people need the support and encouragement of others who understand the extreme difficulty of the battle to reduce food intake. The *best treatment for obesity is appetite re-education* in which the individual learns to eat and be satisfied with nutritious, well-balanced foods that are low in calories. Support groups such as TOPS (Take Off Pounds Sensibly, a nonprofit organization), Weight Watchers, Inc., and other weight loss groups and clinics seek to help the individual by various approaches. In some areas Overeaters Anonymous Groups have organized that imitate the Alcoholics Anonymous approach. Individuals differ in their needs and psychological make-up, so each person should seek the approach that meets his or her needs for support and/or admonishment. Most of these groups seek to educate the individual regarding nutrition as well as encourage adherence to a weight loss diet. Since weight tends to be self-sustaining, vigilance and continued support are needed to maintain losses that are achieved. None of these approaches will work, however, unless the individual is motivated to lose weight.

Surgery. One surgical approach to treating obesity is an attempt to reduce the ability of the body to absorb nutrients that are ingested. This is done by short-circuiting the small bowel. Trial has shown that the best results from this type of surgery are obtained when a shunt is created by severing the jejunum 14 inches from its beginning and anastomosing this end to the terminal ileum 4 inches above the ileocecal valve (Fig. 62–1). This leaves the patient with 18 inches of small bowel. The weight loss after operation averages 11 pounds per month for 6 months and then 6 pounds per month the second 6 months, 4½ pounds per month the second year, and 2 pounds per month the third year.

When an optimal weight is reached, the patient tends to maintain it. When the short circuit has been removed surgically and the bowel returned to normal, patients have regained their former weight.[157] Postoperatively the patient may have diarrhea for a time because of induced malabsorption. Other complications include liver dysfunction, malnutrition, electrolyte imbalance, and kidney stones. These complications have occurred more frequently when the jejunum was attached to the colon (jejunocolostomy). This surgery should be reserved for the extremely obese person, weighing 300 or more pounds, for whom weight loss is essential to the maintenance of health. Reanastomosis has been necessary due to complications in from 20 to 50 per cent of cases. Tapper reports performing a subtotal gastrectomy when he re-anastomoses the bowel to prevent regaining of weight.[186]

Before the surgery is done, a psychiatric evaluation should be made, as patients who have been meeting emotional needs or escaping problems by their excessive weight may have other problems after a weight loss. Degeneration of the marital relationship has occurred quite frequently as one spouse loses weight.[136a]

Another surgical approach that has gained popularity recently is the gastric stapling procedure. In this method, staples are placed across the top part of the stomach, creating a small pouch to receive ingested food. A small opening is left in the line of staples to allow the food to slowly enter the rest of the stomach (Fig. 62–2). Depending upon the size of the pouch created, the patient can only eat about 56 grams of food at one time. Pain is caused by another 30 grams and very little over 100 grams (3.5 ounces) causes vomiting. The advantages of this surgery over the bypass procedures are in the shorter length of time it takes to perform and the lessened chance of infection, since the gut is not opened. To date, no complications have been reported following this procedure.[66a]

Complications. Atherosclerosis and its associated ischemic heart disease are caused by the altered metabolism of obesity. Hypertension and left ventricular hypertrophy occur as a result of pumping blood through an enlarged vascular bed. Diabetes mellitus is four times more common in the obese individual.

INFLAMMATIONS

Acute Gastritis. The acute form of gastritis may be manifested by nausea and vomiting, hemorrhage, pain, malaise, anorexia, or headache and is usually due to ingestion of a corosive, erosive, or infectious substance. Aspirin, acute alcoholism, and food poisoning are common causes. This type of gastritis is usually of short duration unless extensive damage is sustained by the gastric mucosa. Treatment is to remove the cause and treat the condition symptomatically. Vomiting frequently responds to some of the drugs of the phenothiazine group given orally or intramuscularly; pain usually responds to antacids. If hemorrhage is severe enough, a transfusion may be necessary.

Chronic Gastritis. This condition is seen in three different forms:

Superficial gastritis causes a reddened, edematous mucosa with hemorrhages and small erosions.

Atrophic gastritis occurs in all layers of the stomach, with a decreased number of parietal and chief cells. This form of gastritis is seen frequently in association with gastric ulcer and gastric cancer and is invariably present in pernicious anemia.

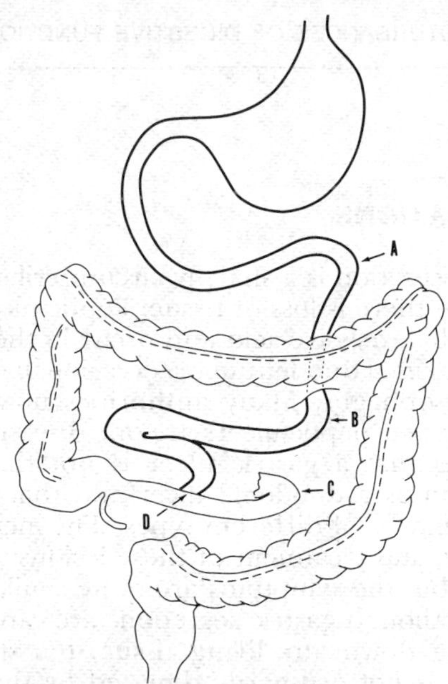

Figure 62–1. Representation of the "14 and 4" surgical procedure for weight reduction for obesity. *A* represents the ligament of Treitz; *B* represents the 14 inches of jejunum beyond the ligament of Treitz which is left in continuity. *C* represents the remainder of the bypassed jejunum and ileum, and *D* represents the end-to-side jejunoileostomy. (From Bockus, H. L.: *Gastroenterology,* 3rd ed, Vol 2. Philadelphia: W. B. Saunders Co., p. 322.)

Hypertrophic gastritis produces a mucosa that is dull and nodular in appearance and has irregular, thickened, or nodular rugae. Hemorrhages are frequent.

Chronic gastritis usually heals without scarring but can go on to hemorrhage and the formation of an ulcer. Symptoms of chronic gastritis are vague and may be absent. The patients are apt to have a loss of appetite, a feeling of fullness, belching, vague epigastric pain, and nausea and vomiting. Most patients learn to avoid foods that cause symptoms. Antacids sometimes give symptomatic relief.

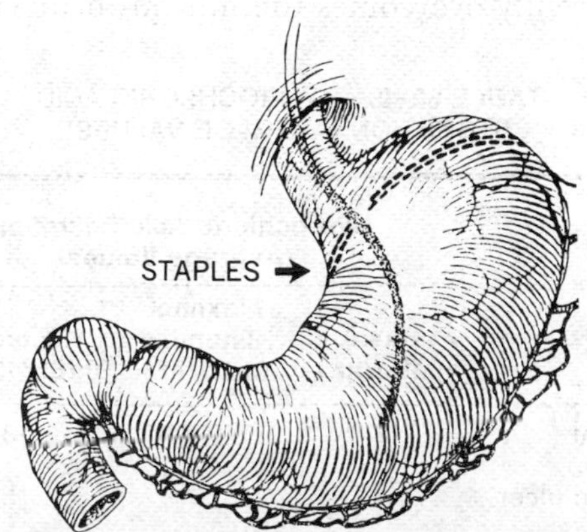

Figure 62–2. In gastric stapling, a row of stainless steel staples is used to seal off top part of stomach. Procedure does not entail reconnection of any parts of intestinal tract. (From Elliott, J.: More help for the morbidly obese: Gastric Stapling. *JAMA,* 240:1941, Oct. 1978.)

ULCERATIONS

An ulceration is a sharply circumscribed area in which there is loss of tissue. Peptic ulcers are caused by excessive acid and occur in the stomach, proximal duodenum or, occasionally, in the lower esophagus. Many authorities now question whether peptic ulcers are one disease entity and feel that a gastric ulcer is not the same condition as a duodenal ulcer and that gastric ulcers may be of different types. The incidence, etiology, and treatment of these lesions are different, but the symptoms are quite similar.

Even though gastric secretions are capable of breaking down any living tissue, the stomach mucosa is not ordinarily digested by them because they are adequately diluted, neutralized, and buffered before they can harm the mucosa; also, the mucosa is thickly covered by a protective layer of mucus. An alteration in either of these defense systems can cause autodigestion to occur. Another protective mechanism is the rapidity with which the gastric mucosa normally heals. In addition to peptic and gastric ulcers, acute gastric erosions, which are frequently called "stress ulcers," occur after an acute medical crisis such as head injury, burn, shock, septic state, or trauma and after ingestion of chemically irritating substances such as aspirin or alcohol.

Types of Ulcers

Peptic, Duodenal, and Gastric Ulcers. Duodenal ulcers and some prepyloric gastric ulcers are caused by an increased quantity or an increased level of acidity of the gastric juice, which apparently overcomes the mucous blanket. Hypersecretion of acid continues between meals when there is no stimulus for secretion. (See Table 62–2.) The cause of this is unknown, but in duodenal ulcer it is thought to be of vagal origin because a vagotomy reduces it.

TABLE 62–2. HYDROCHLORIC ACID SECRETION (AVERAGE VALUES)

	Hydrochloric Acid Secretion (Average Values)		
	Basal (mEq/hr.)	Maximal Histamine (mEq/hr.)	Nocturnal (mEq/12 hr.)
Normal	2	20	18
Gastric ulcer	4	20	8
Duodenal ulcer	8	35	60

Adapted from Beeson, P. B., and W. McDermott: *Cecil-Loeb Textbook of Medicine.* 13th ed, Philadelphia: W. B. Saunders Co., 1971, p. 1262.

Gastric ulcers are not associated with excessive acid levels, and theories as to their origin vary. One theory proposes that excess acid is secreted by the stomach but is resorbed by an abnormal diffusion of hydrogen ions through the mucous membrane, damaging the mucous barrier. Another theory suggests that destruction of the mucous blanket occurs from the reflux of alkaline duodenal contents. There is a variation in the number of parietal cells in relation to the location of the ulcer. The normal stomach is estimated to have 0.92 billion, while the stomach with a gastric ulcer has 0.65 billion, and the one with a duodenal ulcer has 1.72 billion. It is felt that vagal stimulation causes this increase in the parietal cell mass.

Psychogenic influences have been shown to affect the development of peptic ulcers. This is more true for the duodenal than the gastric ulcer. The tensions and strains of life cause an increase in the tonus of the vagus nerves, involving both the motor and secretory fibers. The secretions increase and the friability of the mucosa also increases. Those who live under stress, such as those with responsible managerial positions, are more prone to this disorder. However, prolonged psychotherapy has not proved to be of any help.

Stress and Drug-Induced Ulcers. As mentioned above, acute gastric erosions called stress ulcers occur after major assaults upon the body. The four clinical situations giving rise to gastroduodenal ulcerations are (1) severe trauma or major illness; (2) after severe burns (sometimes called Curling's ulcers); (3) head injury or intracranial disease (frequently called Cushing's ulcers); and (4) ingestion of drugs, e.g., aspirin and alcohol, which act on the gastric mucosa. Critically ill patients are susceptible to stress ulcers if they develop sepsis. Stress gastric mucosal changes develop within 72 hours in 78 per cent of patients with burns of greater than 35 per cent total body surface area. Twenty five per cent of these burned individuals will develop definite stress ulcers, and 11 to 22 per cent will hemorrhage. Cushing's ulcers are associated with excessive acid secretions, which are thought to be stimulated by a rise in intracranial pressure and may involve the esophagus, stomach, or duodenum.[73]

Stress ulcers are manifested by superficial gastric erosions that are frequently accompanied by massive gastric hemorrhage. The patient characteristically has multiple lesions, usually small, which may give the appearance of "oozing blood." The mechanism causing these ulcerations is unknown but thought to be multiple. Experiments with the condition have shown that a low gastric pH (high acidity) is necessary for its development, but acid secretion in patients is frequently low or normal. However, antacids are sometimes given prophylactically to patients with major trauma. Menguy et al.[145] have proposed that the lesions are caused by a decrease in energy metabolism within the gastric mucosa, which causes a rapid cellular necrosis. The proposed basis for this diminished metabolism is ischemia of the mucosa caused by shock, hemorrhage, or cardiac dysfunction. It has been found that gastric ulcerations occur when ischemia of the mucosa occurs in association with a disruption of the mucosal barrier. This decrease in the protective ability of the mucous barrier can occur as a result of a chemical assault from food or drug ingestion, from reflux of bile, or from causes as yet unknown. Much research is being conducted in an effort to understand the precise mechanism by which stress ulcers occur.

Few symptoms accompany stress ulcer. These ulcers are typically painless unless perforation occurs; perforation fortunately is rare. Upper gastrointestinal hemorrhage is the major sign of stress ulcer. About 10 per cent of patients experience dyspepsia prior to hemorrhage.[73]

Treatments are usually directed at stopping the bleeding and include irrigation with ice saline solution, intra-arterial infusion of vasopressors, and administration of steroids, vitamin A, and growth hormone. Romero[164] reports that in 80 per cent of cases bleeding stops with these therapies; the other patients need surgery. Since the advent of flexible gastroscopes, some physicians recommend attempts to stop the bleeding by coagulation through the scope.

Zollinger-Ellison Syndrome. A non-islet cell tumor of the pancreas called a gastrinoma secretes high levels of gastrin without relation to the normal factors that cause the antral cells to secrete gastrin. The abnormal blood level of gastrin increases the volume of gastric secretions and results in multiple ulcers of the duodenum. Recurrent ulcers after a gastrectomy are sometimes caused by this tumor. The diagnosis is made by finding high levels of serum gastrin. Since removal of the tumor is impossible because it is difficult to locate and it tends to metastasize to multiple locations, the only treatment is to remove the acid-secreting ability of the stomach by a total gastrectomy.

Symptoms

The most common and typical symptom is chronic and periodic *pain,* which has been variously described as gnawing, aching, burning, and boring. It occurs from 1 to 4 hours after eating and may also occur in the middle of the night. The pain is sharply localized in the epigastrium to the left of the middle. Sometimes it occurs as heartburn. Periods of remission, which may last from a few months to a period of years, are common. Pain of this nature is pathognomonic of a peptic ulcer.

Weight loss, probably from a reduced intake of food, is typical, but some persons gain weight from excessive eating to neutralize the pain. Other symptoms relate to the development of complications. *Bleeding* from erosion through a blood vessel is common. It may occur as a massive hemorrhage or it may be occult from slow oozing.

Longstanding disease causes scarring from repeated ulcerations and repeated healing. Scarring at the pylorus frequently causes pyloric obstruction, which is manifested most often by pain at night as a result of the retention of acid. Pyloric obstruction can also lead to *vomiting.*

Perforation occurs when an ulcer erodes through the muscularis and is manifested by sudden, sharp, severe pain which begins in the midepigastrium and, as peritonitis develops, spreads over the entire abdomen, which then becomes hard and rigidly board-like. (See discussion of peritonitis in Chapter 63.)

Incidence

Ulcers, particularly duodenal lesions, are more common in men than in women. Both gastric and duodenal ulcers occur at all ages, but peptic ulcers have the highest incidence in the 45 to 55 year old group. The possible presence of a hereditary factor in the development of an ulcer, which has been suspected for years, has recently gained some credence. A relationship has been shown between the individual's ABO blood group and the site of occurrence of an ulcer. For instance, Johnson[112] found an association between blood group A and certain types of gastric ulcer. Also, the parietal cell mass, and consequently the rate of gastric acid secretion, are felt by some workers to be genetically determined.[176] Hereditary factors cannot be considered without also considering other factors that might influence the incidence, such as dietary habits, emotional reactions, and economic and occupational status, which are frequently similar among family members. Gastric ulcers are more apt to occur in the impoverished social groups, in the elderly, and in the poorly nourished

Diagnosis

Ulcers are diagnosed by the symptoms, by x-ray evidence, and by gastroscopy. The differentiation between the types of ulcers is sometimes difficult. The time lapse between eating and the onset of pain may help to pinpoint the location of the ulcer. Pain relieved by antacids or food is typical of duodenal ulcer. Acid determinations may be done on aspirated gastric juices, but the results are frequently not very helpful because individual variations tend to obscure the typical findings in each type of ulcer.

Complications

Hemorrhage varies from minimal, which is manifested by occult blood in the stool, to massive, in which the patient vomits bright red blood — hematemesis. The usual symptoms of GI bleeding are either vomiting coffee-ground material or passing tarry stools. Acid digestion of blood in the stomach results in a granular dark emesis, whereas the complete digestion process results in a black stool. If the patient bleeds rapidly enough, he can be prostrated and go into shock. It is important to locate the area of bleeding so treatment can be started. Observations as to the color, consistency, and quantity of emesis and stools and the time of their passing will help the physician to make this decision. A nasogastric tube may be inserted and lavage with iced water or saline carried out to slow or to stop the bleeding; angiography to identify the site of bleeding or gastroscopy to view the bleeding area may be done. A string test may be performed. In this test the patient swallows a measured string that is viewed for staining after its removal to help to locate the level of the bleeding.

Perforation is usually a surgical emergency, since anterior wall perforation, unless it is walled off by the omentum, causes a chemical peritonitis. Surgical treatment is usually limited to closure of the perforation by patching it with a bit of omentum and cleansing the peritoneal cavity. Mortality is high in this condition, about 10 to 15 per cent. If the perforation occurs on the posterior gastric wall, it may erode through to adjacent organs and be sealed off, causing few symptoms. Pancreatitis usually results when a perforation erodes into that organ.

Obstruction, manifested by vomiting, occurs at the pylorus and is due to scarring, edema, or inflammation, or a combination of these. When vomiting persists, the patient is apt to go into alkalosis as a result of losing large quantities of acid gastric juice in the emesis. A patient who vomits persistently is usually hospitalized to receive intravenous fluids fortified with electrolytes. Before stenosis causes complete obstruction, the patient will probably experience gradually increasing difficulty in emptying the stomach and have feelings of fullness, with a loss of appetite and weight loss. The treatment is surgical release of the scar.

Therapeutic Regimen

The goals of treatment for a patient with an ulceration are to prevent complications and to allow the ulcer to heal. Gastric mucosa has great regenerative powers, and ulcers frequently heal when the etiologic agent is removed. Mental, physical, and gastric rest is frequently sufficient therapy. Since psychogenic influences in the development of this condition are great, patients need emotional support while identifying the stressors in their lives and learning to either eliminate them or cope with them. In many cases the biggest problem is the patient's inability to recognize or admit the causes of stress.

Much of the therapeutic regimen is aimed at relieving symptoms. This means eliminating factors that stimulate secretions or harm the mucous barrier, especially smoking, alcohol, coffee, and ulcerogenic drugs such as aspirin, steroids, and indomethacin. Antacids are administered to neutralize excess acidity; they seem to work even when excess acidity has not been shown to be present.

Medical. Traditionally, diet and antacids have been the principal method of managing an ulcer. Milk and cream formed the basis of the diet and were taken every hour, with antacids given on half hour in between. Currently this has fallen into some disfavor. Many authorities feel that eliminating strong secretagogues, roughage, gas-forming foods, highly seasoned foods and stopping smoking is sufficient. Any food that causes pain should be avoided; these vary with the individual. Some physicians feel that six small meals are desirable, whereas others prefer the normal three-meal routine. In clinical studies a bland or ulcer diet had no detectable effect on a gastric ulcer, whereas bedrest and stopping smoking did have a beneficial effect.[128] This has not yet been investigated with a controlled study for duodenal ulcer. Antacids have been universally accepted as an effective method of relieving ulcer pain. Recently however some doubt has been cast on this universal belief. Studies have shown that antacids do not seem to accelerate ulcer healing.[128]

Medications. The rationale for using drugs in the treatment of peptic ulcers involves several different mechanisms: the reduction of secretions (hyposecretory drugs), the neutralization of acid (antacids), and the protection of the mucous barrier (mucosal barrier fortifiers).

Hyposecretory drugs which cause a reduction in acid secretions include the anticholinergics, prostaglandin analogues, and histamine antagonists.

Anticholinergics interfere with the transmission of nerve impulses at the neuro-effector junctions of the postganglionic nerves. They suppress both vagal and antral secretion mechanisms and produce what is sometimes called a medical vagotomy. The problem with these drugs is that they do not suppress acid secretion in response to food as well as they do the basal flow of secretion, and in order to achieve sufficient suppression of secretion a large enough dosage is necessary to cause intolerable side effects such as dryness of the mouth, blurring of vision, constipation and, sometimes, urinary retention owing to bladder atony. They also reduce the motility of the stomach, causing a feeling of fullness because of slowed emptying. There are many drugs of this nature on the market, but none is used for total therapy.

Prostaglandins are local tissue hormones which are formed from essential fatty acids and seem to be present in various forms in almost every tissue of the body. Two of them, E_1 and E_2 (PGE_1 and PGE_2) inhibit the secretion of gastric acid. Synthetic analogues of these have been developed, and early reports of their use indicate that they inhibit gastric secretions and hasten healing.[128]

Histamine antagonists which block histamine-stimulated gastric secretions have recently been developed. The usual antihistamine drugs such as dyphenhydramine (Benadryl) have no effect upon histamine-stimulated gastric secretions. A new class of antihistamines, called H_2 receptor antagonists, has been developed which block the action of the H_2 histamine receptors. The first drug of this type that is classified as safe for human use is cimetidine (Tagamet). Early results with this drug seems to indicate that it is very effective in healing both gastric and duodenal ulcers.[128]

The ideal *antacid* is one that decreases the acidity, is effective for a prolonged period of time, is pleasant to take orally, is not constipating or cathartic in effect, and is not absorbed to cause systemic effects. There is no perfect antacid. Calcium carbonate is a potent antacid but is constipating, and triggers gastrin release which causes a rebound acid secretion. Magnesium carbonate and magnesium oxide are also potent antacids but are laxative; they are sometimes prescribed to counteract the constipating effects of calcium carbonate. Frequently the patient takes them alternately or balances dosages of each to produce a stool of the desired consistency. Aluminum hydroxide, phosphate, and carbonate are less effective, since they only partially neutralize the acid. The magnesium and aluminum preparations are more palatable. Sodium bicarbonate is a potent antacid, but its effects are very brief and it is absorbed systemically. New products are on the market that are mixtures of aluminum and magnesium products with some calcium carbonate. Pharmaceutical firms have attempted to produce an antacid with ideal qualities by mixing these drugs. Table 62–3 lists the more commonly used antacids.

Mucosal barrier fortifiers are still in the developmental stage, but studies show carbenoxolone to be effective in preventing hydrogen ion back diffusion into the mucosa and in stimulating mucous production that results in accelerated gastric ulcer healing. There are several potential adverse effects from the use of this drug, including salt and water retention and occasionally hypokalemia and elevated blood pressure.[128]

Patient Education. Patient cooperation, which results from patient education, is a cornerstone of treatment. The patient needs and should receive instruction and understanding support from the medical and nursing personnel involved in his or her care. Along with the physician, the nurse can help the patient to:

- Understand the pathogenesis of the ulcer and the significance of the pain.
- Realize that healing takes place rapidly when the irritating effect is removed.
- Understand what caused the condition to develop and what must be done to lessen the stimulation so that a cure can occur and be maintained.
- Discover what substances cause pain by stimulating the secretion of gastric juices and eliminate them from the diet until healing has occurred. (Some substances can probably be consumed in moderation after healing has occurred.)
- Understand the importance of continuing the medical regimen, even though pain is gone, until healing is completed.

Nursing Responsibilities. Nursing management of the patient with an ulcer depends on the physical state of the patient. Both physical and psychosocial assessment of the patient are important nursing functions. Physical assessment includes accurately observing and immediately reporting to the physician symptoms that help pinpoint the diagnosis or symptoms that might indicate the presence of a complication. (Symptoms and complications are discussed in preceding sections.)

The nursing goal is to promote recovery by helping the patient achieve total rest — physically and mentally. This is done by maintaining the medical regimen and by arranging the patient's environment to encourage relaxation. Interacting with the patient and listening attentively allows the nurse to assess how to help the patient accept and maintain the prescribed dietary and drug regimen.

The nursing staff must be alert for factors that interfere with the patient's rest. Certain visitors or telephone calls may cause the patient to become agitated. Some patients attempt to carry on their normal work routine from the hospital bed; patients have been known to move a secretary and typewriter into the hospital room. In many cases the biggest problem is the patient's inability to recognize or admit that he or she is under stress and needs rest. The nurse may need great ingenuity and tact to plan and implement nursing interventions to help these patients meet their needs for physical rest and mental relaxation.

Surgical Treatment of Peptic Ulcer

Surgery of the stomach is done (1) to reduce the acid-secreting ability of the stomach, (2) to remove a malignant or potentially malignant lesion, or (3) to treat a surgical emergency that develops as a complication of peptic ulcer disease.

When medical management of an ulcer fails, surgical intervention is indicated. Most chronic, recurring ulcers are eventually treated surgically.

The possibility of cancer in a gastric lesion is a generally accepted indication for surgery. When an ulcer does not respond to intensive medical therapy and a definite diagnosis cannot be made by x-ray and gastroscopy, surgery is done to remove the lesion and to make certain it is not malignant.

Emergencies such as acute obstruction, perforation, and acute intractable hemorrhage are usually treated by surgical intervention as soon as possible. Hemorrhage, as mentioned, sometimes responds to medical management, but when medical approaches such as cooling and neutralization of the acid do not stop the bleeding, the situation is a surgical emergency, done to save the patient's life. In patients who are poor candidates for surgery, hemorrhage can sometimes be stopped or slowed temporarily by intravenous infusion of a vasoconstricting drug into the vessel nearest the site of bleeding. This is done after localization of the vessel by angiography.

Goals of Therapy. Since excess acidity is the cause of many ulcerations, the goal of surgery is

TABLE 62–3. GASTRIC ANTACIDS

Official Nonproprietary Name	Action*	Properties	Synonyms or Trade Names
Aluminum hydroxide gel	C	Slowly reactive as antacid	Amphojel
Aluminum phosphate gel	C	Slowly reactive as antacid	Phosphajel
Aluminum carbonate gel	C		Basaljel
†Calcium carbonate, precipitated	C	Chalky taste; may produce hypercalcemia, rebound gastric hyperacidity, or systemic alkalosis	Precipitated chalk Titralac
Dihydroxy aluminum aminoacetate	C	Less constipating and faster acting than aluminum hydroxide.	Alglyn, Robalate
Magaldrate	C	Aluminum and magnesium (mild) hydroxide in union as a single chemical	Riopan, monalium hydrate
Magnesium carbonate	L	High neutralizing action forms CO_2	
†Magnesium oxide	L	High neutralizing action	
Magnesium trisilicate	L	Slower onset of action	
Magnesium hydroxide	L	Some systemic action	Milk of magnesia; magnesia magma
Polyamine-methylene resin	L	May cause mild bulk action; low neutralizing action	Resinat, Carboresin
Potassium bicarbonate		Systemic action	
†Sodium bicarbonate		Systemic action; may cause rebound gastric hyperacidity and systemic alkalosis	Baking soda

Note: Magnesium salts should be given with caution to persons with impaired renal function.
*Key: C = constipating action; L... laxative or cathartic action
†Most potent agents

to reduce the acidity and thus allow the ulcer to heal. The surgical procedure may or may not remove the ulcer itself. In the presence of obstruction the second goal is to reestablish the patency of the lumen of the bowel by removing or relaxing the pyloric scar formation or by creating a new exit from the stomach.

Types of Surgery. The approaches for reducing acidity of the stomach surgically are (1) severing nerves that stimulate the acid-secreting cells and (2) removing the acid-secreting portions of the stomach.

A *vagotomy* is done to eliminate the acid-secreting stimulus to gastric cells. Three types of vagotomy might be done: *truncal, selective* (also called total gastric), and *proximal* (sometimes called highly selective or parietal cell) (Fig. 62–3*A*). The *truncal* vagotomy interrupts the parasympathetic innervation to the stomach, bile ducts, liver, pancreas, and small intestine. The *selective* vagotomy eliminates vagal stimulation to the entire stomach. Since the vagus nerve also

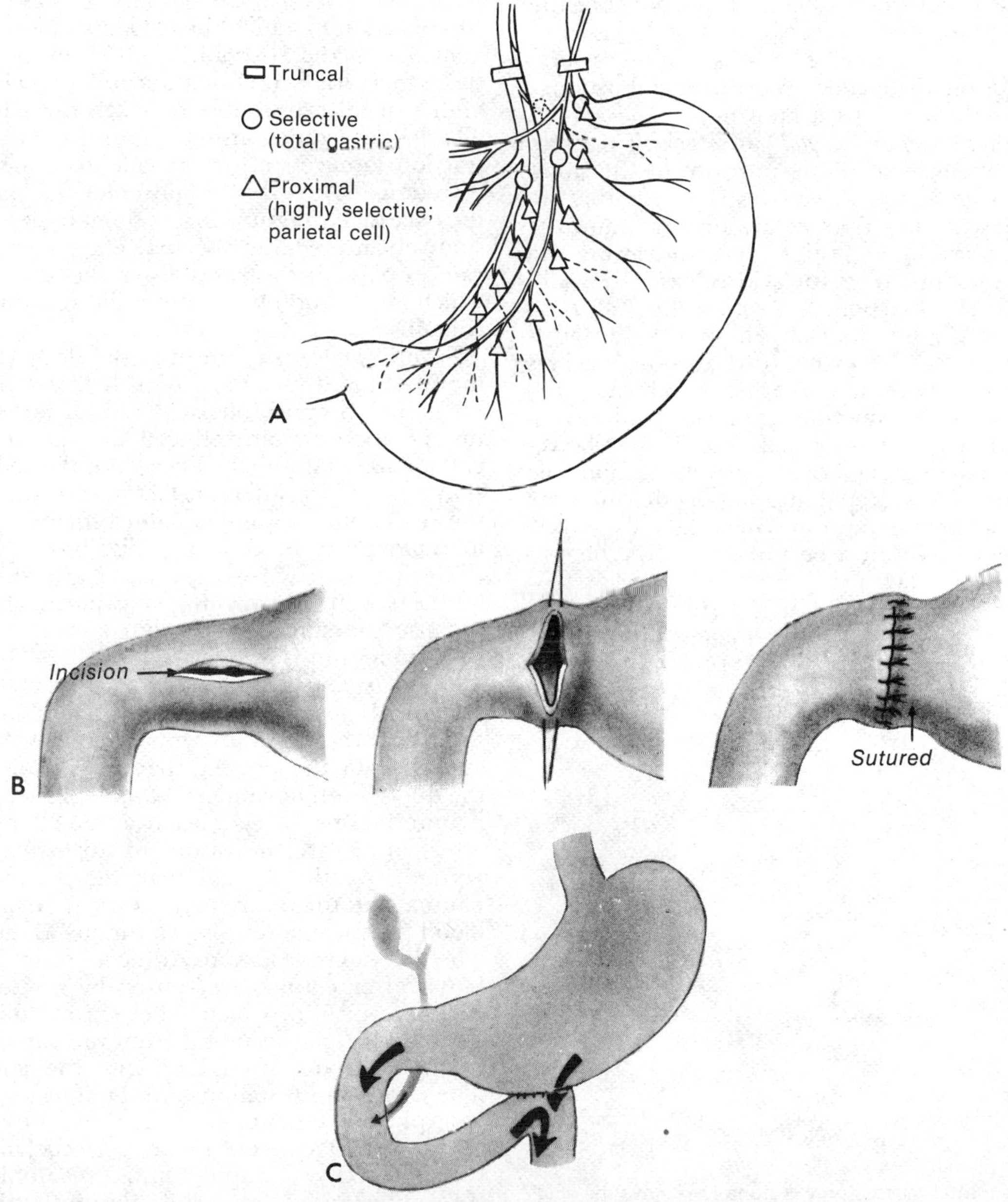

Figure 62–3. Types of vagotomy and associated surgical procedures. **A.** The sites at which the three types of vagotomy are performed. **B.** A *pyloroplasty,* which provides a larger opening from the stomach to the duodenum, may be performed after a vagotomy, to counteract the loss of motility that a vagotomy produces. **C.** Another procedure used to enhance emptying of the stomach after a vagotomy is a *gastroenterostomy,* which is the surgical creation of a passage between the stomach and small intestine.

stimulates motility, the stomach is relatively atonic following these procedures and therefore empties slowly. In order to prevent this and the resultant feeling of fullness, belching, and weight loss, a *pyloroplasty* or *gastroenterostomy* is usually done in conjunction with the surgery to enhance emptying (Fig. 62–3*B* and *C*). In a *highly selective* vagotomy (i.e., parietal cell), branches of the vagus which innervate the fundus and corpus (acid-secreting portions) of the stomach are removed. Since motility is preserved, a gastroenterostomy is not necessary. This is a relatively new procedure, and its long-term results are not yet known.

An *antrectomy* or *subtotal gastrectomy* is done to reduce the acid-secreting portions of the stomach. An antrectomy removes the cells that secrete gastrin and thus delays or eliminates the gastric phase of digestion by withdrawing tha source of stimulation for acid release. In a subtotal gastric resection, the removal of 60 to 80 per cent of the stomach eliminates the acid-secreting cells. The extent of reduction of acid is determined by the amount of stomach removed. A vagotomy is sometimes done in conjunction with either of these procedures. It must be remembered that pancreatic secretions and bile continue to be secreted into the duodenum even after gastrectomy and are necessary for digestion, so a route must be preserved for them to reach the chyme.

Note in Figure 62–4 that a subtotal gastrectomy may be formed by means of either a Billroth I or a Billroth II procedure. In a Billroth I resection, the proximal remnant of the distal stomach is reanastomosed to the duodenum; a Billroth II resection involves reanastomosis of the proximal remnant of the stomach to the proximal jejunum. The Billroth II technique is preferred for treatment of duodenal ulcer because recurrent ulceration develops less frequently.

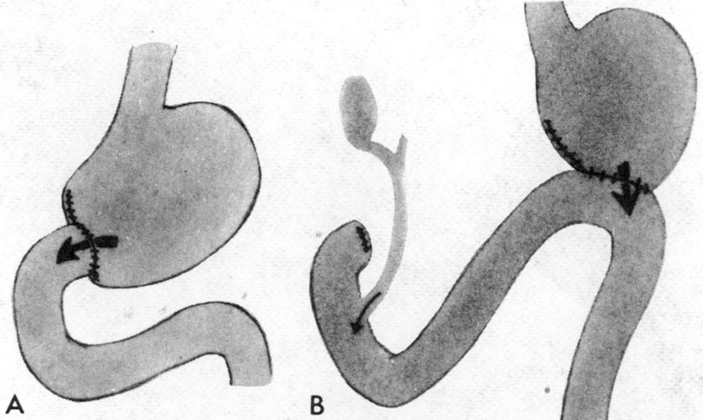

Figure 62–4. A subtotal gastrectomy is done to remove the acid-secreting portions of the stomach. **A.** The Billroth I operation creates an anastomosis of the severed end of the duodenum with the partially closed end of the stomach. **B.** The Billroth II operation closes the duodenal stump and joins the resected stomach to the jejunum.

Complications. When a high level of gastric acid secretions remains after a gastroenterostomy or gastric resection, a *marginal* ulcer can develop where the gastric acids contact the operative site, either at the site of the anastomosis or in the jejunum. This ulceration can cause scarring and obstruction of the passages; hemorrhage and perforation can also occur.

Afferent loop syndrome is the name given to a complication in which the duodenal loop is partially obstructed after a Billroth II resection and the pancreatic secretions and bile which fill it after a meal are unable to reach the jejunum. The loop becomes distended, and painful contractions occur as effort is made to propel these secretions. When they finally enter the jejunum, the excessive pressure forces them back into the stomach and vomiting occurs. The patient experiences pain, nausea, and distention after meals, which is relieved by vomiting; the vomit usually contains bile.

Several *problems of nutrition* develop from removal of the stomach; these include a deficiency in vitamin B_{12} and folic acid, a disordered calcium metabolism, and reduced absorption of calcium and vitamin D. These are caused by a shortage of the intrinsic factor resulting from the resection, and inadequate absorption owing to rapid entry of food into the bowel. In the Billroth II gastric resection there is a reduction in the secretion of pancreatic juices and bile because the stimulus of food passing through the duodenum is missing.

The *dumping syndrome* occurs after gastric resection because of the rapid entry of ingested food into the jejunum without proper mixing and without the normal digestive processes of the duodenum having been accomplished. Early manifestations, which occur 5 to 30 minutes after eating, are the vasomotor disturbances of vertigo, sweating, pallor, palpitation, diarrhea, nausea, and the desire to lie down. The patient's blood pressure and pulse may either rise or fall. The late manifestations, which occur 2 to 3 hours after eating, are caused by a release of excessive insulin, which follows a rapid rise in the blood sugar resulting from the rapid entry of high carbohydrate food into the jejunum. The early manifestations are thought to be due to rapid movement of extracellular fluids into the bowel to convert the hypertonic material that entered very rapidly into an isotonic mixture. This rapid fluid shift decreases the circulating blood volume, causing the symptoms.

The treatment of the dumping syndrome is to decrease the amount of food taken at one time and to give a high-protein, high-fat, low-carbohydrate, dry diet. Gastric emptying can be delayed by not taking fluids with meals and by eating in a recumbent or semirecumbent position or by lying down after meals. Sedatives and antispasmodics are given to delay gastric emptying. This syndrome frequently occurs soon after surgery and subsides in 6 months to a year. When it continues, surgical attempts to relieve the symptoms have included reducing the size of the gastroenterostomy or converting a Billroth II resection to a Billroth I by inserting a short segment of jejunum between the duodenal stump and the stomach.

Nursing Care of the Patient Who Has Gastric Surgery. Since surgical intervention for gastric and duodenal conditions can be either an emergency or a planned procedure, the nursing care will vary. When surgery is an *emergency procedure* required for acute obstruction, perforation, or hemorrhage, the patient is very ill, and both the patient and significant others will probably be very apprehensive. The patient may be too ill to express these apprehensions. The nurse can maintain the patient's sense of security by providing calm, efficient, knowledgeable care and by not saying or doing anything in front of the patient that would undermine the patient's confidence. Reassurance can be given by explanations of what is being done and by noting nonverbal reactions and responding to them. The family's effect upon the patient should be noted, as some patients are better off with family members present, whereas others are more relaxed and calm without them.

If there is a possibility that the diagnosis is cancer, the patient may wish to express fears about this. The nurse should listen to the patient and offer support and understanding. The patient may wish to attend to personal matters before surgery (e.g., check a will, see a minister). The nurse should be alert to cues about the patient's needs.

When surgery is done on an *elective basis,* the patient will probably have an extensive series of preoperative examinations such as gastrointestinal series, gastroscopy, and perhaps acid-secretion studies (Chapter 59). These may be done on an outpatient basis. A patient who has had a peptic ulcer for a number of years is frequently a "veteran" at these procedures. The patient may either easily swallow the nasogastric tube (which is frequently inserted and attached to suction before surgery) or may have developed strong fears of tubes and resist its insertion. When the patient reacts in this manner, it sometimes helps to give a sedative prior to insertion of the tube.

Preoperative teaching includes the same explanations as given to other surgical patients and should also include an explanation that gastric suction will be present after surgery and that fluids will be given by intravenous infusion until the gastric surgical site is healed. Discussing the need for deep breathing is especially important for the patient because of the high abdominal incision, which causes increased discomfort from deep breathing and is an added hazard for the development of respiratory complications.

Postoperative nursing observations, in addition to those made on all surgical patients, include checking drainage from the nasogastric tube. It may be bright red during the early hours after surgery but should become dark by the end of 24 hours. The nurse should note the color and consistency of the drainage and report any occurrence of hemorrhage. The care of this patient is the same as for any patient with an indwelling nasogastric tube. (See details of care in Chapter 58.) The tube should be irrigated only on a specific order, as it is usually placed during surgery and the surgeon knows its position in relation to suture lines and can tell how much and what kind of fluid can safely be instilled through it.

A nonfunctioning gastric suction tube should be reported to the physician, as distension of the operative area by gas and fluids can have drastic sequelae.

The patient must be encouraged to deep breathe and to move, even though this may be difficult because of the location of the incision. Keeping the patient comfortable with the judicious administration of pain medications will allow more cooperation in deep breathing and coughing.

Fluids will be given by intravenous infusion until edema and swelling have diminished enough to allow food and fluids to pass the operative area. A common method of beginning feedings is to give clear water, usually 30 ml. at a time, and aspirate the tube an hour or so later to see if the fluid was retained. When clear water is tolerated, the nasogastric tube will be removed and the patient started on a regimen that starts with a small quantity of fluid given hourly and progresses to soft foods and eventually to a regular diet of five or six small feedings. At first the patient may experience discomfort if too much is taken at one time. The tissues will gradually expand, and within a year or so the patient may be able to eat three normal meals.

Occasionally the diet is begun too rapidly or too soon, and nasogastric suction must be reinstituted. The patient is usually very depressed by this. The nurse can give reassurance that this is not an indication of failure of the surgery but merely an indication that healing is not yet complete.

It should be remembered that some of the patients who have surgery are those same patients who were unable to leave their work at home when hospitalized for medical treatment of peptic ulcer disease. These patients, who are in a hurry for everything, need calm understanding and need to be encouraged to let nature heal them in her time and not to rush the situation. Convalescence after gastric surgery tends to be slow, and it may be 3 months before the patient regains strength and even a partial ability to eat in a more normal manner.

When complications such as the afferent loop syndrome or the dumping syndrome occur, the patient may need to express displeasure at the situation. (Remember the patient probably held high expectations for the surgical result.) Frequently, the patient can be taught how to control these symptoms by the measures mentioned previously.

Postoperative teaching includes helping the patient to:

1. Learn to live with the residual deficiencies resulting from the surgery.
2. Choose an appropriate diet or obtain assistance from a dietician.
3. Understand the need for continued medical supervision.
4. Realize that convalescence may be fairly long.

NEOPLASMS

The incidence of cancer of the stomach has diminished steadily in the United States during the last four decades. The reason for this is unknown. Despite the reduction in incidence, it was the fourth ranked cause of death from cancer among males in the United States in 1975 because of the low cure rate.

Little is known about its etiology, but it is twice as common in men as in women, more common in the American black than in American whites, and it occurs more frequently in persons who have pernicious anemia. It often occurs in conjunction with atrophic gastritis. Other factors that are related to a high incidence of cancer of the stomach include a low socioeconomic status, living in an urban area, having smoked fish in the diet, and the presence of background radiation or trace metals in the soil. Worldwide mortality varies greatly, being high in Japan, Hungary, Portugal and Chile, but low in the United States, El Salvador, Thailand, the Phillipines, Honduras and New Zealand. The reasons for these differences are unknown, but studies are being done of the variations in diet in these countries.

Summarizing what is now known about gastric cancer and drawing what conclusions are possible Kirsner states:[124]

> Gastric carcinoma thus may be regarded as an acquired disease, developing in an abnormal gastric mucosa and probably arising on the basis of cellular reaction to continued injury, presumably from unknown chemical carcinogens.

Symptoms and Diagnosis. Cancer of the stomach is seldom diagnosed in an early stage because the symptoms occur late and then, unless hemorrhage or perforation occurs, are vague and indefinite. They depend upon where in the stomach the tumor occurs. If it is near the cardia, the patient may experience dysphagia from early involvement of the esophagus; if it is near the pylorus, symptoms may occur from obstruction. The major symptoms are weight loss and a vague indigestion or feeling of fullness or mild discomfort that is so insidious that the patient does not recognize it as an abnormality or seek medical aid. Discomfort may be brought on, or relieved, by food. Anemia from blood loss is a common symptom, and occult blood is present in the stools of 45 per cent of persons with this condition. The presence of a palpable mass, ascites, or bone pain from metastasis may be the first symptom.

When the cancer causes ulceration, differentiating it from a benign gastric ulcer can be difficult, but upper gastrointestinal x-rays and fluoroscopy used together with gastroscopy diagnose about 95 per cent of the cases correctly. Cytology as an aid to diagnosing gastric lesions is thought to be valuable by some and worthless by others. Most authorities agree that, to rule out cancer, surgery should be done for any gastric lesion that does not improve after 2 weeks of intensive medical therapy.

Metastasis and Prognosis. Cancer of the stomach is spread by direct extension into the pancreas; by lymphatic spread, which occurs early; or by hematogenous spread to the liver, lungs, and bones, which occurs at varying times. The occurrence of spread by these routes depends upon the location of the tumor and the type of growth it undergoes, since some penetrate, some ulcerate, and some spread along the tissue planes.

The overall prognosis is poor, with a five-year cure rate for all patients of between 5 and 10 per cent. When curative surgery is done at an early stage this five-year survival rate is from 30 to 35 per cent. When surgery is done and metastases are found, the rate is only 9 per cent. This explains the high death rate for this low-incidence cancer.

Treatment. Surgery is the only treatment that affects the progress of the disease favorably. Unfortunately, because of the usually late diagnosis, this is more often palliative than curative. Gastrectomy, either partial or complete, depending upon the location of the tumor, is the usual procedure. Ideally all local growth and the associated lymph nodes are removed. When extensive growth makes resection impractical or impossible and the pylorus is obstructed, palliation is often achieved with a gastroenterostomy. (See Fig. 62–3*C*).

Radiation therapy has not proved helpful, and response to chemotherapy is not consistent. At present best results are achieved with the use of multiple drug combinations. Those giving the best results are 5 FU, mitomycin-C, BCNU, and cytarabine. Nonspecific immunotherapy with BCG is also being tried. See Chapter 23 for a discussion of chemotherapy for cancer.

Postoperative Nursing Care. Patients with cancer of the stomach are frequently malnourished and anemic. They should be protected from secondary infections as well as from the various complications of debilitating conditions. When a total gastrectomy has been done, the patient will probably have chest drainage because the thoracic cavity is usually entered in order to do a total resection. The nasogastric tube will have very little drainage because most secretions normally come from the stomach.

Postoperative progress will be similar to that with a subtotal gastrectomy but is usually much slower. As with other gastric surgery, the first feeding will be clear water. Feedings will be increased gradually until the patient is on five to six small meals a day. The patient should be taught to chew food well, since the mixing and liquefying functions of the stomach have been lost. When a good surgical response is achieved, a high-protein, low-carbohydrate, moderate-fat diet is tolerated well. Some patients are not noticeably improved by surgery and may be unable to tolerate or digest even small amounts of food satisfactorily.

Because of the loss of the intrinsic factor, these patients need injections of vitamin B_{12} to maintain hemoglobin levels. Balanced nutrition is important. The nurse should promote a well-balanced diet that is not too high in bulk, because of the patient's limited capacity. Instructions on what foods to include in the diet may be needed.

Other nursing responsibilities in cancer of the stomach are case-finding by recognizing the vague symptoms and encouraging people to seek medical assistance for vague gastric complaints that persist or for changes from the patient's normal digestive habits. These patients usually undergo many diagnostic tests and need nursing support and instructions concerning these tests.

CHAPTER 63

DISORDERS OF THE LARGE AND SMALL BOWEL

The major function of the small bowel and of the proximal half of the large bowel is digestion of food substances and absorption of the end products, while the function of the left colon is storage of the feces until defecation occurs. The small bowel is narrower in diameter and longer than the large bowel. The arterial supply and venous drainage are so divided that the small bowel and right colon to the midpoint of the transverse colon receive blood from the superior mesenteric artery, whereas the remainder of the colon and the rectum receive blood from the inferior mesenteric artery. The venous drainage is divided the same way, with blood from both the superior and inferior mesenteric veins draining into the portal system. See Figure 64–2. Peristaltic activity in the small bowel is much more active than that in the large bowel, which is relatively inactive except during the mass movements that are stimulated by distention of the rectum.

SYMPTOMS AND PROBLEMS

Symptoms that occur in this area depend upon which function — motility, digestion or absorption — is disturbed and upon the cause of the disturbance. The major symptoms of dysfunction are pain, tenderness, hemorrhage, distention, nausea and vomiting, constipation and diarrhea, abdominal masses, and abnormal constituents in the feces.

Obstruction to the flow of chyme in either portion causes increased peristalsis, pain, and distention, but the symptoms occur sooner and will be more intense in a small bowel blockage than in the large because of the differences in size and normal activity in the two segments. The large volume of secretions from the small bowel add to the distention; the only significant secretion from the large bowel is mucus.

Hemorrhage. Bleeding may be caused by trauma or by ulceration or inflammation or a growth that erodes through a blood vessel (Table 63–1). It is usually manifested by blood in the stools rather than by emesis and varies from a minute quantity that is invisible except by testing (occult blood) to larger quantities that cause the stools to be any gradation of color from bright red to tarry black. Since color comes from the digestive processes acting upon the blood, the amount of color change can be used to determine roughly the level of the bowel in which bleeding occurs. The rapidity with which the chyme passes through the bowel will also affect this. When the patient is passing bloody stools, the nurse should note the number of stools passed in any certain time period and what color changes occur between early and late specimens. For instance, slow bleeding from the duodenum might not increase peristalsis and

TABLE 63–1. RELATIVE FREQUENCIES OF MAJOR CAUSES OF LOWER GI BLEEDING ACCORDING TO EXTENT OF BLEEDING

Minimal	Moderate	Severe*
Local conditions such as hemorrhoids, fissures, or prolapse	Cancer of colon	Diverticular disease
Colonic polyps	Diverticular disease	Vascular malformations
Cancer of colon	Ulcerative colitis	Cancer of colon
Inflammatory bowel disease	Colonic polyps	Duodenal ulcer Small bowel diverticula

*Requiring immediate blood transfusion.

From Steinheber, F. U.: Bleeding from the lower gastrointestinal tract: Diagnostic approach. *Hospital Medicine,* 15:27, Apr. 1979, by permission © 1979 by Hospital Publications, Inc.

could be manifested by a tarry stool; if the rate of bleeding or the rate of peristalsis increased, the patient could have subsequent stools that become brighter. The knowledge that previously black stools have changed to bright bloody ones and are now occurring every half hour is a fact that will help the physician in making a diagnosis or in determining what tests to make to conform the diagnosis.

Pain. Pain is caused by stimulation of the nerve endings in the muscular or submucosal layers of the bowel and by an increase in tension; it may also be influenced by the rate of tension change. It is manifested in various places, including the involved portion of the bowel, another previously diseased area, or a nearby somatic portion of the body. Previous surgical procedures will also influence the location at which pain is felt.

Obstruction of the blood supply to the intestine is another cause for pain. This can be from acute occlusion of the mesenteric artery or from partial occlusion, which causes intermittent pain when digestion is taking place because of the increased need for blood at that time. Acute occlusion can occur in the major artery or one of the smaller branches. Partial occlusion causing intermittent pain is sometimes called intestinal angina.

Nausea and Vomiting. When this symptom originates in the bowel, it is usually due to an obstruction of the forward motility of peristalsis. Nausea occurs from distention of the duodenum.

Constipation and Diarrhea. Usually, fast propulsion of intestinal contents through the bowel results in diarrhea, unless it is compensated by a longer period of residence in the large bowel; however, increased peristalsis in the small bowel usually affects forward motility within the large bowel also.

Irritant action of intestinal contents is the usual cause for increased activity. This can result from the presence of abnormal bacteria or parasites or from highly irritating organic acids that are formed by bacterial actions, made possible by an abnormal absorptive process.

Constipation, a very common symptom, can be caused by something as simple as inadequate fluid or bulk in the diet or lack of attention to the urge to defecate. It can also be the symptom of something that mechanically blocks the passage of intestinal contents or slows peristalsis by inadequate stimulation of mass movements. Constipation due to inadequate neurologic stimulation can be caused by electrolyte or metabolic disturbances as well as neurologic disorders, mental depression, and the ingestion of various drugs. Constipation must always be considered in relation to other symptoms.

Abdominal Masses. Palpation of abdominal masses is more useful in finding lesions in the large bowel than in the small bowel. The amount of abdominal adipose tissue will also affect the ease of palpation.

Abnormalities in Fecal Content. The presence of nonabsorbed factors such as fats in the stool indicates malabsorption. Other abnormal constituents that may aid in diagnosis are bacteria, parasites, pus, blood, and abnormal quantities of mucus from the colon.

INFLAMMATIONS

Inflammations occur in any portion of the bowel and can be caused by an organism, by toxins produced by an organism, by infiltration of the bowel wall by granulomatous processes, by injury from radiation, and by drugs. All types of organisms can be involved, from viruses to large parasites. Almost any abnormal constituent in the bowel can cause an inflammatory process to develop.

Bacterial, Parasitic, and Chemical Irritations

Gastroenteritis. This is a general name for a condition that affects the small bowel predominantly and is manifested by abdominal cramps, diarrhea, and vomiting. It can be caused by various agents, with viruses and bacteria being common causes. Staphylococcal food poisoning, in which the irritating factor is the toxin produced by the organism, may occur when foods such as cream-filled pastries, custard pies, processed meats, and potato salad are allowed to remain at room temperature for a period of time before they are eaten. The staphylococcal organisms multiply and form a toxin which, when ingested, causes a violent gastroenteritis in 2 to 4 hours. Bacterial or viral food poisoning usually develops 10 to 16 hours after ingestion of contaminated food.

Many organisms "pass through" a community during a year, and transitory epidemics of gastroenteritis are common. These infections are temporarily quite disabling, depending upon the intensity of the symptoms, but they are of short duration and usually are not serious, except in infants, the very elderly, and weakened debilitated individuals. Fluid and electrolyte imbalances occur easily in these persons because of the lowered efficiency of their compensatory mechanisms.

Bed rest with nothing by mouth until vomiting has stopped is the best treatment. Fluids such as broth, ginger ale, and lemonade, which contain nutrients and electrolytes, are given as soon as possible to replace losses. Sometimes antibiotics are given if the infecting organism is identified and the condition is persistent.

Dysenteries. The conditions that fall into this category affect the large bowel and are manifested by an intense diarrhea and abdominal cramping. Varying amounts of blood may be present in the stool, and the patient may have a mild to severe temperature elevation, depending upon the causative organism. Most dysenteries are caused by amebic and bacterial organisms such as *Entamoeba histolytica* and shigella bacilli. Cholera also causes dysentery-like symptoms. These organisms are carried in the large bowel by infected individuals and transmitted by ingestion of contaminated foods and drinking water. Dysentery develops commonly in countries where there is crowding, where sanitary conditions are poor, and where the temperature is high enough for the organisms to incubate easily. The major manifestation is a profuse diarrhea, and the resultant fluid and electrolyte loss is the greatest problem. Dysentery can be fatal in the debilitated, the aged, and the very young; it can cause severe fluid imbalances in the generally healthy individual.

Parasitic Infestations. The intestinal tract may be infested with any of several species of parasitic worms. These include the Ascaris (roundworms), the Enterobius (pinworms), the *Trichinella spiralis* (causing trichinosis), and various species of tapeworms. These parasites are found in all parts of the world, and are often encountered in the poorer regions of the United States. Worm infestations can cause serious and even fatal disease if the parasites are not eradicated from the intestinal tract. Fortunately most of these parasites are susceptible to treatment with compounds such as piperazine (Antepar). Trichinosis, formerly the most difficult of the group to treat, is now often effectively treated by thiabendazole.

SCHISTOSOMIASIS. Schistosomiasis is caused by a *blood fluke* (a parasitic worm) that penetrates the skin of a person who wades or bathes in fresh water in which an infected snail resides. Three species infect humans. The disease is prevalent in various parts of the world such as Africa, Japan, China, Egypt, and South America and is frequently found in the United States among Puerto Ricans. The cercariae of the parasite penetrate the skin and migrate to the liver via the lungs and remain in the intrahepatic portal venules while the worm matures. The mature worm, which does not multiply within the human, then moves against the blood flow into its final habitat, the veins of the large or small bowel or bladder depending upon the species involved. Here it lays an estimated 300 to 3500 eggs per day, depending upon the species. These eggs, which form pseudotubercles, are commonly found in the liver and veins of the abdomen and lungs but have been found in every system of the body, including the nervous. Some eggs are excreted in the urine or feces. Without adequate sewage disposal, the eggs may be deposited in water that contains a susceptible snail, thus continuing the cycle.

In the human the disease may have no symptoms, may be mild, or may be severe, depending on the species involved and the number of worms present. The prognosis is usually good. The schistosomes do not multiply within the body, but a large number may be present due to repeated infections. Their life span is probably about 3 to 5 years but may be as high as 30 years.

The disease begins with a dermatitis at the site of penetration. The dermatitis is followed by a fever in 20 to 60 days and later by symptoms from the extrusion of eggs. Different drugs are used to treat the various species. Therefore, the eggs or worms must be examined and the species identified before treatment can begin unless the species is known to be endemic in the local area.

Regional Enteritis (Terminal Ileitis, Granulomatous Jejunoileitis, Crohn's Disease)

This disease was first described in 1932 by Crohn; and the incidence, especially among the young, has increased worldwide since then. Originally it was thought to affect only the terminal ileum, but it has been found in segments of the alimentary tract from the mouth to the anus. It is a chronic, relapsing disease that is characterized by involvement of the whole thickness of the bowel wall. It is typically present in several separated segments and is grossly visible and sharply demarcated from normal tissue. There is an edematous, heavy, reddish-purple area; there may be granular spots. The disease causes a narrowed lumen, ulcerations, abscesses, and fistulas and their complications.

The etiology is unknown, though it has been suggested that there may be some genetic or hereditary basis to the disease or that some new environmental factor may be responsible. It has an equal incidence in the sexes and occurs at all ages, but 50 per cent of the cases occur between the ages of 20 and 30. There is a high incidence of familial occurrence and a high incidence in Jews. There has been a low incidence among blacks, but this is now increasing.

Symptoms results from the inflammatory reaction, the obstructive problems, and dysfunction of the bowel and may include diarrhea, constipation, abdominal discomfort, and cramping as well as abscesses and a low-grade fever. In children growth may be retarded. Treatment is mainly symptomatic and is aimed at maintaining good nutrition so that the patient can lead a productive life. Other therapies include surgery, which is used only to treat the complications (since removal of the diseased portion of the bowel has resulted in a 50 per cent incidence of recurrence), antibiotics to control infectious processes, and anti-inflammatory drugs for patients who fail to respond to general supportive measures. (See Table 63–2.)

Ulcerative Colitis

Ulcerative colitis seems to be related to regional enteritis, or Crohn's disease, in that some cases are difficult to tell apart when regional enteritis affects the colon. They both tend to be familial and frequently patients with one condition have a blood relative with the other.

> A large number of patients have clinical manifestations ranging from what appears to be classical ulcerative colitis involving the entire colon to clear-cut Crohn's Disease of the gut with involvement of esophagus, duodenum, small bowel, and colon . . . There is general agreement not only that Crohn's colitis and ulcerative colitis are difficult to tell apart . . . but in addition that they share the same extraintestinal manifestations, they occur in the same kinds of people, and their immunologic abnormalities and responses seem to be the same.[179]

These observations lead the clinician "to believe that inflammatory bowel disease represents a spectrum of responses to a noxious agent as yet undefined, responses modulated by differing immunologic and idiosyncratically personal bodily reactions."[179]

Ulcerative colitis involves the mucosa and submucosa of the colon and consists of congestion, edema, and minute ulcerations that ooze blood and eventually develop into abscesses. The edema may lead to extreme friability of the mucosa, so that bleeding occurs from any minor trauma. The general manifestations of this disorder are frequent stools that contain pus, blood, and mucus and may or may not contain liquid feces; weight loss; anorexia, and an intermittent mild fever. See Table 63–2 for comparison of the symptoms of chronic ulcerative colitis and Crohn's disease of the colon.

Ulcerative colitis has three typical types of onset: In one it is gradual, beginning with malaise and vague abdominal discomfort which develops into attacks of crampy abdominal pain, with the passage of blood, pus, and mucus. The desire to defecate is great, and the patient experiences severe tenesmus. Stools are apt to be scanty and hard. In another type the onset is abrupt and manifested by bloody diarrhea, fever, anorexia, and weight loss that becomes progressively worse. The stools are sometimes liquid and sometimes hard, depending upon which portion of the colon is involved. The pa-

TABLE 63–2. CROHN'S DISEASE AND ULCERATIVE COLITIS—DIFFERENTIAL DIAGNOSIS

	Crohn's Disease of Colon	Chronic Ulcerative Colitis
Clinical		
Diarrhea	Most common symptom, but usually of moderate severity	Most common symptom but more severe and often of extreme degree
Rectal bleeding	Uncommon and never severe	Almost always during active phase
Abdominal pain	Common	Unusual
Fever	Common and often persistent	Only during acute attack
Abdominal mass	Frequent in right lower quadrant	Absent
Perianal disease	Frequent, often an early feature and persistent	Unusual
Sigmoidoscopy	May be negative, or scattered ulcers	Always reveals diffuse ulcerative disease
Rectal biopsy	May reveal granulomas	Active inflammation, often "crypt abscesses"
Toxic megacolon	Rarely occurs	5–10% of severe cases
Carcinoma	Rarely occurs	Risk increases proportionate to duration of disease; 4–6% in prolonged cases
Radiologic		
Site	Rectum rarely involved, distribution often segmental and discontinuous, right colon a common site	Rectum always involved, extends proximally in continuous pattern into left colon and beyond
Symmetry	Eccentric distribution with unequal involvement of colon circumference	Entire circumference involved
Terminal ileum	Often involved	Usually normal, occasional "backwash ileitis"

From Tumen, H. J.: Crohn's disease. *In* Conn, H. F., and R. B. Conn (Eds.): *Current Diagnosis*. Philadelphia: W. B. Saunders Co., 1977, p. 630.

tient usually has abdominal tenderness, and the rectum and anus are spastic. Signs and symptoms tend to fluctuate, with remissions and exacerbations. The third general type also has an abrupt onset, but the course is rapid and fulminating, and unless successful treatment is achieved, the patient can die of toxicity or shock from the sequelae.

Like Crohn's disease, ulcerative colitis occurs at all ages but is most common among young adults and common among Jews. It is less common among blacks than among whites. A number of theories concerning its etiology exist, including the possibility that the disease is of bacterial origin, since a number of patients have had a history of a bacterial infection prior to the onset of the condition. Allergic reactions have been suspected, because remission sometimes occurs when the patient eliminates milk from the diet. It is thought by some to be due to an altered immunity, because colon antibodies have been found in patients with the condition. These antibodies may cause the disease, perpetuate it, or may result from the tissue damage caused by the disease. A number of the theories of etiology depend upon the assumption of a specific vulnerability of the bowel to certain stimuli. The bowel may be hypersensitive to trauma or other stimuli, and the inflammation of the mucosa may result from the release of histamine or some other substance in response to these stimuli.

Many have implicated emotional instability as a factor in the disease. Patients with ulcerative colitis have been described as dependent, immature, and hypersensitive to criticism; many are known to have different inward feelings than their outward appearance would indicate. One theory states that there is an increased cholinergic stimulation induced by emotional stress or some other agent and an increased tissue vulnerability to this stimulation. This has not been substantiated in all studies. However, *all researchers do agree that emotional stress does influence recurrences of the disease.*

Complications. Local tissue involvement causes rectal complications such as hemorrhoids and anal fissures, and such bowel complications as local abscesses, perforation, and stenosis from healing lesions. As a result of the physical manifestations of the conditions, patients develop anemia and malnutrition owing to malabsorption and iron deficiency. They may also be deficient in vitamin K with resulting bleeding tendencies. They develop weakness, anorexia, weight loss, and sometimes a stomatitis resembling that of vitamin deficiencies. Cancer of the colon is more common among patients with this condition than among the general population; the incidence is greatly increased among those who develop ulcerative colitis before the age of 16 and those who have had the condition more than 10 years. The 5 year survival rate for the colitis patients who undergo surgery is also much lower than for other patients with cancer of the colon.

Treatment. The aims of treatment are to maintain the patient's nutritional status, give symptomatic relief, prevent complications, and restore blood volume.

A high-protein, high-caloric diet is given in an attempt to restore normal nutritional levels. This is not always well ingested or tolerated. Eating tends to increase the diarrhea and the anorexia with nausea and vomiting that are frequently present. These patients tend to have definite ideas about what they want to eat and, probably because of the miserable symptoms of the disease, they tend to vent their aggressions on the diet. If the patient can be given a self-selected diet it will probably be more beneficial than attempting to give the low-residue, bland, high-caloric, high-protein diet that is usually ordered and is accepted so poorly. Foods that patients want tend to be better tolerated than those that are "ordered." Fluids, electrolytes, and blood are replaced as needed to maintain the patient's homeostasis.

Antibiotics may be given to control secondary bowel inflammations.

During acute exacerbations the patient is put on bed rest and given anticholinergic drugs to relieve the abdominal cramps and to help control the diarrhea. In an attempt to control diarrhea, tincture of opium and paregoric are sometimes given on a routine basis, instead of after each stool as in other conditions.

These patients need a great deal of emotional support. The physician usually attempts to establish an open relationship with the patient, and the nurse also should be aware of the patient's reactions and encourage on open expression of feelings. The patient should be encouraged in developing a positive self-image and helped to achieve self-acceptance.

Surgical Treatment. When medical management fails and when the condition proves intractable, surgical treatment is usually indicated. Surgical intervention varies, but the most common procedure is the surgical excision of the entire colon, rectum, and anus and the creation of a permanent ileostomy. The entire colon is usually removed, as toxic products are absorbed from it even when it is nonfunctional and symptoms of general toxicity may continue if it remains.

Another indication for surgical intervention is the probability of the presence of a carcinoma of the colon. Some surgeons recommend colectomy for all patients who have had this condition for more than 10 years because of the high cancer incidence in these persons. Most surgeons do not consider this an adequate indication for surgery, since a permanent ileostomy is such a serious consequence. However, with a long history of ulcerative colitis patients should be examined frequently for cancer even when they are in a period of remission of the disease.

Irritable Colon

An irritable colon is a chronic noninfectious irritation that is thought to be caused by an increased spasticity of the colon. It can be manifested in a number of different ways, including frequent liquid stools, scanty, small hard stools, and abdominal cramps that are brought on by eating coarse or raw foods, since these increase the spasticity. The condition occurs in people who are tense, anxious, and emotionally labile. Its major danger is that it mimics a number of other conditions and the patient may undergo unnecessary surgery, or the presence of a serious illness may not be recognized. Among the disorders simulated are infections of the colon, food allergies, ulcerative colitis, carcinoma of the colon, diverticulitis, gallbladder disease, and even angina pectoris and myocardial infarction.

Nursing Care

Remember: A patient with an inflammatory condition of the bowel is losing fluids at an abnormally rapid rate, and thus electrolyte imbalance and inadequate nutrition are potential problems.

These patients experience a great deal of discomfort from nausea, frequent liquid stools, abdominal cramping, and generalized debility from inadequate intake. The goals of nursing should be to promote the patient's comfort and to maintain adequate nutrition and hydration.

If the condition is caused by or suspected of being caused by a microorganism, nurses should take care to wash their hands, the patient's hands, and all the utensils used if the patient vomits or defecates. Handwashing and preventing contamination of the uniform to avoid taking the organisms to another patient are basic factors of good nursing.

The following discussion of nursing care of patients with diarrhea and nausea is applicable to all patients with these conditions, and not just to persons with an inflammatory bowel condition.

Diarrhea. Prompt emptying of the patient's bedpan or commode is essential, as liquid stools are usually very malodorous. Washing the patient after defecations and gently drying and lightly dusting the area with a nonirritating powder will help to prevent excoriation from the stools, which may be very irritating to the skin about the anus. Sometimes patients have involuntary stools and are unable to position themselves on a commode or bedpan in time. They should not be censured or ridiculed for this; rather, the nurse should by manner and words make patients feel that this is not their fault and that they need not be embarrassed about it. They should, of course, be cleansed immediately and their bed linens changed.

Intake of fluids and foods should be encouraged. Sometimes eating stimulates the gastrocolic reflex and brings on another stool, so many of these patients fear eating. Very small feedings may avoid this problem. Foods should be bland and easily digested to promote absorption during the short period the food remains in the bowel.

Nausea. The patient who is vomiting should be kept as physically comfortable as possible. Removing the emesis basin promptly, giving thorough oral hygiene, and keeping the physical unit attractive, aired, and clean will help to eliminate the psychogenic and physical influences that perpetuate vomiting. Patients especially need to have a clean fresh mouth and to have the odor and sight of the vomitus removed.

Do not force patients to eat, as this frequently promotes more vomiting. Let the patient be the judge of when food can be tolerated. However, sometimes these patients need encouragement because they are afraid to eat.

Broth, ginger ale, and weak tea are frequently the first foods tolerated. Fluids that contain electrolytes are preferred to clear water. The first foods should be bland and easily digested. Strong secretagogues should be avoided. (See Chapter 62 for discussion of peptic ulcers.) When vomiting continues for more than 24 to 48 hours, intravenous fluids will usually be given to maintain fluid balance.

Medications. Antispasmodics, binding agents, sedatives, and antiemetics may be given to help to control the patient's symptoms of nausea and vomiting.

Observations. Included in the observations made on the patient who is vomiting or has diarrhea should be the presence of pain or tenderness in the abdomen, including its location, intensity, duration, type, and timing in relation to the diarrhea or vomiting. The presence of cramping of the bowel and tenesmus, which is the feeling of cramping pain and discomfort that occurs in the lower abdomen when one is straining to defecate, should also be reported. Whether these are relieved by the passage of a stool is also pertinent.

The characteristics of the stool should be reported and recorded and include the color, volume, odor, quantity, and the presence of any abnormal constituents such as mucus, blood, undigested food, foam, pus, oil, and other matter such as worms. The physician may wish to have the stool saved for inspection.

In addition to the volume, emesis should also be described completely as to color, odor, consistency, and the presence of undigested food or drug particles. Other things to observe about the patient who vomits include the nature of the vomiting process. Does the vomitus come up slowly and easily or is it propelled out forcibly? Does the patient have warning that he or she is about to vomit? Is the vomiting accompanied by nausea? Does the emesis relieve the symptoms and for how long? The patient should also be observed for signs of fluid imbalance. (See Chapter 12.)

Inflammations Usually Treated Surgically

APPENDICITIS

Even though today almost all lay people are familiar with the disease entity appendicitis, it was not until 1866 that its cause was identified and surgical removal advocated as the treatment of choice. Prior to this the treatment had been to wait for the appendix to rupture and then to treat the resulting abscess. Remember that this was long before the days of antibiotics; it is small wonder few survived the disease.

The *symptoms* are classic and begin with *acute abdominal pain,* which comes in waves. In the beginning it may be merely a discomfort that makes the patient feel as though passing flatus or having a bowel movement will give relief. Unfortunately many individuals take a laxative during this period. The pain typically starts in the epigastrium or periumbilical region and shifts to the right lower quadrant as the inflammatory process spreads to involve the serosal layers of the bowel and brings the inflammation into contact with the peritoneum. (See the section on peritonitis below.) The pain now becomes steady rather than intermittent, and the patient guards the area by lying still and drawing the leg up to relieve tension on the abdominal muscles. The exact location of pain depends upon the location of the appendix.

Other symptoms include vomiting, which begins after the pain starts, loss of appetite, a low-grade fever, coated tongue, and bad breath. A mild leukocytosis is usually present, with the white blood cell count between 10,000 and 15,000.

There are several causes for inflammation of the appendix, including a fecolith which occludes the lumen. This is the only cause many laymen are aware of, and the stories children are told about not eating cherry pits because they may cause appendicitis have some basis in fact because such foreign objects can occlude the lumen of the appendix. Fibrous disease conditions in the wall of the bowel and external occlusion by an adhesion may also cause appendiceal inflammation.

Treatment is removal of the appendix within 24 to 48 hours of onset of the symptoms; when this is done the mortality rate is less than 0.5 per cent. Delay usually causes rupture of the organ and resulting peritonitis. A frequent cause for delay in surgery is difficulty in diagnosis or the late arrival of the patient for medical aid.

Older people may have very few symptoms and frequently do not seek aid until after perforation has occurred.

In very young children diagnosis can also be difficult. Many diseases mimic appendicitis, including mesenteric adenitis, ovarian cyst, cholelithiasis, renal or ureteral calculi, diverticulitis, Meckel's diverticulum, and pneumonia.

MECKEL'S DIVERTICULUM

This is an outpouching of the bowel, a vestige of embryonic development found on the ileum within 100 cm. of the cecum. It may be lined with gastric mucosa or contain pancreatic tissue and sometimes develops a peptic ulcer that may bleed or perforate, or it may become inflamed and mimic appendicitis. It is sometimes attached to the umbilicus by a fibrous band and may be the focus around which the bowel twists, causing an obstruction. Treatment is surgical excision.

DIVERTICULOSIS; DIVERTICULITIS

A diverticulum is an outpouching of the mucosa and may or may not be covered by muscular tissue (see Fig. 59–1). Diverticula occur at any point in the gastrointestinal tract but are most common in the sigmoid region of the colon. Most colon diverticula are acquired and caused by increased pressure within the lumen, which causes the tissue to balloon out between the muscle fibers. This usually occurs at spots where blood vessels pass through the bowel wall. Some think that lack of bulk in the diet and stress are also factors in their development. The presence of diverticula is referred to as *diverticulosis.*

Unless complications develop, a diverticulum is no problem to the patient. Complications are perforation, hemorrhage, and inflammation (*diverticulitis*). Perforations are frequently walled off by the omentum and heal over without surgical intervention. They can also cause abscess formation resulting in the development of a fistula to the bladder or other adjacent structure. Diverticula are a common cause of bowel bleeding in adults. Patients who have periodic bouts of pain from diverticulitis are usually encouraged to eat a high residue diet and take bulk laxatives and are given antispasmodics to relax the bowel. Many can avoid attacks by this routine. Antibiotics are frequently given during periods of inflammation.

PERITONITIS

The peritoneum covers all the organs in the abdominal cavity and lines the cavity. It is highly permeable, and constituents of the blood pass through it freely. For this reason peritoneal dialysis can be used in renal failure (Unit XIII). Stimulation of the parietal portion that lines the abdominal and pelvic cavities causes sharp, well-localized pain since it is well supplied with somatic nerves. The visceral peritoneum is relatively insensitive.

Peritonitis can be primary or secondary, acute or chronic. The major sources of inflammation are from the gastrointestinal tract, from the external environment, and through the blood stream. In the female the uterine tubes penetrate the peritoneum, providing a potential route from the outside. The peritoneum is able to produce an inflammatory reaction and wall off a localized process to combat an infection, if the stimulus is not too massive or if the source of infection does not continue. For instance, a perforation, as of a gastric ulcer, that continues to drain contaminants into the peritoneal cavity will overcome the ability of the peritoneum to localize and combat the inflammatory process. The causes of peritonitis include the following:[38a]

- Ruptured liver
- Ruptured liver abscess
- Gangrenous cholecystitis
- Ruptured gallbladder
- Perforated carcinoma of the stomach
- Perforated stomach ulcer
- Ruptured spleen
- Acute pancreatitis
- Laceration of pancreas
- Perforation of any part of GI tract by swallowed foreign body
- Penetrating wound of GI tract
- Ulcerative colitis
- Gangrenous obstruction of small bowel
  - Adhesion
  - Carcinoma
  - Volvulus
  - Intussusception
- Perforation of Meckel's diverticulum
- Mesenteric thrombosis
- Perforation of diverticulum
- Regional ileitis
- Appendicitis with perforation
- Ruptured retroperitoneal abscess
- Strangulated hernia
- Puerperal infection
- Salpingitis
- Septic abortion
- Ruptured bladder

Symptoms of peritonitis vary, depending upon the cause. Pain is universal and may be either localized or generalized. A well-localized pain that causes rigidity of the abdominal muscles and increased pain from any pressure or motion of the abdomen is almost pathognomonic of peritonitis. The patient is usually nauseated and vomiting and may have a low-grade fever. Bowel sounds are absent, and respirations are usually shallow because the patient attempts to avoid the pain caused by body movement.

Systemic Effects. The circulatory system undergoes great stress from several sources: The infectious process causes an increased amount of circulating blood volume to be detoured to this area to combat the process. The peristaltic activity of the bowel ceases, with a resultant retention of fluids and air within its lumen and consequent increased pressure that causes increased secretion of fluid into the bowel. The circulating blood volume is thus reduced.

The inflammatory process causes an increase in the oxygen requirements at a time when the patient has a decreased ability to ventilate because of pain and an elevated diaphragm caused by increased abdominal pressure. These fluid shifts and respiratory alterations can pose grave problems in fluid and electrolyte management of the patient.

Treatment. If possible the cause is eliminated surgically, but sometimes the process has progressed so far that the patient is in no condition for surgery. Intravenous fluids for replacement of electrolyte and protein losses are essential. Usually a long tube is inserted through the nose into the intestine to reduce the pressure within the bowel. Positive pressure respiratory treatments may help to achieve adequate ventilation.

The patient may be placed in a semi-Fowler's position or have the head of the bed elevated 4 to 6 inches on blocks to promote the flow of drainage to the pelvic region where it can localize in an abscess and be drained or be resolved by body defenses.

Nursing Care of the Patient with an Acute Surgical Inflammation of the Bowel

The patient who has an acute inflammatory process of the bowel is very ill, usually is in a great deal of pain, frequently is vomiting, and needs expert medical and nursing care. In the early stages, an accurate diagnosis is of prime concern. The nurses' responsibilities therefore, in addition to making the patient comfortable, include making observations that will aid in diagnosis.

Specific nursing measures for the patient in pain, who is vomiting, and who has gastrointestinal decompression are mentioned elsewhere in this text. Patients need gentle handling to avoid increasing their pain, and complete care to conserve their strength and to promote rest. Supportive nursing measures such as bathing, mouth care, and frequent position changes, and comfort measures such as backrubs, if tolerated, are important, as are the therapeutic measures that include careful attention to the maintenance and flow of intravenous fluids, gastrointestinal suction, and catheter drainage. Observations to help the physician include the patient's description of the pain, the vital signs, and other signs of systemic malfunction (e.g., skin condition, the position the patient assumes for comfort, and general patient responses, including alertness and mental perceptiveness). Analgesics are usually not given until the diagnosis is made, because they may mask symptoms that might help in making a diagnosis.

The postoperative care of patients who have undergone surgery to treat these inflammatory conditions has been covered in Unit VIII.

HERNIATIONS

The classic definition of a hernia is a "protrusion of a viscus from its normal cavity through a congenital or acquired aperture." This definition limits a hernia to a situation in which there is a protrusion, but in normal usage a patient who has a weakness in the abdominal musculature through which a viscus or other abdominal structure periodically penetrates is considered to have a hernia, whether or not it is protruding.

Hernias may penetrate through any defect in the abdominal wall, through the diaphragm, or through some internal structure within the abdominal cavity. For this discussion, only the more commonly seen types of hernia will be mentioned.

Causes. Two things must be present for a hernia to occur: a defect in the integrity of the muscular wall, and increased intra-abdominal pressure. Defects in the muscular wall may be developmental, owing to an inherited tendency such as weakened collagen tissues or a wide space at the inguinal ligament, or may be caused by trauma.

Intra-abdominal pressure is most commonly increased from pregnancy or obesity. Heavy lifting also causes increased pressure, as do coughing and traumatic injuries from blunt pressure. When two of these factors coexist, along with some tissue weakness, a hernia can easily occur. Increased pressure without a weakness is not likely to cause a hernia. Weaknesses, in addition to being present from birth, are acquired as part of the aging process as muscular tissues become infiltrated and replaced by adipose and connective tissues.

Terminology. When the contents of the hernia sac can be replaced into the abdominal cavity, the hernia is said to be *reducible. Irreducible* and *incarcerated* are terms used to refer to a hernia that cannot be reduced. When the blood supply to the herniated segment of bowel is cut off by pressure from the hernia ring, the bowel becomes *strangulated.* Incarcerated hernias usually become strangulated sooner or later. This is a surgical emergency, because unless the bowel is released it soon becomes necrotic owing to lack of blood supply. A *hernia ring* is the ring of muscular tissue through which the bowel protrudes.

Types

The most common hernias are the inguinal, both direct and indirect, femoral, incisional, and umbilical. The hiatus hernia was discussed with conditions of the esophagus.

Indirect Inguinal. This herniation occurs through the inguinal ring and follows the spermatic cord through the inguinal canal (Fig. 63–1). It is far more common in males because of the space allowed for the descent of the testes. These hernias have a high incidence among infants and young persons, after which the incidence drops, then rises again among persons in their 50's, and then tapers off. These hernias can become extremely large and frequently descend into the scrotum.

Direct Inguinal. This hernia passes through the abdominal wall in an area of muscular weakness and not through a canal, as do the indirect inguinal and the femoral. It is more common in the elderly and is the result of a gradually developed weakness in an area that is congenitally deficient in the number of fibers present.

Femoral. The femoral hernia occurs through the femoral ring and is more common in females than in males. It begins as a plug of fat in the femoral canal that enlarges and gradually pulls the peritoneum, and almost inevitably the urinary bladder, into the sac. There is a high incidence of incarceration and strangulation in this type of hernia.

Umbilical. There are three kinds of umbilical hernias, two of which occur in infants. One of these is a surgical emergency at the time of birth, because abdominal viscera protrude through the umbilicus with the cord and, unless surgery is done to replace them and repair the associated defect of the abdominal wall, necrosis occurs along with the normal umbilical cord necrosis.

The more common type of umbilical herniation at birth is due to an abnormality of the muscular structures about the cord. It frequently gradually disappears owing to pull of the muscles and fascia across the defect, and heals in the months following birth; the usual treatment has been to keep the herniated area in position with a small strip of adhesive tape during this time. However, some authorities now feel that the hernia will heal whether or not it is kept reduced.

The third type of umbilical hernia, the adult type, is acquired and is more common in women. It is due to increased abdominal pressure and occurs in obese persons and women who have had several pregnancies. It is due to a defect of the umbilicus that has persisted from birth.

Incisional. This type of hernia occurs at the site of a previous surgical incision. It is the result of inadequate healing of the incision because of a postoperative problem such as infection, inadequate nutrition, extreme distention, obesity, or other factors. The incidence of this type of hernia is increasing, probably because of the higher number of surgical procedures being performed.

Nursing Care

The care the patient needs after hernia repair is dependent upon the location of the hernia and the type of anesthesia used. The hernias in the inguinal region are usually repaired under a spinal or local anesthetic, and the patient is allowed to ambulate immediately after recovery from the effects of the anesthesia and the surgical procedure. The patient should be checked to make certain voiding occurs after surgery. A full diet is given as soon as the patient tolerates food, which is usually soon after recovery from the anesthesia. A general anesthesia is commonly used for hernias in the upper abdomen, and the postoperative progress is thus slower.

The patient can be assured that during the immediate postoperative period there is no chance of the hernia breaking open again. Some patients hesitate to become active because of this fear. Obese patients make slower progress, heal more slowly, and may need more encouragement to participate in postoperative activities.

INTESTINAL OBSTRUCTIONS

Any impairment to the forward flow of the intestinal contents, whether by partial or complete stoppage or by a reversal of the flow, is known as an intestinal obstruction. It can be caused by mechanical, vascular, or nervous disorders.

Pathophysiology

With the onset of an obstruction, fluids and air collect proximal to the site of the problem.

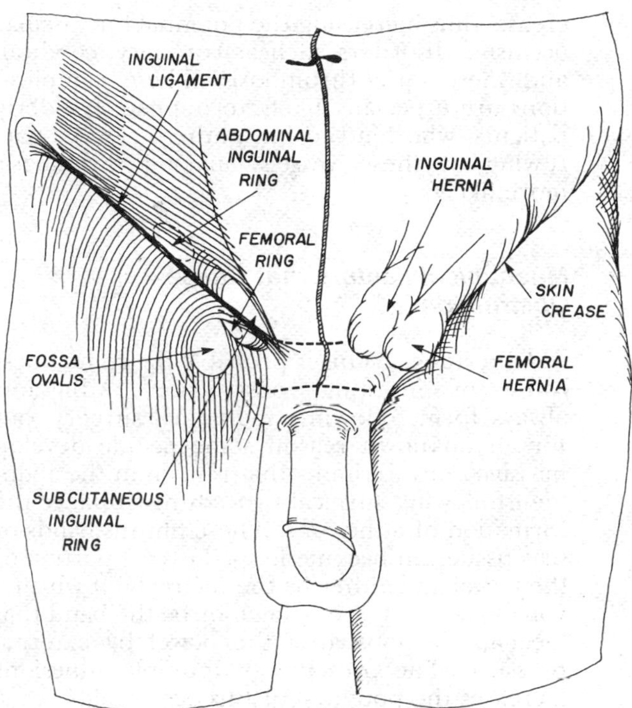

Figure 63–1. Areas involved in femoral and inguinal hernias. (From Artz, C. P., et al.: *Brief Textbook of Surgery.* Philadelphia: W. B. Saunders Co., 1976, p. 365.)

This causes a temporary increase in peristalsis as the bowel attempts to force the material through the obstructed area. Within a few hours the increased peristalsis ends and the bowel becomes flaccid, thus decreasing the pressure within the lumen and slowing the process caused by the obstruction. Increased pressure within the bowel causes a decrease in the absorptive ability of the bowel, which increases the fluid retention still further. Soon the intraluminal pressure causes a reduction in venous return, which increases venous pressure. This, in turn, increases the capillary permeability and allows plasma to extravasate into the bowel lumen and also into the peritoneal cavity. The bowel wall becomes permeable to bacteria, and bowel organisms enter the peritoneal cavity. Increasing pressure in the bowel wall soon slows the arterial blood flow, causing necrosis to develop.

Normally 7 to 8 liters of electrolyte-rich fluid are secreted by the bowel and most of it is resorbed. During an obstruction this fluid is partially retained within the bowel and partially eliminated by vomiting, thus causing a severe reduction in circulating blood volume which results in hypotension and a diminished renal and cerebral blood flow. Since fluid is lost without blood cells, the hematocrit and hemoglobin increase, thus increasing the potential for vascular occlusive disorders such as coronary, cerebral, and mesenteric thrombosis. These complications are especially likely to happen in elderly patients, who tend to have atherosclerotic narrowing of these vessels, making thrombosis more likely.

Mechanical Factors that Cause Obstruction

Adhesions. This is probably the commonest cause of intestinal obstruction. Adhesions always form following abdominal surgery, but for an unknown reason some people develop massive ones. Irritants that remain in the abdomen following surgical procedures enhance the formation of adhesions. These fibrous bands of scar tissue can become looped over a portion of the bowel and either be the focus about which a volvulus occurs (see below), or be the band that mechanically obstructs the bowel by external pressure. The presence of multiple adhesions increases the potential of this occurring.

Hernia. An incarcerated hernia may or may not cause an obstruction, depending upon the size of the hernia ring. However, the potential for obstruction is always present in any hernia. A strangulated hernia is always obstructed, because the bowel is not functional when its blood supply is cut off. See previous section for a description of hernias.

Volvulus. This is a twisting of the bowel that frequently occurs about a stationary focus in the abdominal cavity. It can occur in either the large or small bowel and sometimes releases without surgical intervention. When decompression with a long tube is accomplished successfully, a small bowel volvulus may relax as the pressure against the proximal end of the loop is relieved. A large bowel volvulus sometimes releases when a barium enema is given, as introducing pressure distal to the obstruction equalizes the forces on both sides of the loop.

Intussusception. This is a telescoping of the bowel upon itself and is most common in infants, occurring at the ileocecal junction, with the small bowel telescoping inside the large bowel. In adults it is usually associated with a tumor of the large bowel which telescopes into the bowel distal to it from peristaltic activity. In infants, a barium enema sometimes causes intussusception to release, making surgery unnecessary unless the process was present long enough to cause irreversible damage to the bowel wall.

Tumors. In the large bowel, tumors are the chief cause of obstruction. The process develops slowly and, because of the large lumen of the bowel, may be quite advanced before a fecal mass becomes lodged at the constricted site and precipitates an acute obstructive process. In the small bowel, obstructive symptoms are frequently the first sign of a tumor. Even though the lumen of the bowel is smaller, these symptoms still do not occur early in the process because the intestinal contents are liquid. Tumors of the large and small bowel are discussed on pp. 1453–1457.

Neurogenic Factors that Cause Obstruction

An adynamic (or functional) obstruction, sometimes called a "paralytic ileus," is caused by a lack of peristaltic activity. The propulsive activity of the bowel is inhibited by reflex stimulation which can be due to a number of different pathologic processes. It commonly occurs following abdominal surgery as the bowel ceases to function for a time, ranging from a few hours to several days. Procedures in which the bowel is handled extensively and procedures in the retroperitoneal area are quite apt to cause a postoperative problem. Treatment is aspiration of the secretions by gastric suction until the bowel begins to function.

Infections of the abdomen and sometimes of the thoracic cavity, such as lobar pneumonia, peritonitis, or pancreatitis, are frequent causes of an ileus of infectious origin. The other common cause is electrolyte imbalance, especially hypokalemia.

Vascular Factors that Cause Obstruction

Interruption of blood supply to any body part causes pain to occur and function to cease. Blood is supplied to the bowel by way of the celiac and superior and inferior mesenteric arteries. These vessels have anatomotic intercommunications at the head of the pancreas and along the transverse bowel.

Complete Occlusion (Mesenteric Infarction). Any occlusion of arterial blood supply to the bowel, as in mesenteric thrombosis, will effectively stop bowel function. This is usually caused by an embolus, and the extent of symptoms is determined by the size of the vessel that is occluded, the extent of bowel without blood supply, and the rapidity with which the occlusion occurs. An acute occlusion will, at its onset, cause intense abdominal pain without signs of advanced intestinal obstruction because the pain is caused by ischemic tissue rather than the results of obstruction. As the process advances, symptoms of gangrene of the bowel develop, such as fever, leukocytosis and shock.

Acute mesenteric obstruction is a surgical emergency and has a high mortality rate — approximating 75 per cent. Sometimes an embolectomy can be done to restore circulation. Necrotic segments of the bowel must be resected, so early surgical intervention is essential.

Partial Occlusion (Abdominal Angina). This is usually due to atherosclerosis of the mesenteric arteries, which is quite common though asymptomatic, and is found in 33 per cent of routine autopsies. Pain may develop 15 to 30 minutes after eating, as an increased need for oxygenation occurs during the digestive process. Originally pain may occur only on ingestion of a large meal, but as the arterial process enlarges, it may occur even after ingestion of a small meal and eventually become almost continuous. Symptoms are caused only when the interruption of blood supply is sufficient to compromise the function of the bowel and may include, in addition to pain after eating, a change in bowel habits, nausea and vomiting, and weight loss because the patient restricts intake owing to the discomfort experienced when food is ingested. Vascular or by-pass grafts can sometimes be done to improve the blood supply to the affected portion of the bowel.

Treatment

The major objective in treating bowel obstruction is to relieve the cause and thus eliminate the problem. However, the cause is not always immediately obvious. The diagnosis of the cause of an acute abdominal condition may be quite difficult and frequently is made in surgery. It is important to make as specific observations as possible to aid the physician in the diagnosis. In the vast majority of the vascular and mechanically caused obstructions the only treatment is surgical intervention to remove the cause. In adynamic ileus, drugs are not effective in stimulating bowel activity, and the best treatment is rest and prevention of distention by use of gastric suction. The bowel will respond when recovery from the physical insult is complete.

TUMORS

Both benign and malignant tumors occur in all portions of the bowel, but their incidence varies greatly from one area to another. Malignant tumors are uncommon in the small bowel, being 1 per cent of all malignant neoplasms of the alimentary tract. Few benign tumors are found in this region either, but this may be due mostly to their lack of symptoms. In the large bowel, carcinoma is the most common tumor, and 60 to 70 per cent of these occur in the distal portion, from the sigmoid to the anus.

Benign

In the small bowel various kinds of benign tumors are found. Polyps are the most commonly found benign tumor of the large bowel. A *polyp* is a lesion that projects into the lumen of the bowel. If it has a stem, it is known as *pedunculated;* if there is no stem, it is called *sessile* (Fig. 63–2; see also Fig. 59–1). These lesions can be either benign or malignant, but the term polyp usually refers to the benign form. Some types of polyps are precursors of cancer and can be considered to be premalignant tumors. The symptoms of benign tumors may be quite similar to those of malignant tumors. Also, benign tumors, in both the large and small bowel, may be the cause of an intussusception. The major dangers they present are in masking a malignant tumor and serving as the focus for a bowel obstruction. Some benign tumors bleed profusely and cause symptoms of abdominal discomfort. These are usually removed surgically.

Malignant

SMALL BOWEL

Malignant tumors of the small bowel are rare (about 1 per cent of all gastrointestinal cancers), occur in younger people than do malignant tumors of the large bowel, have an average age of onset of 53 to 58 years, and occur in nearly equal numbers in men and women. Almost half of the tumors reported in medical reviews[203, 175] were in the ileum, with the remainder almost equally divided between the duodenum and jejunum. The low incidence has been variously explained as due to the low bacterial content of the small bowel and to the rapid transit of the chyme or its liquid nature. Recent evidence suggests that an intrinsic protective mechanism may exist, since high levels of immunoglobulins have been found. Symptoms, which include weight loss, pain, anemia, nausea or vomiting, obstruction, palpable mass, and hemorrhage, are vague and nonspecific and usually develop over a period of months before medical care is sought.

Surgery is the only treatment that offers any hope of cure, but even when diagnosis is made early and a resection is done, prognosis for 5 year survival is only about 20 per cent. With late diagnosis or early spread to the liver, the five-year survival rate is about 5 per cent.

LARGE BOWEL

In both men and women cancer of the colon and rectum is the second most frequent cause of

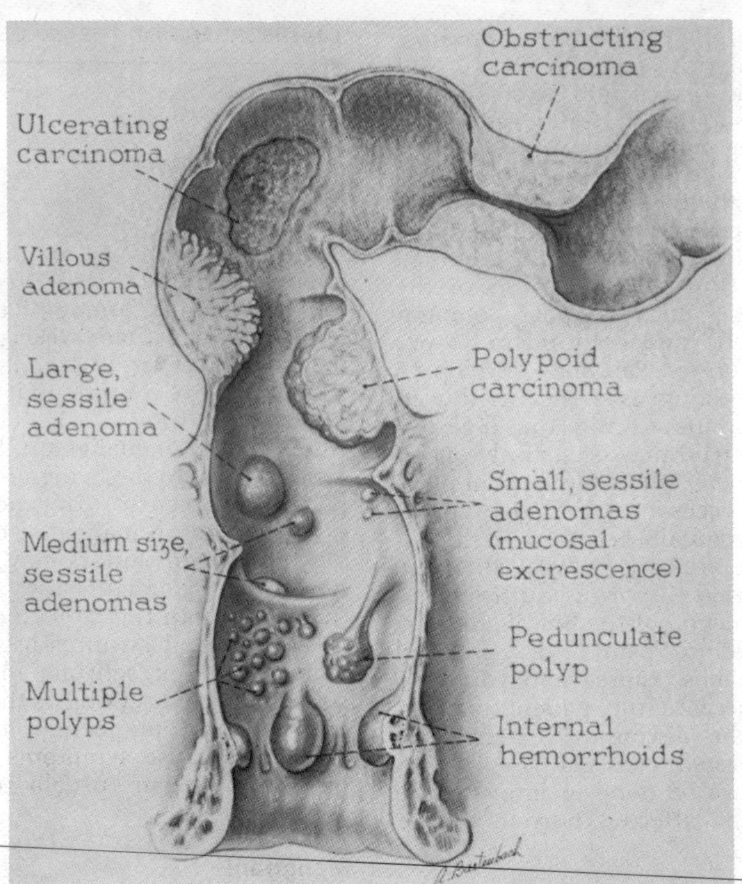

Figure 63–2. Composite drawing illustrating pedunculate and sessile adenomas of the colon and rectum. These, along with carcinoma and internal hemorrhoids, are the three most common lesions that produce bleeding. (From Turell, R. (Ed.): *Diseases of the Colon and Anorectum*, 2nd ed. Vol. I. Philadelphia: W. B. Saunders Co., 1969, page 335.)

death from cancer in the United States, ranking right behind cancer of the lung in men and cancer of the breast in women. The death rate for women has decreased slightly in the last two decades, while for men there has been no change. Males and females are affected in equal numbers, but cancer of the colon is more common in women, whereas cancer of the rectum is more common in men. The incidence of malignant lesions varies from one portion of the bowel to another with the greatest incidence occurring in the portion most accessible to examination. In recent years the incidence of carcinoma of the right colon has increased while there has been a decline in the rectosigmoid cancer incidence. Table 63–3 presents data obtained at New England Deaconess Hospital from 1928 to 1967. Note that the site with the greatest percentage of cases is still the rectosigmoid portion of the colon.

Considering that early diagnosis with a resultant improvement in mortality figures should be possible, it seems that many people still do not avail themselves of the knowledge available con-

TABLE 63–3. CHANGE IN CANCER OF THE COLON

	1928–1937		1938–1947		1948–1957		1958–1967	
	No.	*Percent*	*No.*	*Percent*	*No.*	*Percent*	*No.*	*Percent*
Right colon	39	6.7	191	10.5	258	13.7	316	21.4
Rectosigmoid	462	79.6	1,401	74.6	1,334	70.8	908	61.6
Transverse, left and unspecified	79	13.6	286	15.0	290	15.4	249	16.9
TOTAL	580		1,878		1,882		1,473	

*Significant.
Adapted from Cady, B., et al.: Changing patterns of colorectal carcinoma. *Cancer*, 33:422, 1974.

cerning the diagnosis and treatment of this condition.

Etiology. Research studies indicate that over-nutrition, especially too much fat in the diet, is the major factor in the development of cancer of the large bowel.[206] Studies on bulk in the stool and the rate of transit of fecal matter have so far given mixed results. Some propose that metabolic and bacterial end products are carcinogenic and that constipation allows a longer contact with the bowel wall, thus increasing the probability of cancer developing.

Symptoms. Symptoms vary according to the area in which the tumor is found, but include bleeding, changed bowel habits, abdominal pain, weight loss, anorexia, and nausea and vomiting (Fig. 63–3). In general, tumors in the small bowel and right colon are more likely to cause abdominal pain and nausea and vomiting, while those in the left colon and rectum are more likely to cause an alteration of bowel habits and passage of blood or mucus and a feeling that the bowel is not empty after defecation. The symptoms differ, also depending upon the type of growth that is involved. Polypoid, cirrhous, ulcerating, annular, and colloid growths may occur in the bowel. (See Figure 63–2).

When the tumor occludes the bowel, symptoms of an obstruction result. Tumors in the right colon are unlikely to cause obstruction because of the large lumen of the bowel and the liquid quality of the feces. Tumors in the left colon and rectum frequently cause obstructive symptoms (Fig. 63–3).

Diagnosis. One third of the malignant tumors of the distal colon and rectum can be felt with the examining finger. This makes the digital rectal examination one of the more important diagnostic methods. X-rays of the colon show either a filling defect or a stricture when cancer is present. By use of the sigmoidoscope one half of the tumors can be seen. Many authorities feel that all individuals over 40 should have a sigmoidoscopy done as part of a routine yearly physical examination. The use of fiberoptic flexible scopes for examining the colon is increasing; they can reach even into the right colon, extending the diagnostic capabilities of the physician greatly. Cytologic examination is used in some medical centers, but, as with stomach tissues, authorities do not agree on its usefulness. More than 90 per cent of the patients who have noninvasive lesions and who survive surgery live 5 years following the surgery. This would indicate the importance of early diagnosis in improving the mortality figures for this condition.

Spread. Tumors of the bowel spread by direct extension to a nearby organ, as to the stomach from the transverse colon; by lymphatic and hematogenic channels; and into the peritoneal cavity by seeding or implanting of cells. The urinary bladder, ureters, and reproductive organs are frequently involved by direct extension, and the formation of a fistula between the bladder and the bowel or between the bowel and

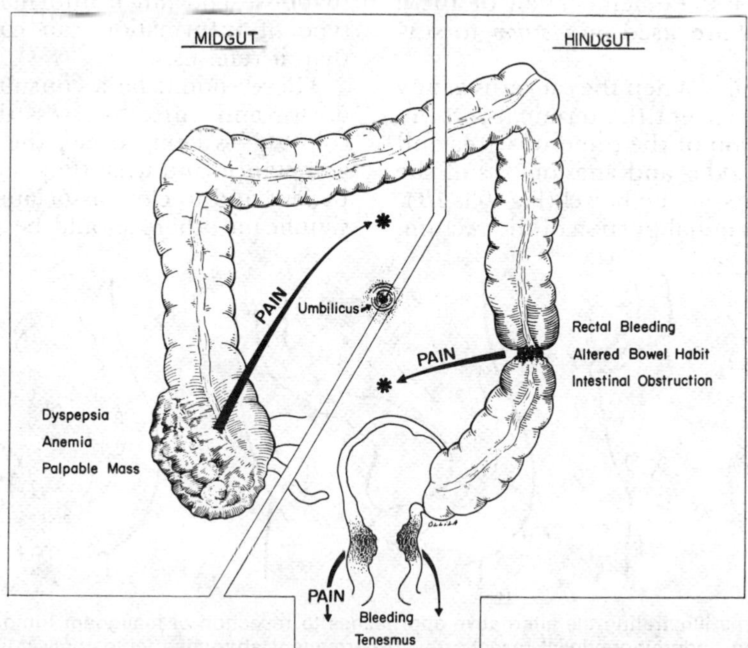

Figure 63–3. Symptoms of carcinoma in the right and left colon. (From Cohn, I., Jr., and F. C. Nance: The colon and rectum. Part VI. Intermediate or precancerous lesions and malignant lesions. *In* Sabiston, D. C. (Ed.): *Davis-Christopher Textbook of Surgery.* Philadelphia: W. B. Saunders Co., 1977, p. 1104.)

vagina is not uncommon. Blood-borne extension goes most frequently to the liver but may also involve the lungs, kidneys, and bones.

Treatment. This depends upon the tumor — its location, the presence of metastases, the grade of differentiation of the cells —and on the patient's general condition. With the present 5 year survival rate at about 50 per cent, surgery is the only treatment that offers hope of cure. Work is currently being done to increase the survival rate by controlling the disseminations that occur. *Radiation therapy* is given before surgery in the hope that it will (a) alter the malignant cells so that those which spread to the lymphatics, blood stream, or locally during surgery will not survive and (b) reduce the size of the tumor and thus make it more resectable. A newer treatment that aims at reducing spread during surgery is *anticoagulation therapy,* usually with streptokinase, to lower the ability of the cancer cells to gain a foothold and grow in some distant site. Local treatments of the tumor site after surgery include the implantation of *isotopes* into the tumor area and *electrocoagulation. Chemotherapy* has not been too successful; 5-FU is the only drug that has produced results, and these have been temporary. Recently work has been done to improve this picture by using combinations of drugs. *Immunotherapy* is also being used and studies so far have shown an increased disease-free interval — especially in patients with liver metastases. Remember, all of these adjuvant therapies are used *in addition* to surgery.[108]

Surgical Treatment. When the cancer is at any point in the bowel except the terminal rectum, treatment is resection of the tumorous area and associated lymph nodes and anastomosis of the remaining segments of the bowel (Fig. 63–4*B*). In the anus and terminal portion of the rectum, the usual surgical procedure is an abdominoperineal resection, sometimes known as anterior-posterior resection, with the formation of a permanent colostomy (Fig. 63–4*A*). When the tumor is in the upper rectum and not of high grade malignancy, it can frequently be resected and the sphincter retained.

Occasionally, in some medical centers, a procedure called a "pull through" is done. This consists of loosening the bowel through an anterior incision and then literally pulling it through the rectal sphincter. Thus, the tumor is eliminated and the sphincter is retained (Fig. 63–4*C*). This is usually employed when the growth is extensive, the hope of cure is small, and the physician does not wish to inflict a colostomy on a patient with so many other problems.

Nursing Care. The patient who is suspected of having cancer of the colon may be admitted to the hospital for x-ray and sigmoidoscopic examinations, or these may be done on an outpatient basis. The patient will probably be apprehensive about both the test procedures and their outcome. If the lesion is in the rectum, the physician may have told the patient of the probability of a colostomy being done. The average patient has had almost no contact with others who have a colostomy and has only vague ideas concerning it. Usually the preconceived ideas patients have are erroneous and include the notion that the colostomy will be "awful." In the preoperative period the nurse should give patients some positive information about a colostomy. However, before telling a patient anything about this condition, learn about how this individual generally accepts life's traumatic situations. Too much information or the wrong type of information can cause more anxiety than it relieves.

There should be a consultation between the doctor and nurse to assess the probability of a colostomy's being done, the patient's probable acceptance, and what they should explain to the patient and to close associates. The patient and significant others should be prepared for a co-

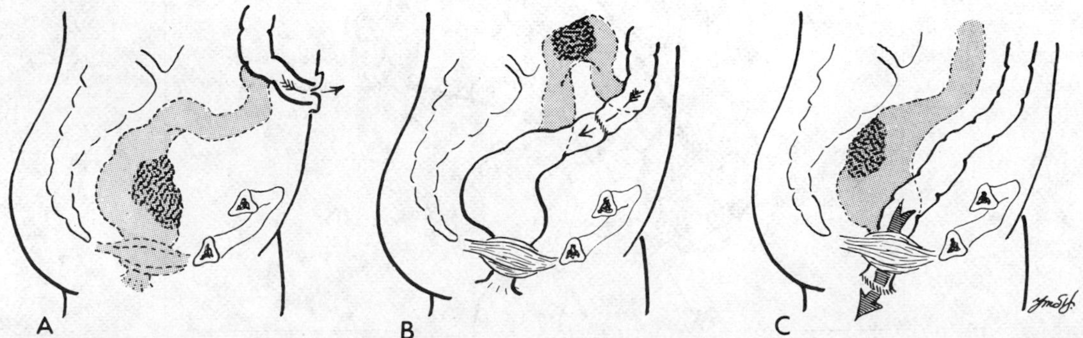

Figure 63–4. Diagrams illustrating the alternative approaches to resection of malignant tumors in the rectosigmoid segment. **A.** Combined abdominoperineal resection with permanent abdominal colostomy (Miles' operation). **B.** Anterior resection with primary anastomosis. **C.** Proctosigmoidectomy with "pull-through" and anastomosis and preservation of external sphincter muscles. (From Block, M. A.: Malignant tumors of the colon and rectum. Part II. Surgical treatment. In Bockus, H. L.: *Gastroenterology,* 3rd ed. Vol. 2. Philadelphia: W. B. Saunders Co., 1976, p. 1050.)

lostomy only if there is a strong possibility that one may have to be done. Always remember that patients may feel that their condition is inoperable if a colostomy is not performed after the physician has discussed the possibility of a colostomy. See Chapter 59 for care of the patient who has a colostomy.

A nursing function, in addition to caring for a patient with potential or diagnosed cancer, is to aid in case finding. Some patients will not go to a physician who routinely performs a sigmoidoscopy during a physical examination. The nurse is in a good position to interpret the importance of the examination in diagnosis and thus cure of debilitating conditions. Much teaching should be done among the general public concerning the importance of the symptoms of rectal bleeding and a change in bowel habits. If more patients sought medical help at the first sign of such symptoms, more patients would survive.

NURSING CARE OF PATIENTS WHO HAVE HAD BOWEL SURGERY

Care of patients with bowel surgery varies according to whether or not the lumen of the bowel was opened during the surgical procedure. The repair of hernias and the release of some types of bowel obstruction do not require that the bowel be opened, whereas the resection of a tumor in the lumen of the bowel or the resection of a portion of the bowel will necessitate its opening.

Preoperative Care. Patients who have the bowel opened will probably enter the hospital a day or so before surgery for bowel preparation. This includes a low-residue or liquid diet to reduce the fecal contents of the bowel and the administration of antibiotics either by mouth, parenterally, or occasionally by means of rectal or colostomy instillation. Enemas to cleanse the bowel are mandatory. The objective is to make the inside of the lumen of the bowel as clean and bacteria-free as possible. When the surgical procedure is done as an emergency, preparation is of necessity brief, and the patient has a higher probability of developing postoperative complications and infection.

Preoperative management may include gastrointestinal decompression with either a long or short tube (See Chapter 59).

The preoperative teaching depends on the nature of the proposed surgery but will always include such things as what to expect postoperatively in the way of therapy, and the various measures such as deep breathing and leg exercises that are designed to prevent complications. The type of anesthetic used and duration or presence of intravenous infusions and gastric suction will vary.

Postoperative Care. Depending upon the extent of the surgical procedure and the type of anesthesia used, patients may be up immediately after surgery and walking down the hall, as in a herniorrhaphy done with a local anesthetic, or they may be severely ill for several days, e.g., patients who have had large portions of the bowel resected.

An important sign of progress in a postoperative bowel surgery patient is the return of bowel function.

The passage of flatus rectally indicates that peristalsis is returning. The presence of peristalsis can also be determined by using a stethoscope to listen for bowel sounds. Gastric suction is frequently used until peristaltic activity returns. It is usually several days before food and fluids are taken orally. Diet is resumed progressively, beginning with liquids and advancing as the patient tolerates food. The presence of abdominal cramps is common, as is distention of the bowel. Distention is uncomfortable for the patient and, if extreme, not good for new suture lines. Some surgeons routinely use a cecostomy when large bowel surgery is done in order to decompress the bowel and prevent tension on sutures (see Chapter 59). The insertion of a rectal tube for 20 to 30 minutes will be of help if there is gas in the rectum.

Insertion of any tube into the rectum should be done only with the surgeon's consent if there is a low suture line which could be traumatized.

The physician may suture or tape a rectal tube in place when rectal sutures are present. Like a cecostomy tube this tube should be kept open; it is usually irrigated periodically with water.

Drains are often left in the incision, and attached to a suction device such as a Hemovac. Frequent dressing changes may be needed if suction is not used. See Chapter 19, Goal 7 "Promotion of Wound Healing." The character and volume of drainage should be noted carefully in addition to the odor. Should the drainage in any way suggest a developing infection, a culture should be taken to identify the organism and thus give information about what antibiotic will be effective and the possible necessity for isolating the patient. Isolation precautions should be used on all dressings from any draining wound, both to protect the wound from infection and to prevent the spread of organisms that may be present (see the discussion of wound infection in Chapter 20).

Chapter 59 discusses the care of a patient who has had a colostomy created. If an abdominoperineal resection was done, the patient will have, in addition to an abdominal incision, a single barrel colostomy and a deep wound where the rectum was resected. A colostomy bag will be used over the stoma; when it is changed or emptied, care must be taken to prevent contamination of the surgical wound by fecal discharges. Return of bowel function can be monitored by observing the type and quantity of discharges from the stoma. In the immediate postoperative period, sump drainage is frequently used for the perineal wound. This is attached to suction and allows the wound to heal from its deepest portion without forming a pocket of drainage. If suction is not used, rectal dressings will need to be changed frequently because the large deep wound drains profusely. It will take several weeks for the wound to heal completely because of its size. Since drainage continues during the healing period, the patient should be prepared to wear a rectal dressing for some time.

It may be several weeks before the patients regain their strength after major bowel surgery. When segments have been removed from the bowel, the patient's bowel habits may be altered until the body readjusts to the situation. Patients probably have many questions, especially after going home. Draining wounds occasionally develop into chronically draining fistulas, and it is not uncommon that dressings must be changed at home. The nurse should make sure that the patient knows how to change dressings correctly and is aware of any dietary or activity restrictions to be followed. The patient should know whom to call if help is needed at home. A public health nurse's visit can add much to the patient's peace of mind and can also identify problems that might not otherwise be known.

CHAPTER 64

DISORDERS OF THE RECTUM AND ANUS

The major function of the rectum is storage of the feces until evacuation takes place. Entry of feces into the rectum distends its walls and causes mass peristaltic movements to occur and, ideally, at this time the patient cooperates and encourages defecation. Many of the disorders that occur in the rectal area result from constipation and failure of the patient to empty the rectum when the mass peristaltic movements occur.

ANATOMY

To understand the pathologic processes that occur in the rectal area, it is necessary to have a clear picture of the normal anatomic landmarks. The distal portion of the rectal walls form longitudinal folds, called rectal or anal columns, which terminate about ½ inch from the anal orifice. These are connected to each other by transverse folds of tissue called *valves*. The pockets formed by the valves are called *sinuses* or *crypts*. Since the external portion of the anal opening is lined with skin that changes at this point to mucosa, this area is sometimes called the *mucocutaneous border*. Other names for this border are the dentate, pectinate, or anorectal line. The venous drainage and the nerve supply also change at this point. Above this line, the venous drainage is into the portal system; below it into the vena cava. The autonomic nervous system supplies innervation above the line, and the central nervous system below (Fig. 64–1).

SYMPTOMS

At the mucocutaneous border of the anal canal, the mucous membrane changes to skin that has cutaneous somatic nerve endings. Because of this, lesions of the external anal canal are exquisitely painful. The two most common symptoms are bleeding and pain. Drainage of mucus and fecal matter and irritation of the skin from organisms can cause intense itching. Hem-

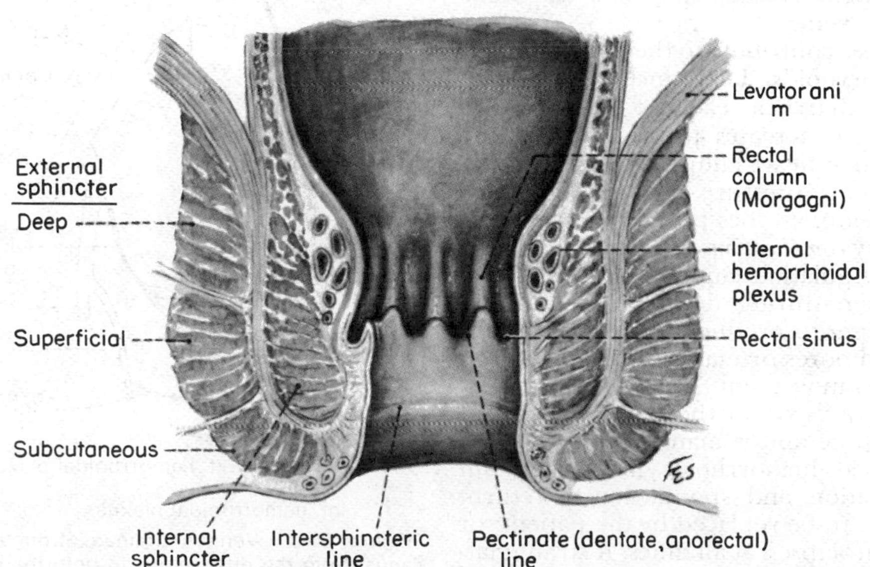

Figure 64–1. Normal anorectal anatomy. (From Corman, M. L.: Rubber band ligation of hemorrhoids. *Archives of Surgery,* 112:1257, Oct. 1977.)

orrhoids and skin tags may protrude from the anal opening, and there may be drainage of pus from abscesses.

DEVELOPMENTAL, STRUCTURAL, AND VASCULAR DISORDERS

Hemorrhoids

Hemorrhoids, sometimes called piles, are a common affliction of mankind. They are probably caused by our upright position, and the pressure it causes on the anorectal veins; they have their greatest incidence during the most active years of adulthood, from 20 to 50 years. Hemorrhoids may be either internal or external; they consist of dilated veins which lie under the mucous membrane. Internal hemorrhoids are varicose dilatations of veins of the superior hemorrhoidal plexus. They occur above the mucocutaneous border and are covered by mucous membrane. External hemorrhoids are dilatations of the inferior hemorrhoidal plexus, are below the mucocutaneous junction, and are covered by anal skin. As these vessels dilate, they stretch the overlying mucous membrane and skin and eventually protrude down the anal canal to prolapse outside. Figure 64–2 illustrates the venous drainage of this area.

Internal hemorrhoids are frequently caused by portal hypertension. Both types can be caused by the many anastomoses between the plexuses and by the lack of valves in the veins of the superior hemorrhoidal plexus which leads into the portal vein.

Several causes contribute to the acute enlargement of hemorrhoids. These include both constipation and diarrhea, each of which causes straining, which increases pressure within the veins. Congestive heart failure and its resultant increased venous pressure can cause hemorrhoids to develop, as does portal hypertension.

The primary *complications* of hemorrhoids are bleeding, strangulation, and thrombosis. Trauma to the vein during defecation can cause enough bleeding to produce an iron deficiency anemia. Blood oozes or may even spurt out following a bowel movement. Thrombosis, or clotting of the blood within the hemorrhoid, can occur at any time and is manifested by intense pain. Prolapsed hemorrhoids may come out during defecation and spontaneously return; they may have to be replaced by the patient; or they may be prolapsed at all times. A strangulated hemorrhoid is a prolapsed one in which the blood supply is cut off by the anal sphincter. The blood within it becomes clotted and thrombosis occurs. This is a very painful condition, with extreme edema and inflammation present. Cold applications and elevation of the buttocks may allow the prolapsed hemorrhoid to reduce itself spontaneously.

Four *treatments* are commonly used for hemorrhoids: medical management, surgical excision of the dilated veins, rubber band ligation, or injection of a sclerosing substance into the tissues at the base of the vein. This last one may be only temporarily effective.

Medical therapy, used only for small hemorrhoids with mild symptoms, includes reducing pressure by treating the constipation and relieving pain with the application of heat and astringent lotions. A recumbent position may be needed if the hemorrhoid is prolapsed or thrombosed.

In *surgical excision* the vein is excised and the area either left open to heal by granulation or sutured closed. The open method is very painful for the patient but has a high rate of success, whereas the sutured method, while far less painful, is more likely to cause infection resulting in poor healing.

Postoperative complications include, other than infection, stricture formation as the lesion heals, and hemorrhage. Hemorrhage, which may occur immediately after surgery or about 10 days after surgery as a result of sloughing of tissue, can be quite extensive and may not be

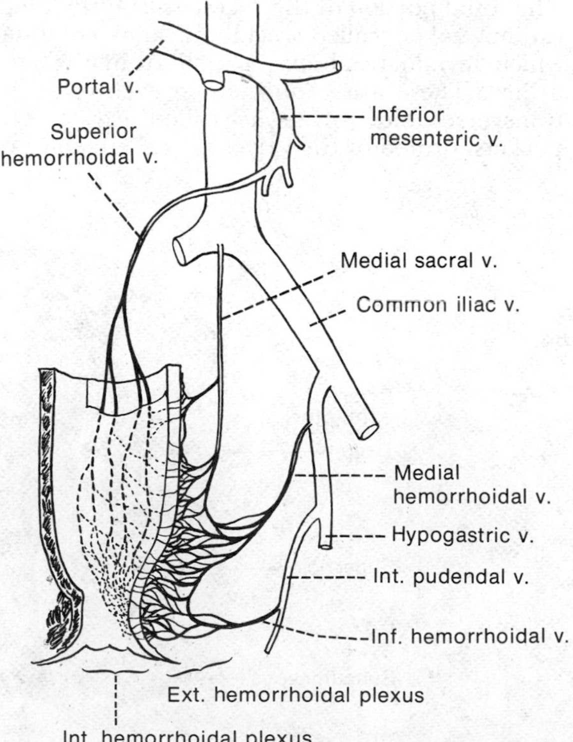

Figure 64–2. Venous drainage from the rectum and anus. Note the dual return to both the portal and caval systems providing for collateral venous circulation through the hemorrhoidal plexuses. (Based on Bockus, H. L.: *Gastroenterology*, 3rd ed. Vol. II, 1974.)

evident since bleeding can occur into the rectum and not be passed to the outside unless a drain was placed in the area. The patient can become quite constipated after the surgery unless measures are taken to avoid it. The area is very painful, and patients may avoid defecating to avoid the pain they are certain will accompany passage of a stool. This can result in the formation of a hard stool (which may traumatize the area) or a fecal impaction. Most surgeons give patients bulk laxatives and order enemas or mineral oil to promote passage of a stool. Patients are usually not allowed to leave the hospital until they have had a bowel movement. The nurse should check the stool, since some patients pass only a very small particle of feces in the first bowel movement. Rectal dilatations are frequently given at intervals after surgery to dilate the area and to prevent stricture formation; however, it is preferable for the patient to have a well-formed stool daily to dilate the area naturally.

Rubber band ligation is gradually becoming a common procedure for treating internal hemorrhoids. The advantages over hemorrhoidectomy are that the procedure is done in the physician's office, and the patient can usually carry on normal activities. It cannot be used for external hemorrhoids because they are below the dentate line and have somatic nerve endings (see section on symptoms).

The procedure is simple. The surgeon inserts a ligator through an anoscope; a ligator is a small double-lumen cylinder with a small rubber band on the inner layer. The hemorrhoid is grasped with a forcep and pulled through the ligator. Then the operator retracts the inner cylinder, forcing the rubber band over the neck of the hemorrhoid (Fig. 64–3). The patient takes a bulk laxative after the procedure to avoid trauma to the area from a hard fecal mass. In 8 to 10 days the rubber band cuts through the neck of tissue, and the tissue sloughs. Complications (pain or bleeding) occur rarely.

Nursing Care. A patient who has a rectal condition is frequently sensitive and embarrassed about the condition and needs matter-of-fact care from the nurse. The importance of keeping the stool soft but formed to help to prevent the formation of strictures should be stressed as well as the importance of keeping the area clean. The patient should be encouraged to wash the anal area after defecation and to pat it dry rather than irritate the tissues by cleansing with dry paper. Local moist heat applied with a washcloth or piece of cotton directly to the anal opening for a few minutes is soothing, cleansing, and healing for a sore area. Patients can do this for themselves by moistening the material under hot water from the tap. Heat should not be applied in the immediate postoperative period because of the possibility of hemorrhage. Most physicians order sitz baths to be taken three or four times a day or as the patient desires, beginning 12 hours after surgery. These

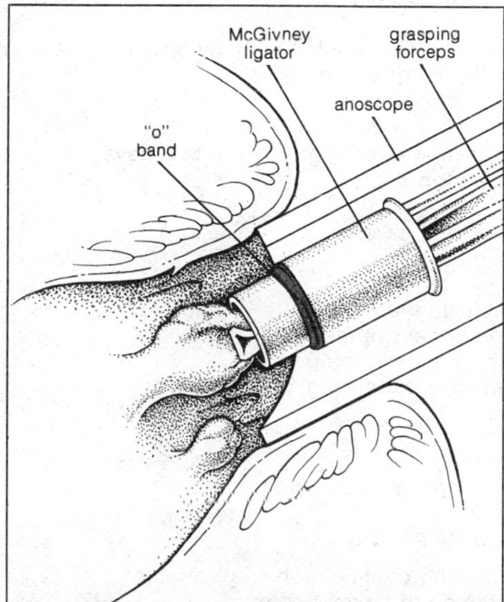

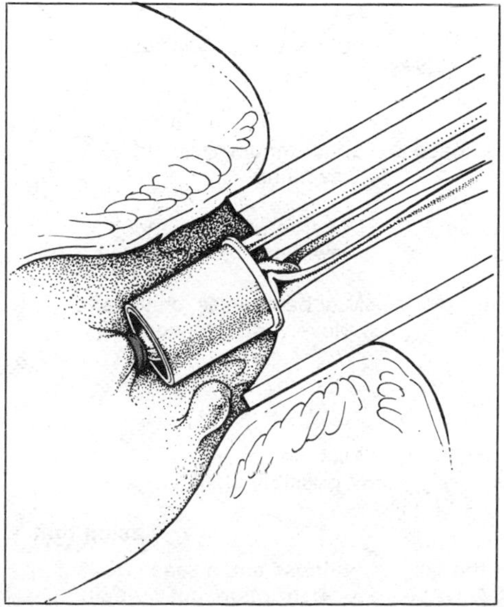

Figure 64–3. Banding a hemorrhoid. The hemorrhoid is grasped with forceps and pulled through the ligator. The size "0" rubber band is released by operating the trigger mechanism, which snaps it over the neck of the hemorrhoid. (From A snap cure for hemorrhoids. *Emergency Medicine,* 9:200, July 1977.)

cleanse the area as well as apply localized heat.

Postoperative complications requiring nursing vigilance include hemorrhage and urinary retention. The proximity of the bladder and the tenderness in the area sometimes make urination difficult.

> *After hemorrhoid surgery, the patient should be checked for hemorrhage and voiding.*

Reestablishing bowel habits is another postoperative problem. A diet high in bulk and including sufficient fluids should be encouraged. This patient may need instruction on the relationship of diet and fluid intake to bowel regularity, the physiology of defecation, and the importance of establishing a routine.

Pilonidal Cyst

This is a cyst usually containing hair, which becomes infected, forms an abscess, and then a sinus tract. It occurs at the base of the sacrum and is most common in young adults, especially males. It has traditionally been though to be caused by abnormal embryologic development, but other theories suggest that it results from hairs that penetrate the skin and cause sinus tracts to form. Rubbing from clothing and from chairs, can cause hairs in this area to become embedded and then infected. Acute pain and swelling result, followed by a discharge.

Treatment is surgical excision of the abscess formation. The period of healing is quite long. If the infectious process is not completely removed the patient may have a recurrence of the condition. Removing the hairs in this area is a

TABLE 64–1. ANORECTAL LESIONS

Lesion	First Symptoms	Later symptoms	Duration of Symptoms
	Lesions Producing Pain*		
Anal fissure	Moderate-to-severe sharp pain	Decreasing severity with soft stools.	Less than one week, if stools are soft.
Anal cryptitis	"Sticking" or irritated sensation	Severe, sharp and throbbing pain.	Symptoms begin with infection, may become chronic.
Thrombosed external hemorrhoid	Sudden pain with defecation or heavy lifting	Continued aching. Firm, tender, bluish mass at an anal margin. May bleed if eroded.	Generally less than 24 hours. Erosion after 3 or 4 days.
Internal hemorrhoids	Fullness, if prolapsed	Severe pain and aching if thrombosis and prolapse occur.	Symptoms date from prolapse.
Cutaneous abscess	Local tenderness and swelling	Increasing severity of symptoms.	2 to 3 days.
Subcutaneous abscess	Local tenderness and swelling	Increasing severity of symptoms.	2 to 3 days.
Ischiorectal abscess	May be malaise, chills, and fever; local tenderness	Localized induration, tenderness, and swelling, with pain of steadily increasing severity.	3 to 5 days.
Superior pelvirectal abscess	Malaise, fever and possibly chills	Dull aching lateral to rectum. Leucocytosis.	4 to 5 days.
	Lesion that May Not Be Painful		
Cancer of the rectum	Fullness and a sense of obstruction, but no pain	Increasing constipation, change of bowel habits, blood in stools.	Variable

*Adapted from Thiele, G.: Anorectal pain. *American Family Physician,* 6:56–7, Aug. 1972.

good measure to help to prevent recurrence after healing has occurred.

INFLAMMATIONS

Rectal Fissure (Fissure-in-Ano). This is an ulceration of the skin of the anal canal that is actually a longitudinal crack in the skin. An acute fissure occurs as a result of stretching of the tissue and possibly from the trauma of a hard or large stool passing through the area. The skin is torn as the mass passes and leaves a long open area which is very tender and which tends to reopen at the time of the next defecation. Chronic fissures are usually secondary to cryptitis. Sharp pain accompanies defecation, followed by burning because of the presence of mucus, fecal matter, and general irritation of the open area. Severe muscle spasm of the sphincter usually accompanies chronic conditions. The patient may try to avoid having a stool, which only aggravates the condition.

If the acute lesion does not heal with local dilatations, cleansing and control of constipation, then the tract is excised surgically. Chronic fissures usually require surgery. The patient should be taught to achieve a soft stool, have a defecation daily, and clean the area after defecation, preferably with warm water. Sitz baths aid healing and may relieve pain. See Table 64–1 for a summary of causes of rectal pain.

Rectal Fistula (Fistula-in-Ano). A fistula is a sinus tract that develops between two body cavities or between a body cavity and the outside. A rectal fistula is a tract that goes from the anal canal to the skin outside the anus or from an abscess to either the anal canal or the perianal area. It is usually preceded by the formation of an abscess.

A fistula may heal over temporarily and then open up periodically to drain. It is a chronic condition for which surgery is the only cure. The tract is surgically excised and the area cleaned and left open to heal by granulation. It may heal very slowly and will be very painful during this time. The patient needs to be encouraged and taught the importance of cleanliness in caring for the wound.

Cryptitis. When particles of stool become lodged in one of the anal crypts and decay, they cause a pocket of infection known as cryptitis. The depth of the crypt determines the ease with which the inflammatory material is cleared away. If it is deep, the infectious material may be retained and may spread through the perianal tissues to form an abscess (Fig. 64–4).

Rectal Abscess. Rectal abscesses form in several positions; Figure 64–4 illustrates the common ones. Most of the abscesses of this area begin as cryptitis, with the formation of cysts that extend through the tubular ducts into the submucosal spaces. These abscesses may also originate from abrasions of the local tissues, with the entry of a virulent organism.

The treatment of these condtions is drainage of the abscess and surgical excision of any associated fistulas. It may take two stages of surgery to accomplish the needed resection.

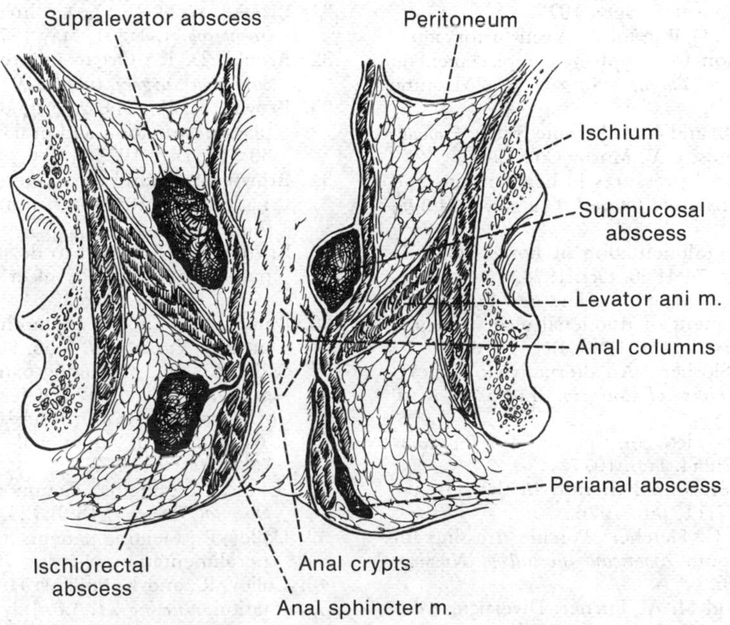

Figure 64–4. Abscesses of the anorectal area.

TUMORS

Carcinoma and melanoma both occur at the anus but both are relatively rare. They spread by local extension into the perirectal spaces and then to the inguinal nodes. Treatment is excision of the anus with an abdominal-perineal resection (see Fig. 63–4).

Cancer of the anal canal or lower rectum can coexist with other rectal conditions, and the patient may falsely attribute bleeding to a hemorrhoid instead of the more serious condition. Many cancers are overlooked until they are quite large and the prognosis is poor. A physician should investigate all cases of rectal bleeding, even though it can easily be attributed to hemorrhoids or some other local rectal condition. The nurse should encourage all persons who experience rectal bleeding to consult a physician and have the origin of the bleeding investigated.

See Chapter 63 for treatment and nursing care of a patient with cancer of the rectum; the treatment for anal cancer is the same.

BIBLIOGRAPHY (Unit XVII)

1. Ackerman, J., and H. delRegato: *Cancer: Diagnosis, Treatment and Prognosis*, 5th ed. St. Louis: C.V. Mosby Co., 1977.
2. American Cancer Society: 1978 *Cancer Facts and Figures*, American Cancer Society, 1977.
3. Anderson, D., and J. G. Randolph: A satisfactory alternative to the colon for esophageal replacement in children. *Annals of Thoracic Surgery*, 25:251, June 1978.
4. Anderson, W. A. D., and J. M. Kissane (Eds.): *Pathology*, 7th ed. St. Louis: C.V. Mosby Co., 1977.
5. Arabi, Y., et al.: Anal pressures in hemorrhoids and anal fissure. *The American Journal of Surgery*, 134:608, Nov. 1977.
6. Baker, D. I.: Hyperalimentation at home. *American Journal of Nursing*, 74:1826, Oct. 1974.
7. Barreras, R. F.: Facts, anecdotes, and new horizons in the medical treatment of duodenal ulcers. *Surgical Clinics of North America*, 56:1243, Dec. 1976.
8. Bartizal, J., and P. Slosberg: An alternative to hemorrhoidectomy. *Archives of Surgery*, 112:534, April 1977.
9 Bass, L.: More fiber — less constipation. *American Journal of Nursing*, 77:254, Feb. 1977.
10. Baum, M. E.: Enterostomal therapy in the hospital. *Supervisor Nurse*, 7:11, Jan. 1976.
11. Baum, M., and J. C. Fletcher: Porcine dressing for ileostomy retraction. *American Journal of Nursing*, 76:760, May 1976.
12. Beachley, M. C., and M. A. Turner: Diverticular disease of the gastrointestinal tract. *Current Concepts in Gastroenterology*, 2:30, Feb. 1978.
13. Beahrs, O., and M. A. Adsen: Ileal pouch with ileostomy rather than ileostomy alone. *American Journal of Surgery*, 125:154, Feb. 1973.
14. Beart, R. W., and F. Curlee: Intestinal stomas: Managing the "unmentionable." *Geriatrics*, 33:45, Nov. 1978.
15. Beeson, P. B., and W. McDermott (Eds.): *Cecil-Loeb Textbook of Medicine*, 15th ed. Philadelphia: W. B. Saunders Co., 1979.
16. Benson, J.: Simple chronic constipation. *Postgraduate Medicine*, 57:55, Jan. 1975.
17. Black, D., et al.: Drug interactions in the G. I. tract. *American Journal of Nursing*, 77:1426, Sept. 1977.
18. Blackwell, A. K., and W. Blackwell: Relieving gas pains. *American Journal of Nursing*, 75:66, Jan. 1975.
19. Block, P. L.: Dental health in hospitalized patients. *American Journal of Nursing*, 76:1162, July 1976.
20. Bloom, S. R.: Gastrointestinal hormones. *International Review of Physiology*, 12:71, 1977.
21. Bockus, H. L.: *Gastroenterology*, 3rd ed. Philadelphia: W. B. Saunders Co., 1974.
22. Borgen, L.: Total parenteral nutrition in adults. *American Journal of Nursing*, 78:224, Feb. 1978.
23. Bosten, A., et al.: Controlling colostomy odor. *American Journal of Nursing*, 77:444, Mar. 1977.
24. Bowen, W. H.: Nature of plaque. *Oral Sciences Review*, 9:3, 1976.
25. Bowen, W. H., et al.: Summary of immunization against dental caries. *Journal of Dental Research*, 55 (Special issue C): C164, Apr. 1976.
26. Boyar, R. M., et al.: Cortisol secretion and metabolism in anorexia nervosa. *New England Journal of Medicine*, 296:190, Jan. 1977.
27. Brantigan, O., and A. E. Cocco: Recognition and management of esophagitis, a pathophysiologic disease. *American Surgeon*, 39:134, Mar. 1973.
28. Brady, P. G.: Small intestinal syndromes: Guide to diagnosis. *Hospital Medicine*, 15:41, May 1979.
29. Bray, G. A., et al.: Surgical treatment of obesity; current status. *American Family Physician*, 15:111, Mar. 1977.
30. Broadwell, D. C., and S. L. Sorells: Loop transverse colostomy. *American Journal of Nursing*, 78:1029, June 1978.
31. Brooke, B. N. (Ed.).: Crohn's disease. *Clinics in Gastroenterology*. 1:261, May 1972.
32. Brooks, D. K.: Organ failure following surgery. *Advances in Surgery*, 6:302, 1972.
33. Brown, A. T.: The role of dietary carbohydrates in plaque formation and oral disease. *Nutrition Review*, 33:353, Dec. 1975.
34. Brown, M. S., and Alexander, M. M.: Physical examination. Part 10: Mouth and throat. *Nursing '74*, 4:57, Aug. 74.
35. Brunner, L. S.: What to do (and what to teach your patient) about peptic ulcer. *Nursing 76*, 6:27, Nov. 1976.
36. Burns, N.: Cancer chemotherapy: A systemic approach. *Nursing 78*, 8:56, Feb. 1978.
37. Cady, B., *et al.*: Changing patterns of colorectal carcinoma. *Cancer*, 33:422, Feb. 1974.
38. Christensen, E., *et al.*: Progress in gastroenterology — treatment of duodenal ulcer. *Gastroenterology*, 73:1170, Nov. 1977.
38a. Clinical highlights: Common causes of peritonitis. *Hospital Medicine*, 13(3):123, Mar. 1977.
39. Colley, R.: Meeting patients nutritional needs with hyperalimentation. Nursing 79, 9:76, May 1979.
40. Colley, R., and K. Phillips: Helping with hyperalimentation. *Nursing 73*, 3:6, July 1973.

41. Conners, M.: Ostomy care: A personal approach. *American Journal of Nursing*, 74:1422, Aug. 1974.
42. Controlling colostomy odor. *American Journal of Nursing*, 77:444, Mar. 1977.
43. Corman, M. L., et al.: Cathartics. *American Journal of Nursing*, 75:273, Feb. 1975.
44. Corrington, C.: Facts about colonoscopy. *Nursing 76*, 6:52, Aug. 1976.
45. Crom, R.: Tumors of the small intestine. *The American Surgeon*, 41:160, Mar. 1975.
46. Crossman, M. I., et al.: A new look at peptic ulcer. *Annals of Internal Medicine*, 84:57, Jan. 1976.
47. Cullen, P. P.: Patients with colorectal cancer: How to assess and meet their needs. *Nursing 76*, 6:42, Sept. 1976.
48. Curtis, C.: Colonoscopy: The nurse's role. *American Journal of Nursing*, 75:420, Mar. 1975.
49. Daly, K. M.: Don't wave good-by. *American Journal of Nursing*, 74:1641, Sept. 1974.
50. Davis, W. D.: Treatment of uncomplicated gastric ulcer. *American Journal of Digestive Diseases*, 21:190, Feb. 1976.
51. Day, N. E.: Some aspects of the epidemiology of esophageal cancer. *Cancer Research*, 35:334, Nov. 1975.
52. Dericks, V. C.: The psychological hurdles of new ostomates: helping them up . . . and over. *Nursing '74*, 4:52, Oct. 1974.
53. Dericks, V. C., and C. T. Donovan: The ostomy patient really needs you. *Nursing 76*, 6:30, Sept. 1976.
54. Dienhart, C. M.: *Basic Human Anatomy and Physiology*, 3rd ed. Philadelphia: W. B. Saunders Co., 1979.
55. Dobie, R. A.: Rehabilitation of swallowing disorders. *American Family Physician*, 17:8495, May 1978.
56. Domenick, N. P.: The methanol extract residue (MER) of Bacillus Calmette-Guerin in cancer immunotherapy. *Nursing Clinics of North America*, 13:369, June 1978.
57. Dousa, T. P., and R. R. Dozois: Interrelationships between histamine, prostaglandins, and cyclic AMP in gastric secretion: A hypothesis. *Gastroenterology*, 73:904, 1977.
58. Doust, B.: The use of ultrasound in the diagnosis of gastroenterological disease. *Gastroenterology*, 70:602, Apr. 1976.
59. Dudrick, S. J.: A patient on I.V. therapy need not starve! *Consultant*, 18:142, Feb. 1978.
60. Dudrick, S. J., and J. E. Rhoads: Total intravenous feeding. *Scientific American*, 226:73, May 1972.
61. Dunphy, E. J., and L. W. Way: *Current Surgical Diagnosis and Treatment*, 3rd ed. Los Altos, Calif.: Lange Medical Publications, 1977.
62. Duodenal ulcer: Important considerations in the pathogenesis. *Hospital Medicine*, 15:20, Feb. 1979.
63. Dyer, E., et al.: Dental health in adults. *American Journal of Nursing*, 76:1156, July 1976.
64. Ebeid, A. M., and J. E. Fischer: Gastrin and ulcer disease: What is known. *Surgical Clinics of North America*, 56:1249, Dec. 1976.
65. Edelstein, B.: *The Woman Doctor's Diet for Women*. New York: Ballatine Books, 1977.
66. Elias, G.: Where we stand with chemotherapy in colorectal cancer. *Consultant*, 18:189, Feb. 1978.
66a. Elliott, J.: More help for the morbidly obese: Gastric stapling. *Journal of the American Medical Association*. 240:1941, Oct. 1978.
67. Esselstyn, C. B.: Surgical management of actively bleeding duodenal ulcer, *Surgical Clinics of North America*, 56:1387, Dec. 1976.
68. Feldtman, R. W., and R. J. Andrassy: Meeting exceptional nutritional needs. 1. Total parenteral nutrition. *Postgraduate Medicine*, 64:64, Aug. 1978.
69. Fleshler, B.: Medical management of bleeding duodenal ulcers. *Surgical Clinics of North America*, 56:1375, Dec. 1976.
70. Fordtran, J. S., et al.: In vivo and in vitro evaulation of liquid antacids. *New England Journal of Medicine*, 288:923, May 1973.
71. Fordtran, J. S.: Placebos, antacids and cimetidine for duodenal ulcer. *New England Journal of Medicine*, 298:1081, May 1978.
72. Freedman, A. M., et al.: *Modern Synopsis of Comprehensive Textbook of Psychiatry/II*, 2nd ed. Baltimore: Williams and Wilkins Co., 1976.
73. Fromm, D.: Stress ulcer. *Hospital Medicine*, 14:58, Nov. 1978.
74. Ganong, W. F.: *Review of Medical Physiology*, 8th ed. Los Altos, Calif.: Lange Medical Publications, 1977.
75. Garfinkel, P. E., et al.: Prognosis in anorexia nervosa as influenced by clinical features, treatment and self-perception. *Canadian Medical Association Journal*, 117:1041, Nov. 1977.
76. Geels, W., et al.: The enterocutaneous fistula: Supplanting surgery with meticulous nursing care. *Nursing 78*, 8:52, Apr. 1978.
77. Gelb, A. M.: Reflux esophagitis: Myths and realities. *Consultant*, 16:44, July 1976.
78. Glickman, L.: Periodontal disease. *New England Journal of Medicine*, 284:1071, May 1971.
79. Grossman, M. I., et al.: A new look at peptic ulcer. *Annals of Internal Medicine*, 84:57, Jan. 1976.
80. Grant, J. A. N.: Patient care in parenteral hyperalimentation. *Nursing Clinics of North America*, 8:165, March 1973.
81. Greenwood, M. R. C., and P. R. Johnson: Adipose tissue cellularity and its relationship to the development of obesity in females. *Current Concepts in Nutrition*. New York: Wiley, 1977.
82. Griffen, W. O.: Management of diverticular disease of the colon. *Hospital Medicine*, 14:108, Nov. 1978.
83. Griggs, B. A., and M. C. Hoppe: Update: Nasogastric tube feeding. *American Journal of Nursing*, 79:481, Mar. 1979.
84. Grossman, M. I., et al.: A new look at peptic ulcer. *Annals of Internal Medicine*, 84:57, Jan. 1976.
85. Guyton, A. C.: *Medical Physiology*, 5th ed. Philadelphia: W. B. Saunders Co., 1976.
86. Hallenbeck, G. A.: The natural history of duodenal ulcer disease. *Surgical Clinics of North America*, 56:1235, Dec. 1976.
87. Halverson, J. D., et al.: Reanastomosis after jejunoileal bypass. *Surgery*, 84:241, Aug. 1978.
88. Hampton, J. M.: Anal fissure. *Consultant*, 17:64, June 1977.
89. Hardie, J. M., and G. H. Bowden: Bacterial flora of dental plaque. *British Medical Bulletin*, 31:131, May 1975.
90. Hartles, R. L., and S. A. Leach: Effect of diet on dental caries. *British Medical Bulletin*, 31:137, May 1975.
91. Heindel, M.: How to protect your ostomy patients from post-op skin problems. *RN*, 41:43, Jan. 1978.
92. Heizer, W. D., and E. P. Orringer: Parenteral nutrition at home for five years. *Gastroenterology*, 72:527, Mar. 1977.
93. Heomlich, H. J., and T. W. O'Connor: Vascular dysphagia: cancer is not always the culprit. *Geriatrics*, 34:93, Mar. 1979.
94. Herrera, A. F.: Medical therapy of colonic diverticular disease. *Postgraduate Medicine*, 60:107, June 1977.

95. Heydman, A. H.: Intestinal bypass for obesity. *American Journal of Nursing*, 74:1102, June 1974.
96. High fiber diets and colonic disease. *American Journal of Nursing*, 77:255, Feb. 1977.
97. Hill, G. L.: *Ileostomy – Surgery, Physiology and Management*. New York: Grune and Stratton, 1976.
98. Hill, M. J., et al.: Aetiology of adenoma — carcinoma sequence in large bowel. *Lancet*, 1:245, Feb. 1978.
99. Hodges, R. E.: Total parenteral nutrition: an important therapeutic advance. *Postgraduate Medicine*, 65:171, Mar. 1979.
100. Holt, R. W., and D. C. Wherry: Why flexible fiberoptic sigmoidoscopy is important in the geriatric patient. *Geriatrics*, 34:85, May 1979.
101. Howard, L.: Obesity: A feasible approach to a formidable problem. *Nursing Digest*, 4:86, Winter 1976.
102. Howard, R. B., and N. H. Herbold: *Nutrition in Clinical Care*. New York: McGraw-Hill Book Co., 1978.
103. Hyman, E., et al.: The pouch ileostomy. *Nursing 77*, 7:44, Sept. 1977.
104. Innovation in Nursing: I.V. hyperalimentation: Now they can get it at home. *Nursing 77*, 7:23, 1977.
105. Ippoliti, A., and J. Walsh: Newer concepts in the pathogenesis of peptic ulcer disease. *Surgical Clinics of North America*, 56:1479, Dec. 1976.
106. Isler, C.: A new ball game for colostomy patients? *RN*, 40:52, Sept. 1977.
107. Isler, C.: If the ileostomy is continent, the benefits are obvious. *RN*, 40:42, Apr. 1977.
108. Jackson, R.: Contemporary management of rectal cancer: An overview. *Cancer*, 40:2365, Nov. 1977.
109. Janici, P., and R. J. Alfidi: Selective visceral angiography in the diagnosis and treatment of gastroduodenal hemorrhage. *Surgical Clinics of North America*, 65:1365, Dec. 1976.
110. Jensen, V.: Better techniques for bagging stomas. Part 2: Colostomies. *Nursing '74*, 4:3, Aug. 1974.
111. Jensen, V.: Better techniques for bagging stomas. Part 3: Ileostomies. *Nursing '74*, 4:60, Sept. 1974.
112. Johnson, J. B.: Gastric ulcers: Classification, blood group characteristics, secretion patterns, and pathogenesis. *Annals of Surgery*, 162:996, Dec. 1965.
113. Johnson, W. D., and A. J. Ballantyne: Prognostic effect of tobacco and alcohol on tongue cancer. *American Journal of Surgery*, 134:444, Oct. 1977.
114. Jonas, A. D., and D. F. Jonas: Obesity: Separating the herbivores from the carnivores. *Modern Medicine*, 44:10, May 1976.
115. Johnston, D.: Highly selective vagotomy. *Progress in Surgery*, 14:1, 1975.
116. Johnston, D., and J. C. Goligher: Selective, highly selective, or truncal vagotomy? *Surgical Clinics of North America*, 56:1313, Dec. 1976.
117. Jubert, A. B., et al.: Correlation of immune responses with Dukes classification in colorectal carcinoma. *Surgery*, 82:452, Oct. 1977.
118. Katz, S.: *Preventive Dentistry in Action*. Upper Montclair, N.J.: D.C.P. Publication, 1972.
119. Kaye, M. D.: 10 questions physicians most often ask about disorders of the esophagus. *Consultant*, 18:31, Dec. 1978.
120. Keithley, K.: Proper nutritional assessment can prevent hospital malnutrition. *Nursing 79*, 9:68, Feb. 1979.
121. Keough, G., and H. N. Niebel: Oral cancer detection — A nursing responsibility. *American Journal of Nursing*, 73:684, Apr. 1973.
122. Keusch, G.: Bacterial diarrheas. *American Journal of Nursing*, 73:1028, June 1973.
123. Kirsh, M., and F. Ritter: Caustic ingestion and subsequent damage to oropharyngeal and digestive passages. *The Annals of Thoracic Surgery*, 21:74, Jan. 1976.
124. Kirsner, J. B.: The stomach. *In* Sodeman, W. A., and W. A. Sodeman, Jr.: *Pathologic Physiology: Mechanisms of Disease*, 5th ed. Philadelphia: W. B. Saunders Co. 1974.
125. Kratzer, J. B., and D. S. Rauschenberger: What to teach your patient about his duodenal ulcer. *Nursing 78*, 8:54, Jan. 1978.
126. Kronborg, O.: Assessment of completeness of vagotomy. *Surgical Clinics of North America*, 56:1421, Dec. 1976.
127. Lamanske, J.: Helping the ileostomy patient to help himself. *Nursing 77* 7:34, Jan. 1977.
128. Langman, M. J. S.: Drugs in the treatment of gastric and duodenal ulcer. *Drugs*, 14:105, 1977.
129. Lee, Yea-Tsu, N.: Carcinoma of the rectum. *Review of Surgery*, 33:75, Mar.–Apr. 1976.
130. Lenneberg, E., and J. L. Rowbotham: *The Ileostomy Patient*: Springfield, Ill.: Charles C. Thomas, 1970.
131. Li, M. C., and S. T. Ross: Chemoprophylaxis for patients with colorectal cancer *JAMA*, 235:2825, June 1976.
132. Literte, J. W.: Nursing care of patients with intestinal obstruction. *American Journal of Nursing*, 77:1003, June 1977.
133. Long, G. D.: G.I. bleeding: What to do and when. *Nursing 78*, 8:44, Mar. 1978.
134. Lupton, M.: Minireview — biological aspects of anorexia nervosa. *Life Sciences*, 18:1341, June 1976.
135. Lynch, M. A. (Ed.): *Burkett's Oral Medicine*, 7th ed. Philadelphia: J. B. Lippincott Co., 1977.
136. Mackety, C. J.: Caring for the cancer patient who has an esophageal endoprosthesis. *RN*, 40:51, Oct. 1977.
136a. MacLean, L. D., and H. R. Shibata: The present status of bypass operations for obesity. *Surgical Annual*, 9:213–230, 1977.
137. Mahoney, J. N.: *Guide to Ostomy Nursing Care*. Boston: Little Brown and Co., 1976.
138. Manson, H.: Exorcising excoriation from fistulae and other draining wounds. *Nursinsg 76*, 6:57, Mar. 1976.
139. McCaffrey, T. D., and J. O. Lilly: Antacids and bleeding prophylaxis. *American Journal of Digestive Diseases*, 21:194, Feb. 1976.
140. McConnell, E. A.: All about gastrointestinal intubation. *Nursing '75*, 5:30, Sept. 1975.
141. McConnell, E. A.: Ensuring safer stomach suctioning with the Salem sump tube. *Nursing '77*, 7:54, Sept. 1977.
142. McConnell, E. A.: Ten problems with nasogastric tubes . . . and how to solve them. *Nursing 79*, 9:78, Apr. 1979.
143. McKechnie, J. C.: Outdated and updated diets for G.I. disease. *Consultant*, 18:82, Sept. 1978.
144. Melton, J. H.: A boy with anorexia nervosa. *American Journal of Nursing*, 74:1649, Sept. 1974.
145. Menguy, R.: Gastric ulceration. *Advances in Surgery*, 6:103, 1972.
146. Menguy, R., et al.: Mechanism of stress ulcer: Influence of hypovolemic shock on energy metabolism in the gastric mucosa. *Gastroenterology*, 66:46, Jan. 1974.
147. Mizroch, S.: Epidemiology of esophageal cancer (Letter). *Journal of the American Medical Association*, 239:2340, June 1978.
148. Moody, F. G., and L. Y. Cheung: Stress ulcers: Their pathogenesis, diagnosis, and treatment. *Surgical Clinics of North America*, 56:1469, Dec. 1976.

149. Moore, C.: Cigarette smoking and cancer of the mouth, pharynx, and larynx. *J.A.M.A.*, 218:533, Oct. 1971.
150. Myer, S.: The chronic threat of Crohn's disease. *RN*, 41:65, Nov. 1978.
151. National Institute of Health: Research findings of potential value to the practitioner, oral cancer. *Journal of the American Medical Assocition*, 237:19, Jan. 1977.
152. Neill, J. R., et al: Marital changes after intestinal bypass surgery. *Journal of the American Medical Association*, 240:447, Aug. 1978.
153. Nizel, A.: Preventing dental caries: The nutritional factors. *Pediatric Clinics of North America*, 24:141, Feb. 1977.
154. Nolte, W. A.: *Oral Microbiology*, 2nd ed. St. Louis: C. V. Mosby Co., 1973.
155. Palmer, E. D.: Gastrointestinal problems in the elderly. *Hospital Medicine*, 18:32, Dec. 1978.
156. Parker, J. B., Jr., et al.: Anorexia nervosa: A combined therapeutic approach. *Southern Medical Journal*, 70:448, April 1977.
157. Payne, J. H., and L. T. DeWind: Surgical treatment of obesity. *American Journal of Surgery*, 118:141, Aug. 1969.
158. Peterson, W. L., et al.: Healing of duodenal ulcer with an antacid regimen. *New England Journal of Medicine*, 297:341, 1977.
159. Poskitt, M. E., and T. J. Cole: Do fat babies stay fat? *British Medical Journal*, 1:7, 1977.
160. Price, J. H.: Oral health care for the geriatric patient. *Journal of Gerontological Nursing*, 5(2):25, Mar.–Apr. 1979.
161. Reitz, M., et al.: Mouth care. *American Journal of Nursing*, 73:1728, Oct. 1973.
162. Rodman, M. J.: Current and coming treatment for peptic ulcers. *RN*, 40:74, Feb. 1977.
163. Rodman, M. J., and D. W. Smith: *Pharmacology and Drug Therapy in Nursing*. Philadelphia: J. B. Lippincott Co., 1968.
164. Romero, R., and W. C. Butterfield: A review of recent therapeutic approaches to treatment of stress ulcers. *Review of Surgery*, 32:379, Nov.–Dec. 1975.
165. Roth, J. L.: Complications of colonic diverticulum. *Postgraduate Medicine*, 60:115, June 1976.
166. Roth, J. L.: Introduction: Colon diverticular disease. *Postgraduate Medicine*, 60:75, June 1976.
166a. Sabiston, D. C., Jr. (Ed.): Davis-Christopher Textbook of Surgery, 11th ed. Philadelphia: W. B. Saunders Co., 1977.
167. Samborsky, V.: Drug therapy for peptic ulcer. *American Journal of Nursing*, 78:2064, Dec. 1978.
168. Schachter, H., and J. B. Kirsner: Definitions of inflammatory bowel disease of unknown etiology. *Gastroenterology*, 68:591, March 1975.
169. Schauder, M. R.: Ostomy care: cone irrigations. *American Journal of Nursing*, 74:1424, Aug. 1974.
170. Schmidt, M., and B. Dundan: Modifying eating behavior in anorexia nervosa. *American Journal of Nursing*, 74:1646, Sept. 1974.
171. Schwartz, S. I., et al.: *Principles of Surgery*, 2nd ed. New York: McGraw-Hill Book Co., 1974.
172. Selkurt, E. E. (Ed.): *Physiology*. Boston: Little, Brown and Co., 1963.
173. Sethbhakdi, S.: Pathogenesis of colonic diverticulosis. *Postgraduate Medicine*, 60:76, June 1976.
174. Shils, M. E.: A program for total parenteral nutrition at home. *American Journal of Clinical Nutrition*, 28:1429, Dec. 1975.
175. Silberman, H., et al.: Neoplasma of the small bowel. *Annals of Surgery*, 180:157, Aug. 1974.
176. Sleisenger, M. H., and J. S. Fordtran: *Gastrointestinal Disease*. Philadelphia: W. B. Saunders Co., 1973.
177. Sodeman, W. A., and W. A. Sodeman, Jr.: *Pathologic Physiology: Mechanisms of Disease*, 5th ed. Philadelphia: W. B. Saunders Co., 1974.
178. Sollow, C., et al.: Psychosocial effects of intestinal bypass for severe obesity. *New England Journal of Medicine*, 290:300, Feb. 1974.
179. Spiro, H.: *Clinical Gastroenterology*, 2nd ed. New York: MacMillian Co. 1977.
180. Stahlgren, L. H., and N. W. Morris: Intestinal obstruction. *American Journal of Nursing*, 77:999, June 1977.
181. Steiger, E., and A. M. Cooperman: Considerations in the management of perforated peptic ulcers. *Surgical Clinics of North America*, 56:6:1395, Dec. 1976.
182. Steinberg, W. M., and P. P. Toskes: A practical approach to evaluation maldigestion and malabsorption. *Geriatrics*, 33:73, July 1978.
183. Steinheber, F. U.: Bleeding from the lower gastrointestinal tract: Diagnostic approach. *Hospital Medicine*, 15:27, Apr. 1979.
184. Steinheber, F. U.: Bleeding from the upper gastrointestinal tract. *Hospital Medicine*, 15:47, Mar. 1979.
185. Sveger, T.: Does overnutrition or obesity during the first year affect weight at age four? *Acta Paediatrica Scandinavica*, 67:465, July 1978.
186. Tapper, D., et al.: Conversion of jejunal bypass to gastric bypass to maintain weight loss. *Surgery, Obstetrics and Gynecology*, 147:353, Sept. 1978.
187. Taylor, T. V., et al.: A non-invasive test of gastric function. *British Journal of Surgery*, 64:702, Mar. 1977.
188. Theilade, E., and J. Theilade: Role of plaque in the etiology of periodontal disease and caries. *Oral Sciences Reviews*, 9:23, 1976.
189. The Living Bible, Paraphrased. Wheaton: Tyndale House Publishers, 1971.
190. Thiele, G.: Anorectal pain. *American Family Physician*, 6:54, Aug. 1972.
191. Travaglini, P., et al.: Some aspects of hypothalamic pituitary function in patients with anorexia nervosa. *Acta Endocrinological*, 81:252, 1976.
192. Trimpi, H. D., et al.: Guide to the management of rectal abscesses. *Hospital Medicine*. 12:79, Sept. 1976.
193. Turell, R. (Ed.): *Diseases of the Colon and Anorectum*. Philadelphia: W. B. Saunders Co., 1969.
194. University of N.Y. at Buffalo School of Dentistry and the National Caries Program. Immunological aspects of dental caries. *Journal of Dental Research*, 55, Special Issue C, Apr. 1976.
195. Valdivieso, M., et al.: Chemoimmunotherapy of metastatic large bowel cancer. *Cancer*, 40:2731, 1977.
196. Watson, P. G.: Applying rehabilitation concepts in the care of persons with ostomies. *ARN Journal*, 1:12, Nov.–Dec. 1976.
197. Watt, R. C.: Colostomy irrigation yes or no? *American Journal of Nursing*, 77:442, Mar. 1977.
198. Webster, D. J. T., et al.: The use of bulk evacuant in patients with haemorrhoids. *British Journal of Surgery*, 65:291, 1978.
199. Welty, M. J., W. P. Graham, III, and R. H. Rosillo: The patient with maxillofacial cancer. I: Surgical treatment and nursing care. *Nursing Clinics of North America*, 8:137, Mar. 1973.
200. Wentworth, A., and B. Cox: Nursing the patient with a continent ileostomy. *American Journal of Nursing*, 76:1424, Sept. 1976.

201. Willacker, J.: Bowel sounds. *American Journal of Nursing*, 73:2100, Dec. 1973.
202. Wiley, L., et al.: The G.I. bleeder — seldom as safe as he seems. *Nursing '75*, 5:48, Sept. 1975.
203. Wilson, M., et al.: Primary malignancies of the small bowel: A report of 96 cases and review of the literature. *Annals of Surgery*, 180:175, Aug. 1974.
204. Wurman, L. H., et. al.: Carcinoma of the lip. *American Journal of Surgery*, 130:470, Oct. 1975.
205. Wynder, E. L.: The epidemiology of large bowel cancer. *Cancer Research*, 35:3388, Nov. 1975.
206. Wynder, E. L., and S. R. Bandaru: Diet and cancer of the colon. *Nutrition and Cancer: Current Concepts in Nutrition*, pp. 55–71, 1977.
207. Zuidema, G. D., and M. K. Klein: A new esophagus. *American Journal of Nursing*, 61:69, Sept. 1961.

UNIT XVIII

NURSING PEOPLE EXPERIENCING DISTURBANCES OF THE LIVER, BILIARY TRACT AND PANCREAS

by Dolores Hilden, R.N., M.S.N.

INTRODUCTION AND STUDY GUIDE

The liver, biliary tract, and pancreas are located together in the upper abdominal cavity. They all function to facilitate digestion and utilization of foods. In addition, the liver is vital to other life processes, e.g., detoxification of chemicals, blood storage. Disease of one organ is often manifested by a sign or symptom in an adjacent organ. This unit explores the functions of each area, identifies problems unique to one or common to all, and discusses medical and nursing care measures that assist persons experiencing alteration in functions.

Severe hepatic and pancreatic damage demands intensive, frequently complex care. Chronic, progressive disorders may produce limitations altering life style and requiring long-term health care and planning. Acute, episodic problems of the gallbladder may necessitate surgery. Intensive care is needed in the immediate postoperative period, but few, if any, long-term difficulties result. In addition, the liver, biliary tract, and pancreas seem to be the first organs affected when drugs or alcohol are abused. In these situations, not only is physiology distorted, but the life style adopted may place the individual in immediate conflict with recommended health care. (See Ch. 94.)

This unit reviews anatomy and physiology, discusses tools and information necessary for assessment, presents a summary of pathophysiologic dynamics and clinical care in problems commonly seen, and discusses in turn the specific disorders of each organ.

Study Guide

1. As you study, familiarize yourself with these terms:

hepatitis
ascites
hepatic encephalopathy
esophageal varices
jaundice
icterus
bilirubin
asterixis
liver flap
Australian antigen
abscess
inflammation
necrosis
peritonitis
diuresis
pancreatitis

exocrine
endocrine
acinar
duct of Wirsung
ampulla of Vater
amylase
lipase
trypsin
chole
cholang
cholecyst
choledocho
lithiasis
ostomy
ectomy
vascular spider
cystic fibrosis
steatorrhea

2. Also, become acquainted with the following concepts and the ways in which they apply to disorders of the liver, biliary tract, and pancreas:

immune process
clotting process
edema formation
vascular shock
renal failure
complications of bedrest
dynamics of pain
function of carbohydrates, fat, and protein
function of fat-soluble vitamins

3. Upon completion of this unit, you should be able to:

a. Describe the normal anatomy and physiology of the liver, biliary system, and pancreas as well as interrelationships of structure and function that exist between these organs.

b. Describe in detail the clinical problems that are most frequently associated with the liver, biliary tract, and pancreas; e.g., jaundice, ascites, altered blood clotting mechanism, hepatic encephalopathy, and hepatic coma.

c. Discuss how alcoholism and drug abuse cause and complicate liver and pancreatic disease.

d. Prepare in detail a plan for complete assessment of a patient's liver, biliary tract, and pancreatic function.

e. Prepare the patient and significant others for specific diagnostic procedures.

f. Interpret results of laboratory and diagnostic tests in terms of their impact upon patient needs and patient care.

g. Design and carry out effective care plans that are based upon identified needs of patients with disorders of the liver, biliary tract, and pancreas.

h. Be thoroughly familiar with the medications and surgical procedures described in this unit. Be prepared to participate in giving effective preoperative and postoperative care.

i. Include the patient and significant others in all aspects of the nursing care process.

CHAPTER 65

NORMAL LIVER, BILIARY, AND PANCREATIC STRUCTURE AND FUNCTION

ANATOMY AND PHYSIOLOGY

Liver

The liver, largest organ in the body, lies in the upper right quadrant of the abdomen and is enclosed by the rib cage, except for the lower margin (see Figure 65–1). This large organ, which represents 2 per cent of body weight, lies just below the diaphragm, with the lungs extending over its upper portion. The lower portion of the liver provides a roof over the stomach and intestines. Most of the liver is blanketed by peritoneum, as is the adjacent gallbladder.

Note in Figure 65–2 that the liver is divided into *lobes.* The two major lobes are the right and left lobes; these two lobes are separated by the falciform ligament. Observe that the right lobe is the largest and that the left lobe extends past the midline of the body (Figure 65–1). The major lobes, in turn, are divided into posterior, anterior, medial, and lateral segments.

Two major *blood vessels* supply the liver. The *hepatic artery* brings oxygenated blood to the liver. The *mesenteric* and *splenic veins* join to become the *portal vein,* which brings blood with nutrients, metabolic substances, and toxins from the stomach and intestine to be processed, detoxified, or assimilated. About one third of the blood coming to the liver travels via the hepatic artery and the other two thirds travels by way of the portal and splenic veins. Once filtered and processed, blood returns to the systemic circulation from the portal circulation by way of the *hepatic vein* into the inferior vena cava, joining near the right atrium. Hence, any process impeding blood flow through the right atrium of the heart causes engorgement of the liver; also, any process impeding blood flow through the liver causes engorgement of vessels draining the

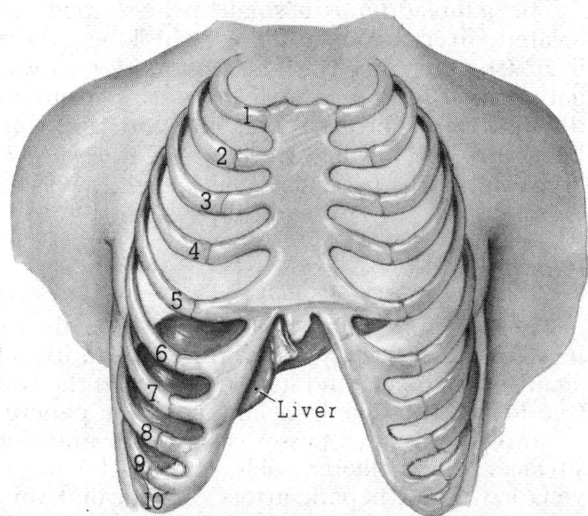

Figure 65–1. Normal location of the liver. (From Jacob, S. W., C. A. Francone, and W. L. Lossow: *Structure and Function in Man.* 4th ed. Philadelphia: W. B. Saunders Co., 1978, p. 467.)

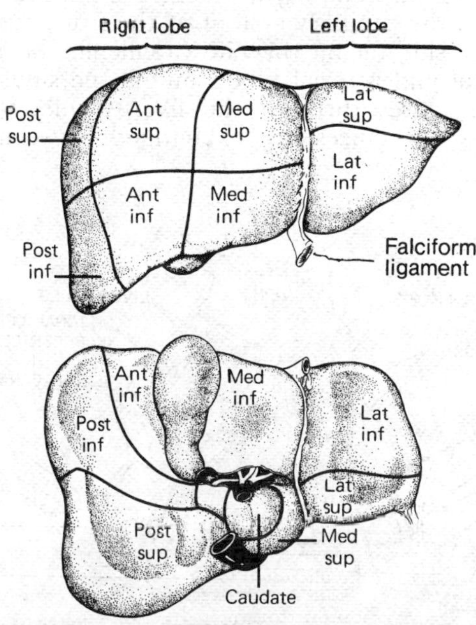

Figure 65–2. Lobes of the liver. (From Way, L. W., and R. C. Lim: Liver. *In* Dunphy, J. E., and L. W. Way (Eds.): *Current Surgical Diagnosis and Treatment.* Los Altos: Lange Medical Publications, 1977.)

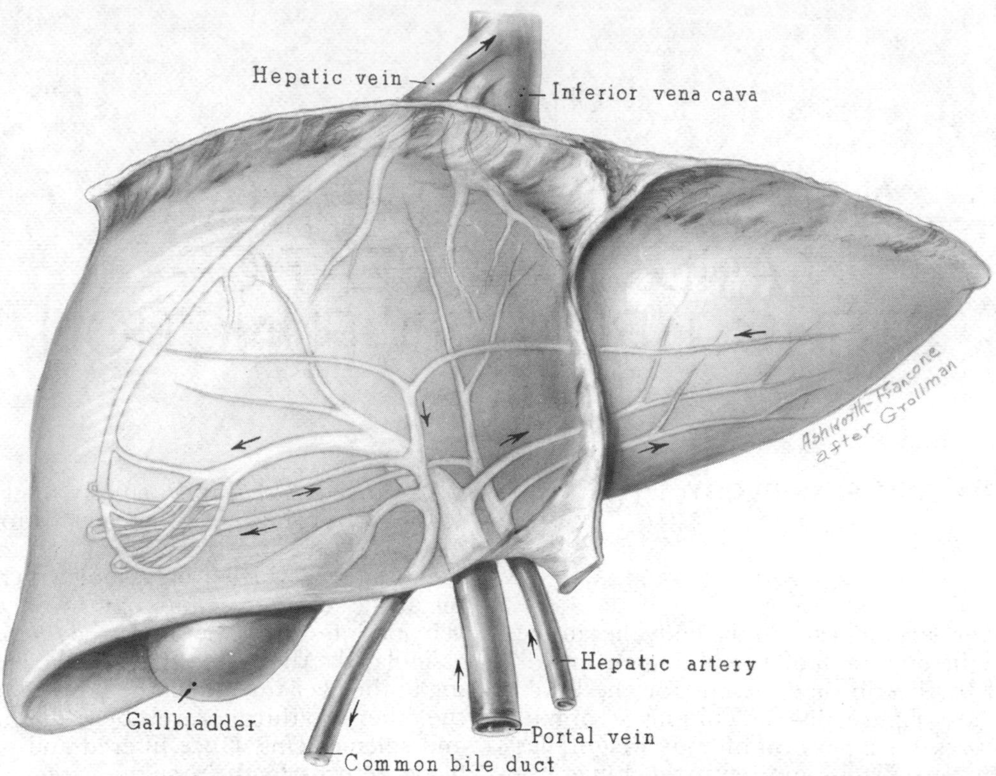

Figure 65–3. Hepatic portal system of the liver. (From Jacobs, S. W., C. A. Francone, and W. L. Lossow: *Structure and Function in Man.* 4th ed., Philadelphia: W. B. Saunders Co., 1978.)

stomach and gut. The hepatic portal system of the liver is depicted in Figure 65–3.

The functional unit of the liver is the *liver lobule,* with the *hepatocyte* being the chief cell. In the liver lobule, these cells are arranged hublike around a central vein, with one side of the polyhedral hepatocyte facing the hepatic sinusoids, the capillary system of the liver, and the other side facing the bile canaliculi. Incoming portal and arterial blood enters the sinusoids, then passes through the liver lobule, where many substances are exchanged between the hepatocytes and the blood, then courses on to the central vein, with special substances filtering into the bile ductules. *Endothelial and Kupffer cells* form the walls of the sinusoids. The basic structure of a liver lobule is illustrated in Figure 65–4.

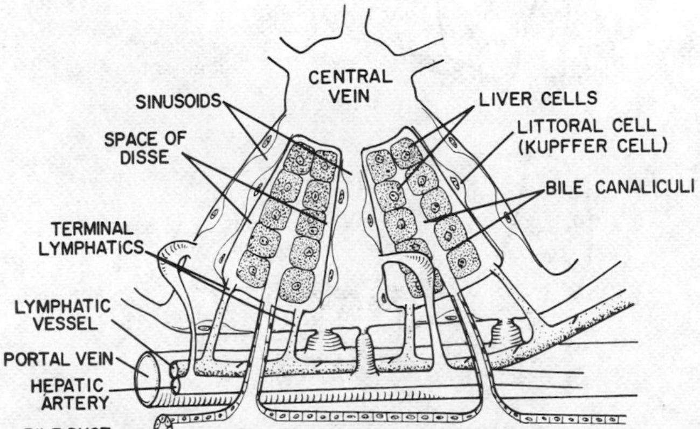

Figure 65–4. Basic structure of a liver lobule. (From Guyton, A. C.: *Textbook of Medical Physiology.* 5th ed., Philadelphia, W. B. Saunders Co., 1976.)

Biliary Tract

The gallbladder is a small, pear-shaped sac located directly beneath the right lobe of the liver (see Fig. 65–3). It serves as a *reservoir,* gathering *bile* from the liver via a system of ductules, concentrating the bile, and releasing bile into the intestinal tract via the *common bile duct* when fat is present in the intestine.

Pancreas

The pancreas is located retroperitoneally, its head in the concavity of the duodenum, its tail against the spleen, and its body between the two (see Fig. 65–5). The liver lies above the pancreas, and the stomach passes close to the anterior surface. Major blood vessels, namely the aorta, vena cava, and hepatic artery, are located very near the head of the pancreas, greatly complicating extensive surgery in this area. The pancreas functions as an *endocrine gland,* secreting *insulin* and *glucagon* directly into the blood stream, and as an *exocrine gland,* secreting multiple *digestive enzymes* into a system of ducts which flow into the *duct of Wirsung* (which extends to the common duct) and thence empty into the duodenum. The site where the duct of Wirsung joins the common bile duct and enters the duodenum is referred to as the *ampulla of Vater* (see Fig. 65–6). The *sphincter of Oddi* controls the release of both pancreatic juices and bile into the duodenum. (The exocrine function of the pancreas is discussed in this unit. Endocrine function and disorders are discussed in Unit XIX.)

METABOLIC FUNCTIONS

The liver, gallbladder, and pancreas function to produce, detoxify, and store many chemical substances in the body. These aid in the digestion, assimilation, and use of carbohydrates, fats, and protein by the body. Major substances and their role in body function are described below.

Liver Functions

Bile Production. The basic components of bile are bilirubin, bile salts, cholesterol, lecithin, fatty acids, electrolytes, and water. The liver uses these substances to create bile. *Bilirubin,* metabolically inert, comes from a breakdown of hemoglobin, and is converted by bacteria in the intestine to *urobilinogen,* some of which acts as the pigment that colors feces and some of which enters the systemic circulation and travels to the kidney, where it colors urine. (Bilirubin metabolism is discussed in more detail in Chapter 66.) *Bile salts* are the metabolically active parts of bile. They increase fat solubility and have a detergent action that breaks up fat into tiny particles that can pass through the intestinal wall. *Cholesterol,* a precursor of bile acid, later serves with *lecithin* to keep bile salts in suspension. When the balance of cholesterol, lecithin, and bile salts is disturbed, precipitation of bile salts may cause the formation of *gallstones.*

The liver continuously secretes bile. Some bile is stored in the gallbladder until fat molecules in the small intestine cause release of the enzyme *cholecystokinin,* which causes both contraction of the gallbladder and relaxation of the sphincter of Oddi. Bile salts are almost totally reabsorbed and returned to the liver for recycling.

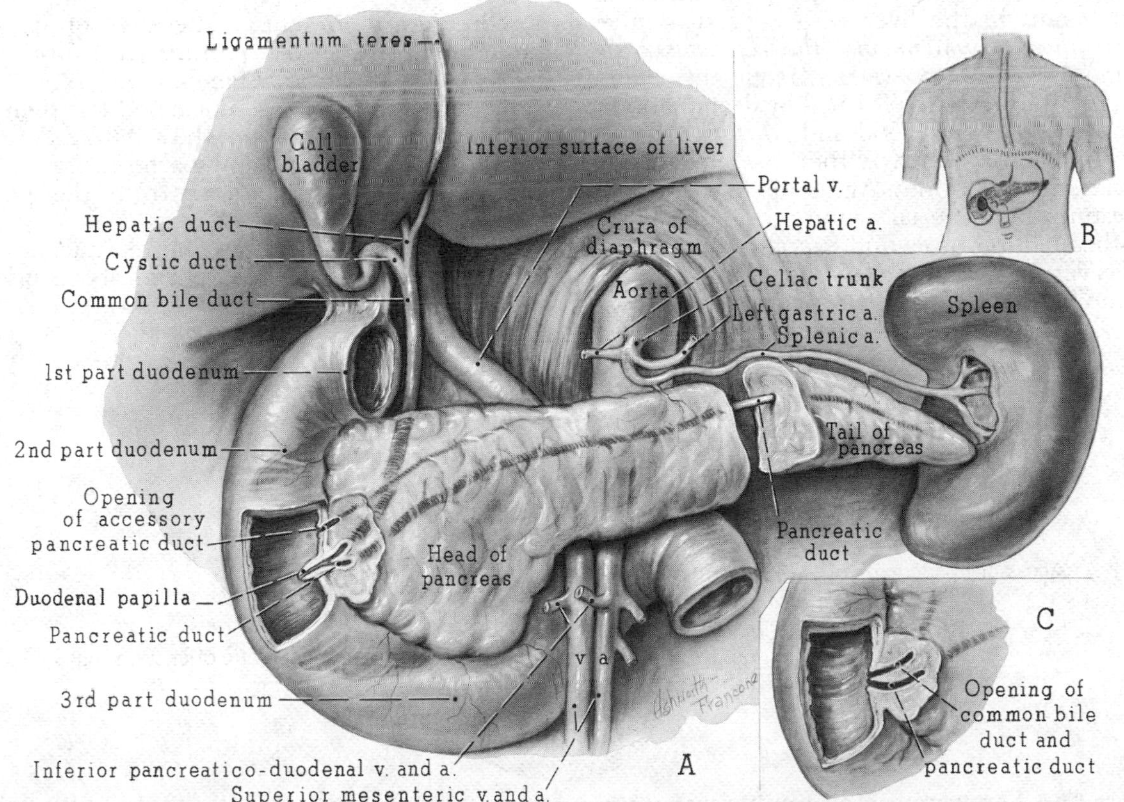

Figure 65–5. **A.** Anatomy of the pancreas and its relationship to adjacent organs. **B.** Anatomic position. **C.** Common variation. (From Jacob, S. W., C. A. Francone, and W. L. Lossow: *Structure and Function in Man.* 4th ed., Philadelphia: W. B. Saunders Co., 1978.)

Carbohydrate Metabolism. The liver performs a major function in carbohydrate metabolism, namely in *producing and releasing glucose* according to body need. When glucose is not needed, it is stored as glycogen. Disturbances in the process of glyconeogenesis (the conversion by the liver of non-carbohydrate precursors first into glucose and then into glycogen) may explain some types of hypoglycemia. (See Chapter 72.)

Lipid (Fat) Metabolism. Neutral fat (triglycerides) is degraded in the liver to be used for energy, or is used to synthesize other lipids. The liver is also able to synthesize fat from protein and carbohydrates.

Protein Metabolism

The liver's role in protein metabolism is needed for survival.

The *degradation of amino acids* occurs almost exclusively in the liver. Degradation is a process by which excess amino acids are catabolized and then used for energy or stored as fat. Degradation begins in the liver with a process called *deamination,* which means "the removal of the amino acid groups (NH_3) from the amino acids."[40] The *ammonia* formed by deamination is removed from the blood and converted by the liver into *urea,* which is then excreted by the kidneys and intestines. Ammonia formed in the intestines by bacterial action on protein is also synthesized into urea and excreted by the liver. However, in severe liver disease or damage, the ammonia that is normally converted to urea and excreted by the liver is allowed to accumulate to dangerously high levels in the blood; as a result, a highly toxic state develops, which can terminate in *hepatic coma.* (See Chapters 66 and 68.)

Plasma proteins, namely albumin, prothrombin, fibrinogen, and clotting proteins (Factors V, VI, VII, IX, and X), are synthesized in the liver. *Albumin* is essential for maintaining *plasma oncotic pressure.* The remainder named above contribute to the *blood clotting mechanism.* (See Chapter 46.) *Vitamin K,* which is fat soluble, must be present along with normal fat metabolism for effective clot formation. For vitamin K to be assimilated, bile must be present in the intestine. Gamma globulin, although a plasma protein, is not synthesized by the liver.

Detoxification Processes. Detoxification processes in the liver relate mainly to *hormones, drugs, and other chemicals.* Some substances may be inactivated by deamination, hydroxylation, oxidation, proteolysis, or reduction. Other substances may be conjugated, i.e., become soluble in water, and then be excreted via bile or urine. Certain substances may require both inactivation and conjugation to detoxify.

When liver function is compromised, prolonged drug action as well as increased potency of drug action may appear. Also, blood levels of certain hormones may be elevated.

Circulatory Function. Because of its size and multiple sinusoid passages, the liver is a *reservoir for storing blood,* keeping it in readiness for use when major systemic blood loss (hemorrhage) occurs. In addition, the *Kupffer cells* serve as *filters* to remove colon bacteria and other debris that enter the liver from the portal vein.

As knowledge increases, more functions of the liver will be identified. The above briefly describe the major functions known today.

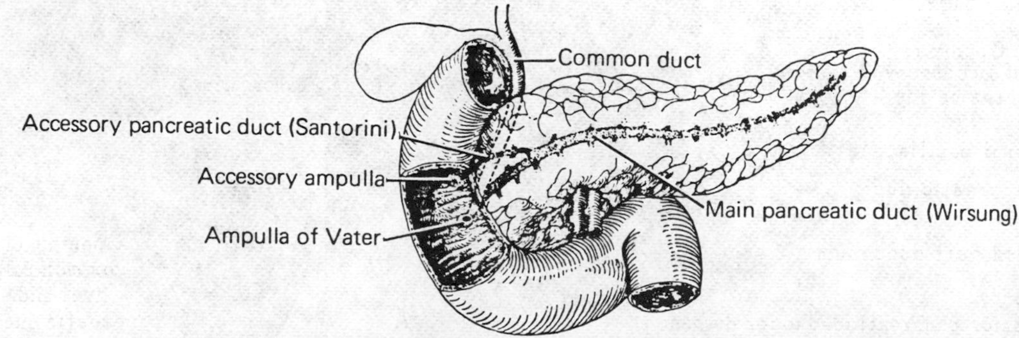

Figure 65–6. Anatomic configuration of pancreatic ductal system. (From Reber, H. A., and L. W. Way: Pancreas. *In* Dunphy, J. E., and L. W. Way: *Current Surgical Diagnosis and Treatment.* Los Altos: Lange Medical Publications, 1977, p. 554.)

Biliary Tract Function

The bile ducts and gallbladder function as a *collecting-concentrating system* and *reservoir for bile.* When the gallbladder is removed, the bile ducts act as reservoirs, and body processes proceed normally.

Pancreatic Function

Normally 1200 to 3000 ml. of *pancreatic juice* is produced daily. It is a clear alkaline solution carrying three major types of digestive enzymes. Pancreatic *amylase* splits carbohydrates to dextrins and maltose; pancreatic *lipase* hydrolyzes fat to yield glycerol and fatty acids; and pancreatic *trypsin* is representative of the group of enzymes that split proteins. Trypsin is activated in the intestine and functions as a *catalyst* to initiate a chain of other proteolytic enzymes. In the pancreas, a special *trypsin inhibitor* is stored to prevent that enzyme from digesting pancreatic tissue. (A dysfunction of the inhibitor is thought to be present in pancreatitis.)

Familiarity with the normal metabolic functions of the liver, biliary tract, and pancreas will aid in understanding (a) the signs and symptoms of dysfunction of these tissues, (b) the particular diagnostic measures used to document pathophysiology, and (c) treatment and nursing care measures.

CHAPTER 66

CLINICAL PROBLEMS COMMONLY ASSOCIATED WITH LIVER, BILIARY, AND PANCREATIC DISORDERS

Because of their close anatomic proximity as well as interrelated metabolic activities, certain disease manifestations may arise as a result of (a) dysfunction of *either* the liver, biliary tract, or pancreas or (b) dysfunctions involving *all* of these organs together. This interrelatedness of organ structure and function complicates the tasks of differential diagnosis, treatment, and nursing care.

The clinical *disorders* most commonly associated with the liver, biliary tract, and pancreas are listed below in Table 66–1, together with a brief definition of each, and some of the typical clinical problems encountered. Pathologic changes in these disorders are multiple and vary widely. They may be broadly categorized into three types: *inflammatory, fibrotic, and neoplastic.* Hepatitis, pancreatitis, and cholecystitis show evidence of acute and chronic inflammation of involved tissues. Fibrotic changes occur with cirrhosis and with inflammatory diseases that have become chronic. Primary tumors, benign or malignant, of these tissues are uncommon. Factors implicated in pathogenesis vary from viruses to alcoholism to gallstone formation.

The clinical problems *most frequently associated with the liver, gallbladder, and pancreas are jaundice, ascites, altered blood clotting mechanism, hepatic encephalopathy, and hepatic coma as well as drug intolerance and drug and alcohol abuse.*

Below we briefly consider these clinical problems and their treatment. The major disorders listed in Table 66–1 are discussed in detail in Chapters 68, 69, and 70.

JAUNDICE

Definition and Causes

Jaundice, or icterus, is the *yellow pigmentation of the skin due to excessive accumulations of bilirubin pigment in the blood serum.* Though bilirubin (bile pigment) is merely a metabolic end-product with no active physiologic role, its tendency to *color* whatever medium it is in makes it an important indicator of a variety of disorders

TABLE 66–1. DISORDERS COMMONLY ASSOCIATED WITH THE LIVER, BILIARY TRACT, AND PANCREAS

Disorder	Definition	Typical Clinical Problems
Hepatitis	Inflammation of liver due to viral infection transmitted by fecal-oral (type A) or blood (type B) route	Fatigue, anorexia, nausea, vomiting, jaundice, pruritus, abdominal pain, bleeding tendencies
Cirrhosis	Chronic liver disease with impaired function due to extensive scar tissue; usually associated with alcoholism	Ascites, bleeding tendencies, ruptured esophageal varices, anemia, alcoholism, malnutrition
Cholecystitis	Inflammation of gallbladder usually associated with presence of gallstones (lithiasis)	Abdominal pain, nausea and vomiting, jaundice, fever, bleeding tendencies
Pancreatitis	Inflammation of pancreas often associated with alcoholism or biliary tract disease	Abdominal pain and vomiting; hypovolemia and shock in acute episodes; hyperglycemia; incomplete digestion and vitamin deficiency; steatorrhea and diarrhea in chronic cases

involving the hepatic cells and the biliary tract. Thus, patients with abnormalities of bilirubin metabolism and excretion (and consequently jaundice) may have yellow sclerae, yellow skin, dark yellow urine, clay-colored stools owing to biliary obstruction), etc. The precise reasons for these color changes are considered below and throughout this unit.

Bilirubin Formation and Excretion. To understand abnormalities of bilirubin metabolism and excretion, one must first review the normal, which is presented in Figure 66–1 and briefly described in Chapter 65. Note in Figure 66–1 that once red blood cells have completed their 120 day sojourn through the circulatory system, they become very fragile. As a result, their cell membranes rupture and the *hemoglobin* that is released is phagocytized by cells of the reticuloendothelial system and thus split into *globin* and *heme.* It is from the heme ring that bile pigments are made. *Biliverdin* is the first pigment to be formed, however, it is soon reduced to *free bilirubin* and released into the plasma. Once in the plasma, free bilirubin combines quickly into a strong union with plasma albumin and becomes *protein-bound free bilirubin.* Protein-bound bilirubin is still termed "free" in order to categorize it separately from *conjugated bilirubin.* Free bilirubin becomes conjugated once it is absorbed through the hepatic cell membrane and combines with other substances inside the hepatic cells. Approximately 80 per cent of protein becomes conjugated with glucuronide acid to form *bilirubin glucuronide;* another 10 per cent conjugates with sulfate to form *bilirubin sulfate;* and the remaining 10 per cent conjugates with still other substances. In these three forms, bilirubin is excreted into the bile and passes through the bile ducts. Note in Figure 66–1 that from this point on, bilirubin may be found in the plasma, intestinal contents, and urine. Observe the following:

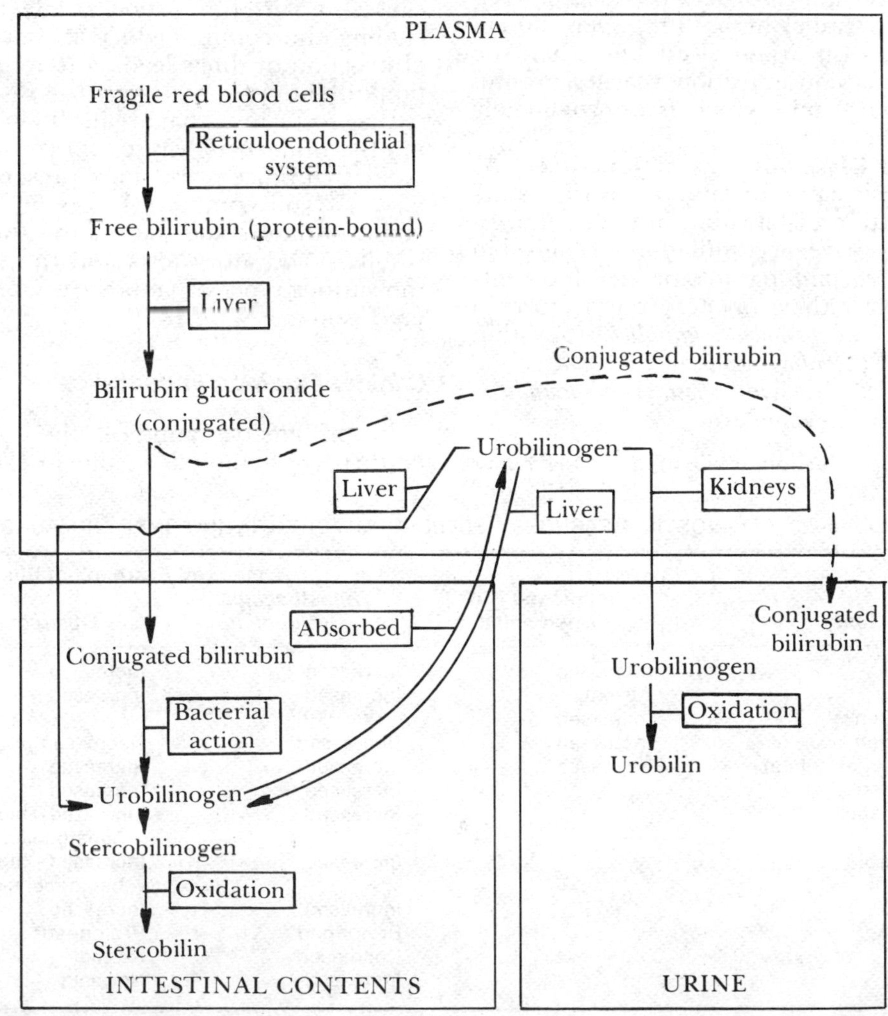

Figure 66–1. Biliary formation and excretion. (From Guyton, A. C.: *Textbook of Medical Physiology.* 5th ed., Philadelphia: W. B. Saunders Co., 1976.)

1. A small amount of conjugated bilirubin formed by the hepatic cells escapes back into the plasma; this means that a small portion of plasma bilirubin is always conjugated rather than free.
2. Most of the bilirubin passes into the intestines, where bacterial action produces *urobilinogen.*
3. Some urobilinogen is reabsorbed by the portal blood and returned to the liver, which, in turn, re-excretes most of this urobilinogen back into the intestines.
4. About 5 per cent of this urobilinogen passes into the urine and is excreted.
5. Urobilinogen oxidized in the feces becomes *stercobilinogen.*
6. Urobilinogen exposed to air in the urine becomes oxidized to *urobilin.*

Normally, the plasma concentration of both the free and conjugated forms of bilirubin is approximately 0.5 mg. per 100 ml. of plasma. However, in certain disorders this plasma concentration may rise as high 40 mg. per 100 ml. The skin takes on a jaundiced hue when the serum bilirubin concentration reaches around 1.5 mg. per 100 ml., which is approximately three times the normal.[40]

Causes and Classifications of Jaundice. As stated, the basic cause of jaundice is the excessive accumulation of bilirubin in the serum. In turn, the excessive accumulation of bilirubin results from certain pathologic developments that take place either: (a) before the bilirubin comes to the liver *(prehepatic jaundice),* (b) within the liver itself *(hepatic jaundice),* or (c) after the bilirubin leaves the liver *(posthepatic jaundice).* These pathologic events are:

1. Excessive production of bilirubin due to *excessive red blood cell destruction.* This problem is a consequence of *hemolytic anemia* and is called *prehepatic jaundice.* Given time and an adequately functioning liver, the jaundice of red blood cell destruction disappears once the destruction of cells ceases and the hemoglobin is conjugated by the liver and excreted in the urine and feces. (See Chapter 45.)
2. Excessive serum bilirubin due to either *defective uptake* of bilirubin by the liver or *defective conjugation* of bilirubin within the liver. Liver cell dysfunction or necrosis is the basis for this problem. The resulting jaundice is termed *hepatic jaundice* because it develops within the liver.
3. Impaired excretion of bile from the liver due to *defective* transport in the *bile canal* and *small bile duct.* This problem is also a form of *hepatic jaundice* and is sometimes called *obstructive jaundice.*
4. Impaired bilirubin excretion and bile flow due to *obstruction of an extrahepatic bile duct.* This form of jaundice is termed *posthepatic* and is an *obstructive* type.

The stagnation of bile in the hepatic cells or in the intrahepatic or extrahepatic bile ducts is called *cholestasis.* Through unknown channels, the pooled bile components are absorbed into the blood stream. *Hepatitis* is a disease that causes impaired excretion of bile. *Gallstones* occluding the common duct are an example of obstruction of ducts leading to impaired excretion of bile.

Diagnostic tests that are useful in differentiating the underlying cause and consequently the type of jaundice present are presented in Table 66–2. If you compare Tables 66–1 and 66–2, you can understand the reasons for certain test results. Laboratory tests and the symptoms of the various types of jaundice are briefly considered below.

Clinical Findings in Jaundice

In prehepatic jaundice, the rapid rate of erythrocyte hemolysis results in excessive accu-

TABLE 66–2. DIAGNOSTIC MEASURES USEFUL IN DIFFERENTIATING TYPE OF JAUNDICE

Laboratory Test	Increased RBC Destruction	Impaired Excretion of Bile: *Hepatocellular Dysfunction*	Impaired Excretion of Bile: *Obstruction of Duct*
Serum bilirubin	Increased	Increased	Increased
Urine bilirubin	Absent	Increased	Increased
Urine urobilinogen	Increased		
Fecal urobilinogen	Increased	Decreased	Decreased or absent
Indirect (unconjugated bile)	Increased	Increased	Increased
Direct (conjugated bile)		Increased	Increased
Alkaline phosphatase		Increased	Increased—higher than hepatocellular
Serum cholesterol		Increased	Increased—higher than hepatocellular
Serum bile salts		Increased	Increased
Prothrombin time		Prolonged*	Prolonged*
Serum protein		Decreased	Normal
Enzyme level		Increased	Normal

*If vitamin K is given parenterally to a person with obstructive jaundice, the prothrombin time will improve within 4 hours, but when given to a person with hepatocellular impairment no such change will be noted.

mulations of unconjugated or free bilirubin. The skin becomes jaundiced and, as the liver conjugates and excretes the excessive amount of pigment, greater than normal quantities of urobilinogen become present in urine and feces. Diagnosis is made on the basis of increased indirect (unconjugated) serum bilirubin values, absence of bilirubin in the urine (unconjugated bilirubin is water insoluble), and increased urobilinogen levels. Hepatic jaundice (seen for example in hepatitis) and posthepatic jaundice (seen in common bile duct obstruction) have many manifestations in common, as well as other manifestations that differentiate the two types. *Common symptoms* include increased levels of direct (conjugated) serum bilirubin, since it returns to the plasma when excretion is blocked; increased indirect serum bilirubin for unclear reasons; increased bilirubin in urine owing to high blood concentrations; reduced fecal urobilinogen, since it does not reach the intestine; increased alkaline phosphatase and cholesterol serum levels, since they cannot be excreted as normal into the bile; increased serum bile salts with consequent deposition in the skin to cause pruritus; and prolonged prothrombin time owing to reduced absorption of fat-soluble vitamin K. Hepatic jaundice is differentiated from extrahepatic blockage by demonstration of reduced hepatic cell function (diminished serum proteins, increased release of enzymes as a result of cellular damage). Extrahepatic obstruction to biliary excretion is more complete and may be differentiated from hepatocellular jaundice by higher alkaline phosphatase and cholesterol levels, more extreme pruritus, and the almost complete absence of fecal urobilinogen. *Percutaneous cholangiography* will visualize the site of obstruction by injection of opaque media directly into the extrahepatic ducts. (See Chapter 67.)

Clinical Interventions to Resolve Jaundice or Alleviate Symptoms

Jaundice can be reduced only by *elimination of the underlying disease.* (See Chapter 45 for discussion of therapy in hemolytic anemia.) *Extrahepatic biliary obstruction* can be treated solely by *surgical removal of obstruction.* Without surgical exploration final differentiation between choledocholithiasis (stone in the common bile duct) and tumor may be difficult. The surgical exploration of the common bile duct is called *choledochostomy.* If carcinoma, most commonly affecting the head of the pancreas, is found, a palliative anastomosis of the gallbladder to the jejunum is done to bypass the common bile duct. Resolution of jaundice in hepatitis relies on time as the prime therapeutic agent. Treatment is symptomatic.

Jaundice is a warning sign of disease, but of itself does not cause physical injury. Therapy will reduce accompanying complaints. *Pruritus,* believed to be caused by accumulation of bile salts in the skin when biliary excretion is obstructed, can be merely irritating or can drive patients to distraction — to tearing at their skin until excoriation develops. Oral cholestyramine resin provides some relief by binding bile salts and promoting intestinal elimination. Antihistamines provide some help.

A highly visible sign of illness, jaundice may have considerable emotional impact and may impair body image. Each day the person may study his or her eyes in hope of improvement, and may ask every staff member who walks in, "Do you think my color is any better?" Jaundice can become a stigma causing patients to feel physically, socially, and emotionally isolated from others. Feelings need acknowledgement, and ongoing explanation reduces unfounded fear. Patients may become preoccupied with physical appearance; their sense of being unattractive may be compensated for by the maintenance of an otherwise satisfying appearance.

ASCITES

Fluid accumulation in the peritoneal cavity (ascites) is the result of interaction of several pathophysiologic changes: namely, portal hypertension, lowered plasma colloidal oncotic (osmotic) pressure, and sodium retention. Disease processes leading to these events include cirrhosis of the liver, right-sided heart failure, tuberculous peritonitis, cancer, and complications of pancreatitis.

Mechanisms of Accumulation

Any process that blocks the flow of blood through the sinusoids to the hepatic vein and vena cava causes an *increase in hydrostatic pressure* in the portal venous system. Most commonly, this occurs in cirrhosis of the liver or right-sided heart failure. As portal pressure increases, *splenic congestion* occurs with subsequent plasma leaks directly from the liver capsule and the portal vein into the peritoneal cavity. *Congestion of lymph channels* also occurs, leading to the leaking of more plasma into the peritoneal cavity. *Loss of plasma proteins* from the portal system reduces oncotic pressure within the circulating blood volume, thus limiting the ability of the vascular tree to hold on to or collect water. In addition, *hepatocellular damage* reduces the liver's ability to synthesize more albumin to replace that being lost in the peritoneal cavity. As circulating blood volume decreases (from loss of oncotic pressure), the secretion of *aldosterone is increased* in order to stimulate the kidneys to retain sodium and water. Once again as a result of hepatocellular damage, the liver is unable to inactivate the hormone aldosterone, and its sodium and water retention effect is prolonged. Hence, more fluid is held and the volume of ascites grows.

> *Remember, the three mechanisms underlying* ascites *formation:*
>
> *1.* Portal hypertension *resulting in increased plasma and lymphatic hydrostatic pressures.*
>
> *2.* Hypoalbuminemia *resulting in decreased oncotic (osmotic) pressure.*
>
> *3.* Hyperaldosteronism *resulting in increased sodium and water retention.*

Diagnosis of Ascites

Ascitic fluid typically produces abdominal distention, bulging flanks, and a protruding umbilicus, which is displaced downward. An extreme example of ascites is depicted in Figure 66–2. While large accumulations of ascitic fluid are fairly obvious, small or moderate amounts may be more difficult to diagnose. Some simple diagnostic methods that can be performed at the bedside are as follows:

- *Percuss* the abdomen; if the patient has ascites, the sound will be dull.
- *Turn* the patient on his or her side and *percuss* the abdomen (see Fig. 66–3). Because ascitic fluid flows to the lowest point in the abdomen, when the patient turns, the ascitic water will flow downward and cause a shift in the area where dullness is heard.
- *Fluid waves* may also be elicited by tapping the abdomen. "A fluid wave is pathognomonic of fluid in the abdominal cavity and, when associated with shifting dullness, confirms the presence of free fluid."[22a] The method for producing a fluid wave is described in Chapter 15.

In addition, *abdominal x-rays* of the person in the supine and erect positions may be helpful if the fluid accumulation approaches 1000 ml. Fluid will cause a dulling or blurring of normal angles and shadows. *Ultrasound* may also locate small amounts of fluid in the peritoneal cavity. *Paracentesis* may be useful to document the presence of ascitic fluid and to provide samples of fluid for analysis. Fluid may be *analyzed* for protein, amylase, blood cells (WBC, RBC), cancer cells, and fat in order to determine the source of the fluid and the presence or absence of infection.

Management

The following goals guide the reduction of symptoms due to ascites:

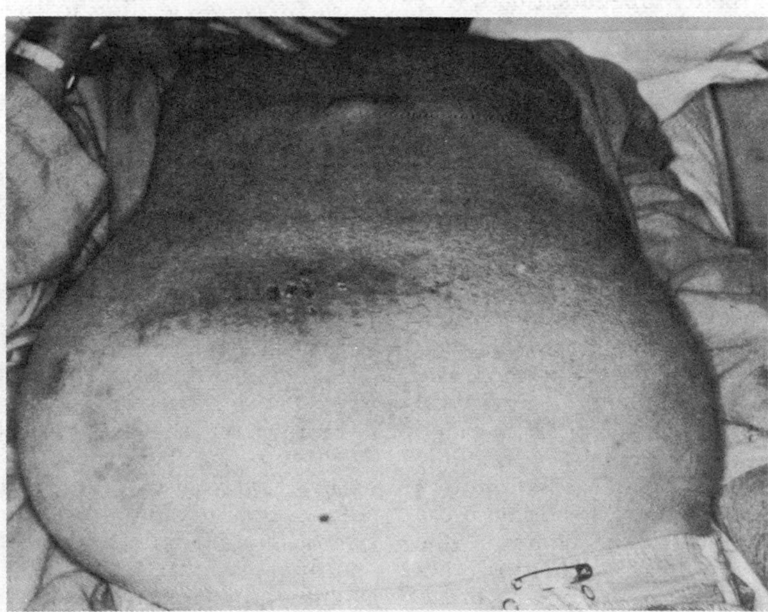

Figure 66–2. Abdominal distention due to excessive fluid. (From Sherman, J. L., and S. K. Fields: *Guide to Patient Evaluation.* 2nd ed., Flushing, N.Y.: Medical Examination Publishing Co., Inc., 1976.)

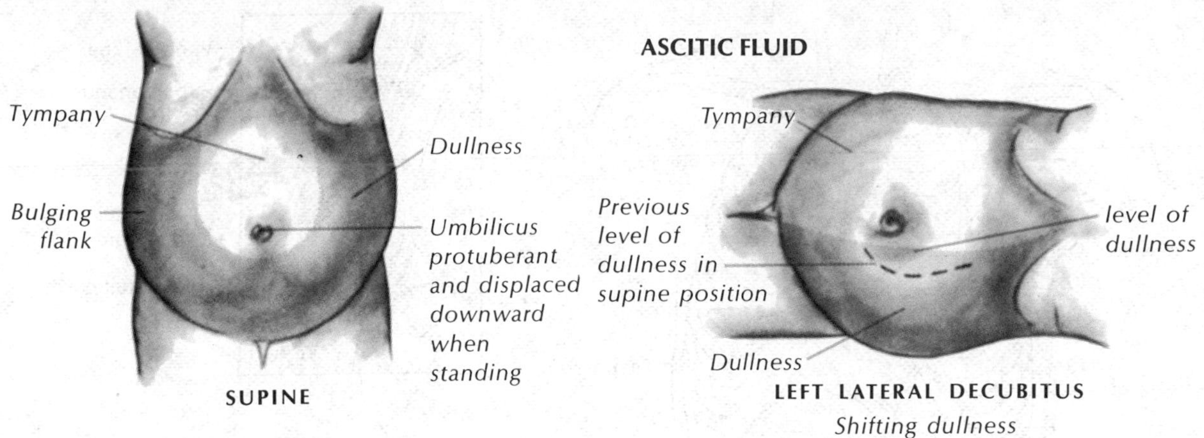

Figure 66–3. Detecting ascites by noting position shifts in fluid level. (From Bates, B.: *A Guide to Physical Examination.* Philadelphia: J. B. Lippincott Co., 1974.)

Evaluate the Extent of Ascites Accumulation. Evaluation is needed to note (a) increases or decreases in the fluid collection; (b) the pathologic course of the condition producing the ascites; and (c) the effectiveness of therapy. Daily weights provide a sensitive monitor of fluid retention and loss. Measurements of *abdominal girth* provide a gross estimate of progress or regression of abdominal swelling. Patients with ascites face long-term medical management and the need for ongoing adjustments in therapy. They must be taught the importance of assessing their weight and measuring abdominal girth and immediately report rapid gain in pounds and inches to the physician. Be sure that the patient will have access to an accurate scale or all your teaching will be in vain!

Control Sodium and Water Retention Through Dietary Restriction and Diuretics. The aim in *sodium restriction* is to create a negative sodium balance, namely, measuring the amount of sodium lost in the urine and allowing only a portion of that amount in the diet for the next day. For example, if the patient's 24-hour urinary output contains 20 mEq of sodium and the person subsequently takes in only 10 mEq in the next 24 hours, in 14 days the individual will have reduced the sodium content in the body by 140 mEq. The concurrent fluid loss will be 1 liter or, in body weight, 1 kg. (As a guide, 23–40 mEq sodium diet is equivalent to 500–1000 mg.) A diet containing 500 mg. or less of sodium may be quite unpalatable and restricted, so ongoing dietary consultation is important. If sodium restriction alone does not cause reduction in ascites, *water* may also be restricted.

Diuretics are added to treat ascites when dietary restriction alone is not providing effective control. This occurs when the primary causal factors in ascites — portal hypertension and hypoalbuminemia — are severe. Poor renal sodium excretion and minimal sodium of a restricted diet results in retention of ascitic fluid. The use of diuretics is based on the fact that they stimulate the kidneys to increase their reduced sodium and water excretion. Potassium-sparing diuretics (spironolactone and triamterene) may be prescribed in conjunction with either thiazides, ethacrynic acid, or furosemide to achieve safe and effective diuresis. These are prescribed with caution, since they may cause further electrolyte imbalances.

Occasionally potassium chloride supplementation is necessary. Fluid and electrolyte levels are watched very carefully during the first few days of diuretic therapy. Hypokalemia, with alkalosis, as well as hyperkalemia, and hyponatremia, are possible. Too rapid diuresis can precipitate oliguria and renal failure from diminished circulatory volume, and the development of hepatic encephalopathy is not unusual. Thus initially diuresis should be slow if it is to be safe. Refer to Chapter 12 to review mechanisms of the fluid and electrolyte imbalances that threaten.

Increase Albumin Levels when Hypoalbuminemia is Severe. When diet and diuretic therapy fail to control ascitic accumulations, intravenous albumin and paracentesis may benefit the patient. *Salt-poor albumin* is given, and expanded blood volume should initiate diuresis, the patient must be observed carefully for concomitant signs of pulmonary edema. Occasionally *ascitic fluid is reinfused* to expand volume.

Control Ascites by Paracentesis or a Peritoneal–Venous Shunt. Though it once was standard therapy, *paracentesis* is now indicated only when fluid accumulations are large and disabling and all else has failed. Usually only amounts up to 1 liter are removed to avoid the risks of fluid shift and protein loss, but multiple complications are still possible. The fluid removed rapidly reforms, and little or nothing is gained. Thus paracentesis is only a temporary palliative procedure. Paracentesis is discussed further in Chapter 67.

If all other measures fail to control ascites, a *peritoneal–venous shunt (the LeVeen shunt)* may be tried. This surgical procedure involves placement of one end of a tube below the peritoneum and the other end into the jugular vein or superior vena cava (see Fig. 66–4). Inclusion of a one-way pressure valve in the shunt controls the direction of fluid flow. When open, this one-way valve allows the peritoneal fluid to pass into a silicone-rubber tube that runs beneath the subcutaneous tissues and empties into the superior vena cava. The action of the shunt is triggered by the patient's breathing in the following manner. When the patient takes in a breath, his or her diaphragm descends, causing a rise in intraperitoneal fluid pressure and a fall in intrathoracic superior vena cava pressure. The resulting pressure differential of approximately 5 cm. H_2O opens the shunt valve and

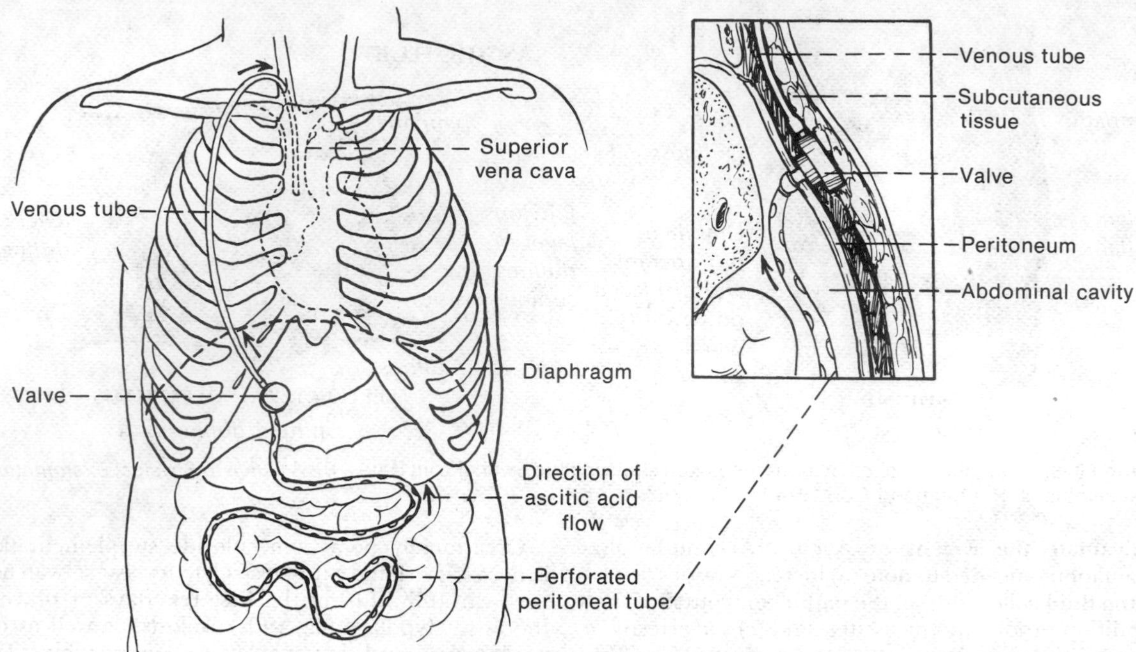

Figure 66–4. The LeVeen shunt.

forces the fluid to flow. However, this procedure is not without risk, such as hemodilution, leakage of ascitic fluid from the incision site, wound infection, shunt occlusion, disseminated intravascular coagulation, gastrointestinal bleeding, and elevated bilirubin.

Relieve Symptoms due to Pressure of Ascites. Gross distention may force the diaphragm upward and restrict lung expansion. High Fowler's position will maximize respiratory effectiveness. Skin circulation is also compromised by pressure within the abdomen and by inadequate cellular perfusion due to interstitial edema. Turning and positioning are vital to prevent prolonged external pressure and skin breakdown.

Give Psychologic Support. Persons with ascites frequently require long-term care. Involving them in activities of care while in the acute care center, helping them to understand *why* certain things are done as well as *what* is being done for them, and providing support persons to whom they can come with questions about their care may enhance their independence and improve their quality of life during this period of time.

BLEEDING

Causative Factors

Bleeding tendencies may be present in viral hepatitis, cirrhosis, and biliary obstruction. There are two fundamental causes of bleeding: (1) reduced clotting factors and (2) intolerable pressure changes in the portal venous system, which can lead to ruptured esophageal varices.

Clotting factors may be reduced because of:

1. *Lack of bile* in the intestine to break down fat-soluble vitamin K.
2. *Ineffective hepatocytes* that are unable to synthesize prothrombin even if vitamin K is available. (Observing prothrombin time after parenteral administration of vitamin K will help differentiate between causes 1 and 2.)
3. *Damaged hepatocytes* unable to synthesize other clotting proteins such as Factors V, VI, VII, IX, and X.
4. *Portal hypertension* causing splenic congestion with increased destruction of platelets.

Hence, alteration in the physiology of the hepatocyte leads to one chain of events predisposing to bleeding. At the same time, hepatocellular damage causes alteration in portal pressure, thereby placing extreme stress on the blood vessels leading to the liver. This stress predisposes the vessels to rupture with immediate loss of significant amounts of blood.

Changes in portal pressure and consequent rupture of vessels occur for these reasons:

1. Obstruction of blood flow through the liver causes an *increase in portal vein pressure* leading to the development of an elaborate system of collateral vessels, all attempting to bypass the liver and deliver blood directly into the hepatic vein or vena cava.
2. These collateral vessels *become engorged* with blood under pressure. (Since portal veins drain the esophagus, stomach, intestines, and rectum, the collateral vessels develop around these organs.) For some reason, the vessels around the esophagus and rectum have a tendency to bleed first.
3. When engorged vessels are strained beyond their ability to withstand, they *perforate*, and *hemorrhage* occurs. Portal pressure, increased intrathoracic pressure (coughing, straining at stool), irritation by

food or alcohol, and erosion by gastric juices may all contribute to the rupturing of the varices.

When bleeding occurs, the blood is usually bright red. The amount varies with the size of the ruptured vessel. If the broken blood vessel is in the stomach or intestine, the blood may appear darker because of its interaction with digestive juices.

Ruptured esophageal varices (swollen, dilated esophageal veins) produce massive hemorrhage as a dreaded complication of cirrhosis. They develop as a consequence of portal hypertension. Rupture of esophageal varices can occur with any increase in portal hydrostatic pressure, such as with increased intrathoracic or intra-abdominal pressure or with increased blood volume. Blood loss under such pressure is rapid and great. Direct trauma by food and irritation by gastric juices have also been implicated.

Diagnosis

Bleeding tendencies due to hypoprothrombinemia or thrombocytopenia are identified through blood tests such as *prothrombin time* or *platelet count.* Prothrombin time is routinely evaluated with patients being worked up for biliary and liver disease, and is included in intermittent evaluations of those with an identified disorder. (See also Ch. 46.)

Clinical Intervention to Restore Hemostasis

Hemostasis in liver and biliary disease is achieved in five ways:

1. *Restore clotting factors.* When hypoprothrombinemia has been identified, parenteral vitamin K is given with the hope that reduced fat absorption owing to reduced bile excretion has been at least a partial cause. When hepatic damage is the sole cause of reduced prothrombin synthesis, vitamin K will not help. In such a case, fresh plasma or whole blood will be effective in replacing clotting factors for short periods. When the problem is reduced platelets, platelet transfusions are possible.

2. *Prevent bleeding.*

> *Because of their prolonged clotting time, it is imperative to* protect patients *with bleeding tendencies from physical injury (falls, bruises, abrasions). Also it is important to astutely* observe *these persons for any signs of bleeding.*

Early sites of bleeding might include the *gums* (from brushing teeth vigorously or with a hard bristled brush), the *nose* (from forceful blowing), the *urine* (from rupturing of blood vessels within a kidney), and the *skin over bony prominences* (from trauma of bone on fragile vessels). Melena and hematemesis may occur in mild bleeding of the *gastrointestinal tract,* which is the most common site for bleeding.

Moreover, teach patients that certain types of behavior will *decrease* the risk of bleeding; e.g., avoiding aspirin and alcohol, which irritate the mucosa; avoiding constipation so that straining at stool will not increase intra-abdominal pressure; avoiding heavy lifting; treating coughs to avoid increased intrathoracic pressure, and avoiding eating large meals, which may temporarily increase portal pressure. Food should be chewed well in small portions to avoid trauma to mucosa. Antacids may be ordered to neutralize irritating gastric acid. Occasionally dietary sodium restrictions and diuretics may be prescribed to keep plasma volume, and therefore portal pressure, low.

Finally, patients and their families or significant others must have a workable emergency plan thought out should the patient begin to bleed. They need to be able to reach a doctor, hospital, emergency clinic, etc. immediately.

3. *Lavage bleeding gastric ulcers using cold fluid.* Ice water or saline is instilled through a nasogastric tube; the resulting vasoconstriction will reduce blood flow from peptic or duodenal ulcers but will have little impact on hemorrhaging varices.

4. *Apply pressure to ruptured varices. A Sengstaken-Blakemore (B-ST) tube* (Fig. 66–5) provides pressure with balloons directly over the bleeding esophageal varices and in the cardia of the stomach to compress supplying veins. The B-ST is a tube with three lumens and two balloons. It is placed in the esophagus and stomach. The distal balloon is inflated and pulled snugly against the esophageal–gastric junction; the second balloon is inflated to place pressure against the walls of the esophagus. Each balloon has its own lumen. The third lumen is patent through the length of the tube and provides means for lavage or gavage of the stomach. Pressure at the end of the B-ST is necessary in order to hold it in place. The B-ST presents a challenge to persons caring for the patient. Special care must be taken to keep the tube in proper position to prevent irritation of the nares, to prevent suffocation or erosion of the esophagus from the balloon, to prevent aspiration of gastric contents if the gag reflex is absent, and to record and describe the amount of gastric drainage. (See p. 1484.)

5. *Lower portal pressure. Temporary* lowering of portal pressure is achieved by the administration of *posterior pituitary hormone* (pituitrin, Pitressin). It is believed to constrict afferent arterioles and thus reduce portal blood flow to cause portal hypotension. Systemic side effects include fluid retention, myocardial ischemia, and stimulation of uterine and gastrointestinal contraction (cramping and diarrhea).

Permanent lowering of portal pressure is achieved by surgical procedures that shunt blood away from the portal system. Most commonly performed are portacaval and splenorenal shunts. *Splenectomy* is necessary to allow splenorenal anastomosis. Portal shunts definitely stop bleeding, but the overall survival of cirrhotic patients is not much enhanced owing to multiple complications. Patients are considered good surgical risks in the *absence* of jaundice, severe ascites, encephalopathy, and severe hypoalbuminemia. Shunts are considered in detail in Chapter 68.

Special Care for Esophageal Varices

Ruptured bleeding esophageal varices comprise an acute physiologic and emotional crisis, and nursing care is intensive and complex. Sixty-seven per cent of patients with ruptured varices die. Around 55 per cent of these patients expire in one year after the initial hemorrhage.[91]

The following discussion indicates the goals of care for the patient with ruptured varices, and the multiple nursing actions needed to meet these goals.

▶ *To achieve hemostasis.* Assist in insertion of deflated B-ST tube. Before insertion, both balloons must be *checked* under water *for leaks.* Also the stomach may be lavaged with iced saline and emptied per Levin tube to prevent aspiration. Final positioning of BS-T tube is checked by x-ray. Traction on the BS-T tube prevents downward movement. Check and maintain ordered balloon manometer pressures. Monitor gastric suction drainage for bleeding; amount indicates effectiveness of therapy. Maintain traction. Perform iced gastric lavage every hour, or more often if ordered. Maintain pump circulating ice water through esophageal balloon if ordered. In case of malfunction, have extra Sengstaken-Blakemore tube on hand.

Pitressin or pituitrin may be given systemically (IV) in doses of 20 to 50 units in 100 to 200 ml. of 5 per cent dextrose in water or by intra-arterial infusion via the superior mesenteric artery. In this case, vasopressin is given by an infusion pump at the rate of 0.05 to 0.1 unit per minute. Results of vasopressin therapy can be monitored by checking samples of aspirated gastric contents for blood, and by serial pulse and blood pressure readings.[91] Possibly assist with paracentesis to decrease pressure on portal collaterals. Maintain transfusions of *fresh* blood to provide clotting factors. Give vitamin K IM, if ordered.

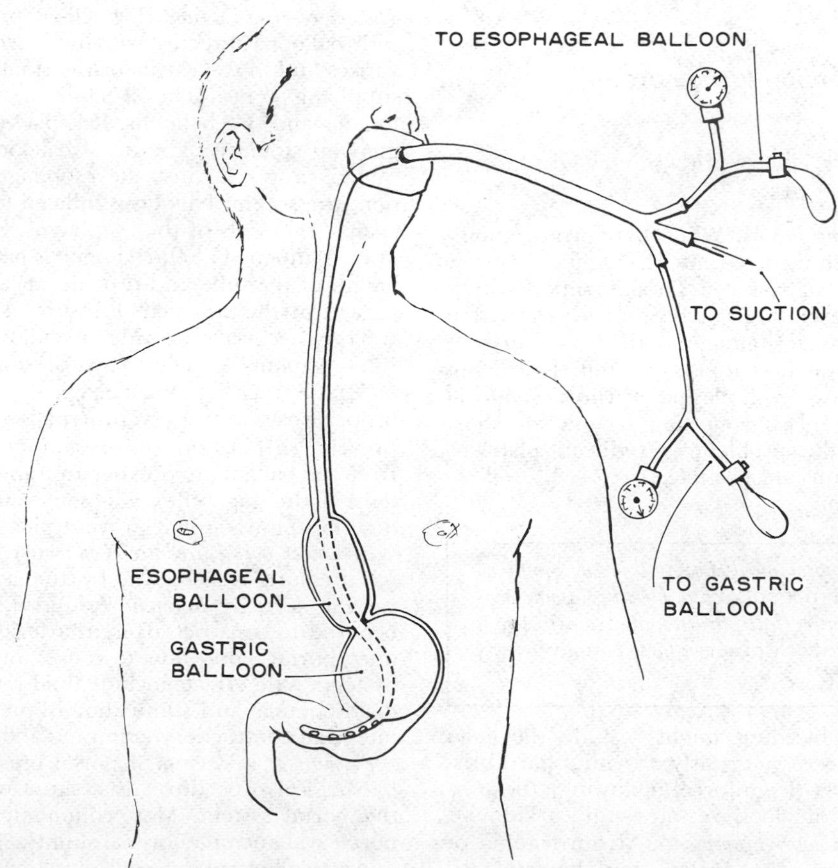

Figure 66–5. Sengstaken-Blakemore tube in place. (From Price, A. P., and L. M. Wilson: *Pathophysiology: Clinical Concepts of Disease Processes.* New York: McGraw Hill Book Co., 1978, p. 276.)

- *To maintain circulatory volume.* Multiple blood transfusions, including packed cells and an occasional unit of fresh blood or plasma. Critical observation, including: CVP and/or intraarterial pressure to monitor blood volume in order to detect possible hemorrhage; vital signs every 15 min.; hematocrit, electrolytes; hourly urines, BUN to detect reduced renal perfusion; evaluation of mental status to detect reduced hepatic perfusion.
- *To prevent respiratory complications.* NPO, patient unable to swallow. Frequent expectoration and mouth care, oral suction of saliva. Frequent tracheal suctioning to prevent aspiration of blood and clear secretions. Have patient turn and move freely to prevent respiratory complications. Oxygen and other respiratory treatments. (See Ch. 54.) Observe for sudden respiratory crisis indicating aspiration or airway obstruction due to upward balloon displacement from pull of traction if gastric balloon ruptures. Check for esophageal balloon in oropharynx and then either deflate or cut the tube at once!

> *A heavy pair of scissors must always be kept at the bedside in case of this emergency.*

Also, *proper labeling* of each lumen of the B-ST tube helps prevent accidental deflation of the gastric balloon and resultant upward movement of the esophageal balloon into the oropharynx.

- *To prevent esophageal erosion.* Periodically deflate balloons every 8 to 12 hours; some physicians will leave balloons fully inflated for 2 to 3 days.
- *To prevent hepatic coma.* Cathartics, enemas, neomycin as ordered. Restraints may be necessary for patients with encephalopathy.
- *To prevent nasal breakdown.* Keep nostrils clean and lubricated. Maintain padding (foam rubber) in position at the external nares.
- *To provide patient and family comfort.* Provide a calm environment. Significant others frequently included in intensive care environment. Ongoing explanation given; touch used. Acknowledge the fact that severe bleeding is very frightening and give reassurance that the B-ST tube does stop bleeding in almost 90 per cent of patients. Judicious use of p.r.n. pain medication with consideration of how drug is detoxified.
- *To prepare patient for emergency portal shunt if indicated.* Measures to improve prothrombin levels, increase platelet levels, reduce ascites, increase albumin levels, reduce hepatic encephalopathy, reduce anemia, and overcome concurrent infection may be necessary.
- *To provide postoperative care after shunt.* Standard postoperative abdominal measures with special attention to respiratory measures and circulatory monitoring. Observe for and prevent hepatic encephalopathy (see below). According to some sources, another problem following a shunt is an increased frequency of *peptic ulcers.* This complication is thought to be caused by the presence of *secretagogue,* a substance produced in the intestines and normally inactivated by the liver. Peptic ulcers are serious for patients with liver disease because of the possibility of gastric bleeding, which, in turn, increases the incidence of hepatic coma. Therefore, take time to teach these persons about the signs and symptoms of peptic ulcers (see Chapter 62) and have them report them to their physicians at once.[2]

Nutrition is also an important post-shunt consideration. Because the esophageal varices are still present, patients must take care to not eat spicy rough foods that may cause esophageal irritation. An adult patient needs between 2500 and 3000 calories a day; furthermore, the diet should provide 100 Gm. of protein, 80 to 110 Gm. of fat, and 400 Gm. of carbohydrate. However, as we discuss below, *protein* must be drastically curtailed if hepatic coma complicates the patient's postoperative course. Finally, if the patient has post-shunt edema or ascites, sodium and fluid intake must be adjusted.[2]

HEPATIC ENCEPHALOPATHY/ HEPATIC COMA

Causative Factors

Hepatic encephalopathy encompasses a *spectrum of CNS disturbances* that may appear with severe liver injury, liver failure, or portal shunt. Changes manifested in hepatic encephalopathy range from reduced mental alertness, confusion, and restlessness in the initial stages to loss of consciousness, convulsions, and irreversible coma in the terminal stage.

The exact cause of hepatic encephalopathy is unknown; however, there is characteristically an *elevated level of ammonia in the blood and cerebrospinal fluid.* Concerning its *etiology,* Price and Wilson explain:[74]

> In simplest terms, hepatic encephalopathy can be described as a form of cerebral intoxication caused by intestinal contents that have not been metabolized by the liver. This condition may occur when there is liver cell damage due to necrosis or shunting (pathological or surgically created), which permit large amounts of portal blood to reach the systemic circulation without transversing the liver.

The exact metabolites responsible for this condition are still not identified. While *ammonia,* a product of protein digestion, has been most extensively studied, biogenic amines, amino acids, certain fatty acids, and infectious organisms may also be causative factors or may interact in some way with ammonia.

The *pathophysiology* of hepatic encephalopathy is also unclear. Apparently ammonia or some other unidentified factors interfere with the metabolism of the brain and thus cause cerebral symptoms. Individuals vary as to the blood level of ammonia that will cause cerebral manifestations.

> Remember:
> *Any process that increases protein in the intestine, such as increased dietary protein or gastrointestinal bleeding, will cause elevated blood ammonia and possibly signs of hepatic encephalopathy.*

Assessment

Manifestations of hepatic encephalopathy progress from early prehepatic coma with mild mental confusion to deep hepatic coma. Critical observation and interviewing are essential in all susceptible patients. Memory, attention, concentration, and rate of response become impaired and worsen with depression of function. Handwriting and speech are evaluated for change. Personality changes with labile feeling states are often seen. As the syndrome progresses, *level of consciousness is slowly depressed,* and confusion becomes more severe. Flapping tremor ("liver flap" or asterixis) is elicited when the patient is asked to dorsiflex his or her hand with the rest of the arm resting on the bed. The skin may be very jaundiced and there may be signs of hemorrhagic phenomena. At this time, delta waves on the electroencephalogram (EEG) are characteristic. Finally, coma follows and may deepen until there is no pain response and the reflexes, including corneal, are completely absent.

Fluctuations in level of depression are common. The nurse, who is with the patient over time, is the best person to see a change in level of mental functioning. Early detection greatly improves the patient's chance of recovery. Nursing progress notes are relevant when they describe behavioral change vividly as raw data ("Patient states pigeons are pecking at his bedclothes") rather than as a vague generalization that has a different meaning for each reader ("Patient seems more confused"). As the patient progresses into coma, ongoing neurologic checks by the nurse are essential to determine level of consciousness. (See Unit X for checks usually performed on comatose patients.)

Some patients develop hyperventilation with *respiratory alkalosis.* A characteristic odor on the breath, *fetor hepaticus,* is attributed to the presence of methyl mercaptan. Throughout the course of this syndrome, serum ammonia levels, electrolytes, blood gases, and hepatic function (bilirubin, albumin, prothrombin, enzymes) are monitored to determine degree of imbalance and extent of hepatic injury and failure to function (see Chapter 67).

Clinical Intervention

Nursing and medical care of persons with hepatic encephalopathy seeks to control or reduce further degenerative processes, correct present metabolic imbalances, and preserve remaining physiologic functioning.

Four principles guide therapy in hepatic encephalopathy, prehepatic coma, and coma:

1. Reduce Protein in Intestine. One way this is done is by *reduction of dietary protein.* If no other precipitating factors are present, this alone may eliminate symptoms. Protein may be eliminated entirely with an intake of fruit juices and intravenous fluids, or it may be restricted to 20 to 40 Gm. In the patient chronically susceptible to coma, a long-term low-protein diet (50 to 60 Gm.) may impose severe strain on self-control. Patient understanding and motivation are essential for cooperation. Also, gastrointestinal bleeding resulting in accumulations of protein in the intestine must be identified and treated to reverse the progression of symptoms. Constipation must be reversed. As behavioral manifestations worsen, *cathartics* and *enemas* will be prescribed to hasten exit of protein material from the intestine. Milk of magnesia, 30 ml. four times daily, or magnesium sulfate by indwelling nasogastric tube may be given.

2. Reduce Bacterial Production of Ammonia. This is commonly done by the administration of *neomycin* in large oral doses. Neomycin is not absorbed into the circulation and therefore exerts a powerful effect on the intestinal bacteria responsible for ammonia production. Undesirable side effects due to the depletion of intestinal flora include diarrhea and vitamin K deficiency. *Neomycin is commonly combined with protein restriction and bowel cleansing in the treatment of prehepatic coma and actual coma.* It may be prescribed in maintenance doses with low-protein diet in the patient with a tendency to chronic recurrence of coma. Lactulose, a combination of galactose and fructose that passes through the intestine unchanged, is sometimes administered in these cases. It has been demonstrated to decrease ammonia by pulling ammonia into the bowel. Lactulose is prescribed in a dosage that causes two to three soft stool evacuations daily. Diarrhea may be a side effect and necessitate reduction of dosage in order to prevent further electrolyte imbalance.

3. Eliminate Fluid and Electrolyte Imbalances, Uremia, Hypoxia, Infection, Sedation. *Hypovolemia* often precipitates hepatic coma by reducing hepatic cellular perfusion, which precipitates poor renal perfusion, leading to retention of urea. Recall that urea eventually breaks down to ammonia in the body. Therapy during coma requires intravenous intake. Therefore, achieving, maintaining, and monitoring fluid balance are essential to prevent further hepatic injury as well as reduced renal perfusion with uremia. Intravenous volume must be delivered evenly over a period of time. Vital signs and central venous pressure are monitored frequently, often hourly urine determinations are essential. *Electrolyte* and *acid-base disturbances* may precipitate hepatic coma or develop during coma. Laboratory tests indicate the replacement therapy necessary.

Hypoxia may precipitate hepatic coma due to hypoxic damage to the hepatic cell; both therapeutic and preventive management of the patient will include attention to respiratory measures such as maintaining a patent airway, oxygenation, and other respiratory measures. Concurrent *infection,* with protein accumulating from tissue catabolism, must also be treated, and the patient is particularly vulnerable to hospital-acquired infections. Careful attention must be paid to the prevention of cross infection. Finally, *depressants* may precipitate coma, and must be avoided during therapy. Sedation during agitation occurring in prehepatic coma must be provided by agents, such as phenobarbital, which are excreted through the kidney instead of the liver.

Remember to administer phenobarbital with caution! Narcotics, tranquilizers, or sedatives excreted by the liver may often be contraindicated in a severe decrease of hepatic function.

4. Maintain Function in the Unconscious Patient. Complications possible in the immobile patient lacking reflexes are numerous, and their prevention requires intensive nursing. To preserve physiologic functioning, patient care measures include preventing pneumonia and skin breakdown by frequent turning, positioning, and lung aeration. In addition, it is important to protect the patient from self-injury should he or she become agitated due to the accumulation of metabolic substances in the body. For further discussion of the comatose patient and individual with neurologic disturbances, see Unit X.

Therapy usually alleviates hepatic coma, though the patient may succumb to circulatory or respiratory complications, infection, or delirium and convulsions. There is a high mortality among patients who progress into coma with hepatic failure. Many dramatic measures, such as peritoneal dialysis and exchange transfusions that remove and then replace approximately 80 per cent of the person's blood, have been developed to reduce toxic levels in hopes of regeneration of cells. Corticosteroids and antimetabolites improve laboratory values, but whether they halt degeneration is questionable. In the most advanced research centers, liver transplant may be tried when there is complete hepatocellular failure in a young, otherwise healthy, patient.

INTOLERANCE TO SEDATION

The patient with hepatic damage responds adversely to sedation. Reasons remain unclear. The explanation is often given that the drug accumulates to toxic levels when the damaged liver cells fail to metabolize and excrete it, but elevated levels may not be demonstrated during drug reactions. It has been postulated that the brain of the patient with hepatic damage is oversensitive to the effects of these drugs; underlying dynamics remain undefined. Precise information on routes of drug metabolism is also lacking. Opiates, short-acting barbiturates, and major tranquilizers are believed to be metabolized primarily in the liver, and are avoided as therapeutic agents. In the absence of drugs, nursing measures become the major means of achieving rest and comfort for these patients. Phenobarbital, believed to be excreted primarily through the kidney, is the agent of choice if medication is indicated. Paraldehyde is another agent used for sedation.

ALCOHOL AND DRUG ABUSE

Alcoholism and parenteral drug abuse precipitate many disorders discussed in this unit. They also become ongoing clinical problems, as therapy is limited and prognosis often poor when the patient is unwilling to give up the cause of disorder. Increasingly, both alcohol and drug abuse are being seen in the same person.

Alcoholism is characterized by physiologic dependency manifested by withdrawal symptoms when ethanol intake is eliminated, development of tolerance to increasing quantities, blackout spells, and psychologic dependency when the person drinks despite social or medical contraindications. Alcoholic hepatitis, Laennec's cirrhosis, and pancreatitis are commonly associated with alcoholism.

Drug abuse may rarely precipitate toxic hepatitis if hepatic toxins are ingested over time, and commonly precipitates viral hepatitis if needles contaminated with infected blood are shared without intervening sterilization. The injected agents that most commonly are involved in producing viral hepatitis are the opiates, amphetamines, and barbiturates. Alcoholism and drug abuse are discussed further in Chapter 94.

CHAPTER 67

ASSESSING PERSONS WITH POSSIBLE DISORDERS OF THE LIVER, BILIARY TRACT, OR PANCREAS

Pathologic changes in the liver, biliary tract, or pancreas are multiple and may vary widely. As stated earlier, changes may be due to inflammation, fibrosis, or neoplastic growths. Exposure to viruses and toxic substances, alcoholism, drug abuse and addiction, dietary habits, working conditions, environmental conditions, and travel to certain locations are all implicated as contributing to pathologic changes. Therefore, when assessing persons with possible dysfunctions of these organs, not only are bacteriologic studies, biochemical studies, radiographic tests, and surgical procedures important but close attention also must be given to the patient's account of life style and behavior patterns.

PATIENT HISTORY

In suspected disease of the liver, gallbladder, and pancreas, special emphasis is placed upon discomforts and manifestations involving the patient's *gastrointestinal tract* and *neurologic system.* Thus it is important to document with the patient or significant others the presence (past or current) of the following: nausea, vomiting, anorexia, melena, clay-colored stools, dark yellow urine, jaundiced eyes or skin, abdominal colic or tenderness, ascites, edema of limbs, nose bleeds or easy bruisability, hemorrhoids, disturbed bowel patterns, fever, chronic indigestion and fatty food intolerance (signs of chronic cholecystitis), and steatorrhea (bulky, foul, fatty stools, which appear in chronic cholecystitis).

Inquiry into the *site and type of pain* is extremely important. Frequently, right upper quadrant discomfort with or without colicky severity accompanies these disorders. Also pain referred to the right shoulder may suggest organ dysfunction.

Eating patterns are another vital area for exploration. Investigate the following: food preferences; amounts of protein, carbohydrates, fat, and sodium consumed daily; changes in eating patterns and when these changes developed; who prepares the patient's meals; and food intolerances that have recently developed.

The *occupational history* might help to identify liver abnormalities in persons working with known hepatotoxins. An individual's use of *alcohol* is a crucial part of the history because alcoholism often accompanies liver and pancreatic disease. If you suspect that the patient's response is unreliable, seek additional information concerning the patient's drinking habits from persons close to the patient. (See Chapter 94 for a discussion of alcoholism.) Ask tactfully about *drug usage,* especially anesthetic agents, oral contraceptives, chlorpromazine, and illicit drugs — all of which may cause liver damage. Explore the individual's recent experiences with *skin or membrane disruption;* e.g., blood tests, transfusions of blood products, dental procedures, piercing of the ears, and tattooing. Note any unexplained puncture holes. Such breaks in the skin may be the cause of infectious hepatitis.

Finally, *environmental factors* may be linked with the patient's condition. Ask about swimming or accidental immersion in polluted water, travel in an area endemic for hepatitis or pancreatitis, eating of raw or steamed clams from polluted water, and contact with hepatitis-infected animals. In regard to any of the historical areas above, try to help the patient recall his or her experiences and the onset of symptoms in a *time sequence,* so that links between events and manifestations of disease can be made and used for diagnostic purposes.

MEDICAL ASSESSMENT

Physical Examination

Physical examination for the purpose of determining the presence of liver, biliary, or pancreatic disease involves exhaustive exploration of the entire body. In particular, *palpation of the abdomen,* especially the liver and spleen, is definitive. The pancreas is not palpable. Deep palpation is essential to evaluate *tenderness,* a common complaint with inflammatory processes of these organs. Since the peritoneum is often involved, the presence of localized peritoneal irritation is determined by rapidly removing the examining hand, which as a consequence rapidly jerks the peritoneum. If it is inflamed, pain is severe with this maneuver and *rebound tenderness* is thus established.

The liver edge is palpated in the right upper quadrant just below the ribs; inhalation and hand pressure over the posterior ribs bring the liver closer to the examiner's hand as he or she evaluates it for tenderness, size, presence of masses, and consistency (scarring or swelling). The spleen is palpated in the left upper quadrant just below the ribs; the same maneuvers as described with the liver bring it closer to the examiner's hand. (The physical examination is discussed in Chapter 15.) Enlargement of the spleen is common in cirrhosis as a result of congestion from portal hypertension.

In addition to palpation, comprehensive *inspection* is essential. Inspection of the abdomen reveals ascites (fluid-filled abdomen) and prominent venous collateral networks common to cirrhosis. Systemic signs such as jaundice, purpura, hair loss, weight loss, and enlarged breasts, spider angiomas, and reddened palms of cirrhosis are among a long list of manifestations to be seen.

Psychosocial Assessment

While taking the patient's history and performing the physical examination, remember to assess the individual's mental alertness and neurologic status. Note whether the patient appears to be confused, disoriented, very tired, etc. A poor self-image may be evident if the patient has a history of drug abuse or alcoholism. Recording a sample of the patient's handwriting for comparison later may be useful if progressive hepatocellular damage is suspected, handwriting steadily deteriorates as the condition worsens. (See also Chapter 14.)

Diagnostic Measures

There is no single laboratory test, radiographic study, or surgical procedure that will answer all the questions needed to aid or confirm the diagnosis and degree of malfunction of the liver, biliary tract, or pancreas. The diagnostic measures are useful to follow the course of the metabolic changes. Some of the tests indicate the presence of dysfunction, but frequently a number of measures are required to isolate the specific disease.

Ultrasound and Doppler techniques are newer noninvasive methods now being used to diagnose gallbladder disorders.

LABORATORY STUDIES

Common laboratory tests of liver, biliary, and pancreatic function are summarized in Table 67–1.

RADIOLOGIC TECHNIQUES

Cholecystogram (Gallbladder Series). This is a test for gallbladder disease done by visualizing the gallbladder. Telepaque or another organic iodine dye is given 12 hours before the test. Be sure to check whether the patient is allergic to iodine or seafood before giving the dye. The allergic effects of the dye may include nausea and vomiting, diarrhea, abdominal pain, and rash; anaphylaxis also is possible.

The patient is given a low-fat evening meal to avoid gallbladder contraction and is NPO or on fluid restriction in the morning. The bowel is cleansed with enemas, and sometimes a cathartic is given.

The dye is conjugated in the liver, excreted into bile as an opaque medium, and outlines the gallbladder. The test takes about an hour; sometimes a high-fat meal is given after the procedure to test gallbladder contraction. Gallbladder disease is indicated by poor or no visualization of the bladder, presumably because biliary obstruction prevents passage of the dye into the gallbladder. Occasionally, stones are visualized as shadows within the opaque medium. The test results are accurate only when gastrointestinal and liver function allows absorption and conjugation of the dye.

Cholangiogram. This procedure is used to visualize the bile ducts. Cholografin or another organic iodine dye is used, and again iodine allergies should be considered. Possible allergic reactions include dyspnea, tachycardia, sweating, nausea and vomiting, and chills. The dye burns intensely on injection. Prior fluid restriction is observed and the bowel is cleansed beforehand.

The dye usually is given intravenously but may be given through percutaneous puncture when obstructive jaundice prevents the flow of dye through the bile. Occasionally the dye is also introduced directly into the ducts during surgery, or into a T-tube postoperatively. Other than drug reactions, the main danger is from bleeding and bile peritonitis, which sometimes complicate percutaneous cholangiography.

Duct obstruction is directly visualized by the failure of the opaque dye to pass a certain point in the bile ducts.

Roentgenogram of Abdomen. Diaphragm elevation or distortion by hepatic enlargement

TABLE 67–1. LABORATORY TESTS OF LIVER, BILIARY, AND PANCREATIC FUNCTION

Measurement	Normal Value*	Procedure	Interpretation
1. Biliary excretion		Blood drawn without special patient preparation	Direct bilirubin increased with impaired biliary excretion, causing conjugated fraction to accumulate in plasma.
a. Serum bilirubin			Indirect bilirubin increased with increased erythrocyte hemolysis.
Direct (conjugated)	< 0.2 mg./100 ml.		Total bilirubin measures direct and indirect.
Indirect (not conjugated)	< 0.8 mg./100 ml.		
Total	< 1 mg./100 ml.		
b. Urine bilirubin	0	Simple urine collection (urine appears smoky or tea-colored)	Urine bilirubin measures conjugated bilirubin only and is increased with impaired bile excretion.
c. Urine urobilinogen	0–4 mg./24 hr.	24 hr. or 2 hr. afternoon collection placed in brown refrigerated bottle with sodium carbonate	Urine urobilinogen decreased with impaired bile excretion. Increased with erythrocyte hemolysis.
d. Fecal urobilinogen	40–280 mg./24 hr.	Entire stool to laboratory	Fecal urobilinogen decreased with impaired bile excretion; increased in erythrocyte hemolysis.
e. Serum cholesterol	150–250 mg./100 ml.	Blood drawn after low cholesterol diet for 12 hr.	Cholesterol elevated when excretion blocked by bile duct obstruction, but reduced when severe liver damage reduces ability to synthesize it.
2. Carbohydrate metabolism			Pancreatic digestive enzyme released with breakdown of acinar cells; serum elevations over 300 U. indicate pancreatitis; elevations not directly correlated with severity; urinary levels elevated longer (about 1 week); over 300 U./hr. indicates pancreatitis.
a. Serum amylase	80–160 U./100 ml.	Blood drawn without special patient preparation	
b. Urine amylase	< 260 U./hr.	2, 12, or 24 hr. urine collection with no preservative unless specified	
3. Protein metabolism			Less plasma proteins synthesized in liver damage; albumin synthesis consequently reduced, but increased serum gamma globulins produced by plasma cells.
a. Total protein	6–8 Gm./100 ml.	Blood drawn without special patient preparation	
b. Serum albumin	3.5–5.5 Gm./100 ml.	Same as above	
c. Serum globulin Include Alpha, Alpha$_2$, Beta, Gamma	2.5–3.5 Gm./100 ml.	Same as above	
d. A/G ratio	1.5:1–2.5:1	Same as above	A change in the ratio may indicate chronic hepatitis or other disease.
e. Blood ammonia	< 75 mcg./100 ml.	Blood drawn without special patient preparation	Reduced synthesis of urea from body ammonia in severe hepatocellular damage produces elevated blood ammonia.
f. Flocculation tests			
Cephalin	0 or 1+	Blood drawn without special patient preparation	Hepatocellular disease indicated when precipitation occurs in sera mixed with thymol or cephalin-cholesterol; alterations in serum protein fraction cause reaction. Not commonly used now.
Thymol turbidity	0–5 U.	Blood drawn on patient with fat restriction 12 hr. beforehand	

TABLE 67–1. LABORATORY TESTS OF LIVER, BILIARY, AND PANCREATIC FUNCTION *(Continued)*

Measurement	Normal Value*	Procedure	Interpretation
g. Serum methemalbumin	Absent	Fluid from peritoneal or pleural tap analyzed	Product of hemoglobin digestion elevated when blood released into body fluids, as in hemorrhagic pancreatitis.
4. Fat metabolism Serum lipase	<1.5 U.	Blood drawn on fasting patient	Pancreatic digestive enzyme released with breakdown of acinar cells.
5. Metabolism of foreign substances			
a. BSP excretion	<0.4 mg./100 ml. <5% retention in 1 hr.	Control blood taken from patient fasting for 12 hr.; Bromsulphalein given, blood drawn at 30 min. and 1 hour or once at 45 min.	Dye retained with diminished hepatocellular ability to remove it from the blood and excrete it. Observe patient carefully for reaction to dye.
b. Indocyanine green excretion	500–800 ml./sq. m. body surface/min.		
6. Serum enzymes			
a. SGOT b. SGPT c. LDH	5–40 U./ml. 5–35 U./ml. Varies with units used	Blood drawn without special patient preparation	Serum glutamic oxaloacetic transaminase, serum glutamic pyruvic transaminase, and lactic acid dehydrogenase released from damaged hepatic, heart, kidney, and muscle cells; levels not directly correlated with degree of damage; elevations above 400 U. accompany acute hepatocellular alteration.
d. Alkaline phosphatase (ALP)	Varies with method	Blood drawn without special patient preparation	Increase in biliary obstruction, probably due to continued hepatic production with excretion blocked. This enzyme is also found in bone, intestine, and placenta.
e. Serum 5′ nucleotidase	0.3–3.2 Bodansky units	Blood drawn without special patient preparation	Enzyme located mainly in liver and confirmation of liver disease occurs if ALP and this both elevated.
f. Serum gamma glutamyl transpeptidase (G6TP)	Varies	Blood drawn without special patient preparation	Enzyme located in liver and kidney. Elevation of G6TP and ALP significant of liver disorders.
7. Tests for Australia antigen including agar gel diffusion, counterelectrophoresis, complement fixation, passive hemagglutination, and radioimmunoassay	Negative	Blood drawn without special patient preparation	Multiple techniques identify Australia antigen (indicating viral hepatitis B (serum).
8. Tests for hemostatic function			
a. Clotting time	6–17 min.	Blood drawn without special patient preparation	Time is greater when there is profound decrease in clotting factors.
b. Partial thromboplastin time (PTT)	30–40 sec.	Blood drawn without special patient preparation	Longer if level of factors needed for intrinsic pathway is decreased (XII, XI, IX, VIII) or if heparin is present.

Table continued on the following page.

TABLE 67-1. LABORATORY TESTS OF LIVER, BILIARY, AND PANCREATIC FUNCTION (*Continued*)

Measurement	Normal Value	Procedure	Interpretation
c. Prothrombin time (PT)	11.5–12.5 sec. or 100%	Blood drawn without special patient preparation	Assesses function of extrinsic pathway in clotting process (Factors I, II, III, V, VII, X). When it reaches 50% there is danger of bleeding. PT prolonged with decreased synthesis owing to liver cell damage or decreased vitamin K absorption due to bile duct obstruction reducing bile in intestine. Vitamin K necessary for liver to synthesize prothrombin.
d. Platelets	150,000–300,000/ cu. mm.	Blood drawn without special patient preparation	May fall when spleen is enlarged in portal hypertension.

*Please refer to normal values used at your particular laboratory, since variance in equipment may yield slight numerical differences.

may be present. This study will also reveal the presence of calcium in the hepatocyte, biliary tree, or gallbladder.

Upper Gastrointestinal Series. This test may demonstrate varices of the esophagus if present; however, there is a 10 to 30 per cent failure rate with this method. Stomach displacement may occur in the presence of cirrhosis, abscess, or tumor.

The upper GI series is discussed in Chapter 59.

Angiography. This x-ray procedure allows visualization of the visceral vessels in order to identify abnormalities of vascular structure and function, to visualize masses, and to note sites of bleeding. Angiography is employed to study the pancreas, spleen, and portal system, recall that it is also used in disorders of the kidneys, lower extremities, and gastrointestinal tract. For injection of contrast media, the femoral artery is usually used for introduction of the needle. Then the needle is exchanged for a catheter, which is passed into the celiac artery or one of its branches (superior mesenteric or hepatic). The contrast media are injected, and rapid sequence films are taken. Following this procedure it is important to observe the needle *insertion point for signs of bleeding,* particularly because patients with liver conditions so often have concurrent clotting disorders.

Other Procedures Using Contrast Media. Procedures in which contrast media are injected into the portal and related vessels include: celiac angiography, hepatoportography, splenoportography, percutaneous splenoportography, portal portography, and umbilical venography. The pancreatic vessels are studied using pancreatic angiography. In all these procedures, Hypaque or another organic iodine dye is injected into a vessel, then flows to the vessels being studied and outlines them. The solution burns intensely for a few seconds after injection. Possible allergic reactions to iodine should be watched for, and the IV site should be observed for edema or thrombosis.

These procedures determine the patency of vessels supplying the organ in question, measure vessel pressures, and disclose the presence of lesions that may distort the vasculature. They are used in cirrhosis to detect esophageal varices.

Radioisotope Scanning of the Liver. This procedure involves the intravenous infusion of gamma-emitting isotopes. Then the area of the liver is scanned by passing a scintillation detector over the abdomen. This procedure is used to investigate liver structure and function (i.e., biliary duct patency). These gamma-emitting isotopes are concentrated in functional liver tissue, with lesions appearing as filling defects. (See Unit IX for details on radioisotope scanning.) The most common scan is the colloid scan, using colloidal gold or sulfur, which the Kupffer cells absorb. The hepatocytes are the major absorption sites of rose bengal, another scanning agent. Hepatomas or liver abscesses will take up less dye. A third agent, gallium, appears to concentrate in neoplastic and inflammatory cells.

Miscellaneous Diagnostic Procedures

MEASURES OF PORTAL PRESSURE AND FLOW

These are minor surgical procedures performed in the operating room or a special studies laboratory. They are often combined with the injection of contrast media and require standard pre- and post-operative care, with special observation of the incisional site for hematoma.

The principal procedures are transhepatic puncture, umbilical-portal or hepatic vein catheterization, and percutaneous splenic pulp manometry. In the last-mentioned procedure, a manometer is inserted into the spleen through a needle placed between two of the lower ribs. It is important that the patient does not breathe during needle insertion or passage. Careful observation for bleeding or pneumothorax is important afterward.

These procedures measure portal vein pressure and flow, indicate the severity of portal hypertension, and guide decisions as to appropriate treatment measures. The indirect calculation of sinusoid pressure helps to determine the location of obstruction and thus identify the underlying disorder.

ANALYSIS OF DIGESTIVE JUICES

Duodenal drainage is done through a nasogastric tube in a fasting patient. For a period of 1 to 6 hours the tube is left in the duodenum. Magnesium sulfate is inserted to stimulate bile flow and the secretions are aspirated. It may be followed by the *secretin test,* in which secretin is given intravenously, possibly followed by pancreozymin, and the secretions are again aspirated.

These procedures are currently reserved for patients allergic to iodine who cannot undergo cholecystography or cholangiography. Disproportions in the bile and pancreatic juice fractions indicate obstruction to ductal flow. The presence of cholesterol crystals indicates lithiasis. The secretions are analyzed for volume, bicarbonate, enzyme, and biliary content.

PERITONEOSCOPY

A peritoneoscope is inserted through an abdominal stab wound to permit direct visualization of the liver and peritoneum. Structural changes can be visualized, thus aiding in the diagnosis of cirrhosis or cancer.

Peritoneoscopy has become more refined over the years; celioscopy and laparoscopy are terms utilized in the past. Since the 1950s, scopes with increased optic quality have aided the refinement of this procedure. Photos and biopsy procedures are also done at the time of peritoneoscopy.

Peritoneoscopy is a relatively safe and simple procedure, with a 90 per cent accuracy. It aids in the diagnosis of metastatic cancer. *Contraindications* for this procedure are infections of the abdominal cavity, clotting disorders, intestinal obstruction, and an uncooperative patient. The test has limited results in ascitic or obese patients and in those who have had a previous cholecystectomy.

The necessary patient preparation for this test includes a signed permit, presence of adequate clotting factors, a patient who is NPO, pre-procedure medication if not contraindicated, a check for sensitivity to local anesthetics, empty bowel and bladder, skin prep, and adequate teaching. Explain to the patient that difficulty in breathing will occur when air is placed in the abdominal cavity. The patient should know how to elevate the anterior abdominal wall to protect the major organs during needle insertion. The procedure may take a half hour if biopsies, photos, or teaching is omitted. The patient is up after the medication effect passes unless a liver biopsy is done; then, 24 hours of bed rest are necessary.

Complications are not very common and more often occur if a liver biopsy is also done. The possible post-procedure complications are shown in the box below.

Post-Peritoneoscopy Complications

Pneumothorax
Subcutaneous emphysema
Air embolism
Bile peritonitis
Viscus perforation
Shoulder/abdominal pain

LIVER BIOPSY

Liver biopsy may be an open or closed procedure. An open liver biopsy necessitates a general anesthetic and a major abdominal incision. A person may have an open liver biopsy at the time of a concurrent procedure. The open biopsy procedure would be too drastic for a patient with an acute process or to follow the course of hepatocellular injury and regeneration.

Open Biopsy. A wedge of liver is removed for study and the remaining edges are sutured together. An advantage of this type of procedure is that visualization of the entire liver allows the biopsy specimen to be removed from the grossly altered tissue area.

Needle Biopsy. Generally, a person is kept fasting the night prior to a needle liver biopsy, in case of hemorrhage and a possible need for surgery to control it. Local anesthesia is used. The person needs to hold his or her breath while the biopsy is done to avoid puncture of the diaphragm. The person is supine or in the right lateral position with the right arm elevated.

Vital signs must be taken every hour for the first 8 to 12 post-biopsy hours. The patient should remain on bedrest for 24 hours. Pre- and post-medications depend on the patient's physical state. Vitamin K is given if necessary. Maintenance of a right lateral position is recommended for about one hour post-procedure.

Contraindications are: an uncooperative person, prothrombin time less than 50 per cent or 3 seconds above control, thrombocytopenia less than 80,000 to 100,000 per mm., local infection of lung base or peritonitis, ascites (intensive) and extrahepatic obstructive jaundice, especially with an enlarged gallbladder. The person with cancer or amyloidosis has an increased risk of post-procedure hemorrhage.

Some typical *reactions* and *complications* the nurse might expect the patient to experience are: pain, hemorrhage, bile peritonitis, ascites into the pleural space, pneumothorax (mild), and shock. The pain may occur in the right hypochondrium owing to a subcapsular accumulation of blood or bile, or at the right shoulder as a result of blood on the undersurface of the diaphragm. Hemorrhage will usually occur within the first 24 hours. The risk is increased when vascular channels are distended or when the patient breathes during needle insertion in the liver. Bile peritonitis is treated with surgical decompression.

PARACENTESIS

Paracentesis or peritoneal tap is performed to analyze fluid accumulations in the peritoneum (ascites). It is usually done at the bedside; the nurse is actively involved in care. The patient is instructed and must give written permission beforehand. To avoid puncture of the bladder, he or she must void immediately prior to the procedure. The patient is then positioned sitting upright on the edge of the bed with feet resting on a stool and back well supported. Following cleansing of the skin and infiltration with local anesthetic, a trocar is inserted aseptically through a small stab wound below the umbilicus and fluid slowly drained through a catheter into a collection bottle.

Many complications threaten with paracentesis. The greatest danger is hypovolemia as circulatory fluid is rapidly altered due to the pressure changes. Vital signs and peripheral circulation are noted frequently during and following the procedure. Other manifestations of reduced systemic circulation, renal failure, and hepatic coma due to reduced tissue perfusion should be anticipated. Because of the high protein concentration of ascitic fluid, salt-poor albumin is often infused over the 24-hour period following the procedure. Infection (peritonitis) and bleeding due to trauma of vessels are occasional complications; complaints of abdominal pain must be carefully assessed.

NURSING ASSESSMENT

Nursing assessment of these patients focuses particularly on gathering complete data on nutrition and elimination, fluid balance and circulation, skin, and comfort status. In conditions associated with alcohol or drug abuse, sensitive psychosocial and environmental assessment is vital. Affording the individual a sense of self-worth and understanding during repeated laboratory, x-ray, and other diagnostic procedures is extremely important, both to gain the person's cooperation and to reduce fear, which frequently accompanies these experiences. Since many tests are performed to document the specific pathology that is occurring, astute observation for mental or physical changes during the process is important. Ongoing evaluation of the status of problems may lead to an ever-changing diagnosis.

CHAPTER 68

DISORDERS OF THE LIVER

HEPATITIS

Simply stated, hepatitis means *inflammation of the liver.* It may be caused by a virus, bacteria, or a toxic substance. *Jaundice* usually occurs, and the liver is tender. Other systemic manifestations occur, but their presence depends on the type of causative agent and the degree of disruption. Hepatitis occurs worldwide.

There are several types of hepatitis. These include viral hepatitis, toxic hepatitis, hepatitis that is a complication of other viral and bacterial illnesses, chronic active hepatitis, and alcoholic hepatitis. We consider each of these forms in this chapter.

Viral Hepatitis

Types of Viral Hepatitis. There are two major types of viral hepatitis: hepatitis A and hepatitis B. The organisms responsible for these conditions are different and discrete viruses, but they both cause inflammation of the liver and other sequelae that are similar. They differ in their incubation periods, major methods of spread, and severity of resultant disease process.

HEPATITIS A. Hepatitis A is *endemic* in some areas of the world, especially those with poor sanitation. But *epidemics* do occur in countries with good sanitation. Epidemics are due to infected water, milk, or food, especially raw shellfish. In the civilian population the *group* most at risk is under 15 years of age and of both sexes. The *incidence* is fairly constant throughout the year.

Hepatitis A has an *incubation period* of about 15 to 45 days. The *fecal-oral route* is the major path of transmission. Type A hepatitis has a low mortality rate: about 2 per 1000 cases. *Immune serum globulin,* if given early, can prevent hepatitis or decrease the severity of symptoms. The person with hepatitis A is a virus carrier through the preicteric stage. The person is thought to be free of virus within seven to nine days after jaundice occurs. Schiff reports a few cases that were thought to be transmitted in nasopharyngeal secretions.[88]

This condition spreads from person to person by close contact. *The carrier is most infectious just before the onset of symptoms.* This places the remaining household members at risk because the first person can be transmitting the virus before precautions can be started. Secondary infections tend to occur in household members about every 20 to 30 days. If this problem spreads in an institution it may take months to control it.

People who work with animals imported from areas where hepatitis A is high are at increased risk, as are individuals who eat raw or steamed shellfish. People who are otherwise healthy usually recover from hepatitis A without major sequela.

New methods and techniques are playing a role in the *identification process* of hepatitis A antigen and antibody. Current information suggests that hepatitis A is an RNA virus of the enterovirus family. Old nomenclature still appears now and again. The previous terms for hepatitis are short incubation, infectious, and MS_1 hepatitis.

HEPATITIS B. Hepatitis B is found *worldwide,* even in remote areas. Its *incidence* increases in areas of high population density and poor hygiene. The major sources of this infection are healthy carriers and people with the acute process.

Hepatitis B has an *incubation period* of 28 to 160 days. Contact with the *serum of an infected person* was thought to be the major source of transmission. While hepatitis is mainly transmitted via the blood, current evidence supports the fact that hepatitis B can be transmitted by semen and respiratory secretions. Health care workers are at high risk for hepatitis B because of their close contact with the blood of carriers. Patients who have multiple transfusions or dialysis are also at high risk.

Hepatitis B antigen has been the focus of intensive study since Blumberg's work with the Australia antigen in 1965. Today, the Dane particle, or hepatitis core antigen, and the surface antigen from the spherical coat and their respective antibodies are detectable. Table 68–1 presents the tests used to detect the presence of HB surface antigen and its antibody.

Tests have also detected the presence of HB_e Ag, anti HB_e, and anti HB_c in the serum of some patients. The persistence of HB_e antigen

TABLE 68–1. TESTS USED TO DETECT THE PRESENCE OF HB_sAg AND ANTI-HB_s

Test	HB_sAg (surface antigen)	Anti-HB_s (antibodies to surface antigens)
Agar gel diffusion AGD	Sensitive	No
Counterelectrophoresis CEP	Sensitive	No
Complement fixation CF	Sensitive	No
Radioimmunoassay* RIA	Very sensitive	Sensitive
Reversed passive hemagglutination RPHA	Very sensitive	
Passive hemagglutination PHA		Very sensitive
Double antibody radio-immunoprecipitation		Very sensitive

*This test is the most sensitive and is preferred when establishing presence of HB_sAg.

in the serum of a patient with HB is highly associated with the development of chronic persistent or chronic active hepatitis.

Pathology of Viral Hepatitis. The physical signs and symptoms that the person with hepatitis experiences are reflections of *cellular damage in the liver.* The hepatocyte has alterations in function resulting from damage caused by the virus and the resultant inflammatory response. The endoplasmic reticulum is the first organelle to undergo change. Since this organelle is responsible for protein and steroid synthesis, glucuronide conjugation, and detoxification, functions that depend on these processes will be altered. The degree of impairment depends on the amount of hepatocellular damage. The mitochondria sustain damage later than the endoplasmic reticulum. The Kupffer cells increase in size and number. The vascular and ductule tissues experience inflammatory changes. In most cases of uncomplicated hepatitis the reticulum framework is not in danger, and excellent healing of the hepatocytes occurs in three to four months.

Clinical Features. Hepatitis A and B have similar clinical courses. The person is not sick immediately after being infected, and the onset of symptoms will vary according to the incubation periods and the degree of infectivity. In *anicteric hepatitis* the person suffers symptoms of hepatitis and has altered laboratory tests but *no jaundice.* This state may precede jaundice or jaundice may never occur. Usually the person notices darker urine and clay-colored stools a few days prior to clinical jaundice. The signs and symptoms, other than jaundice, are systemic and vary from person to person. These might include lethargy, irritability, myalgia, anorexia, nausea, vomiting, abdominal pain, diarrhea or constipation, fever, and other "flulike symptoms." The jaundice is first seen in the eyes and mucous membranes. The symptoms sometimes abate when jaundice is present but at times the symptoms become worse. *Pruritus (itching)* is usually transient and mild and may be more intense at its onset and exit. The jaundice usually starts to disappear in two weeks in children and in four to six weeks in adults. *The return of normal stool color is an indication of resolution.*

If *irritability* and *drowsiness* become severe, the possibility of *hepatic coma* may need to be evaluated. *Asterixis* may also be present if coma is impending. *Mild depression* is not uncommon owing to the nature of the illness (weakness, jaundice, itching, nausea), length of the illness, cost of the illness, and confinement.

Anemia may occur as a result of the decreased life span of the RBC's. This is a result of liver enzyme alterations. A *transient hyperglycemia* may occur, and a diabetic person may need increased levels of insulin at this time. The liver is larger than normal and tender on palpation. Some people will develop spider angioma, palmar erythema, and gynecomastia, which disappear during the recovery period. A small percentage (5 to 15 per cent) of people will experience splenomegaly or enlargement of the posterior cervical lymph nodes.

Major manifestations and their bases are summarized in Table 68–2.

Laboratory Findings. The *serum transaminases* are the first to elevate, and they begin to fall as the bilirubin starts to increase. Jaundice occurs as bilirubin begins to rise above 2.5 mg. per 100 ml. If the bilirubin rises above 20 mg. per 100 ml. and remains elevated for a long period, the possibility of severe liver necrosis with a poor prognosis is probable. Mild prolongation of the prothrombin time may occur. Some people have mild steatorrhea, hypoglycemia from decreased glycogen or decreased oral intake, mild hematuria, and proteinuria. The gamma globulin fraction and alkaline phosphatase elevate in some people. If hepatitis B is responsible, detection of HB_sAg is possible even before the SGOT rises.

VIRAL HEPATITIS VARIANTS

These include the following:

- *Cholestatic viral hepatitis:* In this variant the disease process resembles *mechanical obstruction.* The period of jaundice is longer and the itching is more intense. The serum bilirubin reaches levels of 10 to 15 mg. per 100 ml. The "flulike" and gastrointestinal problems are usually present and similar to hepatitis A or B. Elevations of serum lipoproteins, globulins, cholesterol, and alkaline phosphatase are common. Progressive liver enlargement rarely occurs.

- *Chronic persistent hepatitis:* Clinically, about two thirds of the people with chronic persistent hepatitis manifest the symptoms that are associated with acute viral hepatitis at the onset. Their recurrent episodes are not acute in nature, and extrahepatic involvement rarely occurs. The presence of fibrosis in the liver and the progression to cirrhosis is infrequent.
- *Fulminant viral hepatitis:* This *life-threatening* form of viral hepatitis resembles acute liver failure with signs and symptoms of encephalopathy (increased excitability, irritability, insomnia, somnolence, and impaired mentation). The liver rapidly decreases in size. Laboratory data show a decreased serum aminotransferase and a prolonged prothrombin time. Gastrointestinal bleeding and disseminated intravascular coagulation may be a problem. Fever with leukocytosis and neutrophilia is present. Hepatorenal problems of oliguria and azotemia occur, as do edema and ascites. The person has a low serum bicarbonate value and hyperventilates as a result of the acidosis of hepatic coma. The prognosis is poor and death may occur before the appearance of jaundice.
- *Confluent hepatic necrosis:* This entity also appears under the title of subacute or submassive hepatic necrosis. It occurs more commonly in women over 40 years. Diagnosis depends on the location and degree of hepatocellular necrosis on liver biopsy. The preicteric phase is longer than usual, with greater levels of anorexia, malaise, lassitude, and debilitation. Sometimes ascites is the first overt sign. The spleen enlarges also.

  The laboratory data reflect a decreasing serum albumin and rising gamma globulin, normal or elevated alkaline phosphatase, positive LE, RH, or Wasserman antibody, and fluctuating serum aminotransferase levels.

Treatment for Viral Hepatitis. *Bed rest with bathroom privileges* is usually recommended during the acute phase. The laboratory data are not always valid indicators of the patient's degree of illness or recovery, and it is difficult on the basis of these data to set the time period for bed rest. Often the person who is very ill with hepatitis finds little difficulty adhering to bed rest requirements, but as improvement occurs, confinement to bed may be difficult. Experience demonstrates that most people who feel capable of being up and around can do so without harm if they rest after meals and do not engage in any activity to the point of being overly tired. Since prolonged bed rest in itself can lead to weakness, it is likely that a *reasonable activity level* is more conducive to recovery.

Diet should be considered according to the person's state. Adequate *calories* should be supplied in the daily diet or by intravenous methods. Hard candy, juice, and carbonated drinks can be helpful in supplying calories. *Fat intake as tolerated* is the rule. Fat metabolism alterations will differ according to the degree of interruption in bile production and excretion. *Protein intake* should also be based on the person's condition. If the person has no problems with protein metabolism, a normal intake is helpful for tissue repair. *Vitamin K supplements* are advisable if prothrombin time is longer than normal. The use of *alcohol* is generally to be

TABLE 68–2. MAJOR SIGNS AND SYMPTOMS OF HEPATITIS AND THEIR BASES

Signs and Symptoms	Bases
Jaundice, clay stools (no pigment), darkened urine (bilirubin and urobilinogen)	Impaired excretion of conjugated bilirubin into intestine results in elevated serum levels, staining of skin (jaundice), reduced bile pigment in feces, high levels of conjugated bilirubin excreted into the kidneys, and elevated urinary urobilinogen, because small amount of urobilinogen still produced in intestine and reabsorbed into blood is excreted through kidneys instead of liver
Pruritus	Bile salt accumulation in skin
Abdominal pain in right upper quadrant	Stretching of Glisson's capsule due to swelling of inflamed liver
Fever	Release of pyrogens in inflammatory process
Fatigue and weakness	Reduced energy metabolism by liver
Anorexia, nausea, vomiting	Possibly visceral reflexes reduce peristalsis. Postulated changes in stomach or bowel
Bleeding tendencies in severe cases	Reduced prothrombin synthesis by injured hepatic cell. Reduced fat-soluble vitamin K absorption due to reduced bile in intestine
Anemia	Decreased red blood cell life due to liver enzyme alterations; bleeding and hemorrhage in severe cases

avoided, since it appears to interfere with recovery. The biochemical aspects of alcohol use and hepatitis are unknown at present.

Drug therapy for viral hepatitis is not extensive. Antibiotics are not helpful. Immune serum globulin is not helpful in the treatment of viral hepatitis but its use for a family member is recommended. Antiemetics, such as the phenothiazines, can be helpful in the management of nausea and vomiting.

The *corticosteroids* are not very helpful in uncomplicated cases of acute viral hepatitis. However, they are useful in severe cases and in women over 45. Corticosteroids may decrease the serum aminotransferases and bilirubin levels but they have no effect on liver necrosis or regeneration.

Estrogens are known to raise the serum bilirubin levels; therefore, the use of oral contraceptives during acute viral hepatitis needs to be evaluated. The American Medical Association states that they should be avoided. The World Health Organization and a Swiss study disagree, however.

People with severe *cholestasis* and resultant pruritus can obtain relief by the administration of cholestyramine. This drug acts by binding bile salts.

Reduction of fat intake will also be helpful during this period.

All in all, *drug therapy for persons with hepatitis is reduced to a minimum.* Those drugs known to be toxic to the liver are eliminated. Sedatives and hypnotics are used with caution.

Sequelae of Viral Hepatitis. A *relapse* may occur after the following: ambulation too early in the treatment process, excessive physical activity, alcohol consumption, illicit self-injection, and use of corticosteroid therapy during the acute phase. *Hyperbilirubinemia* that does not interfere with a normal life may occur for months or years after viral hepatitis. *Jaundice* usually follows a period of exertion, and the serum levels rise 4 to 5 mg. per 100 ml. *Chronic active hepatitis* (which will be discussed later) is more common after hepatitis B and predisposes to liver destruction. *Cirrhosis* may follow a severe case of hepatitis B or chronic active hepatitis. Hepatoma occurs in higher frequency when hepatitis B and cirrhosis are present.

Prognosis. Typically, most patients with viral hepatitis completely recover from the illness in 3 to 16 weeks. Overall mortality is less than 1 per cent. However, there is possibly a higher mortality rate among older people—particularly post-menopausal women.[52]

Prevention. To a great extent viral hepatitis can be prevented by means of proper controls within the home, community, and hospital setting. Let us first consider the prevention of hepatitis A.

Because *hepatitis A* transmission is by the oral-fecal route, *good personal hygiene is very important.* Handwashing, especially by food handlers, is essential. In institutions where the disease is present as a result of an inability of the residents to care for themselves properly, supervised handwashing is recommended.

Treatment of *municipal water supplies* is sufficient to prevent transmission of hepatitis virus A, but private water supplies may be sources of contamination. Polluted fishing waters pose a threat. Shellfish that come from these waters could be a major source of hepatitis A. Therefore, local governments play a large role in infection control. The local health authorities also play a role in the *monitoring of eating establishments.* Because the disease can be transmitted when handling food, a person with hepatitis A should not work in food services while he or she is a carrier of the virus.

The incidence of hepatitis A among *people who work with animals* can be reduced by isolating newly imported animals for a two month period. If this is not possible, protective clothing and good handwashing are essential. If the risk of contamination is high, the prophylactic use of immune serum globulin would be a helpful preventive measure.

Passive immunization for hepatitis A in the form of immune serum globulin is possible. Pain, tenderness, and at times hematomas are adverse effects of intramuscular injection. Immune serum globulin is helpful in prophylaxis both before and after exposure. People who are going to visit or live in areas of high risk for hepatitis A can benefit from immune serum administration, but the exact length of protection is unknown at present. The *earlier* in the incubation period that the prophylactic immune serum is given, the greater is the protection.

Turning next to prevention of *hepatitis B,* remember that hepatitis B is mainly in the serum of the infected person. *Therefore blood, blood products, or instruments that pierce the skin and contact the vascular system are all potential sources of contamination.* Some donor-related precautions that would help decrease the incidence of hepatitis B are screening of donors' blood for hepatitis B surface antigen, use of volunteer donors, registration of carriers, and the sharing of accurate records between institutions. It is possible to reduce the transfusion recipient's exposure to hepatitis B by using blood products only when necessary, by cross-checking laboratory data to reduce errors of reported results, and if blood products are needed, to use only the amount necessary.

In addition, many health care institutions use *disposable equipment,* especially needles and syringes, in an attempt to reduce hepatitis transmission. Nondisposable equipment must be *sterilized* to prevent virus transmission.

Toxic Hepatitis

Toxic hepatitis occurs after exposure to certain substances. These *hepatotoxins* cause liver alterations by initiating either a sensitivity response or a toxic response. *Drugs* are usually the causative agents in the *sensitivity responses,* and *industrial chemicals* are usually the causative agents in *toxic* problems, but the categories are not mutually exclusive.

In hepatitis following *toxic exposure* to a hepatotoxin, a specific pattern of liver tissue damage always develops in both animals and people. Furthermore the greater the degree of exposure, the greater the damage. Conversely, hepatitis following a *sensitivity reaction* does *not* exhibit a consistent pattern of liver damage, does not seem to be related to the amount of exposure to the hepatotoxin, and does not appear to affect all persons and animals in a consistent manner.

The exact *mechanisms* that cause the pathogenesis for both toxic and sensitivity reactions are not clearly understood. In *toxic* problems, the hepatocyte and its subcellular structures undergo changes. The questions that need further research relate to (a) the exact agent responsible for alterations (the toxin or its metabolite), (b) the injury process itself (altered blood flows, tissue swelling, disturbances in protein or lipid metabolism of the hepatocyte) and (c) the role of nutrition (starvation, high fat intake, alcohol) in protecting the liver from damage. In *sensitivity* reactions either a cholestatic type of hepatitis with bile stasis and portal inflammation develops, or hepatitis similar to an acute viral process but with more hepatocellular damage occurs. In people at risk for sensitivity reactions, a genetically determined factor is thought to play a role in pathogenesis.

Liver necrosis occurs within two or three days of acute exposure to a *toxic* substance, but two to five weeks may pass before signs and symptoms of *sensitivity* reactions appear. People with either process manifest abnormal liver function tests. Persons who are repeatedly exposed to *toxic* agents in minimal amounts over long periods of time may develop cirrhosis. Individuals experiencing a sensitivity reaction may demonstrate eosinophilia, fever, arthralgia, and sometimes xanthomatosis (an excessive accumulation of lipids brought about by faulty lipid metabolism).

Treatment consists of removing the causative agent, bed rest, supportive care of side effects (e.g., cholestyramine for pruritus), 3000 calorie diet, fats if tolerated, high protein intake if no evidence of impending hepatic coma, and steroids for sensitivity reactions. Should renal failure appear, appropriate measures must be taken. (See Chapter 43.)

Hepatitis as a Complication of Various Other Viral and Bacterial Illnesses

Hepatitis may follow or be a part of the disease process of many viral and bacterial agents. Table 68–3 identifies the more common agents. The exact mechanisms of pathogenesis are unknown at present. The organism may cause alterations by direct liver invasion, by production of toxins harmful to the hepatocyte, or by reactivation of old disease in the liver. Yellow fever and infectious mononucleosis are two rather common pathologic agents that deserve special mention.

Yellow fever is a disease with flulike symptoms, jaundice, and hemorrhagic sequelae, which follows a short incubation period of three to six days. There are two types of yellow fever: the *jungle* variety and the *urban* form. Both are spread by the *Aedes* mosquito. They are group B arboviruses. Laboratory values are typical for hepatitis, and fatty degeneration of the liver occurs. Treatment involves supportive care, and prevention is possible with inoculation.

Infectious mononucleosis has an incubation period of four to seven weeks, and close physical contact, especially oral, is the method of spread. All youngsters are at risk, but the majority of cases occur in the 15 to 25 year age group. The affected person exhibits jaundice (11%), hepatomegaly (17%), splenomegaly (75%), a positive heterophile, lymphocytosis, lymphadenopathy, and exudative pharyngitis. Treatment is supportive, and low dose steroids may be used. Avoidance of a common drinking utensil will help to reduce spread. (See Chapter 46.)

TABLE 68–3. VIRAL OR BACTERIAL AGENTS RELATED TO HEPATITIS

Pneumococcus	Tuberculosis
Staphylococcus	Adenovirus
Streptococcus	Coxsackie virus
Clostridia	Cytomegalic inclusion disease
Gonococcus	
Escherichia coli	Echovirus
Salmonella	Herpesvirus
Typhoid	Infectious mononucleosis
Shigella	Marburg virus
Brucellosis	Psittacosis
Granuloma inguinale	Reovirus
Tularemia	Rubella
	Varicella

Chronic Active Hepatitis

This form of hepatitis leads to hepatic inflammation, hepatic necrosis, and progressive fibrosis. Cirrhosis usually occurs with this variant. In addition to the signs and symptoms of chronic liver disease, seroimmunologic alterations and extrahepatic abnormalities are characteristics of chronic active hepatitis. These associated problems are often the source of the variety of names in use to describe this entity.

Both *chemical* and *viral* agents are causes of chronic active hepatitis. Hepatitis B in a persistent form, and cytomegalovirus infections during immunosuppressed states are common viral causative agents. Alpha-methyldopa, Isoniazid, and oxyphenisatin are drugs that may cause this entity. Altered immune systems in individuals afflicted with this variant are also under investigation.

The clinical features and laboratory findings are not always consistent from patient to patient, and the data may resemble those found in some aspects of chronic persistent hepatitis and biliary cirrhosis. Therefore, liver biopsy is necessary to establish the diagnosis. Women and young adults experience this entity more commonly than others, and the onset is usually slow. Others report the symptoms of acute viral hepatitis, cirrhosis, or extrahepatic problems at the onset. The person may have periods of remission from symptoms but liver necrosis continues.

People who do not seek treatment suffer a high mortality rate, which results from hepatic failure, bleeding varices, hepatic coma, and hepatoma. *Medical treatment* is the administration of *steroids* for a period of one year even though the laboratory values and clinical features resemble normal values much earlier. In some patients who cannot tolerate high doses of steroids, azathioprine and lower steroid doses may be helpful. In addition to drug therapy, general supportive care and bedrest during the active phase are the major methods of treating this process. Treatment in the acute care setting is mainly for liver biopsy and the identification of extrahepatic sequelae.

The laboratory values return to normal within weeks or months following the administration of steroid therapy, while the symptoms of fatigue and anorexia resolve in a few days or weeks. Drug reduction in slow increments is wise, not only to prevent a relapse but also to allow the adrenals time to regain their full level of secretion.

Alcoholic Hepatitis

Alcoholic hepatitis may be either an acute or a chronic inflammation of the liver caused by parenchymal necrosis resulting from alcohol abuse. Although it is sometimes reversible, this condition is the most frequent *cause of cirrhosis.* This fact is important because cirrhosis of the liver is a common cause of death among adults in the United States. The exact incidence of alcoholic hepatitis among alcoholics is unknown, but it is believed to develop in about one third of all chronic heavy drinkers. Women appear to be particularly susceptible.

Symptoms of alcoholic hepatitis usually develop following a recent bout of heavy drinking. Manifestations include anorexia, nausea, abdominal pain, splenomegaly, hepatomegaly, jaundice, ascites, fever, and encephalopathy. The *laboratory* studies typically show anemia, leukocytosis, and an elevated serum bilirubin. Diagnosis of alcoholic hepatitis is confirmed by *liver biopsy.*

Treatment includes a high vitamin, high carbohydrate diet, folic acid supplements, and the administration of parenteral fluids. Steroids may sometimes have a beneficial effect, although their use is controversial.

Hepatitis due to excessive alcohol intake has a poor prognosis, particularly if the individual cannot abstain from drinking or increases his or her use of alcohol. Even if these patients recover from an acute attack of alcoholic hepatitis, they have a 10 times greater mortality rate (over a three year period) than do individuals in the general population.

General Nursing Care for Patients with Hepatitis

The nursing care needs of the person with hepatitis will vary with the type of hepatitis, the degree of affliction, and the presence of other concurrent health problems. Other than those differences related to the route of infection, the nursing care of the person with uncomplicated viral or chemical hepatitis is similar to that of the patient with hepatitis A or B.

The person needs *adequate rest.* Most people with hepatitis experience the greatest amount of fatigue during the anicteric phase and begin to feel stronger during the icteric phase. During the period of severe fatigue, bed rest is necessary. Activities of daily living, such as bathroom privileges, personal hygiene, and feeding, are encouraged unless they cause excessive fatigue. The person should continue to plan rest periods, especially after meals, during the period of jaundice. If excessive activity occurs too early in the recovery phase, a relapse is possible. In very severe cases of hepatitis, in which prolonged bed rest is necessary, the nurse needs to institute measures to prevent the complications of prolonged immobility.

Nutrition may be a problem because of anorexia, nausea, bile stasis, and altered absorption and metabolism of ingested foods. A diet high in protein (75 to 100 Gm.) and carbohydrates

(300 to 400 Gm.) and moderate in fat (100 to 150 Gm.) is optimum to allow recovery of injured liver cells. The amounts of protein and fat need to be decreased only if there is a problem in their digestion and metabolism. People with very severe hepatitis who are in danger of hepatic coma should be on a diet low in proteins. A diet of 2500 to 3000 calories is difficult for a person with anorexia; therefore, multiple small feedings may be helpful. Vitamin supplements are not generally necessary in uncomplicated hepatitis if an adequate diet is tolerated. Severe nausea and vomiting may occur in some individuals, and antiemetics are helpful, but be sure to know how such drugs might affect liver function.

The person with hepatitis may need to express his or her feelings about being ill, about the length and cost of the illness, about the alterations in family life (mother of young children, sole breadwinner), or about the effect on future health problems or maybe death for someone with a severe process.

Patients with severe jaundice may suffer with *pruritus.* Nursing measures to deal with itching are on page 1744 (Chapter 79).

Teaching needs for people with hepatitis will vary with the causative agent. In addition to knowing how to prevent a recurrence and spread, the person will need to return to former activity levels slowly in order to avoid a relapse.

FATTY LIVER

Lipid infiltration is one of the more common types of metabolic disease of the liver. These infiltrations cause decreased liver function, liver enlargement, and increased liver firmness. which might progress to portal hypertension. Liver biopsy is necessary to establish a definite diagnosis.

Chronic alcoholism, protein malnutrition in the early life cycle, diabetes mellitus, obesity, Cushing's syndrome (natural or induced), jejunoileal bypass, prolonged intravenous hyperalimentation, chronic illnesses interfering with normal cell nutrition, and some hepatotoxins (CCl_4, DDT) are the common *causes* of lipid infiltrations. Triglyceride is the major lipid found at biopsy but small amounts of cholesterol and phospholipid are also present.

Symptoms in people with moderate to severe amounts of lipid infiltration are infrequent, but people with massive infiltrations complain of anorexia and abdominal pain. Jaundice may also occur. *Laboratory studies* demonstrate BSP retention and elevated serum alkaline phosphatase and bilirubin levels.

Recovery occurs after restoration of metabolic balance and adequate nutrition. Residual damage, if it occurs, usually follows persistent fatty infiltration and chronic alcoholism. *Fat embolization* is a potential problem and may be responsible for mortality.

Nursing care needs for people with fatty infiltration of the liver are related to use of observational skills and emotional support (allowing verbalization of concerns and fears, preparation for diagnostic procedures), supportive physical care, proper administration of therapeutic regimens, and health teaching related to prevention of a recurrence.

CIRRHOSIS

Cirrhosis of the liver occurs when the regeneration of new hepatocytes, bile ductules, vascular channels, and reticulin substance alters the normal flow of blood, bile, and hepatic metabolites. Any chemical or organism that causes liver destruction and irregular patchy regeneration will predispose to cirrhosis. The more common variations of cirrhosis are Laennec's (alcoholic), post-necrotic (post-hepatitis or toxin induced), biliary, and cardiac. The major clinical problem in cirrhosis, besides that of decreased liver function, is the presence of *portal hypertension,* which develops in severe cirrhosis. This increase of pressure in the portal vein, which receives blood from the intestines and spleen, allows (a) reverse flow of blood and enlargement of the esophageal, umbilical, and rectal veins, (b) formation of ascites, and (c) incomplete clearing of metabolic wastes.

Laennec's Cirrhosis

Laennec's cirrhosis is most commonly found in chronic alcoholics but it is also found in people who don't abuse alcohol. The exact quantity of alcohol that causes the diffuse scarring of Laennec's cirrhosis is currently unknown. Also, the factors of faulty nutrition, individual response to trauma, concurrent infectious agents, metabolic defects, and length of excessive intake all need further study and evaluation before their role in the development of cirrhosis is understood.

Pathology

Cirrhosis is the final stage of many types of liver injury. The cirrhotic liver varies in appearance, but a nodular consistency with bands of fibrosis (scar tissue) and small areas of regen-

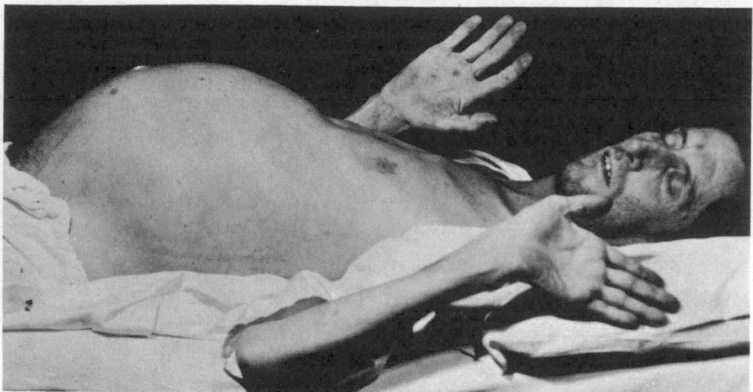

Figure 68–1. Wasting in cirrhosis of the liver (From Delp, M. H., and R. T Manning: *Major's Physical Diagnosis.* 8th ed , Philadelphia: W. B. Saunders Co., 1975.)

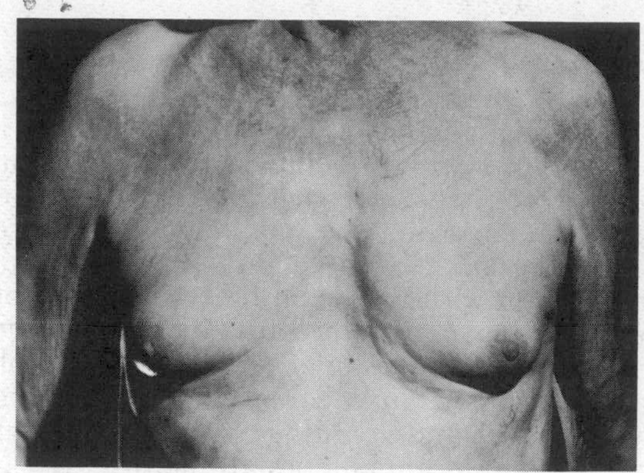

Figure 68–2. Gynecomastia in a patient with cirrhosis. (From Delp, M. H., and R. T. Manning: *Major's Physical Diagnosis,* 8th ed., Philadelphia, W. B. Saunders Co., 1975.)

erating tissue is prominent. Stasis of bile, precipitating jaundice, may occur at periods of acute exacerbations.

Bases of Symptoms

Common manifestations of advanced cirrhosis and their pathophysiologic explanation are identified in Table 68–4.

The wasting, gynecomastia, and edema of the legs seen in severe cirrhosis are illustrated in Figures 68–1, 68–2, and 68–3. Manifestations of cirrhosis will diminish if the process is arrested in an early stage. Continued progression of the process from unknown causes or from alcohol abuse usually results in death from hepatic coma, bacteria (gram negative), peritonitis (bacterial), hepatoma, or complications of portal hypertension.

Diagnosis

The patient with cirrhosis often presents with critical problems such as ascites, gastrointestinal bleeding, or encephalopathy. The disease often progresses quietly until such an emergency occurs. Hepatomegaly (enlarged liver), splenomegaly (enlarged spleen), vascular changes, or abnormal laboratory tests may be the first indicator in the patient who is seen for another problem. The patient may also be seen for hepatitis or other disabling disorders.

Inspection and interview reveal the presence of at least several of the symptoms listed above. Palpation reveals a firm (scarred), lumpy (nodular), usually enlarged liver. Splenomegaly may be present if portal hypertension is severe. Identification of ascites, bleeding with esophageal varices, and hepatic encephalopathy is discussed in Chapter 66. Laboratory tests indicate impaired hepatocellular function: elevated serum enzymes (SGOT, SGPT, LDH), abnormal flocculation tests, reduced BSP dye excretion, hypoalbuminemia, and elevated prothrombin time. Anemia, leukopenia, or thrombocytopenia may be a result of splenomegaly. *Liver biopsy* is considered essential to definitive diagnosis of cirrhosis and its follow-up.

Clinical Intervention

Two goals guide treatment of the patient with cirrhosis:

1. *Maximize liver function.* Though cirrhosis is a progressive degenerative disorder, certain actions will at least minimize trauma and maximize regeneration. Thereby, the course of the illness can possibly be slowed and life prolonged. *Diet* should provide ample protein to rebuild tissue, at least 75 to 100 Gm./day. Enough carbohydrate must be given to sustain weight

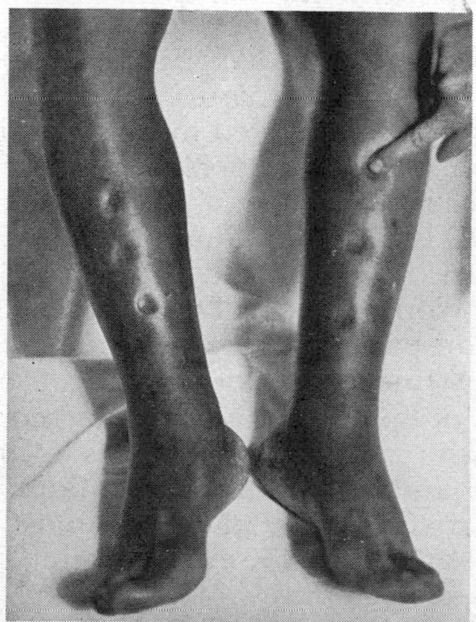

Figure 68–3. Edema of legs in cirrhosis of the liver. (From Delp, M. H., and R. T Manning: *Major's Physical Diagnosis,* 8th ed., Philadelphia, W. B. Saunders Co., 1975.)

TABLE 68–4. SIGNS AND SYMPTOMS OF CIRRHOSIS

Signs and Symptoms	Bases
Emaciation, ascites (Chapter 66)	Malnutrition; portal hypertension hypoalbuminemia, and hyperaldosteronism
Lower leg edema	Hypoalbuminemia, hyperaldosteronism, and pressure of massive ascites obstructing venous return from legs
Prominent abdominal wall veins	Collateral vessels bypass scarred liver to carry portal blood to vena cava
Esophageal varices (Chapter 66)	Collateral veins in esophagus bypass scarred liver to carry portal blood to superior vena cava. Portal hypertension causes dilatation
Hemorrhoids	Internal hemorrhoidal veins dilate with pressure of portal hypertension
Palmar erythema, amenorrhea, atrophy of testicles, enlarged breasts, parotid hypertrophy, spiders (vascular lesions resembling small spiders)	Probable abnormal hormone metabolism in liver, resulting in manifestations of estrogen excess, androgen deficit
Bleeding tendency, especially gastrointestinal (Chapter 66)	Hypoprothrombinemia, thrombocytopenia; portal hypertension and esophageal varices; peptic ulcers common in alcoholics
Anemia	Gastrointestinal blood losses; erythrocyte destruction by pooling in enlarged spleen; folic acid deficiency due to dietary inadequacy
Renal failure	Rapidly failing hepatic function; occasionally precipitated by volume depletions[2]
Infections	Leukopenia due to enlarged overactive spleen. Hypoproteinemia; bacteria in portal blood bypass liver so not removed by Kupffer's cells
Encephalopathy and coma (Chapter 66)	Ammonia, no longer removed by liver, accumulates to levels toxic to brain
Initial or recurrent symptoms of hepatitis	Chronic viral, toxic, or alcoholic hepatitis progressing to cirrhosis may have inflammatory exacerbations

and spare use of protein for energy. Fat restriction is no longer considered necessary. Total calories should range between 2000 and 3000 daily. If the patient has ascites or edema, sodium must be restricted and possibly fluids. Small frequent meals will expedite consumption of sufficient quantities in an anorexic patient. A maintenance multivitamin preparation is usually prescribed, and therapeutic levels are given in severe malnutrition. Vitamins A, D, E, and K are given in cases of fat malabsorption. Severe malabsorption may necessitate intravenous vitamins with calcium gluconate supplemented.

> Intake of all hepatotoxins must be eliminated. *The alcoholic must stop drinking completely or the condition will worsen and progress to a terminal stage.*

All known hepatotoxic drugs must be removed from therapeutic regimens, and the drug abuser must understand that certain drugs may further damage the liver. Dosages of all drugs thought to be metabolized by the liver must be lowered. Sedatives and opiates are avoided.

Infection must be prevented by adequate rest, diet, and environmental control. Prior to antibiotics, infection was the major cause of cirrhosis mortality. *Rest* is often prescribed for the cirrhotic, but the amount is debatable. During periods of acute malfunction, rest will reduce metabolic demands on the liver and increase circulation. Long-term planning should include counseling the patient to rest frequently and to avoid unnecessary fatigue. In postnecrotic and posthepatic cirrhosis, *corticosteroids* may be given to reduce manifestations and improve liver function.

2. *Control disabling symptoms.* Ascites, bleeding esophageal varices, and hepatic encephalopathy progressing to coma are discussed in depth in Chapter 66. These three are the most feared complications of cirrhosis and frequently the cause of death. Renal failure and infection can also be mortal complications. See Unit XIII for identification and care of the person in renal failure.

Nursing Care Needs. Nursing care needs of these patients, while hospitalized, can be guided by the laboratory data. The degree of anemia, leukopenia, and thrombocytopenia reported can be used to determine the patient's (a) *activity level* and (b) need for *oxygen, protective isolation, and protection from trauma,* which can cause bleeding. (See Unit XIV for care of patients with blood dyscrasias.) Remember that bleeding in liver disorders can also occur from a deficiency of other blood-clotting factors. Serum protein studies usually reflect an increase in globulins and a decrease in albumin. This reversal of protein composition may lead to edema, and the person will thus require *special care to prevent skin breakdown.* Skin problems may also develop as a result of elevated bilirubin levels, which can cause itching and scratching. (See p. 1744 for *treatment of pruritus.*) The person's serum glucose levels may be elevated as a result of faulty utilization of insulin; therefore, carefully *observe intake and output* to prevent dehydration. (See Chapter 72, on serum glucose.) Also note and *report signs of electrolyte imbalance.* (See Chapter 12.) For example, high urinary loss may decrease serum potassium. Magnesium might also be decreased as a result of increased urinary output and poor nutritional intake. Sodium imbalance may result from secondary hyperaldosteronism associated with ascites and edema. Bromsulphalein (BSP) retention, elevated alkaline phosphatase and transaminase levels, and increased serum ammonia not only indicate impairment of hepatic function but also may forewarn the nurse that the patient's mentation and judgment will deteriorate. At this stage in their illness, patients need to be protected from falling out of bed, wandering off the ward, etc.

The patient and significant others need *information and teaching* in preparation for care at home. Current statistics indicate a five year survival for 60 per cent of these people if they abstain from alcohol and eat properly. The survival rates decrease when alcohol consumption continues or when variceal hemorrhage develops.

The family must learn about the signs of impending hepatic coma and how to cope with them. This information is presented on p. 1486. The family group may also need some professional counseling services to assist them with their interpersonal relationships.

Other Types of Cirrhosis

Postnecrotic cirrhosis, biliary cirrhosis, and cardiac cirrhosis are presented and compared in Table 68–5. The nursing care needs are similar to those for Laennec's cirrhosis.

TABLE 68–5. COMPARISON OF POSTNECROTIC CIRRHOSIS, BILIARY CIRRHOSIS, AND CARDIAC CIRRHOSIS

Definition	Etiology	Pathology	Clinical Features	Diagnosis and Prognosis	Treatment
Postnecrotic —Most common worldwide form —Massive loss of liver cells, with irregular patterns of regenerating cells	Post-acute viral (type B) hepatitis Post-intoxications with industrial chemicals Some infections and metabolic disorders	Liver small and nodular	Similar to Laennec's except less muscle wasting and more problems of jaundice Serum transaminases —Any gammaglobulins —Elevations occur	Needle biopsy of liver establishes pathology Within 5 years 75% of this group die of complications	Treat complications as needed
Biliary Bile flow is decreased with concurrent cell damage to hepatocytes around bile ductules	1. *Primary* —Chronic stasis of bile in intrahepatic ducts —Cause unknown —Immune process suspected 2. *Secondary* Occurs after obstruction of bile ducts outside of the liver	Early stage biopsy reveals inflammatory process with necrosis of cells in ductule areas —Hepatocytes are lost and scar tissue remains —End stage similar to postnecrotic	—Generalized itching —Dark urine —Pale stools —Jaundice —Impaired bile flow steatorrhea ↓ absorption of fat soluble vitamins —Elevated serum lipids —↑ Cholesterol becomes deposited in subcutaneous tissues —Signs of portal hypertension	—Elevated serum bilirubin levels Early: 3–10 mg./100 ml. Late: ↑ 50 mg./100 ml. —High elevations of alkaline phosphatase —Increase in gamma globulins —Increase in blood lipids —Presence of lipoprotein X —↑ Serum bile salts —Hypoprothrombinemia —Positive mitochondrial antibody test for primary cases —↑ Serum copper in primary cases	Relief of mechanical obstruction is primary choice for secondary biliary cirrhosis Primary biliary relief is treated symptomatically, e.g., —High caloric diet; lower fat 30–40 gm./day if a problem —Cholestyramine for itching —Supplement of fat soluble vitamins
Cardiac cirrhosis Chronic liver disease associated with severe right sided, long-term congestive heart failure Fairly rare	1. Atrioventricular valve disease 2. Prolonged constrictive pericarditis 3. Decompensated cor pulmonale	*Early* Dark colored liver enlarged by blood and edema fluid *Late* Liver capsule thickens and modular scarring occurs in the centrilobular areas	Slight jaundice enlarged liver, ascites, in person with severe cardiac impairment over a ten year span —RUQ pain during acute congestion —Cachexia —Fluid retention —Circulatory problems	—↑ Conjugated bilirubin in serum —↑ BSP —↓ Albumin in serum —↑ Transaminase values —↑ Alkaline phosphatase —Liver biopsy	Treatment of cause for chronic congestive failure if possible

PORTAL HYPERTENSION*

Definition, Etiology, and Pathophysiology

Recall from Chapter 65 that normal blood flow to and from the liver depends upon the proper function of the portal vein (70 per cent of inflow), the hepatic artery (30 per cent of inflow), and the hepatic vein. Disease processes that damage or alter the flow of blood through the liver or its major vessels are responsible for the development of portal hypertension. Table 68–6 identifies other factors that may cause portal hypertension. The majority of cases of portal hypertension in the United States are related to *cirrhosis*. The next most common cause is *obstruction of the portal vein by a thrombus or tumor*. The remaining cases result from obstruction of *hepatic vein outflow*. The amount of liver dysfunction will vary with the initial process, the length of the process, and individual differences.

Normal portal pressure is 5 to 10 mm. Hg. Portal hypertension exists when the *pressures rise above 25 mm. Hg and collaterals form as a result of poor blood flow through major venous channels*. The spleen and other organs that empty into the portal system also begin to undergo the effects of congestion. Eventually, clinical manifestations arise.

TABLE 68–6. FACTORS IN THE PATHOGENESIS OF PORTAL HYPERTENSION

I Increased vascular resistance
- *A* Intrahepatic
  - *1* Cirrhosis
  - *2* Infiltrations (e.g., tumors, sarcoidosis)
  - *3* Polycystic disease
  - *4* Schistosomiasis
  - *5* Noncirrhotic portal fibrosis (hepatic phlebosclerosis)
- *B* Portal vein
  - *1* Thrombosis
  - *2* Tumor
  - *3* Infection (pylephlebitis)
- *C* Hepatic veins
  - *1* Thrombosis (Budd-Chiari syndrome)
  - 2 Veno-occlusive disease

II Sustained high splanchnic inflow
- *A* Splenomegaly
- *B* Diffuse AV shunts(?)
- *C* Major AV fistulas

III Inadequate decompression via venous collaterals
- *A* Esophageal
- *B* Retroperitoneal
- *C* Periumbilical
- *D* Hemorrhoidal

From LaMont, J. T., and K. J. Isselbacher: Cirrhosis. *In* Thorn, G. W., et al. (Eds.): *Harrison's Principles of Internal Medicine,* 8th ed., New York: McGraw-Hill Book Company, 1977, p. 1611.

Clinical Manifestations

Observable manifestations of portal hypertension include the following:

- ► Slightly tortuous epigastric vessels that come off the area of the umbilicus and lead toward the sternum and ribs. This manifestation is termed a *caput medusae*.
- ► An enlarged, palpable spleen.
- ► Hemorrhoids.
- ► Blood in the stool.
- ► Bruits, which may be heard over the area of the upper abdomen.
- ► Ascites, which typically appears when there is concurrent liver disease.

Complications

The major life-threatening complication that accompanies portal hypertension is *hemorrhage*. As portal pressures rise, the rectal veins, abdominal wall veins, and esophagogastric veins attempt to lower portal pressure and become dilated and distended. The exact mechanism that precipitates the actual bleeding is unknown. Veins of the stomach and esophagus are the most subject to rupture.

Other problems involve the *spleen*. The splenic vein merges with the superior mesenteric vein to form the portal vein. When pressure increases in the portal system, the spleen is damaged. The damage to the spleen is not proportional to the amount of portal pressure increase. As the spleen enlarges, it tends to *destroy blood cells,* especially the platelets, which then increases the risk of hemorrhage and anemia.

A third complication of portal hypertension is *hepatic encephalopathy,* which can progress to *coma*. This problem usually arises following a period of internal bleeding. Because blood is a protein substance, its digestion in the intestines increases ammonia in the gut and blood stream, which then disturbs brain function. Hepatic coma is discussed in Chapter 66.

Diagnosis

Direct measurement of portal pressure is only possible at laparotomy; therefore, liver scans, splenoportography, and/or abdominal angiography must be relied upon to establish the

*Portal hypertension is also discussed in Chapter 66.

diagnosis. Liver biopsy and other laboratory data are also helpful. Variceal hemorrhage must be established by radiography and/or endoscopy procedures. This is because these patients may be bleeding from other gastrointestinal areas (e.g., duodenal ulcer).

Medical Treatment

In Chapter 66, we discussed in detail the medical measures used to control bleeding due to portal hypertension and reduction in clotting factors. To quickly review, these measures include: (a) transfusions of whole blood to replace blood losses and losses of clotting factors, (b) vasopressin infusions, which cause vasoconstriction and thus help control bleeding; (c) balloon tamponade (e.g., Sengstaken-Blakemore tube), which exerts pressure against the bleeding points; and (d) gastric cooling. Recall that when these measures fail or if the possibility for further hemorrhage is high, surgical treatment is considered.

Surgical Treatment

Varied operative approaches have been employed to stop or prevent bleeding from varices associated with portal hypertension. *Ligation of the esophageal and gastric veins* is the most direct approach to the problem, while shunting blood from the portal vein or one of its contributing vessels to the systemic circulation (usually the inferior vena cava) is an indirect approach. Variceal ligation usually stops acute bleeding. However, because variceal ligation does nothing to reduce portal pressure, bleeding may recur.

Early shunting procedures to reduce portal hypertension were performed in the mid-1940's. These early approaches to the problem attempted to decrease portal hypertension by diverting the portal vein into the inferior vena cava. The main disadvantage of this procedure was that portal inflow was nonexistent. The liver was deprived of about 70 per cent of its blood supply, and toxic metabolic wastes, especially ammonia, were delivered directly into the systemic veins. As a result the post-shunt person was at risk for episodes of hepatic encephalopathy. Various arteriolization procedures have been tried in attempts to preserve post-shunt liver function by trying to increase the blood supply to the liver. These attempts were not the answer. Bleeding from the gastrointestinal tract in sites other than the variceal areas occurred more frequently following the shunt. Also if ascites was a pre-shunt problem, it was not always relieved after the procedure.

Modifications of this shunt attempt to reduce portal pressure, preserve adequate liver function, and avoid or decrease the complications of encephalopathy and gastrointestinal bleeding. In hopes of maintaining adequate liver perfusion, a side-to-side anastomosis between the portal vein and vena cava was developed to decrease pressure and still allow some flow of blood to the liver. Unfortunately in a large number of instances, the portal vein became an outflow system for the diseased liver after shunting. Thus, other procedures, such as splenorenal shunts, portorenal shunts, and mesocaval shunts, were developed to reduce pressure more distal to the liver and thereby preserve adequate liver perfusion. However, the major problem in creating shunts in vessels that are smaller than the portal vein is the danger of *thrombosis.* If the thrombus is large enough to close the shunt, portal decompression is lost. Figure 68–4 illustrates varieties of portal decompression procedures. Table 68–7 summarizes the advantages and disadvantages of the different types of shunts in common use.

Other factors that are important in shunt choice relate to the patient's physical condition, anatomic structure, whether or not there is fibrosis from previous surgeries, and the surgeon's choice. At the present time a number of institutions use *Child's Classification* for assistance in patient selection (see Table 68–8). Patients are assigned to one of three groups based on five criteria. Those in group A are in a good state of nutrition, without ascites or neurologic disorders, serum bilirubin is below 2 mg. and serum albumin is above 3.5 Gm. This group tolerates the procedure best. Patients in group C are poor operative risks.

The perfect procedure for portal hypertension has not yet been developed. This factor, plus the patient's poor state of health in the majority of cases, leads to high post-shunting mortality. Currently, studies are being done to evaluate shunt surgery and its implications for the future.

Nursing Care

The nursing needs for the person with portal hypertension will depend upon the overall state of health and the presence or absence of a shunt. Besides routine care of the person, the nurse must observe for hemorrhage, encephalopathy, and complications of splenomegaly. If the individual is to be *discharged without surgery,* then the patient and at least one family member

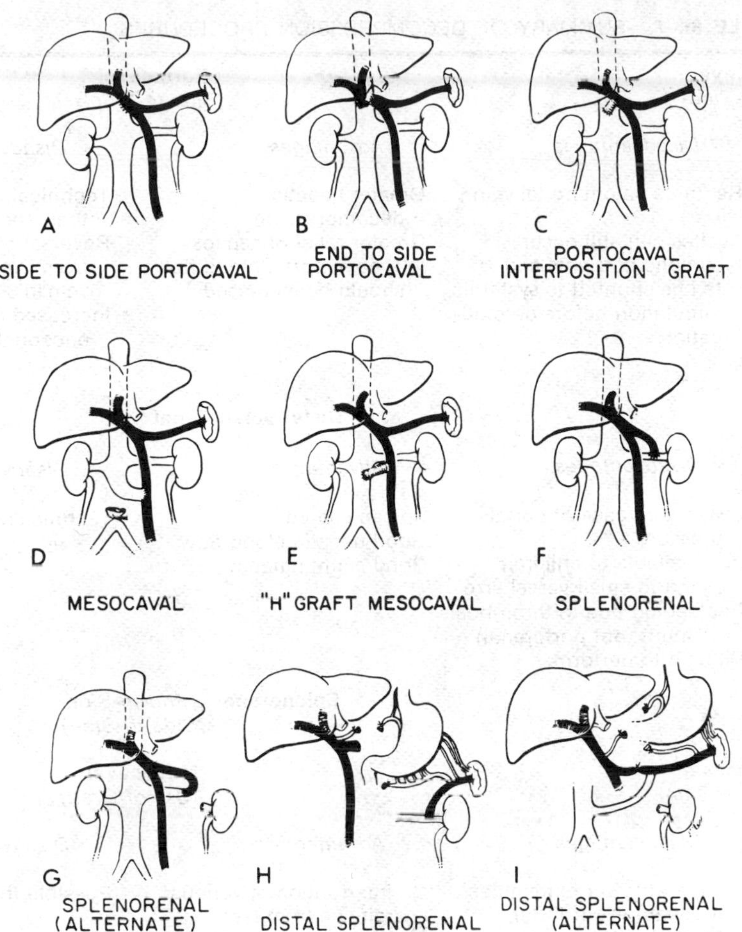

Figure 68–4. Varieties of portal decompression procedures. (From Altshuler, A., and D. Hilden: The patient with portal hypertension. *Nursing Clinics of North America*, 12:317, June 1977.)

should be taught how to observe for the above complications. The importance of adequate follow-up care cannot be overemphasized. In addition, the person may need dietary instruction regarding sodium intake and medication precautions for diuretics if ascites is a problem.

When a *shunt* is performed, the patient will need careful postoperative observation of his or her respiratory and circulatory functions. The disease process and the increased systemic blood flow after the shunt procedure predispose the person to greater stress on these systems. If the patient has very poor liver function, postsurgery clotting may be a problem. Associated damage to the spleen and platelets compounds the situation. Often platelets and fresh frozen plasma are given intraoperatively and postoperatively to aid clotting.

At the time of discharge, the patient and significant others should know how to recognize the complications of encephalopathy, gastrointestinal bleeding, and drug therapy. They should also know what to do if these conditions arise. If the portal hypertension and resultant surgery are a result of alcohol abuse, plans must be made to help the patient quit drinking.

When an *emergency shunt* is performed for severe hemorrhage, the patient and family have little time for preoperative teaching. They need calm interventions and specific instructions relating to present needs. The postoperative care for the emergency patient requires specific communications to assist the patient and significant others to understand the care during this period.

At times, judgmental feelings, statements, and actions may arise from both family and staff, especially if the current situation is precipitated by alcohol abuse. People often forget that alcoholism is a disease and needs treatment. Health team members and family members may also become frustrated with the patient's slow

TABLE 68–7. SUMMARY OF DECOMPRESSION PROCEDURES

Portacaval *(End-to-Side)*		**Portacaval** *(Side-to-Side)*	
Advantages	*Disadvantages*	*Advantages*	*Disadvantages*
Technically easiest	Requires patent portal vein	Greater hepatic decompression	Technically more difficult than end-to-side
Thrombosis rare	Ascites can still occur	Greater relief of ascites	Reversal of blood flow from liver via portal vein in 60–85%
Excellent decompression	Metabolic nutrients and toxins shunted to systemic circulation before detoxification	In theory, portal blood flow should be increased	Increased evidence of encephalopathy
Decreased recurrence of bleeding			
Some decrease in splenomegaly			

Portorenal		**Distal Splenorenal**	
Advantages	*Disadvantages*	*Advantages*	*Disadvantages*
Eliminates hypersplenism	Lesser decrease of portal pressure	Spleen spared	Technically difficult
Maintains some portal blood flow	Not available to children, owing to small vessel size	Good hepatic blood flow	
Decreases encephalopathy	Rebleeding due to thrombosis of shunt (not portorenal)	Good shunt patency	
	Difficult to perform		

		Splenorenal *(End-to-Side, Side-to-Side)*	
Mesocaval *(End-to-Side)*		**Mesocaval** *(Use of Graft)*	
Advantages	*Disadvantages*	*Advantages*	*Disadvantages*
Useful for patients with extrahepatic block where portal and splenic vein is unavailable	Edema of lower extremities if collaterals of lower trunk don't develop	No interruption of venous drainage from legs	Possible thrombosis
Maintains hepatic blood flow		Maintains hepatic blood flow	
		Technically easier	

From Altshuler, A., and D. Hilden: The patient with portal hypertension. *Nursing Clinics of North America,* 12:317, June 1977, p. 323.

recovery or continued drinking after much investment of time, care, supplies, and money. Family and staff may be able to resolve some of these conflicts or they may need the assistance of a resource person.

LIVER NEOPLASMS

Tumors of the liver may be primary or metastatic in origin. *Primary* liver tumors may arise from the hepatocytes, the bile ducts, the connective tissue, or the blood vessels. These tumors may be benign or malignant. A classification of primary liver neoplasms is presented in Table 68–9.

Metastatic tumors arise from the gastrointestinal tract (particularly the colon), the breasts, and the lungs.

Types of Primary Liver Neoplasms

Adenomas. Adenomas are *benign hepatic cell tumors.* The incidence of this type of tumor appears to be increasing. In 1973, Baum[9] re-

TABLE 68–8. CHILD'S CLASSIFICATION FOR PATIENT SELECTION FOR SHUNTING

	Group A	Group B	Group C
Serum bilirubin (mg./100 ml.)	Below 2.0	2.0–3.0	3.0
Serum albumin (Gm./100 ml.)	Over 3.5	3.0–3.5	3.0
Ascites	None	Easily controlled	Poorly controlled
Neurologic disorder	None	Minimal	Advanced coma
Nutrition	Excellent	Good	Poor, "wasting"

From Altshuler, A., and D. Hilden: The patient with portal hypertension. *Nursing Clinics of North America.* 12:317, June 1977, p. 324.

TABLE 68-9. CLASSIFICATION OF PRIMARY LIVER NEOPLASMS

Origin	Benign	Malignant
Hepatic cell	Adenoma	Hepatocellular carcinoma
Connective tissue	Fibroma	Sarcoma
Blood vessels	Hemangioma	Hemangioendothelioma
Bile ducts	Cholangioma	Carcinoma

From Swenson, S.: Benign and malignant liver neoplasms. *Hospital Medicine.* 14:71, May 1978. p. 71. © 1978 by Hospital Publications, Inc.

ported on seven women who had been on *oral contraceptives* and who consequently developed adenomas. This figure is high when compared with a study of 200 autopsies over a 10-year period by Berkheiser.[10a] His review discovered only one case. Studies were initiated to detect the role of different oral contraceptive agents in producing adenomas. Edmondson and his group[26a] reported a higher percentage of adenomas following the taking of mestranol preparations than following the taking of ethinyl estradiol products. Their study also computed the mean usage rate prior to tumor development, it was 73 months. Another interesting finding was the possible relationship between the onset of menstruation and tumor rupture in some women.

Ameriks and associates[3] explored the three modes by which these adenomas were discovered. First, according to their findings, the tumor was found by women or their physicians during a routine visit. These women had not experienced abnormal liver function and reported no symptoms. The second group of women reported right upper quadrant pain of intermittent nature with various amounts of nausea, anorexia, vomiting, and weight loss. This group often received the diagnosis of cholecystitis.

The final group had a mortality figure that resulted from tumor rupture and hemorrhage. This study demonstrates that even though these tumors are classed as benign, they are nevertheless dangerous because of their vascularity. *Hepatic arteriography* is a valuable early diagnostic test for this condition. Liver biopsy is considered dangerous because of the problem of possible hemorrhage. The results of other liver function tests are usually normal in this disorder.

Treatment for benign adenomas depends upon the individual patient. It might consist of *withdrawal of contraceptive drugs* for someone with a tumor that appears to be hormone dependent. Otherwise, *tumor excision* of the involved liver segment is suggested. If acute hemorrhage precipitates surgery, a *hepatic lobectomy* may be necessary. Rudolph[83] suggests that, because the number of current cases of hepatic adenoma is small at the present time, discontinuation of oral contraceptive agents is not necessary. However, women and physicians need to be informed of the potential hazards of these agents.

Malignant Hepatocellular Carcinoma or Hepatoma. This tumor is reported to have greater incidence among men. Alpert and Isselbacher[1] report the following etiological factors that are thought to contribute to hepatomas: hepatitis B, chronic liver disease, hemochromatosis, certain mycotoxins (aflatoxins), and long-term androgen therapy. These substances have also been implicated by different researchers in multiple areas of the world. For example researchers in Africa and Asia have reported a large incidence of hepatomas that may be related to the high incidence of mycotoxins and hepatitis B in those countries. Rudolph[83] reports that in some cases tumors that were associated with androgen therapy have undergone spontaneous regression once hormonal therapy was discontinued.

Angiosarcoma. Angiosarcoma is a relatively rare but fatal tumor of the liver. Recent studies reported by Rudolph[83] link this tumor with persons who have been exposed to vinyl chloride over long periods. This product is extensively used in the furniture and plastics industries. Other chemicals also implicated in Rudolph's report are certain inorganic arsenic products and thorium oxide, or Thorotrast (a radiopaque dye).

Metastatic Tumors

Metastatic tumors are more common than primary tumors in the United States. The liver is at great risk for metastatic tumors, owing to its high rate of blood flow, to its size, and to its portal drainage input from the major abdominal organs. Melanomas and tumors of the gastrointestinal tract, lung, and breast cause greater liver metastases than do tumors of the prostate, skin, or thyroid. These secondary forms of cancer spread to the liver by: (a) direct extension from adjacent organs (stomach, gallbladder); (b) the hepatic arterial system; and (c) the portal venous system. Also, the surface of the liver may be seeded with metastatic cells as a result of peritoneal migration.

Unfortunately, these metastatic tumors may be far advanced before clinical manifestations or laboratory findings indicate their presence. For this reason, the patient's prognosis is almost always poor, and treatment with radiotherapy and chemotherapy is palliative at best.

Clinical Features of Liver Neoplasms

People with primary (benign and malignant) and secondary (metastatic) tumors often present with *similar* signs and symptoms. Early indicators of liver neoplasm are usually vague. The person may complain of right upper quadrant distress and tenderness, nausea, and minor temperature elevation. Medical studies might reveal the presence of hepatomegaly, liver mass, blood-tinged ascites, positive angiographies, decreased liver function, elevated alkaline phosphatase, and a friction rub or bruit over the liver.

In primary hepatocellular cancers the presence of high levels of *alpha-fetoprotein (AFP)* (500–1000 ng./ml.) is fairly common. This substance is sometimes present in people who have metastatic tumors, but the levels rarely match primary tumor levels.

Some patients may also develop metabolic derangements such as polycythemia, blood sugar disorders, and high levels of calcium. Other patients may present with leukocytosis and anemia. Jaundice is more common when the bile ducts are the primary site or the tumor mass obstructs a major outflow duct. Still other signs and symptoms may be present but they vary according to the concurrent pathology. At times, the tumor process may cause elevation of the diaphragm and some respiratory problems.

Although neoplasms of the liver create numerous clinical manifestations, it is important to remember that these manifestations may not occur until the tumors have grown quite large. As Swenson[98] points out: "Symptoms of liver insufficiency may not become evident until up to 90 per cent of normal liver is replaced by tumor cells."

Diagnostic Procedures

Liver biopsy is very helpful in diagnosis. It may be done percutaneously, directly via laparotomy, or by peritoneoscopy. Each method has limitations. *Percutaneous procedures* may cause seeding of tumor cells along the exit pathway. *Laparotomy* may be too dangerous, owing to a need for anesthesia. *Peritoneoscopy* may be impossible if extensive adhesions are present. All of these procedures require membrane puncture; therefore, be sure the person has an acceptable prothrombin time.

Clinical Management

For tumors that are small and confined to one liver segment or lobe, *resection of the segment or lobe* may be possible if the patient is able to withstand the stress of surgery. *Regional perfusion* of the liver via the *hepatic artery* is helpful for pain relief and/or slowing the growth of the tumor. In metastatic growths, *systemic chemotherapy* may be used to reduce tumor size and pain. Post-treatment levels of alpha-fetoprotein in people with primary tumors are monitored to assess progress.

Dearterialization of the liver by ligation or occlusion decreases oxygen supply to the liver; as a result, tumor cells undergo a reduction in number and activity. Although the portal vein carries a sufficient oxygen supply to nourish the hepatocytes, the person must be carefully observed for signs of liver failure. *Chemotherapy* by direct perfusion or systemic infusion may be used with dearterialization.

Liver transplantation for liver tumors has not been successful at this time, owing to tumor recurrence and post-implantation metastases, as well as problems with rejection.

Prognosis

Following the diagnosis of cancer of the liver, the median survival time of patients is four to six months. The administration of systemic chemotherapy may extend the patient's life to six to eight months. When either regional chemotherapy or hepatic dearterialization is employed, survival time increases to 12 to 14 months. Hepatic resection, when feasible, increases life expectancy to 24 months. However, when these various measures fail to terminate the tumor process, the patient usually dies of hepatic failure within months.

Nursing Care

The physiological needs of the patient with liver neoplasms vary according to the amount of liver dysfunction. The nurse will need to assess the client for metabolic malfunctions, bleeding problems, ascites, edema, hypoproteinemia, jaundice, endocrine complications, and inability to detoxify endogenous and exogenous (drug) wastes. The person who is in the diagnostic stages needs adequate preparation for these procedures and careful post-procedure assessment for complications. (See individual diagnostic procedures for more detailed information.)

Psychological care of the person with a terminal process needs to be initiated. Both the patient and significant others need adequate information, time to integrate the information, and the emotional support necessary to cope with terminal illness. The nurse does not have to be the sole provider of support, but he or she should be able to assist the family to identify their best sources of assistance.

If the terminally ill person is going to spend time at home during the last stages, the family will need sufficient knowledge to recognize the problems and complications that require rehospitalization. They will also need information related to drug therapy and availability of nursing services and support for home-care patients.

LIVER INJURIES

Liver injury usually occurs as a result of a penetrating injury or blunt trauma. Both of these injuries may lead to *laceration* and *hemorrhage.*

Penetrating injuries are usually knife or missile wounds (pistol or rifle). A knife wound generally is superficial and leaves a sharp clear edge, while missile wounds cause perforations through the liver tissue (entrance and exit points). The higher the velocity of the missile, the greater the damage. Often, a close range missile injury is fatal because of the large amount of damage.

Blunt trauma (e.g., steering wheel, fall) can have various effects, from small hematomas that remain under the liver capsule to large starlike lacerations from severe impact forces. The major immediate problem after injury is the treatment of *hemorrhage.* The problem is more difficult if the liver's blood vessels or bile ducts are also damaged. Problems that may occur later are *bile peritonitis* and *abscess formation.*

Treatment of liver injuries consists of hemorrhage control, debridement, and drainage. Liver lobes may be removed if necessary, but more often control of hemorrhage is the major consideration. A late problem is hemorrhage after a hepatic segment sloughs as a result of a damaged blood supply. Pulmonary infections and abscess formation are also common postoperative problems.

LIVER ABSCESS

Liver abscess usually develops after one of the following conditions: (a) *bacterial cholangitis,* which results from obstruction of the bile ducts by stone or strictures, or (b) *portal vein bacteremia,* which may develop following bowel inflammation or organ perforation.

The patient commonly reports of right-sided abdominal and right shoulder pain. Liver enlargement, tenderness, nausea, vomiting, weight loss, fever, and sweating are also common. The person's laboratory data will reflect high levels of transaminase, alkaline phosphatase, and bilirubin if a concurrent obstruction is present, otherwise these levels will be slightly elevated. A positive blood culture may be found in some cases. A serum albumin value that is below 2 Gm. per 100 ml. indicates a poor chance for recovery.

Liver scans are extremely valuable in diagnosis. *Ultrasound* and *arteriography* may also be used, especially if the scan's results need further clarification. At times, a right pleural effusion may be present. The liver's close relation to the base of the right lung contributes to this process.

Treatment for hepatic abscesses is either *surgical drainage* of large abscesses with postoperative antibiotic therapy or *antibiotic therapy* for a few months. Any concurrent problem predisposing the person to abscess also needs attention. These patients are very ill, and mortality figures for liver abscess remain in the range of 30 to 50 per cent.

Abscesses due to *amebic infestation (Entamoeba histolytica)* are similar to other liver abscesses. The major difference in treatment is the use of *metronidazole (Flagyl)* or *chloroquine phosphate (Aralen)* instead of the broad-spectrum antibiotics. *Proper disposal of feces* to prevent transmission of this organism is also important.

Nursing care for the person with liver abscess involves careful assessment of *vital signs* because of the danger of general sepsis with a resultant high temperature, pulse, etc. Good *respiratory care* is imperative to prevent or limit pulmonary complications related to hepatic abscess. All the body processes that depend on an adequately functioning liver need to be evaluated (clotting; metabolism of CHO, fats, proteins; detoxification processes; albumin production; etc.) If the patient has hyperpyrexia, *increased fluid intake* and *skin care* are important.

The person's significant others need to be aware of the seriousness of the patient's condition. A supportive environment, which allows close associates to express their fears and concerns, is important.

HEMOCHROMATOSIS

Hemochromatosis is a disorder of *iron metabolism,* but since it is often associated with portal hypertension and causes hepatomegaly, we include it with liver disorders. This process, which is relatively rare, affects men more than women. Two current theories of *causation* are that hemosiderosis (a) results from an *inborn error of metabolism* and/or (b) develops as a *variant of portal hypertension.* A high percentage of people with hemochromatosis manifest concurrent *alcoholism* problems. The exact relationship is unknown at present, but some wines do have a high iron content.

Total body iron in most people ranges from 3 to 5 Gm. People with hemochromatosis often have levels of 20 Gm. or higher. The excess iron travels to parenchymal cells and is deposited as *ferritin* or *hemosiderin.* The *liver* and *pancreas* are most at risk. The heart, spleen, kidney, and skin are damaged to a lesser degree. Fibrosis begins to occur in these organs, and their ability to function is lost. Therefore, the more common problems associated with hemochromatosis are *diabetes, enlarged liver, cardiac disease,* and *increased skin pigmentation.*

Diagnosis depends upon the presence of (a) elevated iron plasma levels (above 150 μg. per 100 ml.), (b) 75 to 100 per cent saturation of iron-binding protein, and (c) signs of specific organ dysfunction. *Liver biopsy* is the most definite method to establish a diagnosis.

The long-term *prognosis* for most people with this condition is less than five years. Death usually results from cardiac failure, liver coma or hepatoma, hematemesis, and pneumonia.

Treatment involves *phlebotomy* on a biweekly or weekly basis over a two year period (2 ml. of blood = 1 mg. of Fe). Chelating agents are not therapeutically useful. Liver disease, cardiac disease, and diabetes are managed as necessary. Hypogonadism, if present, can be treated with testosterone. Hemosiderosis begins with excess absorption of iron, for that reason, dietary intake, drinking patterns, iron supplements, iron content of water, and excess blood transfusions all need to be discussed and evaluated to prevent a recurrence.

AMYLOIDOSIS

Amyloid is another substance that can infiltrate the liver and other organs. This connective tissue material, which is composed mainly of protein with some carbohydrate elements, causes tissues to become waxy and nonfunctioning. Much is unknown about the specifics of this disease — especially its incidence, pathology, and etiology.

Primary amyloidosis is possibly caused by an obscure *metabolic disturbance* that brings about the presence of abnormal protein in the plasma. The tissues most damaged by this abnormal protein material are those of the cardiac, smooth, and skeletal muscles. *Secondary* amyloidosis follows *chronic suppuration* (pus formation) and is linked with such disorders as tuberculosis, lung abscess, osteomyelitis, and bronchiectasis. The tissues most disturbed by secondary amyloidosis are those of the spleen, kidney, liver, and adrenal cortex.

Amyloidosis becomes a problem when it begins to interfere with organ function. Although many organs may be afflicted, emphasis here will be placed on the liver. *Hepatomegaly* is the most noticeable effect of this process. Liver function is minimally reduced. Clinical *jaundice* is uncommon.

Liver biopsy is an excellent diagnostic parameter but the incidence of post-biopsy hemorrhage or liver rupture is high. Bleeding is probably related to the effects of this process on the walls of small blood vessels. Gingival, skin, or rectal biopsies are usually quite satisfactory for diagnosis.

When the kidneys, heart, and/or gastrointestinal tract are involved, the afflicted person usually experiences progressive deterioration. At the present time there is no established treatment for primary amyloidosis; therefore, *supportive care* relating to organ involvement is the major focus of treatment.

Secondary amyloidosis is treated by *removal of the primary cause* and with *antibiotic* therapy to relieve suppuration.

LIVER TRANSPLANTATION

Liver transplantation is now considered a feasible, if imperfect, form of therapy for hepatic malignancy, biliary atresia, cirrhosis, and other forms of end-stage liver disease.

There are two general approaches to transplantation of the liver, *orthotopic homotransplantation* and *auxiliary homotransplantation* at an ectopic site. Although early transplants may have favored the insertion of an extra liver, recent results have shown that homografts (orthotopic homotransplantation) provide the most encouraging results.[84]

As with other transplants, immunosuppressive therapy is necessary to prevent rejection of the transplanted organs. Tissue typing for histocompatibility may also be effective in improving clinical results. Of paramount importance, however, is the procurement of a fresh, functioning, nonischemic liver.

Some of the more common problems associated with the surgical techniques of orthotopic transplantation are vascular anomalies (either in host or graft structures), bile duct problems (anomalies and biliary drainage), derangements in the coagulation mechanism (resulting in either hemorrhage or thrombosis), and the complexity of the anesthetic management.

In the immediate postoperative period the major areas of concern for the nurse are related to the general surgical complications, to immunosuppressive protocols, and to the proper function of drains. In addition, these patients need long-term follow-up and careful patient education.

CHAPTER 69

DISORDERS OF THE GALLBLADDER AND BILE DUCTS

The biliary system is composed of the gallbladder, the bile ducts, and the cystic duct. The cystic duct (from the gallbladder) joins with the hepatic duct (from the liver) to form the common bile duct (see Fig. 65–5). Recall from Chapter 65 that the function of the biliary system is to transport bile (secreted by the liver) from the gallbladder (where it is stored) into the duodenum.

Disorders of the gallbladder and ducts are extremely common. Within the United States alone more than one-half million people every year are hospitalized because of biliary tract disorders. Disorders include gallstones, inflammatory conditions, infections, tumors, and congenital malformations. The two most common conditions are *cholelithiasis* (stone formation) and associated *cholecystitis* (inflammation of the gallbladder). Malignancies of the biliary system are relatively uncommon.

The symptoms of diseases of the biliary system tend to mimic those of a number of other conditions. Some of the more common disorders to be differentiated are renal stones, chronic or acute pancreatitis, hiatal hernia with or without ulceration, angina or MI, peptic ulcer, irritable colon or a right colon cancer, pulmonary inflammation, acute hepatitis or necrotic process of liver, and acute appendicitis.

Before we begin our discussion of biliary tract disorders, note the list of rather confusing terms that are used in association with these conditions (see Table 69–1).

CHOLELITHIASIS, CHOLECYSTITIS, AND CHOLEDOCHOLITHIASIS

Cholelithiasis (Gallstones)

INCIDENCE

The "lowly" gallstone is not such a benign entity. About 10 per cent of the people in the United States are victims of this process, and approximately 6000 people die each year as a result of it. Snodgrass[95] reports that 500,000 people enter the hospital each year for gallstones, and about one-half of this group have a cholecystectomy. Before the age of 50, women have a higher morbidity rate, but the frequency of stones is more evenly distributed among the sexes after the fifth decade.

Kaplan and Ludwig[50] report that gallstones are more common in diabetics, women who have been pregnant, obese people, postvagotomy patients (decreased gallbladder motility), those having ileal disease or resection (bile salts depleted), and persons with chronic hemolytic disorders (increased bile pigments). Snodgrass[95] states that pregnant women with gallstones are more likely to become symptomatic during the pregnancy and that the pregnancy itself does not cause stones. In addition, this author states that when thin, normal weight, and obese patients are reviewed together, no one group has a higher frequency than the others. Female American Indians, however, have higher frequencies of gallstones after the age of 30 (70 per cent).

Composition and Formation of Gallstones. Our knowledge is still incomplete regarding the process of gallstone formation. Stones generally belong to one of the following three groups: (1) cholesterol stones, (2) pigment stones, or (3) a mixed variety. Some authors identify more

TABLE 69–1. BILIARY TRACT TERMINOLOGY

chole – pertaining to bile
cholang – pertaining to bile ducts
cholangiography – x-ray of bile ducts
cholangitis – inflammation of a bile duct
cholecyst – pertaining to gallbladder
cholecystectomy – removal of gallbladder
cholecystitis – inflammation of gallbladder
cholecystography – x-ray of gallbladder
cholecystostomy – incision and drainage of gallbladder
choledocho – pertaining to common bile duct
choledocholithiasis – stones in the common bile duct
choledochostomy – exploration of common bile duct
cholelith – gallstone
cholelithiasis – presence of gallstones

types, usually by subdividing the "mixed group." *Cholesterol stones* are the most common variety and are light-tan to yellow in shading. They have a laminated appearance when viewed from the inner aspect. A stone with a 75 per cent cholesterol composition fits into this group. *Pigment* stones contain calcium bilirubinate and unconjugated bilirubin as their major constituents. Kaplan and Ludwig[50] report that about 10 per cent of gallstones are pigment stones, but others estimate the incidence at about 23 per cent.[95] *Mixed stones* may be a combination of a cholesterol stone and a pigment stone or either of these with some other substance. Calcium carbonate, phosphates, bile salts, and palmitates are the more common minor constituents of stones. The *matrix* for stone growth is composed of an acid mucopolysaccharide substance. The exact mechanism of why or how cholesterol or pigment adheres is unknown. A typical gallstone is depicted in Figure 69–1.

The *etiology* of gallstones is still not understood, although many theories have been proposed. From the various theories, three possible explanations of stone formation are:

- *The bile undergoes changes in composition.* Studies of persons with cholesterol gallstones have indicated that their bile is supersaturated with cholesterol and the amount of bile salts is reduced. In these patients, an enzyme for synthesis of cholesterol is increased (HMG CoA reductase) and an enzyme promoting synthesis of bile salts is reduced (alphahydroxylase). This altered enzyme process is believed to result from a *genetic defect.* However, changes in bile composition, while important, do not completely explain why gallstones form.
- *Gallbladder stasis leads to stasis of bile.* Bile stasis may result in supersaturation of bile with cholesterol, changes in bile composition, and the precipitation of some of the constituents of bile. Gallbladder stasis may be caused by decreased contractility of the gallbladder or spasm of the sphincter of Oddi, or both. Delayed emptying of the gallbladder may be related in some way to hormonal factors, which may, in part, explain why gallstones seem to be associated with pregnancy.
- *Infection may be a causal factor.* It is known that inflammation debris can form a nidus (point of origin) for stone growth and that injury increases the reabsorption of bile salts and lecithin (predisposing to a saturated bile). Particular organisms may be involved in stone formation. For example, *Escherichia coli* increases the amount of free bilirubin available for pigment stones and *Streptococcus faecalis* reduces bile salts, which again allows the bile to supersaturate.

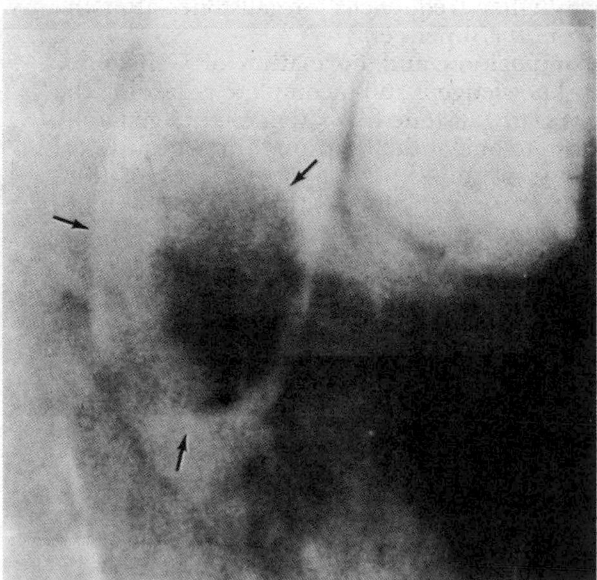

Figure 69–1. Gallstone. (From Price, A. P., and L. M. Wilson: *Pathophysiology: Clinical Concepts of Disease Processes.* New York: McGraw Hill Book Co., 1978.)

Signs and Symptoms. Only half of the people with gallstones report distress. *Pain* (right upper quadrant pain or biliary colic) and *jaundice* are the two most common symptoms. *Chills* and *fever* may also be present. If the stone is blocking the cystic duct, signs of acute cholecystitis might be more evident. (See p. 1515.) If the stone lodges in the common duct, cholangitis and pancreatitis might also be present.

Although the *pain* associated with gallstones is termed colic, it is not as variable in nature as the term suggests; instead, it may be constant with increasing intensity. The pain usually starts in the upper midline area and then centers in the right upper quadrant. The person is often quite restless and changes positions frequently in an attempt to relieve the pain's intensity.

Although flatulence, bloating, dyspepsia, and fatty food intolerance may occur in gallbladder disease, they are not specific for this entity. Often people who experience these problems still have them after cholecystectomy.

Diagnosis. The *cholecystogram* (gallbladder series) is most helpful in establishing the diagnosis of cholelithiasis. (See Chapter 67). Figure 69–1 illustrates a gallstone revealed by cholecystogram. Recovery of cholesterol crystals or granules of bilirubinate via a nasogastric tube is also diagnostic.

Treatment. *Cholecystectomy* is the most common treatment. It will be discussed in more detail later in this chapter. Cholecystectomy for *symptomatic* patients is usually attempted after the acute attack has subsided but before chronic cholecystitis and its potential complications occur. In *asymptomatic* cholelithiasis, the performance of elective cholecystectomy is still debated. About one third of the stones entering the common duct pass into the duodenum without problems. Thus medical treatment is possible for about 40 per cent of patients with cholesterol stones.

Medical management during an acute attack involves monitoring for progression of abdominal complications, maintaining fluid and electrolyte balance, controlling pain, and inserting a nasogastric tube for vomiting patients and for those with suspected pancreatitis. Strong analgesics are commonly used for discomfort. Nitroglycerin is also administered in some institutions to reduce pain.

Longer-term medical management involves teaching the patient to *avoid* those *foods* that seem to precipitate acute attacks. *Chenodeoxycholic acid,* a primary bile salt, may be ordered in some cases. This acid, if given orally daily, dissolves stones in 6 to 30 months. However, stones do recur in some patients after chenodeoxycholic acid administration is discontinued. Also, this drug is currently considered unsafe for administration to women in their childbearing years because it might cause hepatotoxicity in the fetus. The safety of this drug is currently being studied in the United States on a trial basis before possible release to the public for general use.[101]

Cholecystitis

Inflammation of the gallbladder may be an *acute* or a *chronic process.* Each will be discussed below. The major difference manifested by the person with an acute attack is a leukocytosis of about 12,000 and the presence of more localized pain and tenderness upon palpation of the gallbladder.

Acute Cholecystitis. Acute inflammation follows *stone impaction of the cystic duct* in all but 5 to 10 per cent of episodes. *Trauma* and *previous surgery* account for the remaining cases. Stone impaction in the cystic duct precipitates *distention,* which leads to decreased blood supply, decreased lymph drainage, and proliferation of bacteria.

Pain in acute cholecystitis may be in the epigastric area, subscapular area, or right upper quadrant area. Sometimes the pain is referred to the right scapula. When being examined, the patient often attempts to guard the upper right quadrant of the abdomen because it is so tender. Also, when the patient is asked to take a deep breath during palpation in the right subcostal area, he or she may experience extreme tenderness and stop breathing upon inspiration *(Murphy's sign).* The pain usually starts suddenly, steadily increases in intensity, and reaches a peak in around one-half hour. About 75 per cent of patients with an acute attack of cholecystitis have experienced biliary colic in the past due to cholelithiasis.[104] (See Unit XI.)

Jaundice is present in about 20 per cent of these patients. Furthermore, 60 to 70 per cent of patients develop an *elevated temperature,* which ranges between 38 and 38.5°C. (100.4 to 101.3° F.). Also approximately one-half of the patients suffer from *nausea and vomiting.* Many patients experience *intolerance to fatty foods.* Signs and symptoms of cholecystitis and cholelithiasis along with their bases are summarized in Table 69–2.

Diagnostic tests are usually somewhat helpful. The white blood cell count averages between 12,000 and 15,000. The transaminases, alkaline phosphatase, and BSP parameters are slightly abnormal. Upon x-ray of the abdomen, the enlarged gallbladder may occasionally be seen. In 15 per cent of the cases, the gallstones contain enough calcium to be visible on film. An oral cholecystogram is usually not done during

TABLE 69–2. BASES OF SIGNS AND SYMPTOMS OF CHOLECYSTITIS AND CHOLELITHIASIS

Signs and Symptoms	Bases
Abdominal pain, most commonly right upper quadrant or epigastric. Often radiates to back	In cholelithiasis, ductal spasm when a stone moves from gallbladder into ducts may cause waves of pain (biliary colic); in cholecystitis, pain may be steady (owing to inflammation) and increases in severity with peritoneal extension
Nausea and vomiting	Distention of bile ducts initiates impulses to vomiting center
Fat intolerance	Contraction of inflamed gallbladder to release bile to digest fat often precipitates pain
Fever and leukocytosis	Response to inflammation
Jaundice	In cholelithiasis, obstruction to common bile duct causes increased serum bilirubin; in cholecystitis, edema sometimes obstructs the duct enough to increase bilirubin levels

the acute attack because of nonvisualization problems and because approximately one-half of the patients have nausea and vomiting. Intravenous cholangiography may be diagnostic. A gallbladder scan and ultrasound may verify that stones are indeed present in the biliary tract.

Twenty-five per cent of people with acute cholecystitis may develop *complications* necessitating immediate surgery (cholangitis, empyema, gangrene, perforation, or pancreatitis). The remainder either will be hospitalized for observation and medical therapy or will be sent home with analgesics and orders for bed rest. Typically, symptoms will completely abate within one to four days. The doctor may then order follow-up studies.

The treatment may be either conservative or surgical. If surgery is indicated, it may in some cases be done within a few days of the acute attack. In other cases, it may be done within two or three months. The surgery of choice is *cholecystectomy*. In poor-risk patients, *cholecystostomy* may be performed instead of cholecystectomy. Both medical and surgical treatment are discussed in more detail on the following pages.

Chronic Cholecystitis. The signs and symptoms of chronic cholecystitis are similar to those of the acute form except that: (a) the pain is not as severe, (b) the temperature is not as elevated, and (c) the leukocyte count is not as high. Chronic cholecystitis is also accompanied by vague symptoms of dyspepsia, fat intolerance, heartburn, and flatulence—manifestations that the patient states have been troublesome for a long time. The patient with this condition suffers repeated attacks (mild or severe) of acute cholecystitis until at last fibrous tissues begin to replace the normal muscle and mucosal tissues of the gallbladder. As a consequence, the gallbladder eventually loses its biochemical ability to concentrate bile.

Diagnosis of chronic cholecystitis is based upon the oral cholecystogram. When the patient's gallbladder is fibrous as a result of chronic inflammation, it cannot be visualized, even after a double dose of oral contrast medium. Nevertheless, chronic, as well as acute, cholecystitis is sometimes difficult to differentiate from other disorders. The conditions that mimic the manifestations of cholecystitis (acute and chronic) and that must be ruled out during diagnosis are presented in Table 69–3.

Cholecystectomy is the treatment of choice for chronic cholecystitis, and 90 per cent of patients obtain relief of symptoms. All but 5 per cent of gallbladders removed are hard and contain stones.

TABLE 69–3. DIFFERENTIAL DIAGNOSIS OF ACUTE AND CHRONIC CHOLECYSTITIS

Chronic Cholecystitis	Acute Cholecystitis
Angina pectoris	Acute appendicitis
Hiatal hernia	Acute myocardial infarction
Peptic ulcer	Perforated or penetrating ulcer
Irritable colon	Pancreatitis
Renal disease	Right lower lobe pneumonia
Chronic pancreatitis	Intestinal obstruction
	Acute right kidney disease
	Acute hepatitis

Choledocholithiasis

Stones in the *common duct* can arise from the gallbladder or hepatic ducts; therefore, common duct stones can occur in the absence of a gallbladder. At times the force of gallbladder contraction during an episode of biliary colic can clear the cystic and common ducts of stones.

Symptoms of common duct stones include epigastric pain, which may radiate to the back and right hypochondrium, emesis, and jaundice, which is often mild and transient. Chills and spiking fevers are present when cholangitis is a complication. Leukocytosis is present, and BSP retention is increased. The transaminases are elevated but rarely increase above 300 units. Alkaline phosphatase levels can rise markedly, even though jaundice and bilirubin elevations are minimal. If the duct stone is blocking flow from the pancreas, serum amylase elevation occurs, indicating a concurrent pancreatitis.

Intravenous cholangiography is helpful in establishing a diagnosis of common duct stones. However, when the serum bilirubin is rising quickly and the patient has no pain, a percutaneous transhepatic approach is preferred, to rule out a hepatocellular condition. Surgery during an acute hepatocellular process carries a higher mortality rate.

Typically, following a diagnosis of choledocholithiasis, *surgical exploration* and *choledochotomy* are scheduled. If the gallbladder is present, *cholecystectomy* is performed, the common duct is opened and explored, and the stones are removed. Patients with advanced choledocholithiasis may have hundreds of stones in the duct, causing the common duct to be dilated to 3 cm. or more in diameter.[103]

SUMMARY OF TREATMENT MEASURES FOR CHOLELITHIASIS, CHOLECYSTITIS, AND CHOLEDOCHOLITHIASIS

Medical Intervention

Conservative care of the person with these conditions is based on the following:

1. *Relieve pain.* Meperidine (Demerol) in small frequent doses is the drug of choice. Morphine is believed to increase spasm of the sphincter of Oddi. Phenobarbital may be given for sedation and to relax smooth muscle. Nitroglycerin sublingually also reduces pain and may relax smooth muscle. Debate still exists over the usefulness of anticholinergic drugs (e.g., atropine) to reduce spasms of the sphincter of Oddi. Medication is combined with nursing measures to allay discomfort. (See Unit XI.)

2. *Relieve vomiting and reduce gastric stimulus.* A nasogastric tube is usually passed and attached to suction. This relieves distention and vomiting and eliminates the gastric juices that stimulate cholecystokinin.

3. *Maintain fluid and electrolyte balance.* This is achieved by intravenous solutions and careful monitoring of fluid output and serum electrolyte levels.

4. *Eliminate infection.* Some physicians will prescribe broad-spectrum antibiotics, particularly if the acute process does not subside in 24 hours or if cholangitis (inflammation of a bile duct) is suspected. Any infection superimposed on the chemical inflammation will thus be eliminated.

5. *Low fat diet.* A low fat diet may be helpful if the patient's biliary tract condition prevents adequate bile flow for proper digestion of fat. Small frequent meals and restricted use of alcohol may also relieve symptoms.

Administration of bile acid (chenodeoxycholic acid) has been used to restore the proper bile acid:cholesterol ratio to dissolve cholesterol stones in research studies.[30] This may greatly reduce the need for surgery in the future if its adverse effects on the liver can be controlled. As indicated earlier, bile acid is still being studied and is used on a trial basis only.

Surgical Intervention

Cholecystectomy. The treatment of choice for patients with symptomatic cholelithiasis and cholecystitis is cholecystectomy. However, surgeons do not agree upon exactly *when* cholecystectomy should be performed. Those who believe in immediate surgical intervention base their argument upon the fact that early surgery may prevent serious complications (e.g., perforation of the gallbladder, gangrene of the gallbladder, sepsis, etc.). Some surgeons believe that cholecystectomy should be done after an acute attack subsides because they believe that the surgery is less dangerous once the acute inflammation has diminished, also the waiting period can be used for further diagnostic studies and for conservative management, to reduce inflammation.

Whether to operate at all on a patient with asymptomatic cholelithiasis (silent gallstones) is another area under question. Should the gallbladder be removed because the person might develop a serious complication such as acute cholecystitis, choledocholithiasis, or sepsis? Or should only certain high-risk patients undergo elective cholecystectomy? The elderly and the diabetics (not mature onset), who tend to have a high incidence of gallstones, do not tolerate acute conditions or emergency procedures well. Those surgeons who favor medical follow-up for asymptomatic stones point to the operative mortality figures as a reason to follow conservative management. However, since statistics rarely include data regarding patients' additional medical problems, the sophistication of available facilities, and patient support systems, they cannot be relied upon to be the sole indicator for action. Decisions concerning surgery must be shared by the doctor, the informed patient, and the family and significant others.

Cholecystectomy consists of excising the gallbladder from the posterior liver wall and ligating the cystic duct, vein, and artery. The gallbladder is usually approached through a right subcostal incision (Fig. 69–2). Common duct exploration may also be accomplished through this incision site, if necessary. If the common duct is suspected of having stones, an operative cholangiography may be performed if it was not ordered preoperatively. The common duct, if not dilated from pathology, may be dilated before the stones are removed. A fine instrument is inserted into the ducts to collect the stones, either whole or after crushing. After exploration of the common duct, a *T-tube* is generally insert-

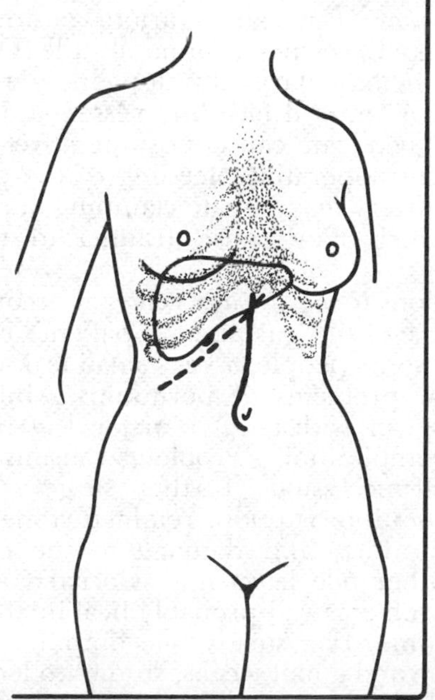

Figure 69–2. Cholecystectomy. Either vertical or subcostal incision may be used. The determining factor is usually the distance between the costal margins. (From Carey, L. C., and P. W. Catalano: Acute cholecystitis. *In* Sabiston, D. C. (Ed.): *Textbook of Surgery.* 11th ed., Philadelphia: W. B. Saunders Co., 1977.)

ed to allow adequate bile drainage during duct healing and to provide a route for postoperative cholangiography, if desired. Stones discovered post-operatively have been successfully dissolved with heparin administered via the T-tube.

In addition to the usual postoperative complications, the following conditions may occur: subhepatic abscess, wound infection, hemorrhage, bile leakage, duct stricture, postoperative jaundice, pancreatitis, and disruption of the ducts.

Subhepatic abscess is more likely to occur if there is (a) surgical damage to the liver, (b) rupture of a small bile ductule along the gallbladder bed, (c) leakage of a common duct repair, or (d) leakage of the cystic duct, possibly due to a lost ligature. To prevent complications from these above possibilities the patient usually returns from surgery with a *Penrose drain.* The drain exits from a stab wound site separate from the incision and stays in place for a few days. Some surgeons prefer to use a drain only when a large amount of inflammatory fluid is expected. If no drainage occurs, the drain will be removed.

Excessive tissue traction, inadequate incision, dead space between tissue layers, excessive suture material, or electrocautery all predispose the person to a possible *wound infection.*

Hemorrhage can cause various postoperative problems. Excessive trauma to the liver can cause a hematoma to develop under the liver capsule. A "missed bleeding vessel" in the gallbladder bed can cause postoperative hemorrhage. Intraoperative bleeding of the cystic or hepatic artery may initiate clamping in a bloody field, which may cause trauma to the bile ducts.

Reactions to *bile leakage* will vary according to the source of the leak and the patient's response to it. In some people, a very small leak will lead to major problems of peritonitis, while other patients can withstand a major leak with no major complications. Problems causing leakage that will necessitate further surgery include cystic duct interruption, retained stones in the common duct, and damage to the common duct. Other bile leaks not associated with the above problems will probably heal in about one week's time. If a steady bile output continues after one and a half weeks, studies to locate and repair the damage are necessary. If the patient is losing large amounts of bile via the fistula (1000 to 1500 ml. daily), this bile is sometimes returned to the patient by feeding tube or in juice.

Postoperative *jaundice* most commonly occurs when stones in the common duct are missed. Other, less common, causes of jaundice are stenosis at the sphincter of Oddi, a missed tumor in the area of the ampulla, and liver necrosis after interruption of the blood supply. Jaundice may occur as a result of a transfusion reaction, hepatitis, or other medical problems that develop following surgery.

Pancreatitis can occur after any surgical procedure; however, common duct exploration increases the chance of occurrence in the postoperative period. This inflammation appears to be related to trauma and fibrosis in the common duct after forceful dilatation of the ampulla. There is often a high mortality rate for patients who develop pancreatitis in the immediate postoperative period.

The most common complication after biliary tract surgery is *disruption of the ducts.* Damage while attempting to clamp a bleeding vessel, anatomical anomalies not properly identified, and closure of the hepatic duct by overzealous ligation of the cystic duct are the most common causes of duct damage. If the damage is recognized during surgery, repair is immediate and a T-tube is placed in the common duct. Bile leakage or fistula formation will signal duct damage not discovered at surgery. The same diagnostic procedures that are used to identify biliary disease can be utilized to determine the extent of duct damage. The problem must be corrected surgically. Note in Figure 69–3 that there are a number of procedures for correction of damaged bile ducts.

Cholecystostomy. This procedure is an alternative when a cholecystectomy will not be tolerated or is not safe for the person with acute cholecystitis. Patients who are very poor operative risks with short life expectancy, patients with severe inflammation limiting anatomical landmarks, and patients with perforated gallbladders and abscess formation or bile peritonitis are good candidates for cholecystostomy. Often, at a later time, a cholecystectomy will be needed to finally resolve the biliary disease.

The cholecystostomy procedure involves (a) making an incision in the fundus of the gallbladder, (b) emptying the gallbladder of all its gallstones, and (c) suturing a large-lumen tube into the gallbladder for drainage during the postoperative period. After the patient has sufficiently recovered, Hypaque is injected into the tube, and x-rays are taken. If stones are still present in the gallbladder or common duct, then elective cholecystectomy will be scheduled for when the patient is stronger and is a better surgical risk. If no stones are discovered upon x-ray, then the tube is removed and the patient is followed for evidence of new stones. In about 50 per cent of cases, stones recur within five years of surgery.

Choledochostomy. This surgical procedure consists of opening the common duct, removing stones from the duct, and inserting a T-tube into the duct for drainage. A cholecystectomy may be necessary at a later date.

NURSING CARE FOR PATIENTS WITH CHOLELITHIASIS, CHOLECYSTITIS, AND CHOLEDOCHOLITHIASIS

Nursing care will vary according to the type of biliary tract disorder present as well as the acuteness of the illness. For example, a patient may complain of vague abdominal symptoms and have diagnostic testing on an out-patient basis, or the patient may arrive at the hospital suffering an acute attack and require immediate diagnostic procedures and medical intervention. If surgical intervention is necessary, the patient will have additional specific pre- and postoperative nursing care needs.

Patients undergoing *diagnostic tests* need help to understand the necessity for the tests, what happens to them during the procedure, their

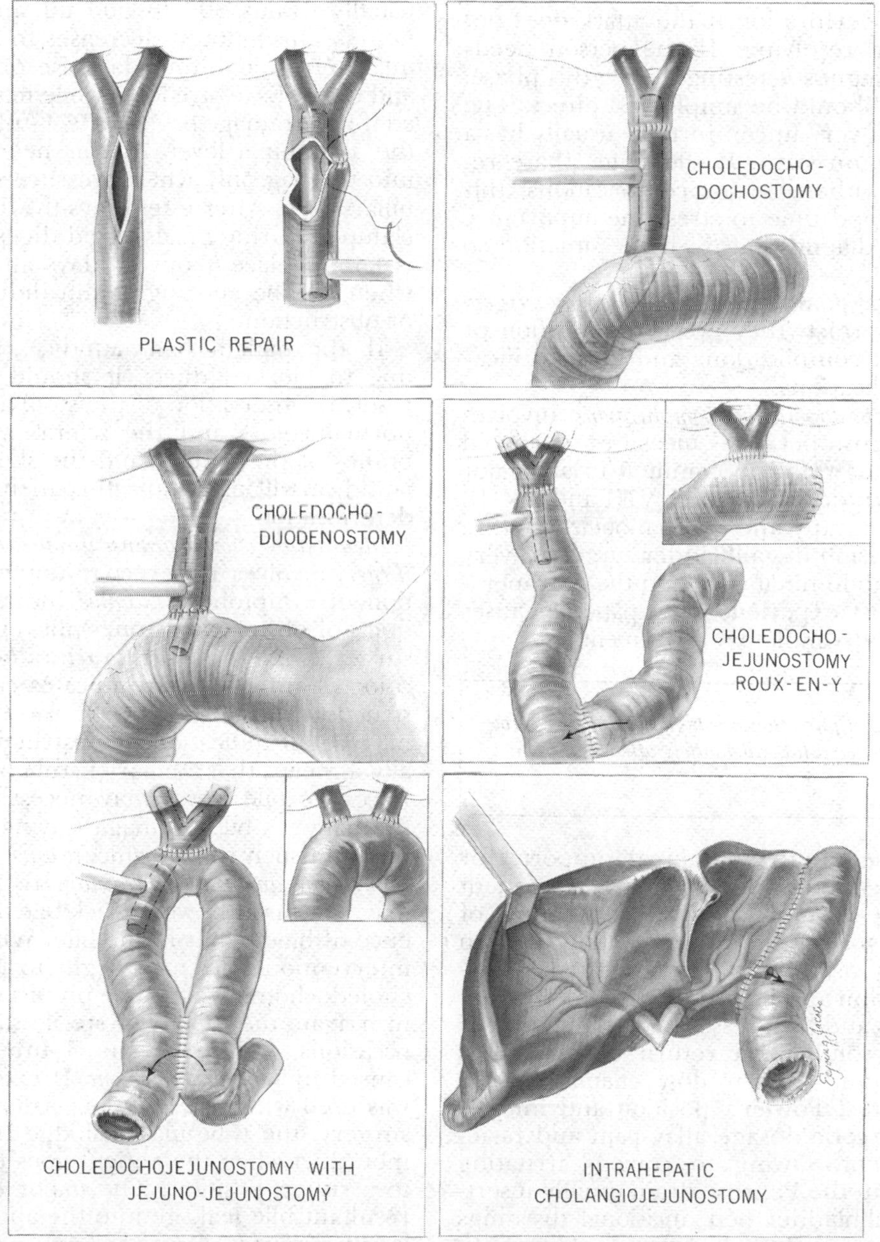

Figure 69–3. Operations for correction of acquired traumatic strictures of the bile ducts. (From Orloff, M. J.: The biliary system. *In* Sabiston, D. C. (Ed.): *Textbook of Surgery.* 11th ed., Philadelphia: W. B. Saunders Co., 1977.)

responsibility for test preparation, and proper aftercare, if indicated. If the patient is going to have diagnostic work outside the hospital or as an out-patient, printed sheets of instructions to reinforce teaching are helpful. (See Ch. 67.)

Nursing care during the *acute phase* involves providing rest and actively assessing the person's need for analgesia. If fluid and electrolyte retention is a problem, assess the patient's response to fluid therapy. Also observe for potential problems of infection, severe inflammation, and possible perforation if the attack does not appear to be resolving. If the person needs emergency diagnostic testing during this phase, explanations should be simple and direct. The person who is very uncomfortable usually has a shorter attention span. If the acute phase resolves itself without major complications, this might be a good time to stress the importance of follow-up diagnostic care if the situation so warrants.

Two general goals guide care *following surgery* of the biliary tract: they are (1) prevention of postoperative complications and (2) identification of complications.

Preventing postoperative complications involves thoughtful postoperative measures to avoid those problems that are common to all major abdominal surgery. (See Units VIII and XVII.) Respiratory therapy and rapid mobilization are vital. The incision in gallbladder surgery is very high on the abdominal wall, and the postoperative discomfort experienced by patients causes them to inhibit ventilatory movement.

The incidence of pneumonia is high if patients are not encouraged to ventilate adequately after biliary tract surgery.

Also, the use of an abdominal support (for example a scultetus binder) helps the patient move and sit up more comfortably. Return of bowel sounds is monitored. Distention is often prevented by use of a nasogastric tube; provision of nutrition and fluids begins with intravenous solutions and progresses to oral ingestion of liquids and solids with return of peristalsis. Ambulation and return flow enemas aid in releasing flatus. Fowler's position and initially generous narcotic dosage allay pain and facilitate movement. Owing to copious irritating drainage from the Penrose drain usually inserted in the gallbladder bed, incisional dressings must be reinforced and changed often, with careful skin care provided. The use of a skin agent (e.g., petrolatum, karaya, aluminum, zinc oxide) and a closed bag over the draining site are usually sufficient to prevent irritation.

After choledochostomy, a T-tube prevents spillage of bile into the peritoneum and maintains ductal patency in the presence of edema from trauma due to surgery or stones. The T-tube is sutured into the common duct, with arms toward the hepatic duct and the duodenum; its length is brought out in a stab wound near the incision and sutured to the skin. T-tubes may be attached to continuous bedside gravity drainage, or collapsible bags may be attached at the dressing site to drain only bile overflow. Tension on long tubing and obstruction by kinking must be avoided. *Drainage* from the T-tube is carefully measured. The T-tube usually drains 300 to 500 ml. in the first 24 hours. This amount decreases to less than 200 ml. after three to four days. Record the volume and color. Excessive loss of bile may be prevented if the drainage bag for the T-tube is placed at the abdominal level. At this height, bile flows into the bag only when pressure is high in the biliary tree. After a few days the T-tube may be clamped during meals to aid digestion of fat. It is left in place about 10 days and is removed when T-tube cholangiogram indicates absence of obstruction.

If the patient had jaundice preoperatively due to blocked ducts, it should not begin to resolve. Observation of the stool and urine (for normal color) and the sclera, mucous membranes of the mouth, and the skin for signs of jaundice will also indicate patient progress or deterioration.

Identifying complications unique to biliary tract surgery involves early recognition of the implication of symptoms. *Jaundice* indicates injury to ducts or obstructing stones not removed during surgery. *Failure of stools to return to normal brown* color of urobilin also indicates continuing obstruction to bile flow. *Excessive T-tube drainage* may be an indication of obstruction; occasionally it means that a biliary fistula has developed. Excessive bile losses may necessitate recycling the patient's bile drainage (giving it orally in a medium such as fruit juice). *Lack of drainage* or *inadequate amounts of drainage* from the T-tube may be caused by very thick bile or by the presence of blood clots in the bile. Without medical intervention, bile may begin to leak from the choledochotomy site. The physician may decide to irrigate the tube with sterile saline. On rare occasions, failure of the T-tube to drain is caused by *tube dislodgement.* If excessive tension was used when the T-tube was inserted during surgery, the tube may dislodge from the common duct when the patient goes from a supine to a sitting position. The major danger of the resultant bile leakage into the abdominal cavity is *bile peritonitis. Fevere and severe abdominal pain* with guarding may indicate bile peritonitis resulting from seepage of bile at the sutures or slippage of the T-tube, or occasionally it may mean that direct trauma to the pancreas has caused pancreatitis. *Bleeding* after cholecystectomy may indicate reduced prothrombin levels as a result of decreased vitamin K absorption.

In the *immediate postoperative period* the person is kept NPO and may have a nasogastric tube. Intravenous therapy with potassium is commonly used to maintain fluid levels until oral feedings begin. In uncomplicated cases, food intake, starting with clear liquids, will begin in 24 to 48 hours. Each day the person moves toward the full diet. The use of fat in the diet postoperatively depends on the patient's tolerance and the physician's preferences. If fat is decreased in the diet, then the necessary calories need to be replaced with CHO or protein.

The majority of patients can expect to go home two weeks postoperatively. They should be informed of activity levels (i.e., Can they go up steps? How many steps? When can they drive?) and of the need for a follow-up visit. They should have adequate knowledge of any special care. Unfortunately, some patients experience *post-cholecystectomy syndrome*—a confusing term because it is not truly a syndrome. These patients, who had nausea, bloating, and dyspepsia before surgery, still have the same problems postoperatively. The cause of these symptoms is often related to other gastrointestinal disorders (hiatal hernia, peptic ulcer, colon disorders). Other causes may be residual stones in the common duct, bile fistula, a missed malignancy, and surgical trauma with a resultant stricture of the ducts.

CANCER OF THE BILIARY TRACT

Cancer of the Gallbladder

Cancer of the gallbladder is quite rare. The most common type is adenocarcinoma associated with chronic gallstones. It is preventable by early cholecystectomy.

Carcinoma of the gallbladder is more commonly found in women aged 50 to 60 years with gallstones, but the exact relationship between gallstones and cancer has not been established. Gallbladder malignancies account for only 1 to 13 per cent of all cancers. The fundus and the neck of the gallbladder are the most common sites for tumors, while only one fifth of the gallbladder tumors grow in the lateral walls. Tumors may be infiltrating or fungating. The *infiltration* type tumor penetrates the gallbladder walls and usually ulcerates on the mucosal surface. It may invade the liver bed directly or cause a fistula into an adjacent organ. The *fungating* group proliferates both above and below the gallbladder wall and can extend into adjacent structures as well as obstruct bile outflow. This form is less common than the infiltrating type.

Both of these tumors may be present for a long time before discovery. Jaundice is a late sign. The more common presenting signs and symptoms are indistinguishable from those of cholecystitis with cholelithiasis. As the tumor grows, weight loss and other signs of a malignant process appear. Average life expectancy after diagnosis is one to one and a half years. Few people have made the 5-year survival period.

Cancer of the Bile Ducts (Extrahepatic)

This process is also more common in the elderly but men are more at risk. These lesions cause obstruction and jaundice and therefore diagnosis is made early. Other symptoms are acute onset of right upper quadrant pain, biliary colic, weight loss, and digestive disorders. Late complications are pruritus, cholangitis, biliary cirrhosis, and hydrops. The average survival rate is 3 to 6 months. The tumor can spread, but the metastatic problems are not usually significant. Surgical excision and reestablishment is not yet an option for this process, except when the tumor is confined to the ampulla. (See Unit IX.)

CONGENITAL ABNORMALITIES

The gallbladder may be absent, present as a double structure, or have an unusual position on the liver. The bile ducts are also prone to defects of atresia, cystic dilation, and intrahepatic duct dilatation. Recognition that these alterations exist and may cause difficulty during surgery should alert the nurse to be extremely observant in the immediate postoperative period for potential complications.

CHAPTER 70

DISORDERS OF THE PANCREAS

INTRODUCTION

The pancreas is a solid, slender organ in the upper retroperitoneal abdominal cavity, traversing the posterior abdominal wall. It consists of a head, neck, body, and tail. The head and neck of the pancreas are just to the right of midline, while the body and tail extend across the abdomen to the spleen. Pancreatic function can be divided into two parts: exocrine and endocrine. The *exocrine pancreas* contains acinar cells that secrete enzymes needed for the digestion of carbohydrates, proteins, and fats, as listed in Table 70–1. The centroacinar cells of the pancreas produce sodium bicarbonate and water, which are important in neutralizing the highly acid pH of chyme as it enters the duodenum from the stomach. The *endocrine function of the pancreas* rests with the alpha and beta cells of the islets of Langerhans, which are located throughout the pancreas. The alpha cells secrete glucagon and the beta cells secrete insulin. Delta cells, which are also located in the islets, secrete gastrin. Glucagon, as you may recall, is the hyperglycemic factor in that it facilitates the conversion of glycogen to glucose, thus raising the blood sugar. Insulin is required for the cellular uptake and metabolism of carbohydrates, proteins, and fats. Gastrin has several functions among which are: (a) to stimulate the release of gastric acid, pepsin, and intrinsic factor by the stomach, (b) to stimulate growth of the stomach, exocrine pancreas, mucosa of the small intestine, and colon, (c) to decrease absorption of nutrients from the gut, and (d) to stimulate pancreatic secretion. Pancreatic exocrine (digestive) and endocrine functions are illustrated in Figure 70–1.

TABLE 70–1. PANCREATIC ENZYMES

Enzyme	Function
Amylase	Catalyzes the hydrolysis of starch and glycogen to maltose or maltotriose. Contains calcium. Excreted in the urine.
Lipase	Hydrolyzes fats into mono-, di-, and triglycerides and free fatty acids.
Proteases: Trypsinogen Chymotrypsinogen Procarboxypeptidase Proaminopeptidase	Splits proteins to peptides and a few amino acids. The proteases are secreted in an inactive form; otherwise they would act on pancreatic tissue and cause destruction. Once in the intestine, intestinal enterokinase acts on trypsinogen, converting it to trypsin. Trypsin then acts on the other proteases to convert them to active enzymes.

Stimulation of pancreatic secretion is predominantly hormonal, although both the sympathetic and parasympathetic nervous systems exert their influence. In general, the sympathetic nervous system inhibits pancreatic secretion, while the parasympathetic nervous system has a stimulating effect. This may be an important consideration when caring for the patient who has had a vagotomy for peptic ulcer disease. Unless a selective vagotomy was done, and the pancreatic innervation maintained, the patient may experience alteration in pancreatic function. Also, parasympatholytic agents (anticholinergics such as atropine and Pro-Banthine) have been used in the past in the management of patients with pancreatitis with the goal of decreasing pancreatic secretions and promoting rest of the organ.

Normal digestive processes have been divided into three phases: (a) cephalic, (b) gastric, and (c) intestinal. Each phase plays a role in the stimulation of pancreatic secretion. The *cephalic phase* of digestion is stimulated by the thought, smell, taste, chewing, and swallowing of food. These stimuli affect the vagus nerve, with resulting stimulation of the stomach to secrete acid and gastrin. Gastrin then stimulates the release of pancreatic enzymes. During the *gastric phase*, when food actually enters the stomach, changes in gastric pH, distention of the stomach, and the presence of chemicals from the food ingested serve to sustain both the vagal stimulation and the release of acid and gastrin. When chyme enters the duodenum, the *intestinal phase* of digestion is initiated. In this phase the major stimuli for pancreatic secretion are secretin and cholecystokinin-pancreozymin (CCK-PZ). These two substances are released by the duodenal mucosa in response to both acid and the by-products of protein and fat digestion. The mechanisms involved in pancreatic stimulation are illustrated in Figure 70–2.

In healthy individuals pancreatic juice is a thin, clear fluid containing a large amount of sodium chloride and bicarbonate as well as enzymes. The average individual produces approximately a liter of pancreatic fluid in 24 hours. During illness or injury the volume of pancreatic fluid usually decreases, and the composition may change. For example, both the volume and bicarbonate concentration of pancreatic fluid are often decreased in the patient with chronic pancreatitis, while the patient with acute pancreatitis may have normal secretion. In cystic fibrosis both the volume and enzyme concentration are diminished.[49]

From the previous discussion one can appreciate that the patient with a pancreatic disorder may have interference with either digestion or glucose utilization, or both. Disorders of the pancreas may be divided into four groups: (a) inflammatory, (b) neoplastic, (c) traumatic, and (d) genetic. The diseases included under each category are listed in Table 70–2 and are discussed in the following section. Laboratory and radiographic studies used in the diagnosis of pancreatic disorders are outlined in Tables 70–3 and 70–4.

PANCREATITIS

Acute pancreatitis is a fairly common and potentially lethal inflammatory process with varying degrees of pancreatic edema, fat necrosis, or hemorrhage. There is a 5 to 10 per cent mortality associated with pancreatic edema, a 20 to 30 per cent mortality with partial necrosis of the pancreas, and a 50 to 80 per cent mortality when hemorrhagic pancreatitis occurs.[95] As shown in Table 70–2, a patient may have a single attack of acute pancreatitis, repeated episodes of acute pancreatitis, chronic pancreatitis with periodic acute pancreatitis, or chronic pan-

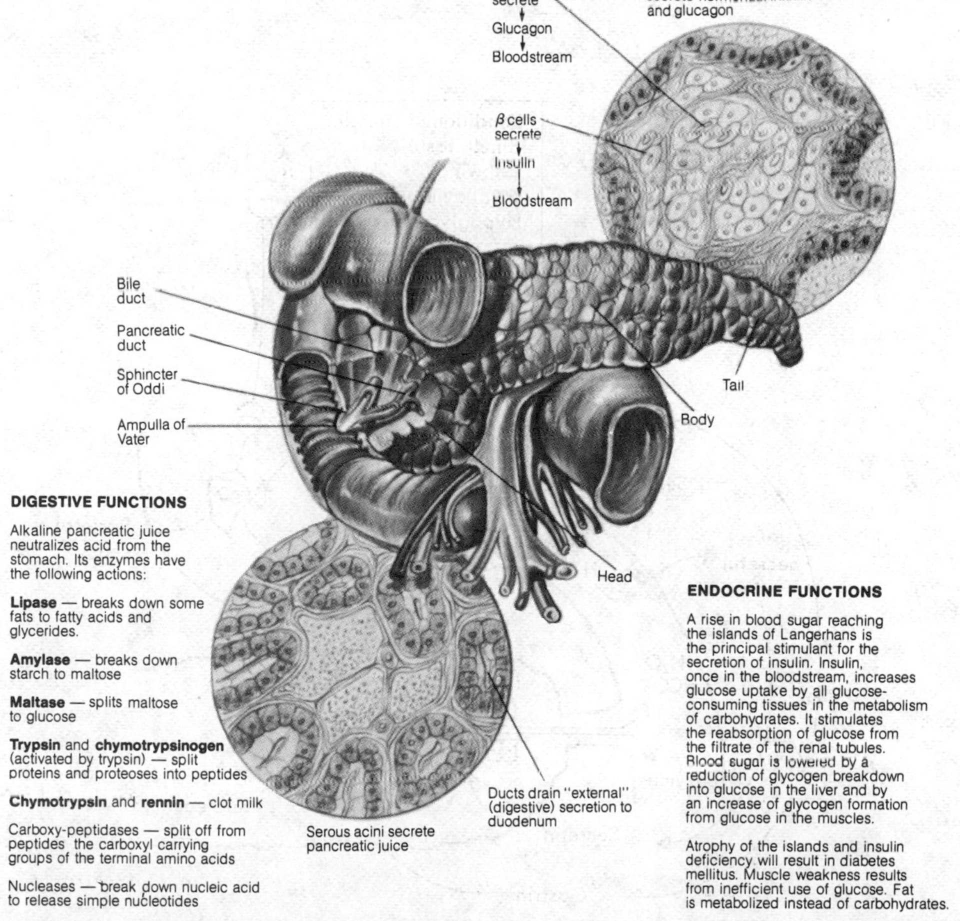

Figure 70–1. Physiology of the pancreas. (From DaCosta, L., et al.: Meeting the challenge of pancreatitis. *Patient Care,* 11:71, Sept. 1977. Reproduced with permission of *Patient Care* magazine. Copyright © 1977, Patient Care Publications, Inc., Darien, Ct. All rights reserved.)

creatitis without exacerbations of an acute process.

Although there is no genetic predisposition to the development of acute pancreatitis, men are more often afflicted. Perhaps this is due to the fact that pancreatitis is associated with alcohol use and abuse, and that there are more male alcoholics in the United States at this time. Pancreatitis is also noted in patients with cholecystitis with stones, a disorder that is more often seen in females than in males. In the past children have had a low incidence of pancreatitis; in general, the pancreatitis seen in children has been associated with hyperlipidemia or ascariasis of the biliary tree, or has been hereditary. However, the recent and most alarming increase in alcoholism among adolescents may result in an increased incidence of pancreatitis among this age group.

As previously mentioned, the most common cause of pancreatitis is alcohol abuse. In addition to gallstones, other conditions that may predispose a person to developing pancreatitis are viral hepatitis, mumps, peptic ulcer, periarteritis, hyperlipidemia, hyperparathyroidism, and hypothermia. Recent research indicates that pancreatitis may develop in patients with anorexia nervosa.[65] Additional causes of pancreatitis include blunt and penetrating trauma, electrical shock, and surgical procedures, including diagnostic procedures. Drugs such as chlorothiazide, azathioprine, sulfonamides, and glucocorticoids may precipitate pancreatitis. It is estimated that a precipitating cause cannot be identified in approximately 20 per cent of the patients with acute pancreatitis.

Pathophysiology

The precise mechanism involved in pancreatic damage has not been established. The pathologic changes occurring in the pancreas are due to proteolytic and lipolytic pancreatic enzymes, which are activated in the pancreas rather than in the duodenum. You will recall from Table 70–1 that pancreatic proteases are normally released in an inactive form. Once in the intestine, pancreatic trypsinogen (one of the proteases) is converted into trypsin through the action of intestinal enterokinase. In pancreatitis, however, the proteases and lipases are activated

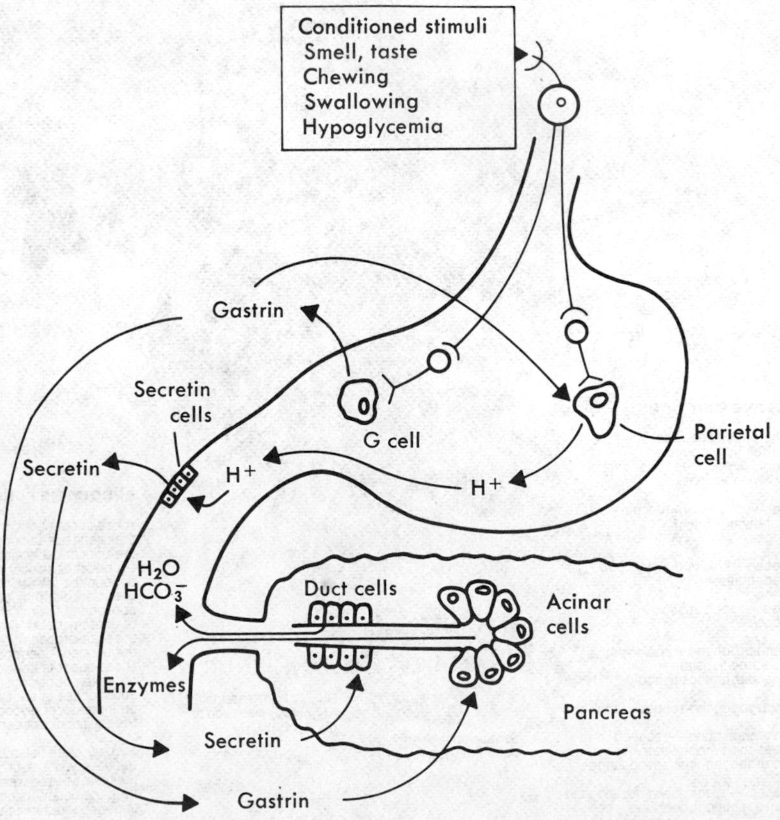

Figure 70–2. Mechanisms involved in the stimulation of pancreatic secretion during the cephalic phase of digestion. (From Johnson, L. R. (Ed.): *Gastrointestinal Physiology.* St. Louis: C. V. Mosby Co., 1977.)

prior to secretion into the intestine. This causes the actual tissue damage in the pancreas. How and why the enzymes are activated in the pancreas is unknown. "The basic mechanism is probably either reflux of some substance into the pancreatic duct or obstruction of the pancreatic duct during outflow of pancreatic juice."[19] The net effect of the enzymatic action is *autodigestion* of the pancreas.

Signs and Symptoms of Acute Pancreatitis

The patient with acute pancreatitis usually presents to the emergency service with severe and impressive pain, which is often located in the left upper quadrant or the epigastric area. Often the pain radiates through to the back. Commonly one can elicit a history of onset of pain associated with food or alcohol intake. Careful questioning of the patient or significant others may reveal a history compatible with pancreatitis; e.g., alcohol use, gallbladder disease, etc. The common manifestations are summarized in Table 70–5.

Symptoms of Chronic Pancreatitis

Chronic pancreatitis involves progressive degeneration of both acinar and islet functions of the pancreas due to scarring and calcification of tissue after repeated attacks of acute pancreatitis. Dull pain alternates with severe pain, vomiting, fever, and jaundice as in acute pancreatitis. Eventually hyperglycemia becomes a clinical problem with manifestations of diabetes. Digestive enzyme secretion is so severely reduced that malnutrition and weight loss, coupled with severe elimination problems, become evident. Abdominal distention with flatus and cramps is accompanied by frequent foul fatty stools (steatorrhea).

Diagnosis

As previously mentioned, the patient with acute pancreatitis usually is first seen in acute pain with the manifestations detailed above. Pain or digestive disturbance may motivate the chronic patient to seek help. The pancreas is never palpable, but a pseudocyst, a pocket created by chronic obstruction to accumulating secretions, may occasionally be felt.

Diagnostic tests are nonspecific. Elevated serum amylase and lipase are cardinal signs, but they may be caused by other acute gastrointestinal disorders, and are not directly correlated with the severity of the disorder. Serum amylase rises in a few hours and lasts about three days; urinary amylase remains elevated longer. Recently, elevation of the amylase-creatinine clearance ratio has been purported to be a more accurate means of assessing acute pancreatitis than either serum or urine amylase values.[5] Lipase rises in 24 hours and lasts up to 10 days. Enzymes may be normal with reduced functioning tissue in chronic pancreatitis. Plain x-rays may show reduced bowel motility, calcifications (see Fig. 70–3), and adhesions. Angiography indicates vascular changes. Cholangiography and/or cholecystography shows biliary changes, which may be either causes or consequences of pancreatic disorder. Paracentesis frequently reveals bloody fluid, high in amylase and methemalbumin from hemoglobin digestion. Other studies that may be indicated, especially when the diagnosis is obscure, are included in Tables 70–3 and 70–4.

TABLE 70–2. CLASSIFICATION OF PANCREATIC DISEASE*

I. Inflammatory
  1. Acute pancreatitis
  2. Relapsing acute pancreatitis
     In acute and relapsing acute pancreatitis, functional and morphological restoration may occur if causes (e.g., alcohol, gallstones) are eliminated.
  3. Relapsing chronic pancreatitis
     Chronic pancreatitis with acute exacerbations.
  4. Chronic pancreatitis
     Permanent structural and functional damage has occurred; may be related to nutritional, metabolic, or endocrine factors.

II. Neoplastic
  A. Parenchymal origin (acinar cells)
    1. Adenoma
    2. Acinar cell adenocarcinoma
  B. Ductal origin
    1. Cystadenoma
    2. Adenocarcinoma
  C. Islet cell origin
    1. Insulinoma
    2. Gastrin-producing tumor
    3. VIP-producing tumor
    4. Glucagonoma
    5. Other tumors derived from APUD cells

III. Traumatic
  1. Nonpenetrating or blunt trauma
  2. Penetrating injuries

IV. Genetic
  1. Cystic fibrosis
  2. Hereditary and familial pancreatitis

*Abbreviations are VIP, vasoactive peptide; APUD, amine precursor uptake and decarboxylation.

From Arvanitakis, C., and A. R. Cooke: Diagnostic tests of exocrine pancreatic function and disease. *Progress in Gastroenterology*, 74:932, May, 1978.

Clinical Intervention in Acute Pancreatitis

Treatment of the milder edematous pancreatitis may require only analgesics, but acute hemorrhagic pancreatitis requires intensive measures. The goals of intervention are discussed here.

TABLE 70–3. LABORATORY TESTS IN ASSESSING PANCREATIC FUNCTION*

I. *Direct tests*
   1. Secretin test
   2. Secretin-CCK test
   3. Caerulein test
   4. Bombesin test

II. *Indirect tests*
   1. Lundh test meal
   2. Duodenal perfusion with essential amino acids
   3. Synthetic peptide Bz-Ty-PABA

III. *Fecal tests*
   1. Microscopic examination for neutral fat and free fatty acids, and for meat fibers
   2. Fecal fat determination (g/72 hours)
   3. Fecal chymotrypsin assay
   4. Fecal nitrogen

IV. *Radioisotope tests*
   1. ^{131}I-labeled triolein
   2. ^{14}C tripalmitate

V. *Amylase, lipase, and methemalbumin levels in body fluids*
   1. Serum amylase
   2. Urinary amylase
   3. Serum lipase
   4. Amylase–creatinine clearance ratio
   5. Amylase in pleural and ascitic fluid
   6. Methemalbumin

*Abbreviations are CCK, cholecystokinin; Bz-Ty-PABA, N-benzoyl-L-tyrosyl-p-aminobenzoic acid.
Modified from Arvanitakis, C., and A. R. Cooke: Diagnostic tests of exocrine pancreatic function and disease. *Progress in Gastroenterology,* 74:932, May 1978.

TABLE 70–4. RADIOGRAPHIC STUDIES USED IN DIAGNOSING PANCREATIC DISEASE

Study	Indications	Diagnostic Value	Comment
Hypotonic duodenography	To investigate suspected lesions in head of pancreas, periampullary region, and duodenum	Improved results (85% accuracy) obtained with injection of barium into duodenum after intubation and administration of spasmolytic agent	1. Effacement of medial duodenal aspect in chronic pancreatitis 2. Radiographic signs in pancreatic carcinoma become apparent in advanced disease; false-negative results approximate 20%
Pancreatic scanning	As adjunct diagnostic study to investigate patients with suspected pancreatic carcinoma and chronic upper abdominal and back pain	Results variable and scintigraphic appearance nonspecific	1. False-positive results may occur in up to 43% 2. False-negative results occur in 15%
Ultrasonography	In cases of suspected pancreatic pseudocyst or carcinoma	Well established in detection of pancreatic pseudocysts	Pancreatic tumor may be detected as space-occupying lesion, if size exceeds 3 cm
Angiography	To detect pancreatic carcinoma, islet cell tumor, and pseudocyst	Helpful in diagnosis of pancreatic tumors	Diagnostic accuracy in pancreatic cancer may be 75%
Computerized total body tomography	Suspected abdominal tumors, pancreatic carcinoma, pseudocyst	May be useful in detection of pancreatic tumor	1. Distinction between inflammatory and neoplastic mass not always possible by CAT scan alone; false-positive results occur 2. Provides accurate localization of tumor for fine needle biopsy of lesion

From Arvanitakis, C., and A. R. Cooke: Diagnostic tests of exocrine pancreatic function and disease. *Progress in Gastroenterology,* 74:932, May 1978.

TABLE 70–5. BASES OF SIGNS AND SYMPTOMS OF ACUTE PANCREATITIS

Signs and Symptoms	Bases
Extreme epigastric or umbilical pain, extending into back and flank	Edematous distention of pancreatic capsule, local peritonitis due to enzyme release into peritoneum, ductal spasm; stimulated by increased secretion of enzymes by eating
Persistent vomiting	Pain induces stimulus to vomiting center; intestinal peristalsis reduced owing to localized peritonitis
Abdominal distention	Paralytic ileus of small bowel loop due to localized peritonitis
Fever	Release of pyrogens by tissue breakdown
Shock	Kinin, a vasodilator, activated by trypsin; inflammatory fluid lost into peritoneum; activated elastase dissolves elastic fibers of blood vessels to cause hemorrhage into peritoneum; multiple other factors implicated
Hypocalcemia, usually mild, though tetany is possible	Calcium may be deposited in areas of fat necrosis
Impaired glucose tolerance	Some degree of islet involvement
Jaundice	Common bile duct obstruction by pancreatic edema
Cardiac dysfunction	Possibly due to a myocardial depressant factor released by the pancreas.

Maintain Circulatory Volume and Replace Fluid and Electrolyte Loss. The fluid losses associated with acute pancreatitis may be massive. Since losses are primarily into areas that are not accessible (e.g., retroperitoneal space), the extent of the volume depletion may not be appreciated. Shock and anuria are the main causes of death. Colloid and large volumes of electrolyte solution are administered; central venous pressure and urine output are carefully monitored hourly. Intravenous mannitol may be given when hourly urine output drops, and the response is noted. Serum electrolytes are monitored and replacements determined accordingly; calcium gluconate is often indicated. The patient should be observed for the increased neural excitability of tetany. (See Chapter 12.)

Alleviate Pain. Frequent doses of meperidine (Demerol) are indicated rather than morphine and its derivatives, which increase sphincter of Oddi spasm. Extensive nursing measures are applied to relieve the severe pain. (See Unit XI.) In extreme cases, morphine may be necessary.

Reduce Pancreatic Stimulus. Multiple approaches are involved here. *Fasting* and insertion of a nasogastric tube connected to intermittent suction reduce acid stimulation of secretin. Nasogastric suction is routine in the management of patients with acute pancreatitis. Several recent studies, however, question its value in the management of mild pancreatitis, and some clinicians reserve it for those with severe forms of pancreatitis.[28] Anticholinergics, such as Pro-Banthine, have also been used to reduce pancreatic secretion and relax the sphincter of Oddi, primarily through their vagolytic action. Their value has also been questioned recently, and there is a trend to eliminate anticholinergics from the therapeutic regimen of pancreatitis patients. Antacids are administered every 2 hours in mild cases. The person convalescing from a severe attack will progress to hourly antacids once he or she is free of pain and has

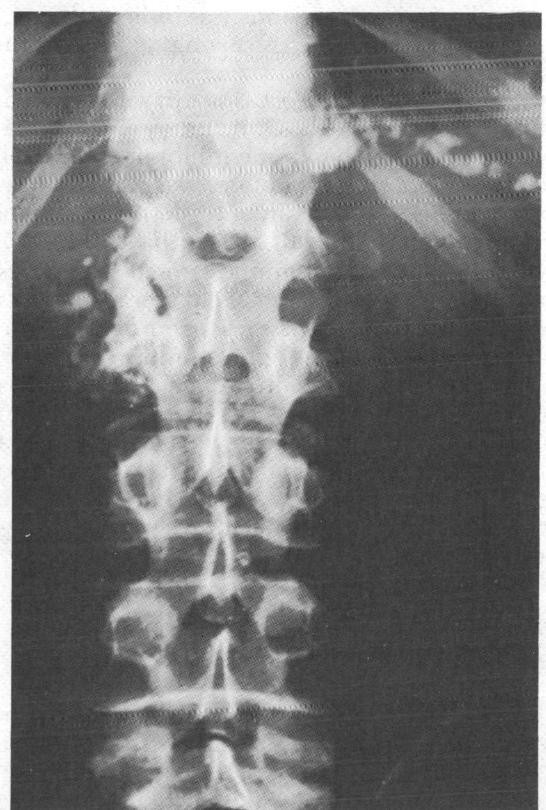

Figure 70–3. Chronic relapsing pancreatitis In this film of the upper abdomen the entire pancreas is shown outlined by extensive calcific deposits. (From Wintrobe, M. M., et al.: *Harrison's Principles of Internal Medicine,* 7th ed., New York: McGraw-Hill Book Company, 1977.)

normal peristalsis. Acetazolamide (Diamox) is occasionally administered to prevent carbonic anhydrase from catalyzing secretion of bicarbonate into pancreatic juice. With regression of symptoms and restoration of normal bowel tones, the patient is gradually started on clear liquids, progressed to an elemental diet, e.g., Vivonex, and given a diet that avoids pancreatic stimulus: low fat, no alcohol, no caffeine to stimulate gastric acid.

Prevent or Treat Infection. The use of prophylactic antibiotics in the hope of preventing pancreatic abscesses has been shown to be ineffective.[6] Associated infections, such as pneumonia, are treated with antibiotics as appropriate. There is controversy over the value of administering prophylactic antibiotics to critically ill patients who will be subjected to multiple invasive procedures. One concern is that infections that do occur in patients previously treated with antibiotics are much more virulent and do not respond to standard antibiotic therapy.

Prevent Hyperglycemia. Blood glucose is determined frequently, and fractional urine specimens may be tested for sugar and acetone. Insulin is given intravenously as indicated, especially if the patient is receiving glucose infusion.

Other measures are occasionally used to treat acute pancreatitis. These include peritoneal lavage and unproven enzyme inhibitors. Trasylol, one of the enzyme inhibitors, was initially purported to be of great value in the management of pancreatitis. Several studies have not supported this claim; and, in the United States, it is not in general use. Glucagon, because of its gastrin-inhibiting effect, has been used in the management of acute pancreatitis; however, its effectiveness is controversial.[6] Surgery is indicated when diagnosis is doubtful, when biliary tract disorder is suspected, or when a pseudocyst requires drainage. In patients who are moribund and when no alternatives are available a total pancreatectomy may be necessary.[19]

Clinical Intervention in Chronic Pancreatitis

Therapy focuses on (1) reducing pancreatic stimulus, (2) alleviating fat indigestion, (3) treating diabetes.

Reducing pancreatic stimulus is accomplished by a low-fat diet with avoidance of alcohol and caffeine; meals should be small. The dietary regimen in itself may prevent recurrence of chronic attacks after the initial acute episode. Oral antacids to reduce gastric acid stimulus to pancreatic juice secretion are frequently taken by the patient with chronic disease.

Alleviating fat indigestion is accomplished by several approaches. Three to 6 Gm. of pancreatic extracts, such as Pancreatin or Viokase, is taken with each meal. Fat losses in stool should diminish. Medium-chain triglyceride (MCT) losses may be replaced. Finally, supplementary fat-soluble vitamins and calcium are given.

Treating diabetes involves dietary and insulin control. See Chapter 72 for care of the patient experiencing diabetes.

Surgery for the patient with chronic disease is occasionally tried to revise the biliary or pancreatic ducts or sphincter of Oddi to reduce pressure and promote free flow of pancreatic juice. Some of the surgical procedures used are illustrated in Figure 70–4.

Efforts to control pain include surgical procedures to eliminate obstruction of the duct, diversion of gastric juices (gastroenterostomy), and division of autonomic nerve fibers when other modalities are unsuccessful. Although not generally mentioned in the literature, pain control techniques such as biofeedback, transcutaneous nerve stimulation, and similar methods may be of value for the patient with chronic pancreatitis. If the patient is relying on large doses of narcotics for pain control, a referral to a pain clinic is probably indicated. (See Unit XI.)

Prognosis in chronic pancreatitis is good if acute attacks decrease in frequency; replacement therapy for chronic fat indigestion permits a fairly normal life. If the patient continues to drink alcohol, prognosis is grim, with repeated attacks eventually causing death from shock or renal failure.

PSEUDOCYSTS

Pseudocyst (see Fig. 70–5) is the term given to accumulations of fluid that result from inflammation, necrosis, or hemorrhage. Pancreatic pseudocysts are a frequent complication of acute pancreatitis but occasionally may result from trauma. Typically, the cysts are located adjacent to the pancreas, rather than within it, and the majority are found in the region of the pancreatic tail. The size of a cyst may vary, but it is usually tender and palpable. Patients may complain of an aching type epigastric or left upper abdominal pain.

The *diagnosis* is aided by a history of pancreatitis, trauma, gallstones, etc. Laboratory and radiographic studies previously mentioned in the diagnosis of pancreatitis are of value in confirming the presence of a pseudocyst.

The major concern is that the pseudocyst will rupture, spilling its contents in the abdominal cavity, causing a chemical peritonitis. *Treatment* is drainage, surgical resection, or oversewing the affected area of the pancreas into a loop of the small bowel or a section of the stomach.

PANCREATIC CARCINOMA

Carcinoma of the exocrine pancreas is often fatal, accounting for 6 per cent of the deaths due to cancer each year in the United States. It is usually diagnosed in persons over the age of 40, with a higher incidence in men. A dramatic increase in the number of persons with pancreatic carcinoma has been noted. An association of pancreatic carcinoma and heavy smoking, industrial chemical carcinogens, and high fat, high calorie diets has been proposed. Robbins notes that heavy smokers have a risk for developing pancreatic cancer that is two to three times that for nonsmokers.[81] Chemists and other workers exposed to industrial chemicals such as beta-naphthylamine and benzidine may have an increased risk for developing pancreatic carcinoma.[81]

The *signs and symptoms* of pancreatic carcinoma largely depend upon the location of the tumor and the extent of metastasis. Sixty to 70 per cent of the tumors are located in the head of the pancreas. Tumors in this area are usually symptomatic, characterized primarily by biliary obstruction. Symptoms due to masses of the body and tail do not usually develop until the mass is quite large. When this occurs, metas

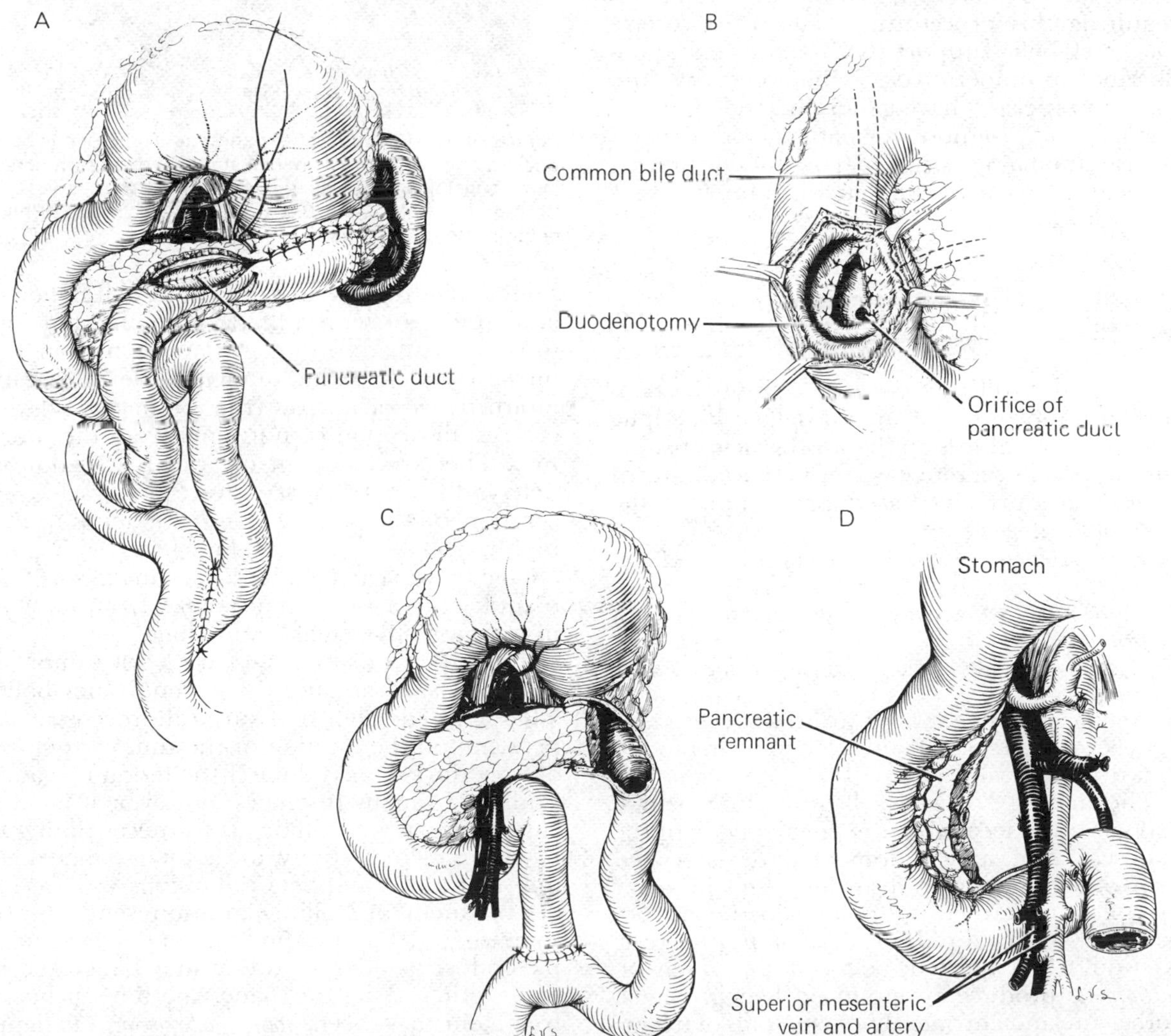

Figure 70–4. Operations for chronic pancreatitis *A:* Longitudinal pancreaticojejunostomy (Puestow). *B:* Sphincteroplasty. *C:* Caudal pancreaticojejunostomy (DuVal). *D:* 95% pancreatectomy. (From Reber, H. A , and L. W. Way: Pancreas. *In* Dunphy, S. E. and L. W. Way (Eds.): *Current Surgical Diagnosis and Therapy.* Los Altos: Lange Medical Publications, 1977.)

tasis to surrounding organs is often noted. The clinical features and laboratory findings associated with cancer of the biliary system and pancreas are outlined in Table 70–6.

Surgical treatment for tumors of the head of the pancreas is most effective; a pancreaticoduodenal resection is commonly performed if there is no evidence of metastasis. Bypass procedures, which will allow drainage of the common bile duct and pancreas, may be indicated in order to decrease symptoms. A partial pancreatectomy for cancer of the pancreatic head or ampulla involves a resection of the stomach, the duodenum, the common duct, and the remaining pancreatic stump. This procedure is often referred to as the Whipple. A total pancreatectomy may be done in selected patients. Persons requiring this procedure usually must receive total metabolic support (both exocrine and endocrine) postoperatively. Chemotherapy and radiation therapy have generally yielded dismal results. The prognosis for patients with pancreatic carcinoma is poor. A majority of the patients die within a year of the diagnosis; the five year survival rate is only 2 per cent.[81]

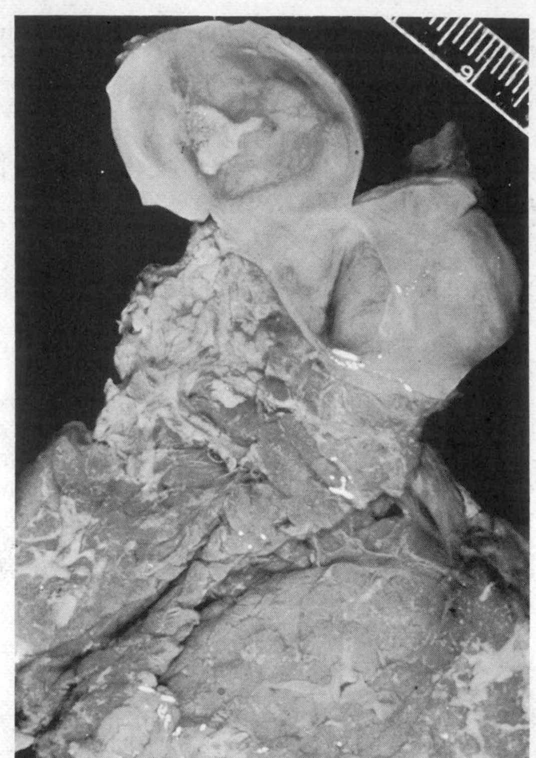

Figure 70–5. Pseudocyst of pancreas The cyst has been opened and contents drained. A small plaque of white calcium is visible in the wall. (From Robbins, S. L., and R. S. Cotran: *The Pathologic Basis of Disease.* 2nd ed., Philadelphia: W. B. Saunders Co., 1979.)

LESIONS OF THE PANCREATIC ISLETS

You will recall that the islet cells of the pancreas are the alpha, beta, and delta cells. Alpha cells produce glucagon, beta cells yield insulin, and delta cells secrete gastrin. Lesions of any of these cells cause increased production of the cell's normal secretion.

- *Hyperinsulinism* results from beta cell hyperfunction.
- Alpha cell overactivity results in *hyperglucagon syndrome.*
- Gastrin-secreting lesions cause *Zollinger-Ellison syndrome.*
- Another disorder, termed "pancreatic cholera," is believed to result from islet cell synthesis of vasoactive intestinal peptide (VIP).

The majority of islet cell tumors are benign and are often located in the tail and body of the pancreas. Metastatic lesions or those associated with other endocrine disorders, e.g., pituitary dysfunction (termed multiple endocrine adenomas), may be scattered throughout the pancreas. As would be expected, beta cell tumors, or *insulinomas,* produce pronounced hypoglycemia, both acute and chronic. The symptoms of hyperinsulinism are discussed in Chapter 72. Glucagon-secreting tumors precipitate hyperglycemia, which is also discussed in Chapter 72. Zollinger-Ellison syndrome, caused by delta cell hypersecretion of gastrin, is a life-threatening, but fortunately rare, disorder. As mentioned in the introduction, gastrin stimulates the release of hydrochloric acid from the stomach and decreases absorption of nutrients from the intestine. The large amount of gastrin secretion in delta cell tumors causes severe, protracted ulceration of the stomach and duodenum. The highly acid environment interferes with pancreatic lipase activity and causes malabsorption of nutrients. Death often results from massive upper gastrointestinal hemorrhage.

Treatment of alpha and beta cell tumors is primarily surgical once the patient is metabolically stabilized. Choice of surgical procedure depends upon the location of the tumor; removal of only the tumor is done if the lesion is readily evident. In many instances, however, it is difficult to isolate a tumor, thus necessitating a partial pancreatectomy or a total pancreatectomy for alpha and beta cell lesions.

Treatment of Zollinger-Ellison syndrome is somewhat different. Many patients have multiple endocrine adenomas that may be located in areas other than the pancreas. The primary treatment has been *total gastrectomy.* Patients having only partial gastrectomies have experienced a return of symptoms. Recently, cimetidine has been used in patients with Zollinger-

TABLE 70-6. CLINICAL FEATURES AND LABORATORY FINDINGS IN CANCER OF THE BILE DUCTS AND PANCREAS*

Clinical Feature	Cancer of Ampulla of Vater	Cancer of Bile Ducts	Cancer of Head of Pancreas	Cancer of Body and Tail of Pancreas
Pain	Absent—60% Moderate—40%	Absent—40% Moderate to severe—60%	Absent to mild—15% Moderate to severe—85%	Almost invariably present. Agonizing and boring. Often worse in back and accentuated when patient is supine.
Jaundice:				
Onset	Early	Early	Variable	Late to terminal.
Character	Progressive and marked—80% Fluctuating—20%	Progressive and marked—90% Fluctuating—10%	Progressive and marked	Mild to moderate.
Weight loss before onset of jaundice†	None to mild	None to moderate	Occasionally none, but often 10 to 20 lb.	Marked, 10 to 60 lb.
Fever and chills	20%	10%	None	May have low-grade fever. No chills.
Hepatomegaly	None to slight	Slight in some cases, but may be extreme	Moderate Marked only if metastases present	None to marked. Size depends on degree of metastatic involvement.
Enlarged gallbladder palpable or visible	50%	20%	50%	0.
Splenomegaly	None	None	None	Occasional.
Bile in stools and urobilinogen in urine	Absent—80% Fluctuating—20%	Absent—90% Fluctuating—10%	Absent	Present.
Occult blood in stools	82%	15%		Rare.

*Because of their anatomic proximity, advanced cancers of the ampulla of Vater, the bile ducts, and the pancreatic head at times cannot be distinguished clinically.

†All these cancers cause impressive weight loss sooner or later.

From Wintrobe, M. M., et al. (Eds.): *Harrison's Principles of Internal Medicine,* 7th ed., New York: McGraw-Hill Book Co., 1977.

Ellison syndrome and the results have been encouraging. Cimetidine is a very effective antacid that can be administered orally or parenterally. Since cimetidine is a fairly new medication, and is recommended primarily for short-term use, problems associated with long-term usage have not been completely identified. Patients with Zollinger-Ellison syndrome who are taking cimetidine must take their medication religiously. The importance of patient/family teaching in this regard cannot be overemphasized. Failure to maintain adequate levels may result in massive ulceration and hemorrhage.

TRAUMA

Both penetrating and blunt trauma of the pancreas are associated with a high mortality rate. Since the pancreas is a solid organ, it is more likely to be injured as a result of blunt trauma than would a hollow organ such as the stomach. Deceleration injuries, such as those associated with high speed automobile accidents, are a common source of pancreatic damage.

Evaluation of the patient with blunt abdominal trauma often includes a diagnostic peritoneal lavage. This involves the insertion of a dialysis catheter into the abdominal cavity and instillation of a liter of normal saline or Ringer's lactate. The patient is moved from side to side, and placed in Trendelenburg's position in order to disseminate the fluid throughout the abdominal cavity. The fluid is then drained from the abdominal cavity by gravity and analyzed for red blood cells, amylase, and bacteria. If the tests are positive, an exploratory laparotomy is usually performed. Because of its location deep in the abdominal cavity, the pancreas is seldom the only organ injured. When pancreatic injury is present in patients with other organ injury the mortaility is approximately 50 per cent. Because of the difficulties associated with repair, and the physiologic importance of its structures, injuries to the head of the pancreas are much more serious.

Initial surgical procedures used in management of pancreatic injury are control of hemorrhage, evacuation of hematomas, and debridement of nonviable tissue. Many patients require a subsequent surgical reconstruction.

CYSTIC FIBROSIS

Cystic fibrosis is a multi-system disorder primarily affecting infants and young children. However, recent improvements in the management of the pulmonary and pancreatic disorders associated with this disease may result in an increase in the number of adults with cystic fibrosis. The cause of cystic fibrosis is unknown; the disease is believed to be inherited as an autosomal recessive trait.

One of the *characteristics* of this disease is the formation of thick mucus, which causes obstruction in many organs. The viscous intestinal mucus may cause a thick meconium mass leading to ileus, intussusception, fecal impaction, and rectal prolapse. The pancreatic involvement includes replacement of acinar cells by cysts, fibrotic tissue, thick mucus, and fat. Obstruction of the biliary ducts from the mucus may cause cirrhosis and portal hypertension. Pulmonary complications such as bronchopneumonia and chronic bronchitis are common. The sweat of patients with cystic fibrosis contains a large amount of sodium, which can result in salt depletion during periods of warm weather.

The *diagnosis* of cystic fibrosis is made by a sweat test, in which the sodium concentration exceeds 60 mEq./liter, by evidence of exocrine insufficiency, and by the general clinical picture of the child, e.g., malnourished, steatorrhea, etc.

Treatment includes administration of pancreatic enzymes, a high protein, high calorie, low fat diet; replacement of fat-soluble vitamins, and a high salt intake. Prophylactic antibiotics and pulmonary support (e.g., expectorants, postural drainage, high humidity tents, etc.) are included in order to prevent pulmonary complications.

POSTOPERATIVE NURSING CARE

The person who returns from pancreatic surgery needs the routine postoperative care of vital sign assessment, pulmonary care, fluid management, wound assessment, and psychological support. In addition, it is important to have a clear idea of the surgical procedure. If there are multiple drains, especially external drains, it is often difficult to assess their proper function when location and purpose are obscure. Tubes or drains that are inserted for decompression need continual assessment for patency. If a T-tube or internal splint becomes non-functional, immediate attention is necessary to prevent leakage at the internal insertion site. Failure to prevent leakage may lead to peritonitis or fistula formation.

When pancreatic excision is done, the nurse needs to know whether the patient has sufficient pancreas left to maintain function, especially endocrine function. Exocrine loss is not an immediate postoperative problem, but this loss will necessitate lifelong enzyme replacement when the person returns to oral food ingestion.

It is important to remember that surgery for the complications of pancreatitis, trauma, and extensive internal shunt insertion may predispose the person to complications that may occur after discharge from the acute care setting. The patient and family need proper instructions for warning signs of complications. Other areas of health teaching that might need to be considered for the patient are home wound care, nutritional needs and diet counseling, knowledge of hyperglycemia (polyuria, polydipsia, polyphagia) and hypoglycemia, drug therapy (pancreatic enzymes), counseling for alcohol abuse, and discussion of supportive services to obtain assistance if necessary.

Newer advances in surgery and the advent of hyperalimentation allow more extensive pancreatic procedures. They also require nurses to develop new skills in assessing and monitoring these patients and to evolve new and creative teaching plans.

BIBLIOGRAPHY

1. Alpert, E., and K. Isselbacher: Tumors of the liver. *In* Thorn, G., et al.: (Eds.): *Harrison's Principles of Internal Medicine*, New York: McGraw-Hill, 1976.
2. Altshuler, A., and D. Hilden: The patient with portal hypertension. *Nursing Clinics of North America*, 12:317, June, 1977.
3. Ameriks, J. A., et al.: Hepatic cell adenomas, spontaneous liver rupture, and oral contraceptives. *Archives of Surgery*, 111:548, 1975.
4. Ammann, R. W., et al.: Pain relief by surgery in chronic pancreatitis? Relationship between pain relief, pancreatic dysfunction, and alcohol withdrawal. *Scandinavian Journal of Gastroenterology*, 14:209, Feb. 1979.
5. Arvanitakis, C., and A. R. Cooke: Diagnostic tests of exocrine pancreatic function and disease. *Progress in Gastroenterology*, 74:932, May, 1978.
6. Auslander, M. O., et al.: Drug therapy of acute pancreatitis. *Clinical Gastroenterology*, 8:219, Jan. 1979.
7. Baranowski, K.: Viral hepatitis. *Nursing 76*, 76:31, May 1976.
8. Barkin, J. S.: Ascites as a complication of chronic pancreatic disease. *Postgraduate Medicine*, 64:195, Sept. 1978.
9. Baum, J. K., et al.: Possible association between benign hepatomas and oral contraceptives. *Lancet*, 2:926, 1973.
10. Berk, J. E.: Facts and fallacies about gallbladder disease. *Consultant*, 17:25, April, 1977.
10a. Berkheiser, S. W.: Recurrent liver cell adenoma. *Gastroenterology*, 37:760, Dec., 1959.
11. Berkow, R., and J. H. Talbott: *The Merck Manual of Diagnosis and Therapy*, 13th ed. Rahway: Merck Sharp & Dohme Research Laboratories, 1977.

12. Bossone, M. C.: The liver: A pharmacologic perspective. *Nursing Clinics of North America,* 12:291, June, 1977.
13. Boyer, C., and S. Oehlberg: Interpretation and clinical relevance of liver function tests. *Nursing Clinics of North America*, 12:275, June, 1977.
14. Burke, M. D.: Hepatic function testing. *Postgraduate Medicine*, 64:177, Sept. 1978.
15. Byrne, J.: Liver function studies. Part 1: Introduction and bilirubin. *Nursing 77,* 7:12, Oct. 1977.
16. Byrne, J.: Tests that measure protein metabolism. *Nursing 77,* 7:13, Oct. 1977.
17. Byrne, J.: Using enzyme levels to assess liver function. *Nursing 78,* 8:50, Jan. 1978.
18. Collin, J.: Current state of transplantation of the pancreas. *Annals of the Royal College of Surgeons of England,* 60:21, Jan. 1978.
19. DaCosta, L., C. Hines, F. G. Moody, and N. A. Natkow: Meeting the challenge of pancreatitis. *Patient Care,* 11:71, September 15, 1977.
20. Daniel, E.: Chronic problems in rehabilitation of patients with Laennec's cirrhosis. *Nursing Clinics of North America*, 12:345, June, 1977.
21. Danzinger, R. G., et al.: Dissolution of cholesterol gallstones by chenodeoxycholic acid. *New England Journal of Medicine*, 286:1, Jan. 1972.
22. Davenport, H. W.: *A Digest of Digestion*, 2nd ed. Chicago: Year Book Medical Publishers, Inc., 1978.
22a. Delp, M. H., and Manning, R. T.: *Major's Physical Diagnosis.* Philadelphia: W. B. Saunders Co., 1975.
23. Detecting a poisoned pancreas. *Emergency Medicine*, 11:162, July, 1979.
24. Douglass, H., et al.: Guide to the diagnosis of pancreatic cancer. *Hospital Medicine*, 14:40, Jan. 1978.
25. Dunphy, J. E., and L. W. Way (Eds.): *Current Surgical Diagnosis and Treatment.* Los Altos: Lange Medical Publications, 1977.
26. Eddy, M. E.: Teaching patients with peripheral vascular disease. *Nursing Clinics of North America*, 12:151, June 1977.
26a. Edmondson, H. A., B. Henderson, B. Benton: Liver cell adenomas associated with the use of oral contraceptives. *New England Journal of Medicine*, 294:470, Feb. 1976.
27. Embolizing a bleeding liver. *Emergency Medicine*, 11:76, July, 1979.
28. Field, B. E., et al.: Nasogastric suction in alcoholic pancreatitis. *Digestive Diseases and Sciences*, 24:339, May, 1979.
29. Frank, D. J., and E. R. Schiff: Chronic hepatitis: Which cases should be treated? *Consultant*, 18:118, Nov. 1978.
30. Freeman, J. B., et al.: Cholecystokinin cholangiography and analysis of duodenal bile in the investigation of pain in the right upper quadrant of the abdomen without gallstones. *Surgery, Gynecology, and Obstetrics,* 140:371, 1975.
31. Gaines, R.: Surgery for gallbladder disease in the elderly. *Geriatrics*, 32:71, June, 1977.
32. Galambos, J. T.: *In* Conn, H. F. (Ed.): *Current Therapy, 1978.* Philadelphia: W. B. Saunders Co., 1978.
33. Ganong, W. F.: *Review of Medical Physiology*. 8th ed. Los Altos: Lange Medical Publications, 1977.
34. Gelfand, M. D.: Gallbladder disease: diagnostic guide. *Hospital Medicine*, 15:8, Jan. 1979.
35. Giacquinta, B.: Helping families face the crisis of cancer. *American Journal of Nursing*, 77:1585, October, 1977.
36. Glenn, F., and C. K. McSherry: Calculous biliary tract disease. *Current Problems Surgery*, 1:38, June, 1975.
37. Goldfarb, R. D., et al.: The chemical nature of a pancreatic cardiodepressant factor. *Circulatory Shock*, 4:95, 1977.
38. Graham, D. Y.: Choosing the best and safest ways to diagnose obstructive jaundice. *Consultant*, 18:80, Oct. 1978.
39. Grosberg, S. J., et al.: Specificity of serum amylase and amylase creatinine clearance ratio in the diagnosis of acute and chronic pancreatitis. *American Journal of Gastroenterology*, 72:41, July, 1979.
40. Guyton, A. C.: *Textbook of Medical Physiology*. 5th ed., Philadelphia: W. B. Saunders Co., 1976.
41. Hepatitis prophylaxis. *Emergency Medicine*, 10:238, Oct. 1978.
42. Hunter, G., and W. Gaisford: Guide to the diagnosis and management of obstructive jaundice. *Hospital Medicine*, 13:82, June, 1977.
43. Iber, F. L.: Axioms on biliary tract disease. *Hospital Medicine*, 15:51, June, 1979.
44. In abdominal trauma, check the pancreas. *Emergency Medicine*, 11:111, May, 1979.
45. Iwatsuki, S., and J. Ray: Hepatic complications. *Surgical Clinics of North America*, 6:57, Dec. 1977.
46. Jacobs, S. W., C. A. Francone, and W. J. Lossow: *Structure and Function in Man,* 4th ed. Philadelphia: W. B. Saunders Co., 1978.
47. Jacox, A. K.: Assessing pain. *American Journal of Nursing*, 79:895, May, 1979.
48. Javitt, N. B.: Hyperbilirubinemic and cholestatic syndromes. *Postgraduate Medicine*, 65:120, Jan. 1979.
49. Johnson, L. R. (Ed.): *Gastrointestinal Physiology*. St. Louis: C.V. Mosby Co., 1977.
50. Kaplan, A., and W. Ludwig: A guide to the diagnosis and management of cholelithiasis. *Hospital Medicine*, 12:111, April, 1976.
51. Kiefer, W. S., and J. C. Scott: Liver neoplasms and the oral contraceptives. *American Journal of Obstetrics and Gynecology*, 128:448, June, 1977.
52. Krupp, M. A. and M. J. Chatton (Eds.): *Current Medical Diagnosis & Treatment*. Los Altos: Lange Medical Publications, 1978.
53. LaVeen, H. H., et al.: Further experience with peritoneo-venous shunting for ascites. *Annals of Surgery*, 184:574, 1976.
54. Lawrence, A. G. and B. C. Ghosh: Total pancreatectomy for carcinoma of the pancreas. *American Journal of Surgery*, 133:244, Feb. 1977.
55. Loebl, S., et al.: *The Nurse's Drug Handbook*. New York: John Wiley & Sons, 1977.
56. Luft, F.: Antimicrobials in kidney and liver failure. *American Family Physician*, 14:92, Aug. 1976.
57. Macy, A. M.: Preventing hepatotoxicity in acetaminophen overdose. *American Journal of Nursing*, 79:301, Feb. 1979.
58. Manning, R. T.: Elevated serum alkaline. *Consultant*, 18:192, Oct. 1978.
59. Mattox, K. L.: Diagnosis and management of hepatic trauma. *Hospital Medicine*, 13:92, March 1977.
60. Mendenhall, C. L.: New hope in chronic active hepatitis. *Consultant*, 17:511, Jan. 1977.
61. McBride, C.: Cancer in the liver. *Hospital Medicine*, 13:32, Nov. 1977.
62. McElroy, D. B.: Nursing care of patients with viral hepatitis. *Nursing Clinics of North America*, 12:305, June, 1977.
63. McSherry, C. K.: Cholecystitis and cholelithiasis. *In* Conn, H. F. (Ed.): *Current Therapy, 1978.* Philadelphia: W. B. Saunders Co., 1978.
64. Motson, R., and L. Way: Differential diagnosis of gall-

bladder disease. *Hospital Medicine*, 13:26, March, 1977.
65. Nordgren, L., et al.: Hepatic and pancreatic dysfunction in anorexia nervosa: A report of 2 cases. *Biological Psychology*, 12:681, October, 1977.
66. *Nurse's Guide to Drugs: Nursing '79 Books Series*. Horsham: Intermed Communications Inc., 1979.
67. O'Connor, P., and H. Greene: Conquering cirrhosis of the liver. *Nursing '76*, 6:44, Nov. 1976.
68. Perez-Stable, E.: How to manage ascites in cirrhosis. *Consultant*, 17:75, Nov. 1977.
69. Peterson, A. M.: Acute viral hepatitis. *Nurse Practitioner*, 4:9, July-Aug. 1979.
70. Pickleman, J. R.: Biliary tract surgery. *Surgical Clinics of North America*, 57:1221, Dec. 1977.
71. Pierce, L.: Anatomy and physiology of the liver in relation to clinical assessment. *Nursing Clinics of North America*, 12:259, June, 1977.
72. Plotkin, S.: Antibiotics for typhoid carrier. *Consultant*, 17:96, April, 1977.
73. Polish, E.: Jaundice: Guide to diagnosis. *Hospital Medicine*, 17:96, April, 1977.
74. Price, A. P., and L. M. Wilson: *Pathophysiology: Clinical Concepts and Disease Processes*. New York: McGraw-Hill Book Co., 1978.
75. Price, H.: Halothane hepatitis. *American Family Physician*, 16:198, Sept. 1977.
76. Reber, H. A., and W. W. Lawrence: Pancreas. *In* Dunphy, J. E., and L. W. Way (Eds.): *Current Surgical Diagnosis and Treatment*, Los Altos: Lange Medical Publications, 1977.
77. Redinger, R. N.: Cholelithiasis — review of advances in research. *Postgraduate Medicine*, 65:56, June, 1979.
78. Regan, P. T.: Acute pancreatitis: diagnosis and treatment. *Hospital Medicine*, 15:30, Aug. 1979.
79. Reynolds, T. B.: Bleeding esophageal varices. *In* Conn, H. F. (Ed.): *Current Therapy, 1978*. Philadelphia: W. B. Saunders Co., 1978.
80. Richman, A.: Infectious hepatitis. *Hospital Medicine*, 14:72, March, 1978.
81. Robbins, S. L., and R. C. Cotran: *The Pathologic Basis of Disease*. Philadelphia: W. B. Saunders Co., 1979.
82. Rodman, M.: Controlling chronic liver disease. *R.N.*, 39:75, Feb. 1976.
83. Rudolph, R.: Benign and malignant liver neoplasms. *Postgraduate Medicine*, 63:56, March, 1978.
84. Sabiston, D. C. (Ed.): *Davis-Christopher Textbook of Surgery: The Biological Basis of Modern Surgical Practice*. Philadelphia: W. B. Saunders Co., 1977.
85. Sampliner, R. E.: How not to get hepatitis from your patients. *Consultant*, 19:49, Feb. 1979.
86. Schaffner, F.: Primary biliary cirrhosis as a collagen disease. *Postgraduate Medicine*, 65:97, June, 1979.
87. Schiff, L.: *Diseases of the Liver*, 4th ed. Philadelphia: J. B. Lippincott, 1975.
88. Schiff, L.: How to examine the jaundiced patient. *Consultant*, 17:64, April, 1977.
89. Seybert, P. L., et al.: New hope for ascites patients. *Nursing 79*, 9:25, Jan. 1979.
90. Seybert, P. L., et al.: The Leveen shunt: New hope for ascites patients. *Nursing 79*, 9:24, Jan. 1979.
91. Shanipour, N: The adult patient with bleeding esophageal varices. *Nursing Clinics of North America*, 12:331, June, 1977.
92. Shear, L.: Answers to questions on refractory ascites. *Hospital Medicine*, 13:25, Feb. 1977.
93. Sherlock, S.: Chronic hepatitis. *Postgraduate Medicine*, 65:81, June, 1979.
94. Sibrack, L. A., and I. H. Gouterman: Cutaneous manifestations of pancreatic diseases. *Cutis*, 21:763, June, 1978.
95. Snodgrass, P.: Diseases of the gallbladder and bile ducts. Thorn, G., et al. (Eds.): *Harrison's Principles of Internal Medicine*, 8th ed. New York: McGraw-Hill, 1976.
96. Snodgrass, P., and A. Americo: Diseases of the pancreas. *In* Thorn, G., et al. (Eds.): *Harrison's Principles of Internal Medicine*, 8th ed. New York: McGraw-Hill, 1976.
97. Stillman, M. J.: Nursing intervention in acute pancreatitis. *R.N.*, 41:67, Dec. 1978.
98. Swenson, S.: Benign and malignant liver neoplasms. *Hospital Medicine*, 14:71, May, 1978.
99. Thorn, G., et al.: *Harrison's Principles of Internal Medicine*, 8th ed. New York: McGraw-Hill, 1976.
100. Vana, J., et al.: Primary liver tumors and oral contraceptives. *Journal of American Medical Association*, 238:2154, 1977.
101. Warren, K., and G. Hoffman: Changing patterns in surgery of the pancreas. *Surgical Clinics of North America*, 56:615, June, 1976.
102. Warshaw, A. L., and A. F. Fuller: Specificity of increased renal clearance of amylase in diagnosis of acute pancreatitis. *New England Journal of Medicine*, 292:325, Feb. 1975.
103. Way, L. W.: Portal hypertension. *In* Dunphy, J. E., and L. W. Way, (Eds.): *Current Surgical Diagnosis and Treatment*. Los Altos: Lange Medical Publications, 1977.
104. Way, L. W., and J. E. Dunphy: Biliary tract. *In* Dunphy, J. E., and L. W. Way (Eds.): *Current Surgical Diagnosis and Treatment*. Los Altos: Lange Medical Publications, 1977.
105. Way, L. W., and R. C. Lim: Liver. *In* Dunphy, J. E. and L. W. Way (Eds.): *Current Surgical Diagnosis and Treatment*. Los Altos: Lange Medical Publications, 1977.
106. Williams, G. R.: Surgery of the aged: management of gastrointestinal problems. *Major Problems Clinical Surgery*, 17:111, June, 1975.
107. Willson, R. A.: Acute fulminant liver failure. *Hospital Medicine*, 13:8, Oct. 1977.
108. Wilson, S., and E. Passaro: Guide to the diagnosis and management of acute pancreatitis. *Hospital Medicine*, 12:64, Dec. 1976.
109. Wortzel, E., and A. Rogers: A hypothetical case of ascites. *Postgraduate Medicine*, 61:246, May, 1977.

UNIT XIX*

NURSING PEOPLE EXPERIENCING DISTURBANCES OF ENDOCRINE AND METABOLIC FUNCTION

INTRODUCTION AND STUDY GUIDE

Only within the last 50 years has endocrinology been regarded as a bona fide part of internal medicine. Before that time the study of glands and hormones appeared more linked with ritual and magic than with science and medicine. Patients with endocrine disorders were regarded as fascinating "oddities" rather than as people with treatable physiologic disturbances.

Today endocrinology is an exciting, highly respected, rapidly expanding area of study and practice. Because of the explosion of knowledge, nursing patients with endocrine disorders is now more challenging than ever. It is the nurse who teaches the patient about his or her disease and how to live successfully with it. Also, nurses often conduct the newest complicated diagnostic studies and administer the latest, potentially dangerous hormonal drugs. In order to succeed in these endeavors, the nurse must be, above all else, knowledgeable. Thus it is essential not only to obtain a basic understanding of the endocrine system and its disorders but also to keep abreast of new discoveries in the field.

As you read this unit, familiarize yourself with the definitions of the following terms:

endocrine gland
exocrine gland
hormone
tropic hormone
target gland
insulin
glucagon
somatostatin
carbohydrate catabolism
carbohydrate anabolism
insulin dependent diabetes
non–insulin dependent diabetes
hyperglycemic
hyperosmolar
nonketotic coma
fractional urines
lipodystrophies
hyperglycemia
hypoglycemia
ketoacidosis
insulin reaction
diabetic retinopathy
thyroxine
triiodothyronine
thyroid-stimulating hormone (TSH)
thyroid-releasing hormone (TRH)
euthyroid
hypothyroidism
hyperthyroidism
goiter

*David Johnson, M.D., critically reviewed and assisted with the revision of this unit. Jean Espenshade, R.N., M.N., critically reviewed the nursing care given to diabetic patients, as discussed in Chapter 72.

thyroiditis
thyrotoxicosis
exophthalmos
hyperparathyroidism
hypoparathyroidism
osteitis fibrosa cystica
nephrocalcinosis
adrenal medulla
adrenal cortex
catecholamines
steroids
corticoids
pheochromocytoma
hypocorticism
hypercorticism
virulism
pseudohermaphroditism
neurohypophysis
adenohypophysis
hyperpituitarism
hypopituitarism
gigantism
acromegaly
dwarfism
hypophysectomy
multiple endocrine abnormalities (MEA)
long-acting thyroid stimulator (LATS)
melanocyte-stimulating hormone (MSH)

After studying this unit, you should be able to do the following:

1. Set up a program of instruction for an insulin-dependent diabetic patient: (a) help the patient draw up a week of menus from the American Diabetes Association food lists, (b) teach the techniques of self-administered insulin, (c) provide guidance concerning foot care and the care of cuts and abrasions; (d) instruct the patient in the techniques of urine testing.

2. Recognize the signs of underdosage and overdosage of the following hormonal drug preparations: insulin, thyroid hormone, corticosteroids, estrogens, androgens, vasopressin tannate.

3. Summarize the preoperative and postoperative nursing care of patients undergoing the following surgeries: thyroidectomy, parathyroid gland resection, unilateral adrenalectomy, bilateral adrenalectomy, hypophysectomy, pancreatectomy.

CHAPTER 71

INTRODUCTORY CONCEPTS

NORMAL ANATOMY AND PHYSIOLOGY OF THE ENDOCRINE SYSTEM

The Endocrine Glands

The word "gland" is derived from the Latin *glans,* meaning "acorn." The word is thus an appropriate symbol of the powerful effect that small organs, such as the pituitary, have on the total function of the body.

There are two types of glands: exocrine glands and endocrine glands. *Exocrine glands* release their secretions through *ducts,* either inside the body or onto the skin. Examples of exocrine glands include the salivary, sebaceous, and sweat glands; the liver, gastric, and intestinal glands; the pancreas (which is also in part an endocrine gland); the prostate; and the mammary and lacrimal glands. In contrast, the *endocrine glands* discharge their secretions (which are called hormones) *directly* into the blood stream rather than through ducts. The endocrine glands include the islets of Langerhans in the pancreas; the gonads; the adrenal, pituitary, thyroid, and parathyroid glands, thymus; and the pineal gland (see Fig. 71–1.) Although each endocrine gland has its own unique independent functions, the various glands are also *interdependent.* Thus the release of hormones from one gland influences the release of hormones from other glands and vice versa. The influence of the endocrine glands upon each other helps to maintain optimum hormonal levels, thereby promoting homeostasis.

Hormones and Their Functions

The term *hormone* is derived from the Greek term *hormon,* which means "to set in motion." Hormones set in motion the various processes that govern our lives — physical and intellectual growth, puberty, reproduction, metabolism, personality development, reactions to stress from both the external and internal milieu, and the maintenance of homeostasis. Although hormones themselves do not initiate the above processes, they act as chemical envoys, creating an intricate chain of communication which links one body system with another, thereby controlling and integrating the body's functions. In its communicative and integrative roles, the endocrine system resembles the nervous system. However, the nervous system sends its messages more swiftly than do the endocrine glands; also neural effects usually are more rapid in onset, shorter-lived, and more localized.

In terms of their *chemical nature,* hormones are classified as follows:

- Biogenic amines (epinephrine, norepinephrine).
- Amino acids (thyroxine).
- Peptides (vasopressin, or antidiuretic hormone).
- Proteins (pituitary growth hormone, parathyroid hormone).
- Steroids (aldosterone, cortisol, androgenic hormones).
- Prostaglandins

The major specific *functions* of each of the endocrine glands and its hormones are delineated in Table 71–1. Note that each of the endocrine glands affects organs and tissues which are far removed from its location in the body; e.g., oxytocin, which is released from the posterior lobe of the pituitary gland located in the brain, causes uterine contractions. Also note that several glands (the thyroid, gonads, and adrenal cortex) are under control of the "master" pituitary gland. The pituitary hormones which govern the secretion of hormones from other glands are called *tropic* hormones. On the other hand, the glands which are influenced by tropic hormones are called *target* glands. As explained later, the target glands also control the secretion of tropic hormones from the pituitary gland by means of negative feedback.

Characteristics of Hormones

Although each endocrine gland possesses its own unique attributes, all endocrine glands share in common the following characteristics:

- Endocrine glands secrete hormones *cyclically* (e.g., circadian) and in response to certain body and environmental rhythms. For example, estrogen levels rise and fall in a predictable fashion during the menstrual cycle. Also, blood levels of adrenocortical hormones are low in the night, rise during the morning, and then drop back to lower levels in the evening.

- Endocrine glands control the *rate* of cellular activities; they do not in themselves initiate biochemical changes.
- Hormones are secreted in *minute* concentrations; however, even tiny amounts of a hormone can have far-reaching effects on body structure and function.

Hormonal Regulation

The release of hormones from their parent glands is controlled by both chemical and neurologic factors.

Chemical Control. Hormonal blood levels are controlled in part by *negative feedback.* Thus a rise or fall in the blood level of one hormone can cause an increase or decrease in the blood level of another hormone. For example, an increased secretion of adrenocorticotropic hormone (ACTH) from the anterior pituitary gland stimulates a rise in the release of cortisol from the adrenal cortex, which in turn causes a decrease in the release of ACTH and so forth. In addition, blood levels of substances *other than hormones* affect hormonal secretion. For example, you recall from Unit V, Chapter 12, that the

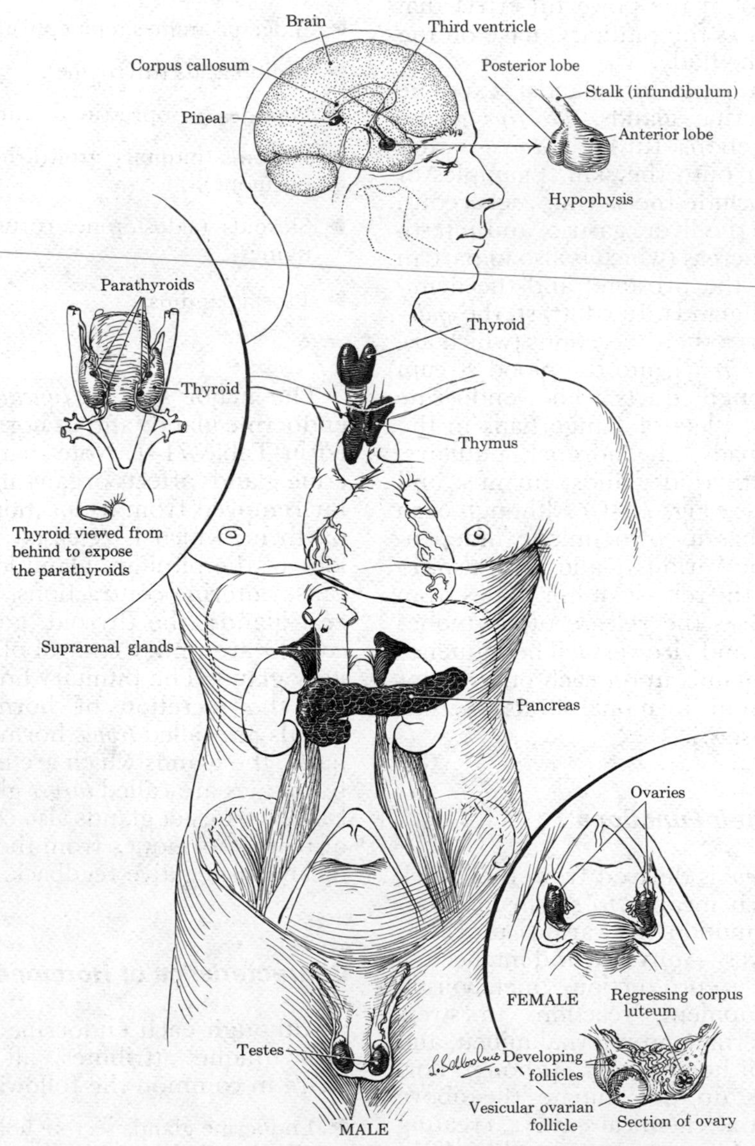

Figure 71–1. Diagram of the endocrine system. (From *Dorland's Illustrated Medical Dictionary,* 25th ed. Philadelphia: W. B Saunders Co., 1974.)

calcium level in the blood regulates the release of parathormone (PTH) from the parathyroid glands. Also, the release of insulin from the islets of Langerhans in the pancreas depends upon blood glucose levels.

Neurologic Control. Both the autonomic nervous system and central nervous system aid in hormonal regulation. The central nervous system reacts to stimuli of all types from both the external and internal milieu. These reactions are transmitted to the hypothalamus (a vital part of the central nervous system), which in turn conveys impulses to the pituitary gland. Pituitary hormonal secretions next stimulate appropriate target glands, which results in the release of more hormones.

In addition, two endocrine glands—the adrenal medulla and the posterior pituitary—are of neural origin. Should these two glands be destroyed or removed, their functions are taken over by the nervous system.

TABLE 71–1. FUNCTIONS OF ENDOCRINE GLANDS

Gland	Hormone	Action of Hormone
Pituitary		
Anterior lobe	Growth hormone (GH)	Stimulates growth of body tissues and bones
	Prolactin	Stimulates mammary tissue growth and lactation
	Thyrotropic hormone (TSH)	Stimulates thyroid gland
	Gonadotropic hormones (LH and FSH)	Affect growth, maturity, and functioning of primary and secondary sex organs
	Adrenocorticotropic hormone (ACTH)	Stimulates steroid production by the adrenal cortex
	Melanocyte-stimulating hormone (MSH)	May stimulate adrenal cortex; may affect pigmentation
Posterior lobe	Antidiuretic hormone (ADH, vasopressin)	Promotes reabsorption of water by the distal tubules and collecting ducts of the kidney, thus decreasing urine output
	Oxytocin	Stimulates ejection of milk from mammary alveoli into the ducts; stimulates uterine contractions; may possibly be involved in the transport of sperm in the reproductive tract of the female
Thyroid	Thyroxin Triiodothyronine	Stimulates metabolism (catabolic phase)
	Thyrocalcitonin	Lowers serum calcium level
Parathyroid	Parathormone (PTH)	Regulates calcium and phosphate levels
Adrenal		
Cortex	Hormones divided into three main groups:	
	Glucocorticoids	Tend to increase the amount of sugar in the blood
	Mineralocorticoids	Tend to increase serum sodium and lower serum potassium
	Androgens (male hormones)	Govern certain secondary sex characteristics
		All corticoids are important for defense against stress or injury
Medulla	Epinephrine (Adrenalin)	Elevates blood pressure; converts glycogen to glucose when needed by muscles for energy; increases heart rate; dilates bronchioles
Ovaries	Estrogens and progesterone	Stimulate development of secondary sex characteristics; effect repair of the endometrium after menstruation
Testes	Testosterone	Essential for normal functioning of male reproductive organs; stimulates development of male secondary sex characteristics
Pancreas		
Islets of Langerhans	Insulin	Promotes metabolism of carbohydrates, protein, and fat
	Glucagon	Mobilizes glycogen stores, thus raising the blood glucose level

ABNORMALITIES OF THE ENDOCRINE SYSTEM: AN OVERVIEW

In essence, endocrine diseases result from hormonal imbalance. Traditionally, endocrine disorders have been classified as arising from either a deficiency or an overabundance of a particular hormone or hormones. However, this way of viewing endocrine disease constitutes a gross oversimplification of a highly complex subject. As Christy points out: "In the light of the discoveries made during the last two decades, it is no longer enough to think of endocrine disease simply as too much or too little hormone."[25] For this reason, Christy suggests using the following comprehensive clinical classification.*

1. *Primary hyperfunction of endocrine glands:* major causes include benign tumors and hyperfunctional states which are not linked with tumor growth. Malignant hormone-secreting tumors are uncommon.
2. *Primary hypofunction of endocrine glands:* causes include congenital absence of the gland, tumor growths which destroy the gland, and infections. In addition, some authorities speculate that certain hypofunctional disorders of the thyroid, parathyroid, and adrenal glands may be autoimmune in nature.
3. *Secondary failure of endocrine glands:* hypofunction of the gonads, thyroid, and adrenal cortex may develop secondary to *pituitary* insufficiency.
4. *Functional disorders of the endocrine glands:* endocrine disease develops not only secondary to pituitary disorders but also as a consequence of nonendocrine disease. For example, hyperparathyroidism may complicate renal failure, and hyperaldosteronism may develop secondary to cirrhosis of the liver.
5. *Failure of an end-organ to respond to a hormone:* for example, the bones may fail (for unknown reasons) to grow linearly despite the administration of human growth hormone.
6. *Production by an endocrine gland of an abnormal or unusual hormone:* these congenital disorders are classified as *inborn errors of metabolism.* Examples include congenital adrenal hyperplasia and goitrous cretinism.
7. *Production of a hormone by a nonendocrine organ:* ectopic secretion of hormones by nonendocrine tumors is a fairly common cause of glandular hyperfunction. Tumors which are most frequently linked with ectopic syndromes are cancers of the lung, thymus, and pancreas.
8. *Prostaglandins.* The status of prostaglandins is as yet obscure. They are 20-carbon, unsaturated, cyclic fatty acids which are found in most tissues and body fluids. The action of the 16 prostaglandins which have been isolated appears to be hormonal. However, it is not clear whether these fatty acids are truly hormones.
9. *Iatrogenic endocrine disease:* causes include (a) the prescribed administration of hormones either for hormonal replacement therapy or as a pharmacologic method for controlling inflammation, obesity, infertility, and so forth; (b) surgical removal of a gland; and (c) destruction of a gland by irradiation.

*Classification adapted from Christy.[25] p. 1663.

Nonspecific Symptoms of Endocrine Disease

The manifestations of endocrine disease are numerous and varied. Nonspecific symptoms which may develop in some endocrine disorders include the following

- Growth abnormalities: growth may be delayed, stunted (dwarfism), excessive (gigantism), or inappropriate (acromegaly).
- Weakness and exhaustion.
- Appetite changes (polyphagia or anorexia).
- Blood pressure abnormalities (hypertension or hypotension).
- Polyuria and polydipsia.
- Renal colic and stones.
- Tetany, paresthesias, and muscle cramps.
- Bone and joint disease.
- Untoward changes in appearance.
- Abnormal skin pigmentation.
- Hirsutism.
- Personality changes (patients may be nervous and restless or lethargic, depending upon the nature of the imbalance).
- Sexual disturbances (impotence, menstrual irregularity, or infertility).

NURSING CARE OF PATIENTS WITH ENDOCRINE DISEASES: AN OVERVIEW

Patients with endocrine disorders endure many problems and experience multiple needs. For example, some suffer from a loss of self-esteem due to an unusual appearance; they may experience family problems and rejection from loved ones due to personality changes; they may feel exhausted, debilitated, disgusted, and totally unable to cope with the stresses of life. Moreover, these persons must endure numerous exacting diagnostic tests, and some face the possibility of undergoing dangerous surgery. Others are faced with the often bitter realization that they must permanently change their diet, activities, and life style. How can the nurse help these patients cope with such serious problems?

First of all, the nurse must *offer genuine emotional support* to both the patient and significant others. This is not always easy to do, because patients with endocrine diseases may be lethargic, agitated, forgetful, depressed, or even frankly psychotic. Patients may also be afraid of the final consequences of their disease, and their fear may be manifested toward others in the guise of anger, hostility, rejection, and so forth. It is important to recognize that the patient's behavior, however bizarre, is probably a symptom of the illness and that the personality and behavior may return to normal with treatment.

Secondly, the nurse is usually responsible for *collecting specimens for laboratory tests.* It is essential to begin and end all tests on time, to preserve specimens correctly, and to instruct the patient and other ward personnel concerning their role in conducting tests.

Thirdly, the nurse is responsible for *administering hormones to patients with hormonal deficiencies.* When giving a particular hormone, always know the symptoms of underdosage and overdosage. The dosage of hormones must often be readjusted to meet the changing needs, tempos, and stresses of a person's life, or serious imbalances occur. For example, a diabetic's insulin dosage must be increased when food intake increases or infection develops.

Finally, the nurse must *act as a teacher.* Many patients with endocrine disorders undergo a lifelong program of therapy. It is the nurse's task to teach patients the basics of self-care, e.g., dietary requirements, self-administration of drugs, personal hygiene, and indications of hormonal imbalance. With help and guidance, the majority of patients with chronic endocrine disorders can learn to regulate their lives and successfully live with their disease.

CHAPTER 72

NURSING PATIENTS WITH ENDOCRINE DISORDERS OF THE PANCREAS

PHYSIOLOGY OF THE PANCREAS

The pancreas, a large, fish-shaped organ which lies behind and inferior to the stomach and liver, is both an exocrine and an endocrine gland. You recall that the *exocrine* role of the pancreas is carried out by cells within the walls of the tubular and acinar units of the gland; these cells secrete enzymes which catabolize the *digestion* of *proteins, carbohydrates,* and *fats* (see Unit XVIII, Chapter 65).

The *endocrine* functions of the pancreas are controlled by the *islets of Langerhans;* the islets, which contain alpha and beta cells, are scattered throughout the pancreatic tissues. The two hormones (insulin and glucagon) secreted by the islets play a vital role in the control of carbohydrate metabolism. *Insulin,* which is synthesized by the beta cells, also plays a role in fat and protein metabolism. It is also a powerful *hypoglycemic* agent; i.e., it acts to lower blood sugar levels by promoting the passage of glucose into the cells. Conversely, *glucagon,* which is synthesized by alpha cells, is a *hyperglycemic* agent; i.e., it raises blood sugar by promoting the conversion of glycogen (the principal form in which carbohydrates are stored in mammals) to glucose within the liver. In the section below and throughout this chapter, we will study the effects of these powerful hormones more closely.

Hormonal Factors Regulating Carbohydrate Metabolism

The hormones which play a role in the regulation of carbohydrate metabolism include the following: (a) insulin, (b) glucagon, (c) adrenocorticotropic hormone (ACTH), (d) corticosteroids, (e) epinephrine, and (f) thyroid hormone. The role of each hormone is considered below.

Insulin and Glucagon. The two principal hormones controlling carbohydrate metabolism are insulin and glucagon, both of which are small proteins. *Insulin,* the hypoglycemic factor, plays a key role in carbohydrate, fat, and protein metabolism; more specifically, it performs the following functions:

- ▶ Stimulates the active transport of glucose into muscle and adipose tissue cells. When insulin levels are inadequate, glucose remains outside of the cells, which in turn causes the blood sugar concentration to rise above normal. The exact means by which insulin promotes intracellular transport remains unknown.
- ▶ Regulates the rate at which carbohydrates are burned by cells for energy.
- ▶ Promotes the conversion of glucose to glycogen for storage, but inhibits the conversion of glycogen to glucose.
- ▶ Promotes the conversion of fatty acids into fat which can be stored as adipose tissue, but inhibits the breakdown of adipose tissue, the mobilization of fats, and the conversion of fat to glucose.
- ▶ Stimulates protein synthesis within the tissues, but inhibits the conversion of protein into glucose.

In sum, insulin actively *promotes* those processes which *lower* blood sugar levels (e.g., the transport of glucose into cells and the conversion of glucose to glycogen) and *inhibits* those processes which *raise* blood sugar levels (e.g., the conversion of glycogen and proteins into glucose).

The *rate* of insulin secretion by the beta cells is regulated by the amount of sugar in the blood. When the blood sugar level *rises,* the islet cells are stimulated to release increased amounts of insulin into the blood, which accelerates glucose transport into the cells and glucose conversion into glycogen. As the blood sugar level *falls,* insulin release from the islets slows until the blood sugar drops below normal. If food is absorbed, the islets again release insulin, and so forth.

When insulin is *deficient,* the blood sugar level remains abnormally high, and *diabetes mellitus* eventually develops. When there is an *excess* of insulin, blood sugar levels drop dangerously low and *insulin-induced hypoglycemia* (so-called "insulin shock") develops.

In contrast to insulin, *glucagon* promotes a *rise*

in blood sugar, whenever glucose levels drop too low. Glucagon causes hyperglycemia by promoting the conversion of glycogen to glucose. Glucagon imbalance (excess or deficiency) is rare.

To illustrate the opposing but complementary roles of insulin and glucagon, consider what happens to the blood sugar after eating a meal. Note in Figure 72–1 that when one eats breakfast at 8:00 in the morning, around 8:15 the blood sugar starts to rise, and insulin release begins. By approximately 9:00 A.M. the blood sugar level will have reached its peak, and insulin secretion will stop shortly afterwards. By 10:00 A.M. the blood sugar will have dropped back to low normal, because insulin will have promoted glucose transport into the cells and glucose conversion into glycogen and fatty deposits. If nothing is eaten again until noon or 1:00 P.M., the body (with the aid of glucagon) will convert glycogen back to glucose, and this glucose will then be used by the cells for in-between meal energy. If no more food is eaten until 8:00 that evening, the body will obtain energy by converting adipose tissue into glucose.

What factors are necessary for the synthesis and release of insulin and glucagon? Production of these essential hormones is dependent upon the following three requirements:

▶ A *healthy pancreas* with actively functioning alpha and beta cells.
▶ A *diet adequate in protein:* remember that both insulin and glucagon are protein substances.
▶ *Normal potassium* (K^+) levels; for unknown reasons, hypokalemia (abnormally low K^+ levels) results in diminished insulin production.

When either insulin or glucagon secretion is inadequate to meet the body's needs, the missing hormone may be administered *parenterally.* These two hormones cannot be given orally because they are both inactivated within the gastrointestinal tract by proteolytic enzymes.

Other Hormonal Factors. Although insulin and glucagon play the predominant roles in carbohydrate regulation, the following hormones also influence blood sugar levels:

▶ *Adrenocorticotropic hormone* (ACTH) and the *glucocorticoids* of the adrenal cortex raise the blood sugar by stimulating the conversion of fat and protein into glucose. These hormones are released whenever the body is subjected to stress or blood sugar levels drop abnormally low.
▶ *Epinephrine,* another hormone released under stress, stimulates a rise in blood sugar by promoting the conversion of glycogen to glucose.
▶ *Thyroid hormone* can raise or lower the blood sugar. Under normal conditions, thyroid hormone (like insulin) promotes the utilization of glucose for energy. However, under starvation conditions, thyroid hormone promotes the conversion of fats and proteins to glucose for energy.

Normal Carbohydrate Metabolism

Carbohydrates (which are compounds of carbon, hydrogen, and oxygen) are the body's *preferred fuel* as well as its most immediate source of energy. The metabolism of carbohydrates involves a number of intricate chemical processes which are dependent upon the presence of insulin, glucagon, and, to a lesser extent, the other hormones discussed above. In review, carbohydrate metabolism, like all forms of metabolism, has a consumption phase (catabolism) and a synthesis phase (anabolism). *Carbohydrate catabolism* is the process by which the body breaks carbohydrates down into smaller molecules and uses the energy which is released in the process. The three major forms of carbohydrate catabolism are listed below.

1. *Glycolysis,* the initial process in carbohydrate catabolism, is the breakdown of sugars into simpler compounds. As a result of glycolysis, a molecule of glucose is split, and its energy is partially released.
2. The *Krebs cycle,* which completes the mechanism of carbohydrate catabolism, is a series of chemical changes which results in the total breakdown of the glucose molecule into carbon dioxide, water, and energy.
3. *Glycogenolysis* — the conversion of glycogen to glucose — takes place whenever blood sugar levels drop abnormally low. As stated earlier, this process depends upon the presence of glucagon.

Carbohydrate anabolism, on the other hand, is a process by which molecules of carbohydrate, fat, or protein are chemically converted into glycogen and stored principally within the liver and muscle. The process of anabolism, unlike catabolism, does not release energy but instead

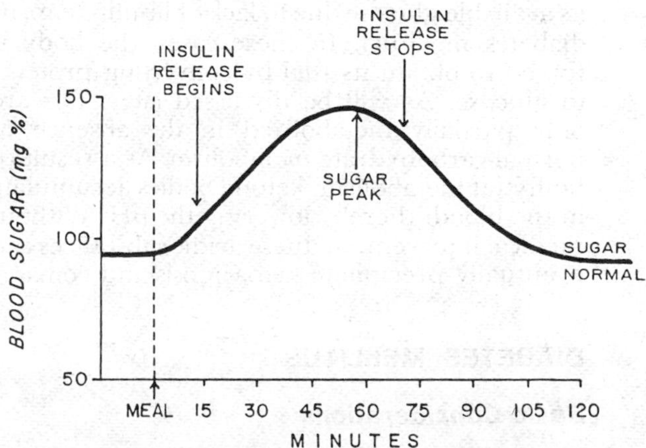

Figure 72–1. The effect of insulin upon blood sugar following meals. (From Crampton, J. H., et al.: *Instructions for the Diabetic Patient,* 9th ed. Seattle: The Mason Clinic.)

uses the body's energy. The two biochemical processes which are involved in carbohydrate anabolism are as follows:

1. *Glycogenesis* (the reverse of glycogenolysis) is the conversion of glucose, fructose, or galactose into glycogen; as you recall, this process depends upon the release of insulin.
2. *Gluconeogenesis* is the transformation of fats and proteins (i.e., noncarbohydrate materials) into glucose or glycogen for use by cells as fuel. This process is employed by the body whenever carbohydrates are not available for use as fuel.

In sum, carbohydrate metabolism involves (a) the active transport of glucose into cells and the release of energy; (b) the storage of that glucose which is not immediately needed for energy as glycogen and as fat; (c) the conversion of glycogen back to glucose whenever blood glucose drops; and (d) the conversion of fats and proteins to glucose or glycogen, whenever these two carbohydrate substances are depleted and energy is needed.

It is apparent from this discussion that carbohydrate metabolism is intricately linked with protein and fat metabolism. Carbohydrates, proteins, and fats can all be burned by the body for energy. However, as we emphasized earlier, carbohydrates are the body's *preferred* source of fuel. This means that the body will metabolize carbohydrates rather than fats and proteins, provided (a) carbohydrate intake is adequate; (b) sufficient insulin is present to promote the passage of glucose into the cells; and (c) reserve stores of glycogen are present. However, carbohydrates *cannot* supply the body's energy needs (a) when the blood glucose is low and glycogen stores have been depleted (e.g., during starvation diets), or (b) when the body is unable to use its available glucose due to lack of insulin (e.g., in diabetes mellitus). In these cases, the body is forced to obtain its fuel by converting proteins to glucose. As will be discussed later, fats are only partially metabolized in the absence of normal carbohydrate metabolism. As a result of faulty fat metabolism, ketone bodies accumulate in the blood, thereby lowering the pH. Without medical intervention, these acidic substances can eventually precipitate ketoacidosis and coma.

DIABETES MELLITUS

Basic Considerations

Diabetes mellitus is a chronic disorder of carbohydrate metabolism. The major feature is an imbalance between insulin supply and insulin demand. Too little insulin is available, either because the pancreas produces subnormal amounts, or because the person's body requires abnormally high amounts (*e.g.,* in the obese person). Thus there is impaired utilization of insulin by body cells, resulting in hyperglycemia. Diabetes mellitus also causes disturbances of protein and fat metabolism, which can lead to symptoms of ketosis and acidosis if not controlled. Diabetic vascular lesions can lead to blindness, heart disease, kidney disease and peripheral vascular disease. Neuropathy may also be a late complication.

The term *diabetes* is derived from a Greek word which means "something which goes through," or a *siphon;* thus the term "diabetes" is applied to diseases which are characterized by *polyuria* (overproduction of urine).* The term *mellitus* is taken from the Latin *mel,* which means "honey," thereby describing the "honeyed" or sweet taste of the urine. The urine is "sweet" in diabetes mellitus because, in the absence of sufficient insulin, sugar accumulates in the blood and eventually spills into the urine.

The exact cause of diabetes mellitus is unknown. There are two common types of diabetes: *insulin dependent* (juvenile diabetes) and *non-insulin dependent* (maturity onset diabetes). These two disease forms are compared and contrasted in Table 72–1.

Diabetes mellitus can also develop as a result of pancreatitis, pancreatic tumors, or hemochromatosis. Therapeutic agents such as thiazide diuretics, steroids or estrogens can cause abnormal glucose tolerance with glycosuria. Similarly, obesity, hyperthyroidism, acromegaly, hyperadrenocorticism, pregnancy, infection, and stress are all conditions which increase the body's need for insulin. If this need cannot be met, hyperglycemia and glycosuria will result.

Incidence and Predisposing Factors

Diabetes mellitus is one of the most common endocrine diseases, affecting several million people in the United States. Diabetes with its complications is the third leading cause of death by disease in the U.S., resulting in more than 300,000 deaths each year. The disease decreases average life expectancy by about one third. Even when diabetes does not kill, it can produce major permanent disabilities. Also, diabetes (with all its complications) in the United States alone costs society billions of dollars annually. Additionally, there are a large number of undiagnosed diabetics as well as potential diabetics. In general, the undiagnosed diabetics are usually non-insulin dependent diabetics who may have few or no major symptoms.

---

*Diabetes *insipidus,* which is characterized by the excretion of large amounts of dilute urine, is described on p. 1619.

TABLE 72–1. A COMPARISON OF INSULIN DEPENDENT AND NON-INSULIN DEPENDENT DIABETES

Factors	Insulin Dependent Diabetes	Non-Insulin Dependent Diabetes
Synonyms	Juvenile diabetes, growth-onset diabetes, labile diabetes	Adult-onset diabetes, maturity-onset diabetes, senile diabetes or mild diabetes
Age at onset	May occur at any age; usually appears before age 15	Usually occurs in persons over the age of 40
Possible etiology	*Absolute* deficiency of insulin caused by inadequacy of pancreatic islets	*Relative* insulin deficiency possibly caused by insulin antagonists, or by excessive demands for insulin due to obesity, persistent stress, etc.
Severity	Usually more severe; little or no circulating insulin may be present	Usually mild; some circulating insulin present
Therapeutic control	Insulin injections and careful planning of diet essential	Insulin administration often unnecessary; may be controlled by diet alone or in combination with oral hypoglycemic agents.
Emergency conditions	Diabetic ketoacidosis; hypoglycemic reactions	Hyperglycemic, hyperosmolar, non-ketotic coma
Sequelae	Vascular disease and neuropathy often develop	Same as insulin dependent diabetes

The risk of developing diabetes is greatly increased when a person has relatives with diabetes. The study of identical twins by Tattersall and Pyke[116a] in Table 72–2 indicates that when one twin has diabetes, the chances of the other twin developing diabetes are very high. However, the hereditary predispostion to developing diabetes is more often associated with non-insulin dependent diabetes. This is seen in the greater incidence of concordance (both twins having diabetes) in cases where diabetes was diagnosed over the age of 40 years.

As shown in Figure 72–2 most people who develop diabetes after the age of 40 are overweight. People who are overweight require more insulin to metabolize the food they eat, regardless of whether they are diabetic. Hyperglycemia develops when the pancreas is unable to produce enough insulin to metabolize the food consumed. If the overweight person achieves a normal body weight, often the blood glucose will lower to within normal limits.

Over the last decades, the incidence of diabetes in the United States has steadily increased. Every year more than 250,000 new cases of diabetes are discovered. Diabetes statistics are on the rise for a number of reasons. People live longer today than in the past, consequently there is a large population of older persons, who are more susceptible to diabetes. Also diagnostic tests for diabetes are improving, and public awareness of the disease is growing. In addition, obesity is increasing in the general population and is known to contribute to the development of diabetes. Finally treatment with insulin has lowered the mortality rate among those people with insulin dependent diabetes. As a result, young diabetics marry and have children, who are predisposed to the development of diabetes.

TABLE 72–2. DIABETES IN IDENTICAL TWINS

Number of pairs in study:	96
Total number of pairs concordant:	65

	Diagnosed Under Age 40	Diagnosed Over Age 40
Concordant	31	34
Discordant	28	3

In study by R. B. Tattersall and D. A. Pyke. Extracted from Ganda, O. P. and S. S. Soeldner: Genetic, Acquired, and Related Factors in the Etiology of Diabetes Mellitus. *Archives of Internal Medicine,* 137:461, Apr. 1977.

OUT OF EVERY **20** DIABETICS OVER 40 YEARS OF AGE,
17 WERE OVERWEIGHT BEFORE ONSET

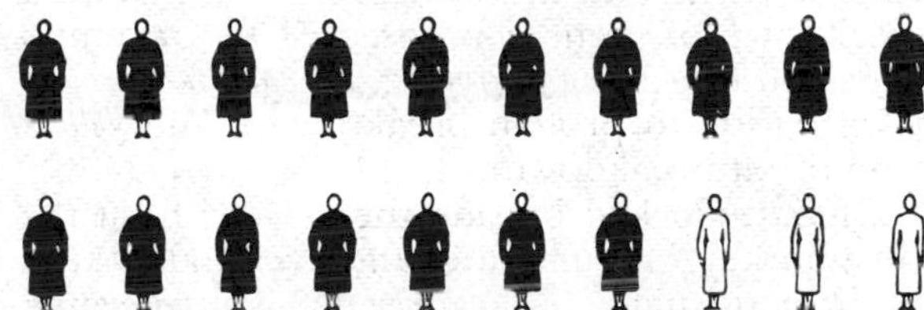

Figure 72–2. Incidence of overweight before onset of diabetes. (Used by permission of Metropolitan Life Insurance Company.)

Pathophysiology and Bases of Symptoms

Insulin regulates the rate of carbohydrate, fat, and protein metabolism, as illustrated in Figure 72–3. Consequently, an insulin deficiency, due to beta cell damage, obesity, overwhelming stress, and so forth, inevitably triggers a chain reaction of untoward events. First of all, glucose is not conveyed from the extracellular fluid to

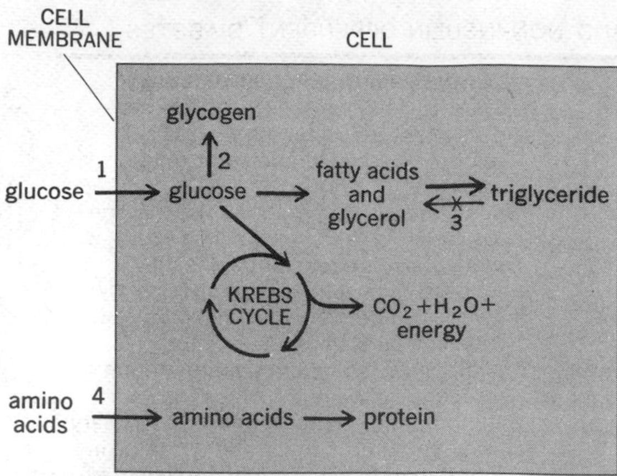

Figure 72–3. Major effects of insulin on organic metabolism. The numbers denote distinct direct effects, the others being the indirect effects of increased glucose and amino acid entry. The X on arrow 3 denotes inhibition of triglyceride breakdown. (From Vander, A. J., J. H. Sherman and D. S. Luciano: *Human Physiology—The Mechanisms of Body Function,* 2nd ed. New York: McGraw-Hill Book Co., 1975, p. 399.)

the intracellular compartment. Without glucose for energy, the cells become *energy-depleted* and must oxidize fats and proteins drawn from adipose tissue and muscle stores. The resultant breakdown of tissue composed of fat or amino acids causes *wasting* of tissue, a *negative nitrogen balance* (due to protein breakdown), and *ketosis* (due to fat breakdown).

Glucose, locked outside the cells without the "insulin key," accumulates and eventually raises the blood sugar (*hyperglycemia*). The elevated blood sugar (which exerts a strong osmotic force) pulls cellular water into the blood, which results in *cellular dehydration* (Chapter 12). As the blood sugar level rises, glucose eventually spills into the urine, causing *glycosuria.* The osmotic load of glucose in the urine prevents the reabsorption of water in the kidney tubules, causing *extracellular dehydration.* Finally, these pathologic developments result in the following *four cardinal symptoms of diabetes:*

Symptom	Bases of Symptoms
Polyuria (frequent urination)	Water is not reabsorbed by the renal tubules because of the osmotic activity of glucose.
Polydipsia (excessive thirst)	Polyuria causes severe dehydration, which in turn causes thirst.
Weight loss (insulin dependent diabetes primarily)	Because glucose is not available to the cells, fat and protein stores are broken down and used for energy.
Polyphagia (excessive hunger)	Tissue breakdown and wasting causes a state of starvation which compels the stricken individual to eat voraciously.

In addition to the four cardinal symptoms, persons with diabetes may develop other distressing problems. One of the most severe acute complications of insulin dependent diabetes is *ketoacidosis,* a form of metabolic acidosis; this condition arises in untreated diabetics and in those patients whose condition remains uncontrolled by insulin and diet (see later in this chapter).

Another serious complication is *hyperglycemic, hyperosmolar, non-ketotic coma (HHNK).* HHNK occurs most often in non-insulin dependent diabetics who are being treated with diet, and possibly with oral hypoglycemic agents. As the term implies, the serum glucose may be markedly elevated, resulting in a hyperosmolar state. However, since these patients often have some circulating insulin, they do not develop ketoacidosis as insulin dependent diabetics do. Profound dehydration may result, and the mortality rate may approach 50 per cent. The high mortality rate may be due to a failure to promptly recognize and treat this disorder. Since HHNK may be precipitated by stresses such as infection, myocardial infarction, or other acute illness, the underlying cause must be identified and treated as well. Patients and significant others need to be aware of this complication as well as hypoglycemia and ketoacidosis.

A third serious complication of diabetes is *chronic hyperlipemia* (excessive fats in the blood). Chronic hyperlipemia coupled with hyperglycemia results in the premature development of vascular lesions both in the coronary arteries and in the peripheral arteries and arterioles (*peripheral obstructive vascular disease*). Vascular degeneration may, in turn, affect the kidneys, causing *nephropathy,* and the eyes, resulting in diabetic *retinopathy* and *blindness.* In addition, diabetes may eventually cause *neuropathy.*

Finally, patients with diabetes are more susceptible to some *microorganisms* and *fungi,* in part because of the high sugar content of their blood and urine. Also diabetics, because of their impaired circulation, suffer from *retarded healing* of infections and wounds.

Diagnostic Tests

Insulin dependent diabetes mellitus is diagnosed on the basis of the following findings:

- ▶Presence of the clinical symptoms of polyphagia, polydipsia, polyuria (the three P's), and weight loss.
- ▶Laboratory findings which may include glucosuria, ketonuria, hyperglycemia, ketonemia, and acidosis.

The two major diagnostic tests for diabetes are blood tests and urine tests for glucose and acetone.

Blood Tests. The major blood tests which are employed to diagnose the presence and severity of diabetes include (a) fasting blood sugar; (b) postprandial blood sugar; and (c) oral glucose tolerance tests (GTT). These blood tests are described in Table 72–3. Instruct the patient taking these tests to ingest only the food and drugs received from the hospital staff. Explain to your patient that food and certain medications can distort test results. Of particular importance, the patient must eat a diet high in carbohydrate-containing foods (sugar and starches) for three days prior to the glucose tolerance test.

Urine Tests. Three common nursing procedures related to diabetic tests are (a) collecting urine specimens at specified times, (b) testing the urine for sugar and acetone, and (c) teaching patients methods for testing their own urine. Let us first consider urine tests for *sugar*.

As stated earlier, when the blood sugar rises to abnormal levels, the excess glucose eventually spills into the urine. There are two simple types of tests available that enable doctors, nurses, and patients to measure roughly the resulting glucosuria. They are *chemical reduction* and *enzyme tests*. Three test materials are commonly used both in the hospital and at home. They are: *Clinitest, Tes-Tape,* and *Diastix*. The Clinitest method may use either two or five drops of urine so it is important that the desired testing method is understood by the patient. Also, in the past, sliding scale insulin dosage orders were written for urine test results of 1+, 2+, 3+, and 4+. Alternatively, patients reported the color of the test. With the newer testing materials, however, relying on reports of color may lead to inaccuracy in insulin dose prescribed. For example, a dark green color indicates a negative test

TABLE 72–3. BLOOD TESTS FOR DIABETES MELLITUS

	Fasting Blood Sugar (FBS)	Postprandial Blood Sugar	Oral Glucose Tolerance Test (GTT)
Measurement and Purpose	Determines amount of glucose in blood when patient fasting	Measures blood sugar following a meal	Determines patient's response to a measured dose of glucose
Restrictions (Food, Water, Activity)	No food for 12 hours prior to test (usually 8 P.M. to 8 A.M.); water allowed	None	No food for 12 hours prior to test or during test; water allowed; no smoking, coffee, or tea allowed during test; these substances alter body's response to carbohydrate. *Minimize activity* (e.g., walking) which alters glucose metabolism; *minimize stress* because epinephrine and cortisone release raise blood sugar by promoting gluconeogenesis
Procedure	Blood drawn from venipuncture and sent to laboratory	Patient given meal with approximately 100 Gm. carbohydrate; venous blood drawn 2 hours after meal	High carbohydrate diet for 3 days prior to test; NPO for 12 hours before test; weigh patient; obtain fasting blood and urine specimens; administer 100 Gm. glucose by mouth diluted in lemon juice; obtain blood and urine specimens ½, 1, 2, 3, 4, and 5 hours after dose of glucose; mark all specimens with time obtained and take to laboratory
Findings	*Normal:* 80–120 mg./100 ml. serum; *abnormal:* 200 mg./100 ml. or more diagnostic of diabetes mellitus	*Normal:* Same as normal findings above	*Normal:* blood glucose climbs to peak of 140 mg./100 ml. in first hour and returns to normal by 2nd or 3rd hour; *abnormal:* blood glucose *does not* return to normal by 2nd or 3rd hour; all urine specimens *positive for glucose*
Untoward Effects	None	None	Transitory weakness, sweating, and dizziness may develop during 2nd and 3rd hour
Precautions	None	None	Diuretics, glucocorticoids, estrogens, and oral contraceptives may distort test findings; these medications should be omitted prior to testing. Test should *not* be performed on patient with initial FBS of over 200 mg./100 ml.

when Clinitest is used, but 2 per cent glucose with Tes-Tape. A 2 per cent report with Tes-Tape is equivalent to 4+ with Clinitest. The values of each test are compared in Table 72–4.

Urine is also tested for the "ketones" (β-hydroxybutyric acid, acetoacetic acid, and acetone) which appear in the urine of insulin dependent diabetics who are poorly controlled. Two simple types of tests are available: the *Ketostix* and *Acetest.* To perform these tests, place a drop of urine on an Acetest tablet or insert a Ketostix stick into the urine specimen. Wait for the time period indicated on the instructions and then compare the color of the tablet or stick with an accompanying color chart.

Urine testing may be ordered for a variety of reasons. There are three different types of *urine specimens*: (1) the single specimen, (2) fractional urine specimens, and (3) 24-hour specimens. Briefly, these tests are used for the following reasons:

1. The *single* specimen of urine for glucose testing is often ordered as a *screening procedure* for diabetes. If sugar is found in the patient's urine, further blood and urine tests will be ordered, to confirm or rule out the diagnosis. Non-insulin dependent diabetics may be asked to test single voided urine specimens in order to determine if sugar is present. If sugar is present, the patient may need to further decrease the number of calories consumed.

2. *Fractional urines* for glucose and acetone are usually performed by nurses or patients every six hours over a 24-hour period. Generally, fractional urines are required only of insulin dependent diabetics. The results of the urine tests are often used to determine the patient's insulin dosage for the day (see p. 1556). Test results also indicate whether or not the diabetic's condition is being adequately controlled by diet and medication. Because accuracy is necessary, the specimen collected for testing should *not* contain urine which has been in the patient's bladder all night or even for several hours. Stagnant urine will *not* accurately reveal the amount of glucose in the urine at the *time of the test.* To assure accuracy, have the patient void 1/2 hour before the test, drink no more than 8 ounces of water (drinking large amounts of water may invalidate the test results), and then void again at the time of the test. Urine from the second voiding can then be used with confidence for testing. This specimen is called a double-voided specimen.

3. *24-hour urine specimens* are ordered to determine *quantitative sugar* or the amount of glucose which a patient loses over a 24-hour period. At the beginning of the 24 hours, the patient is asked to void and the urine is discarded. Thereafter, all urine voided is saved in a gallon jug. At the end of the 24 hours, the patient is again asked to void, the urine is poured into the jug, and the jug is sent to the laboratory.

Prevention and Early Detection of Diabetes

As stated earlier, the number of new diabetics diagnosed yearly is rising. Health agencies (e.g., public health departments, insurance companies, and the American Diabetes Association) are attempting to diagnose and treat diabetes through professional and public educational programs, mass screening tests, and research.

Through educational campaigns, people are gradually becoming aware of the dangers of obesity, diabetes being but one such danger. Persons with prediabetes are being taught to adhere to low-calorie diets in order to prevent the eventual appearance of overt diabetes.

Since diabetes often cannot be prevented, health agencies are striving to diagnose diabetes in its early, less dangerous stages. Persons who should always be examined for diabetes include (a) the obese; (b) anyone suffering from excessive thirst, hunger, urination, and weight loss; (c) persons with abnormal glucose tolerance tests during periods of stress, e.g., pregnancy; (d) mothers who have given birth to several overweight babies; and (e) persons over 40 years of age.

The laboratory tests used for mass screening include (a) the Dextrostix blood test for fasting blood glucose, which uses blood from a pinprick; (b) post-prandial blood sugar; and (c) urine tests for glucose.

Mass testing must be followed by further testing of all persons with suspected diabetes.

TABLE 72–4. RELATIONSHIP BETWEEN GLUCOSE CONCENTRATION AND TEST SYMBOLS IN COMMON URINE TESTS

Testing Method	Concentration of Glucose in the Urine							
	1/10%	*1/4%*	*1/2%*	*3/4%*	1%	2%	3%	5%
Clinitest								
5 drop	neg.	trace	1+	2+	3+	4+	4+	4+
2 drop	neg.	trace	1/2	–	1%	2%	3%	4%
Tes-Tape	1+	2+	3+	–	–	4+	4+	4+
Diastix	trace	1+	1+	–	3+	4+	4+	4+

TABLE 72–5. PRINCIPLES OF DIETARY REGULATION IN DIABETES

Dietary Strategies	Obese Patient Not Requiring Insulin	Non-Obese Patient, Insulin Dependent
Decrease calories	Yes. Reduction of adiposity reduces hyperglycemia and reduces the insulin resistance that attends obesity.	No. Calories should not be restricted below normal levels.
Increase frequency and number of feedings	Usually no.	Yes.
Meal regulation	Desirable, but not crucial if average caloric intake is reduced to provide for weight loss of 1–2 lb/week.	Very important. Three meals with appropriate snacks.
Extra food for unusual exercise	Not usually appropriate.	Usually appropriate.
Use of food to treat or prevent hyperglycemia	Not necessary.	Important.

From DeHoog, S., M. Ishii, J. Karceck, J. Okamoto, and C. Scalesi: *Nutritional Care Manual*. Seattle: University of Washington Affiliated Hospitals, 1977, p. 54.

Individuals with an elevated blood sugar or glycosuria should be referred to their physician for careful evaluation of their health status. It is important to emphasize to possible diabetics that recognition and treatment of this disease prevent some of its serious complications.

Clinical Care

Introduction. To date, there is no cure for diabetes. Consequently, the overall goal of care for diabetic patients is *control* or *regulation* of their disease rather than cure. When diabetes is successfully regulated, the diabetic is able to avoid many complications while continuing to live a normal and useful life. It is important to understand, however, that diabetic patients may develop complications despite their own vigorous efforts at careful control of their disease.

Essentially diabetic control depends upon the proper interaction of the following three factors: (1) diet; (2) insulin or hypoglycemic pills; and (3) exercise. The *diet*, which should avoid concentrated sweets, is prescribed on the basis of the patient's size, weight, age, and occupation (e.g., sedentary, moderately active, very active). *Insulin* is administered when the patient's own secretion of insulin is inadequate. In general, insulin administration is reserved for insulin dependent diabetics. The administration of insulin to non-insulin dependent diabetics may, in fact, make it more difficult for these patients to maintain their normal body weight. Oral hypoglycemic agents are used only for non-insulin dependent diabetics. Ideally, non-insulin dependent diabetics are best treated by dietary control and weight loss.

Finally, the insulin dependent diabetic must regulate exercise and activity so that the rate of energy expenditure is in balance with the amount and kind of insulin injected and the food intake. For instance, if the patient exercises less than usual, a lighter diet or more insulin may be necessary; if exercising more than usual, the diabetic will need to either eat more food or lower the insulin dosage. Thus any variance in one factor will necessitate adjustment of the other two factors. The non-insulin dependent diabetic, on the other hand, should be encouraged to exercise in order to foster weight loss.

What are the major *criteria for good control* of diabetes? Generally diabetes is considered under control when the following conditions are met.

- The fasting blood glucose is normal.
- The blood glucose is no higher than 180 mg./100 ml. 2 hours after breakfast and no more than 200 mg./100 ml. 2 hours after lunch.
- The urine is negative for glucose and acetone before breakfast and dinner.
- 24-hour collections of urine contain below 5 Gm. of glucose.
- The patient has optimal weight and enjoys good health.

While authorities agree that diabetes should be controlled if the diabetic is to avoid complications, exactly what constitutes a workable program of control remains debatable. As in the treatment of all chronic disorders, the patient's age and basic personality patterns must be considered when drawing up a treatment regimen. For example, an adolescent with insulin dependent diabetes may rebel if the diet and activities are too strictly controlled; rebellion, in turn, may result in the patient's self-destructive refusal to comply with *any* restrictions on diet or activity. On the other hand, another person may ritualize the diabetic regimen to the point that it totally dominates life. An anxious individual may worry so much about diabetes that the accumulated stress actually raises the blood sugar! Therefore it is essential to investigate the patient's habits and attitudes toward the illness before deciding on the exact degree of control necessary. The program which is tailored as much as possible to the individual diabetic's personality is most likely to prove successful over the years.

GENERAL PRINCIPLES OF THE DIABETIC DIET

Despite the discovery of insulin in 1921 and oral hypoglycemic agents during the 1950's, *diet* still remains the most important aspect of the diabetic treatment regimen. The twofold purpose of the diabetic diet is to curtail the ingestion of foods with high sugar content and to correct or avoid obesity. The contrasting strategies used to regulate the diet for the two main types of diabetic patients are outlined in Table 72–5.

> *The most important factor in the success of a diabetic diet is the patient's willingness to adhere to a prescribed diet.*

If the non-insulin dependent diabetic follows a diet that results in adequate weight control, there may be no need for insulin or oral hypoglycemic agents. As emphasized earlier, it is ideal to control this type of diabetes mellitus with diet alone, thereby eliminating the need for medication. However, for the following reasons, this ideal is not always attainable:

▶The *older* diabetic may resist dieting. Lifelong food habits are difficult to change. Food is associated in the minds of many persons with love, memories of childhood, religious rituals, ethnic holidays, and special personal occasions, such as birthdays, weddings, and so forth. Adherence to a diet, especially during holidays, may make the patient feel deprived, unhappy and unwilling to continue dieting.

▶The *adolescent* diabetic may resent any diet which makes it necessary to eat differently from peers; for example, a young person may find it difficult to eat low-calorie, low-carbohydrate foods while friends drink endless bottles of soda pop and eat all the candy and potato chips they desire. Adolescence in our culture is already a time of crisis and stress. Needless to say, being a diabetic *and* an adolescent may cause the patient to rebel against parents, doctor, and diet.

▶Highly *neurotic persons* are sometimes compulsive eaters. Satisfying the urge to eat may be more important to such individuals than the need to control their diabetes. To prevent complications, the obese compulsive eater will need to seek psychiatric help.

▶Because diabetes is a chronic disease, weight reduction in the obese patient must be maintained. Many persons (including nondiabetics) do not have the necessary self-discipline for permanent weight maintenance. According to reports from private and public hospitals, only 5 to 40 per cent of diabetic patients are successful in their weight control programs.[58a]

In each of these situations the nurse, through careful assessment and understanding of the goals of therapy, may be of great value in helping develop a dietary plan that is compatible with the patient's life style.

When patients cannot or will not adhere to their prescribed diabetic diets, the doctor may prescribe insulin or oral hypoglycemic agents in order to lower the patient's blood sugar and prevent symptoms. What nurses can do to promote dietary control is discussed on pp. 1551 to 1555.

Types of Diabetic Diets. There are two types of diabetic diets: (1) the qualitative diet, and (2) the quantitative diet. The *qualitative* diet is prescribed for persons with mild diabetes. Patients on the qualitative diet must be taught to (a) avoid adding sugar to their coffee, cereal, and so forth; (b) avoid foods sweetened with sugar, e.g., jellies, jams, cakes, ice cream; (c) test their urine regularly and (d) keep periodic appointments with their health care provider for evaluation of diabetic control. It is also important that the insulin dependent diabetic understand the need for *consistency* in regard to the amount, distribution, and timing of nutrients. The possible need for increased carbohydrate prior to sustained exercise should also be emphasized.

> *Caution patients on a qualitative diet to call their physician should they develop an infection or experience accidental trauma. During these times mild diabetics may need a stricter diet and possibly medication.*

The *quantitative* diet is prescribed when more control is deemed necessary. There are two methods for preparing quantitative diets; they are as follows:

Exchange measured diet. This highly practical diet is followed by many diabetics today, and was developed jointly by the American Diabetes Association (ADA) and the American Dietetic Association. This method is based upon the premise that foods which contain the same food value can be exchanged with one another without altering the patient's basic dietary prescription. For example, note in Table 72–6 that foods are categorized into six basic lists or groups: (1) milk exchanges; (2) vegetable exchanges; (3) fruit exchanges; (4) bread exchanges; (5) meat exchanges; and (6) fat exchanges. Note further that the foods in each list contain the same number of calories, as well as the same amounts of protein, fat, and carbohydrate. Thus a patient may drink 1 cup of skim milk or ½ cup of evaporated skim milk and still receive the same amount of calories, carbohydrate, protein, and fat. As you can see, the exchange diet provides the patient with considerable variety and choice. It is also less cumbersome than the weighed diet because the patient can measure food and liquids with household measures (i.e., measuring cups, tablespoons) and can estimate the size of meat and fruit portions (e.g., 1 slice cold cuts, 1 medium peach).

Fixed weighed diet. This form of quantitative diet may be more accurate than the exchange measured diet, but it is also more cumbersome and tedious. As the name implies, the diabetic weighs all food (drawn from a list of meats, fish, vegetables, and fruit) in grams on a food scale. The diet is "fixed" in that the amounts of milk, fat, bread, and cereal do not vary from day to day. For most diabetics, weighing food is unnecessary and time-consuming.

HIGH CARBOHYDRATE AND FIBER DIET. It has been observed that underdeveloped countries have a much lower incidence of diabetes mellitus than the United States and many European countries. Foods typically consumed in these nations are high in carbohydrate, high in fiber, and low in fat. Whole grains and other fibrous foods constitute a large part of the diet. Some researchers have found that such a diet may be of value in improving glucose tolerance and have prescribed the diet for selected diabetic patients.[41] Many non-insulin dependent diabetics who had previously required small amounts of exogenous insulin (25 units or less per day) were able to decrease or eliminate their daily insulin. An example of the distribution of nutrients in such a diet is: 60 per cent carbohydrate (with three-fourths to be complex carbohydrate), 20 per cent protein, and 20 per cent fat. Some prescriptions may recommend as much as 70 per cent carbohydrate. The use of high fiber foods is important and the amount of animal fat is minimal. A high carbohydrate and low fat diet is currently not the ADA diet, but its value in reducing insulin needs and improving glucose metabolism is being evaluated by several researchers.

Calculating the Diabetic Diet. The balanced diabetic diet should contain the following nutrients: (a) calculated quantities of carbohydrates, proteins, and fats in approximately the same percentage composition as a "typical" normal diet: 20 per cent of total calories as protein, 30 per cent fat, and 50 per cent carbohydrate; and (b) normal amounts of vitamins and minerals. When a diabetic diet is prescribed, the following factors must be considered:

▶ The patient's *ethnic, religious, and cultural background;* e.g., if the patient is Italian, some allowance might be made for eating slightly starchier foods and drinking an occasional glass of wine with dinner. When such allowances are not made, the patient may eventually reject the diet completely.

▶ The patient's *height* and *weight.* If the patient is overweight, the doctor will prescribe a low-calorie reducing diet. If the patient's weight is satisfactory, the doctor will prescribe a maintenance diet. The *basal* caloric *requirement* (i.e., the caloric requirement in the resting state) for the maintenance of one's ideal weight is 10 cal. per lb. or about 23 cal. per kg. (120 lb. equals approximately 55.5 kg.) ideal weight. Thus the woman who ideally weighs 120 lb. will need 120 × 10 or 1200 cal. a day to maintain her weight *when at rest;* note below that calories must be added to the basal calorie requirement to compensate for the patient's activity level.

▶ The patient's *occupation* and *normal activity level.* Patients who have sedentary occupations (e.g., typist) will require fewer calories than a person with a moderately active occupation (e.g., floor nurse) or a strenuous job (e.g., manual laborer). To calculate total daily calories, the physician adds 25 per cent of the basal caloric requirement to the total daily caloric allowance of the sedentary person, and 50 to 75 per cent of the basal requirement for more active patients. For example, a typist who ideally weights 120 lb. and whose basal caloric requirement is 1200 cal. per day will require 300 more calories daily (25 per cent of 1200) and thus a total daily requirement of 1500 calories.

▶ *Distribution of carbohydrate, protein, and fat in the diet.* Using the exchange system, the ADA has developed different diabetic meals which are based upon the patient's daily caloric requirements. For example, a 1200-cal. diet may call for 150 Gm. of carbohydrate or 600 cal. (150 × 4); 60 Gm. of protein or 240 cal. (60 × 4); and 40 Gm. of fat or 360 cal. (40 × 9).*

▶ *Meal distribution.* For a mild diabetic who does not require insulin, the physician usually distributes the food exchanges among three daily meals. However, the diabetic patient who takes insulin often will need mid-afternoon and evening snacks to prevent insulin reactions.

A typical meal plan based upon the exchange method for a hypothetical patient called Ms. L. Jones is shown in Table 72–7.

Note that this diabetic diet is relatively low in calories; note also that the various exchanges are listed for the entire day as well as for each individual meal. Because this patient takes insulin, she requires mid-afternoon and bedtime snacks.

Two possible breakfast menus for Ms. Jones drawn from the ADA exchange lists could include the following foods:

Exchange	Breakfast No. 1	Breakfast No. 2
1 fruit	½ cup orange juice	½ cup blue berries
1 bread	1 muffin	1 slice toast
1 milk	1 cup skim milk	1 cup skim milk
1 medium fat meat	1 egg (hardboiled)	1 poached egg
1 fat	1 teaspoon butter (for muffin)	1 slice crisp bacon

From *Exchange Lists for Meal Planning.* Prepared by American Diabetes Association, Inc., and the American Dietetic Association.

*Recall from Chapter 12 that 1 Gm. of carbohydrate is equivalent to 4 cal., 1 Gm. of protein to 4 cal., and 1 Gm. of fat to 9 cal.

TABLE 72-6. DIABETIC DIET EXCHANGE LISTS

List 1. Milk Exchanges
Carbohydrate: 12 grams, protein: 8 grams, fat: trace, calories: 80

Non-Fat Fortified Milk	
Skim or non-fat milk	1 cup
Powdered (non-fat dry, before adding liquid)	1/3 cup
Canned, evaporated – skim milk	1/2 cup
Buttermilk made from skim milk	1 cup
Yogurt made from skim milk (plain, unflavored)	1 cup
Low-Fat Fortified Milk	
1% fat fortified milk (omit 1/2 fat exchange)	1 cup
2% fat fortified milk (omit 1 fat exchange)	1 cup
Yogurt made from 2% fortified milk (plain, unflavored) (omit 1 fat exchange)	1 cup
Whole Milk (omit 2 fat exchanges)	
Whole milk	1 cup
Canned, evaporated whole milk	1/2 cup
Buttermilk made from whole milk	1 cup
Yogurt made from whole milk (plain, unflavored)	1 cup

List 2. Vegetable Exchanges
Carbohydrate: 5 grams, protein: 2 grams, calories: 25

Cooked Vegetables
(one exchange is 1/2 cup)

Asparagus	eggplant	string beans (green or yellow)
bean sprouts	green pepper	summer squash
beets	greens	tomatoes
broccoli	mushrooms	tomato juice
Brussel sprouts	okra	turnips
cabbage	onions	vegetable juice cocktail
carrots	rhubarb	zucchini
cauliflower	rutabaga	
cucumbers	sauerkraut	

Raw Vegetables
(used as desired)

chicory	Chinese cabbage	endive	escarole
lettuce	parsley	radishes	watercress

Starchy Vegetables
Listed under Bread Exchange

List 3. Fruit Exchanges
Carbohydrate: 10 grams, calories: 40

Apple	1 small
Apple juice	1/3 cup
Applesauce (unsweetened)	1/2 cup
Apricots, fresh	2 medium
Apricots, dried	4 halves
Banana	1 small
Berries	
blackberries	1/2 cup
blueberries	1/2 cup

List 3. Fruit Exchanges *Continued*

raspberries	1/2 cup
strawberries	3/4 cup
Cherries	10 large
Cider	1/3 cup
Dates	2
Figs, fresh or dried	1
Grapefruit	1/2
Grapefruit juice	1/2 cup
Grapes	12
Grape juice	1/4 cup
Mango	1/2 small
Melon	
canteloupe	1/4 small
honeydew	1/8 medium
watermelon	1 cup
Nectarine	1 small
Orange	1 small
Orange juice	1/2 cup
Papaya	3/4 cup
Peach	1 medium
Pear	1 small
Persimmon, native	1 medium
Pineapple	1/2 cup
Pineapple juice	1/3 cup
Plums	2 medium
Prunes	2 medium
Prune juice	1/4 cup
Raisins	1/4 cup
Tangerine	1 medium

Cranberries may be used as desired if no sugar is added.

List 4. Bread Exchanges
Carbohydrate: 15 grams, protein: 2 grams, calories: 70

Bread	
White (including French and Italian)	1 slice
Whole wheat	1 slice
Rye or pumpernickel	1 slice
Raisin	1 slice
Bagel, small	1/2
English muffin, small	1/2
Plain roll, bread	1
Frankfurter roll	1/2
Hamburger bun	1/2
Dried bread crumbs	3 Tablespoons
Tortilla, 6"	1
Cereal	
Bran flakes	1/2 cup
Other ready-to-eat unsweetened cereal	3/4 cup
Puffed cereal (unfrosted)	1 cup
Cereal (cooked)	1/2 cup
Grits (cooked)	1/2 cup
Rice or barley (cooked)	1/2 cup
Pasta (cooked), spaghetti, noodles, macaroni	1/2 cup
Popcorn (popped, no fat added)	3 cups
Cornmeal (dry)	2 Tablespoons
Flour	2 1/2 Tablespoons
Wheat germ	1/4 cup

From American Diabetes Association and The American Dietetic Association: *Exchange Lists for Meal Planning.* 1976.
*Fat content is primarily monosaturated.
**If made with corn, cottonseed, safflower, soy or sunflower oil can be used on fat modified diet.

TABLE 72–6. DIABETIC DIET EXCHANGE LISTS *(Continued)*

List 4. Bread Exchanges *Continued*

Crackers	
Arrowroot	3
Graham, 2½" square	2
Matzoth, 4" × 6"	½
Oyster	20
Pretzels, 3⅛" long × ⅛" diameter	25
Rye wafers, 2" × 3½"	3
Saltines	6
Soda, 2½" square	4
Dried Beans, Peas and Lentils	
Beans, peas, lentils (dried and cooked)	½ cup
Baked beans, no pork (canned)	¼ cup
Starchy Vegetables	
Corn	⅓ cup
Corn on the cob	1 small
Lima beans	½ cup
Parsnips	⅔ cup
Peas, green (canned or frozen)	½ cup
Potato, white	1 small
Potato, mashed	½ cup
Pumpkin	¾ cup
Winter squash, acorn, or butternut	½ cup
Yam or sweet potato	¼ cup
Prepared Foods	
Biscuit, 2" diameter (omit 1 fat exchange)	1
Corn bread, 2" × 2" × 1" (omit 1 fat exchange)	1
Corn muffin, 2" diameter (omit 1 fat exchange)	1
Crackers, round butter type (omit 1 fat exchange)	5
Muffin, plain, small (omit 1 fat exchange)	1
Potatoes, French fried, length 2" to 3½" (omit 1 fat exchange)	8
Potato or corn chips (omit 2 fat exchanges)	15
Pancake, 5" × ½" (omit 1 fat exchange)	1
Waffle, 5" × ½" (omit 1 fat exchange)	1

List 5. Meat Exchanges: Lean Meat
Protein: 7 grams, fat: 3 grams, calories: 55

Beef: Baby beef (very lean), chipped beef, chuck, flank steak, tenderloin, plate ribs, plate skirt steak, round (bottom, top), all cuts rump, spare ribs, tripe	1 ounce
Lamb: Leg, rib, sirloin, loin (roast and chops), shank, shoulder	1 ounce
Pork: Leg (whole rump, center shank), ham, smoked (center slices)	1 ounce
Poultry: Meat without skin of chicken, turkey, Cornish hen, guinea hen, pheasant	1 ounce
Fish: Any fresh or frozen	1 ounce
Canned salmon, tuna, mackerel, crab, or lobster	¼ cup
Clams, oysters, scallops, shrimp	5 or 1 ounce
Sardines, drained	3
Cheeses containing less than 5% butterfat	1 ounce
Cottage cheese, dry or 2% butterfat	¼ cup
Dried beans and peas (omit 1 bread exchange)	½ cup

Medium-Fat Meat

For each exchange of medium-fat meat omit ½ fat exchange

Beef: Ground (15% fat), corned beef (canned), rib eye, round (ground commercial)	1 ounce

List 5. Meat Exchanges: Lean Meat *Continued*

Medium-Fat Meat

Pork: Loin (all cuts tenderloin), shoulder arm (picnic) shoulder blade, Boston butt, canadian bacon, boiled ham	1 ounce
Liver, heart, kidney and sweetbreads (these are high in cholesterol)	1 ounce
Cottage cheese, creamed	¼ cup
Cheese: mozzarella, ricotta, farmer's cheese, Neufchatel, Parmesan	1 ounce 3 tablespoons
Egg (high in cholesterol)	1
Peanut butter (omit 2 additional fat exchanges)	2 tablespoons

High-Fat Meat

For each exchange of high-fat meat omit 1 fat exchange

Beef: Brisket, corned beef, (brisket), ground beef (more than 20% fat), hamburger (commercial), chuck (ground commercial) roasts (rib), steaks (club and rib)	1 ounce
Lamb: breast	1 ounce
Pork: Spare ribs, loin (back ribs), pork (ground), country style ham, deviled ham	1 ounce
Veal: Breast	1 ounce
Poultry: Capon, duck (domestic), goose	1 ounce
Cheese: Cheddar types	1 ounce
Cold cuts 4½" × ⅛" slice	1
Frankfurter	1 small

List 6. Fat Exchanges
Fat: 5 grams, calories: 45

Margarine, soft, tube or stock (made with corn, cottonseed, safflower, soy, or sunflower oil only)	1 teaspoon
Avocado (4" in diameter)*	⅛
Oil, corn, cottonseed, safflower, soy, sunflower	1 teaspoon
Oil, olive*	1 teaspoon
Oil, peanut*	1 teaspoon
Olives*	5 small
Almonds*	10 whole
Pecans*	2 whole
Peanuts*	
Spanish	20 whole
Virginia	10 whole
Walnuts	6 small
Nuts, other*	6 small
Margarine, regular stick	1 teaspoon
Butter	1 teaspoon
Bacon fat	1 teaspoon
Bacon, crisp	1 strip
Cream, light	2 tablespoons
Cream, sour	2 tablespoons
Cream, heavy	1 tablespoon
Cream cheese	1 tablespoon
French dressing**	1 tablespoon
Italian dressing**	1 tablespoon
Lard	1 teaspoon
Mayonnaise**	1 teaspoon
Salad dressing, mayonnaise type**	2 teaspoons
Salt pork	¾" cube

There are many other combinations of breakfast foods which you could plan for this patient, as well as many appetizing lunches and dinners. Remember, the more varied the exchanges, the more enjoyable the patient will find eating and the more likely she will be to adhere to her diet.

Basic Diabetic Dietary Rules. Usually it is either the nurse or dietitian who instructs the diabetic patient concerning diet. When you have this responsibility, be certain to emphasize to your patient the following guidelines:

- ▶ If strict dietary control becomes necessary, the patient should measure all foods with household measures or weigh it.

TABLE 72–7. TYPICAL MEAL PLAN

Your Meal Plan In Exchanges

Must Be Planned With The Assistance Of Your Diet Counselor

Meal Plan For Mr. Jones

Carbohydrate 225 grams Protein 90 grams Fat 60 grams Calories 1800

	1 Milk NON FAT	2 Vegetable	3 Fruit	4 Bread	5 Meat LEAN	6 Fat POLYUNSAT.
Breakfast Time 7 AM	1		1	2	2	2
Snack Time 9 30			1	1		
Lunch or Dinner Time 12		1		2	3	2
Snack Time 2 30			1	1		
Dinner or Supper Time 5 00		1	1	2	3	2
Bedtime Snack Time 10 00	1		1	1		1

NOTE TO DIETITIAN When listing Exchanges Specify:
LIST 1, Non-Fat, Low-Fat or Whole Milk—If Fat Exchange is to be omitted
LIST 4, If Fat Exchange is to be omitted
LIST 5, Lean Meat, Medium-Fat or High-Fat Meat—If Fat Exchange is to be omitted
LIST 6, Polyunsaturated or Saturated Fat

The blank form from American Diabetes Association, Inc., and The American Dietetic Association: *Exchange Lists for Meal Planning*, 1976. American Diabetes Association, 600 Fifth Avenue, New York, N.Y. 10020. American Dietetic Assoc. 430 North Michigan Ave., Chicago, Illinois 60611.

- ▶ Vary the different exchanges so that the daily diet is interesting and palatable.
- ▶ Weigh in at least twice a week, at the same time, in the same amount of clothing and on the same scale. Report to the doctor changes in weight of over 2 kg.
- ▶ Do not add sugar, syrup, honey, jelly, or jam to foods, and do not add sugar when cooking.
- ▶ Do not use fruits which are packed in heavy syrup; use only water-packed fruits, artificially sweetened candies, gelatin desserts, beverages, and so forth. However, it is expensive and unnecessary to buy "dietetic foods."
- ▶ Use only pure canned or frozen fruit juices, and avoid the purchase of fruit "drinks" because these usually contain sugar.
- ▶ Drink only certain approved "diet" pops. Among these are: Canada Dry Low-Calorie Sodas, Fresca, Diet Shasta, Sugar-Free Dr. Pepper, Tab, Pepsi Light and Diet Pepsi. Since the banning of cyclamates by the Federal Food and Drug Administration in the U.S., other diet drinks contain too much sugar for use by diabetics.
- ▶ Do not drink excessive amounts of coffee, because caffeine causes the blood sugar to increase significantly.
- ▶ Alcohol may sometimes be used moderately; however, do not drink more than 2 oz. of liquor a day. If a mix is desired, combine liquor with either water or nonsweetened mixers. However, the opinion of the health care provider should be obtained prior to the ingestion of alcohol.
- ▶ Eat *all* of the food prescribed; this is particularly important when insulin or oral hypoglycemic agents are also prescribed. If unable to finish a meal, always compensate for the uneaten portion of food by eating a comparable amount of calories and nutrients as a snack later in the day.
- ▶ If a meal is delayed, drink a glass of milk or eat a cracker while waiting in order to avoid an insulin reaction.
- ▶ When dining out in restaurants, order standard foods (e.g., a broiled steak, baked potato) and avoid casseroles, gravies, fried foods, and sweetened desserts.
- ▶ Make an effort to use polyunsaturated fats rather than saturated fats whenever possible.

INSULIN THERAPY

The *principal action* of insulin is to lower blood sugar by (a) promoting the transport of glucose into the cells, and (b) inhibiting the conversion of glycogen, fats, and proteins into glucose.

Insulin injections are necessary when either (a) the patient's beta cells are so severely damaged that there is insufficient production of insulin (e.g., in insulin dependent diabetes and cancer of the pancreas) or (b) the patient (usually an obese maturity-onset diabetic) is unwilling to adhere to a low-calorie diet, and consequently needs additional insulin to metabolize the excessive calories.

It is important to remember that any person who takes insulin may develop a hypoglycemic reaction ("insulin shock") to an overdose of insulin or the omission of a meal or part of a meal. Insulin reactions are discussed on p. 1569.

Types of Insulin. There are several different types of insulin which are grouped according to their speed of action in the body: (a) rapid acting; (b) intermediate acting; and (c) long acting. These insulins are compared and contrasted in Table 72–8. While the basic action of all types of insulin is the same (i.e., the reduction of blood sugar), note that the various insulins differ in onset and duration of hypoglycemic effect and thus in the time period during which an insulin reaction is most likely to occur.

For patients whose blood glucose is difficult to control, two different insulins are sometimes mixed together and administered in a single injection. For example, doctors often order NPH insulin mixed with regular insulin in order to provide for both the patient's immediate needs and day-long requirements. Likewise, Lente, Semilente, and Ultralente insulins may be mixed with each other; also Lente insulin and regular insulin can be mixed. In an effort to more effectively control blood glucose levels, some patients may receive two injections of mixed insulin each day.

Insulin Dosage. Insulin dosage is highly variable. It is regulated, first of all, by the *requirements of the individual.* The insulin requirement usually increases when a patient is seriously ill, develops an infection, undergoes surgery, suffers trauma, or during puberty.

Secondly, insulin dosage is based upon the patient's *response* to his insulin injections. The patient's response, in turn, is measured by blood and urine tests for sugar and acetone. Because diabetics vary widely in their response to insulin, the doctor initially determines dosage by trial and error. The process of regulating the patient's insulin dosage may require several weeks. For example, the admitting orders for a newly diagnosed adult patient whose diabetes is not complicated by ketosis or acidosis might be approximately as follows:

Intermediate insulin (either NPH or Lente insulin is often used), 20 units of U-100, a.c.
Fractional urines QID
Fasting blood sugar daily

Daily postprandial blood sugar 2 hours following lunch

Supplemental regular insulin for glycosuria to be given every 6 hours on the following sliding scale schedule according to the fractional urines:

1+ ....no insulin
2+ .... 5 U.
3+ ....10 U.
4+ ....15 U.
Positive acetone, add additional 5 U. insulin

Guided by the patient's blood sugar levels and urine tests, the physician next increases the dosage of NPH insulin until the patient's blood sugar level stabilizes and he no longer requires supplemental doses of regular insulin. In some cases, the doctor may prescribe mixing an intermediate insulin or long-acting insulin with a short-acting insulin for better control. It should be noted that some physicians prefer to regulate stable, newly diagnosed diabetic patients as out-patients, rather than as in-patients, because their metabolic demands may be quite different.

Administration of Insulin. Administered correctly, insulin is a lifesaving drug for the insulin dependent diabetic; administered incorrectly, insulin may cause complications ranging from tissue damage to lethal hypoglycemia (insulin shock). To administer insulin properly, you will need to study the following subject areas: (a) insulin concentrations; (b) insulin syringes; (c) insulin storage; (d) preparation for administration; (e) site selection and rotation; (f) insulin administration; and (g) self-injection of insulin.

Insulin Concentrations. Insulin dosage is always prescribed in *units;* this means that all types of insulin (crystalline, NPH, Lente, and so forth) are commercially prepared in 10-ml. vials which contain either 40, 80, or 100 U./ml. Thus U-80 insulin contains 80 U. of insulin per ml., and is *twice* as concentrated a preparation as U-40 insulin, which contains 40 U. of insulin per ml. U-100 insulin is a new preparation which

TABLE 72–8. A COMPARISON OF INSULIN PREPARATIONS

Action	Preparation[2]	Appearance	Action in Hours[1,3,4,5] Onset	Peak	Duration	Compatible Mixed With
	Insulin Injection					
	Insulin (Regular)	clear				all insulin preparations
	Regular Iletin	clear	½–1	2–4	6–8	
	Regular Iletin U-500	clear				all insulin preparations
RAPID						
	Insulin, Zinc Suspension					
	Semilente Insulin	cloudy	½–1	2–4	8–10	Lente preparations
	Semilente Iletin	cloudy				Lente preparations
	Isophane Insulin Suspension					
	Isophane Insulin (NPH)	cloudy	1–1.5	8–12	24	regular insulin injection
	NPH Iletin	cloudy				regular insulin injection
	Insulin, Zinc Suspension					
	Lente Insulin	cloudy	1–2.5	7–15	24	regular insulin and Semilente preparations
INTERMEDIATE						
	Lente Iletin	cloudy				regular insulin and Semilente preparations
	Globin Zinc Insulin Injection					
	Globin Zinc Insulin	cloudy	2	6–12	18–24	–
	Protamine Zinc Insulin Suspension					
	Protamine Zinc Insulin	cloudy	4–6	18+	36–72	regular insulin injection
	Protamine Zinc and Iletin	cloudy				regular insulin injection
	Extended Insulin Zinc Suspension					
LONG	Ultralente Insulin	cloudy	4–6	8–12	24–36	regular insulin and Semilente preparations
	Ultralente Iletin	cloudy				regular insulin and Semilente preparations

From Fonville, A. M.: Teaching patients to rotate injection sites. *American Journal of Nursing,* 78:880, May 1978.

[1]Figures reported by Burke, E. L.: Insulin. *In* Guthrie, D. W., and Guthrie, R. A. (Eds.): *Nursing Management of Diabetes,* St. Louis, C. V. Mosby Co., 1977, p. 87.

[2]Based on Larner, J., and Maynes, R. C., Jr.: Insulin and oral hypoglycemic drugs: glucagon. *In* Goodman, L. S., and Gilman, A. (Eds.): *Pharmacological Bases of Therapeutics,* 5th edition. New York, Macmillan Co., 1975, p. 1517.

[3]Kastrup, E. K. (ed.): Facts and Comparisons. St. Louis, Facts and Comparisons, Inc., 1981, p. 130.

[4]Reynolds, J. E. (ed.): Martindale: The Extra Pharmacopoeia, 28th ed., London, Pharmaceutical Press, 1982, p. 848.

[5]May, J. R.: (ed.): Drug Information Newsletter, Vol. 9, No. 4, Jul/Aug, 1983.

will eventually replace both U-40 and U-80 insulins. U-500 insulin is also available for selected patients. The concentration of an insulin preparation is always clearly marked on the bottle. The caps on the vials may be color coded and the vials may be shaped differently according to the concentration of insulin.

Insulin Syringes. Administer insulin in an *insulin syringe* which corresponds in calibration to the concentration of insulin in the vial.

> Remember:
> *To prevent dangerous error, administer U-40 insulin in a U-40 syringe, U-80 insulin in a U-80 syringe, and U-100 insulin in a U-100 syringe.*

Needles used to administer insulin include (a) 25 or 26 gauge (½–¾ inch long) stainless steel needles, or (b) 25 to 26 gauge disposable needles. However, Burke points out that an obese diabetic patient may need a 1–1½ inch needle for best results.[18] Teach patients who will give their own insulin to discard any needles which have dull or rough points.

Storage. In the past it was necessary to refrigerate insulin in order to prevent deterioration. Recent improvements in the processing of insulin have eliminated the need for refrigeration. While extremes of temperature are undesirable, regular insulin is stable for 18 months at 75° F., and Lente insulins are stable for 24 months at that temperature. Although refrigeration is not necessary, it is important that patients understand that insulin should not be left in the trunk of a car on a hot day, or stored in the baggage compartment of an airplane. Once opened, insulin vials should be stored in their boxes to protect them from contamination and from exposure to strong light. Discard any bottle of insulin which is older than the expiration date printed on the bottle or contains granules or clumped particles.

Preparation for Administration. Always observe the following safety rules when preparing insulin:

- ▶ Carefully check the label on the insulin bottle against the doctor's order for the *type* of insulin ordered; also check the bottle for the *concentration* of insulin (U-40, U-80, U-100), the *expiration* date, and the *appearance* of the insulin (i.e., clear, cloudy, or containing abnormal precipitation).
- ▶ Prepare insulin at room temperature; the administration of cold insulin may possibly be one factor in the development of lipodystrophy (see p. 1562). Insulin should be removed from the refrigerator several hours before preparation time.
- ▶ Use an insulin syringe which corresponds to the concentration of the insulin you are administering.
- ▶ Before drawing up NPH, Lente, Semilente, Ultralente, or PZI insulins, roll the bottle between the palms of your hands until the insulin is thoroughly mixed. Do not shake the bottle.
- ▶ If you must mix two types of insulin (e.g., NPH or Lente with regular insulin), follow the steps outlined in Table 72–9.
- ▶ On some nursing units it is standard procedure to have two nurses check insulin dosages prior to administration. In some instances it might be preferable to check the dosage with the patient, or have the patient draw up and administer the insulin. Double check the information on the medication card against both the label on the insulin bottle and the amount of insulin in the syringe.

> Remember:
> *Administering an overdose of insulin or the wrong type of insulin could kill the patient.*

TABLE 72–9. STEPS IN PREPARING TWO INSULINS IN ONE SYRINGE

1. Check physician's order and medication card.
2. Check insulin concentration (units/ml.) and expiration date.
3. Wash your hands and obtain the necessary equipment.
4. Turn the vial of cloudy insulin several times to mix the solution; *avoid shaking the vial.**
5. Insure that you are using the proper syringe for the insulin to be administered, e.g., U-100 syringe for U-100 insulin. Insure that the concentrations of both insulins are the same, e.g., both are U-100.
6. Wipe off the rubber stopper of each vial with alcohol.
7. Withdraw air into the syringe equal to the number of units of clear insulin to be administered, and inject the air into the clear vial. Repeat the process for the cloudy insulin. (Note: it matters little which vial is injected with air first, however, it is helpful to do it the same way each time in order to avoid errors.)
8. Withdraw the insulin from the cloudy vial first, then from the clear vial. (Note: While not essential, this order of withdrawing the insulins may be helpful. It is easier to detect inadvertent contamination of regular (clear) insulin with cloudy insulin than it is to detect contamination of cloudy insulin with clear insulin.)
9. Once both insulins have been drawn into the syringe, pull back on the barrel to allow a small air bubble to enter the syringe.
10. Replace the needle cap and rotate the syringe to mix the insulins. Once adequately mixed the insulins may be administered.

*In some cases both long and short acting insulins will be cloudy. Extra care should be taken to avoid confusion.

▶ Before giving insulin, double check the *patient's identity.* Patients are often drowsy in the early morning hours before breakfast and may answer to any name. As an added precaution, ask the patient's name, and check the patient's armband.

▶ Do not give insulin to the patient who is NPO prior to surgery or a special diagnostic procedure without first consulting the physician.

> Remember:
> *If the patient does not eat for a long period but still receives his or her usual dose of insulin, an insulin reaction may develop.*

Site Selection and Rotation. The diabetic patient may need insulin injections all through life. Over time, the repeated use of only a few sites for injection can result in either *atrophy* or *hypertrophy* of the tissues at the injection site. These abnormal tissue changes may result in poor absorption of the injected insulin with consequent loss of control. To prevent tissue changes, it is important to choose the site for injection carefully and *rotate sites systematically.* The sites for injections should be (a) easily accessible (use thighs, abdomen, upper back, buttocks, and upper arms); (b) relatively insensitive to pain (avoid the midline of the body where there are numerous nerve endings); and (c) relatively normal in appearance and to touch (avoid areas already damaged by hypertrophy or atrophy).

Once the sites for injection have been chosen, they are rotated *systematically* so that the same site is not injected more often than once every 6 to 8 weeks. To plan the patient's site rotation, first of all construct a map of the sites you will use. Note in Figure 72–4 the large number of sites available. When you or the patient daily inject each site, check that site off on the map.

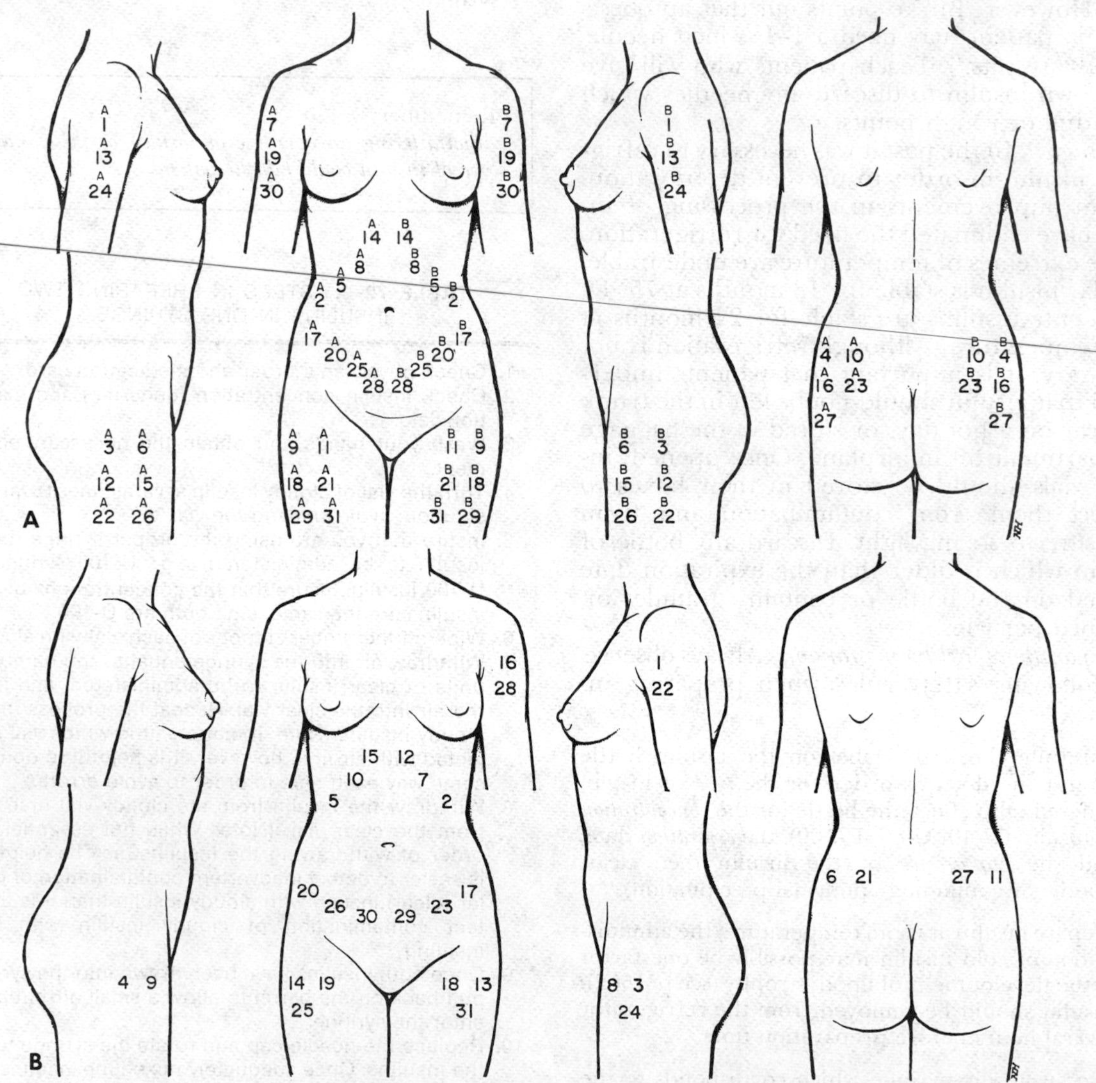

Figure 72–4. Rotation plan for insulin injection sites. Figure *A* is used for patients requiring two injections daily, with sites labeled A used in the morning and B sites used in the evening. Figure *B* is used for patients requiring only one injection per day. This plan eliminates sites on the dominant right arm. The numbers correspond to the day of the month, thus eliminating the need for an injection record. (From Fonville, A. M.: Teaching patients to rotate injection sites. *American Journal of Nursing,* 78:880, May 1978.)

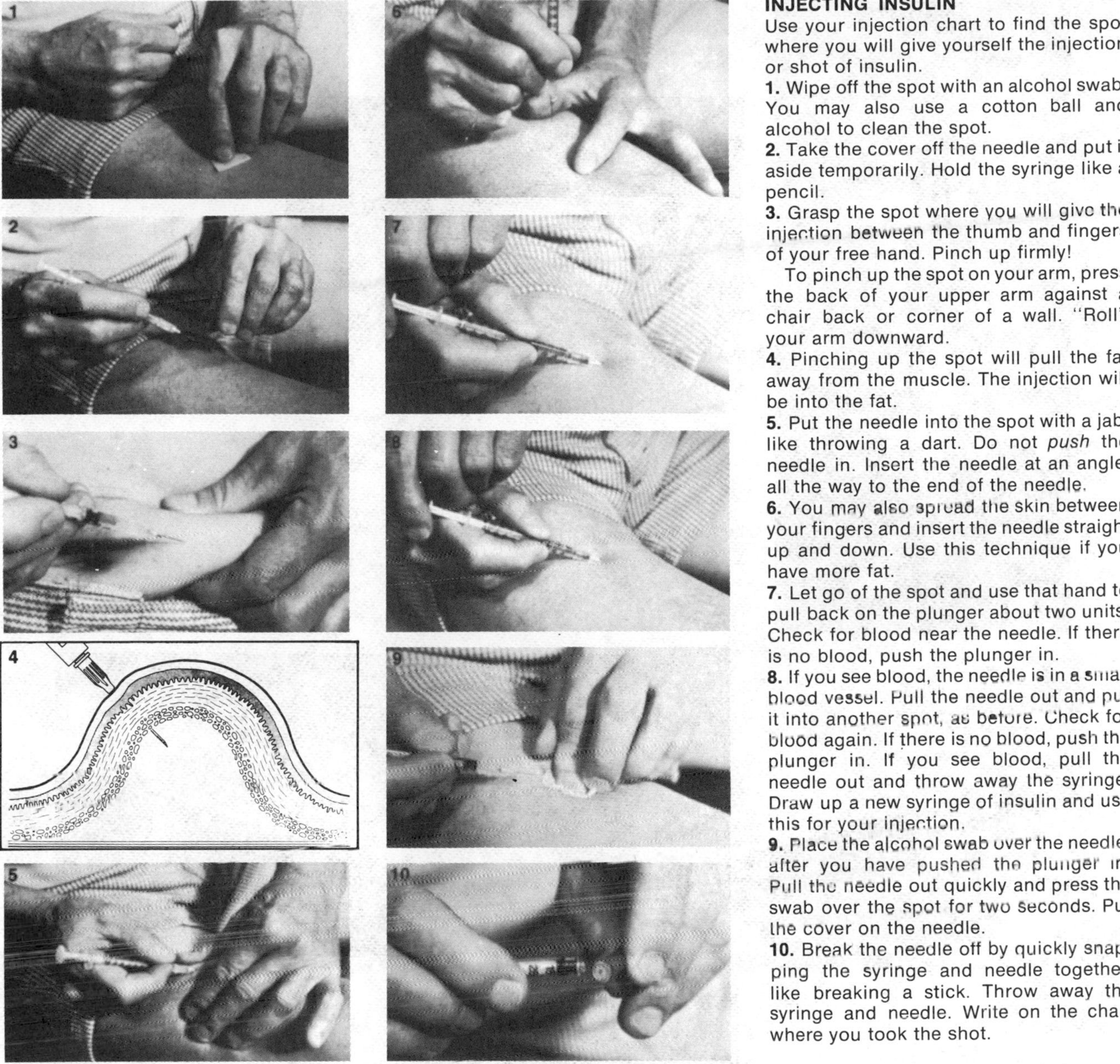

Figure 72–5. Techniques of administering insulin. (From Engle, V., and R. Zelm: Diabetic teaching. How to win your patient's cooperation in his care. *Nursing '75*, December 1975, p. 17.)

Emphasize to the patient the importance of adhering to a definite injection plan to avoid eventual tissue damage.

Insulin Administration. There are two common ways of positioning the skin over the subcutaneous tissue to be injected with insulin: (a) bunching the tissue up or (b) spreading the tissue taut. Both techniques are illustrated in Figure 72–5. While spreading the tissue may be more comfortable, the major factor is the amount of subcutaneous tissue in the area to be injected. If there is a great deal of adipose tissue, it may be desirable to spread the tissues and administer the insulin with the needle and syringe at a 90 degree angle to the skin. When the tissues are bunched, the needle is placed at a 45 to 60 degree angle. In most instances a 25 gauge, ½ inch needle is used.

Self-Injection of Insulin. The majority of patients who take insulin learn to give their own injections. It is principally your responsibility to instruct diabetic patients in the technique of preparing insulin and giving injections to themselves. Teaching patients about insulin and other aspects of diabetic care is described later in this chapter.

Equipment which the diabetic patient will need to purchase for home use includes (a) insulin of the type prescribed, (b) absorbent cotton, (c) approved syringes (may be either glass or

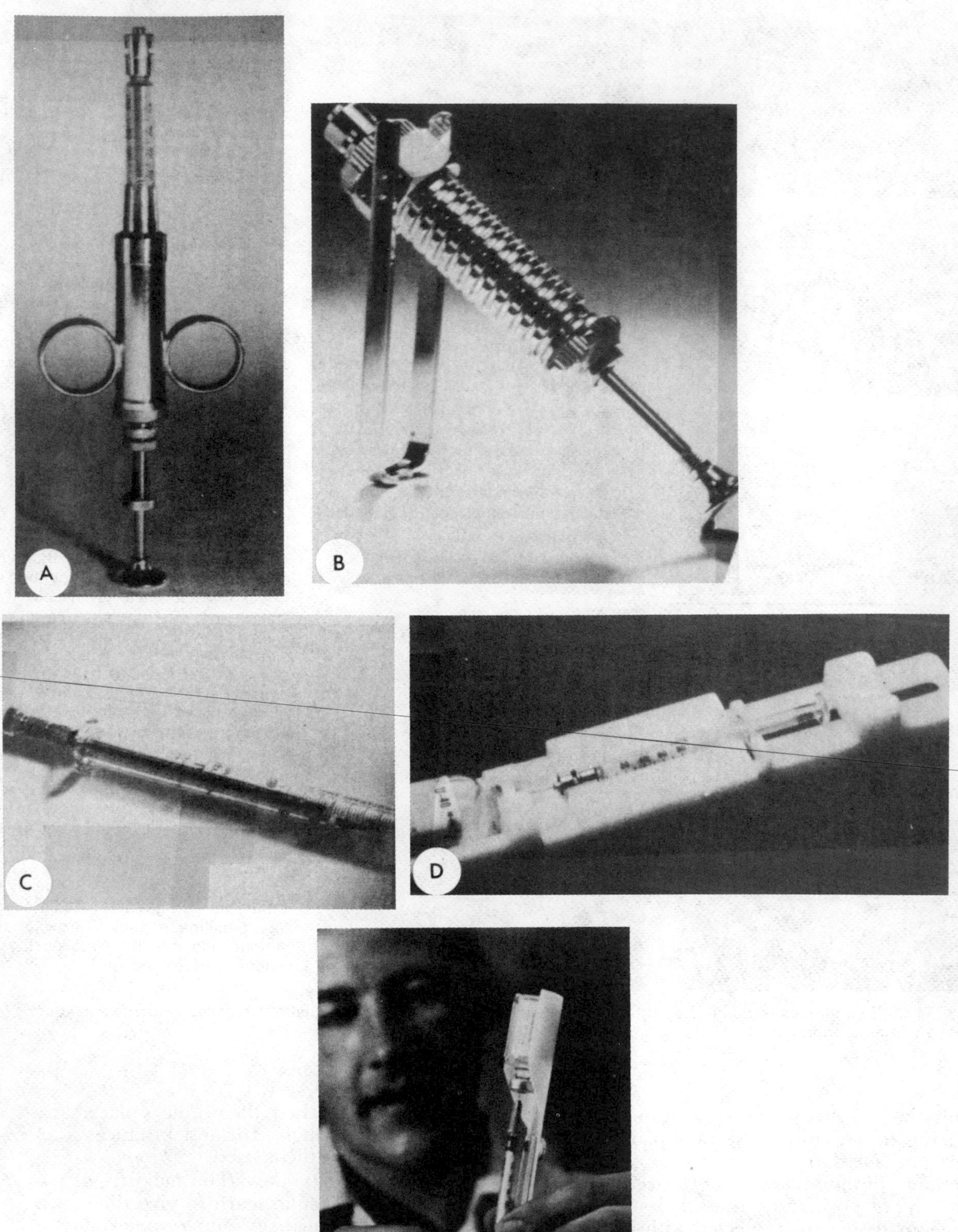

Figure 72–6. Devices used to assist the diabetic in drawing up and administering the correct dosage of insulin. (*A* through *D* from Boyles, V. A.: Injection aids for blind diabetics. *American Journal of Nursing,* 77:1456, Sept. 1977. *E* from George Wright Industries, 82 Lake Shore Drive, Lincoln, Neb. 68528. Picture appeared in *American Journal of Nursing,* 78:287, Feb. 1978.)

disposable), (d) needles (2 rustless 25 gauge hypodermic needles or disposable needles), (e) 70 per cent ethyl or 91 per cent isopropyl alcohol, and (f) a pan and large strainer for boiling and sterilizing nondisposable syringes and needles. Patients with visual or motor impairments may benefit from the use of injection aid devices such as those illustrated in Figure 72–6. The major steps involved in the self-injection technique are shown in Figure 72–5. Note in part 5 the patient is giving himself an injection deep into the pocket between the fat and muscle.

While the prospect of having to give oneself daily injections for life is far from pleasant, the patient's attitude toward this aspect of care may be largely influenced by the way in which patient teaching is approached. A matter-of-fact attitude may be important in assisting the patient to understand and accept responsibility for care. The extent of instruction depends on the individual patient's familiarity with insulin and the injection equipment. Some patients may benefit from advance notice of the instruction, while this may increase anxiety in other patients. In some instances, after you have selected the site and aspirated to check for blood, have the patient push in the plunger and remove the needle as the first step in self-injection.

When instructing patients in self-injection techniques, emphasize the following points to them:

▶ Always purchase an extra bottle of insulin, an extra syringe, and extra needles; extra equipment is needed in case the equipment breaks or is lost.

▶ Wash hands thoroughly before preparing an injection.

▶ Use only sterile syringes and needles. To resterilize equipment following use, boil the syringe, plunger, and needle in a pan of water for 5 minutes. Also it is permissible to sterilize the syringe parts and needle by covering them with alcohol for 5 to 10 minutes. When traveling, use disposable syringes.

▶ Always clean the top of the insulin bottle before inserting the sterile needle and withdrawing the insulin. Alcohol is usually acceptable.

▶ Rotate sites systematically according to a definite plan.

▶ Following the injection, break the needle and syringe when using disposable equipment. When using nondisposable equipment, flush the needle and place in a jar of alcohol to prevent it from becoming plugged. Place some cotton in the bottom of the jar to prevent the needle points from becoming damaged. Also wash the syringe parts in cold clear water.

▶ When taking insulin, carefully follow the diet prescription. Do not alter the diet without consulting the doctor. If for some reason a meal is postponed and the insulin injection has already been given, drink a glass of orange juice. Always have hard candy or lump sugar handy in the event of a hypoglycemic reaction.

▶ Wear a medical alert bracelet or necklace, and carry an identification card (Fig. 72–7).

▶ Consult the physician if nausea, vomiting, fever, or infection develops. Nausea and vomiting may decrease one's need for insulin, whereas fever and infection increase insulin requirements. Additionally, nausea and vomiting may indicate hyperglycemia.

▶ Urine should usually be tested for sugar at least once daily. If there is sugar in the urine you should also test for acetone. When ill, urine should be tested every 3 to 4 hours, and the physician should be consulted concerning the results.

▶ Be thoroughly familiar with the early symptoms of hypoglycemia and hyperglycemia and the treatment for each (see below).

Complications of Insulin Therapy. Insulin therapy may be complicated by one or more of the following six conditions: (1) hypoglycemia, (2) hyperglycemia, (3) tissue hypertrophy or atrophy or both, (4) erratic insulin action, (5) insulin allergy, and (6) insulin resistance. These problems are briefly considered below.

Hypoglycemia. Usually, patients will experience symptoms of hypoglycemia (such as altered consciousness, tachycardia, or increased perspiration) when the blood glucose level drops to 60 mg./100 ml. or less (Folin and Wu method). In diabetes, hypoglycemic reactions are usually caused by an overdose of insulin or overzealous exercise — both of which remove glucose from the blood. Details concerning the symptoms and treatment of hypoglycemia are discussed later in this chapter.

Hyperglycemia. When the blood sugar concentration is too high (greater than 180 mg./100 ml.) sugar usually begins to appear ("spill over") in the urine. This causes symptoms of polyuria and nocturia. When the blood sugar levels rise extremely high (300–800 mg./100 ml.), the patient may develop ketoacidosis or hyperosmolar

I Am a Diabetic and Take Insulin

If I am behaving peculiarly but am conscious and able to swallow, give me sugar or hard candy or orange juice slowly. If I am unconscious, call an ambulance immediately, take me to a physician or a hospital, and notify my physician. **I am not intoxicated.**

My name ______________________

Address ______________________

Telephone ______________________

Physician's name ______________________

Physician's address ______________________

Telephone ______________________

Figure 72–7. Identification card which should be carried by all diabetics who take insulin.

coma. Hyperglycemia and ketoacidosis are discussed later in this chapter.

Tissue Hypertrophy or Atrophy. Tissue *hypertrophy,* which is sometimes termed an "insulin tumor," is a thickening of the subcutaneous tissues at injection sites.[18] On the other hand, *atrophy* is a "loss of subcutaneous fat or depression at the site of injection."[18] A hypertrophied area may feel lumpy and hard, or soft and spongy. Tissue changes due to atrophy may be slight, causing only a dimpling of the tissues, or they may be more extensive, causing the appearance of large craters. Both tissue atrophy and hypertrophy are classified as *lipodystrophies* or localized disturbances of fat metabolism. Lipodystrophy, as summarized in Table 72–10, can alter the absorption of insulin, thus creating difficulty in the control of the patient's blood sugar. Atrophy and hypertrophy may be associated with (a) the use of cold insulin, (b) failure to rotate sites, and (c) injection of the insulin directly into the fat. More commonly these conditions appear to be due to allergic or immune mechanisms and may respond to "purer" kinds of insulin (e.g., pure pork or monocomponent insulin).

> *To help prevent lipodystrophy, remember to (a) use insulin at room temperature; (b) rotate the injection site systematically; and (c) inject insulin into a pocket between the fat and muscle.*

If the patient's tissues have already been damaged by repeated injections, fresh sites must be used for a period of time to allow the damaged areas to heal. Patients who give their own injections normally use their abdomen, thighs, and arms. When these areas are damaged, you will need to teach a neighbor or relative to inject the patient's buttocks and back until the injured sites can be used again. Remember, however, that patients who have consistently used abnormal tissues for injection usually suffer from an inadequate absorption of insulin. In these cases, the patient's doctor may have ordered higher and higher doses of insulin to compensate for the poor absorption and to cover for sugar spillage into the urine. Consequently, when *normal tissues are used for injection,* the patient may develop an *insulin reaction,* because the higher dose of insulin is *completedly absorbed* into the undamaged tissues, and it acts immediately to lower the blood sugar.

> Remember: *When a fresh undamaged site has been used for injection, observe the patient for signs of hypoglycemia (trembling, diaphoresis, headache, and irritability) at the time the insulin has its peak effect. Have orange juice on hand in the event of an insulin reaction.*

Recently, research efforts have been directed at developing an insulin reservoir and pumping device that can be used to pump small amounts of insulin directly into the patient's blood according to need. While the concept seems promising, the effectiveness and practicality of such a device remain to be determined.

Erratic Insulin Action. Some patients respond erratically to insulin (i.e., with periods of hypoglycemia followed by periods of hyperglycemia) for a number of reasons. The important causes of erratic insulin action are listed in Table 72–11.

Insulin Allergy. Patients who develop allergies during insulin therapy are usually sensitive to the protein component of insulin. Some patients may develop allergic reactions because of the alcohol used to sterilize the equipment, while in others the problem may result from failure to inject the insulin deep enough into the subcutaneous tissue. Localized allergic reactions to insulin occur frequently, but systemic allergic reactions are rare.

TABLE 72–10. LIPODYSTROPHY*

	Atrophy	Hypertrophy
Appearance	Small dimpling to extensive pitting at injection site	Mass of fibrous avascular scar tissue at injection site
Incidence	More common in adult females and children	More common in adult females and children
Cause	Undetermined	Undetermined
Significance	Cosmetic only; physiologically harmless	Patients' preferred site due to relative anesthesia; insulin absorption is unpredictable and incomplete, leading to possible misdiagnosis of "insulin resistance"
Treatment	Avoid affected areas with good rotation plan	Avoid affected areas with good rotation plan

*From Fonville, A. M.: Teaching patients to rotate injection sites. *American Journal of Nursing,* 78:880, May 1978.

TABLE 72–11. CAUSES OF ERRATIC INSULIN ACTION*

1. *Dietary dereliction* (surreptitious overeating, free sugar ingestion, irregular feedings, omission of snacks, etc.)

2. *Errors in insulin technique*
   a. Inaccurate measurement (visual ?)
   b. Failure to rotate injection sites
   c. Injecting sites of lipodystrophy
   d. Inadequate mixing
   e. Frozen or outdated insulin
   f. Improper dosage adjustment ("insulin timing")

3. *Emotional or psychiatric conflicts*
   a. Deliberate omission or overdosage of insulin (masochistic or suicidal)
   b. Misplaced affect (indifference or obsessed)
   c. Spurious urine tests ("faked" vs. spoiled tablets)
   d. Feigned insulin reactions (especially children)
   e. Marital or parental tensions

4. *Chronic overdosage of insulin* (Somogyi effect)

5. *Intermittent use of hyper- or hypoglycemic drugs* (Examples:)
   a. Aspirin, Butazolidin, etc.
   b. Steroids
   c. Birth control pills
   d. Alcohol, beer
   e. Cough syrups
   f. Thiazides
   g. Nicotinic acid

6. *Irregular exercise and/or rest periods*

*From Haunz, E. E.; Diabetes mellitus in adults. *In* Conn, H. F. (ed.): *Current Therapy, 1973.* Philadelphia: W. B. Saunders Co., 1973, p. 379.

Symptoms characteristic of local reactions include itching, redness, and burning at the site of injection. Fortunately, the majority of allergic reactions are self-limiting in nature. For example, allergic symptoms may appear during the first day or so of insulin therapy and then disappear 1 to 2 weeks later.

Treatment of local allergic reactions varies with the cause and severity of the reaction. For example, since many insulins contain both pork and beef insulin, if the patient is sensitive to beef insulin, the doctor may prescribe pure porcine (pork) insulin for a period of time; also new monocomponent insulins are now appearing on the market which are hypoallergenic. If the patient is allergic to alcohol, the patient will need to either boil the syringes or use disposable equipment; also Zephiran chloride or povidone-iodine can be used to cleanse the skin prior to injections. When allergy is severe, the doctor may order an *antihistamine* drug such as diphenhydramine (Benadryl) to be given until the allergy disappears. If all the above therapeutic methods fail, the doctor may attempt to *desensitize* the patient to insulin so that insulin can be used both on a daily basis and in emergencies (e.g., diabetic acidosis). The desensitization program involves injecting the patient several times a day with diluted insulin solutions. Over time, the physician increases the amount of insulin in the daily injections until the patient tolerates the prescribed insulin dosage without allergic symptoms.

Insulin Resistance. The patient who is insulin resistant requires more than 100 U. of insulin per day for control of diabetes. The exact etiology of insulin resistance is unknown; it may be caused by specific insulin antagonists within the blood or by circulating antibodies which are destructive to insulin. There is some indication that the diabetic who becomes insulin resistant because of an immunological response is one who has been on insulin intermittently, rather than continually.[3] Some authorities classify the degree of resistance to insulin as follows:[115b]

▶ Mild resistance — 80 to 125 U. required per day.
▶ Moderate resistance — 126 to 200 U. required per day.
▶ Severe resistance — more than 200 U. required per day.

To treat insulin resistance, the doctor may first attempt to give the patient a pork-based insulin; pork insulin is very similar in chemical structure to human insulin, and its use is sometimes sufficient to overcome the patient's insulin resistance. Recently, the use of sulfated insulin, which is regular insulin that has been chemically modified, has been found to be of value in treating insulin resistance in selected patients.[3] If the use of pork insulin or sulfated insulin fails, the physician must then order as high a dosage of insulin as is needed to control the patient's diabetes. Consequently, dosages may range from as low as 80 U. per day to as high as thousands of units per day. There are special preparations of U-500 insulin available for those patients who require 500 or more units daily.

Patients who are being treated for insulin resistance must be carefully watched for signs of either hyperglycemia or hypoglycemia (see below). *Hyperglycemia* is a signal that the patient needs a higher dosage of insulin to overcome insulin resistance. On the other hand, *hypoglycemia* and shock may occur quite suddenly when the insulin resistance is exceeded and the high doses of insulin are abruptly absorbed. For this reason patients being treated for insulin resistance require frequent blood tests and careful nursing observation and supervision.

Insulin resistance, particularly in obese non-insulin dependent diabetics, may be related to an inadequate number of insulin receptors at the cellular level. These patients often have normal or elevated levels of plasma insulin, yet they have hyperglycemia. Hyperglycemia persists in the presence of elevated insulin levels because of a lack of insulin receptors. The number of insulin receptors at the cell is inversely proportional to the plasma insulin level; as the insulin level increases, the number of insulin receptors decreases. The cause of the increase in plasma insulin is excessive food intake. The therapy, then, for the insulin resistant, obese, non-insulin dependent diabetic is restriction of calories and weight reduction. Research has demonstrated that the number of insulin receptors increases as the caloric intake is decreased.

The Somogyi Effect.[59] Certain diabetic patients may exhibit wide swings in blood sugar level, creating difficulty in establishing a routine insulin dosage. The wide variation begins when exogenous insulin administration produces hypoglycemia. The normal bodily response to hypoglycemia is the release of hyperglycemic substrates such as epinephrine and glucagon. These substances prevent the utilization of insulin for glucose metabolism, and the blood sugar becomes seriously elevated. Classically the blood sugar is elevated when tested, but patients may have periods of profound hypoglycemia. If insulin rebound due to the Somogyi effect is suspected, the patient may be advised to test his urine and/or blood at times other than after meals. The treatment is gradual lowering of the insulin dosage, dividing the dosage into smaller increments, or administering insulin at different times throughout the day.

ORAL HYPOGLYCEMIC AGENTS

As mentioned, insulin must be administered parenterally because it is destroyed by gastrointestinal tract enzymes. To date, scientists have never succeeded in developing an oral form of insulin. However, there are oral agents available (called oral hypoglycemic agents) which are capable of lowering the blood sugar. Oral hypoglycemic agents are mainly prescribed for *mild* diabetics who are unable to control their condition with diet alone.

There are two classifications of oral hypoglycemic agents: (1) the sulfonylureas, and (2) the biguanides (see Table 72–12). The *biguanide* agents have been banned recently by the Food and Drug Administration in the United States. The *sulfonylureas* lower the blood sugar in part by stimulating the pancreatic beta cells to release insulin. For this reason the sulfonylureas are useful only for non-insulin dependent diabetics whose beta cells are still capable of producing insulin. Thus the average candidate for the sulfonylureas can be described as follows: (a) is over 40 years old; (b) has been a diabetic for less than 10 years; (c) cannot be controlled by diet alone; and (d) can be controlled with less than 20 U. of insulin daily.

Major sulfonylureas are tolbutamide (Orinase), chlorpropamide (Diabinese), acetohexamide (Dymelor), and tolazamide (Tolinase). These drugs can occasionally produce hypoglycemic reactions. Warn patients not to ingest large amounts of aspirin when taking the sulfonylureas, because aspirin tends to increase the hypoglycemic effect of these agents. Also instruct patients taking oral agents to notify their physician at once should they develop an infection or febrile illness. When ill, the diabetic has a greater need for insulin; consequently temporary insulin injections may be needed as well as the usual oral agent.

The *biguanides,* which are no longer available in the United States, are still being studied for their exact mode of action. These drugs, by some mysterious means, are capable of lowering the patient's blood sugar in the absence of beta cell function. Many theories have been advanced to explain the effectiveness of the biguanides but none have been fully accepted. The biguanide most commonly used is phenformin; phenformin is made in a short-acting form (DBI) and a long-acting capsule (DBI-PT). Phenformin is sometimes given in conjunction with insulin to increase the latter's effectiveness. Instruct patients to always take the biguanides with meals in order to prevent nausea, vomiting, and diarrhea.

While the oral hypoglycemic agents have their place in diabetic therapy, we must emphasize again that adult onset diabetes should ideally be controlled by diet alone. Instruct patients that oral tablets must never be considered a substitute for their prescribed diet.

EXERCISE

A program of planned exercise can be highly beneficial for the diabetic patient, because exercise (like insulin) acts to lower the blood sugar by oxidizing carbohydrates. Also exercise aids in weight reduction and proper weight maintenance. On the other hand, unplanned exercise can cause a dangerous hypoglycemic reaction unless the patient ingests additional food. Unplanned exercise can be particularly dangerous for patients who take insulin or oral agents. When instructing patients concerning exercise, take care to include the following points in your discussion:

▶ While the doctor is initially planning the treatment regimen, the patient should follow a normal activity schedule so that diet and insulin dosage are in balance with activity level.

▶ Once insulin dosage has been determined, the patient should eat additional food if exercising more than usual; the equivalent of a bedtime snack is generally adequate.

TABLE 72-12. ORAL HYPOGLYCEMIC AGENTS

Generic Name	Brand Name	Strength (mg.)	Onset of Action[2] (hrs.)	Action Curve[1] (hrs.)	Dosage[1]
Sulfonylureas					
Tolbutamide	Orinase	500	½	12	500–3000
Chlorpropamide	Diabinase	100, 250	1	60–90	100–500
Acetohexamide	Dymelor	250, 500	½	12–24	250–1500
Tolazamide	Tolinase	100, 250, 500	4–6	14–24	100–1000
*Biguanides**					
Phentormin	DBI	25	1	4–5	25–200
Phenformin TD	DBI TD	10, 50	1	8–14	50–200

[1]Source: Goldner, M. G.: Diabetes mellitus in the adult. *In* Conn, H. F. (Ed.): *Current Therapy*, 1978. Philadelphia: W. B. Saunders Co., 1978.

[2]Source: Adapted from Eliopoulos, C. E.: Diagnosis and management of diabetes in the elderly. *American Journal of Nursing*, 78:884, May 1978.

*Withdrawn from the market in the United States by order of the FDA.

▶ If the patient still experiences a mild hypoglycemic reaction after eating a snack, he or she must consume more food when performing that particular activity. If, on the other hand, a urine test is positive for sugar or acetone, then he or she has eaten more than necessary for a certain activity.

▶ Stress that, with time and practice, the patient will gradually learn how much energy is consumed in various activities, and will be able to regulate the diet accordingly.

▶ Insulin-dependent diabetics should not exercise when they are very hypoglycemic or acidotic.

THE COMPLICATIONS OF DIABETES

Acute Complications

KETOACIDOSIS AND COMA

The two major hallmarks of insulin-dependent diabetes mellitus are *hyperglycemia* and *ketosis*. Hyperglycemia results when glucose cannot be transported to the cells because of a lack of insulin. You will recall that, without available carbohydrates for cellular fuel, the liver converts its glycogen stores back to glucose (glycogenolysis) and biosynthesis of glucose (gluconeogenesis) increases. Unfortunately, however, these maneuvers only aggravate the situation by raising the blood sugar even higher.

As the need for cellular fuel grows more critical, the body begins to draw on its fat and protein stores for energy. Excessive amounts of fatty acids are mobilized from adipose tissue cells and transported to the liver. The liver, in turn, accelerates the rate at which it produces ketone bodies (ketogenesis) for catabolism by the tissue cells. As fat metabolism increases, the liver may produce *too many* ketone bodies resulting in the accumulation of ketone bodies in the blood (ketosis) and the spillage of ketone bodies into the urine (ketonuria). *Metabolic acidosis* develops from the pH-lowering effect of the ketones, acetoacetic acid and B-hydroxybutyrate. When acidosis is severe, the patient may lose consciousness. Loss of consciousness in the diabetic due to metabolic acidosis is termed *diabetic coma*.

Etiology and Prevention of Ketoacidosis. Acidosis is primarily a complication of insulin-dependent diabetes, although non-insulin dependent diabetics can develop acidosis during periods of increased stress. Common precipitating causes of diabetic acidosis include (a) taking too little insulin; (b) omitting doses of insulin; (c) an increased need for insulin due to surgery, trauma, pregnancy, puberty, febrile illness, (d) insulin resistance due to the development of insulin antibodies or severe emotional stress.

The development of this grave complication can be prevented in most cases by careful patient teaching. To prevent diabetic coma, patients must be taught to (a) take their insulin as prescribed; (b) perform fractional urines at least twice daily when in good health and 3 to 4 times daily when ill or under stress; and (c) schedule regular appointments with their physician for urine tests, review of weight gains or losses, and so forth. Remind patients to call their physician should they develop any of the following: (a) an infection or febrile illness; (b) anorexia, nausea, or vomiting; (c) ketonuria which persists for more than 12 hours; or (d) any of the signs and symptoms of acidosis. Emphasize that conscientious adherence to their therapy program and early treatment of mild ketosis are the patient's greatest weapons against development of diabetic coma.

Pathophysiology. When insulin is lacking and carbohydrates cannot be used for energy, ketosis and acidosis represent the final stages in the body's struggle for fuel. The process of burning fats for fuel in the absence of carbohydrates gives rise to four pathologic events:

1. Incomplete lipid metabolism,
2. Dehydration,

3. Ketoacidosis and lactic acidosis,
4. Electrolyte imbalance.

Incomplete Lipid Metabolism. First, let us review a few facts about normal fat metabolism. The three ketone bodies (beta-hydroxybutyric acid, acetoacetic acid, and acetone) are the intermediate products of fat metabolism. In the nondiabetic, ketone bodies are quickly used by cells for energy as needed, swiftly disarmed by the body's buffer systems, oxidized, and finally excreted as CO_2 and water.

In the insulin-dependent diabetic deprived of insulin, however, fat metabolism and the production of ketone bodies are greatly accelerated owing to the unavailability of carbohydrates. As production speeds, the increase in ketone bodies eventually exceeds the body's capacity to oxidize them for energy. When ketone bodies are not oxidized and excreted as CO_2 and water, these intermediate products of fat metabolism soon begin to escape into the urine. Once the numbers of ketone bodies overwhelm the kidney's capacity to excrete them, they accumulate in the blood.

In the meanwhile, to defend itself against the rising ketosis, the body brings into play its three lines of defense against H^+ excess (Chapter 12). As you recall, the first line of defense is *buffering.* Thus acetoacetic acid unites with sodium bicarbonate to form carbonic acid and acetoacetate. The lungs excrete carbonic acid as carbon dioxide, and the kidneys excrete sodium acetoacetate in the urine. The phosphate buffer system is also active in the buffering of other ketone bodies. At the same time the *respiratory system* (the second line of defense) becomes activated, and acetone, as well as carbonic acid in the form of CO_2 and H_2O, are blown off in the breath. Owing to this defense, respirations increase in depth and rate (Kussmaul respirations), and the breath has a "fruity" acetone odor. The *renal* system (the third line of defense) can excrete between 30 and 100 Gm. of ketone bodies every day to control ketoacidosis. Also the ammonia mechanism is activated, which promotes the removal of excess H^+.

Unfortunately, in uncontrolled ketoacidosis, the rising tide of ketone bodies eventually overwhelms the body's defenses against H^+ excess. With depletion of its alkaline reserves and failure of its respiratory and renal defenses, the body finally succumbs to its acid overload, and diabetic coma ensues.

Dehydration. Patients suffering from ketoacidosis lose fluids from several sources. First of all, severely ill diabetics excrete large amounts of urine in an attempt to eliminate excessive amounts of glucose and ketone bodies. Secondly, acidosis causes severe nausea and vomiting, which results in further losses of fluid and electrolytes (notably sodium and chloride). Finally, water is lost in the breath as the patient attempts to blow off excessive acetone and CO_2. Severe dehydration resulting from these fluid losses may be followed by the complications of *hypovolemic shock* and *lactic acidosis.*

Lactic Acidosis. When water losses are critical, the patient's blood volume falls, with resultant *hemoconcentration.* Hemoconcentration, in turn, impedes blood circulation, causing a severe generalized tissue anoxia accompanied by the production of large amounts of lactic acid. The rise in lactic acid within the blood adds more H^+ to the body's already overwhelming acid load.

Electrolyte Imbalance. As the pH of the blood decreases in acidosis, the rapidly accumulating H^+ moves from the extracellular fluid (ECF) to the intracellular fluid (ICF). The movement of H^+ into the cells promotes the movement of K^+ out of the cells into the ECF. This results in severe cellular hypokalemia. Initially the hypokalemia may not be appreciated because the serum potassium levels are often normal or elevated. As the osmotic diuresis continues, however, much potassium is excreted in the urine and hypokalemia becomes apparent. If the patient is severely dehydrated, hemoconcentration coupled with oliguria due to renal involvement causes the serum K^+ levels to rise higher. Hyperkalemia, in turn, results in muscle weakness, paralysis, and respiratory or cardiac arrest.

In addition to K^+ losses, the patient in metabolic acidosis also loses excessive amounts of sodium, phosphate, chloride, and bicarbonate in the urine and vomitus.

Bases of Signs and Symptoms. Diabetic acidosis has many easily recognized symptoms. The major manifestations of this complication and their causes are shown in Table 72–13 and summarized in Figure 72–8.

Clinical Care. *Severe diabetic acidosis is an emergency! The patient must receive immediate intelligent medical and nursing care or death may result.*

The primary goal of care in diabetic ketoacidosis is to shift the metabolism from a state of fat catabolism to a state of carbohydrate utilization by providing exogenous insulin. Secondary goals include (a) restoration of normal circulating blood volume, (b) correction of fluid and electrolyte imbalances, and (c) correction of those factors which precipitated the development of acidosis in the first place.

When the diabetic patient with coma is brought to the emergency department, part of the initial care is directed at determining whether the problem is hypoglycemia or ketoacidosis. A third possibility, seen most often in the non-insulin dependent diabetic, is hypergly-

TABLE 72–13. MANIFESTATIONS OF DIABETIC KETOACIDOSIS

Signs and Symptoms	Bases
Polyuria (early symptom)	Large amounts of glucose, ketone bodies, and protein must be excreted by the kidney; osmotic effect of sugar attracts water and promotes diuresis
Thirst (early symptom)	Polyuria causes loss of ECF, which causes water to be drawn from the cell, thereby promoting cellular dehydration
Nausea and vomiting	Cause of vomiting not known; nausea results from electrolyte imbalance due to glucosuria and ketonuria
Dry mucous membranes and cracked lips; hot, flushed skin	Severe dehydration; flushed appearance is due to acidosis
Weight loss	Dehydration is one cause; also patient is unable to use carbohydrate for energy, and consequently must burn protein and fat reserves
Abdominal pain and abdominal rigidity (similar to "acute abdomen")	No known cause; possibly associated with either dehydration or sodium deficit
Kussmaul respirations (deep rapid breathing)	When the alkaline reserve is depleted and the body can no longer buffer the excessive ketone bodies, the lungs attempt to blow off the overload of acetone as well as excess CO_2, which decreases the amount of carbonic acid in the blood, thereby raising the pH.
Acetone odor of the breath	Excess acetone is being blown off through the lungs
Weakness, paralysis, and paresthesia	Either K^+ deficiency or excess can produce neurologic problems
Soft eyeballs	Dehydration
Hypotension and shock (late signs)	Profound dehydration eventually leads to hypovolemic shock and circulatory collapse
Oliguria or anuria (late signs)	A dreaded complication arising secondary to severe dehydration and shock; decreased circulating fluid volume lessens blood flow to the kidney, resulting in renal shutdown
Coma or stupor (late signs)	Electrolyte imbalances, profound shock, and the rapidly lowering pH all contribute to loss of consciousness

cemic hyperosmolar non-ketotic coma (HHNK). If hypoglycemia, rather than hyperglycemia, is the problem, time is of the essence. Permanent brain damage can occur when the blood sugar is very low. The steps used in evaluating the etiology of the coma, and treating ketoacidosis include:

▶Establish and maintain a patent airway; oxygen may be administered.
▶Start a large bore IV and draw blood for the following studies: CBC, blood sugar, BUN, electrolytes, ketones, osmolarity.
▶Give 50 ml of 50 per cent dextrose IV *after* the bloods have been drawn. (Note: when it is difficult to obtain enough blood for these studies, or when the patient's condition is critical, a drop of blood can be tested with a Dextrostix. This will give you some idea whether the patient is hypoglycemic or hyperglycemic.)
▶Insert a Foley catheter and test the urine for sugar, ketones, and protein; send a sample to the lab for UA and possibly culture and sensitivity. (Note: urinary tract infections such as pyelonephritis may precipitate ketoacidosis.)
▶Obtain arterial blood for blood gas analysis.
▶Obtain a 12 lead electrocardiogram and initiate continuous cardiac monitoring.
▶Keep the patient NPO; an N-G tube may be inserted.
▶Monitor IV fluid administration. Isotonic saline solution or 0.45 per cent sodium chloride are used for the patient with ketoacidosis while a 5 per cent or 10 per cent solution of glucose is used in the patient with hypoglycemia.
▶Arrange for x-ray as indicated (chest and/or abdomen).

Once the patient's preliminary laboratory results are reported, definitive treatment begins. See Table 72–14 for a comparison of the findings in diabetic ketoacidosis; hyperglycemic, hyperosmolar, non-ketotic coma; and hypoglycemia. A fairly standard program of care for the patient in diabetic coma is described below.

Insulinization. Insulin dosages vary, depending upon the patient's condition and the level of the blood sugar. Insulin is usually not given subcutaneously during this period because the patient's subcutaneous tissues are dehydrated and poorly perfused with blood, owing to dehydration and hypovolemic shock. For this reason insulin is often administered IV or IM until the patient's condition improves. When insulin is administered IV, it may be administered IV push or by IV drip. Some of the insulin in an IV infusion may adhere to the walls of the IV container. To prevent this, small amounts of serum albumin may be added to the IV fluid.

Caution: *Only* regular *insulin may be administered intravenously.*

During the period when insulin is being given, laboratory studies are ordered frequently so that insulin is administered on the basis of the patient's current metabolic status.

Correction of Salt and Water Losses. As mentioned, dehydration resulting in hypovolemic shock, acute tubular necrosis, and uremia is a major cause of death in diabetic acidosis. The typical patient in diabetic coma loses an amount of water equivalent to 10 per cent of his body weight, and he also loses approximately 40 Gm. of sodium.[20] Consequently, intravenous infusions of isotonic saline (0.9 per cent sodium chloride) are started immediately upon admission. Typically, 1000 ml. of isotonic solution is

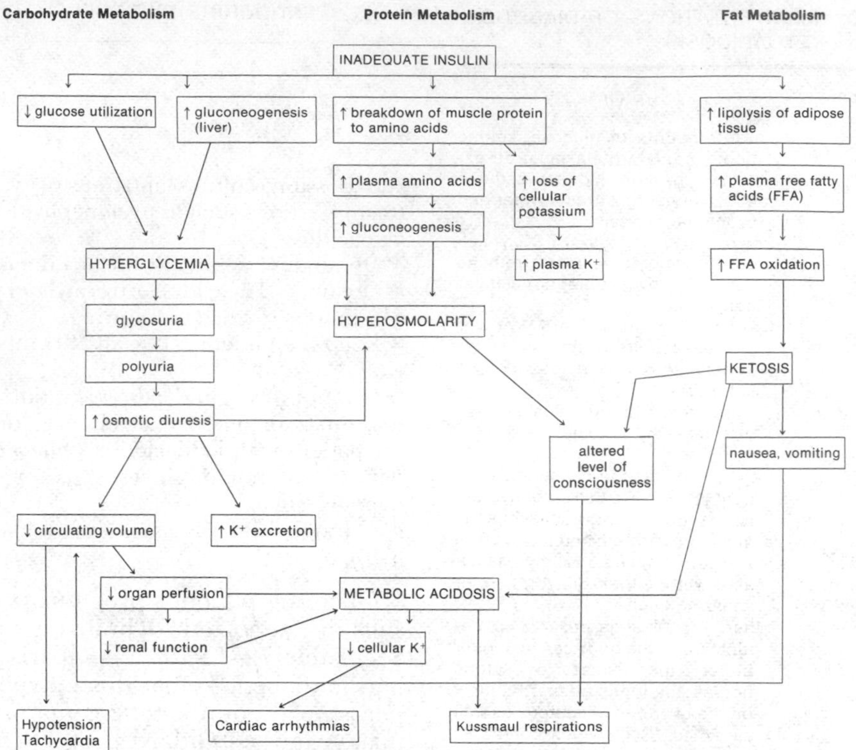

Figure 72–8. Pathophysiology of diabetic ketoacidosis

given IV during the first hour, followed by 2000 to 8000 more ml. of solution over the next 24 hours. Patients with compromised cardiovascular function may require slower intravenous fluid replacement.

Once the patient is fully conscious, encourage as much fluid intake as possible. Drinking broth is quite beneficial because broth contains needed sodium chloride. Remember to record the patient's intake *accurately*.

If the patient is being sufficiently hydrated, skin turgor improves, weight increases, and the hematocrit drops to normal levels.

Reversal of Shock. If the patient is in circulatory collapse, the physician will order either blood, albumin, or other plasma volume expanders, such as dextran, to be administered alternately with normal saline solutions. Also combinations of colloids and saline solution may be administered to raise the serum levels of both sodium chloride and plasma protein.

Correction of pH. Sodium bicarbonate or 1/6 molar lactate is usually administered to patients with a pH of 7.0 or below or a carbon dioxide combining power of 15 mEq. per liter or less. Replacement therapy is designed to partially correct the metabolic acidosis. As the patient's condition improves, normal body mechanisms will restore the blood pH to normal.

Restoration of Potassium Balance. As you recall, K^+ leaves the cells in untreated ketoacidosis, and hyperkalemia develops; however, *once treatment starts*, the patient may develop dangerous *hypokalemia* with weakness, extreme dyspnea, and even cardiac arrest. Hypokalemia develops because (a) K^+ reenters the cells along with glucose once insulin is administered; and (b) K^+ is washed out in the urine once dehydration is relieved and renal function reestablished. General agreement exists on the following points of care:

▶ Frequently assess and measure urine output. Potassium administration to the patient with poor urine output is hazardous since dangerous hyperkalemia may develop. Notify the physician promptly if the urine output falls dramatically or is less than 30 ml./hour.

▶ Observe the patient continuously for signs of hyperkalemia (bradycardia, cardiac arrest, weakness, flaccid paralysis, oliguria) or hypokalemia (weakness, flaccid paralysis, paralytic ileus, cardiac arrest) or both. Hyperkalemia may be present upon admission and approximately during the first 4 hours after the start of therapy. Hypokalemia usually develops during the period of 4 to 24 hours following initiation of therapy.

▶ Carefully monitor the patient's ECG. Flattening or inversion of T waves and prolonged Q-T intervals indicate hypokalemia, while peaking of T waves, loss of P wave, and a disrupted QRS complex indicates hyperkalemia (see Unit XII, Chapter 33).

▶ K^+ administration is usually started 2 or more hours after the patient's admission.

▶ When the patient has recovered sufficiently to resume eating and drinking, foods and liquids high in K^+ should be given.

Prevention of Hypoglycemia. Once insulin therapy is started and the patient's blood sugar has dropped to 300 mg./100 ml. 5 to 10 per cent glucose in water may be given intravenously to prevent hypoglycemia. The blood sugar level usually begins to drop within 4 to 6 hours following insulinization.

Several days of intensive therapy may be needed to correct severe ketoacidosis. Moreover, it may take 10 days or longer to restore fluid, electrolyte, and nitrogen balance in the critically ill patient. Once the patient is fully conscious and alert, it is important to carefully explore the reasons why ketoacidosis developed and to correct any faulty health practices. As we emphasized earlier, ketoacidosis is usually preventable provided the patient is both knowledgeable and willing to adhere to his therapeutic program.

Prevention of Cerebral Edema. Although an uncommon complication of treatment of diabetic ketoacidosis, *cerebral edema* may occur due to sudden fluid shifts as a result of IV fluid administration. The mortality rate is quite high, exceeding 50 per cent. Careful nursing assessment of the level of consciousness and other neurologic signs is essential in preventing this catastrophic event. Normally, patients with DKA become more responsive and alert as treatment progresses. If the patient's neurologic status deteriorates even slightly, the physician should be notified promptly. Treatment of cerebral edema under these circumstances differs little from the treatment used for cerebral edema resulting from other problems, e.g., steroids, mannitol, and/or furosemide (Lasix). The head of the bed may be elevated as well. (See Ch. 26.)

HYPERGLYCEMIC, HYPEROSMOLAR, NON-KETOTIC COMA (HHNK)

Non-insulin dependent diabetics generally have enough insulin, but are unable to use the insulin to combat hyperglycemia. HHNK occurs most often in these people. It is characterized by often extremely elevated blood sugar values, but *no ketosis.* These patients apparently have enough insulin to prevent breakdown of adipose tissue and the subsequent development of ketonemia, but there is inadequate carbohydrate metabolism.

The high glucose levels cause a profound hyperosmolar state which leads to serious volume depletion and shock. Unlike the patient in ketoacidosis, however, the patient with HHNK often is not in metabolic acidosis unless shock is profound and prolonged. In this instance the metabolic acidosis would be a lactic acidosis rather than ketoacidosis.

The symptoms of HHNK are very similar to those noted in the patient with ketoacidosis. However, patients with HHNK often do not have Kussmaul respirations unless they have a significant lactic acidosis. Serum and urine ketones are usually not elevated.

The precipitating factor in the development of HHNK may be the same as that precipitating diabetic ketoacidosis, e.g., infection, cardiovascular problem, stress. It may also be associated with total parenteral nutrition (hyperalimentation) and dialysis when solutions containing large amounts of glucose are used.[126]

HHNK is treated with vigorous fluid replacement with half normal (0.45 per cent sodium chloride) saline and insulin. Since ketosis does not occur, sodium bicarbonate is not usually necessary.

HYPOGLYCEMIA (INSULIN REACTION)

Most diabetics who take insulin experience a hypoglycemic reaction at some time. Because insulin reactions are so common, it is important to instruct your patients concerning (a) why reactions occur; (b) when reactions are most likely to occur; (c) the early symptoms of hypoglycemia; (d) the danger of severe or repeated reactions; and (e) the early treatment and prevention of insulin reactions.

First of all, hypoglycemic reactions result from (a) an overdose of insulin or (rarely) a sulfonurea; (b) omission of meals or eating less food than prescribed; (c) overexertion without compensating with the ingestion of additional carbohydrates; and (d) nutritional and fluid imbalances due to nausea and vomiting.

The *time period* during which an insulin reaction is most likely to occur depends upon the type of insulin given, the individual patient's response to that type of insulin, and on the timing of the insulin injection. You will recall from Table 72–8 that if given in the morning short-acting insulins tend to produce reactions before lunch, intermediate-acting insulins 2 or 3 hours before dinner, and long-acting insulins between 2 A.M. and breakfast.

Early symptoms of an insulin reaction include headache, weakness, irritability, lack of muscular coordination, and apprehension. (Note in Table 72–14 differences in rate of onset, symptoms, signs, and urinalysis between diabetic coma, hyperglycemic hyperosmolar nonketotic coma, and insulin reactions.) Also, because epinephrine is released when the blood sugar drops abnormally low, the patient usually beomes diaphoretic. In addition, patients may behave in a bizarre, even psychotic fashion.

> *When you care for diabetic patients at night, always check your sleeping patients for diaphoresis, because sweating may be the* only *observable symptom of insulin shock. Don't just visually observe the patient; actually feel the bed clothing for moistness.*

When hypoglycemia is allowed to continue unchecked, the patient eventually becomes comatose. If hypoglycemia is severe or attacks are habitual, the patient is in danger of dying. If the patient survives, *permanent brain damage* may be present. Brain damage resulting in memory loss, lessened learning ability, and even paralysis can develop because the brain is deprived of needed glucose when the blood sugar is low. In this respect, hypoglycemic shock is more dangerous than diabetic coma; in ketoacidosis, the brain can still use available glucose, even in the absence of insulin. For this reason, some physicians actually prefer that their patients spill a little sugar into their urine (trace or 1+ sugar) rather than risk repeated insulin reactions.

The *treatment* for hypoglycemia depends upon whether the reaction is mild or severe. To reverse *mild* hypoglycemia, instruct the patient to drink a glass of orange juice or to eat some lump sugar or candy. Instruct patients to carry lump sugar or candy at all times so that they can guard against insulin shock when away from home. Alternatively, a glucose paste packaged in a tube is commercially available. If the patient

TABLE 72–14. A COMPARISON OF DIABETIC KETOACIDOSIS (DKA), HYPERGLYCEMIC HYPEROSMOLAR NON-KETOTIC COMA (HHNK), AND HYPOGLYCEMIA

Factor	Diabetic Ketoacidosis	HHNK	Hypoglycemia
Type of diabetic	Insulin dependent	Non-insulin dependent; non-diabetic person	Insulin dependent
Signs & symptoms	History of nausea, vomiting, warm and dry skin, flushed appearance, dry mucous membranes, soft eyeballs, Kussmaul respirations or tachypnea, abdominal pain, alterations in level of consciousness, hypotension, tachycardia, acetone breath	Same as in DKA except do not have Kussmaul respirations or acetone breath	Nausea, loss of appetite, hunger, malaise, cool and moist skin or diaphoresis, pallor, bradycardia, bradypnea, visual disturbances, alterations in level of consciousness: memory loss, confusion, hallucinations, generalized or focal seizures, status epilepticus, primitive movements (sucking, smacking lips, picking or grasping, Babinski reflex) may be present
Precipitating Factor	Undiagnosed diabetic; neglect of treatment; infection; cardiovascular disorder; other physical or emotional stress	Undiagnosed diabetic; infection, or other stress; medications: dilantin, thiazide diuretics, mannitol steroids; dialysis; hyperalimentation; acute pancreatitis; CNS disorders; major burns treated with high concentrations of sugar	Delay or omission of meal; insulin overdosage; excessive exercise
Onset of symptoms	Slow (hours to days)	Slow (hours to days)	Rapid (minutes to hours)
Lab findings:			
Blood glucose	300–1500 mg./100 ml.	600–3000 mg./100 ml.	60 mg./100 ml. or less
Serum sodium	Normal or decreased	Elevated	Normal
Serum potassium	Normal or elevated at first, then decreased	Same as DKA	Normal
Blood urea nitrogen	Elevated	Elevated	Normal
Serum ketones	Elevated	Normal	Normal
WBC	Elevated	Elevated	Normal or elevated
Hematocrit	Elevated	Elevated	Normal
Urine glucose	Elevated	Elevated	Normal
Urine ketones	Elevated	Normal	Normal
Arterial blood gas	Metabolic acidosis with compensatory respiratory alkalosis	Normal or slight metabolic acidosis	Normal or slight respiratory acidosis
Treatment	Insulin; IV fluids such as normal saline, possibly half normal saline; potassium* when urine output is adequate; sodium bicarbonate if pH is less than 7.0	Insulin; IV fluids such as half normal or 3/4 normal saline; potassium when urine output is adequate	Candy; glucose paste; orange juice if awake; 50% dextrose IV push; 5–10% D/W IV drip; glucagon; epinephrine; steroids; diazoxide in cases of insulinoma

*Potassium phosphate rather than potassium chloride may be used since patients may have hypophosphatemia.[85]

is unconscious or unable to swallow, the paste may be placed under the tongue where it is rapidly absorbed. The paste is also less tempting than candy for certain patients. Recently there has been a trend to provide patients and families with glucagon which can be administered at home in the event of a serious hypoglycemic reaction. Glucagon is administered subcutaneously and may eliminate the need for emergency department treatment. Finally, be certain that the patient obtains a diabetic identification tag or bracelet and an identification card from the doctor or the ADA (see Fig. 72–7). Sometimes diabetics who are suffering an insulin reaction behave as if they are intoxicated or mentally disturbed. By carrying proper identification, the diabetic can avoid being arrested at a time when emergency care is desperately needed.

The patient with *severe* hypoglycemia who is unconscious needs *intravenous glucose immediately*; usually the patient is slowly given 20–50 ml. of 50 per cent glucose IV. Once the patient fully regains consciousness, give sugar water or orange juice to drink to raise the blood sugar.

> *Never attempt to force an unconscious or semiconscious patient to drink liquids, because fluid may be aspirated into the lungs!*

Two other emergency drugs which are used to treat severe hypoglycemia are:

Glucagon, 1 mg. given intravenously or subcutaneously

Epinephrine (Adrenaline), 0.5–1 ml. of 1:1000 solution administered subcutaneously.

Both glucagon and epinephrine help to raise the blood sugar by promoting the conversion of glycogen reserves within the liver back to glucose. Unfortunately, these drugs will reverse hypoglycemia only in those cases in which glycogen reserves are still available. If the patient is critical and has been in coma for some time, he or she will probably have already utilized glycogen stores and therefore will respond only to the administration of IV glucose. Diazoxide (Hyperstat), normally used for hypertensive emergencies, may be administered for refractory hypoglycemia due to insulin-producing tumors. The dosage is 200–600 mg. IV over several hours, or 100–200 mg. orally every 6 hours.[54] Occasionally a patient with hypoglycemia associated with pituitary or adrenal dysfunction may need steroids for initial treatment of the hypoglycemia.[54]

Once the patient fully recovers from the episode of hypoglycemia, it is essential to reassess the program of care. In some cases, insulin reactions develop because the patient is careless about preparing the insulin dosage, fails to eat, or exercises excessively. Talk to patients who are careless about the dangers of repeated insulin reactions and stress the importance of conscientious adherence to the doctor's orders. In other cases, hypoglycemia develops because the prescribed insulin dosage is too large or the patient's dietary intake is too small. Under these circumstances, the doctor will alter the patient's regimen until hypoglycemic reactions cease. As stated earlier, some physicians prefer to lower insulin dosage to the point at which the patient experiences a continuous *mild* hyperglycemia, thereby lessening the possibility of insulin reactions. As with many diseases, self concept and a feeling of control over the situation are important considerations in the care of a diabetic. Patients and their relatives and friends need to understand the complications associated with diabetes, but it is equally important that health care providers assist the patient in developing a plan of therapy that will best meet emotional and social needs as well as physical ones.

Long-Term Complications

Because diabetes is a long-term disease, diabetics can develop a myriad of chronic complications. Major chronic disorders associated with diabetes are degenerative vascular changes, neuropathy, ocular disturbances, kidney diseases, infections, and skin lesions. These complications principally strike the *blood vessels* and *nerves* and mainly damage the heart, extremities (particularly the feet), the eyes, and the kidneys.

Premature Degenerative Vascular Changes. Diabetes is often associated with severe degenerative vascular changes. Lesions of the blood vessels not only strike diabetics at an earlier age than nondiabetics but also tend to produce more severe pathologic changes in diabetics than in the general population. For example, diabetics are twice as likely as nondiabetics to have heart disease and cerebrovascular accidents. Basically diabetics are prone to two types of vascular disease: (1) atherosclerosis, and (2) microangiopathy.

ATHEROSCLEROSIS. As you recall from Unit XII, atherosclerotic lesions cause hardening and degeneration of the walls of the *large* arteries; among diabetics, early atherosclerotic changes are probably caused by the high glucose and lipid levels which are characteristic of diabetes. Atherosclerosis, in turn, may lead to the premature appearance of *coronary artery disease* (i.e., angina pectoris and myocardial infarctions) even among young diabetics. Hypertension is very prevalent. In addition, atherosclerosis results in reduced blood supply to the *feet*, causing intermittent claudication, cold feet, paresthesias, foot infections, inadequate healing of foot lesions, ulceration and gangrene of the extremities. Diabetics are five times more likely than nondiabetics to develop gangrene. Lesions of the extremities may become so severe that the patient faces amputation of the toes, foot, or leg. To decrease the development of foot infections and lesions, it is important to teach diabetics the principles of *good foot care*. Instructions for the care of the feet are outlined on the opposite page.

MICROANGIOPATHY. While atherosclerosis is common among the general population, destruction of the *small blood vessels* is a major hallmark of diabetes. The specific characteristic of microangiopathy in diabetes is thickening of the basement membrane of the capillaries. Moreover, pathology of the capillaries has even been reported to occur at an earlier age than the clinical symptoms of the diabetes itself. There is some evidence to suggest that a major factor in the development of microangiopathy is the metabolic derangement that occurs as a result of high glucose levels, hypoxia, and lactic acidosis at the cellular level, particularly in the eye.[13]

The widespread effects of microangiopathy can be disastrous if not controlled. The two organs which are most seriously affected are the *eyes* and the *kidneys*. Vascular degeneration within the retina can cause microaneurysms, retinal hemorrhages, and eventual blindness. Small vessel changes within the kidney eventually result in intercapillary glomerulosclerosis.

Ocular Disorders. Diabetes is the leading cause of new cases of blindness in the United States today. The most common eye complications affecting diabetics include blurring of vision, cataracts, and diabetic retinopathy.

Blurred vision is usually caused by an abnormally elevated blood sugar; consequently, once the patient's diabetes is brought under control, vision clears. Advise patients to wait until control is established before obtaining new prescription lenses.

Cataracts, the second type of ocular disturbance, strikes a proportionately greater number of diabetics than nondiabetics. (A cataract is a clouding or opacity of the lens of the eyes. See Unit XXIII). Fortunately, surgical removal of the cataracts and the use of glasses or implanted lenses is helpful in restoring vision in the majority of patients.

The third entity, *diabetic retinopathy*, is a major cause of blindness among diabetics. As mentioned, one of the severe complications of diabetes is microangiopathy or vascular degeneration of the small vessels supplying the eyes and kidneys. The *retina*, which is the most essential structure of the eye, has the highest rate of oxygen consumption of any tissue in the body. Consequently, if the retina is deprived of oxygen-carrying blood owing to destruction of its capillaries, tissue anoxia swiftly develops. In addition, the weakened damaged vessels frequently rupture, causing retinal hemorrhage and exudates. Hemorrhage is followed by the growth of new capillaries into the vitreous and by the formation of retinal scar tissue. Finally, contraction of the scar tissue can result in retinal detachment. The common findings associated with diabetic retinopathy are illustrated in Figure 72–9.

While many diabetics develop retinopathy, most do not have visual impairment. The incidence of the development of retinopathy is related to the length of time the patient has been diabetic; of patients with diabetes for more than 15 years, 60 to 70 per cent will have retinopathy.[13] When retinopathy does occur, it tends to develop slowly and insidiously. Diagnosis of this condition is based upon direct ophthalmoscopic observation of vascular changes within the retina and the use of fluorescein angiography.

Unfortunately, no therapy currently exists which is guaranteed to cure this condition; it may progress to permanent blindness — either partial or total. The advance of diabetic retinopathy can sometimes be slowed by instituting and maintaining good diabetic control. Many authorities believe that careful control of the blood sugar is essential in the management of the patient with diabetic retinopathy. Equally important is the control of hypertension, if present. Some researchers believe that platelet aggregation is a major contributing factor in the development of retinopathy and advocate the use of aspirin to decrease platelet aggregation. The use of aspirin is currently being evaluated.[13] The most common modality used is photocoagulation to destroy retinal tissue and/or blood vessels. The photocoagulation is accomplished through the use of a laser beam or xenon arc. Another therapy is the actual removal of vitreous hemorrhages thereby minimizing the tension on the retina. The use of prophylactic vitrectomy in patients with retinopathy but without visual impairment is currently being investigated. Also, a few patients such as those with very rapid progression of retinopathy benefit from hypophysectomy (surgical removal or destruction of the pituitary gland) (Chapter 74). Destruction of the pituitary gland alleviates the secretion of the following four pituitary hormones, all of which act to raise the blood sugar

Instructions in the Care of the Feet
for Persons With Diabetes Mellitus or Vascular Disturbances

Hygiene of the Feet

(1) Wash feet daily with mild soap and lukewarm water. Dry thoroughly between the toes by pressure. Do not rub vigorously, as this is apt to break the delicate skin.

(2) When feet are thoroughly dry, rub well with vegetable oil to keep them soft, prevent excess friction, remove scales, and prevent dryness. Care must be taken to prevent foot tenderness.

(3) If the feet become too soft and tender, rub them with alcohol about once a week.

(4) When rubbing the feet, always rub upward from the tips of the toes. If varicose veins are present, massage the feet very gently; never massage the legs.

(5) If the toenails are brittle and dry, soften them by soaking for ½ hour each night in lukewarm water containing 1 tbsp of powdered sodium borate (borax) per quart. Follow this by rubbing around the nails with vegetable oil. Clean around the nails with an orangewood stick. If the nails become too long, file them with an emery board. File them straight across, and no shorter than the underlying soft tissues of the toe. Never cut the corners of the nails. (If the patient goes to a podiatrist for this attention, he should tell him that he has diabetes.)

(6) Wear low-heeled shoes of soft leather which fit the shape of the feet correctly. The shoes should have wide toes that will cause no pressure, fit close in the arch, and grip the heels snugly. Wear new shoes ½ hour only on the first day and increase by 1 hour each day following. Wear thick, warm, loose stockings.

Treatment of Corns and Calluses

(1) Corns and calluses are due to friction and pressure, most often from improperly fitted shoes and stockings. Wear shoes that fit properly and cause no friction or pressure.

(2) To remove excess calluses or corns, soak the feet in lukewarm (not hot) water, using a mild soap, for about 10 minutes, and then rub off the excess tissue with a towel or file. Do not tear it off. Under no circumstances must the skin become irritated.

(3) Do not cut corns or calluses. If they need attention it is safer to see a podiatrist.

(4) Prevent callus formation under the ball of the foot (a) by exercises, such as curling and stretching the toes several times a day; (b) by finishing each step on the toes and not on the ball of the foot; and (c) by wearing shoes that are not too short and that do not have high heels.

Aids in Treatment of Imperfect Circulation (Cold Feet)

(1) Never use tobacco in any form. Tobacco contracts blood vessels and so reduces circulation.

(2) Keep warm. Wear warm stockings and other clothing. Cold contracts blood vessels and reduces circulation.

(3) Do not wear circular garters, which compress blood vessels and reduce blood flow.

(4) Do not sit with the legs crossed. This may compress the leg arteries and shut off the blood supply to the feet.

(5) If the weight of the bedclothes is uncomfortable, place a pillow under the covers at the foot of the bed.

(6) Do not apply any medication to the feet without directions from a physician. Some medicines are too strong for feet with poor circulation.

(7) Do not apply heat in the form of hot water, hot water bottles, or heating pads without a physician's consent. Even moderate heat can injure the skin if circulation is poor.

(8) If the feet are moist or the patient has a tendency to develop athlete's foot, a prophylactic dusting powder should be used on the feet and in shoes and stockings daily. Change shoes and stockings at least daily or oftener.

(9) Exercises to increase circulation should be prescribed by a physician.

Treatment of Abrasions of the Skin

(1) Proper first-aid treatment is of the utmost importance even in apparently minor injuries. Consult a physician immediately for any redness, blistering, pain, or swelling. Any break in the skin may become ulcerous or gangrenous unless properly treated by a physician.

(2) Dermatophytosis (athlete's foot), which begins with peeling and itching between the toes or discoloration or thickening of the toenails, should be treated immediately by a physician or podiatrist.

(3) Avoid strong irritating antiseptics such as tincture of iodine.

(4) As soon as possible after any injury, cover the area with sterile gauze. Sterile gauze in sealed packets may be purchased at drug stores.

(5) Elevate and, as much as possible until recovery, avoid using the foot.

From Krupp, M. A., and Chatton, M. J.: *Current Diagnosis and Treatment.* Los Altos, California, Lange Medical Publications, 1972, p. 648.

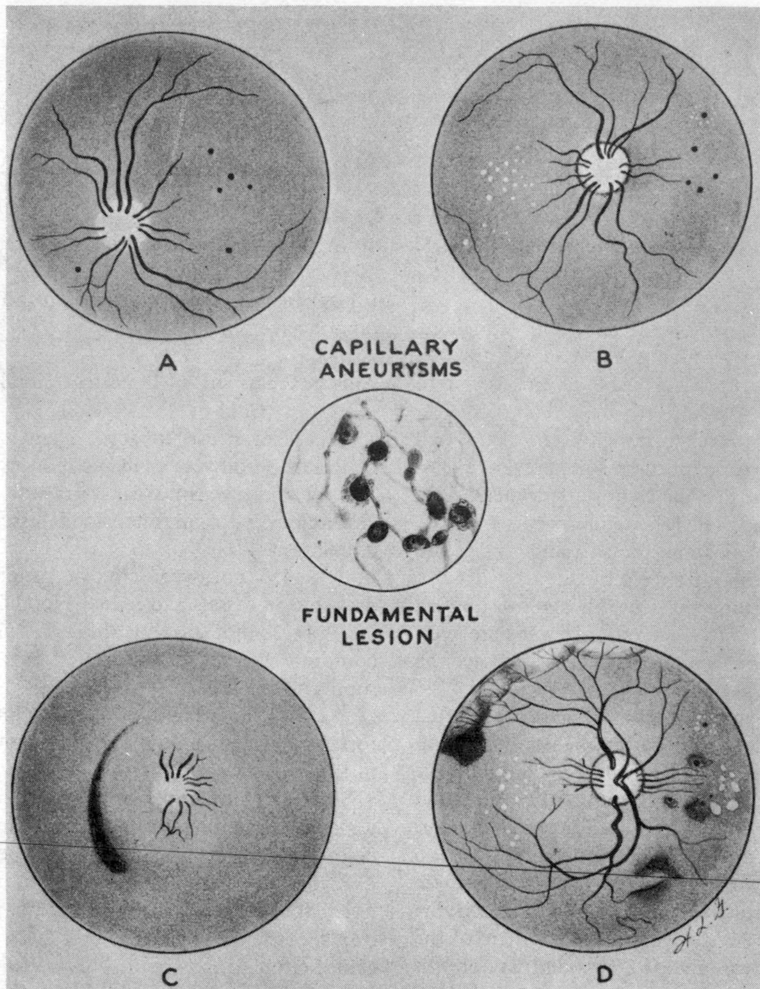

Figure 72–9. Characteristic eyeground changes in diabetic retinopathy as seen by ophthalmoscopic examination. Early punctate hemorrhages, *A* and *B* (right), with waxy, round exudates, *B*, (left). *C*, Vitreous hemorrhage obscuring all but the nerve head. *D*, Retinitis proliferans with fibrosis emanating from the nerve head; retinal detachment (top); flame-shaped hemorrhage and tortuosity of the retinal venules (below the center). The fundamental capillary lesions, the "microaneurysms," are shown in the center as they appear in a high-power microscopic view. (From Williams, R. H. (Ed.): *Textbook of Endocrinology*, 5th ed. Philadelphia: W. B. Saunders Co., 1974.)

and consequently have a diabetogenic effect: growth hormone, corticotropin, thyrotropin, and luteotropin. In the absence of these hormones, diabetes is often easier to control, and the progression of retinopathy may slow or halt. Following hypophysectomy, the patient will need hormonal replacement therapy throughout life.

Kidney Disease. Diabetics are susceptible to kidney infections — particularly *recurrent pyelonephritis*. Female diabetics are far more susceptible to renal infections than are males. One source estimates that one half of all women who have had diabetes for 10 or more years have suffered from at least one kidney or bladder infection during that time.[27a] Fortunately, the majority of diabetics with renal infections are successfully treated with sulfonamides, antibiotics, and the urinary antiseptics.

A second and far more devastating form of kidney disease is diabetic *nephropathy*. A consequence of microangiopathy, nephropathy is characterized by damage and eventual obliteration of the tiny capillaries which supply the glomerulus of the kidney. Damage of the glomerular capillaries, in turn, leads to a complex of pathologic changes and symptoms (intercapillary glomerulosclerosis, nephrosis, gross albuminuria, and hypertension) called *Kimmelstiel-Wilson disease*. With worsening of the nephrosis, chronic renal failure ensues. Unless the patient can be maintained with hemodialysis or receives a renal transplant, *uremia* will eventually cause death.

As in the case of diabetic retinopathy, there is as yet no cure for diabetic nephropathy. However, prompt and adequate treatment of renal and bladder infections can prevent these additional causes of renal failure.

Neuropathy. Diabetics may develop both temporary and permanent neurologic problems during the course of their illness. Identified causes of diabetic neuropathy include vascular insufficiency and high blood sugar levels, both of which can lead to metabolic disturbances within the neuron itself. Patients may present with mononeuropathy or polyneuropathy, and can have sensory and/or motor impairment. The three major forms of diabetic neuropathy are discussed below.

PERIPHERAL NERVE DEGENERATION. This common form of diabetic neuropathy tends to develop in stages. During its earliest stage, the patient usually suffers from temporary episodes of pain and tingling in the extremities (particularly the feet). In later years the pain tends to grow more nagging and constant; also discomfort is particularly troublesome at night. Finally, 10 or 15 years following development of diabetes, the patient may experience a *painless neuropathy* characterized by an *inability to perceive pain*.

> *Painless neuropathy is a dangerous condition. Patients may be totally unaware of injury — particularly of the lower extremities.*

One of the authors (J. L.) once witnessed a dramatic example of the dangers of painless neuropathy. Her patient, a 50-year-old woman with *undiagnosed* diabetes, was admitted to the hospital one evening with a huge ulcerated lesion on her heel. Only that morning, the patient had gone with her family to a county fair where she had walked (without pain) for most of the day. Before she left for the fair, the woman had noted a small blister on her heel but had disregarded it. That evening, when the patient removed her shoe, she was horrified to discover that the tiny blister had grown into a large gaping sore. It took many weeks following admission for the lesion to heal and for the patient to be brought under control. Throughout her hospitalization, the patient faced the definite possibility that her foot might have to be amputated.

You can see from this example how important it is to instruct diabetic patients to visually and manually inspect their feet for blisters, sores, cuts, ingrown nails, and so forth. Emphasize to older diabetics that their ability to perceive pain may be diminishing and that they must rely upon their senses of touch and sight to protect them from injury. Also point out that even trivial injuries (particularly of the feet) require medical care to prevent the development of severe complications.

OTHER NEUROLOGIC LESIONS. Two other forms of diabetic neuropathy include disease of the autonomic nervous system and cranial nerve lesions. Symptoms of autonomic nerve damage include diarrhea or constipation, urinary incontinence or retention, decreased sweating, orthostatic hypotension, and impotence in the male. One of the problems associated with autonomic nerve damage is that patients and their families and friends may be unable to rely on signs of hypoglycemia which depend on an intact autonomic nervous system. Therefore, it is important that this be considered when carrying out patient teaching. Symptoms of cranial nerve lesions include ptosis (drooping eyelid), diplopia (double vision), and pain in the orbit, i.e., behind the eye.

Infections. Diabetics are susceptible to infections of many types, and infections, once they occur, are frequently difficult to treat. Infected areas often heal slowly because the diabetic's vascular system is damaged and unable to carry sufficient oxygen, nutrients, and antibodies to the injured site. Also infections increase the diabetic's need for insulin and predispose to the possibility of ketoacidosis. Areas of the skin which are particularly subject to local infection include the neck, axillae, and groin. In addition, obese diabetic women may develop raw infected areas under their breasts.

Diabetic patients need careful instruction in how to prevent and treat infections and skin injuries. Important points to stress when teaching diabetics skin care include the following:

▶ Even *slight injuries* can become infected; e.g., scratches, small cuts, hangnails, slivers under the skin, and so forth.

▶ Carefully cleanse areas that are slightly injured with soap and water. Do not use antiseptics that contain phenol, bichloride of mercury, oil of mustard, cantharidin, or salicylic acid, because these substances tend to burn the skin. After cleansing, apply a sterile gauze bandage. Avoid using adhesive tape because it irritates the skin.

▶ Report serious injuries and infections to the physician immediately; e.g., boils, carbuncles, ulcers, burns, abscesses, blisters, deep cuts.

▶ Exercise caution when using heat lamps, hot water bottles, and heating pads, particularly in the presence of painless neuropathy.

▶ Avoid the use of irritating household cleaning fluids, powders, and disinfectants unless protective gloves are worn.

NURSING DIABETIC PATIENTS WHO UNDERGO SURGERY

Undergoing surgery is a stressful experience for anybody. For the diabetic patient, surgery imposes several additional stresses. For example, surgery interrupts the patient's usual treatment regimen; the diet must be temporarily changed and insulin dosage readjusted. Furthermore, diabetics are prone to infection, and the surgical incision itself opens a new portal for infectious agents. Also postoperative healing in diabetics may be slow owing to degeneration of the vascular system. (See Unit VIII.)

To offset these problems, diabetic patients require special care both preoperatively and postoperatively. Specific clinical care varies, depending upon whether the patient has insulin dependent or non-insulin dependent diabetes and also upon whether the surgery is elective or emergency.

The goal of *preoperative care* for diabetic patients is to *thoroughly regulate their diabetes* before taking them into the operating room. Patients with insulin dependent diabetes may need to be hospitalized for several days or even weeks prior to elective surgery in order to stabilize their condition and thereby decrease surgical risk. If the insulin dependent diabetic's blood sugar is not well controlled and requires *emergency* surgery, the surgeon must sometimes make the painful choice between operating on a poorly controlled diabetic or postponing an emergency operation while attempting to control the diabetes. In either case, the patient will need constant monitoring of vital signs, frequent laboratory studies, and vigilant nursing care.

In contrast to insulin dependent diabetes, patients with well-controlled non-insulin dependent diabetes usually undergo surgery with only slightly more risk than nondiabetics. Typically, preoperative preparation for these patients includes the following:

- ▶The omission of food, water, insulin, or oral hypoglycemic agents on the morning of surgery.
- ▶Early morning scheduling of the surgery so that the patient's diet and insulin regimen are interrupted as little as possible.
- ▶Preoperative laboratory tests, including fasting and postprandial blood sugars, urine tests for sugar and acetone, CO_2 combining power, and blood urea nitrogen; also an EKG and chest x-ray.
- ▶A blood sugar determination performed and reported to the physician within 1 hour before the operation to prevent the possibility of the patient (who has been NPO since midnight) developing hypoglycemia while in surgery. If the blood sugar level is low, then the patient will require an intravenous infusion of 5 per cent glucose in water prior to the induction of anesthesia.

Once the patient arrives in surgery, management depends, once again, upon the severity of the diabetes and the extensiveness of the surgery. The patient with *mild* diabetes who is undergoing minor surgery usually does not require either insulin or intravenous glucose until returned to the recovery room. If the patient is undergoing major surgery or has moderate or severe diabetes, an intravenous infusion of 1000 ml. 5 per cent glucose in saline or water is given while in surgery. To "cover" the IV glucose, insulin, in approximately half of the patient's normal daily dosage, is usually given.

Following surgery, the goals of *postoperative care* are to stabilize the patient's condition, reestablish control of the diabetes, prevent wound infection, and promote wound healing. Important postoperative clinical measures are as follows:

- ▶Intravenous infusions of 5 per cent dextrose in water and regular insulin are administered until the patient is able to take oral nourishment.
- ▶Once the patient can eat, he or she is usually placed on a normal 3-meals-a-day plan with between-meal snacks as necessary for blood sugar control.
- ▶Blood sugar levels are usually ordered 3 times daily, and fractional urines for sugar and acetone 4 times daily.
- ▶Regular insulin is administered on the basis of urine tests. The patient returns to his preoperative insulin type (i.e., NPH, Lente, and so forth) and dosage once diabetic control is reestablished.
- ▶Catheterization is avoided if at all possible in order to prevent bladder infections.
- ▶Wound dressings are changed with meticulous sterile technique in order to prevent wound infection.

EDUCATING THE DIABETIC PATIENT FOR LIFELONG SELF-CARE

Throughout our discussion of diabetes, we have stressed the importance of patient education. We have indicated strongly that the success of any diabetic regimen depends upon the patient's willingness to adhere to the care plan.

Essentially, learning to live with diabetes is like any other form of learning; it requires that the learner (a) obtain a grasp of unfamiliar factual material (e.g., the nature of diabetes, insulin, and so forth); (b) learn to perform certain procedures (e.g., urine testing); and (c) permanently change certain behavior patterns (e.g., eating habits, recreational activities, and so forth). Like any student, the diabetic needs scheduled classes; planned instruction; reading materials which are geared to educational level; demonstrations of procedures (e.g., urine tests and insulin preparation); and the opportunity to perform these procedures with supervision.

Diabetics may be instructed either individually or in groups, depending upon the policy of the individual hospital or clinic and the number of staff members available for teaching. One advantage of group instruction is that diabetics have an opportunity to meet other diabetics and to discuss mutual problems and feelings.

When it becomes your responsibility to instruct diabetics for lifelong self-care, you will, first of all, want to review the important principles of learning. For instance, we know that students learn more easily when they are rested and alert, when the environment is quiet, when instruction is given at the patient's level of education and new terms are defined, and when assimilation of new knowledge is periodically tested.

Next, you will wish to plan your course of instruction and obtain the necessary teaching aids. In order to insure that all important points are discussed, it is helpful to have a standardized teaching program. Helpful teaching aids for your classes include instructional charts and pamphlets which can be obtained from the ADA; diabetic identification cards, copies of *Diabetes Forecast* and *Diabetes Forecast Reprints*, "A Cookbook for Diabetics"; urine testing apparatus; samples of various types of insulin; insulin syringes calibrated for 40, 80, and 100 unit insulin, alcohol and alcohol sponges, and a pan and strainer for boiling injection equipment.* It is also helpful to give patients a price list, drawn from local pharmacies, for the various items they will need to purchase.

Throughout each session, you will want to test your patient to make certain that all the key points concerning diabetes and its care are being grasped. Ask questions frequently. Have the patient perform urine testing and insulin preparation and injection until these are done with ease. At the end of your course, stress the importance of continued health supervision; emphasize that the patient will need to schedule periodic medical examinations throughout life.

You may wish to close your class with the thought that learning is a continuing process and that your classes have presented only the most basic facts about diabetes. Hopefully, your patients will continue to read and learn about their disorder and to keep abreast of new developments in the field. Knowledge and self-confidence go hand in hand. The more the patient knows about diabetes, the easier it will be to control the disorder and to live a normal, productive life.

HYPERFUNCTION OF THE ISLETS OF LANGERHANS (HYPERINSULINISM)

Hyperinsulinism (excessive secretion of insulin by the pancreas) is classified as either organic or functional. *Organic* hyperinsulinism is usually caused either by *hyperplasia* (overgrowth) of the islets or by an *adenoma* of the pancreas which secretes excessive amounts of insulin.

Because oversecretion of insulin causes an abnormally low blood sugar, the *symptoms* of hyperinsulinism are identical to those of hypoglycemia previously discussed (e.g., hunger, weakness, tremor, sweating, personality changes). Repeated or prolonged attacks of hypoglycemia may ultimately result in progressive and irreversible neuropathy and myelopathy, retinal hemorrhages, cerebral vascular accidents, permanent personality changes, and intellectual damage.

Emergency treatment of acute hypoglycemic attacks is the same as that for an insulin reaction, i.e., immediate administration of sugar in any quickly utilized form (sugar lumps, orange juice). However, to permanently alleviate organic hyperinsulinism, the patient must undergo *surgery*. The operation involves either removal of the insulin-secreting tumor or resection of hyperplastic pancreatic tissue. In a few cases, partial or total pancreatectomy is necessary.

Functional hyperinsulinism develops with far greater frequency than does the organic form. In this case, the exact cause of insulin hypersecretion is unknown. However, functional hyperinsulinism frequently strikes *tense, anxious persons* who also have various manifestations of autonomic nervous dysfunction, e.g., neurocirculatory asthenia and excessive diaphoresis. Secondly, this disorder may possibly be a forerunner of *diabetes mellitus*. According to some investigators, a large majority of persons diagnosed with functional hyperinsulinism later develop diabetes. Finally, functional hyperinsulinism sometimes follows *gastrectomy*. When the stomach is removed, ingested carbohydrates pass directly into the small bowel (the "dumping syndrome") and are absorbed. The sudden resultant hyperglycemia causes excessive insulin release with symptoms of hypoglycemia appearing 1 to 2 hours later (see Unit XVII).

The goal of care in functional hyperinsulinism is to control and prevent the symptoms of hypoglycemia. Methods of treatment include the following:

Psychological counseling: Tense, nervous persons may find relief from symptoms by learning to relax more fully and more frequently. The help of a psychiatrist may be needed in extreme cases.

Diet: Some physicians advise a high-protein, low-carbohydrate diet. Other authorities recommend a diet of normal composition, but with no large meals or concentrated sweets. Carbohydrates ingested should be of the slowly assimilated variety (e.g., bananas and vegetables).

Medications: Sedation may help the anxious person relax. Also anticholinergic drugs may be used to control the "dumping syndrome."

Follow-up: Patients with functional hyperinsulinism should be examined at least every 6 months for the signs of overt diabetes mellitus.

**Diabetes Forecast* is a bimonthly magazine which is published by the ADA for diabetics. Currently a subscription costs $6.00 per year. "A Cookbook for Diabetics" is also published by the ADA and can be purchased for $5.50. The address of the American Diabetes Association is 600 Fifth Avenue, New York, N.Y. 10020.

CHAPTER 73

NURSING PATIENTS WITH DISORDERS OF THE THYROID AND PARATHYROID GLANDS

THE THYROID GLAND

Normal Anatomy and Physiology

The thyroid gland is a shield-shaped organ located in the neck below the larynx. It consists of two lobes, located on either side of the trachea, and connected by a thin isthmus which stretches over the trachea's anterior surface. Each of the lobes is composed of irregular lobules, while the lobules themselves consist of multitudes of tiny sacs called *follicles.* The follicles are filled with a jelly-like, iodine-containing substance called *colloid,* which is mainly composed of *thyroglobulin* — the storage form of the hormone *thyroxine.*

Thyroxine is one of the three hormones secreted by the thyroid gland — triiodothyronine and thyrocalcitonin being the other two. A derivative of the amino acid tyrosine, thyroxine is composed largely of *iodine.* The major role of thyroxine is to *regulate body metabolism* so that oxygen consumption and heat production keep pace with the body's needs and activities. By controlling body metabolism, thyroxine also aids in regulating growth and development (both physical and mental); carbohydrate, fat, and protein metabolism; reproduction; vitamin requirements; and resistance to infection. Too much thyroxine causes a dangerous speeding of metabolism and high rate of oxygen consumption. Conversely, too little thyroxine results in a sluggish metabolism, a slowing of both physical and mental function in the adult, and retardation of growth and development in the child.

> Thyroid secretion appears to act as a general and necessary stimulant without which there can be no health or vigor of the body, no flash and speed of the mind. Someone with a turn for the picturesque has remarked that thyroxine converts the sluggish toad into the lively frog.[14]

Production of this remarkable hormone depends upon the ingestion of sufficient amounts of protein and iodine and upon the release of a vital anterior pituitary hormone called *thyroid-stimulating hormone* (TSH), or thyrotropic hormone. TSH, as the name implies, stimulates the thyroid gland to produce thyroxine from iodine and tyrosine. TSH release is controlled by a *negative feedback system* in which low serum levels of thyroxine stimulate the increased secretion of TSH, and high serum levels of thyroxine inhibit TSH secretion, thereby promoting a steady state of hormonal production and release.

Thyroxine production is also dependent upon a number of environmental factors. Situations which speed thyroxine production are physiologic and psychologic stress and prolonged exposure to cold. Factors which depress thyroxine secretion are excessive intake of dietary goitrogens (see below), ingestion of certain drugs (sulfonamides, salicylates, phenylbutazone, and *para*-amino-salicylic acid), and exposure to prolonged heat.

Thyroxine is stored as part of the *thyroglobulin* molecule in the thyroid follicles. Whenever the body's circulatory thyroxine levels drop too low, thyroxine is released from thyroglobulin into the blood. Within the blood, thyroxine combines with a plasma protein and is carried to organs and tissues in the form of *protein-bound iodine.* The pathways of thyroxine are illustrated in Figure 73–1.

Triiodothyronine, a second thyroid hormone, is much more potent than thyroxine. Thyroxine is converted to triiodothyronine by peripheral target tissues in the body.

Thyrocalcitonin, the third thyroid hormone, is a polypeptide produced by specialized "C" cells in the thyroid. Discovered recently (during the 1960's), thyrocalcitonin is capable of lowering both plasma calcium and phosphates. Apparently it serves no other function.

Abnormalities of Thyroid Function

There are many terms to describe normal and abnormal states of thyroid function. *Euthyroid* is a word which signifies *normal* thyroid function and secretion. Thyroid *abnormalities* are basically of three types: (1) enlargement of the thyroid (goiter), (2) hyperfunction (hyperthyroidism), and (3) hypofunction (hypothyroidism).

Enlargement of the thyroid gland may or may not be associated with abnormalities of hormone secretion. An enlarged thyroid may result from (a) lack of iodine (simple goiter), (b) inflammation (thyroiditis), or (c) benign or malignant tumors. Enlargement may also appear as part of the clinical picture of hyperthyroidism, especially Graves' disease.

Hyperthyroidism is a condition characterized by overactivity of the thyroid gland, hypersecretion of thyroid hormone, and increased body metabolism and heat production. Persons suffering from severe hyperthyroidism may become overactive to the point of mania and psychosis. Conversely, *hypothyroidism* is characterized by *underactivity* of the thyroid, hyposecretion of thyroid hormone, and decreased body metabolism and heat production; in its most extreme form – myxedema coma — body metabolism slows almost to the point of death.

Assessment of Thyroid Function

A number of tests are available for the assessment of thyroid function. They include the following: (1) serum thyroxine; (2) serum triiodothyronine; (3) triiodothyronine (T_3) resin uptake test; (4) radioactive iodine (^{131}I) uptake and excretion tests; (5) serum thyroid-stimulating hormone (TSH); (6) thyrotropin test (TSH), (7) thyrotropin-releasing hormone (TRH) test, (8) serum cholesterol, (9) serologic studies; (10) basal metabolic rate (BMR); and (11) Achilles tendon reflex recording. The purposes of each of these diagnostic studies, as well as of factors which interfere with testing, are briefly considered below. Details concerning patient preparation, the procedure, and normal and abnormal findings for the most important tests are outlined in Table 73–1.

Serum Thyroxine and Triiodothyronine. The serum concentrations of the two thyroid hormones, thyroxine and triiodothyronine, can now be measured by radioimmunoassay. Since thyroxine is transported in the blood largely bound to thyroid-binding globulin, conditions that affect thyroid-binding globulin levels will alter the serum thyroxine concentration. For example, pregnancy and oral contraceptive use both increase serum thyroxine.

Triiodothyronine (T_3) Resin Uptake. Triiodothyronine (like thyroxine) circulates in the blood stream attached to plasma proteins and to red blood cells. However, triiodothyronine tends to bind far more readily to plasma proteins than to erythrocytes; indeed, only when there are few binding sites available on plasma proteins does triiodothyronine link itself to circulating red cells.

In this test a specimen of the patient's serum is incubated with (a) a specific amount of radioactive triiodothyronine, and (b) particles of resin, which act as an absorbent material in place of erythrocytes. If thyroid function is low or if serum protein levels are high, resin uptake of T_3 will be depressed. On the other hand, if

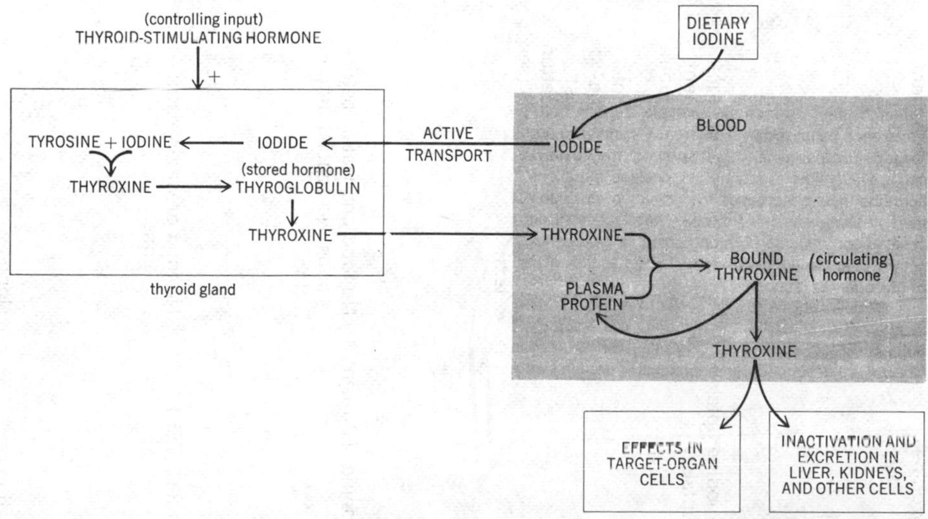

Figure 73–1. Summary of thyroxine pathways. Besides iodine, the diet must also supply the amino acids which are used for the synthesis of tyrosine, colloid globulin, and plasma protein. Thyroid-stimulating hormone is produced by the anterior pituitary. Iodine is converted to iodide in the process of absorption by the gastrointestinal tract. (From Vander, A. J., J. H. Sherman, and D. S. Luciano: *Human Physiology—The Mechanisms of Body Function*, 2nd ed., p. 175. Copyright ©1975 by McGraw-Hill, Inc. Used by permission of McGraw-Hill Book Company.)

TABLE 73–1. THYROID FUNCTION TESTS

Test	Patient Preparation	Procedure	Normal Findings	Significance of Abnormal Findings
Serum thyroxine or triiodothyronine	No food or water restrictions. Question patient concerning drugs recently taken.	Sample of venous blood drawn and sent to laboratory	4.5–11.5 mcg./100 ml. of serum (adults)	Low concentration of thyroxine or triiodothyronine indicates hypothyroidism; excessive concentrations of thyroid hormones indicates hyperthyroidism.
Radioactive iodine uptake test (^{131}I uptake)	No food or water restrictions. Reassure patient that doses of radioiodine used for tests are extremely small and not harmful. Question patient concerning past history of drug ingestion and diagnostic tests (see text).	Patient receives tracer dose of ^{131}I. 24-hour urine specimen is started at time of drug administration. After 24 hours, scintillation counter is placed over thyroid gland to measure exact amount of radioactivity emitting from the gland. 24-Hour urine specimen is labeled and sent to laboratory for analysis.	15–35% uptake. Urine excretion: 40–80% ^{131}I within first 24 hours.	(1) *Uptake results:* early high peak in ^{131}I uptake indicates hyperthyroidism; persistent low ^{131}I uptake indicates hypothyroidism. (2) *Urine excretion:* excretion less than 40% indicates hyperthyroidism; excretion greater than 80% indicates hypothyroidism.
Triiodothyronine (T_3) resin uptake	No food and water restrictions. No special preparation.	Blood sample drawn from patient and sent to laboratory for incubation with T_3 and resin particles.	Standardized in each laboratory.	Depression of resin uptake of T_3 may indicate hypothyroidism; elevation of resin uptake of T_3 may indicate hyperthyroidism.
Thyrotropin test (TSH)	No food or water restrictions.	^{131}I uptake performed. Thyrotropin given by injection. ^{131}I uptake and serum thyroxine repeated 24 hours following TSH administration.	Increase in ^{131}I uptake and serum thyroxin.	If no change in ^{131}I uptake or serum thyroxin, patient has primary hypothyroidism.
TRH stimulation test	None	Patient is given 500 mcg. of TRH intravenously. Serum TSH is measured in serum drawn before and 30 minutes after TRH injection.	Increase in TSH.	No rise in TSH in pituitary disease (secondary hypothyroidism) or hyperthyroidism.

thyroid function is increased above normal or serum protein levels are low, resin uptake of T_3 will be elevated. When compared with the serum thyroxine or triiodothyronine levels, this test can detect abnormal plasma thyroid-binding globulin levels.

Radioiodine ^{131}I Uptake and Excretion Test. This important test for estimating thyroid function and diagnosing thyroid disease was discussed in Unit IX. As you recall, the body cannot distinguish between radioactive or "tagged" atoms of iodine and nonradioactive iodine; consequently the thyroid takes up radioactive iodine and processes it in exactly the same manner as it does regular iodine. Furthermore, radioiodine is excreted in the urine just as is ordinary iodine. Thus by using a scintillation scanner, it is possible to measure the amount of radioactive atoms of iodine which are concentrated in the thyroid following the administration of a radioactive iodine preparation. In addition, the laboratory may measure the patient's urine output of radioactive iodine following the test.

There are many factors which can distort findings. Careful questioning of your patient concerning the following drugs, procedures, and activities will ensure more accurate test results.

- Has the patient taken any iodine containing drugs within the last 30 days? Any estrogens which can cause a false high?
- Has the patient within the last decade or longer undergone x-ray studies of the gallbladder, ureters, bronchi, uterine tubes, or heart?
- Within the last 2 weeks, has the patient been eating principally sea foods? Seafood is so rich in iodine that ^{131}I uptake could show a falsely low reading. Be certain to inform the physician if the patient answers "yes" to any of these questions.

Serum Thyroid-Stimulating Hormone (TSH). The TSH concentration is elevated in hypothyroidism because of the loss of negative feedback control at the pituitary by the low circulating levels of thyroid hormone. If a patient is hypothyroid, but the TSH levels are low, the cause of the hypothyroidism is not due to a primary disease in the thyroid, but rather the pituitary gland. This is called secondary hypothyroidism.

Thyrotropin Test (TSH). The TSH test is also used to make a *differential* diagnosis between *primary* hypothyroidism (a condition originating in malfunction of the thyroid gland itself) and hypothyroidism *secondary* to pituitary malfunction.

You recall that thyrotropin is a hormone, secreted by the anterior pituitary gland, which stimulates the thyroid gland to secrete thyroid hormone. Normally, when a patient receives large doses of TSH, the thyroid gland will function at a higher level in secreting thyroid hormone; consequently serum thyroxine and ^{131}I uptake levels will be elevated. However, if the patient has *primary* hypothyroidism, a dose of TSH will have *no* effect upon thyroxine and ^{131}I uptake test results; i.e., no amount of TSH will be able to increase thyroid function if the gland is in a state of hypofunction due to disease. On the other hand, if the patient suffers from hypothyroidism *secondary* to anterior pituitary gland insufficiency, an injection of TSH *will raise* the serum thyroxine levels and ^{131}I uptake test results, because the thyroid gland is normal and capable of responding to TSH when it is available.

TRH Stimulation Test. Thyrotropin-releasing hormone (TRH) is normally released from the hypothalamus and stimulates release of TSH from the pituitary. In the TRH stimulation test, patients are given TRH intravenously. If the TSH levels rise, the pituitary is functioning normally. In either hyperthyroidism or pituitary disease, there will be no rise in the TSH.

Serum Cholesterol. Serum cholesterol is *not* a specific test of thyroid function, because its levels are influenced by many other factors besides thyroid hormone levels. Nevertheless, the serum cholesterol tends to be relatively elevated in myxedema and hypothyroidism. Possibly this may explain why these conditions are accompanied by a marked tendency toward atherosclerosis. Persons with hyperthyroidism usually have a relatively low serum cholesterol level (see also Chapter 36).

Serologic Tests. Many thyroid disorders are presumed to have an autoimmune basis, e.g., Hashimoto's thyroiditis, myxedema, and Graves' disease (a form of hyperthyroidism). Consequently, serologic tests are performed in order to determine if the patient's blood contains any antithyroid antibodies.

Basal Metabolic Rate (BMR). The basal metabolic rate is an indirect measure of the amount of oxygen which is consumed by the body under basal conditions during a given time, i.e., while the patient is in a state of complete mental and physical relaxation. Factors which can alter test results include inadequate rest prior to the examination, anxiety and emotional stress, a noisy environment, and the prior ingestion of almost any drug. The BMR, once the major test of thyroid function, is now being largely replaced by newer, more sophisticated diagnostic techniques.

Achilles Tendon Reflex Recording. The Achilles tendon reflex test is a measurement of the ankle jerk when the strong tendon at the back of the heel is tapped with a special instrument. Persons with hyperthyroidism tend to experience a more rapid tendon reflex; individuals with underactive thyroid glands, diabetics, and pregnant women have a slower jerking reflex and a prolonged relaxation time.

Enlargement of the Thyroid

Enlargement of the thyroid may be caused by the following three disorders: (1) simple goiter, (2) thyroiditis (inflammation of the goiter), and (3) tumors of the thyroid (benign and malignant). Each of these conditions is briefly considered below.

Simple Goiter (Nontoxic Goiter, Nodular Goiter). As stated earlier, the thyroid gland needs iodine in order to synthesize and secrete its hormones. If an individual fails to ingest sufficient amounts of iodine in his diet or if the production of thyroid hormone is suppressed for any other reason, the thyroid enlarges in an attempt to *compensate* for hormonal deficiency. Thus goiter essentially "is an adaptation to the deficiency of thyroid hormone."[80a] Enlargement of the gland occurs in response to increased pituitary secretion of TSH; as you recall, TSH stimulates the thyroid to secrete more thyroxine when blood thyroxine levels are low. Eventually, in its attempt to respond to TSH and meet the body's needs, the gland may become so large that it compresses structures in the neck and chest, causing respiratory symptoms and dysphagia.

TYPES OF GOITER. There are two major forms of simple goiter: endemic goiter and sporadic goiter. *Endemic goiter* is principally caused by *nutritional iodine deficiency.* It tends to occur in "goiter belts," which are geographic areas characterized by soil and water deficiency in iodine; major "goiter belts" within the United States are the Midwest, Northwest, and Great Lakes Region. Endemic goiter typically occurs in the winter and fall; it is twice as prevalent among women as men. Also, because the need for thyroid hormone is particularly great during growth spurts, pregnancy, and lactation, goiter commonly develops among adolescents, pregnant women, and nursing mothers residing in iodine-deficient regions.

Sporadic goiter is not restricted to any geographic area. Major causes include:

- *Genetic defects* resulting in faulty iodine metabolism.
- Ingestion of large amounts of *nutritional goitrogens* (goiter-producing agents that inhibit thyroxine production), e.g., rutabagas, cabbage, soybeans, peanuts, peaches, peas, strawberries, spinach, and radishes, all of which contain goitrogenic glycosides.
- Ingestion of *medicinal goitrogens,* e.g., thioureas (propylthiouracil), thiocarbamides (aminothiazole, tolbutamide), and iodine in large doses (some persons take iodine-containing solutions as a tonic).

DIAGNOSIS AND TREATMENT. Typically the patient with goiter seeks medical advice when the goiter grows large enough to distort the appearance of the neck, as pictured in Figures 73–2 and 73–3. Also, the patient may complain of respiratory distress and difficulty in swallowing if the goiter is very large. In addition to the patient's appearance and complaints, diagnosis of simple goiter is confirmed by the patient's history (residing in a "goiter belt" or ingesting large amounts of goitrogens) and by laboratory tests (^{131}I uptake is usually high, while the serum thyroxine is normal). Typically the patient with simple goiter is euthyroid; symptoms and laboratory signs of hypothyroidism seldom appear, because the gland enlarges enough to produce normal amounts of thyroxine.

The *goals of treatment* for simple goiter are to halt further enlargement of the thyroid and to promote regression of the gland. When enlargement is a compensatory reaction to iodine deficiency and consequent suppression of thyroxine secretion, patients can be treated with preparations of iodine or thyroid hormone. *Iodine* is administered either in the form of strong iodine solution (Lugol's solution) or saturated solution of potassium iodide (SSKI drops). Dosage is usually 5 drops of iodine solution given daily in ½ glass of water. Drugs of choice for *thyroid hormone replacement* include desiccated thyroid, sodium-L-thyroxine, and L-triiodothyronine. Dosage is based upon the age of the patient; children and elderly patients receive smaller doses than adults.

When administering thyroid preparations, watch the patient carefully for symptoms of *thyrotoxicosis,* i.e., tachycardia, increased appetite, diarrhea, sweating, agitation, tremor, palpitations, shortness of breath. If any of these symptoms develops during thyroid therapy, notify the physician at once so that he can reduce the dosage. Also the patient must be carefully observed for *further enlargement* of the gland, as well as for growth of *nodules* within the thyroid tissues; these signs are particularly dangerous because they may indicate cancer of the thyroid.

While patients with small or moderately large goiters may respond successfully to drug therapy, those with large goiters may need to undergo a subtotal thyroidectomy. In such cases, surgery is indicated for cosmetic reasons and also to alleviate respiratory problems. Surgery is also performed on patients with possible malignancy of the thyroid. Cancer is suspected when-

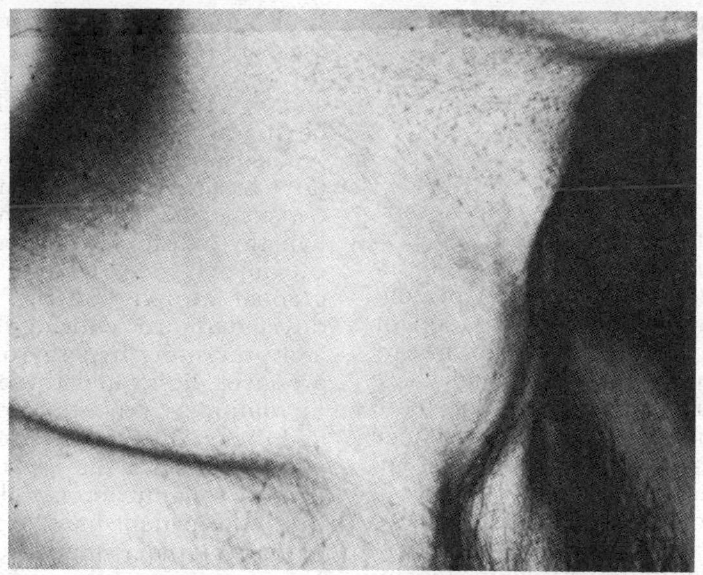

Figure 73–2. Enlargement of the thyroid gland. Note the position of the thyroid gland in relation to the prominence of the thyroid cartilage. (From Sherman, J. L., Jr., and S. K. Fields: *Guide to Patient Evaluation,* 2nd ed. Flushing, N.Y.: Medical Publishing Co., 1976, p. 73.)

ever the thyroid gland contains a single nodule and also when there has been no decrease in the size of the goiter despite 3 to 6 months of thyroid and iodine therapy.

PREVENTION OF SIMPLE GOITER. Endemic goiter can be prevented by the use of *iodized salt.* The minimum adult iodine requirement is 50 μg. iodine per day; however, an adequate iodine intake guaranteed to prevent goiter is 200 to 300 μg. per day. Iodized salt, which has been used in the United States since 1924, contains 1 part iodine per every 100,000 parts of salt. Thus the average person, who ingests approximately 6.2 Gm. of salt a day, is also ingesting 474 μg. of iodine daily *if* the salt is iodized. The problem is that many people are unaware of their need for iodized salt as a goiter preventative; indeed, it is possible that fewer Americans are using iodized salt today than during the 1950's.[80a] Also many modern foods are being processed with the cheaper, noniodized, bag salt rather than with iodized salt. As a result of public misinformation and new food processing methods, the potential for developing simple goiter today is as great or greater than in the past. To correct this problem, Matovinovic suggests that *all* salt to be used for human or animal consumption should be iodized. He points out that

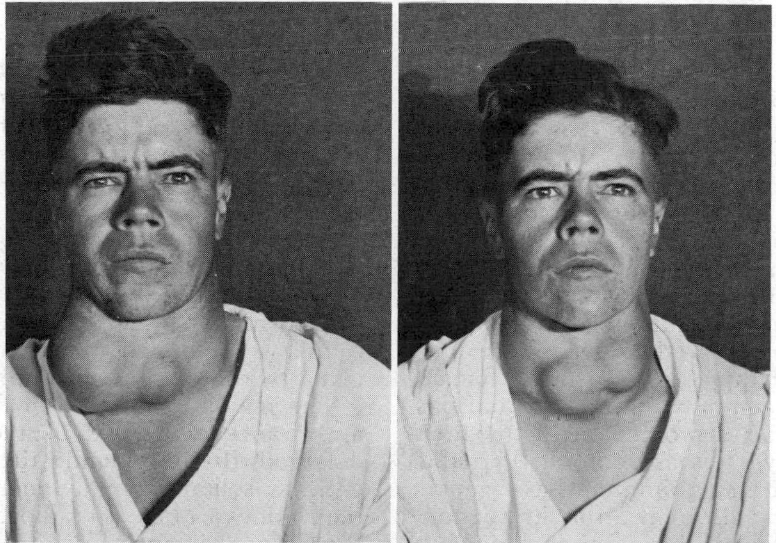

Figure 73–3. Colloid goiter with myxedema in twins. (From Delp, M. H., and R. T. Manning (Eds.): *Major's Physical Diagnosis,* 8th ed. Philadelphia: W. B. Saunders Co., 1975, p. 217.)

the use of iodized salt by persons with normal thyroid glands is not harmful to them.[80a]

Nurses can play an important role in educating the public to use iodized salt. Many persons strongly believe that *any* additive to food or water is harmful; e.g., groups lobbied for years against fluoridation of water even though there was ample evidence that fluorine prevents tooth decay. It is the nurse's task to help change outmoded attitudes and dispel irrational prejudice with scientific facts. The need for iodized salt in the diet as a goiter preventative cannot be overemphasized.

Thyroiditis. Thyroiditis simply means inflammation of the thyroid gland; it appears in three basic forms: (1) acute suppurative thyroiditis, (2) subacute granulomatous thyroiditis, and (3) chronic thyroiditis.

Acute suppurative thyroiditis is a rare condition caused by bacterial invasion of the thyroid gland. This disorder usually responds to antibiotic therapy and to incision and drainage of the infected gland.

Subacute granulomatous thyroiditis is a self-limited inflammatory condition which is believed to be caused by a *virus.* Although no etiologic agent has as yet been identified, subacute thyroiditis often follows in the wake of viral or streptococcal infections. *Symptoms* may include fever, neck pain over the thyroid which sometimes radiates to the jaws and ears, fatigue, and malaise. Thyroid function usually remains normal, although transient hyperthyroidism or hypothyroidism can occur. *Treatment* is based upon the severity of the disease. Patients with *mild* cases usually respond adequately to rest, fluids, and acetylsalicylic acid to relieve pain. *Severe* subacute thyroiditis may be treated with (a) corticosteroids to reduce inflammation, (b) propylthiouracil (see below) to reduce glandular tenderness, and (c) thyroid hormone to suppress TSH secretion and thus shrink the gland. Even without treatment, many patients with subacute thyroiditis experience a spontaneous remission within several months following the appearance of symptoms.

Chronic thyroiditis (Hashimoto's thyroiditis), a long-term inflammatory disorder, is the most common form of thyroiditis. It strikes females 30 times more frequently than males, and particularly tends to affect women during the menopause. Like Graves' disease, chronic thyroiditis is believed to have an autoimmune basis; genetic predisposition may also play a role in its etiology. *Symptoms* of chronic thyroiditis include painless enlargement of the gland, respiratory distress, and dysphagia due to pressure of the swollen gland upon surrounding structures. *Diagnosis* is based upon (a) needle biopsy of the thyroid, which reveals typical tissue changes; and (b) serologic tests, which reveal the presence of circulating antithyroid antibodies.

The course of Hashimoto's thyroiditis varies: (a) a few cases remit spontaneously; (b) many patients' conditions remain stable for years; (c) hypothyroidism and myxedema develop in approximately one third of cases owing to the gradual atrophy of the gland. *Treatment* is directed toward reducing the size of the thyroid and preventing hypothyroidism. Thus patients are given desiccated thyroid to prevent hypothyroidism as well as to suppress TSH secretion and thus reduce gland size. Corticosteroids are also useful on a short-term basis for reducing thyroid inflammation and swelling. In a few cases, the patient may be forced to undergo a partial thyroidectomy for relief of symptoms. However, surgery is used only as a last resort, because removal of part of the thyroid increases the risk of myxedema. If surgery is necessary, the patient may need to take thyroid hormone for life.

Thyroid Tumors. Benign adenomas and malignant thyroid tumors constitute the third cause of thyroid enlargement. Like other benign tumors, most thyroid adenomas are usually well encapsulated and consequently do not spread out or extend into other tissues. When the patient is given tracer doses of ^{131}I, these tumors may take up the radioiodide; consequently these benign adenomas are said to be "hot nodules."

Benign adenomas are usually not dangerous, although they may grow large enough to cause respiratory symptoms by pressing against the trachea. Occasionally, however, *malignant transformation* occurs, and the benign nodules become cancerous. While no one knows the exact incidence of malignant transformation, one study estimates that it occurs in 14 per cent of patients with benign thyroid tumors.[103a]

Malignant tumors of the thyroid are fortunately fairly rare; thyroid cancer accounts for around 0.5 per cent of cancer deaths. It develops mainly in persons between the ages of 40 and 60 and affects twice as many women as men.

Thyroid carcinoma develops frequently in persons who have received large doses of radiation to the head and neck. Also, malignant transformation of benign nodules can apparently follow prolonged stimulation of the thyroid gland by the pituitary hormone TSH.

The major *symptom* of thyroid cancer is the appearance of a hard, painless nodule in an enlarged thyroid gland; the nodule itself is typically solitary, rapidly enlarging, and "cold" (i.e., it does *not* take up radioactive iodine). Also, the patient's lymph nodes are sometimes palpable. In long-standing cases, the patient may suffer from respiratory difficulty and dysphagia due to pressure of the enlarged thyroid against structures in the neck.

There are four major types of thyroid cancer: (1) papillary adenocarcinoma, (2) follicular adenocarcinoma, (3) medullary carcinoma, and (4) anaplastic carcinoma. The incidence, symptoms, treatment, and prognosis of each of these thyroid cancers are compared in Table 73–2.

Disorders of Thyroid Hormone Production

The thyroid gland can produce either too little hormone or too much. The hypometabolic hypoactive state associated with a deficiency of thyroxine or triiodothyronine or both is called *hypothyroidism.* The hypermetabolic, overactive state associated with an excess of thyroxine or triiodothyronine or both is called *hyperthyroidism.* Both conditions affect the heat and energy-producing mechanism, the circulatory system, the muscular system, the nervous system, and other endocrine glands; hyperthyroidism often produces an effect opposite to that of hypothyroidism.

Treatment of these two conditions can also be sharply contrasted. The goal of care in *hypothyroidism* is to increase the patient's metabolism by correcting the thyroid hormone deficiency; thus the major form of treatment is *thyroid hormone administration.* Conversely, the goal of care in *hyperthyroidism* is to slow the patient's racing metabolic state by correcting the thyroid hormone excess. The three methods for reducing thyroid hormone secretion include (1) *surgical removal* of part of the thyroid (subtotal thyroidectomy); (2) *drug therapy* with antithyroid preparations, and (3) *irradiation* of the thyroid with radioiodine. These conditions are now examined in more detail.

HYPOTHYROIDISM

There are two major forms of hypothyroidism: (1) cretinism and (2) myxedema.

Cretinism

Cretinism is a severe hypothyroid condition of infancy which is caused by a deficiency of thyroid hormone synthesis during fetal life or soon after birth. Causes of cretinism include the following:

- Severe iodine deficiency in the diet of the mother; this is particularly common in the Alps and Himalayas.
- Inborn errors of iodine metabolism and of thyroxine or triiodothyronine synthesis or both.
- Congenital absence of the thyroid or anatomic malformation.

The two major hallmarks of cretinism are *defective physical development* and *mental retardation.* As William Osler once wrote of the cretin:

> No type of human transformation is more distressing to look at than an aggravated case of cretinism. The stunted stature, the semi-bestial aspect, the blubber lips, retroussé nose sunken at the root, the wide-open mouth, the lolling tongue, the small eyes half closed with swollen lids, the stolid expressionless face, the squat figure, the muddy dry skin, combine to make the picture of what has been termed "the pariah of nature."[14]

The tragic syndrome of cretinism may be reversed if the infant is treated immediately upon diagnosis with daily doses of desiccated thyroid or thyroxine. It is unfortunate that, even with treatment, the child may be mentally deficient even though physical and sexual development unfold normally.

Myxedema

In contrast to cretinism, *myxedema* results from a deficiency of thyroid hormone synthesis in the adult. Distinguishing features of myxedema are (a) slowed body metabolism due to decreased oxygen consumption by the tissues, (b) pronounced personality changes (lethargy, apathy), and (c) the appearance of generalized interstitial edema — thus the term myxedema. (See Figures 73–3 and 73–4.)

The *etiology* of myxedema may be traced either to pathologic changes within the thyroid gland itself (*primary* hypothyroidism) or to disorders of the pituitary gland which disturb thyroid gland function (*secondary* hypothyroidism). The development of *primary* myxedema may possibly have an autoimmune basis; studies show that 98 per cent of patients with newly diagnosed myxedema and 70 to 80 per cent of patients with myxedema of long duration have circulating thyroid autoantibodies within their blood.[103a] Further, myxedema may appear during the course of chronic (Hashimoto's) thyroiditis, which is also an autoimmune disorder. Finally, primary myxedema sometimes develops as an iatrogenic result of treating hyperthyroidism. Thus myxedema may follow (a) thyroidectomy without sufficient thyroid hormone replacement therapy, (b) destruction of the thyroid gland by overzealous radioiodine therapy, and (c) overuse of antithyroid drugs.

Secondary hypothyroidism may follow (a) the development of destructive pituitary tumors, (b) pituitary insufficiency, and (c) postpartum necrosis of the pituitary gland. Without the stimulating effect of TSH, the thyroid gland atrophies and ceases to function.

Myxedema is principally a disease of older persons and of women. Thus it mainly strikes people in their 60's, and it affects five times as many women as it does men.

TABLE 73–2. TYPES OF THYROID CANCER: INCIDENCE, CHARACTERISTICS, TREATMENT, AND PROGNOSIS

Type	Incidence	Characteristics	Treatment	Prognosis
Papillary adenocarcinoma	Mainly affects persons in their 40's. Comprises 61% of thyroid cancers	Slow-growing tumor. Palpable nodules appear within thyroid. Spreads to regional nodes in approximately 50% of cases.	Some authorities recommend total thyroidectomy. Others recommend lobectomy and isthmusectomy.	Excellent if cancer restricted to thyroid gland. Surgical resection usually curative.
Follicular adenocarcinoma	Comprises 18% of thyroid cancers. Mainly affects persons in their 50's.	Composed of well-developed follicles. Rarely spreads to regional lymph nodes. Tends to adhere to trachea, muscle, skin, and great vessels of neck, causing dyspnea and dysphagia.	Same as for papillary adenocarcinoma.	Prognosis good but inferior to that of papillary adenocarcinoma.
Medullary carcinoma (amyloidic carcinoma)	Comprises 6% of thyroid cancers. Mainly affects persons in their 50's.	Tumor may be hereditary and familial. Tends to secrete calcitonin, ACTH, and serotonin. Tends to invade surrounding structures.	Total thyroidectomy. Radical neck resection necessary if metastasis present.	Poor. Mean survival time approximately 6.6 years.
Anaplastic carcinoma	Comprises 15% of thyroid cancers. Mainly affects persons between 60 and 80 years.	Highly malignant. Grows extremely rapidly. Widespread metastasis within one year.	Surgery to prevent respiratory obstruction.	Extremely poor. Typically results in death within 1 year.

The *symptoms* of myxedema depend upon whether the degree of hypothyroidism is mild or full-blown. Patients with mild myxedema (the most common form) may be asymptomatic; in other cases, they may suffer from vague complaints which are so ordinary that they often escape detection, e.g., mild sensitivity to cold, lethargy, dry skin and hair, forgetfulness, depression, and some weight gain. On the other hand, individuals with the rarer full-blown myxedema develop a multitude of striking symptoms. The patient slows drastically in both physical and mental reactions and appears abnormally fatigued and apathetic; for example, he may sit for hours in one place without moving or responding to persons or things around him. Indeed, the person with myxedema must often be taken to the doctor by a friend or relative because he is too complacent and apathetic to seek help for himself.

The patient's physical appearance also changes (see Fig. 73–4). In many cases, obesity develops; features become coarse; hair grows in dry and sparse; skin feels dry, flaky, and inelastic. The patient also looks puffy and edematous owing to the infiltration of fluid into the interstitial tissues. In addition, the patient suffers from a severe intolerance to cold due to his decreased metabolic rate; ability to sweat diminishes. Constipation and fecal impactions due to slowed peristaltic action and lack of normal physical activity constitute serious problems. Susceptibility to infection increases. Finally, patients with myxedema become dangerously hypersensitive to narcotics, barbiturates, and anesthetics.

> Remember: *Even an average dose of a narcotic, barbiturate, or anesthetic agent may result in the death of a myxedematous patient!*

Diagnostic tests for myxedema confirm the clinical picture of hypometabolism and depressed thyroid activity. Although seldom measured at the present time, BMR is below 30 per cent owing to decreased oxygen utilization by the body tissues. Serum thyroid hormone levels are abnormally low. In addition, the serum cholesterol is markedly elevated — a factor which probably contributes to the later development of cardiac problems.

Complications of myxedema principally affect the heart. Long-term myxedema patients are particularly subject to the rapid development of atherosclerotic coronary heart disease, leading to angina pectoris, myocardial infarction, or congestive heart failure. *Acute organic psychosis* is a second complication of severe hypothyroidism. Patients with "myxedema madness" typically suffer from paranoia and delusions. Finally, a few patients with severe myxedema may develop *myxedema coma.* This critical condition is characterized by hypoventilation, hypothermia, and respiratory acidosis. Without emergency treatment (see Chapter 95) with injectable thyroid hormone preparations, myxedema coma can be fatal.

The *goals of care* in myxedema are to correct thyroid hormone deficiency, reverse symptoms, and prevent further heart and arterial damage. To reverse hypothyroidism permanently, the patient *must usually take thyroid hormone preparations for the rest of his life.* Thyroid drugs available include thyroxine (Synthyroid), triiodothyronine (Cytomel), or desiccated thyroid which is a combination of thyroxine and triiodothyronine. Dosage varies with the severity of the patient's hypothyroidism and the degree of heart disease present.

Persons with cardiac complications must be initially started on *small doses* of thyroid hor-

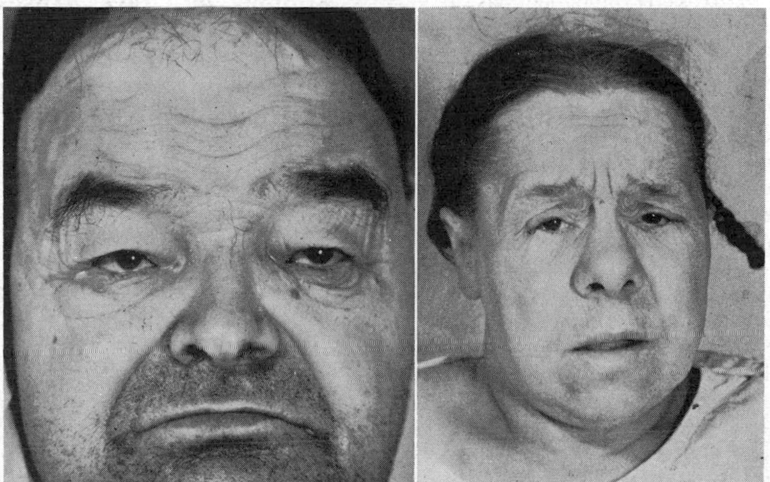

Figure 73–4. Typical facial appearance of myxedematous patients. (From Williams, R. H. (Ed.): *Textbook of Endocrinology,* 5th ed. Philadelphia: W. B. Saunders Co., 1974.)

mone; large doses could precipitate heart failure or myocardial infarction by increasing body metabolism, myocardial oxygen requirements, and consequently the work of the heart. When administering thyroid hormone to a myxedematous patient with heart disease, watch the patient carefully for anginal pain, dyspnea, orthopnea, and so forth. If any new cardiac symptoms appear, notify the physician immediately; *do not* give the hormone until the doctor reappraises the patient's condition.

Once the patient has adequately responded to thyroid hormone therapy, he or she is placed on a maintenance dose equivalent to 0.1–0.3 mg. of thyroxine daily.

Nursing patients with myxedema is very rewarding because these patients respond so dramatically to hormone replacement therapy. To assess the patient's progress and prevent complications, take time to make the following observations and perform the following measures.

▶Observe the patient's level of physical and mental activity. With thyroid hormone therapy, the patient should gradually become more energetic and more interested in the surroundings.

▶Observe daily for a lessening of the patient's edematous, puffy appearance. Note intake and output records; urine output should significantly increase during the course of thyroid therapy. Obtain the patient's daily weight; as activity increases and edema decreases, the patient should experience a significant weight loss.

▶Observe the patient's sacrum, coccyx, elbows, scapula, and so forth for signs of redness or tissue breakdown. Remember that edematous tissues are particularly prone to decubitus ulcer formation. Place the patient on a strict turning schedule and on an alternating pressure mattress. If the patient has cardiac complications, obtain help in moving him or her so that you don't place a greater strain on the already overburdened heart.

▶Avoid sedating the patient if at all possible. If a sedative or narcotic must be given, administer no more than one half to one third the usual dose and then observe the patient carefully for signs of respiratory depression or coma.

▶Provide the patient with a comfortable, warm environment. Remember that hypothyroidism sharply increases sensitivity to cold. If necessary, give the patient extra clothing and warm blankets.

▶Observe the patient's appetite; typically a low calorie diet is prescribed until the patient's weight is stabilized.

▶Prevent constipation and fecal impactions. As the hypothyroidism reverses and cardiac status improves, encourage the patient to be more active. Patients are advised to drink 6 to 8 glasses of water every day and to eat foods which contain roughage, e.g., fresh fruits, vegetables, and grains. If these efforts are ineffective, a stool softener or cathartic may be indicated.

▶Once mentally alert, the patient is taught about the disorder and the importance of taking thyroid hormone *daily* for life. Also, provide a written list of the symptoms of thyroid deficiency or excess so that the patient will know when the medication dosage warrants re-evaluation.

With early thyroid hormone replacement therapy, the prognosis for patients with severe hypothyroidism is excellent. Moreover, as long as the thyroid hormone is taken daily, the patient should never again experience the depressed hypometabolic state of myxedema.

HYPERTHYROIDISM (THYROTOXICOSIS)

Hyperthyroidism is a highly prevalent endocrine disease. Like the majority of thyroid conditions, hyperthyroidism is predominantly a disorder of females; it affects women four times as frequently as it does men. It has a particularly high incidence among young women between the ages of 20 and 40.

Graves' disease (toxic diffuse goiter, exophthalmic goiter) is the major cause of hyperthyroidism. The three principal hallmarks of Graves' disease include (1) hyperthyroidism; (2) enlargement of the thyroid gland (goiter); and (3) exophthalmos (abnormal protrusion of the eyes). Less commonly, hyperthyroidism is caused by either a functioning toxic adenoma, by a single toxic nodule, by thyroid cancer, or by certain medications. Also, overtreatment of myxedema with thyroid hormone may result in hyperthyroidism. Very rarely a pituitary adenoma causes hyperthyroidism by secreting excessive amounts of TSH. Because the most common as well as classic picture of hyperthyroidism is caused by Graves' disease, our discussion will center upon this condition.

Etiology of Graves' Disease. For generations, physicians have linked the appearance of Graves' disease with periods of emotional stress in the patient's life. However, evidence for the theory that psychologic upheavals cause Graves' disease is meager. It is far more likely that Graves' disease, like Hashimoto's thyroiditis and primary myxedema, is an *autoimmune disorder.* Around 60 to 80 per cent of patients with Graves' disease have circulating autoantibodies which react against thyroglobulin.[29] Moreover, "long-acting thyroid stimulator" (LATS), a gamma globulin, has been discovered circulating in the serum of around 80 to 90 per cent of hyperthyroid patients.[103a] There is still much to learn about LATS and its role in the causation of Graves' disease. Evidently LATS is an autoantibody which reacts against a "component of the thyroid cell membranes," somehow stimulating enlargement of the thyroid gland and secretion of excess thyroid hormone. Apparently, LATS is not involved in the development of exophthalmos. Additionally, the severity of the hyperthyroidism cannot be determined by the LATS levels in the serum.

Since the discovery of LATS, several different tests have been developed to test for a thyroid stimulating factor in the serum or patients with Graves' disease. The term *TSI* (thyroid-stimulating immunoglobulins) was originally applied to one specific test, but is gaining popularity as a general term for all of these stimulating substances.

Symptoms and Diagnostic Tests. Because *hyperthyroidism* is caused by an excess secretion of thyroid hormone, the clinical picture of Graves' disease is, in many ways, directly opposite that of myxedema. Thus, the patient is extremely nervous, agitated, and irritable. Despite a ravenous appetite, the patient may lose weight owing to the quickened metabolism. Because of the high levels of circulating thyroid hormone, the patient's bodily processes literally "speed up"; loose bowel movements, heat intolerance, profuse diaphoresis, tachycardia, incoordination due to tremor, and an accelerated circulation to the tissues that causes the skin to become warm, smooth, and silky; also the hair appears smooth and soft.

Moreover, the patient's emotions are adversely affected by the turbulent activity within the body. Moods may be cyclical, ranging from mildly euphoric states to extreme hyperactivity to delirium. The excessive hyperactivity, in turn, leads to extreme fatigue and depression, which is then followed by episodes of overactivity, and so forth. As a result of the patient's chaotic emotional state, family life and social relationships may deteriorate rapidly, which further accentuates the patient's emotional disturbance.

Goiter, the second characteristic of Graves' disease, is due to hyperplasia and hypertrophy of the thyroid cells; cellular overgrowth results in the release of excessive amounts of thyroid hormone into the blood. The gland may enlarge up to three to four times its normal size.

Exophthalmos, the third major manifestation of Graves' disease, has an obscure etiology. The patient who suffers from exophthalmos has protruding eyes and a fixed stare due to the accumulation of fluid in the fat pads which lie behind the eyeballs. Because the eyes are surrounded by unyielding bone, edema of the fat pads forces the eyes forward out of their sockets, producing the typical facies of exophthalmos (Figure 73–5). In severe cases, patients may be unable to close their eyelids and must have their lids taped shut to protect the eyes. Without treatment, severe exophthalmos can progress to corneal ulceration or infection and loss of vision.

Graves' disease is *diagnosed* on the basis of the patient's often striking physical appearance (enlarged neck, protruding eyes, agitated expression); the symptoms of restlessness, weight loss, and so forth; and laboratory findings. The serum thyroid hormone levels, 24-hour radioiodine uptake, and T_3 resin uptake are all elevated, although they may occasionally be within the normal range (so-called "euthyroid Graves' disease"). Serum cholesterol levels are usually depressed.

Specific Treatment Measures. The goals of treatment for patients with Graves' disease are to curtail the excessive secretion of thyroid hormone, to establish a euthyroid (normal thyroid) state, and to prevent and treat complications. The three major forms of therapy include (1) antithyroid drug therapy, (2) radioiodine therapy, and (3) surgery. Choice of treatment is based upon (a) the patient's age, (b) the size of the goiter, and (c) whether or not other medical problems exist. Below, each of these clinical methods is described briefly.

ANTITHYROID DRUG THERAPY. This form of treatment is recommended for patients who are under 18 and for pregnant women. The major drugs used to control hyperthyroidism include (1) propylthiouracil, (2) methimazole (Tapazole), and (3) iodine (Lugol's solution or saturated solution of potassium iodide). Adrenergic blocking agents may also be administered as adjunctive therapy.

Propylthiouracil is the most commonly used antithyroid drug. It corrects hyperthyroidism by blocking thyroid hormone synthesis. The usual dosage of 100 mg. orally every 8 hours ameliorates Graves' disease within 4 to 8 weeks; however, several months may pass before symptoms completely abate. Once euthyroid, the

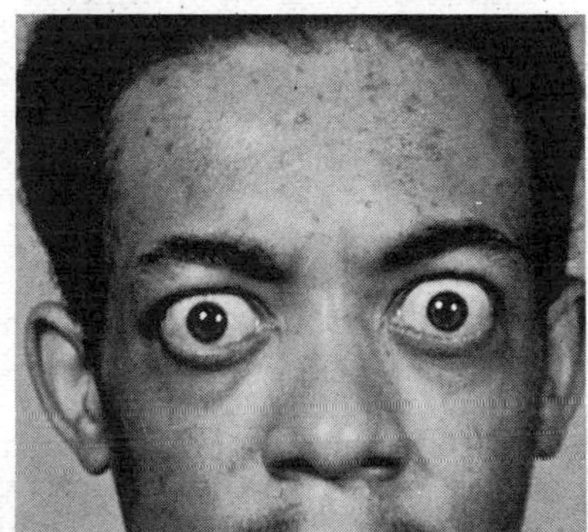

Figure 73–5. Extreme exophthalmos in hyperthyroidism. (From Delp, M. H., and R. T. Manning (Eds.): *Major's Physical Diagnosis,* 8th ed. Philadelphia: W. B. Saunders Co., 1975, p. 266.)

patient is given a maintenance dose of propylthiouracil daily. While propylthiouracil is an ideal drug in many ways, it produces toxic reactions in approximately 9 per cent of patients.

The most serious toxic effect of propylthiouracil is *agranulocytosis* (see Chapter 46). A white blood count should be taken prior to initially administering the drug. Instruct nonhospitalized patients to report a sore throat, fever, or rash immediately to their physician so that further WBC tests can be performed and the patient's condition evaluated. Other less severe drug reactions include mild allergies (rash and pruritus). Rarely, the patient develops hepatitis or drug fever.

Methimazole (Tapazole) acts upon the thyroid gland in a way very similar to propylthiouracil, so that this drug can often be given to patients who are allergic to propylthiouracil. Unfortunately, methimazole also produces agranulocytosis in a small percentage of patients.

Iodine therapy is prescribed for two reasons: (1) to reduce the vascularity of the thyroid gland prior to subtotal or total thyroidectomy; and (2) to treat "thyroid storm" (see complications of Graves' disease, below). Iodine preparations *temporarily* act to prevent release of thyroid hormone into the circulation by increasing the amount of thyroid hormone stored within the gland. However, the stored thyroid hormone is eventually released back into the circulation, once again producing hyperthyroidism. For this reason, iodine preparations are usually only given for a 10- to 14-day period prior to surgery. If iodine is given for a longer period, or if it is given alone (i.e., not in combination with propylthiouracil), the thyroid gland may "escape" prior to thyroidectomy. The term "escape of the thyroid" means that the iodine is no longer capable of maintaining thyroid hormone storage; as a result, thyroid hormone floods the circulation, and hyperthyroidism returns in a more severe form than before.

The iodine drug of choice is saturated solution of potassium iodide (SSKI); the usual dose of SSKI is 5 to 10 drops in water 3 to 4 times daily. Lugol's solution is also used, but it is more expensive than SSKI, and it tends to inactivate antithyroid preparations within the bowel.

Adrenergic blocking agents are sometimes given as adjunctive therapy to control overactivity by the sympathetic nervous system, thereby lessening such distressing symptoms as tachycardia, tremor, and nervousness. These drugs include propranolol and reserpine.

RADIOIODINE THERAPY. Therapy with ^{131}I is principally prescribed for middle-aged and elderly patients. This form of treatment offers many advantages: it is economical, simple to administer, and it can be prescribed on an outpatient basis. Radiotherapy is contraindicated in pregnant women and is rarely used for children.

The rationale behind ^{131}I therapy for Graves' disease is simple. The thyroid gland is unable to distinguish between regular iodine atoms and radioiodine atoms. Consequently, when the patient receives a dose of ^{131}I, the thyroid gland picks up the radioiodine and concentrates it just as it would regular iodine. As a result, some of the cells which concentrate iodine and make thyroxine are destroyed by the local irradiation; thus thyroid hormone secretion diminishes, and the signs of hyperthyroidism and goiter disappear. However, because radioiodine destroys thyroid cells, one of the major possible complications of ^{131}I therapy is *myxedema.*

^{131}I is administered orally in the form of a "radioactive cocktail." Dosage is determined both by the size of the gland and by the thyroid's degree of radiosensitivity (see Chapter 23). After receiving the "cocktail," the patient may then go home unless the dosage is extremely large; in the latter case, the patient must be placed in isolation for several days. The symptoms of hyperthyroidism usually subside within 6 to 8 weeks following the administration of ^{131}I. Sometimes, resistant patients will require a second or (in rare cases) a third dose of radioiodine. Patients should continue to have regular medical check-ups once they become euthyroid, because hypothyroidism may develop several years following radiotherapy. Should the patient become hypothyroid, life-long hormonal replacement with thyroid preparations will be needed.

SURGERY. Surgery has been performed since the early 1880's to treat hyperthyroidism. Ideally, patients selected for surgery are fairly young and free from any condition that would make them poor operative risks (e.g., diabetes, heart disease, renal disease, drug allergies).

Preoperative preparation for a subtotal thyroidectomy is extremely important. The patient should be euthyroid prior to the operation if possible. Thus preoperative care for patients with Graves' disease includes (a) the administration of antithyroid drugs to suppress secretion of thyroid hormone, and (b) the administration of iodine preparations to reduce the size and vascularity of the organ, thereby diminishing the chance of hemorrhage. The patient should be adequately rested, at optimum weight, and in good health before entering the operating room. Adequate preoperative preparation may take as long as 2 to 3 months.

Surgical treatment is effective in the majority of patients with Graves' disease. A small percentage of patients remain hyperthyroid, and some patients develop hypothyroidism. Rarely, vocal cord paralysis or hypoparathyroidism or both develops.

General Symptomatic Care. No matter which treatment is received (drug, surgery, radiotherapy), expert nursing care is needed in order to assist the patient in coping with distressing symptoms. Provide an environment which is *restful* both mentally and physically. Helping patients who are hyperthyroid to relax is a true challenge. Assigning the patient to a private room may promote rest, and it will also prevent the patient from agitating other patients owing to hyperactivity and restlessness. Explain to friends and relatives that the patient's bizarre, difficult behavior is likely to be temporary and should steadily improve with treatment. Caution visitors to avoid discussing upsetting topics until the patient feels better and calmer. Attempt to maintain a quiet, understanding manner when working with the patient; accept irritation and emotional outbursts for what they are — expressions of the disease.

Ask the occupational therapy department for assistance; the occupational therapist may be able to provide the patient with simple activities designed to distract the patient from focusing on the disease, e.g., putting together a puzzle with large pieces, molding clay, watching TV, and so forth. For the very restless patient, obtain an order for a sedative (e.g., phenobarbital) or for one of the adrenergic blocking agents discussed earlier.

Provide a *well-balanced diet.* The patient with Graves' disease is usually extremely hungry owing to increased metabolism. Indeed, six full meals a day may be needed to satisfy the patient's appetite. However, you recall that these patients may lose weight rapidly despite huge meals, also they usually are in a state of negative nitrogen balance. Therefore, encourage patients to eat foods that are highly nutritious and contain ample amounts of protein, carbohydrates, and minerals. Discourage ordering foods which increase peristalsis and resultant diarrhea, e.g., highly seasoned, bulky, or fibrous foods. Weigh the patient daily and report weight losses of more than 2 kg. If the patient continues to appear malnourished despite an ample diet, obtain an order for supplemental vitamins — particularly vitamin B complex.

Provide a *cool environment.* Remember that patients with Graves' disease suffer from heat intolerance. When making the bed, omit the plastic draw sheet, as it tends to cause diaphoresis. Use only a lightweight sheet for the top cover. Provide the patient with light, loose pajamas; if the patient is diaphoretic, frequent changes of bedsheets and night clothes may be needed.

Treating Complications of Graves' Disease. The three major complications of Graves' disease are (1) exophthalmos, (2) heart disease, and (3) thyroid storm.

Unlike the manifestations of goiter and hyperthyroidism, exophthalmos does not necessarily regress with treatment. In fact, occasionally the removal of thyroid secretion seems to worsen exophthalmos. Exophthalmos is generally treated with the following specific drugs and procedures:

▶ *Thyroid hormone* is administered orally if the patient continues to have progressive exophthalmos following treatment.

▶ *Diuretics* may alleviate some of the periorbital edema.

▶ *Glucocorticoids* such as prednisone are given in large doses to reduce inflammation of the periorbital tissues. Unfortunately, steroids produce many undesirable side effects, including acute psychoses.

▶ *Estrogen* therapy is occasionally of value in postmenopausal women.

▶ *Methylcellulose eye drops,* ¼ per cent four times daily, help reduce eye irritation.

▶ *Surgical decompression of the orbits* is performed when all other measures fail to correct the exophthalmos; this procedure may save the patient's vision when eye changes are severe.

There are also a number of general nursing measures which help to reduce eye discomfort and prevent corneal ulceration and infection; they are as follows:

▶ Instruct patients with exophthalmos to wear dark glasses; warn them to avoid getting dust or dirt in their eyes.

▶ When patients cannot close their eyelids easily or at all, have them wear a sleeping mask (which can be bought in drug stores) or lightly tape the eyes shut with non-allergic tape. In severe cases, the physician may be forced to suture the patient's lids closed.

▶ Elevate the head of the bed at night and have the patient restrict salt intake to relieve edema.

▶ Encourage the patient to exercise the extraocular muscles daily by directing eyes from the upper left to the upper right to the lower left to the lower right and so forth several times around. Exercise of the eye muscles seems to improve eye function.

Heart disease, the second complication of Graves' disease, poses a serious threat. Tachycardia almost always accompanies thyrotoxicosis; atrial fibrillation may also appear. Congestive heart failure is found among older persons with longstanding thyrotoxicosis. The treatment of these cardiac complications is discussed in detail in Unit XII.

Thyroid storm is a sometimes fatal, acute episode of thyroid overactivity characterized by high fever, severe tachycardia, delirium, dehydration, and extreme irritability. Once a commonly occurring crisis, thyroid storm seldom develops today, thanks to modern treatment techniques. However, it can develop when a patient with Graves' disease undergoes severe sudden stress, develops an infection, or enters labor, also it strikes patients who have not been adequately prepared for thyroid surgery.

Because it is an emergency, thyroid storm may require heroic treatment measures for control. The high fever is combated with hypothermia or ice packs; dehydration is relieved with intravenous fluids. To block thyroid hormone secretion, the doctor orders an oral or parenteral antithyroid drug, followed 1 hour later by potassium iodide. Corticosteroids are sometimes administered, especially if there is any possibility that the patient is suffering from adrenal insufficiency. Sometimes large doses of propranolol (Inderal) are given to block sympathetic nervous stimulation and relieve cardiac arrhythmias. The steps in emergency management of the patient with thyroid storm are outlined in Chapter 95.

Thyroidectomy

Thyroidectomy (removal of the thyroid gland) may be either total or partial. *Total* thyroidectomy is performed to remove thyroid cancer; patients who undergo this operation must take thyroid hormone on a permanent basis. *Subtotal* thyroidectomy is employed to correct hyperthyroidism and extreme cases of simple goiter. Approximately five-sixths of the gland is removed. Because one-sixth of the functioning thyroid is left intact, hormonal replacements may not be necessary.

Preoperative Care. As emphasized earlier, patients must be carefully prepared for thyroidectomy or complications will ensue (e.g., thyroid storm and hemorrhage). Criteria for successful preparation of patients for thyroid surgery include the following:

- The patient is *euthyroid* before entering the operating room; tests of thyroid function are within the normal range.
- Signs of thyrotoxicosis are greatly diminished or absent; the patient appears rested and relaxed.
- Weight and nutritional status are normal; any weight losses suffered earlier have been regained.
- Cardiac problems are under control; pulse rate is normal; electrocardiogram tracings taken before surgery show no dangerous arrhythmias.

To assist in meeting these four criteria, the patient facing thyroidectomy is treated with antithyroid drugs, iodine preparations, bed rest, nutritious diet, and supplemental vitamins. As we stated earlier, thorough preparation may take months. However, once armed with good health and adequate weight, the patient can undergo surgery with confidence that the operation will be successful and the symptoms will be alleviated. (See Chapter 17.)

Postoperative Care. The immediate goals of postoperative care following thyroidectomy are (a) to decrease strain on the patient's suture line; (b) to relieve discomfort from sore throat and tracheal irritation; (c) to prevent pooling of respiratory secretions; and (d) to prevent and/or relieve the complications of thyroidectomy.

Typical postoperative orders accompanied by rationale and important associated nursing actions are outlined in Table 73–3. Note that you will need to assemble several pieces of equipment at the patient's bedside before he returns from surgery, e.g., blood pressure cuff and stethoscope, sandbags or additional pillows, a suction machine, tracheostomy set, oxygen, humidifier, and rectal thermometer; ampules of calcium gluconate should also be on hand in the medicine cabinet or on the emergency tray.

The major complications which may follow thyroidectomy include: (1) hemorrhage; (2) respiratory obstruction due to edema of the glottis, bilateral laryngeal nerve damage, or tracheal compression from hemorrhage; (3) weakness and hoarseness of the voice due to damage of one laryngeal nerve; (4) hypocalcemia and tetany resulting from accidental removal of one or more of the parathyroid glands; (5) thyroid storm.

Hoarseness and weakness of the voice may occur if there has been unilateral injury of the pharyngeal nerve during surgery; this condition is usually temporary. The patient's voice should be assessed by asking the patient to state his or her name as soon as full recovery from anesthesia occurs. Have the patient speak every 30 to 60 minutes thereafter, and carefully note any voice changes. If hoarseness or voice weakness is present, reassure the patient that the problem will probably subside in a few days. Discourage the patient from unnecessary talking because overuse of vocal cords prolongs hoarseness.

Muscular twitching and hyperirritability of the nervous system indicates *tetany;* hypocalcemia develops if the parathyroid glands are accidentally removed during surgery. Symptoms may develop in from 1 to 7 days after surgery. Report immediately any muscular spasms or twitching; have calcium gluconate ampules on hand. (The care of patients with tetany is discussed in Chapter 12 and later in this unit.)

Once the immediate postoperative period and its dangers have passed, turn your attention next to patient instruction. Important areas to cover are as follows:

TABLE 73-3. POSTOPERATIVE ORDERS, RATIONALE, AND ASSOCIATED NURSING ACTIONS FOLLOWING THYROIDECTOMY

Postoperative Order	Rationale	Associated Nursing Actions
1. Vital signs q. 15 minutes until stable; then q. 30 min. for next 12 hours.	Following thyroidectomy, hemorrhage and respiratory obstruction may develop. Elevated pulse and hypotension indicate hemorrhage and shock. Dyspnea, crowing respirations, and retraction of neck tissues indicate respiratory obstruction.	Check dressing after checking vital signs. Observe for bleeding at front, sides, and *back* of neck. Examine back of patient's neck and shoulders for bleeding because blood tends to drain posteriorly. Check dressing for tightness; uncomfortable tautness may indicate bleeding into tissues. Loosen dressing and call surgeon immediately.
2. Semi-Fowler position when conscious; support head and neck with pillows and sandbags; ambulate second day as tolerated.	Immobilization of head and neck is essential to prevent flexion and hyperextension of neck with resultant strain on suture line; semi-Fowler position is used for comfort.	Place sandbags on either side of patient's head for immobilization and maintenance of good alignment. Warn patient not to extend or hyperextend neck; reassure the patient that sandbags will prevent him or her from moving the head too much. Gently rub back of patient's neck to relieve tension. Support patient's head and neck when moving or changing position.
3. Fluids by mouth as tolerated; if nausea or vomiting, notify surgeon. Soft diet second day PM.	Patient who is nauseated or vomiting is given IV fluids; otherwise, oral fluids are started as soon as patient is fully conscious.	Maintain intake and output record for 2 or 3 days. Observe patient for difficulty in swallowing; normally this problem lasts for only a day or two postoperatively. Weigh patient once a full diet is started; weight lost during early postoperative period should be regained.
4. Meperidine (Demerol), 50–100 mg. q. 3–4 hours p.r.n. for pain in throat area.	Demerol and morphine sulfate are both used during early postoperative period to relieve pain and promote rest.	Do not give narcotics to patients with respirations below 12 per minute or to patients with respiratory congestion; consult physician for further orders.
5. Cough and deep breathe q. ½ hour; suction mouth and trachea if necessary.	Pooling of mucous secretions in trachea, bronchi, and lungs will cause respiratory obstruction with resultant atelectasis and pneumonia. Secretions must be raised to prevent respiratory complications.	Instruct patient to cough and deep breathe as taught during preoperative period. If patient cannot raise secretions, gently suction mouth and trachea. Do not oversedate patients with profuse respiratory secretions; also give narcotics judiciously.
6. Tracheostomy set and oxygen on hand in room.	Acute respiratory obstruction due to hemorrhage, edema of glottis, laryngeal nerve damage, or tetany is an emergency; equipment for establishing an airway and administering oxygen must be available for immediate use.	Continuously observe patient for signs of airway obstruction, e.g., increasing restlessness, tachycardia, apprehension, cyanosis, crowing respirations, and retraction of neck tissues. Report any of these signs to surgeon immediately.
7. Continuous mist inhalation until chest clear.	Humidification of the air promotes easier breathing; moistness of air also helps to liquefy mucous secretions.	Keep patient's door closed so that the moist air is retained in the room.
8. Rectal temperature q. 4 hours for 24 hours, then orally.	One of the first signs of thyroid storm is an elevated temperature.	Carefully observe patient for signs of thyroid storm: elevated temperature, extreme restlessness, agitation, and tachycardia. Report any elevation over 100° rectally or 99° orally.

▶Teach patients how to support the weight of their own head and neck when sitting up in bed. Show them how to place their hands at the back of the head when flexing the neck or moving. Usually the patient is able to perform this maneuver by the second postoperative day.

▶Once sutures have been removed (usually on the second to fourth postoperative day), instruct the patient in range of motion neck exercises to prevent contractures. With the surgeon's permission, teach the patient to flex the head forward and laterally, to hyperextend the neck, and to turn the head from side to side. Have the patient perform these exercises several times every day.

▶To diminish scarring of the neck, have the patient apply cold cream or other lubricant daily to the incision once sutures are removed.

▶If a total thyroidectomy has been performed, instruct the patient concerning the self-administration of thyroid medications.

▶Make an appointment for the patient for a follow-up visit in the hospital clinic or doctor's office following discharge. Emphasize to patients that they must see their physician at least twice a year for the rest of their lives in order to avert any possible complications (e.g., hypothyroidism, hypoparathyroidism, or recurrent hyperthyroidism).

THE PARATHYROID GLANDS

The parathyroid glands are four small glands which are either near to, attached to, or embedded in the thyroid gland. The hormone secreted by the parathyroid gland is a polypeptide substance called parathormone (PTH). The *functions* of PTH are as follows:

- ▶ Controls calcium and phosphate metabolism (see Chapter 12).
- ▶ Increases the breakdown and resorption of bone, thereby maintaining normal serum calcium levels.
- ▶ Maintains an inverse relationship between serum calcium and phosphate levels, thereby fostering normal excitability of nerves and muscles.

The regulation of PTH release depends upon a feedback relationship between the level of serum calcium and the level of PTH in the blood (see Fig. 12–8, p. 203). Note that, when serum calcium is elevated, PTH secretion decreases, resulting in the decreased mobilization of calcium ions from bone and a lowering of the serum calcium. Conversely, when serum calcium levels are low, PTH secretion increases, resulting in increased mobilization of calcium from bone and an increase in the level of serum calcium.

Disorders of the Parathyroid Glands and Their Diagnosis

There are two major disorders of the parathyroid glands. The parathyroid glands may secrete *too much hormone* (hyperparathyroidism), or they may secrete *too little hormone* (hypoparathyroidism). *Hyperparathyroidism* is characterized by the following findings:

Increased bone resorption
Elevated serum calcium levels
Depressed serum phosphate levels
Hypercalciuria and hyperphosphaturia
Decreased neuromuscular irritability

Conversely *hypoparathyroidism* has the following characteristics:

Decreased bone resorption
Depressed serum calcium levels
Elevated serum phosphate levels
Hypocaliuria and hypophosphaturia
Increased neuromuscular activity which may progress to tetany.

Laboratory studies of parathyroid function and malfunction include the following: total serum calcium, qualitative urinary calcium (Sulkowitch test), quantitative urinary calcium, serum phosphorus, serum alkaline phosphatase, and radioimmunoassay of parathormone. In Table 73–4, these tests are briefly characterized and compared.

HYPERSECRETION OF THE PARATHYROID GLANDS (HYPERPARATHYROIDISM)

Hyperparathyroidism is a disorder caused by *overactivity* of one or more of the parathyroid glands. It is classified as either primary or secondary. *Primary* hyperparathyroidism is a rare, potentially curable condition which develops within the parathyroid glands themselves. Ninety per cent of cases of primary hyperparathyroidism arise from a *single adenoma* (a benign epithelial tumor composed of glandular tissue), 8 per cent of cases result from *hyperplasia* and *hypertrophy* of the four glands, while 2 per cent develop from *carcinoma* of a single gland.[73] *Secondary* hyperparathyroidism is caused by a *compensatory oversecretion* of PTH in response to the hypocalcemia caused by chronic renal disease, rickets, osteomalacia, and acromegaly. Hyperparathyroidism is also associated with the ectopic secretion of parathormone by cancerous tumors located in the lungs, kidneys, and so forth.

Pathophysiology and Symptoms. The normal function of PTH is to control and increase bone resorption, thereby maintaining the proper balance of calcium and phosphorus ions within the blood. What happens then when PTH secretion is excessive? Excessive circulating PTH creates the following pathologic changes:

▶*Bone damage:* Oversecretion of PTH causes excessive *osteoclast* growth and activity within the bones. Osteoclasts are large multinuclear cells which are active in promoting resorption of bone. Because of

TABLE 73–4. DIAGNOSTIC TESTS OF PARATHYROID FUNCTION: PURPOSE, PROCEDURE, NORMAL RANGE, AND INTERPRETATION OF ABNORMAL FINDINGS

Test	Purpose	Procedure	Normal Range	Interpretation of Abnormal Findings	Remarks
Total serum calcium	Measures amount of ionized and nonionized calcium in serum.	Venous blood to laboratory.	4.8 to 5.2 mEq./liter or 8–11 mg./100 ml.	Elevated in hyperparathyroidism; depressed in hypoparathyroidism, tetany, rickets, nephrosis, and osteomalacia.	Normally 50% of total serum calcium is ionized. Amount of ionized calcium available decreases in alkalosis.
Qualitative urinary calcium (Sulkowitch test)	Measures roughly amount of calcium in urine. Used as a quick method for diagnosing if tetany is due to hypoparathyroidism.	Collect urine specimen and send to laboratory.	Fine white precipitate should form when Sulkowitch reagent is added to urine specimen.	Absence or decreased density of precipitate indicates low serum calcium and hypoparathyroidism.	Drugs which elevate serum calcium levels include vitamin D, parathyroid injection, and dihydrotachysterol.
Quantitative urinary calcium (calcium deprivation test)	Measures exact amount of calcium in a 24-hour urine specimen.	24-hour urine specimen collected and sent to laboratory	75–175 mg. of calcium per 24 hours.	Elevated in hyperparathyroidism; depressed in hypoparathyroidism.	Foods high in calcium include milk, cheese, molasses, turnip greens, and dandelion greens.
Serum phosphorus	Measures amount of inorganic phosphorus in the serum.	Venous blood to laboratory.	1.3 to 1.75 mEq./liter (2.5 to 4.5 mg./100 ml.) in adults.	Elevated in hypoparathyroidism, uremia, and alkalosis; depressed in hyperparathyroidism, rickets, and osteomalacia.	There is an inverse relationship between serum calcium and serum phosphorus.
Serum alkaline phosphatase	Measures amount of alkaline phosphatase in serum. Aids in diagnosing bone and liver disorders.	Venous blood to laboratory.	2.0–5.0 Bodansky units.	Elevated in hyperparathyroidism, osteomalacia, rickets, healing fractures, pregnancy, and following ingestion of large amounts of vitamin D.	Alkaline phosphatase is an enzyme normally present in small amounts in serum. Some drugs causing false elevations of alkaline phosphatase levels include allopurinol, some androgens, colchicine, erythromycin, methyldopa, some oral contraceptives, procainamide, and tolbutamide.
PTH radioimmunoassay test	Measures level of PTH in serum.	Venous blood to laboratory.	Depends on serum calcium concentration.	High concentrations indicate hyperparathyroidism.	When evaluated together with the serum calcium, this is the most specific test for hyperparathyroidism.

increased bone resorption, calcium drains from the bones into the blood, causing *hypercalcemia.* Thus the bones suffer *demineralization* due to calcium loss. In time, the bones may become so fragile that they break easily with even mild trauma, causing pathologic fractures. Also, as the uncontrolled osteoclast proliferation continues, the skeleton may develop cystic lesions; without treatment of hyperparathyroidism and without replacement of calcium losses through diet and medication, the patient eventually develops a severe bone disease called *osteitis fibrosa cystica* (von Recklinghausen's disease of bone).

▶*Hypercalcemia:* An increased serum calcium level is the consequence of bone resorption due to excessive PTH secretion. Hypercalcemia eventually results in *hypercalciuria* (spillage of excess calcium into the urine). Also, because of the high serum calcium levels, calcium may precipitate as calcium phosphate in the lungs, muscles, heart, and eyes. In addition, hypercalcemia causes gastric ulcers, possibly because excess serum calcium acts to increase gastric secretions.

▶*Kidney damage:* Excessive parathormone levels cause hyperphosphaturia. As serum calcium continues to rise in hyperparathyroidism excessive amounts of both phosphorus and calcium are excreted and lost from the body. Because high amounts of both calcium and phosphate are being excreted by the renal system, calcium phosphate may be deposited within the renal tubules, causing a kidney condition called *nephrocalcinosis.* Also, *kidney stones* composed of calcium phosphate are found in the urine of patients with primary hyperparathyroidism. Stones develop because calcium salts are quite insoluble in urine.

Patients with hyperparathyroidism may be asymptomatic, with the exception of hypercalcemia, as demonstrated by laboratory tests. Other patients suffer from a myriad of symptoms arising from skeletal damage, renal involvement, and hypercalcemia.

Manifestations of *bone disease* range from backache, joint pain, and bone pain to pathologic fractures of the spine, ribs, and long bones. In longstanding cases, deformities and bending of the bones due to osteitis fibrosa cystica develop.

Symptoms of *renal* involvement include polyuria and polydipsia; the appearance of sand, gravel, or stones within the urine; azotemia; and hypertension due to renal damage. Without treatment, renal insufficiency may progress to fatal renal hypertension and uremia.

Hypercalcemia mainly produces gastrointestinal tract symptoms, e.g., thirst, nausea, anorexia, constipation, ileus, and abdominal pain. Often patients have a history of peptic ulcer or gastrointestinal bleeding. Psychiatric symptoms (listlessness, depression, paranoia) are also associated with high levels of serum calcium. Finally, calcium may form calcifications within the eyes, impairing vision.

The diagnosis of hyperparathyroidism mainly rests upon laboratory and x-ray findings. Serum calcium is elevated, while serum phosphate is depressed; urine calcium and phosphate are both high. In addition, alkaline phosphatase is elevated among the 25 per cent of patients who have associated bone disease. Also, patients with skeletal damage have the following characteristic x-ray findings: diffuse demineralization of bones, bone cysts, subperiosteal bone resorption, and loss of the lamina dura surrounding the teeth.

Clinical Care. Primary hyperparathyroidism is always treated *surgically:* the parathyroid tumors which are causing hypersecretion of parathormone are located and removed. Usually only the diseased parathyroid glands are resected. However, if all four glands are hyperplastic, three and a half glands are removed. Fortunately one half of a parathyroid gland is usually sufficient to maintain normal levels of circulating parathormone.

The goals of *preoperative care* for hyperparathyroid patients undergoing surgery are (a) to reduce hypercalcemia, (b) to prevent further renal damage, and (c) to treat and prevent complications, e.g., pathologic fractures, peptic ulcers, and so on. Actions which promote these goals include the following:

▶*Force fluids* to at least 3000 ml. per day. Dehydration is dangerous for these patients, because it both increases the serum calcium level and promotes the formation of renal stones. Encourage the patient to drink cranberry juice and prune juice, because these acid-ash fruit juices make the urine more acidic. Higher urinary acidity helps prevent renal stone formation, because calcium is more soluble in an acid urine than in an alkaline urine.

▶*Phosphate or sodium phytate* (Rencal) may be ordered to lower reabsorption of calcium by the gastrointestinal tract. Also the hormone *calcitonin* is being experimentally used in some cases to lower serum calcium. The benefits of calcitonin therapy are still debatable.

▶Encourage a *low-calcium diet* to correct hypercalcemia. Explain to the patient that the omission of milk and milk products from the menu may help alleviate some of the distressing gastrointestinal symptoms. If the patient suffers from peptic ulcers, he or she will need to take antacids.

▶*Prevent constipation* and *fecal impaction* resulting from hypercalcemia. Help the patient to be as active as possible, depending upon the extent of the bone disease. If constipation continues despite these measures, obtain an order for a stool softener or laxative.

▶If the patient has kidney stones, *strain all urine* to detect gravel and stones. Save any specimens of abnormal urine for the physician to examine. Also observe the urine for blood and the patient for renal colic (see Unit XIII).

▶ *Protect the patient from accidents.* If bone involvement exists, the patient may develop pathologic fractures from even small bumps or minor falls. Keep the patient's bed in the low position and use siderails. If the patient is weak or has joint or skeletal disease, always assist in ambulation.

Individuals with hypercalcemia are hypersensitive to digitalis and may quickly develop toxic symptoms.

During the *postoperative* period, new problems arise, some of which are the reverse of those found preoperatively. During the *immediate* postoperative period, nursing care is similar to that following thyroidectomy; i.e., observe the patient carefully for hemorrhage, airway obstruction, injury to the recurrent laryngeal nerve, tetany, and so forth. In addition, watch the patient for signs of *hormonal imbalance.*

Mild tetany due to the drop in serum calcium is *expected* following removal of parathyroid tissue (see Chapter 12). Typically, the uncomfortable tingling of the hands and around the mouth which follows parathyroid resection usually disappears without problem. However, if tetany persists or is severe, calcium gluconate is administered IV to relieve symptoms.

Patients with *bone disease* require additional therapy following surgery. Because removal of the parathyroid glands reduces bone resorption and because bone rebuilding proceeds at a rapid rate, the patient can develop the "hungry bones" syndrome. This syndrome is characterized by hypocalcemia and severe tetany resulting from the rapid utilization of calcium by the bones. To prevent low serum calcium levels due to bone recalcification, the patient should eat foods high in calcium. Tetany is treated with injections of calcium gluconate. To maintain adequate calcium levels, oral calcium preparations are usually given for months until the skeletal tissues have been rebuilt. Finally, patients are usually encouraged to ambulate as soon as possible following surgery because weight-bearing speeds the recalcification process.

Prognosis. If hyperparathyroidism is surgically treated early in its course, the chance for total recovery is good. Bone pain may disappear within three days following removal of parathyroid tissue, and bone lesions may heal completely. Unfortunately, serious renal disease may not be reversible with surgery.

HYPOSECRETION OF THE PARATHYROID GLANDS (HYPOPARATHYROIDISM)

Hyposecretion of the parathyroid glands produces a syndrome which is opposite that of hyperparathyroidism, thus serum calcium levels are abnormally low, serum phosphate levels are abnormally high, and pronounced neuromuscular irritability (tetany) develops.

The causes of hypoparathyroidism are either iatrogenic or idiopathic. *Iatrogenic causes* of hypoparathyroidism include (a) accidental removal of the parathyroid glands during thyroidectomy, (b) infarction of the parathyroid glands resulting from an inadequate blood supply to the glands during surgery, and (c) strangulation of one or more of the glands by postoperative scar tissue. *Idiopathic* hypoparathyroidism (like myxedema, Graves' disease, and Hashimoto's thyroiditis) may possibly be an *autoimmune* disorder with a genetic basis. This type of hypoparathyroidism is far less common than the post-thyroidectomy form. It strikes children nine times as frequently as adults, and it affects twice as many women as men.

Pathophysiology and Symptoms. As stated before, parathormone normally acts to increase bone resorption, which in turn maintains proper serum calcium levels. The hormone also regulates phosphate clearance by the renal tubules, thereby maintaining the correct inverse balance between serum calcium and serum phosphate. Consequently, when parathyroid secretion is reduced, bone resorption slows, serum calcium levels fall, somewhat paradoxically, calcifications form in varied organs (e.g., eyes, basal ganglia), and severe neuromuscular irritability develops. Also without sufficient PTH fewer phosphorus ions are secreted by the distal tubules of the kidney, renal excretion of phosphate decreases, and serum phosphate levels rise.

The *symptoms* of hypoparathyroidism are mainly caused by low serum calcium levels. *Acute hypoparathyroidism* (caused by accidental damage to parathyroid tissues during thyroidectomy) is characterized by greatly increased neuromuscular irritability, resulting in tetany. You recall from Unit V that patients with tetany experience painful muscle spasm, irritability, grimacing, tingling of fingers, laryngospasm, and arrhythmias. Chvostek's sign (signifying hyperirritability of the facial nerve) and Trousseau's sign (carpal spasms of the fingers and hands following application of a pressure cuff to the arm) are present. In some cases, tetany is so severe that tracheostomy is required to correct acute respiratory obstruction due to laryngospasm.

Chronic hypoparathyroidism (which is usually idiopathic in nature) causes lethargy; thin, patchy hair; brittle nails; dry, scaly skin; and personality changes. Ectopic calcification may appear in the eyes and basal ganglia; thus, the patient may develop cataracts and permanent brain damage accompanied by psychosis or convulsions. In addition, severe persistent hypocalcemia adversely affects the heart, causing arrhythmias and eventual heart failure. When hypoparathyroidism develops in infancy or early childhood, the patient may suffer from malformed teeth, poor physical growth and development, and mental retardation.

The symptoms of hypoparathyroidism are always more severe in patients who have an *elevated serum pH* (alkalosis) due to any cause (e.g., ingesting antacids, hyperventilating from emotional causes). Symptoms worsen because when the pH of the blood rises, the amount of ionized calcium drops, eventhough total serum calcium remains the same. With less ionized calcium available to the body, the symptoms resulting from hypocalcemia become more severe until the alkalosis is corrected.

The *diagnosis* of hypoparathyroidism is based upon the following:

- ▶ Presence of a positive Chvostek's sign and Trousseau's sign
- ▶ Laboratory findings of low serum calcium, high serum phosphate, and a low or absent urinary calcium.
- ▶ X-ray studies which show calcifications of the basal ganglia.
- ▶ Eye examinations which may reveal the early development of cataracts due to the formation of calcifications within the eyes.

Clinical Care in Acute Hypoparathyroidism. Acute hypoparathyroidism (with its major manifestation of acute tetany) is a *life-threatening disorder*. The goals of *emergency* care are (1) to elevate serum calcium levels as rapidly as possible, (2) to prevent or treat convulsions, and (3) to control laryngeal spasm and consequent respiratory obstruction.

First of all, to quickly elevate serum calcium levels, the patient is given 10 per cent calcium gluconate solution in an intravenous infusion (see Chapter 12). While administering calcium gluconate, instruct the patient to inhale his or her own carbon dioxide by breathing into a paper bag. The inhaled carbon dioxide causes a mild respiratory acidosis which serves to elevate the amount of *ionized* calcium in the blood.

> *Always be prepared for the possibility that the patient with tetany may suffer laryngeal spasm and respiratory obstruction. Always have an* endotracheal tube *and* tracheostomy set *close at hand when caring for patients with acute tetany.*

Once the condition has stabilized and the dangers of tetany have passed, the patient is given *oral* calcium salts and vitamin D in order to maintain normal serum calcium levels.

Clinical Care in Chronic Hypoparathyroidism. The goal of maintenance therapy for patients with chronic hypoparathyroidism is to restore the serum calcium level to normal concentrations. To achieve this goal, the following measures are taken:

▶ Instruct the patient to eat a diet high in calcium but low in phosphorus; remind the patient to omit cheese and milk products from the diet because these nutrients have a high phosphorus content.

▶ Administer *oral calcium salts* (either calcium gluconate, calcium lactate, or calcium chloride) as ordered. Calcium supplements may be obtained in either tablet or solution form, depending upon the patient's preference. Oral calcium administration is usually discontinued if the patient responds successfully to the vitamin D preparations described below.

▶ Administer prescribed *vitamin D* preparations. You recall from Chapter 12 that the absorption of calcium is dependent upon the presence of vitamin D. Indeed, vitamin D is capable of raising blood calcium levels to normal. Commercially available forms of vitamin D include calciferol (vitamin D_2), cholecalciferol (vitamin D_3), and dihydrotachysterol (Hytakerol). Although calciferol is a more reliable and less expensive drug than Hytakerol, all three forms of vitamin D are effective in correcting hypocalcemia. They are all obtainable as either tablets or oily liquids. Also all forms are slowly assimilated by the body; therefore, warn the patient that it may take a week or longer for symptoms to improve.

▶ Emphasize to the patient the importance of *lifelong* follow-up medical care. Instruct the patient to have the serum calcium level checked by a physician at least three times a year — *every year.* Normal blood serum calcium levels must be maintained to prevent complications. If either hypercalcemia or hypocalcemia develop, the doctor will have to adjust the patient's treatment regimen to correct the imbalance.

Prognosis. The patient may fully recover from the effects of hypoparathyroidism if the condition is diagnosed *early*, before the advent of serious complications. Unfortunately, cataracts and brain calcifications, once formed, are irreversible.

CHAPTER 74

NURSING PATIENTS WITH DISORDERS OF THE ADRENAL AND PITUITARY GLANDS

THE ADRENAL GLANDS

Normal Anatomy and Physiology

The adrenal glands (or suprarenal glands) are two small but vital endocrine structures which cap the top of the kidneys. Each adrenal gland is composed of two distinct structures, each with its own function, which are merged into one powerful glandular organ. The inner core of the adrenal gland is called the *adrenal medulla* while the outer shell of the gland is called the *adrenal cortex.* Although both structures contribute to the individual's survival and well-being, only the adrenal cortex is essential for life.

The Adrenal Medulla. The adrenal medulla, which is a part of the sympathetic nervous system (sometimes called the sympathoadrenal system), releases two potent hormones called epinephrine and norepinephrine. The secretion of these two *catecholamines* is controlled by the brain, especially from regions of the hypothalamus. (Catecholamines are compounds composed of a catechol and an amine.) The effects of epinephrine and norepinephrine upon the body are similar to those produced by activation of the sympathetic nervous system, in which norepinephrine is the major neurotransmitter; for this reason they are called "sympathomimetic agents." Like the sympathetic nervous system, these medullary hormones enable threatened individuals to either fight or flee when faced with danger.

The primary actions of *epinephrine* during situations of stress are to convert glycogen within the liver into glucose, and to increase cardiac output. It is the release of epinephrine which produces the cold sweat, pounding heart, deep rapid breathing, and wide-eyed, "keyed up" alertness which we all experience in times of emergency.

The primary action of norepinephrine is to produce extensive *vascular constriction,* thereby causing a marked rise in blood pressure. Note, however, in Table 74–1 that norepinephrine has several of the same general effects upon the body as epinephrine, e.g., it dilates the pupils and inhibits the gastrointestinal tract.

Overactivity of the adrenal medulla can be life-threatening. Overactivity is usually caused by a catecholamine-producing tumor called a *pheochromocytoma*, which is usually (but not always) found in or near the adrenal gland. Pheochromocytomas produce marked hypertension, hypermetabolism, and hyperglycemia owing to the oversecretion of epinephrine and norepinephrine. This condition can usually be cured by surgical removal of the tumors.

While overactivity of the adrenal medulla is dangerous, *underactivity* or loss of this gland rarely causes problems. As implied earlier, the adrenal medulla is *not* an essential structure. Should the medulla be destroyed by disease or surgically removed, its loss is compensated for by the sympathetic nervous system.

The Adrenal Cortex. The adrenal cortex, unlike the adrenal medulla, is *essential for survival.* If this vital structure is removed or destroyed, death follows within a few days unless the adrenal cortical hormones are replaced.

The adrenal cortex releases numerous steroid hormones called *corticoids. Steroids* are molecules with a nucleus composed of four interlocking rings containing carbon atoms. Three of the rings hold six carbon atoms apiece, while the fourth ring contains five.

Corticoids may be classified into three groups according to their specific functions: thus one group regulates sodium and electrolyte balance; the second group regulates carbohydrate, fat, and protein metabolism; while the third group is linked with sexual characteristics. As Boyd helpfully reminds us:

> For those of weak memory or mentality, the three functions [of the hormones of the adrenal cortex] may be represented by the letter S: salt, sugar, and

sex. To the more sophisticated they are the mineralocorticoids, the glucocorticoids and the androgens (masculinizing hormones).[13a]

MINERALOCORTICOIDS. The mineralocorticoids (which include aldosterone, desoxycorticosterone, and corticosterone) regulate electrolyte balance by promoting sodium retention, secondary water retention, and potassium excretion. The principal mineralocorticoid is *aldosterone,* which was discussed more fully in Chapter 12. You will recall that the major functions of aldosterone are to conserve sodium and to maintain the blood and extracellular fluid volume, thereby sustaining normal blood pressure and cardiac output. When the mineralocorticoids are deficient (as in Addison's disease), the patient suffers from hyperkalemia, hypotension, decreased cardiac output, and (in acute cases) severe shock. On the other hand, *excessively high levels* of mineralocorticoids (hyperaldosteronism) result in hypertension due to sodium and water retention and hypokalemia.

GLUCOCORTICOIDS. The glucocorticoids derive their name from the fact that they act to regulate blood sugar by conserving body glucose and promoting gluconeogenesis. The major steroids composing the group are cortisol (the principal glucocorticoid), cortisone, and corticosterone, the latter being also a mineralocorticoid. Release of these potent hormones has the following effects upon the body:

▶ *Glucose metabolism:* Protein and fat molecules are

TABLE 74–1. COMPARATIVE EFFECTS OF EPINEPHRINE AND NOREPINEPHRINE

Epinephrine	Norepinephrine
Cardiovascular System	
Constricts superficial blood vessels. In small doses dilates muscle, brain, and coronary vessels, thus shunting blood supply to organs essential for "flight or fight"	Constricts all blood vessels, especially peripherally, causing greatly increased peripheral resistance
Raises blood pressure	Markedly hypertensive
Increases cardiac output	Tends to decrease cardiac output because of increased peripheral resistance
Increases pulse greatly	Increases the pulse, but not greatly
Constricts the spleen, shunting stored red blood cells into general circulation	
Increases coagulability of the blood	
Respiratory System	
Increases rate and depth of respirations	
Dilates bronchi	
Nervous System	
Stimulates the central nervous system, increasing alertness and producing a feeling of fright, excitation, and impending doom	
Dilates the pupil	Dilates the pupil
Inhibits the gastrointestinal tract	Inhibits the gastrointestinal tract
Metabolism	
Increases the nonesterified fatty acid level of the blood	Increases the nonesterified fatty acid level of the blood
Promotes the conversion of glycogen to glucose	
Increases body metabolism	Increases body metabolism slightly

From Spencer, R. T.: *Patient Care in Endocrine Problems.* Philadelphia, W. B. Saunders Company, 1973, p. 52.

converted within the liver to glucose (gluconeogenesis), which raises the blood sugar; for this reason, the glucocorticoids are said to have an "anti-insulin" effect. Indeed, excessive glucocorticoid secretion can produce diabetes mellitus.

▶ *Protein metabolism:* Protein tissue catabolism increases. Amino acids are transported into the extracellular fluid and then to the liver where they are converted to glucose. Excessive secretion of the glucocorticosteroids causes tissue wasting.

▶ *Fluid and electrolyte balance:* Sodium retention, secondary water retention, and potassium excretion all increase. Overabundance of glucocorticoid secretion results in hypervolemia and hypertension due to sodium and water retention. Note that these effects of the glucocorticoids are similar to those of the mineralocorticoids.

▶ *Inflammation and immunity:* The glucocorticoids suppress both the normal inflammatory response to tissue injury and the protective immune response to invasion by infectious agents. As you recall from Unit III, Chapter 5, Selye calls the glucocorticoids *anti-inflammatory corticoids* (A.C.'s) because he evidently believes that the suppression of inflammation as a response to stress is the glucocorticoid's major role. In some cases, the suppression of inflammation can be beneficial. For example, patients with arthritis (inflammation of the joints) obtain relief from severe pain with cortisone injections. On the other hand, too much cortisone or other glucocorticoid impedes healing, decreases antibody formation, lowers the numbers of circulating eosinophils and lymphocytes, and lowers resistance to infection.

▶ *Stress:* Resistance and adjustment to stress of all kinds is dependent upon the presence of glucocorticoids. Selye points out that during the "alarm reaction" to stress (stage 1 of the General Adaptation Syndrome) large amounts of both adrenal and glucocorticoids are released into the blood stream. These hormones, if secreted in sufficient amounts, enable the individual to cope with stress provided the stress is not overwhelming, e.g., severe burns over the majority of the body. Conversely, insufficient production of glucocorticoids (as seen in Addison's disease) *decreases* resistance to stress; such patients may die in profound shock following relatively minor traumas unless they quickly receive an injection of glucocorticoid.

Sex Hormones. The adrenal cortex secretes very small quantities of *androgens* (masculinizing hormones) and *estrogens* (female sex hormones). Normally, adrenal secretion of sex hormones is less than the large amounts of androgens and estrogens secreted by the gonads. However, when production of sex hormones by the adrenal glands is excessive, symptoms result. For example, excessive release of androgens causes virilism, while excessive release of estrogens causes gynecomastia and sodium and water retention (see discussion later in this chapter).

Disorders of the Adrenal Medulla

Two important tumors occur in the adrenal medulla: (1) *pheochromocytoma* — a tumor which results in hyperactivity of the gland, and (2) *neuroblastoma* — a malignant tumor which is a major cause of death in children.*

Pheochromocytoma. The pheochromocytoma is a small tumor (usually less than 200 Gm.) which is composed of chromaffin cells. These cells are named "chromaffin" cells because they stain a dark color with chromium salts. In 80–90 per cent of cases, pheochromocytomas arise within the adrenal medulla; occasionally, however, they develop from the chromaffin tissues forming the sympathetic paraganglia (Fig. 74–1).

These tumors are typically benign; less than 5 per cent of pheochromocytomas are malignant. However, pheochromocytomas can produce severe symptoms and even death owing to the excessive amounts of epinephrine and norepinephrine which they secrete. Fortunately, when pheochromocytomas are discovered early in their development, they are usually curable.

In some cases pheochromocytomas apparently have a hereditary basis. Also, in a small percentage of cases, these tumors appear in association with neuroectodermal diseases and with medullary cancer of the thyroid gland. Two events which apparently precipitate the clinical appearance of pheochromocytoma are pregnancy and stress.

Bases of Symptoms. Symptoms experienced by the patient with pheochromocytoma result from the excessive secretion of epinephrine and norepinephrine by the tumor. The main manifestation of pheochromocytoma is *hypertension*, which may be persistent, fluctuating, intermittent, or paroxysmal in nature. Typically patients suffer from attacks in which they experience not only high blood pressure accompanied by a pounding headache, but numerous other manifestations of sympathetic overactivity; e.g., sweating, apprehension, palpitations, nausea, and vomiting. Moreover, the release of catecholamines results in the conversion of glycogen into glucose within the liver; consequently hyperglycemia and glycosuria may appear during attacks. Such manifestations may develop spontaneously, or they may be precipitated by emotional stress, physical exertion, or change in body position.

When attacks are acute, the patient appears to

*For a description of neuroblastoma, consult a pediatrics textbook.

be in a shocklike state due to the excessive epinephrine released; i.e., diaphoresis is profuse, the pupils are greatly dilated, and the extremities are cold. Also, the patient may develop a cerebral vascular accident or sudden blindness as a result of severe hypertension. Without early treatment (see Chap. 95) permanent cardiovascular damage can develop, and death may follow cerebral hemorrhage or cardiac failure.

DIAGNOSIS. The clinical picture of the patient with pheochromocytoma resembles that of several other disorders; e.g., diabetes mellitus (elevated blood sugar and glycosuria), essential hypertension (elevated blood pressure, headaches), hyperthyroidism (increased metabolic rate, diaphoresis, agitation, rapid pulse, emotional outbursts), and psychoneurosis (emotional instability). Because pheochromocytoma is potentially curable, the importance of early and accurate diagnosis cannot be stressed enough. Current methods of diagnosis include the following:

- *History and physical examination:* The patient may complain that he has suffered attacks of symptoms (such as those just described) for weeks, months, or even years. Upon examination, it may be noted that the patient's blood pressure sharply rises whenever he changes position, exerts himself, or becomes emotionally upset. Also, in long-standing cases, the patient may already have developed the complications of hypertension: e.g., visual disturbances, symptoms of heart disease (dyspnea, exhaustion, edema), and manifestations of kidney damage (albuminuria, proteinuria, and an increased blood urea nitrogen).

- *Chemical tests (hormonal assays):* Chemical tests have replaced the more dangerous and inaccurate pharmacologic tests in the diagnosis of pheochromocytoma. The two hormonal assay tests available are (1) assay of urinary catecholamines and their metabolites (metanephrines and VMA), and (2) concentrations of plasma catecholamines.

  Assays of catecholamines may be performed on a single voided urine specimen, on a 2- to 4-hour specimen, and on a 24-hour urine specimen. The normal range of urinary catecholamines is up to 14 μg./100 ml. of urine. In pheochromocytoma, catecholamine levels are elevated.

  Assays of urinary VMA (vanillylmandelic acid) levels are performed on 24-hour urine specimens only. Prior to testing, advise the patient to avoid chocolate, tea, vanilla, and all fruits for at least 2 days before urine collection begins. Also remind the patient not to take any drugs for 3 days prior to testing. Finally, when collecting urine for 24-hour hormonal assays of VMA or other hormones, proceed with care or test results will be inaccurate. Rules to remember when collecting these specimens are:

  1. Ask laboratory personnel how urine is to be preserved over the 24-hour period (i.e., refrigeration, use of a special collecting bottle, or addition of hydrochloric acid to the collecting prior to beginning the test).
  2. Accurately time collections; have patient begin test with an empty bladder and also empty the bladder just at the end of the test.
  3. Remind the patient to void *before* defecating so that urine is not contaminated by feces.

  Normally, the amount of VMA is under 7 mg./24 hours. Urinary VMA is elevated in pheochromocytoma.

- *Direct assay of catecholamines in the blood:* The normal range of the catecholamines in the blood is as follows:

  Epinephrine, 0.02–0.2 μg./ml.
  Norepinephrine, 0.1–0.5 μg./ml.

  Blood catecholamine levels increase in pheochromocytoma.

- *X-ray examinations:* Presence of an adrenal medullary tumor can often be confirmed by various x-ray techniques; e.g., arteriography, intravenous urogram, venography, retroperitoneal pneumography, and computerized axial tomography (CAT scan).

- *Miscellaneous nonspecific laboratory tests:* In the presence of pheochromocytoma, the basal metabolic rate is elevated, blood sugar is elevated, and glycosuria usually appears.

  A pheochromocytoma noted radiologically is pictured in Figure 74–1.

CLINICAL CARE. There is only one form of treatment for pheochromocytoma — *surgical excision of the tumor.* While surgery may completely cure the patient (provided the growth is discovered before cardiovascular damage becomes permanent), the operation is not without its dangers. Sjoerdsma warns that there are two serious hazards. "First, excessive discharge of pressor hormones may occur during induction of anesthesia or during manipulation of the tumor leading to extreme rises in blood pressure and *cardiac* arrhythmias. Second, following resection, the blood pressure may fall precipitously to shock levels."[115a]

During the *preoperative* period, the goal is to prevent further attacks of acute paroxysmal hypertension, thereby decreasing the risk of further damaging the cardiovascular system. Important general measures include (a) promotion of rest and relief from emotional tension; (b) sedation; (c) high vitamin, mineral, and caloric diet; (d) the omission of such stimulating beverages as coffee and tea; and (e) frequent monitoring of vital signs. In most cases, the doctor will order the administration of adrenergic blocking drugs, such as phenoxybenzamine or propranolol.

Following surgery, the patient enters a critical period ranging from 24 to 48 hours, during which time constant nursing observation and care is needed. During the *immediate postoperative period,* observe the patient closely for signs of *shock* and *hemorrhage.* Following removal of the tumor, profound shock may develop because catecholamine blood levels drop dramatically; hypotension may persist for 24 to 48 hours postoperatively. Also hemorrhage can occur because the adrenal glands are highly vascular organs.

To combat postoperative shock, take the following actions:

- Give intravenous fluids as ordered to maintain the blood volume and combat shock. Blood, plasma, dextran, and glucose in water are all employed for this purpose.
- Administer pressors as ordered intravenously at a rate sufficient to maintain the patient's blood pressure within a safe range. Check the patient's blood pressure as frequently as is necessary to regulate the drug.
- Carefully measure the patient's hourly urinary output. If the patient excretes less than 15 ml. in one half hour or 30 ml. in an hour, notify the physician. Oliguria may signify the development of profound shock and consequent renal shutdown.
- Observe the patient for signs of hemorrhage. Check the dressing every half hour for bloody drainage. If the patient is bleeding internally, he may develop an abdominal hematoma with resultant paralytic ileus. Symptoms of paralytic ileus include abdominal pain, distention, severe nausea, and vomiting.
- When administering medication for incisional pain, monitor the patient's blood pressure frequently. Remember that narcotics, particularly Demerol, produce hypotension as a side effect.
- If cortical tissue was resected during surgery, observe the patient closely for signs of adrenal cortical insufficiency (see below). If *both* adrenals have been removed, the patient must take corticosteroids for life.

Once the critical immediate postoperative period is over, the majority of patients pass through an uneventful convalescence. Patients who will be taking corticosteroids upon discharge will need instruction concerning their administration and side effects (see p. 1606).

Disorders of the Adrenal Cortex

The major disorders of the adrenal cortex are characterized by either glandular hypofunction or hyperfunction. Underactivity of the adrenal cortex *(hypocorticism)* results in a deficiency of glucocorticoids, mineralocorticoids, and adrenal androgens, while overactivity *(hypercorticism)* results in excessive production of the corticosteroids. The majority of conditions arise because of the excessive secretion of mainly one of the three classes of cortical hormones.

Adrenal Cortical Hypofunction (Hypocorticism. Hypofunction of the adrenal cortex is usually caused by a disorder originating within the adrenal gland itself (primarily adrenal cortical insufficiency). However, in other cases, adrenocortical insufficiency develops *secondary* to hypopituitarism, or prolonged administration of corticosteroids, (secondary adrenocortical insufficiency). Primary adrenocortical insufficiency may be either chronic or acute.

Chronic Primary Adrenocortical Insufficiency (Addison's Disease)

Incidence and etiology. Chronic primary adrenocortical insufficiency was named Addison's disease in honor of Thomas Addison who first described this condition more than a hundred years ago. A clinically rare disorder, Addison's disease strikes only four out of every 100,000 persons.

The causative factors in Addison's disease have changed in recent years. At one time, the

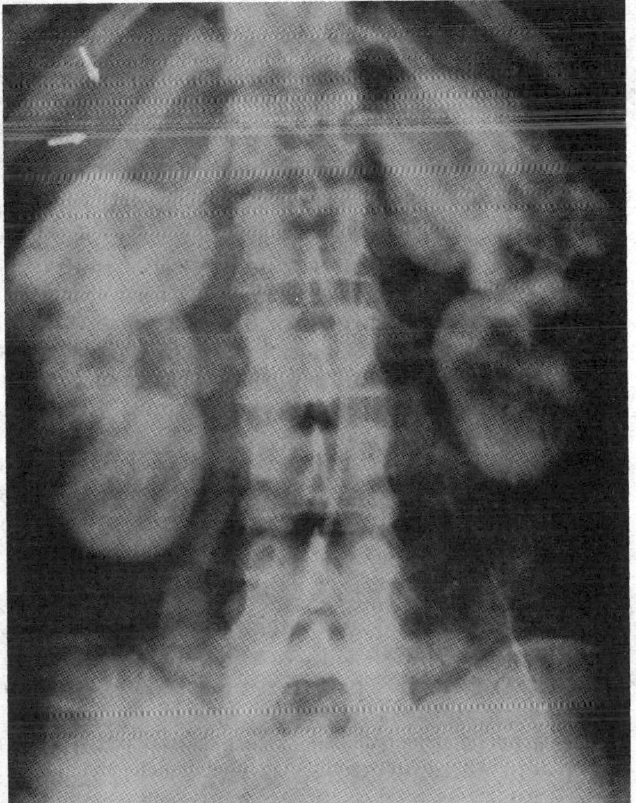

Figure 74–1. Mass above the right kidney (arrows) due to hemorrhagic pheochromocytoma. (From Bissada, N. K.: Surgical diseases of the adrenal gland. *American Family Physician,* 15:130, June 1977.)

majority of cases developed as a complication of chronic tuberculosis. Today, less than half of cases are caused by tuberculosis, and approximately 70 per cent of cases are considered *idiopathic* in origin. However, since 50 to 67 per cent of patients with idiopathic Addison's disease have circulating autoantibodies which react specifically against adrenal tissues, it is possible that this condition may have an *autoimmune* basis. Also, a few cases of Addison's disease are caused by neoplasm, amyloidosis, and systemic fungal infections.

All age groups and both sexes are susceptible to adrenal insufficiency.

Bases of symptoms. As stated earlier, the adrenal cortex is essential to life. Untreated Addison's disease is ultimately fatal because it destroys the adrenal cortex, thereby causing severe deficiencies of vital adrenocortical hormones. As a result of this condition, the adrenal glands become shrunken and contracted. Although the adrenal medulla continues to function normally, the cortex becomes a mass of fibrous nonfunctioning scar tissue. Finally, the cortex no longer produces adequate amounts of aldosterone, cortisol, and androgens, and symptoms appear.

Aldosterone deficiency causes numerous *fluid and electrolyte* imbalances. Aldosterone *normally* promotes the conservation of sodium (and consequently water) and the excretion of potassium. When aldosterone is deficient, *sodium excretion increases,* which results in the following unfortunate chain of events: (a) water excretion increases, (b) extracellular fluid volume becomes depleted (dehydration), (c) hypotension develops, (d) cardiac output decreases, and (e) the heart becomes smaller owing to its diminished work load. Eventually hypotension may become so severe and heart action so weak that the patient dies in circulatory collapse and shock. Secondly, while excessive sodium ions are being excreted, excessive potassium ions are being retained in the body. Potassium levels of more than 7 mEq./liter result in arrhythmias and possibly cardiac standstill.

Glucocorticoid deficiencies cause widespread *metabolic disturbances.* Remember that the glucocorticoids promote gluconeogenesis (the conversion of fat and proteins into glucose within the liver) and are thus said to have an "anti-insulin" effect. Consequently, when glucocorticoids are deficient, gluconeogenesis decreases with resultant *hypoglycemia* and liver glycogen deficiency. The patient grows weak and exhausted and suffers from anorexia, weight loss, nausea, and vomiting. Secondly, *emotional disturbances* develop, ranging from mild neurotic symptoms to deep depression. In addition, *resistance to even minor stress diminishes* when glucocorticoids are deficient. Surgery, pregnancy, injury, infection, or salt loss due to profuse diaphoresis during hot weather can cause the patient to go into Addisonian crisis. Finally, cortisol deficiency stimulates the pituitary gland to secrete greater amounts of ACTH and melanocyte-stimulating hormone (MSH)* (see Fig. 74–2). Increased MSH secretion results in *increased pigmentation* of the skin and mucous membranes. As a result, patients with Addison's disease have an "eternal tan" and a peculiar bronzed appearance.

Androgen deficiency fails to produce symptoms in men because the testes supply the male with adequate amounts of sex hormones. However, females are dependent upon the adrenal cortex for an adequate secretion of androgens. For this reason, women with Addison's disease have less axillary and pubic hair growth than do women with normal adrenal function.

The *onset* of Addison's disease is usually insidious, and the patient experiences mild fatigue, languor, irritability, weight loss, nausea, vomiting, and postural hypotension weeks or months before the disease is diagnosed. As the disease progresses, symptoms intensify. Addison himself vividly describes the manifestations of this debilitating and potentially fatal condition:

> The patient in most of the cases I have seen, has been observed gradually to fall off in general health; he becomes languid and weak, indisposed to either bodily or mental exertion; the appetite is impaired or entirely lost; . . . the pulse small and feeble . . . excessively soft and compressible; the body wastes . . . slight pain or uneasiness is from time to time referred to the region of the stomach, and there is occasionally actual vomiting . . . it is by no means uncommon for the patient to manifest indications of disturbed cerebral circulation . . . We discover a most remarkable, and, so far as I know, characteristic discoloration taking place in the skin, — sufficiently marked indeed as generally to have attracted the attention of the patient himself, or of the patient's friends . . . It may be said to present a dingy or smoky appearance, or various tints or shades of deep amber or chestnut brown . . . The body wastes . . . the pulse becomes smaller and weaker, and . . . the patient at length gradually sinks and expires.[76]

Without early diagnosis and treatment, the patient with Addison's disease lives in the constant (often unrecognized) danger of fatal addisonian crisis should he or she be subjected to any stress. Acute addisonian crisis is characterized by sudden profound asthenia; severe abdominal, back, and leg pain; hyperpyrexia fol-

*Melanocytes are epidermal cells which synthesize melanin — the dark pigment which colors the hair, skin, and parts of the eye.

lowed by hypothermia; peripheral vascular collapse; coma; and finally renal shutdown.

Diagnostic studies. Addison's disease is primarily diagnosed on the basis of blood and urine hormonal assays. Dangerous provocative tests such as the *salt withdrawal test* are no longer used. Modern definitive tests of adrenocortical hypofunction include the following:

1. *The 8-hour intravenous ACTH test:* This is the most reliable diagnostic test for Addison's disease. The procedure is as follows:

Day one: (a) Start 24-hour urine specimen for measurement of 17-ketosteroids (17-KS) and 17-hydroxycorticosteroids (17-OHCS) or 17-ketogenic steroids (17-KGS). The *17-ketosteroids* (17-KS) are the excretory metabolites of the *androgenic* (male) *hormone.* In men two thirds of 17-KS are derived from the adrenals and one third from the testes; in women, 17-KS are derived almost exclusively from the adrenals. The *17-hydroxy corticosteroids* (17-OHCS) are excretory metabolites of *cortisol, corticosterone, cortisone,* and *11-hydroxycorticosterone.* The *17-ketogenic steroids* (17-KGS) are 17-OHCS which have been artificially converted within the laboratory to 17-ketosteroids. Conversion is helpful because 17-KGS are more stable than 17-OHCS and therefore more easily analyzed. (b) Administer dexamethasone, 0.5 mg. orally t.i.d. Dexamethasone is an adrenocortical steroid; it is given to patients to prevent toxic reactions to ACTH. Dexamethasone does not seriously alter urinary steroid levels.

Day two: (a) Administer 25 units of ACTH dissolved in 500 ml. of saline over exactly 8 hours. (b) Collect a second 24-hour urine specimen. (c) Continue to administer dexamethasone as ordered.

Results: Normally, urinary steroid output increases three- to fivefold following the administration of ACTH. In *primary* Addison's disease, urinary steroid output *does not* rise following ACTH stimulation because of permanent adrenal gland atrophy. In Addison's disease *secondary* to pituitary insufficiency, 17-OHCS and 17-KS gradually rise if the test is repeated over several days. Steroid levels are slow to rise because temporary adrenal atrophy always occurs in the face of pituitary hyposecretion of ACTH.

2. *Plasma cortisol response to ACTH:* This test is reliable and can be performed more rapidly than the 8-hour I.V. ACTH test. First of all, the patient's blood is drawn in the fasting state and examined for plasma cortisol levels. Next, 25 U. of ACTH is given I.M. Thirty minutes later a second blood sample is drawn. If the plasma

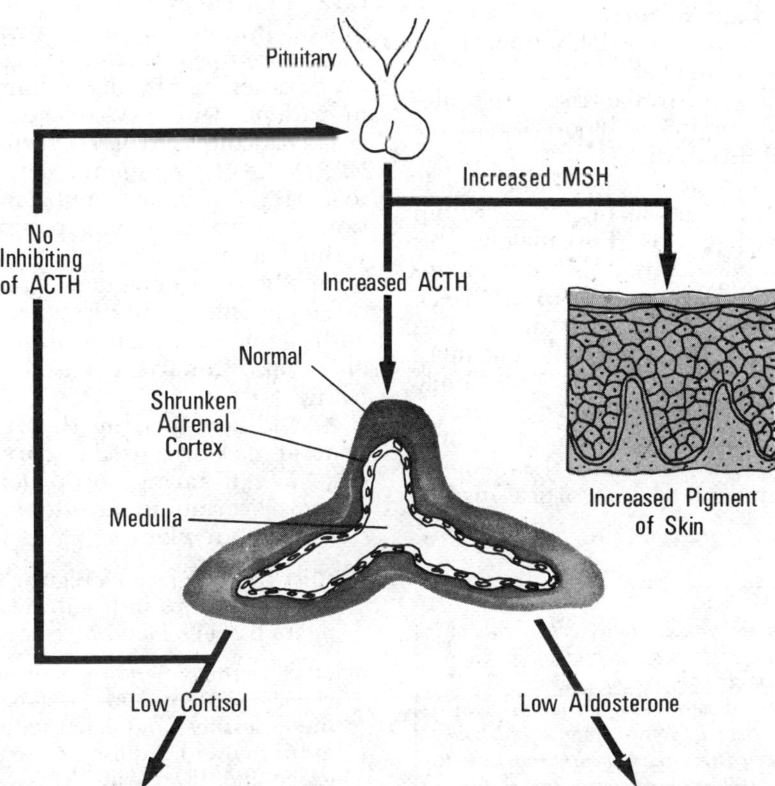

Figure 74–2. Causation of increased skin pigmentation in Addison's disease. (From Snively, W. D., and D. R. Beshear: *Textbook of Pathophysiology.* Philadelphia: J. B. Lippincott Co., 1972, p. 192.)

cortisol level in the second blood specimen fails to rise by at least 10 μg./100 ml., Addison's disease is probably present.

3. *Thorn test* (4-hour corticotropin test): Today the Thorn test has been largely replaced by the two tests which we just described. The object of the Thorn test is to measure the *eosinophil count* following an I.M. injection of ACTH. Normally, glucocorticoids owing to their immunosuppressive action, cause the eosinophil count to fall to 20 to 30 per cent of the initial count of 200 per cu. mm. If the patient has Addison's disease, the injection of ACTH does not stimulate glucocorticoid secretion, and it consequently fails to cause the expected decrease in the eosinophil count.

4. *Water excretion test (Robinson-Kepler-Power):* This test of diuresis following ingestion of a large amount of water is sometimes used as a screening procedure. First ask the patient, who is NPO for 16 hours, to void and discard the urine. Next, give 1500 ml. of tap water and ask the patient to drink it within 15 to 30 minutes. Finally, collect all the patient's urine for the next 5 hours and send it to the laboratory. Normally, the patient will void more than 1000 ml. following the water ingestion and the urine specific gravity is low. Patients with Addison's disease excrete less than 800 ml. because adrenocortical insufficiency reduces the body's ability to handle the stress of an additional water load.

5. *Laboratory findings:* Addison's disease is characterized by a low serum sodium (< 130 mEq./liter) and a high serum potassium (> 5 mEq./liter). Other important laboratory findings are summarized in Table 74–2. Also autoimmune antibodies to adrenal tissue are sometimes found circulating in the blood of patients with idiopathic Addison's disease.

Clinical care in chronic adrenocortical insufficiency. Addison's disease was once fatal within months following diagnosis. Fortunately, this grim outlook has totally changed since the manufacture of synthetic corticosteroid drugs. Today, the patient with Addison's disease can hope to live a normal active life *provided* he takes his steroid medications (see Table 74–3) daily without exception.

Cortisone or *hydrocortisone* (both glucocorticoids) is prescribed daily to correct the metabolic imbalances created by adrenocortical insufficiency.

> *Administer oral cortisol preparations with meals or antacids to lessen gastric irritation and the possible development of peptic ulcer.*
> *Administer* parenteral *cortisol preparations* deep *into the gluteal muscle and* not *into the deltoid muscle; cortisol injected into the subcutaneous tissue can cause sterile abscesses, atrophy of tissues, and abnormalities of pigmentation.*

TABLE 74–2. LABORATORY FINDINGS SUGGESTING ADDISON'S DISEASE*

Blood chemistry	Low serum Na† (< 130 mEq./liter)
	High serum K (> 5 mEq./liter)
	Ratio of serum Na:K (< 30:1)
	Low fasting blood sugar (< 50 mg./100 ml.)
	Decrease in CO_2 combining power (< 28 mEq./liter)
	Elevated BUN (> 20 mg./100 ml.)
Hematology	Elevated hematocrit
	Low WBC count
	Relative lymphocytosis
	Increased eosinophils
X-ray	Evidence of:
	Small heart
	Calcifications in the adrenal areas
	Renal tuberculosis
	Pulmonary tuberculosis

*From Holvey, D. N., et al. (eds.): *The Merck Manual of Diagnosis and Therapy,* 13th ed. West Point, Pa., Merck Sharp & Dohme Research Laboratories, 1977, p. 1268.

†Na = sodium; K = potassium.

Carefully observe the patient for signs of Cushing's syndrome — the consequence of excessive long-term cortisol therapy. Also incorporate the nursing actions described in the section on Cushing's syndrome into your plan of daily care; e.g., check daily weight, blood pressure, intake, and output (see below).

Fludrocortisone acetate (Florinef) is given daily or every other day for its sodium-retaining action in patients with evidence of insufficient mineralocorticoid activity. *Deoxycorticosterone (Cortate, DOCA-A),* a mineralocorticoid, is also used to correct electrolyte imbalance and hypotension and to maintain plasma volume levels within the normal range.

Finally, the debilitated, malnourished patient often benefits from injections of *testosterone;* this androgenic agent has a protein anabolic effect, and it also imparts a sense of vitality and well-being.

In addition to drug therapy, there are also general measures used to correct Addison's disease. When caring for patients with this disorder, be certain to include the following procedures in your plan:

- ▶ Check vital signs on a regular basis. Report to the physician drops in blood pressure below the patient's baseline blood pressure.
- ▶ Observe the patient for signs of increased physical vitality and emotional well-being. With therapy, the listlessness and exhaustion which shadow the individual with Addison's disease should gradually lessen and disappear.
- ▶ Prevent exposure to infection. Report "sniffles," sore throats, bladder infections, and so forth at

once to the physician. Remember that the person with Addison's disease cannot tolerate stress. Because infection always imposes additional stress upon the body, the dosage of steroids should be increased during infectious illnesses.

- ▶ Weigh the patient regularly. Weight gain usually occurs as a result of sodium and water retention due to the steroid drugs.
- ▶ Observe carefully for signs of sodium and potassium imbalance (see Ch. 12). If steroid replacement therapy is inadequate, sodium loss and potassium retention will continue. If the dosage of steroids is too high, excessive amounts of sodium and water will be retained, and potassium will be excreted in inordinate amounts.
- ▶ Encourage a high-carbohydrate, high-protein diet.
- ▶ Contruct a plan for teaching the patient self-administration of steroid drugs. Your plan should include the following points: (a) oral administration of drugs; (b) the action of the prescribed hormones; and (c) signs of overdosage and underdosage. Emphasize to the patient who takes glucocorticoids that he must call his doctor for an increase in dosage when undergoing situations involving stress; e.g., emotional upheavals, dental extractions, minor surgery, or upper respiratory tract infections. In addition, dosages of mineralocorticoids may need to be temporarily raised if the patient is diaphoresing profusely for any reason; e.g., as a result of "heat spells," strenuous physical exertion, fever. Finally, while steroids are usually administered orally, remind the patient that he will need to give the drugs intramuscularly if he is nauseated or vomiting.
- ▶ Prior to discharge, obtain for the patient an identification bracelet and an emergency kit which he must carry with him at all times. The identification bracelet should carry the patient's name as well as the names and telephone numbers of his doctor and emergency contact. Also, on the bracelet, Liddle recommends engraving the following inscription:[26] I have adrenal insufficiency. In any emergency involving injury, vomiting, or loss of consciousness, the hydrocortisone in my possession should be injected under my skin, and my physician notified. The hydrocortisone (100 mg. of hydrocortisone phosphate solution) is kept in a prepared syringe within the emergency kit along with sterile alcohol sponges. Also the emergency kit may contain notes concerning the patient's drug prescription, dosage schedules, and so forth.
- ▶ Remind the patient to make biyearly appointments with his doctor, even when he is in good

TABLE 74–3. MAJOR ADRENOCORTICAL DRUG PREPARATIONS: ACTION, USES, SIDE EFFECTS

Drug	Action	Uses	Side Effects
Cortisone acetate	Glucocorticoid, mineralocorticoid, anti-inflammatory, anti-immunologic, antianabolic.	Replacement therapy for Addison's disease. Control allergic reactions. Suppress inflammatory reactions. Treat mesenchymal or collagen disorders.	Overdosage produces Cushing's syndrome and its symptoms (see p. 1608). Abrupt withdrawal of drug may cause headache, nausea, and vomiting, and papilledema.
Hydrocortisone	Similar to cortisone.	Replacement therapy for Addison's disease. Management of inflammatory skin, joint, and eye conditions.	Same as cortisone acetate.
Prednisone methylprednisolone	Similar to cortisone but 4–5 times more potent glucocorticoid activity.	For anti-inflammatory action and to suppress the immune system, e.g. following organ transplants.	Similar to cortisone but less mineralocorticoid activity.
Dexamethasone	Similar to cortisone but 20–25 times more potent glucocorticoid activity.	For very potent glucocorticoid effects	Similar to prednisone.
Fludrocortisone acetate (Florinef)	Mineralocorticoid action.	Replacement therapy for Addison's disease.	*Mineralocorticoid effects:* hypertension, edema due to sodium retention, muscle weakness, and arrhythmias due to hypokalemia.
Deoxycorticosterone (cortate, DOCA-A)	Mineralocorticoid.	Replacement therapy for Addison's disease and Simmond's disease.	*Mineralocorticoid* effects: same as for Florinef.

health. Like diabetes mellitus, the control of Addison's disease is a lifelong responsibility.

Clinical care in acute adrenal insufficiency (Addisonian crisis). Acute adrenal insufficiency is characterized by a critical deficiency of glucocorticoids, severe hypotension, hyperkalemia, and vascular collapse. Thus the development of Addisonian crisis constitutes a medical emergency which must be treated rapidly and vigorously. Three three major goals of care are to (1) reverse shock, (2) restore blood circulation (the patient usually suffers from a deficit of at least 20 per cent of the extracellular fluid volume), and (3) replenish the body with needed steroids.

Upon admission, the patient is rapidly infused with 1000 ml. of physiologic saline to which has been added 100 mg. of a water-soluble glucocorticoid (hydrocortisone phosphate or hydrocortisone sodium succinate). The dosage of the prescribed glucocorticoid is then often lowered to 50 mg., and it is administered (either I.M. or I.V.) every 6 hours during the first day of the crisis, every 8 hours of the second day, and gradually reduced thereafter. In addition, the doctor may order plasma, oxygen, and vasopressor drugs to counteract persisting hypotension. Also, if an infection triggered the crisis, antibiotics are given. Throughout this emergency period, the nurse is responsible for (a) monitoring blood pressure, (b) administering the intravenous infusions and medications, (c) measuring hourly urinary output and reporting oliguria (a sign of shock), and (d) guarding the patient from further emotional and physical stress. In addition to observing for signs of shock, you must also watch for symptoms of overhydration and overdosage with glucocorticoids, e.g., generalized edema due to fluid retention, hypertension, flaccid paralysis resulting from hypokalemia, psychoses, and loss of consciousness.

With rapid, efficient treatment, Addisonian crisis usually passes within a few hours; the patient's condition stabilizes, and the convalescent period begins. While convalescing, the patient begins to take water and food by mouth. Also corticosteroids are given orally and the dosage is gradually reduced to maintenance levels.

OTHER CAUSES OF ADRENOCORTICAL INSUFFICIENCY. Adrenocortical insufficiency develops in response to the following four conditions:

- Bilateral adrenalectomy.
- Hemorrhagic infarction and necrosis of the adrenal glands; adrenal apoplexy may develop as a complication of meningococcal septicemia or anticoagulant therapy.
- Hypopituitarism resulting in a decreased secretion of ACTH by the pituitary gland, which in turn results in the decreased secretion of cortisol and androgens by the adrenal gland (secondary adrenocortical insufficiency).
- Suppression of the hypothalamic-pituitary secretion of ACTH due to either (a) the pharmacologic administration of corticosteroids, or (b) the oversecretion of corticosteroids by an adrenal tumor. In both these cases the adrenal glands shrink, atrophy, and become filled with lipids. However, because the level of circulating corticosteroids is high, these patients do not develop symptoms of adrenocortical insufficiency *unless* steroid therapy is discontinued suddenly or the tumor is resected. Fortunately, if corticosteroid drug therapy is terminated gradually and if the dosage of medication is slowly reduced each day, the adrenal glands usually return to normal function.

Clinically, patients with secondary adrenocortical insufficiency suffer from the symptoms of cortisol and androgen deficiency; aldosterone continues to be secreted in sufficient amounts. Also, as in Addison's disease, these persons are subject to the development of acute crises when exposed to various stresses.

Treatment involves the administration of glucocorticoids in the same manner as for Addison's disease. Mineralocorticoids are not given except if the patient develops signs or symptoms of mineralocorticoid deficiency. The patient, as in Addison's disease, should be instructed to carry an identification card and emergency kit at all times in the event of an acute crisis.

Adrenocortical Hyperfunction (Hypercorticism). Hyperfunction of the adrenal cortex results in the excessive production of either glucocorticoids, mineralocorticords, or androgenic steroids. The three major conditions classified under hypercorticism and the type of steroid overproduction which predominates are as follows: (1) Cushing's syndrome (glucocorticoid oversecretion), aldosteronism (aldosterone oversecretion), and (3) adrenogenital syndrome (adrenal androgen oversecretion). All three of these conditions appear more frequently in women than in men.

CUSHING'S SYNDROME

Etiology and incidence. Cushing's syndrome was first described by Dr. Harvey Cushing in 1932. It results from overactivity of the adrenal gland with consequent *hypersecretion* of *glucocorticoids.* Hypersecretion of glucocorticoids is caused by one of the following pathologic conditions:

1. A cortisol secreting *adrenal tumor.* Adrenal tumors are responsible for approximately 30 per cent of cases of Cushing's syndrome. The

majority of tumors (85 per cent) are benign, while 15 per cent are malignant. These tumors are found in approximately one out of every 10,000 hospital admissions.

2. *Hyperplasia* of the *adrenal cortex* caused by overproduction of adrenocortical-stimulating hormone. Bilateral adrenal hyperplasia due to excessive ACTH stimulation accounts for approximately 60 per cent of cases of Cushing's syndrome. Sources of excessive ACTH secretion are two in number:

1. *Pituitary hypersecretion:* Pituitary tumors cause approximately 10 per cent of cases of Cushing's syndrome.[76] The tumors, which are usually benign, are either small basophil adenomas or large chromophobe adenomas. However, there are numerous cases of pituitary hypersecretion of ACTH in which no tumor can be located; to date there is no satisfactory explanation for this phenomenon. In any case, when pituitary hypersecretion of ACTH (due to either a tumor or unknown causes) results in excessive secretion of glucocorticoids, the condition is usually referred to as *Cushing's disease* rather than Cushing's syndrome. Cushing's disease is discovered in approximately one patient out of every 2000 patients admitted to the hospital.

2. *Ectopic hypersecretion of ACTH:* ACTH-secreting tumors located in organs far removed from the pituitary gland are a major cause of Cushing's syndrome. This particular form of the syndrome is sometimes called the *ectopic ACTH syndrome*. The tumor which is most frequently linked with ectopic ACTH syndrome is the bronchogenic oat-cell carcinoma.

In addition to being caused by adrenal tumors, pituitary hyperfunction (Cushing's disease), and ectopic ACTH-secreting tumors (ectopic ACTH syndrome), Cushing's syndrome also results from the prescribed administration of synthetic glucocorticoids; this complication is called *iatrogenic Cushing's syndrome*. Prolonged administration of cortisone results in temporary atrophy of the adrenal glands and in the typical symptoms of Cushing's syndrome.

Bases of symptoms. The function of the glucocorticoids was described at the beginning of this chapter. When Cushing's syndrome develops, all the normal functions of the glucocorticoids become exaggerated, and the classic picture of the patient with Cushing's syndrome emerges (see Fig. 74–3). Exaggeration of the normal functions of the glucocorticoids results in the following problems:

- *Persistent hyperglycemia* which may result in the development of diabetes mellitus.
- *Protein tissue wasting* and the excessive deamination of amino acids which results in (a) the stunting of linear growth in children, (b) weakness due to wasting of muscle, (c) capillary fragility resulting in ecchymosis, and (d) osteoporosis due to wasting of the bone matrix. Osteoporosis may grow so severe that the patient develops pathologic fractures upon even mild trauma. Also compression fractures of the osteoporotic spine leading to kyphosis and height loss are not uncommon.
- *Potassium depletion* leading to hypokalemia, arrhythmias, muscle weakness, and renal disorders.
- *Sodium and water retention* which causes edema and hypertension. Hypertension, in turn, eventually predisposes the patient to left ventricular hypertrophy, congestive heart failure, and strokes.
- *Abnormal fat distribution* (in conjunction with

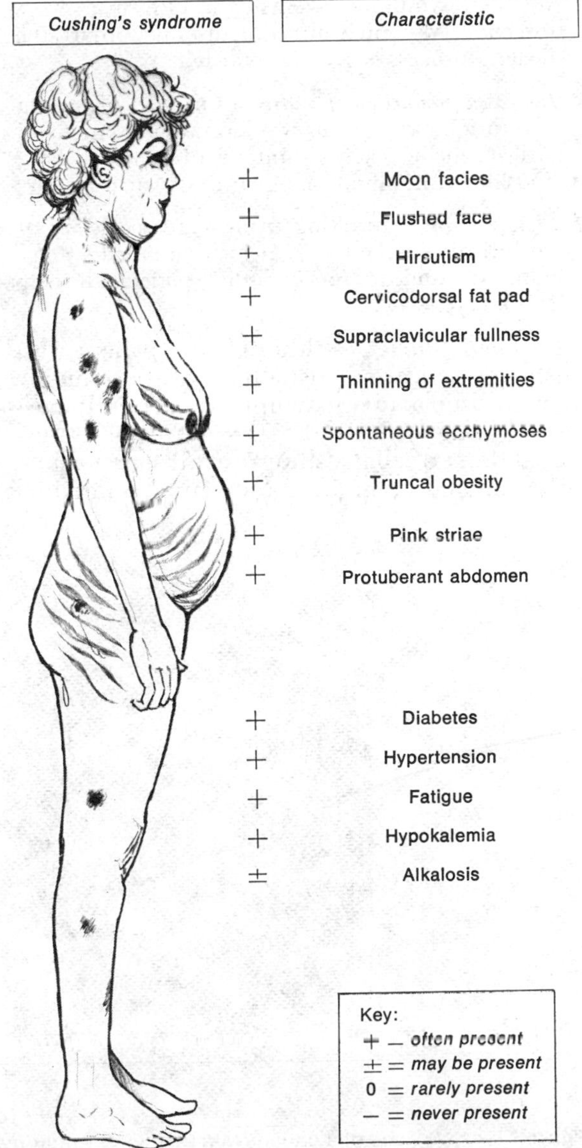

Figure 74–3. Findings in Cushing's syndrome. (From Meloni, R. C.: Obesity or Cushing's disease? *American Family Physician* 5:93, 1972.)

edema) which results in a moon face, cervical-dorsal fat pad on the patient's neck (called a "buffalo hump"), and truncal obesity with slender limbs. Also pink striae appear on the breasts, axillary areas, and legs. Striae develop when the skin in a particular area is unduly stretched by large accumulations of fatty tissue. Changes in appearance following the development of Cushing's syndrome as well as after therapy are striking.

- *Increased susceptibility to infection* and *lowered resistance to stress* make the patient vulnerable to microorganisms of all types. Because the inflammatory response is suppressed, the patient may develop very few symptoms even in the face of a severe infection. Also, once infection or injury occurs, the healing process is greatly retarded.
- *Increased production of androgens* may occur, giving rise to mild virilism in women. Manifestations of virilism include acne, thinning of the scalp hair, and hirsutism (abnormal growth of hair).
- *Mental changes* resulting from increased levels of glucocorticoids and ACTH include mood swings, euphoria, and depression; some patients develop frank psychosis.

Diagnostic studies. Although the patient with Cushing's syndrome usually displays a highly characteristic array of symptoms, precisely performed diagnostic studies are nevertheless essential. First of all, Cushing's syndrome must be differentiated from (a) obesity compounded by diabetes mellitus and hypertension, and (b) the adrenogenital syndrome (see below). Secondly, once a diagnosis of Cushing's syndrome is established, then the physician must decide whether the causative factor is hyperplasia of the adrenal glands or an adrenal tumor. Important diagnostic measures are listed below.

Laboratory tests. Laboratory data diagnostic of Cushing's syndrome reflect the hyperglycemia, fluid and electrolyte disturbances, and immunosuppressive actions which are so characteristic of excessive glucocorticoid secretion. Thus, in Cushing's syndrome, *glucose tolerance* is lowered and *glycosuria* may be present. The *white count* is often elevated over 10,000, but the total eosinophil count is depressed to less than 50 cells per cu. mm. and lymphocytes are reduced to fewer than 20 per cent. *Urinary 17-hydroxycorticosteroids* are elevated and *blood corticosteroids* are high.

Special diagnostic tests. Three special tests which are extremely valuable in confirming a diagnosis of Cushing's disease are as follows:

1. *Plasma cortisol:* Normally the diurnal pattern for plasma cortisol is an elevated level in the early morning (10 to 25 μg./100 ml.), followed by a gradual decline until evening, at which time, the level is less than 10 μg./100 ml. Individuals with Cushing's syndrome have elevated plasma cortisol levels in the morning, and furthermore they do not experience a normal decline in cortisol levels as the day proceeds. A useful screening test is to give the patient 1.0 mg. of dexamethasone at 11 P.M. and draw a plasma cortisol the next morning at 8 A.M. Normally the level is less than 5 μg./100 ml.

2. *Cortisone suppression test:* This test is mainly employed to differentiate between Cushing's

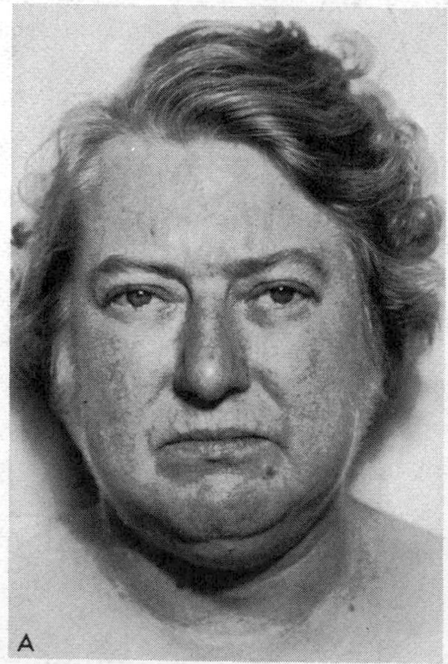

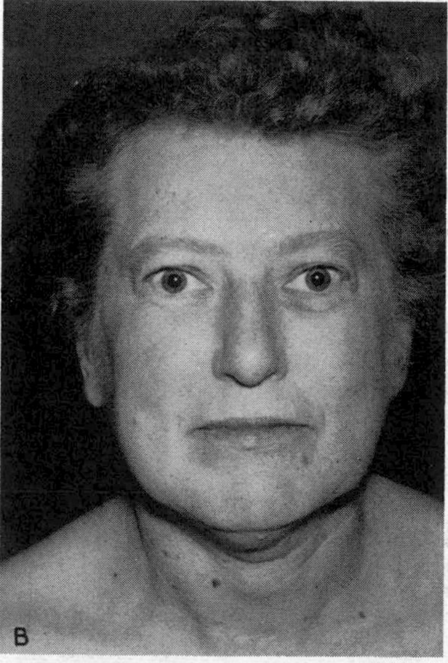

Figure 74–4. *A*, Face of a patient with Cushing's syndrome due to bilateral hyperplasia of the adrenals. This 45-year-old patient underwent a two-stage bilateral total adrenalectomy. *B*, Disappearance of all signs and symptoms 8 months after the second adrenalectomy, during which patient received complete substitution therapy. (From Williams, R. H.: *Textbook of Endocrinology*, 5th ed. Philadelphia: W. B. Saunders Co., 1974.)

syndrome (caused by an adrenal tumor), Cushing's disease (caused by pituitary oversecretion of ACTH), and ectopic ACTH syndrome (caused by ectopic ACTH-secreting tumor).

Steps in the suppression test are as follows: (a) 24-hour urine specimens (used to establish a baseline) are collected for 2 days and are examined for urinary steroids; (b) on the third and fourth days, the patient is given 0.5 mg. dexamethasone (a derivative of fludrocortisone) every 6 hours for 2 days; (c) during the two days of dexamethasone administration, 24-hour urine specimens are again collected and examined for steroid content.

The action of dexamethasone is to *suppress* the *pituitary secretion of ACTH*. Thus, normally by the second day of dexamethasone administration, the levels of urinary ketogenic steroids and hydroxycorticoids drop more than 50 per cent below those of the baseline urine specimen. However, if the patient has Cushing's disease (which is a *pituitary* disorder), urinary 17-OHCS will decrease, but *less* than the normal 50 per cent below baseline until the dosage of dexamethasone is raised to 2 mg. every 6 hours. This is because the diseased pituitary tends to be relatively resistant to the action of dexamethasone unless dosage is high. On the other hand, patients with either Cushing's syndrome (due to an adrenal tumor) or ectopic ACTH syndrome *fail to respond at all* to dexamethasone; i.e., levels of 17-OHCS do not decrease during the test because dexamethasone has no effect upon the adrenals or upon ectopic ACTH-secreting tumors.

Clinical care. Liddle states:

The prime therapeutic objectives in Cushing's syndrome are to reduce cortisol levels to normal and to eradicate any associated tumors. Secondary objectives are to avoid producing hormonal deficiencies and to avoid making the patient chronically dependent upon medication.[76]

The form of therapy prescribed depends, first of all, upon whether the patient has an adrenal tumor. Cushing's disease, or ectopic ACTH syndrome. Secondly, therapies differ, depending upon whether the causative lesion is benign or malignant.

As you can see in Table 74–4, the most common form of therapy for all three subvarieties of Cushing's syndrome is *surgery*. Pituitary irradiation is used to treat Cushing's disease in some medical centers. Drugs are prescribed

TABLE 74–4. THERAPIES PRESCRIBED FOR CUSHING'S SYNDROME

Condition	Responsible Lesion	Therapies	Remarks
Cushing's syndrome	Unilateral adrenal tumors (benign or malignant); bilateral adrenal tumors	*Adrenalectomy* (surgical excision of the adrenal gland containing the tumor); total bilateral adrenalectomy (surgical incision of both adrenal glands)	Adrenalectomy for a benign unilateral tumor usually curative Bilateral adrenalectomy must be followed by lifelong administration of *cortisteroids* to prevent Addison's Disease
	Adrenal carcinoma with widespread metastases	Chemotherapy: *o,p'*-DDD, aminoglutethimide, and metyrapone used to promote remission in patients with inoperable cancer	Chemotherapy largely unsuccessful; drugs used highly toxic
Cushing's disease	Pituitary tumor (or unidentified lesion) which secretes excessive amounts of ACTH	Irradiation of the pituitary gland	Irradiation successful in 25% of cases; therapeutic effects not apparent for months following initiation of therapy
		Total bilateral adrenalectomy (corrects adrenal hyperplasia due to excessive ACTH stimulation)	Total bilateral adrenalectomy must be followed by lifelong replacement therapy with a glucocorticoid and mineralocorticoid
		Hypophysectomy or subtotal destruction of the pituitary by microsurgical resection, cryosurgery, yttrium implant, proton beam, or localized high-dosage irradiation (see p. 1621)	Hypophysectomy results in panhypopituitarism; all hormonal secretions dependent upon pituitary stimulation must be replaced for rest of patient's life (i.e., glucocorticoids, thyroid hormone, gonadal steroids, antidiuretic hormone)
Ectopic ACTH syndrome	Extra-adrenal malignant tumor	Surgical removal of the ectopic malignant tumor. Chemotherapy: used to control hypercorticism and promote remission in patients with inoperable cancer	Surgery rarely successful because metastasis usually occurs prior to diagnosis; chemotherapy purely palliative.

only as palliative measures for the treatment of inoperable cancer. Current drugs in use are as follows:

- ▶ *o,p'*-DDD[2.2-bis(2-chlorophenyl-4-chlorophenyl)-1,1-dichloroethane]* This cytotoxic agent is still under investigation. It acts to inhibit the production of glucocorticoids by the adrenal glands, but leaves aldosterone production intact. Side effects include minor gastrointestinal tract disturbances, skin rash, lethargy, and ataxia. *o,p'*-DDD is the least toxic of all the adrenocorticolytic drugs.

- ▶ *Aminoglutethimide* (Elipten): Like *o,p'*-DDD, aminoglutethimide is a drug which decreases cortisol production; it is also an anticonvulsant. Side effects include transient leukopenia, mild respiratory depression, drowsiness, ataxia, gastrointestinal disturbances, and skin rashes.

- ▶ *Metyrapone* (Metapirone): This drug acts to decrease cortisol production by selectively inhibiting 11-beta-hydroxylation in the adrenal cortex. It is rapid-acting and may produce therapeutic effects in one day. Side effects are transient vertigo and nausea. Metyrapone is not effective for long-term therapy.

Care of the patient undergoing adrenocortical surgery. During the *preoperative* period, the patient with Cushing's syndrome needs expert nursing care. The crucial problems of hypertension, edema, possible heart disease, diabetes mellitus, increased susceptibility to infection, decreased resistance to stress, and emotional lability must all be brought under control. Important nursing actions during this time include the following:

- ▶ Promote mental and physical rest. Obtain orders for sedatives or hypnotics as necessary.

- ▶ Encourage a diet which is low in calories, carbohydrates, and sodium, but has ample protein and potassium content. Such a diet will promote weight loss, reduction of edema and hypertension, control of hypokalemia, and rebuilding of wasted tissue. Special diets are required for the patient with frank diabetic mellitus (Chapter 72) or gastric ulcers (Unit XVII).

- ▶ Check vital signs on a scheduled basis. Observe the patient carefully for signs of severe hypertension, e.g., elevated blood pressure readings, headache, failing vision, irritability, and dyspnea.

- ▶ Weigh the patient daily at the same time and on the same scales. If sodium intake is decreased, the patient's weight should decrease and edema lessen.

- ▶ Test the patient's urine for sugar and acetone daily. Positive urine specimens may indicate the development of overt diabetes mellitus.

- ▶ Protect the patient from exposure to infectious organisms. Isolate the patient from hospital personnel, family members, or other visitors with contagious disorders.

> Remember:
> *Because glucocorticoids suppress the immune and inflammatory reactions, the patient with Cushing's syndrome may experience only mild symptoms even though there is actually a severe infection.*

For this reason, even a slight temperature or a little drainage from a cut or wound must be considered serious. Almost without warning, it is possible for a superficial or minor bacterial infection to develop into a severe infection.

- ▶ Guard the patient from falls and other accidents. Remember that individuals with Cushing's syndrome have osteoporosis and a resultant tendency to develop fractures even upon mild trauma. Therefore be careful to keep the patient in a low bed. Also raise the siderails if the patient is restless or mentally disturbed. Steady the patient (who is obese and often uncoordinated) when he ambulates.

- ▶ Attempt to understand the patient's mood swings and depressions. Most people with Cushing's syndrome are understandably upset by the rather grotesque changes in their appearance due to the disease; they may also be alarmed by the bizarre emotional feelings which they experience. It helps to explain to the patient that his appearance and moods should gradually return to normal with treatment.

- ▶ On the morning of surgery, administer a glucocorticoid preparation (usually intramuscularly) as ordered. A water-soluble cortisol preparation (diluted in an I.V. infusion) is also administered throughout the surgical procedure. Cortisol protects the patient from developing acute adrenal insufficiency during adrenalectomy. Even if only one adrenal gland is being removed, temporary support with glucocorticoids may be necessary; this is because the "normal" gland may have atrophied in response to the excessive secretion of glucocorticoids by the tumorous gland. Usually the normal remaining adrenal gland begins to secrete corticosteroids again at some point following surgery.

During the immediate *postoperative* period, major goals are to (a) prevent shock, (b) prevent infection, (c) sustain adequate cortisol levels, and (d) control pain and abdominal discomfort. Important nursing actions include (a) observing for signs of shock (hypotension, rapid weak

---

*Cytotoxic agents and cancer chemotherapy are discussed in Unit IX, Chapter 23.

pulse); (b) taking and recording vital signs at least every 10 to 15 minutes; (c) measuring the patient's urine hourly and observing for oliguria (a sign of shock and renal shutdown); (d) administering intravenous fluids, pressor amines, and corticosteroid preparations as ordered; (e) encouraging coughing, turning, and deep breathing to prevent dangerous respiratory infections; and (f) employing meticulous sterile technique when changing or reinforcing the dressing in order to prevent wound infection.

Because the abdominal approach is usually preferred, some patients will also require nasogastric suction until peristalsis returns to normal and nausea and vomiting diminish.

Once the patient becomes a convalescent, he or she will then need instruction in the self-administration of replacement hormones. As stated earlier in Table 74–4, the patient who undergoes either total bilateral adrenalectomy or hypophysectomy will need to take cortisol preparations for the remainder of his life. On the other hand, if only one adrenal gland has been removed, 15 to 20 mg. of cortisone is given daily until the remaining adrenal gland begins to function normally. Usually the maintenance dose of cortisone can be discontinued within 6 to 12 months.

PRIMARY HYPERALDOSTERONISM (CONN'S SYNDROME). Aldosterone is the most powerful of the mineralocorticoids. Its primary role is the conservation of sodium. Important secondary roles are water conservation and promotion of potassium excretion.

Hypersecretion of aldosterone due to an adrenal lesion results in *primary* hyperaldosteronism. In contrast, *secondary* hyperaldosteronism arises as a consequence of edematous disorders (cardiac failure, cirrhosis of the liver with ascites, the nephrotic syndrome); it also develops in hypertension due to destructive renal artery disease.

The major cause of primary hyperaldosteronism is a *benign aldosterone-secreting adrenal tumor* called an *aldosteronoma.* Although multiple tumors are sometimes found, the causative factor in 90 per cent of cases in a *single* adenoma. Rarely, Conn's syndrome develops as a consequence of adrenocortical carcinoma.

The exact incidence of Conn's syndrome is unknown. However, some authorities maintain that the aldosteronoma is the most frequently diagnosed functioning adrenal tumor. Conn's syndrome strikes females twice as often as males, and it appears most frequently among middle-aged individuals.

Hypersecretion of aldosterone results in sodium and water retention and excessive potassium excretion. The two major hallmarks of primary hyperaldosteronism are *hypertension* and *hypokalemia.* Without treatment, the patient can develop all of the complications of chronic hypertension, e.g., visual disturbances, heart failure, renal damage, and cerebral vascular accidents.

Hypokalemia, the second major manifestation of Conn's syndrome, results from excessive urinary excretion of potassium (see Chapter 12). Hypokalemia, in turn, causes *muscle weakness* because potassium loss reduces normal neuromuscular irritability. In addition, the excessive excretion of K^+ causes *polyuria.* The large urinary output results in *polydipsia* (excessive thirst). Finally, hypokalemia leads to *metabolic alkalosis* due to (a) the shifting of H^+ into the cells in exchange of K^+ and (b) the exchange of hydrogen ions within the tubular cells for sodium ions from the tubular urine (see Fig. 74–5). Metabolic alkalosis causes a decrease in ionized calcium levels, which may result in tetany and respiratory suppression (Chapter 12).

Oddly enough, despite sodium retention, patients rarely develop overt edema. Although extracellular fluid increases moderately, excessive water is usually excreted in the urine along with the potassium ions. Also the kidneys, over a period of time, tend to physiologically "adjust" to the excessive secretion of aldosterone, so that water excretion reaches an equilibrium with sodium intake. The ability of the kidneys to eventually "escape" from the sodium- and water-retaining action of aldosterone is sometimes referred to as the "renal escape phenomenon."[76]

Diagnosis of primary hyperaldosteronism is based upon the following laboratory findings: low serum potassium, alkalosis, and elevated urinary aldosterone levels. In addition, x-ray studies may reveal cardiac hypertrophy resulting from chronic hypertension. The tumors may be visualized by radionuclide scanning techniques using labeled iodocholesterol.

The three *goals of treatment* for patients with primary hyperaldosteronism are to (1) reverse hypertension, (2) correct hypokalemia, and (3) prevent kidney damage. In two thirds of cases, hypertension is completely reversed by removal of the aldosterone-secreting tumor. Indeed, the majority of patients have normal blood pressure readings by the third postoperative month. *Hypokalemia* is corrected by the administration of potassium salts. Unfortunately the *renal complications* resulting from long-term hypertension tend to be progressive. For this reason, it is important for patients with primary hyperaldosteronism to be diagnosed and treated *early* in the course of the disease.

ADRENOGENITAL SYNDROME. The adrenogenital syndrome is a rare condition which is characterized by *virilism* resulting from the excessive secretion of *androgenic steroids* from the adrenal cortex.

In the majority of cases, the androgenic syndrome is a *congenital* disorder. In essence, the cause of prenatal androgenic syndrome is an inherited enzyme deficiency which leads to a number of pathologic consequences. Note in Figure 74–6 that, without the missing enzyme, adequate amounts of cortisol cannot be synthesized. Cortisol, by means of negative feedback, normally acts to regulate the secretion of ACTH from the anterior pituitary gland (see Ch. 3). Thus, without the inhibitory effects of cortisol, pituitary secretion of ACTH is not suppressed, and blood levels of ACTH are consequently elevated. Excessive secretion of ACTH results in hyperplasia of the adrenal glands and the hypersecretion of sex steroids. Finally, the excessive production of androgenic steroids results in *masculinization* of the afflicted individual.

While the adrenogenital syndrome is primarily a congenital syndrome, it does occasionally first present symptoms during adulthood.

The symptoms of the adrenogenital syndrome differ, depending upon the age and sex of the patient. The female infant may be born with *pseudohermaphroditism* ("masculinization of the female external genitalia"). Older girls and women with adrenal tumors may develop hirsutism, enlargement of the clitoris (see Figure 74–7), balding, atrophy of the breasts, and a masculine body build. Masculinizing changes in boys and men are not nearly as dramatic as they are in females. Young male children may be sexually precocious for their age.

Other manifestations (depending upon the specific type of enzyme deficiency) may include either *salt wasting* accompanied by hypotension and dehydration or *excessive salt and water retention* accompanied by hypertension. In addition, many patients (particularly women) suffer from mental disturbances due to their abnormal appearance.

Diagnostic findings which confirm the adrenogenital syndrome include elevated 17-ketosteroids that can be suppressed by administration of glucocorticoids. If the urinary 17-ketosteroids are not decreased by glucocorticoid replacement, the patient probably has an androgen-producing tumor.

Treatment of the adrenogenital syndrome involves giving cortisol preparations in order to (a)

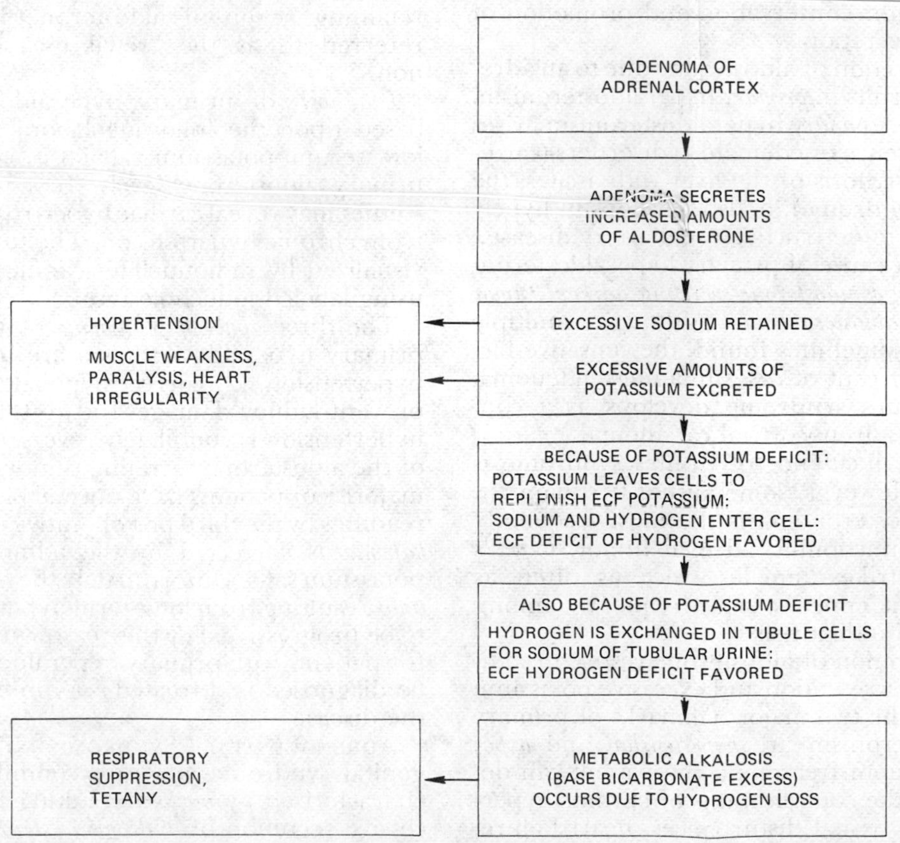

Figure 74–5. Sequence of events: primary aldosteronism. (From Snively, W. D., and D. R. Beshear: *Textbook of Pathophysiology.* Philadelphia: J. B. Lippincott Company, 1972, p. 194.)

correct the cortisol deficiency, and (b) inhibit the production of ACTH by the anterior pituitary gland which, in turn, reverses adrenal hypertrophy and overproduction of androgenic steroids. In addition, these patients should take the same precautions as persons with Addison's disease, i.e., wear an identification bracelet and carry an emergency kit which contains an ampule of hydrocortisone. On the other hand, if an adrenal tumor is causing masculinization, the tumor must be removed surgically. Malignant tumors must be discovered early and removed before metastasis occurs.

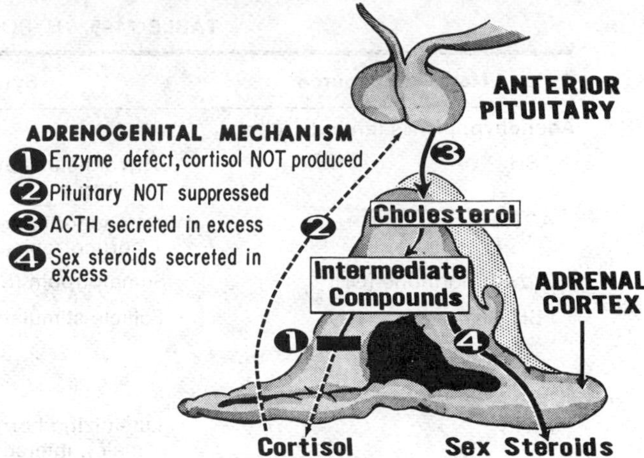

Figure 74–6. Mechanism of the adrenogenital syndrome. (From Liechty, R. D., and R. T. Soper: *Synopsis of Surgery,* 2nd ed. St. Louis: C. V. Mosby Co., 1972, p. 213.)

THE PITUITARY GLAND

Normal Anatomy and Physiology

The pituitary gland (also called the hypophysis cerebri) is a tiny organ which is securely cradled within a small recess in the sphenoid bone called the *sella turcica* (Turk's saddle). It is composed of a posterior and an anterior lobe which are separated and connected by a small, rather poorly developed, intermediate lobe.

The *posterior* lobe is called the *neurohypophysis* because it is of *neural* origin rather than glandular origin. An extension of the hypothalamus, the posterior lobe evidently does not produce any hormones itself; instead it simply stores and releases antidiuretic hormone (ADH) and oxytocin (a hormone which stimulates uterine contractions). Both these hormones are manufactured by the hypothalamus.

In contrast, the *anterior* lobe (called the adenohypophysis) is a *glandular* structure.* It is composed of three basic cell types: (1) eosinophils, (2) basophils, and (3) chromophobes. As a gland, the adenohypophysis synthesizes and releases vital hormones (see Table 74–5). Of the seven hormones, only *growth* hormone, MSH, and prolactin can act directly upon the body's non-endocrine target tissues. Even the effects of

**Adeno* is a Greek word element meaning *gland.*

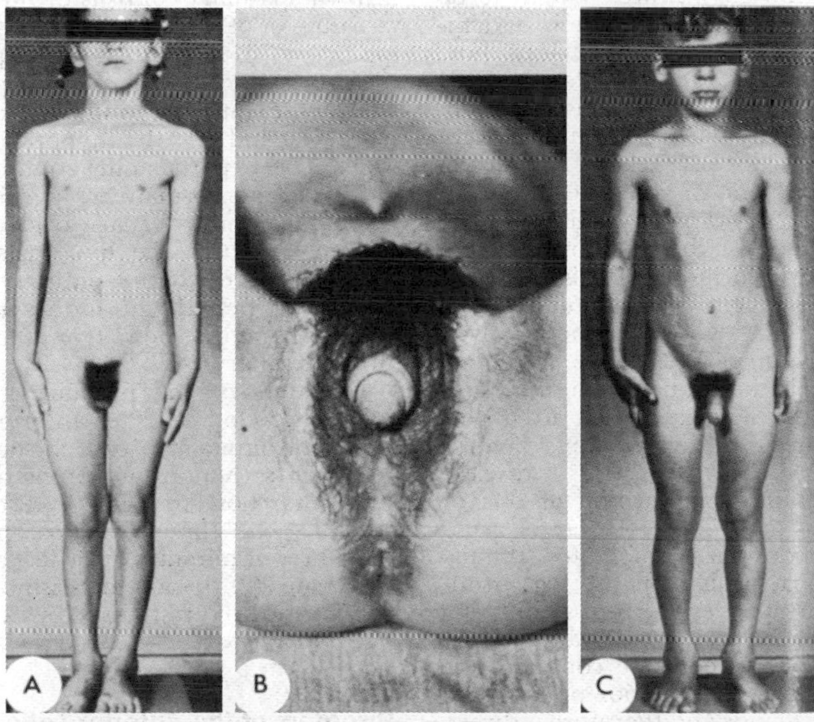

Figure 74–7. Congenital adrenal hyperplasia in a six-year-old girl (*A*) and her five-year-old brother (*C*). Masculinization is manifested by enlargement of clitoris and labial fusion (*B*). Boys look normal at birth but virilization is rapid. Rapid bone growth also results. Her height age is 8½ and bone age is 13 years. His height age is 8 and bone age is 12½. (From McFarlane, J.: Congenital adrenal hyperplasia. *American Journal of Nursing,* 76:1290, Aug. 1976.)

TABLE 74–5. HYPOPHYSEAL HORMONES

Name and Source	Synonyms	Function
Adenohypophysis (anterior lobe)		
TSH	Thyroid-stimulating hormone; thyrotropin	Stimulates thyroid growth and secretion
ACTH	Adrenocorticotropic hormone; corticotropin	Stimulates adrenocortical growth and secretion
Growth hormone (GH)	Somatotropin (STH)	Accelerates body growth
FSH	Follicle-stimulating hormone	Stimulates growth of ovarian follicle and estrogen secretion in the female and spermatogenesis in the male
LH	Luteinizing hormone (in the female); interstitial cell-stimulating hormone, ICSH (in the male)	Stimulates ovulation and luteinization of ovarian follicles in the female and production of testosterone in the male
Prolactin	Mammotropin, lactogenic hormone	Stimulates synthesis of milk
MSH	Melanocyte-stimulating hormone	Stimulates melanocytes causing pigmentation
Neurohypophysis (posterior lobe)		
Antidiuretic hormone (ADH)	Vasopressin	Promotes water retention by way of the renal tubules and stimulates smooth muscle of blood vessels and digestive tract
Oxytocin		Stimulates release of milk and contraction of smooth muscle in the uterus

From Jacob, S. W., C. A. Francone, and W. J. Lossow: *Structure and Function in Man,* 4th ed. Philadelphia: W. B. Saunders Co., 1978.

growth hormone on growth are thought to be due to its stimulation of the synthesis and release of somatomedins. The other four hormones stimulate the "target" glands governed by the pituitary (thyroid, adrenals, gonads), thereby *indirectly* influencing body growth, structure, and function as well as intellectual and sexual development. As you have learned in earlier chapters, the "target glands" depend upon the stimulation of the pituitary gland to synthesize their own hormones. If stimulation is excessive and too much of one pituitary hormone is released, the "target" gland involved becomes overactive in response; e.g., too much adrenocorticotropic hormone from the pituitary stimulates the adrenal cortex to hypertrophy and produce excessive amounts of cortisol, thereby causing Cushing's disease. Conversely, if pituitary production of one or more hormones is inadequate, the target gland which depends upon that hormone for stimulation becomes hypoactive in response; e.g., insufficient production of adrenocortical-stimulating hormone (ACTH) can cause secondary adrenocortical insufficiency. When one considers the powerful influence of the anterior pituitary directly upon other glands and therefore indirectly upon the body as a whole, it is no wonder that the pituitary gland is often described as the "master gland."

If the pituitary controls growth as well as the activities of other glands, what then controls the pituitary? To help answer that question, review Figure 74–8. Note that the hypothalamus lies above the pituitary and is connected to the master gland by the hypophyseal (pituitary) stalk. The hypothalamus continuously receives or monitors information regarding the internal milieu and the external world via the nervous system. In turn, the hypothalamus transmits these messages to the pituitary gland via the release of peptide hormones into the portal blood stream that flows from the hypothalamus to the pituitary.

Disorders of the pituitary gland predominantly develop in the anterior lobe. Major causes of pituitary disease include (a) functioning tumors, (b) nonfunctioning tumors, (c) pituitary infarction, (d) genetic disorders, and (e) trauma. The three principal pathologic consequences of pituitary disorders are (1) hyperpituitarism, (2) hypopituitarism, and (3) local compression of brain tissue by expanding tumor masses.

Disorders of the Anterior Lobe

Hyperpituitarism. Hyperpituitarism is defined as the oversecretion of one or more of the hormones secreted by the pituitary gland. The major cause of hyperpituitarism is a *secreting pituitary tumor,* which is typically a benign adenoma. More specifically, there are three major types of pituitary tumors, each of which represents an overgrowth of one of the basic cell types composing the anterior pituitary gland, i.e., eosinophils, basophils, and chromophobes. Important characteristics of each type of tumor are as follows:

- *Eosinophilic tumor:* a secreting tumor which produces excessive amounts of growth hormone (GH) and possibly prolactin (LTH). Eosinophilic tumors tend to develop in males who are between the ages of 20 and 50. Although they are rarely malignant, these benign adenomas can produce gigantism in children and acromegaly in adults.
- *Basophilic tumor:* a secreting tumor which can produce excessive amounts of adrenocortical-stimulating hormone (ACTH), thyroid-stimulating hormone (TSH), follicle-stimulating hormone (FSH), luteinizing hormone (LH), and possibly melanocyte-stimulating hormone (MSH). Typically only ACTH is synthesized in excessive amounts. As you recall, excessive secretion of ACTH by the pituitary causes *Cushing's disease.* Like the eosinophilic tumors, basophilic tumors are rarely malignant.
- *Chromophobe tumor:* most common of the pituitary tumors. This benign adenoma may or may not secrete hormones. Secreting chromophobe tumors probably elaborate ACTH and growth hormone, thereby causing hyperpituitarism. On the other hand, nonsecreting tumors may cause hypopituitarism by growing so large in size that they eventually obliterate the pituitary gland (see Hypopituitarism.)

Pituitary tumors produce both systemic effects and local manifestations. *Systemic* effects include (a) excessive or abnormal growth patterns (due to overproduction of growth hormone), and/or (b) overstimulation of one (or more) of the target glands, which results in the release of excessive thyroid, sex, or adrenocortical hormones. *Locally,* pituitary tumors produce symptoms because the bony cranium which houses the tumor cannot expand to accommodate a growing space-occupying mass. Local manifestations include blindness due to pressure on the optic chiasma, headaches, and somnolence.

Major disorders arising from hypersecretion of one or more of the pituitary hormones include the following:

- *Gigantism and acromegaly:* Both of these disturbances of growth arise from an oversecretion of *growth hormone* (GH). Gigantism, which is an overgrowth of the *long bones,* develops in *children* before the age at which the epiphyses of the bones close. Individuals suffering gigantism may grow as tall as 8 or 9 feet. On the other hand, *acromegaly* is a disease of *adults* which develops following *closure* of the epiphyses of the long bones. As implied by its name, acromegaly (*acro* is the Greek word element for "extremity") is marked by both increases in bone thickness and hypertrophy of the soft tissues. Victims of full-blown acromegaly have a grotesque appearance; note in Figure 74–9 the gradual coarsening of the patient's features over the years, as well as the prognathism (protrusion of the jaw), wide hands, and broad, spadelike fingers which characterize the final stages of the disease. In addition, persons with acromegaly de-

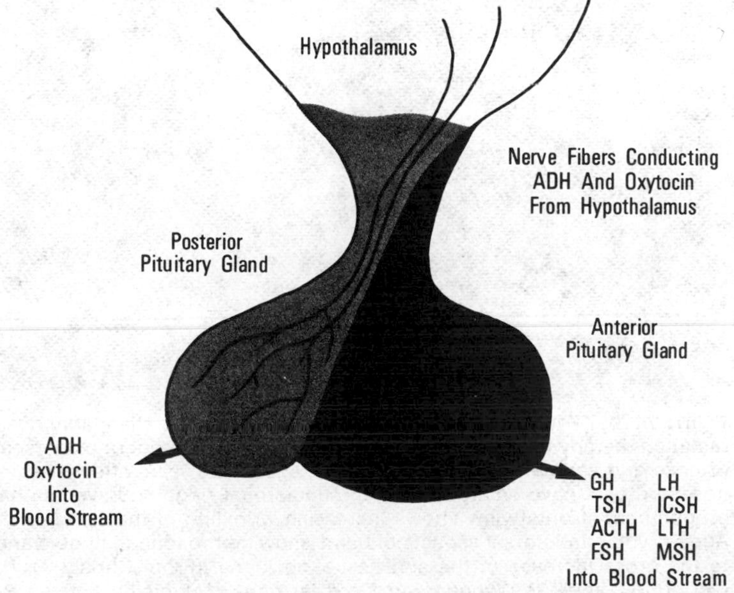

Figure 74–8. The relationship between the hypothalamus and the pituitary gland. The posterior pituitary gland (neurohypophysis) stores antidiuretic hormone (ADH) and oxytocin. The anterior pituitary gland (adenohypophysis) secretes hormones to stimulate growth (GH), the adrenal cortex (ACTH), ovarian follicles (FSH), corpus luteum (LH), testicular interstitial cells (ICSH), milk production (LTH), and melanocytes (MSH). (From Snively, W. D., and D. R. Beshear: *Textbook of Pathophysiology.* Philadelphia: J. B. Lippincott Co., 1972, p. 184.)

velop local manifestations due to compression of brain tissues by the causative tumor; e.g., headache, diplopia, blindness, and lethargy. In far-advanced cases, victims may suffer from associated hormonal disturbances, e.g., diabetes mellitus, goiter, Cushing's disease, disturbances of libido, and menstrual disorders. The treatments of choice for both gigantism and acromegaly are either surgical hypophysectomy or supervoltage irradiation of the pituitary. Prognosis depends upon the age at which oversecretion of GH develops and is diagnosed. Obviously, because many of the somatic changes are irreversible, the earlier the problem is discovered, the more likely the patient is to benefit from therapy.

- *Cushing's disease:* As you recall, Cushing's disease is one form of Cushing's syndrome. It results from oversecretion of ACTH by a basophilic tumor, which in turn results in the oversecretion of adrenocortical hormones.

- *Sexual disturbances:* Excess secretion of gonadotropic hormones from pituitary tumors produces sexual precocity in children. Excess prolactin secretion causes amenorrhea/galactorrhea in women. Treatment of choice is surgical removal of the tumor. Patients with increased prolactin secretion and no evidence of a pituitary tumor often respond to treatment with bromo-ergokryptine, an ergot-like compound.

Hypopituitarism. In contrast to hyperpituitarism, *hypopituitarism* is a *deficiency* of one or more of the hormones produced by the anterior lobe of the pituitary. When both the anterior *and* posterior lobes are failing to secrete hormones, the condition is referred to as *panhypopituitarism.*

The five important *causes* of hypopituitarism are as follows:

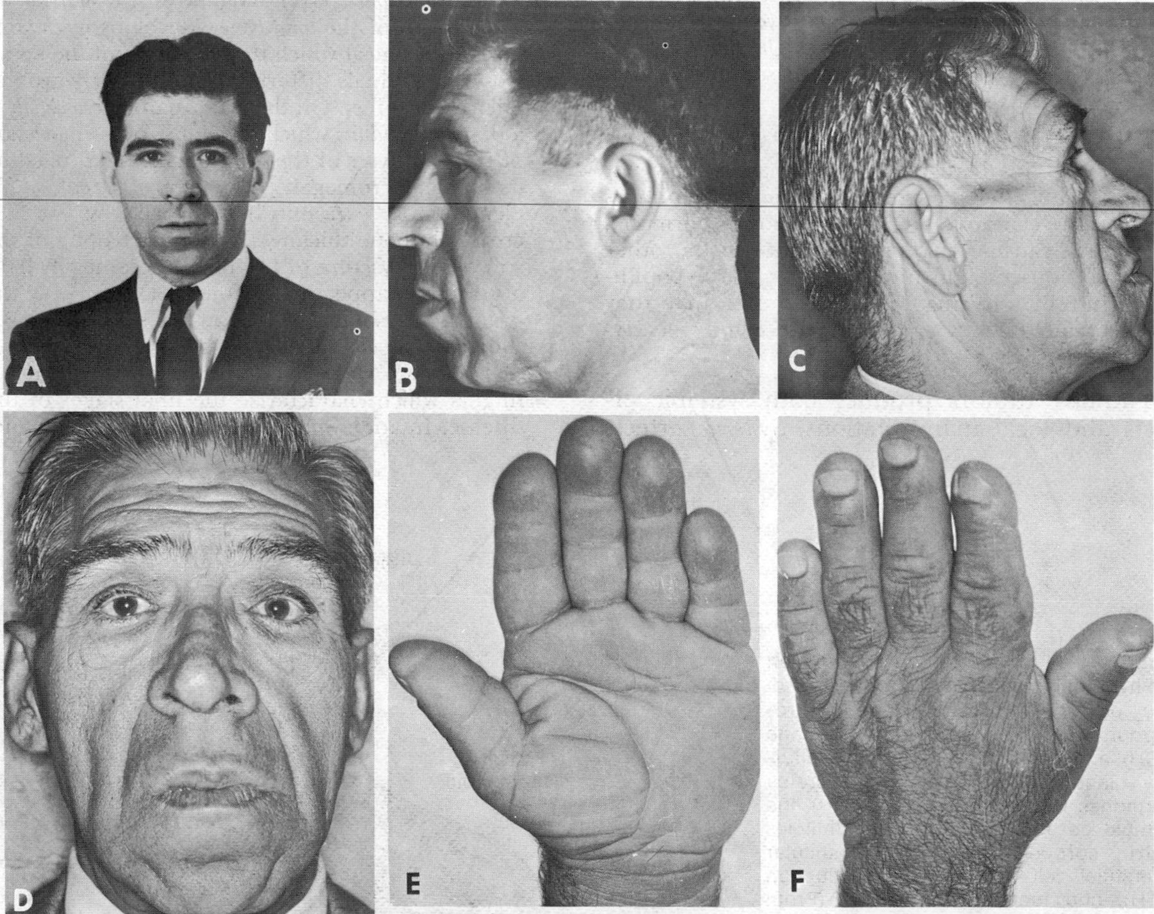

Figure 74–9. Evolution of acromegaly. *A,* Age 38, within a year after onset of the disease. *B,* Age 55, after two courses of radiation therapy to sella; disease has progressed with moderate coarsening of features: thickening of lips, enlargement of nose and ears, and prognathism. *C, D,* Age 64, 26 years after onset, after a third series of x-ray treatments to sella; nose and ears have enlarged further, supraorbital ridge and zygoma have become more prominent, and jaw is more prognathous, frontal view shows increasing wrinkling of the skin (temporary atrophy is a result of x-irradiation). *E, F,* Age 64, volar and dorsal aspects of hand, showing broadened fingers and characteristically "meaty" appearance owing to the gross increase in the soft tissue, not bone. (From Christy, N. P.: The anterior pituitary. *In* Beeson, P. B., W. McDermott, and J. B. Wyngaarden: *Cecil Textbook of Medicine,* 15th ed. Philadelphia: W. B. Saunders Co., 1979, p. 2107.)

- *Hypophysectomy* (removal or destruction of the pituitary): This procedure is sometimes performed as a palliative measure for persons with diabetic retinopathy or cancer of the breast.
- *Nonsecreting pituitary tumors:* There are two types of nonsecreting pituitary tumors which cause hypopituitarism: the *nonfunctioning chromophobe adenoma* and the *craniopharyngioma.* Because these tumors expand and therefore occupy space, they eventually compress and obliterate pituitary tissues, thereby diminishing the secretion of pituitary hormones.
- *Pituitary dwarfism:* When a child is born with a deficiency of growth hormone he will become dwarfed in stature, unless he is given injections of human growth hormone. Victims of *hypophyseal dwarfism* are normally proportioned and have normal intelligence.
- *Postpartum pituitary necrosis:* Hypopituitarism can develop following postpartum hemorrhage and circulatory collapse. The fall in blood pressure following the baby's delivery evidently causes necrosis of the gland due to tissue anoxia.
- *Functional disorders:* Functional hypopituitarism develops whenever the pituitary gland is inadequately nourished. Causes of this problem include starvation, anorexia nervosa, severe anemia, and gastrointestinal tract disorders which reduce the absorption of nutrients.

Because of the pituitary's enormous functional reserve, manifestations of hypopituitarism usually do not appear until almost 75 per cent of the pituitary has been obliterated by tumors, thromboses, and so forth. Symptoms depend upon the age at onset of the disorder as well as upon the hormones which are deficient. Specific disorders resulting from pituitary hyposecretion include the following:

- *Dwarfism:* Severely stunted growth results from either (a) congenital lack of growth hormone, or (b) the development of space-occupying intracranial tumors, meningitis, or brain injury during early childhood. Dwarfism, if diagnosed early, can be successfully treated with injections of human growth hormone. Unfortunately human growth hormone is currently available for only a few patients. Methods of commercially producing synthetic growth hormone are under investigation.

  Secondary adrenocortical insufficiency: Adrenocortical insufficiency can follow diminished synthesis of ACTH by the pituitary gland, which in turn causes diminished secretion of adrenocortical hormones by the adrenal cortex.
- *Myxedema:* Because the synthesis of thyroid hormone is dependent upon the production of thyroid stimulating hormone (TSH) by the pituitary, therapeutic ablation or pathologic destruction of the pituitary can cause myxedema unless the patient is treated with thyroid hormone (see Chapter 73).
- *Sexual and reproductive disorders:* Deficiencies of the gonadotropins (LH and FSH) can produce sterility, diminished sexual drive, and decreased secondary sexual characteristics. Women who suffer from lessened FSH and LH synthesis develop infertility and amenorrhea. Men who lack FSH and LH experience diminished spermatogenesis and testicular atrophy. The hypogonadism which follows hypophysectomy or destruction of the pituitary gland by disease leads to permanent sterility which cannot be corrected by hormonal replacement therapy.

The *treatment* of hypopituitarism is based upon (a) removal, if possible, of the causative factor (e.g., tumors), and (b) permanent replacement of the hormones secreted by the target organs.

Drugs used for hormonal replacement include (a) corticosteroids for correction of secondary adrenocortical insufficiency, (b) thyroid hormone for treatment of myxedema, and (c) sex hormones to correct hypogonadism. To date, tropic hormones are seldom used because of their expense and ineffectiveness when used on a long-term basis. Also, as stated earlier, human growth hormone (HGH) is used to correct hypophyseal dwarfism.

Disorders of the Posterior Lobe (Neurohypophysis)

Unlike the adenohypophysis, the neurohypophysis is rarely destroyed by disease. Even if the posterior lobe becomes damaged or is surgically destroyed along with the anterior lobe, hormonal deficiencies do not develop because oxytocin and ADH continue to be synthesized by the hypothalamus. On the other hand, if the hypothalamus is damaged, deficiencies of oxytocin and ADH will develop even if the neurohypophysis is healthy and intact.

The major posterior lobe disorder is *ADH deficiency* (diabetes insipidus). In addition, inappropriate secretion of ADH may occur in conjunction with lung cancer, head injuries, pituitary tumors, encephalitis, poliomyelitis, and myxedema. Oxytocin imbalances have not been documented; for further information concerning oxytocin, consult an obstetrics textbook.

Diabetes Insipidus. Diabetes insipidus, like diabetes mellitus, is characterized by the passage of excessive amounts of urine. However, the urine of patients with diabetes mellitus contains large amounts of sugar, whereas the urine in diabetes insipidus is highly dilute and contains no sugar. The fundamental cause of diabetes insipidus is a *deficiency* of *antidiuretic hormone*

(*ADH*). You recall from Chapter 12, that the major functions of ADH are to: (a) promote water reabsorption by the kidney, and (b) control the osmotic pressure of the extracellular fluid. Thus, when ADH production decreases excessively, water is *not* reabsorbed by the kidney tubules, and consequently the stricken individual secretes large amounts of dilute urine.

Causes of ADH deficiency are categorized in the following way:[73]

A. *Vasopressin deficiency*
   1. The hypothalamus and pituitary gland are defective due to familial or idiopathic causes (primary diabetes insipidus).
   2. The gland is destroyed by tumors in the hypothalamopituitary region, trauma, infectious processes, vascular accidents, or metastatic tumors from the breast or lung (secondary diabetes insipidus).

B. *"Nephrogenic" diabetes insipidus:* Due to an inherited defect, the kidney tubules are unable to reabsorb water. Also this condition may develop secondary to potassium depletion or pyelonephritis.

Diabetes insipidus may arise slowly, or it may appear suddenly following injury or infectious disease.

> *The two major manifestations of diabetes insipidus are polyuria and polydipsia.*

The patient may drink and excrete from 5 to 40 liters of fluid per day! Because it is so dilute, the urine has a low specific gravity of between 1.001 and 1.006 (normal:1.003 — 1.030). Unless the patient continues to drink fluid almost continuously, he is in danger of developing severe dehydration and hypovolemic shock.

Persons with diabetes insipidus often benefit from treatment with the *benzothiadiazine diuretics,* either alone or in combination with the sulfonylurea chlorpropamide. Individuals with diabetes insipidus secondary to a known causative factor (e.g., a tumor) may be cured by *surgical resection* of the tumor.

The symptoms of hypothalamic diabetes insipidus can also be controlled in most cases by the administration of *vasopressin tannate* (Pitressin tannate). Pitressin typically alleviates polyuria and usually polydipsia for 24–72 hours.

> *When administering vasopressin tannate, always shake the bottle well before drawing up the drug to ensure adequate suspension of the hormone in the oil.*

In addition to parenteral preparations, posterior pituitary hormone or related synthetic analogs are also available in the form of a *snuff* which the patient can inhale two or three times daily. The snuff is sometimes irritating to the nasal mucosa.

Syndrome of Inappropriate Antidiuretic Hormone (SIADH). The syndrome of inappropriate antidiuretic hormone is quite the opposite of diabetes insipidus. Rather than having large fluid losses, patients with SIADH may have water intoxication due to the retention of fluid. As previously mentioned, the cause of SIADH may vary; however, the syndrome is seemingly becoming more common, especially among patients critically ill from other causes. Some of the factors which affect ADH secretion are summarized in Table 74–6.

Under normal circumstances the osmolality of the serum is regulated by ADH; when the serum osmolality falls, a feedback mechanism causes the inhibition of ADH. This promotes increased excretion of water by the kidneys in order to raise the serum osmolality to normal. When this feedback mechanism fails, and ADH levels are sustained, there is fluid retention. Ultimately, the serum sodium falls, resulting in hyponatremia and water intoxication. Central nervous system dysfunction, characterized by alterations in level of consciousness, seizures,

TABLE 74–6. FACTORS AFFECTING ADH SECRETION

Factors which increase ADH secretion:

A. Increased plasma osmolality and decreased blood volume
   1. Hemorrhage
   2. Decreased cardiac output
   3. Dehydration
   4. Hypoalbuminemia
B. Limbic stimulation
   1. Pain
   2. Fear
   3. Major trauma
C. Pharmacologic agents
   1. Nicotine
   2. Morphine
   3. Barbiturates
   4. General anesthetics
   5. Beta-adrenergic agents
   6. Clofibrate (Atromid S.)
   7. Vincristine
   8. Cyclophosphamide (Cytoxan)
   9. Carbamazepine (Tegretol)
   10. Chlorpropamide

Factors which decrease ADH secretion:

A. Ethanol
B. Diphenylhydantoin
C. Hypoosmolality
D. Beta-adrenergic agents
E. Morphine antagonists
F. Total body immersion
G. Hypervolemia

From Kubo, W. M., and M. M. Grant: The syndrome of inappropriate secretion of antidiuretic hormone. *Heart and Lung,* 7:469, May-June, 1978.

and coma may become evident when the serum sodium is 120 mEq/ liter or less.

The treatment of SIADH includes fluid restriction, replacement of sodium chloride, diuretics, demeclocycline (a tetracycline that increases free water clearance), and treating the cause if possible.

The nursing care of patients prone to develop SIADH includes: (a) accurate and frequent monitoring of fluid balance, (b) daily taking of weights, (c) careful and frequent assessment of neurological status, (d) positioning the head of the patient so that it is flat or raised no more than 5° , unless contraindicated because of the possibility of developing or worsening of cerebral edema (e.g., neurosurgical patients). The rationale for positioning the patient flat is that receptors in the atrium which are sensitive to changes in volume, and which stimulate ADH secretion when volume is decreased, are not stimulated by this position. In addition, assessment of gastrointestinal function is important. Hyponatremia may result in diminished GI function, and this is further complicated by the need for fluid restriction. Cathartics or low volume, hyperosmolar fluid enemas may be indicated in selected patients. Tap water or saline enemas are generally contraindicated because the fluid may be absorbed from the bowel and contribute to water intoxication.

Nursing Care of the Patient Undergoing Hypophysectomy

Partial or complete ablation of the pituitary gland is performed for the following reasons:

- To slow the growth and expansion of endocrine-dependent malignant neoplasms of the breast and ovaries.
- To halt the advance of diabetic retinopathy (see Chapter 72).
- To correct Cushing's disease (which is caused by a pituitary tumor).

Methods used for ablating the pituitary gland include (a) yttrium-90 implantation, (b) irradiation, (c) cryohypophysectomy (destruction of the pituitary by the use of extreme cold), (d) pituitary coagulation with radiofrequency, (e) transphenoidal microsurgical hypophysectomy, and (f) total or partial surgical removal of the gland.

Surgical removal of the pituitary is a frightening prospect for patients and their families because it involves manipulation of tissues near the brain. Consequently it is essential to provide the patient with emotional support and comfort throughout the preoperative period. Let the patient know what he can expect to experience following surgery. Tell him that his vital signs will be checked frequently immediately following the operation. Advise him that he will have an indwelling catheter and an I.V. needle in his arm, and his head may be wrapped in dressings which may feel tight and uncomfortable; also his eyes may be swollen and black due to ecchymosis.

On the day prior to surgery, the patient usually receives his first injection of cortisol. A glucocorticoid is given to help the patient better endure an operation which will result in loss of adrenocortical function. Also at this time the patient's head is prepared for brain surgery according to the surgeon's instructions. Usually it is necessary to shave only a small area at the front of the head.

Postoperative care following hypophysectomy performed through a cranial approach is similar to that done for any craniotomy (see Chapter 28). Immediately following surgery, remember to check for the signs of cerebral edema and rising intracranial pressure (elevated blood pressure, low pulse rate, pupil changes). Also, because tropic hormones are no longer being produced, watch for signs of target gland deficiencies, e.g., adrenal insufficiency and hypothyroidism. In addition, the patient may temporarily suffer from diabetes insipidus due to ADH deficiency. Finally, observe the patient carefully for the signs of *meningitis* — a complication of brain surgery. Report any elevation of temperature, severe headache, irritability, and so forth.

Drug replacement of cortisone is started during surgery and is continued in replacement doses for the rest of the individual's life. Some patients may also require thyroid hormone replacement as well as the administration of sex hormones. Also, a few patients will require posterior pituitary hormone replacements to control polyuria. It is a major nursing responsibility to educate the patient who has undergone hypophysectomy in the technique of safe self-administration of hormones. Also, because of the many hormonal imbalances which can potentially develop due to hypophysectomy, be certain to advise the postoperative patient to obtain a medical check-up at least every 6 months and whenever symptoms of imbalance appear.

BIBLIOGRAPHY (Unit XIX)

1. American Diabetes Association, Inc.: *Recognition and Care of Hypoglycemic Reactions.* New York: ADA, 1977.
2. American Diabetes Association, Inc.: *The Effective Application of "Exchange Lists for Meal Planning."* New York: ADA, 1977.

3. An insulin they just can't resist. *Emergency Medicine*, 10:240, Oct. 1978.
4. Arky, R. A.: Diet and diabetes mellitus. Concepts and objectives. *Postgraduate Medicine*, 63:72, June 1978.
5. Ashkar, F. S.: A better outlook in thyroid cancer. *Consultant*, 12:148, Jan. 1972.
6. Asimov, I.: *Words of Science and the History Behind Them*. New York: New American Library, 1969.
7. Askew, G. B., and K. I. Letcher: Oral hypoglycemic agents. *Nursing '75*, 5:45, Aug. 1975.
8. Aurbach, D. G.: Parathyroid. *In* Beeson, P. B., W. McDermott, and J. B. Wyngaarden (Eds.): *Cecil Textbook of Medicine*, 15th ed. Philadelphia: W. B. Saunders Co., 1979.
9. Bacchus, H. (Ed.): *Metabolic and Endocrine Emergencies. Recognition and Management*. Baltimore: University Park Press, 1977.
10. Bavli, S. Z., and P. R. Larsen: Hyperthyroidism. *In* Conn, H. F. (Ed.): *Current Therapy*. Philadelphia: W. B. Saunders Co., 1978.
11. Bennett, M.: *The Peripatetic Diabetic*. New York: Hawthorne Books, Inc., 1961.
12. Berg, D. L. (Ed.): Insulin defect in adult diabetes reversed with I.V. "aspirin." *RN*, 40:28, Sept. 1977.
13. Blankenship, G. W., and J. S. Skyler: Diabetic retinopathy: A general survey. *Diabetes Care*, 1:127, Mar.-Apr. 1978.
13a. Boyd, W.: *An Introduction to the Study of Disease*, 5th ed. Philadelphia: Lea and Febiger, 1962.
14. Boyd, W., and H. Sheldon: *An Introduction to the Study of Disease*, 7th ed. Philadelphia: Lea and Febiger, 1977.
15. Brown, J. R.: New approach to diabetic coma. *Consultant,* 16:190, Sept. 1976.
16. Bruce, G. L.: The Somogyi phenomenon: Insulin-induced posthypoglycemic hyperglycemia. *Heart and Lung*, 7:463, May-June 1978.
17. Bruhn, J. G.: Self-concept and the control of diabetes. *American Family Physician*, 15:93, Mar., 1977.
18. Burke, E. L.: Insulin injection: The site and technique. *American Journal of Nursing*, 72:2194, Dec. 1972.
19. Caplan, R. H.: Answers to questions on "disguised" hyperthyroidism. *Hospital Medicine*, 14:51, Oct. 1978.
20. Carozza, V.: Ketoacidotic crisis: Mechanism and management. *Nursing '73,* 3:13, May 1973.
21. Chandler, P. T.: An update on reactive hypoglycemia. *American Family Physician*, 16:113, Nov. 1977.
22. Chandler, P. T.: Diabetic foot care. Problems and practical suggestions. *Postgraduate Medicine*, 60:59, Dec. 1976.
23. Chandler, P. T.: Diabetic vascular disease: An update. *Consultant*, 19:43, June 1979.
24. Cherner, R.: 10 pitfalls to avoid in managing diabetic ketoacidosis. *Consultant*, 17:21, Jan. 1977.
25. Christy, N. P.: Diseases of the endocrine system: General considerations. *In* Beeson, P. B., and W. McDermott, (Eds.): *Cecil-Loeb Textbook of Medicine*, 14th ed. Philadelphia: W. B. Saunders Co., 1975.
26. Cooperman, D., and W. B. Malarkey: Pituitary apoplexy. *Heart and Lung*, 7:450, May-June 1978.
27. Cox, M.: Diabetes insipidus. *In* Conn, H. F. (Ed.): *1978 Current Therapy*. Philadelphia: W. B. Saunders Co., 1978.
27a. Crampton, J. H., et al.: *Instructions for the Diabetic Patient,* 9th ed. Seattle: The Mason Clinic, 1966.
28. Daniels, G. H.: Simple (nontoxic) goiter. *In* Conn, H. F. (Ed.): *1978 Current Therapy*. Philadelphia: W. B. Saunders Co., 1978.
29. DeGroot, L. J.: Diseases of the thyroid. *In* Beeson, P. B., W. McDermott, and J. B. Wyngaarden (Eds.): *Cecil Textbook of Medicine*, 15th ed. Philadelphia: W. B. Saunders Co., 1979.
30. DeJong, R. N.: CNS manifestations of diabetes mellitus. *Postgraduate Medicine,* 61:101, Jan, 1977.
31. deShazo, R. D.: Insulin allergy and insulin resistance. Two immunologic reactions. *Postgraduate Medicine*, 63:85, Jan. 1978.
32. Diabetic ketoacidosis. *Emergency Medicine*, 5:103, Feb. 1973.
33. Drash, A. L.: Managing the child with diabetes mellitus — Practical aspects. *Postgraduate Medicine*, 63:85, June 1978.
34. Ellenberg, M.: Evaluating sexual impairment in your diabetic patients today. *Consultant,* 19:125, April 1979.
35. Engelman, K.: The adrenal medulla and sympathetic nervous system. *In* Beeson, P. B., W. McDermott, and J. B. Wyngaarden (Eds.): *Cecil Textbook of Medicine*, 15th ed. Philadelphia: W. B. Saunders Co., 1979.
36. *Exchange Lists for Meal Planning*. Pamphlet. American Diabetes Association, Inc., and The American Dietetic Association, 1976.
37. Fagan, J. E., and R. G. McArthur: Maximizing diabetic control in children — An improved method for monitoring. *Postgraduate Medicine*, 63:58, Feb. 1978.
38. Feldman, J. M.: The practical use of thyroid function tests. *American Family Physician*, 16:159, Sept. 1977.
39. Feustel, D. E.: Nursing students' knowledge about diabetes mellitus. *Nursing Research,* 76:4, Jan.-Feb. 1976.
40. Finby, N., et al.: Diabetic osteopathy of the foot and ankle. *American Family Physician*, 14:90, Sept. 1976.
41. For diabetes, a return to innocence. *Emergency Medicine*, 11:24, Sept. 1979.
42. Frantz, A., et al.: Pituitary workup: When, why, and how. *Patient Care,* 12:80, Nov. 1978.
43. Fredlund, P. N., and R. S. Mecklenburg: Acute adrenal insufficiency: Diagnosis and management. *Hospital Medicine*, 15:28, June 1979.
44. French, R. M.: *Nurses' Guide to Diagnostic Procedures*, 4th ed. New York: McGraw-Hill Book Co., 1975.
45. Frykberg, R. G., and G. P. Kozak: Neuropathic arthropathy in the diabetic foot. *American Family Physician*, 17:105, May 1978.
46. Garber, R.: The use of standardized teaching program in diabetes education. *Nursing Clinics of North America*, 12:375, Sept. 1977.
47. Garofano, C.: Deliver facts to help diabetics plan parenthood. *Nursing '77*, 7:13, April 1977.
48. Garofano, C.: Travel tips for the peripatetic diabetic. *Nursing '77*, 7:44, Aug. 1977.
49. Gerich, J. E.: Diabetic control and the late complications of diabetes. *American Family Physician*, 16:85, Aug. 1977.
50. Gerich, J. E.: Somatostatin. *American Family Physician*, 15:149, Mar. 1977.
51. Gillies, D. A., and I. Barrett: Caring for patients with thyroid disorders: How good are your skills? *Nursing '77*, 7:71, Oct. 1977.
52. Gold, E. M.: Hypothalamic-pituitary function tests. *Postgraduate Medicine*, 62:105, Nov. 1977.
53. Goldner, M.: Diabetes mellitus in the adult. *In* Conn, H. F. (Ed.): *1978 Current Therapy*. Philadelphia: W. B. Saunders Co., 1978.
54. Gross, R. C.: Emergency management of diabetes mellitus and hypoglycemia. *In* Warner, C. G. (Ed.):

Emergency Care Assessment and Intervention, 2nd ed. St. Louis: C. V. Mosby Co., 1978.
55. Guimond, J. H., and S. G. Wilson: Postirradiation thyroid disorders. *American Journal of Nursing*, 79:1256, July 1979.
56. Guthrie, D. W.: Exercise, diets and insulin for children with diabetes. *Nursing '77* 7:48, Feb. 1977.
57. Guthrie, D. W., and R. A. Guthrie: DKA — Breaking a vicious cycle. *Nursing '78*, 8:52, June 1978.
58. Hallal, J. C.: Thyroid disorders. *American Journal of Nursing*, 77:418, Mar. 1977.
58a. Haunz, E. A.: Diabetes mellitus in adults. *In Current Therapy, 1973*. Conn, H. F. (Ed.): Philadelphia: W. B. Saunders Co., 1973.
59. Hite, A. F., and J. P. Humphrey: How to spot the vicious cycle of insulin "rebound." *RN*, 42:44, July 1979.
60. Hunter, D. J.: Normoglycemia: Essential in pregnant diabetic women. *Consultant*, 17:162, Nov. 1977.
61. In diabetes, screen for UTI. *Emergency Medicine*, 10:196, June 1978.
62. James, R. C., and D. W. Guthrie: 1 out of 20 will develop diabetes. *A Guide to the Better Understanding of Diabetes Mellitus for Patients and Their Families*. Columbia, Mo.: University of Missouri Medical Center and the Veterans Administration Hospital, 1973.
63. Kaufmann, S. J.: In diabetic diets, realism gets results. *Nursing '76*, 6:75, Nov. 1976.
64. Kent, S.: Is diabetes a form of accelerated aging? *Geriatrics*, 31:140, Nov. 1976.
65. Kern, E. B., et al.: A transseptal, transsphenoidal approach to the pituitary. *Postgraduate Medicine*, 63:97, June 1978.
66. Khokhar, N.: Inappropriate secretion of antidiuretic hormone. *Postgraduate Medicine*, 62:73, Oct. 1977.
67. Kissebah, A. H.: Management of hyperlipidemia in diabetes. *American Family Physician*, 19:144, Apr. 1979.
68. Kolin, M.: A third diabetic shock syndrome. Hyperosmolar hyperglycemic nonketotic coma. *Journal of Emergency Nursing*, 3:19, Jan. Feb. 1977.
69. Konishi, F.: *Exercise Equivalence of Foods*. Carbondale, Ill.: Southern Illinois University Press, 1973.
70. Kozak, G. P.: Primary adrenocortical insufficiency (Addison's disease). *American Family Physician*, 15:124, May 1977.
71. Kozak, G. P., et al.: Diabetic neuropathies. *American Family Physician*, 15:112, April 1977.
72. Krieger, D.: Cushing's syndrome. *In* Conn, H. F. (Ed.): *1978 Current Therapy*. Philadelphia: W. B. Saunders Co., 1978.
73. Krupp, M. A., and M. J. Chatton: *Current Medical Diagnosis and Treatment*. Los Altos, Calif.: Lange Medical Publications, 1978.
74. Kubo, W. M., and M. M. Grant: The syndrome of inappropriate antidiuretic hormone. *Heart and Lung*, 7:469, May-June 1978.
75. Lavine, R. L.: How to recognize . . . and what to do about . . . hypoglycemia. *Nursing '79*, 9:52, Apr. 1979.
76. Liddle, G. W.: Adrenal cortex. *In* Beeson, P. B., W. McDermott, and J. B. Wyngaarden (Eds.): *Cecil Textbook of Medicine*, 15th ed. Philadelphia: W. B. Saunders Co., 1979.
77. Liechty, R. D., and R. T. Soper: *Synopsis of Surgery*, 3rd ed. St. Louis: C. V. Mosby Co., 1976.
78. Macaron, C., and L. Yuk-Pui: What not to do in pheochromocytoma. *American Family Physician*, 17:120, Apr. 1978.
79. Marshall, M. D., Jr., and B. Weintraub: Hypothyroidism. *In* Conn, H. F. (Ed.): *1978 Current Therapy*, Philadelphia: W. B. Saunders Co., 1978.
80. Martin, P.: It is ketoacidosis. *Journal of Emergency Nursing*, 3:11, Jan.-Feb. 1977.
80a. Matovinovic, J.: Simple goiter. *In* Conn, H. F. (Ed.): *Current Therapy, 1973*. Philadelphia: W. B. Saunders Co., 1973.
81. McConnell, E. A.: Meeting the special needs of diabetics facing surgery. *Nursing '76*, 6:30, June 1976.
82. McFarlane, J.: Congenital adrenal hyperplasia. *American Journal of Nursing*, 76:1290, Aug. 1976.
83. McKenna, T. J.: Acute adrenal insufficiency. *Hospital Medicine*, 12:77, June 1976.
84. Meloni, R. C.: Obesity or Cushing's disease? *American Family Physician*, 5:93, June 1972.
85. Miller, E. C.: Diabetic emergencies. *American Family Physician*, 18:115, Sept. 1978.
86. Myers, S. A.: Diabetes management by the patient and a nurse practitioner. *Nursing Clinics of North America*, 12:415, Sept. 1977.
87. Newmark, S. R.: Axioms on hyperthyroidism. *Hospital Medicine*, 13:6, Nov. 1977.
88. Newton, D. W., et al.: Corticosteroids. *Nursing '77*, 7:26, June 1977.
89. Nickerson, D.: Teaching the hospitalized diabetic. *American Journal of Nursing*, 72:935, May 1972.
90. O'Connor, M. L.: Glucose tolerance test. How you can make it more reliable. *Nursing '75*, 5:10, July 1975.
91. O'Dorisio, T. M.: Hypercalcemic crisis. *Heart and Lung*, 7:425, May-June 1978.
92. Palumbo, P. J.: How to treat maturity-onset diabetes mellitus. *Geriatrics*, 32:57, Dec. 1977.
93. Peake, R.: Thyroiditis. *In* Conn. H. F. (Ed.): *1978 Current Therapy*. Philadelphia: W. B. Saunders Co., 1978.
94. Peters, P. C., and J. M. Gazak: Guide to detection and management of genitourinary tumors in children. *Hospital Medicine*, 14:58, Dec. 1978.
95. Petrlik, J. C.: Diabetic peripheral neuropathy. *American Journal of Nursing*, 76:1794, Nov. 1976.
96. Petrokas, J. C.: Commonsense guidelines for controlling diabetes during illness. *Nursing '77*, 77:36, Dec. 1977.
97. Porter, S. F.: Diabetic education: A role for the inservice instructor. *Supervisor Nurse*, 8:49, May 1977.
98. Prescribing high fiber. *Emergency Medicine*, 11:29, Sept. 1979.
99. Prout, T. E.: The use of screening and diagnostic procedures: The oral glucose tolerance test. *In* Sussman, K. E., and R. J. S. Metz (Eds.): *Diabetes Mellitus*, 4th ed. New York: American Diabetes Association, 1975.
100. Raiti, S.: Endocrine causes of short stature. *Postgraduate Medicine*, 62:81, Dec. 1977.
101. Rancillio, N.: When a pregnant woman is diabetic: Postpartal care. *American Journal of Nursing*, 79:453, Mar. 1979.
102. Randall, R. V.: Acromegaly. *In* Conn, H. F. (Ed.): *1978 Current Therapy*. Philadelphia: W. B. Saunders Co., 1978.
103. Reichlin, S.: The control of anterior pituitary secretion. *In* Beeson, P. B., W. McDermott, and J. B. Wyngaarden (Eds.): *Cecil Textbook of Medicine*, 15th ed. Philadelphia: W. B. Saunders Co., 1979.
103a. Robbins, S. L., and M. Angell: *Basic Pathology*, 2nd ed. Philadelphia: W. B. Saunders Co., 1976.
104. Robbins, S. L., and R. C. Cotran: *The Pathologic Basis of Disease*. Philadelphia: W. B. Saunders Co., 1979.
105. Rosenberg, I. N.: Euthyroid Graves's disease. *The New England Journal of Medicine*, 226:223, Jan. 1977.
106. Rosenthal, H., and J. Rosenthal: *Diabetic Care in Pic-*

tures, 4th ed. Philadelphia: J. B. Lippincott Co., 1968.

107. Ryan, A. J.: Diabetes and therapeutic self-control. *Postgraduate Medicine*, 65:23, Feb. 1979.
108. Schneeberg, N. G.: Hyperparathyroidism: Early diagnosis now possible. *Consultant*, 19:58, Jan. 1979.
109. Schulz, J. M., and M. Williams: Encouragement breeds independence in the blind diabetic. *Nursing '76*, 6:19, Dec. 1976.
110. Schumann, D.: Assessing the diabetic. *Nursing '76*, 6:62, Mar. 1976.
111. Schumann, D.: Doing it better: Tips for improving urine-testing techniques. *Nursing '76*, 6:23, Feb. 1976.
112. Scribner, B. H. (Ed.): *Teaching Syllabus for the Course on Fluid and Electrolyte Balance*, 7th revision. Seattle: University of Washington School of Medicine, 1969.
113. Seltzer, H. S.: Urinary glucose tests: A consumer's guide. *Diabetes Forecast*, 30:25, May-June 1977.
114. Shen, S. W., and R. Bressler: Clinical pharmacology of oral antidiabetic agents. *New England Journal of Medicine*, 296:787, Apr. 1977.
115. Singer, F. R.: Hyper- and hypoparathyroidism. *In* Conn. H. F. (Ed.): *1978 Current Therapy*. Philadelphia: W. B. Saunders Co., 1978.

115a. Sjoerdsma, A.: Sympatho-adrenal system. *In* Beeson, P. B., and W. McDermott (Eds.): *Cecil-Loeb Textbook of Medicine*, 13th ed. Philadelphia: W. B. Saunders Co., 1971.

115b. Spencer, R. T.: *Patient Care in Endocrine Problems.* Saunders Monograph in Clinical Nursing — 4. Philadelphia: W. B. Saunders Co., 1973.

116. The hypoglycemia dilemma. *Emergency Medicine*, 9:133, Dec. 1977.

116a. Tattersall, R. B., and D. A. Pyke: Diabetes in identical twins. *Lancet*, 2:1120–1125, 1972.

117. Travis, L. B.: *An Instructional Aid on Juvenile Diabetes Mellitus*, 4th ed. Galveston, Tex.: University of Texas Medical Branch, 1975.
118. Tzagournis, M.: Hypoglycemia: Be sure. *Consultant*, 16:59, Nov. 1976.
119. U 100 Insulin. *Nursing Clinics of North America*, 8:369, June 1973.
120. Urbanic, R. C., and E. L. Mazzaferri: Thyrotoxic crisis and myxedema coma. *Heart and Lung*, 7:435, May-June, 1978.
121. Van Herle, A. J.: Thyroid gland malignancies. *In* Conn, H. F. (Ed.): *1978 Current Therapy*. Philadelphia: W. B. Saunders Co., 1978.
122. Weathering thyroid storm. *Emergency Medicine*, 11:74, Sept. 1979.
123. Williams, R. H.: *Textbook of Endocrinology*, 5th ed. Philadelphia: W. B. Saunders Co., 1974.
124. Williams, S. R.: *Nutrition and Diet Therapy*, 3rd ed. St. Louis: C. V. Mosby Co., 1977.
125. Wimberley, D.: When a pregnant woman is diabetic: Intrapartal care. *American Journal of Nursing*, 79:451, Mar. 1979.
126. Witt, K.: HHNK — A newly recognized syndrome to watch for. *Nursing '76*, 76:66, Feb. 1976.
127. Zonana, J., and D. L. Rimoin: Current concepts in genetics: Inheritance of diabetes mellitus. *New England Journal of Medicine*, 295:603, Sept. 1976.

UNIT XX*

NURSING PEOPLE EXPERIENCING DISTURBANCES OF MUSCULOSKELETAL FUNCTION

INTRODUCTION AND STUDY GUIDE

Caring for people experiencing musculoskeletal disorders requires a team approach directed at identifying and meeting individual patient needs, preventing complications, and minimizing any disabling effects. Nurses caring for patients with these disorders not only must be familiar with the anatomy and physiology of bones and muscles but also must be knowledgeable about which nerves and blood vessels are located near specific bones and the muscles they supply. Such knowledge is essential to identifying nerve and blood vessel injuries which may coincide with musculoskeletal injuries or which can develop as a complication of treatment procedures, e.g., casting.

Surgical treatment of bone, muscle, and joint disorders may involve the combined efforts of an orthopedic surgeon, a vascular surgeon, a neurosurgeon, and a plastic surgeon. For example, in the treatment of an open (compound) fracture, in which the broken bone protrudes through the skin, the orthopedic surgeon realigns the bone, while a vascular surgeon may reconstruct the limb's blood supply. A neurosurgeon may also be necessary if the broken bone has torn or otherwise severely traumatized nearby nerves. A fractured or dislocated limb may be correctly realigned and heal without deformity, but the limb will be useless if its nerve supply is not restored, and it will be lost if it is not adequately perfused with blood. Amputation may be necessary if a dislocated knee is not reduced early, because the arterial blood supply may be irreparably compromised. The successful reimplantation of extremities which are traumatically severed is sometimes possible with the coordinated efforts of a surgical team. A plastic surgeon may also participate, e.g., by performing necessary skin grafting, cosmetic surgery, or hand surgery.

Advances are constantly being made in the diagnosis and treatment of musculoskeletal disorders. It is now possible to perform endoscopic examination of some joints, e.g., the knee, by inserting an instrument (arthroscope) through which the interior of the joint can be visualized and photographed. A porous ceramic material ("ceramic bone") is being tested for possible use in the surgical replacement of bone. Experiments are being made to determine whether heating fractured bones hastens the healing

*Colleen F. Johnson, R.N., critically reviewed and assisted in the revision of this unit.

process.[75] Recently it has become possible to totally replace hips, knees, and elbows which are seriously damaged, e.g., because of arthritic or degenerative changes. Silicone joint implants can also be made in the hands or feet to replace diseased or destroyed joints. New and innovative materials have made casted extremities more adaptable for mobilization and use, e.g., the "waterproof casts."

Musculoskeletal disorders may cause short-term or long-term periods of illness. However, with the exception of simple uncomplicated injuries, many musculoskeletal problems are of a chronic nature that require long-term care. Rehabilitative care may be implemented by a team consisting of doctors and nurses specializing in physical medicine, as well as a physical therapist, occupational therapist, social worker, psychiatrist, and prosthetist (a specialist who constructs and applies prostheses). Spiritual help is obtained according to an individual patient's expressed preferences. Nurses who specialize in orthopedic care are active in providing patient care in clinics and hospitals. Community health nurses bring nursing care into the home setting when appropriate.

Some patients require several surgical procedures. Pain, immobility, and changes in self-image often cause patients with musculoskeletal disorders to become discouraged and depressed. Patients may be hospitalized for extended periods of time, putting additional stress on family and social structures. Patients may develop guilt feelings because of this. Because of prolonged contact with patients, nurses can frequently be of assistance during periods of distress and can help keep hope and motivation at high levels. Occupational therapy not only helps patients occupy time meaningfully during recovery-rehabilitation periods but also enables patients with musculoskeletal disorders to improve or maintain muscle strength, coordination, and dexterity. Successful rehabilitation is not possible without careful planning and scheduling of activities. Rehabilitation cannot be a haphazard process which one simply "hopes" will occur.

It is necessary for nurses to have some "mechanical know-how" and knowledge of basic physics. Of necessity, orthopedic settings contain a multitude of equipment. In addition to the equipment routinely found on hospital wards (e.g., dressings, catheters, gloves, medications, bath basins, linens), orthopedic wards commonly require special linens and an abundance of pillows, cushions, sandbags, padding, binders, elastic bandages, elastic stockings, and tape. Other equipment includes:

- *Casting equipment,* e.g., casting materials, cast dryer, cast cutter, cast spreader
- *Bracing and splinting equipment,* e.g., leg braces, padded foot splints, Velcro splints
- *Traction equipment,* e.g., metal bars, ropes, pulleys, weights, and appropriate halters and belts
- *Transfer equipment,* e.g., sliding board, mechanical lift, overhead sling, Davis roller
- *Recreational equipment* for occupational therapy
- *Transportation equipment,* e.g., wheelchairs, crutches, canes, walkers, stretchers

Because musculoskeletal disorders affect the locomotor and structural systems of the body, they often make it difficult for the affected individuals to support themselves and move about. It is therefore necessary for orthopedic settings to be amply equipped with devices to help patients, e.g., handrails in the hallways, grab bars by toilets. Mirrors in hallways help patients observe their posture and walking habits and learn correct habits. Special frames (e.g., Foster frame, Stryker frame) or CircOlectric beds are sometimes employed to more effectively care for a patient with a musculoskeletal impairment (See Unit X for discussions of special frames, CircOlectric beds, and wheelchairs.)

Similarities exist between some neurologic disorders (see Unit X) and some musculoskeletal disorders. For example, both can cause impairment or loss of body motion; both are commonly long-term illnesses; and both require prevention of the complications of immobility in their treatment and extensive rehabilitative services.

Impaired or lost musculoskeletal abilities must be regained or compensated for whenever possible. Orthopedic nurses patiently assist patients working to regain musculoskeletal function, e.g., to bend the knees, to use fingers, to stand up and walk. It is difficult to be dependent and unable to move. Relearning processes are time-consuming. However, learning musculoskeletal activities can take place only if the patient is given the supervised opportunity to "try" alone. These patients take a lot of time to care for and may require additional nurses and physical therapists. It is imperative that patients have confidence in persons caring for them and that accidents, e.g., falls, be prevented. As in any setting, nurses must constantly be safety conscious. Also, when handling or supporting a patient who has a musculoskeletal disorder, nurses need to remember to (1) be gentle, (2) provide adequate support, and (3) avoid sudden movements. Handle the patient as carefully as you can. Also, always keep in mind positions and movements which are contraindicated for a specific patient. Careless or contraindicated movements or positioning may cause unnecessary pain, tissue trauma, and the disruption of delicate bone, nerve, or blood vessel healing processes. Once you cause a patient unnecessary or unexpected discomfort, it is difficult (perhaps impossible) to regain his or her confidence. To assist most effectively a disabled person (e.g., to sit up, walk, get into bed), offer help from the person's affected side. You can thus best contribute to the person's strength and you will avoid traumatizing affected tissues, e.g., by grasping or pulling on them.

The successful orthopedic nurse is a good teacher who helps a patient and significant others learn about the condition and its treatment. Additionally, the nurse teaches the patient how to live most effectively with the disorder during the recovery-rehabilitation period of illness. The patient is helped to understand and correctly use and care for equipment which is to be part of self-care. Also, the patient is helped to accept a need for the equipment and the benefits of using assistive devices. Assistive devices used on or by a patient should (1) help, not hinder, the patient; (2) be physiologically tolerated; (3) permit function with reasonable body alignment; and (4) be cosmetically as acceptable as possible. In situations in which assistive devices may be permanently necessary, e.g., wearing of a brace, or when a patient must adapt to permanent cosmetic deformity, it may take a substantial period of time for the patient to adjust to changes in body image. In the home setting, a community health nurse may work with the patient and significant others to help the patient continue to return to or maintain a maximum level of function and to make necessary adaptations in the home environment.

The nurse caring for patients with disorders of bones, joints, and muscles must be highly observant and diligently attentive to details of patient care. *Much orthopedic nursing care is of a preventive nature.* Activities of special importance include:

- Maintaining proper body alignment during periods of bedrest to promote correct posture and the return of effective balance once bedrest is no longer needed.
- Performing or supervising range-of-motion exercises to maintain joint mobility and other exercises to maintain muscle strength.
- Ensuring correct positioning and support to prevent ischemia, nerve damage, muscle spasms, contractures, atrophy, and other deformities, e.g., foot drop. While deformities may be easily prevented, often they are extremely difficult or impossible to correct. Support must be given to painful, weak, or casted body areas.
- Performing periodic neurovascular checks to observe for indications of nerve or circulatory impairment.
- Giving frequent skin care to prevent skin breakdown.

- ▶ Checking traction set-ups to be certain that traction is being correctly applied.
- ▶ Observing indications of special complications, e.g., fat embolism, shock lung. Observing patients in casts for indications of complications, e.g., infection, pressure.
- ▶ Assisting with ambulation and other self-care activities.
- ▶ Relieving pain.

As discussed previously, because many patients with musculoskeletal disorders are limited in their ability to move or to support themselves, nurses often help with positioning and transporting activities. Nurses on the orthopedic service must practice good body mechanics or they may injure themselves while performing assistive services. Casts and braces can be very heavy, thus adding to a patient's total weight and easily throwing him or her off balance.

This unit consists of four chapters. Chapter 75 presents a brief overview of musculoskeletal anatomy and physiology and musculoskeletal disorders. Chapter 76 focuses on diagnostic procedures used to investigate the musculoskeletal system and clinical problems and therapeutic measures common with musculoskeletal disorders. In Chapter 77 musculoskeletal injuries are discussed. The final chapter, Chapter 78, presents other musculoskeletal disorders. Neuromuscular disorders and spinal and skull injuries and their treatment are discussed in Unit X. Amputations are discussed in Unit XV. Mandibular fractures are considered in Chapter 60 of Unit XVII and fractures of the ribs in Unit XVI.

Objectives

After carefully studying the material presented in this unit along with additional study suggested, you can expect to be able to:

1. Demonstrate a thorough and accurate understanding of the anatomy and physiology of the musculoskeletal system.
2. Understand the basic elements of patient history, physical examination, and diagnostic procedures of people experiencing musculoskeletal problems.
3. Appreciate the physical and psychosocial stress experienced by people who have musculoskeletal problems or disorders.
4. Understand the purposes and processes of various therapeutic measures used in the treatment of musculoskeletal problems.
5. Support patients skillfully and sensitively throughout medical and/or surgical procedures in such a way that patient comfort is maximized and potential complications are avoided.
6. Observe patients for the signs and symptoms of musculoskeletal and neurovascular complications and interpret such observations accurately and appropriately.
7. Know the usual clinical care, surgical treatment and biomechanical procedures appropriate for musculoskeletal problems.
8. Communicate relevant and accurate information concerning anatomy and physiology, pathology, diagnostic procedures, treatment regimes, and rehabilitative processes to patients and their significant others.
9. Plan, with the assistance of a professional nurse, personalized nursing care with people experiencing musculoskeletal problems.

Study Guide

Answering the following *study questions* and performing the activities suggested below will help you achieve the objectives of this unit.

I. On separate blank cards (or small pieces of paper) define each of the following terms as you study the unit. Use the completed cards for review purposes.

abduction
adduction
amphiarthroses
ankylosis
arthritis
arthrodesis
arthrograms
arthroplasty
arthroscope
arthrotomy
articular
bursa
bursitis
Bryant's traction
"cast syndrome"
closed reduction
compound fracture
crutch palsy
diarthroses
dislocation
eversion
extension
fat embolism
flexion
fracture
genu varus
genu valgus
haversian system
internal fixation
inversion
kyphosis
laminograms
lordosis
lupus erythematosus
multiple myeloma
"muscle splinting"
myositis
open reduction
orthopedics
osteoblasts
osteomalacia
osteomyelitis
osteoporosis
periarteritis nodosa
pronation
scleroderma
scoliosis
simple fracture
sprain
strain
striated muscle
subluxation
supination
synarthroses
synovectomy
synovial fluid
synovitis
tendon
tendinitis
tomograms
Volkmann's ischemic contracture

II. Answer the following questions:

1. Where does hematopoiesis occur in the bones?
2. Where is yellow marrow located in bones?
3. How can flexion contractures be prevented?
4. What are some physiologic benefits of heat, cold, and massage in the treatment of musculoskeletal disorders?
5. What is the difference between active and passive exercises?
6. During correct usage of crutches, where should the patient's weight rest, i.e., on the handbars or axillary bars of the crutches?
7. What are the "Five P's" and what is their significance in the care of patients with postoperative or casted extremities?
8. What is the difference between skin traction and skeletal traction?
9. What are the symptoms of fat embolism?
10. Why is it important to prevent external rotation of the hip following hip surgeries such as pinnings or arthroplasties?

III. Perform the following activities:

1. Use a textbook of nursing fundamentals (for example, Sorensen and Luckmann, *Basic Nursing: A Psychophysiologic Approach*) to review (1) basic principles of body mechanics, (2) basic techniques for lifting and moving patients and assisting with ambulation, (3) principles of bandaging and massage, (4) range-of-motion exercises and hot and cold applications, (5) principles of a therapeutic nurse-patient relationship, and (6) the effects of stress and a change in body image on a person.
2. Identify the major bones of the upper and lower extremities. While studying the unit, review individual bones, muscles, and other anatomic structures as necessary. Give examples of a hinge joint, ball and socket joint, and gliding joint.
3. Review the evaluation of pain and clinical care of patients in pain as discussed in Unit XI. Also, review as necessary Units VIII and IX and Sections One and Two of this text.
4. Use a textbook of pharmacology to review medications used in the treatment of musculoskeletal disorders, e.g., muscle relaxants, analgesics.
5. Review the following diets: (1) high-protein, (2) high-vitamin, and (3) low-purine.

6. List some specific effects of prolonged musculoskeletal pain on bones, muscles, tendons, and joints.
7. List some physiologic effects of heat, cold, massage, and exercises.
8. Summarize general observations of importance when inspecting a patient's traction set-up.
9. List potential complications which may occur postoperatively following orthopedic surgery.
10. Identify factors of importance in first aid for a fracture victim. (See also Chapter 95.)
11. Summarize factors of importance in the clinical care of patients with the following disorders: (1) fractured femur, (2) cancer of the bone, (3) rheumatoid arthritis, (4) gout, and (5) collagen diseases.

CHAPTER 75

INTRODUCTORY CONCEPTS

OVERVIEW OF NORMAL ANATOMY AND PHYSIOLOGY OF THE MUSCULOSKELETAL SYSTEM

This chapter is not intended as a detailed review of the normal structure and function of the musculoskeletal system. Our summary in outline form will help orient you to material presented in this unit. Consult textbooks of anatomy and physiology for additional detail as required.

I. *Musculoskeletal System:* Includes bones, joints, muscles, and related connective tissue. Can be divided into (1) skeletal system (bones), (2) articular system (joints), and (3) muscular system (muscles).

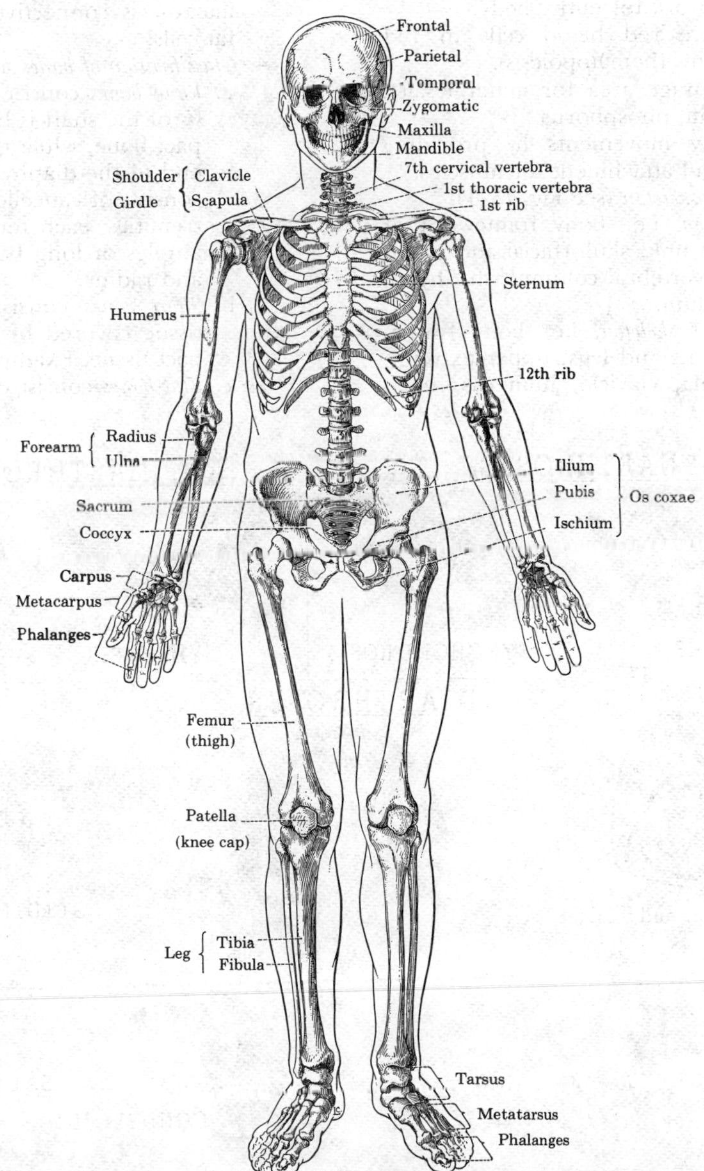

Figure 75–1. Anterior view of human skeleton. (From *Dorland's Illustrated Medical Dictionary*, 25th ed. Philadelphia: W. B Saunders Co., 1974.)

A. *Skeletal System.* Bone tissue is nourished by the *haversian system,* a network of minute canals traversed with blood vessels. Bone tissue is constantly being created and reabsorbed. The rate of activity of these two processes (i.e., the *deposition* of new bone by osteoblasts and the *reabsorption* of bone) determines skeletal bone size and strength.
   1. *Functions* of the skeleton (a joined framework of 206 bones).
      a. Protect vital organs and other soft tissues.
      b. Support surrounding tissues and serve as a framework for entire body.
      c. Manufacture red blood cells in red bone marrow (hematopoiesis).
      d. Provide storage area for mineral salts, e.g., calcium, phosphorus.
      e. Assist body movements by providing leverage and attachment for muscles.
   2. *Divisions of the skeleton* (see Fig. 75–1).
      a. *Axial skeleton,* i.e., bony framework of head and trunk: skull (facial and cranial bones); vertebral column; ribs, hyoid bone; sternum.
      b. *Appendicular skeleton,* i.e., bony framework of arms and legs: upper extremities (scapula, clavicle, humerus, ulna, radius, hand, i.e., carpals, metacarpals, phalanges); lower extremities (pelvic bone, femur, patella, tibia, fibula, foot, i.e., tarsals, metatarsals, and phalanges).
   3. *Histology of bone.* Histologically bone is of two types: (1) *compact,* i.e., strong and dense with closely spaced lamellae (concentric layers of mineral deposits); or (2) *cancellous,* i.e., spongy in appearance with more widely spaced lamellae. Between layers of lamellae are small cavities, i.e., *"lacunae."* Suspended in tissue fluid within each lacuna is an *osteocyte,* busy making new bone. Osteocytes are mature, bone-forming cells. *Red marrow,* which has a hematopoietic function (manufactures red and white blood cells), is located in the spaces of cancellous bone. *Yellow marrow* occurs within the shafts of long bones and extends into the haversian systems. Yellow marrow is connective tissue composed of fat cells.
   4. *Classification of bones* according to shape.
      a. *Long bones* consist of a *shaft* (the *diaphysis* of the shaft is basically made of compact bone, while the flared part at each end of the diaphysis, i.e., the *metaphysis,* consists of cancellous bone) and two extremities, each termed an *epiphysis.* Examples of long bones are the humerus and radius.
      b. *Short bones* consist of cancellous bone tissue covered by a thin layer of compact tissue. Examples: carpals, tarsals.
      c. *Flat bones* consist of cancellous bone en-

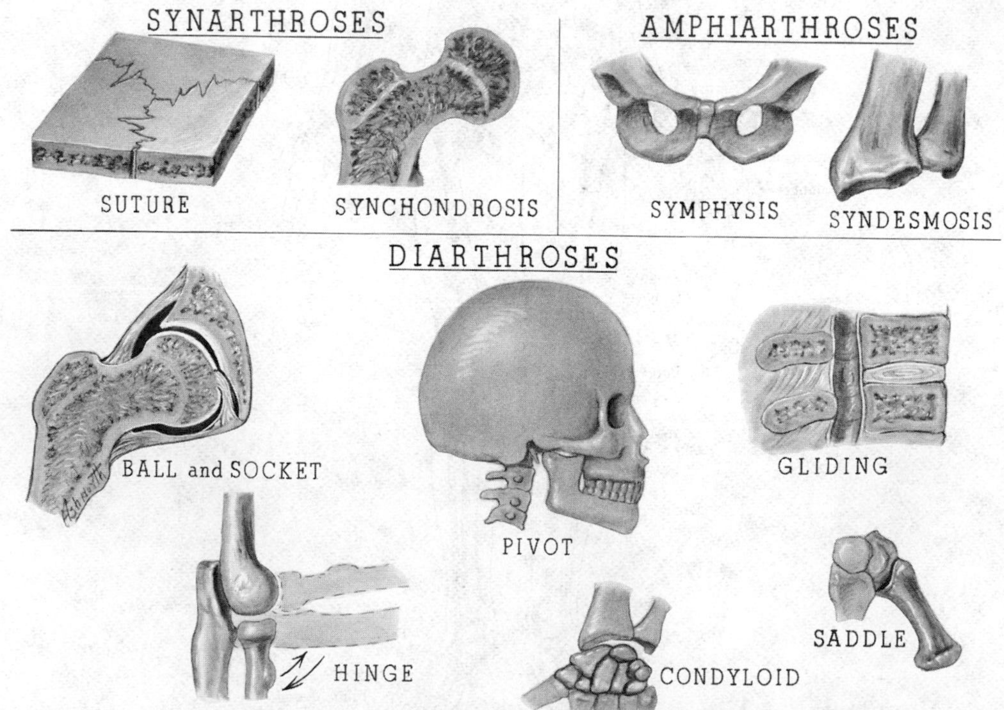

Figure 75–2. Joints are categorized into three groups, according to the degree of movement permitted. Each of these groups is, in turn, subdivided with respect to the structural components of individual joints. (From Jacob, S. W., C. A. Francone, and W. J. Lossow: *Structure and Function in Man,* 4th ed. Philadelphia: W. B. Saunders Co., 1978.)

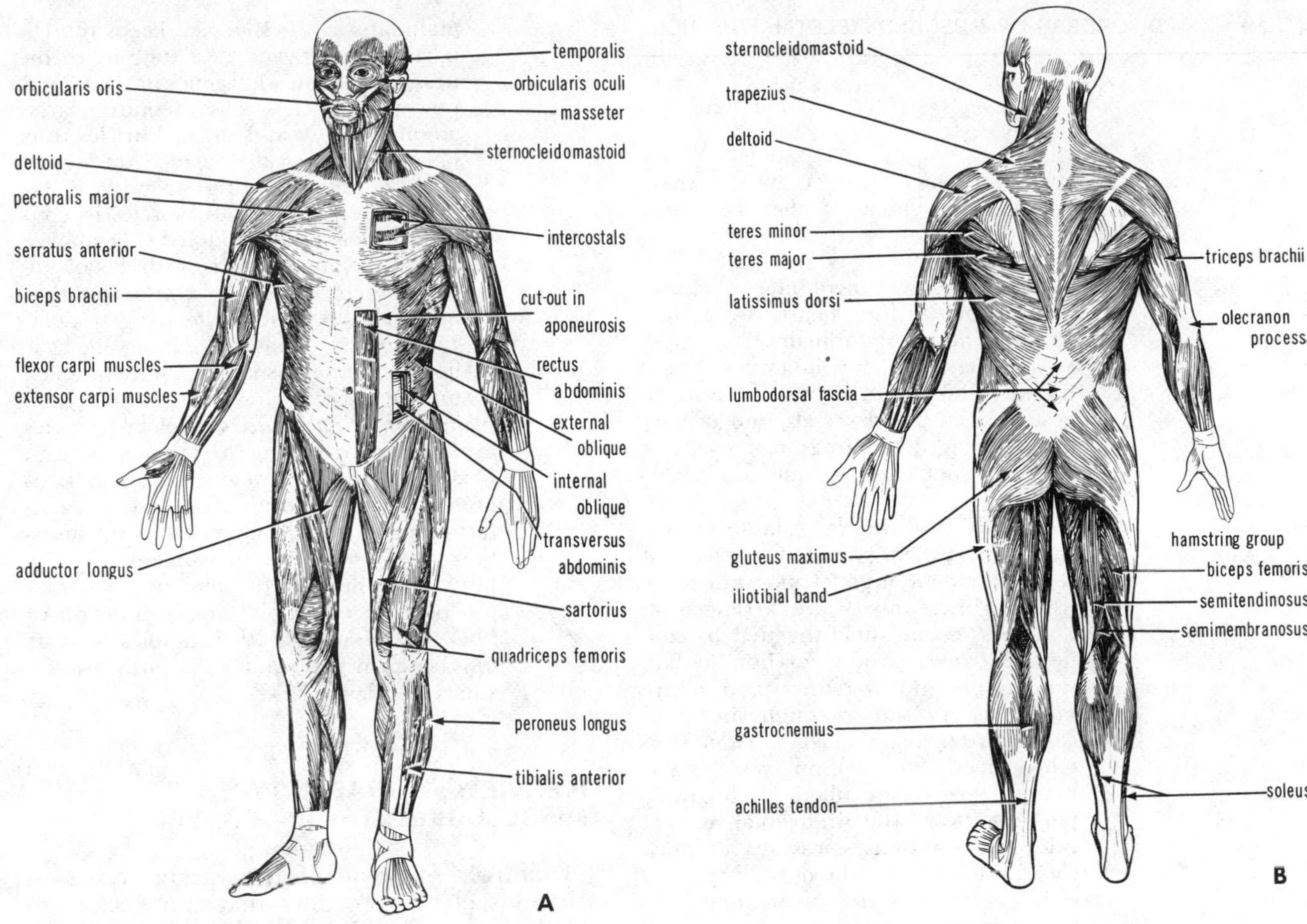

Figure 75–3. Principal muscles. **A.** Anterior view. **B.** Posterior view. (From Memmler, R. L., and R. B. Rada: *The Human Body in Health and Disease,* 3rd ed. Philadelphia: J. B. Lippincott Co., 1970.)

cased in two flat plates of compact bone. Flat bones protect soft body parts or provide large surfaces for muscle attachments, e.g., ribs, skull, scapula, portions of pelvic girdle.

d. *Irregular bones* are of differing peculiar shapes, e.g., vertebrae, ossicles of the ear. Irregular bones are similar in structure and composition to other groups of bones.

e. *Sesamoid bones* are small, rounded bones located adjacent to joints and encased in tendon and fascial tissue, e.g., patella ("knee cap"). Sesamoid bones increase the lever-function of muscles.

B. *Articular System.* Articulations, i.e., joints, are places of union of two or more bones. Movement does not necessarily occur at such junctions.

1. *Groups of joints.* Categorized according to the degree of movement permitted (see Fig. 75–2).

a. *Synarthroses:* no movement, e.g., suture joints of the skull and the temporary cartilage connection between the epiphysis and diaphysis of long bone (replaced by bone with maturation).

b. *Amphiarthroses:* slight movement, e.g., pubic symphysis and connection of ligaments where radius articulates with ulna.

c. *Diarthroses* (synovial joints): freely movable to permit changes of position and motion. Consist of (1) an articular cavity (lined with synovial membrane which produces synovial fluid for joint lubrication and cartilage nourishment) enclosed by a capsule of fibrous articular cartilage; (2) ligaments reinforcing the capsule and helping to limit motion; and (3) cartilage covering the ends of opposing bones (cartilage makes a smooth surface so bone ends can glide over one another). Articular disks are located between the articular cartilage of some synovial joints to help buffer forceful impacts. Muscles help stabilize joints and maintain firm contact of articular surfaces. Synovial joints are classified by the shape of the articulating end of the involved bones (see Fig. 75–2 for types of joints).

Some kinds of movements occurring at synovial joints include protraction, retraction, eversion, inversion, flexion, extension, abduction, adduction, rotation, supination, and pronation.

C. *Muscular System:* Muscles make up 40 to 50

per cent of the body's weight. By *contraction* they produce movement of the body as a whole or of its parts.

1. *Types of muscle.*
   a. *Cardiac muscle:* involuntary muscle found only in the heart. Is striated crosswise and longitudinally.
   b. *Smooth muscle:* involuntary muscle found in hollow structures (such as digestive tract, blood vessels, and urinary bladder) and other areas, e.g., eye. Not striated. Controlled by autonomic nervous system.
   c. *Striated (skeletal) muscle:* voluntary muscle of the skeletal system. Composed of combination of muscle and connective tissue. Muscle fibers are arranged in bundles *(fasciculi)* held together by connective tissue. Groups of bundles are similarly bound together, and entire muscle is encased in tough sheath of connective tissue. The *muscle sheath* contains blood and lymph vessels and nerve fibers. Nerve fibers (each supply perhaps over 100 individual muscle cells) carry impulse-messages to muscles. Endings of motor nerve fibers are called *motor end plates or myoneural junctions.* A continuous flow of stimuli maintains *muscle tone,* i.e., keeps muscle partially contracted in a state of readiness for action. To generate heat and power, muscle cells require large amounts of O_2 and sugar. Muscles thus have a rich *vascular supply.* An *"oxygen debt"* develops during exercise if O_2 cannot be delivered to muscles in concentrations great enough to metabolize accumulations of lactic acid. Following exercise, increased O_2 consumption is necessary to relieve the oxygen debt. *Tendons* (i.e., bands of strong inelastic fibrous tissue) usually indirectly attach muscle to bone.
2. *Individual skeletal muscles.* Skeletal muscles are named according to (1) action, e.g., flexor, extensor; (2) shape, e.g., quadrilateral, pennate; (3) origin, i.e., stationary attachment of muscle to skeleton; (4) insertion, i.e., movable attachment of the muscle; (5) number of divisions, e.g., "tri", (6) location, e.g., tibia; or (7) direction of fibers, i.e., transverse.[126] Examples of some of the principal individual muscles are shown in Figure 75–3.

OVERVIEW OF BASIC TYPES OF MUSCULOSKELETAL DISORDERS

Examples of some of the various types of musculoskeletal disorders that can occur are briefly summarized in the accompanying chart.

Causative Factors	Examples of Disorders
Infection	Osteomyelitis (bone infection); tuberculosis of bones and joints.
Inflammation	Arthritis (joint inflammation); bursitis (bursa inflammation); osteitis (bone inflammation); myositis (muscle inflammation); synovitis (synovial membrane inflammation).
Trauma	Fractures; sprains; strains; dislocations; traumatic arthritis.
Tumors	Multiple myeloma; osteogenic sarcoma; giant-cell tumor; metastatic bone tumors (tumors arising from tissues other than bone).
Degeneration	Osteoarthritis (hypertrophic degeneration of joints).
Neurogenic muscular impairments	Myasthenia gravis and muscular dystrophies (see Unit X).
Metabolic	Arthritis associated with gout; osteoporosis.
Vitamin deficiency	Osteomalacia (vitamin D deficiency in adults results in softening of bones due to impaired calcium and phosphorus metabolism).
Autoimmune	Rheumatoid arthritis; collagen or "connective tissue" diseases (e.g., systemic lupus erythematosus, periarteritis nodosa, scleroderma).
Unknown	Osteitis deformans, i.e., Paget's disease (chronic bone disease characterized by enlargement, softening, and deformity of certain bones).

CHAPTER 76

COMMON MUSCULOSKELETAL DIAGNOSTIC PROCEDURES, CLINICAL PROBLEMS, AND THERAPEUTIC MEASURES

DIAGNOSIS AND ASSESSMENT OF ORTHOPEDIC DISORDERS

ORTHOPEDIC HISTORY

Taking an *orthopedic history* includes gathering information about the onset and course of the presenting problem as well as collecting more general information about the patient. Past history, family history, and social history are also included. Important factors include previous symptoms, onset and duration of present symptoms, progression of symptoms, and extent of disability. Musculoskeletal disorders may produce symptoms of neurologic involvement, deformity, pain, or loss of joint motion. Some musculoskeletal disorders are aggravated by motion of the part, weather change, or weight-bearing. These factors are considered, along with the effect of rest on the ailment. It is important to try to find out not only what aggravates the disorder but also what relieves it. Previous treatments and their effects are carefully scrutinized. A nurse's descriptive charting of symptoms may be helpful in the diagnostic process.

ORTHOPEDIC EXAMINATION

During the orthopedic examination *subjective* physical findings are considered (e.g., tenderness to palpation, presence of muscle weakness) as well as *objective* observations (e.g., signs of redness, and limb lengths and circumferences). Subjective findings may be under the patient's voluntary control; because these findings may be feigned by some patients, subjective findings must be carefully evaluated.[207]

Both a general and a local orthopedic examination may be given. During the *general orthopedic examination,* the examiner inspects general appearance; posture; gait and body mobility; body alignment; body contours; body attitude; carriage; muscle strengths; limb lengths and circumferences; joint motion; cervical, thoracic, and lumbar spines; and the relationships of various body parts to one another, e.g., relationship of feet to legs and hips to pelvis.

While observing a patient's movements and gait, the physician watches for *gait patterns* associated with specific disorders, objective evidence of *discomfort,* evidence of *joint stiffness* or *muscle weakness, lack of coordination,* and *deformities.*

Observation of a patient's stance may reveal *spinal deformities:* (1) *kyphosis,* i.e., abnormally increased roundness of the thoracic curve; (2) *scoliosis,* i.e., an obvious lateral deformity of the spine; and (3) *lordosis,* i.e., abnormal increase in the lumbar curve. Other abnormalities which may be noted are *genu varus,* i.e., "bowed" legs, and *genu valgus,* i.e., "knock-knees" (see Fig. 76–1). (Note: The terms *varus* and *valgus* refer to the direction in which the apex of a deformity lies in relationship to the midline, i.e., in a *varus deformity* the apex of the deformity points away from the midline, while in a *valgus deformity* it points toward the midline. These terms may be used in any body region to describe the direction of a deformity.)

Other deformities that may be detected during orthopedic examinations are (1) equinus and calcaneal deformities of the foot; (2) claw hammer, or mallet toes (see Fig. 76–2); (3) finger deformities, such as mallet finger, boutonniere deformity, swan-neck deformity, or claw-finger deformity. Many orthopedic deformities can be surgically corrected.

The *local orthopedic examination* focuses primarily on the site of the specific complaint. Comparisons are made between the affected and nonaffected sides of the body. For example, if the patient's disorder is in the right arm, the

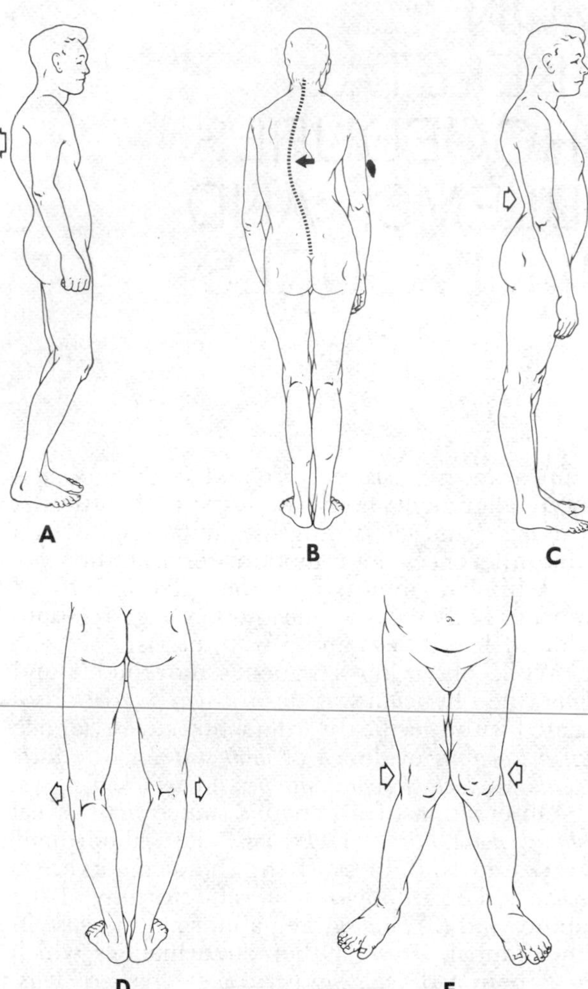

Figure 76–1. A. Kyphosis B. Scoliosis. C. Lordosis. D. Genu varus. E. Genu valgus. (From *Manual of Orthopaedic Surgery.* Chicago: American Orthopaedic Association, 1972.)

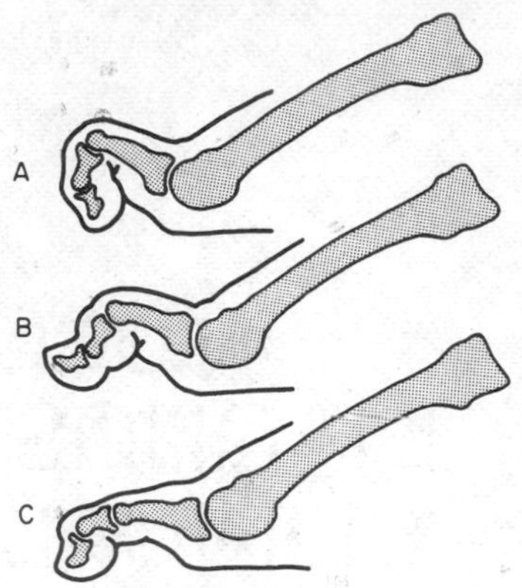

Figure 76–2. Common toe deformities. A, Claw toe; B, hammer toe; C, mallet toe. (From *Manual of Orthopaedic Surgery.* Chicago, American Orthopaedic Association, 1972.)

examiner compares the right arm with the left arm. The local orthopedic examination utilizes inspection and palpation and evaluation of range of motion and joint position. Joint motion is measured in degrees of a circle (see Fig. 76–3). Also, measurements are made (with a tape measure) of limb circumference to identify hypertrophy or atrophy of a part.

Aspects of *neurologic examination* which may be included in the local orthopedic examination are evaluation of (1) the integrity of cutaneous sensation, (2) strength of muscle power, and (3) quality of superficial and deep tendon reflexes.[98] (Assessment of cutaneous sensation and tendon reflexes has been discussed in Unit X.) Two methods of grading muscle power are commonly used. One method is to grade numerically from "0" through "5"; 0 represents the weakest end of the scale, while 5 is the strongest. The second method is to use the following grades (comparable to grades 0–5): (a) zero, (b) trace, (c) poor, (d) fair, (e) good, and (f) normal.

Examination of patients following musculoskeletal trauma is discussed in Chapter 77. Physical and psychosocial assessment is discussed in Chapters 14 and 15.

X-RAY FILMS

Roentgenography is the technique most commonly used to help establish the diagnosis of musculoskeletal disorders. X-ray films are often viewed not only by the attending physician but also by a radiologist. *Anteroposterior* and *lateral* films are commonly ordered. Oblique, notch, and some other views are also useful. Some special x-ray studies which may be used with orthopedic patients include:

- *myelograms* (see Unit X);
- *arthrograms* (see Fig. 76–4), films taken following

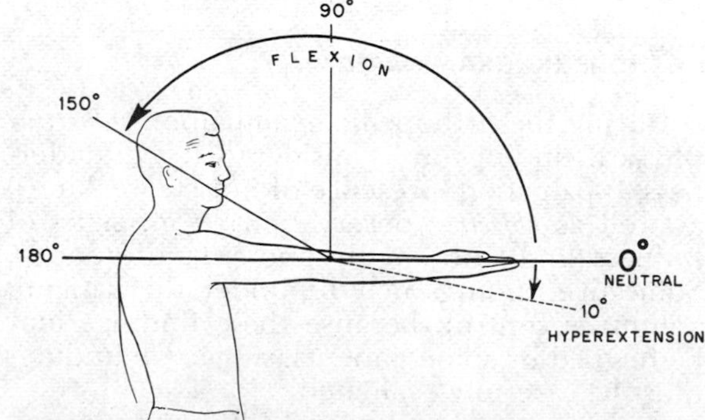

Figure 76–3. Joint motion is measured in degrees of a circle. (From Gartland, J. J.: *Fundamentals of Orthopaedics*, 3rd ed. Philadelphia: W. B. Saunders Co., 1979.)

the injection of radiolucent gases or radiopaque dyes into joints (used to outline masses or soft tissue defects);

- *sinograms,* x-ray films taken after sinuses are injected with radiopaque dyes (to delineate the course of the sinuses and tissues involved);
- *laminograms (planograms),* x-ray films which clarify details of structures which are otherwise hidden by overlying radiopaque bone. Laminography or planography is also called *body section roentgenography.* Special techniques used in this type of roentgenography permit detailed visualization of images of structures which lie in a predetermined plane of tissue, while images of structures lying in other planes are blurred or detail is otherwise eliminated. Body section roentgenography is useful in locating small cavities, foreign bodies, and lesions which are overshadowed by opaque structures;
- *scanography,* a special x-ray technique by which the lengths of long bones can accurately be measured;
- *arteriography,* x-ray films of arteries following injection of radiopaque material into the blood stream, may be performed if an extremity remains pulseless following realignment and stabilization of fractures.

BIOPSY

A biopsy, i.e., *removal and examination of tissue for diagnostic purposes,* may be performed at the time of open surgery or through a special needle or bore which does not necessitate a surgical incision. The latter types are called *aspiration, punch,* or *needle biopsies.* Special needles which may be used for needle biopsies in diagnosing musculoskeletal disorders include the Craig needle for bone and the Vim-Silverman needle for soft tissue lesions. Once tissue is obtained by biopsy, it is histologically examined by a pathologist.

ARTHROSCOPY

As mentioned in the unit introduction, some joints (e.g., knee) may be examined endoscopically by inserting an instrument (*arthroscope*) into them. A trochar is inserted through a small incision and the joint is flushed with normal saline. Trochars are available in two sizes, i,e, a small needle scope and a slightly larger size. Through the 'scope the interior of the knee can be visualized. Photographs of the inside of the joint may also be taken by attaching a camera to the 'scope. Arthroscopy is useful in establishing diagnosis, and in some cases it eliminates the need for open exploratory surgery. Loose bodies may be "sucked out" through the 'scope if they are small. During arthroscopy, aseptic technique must be closely observed. (See Figure 76–5.)

LABORATORY TESTS

Laboratory tests may be employed in orthopedic patients[4] (1) to help establish diagnosis, (2) to preoperatively screen the functional capacity of other body systems, and (3) to monitor various physiologic processes following injury or surgery. *Post-traumatic* and *postoperative* laboratory monitoring is extremely valuable in the prevention or early detection and treatment of complications, e.g., shock, acidosis, alkalosis, dehydration, pulmonary embolism, pulmonary edema. Serial determinations may be made of glucose levels or prothrombin times, and determinations may be made of electrolyte balance, blood volume, and fluid balance. *Preoperative* laboratory studies are discussed briefly later in this chapter.

Diagnostic laboratory tests[4] in orthopedic patients may include analysis of (1) cerebrospinal fluid (to identify infections, neoplasms, and de-

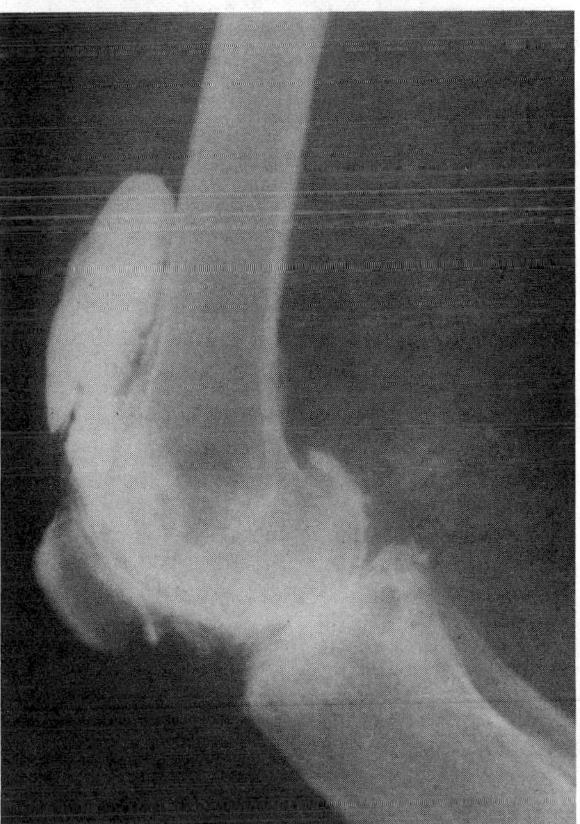

Figure 76–4. Arthrogram of knee showing a large suprapatellar pouch with many nodular filling defects. (From Taylor, A R., and Ansell, B. M.: *Journal of Bone and Joint Surgery,* 54-B:110, 1972.)

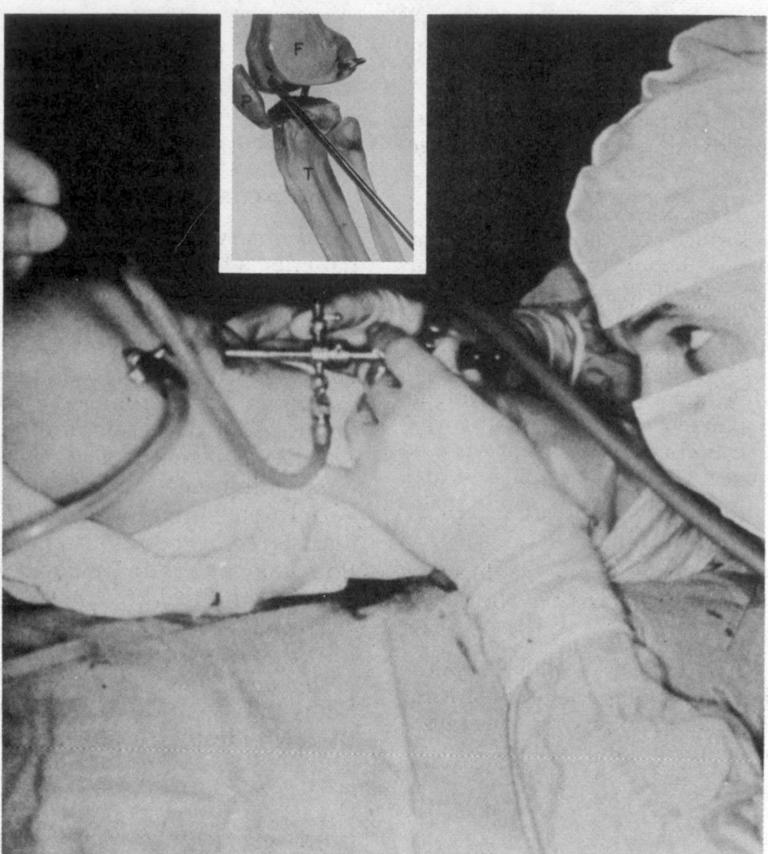

Figure 76–5. The arthroscope is in position. *Inset*, Position of the arthroscope for examination of the articular surfaces of the patella. (From Janecki, C. J., D. H. Hill, and R. G. Eubanks: Arthroscopy of the knee. *American Family Physician*, 17:109, Mar. 1978.)

generative processes); (2) synovial fluid (to distinguish inflammatory from degenerative types of arthritis); (3) muscle enzymes (to distinguish between muscle weakness due to atrophic results of denervation and dystrophic diseases of the muscle itself; and (4) mineral metabolism (levels of calcium, phosphorus, and alkaline phosphates are measured to establish or rule out various specific musculoskeletal disorders).

The most important inorganic constituents of bone are calcium and phosphorus, so that *calcium and phosphorus ion levels* in the serum and urine reflect skeletal metabolic activity. The normal blood value for calcium is 8.5 to 10.5 mg./dl. and for phosphorus 3.0 to 4.5 mg./dl. The average adult urinary excretion of calcium is between 100 and 200 mg./day. About 600 mg./day of phosphorus is excreted in the urine with an ordinary intake. Plasma levels of phosphorus and the daily urinary excretion of phosphorus are both more variable than values for calcium; phosphorus levels vary depending upon time of day and intake.

Assessments of calcium and phosphorus are useful in differentiating diseases which cause changes in skeletal density, e.g., osteoporosis, renal disease, osteomalacia, rickets, parathyroid, or thyroid hyperactivity. *Alkaline phosphatase* levels are used to assess osteoblastic activity, i.e., formation of new bone. Alkaline phosphatase is an enzyme necessary for mineralization of the organic bone matrix.

In addition to the laboratory tests discussed above, *bacteriologic studies* (e.g., smears and cultures) may be employed to identify bacteria that are causing infections.

OTHER DIAGNOSTIC TESTS

Joint aspiration, electromyography, and radioisotope skeletal surveys are other tests that may be of value in diagnosing some musculoskeletal disorders.

- *Aspiration,* e.g., of the knee joint, may be performed to obtain a specimen for diagnostic purposes as well as to instill medications or relieve pain. Blood, synovial fluid, or pus may be aspirated from joints. Blood aspirated from a knee joint usually indicates something has been torn. This leads to further investigation; e.g., arthrograms to accurately diagnose the problem. Local anesthesia may be used for the aspiration. Aseptic technique is imperative. (See Table 76–1 for synovial fluid findings.)
- *Electromyography* is of value in evaluating lower motor neuron lesions. This procedure, which

measures the electrical potential change associated with skeletal muscle contraction, is discussed in Unit X.

- *Radioisotope skeletal surveys,* e.g., with a whole-body profile scanner using radioactive strontium (^{85}Sr), are useful in detecting localized bone disease, e.g., bone cancer and stress fractures.

COMMON CLINICAL PROBLEMS WITH ORTHOPEDIC DISORDERS

PAIN

Disorders of the bones, joints, and muscles commonly produce discomfort and pain. Because of the chronicity of many of these disorders, the management of pain by drug therapy must be carefully planned to prevent drug dependency. Whenever possible, in lieu of administering analgesics and other medications, a wide variety of activities to relieve or prevent pain should be used, e.g., changes of position, applications of heat or cold, massage, relief of pressure from casts or traction, and spending time with patients reassuring them and giving emotional support.

When making assessments of a person with a history of *joint pain* it is important to include the following points:[120]

- circumstances preceding the onset of pain;
- nature of the onset: insidious, subacute, acute;
- spread of joint involvement: original joint, to other joints, changing from one joint to another;
- timing of pain;
- pain intensity, e.g., sharp, aching, dull, stabbing, present on movement and/or strain;
- pain location;
- reference of pain;
- measures that give relief, e.g., rest, gentle exercise, heat, liniment.

General measures used to reduce pain and inflammation associated with *rheumatic disorders*

TABLE 76–1. SYNOVIAL FLUID FINDINGS IN HEALTH AND IN DISEASES AFFECTING THE JOINTS

Condition	Appearance	Viscosity	Mucin Clot	WBC's/mm.³	Poly* (%)	Specific Findings
Normal	Clear, yellow	High	Firm	100 to 200	10	Scanty fluid; no debris
Traumatic arthritis	Red-tinged to bloody	High	Firm	2000+	<20	Few cartilage fragments; many RBC's
Osteoarthritis	Clear, yellow	High	Firm	1000 to 3000	<20	Few to many cartilage fragments; debris
Systemic lupus erythematosus	Slightly cloudy	Slightly decreased	Firm	3000 to 5000	<30	LE cells on Wright's stained smear
Rheumatic fever	Slightly cloudy	Decreased	Firm	7000 to 10,000	<50	Few inclusion bodies among WBC's
Reiter's syndrome	Cloudy	Decreased	Friable	15,000	60+	Hemolytic complement increased; polys in macrophages
Pseudogout	Slightly cloudy to cloudy	Decreased	Fairly firm	10,000+	60+	Rhomboid positively birefringent crystals in WBC's or cartilage fragments
Gouty arthritis	Cloudy to milky	Decreased	Fairly firm	15,000+	75+	Needle-like negatively birefringent crystals in WBC's or free
Rheumatoid arthritis (active)	Cloudy, greenish	Low	Friable	10,000 to 30,000	80+	Many WBC's containing cytoplasmic inclusions; hemolytic complement low; latex fixation test positive
Tuberculous arthritis	Cloudy	Low	Friable	25,000	50	Acid-fast bacilli may be found on smear; culture may be positive; glucose level lower than in blood
Septic arthritis (acute)	Turbid to purulent	Low	Friable	Over 75,000	90+	Glucose level much lower than that in blood; culture positive; hemolytic complement low

*Polys, polymorphonuclear leukocytes.
From Hollander, J. L.: Painful joints: Clues to early diagnosis. *Postgraduate Medicine,* 64:50, Sept. 1978.

include (1) resting the affected joint or extremity, e.g., by bed rest or the application of splints or casts, (2) employing physical measures, e.g., heat (dry or moist), massage, therapeutic exercises, and (3) drug therapy, e.g., aspirin (analgesic, anti-inflammatory), phenylbutazone (Butazolidin), oxyphenbutazone (Tandearil), indomethacin (Indocin), corticosteroids (administered systemically or injected intra-articularly, i.e., into the joint), muscle relaxants. Specific management of various rheumatic disorders is discussed as appropriate in other sections of this unit.

Not only may *orthopedic disorders* cause pain, but also *pain may result from some treatment procedures.* For example, prolonged pressure over bony prominences (e.g., from a cast, traction, or malpositioning) may cause "burning" pain which should be immediately relieved by appropriate measures, e.g., cutting the cast to relieve pressure over the painful area, or correcting the traction set-up or the patient's position to relieve the pain-producing, skin-damaging pressure.

Areas especially susceptible to prolonged pressure include the tuberosity of the tibia, the heel, and the head of the fibula on the lateral side.

Following *musculoskeletal surgery,* pain management is a priority in postoperative clinical care. Orthopedic surgical procedures can be extremely painful. Causes of pain and discomfort must be carefully evaluated so that appropriate relief can be given. Careful assessment of postoperative pain must be made to be sure a complication is not occurring, e.g., compartment syndrome or pulmonary emboli. Pain-relieving measures are similar to those mentioned above.

Generally severe musculoskeletal pain causes a patient to be restless and to frequently change position. Also, the patient attempts to protect the anatomic region from which the pain arises by (1) *muscle splinting,* i.e., active (often involuntary) muscle contraction which immobilizes the part; and (2) *pseudoparalysis* of the part not accompanied by loss of sensation. Muscle splinting differs from muscle spasm in that relaxation of the affected muscles occurs at rest (see below). Prolonged pain in bone, muscle, tendons, or joints, with resultant muscle splinting and pseudoparalysis, may lead eventually to osteoporosis in the affected bone and possibly in adjacent bones. Joint contractures also may develop. Tables 76–2 and 76–3 summarize the characteristics of pain in musculoskeletal tissues, and also the patterns of pain experienced in various types of joint disorders (see also Unit XI).

TABLE 76–2. CHARACTERISTICS OF PAIN IN MUSCULOSKELETAL TISSUES

Tissue	Characteristics
Bone	Slow pain; ache; poorly localized; often throbbing Aggravated by forces of all attached muscles, aggravated by torque (applied manually) and percussion Causes pseudoparalysis of all attached muscles Tenderness, but localization of tenderness mediocre
Muscle belly	Mostly slow pain at rest; aching, some fast pain on contraction Aggravated directly by contraction of affected muscle and by passive stretch Poor subjective localization Affected muscle protected by pseudoparalysis Tenderness with good localization Wasting in pain of long duration, plus osteoporosis in activated bones, plus joint contracture.
Tendon, ligament, fascia	Mostly slow pain at rest; some fast pain on contractile force; localization poor; tender, and localization of tenderness is good
Bony attachments of tendon, ligament, fascia	Mixed slow and fast pain; localization good; protected by pseudoparesis or pseudoparalysis; tenderness accurately localized
Hyaline cartilage	Totally insensitive
Synovia	Slow pain; ache; poorly localized May produce the gelation phenomenon.

From Frost, H. M.: Musculoskeletal pain. *In* Alling, C. C., III (ed.): *Facial Pain.* Philadelphia: Lea and Febiger, 1968, p. 159.

TABLE 76–3. SOME JOINT PAIN PATTERNS

Lesion	Pattern
Acute distention by fluid	Slow pain; ache; mediocre localization; joint held in attitude of greatest fluid volume; pronounced splinting of motion by active muscle contraction; active and passive motion markedly limited; tenderness pronounced and well localized; dramatic relief by aspiration or drainage of joint
Hypersensitive synovia and/or capsule	Splinting of motion by active muscle contraction; comfortable at rest in any attitude once it is produced; gelation phenomenon exists Slow pain, ache, poor localization Synovia usually tender Always pain with motion; usually no pain under load without motion Relieved by intra-articular local anesthetic
Bone pain due to irregular joint surface	Comfortable at rest in any attitude Motion under major load much more painful than motion while free of load Load without motion is painless No tenderness Slow pain; ache; poorly localized Referral and radiation are common Usually not relieved by intra-articular local anesthetic
Bone pain due to subchondral expansile noxious lesion	Worse at night; aggravated by load but not by motion without load; often helped temporarily by motion without load
Gelation	"Stiffens" at rest, hurts for a few minutes when activity resumes but then improves as long as activity is maintained
Prolonged pain	Muscle wasting; local osteoporosis; joint contracture or diminished range of passive motion

From Frost, H. M.: Musculoskeletal pain. *In* Alling, C. C., III (ed.): *Facial Pain.* Philadelphia: Lea and Febiger, 1968, p. 161.

MUSCLE SPASMS

Muscle cramps or spasms often produce discomfort and pain in persons with musculoskeletal disorders. Powerful involuntary muscular contractions shorten the flexor muscles and cause extreme pain which may be incapacitating. These contractions may be stimulated by ischemia and hypoxia of muscle tissue, e.g., due to mechanical compression of blood vessels.

Muscle spasms are a prominent and distressing symptom of *myositic-fibrositic disorders* and many *articular disorders.* In an attempt to relieve skeletal muscle spasms, the physician may order heat applications and massage and may prescribe muscle relaxants, e.g., carisoprodol (Rela, Soma), methocarbamol (Robaxin), orphenadrine (Norflex), diazepam (Valium), and cyclobenzaprine (Flexeril). Usually muscle relaxants are not very potent.

Patients confined to bed commonly experience muscle spasms in the calves of their legs which cause the toes to plantar flex and the feet to forcefully extend and invert. Muscle spasms of this nature are frequently experienced by persons with *advanced arteriosclerosis* and usually occur in positions that create pressure in the popliteal space.

Nursing care activities that may prevent leg cramps include:

- frequent position changes;
- use of a bed cradle to prevent the weight of bed linens on the feet and legs;
- insuring adequate warmth;
- avoidance of heavy sedation (sedation reduces spontaneous movements during sleep);
- positioning which prevents pressure on the popliteal space and minimizes external compression of calf muscles;
- active or passive exercise as recommended by the physician.

Medications which may be prescribed to treat benign muscular cramps may include Benadryl, quinine sulfate, and Myanesin. When a muscle cramp does occur in the calf of the leg, it may be relaxed by causing the vigorous contraction of the opposing muscle group. This maneuver, called *reflex inhibition,* involves forcefully dorsiflexing the foot and toes while pressing downward on the top of the foot (e.g., with the heel of the opposite foot or the hand). When correctly performed, the ankle of the affected leg should be at an angle of about 90°. Motor nerve impulse transmission is thus prevented to the calf muscles.

CONTRACTURES

As mentioned previously, joint contractures may develop in painful limbs if these extremities are maintained for long periods of time in pain-reducing positions. The patient with a painful limb, e.g., arthritic shoulder and arm, must be encouraged to exercise the affected extremity as prescribed by the physician to maintain maximum range of motion. A patient's natural tendency in such a situation is not to move the limb (since movement may produce pain) but rather to hold it in the position which causes the least discomfort, e.g., a painful arm may be held flexed close to the body.

> *Prolonged inactivity may cause positional deformities and stiffness, not only in affected limbs but also in uninvolved parts of the body, unless frequent position changes, correct repositioning, and exercises are faithfully carried out.*

In *flexion contractures* the patient cannot extend the affected extremity. Flexion contractures will develop in people confined to bed who are not given proper preventive care. Poor posture in bed and a sagging mattress contribute to the development of joint contractures, particularly *hip flexion contractures.* Following fracture of the hip, contractures may develop if the patient is permitted to (a) flex and adduct the hips, (b) flex the knees, or (c) maintain an equinus position of the feet for prolonged periods of time. Continuous support of the knees of any patient in a flexed position causes *knee flexion contractures.* The hamstring muscles of the posterior thigh (whose tendons pass under the knee) contract over a relatively short period if the knee is continuously flexed.

Absence of proper foot support, e.g., against a padded footboard, encourages *foot drop,* especially in patients with muscular weakness. If the foot is permitted to rest unsupported, the muscles in the anterior leg stretch, and the tendon of the calf muscles shortens.

Contractures will develop in the *pectoral muscles* and other muscles close to the *axilla* if a patient is permitted to assume a posture for prolonged periods in which arms are held close to the person's sides, elbows flexed at right angles, and wrists dropped. Contractures in these positions may develop following cerebrovascular accidents or in any patient who lies in bed for long periods.

Kerr[137] observes: "We all tend to allow the desperately ill patient to remain in any position in which he appears comfortable because it seems a waste of his limited strength to disturb or move him. . . . Such mistaken kindness and consideration may permanently deform the patient if he survives." There is commonly a tendency not to "disturb" patients who are desperately ill, and also not to require patients who are in pain to move about or change their positions. These tendencies are not generally in the best long-range interests of persons who are ill and suffering. The skillful nurse can, with compassion and understanding, achieve necessary position changes and exercises even for persons who have a natural reluctance to move about. It is indeed tragic when preventable contractures are allowed to develop, since contractures may seriously interfere with successful rehabilitation. For example, postamputation contractures may prevent the use of a prosthesis.

Volkmann's ischemic contracture (see Fig. 76–6) is a serious, deforming, crippling condition of the hand and forearm which may develop as a complication of a fracture about the elbow joint or forearm bones. Vascular obstruction following reduction of the fracture may result from a position of extreme flexion or tight bandages. Vascular obstruction in this instance is indicated by absence of a radial pulse, and this finding should be immediately reported, before massive infarction of muscle tissue can occur. After such infarction, muscle is slowly replaced with fibrous tissue, and tendons and nerves become restricted by scar tissue. Although it most commonly involves the arms, Volkmann's ischemic contracture may also develop in the lower extremities as a complication of fractures of the femur and tibia. Immediate treatment of suspected ischemia includes the release of constricting bandages and the elevation of the extremity. Emergency surgery may be necessary if relief of the ischemia does not occur within 1 to 2 hours.

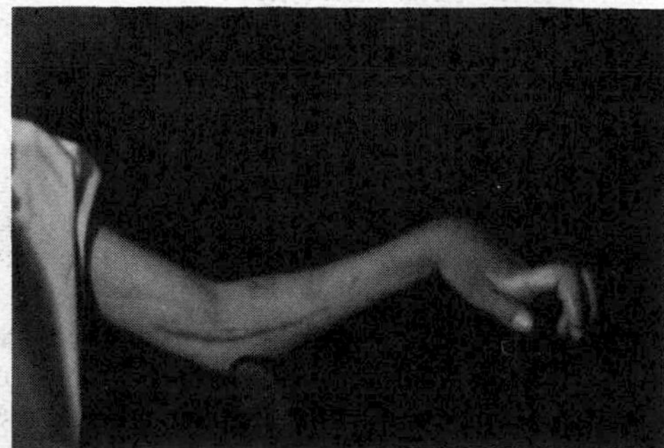

Figure 76–6. Volkmann's contracture after fracture of the elbow. (From O'Donoghue, D. H.: *Treatment of Injuries to Athletes,* 3rd ed. Philadelphia: W. B. Saunders Co., 1976.)

THERAPEUTIC MEASURES COMMONLY USED IN THE TREATMENT OF ORTHOPEDIC DISORDERS

REST

Rest is an important aspect of the treatment of many musculoskeletal disorders. Following trauma, a period of rest promotes healing and minimizes inflammation, swelling, and pain. In the management of rheumatic diseases, rest of the affected joints or extremities helps reduce pain and inflammation. At times bed rest is advisable. Immobilization of affected joints may be achieved by the application of splints or casts. Splints prevent joint deformities in addition to minimizing pain by relieving muscle spasms.

PHYSICAL THERAPY

Physical therapy is an integral part of the total care of persons with musculoskeletal disorders. The goals of physical therapy are variable but may include maintenance or improvement of range of joint motion, dexterity, and muscle strength; reduction or relief of pain and swelling; relief of muscle spasms; prevention of complications of inactivity; and teaching of self-care and ambulation techniques. In many settings specially trained physical therapists are available to implement physical therapy. Nurses assume the responsibility for performing many aspects of physical therapy in the absence of registered physical therapists.

Some of the more common techniques of physical therapy employed in the care of patients with musculoskeletal disorders include application of heat, administration of massage, and assistance with exercises. Space does not permit detailed discussions of these physical therapy processes; however, they are discussed briefly in following pages.

Heat. Heat may be applied in several ways, e.g., hot packs, hot soaks, hot paraffin applications, infrared radiation, whirlpool baths, diathermy. Commonly the application of heat is followed by exercise or massage. Among the physiologic effects of heat are softening of fibrous tissue, sedation, increased edema and arterial blood supply, and reduction or relief of pain.[137] Heat may relax muscle, relieve pain, and induce vasodilation (this, in turn, improves local blood supply and nutrition). Heat may be applied either dry or moist and may be directed *locally* (e.g., at a single joint) or *systemically.*

Methods of applying *moist heat* include the Hubbard tank (for application to multiple joints) and whirlpool baths, hot compresses, or hot paraffin (wax) applications (for local applications). Diathermy and ultrasound may be used in treating nonarticular rheumatic disorders, but generally they are not applied to acutely inflamed joints. Most commonly *dry heat* is applied by using hot air, heat lamps, or heating pads.*

Massage. Massage may relieve pain, stretch fibrous tissue, and reduce edema (because the massage stroke is toward the heart with the hand, thus improving return circulation)[145] Massage relaxes muscles, improves muscle tone, and increases blood flow. It may relieve muscle spasms in many muscular and fibrotic inflammations. *Note that acutely inflamed joints should never be massaged.*

Exercises. Prescribed exercise varies in type, depending upon an individual patient's needs. It may be (1) *active* (the motion is performed by the patient); (2) *passive* (the motion is performed by another person for the patient); or (3) *active-assistive* (the patient actively performs as much of the motion as possible with the help of another person as needed).

Exercises are often categorized according to the type of muscular activity required.

- *Isotonic* exercises are the "normal" type of exercise in which motion of a part takes place, involving shortening of the muscle and muscle contraction.
- *Isometric exercise* (also called static exercise or muscle-setting exercise) involves active contraction and relaxation of muscles without movement of the joint that is normally mobilized by these muscles.
- *Resistive* exercises are those in which motion of a part takes place against the resistance of another person or of the person's own antagonistic muscles. Pulleys and ropes may be used for resistive exercises.
- *Range-of-motion* (ROM) exercises are those in which a joint is moved through its full range of motion, e.g., the full extent to which it is capable of being moved. ROM exercises may be active, passive, or active-assistive.

Therapeutic exercises have numerous benefits. Among these are maintenance or restoration of adequate joint activity, prevention of muscular atrophy and other deformities, building or maintaining muscular bulk and strength, maintaining or improving joint range of motion, building endurance, and stimulating circulation.

In some instances exercises are directed specifically at "building up" those muscles necessary for use with ambulation, e.g., the quadriceps muscles may be strengthened by having the patient straighten the knee while sitting. Bed exercises help prepare a patient for ambulation.

*More detailed discussion about the therapeutic application of heat and cold is in Sorensen and Luckmann, *Basic Nursing: A Psychophysiologic Approach.*

These exercises may include (a) joint ROM exercises, active or passive, to preserve joint motion; (b) deep breathing exercises (see Unit XVI) to stimulate circulation and promote effective lung function; (c) quadriceps setting to stabilize the knees; (d) gluteal and abdominal muscle tightening to improve trunk stability; (e) lifting exercises to increase strength in the biceps; and (f) push-up exercises to increase strength in the triceps.

In addition to the previously discussed activities, the physical therapist (or nurse) may teach patients: *transfer techniques,* e.g., bed to wheelchair; *wheelchair usage;* application of *braces* or other appliances; usage of *crutches, canes,* or *walkers;* or usage of other self-care equipment. Some of these activities are discussed in Unit X.

Crutches. The selection, fitting, and use of crutches is described in detail in Sorensen and Luckmann, *Basic Nursing: A Psychophysiologic Approach,* Chapter 43.

Exercises are taught to strengthen arm and shoulder muscles in preparation for crutch usage. Patients may lift sandbags while lying supine (on the back) and/or push-ups may be done while lying prone (on the abdomen). These exercises strengthen the triceps (extensor muscles of the upper arm). Also, straight-elbow push-ups help the patient learn how to bear weight on the palms of the hands. While standing between *parallel bars,* the patient learns to stand erect and swing forward by pushing down on the hands and swinging the body.

Some of the most important points to remember about the fitting and use of crutches are:

- ▶ Crutches must be of proper length for the individual patient. If too long, they can cause excessive pressure and rubbing in the axilla. *Excessive axillary pressure from crutches may cause nerve damage (to branches of the brachial plexus) and arm paralysis or numbness, i.e., crutch palsy or crutch paralysis. If too short,* crutches can slip and the patient may fall.
- ▶ People on crutches are vulnerable to accidents. No one should crutch walk in stocking feet, slippers, or high heeled shoes. Accidents can be prevented (a) by teaching patients proper crutch walking and making them aware of the possible hazards involved and (b) by constant safety-consciousness on the part of staff members, e.g., keeping floors litter-free and dry, opening doors in patient areas carefully (to avoid toppling over a patient on crutches on the other side of the door).

Canes. A cane is used on the side opposite the impaired leg. Body weight is thus maintained by the weak leg and cane while the strong leg is moved forward. The cane should be of such a length that the patient can extend the elbow and bear weight on the hand grasping the cane. In addition to having a pure rubber suction tip, the cane should have a curved handle with a comfortable grip.

Walkers. Walkers of various kinds are available to help patients ambulate. Walkers may be used prior to crutches for some persons. In preparation for using a walker, patients may practice resistance exercises while in bed to strengthen the triceps muscles. Some walkers have underarm supports similar to those found on crutches. As with crutch walking, to prevent accidents while patients are using walkers be certain floors are dry and free of litter and that supportive shoes are worn. It is desirable for patients to be dressed while using walkers, since bathrobes may easily become entangled and cause falls.

Braces. Braces and other orthopedic devices, e.g., *corsets,* may be worn as part of the treatment of musculoskeletal disorders. Orthopedic appliances are made by an *orthotist* (also spelled "orthetist") and are individually designed for each patient. Often a physical therapist helps a patient learn to apply, use, and care for braces. A patient may have difficulty adjusting to new braces because they may rub, pinch, or otherwise not fit correctly. Additionally, braces are often heavy and may cause a person unaccustomed to them to feel clumsy or off balance. It is not uncommon for a patient to initially dislike the change in appearance which is caused by wearing a brace (see also p. 572).

Braces must be correctly applied and cared for. It is essential that braces fit correctly and comfortably. Braces must not rub or chafe the skin or cause other irritations by excessive pressure. The patient who wears braces is taught to make frequent skin inspections to be certain that no skin damage is being caused by the appliances. Encourage the patient who wears braces to report areas of discomfort to a health professional. It is important that patients not feel they are "unnecessarily complaining." If they do, they will avoid reporting such important symptoms. A mirror should be used to visualize those areas which could not otherwise be seen. If the patient has impaired sensation (e.g., numbness to pain and pressure) in the braced portion of the body, these visual self-inspections of the skin are of particular importance, since they are the primary means by which the patient can detect problems caused by braces. In the hospital nurses make these skin inspections at first, and chart and report indications of skin damage. Poorly fitting appliances are then padded (perhaps with lamb's wool or felt pads), or other adjustments are made, e.g., a strap may be loosened.

The apron, ties, or belts of a brace (or corset) must be smooth when the appliance is being worn, and not wrinkled or twisted next to the skin. Buckles, stays, or hinges should not poke against the skin or cause excessive pressure. (See Figure 76–7.) Often it is necessary initially for the orthotist to redesign and refit new braces. Periodic adjustments in braces may also be necessary later, e.g., if the patient loses or gains weight, or regains function, or if the structure of the braces changes with long-term use.

If a brace does not fit comfortably and cor-

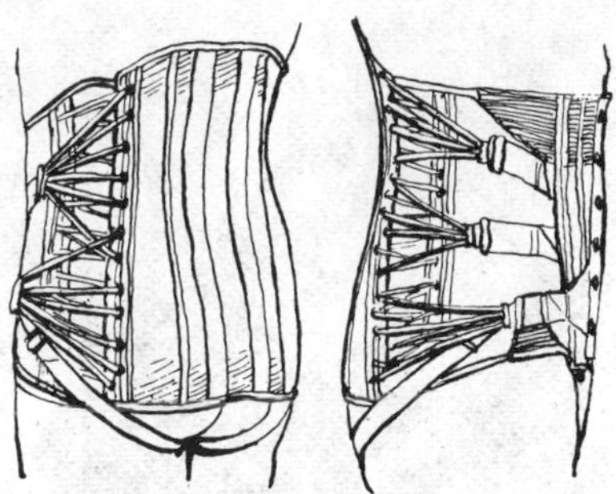

Figure 76–7. A lumbosacral corset. (From The Hip: Proceedings of the Fourth Open Scientific Meeting of the Hip Society, 1976. St. Louis: C. V. Mosby Co., 1976.)

rectly, the patient will become discouraged and his or her condition may be worsened. When patients are capable of taking care of themselves and their braces they are taught how to do so correctly. Such teaching includes that care already mentioned as well as care of the brace, e.g., oiling joints, applying saddle soap to leather parts, replacing worn ties. Injury may be prevented by carefully inspecting the brace at regular intervals for indications of the need for service.

Nurses may be of great assistance to patients and their significant others during the time necessary for them to learn how to use a brace. By maintaining a helpful, encouraging, enthusiastic attitude during this time, nurses can help patients to view a brace as a device which is of benefit, rather than as an uncomfortable, unsightly encumbrance.

CASTS

Purposes. The major purposes of casting include:

- Immobilization, support, and protection of a part during healing processes (e.g., healing of fractures once they are reduced and properly aligned or healing following surgery)
- Prevention of deformities (e.g., with arthritis)
- Correction of deformities (e.g., scoliosis)

The ideal plaster cast, used for immobilization, should be meticulously molded "like a glove" to the contour of the casted part and include "the joint above and the joint below" the affected part. Use of a cast following surgery or in the treatment of a fracture often makes it possible for a patient to be more active during the healing process than would be possible if the disabled part were immobilized by traction. While several types of casting materials are available, plaster of Paris is commonly used.

Plaster of Paris. Plaster of Paris (anhydrous calcium sulfate) is a chalky white powder made by a process that removes water from gypsum. In the process of making plaster of Paris, crystals of gypsum are broken up and reduced to powder form, and intense heat is applied to remove the water from the crystals. A chemical process of rehydration occurs when plaster of Paris is placed in water. The exothermic reaction that takes place during this recrystallization or "setting" period generates heat which can be felt in the newly applied cast. It is important that the heat generated in a newly applied cast be permitted to dissipate into circulating air. If the cast is covered with blankets or placed on a pillow or mattress during the period of most intense heat formation (e.g., the first 10 to 15 minutes following cast application), the patient could be burned, or (if the cast is large, e.g., a body cast) experience symptoms of heat prostration. The amount of heat given off by a setting cast is affected by factors such as the temperature of the water in which the plaster is immersed for rehydration and the amount of plaster used.

Plaster of Paris *bandages* come in individually wrapped, precut rolls of crinoline impregnated with plaster. The bandages are available in varying widths from 2 inches to 8 inches. Plaster is available in various setting speeds: extra fast (2 to 4 minutes), fast (5 to 8 minutes), and slow (10 to 18 minutes). The strength of a completed cast is determined by the number of layers of plaster used. Commonly a cast consists of 5 to 7 layers of plaster bandage in unreinforced areas. Plaster of Paris *splints* of varying sizes are also available. Splints may be applied by themselves (and held in place with elastic or other bandages when dry), or they may be used to strengthen and reinforce areas of casts which require additional support, e.g., areas of stress, such as the axilla, groin, back of knee.

A plaster cast becomes firm (i.e., "sets") rapidly, but takes a while to actually dry. During the setting process, the plaster reacts with water, and long slender crystals develop which interlock through the layers of gauze. *Movement during the setting process disrupts these formations and weakens the cast.* A newly set plaster cast is called a *green* cast. In a green cast, excess unbound water accumulates in pockets in the crystalline lattice work. This water adds to the weight of the cast during the green stage. Eventually the unbound water evaporates, leaving a mature cast. A cast attains its full strength once evaporation occurs of all the water in the cast in excess of that water needed for crystallization. Within mature plaster are numerous pockets of air which lighten the weight of the cast, make the cast permeable, and permit the skin to "breathe."[207]

Preparation for Casting. Prior to cast application, the procedure is explained to the patient, and the skin is prepared over the part of the body to be casted. If a fracture is to be reduced before the cast is applied, the patient may be given a narcotic; a general or local anesthetic may then be administered. *Skin preparation* may include cleansing with soap and water; gentle but thorough drying; application of alcohol; or dusting with a borate or stearate of zinc talcum powder. Some physicians recommend gently rubbing the skin with alcohol to increase skin tone. The skin is closely examined while it is prepared, and lesions, unremovable dirt, or foreign particles are noted and called to the physician's attention.

After the skin is prepared to receive the cast, it may be protectively covered with stockinette or padding. *Stockinette* is a soft knit material which is available in bias-cut (for circumferential wrapping) or tubular form (to completely encircle a body part, like a footless stocking, without seams). Stockinette comes in rolls of various widths, to cover an arm, leg, or body. Tubular stockinette is always cut longer than the expected finished cast length, so the excess portions can be pulled over the rough cast edges.

Materials which may be used for *padding* under a cast include sheet wadding, Webril, sponge rubber, or felt. The skin may be treated with a liquid adhesive, e.g., tincture of benzoin, prior to the application of padding, or padding may be applied directly over the skin or over a covering of stockinette. When used, padding is commonly placed over bony prominences, and may be held in place with crepe paper bandage or narrow strips of adhesive to give better conformation to body structures.

> *When stockinette or padding is applied under a cast, it* must be smooth *on the skin before the plaster cast material is applied. Wrinkled or wadded material under a cast invites trouble, e.g., pressure areas and skin breakdown.*

Casting Equipment. A cast may be applied in a physician's office, clinic, or emergency room, or at a patient's bedside. Portable carts (*cast carts*) are usually available in hospitals and clinics. These carts contain equipment necessary for casting and are taken to wherever the patient is when the cast is to be applied. However, in a hospital the more common procedure is to take the patient to a specially equipped *cast room* for cast application.

Equipment which may be used during casting includes buckets; plaster of Paris splints and bandages, walking heels or irons (see Fig. 76–8), metallic splints; stockinette, sponge rubber, sheet wadding, or Webril; a plaster knife; cast saw; bandage scissors; tape; lubricant; and plaster shears. Sterile dressings (for wounds) may also be needed.

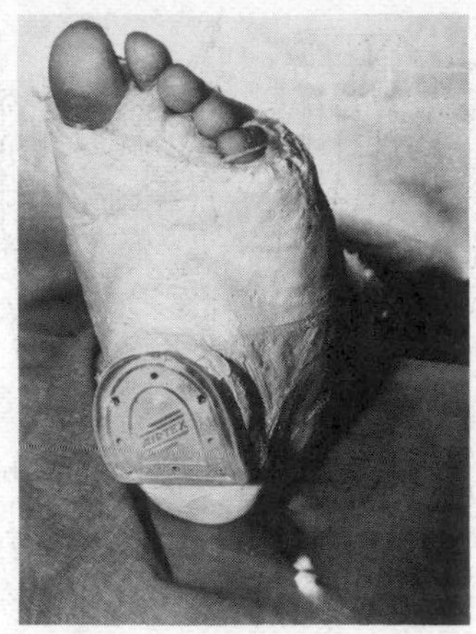

Figure 76–8. Plaster of Paris shoe with walking rubber heel. In this instance the cast was applied following surgery of the forefoot. (From Joplin, R. J.: *Surgical Clinics of North America, 49*:861, 1969.)

Lining water buckets with plastic liners helps keep the buckets clean and makes it easier to dispose of plaster sediment in the water after the casting is completed. *Never empty plaster-laden water into an ordinary sink,* because the plaster sediment will solidify and plug the plumbing. If a sink with a plaster trap is not available, wait for sediment to settle into the bottom of the plastic-lined bucket, then carefully drain off the water from the top of the bucket while flushing the drain with large quantities of water. Dispose of the plastic bag with its plaster sediment into trash containers. The physician and assistants need to be protectively covered so their clothing will not be soiled with plaster. The patient's clothing should also be covered.

Applying a Plaster Cast. A bucket containing tepid water is necessary to saturate the plaster bandages. Setting time is influenced by the type of plaster used and the temperature of the water. Warmer temperatures speed up the setting time, while colder water slows down the setting time.

Submerge the plaster bandages in a bucket of water. Once the air bubbles stop coming from the rolls, the plaster is ready to be rolled. It is gently squeezed out and rolled on the patient slightly "sloppy wet." Never submerge more than two rolls in water at one time, as the plaster is ruined if prepared too far in advance.

If a large cast is being applied, it may be necessary to change the water in the cast buckets if excessive sediment accumulates and begins to adhere to new rolls of plaster. Plaster residue in the dipping water (from previous use) causes the freshly dipped plaster to set too slowly and produces lamination and weakness of the cast.

During application of a cast, the physician positions the patient, and assistants help hold the patient in the desired position until the cast has started to set. It is important to hold the patient precisely as the doctor wishes so the casted structures will remain properly aligned. When supporting newly casted areas for the physician, hold the cast on open palms. *Never grasp or pinch the wet cast with your fingertips because they will make indentations in the cast.*

Throughout the casting procedure the physician works to apply a smooth, strong, correctly positioned cast. The cast is continuously rubbed with moderate pressure exerted by an open hand and molded during application, until the cast is completely set. (See Figure 76–9.) To function effectively and safely, the cast can be neither too loose nor too tight. Because the patient will live in the cast for some time, every effort is made to apply a cast that will be comfortable as well as therapeutic.

Because casting must be done in an uninterrupted, fairly rapid manner, it is easy for the patient to be overlooked while everyone concentrates on properly applying the cast. The nurse can be helpful during the casting process by periodically talking with the conscious patient and providing minor comforts, e.g., making certain the patient is not unnecessarily exposed and is kept as warm as possible. Reassurances that "all is going well" help to relax the patient. The nurse encourages the patient to relax and hold still during application of the cast. If the patient tenses muscles, the cast will not fit properly once the person relaxes. Patients should be informed that the heat they feel during the setting process of the cast is normal and will subside after 10 to 15 minutes.

If a leg cast is to be used for bearing the patient's weight during ambulation, it is fitted (during the green stage) with a *walking heel* or *walking iron* on the plantar surface (see Fig. 76–8). The "walker" bears the patient's weight and prevents wear on the bottom of the cast.

Early in the green stage of the cast the physician trims off excess plaster with a knife. Also, if excessive swelling following application of the cast is expected the physician may split the completed cast longitudinally through all layers to relieve pressure that would otherwise dangerously accumulate within the confines of the cast (see below). As soon as casting is complete, the patient's skin is cleaned to remove excess plaster while it is still damp. Unless removed, these pieces of plaster will dry and may fall under the cast and cause skin damage. Following application of a cast, an x-ray film is commonly taken to verify correct bone alignment. Subsequent films are taken whenever a cast is removed or applied.

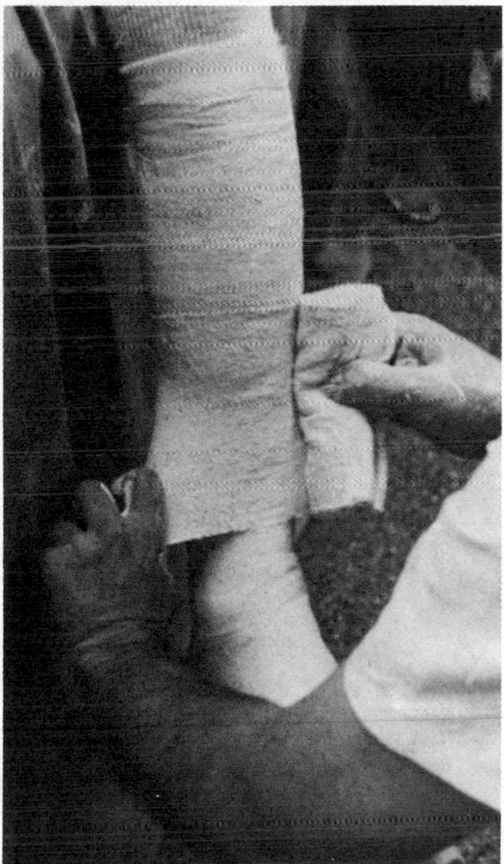

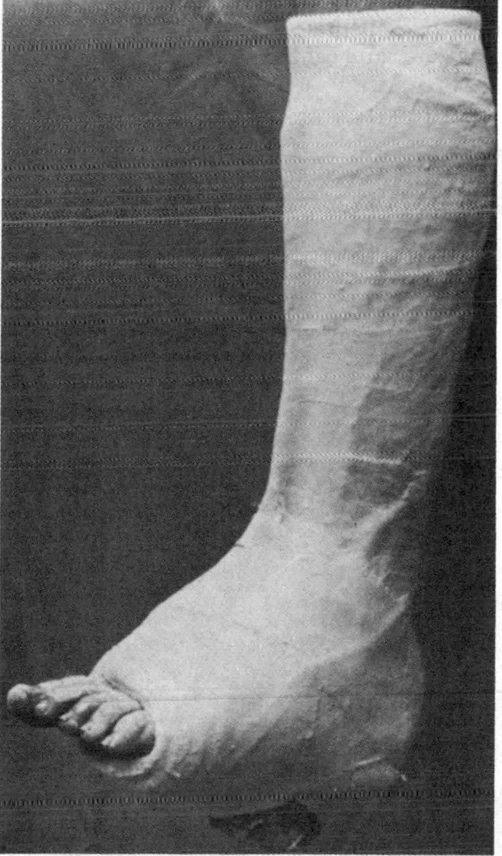

Figure 76–9. The plaster of Paris bandage should be applied in the same direction as the wadding. The roll should be applied with the fingertips and must never be removed from the extremity. In order to make the bandage conform to the varying circumferences of the arm or leg, tucks should be taken in it with the left hand. (From Rockwood, C., and D. Green: Fractures. Vol. I. Philadelphia: J. B. Lippincott Co., 1975.)

"Windowing" and Bivalving a Cast. Cutting "windows" in casts and bivalving casts are two techniques commonly used to relieve or prevent excessive accumulations of pressure in casted body areas, or to permit access to or visualization of certain body areas. *Windows* may be cut (in dried casts) for any of the following reasons: (a) to prevent uncomfortable abdominal distention (e.g., in a body cast or hip spica); (b) to permit taking of the radial pulse (e.g., with an arm cast to check circulation in the involved arm); (c) to inspect areas of discomfort or areas in which tissue damage is suspected; or (d) to remove drains postoperatively or otherwise tend a surgical wound. (When a window is present observe the skin exposed for indications of complications, e.g., edema, discoloration.)

Bivalving a cast means splitting it along both sides. A cast may be bivalved (a) to permit room for tissue swelling; (b) so half of it can be removed to facilitate giving care and during the taking of x-ray films; (c) during the time a patient is learning to gradually adjust to being without a cast; or (d) to make a half-cast which can be used as an intermittent splint (e.g., to prevent deformities). Once a cast is bivalved, either half of it can be removed easily (without disturbing alignment) to inspect the body surface and give necessary care, e.g., the "top half" of the cast may be removed while the patient lies supine and remains in the "bottom half" of the cast, and vice versa. The doctor may order both halves of the cast removed periodically, e.g., to permit exercising. When reapplying a bivalved cast, be certain to handle the patient carefully and take care not to pinch skin between the two cast halves. Once the halves of the cast are properly fitted on the patient, they are secured in place with a wrap. Whenever a patient mentions a pressure point or the cast "not feeling right," assessment should be made by windowing or bivalving the cast.

Types of Casts. The body and extremities can be casted in numerous different ways. In this section some of the more common types of casts are described and illustrated. A short arm cast, a long arm cast, and a hanging arm cast are illustrated in Figure 76–10, along with potential pressure points in a casted arm.

Short arm casts may be used in the treatment of stable fractures of the finger metacarpals, carpals, or distal radius and stable wrist sprains. *Finger splints* may be attached to short arm casts, extending from the plaster in the palm. Finger splints are used to stabilize ligamentous injuries of phalangeal and metacarpal phalangeal joints, phalangeal fractures, and unstable finger metacarpal fractures. A *long arm cast* may be used to treat stable injuries of the elbow joint; stable fractures of the distal humerus; fractures of one or both bones of the forearm; unstable ligamentous injuries of the wrist joint; and unstable fractures of the carpal bones.

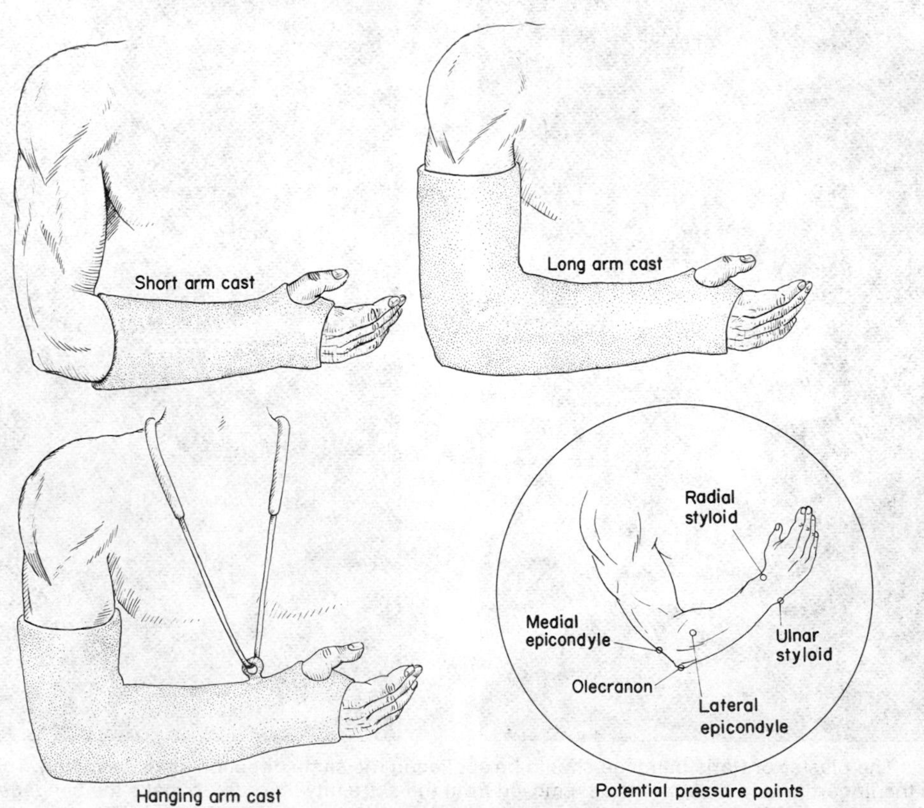

Figure 76–10. Some types of arm casts and potential pressure points in a casted arm. (Drawn by K. C. Sorensen.)

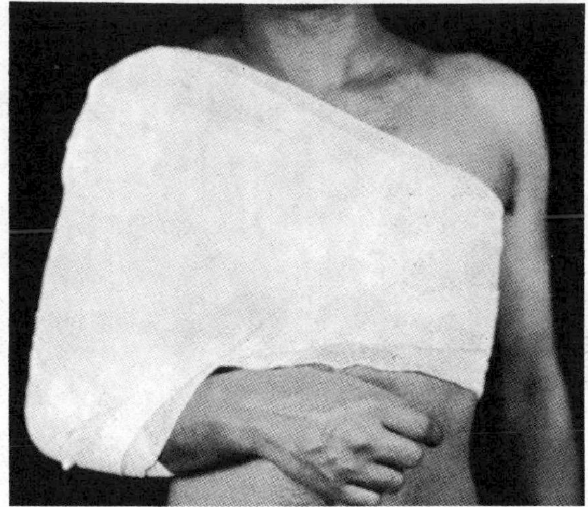

Figure 76–11. Velpeau dressing. Plaster of Paris is applied over the dressing for the treatment of some conditions. (From Gartland, J. J.: *Fundamentals of Orthopaedics,* 3rd ed. Philadelphia: W. B Saunders Co., 1979.)

The purpose of a *hanging arm cast* is for the weight of the hanging cast to exert gentle traction on the humerus while the patient is upright. To accomplish this, the patient should remain erect or semi-erect with the casted arm hanging in position at *all* times. This includes sleeping while sitting upright. A hanging arm cast may be used to treat some shoulder injuries, displaced fractures of the surgical neck of the humerus, or spiral or comminuted fractures of the humeral shaft. The joints above or below the fractured humerus are not immobilized with a hanging cast.

A *Velpeau dressing* is made of plaster bandage or cloth, and splints the arm to the chest (see Fig. 76–11). The elbow is flexed, the forearm is against the abdomen, and the forearm is supported in a sling type of support. Skin-to-skin contact must be avoided, e.g., between the trunk and arm, to prevent skin irritation and maceration. Because skin care is impossible under the dressing, the dressing needs to be changed frequently. Superficial skin irritation often occurs. The dressing is seldom left on continuously for longer than 3 to 4 weeks. The Velpeau dressing immobilizes the shoulder girdle (including the scapula, clavicle, and humerus and their mutual joints) and is used to treat ligamentous injuries to the shoulder joint or acromioclavicular joint, and fractures of the scapula, clavicle, or humerus.

Figure 76–12 illustrates a short leg cast, a long leg cast, and a long leg cylinder cast, as well as areas of the leg especially vulnerable to pressure when casted.

A *short leg cast* (SLC) may be either non–weight-bearing or weight-bearing. All toes should be visible to check for complications and to permit movement. The knee joint is freely moveable. The ankle joint is at 90°, and the heel is neither inverted nor everted. Compression of the peroneal nerve may cause serious complications (e.g., foot drop) in any leg cast and must be prevented. If the cast is to be weight-bearing, a walking heel or iron is applied.

The *patellar tendon weight-bearing cast* is a special type of short leg weight-bearing cast which extends higher on the leg than the typical SLC. This cast is used to treat unstable fractures of the tibia and fibula (see Fig. 76–13).

A *long leg cast* (LLC) is similar to a short leg cast on the bottom but extends over the knee joint to terminate at the groin. If the LLC is to be weight-bearing, a walking heel or iron is incorporated into the cast. Long leg casts are used to treat stable injuries to the knee joint and distal femur and unstable fractures of the tibia, fibula, and ankle joint. A *long leg cylinder cast* (LLCC) is similar to an LLC except that the foot and

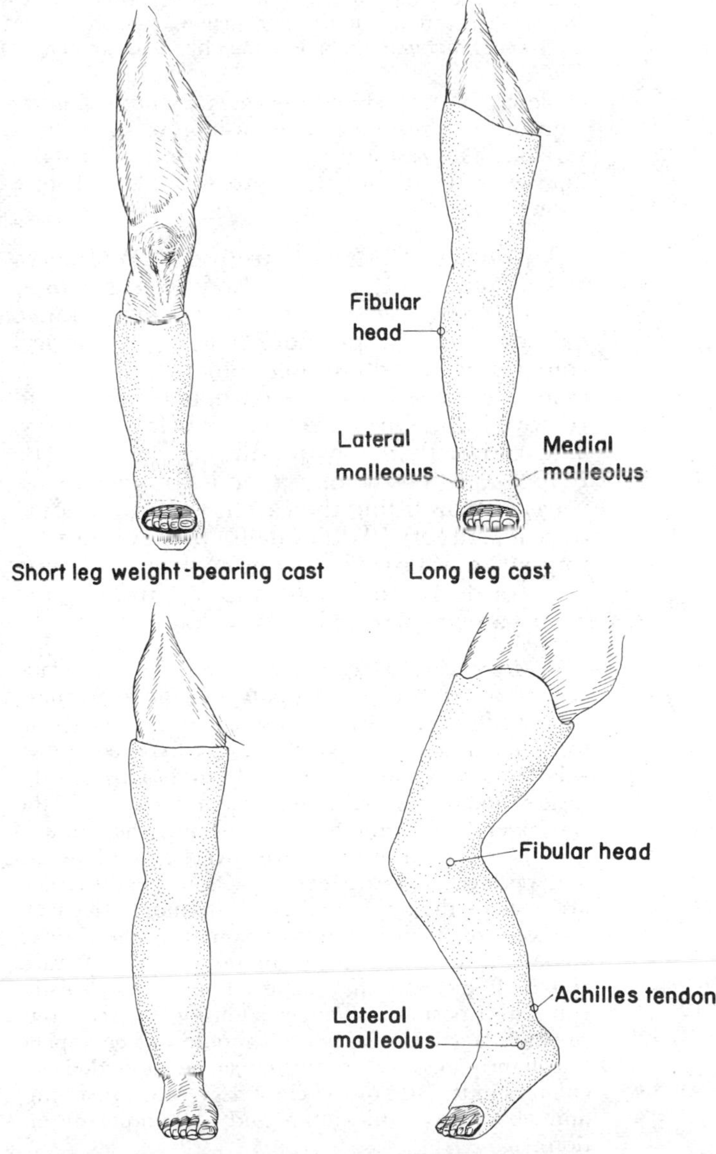

Figure 76–12. Some types of leg casts and potential pressure points in a casted leg. (Drawn by K. C. Sorensen.)

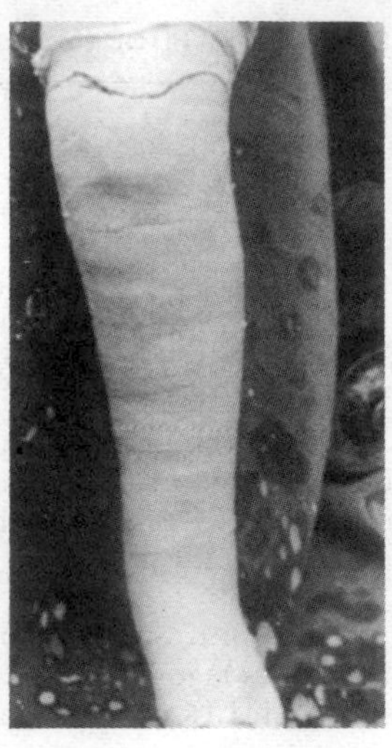

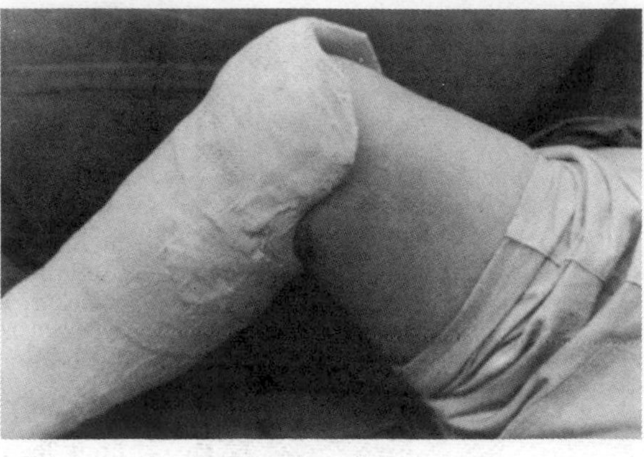

Figure 76–13. The patellar tendon-bearing cast should be cut out to resemble a patellar tendon-bearing prosthesis, and it is particularly important to trim the lateral portion like a wingback chair. When the knee is flexed, pressure is taken from the patellar tendon, but in full extension, pressure is exerted on the thick skin over the tendon. (From Rockwood, C., and D. Green: *Fractures.* Vol. I. Philadelphia: J. B. Lippincott Co., 1975.)

ankle are not casted and the cast may not extend as high on the upper leg. The position of the knee is variable. This cast is used in the treatment of stable injuries of the distal femur, proximal tibia, or knee joint.

Two types of *body casts* are used: (1) Minerva jacket, and (2) body jacket. Body casts are used to immobilize the spine to relieve degenerative disorders and to promote healing of surgical spinal fusions and unstable spinal injuries. Body casts are sometimes fitted (then bivalved and removed when dry) several days before surgery. The cast is then sent to surgery so it can be reapplied when the operation is complete. This is easier than fitting the cast at the end of long, delicate surgery. Additionally, preoperative fitting makes it possible for the patient to identify areas of discomfort in advance of surgery, and these can be corrected.

A *Minerva jacket* covers the frontal and occipital regions of the skull and extends over the neck, chest, back, abdomen, and iliac crests. The face, ears, buttocks, pubic area, and extremities are exposed or they will develop pressure necrosis. With a *body jacket* the head, shoulders, and extremities are free, and the cast extends from the upper chest over the trunk to the pubis. The iliac crests are covered; the buttocks and perineal area are exposed. Some body jackets also include the thighs and pelvis (to more effectively reduce motion in the lumbar spine) or the cervical spine (to more completely immobilize the thoracic spine). Body casts may be used to immobilize the spine in a position of hyperextension to treat compression fractures. Body casts should not be applied too tightly because room must be provided for changes in the size of the chest cage (with breathing) and abdomen (with eating and abdominal distention).

A *turnbuckle cast* is a type of cast that has been commonly used to correct lateral spinal curvatures, e.g., scoliosis. Whenever possible these patients are placed in braces, however, and with the advent of modern technology the turnbuckle cast is almost obsolete.

Spica casts may be applied to the hip, shoulder, or thumb joints. The word "spica" refers to a figure-eight or spiral, having turns that cross one another. With a spica cast, the casted appendage is immobilized to the main part of the body or extremity. To immobilize the affected joint, the bandages are applied in a spiral manner, e.g., around the thumb and the hand or an extremity and the trunk.

A *shoulder spica cast* (see Fig. 76–14) is a combination of a body jacket and long arm cast joined together. Indications for use of a

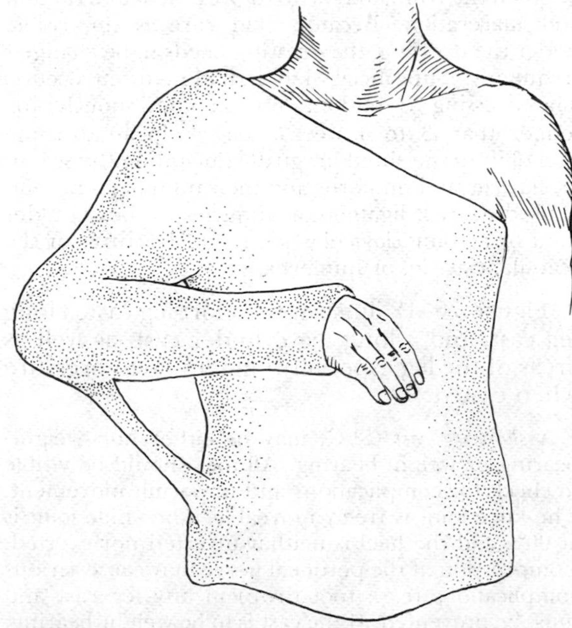

Figure 76–14. Shoulder spica cast. (Drawn by K. C Sorensen.)

shoulder spica include unstable fractures of the shoulder girdle and humerus, unstable elbow joint injuries, and dislocations of the shoulder girdle.

A *hip spica* extends from midtrunk (just below the nipple line) down the entire length of one leg on the affected side (often including the foot). The cast has an opening around the buttocks and perineal region for purposes of elimination and cleanliness. Hip spica casts may be (a) single (includes trunk and one complete extremity); (b) one and one-half (includes trunk, one lower complete extremity, and the other lower extremity to the knee); or (c) double (includes trunk and both complete lower extremities, i.e., a body jacket and two long leg casts). Hip spica casts may be used to treat congenital dislocation of the hip or to immobilize reconstructive surgeries (e.g., following hip fusions or osteotomy of the knee) or injuries to the pelvis, hip joint, or femur. Shoulder or hip spica casts may be reinforced by plastering a stick or bar (abduction bar) between the extended portion of the cast (e.g., leg or arm) and the main body of the cast (e.g., trunk). Never lift a spica cast by these reinforcing devices.

A *thumb spica* is a short (below the elbow) arm cast which includes the thumb. The spiral bandaging is between the thumb and hand. Only the tip of the thumb is exposed. Thumb spica casts are indicated in treatment of fractures of the carpal navicular, fractures of the thumb metacarpal and phalanges, and ligamentous thumb joint injuries.

Drying Casts. Casts take variable lengths of time to dry. While some casts dry completely in only a few hours, others may take several days. Factors influencing drying time include:

- Type of material used for casting.
- Amount of water to be evaporated from the cast.
- Thickness of the cast, e.g., number of layers of plaster bandage, use of plaster splints.
- Condition of the surrounding environment, e.g., humidity, temperature, air circulation. A damp, humid environment delays drying. The circulation of warm, dry air around a cast enhances moisture evaporation from a wet cast and hence speeds up the drying process.

Sometimes a *cast dryer* (a mechanical device which circulates heated air like a hair dryer) is used to promote drying of a cast, but more commonly the cast is simply left uncovered so it is exposed to room air. A cast should dry from the inside out. It is important that a cast not be dried out too quickly with excessive heat, or the inner portions of the cast may remain damp and become moldy. Also, rapid drying may burn the skin beneath the cast or cause the cast to crack. If a cast dryer is used, it should be placed about 18 inches away from the cast and moved frequently so the entire surface area of the cast is gradually dried. A cast dryer should not be used without an order. Hemorrhage may be caused by applying heat to a freshly operated area.[137] *Never use a heat lamp to dry a cast.*

Excessive heat or prolonged exposure to heat may cause skin to burn under a cast.

As mentioned earlier, heat is generated during the initial setting period of a cast (i.e., the period of recrystallization). This heat formation typically causes anxiety. However, anxiety may be reduced if the patient understands why heat is developing and is prepared to expect this "normal" reaction. If the patient with a large body cast or hip spica cast is acutely uncomfortable during this period, an ice bag may be applied to the head or a fan may be used to circulate air around the head. Do not direct the fan on the cast. In extremely warm weather the patient may be made more comfortable with cooling sponges or if circulation of room air can be improved. It is necessary, however, to protect the patient from direct exposure to drafts.

During the green period of the cast (while the cast is still damp and water is evaporating from it), the patient may feel cold and chill easily. Be certain to provide adequate covering for the patient at this time, while leaving the casted area exposed. If a patient is in shock and has a large cast, it may be desirable to avoid excessive chilling by covering some portions of the cast and rotating the exposed portions during the drying process.

A dry cast (a) is odorless, (b) is resonant when percussed, (c) is white and somewhat shiny in appearance, and (d) feels similar to the surrounding room temperature. A cast which still retains moisture (a) is musty smelling, (b) is dull on percussion, (c) is gray and lusterless in appearance; and (d) feels cool to the touch (except during the early period of intense heat formation).

"Finishing" Cast Edges. One of the first activities performed once a cast is completely dry is to make certain *all* edges of the cast are "finished," i.e., protectively covered. Some physicians finish the edges of a cast (while applying it) by pulling the stockinette lining out over the edges of the cast and securing the stockinette against the outer portion of the cast with plaster. If this is not done at the time of applying the cast, adhesive moleskin strips or "petals" should be put around the cast edge, using care not to have the "petals" stick to the skin.

With body casts, hip spica casts, or long leg

casts, it is necessary to protectively cover those areas of the cast near the buttocks and perineal region to prevent dampness and soilage. Waterproof material (e.g., 4-inch strips of thin plastic material) can be *smoothly* placed under the cast edges and taped to the exterior surface of a dry cast. The material must be smoothly applied because wrinkles will promote pressure damage of the skin. Some sources recommend waterproofing the cast by painting it (when thoroughly dry) with shellac, varnish, white lacquer, or cellulose acetate, or by applying a plastic spray. When painting or spraying a cast, be certain to protectively cover exposed body surfaces, e.g., perineal areas, with a towel. The *entire surface of a cast should not be coated with an air-impervious substance* or the skin beneath cannot properly "breathe" and may macerate. Remember that the porous nature of plaster permits the evaporation of moisture from the skin.

Skin and Cast Care. Skin care (e.g., washing and drying the skin, applying emollient lotions, inspecting the skin, turning the patient frequently) is an extremely important part of caring for any patient wearing a cast. The nurse not only *provides* skin care but also *teaches* any patient who is able how to care for the skin and avoid skin damage. Areas of skin subjected to irritation or pressure can easily develop into decubitus ulcers and therefore require prompt, special attention. Notify the physician of the development of areas of skin irritation or pressure.

It is essential that the buttocks be adequately exposed with a hip spica or body cast so the patient will not become soiled or damp while using the bedpan, and so that adequate skin care can be given. The patient must be carefully and comfortably positioned on the bedpan. "Fracture bedpans" are designed with the body cast or hip spica in mind. Slightly raise the head of the bed (to prevent expelled fluids from running up under the back of the cast), but do not raise the head of the bed so far that the front edge of the cast causes abdominal discomfort. Elevation of the head and shoulders to use the bedpan is generally permissible unless the patient is in shock, hemorrhaging, or has a spinal injury. Damp, soiled casts become malodorous and may mold or break. Dampness also causes skin irritation.

Frequently inspect *all* exposed areas of skin, especially around the edges of the cast, and all body pressure areas, e.g., back of the head, ears, elbows, iliac crests, sacrum, heels. Look for friction rubs, swelling, and discoloration, e.g., redness, blanching, cyanosis. A mirror can be used to look inside the cast as far as possible. When using a mirror, pull the skin taut away from the cast and shine a light down inside the cast. Teach the patient how to inspect the skin, and the importance of these observations.

Each time the patient is turned, make certain to (a) brush away loose pieces of plaster; (b) inspect the exposed skin on which the patient has been lying; (c) give appropriate skin care to those areas; (d) smooth out linens on which the patient will be lying; and (e) inspect exposed cast edges. When giving skin care, dip your fingers in alcohol and reach up under the edges of the cast as far as you can. While inspecting the cast edges (for rough places or plaster breakdown), reach up under the edges of the cast as far as you can and remove plaster crumbs.

It is not safe to insert any foreign object under a cast or to scratch the skin under a cast.

Instruct the patient not to poke *any* objects or scratch vigorously under a cast. Rigid objects placed under a cast create pressure areas and therefore predispose to skin breakdown, infection, and decubitus ulcers. Children are particularly likely to poke objects (e.g., coins, buttons, toothbrushes, small toys) under their casts. Often itching under a cast is extremely uncomfortable (especially in hot weather), and a patient is tempted to slip a knitting needle, wooden back scratcher, pencil, or some other object under the cast to scratch. Explain to the patient that scratching under a cast is unsafe because (a) the skin may be broken and infection develop; (b) the scratching movements disturb the smooth padded surface under the cast and make wrinkles that may contribute to skin breakdown; and (c) the "scratcher" may become lost under the cast and cause pressure and skin breakdown. Also, explain that scratching the skin when it itches usually provides only temporary relief and often causes itching and discomfort to worsen. *If a foreign object becomes caught under the surface of a cast, the physician should be immediately notified.*

Tell the patient not to pull stockinette or padding out of the cast. Explain that these materials are placed under the cast to protect the skin and that their removal not only exposes the skin to the plaster surface but also loosens the cast. Petaling a cast or fixing the turned-back stockinette to the outside of the cast helps secure the inner lining and padding.

Keep the fingers or toes (and their nails) clean in a casted extremity. This can most easily be accomplished by using an applicator dipped in alcohol. Cleanliness not only is refreshing to the patient but also permits better visualization of the toes and fingers and removes potentially infectious materials. To prevent drying and scaling of the fingers or toes on a casted extremity, they should be bathed, covered lightly with oil, and massaged at least daily.

It is important to maintain in good condition the skin of *uncasted* body areas as well as those regions which are casted. As a patient moves about in bed, the skin may become irritated on exposed elbows and heels. These and other exposed pressure areas should be inspected regularly for indications of skin breakdown and appropriate skin care should be frequently given. Powdering the skin is generally not advisable, since powder tends to cake and produce skin irritation.

While giving skin care, *inspect the condition of the cast* and *check its fit.* Excessively loose casts usually need replacing. Sometimes casts are somewhat loose in the morning but fit more securely later in the day, e.g., after a casted leg has been dependent during ambulation. Call to the physician's attention areas of a cast that are deteriorated, cracked, molding, soft, or broken. Loose bracing bars should also be reported. The physician may reinforce weakened or soiled areas of the cast by applying fresh plaster at the bedside.

Positioning the Patient. A patient with a cast can easily become off balance and fall off a stretcher. When a casted patient is being transported on a stretcher, make certain the person is secured to the cart with safety straps. Supervise transfer procedures, e.g., from stretcher to cart, to make certain the transfer team exercises care when moving a newly casted patient. Post a sign on the patient's bed stating that he or she has a damp cast and must be handled and positioned cautiously. Once in bed, make sure the patient is positioned in correct alignment.

Handle a damp cast carefully so that you do not accidentally make finger or thumb impressions in the cast. Lift the cast by cupping your hands and sliding them, palms up, under the cast rather than by grasping the cast with a pinching motion. Unwanted indentations in a cast can cause pressure and decubitus formation on the underlying skin once the cast dries.

A casted extremity should be elevated to minimize swelling. Elevation of a casted limb is especially important for the first 24 to 48 hours after casting.

By promoting drainage, elevation of a dependent part stimulates circulation and reduces edema (and thus pressure within the cast). Elevation of casted extremities often may be done with pillows, but sometimes ropes, weights and pulleys, or slings are used. Placing the newly casted area on pillows also protects the cast from pressure and flattening while drying. Support a damp cast on pillows with rubber or plastic undercovers. A cast should not rest on a hard surface while drying, or continuous pressure will cause it to adapt itself to the contour of the surface, e.g., become flattened. Once a cast is completely dry, it can safely be placed on a hard surface if the patient so desires (e.g., a casted arm may rest on a table), but generally it is still most comfortable if the casted area rests on pillows.

Place supportive pillows along the entire length of a casted area. This is of special importance while the cast is drying. To prepare a bed to receive a patient with a green body cast, place three pillows crosswise on the bed. Make certain the pillows are placed side by side touching each other so that no spaces occur between them; i.e., make certain the cast is completely supported so areas of weakness will not develop during the drying period. To prepare a bed for a patient with a wet hip spica cast, place one pillow crosswise at the waist and two pillows lengthwise under the casted leg. If both legs are casted, use two pillows for each leg. It is generally desirable to place a small pillow or folded flannelette sheet under areas such as the popliteal space or lumbar region to maintain the desired body contour of the cast. Be careful that excessive pressure is not applied over bony prominences and weight-bearing areas, e.g., shoulders, buttocks, hips, heels, during the drying process.

Place pillows in such a way that they help the patient to feel "securely" rather than "precariously" positioned. To prevent a casted limb from rolling off a pillow, e.g., while the patient is up in a wheelchair, it is generally wise to secure the limb to the pillow by pinning a towel across the limb and onto the pillow, or by placing a tie around the limb and pillow. If a casted extremity falls off a pillow, it not only may cause unnecessary pain, but also may break the cast. A damp cast may be moved by pulling gently on the pillows on which the cast rests, with the cast lightly supported while being moved.

Firm orthopedic mattresses or mattresses with fracture boards beneath them are generally used for persons wearing casts. A sagging mattress will tend to deform a green cast and may crack a dry cast.

If a body or spica cast is still green, do not place pillows under the shoulders and head, because the pillows push the patient forward against the front of the cast, deforming the cast and producing pressure on the chest and abdomen.

A casted leg should not remain dependent. Keep the leg elevated to the level of the body to avoid swelling. If swelling is already present, it is necessary to elevate the leg higher than the heart: the foot higher than the knee, the knee higher than the hip, to reduce swelling. To avoid placing excessive pressure on the back of the heel, a patient with a leg cast should be positioned with the foot extending over the edge of the pillow. To prevent foot drop, make certain the plantar surface of an uncasted foot has adequate support while the patient is supine. Protect the toes of a casted foot from pressure caused by bed clothing when the patient is supine. Also, prevent outward rotation of the casted leg. Correct body alignment must be maintained. When a patient with a leg cast (or hip spica cast) is lying prone, a pillow should be placed beneath the casted leg under the dorsum of the foot to prevent pressure on the toes. An alternative method of preventing pressure on the toes is to position the prone patient with the foot over the end of the mattress.

Turning the Patient. Unless it is contraindicated, the patient with a green cast is turned periodically so that more of the casted area is exposed to air during the drying process. The physician may specify when and how often a patient can be turned. When a large cast has been applied (e.g., body cast), the physician may specify that the patient is not to be turned until the evening of the day the cast was applied. Thereafter the turning orders may specify that the patient is to be turned from front to back and vice versa every two hours. Position changes are important during the drying period not only to promote drying but also to prevent pressure damage in structures immobilized in the cast. However, if a patient is turned too soon, a wet cast may be bent or otherwise damaged.

Turning is made easier (for patient and staff members) if the patient was given turning instructions and was able to practice turning with help *prior to* application of the cast. This patient teaching should be given again when the patient is first turned in the cast. Frequent position changes are essential while a patient is in bed to prevent complications of immobility.

Plaster casts are heavy and inflexible. Thus, they not only may limit a patient's activities but also cause serious accidents. Someone wearing a cast is naturally more clumsy and therefore more susceptible to accidents, e.g., falls. Keep the patient's environment as safe as possible, e.g., keep bed wheels locked so patients will not slip and fall as they get out of bed. Straps are placed around a bivalved cast when the patient is being turned, to secure the two sides of the cast together.

Have adequate help to move and position the casted patient. Do not attempt to turn a patient with a heavy cast by yourself. *Always* have at least one other person to help you, and always have someone on each side of the bed. Three or four persons may be needed to turn a patient in a body or hip spica cast. Wet casts are particularly heavy.

The weight of a cast may throw a patient off balance while turning over in bed or starting to sit up; therefore side rails should be kept up. Side rails give the patient something to grasp and so make turning and moving in bed easier. An overhead frame with a trapeze bar often helps a casted patient to be more active and self-sufficient. For example, the patient with a large cast may be able to lift his or her body up (by grasping the trapeze bar) so the bedpan can be slid underneath more comfortably or so that skin care can be given or bed linens smoothed out or changed. Use of a trapeze also helps prevent the patient from chafing the skin on the elbows.

Never *use cast braces or turnbuckles to lift a casted patient. These devices are not placed in casts to serve as handles. They may easily be broken, dislocated, or pulled out of casts.*

Never lift hip spica casts by the ankle, foot, or abduction bar (between the legs). This is true not only while the cast is damp but also when it is dry. *To correctly turn a patient in a hip spica cast,* do as follows. Move the patient to the side of the bed. Slide him or her on the bed or on pillows toward the side of the fractured or operated limb. Move the patient by slipping your hands beneath the buttocks and pulling the person toward you. At the same time, have another person slide and support the patient's shoulders and head, while a third person does the same with the legs. (All upper bed linens should be fanfolded to the foot of the bed and the patient protectively draped. If a head pillow is present, it should be removed before turning the patient.) While the patient is on one side of the bed, prepare the unoccupied side: smooth or change sheets and place pillows. When ready to be turned, the patient places arms at the sides or over the head. The arms should *never* be placed over the head if the patient has a dorsal or cervical spinal injury. If the patient keeps the arms at the side when being turned, place a folded towel between the arm and cast (on the side toward which the person will be turned) so the arm will not be pinched when the weight of the cast rolls over it. Then roll the patient onto the freshly prepared pillows and pull the person back to the center of the bed. The patient rolls to the uninvolved side. During the turning process the casted limb is supported in the air.

As a general rule, always turn a casted patient away from the injured or operated side, i.e., keep weight off the fractured or operated side.

The turning process should occur with one smooth movement, rather than in piecemeal jerks, and the patient should feel securely supported. When turning a patient with a hip spica, be certain to support the casted limb inside the thigh and at the knee and ankle. Provide adequate support along the entire length of a cast so excessive strain does not occur on the casted area. Always support the areas of greatest strain, the joints. Once turned, position the patient comfortably in good body alignment and place pillows along the length of the cast to provide support.

Weight-Bearing and Ambulation. Extremity casts set rapidly, in 10 minutes, but may not be completely dry for two days. Weight-bearing is typically not permitted for at least 24 hours after application of the cast. Pain may be experienced when a casted leg is lowered into a dependent position for the first few times and the patient first begins to stand up and walk. Prepare the patient for this. Explain that the pain is not unusual and that it results from blood rushing into the leg as the leg is lowered. Lower the leg for only short periods of time at first and then gradually lengthen the periods of dependency. Once the leg becomes accustomed to complete circulation the pain subsides. Weak, aged, and debilitated patients often find the weight of a cast to be extremely fatiguing and may tire rapidly when up for the first few times. Observe such patients closely and avoid excessive fatigue and accidents.

If a patient has a walking cast, the leg should be kept elevated when not ambulatory. The leg may not swell while the patient is walking because intermittent weight-bearing that occurs with walking acts as a pump, circulating the blood and forcing venous return. However, once the patient stops walking and stands still, or sits down with the leg dependent, it will swell.[137]

A casted arm should be kept elevated when the patient is out of bed. Most commonly this elevation is achieved by placing the arm in a *sling*. Remember the following points:

- Support the entire arm, including the elbow, wrist and hand (permitting wrist drop encourages neurovascular complications).
- When the arm rests in the sling, the fingers should be higher than the elbow (to minimize edema).
- Secure the sling at the back of the neck with two pins (do not tie a knot over the cervical vertebrae; do not place pins over the cervical vertebrae; use two pins to ensure secure fastening of the sling).
- Secure the elbow flap with pins so the elbow is well supported and the arm will not slip out of the sling.

Periodically inspect and readjust the sling so it is comfortable and correctly positioned. Placement of a pad at the back of the neck between the sling and the skin may prevent skin irritation and pressure.

If a sling is awkward while the patient is sitting up, the arm may be elvated on a pillow. To prevent the arm from falling off the pillow place a tie around both arm and pillow. Precautions such as these take but a moment to observe and may spare the patient further pain and injury. Also, they contribute to the patient's feelings of security and thereby promote mental relaxation (an important component in the recovery process).

Exercises. Exercising is important while a patient is in a cast. Appropriate exercises help prevent complications during periods of immobility, enhance healing, and facilitate the rehabilitation process following cast removal. Typically the patient is taught to *exercise the joints above and below the cast*. Thus the patient in a long arm cast is usually advised to exercise the shoulder, thumb, and fingers. With a casted arm it is generally important to exercise the shoulder (if it is outside the cast) because (a) the shoulder joint can rapidly become stiff or "frozen"; and (b) the shoulder must support the weight of the cast. Often there is a tendency to hold the shoulder immobile on the affected side even though it is not casted. Teach the patient to periodically lift the casted arm up over the head. Also, teach the patient with an arm cast to frequently move each finger, which stimulates circulation and increases venous return.

A patient with injury to the shoulder or humerus should *not* exercise the involved arm or shoulder unless specifically directed to do so by the doctor. Shoulder motion should be limited with a hanging arm cast. Maintain the hanging position of this cast at all times.

The patient in a long leg cast should exercise the hip joint and toes. Exercising toes stimulates circulation and increases venous return.

Isometric exercises (isometric muscle contractions) of the muscles immobilized by the cast usually are not routinely performed without the physician's approval. However, when the physician permits, the patient learns isometric exercises and may be advised to practice them at least hourly while awake.[207] Explain that these exercises do not actually cause the limb to move or joints to bend, but they cause muscles to contract.

Teach the patient isometric exercises first on the unaffected limbs. The patient with a casted knee may be taught to try to push down with the knee inside the cast. This exercise (quadriceps setting) tightens the leg muscles and the patient can observe how the muscles contract without moving the limb. It may be helpful, when teaching the patient this exercise, if you place your hand beneath the knee and instruct the patient to try to push the knee down onto your hand. In a casted arm, opening and closing the hand (to make a fist) provides isometric exercising of the arm muscles.

Isometric muscle exercises help to maintain muscle strength and muscle mass. Thus they combat the weakness and disuse atrophy which tend to develop in unused muscles. All forms of exercise help a patient to retain command of muscles, i.e., help the person to remember how to send nerve impulse messages through the central nervous system to control movements.

The patient confined to bed may be taught other exercises to prevent complications and to prepare for future activities, e.g., crutch walking. These exercises may include gluteal setting, abdominal tightening, and deep breathing.

To maintain the muscle tone and mobility of uncasted structures, the unaffected joints should be put through their full range of motion several times daily. Uncasted structures often have to perform "extra duties" to relieve casted areas, and therefore they should be maintained in optimum condition. Encourage the patient to actively exercise. Participation in self-care activities indirectly provides additional exercise for a patient.

Complications. A patient wearing a cast requires professional observation and care, particularly for the first day or two following cast application. A cast does not surround a patient in a haven of protective safety. Although a cast may provide protective and therapeutic functions, it may also create and then hide from view serious complications. Complications in a casted part may be caused by such factors as

- swelling of the casted part;
- application of a cast that is too tight;
- indentations in the plaster;
- wrinkles in underlying padding;
- foreign objects pushed under the cast;
- vascular or nerve damage sustained during injury or treatment, e.g., surgery, fracture reduction, or the formation of vascular emboli or thrombi.

Pressure upon casted structures can cause irreparable damage to skin, muscles, blood vessels, or nerves (see Fig. 76–15). Because a cast is inflexible, it makes certain movements impossible and can dangerously cause pressure on and constriction of underlying structures. Serious complications can develop quite rapidly in a casted limb. As a result of the development of complications, a limb may be paralyzed or anesthetized for life. Loss of blood supply or innervation jeopardizes a limb, and in some instances amputation of the limb is necessary. The development of "cast syndrome" (see below) in a patient with a body cast can be fatal if untreated.

Below are summarized some of the complications most frequently seen in a casted patient, and the symptoms indicative of these complications. These symptoms and their detection and evaluation are discussed further in following paragraphs.

1. *Impaired blood flow* producing soft tissue ischemia, e.g., due to pressure in casted extremity. Possible symptoms include:

   Pulselessness in extremity
   Inadequate capillary refill in nail beds
   Pallor, blanching, or cyanosis of skin
   Pain of various types
   Coldness of skin
   Swelling; painful edema peripheral to cast
   Paresthesias
   Hypesthesia

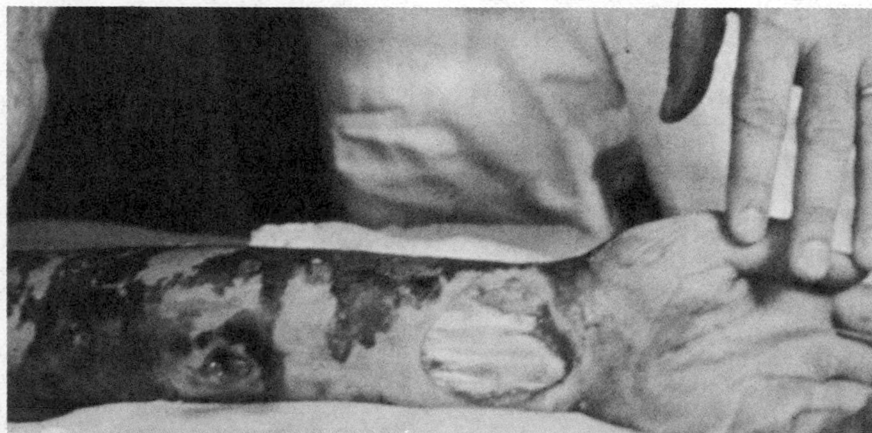

Figure 76–15. This young man had an open fracture of his left forearm treated by a plaster of Paris cast. When, subsequently, the arm became infected and swollen, his complaints of pain were disregarded. Ultimately, his entire arm became necrotic. This is how it looked immediately prior to amputation. (From Rockwood, C., and D. Green: Fractures. Vol. I. Philadelphia: J. B. Lippincott Co., 1975.)

Anesthesia (numbness)
Motor paralysis of previously functioning member

2. *Nerve damage,* e.g., due to pressure on a nerve as it passes over a bony prominence. Possible symptoms include:

Pain, increasing, persistent, and localized
Hypesthesia
Anesthesia (numbness)
Feelings of deep pressure
Paresthesias
Motor weakness or paralysis not previously present

3. *Infection, tissue necrosis,* e.g., due to skin breakdown. Possible symptoms include:

Musty, unpleasant odor over cast and/or at ends of cast
Drainage through cast or cast opening
Sudden unexplained body temperature elevation
"Hot spot" felt on cast over lesion

4. *Cast syndrome,* occurs with body casts. Possible symptoms include:

Prolonged nausea
Repeated vomiting
Abdominal distention
Vague abdominal pain

Constriction of a casted limb may reduce or prevent arterial and venous circulation. *Gangrene* may develop in an ischemic limb which has inadequate arterial blood flow. *Swelling* and *vascular engorgement* typically develop in a limb in which venous return is impaired but the arterial blood flow continues. Blood flow may also be obstructed by the presence of an embolus or thrombus within a blood vessel (e.g., from thrombophlebitis or fat embolism).

A limb may have its arterial blood flow completely interrupted for 2 to 4 hours without residual effects.[207] Therefore, with early treatment, circulatory embarrassment to a limb need not cause irreversible damage. However, *early* recognition and treatment are essential.

Volkmann's ischemic contracture (discussed earlier in this chapter, see Fig. 76–6) is a permanent deformity that can develop in a casted arm unless vigilant preventive care is given. Indications of developing Volkmann's contracture include diminished or absent radial pulse; swelling of the hand and fingers; and bluish discoloration of the hand, fingers, and fingernails. Observe a patient with a casted arm closely for these symptoms and report them immediately if they begin to develop so the cast can be cut and blood flow can be restored to the ischemic tissues before irreparable damage occurs.

A cast can cause *nerve damage* by compressing a superficial peripheral nerve (e.g., the common peroneal nerve in the region of the knee) against underlying bone (e.g., the neck of the fibula). Nerve damage disrupts the transmission of nerve impulse messages back and forth through the nerve. As a result, structures distal to the damage are not adequately innervated, and their function is impaired, i.e., they develop *anesthesia* and *paralysis.* For example, destruction of the common peroneal nerve (located on the lateral side of the leg below the head of the fibula) causes loss of sensation on the foot's dorsolateral aspect and paralysis (loss of ability to extend the toes or dorsiflex the foot, i.e., foot drop). While nerve damage is sometimes reversible (incomplete), in other cases the damage is irreversible. Skin necrosis and irreversible paralysis may develop within 24 hours.

Bony prominences are subcutaneous and have only minimal protection from overly soft tissues. Pressure from a cast over these prominences produces localized *tissue ischemia* by compressing the skin and subcutaneous tissue (with their local veins and arterioles) against the bone. If this pressure continues, the ischemic tissue eventually breaks down and becomes necrotic, i.e., a *decubitus ulcer* (pressure sore) develops. While pressure areas may be painful initially, the pain subsides once death of the tissue devitalizes the nerves in the region. Areas of skin slough thus become anesthetic (i.e., without pain or other sensations) soon after the local sensory nerve endings are destroyed. Pain may last only a few days. While it is present the pain is typically of a localized burning nature. *Remember:* cessation of pain does not mean "all is well." Instead it often means that a lesion has developed which is anesthetized but worsening.

NERVE FUNCTION TESTS

Nerve	Action By The Nurse: Test For Sensory Function	Action By The Patient: Test For Motor Function
Radial	Prick web space between thumb and index finger	Hyperextend thumb or wrist
Median	Prick distal surface of index finger	Oppose thumb and little finger; flex wrist
Ulnar	Prick distal end of small finger	Abduct all fingers
Peroneal	Prick lateral surface of great toe and medial surface of second toe	Dorsiflex ankle; extend toes
Tibial	Prick medial and lateral surfaces of sole of foot	Plantarflex ankle and flex toes

From Farrell, J.: *Illustrated Guide to Orthopedic Nursing.* Philadelphia: J. B. Lippincott Co., 1977, p. 17.

Cast-related complications (e.g., paralysis, pressure sores, and the results of ischemia) are all preventable. *Nurses play an important role in the prevention of these disabling disorders.*

Because nurses are most commonly the professional people who are with a newly casted patient, it is their responsibility to observe the patient closely, report early indications of complications at once, and evaluate the patient's general condition. Report nausea, chills, vomiting, rash, and fever. These symptoms may indicate complications under the plaster. If the patient has been given an anesthetic or has had surgery, give appropriate postanesthesia and postoperative care (see Unit VIII and the last section of this chapter). Watch for symptoms of delayed shock, e.g., sudden weakness, faintness, pallor, dizziness, diaphoresis, alterations in pulse and blood pressure (see Chapter 13).

Evaluation of a casted patient for indications of cast-related complications should be conducted in a planned, orderly manner so that significant findings are not missed.

Establish a pattern for observations and always carry observations out sequentially. For example, in a casted extremity assess (1) skin color, (2) skin temperature, (3) vascular return, (4) sensation, (5) swelling, and (6) active motion. One helpful way of remembering some of the significant symptoms of cast-related complications is the mnemonic of the "*5 P's*": *P*ain, *P*allor, *P*ulselessness, *P*aresthesia, and *P*aralysis.

Every toe or finger should be observable on casted limbs, i.e., not inadvertently covered with plaster. Observe *each* toe and finger separately.

Nurses use the senses of touch, sight, smell, and hearing to assess a patient with a cast. The observations made should be explained to the patient. Patients who are sent home with casts must be taught how to make routine observations for developing complications. They should be instructed to contact their physician immediately if untoward symptoms begin to develop.

Tactile Observations. Feel the *temperature of the skin* in areas distal to a cast, e.g., hand, foot, fingers, toes. Compare the patient's skin temperature on the casted side with the other side of the body. Abnormal skin temperatures should be immediately reported. Remember that ice bags applied to the sides of the cast will contribute to coolness in the casted limb. Arterial insufficiency causes coolness (and pallor) in exposed fingers and toes.

Check *peripheral pulses* and compare the pulse in the casted arm with that in the opposite normal limb. Impaired arterial blood flow to a limb causes loss of the peripheral pulses. Check the radial pulse at the wrist (of a casted arm) or the dorsalis pedis pulse on the dorsum of the foot (of a casted leg). Casts may be windowed over these areas to permit palpation of the pulse. Notify the doctor at once of pulselessness.

Evaluate the patient's awareness of *pinpricks* and *light touch*. Hypesthesia (hypoesthesia) and anesthesia are indications of serious damage to the limb. Hypesthesia means an abnormally reduced sensitiveness of the skin; anesthesia refers to total loss of feeling or sensation.

Have patients shut their eyes while you touch each finger or toe on a casted extremity. Ask them to tell you when they can feel the touch and have them identify which finger or toe they think you are touching. With a pin, gently touch the surface of the skin to identify areas of numbness. Specifically search for indications of damage to the peroneal nerve (in a casted leg) and the median, ulnar, and radial nerves (in a casted arm).

- *Peroneal nerve:* check for sensation in the web space dorsally between the great and second toes. Report loss of sensation immediately. As stated previously, peroneal nerve damage can result in foot drop.
- *Median, ulnar, and radial nerves:* check volar surface of index finger for innervation by the median nerve; test volar surface of little finger for ulnar innervation, and dorsal surface of web space between thumb and index finger for radial innervation.

When assessing sensory losses, review the patient's records to see if these losses were present before the cast was applied.

Feel the *surface* of the cast. Place the palm of your hand on the cast and move it over the entire surface of the cast. This inspection is made to identify areas of the cast that feel appreciably warmer than other areas—"hot spots." Often areas of tissue necrosis or infection will cause the overlying area of cast to feel warmer. Evaluate with particular care the cast sections which are over pressure points.

Visual Observations. Note the *color of the skin* distal to the cast. Observe for indications of circulatory impairment, e.g., pallor, blanching, cyanosis. Compare the skin color around casted areas with skin color in other parts of the body. Compare the color of the skin in the casted extremity with the opposite extremity (when held in the same position). Cyanosis results from impaired venous return (e.g., due to soft tissue constriction) and may be a late indication of impaired circulation. Increasing cyanosis, accompanied by persistent pain or paresthesias, requires immediate relief. Pallor or blanching may indicate arterial insufficiency, e.g., due to thrombosis or vasospasm. Freshly oxygenated blood is not reaching the part when arterial blood flow is impaired.

► The *blanching test* is a useful measurement of circulatory effectiveness of particular importance in evaluating a patient with an extremity cast. The test evaluates capillary refill in the nailbed of a casted limb. With your thumbnail briefly (and gently) compress the nail of the patient's thumb (on the casted arm) or the great toe (on the casted leg). You will be able to see color leave the compressed area. Then quickly release the pressure and observe the speed with which color returns to the blanched area (as the capillaries, which had blood squeezed out of them, refill with blood). Compare the capillary refilling on the casted limb with that on the patient's unaffected side. If color returns too rapidly, it may indicate venous congestion. Sluggish return of color may be indicative of circulatory obstruction producing arterial insufficiency.[135] However, it is possible for capillary refill to be relatively normal in the nailbeds even though a limb is pulseless.

Ask the patient to *move the fingers or toes* on the casted limb. Movement should typically be easy and painless, unless the patient has an injury to the hand or foot that restricts motion. Motor paralysis of the fingers or toes may be present owing to primary nerve damage, or the patient may be unable to move because of pain. Painful motion usually indicates an excessive degree of swelling and should be reported. Even gentle passive motion of the fingers or toes of an ischemic limb produces extreme pain. Motor paralysis is a late symptom of ischemia. When motor paralysis results from primary nerve injury, other symptoms of vascular insufficiency are not present.[207]

Inspect the skin all around the cast edges for evidence of *skin damage or swelling.* Injury to an extremity and the subsequent treatment of the injury (e.g., reduction, surgery) usually produce swelling which progresses for the first 12 to 24 postinjury or postoperative hours and may be greatest for the first 24 to 48 hours. While mild swelling, i.e., edema, of exposed fingers and toes is not unusual (particularly if the cast limb is in a dependent position), moderate or severe swelling associated with pain and discoloration is abnormal. Edema should not be painful and should not be greater than plus 2. When a casted part swells markedly, mechanical constriction of the structures within the cast occurs, and severe complications result. Swelling causes the cast to feel tight. Edema may obstruct blood flow so much that blood moves ahead in vessels only when the heart contracts. This may cause a throbbing sensation which may be painful. Report increasing edema, accompanied by pain or other symptoms, e.g., paresthesia, numbness.

Measures effective in preventing or relieving excessive swelling include[135] (a) elevating the full length of the cast higher than the heart, (b) exercising the fingers and toes to stimulate circulation, and (c) placing ice bags beside (not on) the cast. If excessive swelling and pressure persist in spite of therapeutic measures, notify the physician immediately. Pressure caused from edema must be relieved by cutting the cast before irreversible damage occurs. In the absence of edema, pressure against the skin caused by the edge of a cast may be relieved by changing the patient's position or by loosely padding the area which is causing the patient discomfort.

Observe the surface of the cast for indications of *wound drainage* (stains) or *bleeding.* Inspect the cast closely at areas covering known wounds (e.g., surgical incisions or accidental wounds) and over all pressure points (for indications of damage to underlying skin). When an area of drainage or bleeding becomes visible, a notation should be made of the time and date of the observation. Charting should include the size of the drainage area and the character of the drainage. Repeated observations are made to determine whether the area of drainage is enlarging. Always call areas of drainage or bleeding to the physician's attention. The physician may decide to "window" the cast to examine the wound directly. Complete cast removal may be necessary if excessive hemorrhage occurs.

Observe the patient wearing a body cast for *abdominal distention.* It may be necessary to have an opening cut over the patient's abdomen to relieve pressure from distention and listen for bowel sounds. Additionally, if ordered, a nasogastric tube may be inserted for decompression. *Cast syndrome*[178] is a potentially fatal complication that can develop in a patient with a body cast. The syndrome is characterized by prolonged nausea and repeated vomiting secondary to gastric and duodenal dilatation. Abdominal distention and vague abdominal pain may also occur. If untreated, the patient develops severe hypokalemic alkalosis and hypovolemia and eventually dies. While gastrointestinal dilatation may have various causes, when it occurs as part of the cast syndrome the pathogenesis is mechanical compression of the fourth portion of the duodenum by the superior mesenteric artery. Total bowel obstruction may develop once the edematous duodenum dilates so much that it cannot continue to propel its contents into the jejunum. Treatment includes intestinal decompression, fluid and electrolyte replenishment, and removal of the cast. In some cases surgical intestinal anastomosis is necessary.

Olfactory Observations. Place your nose close to the cast and smell for odors indicative of tissue necrosis and infection. It is not unusual for casts to develop a somewhat "sour" smell after a period of time. This odor is produced by perspiration and the normal amount of sloughing of the skin's outer layers. Pathologic tissue necrosis emits a musty offensive odor which can easily be detected and which is much more unpleasant and strong than the typical odor of a cast which has been on for some time. With experience, nurses can easily identify abnormal odors *if* they take the time to smell the cast each day. Cast odor may take several days to appear. Areas of the cast which must be evaluated especially carefully in this manner are around the edges of the cast and over any "hot spots" or areas of discoloration on the cast. A musty odor may be the only indication of skin necrosis or infection (e.g., gas bacillus infection) beneath a cast. However, also assess the patient for other indications of infection, e.g., elevated temperature, elevated white blood count.

Auditory Observations. *Listen, listen, listen* to patients' comments about how they feel, and investigate *all* reports indicative of developing complications!

> *Many patients have suffered serious irreversible complications from casts because no one listened and appropriately responded to their "complaints."*

Negligence of this sort is inexcusable. Pay attention to what patients tell you and evaluate what they say. Make additional observations of your own and make appropriate responses.

Pain is the main symptom of circulatory impairment from a cast.[207] The pain is not localized and is usually burning or cramping in nature. The amount of pain is greater than that expected to occur from the surgery or injury. A fractured extremity typically becomes progressively painless once it is properly immobilized. Constant, undiminished pain which is present for as long as *four* hours after a patient recovers from anesthesia should be viewed with suspicion. If the pain remains unchanged after *six* hours the physician is notified and an immediate investigation is made of the cause of the pain. The patient is not given narcotics until the safety of the extremity is established. Pain is an important diagnostic symptom in this situation, and should not be suppressed or masked until a thorough assessment is made of the patient's condition.

> *Do not administer pain medication to a patient wearing a cast until the cause of the pain has been evaluated.*

All personnel working with casted patients should be knowledgeable about potential complications of casts and should see that indications of these complications are reported at once to persons who will provide help to the patient. *All* patients wearing casts should be encouraged to report any abnormal symptoms, and each patient should be given a *complete* cast inspection at least once each day (more often in the newly casted patient). Findings from these inspections should be charted. These records not only serve as guides for future care but also may provide useful evidence in court in malpractice or negligence suits.

Notify the physician *immediately* of any indications of complications in a casted patient so appropriate action can be taken immediately. Waiting to tell the doctor may cause the patient to suffer serious complications which could have been prevented by prompt therapy.

Often when symptoms of complications are present the physician decides to bivalve (split) the patient's cast to relieve pressure or to inspect the limb. *The cast and underlying padding must be cut completely down to the skin to properly bivalve a cast.* It is not sufficient to merely cut through the top layers of the cast, because the pressure is being exerted by those layers of bandages and casts which are directly against the skin. If cast pressure was the cause of a patient's symptoms, immediate relief of pain will be experienced when the cast is opened. If pain persists, the physician continues assessment to determine the cause of the pain. It may be necessary to return the patient to surgery. When bivalving is performed to relieve pressure, be certain to elevate the limb after bivalving is accomplished to aid in the reduction of swelling.

Nutrition. Increased roughage content in the diet of a patient with limited activity may help maintain normal bowel elimination. The patient in a body cast or hip spica cast may need to avoid gas-forming foods if they tend to create abdominal distention. A general, well-balanced diet promotes wound healing.

Psychosocial Adjustments. Patients wearing casts frequently find it difficult to become accustomed to the physical restraint imposed by confinement in plaster. In addition to restricting mobility and natural movements, casts often create other discomforts, e.g., itching, fatigue (from the weight of the cast). It is not unusual for persons with casts (especially large casts, such as body casts, hip spicas, etc.) to become irritable, tense, discouraged, or depressed.

Physical tension may be relieved by activity and massage. Patients should be encouraged to practice self-care as much as possible and to follow their physician's orders for exercises and activity. Nurses, occupational therapists, and physical therapists combine their professional efforts to help patients engage in meaningful activities during the rehabilitative-recovery period. Activities are individually selected to meet a given patient's needs and life style. When a nurse understands the problems which a patient may be experiencing during recovery, it is possible to more accurately interpret behavior and help significant others so they do not unnecessarily contribute to the patient's burdens.

It is desirable for a casted patient to perform as much self-care as possible so that the person will not only move about (indirectly exercise) but also maintain feelings of independence and self-esteem. Remember that a cast limits motion. Thus, if you want patients to be able to perform various self-care activities, you must make certain they are able to reach the items they need. Attempt to anticipate the patient's needs and

PATIENT-FAMILY TEACHING GUIDE TIPS IN CARING FOR YOUR CAST

If it becomes soiled, clean with a cloth dampened with dry cleanser. If still soiled, use white shoe polish, but *sparingly;* too much may saturate and soften cast.
Avoid getting water on or in your cast. If it becomes damp, use a hair dryer to dry area.
Plastic bags are good covering in wet weather.
If cast becomes rough on edges, cover rough area with tape.

Caring For Your Skin While Wearing Your Cast

Wash skin area around cast taking care not to saturate cast in the process.
Rub the areas around the cast frequently with alcohol. Lotion has a tendency to build up on the inside of the cast and becomes sticky, so it should never be used around the cast or under it.
If edges are causing irritation to the skin, pad with some soft materials such as cotton or foam. Be sure the padding is well anchored to the cast, as loose material slipping into the cast will cause even more irritation.

Important Things to Watch For and Do While You Are Wearing Your Cast

Twice a day check your fingers, if the cast is on your arm; and toes, if the cast is on your leg.
Are they pink in color? Squeeze the nails till white; when released, they should have an immediate return to their pink color. If return is slow, call your doctor.
Do not be alarmed if your foot appears darker when it is down. This is normal.
Watch for swelling. Compare it to the other hand or foot. Are they about the same?
Move fingers or toes, NOT JUST WIGGLE, but fully extend the fingers or toes. If any loss of motion or any increased pain, call your doctor.
Make sure there is feeling on all surfaces of the hand and fingers, or foot and toes. If *any* numbness, tingling, or pinprick pain develops, call your doctor.
Check around cast for any odors other than those that may be from something spilled on or around the cast. Ordinarily, casts won't smell. Be especially conscious of odors if there are stitches under the cast. If any smell is noticed, don't delay, call your doctor. Also watch for any staining of, or discharge from, the cast.
If swelling is noted after activity, elevate the extremity, the higher the better.
Arm casts are most comfortable with a sling support.

If Your Doctor Permits—Then—

To keep shoulder from becoming stiff, EACH DAY, four times a day, remove the sling and exercise the arm by putting it through its full range of motion. In other words, move it the way it normally goes.
For the leg in a cast, if possible, work at "setting," that is, tightening, then relaxing the thigh muscles, doing this frequently, or every two hours while awake. You should discuss this with your doctor FIRST, but some exercise is essential.
If skin under the cast begins to itch, DO NOT try to stick anything inside the cast to scratch, especially if there is an area with stitches. Parents: especially be alert to children sticking forks, sticks, or other ingenious objects inside the cast.

Remember:
Cast Care Must Continue As Long As Your Cast Is On

If you undergo a cast change, the whole process of observation and care begins anew.

From Farrell, J.: *Illustrated Guide to Orthopedic Nursing.* Philadelphia: J. B. Lippincott Co., 1977, p. 23.

then unobtrusively perform activities the patient cannot manage, e.g., cutting meat. Have a call bell within easy reach at all times. When the patient with a cast is able to be dressed, instruction may be required about how to put on clothes most easily. Some casts restrict the wearing of certain types of clothing, and clothing must be modified to be worn over the cast.

Discharge. Some patients are sent home with green casts. Others are kept in the hospital until their casts are dry and then are discharged if no symptoms of complications have appeared. Still others remain hospitalized as long as they are casted.

The patient who is sent home with a cast should be provided with explanations of proper cast care and cast observations. Include significant others in these teaching sessions when possible. Printed instructions will give them something accurate to refer to. Anxious persons often have difficulty remembering details, and if sent home soon after the cast is applied, the patient may be too overwhelmed by the injury and its treatment to remember detailed instructions. Illustrations can be valuable teaching aids for both literate and nonliterate persons.

Instructions should include not only details of immediate cast care during the drying period (if the cast is wet) but also information about care of the dry cast. Tell the patient to keep the casted extremity elevated and to keep the cast dry and protected. A stocking or piece of stockinette may be worn to keep the exterior of the cast clean and to keep toes or fingers warm. If the cast is to be worn for some time, the exterior sometimes may be painted with shellac, plastic spray, or varnish (once it is dry) to help keep the surface clean. If the cast surface becomes soiled, it may be cleaned by using a damp (not soaking wet) cloth and some scouring powder.

The patient with a casted leg should be told whether weight-bearing on the affected side is possible. A weight-bearing cast must be completely dry before weight is placed on it. Crutches, when necessary, are fitted to the patient, who is given instruction in their use before discharge.

Make certain patients understand the symptoms of complications that should be watched for and that they know how to notify the doctor if any complications appear to be developing. Emphasize that symptoms such as severe pain, burning, numbness, tingling, swelling, skin discoloration (e.g., blueness), paralysis, and pallor should be reported *immediately* day or night. Provide instruction for activity, e.g., move toes and fingers for several minutes every one-half hour. Also, supply the patient with information about when and where to see the doctor for the next scheduled appointment. Between appointments the patient should report by telephone indications of deterioration of the cast, e.g., cracking or softening.

Cast Changes. Changes are commonly necessary when a cast no longer fits, owing to weight loss, weight gain, or muscular atrophy. Sometimes it is necessary to change a patient's cast more than once, to provide additional treatment or to inspect the involved area. Between changes the patient's skin is cared for according to the physician's specifications. Sometimes the doctor orders calamine lotion with Benadryl to be applied before recasting to relieve or prevent itching. Frequent observations should be made for the first day or two following cast changes, just as with a newly casted patient. These observations are especially important if the angle of the cast has been changed (e.g., with a body cast or turnbuckle cast) because new pressure areas may appear and rapidly cause severe neurovascular damage.

Cast Removal. The length of time a patient continues to wear a cast varies depending upon the type and extent of injury, disease, or surgery and the rate of healing.

Removal of a cast is usually accomplished with an *electric cast cutter,* which resembles a small electric saw with a circular blade (See Figure 76–16*A*.) Because of its appearance and the noise it produces, a cast cutter is often frightening to the patient. Explain to the patient that the fine toothed blade does not whirl around and cut like a saw blade, but rather the blade breaks the plaster by oscillating or vibrating rapidly back and forth. The vibrations separate the plaster by shaking it. Reassure the patient that he or she will not be cut by the blade. Bandage scissors are used to cut open the final padded layers of the cast. When a cast cutter is used, the patient may feel sensations of heat, vibrations, or pressure, but no pain. Instruct the patient to hold still while the cutter is being used. Cast cutters usually have a vacuum apparatus on them that will vacuum the plaster dustings.

A cast may also be removed manually by drawing the blade of a *plaster knife* or *hand saw* along the outside of the cast and then cutting the cast with *heavy plaster shears* or wedging the cut open with a *spreader* (See Figure 76–16*B*). Cast cutting is sometimes made easier by applying acetic acid (vinegar) along the cutting line to soften the plaster.

The time of cast removal is frequently a time of mixed anxiety and anticipation for the patient. To keep expectations realistic, the patient should be told before the cast is removed generally how the casted area will look and feel. The skin under a casted area is commonly mottled and covered with yellow-brown scales or crusts of dead skin, oil, and exudate. The muscles may appear flabby and slightly atrophied (disuse atrophy). If an incision underlies the cast, it will be exposed, possibly for the first time. Additionally, a cast extremity will not "feel like new" when the cast is removed, but rather it will be stiff and weakened from inactivity. New aches and pains may appear with movement following cast removal as muscles and tissues are subjected to new stresses and strains. Finally, removal of the weight of the cast will cause the body to feel lighter.

Handle the limb gently when removing it from the cast. The patient may be physically quite tense and fearful of motion and pain. Provide adequate support, especially under joints, and avoid quick or jerky movements. Joints tend to be unstable initially when the rigid support of a cast is removed. It is necessary to continue to protect and support the weakened limb for a while. This may be accomplished in various ways, e.g., by the use of pillows, elastic bandages, crutches, or a splint, brace, sling, or cane. The patient will initially be most comfortable if positioned similar to the position maintained while casted.

Opinion varies concerning management of the skin following removal of a cast. Some physicians believe that the caked exudate on the skin serves a protective function, and they recommend gradually cleansing the skin over a period of several days by general soaking. Other physicians recommend scrubbing off the exudate, e.g., with pHisoHex or Betadine. If scrubs are ordered, they should be gently performed so as not to traumatize the skin or be painful to the patient. The underlying new skin is highly sensitive. Whether or not the exudate is removed, the skin is lubricated with cocoa butter, a lanolin solution, mineral oil, A & D ointment, or some other emollient to help soften and remove the crusts. A soft cotton wrap or elastic bandage may then be applied. If Ace bandages are recommended, they should be used only during the daytime. During the day the bandages need to be periodically removed and reapplied to prevent excessive constriction. Care must be taken not to pull the bandages taut when applying them. Advise the patient not to pick at or scratch the skin.

Rehabilitation. Rehabilitative instructions are given by the physician and should be individualized according to the patient's condition. If a leg has been casted, the patient is told if he or she can be weight-bearing and how much ambulation is permitted. If an arm has been casted, the patient is instructed as to how to use the arm, e.g., how much weight can be safelty lifted. Reassure the patient that with exercise and use muscle atrophy will be overcome and the weakness and stiffness present when the cast is removed.

The physical therapist often participates in rehabilitative care following cast removal, e.g., by teaching and supervising graded active exercises (to stimulate circulation and increase muscle strength and joint range of motion) and by carrying out other prescribed activities like

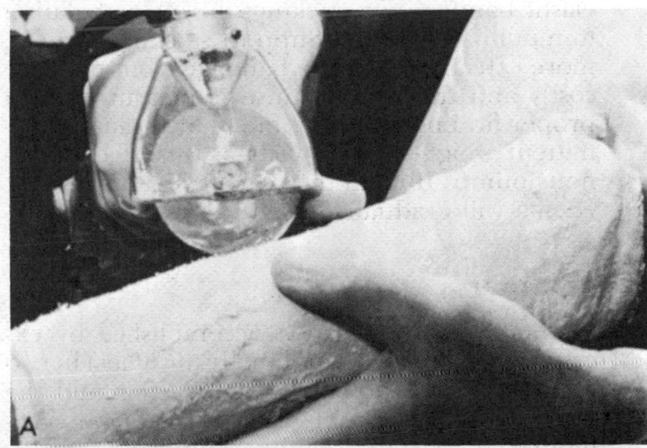

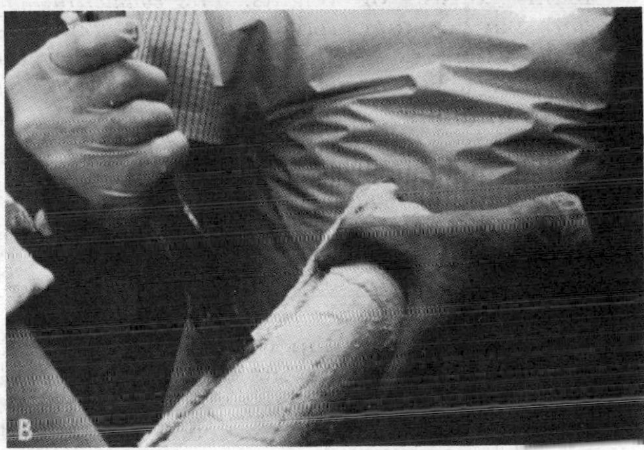

Figure 76 10. Cast removal. A, An oscillating saw (cast cutter) is used first. B, The cast edges are then slightly separated, using a spreader. (From Farrell, J.: Illustrated Guide to Orthopedic Nursing. Philadelphia: J. B. Lippincott Co., 1977.)

whirlpool baths and massage. It is undesirable to force joints and muscles during the period of recovery (by passive stretching exercises, resistive exercises, or forced movements) because placing excessive demands on stiff, weakened limbs will only cause further impairment of motion by increasing fibrosis and excessively engorging the area with blood. Commonly the patient is advised to move the limb actively within limits of stiffness or pain, but not to force movement.

Following cast removal, edema and swelling tend to occur for a while when the involved limb is placed in a dependent position. With increased activity and improvement in muscle tone and circulation, these problems will gradually lessen. However, until they subside the limb should be kept elevated most of the time (higher than the heart) while the patient sits or lies down. Sometimes the physician recommends the use of elastic bandages or stockings during ambulation to minimize swelling. Support stockings may be more effective than the bandages, but they are costly and the patient must be measured for a proper fit. Encourage ambulation because intermittent weight-bearing acts as an effective venous pump. Inform the patient that dependent edema will gradually lessen.

TRACTION

Therapeutic traction is accomplished by exerting a pull (on the head, body, or limbs) in two directions, i.e., the pull of the traction and the pull of countertraction. The *traction force* commonly consists of weights. The *countertraction force* may be either (a) the weight of the patient's body (as it rests on and tends to slide down an inclined surface, such as a tilted bed); or (b) other weights.

> *When traction (pull) is applied in one direction it is necessary to have an equal traction (countertraction) in the opposite direction.*

When traction is properly applied, the patient is centered in a bed and the affected part is held properly aligned by a constant pull. The patient will be immobilized in the center of the bed when traction and countertraction are equal. The direction of pull when applied to long bones is in line with the bones' long axes; it is in line with the spinal column when applied to the head or pelvis. As indicated, countertraction may be obtained by elevating the bed in such a way that the patient's body weight opposes the pull of the traction. Commonly the bed is elevated or tilted under the part which is in traction; e.g., the foot of the bed may be elevated when traction is applied to the lower extremities. If the bed is not properly tilted, the countertraction achieved is inadequate and the patient tends to slide in the direction of the traction force rather than away from it. This defeats the purpose of the traction apparatus, and an effective stretch cannot be obtained on the injured part. With some types of traction, countertraction can be applied with ropes, pulleys, and weights pulling in a direction opposite to that of the traction (see below).

Methods of Applying Traction. Traction may be applied (a) *manually,* by pulling on the part with the hands; (b) *mechanically,* by exerting a pull on the part with ropes and pulleys; (c) with special devices inserted in *casts* (plaster traction); or (d) with *braces.*

- *Manual traction* may be applied for various therapeutic purposes, e.g., correction of a dislocation or reduction of a fracture. With the physician's permission and direction, nurses may apply manual traction (a) when a patient with an injury requiring continuous traction is being transported or repositioned in bed or (b) when casts or traction are being initially applied or changed. Manual traction is applied with a firm steady pull rather than a sudden jerking motion. Manual traction may be used when giving emergency care to an injured person.
- *Mechanical traction* can be applied (e.g., with special halters, splints, bandages, ropes, pulleys, and weights) to either the skin (*skin traction*) or bones (*skeletal traction*).
- *Plaster traction* may be accomplished by the use of turnbuckle casts or hyperextension casts. Also, *skeletal traction* can be applied by fixing the ends of Kirschner wires or Steinmann pins in plaster when applying a cast. Skeletal traction obtained in this way provides a fixed type of traction which maintains the position of the extremity and yet permits the patient to move around without disturbing the alignment of the traction.[137] (Turnbuckle casts and body casts were discussed in the previous section.)
- Traction may also be applied with special *braces,* e.g., hyperextension braces. (Braces were discussed earlier in this section.)

Uses. Therapeutic traction may be applied to the neck, extremities, or pelvis. *It is most commonly used to align fragments of broken bones and to maintain proper alignment until bone union develops.* Traction used to reduce fractures is most frequently used on the extremities. The application of traction overcomes the injured limb's tendency to shorten (due to muscle spasm) and holds the limb constantly in a position of corrective extension with the ends of the fractured bone aligned. Other uses of therapeutic traction include

- Relief of painful muscle spasms;
- Correction and prevention of deformities;
- Stretching adhesions;
- Immobilization or distraction (e.g., pulling apart) of disease or painful joints;
- Treatment of painful arthritis, sore muscles and ligaments, dislocations, degenerated or ruptured intervertebral disks, and spinal cord compression.

General Care of the Patient in Traction. The major *disadvantage*[206] of traction is that it requires a long period of recumbency, and the patient typically must remain hospitalized during treatment. *Advantages* of traction include (a) greater potential for exercising joints and muscles than is possible with casting; and (b) avoidance of surgically induced bone devascularization and infection (if surgery is not required prior to application of traction). Any type of traction must permit some movement of the patient in bed and be only minimally uncomfortable.

The nurse caring for a patient in traction should know (a) the nature of the patient's injury; (b) the purpose of the traction; (c) how the traction device accomplishes its purpose; (d) movements and positions which are permitted and those which are contraindicated; and (e) potential complications associated with the use of traction and their prevention.

When caring for a patient in traction remember to maintain

(a) alignment of the injured part;
(b) general body alignment (the pull of the traction tends to move the patient out of positions of good alignment);
(c) alignment of the traction apparatus; and
(d) range of motion in as many joints as possible.

Before a patient is placed in traction, physical and psychologic preparation should be given. Because of its formidable appearance, a traction set-up may look to lay persons like an implement of torture rather than a helpful, therapeutic device. Explain to the patient and significant others the purposes of traction and reasons why certain body positions must be maintained for long periods of time. Make sure the patient is informed of contraindicated movements or positions. Explain to the patient that moving into contraindicated positions will defeat the purposes of the traction and may disrupt healing processes. When first placed in traction the patient should be told that traction will help the muscles begin to relax after a few hours and that he or she will begin to feel more comfortable. A patient placed in traction to treat a fracture should feel progressively better after traction is applied. The doctor should tell the patient how long traction will be maintained.

Three factors of importance in therapeutic reduction traction are[206] (1) the extremity should be supported and stretched in a direction that will properly align bone fragments (traction is exerted on the distal fragment to align it with the proximal fragment); (2) the extremity should not be overstretched (overstretching results in excessive distraction of bone fragments); and (3) stretching forces must remain constant (in amount and direction) until bone union occurs. The amount of weight applied in treating a fracture with traction may be gradually reduced by the physician as the injured bone heals.

In order to conserve space, only some of the more commonly used types of mechanical traction will be discussed and illustrated here. Traction techniques for the arm, hand, and forefoot are omitted entirely. The intricacies of actually setting up specific types of traction are not discussed. Commonly, persons with special training in setting up traction are available in hospital settings, or the physician assists with setting up the equipment. Detailed manuals discussing specific pieces of traction equipment and various traction set-ups are provided by manufacturers. Additionally, it is helpful to consult books on traction or orthopedics for details.

Equipment. Bed boards and firm mattresses are necessary components of any traction bed in order to prevent uncomfortable and incorrect positioning of the patient. A *Balkan frame* is used with some traction set-ups. The metal frame is fastened to the corners of the bed and consists of an overhead rectangular structure (about the size of the edges of the bed) which is supported by uprights. This frame serves as the basic overhead structure from which other parts of the traction set-up may be suspended or to which they may be attached, e.g., crossbars, clamps, pulleys. Octagonal poles are preferable to round poles because the latter tend to slip at clamped joints under stress.

Traction carts are available in most hospitals. These carts contain basic equipment necessary to position and care for a patient in traction. The large pieces of traction equipment, e.g., splints, trapezes, frames, poles, pulleys, are commonly stored in a *traction room.*

Periodically inspect a patient's traction set-up to ensure that the apparatus is accomplishing its purpose and that the equipment is as safe as possible. Some factors of importance to note during inspection of a traction apparatus are summarized below:

▶ *Ropes, knots,* and *pulleys:* Braided nylon cord (1/8 inch thick) is commonly used as a traction rope. Traction ropes must be of adequate strength to support the weights without breaking. The rope should be discarded after use. Prior to cutting lengths of traction rope, wrap the rope with adhesive tape where the cut is to be made. Then cut through the rope. The tape prevents raveling of the rope ends. Traction ropes must be of proper length and contain no unnecessary knots which can catch in the pulleys. If the ropes are too short, the weights may be pulled up against the pulleys; if the ropes are too long, the weights may rest on the floor.

Traction ropes should be kept free of the bed and bedding. The ropes should feel taut and ride easily over pulleys. Traction ropes should not touch the patient or rub together. Ropes passing over the foot of the bed should not touch the mattress or the bed. Make certain the ropes do not slip out of the wheel grooves of pulleys. See that frayed rope is replaced with fresh rope to prevent accidental breakage of the rope.

Ropes and pulleys should be unobstructed, freely movable, and in straight alignment. Pulleys should not squeak. All pulleys should be lubricated with silicone spray or a small amount of mineral oil *before* they are threaded with ropes. Once the traction is set up, the pulleys should not be lubricated unless the physician is present to readjust the amount of traction weight. Lubrication changes the balancing forces because it alters the friction.[238]

Pulleys should be free of the supporting equipment. They should be placed out on traction arms far enough that weights hang free of the bed.

Examine knots frequently to make certain they are secure. Knots used with traction equipment should not slip. Three types of knots which may be used are illustrated in Figure 76–17. The *bowline* may be used to hang some weight carriers. It makes a loop which will not slip. *Two half-hitches* may be used to secure a rope to a pole or a ring. *Square knots* will firmly hold two pieces of rope together.

▶ *Clamps* and *weights:* Check clamps to make certain they are tightened securely. Traction weights may be made of metal or bags of sand or shot. Weights should hang free so they will maintain an even, constant pulling force in a straight line. Weights should not rest on the bed, floor, a chair, or other weight systems. Also, they should not have added weight placed on them by bed linens. If weights are resting on the floor, it is because the rope is too long or the patient has slipped too far in the direction of the pull. Keep weights visible so they are not displaced. Weights should be securely fastened to the rope (e.g., knots should be covered with adhesive tape) so they will not slip off or accidentally be jarred off.

Weights should not hang over any part of the patient. If necessary, the traction apparatus should be modified so the weights will hang freely away from the patient.

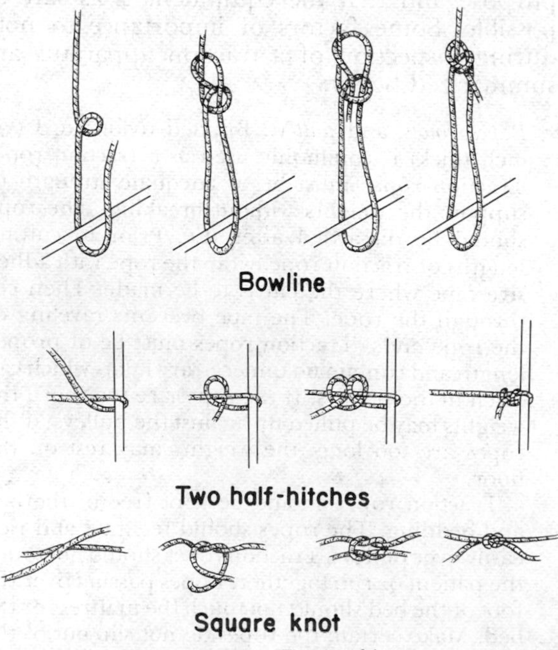

Figure 76–17. Types of knots

Do not bump or jar the bed or traction equipment, thus causing weights to swing. This can easily happen when equipment projects beyond the edges of the bed and not only is uncomfortable and disturbing to the patient but also can injure you.

If you detect adjustments that need to be made on the traction equipment (e.g., changing a frayed rope) and you know how to make the necessary adjustments, ask the physician's permission to do so. Also, ask the physician if traction is to be maintained manually until the mechanical traction is reapplied.

Continuous or Intermittent Traction. The physician specifies whether a patient's traction is to be *continuous* (i.e., pull constantly applied) or *intermittent* (i.e., pull may be relieved periodically). The pull of traction is relieved by lifting the traction weights. Typically, continuous traction is necessary in the treatment of fractures or dislocations. Traction may be applied intermittently in arthritis (e.g., to reduce flexion contractures) or in the treatment of low back disorders (e.g., to reduce pain and muscle spasm). *Traction is always assumed to be continuous unless the physician specifies that the traction may be relieved periodically.* Orders for intermittent traction should state precisely the length of time traction may be removed.

Running or Suspension Traction. *Running traction* (also called "straight" traction) exerts a direct pull on the affected part without a hammock or splint to give balanced support. Running traction exerts a pull in one plane and may be unilateral or bilateral. There are both skin and skeletal types of running traction. Buck's extension and Bryant's traction are examples.

Suspension traction (also called "balanced" traction) exerts a pull on the affected part and also supports the extremity in a hammock or splint which is held in place by balanced weights attached to an overhead bar (see Fig. 76–18). With suspension traction the countertraction is supplied by a system of ropes, pulleys, and weights rather than by the patient's body. With this form of traction the pull of the traction remains the same even when the patient moves. The suspension apparatus gives countertraction which takes up any slack caused in the traction by the patient's movements. As the patient lifts up off the bed, the weights attached to the traction apparatus move down (thus maintaining the original line of pull). For example, when suspension traction is applied to a leg, the leg and splints should rise when the patient elevates the hips. Thus, an extremity placed in suspension traction "floats," suspended (or balanced) in the traction apparatus.

Suspension traction permits greater range of motion and activity than standard running traction. It makes it easier to care for a patient and improves the patient's comfort and general well-being. By increasing circulation to the affected part and by decreasing prolonged pressure on weight-bearing areas, suspension traction reduces the possibilities of complications developing.

Suspension traction may be used with either skeletal or skin traction, and with any splint or hammock type of traction. Examples of suspension traction are Russell's traction and the use of a Thomas splint with a Pearson attachment. Suspension traction may be set up on a CircOlectric bed or from a Balkan frame. The traction must be maintained continuously to be effective.

Skin Traction. Skin traction is a nonsurgical procedure which indirectly applies traction on the underlying skeletal system and other structures, e.g., muscles. Skin traction may be applied (a) by fastening traction strips (e.g., strips of moleskin or adhesive tapes) to the extremities with woven bandage or bias-cut stockinette; or (b) by encircling a part with a special halter, corset, or sling. Traction strips are used with Buck's extension, Bryant's traction, and Russell's skin traction (see below). (Russell's traction may also be applied directly to the skeleton.) A halter may be used to apply traction to the head, and a corset or sling may be used to exert traction on the pelvis. A special anklet or bandage may be used with a splint to apply temporary traction to an ankle. If countertraction is needed with skin traction, it is achieved by using the patient's weight on the tilted surface of the bed. (Specific examples of various types of skin traction are presented throughout the text, particularly in this chapter.)

> *Skin traction cannot be used for prolonged periods of time and cannot be used with heavy weights.*

Skin traction may be used to partially or temporarily immobilize a part. Some stable fractures in adults can be treated with skin traction. However, most adult fractures cannot be treated by this type of traction because it (a) does not adequately control rotation; (b) cannot be applied with sufficient force to reduce and maintain the fracture; and (c) cannot be maintained continuously for the length of time necessary for adult bone healing.[207] Skin traction may be temporarily applied in the treatment of adult fractures before definitive treatment is undertaken, e.g., prior to surgical fixation of a fractured hip. Occasionally skin traction is used intermittently on an arthritic patient to help stretch out flexion contractures of the knee or hip. Other uses of skin traction are discussed as appropriate throughout the text.

A variety of tapes for skin traction are available commercially, under such names as Fas-

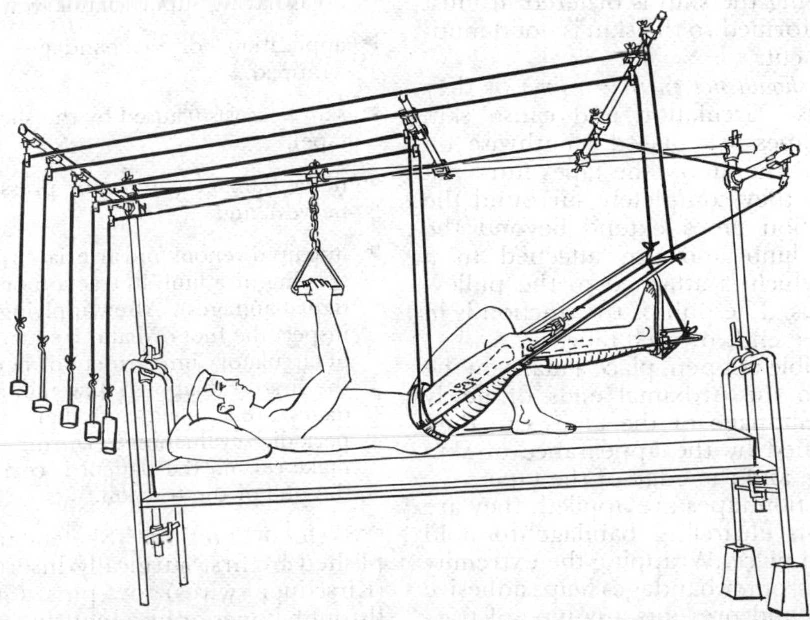

Figure 76–18. Proximal tibial traction with balanced suspension. (From Schmeisser, G., Jr.: *A Clinical Manual of Orthopedic Traction Techniques.* 1963)

trac, Flex-foam, Foam-trac, and Trac-grip. These products are usually accompanied by information about recommended skin preparation and use of the tapes.[137] Some physicians use strips of moleskin or adhesive tape instead of commercial products for skin traction tapes.

Traction tapes cannot be applied to skin which is irritated or damaged; otherwise skin breakdown may occur under the tape. Also, skin tapes cannot be applied over areas which may subsequently be operated on, because skin damage from the tape increases the possibility of postoperative infection.

Opinions differ concerning *skin preparation* for the application of skin traction. Some authorities believe the skin should be shaved (especially if the patient is quite hirsute) or that tincture of benzoin should be applied or both. Others believe that shaving the skin denudes it (inviting skin damage when the traction strips and overlying bandage are applied) and that the application of tincture of benzoin is unnecessary or undesirable. Still others paint the extremity with an Ace adherent and cover it with stockinette before applying the traction strips and covering bandage. It is necessary to check skin preparation orders carefully to comply with these varying practices. Proponents of benzoin claim that it is helpful because it minimizes itching of the skin, promotes the adhesion of materials to the skin, disinfects the skin, and generally keeps the skin in better shape and the patient more comfortable when skin traction is applied. If shaving the skin is ordered, it must be carefully performed so the skin is not denuded, irritated, or cut.

Traction tapes should not encircle a limb or they may compromise circulation and cause skin damage. The tapes are placed lengthwise on opposite sides of the limb. The tapes must not be so wide that they completely surround the limb. The traction tapes extend beyond the length of the limb and are attached to a spreader bar, which is attached to the pulley-weight apparatus. The pull of the traction is in line with the free ends of each tape.

With an indelible felt pen, place a mark on the skin adjacent to the proximal ends of newly applied tapes. Slippage of the tapes can then easily be identified by the appearance of skin between the line and the edge of the tape.

After the traction tapes are applied, they are covered with an encircling bandage to hold them securely in place. Wrapping the extremity in elastic or other outer bandages helps adhesive strips to adhere and prevents any type of traction tape (adhesive or nonadhesive) from slipping out of place. Limbs must be adequately supported once skin traction is applied.

The amount of traction that can safely be applied is determined by the *skin's tolerance to traction and friction* rather than by the strength of the traction tape material. Only 5 to 7 pounds of longitudinal force can safely be applied to the skin. Three to four weeks is the maximum length of time for which skin traction can be applied.[207]

Skin traction applied to the leg may cause pressure on the Achilles tendon at the back of the ankle or over the malleoli or the peroneal nerve below the knee (at the neck of the fibula) on the lateral side of the leg or both. Skin traction applied to the arm may cause pressure damage to the ulnar nerve at the elbow. *Bony prominences must be protectively padded* prior to the application of skin tapes or the traction force will rapidly cause skin breakdown or damage to superficial nerves or both. Prominences which should be padded on the arm include the lateral and medial epicondyles, the olecranon, and the styloid process of the ulna. On the leg the head of the fibula and the lateral and medial malleoli should be padded.

Bandages and tapes must be smoothly applied. Wrinkles irritate the skin and cause pressure damage. Some physicians request that the outer bandages be rewrapped periodically. Frequently inspect the condition of the skin around the tape and bandage edges. Look for and report pimples, irritation, abrasions, reddened areas, maceration, and purulent discharge. Also, check the condition of tapes and bandages.

Complications could arise from:

- application of excessive weights,
- failure to adequately pad bony prominences and areas having superficial nerves,
- application of a bandage which is tightly wrapped,
- skin necrosis (caused by the shearing force of the tape),
- nerve damage (caused by pressure on superficial nerves), and
- impaired venous and arterial circulation (caused by twisting of a limb in traction or constriction from tight bandages). After applying elastic bandages, inspect the foot or hand frequently for indications of circulatory impairment or nerve damage. Make the first evaluation a few minutes after the bandages are applied and then subsequently make periodic evaluations. During your evaluations make certain the patient is correctly aligned with the pull of the traction.

Skeletal Traction. Skeletal traction is accomplished by first surgically inserting metal wires (Kirschner wires) or pins (Steinmann pins) through bones or by anchoring metal tongs (e.g., Crutchfield, Barton, or Vinke tongs) in the skull.

The traction apparatus is then attached to the metal insertion. Skeletal traction applied to the skull is discussed in Unit X.

Kirschner wires and Steinmann pins are round stainless steel rods which are typically inserted (with a drill) perpendicular to and completely through bones. A traction bow is then attached to the wire or pin and the traction force is applied to the bow (also called spreader, stirrups, or calipers). Figure 76–19 shows common sites of insertion of skeletal traction. The site of insertion of the pins, wires, or tongs determines precisely the location to which the traction force will be applied.

Note that wires and pins are not inserted through joints. The physician attempts to place the wire or pin in such a way that only skin, subcutaneous tissue, and bone are penetrated, avoiding muscles, tendons, arteries, and nerves. Skeletal pins should not pass through a fracture hematoma. Also, the pins cannot be inserted through skin which is infected or abraded or has a rash.

Bone infection (osteomyelitis) can develop with skeletal traction. This is a serious complication.

The procedure of inserting skeletal pins or wires must be performed with aseptic technique to prevent postoperative infection. Skin preparation for skeletal traction is the same as that prior to any orthopedic surgical procedure (see below). Skeletal pins or wires are inserted under either local or general anesthesia. The procedure requires a signed surgical consent from the patient.

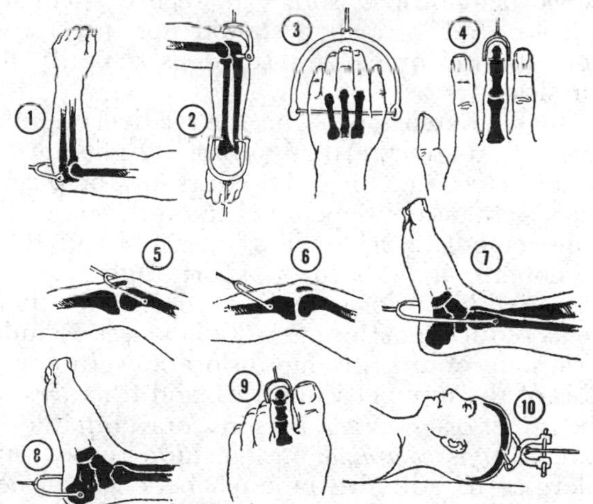

Figure 76–19. Sites for skeletal traction. 1, Below the olecranon; 2, below the olecranon together with a pin through the distal ends of the radius and the ulna; 3, through the middle three metacarpals; 4, through the distal phalanx of the fingers; 5, through the supracondylar area of the femur; 6, through the upper end of the tibia; 7, through the lower end of the tibia and fibula; 8, through the os calcis; 9, through the distal phalanx of the toes; 10, skull traction. (From DePalma, A. F.: *The Management of Fractures and Dislocations,* 2nd ed., Vol. I. Philadelphia, W. B. Saunders Co., 1970.)

Skeletal traction can be used for relatively long periods of time and can be used with heavier weights than skin traction. It is highly effective in treating fractures in bones surrounded by large muscle masses (e.g., femur) and in reducing unstable dislocations and fracture-dislocations. Other disorders which are commonly treated with skeletal traction are unstable spinal cord injuries and displaced fractures of the pelvis. The proper application of skeletal traction typically causes the patient with a fracture to become increasingly comfortable as it reduces muscular spasms and holds fractured bones in alignment.

Skeletal traction provides excellent traction because it applies force directly to the bone, making it possible not only to exert a longitudinal pull on the bone, but also to control rotation.[207] With skeletal traction, as much as 20 to 30 pounds of pull may be exerted, and the traction may safely be applied for several months. The pull is exerted via a fixed system of ropes, pulleys, weight carriers, and weights. Special equipment which may be used to apply skeletal traction to the lower extremities may include a Thomas splint (or a variation of this splint), with or without a Pearson attachment or Böhler-Braun frame.

During application of skeletal traction, neurovascular evaluations should be made frequently. The neurovascular status of the part should be evaluated and recorded prior to pin insertion so that a basis of comparison between the pre- and postinsertion is available.

Periodic inspections of the skeletal traction apparatus are essential. Sometimes the sharp ends of the wires or pins extend beyond the bow. Place corks or adhesive over these protruding ends to prevent bed linens from catching on the sharp points and to prevent scratching of the patient's skin or that of persons giving care. If a tong becomes accidentally displaced and it catches soft tissue, the patient experiences severe pain. The physician should be notified immediately. Loose wires or pins should also be called to the attention of the physician at once because movement of the extremity causes the wire or pin to cut into the bone and may introduce infection from outside (into the pin tract and along the tract into the bone).[137]

The insertion points of skeletal wires, pins, or tongs may become infected. Observe skin around these sites frequently for indications of infection, e.g., odor, redness, drainage. Take care that these stab wounds do not get wet, e.g., when bathing the patient. Opinions vary about the management of the insertion points. Some doctors cover the stab wounds with small sterile dressings and do not want the dressings to be disturbed unless there is evidence of infection. Therefore, do not change dressings or otherwise tend the wounds without specific orders. Some[149] state that infections may result from overzealous dressing and cleansing of these wounds and that daily wound inspections are not necessary. Others[137] emphasize that the areas around pins, wires, and tongs should be kept clean and dry and not be covered with collodion, dressings, or accumulations of serum exudate. Several sources recommend that each insertion point should be inspected daily and drainage should be aseptically removed by cleaning the site with solutions as specified by the surgeon. They maintain that if the opening to the insertion tract becomes sealed off (e.g., with accumulations of drainage), an ideal medium is developed within the tract for the growth of bacteria. Infection may then proceed inward internally along the tract and affect the bone.

Also, to prevent infection, instruct the patient who has skeletal traction not to touch the skin around the insertion points of wires, pins, or tongs.

When a skeletal wire (or pin) is to be removed, prepare the surrounding skin according to the physician's instructions. Iodine, alcohol, and ether may be used to sterilize the exposed wire end on the outer portion of the limb. The physician then removes the wire by (a) depressing the skin around that end of the wire and cutting the wire beneath the surface of the skin; and then (b) pulling the wire through from the opposite side of the limb. The insertion and exit incisions on the skin may then be covered with small sterile dressings.

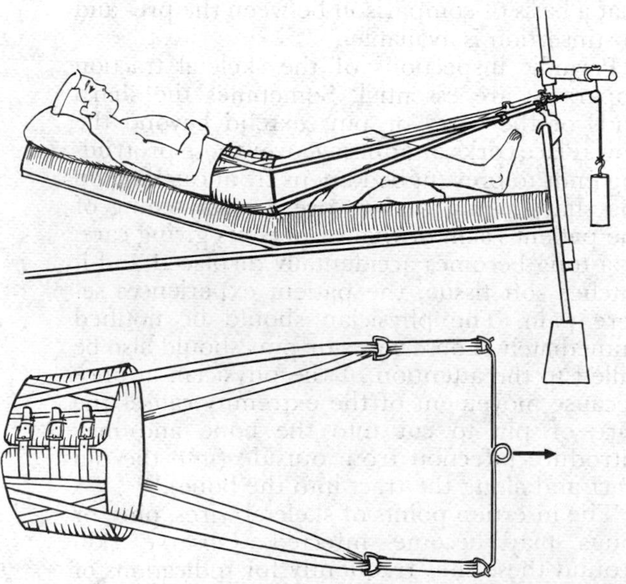

Figure 76–20. Pelvic traction belt. (From Schmeisser, G., Jr : *A Clinical Manual of Orthopedic Traction Techniques.* 1963.)

SPECIFIC TYPES OF TRACTION

Pelvic Traction. A pelvic traction belt or bilateral Buck's extension (see below) may be used to relieve low back pain which is not caused by spinal fracture or dislocation. (Spinal injuries are discussed in Unit X.) While these forms of traction do not apply adequate force to directly affect the paravertebral muscles or the vertebral articulations, they may bring relief from pain by keeping the patient recumbent and relatively inactive through enforced bed rest. The patient must be kept in straight alignment with the traction so the force will be effectively applied.

Pelvic traction (see Fig. 76–20) is accomplished with an encircling device, i.e., a belt applied just above and surrounding the iliac crests. The belt is attached to a spreader bar and pulley system. Traction is applied to the lumbar spine. Note in Figure 76–20 that the backrest is slightly elevated and the hamstring muscles are relaxed by placing pillows beneath the knees. Some physicians do not use pillows beneath the legs, but instead elevate the foot of the bed in a gatch position. If the backrest is excessively elevated, the patient will slide down in bed. An overhead trapeze is generally provided so the patient can lift up. The pelvic belt must fit snugly to secure adequate traction. Pelvic traction should not increase a patient's back or leg pain. If it does so, notify the physician.

Buck's Extension. This is a relatively simple form of skin traction that exerts a straight pull on the affected leg. One or both legs may be put in Buck's extension, depending upon the patient's requirements. Buck's extension may be used to immobilize a limb for a short time (e.g., a fractured hip prior to internal surgical fixation) or to reduce muscle spasm. Other uses include treatment of arthritis, hip dislocations, tuberculosis of the hip, pelvic injuries, and fractures of the upper or lower leg. Persons for whom Buck's extension is *contraindicated* include those with allergies to adhesive tape, diabetic gangrene, stasis dermatitis, arteriosclerosis, or serious varicosities or varicose ulcers. Buck's extension can be applied only in amounts of traction which the skin can safely tolerate. These relatively small amounts of weight are inadequate to treat some conditions, e.g., fractures with extensive overriding of bone fragments. In such situations, the patient must be treated by other means, e.g., another form of traction (skeletal traction) which can exert greater amounts of force.

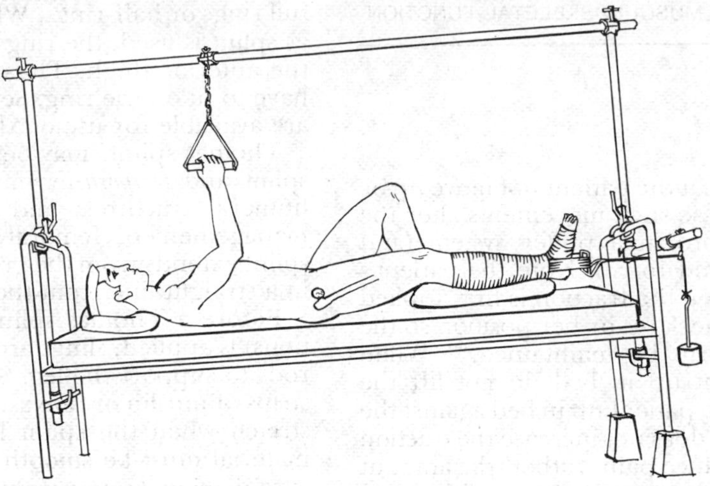

Figure 76–21. Buck's extension with overhead trapeze. (From Schmeisser, G., Jr.: *A Clinical Manual of Orthopedic Traction Techniques.* 1963)

Buck's extension (see Fig. 76–21) can be applied in varying ways. Details of application can be found in many of the reference sources listed at the end of this unit. Essentially the application of Buck's extension is as follows: (a) the skin is prepared according to the physician's instruction; (b) traction strips are smoothly applied to the lateral and medial aspects of the thigh and leg; (c) the strips are secured in place by smoothly bandaging the leg with elastic bandage or circular gauze; (d) the ends of the strips (which extend beyond the foot) are attached to a spreader or footplate; and (e) the traction rope (with its system of pulleys and weights) is attached to the spreader or footplate. Countertraction may be obtained by elevating the foot of the bed.

During application of the traction strips, the knee may be held slightly flexed to prevent hyperextension when the traction is applied. If the strip or bandages cover the head of the fibula (on the lateral side of the leg), the area is protectively padded before it is covered to prevent damage to the peroneal nerve.

The traction strips are not attached to the skin over the malleoli or the foot, but rather they extend unattached from a point above the malleoli on down past the foot to the spreader. If the traction strips are made of an adhesive substance, the sticky side of the tape is covered with another piece of the material (sticky side to sticky side) to prevent the strip from adhering to the malleolar region or the foot.

Spreader bars or blocks (sometimes blocks of wood are used for spreaders) must be of correct width. If spreaders are too narrow, the traction tapes will rub against adjacent areas of skin, e.g., malleoli. If spreaders are too wide, they will pull the traction tapes away from the skin.

Bryant's Traction. This form of skin traction is occasionally used to reduce fractured femurs or to reduce hip dislocations in very young children. Bryant's traction (also called "gallows traction") is a *dangerous* type of traction in which both of the child's legs are suspended vertically, with the hip flexed at 90° and the knees extended. The buttocks just clear the bed. Owing to the hazards associated with Bryant's traction, it is seldom used today. Because of the position of the legs, Bryant's traction compromises circulation, and also it may damage the popliteal vessels (posterior to the knee) by hyperextending the knees. Currently Bryant's traction is sometimes used in very young infants as a primary stage of reducing dislocated hips. (Management of hip dislocations and other orthopedic disorders affecting children is discussed in pediatric nursing textbooks.)

Russell's Traction. This form of traction may be used in treatment of fracture of the shaft of the femur. Also, it is sometimes applied bilaterally to treat low back pain. It may be applied as either skin or skeletal traction. Skin traction may adequately treat femoral fractures in children; however, adults usually require skeletal traction. Russell's traction creates a forward and upward pull on the leg by applying vertical traction at the knee at the same time a horizontal force is exerted on the tibia and fibula. The knee joint can be bent and the patient can move about with relative ease with Russell's traction.

With Russell's traction the peroneal area is exposed, but the popliteal area may be subjected to pressure. If the sling is applied behind the knee or if it impinges on the popliteal area, precautions must be taken to prevent pressure damage. A heavy piece of felt (covered with stockinette) may be placed in the sling as protective padding. Check the popliteal area daily for indications of skin damage, and report abnormal findings to the physician. Also, pressure on the popliteal vessels and immobility can cause thrombophlebitis. Notify the physician immediately of indications of this complication. Provide a foot support to prevent foot drop.

It is important that the patient not move up or down in bed because such movements alter the direction of the proximal pulley system (and hence the result and force). Note the patient's position in bed when the traction is first applied and periodically check his or her position so the original position can be maintained.[207] When moving the patient up in bed do not lift the weights. Pulling the patient up in bed against the pull of the traction does not increase the traction on the legs or produce pain; rather, the amount of pull remains constant.[137] Elevation of the head of the bed reduces the amount of traction; however, the physician may give permission for the head of the bed to be slightly elevated. Find out precisely the maximum amount of elevation permitted.

Ring Leg Splints; Pearson Attachment. Various ring leg spints are available, e.g., Thomas, Hodgen, Keller-Blake. The original ring leg splint was the *Thomas splint.* A Thomas splint in balanced traction with a Pearson attachment is illustrated in Figure 76–22.

The Thomas splint may be applied either in balanced or fixed traction, and may be used alone or in combination with a Pearson attachment. A Thomas splint consists of (a) two rods on either side of the limb, which converge distally to conform to the limb; (b) a large ring which connects the two rods proximally and encircles the upper thigh when in place; and (c) a crossbar which connects the two rods distally. The crossbar is located beyond the foot when the splint is in place. Thomas splints are available with either full rings or half-rings. When a half-ring Thomas splint is used, the ring portion is placed over the anterior thigh. Thus, the patient does not have to sit on the ring. Separate Thomas splints are available for use on the right or left legs.

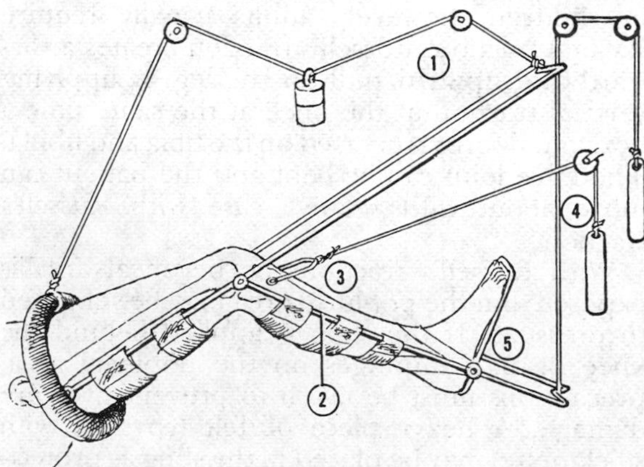

Figure 76–22. Thomas splint with Pearson attachment using balanced suspension traction. 1, The limb is suspended in balance in a Thomas splint by a system of cords and weights. 2, A Pearson attachment permits motion of cords and weights designed to exert continuous traction in the line of the femur. 5, Foot plate (this is essential to prevent footdrop). (From DePalma, A. F.: *The Management of Fractures and Dislocations,* 2nd ed. Vol. I. Philadelphia, W. B. Saunders Co., 1970.)

Thomas splints may be used (a) to *immediately* splint and *temporarily* immobilize femoral and humeral fractures; and (b) for the *long-term* management of femoral fractures. A Thomas splint extends from the groin to beyond the foot, in a straight line from the femur.

Before a Thomas splint (or one of its variations) is applied, slings are attached to the splint rods to support the leg. Slings may be made of strips of muslin or canvas; they must not slide or stretch when the splint is in place. The sling material must be smooth to prevent skin pressure damage from wrinkles.

A Thomas splint makes it possible to maintain two separate lines of pull on the same extremity, e.g., fractures can be aligned in the femur as well as the lower leg of the same extremity. With "fixed" traction, the distal end of the Thomas (or Keller-Blake splint) is attached to a fixed point at the foot of the bed and does not move with the patient.

A *Pearson attachment* to a straight ring splint makes it possible to flex the knee and move the lower leg if desirable. The Pearson attachment can move independently of the long leg splint. Slight flexion of the knee prevents subsequent joint instability by preventing stretching of the posterior knee capsule and ligaments. With balanced suspension traction, the knee can be moved actively and passively if the physician desires.

Typically the Thomas splint is elevated at a 45° angle to the bed and the leg is flexed at 45°.[149] The lower leg rests horizontal to the mattress in the Pearson attachment. A Thomas splint with a Pearson attachment may be used with either skin or skeletal traction. Sometimes Buck's extension is applied below the knee. The ring of a Thomas splint must fit snugly in the perineum (against the ischium); however, it should not cause excessive pressure in the groin. The ring makes it difficult for the patient to use a bedpan and keep the ring dry. Frequent skin care is necessary. Some sources recommend protectively padding the ring before the splint is applied; however, most do not. Padding holds moisture and thus promotes skin irritation. Inspect the adductor regions of the thigh frequently for indications of skin irritation. Notify the physician of indications of skin breakdown or if the patient reports excessive pressure in the groin.

The *Keller-Blake splint* has a half-ring at the proximal end of the splint, instead of a full ring. The half-ring portion of the splint is most commonly placed in front of the thigh and is secured posteriorly with a strap. However, at times the splint is positioned with the ring portion behind the thigh. Keller-Blake leg splints have neoprene-padded half-rings. The splints are reversible for use on either leg.

Prime goals in the care of any patient in traction are to prevent complications which (a) can develop from prolonged immobility and recumbency and (b) can result from the traction equipment being used. Traction equipment can produce complications similar to those which may result from casting, e.g., skin breakdown, neurovascular damage. These complications and their recognition are discusssed in detail earlier in this chapter. The patient in traction requires frequent inspections to identify skin breakdown or neurovascular damage or both. Skin care is discussed below. Extremities in either skin or skeletal traction are particularly vulnerable to neurovascular damage. To detect neurovascular damage, examine distal portions of extremities in traction for symptoms such as coolness, swelling, discoloration, paralysis, or anesthesia. Ask if pain or paresthesia is experienced.

Summarized below are some of the potential complications which may develop in a patient immobilized by traction:

- ▶ Hypostatic pneumonia; atelectasis.
- ▶ Constipation; fecal impaction; abdominal distention.
- ▶ Urine retention; kidney stones.
- ▶ Impaired circulation; edema; thrombophlebitis; phlebothrombosis; emboli, e.g., pulmonary embolism, fat embolism (see below).
- ▶ Disorientation.
- ▶ Nerve damage; motor weakness or paralysis; foot drop; wrist drop.
- ▶ Hyperextension of the knee; outward rotation of the leg.
- ▶ Disuse osteoporosis; muscle atrophy; contractures; joint stiffness.
- ▶ Wound infection, e.g., with skeletal traction, infected decubitus ulcers, or infection in traumatic open wounds or surgical incisions.

The patient in traction is given intensive *preventive care* and is *evaluated frequently* for indications of developing complications. Symptoms indicative of complications are promptly reported to the physician, so that *early* treatment can be started.

> *Investigate* all *symptoms indicative of developing complications and all complaints stated by a patient in traction.*

Various techniques of pulmonary physiotherapy and respiratory therapy are used to prevent respiratory complications in the patient immobilized by traction (see Unit XVI). These activities, e.g., breathing exercises, IPPB treatments, are basically directed at promoting lung expansion and keeping the tracheobronchial tree free of secretion accumulation. Maintaining a high fluid intake helps prevent problems with elimination. Some physicians have their patients wear elastic stockings while in traction to help prevent problems of venous stasis in the legs. Therapeutic exercises help minimize disuse osteoporosis and stimulate circulation. Additionally, exercises combat muscle atrophy, contractures, and joint stiffness.

Some areas which may be subjected to pressure (and hence develop pressure damage to skin or nerves) during therapeutic traction of particular extremities or body areas:

▶ *Pressure areas in traction of arm:*
- Axilla
- Anterior soft tissues of elbow joint
- Bony prominences around elbow, e.g., olecranon, lateral epicondyle, medial epicondyle
- Bony prominences around wrist, e.g., styloid process of ulna
- Dorsum of hand
- Volar palm surface at base of hand

▶ *Pressure areas in traction of leg:*
- Greater trochanter (upper outer thighs)
- Popliteal space; hamstring tendons at back of knee
- Outer aspect of head of fibula (lateral upper calf) where peroneal nerve is superficial
- Bony prominences around ankle, e.g., lateral malleolus, medial malleolus, Achilles tendon
- Back of heels
- Soft tissues at front of ankle and top of foot

▶ *Pressure areas in traction of trunk:*
- Borders of scapulae (shoulder blades)
- Prominences of spine
- Iliac crests (upper edges of pelvic bones)
- Sacral areas (tail bone)

If symptoms of neurovascular damage appear in an extremity in skin traction (see previous discussion of cast complications) and you cannot contact the doctor and do not have permission to unwrap the bandages, do as follows: (a) snip the bandage at the point of pressure, (b) anchor the traction above (to maintain the pull of traction), and (c) notify the doctor of the situation and your actions as soon as possible.[137]

Observe wrapped extremities for indications of constriction due to swelling. Swelling is most likely to occur during the first 24 to 48 hours following fracture. The toes or fingers should be visible for observation. Indications of constriction were discussed in detail in the section on cast complications.

NURSING CARE

Skin Care. The patient in traction is highly susceptible to skin breakdown because such a person cannot usually turn off the back or have traction released. The underside of the body is thus subjected to sustained pressure for a prolonged period, and skin care is difficult to administer effectively. *Skin care must be given frequently.* Check with the physician concerning the positions which a given patient may safely assume for skin care. If the patient is permitted to turn slightly, this facilitates giving skin care. If the patient cannot turn, skin care may be given while the patient raises up for brief periods by using an overhead trapeze.

Patients must take care not to become fatigued by holding up on the trapeze for too long. Instruct them to lift up periodically merely to "rest" the buttocks and permit circulation to enter the compressed areas of skin on which they are lying most of the time. Remember it will take a while for some patients (e.g., elderly persons) to learn how to use trapezes effectively. They will gradually develop the muscular skills, strength, and coordination needed to lift themselves up with their arms. Some patients need assistance and support while lifting themselves.

Instruct a patient who is first learning to use a trapeze to grasp the bar firmly and lift *straight up off* the bed. Teach the patient to place the feet (or uninjured foot) *flat* on the bed to help push up while pulling on the trapeze. Discourage pushing with the back of the heels, since these areas can develop pressure and friction damage. Synchronize your movements to those made by the patient, e.g., when the person raises up, reach under the buttocks and give skin care.

Often skin care can most effectively be given to a patient in traction by two persons working together. One person may help the patient lift up on a trapeze and help keep an elevated position, while the other gives skin care. If a patient cannot use a trapeze, one person presses down on the mattress while the other gives skin care by sliding hands under the patient.

Periodically use a flashlight to inspect the skin on the back and buttocks while the patient lifts up. A mirror will help you inspect areas difficult to view directly. Give extra skin care to areas which show indications of developing complications. While giving care inspect the patient's skin carefully with your hands. Development of an increased acuteness of your sense of touch will help you to locate lesions which you cannot see and to detect crumbs and wrinkles in bed linens. Ask the patient to report wrinkles or other sources of irritation and pressure.

Immediately report if the patient notices paresthesias, burning, or pain under skin traction bandages.

Skin breakdown may result from contact of the skin with the traction equipment (e.g., bows, spreader blocks, ropes) or may result from irritation caused by friction against bedding, traction tapes, or bandages. Pressure necrosis may develop rapidly. Inspect skin at the edges of traction strips. Examine areas covered with adhesive materials or bandages for indications of skin necrosis or infection. Look for drainage through adhesive dressings and elastic bandages and smell the areas to detect odors indicative of infection and drainage. The skin under *encircling devices* is especially prone to breakdown from pressure and friction.

Meticulous preventive skin care is required for areas of skin which are in contact with adhesive bandages or other pieces of traction equipment, especially when contact occurs over pressure points. Nurses should be aware of areas of potential skin damage associated with specific types of traction. For example, the ring of a Thomas splint may traumatize skin in the groin and gluteal fold. Skin traction applied to the lower leg may cause damage to skin on the ankle malleoli. When skin traction is applied to the leg, look for pressure over the dorsum of the foot and the heel if bandages or tapes appear loose. The traction weights may pull the bandages or tapes down in these areas and cause pressure damage to the skin.

Skin breakdown on the heel of the unaffected foot may develop if the patient pushes with this heel when lifting up in bed. Also, the elbows may become sore from rubbing on the sheets during attempts to push up. Use of an overhead trapeze helps the patient lift up without pushing on the elbows. Remember to frequently examine and give appropriate skin care to *all* pressure points upon which the patient rests while recumbent, e.g., back of the head, shoulder blades, elbows, iliac crests, sacrum, back of the heels. Cleanse the fingers or toes of extremities which are in traction.

Bedding. Without interfering with the effectiveness of the traction it is often desirable to cover an affected limb (or limbs) to prevent chilling. This may be accomplished in various ways, e.g., wrapping the limb in cotton batting or a lightweight blanket. Coverings should not press on the footplate with leg traction. Make certain that ropes and pulleys are free of bedclothes. Split linens, which fit around the top of an extremity in traction, can be used to keep the rest of the patient's body warm. Linen changes can be made either by working from the top toward the bottom of the bed or by working from the unaffected side toward the affected side. Be careful not to jerk the patient by catching linens on the traction equipment.

Positioning; Turning; Release of Traction. Check the doctor's orders to determine whether a patient can turn or if traction can be removed periodically. Also, identify contraindicated positions.

Never lift or change traction weights without a doctor's orders. Do not remove traction or increase or decrease the amount of the weights without specific orders.

When the physician gives permission, some patients, e.g., with arthritis or low back pain, are permitted to be relieved of traction for short periods. Patients with pelvic traction, for example, may have bathroom privileges. However, continuous traction is necessary with other disorders, e.g., when traction is being employed to immobilize a new fracture. If the doctor states that the traction may be removed periodically, lift and reapply weights gently so the patient is not subjected to the sudden release from traction or to the sudden reapplication of tension. Always tell the patient when you are going to remove or reapply the tension. Never "drop" a weight when reapplying traction, but gradually lower the weight so the patient does not undergo sudden, extreme stress.

Never change the heights of elevating blocks ("shock blocks"), knee rests, or backrests of patients in traction without the physician's permission.

A patient in traction should not roll laterally or have the position of the bed changed without the physician's permission. Turning on the side changes the line of pull even with balanced traction.

Some patients in traction are restricted in the amount the headrest can be elevated, since raising the head of the bed disrupts the line of pull in arm and cervical traction and the amount of pull in leg traction. Changing the position of the bed (e.g., elevating the backrest of a patient who has been kept in a flat position) may make effective traction impossible by disrupting the line of the pull. If elevation of the headrest is permitted, the physician should specify how far the bed can be elevated and still maintain adequate countertraction. Raising and lowering the headrest (when permitted) not only increases the patient's comfort but also minimizes pulmonary complications by promoting drainage of the tracheobronchial tree. A patient who may have the headrest up and down should be positioned *completely flat* at least half the time to prevent hip flexion contractures. Explain the importance of this positioning to the patient. With many types of traction, hip flexion contractures are also prevented by maintaining 20° of hip flexion between the thigh and the bed.

If the doctor gives permission for the patient to turn slightly (e.g., for back care and linen changes), make certain you know which side the patient may turn toward, e.g., the patient with a fracture may be permitted to turn slightly toward the side of the fracture. With the physician's permission a patient with a limb in traction may be turned slightly toward the limb which is in traction. Turning away from the traction set-up would obviously not be possible. A patient in traction cannot assume a prone position unless on an orthopedic frame or Circ-Olectric bed.

When the patient moves about (e.g., lifts up by the trapeze, turns for back care, or slides up in bed), someone should steady the traction equipment while another person assists the patient or provides other care, e.g., places a bedpan or gives skin care. In some cases it is advisable to manually exert a slight pull on the traction during these times.

Help the patient to be as comfortable as possible while on the back. Even slight changes of position can be relaxing. Make frequent evaluations of the patient's position in bed and the body alignment. The patient should be centered in the bed. If the patient slips toward the pull of the traction, repositioning is necessary or the effectiveness of the traction may be compromised, e.g., footplates or spreaders may be pulled against the foot of the bed or against pulleys.

Some patients in traction should not be pulled up in bed since movement alters the traction pull. For example, a patient with arm traction cannot be moved up in bed once traction is applied. Thus, the person must be properly centered in the bed (e.g., so hips and knees fit the gatched areas of the bed) *before* traction is applied. Position must subsequently be checked periodically. If repositioning in the bed is necessary, it must be done with the physician's help.

Maintain correct body alignment and effective traction. Exercise special precautions to prevent foot drop. When traction is applied to a leg, a footplate may be applied to prevent foot drop. An alternative method of preventing the equinus position is the application of a wide strip of adhesive tape to the bottom of the foot. The free end of the tape extends beyond the toes and may then be attached to a small rope, pulley, and weight (or to another peice of the traction apparatus) to hold the foot upright. Prevent rotation of the leg and splint. The leg should not rub against the rods of the splint. The heel should not rest on the bed or pressure necrosis will develop. Sometimes the foot is left free for exercising.

Remember to care properly for extremities which are *not* in traction as well as those which are immobilized. For example, keep *both* legs in straight alignment; prevent hyperextension in *both* knees, and maintain *both* feet in a natural position (without inward or outward rotation). If the patient appears to be developing abnormalities (e.g., hip flexion contractures, hyperextension of the knee, foot drop, wrist drop), take appropriate corrective action and call the defect to the attention of the doctor. If a patient's leg is in traction, the foot should never rest against the foot of the bed. This prevents effective traction.

Often it is difficult to place a patient on the bedpan while in traction. As discussed, the foot of the bed may be elevated for countertraction. This elevation causes urine to tend to run up beneath the patient while on a bedpan. Another problem is that the patient must be kept in proper alignment while on the bedpan and while moving off the bedpan.

When possible, a *fracture bedpan* (i.e., a small, flat bedpan with a tapering slope from front to back) is used for a patient in traction. However, a large bedpan is necessary for enemas. Some women can void into a female urinal or kidney basin. When permitted, placing a pillow under the back and shoulders keeps the patient more level with the bedpan. The physician may permit the backrest to be elevated slightly for bedpan use.

Patients with injuries that prevent use of an overhead trapeze (e.g., upper extremity injuries, spinal injuries) or make it difficult to place a bedpan (e.g., unstable pelvic fractures) may be placed on special orthopedic frames (Bradford frames) which have an opening for placement of a bedpan beneath the patient without lifting. If the patient can use a trapeze, the bedpan is placed and removed while the patient raises the hips off the mattress.

Do not place any pillows under a limb in traction without the permission of the physician.

If pillows are permitted, the doctor should place them the first time so the limb is positioned as desired, with effective traction. Some physicians do not want *any* pillows placed under a limb in traction because they believe it increases the chances of thrombosis. If pillows are used they should be firm so they will provide adequate support and will maintain alignment of the limb with the traction apparatus. Do not support just a portion of an extremity, but rather provide support along its entire length. When placing a pillow under the lower leg, make certain the heel is free of the bed. Elevation of the heel should not hyperextend the knee.

Exercises. Consult with the physician concerning exercises for a patient in traction. Maintenance of general muscle tone and joint mobility not only prevents complications but also speeds up the patient's rehabilitative progress once the traction is removed and mobility is permitted. Commonly the physician advises the patient to put every joint (except those immediately above and below fractures) through a full *range of motion* several times each day. *Deep breathing exercises* and *abdominal setting exercises* are routinely instituted as soon as the patient is placed in traction. The patient is often placed on an exercise program that will prepare for crutch walking if indicated. (See discussions of exercises and of crutches earlier in this chapter.) Typically when pain and swelling are sufficiently reduced, the physician permits *muscle setting exercises* (e.g., quadriceps setting) over the injured part of an extremity, and once callus formation is visible by radiology, limited range of motion exercises are initiated in the joints immediately above and below fractures. Since one advantage of traction is that it may permit greater movement of the affected limb, the amount of exercise advised by the physician should be performed.

Self-Care and Diversion. Lying on one's back in traction is tiring, and the patient usually welcomes diversion, e.g., visitors, occupational therapy projects, visits from the staff or patients. The use of prism glasses may enable the patient to read more easily while flat. Also, mirrors may be placed in ways which help enlarge the patient's view of the surroundings. The patient's immediate environment should be kept neat and attractive.

Prolonged immobilization may induce disorientation in some patients, especially older persons. Prolonged immobilization also fosters discouragement, depression, and difficulty in sleeping at night. Evaluate the patient's mental attitude and sensorium periodically. Inform the physician if a patient appears disoriented or seriously depressed, or is sleeping poorly. Make every attempt to keep the patient meaningfully involved in daily activities. If the patient remains awake during the day, he or she may be able to sleep for longer periods at night.

Encourage self-care as much as possible for a patient in traction, since it provides stimulation and exercise. The patient should do as much of hygiene care as possible and any other self-care activities, e.g., feeding, exercises. Explain to patients that self-care is an important part of treatment and that you are not having them do things for themselves simply to reduce the work load of the staff. Place items which the patient may require within easy reach and make sure of a call bell at all times to summon help as needed. Consciously strive to minimize the discomforts of the dependency that traction imposes on a person. Attempt to anticipate the patient's needs, e.g., it may be difficult to cut food while lying flat.

Removal from Traction. When patients are finally removed from traction they will probably find that they are quite weak and possibly unsteady. If a limb has been immobilized in traction, it may show some muscle atrophy (appear thin) and be weak and unstable. Additionally, orthostatic hypotension is commonly present if the patient has been in a head-lowered position.

To combat hypotension the patient is helped to gradually resume a sitting (and later standing) position. The head of the bed is elevated progressively higher. Raising the bed to a full sitting position may require several sessions. Physical support is given when the patient first sits on the edge of the bed or moves out of bed. Safety precautions, such as supporting the patient, are imperative to prevent falls until you are sure the person has secure balance and support.

Patients should be told how they might expect to feel once the traction is released. Explanations should be given about why they may feel faint or weak, and why joints may be stiff or unstable. Plans for rehabilitative activities (to help regain strength and function) are discussed with patients and their significant others. The physician should talk with patients about activities and movements which are permitted and those which are contraindicated. Weakened limbs may require support at the joints. Crutches may be required for a while. Reassure the patient and significant others that after following the prescribed exercise activity program muscles will become stronger.

ORTHOPEDIC SURGERY

While the majority of orthopedic patients can be treated successfully without surgery, it is needed for some. Orthopedic surgical procedures are usually not emergency surgeries but rather are performed electively. Thus, there is usually time to prepare patients physically and psychologically for surgical experiences.

Giving patients and their significant others appropriate *psychologic support* pre- and postoperatively is an integral aspect of the clinical care provided with orthopedic surgery. Prior to surgery some patients have had long, fatiguing, painful periods of illness. Some patients with degenerative joint diseases may be ill for long periods before reconstructive surgery is performed. Commonly such persons face surgery with mixed feelings of hope and dread. They are hopeful that surgery will reduce their pains and increase their mobility; they are fearful that surgery will merely add to their burdens of suffering and disability.

Physician and nurse attempt to realistically discuss with patients the expectations of surgical procedures and to help patients adjust their lifestyles to accommodate permanent disabilities when necessary. Patients who have required numerous operations may well be discouraged and depressed as they face still other procedures. Financial concerns may also be overwhelming. Some orthopedic surgical procedures cause significant *changes in body image* which may be difficult for patients to accept. In addition to providing direct patient care services during pre- and postoperative periods, nurses also provide indirect services by helping to refer patients to other persons who are qualified to give specialized help, like social workers, psychiatrists, clergy.

As with any surgery, patients should be told preoperatively how they can expect to feel and where they can expect to be when they awaken from general anesthesia, e.g., "You will awaken in a recovery room with a cast on your arm. A nurse will be nearby to help you as you need it."

Preoperative Preparation. The general preparation of a patient for surgery is discussed in Unit VIII. This discussion focuses specifically on preparation for orthopedic surgery.

Pre- and postoperatively it is important to maintain adequate levels of hydration in patients immobilized for prolonged periods. Adequate hydration helps prevent some complications of immobility, e.g., renal complications.

Preoperatively, antibiotics may be ordered for some patients, e.g., those with a history of osteomyelitis. Other preoperative orders typically include orders to increase fluid and carbohydrate intake and orders for preoperative skin preparation and sedation. Barbiturates may be ordered the evening before surgery or the morning of surgery. Breakfast is withheld prior to general anesthesia. While inhalation anesthesia is commonly used for orthopedic procedures, in some cases spinal, rectal, or local anesthesia may be employed. A mild cathartic or enema may or may not be ordered preoperatively.

In addition to ordering routine preoperative laboratory tests (e.g., urinalysis, bleeding and clotting time, blood count, Hgb estimation), the orthopedic surgeon may also order evaluations of the blood sedimentation rate and serum calcium, phosphorus, and phosphatase.[149] The latter tests are useful in evaluating metabolic bone changes. Many diseases of coagulation cause joint disorders. Bleeding tendencies must be carefully evaluated preoperatively in the presence of such joint disorders.

Prior to orthopedic surgery special precautions are taken to minimize the possibility of postoperative infection. Bone is more susceptible to infection than soft tissue. If infection of the bone, i.e., osteomyelitis, develops, it is difficult to treat and may result in permanent disability, e.g., chronic infection or stiffness of the joint. Also, in the presence of infection, bone union will not occur. To prevent infection, careful attention must be given to preoperative skin preparation, operating room technique, and postoperative dressing changes and reinforcements.

While specific operative skin preparation procedures for orthopedic surgery may vary from place to place, the underlying principles are similar. Orthopedic skin "preps" are meticulously performed in a nontraumatic manner. If ordered, cleansing enemas are given prior to skin preparation. Skin "preps" may be performed in the patient's room, emergency room, or operating room. Final preparation of the operative site is always carried out in the operative suite.

Specific procedures for preparing the operative site and the antiseptic solutions vary, depending upon the surgeon's preferences and hospital policies.

When casted areas are to be operated on, it is usual for the cast to be removed several days before surgery. This allows adequate time for skin inspection and preparation. If there are skin infections, the surgeon may postpone surgery until the infection has been adequately treated. Hair is difficult to disinfect. Time is spent removing grime from the hand or foot and thoroughly cleaning and then clipping the fingernails or toenails. It may be necessary to soak the hand or foot to clean it thoroughly.

In surgery, open traumatic wounds, e.g., compound fractures, are carefully cleansed since each is potentially contaminated. The prep is carried out under aseptic conditions (masks, sterile gowns, gloves) and is commonly performed by the surgeon. During the prep the open wound is covered with sterile gauze while the area surrounding the wound is cleansed with solutions. Care is taken to prevent the solutions used during this time from entering the open wound. After the surrounding area has been cleansed, the dressing is removed from the open wound, and fresh sterile solutions are used to flush the open wound of dirt, debris, and bacteria. Following preparation of the wound it is debrided, i.e., "dead" or devitalized tissue is removed. Thorough wound debridement and removal of every particle of foreign material is imperative to prevent postoperative infection.

Orthopedic Surgical Procedures. Orthopedic surgical procedures may be performed to reconstruct or replace diseased or injured structures or to correct deformities. Orthopedic surgery encompasses a variety of specific surgical procedures, including reduction of fractures, reconstructive procedures, replacement procedures, tendon repair (realigning severed ends, lengthening, shortening, transferring). Orthopedic surgical procedures may be performed on bone or soft tissues. Examples of orthopedic bone procedures include arthrodesis, arthroplasty, arthrotomy, bone grafting, and osteotomy. Soft tissue surgical procedures include tendon transplantation, tendon lengthening, tenotomy, and capsulotomy.

Some of the more common orthopedic procedures are:

- *Tenotomy:* the cutting of a tendon, for example, to correct club foot.
- *Tendon lengthening:* procedure to lengthen a tendon without disrupting its continuity.
- *Tendon transplantation:* procedure by which a tendon from a normal muscle is moved to another location so it can assume the function of a damaged muscle.
- *Capsulotomy:* surgically incising a joint capsule.
- *Synovectomy:* excision of a synovial membrane, e.g., at the knee. May be used to treat arthritic joints.
- *Osteotomy:* cutting bone to correct bone or joint deformities.
- *Arthrotomy:* incising a joint for exploration or removal of diseased tissue.
- *Arthrodesis* (artificial ankylosis or fusion): repairing a joint by fusing the joint's surfaces. Fusing the bones together makes the joint permanently immobile. Such procedures may be used to treat spinal disorders, i.e., spinal fusion (see Unit X), or to stabilize painful joints or knee and ankle joints that have become unable to support weight. In the latter instances, arthrodesis minimizes pain caused by rubbing together of irritated joint surfaces, and it facilitates weight-bearing. Thus, arthrodesis commonly produces a stiff but stable and painless joint once the bones of the joint have fused, i.e., grown together. Frequently arthrodesis is accomplished surgically by removing the articular hyaline cartilage and placing bone grafts across the surface of the joint. In some instances metallic internal fixation devices are placed.
- *Arthrolysis:* loosening adhesions in an ankylosed (i.e., abnormally immobile) joint.
- *Arthroplasty:* plastic surgery on injured or diseased joints to reestablish a movable joint. Arthroplasties may be performed in differing ways, e.g., the bones of the joint may be surgically reshaped, and soft tissue or a metallic interposition device may be placed between the reshaped bone ends to help reestablish motion, or joints or parts of joints may be replaced with prostheses made of metal or other materials (see below).
- *Bone grafting:* pieces of cancellous or compact bone are surgically transplanted to other locations in the body. Grafts or transplants of bone may be (a) *autogenous,* i.e., obtained from the person into whom they are being transplanted; (b) *homogenous,* i.e., obtained from another individual of the same species; or (c) *heterogenous,* i.e., obtained from an animal of another species. Autogenous bone transplants are the most successful. Bone transplants or grafts may be used to (a) establish bony joint fusion; (b) fill in gaps or defects in bone; or (c) facilitate the healing of fractures which are difficult to heal otherwise.[98]

A variety of other surgical procedures may be used in orthopedic practice, e.g., *excision of calcium deposits* from joints, *removal of tophi* (i.e., chalky deposits of urates) produced by gout, *excision of rheumatic nodules,* and surgical *removal of exostoses,* i.e., bony growths projecting outward from bone surfaces.

Reconstructive surgical procedures are commonly performed on persons beyond middle age. Degenerative bone and joint diseases, e.g., arthritis, cause pain and deformity by eliminating the smooth surfaces of bones inside joints. *Silastic implants* may be used to replace diseased knuckles. In the *hip* joint the head of a diseased femur may be replaced with a *prosthetic device.* Recently it has become possible to *replace the total hip,* i.e., the acetabulum as well as the head of the femur, with a Vitallium or other prosthesis. *Total knee and shoulder replacements* are also becoming more common orthopedic procedures. Procedures such as these restore useful function and relieve pain.

During surgery implants are handled carefully. Implants are subject to erosion postoperatively if they are marred or scratched when implanted.

Postoperative Care. General postoperative care is discussed in Unit VIII. Following bone and joint surgery a prolonged period of immobilization is usually necessary to permit adequate healing. Immobilization may be achieved in various ways, e.g., special orthopedic frames (Stryker, Foster, CircOlectric beds), casts, or traction. Care of patients in casts and traction has been discussed in the preceding sections of this chapter. Management of pain following orthopedic surgery was discussed earlier in this unit. Muscle spasms may occur postoperatively following orthopedic procedures; see discussion earlier in this chapter.

As with any postoperative patient, much of the clinical care given the postoperative orthopedic patient is directed at *preventing complications* which may result from (a) the surgical procedure; (b) pre-illness pathology; or (c) immobilization. Since complications cannot always be prevented, the patient is closely observed for *early* indications of developing complications so that prompt treatment may be instituted. *Postoperative complications* to be watched for following orthopedic surgery include the following:

- *Shock.* As with other surgery, shock may occur during the early postoperative period. Patients especially prone to shock during surgery include (a) elderly hypertensive patients who have been on prolonged antihypertensive drug therapy; and (b) patients who have received corticosteroid therapy, e.g., persons with arthritis who are undergoing reconstructive joint procedures. It is important that a complete drug history be obtained preoperatively so adequate preventative precautions can be taken to ensure safety during and following surgery. (Shock is discussed in Chapter 13.)

- *Thrombophlebitis* is indicated by such symptoms as pain, swelling, redness or heat in the extremity, e.g., calf of the leg. The common necessity for prolonged periods of immobilization, plus the nature of orthopedic surgical procedures, makes thrombophlebitis with subsequent pulmonary embolization a particularly common complication in postoperative orthopedic patients. Preventative actions are indicated pre- and postoperatively to reduce the likelihood of these serious complications. (Thrombophlebitis and pulmonary embolism are discussed in Unit XV.)

- *Pulmonary embolism and fat embolism.* Fat embolism, i.e., embolism of a globule of fat, may follow bone surgery or bone injuries, e.g., multiple long bone fractures. (Fat embolism following fracture is discussed in Chapter 77. Treatment is also briefly discussed in that section. See also Unit XV.) Symptoms of fat embolism vary depending upon the area in which the embolus lodges, whether in the brain or lung or peripherally. Indications of cerebral fat embolism may include pupillary changes, muscular twitching, and altered states of consciousness (see Unit XV). Among the symptoms of fat embolism in the lungs are tachycardia; pallor followed by cyanosis; hypoxia; petechiae over the chest and shoulders; disorientation; and rapid, dyspneic breathing. When an embolus lodges in an extremity, the affected area typically becomes pale and numb and feels cold to touch. The patient may become faint and experience nausea and vomiting. Shock may develop. Gangrene of the extremity may develop unless the vascular obstruction caused by the embolus can be relieved. *Pulmonary embolism* typically develops much later in the postoperative period than fat embolism, perhaps as much as 10 to 24 days postoperatively. Indications of pulmonary embolism include sudden severe chest pain. Sudden death may occur. Fat embolism and pulmonary embolism, e.g., from blood clots or air, are serious complications which must be given emergency treatment. The alert, competent nurse who recognizes early indications of these complications and who participates effectively in obtaining and initiating emergency care can play a significant role in saving the lives of patients with these complications.

- *Urine retention* or *abdominal distention* or both are other complications which may develop following orthopedic surgery. Treatment of these disorders has been discussed in other sections of this text.

While observing for indications of the above complications, the nurse also evaluates the postoperative orthopedic patient for early symptoms of other potential complications, e.g., infection, hemorrhage, pneumonia, atelectasis, mechanical obstruction of circulation (e.g., from a tight cast), or neurologic damage.

Neurovascular complications are most likely to develop following the reduction of open fractures, but they may also occur postoperatively with other disorders. Neurovascular damage may be indicated by the presence of any of the following *"five P's":* Pain, Pallor, Pulselessness, Paresthesia, and Paralysis. The presence of any of these previously discussed symptoms in an operated extremity should be immediately reported. (Neurovascular complications are discussed in detail in the earlier discussion of casts.)

Orthopedic surgeries are often lengthy procedures. Therefore postoperatively it is not uncommon for a patient to feel stiff and sore from lying relaxed on the operating table for a long period. During surgery care is taken to prevent neurovascular injuries by correctly aligning and supporting the patient's body and extremities.

Postoperatively, periodic back care (including massage) can greatly contribute to the patient's comfort.

> *Following orthopedic surgery it is important to know (and hence avoid) contraindicated positions, movements, or activities for individual patients.*

Position, turn, and exercise the patient as ordered during the postoperative period. To ensure healing in correct alignment and to prevent musculoskeletal complications, frequently check the posture and positioning of orthopedic patients while they are confined to bed. Often beds on orthopedic services are equipped with special firm mattresses to promote comfort and correct body alignment during periods of prolonged immobilization. If orthopedic mattresses are not available, bed boards may be placed under the mattress.

Operated extremities are typically elevated during the postoperative period to minimize or prevent edema. Remember to support extremities along their entire length. Do not simply place a pillow under the heel or knee, for example. Do not assume that adequate pillow support is unimportant because the leg or arm is in a cast. Unless casted body areas are properly supported, excessive strain is placed on the cast and it may crack, and also the patient may feel extremely uncomfortable.

Check *dressings* frequently during the postoperative period. Report postoperative drainage when it occurs in previously sterile wounds. Use sterile forceps and sterile dressings to reinforce saturated dressings; use of these sterile techniques minimizes the chance of infection being introduced into the wound via capillary action. Dressing changes must be done carefully on orthopedic surgical wounds to prevent introduction of infection. Principles of asepsis are meticulously followed: (a) each patient should have an individual dressing tray, (b) clean wounds should be dressed before contaminated wounds, (c) dusting or sweeping or bed linen changes should never be performed during dressing periods, and (d) the patient and attendants should be masked during dressing changes.[149] Infected patients should always be segregated from those who are free of infection. Chart and report staining of casts, e.g., from seepage of blood, or serous or purulent drainage. Include in your charting measurements of the dimensions of the stained area (e.g., "a circle of drainage about 1 inch in diameter") so these measurements can be used as a baseline when future observations are made to determine whether drainage has stabilized or is increasing.

Mobilization during the postoperative period is of special importance following surgery on patients with joint disease. Without adequate mobilization the affected joints will rapidly become stiff and immobile. Postoperative orders for activity must be conscientiously followed. The skillful nurse uses resourcefulness to encourage self-care following orthopedic surgery. Often patients with orthopedic disorders are reluctant to move because they are fearful that movement will be painful or damaging. Gently and patiently the nurse helps the patient to learn activities which can safely be performed with a minimum of discomfort. The nurse helps the patient to understand the importance of moving as the doctor has ordered. Point out that while some discomfort is necessary during the postoperative period, the immediate discomfort caused while moving is only temporary and will prevent later problems of greater disability and discomfort, e.g., loss of movement and painful contractures.

Early *ambulation* is desirable postoperatively but sometimes cannot be started until the physician determines that adequate bone healing has occurred. Soft tissues heal more rapidly than bone. Thus, while a patient's skin incision may be healed, it must be remembered that underlying bone may not be healed. It is not uncommon for periods of convalescence to be prolonged following bone injury or bone surgery. A long period of healing is especially necessary for weight-bearing structures. Check the physician's orders carefully to determine if weight may be placed on the affected limb while standing or walking. Commonly the patient is to stand (rather than sit) when first getting out of bed postoperatively. Be certain to have adequate help when getting the patient out of bed. Acutely aware that the musculoskeletal structure is impaired, the patient is fearful of falling and being without protection from injury.

Postoperative *rehabilitation* programs for orthopedic patients may include occupational therapy, prosthetics (for amputees), bracing, and physical therapy, e.g., gait training, muscle re-education, exercises, heat applications, massage. During convalescence it is of prime importance to keep the patient mobilized and engaged in safe self-care practices. Patients must realize that they share responsibility for progress and recovery with others. Others are not able to rehabilitate them, but rather they work with others to rehabilitate themselves. The patient role is active rather than passive. By participating meaningfully in the treatment-recovery program, patients actively influence their levels of motivation and performance. Of course, it is necessary for them to be taught those self-care activities which they are expected to perform.

After hospital *discharge* patients continue to be seen by the physician and other members of the health care team as necessary. Home visits may be made by a community health nurse. Patients should be familiar with self-care activities which they are to perform and they should also be informed of contraindicated activities and indications of complications.

CHAPTER 77

MUSCULOSKELETAL INJURIES

INTRODUCTION

Musculoskeletal injuries are relatively common occurrences. Nurses frequently care for patients who have sustained such injuries.

Many musculoskeletal injuries result from *home accidents.* Examples of home accidents include (a) dropping or lifting heavy objects; (b) slipping in a wet bathtub, or on a wet or highly polished floor; (c) tripping over hoses, rugs, pets, telephone cords, or light cords; and (d) falling from ladders or chairs, down stairs, or when getting out of bed.

Accidents with *motor-driven vehicles* greatly increase the incidence of musculoskeletal injuries, particularly whiplash injuries to the neck and fractures (sustained by pedestrians, cyclists, and automobile occupants). High-impact accidents (which throw a pedestrian some distance or which forcibly hurl automobile occupants against the steering wheel, ceiling, floor, or dashboard of the car) often cause multiple system injuries in addition to musculoskeletal injuries.

Musculoskeletal injuries may occur with *sport* and *recreational activities.* Because organized athletics are now available to boys and girls of almost any age, the potential patient population at risk for musculoskeletal injuries is a very large one. Most athletic injuries are accompanied by a sense of urgency by either the parent, coach, or child. Although the injury may not be a true emergency, it may have a strong psychologic impact. The individuals involved may feel that the injury will influence the child's emotional well-being or may destroy the chance for an athletic scholarship or even a professional athletic career.

Each sport may have its own unique injuries, e.g., tennis elbow, jogger's heel.[211] The knee is highly susceptible to sports injuries (see article by Drain[71]). Persons practicing karate may suffer from the HIT syndrome of the hand ("HIT" stands for hypertrophic infiltrative tendinitis).

Some *occupations* are associated with various possible musculoskeletal injuries. Nurses, for example, can injure their backs if they lift patients incorrectly (see article by Davis[60]). Infantry soldiers may suffer fractures in the metatarsals of their feet as a result of long hikes or marches. (These fractures are called fatigue, stress, or march fractures.)

Some forms of musculoskeletal trauma occur quite *unexpectedly* during relatively "normal" activities. For example, during a wide yawn the jaw may dislocate, or during violent coughing a rib may fracture. Persons with some diseases (e.g., cancer of the bone, osteoporosis) may sustain fractures spontaneously in the absence of preceding trauma. These fractures (called "pathologic fractures") are discussed later.

Age may also be a factor in musculoskeletal injuries. As a group, older persons are susceptible to fractures. Their vision and hearing may be impaired, increasing the possibilities of accidents. Atrophy of bone, occurring as part of the aging process, may also increase susceptibility to fracture, e.g., fracture of the femur (commonly referred to as "hip fracture"). Additionally, aged persons may be poorly coordinated, have a decline in postural ability, and have difficulty walking. The abilities to stand erect and walk are learned abilities in human beings, i.e., they are not governed by built-in neural mechanisms. A newly hatched bird may walk out of its eggshell, but a human being does not attain full control of stance until adulthood. With age the level of proficiency progressively deteriorates.

Finally, aged persons may have disorders which predispose them to musculoskeletal injuries, e.g., "drop attacks," cerebral ischemia, osteoporosis, cancer of the bone, arthritis, "dizziness," postural hypotension, muscular weakness, or neurologic disorders that affect locomotion. While disorders such as these predispose a person of any age to injury, the elderly person may be particularly at risk because of concomitant factors already discussed, e.g., processes that accompany aging. Older women are especially prone to fractures, e.g., Colles' fracture or fractured femur. Men most commonly sustain fractures in their younger years, up to age 45.

Musculoskeletal injuries range in severity from relatively minor soft tissue injuries to severe, crushing fractures.

EXAMINATION OF THE PATIENT WITH MUSCULOSKELETAL TRAUMA

Injured extremities are routinely kept elevated and are observed frequently for indications of complications, e.g., neurovascular damage. (Observations were discussed in the section on cast complications, Chapter 76.) Temporary splints should not be removed until the physician orders their removal.

Patients with suspected musculoskeletal trauma are examined thoroughly by the physician for evidence of injury. Commonly missed orthopedic injuries include shoulder dislocations; torn supraspinatus tendon (in shoulder); fractured medial epicondyle (in elbow); fracture-dislocation of forearm (fracture is easily identified, but dislocation may be missed); fractured scaphoid (associated with wrist injury); dislocated lunate (wrist); fractured neck of femur (hip); slipped upper femoral epiphysis (associated with hip injury); locked knee (i.e., a knee which may bend fully but lacks some normal extension, e.g., the last 3 to 4° of extension); dislocated patella; and ruptured Achilles tendon.[5a]

A brief history which gives some details of a patient's accident can be extremely helpful to the physician examining a patient. Nurses can help obtain such a history from the patient or from persons bringing the patient to the hospital, office, or clinic. If possible, persons who witnessed the accident should wait to talk with the physician. Details of how an injury was sustained can help the physician identify possible injuries on the basis of knowledge about structures commonly injured as a result of specific traumatic forces. For example, a fall on an outstretched hand may transmit stress to the clavicle, humerus, radius, or ulna.

Indications of traumatic damage to the musculoskeletal system include swelling, subcutaneous bleeding (ecchymosis), instability of an extremity, crepitation (the sensation felt or heard by the examiner when two ends of fractured bone move against one another, like the sound of loose gravel), and indications of neurologic or circulatory impairment or both.

Injured extremities are gently and thoroughly examined. Commonly *swelling* appears 15 to 30 minutes following injury. Initially the edema is soft and compressible. Once examination of the extremity is completed, continued swelling is treated by applying continuous external pressure, e.g., with an air splint. *Ecchymoses* ("black-and-blue" marks) reflect bleeding subcutaneously. Depending upon the depth of the bleeding, ecchymoses may appear soon after injury or perhaps not for several days. Ecchymoses usually indicate major tissue damage or fracture. Bleeding within a joint *(hemarthrosis)* commonly occurs following tearing of intra-articular structures. After several days the blood may seep from the injured joint into subcutaneous tissues. Joint swelling that develops more slowly is generally due to a reactive synovial effusion. Joint aspiration may be performed to determine whether blood is present.

When the initial examination of an injured limb reveals swelling and ecchymosis, the physician gently moves the limb to determine the presence or absence of *instability.* Instability indicates either a fracture or significant ligament rupture. While examining the unstable, swollen, ecchymotic limb, the physician attempts to elicit localized *crepitation.*

As a final part of the initial examination of the injured limb, the examiner rapidly evaluates the *neurologic and circulatory status* of the extremity, e.g., for evidence of injury to major arteries and nerves. It is important that this evaluation be made *before* any treatment (even splinting) is given. Thus, it can accurately be determined in the future whether neurocirculatory damage resulted from the injury or occurred later as a result of treatment, possibly during reduction of the fracture or as a result of the application of a splint or cast.

Upon completion of the examination, the unstable limb is temporarily splinted until more complete care can be given. Temporary splinting of the limb is important because it enhances the patient's comfort and immobilizes the fracture. Splinting prevents additional soft tissue damage, rubbing together of the ends of the fracture, and poking through the skin of the ends of the fractured bone. Splinting also helps reduce muscle spasms.[14] (See also first aid treatment of fractures later in this chapter.)

Pain medication (morphine, Demerol) is usually ordered promptly once the physician sees the patient with a musculoskeletal injury. Fractures often cause severe pain, and pain medications may have to be given intravenously. Cold, local application (ice bags) may also be ordered.

CONTUSIONS

A contusion is a soft tissue injury resulting from a blunt force or blow. Local hemorrhage occurs and the skin, subcutaneous tissue, and deep soft tissues may also be damaged. Several days after injury the affected area develops ecchymosis. As the blood in the bruised area is absorbed, the discoloration changes to brown, then yellow, and finally the skin regains its normal color. In addition to discoloration, a contusion typically produces well-localized tenderness and swelling.

Sometimes a *hematoma* develops, i.e., a sac filled with effused blood. This may occur when a major blood vessel in a muscle is injured; brisk bleeding results. The blood in the hematoma eventually clots and may then be gradually resorbed. It may take several months for the hematoma to appear. Occasionally the physician may decide to evacuate the hematoma by aspiration or to remove the sac surgically.

Proper treatment of a contused area includes application of cold and a pressure bandage. The area needs to be immobilized to prevent further injury. After approximately 48 hours, measures to encourage healing need to be instituted. Local heat will be of value in this stage. Rehabilitation needs to be started slowly within the limitations of pain and should progress according to the healing process. In extensive contusions, systemic medications with enzyme preparations may be of value.

STRAINS

Strains are produced by overstretching of tendons or overuse of muscles. Strains may be *acute* (e.g., occurring during unaccustomed vigorous exercise) or *chronic* (e.g., developing after the repetitive overuse of muscles). The terms "strain" and "sprain" should not be used interchangeably, since they refer to two different types of injuries. The Subcommittee on Athletic Nomenclature of the A.M.A. Committee on Sports Medicine has confirmed that strains should apply to the muscle-tendon unit and sprain to the ligament injury.[187] These structures are quite distinct: the muscle-tendon units include a motor element whereas the ligament is primarily a stabilizer.

With an acute strain the patient experiences sudden, severe, incapacitating pain (e.g., while running). The acute pain subsides, but the area remains locally tender. Discomfort may be elicited by passively stretching the affected part. Swelling occurs rapidly. Ecchymosis may appear after several days.

With a chronic strain symptoms do not appear for several hours following the overactivity. Onset of symptoms is gradual. Commonly the affected parts feel stiff and sore and may exhibit diffuse generalized tenderness when palpated. Swelling, ecchymosis, and loss of function do not occur.

Chronic strains require no specific *treatment,* but the patient may be made more comfortable by local applications of heat. Acute strains require rest and possibly splinting. Immediately following injury, ice packs may be applied for 24 to 48 hours to reduce swelling. Heat may then be used if it enhances the patient's comfort. Surgical repair may be necessary if a muscle is completely ruptured. During the healing process (which takes 4 to 6 weeks) movement of the injured part should be minimal. Activity should never be so great that it produces symptoms, e.g., swelling, pain. After mature scar tissue has formed, the part is gradually and progressively exercised. During rehabilitation overactivity must be avoided.

SPRAINS

A sprain may be defined as an injury to a ligament resulting from overstress which causes some degree of damage to the ligament fibers or their attachment.[187] Sprains are divided into mild (Grade 1), moderate (Grade 2), or severe (Grade 3) categories for clarity's sake. In a mild sprain, a few fibers of the ligament have been torn, but there is no functional loss and the ligament is not weakened. Because of this, protection of the ligament is not vital. In a moderate sprain, a portion of the ligament is torn, resulting in some functional loss. Protection is vital at this stage to prevent further tearing of the ligament owing to lack of ligamentous strength. In the severe sprain, the ligament is torn completely either from its attachment or in the ligament body itself. Many cases of complete rupture necessitate surgical repair. Approximation of the ligament ends is important to insure strength and stability of the ligament. (See Figure 77–1.)

Following injury, tenderness to palpation develops, well localized at first and later more diffuse. Other symptoms include swelling, severe pain, discoloration, decreased motion (limitation of joint motion and function), and disability. Disability may not be very severe initially after the injury occurs, but may be extensive 2 to 3 hours later. X-ray films may demonstrate soft tissue swelling but no evidence of bone or joint injury.

Immediate *treatment* includes elevation of the injured joint and the application of ice. (Do not have the patient hold the affected part in a dependent position or soak it in hot water.) The joint may then be immobilized by either (a) splinting the joint in a position of comfort and applying a compressive bandage, e.g., Ace bandage; or (b) application of a plaster cast (if the sprain is severe). Casting aids in the approximation of the ligament ends and alleviates pain. If an Ace bandage is used, it is applied gently, not tightly. A mature scar forms in connective fibrous tissue in 4 to 6 weeks. Immobilization of the injured part for 3 to 4 weeks is usually adequate. Following complete healing the patient will need a good rehabilitation program.

A *"whiplash" injury* of the cervical spine is a

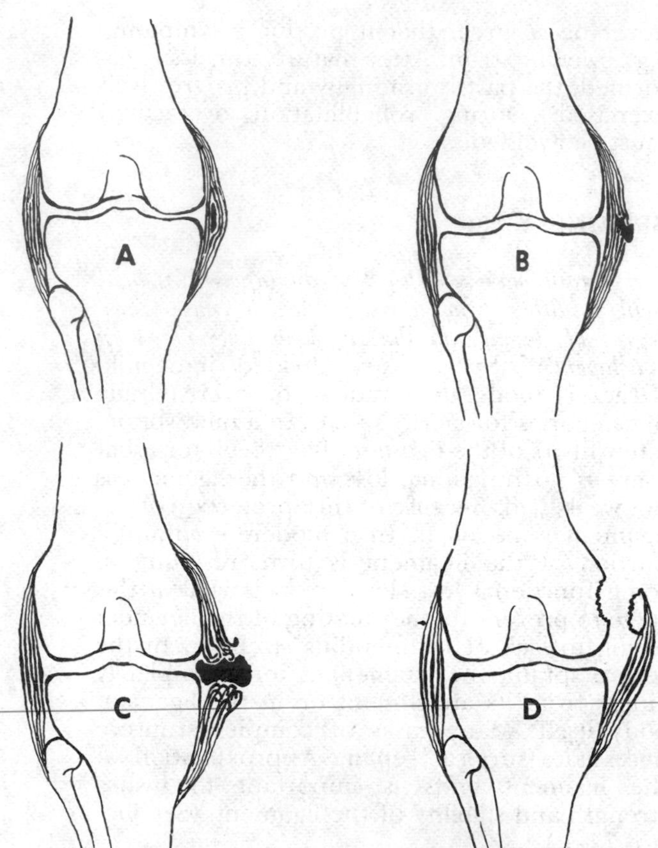

Figure 77–1. Various types of sprain. **A,** Mild (first degree) sprain, in which there is a little hematoma in a very localized area in the ligament with only a few fibers separated. **B,** Moderate (second degree) sprain, a more severe tear of the ligament but with at least half of the fibers remaining intact. **C,** Severe (third degree) sprain. Complete tear through the ligament with separation of the ends. **D,** Sprain-fracture. The ligament is torn off bone with a fragment of bone. (From O'Donoghue, D. H.: *Treatment of Injuries to Athletes*, 3rd ed. Philadelphia: W. B. Saunders Co., 1976.)

sprain of ligamentous tissue around bones and joints in the neck. Commonly the injury results when the auto in which the person was riding was struck from the rear. The impact (rapid acceleration) suddenly and forcibly hyperextends the spine. Then the spine is acutely flexed during rapid deceleration (when the force of the impact ceases). A cervical sprain is treated by immobilizing the neck with a cervical collar.

DISLOCATIONS; SUBLUXATIONS

A dislocation is present when a bone is displaced from its normal joint position and the articulating surfaces lose contact. The displaced bone may impede blood supply, tear ligaments, rupture blood vessels, damage nerves, and rupture muscle attachments. With a *subluxation* the joint's articulating surfaces are only partially separated. Dislocations and subluxations disrupt the joint by tearing the capsule and ligaments. Often these disorders are accompanied by a fracture of the joint surface.

Dislocations may result from trauma or may occur spontaneously as a result of diseases affecting joints. Some dislocations, especially of the hip, may be present at birth.

Deformity may or may not be visible with dislocations or subluxations. Dislocation may change the length of the affected extremity. Localized joint pain and loss of function (i.e., mobility) may be present. A dislocation partially immobilizes a joint, and thus differs from a fracture. (A fracture site typically has abnormal free movement.) X-ray films demonstrate the abnormality, i.e., complete or partial separation of the articulating surfaces (Fig. 77–2.)

Some dislocations reduce themselves, leaving a sprain. Others must be therapeutically reduced by a physician. Prior to treatment the neurovascular supply to parts distal to the injury must be carefully evaluated and deficits noted. Once radiology establishes the diagnosis, the dislocation or subluxation is reduced.

Prompt treatment is necessary to prevent complications, which include (a) ischemia or aseptic necrosis (resulting from impaired blood supply to parts distal to the dislocation); and (b) impaired nourishment of the hyaline cartilage on the articulating surfaces of the injured joint (normally this tissue is nourished by synovial fluid, but disruption of the joint impairs the nourishment process).

Reduction is most often accomplished without surgery ("closed reduction"), but in some cases surgery ("open reduction") is indicated, e.g., with some knee injuries that completely rupture ligaments. When reduction is accomplished by closed manipulation, the physician pulls on the joint with a gradual steady pull rather than a quick forceful jerk. Anesthesia may consist of a local or regional block or a general anesthetic.

Following reduction of a dislocation or subluxation, the joint is immobilized by application of a splint or cast or by placing the patient in mild traction. Immobilization may be maintained for 3 to 6 weeks. Adjacent joints which are not immobilized are actively exercised during the period of healing. Once the affected joint is removed from immobilization, active motion is encouraged, e.g., voluntary muscle contraction. Passive stretching can be harmful.

FRACTURES

A fracture is a disruption of the normal continuity of bone. Commonly a fracture is accompanied by soft tissue injury in surrounding tissues. While some fractures are life-threatening (because of associated hemorrhage and shock), most are not.

CAUSES

Most fractures result from accidents, e.g., automobile accidents, blows, falls, twisting, crushing injuries. As discussed below, some fractures result from disease processes that weaken bone.

Fractures may result from:[137]

- *Direct force,* in which the fracture occurs at the point of contact.
- *Torsion,* in which the fracture occurs at a point remote from the location of the force (e.g., a forceful twisting of the foot may break bones in the leg);
- *Violent contractions* of highly developed muscles (e.g., forcibly throwing an object produces powerful muscle contractions which can fracture the humerus); and
- *Various disease processes* that cause fractures, in the absence of trauma, by weakening bone structure. These fractures are termed *pathologic* or *spontaneous fractures.* They result from disorders such osteoporosis (increased porosity of bone), particularly in the lumbar spine or hip; Cushing's syndrome; malnutrition; complications of cortisone or ACTH therapy; osteogenesis imperfecta (congenital disorder affecting formation of osteoblasts); or metastatic or primary bone tumors (tumors decalcify bone). These various disorders cause bone tissue to collapse or break easily.

TYPES

There are more than 150 different types of fractures which are classified in various ways. Some of the more common types of fractures are described briefly in following paragraphs. (Refer to Fig. 77–3).

The following terms are useful in establishing generally the *severity* of a fracture:

- *Open (compound) fracture:* A break in the skin is present over the fracture site and the wound communicates from the skin (externally) to the fractured bone (internally). Because of this communication with the external environment, an open fracture is potentially infected. The wound may result (a) from external trauma (e.g., bullet) which penetrated through the skin and fractured underlying bone (direction of the injuring force was from outside the body moving inward); or (b) from the ends of a broken bone penetrating out through the skin when the fracture occurred (see Fig. 77–3). The ends of the broken bones may or may not be visible in the skin wound. Sometimes they push through the skin at the time of impact and then are withdrawn back under the surface of the skin.
- *Closed (simple) fracture:* An uncomplicated fracture in which the skin is intact over the fracture site, e.g., broken bone does not protrude through the skin (Fig. 77–3). Because there is no communicating wound, infection is not introduced into the fracture at the time of injury.
- *Complete fracture:* The fracture line extends entirely through the bone substance; i.e., the periosteum is disrupted on both sides of the bone. Two fragments of bone are present on either side of the fracture line.
- *Incomplete (partial) fracture:* The fracture line extends only part way through the bone substance, i.e., the bone continuity is not completely disrupted. Also sometimes called a *willow, greenstick,* or *hickory stick* fracture (Fig. 77–3). Like bending a green stick to the breaking point, one side breaks but the other merely bends.
- *Impacted fracture* (also called *"telescoped fracture"*):

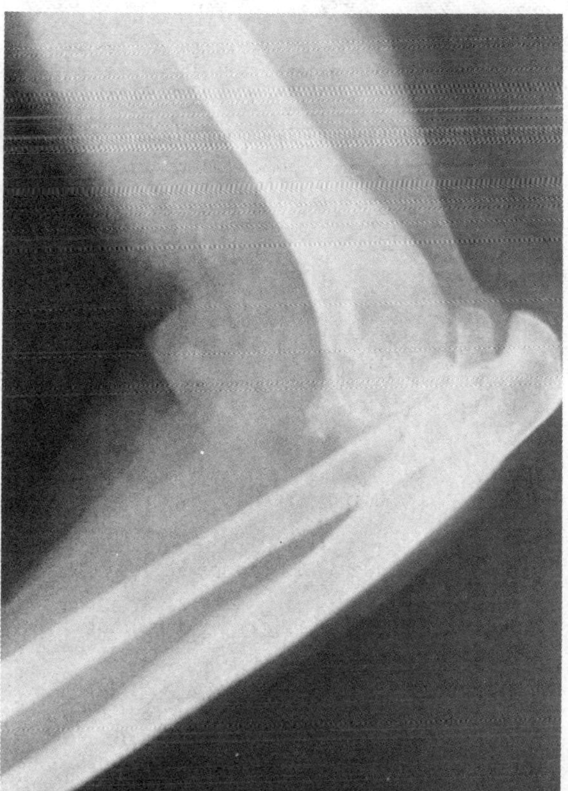

Figure 77–2. Elbow dislocation complicated by fracture of head of radius. (From Huffer, J. M.: Traumatic injuries: Office treatment of dislocations. *Postgraduate Medicine,* 62:223, Nov. 1977.)

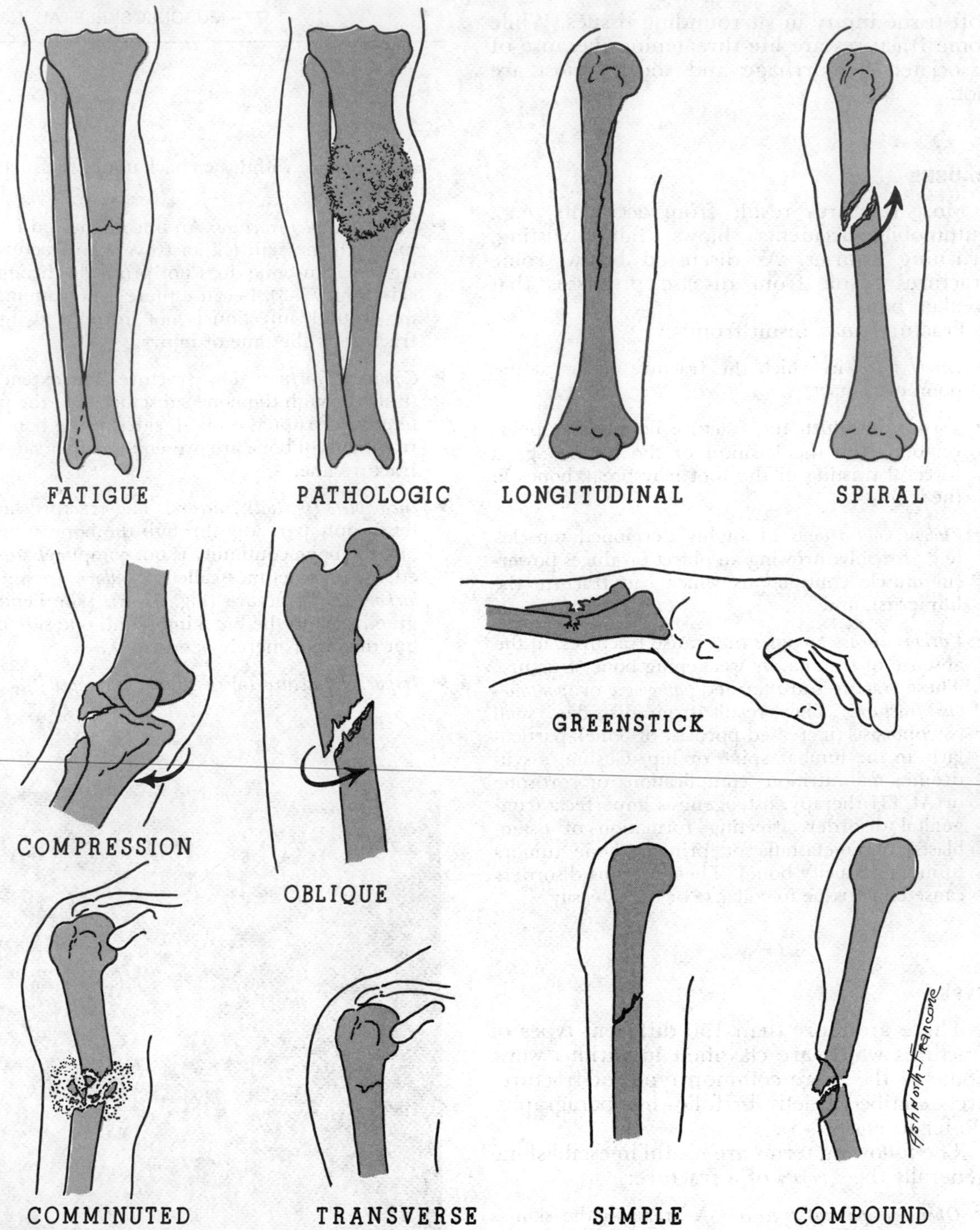

Figure 77–3. Types of fractures. (From Jacob, S. W., C. A. Francone, and W. J. Lossow: *Structure and Function in Man*, 4th ed. Philadelphia: W. B. Saunders Co., 1978.)

One bone fragment is forcibly driven into another adjacent bone fragment.

- *Comminuted fracture:* There is more than one fracture line, and the bone fragments are crushed or broken into several pieces. A *butterfly fracture* is a type of comminuted fracture in which the fragments resemble a butterfly, i.e., on each side of the main fragment are two fragments resembling wings.

- *Displaced fracture:* The bone fragments are separated at the fracture line.

- *Complicated fracture:* The fracture is associated with injury to surrounding structures, e.g., adjacent organs, nerves, blood vessels, joints. For example, a fractured rib may penetrate adjacent lung tissue.

Terms used to describe fractures may be used in combination to provide a more complete description. For example, a patient may have a "closed, complete fracture which is displaced."

When a fracture of an extremity divides a bone into two fragments, the fragments are referred to as the *proximal (uncontrollable) fragment* and the *distal (controllable) fragment.* The proximal fragment is that section of the bone which is nearest to the body. This fragment cannot be manipulated or moved when the fractured bones are being "set" (i.e., correctly aligned) because of its muscle attachments and location. The distal fragment (farthest away from the body) can be manipulated or moved therapeutically to realign it with the proximal fragment.

Summarized below are some terms used to describe the *direction of fracture line* in relation to the affected bone's longitudinal axis.

- *Linear fracture:* line of the fracture runs parallel to the bone's long axis.
- *Longitudinal fracture:* line of the fracture extends in a longitudinal direction.
- *Oblique fracture:* line of the fracture is at an oblique angle (about a 45° angle) to the shaft (axis) of the bone.
- *Spiral fracture* (also called a *"torsion fracture"*): line of the fracture forms a spiral which encircles the bone. Results from the twisting force, e.g., in sports such as football or skiing.
- *Transverse fracture:* line of the fracture is straight across the bone, i.e., at a right angle to the bone's axis.

Fractures are also classified according to the *force* that produces the fracture. Some of these terms include angulation fracture, avulsion fracture, blowout fracture (results from blow that fractures the floor of the orbit of the eye). compression fracture, fatigue or march fracture (fracture of metatarsals due to long marches), and missile fracture.

Fractures are often named for the *physician* who first described them. Two common examples are:

- *Colles' fracture:* A common type of fracture in which the distal portion of the radius is fractured within one inch of the articular surface. Colles' fracture is typically characterized by a "silver fork" deformity (see Fig. 77–4) caused by dorsal displacement of the distal fragment with dorsal and radial deviation of the wrist and an abnormal radioulnar articulation.
- *Pott's fracture:* This fracture occurs at the distal end of the fibula and often is associated with rupture of the internal lateral ligament or chipping off of a piece of the medial malleolus or both. The tibiofibular articulation is seriously disrupted. Frequently the foot is displaced outward.

Another method of classifying fractures is in terms of their *anatomic location.* The site of *long bone fractures* is indicated by visualizing the bone as divided into thirds and then stating the location of the fracture, e.g., in the proximal, middle, or distal third.

Fractures involving or close to *joints* are described as:

- *Articular fractures* (also called *"joint fracture"*): The fracture involves the surface of a joint.
- *Extracapsular fracture:* The fracture is near a joint but does not enter the joint capsule.
- *Intracapsular fracture:* The fracture is within a joint's capsule.

Fractures involving *major bones* may be classified in special terms. For example, fractures of the *humerus* may be identified as follows:

- *Condylar fracture:* A small fragment of bone (including the condyle) is separated from the inner and outer aspect of the humerus.
- *Supracondylar fracture:* The fracture is at the distal end of the humerus.
- *Transcondylar fracture:* The fracture is at the level of the condyles of the humerus (or just above or below the condyles) and partially within the capsule.

Finally, fractures may also be classified according to their causes. For example a *stress fracture* may occur in a bone that is subjected to

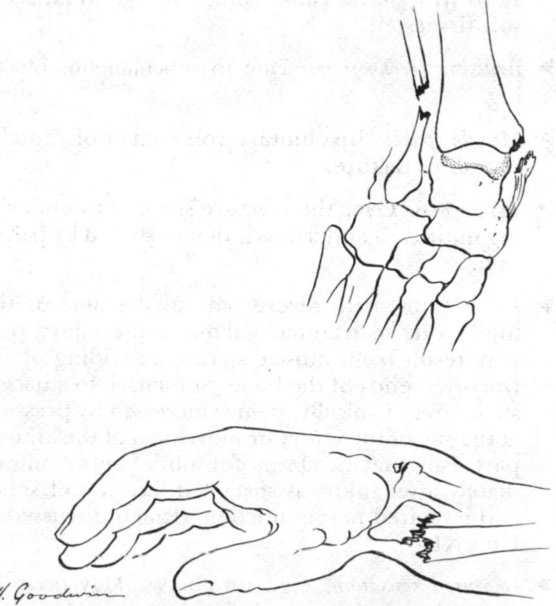

Figure 77–4. Above, Pott's fracture. Below, Colles' fracture. (From *Dorland's Illustrated Medical Dictionary, 25th ed.* Philadelphia: W. B. Saunders Co., 1974.)

prolonged muscular action when it is unaccustomed to it. Such fractures may occur in normal bones.[115] *Pathologic fractures* are those fractures that occur in already diseased bones.

SYMPTOMS

Numerous factors influence the symptoms which a given fracture may produce, e.g., the site, severity, and type of fracture and the amount of damage to other structures. Some fractures produce almost no symptoms and would not be detected if routine x-ray films were not taken to evaluate injuries. Symptoms which may occur with a fracture are briefly summarized below. Various combinations of symptoms may be present.

- *Deformity:* Changes in alignment and contour, such as (a) angulation, rotation, or shortening of a limb; (b) depression of bone; or (c) altered curves. To identify subtle deformities, compare the injured limb with its uninjured counterpart on the opposite side. Shortening of the injured limb occurs with fractures of long bones (e.g., humerus) because the muscles attached above and below the fracture site contract in a state of muscle spasm. Strong muscle pull may cause overriding of the bone fragments.
- *Swelling:* Edema may appear rapidly as a result of localization of serous fluid at the site of fracture and extravasation of blood into adjacent tissues. Fractures always cause some damage to adjacent soft tissues.
- *Bruising (ecchymosis):* Due to subcutaneous bleeding.
- *Muscle spasm:* Involuntary contraction of muscles near the fracture.
- *Tenderness:* Over the fracture site due to underlying injuries. Tenderness is demonstrated by palpation.
- *Pain:* Immediate severe pain at the time of the injury due to trauma. Following the injury pain may result from muscle spasm, overriding of the fractured ends of the bone, or damage to adjacent structures. Typically, pain is increased by pressure at the site of the injury or movement of the injured part. Pain may be absent for a brief period immediately after injury is sustained, because of shock and impaired nerve function. (Pain is discussed in Unit XI.)
- *Imapired sensation,* e.g., numbness: May occur if nerve damage is present. A nerve may be pinched or severed by bone fragments.
- *Loss of normal function:* May result from instability of the fractured bone or from pain or muscle spasm or both. Paralysis may be caused by nerve damage.
- *Abnormal mobility:* Movement of a part which is normally immobile may occur due to instability when long bones are fractured.
- *Crepitus:* Grating sensations or grating sounds may be felt or heard if the injured part is moved. Crepitus results from broken bone ends rubbing together.
- *Shock:* May result from blood loss, i.e., hypovolemic shock, or other factors such as severe pain or extensive soft tissue damage. (Shock is discussed in Chapter 13.)
- *Abnormal x-ray or fluoroscopic findings:* Radiology or fluoroscopy is used to confirm the diagnosis by showing the location of the fracture and the direction of the fracture line. Findings vary according to the site and type of fracture.

If a fracture is suspected the injured part should be kept at rest until a physician can assess the condition. Do not attempt to elicit symptoms (e.g., crepitus, abnormal mobility) by moving the injured part. Movement can cause additional damage, such as displacement of fragments, injury to adjacent structures, or establishment of an open fracture.

X-ray films of fractured bones should be taken in two planes and should include the joint above and the joint below (so dislocations or subluxations can be identified if present). X-ray films are typically taken in anteroposterior and lateral projections. They are commonly taken prior to reduction, following reduction, and then periodically during the healing process. The physician may show the patient the films of the fracture while discussing the treatment plan. It is helpful to the patient to know about how long the injury will be incapacitating so that realistic plans concerning transportation, work, and finances can be made.

Fracture Healing

The body's general responses to injury and infection are discussed in Chapter 10. The following discussion focuses on physiologic processes active in bone healing. Unlike many specialized tissues, bone can regenerate. Healing of fractures thus takes place by the formation of new bone tissue (to reunite bone fragments) rather than by the formation of nonspecialized fibrous scar tissue. Fractures usually heal by passing through the following stages (Fig. 77–5):

- *Hematoma formation:* Bleeding occurs into the fracture site immediately following the fracture. Inflammatory exudate also appears. The blood comes from vessels ruptured within the bone as well as from tears in the periosteum (covering the bone) and adjacent soft tissues. A hematoma forms surrounding the area of the injured bone

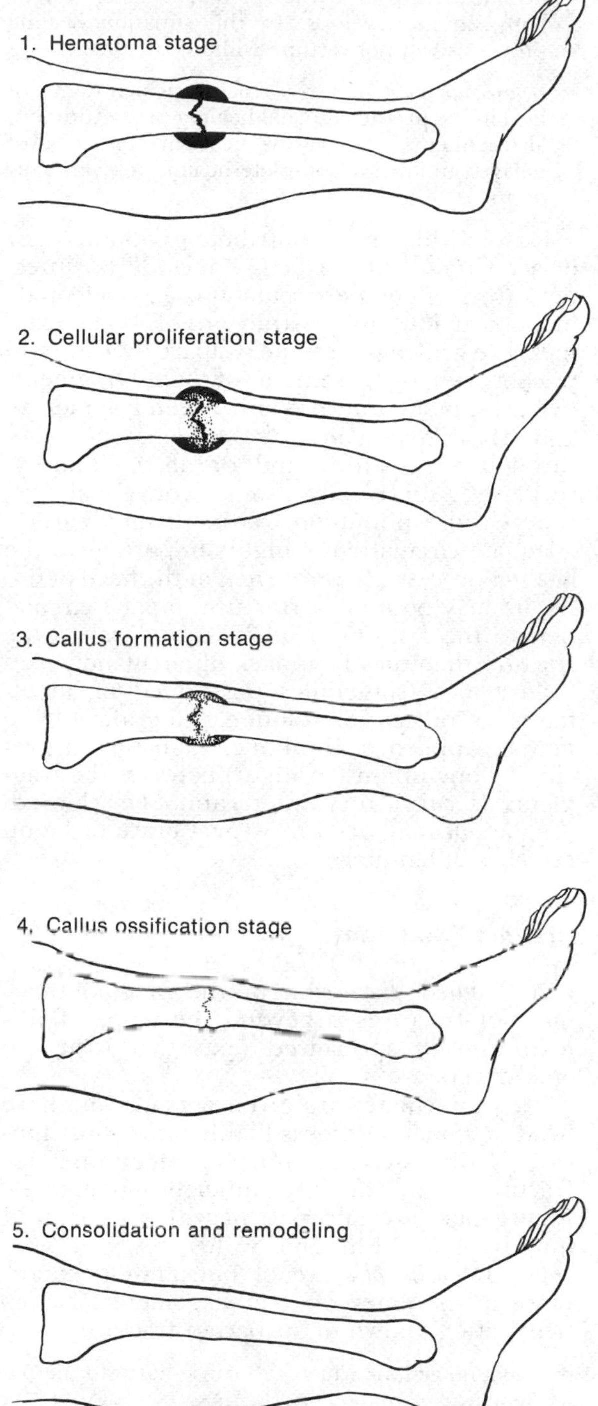

Figure 77–5. Stages of fracture healing. Possible complications during *hematoma stage* include prevention of coagulation and loss of hematoma through (a) open fracture, (b) debridement or (c) action of fibrinolytic synovial fluid. Possible complications during *cellular proliferation stage* include interruption of vascular network by (a) motion or infection, (b) a hostile environment because of an inadequate blood supply, (c) unbridgeable gaps between bone ends or (d) devitalization of periosteal, intramedullary or extraosseous mesenchymal tissues from which red cells originate. A possible complication during *callus formation stage* is that the collagen matrix may be rendered nonossifiable by hypercortisonism or scurvy.

and filling the cleft of the fracture. After 24 hours the main blood supply increases to the fractured bone ends. Also, new capillaries are starting to grow into the blood clot. The clot becomes bound together by fibroblasts. As the blood in the hematoma clots (coagulates), a loose, delicate mesh of fibrin forms around the fracture site. The fibrin mesh protectively encloses the damaged area of bone and also acts as a scaffold for the ingrowth of capillary buds and fibroblasts. Within 24 hours the blood clot begins to organize. Unlike most hematomas, the hematoma which surrounds a fracture is not resorbed during healing. Instead it undergoes changes and develops into granulation tissue.

- *Granulation tissue formation* (also called cellular proliferation stage): Gradually cells and new capillaries invade the hematoma. Within a few days the blood clot is replaced by granulation tissue. Two days after the injury, red blood cell and tissue debris is being removed by phagocytosis. Simultaneously the periphery of the clot is invaded with fibroblasts (from the medullary cavity, periosteum, and adjacent connective tissue). Thus the reparative process is started as fibroblasts form a *soft tissue callus* surrounding the fracture site.
- *Callus formation:* Six to 10 days after the injury the granulation tissue changes and a *provisional callus* or *procallus* is formed. Newly formed cartilage and bone matrix (derived in part from the periosteum and endosteum of the adjacent bone margins) disperse through the soft tissue callus and increase in numbers until the provisional callus is established. The provisional callus is a large, loosely woven mass of bone and cartilage which is considerably wider than the bone's normal diameter. The provisional callus extends beyond the fracture line for some distance, thus serving as a temporary splint to the injury. The provisional callus usually reaches its maximal size at about 14 to 21 days in an uncomplicated fracture. This mass is subsequently remodeled according to Wolff's law, which basically states that the structure of a bone is determined by its function, e.g., the stresses and strains placed upon it.
- *Ossification:* With the deposition of calcium salts, a permanent callus of rigid bone eventually forms. Calcification first forms an external callus (between the periosteum and cortex), next an internal callus (medullary plug), and finally an intermediate callus (between the cortical fragments). During the third to tenth weeks of healing, callus is converted into bone. The formation of bone firmly binds together the fractured ends and healing is complete. While the provisional callus can effectively hold the bone fragments together temporarily, it is not strong enough to hold up if subjected to strains or if made to bear weight.

- *Consolidation and remodeling:* Gradually the provisional callus is increasingly strengthened by the formation of true bone as calcium salts are deposited. At the same time, the callus is remodeled by osteoblastic and osteoclastic activity. In effect, excess bone is chiseled away from the callus and the excess bone is absorbed. Muscle and weight-bearing stresses imposed on the bone govern the remodeling process. During the healing process the external callus is absorbed (by rarefying osteitis), and the intermediate callus consolidates into hard sclerosing osteitis and becomes permanent callus.[168]

Effective bone healing is facilitated by achieving close, accurate approximation of the fractured ends and then immobilizing the structure in this position of proper alignment, by pinning, traction, or casts, until healing occurs. Movement and irritation at the fracture site impair callus formation. During the healing process it is important for the injured part to have adequate circulation. Circulation not only brings oxygen, nutrients, and calcium to the callus but also removes debris from the callus. To promote effective circulation the limb may be elevated (to reduce edema), and the patient is mobilized as soon as possible. Early mobilization promotes not only effective circulation but also a favorable nitrogen balance. A callus must be protected from strain or the delicate healing processes will be interrupted and the bone may refracture.

Fractures normally heal more rapidly in children than adults. Bone union typically occurs in 4 to 6 weeks in children, 6 to 8 weeks in adolescents, and 10 to 18 weeks in adults. Some healing processes may continue for as long as a year. With successful healing the bone is eventually well consolidated, as strong as it was before injury, and contains fat and marrow cells. The healing process is monitored by periodic x-ray films. Healing time is affected by the type of bone injured and the specific nature of an injury. Non–weight-bearing bones may heal more rapidly than weight-bearing bones. Larger bones heal more slowly than smaller bones. Dense bone (which is not highly vascularized) heals more slowly than cancellous, vascular portions of bone, e.g., ends of long bones. Flat bones typically heal rapidly. The patient's general physical condition may also influence healing, e.g., a poor general condition or malnutrition impairs healing. To facilitate healing the patient's diet should be high in vitamins, protein, iron, and calcium.

Unfortunately all fractures do not heal in the usual sequential manner described above.

- *Nonunion* of a fracture is said to exist when the healing processes at the fracture site stop before bony union develops. In this situation healing processes will not resume without treatment.
- *Delayed union* refers to a fracture which does not heal in the predicted usual healing time. Additional treatment is not always necessary in a case of delayed union for complete healing to eventually occur.

Factors which may contribute to nonunion or delayed union of a fracture include (a) infection, (b) inadequate circulation, (c) inadequate immobilization, (d) distraction of bone fragments (e.g., fragments held apart by excessive traction, (e) displacement of bone fragments (e.g., soft tissue interposed between fragments), and (f) accidental loss of the hematoma, e.g., through an open wound or at the time of surgery. Additionally, some congenital disorders cause nonunion. As mentioned earlier, adequate circulation is highly important in the healing process. *Aseptic necrosis* of the head of the femur may occur if a fracture impairs circulation to the femur's head. Tissue distal to the fracture then dies from lack of circulation.

Surgery is sometimes performed in an attempt to correct nonunion, e.g., a graft of bone may be applied to the bone fragments to provide a bony union ("bridge") between the fragments. If satisfactory union cannot be achieved, the patient may need to wear a brace or be on crutches indefinitely.

First-Aid Treatment

A detailed discussion of the first-aid treatment of fractures is beyond the scope of this text. Consult specialized texts that focus on emergency care.

The immediate care given persons who have head or spinal injuries is highly important. This care is discussed in Unit X. Penetrating rib fractures may be life-endangering injuries. Emergency care of a patient with a punctured lung is discussed in Unit XVI.

Several *principles* are of outstanding importance in the emergency management of a patient with a known or suspected fracture:

- Take no actions which can cause harm to the patient.
- Organize bystanders, e.g., direct someone to call for help, ask others to direct traffic around the scene of the accident, and keep crowds back, away from the patient.
- Move the patient no more than absolutely necessary. Do not move the patient unless in danger, until he or she has received the necessary care at the scene of the accident.
- If a fracture is suspected but is not obvious, treat the patient as if a fracture had occurred.
- Consider the patient's total condition, i.e., do not

focus only on the fracture site and overlook other disorders such as shock.

- ▶ Keep the patient as comfortable as possible while giving emergency care.
- ▶ Do what you safely can, but do not act beyond your qualifications, e.g., do not try to reduce a fracture or dislocation.
- ▶ Expose the fracture site to search for evidence of skin breakage.
- ▶ Dress open wounds, e.g., compound fractures, before applying a splint.
- ▶ Splint the injured site *before* permitting the patient to be moved (no matter how short the distance is). Remember the motto: "Splint them where they lie."
- ▶ Inspect and carefully prepare a splint *before* it is applied (e.g., apply padding if necessary) to make certain the application of the splint will not cause additional damage, e.g., pressure damage.
- ▶ Do not try to "push back" any exposed portions of bone, e.g., ends, fragments, or splinters of bone.
- ▶ Elevate the injured extremity when possible (a) to minimize circulatory congestion and edema (swelling); and (b) to control hemorrhage.
- ▶ Make certain the patient is taken directly to a facility where prompt definitive treatment is available.

Movement of a fractured limb before the limb is immobilized may cause irreparable damage, e.g., bone fragments may move out and sever a nerve or blood vessel. If it is *absolutely* necessary to move the patient before a splint can be applied (e.g., to move the person to safety), support the injured extremity both above and below the site of the fracture and have someone apply gentle traction during transportation (i.e., maintain a slow, steady pull on each side of the fracture site while moving the patient).

Do not allow the patient to try to get up or sit up until he or she has been assessed for possible injuries. Also, do not permit other persons to hastily move the patient. When it is time to move the patient make certain that persons helping know the actions they should (and should not) take *before* starting to move the patient. Coordinated, safe movements are imperative. One person should control the injured (splinted) extremity while the patient is moved.

Do not focus exclusively on the fracture and neglect to care for other disorders, e. g., shock, hemorrhage. Remember to evaluate the patient's mental-emotional status and give appropriate care. The person who has suffered a traumatic injury may be highly anxious or in a state of emotional shock.

Fractures may elicit fears of permanent deformity or crippling. Emotional shock (resulting from the impact of the injury process) may be greatly intensified if the patient sees, for example, the badly deformed limb. The nurse who is unaccustomed to seeing fractures also may initially find it distressing to view the disfigurement caused by injuries such as fractures. Such a nurse must take care not to convey his or her own discomfort to the patient.

Expose the site of the injury. If necessary, gently cut or tear away overlying clothing without moving the limb. If it is necessary to cut clothing, try to do so along a seam, so the clothing can later be repaired if the patient desires. Remove rings, bracelets, watches, and so forth from an injured arm as soon as possible before swelling prohibits their removal.

Splinting. Immobilization of a fractured limb is highly important. Prompt application of a splint is useful because immobilization accomplishes the following:

- ▶ Prevents additional damage, by preventing movement of bone fragments. Movement of fragments can damage adjacent structures or can convert a closed fracture into an open fracture. Bones in the arms and legs lie very close to the surface of the skin. Rough, splintered bone ends can easily penetrate the skin if carelessly handled. Movement of the fracture can also convert a simple fracture into a comminuted fracture, and can sever nerves or blood vessels and injure other soft tissues.
- ▶ Minimizes and/or prevents pain, muscle spasm, shock, and hemorrhage. Fractures are often extremely painful. A patient may feel much more comfortable after a splint is applied and muscle spasm is overcome. Severe, unrelieved pain can contribute to shock.
- ▶ Minimizes deformity (e.g., angulation or overriding of the injured limb) which severe muscle spasm causes.
- ▶ Permits blood to clot at the fracture site. As discussed, clotting and formation of a hematoma is of importance in the body's natural healing process.

A variety of commercial splints are available, e.g., inflatable plastic (air) splints, wooden splints, molded aluminum splints, soft wire splints, scored cardboard splints, and special metal splints (e.g., Thomas splints). If commercial splints are not available, splints can be *improvised* from numerous materials, such as pillows, folded blankets, rolled-up newspapers, padded boards or sticks, golf clubs, heavy magazines, baseball bats, or tongue depressors.

Rigid splints should always be long enough that they immobilize the entire bone and can be secured well above and below the fracture site. When applying a splint, apply slight traction. A splint should be securely applied but should not be so tight that it impedes circulation. The splint should immobilize the joints above and below the fracture. Also, a splint should be properly padded (if necessary) before application to protect soft tissues.

Air splints (i.e., plastic inflatable splints or pneumatic splints) are useful because the clear plastic permits visualization of underlying structures to note skin condition and color of the limb, and x-ray films can be taken through the splint. A bulky, absorptive sterile dressing should be applied over compound fractures before application of the splint. Air splints are usually a temporary method of immobilization.

Air splints are available in various shapes; some are rectangular, others are boot-shaped. Some have zippers or other fasteners. Air splints cannot be used to immobilize fractures of the femur or humerus, since they would not immobilize the joint above the fracture. However, they are of value in splinting fractures of the forearm or lower leg.

If an air splint is applied outside in cold weather and the patient is then transferred into a warm area, the air in the splint expands. To prevent excessive pressures from forming in the splint, it may be necessary to remove some air.[105] The proper amount of pressure in an air splint should be about 30 mm. Hg. When firm manual pressure is applied to the plastic of an inflated splint, the tension of air should be such that the plastic can be dimpled about ½ inch.

When indicated, *traction splints* are extremely useful because they can overcome the severe muscle spasms that fractures produce in some large muscles. Hip, femur, and lower leg injuries should be traction splinted if possible. The immediate application of traction may prevent muscle spasm and relieve pain.

> *For a fracture in the shaft of a long bone, traction may be applied manually until the splint is securely positioned.*

When applying traction, remember that it is being applied to align the fracture and immobilize the bone fragments, not to reduce the fracture. To apply traction, grasp the extremity firmly with one hand over the break and the other further down the limb (e.g., grasping the hand or foot). Ask another person to apply countertraction by holding the patient firmly, e.g., grasping the joint above the fracture site. Then pull with a slow, steady motion on the part distal to the fracture. Do not pull quickly and forcibly and do not attempt to overcome firm resistance if it is encountered. Sudden jerks can damage blood vessels, nerves, or soft tissue. Do not apply excessive traction; apply just enough to support and immobilize the fracture in a position of proper alignment. *Once you initiate traction do not release it.* Maintain traction until the splint is secured or until the patient receives appropriate care.

When traction is indicated it can best be applied before muscles in the injured limb go into spasm, i.e., involuntarily contract. It is difficult to apply traction to a spastic limb. Immediately following a fracture the surrounding muscles are flaccid for 10 to 40 minutes. The muscles then go into spasm. Muscular spasms may interfere with circulation of blood and lymph. Additionally, they are painful and may increase deformity by pulling bone fragments further out of alignment.

Space does not permit discussion of the application of splints to various sites. Fractures of the foot or ankle can be immobilized by securing a pillow around the back of the ankle and bottom of the foot.

Compound Fractures. Apply a sterile dressing (if available) to the site of a compound fracture. If a sterile dressing is not available, cover the wound with a piece of clean white cloth if possible. Control bleeding by applying local pressure over the dressing. Remember that even though bone is not exposed, a compound fracture may be present if the skin is open over the fracture site. If bone is initially visible but later pulls back under the skin (e.g., due to muscle spasm or during application of a splint), pin a note on the patient's clothing which tells the doctor that the bone was exposed.

It is generally agreed that compound fractures should not have traction applied to them, since with traction any exposed bone fragments may be pulled back under the skin. This could damage underlying structures; cause the interposition of muscle, nerve, or blood vessels between fragment ends; and/or introduce contaminated material (e.g., hairs, pieces of dirt) into the wound. *Splint the limb in the position in which it is found.*

Angulated Fractures; Joint Injuries. "Angulation" of a fractured limb refers to deformity of the limb caused by the injury displacing the extremity into an unnatural position. Opinion varies about the emergency management of angulated fractures. While some surgeons prefer that the limb be splinted in the position of angulation, others believe it is desirable for the limb to be gently moved into more normal alignment.[137] Fractures of the extremities which are only slightly angulated may easily be immobilized in place. Severely angulated fractures (e.g., in which a limb is at a right angle to its normal position) may make it difficult to transport the patient.

If a joint is injured do not attempt to straighten the injured part. Immobilize the limb as found.

Some sources[105] recommend straightening any severely angulated fracture which can be safely straightened, e.g., fractures of the upper and lower extremities *except* for fractures of the shoulders, elbows, wrists, or knees. Straightening fractures involving joints may cause permanent nerve damage because of the close proximity of major nerves and blood vessels.

A word about *dislocated joints*. They should be immobilized when giving emergency care, but do not attempt to straighten or reduce any dislocation. To do so may damage nerves and blood vessels adjacent to the joint.

Treatment of Fractures

The *goals* of fracture treatment are to return the injured limb to maximum function to prevent complications, and to obtain the best possible cosmetic result. The expected outcomes of the treatment-rehabilitation program should be discussed realistically with the patient by the physician.

Most fractures are treated by *reduction* and *immobilization. Physical therapy* is an important part of the recovery-rehabilitation program.

Fracture reduction is performed in an attempt to restore the injured bone's normal anatomic alignment, position, and length and to bring the fracture fragments into close approximation to one another so that healing will be promoted. Reduction of a fracture is sometimes called "setting" the bone. It is not always possible to bring fracture fragments back into near-perfect anatomic alignment for healing. In some instances the bone fragments must heal with minor shortening or angulation. Repeated attempts at reduction are undesirable.[207]

Fractures may be reduced in three basic ways:

(1) by *reduction traction,*
(2) by *manipulation* ("closed reduction"); or
(3) by *operative procedures* ("open reduction").

These techniques are described further on. Some fractures are treated with a combination of procedures, e.g., traction may be applied for a while before open reduction is performed. Early reduction is important. Reduction minimizes pain and muscle spasm and promotes healing.

Both closed and open reduction procedures are painful. Therefore, anesthesia is administered. Anesthesia also helps muscles relax. Reduction procedures may be performed under local anesthesia, nerve blocks (e.g., spinal anesthesia or brachial or axillary nerve blocks), or general anesthesia. (See discussion of nursing patients experiencing surgery, Unit VIII.)

Not all fractures require reduction. For example, an undisplaced fracture does not require reduction (because the bone fragments are already correctly aligned). In such a case splinting may be advisable to prevent future displacement. A few fractures, such as those of the distal phalanges, cannot even be adequately splinted and are treated by simply keeping the part at rest until adequate healing occurs.

As we have emphasized throughout this chapter, fractures often injure adjacent soft tissues, e.g., nerves, tendons, muscles, blood vessels, subcutaneous tissue, fat, skin. The treatment of a fracture thus includes the treatment of related injuries. For example, seriously injured major nerves and vessels require surgical repair. Laceration of an artery and severance of a major nerve are surgical emergencies. Injured soft tissues become swollen and edematous. If edema fluid is allowed to solidify, it causes pain, adhesions, and stiffness. Edema can be reduced by elevation of the injured extremity, application of cold, activity, and compression bandaging. Uninjured joints which are not immobilized should be actively exercised. Muscular activity helps to pump away edema fluid. Active function helps to prevent fibrosis and stiffness in injured muscles and affected joints. Various techniques of physical therapy enhance recovery.

Reduction Traction. Traction techniques have been discussed in detail in Chapter 76. With reduction traction considerable pull is exerted on the distal fragment of the fracture to align it with the proximal fragment (which is less manageable). The amount of traction needed to achieve alignment is usually quite intense and it is applied for only a short period of time. Once the fracture has been reduced, the amount of weight applied with the traction set-up is reduced to the smallest amount that will maintain proper alignment and apposition of the bone fragments.

It is desirable for traction to be applied to the injured limb *before* muscle spasm begins. Prompt application of therapeutic traction may prevent muscle spasm and pain, in addition to maintaining alignment of the fractured bones.

Closed Reduction (Manipulation). The physician performs closed reduction by manually applying traction to lock the ends of the fragments together and thus restore normal bone alignment (see Fig. 77–6). A surgical incision is not performed. The three basic maneuvers used during manipulation are (1) traction

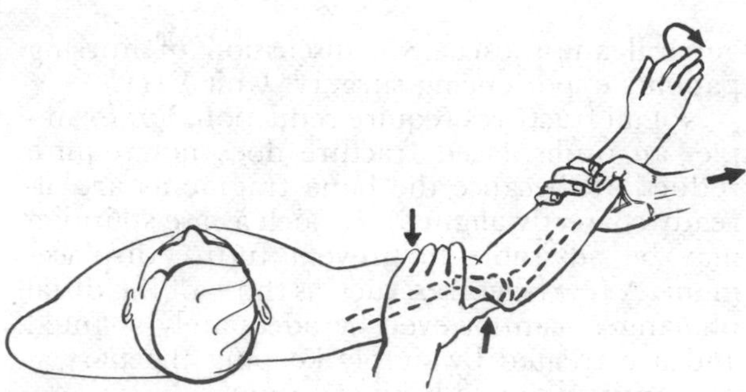

Figure 77–6. Closed reduction. Manipulative reduction of supracondylar fracture. (From Schmeisser, G., Jr.: *A Clinical Manual of Orthopedic Traction Techniques.* 1963.)

and countertraction; (2) angulation; and (3) rotation. Manipulation requires skill and tactile sensitivity. It is a scientific process which reverses the causal force of the fracture. Following a closed reduction x-ray films are taken and a cast is usually applied.

Open Reduction. After a surgical incision is made, the fracture is aligned under direct vision. At the time of surgery various *internal fixation devices* may be applied to the bone to maintain alignment. These devices consist of metallic screws, plates, pins, wires, nails, or rods which may be placed through bone fragments, fixed to the sides of the bone, or (with rods) inserted directly into the bone's medullary cavity. When both screws and a plate are inserted, they must be made of the same metal to avoid a possible electrolytic reaction. The insertion of skeletal pins and wires for use in maintaining skeletal traction has been discussed earlier in this unit.

While internal fixation devices initially help immobilize a fracture and prevent deformity, they are not a substitute for bone healing. Thus, if proper bone healing does not occur, the metallic structures eventually succumb to stress and they loosen or break, thereby failing to rigidly support the weakened bone.

The major *disadvantage* of open reduction is the possible introduction of infection into the bone because surgery converts a closed fracture into an open fracture.[98] Other *potential hazards* include:[207] (a) impaired circulation (open reduction reduces blood supply to the bone, because dissection divides small blood vessels around the bone, and periosteal elevation damages periosteal vessels); (b) accidental injury to major nerves or blood vessels during surgery; and (c) additional damage to bone or adjacent structures caused by the metallic fixation devices implanted during surgery. Because open reduction is not without potential problems, the decision to treat a fracture by this procedure is carefully made.

For some fractures, open reduction is the treatment of choice. For example, *surgery is necessary to treat* compound fractures, fractures accompanied by serious neurovascular injuries, fractures with widely separated fragments, and fractures which have soft tissue interposed between bone fragments. Also, open reduction is typically performed with fractures of the femur and fractured joints. Comminuted fractures may be treated by internal fixation. However, severely comminuted fractures usually do not respond well to internal fixation because enough firm bone is not available to hold the metallic devices, or because the extensive dissection necessary to perform the surgery compromises blood supply to the injured site. Additionally, bone which has a lot of osteoporosis does not respond well to treatment by internal fixation.

To accomplish reduction the patient may be placed on a special fracture table rather than a standard operating table. Fracture tables help hold the patient in position and are particularly useful in procedures such as hip nailing and procedures to be followed by cast application.

X-ray films may be taken during and following open reduction to evaluate alignment of the fractured bone. Upon completion of surgery the patient may be placed in traction or a cast may be applied.

Care of the patient undergoing surgical treatment is discussed in Unit VIII.

Immobilization. Healing fractures must be immobilized until the physician decides that adequate clinical union of the bones has developed. Immobilization prevents movement of the fragments and thus promotes healing, prevents possible overriding or displacement of fragments due to muscle spasm, minimizes pain, and prevents the interposition of soft tissue between the fragments. Immobilization may be accomplished by application of casts, splints, or bandages, or by application of traction. Casts and traction (their uses, applications, complications, and appropriate clinical care) are discussed in Chapter 76.

Excessive immobilization in the treatment of fractures is undesirable since it contributes to muscle atrophy and impaired circulation. It is therefore important that the movement of adjacent structures (joints, muscles) not be unnecessarily restricted when immobilizing a fractured part.

Compound Fractures. The treatment of compound fractures presents special problems because of the possibility that bacteria and foreign objects may have been introduced when the injury was sustained. Every attempt must therefore be made to prevent subsequent infection. With prompt aseptic cleansing of the wound and surgical treatment, infection can frequently be prevented. Antibiotics are commonly prescribed.

Because an open fracture predisposes the patient to possible *tetanus*, the patient may immediately be given hyperimmune serum (Hyper-Tet) (unless previously immunized) or a booster dose of tetanus toxoid (if immunized).

Compound fractures are surgical emergencies. The patient should be operated upon within 4 to 6 hours after injury. The sooner surgery can be performed, the better it is for the patient. During surgery the surgeon removes or flushes away (with sterile solutions) bacteria and foreign particles. Surgical treatment also includes cutting away (debridement) of all devitalized tissue. After reducing the fracture and repairing soft tissue injuries the surgeon either closes the wound primarily (with sutures) or leaves the wound unsutured to be closed several days later with secondary sutures or skin grafts. The latter procedure may be the treatment of choice if treatment has been delayed or when a wound is grossly contaminated. The open wound may be loosely packed, as with petrolatum gauze, and covered with a compression dressing. The surgeon subsequently tends the wound and may leave orders for treatments. At times extremities with compound fractures are damaged so severely that it is necessary to perform amputation.

Complications

Complications of fractures may include arterial damage, peripheral nerve damage, fat embolism, infection, shock, nonunion, and avascular necrosis. Other complications are shown in Table 77–1.

Arterial damage may consist of contused, thrombosed, lacerated, severed, or spastic vessels, as a result of injury associated with the fracture. Vessels may also be constricted by bandages or casts that are excessively tight. Vessels that are highly vulnerable are the popliteal artery (with fractures near the knee joint or dislocations of the knee) and the brachial artery (with supracondylar fractures of the humerus). Impairment of circulation in the brachial artery can produce Volkmann's ischemic contracture. Indications of arterial damage include variable or absent pulse, swelling, pallor or patchy cyanosis distal to the fracture, continuing blood loss, pain, a large fracture hematoma, poor capillary return, poorly filled veins in a cold extremity, and paralysis or anesthesia distal to the fracture (in the absence of known neurologic injury). The nurse observes the fractured extremity closely for indications of these complications and reports symptoms promptly. Emergency treatment may involve splitting or removing tight encircling casts or bandages, elevation or change of position of the part, reduction of fractures or dislocations, or explorative surgery.

Peripheral nerve damage may result from the injury or from pressure over nerves by casts, bandages, or traction equipment. Indications of peripheral nerve damage and the detection of this complication have been previously discussed. Nerves which are particularly susceptible to injury by broken bones or dislocations include

TABLE 77–1. POSSIBLE COMPLICATIONS FROM FRACTURES

Complication	Early Clinical Features	Recommended Nursing Action	Most Common Fracture Type—Location
Pulmonary Embolism (may occur *without* clinical symptoms)	*Sub-sternal pain* Dyspnea Rapid weak pulse	Administer oxygen. Notify physician immediately—as to pain and vital signs.	Lower extremities
Fat Embolism	*Mental confusion,* apprehension, restlessness *due to hypoxia* Followed by fever, tachycardia, tachypnea, dyspnea	It is advisable to have a standing order to draw blood gases at first sign of mental confusion. Notify physician immediately. Administer oxygen.	Lower extremities and/or multiple fractures
Gas Gangrene	*Mental aberration* followed by signs of infection	Notify physician immediately of mental status, vital signs, and appearance of wound.	Compound (especially with small open area)
Tetanus	*May be none* until: patient has tonic twitchings and difficulty opening mouth	Notify physician immediately. Check to see if patient is getting compazine.*	Compound

*One of the side effects of the normal therapeutic dose of compazine *is* hypertonia.
From Farrell, J.: *Illustrated Guide to Orthopedic Nursing.* Philadelphia: J. B. Lippincott Co., 1977.

the ulnar nerve in medial epicondylar injuries of the elbow; the radial nerve in fractures of the middle and lower humeral shaft; the circumflex nerve in shoulder dislocations; the sciatic nerve in posterior hip dislocations; and popliteal nerves in knee dislocations. When nerves are severed in association with open fractures, immediate surgery is indicated. Commonly nerves recover following reduction if they are merely temporarily stretched, compressed, or contused at the time of fracture or dislocation.

Symptoms of *fat embolism*[117, 180, 192] have been described earlier in this unit. See also Table 77–2. The patient may be treated in the high Fowler's position. Oxygen is given at once to reduce local anoxia and reduce the surface tension of the fat globules. Other respiratory support may be indicated, e.g., intracheal tube, tracheostomy, respirator. Oxygen therapy is governed by monitoring the arterial oxygen tension. Various other treatments may be employed, directed at treating or preventing shock and heart failure. Opinion varies concerning management of fat embolism. Treatment may include the administration of alcohol intravenously (5 per cent dextrose–5 per cent ethanol solution); corticosteroid hormones; blood and fluid replacements (to treat shock); digitalis; aminophylline, heparin; and low molecular weight (40,000) dextran.

Laboratory tests in the presence of fat embolism may show a sudden drop in hemoglobin, fat in the urine or in sputum, a low arterial oxygen tension, and elevated free fatty acids. The most valuable single diagnostic test is a cryostat test which demonstrates fat droplets in frozen sections of blood clots.

Fat embolism can occur at the scene of an accident, in the emergency room, in surgery, or at the bedside, precipitating cardiorespiratory insufficiency and cardiac arrest. Most frequently it occurs with multiple fractures of long bones, but may also occur with some other disorders (e.g., fatty liver, burns, diabetes, pneumonia) and poisonings. Sometimes it develops in injuries without fractures. Emboli may lodge in the brain, heart, or lung, producing life-threatening situations.

Some physicians believe that fat emboli may be prevented by proper splinting, careful transportation, and gentle handling of patients with fractures. These actions also reduce shock in persons with fractures.

Infection may result from contamination of open fractures or can be introduced at the time of surgery. Compound fractures may be compli-

TABLE 77–2. FAT EMBOLISM

Possible Symptoms and Signs in Fat Embolism Syndrome

- Tachycardia
- Tachypnea; dyspnea
- Neurologic dysfunction; retinopathy
- Petechiae
- Noncardiogenic pulmonary edema
- Anemia; thrombocytopenia
- Elevated serum lipase level
- Hypocalcemia
- Positive cryostat test; presence of relatively large fat particles
- Fat in urine, CSF, and sputum
- Pulmonary dysfunction
  - Hypoxemia; hypocarbia
  - Increased wasted ventilation
  - Reduced compliance
  - Reduced carbon monoxide–diffusing capacity

Possible Causes of Post-traumatic Respiratory Insufficiency

- Chest trauma
- Pneumonia
- Aspiration
- Atelectasis
- Adult respiratory distress syndrome
  - Fat embolism syndrome
  - Other
- Fluid overload
- Oxygen toxicity
- Pulmonary thromboembolism
- Transfusion reaction

Management of Fat Embolism Syndrome

- Insurance of adequate airway
- Maintenance of bronchial toilet
- Administration of appropriate oxygen therapy (mechanical ventilation,* positive end-expiratory pressure*)
- Maintenance of negative fluid balance; use of diuretics*
- Administration of digitalis (in cardiac failure)
- Administration of corticosteroids

Clinical States Associated with Fat Embolism Syndrome

- Trauma, especially with fracture
- Burn
- Abdominal surgery
- Cardiac massage
- Extracorporeal circulation
- Poisoning
- Chronic alcoholism
- Diabetes mellitus
- Sickle cell anemia
- Infection
- Collagen vascular disease
- Eclampsia
- Iatrogenic causes, e.g., overhydration

**In severe cases.*
From Gong, H., Jr.: Fat embolism syndrome. *Postgraduate Medicine,* 62:42, Dec. 1977.

cated by the development of *tetanus* or *gas gangrene.* Gas gangrene infections may develop in deep, grossly contaminated wounds. Gas gangrene is caused by anaerobic bacteria (various species of *Clostridia*). These organisms produce a characteristic cellulitis in which gas is present under the skin. Indications of infection with this contagious organism are precipitous drop in hemoglobin, temperature elevation, rapid pulse, pain, sudden local puffiness (with discoloration of tissues), and a thin, watery exudate which is extremely foul smelling. Crepitation may be felt, upon palpation of the skin, due to the presence of gas bubbles in muscles and subcutaneous tissues.

Treatment of gas gangrene involves opening the wound widely to admit air and permit drainage. Generous and multiple incisions are made through the skin and fascia. Sutures and any gangrenous material are removed and the wound is irrigated. Transfusions may be indicated. Anti-infective agents are administered, e.g., antitoxin with penicillin G or a tetracycline. If massive gangrene develops amputation is necessary.

Shock is another potential complication of fractures. As stated previously, most musculoskeletal injuries are not life-threatening. However, some are because of shock resulting from the injury. A fractured femur can be a life-threatening injury because severe shock can result from the amount of blood lost from the circulation into tissues. Fractures of the tibia and fibula may also be serious injuries. With open fractures of these bones as much as half of the blood supply may be lost. Traumatic or hypovolemic shock may also occur with fractures of the spine, thorax, and pelvis.

Nonunion and *avascular necrosis* of fractured bone are complications which were discussed previously in relation to healing.

Fractures of the Femur

Space does not permit discussion of the specific treatments of various types of fractures. Most fractures are treated by the application of casts or traction, and details of these methods of treatment have been presented in Chapter 76. Treatment of fractures of the femur has been selected for additional discussion for the following reasons: (a) fractures of the adult femur require treatment by hospitalization (nursing care is therefore important); (b) fractures of the femur commonly occur in older persons (nurses

PATIENT–FAMILY TEACHING GUIDE
PATIENT INFORMATION ON FRACTURES

A fracture is a break in the hard substance of a bone. X-rays usually show such a break but the crack may be so small as not to show until some healing starts. That is why repeat x-rays a week or two later may show a break that could not be seen immediately after injury.

Most fractures require some support to permit proper healing of the bones, such as a cast, splint, or brace; some must be fixed inside with metal. A fracture may need reduction (putting the bones back together in the right position after the break) before the cast is applied.

Nature determines the length of time needed for each fracture to heal. It is usually longer when the bone is big, long, or badly shattered and when the patient is an older person. Following these instructions will improve the likelihood of healing; failing to do so can cause improper healing, resulting in a deformity or disability. Fractures need *time* and *support* to heal properly.

After the Fracture Has Been Treated:

- Elevate the injured extremity to reduce swelling and pain.
- Exercise the free joints above and below the cast to keep them from getting stiff.
- Keep the cast dry because water will weaken and dissolve it.
- Do not walk on a cast unless instructed to do so. If you are told you can walk, wait until 48 hours have passed to give the cast a chance to dry and harden.
- Report any severe pain, blueness, coldness, or numbing ("pins and needles") sensation in the toes or fingers, which could indicate a problem with circulation.
- If you are given a clinic appointment, keep it because severe breaks need close attention and frequent visits.

(From McMicken, D. B.: After the emergency. *Emergency Medicine,* 11:63, Apr. 1979.)

thus frequently care for patients with these disorders); and (c) fractures of the femur are often treated by open reduction with internal fixation (care of patients undergoing internal fixation has not been discussed).

Fractures of the Proximal End of the Femur. Fractures of the proximal end of the femur (the end of the femur that engages with the acetabulum in the innominate bone to form the "hip joint") are classified as either intracapsular or extracapsular.

- *Intracapsular* fractures are those occurring within the "hip" joint and capsule (a) through the head of the femur (capital fracture); (b) just below the head of the femur (subcapital); and (c) through the neck of the femur (transcervical).
- *Extracapsular* fractures are those outside of the joint and capsule, occurring through the femur's greater or lesser trochanter or in the intertrochanteric area, i.e., pertrochanteric and intertrochanteric fractures. Extracapsular fractures are located in that portion of the femur which is distal to the neck of the femur and which extends about 2 inches below the lesser trochanter.

Figure 77–7 illustrates an intracapsular fracture of the femur and an intertrochanteric fracture of the femur.

Elderly women with osteoporosis are especially prone to fractures of the proximal end of the femur sustained during a fall. Even accidents which appear relatively minor can fracture the femurs of elderly persons. Because these injuries are common among the elderly, x-ray films of the hip are routinely taken when a person of advanced age falls or is in an accident. With impacted fractures of the hip a patient may be able to bear weight and perhaps even walk for a short time after injury. However, the more typical fracture of the femur, with displacement, immediately incapacitates the patient, who lies with the painful injured leg shortened, adducted, and in a position of external rotation. The greater trochanter may be felt, displaced in the buttock.

Clinical management of hip fractures in an elderly patient is often complicated by the presence of other coexisting medical disorders which are common among the aged, such as diabetes or cardiac, peripheral vascular, or neurologic disorders. In order to give effective "total patient care," nurses must be aware of these coexisting problems as well as the location (type) of fracture and methods being employed to treat the fracture.

Treatment

Treatment programs vary, depending upon the patient's general condition, length of time since the fracture was sustained, and the type of fracture. Some patients are placed in traction for short periods of time prior to open reduction of the fracture. Temporary distraction, via traction, disengages bone fragments and prevents muscle spasm until the patient is ready for surgery. Elderly patients often cannot tolerate prolonged immobilization and therefore may not be able to withstand methods of treatment which require long-term immobilization in traction or hip spica casts. Fractures of the femur are commonly treated by various surgical methods of *internal fixation*, e.g., insertion of pins or nails; fixation of screw plates; or implantation of a prosthesis to replace the head and neck of the femur. Internal fixation generally makes early mobilization possible soon after surgery. This is especially important for older persons who are susceptible to the complications of immobility. Some patients with femoral fractures are treated by the application of *traction* (e.g., *Russell's traction*) or *casts* (e.g., *hip spica casts*). These procedures and related care are discussed in

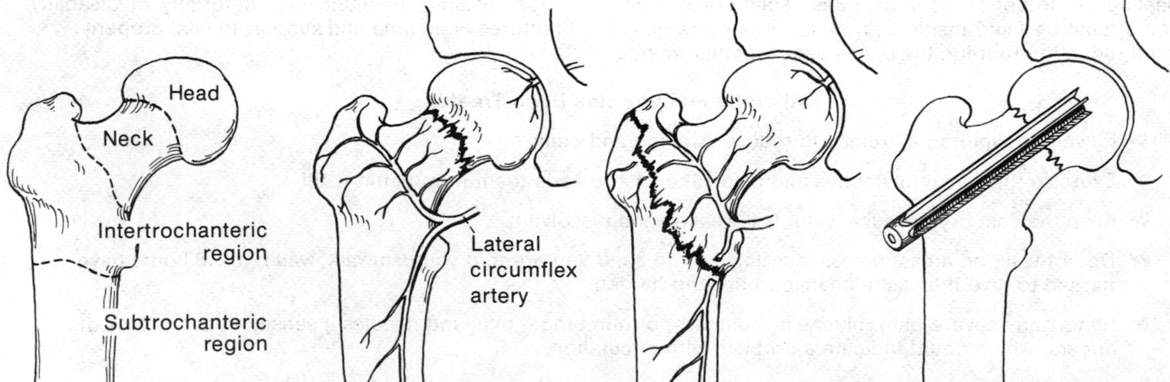

Figure 77–7. **A.** Normal proximal end of femur. **B.** Intracapsular fracture of proximal end of femur. Note blood supply. **C.** Extracapsular intertrochanteric fracture. Note effect of fracture on blood supply. **D.** Intracapsular fracture with nail inserted for reduction.

Chapter 76. Discussion here focuses on treatment by *internal fixation.*

The surgeon performing internal fixation of a femoral fracture has a variety of metallic fixation devices to choose from. In deciding upon the best method of fixing a given fracture, the surgeon considers the angle and location of the line of the fracture. A fixation device is then selected which will most securely hold the fragments of the fracture and which will cause the least disruption of the bone. Fixation devices are made of metals such as stainless steel or Vitallium.

Pins and nails are inserted through the trochanter and femoral neck and then on into the head of the femur (Fig. 77–7*D*). Plates may be fixed with screws of the shaft of the femur. A *hip prosthesis* consists of a ball and intramedullary stem. The head and neck of the femur is surgically removed, and the stem of the prosthesis is then inserted into the shaft of the femur. The ball portion of the prosthesis then replaces the head of the femur in the acetabulum. Prostheses may be used in treating intracapsular fractures which are difficult to reduce, comminuted or prone to nonunion or the development of aseptic necrosis.

During surgery, when internal fixation is being performed, x-ray films or fluoroscopy may be used periodically to guide in placement of the fixating devices. Also, sometimes the surgeon places bone grafts around the fracture line in an attempt to facilitate healing by stimulating bone growth. The grafts may be taken from the patient's tibia or iliac bones.

Complications

Among the *complications* which may occur with fractures of the proximal portion of the femur are the following:

- *Shock and hemorrhage:* May occur immediately following injury or during the early postoperative period.
- *Complications of immobility:* In spite of attempts to prevent these complications, they may rapidly develop, especially among the elderly. Some can be fatal, e.g., pneumonia, thrombophlebitis, pulmonary embolism.
- *Delayed healing, nonunion:* Commonly intracapsular fractures heal more slowly than extracapsular fractures because they may have an impaired blood supply. Nonunion frequently occurs with subcapital fractures treated by nailing. Nonunion may result from poor approximation of the fragments, movement of the fragments, or impaired blood supply.
- *Aseptic necrosis of the head of the femur:* This is a frequent complication following fractures of the proximal femur and traumatic dislocation of the hip. These injuries may jeopardize the blood supply which is delivered to the head of the femur primarily by the posterior retinacular arteries.
- *Deformities; malposition of the femur; secondary arthritis:* Displacement of fragments can produce deformities. Some fractures are difficult to align correctly, and the femur may be malpositioned. The trauma of the injury and surgery may produce secondary arthritic changes in the joint.
- *Postoperative problems with the internal fixation devices:* Internal fixation devices may weaken and break or migrate out of position, causing soft tissue damage. It is therefore sometimes necessary to again perform surgery to remove or replace the damaged or deviant structure.

Postoperative Care

Postoperative care can be adequately given only when the nurse is familiar with the type of operative procedure performed, the presence of coexisting disorders, and the physician's specific orders for the patient. Because postoperative management is variable from patient to patient, it is necessary to check orders carefully to be certain that nursing care given a specific patient conforms with that prescribed.

General postoperative care is discussed in Unit VIII. See Chapter 76 for a discussion of general postoperative care following orthopedic surgery. Discussion here focuses on aspects of care of special importance following insertion of internal fixation devices in the hip. Some patients are placed in casts or traction for a while following surgery. The application of traction for a few days may help overcome muscle spasm. Care of patients in casts and traction is discussed in Chapter 76.

Early in the postoperative period, dressings and linens are checked frequently for drainage and bleeding. Remember to check not only the hip dressing but also dressings over other areas if bone grafts were taken. A Hemovac (low suction drainage device) may be present to prevent fluid accumulation in the operative wound. Injections of narcotics may be required at first to control pain. Later the patient may be given non-narcotic analgesics. A light sedative may be prescribed to facilitate sleep. Respiratory therapy treatments are commonly administered to stimulate coughing. To prevent thrombophlebitis the doctor may have the patient's legs wrapped with elastic compression bandages to minimize venous stasis and dependent edema and to support venous circulation.

The patient often not only is weakened (from the trauma of surgery) but also is commonly elderly. Therefore it is frequently necessary for nurses to consider special aspects of geriatric care for a patient with a fractured hip. Caution is exercised to prevent oversedation or excessive doses of pain medications. It may be advisable to run IV's more slowly to prevent overloading the circulation and straining the heart. Overloading the circulation is dangerous in a patient with limited cardiac reserve. An elderly patient may be more prone to the development of cardiac failure, shock, respiratory depression, and such complications of immobility as disorientation, urinary stasis, skin breakdown, hypostatic pneumonia, thrombophlebitis, and contractures. *Prevention of the complications of immobility* (e.g., by helping the patient to frequently turn, cough, deep breathe, exercise, and take fluids) *is particularly important in an aged patient.* Skin breakdown can rapidly develop. Nutritional problems are common with an elderly patient. Healing is retarded if the patient does not eat adequate protein, vitamins (e.g., B,C,D), and calcium. Supplements may be indicated. Siderails help the disabled older person to move about in bed, and they are a protection for a patient who can easily become confused.

As you care for the patient postoperatively, observe closely for indications of shock, hemorrhage, infection, paralytic ileus, confusion, fat embolism, thrombosis, dislocation of the hip joint, aseptic necrosis, and nonunion. Watch for indications of *dislocation of the hip,* e.g., sharp hip pain or "abnormal" positions of the operated leg (leg shortened and externally rotated). Report these symptoms at once. If dislocation has occurred, as determined by x-ray and physical examination, the patient must be returned to surgery. Also, report excessive *temperature elevations.* They may indicate wound infection, urinary tract infection, pneumonia, or other complications. *Thrombophlebitis* is another possible complication; report lower quadrant pain or pain or tenderness in the calf. *Inadequate reduction* or *avascular necrosis of the head of the femur* may produce pain or muscle spasm during the postoperative period. Report these symptoms if they seem excessively prolonged. Avascular (aseptic) necrosis following hip pinning causes pain, muscle spasm, and limping. Continued weight-bearing can crumble the bone. Early treatment is important. The patient may be taken to surgery where the pins and head of the femur may be removed and replaced with a prosthesis. *Nonunion* may be treated with insertion of bone grafts.

> *Following hip surgery check the physician's orders carefully concerning position and activity restrictions. Usually it is necessary to* prevent *adduction and external rotation of the leg and acute hip flexion.*

The nurse caring for a patient with a hip injury or hip surgery *must* be familiar with the following terms:

- *Adduction:* to "bring toward," drawing toward a center or median line. For example, moving one leg toward the midline of the body while the patient lies flat with both legs straight together, i.e., swinging the leg inward across the other leg.
- *Abduction:* to "take away,'" drawing away from a center or median line. For example, moving one leg out away from the midline of the body while the patient lies flat with both legs straight together, i.e., swinging the leg out, away from the other leg.
- *Internal rotation:* to twist, or rotate toward the midline of the body.
- *External rotation:* to twist, or rotate away from the midline.

While the terms "adduction" and "abduction" are very similar in their spellings, their meanings are completely different. These differences are extremely important when applied to patient care. *Adduction, external rotation, or acute flexion of the hip can dislocate a hip before it is healed.* Check the position of the operated leg frequently to make sure the hip, knee, and foot are aligned as ordered. Know the restrictions of position and activity for a given patient. Teach the patient activities and positions which are desirable and undesirable. Tell the patient *why* some positions are contraindicated.

Handle the operated leg gently. Explain what you are going to do and how the patient can be of help. A *trapeze* is usually placed on the patient's bed to help with moving. Teach the patient how to correctly use the trapeze.

As a general rule, *avoid extremes of position* for a patient following hip surgery. Keep the leg *abducted*, i.e., out to the side, at all times — when the patient lies flat, while turning, and when the patient lies on the side. *Never* adduct the leg past the neutral point or you may dislocate the head of the femur or prosthesis out of the acetabulum. To help maintain abduction a pillow is sometimes placed between the legs when the patient is supine. This serves as a reminder not to cross the legs.

Check to see if the head of the bed can be elevated. If this is permitted, find out how high it can be safely raised. Some patients can have the bed raised 35 to 40°. *Avoid acute flexion of the hip.* This would be caused by excessive elevation of the head of the bed. If the head of the bed can be elevated, instruct the patient not to lean further forward, e.g., to reach for something lying on the foot of the bed. This would additionally increase flexion of the hip.

Often the operated leg tends to lie in slight external rotation when the patient is supine. To *prevent external rotation* while the patient is supine, place a trochanter roll beside the external aspect of the thigh. Also, a covered sandbag may be placed beside the outer aspect of the lower leg. The sandbag should not press against the neck of the fibula (location of the peroneal nerve) or against the external malleolus. To prevent external rotation teach the patient to "toe in" or keep the toes pointed "straight up at the ceiling" while lying on the back.

Turn the patient only with a doctor's order. More commonly following hip surgery the patient is permitted to be turned to the unoperated side. Some patients following hip pinning are permitted to turn to either side. After some types of hip surgery (e.g., total hip replacement, discussed in Chapter 78), no turning is permitted for several days. Checking orders is of obvious importance.

When helping a patient to turn following insertion of an internal fixation device in the hip, remember to avoid adduction and extremes of motion, prevent strain on the hip, and maintain proper alignment of the leg and hip.

Never turn a patient onto the operated hip unless you have a specific order. Typically the patient is turned every two hours during the postoperative period, from back to unaffected side, then onto the back again. When turning the patient onto the unoperated side place one pillow between the patient's thighs and another between the lower legs and feet. The pillows help keep the operated leg in a position of abduction and in a straight line with the trunk. One nurse gently rolls the patient toward the bedside, onto the unaffected side. This is done by reaching across the patient and holding the shoulder and buttock on the operated side. Another nurse supports the operated leg in abduction during the turning by supporting the leg full length (on the pillows) at the same level as the trunk. Once the patient is on the side, keep the hip and knee in the same plane elevated on pillows. Unless pillows are between the legs, the operated leg (uppermost leg) will drop down into adduction. While the patient is lateral the physician may permit the knee of the operated leg to be flexed at right angles to the hip. Before leaving the patient make certain the leg is securely positioned so it will not accidentally become misplaced by falling off the pillows.

If permitted to turn onto the operated side, roll the patient gently toward you after placing pillows between the legs. The bed acts as a splint for the injured leg. If not allowed to turn on either side, the patient may be able to lift straight up on the trapeze periodically for back care and linen changes.

Check with the surgeon to see if the operated limb should be elevated on a pillow. If elevation is ordered, support the entire leg. Sometimes the leg is elevated in traction. When traction is not used the leg is always supported when the patient is turned (as discussed), and is not elevated when the patient is lying on the back.

Postoperative orders following the insertion of a prosthesis usually depend upon the operative approach taken through the joint capsule. Positioning must prevent straining this incision line. Strain on the joint capsule incision can cause the prosthesis to dislocate and push out through the weakened capsule. Commonly with an *anterior* surgical approach the operated limb is rotated internally and is either in a neutral or an abducted position. The patient may be permitted to sit up unless the capsule was removed. With a *posterior* approach the leg is positioned in slight abduction and external rotation. (Yes, *external* rotation — a change from the "typical" positioning.) Also, with the posterior approach the patient is kept relatively flat.

Help the patient to *get out of bed* and *sit in a chair* as soon as the doctor permits. This may be on the first postoperative day. Do not rush or hurry the patient during this activity. Remember an elderly patient may become confused if hurried. Give directions slowly and tell the patient what he or she can do to help. It is important for the patient to know whether or not weight-bearing is permitted on the operated leg. Commonly, weight-bearing is not permitted early in the postoperative course. If the patient experiences postural hypotension a tilt table may be useful in helping the person gradually resume an upright position.

When helping the patient get up in a chair, first select a proper chair. A straight-back, relatively high chair with arms is best. Do not select a low, soft chair. Place the chair on the patient's unoperated side. The chair should be facing the head of the bed and parallel to the bed. To help get up, roll the patient onto the unoperated side and flex the leg. (The patient may be unable to flex the operated leg's knee.) Then gently swing the patient around into a dangling position. Support the injured leg while swiveling the patient. Let the patient rest a moment sitting up. Then, if weight-bearing is not permitted on the operated leg, have the person stand up on the unaffected leg and pivot on that leg and sit down. Support the patient during this transfer and remind him or her not to put weight on the operated leg. Weight-bearing before it is permitted can refracture bone, or displace or break the internal fixation device. Elderly patients often forget easily and tend to bear weight on both legs unless frequently reminded not to do so. Some patients need to be lifted from their beds to chairs. If there is a choice, it is better for a patient to stand and pivot rather than be lifted.

The position of a patient's bed should not be too low when getting up following hip surgery. Less strain and less bending of the hip occurs if the bed is somewhat elevated. Make certain that casters on the bed are locked so the bed will not slip away from under the patient while getting up. Likewise, elevated toilet seats are desirable when the patient has bathroom privileges.

Commonly when a patient first gets up in a chair, the operated leg is extended and supported (elevated). Make certain the leg is securely supported. Later, when the physician permits, the leg is lowered into a dependent position. The first few times the leg is lowered, observe it for swelling and discoloration. Once the operated leg is lowered, the patient should sit with hips even with knees. Tell the patient not to cross legs but to remember to "keep both feet on the floor." Crossing the legs adducts the operated leg and can dislocate the hip.

Assist with *exercises* as soon as they are ordered. Exercises may include quadriceps-setting, gluteal-setting, breathing exercises, exercises for the upper extremities (to prepare the patient for crutch walking), and exercises for unoperated extremities, e.g., to flex and extend the knee and ankle of the unoperated leg to stimulate circulation. Most exercises are started on the day following surgery. The patient may also be instructed to flex and dorsiflex the foot on the operated leg and to begin moving the knee on the operated leg. Moving the knee is done with the patient lying on the side so the knee can be flexed while keeping the hip extended. Other specific exercises may be prescribed as the patient progresses.

Patient-Family Teaching

Follow-up care is important after discharge. The physician continues to evaulate the patient's progress via x-ray films and physical examinations. Visiting nurse services provide valuable home services for the elderly patient living alone.

Patient-family teaching facilitates the recovery process. The patient may become discouraged with the slow rate of healing which occurs in some persons. Encouragement, emotional support, diversion, and self-care can help the patient pass through periods of discouragement. Elderly patients may feel they will not recover. Many fear hip fractures because they know of friends or family members who suffered these accidents and have died. These deep, real concerns should be discussed if the patient wishes to do so. Teaching positive actions a patient can take may help the person feel less dependent and have motivation to recover.

Instruct the patient about how to correctly use a trapeze and siderails to move about. Also, teach the patient exercises that can be done. Be sure you remember to tell the patient when and how many times specific exercises should be performed. Once the patient can get up, teach the person to stand and pivot on the uninjured leg when transferring to a chair. Giving praise and recognition of progress can greatly help lift the patient's spirits. Teach significant others methods of helping the patient; they can be helpful by reminding the patient to cough, deep breathe, take fluids, and exercise. Also, talk with significant others about positions contraindicated for the patient. Instruct the patient not only about actions that can be taken to enhance recovery but also about actions that will be harmful. For example, the patient should know which positions it is unsafe to assume, and *why* these positions are undesirable.

The doctor determines when the bone is healed enough for *ambulation* to begin. The doctor also specifies when the patient can begin to bear weight on the injured leg. Progress of bone healing is carefully followed by periodic x-ray films. Parallel bars and a walker may be used before crutches. Walkers are especially helpful for elderly persons. Some older patients are not taught crutch walking because they are not strong enough or well enough coordinated to safely use crutches.

Fractures of the Shaft of the Femur. This type of fracture most often results from severe violence and occurs in a young or middle-aged person. The injury commonly produces marked displacement and deformity, and extensive soft tissue damage with swelling. It is of extreme importance that the leg be protectively immobilized during transportation of the patient, as with a Thomas splint. Often blood loss at the time of injury is considerable and the patient goes into shock.

If the fracture is relatively simple and the patient is in good general condition with no skin damage, the fracture may be treated by open reduction and insertion of an intramedullary rod to maintain fixation. This technique enables early ambulation (with guarded weight-bearing) and early discharge.

Intramedullary fixation of the shaft of the femur by the insertion of an *intramedullary nail* is illustrated in Figure 77–8. Postoperatively a compression dressing is applied. X-ray studies of the femur are taken on the first postoperative day to evaluate the fixation. The patient is mobilized in bed, and gradual movement of the knee and hip joints is encouraged. After several days (when the physician believes fixation is adequate), the patient begins to ambulate on crutches. If the patient has a transverse fracture

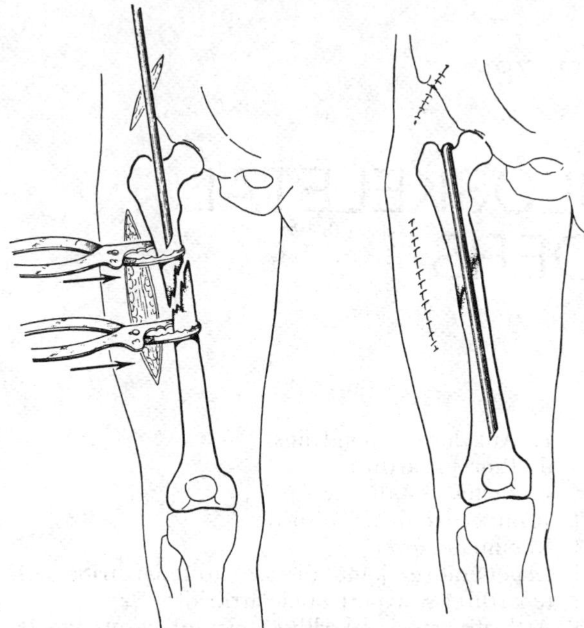

Figure 77–8. Treatment of fracture of midshaft of femur by fixation with intramedullary nail. (From Warren, R., et al.: *Surgery.* 1963.)

that demonstrates adequate fixation, partial weight bearing on the fractured leg may be permitted early in the recovery period. Sutures are usually removed about 8 days after surgery.

Persons with fractures of the shaft of the femur often are placed in *traction* (e.g., Russell's traction or ring leg splints) to counteract muscle spasms in the powerful thigh muscles. Spasm of these strong muscles can cause the bone fragments to become displaced and override each other. Traction may be used *temporarily* prior to intramedullary nailing. *Continuous* skeletal traction (for 10 to 16 weeks) may be necessary to treat complicated fractures, fractures occurring in a patient whose general condition is poor, or fractures in a leg which has other injuries. Frequent x-ray films are taken to check alignment of the fragments. It is important to prevent overpull with traction because this distracts the fragments and impairs healing. The joints and quadriceps are actively exercised early. After 16 to 20 weeks, partial weight-bearing on crutches is usually permitted, and full weight-bearing is permitted after about 6 months.

Supracondylar and Condylar Fractures of the Femur. These fractures of the distal end of the femur may be treated by reduction with continuous skeletal traction and manipulation, or by internal fixation with rods, nails and plates, or screws. These fractures can tear or compress the sciatic nerve or popliteal artery.

CHAPTER 78

OTHER MUSCULOSKELETAL DISORDERS

ARTHRITIS

The terms *rheumatism* and *rheumatic diseases* embrace a variety of disorders, all of which are characterized by pain and stiffness of the musculoskeletal system. *Arthritis* refers to those types of rheumatic disease in which an abnormality of the joint itself is producing the symptoms.

Nonarticular rheumatic diseases are those in which symptoms result from pathologic changes in structures related to or contiguous to the joints (not within the joint itself). These structures include fibrous tissue, muscles, tendons, tendon sheaths, bursae, and nerves. Some of these disorders are described briefly below:

- *Fibrositis* (also called "muscular rheumatism"): inflammation of connective tissue in any location, but especially of that around joints and in or near tendons, muscle sheaths, or other fascial layers of the locomotor system.
- *Bursitis:* inflammation of a bursa, a fluid-filled small sac which facilitates joint movements by making it possible for muscles and tendons to glide over ligaments or bones. Major bursae are located in the shoulder, elbow, knee, and hip; smaller joints also have bursae
- *Tendinitis:* inflammation of a tendon
- *Myositis:* inflammation of voluntary muscle tissue
- *Peritendinitis:* inflammation of a tendon sheath
- *Synovitis:* inflammation of a synovial membrane
- *Tenosynovitis:* inflammation of a tendon and the tendon sheath; most commonly of the hands, wrists, ankles, or feet

Discussion in this section focuses on diseases of the joints. The American Rheumatism Association publishes a detailed classification of diseases of the joints. The following classification by Robinson[198] is somewhat abbreviated and modified from the more detailed classification but it is adequate for our purposes:

1. Polyarthritis of unknown etiology.
   a. Rheumatoid arthritis (atrophic arthritis)
   b. Juvenile rheumatoid arthritis (Still's disease)
   c. Ankylosing spondylitis
   d. Psoriatic arthritis
   e. Reiter's syndrome
2. "Connective tissue" disorders
3. Rheumatic fever
4. Degenerative joint disease (osteoarthritis, osteoarthrosis, hypertrophic arthritis)
5. Arthritis associated with known infectious agents
6. Traumatic and/or neurogenic disorders
7. Gout and pseudogout
8. Tumor and tumor-like conditions

Space does not permit discussion of all of these disorders. Included in the following pages are discussions of rheumatoid arthritis, osteoarthritis, gout, and certain connective tissue disorders (systemic lupus erythematosus, polyarteritis nodosa, scleroderma, polymyositis, and dermatomyositis).

Joint diseases have occurred in human beings and other animals for millions of years. Evidence of degenerative joint disease or osteoarthritis has been identified in the skeletal remains of dinosaurs living 100 million years ago. Signs of arthritis have been found in skeletons of prehistoric people and in Egyptian mummies.

Arthritis is a very common crippling disease. Many people suffering from arthritis seek and receive medical help. Still, many more experience long-term symptoms and do not seek medical help. Arthritis in some form affects more than 18 million people in the United States and causes immeasurable suffering. Some arthritis develops in almost anyone who lives long enough. Some victims of arthritis do not have the money or insurance to afford the necessary periods of long hospitalization, surgery, medications, and physical therapy which are of importance in the treatment of crippling types of arthritis.

It is still not known what causes arthritis or how to cure it, but it is possible in many cases to prevent or correct its crippling effects. A variety of medications may be used to treat arthritis, and recently developed surgical techniques can restore function and relieve pain in many cases. Physical therapy is valuable in the treatment of arthritis as a means of relieving pain and preventing deformity. All of these treatment techniques are discussed in detail further on.

Both *acute* and *chronic* forms of arthritis occur. Acute exacerbations may occur with chronic forms, and acute types of arthritis may progress into subacute or chronic stages. Two basic pathologic processes affect the joints with any arthritic disorder: *inflammation* and *degenerative changes.* Inflammation may be exudative or proliferative or a combination of both types. The degenerative changes that take place within involved joints depend essentially on the ability of articular cartilage to repair itself. In any given patient, varying degrees of inflammation and degeneration may be present.[198]

Rheumatoid Arthritis

Rheumatoid arthritis is the most virulent form of arthritis. Women are affected two to three times more frequently than men. While rheumatoid arthritis can occur at any age, it most commonly affects people between the ages of 35 and 45. It is a chronic, systemic disease in which inflammatory changes occur throughout the body's connective tissues. Commonly the smaller, peripheral joints are involved in a pattern of symmetric distribution. The articular and periarticular structures are progressively destroyed by a chronic proliferative inflammation which replaces involved structures with granulation tissue. As the disease destroys the joints internally, the patient suffers with pain, stiffness, and swelling. Unexplainable remissions and excerbations occur. Physical and emotional stresses are often associated with the onset of rheumatoid arthritis.

An estimated 5 million persons in the United States have rheumatoid arthritis. The incidence of rheumatoid arthritis appears to be about the same in the United States and Canada; the disease is relatively rare in tropical climates. Arthritis is even more common in Great Britain than in the United States.

Etiology. In spite of intensive research efforts, the etiology of rheumatoid arthritis currently remains unknown. Hypotheses are many and varied. Among theories under investigation are those which speculate that the disease may be caused by an undefined virus or some other microorganism (e.g., *Mycoplasma*), by metabolic aberrations, or by immunologic mechanisms. The role of the immune response in the mediation of tissue injury is being given careful consideration (see Chapter 11). Possibly there is a genetic basis for a predisposition to rheumatoid arthritis. It is possible that this disease is caused by several factors.

Pathology. If unarrested, the joint pathology in rheumatoid arthritis passes through four stages: (1) synovitis, (2) pannus formation, (3) fibrous ankylosis, and (4) bony ankylosis (see Fig. 78–1). The involved joint(s) becomes inflamed with a proliferative type of inflammation that is initially localized in the joint capsule, primarily in the synovial membrane *(synovitis).* Edema and congestion thicken the tissue. A *pannus* is a layer of granulation inflammatory tissue which eventually develops, derived from the synovial membrane. The pannus extends over the surface of the articular cartilage into the interior of the joint. It appears reddish and rough and adheres tightly to the underlying cartilage. The pannus formation erodes and destroys the cartilage by interfering with cartilage nutrition. The articular cartilage is then slowly destroyed by invasion, lysis, and starvation. Additional destruction may occur as granulations from the pannus develop on contiguous areas and in subchondral bone. The joint capsule and subchondral bone are thus progressively damaged. *Fibrous ankylosis* (with subluxation and distortion of the affected joint) then occurs as the granulation tissue becomes invad-

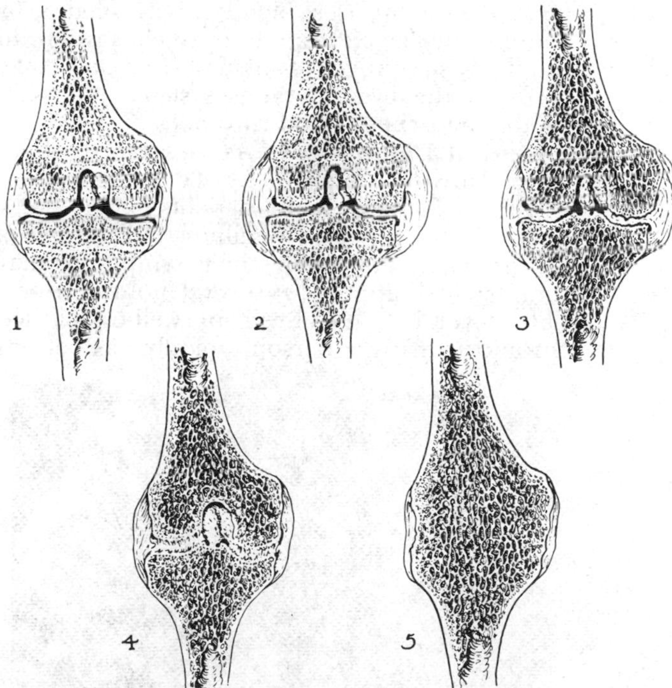

Figure 78–1. Sketches showing the joint pathology in rheumatoid arthritis. (1) Inflammation of the joint capsule with synovitis; beginning proliferative changes. (2) Progression of inflammation with pannus formation; beginning destruction of cartilage and mild osteoporosis. (3) Advanced synovitis with extensive pannus, cartilage destruction, and osteoporosis. (4) Inflammation subsided; fibrous ankylosis. (5) Bony ankylosis. (From Sodeman, W. A., and Sodeman, W. A., Jr.: *Pathologic Physiology: Mechanisms of Disease,* 5th ed. Philadelphia: W. B. Saunders Co., 1974.)

ed with tough fibrous tissue and is converted to scar tissue (which inhibits or prevents joint motion). *Bony ankylosis* (firm bony union) may then develop as the fibrous tissue becomes calcified and changes into osseous tissue.

Other changes occur in additon to the above described joint changes. The muscles, bones, and skin adjacent to an affected joint become somewhat atrophic, and the skin becomes tight, thin, and glossy in appearance. The most characteristic histologic lesions of rheumatoid arthritis are *subcutaneous nodules.* These nodules, which may be present for weeks or months, most commonly develop over bony prominences, especially near the elbow (see Fig. 78–2).

While joint involvement is the most obvious manifestation of rheumatoid arthritis, other body tissues are also affected. Rheumatoid arthritis is a *systemic* disease, attacking connective tissues throughout the body. Nonarticular connective tissue may be diffusely involved. Degenerative lesions may be present in *collagen* in the lungs, heart, muscles, blood vessels, pleura, or tendons. (Collagen is a scleroprotein present in the body's connective tissue.) *Vasculitis* may occur in the eyes, nervous system, and skin, producing ischemia and thrombosis.

Clinical Description. As mentioned, rheumatoid arthritis is characterized by remissions and exacerbations. Some patients experience a relatively brief period of illness lasting only a few months, and then their symptoms may completely disappear for several months or possibly several years. Even in well-established chronic arthritis, a person typically has periods in which the disease activity is heightened and other periods of relative comfort. Tendencies toward remission tend to be greatest, however, early in the course of the disease. Each attack tends to be more stubborn than that which preceded it. Occasionally permanent spontaneous remission occurs, but this is not usual. Generally rheumatoid arthritis progresses, producing some degree of deformity. According to one source,[77] 10 years after onset 15 per cent of patients are likely to be bedridden, 35 per cent may be ambulatory but unable to earn a living, and 50 per cent may be capable of self-care and be employable.

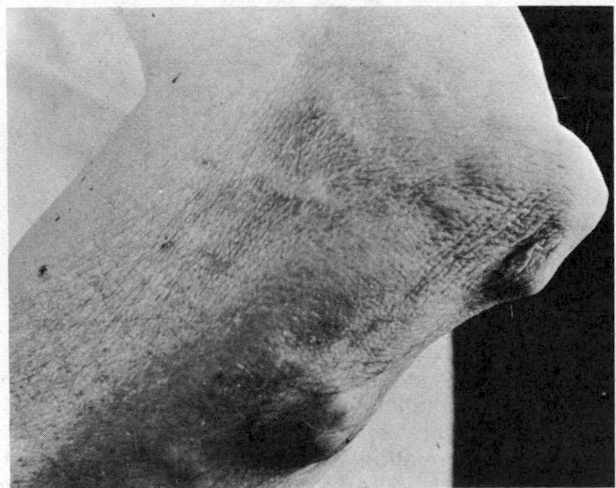

Figure 78–2. Rheumatoid nodules in olecranon bursa and over upper portion of ulna in a patient with classic rheumatoid arthritis. (From Beeson, P. B., and McDermott, W. (eds.): *Cecil-Loeb Textbook of Medicine,* 13th ed. Philadelphia: W. B. Saunders Co., 1975.)

Rheumatoid arthritis may begin abruptly, but more commonly develops insidiously. *Prodromal symptoms* include vague articular pain and stiffness, malaise, weight loss, and vasomotor disturbances such as paresthesias (numbness and tingling of the hands and feet). Typically pain and stiffness worsen markedly following strenuous activity. These symptoms are usually most prominent in the morning and subside during a day of moderate activity. Affected joints not only are stiff and painful, but also may be swollen, red, tender, and warm.

Other findings which may occur with rheumatoid arthritis include: subcutaneous nodules, enlarged spleen, enlarged lymph nodes, anorexia, low-grade fever, weakness, mental depression, and early afternoon fatigue. With advanced disease, ocular manifestations and joint deformities may be present. Atrophy of the muscles and skin around the involved joints may be noticeable. Flexion contractures result from spasm of flexor muscles around inflammed joints and reflex relaxation and atrophy of the antagonistic extensor muscles.

The onset of rheumatoid arthritis often coincides with disturbances which tend to deplete physical or emotional reserves or both, e.g., emotional strain or worry, exposure, overwork, or acute infections.

When rheumatoid arthritis develops *insidiously,* the patient usually experiences pain (on use) and stiffness in one or several joints, followed by swelling. Muscle aching may be present in any part of the body. The temperature may be normal or only slightly elevated. While almost any joint of the body may be initially affected, within several weeks the smaller joints of the hands and feet are typically involved. With an *acute onset* of rheumatoid arthritis, numerous joints suddenly become painful and swollen. The patient experiences chills, prostration, and fever.

Pain produced by rheumatoid arthritis is variable in intensity and tends to be most persistent upon use of the involved joint. Stiffness is often the most constant symptom, tending to be greatest upon arising in the morning. The patient may be most limber in the late morning or early afternoon.

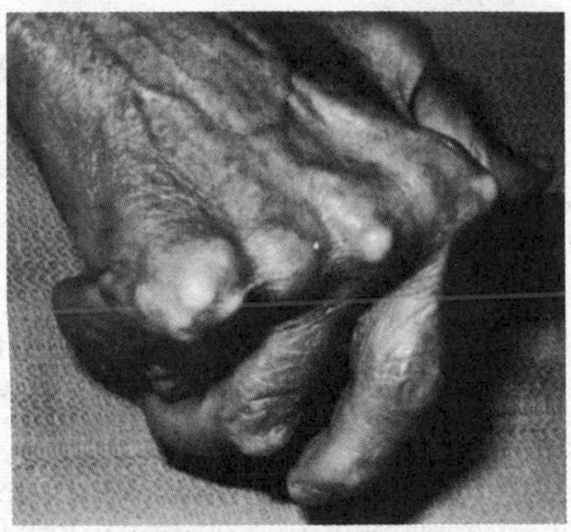

Figure 78–3. Metacarpophalangeal deformity in rheumatoid arthritis. Advanced ulnar drift with volar dislocation of the proximal phalanges. (From Nalebuff, E. A.: Metacarpophalangeal surgery in rheumatoid arthritis. *Surgical Clinics of North America,* 49:825, 1969.)

The joints of the hands, knees, elbows, and ankles are most commonly involved. The characteristic appearance of the hands is shown in Figure 78–3. Usually the patient has a weakened grip and is unable to make a tight fist.

The typical patient with rheumatoid arthritis appears undernourished, chronically ill, and possibly anemic. Eighty percent of patients have a hypochromic, normocytic anemia because of the effect of rheumatoid arthritis upon blood-forming organs.

In addition to a physical examination, *laboratory findings* help establish a diagnosis of rheumatoid arthritis. Frequently serum protein abnormalities are present. Many patients with rheumatoid arthritis have in the serum of their blood, *rheumatoid factors* (RF), which are large antibody-like protein molecules. In 90 per cent of cases of rheumatoid arthritis, the erythrocyte sedimentation rate (ESR) is elevated. The ESR and C-reactive protein are elevated during both acute and chronic phases. As noted, a hypochromic, normocytic anemia is common. Usually the WBC count is slightly elevated or normal; however, leukopenia may be present (e.g., with splenomegaly).

The presence of RF supports the theory that rheumatoid arthritis is a disorder of immunity. It is believed that RF are produced in response to alterations in the connective tissues' gamma globulin. While RF are not specific for rheumatoid arthritis (they are found in numerous granulomatous and infectious diseases), a high RF titer helps confirm the diagnosis of rheumatoid arthritis when symptoms and history of the typical clinical syndrome are present. Treatment influences the RF titer, which commonly falls as inflammatory activity in joints decreases. Typically a high RF titer is indicative of a poor prognosis and is associated with progressive disease, vasculitis, nodules, and pulmonary involvement.[121] A variety of serologic techniques are used to assess the RF titer. The *F2 latex fixation test* is one such test, usually it is positive in 60 to 75 per cent of cases. Even higher percentages of positive reactions occur with tests which are more sensitive. False-positive reactions may occur.

It is helpful for the physician to *aspirate* some *synovial fluid* ("joint fluid") for examination. The fluid is always abnormal in rheumatoid arthritis. The abnormalities reflect the varying degrees of inflammation within the joint. The fluid is generally opaque and sterile with reduced viscosity. From 3000 to over 50,000 WBC's/mm.^{3} are present.

X-ray films may show only soft tissue swelling early in the course of rheumatoid arthritis. Other changes appear later with progression. These changes include osteoporosis around the involved joint, erosion of the cartilage at the periphery of the joint surface, joint space narrowing (due to erosion of cartilage), and bony cysts (from invasion of granulation tissue). After several years the degenerative changes of secondary osteoporosis are apparent.

Because of its chronic and sometimes crippling nature, rheumatoid arthritis is a *difficult diagnosis for a person to accept.* At the time that the physician discusses the diagnosis with the patient, attempts should be made to discuss realistically how the illness may affect the patient's life. Because of the variable nature of rheumatoid arthritis, it is difficult to discuss with accuracy the expected rate of progress. It should be emphasized to the patient that many persons with rheumatoid arthritis continue to lead active productive lives and that with early, intensive treatment only slight modifications in life style may be necessary. Patients who cannot or will not accept their limitations and modify their lives accordingly do more poorly than those who are able to do so. Arthritis does not need to be a "hopeless" disease; however, if treatment is delayed or avoided it typically progressively worsens. A relatively small number of persons with rheumatoid arthritis (10 to 15 per cent) are completely incapacitated, i.e., confined to a bed or wheelchair, in spite of treatment.

Treatment. Rheumatoid arthritis is usually best treated by a conservative approach, e.g., with salicylates, rest, and physical therapy. Some patients are treated initially with a period of hospitalization. An important part of a successful treatment program involves *teaching* the patient about the nature of the illness and about the best methods of treatment. Victims of arthritis often tend to try "quack" cures in hopes of obtaining relief. Patients who do not understand the nature of rheumatoid arthritis are especially vulnerable to claims made by manufacturers of "quack remedies." According to the Arthritis Foundation, more than $400,000,000 per year is spent by arthritics on worthless or harmful treatments, devices, or "cures."

Early, active therapy before the establishment of fibrosis or bony ankylosis is most successful. *Treatment goals* include preservation of function, reduction of pain and inflammation, and prevention or correction of deformities. It is desirable if the patient with rheumatoid arthritis can be seen by both a rheumatologist and an orthopedic surgeon. Preventive surgery can be highly beneficial when performed in earlier stages of the disease.

Treatment-rehabilitation programs are individually prescribed in the treatment of rheumatoid arthritis. Because rheumatoid arthritis is a chronic disorder, the patient requires long-term medical supervision. Prescriptions are changed from time to time as the patient's condition varies. In addition to receiving prescriptions for medications, the patient should be given *written* prescriptions concerning rest and activity (e.g., exercises).

The central figures in any treatment-rehabilitation program are the patient and significant others. Accurate advice about self-help activities is important. For example, exercises should be supervised until it is clear that the patient can correctly perform them without causing additional trauma to involved joints. The patient must also be able to take medications as ordered and to use applications of heat or cold therapeutically if ordered. The importance of exercising, taking medications, resting, and performing other aspects of treatment on a *regular* basis, as advised by the physician, is emphasized during *patient-family education* sessions. The patient needs to be familiar with reportable side effects of prescribed medications.

Patient education should include discussion of factors which will not be curative so the person will not waste money and energy on ineffective "quack" cures (e.g., tonics, diets, vibrators). Also, the patient should be informed of local assistance programs which may be of help. For example, the American Arthritis Foundation provides clinical research and treatment centers, information services, group physical/hydrotherapy programs, home living assistance programs, and a limited number of patient care grants.

A nurse working in the community can help a patient plan modifications in activities and home environment which make it easier to perform activities of daily living. Physical therapists have many helpful suggestions about work simplification techniques. Social workers can help the patient meet problems created by reduced income and high medical expenses. Psychiatric and religious counseling may be of benefit. A person who develops rheumatoid arthritis may well need considerable support while adjusting to the chronicity and disabilities of the illness.

While some persons with rheumatoid arthritis find it necessary to change their type of employment, many are able to continue their jobs. Those individuals living in the United States who need to make job changes may be helped by the State Department of Vocational Rehabilitation if vocational retraining is needed.

Significant others need to be included in the treatment-rehabilitation program so they understand the nature of a patient's illness and so they can participate in the person's care. Both the patient and significant others should understand that much disability and deformity can be prevented with vigorous, early therapy and adherence to prescribed treatment programs.

In the following discussion, methods of treatment are divided into six sections:

- ▶ Rest
- ▶ Activity
- ▶ Heat and cold
- ▶ Diet
- ▶ Medications
- ▶ Surgery

Rest. Both systemic and emotional rest are part of the basic treatment of people experiencing rheumatoid arthritis. It is important to remember that rheumatoid arthritis is not merely a disorder of the joints, but rather it is a systemic disease. It is equally important to remember that illnesses must be approached as somatopsychic disorders (see Unit IV).

The amount of *systemic rest* necessary varies, depending upon the severity of the patient's disease at any given time. With extensive systemic and articular involvement, complete bedrest is indicated. Complete bedrest is anti-inflammatory. As a general rule, the more acute the disease or the greater the number of joints involved, the greater is the benefit of bedrest. With mild rheumatoid arthritis, 2 to 4 hours of rest daily (in addition, of course, to the usual amount of rest at night) may be adequate. Commonly the prescribed amount of rest is continued until the patient has maintained a level of significant improvement for at least 2 weeks. The physician may then modify the prescription.

In order for *bedrest* to be effective, the bed must be firm and the patient must be correctly positioned to prevent deformities (foot drop, fixation of the joints in extension, flexion contractures). Foot boards, splints, sandbags, and other devices are used to maintain proper body alignment.

The patient with rheumatoid arthritis should not be positioned in such a manner that hip and knee flexion contractures are encouraged. For example, pillows should not be placed under the knees, and the patient should not be permitted to remain for long periods of time with head and knee rests elevated. Frequent position changes are important. To prevent hip flexion contractures at least 2 to 3 times per day the patient should lie prone for a half hour. To prevent flexion deformities of the neck, the patient should be advised to use only a small pillow beneath the head if required at all.

During periods of bedrest the patient should be positioned flat on the back much of the time with affected joints in positions of extension. Extension is important to combat the joints' tendencies to be pulled into flexion contractures. Only a small pillow or folded towel should be under the patient's head. A small pillow may be placed under the ankles to straighten the knees. The arms should be positioned (palms upward) with small pillows or folded towels under the elbows or wrists to maintain extension. Sandbags and trochanter rolls are used as necessary to maintain proper body alignment. This supine position should be maintained periodically for at least 10 hours each day while the patient is on complete bedrest. Because it is not the position of greatest comfort, the patient must be helped to realize the reasons for maintaining a position of extension.

Attention must be intensively directed at *preventing complications of immobility* when a patient's activities are reduced, e.g., during bedrest, and if the patient is confined to a wheelchair.

Emotional factors are of paramount importance in rheumatoid arthritis, although current thinking tends to place less emphasis than formerly on emotional factors in the basic etiology.[17] Once the disease is established, emotional problems can trigger exacerbations. The patient requires emotional support from all persons involved in care and from significant others. The physician attempts to help the patient understand the importance of *emotional rest.* It is helpful to evaluate the patient's emotional reactions to diagnosis and illness. It is also necessary to try to understand a given patient's personality. Nurses offering care during a person's hospitalization can provide significant insights into these factors because of the length of time they may spend with the patient. Additionally, persons working with the patient at home (visiting nurse, or visiting occupational or physical therapist) can evaluate the home situation and family relationships and offer appropriate assistance.

Providing *rest for joints* involved with rheumatoid arthritis helps reduce articular inflammation. Weight-bearing joints may be rested by complete bed rest. *Splints* may also be applied to more completely rest inflamed joints. Splints also relieve pain (by relieving spasm) and prevent or reduce deformities. For example, a posterior knee extension splint not only keeps the knees in full extension but also properly positions the ankles. Plaster is the least expensive material for making these splints. Plastic materials of various sorts (e.g., Plastazote) are easier to use for making small splints, e.g., for the hands and wrists. Some physicians use dynamic splinting (see Fig. 78–4), with rubber bands and springs, in an attempt to reduce deformity and increase function. Splints commonly require frequent periodic adjustments to keep them fitting comfortably (they must not damage the skin) and effectively.

Splints must be removable for exercises and other treatments, such as heat applications. To prevent fibrous ankylosis the joints are periodically exercised; for example, splinted joints may be carried through a full range of motion once or twice daily. With improvement, some patients require splints only at night or perhaps not at all for a while.

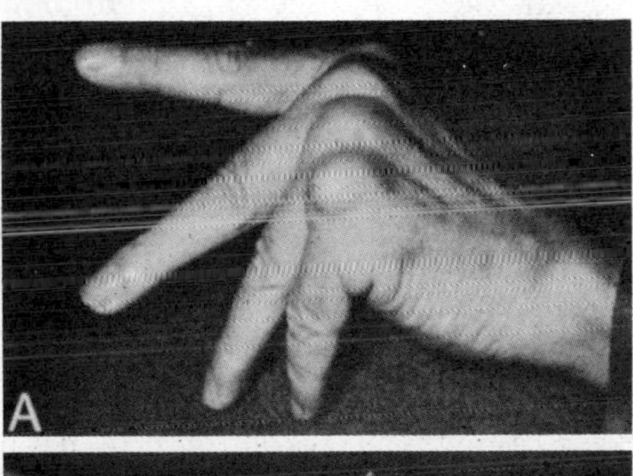

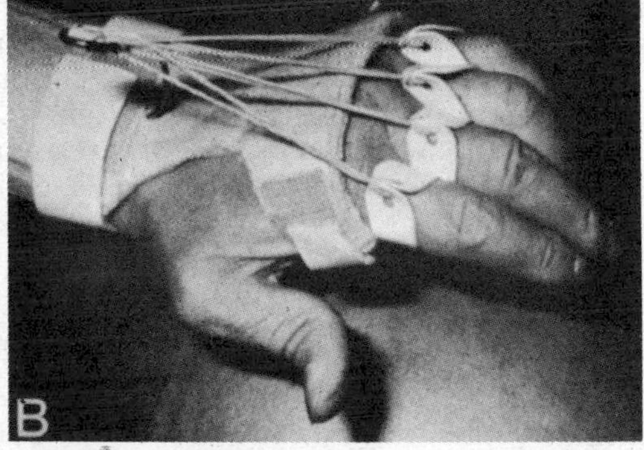

Figure 78–4. Dynamic splints are useful in both the preoperative and postoperative care of the rheumatoid hand. **A,** Patient with loss of active finger extension secondary to displacement of extensor tendons. **B,** Note improved postoperative posture of hand with dynamic splint. (From Nalebuff, E. A.: Metacarpophalangeal surgery in rheumatoid arthritis. *Surgical Clinics of North America,* 49:796, 1969.)

Activity. Prescribed amounts of activity help the patient with rheumatoid arthritis to attain and maintain optimum levels of function and independence. Activity also helps the patient to feel more comfortable mentally.

People with chronic illnesses often tend to think more about their bodies than they would if they were well. While paying attention to physical needs can be helpful during illness, excessive preocupation with themselves can be unhealthy. Becoming involved in interests and activities such as self-care and occupational therapy can be helpful for the patient. The physician should be informed if a patient shows a sustained tendency toward excessive self-preoccupation. Psychiatric counseling may help relieve anxieties.

Acutely inflamed joints are extremely painful when moved. Patients are thus often reluctant to move even though they may know that they require some activity. *Occupational therapy* provides an excellent means of encouraging purposeful movements and makes "exercising" seem less burdensome.

Encourage *self-care* and activity as permitted by the physician. Do not attempt to rush or hurry patients. Remember they may be experiencing pain with every movement and their joints may be stiff and difficult to move.

Physical Therapy. This is important in the treatment of rheumatoid arthritis[183] because it prevents and corrects deformities, controls pain, strengthens weakened muscles, and improves function. Deformities are prevented and corrected by a vigorous positioning program and an active exercise program. Knee and elbow deformities are sometimes corrected by progressive casting. Pain is controlled by teaching patients methods of regulating activities in ways which will not increase pain. Psychologic support is often necessary to help patients continue with treatment programs in spite of some pain. Isometric exercises and progressive resistance methods of isotonic strengthening exercises against maximal force are employed to strengthen weakened muscles. Function is improved by identifying individual patient needs and helping each person to learn more effective methods of daily living.[183] A variety of *self-care appliances* are available to help people experiencing rheumatoid arthritis maintain a maximum level of independence. These include such things as eating utensils with special handles, long-handled "reachers" and combs, specially elevated chairs and toilet seats, and so forth.

Continuous immobilization can cause increasing pain in the patient with rheumatoid arthritis. Exercise (moving the painful joints) can actually relieve pain. This important fact should be emphasized to the patient. Often patients hesitate to move because they fear that movement will intensify pain. It may be helpful to take aspirin ½ hour before exercising, provided the person does not overexercise because aspirin raises the pain threashold.

Isometric exercises are important in maintaining muscle function even when splints are applied. When there is only slight joint activity, *isotonic* exercises are best performed. *Exercises are the most important single part of the physical therapy program* for a patient with rheumatoid arthritis. Rest and therapeutic exercise must always be kept in proper balance. Because fatigue is a common symptom, the patient's tolerance to exercise must be carefully evaluated. Overactivity can inflame affected joints. Exercises should be performed within the limits of pain tolerance. Some specific exercises which the physician may instruct the patient to learn are illustrated in the booklet "Home Care Programs in Arthritis."[9] Deep breathing exercises are also helpful to the patient with rheumatoid arthritis. These are discussed in Unit XVI.

During exercises the patient may experience some pain which persists for a short time. This is not unusual; however, pain which lasts for several hours following exercises may indicate that the exercises are excessive and need to be modified. The patient's reaction to exercises is carefully evaluated, as mentioned, and increased pain or excessive fatigue is reported.

Knapp[144] observes that resistance exercises to strengthen finger flexors (e.g., squeezing a rubber ball) should not be prescribed for persons with rheumatoid arthritis, since these exercises only increase the deformities commonly found in arthritic hands, e.g., ulnar drift of the fingers.

When correctly performed, *massage* may help relieve pain and muscle aching. Joints which are actively inflamed should *not* be massaged, because massage may aggravate inflammation. Patients should be told this because they may have a tendency to "rub" inflamed, aching joints. Massage should be given over surrounding muscles, not over the joints. Most significant others cannot be taught to skillfully perform massage so, if massage is necessary to relieve pain, it is best performed by a skilled physical therapist.

Emphasize the importance of *proper posture.* Teach patients to look at their posture in a mirror and to make conscious attempts to sit and stand erect, to "think good posture." Use illustrations of correct and incorrect posture when teaching patients.

When the patient begins *ambulation,* care is taken to avoid aggravation of flexion deformities by weight-bearing. Until these contractures are corrected, the patient may require supports (crutches, braces) during ambulation. Supportive shoes are of importance when the patient is out of bed. Properly fitted shoes help support the feet and also make ambulation safer. Some patients require corrective shoes or molded shoes. The patient with arthritis should not be permitted to wear soft slippers while out of bed.

The arthritic person with involvement of the hips or knees or both is most comfortable when sitting on a straight-backed armchair which is elevated 3 to 4 inches more than ordinary chairs. This added height prevents excessive hip and knee flexion and makes it easier for the patient to get up and down. Similarly, elevation of the toilet seat may also help the patient to get up and down more easily. "Grab bars" placed on or beside the toilet provide additional help. It is also best if the patient's bed is somewhat raised. For example, if the patient must transfer from bed to a wheelchair the bed should be elevated to the height of the wheelchair.

It is not unusual for a person with arthritis to find that knees become stiff after sitting for a while. Instruct the person to flex and extend the knees several times before trying to stand up. This "limbering up" will help the patient to arise more easily and to feel steadier when doing so. Similar periodic flexions and extension of the knees while seated may make prolonged periods of sitting more comfortable.

Heat and Cold. Applications of heat are frequently used in the treatment of rheumatoid arthritis. *Heat applications* have an analgesic effect and help relax muscles. Heat may also relieve joint stiffness and swelling. Exercises can usually be performed more effectively if preceded by the application of heat. Various forms of heat therapy may be used: moist heat, dry heat, diathermy, ultrasound.

Whirlpool baths are quite effective. They permit active exercising in the bath with minimal resistance. Home models are available (e.g., Jacuzzi or Vibrabath) and may be useful when prolonged treatment is indicated. Hot packs and warm tub baths or showers are commonly used methods of applying heat in the treatment of rheumatoid arthritis. Hot towels can be wrung out and wrapped around painful knees.

The physician may advise some patients to use *dry heat* from an electric heating pad, hot water bottle, or infrared heat lamp. Infrared radiation is an effective method of applying heat therapeutically.

Some patients with rheumatoid arthritis obtain relief from *cold applications* (e.g., crushed ice packs) which induce local anesthesia. Regardless of the manner in which heat or cold is applied, the skin must be protected appropriately from possible trauma. (Details of the application of hot and cold treatments can be found in Sorensen and Luckmann: *Basic Nursing: A Psychophysiologic Approach.*)

Diet. No specific dietary measures have been identified which are effective in the treatment of rheumatoid arthritis. A well-balanced general diet is therefore usually indicated. If a patient is over-weight a weight-reducing diet may help to relieve joints from the need to support excessive amounts of weight. Also, the overweight patient is less likely to exercise effectively.

Medications. No medication is available which will cure rheumatoid arthritis. The patient should be informed that during the course of treatment the doctor may prescribe various medications. It is best when patient and physician work together to identify which medications are most effective in treating the patient's disease process. The patient needs to be informed of side effects which should be reported. Detailed descriptions of medications used with rheumatoid arthritis are presented in textbooks of pharmacology.

▶ *Aspirin or sodium salicylate.* Salicylates form the backbone of drug therapy in rheumatoid arthritis. These medications have analgesic and anti-inflammatory properties. Additionally they are relatively safe and inexpensive. Aspirin is available in various forms: plain tablet, soluble tablet, enteric-coated (Enseal or Ecotrin), with buffer added, and as a suppository. Commonly the patient is allowed to take the type which he or she considers most helpful.

Aspirin should be taken with food because of its possible irritating effects on the stomach. Aspirin may be prescribed after meals with an antacid, or with milk. Usually the medication is prescribed (in writing) in doses sufficient to produce mild symptoms of drug intoxication, e.g., reduced hearing, tinnitus, or gastrointestinal upset. Once those symptoms are produced, the dose may then be reduced slightly. The physician works closely with the patient in an attempt to get the patient to take as much aspirin as can be tolerated. Toxic doses in elderly patients produce acidosis with ataxia and slurred speech. When toxic doses are suspected, a serum salicylate level is obtained.

▶ *Indomethacin (Indocin).* This is an analgesic, anti-inflammatory medication which may be helpful although it appears to be no more effective in treating rheumatoid arthritis than the salicylates. Its efficacy is believed to be similar to that of phenylbutazone. Numerous untoward effects may occur with indomethacin, e.g., headache, nausea, vomiting, anorexia, peptic ulcer, abdominal pain, diarrhea, depression, giddiness, mental confusion, psychosis. Possibly this medication is less toxic than the butazones. Indomethacin shows some antipyretic activity. If gastrointestinal bleeding occurs, medication must be stopped. Patients with significant central nervous system symptoms should be warned not to engage in hazardous occupations or drive. Indomethacin should be taken with food.

▶ *Phenylbutazone (Butazolidin) and oxyphenbutazone (Tandearil).* These drugs have anti-inflammatory and analgesic properties but are not used as major drugs in treating rheumatoid arthritis because of their serious toxic effects and because their usefulness in treating this disorder appears limited. Toxic effects include peptic ulcer, agranulocytosis (bone marrow depression), dermatitis, stomatitis, and sodium and water retention. Weekly white blood counts and hemoglobin determinations are made for the first few months and thereafter at monthly intervals. The patient is advised to stop taking the medication and see the physician if symptoms such as sore throat, melena (darkening of the feces due to blood pigments), or skin rash develop.

▶ *Pure analgesics.* These medications may be necessary (in addition to analgesic anti-inflammatory drugs) to control pain. Analgesics which may be prescribed include propoxyphene hydrochloride (Darvon); acetaminophen (Tylenol); and codeine. Narcotics are commonly not used because of addicting properties. (See Unit XI for discussion of pain.)

▶ *Gold compounds.* The mode of action of gold salts *(chrysotherapy)* in the treatment of rheumatoid arthritis is not known; however, they are used in treating selected patients. Commonly they are given with salicylates to patients who (a) are not favorably responding to conservative treatment; and/or (b) should not be given corticosteroids. Gold compounds are believed to be most effective when given early during the acute stage of rheumatoid arthritis; however, they may also be given to some patients with long-standing disease. Colloidal gold has proved to be ineffective; water-soluble gold compounds are used. Gold compounds do not produce a dramatic effect, but rather are slow acting. They are relatively safe if given cautiously with supervision. This form of treatment is contraindicated in patients with past or present renal or hepatic disease, acute systemic lupus erythematosus, blood dyscrasias, or drug allergies. Toxic reactions include dermatitis, purpura, stomatitis, agranulocytosis, bronchitis, hepatitis, aplastic anemia, nephritis, photosensitization, and nitroid reaction, i.e., acute sensitivity reaction similar to that which can occur after the ingestion of nitroglycerin (flushing, dizziness, sweating, weakness, nausea, vomiting, syncope). Medication is stopped if any of these symptoms appear. The patient should be warned against exposure to strong light, and the skin and mucous membranes should be inspected (before each injection) for dermatitis or purpura. The urine is examined for protein and microscopic hematuria, and every two weeks evaluations are made of the WBC, hemoglobin, and differential white count. If indicated, the physician also orders liver function tests or platelet counts.

Aqueous preparations of gold compounds used in treating rheumatoid arthritis are gold sodium thiomalate (Myochrysine) and gold sodium thiosulfate. Myochrysine is most commonly used and is given intramuscularly at weekly intervals.

▶ *Antimalarials.* Chloroquine (Aralen) and hydroxychloroquine (Plaquenil) are antimalarials sometimes used in treating rheumatoid arthritis. Like gold compounds, these medications are slow acting. Antimalarials can be administered orally, but many physicians believe their toxic effects outweigh possible beneficial effects. Accumulations of these agents in pigmented tissues, particularly the eye, may produce partial or complete loss of vision. When antimalarials are used, the patient should have ophthalmologic examinations 3 or 4 times a year to detect early retinopathy. If detected early, ocular damage is usually reversible. However, some patients have developed irreversible retinal degeneration. Other possible toxic reactions are blanching of hair, nausea, vomiting, rash, leukopenia, and toxic psychosis.

▶ *Adrenocorticosteroids.* These anti-inflammatory medications are important in the treatment of rheumatoid arthritis, but are not a substitute for other forms of comprehensive treatment. Adrenocorticosteroids do not change the natural progression of the disease, even though they often produce dramatic and immediate symptomatic relief. Examples of these medications are cortisone, prednisone, hydrocortisone, prednisolone, triamcinolone, methylprednisolone, and dexamethasone. Side effects of adrenocorticosteroids can worsen some features of rheumatoid arthritis. Prolonged usage can create toxic side effects which are more problematic to treat than the rheumatoid arthritis. Severe rebound phenomena may follow withdrawal of these drugs.

Adrenocorticosteroids may be given after a thorough, sometimes prolonged evaluation of less hazardous medications. They may then be prescribed for patients (a) who should not be given gold compounds; and/or (b) have active progressive disease which has not favorably responded to conservative treatment. The medication is given in the smallest amount that will permit functional improvement. Efforts are made after several weeks to reduce the dose. Morning stiffness may be relieved by giving prednisone orally at bedtime.

Adrenocorticosteroid dosage must be increased during major stressful situations, e.g., surgery. Patients should, therefore, carry a card which states that they are receiving steroid therapy. Such a card will advise medical personnel of the person's condition if ever emergency treatment is required.

- ▶ *Intra-articular injections of corticosteroids* are helpful in temporarily suppressing inflammation in specific joints. These treatments are most effective with acute inflammations of smaller joints. Fluid is removed from the joint prior to injecting the medication. If there is suspicion that a joint is infected, corticosteroids are never injected. Frequent injections cannot safely be made into the same joint because of the possible development of a Charcot joint-like syndrome. Prior to injection the site is sprayed with ethyl chloride or is injected with lidocaine (Xylocaine). Hydrocortisone has commonly been used for intra-articular injections, although longer-acting intra-articular steroids are available. Some long-acting preparations may suppress inflammation for as long as 12 months.
- ▶ Recently some *proprionic acid derivative drugs* are being used. These include ibuprofen (Motrin), naproxen (Naprosyn) and fenoprofen (Nalfon). All these drugs inhibit prostaglandins and thus are similar to aspirin, but they are better than aspirin because less gastric ulceration and bleeding is noted. (It is not known however, whether this advantage will continue with long-term usage.)[67]
- ▶ *Cytotoxic agents,* e.g., cyclophosphamide (Cytoxan), are also being used in the treatment of rheumatoid arthritis for people who do not respond to conventional therapies. These medications may be highly toxic, producing gastrointestinal disturbances, alopecia, bone marrow suppression, blood dyscrasias, dermatitis, and oral lesions. They should not be used for children or women of childbearing age. (See also Unit IX.)[30]
- ▶ *Immunosuppressive drugs* are also being used in a limited way for people who do not respond to conventional therapies. An example is azathioprine (Imuran). These drugs are also highly toxic, producing the same side effects described above for cytotoxic agents. They should not be used for children or women of childbearing age. CBC and urine should be monitored weekly. (See also Unit V, Chapter 11.)[30]
- ▶ An *investigative drug, penicillamine* (Cuprimine), is being tried. It appears to reduce the activity of the disease although the mechanism is unknown. It may produce blood dyscraias or glomerulonephropathy. It should be given before meals when the patient has an empty stomach.[30]

Surgery. Many excellent surgical procedures can be implemented to correct ankylosed and deformed joints. (See pp. 1714–1719.)

Osteoarthritis

Osteoarthritis is also known as *degenerative* or *senescent arthritis.* This is a common disorder of unknown etiology. Predisposing factors appear to include aging, joint trauma, and obesity. Women are affected more often than men. Osteoarthritis may first appear in women at the time of menopause, or symptoms may be markedly accentuated at this time if they have previously been present. Certain forms appear to be familial. Older persons are most commonly affected. The weight-bearing joints and terminal interphalangeal joints of the fingers are characteristically involved. Almost all persons over age 45 have some form of osteoarthritis. It is, therefore, the most common joint disorder.

Figure 78–5 illustrates the progression of joint abnormalities in osteoarthritis. The process is initiated by loss of matrix components from the cartilage. Erosion of the cartilage follows. A proliferative response at the joint margins then produces an outgrowth of cartilage and bone. These outgrowths are called *osteophytes* or *spurs.* The earliest and more severe degenerative changes most typically appear in the spine and weight-bearing joints of the lower extremities. Characteristic hypertrophic spurs cause swellings called *Heberden's nodes* in the terminal interphalangeal finger joints.

Unlike rheumatoid arthritis, osteoarthritis is *not* a systemic disease, but rather a local joint disorder. Also, osteoarthritis is not deforming and is not crippling unless the hip joint is involved. It is important that patients understand which type of arthritis they have.

The patient with osteoarthritis usually does not appear ill and is commonly obese. *Symptoms* usually do not appear before age 40 unless involved joints have been subjected to trauma. Commonly the onset is insidious and gradual Aching pain is the most common symptom.

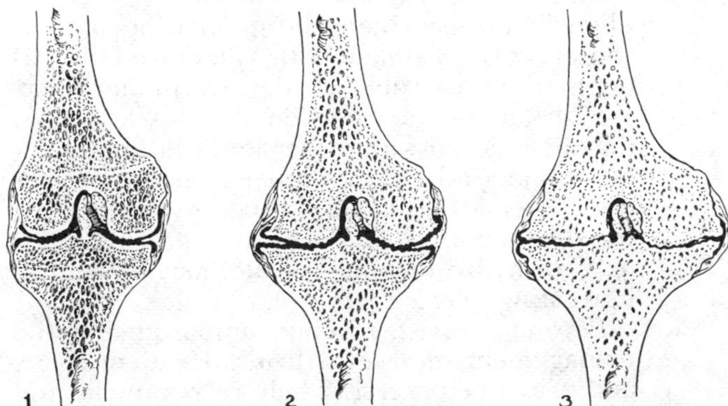

Figure 78–5. Progression of the joint abnormalities in osteoarthritis. (1) Early degenerative changes in cartilage. (2) More extensive cartilage degeneration and early hypertrophic changes of bone at joint edges. (3) Late stage with almost complete destruction of articular cartilages, irregular subchondral bone surfaces, underlying eburnated bone, and extensive hypertrophic spur formation at margins of the joint. (From Sodeman, W. A., and Sodeman, W. A., Jr.: *Pathologic Physiology: Mechanisms of Disease,* 5th ed. Philadelphia: W. B. Saunders Co., 1974.)

Other symptoms are limitation of motion or contractures, and muscle spasm. Unlike rheumatoid arthritis, pain is most pronounced after exercise. Pain may occur with use; however, night pain and morning stiffness may also occur. Constitutional symptoms do not occur. Flexion contraction of the hip and loss of ability to extend the knee may be disabling symptoms. Pain at rest may be caused by muscle spasm. The severity of symptoms and the degree of degenerative joint changes are often not correlated. Therefore a patient with minor degenerative changes may be quite uncomfortable, while a patient with advanced changes may have few or no symptoms. Affected joints may appear normal but may be locally tender. Creaking, grating, and crepitus are often detectable in osteoarthritic joints. Occasionally bony enlargement is prominent. Ankylosis does not occur; however, limitation of motion is common.

X-ray abnormalities are commonly apparent, but laboratory findings indicative of inflammation are absent, e.g., the erythrocyte sedimentation rate is normal.

Osteoarthritis progresses slowly; therefore, even though there is no "cure" for this disorder, joint function may be maintained more effectively than with other types of arthritis. Treatments such as weight reduction, medications, physical therapy, and orthopedic procedures may completely relieve the discomforts of osteoarthritis for some patients.

Weight reduction relieves the strain on affected joints (weight-bearing joints) in obese patients. Acetylsalicylic acid (aspirin) is the most effective *medication.* Indomethacin (Indocin) or phenylbutazone (Butazolidin) may be used if conservative treatment with salicylates fails. Patients who are unable to take aspirin may tolerate acetaminophen (Tylenol). Muscle spasm may be relieved with diazepam (Valium), methocarbamol (Robaxin), or other such antispasmotics. Systemic corticosteroid therapy is not given for osteoarthritis, but intra-articular injections (e.g., of hydrocortisone acetate) may be helpful in treating selected joints (e.g., knee).

Physical therapy is of major importance in the management of osteoarthritis. Heat, massage, and prescribed exercises help relax muscles and relieve aching and stiffness. Moist heat tends to be more effective than dry. Sometimes involved extremities are splinted. Overactivity must be avoided. Good posture is stressed. Pain in the hands may be relieved by contrast baths, e.g., the hands are submerged in warm water for 4 minutes, then in cold water for 1 minute. The process is repeated for 15 minutes two or three times daily. Nerve root pressure in the neck may be relieved by a cervical collar or traction. Progression of osteoarthritis may be delayed by minimizing use of involved joints; however, total rest produces muscle atrophy and must be avoided.

Surgical Treatment of Arthritis

Surgical procedures are becoming more important as part of the treatment-rehabilitation programs for people experiencing arthritis. A variety of different procedures may be performed to relieve general symptoms (e.g., pain), improve function, and correct deformities. Not too many years ago surgery was used only late in the course of arthritis, after severe joint destruction or deformity had developed. Preventive surgery (e.g., to prevent deformities) is now used during early phases of treatment. Surgery may be performed when there is active arthritis. (Orthopedic surgery was discussed generally in Chapter 76 of this unit.)

Among the numerous types of surgical procedures which may be used in the treatment of arthritis are tendon transfers and osteotomy. (See definitions in Chapter 76.) *Tendon transfers* can prevent progressive deformity which would be caused by muscle spasm. Nodules or bony tumors (exostoses) may be surgically removed, and established flexion contractures may be surgically relieved. *Osteotomy* may improve the function of deformed joints or limbs. For example, osteotomy of the femoral neck may give symptomatic relief by changing the position of the head of the femur (when it is being subjected to impact stress against the acetabulum). Femoral osteotomy performed for rheumatoid arthritis of the hip has been less successful than with osteoarthritis. With rheumatoid arthritis the femoral head frequently collapses.[221]

Synovectomy (e.g., of the elbows, wrists, fingers, knees) has proved of value in treating rheumatoid arthritis by helping to maintain joint function. Early surgical removal of the synovium helps prevent recurrent inflammation. With rheumatoid arthritis, joint destruction begins in the synovial tissue and then proceeds to involve bone, cartilage, and other structures.

Surgical correction of problems due to osteoarthritis may reduce abnormal stresses within joints and delay the progression of early disease. Joint instability or malalignment may be corrected, or loose bodies or torn cartilages may be removed. Persons with advanced joint destruction and intractable pain may benefit greatly from surgical procedures such as *arthrodesis* or *arthroplasty* (with or without replacement of joint parts with prostheses). The development of effective, nontoxic adhesive substances has made new arthroplasty and prosthetic replacement procedures possible. Instead of partial joint replacements, "total hip" and "total knee" joint replacements are being performed on selected patients. Arthrodesis (fusion) sacrifices function of the joint but relieves pain in severely damaged joints. Some patients are treated by fusion of the hip, knee, or other joints. Fusion may be performed on the wrists to fix the affected part in a functional position so it can be used more effectively. Some patients (with arthritic involvement of the hip) who cannot withstand extensive surgery are benefited by cutting of the muscles that move the hip joint. This "hanging hip" procedure maintains reasonable function while providing symptomatic relief.

Numerous silicone rubber implants have been developed for use in reconstructive surgery of the extremities in treating deformed hands and feet. Such implants are used to replace finger joints and the great toe, ranging up to implants to replace joints as large as the shoulder joint.

Arthroplasties of the hip and knee have been selected for further discussion because these procedures are gaining increasing importance and require comprehensive nursing care.

Following surgery on joints or bones, orders given for postoperative positioning and exercises must be precisely followed.

Hip Arthroplasty. A severely involved arthritic hip can be the most disabling joint disorder for a person to experience. Severe hip pain can interfere with sleep, prevent walking, produce narcotic addiction, and impair or totally prevent sexual function. The most common resultant hip deformity is that of adduction and flexion which, in turn, produces or worsens deformity of the knee.[45] As indicated previously, disabling osteoarthritis of the hip may be surgically treated by major procedures such as arthrodesis (fusion) or arthroplasty. Arthrodesis of the hip is contraindicated with rheumatoid arthritis because (a) the disease is generalized, and (b) often the other hip becomes involved. Arthroplasty may be performed for rheumatoid arthritis or osteoarthritis to relieve pain and restore joint motion.

Two types of arthroplasties of the hip can be performed: (1) *hemiarthroplasty,* in which only one joint component is replaced; and (2) *total hip replacement,* in which both components of the joint are surgically replaced. (Postoperative care following hip surgery was discussed in detail in the section on fractures of the femur, Chapter 77.)

Hemiarthroplasty. Hemiarthroplasty may be performed not only to treat arthritic joints but also in the early stages of necrosis of the head of the femur or in the presence of post-traumatic pseudarthrosis of the femoral neck. Either the head of the femur or the acetabulum may be separately replaced. *Replacement of the head of the femur* with a metal prosthesis has been discussed in Chapter 77.

Another technique involves *remodeling the head of the femur and the acetabulum* and positioning a movable metal (Vitallium) cup between them. During surgery, ankylosed spongy bone is removed. The interposition of the metal between the newly shaped joint surfaces prevents ankylosis of the joint. Postoperatively, following *cup (mold) arthroplasty,* the patient is often placed in suspension traction to maintain abduction. (Suspension traction was discussed in Chapter 76.) Abduction and internal rotation of the operated leg are important following cup arthroplasty because they help maintain the head of the femur and the cup in the acetabulum. Continuous abduction may be necessary for about 6 weeks. (When the head of the femur is replaced with a prosthesis, continued abduction is usually necessary for only 3 weeks.)[137]

Permitting the operated leg to move into adduction before adequate healing has occurred can ruin the arthroplasty.

Total Hip Replacement. Cup arthroplasty is being rapidly replaced by total hip arthroplasty in the treatment of rheumatoid arthritis and osteoarthritis (except in treating very young patients). Total hip replacements are typically used if the destructive process involves both the acetabulum and femoral head. Bilateral surgery may be performed during the same procedure or several weeks apart. Infection is a contraindication to total hip replacement.

With total hip arthroplasty the femoral head and acetabulum are both replaced by prostheses (see Fig. 78–6.) The prostheses are cemented into the bone with a plastic cement called methyl methacrylate. Total hip replacements were widely used in Great Britain and Canada but were slower in coming into use in the United States because the use of acrylic bone cement was restricted by the Food and Drug Administration (FDA).

Several different total hip prostheses are available, e.g., Charnley-Müller, Bechtol, McKee-Farrar, Ring, and Trapezoidal-28. Com-

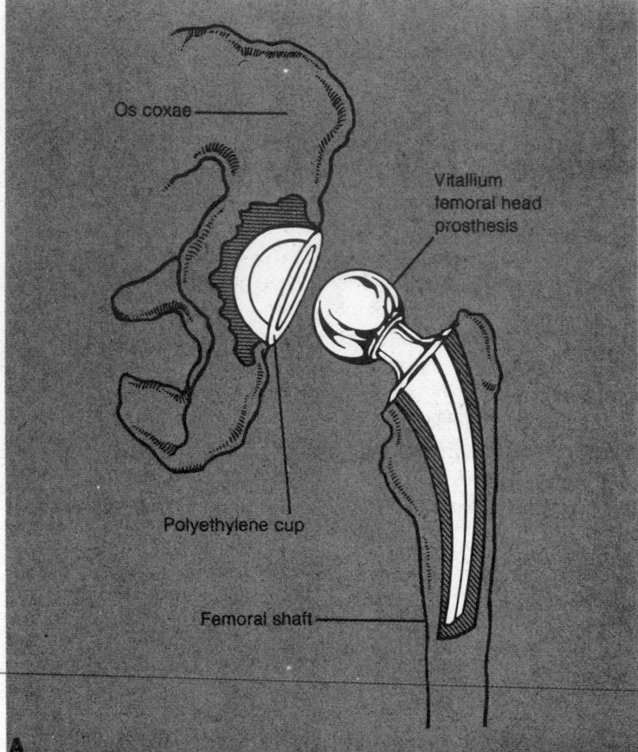

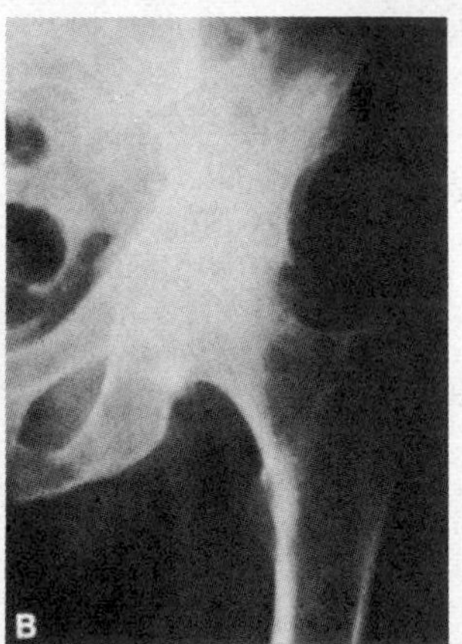

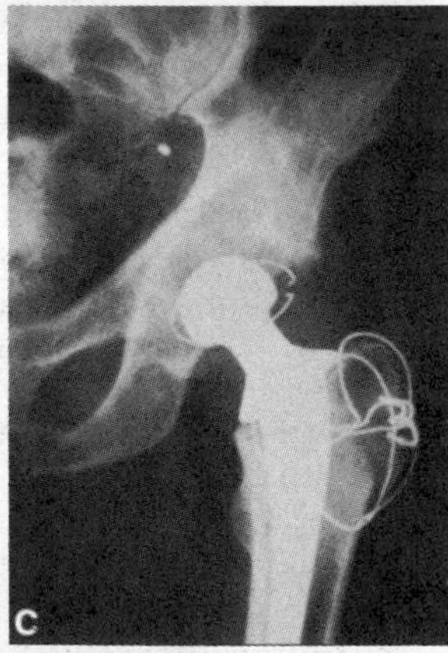

Figure 78–6. Total hip replacement has afforded a new lease on life to 90 per cent of all recipients, many of whom had been severely crippled by severe arthritis. **A,** prosthetic components; **B,** X-ray film before implantation; **C,** after. (From Testa, N. N.: Surgery for arthritis: What can — and cannot — be done. *Consultant,* 18:142. Nov. 1978.)

monly the acetabulum is implanted first during the operative procedure. The location and degree of angulation of this part of the prosthesis are precisely determined, since these factors decide the position of the femoral head and neck piece. The acetabular prosthesis may be made of high-density polyethylene plastic, while the femoral prosthesis is made of metal, usually stainless steel. The bone cement has been used for many years as a dental filling material now evolving for use in orthopedics. Bone cement is not an adhesive or glue, but instead acts as a filler, filling in all the tiny irregularities in the prepared surfaces of the bone. The cement thus securely locks the parts of the prosthesis in place.

Preoperative teaching is highly important when total hip replacement is to be performed. During this time of preoperative education, patients are told that they may need to remain on the back for several days. Also, they are taught how to correctly use a trapeze to lift up for back care during the period of recumbency. The operative procedure and its goals are discussed, and patients are taught exercises they will do postoperatively, e.g., quadriceps-setting exercises, gluteal-setting exercises, and isometric hip extension and abduction exercises. Upper extremity strengthening exercises may also be taught, in preparation for crutch walking or use of a walker.

Postoperative care is discussed generally in Unit VIII and in Chapter 76 of this unit, and postoperative care following hip surgery is discussed in Chapter 77. Care of patients in casts or traction also is discussed in Chapter 76. The following discussion emphasizes only selected aspects of postoperative care which are important following total hip replacement. For detailed discussions of nursing care with these procedures, refer to Eyre[80] and Johnson and Convery.[130]

Postoperatively following total hip replacement the patient is usually placed immediately in bed, and Buck's extension or Russell's traction is applied (Chapter 76). During turning hip abduction *must* be maintained with pillows. Turning following hip surgery has been previously discussed.

Postoperatively the affected leg is maintained in an abducted position in straight alignment while the patient is recumbent. The surgeon may order the patient to wear support hose or the legs to be wrapped with Ace bandages to prevent thrombosis. A hip spica dressing may be applied in the operating room to provide compression and help prevent tissue separation and hematoma formation. Hemovacs are usually in place in the wound immediately following surgery for wound drainage. Some surgeons routinely give antibiotics and dextran therapy. Many patients wear an abduction splint postoperatively and most of the newer splints can be adjusted for the amount of abduction desired.

Exercises, e.g., quadriceps-setting, are encouraged as ordered during the early postoperative period. Muscle strengthening, as of the gluteal muscles, helps prevent dislocation since muscular control replaces the function of the hip capsule. Dislocation of the prosthesis and infection are major possible complications during the early postoperative period. Indications of these complications are immediately reported.

With some procedures the greater trochanter (with the attachment of the abductor muscles) is transferred, e.g., moved distally on the femur to increase the efficiency of the abductor mechanism. When such a transfer is made the greater trochanter is usually held in its new position by wires. The transfer must be protected until it heals in place (e.g., 4 to 6 weeks). In this situation, progressive abduction exercises are limited by the transfer. Excessive exercise may cause nonunion or fracture of the osteotomy site. *The surgeon's orders concerning movement and positioning must be precisely followed.*

Patients were kept flat for several days following total hip replacement a few years ago, but now most patients are carefully ambulated at the bedside the second or third postoperative day. This may be nothing more than standing at the bedside briefly or being assisted to a chair, using care not to excessively flex the hip joint beyond the limits set by the physician, and maintaining abduction of the legs. During the time the patient is supine back care should be given every two hours. Back care is given while the patient turns gently or while the patient raises straight up on an overbed trapeze (if turning is prohibited). It is helpful if the patient lies on a sheepskin and wears sheepskin booties to protect the skin while supine.

Nerve function and circulation checks are made routinely the first day or so, then as frequently as the patient's condition warrants. Pink-tinged sputum may appear postoperatively and is believed to result from some part of the cement being excreted through pulmonary alveoli. This is not considered to be dangerous but should be noted in charting.

Position checks are made frequently while the patient is in bed. External rotation of the leg needs to be prevented. Progressive ambulation follows, e.g., use of parallel bars, crutches or walker, and finally a cane. The surgeon may recommend partial weight-bearing initially or may permit full weight-bearing on the operated leg.

Physical therapy may be started on the fifth or sixth postoperative day. In addition to helping the patient ambulate, physical therapy may include Hubbard baths, use of powder boards, and gentle, active, assisted range-of-motion exercises in sling suspension (within the pain-free range). Until discharge, the patient continues to work on exercises that increase range of motion and muscle strengthening of the hip.

On the fifth or sixth postoperative day, the physician may order the patient to lie prone twice a day for 20 to 30 minutes to prevent hip flexion contractures. This practice may be continued at home after discharge.

The total period of hospitalization for total hip replacement varies from 7 to 10 days or may extend up to 3 weeks depending on the patient's progress. The patient is often discharged with the assistance of only a light cane while walking. Total hip replacement produces dramatic results. Patients are commonly surprised to find their pain relieved and movement increased so markedly and rapidly.

Prior to discharge patients should be given written instructions for home care, including detailed exercise prescriptions and activity limitations. Patients may be advised to continue to place a pillow between the knees (while lying down) for several weeks, to prevent adduction while turning. They may be advised never to sit for longer than one hour continuously; they should stand, stretch, and take a few steps periodically to prevent hip flexion contractures. Hip flexion should not exceed 90° or the operated hip may dislocate. Therefore, patients must learn to put on shoes and stockings without acutely flexing. Additionally they should sit in a straight chair with a straight back and use a raised toilet seat. Rocking or reclining chairs and low toilet seats are contraindicated following total hip replacement because they put the patient in an awkward position usually requiring more than 90° of hip flexion to get out of these chairs/positions. Bicycle exercises may be used to supplement the home program once the patient has gained adequate hip flexion range.

Additional instructions which the physician may give at the time of discharge may include the following: (a) avoid crossing the legs for 3 months; (b) continue to wear support hose for 6 weeks following surgery; and (c) sexual activity and driving may be resumed in 6 weeks. Extremes of flexion, adduction, and internal rotation must be permanently avoided.

Knee Arthroplasty. Like the hip joint, the knee joint may be partially replaced *(hemiarthroplasty)* or totally replaced. Hemiarthroplasty may consist of the replacement of the femoral condyles or tibial plateau, using McKeever and MacIntosh prostheses. This discussion focuses on total knee replacement.

Total knee replacement has been under development for over 25 years (see Fig. 78–7). Over the years the design of the total knee prosthesis has undergone tremendous change. Two piece prostheses are common.

The recent use of methyl methacrylate (acrylic bone cement) in reconstruction of the knee has helped resolve many technical problems by making it possible to securely fix prosthetic components into bone tissue. Acrylic bone ce-

PATIENT-FAMILY TEACHING GUIDE FOR TOTAL HIP PATIENTS AT HOME

1. Don't try to force your hip into more than 90 degree flexion (this is a right angle). This increased motion may cause dislocation.
2. Don't cross your legs when lying, sitting or standing. Be particularly cautious of crossing your involved leg over the non-involved leg.
3. Don't sit on low stools, low chairs, low toilets; but rather, have them up high enough so that your hip doesn't bend more than 90 degrees. You may decide to purchase a raised toilet seat, or place an extra cushion or pillow in your favorite chair.
4. Don't sit on armless chairs. Chair arms are needed to aid in rising to a standing position.
5. Don't get up from a chair until you have first moved to the edge of the chair. Place your involved leg in front of your noninvolved leg, which should be well under the chair. Keep your involved leg in front while getting up.
6. Don't rotate (turn in or out) your hip, but keep it in a neutral straight position when you're sitting, when you're lying in bed, and when you're walking.
7. Don't lie on your "good" side without a pillow between your legs.
8. Don't try to put on your own shoes or stockings.
9. Don't pick up any objects from the floor or reach into lower cupboards or drawers.

Courtesy of Bellin Memorial Hospital, Green Bay, Wisconsin.

ment is now used during the implantation of numerous types of knee prostheses. Two such procedures are the geometric total knee arthroplasty and the polycentric total knee arthroplasty. In these procedures diseased arthritic surfaces of the femoral condyles and tibial plateaus are removed and replaced by durable prosthetic components that are firmly fixed to the bone. Once in place, the components permit simulation of normal knee motions.

Space does not permit detailed discussions of the various techniques of total knee replacement and the postoperative care necessary following each technique. The nurse is advised to consult specific postoperative orders carefully and clarify any questions with the surgeon. Discussed briefly below is postoperative care related to the Walldius knee hinge and the polycentric type total knee arthroplasty.

The Walldius knee hinge was designed for use without bone cement but now may be cemented into the medullary cavities of the femur and tibia. Originally the prosthesis was made of acrylic, but this proved to be not strong enough. The prosthesis was later modified in stainless steel and is now constructed of a cobalt-chrome alloy. *Postoperatively* Walldius uses a full-leg padded plaster cast with the knee in extension for 3 weeks. Then sutures are removed and exercises started. Once the patient can perform a straight leg raise, walking with full weight-bearing may begin.

Other surgeons using the Walldius prosthesis prefer changing plaster at two weeks (to remove sutures) and then applying a groin to ankle cast with the foot free. The patient is permitted weight-bearing at this time to combat osteoporosis. At the sixth week postoperatively the cast is split for exercises and discarded at 8 weeks. While some patients rapidly regain movement it may take others as long as 12 months to reach maximum range. *Physical therapy is highly important* in reconstructive surgery of the knee.

Possible postoperative *complications* include infection, fat embolism, peroneal nerve palsy, skin breakdown, medical complications, technical failure, synovial herniation, loosening of the prosthesis, and stress fracture.

Postoperative care following the *polycentric type of total knee arthroplasty* is essentially as follows:[51]

- A compression dressing immobilizes the knee in maximum extension immediately following surgery. On the third postoperative day the dressing is removed and a posterior plaster shell is applied for use during ambulation and as a resting splint at night.
- Re-education of the quadriceps muscles begins with isometric quadriceps-setting on the first postoperative day. As pain decreases and voluntary muscle control improves, exercising progresses to active straight leg raising. Both ankles are actively exercised to prevent thrombophlebitis.
- After the compression dressing is removed, gentle active assistive range-of-motion exercises are started and a progressive exercise program is continued until discharge to increase muscle strength and range of motion in the operated knee.
- Once the patient has 90° of knee flexion and good voluntary control of the quadriceps muscle (the person can actively straight-leg raise and initiate active knee extension against gravity), ambulation is started.
- A posterior splint may be used during early gait training, e.g., in parallel bars and on crutches. Weight-bearing on the operated leg may be permitted to tolerance or the point of pain.
- The patient is discharged with detailed instructions for a home exercise program.

Flexion contractures can develop with total knee replacement. To prevent this complication the knee is kept extended at all times while the patient is in bed. A trochanter roll is used in bed to prevent external rotation. Swelling can also be a problem; therefore the leg is usually kept elevated with a pillow under the ankle. This position also promotes full extension with the aid of gravity. Whirlpool baths may help the patient obtain adequate flexion and full extension of the knee.

Gouty Arthritis

Primary gout is a familial metabolic disorder of purine metabolism which results in abnormal amounts of urates in the body. Purines are products of the digestion of certain proteins. Inability to properly metabolize purines results in an excessive accumulation of uric acid in the blood's plasma (i.e., hyperuricemia). As a result of this, urate crystals may be precipitated and deposited throughout the body. These deposits of crystals then initiate local irritation and an inflammatory response. Hyperuricemia may result from[215] (a) increased production of urates caused by the abnormal metabolic degradation of purines; (b) a reduced excretion of urates; or (c) a combination of both of these factors. Hyperuricemia may occur without gout.

Acute attacks of gouty arthritis may accompany other disorders (e.g., disorders of the hematopoietic system such as polycythemia or leukemia). These attacks are called *secondary gout* and usually do not have tophi (see below) or a familial history of gout.

The main clinical problem with gout is arthritis. Early in the course of the illness, a recurring, acute arthritis occurs which is usually monarticular, i.e., involves one joint. Later a chronic, deforming arthritis develops. About 95 per cent of patients with gout are men over age 30. If gout develops in women it usually does so after the menopause.

Gout is characterized clinically by acute periodic episodes of pain, swelling, and inflammation in a joint. The joints of the foot (great toe, instep, or ankle) are most often affected; however, any joint may be involved. (See Figure 78–8.)

Histologically, gout is characterized by the formation of *tophi.* A tophus is a nodular deposit of sodium acid urate crystals with an associated foreign body reaction. Tophi may occur in various regions of the body, such as periarticular tissue, bone, tendon, cartilage, kidneys, and subcutaneous tissue. About 10 to 20 per cent of patients with gouty arthritis have uric acid kidney stones.

During acute gouty arthritis, urates may be demonstrated in synovial tissues, producing synovitis. It is this severe joint synovitis that causes the functional disturbances characteristic of an acute attack of gouty arthritis. The attack usually occurs suddenly, most often involving the great toe's metatarsophalangeal joint. However, other joints may be affected. While the attack typically involves only one joint, at times several joints may be involved during the same attack.

The involved joint(s) is usually intensely painful, swollen, and extremely tender. The skin

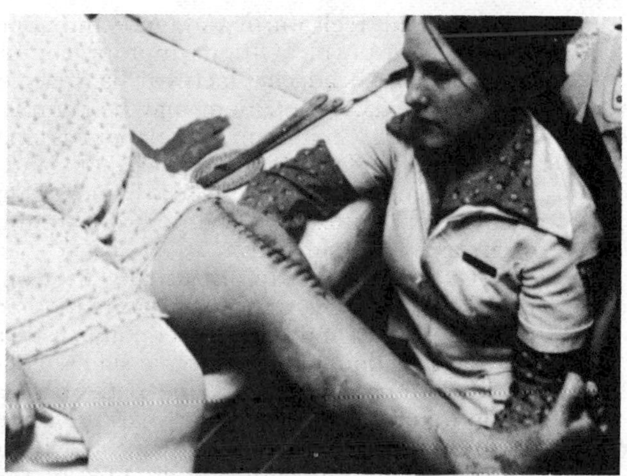

Figure 78–7. This woman has had a total knee replacement and is being helped with postoperative exercises. Individual exercise programs are developed for each patient. Note the position and length of the incision. (From Farrell, J.: *Illustrated Guide to Orthopedic Nursing.* Philadelphia: J. B. Lippincott Co., 1977, p. 186.)

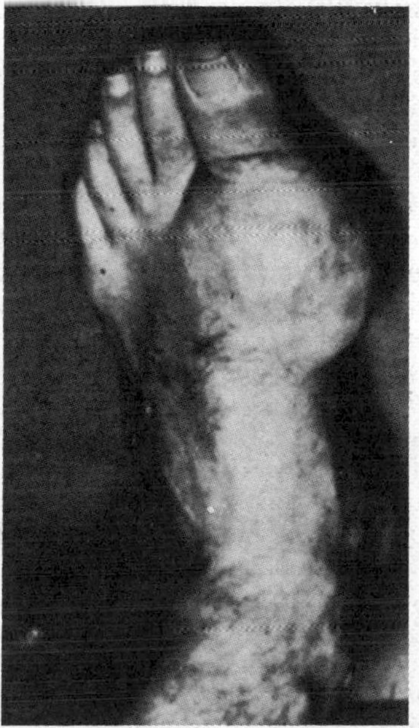

Figure 78–8. Large tophus of left foot. (From Talbott, J. H.: Treating gout. *Postgraduate Medicine,* 63:175, May, 1978.)

over the joint feels warm and tense and appears dusky red or purple. Other symptoms commonly occur, e.g., headache, tachycardia, fever, malaise, anorexia. The patient may be completely incapacitated. Commonly the patient is unable to move the inflamed joint and cannot stand the weight of linens over the affected part. During recovery, pruritus and local desquamation may occur as edema subsides.

Early attacks end rapidly, usually after only a few days or a week or two. Inflammation completely subsides and the affected joints return to normal functional and anatomic states. Following the initial acute attack the patient may be asymptomatic for months or years. Eventually other attacks occur. Gouty arthritis may become chronic so that the patient is disabled by symptoms and progressive loss of function. Gross deformities are then apparent, and x-ray studies reveal punched-out areas in the bone called "radiolucent urate tophi."

Following repeated acute attacks of gouty arthritis tophi may be detected in the cartilage of the ears and on the hands, olecranon, feet, and prepatellar bursae. Large urate deposits develop in and around joint structures. These deposits and the accompanying inflammatory changes may severely damage articular cartilage and subchondral bone; fibrous or bony ankylosis of the joint may develop.

Laboratory findings with gout include (a) elevated WBC and sedimentation rate during acute attacks; (b) elevated blood uric acid (unless uricosuric medications are being taken); and (c) presence of crystals of sodium urate in material aspirated from a tophus or in joint fluid.

Early diagnosis and treatment of gout are important. The emphasis has shifted from the simple treatment of recurrent attacks to permanent medical supervision and treatment directed at preventing not only acute attacks but also progressive disability (e.g., from erosion of bone and joint cartilage and progressive renal dysfunction). *Progressive renal dysfunction is the greatest threat to life.* With early, sustained treatment almost all patients can live full productive lives without disability. Treatment is also beneficial to persons with advanced disease, e.g., joint function can be improved, tophi can be resolved, and renal dysfunction may be improved or arrested. The severity of gout is greatest in patients whose clinical symptoms first appear before age 30.

Acute attacks may be terminated by administering medications such as colchicine, phenylbutazone (Butazolidin), indomethacin (Indocin), or corticotropin (ACTH). Additionally, the treatment of acute attacks includes bedrest (continued for at least 24 hours following subsidence of the attack) and analgesics, e.g., codeine. Some patients receive added relief from hot or cold compresses; others find compresses intolerable. Fluids are forced, to reduce precipitation of urate in the kidneys and to combat dehydration. A soft diet is usually prescribed.

Between attacks treatment is directed at (a) reducing the frequency and severity of recurrent acute attacks, and (b) minimizing the deposition of urate in tissues, i.e., by lowering the serum urate level to a range that will resolve any crystalline deposits of monosodium urate which are present and will prevent further deposition of these crystals.

Therapeutic factors of importance in obtaining the above goals include:

- **Medical Management.** Daily administrations of colchicine have preventive actions (i.e., reduce frequency of acute attacks) and may be continued indefinitely. Also, uricosuric drugs may be given, e.g., probenecid (Benemid), sulfinpyrazone (Anturane), or salicylates. Uricosuric medications block the tubular reabsoprtion of filtered urate in the kidneys and thus reduce the metabolic pool of urates by increasing uric acid excretion. *Salicylates cannot be given with any other uricosuric drug because they antagonize the action of other uricosuric agents.* The patient should be told not to take salicylates while taking other uricosuric drugs.

  Another method of ongoing treatment is the administration of the xanthine oxidase inhibitor allopurinol (Zyloprim). This drug inhibits uric acid formation. In selected patients allopurinol is used in conjunction with uricosuric drugs. Fluid intake should be at leat 3 L. per day when uricosuric drugs are being taken, and attempts are made to keep the urine alkaline (to prevent formation of urinary calculi). The patient is taught to test urine and may be advised to take sodium bicarbonate tablets and ingest alkaline-producing foods and liquids.

- **Dietary Management.** Rigid dietary restrictions are emphasized less than the proper ingestion of uricosuric medications with increased amounts of fluids. The patient is informed of the importance of avoiding acidity and dehydration. Restriction of the purine content of the diet may be temporarily recommended until the serum urate concentration returns to normal. Then dietary restrictions are usually no longer necessary because drugs are effective. Foods high in purine include liver, kidney, sweetbreads, anchovies, sardines, and meat extracts. A moderate ingestion of alcohol does not appear to precipitate acute attacks of gout or be otherwise harmful. However, the patient should avoid foods or alcoholic beverages which precipitate attacks and should practice moderation.

- **Other Management.** With advanced gout large tophi may be removed surgically to correct deformity and reduce the load on renal function. Some patients with renal involvement require hemodialysis. (See Unit XIII.)

CONNECTIVE TISSUE DISORDERS

Connective tissue disorders are commonly called *collagen diseases.* These diffuse diseases are discussed generally in Chapter 11. A variety of disorders are referred to as collagen diseases. Rheumatoid arthritis is a member of this group and has been discussed earlier in this chapter. Other possible collagen diseases are rheumatic fever, nonthrombocytopenic purpuras, glomerulonephritis, systemic lupus erythematosus, polyarteritis nodosa, scleroderma, and dermatomyositis. The last four of these disorders are discussed briefly in following sections.

As a group, collagen diseases (a) produce widespread changes in collagenous connective tissue; (b) cause a wide variety of symptoms referable to almost every organ; (c) may be autoimmune in etiology; (d) are difficult to diagnose; (e) have no cure; and (f) cannot be prevented. General treatment measures used for autoimmune conditions include corticosteroids, ionizing radiation, and salicylates.

Frequently with collagen diseases the anatomic, immunologic, and histologic findings overlap from one disease to another. While serologic tests may help in the process of establishing the differential diagnosis of the various collagen diseases, these tests are not specific. The diseases do tend to differ in their prognosis, clinical patterns, and response to treatment.

Systemic Lupus Erythematosus (SLE). This serious inflammatory disease of unknown etiology occurs mainly in young women and produces symptoms referable to multiple organ systems. SLE diffusely involves the vascular and connective tissues of multiple organs, producing inflammation and biochemical and structural changes. Usually the most important abnormalities occur in the viscera; however, pathologic changes exactly like those with rheumatoid arthritis may also occur in the joints, fascia, tendons, and bursae. The rheumatic symptoms are commonly less severe than with classic rheumatoid arthritis. Also, the prognosis of SLE is poorer than that of rheumatoid arthritis because of the greater visceral pathology.[215] Commonly, death results from failure of a vital organ, e.g., renal failure.

Several abnormal serum protein fractions and antinuclear antibodies may be found with SLE; these findings suggest that an autoimmune mechanism occurs with this disease. Characteristic histologic findings are the so-called lupus erythematosus (LE) cells and extracellular masses called "hematoxylin bodies." However, the LE cell may be found in many diseases and may or may not be demonstrated with SLE. Most patients with SLE have a mild to moderate normochromic, normocytic anemia. The sedimentation rate is usually high, a mild leukopenia is often present, and the serum globulin may be increased.

The clinical pattern and prognosis with SLE are highly variable. The illness may develop rapidly with an acute fulminant course which may produce death within a few weeks, or it may develop insidiously and become a chronic illness subject to remissions and exacerbations. The chronic pattern is more common and with proper steroid therapy the patient may live for many years.

Acute clinical findings may include[77] fever, prostration, delirium, convulsions, psychosis, coma, musculoskeletal aches and pains, "butterfly rash" on the face, pleural effusion, basilar pneumonia, generalized lymphadenopathy, pericarditis, tachycardia, gallop rhythm, hepatosplenomegaly, and nephritis.

Clinical findings that may occur with *chronic* SLE are variable, depending upon the organ systems involved, but may include[77] fever, malaise, weight loss, cutaneous discoid LE lesions, erythema of exposed surfaces, generalized lymphadenopathy, severe hemolytic anemia, thrombocytopenic purpura, hypersplenism, pericarditis, tachycardia, gallop rhythm, peripheral vascular sydromes (e.g., Raynaud's phenomenon, gangrene), ulcerative lesions of the mucous membranes, abdominal pains, nausea, vomiting, anorexia, bloody stools, hepatic dysfunction, hepatomegaly, focal glomerulitis progressing to glomerulonephritis, myalgia, arthralgia, neuritis, hemiplegia, psychosis, convulsions, and coma.

Nursing care is supportive and is determined by the organ systems involved and the pre-

PATIENT-FAMILY TEACHING GUIDE FOR PERSONS WITH SLE

1. Avoid direct rays of the sun. Wear a hat and other protective clothing.
2. Avoid stress as much as possible.
3. Rest a lot.
4. Eat regular, nutritious meals.
5. Follow prescribed treatment regimen carefully.
6. Do not take any other drugs without consulting physician.
7. Contact physician if the condition worsens, i.e., fever, cough, skin rash, or increased joint pain.

Adapted from Davis, J. S.: A summary of systemic lupus erythematosus. *Consultant,* 14:39, Aug. 1974.

scribed medical therapy. Corticosteroids or corticotropin are commonly prescribed in the treatment of SLE. These medications produce variable, sometimes highly favorable effects. If corticosteroid therapy does not produce an adequate response, purine antagonists (e.g., mercaptopurine) or alkylating agents (e.g., nitrogen mustards, cyclophosphamide) may be tried. These drugs are immunosuppressive agents. Physical therapy, salicylates, and other analgesics may be prescribed to reduce musculoskeletal discomforts. Other disorders, e.g., anemia, pneumonia, renal disease, are given appropriate treatment. Commonly a high-calorie, high-vitamin diet is prescribed. The patient is advised to avoid excessive exposure to ultraviolet radiation (e.g., sunlight) and excessive fatigue. Bedrest is necessary during exacerbations.

Polyarteritis Nodosa. This collagen disease produces diffuse inflammation and necrosis in the walls of small to medium-sized arteries. While arterial lesions may occur in any organ, the structures most often involved are muscles, kidneys, heart, liver, gastrointestinal tract, and peripheral nerves. Aneurysms or thrombosis may develop. Muscle biopsy of painful areas demonstrates vasculitis. *Laboratory findings* may include leukocytosis, mild normocytic anemia, eosinophilia, and an elevated sedimentation rate and serum globulin level. Urinary findings may include hematuria, proteinuria, pyuria, and casts.

Like SLE, the symptoms and course of polyarteritis nodosa are highly variable. It is not uncommon, however, for polyarteritis nodosa to run a fulminating course which proves fatal within a few months. *Clinical findings* may include fever, weakness, malaise, weight loss, hypertension, renal disease, musculoskeletal aches and pains, peripheral neuritis, variable skin lesions, angina, congestive heart failure, nausea, melena, abdominal pain, hematemesis, bronchial asthma, and bronchial pneumonia.

Treatment of polyarteritis nodosa is mainly supportive and symptomatic. Corticosteroids may be helpful.

Scleroderma. This collagen disorder is also called "diffuse scleroderma" or "systemic sclerosis." The word scleroderma means "hard skin." In this chronic disorder the connective tissue proliferates in the skin and in numerous internal structures. Insidious symptoms may be present for years (e.g., sweating of the hands and feet, stiffness of the hands), and eventually the toes and fingers become fixed in position and the skin becomes thick and hard. As areas of skin become increasingly involved, ulceration, calcification, pigmentation, or depigmentation may occur. Eventually skin over the entire body may be involved, producing a variety of disorders. For example, sclerodermatous constriction of the thorax may impair effective breathing and, as a result, pulmonary complications may develop. Numerous other disorders may occur, such as difficulty in swallowing, impaired gastrointestinal mobility, cardiac and renal disorders, osteoporosis of bone, and destruction of distal phalanges.

Scleroderma typically progresses slowly. When death occurs it often results from infection or renal or cardiac failure. Supportive, symptomatic treatment is given. Low molecular weight dextran may be administered. Corticosteroids are typically not helpful.

Dermatomyositis; Polymyositis. These collagen diseases affect mainly the skin and voluntary (striated) muscles. When skin changes are the prominent feature, the illness is called "dermatomyositis"; when muscle weakness is the principal clinical feature, it is termed "polymyositis.[240] With either form, the onset is most commonly insidious, and the disease may progress over a period of years, crippling the patient. *Treatment* is basically symptomatic and supportive. Corticosteroids may be quite helpful. Biopsies may demonstrate inflammatory, degenerative muscular changes and variable dermatitis. Serum enzyme levels, e.g., SGOT, are elevated. Creatinuria parallels muscle destruction. Creatine is formed in the muscle, passes into the blood, and is excreted by the kidneys. The serum globulin level and sedimentation rate may be increased, and a mild, normocytic anemia may be present.

The *symptoms* of dermatomyositis and polymyositis are variable but among them are desquamation, pigmentary changes, diffuse erythema, calcification, weakness, fatigue, weight loss, mild fever, multiple gastrointestinal ulcers, muscular tenderness, and aching. Muscular involvement may cause dysphagia or respiratory embarrassment. Emergency restoration of the airway may be necessary. The proximal muscles of the upper and lower extremities and the flexor muscles of the neck are most commonly affected. Muscle contractures and loss of function may occur. During the active inflammatory phase of the disease, range-of-motion exercises are important to prevent these complications. (See Table 78–1.)

OTHER MUSCULOSKELETAL DISORDERS

Bone Tumors

Primary bone tumors (originating in the bone) may be benign or malignant. Primary *malignant* bone tumors are rare. *Benign* tumors of bone

TABLE 78–1. TYPES OF POLYMYOSITIS-DERMATOMYOSITIS

Type I—Typical Polymyositis	The most common form, usually comes on slowly in third to fifth decades, and occurs more frequently in females
Type II—Typical Dermatomyositis	More common in women, occurs in the second to seventh decades. The typical skin rashes are seen in conjunction with progressive muscular weakness and, occasionally, with muscle tenderness. Onset can be acute or subacute and may be associated with joint symptoms
Type III—Inflammatory Myositis Associated with Malignancy	Occurs almost equally in men and women, and may or may not be accompanied by a skin rash
Type IV—Childhood Myositis	Usually a chronic disease but may occur in an acute intermittent form. Rash may be present. Sometimes the disease in children is transient. In the past, the underlying pathology of this childhood form was thought to be vasculitis with ischemic necrosis of segments of muscle, but some recent clinical investigation has not upheld this theory
Type V—Myositis Associated with Overlap Syndromes	Similar to type I (typical polymyositis) but usually associated with one or more other connective tissue disorders (overlap syndromes)

From Janul, L. C.: Polymyositis-dermatomyositis: A perplexing disorder. *American Journal of Nursing,* 77: 1184, July 1977. Based on Pearson, C. M., and A. Bohan: The spectrum of polymyositis and dermatomyositis. *Medical Clinics of North America,* 61:440, Mar. 1977.

most commonly include osteomas, chondromas, giant-cell tumors, cysts, and osteoid osteomas. Benign tumors are usually well circumscribed, grow slowly, and seldom spread. Primary malignant bone tumors tend to be extremely malignant and metastasize early, often to the lung. Examples of primary malignant bone tumors are osteogenic sarcoma (most common), Ewing's sarcoma, multiple myeloma (also called plasma cell myeloma or plasma cell leukemia), reticulum cell sarcoma, and angiosarcoma. Some authorities consider multiple myeloma to be a disorder of the blood-forming organs (bone marrow) rather than a primary tumor of the bone (see Unit XIV).

Certain tumors tend to occur at certain ages. For example, osteogenic sarcomas appear in children, adolescents, and young adults (below age 25); giant cell tumors occur between ages 21 and 35; and multiple myeloma most commonly occurs between ages 50 and 70.

Metastatic (secondary) bone tumors are relatively common, and may come from primary lesions in the breast, lungs, prostate, kidney, ovary, or thyroid. Carcinomas tend to metastasize to bone more commonly than sarcomas. Prognosis with metastatic bone lesions is poor.

Symptoms of bone tumors are swelling, pain, restricted motion, aching, and fracture (due to weakening of the bone). Bone pain may be quite severe and is commonly persistent. Pain may occur before metastases become detectable on x-ray films. Diagnosis may be made by using x-rays, biopsies, or frozen sections. Many bone tumors produce characteristic radiologic appearances. Whenever malignant tumors are suspected, chest films are routinely taken to look for pulmonary metastases and a skeletal radiologic survey is conducted to locate additional bone lesions. The precise identification of tumor type is extremely important. Therefore, biopsy (via aspiration needle or incision) is mandatory.

Bone tumors may be *treated* by chemotherapy, irradiation, and surgery. (Treatment of cancer is discussed in Unit IX.) Radical surgery may be required for primary malignant bone tumors. A major portion of an involved limb may be amputated or possibly completely disarticulated. In some cases an interscapulothoracic amputation is required for upper extremity lesions or a hemipelvectomy for lesions involving the lower limbs. (Amputation is discussed in Chapter 50.) Metastatic bone lesions are treated by palliative measures. Symptomatic relief may be obtained from irradiation and chemotherapy.

Osteoporosis

Osteoporosis is a common disorder of bone metabolism in which the mass of bone is decreased. Both mineral and protein matrix components are reduced. This reduction in bone density occurs in approximately one fourth of all elderly persons, most frequently in women between the ages of 50 and 70. In this disorder bone resorption occurs faster than bone formation takes place over a prolonged period. Osteoporosis may occur (a) with a deficit of estrogen (in postmenopausal women); (b) with catabolic hormone excess (e.g., with Cushing's disease); (c) with long-term administration of high amounts of corticosteroids; (d) with prolonged immobilization; and (e) as a result of other disorders such as liver disease. Osteoporosis is most common in fair-skinned, light-weight, postmenopausal women.

Osteoporosis can be detected with x-ray studies. Blood calcium, phosphorus, and phosphatase are normal.

Symptoms, particularly with postmenopausal women, usually begin with pain in the weight-bearing vertebrae. Because the involved bone tissue loses its density and tensile strength, fractures and kyphosis may occur. Even slight trauma may fracture brittle, osteoporetic bone. Multiple vertebral fractures may cause a loss of height.

Physical activity and exercises are important in the *treatment* of osteoporosis. Postmenopausal women may be treated with cyclic estrogen administration. Large doses of calcium, vitamin D, or fluoride have been tried, as well as calcitonin (which inhibits bone resorption). Currently high doses of calcium and treatment with fluoride are considered to be investigational, and calcitonin has not been adequately evaluated. Androgen and other anabolic steroid therapy is not advised.

Osteomyelitis

Osteomyelitis, i.e., bone infection caused by pyogenic microorganisms, is most commonly produced by *Staphylococcus aureus.* Infection may reach the bone directly (e.g., via compound fracture), through the blood stream, or by direct extension from infections in adjacent structures.

Local *symptoms* of acute bone infection are sudden pain in the affected bone, tenderness over the bone, heat, redness, swelling, painful movement, and involuntary restriction of movement. General symptoms with acute severe bone infection may include sharp rise in temperature, chills, rapid pulse, marked leukocytosis, elevated ESR, and possibly positive blood cultures. Evidence of bone infection may not appear for some time on x-ray films.

Early diagnosis of osteomyelitis is extremely important because chronic osteomyelitis can be a serious, disabling disorder. With early *treatment,* the chances of effectively controlling acute osteomyelitis are quite good. Once osteomyelitis is suspected, an antibiotic is given as soon as blood count results are available. The physician does not wait for other laboratory or x-ray evidence. A penicillinase-resistant penicillin is usually given initially. Later, after laboratory reports are obtained and the causative organism identified, medication may be changed. It is important that the medication reach the bone before necrosis occurs. With delayed treatment, bone necrosis develops and the antibiotic cannot enter the dead bone to combat the infectious organisms effectively.

Infected bone is placed at rest by cast or traction, and the patient is maintained on bedrest until evidence of active infection disappears. If an abscess is present it is evacuated and an appropriate antibiotic is instilled into the cavity daily. The medication is also given systemically. Sometimes a catheter is placed in the wound and is used for continuous drip instillation of an antibiotic solution or for irrigation of the wound. A closed irrigation and drainage system with low pressure suction is another procedure that may be used in treating osteomyelitis. If chronic bone infection develops, the wound is widely exposed and all infected dead bone is carefully removed. Immobilization and antibiotics are also used as discussed above. Drug-resistant organisms can develop which make treatment exceedingly difficult. Fortunately, chronic osteomyelitis is now much less common than in previous years.

Refractory osteomyelitis (not responding readily to treatment) may improve with *hyperbaric oxygen* treatment. This treatment is supplemental to properly timed antibiotic therapy and surgery.[21]

Strict aseptic technique must be practiced when changing dressings over open wounds. If a patient is placed in isolation the nurse must meticulously follow isolation technique. Because infected bone may be extremely painful, the patient must be handled gently.

Every attempt is made in orthopedic practice to *prevent* osteomyelitis. If indications of bone infection do appear, they are immediately reported.

Osteomalacia

Osteomalacia is a disorder in which adult bone becomes softened as a result of disturbed calcium and phosphorus metabolism. These metabolic disturbances result from a vitamin D deficiency due to inadequate dietary intake of vitamin D, to the body's failure to absorb or use vitamin D, or lack of exposure to ultraviolet rays. With inadequate vitamin D, the effect of the parathyroid hormone on bone resorption is decreased, and calcium absorption is decreased. Secondary hyperparathyroidism occurs in response to the resultant hypocalcemia. This has little effect on calcium absorption but does increase the kidney's phosphate loss. Both calcium and phosphorus are consequently low. Parathyroid hormone is believed to stimulate osteoblastic differentiation. The increased number of osteoblasts increases alkaline phosphatase. However, the osteoblasts do not form large amounts of bone, and mineralization is defective in the bone that is formed.

Osteomalacia is characterized by widespread decalcification and softening of the bones, especially those in the spine, pelvis, and lower extremities. The bones become deformed (bent, flattened) as they soften. Osteomalacia develops insidiously and may be identified by reduced calcium and phosphorus levels, rachitic bone deformities, bone pain and tenderness, and x-ray changes (such as pseudo-fractures or possibly cyst formation). Biopsy may help establish diagnosis. A similar disorder occurs in children and is called *rickets.*

Treatment of osteomalacia may involve large amounts of vitamin D and dietary measures to insure adequate intakes of calcium and phosphorus, e.g., eggs, milk, vegetables, fish. Calcium salts and phosphate supplements may also be given.

Scoliosis

"Scoliosis" means a lateral curvature of the spinal column from its normal vertical anatomic position. Scoliosis may develop from various disorders (e.g., rickets, neuromuscular disorders, vertebral disorders), but 90 per cent of the time it is idiopathic (without known cause). While scoliosis may develop at any age, it most frequently develops in children 10 to 12 years of age. With idiopathic scoliosis, girls are affected 10 times more frequently than boys. The type of treatment used depends upon the cause and the severity of the deformity. Corrective exercises may be used. Other treatment methods include use of braces (Milwaukee brace), casts (Risser localizer cast, turnbuckle cast), plastic body jackets, or surgery (the Harrington operation which consists of spinal instrumentation and fusion). Casts and braces are discussed in Chapter 76. For a discussion of the Harrington operation, refer to Boegli and Steele.[25] Detailed discussions of scoliosis may be found in pediatric texts and orthopedic texts. (See Fig. 76–1*B*.)

BIBLIOGRAPHY (Unit XX)

1. Ainsworth, T. H.: Immediate full weight-bearing in the treatment of hip fractures. *Journal of Trauma,* 11:1031, Dec. 1971.
2. Albanese, A. A., E. J. Lorenze, Jr., and E. H. Wein: Osteoporosis: Effects of calcium. *American Family Physician,* 18:160, Oct. 1978.
3. Altemeier, W. A.: The significance of infection in trauma. *AORN Journal,* 15:92, Mar. 1972.
4. American Orthopaedic Association: *Manual of Orthopaedic Surgery.* Chicago: 1972.
5. Anderson, B.: Carole, a girl treated with bracing. *American Journal of Nursing,* 79:1592, Sept. 1979.

5a. Apley, A. G.: Commonly missed orthopaedic injuries. *Journal of Postgraduate Medicine,* 43:568, Sept. 1967.

6. Arden, G. P.: Total knee replacement. *Clinical Orthopaedics and Related Research,* 94:92, July-Aug. 1973.
7. Armstrong, M., and R. Patterson: Arthroscopy: A new approach to knee surgery that affects patient care. *RN,* 41:35, Jan. 1978.
8. Aronoff, P. M., P. M. Davis, Jr., and J. K. Wickstrom: Intramedullary nail fixation as treatment of subtrochanteric fractures of the femur. *Journal of Trauma,* 11:637, Aug. 1971.
9. Arthritis Foundation: *Home Care Programs in Arthritis: A Manual for Patients.* New York: The Arthritis Foundation, 1969.
10. Arthritis Foundation: *Arthritis —The Basic Facts.* New York: The Arthritis Foundation, 1970.
11. Arthritis Foundation: *Arthritis Quackery.* New York: The Arthritis Foundation, 1970.
12. Arthritis Foundation: *The Truth about Aspirin for Arthritis.* New York: The Arthritis Foundation, 1970.
13. Austen, K. F.: Connective tissue diseases ("collagen diseases") other than rheumatoid arthritis: Introduction. *In* Beeson, P. B., W. McDermott, and J. B. Wyngaarden (Eds.): *Cecil Textbook of Medicine,* 15th ed. Philadelphia, W. B. Saunders Co., 1979.
14. Austen, K. F.: Periarteritis nodosa (polyarteritis nodosa). *In* Beeson, P. B., W. McDermott, and J. B. Wyngaarden (Eds.): *Cecil Textbook of Medicine,* 15th ed. Philadelphia, W. B. Saunders Co., 1979.
15. Ballinger, W. F., J. C. Treybal, and A. B. Vose: *Alexander's Care of the Patient in Surgery,* 5th ed. St. Louis: C. V. Mosby Co., 1972.
16. Baum, J.: When to prescribe nonsteroidal anti-inflammatory drugs. *Geriatrics,* 34:51, June 1979.
17. Baum, J.: Rheumatoid arthritis. *In* Conn, H. F. (Ed.): *Current Therapy 1973.* Philadelphia, W. B. Saunders Co., 1973.
18. Beaumont, E.: Wheelchairs. *Nursing '73,* 3:49, Nov. 1973.
19. Bently, G.: Disorganization of the knee following intraarticular hydrocortisone injections. *Journal of Bone and Joint Surgery,* 51:B, 1969.
20. Berens, D. L.: Roentgenographic changes in gout. *Postgraduate Medicine,* 63:154, May 1978.
21. Bingham, E. L., and G. B. Hart: Hyperbaric oxygen treatment of refractory osteomyelitis. *Postgraduate Medicine,* 61:70, June 1977
22. Bisla, R. S., C. S. Ranawat, and A. E. Inglis: Total hip replacement with ankylosing spondylitis with involvement of the hip. *Journal of Bone and Joint Surgery,* 58A:233, 1976.
23. Blechman, W., et al.: Experience with naproxen in treating osteoarthritis. *Geriatrics,* 32:72, July 1977.
24. Bluestone, R.: Physical diagnosis of rheumatic disease. *Consultant,* 17:66, Sept. 1977.
25. Boegli, E. H., and M. S. Steele: Scoliosis: Spinal instrumentation and fusion. *American Journal of Nursing,* 68:2399, Nov. 1968.
26. Bonamo, J. J.: More than just a sprained ankle. *Emergency Medicine,* 9:97, Nov. 1977.
27. Boyes, J. G., Jr.: Wrist sprain with subluxation of the scaphoid. *American Family Physician,* 15:149, Jan. 1977.
28. Boyes, J. H.: *Suture Technics for Wounds of the Hand.* Somerville, N.J.: Ethicon, Inc., 1970.
29. Browler, P., and D. Hicks: Maintaining muscle function in patients on bed rest. *American Journal of Nursing,* 72:1250, July 1972.
30. Brown-Skeers, V.: How the nurse practitioner manages the rheumatoid arthritis patient. *Nursing '79,* 9:26, June 1979.
31. Brunner, N. A.: *Orthopedic Nursing: A Programmed Approach.* St. Louis: C. V. Mosby Co., 1970.

32. Bunker, R. H.: Thoracic outlet compression syndrome: Diagnosis and treatment. *Hospital Medicine,* 12:46, Sept. 1976.
33. Calabro, J. J., and B. A. Maltz: Current concepts on ankylosing spondylitis. *New England Journal of Medicine,* 282:606, Mar. 1970.
34. Calin, A.: Rheumatoid arthritis. *American Family Physician,* 18:89, July 1978.
35. Calin, A.: Back pain: Mechanical or inflammatory? *American Family Physician,* 20:97, Aug. 1979.
36. Capello, W. N., and R. O. Pierce: Soft tissue injuries to the ankle. *American Family Physician,* 15:152, Feb. 1977.
37. Casagrande, P. A., and R. Turner: Total knee replacement. *Clinical Orthopaedics and Related Research,* 89:150, Nov.-Dec. 1972.
38. Casscells, S. W.: Arthroscopy of the knee joint: A review of 150 cases. *Journal of Bone and Joint Surgery,* 53-A:287, Mar. 1971.
39. Charnley, J.: Postoperative infection after total hip replacement with special reference to air contamination in the operating room. *Clinical Orthopaedics and Related Research,* 87:167, Sept. 1972.
40. Charosky, C., P. Bullough, and P. Wilson: Total hip replacement failures. *Journal of Bone and Joint Surgery,* 55-A:49, Jan. 1973.
41. A checklist for venereal arthritis. *Emergency Medicine,* 10:105, Jan. 1978.
42. Chiroff, R. T.: An overview of osteoarthritis. *Geriatrics,* 32:57, June 1977.
43. Ciuca, R., J. Bradish, and S. M. Trombley: Range-of-motion exercises, active and passive: A handbook. *Nursing '73,* 3:25, Dec. 1973.
44. Clary, B. B., and D. E. Couk: Experience with the MacIntosh knee prosthesis. *Southern Medical Journal,* 65:265, Mar. 1972.
45. Clayton, M. L.: Care of the rheumatoid hip. *Clinical Orthopaedics and Related Research,* 90:70, Jan.-Feb. 1973.
46. Cole, W. H., and C. B. Puestow: *Emergency Care,* 7th ed. New York: Appleton-Century-Crofts, 1972.
47. Collins, D. K., and R. C. Johnston: Comparative evaluation of the results of cup arthroplasty and total hip replacement. *Clinical Orthopaedics and Related Research,* 86:102, July-Aug. 1972.
48. Committee on Injuries, American Academy of Orthopaedic Surgeons: *Emergency Care and Transportation of the Sick and Injured.* Menasha, Wis.: George Banta Co., Inc., 1971.
49. Conaty, J. P., and V. L. Nickel: Functional incapacitation in rheumatoid arthritis: A rehabilitation challenge. *Journal of Bone and Joint Surgery,* 53-A:624, June 1971.
50. Conlee, R. K., and A. G. Fisher: Skeletal muscle adaptations to growth and exercise. *Nurse-Practitioner,* 3:34, May-June 1979.
51. Convery, F. R., and C. A. Beber: Total knee arthroplasty. *Clinical Orthopaedics and Related Research* 94:42, July-Aug. 1973.
52. Cooper, D. L.: This sporting life. *Emergency Medicine,* 10:24, Aug. 1978.
53. Coventry, M. B.: The treatment of fracture dislocation of the hip by total hip arthroplasty. *Journal of Bone and Surgery,* 56A:1128, 1974.
54. Cracchiolo, A., III, and E. D. Schmitter: Orthopedics in the office. *Emergency Medicine,* 10:25, Oct. 1978.
55. Current surgical nursing: Symposium. *Nursing Clinics of North America,* 8:107, Mar. 1973.
56. Dandy, D. J.: Fat embolism following prosthetic replacement of the femoral head. *Injury,* 3:85, 1971.
57. Darst, B. J.: "I have a new hip." *American Journal of Nursing,* 78:1489, Sept. 1978.
58. Davie, B.: Arthroscopy of the knee. *Australia-New Zealand Journal of Surgery,* 48:107, Feb. 1978.
59. Davis, J. S., IV: A summary of systemic lupus erythematosus. *Consultant,* 14:39, Aug. 1974.
60. Davis, P. R.: The nurse and her back. *Nursing Times,* 63:1403, Oct. 1967.
61. Dee, R.: Total replacement arthroplasty of the elbow for rheumatoid arthritis. *Journal of Bone and Joint Surgery,* 54-B:88, Feb. 1972.
62. Dehne, E.: The weight-bearing principle in treatment of lower-extremity fractures, 1885–1972. *Journal of Trauma,* 12:539, June 1972.
63. del Bueno, D. J.: Recognizing fat embolism in patients with multiple injuries. *RN,* 36:48, Jan. 1973.
64. De Toledo, C. H.: The patient with scoliosis. The defect: Classification and detection. *American Journal of Nursing,* 79:1588, Sept. 1979.
65. De Vries, H. A.: Tips on prescribing exercise regimens for your older patient. *Geriatrics,* 34:75, April 1979.
66. Deyerle, W. M., and S. A. Crossland: Broken legs are to be walked on. *American Journal of Nursing,* 77:1927, Dec. 1977.
67. DiPalma, J. R.: Rheumatoid arthritis: Picking the right nonsteroid drug. *RN,* 40:63, Dec. 1977.
68. DiStefano, V., and J. E. Nixon: Steroid-induced skin changes following local injection. *Clinical Orthopaedics and Related Research,* 87:254, Sept. 1972.
69. Dobyns, J. H., et al.: The special problems of total elbow arthroplasty. *Geriatrics,* 31:57, April 1976.
70. Donahoo, C.: Bicentennial forecast: Orthopedic nursing. *RN,* 39:19, Oct. 1976.
71. Drain, C. B.: The athletic knee injury. *American Journal of Nursing,* 71:536, Mar. 1971.
72. Drury, J. H., Jr.: Handbook of range-of-motion exercises. *Nursing '72,* 2:19, April 1972.
73. Dukes-Dubos, F.: What is the best way to lift and carry? *Occupational Health Safety,* 46:16, Jan.-Feb. 1977.
74. Dupont, J. A., and J. Charnley, Jr.: Low-friction arthroplasty of the hip for the failures of previous operations. *Journal of Bone and Joint Surgery,* 54-B:77, Feb. 1972.
75. Eagleson, W. M., et al.: The effect of heat on the healing of fractures. *Canadian Medical Association Journal,* 97:274, Aug. 1967.
76. Eftekhar, N. S., and F. E. Stinchfield: Experience with low friction arthroplasty. A statistical review of early results and complications. *Clinical Orthopaedics,* 95:60, 1973.
77. Engleman, E. P., J. E. Giansiricusa, and M. J. Chatton: Arthritis and allied rheumatic disorders. *In* Brainerd, H., S. Margen, and M. J. Chatton: *Current Diagnosis and Treatment.* Los Altos, Cal.: Lange Medical Publications, 1969.
78. Evarts, C. M. (Ed.): Symposium on interposition and implant arthroplasty. *Orthopedic Clinics of North America,* 4:233, April 1973.
79. Eversmann, W. W., Jr.: Ankle fractures in adults. *Hospital Medicine,* 14:84, April 1978.
80. Eyre, M. K.: Total hip replacement. *American Journal of Nursing,* 71:1384, July 1971.
81. Falconer, M. W., et al.: *The Drug, The Nurse, The Patient,* 5th ed. Philadelphia, W. B. Saunders Co., 1974.
82. Farrell, J.: Casts, your patients, and you. Part 1: A review of basic procedures. *Nursing '78,* 8:65, Oct. 1978.

83. Farrell, J.: Part 2: A review of arm and leg cast procedures. *Nursing '78,* 8:57, Nov. 1978.
84. Farrell, J.: Part 3: A review of hip-spica procedures. *Nursing '78,* 8:53, Dec. 1978.
85. Ferguson, R. H.: Connective tissue disease: When to suspect malignancies. *Geriatrics,* 33:26, Sept. 1978.
86. Fessel, W. J.: Distinguishing gout from other types of arthritis. *Postgraduate Medicine,* 63:134, May 1978.
87. Fighting fat after fracture. *Emergency Medicine,* 10:221, Jan. 1978.
88. Finsterbush, A., et al.: Recent experiences with intravenous regional anesthesia in limbs. *Journal of Trauma,* 12:81, Jan. 1972.
89. Foss, G.: Body mechanics: Use your head and save your back. *Nursing '73,* 3:25, May 1973.
90. Foss, G.: Breaking the architectural barrier with crutches, wheelchairs and walkers. *Nursing '73,* 3:17, Oct. 1973.
91. Foss, G.: The "how to's" of bed positioning. *Nursing '72,* 2:14, Aug. 1972.
92. Foss, M., and Garrick, J. G.: *Ski Conditioning.* New York: John Wiley & Sons, 1978.
93. Frankel, V. H., and Burstein, A. H.: Orthopaedic biomechanics. Philadelphia: Lea and Febiger, 1970.
94. Gardner, R. C.: Hypertrophic infiltrative tendinitis (HIT syndrome) of the long extensor. *Journal of the American Medical Association,* 211:1009, Feb. 1970.
95. Gardner, R. C.: A pictorial survey of back problems. *Consultant,* 17:71, Jan. 1977.
96. Gardner, R. C.: What to do about tennis elbow. *Consultant,* 17:135, Sept. 1977.
97. Garrick, J. G., et al.: Injuries in high school sports. *Pediatrics,* 6:465, Mar. 1978.
98. Gartland, J. J.: *Fundamentals of Orthopaedics,* 4th ed. Philadelphia: W. B. Saunders Co., 1978.
99. Gong, H., Jr.: Fat embolism syndrome: A puzzling phenomenon. *Postgraduate Medicine,* 62:40, Dec 1977.
100. Gooch, M. A.: Thoracic outlet syndrome. *American Journal of Nursing,* 78:1328, Aug. 1978.
101. Good, A. E.: Reiter's disease. *Postgraduate Medicine,* 61:153, Jan. 1977.
102. Gordan, G. S., and C. Vaughan: The role of estrogens in osteoporosis. Geriatrics, 32:42, Sept. 1977.
103. Gordon, G. V., and H. R. Schumacher: Management of gout. *American Family Physician,* 19:91, Jan 1979.
104. Gordon, P. C.: The probability of death following a fracture of the hip. *Canadian Medical Association Journal,* 105:47, July 1971.
105. Grant, H., and R. Murray; *Emergency Care.* Washington, D. C.: Robert J. Brady Company, 1971.
106. Grattan, E., and J. A. Hobbs: Injuries to hip joint in car occupants. *British Medical Journal,* 1:71, Jan. 1969.
108. Graves, S., and S. Vincent: Total hip replacement is a family affair. *RN,* 34:35, June 1971.
109. Gray, K. D.: O.R. sterility for total hip replacement. *AORN Journal,* 16:72, Oct. 1972.
110. Green, D. P.: The "sprained" wrist. *American Family Physician,* 19:114, April 1979.
111. Griffin, W., S. J. Anderson, and J. Y. Passos: Group exercises for patients with limited motion. *American Journal of Nursing,* 71:1742, Sept. 1971.
112. Hagberg, L., and B. E. Nilsson: Can fracture of the femoral neck be predicted? *Geriatrics,* 32:55, April 1977.
113. Hamdy, R.: The signs and treatment of Paget's disease. *Geriatrics,* 32:89, June 1977.
114. Harris, E. D., Jr.: Systemic sclerosis (scleroderma). *In* Beeson, P. B., W. McDermott, and J. B. Wyngaarden (Eds.): *Cecil Textbook of Medicine,* 15th ed. Philadelphia, W. B. Saunders Co., 1979.
115. Harvey-Smith, W.: Stress fractures. *Nurse-Practitioner,* 3:46, May-June 1979.
116. Heaney, R. P.: Diseases of bone. *In* Beeson, P. B., and W. McDermott, (Eds.): *Cecil-Loeb Textbook of Medicine,* 13th ed. Philadelphia, W. B. Saunders Company, 1971.
117. Herfort, R. A.: *The Surgical Relief of Pain in Arthritic Disease.* Springfield, Ill.: Charles C Thomas, 1967.
118. Herndon, J. H., E. J. Riseborough, and J. E. Fischer: Fat embolism: A review of current concepts. *Journal of Trauma,* 11:673, Aug. 1971.
119. Higgs, S. L.: For better female athletes, it's all in the training. *Physician and Sportsmedicine,* 2:47, 1974.
120. Hollander, J. L.: Painful joints: Clues to early diagnosis. *Postgraduate Medicine,* 64:50, Sept. 1978.
121. Holvey, D. N. (Ed.): *The Merck Manual,* 12th ed. Rahway, N. J., Merck & Company, Inc., 1972.
122. Huffer, J. M.: Traumatic injuries: Office treatment of dislocations. *Postgraduate Medicine,* 62:223, Nov. 1977.
123. Huffer, J. M.: Traumatic injuries: Office treatment of fractures. *Postgraduate Medicine,* 62:199, Sept. 1977.
124. Irby, R.: Diagnostic tests that identify connective tissue diseases. *Consultant,* 18:157, Oct. 1978.
125. Jackson, R. W., and I. Abe: The role of arthroscopy in the management of disorders of the knee. *Journal of Bone and Joint Surgery,* 54-B:310, May 1972.
126. Jacob, S. W., C. A. Francone, and J. W. Lossow: *Structure and Function in Man.* 4th ed. Philadelphia, W. B. Saunders Company, 1978.
127. Jacobs, D., et al.: Comparison of conservative and operative treatment of achilles tendon rupture. *American Journal of Sports Medicine,* 6:107, May-June 1978.
128. James, S. L., et al.: Injuries to runners. *American Journal of Sports Medicine,* 6:40, Mar.-April 1978.
129. Janecki, C. J., Jr., D. H. Hill, and R. G. Eubanks: Arthroscopy of the knees. *American Family Physician,* 17:109, Mar. 1978.
130. Johnson, C. F., and F. R. Convery: Preventing emboli after total hip replacement. *American Journal of Nursing,* 75:5 806, 1975.
131. Jowsey, J.: Osteoporosis: Dealing with a crippling bone disease of the elderly. *Geriatrics,* 32:41, July 1977.
132. Jowsey, J.: Why is mineral nutrition important in osteoporosis? *Geriatrics,* 33:39, Aug. 1978.
133. Kane, W. J., et al.: Scoliosis and school screening for spinal deformity. *American Family Physician,* 17:123, May 1978.
134. Katler, E. I.: Diagnostics. Laboratory tests for rheumatic diseases. *Consultant,* 18:64, Mar. 1978.
135. Keim, H. A.: Scoliosis. *Ciba Clinical Symposia* 24:No. 1, 1972.
136. Kern, F. C., and L. Poole: Transfer techniques. *Nursing '72,* 2:25, July 1972.
137. Kerr, A. H.: *Orthopedic Nursing Procedures,* 2nd ed. New York: Springer Publishing Co., 1969.
138. Kessler, F. B.: The nurse in hand surgery. *AORN Journal,* 15:44, June 1972.
139. Kessler, I.: Silicone arthroplasty of the trapeziometacarpal joint. *Journal of Bone and Joint Surgery,* 55-B:285, May 1973.
140. Kettelkamp, D. B., and R. B. Leach, (Guest Eds.): Symposium: Total knee replacement. *Clinical Orthopaedics and Related Research,* 94:2, July-Aug. 1973.

141. Khairi, M. R. A., and C. C. Johnston: What we know — and don't know — about bone loss in the elderly. *Geriatrics,* 33:67, Nov. 1978.
142. King, L. S.: Sports medicine. *Journal of the American Medical Association,* 227:1425, Mar. 1974.
143. Klineberg, J. R.: Role of the kidneys in the pathogenesis of gout. *Postgraduate Medicine,* 63:145, May 1978.
144. Knapp, M.: Rheumatoid arthritis. *Postgraduate Medicine,* 42:A-99, Nov. 1967.
145. Knapp, M.: Aftercare of fractures. *In* Krusen, F. H., F. J. Kottke, and P. M. Ellwood, Jr.: *Handbook of Physical Medicine and Rehabilitation,* 2nd ed. Philadelphia, W. B. Saunders Company, 1971.
146. Krusen, F. H., F. J. Kottke, and P. Ellwood, (Eds.): *Handbook of Physical Medicine and Rehabilitation,* 2nd ed. Philadelphia, W. B. Saunders Company, 1971.
147. Kurth, J. S.: Correct application of the Thomas splint and Pearson attachment. *Nursing '73,* 3:20, July 1973.
148. Lane, P.: A mother's confession: Home care of a toddler in a spica cast. What it's really like. *American Journal of Nursing,* 71:2141, Nov. 1971.
149. Larson, C. B., and M. Gould: *Orthopedic Nursing,* 7th ed. St. Louis: C. V. Mosby Co., 1970.
150. Larson, R. L.: Knee injuries in sports. *Hospital Medicine,* 14:57, Feb. 1978.
151. Leadbetter, W. B.: Getting Ahead of the Injury. *Emergency Medicine,* 11:27, June 1979.
152. Leddy, J. P., S. A. Grantham, and F. E. Stinchfield: Hip-mold arthroplasty and postoperative infection. *Journal of Bone and Joint Surgery.* 53-A:37, Jan. 1971.
153. Lichtenstein, L.: *Bone Tumors,* 4th ed. St. Louis: C. V. Mosby Company, 1972.
154. Lienohn, W.: Factors related to hamstring strains. *Journal of Sports Medicine and Physical Fitness,* 18:71, Mar. 1978.
155. Lightfoot, R. W., Jr.: Therapy of rheumatoid disease. *American Family Physician,* 19:186, Mar. 1979.
156. Linscheid, R. L., and R. H. Cofield: Total shoulder arthoplasty: Experimental but promising. *Geriatrics,* 31:64, Apr. 1976.
157. Lockie, L. M.: Gout: A look at current therapy. *Consultant,* 18:27, June 1977.
158. Love-Mignogna, S.: Scoliosis. *Nursing '77,* 7:50, May 1977.
159. Lowell, J. L.: Complications of total hip replacement. *From* Proceedings of the Hip Society: *The Hip.* St. Louis: C. V. Mosby Company, 1976.
160. Lowman, E.: Connective tissue diseases. *In* Krusen, F. H., F. J. Kottke, and P. M. Ellwood, Jr.: *Handbook of Physical Medicine and Rehabilitation,* 2nd ed. Philadelphia, W. B. Saunders Company, 1971.
161. Marmor, L., and J. Treace: A new balanced suspension. *Clinical Orthopaedics and Related Research,* 85:146, June 1972.
162. May, C. M.: Wheelchair patient for a day. *American Journal of Nursing,* 73:650, April 1973.
163. McCarthy, B., et al.: Subclinical fat embolism: A prospective study of 50 patients with extremity fractures. *The Journal of Trauma,* 13:9, Jan. 1973.
164. McEwen, C.: Editorial: Synovectomy and the rehabilitation of the patient with rheumatoid arthritis. *Journal of Bone and Joint Surgery,* 53-A:621, June 1971.
165. McMicken, D. B.: After the emergency. *Emergency Medicine,* 11:63, April 1979.
166. McNamee, J.: Everuse injury of the legs. *Medical Journal of Australia,* 1:426, April 1978.
167. Meek, R. N., B. Woodruff, and D. B. Allardyce: Source of fat macroglobules in fractures of the lower extremity. *The Journal of Trauma,* 12:432, May 1972.
168. Memmler, R. L., and R. B. Rada: *The Human Body in Health and Disease,* 3rd ed. Philadelphia: J. B. Lippincott Company, 1970.
169. Meyers, M. H., D. B. McNelly, and K. Nelson: Total hip replacement — a team effort. *American Journal of Nursing,* 78:1485, Sept. 1978.
170. Micheli, L. J., M. A. Magim, and R. Rouvales: The patient with scoliosis. Surgical management and nursing care. *American Journal of Nursing,* 79:1599, Sept. 1979
171. Micheli, L. J., M. D. Skolnick and J. E. Hall: Supracondylar fractures of the humerus in children. *American Family Physician,* 19:100, Mar. 1979.
172. Millar, A. P.: Acute muscle injuries of the leg. *Medical Journal of Australia,* 1:264, Mar. 1978.
173. Millar, A. P.: Acute recreational injuries. *Australia Family Physician,* 7:379, April 1978.
174. Miller, B. F., and C. B. Keane: *Encyclopedia and Dictionary of Medicine and Nursing,* 2nd ed. Philadelphia. W. B. Saunders Company, 1978.
175. Myskiu, P. M., et al.: The attachment of tendon to bone. *Journal of the American Podiatry Association,* 68:308, May 1978.
176. Nagler, W.: Tennis elbow. *American Family Physician,* 16:95, July 1977.
177. Naylor, R., R. Hamdy, and J. Paul: Detecting the early stages of osteomalacia with the intravenous vitamin D test. *Geriatrics,* 32:52, Jan. 1977.
178. Nelson, J. P., D. O. Ferris, and J. C. Ivins: The cast syndrome. *Postgraduate Medicine,* 42:457, Dec. 1967.
179. Neustadt, D. H.: Ankylosing spondylitis. *Postgraduate Medicine,* 61:124, Jan. 1977.
180. Nice, W.: An increasing problem — fat embolism syndrome: Diagnosis and treatment. *Journal of the Kansas Medical Society,* 69:45, Feb. 1968.
181. Nice, W., A. Huaman, and I. Young: Fat embolism syndrome: Diagnosis and treatment. *AORN Journal,* 17:197, Jan. 1973.
182. Nicholas, J. A.: Ankle injuries in athletes. *Orthopedic Clinics of North America,* 5:153, Jan. 1974.
183. Nickel, V., J. Kristy, and L. McDaniel: Physical Therapy for rheumatoid arthritis. *Physical Therapy,* 45:198, Mar. 1965.
184. Norwood, L. A., et al.: Anterior shoulder pain in baseball pitchers. *American Journal of Sports Medicine,* 6:103, May-June 1978.
185. Nursing Care of the Patient in the O. R. Sommerville, N. J.: Ethicon, Inc., 1973.
186. O'Brien, J. P., et al.: Halo pelvic traction. *Journal of Bone and Joint Surgery,* 53-B:217, May 1971.
187. O'Donoghue, D. H.: *Treatment of Injuries to Athletes,* 3rd ed. Philadelphia: W. B. Saunders Co., 1976.
188. O'Duffy, J. D.: Psoriatic arthritis. *Postgraduate Medicine,* 61:165, Jan. 1977.
189. Orava, S., et al.: Stress fractures caused by physical exercise. *Acta Orthopaedic Scandinavica,* 49:19, Feb. 1978.
190. O'Riordan, C., et al.: A prospective study of wound infections on an orthopedic service. *Clinical Orthopaedics and Related Research,* 87:188, Sept. 1972.
191. Peck, B.: Malignancy that looks like arthritis: How to tell the difference. *Consultant,* 18:136, Oct. 1978.
192. Peltier, L.: The diagnosis and treatment of fat embolism. *Journal of Trauma,* 11:661, Aug. 1971.
193. Perez, C. A., J. S. Bradfield, and H. C. Morgan: Management of pathologic features. *Cancer,* 29:684, Mar. 1972.
194. Programmed instruction. Teaching a patient how to use crutches. *American Journal of Nursing,* 79:1111, June 1979.
195. Ramer, S., and R. Bluestone: Colitic arthropathies. *Postgraduate Medicine,* 61:141, Jan. 1977.

196. Ranalls, J.: Crutches and walkers. *Nursing '72,* 2:21, Dec. 1972.
197. Ring, P. A.: Replacement of the hip joint. *Annals of the Royal College of Surgeons of England,* 48:344, June 1971.
198. Robinson, W. D.: Diseases of the joints. *In* Beeson, P. B., and W. McDermott, (Eds.): *Cecil-Loeb Textbook of Medicine,* 13th ed. Philadelphia, W. B. Saunders Co., 1971.
199. Roe, R. L.: Some guidelines to the new drugs for rheumatic diseases. *Consultant,* 17:21, July 1977.
200. Ryan, A. J.: Traumatic injuries: Office treatment of strain. *Postgraduate Medicine,* 61:215, Mar. 1977.
201. Salter, R. B.: *Textbook of Disorders and Injuries of the Musculoskeletal Ssystem.* Baltimore: Williams and Wilkins, 1970.
202. Schaller, J.: Juvenile rheumatoid arthritis. *Postgraduate Medicine,* 61:177, Jan. 1977.
203. Schatzinger, L. H., E. M. Brower, and C. L. Nash, Jr.: Spinal fusion: Emotional stress and adjustment. *American Journal of Nursing,* 79:1608, Sept. 1979.
204. Scher, A. T.: Spinal cord injuries due to diving accidents. *Journal of Sports Medicine and Physical Fitness,* 18:67, Mar. 1978.
205. Scherbel, A. L.: Nonsteroidal antiinflammatory drugs. *Postgraduate Medicine,* 63:69, Mar. 1978.
206. Schmeisser, G. J.: *A Clinical Manual of Orthopedic Traction Techniques.* Philadelphia: W. B. Saunders Co., 1963.
207. Schneider, F. R.: *Handbook for the Orthopaedic Assistant.* St. Louis: C. V. Mosby Co., 1972.
208. Schur, P. H.: Systemic lupus erythematosus. *In* Beeson, P. B., W. McDermott, and J. B. Wyngaarden (Eds.): *Cecil Textbook of Medicine,* 15th ed. Philadelphia, W. B. Saunders Co., 1979.
209. Schwaid, M. C.: Advice to Arthritics: Keep Moving. *American Journal of Nursing,* 78:1708, Oct. 1978.
210. Sheridan, R., R. Chiroff, and E. Freedman: Operative and Non operative treatment of rachitic lower extremity deformities. *Clinical Orthopedics,* 116:66, 1976.
211. Siegel, I. M.: Jogger's heel. *Journal of the American Medical Association,* 206:2899, Dec. 1968.
212. Sim, F. H.: Replacement of tumor-destroyed bone with joint implants. *Geriatrics,* 31:73, April 1976.
213. Simon, D. J.: Muscle pain syndromes. Part II. *American Journal of Physical Medicine,* 55:15, 1976.
214. Smith, N. J.: The pediatrician and sports medicine. *Pediatrics,* 61:497, Mar. 1978.
215. Sodeman, W. A., and Sodeman, W. A., Jr.: *Pathologic Physiology: Mechanisms of Disease,* 5th ed. Philadelphia: W. B. Saunders Co., 1974.
216. Soika, C. V.: Combatting osteoporosis. *American Journal of Nursing,* 73:1193, July 1973.
217. Spruck, M.: Gold therapy. *American Journal of Nursing,* 79:1246, July 1979.
218. Stauffer, R. N.: Total hip replacement: First year's experience. *Archives of Surgery,* 103:668, Dec. 1971.
219. Steinbrocker, O., and D. Neustadt: *Aspiration and Injection Therapy in Arthritis and Musculoskeletal Disorders.* New York: Harper and Row, 1972.
220. Stern, M., and S. S. Grant: Fifty total hip replacements. *Clinical Orthopaedics and Related Research,* 86:79, July-Aug. 1972.
221. Stiles, P. J.: Surgical treatment of rheumatoid arthritis. *Nursing Mirror,* 126:20, June 1968.
222. Stillman, M. J.: Experiences in clinical problem solving. Mike J.: A young man with a fractured femur. Part 1: Traction. *RN,* 41:63, July 1978.
223. Stillman, M. J.: Part II: Spica cast. *RN,* 41:61, Aug. 1978.
224. Stillwell, G. K.: Therapeutic heat and cold. *In* Krusen, F. H., F. J. Kottke, and P. M. Ellwood, Jr.: *Handbook of Physical Medicine and Rehabilitation,* 2nd ed. Philadelphia, W. B. Saunders Co., 1971.
225. Stright, P. A.: How to help the patient with a dislocated shoulder. *American Journal of Nursing,* 79:666, April 1979.
226. Suiter, R. D., and A. J. Bianco, Jr.: Fractures of the femoral shaft. *Journal of Trauma,* 11:238, Mar. 1971.
227. Swanson, A. B.: Disabling arthritis at the base of the thumb. *Journal of Bone and Joint Surgery,* 54-A:456, April 1972.
228. Swanson, A. B.: Flexible implant arthroplasty for arthritic finger joints. *Journal of Bone and Joint Surgery,* 54-A:435, April 1972.
229. Swanson, A. B.: Implant arthroplasty for the great toe. *Clinical Orthopaedics and Related Research,* 85:75, June 1972.
230. Swezey, R. L., and T. M. Spiegel: Evaluation and treatment of local musculoskeletal disorders in elderly patients. *Geriatrics,* 34:56, Jan. 1979.
231. Talbott, J. H.: Gout. *Medical Clinics of North America,* 54:431, Mar. 1970.
232. Talbott, J. H.: Gouty arthritis and hyperuricemia. *Hospital Medicine,* 13:44, June 1977.
233. Talbott, J. H.: Treating gout. Successful methods of prevention and control. *Postgraduate Medicine,* 63:175, May 1978.
234. Taylor, A. R., and B. M. Ansell: Arthrography of the knee before and after synovectomy for rheumatoid arthritis. *Journal of Bone and Joint Surgery,* 54-B:110, Feb. 1972.
235. Testa, N. N.: The troubles with tendons and bursae. *Emergency Medicine,* 9:84, Nov. 1977.
236. Testa, N. N.: Surgery for arthritis: What can — and cannot — be done. *Consultant,* 18:142, Nov. 1978.
237. Thomas, B. J., and C. Alexander: Psychological aspects of physical trauma. *AORN Journal,* 15.45, Feb. 1972.
238. *The Traction Handbook.* Warsaw, Ind.: Zimmer Manufacturing Company, 1971.
239. Turner, R.: Aspirin and newer anti-inflammatory agents in rheumatoid arthritis. *American Family Physician,* 16:111, July 1977.
240. Tyler, H. R.: Polymyositis and dermatomyositis. *In* Beeson, P. B., W. McDermott, and J. B. Wyngaarden (Eds.): *Cecil Textbook of Medicine,* 15th ed. Philadelphia, W. B. Saunders Co., 1979.
241. Urist, M. R.: Bone morphodifferentiation and tumorigenesis. *Perspectives in Biology and Medicine,* 22:S89, Winter 1979, Part 2.
242. Vidt, L., et al.: Fatigue fractures; A literature review. *Journal of the American Podiatry Association,* 68:326, May 1978.
243. Wagner, M. M.: Assessment of patients with multiple injuries. *American Journal of Nursing,* 72:1882, Oct. 1972.
244. Wanacukapunt, S., Y. Lertratanakul, and H. M. Rubinstein: Effect of fenoprofen calcium on acute gouty arthritis. *Arthritis Rheumatism,* 19:933, 1976.
245. Webb, J. K.: The orthopedic management and rehabilitation of patients with multiple skeletal injuries. *Orthopedic Clinics of North America,* 9:569, April 1978.
246. Wiesman, H. J., Jr., et al.: Total hip replacement with and without osteotomy of greater trochanter. Clinical and biomechanical comparisons in the same pa-

tients. *Journal of Bone Joint Surgery,* 60:203, Mar. 1978.

247. Wilkins, K. E.: Youthful bone and muscle. *Emergency Medicine,* 11:235, Mar. 1979.

248. Yoslow, W.: The painful hip — helping the handicapped cope. *Geriatrics,* 34:27, Aug. 1979.

249. Yü, T.: Nephrolithiasis in patients with gout. *Postgraduate Medicine,* 63:164, May 1978.

UNIT XXI

NURSING PEOPLE EXPERIENCING DISTURBANCES OF THE INTEGUMENTARY SYSTEM

INTRODUCTION AND STUDY GUIDE

The integumentary system is the exterior organ that is commonly taken for granted, but is vital to our emotional and physical health. Skin care has long been the responsibility of nurses, and prevention of skin disease and maintenance of its integrity are important functions that the nurse may assume. In this unit, major problems of the skin and its appendages are presented, including major and minor skin disorders. Trauma is only briefly discussed, except for burns. (See discussions of skin trauma in Chapter 95.) The breast as a modified sebaceous gland is considered part of this system, and carcinoma of the breast is presented in some detail.

Basically, this unit covers:

- Review of the pertinent anatomy and physiology
- The natural history of the presenting disturbances
- Common treatments
- Nursing concerns

The nurse's role involves understanding the above aspects, for the purpose of referring patients to a doctor for early care if indicated by thorough assessment; preventing complications or recurrences; assisting patients in understanding and following the medical regimen; and helping plan personalized care. Nurses in schools, industry, emergency rooms, doctors' offices, and outpatient clinics and those on home visits are particularly likely to be a patient's first contact with the health care system. Many patients present minor concerns to a nurse, which they do not believe are "important enough" to take up a doctor's time. The nurse, therefore, must be knowledgeable in this early assessment.

As well as assessment, nurses are involved in (a) promoting comfort and relief for those experiencing skin disorders, e.g., reducing itching; (b) avoiding and eliminating preventable skin conditions, e.g., decubitus ulcers and venereal disease–related skin problems; (c) encouraging and supporting patients through sometimes lengthy treatments for skin disorders; and (d) offering understanding and support to those for whom skin problems are of emotional concern; e.g., for patients who consider their disorders dirty, embarrassing, or as reflecting on personal hygiene.

Nurses assuming *expanded roles* may have more responsibility for management in selected areas or settings.

While studying this unit, you will be working toward achieving the objectives in the following four topics:

Skin Disorders

1. Explain to others the following facts about how skin integrity is maintained:

   a. that the skin has a normal ecologic flora
   b. that there is more flora in moist intertriginous areas
   c. that bacteria grow less readily on a dry surface
   d. that any break in skin integrity results in proliferation of organisms

2. Adjust skin cleaning to each patient's age and condition; realize that excessive soap destroys the protective film of the skin.
3. Explain to others the causes, symptoms, course, and common treatment of skin disorders.
4. Explain to others proper care of hair and nails.
5. Counsel others about the need for early, gentle, meticulous attention to any skin condition, about the reasons for not using other people's medications, and about the reasons for not switching treatments rapidly.
6. Assess skin disorders and refer a potentially serious condition for early medical care.
7. Help patients understand and follow treatment.
8. Involve patients in self-care and teach them how to monitor their own disorders.
9. Assist patients with problems of discomfort and disfigurement.
10. Describe skin conditions in appropriate, precise medical terms.
11. Manage selected conditions, with specialized preparation in this role.
12. Recognize special dermatologic problems influenced by age, race, sex, and environmental conditions.

Trauma

1. Assess wounds for further referral.
2. Suture minor wounds or assist a doctor with suturing.

Burns

1. Understand major problems of emergency care for burns.
2. Describe to others the rationale for burn wound care, prevention of infection, and skin grafting.
3. Observe early signs of complications such as burn shock, acidosis, Curling's ulcers, and infection.
4. Establish a nursing regimen for caring for people with burns.
5. Realize the importance of involving significant others and the care team in the care of severely burned patients.

Cancer of the Breasts

1. Recognize risk factors contributing to breast cancer and utilize this information in patient and public education.
2. Realize the importance of early detection of lumps and utilize every opportunity to teach women about breast self-examination.
3. Recognize and assist with the profound psychologic problems that may arise in connection with breast cancer — from breast biopsy through terminal cancer.
4. Realize the importance of arm edema following breast surgery and be able to prevent this complication.
5. Explain rationale for treating advanced mammary cancer.

CHAPTER 79

DISORDERS OF THE SKIN AND ITS APPENDAGES

by Rosemary Pittman, M.S., C.R.N., F.N.P.

INTRODUCTION

The extent of skin disorders is difficult to determine, because many people with skin disease do not seek medical care but rather treat their problems with home remedies and patent medicine. Because of their chronicity and lack of dramatic complications, disorders of the integumentary system may go relatively unnoticed except by the person who has them.

Skin disorders are common. About 10 to 15 per cent of all patients seen by physicians are seeking relief from skin disorders. An estimated 60.6 million people between the ages of 1 and 74 years have one or more significant skin diseases.[114] Common skin disorders are allergic skin reaction, acne, warts, and moles.[75, 110] Skin diseases account for 0.51 per cent of deaths from all causes, and neoplastic conditions account for roughly half these deaths. Infectious skin diseases account for the bulk of the rest. Dermatitis causes considerable occupational disability, a high percentage of workmen's compensations claims are awarded for skin disease. The economic cost of skin disease is considerable.

Consultation for acne is one of the most common reasons for seeking medical care. Having a smooth unblemished skin is valued in our culture. Millions of dollars are spent every year on cosmetic preparations. Cutaneous stimulation may play an important part in psychologic development, and the individual with a chronic skin disease may be deprived of this means of human relating.

Many skin diseases are overtreated and mistreated. Nurses must be aware of those conditions that are best treated by a dermatologist. Minor vesicular eruptions between the toes and scabies are examples of conditions that can safely be treated by nurses with a doctor's approval or consultation. Increasingly, paraprofessionals work with patients. Nurses may spend considerable time teaching these individuals about the care and treatment of minor skin disorders, prevention and first aid.

People are frequently concerned about the causes of rashes and eruptions and the handling of insect bites, sunburn, "cold" sores, acne, damaged nails, falling hair, etc. Often nurses have to decide when cuts should be referred for suturing. Some nurses do minor suturing in health stations and outpatient clinics and in isolated areas.

Important areas to be remembered in the care of skin disease are the following:

1. The importance of seeking early referral to a dermatologist in order to get started on a good management program if the disease is chronic or if the condition does not improve under minor simple treatment.
2. The individual with a skin condition needs careful directions and reinforcement concerning the importance of using the recommended treatment as directed, and promptly returning or reporting to the nurse or doctor if the expected progress does not ensue. It is a good idea to have the patient repeat to you exactly how to manage the treatment to be sure the directions are understood, and to caution the patient not to try anything else. It is also necessary to find out whether the patient will have all the necessary ingredients for carrying out the treatment. Help the patient with any emotional feelings connected with the treatment. Demonstration is always desirable.
3. Serious skin diseases are frequently chronic problems, and principles of chronic disease management apply to these diseases. The management has to be integrated into the total life pattern, and patients need to find their own unique ways of managing their disorders.
4. Nurses are in an especially favorable position to teach the importance of good skin care.

OVERVIEW OF THE INTEGUMENTARY SYSTEM

To understand the numerous disorders of the integumentary system and the rationale for nursing actions related to them it is important to understand the anatomy and physiology of the skin and its appendages (Fig. 79–1.)

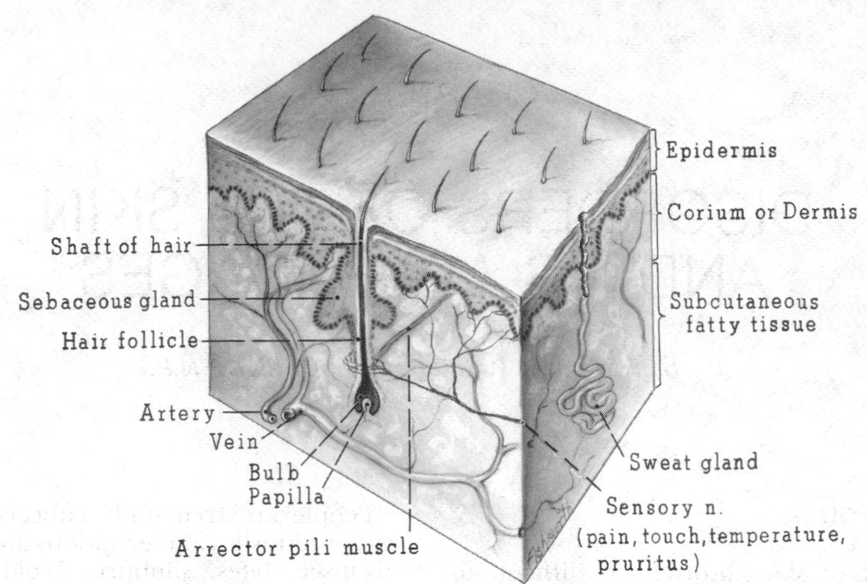

Figure 79–1. Three-dimensional view of the skin. (From Jacob, S. W., C. A. Francone, and W. J. Lossow: *Structure and Function in Man*, 4th ed. Philadelphia: W. B. Saunders Co., 1978, p. 77.)

Anatomy and Physiology

The skin consists of two main parts — the *epidermis* and the *dermis*. The dermis is bound to underlying organs by a layer of loose connective and fatty tissues, called the *subcutaneous tissue*. The skin of an average adult weighs about 6 to 9 pounds, is 0.5 to 5.0 mm. thick, and covers about 18 square feet of surface area.[3, 50]

THE EPIDERMIS

The epidermis is a dry stratified squamous epithelium. The epidermis, the outer layer of the skin, is uniformly thin (0.06 to 0.1 mm.) over most of the body, except on the scalp, the palms, and the soles.[78] Two cell types, *melanocytes* and *keratinocytes*, make up the majority of the epidermal cells. The epidermis consists of four or five layers, although the names of the layers differ slightly among various classification systems. Basically, from superficial to deepest, the following layers can be identified.

Stratum corneum (also termed *horny* or *cornified* layer). The outermost layer of the epidermis, consisting of dead, keratinized cells.

Stratum lucidum. A thin, transparent layer seen in the thicker skin of the palms and soles.

Stratum granulosum (the *granular cell* layer).

Stratum spinosum (the *prickle* layer). In some classifications, this layer is included with the next deeper layer and called the *stratum malpighii*.

Stratum germinativum (the *basal cell* layer). The deepest layer of the skin, which must remain intact for the epidermis to be able to regenerate.

The cells in the basal layer evolve into cells of the cornified layer as they make their way to the surface. Basal keratinocytes are the only cells able to synthesize DNA and are responsible for mitotic turnover.

The skin is a tough protective covering. It acts as a barrier to the loss of water and electrolytes, providing a homeostatic internal environment for other organs. It is resistant to electrical current and corrosive chemicals. Normal mitotic activity and desquamation insure replacement of the epidermis about every 28 days.

It is important for the stratum corneum to maintain plasticity. The ability of the outer layer of the epidermis to absorb water varies directly with the humidity. This layer can absorb four times its weight when submerged in water. The flexibility of the skin depends on maintenance of a proper water content in the outer layer. Fluctuations in the water content of the outer layers are compensated for by changes in interstitial water content of underlying tissues. Water continually moves through the skin to the environment; this is called *insensible perspiration.* In a 24-hour period, 500 to 600 ml. of body water will escape in this way.

The skin barrier is easily permeated by gases, with the exception of carbon monoxide. Substances penetrate the skin more easily with increased skin temperature, in lipid solutions, and with increased water content of the epidermis. These facts can be applied by the nurse to enhance penetration of the skin by topical drugs.

Differences in the amount of *pigment* in the skin of various groups of people result from the rate and quality of production of melanin. A melanocyte-stimulating hormone (MSH) has been isolated from the pituitary gland.

The epidermis invaginates into the dermis and forms the following appendages (Fig. 79–

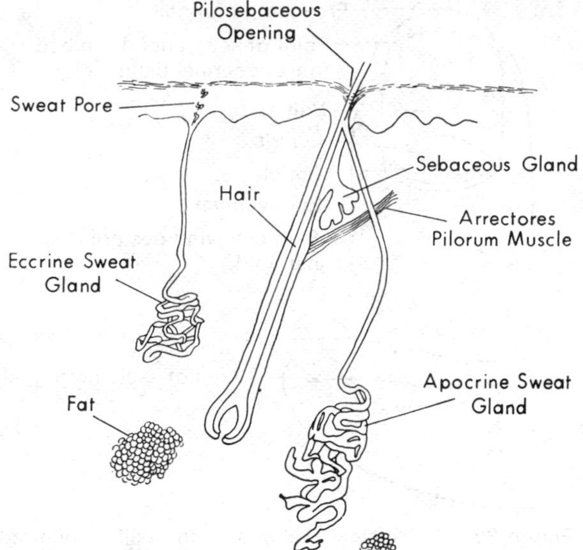

Figure 79–2. Diagram of skin and epidermal appendages. (From Lewis, G. M., and Wheeler, C. E., Jr.: *Practical Dermatology,* 3rd ed. Philadelphia: W. B. Saunders Co., 1967.)

2): (1) the eccrine glands, (2) the apocrine glands, (3) the sebaceous glands, (4) the hair, and (5) the nails.

Eccrine Sweat Glands. The eccrine sweat glands are peculiar to humans. They are found in all areas of the skin except the inner surface of the prepuce, the glans penis, the nail beds, the ear drums, and the margin of the lips. These glands are most numerous on the palms and soles, about 3000 per square inch, and decrease in concentration from the head and neck to the extremities. They are more abundant than sebaceous glands or hair. The total number of eccrine sweat glands on the human body is estimated to be several million.

The chief components of sweat are the following: water, sodium, potassium, chloride, glucose, urea, and lactate. Their concentrations vary among individuals and change with a person's rate of perspiration. Sweat glands are under sympathetic control and are brought into activity by the heat-regulating center. Eccrine glands in hands and palms do not ordinarily produce sweat except with emotional stimulation, although with intense heat even they will sweat.[111]

Sweating is a major function of the skin because of its role in the regulation of body temperature by evaporative cooling. Each liter of evaporated sweat is capable of removing 540 cal. of heat from the body.[64] Under dry hot conditions, a man may lose 6 liters of sweat in 24 hours (average 1.5 liters).[111] Abnormality of sweating plays an important role in cystic fibrosis. These patients cannot tolerate salt restriction or periods of excessive sweating, because of the high concentration of sodium in the sweat.[64]

Apocrine Glands. The *apocrine glands* are large sweat glands whose ducts open into hair follicles to which they are attached and rarely open onto the surface of the skin, as do the eccrine glands. They are found in the axillae, anogenital areas, nipple, and areola, but do not develop fully until puberty. Apocrine glands in the axilla have no known function. They are also found in the external ear, producing wax, and on the eyelids, where cystic blockage may occur.[105] They are adrenergic, respond to emotional stimulation, and produce milky and distinctly alkaline sweat.

Sebaceous Glands. *Sebaceous glands* develop from, and are continuous with, hair follicles which may or may not possess a hair (Fig. 79–3). Occasionally they open directly onto the skin surface. Their secretion, *sebum,* is lipid-rich and probably functions as a coating for the skin and nails. The activity of sebaceous glands is probably under hormonal control, being increased by androgens and suppressed by estrogens. *Vernix caseosa,* present at birth, is a sebaceous gland secretion. There are natural changes in the activity of the sebaceous glands during the life cycle. At birth the sebaceous glands are small, whereas by puberty there is an increase in the size of the glands, especially those of the face, chest, and back. After puberty, sebum output remains at a high level until menopause and old age, when the skin tends to return to a preadolescent level. In males, the androgenic hormones of the testes are responsi

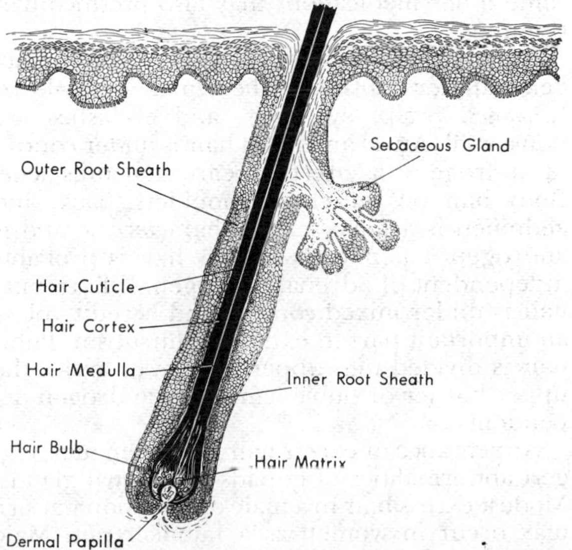

Figure 79–3. Diagram of pilosebaceous apparatus. (From Lewis, G. M., and C. E. Wheeler, Jr.: *Practical Dermatology,* 3rd ed.)

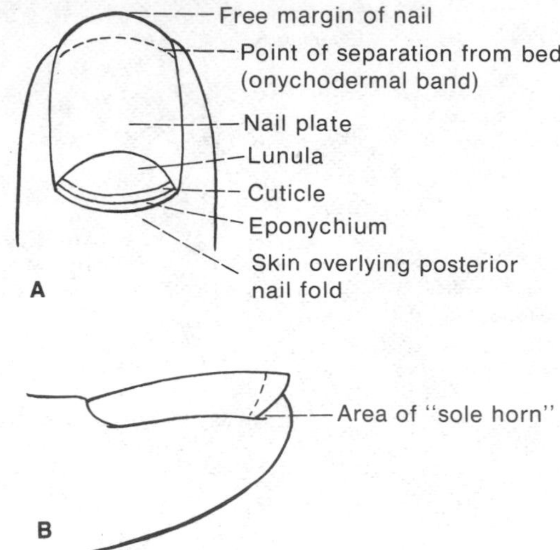

Figure 79–4. Principal features of the nail. A. Viewed from above. B. Viewed from the side. (Redrawn from Samman, P. D.: *The Nails in Disease.* Springfield, Ill.: Charles C Thomas, 1972, p. 6.)

ble for the increase of sebum at puberty. With increasing age, the androgenic output continues to fall and the production of sebum decreases. In females, androgenic hormones are produced by both the ovaries and the adrenals.[51]

Hair. Hair is a keratinized structure that grows out of a tubular invagination of the epidermis called a *hair follicle.* Most of the hair is associated with sebaceous glands; this combination is spoken of as the *pilosebaceous unit.* (Refer to Fig. 79–3.) Hair goes through cyclic changes: growth (anagen), atrophy (catagen), and rest (telogen).[51] Healthy human hair on the scalp has a growth period of 2 to 5 years. Cutting or shaving has no effect on coarseness or growth of the hair. Melanocytes are present in the bulb of the hair and are responsible for its *pigmentation.* Whitening of the hair is due to failure of pigment formation in replacement hairs. Sudden whitening through fear is not proved. Hair follicle muscles are immediately beneath the sebaceous glands and, when innervated by adrenergic fibers, cause "*goose bumps.*" This is a vestigial function, which serves fur-bearing animals by increasing their thermal insulation. There are about 100,000 follicles on the human scalp; they grow in a mosaic pattern. Old hairs are lost at the rate of about 50 to 100 a day. The health of the hair depends on the health of the individual. The visible hair is a dead structure.

After pregnancy, a shortening of the active growing cycle occurs, and the hair returns to the resting stage, which results in temporary thinning of the scalp hair. Oral contraceptives and some other medications may also produce hair thinning.

Hair may be classified as either being or not being under control of the female or male *sex hormones.* Scalp, eyebrows, and eyelashes are nonsexual. Aural and nasal hair is under control of androgens, as are the beard and mustache. Body hair on the chest, shoulders, back, and abdomen is a male sexual characteristic and is androgen dependent. Axillary hair is probably independent of adrenal androgen.[111] Extremity hair is under mixed control, and heredity plays an important part in extremity hirsutism. Pubic hair is divided into upper and lower areas, the upper border of pubic hair being androgen dependent.

Appearance of excess hair in women may suggest abnormalities of gonads or adrenal glands. Modest excess hair in a male distribution pattern may occur in women as a familial trait. Male pattern baldness (notable decrease in the number of hairs) is a sex-linked dominant trait. The typical distribution of loss of hair on the crown and recession at the sides in front may also occur in women as a normal part of the aging process, although it seldom leads to baldness.

Nails. Human *nails* are hard keratinized epidermal structures. The *nail plate* grows continuously and, under normal conditions, persists through life. It is usually replaced if injured, unless matrix is destroyed, in which case it is permanently lost and replaced by the stratum corneum of the epidermis. If the *matrix* is damaged, the nail grows in a distorted manner or is split. The body of the nail, the nail plate, grows forward from the *nail fold* and covers the *nail bed.* (See Figs. 79–4 and 79–5.)

The average growth rate of nails is 0.1 mm. daily. It takes 100 to 150 days for a fingernail to reproduce itself and about three times as long for a toenail to do so.

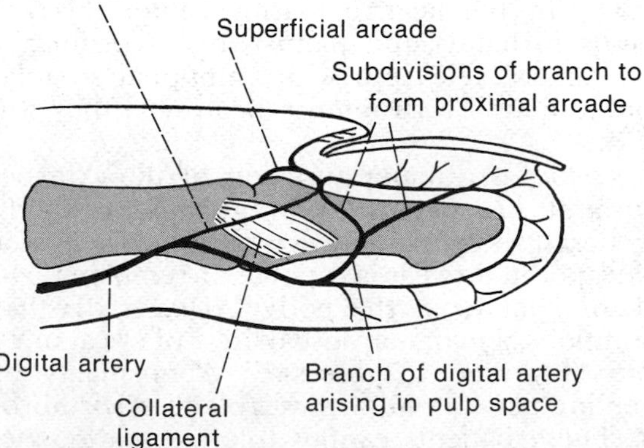

Figure 79–5. Arterial blood supply to nail and nail bed. (Redrawn from Samman, P. D.: *The Nails in Disease.* Springfield, Ill.: Charles C Thomas, 1972, p. 7.)

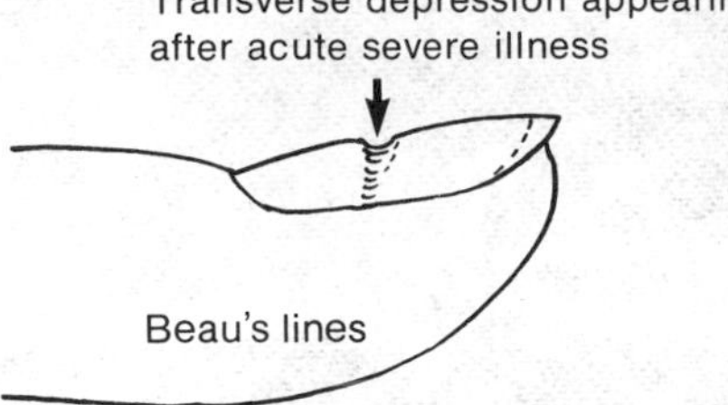

Figure 79–6. Beau's lines. (Redrawn from Bates, B.: *A Guide to Physical Examination.* Philadelphia: J. B. Lippincott Co., 1974.)

There is individual variation in nail growth. Growth may be temporarily halted by many systemic disorders, which may result in transverse grooves or *Beau's lines* (Fig. 79–6).

Nails function to protect the toes and fingers, especially to protect the delicate sense of touch in the ends of the fingers. Also, nails help a person pick up small objects, and they provide clues to internal disorders.

DERMIS

The *dermis* is the connective tissue layer of the skin, which supports the epidermis and separates it from the cutaneous adipose tissue. The dermis is divided into papillary and reticular areas. It serves as a source of nutrition for the epidermis. The *papillary part* interdigitates with the epidermis and contains blood vessels and some nerve elements. The *reticular part* contains connective tissue fibers (elastin and collagen), cellular elements, blood vessels, nerves and lymphatics. Collagen, a fibrous protein, forms the greatest part of the substance of the dermis. Although it is present in every organ system, approximately one half of the total collagen in the body is in the skin.[64, 105]

Apart from sensory information derived from sight and hearing, the major part of our *sensory apparatus* is in the skin. The sensory fibers responsible for pain, touch, and temperature form a complex dermal network. There are four types of sensation: pain, touch, cold and warmth. *Pain* may be caused by physical, chemical, or mechanical stimulation. (See Unit XI.) *Touch* stimuli are received from hair follicles and intervening skin. *Itching* arises from terminal nerve endings close to the skin surface. (Itching does not occur when the epidermis is absent.) *Temperature* sense is probably gained through the free sensory nerve endings in the epidermis.

Bacterial Flora

The human skin harbors various normal bacteria.

> *A damaged area of skin can be a source of entry for infection.*

Some persons have large numbers of resident bacteria on the skin and others have small numbers. The number for the individual remains relatively constant from month to month unless disturbed. The axillae, groin, perineum, and areas of occlusion and intertrigo constantly harbor large numbers. Persons with oily moist skin have a large number of organisms, and more are present on the skin in warm wet weather than in cold dry weather. Body odor is influenced by bacterial flora. Resident gram-positive bacteria operate on apocrine sweat to produce the characteristic odor of the axillae.

Although the skin is constantly bombarded by potentially pathogenic bacteria, infection seldom occurs. Continuous exfoliation of the skin removes organisms. Bathing and rubbing may also remove organisms, as may drying. The normal pH of the skin, which is 4.2 to 5.6, retards the growth of some organisms. Streptococci are more affected than staphylococci by acid pH. Fatty acids in the surface film are fungostatic or bacteriostatic for certain organisms. Certain organisms may exert an inhibitory defense on other organisms, and leukocytes in the epidermis may contribute to defense against invasion by microbes.[64]

*Classification of Skin Lesions**

As nurses assume more responsibility in the primary care setting as being first to see the patient, they need to become increasingly skillful in observing and describing dermatologic conditions. One method of describing lesions is to classify them according to size.[121]

Primary Lesions

1. *Macule:* A flat circumscribed discoloration of the skin or mucous membrane up to 1 cm. in the largest diameter. A macule is not raised above the skin and cannot be felt. If the lesion is greater than 1 cm., it is called a "patch."
2. *Papule:* A raised solid lesion up to 1 cm. in size. Lesions that are greater than 1 cm. in their longest diameter are called "plaques."
3. *Nodule:* A raised solid lesion that can be felt to be deeper in the skin than a papule. If greater than 1 cm. in its longer diameter, it is called a "tumor."
4. *Vesicle:* A fluid-filled superficial elevated lesion of the skin or mucous membrane less than 1 cm. in diameter. If it is larger, it is called a "bulla."

Vesicles may be *unilocular* or *multilocular.* Vesicles from viral diseases tend to have more than one

*Refer also to chapter 15, especially Figure 15–31.

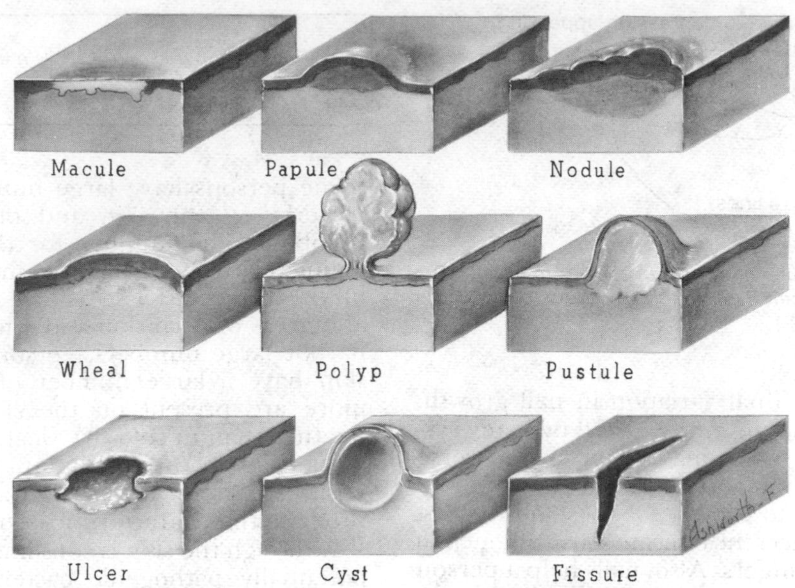

Terms used in connection with abnormalities of the skin:

Macule	A discolored (especially reddened), unelevated spot, on the skin
Papule	A solid elevation of the skin
Nodule	A small node, solid and irregular in form
Wheal	A flat edematous elevation, frequently accompanied by itching
Polyp	A pedunculated or sessile growth
Pustule	An elevation filled with pus
Ulcer	A loss of substance on a cutaneous or mucous surface
Cyst	Any sac, normal or otherwise, especially filled with liquid or semisolid substance—without pus
Fissure	Any cleft or groove

(From Jacob, J. W., C. A. Francone, and J. W. Lossow: *Structure and Function in Man*, 4th ed. Philadelphia: W. B. Saunders Co., 1978, p. 81.)

compartment, e.g., cold sores and chicken pox. When the blister lies within the epidermis, it is said to be *intraepidermal.* When the epidermis is above the blister cavity, the lesion is referred to as *subepidermal.*

5. *Pustule:* A vesicle or bulla containing pus.

6. *Wheal:* Irregularly shaped, elevated, changing lesion of the skin or mucous membrane due to edema.

7. *Telangiectasia:* A fine, often irregular, red line produced by a dilatation of a normally invisible capillary.

Secondary Lesions

1. *Plaques:* Usually result from a confluence of papules developing into flat-topped elevated layers, e.g., psoriasis.

2. *Scales:* Dry or greasy masses of dead tissue from the horny layer. They may be dry and silvery, as in psoriasis, or greasy and yellow as in seborrheic dermatitis.

3. *Erosion:* Frequently a ruptured bulla or vesicle. A moist demarcated depressed area due to loss of partial or full thickness of epidermis.

4. *Ulcer:* Irregularly shaped excavation resulting from necrosis of tissue, including complete loss of dermis. Each ulcer has a shape, floor, base, edge, or secretion. All ulcers leave a scar when they heal.

5. *Scars:* Scars are the result of damage to the dermis.

6. *Lichenification:* A dry leathery thickening of the skin, with increased skin markings. The thickening of the epidermis is a result of excessive rubbing of the skin in chronic dermatitis.

7. *Fissure:* A deep linear split through the epidermis into the dermis.

8. *Atrophy:* Wasting of the epidermis, its appendages, and the dermis.

9. *Hyperkeratosis:* Thickening of the keratin layer of the epidermis.

Diagnosis by Groupings and Characteristics. Lesions may be grouped into classifications in order to assist in diagnosis. Various classification systems may be used. One example would be the following:

1. Eczematous
2. Maculopapular
3. Papulosquamous
4. Pustular
5. Urticarial erythematous
6. Nodular
7. Telangiectatic
8. Atrophic
9. Ulcerative.

After determining which group the lesion belongs to, one can consider the specific disease possibilities within the group. Pustular lesions, for example, might include acne vulgaris, acne rosacea, pyodermas, or pustular psoriasis. Some diseases, of course, may present in several different ways.

Configuration refers to the general form of lesions (Fig. 79–7). The following terms are frequently used in describing configurations:

▶ *Annular, circinate, polycyclic, arciform:* Lesions arranged in rings, circles, arcs or partial rings, e.g., tinea corporis and erythema multiforme.
▶ *Iris lesions:* Concentric rings, typically seen in erythema multiforme.
▶ *Groupings:* Lesions may be grouped, isolated, discrete, solitary, or satellite.
▶ *Borders:* Terms describing a lesion's borders include: irregular, circumscribed, distinct, raised, firm, diffuse, and sharply marginated.
▶ *Linear or striate:* Lesions are in a line, e.g., as in poison ivy. Insect bites may be linear or grouped.
▶ *Zosteriform:* A broad band-like distribution of lesions along a dermatome area.
▶ *Halo effect:* Erythematous area around a central lesion. Lesions may be described as being located on an erythematous or edematous base, e.g., follicular impetigo or sycosis barbae.
▶ *Gyrate:* Twisted in a ring or spiral shape. Urticaria may be annular or gyrate. A *serpiginous* lesion has a much-indented, wavy margin.
▶ *Punctate:* Resembling or marked with points or dots. Bites frequently have a central punctum.
▶ *Reticulated or retiform:* Resembling a network, e.g., livedo reticularis.
▶ *Nummular:* Coinlike. A clinical variety of eczematous dermatitis.
▶ *Polymorphous:* Occurring in several forms.
▶ *Symmetrical or asymmetrical:* Lesion may be located on one extremity only or on one side of the body, or on both.
▶ *Vegetating lesions:* Those growing on the skin in uneven, fleshy, soft tufts.

NURSING FUNCTIONS IN SKIN DISEASES

The extent of nursing actions depends on the setting. In occupational health, school nursing, community health, and in those settings where nurses assume the triage role, their judgments and actions may be very independent. In a dermatologist's office and in the hospital, where the more acute and serious conditions are seen, nurses' functions are more a part of a team therapy effort.

Many skin diseases are chronic, and the knowledgeable concern for and support of patients with these diseases extends over a considerable period of time. In this day of increasing specialization, it is easy to focus on the primary disorder and difficult to maintain an awareness of the person as a whole, experiencing the problem and interacting with the environment.

Assessment

Observation and history are the main tools of assessment. Effective observation requires edu-

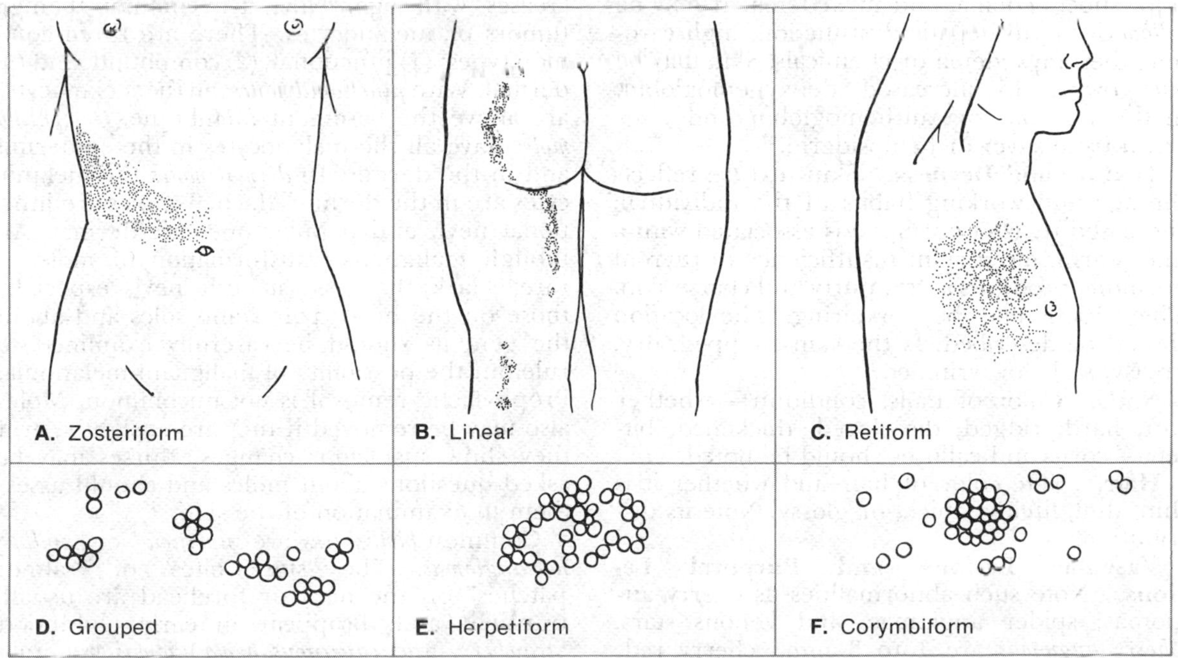

Figure 79–7. Diagnosis of skin lesions by configuration. (Redrawn from Fitzpatrick, T. B., and Walker, S. A.: *Dermatological Differential Diagnosis.*)

cation, awareness, and practice in describing the skin of patients of different ages and with different conditions.

During observation or inspection, explain to the patient the need to inspect the entire skin. Draping can be done sequentially, as you proceed from the patient's head to toes. Skin flexures, intertriginous areas, mucous membranes, hair, and nails are all examined. The importance of good lighting (daylight or adequate artificial lighting) during examination cannot be overemphasized. Have available a flexible clear plastic ruler for measuring the size of the lesion and a small hand lens for closer inspection of individual lesions. Compare each body area with its opposite to determine if lesions are symmetrical. Compare sun-exposed skin areas with non–sun-exposed areas. (Psychosocial and physical assessment is discussed in Chapters 14 and 15.)

OBSERVATIONS

Color of Skin. Skin color depends on skin thickness and on the amount of melanin present in the epidermis. In disease, it is affected by the amount of edema or fibrosis and by either endogenous or exogenous pigmentary substances. Skin appears *reddened* if there is cutaneous vasodilatation or increased hemoglobin concentration. It may appear *white* with anemia, cold, shock, edema, and myxedema. It may be *yellow* owing to hepatic dysfunction, high carotene diet, myxedema or chemicals. Skin may be *blue* owing to increased deoxyhemoglobin, methemoglobin or sulfhemoglobin and *gray-brown* from silver or hemosiderin.[27]

Texture and Dryness. Skin texture reflects the age and working habits of the individual. Increased thyroid hormone is associated with a fine, warm, moist skin; insufficiency of thyroid hormone produces a dry, puffy and coarse skin. The patient may be perspiring. The location should be described. Is the skin chapped, dry, greasy, scaly, or wrinkled?

Nails. Color of nails, condition — whether soft, hard, ridged, discolored, thickened, bitten — corns and calluses should be noted.

Hair. Note color of hair and whether it is thin, dull, lifeless, thick, or glossy. Note its distribution.

Vascular Lesions and Purpural Lesions. Note such abnormalities as cherry angiomas, spider angiomas, and venous stars. *Cherry angiomas* are 1 to 3 mm., cherry red, round, raised areas distributed over the trunk and extremities. While these lesions have no special significance, they may become browner and increase in size and numbers with aging. *Spider angiomas* are small, fiery red, pulsating, arterioles, from which small vessels radiate in a "spider-like" fashion over a reddened area. They blanch on pressure and are generally found in areas drained by the superior vena cava. Spider angiomas most frequently occur with chronic liver disease, although they may also be found in normal individuals and during pregnancy. *Venous stars* are blue lesions resembling a spider. They are not pulsatile, and pressure does not cause blanching. Venous stars are frequently found with varicose veins or on the anterior chest.

Purpura are disorders resulting from bleeding into the skin. The individual tiny red hemorrhages are known as *petechiae.* Petechiae are less than 0.5 mm. in diameter. They may occur because of capillary fragility, vitamin deficiency, severe infection, or blood abnormalities. Petechiae do not disappear with pressure. Larger hemorrhages are referred to as *bruises* or *ecchymoses* and may be due to trauma or to blood abnormalities.

Senile purpura, frequently seen in older persons, usually appear as large ecchymoses on the back of the hands and backs of forearms. Areas also occur on the sides of the face and neck. Senile purpura is a benign phenomenon, probably more often seen on persons having associated diseases, (e.g., rheumatoid arthritis) or on persons who have been on steroid therapy.

Nevi, Scars, and Birthmarks. Nevi, or moles, of all types are very common. Nevi are present in over 95 per cent of all adults, with an average of more than 10 per person.[88, 119] Few nevi are present at birth; their incidence increases with age. Nevi are common benign tumors or melanocytes. There are three common types: (1) junctional, (2) compound, and (3) dermal. With *junctional moles,* all the melanocytes are above the basement membrane. *Compound moles* have all the melanocytes in the epidermis and in the dermis. In *dermal moles* the melanocytes are in the dermis. Macular moles are junctional nevi, and papular ones are dermal. Although malignant transformation of moles is rare, black, hairless, smooth nevi, especially those on the head, palms and soles and about the genitals should be carefully examined to rule out the possibility of malignant melanoma. Prophylactic removal is not uncommon. Moles also may be removed if they are unsightly, or if they show suspicious changes. Nurses may be asked questions about moles and should assess them in examination of the skin.

Common *birthmarks* are *superficial* or *capillary hemangiomas.* The "stork bites" or "salmon patches" on the neck or forehead are usually transient and disappear in early childhood. *Strawberry* and *cavernous hemangiomas* generally grow during the first few months or a year following birth; most of them then slowly regress until they disappear around 6 years of age. Hemangiomas are best treated when the patient is young, because old hemangiomas are recalcitrant to treatment. *Port wine stains* are broad, flat, vascular nevi that are either purplish and thick, or superficial and red. Although they may disappear in the first few months after birth, they ordinarily do not. Often this type of hemangioma may cover one side of the face. No treatment of port wine stains is satisfactory. The affected person may choose to wear some covering cosmetic.

Scars should always be noted and measured. A drawing of the location in the patient's record is sometimes helpful. Be alert to the possibility of malignant changes in old wounds, especially in burn wounds. (Fig. 79–8). Typically, carcinomatous changes in burn wounds appear 20 to 30 years after the original injury. These changes usually occur in lower extremity wounds that have been allowed to heal secondarily without skin grafting. *Scar carcinoma* can also arise in areas of chronic osteomyelitis, chronic cutaneous ulceration of the lower extremity from any cause, and other sinuses or fistula that may have been present for a long time.

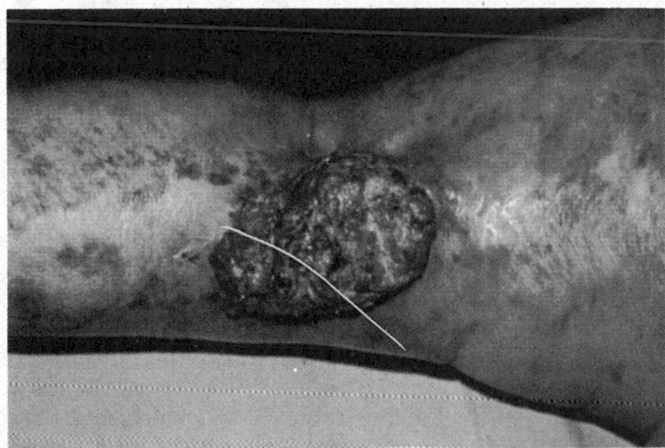

Figure 79–8. Fungating carcinoma of popliteal fossa following a burn 35 years previously. (From Kennedy, T., et al.: Carcinomatous change in old scars. *American Family Physician,* 16:106, July 1977.)

HISTORY

After the description of the current disorder, further history will need to be taken:

Has the patient seen a doctor for the condition and how recently? Was the doctor a dermatologist? What did the doctor say the skin condition was, and what should be done? Did it help?

If the answer to the last question is no, inquire how the patient carried out the doctor's recommendation, and assess a tentative reason for treatment failure. Of course, some patients who do not follow the prescribed medical regimen get better.

Find out what home remedies or other treatments have been used. Many people have items in the medicine cabinet that were used for other conditions, or have gotten some neighborly or drugstore advice. Patients often under- or overtreat skin conditions.

If the diagnosis of the condition is known and the condition is chronic, the nurse assesses the patient's knowledge about the condition and its management, and how the patient feels about the skin disease and treatment. What do the patient's actions concerning treatment imply? Does the patient have any other serious systemic diseases? What tensions are there at home and work? Are there financial problems?

> *Research indicates a relationship between severe skin disease and anxiety.*[33]

It is probably best to elicit the history by following the patient's leads, and then later comparing information obtained with a systematic guide (see Table 79–1) to see if all necessary information has been obtained. Listening carefully to the patient and following tangential leads may give more relevant information than a systematic interview in which the nurse's eyes are on a form rather than on the patient.

TABLE 79–1. DERMATOLOGIC ASSESSMENT HISTORY

Name:

Presenting complaint (Use patient's words):

How does it bother you? (Elicit symptoms and their duration. Use questions such as: When did it start? Does it come and go? Is it wet or dry? Does it itch? Did it spread?)

What have you done for it? (Has the patient seen a doctor? What kind? What did the doctor say the condition was, and what was prescribed? Did it help? If it did not, what did the patient do? Were the doctor's recommendations carried out? What drugstore or home remedies have been used and with what effect? If a doctor has not been seen, what are the reasons?)

Observation of the lesion (Describe distribution, character, and configuration):

General history:

Tensions (Clues may be elicited from the following questions): How do you sleep? Eat? What is your job and how has it been going? How are your relations with the people close to you? What do you do when you aren't working?

General: Do you, your family, or other people close to you have any serious systemic diseases? Record general observations concerning skin, hair, nails.

Always include in the history of a woman whether she regularly practices breast self-examination, and always take time to explain its importance.

Special Diagnostic Techniques

Certain special techniques assist in diagnosing skin lesions. Depending on the clinical situation, nurses may participate in or be responsible for expanding these diagnostic procedures to patients. Infected skin, hair, and nail specimens may be examined under the *microscope* and *cultured* to demonstrate the presence of fungi. The material for direct examination may be placed on a glass slide and covered with a cover slip. A drop of 10 to 40 per cent potassium hydroxide may be added to the specimen. If no fungi can be seen, the slide may be warmed slightly over a low flame in an attempt to make the keratin more transparent. In scrapings from the skin or nails, fungi appear as segmented, branching, threadlike elements — called *myceliae* or *hyphae.* Fungi are best identified by culture. A new dermatologic test medium (DTM) for culturing inhibits the growth of bacteria and nonpathogenic molds and turns red when disease-causing fungi grow in it.[113]

A *Wood's light* may be used to demonstrate the presence of certain fungi. A Wood's light is a source of ultraviolet radiation, and certain disease-producing fungi and bacteria show a characteristic color when viewed under a Wood's light.

Scabies may be identified by scraping or shaving an unopened burrow and examining the specimen under a microscope.

A *punch biopsy* is frequently used to secure tissue for diagnostic examination. The lesion is marked, and the area infiltrated with lidocaine. A small circular punch instrument is used to obtain the tissue sample. Generally, the post-biopsy bleeding stops with the application of local pressure, and the wound does not need to be sutured.

Encouraging Patient Participation in Care

Following assessment, an important nursing activity is to obtain the patient's participation as an equal in planning care. The nurse and doctor, of course, contribute special knowledge and skills; however, the patient should exercise decision-making and responsibility for his or her own care. This means that the patient needs information about the condition and the possible treatments. Patients can learn to monitor their own symptoms and treatment by learning what exacerbates or improves their condition. Many skin diseases are chronic, and the patient is usually hospitalized only if the on-going management fails.

Education. Effective education of the patient requires that a nurse assume the role of learner, since every patient has much to teach the nurse about her or his own condition. With maximum patient input, the nurse can better gauge the patient's needs and provide individualized nursing care. Patients need to know the rationale for treatments and their own role in making the treatments effective.

Realism is always the best policy in dealing with a patient. Giving a patient information about the disease helps eliminate misconceptions — the patient may need to know what the disease is *not,* as well as what it *is.* (For example, a patient may fear that a skin lesion is cancerous, but may be afraid to directly ask whether it is.) Specific directions about self-care are essential. With chronic skin disorders, a patient can easily become discouraged with treatment and may want to change treatments. Part of the nurse's role in education, then, is to explain how long treatment will continue and what results can be reasonably expected.

Psychologic Needs of the Patient. Awareness of the psychologic needs of the patient is particularly important with disorders of the skin, given the values associated with a smooth unblemished skin in our society. A nurse needs to maintain an open mind about the meaning of a patient's behavior. Behavior is meaningful, and inferences must be confirmed with the patient and supported by recorded observation. If patients fail to follow through with treatments, there is a reason or reasons, and these may be tangential to the immediate skin disorder. *Many skin diseases are aggravated by psychologic factors, and some decision must be made as to the importance of these factors to the skin condition, and the possibility of change.* Again change is the prerogative of the patient, upon becoming aware of the possible contributing factors. Slow progress and discouragement with a chronic condition are commonly experienced by people with skin disorders. Encouragement and support from a nurse may help the patient continue treatment.

Serious skin diseases can pose severe psychologic handicaps. The individual who focuses attention excessively upon a chronic skin problem has less energy and desire to invest in relations with other people. An accepting, sympathetic attitude on the part of nurse and doctor is important in assisting such a person with social contacts.

Self-inflicted injuries to the skin, *compulsive ex-*

coriations, and *delusions of parasitosis* (acarophobia) are conditions that generally need psychiatric care. Other conditions such as pruritus vulvae may have a large functional component.

Nursing activities planned to relieve anxiety and reduce stress are highly important in a patient with skin disease. Seeing that the room is cool with the proper amount of humidity, that the patient has sufficient (not excessive) covering is important. It is necessary to find out usual sleep patterns, and to see they are provided. TV or reading material at bedtime may assist with falling asleep. If a patient wishes to talk, the nurse may be able to help the patient work out some stress situation. In all situations, observation as to when scratching occurs or is aggravated is essential.

Disfigurement. The person with a chronic noticeable skin disease may be acutely sensitive and may wish to "hide" or seek isolation. In the hospital, it is advisable to inform roommates, if any, that the disease is not contagious. It may be helpful to have the "right kind" of roommate, e.g., one with hordes of staring visitors would not be acceptable. The nurse needs to be keenly aware of the effect of a roommate on a patient with skin disease. Mutual temperature requirements need to be ascertained. For example, if a patient with a skin disorder is getting cool compresses, a warm room is necessary. A cool environment helps relieve itching. Patients can be therapeutic for each other, and this needs to be carefully considered.

If a patient has severe problems of disfigurement, the nurse needs to be aware of the patient's tendency to seek isolation and avoid others. The nurse thus needs to prepare and provide adequate staffing. Planned friendly interaction cannot be taken for granted. Some staff may provide only essential services. A person who has the expectation of being rejected may behave in a way that causes this to take place. It is important to provide a therapeutic milieu. Seriously disfigured people may benefit from an interactive group or referral to a psychosocial professional. These individuals are going to be stared at, and they have to learn to deal with this problem.

Commercially available opaque coverings may be used to cover some areas of disfigurement. Use of these products should be checked with the physician.

The nurse, faced with the problem of assisting people with a visible disability, may help them realize the existence of other values. Devaluations due to damaged appearance will be lessened to the extent that the person feels surface appearance to be less important than other factors such as kindness, wisdom, effort and cooperativeness. Individuals may be encouraged to recognize their remaining assets and values rather than comparing themselves to others.

Special Nursing Care Problems

Dryness. *Dry skin* is a common problem. Excessive loss of water, not of oil, causes this problem. Fair skin and advancing age predispose to skin dryness. Contributing factors include: excessive bathing, long exposure to low humidity, excessive use of strong soap or solvents, exposure to ultraviolet light, and swimming. In winter months, persons with dry skin should limit baths to only one a week or less. During the summer, bathing twice a week or less is recommended for such persons. Additionally, home heating systems for persons with dry skin should include central humidifiers. Almost all types of air conditioners dehumidify air, and practically all soaps contribute to dry skin. Oil-containing cream or lotion applied to moist skin is likely to be helpful. Tallow and vegetable shortening can also be used for lubricating dry skin. These substances are less expensive than commercial skin lubricating products, and they reduce the chance of an allergic reaction to the perfumes which oils or lotions may contain.

Pruritus. Pruritus is defined as an *unpleasant* cutaneous sensation that produces the desire to scratch. Itching is a common problem of individuals with skin disease.

Stimulation of the nerve endings is brought about by chemical, thermal, mechanical and electrical stimuli, both internal and external. *Even after the initial itching stimuli have subsided, the area seems to remain in a state of increased excitability, and cycles of increasingly violent itching and scratching may develop.* The nerve endings mediating the itching sensation are made more sensitive by increased capillary dilatation. Heat thus increases the symptoms, while cold and vasoconstriction decrease it. Corticotropin and adrenal corticoids have a dramatic effect on itching because of their anti-inflammatory action.

Tissue anoxia due to venous stasis results in itching and is relieved when blood flow becomes adequate. The perception of itching may be elicited not only by peripheral mechanisms but centrally. The perception of itching has an integrating center in the hypothalamus, and the excitability of this center can be influenced by drugs. Itching may be due to the release of histamines or a histamine-like substance, whatever the stimulus may be.

Noting the presence or absence of itching may provide additional information about the presence or absence of certain diseases. Itching may be established when scratch marks are present. Patients' statements need to be evaluated objectively. Like the absence of sleep, the presence of itching may be exaggerated.

Questions useful in assessing itching include: Is your sleep disturbed by itching? Do you wake up at night and find yourself scratching? Can you forget your itching in the daytime when your attention is distracted? Can you stop scratching easily when you make up your mind to do so? Does itching arise only in certain situations, such as warm environment or cold weather?

Itching may be classified as *obligate itching* only if it disturbs the patient's sleep.

Classification of Obligate, Facultative and Non-itching Disorders[100]

A. *Obligate Itching Disorders*
   1. Pediculosis, scabies and related mite infestations, insect bites and other external injuries resulting in urticarial wheals
   2. Contact dermatitis (both primarily toxic and allergic) caused by exposure to chemical or physical agents
   3. Urticaria and toxic eruptions
   4. Neurodermatitis, prurigo, strophulus (miliaria)
   5. Pruritus due to pregnancy, liver diseases, lymphoblastoma, malignant internal neoplasms, kidney insufficiency
   6. Dermatitis herpetiformis
   7. Lichen planus

B. *Facultative Itching Disorders* (with great variety in intensity, largely depending upon the degree of inflammation):
   1. Asteatosis (xerosis, dry skin)
   2. Pruritus due to diabetes
   3. Psoriasis
   4. Seborrheic dermatitis
   5. Pityriasis rosea
   6. Skin infections due to pyogenic organisms and fungi
   7. Local anoxia due to varicose veins, tight clothing, etc.
   8. Mechanical irritation

C. *Non-itching Disorders*
   1. Developmental anomalies
   2. Atrophies, degenerations and hyperplasias
   3. Benign neoplasms
   4. Malignant neoplasms
   5. Dermotropic virus infections
   6. Chronic infectious granulomas (tuberculosis, syphilis, etc.)
   7. Lupus erythematosus
   8. Pigmentary anomalies
   9. Trophic and deficiency diseases
   10. Diseases of sweat glands, sebaceous glands, hair follicles and nails

Of importance for a nurse to remember are the following:

1. There is a marked variation from individual to individual in response to the itch stimulus, as there is to the pain stimulus (see Unit XI).
2. Some skin diseases produce itching and others do not.
3. Itching is worse at night.
4. Areas most frequently affected by itching are around body openings. Pruritus ani, pruritus vulvae, and otitis externa are the most common.
5. The epidermis becomes dry and brittle with age. Most cases of dermatitis in the aged are due to irritants superimposed on dry, already itchy skin. Aged skin dehydrates and chaps more readily than younger skin; the alkalinizing effects of soap aggravate this condition.

General nursing activities to relieve itching fall into the areas of: temperature control, diversionary activities, alleviation of anxiety and stress, and carrying out the treatment regimen. Observation of when a patient scratches, how long and the way he or she scratches may be helpful in setting up some kind of a plan with the patient to reduce trauma from itching. The patient should have nails cut short, and could use a soft brush for stroking, or gentle firm pressure on the itching area if this relieves it.

BATHS. Baths of various kinds may relieve itching:

1. Two tablespoons of liquor carbonis detergens, Zetar, Alma-Tar, Balnetar or Dometar may be added to a tub of water. Tar baths are used chiefly in the treatment of psoriasis.
2. Potassium permanganate bath solution 1:10,000 may be used in infected weeping dermatoses. However, it stains the skin, so it is infrequently used as a general measure.
3. Dial or pHisoHex baths may be used for pyodermas.
4. Oil baths are often helpful if the skin is dry. These can be prepared by adding ½ to 1 oz. of Lubath, Alpha-Keri, Geri bath or Nivea oil to the tub. Eczematous skin may be relieved by mixing ½ cup oilated Aveeno with a bath oil. Mineral oil, olive oil, or peanut oil will also work. One must be careful that the patient is not allergic to any of these mixtures. Bath water should be at body temperature, and the patient should not stay in the tub too long. With oil and colloidal baths, one must be extremely careful that the patient does not slip.
5. Cornstarch baths may be used — ½ to 1 lb. of starch to a pot of very hot water. This makes a gel which is then put into a tub of water in which the patient soaks for about 15 minutes. The bath should be body temperature.
6. Oatmeal bath: Put old-fashioned cereal in a cloth bag and cook it in boiling water for a half hour. Put

cooking water and bag in tub of water. Squeezing the bag presses out soothing gelatinous starches. The commercial preparation Aveeno oatmeal (½ to 1 cup to a tub of water) is much easier to use.

7. Soyaloid is a preparation made from soybeans and is used for soothing baths. Aveeno and Soyaloid can be used to both soothe and clean.

Baths have the advantage of not cooling the patient as much as extensive *wet dressings.* However, they are often not used because of the amount of time required for supervision. *Antipruritic lotions,* creams or ointment may be applied after the bath.

ANTIPRURITIC LOTIONS, CREAMS AND OINTMENTS. *Antipruritic lotions* include:

- ▶ Quotane lotion contains menthol and quotane, a relatively nonsensitizing topical anesthetic.
- ▶ Cetaphil lotion, 0.125 to 0.5 per cent menthol, may be added for antipruritic effect.
- ▶ Hydrocortisone lotion: Hydrocortisone in 0.125 to 0.5 per cent concentration may be added to lotions for its anti-inflammatory effect.
- ▶ Phenol: 0.5 to 1 per cent can be added to calamine lotion or calamine liniment, Schamberg's lotion or Wises' lotion.

Shake lotions are aqueous suspensions of powdered solids which, on evaporation of water, leave a thick deposit of powder on the surface of the skin. These are applied to vesicular or slightly exudative surfaces, and may be applied with a soft paintbrush or the bare hand. An *emulsion,* which is a shake lotion containing oil, is less drying and has less tendency to cake on the surface.

Ointments and *creams* are in water-washable ointment bases or are not freely water-washable. Some examples of water base ointment bases are Unibase, Acid Mantle, Cetaphil and Neobase. Examples of water in oil bases are yellow and white petrolatum, lanolin, cold cream, Nivea Cream, Aquaphor and Eucerin. Phenol, 0.5 to 1 per cent, or menthol, 0.125 to 1 per cent, may be added to almost any base. Boric acid ointment (2.6 to 5 per cent) is mildly bacteriostatic and fungistatic. Its use over extensive areas is contraindicated because of the danger of possible absorption and renal damage.

COMPRESSES AND SOAKS. Cool *wet compresses* may be used for localized itching. If the area becomes dry from the compresses, a teaspoonful of Alpha-Keri or other oil may be added to the compress fluid. Acute eczematous eruptions are frequently treated with *wet compresses* for their soothing and anti-inflammatory effects. These are often helpful in cleaning the skin as well as in getting rid of old crusts. Solutions used could be normal saline, Burow's solution (aluminum acetate) diluted 1:10 or 1:20, or milk of magnesia diluted equally with water. These should be applied to light coverings of gauze (four to eight layers) at body temperature, and are not to be covered with other materials to prevent maceration. A schedule is useful, e.g., compresses should be applied for a half hour, and removed for a half hour the first day or two. As the acute eruptions subside, the intervals can be decreased to several times a day. Handy packets of Burow's solution available commercially are Bluboro and Domeboro, each diluted in 8 to 16 oz. of water.

Soaks of mild antiseptic solutions may be used for acute or weeping conditions or infections in the extremities for 15 minutes or so several times a day. Soaks may be used for acute athlete's foot. Between soaks, drying lotions (suspensions of inert powders in water) are helpful in drying weeping eruptions as well as being soothing and antipruritic.

DRUG MANAGEMENT OF SKIN DISORDERS

Because of the epidermal barrier, topical application to the skin is an inefficient method of introducing most drugs into the body. However, topical *corticosteroids* have made a great change in management of skin disease because of their anti-inflammatory activity.

Probably half of the prescriptions written by dermatologists today are for topical *glucocorticosteroids.*

> *The more potent a topical drug is, the more likely it is to produce undesirable side effects.*

Although not common, the systemic effects of the stronger steroids are thought to include: (1) purpura, (2) rosacea-like eruption of the face, (3) severe exacerbation of acne, (4) epidermal and dermal atrophy, (5) striae, (6) glaucoma (suspected but not proven), and/or (7) exacerbation of dermatophyte infections. Low daily doses of corticosteroid therapy over a period of time result in greater improvement in skin diseases than large doses for a short period. Steroid ointments are contraindicated in herpes, viral, or fungal infections. Effectiveness of topical steroids is enhanced when they are applied under a transparent plastic wrap. However, this technique also enhances systemic absorption, occasionally resulting in suppression of natural hormone production by the adrenal cortex.[113]

Kligman and Kaidbey state that it is irrational to prescribe potent steroids for diseases that can be managed with weaker steroids. Stubborn, chronic dermatoses such as psoriasis may require potent steroids; however, disorders such as atopic dermatitis in children and seborrheic dermatitis in adults can generally be managed with hydrocortisone. Steroids must be used with caution. For example in patients with adverse effects from long-term use of potent steroids, steroid use must be gradually reduced to avoid a "rebound reaction" that results from sudden steroid withdrawal. This may take months. Hydrocortisone may be used to maintain steroid-sensitive dermatoses in remission after they have been brought under control with a potent steroid.[60]

Certain *cancer therapeutic agents* are also used topically in selected skin disorders. Those most widely used are 5FU, and nitrogen mustard. Nitrogen mustard is used in treating mycosis fungoides and in psoriasis. 5FU is used in treating actinic keratoses. Methotrexate has been widely used as a systemic treatment of psoriasis. The potential benefit of cancer therapeutic drugs must be balanced against toxicity of these agents.

Topical *antibiotics* are not usually used in bacterial pyodermas. The use of systemic antibiotics is recommended because of rapid clinical response and the reduction of risk of spread of infection.

Topical *antifungal agents* have been found to be effective in the management of selected cutaneous fungal and yeast infections. Griseofulvin has been shown to be an effective and relatively safe drug for superficial skin mycoses. It is less effective in fungus infection of the toenails. In this situation long-term treatment is required, and in many cases the nails fail to respond to therapy.

Antihistamines are nonspecific anti-inflammatory agents used in urticaria and in a number of pruritic dermatoses. The relief they provide is likely due to sedative effect produced by these agents rather than to any peripheral antihistamine effects.

Antimalarial agents have been used in management of discoid lupus erythematosus and polymorphic light eruption. Sulfones are most frequently used in the treatment of leprosy and in dermatitis herpetiformis. The latter disease responds so well that failure of the disease to improve indicates that the original diagnosis should be reconsidered.

DISEASES OF THE APPENDAGES

Diseases of the Nails

Paronychia. This is an inflammation of the tissue surrounding the nail plate. *Acute paronychia (whitlow)* is a rapidly developing, painful red swelling around the nail. Acute infection usually follows an injury or a "hangnail." It may spread around the nail, and, if neglected, a cellulitis or lymphangitis may develop. Approximately half the cases are due to *Candida albicans. Chronic paronychia* is frequently found in middleaged women who have their hands continually in water. It is approximately three times as common in persons with diabetes as in the general population.

If neglected, the lesion may have to be incised surgically, cultured, and the patient given antibiotics and warm wet packs. The most important point in preventing recurrence is to keep the area scupulously dry. Squeezing the affected area aggravates the condition. Treatment includes amphotericin B lotion or nystatin cream, lotion, or ointment. It usually takes some weeks to clear completely.

The nurse should urge attention to any injury around the nail and stress the importance of gentleness in manicuring. If a hangnail is not infected, the filament may be flattened and secured with flexible collodion. If an infection occurs or a person is prone to chronic paronychia, a finger cot or gloves should be used to keep hands dry.

Ingrown Toenails (Unguis Incarnatus). This condition occurs when a fragment of nail pierces the skin of the nail lip. Painful inflammation and infection may develop. *Ingrown toenails* may be the result of improper self-treatment or external pressure. They are more likely to occur if there is a curvature of the nails. Ingrown toenails usually have two etiologic factors, a special familial configuration of the nail and use of tight, ill-fitting shoes. Obesity, flat feet, and short nails also favor development.

Initial care of infected ingrown toenails consists of: (1) drainage of the abscess by partial excision of the penetrating nail and (2) intermittent saline soaks and antibiotic therapy.

Development of ingrown toenails can be stopped by raising the toenail from its bed by means of a small pledget of cotton under the free edge of the nail, thus relieving pressure on the lateral edge. The nail should be trimmed to allow the lateral part to grow forward. The elderly have difficulty in reaching their toes, in seeing them, and in handling the trimming instruments. Therefore, a nurse with special training or a podiatrist should trim the toenails if there is any problem. Nursing observation of predisposing factors and education of the patient concerning prevention are desirable.

Hypertrophy of the Nails (Onychauxis). Onychauxis is a thickening of the nail associated with: aging, nutritional disturbances, repeated trauma, inflammation, local infection, or various degenerative diseases. The nail plate becomes thickened and discolored, callous nail groove, subungual hyperkeratoses, and debris are common. The distal portion of the nail becomes loose, which adds to the collection of debris. *Onychogryphosis (ram's horn nail)* is an unusually large and curved nail plate, resulting from neglect and lack of treatment. A good way to prepare nails for thinning is to have the patient cover them with a softening agent such as petroleum jelly or Whitfield's ointment for a week before treatment. Then the nail may be thinned with a surgical knife or an electric bur. At times, total and permanent removal of the nail plate is the treatment of choice. *Onychoposis (callus nail groove)* is usually the result of repeated trauma on the nail plate from some external pressure or curvature of the nail. Removal of the cause is desirable. A massage with warm olive oil induces some improvement in patients with hypertrophied nails. Nurses can teach patients about care of the feet, urging physical examination and referral to a podiatrist.

Brittleness of the Nails. This is a common disorder of the nails, in which they are soft and split. The exact etiology is not known. Individuals are commonly concerned about this and wish to know what to do about it. Evidence is somewhat controversial, but one dermatologist recommends 7 gm. daily of gelatine for about 15 weeks as a result of a controlled experimental trial.[42]

Clubbing. This is a secondary condition that may be observed in patients with chronic cardiac and pulmonary conditons.

Clubbing is characterized by the diffuse bulbous enlargement of the fingers and toes. The obvious changes are the loss of the angle between the base of the nail and the dorsal surface of the finger (Fig. 79–9). This finding is best viewed from the side. The end of the finger also flattens and widens. The nails may appear lustrous and are curved but without a change in color.

Disorders Associated with the Sebaceous Glands, Hair, and Scalp.

SEBORRHEIC DERMATITIS

Seborrheic dermatitis is a common, chronic, recurrent condition frequently associated with an oily skin and scalp. Seborrheic dermatitis is a term employed for a number of clinical conditions and probably does not represent a single problem. It is often seen in patients with acne vulgaris and rosacea. Tension and diet may be associated with flareups, although the cause of this disorder is not known. The lesions are greasy, scaly red patches affecting the scalp, the eyebrows, the nasolabial and postauricular areas, the chest and skin folds. The lesions may become secondarily infected and show eczematous changes.

For mild cases, shampooing with a detergent shampoo several times weekly and application of scalp lotion for slight scaling are recommended. With heavier scaling, an ointment or steroid lotions and creams may be applied. Mild bland baths daily for 15 minutes may be helpful in widespread eruptions. All external irritants, excess heat and excess perspiration will aggravate the disorder. Rubbing and scratching also aggravate the condition and may produce infection. If a patient has oily skin or hair, urge frequent shampooing and reassure the patient that the condition can be controlled with care. The patient should be cautioned about overtreatment.

ROSACEA

This is a chronic disorder which usually occurs in middle age or later. It tends to localize

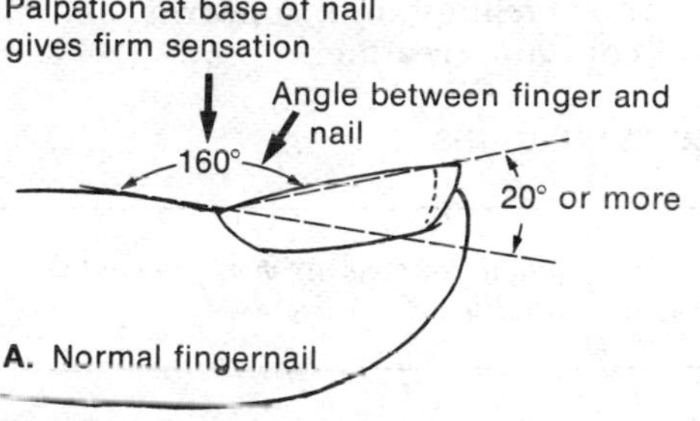

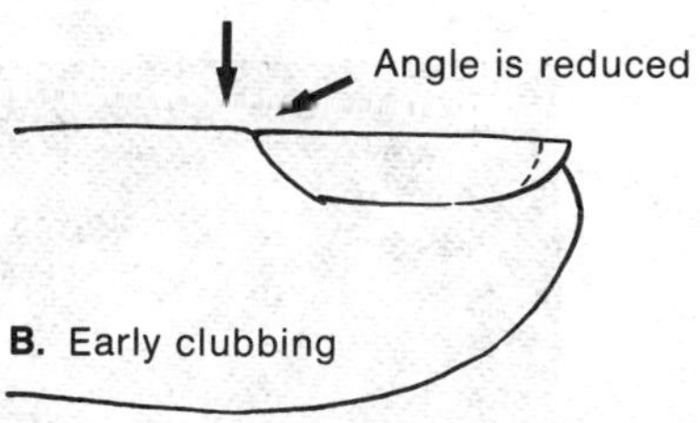

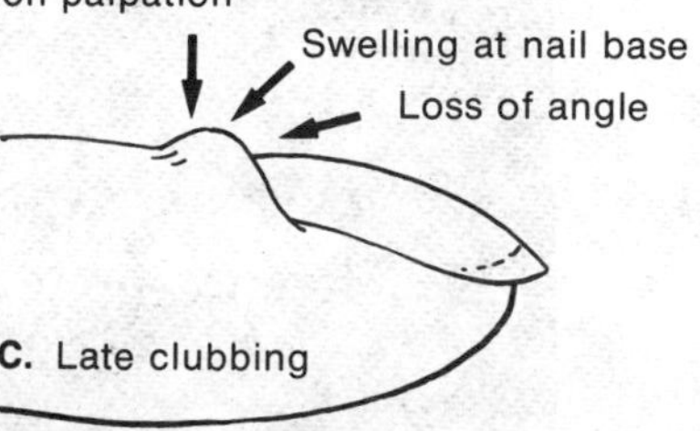

Figure 79–9. The normal nail and indications of clubbing. (Redrawn from Bates, B.: *A Guide to Physical Examination.* Philadelphia: J. B. Lippincott Co., 1974.)

in the middle third of the face (the flush area). In mild cases there is vasodilatation of the capillaries of the cheek and nose but, in more severe cases, papules and pustules may appear as well. The condition can be quite disfiguring. When there is a gross hyperplasia of the sebaceous glands of the nose, the person's appearance may be wrongly interpreted as indicative of excessive drinking. The conditon affects females in the fourth and fifth decades who have a labile vasomotor system. Enlargement of the nose is seen more often in males.

Treatment is directed toward avoiding anything that contributes to facial hyperemia, such as alcohol, hot foods, or excessive sun exposure. Hair should be shampooed frequently to reduce oiliness. The pustule formation with rosacea is found to respond to a regimen of tetracycline. Treatment does not affect the erythema. Topical corticosteroids should be avoided because of worsening when they are discontinued and because they may cause increased redness and telangiectasis. Cosmetic surgery may be of benefit if there is rhinophyma. Since the disease may be somewhat embarrassing and disfiguring, the nurse needs to encourage the patient to express feelings and concerns and to obtain and continue treatment.

ACNE VULGARIS

Consultations for acne are more frequent than for any other skin disease.

Acne is a disorder of the pilosebaceous follicles that primarily affects adolescents and young adults. It may be divided into noninflammatory and inflammatory types. *Noninflammatory acne* is characterized by open and closed whiteheads and blackheads (comedones), consisting of compact masses of keratin, sebum, and bacteria dilating the follicular duct. In *inflammatory acne*, the skin is inflamed, and there are papules, pustules, and nodulocystic lesions with a tendency for destructiveness and scarring (Fig. 79–10). The lesions are found in areas of greatest concentration of the sebaceous glands — the face, neck, and upper trunk.

Causal Factors. A convenient working hypothesis for the production of acne lesions is as follows:

> Increased androgenic influence (or perhaps increased end-organ responsiveness) produces sebaceous gland hyperplasia and seborrhea. Comedo formation results from an abnormality of the keratinization of the follicular mouth. Follicular damage occurs mainly in follicles with large sebaceous glands and weak hair growth and in follicles that have small blocked openings. Fatty acids are freed by hydrolysis from triglycerides in the sebum along with bacterial esterases from *Propionibacterium acnes* high in the follicles. (It is possible that *Staphylococcus epidermidis* contributes to the lipolysis.) The fatty acids diffuse through the follicular walls and cause inflammation and follicular destruction. Keratin freed from the injured follicles produces a granulomatous response in the dermis.[23]

Treatment. Since acne vulgaris is associated with increased sebum excretion, obstruction of the pilosebaceous duct, and alteration of the lipid composition of the skin surface, *treatment* generally attacks one or more of these areas.

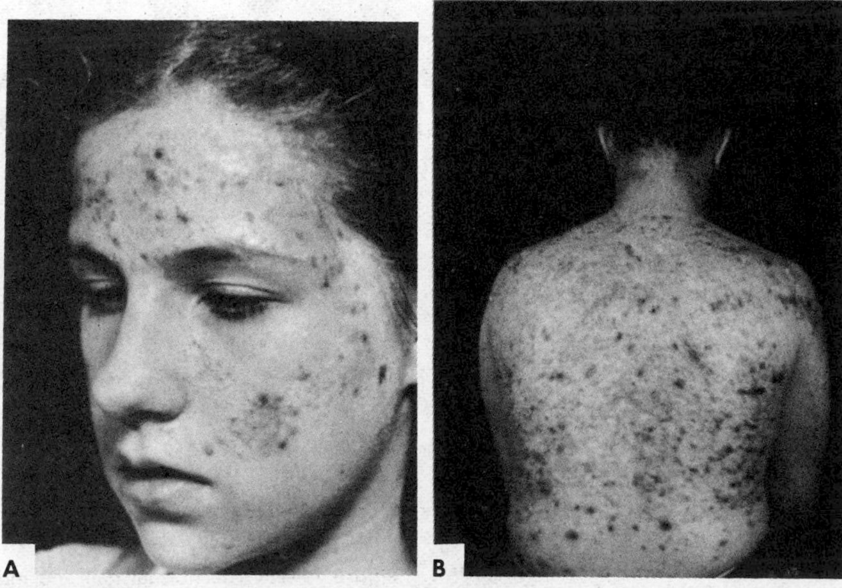

Figure 79–10. Acne vulgaris. **A.** Moderately severe, with comedones, papules, and pustules. **B.** Extensive distribution of cysts, pustules, and scars. (From Lewis, G. M., and C. E. Wheeler, Jr.: *Practical Dermatology*, 3rd ed.)

Oral contraceptives may be of use in very severe or otherwise unresponsive cases in young women. This is effective because of the medication's estrogen content. Some researchers have found oral contraceptive therapy to be particularly effective in preventing the common premenstrual flare of acne. Oral contraceptive therapy is particularly helpful for treating acne in women in their twenties and thirties. It is important to continue the pill for a minimum of three to four cycles and to explain that there may be an increase in pustule formation initially. It is not known whether the new low-dose estrogen pills have enough estrogen to reduce acne. The use of anti-androgens in a topical medication base is a possible helpful future development. Topical corticosteroids are not helpful in treating acne and may, in fact, make it worse. X-ray therapy may be tried when other forms of therapy have failed, even though there is little evidence that it is helpful.

Other treatments for acne vulgaris try to reduce obstruction of the pilosebaceous duct. In most patients undergoing treatment for acne, exposure to sunlight or artificial ultraviolet light is very effective. During treatment, the patient's eyes should be screened, and the patient should be carefully supervised for graduated exposure.

Retin-A seems to be a useful preparation for patients affected by comedones and early inflammatory lesions. Patient cooperation is vital in the use of this medication. The patient is instructed to avoid excessive exposure to ultraviolet light, excessive face washing, and excessive use of the Retin A. Care must be taken that the Retin-A does not come in contact with the corners of the mouth, nose, eyes, and mucous membrane. No other topically applied agent should be used at the same time. The patient should be told that the acne may appear to get worse before it gets better and that at least 6 weeks of application may be necessary before any clinical improvement occurs. Treatment is regulated to produce a mild erythema. Benzyl peroxide gel therapy has also been found to be effective in treating inflammatory acne.[35]

A wide variety of therapeutic agents have been used in the hope of modifying the skin flora. Tetracycline is widely used and is often effective. Treatment with tetracycline for a period of 2 to 3 months is effective in about 80 per cent of patients with moderate and severe pustular acne. It is important not to give tetracycline to patients with impaired renal function or to pregnant women or children under age 8 years. Clindamycin seems to be an effective drug. Because of the risk of severe colitis, however, it should be reserved for persons with severe pustular and cystic acne that has remained resistant to other types of therapy.[15, 66, 73]

Topical application of antibiotics in treatment of acne is a field of experimentation. Some persons believe that antibiotics (tetracycline, erythromycin, and clindamycin) can be prepared in lotion form for topical application in vehicles capable of carrying the antibiotics into the follicular canal where the primary lesion occurs. This avoids the possible adverse effects of systemic treatment and also avoids the drying and scaling of the skin that occurs with most other topical treatment.[29]

Nursing Implications. Young people benefit from being taught in their preadolescent years about the natural course and care of acne. School, office, and clinic nurses are in strategic positions to assist in the management and prevention of severe acne. Frequent washing of oily hair and skin is desirable, as is a hairdo in which the hair is not touching the face. Patients and their parents may be taught the use of the comedo extractor, extracting only those blackheads that come out easily and doing about 10 at one sitting. Squeezing, rubbing, and picking should be discouraged. Encourage the person affected with acne to eat a balanced diet; avoid undue stress, fatigue, and perspiration; and get out into the sunlight.

When an ultraviolet light is prescribed for home use, the client's understanding of the use of the ultraviolet lamp requires careful review. Teach the patient to: (a) always wear dark glasses; (b) always have someone else time the exposure, in case the timing mechanism does not work or the patient falls asleep; (c) actually measure the distance from the lamp with a yardstick so that a uniform distance is always maintained. The amount of ultraviolet light recommended is the amount that will produce a mild erythema in 24 hours.

Nurses often need to give psychologic support to young people with acne, since they are particularly sensitive about their body image at this time. Acne may disturb relationships with the adolescent's peer group and undermine a person's self-confidence, because of concern about personal appearance. Although acne is connected with sexual development, in that the sebaceous glands become more active at puberty, acne is not associated with masturbation or other sexual activity. An adolescent may use acne as an excuse to avoid anxiety-arousing social relationships, A sympathetic and understanding relationship with a health professional can help a vulnerable young person through this difficult time.

ALOPECIA

Comments about hair loss may be brought to the attention of the nurse. The presenting signs of diffuse hair loss are thinning of the scalp hair, with associated receding of frontal and temporal hairlines.

Hints for keeping your acne under control

1. **Keep your hands away from your face.** Squeezing blackheads and pimples can make them worse.
2. **Keep your hair off your face.** Cut, tie, or comb it as you please, but don't let it add to your acne by spreading oil and bacteria.
3. **Avoid oily soaps,** moisturizing creams, oily hair preparations, and all heavy makeup.
4. **If you use makeup,** be sure to use water-base preparations.
5. **Within the limits of a healthy diet,** eat whatever you like. There is no evidence that diet affects acne. If you believe that you react to certain foods, keep a record of what happens each time you eat the food and eliminate that food if you are convinced that it flares your acne.
6. **If tetracycline is prescribed,** be sure to take it at least one hour before or two hours after mealtime. Never take milk, ice cream, or other dairy products within two hours before or after taking medicine. It's best to take medicine at bedtime with a glass of water. Other antibiotics can be taken with meals. Please ask for instructions.
7. **Be patient.** There is no quick or magic cure for acne, but following the treatment prescribed for you should bring real improvement after about two months.
8. **Remember, treatment only *controls* acne;** it doesn't cure it. Don't stop treatment because your skin clears up. Acne lesions begin at least a month before you can see them.
9. **Learn to accept** the ups and downs of acne activity. With persistence, you will ultimately see real improvement.

Figure 79–11. Patient teaching guidelines for acne. (Reproduced with permission of *Patient Care* magazine. Copyright © 1975, Patient Care Publications, Inc., Darien, Conn. All rights reserved.)

Four major types of hair loss are: male pattern hair loss, female pattern hair loss, alopecia areata, and traumatic alopecia. *Male pattern hair loss* characteristically shows bilateral frontal recession with short hairs. *Female pattern* hair loss is diffuse, except in the occipital region; it usually occurs in women over 40 years. *Alopecia areata* is potentially reversible and can occur at any age. *Traumatic alopecia* may be from damage due to grooming.[5]

The *cause* of the hair loss might be due to hereditary, hormonal or systemic disorders, drugs, nutritional deficits, neoplasms, physical and chemical trauma, or psychologic disorders. A careful history is needed in all cases of hair loss (Table 79–2).

Treatment is dependent on the etiology. In women with hair loss related to postpartum conditions, menopause, use of birth control pills or synthetic female hormones, the disorder tends to be self-limited, with a recovery in 6 to 12 months. Persons with systemic disease may have a decrease in daily hair shedding after therapy for their disease. Good nutrition and correction of borderline iron deficiency anemia generally results in correction of the problem. Patients with hair loss associated with a surgery, extreme stress, or drugs might recover in 6 to 24 months. Idiopathic alopecia may do best with reassurance and a followup evaluation every 4 to 6 months.[9]

HIRSUTISM (HYPERTRICHOSIS)

Essential hirsutism is usually due to heredity rather than disease. Hormonal imbalance should be considered in all but the mildest cases. This condition is marked by an increase in the amount of coarseness or darkness of body or facial hair. It causes greatest worry when the hair is on the face.

Normal menstrual history is important in ruling out *endocrine hirsutism*.

When endocrinopathy is suspected, the client is often referred to an endocrinologist. Hair can be removed by root destruction with an electric needle inserted into the hair follicle. This procedure is called electrolysis. Most states require electrologists to be licensed. To bleach hair, a 6 per cent hydrogen peroxide solution alkalinized with ammonia (20 gtts. ammonia for each ounce of peroxide) may be used 30 minutes at a time as needed. Shaving causes stubble, and tweezing and use of hot wax for epilation can cause ingrown hairs.[19]

Changes in hair are evident in aging, and scalp hair is lost with increasing maturity in both sexes. Axillary, pubic and eyebrow hair also change, generally decreasing. Hormonal changes are more important in the study of hair distribution than aging as such. All areas that are hairy in men may become hairy in women under pathologic conditions.

CYSTS

Sebaceous cysts are round, smooth, globular, cutaneous or subcutaneous tumors arising from the sebaceous glands and are found on the face, neck, scalp, back and genitalia. They are caused by occlusion of a sebaceous gland or cystic dilatation of a sebaceous gland. *Treatment* is excision to include the epithelial wall; otherwise the cyst will probably re-form.

Epidermoid cysts (wens) are difficult to distinguish from sebaceous cysts, but they are nevoid structures with an epidermal lining. *Treatment* is the same. It appears to be an inherited disorder, transmitted as an incomplete dominant trait.

TABLE 79–2. HAIR LOSS HISTORY

Patient's age, sex, race
Hair loss
  Onset
  Duration
  Daily shedding
Altered growth cycle?
Damaged hair shaft?
Family history (male and female)
Menstrual history
  Menarche
  Menstrual periods
  Pregnancy
  Menopause
Medical illness
  Endocrine
  Infections
  Neoplasm
  Others
Surgery
  Anesthesia
Drugs
  Estrogen
  Corticosteroids
  Antimetabolites
Hair care history
  Local
    Shampoo
    Oils, creams, conditioners
    Chemicals (rinses, bleaches, dyes, straighteners, permanents)
    Holding preparations (sprays, setting lotions, etc.)
  Physical
    Heat (electric rollers, dryers, hot combs and curlers)
  Mechanical
    Setting technique (pincurlers, rollers, etc.)
    Teasing
    Type of brush and roller
    Rubber bands
    Frequency of hair care programs, including beauty salon

From Bergfeld, W. F.: Diffuse hair loss in women. *Cutis,* 22:190, Aug 1978.

Disorders of the Sweat Glands

Hyperhidrosis (Excessive Perspiration). An abnormal increase in perspiration is seen most frequently during stress situations in predisposed individuals. Most frequently affected are the axillae, palms, soles, and face. The condition most frequently occurs in adolescents and young adults. Other signs may point to a labile sympathetic nervous system, e.g., tachycardia, vasomotor instability, and cold, clammy hands.

Treatment includes soaking the feet in 1:1000 solution of potassium permanganate 20 minutes daily. Antiperspiration powders are used several times daily, as well as antiperspirants. Successful use of a 10 per cent solution of glutaraldehyde, a tanning agent, has been reported.

Patients are embarrassed by this condition and may withdraw from physical contact and be less socially active. The nurse needs to assist the person in coping with this condition and in not withdrawing from social contact. The patient may wear cotton underwear and socks and change these daily.

DISEASES DUE TO PARASITES AND INSECTS

Nurses in any setting may frequently meet patients with insect bites or parasitic infections. *The second most common source of referrals to school nurses (after upper respiratory infections) is skin disease.*

Infestations of scabies or lice occur in all social and economic classes and "epidemics" often sweep through schools. All persons who are in contact with an infected individual usually become infected. No stigma or embarrassment should be associated with these infestations.

SCABIES

Scabies is an irritation of the skin caused by a crab-shaped mite whose penetrations into the skin are visible as papules and vesicles, housing males and nymphs, or as tiny linear burrows, containing females and their eggs. A fertile female mite burrows promptly and lays one egg after another. These hatch after 7 days; the larvae leave the burrow, residing on the skin surface to make several molts, mature by the twenty-eighth day, and make their own burrows. A burrow or papule may be scraped off the skin with a razor blade. However, the ova or feces may be found in the absence of a living recognizable mite. The female mite can survive 2 to 3 days away from human beings.

Diagnosis of scabies is indicated by itching at night, distribution of the rash, and presence of the disease among associates. The itching is at first intermittent, then continuous, and may persist for days after treatment. The lesions appear between the fingers, in the flexures of the wrist and anterior axillary folds, on the penis and the buttocks, and around the waist, lower abdomen and areolae of the nipples (Fig. 79–12). The skin above the neckline is rarely affected in adults, because the mite avoids the cold. Transmission is by direct contact and, to a limited extent, from soiled sheets and undergarments.

Treatment. The preferred treatment is application of 1% gamma benzene hexachloride cream or lotion to the whole body. If the skin is crusted, a warm bath before application is helpful. After a bath, allow the skin to dry and cool before applying medication. The cream or lotion is applied in a thin layer and rubbed in thoroughly. The entire body is covered, from the neck down. The medication is left on for 8 to 12 hours and then thoroughly washed off. *One application is usually curative.*

It is important not to overtreat. Individuals are likely to itch and be uncomfortable for some weeks; this is not an indication that the mites are still active. Caution patients to follow medication directions and *not* to apply the lotion a second time without consulting their physician.

Clothing, linens, and towels should be thoroughly washed. Outer clothing may be dry cleaned. All potential cases among significant others should be treated at the same time.

Nursing Implications. School nurses need to remember that some people may still consider scabies a stigma. Reassurance may be given that it is common and can easily be eliminated.

PEDICULOSIS

Pediculosis means infestation by lice. There are three types: (1) pediculosis capitis (head louse), (2) pediculosis corporis (body louse), and (3) phthirus pubis (pubic louse).

Lice are oval and gray, about 2 to 4 mm. long, and wingless with six legs. Pubic lice are the smallest, and body lice the largest. The female lays several eggs called "nits," each one being glued to hair. A larva is hatched in 6 to 10 days and becomes a fully grown louse in 1 or 2 weeks. Lice live on blood which they suck from the skin.[94]

Nursing Implications. School nurses should have witnesses to identify lice, since an occasional parent becomes highly indignant. The nurse needs to be aware that any person who has been in contact with a person with lice may also be infested. Teaching the individual how to clean clothing and surroundings, as well as the importance of getting contacts examined and treated, is the usual role of the nurse.

Pediculosis Capitis. Examination of the hair will disclose the nits. They are firmly fastened to the hair and cannot be removed with the fingers but can, with difficulty, be removed with the nails or a fine comb.

Gamma benzene hexachloride shampoo is the most widely used treatment in the United States for head lice. Teach patients to follow product directions carefully. The hair need not be cut. Significant others should be examined, especially if they share hats, combs or beds.

Pediculosis Corporis. The louse lives in clothes and leaves them only to "have a meal" off the skin. Scratch marks that are secondarily infected and pruritus may be the only signs. Pediculosis corporis is generally associated with unhygienic living conditions. It is sometimes called "vagabond's disease" (Fig. 79–13).

Treatment consists of sterilization of the clothing by laundering and pressing with a hot iron. Gamma benzene hexachloride or 1% malathion

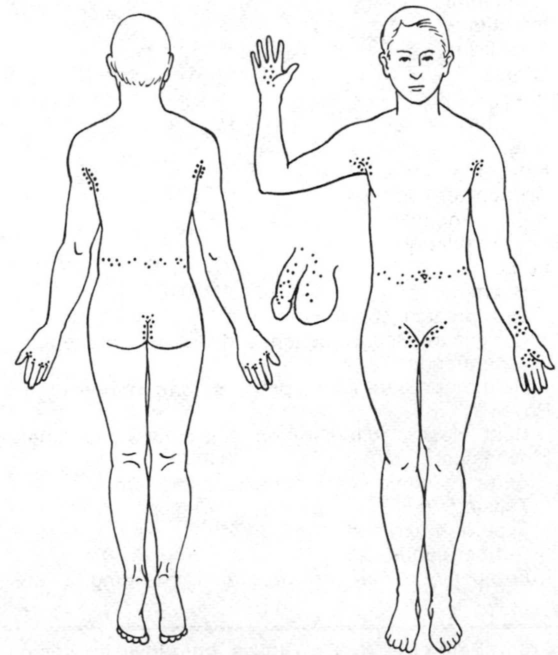

Figure 79–12. Scabies. (Redrawn from Fitzpatrick, T. B., and Walker, S. A.: *Dermatological Differential Diagnosis.*)

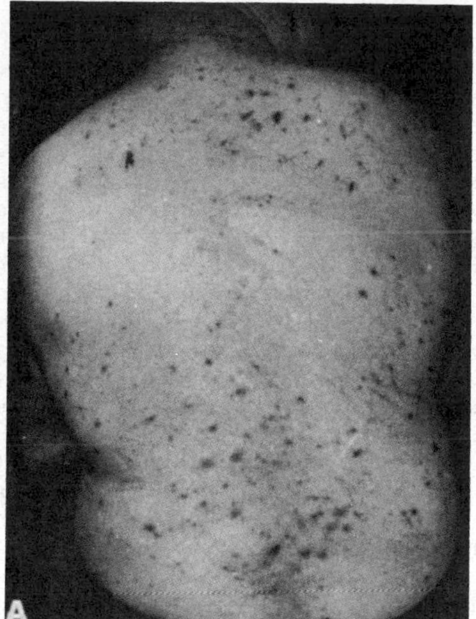

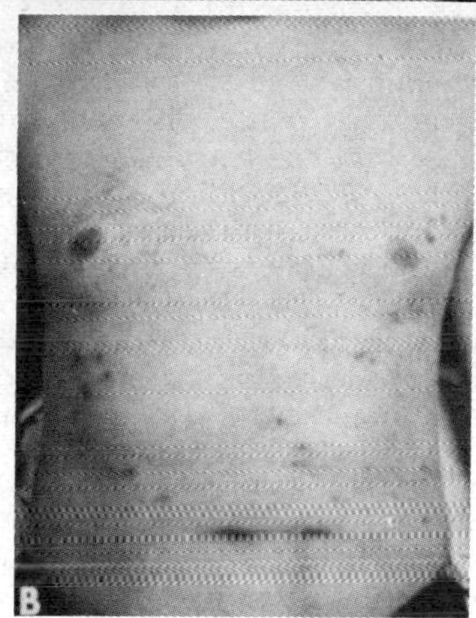

Figure 79–13. Infestations. **A.** *Pediculosis corporis.* The linear, parallel scratch marks indicate the severe associated pruritus. **B.** Bedbug bites. The erythematous wheals have a central punctum and tend to be grouped (occurrence of three lesions in proximity is especially diagnostic). (From Lewis, G. M., and C. E. Wheeler, Jr.: *Practical Dermatology,* 3rd ed.)

or dusts containing either 0.2% pyrethrin or 0.3% allelthrin synergized with pipironyl butoxide are recommended. The insecticide Abate, which is nontoxic to man, is also effective and is recommended by WHO for use in areas where strains of pediculi are resistant to malathion.[8] Unless vigorous action is taken, the condition will return.

Pediculosis Pubis. Transmission is generally by close personal contact, usually sexual contact. It should be looked for in cases of pruritus ani and vulvae. There may be reddish brown dust on the underclothing from the excreta of the insects. Dusky gray macules 1 to 3 cm. in diameter may be observed on the thighs, trunk and axillae, as a result of the insect's saliva.

Pubic lice (sometimes called "crabs") may be treated by shampooing with gamma benzene hexachloride or by application of the cream or lotion. Ophthalmic ointment with 0.25% physostigmine will eliminate crab lice from the eyelashes.

INSECTS

Nurses are frequently queried concerning the bites or stings of insects. Bedbugs, fleas, spiders, mosquitoes, bees, wasps and chiggers are common problems.[39] Emergency care of spider bites and bee stings is discussed in Chapter 95.

Fleas. Humans may be attacked by dog and cat fleas. Many people are relatively immune or become so. The legs are chiefly attacked. The bite produces a hemorrhagic spot surrounded by an itchy wheal. It is necessary to get rid of the fleas by spraying with commercially available agents. Carpets, upholstered furniture, sleeping places of pets should be treated. A lotion for itching may be applied to the legs several times a day. Pets should be treated as advised by a veterinarian.

Bedbugs. The bedbug (*Cimex lectularius*) lives in cracks and crevices in the room and usually comes out at night to acquire food. The bugs may be picked up in motion picture theaters. The bedbug has a disagreeable strong odor if squashed. Bites are usually found in the morning, grouped in twos or threes (see Fig. 79–13*B*). There is a wheal with a central punctum. Local antipruritic treatment may be given, and the environment should be rid of bedbugs.

Chiggers. Several species of reddish mites are found throughout the world. They are common in the southern United States but extend at least to the Canadian border. Mites are found on grass and bushes. The mite attaches itself to the legs or thighs and punctures the skin to obtain blood. Dermatitis consists of papules with surrounding urticaria, excoriations and subsequent pustules. There may be marked erythema and itching. The mite leaves the skin of its own accord, so treatment is directed toward relief of itching. Insect repellent on wrists and ankles may help in prevention.

BACTERIAL DISEASES

The skin is normally colonized with many potentially pathogenic organisms. A local area of infection is accompanied by a rapid increase in number of bacteria on the skin which serve as a source of continuing infection.

Pyoderma

A pyoderma is a purulent infection of the skin. Most are caused by streptococci or staphylococci.

Pyoderma includes impetigo, ecthyma, folliculitis, furuncles and carbuncles, cellulitis, and erysipelas.

IMPETIGO. Impetigo occurs primarily in children. The disease is characterized by intraepidermal vesicles that progress to pustules and are soon overlain with gummy, honey-colored crusts (Fig. 79–14). The size of lesions varies; they are roughly circular. The lesions enlarge peripherally as well as spread by satellite lesions. Impetigo usually appears in the central facial area and is produced by coagulase-positive staphylococci and by beta-hemolytic streptococci. Acute glomerulonephritis appears in 1 to 5 per cent of patients.[68, 114]

Treatment. Experimental and epidemiological data suggest that a single injection of benzathene penicillin G is the best treatment for typical uncomplicated impetigo in a nonatopic patient.[58] Some dermatologists believe that it is best not to manipulate the lesion by aggressive debridement and that topical antibiotics may sensitize the patient or may not be effective.

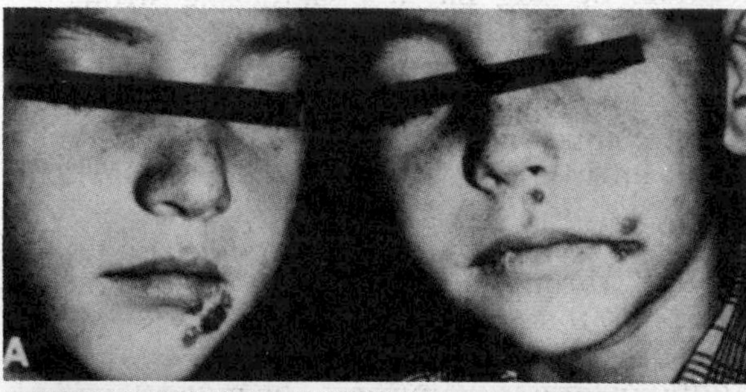

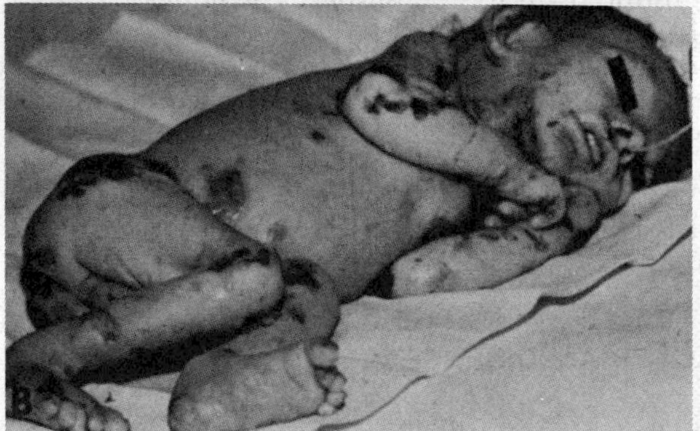

Figure 79–14. Impetigo. **A.** Impetigo in twin brothers. **B.** Bullous impetigo in a newborn, the so-called pemphigus neonatorum, a serious disease at this age.) (From Lewis, G. M., and C. E. Wheeler, Jr.: *Practical Dermatology*, 3rd ed.)

FOLLICULITIS. Folliculitis is a variable disease that ranges from tiny white pustules in infants to large, yellow, pus-containing tender lesions in the scalp, beard, or nose. Staphylococci rapidly take advantage of any damaged or blocked follicle to colonize in those areas. Multiple lesions on forehead, face and neck of infants respond well to treatment. In adults these lesions are found in hairy areas such as thigh, face, scalp, groin, or axillae. If the lesions persist, the condition can become chronic and difficult to get rid of. Infection of beard follicles is known as "barber's itch" or *sycosis barbae.* Infection may also occur in the follicles of the nasal vibrissae. Many people with this condition are nose manipulators.

Treatment. Thorough cleansing with a mild soap followed by 70 per cent alcohol may be all that is necessary in non-erythematous lesions in infants. For adults with sycosis barbae, an effective systemic antibiotic such as sodium cloxacillin may be used.[43]

FURUNCLES (BOILS) AND CARBUNCLES. A *boil* or *furuncle* is an acute painful infection of a hair follicle, caused by *Staphylococcus aureus.* A *carbuncle* may involve many pilosebaceous units and may cause regional lymphadenopathy. The onset is quite sudden, with the skin becoming red, tender, and hot around a hair follicle. The center becomes yellow with pus and forms a core that may be extruded spontaneously or with gentle manipulation.

Treatment. Recurrent boils are sometimes a symptom of underlying disease, such as glycosuria. If patients have repeated episodes, antibiotic therapy should be delayed until the lesion is cultured and sensitivity tests are performed. After this, a 14 day course of treatment of the appropriate antibiotic may be prescribed. Patients are advised to bathe with mild soaps, e.g., Dove, Palmolive Green, Ivory or Castile. A bandage is useful only to protect the boil from trauma, unless it is draining. The patient must take precautions to avoid passing the infection to significant others, by using separate towels, linens and clothing, by burning dressings, and washing hands with soap after touching the site. Significant others should also use a mild soap. The patient should keep moist skin areas dry with antiperspirants or alcohol lotion, since dryness inhibits growth of bacteria.

CELLULITIS. Cellulitis is a more serious infection of the dermis and subcutaneous tissue by streptococci. Red streaks and regional nodes are indications of the infection. Pronounced constitutional symptoms are common. If the infection is recurrent, permanent lymphedema may result. Treatment includes immobilization of the infected area and rest for the patient. Systemic antibiotics are prescribed. If there are constitutional symptoms, the patient should be hospitalized.

ERYSIPELAS. Erysipelas is an acute streptococcal cellulitis that usually occurs on the face, although it may occur elsewhere. The lesion is warm, with an advancing area of erythema and a definite border. Elderly persons are particularly susceptible. Constitutional symptoms accompany the disease and systemic treatment is necessary.

ERYTHRASMA. Erythrasma is a low-grade infection involving the intertriginous and moist areas of the body. Recent studies show the causative organism to be a diphtheroid, causing slightly inflamed, dry, slowly spreading, slightly scaling, circumscribed macular patches.

Erythrasma may be diagnosed by the coral red fluorescence under the Wood's lamp. Safeguard soap is effective against the condition. Erythromycin or tetracycline may be prescribed. Recurrence is not uncommon. About 10 per cent of older people may be found to have the condition.

Nursing Implications and Prevention in Pyoderma. Nurses need to recognize and teach to patients the importance of maintaining the integrity of the skin and methods of doing this. Environmental changes to promote drying and to aerate the body folds are essential. Climate of living and working areas should be cool and dry. It is advisable for clothing to be light, nonconstricting, and absorbent. Wool, nylon, and synthetic fibers should be avoided. Intertriginous areas should be washed, rinsed, dried, and powdered with a baby powder at least twice daily. Care must be used to prevent spread of a pyoderma to significant others. Careful separation of towels and personal articles is necessary. Handwashing after handling lesions is essential. Lesions near the nose are dangerous in adults and need systemic treatment to avoid spread. Soaps with chemicals added should be avoided, as they may interfere with the normal colonization and acidity of the skin. Dove, for example, is a neutral soap, with a pH of 7.5 or less.

VIRAL DISEASES

Introduction. A virus is an ultramicroscopic organism. Viruses are often divided into those containing ribonucleic acid (RNA) and those containing deoxyribonucleic acid (DNA). The RNA viruses are of less importance to the dermatologist. The epidermal viruses are all DNA viruses. They invade the nucleus of the keratinocyte and cause cellular proliferation or cellular destruction by lysis. (See Table 79–3.)

Useful *antiviral agents* include the following:[111]

Idoxuridine (IDU, Stoxil) and cytosine arabinoside. By preventing certain aspects of DNA synthesis, these agents inhibit propagation of the virus without interfering with normal cellular activity.

Thiosemicarbazones (methisazone). These agents inhibit replication of the virus and prevent its maturation. This is useful in vaccinia and early smallpox.

Interferon. Interferon is a protein produced by cells that have harbored viruses. This agent is active against all known viruses.

Amantadine. An amine that is useful in influenza, rubella, and some tumor viruses. It probably inhibits viral penetration into susceptible cells.

The present epidemiologic situation regarding viral skin disease is being influenced by:

1. World-wide use of contraceptive medication, which can have immunosuppressive reactions and thus heighten vulnerability to infection.
2. Increased use of steroids systemically and locally. Corticosteroids should never be applied in early stages of viral infection, since they decrease both toxin clearance by the reticuloendothelial system and antibody formation. Virus multiplication may thereby be enhanced, while clinical symptoms are masked.
3. Suppression of bacterial infections by massive use of antibiotics. Viral infections seem to be increasing all over the world relative to bacterial diseases.[74]

Molluscum Contagiosum. Molluscum contagiosum is a virus-induced, wart-like epitheliosis. It occurs world-wide and in all races. It can be transmitted indirectly by towels or washcloths or directly from human to human. Recently, an

TABLE 79–3. EPIDERMAL VIRUSES

Virus Class	Virus Species	Clinical Disease	Pathologic Mechanism
Herpesvirus	H. hominis Type I	Herpes labialis	Cellular destruction
	H. hominis Type II	Herpes progenitalis	
	H. varicellae	Chicken pox and H. zoster	
Poxvirus	Molluscum contagiosum	Molluscum contagiosum	Cellular destruction
Papoavirus	Papoavirus hominis	Verruca vulgaris	Cellular proliferation
		Condyloma acuminatum	

From Mims, C. A.: Pathogenesis of rashes in viral diseases. *Bact. Review, 30*:739, 1966.

increase has been seen in patients on long-term corticosteroid treatment.[33] Molluscum contagiosum is characterized by single or multiple, rounded, dome-shaped, waxy, occasionally pink papules 2 to 5 mm. in diameter, with a typical slight central umbilication. The central core of the lesion, when expressed, is a soft grayish mass. Principal areas involved are face, neck, eyelids, genitalia, and axillae. Children and adolescents are most commonly affected. The disease is self-limiting and the prognosis favorable. The lesions may be removed by a curette, light desiccation, or cryosurgery. They may disappear in several months if left alone, or they may spread on the patient or to others.

Herpes Simplex. This lesion, often called *cold sore* or *fever blister,* is caused by two types of herpes virus, hominis types I and II. Type I is the more common and causes most of the common herpes lesions. Most of the primary infections occur in childhood and are subclinical. It is commonly transmitted by air and direct contact, and the lesion usually appears at the mucocutaneous junction.

Herpes is characterized by a cutaneous viral infection, which starts out with burning, tingling and itching in the area, soon followed by multiple grouped tiny vesicles on an erythematous base. Generally after 48 hours, crusting occurs. The lesion most frequently occurs on the lips and face and around the mouth. It normally runs a course of about 7 to 10 days and is troublesome to the 1 per cent of individuals in whom it is recurrent. It is probably not an actual reinfection but an exacerbation of a latent permanent infection triggered by exogenous factors such as sunlight, fever, or menses. Basically there are two different forms of herpes simplex; one recurs at the same location, and the other recurs at a different location. The recurrences at the same location seem to be influenced more easily by such treatment as phototherapy with neutral red or soft x-ray treatment. Treatments only shorten the episode but do not change the frequency of recurrence.

Local application of ointments containing 5% IDU and desiccating procedures may help symptoms and shorten the course. In pronounced bacterial infection, antibiotic ointment should be added. Immunization with inactivated herpes type I vaccine (Lupidon H) is successful if the virology match is correct.[32] During the acute stages, cold compresses may help. If applied frequently, 70 per cent alcohol will dry the lesion. Very potent glucocorticoids will abort most common cutaneous cold sores, but systemic glucocorticoid therapy suppresses host defenses and is generally undesirable in viral infections. It should not be utilized in the eyes for herpetic lesions.

Herpes Zoster. Herpes Zoster or *shingles,* an acute virus infection of the central nervous system which causes cutaneous lesions, is discussed in Chapter 27.

Warts (Verrucae). *Warts* are caused by papovavirus hominis. They are moderately contagious and autoinoculable and may affect any part of the body. Warts can occur in a variety of forms on any part of the skin or mucous membrane. There appears to be tremendous individual variation in susceptibility. Warts have an unpredictable course and may eventually disappear without any treatment.

Among the *varieties of warts* are the *common wart (verruca vulgaris),* usually occurring on the hands and the fingers; the *plantar wart,* which appears on the sole of the foot; and the *venereal wart (condyloma acuminatum)* seen in the mucous membranes or skin of the genital organs and the perianal region (Fig. 79–15).

TREATMENT. Ninety-five per cent of warts go away in 5 years. Small warts can be treated with caustics like phenol, podophyllin, or silver nitrate. Other treatments are cryotherapy with solid carbon dioxide or liquid nitrogen and electrodesiccation and subsequent curettage. Salicylic acid preparations are helpful but probably less so than the previously mentioned treatments. For plantar warts, in addition to curettage and freezing, salicylic acid or cantharidin may be applied to the wart. Simple excision of a

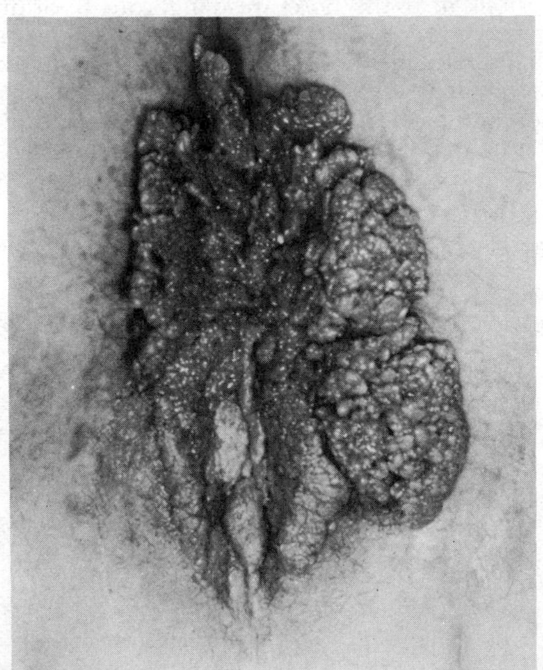

Figure 79–15. Numerous condylomas of the vulva. (Courtesy of Dr. Arthur Hertig, from Robbins, S. L. and R. S. Cotran: *Pathologic Basis of Disease,* Second ed., Philadelphia, W. B. Saunders Co., 1979.)

plantar wart may result in a painful scar that is far worse than the original lesion. Venereal warts are treated by podophyllin, 20 to 25 per cent in tincture of benzoin, applied to the warts and washed off in 4 to 6 hours. Patients should be warned about transfer to the eyes, as it causes severe conjunctivitis. Patients should be instructed to return promptly if new warts appear and told that the incubation period may be as long as a year. All persons living together should have warts treated at the same time.[55, 58, 78, 82]

COMMON COMMUNICABLE VIRAL DISEASE WITH EXANTHEMS

Viral diseases with exanthems commonly affecting children are: German measles (rubella), measles (rubeola), erythema infectiosum (fifth disease), and hand-foot-and-mouth disease. Many people do not realize the extent to which different viruses produce rashes and thus mistakenly think they have had measles several times. For discussion of communicable diseases affecting children, consult specialized pediatrics texts.

FUNGUS DISEASES

A fungus is a saprophytic or parasitic plant that possesses cells lacking true chlorophyll. *Ringworm* is a general term applied to fungus, or mycotic, infections of keratinized areas of the body, hair, skin and nails. Various genera and species of fungi known collectively as the dermatophytes are causative agents. Microsporum, Epidermophyton and Trichophyton are the three important genera. Contraction of an infection depends a great deal on individual susceptibility and individual factors such as moisture and warmth.

For discussion of ringworm of the scalp (tinea capitis) and ringworm of the body (tinea corporis), consult specialized texts dealing with children's disorders.

Ringworm of the Foot (Tinea Pedis). Scaling or cracking of the skin, especially between the toes, or blisters containing a thin watery fluid, are so characteristic that most people recognize *athlete's foot.* In severe cases, vesicular lesions appear on various parts of the body, especially the hands. These dermatophytids ("*id*" *reaction*) do not contain the fungus and constitute an allergic reaction to fungus and spores. Leyden and Klegman state that fungi are not the sole cause of tinea pedis and have categorized the disease as dermatophytosis simplex and dermatophytosis complex. The former refers to the dry scaly type and the latter to the soggy macerated type.[63]

Treatment. Suppression of bacteria is essential in treating symptomatic athlete's foot. Exposing the feet to air and using topical antibiotics with both broad-spectrum antibacterial and antifungal activity may be recommended. The agent of choice may be aluminum chloride, which combines broad-spectrum antimicrobial activity with chemical drying. The use of topical imidazoles is recommended, because an accurate mycological diagnosis need not be made since the agents have a wide spectrum of usefulness.[63]

Prevention. Plenty of ventilation should be given the feet, and being barefoot on the beach for an extended vacation may help clear up the condition. The person should wear well ventilated shoes and clean lightweight socks. Dusting between the toes with antifungal powder may help prevent a recurrence. The "id" reaction on the hands may clear up when the infection on the feet has been cured, or it may not.

Ringworm of the Nails (Tinea Unguium). This is a chronic infection involving one or more nails on the hand or foot. The nail gradually thickens, becomes discolored and brittle, and an accumulation of caseous-appearing material forms beneath the nail, or the nail becomes chalky and disintegrated. It is treated by scraping off as much of the affected nail as possible and applying an ointment containing salicylic acid or one of the higher fatty acids, propionic acid or undecylenic acid. Griseofulvin by mouth is the treatment of choice.

Tinea versicolor is a very superficial infection of the skin caused by *Malassezia furfur.* The lesions consist of asymptomatic patches which filter out the sunlight, producing white or light patches on a tanned skin. Almost any type of mild antifungal preparation is temporarily effective, but recurrences are common. The infection fluoresces under a Wood's lamp, giving a whitish, yellow or brown color. The patient should be examined under a Wood's lamp both before and after treatment.

Fungus infections among the *elderly* usually occur in the diabetic. Tinactin, which is not irritating like the peeling agents, can often be helpful with applications two to three times a week. Yeast infections or moniliasis between the toes can cause problems. Mycolog cream is effective in most cases. Good cleansing and careful drying are important.

ECZEMA AND DERMATITIS

More than half of all skin diseases are included in this heading. Both terms are used to describe a condition that exhibits some of the following symptoms: (1) edema and swelling; (2)

TABLE 79–4. SUMMARY OF NURSING CARE IN DERMATITIS

Acute		Chronic	
Signs and Symptoms	*Treatment*	*Signs and Symptoms*	*Treatment*
Erythema	Intermittent compresses	Erythema	Topical steroids sparingly
Pruritus	Intermittent compresses plus oral antihistamines	Pruritus	Topical steroids sparingly; oral antihistamines
Infection	Appropriate oral antibiotics	Infection	Appropriate oral antibiotics
Vesicles/weeping	Intermittent compresses	Lichenification/dryness	Emollients frequently

From Scotvold, M. J.: The management of dermatitis. Mimeographed lecture notes, University of Washington, Seattle.

discrete or grouped vesicles, changing to weeping and crusted lesions and/or papules and scaling; and (3) itching or burning with scratching or rubbing leading to lichenification of the skin.

General Nursing Care in Dermatitis. Dermatitis may be acute or chronic.

In *acute* dermatitis, one sees erythema, pruritus or burning, edema, bullae, and/or weeping. In *chronic* dermatitis, erythema, lichenification, dryness, scaling, fissuring and a feeling of roughness may be present. Both conditions may be secondarily infected. Treatment is based on whether the condition is chronic or acute (see Table 79–4).

Acute dermatitis is generally treated with intermittent moist compresses which produce evaporation. This results in cooling, thus reducing itching, burning and redness, and produces drying. Intermittent compressing results in effective debridement. After the acute symptoms have subsided, the lesion can be treated as a chronic dermatitis.

Chronic dermatitis is commonly treated by a topical application of a dilute concentration of a fluorinated steroid sparingly applied several times a day to reduce inflammation and diminish itching and dryness. In some patients, an oral antihistamine will help with the itching. If the specific cause can be found and eliminated, this will of course aid in patient recovery, but since in many cases no specific cause is discovered, care must be consistent, gentle and persistent.

Some specific forms of dermatitis will be discussed below.

Atopic Dermatitis (Allergic Eczema, Neurodermatitis). Atopy is used to describe the following: (1) a history of infantile atopic eczema; (2) a familial tendency for asthma, hay fever, rhinitis and urticaria; (3) hypersensitivity to protein; and (4) unusual reaction to heat, cold and emotional tensions. (See Fig. 79–16.)

Atopic dermatitis may appear soon after birth with skin lesions on face, neck, scalp and diaper area. The disease may clear at about 4 years of age but may become clinically apparent as the person gets older. The antecubital and popliteal areas are commonly involved. Pruritus is the main complaint. The involved sites are usually dry, excoriated and erythematous, and the skin exhibits lichenification. The disease tends to improve in the summer and generally disappears around the age of 30.

TREATMENT. The most important treatment principle is control of the pruritus. If the process is acute and *localized,* wet compresses of Burow's solution (1 tablespoon to 1 pint of water) may be used three times daily for 10 minutes. If the process is *generalized,* a cool brief tar or colloidal bath may be advised. Regular application of an adrenocorticosteroid cream three times daily is one of the most effective treatments. For localized areas, steroid creams may be used every 3 to 4 hours under occlusive pliable dressings. Alternative topical medication is a vioform or coal tar ointment under a dressing at night. Since this is a chronic disease, dermatologists are reluctant to use systemic steroids.

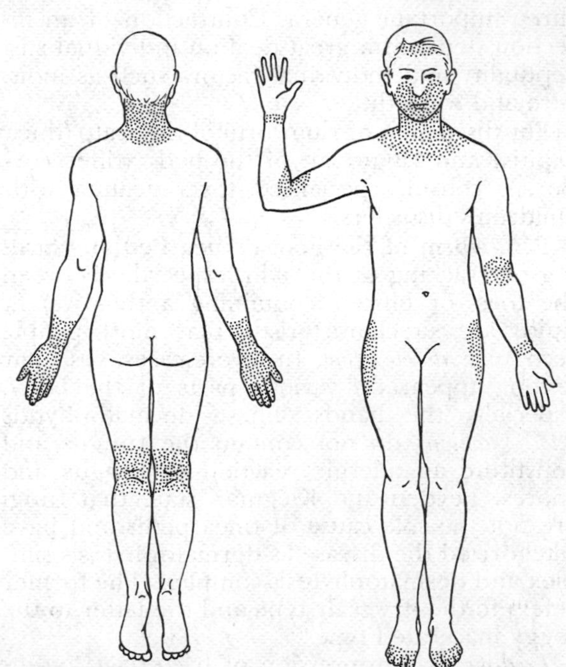

Figure 79–16. Atopic dermatitis. (Redrawn from Fitzpatrick, T. B., and S. A. Walker: *Dermatological Differential Diagnosis.*)

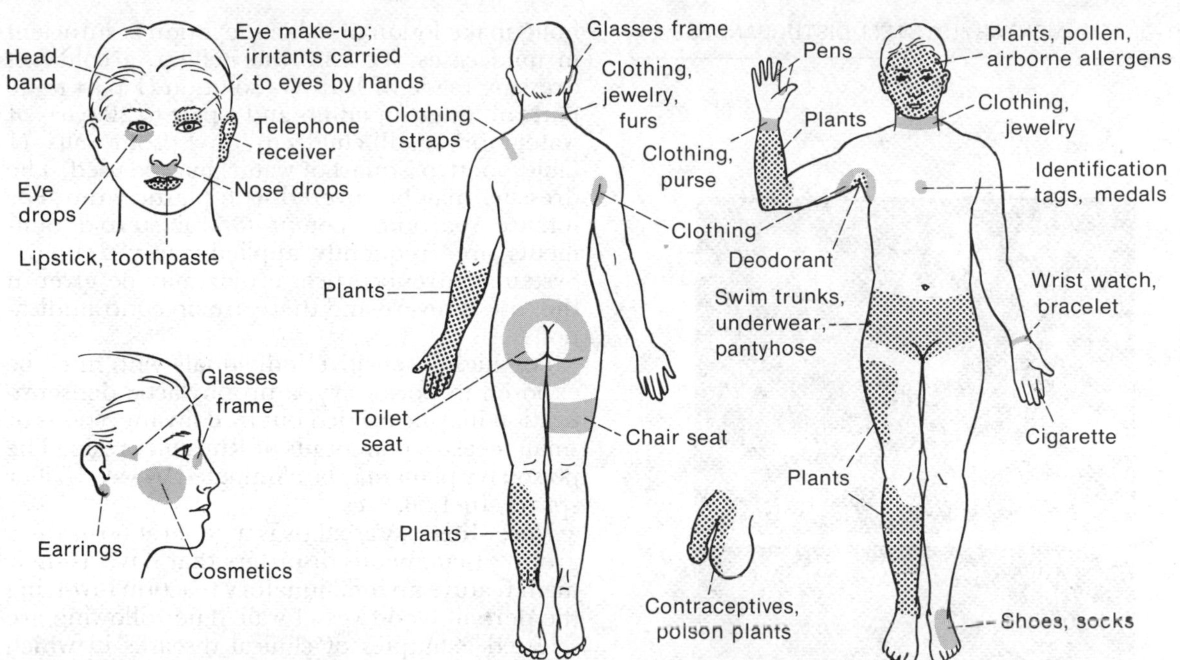

Figure 79–17. Contact dermatitis—representative sites. (Redrawn from Fitzpatrick, T. B., and S. A. Walker: *Dermatological Differential Diagnosis.*)

Nursing Implications. (1) General measures for pruritus. (2) Encourage the individual to get adequate rest and relief from nervous tensions and pressure. (3) The person should avoid vaccination or any person with a vaccination or with herpes simplex to avoid Kaposi's varicelliform eruption. This is a generalized infection and, if the infection is due to smallpox vaccine, early administration of hyperimmune gamma globulin may be necessary and may be obtained through local health departments. School nurses or nurses working in immunization clinics need to be especially mindful of the total family and should inquire if any other children have eczema. (4) Irritating clothing such as woollens should be avoided. Nothing must be applied that will irritate the skin. Detergents and household cleaners should be avoided. The patient should avoid being chilled or overheated. Emotional support and encouragement are necessary because of the disfigurement and the smelly ointments necessary to control the itching.[45]

Contact Dermatitis. This condition is characterized by redness, edema, vesicles, bullae and itching. There are two types of contact dermatitis: irritant dermatitis and allergic dermatitis. An *irritant contact dermatitis* is caused by a substance capable of producing a dermatitis in almost any skin. Prevention of recurrence is by avoiding the irritant by means of special clothing, washing after exposure or barrier creams. Typical sites are shown in Figure 79–17.

Allergic contact dermatitis is caused by sensitizers. The number of exposures to substances which will produce the rash varies from a few to many. The cause is an allergen to which the patient is specifically and often highly sensitive. There is a wide variety of possible agents, but generally a few for each patient.

The most common agents implicated in contact dermatitis include:

- *Clothing.* The first location of the eruption is important. Offending clothing will cause dermatitis in the area covered by it. The irritation is generally caused by a dye in the clothing. The feet may be affected by dye, glue or leather in shoes (Fig. 79–18*A*). After a time, the acute infection tends to spread to other areas, even without additional exposure to the causal agent. The exact mechanism of this spread is not known.
- *Cosmetics.* Perfume, deodorants, nail polish, lipstick, hair dyes, shampoos and hair sprays may all cause dermatitis. The causal agent can usually be determined from the site and history of use of any new product.
- *Household products.* Detergents are a common cause of irritant, nonallergic dermatitis. They defat the skin and may cause a persistent rash that is hard to treat, since it is difficult to keep the hands out of water.
- *Occupational substances.* Almost any substance used in industry, such as paints, dyes, cement, can cause dermatitis. Industry, however, usually requires protective clothing, etc.
- *Plants. Poison ivy dermatitis is probably the most common allergic eczema in the United States.* Common antigens are also present in poison oak, poison sumac, Japanese lacquer tree, cashew nut, mango fruit and Ginkgo tree. A resinous, sticky, saplike substance in all parts of the plant from roots to leaves is the source of the reaction. No one is immune to it and,

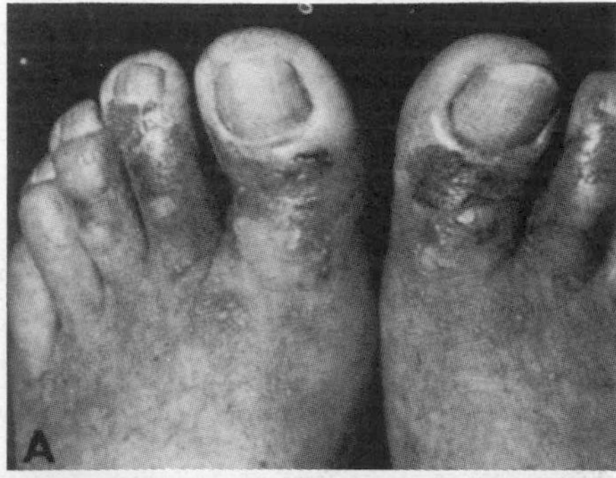

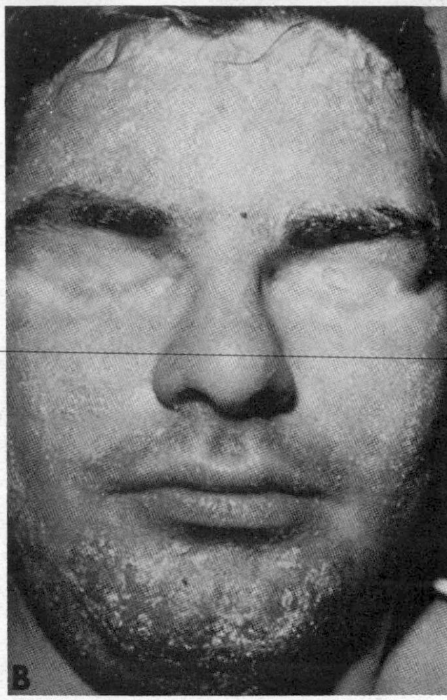

Figure 79–18. Contact dermatitis. **A.** Dermatitis due to a yellow dye in cloth lining of shoes. **B.** Subsiding plant dermatitis. (From Lewis, G. M., and C. E. Wheeler, Jr.: *Practical Dermatology,* 3rd ed.)

although a person does not react on the first exposure, he or she may become sensitized and have a reaction the next time. The individual can become affected by directly touching the stem or leaves or by touching trails of the sap that have adhered to clothing, tools, the fur of pets, or from particles in the air. The diagnosis is made on the basis of history of exposure, and the finding of linear arrangement of the eczematous vesicles. This linearity is due to a brushing motion over the extremely antigenic plant. The way to cope with these plants is to learn to recognize and avoid them. (See Fig. 79–19*B*).

Treatment. If exposure has occurred, the oil can be washed off with soap and water if this is done immediately. Application of a drying alcoholic shake lotion or calamine lotion is sufficient in mild cases. To ease the itching, a cold wet dressing made of Burow's solution (1 part to 10 parts of water for adults and 1 part to 20 parts of water for small children) or Epsom salts (1 tablespoon to a quart of water) may be used. The dressing may be covered with plastic wrap. For intense reactions, potent topical steroid ointments are frequently applied every 2 hours. Systemic adrenocorticosteroids may be given if the case is severe and there are no contraindications.

For highly sensitive individuals who must be exposed to poison ivy, a prophylactic densensitization may be carried out by daily ingestions of small measured amounts of Rhus oleoresin. The poison ivy plant may be eliminated by weed-killer sprays, fuel oil, etc.

Vasculitis. Vasculitis is a general term for a group of cutaneous disorders that have as their main feature an inflammatory reaction involving the dermal blood vessel wall. The following are selected examples of clinical diseases in which vasculitis is the major pathologic process: *Pigmented purpuric dermatoses, erythema multiforme, acute parapsoriasis, nodular vasculitis, Henoch-Schönlein purpura; hypersensitivity angiitis, Wegener's granulomatoses,* and *polyarteritis nodosa.* Recent studies indicate that immunologic processes are at work in this group of diseases. This disorder is characterized by damage to superficial blood vessels, with small infarcts of the skin. Purpura invariably occurs, associated with necrotic blisters and ulcers. The lesions usually come in crops and may recur, mostly in the legs and feet. *Henoch-Schönlein purpura* is associated with gut, renal, joint and other lesions. It is necessary to explore the history for possible sources of drug allergy, visceral or joint involvement, collagen disease, or presence of bacterial infection.

Tests might include:

1. Hgb, WBC, sedimentation rate, for estimates of systemic involvement
2. Microscopic urinalysis for red cells and casts
3. X-ray films of the chest, sinus tract, and teeth
4. X-ray films of the GI tract if indicated
5. Blood culture and antistreptolysin titer
6. Antinuclear factor and serum proteins, rheumatoid factor, and STS to see if collagen disease is present.
7. Serum complement, cryoglobulins
8. Biopsy
9. Determination of serum fibrinolytic activity

Treatment. Systemic glucocorticoids appear to produce the most satisfactory response in these disorders, although all therapy may be inadequate. Early signs of the diseases may be very subtle and may initially be brought to the attention of the nurse.[32, 111]

Erythema Multiforme. This is a toxic eruption characterized by symmetrical distribution of macules, papules and vesicles (Fig. 79–19). The lesions may have elevated circular borders, a

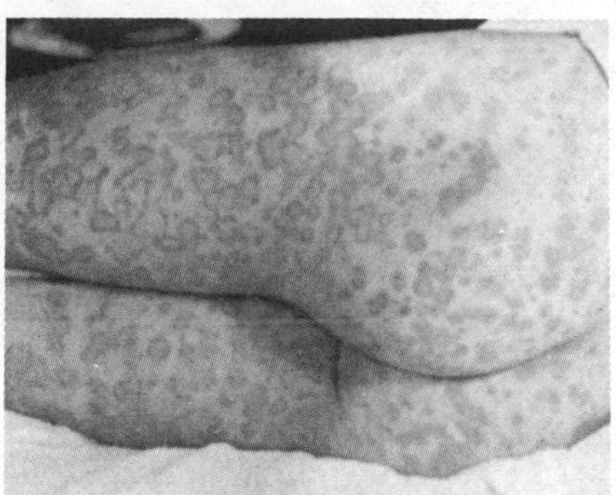

Figure 79–19. Erythema multiforme. The clinical appearance varies in location, form, and chief presenting component. Here are shown multiple erythematous plaques with a tendency to coalescence. (From Lewis, G. M., and C. E. Wheeler, Jr.: *Practical Dermatology,* 3rd ed.)

depressed inner ring and central erythema or fluid-filled bullae. The disease varies in severity from a mild form without symptoms to a generalized serious bullous disease accompanied by fever and prostration. The etiology is unknown but appears to be a reaction to various causes.

The disease may follow any of five general patterns. It may be idiopathic and self-limited, lasting from 4 to 6 weeks. It may result from drug eruptions. It may be associated with the last half of pregnancy, with internal disease or viral infections, or rarely with various kinds of internal cancer.

TREATMENT. Systemic adrenocorticosteroids will relieve the disease or shorten the course if no infection or underlying cause is found. Local treatment depends on the cause of the eruptions.

Erythema Nodosum. Erythema nodosum is a cutaneous manifestation of underlying disorder, probably due to a hypersensitivity reaction. This is an acute inflammatory condition characterized by red tender nodules on the anterior portion of the legs and thighs, usually 6 to 8 mm. in size or larger. There may be associated malaise, fever and joint pain. Sixty to 80 per cent of patients have some form of joint involvement.[111] The lesions appear in crops, and there are frequent recurrences. The disease is much more frequently diagnosed in winter and spring, coinciding with the higher incidence of infectious diseases. As the lesions fade, they begin to resemble old bruises. In a large number of cases, the cause remains undetermined. Erythema nodosum occurs more often among women than men. Historically, the disease has been associated with tuberculosis and streptococcal infections. Sarcoidosis ranks third among systemically associated diseases. Oral contraceptives lead the list of drugs associated with erythema nodosum. A dermatologist has found an association with fungus infection of the feet or nails and states the skin nodules disappeared when the fungus infection was eradicated.[41] The following information is included in a diagnostic workup:

1. History of drugs, recent travel, exposure to pets or venereal disease
2. Complete blood count
3. Urinalysis
4. Chest x-ray
5. Intermediate-strength PPD tuberculin test
6. Histoplasmin skin test
7. Coccidioidin skin test
8. Throat culture
9. Antistreptolysin titers or streptozyme test
10. Serum and urinary calcium determination.

TREATMENT. Diagnosis and treatment of the underlying disease is the keystone of therapy. For the nodules, oral salicylates have mainly been used. Steroids are not advised, because they may compromise the body's ability to deal with the underlying disease processes.[34, 86]

Exfoliative Dermatitis. This condition is characterized by a more or less sudden episode of generalized erythema with a scaling of the cutaneous surface in either fine scales or larger sheets. It may begin without obvious cause, or may occur secondarily to some other skin disorder or follow administration of a drug. Itching may be severe. This is a severe disease and can have a fatal outcome. The patient is in acute distress since the total skin area is affected, and there is considerable water and protein loss from the skin. Control of heat regulation is poor, and the patient is susceptible to infection.

TREATMENT. The patient is taken off any drugs being taken. Fluid and electrolyte balance must be maintained and infection prevented, necessitating nursing care similar to that given in burn cases. Anti-inflammatory agents may be applied externally, and adrenocorticosteroids given as a lifesaving procedure.

Urticaria (Hives). This is a common pruritic condition produced by toxic or allergic mechanisms and characterized by transient wheals or welts of varying size. The trunk is the usual site of involvement, although they may appear anywhere on the body. Contact with certain plants or insects produces a local reaction, whereas drugs or ingestants usually produce a symmetrical distribution over the entire skin. The initial lesions are usually pink, turn white and then turn pink again. They may disappear in minutes to hours and are followed by new lesions. Central healing or coalescence may produce annular or gyrate forms.[26] If they involve the lips or eyes, there may be just a generalized swelling. Hives develop quickly, often in large numbers, and typically disappear in a few hours without sequelae. Severe allergic responses may be life-threatening.

Many experts believe that acute and chronic urticaria are no different except for duration. When the cause is discovered and eliminated, it is considered to be *acute.* Discovering the possible food source may be done by putting the patient on a lamb and rice diet for 2 weeks and adding one food at a time. An offending food usually produces urticaria in 2 days, so a new food can be added every 3 days. Possible causes of *chronic* urticaria are many, including cold, animal danders, infections, exposure to sunlight, malignancy, drugs, foods, insect bites, vaccinations, insulin, pregnancy, and psychosomatic cause.

Chronic urticaria requires detective work to identify and remove the cause.[26]

TREATMENT. It is important to eliminate the cause. Skin tests are not very helpful, because the patient's skin is very reactive. Antihistamine drugs may be helpful. Colloidal baths or some lotion such as Cetaphil or any oil-in-water type that can be easily washed off, with 0.025 to 0.050 per cent menthol, may be soothing. Epinephrine (0.3 ml. of 1:1000 solution) may be lifesaving in an emergency and may relieve the urticaria in any situation.

Pityriasis Rosea. This is a self-limiting disease of unknown etiology that peaks in the spring and fall. Characteristically, a single oval lesion develops first, called a *herald patch.* From several days to 2 to 3 weeks later, an eruption develops on the trunk and extremities in the direction of lines of cleavage of the skin. Lesions are rarely seen on exposed areas and they are usually confined to the trunk. Individual lesions are fawn colored with a pink or reddish edge. Each lesion is covered by a fine scale attached at the edge. Itching varies from severe to pratically none. Spontaneous cure regularly occurs in 6 to 8 weeks. Ultraviolet exposure usually shortens the disease course. Treatment is ordinarily unnecessary, unless there is severe itching.

Drug Reactions.

> *Adverse reactions to drugs occur more often in the skin than in any other organ, and are most common in patients with serious illness who receive a number of drugs.*

The following considerations regarding drug allergy are important:

- ▶ The drug may have been used before without untoward reaction.
- ▶ After the first reaction to the drug only a small dose is required to cause a recurrence.
- ▶ Drugs may produce different reactions in different people and many drugs produce similar reactions.
- ▶ The risk is directly related to the number of drugs the patient is taking.
- ▶ Drug reactions persist.

Some drug may produce an inflammatory reaction in the skin when light is present. These may include the sulfonamides, phenothiazine and some tetracyclines. *Fixed drug reactions* recur specifically at previously affected areas. The eruption is usually a purplish red, round or oval plaque with a sharply defined border. They are more common in the extremities. Some drugs likely to produce fixed eruptions are barbiturates, salicylates and antipyrine.

TREATMENT. Most drug eruptions disappear when the causal agent is discontinued. A relapse may be caused by taking a very small amount of drug. Fluids should be encouraged to speed up the elimination of the drug. The patient should be advised of the drug sensitivity and the necessity of informing any physician who may be prescribing medication of this sensitivity.

Lichen Planus. *Lichen planus* is a chronic, pruritic, inflammatory, papular eruption of the skin and mucous membranes of unknown etiology. The disease begins insidiously with the individual appearance of a discrete shiny flat-topped papule. Lesions are usually found on the front of the wrists or forearms, ankles, thighs, and abdomen. They are seldom found on the scalp, face, palms and soles. Mucous membranes may be affected, and sometimes the nails will be involved, with thinning or increased longitudinal ridging. Most cases occur in adult life. Women are more likely to develop the disease than men. Nervous strain is regarded as a secondary factor.

TREATMENT. The patient is generally taken off all drugs, and a substitute given for essential drugs. Adrenocorticosteroid cream under occlusive dressings may be used for localized lichen planus. In cases of hypertrophic lichen planus of the legs, a firm occlusive dressing of an Unna boot type, changed weekly, relieves the pruritus and flattens the lesions over a period of weeks. Grenz radiation may be prescribed. Systemic administration of adrenocorticosteroids may be helpful in suppressing the disease when patients have generalized disease. A lotion for itching may be advised.

NURSING IMPLICATIONS. The nurse may be the first professional to notice or be told about the first lesions of lichen planus. Since early care and discontinuation of medication are important, a high level of awareness of skin lesions is necessary.

Psoriasis. Psoriasis is a common skin disease found in people in good health. The disease

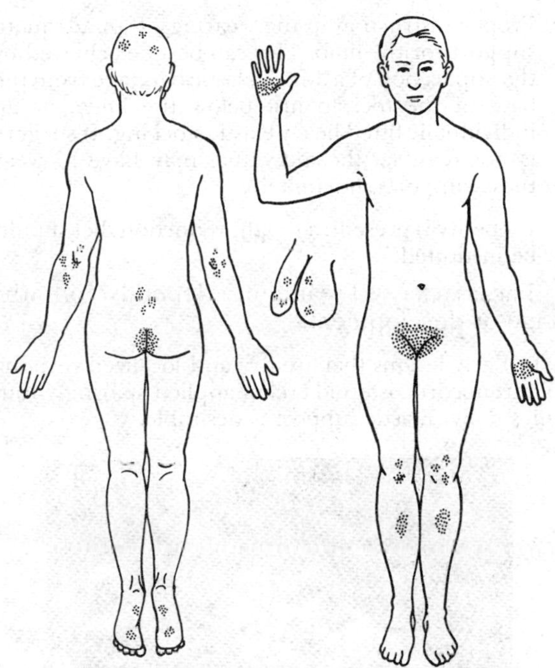

Figure 79–20. Psoriasis. (Redrawn from Fitzpatrick, T. B., and S. A. Walker: *Dermatological Differential Diagnosis.*)

affects about 5 per cent of the population. It commonly begins in the second and third decades and runs a variable course. Psoriasis is definitely familial and is classified genetically as an irregularly autosomal dominant trait with incomplete penetrance.

The basic problem in psoriasis is loss of control of epidermal cells, which leads to marked epidermal hyperplasia and rapid cell turnover. Normal epidermal cell turnover is 457 hours. Normal cells take 13 days to arrive at surface and 13 to 14 more days to slough off. In psoriasis cell cycling occurs in 37.5 hours. This rapid turnover results in the formation of thick scaling plaques. Biochemical factors are unknown but recent studies have implicated deficiency of cyclic nucleotides and prostaglandins. Association with HLA antigens raises the question of immunologic susceptibility.

This is a chronic disease characterized by sharply demarcated lesions of a deep red color covered by thick overlying silvery scales. Two observable signs of psoriasis are *Auspitz's sign* and *Koebner's isomorphic phenomenon.* In the former, when the scale is removed manually punctate bleeding points may be seen underneath; the latter phenomenon refers to the spreading of psoriasis along scratch marks and other trauma sites. There is a marked frequency of lesions in certain areas of the body, such as the scalp, regions over the elbows and knees, and the lower part of the back. These lesions most often have striking symmetrical distribution. Pruritus is a main complaint. No portion of the skin is free from the disease. It is common to observe pitting and discoloration of the nails with an accumulation of detritus under the free edge of the nails (Fig. 79–20).

Psoriasis is extremely variable in its duration and course. A single lesion may persist for a lifetime, or many lesions may be present. Some patients are never free of the disease, whereas others have long remissions. Most patients are better in the summer.

Warm weather, sunlight and humidity usually have a beneficial effect on psoriasis. Persons with psoriasis tend to fare badly in cold weather.

Acute guttate (drop-like) forms of psoriasis in children and young adults commonly follow upper respiratory infection with beta hemolytic streptococcus. Almost one half of psoriatic patients note that emotional stress and anxiety cause exacerbations.[101]

TREATMENT. General principles of the treatment of psoriasis are:

- The physician has to establish the necessity of continual adherence to the treatment plan.
- No treatment should produce trauma to the skin, as this may result in new psoriatic lesions, since they tend to form in the area of skin trauma.
- Slow inactive thick lesions should be treated aggressively.
- Acute recent spreading lesions should be treated gently.
- Tar and dithranol compounds should be used very cautiously in flexural and anogenital areas because of the irritating potential.
- When topical steroids are discontinued, some other preparation should be used to maintain therapeutic effect because of possible rebound.

Therapy is directed at slowing down epidermal turnover time and reducing pruritus. Skin dryness may be relieved by daily emollient baths using tar-containing bath oils. Topical white petrolatum is a good treatment. Three to five per cent salicylic acid combined with other therapies is a major kerolytic agent.

Fluorinated topical corticosteriods are most widely prescribed in treating psoriasis. They are effective in resolving psoriatic plaques, particularly if used with occlusive dressings. The long-term continued use of corticosteroid preparations is undesirable because of adverse reactions such as skin atrophy, telangectasia, and striae or depression of adrenocortical function. Topical preparations containing coal tar are especially effective when used with ultraviolet light. Recently, coal tar has been incorporated into a cosmetically acceptable gel base (Estargel).

Regular exposure to ultraviolet light (one to three times weekly), avoiding production of erythema or burning, is desirable. Grenz ray therapy may be used for lesions that are difficult to control by local therapy alone. Grenz radiation is a form of ionizing radiation with a spectrum between ultraviolet and roentgen rays. It has no permanent effects when used correctly and has a beneficial effect on superficial psoriatic lesions. Patients whose psoriasis is refractory or severe may respond to a new technique in which the patient is treated with PUVA systemic 9-methoxypsoralen followed by irradiation of the skin with long wave ultraviolet light.[101, 104]

Methotrexate, an antifolic acid drug, is one of the most important and effective new agents to be used in severe psoriasis. It is applied under occlusion as indicated for steroids.

Many different drugs and treatment are used in the treatment of psoriasis, but because it is a long-term, chronic condition, caution is emphasized.[77, 101, 104]

Stasis Dermatitis and Ulceration. Stasis dermatitis is a very common problem related to an underlying venous insufficiency. It is identified with varicose veins with or without varicose ulcers (Fig. 79–21). (See also p. 1121.)

One of the earliest indications of chronic venous insufficiency is ankle edema, usually occurring at the end of the day. After a time, patches of tan pigmentation appear on the lower third of the leg. The pigment is hemosiderin resulting from extravasation of blood through capillary walls due to increased venous pressure. A patchy erythema may develop which may be dry or oozing and vesicular. Secondary infections may occur and a characteristic subcutaneous induration may develop. The final stage is associated with atrophy and fibrous scarring of the area. At any stage of this process, an ulcer may develop in the devitalized area.

Hypostatic ulcers are very slow in healing and, since the skin is easily irritated, bland nonsensitizing applications must be used. The basis of treatment of venous insufficiency is the prevention of orthostatic edema. The following suggestions are offered for people who must be managed conservatively:

- Strict avoidance of standing or sitting in one position for a long period of time.
- Regular 15- to 20-minute rest periods during the day when the legs can be maintained at a level well above the heart. The foot of the bed should be raised 6 inches or more.
- Proper instruction in the wearing of an adequate support for the limb. This can best be achieved by the application of a 3-inch elastic bandage from the base of the toes to just below the knee, or an individually fitted heavy elastic stocking. If surgery is not feasible, the individual may have to wear these supports indefinitely.
- If obesity is present, a weight reduction diet should be instituted.

Treatment. Treatment depends on the stage of development.

1. Early lesions that are dry and localized respond to adrenocorticosteroid cream applied sparingly four times daily. Elastic support is desirable.

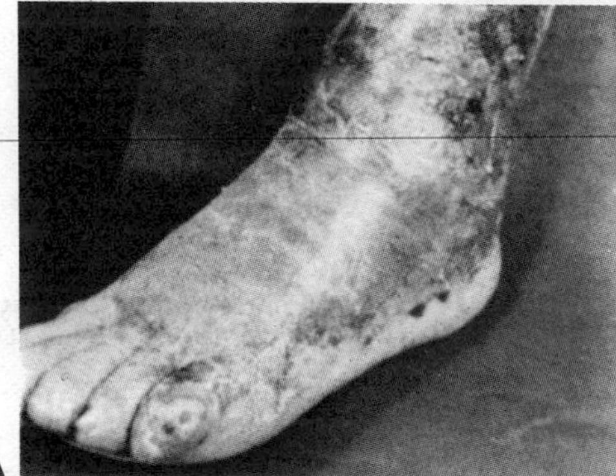

A

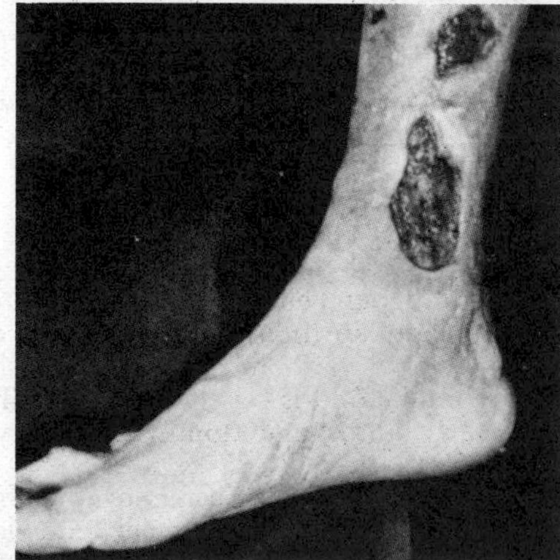

B

Figure 79–21. Stasis dermatitis (eczema) and stasis ulcers. **A.** Diffuse eczematous eruption; varicosities, heredity, middle age, and occupation (standing) are usual etiologic factors. **B.** Ulcers are often furthered by trauma and infection in a setting of stasis dermatitis. (From Lewis, G. M., and C. E. Wheeler, Jr.: *Practical Dermatology,* 3rd ed.)

2. Subacute (moist) lesions are treated with cool compresses of Burow's solution 1:20 dilution for 15 minutes three times daily followed by air drying, and steroid ointment. Elevation of the leg for 15 minutes three times daily and use of elastic stockings are advised.

3. Severe lesions require bedrest with the foot of the bed elevated, and the compresses and cream. The patient should wear the elastic support only after ambulation is allowed. Systemic drugs may be indicated, depending on whether there is generalized dermatitis or secondary infection.

Treatment of Varicose Ulcer. Varicose ulcers are far more satisfactorily prevented than treated. Bedrest is recommended. Steps are taken to eliminate infection. After infection is eliminated, the leg may be covered with a commercially available gelatin-zinc oxide paste (modified Unna's boot), allowing for some shrinkage when dry. This is replaced at weekly intervals at first, and then at longer intervals as the ulcer heals.

Other treatments used have been high oxygen concentrations in the immediate region of ulcer, topical application of gold leaf, oral zinc sulfate, etc. Surgical consultation is recommended, since the earlier the chronic venous insufficiency of the limb is corrected, the more satisfactory is the operative result.[21, 22, 88, 126]

LUPUS ERYTHEMATOSUS

Lupus erythematosus is usually classified as one of the *collagen diseases* and is discussed in Chapters 10 and 78. Lupus erythematosus takes two forms: localized (or discoid) and systemic. The disease is considered here because both forms have skin manifestations.

Discoid Lupus Erythematosus. This term refers to a chronic skin eruption which is not life-threatening, whereas systemic lupus erythematosus is a serious disease often terminating fatally. Views differ as to whether these are two different diseases or whether the discoid type is the benign end of the disease spectrum.

Discoid lupus begins with scaling erythematous macules over the nose, cheeks, forehead and temples, the so-called "butterfly" distribution. It may start with a small lesion and gradually involve more areas of the neck, ears and scalp. Exposure to sunlight may precipitate the appearance of new lesions and aggravate those already present. Antibiotics should be avoided, since they disseminate the disease process.[105]

Treatment. Fluorinated adrenocorticosteroid under a plastic dressing may be used; chloroquine, an antimalarial drug, also has been found to be a satisfactory treatment. Patients may need to avoid sunlight and use a sunscreening agent.

Systemic Lupus Erythematosus. This is an autoimmune disease. Patients with this condition have a very reactive antibody system. Antigen-antibody reactions lead to petechial skin lesions, skin ulcers, glomerulitis or widespread vasculitis, arthritis, pericarditis and pleuritis.

Glucocorticosteroids are effective in reducing systemic symptoms but frequently produce side effects. Other drugs are presently being studied for their action in suppressing the inflammatory response.

SKIN CONDITIONS DUE TO HEAT AND SUNLIGHT

Prickly Heat (Miliaria Rubra). This condition is characterized by pinpoint or pinhead-sized vesicles and papules with pricking and burning sensations, generally occurring under clothing and in individuals working in tropical climates or in conditions of excessive heat. Obstruction of outflow of sweat occurs at the sweat pore. Continued secretion of sweat results in its escape into the epidermis. This condition is frequently seen in infants.

Treatment is by avoiding sweating and by allowing circulation of air with looser, cooler clothing. Air conditioners and fans should be used when available. Cool baths and steroid sprays may be helpful. Topical ointments that are occlusive should be avoided. Once the tendency to prickly heat is established, it persists.

Skin Conditions Due to Sunlight. Exposure to sunlight is not an unmixed blessing. Although sun is necessary for life on this planet, exposure to ultraviolet radiation is potentially dangerous to people with white skin.

Sunburn is an inflammatory response of the skin to the ultraviolet radiation. The skin defends itself against this by producing more melanin. Tanning therefore provides the best protection against sunburn. Ultraviolet radiation can be reduced by as much as 90 per cent by a good tan.[78] Individuals incur more ultraviolet radiation at the mountains or beach because of the reflected radiation from water or snow. The longer the pathway through the atmosphere, the less ultraviolet radiation. Sunbathing is therefore safer in the early morning and late afternoon.

Long-term exposure to ultraviolet radiation can cause damage to the skin. The damage in the dermis attributed to aging is in reality the result of chronic exposure to the sun and to short-wave-length ultraviolet light, as can be evidenced by comparing aging skin from the buttocks with skin from exposed areas. The alterations in connective tissue give the skin the coarse wrinkled appearance of aging. Undue exposure to the sun undoubtedly predisposes

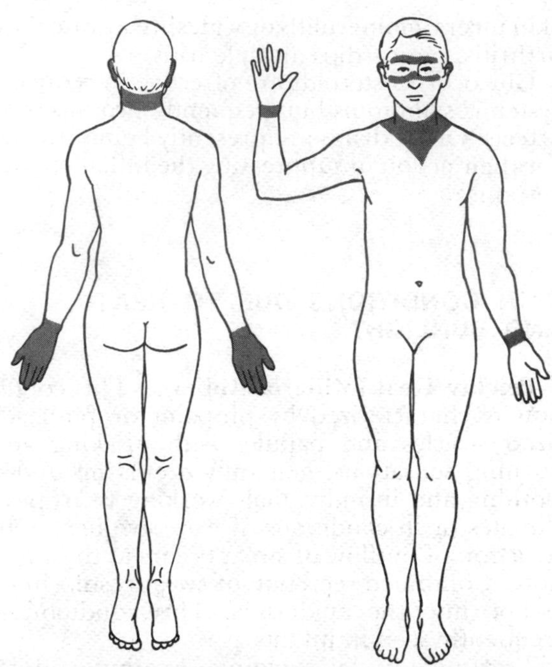

Figure 79–22. Dermatoses related to sunlight. (Redrawn from Fitzpatrick, T. B., and S. A. Walker: *Dermatological Differential Diagnosis.*)

the skin to cancerous and precancerous growth. Typical sites of dermatoses related to sunlight are shown in Figure 79–22.

Retinoic acid may enhance the cancer-causing effects of the sun on skin according to preliminary results of a study in animals. Especially in summer, FDA recommends that people be warned about using topical retinoic acid gel, cream, or liquid preparations and to avoid or minimize exposure of treated areas to sun. Patients with a family history of sunlight-induced skin cancer or who show unusual susceptibility to skin damage from sunlight should be particularly cautious when using retinoic acid.[31]

Lentigo Senilis. This common skin condition called "liver spots" seldom occurs before the fourth or fifth decade. The spots increase in numbers with advanced age. It is felt that chronic sunlight exposure is an important factor in their development. They have no relation to internal disease.

Cheilitis. Because of the prominence of the lower lip, people with chronic sun damage may have lesions confined to the lower lip. These appear in the warm season as a result of exposure to the sun. A sunscreen containing para-aminobenzoic acid (PABA) and certain of its esters should always be used by sun-sensitive people when outdoors.[125]

Topical or systemic photosensitizers produce abnormal reactions to sunlight or artificial light. A number of internal diseases are characterized by abnormal reactions to light. In diagnosing dermatitis that is first affected or is limited to exposed areas, and that worsens in summer with outdoor exposure and is intensely pruritic, the possibility of photosensitivity must be considered (see Tables 79–5 and 79–6).

Sunburn. Varied burns of the skin result from intense and prolonged exposure to ultraviolet rays. First, second or third degree burns may occur, although the first two are more common. (Burns are discussed in Chapter 80.)

TREATMENT. For mild first degree burns, bland creams or corticosteroid creams may be applied several times daily. Second degree burns characterized by blister formation should be treated by a doctor if extensive. A prolonged soak in a tub of cold water can be tried. Cold wet compresses or a water-miscible ointment can be applied to the affected areas. Aspirin may reduce the general discomfort. Increase fluid intake.

PREVENTION.

> *Avoidance of sun exposure during the hours of intense short-wavelength untraviolet light, that is, between 10* A.M. *and 3* P.M., *is important in all ages.*

Whenever possible, one should wear adequate clothing and gradually develop a tan. If untanned skins must be exposed to sun rays,

TABLE 79–5. CHEMICAL AGENTS CAUSING PHOTOSENSITIZATION

Substance	Reaction
Topical Photosensitizers and Usual Types of Reactions	
Bithionol	Erythema
Tetrachlorosalicylanilide	Erythema
Coal tar preparations	Erythema and pigmentation
Perfumes	Pigmentation
Laundry whiteners	Erythema
Parsnips and celery	Vesiculation and bullae
Lime and citrus fruits	Erythema and vesiculation
Ingested Chemicals Producing Photosensitivity	
Phenothiazines	Chloroquine
Tetracyclines	Quinine
Griseofulvin	Psoralens
Sulfonamides	Sulfonylureas
Chlorothiazide	Gold
Barbiturates	

Modified from Stewart, W. D., J. L. Danto, and S. Maddin: *Synopsis of Dermatology,* 2nd ed. St. Louis: C. V. Mosby Co. 1970.

TABLE 79–6. SKIN DISEASES ADVERSELY AFFECTED BY SUNLIGHT

Albinism and vitiligo	Porphyria
Hartnup syndrome, a rare genodermatosis	Psoriasis (benefited by moderate sun exposure but made worse by sunburn)
Herpes simplex	
Lupus erythematosus	
Pellagra	Xeroderma pigmentosum

Modified from Stewart, W. D., J. L. Danto, and S. Maddin: *Synopsis of Dermatology*, 2nd ed. St. Louis: C. V. Mosby Co. 1970.

sunscreen preparations with para-aminobenzoic acid (PABA) are usually effective.

Precancerous Conditions.

> *There is a direct relationship between the changes of chronic sun exposure and the development of precancerous or cancerous growths on the skin.*

Premalignant lesions are usually flat or raised, hard, dry adherent scales on a red base. In 25 per cent of persons with these senile or actinic keratoses, squamous cell carcinoma develops in one or more of these lesions. The use of sun screens by individuals with marked skin change can be helpful. Topical chemotherapeutic agents are being used. One of the most often used is 5-fluorouracil. This topically applied antimetabolite has been used by persons with actinic keratoses. The individual applies the medication with the fingers to the entire face and neck twice daily after washing, taking care to avoid the eyelids and lips. Erythema develops. The application is generally continued for 2 to 3 weeks on the face and for 6 to 8 weeks on the hands and arms. The patient needs to be seen by the doctor every 7 to 10 days. This treatment produces photosensitivity and the patient has an unsightly appearance and some local discomfort during treatment, but it has been fairly successful in clearing the skin of precancerous lesions.

MALIGNANT TUMORS OF THE SKIN

Basal Cell Epithelioma. *This is the most common type of skin cancer.* The mid-fifties is the average age of onset. Typical appearance of the lesions is shown in Figure 79–23.

The most common variety begins as a papule

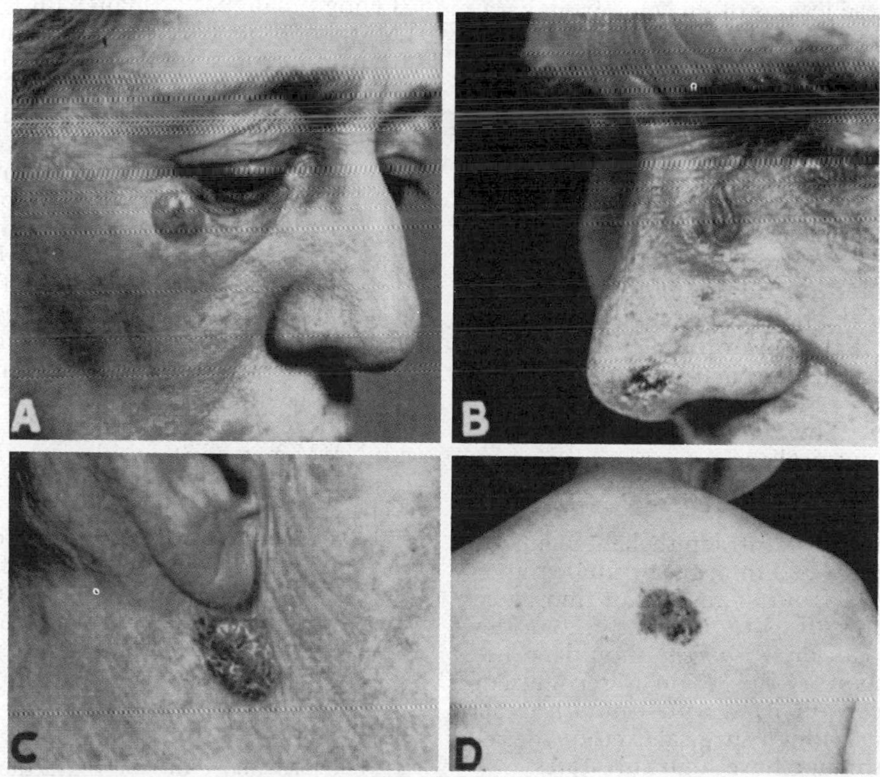

Figure 79–23. Basal cell epithelioma. **A.** Nodule on the right lower eyelid; treated by electrodesiccation and curettage, with an excellent cosmetic result. **B.** In this location neglect will allow sufficient destruction so that a noticeable scar will result; x-ray therapy was successful. **C.** Rapidly developing anaplastic type. **D.** Superficial variety; the clinical appearance may resemble psoriasis. (From Lewis, G. M., and C. E. Wheeler, Jr.: *Practical Dermatology*, 3rd ed.)

that enlarges peripherally. It soon develops a central depression, becomes crusted and may bleed easily. The central area may become depressed, leading to ulceration and the classic *rodent ulcer.* The border may be translucent and elevated with a smooth shiny appearance on which fine telangiectatic vessels may be found. The lesion tends to be asymptomatic. Ninety per cent of the cases occur between the hairline and the upper lip. This locally invasive cancer destroys underlying and adjacent tissue. It rarely metastasizes.

The major causative factor is prolonged sun exposure. The greatest natural protection is pigmentation. The tumor occurs more frequently in males, blonds and redheads. The incidence is increasing in the younger age group because of greater sun exposure.

TREATMENT. The three equally effective treatment modalities are (1) electrodesiccation and curettage; (2) x-ray therapy; and (3) surgical excision. The initial treatment of the lesion should be aggressive enough to be curative, and patients should be checked at 6-month intervals for evidence of recurrence.[39, 49, 83, 90, 120, 125, 127]

Squamous Cell Carcinoma (Epidermoid Carcinoma). These lesions often come from keratoses due to exposure to ultraviolet, but may lack the pearly border of the basal cell epithelioma. Instead, one sees a flesh-colored nodule that may ulcerate. It enlarges more rapidly and can produce metastases. Squamous cell carcinomas arise on the mucous membrane from the chronic irritation of pipe smoking, dentures and teeth, and on the glans penis in uncircumcised males. However, squamous cell carcinomas are most often found on the lower lip, ears, neck and dorsum of the hands. They are more likely to metastasize if they are on the ears, cheek or temple areas, and particularly on the mucous membranes.

TREATMENT. The most satisfactory treatment includes surgical excision or irradiation by superficial or deep x-ray, radium or cobalt therapy.

Bowen's Disease. Intraepithelial squamous cell carcinoma can be a multiple or single tumor and may result from ingestion of inorganic arsenic. Bowen's disease frequently coincides with systemic cancer. *Treatment* should be undertaken as soon as the lesion is recognized. Success has been reported with 1-month treatment of 5 FU, although surgical excision, desiccation, and curettage have high cure rates.

Melanoma. Melanoma is the most malignant primary cutaneous cancer. This tumor is increasing among populations with the greatest exposure of light-skinned persons to sunlight.

Most melanomas arise de novo, although some appear to arise in association with a preexisting benign nevus. (See also discussion on p. 1740.) The incidence of the tumor is higher in females than in males and hits a peak around the menopausal years. One third of the lesions occur on the face and neck and one third on the lower extremities.

A biopsy of a potentially malignant melanoma should consist of total excision and microscopic examination of the whole lesion. Treatment of a malignant melanoma consists of adequate surgical excision with removal of regional lymph nodes. Arterial regional perfusion with new cytotoxic agents shows some promise in treatment.

Melanoma can be classified into *three types:* (1) *superficial spreading melanoma,* (2) *lentigo-maligna malignant melanoma,* and (3) *nodular malignant melanoma.*

Superficial spreading melanoma (SSM) is the most common type of melanoma, accounting for about 70 per cent of diagnosed cases. SSM is not related directly to exposure to sunlight, as it may also occur on unexposed skin. However, SSM may be related indirectly to exposure to sunlight, since these lesions are more common in those areas that have more sunlight exposure and in lighter skinned persons. SSM is most common in the 40 to 45 year old age group.

Lentigo-maligna malignant melanoma (LMM) is definitely related to chronic overexposure to sunlight; and, as a result, tends to most commonly affect older people. Diagnosis of this type of melanoma is usually made in patients in their 50's or 60's, although malignant changes do not usually start until these patients are in their 70's. While LMM generally appears on the head and neck, it may occur on other sun exposed areas, e.g., the back of the hands. LMM accounts for about 15 per cent of all cases of melanoma and has a better prognosis than nodular malignant melanoma (NMM) lesions.

NMM lesions tend to spring up suddenly from a mole or clear skin, and these lesions tend to penetrate deeply into the epidermis. Patients with NMM may be 30 or 40 years of age or even younger.

The nurse is in a good position to conduct a total skin examination and ask about previous melanomas and a family history of the disease. One should confirm whether any suspect moles have been present since birth. Any patient's suspicion of recent changes in moles or the skin should be investigated. Color, size, configuration, and texture should be noted. It is important to examine:

1. The back above the waist; this site is least often examined.
2. Toe webs and soles in deeply pigmented per-

sons. These are the most common sites of SSM growth in orientals and blacks.

3. Leg skin between the knees and ankles in women. This is the most common site for development of SSM in females.

4. Fingernails, because LMM lesions have a tendency to develop in periungual skin.

5. Face and the back of the hands, as most LMM lesions occur in these areas.

6. Body orifices and under the arms; lesions can remain hidden for years in these areas.

It is particularly important to note color change. Early SSM lesions have a haphazard collection of colors, e.g., tan, brown, blue and black. Late SSM lesions have a characteristic red, white, and blue coloration. Early LMM lesions are primarily brown and do not fade in the winter. Late LMM lesions show a haphazard combination of colors, but tans and browns continue to dominate, and one does not see pink or rose tones. NMM lesions may be forming when pigmented nevi begin to turn darker, then bluish black.

In addition to color change and irregular border, a sizable notch in the border of a pigmented lesion may be a sign of malignant change. Uneven skin elevations, loss of skin markings and irregular borders are also suspicious signs. Lethality of melanoma lesion varies directly with the depth of the primary lesion. Lesions of less than one mm. in thickness are cured by incision alone.[11, 20, 53, 89]

THE BLACK SKIN

Variation in pigmentation among different groups of people is the consequence of varying productions of melanin by melanocyte cells in the epidermis, dermis, hair follicles and ocular retina. There are no sexual or racial differences in the number of melanocytes. The difference in color is accounted for by the rate and quantity of production of melanin. Pigmentation is affected by genetic mechanisms, hormones, and environment. White skinned individuals are less efficient than darker skinned persons in producing melanin. One of the results of this is that skin cancer occurs more often in persons with white skins.

Because of the greater amount of pigment in black skins, pathologic signs have a different appearance than with white skin. For example, in a black skinned person an increase in pallor gives a gray appearance, and cyanosis may be difficult to observe except in the fingernails and under the tongue. Mild jaundice may be difficult to determine, but one can look for indications under the patient's tongue and in the sclera of the eyes.

One of the first differences observed in Black American, American Indian, and Oriental infants is the *Mongolian Spot.* This is a benign hyperpigmented macula to patch size lesion, located in the lumbosacral area and present at

birth. These spots are blue to black. In most cases, only a single lesion is present although they may be found on the buttocks, abdomen, back arms and thighs. They usually disappear in early childhood, but occasionally persist to adulthood.[57]

Pigmentary disorders are commonly encountered in black clients. *Vitiligo* is a noticeable disease of *hypopigmentation* (Fig. 79–24). This is a genetically determined, focal, complete loss of pigment of unknown etiology. Vitiligo occurs in 1 per cent of the human race and varies from barely noticeable lesions of the hands, face, and genitalia to the extensive absence of pigment over the entire body. In about 50 per cent of patients, vitiligo starts before the age of 20 years of life; in about 20 to 30 per cent of cases, there is a familial incidence. Vitiligo leaves the skin white and is, therefore, more noticeable in dark people. Pigment loss is usually symmetrical, slowly progressive, and permanent. Erythema or itching may precede the disappearance of pigment. Vitiligo may also occur at the site of trauma. Most patients with vitiligo are otherwise "normal," however, vitiligo is seen with increased frequency among patients with hyperthyroidism, achlorhydria, Addison's disease, pernicious anemia, adult onset diabetes, alopecia areata, and autoimmune disorders.

Three *therapeutic choices* are usually available to patients with vitiligo:

1. Bleaching of the surrounding skin in order to blur the margins of the lesions or removing all pigmentation in severe cases. Benoquin may cause irreversible depigmentation and should only be used in patients with extensive vitiligo.

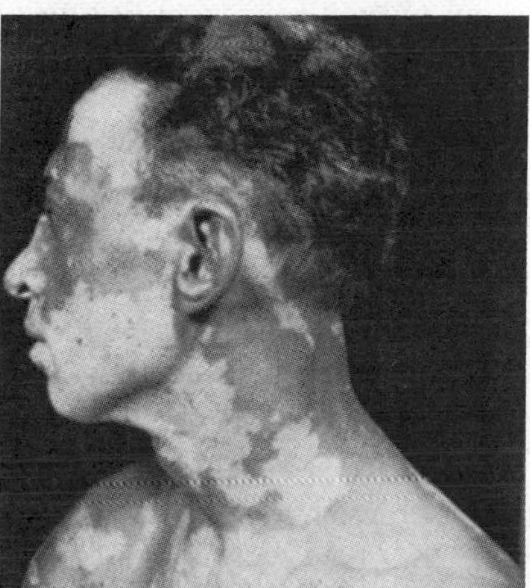

Figure 79–24. Vitiligo: a complete absence of pigment in patches, without other findings. (From Lewis, G. M., and C. E. Wheeler, Jr.: *Practical Dermatology,* 3rd ed.)

2. Attempts to repigment the skin through the topical or systemic use of Psoralen compounds plus exposure to sunlight or long-wave ultraviolet light. Psoralen compounds are found naturally in various plants and are also produced synthetically. Psoralen compounds radically increase the response of the skin to light after either topical application or systemic administration. Pigment first appears around hair follicles and then slowly spreads. To be successful, the therapy must continue for 3 to 8 months and often through several summers.

3. Lesions may be covered with stains or cosmetics, e.g., Cover-Mark, Neo-Dyoderm, a stain that contains aniline dyes and dihydroxyacetone or Walnut Stain Depelle.

Depigmentation can also occur in blacks with nonpigmenting skin diseases such as *tinea versicolor* and *atopic dermatitis.* This disorder is usually corrected after treatment with steroid creams.

Hyperpigmentation. Acne, drug eruptions, neurodermatitis, and pityriasis rosea can all leave clients with persistent hyperpigmented areas. These areas usually fade gradually but are so upsetting to some persons that they seek therapy. One treatment used is hydroquinone combined with an epidermal turnover stimulating agent. Skin sensitivity to the therapeutic agents should be tested. If there is no reaction, the client may massage the preparation into the dark spots twice a day. A sun screen lotion should be used to cut down on further stimulation of pigmentation.

Hair Problems. *Traction alopecia* is a condition seen in blacks, owing to trauma to hair which is tightly pinned into elaborate styles for prolonged periods of time. Corn-row, pick combing, or hot combing can produce hair damage. If the client gives up the aggravating practice, normal hair growth will usually occur.

Pseudofolliculitis Barbae. Ingrown hair is a special problem in blacks. Shaving with a straight razor is the cause of this disorder. Hair follicles in black people are curved. A razor cuts the hair obliquely, giving it a sharp point; when the hair emerges from a curved follicle, it reenters the skin and causes an inflammatory reaction, predisposing the patient to chronic folliculitis or possibly even keloids. Growing a beard is one solution to this problem.

Keloid folliculitis is characterized by development of pustules and hard follicular papules. They most often begin at the nape of the neck and extend upward into the occipital region of the scalp. Eventually these papules fuse into hard keloid plaques. Early, the condition can usually be controlled by the intralesional or sublesional injection of steroids plus oral administration of antibiotics. More difficult cases may require excision of the papules to skin level; epilation of involved hairs; intralesional steroid injection and the use of antibiotics and steroid cream.[43, 57]

Keloids. Keloids are more common in black people than in lighter skinned persons. There seems to be a genetic transmission of this tendency. A keloid is an abnormal scar — a hard, smooth, rounded lump of broad interwoven bundles of dense fibrotic tissue. A keloid is dome-shaped, circular, linear or irregular in outline and has claw-like projections. Locations prone to scarring are the ear lobe, shoulders, upper chest, neck, back, and abdomen. Keloids tend to recur if excised and often appear following burns. Keloids respond satisfactorily to x-ray treatments given within the first few months. If a keloid-prone person requires surgery or if an established keloid is to be excised, triamcinolone suspension injected into the new wound or x-ray treatments given immediately after the new wound heals, usually prevent recurrence. Dry ice with moderate pressure at 2 week intervals is safe and usually effective for small keloids.[108] (See Fig. 10–3, p. 128.)

Congenital Ichthyosis. This "fish skin" disease may be more common in blacks. The epidermis is diffusely thick, dry, and harsh; its extra keratin is broken up in areas similar to fish scales. Ichthyosis vulgaris is the common form. It is familial, is transmitted as an autosomal trait, and is often associated with atopy. The ichthyotic skin is intolerant of hot water and soap. Dryness and scaliness are troublesome, especially in the winter when the humidity is low. Plain water baths with a teaspoon of bath oil or cool soaks with a cupful of salt to the tub, may cleanse, improve hydration, and afford some relief. Mineral oil is a suitable emollient to apply immediately after bathing. An emulsion incorporating 20 to 42 per cent urea may help to soften the keratin. A 50 per cent aqueous solution of propylene glycol with plastic film occlusion at night may be effective.

Dermatitis papulosis nigra are small black warty growths commonly seen on the face of blacks. Affected persons regard these growths as moles; however, they are a variety of seborrheic keratoses and may be removed by any method of separating the epidermis from the dermis, e.g., liquid nitrogen, electrodesiccation, cautery, or curette.

Sarcoidosis and *systemic sarcoid* are much more common among Afro-American adults, particularly females, than among caucasians. The cause of sarcoid is unknown and it can be anywhere on the body. Skin treatment must be coordinated with the management of the whole disease. (See Unit XVI.)

SKIN IN THE ELDERLY PERSON[88, 91, 120, 125]

Summary of Changes in Skin in Aging. The so-called "aged skin" is not the direct result of the natural aging process, but rather of exposure to sunlight.

1. Elasticity of skin lessens with age.
2. Progressive impairment of peripheral vascular circulation alters cutaneous response to physical trauma, cold, or infection.
3. Changes in central nervous system, often a consequence of atherosclerosis, modify perception of itching and pain.
4. Atrophy of the reticuloendothelial system may impair immune responses.
5. Skin tends to be thinned, dry and sometimes scaly, rough, lax, and wrinkled.
6. There is a gradual loss of subcutaneous fat.
7. The number of eccrine sweat glands is reduced, as well as output per gland.
8. Apocrine glands atrophy.
9. Sebaceous gland secretion commonly decreases.
10. There is diffuse reduction in density of hair follicles, resulting in widespread scalp hair thinning.
11. Pigmentary changes occur, especially in exposed areas.
12. Small dermal blood vessels become fragile and easily tear, even without trauma. This gives rise to purpura, especially over the back of the hands and the arms.
13. Telangiectases on aging, light-exposed skin are very common.
14. Nails become more brittle, and their rate of growth is increased.
15. Seborrheic warts, senile hemangiomata, and senile lentigines are very common.

General factors about skin in elderly people:

a. When elderly persons develop skin infections, they may well have one or more systemic diseases in addition to the skin problem. Many systemic diseases show skin manifestations, e.g., cancer, diabetes.

b. Emotional factors, e.g., grief or depression, may set off a skin condition or cause delay in seeking treatment.

c. Humidity in the living environment should be 60 per cent or higher. Lubrication of moist skin after bathing helps seal in the water and prolongs the beneficial effect. Itching is extremely common in the elderly and is usually related to dry skin. It is necessary, however, to exclude organic causes. Conditions that may give rise to generalized itching include: uremia, myxedema, polycythemia rubra vara, and the reticuloses. Dry skin is more vulnerable to irritant dermatitis.

d. Dermatitis in aged persons may be slow to respond to treatment and may be very distressful to experience, so the nurse must encourage the patient to continue treatment and not expect quick results.

e. Since elderly people may take a lot of drugs, iatrogenic skin disorders must be ruled out when there is a skin condition.

f. It is necessary to inquire about any changes in all pigmented lesions. New growths, especially those with variations in pigmentation, those that bleed easily, and those with small satellite lesions, should be removed and submitted for pathologic examination.

g. People with actinically damaged skin should: use sun screens; avoid direct sunlight between 10:00 and 3:00 P.M., and watch for skin lesions or changes.

h. The ability to differentiate normal skin from abnormal skin is more difficult in older persons, because of the physical changes that occur with aging.

Common Skin Diseases in Elderly Persons

Common skin disorders in elderly persons include: basal cell epithelioma, squamous cell carcinoma, seborrheic keratoses, herpes zoster, statis dermatitis and ulcerations and various blistering lesions.

Leukoplakia. This is a white hyperkeratotic plaque affecting the mucosal or mucocutaneous tissue. The lips (usually the lower), hard palate, vulva, and labia are the most common sites of involvement. Clinically the disease appears as discrete, white rough patches with moderately defined borders. Diagnosis is confirmed by biopsy and since the lesions are premalignant, treatment is indicated.

Lichen Sclerosus et Atrophicus. This disease is characterized by pinkish papules that in time become white atrophic spots. They commonly involve the external genitalia in middle-aged women, causing severe itching and dyspareunia. Since there is a 3 per cent incidence of squamous cell neoplasia occurring in these patches, a long period of follow-up is necessary.

Venous Lakes. These soft asymptomatic dark papules occur most commonly on the ear, but are also frequently seen on the face, neck, and lower lip. They are persistent and solitary and seldom become larger than a few mm. They occur on sun-exposed areas. They are more common in older men and are seldom seen in women. They are not related to cancer or internal illness.

Senile Telangiectasia. This condition is characterized by dilated superficial blood vessels. They are often small and almost unnoticeable on the face and necks of older people who have cumulative actinic damage. They produce no symptoms, but the changes are permanent. Such lesions disappear when you empty the blood vessels by pressure.

Other Skin Problems in the Elderly. Stasis Dermatitis and Ulceration. These are common problems in the elderly, involving the lower legs. *Blistering lesions* may occur in a number of generalized skin conditions, such as dermatitis herpetiformis and erythema multiforme, but two skin diseases are important in old age — pemphigus and pemphigoid. Both have blisters as their most common presentation and are relatively common in the elderly.

BIBLIOGRAPHY (Chapter 79)

1. A look at Steven-Johnson syndrome. *Consultant* 18:156, Sept. 1978.
2. A new approach to herpes zoster. *Consultant*, 17:39, Aug. 1977.
3. Arey, L. B.: *Human Histology*. Philadelphia: W.B. Saunders Co., 1974.
4. Arnold, V., and S. Rose: Photochemotherapy for psoriasis. *American Journal of Nursing*, 79:466, Mar. 1979.
5. Baden, H.P.: Hair loss: Finding out why. *Consultant*, 17:29, Aug. 1977.
6. Basler, R.S.W., and P.J. Lynch: Can you recognize and treat mycosis fungoides? *Geriatrics*, 33:55, Nov. 1978.
7. Bean, S. F.: Immunofluorescent techniques and blistering diseases. *Consultant*, 18:49, Feb. 1978.
8. Benesen, A.S. (Ed.): *Control of Communicable Disease in Man*. Washington D.C., American Public Health Association, 1975.
9. Bergfield, W.F.: Diffuse hair loss in women. *Cutis*, 22:190, Aug. 1978.
10. Bielan, B.: Honing your assessment skills: What that rash really means. *RN*, 42:58, Feb. 1979.
11. Blois, S. M., and W. L. Epstein: Melanoma: Value of early detection and treatment. *Postgraduate Medicine*, 61(5):82, June 1977.
12. Botero, F.: Pruritus as manifestation of systemic disorders. *Cutis*, 21:873, June 1978.
13. Breaking the skin barrier. *Emergency Medicine*, 9:175, Jan. 1977.
14. Brodin, M.B.: The diagnosis of difficult dermatologic disorders. *Resident and Staff Physician*, 23:54, Apr. 1977.
15. Brown, M.S.: Over-the-counter drugs for skin disorders. Part 1: Anti-acne aids. *Nurse Practitioner*, 2:23, Mar.–Apr. 1977.
16. Cameron, G.: Pressure sores: What to do when prevention fails. *Nursing 79*, 9:42, Jan. 1979.
17. Carpenter, C. Jr., et al.: Coping with warts and calluses. *Patient Care*, 2(16):90, Sept. 1977.
18. Carpenter, C. Jr., et al.: Minding moisture stores of the skin. *Patient Care*, 2(18):90, Oct. 1977.
19. Castrow, F.F., II, et al.: Hirsutism. When a woman wants epilation. *Patient Care*, 71(16):60, Sept. 1977.
20. Clark, W. A., et al.: Skin cancer: Spotting changes that signal melanoma. *Patient Care*, 8:132, Aug. 1974.
21. Cobey, J.C., and J.H. Cobey: Chronic leg ulcer. *American Journal of Nursing*, 74:258, Feb. 1974.
22. Connors, P.: Treating leg ulcers. *Nursing 77*, 77(5):66, May 1977.
23. Cunliffe, W.J., and J.A. Cotterill: The acnes. *Major Problems in Dermatology*. Philadelphia: W.B. Saunders Co., 1975.
24. Di Mascio, S.: Debrisan for decubitus ulcers. *American Journal of Nursing*, 79:684, Apr. 1979.
25. Epstein, J.H.: Photosensitivity and skin disease. *Consultant*, 18:73, June 1978.
26. Fellner, M.J.: Tracking down the cause of urticaria. *Consultant*, 16:55, Oct. 1976.
27. Finch, C.: *A Patient Oriented Approach to General Medicine*. University of Washington School of Medicine, Seattle, 1972.
28. Fisher, A.A.: Drug-induced skin eruptions: Typical treatments for topical problems. *Geriatrics*. 34:45, Mar. 1979.
29. Frank, S.B.: Treatment of acne with topical antibiotics. *Postgraduate Medicine*, 61:92, June 1977.
30. Frank, S.B., and H.J. Cohen: A case of foot rash. *Consultant*, 18:183, Oct. 1978.
31. FDA Drug Bulletin: Retinoic acid and sun-caused skin cancer. Aug–Sept, 1978, p. 26.
32. Fry, L.N., and P.P. Leah: *Immunologic Aspects of Skin Disease*. Lancaster, England: MTP Medical and Technical Publishing Company, 1974.
33. Garrie, S.A., and E. Garrie: Anxiety and skin diseases. *Cutis*, 22:205, Aug. 1978.
34. Getting to the foot of erythema nodosum. *Emergency Medicine*. 9:64, July 1977.
35. Goldman, L.: Acne prevention in the family. *American Family Physician*, 16:68, Aug. 1977.
36. Hanifin, J.M.: Eczematous conditions in the elderly: Common and curable. *Geriatrics*, 34:29, Jan. 1979.
37. Hawkins, K.: Wet dressings: Putting the damper on dermatitis. *Nursing 78*, 8:64, Feb. 1978.
38. Hawkins, K.: What's troubling Brian? *Nursing 79*, 9:31, May 1979.
39. Haynes, H.: The front line on skin cancers. *Emergency Medicine*, 10:131, Oct. 1978.
40. Help for herpes encephalitis. *Emergency Medicine*, 10:121, Aug. 1978.
41. Hicks, J.H.: Erythema nodosum in patients with tinea pedis and onychomycosis. *Southern Medical Journal*, 70:27, Jan. 1977.
43. Honeycutt, W.M.: Follicular infections. *Consultant*, 18:108, May 1978.
44. Hughes, J.H., and D.B. Stoll: Kaposi sarcoma. *American Family Physician*, 17:181, April 1978.
45. Huntley, C.C.: Atopic dermatitis and contact dermatitis in children. *American Family Physician*, 16:111, Aug. 1977.
46. Hurwitz, S.: Congenital nevi — When to remove them. *Consultant*, 18:171, Jan. 1978.
47. Hutchinson, R.: What to do . . . and what to worry about . . . when treating stings and bites. *Nursing 77*, 7:69, June 1977.
48. It's only acne. . . . *Emergency Medicine*, 9:169, Jan. 1977.
49. Jackson, R.: Some reminders about skin cancer. *Consultant*, 16:34, Dec. 1976.
50. Jacob, S.W., C.A. Francone, and W.J. Lossow: *Structure and Function in Man*, 4th ed. Philadelphia: W.B. Saunders Co., 1978.
51. Jarrett, A., R.I.C. Spearman, P.A. Riley: *Functional Dermatology*. Philadelphia: J.B. Lippincott Co., 1966.
52. Jessen, R.T., and C.F. Merwin: Identifying and treating skin malignancies. *Geriatrics*, 34:71, June 1979.
53. Jepsen, L.: Malignant melanoma: Rare cancer. Unique problems. *Nursing 77*, 7:38, Dec. 1977.
54. Kahn, G.: Skin problems of pregnancy. Part 3: Effects of pregnancy on pre-existing skin disease. *Consultant*, 17:116, Jan. 1977.
55. Kaminester, L.H.: Warts: Another look at a nuisance. *Consultant*, 18:223, Sept. 1978.
56. Kennedy, T., Jr., et al.: Carcinomatous changes in old scars. *American Family Practice*, 16:106, July 1977.
57. Kenney, J.A., Jr.: Dermatoses common in blacks. *Postgraduate Medicine*, 61(6):122, June 1977.
58. Kern, A.B.: Warts: How to tell them apart and what to do about them. *Consultant*, 17:37, June 1977.
59. Klaus, S.N., and R.R. Kierland: When primary cancer spreads to the skin. *Geriatrics*, 31:39, Dec. 1976.
60. Kligman, A.M., and H. Kaidbey: Hydrocortisone revisited. *Cutis*, 22:232, Aug. 1978.
61. Knox, J.M.: Taking the sting out of suntan. *Consultant*, 14:93, July, 1974.
62. Leyden, J.J.: Getting to the root of the dandruff problem. *Consultant*, 16:32, Nov. 1976.
63. Leyden, J.J., and A.M. Kligman: Interdigital athletes foot. New concepts in pathogenesis. *Postgraduate Medicine*, 61(6):113, June 1977.

64. Lewis, G.M., and C.E. Wheeler: *Practical Dermatology*. Philadelphia: W.B. Saunders Co., 1967.
65. Living with leprosy. *Emergency Medicine*, 10:81, Aug. 1978.
66. Lumpkin, L.R.: Simple treatment for common acne. *Consultant*, 18:29, Jan. 1978.
67. Magnus, I.A.: *Dermatological Photobiology*. Oxford: Blackwell Scientific Publications, 1976.
68. Marks, R.: *Common Facial Dermatoses*. Bristol: John Wright & Sons Ltd., 1976.
69. Matus, N.R.: Topical therapy: Choosing and using the proper vehicle. *Nursing 77*, 7:8, Nov. 1977.
70. Michaelssen, G., et al.: Effect of oral zinc and vitamin A on acne. *Archives of Dermatology*, 13:31, Jan. 1977.
71. Michiyuki, K.: Vitiligo, a new classification and therapy. *British Journal of Dermatology*, 97:255, Sept. 1977.
72. Montgomery, R.M.: Painful plantar problems. *Consultant*, 17:45, Oct. 1977.
73. Mysliborski, J.A.: and L.R. Lumpkin: Treating acne vulgaris. *American Family Physician*, 15:86, Feb. 1977.
74. Nasemann, T.: *Viral Diseases of the Skin, Mucous Membrane, and Genitalia*. Philadelphia: W.B. Saunders Co., 1977.
75. National Center of Health Statistics *Advanced Data*. 4:26, Jan. 1977.
76. Nickel, W.R.: Neurodermatitis — A concept. *Cutis*, 21:677, May 1978.
77. North, C., and G.D. Weinstein: Treatment of psoriasis. *American Journal of Nursing*, 76:410, Mar. 1976.
78. Odland, G.F.: *The Skin*. A description of the external organ and its common afflictions. Seattle: University of Washington School of Medicine, 1971.
78a. O'Donoghue, M.N., and R.E. Melcher.: Methotrexate for psoriasis — Revisited. *American Family Physician*, 19:99, Apr. 1979.
79. Pardo-Costello, V., and O.A. Pardo: *Diseases of the Nails*, 3rd ed. Springfield, Ill.: Charles C Thomas, 1960.
80. Parrish, J.A.: *Dermatology and Skin Care*. New York: McGraw-Hill Book Co., Inc., 1975.
81. Pearson, L.B. (Ed.): Contact dermatitis as a clinical entity for the nurse practitioner. *Nurse Practitioner*, 2:27, Mar.–Apr., 1977.
82. Perel, M., and L.R. Lumpkin: Management of warts. *American Family Physician*, 14:96, Oct. 1976.
83. Ploch, F.H., and T.S. Meyler: Radiotherapy for facial epithelial cancer. *American Family Physician*, 15:96, Jan. 1977.
84. Ploeg, D.E.V.: A summary of skin signs of systemic disease. *Consultant*, 18:31, Mar. 1978.
85. Programmed instruction: Skin rashes in infants and children. *American Journal of Nursing*, 78:P.I. 1, June 1978.
86. Reece, R.M.: Erythema nodosum. *American Family Physician*, 13:99, Mar. 1976.
87. Rees, B.: Newest treatments in dermatology–1977. *Medical Times*, Mar. 1977, p. 43.
88. Reichel, W.: *Clinical Aspects of Aging*. Baltimore: Williams and Wilkins, 1978.
89. Rice, I., and L. Zimmerman: A case of malignant melanoma. *Nursing 76*, 6:46, Dec. 1976.
90. Richardson, D., and L.R. Lumpkin: Common skin cancers. *American Family Physician*, 5:114, June 1977.
91. Ridgway, H.B.: Skin signs of internal malignancy. *American Family Physician*, 17:123, Mar. 1978.
92. Roach, L.B.: Assessing skin changes: The subtle and the obvious. *Nursing 74*, 4:65, Mar. 1974.
93. Roberts, S.L.: Skin assessment for color and temperature. *American Journal of Nursing*, 75:610, Apr. 1975.
94. Rogers, R.E., et al.: Dermatoses and pregnancy. *Hospital Medicine*, 8:29, Jan. 1972.
95. Rosen, T., and A.H. Rudolph: Identifying and treating bacterial and fungal infections of the skin. *Geriatrics*, 33:71, Oct. 1978.
96. Rostas, A. et al: Management of recurrent aphthous stomatitis. *Cutis*, 22:183, Aug. 1978.
97. Rubin, B.A.: Black skin: Here's how to adjust your assessment and care. *RN*, 42:31, Mar. 1979.
98. Sauer, G.C.: Say, doctor what can you do. . . ? *Consultant*, 17:64, Jan. 1977.
99. Scher, R.K.: Common nail disorders: Not always fungal. *Consultant*, 17:41, Nov. 1977.
100. Shapiro, A.L.: Itching (pruritus). In MacBryde, C.M. (Ed.): *Signs and Symptoms*, 5th ed. Philadelphia: J.B. Lippincott Co., 1970.
101. Shason, R.G., and L.R. Lumpkin: Current therapy of psoriasis. *American Family Physician*, June 1977.
102. Shelley, W.B.: Now you can really help the patient with hyperhidrosis. *Consultant*, 16:43, Sept. 1976.
103. Shelley, W.B., and R.P. Arthur: Neurohistology and neurophysiology of itch sensation in man. *Archives of Dermatology*, 76:296, Sept. 1957.
104. Shoss, R.G., and L.R. Lumpkin: Current therapy of psoriasis. *American Family Physician*, 15:114, Jan. 1977.
105. Solomons, B.: *Lecture Notes on Dermatology*, 3rd ed. Philadelphia: F.A. Davis Co., 1967.
106. Steck, W.D.: PUVA in severe psoriasis. *Consultant*, 17:130, Apr. 1977.
107. Steck, W.D.: The ubiquitous louse. *Consultant*, 16:232, Oct. 1976.
108. Stegman, S.J.: Successful treatment of keloids. *Consultant*, 17:79, Sept. 1977.
109. Stengel, F., and A.B. Acherman: Diagnosing the common alopecias. *American Family Physician*, 18:76, Nov. 1978.
110. Stern, R.A., et al.: Utilization of physician services for dermatologic complaints. *Archives of Dermatology*, 113:1062, July 1977.
111. Stewart, W., et al.: *Synopsis of Dermatology*. St. Louis: C.V. Mosby Co., 1974.
112. Stone, S.P.: Scabies. *American Family Physician*, 15:5, May 1977.
113. Stoughton, R.: Evaluation of new potent steroids. *In* Frost, P., and E.G. Gomez, and N. Zaias: *Recent Advances in Dermatopharmocology*. New York: Spectrum Publications, 1978.
114. Sulzberger, M.B.: *A Brief Course in Dermatology*. American College of Physicians, Dec. 1977.
115. Sulzberger, M.B.: Selected dermatologic problems: Introduction. *Postgraduate Medicine*, 61:81, June 1977.
116. Ten plus ten = Scalded skin syndrome. *Emergency Medicine*, 9:255, Apr. 1977.
117. The cutaneous tip of the fungus. *Emergency Medicine*, 9:214, June 1977.
118. The other edge of podophyllin. *Emergency Medicine*, 11:219, Jan. 1979.
119. Thorne, E.G.: Coping with pruritus — a common geriatric complaint. *Geriatrics*, 33:47, July 1978.
120. Uhler, D.M.: Common skin changes in the elderly. *American Journal of Nursing*, 78:1342, Aug. 1978.
121. Watson, W., and E.M. Farber: Controlling psoriasis. *Postgraduate Medicine*, 61:103, June 1977.
122. Watt, T.L., and O.F. Jillson: On standard definitions. *Archives of Dermatology*, 90:454, 1964.
123. Webb, D.R.: Understanding urticaria. *Consultant* 18:83, Feb., 1978.
124. Williams, R.A. (Ed.): *Textbook of Black-Related Diseases*. New York: McGraw-Hill Book Co., Inc. 1975.
125. Willis, I.: Sunlight, aging and skin cancer. *Geriatrics*, 33:33, Aug. 1978.
126. Witkowski, J.A. and L.C. Parish: Leg ulcer: Treat the cause, too. *Consultant*, 16:83, Aug. 1976.
127. Woolridge, W.E.: A freeze on skin cancer. *Consultant*, 17:184, Jan. 1977.
128. Word of mouth on herpes. *Emergency Medicine*, 9:179, Oct. 1977.
129. Wright, E.T.: Identifying and treating common benign skin tumors. *Geriatrics*, 18:37, June 1978.

CHAPTER 80

SKIN TRAUMA AND BURNS*

by Rosemary Pittman, M.S., C.R.N., F.N.P., and Patti Sullivan Fenton, R.N.

Trauma is one of the most frequent problems for humans, and the skin is the recipient of a major portion of this buffeting. It is fortunate that, generally, those tissues most likely to be injured also have the greatest power of repair. The epidermis, for example, regenerates very well, probably better than any other tissue in the body. In most superficial wounds, such as minor burns and abrasions, the only tissue lost is the superficial layer of the epidermis. This is healed by acceleration of the normal process of maturation of basal cells. (Wound healing is also discussed in Chapters 10 and 95.) The phenomenon of blistering, unique to humans, may have a protective function for this rapid multiplication of basal cells. The fluid from the blister, if left alone, is absorbed quite rapidly. When there is a large patch of epidermis lost, repair is by a process of epithelial migration from the edges of the wound and from any epithelial remnants left in the dermis.

WOUND ASSESSMENT†

Thorough wound assessment is essential both before initiating wound treatment and *after treatment* (during the healing phase). Such assessment includes: obtaining a history, assessing present characteristics of the wound, assessing for associated injury or complications, evaluating healing potential prior to initiating treatment, and post-treatment assessment during the healing period.

Immediate assessment is made of the severely wounded person's A, B, C's, i.e., airway, breathing and circulation. Resuscitative measures are begun if needed. General physical evaluation and wound assessment are then usually done concurrently with reviewing the history. If the wounded person is unable to give a history, consult witnesses, significant others and/or records.

Presented below are some key points you will want to consider as you obtain a *history of the wounding event and the wounded person:*

- *Circumstances* under which the wound was produced and evaluation of the possibility of wound *contamination* by the offending object or environment. Give careful attention to information suggesting *additional or multiple injuries.*
- *Nature of the wounding object* (e.g., blunt, sharp, ragged, explosive) and the *assumed depth of penetration* of the object, Puncture wounds may be difficult to identify and may appear innocuous. This is especially true if surface blood has been cleaned away and bleeding has stopped. If the penetrating object is believed to be a bullet, be sure to look for an *exit wound*, e.g., opposite the *entrance wound.* Palpation opposite the puncture wound may identify a bullet that lacked sufficient force to exit the body.
- *Duration of time since the injury.* It is generally recommended that primary closure of routine wounds be made within the first 6 to 10 hours after injury.
- *Prior healing history.* Has the injured person typically healed rapidly? Have there been difficulties associated with healing? If the latter is true, record the difficulties, e.g., prolonged wound bleeding, abnormally long healing time, failure of wounds to close, formation of excessive scar tissue.
- *Presence of existing diseases* that could adversely influence healing, e.g., diabetes and *general state of health.*
- *Drugs* the injured person has been taking, e.g., steroids, antimetabolites, and/or medications administered at the scene of the accident.
- *Allergic response history.* Has the individual ever shown indications of an allergic reaction to local anesthetics or other medications?
- Date of most recent *tetanus immunization.* (Importance of this is discussed later.)
- *Previous injury* to the involved area.

*For detailed discussion of caring for persons with wounds, see Sorensen and Luckmann, *Basic Nursing: A Psychophysiologic Approach,* Chapter 42.

†This discussion was written by Karen Creason Sorensen.

One point to remember when you are taking a wound history is that *the information you are given may not be accurate.* For example, the injured person may not actually know what caused the wound, whether or not the object was removed intact, or the depth of penetration. Also, in some instances, the person giving the history may deliberately lie.

Dr. A. J. Ryan[109] reports removing a 2-inch-long sewing needle from the buttock of a woman who said she was unable to see what the object was but "something pricked her" as she sat down in a chair. He also recalls a man who described his wound as "very superficial"; however, it was found to be a stab wound of his abdomen that lacerated his spleen and penetrated his diaphragm. Another interesting case history follows:

> I remember the case of an elderly man who was admitted to an emergency room in deep shock and who died shortly thereafter. A tiny puncture wound was present over the interspace between the second and third ribs, just to the left of the sternum. The woman who accompanied him (and who turned out to be his common-law wife) stated that it had resulted from his turning over on a loose bedspring. Postmortem examination showed a tract beneath the wound leading to a massive hemorrhage from puncture of the aorta. The police recovered a bloody ice pick, and the woman went to jail.[109]

Present characteristics of the wound also assessed include:

- *Wound location and type.* The hands and the neck are well-supplied with blood, whereas the lower legs and feet are less vascular. Treatment varies depending upon the type of wound. Wounds may be classified as *open* or *closed.* Wound types and wound care are discussed in following sections.
- *Wound contamination,* e.g., obvious presence of dirt, debris, feces, or other materials. Remember that puncture wounds may contain pieces of the penetrating object (e.g., tip of a broken needle) that may not be visible on the skin surface.
- *Presence of penetrating object in wound.* Do *not* disturb a penetrating object if it remains in the wound, e.g., do *not* break it off, push it in further, or pull it out during initial assessment. Later, wound exploration and x-rays will help identify the presence of previously undectected foreign bodies in the wound.
- *Presence of devitalized tissue.* Does the wound contain necrotic tissue ("dead tissue")? This must be removed with a scalpel or sharp scissors prior to wound closure. (Debridement is discussed later.)
- *Wound depth and length.* Generally, wounds that completely lacerate the dermis benefit from suture approximation, while lacerations that are only partial may not. (Suturing is discussed later.) Deep puncture wounds tend to heal over at the skin surface and may develop such complications as an underlying soft-tissue infection, tetanus, and septicemia.
- *Wound bleeding.* Although some free bleeding helps remove contamination, excessive bleeding must be controlled, e.g., if a major vessel is severed. Bleeding can generally be stopped in simple cuts by placing gauze pads directly over the wound and applying pressure. Ice packs may help control persistent bleeding. Occasionally, tourniquet application is necessary for vigorously spurting wounds. (*Remember that tourniquets are potentially dangerous and must be carefully managed.)*

It is also important to *assess for complications* (e.g., airway obstruction, shock) or *associated injury* (e.g., skeletal or musculoskeletal injuries). Questions important to consider in this assessment include: Is the patient able to move the injured part? Is there an obvious grossly deformed part or possible compound fracture? Does the patient have normal sensation? Is breathing difficult? Are vital signs abnormal? Assess level of consciousness (especially following head or face injuries). Determine the need for x-rays by considering factors such as the possibility of underlying fractures and the possible legal considerations.

> *Always examine the injured person for associated injuries – which may be less obvious but potentially more serious than the observable injury.*

As previously mentioned, all traumatic lesions must be considered to be potentially infected. Soft-tissue infection or more serious *complica-* may develop. Thorough and repeated wound assessment and appropriate *preventative measures* are thus imperative, e.g., wound cleaning, tetanus immunization.

> *Persons with "dirty" wounds should be given prophylactic treatment against tetanus.**

Assessment of *healing potential* and healing outcomes is necessary in deciding upon treatment. Some wounds are best left to heal by contraction; in others, the best functional and cosmetic effects may be achieved through suturing. Consider whether or not impaired function, distortion, or excessive scarring may result from natural closure.

Persons with the following injuries should be seen by a doctor (possibly a specialist) for repair:

---

*See Chapter 95.

(a) face or hand lacerations or any wounds with potential cosmetic or functional problems, (b) wounds penetrating fascial compartments, and (c) wounds involving repair of nerves, blood vessels, muscles, or tendons.

CARE OF CLOSED WOUNDS*

A closed wound has no free outward opening, i.e., the skin is not broken. The most common type of closed wound is a *contusion,* a bruise from a direct blow causing injury to the skin and underlying tissue. A common painful example of a contusion is hitting the fingertip with a hammer. The degree or extent of the injury is in direct proportion to the force of the blow or degree of violence exerted against the tissue. Contusions are diagnosed by presence of swelling and tenderness.

Treatment consists initially of cold wet compresses. An ice bag or fresh water aids in preventing further leakage of blood into the tissue from the broken blood vessels. The injured part should be rested. After 24 hours, periodic heat may be applied to enhance absorption. If the contusion does not begin to improve within 24 hours or increases in size, the individual should see a physician.

CARE OF OPEN WOUNDS*

Open wounds have free outward openings.

Abrasions (Scrapes). An abrasion is an irregular superficial open wound of the skin in which the outer layers are scraped off. There is usually not much bleeding, but many nerve endings are exposed, making the wound painful and prone to infection. If grease, gravel, or other foreign matter is ground into the wound at the time of the accident, the injured person may get a permanent tattoo as well as infection if the foreign material is not removed.

Abrasions require careful tedious cleaning. A petroleum jelly dressing can be applied for comfort. If left exposed to the air, an eschar (slough) will form and provide proper protection.

Incised Wound. This is a wound cleanly cut by a sharp instrument. This tidy wound has no bruising or crushing of the wound margin. It tends to gape open and bleed freely.

Stab or Puncture Wound. This wound, deeper than it is long, is caused by objects such as knives, pins, and spikes. While the wound entrance may be surprisingly small, there may be damage to important underlying deep structures and concealed blood loss may occur. Foreign bodies may be concealed within puncture wounds.

Puncture wounds should each be explored to their full depth. (Possible exceptions are pleural and abdominal wounds.) This exploration cannot be satisfactorily achieved with a probe or hemostat. Direct tissue inspection is necessary to accurately determine the depth of the puncture wound. In this manner it is possible to see where bleeding and tissue disruption stop and intact tissue begins. Usually, puncture wounds must be enlarged for adequate exploration. It may be helpful to make a new incision adjacent to the wound, e.g., an incision in the form of a semicircle around the wound. Thus, the tract may be isolated by dissection through intact tissue. Exploration may demonstrate the laceration or complete division of significant structures. Following exploration, removal of foreign bodies, and necessary tissue repairs, the wound is thoroughly irrigated with sterile saline solution. Sutures are placed in any incision made to explore the original wound, and a small tissue drain may be brought out through the puncture wound. The puncture wound should *not* be closed with sutures.[109]

> *In treating puncture wounds, the first priority is to control bleeding. Subsequent activities are exploration, repair, irrigation, and drainage.*

Perforated or Penetrating Wound. These are puncture wounds caused by forcing bodies, which may lodge in or pass through the tissue.

Laceration. This is an untidy wound caused by tearing, destruction, and disruption of the tissues. A lacerated wound is unlikely to heal well. Immediate management is directed toward control of bleeding and the prevention of infection. See Chapter 95, p. 2187.

Superficial lacerations that are not large or deep can be drawn together with a "butterfly" strip. A strip of ½ inch wide adhesive tape may be folded back on itself, and broad nicks cut at the folded end on each side to make the butterfly.

Treatment of a laceration is based upon the following major principles: (1) If the skin edges are brought together (approximated), they will heal more rapidly and with less scar formation than if the wound is left to heal on its own. (2) All traumatic lesions must be considered to be as possibly infected. (3) Hemostasis must be achieved to prevent excessive blood loss.

SUTURING SIMPLE LACERATIONS*

Simple lacerations are wounds less than 12 hours old, without gross contamination. Such wounds do not penetrate deeper than subcutaneous tissue. In some areas, nurses who have been prepared and are supervised by physicians

*See also Chapter 95.

*This section was written by Karen Creason Sorenson in consultation with Rosemary Pittman and Margaret M. McMahon.

have the option of doing minor suturing. It is important to be aware of the side effects and toxic effects of anesthetic agents. Use the lowest concentration (e.g., 0.5% lidocaine) and smallest amount necessary. Consider the maximum amounts that can safely be used. Do not use lidocaine with epinephrine on fingers, toes, ears, nose, or penis, or for elderly persons, with thin skin.

Common practices in *caring for simple cuts* are summarized below.[75, 109, 129]

Step 1: Inform the patient of necessary treatment. Explain what you are going to do and why. Obtain patient agreement. Carefully assess the wound as previously discussed, e.g., assess nerve, tendon, or bone damage.

Step 2: Prepare wound area. If necessary, shave hairy regions. (Keep hair removal minimal and never shave eyebrows.) Thoroughly clean surrounding skin with soap and water or a mild antiseptic solution. Place a sterile gauze sponge in the wound to prevent antiseptic solutions or detergents from entering the wound.

Step 3: Position the patient and yourself so that you are both comfortable.

Step 4: Wear sterile gloves and drape area with sterile towels to *minimize contamination.* When possible, *hemostatis* is obtained by exerting pressure, rather than by tying or clamping bleeding vessels.

Step 5: Prepare to *anesthetize the area.* First question the patient about any known allergies to anesthetic agents. Inform the patient that some discomfort will be experienced during the process of "numbing" the area. If necessary, restrain injured part. An anesthetic jelly or spray may be placed on the wound to minimize discomfort prior to injecting the area. Then, insert a small-gauge needle (e.g., 25 or 27 gauge) gently into the margin of the wound. Make this insertion under the dermis, where there may be a clear plane of cleavage. Aspirate, to prevent accidental injection of the anesthetic agent into a blood vessel. Inject the anesthetic slowly into the wound margin. Proceed to raise a ring of confluent wheals. (Fig. 80–1.)

Step 6: After evaluating the effectiveness of the anesthetic, thoroughly *clean the wound* by irrigating it with copious amounts of saline solution or other physiologic solution, e.g., Tissusol. A 30 to 50 ml. syringe with a 14 to 18 gauge blunt-tipped needle is effective for wound irrigation. Bulb syringes, catheter irrigating syringes, and IV tubing are less effective. With the use of gloved fingers or non-toothed forceps, the wound is opened gently and tissue is manipulated to locate and remove all foreign bodies. Additional wound assessment is made at this time, e.g., looking for damaged bone or tendons. (Although extensive wounds require further treatment, minor cuts may be cleaned, sutured, dressed, and bandaged at this point.)

Step 7: Debride and trim the wound. Severely contused or frayed skin edges must be pared or trimmed to provide optimal surfaces for wound apposition. Sharp scissors or a scalpel may be used to remove any necrotic tissue, while preserving as much tissue as possible. With the exception of hair-bearing areas, e.g., eyebrow and scalp, beveled wound edges are converted to straight edges. *Undermining* of tissue is sometimes necessary to minimize tension on the suture line or to avoid the edema and thickening of skin flaps that can occur in some wounds, e.g., avulsed wounds or tangential lacerations or skin flaps (Fig. 80–2). It is important to remember the location of major nerves and vessels during undermining to prevent injury. Using sterile saline solution, the wound is *again irrigated.*

Tailoring the jagged edges of a wound (to form straight edges) may not always be advisable. Sometimes a better cosmetic result is possible by closing the wound in its initial form, i.e., an irregular closure line may be less obvious when some surfaces heal.

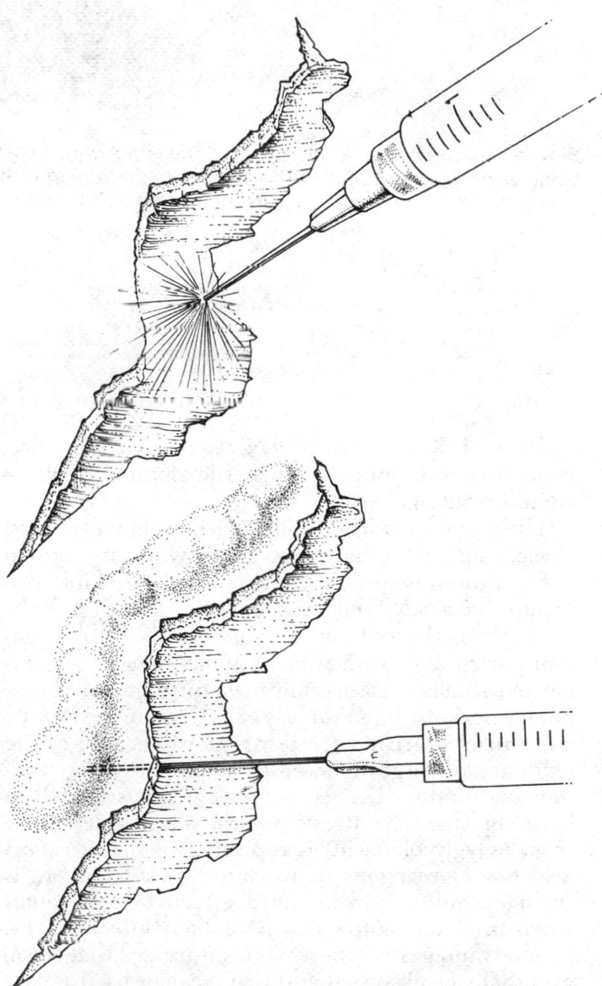

Figure 80–1. Anesthetizing a wound area in preparation for suturing. Spray the wound with anesthetic and then inject into the wound margins under the dermis, where there is often a clear plane of cleavage. (From Larsen, G. K., and C. W. Linder: Caring for simple cuts. *Emergency Medicine,* 10:206, Sept. 1978, p. 211.)

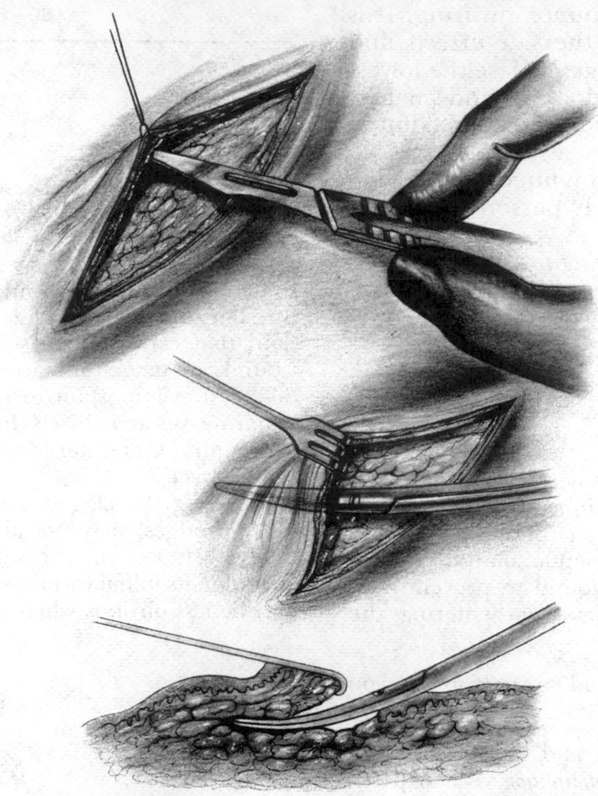

Figure 80–2. Undermining can be done either with a scalpel or with scissors. Remember that a scalpel *makes a plane,* while scissors *find a plane.* The level of undermining of the face is usually at a much more superficial level than on the trunk. (From Yarington, C. T., Jr.: Managing soft tissue injuries. *American Family Physician,* 16:109, Oct. 1977.)

Step 8: Proceed with *wound closure.* To minimize contamination, put on fresh sterile gloves and add to wound draping.

The *objectives* of using sutures are to obliterate dead space, stop hemorrhage, and give physical strength to a discontinuous surface. Sutures are divided into two groups, *absorbable* and *nonabsorbable.*

Catgut is the only absorbable *natural* suture generally used and is plain or chromic. *Chromic catgut* is treated to allow absorption over different predetermined periods. *Plain catgut* is absorbed more rapidly and causes a greater tissue reaction. Because of the tendency of catgut to swell by absorbing water from the surrounding tissues, longer ends must be left in knots in catgut sutures. *Synthetic* absorbable suture (e.g., polyglycolic acid) is replacing catgut. It causes less tissue reaction than catgut, lasts longer, is stronger, and may be more effective than catgut when used in a known or potentially infected area. The advantages of absorbable suture are that it will eventually be absorbed and that it can be used as continuous suture when desired.

The most commonly used nonabsorbable suture materials are silk, cotton, stainless steel, dermal, and synthetics such as nylon. Nonabsorbable suture has the advantages of having a known strength that will not change in a few days. It produces less tissue reaction, and knots of this material will not slip. The suture material should never be stronger than the tissue it is expected to hold together.

When suturing in a deep field, the tissue is grasped with a forceps. While holding the tissue, insert the needle — a *curved (half circle) needle. Round point needles* are used for subcutaneous tissue and *cutting-edge needles* for skin. *Swaged needles* (with suture material fused to the needle) minimize tissue trauma and hence may be preferable to *threaded needles.* Using a needle holder, grasp the needle in the middle of the needle, or a quarter of the distance from the eye end of the needle. Grasping the needle where it is swaged to the suture will cause the needle to bend, resulting in inaccurate suture placement. While holding the tissue, insert the needle.

To insert a curved needle, a turning force may be exerted on the needle holder. The insertion and pull-through of a curved needle should be in the same line as the curve of the needle. Everting the wound edge may facilitate needle insertion (Fig. 80–3). The needle should enter and leave the skin at right angles to the surface. Entrance and exit points should be close to the wound margin, but not so near the edge that the stitch could tear or pull out.

The wound is closed layer by layer as exactly as possible. Dead space must be obliterated if possible. To prevent entrapping dead space, *subcutaneous tissue* is first closed with a loose running stitch. Each subcutaneous layer may be closed with absorbable suture in a size appropriate for the tissue.

Next, *wound margins* are carefully brought together (approximated). When approximated, the wound edges should be everted to prevent a *dermal dent*. Visible skin marks (e.g., creases) are lined up. The first external stitches are placed to anchor these visible marks in place. Nonabsorbable 4–0 sutures are used on most skin surfaces. (On the face and neck 6–0 is recommended; sometimes absorbable suture is used for deeper layers, and the skin is closed with adhesive strips, e.g., Steri-Strips. Monofilament suture, e.g., nylon, may slip but may be preferable since it causes less tissue irritation than natural materials. Skin edges are opposed by sutures placed very close together and as near the edge of the skin as possible. *Stitch depth should equal stitch width. Stitch width should equal the distance between stitiches.*

Simple interrupted sutures are used, tied with a square knot (Fig. 80–4). Sutures should be firm, but not tied with excess tension, which would cause necrosis and scarring.

A no-touch technique may be achieved by using a sterile towel and by placing those parts of the instruments that touch the wound on the towel.

Instruments necessary:

Dissecting forceps, one with and one without teeth
Suture scissors
Straight and curved Iris scissors
Gillies skin hooks
Needle holder

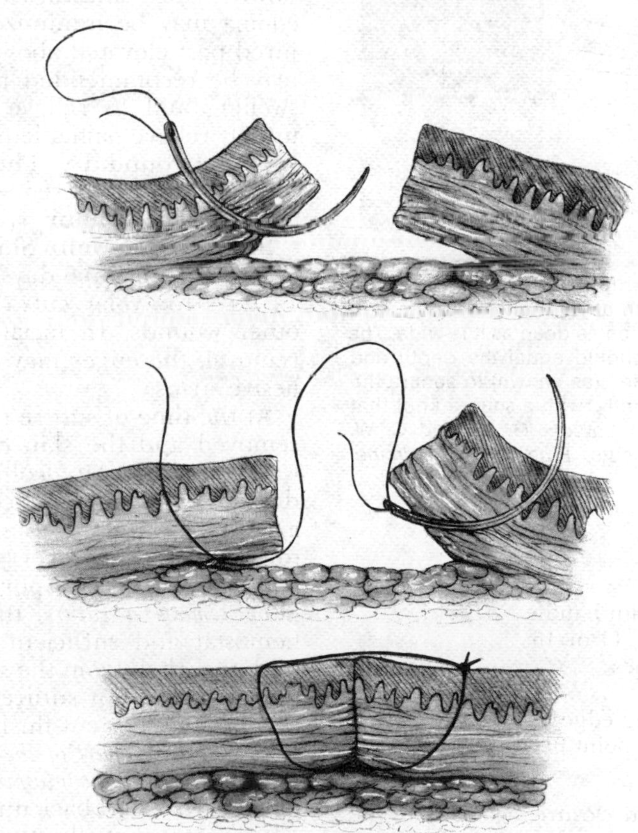

Figure 80–3. The insertion and pull-through of the needle should be in the same line as the curve of the needle. This is best accomplished by everting the wound edge for more accurate needle insertion. A swaged needle is preferred in some instances. (From Yarington, C. T., Jr.: Managing soft tissue injuries. *American Family Physician*, 16:109, Oct. 1977, p. 111.)

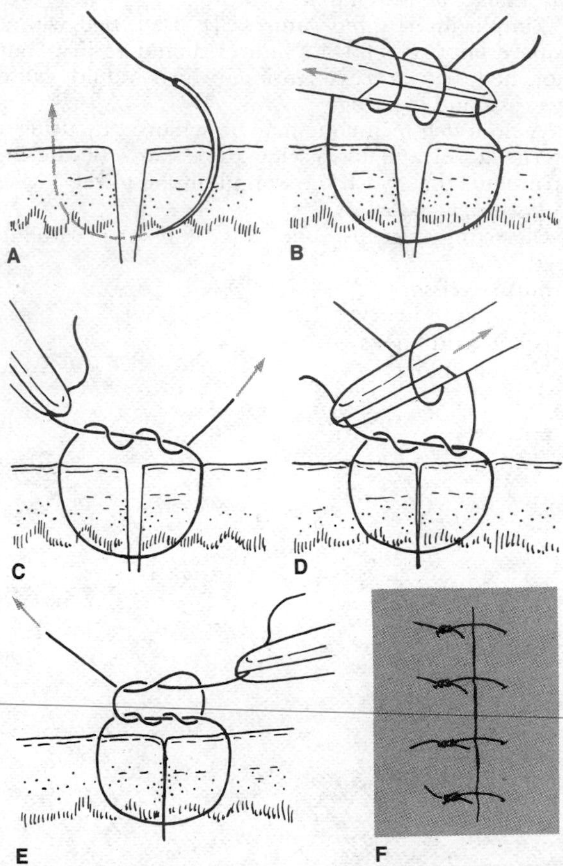

Figure 80–4. Simple interrupted sutures. Insert the needle and bring it out again at right angles to the skin surface. Each suture should be as deep as it is wide. The distance between sutures should equal the depth and width. Use an "instrument tie" (as shown) to secure the suture, firmly but not too tightly, with a square knot that will lie flat. (Redrawn from Larsen, G. K., and C. W. Linder: Caring for simple cuts. *Emergency Medicine*, 10:206, Sept. 1978, p. 213.)

1 Bard-Parker scalpel with handle No. 3
2 scalpel blades Nos. 10, 11 or 15
1 tissue forceps 4½ inches
1 straight skin needle
1 medium curved cutting edge needle
1 medium curved taper point needle
Suture material

Step 9: Following wound closure, again clean the area, and apply a layered dressing. The first layer should be of a material that will promote drainage, yet will not adhere to the wound. Owen's silk or fine mesh gauze are commonly used. The second layer is used to promote absorption; gauze sponges are ideal. The third layer is to minimize dead space in the dressing and to provide slight pressure. A woven roller gauze such as Kling or Kerlix is ideal. The roller gauze may be held in place by either adhesive tape or elastic net. Avoid placing adhesive tape over the wound area, because occlusive tape may foster moisture accumulation and subsequent maceration of wound edges. Some physicians use a petroleum based ointment applied directly to wound edges to minimize crusting and promote a thinner scar.

Follow-Up Care. If sutured wound edges are perfectly opposed and not disturbed or manipulated, adhesion of wound edges occurs in about 6 hours, and infection cannot enter. Dry skin is more resistant to infection than moist, and friction increases the possibility of infection. Unless signs of infection occur, the dressing should be left alone until time for suture removal. Dressings should be removed only if there is excessive bleeding or drainage, unexplained fever, or other indications of infection.

Following insertion of sutures, discuss the condition of the wound with the patient and give instructions concerning home care and a return visit. To prevent fainting, permit the patient to rest following suturing and to rise slowly. Once anesthesia wears off, pain and edema may be minimized by keeping the injured part elevated above heart level. Ice packs may be recommended to decrease or prevent swelling and to relieve pain. Mild analgesics usually relieve pain adequately. It is advisable to keep the wound dry. The patient should return for evaluation if there is evidence of infection or excessive bleeding or pain.

Suture Removal. Skin sutures are usually *left in place* for: (a) 3 days for a facial wound, (b) 14 days for volar cuts, and (c) 7–10 days for other wounds. In facial wounds, after suture removal, the edges may be reinforced with adhesive strips.

At the time of suture removal, the dressing is removed and the skin cleaned with soap and water, followed by alcohol. Adhesive tape residue is removed with acetone or other similar agent. If wound edges appear to be separating (or likely to do so), every other stitch is removed and the wound is supported with Steri-Strips.

To remove a suture, the knot is seized in a hemostat and sufficient traction is exerted to raise the stitch from the skin. Then, using a fine pointed scalpel or suture removal scissors (sterile) the suture is cut flush with the skin. *It is important that no part of the stitch which is above the skin level enter and contaminate the skin tract,* i.e., do not pull that part back under the wound or skin. After removal of all sutures, it is not necessary to do special wound cleansing. However, crusts or other material may be removed. Leave the wound dry and apply a vapor-permeable dressing.

BURNS

What makes nursing the burned patient different from other nursing? Nothing and a lot! Nothing, because what is done for a burned patient is not unique to burn care. A lot, because in burn care all *nursing skills may become specialized.*[7]

INTRODUCTION

In recent decades major strides have been made in the management of burn injuries. Survival rates have dramatically increased for persons with burns that cover 30 to 50 per cent of their body surface. Burn shock has been almost eliminated as a cause of death. The mortality rate of victims of severe smoke inhalation has markedly decreased with sophisticated techniques of respiratory support. Invasive wound sepsis can be more effectively controlled through the use of topical antimicrobials on burn wounds. Burn hypercatabolism can be more effectively managed through the use of occlusive dressings, topical antimicrobial agents, improved control of the ambient temperature and improved nutrition, particularly intravenous routes of nutrition. However, in spite of advances in providing care to burned persons, many patients with major burns die . . . frequently just short of the point where their survival should be possible. Such late deaths are typically due to a combination of sepsis, suppressed immunity, negative nitrogen balance, and a general depletion of the reserves of the burned individual.[79]

Incidence. Burns are usually acquired in one of two ways: (1) by involvement in an uncontrolled fire or explosion or (2) through contact of some part of the body with a hot object, liquid, acid, or other substance with a flame. The former is the more common cause of death, and the latter of nonfatal injury.

The magnitude of suffering, disfigurement, and death from burn injuries to humans is beyond comprehension. Complete worldwide statistics on burn incidence are not available. However, burns are the third leading cause of accidental deaths in the United States, exceeded only by motor vehicle accidents and falls. Fires and burns are the leading cause of deaths in children from birth to 5 years. Almost 2.2 million persons, in the United States alone, seek medical attention each year because of burns. Of these, some 75,000 are hospitalized and 9,000 die from their burns. Two-thirds of all burn injuries are caused by flame (fire). And, 85 per cent of all flame burns involve the ignition of fabrics. The home is the site of 85 per cent of all burn injuries.*[7]

Figure 80–5 shows the relationship between expected survival rate and patient's age and extent of burn.

Causes. Burn injuries may be caused by: heat from flame, hot liquids or hot surfaces; chemicals; radiation, or electrical currents. Frostbite or freezing caused by extreme cold temperatures causes injuries requiring treatment similar to burn injuries. Deaths and injuries from fires and explosions are usually caused by one of the following:

- Fire from cooking or heating sources
- Smoking and the use of matches
- Electrical deficiencies or improper use of electrical equipment or utilities
- Fire in rubbish or trash
- Flammable liquids or grease

Prevention. Severe burns are particularly tragic because most injuries can be avoided. Some injuries are deliberately inflicted, e.g., children intentionally burned as punishment. (See Chapter 95 for discussion of child abuse.) Burn prevention is, thus, an extremely important function of health professionals.

The causes of burns are complex. Frequently they happen to young children who are inadequately supervised. There are statistical indications that burn incidence has a relationship with poverty. Parents who are emotionally disturbed or who lack money for child care (and might have to leave children by themselves) need emergency resources where help can be secured. Nurses working with parents or children can be alert to cues indicating inability to adequately protect children. In home settings, community health nurses have an even better opportunity to help families "burn-proof" their homes and to establish family escape plans in case of fire.

*Statistics concerning burns in the United States are available from the National Burn Information Exchange (NBIE), National Institute for Burn Medicine, Ann Arbor, Michigan.

Education about the first aid care of burns may also be helpful. (See Chapter 95.) School nurses can promote the incorporation of fire prevention and first aid in the school curriculum. As citizens, nurses can bring dangerous appliances, clothing, etc., to the public attention and encourage citizen action. The elderly need to take special safety precautions. Persons who smoke, drink alcoholic beverages, or abuse drugs present difficult problems in burn prevention because of the dangers associated with these habits, e.g., impaired judgment.

BURNS: AN OVERVIEW

The skin has many important *functions.* Among these are:

1. Protects against infection
2. Prevents loss of body fluids
3. Controls body temperature
4. Functions as an excretory organ
5. Functions as a sensory organ
6. Produces vitamin D
7. Determines identity

When the skin is burned, these functions are either diminished or totally eliminated, depending upon various aspects of the burn.

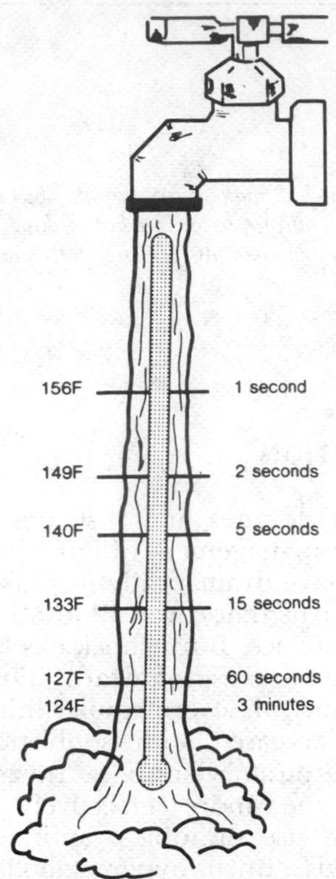

Length of time needed to receive a third-degree burn. (From McGuire, A.: Prevention of burns. *Critical Care Quarterly,* 1:1, Dec. 1978, p. 8.)

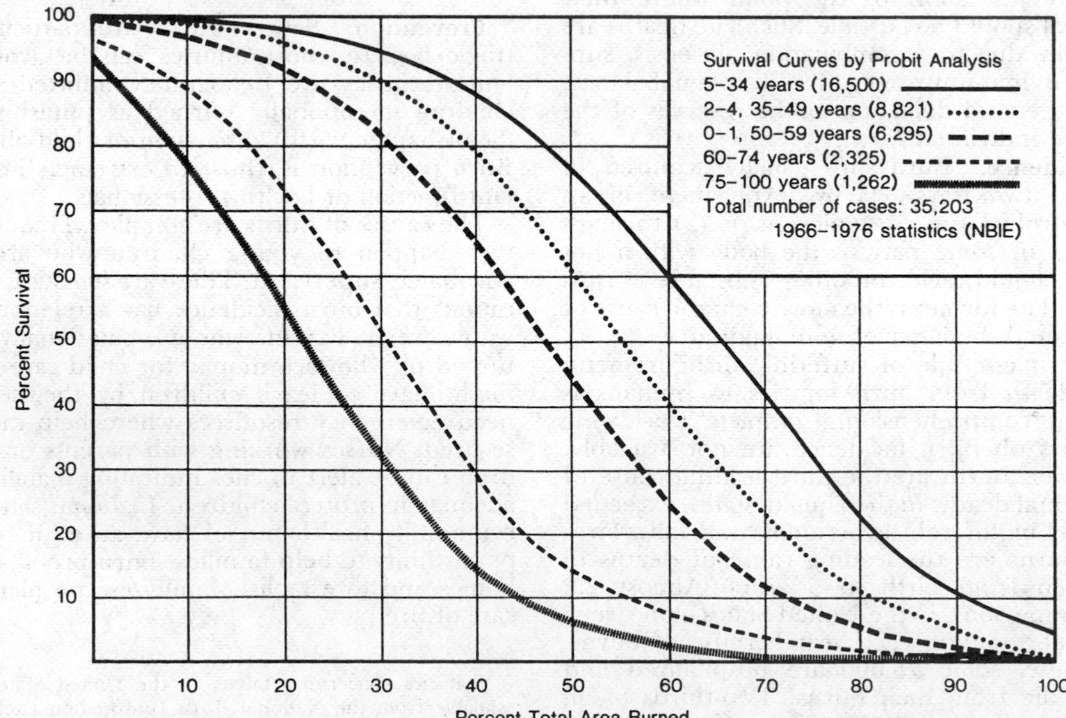

Figure 80–5. Relationship between expected survival rate and patient's age and extent of burn. (Reproduced with permission from the National Burn Information Exchange, National Institute for Burn Medicine, Ann Arbor, Michigan, Irving Feller, M. D., Director.)

FACTORS DETERMINING THE SEVERITY OF A BURN

The *severity of a burn* is determined by many factors. Among these are:

- Depth of burn
- Size of burn (percentage of body surface area)
- Part of body burned (location)
- Age
- Past medical history
- Cause of burn

Burn Depth. The depth of a burn is typically divided into three major categories: superficial, partial-thickness, and full-thickness injuries (Fig. 80–6). Sometimes a fourth category (fourth degree burns) is used.

1. A *superficial burn,* or *first degree burn,* affects only the epidermis. The skin appears pink and red and may form small thin blisters. Often, mild to severe erythema accompanies this type of burn. A good example of a superficial burn is a sunburn, which will usually heal by itself in 3 to 7 days.

2. A *partial thickness burn,* or *second degree burn,* is one in which only a part of the skin has been damaged or destroyed. This type of burn affects both the epidermis and the dermis. It has large, thick-walled blisters, often covering the entire burned area. The underlying tissue is deep red in color and is usually wet and shiny in appearance. In a partial-thickness burn, healing is accomplished through the evolution of the undamaged basal cells, usually requiring from 21 to 28 days.

3. In a *full-thickness burn,* or *third degree burn,* all of the skin (epidermis and dermis) is destroyed, and underlying structures (e.g., subcutaneous tissues, muscle, bone) may be involved. The appearance of a full-thickness burn may vary. The color may be deep red, white, black, or brown. Usually this type of burn appears dry. A full-thickness burn requires grafting procedures, since it will not heal spontaneously.

4. A *fourth degree burn* is a type of full-thickness burn in which structures beneath the

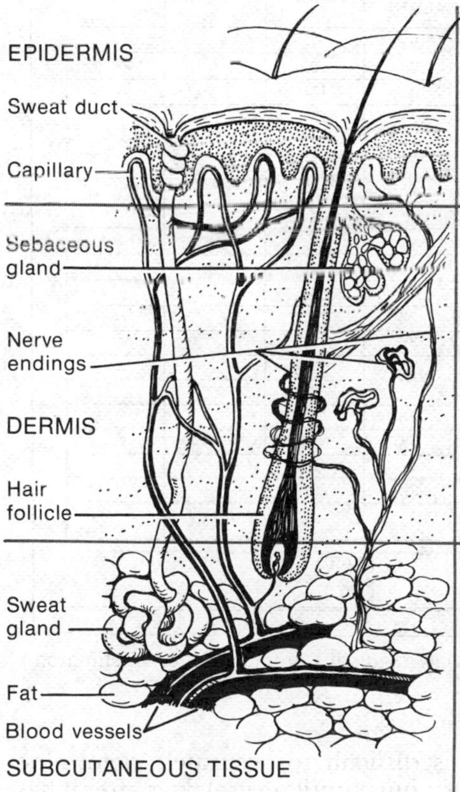

EPIDERMIS
Sweat duct
Capillary
Sebaceous gland
Nerve endings
DERMIS
Hair follicle
Sweat gland
Fat
Blood vessels
SUBCUTANEOUS TISSUE

	APPEARANCE	SENSATION	COURSE
FIRST DEGREE	Mild to severe erythema; skin blanches with pressure Skin dry Small, thin-walled blisters	Painful Hyperesthetic Tingling Pain eased by cooling	Discomfort lasts about 48 hours Desquamation in 3 to 7 days
SECOND DEGREE	Large thick-walled blisters covering extensive area (vesiculation) Edema; mottled red base; broken epidermis; wet, shiny, weeping surface	Painful Hyperesthetic Sensitive to cold air	Superficial partial thickness burn heals in 10 to 14 days Deep partial-thickness burn requires 21 to 28 days for healing Healing rate varies with burn depth and presence or absence of infection
THIRD DEGREE	Variable, e.g., deep red, black, white, brown Dry surface Edema Fat exposed Tissue disrupted	Little pain Anesthetic	Full-thickness dead skin suppurates and liquefies after 2 to 3 weeks. Spontaneous healing impossible Requires removal of eschar and skin grafting Scarring deformities and function loss Beneath eschar capillary tufts and fibroblasts organize into granulating tissue

Figure 80–6. Note that first and second degree burns affect areas containing nerve endings and are thus painful. First degree burns involve epidermis. Second degree burns involve epidermis and dermis. Third degree burns involve epidermis, dermis, and varying degrees of subcutaneous tissue.

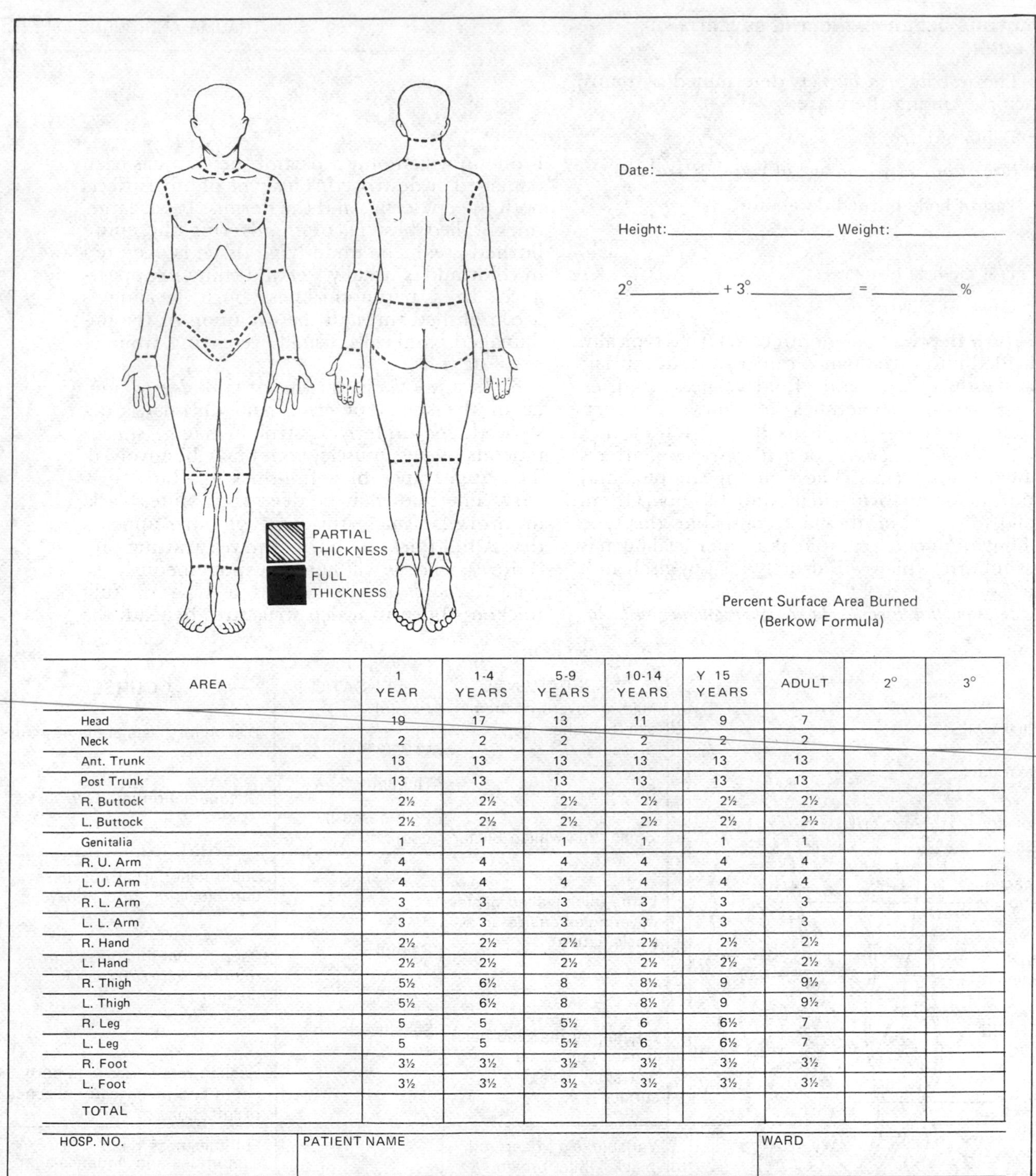

Date: ____________

Height: ____________ Weight: ____________

2° ________ + 3° ________ = ________ %

Percent Surface Area Burned
(Berkow Formula)

AREA	1 YEAR	1-4 YEARS	5-9 YEARS	10-14 YEARS	Y 15 YEARS	ADULT	2°	3°
Head	19	17	13	11	9	7		
Neck	2	2	2	2	2	2		
Ant. Trunk	13	13	13	13	13	13		
Post Trunk	13	13	13	13	13	13		
R. Buttock	2½	2½	2½	2½	2½	2½		
L. Buttock	2½	2½	2½	2½	2½	2½		
Genitalia	1	1	1	1	1	1		
R. U. Arm	4	4	4	4	4	4		
L. U. Arm	4	4	4	4	4	4		
R. L. Arm	3	3	3	3	3	3		
L. L. Arm	3	3	3	3	3	3		
R. Hand	2½	2½	2½	2½	2½	2½		
L. Hand	2½	2½	2½	2½	2½	2½		
R. Thigh	5½	6½	8	8½	9	9½		
L. Thigh	5½	6½	8	8½	9	9½		
R. Leg	5	5	5½	6	6½	7		
L. Leg	5	5	5½	6	6½	7		
R. Foot	3½	3½	3½	3½	3½	3½		
L. Foot	3½	3½	3½	3½	3½	3½		
TOTAL								

HOSP. NO.	PATIENT NAME	WARD

Figure 80–7. Sample burn chart for recording extent of burns. (Courtesy Harborview Medical Center, Seattle, Washington.)

skin are definitely affected. Charring is commonly seen with this type of burn.

> *Most burn injuries are a combination of partial- and full-thickness burns.*

Often it is difficult to accurately determine the depth of a burn until several days after it has occurred; there are some assessments that help to estimate the depth. One method of assessing burn depth is to lightly touch the burned area, while wearing sterile gloves. This is done to assess capillary refill. Erythematous areas that

TABLE 80–1. CLASSIFICATION OF BURN INJURIES

Rule of Nines	
Head and neck	9%
Right upper extremity	9%
Left upper extremity	9%
Anterior trunk	18%
Posterior trunk	18%
Right lower extremity	18%
Left lower extremity	18%
Perineum	1%

From Luterman, A. Burn injuries. Initial evaluation and treatment. *Cutis,* 22:437, Oct. 1978.

blanch with fingertip pressure and then refill are shallow partial-thickness burns. The erythema indicates tissue damage where viability remains, i.e., the tissue has been damaged, but is still viable and may heal. Large blisters usually indicate a deeper partial-thickess burn and are not palpated. Full-thickness burns are characterized by their leather-like surface and the absence of pain response, owing to destruction of the nerves.

Burn Size. The *size of a burn* may be determined fairly accurately by using one of several techniques, requiring the use of diagrams. The body areas affected are shaded anteriorly and posteriorly. (See top of Fig. 80–7.) From these charts, the size of the burn is calculated and expressed as a *per cent of the total body surface area (TBSA).* Two of the most common methods used for such calculations are the "Rule of Nines" and the Berkow formula.

According to the Rule of Nines, the body is divided into areas, each of which represents 9 per cent (or multiples of 9) of the total body surface. (Table 80–1). This formula is easy and quick to use, for an initial assessment; however, it is often inaccurate and does not allow for differences in proportion in infants, children, and adults.

The *Berkow formula* is accurate for all ages, although it requires more time to calcualte. This method consists of a diagram of the body, divided into sections, and a grid containing corresponding sections along with the percentage of body surface area they represent for ages 1 year through adult. The diagram is shaded according to partial- or full-thickness, and then the grid is used to calculate each area and the total per cent of the burned area. (An example of the use of Berkow formula appears in the lower half of Figure 80–7.)

Burn Location. The location of a burn is considered when determining burn severity. Burns of the upper part of the body have the highest mortality rate. Burns involving the head, neck, and chest often result in pulmonary complications. Burns of the head and face should be carefully assessed, to identify burns or abrasions to the eyes and ears. Ear burns may lead to chondritis or the deterioration or loss of cartilage, owing to infection.[70] The perineum requires special care because it is highly prone to infection due to contamination from urine and stool.

Patient Age. The *age of a patient* not only determines the severity of a burn, but often its outcome. Children under 2 and adults over 60 have a markedly higher mortality rate than those in other age groups with similar burns.

Minor Burn—Outpatient Care

It is a minor burn if:

- the injury is less than 10% of the total body area;
- the patient is less than 35 years old or more than 4 years old;
- the medical history is negative for chronic and severe illness;
- the burn does not include the face, hands, feet or perineum and is not circumferential;
- there are no significant concurrent injuries (i.e., respiratory damage, fracture, etc.);
- it is not an electrical injury;
- individual considerations permit (i.e., patient is capable of managing own outpatient care and there is no evidence of neglect or abuse).

Major Burn—Inpatient Care

It is a major burn if:

- the injury is greater than 10% of the total body area;
- the patient is more than 35 years old or less than 4 years old;
- the medical history is positive for chronic or severe illness;
- there are burns of the face, hands, feet or perineum, or there are circumferential burns;
- there are significant concurrent injuries (i.e., respiratory damage, fracture, etc.);
- it is an electrical injury;
- individual considerations permit (i.e., patient is unable to manage own care or there is evidence of neglect or abuse).

Source: Taken with permission from the "EMS Burn Care Poster," Irving Feller, M.D., Director, National Institute for Burn Medicine, Ann Arbor, Michigan, 1975.

Minor and major burn definitions (From Archambeault-Jones, C., and I. Feller: Burn nursing is nursing. *Critical Care Quarterly,* 1:77, Dec. 1978, p. 82.)

The skin of the very young and the very old is thin and translucent, making an accurate assessment of burn depth difficult. Usually burns of persons in these extremes of age are deeper than initially estimated. Since infants have poor antibody response to infection, their resistance is low and septicemia may occur. "In the older patient exacerbation of latent degenerative processes may be fatal."[47]

Patient History. Severely burned patients initially are often clear mentally and cooperative, therefore as much history should be obtained as possible from the patient and observers at this time. An adequate account of the present burn, and past medical and allergic history may be difficult to obtain later. All patients with *history* of cardiovascular, pulmonary, renal metabolic, or neurologic problems must be carefully followed, as the stress of a burn may exacerbate or worsen these conditions. Patients with know drug or alcohol addiction should also be considered as being high risk, i.e., having an increased mortality rate. "Almost any chronic or debilitating systemic diseases convert even a minor burn injury into a potentially lethal disease."[47]

Cause of Burn. The final factor in determining the severity of a burn is knowing its *cause.* Regardless of the etiology of the burn, the principles for care are the same. Some types of burns, however, require special initial care or continuing observation.

An *electrical burn,* which is not seen as frequently as flame or scald burns, is in some ways more devastating. An electrical burn courses through the body, following the path of least resistance. *Observable injuries* from an electric burn may be minimal, e.g., a small burn at the point of entry in a patient's hand and a larger burn at the exit site in the foot. The current may appear to have "exploded" from the exit site, e.g., a crater-like wound may be left. However, although injuries may appear minimal, extensive *internal damage* may have occurred in those body structures that conducted the electrical energy through the body, e.g., nerves, muscles, blood vessels, bone. Such damage may not become evident for days or months afterwards. For example, some persons develop eye damage, e.g., cataracts, years after sustaining an electrical injury.

A *fasciotomy* may be performed a day or so following the initial injury to check for viable tissue and thus assess damage to underlying structures. A fasciotomy is a surgical procedure in which an incision is made, and underlying tissue (e.g., muscle) explored and tested for viability. The incision may be left open for further exploration.

Depending on the course of the electricity and the amount of tissue damage, persons with electrical burns may require one or often multiple amputations. (Amputations are discussed in Chapter 50.)

FIRST AID AND IMMEDIATE TREATMENT

On Site Burn Management.

> *The major goals of first aid for a burn victim are:*
>
> 1. *Provide relief from pain*
> 2. *Minimize contamination of the wound*
> 3. *Transport quickly*

Since the person with a burn has lost a part of the protective layer of skin, the following may occur: (1) *pain* due to exposed nerve ending, (2) *chilling* due to loss of skin, and (3) wound *contamination.*

All of these factors may be minimized by wrapping the affected area with a clean, moist towel or sheet. This decreases the pain caused by air touching the exposed nerve endings, e.g., the covering used substitutes for skin in this way. The covering also decreases the possibilities of infection or contamination, and decreases loss of body heat.

The patient will often be cold, even on a warm day, owing to loss of body heat through the burn. Keep the injured person as warm as possible while he or she is being transported.

In the event of a *chemical burn,* clothing which has been soaked or splattered by the chemical agent must be removed immediately! Prolonged contact of the chemical with the skin will increase burn severity. The affected area should be rinsed with clean cool water — for 10 to 15 minutes — to remove the chemical agent.

In all other types of burns, the rescuer should not attempt to remove the victims' clothing, with the exception of removing metal objects (jewelry, belt buckles), which will retain heat.

> *Never apply any topical home remedies or creams to a newly burned area.*

Topical creams should never be applied by the rescuer. This activity can be time consuming as well as painful to the patient since the substance used will have to be removed in the emergency room in order to see the wound. Many "home remedies" can have devastating effects when applied to a burn wound.

Emergency Room Management of Outpatients. Minor burns not requiring hospitalization are typically first degree burns and superficial second degree burns covering less than 10 per cent of an adult's body, less than 5 per cent of a child, or not involving hands, face, or feet. An extensive first degree burn may be treated in a doctor's office or in an emergency room by cleaning with Betadine, debriding ruptured blisters and those that might rupture, applying a topical cream, and wrapping with sterile gauze. Individuals with such burns should have tetanus prophylaxis, and antibiotics will probably be prescribed for several days. The patient should keep a daily temperature record and notify the physician of any rise in temperature or any wound changes, such as swelling, redness, increased tenderness, or exudate.

Persons treated on an outpatient basis should return within a week of initial treatment for a follow-up visit, allowing a physician to check on progress. Individual instructions concerning wound management should be followed.

Hospital Admission. It is of utmost importance to transport a patient with a major burn immediately to the nearest hospital. Many hospitals are not adequately equipped or staffed to care for persons with major burns. In this event, the patient may be transferred by helicopter, plane, or ambulance to a hospital with the needed facilities — often a special burn center.

Communication. Telephone communication plays an important role in transferring a patient with burns from one hospital to another. Many hospitals use a *transfer check list* (Fig. 80–8) or a similar patient referral form. These forms provide physicians with vital information concerning a patient's injury. Also, they enable

BURN TRANSFER CHECK LIST

ALBERT EINSTEIN COLLEGE OF MEDICINE - BRONX MUNICIPAL HOSPITAL CENTER

DATE______ TIME OF CALL______ a.m. p.m.

REFERRING DOCTOR______

REFERRING HOSPITAL______

PHONE#______

CLOSED SPACE YES NO
ENDOTRACHEAL TUBE YES NO
VENTILATOR YES NO
I.V. LINES YES NO
(size & site)______
ALCOHOLIC YES NO
NOW DRUNK YES NO
NARCOTIC USER YES NO
CONSCIOUS NOW YES NO
DIABETES YES NO
HEART DISEASE YES NO
Type______
ALLERGIES? YES NO
To What?______

ASSOCIATED INJURIES: (Fractures, abdominal or chest injury, head trauma, etc.)______

THERAPY GIVEN THUS FAR
IV's______cc Normal Saline
______cc Ringers
______cc D_5W
Foley______cc urine total
______cc urine last hour

IF PATIENT IS ACCEPTED SUGGEST:
1. M. D. accompany (if needed but must come with patient with endotracheal tube.)
2. I. V. Morphine for sedation if needed.
3. N.G. tube for burns over 30% or if drunk or intubated - DON'T CLAMP TUBE.
4. I. V. fluids - Ringers fast enough to produce urine output
5. NO topical cream, antibiotics IM meds of any kind. Debridement of burn wound to be discussed.
6. Escharotomy if needed.
7. Does family know about transfer?

PATIENT NAME______

AGE______ DATE & TIME OF BURN______

TYPE OF BURN: FLAME SCALD ELECTRICAL CHEMICAL RADIATION

LAB RESULTS: Na____, K____, Cl____,
CO_2____, BUN____, Sugar____,
pH____, PO_2____, PCO_2____,
Is there blood in urine______
Chest X-ray______

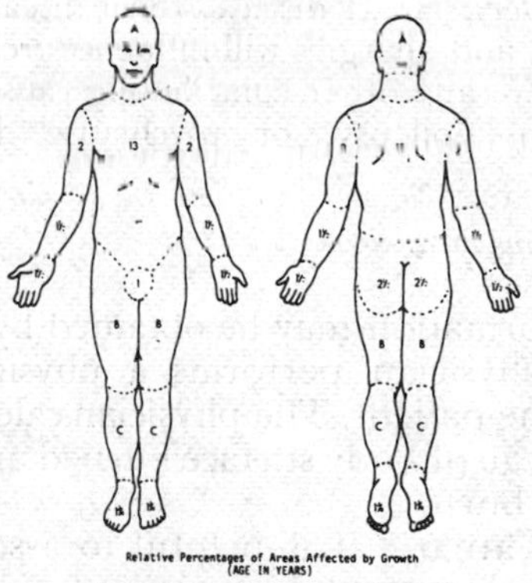

Relative Percentages of Areas Affected by Growth (AGE IN YEARS)

TOTAL PER CENT BURNED____2 +____3 =____

INSURANCE DATA:
Type:______
Policy#______
Workman's Compensation? YES NO

Resident making report______
Senior resident notified______
Attending notified______
Accept patient______
Refer to______

Figure 80–8. Sample check list used for discussing by telephone the transfer of burned patient to special facilities. Note the specific types of information requested. This type of information helps the staff at the receiving facility know exactly how to prepare for the patient's arrival and what care the patient will need. (From Stein, J. M., and Stein, E. D.: Safe transfer of civilian burn casualties. *JAMA*, 238:490, Aug. 1977.)

hospital staff to prepare necessary equipment for an incoming patient, thus saving valuable time when the patient arrives in the emergency room.

ASSESSMENT — DATA BASELINE. Upon arrival at the emergency room, the person with burns is carefully assessed. As mentioned previously, severely burned people are often *initially* mentally clear and cooperative, therefore as much information should be obtained as possible from the patient and observers at this time. An adequate account of the present burn and past medical and allergic history may be difficult to obtain later. The following information should be obtained as soon as possible:

- *When and how the burn occurred:* Fluid therapy for the first 24 hours is based on the number of hours after the injury. Associated injuries must also be considered. A person burned in an automobile accident may have other injuries.
- *Identification of cause and circumstances of burn:* Was it a flash explosion, scald, chemical, or electrical burn? Was it accidental or intentional?
- *Prior treatment:* What kind of first aid was given? Has patient been given medication or fluids? (If so, record amount and kind.) Has tetanus prophylaxis been given?
- *Relevant past history:* Heart disease, renal disease, diabetes, ulcers, and allergies will influence treatment. Were there any other contributing causes, e.g., alcoholism, epilepsy, or psychiatric disorders?
- *Current medications or drugs*

The above information may be obtained by a nurse while a physician performs a physical examination of the patient. The physician calculates the percentage of body surface burned and the depth of the burn.

THE INJURED CHILD. It is helpful to assess the developmental status of an *injured child.* Also, the sensitive nurse observes interactions within the family in order to help meet the needs of the family and a burned child. Burn injury is a more prevalent form of child abuse than is generally recognized. It is necessary for the burn staff to keep this in mind.[80]

Children with burns have a higher mortality rate than adults. An entire family is affected when a child is burned and hospitalized. Parents' work hours, the need for baby sitting at home, and transportation may present problems in working out visiting hours. Siblings may be acutely affected by the sudden removal of the injured child from the home.

EARLY TREATMENT OF MAJOR BURNS

The following is typical of early burn management. Some procedures may be done in the emergency room and others on the unit.

▶ Institute and maintain *strict isolation,* i.e., personnel must use gowns and masks and wash their hands scrupulously for those procedures not requiring sterile gloves.

▶ Institute *route for fluid therapy,* e.g., two large-bore catheters, cutdown, arterial catheter. Two useful insertion sites are the cephalic vein in the shoulder area or the subclavian vein.

▶ Begin *individualized fluid therapy,* using chosen formula.

▶ *Medicate for pain alleviation.* Morphine sulfate, 0.1 mg/lb. for children and 10 mg. total for adults diluted in 3 to 5 ml. of saline, may be injected into the vein over a period of 2 to 3 minutes.

> *Extreme restlessness in burn patients may be due to hypovolemia and hypoxia rather than pain from severe burn injury, and gastric dilatation may occur.*

▶ Insert *nasogastric tube* and maintain patient on *nothing by mouth* (paralytic ileus commonly occurs as a complication). Typically, suction is low intermittent and *gastric secretion pH* is checked hourly. The pH is tested to identify the presence of Curling's ulcer (stress ulcer) (see p. 1795).

▶ Insert *Foley catheter.* Measure urine output hourly. Fluid therapy is titrated to urine output, e.g., if urine output is low for 1 hour, the IV rate may be increased during the next hour. Schedules for IV replacement vary according to formula used and are adjusted to each patient's needs. (Fluid resuscitation is discussed later in this chapter.)

▶ Administer *tetanus prophylaxis.* Tetanus is always a potential danger in patients who have a large amount of dead tissue present. In unimmunized persons, hyperimmune tetanus globulin is used. Anyone who has had tetanus toxoid within 5 years should receive a booster dose of toxoid. If more than 5 years have passed, hyperimmune human tetanus globulin should be used. (See Chapter 95.)

▶ *Obtain specimens* for clinical laboratory analysis. Typically a blood chemistry, blood count, blood gas, urinalysis, and myoglobin (indicative of cell and muscle destruction) are obtained. Blood is typed and cross-matched. A chest x-ray and ECG are also performed.

▶ Obtain *wound cultures* prior to administering antibiotics. This culture provides base line information about organisms present at the time of the patient's admission.

▶ Begin *prophylactic antibiotics* if ordered. Some hospitals do not use any prophylactic drugs for fear of making organisms drug-resistant.
▶ *Bathe* the patient (discussed in a later section). Explain the procedure to the patient and premedicate as ordered to minimize pain or discomfort. The entire body should be bathed, and body hair cut back from around burned areas. Hair is also shaved from the surrounding area. Follow agency policy concerning nail trimming and clipping eyelashes or eyebrows. Gently wash burned areas with Betadine solution. Examine eyes and ears for burn damage, to determine if special treatment is necessary. Take *photographs,* if permitted by the patient. These are used as a record of the patient's injury. Bathing may also be referred to as hydrotherapy, "tanking," or "tubbing."
▶ *Weigh* the patient. Fluid and diet therapy is based on the patient's weight upon admission. Typically, daily weights are recorded.
▶ *Transfer patient to bed* on clean sheets. Use heat shield to *maintain comfortable body warmth* (Fig. 80–9) or place top sheet over bed cradle if heat shield is not available. Special bed linens may be used to help maintain patient comfort.
▶ Apply *topical cream* or *biological dressing* to burn. These agents, discussed later, enhance patient comfort and facilitate healing.
▶ Check the patient's *vital signs* and *urine output* as indicated, e.g., hourly if patient appears stable, and every 15 minutes on the unstable patient. Every hour, check urine fractionals and specific gravity. Observe urine for blood.

Escharotomy. A burned person is checked for *circumferential third degree burns* to the extremities, trunk, or neck, i.e., burns totally encircling an area. Pulses in the extremities should be checked hourly with a *doppler,* and the extremities observed for color, temperature, and capillary refill.

Edema forming beneath the thick eschar (devitalized skin) will impede blood flow or may inhibit respirations.

A circumferential burn may require an *escharotomy,* i.e., a lengthwise incision through the tight eschar, which allows expansion of the skin as edema forms (Fig. 80–10). Since the incision is made only through the tight dead eschar, no anesthesia is required. If there is a large amount of bleeding, the incision may be packed with Avitene. Sometimes cautery or sutures may also be required.

An escharotomy is quite dramatic to observe and often provides great relief for the patient. Prepare significant others for the patient's appearance and reassure them that the procedure is not painful to the patient.

In the presence of circumferential burns to the trunk or neck, the patient must be moni-

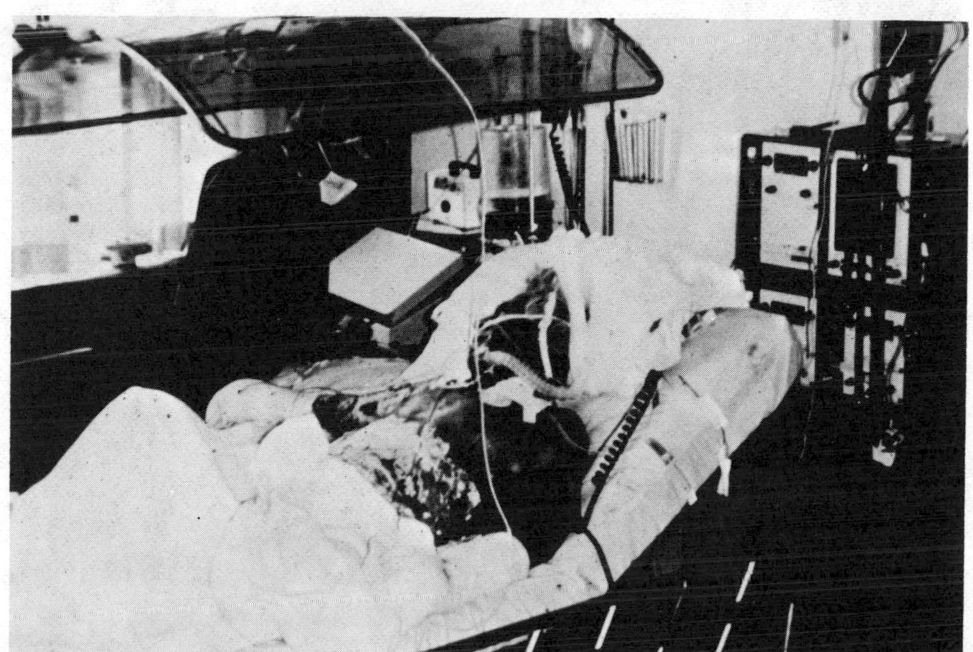

Figure 80–9. Heat shield used to maintain comfortable level of body warmth for a burned person. (Courtesy of Harborview Medical Center Burn Unit, Seattle, Washington.)

tored for signs of respiratory distress. Often, patients with severe burns to the face and neck are *prophylactically intubated* before edema begins to occlude the airway. Such edema makes intubation difficult.

Care of Special Areas. Several parts of the body, when burned, require special treatment and observation.

▶ HANDS. Fingers should be covered with a topical ointment for comfort. Strips of gauze or gauze 4 × 4's are placed between the fingers to *prevent webbing,* i.e., the growing together of burned body parts. The hand should be placed on a hand splint and wrapped with Kling gauze, e.g., Kling or Kerlix to *maintain a functional position.*

The arm is elevated above heart level on pillows or by using Stockinette (Fig. 80–11) or pillow case slings attached to IV poles to decrease edema. Radial, palmar, and digital pulses are checked with a doppler each hour. *If absent pulses are not recognized in time, ischemia and necrosis may occur.* Eschartomy may be required.

▶ LEGS. Burns to toes should be treated as those on fingers, using gauze or 4 × 4's to prevent webbing. Long leg splints may be used to *keep legs extended and to prevent external or internal rotation or foot drop.* The legs should be elevated above heart level.

▶ NECK. The neck should be *hyperextended* as far as possible to prevent contractures. This can be done by using a split thickness mattress or traction. Do *not* permit a head pillow.

▶ EYE. Any patient with a facial burn requires an *initial ophthalmology consultation,* which will give specific orders for care, e.g., drops or ointments. Additional follow-up care may be indicated.

▶ EARS. Persons with ear burns must be protected to prevent *further damage or loss of cartilage.* Great care must be taken in washing and applying a topical ointment to the ear. Head pillows are *not* given to a patient with ear burns.

▶ PERINEUM. Since this area is often contaminated by urine and feces, it is prone to infection. A Foley catheter helps decrease this contamination. Upon voiding, the patient should *always* be thoroughly cleansed, dried, and given a clean sheet.

POSITIONING OF THE BURN-INJURED PATIENT

Burn-Injured Area	Description of Position
Ear	No pillow: A small foam pad may be placed under the head
Neck	No pillow: A small foam pad may be placed under the head
Shoulder	90° abduction, neutral rotation, elbow splint may be used to aid in maintaining position
Elbow	Extended, forearm in neutral position
Wrist	10–20° dorsiflexion
Metacarpophalangeal Joints	45–65° flexion
Interphalangeal Joints	Extended
Hips	Extended, abducted 10–15°, neutral rotation
Knees	Extended
Ankles and Feet	90° dorsiflexion at ankles

From Stoddard, J. E.: Rehabilitation of the burn-injured patient. *Critical Care Quarterly,* 1:63, Dec. 1978.

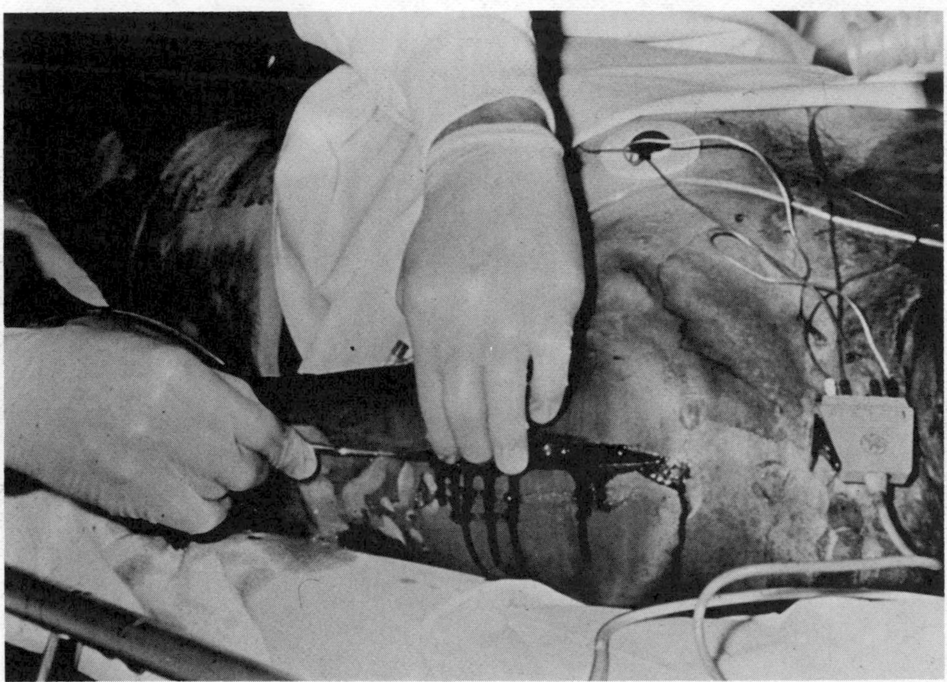

Figure 80–10. Escharotomy. Incision through tight burn eschar to permit expansion of skin as edema forms. (Courtesy of Harborview Medical Center Burn Unit, Seattle, Washington.)

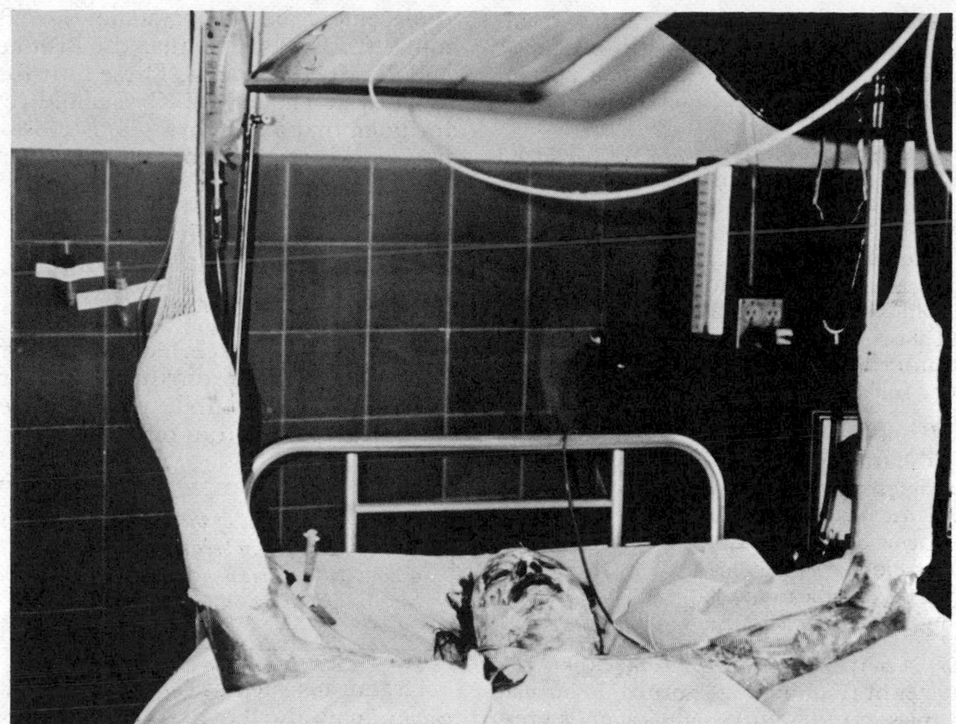

Figure 80–11. Use of Stockinette to elevate arms of burned person above heart level. (Courtesy of Harborview Medical Center Burn Unit, Seattle, Washington.)

FLUID THERAPY

Burn shock is characterized primarily by the slowness with which it develops. As stated, an adult patient is frequently alert when admitted. When a patient is initially obtunded, suspect related injuries, e.g., head trauma.

Symptoms of Shock. The nurse is an important member of the team in observing and managing patients with burns and must be alert to indications of shock. (See also Chapter 13.) The body can respond initially to burn fluid losses. It is only after the body has exhausted its protective defenses that shock occurs.

The body is quick to preserve the blood volume and its constituents by vasoconstriction, increased heart rate, decreased cardiac output, decreased blood flow, oliguria, and output of protective stress hormones, e.g., epinephrine, antidiuretic hormones, and aldosterone.

Wound edema is caused by damaged capillaries that have lost water, sodium chloride, and plasma into the damaged areas. Large quantities of fluid replacement solutions must be given *before* shock sets in.

Symptoms of shock include:

- *Thirst.* Nearly every burned person experiences thirst. However, a person is *not* permitted to drink anything for the first 48 hours when burns are severe or undetermined in extent. Renal excretion of water is drastically decreased shortly after burning, so that water intoxication can easily occur. Clinically, water intoxication shows itself by apathy, tremors, loss of visual acuity, headache, diarrhea, oliguria, vomiting, and, finally, generalized seizures and death. (See also Chapter 12.)
- *Restlessness.* Restlessness is likely to be present in severely burned patients. It is important to observe whether restlessness increases or regresses as treatment continues. Increasing restlessness is likely to be a sign of inadequate fluid resuscitation.
- *Delirium, Coma, or Seizures.* Delirium or coma is an especially serious sign within the first 96 hours if there has been no head injury, since it probably results from inadequate cerebral blood flow. Seizures can result from cerebral ischemia and may be a sign of increasing shock. Alcoholic persons can be expected to develop delirium tremens during the first hours after burning. Many patients are intoxicated when they are burned, and it is helpful to elicit this information from observers or from the patient's history. (Management of delirium tremens is discussed in Chapter 94.)
- *Blood Pressure and Pulse.* A badly burned patient should be left supine for at least 48 to 72 hours to eliminate unnecessary postural stress. The supine person can tolerate a deficit of 20 to 25 per cent of blood volume with little or no change in pulse or blood pressure. Blood pressure may be unobtainable with a pneumatic cuff, since there frequently are burns on all limbs. Central venous pressure is sometimes monitored; however, cardiac output or pulmonary wedge pressure may give a more accurate indication. Blood pressure and pulse should approach normal as treatment progresses.
- *Cyanosis.* Unburned skin should be pressed to test capillary filling. In white persons, a warm pink skin

with normal capillary filling time indicates a circulation that is physiologically intact. It is difficult to assess capillary filling in a dark-skinned person. Other signs of shock must then be observed carefully.

Most patients with severe burns have pale, cool skin for some hours because of compensatory cutaneous vasoconstriction. This is not a serious symptom unless it persists. Cyanosis in an acutely burned patient may be due to: (1) a circumferential eschar (if it is thoracic or abdominal, it may cause general cyanosis); (2) cardiovascular decompensation, with stasis of blood in the peripheral tissues; (3) ventilatory insufficiency due to injury to the respiratory tract.

- *Oliguria.* Urine flow is scanty or absent following any major burn, and indicates shock. The first urine specimen may be chocolate brown or red in color, because of hemoglobin pigment released into the plasma by the destroyed red blood cells. In adults, a urine flow of at least 30 ml./hour is a reasonably safe indication that the kidneys are functioning. *Renal shutdown is a serious problem.*
- *Respiration.* Tachypnea may be present. Otherwise, the character of respiration is "normal" in burned persons unless a respiratory complication is present, e.g., inhalation injury.

Fluid Replacement Formulas. Burned body parts immediately and inevitably swell. Although blisters may contain fluid and fluid may ooze from debrided areas, most of the fluid is in the tissues around and beneath the wound. These factors may cause severe fluid and electrolyte imbalance, requiring immediate attention (See Chapter 12.)

The ideal fluid resuscitation formula must rapidly restore normal homeostasis. *Body response* is related to: (1) the rate at which fluid is lost from the extracellular fluid compartment, (2) the fluid composition, and (3) the ability of replacement solutions to restore an effective circulating extracellular volume.

Indications of adequate fluid resuscitation *are*[84]:
Blood pressure
Systolic > 90–100 (age dependent)
Pulse Rate
< 120 (children)
< 100 (adults)
CVP or PCWP
CVP < 12 cm. of H_2O
PCWP < 18 mm. Hg
Hourly urine
10–20 cc./hr. (infant)
20–50 cc./hr. (child)
30–70 cc./hr. (adult)
Sensorium — clear
Gastrointestinal function
Absence of ileus or nausea

Additionally, acidosis is usually corrected in 18 to 24 hours. Four popular formulas for fluid replacement are: (1) crystalloid, or Baxter formula, (2) Evans formula, (3) Brooke formula, and (4) MGM formula. These four formulas are detailed in Table 80–2. Crystalloid resuscitation formula, or Baxter formula, is most commonly used and is recommended by the Committee of Trauma of the American College of Surgeons.

BURN MANAGEMENT AND COMPLICATIONS

The skin is an effective barrier between humans and their environment. Until a new skin cover is provided, a burned person is in serious jeopardy from overwhelming infection.

Effective treatment of the wound is just as important as shock prevention because, after 18 to 24 hours, the wound will become densely colonized with pathogenic bacteria if untreated.

Organisms such as *Candida albicans or Pseudomonas* may also be present. The resistance to bacterial infection is decreased markedly for the first week after injury.

BURN INFECTION

Infection is controlled by: (a) removal of the eschar and necrotic material, (b) by wound cleaning, and (c) by the use of topical agents to inhibit bacterial growth. Except for *Staphylococcus aureus* and β-hemolytic streptococcus, the majority of wound organisms are gram-negative *(E. coli,* and *Proteus, Enterobacter, Klebsiella, Aerobacter,* and *Pseudomonas* organisms). The bacteria of the normal flora do not cause disease unless accidentally introduced into normally protected body regions.

Each region of the body has a characteristic flora. The bacteria that populate the skin include mainly corynbacteria, micrococci, nonhemolytic streptococci, and mycobacteria. Moist areas harbor yeasts and other fungi. *Pseudomonas aeruginosa,* an anaerobic gram-negative organism, requires organic compounds as an energy source and is able to establish infection only in individuals with severely lowered natural resistance. Yeasts and *Candida albicans* are dominant and important when more susceptible bacteria of the normal flora are suppressed. They may invade the blood and result in a fatal sepsis (Table 80–3). Infections that typically occur during various stages of a burn are summarized in Table 80–4.

Patients with burns are almost twice as likely to get infections from cross-contamination as from autocontamination.

Personnel must use every possible means of preventing cross-contamination between patients. Numbers of people permitted access to a

TABLE 80–2. FLUID RESUSCITATION FORMULAS

Baxter Formula[84]

First 24 hours

Ringer's lactate: 4 ml./kg./% TBSA
No plasma or plasma substitutes
No dextrose-containing solutions
Administered:
½ of 24-hour total in first 8 hours
¼ of 24-hour total in second 8 hours
¼ of 24-hour total in third 8 hours

Second 24 hours

In fourth 8-hour period, plasma is given according to % TBSA burned. Amount of plasma given is usually 0.3 to 0.5 ml./kg./ %TBSA. By this time, the capillary leak should have sealed, and plasma will remain in the intravascular space

Glucose in water (2000 to 6000 ml.) given according to serum sodium level.

Evans Formula

First 24 hours

Colloids: 1 ml./kg./ %TBSA
Physiologic saline solution: 1 ml./kg./ %TBSA
Nonelectrolytes: 2000 ml. of 5% dextrose in water, or correspondingly less in children

Second 24 hours

½ of amounts of colloids and electrolytes administered in first 24 hours.

Notes

Evans was first to warn that when a burn involves more than 50% of body surface area, fluid requirements should be estimated as though only 50% of the body surface had been burned.

Brooke Formula

First 24 hours

Colloids (blood, dextran, or plasma): 0.5 ml./kg./ %TBSA
Ringer's lactate: 1.5 ml./kg./%TBSA
Water requirement (dextrose in water): 2000 ml. for adults; children correspondingly less

Brooke Formula (*Continued*)

Administered:
½ of 24-hour total in 1st 8 hours
¼ of 24-hour total in 2nd 8 hours
¼ of 24-hour total in 3rd 8 hours

Second 24 hours

Colloids and Ringer's lactate: about ½ of amount given in first 24 hours

Notes

If burns cover more than 50% of TBSA, requirements must be calculated as though only 50% had been burned. Usually not necessary to give more than 10 liters of fluid during first 24 hours to any patient regardless of extent of burn.

If, in a burn of more than 50% in a large patient, fluid therapy based on a 50% calculation fails to prevent signs and symptoms of circulatory failure, therapy is cautiously increased.

Massachusetts General Hospital (MGH) Formula

First 24 hours

125 ml. plasma/percent burn
15 ml. saline/percent burn
2000 ml. 5% dextrose in water

Second 24 hours

½ of the first 24-hour requirement of plasma and saline
2000 ml. 5% dextrose in water

Notes

1. The principle in this formula is to use plasma with only a very small amount of added saline.
2. For children, a more precise allowance for surface area is necessary. It is recommended that 90 ml. of plasma and 10 ml. of saline for each per cent of burn times the surface area in square meters be used to calculate the colloid and electrolyte requirements. In addition, an amount of 5% dextrose in water is given, according to the calculated normal fluid needs of the child.

patient must be kept minimal, and no one should be allowed into a patient's room without carefully following specific isolation procedures. Specific measures that nurses can take to decrease infection are:

1. Avoid undue contamination
2. Use strict handwashing procedures
3. Use protective clothing and masks
4. Use sterile instruments and gloves when touching the wound
5. Thoroughly clean *all* equipment, e.g., tanks

The moist warm environment of a burn wound promotes bacterial growth. However, covering the wound with a biological dressing (discussed later) may eliminate virtually all bacteria within 24 hours.

The use of *exposure treatment* in an environment of 32° C. (90° F.) and 20 to 30 per cent relative humidity without systemic antibiotic seems to be strikingly successful. The method seems to dramatically decrease mortality and provide rapid drying of the burn and a smaller weight loss.[62]

Burke et al.[20] report on a system (Bacteria Controlled Nursing Unit) developed to protect highly susceptible, seriously burned patients from cross-contamination — at a reasonable cost. The system is based on two principles: (1) *environmental control* of the area immediately surrounding the patient's bed, rather than isolating a whole room or ward and (2) delivering the medical care, monitoring life support, and locating intravenous equipment outside the *controlled sterile environment.* This study indicates that rates of bacterial cross-contamination and infection were markedly reduced for patients in the experimental unit. The system was not only a benefit to the individual patient but also a long-term advantage to the entire population of the burn unit. In Burke's experience, the method allowed prompt eschar excision and immediate wound closure. These activities have been shown to reduce burn mortality and increase the effectiveness of treatment, as judged by shortening the length of hospital stay. Control of the patient's immediate environment allows such techniques as temporary allograft

TABLE 80-3. CHARACTERISTICS OF BURN INFECTIONS

	Staphylococcus aureus	Pseudomonas	Candida albicans
Appearance of wound	Dissolution of granulation	Patchy black necrosis	Dry, flat, yellow or orange, granular
Course	Insidious, 2–6 days	Rapid, 12–36 hours	Chronic
Disorientation	Severe	Mild or absent	None
Temperature	Hyperpyrexia	Hypothermia	Normal to low
WBC	Usually increased	Usually depressed	Normal to increased
Ileus	Severe	Severe	None
Hypotension	Insidious, followed by oliguria	Sudden, with oliguria	None
Mortality	0–10%	50–60%	90%

transplantation and immunosuppression to be carried out without the threat of bacterial infection in the immunologically modified burn patient.

BURN COMPLICATIONS

All severe burns result in complications—"Complications are the rule rather than the exception."[42]

For a burned person, *any complication* can be a potential cause of death. A severely burned patient will "experience from four to six major complications, often at the same time — and one or a combination of several may be fatal."[42] These complications involve almost every system in the body.

Some of the *leading causes of death in burn patients* are: septicemia, pneumonia, renal failure, heart disease, Curling ulcer, and brain damage.

Sepsis. Of the causes of death, *sepsis is probably the leading one.* Sepsis is caused when bacteria, often from the burn wound itself, enter the blood stream, and the body's weakened defenses are unable to adequately remove the bacteria. Any invasive procedure (e.g., Foley or IV catheters, respirators, or chest tubes) increase the possibilities of infection. Often, manipulation of the burn wound — such as through tanking or surgery — can seed the bacteria into the blood stream.

TABLE 80-4. COURSE OF BURN INFECTION AND ITS TREATMENT

Initial 0–7 days	β-hemolytic streptococcus	Penicillin
Autolytic 8–21 days	*Staphylococcus aureus*	Staphcillin Erythromycin Novobiocin
Granulating 22–30 days	Pseudomonas	Gentamicin Colymycin Carbenicillin
Grafting 31 days to coverage	β-hemolytic streptococcus	Penicillin Chloramphenicol
	Yeast	Nystatin Amphotericin B

Early signs of sepsis include:

Rise in heart rate
Temperature greater than 38.3° C. (101° F.) or less than 37° C. (98.6°F.)
Increase in depth and number of respirations
Insidious decrease in blood pressure
Insidious decrease in urine output
Change in orientation
Chills
Glucose intolerance
Decreased platelet count

Management of patients with sepsis is difficult. Since their bodies are in a hypermetabolic state in response to the burn itself, some have already reached their optimal response and are unable to meet the further demand caused by sepsis. The body tries to compensate by: dilatation of the vascular tree; hypovolemia; decreased cardiac output; and decreased myocardial, cerebral, renal, and intestinal perfusion.

Treatment of sepsis includes the following: drainage of the seeding source, antibiotics specific for the infecting organism, fluid replacement, glucocorticosteroids, and a vasodilator. These patients must be closely monitored, since their condition is likely to change rapidly.

Respiratory Complications.[57] In at least 20 to 25 per cent of all hospitalized burn patients, some pulmonary complication will develop, with an attendant mortality rate of about 50 per cent. Thus, it is important to *identify early* those patients in whom respiratory complications may be expected. Respiratory complications arise from any burn that:

- ▶ Occurred within a closed space
- ▶ Involved electrical shock or chemical inhalant
- ▶ Involves the face, neck, or chest

When making the *initial assessment* of a burned patient, watch for: singed nasal hairs, red swollen mouth, darkened mucosa, hoarseness, use of accessory muscles to breathe, smoky smell on the breath, inspiratory wheezes, carbon particles in the sputum, and blood-tinged mucus. These are all signs that the patient probably has a respiratory involvement.

Possible respiratory complications with burns include:
A. Early
  1. Primary pulmonary irritants and direct burn of the respiratory tract
  2. Pulmonary edema
  3. Constriction caused by eschar of the neck and trunk
B. Later
  1. Pneumonia
  2. Atelectasis
  3. Pulmonary emboli
  4. Tension pneumothorax, hemothorax
  5. Respiratory alkalosis or acidosis

Smoke inhalation is a common cause of respiratory complications. The severity varies with the amount of smoke inhaled and its constituents. Two types of pulmonary complications are: (1) *Asphyxia/obtundation* and (2) *chemical tracheobronchitis* (airway obstruction) and pulmonary alveolar disease.[57]

Persons with *asphyxia/obtundation* may be those subjected to smoke inhalation in an enclosed space after ingesting large amounts of alcohol or drugs. Patients who are significantly obtunded on admission require immediate control of the airway by insertion of an endotracheal tube. Pure oxygen (100%) is the treatment of choice for patients with an elevated carboxyhemoglobin level. Arterial blood gas analysis and COHb levels are guides to the management of these patients.[57]

In patients with *chemical tracheobronchitis,* high incidences of bronchospasm, irritative conjunctivitis, and carbonaceous sputum (i.e., sputum flecked with carbon) may be noted. The most significant procedure for diagnosis of upper airway inhalation disease is fiberoptic bronchoscopy. The vast majority of patients who show significant compromise of the upper airways can be adequately treated by endotracheal intubation and the inhalation of moist humidified air. If significant bronchospasm is present, a bronchodilator such as aminophylline may be added to the treatment. Abnormalities will be indicated on arterial blood gas analysis. Most patients with upper airway obstructive problems can be managed by attention to bronchopulmonary toilet. Occasionally, persistent abnormalities such as bronchiectasis may result from a smoke inhalation injury.[57]

Small airway/alveolar disease may also result from smoke inhalation. *Adult respiratory distress syndrome* (ARDS) has the following characteristics: (1) Hypoxemia, resistant to elevations of the inspired oxygen concentration; (2) progressive decrease in pulmonary compliance; (3) characteristic x-ray changes of interstitial edema, with diffuse fluffy infiltrates that appear on the second or third day and progress to widespread areas of consolidation.[57]

Since persons with burns often require prolonged hospitalization, it is important to implement good respiratory care *early* (See Unit XVI). Most severely burned patients require:

- ▶ Oxygen therapy (respirator, nebulizer, etc.)
- ▶ Frequent coughing and deep breathing or suctioning
- ▶ Frequent turning or postural drainage

These patients should also be followed up with daily chest x-ray and arterial blood gases as indicated by the physician.

Curling's (Stress) Ulcer.[48, 98] *Curling's ulcer* or *stress ulcer* is a complication of severe burns. (See also Chapter 62.) Curling's ulcer, a symptom of stress, occurs in about one half of severely burned persons. The incidence increases with increasing burn size. Occult blood in the stool is present in about half of those persons who have sustained severe burns. Pre-existing sepsis has been shown to be an additive stress, predisposing the burned individual to Curling's ulcer. Almost all patients with a positive blood culture show mucosal disease. Sepsis control reverses mucosal pathology.[48]

High risk factors for hemorrhage in persons with stress ulcer include: hypotension, peritonitis, renal failure, respiratory failure, jaundice, and sepsis. When three or more of these risk factors are present, there is a 40 per cent chance that bleeding will occur. Mortality ranges from 20 to 70 per cent once hemorrhage occurs.[48]

Curling's ulcer usually begins with interspersed areas of pallor and hyperemia in the gastric wall, appearing within a few hours after the burn. Within 24 hours after the burn occurs, superficial mucosal necrosis develops, i.e., erosions are present. By 48 hours, the lesions have eroded the gastric wall, through the muscularis mucosae. The lesions are now ulcers.[48]

Typically, the stress lesions first appear in the proximal stomach and then spread distally to the junction of the stomach's body and antrum. Duodenal stress ulcers may develop; however, they usually do not occur within the first 72 hours.[48]

Signs and symptoms of Curling's ulcer include:
Early
1. *Gastric distention*
2. *Blood flecks in nasogastric residua*
3. *Pallor and sweat*

Later
1. *Ileus*
2. *Decreased hematocrit*
3. *Brisk bleeding*

Prophylactic antacid therapy helps prevent hemorrhage from Curling's ulcer. Thus, many patients with burns are started on prophylactic antacids upon admission to the hospital. Commonly, 30 ml. of a magnesium-containing antacid is put down the nasogastric tube every hour. Tube is clamped for 15 to 30 minutes, then returned to intermittent suction. The pH of the gastric residual is checked every hour to determine acidity levels. A treatment regimen may be written specifying that additional antacid is to be given if pH drops to 5 or below.

Cimetidine is another effective prophylactic used for Curling's ulcer. Since cimetidine is a histamine H_2 receptor antagonist, it inhibits acid secretion; it usually is given IV or orally every 4 to 6 hours.

In the case of hemorrhage, *iced lavage, Pitressin, catecholamines,* or *surgical intervention* may be indicated.

THERAPY

Hydrotherapy ("Tanking").*[67] At least once a day the patient with burns is bathed, or tanked, to remove the topical agent and clean the burned area. Various types of tubs or tanks may be used, depending largely upon available facilities. Types vary, including regular bath tubs, Hubbard tanks, and a flat steel table equipped with a long flexible shower hose (Fig. 80–12).

Hydrotherapy has several *advantages,* the most important of which are:

- Allows for easier removal of the topical agent
- Softens the eschar, thus permitting easier, less painful ROM (range of motion)

The *disadvantages* of hydrotherapy include:

- Loss of body heat
- Stress and pain
- Sodium loss in the water
- Possible cross-contamination

For the patient, hydrotherapy is a very stressful, painful time. Every effort should be made to promote patient relaxation and comfort.

If possible, it may help to have a specific time each day reserved for hydrotherapy. The patient should participate in selecting the time if possible. Often this helps to lower the patient's anxiety about the procedure and gives the pa-

*Hydrotherapy may also be called bathing, tanking, or tubbing.

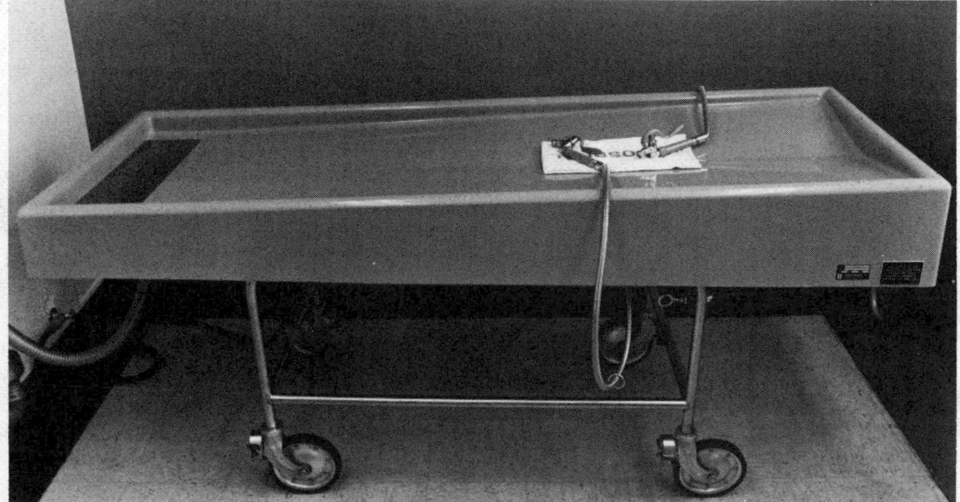

Figure 80–12. Table equipped with long flexible shower hose, used for hydrotherapy ("tanking") of persons with burns. (Courtesy Harborview Medical Center Burn Unit, Seattle, Washington.)

tient some control in decision-making. Prescribed pain medication is given prior to going to the tub or tank. IM injections are given 15 to 30 minutes prior to the treatment, or an IV medication may be given immediately before.

The nurse should thoroughly explain the hydrotherapy procedure to the patient before beginning. It is important to let the patient know that you realize that the procedure is very painful and that it is all right to verbalize the pain. The patient should be encouraged to "let it out."

During hydrotherapy, blisters are broken and devitalized skin (eschar) is removed (i.e., debrided). Sterile scissors and forceps are used. Initially, patients have all of the hair on and around the burn shaved. Shaving is repeated during tanking at least once a week to decrease the growth of bacteria around the burn. It is important not to nick the skin during shaving, since this would provide a portal of entry for bacteria.

Hydrotherapy time is typically limited to 30 minutes to minimize sodium loss (since the water is hypotonic) and loss of body heat, and to keep stress and pain minimal.

The patient is typically weighed each day on the way back to the room. Following these activities, patients may be extremely cold and may be shaking. The thoughtful nurse thus plans for the heat shield to be on prior to the patient's return to bed.

Tanks or other bathing equipment *must* be thoroughly cleaned with an antibacterial agent between uses by patients, to lower the possibility of infection by cross-contamination.

Topical Therapy. Bacteria are typically present within a burn wound. Thus it is not unexpected to culture them from the wound, and a positive culture does not constitute burn wound sepsis. Tissue biopsy must be done in order to demonstrate burn wound sepsis.

During the first 24 hours, there is only a scant growth of organisms in a burn wound. However, within the next 24 hours colonization of the wound is quite extensive and penetrates through the openings of the hair follicles. At this time, gram-positive organisms predominate, with smaller numbers of gram-negative organisms. Near the end of the first week the eschar has extensive bacterial growth. If control is not established by this time, the organisms increase in numbers and invade the adjacent unburned tissue.

> *Topical antibiotic therapy of a burn wound is effective only in controlling or lessening the numbers of organisms present within the wound and does not result in eradication of infection.*

There are many effective *types of topical agents* in use for burn therapy. Some of the most popular are: silver sulfadiazine (Silvadene Cream), mafenide acetate (Sulfamylon), silver nitrate ($AgNO_3$), povidone-iodine (Betadine Ointment), sutilains ointment (Travase).

There are many advantages and disadvantages to each of these types of therapy.

Silver Sulfadiazine. Silver sulfadiazine, or *Silvadene,*[88] is now used as a 15 per cent ointment in a water soluble base. Its appearance is creamy white. It spreads easily over a burn with a gloved hand and is easily removed with water. Silvadene is effective against a wide range of gram-negative and gram-positive bacteria, as well as yeast. Silvadene acts only on the cell wall and membrane. It is applied directly to the burned area, using sterile gloves, immediately following tanking and may be reapplied as needed.

Advantages of Silvadene include:

1. Has antimicrobial action against gram-negative and gram-positive organisms.
2. Does not cause electrolyte imbalance or kidney disease.
3. Delays separation of eschar less than many other topical agents.
4. Has a long shelf life.
5. Is easy and fast to apply.
6. Application is painless.
7. Softens eschar, giving increased ROM.

Disadvantages of Silvadene include:

1. On occasion causes rash, burning, and pruritus.
2. Is absorbed into eschar less than other topical agents.
3. Not consistently effective in large burns, or against some bacteria and yeast.
4. Tends to depress granulocyte formation.

Mafenide Acetate. Mafenide acetate, or *Sulfamylon,*[113] is a topical sulfonamide drug intended to prevent burn wound sepsis. In patients with intact subcutaneous vasculature, peak concentrations occur two hours after application, or up to 4 hours in avascular areas. Sulfamylon is effective against *Pseudomonas aeruginosa, Staphylococcus aureus,* and *Aerobacter aerogenes.*

Sulfamylon is applied in cream form once or twice daily with a gloved hand. (Fig. 80–13). It has the consistency of soft butter and burns and stings for 15 minutes to an hour following application because it is hydroscopic and draws water out of the tissues.

Advantages of Sulfamylon include:

1. Penetrates through thick eschar.
2. Easily applied.
3. Has a long shelf life.
4. Effective against Pseudomonas.

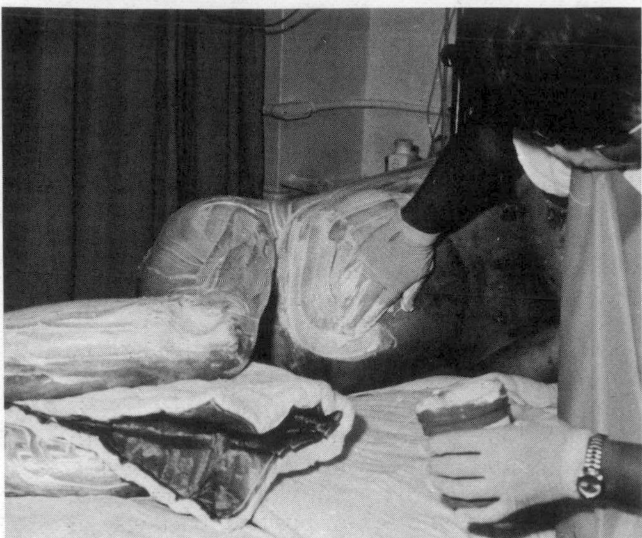

Figure 80–13. The topical antimicrobial of choice is applied to the burn wound with the sterile gloved hand. (From Artz, C. P., J. A. Moncrief, and B. A. Pruitt: *Burns—A Team Approach.* Philadelphia: W. B. Saunders Co., 1979, p. 373.)

Disadvantages of Sulfamylon include:

1. In some cases causes hyperpnea, rash, and metabolic acidosis.
2. Is painful when applied.
3. Tends to slow eschar separation.

Silver Nitrate. Silver Nitrate ($AgNO_3$),[113] has been used as a burn treatment for many years. When used properly, it controls the wound's bacterial population and reduces water evaporation. Therapeutic effects are limited to the more superficial tissues. Biochemical abnormalities are the major problem in the use of silver nitrate. The hypotonicity of the distilled water used to carry the silver nitrate produces large absorption of distilled water into the body and large quantities of body minerals (sodium, potassium, chloride, magnesium, and calcium) are leeched from the tissues. If patients have more than 20 per cent TBSA burns, they are likely to have a mineral deficiency, unless regular electrolyte replacement takes place. Monitoring of serum and urinary electrolytes daily may be necessary. Experience indicates that if the urinary sodium concentration falls below 40 mEq/L., the serum sodium concentration will fall within 24 hours. It is important to recognize that in infants and children and in some adults these deficiencies can occur within 6 to 8 hours of beginning therapy, so that careful monitoring is essential.[92]

Advantages of Silver Nitrate include:

1. Inexpensive to the patient.
2. Painless to the patient.

Disadvantages of Silver Nitrate include:

1. Since it penetrates into the wound only 1 to 2 mm., it acts only on surface organisms.
2. May cause hypocalcemia, hypochloremia, and hyponatremia.
3. Messy and time-consuming to apply.
4. Decreases ROM owing to bulky wet dressings.
5. If dressings are not kept continually wet, the burn may be converted to third degree.

To apply *Silver Nitrate dressings,* a plastic wash basin is filled with warmed 0.5 per cent silver nitrate solution. Precut and rolled dressings are soaked in the solution and then applied to all burned areas. The dressings are held in place with bias-cut stockinette, secured with safety pins; and the patient is covered with dry sheets and at least one dry cotton blanket. The dry covers are important and *must* be changed when they become wet. *The dressings must be kept soaking wet.* If kept wet, reepithelialization will take place between the 15th and 40th days.

During the first 7 to 14 days, the dressings need be changed only once daily. After the eschar begins to liquefy and separate, three or four daily dressings may be necessary. As soon as treated parts are exposed to sunlight, the eschar darkens and turns brown or black or blue, depending on the depth of the burn and the amount of sunlight. Hard blue-black eschars on wounds dressed with solution for more than a week indicate a probable subdermal burn. If infection is controlled, these will remain in place for weeks, until they finally separate from the granulating adipose tissue. If the adipose tissue is burned, the eschars will begin to separate a few days after the injury. If this occurs, they must be removed promptly because liquefied fat is an excellent medium for bacterial growth. Eschars of intradermal burns are brown or black and begin to separate after 7 to 10 days.

Povidone-Iodine. Povidone-iodine (*Betadine*)[16a] is also used to help prevent burn wound sepsis. It is effective against gram-negative and gram-positive organisms. Betadine is available in solution, foam, and ointment. It is easily applied to the burn wound with a sterile gloved hand. Gauze dressings are applied over the Betadine and are kept moist with Betadine solution every 6 hours or as necessary. Betadine has a tendency to build up a crust, thus special care must be given in the tank to thoroughly clean the wound.

Advantages of Betadine include:

1. Effective against gram-negative and positive organisms, yeast, fungi, viruses, and protozoa.
2. Wide assortment of forms available.
3. Long shelf life.

Disadvantages of Betadine include:

1. May cause metabolic acidosis.
2. May cause irritations, swelling, and redness in persons with allergies to iodine.
3. Bulky dressings impair ROM.
4. Crusts may form if not properly cleaned.
5. Stains bed linens.
6. May burn or sting when applied.

Sutilains Ointment. Sutilains ointment (*Travase*)[21] is a topical enzymatic agent. Travase is used on second and third degree burns to dissolve and remove necrotic tissue. It acts by selectively digesting necrotic tissue, thus helping debride the burn wound. Its effectiveness is usually noted within 24 to 48 hours after treatment has begun.

The enzyme action of Travase may be inactivated if it is used in conjunction with iodine, Furacin, or hexachlorophene. Neomycin, Sulfamylon, streptomycin, and penicillin do not affect the enzyme activity. It should be used on no greater than 15 per cent of the total burn wound at a time.

Travase should be applied in a thin layer over the wound with a sterile, gloved hand. The Travase should overlap onto the unburned skin by about 1/4 inch. A wet saline dressing is then applied over the enzyme. *This dressing must be kept moist at all times.* Travase may be applied from one to four times daily.

Advantages of Travase include:

1. Begins initial debridement of the wound.
2. Easily applied.

Disadvantages of Travase include:

1. May cause bleeding.
2. Must be refrigerated.
3. Is not bactericidal.
4. Increases body fluid loss.
5. Is often irritating to the wound and sometimes to surrounding skin.

Subeschar Clysis. *Subeschar clysis* is a valuable adjunct to effective topical therapy. With this technique, appropriate antibiotics are infused directly into the subeschar space. A physician determines the area to be clysed, as well as the antibiotic and the amount and type of carrier fluid to be used.

The nurse will fill a Buretrol (with IV tubing attached) with 100 ml. of this fluid. Several Buretrols may be needed, depending on the amount of fluid being used. A 21-gauge needle is attached to the end of the IV tubing. After the area is cleaned with an alcohol swab, the needle is inserted into the subeschar space at a 45-degree angle. Twenty-five ml. of fluid is infused into each 7.5 cm.-square area (roughly the size of a softball). A new needle is used for each insertion site. This technique is often used in burns of greater than 40 per cent TBSA burn.

Biologic Dressings. A frequently used way to clean up a burn site and prepare it for grafting is to use biologic dressings, which are changed every 2 to 3 days.

> *Biologic dressings prevent loss of water and protein from the wound. They decrease pain in open wounds, permit increased mobility of the area, decrease bacterial growth on the wound surface, and appear to enhance growth of epithelium.*

Some commonly used biologic dressings are:

- *Xenograft or heterograft* — skin from another species
- *Homograft or allograft* — skin taken from cadavers of the same species
- *Synthetic dressings*
- *Amnion* — human amniotic membrane

XENOGRAFTS. Xenografts, or heterografts, are suitable temporary dressings for early noncontaminated second degree wounds if they can be applied within several hours of injury. The most common type of heterograft is *porcine,* or *pig skin* (Fig. 80–14). With this treatment, there is marked reduction in pain and loss of wound exudate. Superficial, second degree burns generally heal under the heterografts and do not require subsequent grafting. The wound must be inspected frequently for indications of infection.

Porcine dressings are used in full-thickness injuries to clean up (help debride) areas of granulation tissue in preparation for autografting. Heterografts may be used temporarily to cover burn wounds following eschar excision until autografting (grafting with patient's own skin) can be carried out. Porcine grafts have been shown to have no immunologic properties. Heterografts are applied carefully to the wounds, with the dermal side in apposition to the wound surface. Wrinkles are smoothed out, and the graft is trimmed to fit the area of the burn wound. The grafts are ordinarily changed at 3-day intervals. If fluid collects under the grafts, they may be changed daily or as indicated by the physician. If fever develops, the grafts may be discontinued entirely and the patient put on antibiotics.[118]

Porcine xenograft is readily available in most areas, is relatively inexpensive and is easy, although time-consuming, for the nurse to apply. It is available by the square or by the roll and must be refrigerated.

HOMOGRAFTS. Homografts are frequently used as a dressing for the wound. The graft is taken off before tissue rejection occurs; and another homograft is applied, or an autograft if available. Homograft is usually reapplied every 3 to 7 days, or as necessary, if fluid accumulates beneath the graft. In many cases, a physician applies the homograft to the burn wound.

Homografts are not as readily available in some areas as heterografts, often owing to a shortage of donors. In the United States, there are now several *human cadaver skin banks* with facilities for freezer preservation and storage of

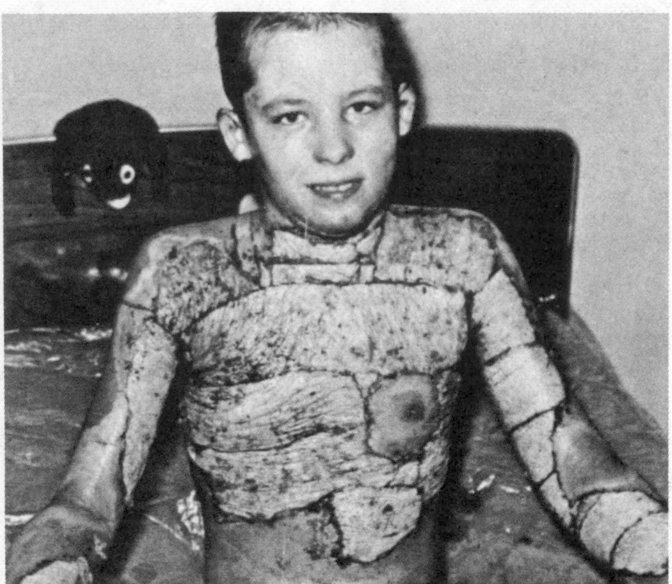

Figure 80–14. Porcine skin dressing. This biologic dressing is a heterograft (xenograft) of pigskin. (From Stinson, V.: Porcine skin dressings for burns. *American Journal of Nursing,* 74:111, Jan. 1974.)

viable human skin for as long as several months. Homografts have been most widely used on patients with massive thermal injuries and limited donor sites, who undergo primary wound excision.

SYNTHETIC DRESSINGS. Yarborough[128] recommends a synthetic dressing called Hydron. Hydron has been used primarily on small second degree burns and on donor sites. When used on such areas, Hydron may reduce pain and adhere well to the wound surface. It is fairly flexible and may prevent infection. However, this synthetic dressing washes off rather easily, cracks frequently over joints, somewhat reduces mobility, and enhances bacterial growth if applied to a contaminated wound. Hydron is applied by spraying. It should be maintained intact over the entire wound until the wound has healed and should be inspected frequently for signs of infection.

AMNION. Human amniotic membranes may also be suitable biologic dressings for burns. Amniotic membrane may be obtained without cost to patient or hospital. One amnion will cover a large area and adhere more rapidly than other dressings since it is structurally similar to skin. The membranes are sterilized with sodium hypochlorite solution. Amnion is effective in preventing infections. Amniotic membrane consists of two distinct membranes: the *inner amnion* and the *outer chorion*. Either membrane or a combination of the two can be used on the burn wound, depending on whether the wound is a partial- or full-thickness burn. Since vascular penetration is more desirable in full-thickness wounds, for these the more vascular chorion may be placed directly on the granulation tissue. Both membranes may be used in weight-bearing areas.

The granulation tissue to which the amniotic membrane is applied should be free from exudate and topical agents. The membranes are placed over the granulation tissue so they adhere closely, without any air pockets or wrinkles. If possible, the area should then be left open to the air so that the dressings can be observed closely for exudate. The membranes should be changed no later than 48 hours after being applied to the wound, or sooner if infection begins to develop.[94, 127]

Methods of Debridement. In any form of trauma, the sooner wound closure is achieved, the better. A burn wound presents special problems. Rapid wound closure is often not possible because of massiveness of injury and lack of donor sites (autografting is discussed in the following section) to provide adequate skin coverage.

> *There is general agreement that rapid removal of eschar is essential to prevent multiplication of bacteria.*

There are four commonly used *methods of removing eschar*: (1) primary, (2) surgical, (3) mechanical, and (4) enzymatic.

Primary Excision. Primary excision means the burn wound is excised down to fascia and a skin graft applied. The removal of large amounts of devitalized tissue by excisional therapy has been shown to reduce morbidity and mortality. The greatest success has been shown when large areas of full-thickness burns have been removed down to the deep fascia by using either the *cold knife, avulsion techniques*, or the *laser scalpel*. Excisional therapy is not advised for children under 1 year of age or adults over 60 years. Nutritional supplements are important to minimize weight loss in patients who are undergoing excisional therapy. If weight loss can be kept to no more than 5 to 10 per cent of the preburn weight, septic complications during excisional therapy are reduced. The optimal time for performing an excisional procedure has been found to be between the second and fifth days after the burn. Excisional procedures should be carried out on only one side of the body at a time. The excised burn wound should be resurfaced with skin grafts.[83]

Surgical Debridement. Surgical debridement consists of removing the top layers of the eschar in a limited area, usually no more than 15 per cent of the body surface area at one time.

Surgical debridement is referred to as *tangential excision* and is done with a *dermatome* (see Fig. 80–15) or *freehand knife*. The purpose of this procedure is to remove areas of necrotic tissue that have not sloughed on their own. It allows rapid removal from critical areas, such as joints where contractures may develop. The resulting wound is then treated as a conventional wound. Disadvantages of surgical debridement are: cost, multiple trips to the operating room, dangers of anesthesia, difficulty in differentiating viable tissue from necrotic tissue, and the need for multiple transfusions.

Mechanical Debridement. Several methods of mechanical debridement may be used. The most common are wet to dry dressings, or continuous wet dressings (soaks) with frequent changes. For *wet to dry dressings*, fine mesh gauze is soaked in saline or in some type of antimicrobial agent in solution and placed on the wound and allowed to dry. As the dry dressings are removed, necrotic tissue that has stuck to the gauze is pulled off. The *continuous wet dressings* do not remove as much dead tissue as the wet to dry dressing.

Major disadvantages of mechanical debridement are that eschar removal is very painful, the process must be done frequently, and some epithelialization may be destroyed in the process. More time is required from support personnel than with some other types of treatment. This type of debridement is generally used for small areas of the burn where a minimal amount of eschar remains.

Loose necrotic tissue may also be removed while the patient is receiving *hydrotherapy*. The patient is placed in a hydrotherapy tank once or twice a day and any residue from antimicrobial creams is gently washed away. Forceps are then used to lift any loose necrotic tissue so that it can be cut away with scissors or scalpel. This process is tedious and lengthy. However, since only loose dead tissue is removed, there is no bleeding or additional trauma to the patient. Any qualified member of a burn team can do mechanical debridement, and evaluation of the burn wound is assured daily.

Enzymatic Debridement. The final type of debridement includes the use of an enzymatic debriding agent such as Travase (sutilains) ointment. This proteolytic enzyme will digest necrotic tissue without harming viable tissue. Enzymatic debridement can be used on any type of burn and on any part of the body except the face. *It is essential to keep the chemical out of the eyes.*

This treatment method is *contraindicated*: if the wound communicates with a major body cavity; if major nerves or tendons are exposed, or if the patient is pregnant. The enzyme causes increased fluid drainage through the excised area; therefore, no more than 20 per cent of the body area should be treated at any one time. Generally, sutilains ointment is applied on the day of admission unless the patient has complicating medical problems, in which case the use of the enzyme is postponed until the patient's condition is stabilized.

Patients undergoing enzymatic debridement are taken to a Hubbard tank where they are placed in plain tap water. Dressings are removed and the burn wound cleaned using sterile technique. The patient is then removed from the tank, covered with a sterile sheet, and transferred to the dressing room. The area to be treated is covered with a thick layer of the enzyme, applied with a gloved hand. Wet dressings are applied directly over the sutilains ointment. Then a layer of Kerlix gauze is applied, followed by a layer of Kling gauze.

As the enzyme begins to liquefy the eschar, fluid is lost. During this period the patient should be monitored closely to insure adequate fluid resuscitation. Another side effect is some bleeding, as small capillaries that were thrombosed by the thermal injury may open and cause oozing. There may also be an elevation in body temperature; a spike to 38.8°C. (102°F.) or 39.4°C. (103°F.) is not unusual. There is no concern if the temperature returns to baseline in a few hours. If it goes higher or remains elevated, there is the possibility of invasive infection and broad-spectrum antibiotics should be given.

With second degree burns, sutilains ointment may be painful. The pain usually does not last more than an hour and can be lessened by the administration of a mild analgesic. The cooling of the topical antibiotic ointment used with the ointment often relieves the burning sensation.

Enzyme debridement works most effectively if used 28 to 48 hours postburn. The debriding agent is used on the burn wound for an average of 5 to 6 days. At that time the wound is usually free of loose necrotic tissue and ready for surgery. If it is a deep full-thickness injury, the enzyme will debride only down to the subcutaneous fat area. Some physicians take the patient to surgery, debride the fat and apply a skin graft at that time.[34]

Chemical debridement produces a white stringy material called *collagen moss* in the wound, giving it a slimy appearance. In this situation a 4 × 4 inch gauze sponge is opened up and applied directly to the wound. The ointment is applied to the gauze, which is then covered by gauze impregnated with silver sulfadiazine. The use of the enzyme has resulted in a decrease in hospital stay and a higher incidence of graft take, although average survival rate and incidence of sepsis has not changed.[34]

Grafting. Since full-thickness burns will not

heal by themselves, they will require *autografting*. An autograft is a piece of skin taken from the burned patient's own body. A patient may be autografted as soon as the physician believes the granulation bed is clean and ready to accept a graft.

Skin may be transferred from one part of the body to another either as a *free graft* or as a *flap*. A free graft is a piece of skin which is completely detached from its donor area and placed on the area to be grafted. It depends for its survival on the blood supply and nutrition of the recipient area. The graft will not survive if placed on compact bone, bare cartilage, tendons, or on heavily irradiated tissue.

> *When a free graft is placed on a raw surface, it usually adheres in a few minutes, but this adhesion is easily broken by any moving of the graft sideways.*

After 72 hours, the graft will have "taken" and will survive unless a severe infection or shearing force occurs. Free grafts can be left exposed to the air as long as nothing is allowed to rub them off. A thick graft is more likely to maintain its normal color and is more durable. A thin graft is more likely to contract, but it also is more likely to survive because it is easily permeated by tissue fluid. There is usually pain and temperature sensation within 3 months.

Free grafts are classified as follows: (1) Thiersch grafts; (2) split-thickness grafts; (3) Wolfe full-thickness grafts; (4) pinch grafts, and (5) Tanner Vanderput mesh graft.

- A *Thiersch graft* is a thin sheet of skin consisting of the epidermis and the superficial part of the dermis. This term is applied only to the thinnest type of grafts. The donor areas will usually heal in 7 to 10 days.
- *Split-thickness grafts* are grafts that take more dermis than a Thiersch graft but less than a Wolfe graft. When cut into small squares, they are known as "postage stamp" or patch grafts, and are used to cover extensive granulating surfaces. The donor area will usually heal in 10 to 14 days.
- A *Wolfe graft* consists of the full thickness of the skin with no subcutaneous fat. The donor area does not heal spontaneously.
- *Pinch grafts* are small, full-thickness pieces of skin. They are particularly resistant to infection and grow in areas of poor blood supply. However, pinch grafts leave an unsightly pitted donor area that cannot be used again.
- The *Tanner Vanderput mesh graft* has multiple slices in the graft, allowing it to be opened to three times its original size.

The Grafting Procedure. In a general hospital, a grafting procedure is done in the operating room. When large amounts of skin are needed, as for a burn, any surface of the limbs and trunk may be used as a *donor area*. The largest surface available is the medial aspect of the thigh. The physician gives priority to grafting of the hands and face and areas that will help the patient to be self-sufficient.

Skin for burn coverage is usually cut with a *dermatome.* (See Fig. 80–15.) The greatest care should be taken to prevent infection, so rigorous

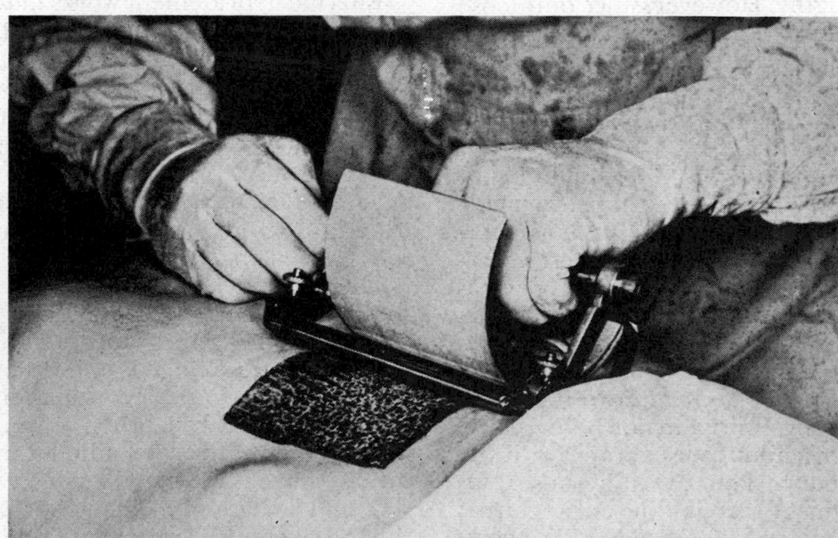

Figure 80–15. The Padgett dermatome in action. A full drum of skin measures 10 by 20 cm. This dermatome is particularly useful in removing skin for coverage of areas of motion. (From Artz, C. P., J. A. Moncrief, and B. A. Pruitt: *Burns—A Team Approach.* Philadelphia: W. B. Saunders Co., 1979, p. 279.)

skin preparation is usually prescribed. The Padgett dermatome depends on the efficiency of an adhesive cement for successful skin cutting. For successful adhesion of the cement, no moisture or grease can be allowed near the dermatome or drum. Both skin and drum are cleaned with ether. The cement is painted onto the skin and onto the drum and allowed to become tacky. The skin adheres to the drum, which is slowly rotated as the graft is cut by to-and-fro movements of the blade. The electric dermatome permits removal of calibrated skin grafts without requiring use of adhesive cement.

The donor site is draped aseptically and is anesthetized with lidocaine injected intradermally and subcutaneously. After 10 to 20 minutes, the skin grafts are cut with the dermatome. An assistant provides appropriate traction and positioning of the skin. The grafts are placed in a basin of balanced solution after they are cut. The grafts are then smoothed out, epidermal side down, on sterile wrapping paper. A paper template is cut out leaving a few millimeters of paper beyond the graft edge, and the graft is laid on the wound at the selected site using the edge of the paper as a handle. If there is not enough skin for autographs, homografts are used.

Some physicians believe that the donor area should be dressed before the graft is applied, and others favor putting wet sterile saline dressings on the donor wound and dressing this site later in surgery after the oozing stops. The donor site may be covered with fine meshed hot packs. These large packs are later removed, leaving only the fine mesh gauze as a covering for the donor area. The gauze is allowed to remain in place until it detaches by itself, usually between 2 and 3 weeks later. Monafo[91] applies a single layer of porous polyurethane foam $^1/_{16}$ inch in thickness. The site may be treated with wet silver nitrate dressings, as is the burn wound, or topical antiseptic cream may be smeared over the polyurethane and renewed as needed.

Depending on hospital policy, nurses on the unit may be responsible for rolling over the top of the graft regularly with a sterile applicator to express any fluid to the edge of the graft. This promotes adhesion. With a sheet graft a nick may be made in the graft's center and the fluid expressed through the opening. If the patient is being treated by the *open method*, hydrotherapy may be started within 72 hours after grafting. If the graft is washed off by the water agitation, it is already dead. Additional grafting is then subsequently necessary. Grafts may also be cared for by the *closed method* using dressings. Dressings are changed in 18 to 24 hours. Agency policies vary concerning graft care.

Nutrition in Burn Patients. Good nutrition and maintaining weight are important for the successful treatment of a burned person. A burned patient's weight will usually sharply increase postburn because of edema. This is reabsorbed 3 to 12 days later; at this time the person should return to a preburn weight. After this time, the person usually loses weight gradually, owing to the increased energy and protein requirements of hypermetabolism and hypercatabolism. The basal metabolic rate may be doubled or more.

> *Caloric intake may be determined by the following equation:*
> *Adult (25 Kcal × kg, body weight)*
> *plus (40 Kcal × % burn)*
> *Child (60 Kcal × kg, body weight)*
> *plus (35 Kcal × % burn)*[30a]

A burned person requires food that will provide carbohydrates, proteins, fats, vitamins, salts, water, minerals, and a sufficient amount of energy.

In most hospitals, a dietitian works with the nursing staff and the patient to prepare a diet that will meet individual needs. When possible, the burned person should be encouraged to express food and beverage likes and dislikes to the dietitian, thus participating in this aspect of care.

The extensively burned patient presents dietary problems that do not stop until skin grafting is complete. The continuous discomfort of extensive burns and daily dressings or treatment may ruin the patient's appetite. Frequent small feedings are often required. High calorie drinks may be given between meals to help meet caloric needs. It is important to keep an accurate daily account of the person's weight and caloric intake. The caloric intake is often computed daily by the dietitian.

Polyunsaturated fat is necessary to prevent essential fatty acid deficiency. Multivitamins should be given daily. Iron and potassium supplements may also be needed. In order to compensate for fluid loss, a high fluid intake is needed. Commonly the postburn patient may remain on clear fluids for 3 to 4 days and then move to a full diet as soon as tolerated. The patient should be weighed daily after removal of wound dressings. If a patient's food intake is insufficient to meet caloric needs, a *tube feeding* or *hyperalimentation* regimen may be necessary. These procedures should be discontinued as soon as possible. A form of hyperalimentation is provided by an IV fat preparation (see Chapter 59). This preparation can be given through a peripheral intravenous line, which means fewer infectious complications.[47]

PSYCHOSOCIAL IMPACT OF SERIOUS BURNS*

A seriously burned person may behave in ways that are simultaneously familiar and perplexing. The behavior is familiar because it reflects feelings that we have all had when we have experienced an accident, however small. It is perplexing, and maybe even frightening, in that the behavior may have an energy force behind it that — although similar in nature — is greater in degree than we have ever experienced.

> *A person who has been seriously burned experiences extreme physiologic and psychosocial stresses at the same time.*

Burned people usually suffer because of accidents which, in different circumstances, might not have happened. This in itself is enough to evoke such feelings as anger, guilt, regret, resentment.

Consider the following statistics:[7] 70 per cent of burned persons cause the accident by their own actions; 20 per cent are burned because they are "innocent bystanders"; 4 per cent have a medical condition predisposing them to an accident; 4 per cent are victims of another person, and 1 per cent are rescue workers. A person in any of these categories can be expected to be *angry* about being burned. For example, people burned because of their own carelessness may well be angry at themselves; persons burned through the intentional or unintentional actions of others are likely to be angry at those viewed as "responsible" for the burning; people whose medical condition predisposes them to burns may be angry at more nebulous figures, e.g., "doctors," "scientists," God. Given this information, can we be surprised if burned people and their significant others are angry and behave in angry ways?

People affected by burn accidents may feel *guilty* and *ashamed*. "If only I had been more careful!" "I should not have left my child alone!" "I am being punished by God."

Likewise, burned people and their loved ones may be *afraid* of experiences such as death; disfigurement and its personal and social implications; pain and prolonged discomfort; and lengthy and costly treatment and rehabilitation. Wouldn't *you* be afraid if you found yourself severely and suddenly burned?

Burned people may feel *resentful*. "Why me? I have always been careful. I always anticipate potential danger and try to warn everyone of it. I do not deserve to suffer this way."

Additionally, burned people and their significant others have to cope with the stress of undergoing emergency treatment at a time when their physical and emotional resources are reduced. They have to adapt to unknown people, unfamiliar surroundings, and frightening, often painful procedures. It is not surprising then that such people may show behavioral signs of stress. (See Unit III.)

While factors such as these contribute to a patient's behavior, the patient is usually not aware of the dynamics underlying his or her behaviors or feelings. Knowledge of possible underlying emotions can help nurses to better understand emotional responses made by stressed people, even though the responses may be quite difficult to deal with, e.g., depression, anger, resentment, "contrariness." Excellent nurses know that a burned person and significant others are responding out of personal loss, pain and sorrow, and the nurse accepts this as a natural occurrence.

You would do well to review Chapter 1 to consider the nursing approach to a "whole" person; Unit III to rethink the effects of stress on an individual; and pp. 521–524 and p. 527, where the psychosocial impact of serious spinal injuries are discussed. (The psychosocial impact of burns is similar to that of disabling spinal injuries in that both involve multiple losses.) Review the relaxation exercises described in Chapter 7. Treatments, especially dressing changes, for a burned person are often extremely painful, and you may be able to help a burned person by teaching relaxation exercises to be done during these procedures. You are also referred to the chapters in Sorensen and Luckmann, *Basic Nursing: A Psychophysiologic Approach*, that consider the therapeutic nurse-patient relationship; nursing people who are grieving and those experiencing disturbances of body image. Persons who have been burned and their significant others are *stressed and grieving* and require the expert care and support of skilled nurses.

> *The most useful things a nurse can do for an emotionally upset person are to accept the person's behavior without judgment, to communicate genuine caring and empathetic understanding, and to encourage the person to express feelings – whatever they are – in words.*

Physical recovery from burns takes some time. So does psychosocial recovery. Dr. Hans

*This section was written by Margaret Helen Parkinson, R.N., M.N.

Steiner explains that "after all, if we're honest about it, most of us feel that we're essentially invulnerable. Then, if something happens to us, and particularly if something happens suddenly, as it does to burn victims, there's no rapid way to handle that feeling of having lost the sense of wholeness and invulnerability."[107]

A burned person is recovering from multiple losses. There are a number of schematic descriptions of typical responses to loss. Many are useful when used to help us understand. They are not useful if they replace specific assessment and care planning for individual patients. We briefly discuss a schema described by Steiner and Clark based on their research study of 35 people who had suffered burns over 7.5 to 90 per cent of their bodies.[117]

Stage 1. Physiologic Emergency. This stage occurs for 2 to 4 weeks postburn, during which time a patient struggles with an enormous variety of stresses. *Delirium* may occur, including hallucinations, delusions, confabulations, apathy, agitation, and withdrawal. *The cause of the delirium must be found.* Possible causes include: (a) physiologic causes, e.g., toxins, infection, anoxia, metabolic and electrolyte imbalances, cardiovascular insufficiency and immobility, (b) isolation from significant others physically and/or emotionally, (c) being surrounded by frightened, unsupportive health professionals and their assistants, and (d) sensory deprivation.

- ▶ Physiologic causes of delirium must be identified and treated.
- ▶ Supportive nonjudgmental nursing care must be offered continuously to the patient and significant others.
- ▶ Patient and significant others must be kept informed of what is happening and what is about to happen to them.
- ▶ Whenever patients and any of their significant others wish to express concerns and feelings they must be allowed and helped to do so. This kind of grieving — as with all kinds of grieving — is done at least in part by talking.

Stage 2. Psychologic Emergency. This stage occurs from about 2 to 8 weeks postburn. The possibility of death is probably past and the burned person now begins to contemplate living with a deformity. The person gradually becomes aware of losses and the possibility of facing months of treatment. Patients who are having difficulty accepting the changes that have occurred in their lives may become at times demanding, irritable, rebellious, and uncooperative. They may be emotionally labile, alternating between emotional highs and emotional lows. They may be anorexic, hypersensitive, and insomniac and may have "night terrors." Vague physical symptoms may develop.

The reaction of persons around them during this time is very important to the long-term outcome for patients. If health professionals, family and friends respond to the patient's "difficult" behavior with irritation and take personal offense, the patient is less likely to mourn satisfactorily than if all concerned can deal with the patient's irritating behavior with understanding and calmness.

> *It is important to remember that a patient's anger is more often an expression of personal grief and sorrow than a direct attack on another person.*

- ▶ Pain relief is important, as a patient may not have additional strength to tolerate pain.
- ▶ Brief crisis-oriented psychotherapeutic intervention may be helpful during this time. This may be offered by skilled psychosocial nurses or psychiatrists.
- ▶ Long-term, untiring supportive nursing care that emphasizes the patient's strengths and abilities is essential.

Stage 3. Social Emergency. This stage occurs from the time of discharge from a hospital until about 1 year postburn. During this time, patients are often worried about (a) physical limitations brought about by disability and (b) the reactions of others to their disfigurements. Continued support is essential for the patient and significant others. The most important support for burned people can come through the most intimate personal relationships in their lives. Both patients and their most significant others will probably need the ongoing support of a health professional until the difficult adjustment period is over.

The effects of disfigurement from burns must never be taken lightly. Burns are among the most severely disfiguring of all injuries. Severe, unpleasant changes in a person's appearance can precipitate serious psychiatric crises. People especially prone to psychiatric complications of burns include people with:

- ▶ Disfigurement of face and hands
- ▶ A history of previous psychiatric symptoms
- ▶ Limited or inadequate social support systems
- ▶ Extensive burns and disfigurement and residual disability

Psychiatric consultation and intervention may be helpful for some patients. This must never, however, substitute for the genuine empathetic and realistic support of an excellent nurse.

Choice of Living or Dying:[12] It has been noted that the most severely burned patient is usually alert and mentally competent during the first few hours following injury. Certain professionals feel that a patient has the right to know when the injuries are so severe that others with similar injuries have *not* been saved, and that the patient should make the decision as to whether aggressive therapy or ordinary care should be given. At the Los Angeles County-University of Southern California Medical Center, 24 cases were diagnosed during 1975 and 1976 as being without precedented survival. When given the information, only three burned persons chose heroic measures. The 21 who chose ordinary care became amazingly peaceful and gave their full attention to the things they wanted to get done before they died. Warmth and support are provided for all patients no matter what their decision; and the chaplain, nurse, physician and all members of the team do whatever they can to help the patient.

RECONSTRUCTIVE AND PLASTIC PROCEDURES

Persistent attention to preserving the range of motion and to splinting in functional positions are important in preventing significant contractures. Much less effort and expense are required to prevent contractures than to correct them surgically.

Reconstructive surgery may be either functional or cosmetic. Plastic surgery is generally one of the following procedures:

▶*Z-plasty*. This procedure elongates the line of contracture and distributes the tension in the scar. Adjacent soft tissue must be sufficiently pliable. If the underlying muscle and tendon are contracted, prolonged immobilization in extension in a plaster cast may be necessary.

▶*Thick, split-thickness skin grafts*. If Z-plasty is not applicable, thick, split-thickness grafts are probably best. These should be a thick as possible to prevent recurrent postoperative contracture. Physical therapy and splinting may be necessary in the extremities.

▶*Full-thickness free skin grafts*. These are used at times on the face and on the hands in small areas, e.g., resurfacing of the eyelids.

▶*Adjacent flaps and distant flaps*. These are occasionally used in reconstruction of the axilla and in coverage of exposed bone. Cosmetic surgery is done to restore destroyed parts such as ear, nose, mouth or eyebrows, or to remove disfiguring scars. A *pedicle flap* takes in the full thickness of the skin and subcutaneous fat. It is left attached to both the recipient and donor areas until a sufficient blood supply to the recipient site is established. This graft is used in areas where a free graft could not be used, and to restore lost features, contour, or bulk. These may be local flaps rotated to the wound from a near area or flaps may be brought from a more distant area in stages. A *sliding graft* is a single stage graft, in which the skin flap is rotated over the recipient area and sutured to it. The donor area may be covered with a split-thickness graft. Flap grafts are done in two stages, and pedicle flap grafts require a three-stage procedure.

The immobilization necessary for these extensive procedures is distressing for the patient, and the nurse must be ingenious in creating distractions or comfort devices. Of course, it is necessary to be alert to the condition of the graft, e.g., note color, signs of infection.

BIBLIOGRAPHY (Chapter 80)

1. Allyn, P.: Inhalation injuries. *Critical Care Quarterly,* 1:37, Dec. 1978.
2. American Burn Association. Where burns get special care. (List of Burn Centers). *Emergency Medicine,* 10:94, Oct. 1978.
3. Andreasen, N. J. C., and A. S. Norris: Long-term adjustment and adaptation mechanisms in severely burned adults. *in* Moos, R. H. (Ed.): *Coping with Physical Illness.* New York: Plenum Publishing Corporation, 1977.
4. Andreasen, N. J. C., A. S. Norris, and C. E. Hartford: Incidence of long-term psychiatric complications in severely burned adults. *Annals of Surgery,* 174:785, Nov. 1971.
5. Andersen, H. W.: An open wound is a whole patient. *Emergency Medicine,* 9:127, Nov. 1977.
6. Another chance for a severed foot. *Emergency Medicine,* 9:100, June 1977.
7. Archambeault-Jones, C., and I. Feller: Burn nursing is nursing. *Critical Care Quarterly,* 1:77, Dec. 1978.
8. Archambeault-Jones, C. and I. Feller: *Procedures for Nursing the Burned Patient.* Ann Arbor, Mich.: The National Institute for Burn Medicine, 1975.
9. Artz, C. P.: Guide to assessment and management of burns. *Hospital Medicine,* 13:105, March 1977.
10. Artz, C. P., J. A. Moncrief, and B. A. Pruitt: *Burns—A Team Approach.* Philadelphia: W. B. Saunders Co., 1979.
11. Artz, C. P., M. S. Rittenbury, and D. R. Yarbrough, 3rd: An appraisal of allografts and xenografts as biological dressings for wounds and burns. *Annals of Surgery,* 175:934, June 1972.
12. Autonomy, authenticity, ethics and death. *Emergency Medicine,* 10:148, Feb. 1978.
13. Ballinger, W. F., R. B. Rutherford, and G. D. Zuidema: *The Management of Trauma,* 2nd Ed. Philadelphia: W. B. Saunders Co., 1973.
14. Beal, J. D., and J. E. Eckenhoff: *Intensive and Recovery Room Care.* New York: The Macmillan Company, 1969.
15. Bell, J. G.: Bitsy was so little. . . and her problems so big. *Nursing 77,* 7:34, June 1977.
16. Betadine — Yes and no. *Emergency Medicine,* 8:238, May 1976.
17. Blakemore, W. S., and W. T. Fitts, Jr. (Eds.): *Management of the Injured Patient.* New York: Harper and Row, 1969.
18. Bowden, M. L., and I. Feller: Family reaction to a severe burn. *American Journal of Nursing,* 73:317, Feb. 1973.
19. Burke, J. F.: Use of antibiotics in management of the burn patient. Part II. *Journal of Surgical Practice,* 7(3):12, May–June 1978.
20. Burke, J. F., et al.: Isolated environment for burns. *Annals of Surgery,* 186(3):376, Sept. 1977.

21. Burn update. *The Canadian Nurse,* Aug. 1977, pp. 24–25.
22. Calabretta, A. M.: The how and why of skin grafting. *Consultant,* 18:69, Jan. 1978.
22a. Campbell, L.: Special behavioral problems of the burned child. *American Journal of Nursing,* 76:220, Jan. 1976.
23. Castle, M.: Consultation: How to clean an infected wound. *Nursing 78,* 8:17, Aug. 1978.
24. Chang, L. F.: How to succeed with wet-to-dry dressings. *RN,* 42:63, Jan. 1979.
25. Chouinard, F., N. Foley, and K. Millar: Vigilant nursing care after reconstructive microsurgery. *Nursing 79,* 9:18, June 1979.
26. Christoferson, B. A., and M. L. Piercey: The role of the nurse practitioner in early management of thermal burns. *Nurse Practitioner,* 2:20, September-October 1976.
27. Clarke, A. M.: Burns in childhood. *World Journal Surgery,* 2:175, Mar. 1978.
28. Cosman, B.: Management of the patient with burns. Part 1. Differentiating between serious and nonserious burns and their initial care. *Hospital Medicine.* 7:55, Oct. 1971.
29. Cosman, B.: Management of the patient with burns. Part 2. Treatment and coverage of burn wounds, and subsequent rehabilitation of the patient. *Hospital Medicine,*7:29, Oct. 1971.
30. Crews, E. R.: *A Practical Manual for the Treatment of Burns.* Springfield, Ill.: Charles C Thomas, Publisher, 1964.
30a. Curreri, P. W., D. Richmond, J. A. Marvin, et al.: Dietary requirements of patients with major burns. *Journal of American Dietetic Association,* 65:415, 1974.
31. Cuzzell, J.: Guidelines for the development of nursing goals for the patient with a major burn. *Cutis,* 22:509, Oct. 1978.
32. Delayed closure, less infection. *Emergency Medicine,* 9:77, Aug. 1977.
33. Delayed reactions to celestial flashes. *Emergency Medicine,* 11:63, May 15, 1979.
34. Dimmick, A. R.: Debridement, mechanical and biochemical. *Cutis,* 22:480, Oct. 1978.
35. Dimmick, A. R.: Be aggressive with burns. *Emergency Medicine,* 6:217, Apr. 1974.
36. Douglas, D. M.: *Wound Healing.* Baltimore: Williams and Wilkins Co., 1963.
37. Do we need a burn severity grading system? *The Journal of Trauma,* 13(3):376, Mar. 1977.
38. Emig, E., and J. R. Lloyd: How to get burned children home sooner. *RN,* 40:37, July 1977.
39. Epstein, E. H. (Ed.): *Skin Surgery,* 3rd Ed. Springfield, Ill.: Charles C Thomas, 1970.
40. Falkner, B., et al.: Hypertension in children with burns. *Journal of Trauma,* 18(3):213, Mar. 1978.
41. Faster clean up for burns. *Emergency Medicine,* 10:63, May 1978.
42. Feller, I., and C. Archambeault-Jones: *Nursing the Burned Patient.* Ann Arbor, Mich.: The National Institute for Burn Medicine, 1973.
43. Feller, I., and C. Archambeault-Jones: *Teaching Basic Burn Care.* Ann Arbor, Mich.: The National Institute for Burn Medicine, 1975.
44. Finn, K. L: Rebuilding skin. Part 1: A successful graft may be up to you. *RN,* 40:41, Oct. 1977.
45. Finn, K. L.: Rebuilding skin. Part 2: Meeting the challenges of flap care. *RN,* 40:47, Nov. 1977.
46. Fitzgerald, R. T.: Prehospital care of burned patients. *Critical Care Quarterly,* 1:13, Dec. 1978.
47. Fortier, R. R.: Nutrition and the burn patient. *Canadian Nurse.,* p. 30, Aug. 1977.
48. Fromm, D.: Stress ulcer, *Hospital Medicine,* 14:58, Nov. 78.
49. Furste, W., and A. Aguirre: Preventing tetanus. *American Journal of Nursing,* 78:834, May 1978.
50. Garrison, A. F., and C. Jelenko, 3rd: Management of the acute burn patient. *Postgraduate Medicine,* 54:43, Aug. 1973.
51. Gaul, A. L., and G. B. Hart: Baromedical nursing combines critical, acute, chronic care. *AORN Journal,* 21:1038, May 1975.
52. Graham, W. P., 3rd, et al.: Chain saw injuries. *American Family Physician,* 16:89, Dec. 1977.
53. Graham, W. P. 3rd, et al.: Injuries from rotary power lawnmowers. *American Family Physician,* 13:75, May 1976.
54. Hartford, C. E.: The early treatment of burns. *Nursing Clinics of North America,* 8:447, Sept. 1973.
55. Hayter, J.: Emergency nursing care of the burned patient. *Nursing Clinics of North America,* 13:223, June 1978.
56. Hersperger, J. A., and L. M. Dahl: Electrical and chemical injuries. *Critical Care Quarterly,* 1:43, Dec. 1978.
57. Horowitz, J. H.: Pulmonary complications in the burn patient. *Cutis,* 22:48, Oct. 1978.
58. Hughes, J. H., E. H. Freimer, and J. K. Mantis: Tetanus. *American Family Physician,* 13:76, March 1976.
59. Hummel, R. P., H. C. MacMillan, and W. A. Altemeier: Topical and systemic antibacterial agents in the treatment of burns. *Annals of Surgery,* 172:370, Sept. 1970.
60. Iskrant, A. P., and P. V. Joliet: *Accidents and Homicide.* Cambridge: Harvard University Press, 1968.
61. Isler, C.: Don't act thunderstruck: Save victims of lightening: *RN,* 39:37, Aug. 1976.
62. Jackson, D. M.: Burns as a special problem in trauma. *Journal of Trauma,* 10:991, Nov. 1970.
63. Jacoby, F. G.: Current nursing care of the burned patient. A review. *Nursing Clinics of North America,* 5:563, Dec. 1970.
64. Jacoby, F. G.: *Nursing Care of the Patient with Burns.* St Louis: C. V. Mosby Co., 1976.
65. Jacoby, F. G.: Individualized burn wound dressing. *Nursing 77,* 7:62, June 1977.
66. Jelenko, C. III, et al.: Respiratory problems complicating burn injury: Recognition, assessment and treatment. *Nursing Digest,* 5:35, Spring 1977.
67. Jones, C. A., and I. Feller: Burns, what to do during the first crucial hours. *Nursing 77,* 7:22, Mar. 1977.
68. Jones, C. A., and I. Feller: Burns: Avoiding and coping with complications before and after grafting. *Nursing 77,* 7:72, Nov., 1977.
69. Jones, C. A., and I. Feller: Burns: The home stretch. Rehabilitation. *Nursing 77,* 7:54, Dec. 1977.
70. Jones, C. A., and I. Feller: Caring for burned eyes and ears. (From *Nursing the Burned Patient). Nursing 76,* Feb. 76.
71. Jones, C. A., and K. E. Richards: Burns: Fluids resuscitate. In *Nursing Skillbook: Monitoring Fluid and Electrolytes Precisely.* Nursing 78 Books, Horsham, Penn.: Intermed Communications, Inc. 1978.
72. Kenner, C.: Patients with thermal injuries. *In* Beyers, M., and S. Dudas: *Clinical Practice of Medical-Surgical Nursing.* Boston: Little, Brown and Company, 1977.
73. Krizek, T. J., et al.: Surgical Decompression of the Burned Extremity. *Cutis,* 22:457, Oct. 1978.
74. Krupp, N. E.: Psychiatric implications of chronic and crippling illness. *Psychosomatics,* 9:109, March–April 1968.

75. Larsen, G. K., and C. W. Linder: Caring for simple cuts. *Emergency Medicine,* 10:206, Sept. 1978.
76. Leavitt, M.: Andy was a fighter — in more ways than one. *Nursing 79,* 9:64, Apr. 1979.
77. Levine, M. S., and E. P. Radford: Fire victims: Medical outcomes and demographic characteristics. *American Journal of Public Health,* 67:1077 Nov. 1977.
78. Lewis, S. R., and J. B. Lynch, (eds.): *Symposium on the Treatment of Burns,* St. Louis: C. V. Mosby Co., 1973.
79. Lloyd, J. R., and K. Imamoglu: Thermal injuries. *In* Walt, A. J., and R. F. Wilson: *Management of Trauma: Pitfalls and Practice.* Philadelphia: Lea and Febiger, 1975.
80. Lung, R. J., et al.: Recognizing burn injuries as child abuse. *American Family Physician,* 15:134, Apr. 1977.
81. Luterman, A.: Burn injuries. Initial evaluation and treatment. *Cutis,* 22:437, Oct. 1978.
82. Lynch, J. B.: Thermal burns. *In* Grabb, W., and J. Smith (Eds.): *Plastic Surgery.* Boston: Little, Brown and Co., 1973.
83. MacMillan, B. G.: Primary excision. *Cutis,* 22:464, Oct. 1978.
84. Marvin, J.: Acute care of the burn patient. *Critical Care Quarterly,* 1:25, Dec. 1978.
85. McGuire, A.: Prevention of burns. *Critical Care Quarterly,* 1:1, Dec. 1978.
86. Mieszala, P: Postburn psychological adaptation: An overview. *Critical Care Quarterly,* 1:93, Dec. 1978.
87. Mieszala, P., and R. Hartmann: Burn prevention group teaching for victims. *Supervisor Nurse,* 7:66, June 1976.
88. Miller, S. F.: Outpatient management of minor burns. *American Family Physician,* 16:267, Nov. 1977.
89. Mills, W. J., Jr.: Out in the cold. *Emergency Medicine,* 11:211, Mar. 1979.
90. Minckley, B.: Expert nursing care for burned patients. *American Journal of Nursing,* 70:1888, Sept. 1970.
91. Monafo, W. W.: *The Treatment of Burns, Principles and Practice.* St. Louis: Warren H. Green, Inc., 1971.
92. Moncrief, J. A.: Topical therapy for control of bacteria in the burn wound. *World Journal of Surgery,* 2:151, Mar. 1978.
93. Nealon, T. V.: *Fundamental Skills in Surgery.* Philadelphia: W. B. Saunders Co., 1971.
94. Ninman, C., and P. Shoemaker: Human amniotic membranes for burns. *American Journal of Nursing,* 75:1468, Sept. 1975.
95. O'Malley, P., et al.: Septic shock in a burn patient. *Nursing 76,* 6:39, Jan. 1976.
96. Peacock, E. E., Jr., and W. Van Winkle, Jr.: *Wound Repair,* 2nd Ed. Philadelphia: W. B. Saunders Co., 1976.
97. Pietsch, J., and J. L. Meakins: Complications of providone-iodine absorption in topically treated burn patients. *Lancet,* 1:280, Feb. 1976.
98. Pruitt, B. A., Jr., et al.: Curling's ulcer: A clinical study of 323 cases. *Annals of Surgery,* 72:525, Oct. 1970.
99. Pruitt, B. A., Jr., et al.: Progressive pulmonary insufficiency and other pulmonary complications of thermal injury. *Journal of Trauma,* 15:369, 1975.
100. Psychic survival after the burn. *Emergency Medicine,* 10:197, Jan. 1978.
101. Quinn, E. L., et al.: Pseudomonas infections. *American Family Physician,* 14:84, Nov. 1976.
102. Rinear, C., and E. Rinar: Emergency: On the spot care for aspiration, burns and poisoning. *Nursing 75,* 5:43, Apr. 1975.
103. Roffa, J., and D. D. Trunkey: Myocardial depression in acute thermal injury. *Journal of Trauma,* 18:(2):90, Feb. 1978.
104. Rogenes, P. R., and J. A. Moyland: Restoring fluid balance in the patient with severe burns. *American Journal of Nursing,* 76:1952, Dec. 1976.
105. Rosello, R. H., and M. L. Fogel: Emotional support. *Psychosomatics,* May–June, 1970.
106. Rosenthal, A.: Pulmonary problems associated with burn injury. *Hospital Medicine,* 13:108, Feb. 1977.
107. Rouse, R. G., and A. Dimick: The treatment of electrical injury compared to burn injury. A review of pathophysiology and comparison of patient management protocols. *Journal of Trauma,* 18:43, Jan. 1978.
108. Rudowski, W.: *Burn Therapy and Research.* Baltimore: Johns Hopkins University Press, 1976.
109. Ryan, A. J.: Traumatic injuries: Office treatment of puncture wounds. *Postgraduate Medicine,* 60:165, Aug. 1976.
110. Sato, R. M., et al.: Early wound excision and closure of the burn wound. *Critical Care Quarterly,* 1:51, Dec. 1978.
111. Scan for a scorched lung. *Emergency Medicine,* 11:87, June 1979.
112. Schuck, J. M., and T. L. Wachtel: Burned, but not too badly. *Emergency Medicine,* 9:24, Aug. 1977.
113. Schumann, L., and S. Gaston: Commonsense guide to topical burn therapy. *Nursing 79,* 9:34, Mar. 1979.
114. Skin puncture. . . bone disease. *Emergency Medicine,* 9:187, May 1977.
115. Stahl, W. M.: The superficial burn and beyond. *Emergency Medicine,* 9:113, Nov. 1977.
116. Stein, J. M., and E. D. Stein: Safe transfer of civilian burn casualties. *JAMA,* 238:(6):489, Aug. 1977.
117. Steiner, H., and W. R. Clark, Jr.: Psychiatric complications of burned adults: A classification. *The Journal of Trauma,* 17:134, Feb. 1977.
118. Stinson, V.: Porcine skin dressing for burns. *American Journal of Nursing,* 74:11, Jan. 1974.
119. Stoddard, J. E.: Rehabilitation of the burn-injured patient. *Critical Care Quarterly,* 1:63, Dec. 1978.
120. Talabere, L., and Graves, P.: A tool for assessing families of burned children. *American Journal of Nursing,* 76:225, Feb. 1976.
121. Wagner, D. K.: Trauma rounds. Problem: A puncture wound of the axilla. *Emergency Medicine,* 11:189, Jan. 1979.
122. Wagner, D. K.: Trauma rounds. Problem: windshield injury with facial cut. *Emergency Medicine,* 10:226, Sept. 1978.
123. Wagner, M. M.: Emergency care of the burned patient. *American Journal of Nursing,* 77:1788, Nov. 1977.
124. When trauma tatoos. *Emergency Medicine,* 9:181, May 1977.
125. White, C. E.: Looking beyond the obvious. *Emergency Medicine,* 10:58, Nov. 1978.
126. Wiley, L. (Ed.): Realistic goals don't mean failure. *Nursing 79,* 9:55, May 1979.
127. Wound care: An amniotic alternative. *Emergency Medicine,* 10:177, Sept. 1978.
128. Yarborough, M. F.: Care of the burn wound. *Cutis,* 22:447, Oct. 1978.
129. Yarrington, C. T., Jr.: Managing soft tissue injuries. *American Family Physician,* 16:109, Oct. 1977.
130. Zawacki, B., et al.: Multifactorial prohibit analysis of mortality in burned patients. *Annals of Surgery,* 189:1, Jan. 1979.

CHAPTER 81

DISORDERS OF THE BREAST

by Rosemary Pittman, M.S., C.R.N., F.N.P., and Karen Creason Sorensen, R.N., M.N.

INTRODUCTION

For both men and women the breasts are body areas highly invested with emotional feelings. Breast size is commonly viewed in terms of masculinity, femininity and attractiveness. Persons who are uncomfortable about the size of their breasts may feel distressed. Breasts are erogenous zones (responsive to sexual stimuli) and, as such, are usually considered to be private body parts. Many people are reluctant to have their breasts touched by others; some are unable to comfortably touch their own breasts. Thus, it is not surprising that some individuals hesitate before seeking or performing breast examinations. It is not uncommon for some individuals to also be uncomfortable in talking with others about breasts. All of these factors make it difficult to get people to develop habits of regular breast examinations. Nurses are frequently in situations where they can teach others about the importance of the early detection of breast disorders and the technique of performing breast self-examination (BSE).

Some people do not seek professional advice even when they discover something unusual about their breasts. The reasons for such delays are no doubt varied and compounded and may include factors such as: (a) attempts to deny the presence of the abnormality; (b) lack of education about breast disorders, their recognition and treatment; (c) fear of mutilating surgery and its associated changes in body image and possible related changes in relationships with significant others, e.g., one's sexual partner; and/or (d) reluctance to submit to diagnostic examinations and procedures.

> *It is vital that individuals perform* regular *breast self-examinations and that those who identify abnormal breast changes* promptly *seek professional assessment. Early diagnosis of cancer is important. Patients with the smallest cancers and the least spread to the lymph nodes have the best prognosis.*

A substantial number of breast abnormalities are not cancer. Table 81–1 summarizes the most frequent causes of breast masses for three age groups, ranked in order of frequency.

Most cancers of the breast are first discovered by the patient during self-examination. While most disorders of the breast are benign, they nonetheless generate great concern. Most women experience some kind of breast disorder at some time in their lives. Breast cancer is a concern of most women because it is extremely common and serious. About 1 out of 14 women will at some time in life develop breast cancer. (Carcinoma arising in the male breast is rare.) In

TABLE 81–1. MOST FREQUENT CAUSES OF BREAST MASSES FOR THREE AGE GROUPS, RANKED IN ORDER OF FREQUENCY

Under 35 Years
1. Fibrocystic disease (masses may be multifocal and bilateral)
2. Fibroadenoma (solitary benign tumor)
3. Mastitis (often during pregnancy or nursing, associated with pain and systemic signs)
4. Carcinoma (infrequent in this group)
5. Traumatic fat necrosis (rare; history of trauma in about 50 per cent of cases)

Between 35 and 50 Years
1. Fibrocystic disease
2. Carcinoma (usually invasive scirrhous type)
3. Fibroadenoma
4. Mastitis
5. Traumatic fat necrosis (rare)
6. Papilloma (rare as cause of palpable mass)

Over 50 Years
1. Carcinoma
2. Fibrocystic disease
3. Traumatic fat necrosis
4. Mastitis (rare in this group)

From this list it will be seen that, overall, the two most important entities are carcinoma and fibrocystic disease.

From Robbins, S. L., and M. Angell: *Basic Pathology*, 2nd ed. Philadelphia: W. B. Saunders Co., 1976, p. 582.

It is a truism of medicine that the availability of many different treatments for a given condition reflects the inadequacy of any single modality. Such is the case in breast cancer at the present time.[109]

the United States, cancer of the breast kills more women than any other cancer each year.

The skilled health professional keeps in mind that the identification and treatment of disorders of the breast involves psychosocial as well as physiologic factors.

A study[71] in Australia attempted to determine psychosocial factors affecting why only one-eighth of women regularly examine their breasts and more than one-fourth of women with breast symptoms delay longer than 3 months in seeking treatment. In the study, persons who performed regular breast self-examination (BSE) tended to not use denial and reaction formation as defense mechanisms as often as persons who did not practice BSE. Also, performers of BSE tended to more often discuss breast symptoms and breast loss with their sexual partners. Women not doing BSE seemed more likely to have a malignant tumor. Delay in seeking treatment was determined by unconscious psychologic processes, including the use of the ego-defenses of denial and suppression, nonverbal anxiety, presence of depression reported verbally, and the non-use of defenses of intellectualization and isolation. These researchers suggest that women presenting with a bland, indifferent attitude towards breast examination and breast symptoms, and women who show nonverbal signs of anxiety and are prone to depression might be considered as a high risk group. since they do not do breast screening. It is among women with these characteristics that the longest delay in seeking treatment occurred.

Breast size and shape may be important factors in an individual's body image and self-concept. These factors may also contribute to the way in which the individual is perceived by others. Hence, cosmetic surgical procedures on the breast (e.g., augmentation mammoplasty) are sought by some persons wishing to alter their appearance — to increase their attractiveness as perceived by themselves or others.

Some breast surgeries performed to treat breast cancer are highly disfiguring, e.g., radical mastectomy. This disfigurement, coupled with the fear of having a possibly terminal disease, deals severe blows to the patient and her significant others. The excellent nurse knows that caring for people who are experiencing such extreme stresses involves consideration of emotional, social, intellectual, and physical factors. (See Chapter 1.) Currently, less extensive surgical procedures may be performed than were formerly. Also, new surgical techniques for rebuilding breasts or creating new nipples are becoming more widely available. Breast reconstruction helps some women adjust to mastectomy more easily.

The detection and treatment of breast cancer are highly important activities for health professionals — and, they are activities surrounded by controversy. Current controversies involve the etiology of breast cancer, and the question of whether or not to use mammography as a routine screening device for asymptomatic women under age 50. Other controversies involve the selection of patients for the various therapeutic modalities available. The four major methods of treatment are: surgery, radiotherapy, endocrine manipulation, and chemoimmunotherapy with cytotoxic agents. Nurses often find themselves in a position of trying to help lead patients through these controversial mazes and trying to help them make sense out of conflicting opinions, so that a path of action can be determined.

The Nurse's Responsibility in Breast Cancer Detection

Cancer of the breast is a major concern to women and health professionals. Breast self-examination can be taught to all women at some time during their stay in the hospital, as well as to individuals in other settings, e.g., home and clinic visits. Teaching needs frequent reinforcement for breast self-examination to become a monthly, routine pattern with the individual. After a suspicious lump is detected, a woman may still delay going to a doctor. Women who are upset or depressed or who have serious problems may neglect medical attention for various reasons. Increasing attention must be given to the routine inclusion of breast examination by health professionals in their contacts with patients. High-risk individuals should be especially attentive to the possibility of cancer. Since at the present time, getting the patient under care at the earliest possible time offers the best chance of cure, every avenue should be used to insure regular breast examination, both self-examination and professional examination.

ANATOMY AND PHYSIOLOGY

The *breast* is a modified sebaceous gland, an appendage of the skin. The *mammary gland* extends vertically from the 2nd to the 6th rib and horizontally from the sternum to the midaxillary line. It lies entirely within the superficial fascia of the anterior chest wall. The largest part of the breast rests on the fascia of the pectoralis major fascia and the rest on the fascia of the serratus anterior. The nonlactating breast weighs about 150 to 250 gm., and the lactating breast weight may be between 400 and 500 gm.

The mammary gland is made up of 12 to 20 lobes subdivided into *lobules* and these in turn are composed of *acini*. The lobes are arranged like the spokes of a wheel around the *nipple*. Each lobe is drained by a *duct*, 12 to 20 of which open on the nipple. Each duct opens independently of each other on the surface of the nipple and has a dilated ampulla just before its opening (Fig. 81–1).

The breast is fixed to the overlying skin and underlying pectoral fascia with fibrous bands (*Cooper's ligaments*). A fascial cleft on the undersurface of the breast allows for mobility of the breast.

The nipple is located in the 4th intercostal space. Its base is surrounded by a circular pigmented area called the *areola*. Pigmentation at any age is increased by the administration of estrogen. The *areolar epithelium* contains some small hairs and three types of glands — *sebaceous glands, sweat glands* and *accessory mammary glands*. The sebaceous glands (*Montgomery's glands*) enlarge during pregnancy and lactation to lubricate the nipple.

The *parenchyma* of the breast consists of the ductular, lobular, and acinar epithelial structures. The *stroma* of the breast is made up of fibrous and fatty tissue. The central and upper portion is mostly glandular and the periphery mostly fatty.

The large amount of glandular tissue in the upper outer quadrant probably accounts for more cancer occurring in that area.

The two main sources of *blood supply* to the breast are the lateral mammary artery and the lateral thoracic artery. These arteries form an extensive network of anastomoses over the breast. The main veins follow the arterial pattern. The veins are a key to the lymphatic pathways which, in general, follow the pathways of the veins.

The superficial veins over the breast are often dilated over an area which contains disease. Tumors, malignant or benign, need an increased blood supply, and the prominent superficial veins are indicative of the need.

The *lymph drainage* of the breast consists of three parts: (1) cutaneous or superficial; (2) areolar; and (3) glandular or deep. Figure 81–2 shows the principal routes of lymphatic drainage from the breast.

The *nerve supply* is derived from the anterior and lateral branches of the 4th to 6th intercostal nerves.

There are three types of physiologic changes affecting the breast — those related to growth and development, to the menstrual cycle, and to pregnancy and lactation.

Estrogen and *progesterone* act synergistically with the pituitary growth hormones, prolactin and corticotropin, to produce the development and function of the mammary gland. Estrogens are responsible for the growth of the mammary gland and of the periductal

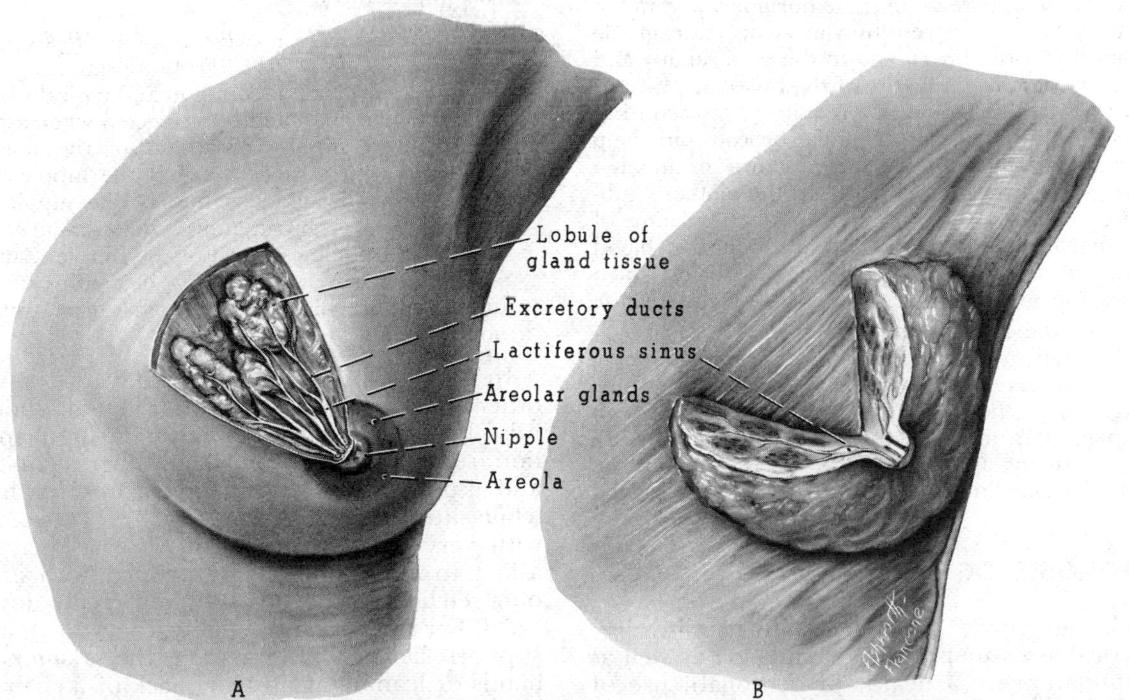

Figure 81–1. The female breast. **A,** The skin has been partly removed to show the underlying structures. **B,** A section has been removed to show the internal structures in relation to the muscles. (From Jacob, S. W., C. A. Francone, and W. J. Lossow: *Structure and Function in Man,* 4th ed. 1978, p. 579.)

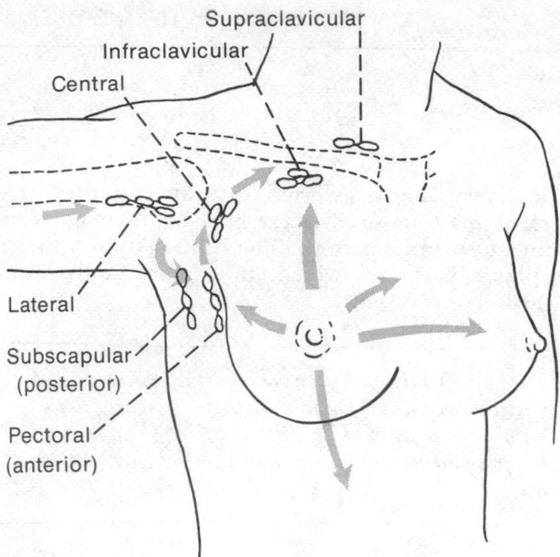

Figure 81–2. Principal routes of lymphatic drainage from the breast. Central axillary nodes are located high in the axilla, close to the ribs. Into these nodes drains lymph from three other groups of lymph nodes: the pectoral (anterior); the subscapular (posterior), and lateral groups. Lymph drains from the central axillary nodes to the infraclavicular and supraclavicular nodes. (Adapted from Bates, B.: *A Guide to Physical Examination.* Philadelphia: J. B. Lippincott Co., 1974, p. 147.)

stroma, whereas progesterone promotes the development of the lobular and acinar structures.

In women with normal menstrual cycles, the cyclic secretion of estrogen and progesterone is responsible for the female breast structure. During *pregnancy* there is a high increase in these hormones and in the pituitary hormones, resulting in an increase in the vascularity of the breast and in the permeability and dilatation of the lymphatics of the breast.

With the termination of pregnancy, prolactin initiates lactation. Prolactin and corticotropin help maintain lactation, but the "letting down" of milk is a more complex response involving the mother's subjective response and the mechanical stimulation of suckling. Suckling causes release into the blood stream of the pituitary hormone, oxytocin, which causes the mammary acini to contract and release milk into the duct system.

After the *menopause*, the ovaries cease producing the cyclic secretion of estrogen and progesterone. Estrogens are then produced by the adrenals through stimulation from the anterior pituitary. There is a continuous involution of the breast with loss of the glandular elements and atrophy.

DIAGNOSIS OF BREAST LESIONS

The diagnosis of breast lesions may involve: physical assessment (self-examination as well as examination by a health professional); use of special radiographic techniques (e.g., mammography); laboratory studies; and biopsy (needle and open).

*Physical Assessment of Breasts**

Breast examination should be included in the *regular health checkup given by health professionals*. Annual examination by a qualified health professional is typically recommended. Some women (e.g., women with a family history of breast cancer) may be advised to seek a breast examination at least twice a year. *Breast self-examination (BSE)* should be performed on a regular monthly basis about one week after each menstrual period and on a regular monthly basis after the menopause. (BSE is discussed later.)

Technique of Examining the Female Breast.[14] The patient should be undressed to the waist. The examination begins with the patient sitting upright in a relaxed position with arms at her sides. The examiner looks at the breasts individually and in comparison with each other. Note the following:

- *Breast size and symmetry*. It is not unusual for there to be some difference in size. Look for abnormal *contours*.
- *Masses, dimpling or flattenings*. When a mass is suspected, watch for dimpling while gently compressing or moving the breast. Skin dimpling or flattening or deviation of the nipple suggests an underlying malignancy.
- *Skin color, thickening or edema, and venous patterns* (increased venous prominence). Blocked lymphatic drainage causes skin edema, manifested by thickened skin with enlarged pores. Such skin is sometimes called *pig skin* or *peau d'orange* (orange peel appearance).
- *Nipple size and shape, direction in which nipples point, rashes, ulcerations or discharge.* Long-standing simple nipple inversion is common and typically normal. Malignancy should be suspected when a previously erect nipple inverts. Also, the fibrosis associated with a cancer behind the nipple may cause the following: deviation of the nipple towards the cancer; broadening and flattening of the nipple, and pulling inward of the nipple. Cancer should be suspected with any dermatitis of the nipple and areola. Nipple discharge is usually nonmalignant in origin.

In order to bring out dimpling, retraction or other changes in contour, the woman should raise her hands above her head during inspection (see Fig. 81–5, *B* and *D*, and Figure 15–22) and also press her hands firmly against her hips while sitting down (see Fig. 15–23). The woman with very large or pendulous breasts may be asked to stand and bend forward with arms outstretched so the breasts hang freely downward. For comfort and stability, the woman may support herself by grasping the examiner's hands or leaning against the back of a chair or against a firm examining table.

*See also pp. 342–344 (Chapter 15).

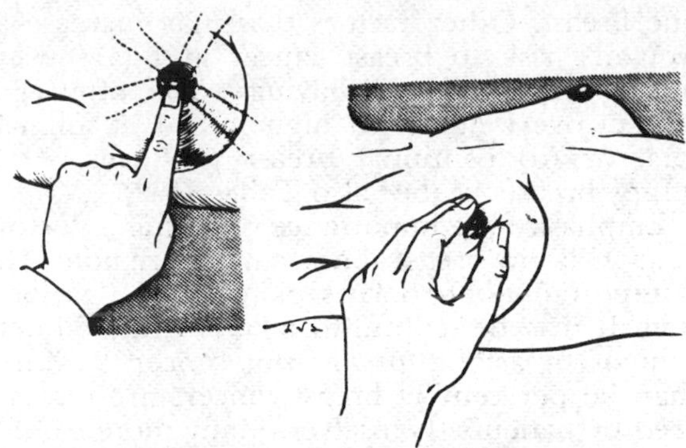

Figure 81–3. In patients with nipple discharge, the involved duct can usually be localized by fingertip pressure at successive points around the areola. (From Dunphy, J. E., and L. W. Way: *Current Surgical Diagnosis and Treatment*, 3rd ed. Los Altos, Calif.: Lange Medical Publications, 1977, p. 297.)

To palpate the breast, ask the patient to lie down on her back. A small pillow or folded towel placed under the side being examined may facilitate examination (except for very small breasts) by spreading the breast tissue across the chest more evenly. (See Fig. 81–5*G*) Using the pads of three fingers, compress the breast tissue gently against the breast wall in a rotary (circular) motion. Examine each breast systematically and completely, including the periphery, tail, and areola. It is helpful to develop and follow a systematic pattern of examination to ensure a thorough assessment, e.g., proceed in a clockwise pattern.

- ▶ *Palpate each nipple*, noting discharge and elasticity. Compress the nipple between your thumb and index finger. Note color of any discharge and try to determine its source by compressing the areola with your index finger placed in radial positions around the nipple. During compression, watch for discharge through one of the duct openings on the nipple's surface (Fig. 81–3).
- ▶ Try to *palpate regional lymph nodes* by compressing them against underlying structures. *Examine axillae.** The axillary, pectoral, infraclavicular, and subscapular nodes on both sides should be palpated. (*Note*: These should also be palpated by persons doing breast self-examinations.) Axillae are best examined with the patient sitting up, with the arms relaxed at the sides. (For location of nodes, refer to Fig. 81–4).

During examination of the breast the following *characteristics of the breast* should be remembered. Normally one may feel firm elasticity in the breast tissue of a young person. Lobules of glandular tissue may be present in breasts. In older breasts, the tissue may feel granular or stringy. A firm transverse ridge of compressed tissue may be present along the lower edge of the breast, especially in large breasts. This is a normal inframammary ridge. Premenstrual tenderness, fullness and nodularity are common.

Abnormalities should be noted, carefully described and properly reported. Nodules should be described according to location, size in centimeters, shape, consistency, mobility on underlying tissues, and tenderness. Also, note if the border is well defined.

Tumors due to cancer are more likely to be solitary and unilateral, while benign breast lesions are likely to be multiple and bilateral. Cancers tend to be irregular and poorly outlined. Tenderness is common in benign lesions but uncommon in cancers. Cysts are clear on transillumination but cancers are always opaque.

Mobility, attachment and fixation are terms used to describe certain physical signs.

Mobility indicates movement of a lesion within the breast (especially characteristic of fibroadenoma). Mobility is not typical of tumors due to cancer, but is a common symptom in benign disease.

Attachment means adherence to skin or nipple with skin dimpling, edema or nipple retraction or elevation.

Fixation is used to indicate inability to move the tumor on the chest wall. Nipple changes such as retraction, elevation, and ulceration are very uncommon in benign lesions. Although discharge is usually due to intraductal papilloma, it can be due to cancer.

Skin changes such as dimpling, color change, and ulceration are commonly due to cancer.

> *Breast cancer is typically indicated by a nontender, firm or hard lump with poorly delimited margins (caused by local infiltration). Slight skin or nipple retraction is an important finding. Minimal breast asymmetry may be present.*

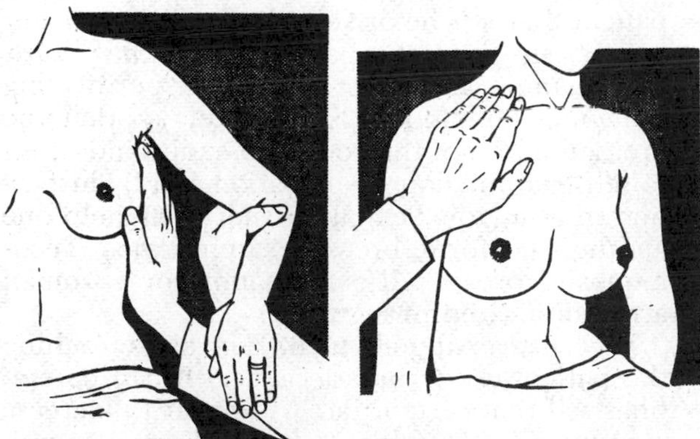

Figure 81–4. Palpation of axillary and supraclavicular regions for enlarged lymph nodes. Assessment of axillary nodes by palpation is not always accurate. Firm or hard nodes larger than 5 mm. in diameter must be assumed to contain metastases until proved otherwise. An advanced stage of breast cancer (at least stage III) is indicated by axillary nodes matted or fixed to skin or deep structures. (From Dunphy, J. E., and L. W. Way: *Current Surgical Diagnosis and Treatment*, 3rd ed. Los Altos, Calif.: Lange Medical Publications, 1977, p. 275.)

*See Figure 15–24, p. 344.

Technique of Examining the Male Breast. Men's breasts should also be examined by health professionals for abnormalities, and men should be taught the importance of breast self-examination (BSE) in detecting indications of cancer, even though cancer of the male breast is rare.

Examination of the male breast is less complex than examination of the female breast. In the male, *inspection* is made of the nipple and areola for swelling, ulceration, or nodules. The aerola is then *palpated* to identify any nodules. An assessment is made of breast size and symmetry. As with a female patient, the male's breasts are assessed individually as well as by comparison with each other. Obesity may cause soft fatty enlargement of breast tissue. Glandular enlargement produces a firm disc.[14]

Teaching Breast Self-Examination (BSE). Many situations may be used for teaching breast self-examination. For example, while performing breast examination on a patient, the health professional teaches the patient techniques of breast self-examination. It is desirable, as with the teaching of any procedure, to have the patient do a return demonstration and allow time for discussion of any questions.

> *Teaching BSE is one of the most important activities any health professional performs. Teaching a patient the skills of BSE can be a life-saving activity, because through regular BSE a patient may discover* early *a malignancy that can then be effectively treated.*

When teaching the BSE, emphasize to the patient that it is he or she who knows his or her body best. Thus the patient can identify *early* any changes in breast tissue, by performing *regular* examinations. Emphasize also that the breast is a part of the body that easily lends itself to self-examination by palpation and by inspection in a mirror. Sexual partners may help one another perform breast examinations. Techniques of breast self-examination for a woman are summarized in Figure 81–5.

Part of teaching about BSE involves teaching the patient about breast cancer. It can be emphasized that certain factors appear to increase a woman's *risk of breast cancer.* Women at risk need to be particularly careful to identify changes in their breasts, i.e., to perform regular BSE. Women believed to be at *highest risk* to breast cancer are those who: (a) are over 50 years of age; (b) have mothers or sisters who have had breast cancer, or (c) have had cancer in one breast. Other factors that may increase a woman's risk to breast cancer are: (a) never having had a child; (b) having a child after age 30; (c) overweight; (d) high intake of animal fats; or (d) continual breast problems, e.g., lumpy breasts.[114] (See also Table 81–2).

Emphasize the importance of seeing a doctor as soon as any breast abnormalities are noted. It is important not to delay seeking further evaluation. It may be helpful to mention that 80 per cent of breast lumps are not cancer.[114] More than 90 per cent of breast cancers are discovered by patients themselves. Many more would be detected earlier if regular breast self-examination were practiced. Individual's familiar with their own "normal" breast characteristics can easily note the early development of abnormalities. Nurses have many special opportunities to encourage and educate people concerning this important health maintenance procedure.

> *Regular breast self-examination (BSE) is essential.*

Radiographic Techniques

Various techniques have been tried experimentally in an effort to accurately and safely identify breast cancer in a preclinical stage. Among these techniques are: *ultrasonography, angiography, isotope scanning,* and *thermography*. Thermography has been extensively studied. However, none of these techniques has proven to be reliable enough to warrant general use. Continued study is necessary to determine the relative risks and benefits of using mammography to routinely screen asymptomatic women under age 50. It must be remembered that mammography by itself cannot replace physical examination for the detection of breast cancer or the need for surgical biopsy to establish a diagnosis.[37, 118]

Mammography.[18, 118] Mammograms are soft tissue radiologic examinations of the breast (Fig. 81–6). Two methods commonly used for obtaining mammograms are: (1) *ordinary film radiography* and (2) *xeroradiography (xeromammography)*. In the first method, a roentgen film is used. The second method, xerography, is a photographic process by which an aluminum plate with an electrically charged selenium layer is exposed to x-rays and the electrostatic image is transferred to paper by a special process. The areas on the plate change their charge when exposed to radiation. The exposed plate is then put into a processor, and the image is eventually transferred to a plastic-coated paper.

Both methods described above seem to have the same degree of diagnostic accuracy. Carcinoma can be identified with about 90 to 95 per cent accuracy, although false-positive and false-negative results sometimes occur. With mammography it is possible to identify some breast cancers as long as 2 years before they reach a size that can be detected by palpation. Mammography is the only reliable method of detecting breast cancer before it becomes palpable in the breast.

Mammography would appear to be ideal for use in the early detection of breast cancer through screening programs. There are prob-

lems, however, because the effects of exposure to radiation are known to be both cumulative and carcinogenic. Evidence has been presented suggesting that the amount of ionizing radiation delivered within a few years by use of annual

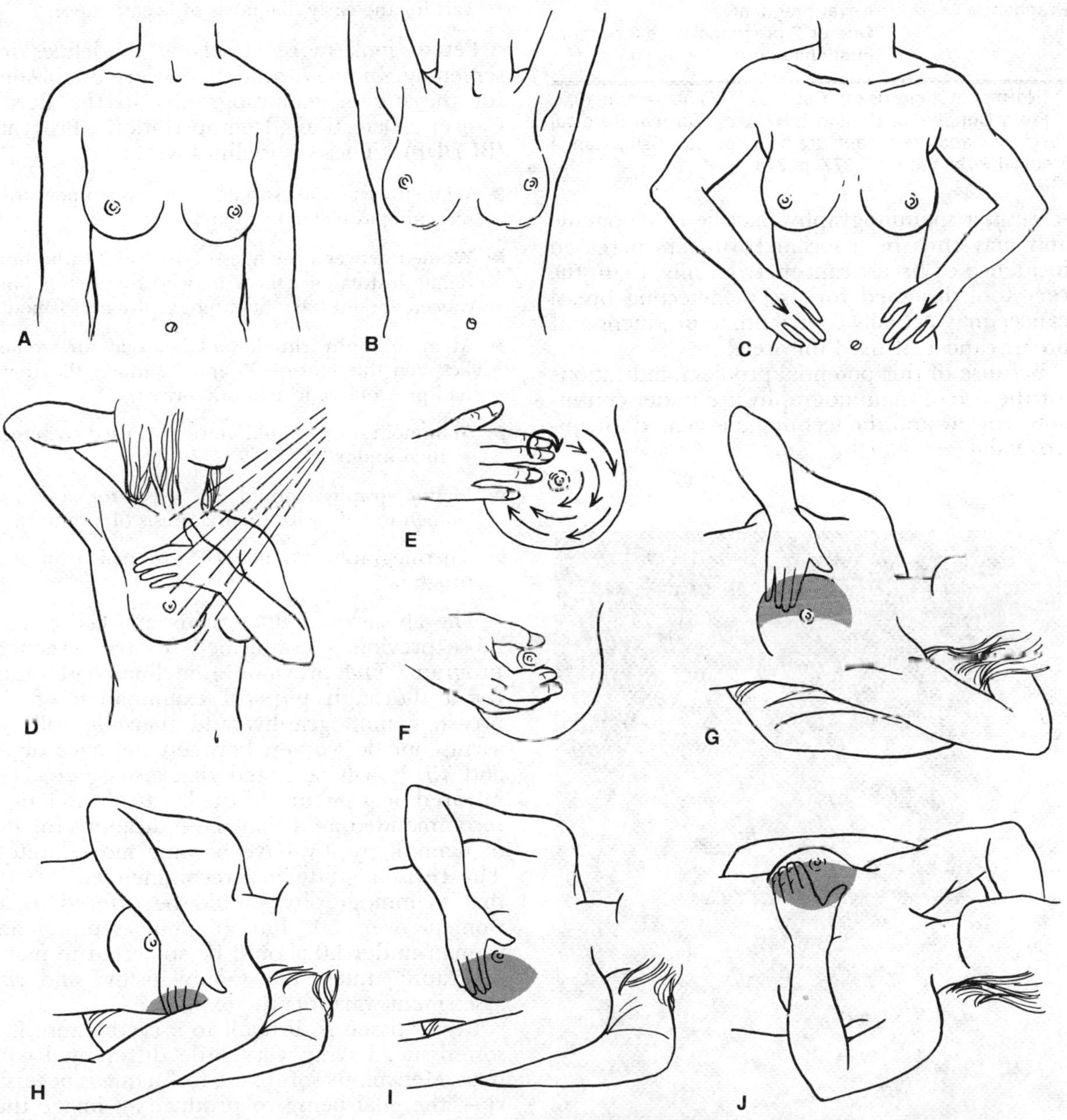

Figure 81–5. Self-examination of female breasts and axillae. Accomplished by observation and palpation. Various positions are assumed for *observation* while standing in front of a mirror. *A.* Arms relaxed at sides. Next, lean forward. *B.* Raise arms high overhead. Press arms behind head. *C.* Rest palms on hips and firmly press inward to flex chest muscles. *D.* In shower, examine breast contours. *E.* Method of palpating breast. With fingers flat, gently press in small circular motions around an imaginary clock face, i.e., begin at 12 o'clock. Move an inch at a time toward nipple. *F.* As a final step, squeeze nipple gently between thumb and index finger. Palpation of breast is accomplished while lying down. *G.* Position to examine inner breast. *H.* Position to examine axilla. *I.* Position to examine outer breast. *J.* Entire process is repeated for opposite breast and axilla. (See text for discussion of technique and observations.)

TABLE 81–2. RISK FACTORS ASSOCIATED WITH INCREASED INCIDENCE OF BREAST CANCER*

Race	Caucasian vs black or Oriental
Age	Over 50
Family history	Breast cancer in grandmother, aunt, mother, sister
Previous medical history	Endometrial cancer
	Mammary dysplasia
	Cancer in other breast
Menstrual history	Early menarche (under age 12)
	Late menopause (after age 50)
	Aggregate years of menstrual activity greater than 30
Marital history	Never married vs married
Pregnancy	Never pregnant
	One or 2 pregnancies vs 3 or more
	First child born after age 30

*Normal lifetime risk in Caucasian women = 1 in 13.
From Dunphy, J. E., and L. W. Way: *Current Surgical Diagnosis and Treatment*, 3rd ed. Los Altos, Calif.: Lange Medical Publications, 1977, p. 273.

screening mammography may be carcinogenic and may thus be associated with an increased incidence of breast cancer. Ironically, then, the very tool designed for use in detecting breast cancer may actually contribute to production of breast cancer, if used unwisely!

Because of this potential problem, indications for the use of mammography are under continuous review and the technique is viewed as controversial.

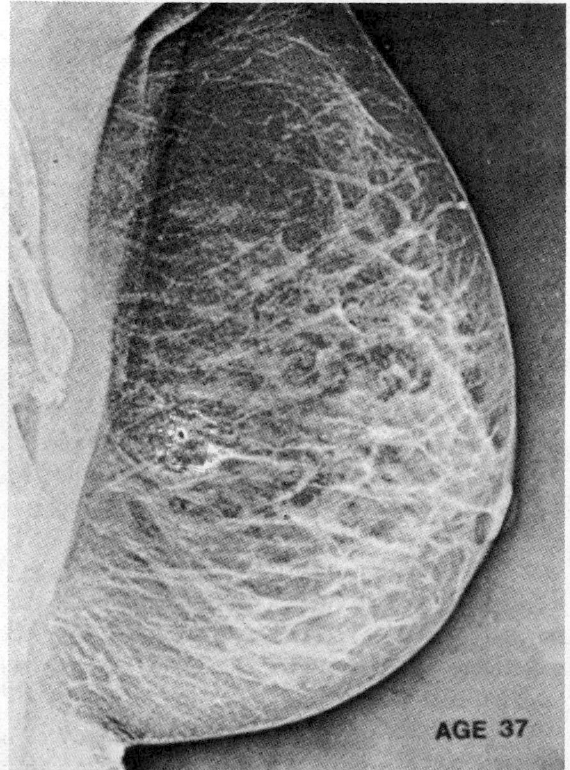

Figure 81–6. Normal mammogram shows breast composed primarily of fat. Note the characteristic trabeculated appearance. (From Prognostic patterns in breast cancer. *Emergency Medicine*, 9:59, Feb. 1977, p. 60.)

Current *general indications* for mammography are:[118]

- To assess the opposite breast when diagnosis of breast cancer is made, and periodically thereafter
- To assess questionable or ill-defined breast masses, nipple discharge, erosion, or retraction, skin dimpling or other suspicious change, or breast pain
- To search for occult breast cancer in women with metastatic disease from an unknown primary
- To screen asymptomatic women at regular intervals for the early diagnosis of breast cancer.

Let us look more closely at guidelines for screening. In 1977, guidelines were established for the use of mammography in the Breast Cancer Detection Demonstration Program (BCDDP).* These guidelines were:[29, 30]

- Women over 50 should have mammography screening available to them.
- Women between the ages of 40 and 49 who have family history of cancer or who themselves have cancer, should have mammography performed.
- Mammography should not be used for women between the ages of 35 and 39 unless they have had previous cancer in one breast.
- Mammography should never be used to screen women under 35.
- Mammography should be used for any age women to help with the diagnosis of a tumor.
- Thermography should be dropped from the program.

The above guidelines differ markedly from those previously established for the screening program. The previous guidelines had called for a thorough physical examination of the breast, mammography, and thermography of asymptomatic women between the ages of 35 and 75. It will be noted that *thermography* (an infrared heat picture of the breast) is no longer recommended, and that the indications for use of mammography have become more limited. The revised guidelines recommended:[29, 30] (a) that mammography should be offered to all women over 50, but (b) no asymptomatic woman under 50 should be subjected to mammography unless her family history and risk assessment warrants the exposure.

Breast tissue is difficult to x-ray because it is soft tissue, having very little differential contrast. Meticulous soft tissue technique is necessary — the goal being to produce an image that can be readily assessed by using the lowest possible rads. Accurate diagnosis is difficult because of the degree of density of breast tissue. Mammography is thus not generally useful in the diagnostic screening of younger women

*The BCDDP is jointly sponsored by the American Cancer Society and the National Cancer Institute in the United States.

because their breasts are too dense and would require high doses of radiation for adequate x-ray penetration.[37]

Xeromammography has an advantage over ordinary film (conventional) mammography, because xeromammography subjects the patient to a lower radiation exposure. With xeromammography, the skin dose is only 1.2 rads per exposure, compared with 8 rads per exposure for conventional mammography and about 2 rads for low-dose techniques.

As a nurse, it is not uncommon to be approached by a woman who asks, "Should I have mammography?" Think about how you would answer this important question. Women need to know not only the risk factors associated with the development of breast cancer (discussed later), but also the risks and benefits of procedures used on them for screening and detection purposes. Some *common questions and answers about mammography include:*[37]

- *How often should one have a mammogram?* When indicated, mammography is recommended every 6 to 12 months to fulfill its purpose in screening programs.
- *Cost?* Approximately $40 to $60 for a complete set of x-rays.
- *Time Involved?* About 45 to 60 minutes to complete the procedure. Results may be available within 1 to 21 days, depending upon the agency.
- *Is there pain?* Some discomfort may be experienced. The use of a balloon attachment to the equipment has reduced the pain associated with the pressure necessary to flatten the breast.
- *Where available?* Mammography is available at most health care centers.

Analysis of the 2-year results of a project screening asymptomatic women for breast cancer found that of 10,008 women examined and 490 breast biopsies, 97 were cancerous. Of these 97 cancerous lesions, 55 were *nonpalpable*. Thirty-six of the 97 were in women under 50 years of age. The incidence of axillary metastases was 7 per cent in the nonpalpable lesions. Sayler et al. conclude that *palpation is not a reliable method for finding early breast cancer and that women at high risk must be better defined and followed more closely.*[94]

Laboratory Studies

Some laboratory studies are being done in an attempt to find a practical way of detecting breast cancer in a preclinical stage in high-risk individuals. Such studies include: (a) determination of certain steroids in the urine, (b) sex chromatin status of the buccal mucosa; (c) determination of the estriol urinary excretion quotient and (d) studies of serum glycoproteins.

Monitoring of *carcinoembryonic antigen*[64] (CEA) seems to be a useful way of evaluating therapy and estimating prognosis in certain cancers, including breast cancer. CEA is a complex protein detectable in serum or plasma, urine, ascitic effusions, and cerebrospinal fluid. An elevation of CEA seems to be associated with tumor recurrence and progression, especially in the breast, gastrointestinal tract, ovaries, prostate, and bladder.

Biopsy[118]

Biopsy is an essential step in the diagnosis of breast cancer. No treatment should be undertaken without an unequivocal histologic diagnosis of cancer. About 30 per cent of lesions that are thought to be malignant by other examinations prove to be benign with biopsy. Likewise about 15 per cent of lesions thought to be benign on other examinations are found to be malignant on biopsy. Indications for breast biopsy include:

- A persistent mass
- A bloody nipple discharge
- An eczematoid nipple
- Positive mammogram

Some authorities recommend biopsy of the opposite breast when operable cancer is found in one breast.

Needle biopsy (aspiration cytology) is done by obtaining a small core of tissue via a needle (e.g., a Vim-Silverman needle). This procedure is usually done in a doctor's office for easily accessible lesions. *If a negative result is found on a needle biopsy an open biopsy should be done.*

Open biopsy is the widely favored procedure currently. It is done in an operating room with either general or local anesthesia. Only about 35 per cent of the people who require an open biopsy for a breast lesion are found to have a malignancy.

A *frozen section* is sometimes done as a way of taking an open biopsy. This involves taking an open biopsy while the patient is under general anesthesia. A frozen section examination is done while the patient and operating team wait for the result. If it is positive, an mastectomy is immediately done.

> *It is very important that the patient understand fully what is to happen before this kind of procedure is done. The patient does not know before surgery whether a mastectomy is to be done or not.*

BENIGN DISORDERS OF THE BREAST

Fibrocystic Disease. *Fibrocystic* disease is the most frequent lesion of the female breast. The exact cause of this disease remains unknown, although some evidence indicates a hormonal imbalance. Fibrocystic disease typically improves during pregnancy and lactation. The disease occurs during the reproductive years and disappears with the menopause. Nodularity, tenderness, and cysts may be present. The lesions may change in size and are much more labile than carcinomas or adenofibromas. Cysts are generally aspirated rather than surgically biopsied. Howver, if there is any question, a biopsy is done.

Adenofibroma. *Adenofibroma* is the third most common tumor of the breast, exceeded only by carcinoma and cystic disease. Adenofibroma is a disease of young women. These tumors are usually well outlined, rounded, discoid or lobulated, and may be soft but more often have a rubbery firmness. Relative movability of the adenoma in the breast tissues is one of its most distinctive characteristics. Excision is the only effective treatment.

Papilloma. *Intraductal papillomas* are neoplasms growing in the terminal portion of a duct (*solitary*) or throughout the duct system of a sector of the breast (*multiple*). Most are of the solitary type. Papillomas within the nipple itself are rare. With few exceptions, solitary intraductal papillomas are not precancerous lesions.

Intraductal papilloma is usually indicated by a serous, serosanguineous or bloody discharge from the nipple. Secretions from only one nipple may signify pathologic changes in that breast. Discharge may be tested for blood with a Hemocult. The usual cause is papilloma, which is typically benign, however, low-grade carcinomas can be present. Frequently, no tumor mass is palpable, although a small soft tumor in a central or periareolar portion of the breast is usually present. It is necessary to excise the lesion and have the tissues examined. Some doctors recommend doing this on a permanent paraffin section rather than on a frozen section, because of the difficulty in determining whether the lesion is benign or malignant.

Duct Ectasia (Comedomastitis). *Duct ectasia* or *comedomastitis* is a disease of the ducts in the subareolar zone. It is a disease of the aging breast and is most common in or near the menopause. It usually occurs in women who have had children and who have nursed them. The patient may have a thick, sticky nipple discharge, and burning pain, itching, and inflammation. Some doctors treat this conservatively at first; but if indicated, the major central ducts of the breast may be excised. There is no demonstrated association with carcinoma.

CARCINOMA OF THE BREAST*

> *Breast cancer claims the lives of more American women than cancer in any other body site. Breast cancer is the leading* cause of death *in women between ages 39 to 44.*[37] *Breast cancer is also the leading* cause of cancer deaths *in women between ages 35 to 74.*

In 1979 the estimated number of new breast cancer cases in the United States was 106,000. It was also estimated in that year that about 39,000 cancer deaths would occur from breast cancer in the United States. One in 14 women will acquire breast cancer at some time, and there has been no reduction in mortality over the last 30 years.

It is extremely important that breast cancer be detected in its early development, prior to metastases. Early detection improves treatment results, as we shall discuss. Also, it will become clear that early detection is difficult. It is best to identify breast cancer *before* they have become large enough to palpate.

Risk Factors. Nurses have a responsibility in finding individuals at high risk of developing breast cancer and of convincing them of the necessity for careful follow-up. Most breast cancers are found in women over age 40, and the incidence increases with age.

The overall group with *increased risk* of breast cancer includes women: over age 40; with fewer offspring or a late first childbirth (after age 30); who have not nursed; with an early menarche and prolonged menstrual history; with a negative history of artificial menopause[75]; with fibrocystic disease, lumps or thickening of the breasts; with nipple discharge or abnormality; who have had cancer of the uterus, colon, ovary, or contralateral breast; with a positive family history for breast cancer (especially in a mother or sister); who are obese and hypothyroid; Caucasian; living in the western world in highly developed countries and in the upper socioeconomic group; Jewish, or women of certain races and countries (incidence is highest in Denmark and lowest in Japan).

Exposure to radiation increases risk. Also, there seems to be an autosomal dominant inheritance pattern and women with mothers having other malignant neoplasms may be at higher risk.[66] Milk-rejection by nursing infants may be a sign of breast cancer in the lactating mother. It is inaccurate to assume that all breast masses in a nursing mother are due to the lactational process.[36]

It is difficult to identify women at risk for

*For a detailed discussion of cancer, refer to Unit IX.

breast cancer. As you will note, there are many factors believed to be associated with high risk. It has been pointed out that 80 per cent of all women are at high risk.[46]

Etiology. Clearly, the *cause of breast cancer* has not been definitely established. However, recent breakthroughs have occurred. The most reasonable current hypothesis is that an oncogenic RNA virus, possibly identical to the MMTV (mouse mammary tumor virus), initiates the tumor. Then tumor development is promoted by hormones over a long latent period. It is less clear whether genetic predisposition is necessary as a possible determinant of immune response or of hormonal imbalance.[87]

Possible dietary influences on the development of breast cancer are interesting. Growing evidence indicates that dietary fat promotes carcinogenesis because of its effect on hormone activity. Reducing dietary fats may protect against breast cancer by altering prolactin levels. Women in the United States have a breast cancer rate almost six times that of Japanese women. Apparently these two groups differ very little, except for the types of food they eat. The average woman in the continental United States consumes 300 per cent more fat than her Japanese counterpart. Some subpopulations within the United States (e.g., Mormons, Seventh Day Adventists) have a risk of breast cancer somewhat lower than the national average. This is probably because some of these groups are vegetarian and others encourage limited meat-eating, which reduces their fat intake. It has been proposed that a high ratio of prolactin to estrogen stimulates the growth of mammary tumor cells, whereas a low prolactin/estrogen ratio inhibits mammary tumor cell growth. Additionally, it is suggested that chronic high fat intake (which has been linked in humans to breast cancer), elevates serum prolactin levels, thereby raising the prolactin/estrogen ratio to promote the growth of mammary tumor cells.[50]

Description. Curiously, carcinoma is somewhat more common in the left breast than in the right. More than 90 per cent of breast cancers arise in the *ductal epithelium* and about 10 per cent in the mammary lobules. Both ductal and lobular cancers are divided into two categories: (1) those that have not penetrated the limiting basement membranes (*noninfiltrating*) and (2) those that have done so (*infiltrating*). Infiltrating duct carcinoma is the most common type of breast cancer. Breast cancers usually first appear as a solitary, painless mass in the breast. Differential diagnosis may be difficult. When first found, approximately two-thirds of breast cancers have already spread to axillary and other nodes. Approximately 25 per cent of breast cancers are inoperable at the time of discovery. This fact heavily influences the overall 5-year survival rate for breast cancer, making it about 50 per cent. Among those breast carcinomas small enough to allow identification of their areas of origin, about 50 per cent arise in the upper outer quadrant; 10 per cent in each of the remaining quadrants, and about 20 per cent in the central or subareolar region.[88]

Breast cancer is popularly believed to be a more aggressive disease among younger women than among those who are older. However, recent evidence refutes this idea and strongly suggests that breast cancer is more aggressive among older women.[4]

Metastases. *Metastases* from cancer of the breast may follow several different lymphatic pathways, depending upon the site of tumor origin within the breast. Patterns of nodal metastases through lymphatic drainage of the breast are: (a) *upper outer quadrant* to the axillary, infraclavicular, supraclavicular nodes, etc.; (b) *upper inner quadrant* to the intercostal and parasternal nodes, directly to parasternal nodes, and directly across mid-line to the opposite breast; and (c) *lower quadrants,* particularly inner aspect, through pectoralis major, external oblique and linea alba, to subperitoneal lymphatic plexus, followed by abdominal and pelvic spread.[67] (Refer to Fig. 81–2.)

Attiyeh has defined *axillary metastases* as "micro" and "macro." Micrometastases refers to nodes less than 2 mm. in diameter and macro as more than 2 mm. Patients with four or more nodes do poorly and may need to be treated with adjuvant therapy. Macrometastases at any level has a poor prognosis.[8]

Breast Cancer and Pregnancy. Since breast cancer most commonly occurs in women over age 40, it is not usual for breast cancer and pregnancy to occur together. When they do, however, there are some additional factors to consider. These include:

1. The advisability of *termination of pregnancy.*[118] Although there is some disagreement among authorities about this issue, current evidence seems to support advising abortion if breast cancer occurs in the first trimester but not if it occurs during later stages of the pregnancy. The rationale for this is that high levels of estrogen produced by the placenta would be harmful to the women with an estrogen-dependent tumor. The actual decision, of course, is made by the patient.
2. The advisability of *future pregnancies*[118] for women who have had breast cancer. Although this question is controversial also, the tendency at the present time is to advise against pregnancy until a woman has been free of cancer for 10 years.

Pregnant women, of course, should have the same kinds of preventive and early detection

TABLE 81–3. INITIAL SYMPTOMS OF MAMMARY CARCINOMA*

Symptom	Percentage of All Cases
Painless breast mass	66
Painful breast mass	11
Nipple discharge	9
Local edema	4
Nipple retraction	3
Nipple crusting	2
Miscellaneous symptoms	5

*Adapted from report of initial symptoms in 774 patients treated for breast cancer at Ellis Fischel State Cancer Hospital, Columbia, Missouri.

From Dunphy, J. E., and L. W. Way: *Current Surgical Diagnosis and Treatment,* 3rd ed. Los Altos, Calif.: Lange Medical Publications, 1977, p. 274.

attention as do any other women. That is, breast self-examinations should be encouraged, breast examinations should be done during antenatal checkups, and any three-dimensional breast lumps should be biopsied.

Symptoms. Table 81–3 summarizes *initial symptoms* of mammary cancer. *Advanced* breast cancer is characterized by:[118] redness, edema, nodularity or ulceration of the skin; enlargement, shrinkage or retraction of the breast; presence of large primary tumor; marked axillary lymphadenopathy; supraclavicular lymphadenopathy, edema of the ipsilateral arm, and distant metastases.

GRADING AND STAGING OF BREAST CANCER[88, 114]

Numerous, often confusing, grading and staging systems have been developed for cancer. The *staging* of a cancer is based upon: (a) the size of the primary lesion; (b) the extent of spread to regional lymph nodes, and (c) the presence or absence of metastases.

A common method of staging is the *TNM staging system* (Table 81–4). This system groups patients according to characteristics of the primary tumor (T), regional lymph nodes (N), and distant metastases (M). In breast cancer, subgroup assignments are made according to tumor size, tumor attachment to underlying structures and other characteristics, e.g., edema.

Two other staging systems are: (1) the *Columbia Clinical Classification* devised by Haagensen and (2) the *Manchester System* (Table 81–5). The latter system is used in many British and European and some American reports of treatment of breast cancer. Stages A, B, C, and D of the Columbia Classification are broadly equivalent to stages I, II, III and IV of the TNM system. The Columbia Classification is the system most frequently used in the United States today for classifying breast cancer.

The *grading* of a cancer is based on the cytologic differentiation of tumor cells and the number of mitoses within the tumor. Grading tries to identify some degree of a tumor's malignancy or estimate its aggressiveness. Pathologically, four grades of breast cancer can be identified on the basis of cellular differentiation and invasiveness (Table 81–6). Information about the microscopic characteristics (histologic appearance) of a given tumor can be correlated with the expected behavior of the cancer, and may thus be useful in deciding upon therapeutic management and predicting prognosis. Various grading systems have been developed, based on the histology of breast cancer.

As yet, a completely satisfactory system has not been developed for grading. However, a more satisfactory level of objectivity and international agreement has been reached for staging.

Breast cancer may be roughly classified as follows:[59]

- *Early.* Solitary, unilateral hard, painless, solid, irregular, poorly outlined, nonmobile lump usually located in the upper outer quadrant of the breast, and opaque to transillumination.
- *Moderately advanced locally.* Axillary nodes, nipple retraction or elevation, skin dimpling, nipple discharge.
- *Far advanced locally.* Signs of local inoperability. Superclavicular nodes, fixation of axillary nodes, fixation of tumor to chest wall, edema (peau d'orange or redness over more than a third of the breast), edema of the arm, ulceration of the skin, satellite nodules.
- *Distant metastases.* Inoperable. Parietal, osseous or visceral.

TREATMENT OF BREAST CANCER: AN OVERVIEW

The diagnosis and staging of breast cancer have been discussed. The selection of the best therapeutic procedure for a patient with breast cancer is based on the stage of the disease and knowledge of the individual patient. Survival appears more closely related to earlier diagnosis (before spreading) rather than to more extensive therapy.

It is impossible to summarize a consensus of the most effective methods of treating the various stages of breast cancer. There is diversity of opinion and, at times, open controversy among specialists. Because of this, the nurse must become informed of the most recent advances in treatment by reading current journals and through other educational activities.

TABLE 81–4. TNM STAGING SYSTEM FOR CARCINOMA OF THE BREAST.

The Definitions of T, N, and M Categories for Carcinoma of the Breast

T Primary Tumors

TIS Preinvasive carcinoma (carcinoma in situ), noninfiltrating intraductal carcinoma, or Paget's disease of the nipple with no demonstrable tumor.
Note: Paget's disease associated with a demonstrable tumor is classified according to the size of the tumor.
T0 No demonstrable tumor in the breast.
T1* Tumor 2 cm. or less in its greatest dimension.
T1a With no fixation to underlying pectoral fascia and/or muscle.
T1b With fixation to underlying pectoral fascia or muscle.
T2* Tumor more than 2 cm. but not more than 5 cm. in its greatest dimension.
T2a With no fixation to underlying pectoral fascia and/or muscle.
T2b With fixation to underlying pectoral fascia and/or muscle.
T3* Tumor more than 5 cm. in its greatest dimension.
T3a With no fixation to underlying pectoral fascia and/or muscle.
T3b With fixation to underlying pectoral fascia and/or muscle.
T4 Tumor of any size with direct extension to chest wall or skin.
Note: Chest wall includes ribs, intercostal muscles, and serratus anterior muscle but not pectoral muscle.
T4a With fixation to chest wall.
T4b With edema (including peau d'orange), ulceration of the skin of the breast, or satellite skin nodules confined to the same breast.
T4c Both of above.

N Regional Lymph Nodes

N0 No palpable homolateral axillary nodes.
N1 Movable homolateral axillary nodes.
$N1_a$ Nodes not considered to contain growth.
$N1_b$ Nodes considered to contain growth.
N2 Homolateral axillary nodes considered to contain growth and fixed to one another or to other structures.
N3 Homolateral supraclavicular or infraclavicular nodes considered to contain growth or edema of the arm.†
Note: Edema of the arm may be caused by lymphatic obstruction; lymph nodes may not then be palpable.

M Distant Metastases

M0 No evidence of distant metastases.
M1 Distant metastases present, including skin involvement beyond the breast area.

Clinical Stage Grouping in Carcinoma of the Breast

TIS Carcinoma in situ.
Invasive carcinoma

Stage I	T1a N0 or $N1_a$	MO
	T1b N0 or $N1_a$	
Stage II	T0 $N1_b$	M0
	T1a $N1_b$	
	T1b $N1_b$	
	T2a or T2b N0, $N1_a$ or $N1_b$	
Stage III	Any T3 with any N	M0
	Any T4 with any N	
	Any T with N2	
	Any T with N3	
Stage IV	Any T any N with M1	

*Dimpling of the skin, nipple retraction, or any other skin changes except those in T4b may occur in T1, T2, or T3 without affecting the classification.

†Homolateral internal mammary nodes considered to contain growth are included in N3 for surgical evaluation classification of postsurgical treatment classification.

From Dunphy, J. E., and L. W. Way, *Current Surgical Diagnosis and Treatment,* 3rd ed. Los Altos, Calif.. Lange Medical Publications, 1977.

TABLE 81–5. CLASSIFICATIONS OF BREAST CANCER

Columbia Clinical Classification

Stage	Clinical Criteria
A	No skin edema, ulceration, or solid fixation of tumor to chest wall; axillary nodes not clinically involved.
B	No skin edema, ulceration, or solid fixation of tumor to chest wall; clinically involved axillary nodes, but less than 2.5 cm in transverse diameter and not fixed to overlying skin or deeper structures of axilla.
C	Any one of 5 grave signs of advanced breast carcinoma: 1. Edema of skin of limited extent (involving less than one-third of the skin over the breast). 2. Skin ulceration. 3. Solid fixation of tumor to chest wall. 4. Massive involvement of axillary lymph nodes; a single node, or group of fused nodes, measuring 2.5 cm or more in transverse diameter. 5. Fixation of the axillary nodes to overlying skin or deeper structures of the axilla.
D	More advanced breast carcinoma, including— 1. A combination of any 2 or more of the 5 grave signs listed in stage C. 2. Extensive edema of skin (involving more than one-third of the skin over the breast). 3. Satellite skin nodules. 4. The inflammatory type of carcinoma. 5. Clinically involved supraclavicular lymph nodes. 6. Internal mammary metastases as evidenced by a parasternal tumor. 7. Edema of the arm. 8. Distant metastases.

The Manchester System

Stage	Criteria
I	The growth is confined to the breast. Involvement of the skin directly over and in continuity with the tumor does not affect staging provided that the area involved is small in relation to the size of the breast.
II	As in stage I, but there are palpable mobile nodes in the axilla.
III	The growth is extending beyond the corpus mammae, as shown by— (a) invasion of the skin, or fixation over an area large in relation to the size of the breast, or skin ulceration; (b) fixation of the tumor to the underlying muscle or fascia. Axillary nodes may or may not be palpable, but if nodes are present they must be mobile.
IV	The growth has extended beyond the breast area as shown by— (a) fixation or matting of the axillary nodes; (b) complete fixation of tumor to chest wall; (c) secondaries in supraclavicular nodes; (d) secondaries in opposite breast; (e) secondaries in the skin wide of tumor; (f) distant metastases, e.g., bone, liver, lung.

From Dunphy, J. E., and L. W. Way: *Current Surgical Diagnosis and Treatment,* 3rd ed. Los Altos, Calif.: Lange Medical Publications, 1977, p. 280.

Four major methods of treatment may be used for cancer of the breast: surgery, radiotherapy, endocrine manipulation, and chemoimmunotherapy. Numerous variables characterize breast cancer. Although advances in treatment are being constantly made, no doubt improved results would occur with more precise classification of patients and revised staging procedures, so that patients could more effectively be selected for the various therapeutic modalities available.[109]

Summarized below are *initial treatment methods:*[109]

▶ *Surgery: Surgical approaches* currently used are local incision, simple mastectomy, modified radical mastectomy, the Halsted radical mastectomy, and extended radical mastectomy. Many would agree that the Halsted radical mastectomy is the best treatment for breast cancer (with certain exceptions) when the cancer is limited in such a manner that cure is possible.

▶ *Radiotherapy:* Radiotherapy may be used either *in combination with surgery or alone* for curative or prophylactic reasons. Usually radiotherapy supplements surgical procedures that are less extensive than radical mastectomy. When dissection is considered and adequate, the axilla is usually not irradiated. The chest wall is irradiated when there is significant risk of recurrent disease in the area.

▶ *Endocrine manipulation:* In the presence of early breast cancer, endocrine manipulation may in-

TABLE 81–6. CLASSIFICATION OF MAMMARY CARCINOMA ACCORDING TO THE CELLULAR GROWTH PATTERN AND RELATIVE FREQUENCY OF TYPES

Type I:	Rarely metastasizing (not invasive) *5% of total cases* 1. Intraductal or comedocarcinoma without stromal invasion. Paget's disease of the breast may exist if the epithelium of the nipple is involved. 2. Papillary carcinoma confined to the ducts. 3. Lobular carcinoma in situ.
Type II:	Rarely metastasizing (always invasive) *15% of total cases* 1. Well-differentiated adenocarcinoma. 2. Medullary carcinoma with lymphocytic infiltration. 3. Pure colloid or mucinous carcinoma. 4. Papillary carcinoma.
Type III:	Moderately metastasizing (always invasive) *65% of total cases* 1. Infiltrating adenocarcinoma. 2. Intraductal carcinoma with stromal invasion. 3. Infiltrating lobular carcinoma.* 4. All tumors not classified as types I, II, or IV.
Type IV:	Highly metastasizing (always invasive) 15% of total cases 1. Undifferentiated carcinoma having cells without ductal or tubular arrangement. 2. All types of tumors indisputably invading blood vessels.

*Infiltrating lobular carcinoma has been moved from type II to type III because of growing experience with its metastasizing potential.

Adapted from Dunphy, J. E., and L. W. Way: *Current Surgical Diagnosis and Treatment,* 3rd ed. Los Altos, Calif.: Lange Medical Publications, 1977.

volve surgical or chemical ablative therapy (castration) and hormone therapy. Formerly prophylactic castration was employed; however, it is currently not used as frequently as in the past. It has not been demonstrated to improve survival, although it may delay recurrence.

- *Chemoimmunotherapy:* A variety of *cytotoxic agents* are of use in treating breast cancer. The best response rate of the *single-drug* regimens has been produced by doxorubicin hydrochloride (Adriamycin). Numerous *combinations* of drugs have been used. One combination is: 5-fluorouracil, Adriamycin, and cyclophosphamide (Cytoxan) (FAC). *Immunotherapy* is of rapidly expanding interest in treating breast cancer. Agents being tried include BCG (bacille Calmette-Guérin vaccination) (see p. 470 for discussion of BCG therapy), MER (methanol extracted residue of BCG), and levamisole. *Drug adjuvant programs* (e.g., FAC-BCG for metastatic breast cancer) show promise in improving survival rates. Cytotoxic drugs seem to compare favorably with endocrine therapy when used singly, and appear to be superior when used in combination.

Treatment of Metastatic Breast Cancer

Metastatic disease from breast cancer usually develops in one or more of the following *sites:*

- Adjacent or distant soft tissue sites (spread via lymphatics)
- Bones, lungs, pleura, peritoneum, liver, and central nervous system.

Patients with metastatic cancer to the central nervous system, liver, and peritoneum have a median survival time of only 6 months. The major clinical variables affecting the probability of *response to any palliative therapy* include:[55]

- Anatomic site of metastasis
- Free interval between initial treatment and the detection of metastasis
- Appearance of recurrent or metastatic disease
- Age and menopausal status of patient

Treatment of metastatic disease may involve radiation therapy, alteration of hormone status surgically or with endocrine treatment, administration of chemotherapy and/or additional surgery. A combination of treatments is typically employed.

No Treatment.[109] Some persons with metastatic disease are best managed by withholding any treatment measures, i.e., by administering no specific therapies. These persons are carefully selected. For example, occasionally, a patient remains asymptomatic in spite of having many known metastases for a number of years. It appears that these individuals have an adequate defense against the tumor, and treatment may even be deleterious for them.

Of course, it must always be recognized that therapy has side effects and risks. Patients have the right to know that the risks are for them before they agree to undergo treatments. Once given information about the possible benefits and the potential hazards of specific therapies, some persons decide they do not wish to submit to a particular treatment. This difficult decision must be respected. Naturally, it is important to continue to *care* for patients even though they are not receiving specific therapies. (See Chapter 1.)

SURGICAL TREATMENT

> *Controversy exists about several aspects of surgical treatment for breast cancer:*
>
> *1. Whether or not surgical treatment is the treatment of choice.*
>
> *2. When surgery is employed, how much tissue should be removed.*
>
> *3. Whether removal of lymph nodes has a therapeutic benefit or provides only prognostic information.*

Present data indicate that the results of partial mastectomy are equal to the results of more radical operations performed on patients with the same stage of cancer.[25] Until recently in most centers throughout the world, a standard radical mastectomy was the treatment of choice for operating on invasive breast cancer.

The selection of a surgical procedure for persons with potentially curable invasive breast carcinoma must be individualized and is related to the natural history of breast cancer; the histology, location, and extent of disease; and the patient's emotional and medical status. Undetectable systemic spread of cancer often exists prior to treatment and results in many treatment failures. Surgical resection is most effective when the cancer is limited to a localized anatomic area. In an attempt to ensure complete removal of cancerous tissue, the tumor and an adequate margin of surrounding breast tissue is typically removed.

Summarized below are *surgical procedures* directed at breast tissue and lymph nodes that may be used in treating breast cancer:[88, 118]

- *Standard radical mastectomy:* En bloc removal of breast, pectoral muscles, and axillary nodes. Removes the local lesion and the axillary nodes with a wide "safety margin" of surrounding tissue. Various incisions are used, depending upon surgeon preference and location of the primary tumor.

Radical mastectomy alone is not curative if the cancer has spread to the internal mammary or supraclavicular nodes or to more distant sites.

- *Supraradical mastectomy:* In addition to the standard radical mastectomy, the internal mammary and supraclavicular nodes are removed (usually following node biopsy).
- *Extended radical mastectomy:* In addition to the standard radical mastectomy described above, this procedure involves removal of the internal mammary nodes. This procedure currently has a few advocates, since it does not seem to be significantly more effective than irradiation in preventing recurrence from internal mammary metastases.
- *Modified radical mastectomy* (Fig. 81–7): Many different techniques are covered by this term. They all include removal of the breast and preservation of the pectoralis major muscle. The extent of axillary dissection varies, and the pectoralis minor muscle may or may not be removed. A modified radical mastectomy has cosmetic and functional advantages over the standard procedure. Preservation of the pectoralis major muscle prevents formation of a hollow beneath the clavicle and also seems to be associated with a lower incidence of arm edema and shoulder dysfunction. A shift has occurred in major centers to the use of modified radical mastectomies (instead of the standard more radical procedure) since considerable evidence now shows not much difference between the morbidity, mortality, local recurrence, and survival rates for standard and modified radical mastectomies for stage I and II breast cancers.

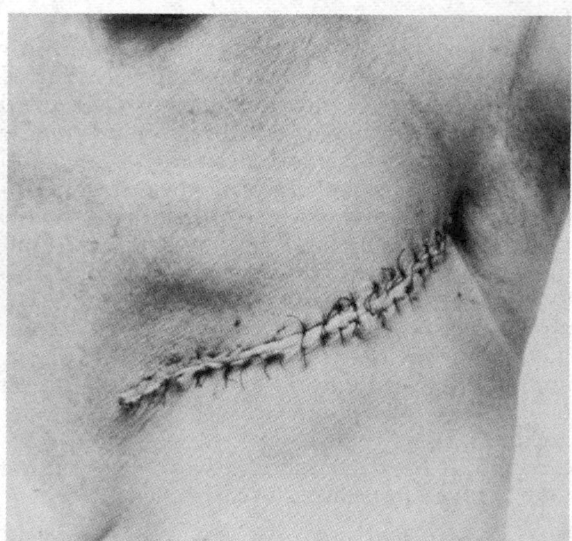

Figure 81–7. Scar from a modified radical mastectomy, two weeks postoperatively. (From Winkler, W. A.: Confronting one's changed image: Choosing the prosthesis and clothing. *American Journal of Nursing,* 77:1433, Sept. 1977.)

- *Simple mastectomy with axillary lymph node dissection:* Simple mastectomy removes only the breast. It may be accompanied with lymph node removal. Some simple mastectomies are followed either by radiation treatment or removal of lymph nodes if they become involved.
- *Simple mastectomy:* Simple mastectomy or even wide local excision may be used if it is known that the cancer is clearly confined to the breast without spread to the adjacent muscles or to the regional nodes or beyond. In other words, it can be used only for certain carefully selected persons with noninvasive (Type I) carcinoma. It is difficult, however, to determine clearly prior to resection and pathologic examination whether the axillary nodes are free of disease. (Physical examination is not a reliable method of detecting axillary metastases.) Crile has taken a controversial position by advocating leaving the axillary nodes until they become clinically positive and performing simple mastectomy for stage I breast cancer, with axillary dissection only if the axillary nodes are suspicious when palpated through the surgical wound or if they later become clinically active. This argument is based on the rationale that the regional lymph nodes may prevent the spread of early cancer by serving as repositories of systemic immunity.
- *Local excision:* Limited surgical procedures have been advocated by some (e.g., Crile) as definitive treatment for early breast cancers, e.g., small stage I nodules at the breast's lateral periphery, especially if the tumor is of histologic type I. Examples of limited procedures are: local excision ("lumpectomy"), quadrant excision, partial mastectomy, and subcutaneous mastectomy. The general position, however, appears to be that limited surgery is not recommended for operable breast cancer. There are serious potential hazards of local recurrence and of leaving unsuspected metastases in axillary nodes. Limited procedures that remove less than the whole breast have been proven to not be as effective as mastectomy.

Radical mastectomy results in the 10-year survival of 80 per cent of patients who have a small primary tumor and uninvolved axillary nodes. Thus, neither radiotherapy or adjuvant chemotherapy may be administered to these persons.[109]

With the increase in the number of women presenting with noninvasive carcinomas or preclinical invasive carcinomas (less than 0.5 cm. and lesions less than 2 cm. in diameter) a *modified radical mastectomy* is an acceptable and adequate method for obtaining local control of the disease. When the original lesion is deep seated or greater than 1 cm. in diameter some believe it is wise to resect the inferior portion of the pectoralis major muscle as part of the modified radical mastectomy. A *standard radical mastectomy* is thought by some to be indicated when patients have large primary lesions and/or extensive axillary node involvement. An *extended radical mastectomy* is often recommended for women with inner quadrant and centrally located primary lesions in order to remove the internal mammary nodes. If this is not possible, radiation therapy is thought to be an acceptable alternative.[86]

Even those persons whose axillary lymph nodes are histologically negative after biopsy (i.e., apparently free of cancer) cannot be assumed to have localized cancer. Breast cancer frequently appears to be a systemic disease at the time of surgery.[88]

When breast cancer is treated with radical mastectomy alone, there is at least a 24 per cent treatment failure after 10 years. Hence, in an attempt to treat any systemic cancer, *prophylactic postoperative chemotherapy* with cytotoxic chemotherapeutic agents (*adjuvant therapy*) has been advocated.[88] Endocrine manipulation (p. 1831) may also be employed (Table 81–7).

In addition to operations on the breast and surrounding lymph nodes, other surgical procedures may be performed in treating breast cancer. In an attempt to reduce levels of circulating estrogens in premenopausal women, *ovariectomy* may be performed. Other measures that may also be used are *adrenalectomy* and *hypophysectomy*. The latter procedures may be employed in an attempt to prolong the life of persons with pain (most often from bone metastases) and progressive disease. (See discussion under *endocrine manipulation*).

Currently some physicians are recommending *prophylactic mastectomy* for some carefully selected high-risk women. (See p. 1830).

TABLE 81–7. TREATMENT OF BREAST CANCER: ALTERNATIVE METHODS FOLLOWING SURGERY

Stage I-no apparent metastasis	Observe
Stage II-axillary metastasis only	Chemotherapy (more aggressive therapy would add prednisone treatment or oophorectomy and adrenalectomy)
Stage III-distant metastasis (skin, bone, lung parenchyma)	Chemotherapy plus oophorectomy and adrenalectomy; androgens for premenopausal patients and estrogens for postmenopausal patients (when ablative procedures are unavailable or unacceptable)
Stage IV-visceral metastasis (brain, liver, pulmonary lymphatics)	Chemotherapy plus prednisone; estrogens (when ablative procedures are unavailable or unacceptable); surgery if patient's condition allows

From Thorn, G. W., et al.: *Harrison's Principles of Internal Medicine.* New York: McGraw-Hill Book Co., 1977, p. 621.

Mastectomy

PREOPERATIVE CARE*

Cancerphobia (fear of cancer) is a prevalent condition. Persons with cancer often die of other causes, however, many continue to associate pain and early death with cancer. Cancer of the breast is doubly threatening to women in this culture, since the breast is a symbol of sexuality and femininity. Even the failure to exercise self-examination may be related to latent fears.

The nurse who first is in contact with a patient assesses the patient's reaction to this potentially frightening experience. Supportive significant others and health professionals are of great help to any person undergoing this crisis, but there are many individuals who do not have ideal support. The patient undergoing breast surgery may need a person with whom she can discuss her concerns, some of which may be of an intimate nature. "Assembly line" hospital care—with many people going in and out of the room—is not conducive to meeting the emotional needs of any patient.

The nursing staff should not leave the emotional preparation of patients to chance, but should plan so that each patient has the opportunity to talk about her surgery and to feel that someone cares about her.

Health professionals share the dread of cancer with the rest of society. Nurses must have an opportunity to explore their personal feelings about cancer of the breast before they can most satisfactorily help patients. The nurse also needs to be as knowledgeable as possible about all aspects of care and of each particular doctor's plan so that the patient's questions can be accurately answered.

The patient must be informed of the total care plan and the rehabilitative efforts that she will be undertaking. The preoperative physical preparation will be in accordance with the guidelines of the particular physician. The general preoperative routine is similar to that for most operations except for the fact that the patient may not know when she goes to surgery how extensive the operation will be. This is true

*For a general discussion of preoperative care see Chapter 17. Review Unit VIII as necessary.

of those women who have given permission for mastectomy to be performed immediately if the biopsy performed during surgery reveals cancer. In some cases, the surgeon does the biopsy of the lesion and the nodes and then does the surgery later if necessary, after receiving a complete pathology report.

Skin preparation may involve having the operative area washed with pHisoHex several days before admission to the hospital, and later, shaving, along with the usual preparation. If a skin graft is to be done, the donor areas will also have to be prepared.

POSTOPERATIVE CARE*

Promoting rest and early food and fluid intake are immediate objectives. Upon awakening, the patient is anxious to learn if the breast has been removed. The possibility of a cure and the fact that there was no spread, if this is true, should be emphasized. Early ambulation and resumption of activity is the usual procedure following mastectomy. Exercises will be prescribed by the physician. The American Cancer Society (ACS) provides a book, *Help Yourself to Recovery,* which illustrates exercises that the physician may prescribe.

The "Reach to Recovery" program of the American Cancer Society is a rehabilitation program for women who have had breast surgery. The program is designed to help these women meet their psychologic, physical and cosmetic needs. Upon authorization of the doctor, volunteers from this program visit the hospital and give the patient information and help as follows:

1. Reach to Recovery kit, ball, book, rope and a temporary prosthesis.
2. Explanation and demonstration of the exercises prescribed.
3. Suggestions for bra comfort.
4. Explanation of various breast prostheses.
5. Suggestions for clothing adjustment.
6. Where indicated, discussions of personal problems. A volunteer who has experienced similar problems can be very helpful.
7. The volunteer's phone number is left with the patient so that help is always available.

When told by the doctor that she is ready to be fitted with a prosthesis, the patient may visit the ACS office, and obtain further information concerning clothing, particularly bathing suits. Mastectomy bras now may be obtained in foundation departments in most large stores. The glycerin filled form is guaranteed for 10 years. It will not evaporate, does not change shape or size, and seals itself if the form is punctured. It does not ride up and even spreads naturally when the patient is lying down.

Edema. Nearly all patients have some degree of arm edema following radical mastectomy. It is the only significant postoperative complication of this operation.

Mobility of the arm on the operative side is important following radical mastectomy and is enhanced if the surgeon never allows any bandages or tapes to fix the arm to the chest wall. In the recovery room, the arm on the side of the operation is placed at right angles to the chest wall and a small towel is placed around the arm and pinned to the bed sheet leaving the elbow free (Fig. 81–8). The arm is kept in this position for 24 to 48 hours.

Early postoperative *arm exercises* are recommended. Bed exercises should be started within 24 hours. The patient is instructed in hand and wrist movements and in flexion and extension of the elbow at hourly intervals. She is encouraged to feed herself, comb her hair and wash her face, being careful not to abduct the arm. (See boxed discussion of exercises.)

When wound healing is well established, abduction and external rotation of the upper arm are begun in the recumbent position. At about the 10th to 12th day, the patient is started on exercises in the erect position, consisting of pendulum swings to improve shoulder function (Fig. 81–9), forward and lateral elevation of the arms, overhead pulley suspension to obtain full elevation, and wall climbing (Fig. 81–10).

The arm should be compressed postoperatively with an *elastic bandage,* to be followed by a custom-fitted *pressure gradient elastic sleeve* to avoid the changes of edema during the period

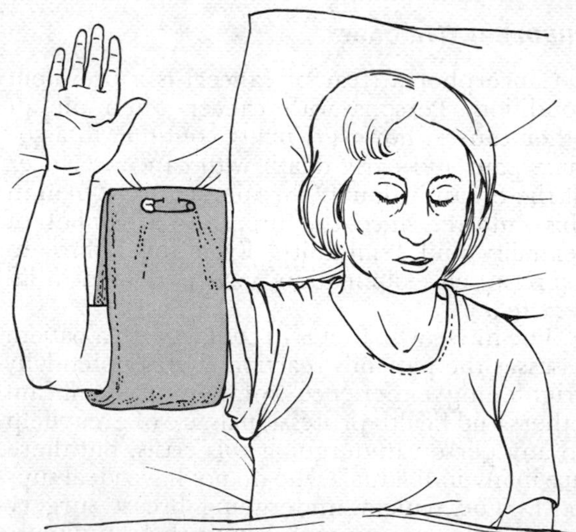

Figure 81–8. Position of the arm on the operated side in the early postoperative course following radical mastectomy. (Redrawn from Degenhein, G.: Mobility of the arm following radical mastectomy. *Surgery, Gynecology, and Obstetrics,* 145:77, July 1977.)

*See Chapters 19 and 20 for a complete discussion of postoperative care.

HAND CARE

After a radical mastectomy, an arm may swell because lymph nodes and lymph vessels were necessarily removed and the body is therefore less able to combat infection in this extremity.

Make every effort to avoid all cuts, scratches, pin pricks, hangnails, insect bites, burns, and the use of strong detergents as these can lead to serious infection with increased swelling.

Some "DO NOT'S":
DO NOT hold a cigarette in this hand
DO NOT carry your purse or anything heavy with this arm
DO NOT wear a wristwatch or other jewelry on this arm
DO NOT cut or pick at cuticles or hangnails on this hand
DO NOT work near thorny plants or dig in the garden
DO NOT reach into a hot oven with this arm
DO NOT permit injection in this arm
DO NOT permit blood to be drawn from this arm
DO NOT allow your blood pressure to be taken on this arm

Some "DO'S":
DO wear a loose rubber glove on this hand when washing dishes
DO wear a thimble when sewing
DO apply a good lanolin hand cream several times daily
DO wear your "Life-Guard Medical Aid" tag engraved with "CAUTION – LYMPHEDEMA ARM – NO TESTS – NO HYPOS"
DO contact your doctor if your arm gets red, warm or unusually hard or swollen
DO return for a check-up and re-measurement for a new sleeve in two months
DO show this Hand Care Sheet to your surgeon

Reprinted through the courtesy of the CLEVELAND CLINIC Department of Physical Medicine and Rehabilitation.

needed for regrowth of lymphatic pathways. Ordinarily, patients have a transient slight increase in diameter of the arm following surgery. This kind of edema usually produces an increase of less than 3 cm. and ordinarily disappears wtih the restoration of arm function. Edema is considered a true complication when it is severe enough to make the patient socially unpresentable and gives her a feeling of tension and discomfort.

Secondary edema resulting from infection in the arm is more frequent, and patients may have some permanent edema following an infection. If wound healing is normal, adequate collateral lymphatic circulation usually develops within a month. Common sources of infection are necrosis of skin flaps or imperfectly obliterated dead space in the axilla. Postoperatively radiation to the axilla often increases the frequency and degree of edema of the arm.

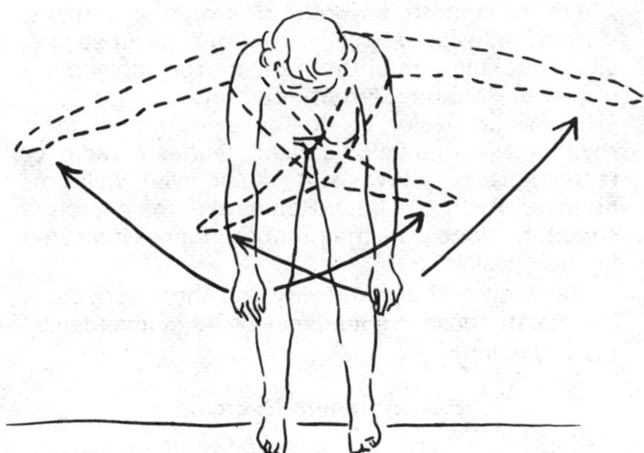

Figure 81–9. Stand with feet 8 inches apart. Bend forward from the waist allowing arms to hang toward the floor by gravity. Swing both arms together describing an arc from one shoulder to the other. Do not bend elbows. Stand and allow arms to fall to side. (Wolf, E. S.: *Nursing Clinics of North America,* 2:587, Dec. 1967.)

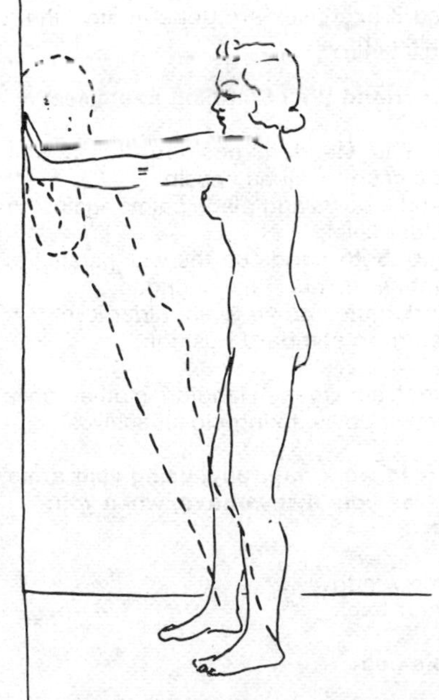

Figure 81–10. Stand facing the wall at arm's length with feet 8 inches apart. Place hands against the wall at shoulder level parallel to each other. Slowly flex the elbow, bending the trunk forward until forehead touches wall. Straighten elbows slowly until body is upright. Repeat. Note: Keep head, trunk, and legs in straight line. (Wolf, E. S.: *Nursing Clinics of North America,* 2:587, Dec. 1967.)

General Rules for Exercises

"Easy does it," so try to relax. Use both arms whenever possible, or place one hand on hip for balance and support.

Aim for smooth, swinging or sweeping motions.

Do as many exercises in front of a mirror as possible. Looking straight into the mirror with shoulders level. Hold head erect—chin in.

It may be easier to do the exercises at home rhythmically if music is used, either a radio or record player. Slow, soft music with well-pronounced rhythm is best. Remember, the exercises should be done only the number of times indicated by the physician.

Starts all exercises slowly for short periods. A gradual increase in speed may be recommended by the physician.

Hair Brushing Exercise

This Exercise Is Frequently Started Before the Patient Leaves the Hospital

1. Sit beside a night table. In the beginning rest the arm (on the operated side) on a few books. Comb and brush the hair keeping the head erect.
2. One side will do to start. Little by little, release the arm from its resting position and work the brush around the head until the entire scalp is covered.
3. Rest whenever needed, but be persistent.

Standard Position for Hand Wall Climbing and Other Recommended Exercises

Stand erect with head high and arms at sides. Place feet hip width apart for balance. Flatten abdomen—avoid hollow back. Better balance is achieved if exercises are done in stocking feet or low heeled shoes.

Hand Wall Climbing Exercises

1. Start in standard position, facing wall, with toes as close to wall as possible.
2. Bend elbows and place palms against the wall at shoulder level.
3. Work both hands up the wall parallel to each other until arms are fully extended.
4. Work hands down to shoulder level.
5. Return to standard position.

Equivalent activities—Hanging clothes on a line, washing windows, fixing closet shelves.

Try to work naturally, using your arms as you always have, when you:

Teach
Type
Wash a window
Dry your back
Cook
Make a bed

Adapted with permission from the American Cancer Society publication, *Help Yourself To Recovery*, 1957. *In* Fitzpatrick, G.: Caring for the patient with cancer of the breast, *Bedside Nurse*, Mar. 1970.

The patient needs to understand that she is vulnerable to secondary edema for the rest of her life and that trauma may lead to infection and edema.

Burns, cuts, abrasions and paronychia (inflammation around fingernails) are the most frequent sources of infection. Controlling obesity is an important factor in reducing edema. "Wearing a custom-made elastic sleeve extending from the wrist to the shoulder during the day, when the patient is up and about, is the most useful method of limiting and improving edema of the arm in its chronic stage."[42] Haagensen also advises that spironolactone, a diuretic, may be tried in moderate doses in combination with the elastic sleeve. He also advocates skin grafting and meticulous aftercare in securing wound healing and avoiding the triad of tension on the skin flaps, necrosis, and infection.[42]

Note the sample instruction sheet that may be given to patients following mastectomy. Additionally the patient is advised to not pull or drag objects and to use the unaffected arm to carry heavy packages or handbag. Hormone beauty creams or hormone drugs should not be used without first consulting with the physician. Tight sleeves should be avoided in clothing. Avoid sunburn.

PSYCHOSOCIAL CONSIDERATIONS AFTER MASTECTOMY

It is important to obtain a complete history on every woman admitted to the hospital for breast cancer biopsy, and to attempt to assess the woman's adjustment and pertinent preexisting problems. Such questions as "Tell me about your home" and "Who is taking care of things while you are in the hospital?" are nonthreatening and may help the nurse better understand the patient. The nurse needs to know who the patient's significant others are in order to talk with them about their feelings, about the crisis, and about plans for supporting the patient.

The sexual history of the patient is most appropriately handled when the nurse has the confidence of the patient. However, since the breast is an important aspect of sexuality in our culture, someone needs to consider its importance in this context, preferably the whole team.

One study has shown that clinically depressed persons, the emotionally labile, and those going through the menopause are more likely to have difficulty in marital, sexual, interpersonal and work adjustments following mastectomy.[74] These patients may benefit from increased opportunities to interact with nurses in such ways that they feel comfortable in expressing their fears and problems and that they receive appropriate information and support.

The patient who has a mastectomy may use a number of defense patterns in adapting to *stress.* Not all patients perceive or handle stress in the same way. Displacement, projection, denial, hope and prayer, stoicism-fatalism, or a combination of these defenses may be used. Patients who lose a breast may adapt in the same way they would to any *loss. Phantom breast symptoms* are not uncommon in the missing breast.

Losing a breast may not make its full impact until the patient goes home. Many women are surprised by the amount of pain and discomfort, marked fatigue, slow healing of the incision, their swollen arm, and jittery feelings. Such "ordinary" things as how to find a comfortable position in bed may be a problem. The patient has to decide whether to hide the lesion from significant others or to let them see it. The defect may be camouflaged by an appropriately fitted brassiere or a special bathing suit or evening dress, but doubts and fears about her attractiveness may affect even the most secure woman.

The patient may relax from one check-up to the next, but in many instances new symptoms cause the patient to realize she is suffering from advanced cancer. Anxiety and depression are common among persons with fatal cancer. Financial and family problems may be precipitated by the disease.

To give the patient hope, the nurse must understand and appreciate the patient's difficulties. By setting short-term goals, the patient may see that she has a choice as to how she faces each small crisis. If she feels that she will not be abandoned and that she will have help in avoiding excessive pain and in "working through" dying, the patient may be better able to live and enjoy each day. Social workers, if available, and pastors can also be sources of ongoing strength for some patients and their significant others. Certainly, the patient's ongoing adjustment will be facilitated by significant others and health professonals who understand and care.

Each new development may precipitate aspects of the *grieving process* such as anger, depression and regression. New symptoms may become magnified in the patient's mind, and every new pain may set off the alarm button. The patient needs someone with whom she can talk about these fears. Ideally, the public health nurse or the nurse in the doctor's office or cancer unit will be a person who can help the patient to realistically handle the new symptoms. *Mastectomy support groups* also can provide a place where patients can talk about their shared and individual problems. When the disease becomes terminal, the patient needs to be encouraged in self-help as long as possible to enhance feelings of worth and self-control. Nurses and others working on a cancer unit need a great deal of help in handling their own feelings and in learning how to interact in a supporting and realistic way with the patient.

It may be helpful to realize that the major emotional stresses associated wtih mastectomy may be short-term for many women. Morris et al.[74] , for example, found in their study that 70 per cent of 160 women studied were no longer stressed by mastectomy after 1 year had passed following surgery.

Breast Reconstruction[118]

Following standard or modified radical mastectomy, breast reconstruction may be technically feasible, provided that there has been no skin grafting or radiotherapy to the chest wall. Typically, breast reconstruction involves several operations and implantation of a prosthesis (Fig. 81–11). It is not unusual for patients to be initially interested in reconstructive surgery and then to subsequently decide against such a procedure after they have experienced a period of adjustment and use of an external prosthesis.

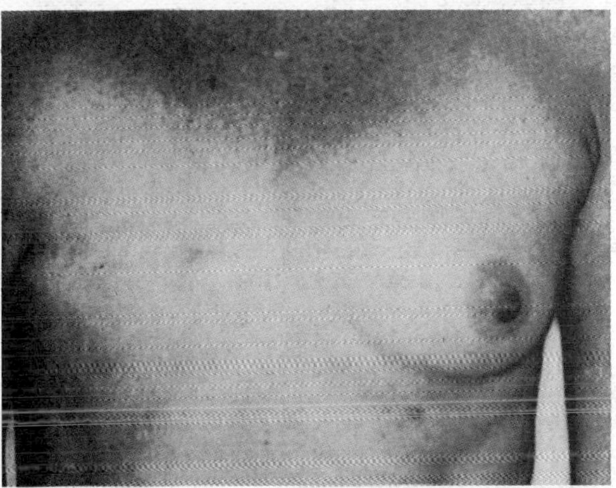

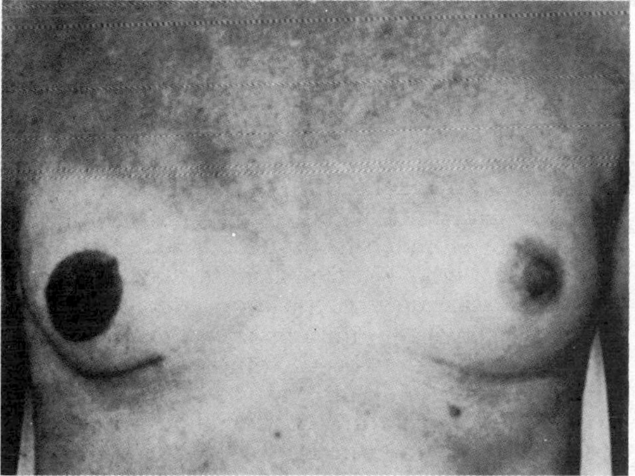

Figure 81–11. A. The chest wall after a modified right radical mastectomy with preservation of pectoralis muscle and anterior fold. **B.** Same patient after Silastic breast implant and reconstruction of nipple-areolar complex with free labial graft. (From Thomas, S. G., and M. M. Yates: Confronting one's changed image: Breast reconstruction after mastectomy. *American Journal of Nursing,* 77:1438, Sept. 1977.)

Breast reconstruction should be performed only when there is very little possibility of recurrence of cancer.

Prophylactic Mastectomy[111]

Prophylactic subcutaneous mastectomies are now being performed on some women who are in a high-risk group for developing breast cancer. This surgical procedure involves removing as much breast tissue as possible, leaving the skin and nipple. Silastic implants are then either immediately inserted, or they are inserted about 3 to 6 weeks later. This procedure is performed in hopes of decreasing the likelihood of breast cancer and reducing the anxieties of women in a high-risk group. Candidates for prophylactic mastectomy are carefully selected. *This procedure is done to reduce the patient's chances of having breast cancer—not for cosmetic reasons.*

Prophylactic mastectomy is a major surgical procedure, requiring healthy subcutaneous tissue for a good surgical result. During the surgery more than 95 per cent of the breast tissue is removed, leaving the nipple, axillary tissue, and subclavicular tissue. The three types of incision used are: breast-halving incision, inframammary or submammary incision, or lateral incision. Drains are inserted in lateral stab wounds. Blood loss can be extensive. Some surgeons prefer that the patient donate her own blood for autotransfusion a week before surgery.

A major postoperative concern is to maintain survival of the skin covering the implants, hence it is essential that *no strain* be placed on the chest. The patient is positioned in bed on her back with the head elevated about 30 degrees. The patient must keep her elbows at her sides *at all* times for about 2 to 4 weeks. Naturally this is difficult, and means that assistance is required in many activities of daily living. Turning onto the side or stomach is not permitted for at least 4 weeks. Light wrist restraints may serve as reminders at night of position limitations. Because of activity limitations in bed, every effort must be made to prevent complications of inactivity, e.g., antiembolic elastic stockings may be worn, deep breathing and coughing are encouraged to aerate the lungs. Dehydration must be prevented. Intake and output are recorded. Since excessive bleeding is a potential problem, frequent checks are made of the suction drains and dressings for evidence of frank bleeding. Frequent dressing changes may be required during the early postoperative days. Because of the potential danger of skin necrosis, absolutely no pressure can be applied when replacing dressings. Properly functioning wound suction can usually prevent hematomas and edema. Because wound infection would be a serious complication, prophylactic antibiotics are typically given. Displacement of the implant (causing the "skin brassiere" to wrinkle and the nipple to point downward) is another potential postoperative complication.

Prior to prophylactic mastectomy, the surgery, its purposes, and potential benefits as well as complications must be carefully discussed. The patient should understand the necessary postoperative course and its limitations. Also, it is imperative that the patient know that her breast appearance will be changed after surgery. For some women the change is distressing even though expected. Initially the breast typically feels hard and firm. Although this sensation usually decreases, at times it persists and is most annoying. It is not unusual for continued discomfort to be experienced. Nipple sensitivity is decreased and some women experience increased sensitivity to changes in the skin covering the breast prosthesis. Naturally, it is extremely difficult for many patients to decide whether or not to undergo this extensive major surgery. Ultimately the woman must be allowed to make the decision herself, given as much information as possible.

OTHER TREATMENTS FOR BREAST CANCER

RADIOTHERAPY

Radiotherapy has been discussed in Chapter 23. Recently, early breast cancer (Stages I and II) has been effectively treated by biopsy or local excision of the primary tumor followed by external beam irradiation and then possibly radioactive implants. This technique has produced results comparable to those with extensive surgery.

Supervoltage irradiation is used for the primary or adjunctive treatment of breast cancer. When used following surgery (i.e., removal of the primary breast mass by biopsy), *external beam irradiation* using 4 million volt x-rays is directed at: (a) the breast and (b) regional lymph nodes in the axillary, supraclavicular, and internal mammary chains. A typical dose is 4500 to 5000 rads delivered via treatments 5 days a week over a period of 4 to 5 weeks. When gross residual disease remains after biopsy (i.e., the mass was not totally excised), additional treatment is given 2 to 3 weeks later. Such treatment consists of a dose of 1500 to 3000 rads delivered to a local area in the breast by the temporary *implantation* of radioactive iridium-192 (Ir-192). When these doses are not exceeded, it is possible to achieve excellent cosmetic results, i.e., normal breast appearance and textures are maintained.

The Ir-192 implantation is made under general anesthesia. First, long needles are inserted through breast tissue, e.g., five needles are inserted in parallel rows one centimeter apart. These needles serve as guides for plastic tubing, which is introduced next. The hollow needles are then removed, leaving the tubing in place. After the patient is returned to her room, the radioactive iridium, loaded into smaller-caliber tubing, is inserted into the implanted plastic tubes. The implant usually remains in the breast 2 to 3 days. Mild local discomfort occurs; however, there are usually no side effects.

While radiation helps achieve *local* control of breast cancer, it must be remembered that cancer has to be viewed as a *systemic* disease even in its early clinical stages. Thus, local treatment alone is not sufficient and consideration must also be given to adjuvant chemotherapy. (See p. 1833).

External beam irradiation typically produces minimal *side effects* during therapy, e.g., loss of appetite, occasional mild nausea, skin reactions such as erythema followed by desquamation of the treated area. The skin gradually regains its normal color after irradiation is completed. Other side effects are possible, since radiation affects all tissues through which it passes. Such side effects include radiation tracheitis (manifested by cough) and radiation esophagitis (indicated by discomfort when swallowing). These disorders are symptomatically treated and rapidly subside when irradiation is completed.

Since advanced cancer therapy is on an outpatient basis, the nurse in the doctor's office, clinic or cancer treatment unit will have opportunity to talk with the patient about her fears and to attempt to help her to see cancer as similar to other chronic diseases that one must learn to live with and treat as symptoms arise.

The patient needs to know about the effects of radiation therapy. Skin changes may vary from a mild erythema to a severe reaction, with pain and weeping. Strong soaps and ointments or creams should not be used, and the skin should not be exposed to the sun. Cornstarch may be used several times a day to keep the skin dry. Vitamins A and D ointment or plain lanolin might be applied. If the skin has broken down or is painful, the doctor will prescribe appropriate treatment. For systemic effects of fatigue or lethargy, nausea, and digestive upsets, patients should eat frequent small meals and get plenty of rest.

ENDOCRINE MANIPULATION THERAPY

Hormone manipulation as a therapeutic approach to breast cancer (either through ablative surgery or endocrine chemotherapy) has received considerable attention over recent years. Considerable research is currently being undertaken, knowledge is being expanded, and many unanswered questions remain.

It is well known, of course, that breast tissue responds to hormonal influence. *Cytoplasmic* or *membrane receptor sites* exist in *normal mammary cells* for the hormones that affect them, e.g., estrogen, progesterone, prolactin, and testosterone. Figure 81–12 shows in simplified form the path of the biochemical reaction that occurs when hormones affect a mammary cell.

When a malignancy occurs in the breast, *a change may occur in the number of receptor sites in cells.* Sometimes all the receptor sites remain in the cells; sometimes the number is reduced. Such changes in the number of receptor sites remaining in the mammary cells affects the hormonal influence upon the growth and function of the breast tissue: e.g., if all the receptor sites remain, hormonal regulation is retained as in the normal breast cell; if the receptors are lost, circulating hormones no longer affect the breast cells.

Those patients who have breast cancers and do retain receptor sites for estrogen in the mammary cells (i.e., whose breast tumors are "estrogen-dependent") are more likely to respond to treatment involving endocrine manipulation than those people who do not retain receptor sites for estrogen in the mammary cells.

It is useful then, when planning treatment regimens for people with breast cancer, to know whether the cancer cells have estrogen receptor sites or not. (Estrogen receptor sites may be abbreviated to ER or ERP [estrogen receptor protein].) Such information helps the physician to decide whether hormonal therapy is likely to be helpful for a particular patient. Laboratory tests are now possible to make such determinations—*Hormone Receptor Assay.* This is most commonly done for estrogen receptors, although it is also possible for progesterone and androgen receptors. The highest success rate of hormonal treatment for breast cancer occurs in those patients with tumors retaining both estrogen and progesterone receptors.

An *estrogen receptor assay* involves an expensive laboratory examination of the tumor tissue taken at the time of a frozen section. Very careful care must be taken of the tissue, as estrogen receptor protein (ERP) is very sensitive to heat. The tissue is placed immediately into a cold environment (−70° C.) to avoid inaccurate results.

Osborne and McGuire[77] have developed a system of grouping patients according to risk, based on the ER status and the status of axillary node involvement. This system can be used as a guide for treatment.

Serum calcium levels are an added factor affecting the decision to use endocrine manipulation in the treatment of breast cancer. Hormones are contraindicated in patients with elevated serum calcium, since both estrogens and androgens are thought to initiate or aggravate hypercalcemia in some patients with bony metastasis.[55] Hypercalcemia can have fatal consequences, as the kidneys, heart, and lungs may be damaged by deposits of calcium.

If endocrine manipulation is indicated and decided upon by both patient and physician, treatment choices include: (1) *ablative surgery* — ovariectomy (also called castration), adrenalectomy or hypophysectomy; (b) *chemical ablative methods* — chemically inhibiting ovaries, adrenals, or pituitary glands; and (c) *hormone additive therapy* — administration of exogenous estrogens and androgens. At the present time, the surgical approaches seem to be the most effective, although with further research it is expected that the medical treatments will replace the surgical treatments altogether.

Ablative Surgery. (See also Unit XIX.) In the premenopausal woman, the cancer develops in an environment of estrogen and progesterone from the ovaries. Surgical (or radiation) *castration* is the procedure generally used in this group of patients. Most clinicians prefer to use castration as a therapeutic approach in premenopausal women with stage I and II breast cancers.

In the menopausal woman, the cancer develops in an unbalanced hormonal environment of estrogen from the adrenals and, in some cases, from the ovaries. *Bilateral adrenalectomy* may be performed to remove another source of endogenous estrogens. *Hypophysectomy,* the removal of the anterior pituitary, removes the source of the adrenocorticotropic hormones as well as hormones that may directly stimulate the breast.

Patients with these operations require daily cortisone replacement to maintain life. Any lapse in the administration of cortisone may cause the patient to go into adrenal crisis, manifested by hypotension, elevated temperature, nausea, vomiting, diarrhea, abdominal pain, and weakness.

There may be mood swings as the cortisone is being regulated. The patient and those providing care need to be aware of the need for cortisone replacement and the need for increased dosage in stress, infection, accidents, etc. Replacement of the adrenal salt-regulating hormone may also be required. Florinef acetate is usually prescribed.

A woman should carry identification papers indicating the type of surgery she has had and the type of replacement therapy required. An identification emblem bracelet to alert others to the medical problem can be purchased from Medic Alert Foundation International, Turlock, California.

Chemical Ablative Methods.[93] These therapies are currently still mainly experimental. The aim is to create the same effect as surgical ablation by administration of medication, e.g., administration of *glucocorticoids* and *aminoglutethimide* are being studied as a way of inhibiting adrenal activity; *antiestrogens* as a way of inhibiting ovarian function, and *bromergocryptine* for inhibiting pituitary function.

Hormone Additive Therapy.[93] This in-

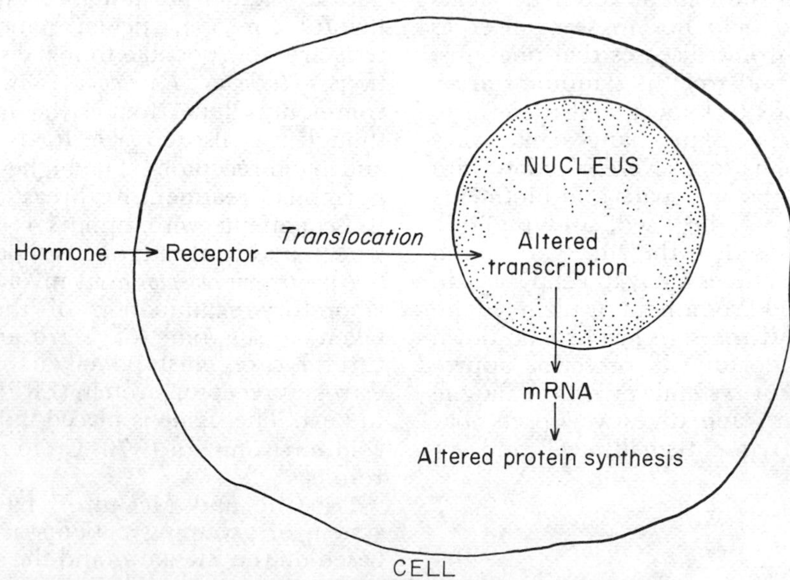

Figure 81–12. A simplified representation of the path of the biochemical reaction that occurs as a hormone (estrogen, progesterone) enters an ER positive cell. The hormone combines with the receptor, which then enters the nucleus and binds with DNA and other proteins. This alters gene expression patterns and induces transcription of specific mRNA's, thus affecting the basic behavior of the cell. This is a generalized figure. Each hormone has a characteristic biochemical reaction of its own.

TABLE 81–8. CHEMOTHERAPEUTIC AGENTS MOST COMMONLY USED IN THE TREATMENT OF BREAST CANCER

	Brand Name	Generic Name	Route of Administration	Toxicity
Alkylating agents	Thiotepa	Triethylenethiophosporamide	IV	Bone marrow depression
	Cytoxan	Cyclophosphamide	PO	Bone marrow depression, alopecia, cystitis, jaundice
	Melphalan	Phenylalanine mustard	PO	Bone marrow depression
Antimetabolites	Fluorouracil, 5-FU	5-Fluorouracil	IV	Gastrointestinal, bone marrow depression, alopecia
	Methotrexate	Methotrexate	PO	Gastrointestinal, liver damage, bone marrow depression
Others	Oncovin	Vincristine	IV	Gastrointestinal, peripheral neuritis, bone marrow depression
	Velban	Vinblastine	IV	Gastrointestinal, bone marrow depression, alopecia

From Haagensen, C. D.: *Diseases of the Breast,* 2nd ed.-Revised Reprint. Philadelphia: W. B. Saunders Company, 1971, p. 770.

volves the administration of several hormones, including estrogens, progesterone, synthetic androgens, and glucocorticoids to *estrogen receptor positive people.* As with chemical ablative methods, hormone additive therapy has not as yet been as successful as surgical ablation. A nonsurgical alternative is a very attractive possibility, however, and is receiving a great deal of research attention at the present time.

If nurses are thoroughly familiar with the rationale for treatment, they can be much more effective in assisting the patient and significant others in their problems.

CHEMOIMMUNOTHERAPY

Chemotherapy of breast cancer is a nonspecific treatment. Therefore, it has an effect on normally functioning cells such as those of the bone marrow and the epithelium of the gastrointestinal tract. It is important that the nurse be aware of the potentially serious side effects of such treatment.

See Chapter 23 for additional discussion of chemotherapy.

The principal types of chemotherapeutic agents used are alkylating agents and antimetabolites, but other drugs such as antibiotics and various alkaloids are also used. The most common agents currently employed are listed in Table 81–8, along with information about side effects. For detailed information about the nursing care of patients receiving these chemotherapeutic agents, see Chapter 23. Various combinations of drugs are used in treating metastatic breast cancer. Some combinations are presented in Table 81–9.

All of the chemical agents used today are toxic to the patient and are generally used after hormonal manipulations, except when life-threatening metastases occur. Six to 12 weeks are required before maximum benefits are apparent from hormonal therapy, but hormonal therapy offers a higher rate of remissions which last longer. An objective remission rate in 20 to 30 per cent of cases with disseminated mammary cancer may result from use of antitumor agents. 5-FU is a current drug of choice.

In the administration of drugs, an initial loading of the system is given to the level of mild

TABLE 81–9. CHEMOTHERAPY COMBINATIONS EMPLOYED FOR BREAST CANCER

Five-drug combinations:

5-Fluorouracil
Methotrexate
Cyclophosphamide
Prednisone
Testosterone

5-Fluorouracil
Methotrexate
Cyclophosphamide
Vincristine
Prednisone

Four-drug combinations:

5-Fluorouracil
Methotrexate
Cyclophosphamide
Vincristine

Three-drug combinations:

5-Fluorouracil
Vincristine
Prednisone

5-Fluorouracil
Cyclophosphamide
Prednisone

5-Fluorouracil
Methotrexate
Cyclophosphamide

From Lawrence, W. Jr., et al.: Management of metastatic carcinoma. *Surgery,* 82:173, 1977, p. 179.

toxicity. From this point, maintenance dosage is given. If the WBC falls below 3000 or other toxic effects develop, the drug is discontinued. Gastrointestinal symptoms, bleeding, dermatitis and alopecia may occur. Death can occur from bone marrow and liver failure.

The nurse is largely responsible for educating the patient concerning the correct dosage and administration of the drug, and for helping the patient to tolerate the distress of milder side effects while being alert for more serious symptoms.

The knowledge of immunologic processes in cancer is still inadequate. Markers such as carcinoembryonic antigen (CEA), ferritin, immune complexes, and especially estrogen receptors have strong potential as prognostic indicators. As a group, breast cancer patients portray reduced immunologic capacity, as do other cancer patients. *Immunotherapy* of breast cancer is relatively recent and may be classified as passive or active-specific or nonspecific. Nonspecific immunotherapy consists of such agents as BCG, Corynebacterium parvum, a methanol extractable residue of BCG or levamisole. Passive immunotherapy consists of transfer factor from leucocytes of healthy adult donors. No conclusive data about these methods are yet available.[13]

AUGMENTATION MAMMOPLASTY[33]

Augmentation mammoplasty (also spelled mammaplasty) has become an increasingly popular cosmetic surgical procedure performed on women's breasts. The procedure involves using implants to either: (a) enlarge underdeveloped breasts (micromastia), or (b) reconstruct breasts following removal of benign lesions. While reconstruction following surgical removal of malignant lesions has been performed, the procedure is still experimental. As with other cosmetic procedures, it is not uncommon for nurses to be asked about the procedure by persons interested in having it performed.

Implants typically consist of a thin, seamless, Silastic envelope filled with an inert dextran, saline, or silicone fluid. Silicone fluid is commonly used because it gives the most realistic result. The implant is placed in a surgically created pocket between the breast tissue and the pectoral fascia. The most common surgical approach is an inframammary approach, at the base of the breast.

Augmentation mammoplasty is most often performed in a hospital's surgical day-care unit under short-term general anesthesia. Upon completion of the surgery, the patient is dressed in a bulky, circumferential, figure-8 bandage that leaves the nipples exposed, to check for swelling or hematomas. Tight bandages, unusual bruises, overt bleeding, and excessive pain or swelling should be immediately reported to the surgeon. Exercises may be prescribed postoperatively and the patient is given instructions about activity limitations. Typically, the patient is advised to also wear an unwired bra night and day for several weeks.

Because the implant is a foreign substance, the body forms a fibrous capsule to wall it off. This capsule of scar tissue sometimes contracts excessively, then requiring either *surgical* or *manual capsulotomy. Infection* and *hematomas* may contribute to *excessive capsular contraction,* and thus every attempt is made to prevent these complications.

BIBLIOGRAPHY (Chapter 81)

1. A better way to check a breast. *Emergency Medicine,* 10:87, Oct. 1978.
2. A real pain in the breast. *Emergency Medicine,* 11:197, Jan. 1979.
3. Achterberg, J., I. Collerain, and P. Craig: A possible relationship between cancer, mental retardation and mental disorders. *Social Science and Medicine,* 12:155, May 1978.
4. Ackerman, L. A., and J. A. Regato: *Cancer, Diagnosis, Treatment and Prognosis,* St. Louis: C. V. Mosby Company, 1970.
5. Age and death in breast cancer. *British Medical Journal,* 1:211, Jan. 1979.
6. American Cancer Society. *1979 Cancer Facts and Figures.* American Cancer Society, 1978.
7. Anthony, C. J.: Risk factors associated with breast cancer. *Nurse Practitioner,* 3:31, July–Aug. 1978.
8. Attiyeh, F. F., et al.: Axillary micrometastases and macrometastases in carcinoma of the breast. *Surgery in Obstetrics and Gynecology,* June 1977, p. 839.
9. Baker, R. R.: Preoperative assessment of the patient with breast cancer. *Surgical Clinics of North America,* 58:681, Aug. 1978.
10. Bailar, J. C.: Mammography: A contrary view. *Annals of Internal Medicine,* 84:77, 1976.
11. Baltruch, H. J. F.: Einige Psychosomatische Aspekte der Krebskrankheit unter Berucksichtigung Psychotherapeutischer Gesichtspunkte. *Zeitschrift fur Psycosomatische Medizin und Psychoanalyse,* 15(1):31, January 1969.
12. Barckley, V.: Enough time for good nursing. *Nursing Outlook,* 12:44, Apr. 1964.
13. Barna, B. P., and S. D. Deodhar: Immunology tumor markers and breast cancer. *Surgical Clinics of North America,* 58:693, Aug. 1978.
14. Bates, B.: *A Guide to Physical Examination.* Philadelphia: J. B. Lippincott Co., 1974.
15. Black, M. M., H. P. Leis, and C. S. Kwon: The breast cancer controversy. *JAMA,* 237(10):970, 1977.
16. Bloom, J. R., R. D. Ross, and G. Burnell: The effect of social support on patient adjustment after breast surgery. *Patient Counseling and Health Education,* 1:50, Fall 1978.
17. Bonadonna, G., et al.: Combination chemotherapy as an adjuvant treatment in operable breast cancer. *New England Journal of Medicine,* 294:405, Feb. 1976.
18. Branda, J. F., Cigtay, O. S., and Powell, D. E.: Xeromammography and histology of common breast lesions. *American Family Physician,* 15:102, Feb. 1977.

18a. Breast cancer, fear and facts. *Time,* November 4, 1974, pp. 107–110,

19. Bross, I. D. J.: Possible hazards of radiologic surveillance of high risk groups. *New England Journal of Medicine,* 296:232, 1977.
20. Burdick, D.: Breast cancer: Patient rehabilitation. *Consultant,* 16:141, Aug. 1976.
21. Busehke, F., and R. G. Parker: *Radiation Therapy in Cancer Management.* New York, Grune and Stratton, 1972.
22. Bush, D. J.: Appraising current therapy for breast cancer. 2. Irradiation. *Postgraduate Medicine,* 60:151, Aug. 1976.
23. Clinical capsules: How diet can promote cancer. *RN,* 42:113, Jan. 1979.
24. Clinical highlights: Only diligent and thorough breast examinations are adequate. *Hospital Medicine,* 14:122, May 1978.
25. Cooperman, A. M., et al.: Partial mastectomy. *Surgical Clinics of North America,* 58:737, Aug. 1978.
26. Cooperman, A. M., and C. B. Esselstyn: Breast cancer: An overview. *Surgical Clinics of North America,* 58:659, Aug. 1978.
27. Crile, G., Jr.: Axioms on cysts and benign tumors of the breast. *Hospital Medicine,* 13:56, May 1977.
28. Crile, G., Jr.: Nipple discharge: Diagnostic guidelines. *Hospital Medicine,* 14:82, July 1978.
29. Culliton, B. J.: Cancer Institute unilaterally issues new restrictions on mammography. *Science,* 196:853, 1977.
30. Culliton, B. J.: Mammography controversy: NIH's entree into evaluating technology. *Science,* 198:171, 1977.
31. Dinner, M. I., and C. R. Peters: Breast reconstruction following mastectomy. *Surgical Clinics of North America,* 58:851, Aug. 1978.
31a. Dunphy, J. E., and L. W. Way: *Current Surgical Diagnosis and Treatment,* 3rd ed. Los Altos, Calif. Lange Medical Publications, 1977.
32. Egan, R. L.: Mammography. *American Journal of Nursing,* 66:108, Jan. 1966.
33. Finn, K. L.: Augmentation mammoplasty: The cosmetic surgery with a lift. *Nursing 79:* 9:60, Feb. 1979.
33a. Fisher, B., et al.: L-phenylalanine mustard (L-Pam) in the management of primary breast cancer. *New England Journal of Medicine,* 292:117, Jan. 1975.
34. Fitzpatrick, G.: Caring for the patient with cancer of the breast. *Bedside Nursing,* Feb. 1970.
35. Francis, G. M.: Cancer: The emotional component. *American Journal of Nursing,* 69:1677, Aug. 1969.
36. Goldsmith, H. S.: Milk-rejection sign of breast cancer. *Nursing Digest,* 4:37, Jan.–Feb. 1976.
37. Gorringe, R., M. M. Lee, and A. Voda: The mammography controversy: A case for breast self-examination. *Journal of Obstetric, Gynecologic and Neonatal Nursing,* 7:7, July–Aug. 1978.
38. Greenberg, D. S.: X-ray mammography — Background to a decision. *The New England Journal of Medicine,* 295:739, Sept. 1976.
39. Greer, S., and T. Morris: The study of psychological factors in breast cancer: Problems of method. *Social Science and Medicine,* 12A:129, May 1978.
40. Gribbons, C. A., and M. A. Aliapoulios: Treatment for advanced breast carcinoma. *American Journal of Nursing,* 72:678, Apr. 1972.
41. Gros, C., et al.: Approche Psychosomatique des Affections Mammaires. *Revue de Medecine Psychosomatique* et de Psychologie Medical. 11(2):239–240, 1969.
42. Haagensen, C. D.: *Diseases of the Breast,* 2nd ed. Philadelphia: W. B. Saunders Co., 1971.
43. Harrell, H. C.: To lose a breast. *American Journal of Nursing,* 72:676, Apr. 1972.
44. Hermann, R. E., and E. Steiger: Modified radical mastectomy. *Surgical Clinics of North America,* 58:743, Aug. 1978.
45. Hermel, M. B., and M. G. Murdock.: Microdose mammography. *Cancer,* 38:1947, 1976.
46. Holleb, A. I.: Restoring confidence in mammography. *Cancer,* 26:376, 1976.
47. Hoover, R., et al.: Menopausal estrogens and breast cancer. *The New England Journal of Medicine,* 295:401, Aug. 1976.
48. Hubay, C. A., et al.: Pregnancy and breast cancer. *Surgical Clinics of North America,* 58:819, Aug. 1978.
49. Kemmerly, S. L.: Breast cancer, confronting one's changed image. What I've learned about mastectomy. *American Journal of Nursing,* 77:1430, Sept. 1977.
50. Kent, S.: Diet, hormones, and breast cancer. *Geriatrics,* 34:83, Jan. 1979.
51. Kern, W. H.: Morphologic and clinical aspects of estrogen receptors in carcinoma of the breast. *Surgery, Gynecology and Obstetrics,* 148:240, Feb. 1979.
52. Klagsbrun, S. C.: Cancer, emotions and nurses. *American Journal of Psychiatry,* 126(9):1237, 1970.
53. Klagsbrun, S. C.: Communications in the treatment of cancer. *American Journal of Nursing,* 71:944, May 1971.
54. Koenig, R. R.: Fatal illness: A study of social service needs. *Social Work,* 4:85, 1968.
55. Lawrence, W. Jr., et al.: Clinical management of metastatic breast carcinoma. *Surgery,* 82:173, Aug. 1977.
56. Leis, H. P., Jr.: Bilateral breast cancer. *Surgical Clinics of North America,* 58:833, Aug. 1978.
57. Leis, H. P.: Breast cancer, patients at risk. *Cancer Detection and Prevention,* 1:311, 1976.
58. Leis, H. P., Jr.: Diagnosis of breast cancer. *Cancer Journal for Clinicians,* 27:209, July–Aug. 1977.
59. Leis, H. P., Jr.: Surgical approach to breast cancer. *New York State Journal of Medicine,* August 1, 1973.
60. Lesnick, G. J.: Detection of breast cancer in young women. *J.A.M.A.,* 237(10):967, 1977.
61. Leven, M. B., et al.: Primary radiation therapy for operable carcinoma of the breast. *Surgical Clinics of North America,* 58:767, Aug. 1978.
62. Levene, M. D.: Breast cancer. Alternative therapy. A new role for radiation therapy. *American Journal of Nursing,* 77:1443, Sept. 1977.
63. Livingston, R. B., and S. K. Carter: *Single Agents in Cancer Chemotherapy.* New York: IFI/Plenum.
64. Lokich, J. J.: CEA: A monitor of therapy for breast and colon cancer. *American Family Physician,* 17:173, Apr. 1978.
65. Lyman, M.: Routine breast biopsy? Not when it's for me! *RN,* 40:61, Aug. 1977.
66. Lynch, H. T., et al.: Familial cancer: Implications for surgical management of high risk patients. *Surgery,* 83:104, Jan. 1978.
67. MacBryde, C. M., and R. S. Blacklow: *Signs and Symptoms: Applied Pathologic Physiology and Clinical Interpretation,* 5th ed. Philadelphia: J. B. Lippincott Co., 1970.
68. Mahoney, L. J., et al.: Early diagnosis of breast cancer. *Canadian Medical Association Journal,* 116:1127, 1977.
69. Mamaril, A. P.: Preventing complications after radical mastectomy. *American Journal of Nursing,* 74:2000, Nov. 1974.
70. Marcus, S. L., and C. C. Marcus, (Eds.): *Advances in Obstetrics and Gynecology.* Baltimore: Williams and Wilkins Co., 1967.
71. Margarey, C. J., P. B. Todd and P. J. Blizard: Psychosocial factors influencing delay in breast self-examination in women with symptoms of breast cancer. *Social Science and Medicine,* 11:229, Pergamon Press, 1977.
72. McCorkle, M. R.: Coping with physical symptoms in metastatic breast cancer. *American Journal of Nursing,* 73:1034, June 1973.

73. McGuire, W.: Current status of estrogen receptors in human breast cancer. *Cancer,* 36:638, Aug. 1975.
74. Morris, T. B., H. S. Green, and P. White: Psychological and social adjustment to cancer. A two year follow-up study. *Cancer,* 40:2381, 1977.
75. Nomura, A., et al: Epidemiologic characteristics of benign breast disease. *American Journal of Epidemiology,* 105:505, June 1977.
76. Ochsner, A.: Diseases of the breast. *Nursing Digest,* 4:5, Mar.–Apr. 1976.
77. Osborne, C. K. and W. L. McGuire: Current use of steroid hormone receptor assays in the treatment of breast cancer. *Surgical Clinics of North America,* 58:777, Aug. 1978.
78. Peck, D. R., and R. M. Lowman: Mammography, Current Application. *JAMA,* 236:1886, 1976.
79. Pennisi, V. R., and A. Capozzi: The incidence of obscure cancer in subcutaneous mastectomy: Results of a national survey. *Plastic and Reconstructive Surgery,* 56:9, July 1975.
80. Pennisi, V. R.: Subcutaneous mastectomy and fibrocystic disease of the breast. *Clinics in Plastic Surgery,* 3:205, Apr. 1976.
81. Pennisi, V. R., et al.: Subcutaneous mastectomy data: A preliminary report. *Plastic and Reconstructive Surgery,* 59:53, Jan. 1977.
82. Prognostic patterns in breast cancer. *Emergency Medicine,* 9:59, Feb., 1977.
83. Puhaty, H. D.: Breast cancer. Confronting one's changed image: Two rehabilitative approaches. *American Journal of Nursing,* 77:1437, Sept., 1977.
84. Quint, J. C.: The impact of Mastectomy. *American Journal of Nursing,* 63:88, Nov. 1963.
85. Reimer, R. R.: Chemotherapy of recurrent breast cancer. *Surgical Clinics of North America,* 58:843, Aug. 1978.
86. Robbins, G. F.: Indications for radical and extended mastectomy. *Surgical Clinics of North America,* 58:755, Aug. 1978.
87. Robbins, S. L., and M. Angell: *Basic Pathology,* 2nd ed. Philadelphia: W. B. Saunders Co., 1976.
88. Robbins, S. L., and R. S. Cotran: *Pathologic Basis of Disease,* 2nd ed. Philadelphia: W. B. Saunders Co., 1979.
89. Rubens, R. D.: The current status of adjuvant chemotherapy. *Surgical Clinics of North America,* 58:789, Aug. 1978.
90. Rubin, P.: Current cancer concepts, carcinoma of the breast. Stage 1: Surgical spectrum. American Cancer Society, 1967.
91. Rosenblatt, R.: Mammography and other procedures in breast cancer diagnosis. *Consultant,* 18:121, Jan. 1978.
92. Sadowsky, N. L., L. Kalisher, G. White, et al.: Radiologic detection of breast cancer. *New England Journal of Medicine,* 294:370, 1976.
93. Santen, R. J.: Hormone responsiveness in breast cancer. *Consultant,* 18:47, May 1978.
94. Sayler, C., J. F. Eagan, and R. Raines: Mammographic screening. Value in diagnosis of early breast cancer. *JAMA,* Aug. 22, 1977, p. 872.
95. Schneiderman, M. A., and L. M. Axtell: Deaths among female patients with carcinoma of the breast treated by a surgical procedure only. *Surgery, Gynecology and Obstetrics,* 148:193, Feb. 1979.
96. Schwartz, M. R.: Breast cancer. Alternative therapy: Hormone receptor assay. *American Journal of Nursing,* 77:1445, Sept., 1977.
97. Screening for breast cancer. Report from Edinburgh breast screening clinic. *British Journal of Medicine,* July 1978, p. 175.
98. Shaper, S.: New York health insurance plan. *Cancer,* 39:2772, 1977.
99. Shipp, R. H.: Breast examination with pap smears. *American Family Physician,* 14:119, Oct. 1976.
100. Shirley, R. L.: Questions and answers: Hormones and breast cancer. *Consultant,* 17:17, December, 1977.
101. Shukla, H. S., et al.: The significance of mammary skin edema in non-inflammatory breast cancer. *Annals of Surgery,* 189:53, Jan. 1979.
102. Sickles, E. A.: Radiation risks of mammography. *Western Journal of Medicine,* 125:493, 1976.
103. Simon, N.: Breast cancer induced by radiation. *JAMA,* 237:789, 1977.
104. Spence, D. P., et al.: Lexical correlates of cervical cancer. *Social Science and Medicine,* 12:141, May 1978.
105. Spingarn, N. D.: Breast cancer: New choices. *Nursing Digest,* 4:33, Jan.–Feb. 1976.
106. Strax, P.: Results of mass screening for breast cancer in 50,000 examinations. *Cancer,* 37:30, 1976.
107. Strax, P.: Evaluation of screening programs for the early diagnosis of breast cancer. *Surgical Clinics of North America,* 58:667, Aug. 1978.
108. Swartz, H. M., and B. A. Reichling: The risks of mammograms. *JAMA,* 237:965, 1977.
109. Tashima, C. K.: The many opinions in management of breast cancer. *Geriatrics* 31:97, June 1976.
110. Thomas, S. G., and M. M. Yates: Breast cancer. Confronting one's changed image: Breast reconstruction after mastectomy. *American Journal of Nursing,* 77:1438, Sept. 1977.
111. Todd, A.: Breast cancer, prevention: Prophylactic mastectomy. *American Journal of Nursing,* 77:1447, Sept. 1977.
112. Tully, J. P., and B. Wagner: Breast cancer: Helping the mastectomy patient live life fully. *Nursing 78,* 8:18, Jan. 1978.
113. Turnbull, E.: Breast cancer: Prevention: Breast examination practices. *American Journal of Nursing,* 77:1450, Sept. 1977.
114. U.S. Department of Health, Education, and Welfare: Progress against breast cancer (Pamphlet). DHEW Publication No. (NIH) 78–1621. National Cancer Institute.
115. U.S. Department of Health, Education, and Welfare: Breast Cancer: Annotated Bibliography of Public, Patient, and Professional Information and Educational Materials (Booklet). NIH Publication # 79–2002. National Cancer Institute.
116. Venet, L.: The clinical examination in mass screening for breast cancer. *Cancer Detection and Prevention,* 1:365, 1976.
117. Weinstein, S., et al.: Phantoms following breast amputation. *Neuropsychologica,* 8(2):185, Apr. 1970.
118. Wilson, J. L.: Breast. *In* Dunphy, J. E., and L. W. Way: *Current Surgical Diagnosis and Treatment,* 3rd ed. Los Altos, Calif.: Lange Medical Publications, 1977.
119. Winkler, W. A.: Breast cancer: Confronting one's changed image: Choosing the prosthesis and clothing. *American Journal of Nursing,* 77:1433, Sept. 1977.
120. Wolfe, J. N.: Value of mammography for breast cancer. *Postgraduate Medicine,* 61:21, Jan. 1977.
121. Woods, J. E.: Experience with subcutaneous mastectomy. *Surgery,* 80:422, Oct. 1976.
122. Zislis, J. N.: Rehabilitation of the cancer patient. *Geriatrics,* 25(3):150, 1970.

UNIT XXII

NURSING PEOPLE EXPERIENCING DISTURBANCES OF THE REPRODUCTIVE SYSTEM

INTRODUCTION AND STUDY GUIDE

People experiencing disorders of the reproductive system and the closely related (especially in the male) urinary system are often reluctant to tell anyone about their problems because of embarrassment and possibly fear that the private sexual aspects of their lives will be discussed. They may be worried that they will have to disclose more of themselves than they want to. Thus, often, unless symptoms become acute, disorders of the reproductive system may not be brought to the early attention of health professionals.

In helping people who are experiencing disturbances of the reproductive system, nurses are concerned with the physical components of the problem as well as the emotional and social components that are inevitably involved. Special care and respect need be given to patients who are seeking medical attention for disorders that involve the genitalia. These patients are likely to feel somewhat embarrassed and threatened by this invasion of what may be the most private aspect of their lives. Encouraging decision making and showing interest in the patient as a person, while always important, are especially necessary in this situation. As always, it is helpful for a patient to maintain as much control as possible over the environment and experiences.

Competence in management of the technical aspects of care and scrupulous attention to asepsis, combined with preparation and instruction concerning tests, routines, and upcoming procedures or treatments, give the patient added reassurance in these awkward circumstances.

Health professionals are often required to discuss reproduction and sexual concerns with clients. If they are unable to do this openly, comfortably, and nonjudgmentally, they should make an appropriate referral to someone who can. At the same time, such individuals would do well to find ways to clarify their own feelings and attitudes concerning sexuality and thus increase their professional competency. We, as nurses, are not in the business of evaluating others' behavior. Instead, our purpose is to assist others to achieve life satisfactions in ways comfortable and desirable for each individual. This unit is designed to help you provide such integrated nursing care.

Chapter 82 includes an overview of the anatomy and physiology of the normal male reproductive system; discussions of common dysfunctions of the male reproductive system; their diagnosis and treatment; and typical nursing care. Bibliography for this chapter is located at the end of the chapter.

Chapter 83 reviews anatomy of the female reproductive system and the physiology of menstruation and discusses the menopause, menstrual abnormalities, and their management. Bibliography for Chapters 83 through 88 is located at the end of Chapter 88.

Chapter 84 discusses diagnostic and treatment modalities used for dysfunctions of the female reproductive system and presents nursing care appropriate for women experiencing such problems.

Chapter 85 considers inflammatory and infectious problems such as leukorrhea, vaginitis, vulvitis, cervicitis, pelvic inflammatory disease, and venereal diseases.

Chapter 86 reviews benign gynecologic problems including tumors of the lower genital tract, fistulas, uterine displacements, and relaxation of the pelvic organs.

Chapter 87 discusses malignancy of the lower genital tract.

Finally, *Chapter 88* discusses birth control and related issues and disorders such as ectopic pregnancy, infertility, contraception, birth control measures, sterilization, abortion, and sexual assault.

After studying the material presented in this unit you can expect to be able to:

- ▶ Identify the anatomic features of the male and female reproductive systems
- ▶ Identify signs and symptoms of common dysfunctions of male and female reproductive systems
- ▶ Interpret the rationale for diagnostic tests and treatment of reproductive systems to patients and their significant others
- ▶ Teach patients and their significant others appropriate self-examination techniques and the early warning signs of health problems of the reproductive systems
- ▶ Use knowledge of the normal and abnormal function of the reproductive systems in teaching health care concerning reproductive systems to patients and their significant others
- ▶ Examine the psychosocial aspects of dysfunction of the reproductive systems and provide opportunity for patients and their significant others to receive appropriate counseling
- ▶ Plan nursing care for people experiencing problems of the reproductive systems

While working to achieve the above objectives, you may find it useful to use the following *study suggestions*.

1. Make a list of all the specific terms used in this unit and in your own words write a definition for each one. Perhaps you would prefer to use a small card for each term.

2. Since the material presented in this chapter is associated with human sexuality and because sexuality is an area associated with strong opinions and beliefs, spend some time considering your own knowledge, attitudes, and beliefs about sexuality. For example,

a. Do you know what physiologic changes occur during human "love making"?

b. What is your *first* response when considering, for example:

premarital sex	pregnancy
multiple sexual partners	extramarital sex
intercourse	frigidity
oral sex	impotence
homosexuality	orgasm
abortion	rape
contraception	prostitution
vasectomy	tubal ligation
venereal disease	"love shops"
heterosexuality	masturbation

Your *first* response will give you some idea of what *your* basic attitudes are. While these topics are not discussed in this unit specifically, they may affect the people you care for. Your attitudes about these issues will, unless you are aware of them, influence the nursing care you are able to offer. Remember that the moral code you choose to follow in expressing your own sexuality may differ from those chosen by others. If you recognize in your initial reactions a lack of knowledge about any of these topics, perhaps extra reading about them is indicated.

3. Consider each of the procedures (diagnostic and therapeutic) described in this unit. Write down *all* the questions you would want answered if *you* were undergoing each procedure, *but which you would be rather reluctant to ask*. This may give you some idea of what your patients may feel.

CHAPTER 82

DISORDERS OF THE MALE REPRODUCTIVE SYSTEM

by Rosemary Pittman, M.S., C.R.N., F.N.P.*

The structures of the male reproductive system include the penis, the prostate, the scrotum, the testis, the epididymis, the vas deferens, the seminal vesicles and the ejaculatory ducts (Fig. 82–1).

THE PENIS

Anatomy and Function

The penis is primarily a sexual organ with a urethral pathway for elimination of urine and the ejaculate through the urethral meatus. The penis is composed of the two corpora cavernosa and the corpus spongiosum, which contains the urethra, whose diameter is 8 to 9 mm. Each corpus is enclosed in a fascial sheath (tunica albuginea), and all are surrounded by a thick fibrous envelope known as Buck's fascia. The phenomenon of erection is caused by engorgement of the cavernous structures with blood as a result of varied stimuli. The distal portion of the corpus spongiosum forms the *glans penis*. The expanded proximal portion of the glans is known as the corona and its junction with the corpora cavernosa is the coronal sulcus; a flap of skin, the prepuce or foreskin, covers the glans. The skin of the penis is dark, nonhair-bearing, thin and loose, allowing considerable distention (Fig. 82–1).

There is wide variation in the normal size of the penis. Striking discrepancies between penile size and age may indicate hypoplasia or hyperplasia. Penile hypoplasia is a manifestation of eunuchoidism occurring before puberty, or a feature of intersexuality. The distinction between a hypoplastic penis with hypospadias and a hyperplastic clitoris may be difficult to make without surgical or histologic examination. Usually, penile hyperplasia is seen only before normal puberty and is commonly caused by tumors of the pineal gland or hypothalamus, tumors arising from the Leydig cells of the testis, or tumors of the adrenal gland.

Inspection and Palpation†

Inspection and palpation will reveal the most common disorders of the penis. In boys, these are redundancy, adhesions, phimosis, paraphimosis, posthitis and balanitis, stenosis or stricture, ulceration of the external meatus, herpes, chafing, scabies, pediculi, verrucae, and syphilis. Early circumcision eliminates the problem of redundancy of the prepuce. If circumcision is not performed, the parents should be taught to retract the prepuce at an early age. The condition is important only when the prepuce cannot be retracted. It has been believed that irritant debris may cause penile cancer, since Jews who have been neonatally circumcised almost never have penile cancer. However, many practicing pediatricians are not convinced that past research indicates the need for circumcision for other than religious reasons. Adhesions existing at birth may be separated by preputial retraction or by stretching so that the prepuce can be freely retracted.

Dysfunctions

Paraphimosis. A tight foreskin, once retracted, may become edematous thus impeding the circulation of the glans, with resultant swelling. Manual replacement may be attempted but surgical incision may be necessary.

---

*Margaret H. Parkinson and Karen C. Sorensen prepared discussions of the following topics in this chapter: penile prostheses, BPH (treatment section), prostatic cancer, testicular tumors, testicular self-examination, catheterization and catheter care, and nursing concerns in human reproductive dysfunction.

†Refer to Chapter 15 (p. 365) for the techniques of examining the male genitalia.

Herpes Progenitalis. Today, sexually transmitted diseases are known to include candidiasis, herpes I or II, cytomegalic inclusion diseases, venereal warts, infection of Chlamydia and ureaplasma (formerly called T. Mycoplasma), trichomoniasis, scabies, and pediculosis.[3] A small group of vesicles with an erythematous base is frequently found on the glans or prepuce. These may rupture, producing superficial ulcers, heal in about a week or serve as a point of entry for other organisms. Treatment consists of local cleanliness, although tetracycline has sometimes been used.

Herpesvirus Hominis Type II. This may produce a penile lesion of clear vesicles much like a cold sore. If a man with the lesion has sexual contact, the woman may become infected. There is no known cure and, during the acute stage, the disease is very painful. Symptomatic treatment with pain medicine and local cortisone may be used. If a child is delivered when the woman has the disease, it definitely will not survive. Because of the severity of the infection in women, men with a herpes infection on the penis should abstain from intercourse.

Cytomegalic Inclusion Disease. Cytomegalic inclusion disease is a disease of the neonatal period, characterized by hepatosplenomegaly and often by microcephaly and mental or motor retardation. Candidiasis and trichomoniasis are discussed in Chapter 85.

Penile Ulcers. *Syphilitic Chancre*. This is the

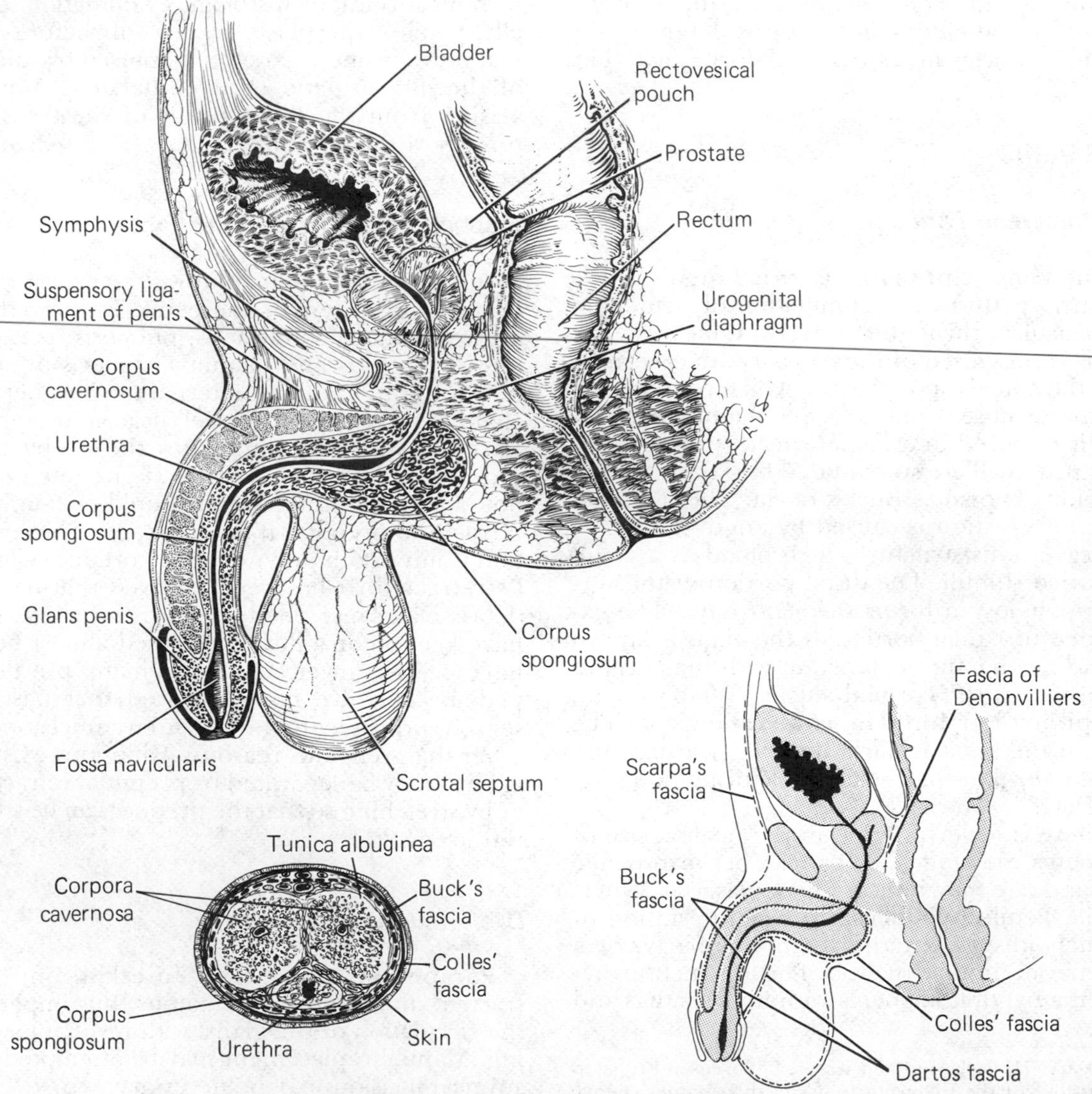

Figure 82-1. Male anatomy. Fascial planes of the lower genitourinary tract. *Bottom right*: Relations of the bladder, prostate, seminal vesicles, penis, urethra, and scrotal contents. *Bottom left*: Transverse section through the penis. The paired upper structures are the corpora cavernosa. The single lower body surrounding the urethra is the corpus spongiosum. (From Smith, D. R.: *General Urology,* 9th ed. Los Altos, Calif.: Lange Medical Publications, 1978, p. 9.)

primary lesion of syphilis and commonly occurs on the corona or the inner side of the prepuce. It begins as a silvery papule that gradually becomes a superficial ulcer containing the treponema pallidum. The chancre is painless, usually round and with a smooth, slightly raised border. The regional lymph nodes may also be moderately enlarged. The ulcer is extremely contagious and the organisms may penetrate the unbroken skin. The diagnosis may be confirmed by a dark-field microscopic examination, since the lesion appears before the serology becomes positive. (Syphilis is discussed in more detail on pp. 1896–1900.)

Chancroid. Another type of lesion producing a penile ulcer is the chancroid or soft chancre caused by the bacillus *Hemophilus ducreyi*. The border is irregular, the center is necrotic, and there is profuse suppuration. In some cases, the regional lymph nodes become swollen, tender and suppurative. Chancroid is much more universally prevalent than syphilis. It is a predominantly local and regional disease of rather superficial nature, contacted generally during coitus and fostered by poor genital hygiene. Most cases are adequately treated by cleansing, by protecting the lesions and by using sulfonamides that have no masking effect on the appearance of syphilis.

Lymphogranuloma Venereum. This is caused by a rickettsia-like organism, *Miyagawanella lymphogranulomatosis*, and is another venereal disease involving the lymphatic system. The initial lesion on the penis is frequently overlooked. This infection manifests itself in a variety of ways: bubo formation, ulceration, elephantiasis of the genitalia, and rectal stricture. Diagnosis is aided by a skin test with Frei antigen. The disease, which occurs throughout the world, especially in tropical and subtropical areas, is endemic in the southern United States and affects the most sexually promiscuous. The course of the disease is often long and disability is great, but the disease is essentially nonfatal. It is communicable when active lesions are present. Specific treatment varies with the stage of the disease. Sulfadiazine is the drug of choice in the bubo phase; tetracyclines may be orally administered for proctitis and other ulcerative lesions.

Condyloma Accuminatum. Venereal warts occur on the corona or in the retroglandular sulcus. In the presence of moisture, secondary infection results in ulceration. Excessive growth and ulceration must be distinguished from carcinoma by biopsy. *Condyloma latum*, a flat and warty growth, is a secondary syphilid and is highly contagious. Treatment consists of proper hygienic measures. Circumcision may be required and, for the smaller clusters, local cauterization by either electrocoagulation or the application of a 2 per cent alcoholic solution of podophyllin may be necessary.

Gonorrhea. In North America, gonorrhea is presently an epidemic disease affecting 2,000,000 Americans each year. A man has a 20 to 50 per cent chance of contracting gonorrhea from a single sexual exposure to an infected partner. The risks of gonorrhea transmission during oral-genital or anal intercourse are not known exactly but they probably are the same as with vaginal intercourse. Chances of getting an infection increase with repeated exposure to an infected partner.

There is a newly recognized type of gonorrhea that cannot be cured by ampicillin or penicillin because it produces a penicillin-destroying enzyme. It is called *Penicillinase Producing Neisseria Gonorrheae*. The treatment of choice is spectinomycin. This drug should be reserved for patients with this strain of gonorrhea so that resistance does not develop. The patient should be reassessed by culture 2 weeks after the initial treatment. This strain of gonorrhea is not prevalent, but it should be suspected whenever the more usual treatment fails.[3]

Symptoms. Most men notice symptoms 3 to 5 days after the infecting sexual contact. It may be up to 17 days, however, before symptoms occur. At first, a thin clear mucus appears at the meatal opening. Within a day or two, the discharge becomes heavy, thick and creamy. It is usually white but may be yellow or green. The lips of the meatus become swollen and stand out from the glans. Most men feel pain and a burning sensation in the penis or at the meatus during urination. The pain can be quite severe and urinating may be difficult. There may be pus and blood in the urine. About 30 to 40 per cent of infected men also have enlarged and tender lymph glands in the groin. Gonorrheal infection of the anus and rectum, called gonorrheal proctitis, can develop in homosexual men who have anal intercourse with an infected male partner. Most men who have gonococcal proctitis do not have symptoms and can unknowingly give the infection to their male partners. From 10 to 22 per cent of males who have gonorrhea may be asymptomatic.

Complications. If treatment of gonococcal urethritis is delayed after symptoms appear, the infection spreads up the urethra and pain on urination becomes more severe and is felt in the whole penis.

After about 2 weeks, symptoms of urethritis begin to disappear on their own. However, the man can still infect his sexual partner. After 2 to 3 weeks of untreated infection, the bacteria invade the posterior urethra and the prostate gland and a prostatic abscess may develop. In about 20 per cent of men who remain untreated for more than a month, the bacteria spread down the vas deferens and reach the epididymis, causing gonococcal epididymitis. If the infection is not treated, testicles will become involved and the man will become sterile.

Arthritis is occasionally a complication of gonorrhea. In about 75 per cent of patients with gonococcal arthritis, skin lesions appear at the onset of bacteremia as papules, then become hemorrhagic pustules, principally in the extremities. Of these patients, 40 per cent have positive blood cultures. If gonococcal arthritis is suspected, cervical cultures from women and urethral cultures from men should be obtained. Pharyngeal cultures should be obtained from both sexes.[2]

Female sex partners should always be treated and male sex partners of persons with gonorrhea must be examined and treated because of the high prevalence of nonspecific urethritis in such men.

Treatment. The regular treatment is with 4.8 million units aqueous procaine penicillin G intramuscularly, with 1.0 Gm. probenecid orally, preferably given 30 minutes prior to injection. The injection is divided into two doses and given in different sites. Oral treatment is with ampicillin 3.5 Gm. orally with 1.0 Gm. probenecid orally at the same time.

For patients in whom penicillin is contraindicated because of allergy or in whom penicillin or ampicillin has been ineffective, spectinomycin 2.0 Gm. intramuscularly may be given in males or tetracycline 1.5 Gm. orally, then 0.5 Gm. orally four times daily for four days (a total of 9.5 Gm.) may be administered.

Posthitis and Balanitis. These are inflammations of the prepuce and glans penis, caused by irritation and invasion by some organism. The initial treatment is cleansing with mild soap and water, followed by application of a drying powder to minimize moisture. Antibiotic therapy will help to control local infection. Circumcision may be necessary.

Stricture of the urethral meatus is usually a congenital malformation.

Stenosis of the external meatus is common and should be sought in all newborn males. It may be congenital or may be acquired after circumcision. The initial symptoms are bloody spotting and crusting of the meatus, which is caused by infection and ulceration just within the opening. Meatotomy is indicated, after which the parents must be taught to carefully dilate the urethra once every day for 2 weeks and at lengthening intervals for 2 more weeks.

Congenital urethral stricture occurs occasionally in male infants. Symptoms may be those of obstruction (small caliber urinary stream, hyperdistended bladder or secondary infection, fever, dysuria). Every child with these symptoms should be examined cystoscopically. Surgical repair is usually necessary.

Urethritis. This is manifested by redness, edema and eversion of the edges of the meatus. A variable amount of pus may be discharged from the urethra. Lymph channels in the dorsum of the penis, as well as the inguinal lymph glands, may be tender and palpable. Micturition and erection may be painful. The cause is difficult to determine. Gonorrhea must be excluded by slide and culture, as it is the most common cause. Urethritis may be demonstrated by increased urethral discharge, or in its absence, discharge in the morning and increased leukocytes in the morning's first urine or in the urethral smear. The presence of 15 or more leukocytes per high power field indicates the need for treatment. A gram stain can be done to rule out gonorrhea.[3,2] Nonspecific urethritis may be part of a triad, along with conjunctivitis and arthritis in Reiter's disease. Fifty per cent of nonspecific urethritis has been found to be associated with *Chlamydia trachomatis*. Treatment is with tetracycline. Sex partners should also be treated. If symptoms recur, the individual should be treated again with tetracycline.

Common Congenital Defects. *Hypospadias*. In the fetus, the urethral meatus may develop so that it occurs on the ventral surface of the glans, on the shaft or at the penoscrotal junction. This is one of the most common urogenital anomalies and requires early attention, the treatment depending on the location. In *epispadias*, the urethral meatus opens dorsally on the glans, on the shaft or at the penoscrotal junction.

Priapism. This is a prolonged, persistent penile erection without sexual desire, usually accompanied by pain. Local mechanical factors such as thrombosis, hemorrhage, neoplasm or inflammation in the penis may be the causes. It is associated with leukemia and sickle cell anemia. Treatment is difficult and frequently unsuccessful.

Impotence. Impotence is the inability to achieve and maintain erection necessary in the performance of coitus. The two main mechanisms connected with erection are vascular and neurologic. There are various etiologic factors, although the most frequent seems to be psychogenic. The following types of causes have been cited: congenital; inflammatory: prostatitis, seminal vesiculitis, peripheral neuritis; neurologic; endocrinologic: diabetic neuropathy, bilateral testicular failure; vascular aortic obstruction; neoplastic; traumatic, iatrogenic (radical perineal prostatectomy) accidental injury; and psychogenic. Impotence is common in diabetes and may manifest itself preclinically. Drugs may have an effect on potency, such as ganglionic blocking agents in hypertension; reserpine, alcohol, narcotics and tranquilizers may all interfere.

In any case of impotence, it is important to obtain a comprehensive history and do a physical examination to exclude other than psychogenic causes. Problems of sexual performance contribute largely to the anxiety states of the elderly male. Impotent males are susceptible to quack medication and therapies advertised by word of mouth or in magazines so oriented. Our culture tends to deprecate sexual activity in the aged; an elderly man is likely to be thought perverse or at best comic if he is interested in satisfying his sexual needs, and an elderly woman even more so. Poor health may reduce sexual activity but does not necessarily eliminate it.

A patient and his significant others need accurate information concerning the likelihood of any complications occurring that may affect sexual activity following surgery or any procedure that involves the genitalia. Such complications include impotence and incontinence. It is the primary responsibility of the doctor to give the *facts* to clients. Nurses can offer support and the opportunity for discussion while patients and their significant others are considering the information they have received. The term impotence should probably be avoided unless there is no doubt that it either has or will occur, as mere mention of the possibility may contribute to its subsequent occurrence. Clients may be told that sexual functioning may be reduced for a time and that that does not necessarily mean the person is permanently impotent.

When impotence occurs to a significant degree, the man and his sexual partner must be treated simultaneously. The secret of successful management is not to treat the symptoms at all, since an erection cannot be voluntarily obtained. The three principal goals are: (1) removal of the man's fears and his partner's fears about sexual performance and (2) reorienting of his involuntary behavioral pattern so that he becomes an active participant. It is necessary to reestablish communication between the partners and to treat the relationship.[29A]

Men experiencing impotence with an organic basis may be helped by the use of *penile prostheses*—a rather recent method of treatment. The most popular technique is the placement of *Small-Carrion prostheses* (Fig. 82–2*A*). These consist of plastic rods introduced into the bodies of the corpora cavernosa through a perineal incision. One disadvantage of these implants is that the penis remains in a state of semi-erection. Although the erection is not painful and does not interfere with daily activities, it is sometimes unacceptable to either patients or their sexual partners.

Another device is the *inflatable penile prothesis*. Two hollow plastic tubes are surgically placed in the corpora cavernosa. A silicone reservoir containing radiopaque fluid is sutured into abdominal fascia. A bulb is implanted in one scrotal sac. These various parts are all connected with silicone tubing in such a way that the fluid can be pumped into the penile prosthesis by

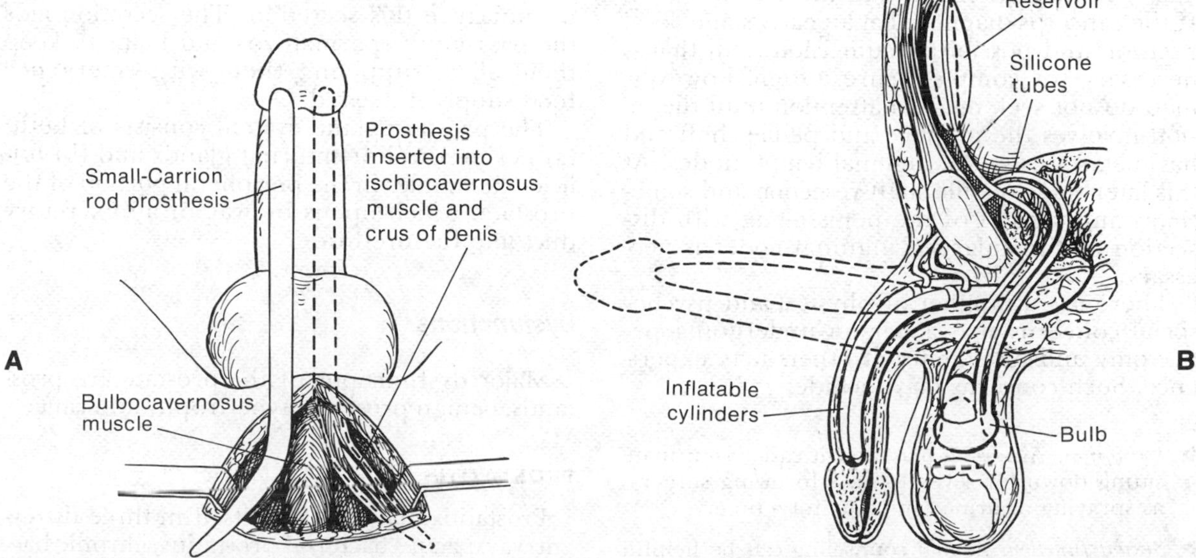

Figure 82–2. Penile prostheses. **A.** Small-Carrion prosthesis consisting of plastic rods. **B.** Inflatable penile prosthesis. (See text for discussion.)

squeezing the scrotal bulb, thus causing an erection. The erection will subside when the release valve in the lower part of the scotal bulb is compressed. The fluid then returns to the reservoir (Fig. 82–2*B*). Mechanical failure may occur.

A person wishing to have a penile implant must meet certain criteria before the surgery is performed. These include:[41] (a) a strong desire for satisfying sexual activity; (b) the presence of some penile sensation; (c) a willing sexual partner; and (d) freedom from other genitourinary problems. In addition, the patient is often required to take a number of psychologic tests.

The patient with an implant may be anxious and embarrassed. Both the patient and his most significant others may be helped by being given the opportunity to express their fears and concerns. It may be helpful if a person who has already adjusted to this procedure can spend some time speaking with the patient. Sexual counseling may be useful for patients and their sexual partners in the months following surgery.

Although these procedures are usually reserved for people experiencing impotence from an organic basis, it is sometimes considered when intensive psychotherapy is unable to relieve psychogenic impotence.

Cancer.[31] Cancer of the penis is essentially skin cancer. The glans and the prepuce are usually the parts affected. Carcinoma of the penis is often related to the presence of chronic infection in the area. Circumcision seems to help in preventing the development of cancer. The treatment is excision of the affected area. If the cancer is diagnosed at an early stage, local excision and possibly circumcision is all that is necessary for complete cure. Often, however, men do not seek medical attention until the lesion involves the prepuce and penile shaft and has metastases in the inguinal lymph nodes. At this later stage, penile shaft resection and sometimes amputation of the penis along with dissection of the enlarged inguinal nodes is necessary.

There are a number of physical and psychosocial concerns that a person undergoing penectomy and his significant others may experience. Such concerns may include:

- *Urination.* A person may find it easier to urinate sitting down for several weeks following surgery, as spraying of urine can occur for a time.
- *Sexual function.* Sexual counseling can be helpful for patients and their sexual partners both before and after surgery.
- *Body image changes.* Adjustment to a change in the appearance of the genitals can take some time. Understanding and support is necessary for both the patient and his significant others.

THE PROSTATE

Anatomy and Function

In childhood the prostate is a small gland, but with puberty, it grows to the size of a walnut. In the adult the prostate gland lies like a flattened cone in the pelvis about 2 cm. posterior to the symphysis pubis (Fig. 82–3). The prostate is inverted so that the base is superior and the apex inferior. The base of the prostate is located at the neck of the bladder, in front of the rectum; its apex is suspended by the urogenital diaphragm. The basal surface is overlain by the bladder, and the posterior prostatic surface is in close contact with the rectal wall and is the only surface of the prostate subject to palpation.

The prostate is enclosed in a firm fibrous capsule and is pierced by the urethra and ejaculatory ducts. The prostate urethra runs through the prostate. A shallow median furrow divides the lower part of the prostate into the right and left lateral lobes. The middle lobe is created by the ejaculatory ducts from either side, which pierce the prostate and converge in the urethra.

In the normal adult male, the prostate measures about 4 to 6 cm. long and weighs 15 Gr. The structure is a network of branching glands, which manufacture a prostatic secretion. The glands are embedded in muscles that contract during ejaculation to eject prostatic secretion. The secretion goes through the ejaculatory ducts. The sole function of the prostate is to manufacture this secretion. The secretion aids the passage of spermatozoa and helps to keep them alive, supplying them with emergency food supply if needed.

The prostate gland system consists of both: (a) periurethral or internal glands and (b) follicle-like tubules in the peripheral portion of the prostate, which opens by way of an excretory duct into the urethra.

Dysfunctions

Major dysfunctions of the prostate are prostatitis, benign prostatic hypertrophy and cancer.

PROSTATITIS

Prostatitis may manifest itself in three different ways: acute bacterial prostatitis, chronic bacterial prostatitis, or prostatosis (abacterial chronic prostatitis).

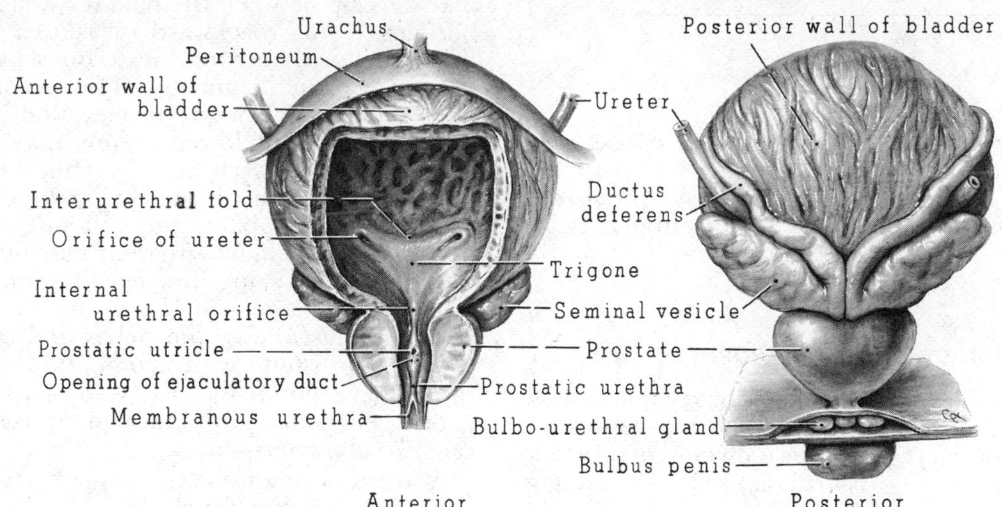

Figure 82–3. Internal and external aspects of the urinary bladder and related structures. (From Jacob, S. W., C. A. Francone, and W. J. Lossow: *Structure and Function in Man*, 4th ed. Philadelphia: W. B. Saunders Co., 1978, p. 508.)

Acute bacterial prostatitis is characterized by the sudden onset of chills and fever. The patient may have symptoms of frequency, urgency, dysuria and pain in the suprapubic, perineal, and scrotal areas. There may be hematuria and a degree of bladder outlet obstruction. The prostate will be swollen and tender. Therapy includes rest, analgesics and antimicrobial therapy. The main purpose of the antibiotic is to control the cystitis and urethritis that accompany prostatitis. It has been reported that 35 per cent of all men over 50 years have chronic prostatitis. In the prostatic secretion, staphylococci are the most frequently found organisms. Chronic infection of the seminal vesicles accompanies prostatitis. It is generally a nonspecific infection and has an extremely varied symptomatology.

Many patients with a mild infection have no *symptoms*. There may be a persistent urethral discharge, usually appearing at the meatus in the morning or during the day when a long time elapses between voidings. There is frequency of urination with mild urgency, dysuria and burning on voiding. A dull ache may be felt; referred pain may occur anywhere below the diaphragm. It is often felt when the patient first arises in the morning and may wear off during the day. There is frequently sexual dysfunction.

Treatment consists of general hygienic measures, chemotherapy, attack on the distant primary focus of infection, eradication of complications, and local therapy. Prostate massage is accomplished by stroking the posterior surface of the prostate toward the midline. The fluid is milked from the urethra and examined under the microscope. In prostatitis, the fluid contains many leukocytes.

The *prognosis* is not very encouraging, although approximately 50 per cent of cases will be cured and 25 per cent will markedly improve.

Prostatosis (*or abacterial chronic prostatitis*) is the most common form of prostatitis. Congestion of the prostate is the main finding. The symptoms are mild frequency and urgency, low back pain, and discomfort in the rectum, urethra or perineal area. The patient may experience a moderate loss of libido. On physical exam the prostate is usually nontender and of normal consistency. The urinalysis and prostatic fluid examination are normal. Prostatosis may be a psychologic problem in a man who is on the borderline of being sexually unable to function;

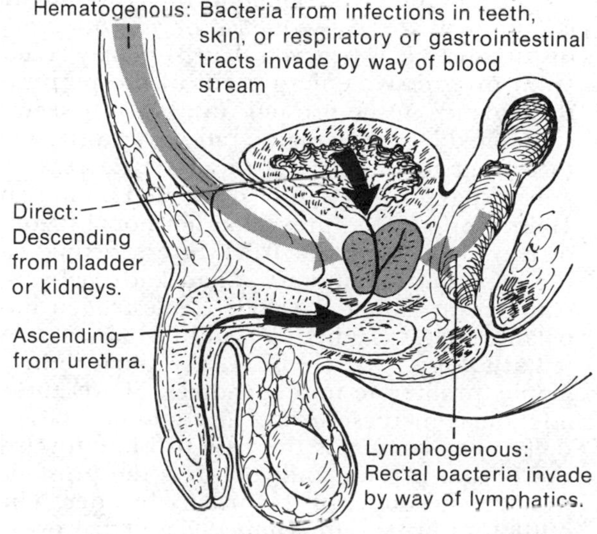

Figure 82–4. Postulated pathways of infection to the prostate gland.

in other cases, it may be due to excess consumption of alcohol or caffeine. No treatment may be necessary, because the symptoms are commonly self-limiting. Counseling may be helpful.

BENIGN PROSTATIC HYPERTROPHY

The prostate is the urologic organ that is most frequently affected by neoplasms—benign or malignant. Here our focus is on benign prostatic hypertrophy (or hyperplasia). This disorder is commonly abbreviated "BPH".

Benign prostatic enlargement develops in one out of ten 40-year-old men and increases in frequency with advancing age. Most men develop some prostatic enlargement by age 50 and by age 60 most have evidence of prostatic hyperplasia that can be palpated by rectal exam. However, the hyperplasia is not always progressive, and surgical treatment is not necessary for most men with prostatic hypertrophy. Not all men with BPH develop symptoms of urinary obstruction or other complications; many do not require treatment.

When treatment is necessary, it may employ conservative or surgical measures. Currently there are no medications to specifically treat BPH when it is present, nor are there therapies to prevent or control the onset or progression of this disorder.

Etiology. The cause of BPH is not exactly known although it is commonly thought that the condition is the consequence of an endocrine disturbance. It is believed that BPH may result from progressive enlargement of the periurethral glands in the prostatic urethra. These are stimulated by the changing ratio of testosterone to estrogen. With aging, this ratio decreases.[3]

Findings of one study done in London in 1976[37] support the prevailing hormonal theory of the pathogenesis of BPH. Stress, acting via the hypothalamopituitary gonadal adrenal axis, could bring about the androgen/estrogen imbalance that is claimed to lead to BPH.

Pathology.[3] With BPH, the periurethral glands proliferate into adenomas. Slowly these adenomas increase in size and number. Gradually, they compress the true prostate toward the fibrous capsule and compress the prostatic urethra and outlet of the urinary bladder. The outflow of urine is thus impeded and may eventually become totally obstructed.

Enlargement of the prostate may produce various *complications* (Fig. 82–5). The bladder muscles thicken and hypertrophy as the *obstruction* gradually develops. Herniations (*diverticula*) may develop between the bladder wall's muscle bundles. *Reflux* (backward or return flow) of urine may occur because of decompensation of the urethrovesical junction. This decompensation results from long-term elevations of bladder pressure. The lower ureters may be compressed and obstructed by the thickened bladder wall. As a result, *hydroureter* develops, i.e., the ureter is abnormally distended with urine. In turn, a similar situation may develop in the kidneys, as urine flow becomes obstructed in the ureters and urine backs up. In this situation (*hydronephrosis*), the pelvis and calices of the kidney distend with urine, and atrophy of the kidney's parenchyma develops. Ultimately, prolonged urinary obstruction or reflux can cause *renal insufficiency*.

Additional complications may occur with BPH. A pouch may form in the bladder and the urine in the pouch may not empty during voiding. This *residual urine* may become a site for *infection*, i.e., *cystitis*. Also, *calculi* ("stones") may develop.

Symptoms. Most patients present with varying degrees of urinary obstruction, although benign hypertrophy is usually slow in developing and may persist for a long time without creating a major problem. As the person becomes older, he may assume that his frequency of urination will increase. However, reduction in both the size and force of the urinary stream is abnormal and necessitates an examination. The urinary stream first lacks force, then becomes weak and dribbling. The individual feels unable to empty his bladder and has to strain to urinate or has to urinate more frequently. Blood in the urine may be another symptom and is more common in benign hypertrophy than in cancer.

As the prostate enlarges, there is a danger of complete obstruction of urination, which may be precipitated by the person's being chilled and/or by his drinking alcoholic beverages. *Obstruction is a painful emergency*, which can be treated by insertion of a catheter. If the retention is of long standing and there is over 1000 ml. of urine in the bladder, it is wise to remove the urine gradually, about 100 ml. an hour.

Infection in an enlarged prostate causes exacerbation of the symptoms in addition to the problems of urinary infection. During the later stages of prostatic disease, the kidneys may be damaged owing to the backing up of urine into the kidney, causing uremic poisoning.

Diagnosis. The disorder is diagnosed by: (1) general physical examination, including a rectal examination; (2) laboratory examination of blood, urine and renal functions; (3) x-ray examination, including intravenous pyelography and excretory cystography; and (4) instrumental examination, including catheterization, cystourethroscopy, and biopsy.

Most patients are vague and unsure about

what an enlarged prostate is and may be afraid of the tests and their results. A complete explanation of each step of diagnostic procedures is helpful. The patient may be shown a picture of the reproductive organs and prostate, and the effects of enlargement upon the excretion of urine can be explained. (Refer to Figs. 82–1 and 82–5). If the patient sees such a picture, he can better understand how the doctor can determine the size and consistency of the glands and the seminal vesicles.

For rectal examination the patient may be placed in the knee-chest position or bent over the table. The nurse may explain that relaxing and taking slow deep breaths may make rectal examination more comfortable and easier. (Rectal examination is discussed in Chapter 15. Also see p. 1855 of this chapter). Prostatic secretion may be obtained during the rectal examination and examined under the microscope for pus cells, which indicate infection. The urine may be normal in asymptomatic cases or may show infection by the presence of red or white cells, albumin and bacteria, or an alkaline reaction. Obtain the urine specimen before prostatic massage.

Renal function tests may be done to assess the patient's renal reserve and to determine if the urinary back pressure (created by the enlarged prostate) has damaged the kidneys. Normal ranges in blood chemistry tests most often used in urology are shown in Table 82–1. Excretory urography, phenosulfophthalein excretory tests, specific gravity test, radioisotope renograms, and renal radioscintillation scanning are tests used in further diagnosis.

The instruments used in urology include urethral catheters and sounds (Fig. 82–6). The catheters are used to (1) relieve urinary obstruction, (2) obtain urine for diagnosis and (3) test for residual urine and bladder lavage or medication. If a catheter is to be left indwelling, a retention catheter of the Foley type is generally used. This catheter is kept in the bladder by an inflatable balloon filled with 5 ml. of water. Sounds are slender, long instruments used to explore and dilate the urethra.

The cystoscope is indispensable in both the diagnosis and treatment of urologic disease. It is a metal instrument with optical systems that provide a magnified illuminated image of the bladder. The cystoscopic examination is a valuable diagnostic procedure. Some indications for cystocopy are: (1) to determine the source of urinary bleeding; (2) to determine the cause of unexplained urinary symptoms; (3) to determine the source of pyuria; (4) to catheterize the ureters for the purpose of localizing the infection and therapy; (5) to obtain biopsy specimens; and (6) for follow-up examinations. The nurse may assist the patient by explaining the procedure and the fact that it will be done under local or general anesthesia.

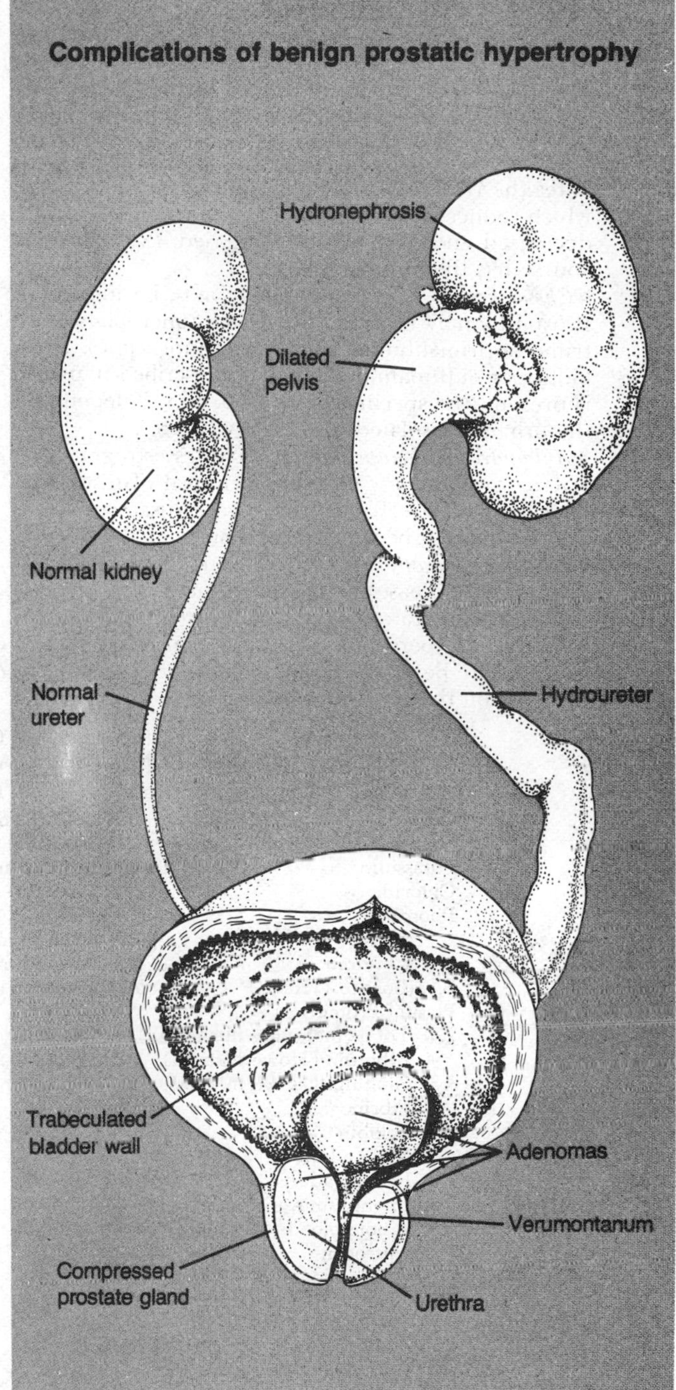

Figure 82–5. Complications of benign prostatic hypertrophy include obstruction of the upper tracts, producing hydroureters and renal insufficiency. (From Brosman, S. A.: Benign prostatic hypertrophy: When should you consider a prostatectomy for your patient? *Geriatrics,* 34:25, Apr. 1979.)

Treatment

CONSERVATIVE TREATMENT. Hypertrophy of the prostate alone is not an indication for surgery. Many people experience considerable relief from some conservative treatment directed toward relieving symptoms. Conservative measures include:[43]

▶*Prostatic massage*, along with *hot sitz baths*. This facilitates the release of small amounts of prostatic fluid, which reduces edema. Frequency of urination is then decreased and stream flow increased. (Sexual intercourse has the same effect.)

▶*Chemotherapy* of various kinds may be indicated. Prostatitis may be treated with antimicrobials (e.g., trimethoprimsulfamethoxazole, minocycline). Antibiotics or sulfonamides may be prescribed if pyuria is present (the specific choice of drug will depend on the organism isolated).

▶*Antiandrogen therapy*, which includes estrogen therapy or orchiectomy (surgical removal of testis) can have beneficial effects. The severe disadvantage is that the patient becomes impotent.

▶*Androgen therapy*. Sometimes drugs such as testosterone can increase the bladder tone and so increase the urine flow rate. Great care must be taken to ensure that the person does not have a malignancy in the prostate before androgens are used, however, as they hasten the growth of cancer.

Patient teaching is very important. It is especially helpful to explain to the patient that if his bladder is distended rapidly it can increase his symptoms considerably and may even precipitate acute retention. This occurs because the hypertrophic muscle of the bladder can lose its tone if it is distended quickly. Patients can reduce the possibility of this happening by: (a) voiding *whenever* the urge to do so is felt; (b) avoiding excessive intake of fluids over a short period of time, and (c) avoid alcohol intake, as its diuretic effect along with volume of fluid intake increases bladder distention (alcohol intake is the most common precipitating factor for acute urinary retention).

Whenever a patient and his significant others have to manage an *indwelling urinary catheter at home*, careful teaching must be offered to them. Repeated explanations may be needed and the opportunity for questions and discussion must, of course, always be given. Remember that procedures and equipment familiar to you can be very frightening to others to whom they are not routine. In fact, you may be so familiar with urinary catheterization and all that it involves, that you may overlook things that may be of concern to patients and significant others. The following information may be included in the

TABLE 82-1. NORMAL RANGE OF BLOOD CONCENTRATIONS OF FUNCTIONAL CONSTITUENTS AND EXCRETORY SUBSTANCES*†

Calcium	9.5–10.5 (10) mg./100 cc.	4.8–5.2 (5.0) mEq./L.
Sodium	317–340 (329) mg./100 cc.	138–148 (143) mEq./L.
Potassium	16–21 (18.2) mg./100 cc.	4.0–5.4 (4.7) mEq./L.
Chloride	355–390 (370) mg. Cl/100 cc.	100–110 (104) mEq./L.
Phosphate		
Adults	3.0–4.5 (3.8) mg. P/100 cc.	1.7–2.6 (2.2) mEq./L.
Children	5.0–8.0 (6.5) mg. P/100 cc.	2.9–4.6 (3.8) mEq./L.
Bicarbonate (HCO_3)	57–62 (60) cc.	25–28 (27) mEq./L.
Plasma Proteins		
Total (including fibrinogen)		6.5–8.0 (7.3) gm./100 cc.
Albumin (Howe method)		4.0–5.5 (4.5) gm./100 cc.
Globulin (Howe method)		2.0–3.0 (2.5) gm./100 cc.
Fibrinogen		0.2–0.4 (0.3) gm./100 cc.
Hemoglobin		
Male adults		14–18 (16) gm./100 cc.
Female adults		12–16 (14) gm./100 cc.
Total nonprotein nitrogen		10–30 (20)
Whole blood		20–40 (32)
Urea nitrogen		8–28 (12)
Whole blood		5–23 (11)
Uric acid		3.0–5.0 (4.0)
Whole blood		3.0–5.9 (4.5)
Creatinine		0.6–1.1 (0.8)
Whole blood		0.7–1.5 (1.2)
Serum Enzymes		
Alkaline phosphatase—Bodansky		
Adults		2.0–4.9 units/100 cc.
Children		5–15 units/100 cc.
Prematures		10–20 units/100 cc.
Acid phosphatase—Bodansky		0.0–1.0 units/100 cc.
Acid phosphatase—King and Armstrong		1.0–5.0 units/100 cc.
Glucose (Folin-Wu method)		80–120 (100)

*Average value is in parentheses; values are for plasma and in terms of mg./100 cc. unless otherwise specified.

†From Leader, A. J., and Carlton, C. E.: Urologic diagnosis and the urologic examination. *In* Campbell, M. F., and Harrison, H.: *Urology*. 3rd. ed. Philadelphia, W. B. Saunders Company, 1970.

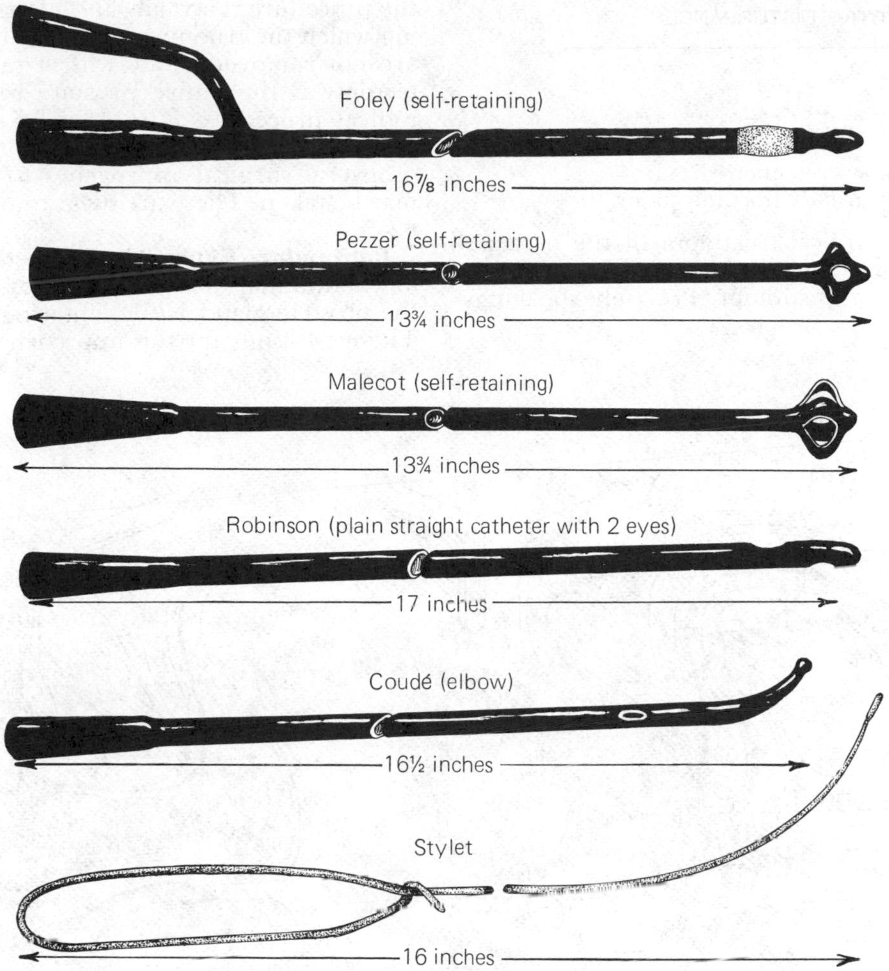

Figure 82–6. Types of catheters: catheter stylet. (From Smith, D. R.: *General Urology*. 9th ed. Los Altos, Calif.: Lange Medical Publications 1978, p. 110.)

teaching. Information may be given both verbally and in writing.

- Explanations, using diagrams, of the anatomy and physiology of the urinary tract along with a description of how the catheter functions.
- Discussion about the danger of infection and the ways this danger can be reduced by careful maintenance of a sterile closed system for urinary drainage; fluid intake of at least 3000 ml./24 hours; careful hygiene, including cleaning around the catheter and urinary meatus and daily showering.
- Demonstration and practice in handling the collecting devices they are to use. This includes changing the bags; securing the tubing, using a leg bag during the day and a bedside gravity drainage system during the night (to avoid reflux).
- Problems that require medical attention include pain, reduced urinary output, catheter displacement or loss, leakage of urine around the catheter, and any discharge from around the catheter. While this list may be given, the patient and significant others should be encouraged to seek professional advice for anything that causes them anxiety. We cannot always anticipate what will be of concern to clients

Surgical Treatment. Surgery sometimes becomes necessary. The indications for surgery vary. Many patients experiencing BPH symptoms are over age 50 years; therefore the risks of surgery may be increased. The decision to operate is made carefully, based on indications such as:

a. The presence of upper urinary tract dilation (hydroureter, hydronephrosis) and impaired renal function. This is usually confirmed by excretory urography.

b. The degree of discomfort and inconvenience the patient is experiencing.

c. The presence of a non-emptying bladder diverticulum.

d. Vesical (urinary bladder) calculus, indicative of longstanding vesical neck obstruction that results in vesical decompensation.

e. Residual urine of 60 ml. or more which is also indicative of longstanding obstruction and vesical detrusor complication.

f. Severe and prolonged hematuria (recurrent bleeding) from congested prostatic vessels.

g. Acute urinary retention.
h. Recurrent urinary tract infections.

While the surgical treatment of the prostate is commonly referred to as "prostatectomy," this term is really a misnomer. Precisely speaking, the procedure is actually an "adenectomy," during which the true prostate and fibrous capsule are not removed. Only with a radical prostatectomy is the entire prostate removed. The radical procedure is performed only for the treatment of some prostatic cancers.

Several surgical approaches to the prostate may be taken. These are diagrammed in Figure 82–7.

Retropubic (Extravesical) Prostatectomy. A low abdominal incision facilitates approaching the prostate gland *without* entering the bladder. The indications for this approach are the same

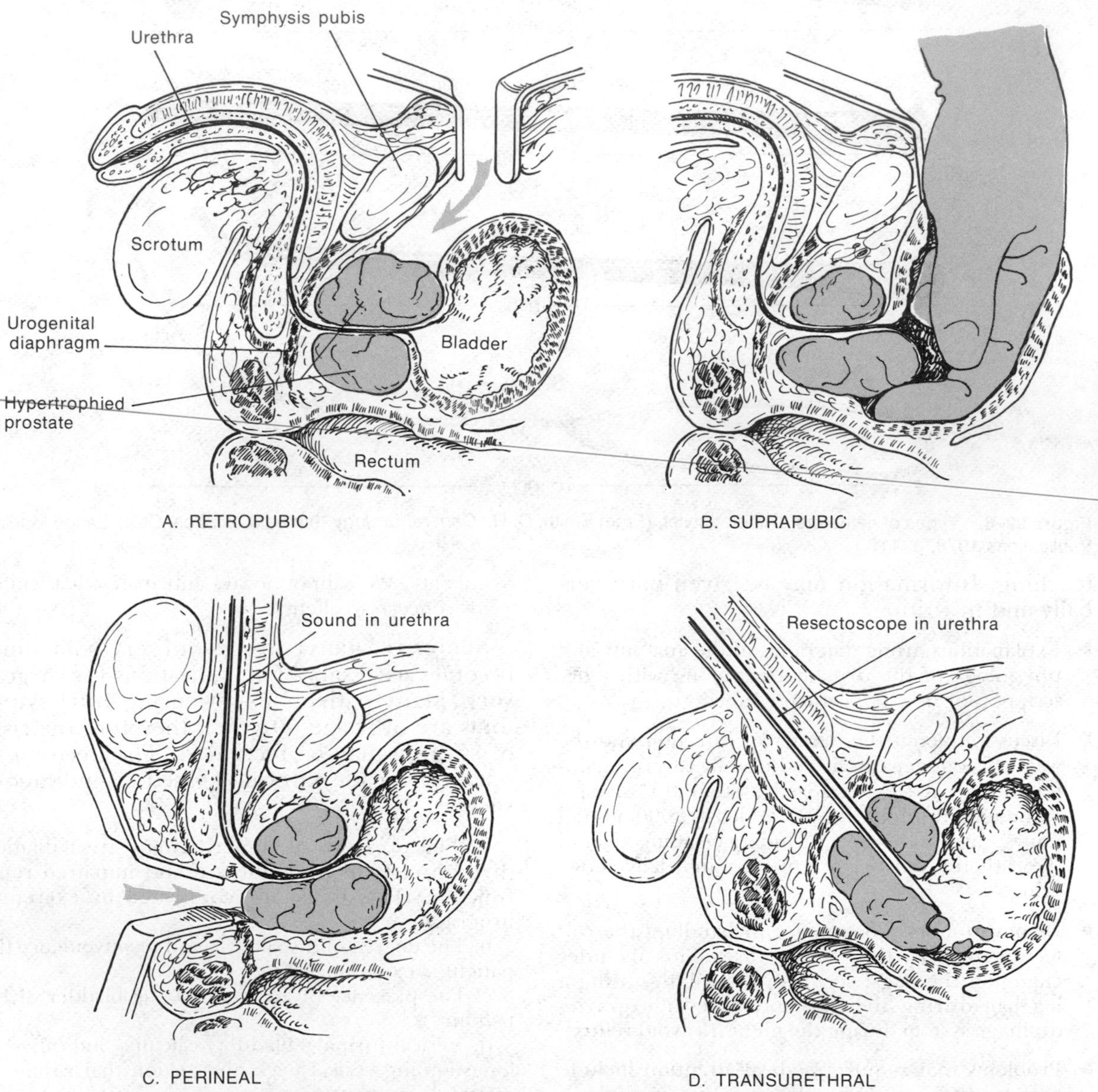

Figure 82–7. Surgical approaches to the prostate. **A.** *Retropubic (extravesical) prostatectomy* is an open method, in which a low abdominal incision is made between the pubic arch and the bladder. **B.** *Suprapubic (transvesical) prostatectomy* is an open method of treatment in which the hyperplastic prostatic tissue is enucleated through the anterior walls of the abdomen and bladder. **C.** *Perineal prostatectomy* is an open method involving an incision between the anus and the scrotum. **D.** *Transurethral resection prostatectomy* (TUR) is a closed method of treatment, i.e., no incision is made and the hyperplastic prostate tissue is removed through a resectoscope (like a cystoscope) inserted through the patient's penis.

as for the suprapubic approach. Advantages include direct visualization of the prostate and direct hemostasis in the posterior fossa. A disadvantage is that associated bladder pathology cannot be treated since the bladder is not entered. Also osteitis pubis (pubic bone inflammation) may occur. Incontinence and impotence are infrequent complications although after the catheter is removed some urinary leakage may occur for a few days.

Suprapubic (Transvesical) Prostatectomy. This surgical approach through a lower abdominal incision may be used in the presence of: (a) large prostate (over 40 Gm.), (b) bladder abnormality (diverticula or stone), or (c) large pedunculated middle lobe. An advantage of this procedure is that bladder abnormalities can be treated concurrently because an incision is made into the urinary bladder. This "open" procedure facilitates thorough exploration and more complete tissue removal than "closed" procedures, i.e., those not requiring an incision. Disadvantages include: (a) difficulty in obtaining hemostasis (watch for shock and hemorrhage), (b) bladder spasms, (c) urinary leakage into abdominal wound around suprapubic catheter, and (d) relatively prolonged, uncomfortable convalescence for the patient. The incidence of postoperative incontinence and/or impotence is relatively low.

Perineal Prostatectomy. This is used in suspected early carcinoma of the prostate, when open biopsy is needed or for removal of prostatic calculi. Other indications include presence of severe cardiovascular or pulmonary disease and/or when TUR (see next paragraph) and abdominal incision are contraindicated. The gland is removed through a V-shaped incision in the perineum above the rectum. This procedure permits good hemostasis and gravity drainage. Also, because of its direct approach, radical surgery is facilitated if malignancy is found. Wound pain is minimal and recovery rapid.

This approach has several possible complications, including infection, sexual impotence, and urinary and fecal incontinence from sphincter injury. To accomplish the surgery the patient is placed in a lithotomy position (this is not recommended for people also suffering from arthritis).

Transurethral Resection. The TUR is generally accepted as the method for removing minor obstructive lesions. TUR is the most widely used of all prostatic surgical techniques. The prostate is small enough in most patients requiring surgery for BPH for the transurethral approach to be used. TUR is especially suitable for patients who are poor surgical risks and have relatively small glands, as no incision is made. Repeated TUR may be necessary, however, because postoperative urethral strictures frequently occur.

In performing TUR a resectoscope is inserted through the urethra and the prostatic tissue enlargement is scraped out. A resectoscope has an insulated sheath which prevents damage to the urethra after the instrument is inserted, and a working element, a movable loop of tungsten wire that cuts tissue with a high frequency current turned on by a foot pedal. The surgeon operates the cutting loop by looking through a telescope. The field is illuminated by a bright electric light. The cutting loop shaves off prostatic tissue at the bladder's opening. Irrigating fluid can be passed in and out of the area through the instrument, and the tissue debris falls back into the bladder and is washed out. Hospitalization is usually short following TUR and convalescence more rapid than with other types of prostatectomy. TUR affords good hemostasis and a relatively pain-free postoperative experience. Incontinence secondary to surgical trauma may occur.

In *punch prostatectomy*, a cold knife is used to remove the enlargement. Tissue is punched out piece by piece with a circular hollow blade. Healing is more satisfactory than when the tissue is burned. Bleeding is controlled by electric current.

Cryosurgery is sometimes used for very poor risk patients. This procedure involves passing an instrument through the urethra. Liquid nitrogen, circulated through a probe, destroys tissue by freezing. Relatively low blood loss occurs.

NURSING CARE AND DELEGATED MEDICAL CARE FOR PATIENTS EXPERIENCING PROSTATIC SURGERY

Prostatic surgery is a stressful event in the lives of patients and their significant others. Such people require excellent and knowledgeable nursing care that attends to their daily basic human needs; thorough explanation of all procedures and treatment options; along with sensitive support during the stressful experience. This is best achieved by a careful application of the nursing process. Information that may help you in this task is discussed below. (For detailed discussion of caring for a person undergoing surgery, see Unit VIII.)

Preoperative Care

- *Anxiety reduction*. Facilitate expression of concerns; give clear information, according to need.
- Establishment of optimum nutritional status. Patients may be malnourished and/or dehydrated because of the distressing symptoms they may

have experienced prior to hospitalization, e.g., urinary frequency, obstruction, pain. Encourage a balanced diet and appropriate fluid intake, based on assessment of the patient's cardiac reserve. When no underlying condition contraindicates, liberal fluid intake is desirable (2500 to 3000 ml. per 24 hours). This helps to correct dehydration and azotemia (presence of nitrogen-containing compounds in the blood).

- *Promotion of optimum urinary flow.* This may be necessary because the patient may have some urinary difficulties on admission to hospital, e.g., obstruction, urinary retention, diminished renal function. Corrective measures may include insertion of an indwelling urethral catheter or drainage by cystostomy. *Gradual* bladder decompression may be advisable. This may take place over several days and requires careful assessment of the patient for indications of shock, e.g., evaluate blood pressure and renal function (see also Chapter 13). Emergency catheterization of the totally obstructed patient requires a urologist's skills and possibly special instruments, e.g., insertion of a stylet (thin wire) into the catheter lumen, metal catheters, or other firm, specially angled catheters.

- *Preparation for surgery.* It is important to have the patient in as good a condition for surgery as possible. Carefully assess the patient's ability to meet his basic human needs. Identify areas in which your assistance may be needed both now and postoperatively. Because patients with prostatic disorders are often over 50 years of age, look carefully for signs of respiratory and cardiovascular disorders.

Postoperative Care. Nursing and delegated medical care common to all postoperative periods is presented in Unit VIII. Specific factors concerning the person experiencing prostatic surgery are discussed here. For a detailed discussion of the care of persons with urinary catheters and irrigation systems, refer to a text such as Sorensen and Luckmann, *Basic Nursing: A Psychophysiologic Approach*.

> *Possible complications* following prostatectomy include:
> *Hemorrhage* and *shock* during or following surgery
> *Urinary tract infection* and/or *wound infection*
> *Urinary obstruction*, e.g., catheter blocked
> *Displacement or accidental removal of catheters*, e.g., patient pulls out catheter
> *Urethral stricture* resulting from instrumentation (e.g., resectoscope) or presence of catheter
> *Urinary incontinence*, e.g., from urethral injury or perineal muscle trauma
> *Impotence* from surgical trauma (see discussion, p. 1842)

Excellent nursing care is of particular importance in preventing postoperative complications and in detecting *early* indications of these problems.

Hemorrhagic shock is discussed in detail in Chapter 13. Assess a patient for evidence of hemorrhage by: (a) making physical assessments, (b) observing the operative site, and (c) observing wound drains and catheter drainage.

Wound drains may be in place following perineal or suprapubic prostatectomies. Additionally, following a suprapubic approach a *suprapubic tube* (catheter) is positioned directly into the bladder through the abdomen. Wound drains are typically removed earlier than suprapubic tubes. At the time of surgery the surgeon may place packing in the wound to control bleeding.

The surgeon may prefer to do initial *dressing changes* and then delegate subsequent changes to nurses. When a perineal incision is present, a double-tailed T-binder may be used to secure the dressings. The tails are crossed over the incision area and then one tail is positioned on each side of the scrotum. Finally, the tails are pulled up to the waist band and secured.

Heat applications (e.g., via sitz bath or heat lamp) may be employed to promote the healing of perineal wounds following suture removal. During the application of heat from a heat lamp, the scrotum should be protectively covered with a towel.

Indwelling urethral catheters are typically used following all types of prostatectomies (Fig. 82–8). Hematuria (presence of blood in the urine) is usual for a few days postoperatively.

Frank bleeding may occur during the first day following surgery. Bleeding may be arterial or venous. *Arterial bleeding* is bright red, has numerous clots and an increased viscosity; with arterial bleeding, a falling blood pressure often occurs, and emergency surgical intervention is frequently required. *Venous bleeding* is more common. It is darker and less viscous than arterial bleeding. Venous bleeding in the prostatic area may be controlled by increasing the pressure in the ballooned end of the urethral cath-

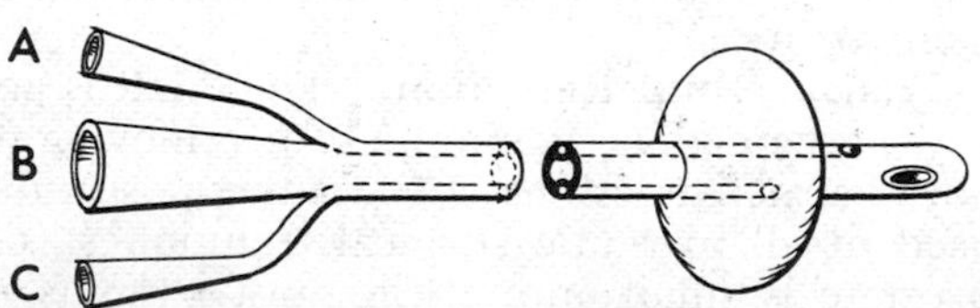

Figure 82–8. The Foley-Alcock three-way catheter. Each catheter lumen has a specific purpose: *A* for inflow of solution; *B* for outflow of urine and solution, and *C* to inflate catheter balloon. Balloon is inflated after insertion and thus holds catheter in position. Balloon is deflated prior to removal of catheter. (From Sutton, A. L.: *Bedside Nursing Techniques in Medicine and Surgery.* 2nd ed. Philadelphia: W. B. Saunders Co., 1969).

eter (this is sometimes referred to as "applying traction").

Various types of catheter irrigation systems may be used after prostatectomy. *Closed irrigation* permits either the *constant or intermittent* flow of irrigating fluid without the hazard of breaking aseptic technique. It is important to prevent overdistention of the bladder, e.g., during irrigation or due to obstruction of urine outflow. Such overdistention can cause secondary hemorrhage by placing undue strain on freshly coagulated blood vessels.

Observe the patient carefully for local or systemic indications of infection. Catheters, drainage apparatus, and urine collecting bags must be carefully tended to prevent the introduction of *infection into the urinary tract*. Following perineal prostatectomy, aseptic technique must be closely maintained because of a high possibility of *wound infection* owing to the location of the incision. Meticulous aseptic technique is also necessary in the area of a suprapubic tube's insertion.

Prevent *wound trauma* following perineal surgery by avoiding enemas, rectal tubes, or the use of rectal thermometers. Also, following prostatectomy via any route, closely supervise confused patients to prevent them from accidentally pulling out their catheters.

The *accidental displacement or removal of a urinary catheter* following prostatic surgery can not only be painful for a patient but also can disrupt recovery. The surgeon assesses such a situation and determines whether or not it is necessary to mechanically reestablish a urinary drainage pathway. With a perineal prostatectomy, a urethral catheter is not only necessary for urinary drainage, but it also serves as a splint for urethral anastomosis. Clearly it is important that the catheter remain properly positioned for as long as it is needed.

While a urinary catheter is in place, it must be kept *patent* (open, clear or unobstructed). *Maintaining catheter patency* is an important, often challenging nursing activity. Urine flow may be obstructed in various ways, e.g., blood clots, mucous plugs, kinked tubing, tube displacement. *Obstruction may produce pain*. Thus, if a patient is experiencing pain following prostatectomy, be certain to assess his drainage apparatus for patency. Relief of obstruction often alleviates pain without the need for analgesics. (Assessment of pain is discussed in Unit XI.)

Blocked catheters can lead to complications such as infections, bladder distention and painful bladder spasms. Some bladder spasms occur with bladder distention while others are a response to irritation from the catheter balloon. Bladder distention may be identified by shutting off continuous irrigation and palpating the lower abdomen. If distention is present, irrigation of the catheter may clear any clots or plugs and thus facilitate urinary drainage. If a catheter cannot be cleared, it may have to be removed and a new one inserted. This is usually done by the urologist attending the patient.

Sometimes antispasmodic drugs are ordered prophylactically to help prevent *bladder spasms*. This is especially true for patients who require "traction." There are some complications that can occur, however, with these drugs. *Persons with severe cardiac disease or glaucoma should not be given antispasmodic drugs*. Constipation can be a problem with these drugs, since they cause diminished bowel function. The patient may be advised not to strain during defecation for at least 6 weeks postoperatively, as straining can lead to bleeding from the operative site. Colace, prune juice, and milk of magnesia are generally satisfactory bowel stimulants to assist the patient during this time.

After TUR and following catheter removal, watch closely for indications of *urethral stricture*, e.g., small urinary stream, dysuria, straining.

Guidelines vary concerning the length of time to leave urethral catheters in place. Factors influencing this decision include: surgeon preference, patient tolerance, and type of surgery performed. A uretheral catheter usually remains in place for as long as 12 to 14 days following perineal prostatectomy. However, following a simple TUR the catheter may be removed after 2 to 3 days, when the urine remains clear. The surgeon determines the appropriate time for *catheter removal*. Sometimes relatively early removal is performed if the catheter is creating excessive problems, e.g., bladder spasms.

Following catheter removal, observe the patient closely for indications of urine retention, e.g., inability to void, bladder overdistention. Teach the patient that it is important to urinate at his *first desire* to do so, i.e., not to delay. Temporary urinary frequency and/or urine incontinence may occur following catheter removal. Of course these problems are distressing and they should be discussed with the patient. It may be reassuring for all concerned to know that urinary control is not expected to return rapidly, and hence a period of "dribbling" is not unusual.

Remember that the removal of tubes from one's body is anxiety provoking (as is their insertion). Hence, patients may worry when they are told their catheters or wound drainage tubes are to be removed. Such concerns should be expressed and discussed. This will happen in the presence of an effective therapeutic nurse-patient relationship.

Penile implants may sometimes be used in the management of *impotence* if it occurs following prostatectomy. (Impotence is discussed on p. 1842). Postprostatectomy *urinary incontinence* may be managed by using a combined program of sphincter exercises (discussed in the teaching section below) and surgery. One surgical approach involves placing a device under the urethral bulb to increase urethral resistance just below the external sphincter.

The thoughtful nurse recognizes how profoundly disturbing sexual dysfunction and/or incontinence usually is for affected persons. Sensitive, supportive care of patients and their significant others is a vital aspect of the nursing care of persons experiencing prostatectomy. A central aspect of such care is the provision of *planned, individualized patient–significant other* education. Common areas of discussion in an education plan may include:

- *Purposes of catheters, wound drains, and urinary drainage and irrigation apparatus.* Discussion of related procedures. Techniques of specimen collection.
- *Ways of protecting catheters* to prevent their accidental displacement, e.g., teach the patient ways of turning in bed and getting out of bed without "pulling" on the catheter or kinking the drainage tubing.
- *Common sensations* experienced by persons following prostatectomy. For example: the presence of an urethral catheter may cause bladder spasms and a sensation of needing to void; following removal of a catheter some dribbling of urine and a sense of urgency (urgent need to void).
- *Expected types of urinary and wound drainage*, e.g., bloody urine is not unusual early in the postoperative course.
- *Reportable symptoms and their management*, e.g., pain, bladder spasms.
- *Self-help activities*, e.g., drinking a lot of fluids while a catheter is in place, bed exercises, general relaxation exercises, early ambulation, measuring fluid intake and urinary output. Prolonged sitting increases intra-abdominal pressure and fosters bleeding. Therefore, a sitting position should be avoided except during meals. Upon discharge, prolonged automobile rides should be avoided until all danger of bleeding has passed. Strenuous exercise is also contraindicated.
- *Post-discharge instructions*. Areas of teaching may include: Indications of secondary complications (e.g., bleeding, infection, obstructed urine flow); procedure for obtaining professional help if needed; program of rest, activity, exercises; recommendations concerning any restrictions of sexual activity; need for continued intake of large amounts of non-alcoholic fluids to minimize clot formation; and follow-up appointment time and place. If a patient is discharged home with an indwelling catheter, prepare the patient for home care (see p. 1848).
- *Perineal exercises* to help the patient regain urinary sphincter control, e.g., contraction of the abdominal, gluteal, and perineal muscles about 12 to 25 times per hour from the second or third postoperative day. Suggest to the patient that he contract his muscles "as if he had to urinate urgently and there were no place to relieve himself" and to breathe normally. Another helpful exercise consists of tensing or squeezing the rectal sphincter while relaxing other body muscles. The patient is taught to keep his hands placed on his abdomen to assess abdominal tension. The abdomen should *not* tense and a Valsalva maneuver should *not* occur when the exercise is correctly performed. While exercising, the patient may be helped to concentrate by saying out loud words such as "relax—squeeze." Perineal exercises should be continued until complete urinary control is achieved. A planned schedule of exercising during waking hours should be established.
- *Additional treatment recommendations* and *plans for management of complications*, e.g., sexual dysfunction, loss of bladder control.

PROSTATIC CANCER

Prostatic cancer is the second most common cause of death from cancer in the male. In men over age 55 years, it is the third most common cause of death and the main cause of death in men over age 75. There has been an increase in the incidence of prostatic cancer over the last few decades, most markedly among black men. While this disease is rare among Oriental men, the incidence is increasing among Japanese migrants to the United States. The U.S. has an estimated 18,000 diagnosed cases annually—the ninth highest rate among Western countries.[41]

Etiology. There is disagreement regarding *etiology*. There are a number of factors that *may* be significant, however. These include:[41]

- Familial tendency—especially son and grandson relationships
- History of multiple sexual partners
- Numerous episodes of venereal disease
- Delayed sexual drive
- Early repression of sexuality
- Premature cessation of sexuality

Although the reasons are quite unknown, it appears that the younger the patient is, the more aggressive the cancer is.

Presenting Symptoms. The presenting

symptoms are most often those of prostatitis—infectious or obstructing. Obstructive symptoms that may indicate a neoplasm include: urinary frequency, slow stream, dysuria, and complete retention. Unfortunately, the presenting symptoms are sometimes symptoms which occur late in the disease and are caused by metastasis, e.g., hip or back bone pain.

Diagnosis. Early *diagnosis* is essential, since prognosis for cure is extremely low once prostatic carcinoma becomes symptomatic. Most prostatic cancers are adenocarcinomas. Evidence of prostatic cancer can be found during rectal examination. Late findings include a large, hard, fixed prostate. Any induration (e.g., nodule) is suspicious—especially if unilateral. About 50 per cent of such nodules are malignant. The cancer is often unoperable when symptoms of bladder neck obstruction and urinary retention from cancer of the prostate are present.

Health teaching geared toward the early detection of prostatic cancer is therefore very important. Men must be encouraged to seek routine examination of the prostate gland. It may be uncomfortable and embarrassing for men to have rectal examinations, and they are unlikely to seek such procedures unless the prophylactic importance is well understood. Nurses need to be as diligent in teaching men about the importance of routine rectal examinations as they often are in teaching systematic breast examinations to women. During such teaching it is helpful to emphasize that prostatic cancer is easily diagnosed, readily treated, and potentially curable. Some sources even recommend regular *self-examination of the prostate* as an addition (*not* a substitute) to examination by a clinician. This can be useful if the man is taught what to feel for and how to go about making the examination.[4]

Rectal-Prostatic Examination

> *Rectal examination of the prostate in every man over age 40 is an essential part of his annual routine checkup.*

Rectal examination every 6 months is advisable if the patient has a history of continuing urinary symptoms, especially if a relative has had prostatic cancer. This is also true if the patient has BPH or has had subtotal prostatectomy.[41]

Just prior to rectal examination, ask the patient to empty his bladder. Explain that this makes the examination more comfortable and more accurate. The base of the prostate is difficult to identify if the bladder is full.

Two possible positions for the patient during rectal examination of the prostate are: (1) buttocks elevated in a knee-chest position on the examining table and (2) bending over from the hips, with elbows placed either on the examining table or on the knees.

The examiner asks the patient to "bear down," explaining that this helps relax the anus and makes it easier to insert a finger for examination. If the anus is tightened, the insertion could be painful. The examining finger should be gloved and well lubricated.

It is recommended[41] that the examiner imagine the prostate as heart shaped (see Figure 82–9). Then identify the median sulcus and proceed to systematically and carefully examine *every* portion of the gland with the examining finger. Each lateral lobe should be palpated, beginning at the median sulcus and moving out to the lateral border. Compare both sides of the prostate; they should be symmetric. During examination of the prostate for cancer, concentrate on symmetry, consistency, and the presence of indurations rather than on the gland's size. Take care *not* to massage the gland during the examination. This could occur if examination is too vigorous. Because the superior notch is the most sensitive region of the prostate, it is palpated last.

The following guidelines provide helpful descriptions of how various prostatic findings feel to an experienced examiner during rectal examination.[39,41]

- *Normal prostate*: feels similar to a normal cervix, i.e., like the tip of the nose or base of the thumb while opposing the little finger. Normal consistency is smooth, rubbery, and firm.

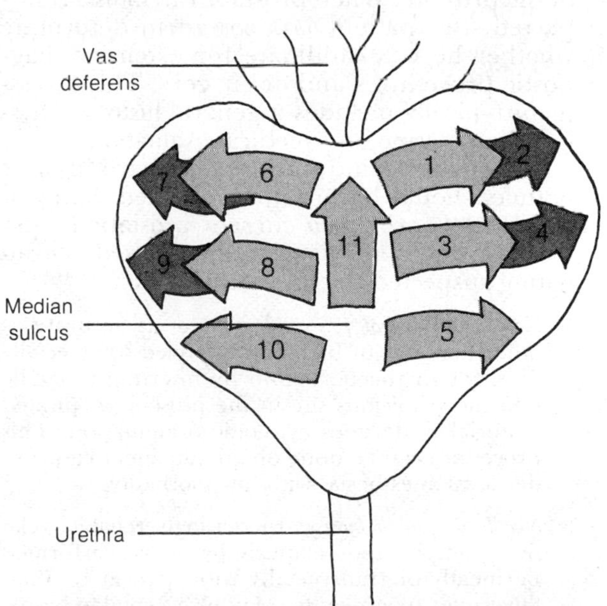

Figure 82–9. Recommended sequence for prostatic palpation during rectal exam. (From Shortridge, L. M., and B. R. McLain: Primary care and prostate cancer. *Nurse Practitioner,* 4:26, Jan.–Feb. 1979.)

- *Prostatitis*: feels like the cheek of the face or "boggy"
- *Abscess of the prostate*: feels like a "puffed out" cheek
- *Benign prostatic hypertrophy (BPH)*: feels like the chin
- *Carcinoma*: feels similar to the forehead of the face. Classic descriptions are "stony hard" or a "hard nodule," i.e., a grossly circumscribed area of induration. Any area of induration is a suspicious finding. During the rectal examination, the degree of fixation of the prostate should be determined as well as whether the process has extended beyond the prostatic capsule to the lateral wall of the pelvis and into the seminal vesicle.

Hard areas and nodules in the prostate may be caused by disorders other than cancer such as (a) *inflammation* (seldom as hard as cancer and commonly preceded by other indications of inflammation such as prostatitis, pyuria, tenderness, white cells in massaged secretion); (b) *prostatic calculi* (easily established by x-ray); and (c) *tuberculosis, syphilis*, and other rarer causes of nodules.

Other Diagnostic Processes

While actual diagnosis is made through biopsy, no x-ray or laboratory examination can substitute for a careful rectal examination in assessing a patient for the presence of carcinoma of the prostate. When prostatic carcinoma is suspected, the patient is assessed to determine whether he is a candidate for extensive diagnostic procedures and/or surgery. This assessment typically includes a general history, physical examination and medical evaluation.

Any prostatic induration, e.g., hard area or nodule, should be promptly biopsied. Summarized below are some current prostatic biopsy methods and other diagnostic tests used in evaluating suspected prostatic carcinoma:[38,39,41]

- *Needle aspiration for cytology*: Not as accurate as other methods of biopsy. Performed transrectally or through the perineum by inserting a needle into the suspicious site in the prostate. Aspirated material undergoes cytologic examination. This procedure can be done on an outpatient basis under local anesthesia, with low morbidity.
- *Needle or punch biopsy*: Increasingly reliable, relatively simple, and relatively harmless. Performed perineally or transrectally with a trocar or Vim-Silverman type needle. May be acceptable by patients who refuse more invasive, extensive procedures. Disadvantages are that the specimen obtained is very small, making precise pathologic diagnosis difficult. Transrectal route has higher morbidity than perineal route. Disadvantages of the transrectal route are (a) the insertion violates a natural barrier (Denonvillier's fascia) and (b) possible contamination of the prostate with rectal contents and subsequent infection. Antibiotics may be given and an indwelling Foley catheter may be kept in place for at least 12 hours following biopsy to minimize the likelihood of extravasated urine leaking along the biopsy site tract. It is not uncommon for the biopsy needle to enter the bladder.
- *Transurethral resection biopsy*: Usually provides a satisfactory specimen; however, at times malignant tissue may not be reached. Performed by excising tissue with a resectoscope loop.
- *Open perineal biopsy*: Facilitates the most complete diagnosis; this method is chosen after extensive work-up demonstrates the patient is suitable for curative surgery. The operation, objected to by some patients, involves entry into the perineum and examination of frozen tissue. With evidence of cancer, the entire prostate is removed immediately. If the pathologic diagnosis is initially unclear (equivocal), the wound may be closed awaiting report from a completely stained specimen. This method of biopsy does not permit evaluation of regional lymph nodes for possible extension of the cancer. Also, as with any perineal surgery, there is risk of impotence.
- *Serum and prostatic acid phosphatase*: Too variable to be highly significant by itself for primary diagnosis. Excessively high values indicate need for further confirmatory tests. A false positive can occur if examination or massage of the prostate has occurred within 48 hours of drawing the blood sample. Prostatic secretions normally remove acid phosphatase (abbreviated as "ac phos") from the body. However, in the presence of metastatic carcinoma of the prostate, the cells producing the enzyme become walled off from the ducts that normally drain the secretion to the exterior. Hence, the level of serum acid phosphatase rises. The normal acid phosphatase range is 1.0-4.0 King-Armstrong units. Serum acid phosphatase determination, although variable, aids in finding whether or not the cancer has spread beyond the confines of the prostate, since the value is frequently elevated in metastatic carcinoma from a prostate malignancy. This elevation may be present even when the osteoblastic metastases cannot be seen on plain x-ray films. It is almost never elevated in benign prostatic hypertrophy (BPH), i.e., noncancerous hypertrophy of the prostate.
- *Bone marrow aspiration:* May be used for *cytologic examination* and determination of *bone marrow acid phosphatase*. Presence of metastatic cells shows disease has obviously spread beyond the prostate and the patient is not eligible for radical surgery.
- *Lymphangiography of pelvic and periaortic nodes:* May prove the presence of cancer in these common

routes of metastases and clarify the likelihood of cure by radical lymphangiectomy.

- *X-ray examination* is essential, since the bones of the pelvis and spine are the most frequent sites of metastasis. Metastasis may be detected by surveying the bones by conventional radiologic methods or by scanning with radioactive uptake methods.
- *Cystoscopy* may help determine local extent of prostatic cancer. It is not necessary for diagnosis, however. An intravenous pyelogram can be a helpful screening procedure for assessing the condition of the bladder and kidneys; evaluating obstructive processes, and surveying the pelvis and spine (common sites of metastasis from prostatic carcinoma).

A physician's personal preferences and treatment philosophy influence the choice of biopsy procedure and possibly other diagnostic tests.

Grading and Staging. *Grading* of carcinoma of the prostate tries to establish the activity and/or virulence of the disease. Generally the disease may be more virulent, the younger the patient is when he develops the disease. *Staging* is an attempt to define the extent to which the carcinoma has developed. There are several different methods of classification; at present there is no consensus for defining each stage. One possible classification of prostatic cancer into four stages is:

Stage A or I: Lesion is occult, with microscopic foci not detectable by rectal examination, possibly well differentiated and located completely within the gland. Found during prostatectomy for a benign condition.

Stage B or II: Lesion is palpable by rectal examination, completely confined within the capsule to the prostate, may be large or small (considered curable).

Stage C or III: Lesion is extracapsular, locally extending to the seminal vesicle or pelvic wall. No evidence of distant metastases.

Stage D or IV: Lesion has distant vascular and/or lymphatic metastases, e.g., bone, liver, lung, skull, nodes.

Treatment.[30,38,39,41] It must be recognized that treatment philosophies and approaches to prostatic carcinoma vary widely for all stages and are intensely debated. Various treatment combinations may be employed for various stages, depending upon physician and patient preferences.

Four major treatment modalities for prostatic cancer are discussed here: (1) surgery, (2) radiation, (3) endocrine therapy, and (4) chemotherapy with cytotoxic agents.

Surgery. Radical prostatectomy is considered by many to be the treatment of choice for stage B prostatic carcinomas. This procedure may be used for selected persons with stage C disease; however, it is rarely performed for stage D. Pelvic node dissection may be performed with radical prostatectomy.

> *Common side effects of radical prostatectomy are impotence (90 to 100 per cent) and incontinence (10 to 15 per cent).*[30,41]

Both these side effects are extremely difficult for a patient to experience and may also be difficult for him to discuss. Improved surgical techniques and advances in treating impotence and incontinence help many men to overcome these difficulties. For example *sphincter control devices* are a relatively recent surgical advance for the treatment of surgically caused incontinence, which can be very helpful for carefully selected patients. Selectivity is essential because the risks involved in such procedures are considerable. Inability to achieve an erection can be surgically corrected by penile prosthesis, along with careful counseling in selected patients (see p. 1842). Refer to p. 1850 for discussion of prostatectomy approaches and care.

Transurethral resection (TUR) may be the treatment of choice in the *obstructed patient* who is not a candidate for radical surgery. Repeated TUR may be necessary to maintain an adequate channel through the prostatic urethra, i.e., to treat or prevent urinary obstruction. If TUR fails, a cystotomy may be performed.

Orchiectomy (removal of the testis) may be performed to relieve obstruction or for persons who either are unreliable about taking medication or who cannot tolerate estrogenic substances (see discussion below about endocrine therapy). Bilateral orchiectomy removes all testicular stimuli to continued prostatic growth.

Radiation. Impressive advances have recently been made in treating prostatic cancer with radiation. Morbidity has been reduced and results improved. The incidence of incontinence with radiation is only half that associated with radical surgical intervention, and potency is maintained in about half the patients. Radiation does not have the psychologic implications of castration, nor is there the likelihood of increased risk of death due to cardiovascular complications. Radiation may be used not only for persons unwilling to have radical surgery but also for those with locally confined adenocarcinoma.

Radiation treatment may employ either (a) *external beam therapy* or (b) *interstitial irradiation* accomplished by implanting radioactive metals such as chromium, gold (^{198}Au), or iodine (^{125}I) to destroy tumors at their original sites. Metastases cannot always be reached and treated by the latter method. However, with implantation, potency is more likely to be maintained and higher doses of local radiation can be delivered safely.

The technique of retropubic implantation of ^{125}I

seeds (Iodine 125) combined with *pelvic lymphadenectomy* has been found by some to be a reliable alternative to radical surgery. This technique effectively controls the tumor and causes minor urinary, rectal, and sexual disturbances. Page and Mathes[30] have found implantation most effective in patients with stage A, B or small C lesions who have negative bone scans. The ^{125}I seeds are implanted in the prostate through needles. The long half life of the seeds allows delivery of an effective radiation dose for 1 year. Since radiation intensity falls off a short distance from the seeds, normal tissues are protected. The technique offers more radiation and fewer side effects than external cobalt radiation. Following lymphadenectomy, edema of the penis occurs. Gradually this edema subsides. Lymphadenectomy is performed through a suprapubic incision. A Penrose drain is left in the incision.

Endocrine therapy. Some sources recommend estrogen therapy for *asymptomatic* clients, while others reserve estrogens and bilateral orchiectomy for late therapy if and when *symptoms* develop. It also appears controversial about what stage of cancer of the prostate should be treated with estrogens, i.e., early or late.

Side effects of estrogen therapy include: (a) gynecomastia (may be prevented by administering one dose of radiation to both breasts before giving any estrogen) and (b) impotence (100 per cent). The estrogen usually used is diethylstilbestrol (DES). Generally, testosterone values are lowered to castration level by a daily dose of 3 mg. The nurse needs to be alert for serious complications affecting the cardiovascular system, e.g., observing closely for indications of fluid retention.

Estramustine phosphate, a combination estrogen and alkylating agent, affects estrogen-resistant prostatic cells. This new drug does not cause impotence and has few side effects except anorexia and nausea.

Chemotherapy with Cytotoxic Agents. Various anticancer drugs show promise, e.g., adriamycin, 5-fluorouracil, cyclophosphamide and doxorubicin hydrochloride. For end-stage cancer of the prostate varying results occur when cytotoxic agents are used singly and in combination.

Treatment of early prostatic cancer may consist of: (a) complete removal via total prostatectomy and seminal vesiculectomy (performed perineally or retropubically or by combining these approaches) or (b) a more conservative approach of transurethral resection plus estrogens with or without bilateral orchiectomy. Some believe that the early use of estrogens is contraindicated since they seem to increase the frequency of heart disease.[38] Radiation is an alternative for persons unwilling to undergo radical surgery. Follow-up x-rays of the chest, lumbar spine, and pelvis may be recommended every 6 months.

Treatment of advanced, late prostatic cancer that has spread beyond the prostatic capsule may provide some symptomatic relief and extension of life for a few more years. In the presence of painful wide-spread metastases, appetite improvement, and a transient sense of well being may be produced by intravenous diethylstilbestrol (DES) or oral testosterone. Palliative measures that may help relieve intractable pain include local radiation, hypophysectomy, and medical or surgical adrenalectomy.

Hopefully, advanced, late prostatic cancer will become rare as increasing emphasis is placed on *early* diagnosis through routine rectal examinations and prompt intervention. Patients with prostatic cancer and their significant others require sensitive support and counseling and accurate information while making the many decisions required of them. Their concerns are often considerable and may include the choices of available treatments, fear of death, anxiety about residual disability and ongoing illness, and the possible effects of the illness on the people included in their social network. For a more complete discussion on the experience of cancer, see Unit IX.

THE SCROTUM

Anatomy and Function

The scrotum is a bilocular sac containing the testicles and portions of the duct system of the male genital tract. The sac hangs from the root of the penis, the left side being lower than the right because the left spermatic cord is longer. The skin of the pouch is bisected by a median raphe extending from the ventral aspect of the penile shaft under the entire sac to the anus. Internally, the two halves of the pouch are separated by a dartos tunic. Each half contains a testis with its epididymis and spermatic cord.

The testis is a smooth, solid, oval structure suspended in the scrotum by the spermatic cord. The testis has 600 to 1200 seminiferous tubules with a combined length of almost a mile. The upper end of the testis is capped by the head of the epididymis and the body of the epididymis is attached to the posterior surface of the testis. The apex of the epididymis at the lower end of the testis becomes continuous with the vas deferens that joins other vessels to form the spermatic cord. The spermatic cord consists of the vas deferens, arteries, veins, nerves and lymphatic vessels held together by spermatic fascia. The cord goes through the inguinal canal, and the vas deferens continues in the abdominal cavity, passing behind the bladder and anterior to the rectum to join the duct of the seminal vesicle and becoming the ejaculatory duct. The spermatic cord is movable for protection from trauma and facilitates optimum spermatogenesis.

The scrotum is examined by inspection and palpation. Because of the rugae, the walls may be inspected by spreading the layers between the fingers. Transillumination will help to distinguish most structures in the scrotal sac.

The seminal vesicles are paired 5 cm. long structures that are closely parallel to the bladder. The ejaculatory ducts separate the posterior and median lobes of the prostate and empty into the urethra. The seminal vesicles secrete a portion of the ejaculate and may contribute to the nutrition and activation of the sperm. Surgically, the seminal vesicles seldom require consideration without simultaneous removal of the prostate. Tumors of the vesicles are rare.

Dysfunctions

External Conditions. The scrotal skin is very thin and contains a large number of apocrine glands that tend to form cysts. It is in constant contact with the clothes and the skin of the thighs. It has many rugae that inhibit proper ventilation and so is subject to collecting moisture and to rubbing. The scrotum is prone to many infections by all organisms as well as to diseases indigenous to tropical areas. Nonvenereal disorders such as erysipelas, abscesses, fistulas and gangrene may occur in the scrotum. Venereal diseases such as chancroid, granuloma inguinale, lymphogranuloma venereum and syphilis may all manifest symptoms in this area. Parasites such as scabies and lice may also infect the scrotum. Many of the common skin diseases such as fungal infections, contact dermatitis, drug eruptions, eczema, lichen planus, herpes progenitales, and psoriasis may spread to the scrotum. Cancer of the scrotum does occur but is rare.

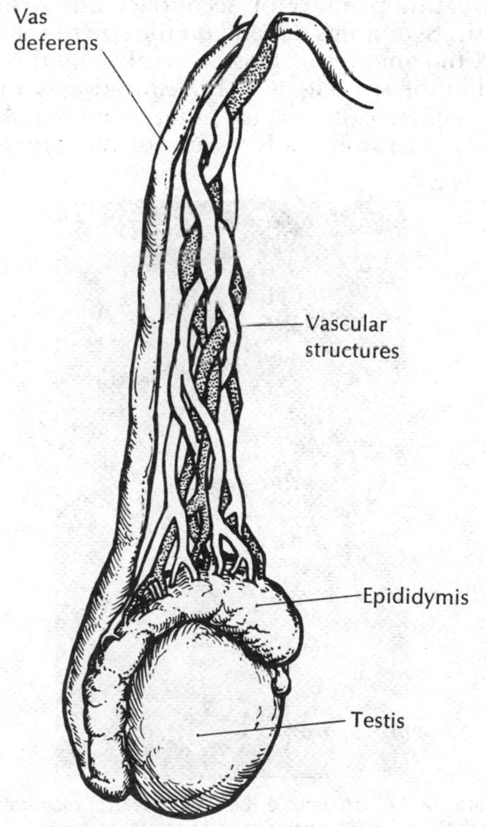

Figure 82–10. The four basic structures in the scrotum. (From Gott, L. J.: Common scrotal pathology. *American Family Physician,* 15:165, May 1977.)

Itching and intertrigo may be severe if the genitalia are affected because of heat, friction and moisture. Obesity and tight clothing aggravate the condition. The cause of the condition must be found and good local hygiene and use of dusting powder such as cornstarch may improve the condition.

The five most common disorders that give rise to a scrotal mass of short duration are (1) mumps orchitis, (2) epididymitis, (3) tumor, (4) tuberculosis and (5) torsion. Scrotal masses may or may not be associated with pain. For example, hydrocele, spermatocele, varicocele, and hernia are usually not painful, whereas strangulated hernia, orchitis, acute epididymitis, and hematocele are painful.

Mumps Orchitis. This is a complication of mumps in about 18 per cent of cases, which rarely occurs before puberty. Onset of the orchitis is usually 4 to 6 days after the appearance of the parotitis, although it may occur without it. In about 70 per cent of the cases, it is unilateral. Impotence and sterility are frequent sequelae. Signs and symptoms are nausea, vomiting and chills, followed by some testicular swelling. The gland is swollen, tender and usually extremely painful. Treatment includes bed rest, scrotal support and hot or cold applications. Mumps orchitis usually subsides in 7 to 10 days.

Epididymitis. Epididymitis is the most common of all the intrascrotal infections. Organisms usually reach the epididymis from established infection in the urine, urethra, prostate, or seminal vesicles. A recent study[20] of the etiology of acute epididymitis revealed that in young men the organism might be a sexually transmitted organism, such as *Neisseria gonorrhoeae* or *Chlamydia trachomatis*.

Urethritis is more common in a chlamydial infection. Inguinal pain occurs more frequently in chlamydial epididymitis. Tenderness over the spermatic cord is common with both chlamydial and coliform epididymitis. Scrotal edema and erythema and midstream pyuria tend to occur more with a coliform infection.

Treatment for epididymitis consists of bed rest, scrotal elevation, and antibiotics. Chlamydial infection is treated with tetracycline. Since chlamydial epididymitis is a sexually transmitted disease, patients' sexual partners must also be treated. Coliform bacteria are generally sensitive to ampicillin. A chlamydial infection can cause obstruction of the vas deferens and infertility.[20] Postoperative epididymitis may complicate all varieties of prostatectomy and urethral catheterization weeks or months after an operation, with recurrent episodes. In cases not responding to antibiotics, removal of the epididymis under local anesthetic is advised in the older age group. Routine use of modern antibiotics and improved surgical technique have reduced the incidence from 20 to 4 per cent.

Torsion of the Spermatic Cord. The peak incidence of torsion is in puberty, although it may occur at any age. Most patients, just before the onset of symptoms, have engaged in some physical exercise such as playing basketball, shoveling snow or riding a bicycle. The presenting symptom is intrascrotal pain radiating to the corresponding groin area. Palpation reveals a tender irregular edematous mass in the scrotum. There is pain only during the first hour or two, followed by marked tenderness of the testicle, nausea, vomiting and scrotal edema. One testicle may be twisted and drawn up much higher. Elevation and support of the scrotum for an hour does not help the pain in torsion, although it relieves it in epididymitis. The leg of the involved side is often held in flexion. This is an emergency and, if surgery is performed within 6 to 10 hours, a 70 per cent salvage rate is achieved. Only 20 per cent of testes are preserved if more than 10 hours have elapsed.

Inflammation of the spermatic cord may involve primarily the vas deferens or one of the other major structures of the cord. The vast majority of infections occur as a result of complications of prostatitis and especially involve the prostate and seminal vesicles.

Varicocele. Varicocele refers to any abnormal dilatation and tortuosity of the veins of the pamponiform plexus within the scrotum. A varicocele is secondary to an altered venous physiology of the blood supply of the testicle. It is generally believed that 10 per cent of young men have a varicocele. The age incidence is usually between 15 and 25 years of age at the time of onset and generally occurs on the left side. Varicoceles often disappear or become asymptomatic after sexual intercourse.

The most distressing disturbance associated with varicoceles is subfertility, with regard to the motility and number of the sperm. This effect on spermatogenesis is due to vascular changes. The symptoms vary according to individual toleration of discomfort, but the main complaint is a dragging, pulling or dull pain in the area of the scrotum. The diagnosis is made by physical examination of the scrotum where the dilated and tortuous veins are readily palpable in the standing position (usually likened to feeling a bag of worms). If the onset is sudden or if the lesion is present on the right side, a complete study is indicated because of the possibility of retroperitoneal disease or pathologic obstructive lesions affecting the venous drainage of that area. The treatment of varicocele is usually conservative, with surgery reserved for more severe cases. Surgical ligation is superior to other types of surgery for varicocele and can restore fertility.

Cystic Diseases of the Scrotum. Sebaceous cysts of the scrotal skin are not uncommon. The tunica vaginalis may be distended with fluid under several conditions. If the contents are straw colored and uninfected, the lesion is called a *hydrocele*. A hydrocele is a common urologic finding, usually secondary to an abnormality in the lymphatic drainage of the testicle, and is said to be present in 1 per cent of all male admissions to general hospitals. Ninety per cent occur after the age of 21. The hydrocele may be chronic, idiopathic primary or secondary and symptomatic. Symptoms depend on the size of the mass and the amount of tension created by the fluid within the sac (Fig. 82–11). Aspiration is a helpful palliative in certain elderly, poor-risk patients but rarely leads to cure of the hydrocele.

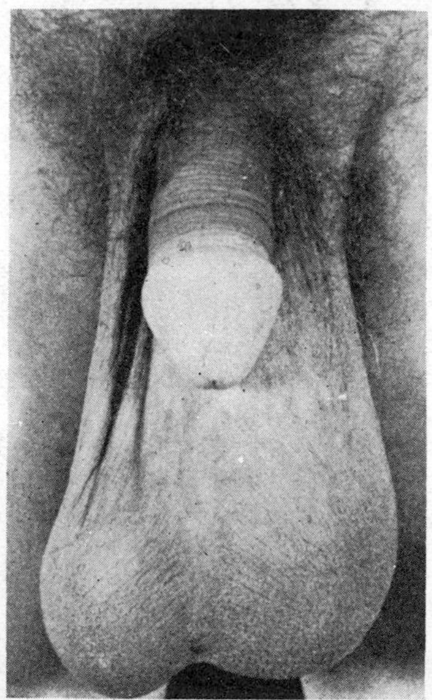

Figure 82–11. Hydrocele. Left hydrocele of moderate size with the testicle in a posterior and somewhat inferior position. The cystic hydrocele mass above the testicle was translucent to light. (From Campbell, M. F., and Harrison, J. H.: *Urology*, 3rd ed. 1970.)

Surgical incision is popular today and present-day technique is successful in probably all cases of primary hydrocele.

Treatment of acute secondary or symptomatic hydrocele is generally conservative, either for relief of symptoms or for aspiration. The patient is prescribed bed rest, with the scrotum elevated. Aspiration is used for the relief of pain or to obtain fluid and to clarify the diagnosis by allowing the scrotal contents to be palpated. Treatment is aimed at the underlying disease which may be orchitis or epididymitis. A spermatocele is an intrascrotal cyst resulting from a partial obstruction of the tubular system that transports sperm. Treatment is unnecessary for smaller cysts, although they may cause discomfort.

Disorders of The Testis, Epididymis and Their Adnexa and Tunic

The testes' role in the propagation of the species is producing spermatozoa and elaborating hormones, whereas the rest of the genital tract is concerned with the maturation, protection, nutrition and reactivity of the sperm. The scrotum regulates the environmental temperature around the testes.

During fetal development, either or both of the testes may be arrested in the abdomen, in the inguinal canal or at the puboscrotal ring, a condition known as *cryptorchism*. When the testis remains in the abdomen, it cannot be palpated. In the inguinal canal or at the puboscrotal junction, the testis can be felt but is frequently smaller than might be expected. A maldescended testis is frequently associated with a congenital inguinal hernia on the same side. Bilateral maldescent may result in sterility. In bilateral cryptorchism, steps to correct the condition should be begun by 3 or 4 years of age. The administration of chorionic gonadotropin makes it unnecessary to wait until puberty to see if the testicle will descend. Early surgery is preferred, since maturation of the testis starts at about 5 years of age.

A malignancy is much more common in undescended testicles than in normal testicles. Even testes that have been moved into the scrotom surgically at an early age may become malignant. When there is nondescent of only one testicle, malignancy may occur in either the descended or the undescended testicle.[8]

When the testes fail to secrete testosterone, puberty does not occur and *eunuchoidism* develops. The genitals and prostate remain infantile, the voice is high-pitched, axillary and pubic hair are scanty and no beard hair develops. Skeletal proportions are abnormal. Medical advice should be sought if puberty seems delayed and secondary sexual characteristics are not developing.

Cancer. Both benign and malignant neoplasms that are found in the testis are diagnosed only by biopsy. The testis is usually enlarged, harder with softer cystic regions, and heavier than with orchitis or a hydrocele (Fig. 82–12). The presence of metastatic lesions elsewhere would indicate that a nodule in the testis might be malignant. The rarity of testis tumor is the greatest obstacle to early diagnosis.

Testicular tumors are predominantly malignant and often have metastasized before the primary lesion is detected. They can be found on palpation, however, which is the reason self-examination of the testes is so important. In the United States, testicular malignancies affect 2.3 males per 100,000 and about 80 per cent of these people are less than 40 years of age. Testicular tumors do occur, however, from infancy through old age. The most common sites are on the testicular anterior and lateral surfaces.[10,34]

Some of the clinical findings are hepatomegaly (from metastases to the liver), possible epigastric mass, palpable Virchow's node (sometimes), pulmonary metastases (on chest film) and possible development of gynecomastia.

X-rays are usually taken to determine whether a malignancy is present. Urine may be tested to determine the presence of chorionic gonadotropins, since some malignant testicular tumors form these hormones. A negative test does not rule out testicular tumors, however. It is now possible to check for serum gonadotropins also. An intravenous pyelogram is often combined with a 24-hour lymphangiogram as part of a work-up. Surgical biopsy, of course, is

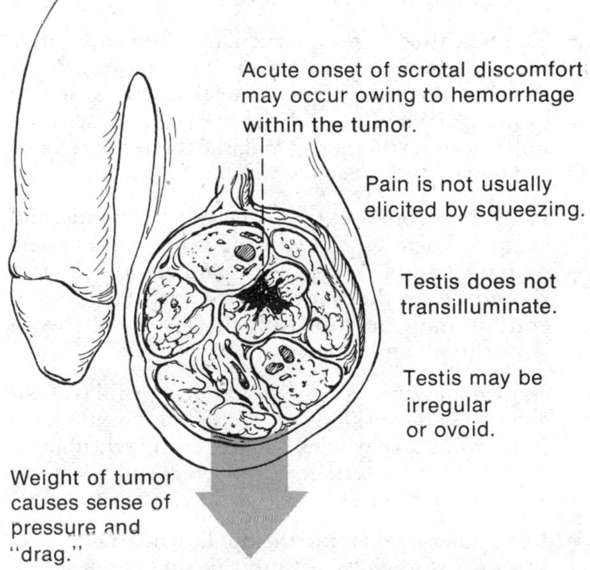

Figure 82–12. Some characteristics of malignant tumors of the testes.

the only sure way to determine malignancy. This is done through a groin incision, and pathological analysis is made on a frozen section.[10,34]

Orchiectomy (surgical removal of the testicle) is usually the first step in treating a malignant testicular tumor. Removal of the iliac and lumbar lymph nodes may also be done. Patients may experience ejaculatory impotence following the removal of these nodes, because of sympathetic nerve damage. Radiation therapy and chemotherapy are also used quite frequently in the treatment of testicular carcinoma.[43]

Testicular Self-Examination. Self-examination of the testes is an important part of self health care and should be included in health maintenance patient teaching. Men may find the idea of examining their own genitals rather difficult at first. Most men are used to touching their own genitals when urinating, bathing, or masturbating. It may take a little while for them to "get used to" touching their scrotum for routine health examinations. They need to (a) have the procedure explained carefully, (b) be given the opportunity to ask questions and express their concerns and (c) be referred to literature for their repeated consultation. (The American Cancer Society publishes a useful pamphlet on testicular self-examination.)

The following points may be mentioned when teaching a person about testicular self-exam (Fig. 82–13).

- ▶ When doing testicular self-exam, look for any deviations from normal in your scrotal structure, especially any hard, small lumps.
- ▶ The best time to do a testicular self-exam is after a bath, when you are warm. The scrotum is relaxed at this time, and the testicles are easier to examine. (When the testicles are cold, the scrotum pulls close to the body, making the testicles hard to feel.)
- ▶ Hold the scrotum in the palms of your hands, and examine each testicle with the thumb and fingers of both hands. Your index and middle fingers should be on the underside of each testicle and your thumbs on top. Roll the testicles between your thumb and fingers.
- ▶ A normal testicle is shaped like an egg and is about 4 cm. (1⅝ inches) long. It feels firm, but not hard (rather like an ear lobe). It may even feel rubbery. Normally your testicle should feel quite smooth and have no lumps.
- ▶ Remember to examine the epididymis. This structure is a storage tube found behind the testicles. Each epididymis should feel soft, and may be spongy and perhaps slightly tender.
- ▶ Examine the spermatic cords, which ascend from the epididymis and behind the testicles. They are normally firm, smooth tubular structures.

It takes some practice before a man feels confident in doing self-testicular examinations. After a time, each person becomes quite familiar with his own genital anatomy and can identify any abnormal changes. A person should consult a urologist about anything unusual or anything that concerns him during the examination.

Nurses who are male do well to regularly examine their own testicles, epididymis and spermatic cords. This is important not only for their own health care but also so that they will become quite familiar with the procedure and the anatomic structures in the male genital areas. This knowledge can then be used when examining, teaching, and advising patients.

Catheterization and Catheter Care

The use of urethral catheters is frequently part of the treatment of disorders of the male reproductive system. Hence, in caring for persons with such disorders, nursing technical skills related to catheterization and catheter care are often required. These skills are highly impor-

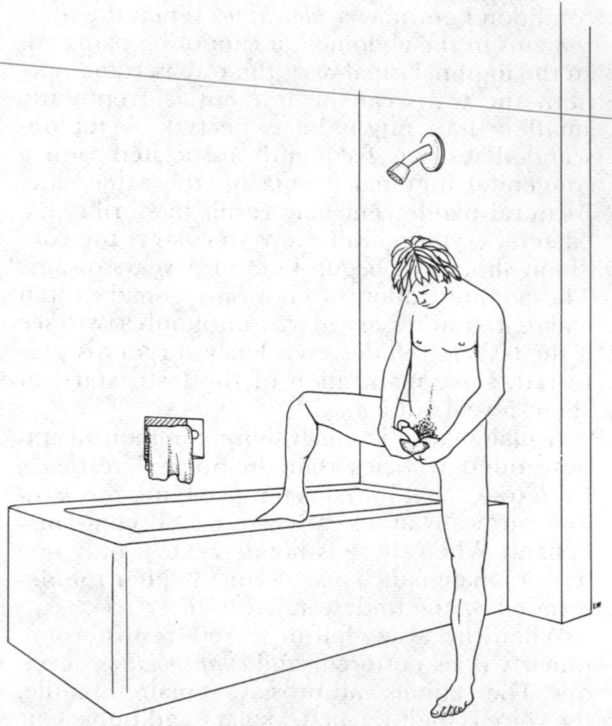

Figure 82–13. *Testicular self-examination* is important for men in early cancer detection in the same way that breast and vaginal self-examination is for women. Increasing emphasis is being given to helping men learn this health maintenance activity. It is recommended that testicular self-exam be performed while the body is warm following bathing.

tant, contributing immeasurably to patient safety, comfort, and recovery.

Space does not permit discussion of the knowledge base necessary for skillfully providing nursing care to a catheterized patient. Such a discussion would cover topics like the following: types of catheters, routes of catheterization, suggested procedures for catheterization, intermittent catheterization, physical hazards of catheterization, psychosocial implications of catheterization, care of the patient with an indwelling catheter (including factors such as perineal care, preventing infection, maintaining patency, comfort and safety), bladder and catheter irrigation and instillation, collecting urine specimens from an indwelling urethral catheter, removal of an indwelling urethral catheter and going home with an indwelling catheter. Refer as necessary to a textbook of basic nursing for discussion of the above topics.*

A brief summary of *male catheterization* follows: The perineum is washed and dried. If the patient is uncircumcised, the foreskin is retracted during cleansing. The distal end of the catheter should be covered with a water-soluble lubricant. The catheter is gently inserted and pushed forward while the patient "bears down," as if trying to urinate. (Bearing down opens the sphincters and allows easier passage.) Once past the sphincter, the catheter usually passes into the bladder. The catheter is usually inserted about 17.5 to 20 cm. (7 to 8 inches). The person inserting the catheter should wear sterile gloves. Absolute asepsis is necessary in the catheterization. Prepackaged sterile packs are generally used for the procedure and contain sterile drapes, cotton balls, lubricating jelly, and catheters. While a self-retaining (balloon-type) catheter is most commonly inserted when a catheter is to remain within the bladder, it is occasionally necessary or advantageous to leave a plain catheter in the bladder. When this is done the catheter must be taped in place or else it will readily slip out.

Conclusion

The nursing responsibilities in disorders of the male reproductive system demand that the nurse be aware of symptoms and psychologic problems resulting from dysfunction of the reproductive system, and thus encourage the patient and his significant others to seek early diagnosis and treatment. The excellent nurse appreciates the need for rectal examination of all men over age 40 in order to help prevent the high death rates from cancer of the prostate. The nurse can help the individual and his significant others to differentiate between the normal impairments of age and signs of dysfunction. Frankness concerning sexual history may be important in discussing with the patient and his significant others what may be expected after surgery. Sexual partners may need to speak openly with the doctor or the nurse concerning sexuality. This may be an area of history taking that may be embarrassing and difficult for clients. (Refer to Chapters 26 and 14 for other discussions of the nursing implications of sexuality.) The skill of the clinician in creating a nonjudgmental and safe environment will have a considerable effect on the accuracy and extent of the sexual history obtained and, in turn, on the quality of nursing care it will be possible to offer.

*A detailed presentation of catheterization and catheter care may be found in Sorensen and Luckmann, *Basic Nursing: A Psychophysiologic Approach*.

BIBLIOGRAPHY

1. Baumrucker, G. O.: *Transurethral Prostatectomy. Techniques, Hazards and Pitfalls*. Baltimore: Williams and Wilkins Co., 1968.

1a. Bias, H. I., C. L. Leverett, W. L. Parry, and D. B. Halverstadt: Implantable penile prosthesis in impotent males. *Urology*, 5:224, Feb. 1975.

2. Bowie, W. R., et al.: Round table venereology for primary physicians. *Patient Care*, 12:88, Jan. 30, 1978.

2a. Bracken, R. D., and D. E. Johnson: Sexual function and fecundity after treatment for testicular tumors. *Urology*, 7:37, Jan. 1976.

3. Brosman, S. A.: Benign prostatic hypertrophy: When should you consider prostatectomy for your patient? *Geriatrics*, 34:25, Apr. 1979.

4. Campbell, M. F., and J. H. Harrison: *Urology*, 3rd ed. Vols. I and II. Philadelphia: W. B. Saunders Co., 1970

5. Castleman, M.: A field guide to men's reproductive health. *Medical Self-Care*, No. 5, 1978.

6. Clinical Highlights: Acute prostatitis. *Hospital Medicine*, 14:144, March 1978.

7. Clinical Highlights: Clinical features of urethral stricture. *Hospital Medicine*, 14:108, Jan. 1978.

8. Clinical Highlights: Important considerations in diagnostic prostatic cancer. *Hospital Medicine*, 14:57, June 1978.

9. Cohen, S.: Patient assessment: Examination of the male genitalia. Programmed instruction. *American Journal of Nursing*, 79:689, Apr. 1979.

10. Conklin, M., K. Klint, K. Morway, et al.: Should health teaching include self-examination of the testes? *American Journal of Nursing*, 78:2073, Dec. 1978.

10a. Culp, D. A.: Benign prostatic hyperplasia. *Urology Clinics of North America*, 2:29, Feb. 1975.

11. Davis, J. E.: The significance and challenges of the vasectomy revolution. *Medical Counterpoint*, 33:55, Dec. 1971.

12. DeGowin, E. L., and R. L. DeGowin: *Bedside Diagnostic Examination*, 2nd ed. London: Macmillan Co., 1971.

13. Finebeiner, A. E., et al.: Complications of vasectomies. *American Journal of Nursing*, 15:86, Mar. 1977.

14. Gault, P. L.: The prostate. Coping with dangerous and distressing complications. *Nursing 77*, 7:34, Apr. 1977.

14a. Flocks, R.: Radiation therapy for prostatic cancer. *Urology Clinics of North America*, 2:183, Feb. 1975.

15. Geller, J. et al.: Using antiandrogen therapy in benign prostatic hypertrophy. *Geriatrics,* 32:63, April 1977.
16. Geriatric Abstracts: Antibiotics do not lessen morbidity after TURP. *Geriatrics,* 29:170, Mar. 1974.
17. Gott, L. J.: Common scrotal pathology. *American Journal of Nursing,* 15:165, May 1977.
18. Greene, L. F.: Selecting patients for transurethral resection. *Geriatrics,* 33:55, May 1978.
19. Gurevich, I.: Selected criteria for closed urinary drainage systems. *Supervisor Nurse,* 10:39, Feb. 1979.
20. Harnisch, J. P. et al.: Etiology of acute epididymitis. *Lancet,* 2:819, Apr. 1977.
21. Infamous anaerobes and the prostate. *Emergency Medicine,* 11:201, Jan. 1979.
22. Jaffe, J. W.: Common lower urinary tract problems in older people. *Working with Older People,* Vol. IV Clinical Aspects of Aging. U.S. Department of Health, Education, and Welfare, July 1971.
23. Kaufman, J. J.: Urologic factors in impotence and premature ejaculation. *Medical Aspects of Human Sexuality,* 1:43, Sept. 1967.
24. Knowing the unknown in epididymitis. *Emergency Medicine,* 10:83, July 1978.
25. Krain, L. S.: Epidemiologic variables in prostatic cancer. *Geriatrics,* 28:93, May 1973.
25a. Krauss, D. J., G. J. Schoenrock, and O. M. Lilien: Reeducation of urethral sphincter mechanism in post-prostatectomy incontinence. *Urology,* 5:533, Apr. 1975.
26. Kunin, C. M.: *Detection, Prevention and Management of Urinary Tract Infections.* Philadelphia: Lea and Febiger, 1972.
27. Logan, D. J.: Office management of prostatitis. *Consultant,* 17:141, Nov. 1977.
28. Logan, D. J.: What to do about impotence. *Consultant,* 17:131, Aug. 1977.
29. Masters, W. H., and V. Johnson: *Human Sexual Inadequacy.* Boston: Little, Brown and Company, 1970.
30. Mathes, G. L., and R. C. Page: An alternative to radical surgery for cancer of the prostate. *Geriatrics,* 33:53, Aug. 1978.
31. Mathews, D. et al.: Counseling after resection of the penis. *American Family Physician,* 19:127, Apr. 1979.
32. Mellinger, G. T. (ed): Urologic surgery. *Surgical Clinics of North America.* 45, Dec. 1965.
33. Mitchell, J. P.: *Urology for Nurses.* Bristol: John Wright and Sons, Ltd., 1965.
34. Murray, B. L. S., and L. J. Wilcox: Testicular self-examination. *American Journal of Nursing,* 79:286, Feb. 1979.
35. Nannings, J. B.: Chronic prostatitis: Two forms of one disease. *Consultant,* 17:147, Sept. 1977.
36. Orandi, A.: A new method for treating prostatic hypertrophy. *Geriatrics,* 33:58, June 1978.
37. Pond, D. A., and J. Maratos: Psychosocial inter-relations and benign prostatic hypertrophy. *Journal of Psychosomatic Research,* 21:201, 1977.
38. Raines, S. L.: Prostatic cancer—More cures with earlier detection. *Consultant,* 17:107, May 1977.
39. Rosenblum, R.: Practical guide to the diagnosis of carcinoma of the prostate. *Hospital Medicine,* 12:31, Jan. 1976.
40. Scott, R. (ed.): *Current Controversies in Urologic Management.* Philadelphia: W. B. Saunders Co., 1972.
41. Shortridge, L. M., and B. R. McLain: Primary care and prostate care. *Nurse Practitioner,* 4:25, Jan.-Feb. 1979.
42. Simone, C. M.: The transsexual patient: How you can help toward a successful outcome. *RN,* 40:37, Mar. 1977.
43. Smith, D. R.: *General Urology.* Los Altos, Calif.: Lange Medical Publishers, 1978.
44. Tobiason, S. J.: Benign prostatic hypertrophy. *American Journal of Nursing,* 79:286, Feb. 1979.
45. Tucker, E. C.: Clinical evaluation and management of the impotent. *Journal of the American Geriatric Society,* 19:180, Feb. 1971.
46. Wagner, D. K.: Trauma rounds. Problem: scrotal swelling and pain. *Emergency Medicine,* 9:62, Dec. 1977.
46a. Walsh, P.: Physiologic basis for hormonal therapy in carcinoma of the prostate. *Urology Clinics of North America,* 2:125, Feb. 1975.
47. Weyrauch, H.: *Life After Fifty. The Prostatic Age.* Los Angeles, The Ward Ritchie Press, 1967.
48. Wiggishoff, C. C, and T. C. Malvar: Acute and chronic bacterial prostatitis. *Hospital Medicine,* 13:64, May 1977.
49. Winter, C. C., and M. R. Barker: *Nursing Care of Patients with Urologic Disease,* 3rd ed. St. Louis: C. V. Mosby Co., 1972.
50. Wood, R. Y., and K. Rose: Penile implants for impotence. *American Journal of Nursing,* 78:234, Feb. 1978.

CHAPTER 83

THE MENSTRUAL CYCLE AND RELATED DISORDERS

by Judith Atwood R.N., M.N., and Judy Johnson R.N., M.A.

A thorough understanding of the anatomy and physiology of the female reproductive tract is essential for nurses giving care to a variety of female clients. Nurses have the opportunity to use this knowledge both in helping patients with problems in this area and in teaching the prevention of disorders of the reproductive tract. In addition, nurses may provide health education about the female reproductive system to students and various other groups.

This chapter provides a review of anatomy, a review of the menstrual cycle, a discussion of the menopause, and consideration of some menstrual abnormalities.

ANATOMIC AND FUNCTIONAL CONSIDERATIONS

INTERNAL FEMALE GENITAL ORGANS

Ovaries. The *ovaries* are located in the posterior lower pelvis, on both sides of the uterus, below the fallopian tubes (Fig. 83–1). They are contained in the posterior surface of the broad ligaments and are supported by several other ligaments that connect to the abdominal wall and to the uterus. The ovaries are approximately the size, shape and weight of an almond. Their surfaces are slightly lobulated and pale. Each ovary is composed of a *cortex* (the outer portion) and a *medulla* (inner portion).

Follicles, each containing a developing ovum, grow and mature in the stromal part of the medulla, close to the abundant blood supply and the lymphatics. Mature follicles (those which are ready to erupt and discharge mature ova) and primary follicles (those which have not yet started growing) are found in the cortex. At birth, there are some 200,000 to 400,000 follicles, each of which contains an *oocyte* (early stage ovum). They decrease in number as puberty approaches and gradually disappear at about the time of menopause.

The ovaries manufacture *hormones* that stimulate sexual desire, prepare and maintain the uterus for implantation, and have additional effects elsewhere in the body.

Fallopian Tubes. The *fallopian tubes* (uterine tubes) connect the uterus to the ovaries. They are the usual site of fertilization (if it occurs) and convey either the fertilized or the unfertilized *ovum* to the uterus. The tubes are approximately 4 inches long and are relatively thin. Each fallopian tube has four subdivisions: (1) Nearest to the ovary is the *fimbriated end*, which has small fingerlike projections that "cup" over the ovary like a funnel. (2) Next to this is the *ampulla*, which makes up the major portion of the length of the tube and is where fertilization usually occurs. (3) Following this is the *isthmus*, a narrow, short, wavy portion of the tube adjacent to the uterus. (4) Last is the straight *intramural (interstitial) portion*, which passes through the uterine wall.

Cilia, or hairlike structures, which are part of the interior of the fallopian tubes, undulate to sweep the ovum toward the uterus. The walls of the tubes have a serosal covering, a muscular layer and a mucus lining; the latter contains the cilia. The tubes are supported by ligaments and supplied by blood from the uterine and ovarian vessels.

Uterus. The *uterus* is a hollow, thick-walled, muscular organ that looks like an inverted pear. It is about 2 inches long, 2 inches at the widest portion, 1 inch wide at the cervix, and between 1 and 2 inches thick. The uterus is situated in the pelvic cavity slightly below and between the fallopian tubes, almost at right angles to the vagina. The bladder is above and in front of it, and the rectum behind it. The uterus is attached to the bladder in front. It is separated from the rectum behind by a pouch (the "cul-de-sac of Douglas") which normally maintains the integrity of the two organs. The uterus is normally movable in all directions.

The uterus is divided into three *anatomic areas*: (1) the fundus, (2) the corpus, and (3) the cervix. The *fundus* or dome is the area between the insertion of the tubes. The *corpus* or body is the largest portion and is separated from the cervix by a slight constriction called the isthmus. The corpus is normally two times larger than the cervix in the adult, whereas in the newborn this relationship is reversed. The *cervix* attaches to and projects into the vagina for a short distance. The cervical opening into the vagina is termed the *"external os"* while the opening into the uterus is called the *"internal os."* The canal itself contains, among other things, glands that produce a mucin secretion.

The uterus has three *functional layers:* (1) the parametrium, (2) the myometrium, and (3) the endometrium. The *parametrium* is the thin peritoneal and fascial covering of the uterus. The *myometrium*, which makes up the bulk of the uterus, is the muscular portion and is itself composed of three layers of mostly involuntary muscles. Blood supply to the myometrium comes from the uterine branch of the hypogastric artery and from collaterals from the ovarian and vaginal arteries; it is then distributed to the rest of the uterus but particularly to the endometrium. The *endometrium* has a type of epithelium, the superior two-thirds of which has a cyclic response to hormones, whereas the basal one-third does not. Menstrual flow begins at the endometium, and it is in the endometrium that the fertilized ovum is implanted.

The uterus assumes its position in the body cavity through the action of *six ligaments* and the *pelvic floor*. Innervation to the uterus is provided by both the sympathetic and the parasympathetic divisions of the *autonomic nervous system*.

Vagina. The *vagina* is a musculomembranous canal that connects the uterus, through the cervical opening, with the external genitalia. The vagina has three layers: (1) the *epithelium*, (2) the *fibrous connective tissue*, and (3) the *muscular layer*. The upper third of the vagina is attached to the cervix. At the level of attachment, there is a shallow space in front called the "anterior fornix." In addition, there are two "lateral fornices" and a deep "posterior fornix." The mucosa of the vaginal wall folds over in a rugal pattern. This, in addition to the elasticity of the vagina allows the vagina to be very distensible. The vagina's rugal pattern and elasticity diminish with age during the menopausal and postmenopausal years. The bladder and the urethra are anterior to the vagina,

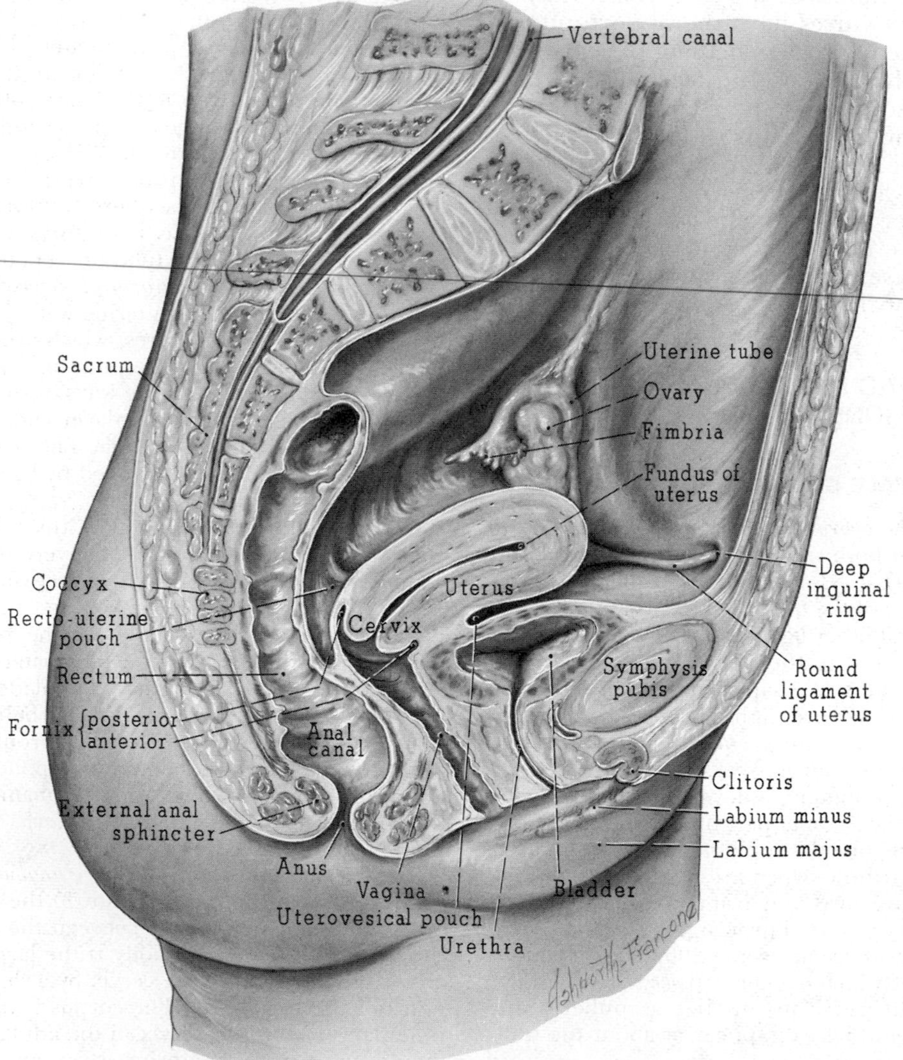

Figure 83–1. Mid-sagittal section of female pelvis. (From Jacob, S. W., C. A. Francone, and W. J. Lassow: *Structure and Function in Man,* 4th ed. Philadelphia: W. B. Saunders Co., 1978, p. 572.)

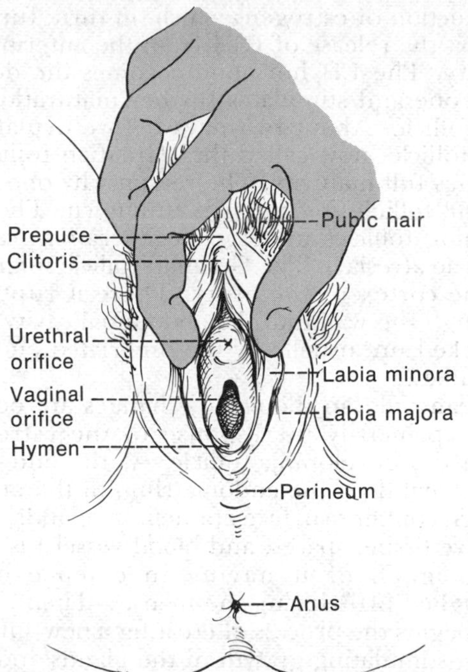

Figure 83–2. Anatomic landmarks of the external female genitalia.

and the rectum is posterior to its lower two-thirds. Thus, the vagina can easily become infected from urethral or rectal secretions, and vice versa.

EXTERNAL FEMALE GENITAL ORGANS

The female *perineum* refers to the area containing the external female genital organs. It is located between the thighs, below the pelvic diaphragm and in front of the rectum and anus. The organs contained in this area play a role in sexual stimulation and in maintaining the integrity of the body from foreign materials.

The *vulva* contains the labia majora, the labia minora, the clitoris, the vaginal opening (with the hymen), sebaceous glands, the urethra, Skenes' ducts, and Bartholin glands. The "vestibule" is the area of mucous membrane containing the urethral and vaginal openings, and is bounded by the labia minora. The anal region is posterior to this and is separated from the vulva by the perineal body (Fig. 83–2).

PELVIC BLOOD SUPPLY, INNERVATION, AND LYMPHATIC DRAINAGE

The most important *blood supply* to the external genitalia comes from the internal iliac artery (the hypogastric), a division of the common iliac artery. This artery branches to supply the pelvic floor, the pelvic walls and the pelvic viscera. The two branches of primary relevance to this discussion are (1) the uterine artery and (2) the vaginal artery. The former provides a rich, anastomotic network to the uterus, and the latter to the vaginal walls. In addition to the hypogastric artery, the ovarian artery (which arises at the level of the renal artery) supplies blood to the ovaries, the fallopian tubes, and the body of the uterus (where it joins the uterine artery to contribute to the uterine blood supply). In both instances, the venous drainage roughly parallels the arterial supply (Fig. 83–3).

Innervation to the pelvic structures is from both the *sympathetic* and *parasympathetic* autonomic nervous systems. The parasympathetic division of the system supplies the majority of the organs but does not seem to supply the uterus itself. The sympathetic system supplies most of the organs through a complex series of plexuses and branches. The perineum is principally supplied by the pudendal nerve.

The *lymphatic system* of the pelvis is divided into a superficial and a deep system. This is a richly anastomotic network, and again, the drainage system roughly parallels the blood supply.

> *There is a definite intermingling of the drainage from both the pelvic lymphatics and the blood vessels. This is important to recognize, as it plays a definite role in the spread of cancer.*

DISTANT STRUCTURES

The hypothalamus (in the brain), the pituitary gland (also in the brain) and a variety of other brain structures play roles in the regulation of the reproductive function of the genital organs and, more particularly, in the menstrual cycle. The thyroid gland and the adrenals may be involved, particularly in dys-

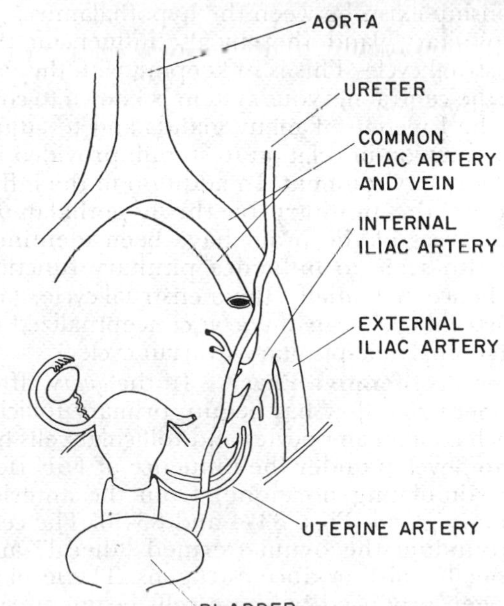

Figure 83–3. Major pelvic blood supply. (From Dilts, P. V., J. W. Greene, and J. W. Roddick: *Core Studies in Obstetrics and Gynecology.* Baltimore, The Williams & Wilkins Company, 1971.)

TABLE 83–1. EVENTS OF PUBERTY

Variable	Average Age (years)	Range (years)
Breast growth	11	8-14
Growth of pubic and axillary hair	11	8-14
Growth spurt	12	9½-14½
Menarche	13½	10-16

From Dickey, R. P.: Reproductive anatomy, physiology, and endocrinology. *In* Esinman, A. W., Knox, E. G., Tyrer, L. (Eds.): *Seminar in Family Planning,* 2nd ed. Chicago, American College of Obstetrics and Gynecology, 1974.

function of the menstrual cycle. These structures are discussed in other units of this book.

THE MENSTRUAL CYCLE

The menstrual cycle of an adult female can be divided into two phases: (1) the proliferative phase and (2) the secretory phase. These phases are separated by the event of ovulation. Both phases are controlled by hormones secreted by the pituitary gland and those secreted by the ovary itself. It is the interaction between these hormones that produces the "typical, normal menstrual cycle." Also, there is experimental evidence, suggesting that an interdependent relationship exists between the hypothalamus and the pituitary gland, thereby also influencing the menstrual cycle. This is in keeping with the fact that the central nervous system is known to control the function of many glands and to adjust their function in relation to stimuli provided by the body environment. In addition to the influence on the pituitary by the hypothalamus, other areas of the brain have been identified that also seem to influence pituitary function and hence, potentially, the menstrual cycle. The menstrual cycle can then be conceptualized as a "hypothalamic-pituitary-ovarian cycle."

The Proliferative Phase. In the *ovary,* after the menstrual flow has begun, primary follicles (which contain an oocyte) and follicular cells begin to develop under the influence of FSH (follicle stimulating hormone) from the anterior pituitary gland (Figs. 83–4 and 83–5). The cells surrounding the ovum (termed "thecal" and "stromal" cells) produce estrogens. The level of estrogen produced by these cells begins to rise and signals the pituitary to inhibit further production of FHS and to stimulate secretion of LH (luteinizing hormone). Then the two pituitary hormones act together to stimulate the further production of estrogens which, in turn, further inhibit the release of FSH from the anterior pituitary. The LH hormone becomes the dominant one and stimulates further maturation of the follicle. About two days before ovulation, one follicle, now called the "Graafian follicle," reaches full maturity. The reason why one particular follicle is chosen is unknown. The remaining follicles undergo degeneration (called "follicle atresia"). The Graafian follicle migrates to the cortex of the ovary. There it ruptures through the wall into the abdominal cavity and is picked up, usually by the fimbriated ends of the tubes.

Meanwhile, in the *uterus,* changes are occurring—primarily in response to the estrogen from the developing follicle. At the end of a menstrual flow, the endometrium of the uterus (which contains surface epithelium, glands, connective tissue, spaces, and blood vessels) is very thin, much of it having in essence been "sloughed off" during the menses. Then estrogen begins the process of creating a new surface layer, stimulating growth of the glands and the stroma and changing the blood vessels, which become progressively more coiled.

The *cervix* also undergoes changes, the most important being that mucus secretion greatly increases just prior to ovulation. At the time of

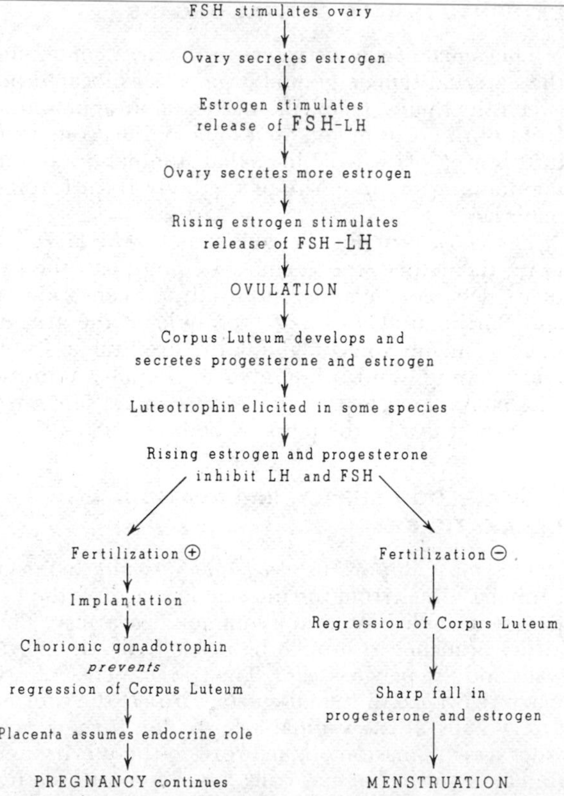

Figure 83–4. Diagram of the menstrual cycle. (From Tepperman: *Metabolic and Endocrine Physiology.* Year Book Medical Publishers, 1962.)

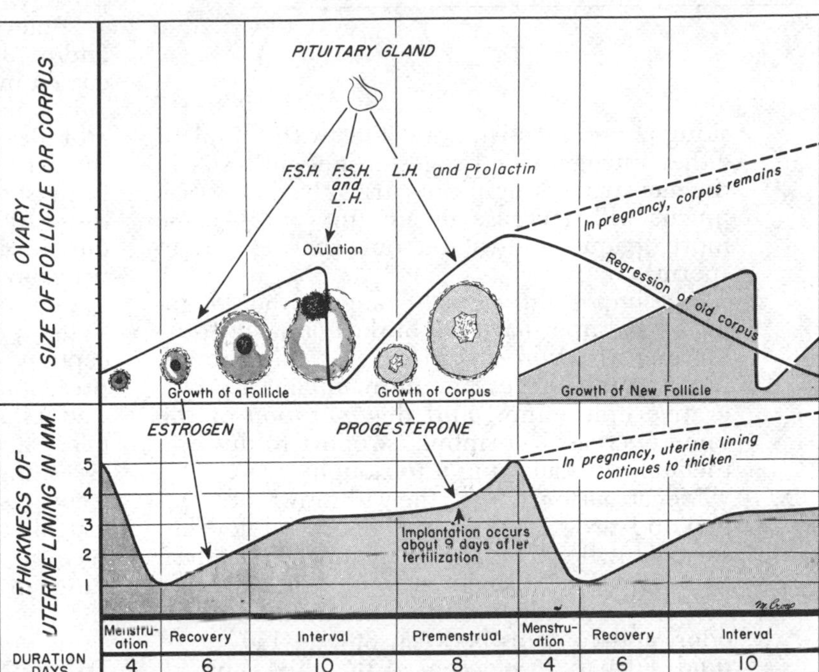

Figure 83–5. Average 28-day menstrual cycle. The cycle begins when hormones from the pituitary gland stimulate the development of an egg in a follicle inside one of the ovaries. About the fourteenth day, ovulation occurs. The follicle bursts, and the egg is discharged from the ovary. If the egg is not fertilized, the cycle ends in menstruation on the twenty-eighth day. If the egg is fertilized, pregnancy begins. (*Note*: Solid lines indicate course of events when ovum is not fertilized; dotted lines indicate course of events when fertilization occurs. Actions of hormones of pituitary and ovary in regulating the cycle are indicated by arrows.) (Villee.) From *Dorland's Illustrated Medical Dictionary,* 25th ed. Philadelphia: W.B. Saunders Co., 1974, p. 394.)

ovulation, mucus secretion is maximal, and the mucus is a clear fluid that is receptive to sperm.

The *vagina* also undergoes changes. Estrogen causes proliferation and thickening of the vaginal epithelium, a change that is greatest at the time of ovulation. This whole phase of the cycle is thus dependent on the ratio of FSH to LH.

Ovulation. Increasing levels of estrogen cause a decrease in the secretion of FSH, thus allowing an LH flood which occurs over a 24-hour period and produces ovulation as well as begins the luteinizing process of the follicle cells. *Ovulation* occurs between 12 and 15 days before the onset of the next menstrual period.

The Secretory Phase. During ovulation, the ovarian follicle collapses and there is a temporary drop in the production of estrogens. Some hemorrhage occurs into the center of the ruptured follicle (where a clot forms quickly) and also occasionally into the abdomen where it irritates the wall and produces the characteristic transient pain that some women experience with ovulation ("mittelschmerz"). Occasionally this pain is mistaken for appendicitis.

Shortly before ovulation, the thecal and granulosa cells that line the follicle begin to hypertrophy and proliferate. This process is enhanced by the LH flood that occurs with ovulation. The clot, which formed in response to the hemorrhage when the follicle ruptured, is replaced with yellowish luteal cells containing lipids. These cells produce progesterone and eventually form the *corpus luteum*, or "yellow body," in response to stimulation from LH. As the corpus luteum is formed, increasing amounts of progesterone and some estrogen are produced.

Full maturity of the corpus luteum is attained about 9 days after ovulation. If pregnancy does not occur, the corpus luteum begins to degenerate on or about the fourth or fifth day before the onset of the next menstrual period, with a concurrent drop in progesterone and estrogen production. The LH and FSH ratio is changed again, and the pituitary is stimulated to increase its production of FSH to begin the cycle again.

The changes occurring in the uterus are intimately associated with and dependent on those occurring in the ovaries. Primarily under the influence of estrogens, proliferation of the endometrium peaks about 2 days before ovulation. During the secretory phase, the progesterone, in addition to the estrogen, promotes the secretory activity of the endometrium. This is characterized by edema of the stromal part of the endometrium, changes and enlargement of the glands, coiling and tortuosity of the arteries, and hypertrophy of the connective tissue. The endometrium is ready then for implantation of the fertilized ovum. This development peaks about 7 or 8 days after ovulation, which is the most favorable time for implantation.

If implantation does not occur, degeneration of the corpus luteum, with its concurrent decline in progesterone and estrogen production, causes retraction and degeneration of the endometrium. Two to 3 days before the menses, there is a heavy infiltration of the endometrium with leukocytes. The blood vessels constrict and ischemia results, leading to the endometrial slough, or menstruation. The withdrawal of either estrogens or progesterone will result in the menstrual slough. Concurrently, the cervical mucus will decrease in amount, will become more opaque, and will be somewhat resistant to sperm.

The important vaginal change is the sloughing of the superficial cells of the epithelium during menstruation. Again, this is related to the fact that the corpus luteum maintains a proliferative epithelium, and degeneration of the same decreases hormonal support to this epithelium, thus allowing it to slough.

Menstruation. With the withdrawal of estrogen and progesterone, the menstrual flow ensues. This flow consists of mucus, endometrial tissue fragments, vaginal epithelial cells, and blood. It is usually dark red, has a characteristic odor, and contains between 60 and 150 ml. of fluid. Fifty to 75 per cent of this fluid is blood, which does not usually clot, although some small clots may occur and be normal. The usual duration of the menses is about 5 days, although durations of 1 to 10 days may be normal for a given individual. The interval between periods, about 25 to 32 days, can also vary considerably and be normal. Most women develop a characteristic pattern, although there are women whose patterns are unpredictable, yet normal. The menstrual pattern can be altered by climate changes, emotionally traumatic experiences, stress, and acute or chronic illness.

Important menstrual abnormalities to be suspicious of are intermenstrual bleeding and prolonged, heavy bleeding. Either of these two problems should be investigated by a physician.

Although these problems may not indicate an abnormality, they can be symptoms of more serious disorders, e.g., cancer.

The amount of bleeding can be assessed approximately by knowing that the average saturated perineal pad contains between 30 and 50 ml. of fluid and by keeping track of the number of pads used in 24 hours.

Normally the blood lost during the menstrual flow slightly decreases the hemoglobin level. However, if a woman already has iron-deficiency anemia, this loss aggravates the anemia. In addition to the medical therapy which a physician may prescribe in such a situation, the nurse should assess the nutritional status and patterns of the woman and counsel her appropriately. (Anemias are discussed in Unit XIV.)

Some women experience discomfort before and/or during the menstrual flow; this is discussed more fully later in this chapter.

It is important for nurses to remember that attitudes about menstruation are formed during the early years of life. The nurse may be asked to present information to young people during these formative years. Two factors are important in giving such a presentation. One, and probably most important, is consideration of the nurse's own attitudes, beliefs and background so that personal prejudices and possibly misconceptions do not inappropriately influence the presentation. The second is the awareness and understanding of the myriad of "old wives' tales" about menstruation. Questions may be asked that reflect individual cultural and familial beliefs and practices. These questions require tactful but honest answers by the nurse. In any such presentation, the naturalness of menstrual function should be stressed.

THE SEX HORMONES: OTHER FUNCTIONS

Before consideration of the menopause, some of the additional roles of the sex hormones should be discussed. Estrogen and (to a lesser extent) progesterone both have effects on the body besides those associated with the normal adult menstrual cycle. In fact, the menopause is often viewed as an "estrogen deficient state."

Estrogens (steroids) are manufactured primarily by the ovarian follicular cells, but a small amount is produced by the adrenal glands. The additional effects produced by estrogenic stimulation are primarily those seen at the time of puberty. These include: growth of the breasts, particularly fatty tissue deposition and pigmentation; fat deposition in the vulva; growth of pubic and axillary hair; growth and broadening of the bony pelvis; vaginal epithelial changes; and growth of the internal and external genitalia. Thus, the typical contours of the adult female are acquired.

In addition to the effects cited above, estrogens have an influence on (a) maintaining positive nitrogen balance; (b) calcium and phosphorus metabolism and retention of calcium in the bones; (c) retention of sodium chloride and, hence, sodium and water balance; (d) the control of blood proteins and lipids; (e) the vascular and skeletal systems; and (f) thyroid function, insulin production, and adrenal function. Because the exact nature of all these relationships is not always clear, there is some controversy regarding treatment with estrogen supplementation during the menopausal and postmenopausal years.

Progesterone also plays a role in sodium and

water balance, although a minor one. It also influences nitrogen balance as well as breast function and body temperature during the menstrual cycle.

THE MENOPAUSE

A transitional phase called *the climacteric* heralds the onset of the menopause, some time between the ages of 45 and 50. Over a period of one to two years during the climacteric, the monthly menstrual flow occurs less frequently, is irregular, and the flow is diminished in amount. After there have been no periods for one year, the *menopause* is said to have occurred. (Many people refer to the climacteric as the menopause.) During this transitional time, both ovulatory and anovulatory periods occur. Occasionally unplanned pregnancy results if women are not informed that contraception should be continued until the menses have been absent for at least 6 months.

The climacteric may be induced by surgical removal of the reproductive organs (including the ovaries) or pelvic irradiation in a woman of any age. In these instances, because of the rapidity of onset, unless replacement hormones are given, many women have a greater tendency for the accompanying signs and symptoms to be severe. Delayed onset of the climacteric (occurring about ages 55 to 60) is associated with a higher incidence of pathologic conditions and should be investigated by a physician.

The climacteric, with its gradual decline in ovarian function, leads to a relative estrogen deficiency state. This is only a "relative" deficiency state because, in addition to the estrogen produced by the adrenals, the ovaries apparently continue to produce estrogens in diminished amounts for up to 10 years. The pituitary gland, in response to the lowered estrogens, secretes gonadotropins, leading to a continuous elevation of the blood gonadotropin level. Therefore, the menopause is sometimes also referred to as an *excess gonadotropin period* rather than an "estrogen deficiency state." In any event many changes occur during this time of life that are related to a rebalancing of physical, hormonal, and chemical patterns.

Symptoms and Body Changes. Approximately 85 per cent of all women experience some symptoms during the climacteric. However, only about one-fourth of these women are distressed enough to consult a physician. Physicians are most often consulted about vasomotor symptoms. Vasomotor symptoms associated with menopause are probably caused by hormonal imbalances. Estrogen appears to exert a protective effect on subcutaneous blood vessels. Lowered estrogen levels render many women more sensitive to stimuli that precipitate sweating, skin discoloration, and the sensation of heat loss. Hot flushes (involving the head, neck and upper thorax) and excessive perspiration, especially at night, are the primary vasomotor symptoms. Combined with the irregularity and final cessation of the menses, these represent the classic symptoms of the climacteric.

A myriad of other symptoms can occur that may or may not be related to the climacteric changes. These include insomnia, headaches, palpitations, nervousness, apprehension, depression and other emotional symptoms, e.g., feelings of futility and uselessness. Emotional problems are severe in a small number of women; some of these women develop involutional melancholia and require psychotherapy.

Estrogen deficiency leads to other changes, in many instances a reversal of the changes which began at puberty. These do not all occur at the time of the climacteric; in fact, they often become evident many years later. These changes include: a redistribution of fat; a tendency to gain weight more readily; arthralgias and muscle pain; loss of elasticity in the skin; atrophy of the external genitalia; loss of subcutaneous fat within the labial folds; thinning of vaginal and vulvar mucosa; and atrophy of breast tissues. The vaginal changes may cause atrophic vaginitis (discussed in Chapter 85). One of the last changes may lead to the development of osteoporosis, with the presence of the "dowager hump" and loss of height. Osteoporosis can also contribute to the higher incidence of fractures, such as those of the hip, in this stage of life. (Osteoporosis is discussed in Chapter 78.) A tendency toward hypothyroidism (and less frequently, to hyperthyroidism) may result from the changes in glandular interrelationships.

Additionally, increasing evidence supports a relationship between estrogens and the function of the cardiovascular system. The statistical incidence of atherosclerotic vascular disease and its sequelae (coronary artery disease, stroke and hypertension) is much higher in postmenopausal women than prior to the menopause.

Clinical Management. Clinical management of women who are having difficulty with the menopause is highly individualized and is based on an accurate assessment of each woman and her needs. Several types of drugs may be used, but regardless of what else is done, *patient education* and *reassurance* are always indicated.

Nurses can assist a woman in menopause to develop an accurate awareness of herself, both physically and psychologically, by encouraging the patient to keep a journal of her symptoms, the times she usually experiences them, and any possible preceding stressors. This valuable information may assist the physician in a medical-pharmacological regimen as well as give the patient a feeling of increased control over an important change in her life. In this way, the patient assumes an active and valued role in her nursing care planning. Review of the written material by both nurse and patient may be an important step in helping the patient expand her style of coping with her symptoms.

Sedatives and *tranquilizers* may be prescribed and can be helpful with some of the symptoms, e.g., insomnia, nervousness, and other emotional manifestations. *Hormonal substitution* with estrogens may also be used on a short-term basis to relieve the classic vasomotor symptoms of hot flushes and excessive perspiration (Table 83–2). In some cases, these hormones also give some relief from other symptoms, including palpitations, nervousness, and other more typically emotional manifestations. Estrogens also help to relieve the pains and discomforts of climacteric arthralgias and arthritis.

It is possible for a physician to demonstrate that a woman is estrogen deficient by doing a "maturation index." This is a test done on a smear of cells from the vaginal wall. Estrogen deficiency causes a shift in the types of predominant cells. Substitution therapy, lasting anywhere from a few months to 2 years, is frequently undertaken with satisfactory relief of the symptoms. Therapy is discontinued gradually after the transitional phase of climateric has ended.

There is evidence accumulating that demonstrates a link between long-term, high-dose exogenous estrogen use and both endometrial and breast cancer. Therefore, many physicians are advocating low-dose cyclic usage of the hormone for between 6 months to 2 years, the usual duration of primary symptoms of menopause.

TABLE 83–2. REPRESENTATIVE PREPARATIONS OF THE THREE MAJOR GROUPS OF ORAL ESTROGENS

Type	Generic Name	Tradename
Conjugated estrogens	Conjugated estrogens (USP)	Premarin
	Esterified estrogens (USP)	Amnestrogen
	Esterified estrogens (USP)	Estratab
	Esterified estrogens (USP)	Evex
	Piperazine estrone sulfate	Ogen
Nonsteroidal estrogens	Diethylstilbestrol	Stilbestrol
Chemically altered estrogens	Ethinyl estradiol	Estinyl
	Ethinyl estradiol	Feminone

From Easterling, W. E., Jr.: Managing the menopause. *American Family Physician*, 7:137, Mar. 1973.

Estrogen may at times be used to treat late manifestations of estrogen deficiency in some patients. These can include osteoporosis and atrophic vaginitis with or without urethritis. In osteoporosis, the estrogens seem to help maintain calcium in the bones, preventing further collapse of the vertebral column and further reduction in the patient's height. The latter is a good index of the success of therapy. With atrophic vaginitis and its attendant symptoms of burning, pruritus, and discharge, a short course of estrogens will cause reepithelialization of the mucosa and, combined with other measures, may relieve the problem.

Currently however, there is controversy and concern about the role of estrogen replacement therapy in menopause and postmenopause. As early as 1947 some medical writers cautioned against the indiscriminate use of estrogen. Today, estrogen is the third largest-selling prescription drug in the United States. Women using the medication for menopausal symptoms may also believe that estrogen can prevent or retard the aging process in all body tissues. With recent studies pointing to an increased association of long-term estrogen use with development of breast and endometrial cancer, more consideration is now given to family histories and thorough and frequent physical monitoring, with the risks of therapy weighed against the benefits for each individual.

One of the more important aspects of the treatment of a menopausal woman is patient education and reassurance. The nurse can play a substantial role in both of these areas. In order to do so, it is important to spend time with the patient both as a sympathetic listener and to gather information about the woman's life style and interests. In this way, the nurse may help the patient to make realistic plans for the future. Some women may be afraid of information about the menopause, because they hold the common misconception that menopause is a time of potential psychologic instability. Such women then have to cope with a major life change without accurate information. Unexamined anxiety then develops that may feed on itself, contributing to greater levels of free-floating anxiety. Depending on the individual, menopause can *symbolize* aging, loss of social role (through loss of fertility), loss of femininity, waning mental and emotional stability, and ultimately death. It must be remembered that women have a life expectancy of approximately 25 years after menopause. It is important to help women express their fears and concerns about the changes that are happening to them, because fear may prevent a woman from assimilating or using the information a nurse gives.

Among the considerations to keep in mind in both assessment and teaching are:

- Unpleasant symptoms of the climacteric can be managed.
- It is helpful for women to understand the physiology of the menopause and to have misconceptions clarified.
- The climacteric and its more common symptoms are normal and limited to the transitional phase.
- Overfatigue and other environmental factors can aggravate the symptoms.
- Satisfying, comfortable sexual activity is possible during menopausal and postmenopausal years.
- Physical activity (including participation in sports) and development of new interests may help to alleviate tension and anxiety.
- Attention to nutrition and diet can prevent weight problems and feelings of fatigue.
- Annual medical check-ups, including a "Pap test," are important for the early detection and treatment of medical problems.
- Good general health habits can help the woman undergoing menopause to feel better and to have an optimistic outlook.

Regardless of the treatment plan devised, it is important for nurses to help the patient to understand the plan and to adapt it to her needs. If drugs are prescribed, a nurse may be the one who teaches the patient about the drugs and their side effects. Special emphasis should be placed on the need for the patient on estrogen therapy to check with her physician should she experience vaginal spotting and/or bleeding. Although withdrawal bleeding can occur, postmenopausal bleeding may also be a sign of cancer and should be investigated.

Withdrawal bleeding can best be described as vaginal bleeding unrelated to menstruation. Women taking exogenous estrogens for menopausal symptoms usually take the medication in a cyclic dosage, often 25 days of the month. Withdrawal bleeding occurs during the days estrogen is not taken, resulting in uterine lining instability. Withdrawal bleeding can be considered abnormal in the sense that no bleeding should occur if the right amount of hormone is prescribed and taken. Should this symptom occur, the health care provider needs to be informed to reevaluate both the dosage of exogenous estrogens and the state of the endometrial tissue.

MENSTRUAL ABNORMALITIES

Commonly encountered menstrual disorders include abnormal uterine bleeding, premenstrual tension syndrome, and dysmenorrhea. These topics are discussed in following sections.

Dysmenorrhea

"Dysmenorrhea" literally means "pain with menses" and should be considered in two categories: primary and secondary. *Primary dysmenorrhea* is essential in nature. The etiology is not known, although there are many theories as to the cause. Among the factors implicated are constitutional factors such as anemia or diabetes; endocrine factors; anatomical factors such as acute anteflexion of the uterus or cervical stenosis; and psychological factors. *Secondary or acquired dysmenorrhea* is associated with pelvic disease; however, a cause-and-effect relationship cannot always be demonstrated.

The incidence of pain with menstruation varies widely, but some form of pain occurs in about one-third of all women. Not all of these women have symptoms severe enough that they consult a physician. However, *dysmenorrhea still remains one of the most common symptoms prompting women to seek gynecologic help.* Additionally, it is an economic problem, as it is one of the most common causes of absenteeism for women.

Primary (Idiopathic) Dysmenorrhea. Primary or idiopathic dysmenorrhea usually does not occur until several years after the menarche, when ovulatory cycles occur more regularly. Anovulatory cycles rarely, if ever, cause primary dysmenorrhea. Usually the pain has its onset at the beginning of the menstrual flow or a few hours before. It may last for a few hours or up to 1 or 2 days. It generally is most severe during the first day and gradually tapers off. During the maximal pain, the menstrual flow is scanty; the flow increases as the pain diminishes. The pain is spasmodic and cramping in nature and is compared by some with the pain of labor. The pain of dysmenorrhea typically occurs in the lower abdomen and occasionally may radiate into the groin, thighs, and vulva. It may be accompanied by malaise, nausea and vomiting, chills, headache, diarrhea, flushing, and the premenstrual tension syndrome. The pain occurs most commonly in the younger reproductive years, although it may persist into later years, particularly in the absence of delivery of an infant. In any event, dysmenorrhea is self-limited in nature, a fact that should be considered when treating a woman with this problem.

Despite the lack of specific knowledge about the *etiology* of primary dysmenorrhea, several factors are related. These include: psychologic factors, a low pain threshold; obstruction of the menstrual flow (as seen with cervical stenosis); vascular ischemia to the uterine musculature; and probably some hormonal imbalance. Recently, prostaglandins have been implicated as possible contributors to menstrual cramps. These biologically active lipids secreted in the endometrium can cause painful uterine contractions in some women.

There are several new medications (such as indomethacin, Naprosyn, and Motrin) now being prescribed that inhibit prostaglandin synthesis. The medications appear to affect the higher levels of prostaglandins during the proliferative phase of the menstrual cycle and also at the onset of menstruation. They decrease myometrial contractility and, therefore, pain. The nurse assumes a teaching role when patients are prescribed these medications, as various side effects may occur. Patients may experience gastrointestinal difficulties such as epigastric pain, nausea, and vomiting. Other adverse effects are headache, pruritus, and fluid retention. As widespread use of these medications is fairly recent, nursing knowledge of uses and side effects is necessary for monitoring patient care plans.

Factors which may aggravate primary dysmenorrhea include: a sedentary occupation, poor posture, poor personal hygiene, and constitutional illnesses such as anemia. Therefore, improving the health status and health habits is always indicated, and the nurse can be most helpful to the patient with regard to the latter.

There appears to be a higher incidence of pain in high-strung, sensitive young women. It is not uncommon to find that these people feel that menstruation is unhealthy or dirty. Although difficult to assess, fear and ignorance seem to contribute to enhancing the pain. The nurse, when assessing the health status of an individual, may observe clues which may clarify the part that these various elements play in pain, and may be able to cautiously instruct such an individual. It is easy to assign the psyche total responsibility for pain with menses. However, this leaves too many factors unexplained. While the psyche cannot be considered the sole cause of menstrual pain, it is equally wrong to ignore its contribution. In treating the patient, the psychologic health status of the individual must be considered.

Treatment of primary dysmenorrhea presupposes that organic disease has been ruled out. Clinical care must be tailored to fit the individual. However, empathy and an understanding attitude on the part of the health care team members are always indicated.

Immediate treatment of a mild to moderate attack includes resting for 1 or 2 hours, aspirin, hot beverages, and the application of heat to the lower abdomen. This regimen suffices for many women and allows them to soon continue their usual activities. The nurse may assist the patient who finds this regimen satisfactory by suggesting that taking aspirin and perhaps hot beverages *before* the attack becomes acute may abort the attack. Therefore, at the first sign of pain or discomfort, the woman may be able to prevent further problems.

Indomethacin, a medication that inhibits prostaglandin production, is one method of treatment available for primary dysmenorrhea. Oral contraceptives may also be prescribed if the dysmenorrhea is not of a congestive nature, as estrogen can contribute to uterine congestion.

Other drugs that may be prescribed by a physician include: antispasmodics; vasodilators; tranquilizers; mild doses of psychic energizers; and occasionally, for very severe pain, narcotics in the form of codeine. Careful management is necessary with some of these drugs because of their addictive potential. The nurse who teaches patients about the drugs should stress that the drugs alone should not be relied on, but that other measures designed to decrease or prevent the pain should also be continued. These include: (a) regular exercise for persons with sedentary occupations; (b) waist-bending types of exercises just before the onset of the period; (c) improving posture when indicated; (d) improving dietary habits when indicated; (e) avoiding constipation; and (f) avoiding overfatigue and overexertion during the period preceding the flow itself. If the pain is mild, remaining active and interested in one's activities may also help.

Hormones, in the form of oral contraceptives are sometimes prescribed to induce anovulatory cycles to treat dysmenorrhea. Therapeutic trials of 3 to 6 cycles with the drug may be used to see if the pattern of dysmenorrhea can be broken. If pain persists while the patient is following this treatment regimen (i.e., is "on the pill") it may mean that some underlying disease is responsible. In any event, after the therapeutic trial has been discontinued, caution should be exercised in evaluating the results, as ovulatory and anovulatory cycles coexist in some patients.

Additional treatment measures that may be employed to stop dysmenorrhea are: (a) dilatation of the cervix (which may give up to 6 months' relief in some patients) and (b) presacral neurectomy (employed very rarely but helpful in some patients).

Secondary Dysmenorrhea. Secondary dysmenorrhea characteristically appears somewhat suddenly, with the patient having a history of previously painless periods. The pain often starts 2 to 3 days before the menses appear and radiates into the entire abdomen, the small of the back and down the legs. It tends to be more constant and congestive in nature, without sharp cramps, and continues throughout the period and even for a short time thereafter.

Secondary dysmenorrhea usually is associated with pelvic disease such as tumors, inflammatory problems, endometriosis, a fixed malpositioned uterus and other problems. When possible, it is treated by removing the cause either medically or surgically. Sometimes treatment must be merely palliative. In all situations the nurse's role is to see that the patient receives medical attention and to provide supportive care based on the treatment plan designed by the physician.

Premenstrual Tension Syndrome

This syndrome not uncommonly occurs in women who also have dysmenorrhea. However, it can also occur as a separate entity, as can dysmenorrhea. In either case, for treatment purposes, it is more helpful to consider premenstrual tension syndrome separately.

The syndrome is characterized by some combination of the following symptoms: backache, abdominal distention, edema, headache, painful breasts, nervousness, restlessness, tremors, irritability, faintness, and insomnia. The symptoms may be mild. In its severest form, however, the patient may closely approach a psychotic state with striking personality changes, and may be suicidal.

Premenstrual tension syndrome may be difficult to recognize, and its etiology is not well understood. Hormonal imbalances leading to fluid retention combined with emotional tension and disturbances have, however, been implicated in the etiology. With these hormonal imbalances, the woman may become somewhat hypoglycemic and feel weak and faint. This is exacerbated by poor diet. One clue that frequently helps establish the diagnosis is the appearance of a significant weight gain 2 to 10 days before the onset of menstruation.

Assessment and treatment are again aimed at the general health habits of the individual, the specific symptoms, and the psychologic health of the individual.

General health habits, such as the consumption of excess coffee, alcohol, salt and nicotine, may exacerbate some of the symptoms. These agents should be decreased or eliminated during the latter half of the menstrual cycle.

Psychologic health problems and environmental stresses may respond to mild pharmacologic agents such as tranquilizers and/or energizers; however, these should be used *only* in conjunction with spending time with the patient for the purpose of listening to and trying to help the patient to find ways to modify the environment appropriately. There is some reported success with the use of pure progesterone in the treatment of premenstrual symptoms.

The premenstrual edema, abdominal bloating, headaches, breast tenderness, irritability and depression may respond to diuretic therapy during the second half of the cycle. This may be accompanied by a mild sodium restriction, or sodium restriction alone may suffice. The nurse can help the patient work out a diet plan with the sodium restriction and help her recognize the need for potassium supplementation with many of the diuretics. Potassium supplementation almost always can be accomplished with increased dietary intake by eating bananas, drinking orange juice, and the like.

Abnormal Uterine Bleeding

Abnormal uterine bleeding includes a variety of menstrual disorders, which are always symptomatic of underlying disease. All women with any of the following symptoms should be seen by a physician for diagnosis and treatment. (See Table 83–3.)

Amenorrhea. The *absence of menses* can be either primary amenorrhea or secondary amenorrhea. *Primary amenorrhea* refers to failure of

TABLE 83–3. ETIOLOGY OF ABNORMAL UTERINE BLEEDING

Pathology of the Cervix, Endometrium or Endosalpinx
- Cervical erosion
- Endocervical polyp
- Cancer of the cervix
- Endometrial polyp
- Submucous leiomyoma
- Chronic endometritis (tuberculosis)
- Adenomyosis
- Cancer of the endometrium
- Cancer of the fallopian tube

Complications of Pregnancy
- Threatened abortion
- Ectopic pregnancy
- Hydatidiform mole

Systemic Disorders
- Blood dyscrasias
- Anticoagulant therapy
- Metabolic abnormality
- Endometriosis
- Pelvic inflammatory disease

Dysfunctional Uterine Bleeding
- Postmenarcho
  - Polycystic ovarian disease
  - Stress-induced menstrual abnormalities
- Perimenopause
  - Declining ovarian function
- Postmenopause
  - Extraglandular formation of estrone

From Cleary, R. E., and L. Green: Dysfunctional uterine bleeding. *American Family Physician*, 15:130, Mar. 1977.

menstrual periods to appear by the age of 18. Further discussion of this topic is beyond the scope of this book, and the interested reader is referred to books and articles dealing specifically with congenital abnormalities and sterility.

Secondary amenorrhea refers to failure to menstruate after regular menstrual cycles have been established. The most frequent causes of secondary amenorrhea in the young female of reproductive age are physiologic and include pregnancy and breast feeding. The other two instances in which amenorrhea is normal are before menarche and after menopause.

With these exceptions, amenorrhea presents a diagnostic challenge because of the numerous potential causes. It can be related to tumors or other abnormalities of the endocrine glands including the adrenal, the thyroid, the pituitary gland and the ovaries. Disease of the vagina and uterus can cause secondary amenorrhea, as can the so-called "hypothalamic causes" such as emotional stress, psychoses or fear of pregnancy. Chronic debilitating diseases, severe anemias, uncontrolled diabetes mellitus, tuberculosis, chronic nephritis, malnutrition and obesity may also cause or worsen secondary amenorrhea. Some drugs, including the contraceptive agents and phenothiazines, may cause either scanty or absent menses.

Thus, the primary nursing role is to assist the woman experiencing amenorrhea in procuring the needed medical attention. In addition, the nurse may wish to assess recent changes in the patient's life style or general health picture, so that appropriate counseling and teaching can be offered once the diagnosis has been established. It is important for the nurse to remember that dietary and general hygienic factors may be overlooked in the therapeutic plan. Assessment of these areas with appropriate intervention may help to ensure success of the medical therapeutic plan.

Dysfunctional Uterine Bleeding (DUB). Use of this term implies that there is *an endocrine abnormality which causes improper regulation of the menses*. Unfortunately, DUB has been used by some to imply any abnormal bleeding associated with menstruation. Therefore, the nurse will need to pay close attention to how the term is being used in particular situations.

Dysfunctional uterine bleeding is commonly manifested by an episode of profuse bleeding, but may also present as chronic hypermenorrhea (prolonged, excessive menses) or chronic polymenorrhea (excessive menses). Blood loss, both acute and chronic, is frequently a concurrent problem and requires evaluation and treatment as needed.

Other causes of abnormal uterine bleeding, in addition to dysfunctional uterine bleeding, include: (a) reproductive problems, e.g., ectopic pregnancy and incomplete abortions; (b) diseases of the pelvic organs, e.g., tumors and inflammatory processes; and (c) disease of other body systems, e.g., blood dyscrasias and hypertension. Some of these problems are discussed in following chapters, while others have been covered elsewhere in this text.

Menorrhagia. This term means *excessive bleeding at the time of a normal period.* In the early reproductive years, menorrhagia is commonly associated with endocrine problems and blood dyscrasias. Later, it is more commonly associated with tumors (including carcinoma) or inflammation of the uterus or ovaries. As has been pointed out, assessing the actual amount of blood loss can be a problem, especially because many women are unable to give a reliable history of loss and tend to either minimize or exaggerate it. Asking them to compare the number of pads used during the abnormal period with the number used during a normal cycle can be helpful. In a more controlled setting, it may be valuable to weigh the pads before and after use to estimate the blood loss. In addition, the usual tests for anemia may be performed.

Metrorrhagia. *Bleeding between periods* may occur in the form of spotting or as outright bleeding. The common causes are similar to those responsible for menorrhagia. Additionally, ectopic pregnancy, spotting with ovulation and "breakthrough bleeding," (which sometimes occurs with contraceptive pills) may be considered. In the latter instance, the dosage needs to be adjusted.

The nurse should remember that irregular spotting may be the only early sign of cervical cancer.

Summary

Each of the above problems can indicate serious diseases and should be investigated. *In the older woman, menstrual symptoms are not uncommonly associated with malignancy of the reproductive tract and, with early diagnosis and therapy, the results can be quite favorable*. The specific treatment is related to the cause and, in many instances, will be discussed in succeeding chapters.

CHAPTER 84

DIAGNOSTIC AND TREATMENT MODALITIES AND RELATED NURSING CARE

by Judith Atwood R.N., M.N., and Judy Johnson, R.N., M.A.

We have stressed the importance of early diagnosis and treatment of gynecologic problems. This chapter discusses some of the more common diagnostic and treatment modalities used. However, it is pertinent first to consider the psychologic impact of disorders of the genital and reproductive organs and the manipulation of these private body regions during diagnostic testing and treatment.

PSYCHOLOGIC IMPACT OF GYNECOLOGIC PROBLEMS

The functions of the genital organs are symbolic to many people in a wide variety of ways. In addition to sexual and reproductive functions, some women associate normalcy of these organs with femininity. For these women, disorders of the reproductive system and their diagnosis and treatment may have a major impact on self-concept. Such women may experience great difficulty in accepting care. For others, the whole process may be an inconvenience, but if the disease is relatively minor, no major psychologic impact is felt. However, the outward reaction of the woman does not necessarily correlate with either her intimate feelings or the seriousness of the condition. For this reason, it is important for the nurse to assess the patient's psychologic status and reaction. In doing so, however, the nurse must be sensitive and be careful not to press the patient into disclosing information that she might later wish she had not revealed. Moreover, it is important to remember that the patient herself may not understand her own response. In any event, the nurse, by being a sensitive listener, may be able to provide support for the patient, and thus lessen the trauma of the experience. This is particularly true if the patient feels that her physician does not or is unable to understand her.

Some of the specific feelings that patients may experience include fear, humiliation, guilt, embarrassment, and anger. These feelings are given by many women as part of the reason they fail to have yearly examinations. The opportunity to ventilate these feelings to an empathetic listener may help the patient to cope with the situation. Moreover, aiding a patient in this manner may encourage her to come in for care or insure that she will seek adequate follow-up or preventive care. "Ventilation" sessions may also provide the nurse with an opportunity to clarify misconceptions the patient may have either about her diagnosis or proposed treatment. Many women have never had an opportunity to acquire reliable information about the reproductive organs and possible problems. Some examples of the more *common misconceptions* the nurse may encounter include:

1. Removal of the uterus means induction of the menopause.
2. A radical hysterectomy (without vaginectomy) means that one's sex life is terminated.
3. Removal of reproductive organs makes a woman less womanly.
4. Removal of one ovary produces sterility.
5. A suspicious Pap test positively establishes the diagnosis of malignancy.

Although reassurance that the above statements are incorrect may help the woman, such reassurance does not necessarily terminate the patient's need to talk to someone, nor does it necessarily correct the patient's misinformation. The nurse must continue to assess the patient's needs and may find that repetition of factual information is necessary. In addition, every effort to maintain the patient's privacy, to understand her emotional lability and to listen to her expression of her needs must continue. The nurse should remember that the goal for the patient who is having difficulty in handling her feelings is to help her to cope in the most healthy manner possible. This is a continuous process attended with ups and downs and does not mean that the patient should remain tranquil and not express her feelings.

THE GYNECOLOGIC EXAMINATION

The gynecologic history and pelvic examination are two major screening modalities used by physicians to detect problems involving the genital tract of women. Currently, nurses are also being trained to use these modalities to screen patients and identify those who need a physician's special attention. These nurse practitioners or clinical specialists provide important health care services.

The focus of this discussion is on the more traditional nursing roles. It is important to recognize that a specialized examination is only a portion of a total health assessment of a woman. This fact should be stressed, since many women do not recognize this. (Physical assessment is discussed in detail in Chapter 15. Psychosocial assessment is discussed in Chapter 14.)

The History. The gynecologic history has traditionally been designed to provide information for the physician as to potential problems the patient may have. In this way it guides the physical examination. Its components are listed in Table 84–1.

Today's nurse practitioner, with special education in the health care of women, also uses the history and physical examination as tools for identifying problems. Women requiring definitive medical treatment are referred to physicians. Problems requiring counseling, teaching, monitoring of therapy, or routine health status surveys may be managed by nurse practitioners.

The Pelvic Examination. The pelvic examination is described in detail in Chapter 15 (p. 362); a brief review of major points is given here. When a woman makes an appointment for a pelvic examination, she should be instructed to not douche for 24 hours before the examination. Just before the examination, she should be instructed to void and to empty her bowels. Explain that this will make the examination more comfortable and more accurate. Often, the urine is to be examined, so she should be instructed in how to collect a specimen. Instruct the woman to remove enough clothing to allow examination of both the abdomen and the perineal structures. If a breast exam is also going to be performed, ask the patient to disrobe completely and to put on a gown.

TABLE 84–1. COMPONENTS OF A GYNECOLOGIC HISTORY

- The Menstrual Cycle
  - Age at onset of menarche
  - Length of cycle
  - Interval between cycles
  - Regularity of cycle
  - Amount and type of flow
  - Date of last menstrual period (L.M.P.)
  - Associated symptoms (e.g., pain, intermenstrual bleeding, etc.)
- Sexual History
- Medications
  - Contraceptives
  - Hormones
  - Others
- Obstetric History
  - Number of pregnancies and outcome of each
  - Complications of pregnancy and delivery and/or abortion
- Previous Surgery and Illness
  - Gynecologic
  - Other major surgery or illness
- Bowel and Urinary Assessment
- Associated Organ Review (e.g., endocrine)
- Presenting Problem

Adapted from Behrman, S. J., and J. R. G. Gosling: *Fundamentals of Gynecology,* 2nd ed. New York: Oxford University Press, 1966.

Help the woman assume the desired position on the examining table. Generally, this is the dorsal recumbent or lithotomy position (Fig. 84–1), although either the Sims' (side lying) or knee chest position may be used. In the lithotomy position, the woman's buttocks should be flush with the end of the table (or end of the table leaf if there is one), and the legs should be placed in and taken out of the stirrups simultaneously.

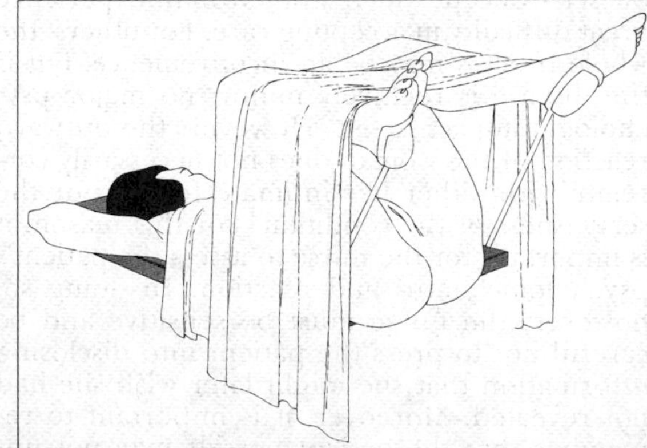

Figure 84–1. Patient positioned for pelvic examination and draped for breast examination. Note that patient's buttocks are positioned well over the edge of the table. (From Haynes, D. M.: *Essentials of the Gynecologic History and Examination.* Philadelphia: Smith, Kline & French Laboratories, 1965, p. 13.)

A drape is used, and the legs should be well protected. (Consult a basic nursing text for a discussion of this type of drape.) The following equipment should be ready for use during the examination:

1. An appropriate size speculum
2. Materials with which to obtain smears and cultures, e.g., Papanicolaou (Pap) smear
3. Long forceps and cotton balls
4. A good light source
5. Water-soluble lubricant
6. Appropriate size gloves

Additionally, biopsy and cauterization equipment should be in the room, so that the nurse does not have to leave the room to get it if these procedures should be performed. (Special tests and procedures are discussed in a later section.)

A pelvic examination consists of four parts:

- *Inspection of the external genitalia* is usually carried out first. Abnormalities such as discharge, areas of inflammation, or outlet relaxation are noted.
- *The speculum examination.* After inspecting the external organs, the examiner puts on gloves and inserts the speculum (see Fig. 15–33), without lubricant, because it would interfere with the accuracy of the various smears. Insertion is easier and more comfortable for the patient if warm water is run over the speculum first. Through the speculum, the vaginal walls and the cervix are inspected. Smears (the Pap smear and others) are obtained. The speculum is then removed slowly, and the vaginal surfaces are observed during removal.
- A *bimanual examination* is usually conducted next. One or two fingers of one hand are inserted into the vagina, and the other hand is placed on the abdomen. The organs are palpated between the fingers and the abdominal hand (see Fig. 15–34).
- Finally, a *rectovaginal examination* is typically performed. By insertion of one finger into the rectum, the rectal tissues can be evaluated for abnormalities such as hemorrhoids, and the posterior aspect of the genital organs can be evaluated between the vaginal finger and the rectal one (Fig. 84–2).

For the most part, the examination in women who have no pathologic conditions causes no discomfort or only minimal discomfort. Exceptions that may produce some discomfort include palpation of the tender ovaries during the bimanual examination, and the rectal examination. The nurse should anticipate this and ask the woman to bear down during the rectal examination and to breathe deeply through her mouth during the palpation of the ovaries. The latter helps to relax the abdominal muscles and may facilitate the whole examination if the patient is tense. After the examination is completed, any indicated instructions should be given and appropriate health teaching conducted. In many instances, these activities are the nurse's responsibility.

Although a pelvic examination is done quickly, and usually with minimal patient discomfort, it is quite common to hear women discuss this type of examination in a manner which points out how much they dread this procedure. Fear and embarrassment regarding the necessary exposure of private body areas and discussion of private matters, as well as fear of what may be found, may make some women reluctant to submit to such an examination. Even those who undergo the examination may fail to give a completely frank history. A kind and matter-of-fact attitude on the part of the nurse and physician may help alleviate part of this distress. Proper draping, explanation of the examination, and explanation of the types of questions asked may also help. In any event, failure to attain a satisfactory patient relationship can hinder obtaining a satisfactory examination.

On occasion, a suspicious mass or other problem may be found during the office examination. In some instances, the patient may then be admitted to the hospital for an examination under anesthesia in the operating room. The examination is then conducted mostly as described, with the addition of anesthesia and sterile conditions. Such an examination is also conducted before various special tests done in

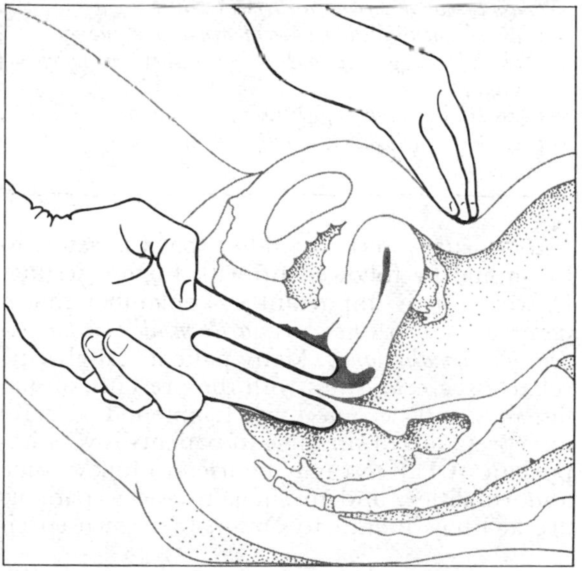

Figure 84–2. Rectovaginal examination. This drawing illustrates combined bimanual examination with the examiner's index finger in the patient's vagina and middle finger rectum. (From Haynes, D. M.: *Essentials of the Gynecologic History and Examination.* Philadelphia: Smith, Kline & French Laboratories, 1965, p. 23.)

the operating room and before some types of surgery.

SPECIAL TESTS AND PROCEDURES

Cytology. Most frequently, "cytology" refers to a *Papanicolaou smear* when the term is used in gynecologic testing. However, this is not a strict definition, as "clinical cytopathology" is the study of cells obtained from a variety of sources. Therefore, there are many different types of specific studies used.

Papanicolaou Smear. This test is based on the fact that both normal and abnormal cells from the lining of the various organs (e.g., uterus, cervix) exfoliate and pass into both cervical and vaginal secretions. By making a smear of these secretions, early cellular changes may be detected before they become clinically apparent. The Pap test is the most useful in diagnosing cervical carcinoma and may be up to 95 per cent accurate in detecting this lesion in its early stages. It is much less accurate (about 40 per cent) in detecting endometrial carcinoma.

The smears are read by a clinical cytologist and frequently reported as follows:

Class I—no abnormal or atypical cells present
Class II—atypical, but no evidence of malignancy
Class III—suggestive, but not conclusive for malignancy
Class IV—strongly suggestive of malignancy
Class V—conclusive for malignancy

It is usually recommended that Classes II to IV should be followed up with further testing. However, it is important to remember that *a suspicious test does not necessarily mean that the patient has a malignancy*. Many patients falsely correlate a suspicious test with the presence of malignancy and become quite frightened. Careful interpretation of findings to patients is very important. A Pap test may be used to follow some abnormalities; and in such instances, patients are at times taught to obtain their own specimens.

The technique for obtaining a smear varies with the desires of the physician performing the test and with those of the cytologist reading it.

Smears are taken when the woman is midcycle and has refrained from douching during the previous 24 hours. A small amount of the secretions found in the vaginal pool located in the posterior fornix and of the secretions extruding from the cervix are obtained using an Ayre spatula. These secretions are smeared separately on clean and dry slides. The slides are marked with "C" for cervix and "V" for vaginal pool. Immediately after the smears are made they are fixed, using either a commercial spray or fixative solution. It is important to fix the secretions before any drying occurs, as drying will distort the cells and make the reading either difficult or impossible. Lubricant is not used on the speculum for the same reason. The procedure is usually painless. After the examination is completed, the nurse should inform the patient how to obtain the test results. A Pap test should be done yearly on all women over the age of 18 years. Sexually active women under 18, those with a family history of cancer, those with venereal infections, especially herpes, and those whose mother ingested stilbestrol during her pregnancy are some of the patients at higher risk. They may require earlier and more frequent testing. Specimens may also be taken from the vulva, vaginal wall, cervix, and endometrium.

Endometrial Smear. Many of the above principles apply in obtaining an *endometrial smear*. The test differs in that the cervix must be dilated under sterile conditions to obtain the specimen. The procedure is usually done during the first 12 hours following the onset of the menses. At this time, the cervix is somewhat easier to enter. Dilatation of the cervix may cause some cramping, which is usually relieved by analgesics and heat application to the lower abdomen.

Cervical Biopsy and Cautery. These procedures are frequently performed on an outpatient basis. A biopsy may be done at the time when a cervical lesion is first noted or delayed until about 1 week after the menstrual period, when the cervix is least vascular. Multiple biopsies are usually obtained at specified sites (frequently those identified by doing a Schiller test) with special biopsy forceps (Fig 84–3). The biopsied tissue is "fixed" appropriately, and then attention is directed toward achieving hemostasis. This may be accomplished by using cautery in the following manner. A lubricated lead plate is placed beneath the patient, in contact with her skin. The actual cauterization is then performed. An unpleasant odor results from the burning tissue, and the patient may experience some discomfort. After the procedure, vaginal packing is inserted and the patient rests for a short time before going home. She should be instructed to avoid any strenuous activity for the next 24 hours. Additional instructions often include: (1) leave the packing in until the physician gives permission for it to be removed (usually 12 to 24 hours), (2) report excessive bleeding to the physician immediately, (3) ab-

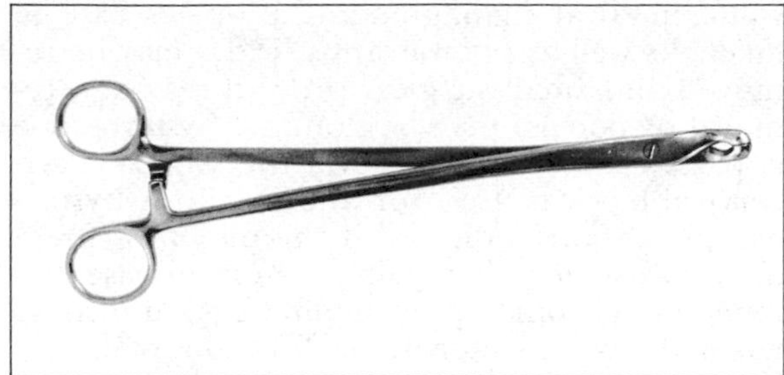

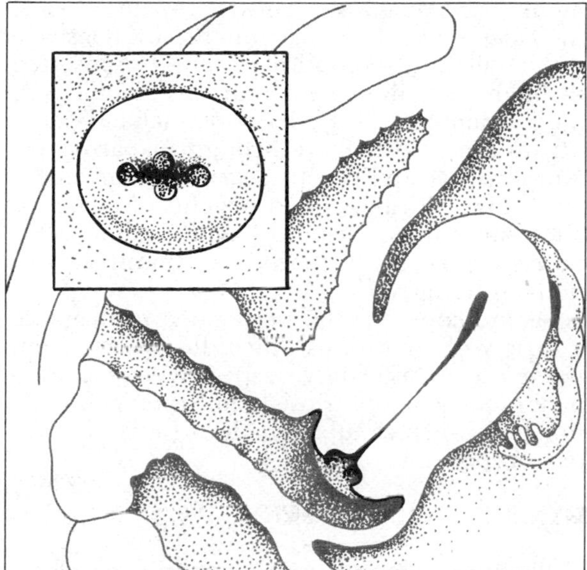

Figure 84–3. A. Gaylor uterine (cervical) biopsy forceps. B. Cervical biopsy sites. Insert shows one recommended pattern of biopsy sites; specimens are also taken from any abnormal appearing cervical area. (From Haynes, D. M.: *Essentials of the Gynecologic History and Examination.* Philadelphia: Smith, Kline & French Laboratories, 1965, p. 19.)

stain from coital activity and douching until otherwise instructed by the physician, and (4) avoid using tampons until the physician gives permission. The patient should also be made aware of the fact that she may have a foul smelling, grey-green discharge beginning about 4 days after the procedure and lasting for about 3 weeks.

Cervical Conization. *Conization* is the removal of the diseased part of the cervix by taking a cone-shaped section of the structure. (Cryosurgery, discussed later in this chapter, may also be used for this purpose.) A special knife is used, and the procedure is generally done in the operating room under anesthesia. The postoperative care is similar to that employed after dilatation and curettage. (Discussed on p. 1883.) A discharge may be expected after about four days and is frequently blood tinged.

Culdoscopy. This procedure is usually done in an operating room with the patient in a knee-chest position. Instrumental visualization of the structures in the cul-de-sac is accomplished through an incision in the posterior fornix of the vagina. Through this incision, a tubular instrument with an attached light source is passed into the cul-de-sac (Fig. 84–4). Preparation for the procedure is similar to that done for minor vaginal surgery, and post-procedure care is usually minimal, since the incision heals rapidly. Douching and sexual activity are avoided for about one week (until the physician tells the patient that these activities may be resumed). Com-

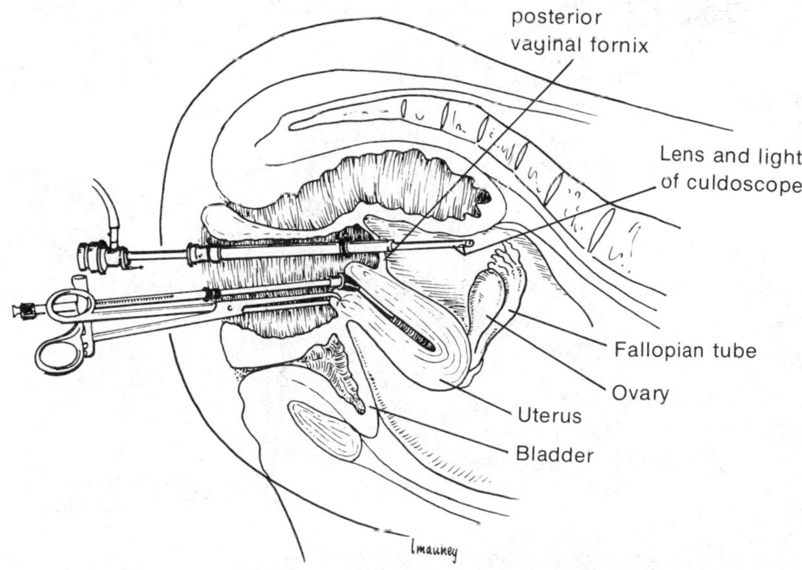

Figure 84–4. Diagrammatic representations of culdoscopy. Patient is in knee-chest position. (From Reid, D. E., and C. D. Christian (Eds.): *Controversy in Obstetrics and Gynecology II.* Philadelphia: W.B. Saunders Co., 1974, p. 601.)

plications can include infection, hemorrhage and, rarely, air embolism.

Culdocentesis. This procedure may be performed in the office or in the operating room. It is similar to culdoscopy except that a needle is inserted through the posterior fornix into the cul-de-sac to drain this area.

Posterior Culpotomy. Similar to culdoscopy, this procedure involves making a horizontal incision into the posterior fornix for the purpose of allowing an examining finger to be slipped into the cul-de-sac. In this manner the various structures can be palpated.

Culposcopy or Culpomicroscopy. This procedure involves the use of a magnifying instrument for examination of the cervical epithelium, the vulva, and the vagina. No incision is made. Epithelial abnormalities are readily identified by an expert. Commonly, visible cervical lesions or the cervix of a patient with an abnormal Pap smear are examined with the culposcope and biopsied as an office procedure. The procedure is safe, painless, and can be done on pregnant women.

Hysteroscopy. In this technique an endoscope (called a hysteroscope) is used to allow direct visual examination of the intrauterine cavity (Fig. 84–5). It is used for diagnosis and some medical management. Biopsies can be taken, as well as photographs. IUDs may be removed and small surgical procedures (e.g., removal of polyps) may be done. A hysteroscope is passed into the uterus via the vagina. Pericervical block is used for anesthesia. A hysteroscopy is contraindicated if the patient is pregnant, has acute pelvic inflammatory disease, has recurrent chronic upper genital tract infection, has had a recent uterine perforation, or has or is suspected of having a cervical malignancy.

Laparoscopy. A relatively new but commonly used diagnostic and therapeutic tool is the *laparoscope*. This instrument is a telescope with an illuminated optical system. It is inserted through a small incision near the umbilicus in the abdominal wall. Both abdominal and pelvic organs can be visualized through a laparoscope. Moreover, a laparoscopy is a safe, convenient procedure with the added benefits of being usable with outpatients and having a short post-procedure recovery period and minimal incisional scarring.

Laparoscopy may be performed to diagnose a variety of conditions—including pelvic pain, pelvic masses, infertility, suspected ectopic pregnancy, and endometriosis—and therapeutically for things such as tubal ligations for contraceptive purposes.

GYNECOLOGIC SURGERY

There are a number of types of gynecologic surgery procedures. Several different ones have

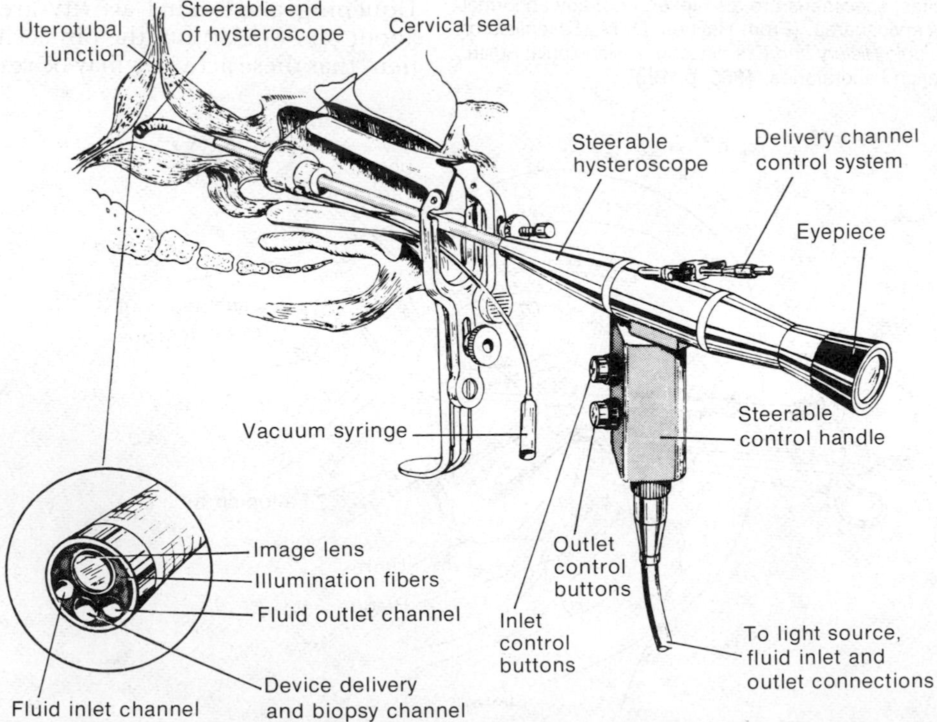

Figure 84–5. Hysteroscopy. (From Brueschlee, E. E., J. T. Archie, and G. D. Wilbanks: Hysteroscopy. *American Family Physician,* 15:126, Apr. 1977).

been chosen for discussion. By consolidating the information discussed here with that presented in the unit on surgery (Unit VIII), the student should be able to identify the type of nursing care required for persons undergoing procedures that are not specifically discussed. Moreover, general pre- and postoperative care considerations are not included here in order to avoid repeating the information discussed in Unit VIII. An example of a surgical procedure involving each of the major genital organs or areas is described.

Vulvectomy. Radical vulvectomy involves the extensive removal of numerous structures including the clitoris, the labia, the perineal subcutaneous tissues, vulvar glands, and extensive dissection of the femoral and inguinal lymphatics.

Preoperatively, preparation of the skin in the perineal and lower abdominal areas is done, and the patient herself should be prepared to face a prolonged healing period with an unpleasant appearing and uncomfortable wound. After healing has progressed, skin grafts may be performed and usually produce a somewhat more aesthetic long-term result. Moreover, sexual function is often retained.

Naturally this radical surgical procedure produces serious body image changes and may be psychologically devastating initially.

Clearly, vulvectomy is a very difficult experience for a woman, both physically and emotionally. She needs to be given (a) accurate information about the surgery and postoperative expectations, (b) repeated opportunities to ask questions and to express concerns to health professionals, and (c) understanding support from people who appreciate the stress the woman and her significant others are experiencing.

There are several operative approaches with vulvectomy, and the procedure is done in either one or two stages, depending on the patient's preoperative condition. After surgery, there are also several approaches to care. The patient has essentially two wounds, one in the perineal area, and one in the groin. The *perineal wound* may be covered with a bulky pressure dressing, which should be secured with a T-binder, or the area may be left without a dressing. The *groin wound* may also be covered or left uncovered. In the latter situation, drains in the wound are usually connected to suction. In both instances the wounds frequently have drains, and care must be exercised to avoid dislodging them. Wound care is done with either hydrogen peroxide or sterile saline and is usually followed by a heat lamp treatment or sitz bath after the sutures are removed. Wound care must be meticulous in order to avoid infection, with delayed healing. Because drainage may be extensive, dressings should be changed frequently.

Bowel and bladder care is important for women following vulvectomy. Feces from the bowel may contaminate the wound; both constipation and diarrhea should be prevented. A retention catheter is inserted into the bladder at the time of surgery, since the surgery involves the area of the urinary meatus. If this catheter is dislodged postoperatively, the extensive edema in the area makes it extremely difficult to replace. Some patients also have a suprapubic catheter. Even when the surgeon orders the catheter removed, the patient may experience difficulty in voiding. Postoperative bladder infections may occur since the catheter is usually left in place for an extended period. Every nursing effort should be made to avoid this complication.

Pain is another problem in the postoperative stage. Heavy, taut sutures are used to close the wounds and are left in place for 2 to 3 weeks. Therefore, many patients require longer periods of analgesics to control the pain. Additionally, pain may be alleviated by careful positioning of the patient in bed. Frequently, a low Fowler's position or a side-lying position with pillow support of the lumbar area and between the legs helps to decrease discomfort in the patient. The upper leg should be bent and kept slightly forward. *The knees should not be gatched, in order to avoid stasis in the perineal area and thrombophlebitis, one of the complications of this procedure.* Hourly leg exercises and frequent position changes will also help to avoid thrombophlebitis and other complications. The patient is usually ambulated 2 or 3 days after surgery. Standing in one position for prolonged periods should be avoided, both in the hospital and at home, because of the potential for pelvic congestion.

Vulvectomy causes mutilation of the perineal area and is accompanied by a high incidence of complications in the postoperative period. The patient usually requires extensive care and psychologic support. After discharge, the patient generally still has not completed her recovery phase and therefore needs instructions in self-care. Women experiencing vulvectomy can benefit from follow-up in the community by a public health nurse.

Vaginal Surgery. Several types of vaginal surgery have been discussed previously, including such vaginal repair procedures as those done for prolapse and fistulas. These discussions presented the major points to be considered in caring for patients who have undergone vaginal surgery.

Dilatation and Curettage ("D&C"). *Dila-*

tation refers to widening the cervical opening with a dilator, and *curettage*, to scraping the lining of the uterine cavity with a curette. The most typical indication for the operation is abnormal bleeding. This is an extremely common gynecologic procedure which, without complications, is relatively minor in nature. In many instances, dilatation and curettage is done as an outpatient procedure, with light general anesthesia.

Preoperatively, the patient should restrict her food and fluid intake. The perineal area is prepared for surgery, and a perineal shave may or may not be done, depending on the judgment of the surgeon. Some surgeons also order an enema before surgery.

Postoperatively, the patient returns to the ward with a sterile perineal pad in place, which should be changed as needed. She may also have vaginal and cervical packing in place, which is usually removed within the first 24 hours.

During the first few hours after surgery, the patient should be watched for excessive vaginal bleeding. Voiding should be assessed; it may be difficult, particularly if the patient has vaginal packing which exerts pressure on the urethra. The patient is usually only somewhat uncomfortable, with cramping being the major source of discomfort, especially if a pack is left in the cervical canal. Mild analgesics such as aspirin and codeine usually relieve this discomfort. Pain which is not relieved with these measures should be reported to the physician, since occasionally the uterus is accidentally perforated by the curette during the procedure.

The patient is most commonly discharged the day after D&C and instructed to: (a) avoid strenuous activity for about one week, (2) avoid douching and sexual activity until the physician gives consent, and (3) expect a vaginal discharge during the healing phase after the procedure. The subsequent menstrual period may or may not be affected.

Cryosurgery. *Cryosurgery* involves the local freezing of cells and tissues. These tissues then "flake off" and are discarded by the body. This type of treatment is used for a variety of gynecologic conditions, including chronic cervical erosion. Cervical polyps, condyloma acuminata, and benign leucoplakia are other commonly treated disorders. The procedure is commonly performed in a physician's office.

Volatile gases such as nitrous oxide, freon, or carbon dioxide are used to freeze the cells. Cell death results from dehydration and destruction of the cell membrane. The procedure is most usually performed one week after a patient's menstrual period. Care is taken to avoid freezing too large an area of the cervix at one time to avoid cervical stenosis. Postoperative healing takes about 10 weeks.

Approximately 80 per cent of the patients so treated for cervicitis require only a single treatment.

Nursing care during and after the procedure involves assessing and treating pain with the prescribed analgesic and teaching the patient what to expect after the treatment. During the procedure a small number of patients experience headaches, dizziness, and flushing. Postprocedure mild pain may continue for several days. A clear, watery discharge and then one that contains debris (e.g., cells) and possibly is malodorous may be present for about 14 days. Should the discharge persist beyond 8 weeks, an infection should be suspected, diagnosed and treated. Meticulous perineal hygiene both minimizes the risk of infection and makes the woman more comfortable.

It is important to explain to patients who are to undergo cryosurgery that the procedure is not actually a "surgical" procedure in that no incision is made.

Hysterectomy. Hysterectomy, or removal of the uterus, is done either through the vagina or through the abdominal wall. Typically, the *vaginal approach* is used when vaginal repair is to be done at the same time, while the *abdominal approach* is used in the presence of large tumors, or if the ovaries and fallopian tubes are to be removed at the same time as the uterus. In the past, a *partial hysterectomy* was done and involved leaving the cervix in place. However, except in rare instances today, only *total hysterectomy* (or removal of the uterus and the cervix) is performed.

Preoperative preparation includes either a standard perineal or abdominal preparation and shave. A vaginal douche and enemas may or may not be given. Postoperatively the patient has either an abdominal dressing and perineal pad or a sterile perineal dressing (pad). These dressings should be checked frequently for bleeding during the early postoperative phase. The perineal pad will normally have a moderate amount of serosanguineous drainage on it postoperatively.

Fluids and foods are restricted for a time and then resumed cautiously, since patients may be nauseated or may vomit early. If extensive handling of the viscera has been necessary, some physicians order a nasogastric tube to be inserted and left in for several days or until the bowel sounds return to normal. A rectal tube may help to relieve "gas pains." Frequently a Fleet enema is given several days postoperatively, as the patient may have difficulty defecating.

Abdominal distention may be present, particularly if a large tumor was removed or if the surgery was extensive. Some physicians will order a scultetus binder for this distention.

If the circulation has been interfered with, the patient may develop the complication of thrombophlebitis. Precautions, as discussed under vulvectomy, should be taken to avoid this sequela. Most patients are ambulated the day following surgery.

> *A serious complication to observe for following hysterectomy is accidental ligation of the ureter during surgery. Any low back pain or decrease in output should be reported to the surgeon.*

Many patients have an indwelling bladder catheter for the first few days postoperatively, as operative handling of the bladder and associated structures can predispose to postoperative problems with voiding. In any event, postoperative voiding should be checked, as retention is rather frequent. Other bladder complications including development of fistulas and infection are not uncommon. Other potential complications include (1) embolism, (2) lung complications, (3) incisional or peritoneal infections and pelvic abscesses, (4) evisceration, and (5) late hemorrhage (about 10 to 14 days after surgery).

At the time of *discharge*, the patient should be instructed to:

1. Avoid sexual activity and douching until further notice.
2. Do abdominal strengthening exercises.
3. Avoid heavy lifting for about 2 months.
4. Avoid any activities that increase pelvic congestion for several months, e.g., dancing, horseback riding.
5. Avoid constrictive clothing for several months.
6. Report any bleeding to the physician.
7. Return for follow-up care at a specified interval.

The effects of surgery upon a patient's menstruation should be understood by her before surgery. She should know that removal of both the uterus and cervix, i.e., total hysterectomy, will result in the cessation of menstruation. However, if the ovaries are still present, those menopausal symptoms related to a changed hormone state should not occur.

A hysterectomy is a major operation and may be associated with a great deal of anxiety for some patients. All patients have the right to receive supportive care; however, those who are extremely distressed may require more extensive care. It is important for the nurse to continually assess the patient's psychologic responses and to help her cope in a healthy manner with her own feelings. As always, patients are helped a lot when nurses can communicate understanding of the stress being experienced and are not critical of the patient's behavior. It is not unusual for women who have had a hysterectomy to experience periodic "crying spells;" these periods are often helpful for the woman. It is important for the woman to recognize that a hysterectomy is a major abdominal procedure. Hence, full recovery takes several months. Nurses should be alert to signs and symptoms that the woman is having more than a usual amount of difficulty in coping. Occasionally a psychiatric referral is necessary.

Removal of the Ovaries and Fallopian Tubes. *Bilateral salpingectomy* (removal of the fallopian tubes) and *oophorectomy* (removal of the ovaries) are often done in conjunction with a hysterectomy. The procedure is abbreviated "BSO" in many institutions, and if the menopause has not already occurred, this procedure will induce it. (Menopause is discussed on p. 1871.) With the exception of care directed toward treating the unpleasant side effects of abrupt induction of the menopause, the postoperative care is similar to that given after abdominal hysterectomy or other abdominal procedures. An important fact the nurse should keep in mind is that this procedure is attended by abrupt hormonal changes which may be manifested by unusual (psychologic) behavior by the patient. Supportive, understanding nursing care is vital.

RADIATION THERAPY

In general, irradiation of the pelvic organs is similar to irradiation done elsewhere in the body. The pertinent nursing care is discussed extensively in Unit IX. It is important, however, to remember that some of the pelvic tissues, e.g., vulvar tissues, heal less readily than tissues in other areas of the body. Hence, wound care must be done more meticulously. Other aspects of care are discussed under the appropriate disease classifications.

CHEMOTHERAPY

Chemotherapy is discussed in Unit IX. That discussion applies to the care of the gynecologic patient who is receiving chemotherapy. With the exception of the patient with trophoblastic disease who receives chemotherapy as a primary form of treatment, most types of chemotherapy have proved to be less useful as primary treatment for gynecologic illness. Thus, chemotherapy is more commonly used as adjunctive treatment or to assist the terminally ill patient to live comfortably for a longer period of time. In the latter instance, the care is complicated by the fact that the patient is often quite ill and debilitated.

TERMINAL CARE

A person can live with terminal gynecologic tumors for quite a long period of time because many of the tumors do not metastasize to vital organs early. Eventual death may be caused by renal failure. Therefore, nursing care of these patients must be carefully planned and must take into account the relative longevity of the patient. (A thorough discussion of terminal care, grief, and death is presented in Sorensen and Luckmann, *Basic Nursing: A Psychophysiologic Approach*.)

Summary

This chapter discussion has focused on some of the diagnostic and treatment modalities used in treating problems involving the female genital tract. It should be noted that the associated individualized care can frequently be predicted if the nurse has a sound knowledge of principles discussed in this Unit.

CHAPTER 85

INFLAMMATORY AND INFECTIOUS PROBLEMS

by Judith Atwood, R.N., M.N. and Judy Johnson, R.N., M.A.

The female reproductive tract maintains its integrity through a variety of natural defense mechanisms. Inflammation and infection of the genital tract occur when organisms disrupt or overcome these natural defenses. The usual treatment of inflammatory and infectious problems is based not only on *elimination of the cause*, but also on *increasing the resistance of the host*. While nurses may assist in the former by administering antibiotics and the like, they can play a particularly important role in improving host resistance by assessing the health habits of individual patients and encouraging modification of those that may predispose to future problems.

The topics presented in this chapter include leukorrhea, the most common symptom of inflammatory and infectious disorders; vaginitis and its more common causes; vulvitis and related causes; cervicitis; pelvic inflammatory disease (venereal and nonvenereal); and venereal diseases.

> *The most common causes of pelvic inflammatory disease (PID) today are venereal diseases.*

For this reason, this chapter ends with a presentation of the various types of common venereal diseases, emphasizing those that are major public health problems. (It may be useful to review Chapter 11 before studying this chapter.)

LEUKORRHEA

Leukorrhea refers to any discharge from the vagina that is not bloody. All women have normally asymptomatic leukorrhea. The endocervical glands secrete a clear exudate that keeps the vaginal mucous membranes moist and clear. As it passes through the vagina, it may become cloudy and acquire a slight odor because of the addition of desquamated epithelial cells, leukocytes, and normal vaginal flora.

The amount of discharge normally varies among different women in relation to the menstrual cycle. Discharge is greatest at ovulation and just before the menses begin. Pregnancy, sexual stimulation, and oral contraceptives also tend to increase the amount of discharge.

Other changes in the amount or changes in color, character, or odor of vaginal discharge may indicate a problem. Most of the inflammatory and infectious problems discussed in this chapter are accompanied by a pathologic leukorrhea. Abnormal leukorrhea can be copious, malodorous, and an abnormal color. It frequently leaks from the vagina, causing irritation and/or redness of the vulva and surrounding areas. It may also be accompanied by burning and frequency of urination, anal discomfort and pain in the lower abdominal region.

VAGINITIS

Vaginitis means inflammation of the vagina. Before discussing vaginitis and its causes, it is important to review the defense mechanisms that protect the vagina. A potential cavity, the vagina has normal flora population that includes various bacteria. Doderleins' bacillus, characteristically found, apparenty helps maintain normal vaginal pH. The normal pH of the adult vagina is acidic because of lactic acid formed from glycogen contained in desquamating epithelial cells of the vagina. The acidic environment of the vagina is an important defense mechanism.

Vaginitis occurs when (a) there is a change in normal flora, (b) the pH becomes more alkaline, (c) the invading organism is virulent, or (d) some combination of these three conditions occurs. Vaginitis is a common problem, experienced by most women at some time in their lives. It can be caused by a variety of insults, including congestion of the pelvic organs; mechanical irritation (foreign objects, e.g., tampons); chemical irritation (e.g., strong douches); vaginal infections; overmedication, especially with antibiotics (destruction of flora); and long-term steroid therapy.

Vaginitis is almost inevitably characterized by a change in the normal vaginal discharge, e.g., it becomes profuse, odoriferous, and purulent. Vaginitis can be a stubborn, discouraging problem and should be treated early and vigorously to avoid chronicity.

A pelvic examination is performed to diagnose vaginitis. Because of the infection, the examination may be painful for the patient. Also, there may be some bleeding during or after the examination. The patient should be told this and provided with a perineal pad. Of course, the examiner must be as gentle as possible.

Treatment is aimed at the cause, but attention to the overall health status of the individual is mandatory to ensure complete success. Rest and sleep, good nutrition and exercise, and meticulous personal (particularly perineal) hygiene all can affect the success of the treatment program.

Nonspecific or Simple Vaginitis. Vaginitis may result from any of the various organisms discussed in the following sections. If the common etiologic factors are ruled out, a patient may be diagnosed as having nonspecific or simple vaginitis. The host resistance is low, and the normal vaginal flora changes. Overgrowth of staphylococci or streptococci or contamination of the vagina with *Escherichia coli* may result. The symptoms commonly include a profuse vaginal discharge with vulvar irritation and urethritis. Some researchers maintain that most "nonspecific" vaginitis is caused by the organism *Hemophilus vaginalis*.[136]

Treatment of simple vaginitis may include: systemic or local antibiotics, restoration of the normal vaginal environment with douches of a weak acid (one tablespoon of white vinegar in one quart of warm water), and beta lactose in the form of a suppository to stimulate the growth of bacilli. Sulfonamide creams may also help. In addition, after every elimination, thorough gentle cleansing of the perineum from front to back should be done. The patient should be instructed about this cleansing pattern and told the reason for cleaning from the front of the perineum in a direction toward the rectum, i.e., to prevent contamination of the vagina and urinary meatus with feces. Sitz baths may relieve local irritation.

Atrophic (Senile) Vaginitis. Atrophic vaginitis occurs in the postmenopausal years when the atrophic, thin mucosa and thin alkaline, vaginal secretions provide an environment conducive to invasion by pyogenic bacteria (as in simple vaginitis). The symptoms include a discharge that may be blood-flecked, a burning in the vagina, itching of the vagina and vulva, and dyspareunia (painful intercourse). If secondary infection is present, burning with urination and vulvar excoriation typically occur.

Short-term use of stilbesterol suppositories or estrogenic creams is the usual *treatment*. If a secondary infection is present, additional therapy with an appropriate drug is added.

Trichomonas Vaginitis. Trichomoniasis is a common minor disorder that affects 25 per cent of all women and is caused by a protozoan, *Trichomonas vaginalis*. The initial source of the infection is unknown; however, it is known that the organism prefers an alkaline climate and that changes in the vaginal flora make the woman more susceptible., The organism is transmitted sexually from one partner to another, making treatment of both partners necessary to effect a cure. The organism does not affect the uterus and tubes.

The symptoms may be minor and are usually so in the male. In the female, they include a heavy greenish white or yellow, frothy, slightly malodorous discharge which is moderately irritating to the vulva, causing itching, burning, and excoriation and maceration of the vulvar tissues. The vaginal mucosa is reddened and slightly edematous, and some women may experience dyspareunia. If the infection extends to involve the urethra, the woman may experience frequency and burning with urination. Anal involvement also may occur either asymptomatically or with a slight discharge. The cervix may occasionally be covered with punctate hemorrhages ("strawberry cervix"). Bladder and anal involvement are more common when the infection has become chronic. Symptoms during the chronic phase tend to be minimal. The infection may be difficult to cure, and recurrence is not uncommon.

The diagnosis is established by obtaining a fresh wet mount on a slide and looking for the organism under the microscope (Fig. 85–2). Cultures can be obtained to establish the diagnosis, but are rarely necessary. The speculum used to perform the examination should be inserted without lubrication, to avoid destroying the organism. The patient should be instructed not to douche before the examination and told that the examination may be uncomfortable or painful. Reassurance and a calm attitude may help to allay the patient's anxiety and minimize the discomfort of the examination. Several infections may occur simultaneously, so other specimens may be obtained at the time of examination.

Various vaginal suppositories and types of douches have been used in treating *Trichomonas* vaginitis. Today, with some exceptions, however, these have been largely replaced with the oral agent metronidazole (Flagyl), which is usually given for 10 days. Some physicians also treat the woman's sexual partner concurrently. *Flagyl may affect fetal development and is therefore generally not used in early pregnancy.* Alternative therapy with Floraquin vaginal tablets, while less specific, is safer and thus is commonly used. Patients taking Flagyl should be advised not to drink alcoholic beverages since Flagyl and alcohol together may cause vomiting. Recently, consumer groups have questioned the safety of Flagyl because it is reported to be carcinogenic in laboratory animals and alternative forms of therapy, although less effective, can be used. However, at this time, in the United States no action has been taken by the Federal Drug Administration.

Treatment designed to increase host resistance to the organisms may also be indicated. This can include sexual abstinence or the use of condoms; douches; sunshine, rest, good nutrition; tampons to absorb the discharge; good perineal hygiene; and proper douche technique.

Treatment should be continued through the menstrual period, as the vagina is more alkaline during this time of the cycle. With extensive cervical involvement, especially due to chronic or repeated infections, conization or removal of part of the cervix may be necessary. After therapy has been completed, both sexual partners should be reevaluated and treated again if necessary.

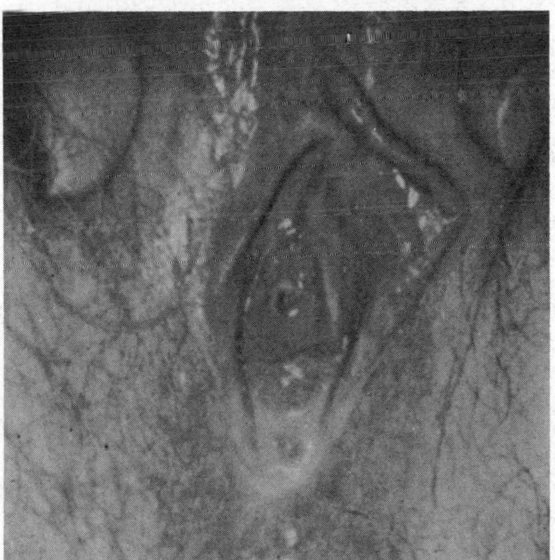

Figure 85–1. The vaginal discharge of trichomoniasis is thin and green, yellow or whitish. The reddening and granular appearance of the inflamed mucous membrane are evident. (From Parsons, L., and S. C. Sommers: *Gynecology,* 2nd ed. Philadelphia: W.B. Saunders Co., 1978, p. 766.)

Monilial Vaginitis. Moniliasis is caused by a fungus, usually *Candida albicans*. (The term "candidiasis" is also used and is preferred by some professionals.[136]) It has a higher incidence in pregnant women, in women with uncontrolled diabetes mellitus, in those taking oral contraceptives, and in those who have taken long-term steroids or antibiotics. It also occurs in others.

The incidence of moniliasis is increasing, making it as common as Trichomonas vaginitis. The source of the infection is unknown, but changes in the vaginal pH seem to allow overgrowth of yeast. In addition to the above mentioned factors, vaginal pH may be changed by tap water and some commercial douches, and by tub baths and some of the preparations used in them.

The symptoms are similar to those of trichomoniasis. The discharge is characteristically thick, white or yellowish, curd-like, and moderate in amount. The vaginal mucosa is diffusely reddened. Thrush-like patches may be seen in the vagina or on the vulva. Vulvar irritation is usually severe, causing the patient much discomfort.

Diagnosis is made by examining a smear of the patches or exudate under the microscope. Cultures may also be obtained if indicated.

Treatment of moniliasis is with topical agents such as nystatin cream or suppositories. The initial treatment is vigorous and is continued through the menstrual period. Treatment is

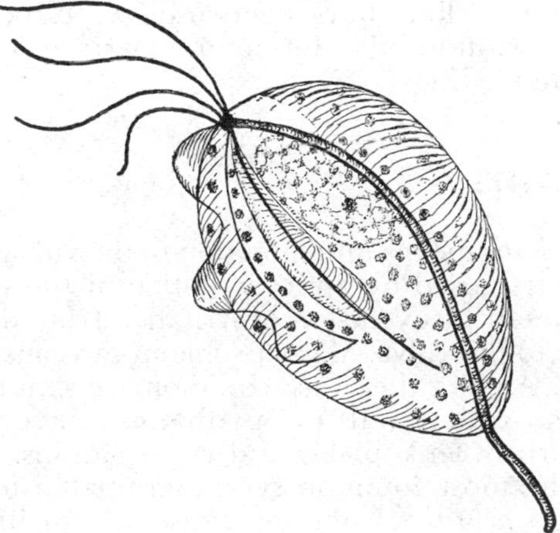

Figure 85–2. Schematic drawing of *Trichomonas vaginalis.* The organism, if present in vaginal discharge, can be readily identified by microscopic examination, and diagnosis is rarely difficult. (From Parsons, L., and S. C. Sommers: *Gynecology,* 2nd ed.)

then generally continued for up to 6 months. Some physicians advocate discontinuing oral contraceptives. Therefore, the nurse needs to be prepared to discuss alternative methods of contraception with the interested patient. Condoms may be suggested for both their contraceptive properties and as protection against infection of or reinfection by a male sexual partner.

Other strict perineal hygiene measures to avoid recontamination are also indicated. In some instances, jellies, acid gels and/or gentian violet may be used locally in conjunction with, or instead of, nystatin. The gentian violet causes staining of the clothing, so perineal pads should be used and old clothing worn. The organism can lie dormant in the vagina until the environment is appropriate, thereby making the infection difficult to cure and tending to recur readily.

Hemophilus Vaginitis. This type of vaginitis is caused by a gram-negative, rod-shaped organism, *Hemophilus (Corynebacterium) vaginalis*. The vaginitis is characterized by a gray, malodorous discharge which, although profuse, is less irritating than those discussed before. The diagnosis is usually established by combining the clinical characteristics of the discharge with a microscopic examination of a fresh wet mount or gram stained smear. There is a specific culture medium that can be used in establishing a definitive diagnosis, but it is not readily available.

Treatment is most often symptomatic, with triple sulfa cream frequently prescribed. More recently, various antibiotics, commonly ampicillin or tetracycline, have been used with good results. Commonly the sexual partner is also treated.

VULVITIS

Vulvitis means inflammation of the vulva. Vulvitis is caused by direct irritation of the vulvar tissues or by extension of irritation from the vagina to the vulva. Many problems can cause vulvitis. Among the more common are skin disorders, inflammatory problems, infection, kraurosis, leukoplakia and vulvovaginitis.

The most common symptom related to vulvitis is *pruritus*. Common causes of vulvitis can include: senile atrophy; irritation secondary to vaginitis; uncontrolled diabetes mellitus (with high urine sugar); pediculosis and scabies; allergies; psychologic problems; cancer; ulcerative, glandular or skin lesions; systemic conditions; urinary incontinence; and poor perineal hygiene.

Treatment is based on determination of the specific cause when possible. If the cause cannot be determined or if the itching is severe, the following may provide some relief:

Calamine lotion
Hot compresses
Sitz baths
Wearing light, nonrestrictive clothing
Wearing well washed and rinsed *cotton* underclothing (Synthetic underpants tend to keep the vulvar area warm and moist.)
Avoiding feminine hygiene sprays
Cleansing the vulva well, especially after elimination
Keeping the vulva dry with cornstarch, hydrocortisone ointment and anesthetic sprays

Nurses can play an important role in teaching the elements of good hygiene, to prevent further vulvar irritation.

Heavy sedation may be prescribed and/or a vulvectomy may be necessary in severe cases. (Vulvectomy is a radical surgical excision of the vulva.)

Skin disorders involving the vulva include many of those mentioned previously as well as chemical burns, irritation with harsh soaps, herpes, psoriasis, folliculitis and eczema. All are treated by removing the cause when possible and by promoting excellent perineal hygiene. Two causes deserving special consideration include the mite *Sarcoptes scabiei*, and the louse *Phthirus pubis*. Both cause vulvar irritation and are transmitted through sexual contact, through infested bedding, and from toilets. Both patient and environment must be treated to get rid of the organisms and their eggs.

Inflammation of the glandular structures of the vulva (e.g., *Bartholinitis*) and of the cervix can be caused by a variety of organisms including the gonococcus, streptococci, staphylococci and *E. coli*. The infection moves in a retrograde fashion and involves the duct, resulting in edema and eventually in obstruction. The drainage from the inflamed gland cannot escape, causing swelling and abscess formation. Cellulitis develops in the surrounding tissues, producing more pain and systemic symptoms. The abscess may rupture spontaneously or may require incision and drainage to relieve the symptoms. After the acute episode, occlusion of the duct due to fibrosis and scarring will lead to retention of the secretions and dilatation of the duct, which then becomes a cyst. The cyst is palpable, mobile and usually not painful. It is usually asymptomatic, except for symptoms related to its size, e.g., dyspareunia or pain on walking.

In addition to drainage of the abscess, *treatment* is with systemic antibiotics specific for the causative organism. Local heat may be helpful in promoting drainage. A cyst may require removal of the entire gland or marsupialization of the cystic duct.

The last two vulvar conditions discussed are *leukoplakia vulvae* and *kraurosis vulvae*, both of which affect the vulvar epithelium. The former is characterized by areas of thickened gray patches of epithelium scattered over the vulva and the perineum. Cracked areas in these patches set up an ideal medium for infection that can lead to ulceration and maceration of the involved areas. Eventually these areas may become malignant. Kraurosis can also become secondarily infected and is characterized by bright red, smooth, almost transparent, vulvar epithelium. It is most common in postmenopausal women and, with progression of the condition, the vulvar tissues shrink with constriction of the vaginal opening. Both disorders cause itching and soreness or pain, or may be asymptomatic. Both are diagnosed according to their appearance; but, in the case of leukoplakia, a biopsy should be done to rule out cancer. Infection in both disorders is treated with the appropriate systemic antibiotic, and other manifestations are treated symptomatically as previously discussed.

CERVICITIS

The cervix serves as a barrier that prevents the spread of infection from the lower to the upper genital tract. Constant exposure to potential pathogens introduced at intercourse, by douching, by trauma from instruments, surgical procedures, childbirth, and other sources may result in inflammation of the cervix, i.e., *cervicitis*. This, in turn, can serve as a focus for the development of infection, both acute and chronic. If the infection is chronic, erosion will occur; repeated insults may lead to an abnormal healing process which is potentially malignant. Thus, evaluation of chronic cervicitis includes looking for a cancerous lesion.

Acute (and ultimately chronic) cervicitis is usually caused by streptococci, staphylococci, *E. coli*, or the gonococcus. These organisms invade the inflamed cervical face or lacerated areas and spread from the epithelium to the endocervical glands. Here congestion and edema occur, and later a discharge may be present. This is usually thick, viscid and white. When the vaginal pH becomes more alkaline, propagation of the infection occurs readily. If the infection is minor or chronic, the patient may be asymptomatic or may have minimal symptoms.

If infection is acute, *treatment* should be prompt and vigorous to prevent spread (see PID) or chronicity. Identification of the organism from cultures or smears will allow appropriate antibiotic administration to begin.

Chronic cervicitis is frequently a chronic infection accompanied by significant inflammatory changes in the cervix. This latter process may require treatment also, in the form of cervical cautery, electrocoagulation, or freezing (cryotherapy with a probe and liquid nitrogen or other agent). This treatment is frequently done on an outpatient basis. A grayish green slough of the destroyed tissue may result, lasting for about 2 weeks. Full healing of the cervix may take 7 to 8 weeks. During this time, topical antiseptic creams or jellies may be prescribed. The patient should be apprised of these expected outcomes and also told that minor bleeding and pelvic discomfort will be present for a short time.

Nursing Care. In addition to the nursing care already discussed, the nurse's primary role in helping women who have vaginitis or vulvitis is that of a teacher. As a teacher, the nurse should assess patients' understanding of the measures prescribed and hence their ability to carry them out. Many women have never been taught to give themselves intravaginal medications, to use the bathtub to take Sitz baths, or to douche properly. Particular attention should be paid to the latter, as many women douch or use feminine hygiene sprays to get rid of the unpleasant symptoms of a vaginal disorder that, in fact, should be treated. The nurse can help women to understand the importance of gynecologic symptoms. Overzealous douching can be harmful as it can destroy the vagina's natural resistance, thus increasing susceptibility to infection. Feminine hygiene sprays can be dangerous, as they are frequently irritating. All of these teaching points are important. Lastly, the nurse can help individual patients to understand the relationship between their general health and gynecologic problems.

PELVIC INFLAMMATORY DISEASE

Pelvic inflammatory disease (PID) refers to ascending pelvic infections i.e., those involving the upper genital tract (beyond the cervix). The gonococcus, staphylococci, streptococci, and other pyogenic organisms are common causes of PID. Moreover, mixed infections involving these organisms and anaerobes may be present. The symptoms are those of a generalized infection. They include: general malaise, fever, chills, anorexia, nausea, vomiting, general aching, tachycardia, and occasionally vaginal bleeding. In addition, the patient usually experiences acute, sharp and severe aching on both sides of the abdomen or pelvis. This pain is aggravated by defecation, and is accompanied by a heavy, purulent discharge which has a foul odor (the latter depends on the organism). The rapidity of onset of PID depends on the virulence of the infecting organism, the status of the pelvic organs, and the general health status of the woman.

Other helpful clues to PID are obtained from the history. A history of an acute lower genital tract infection is significant. It is helpful to know if the pain accompanying the current illness began during menses (typically indicating gonococcal PID) or between periods (usually nongonococcal infections). A variety of other data, including a thorough sexual history, are gathered. Included in the latter is a contraceptive history because the presence of an IUD (intrauterine device) correlates with a higher incidence of PID. (Contraceptive devices are discussed in Chapter 88.)

The usual laboratory tests for infection are ordered, including multiple cultures. Some physicians culture any evident drainage, specimens from various organs such as the cervix, and also do a culdocentesis (see Chapter 84). A sample of peritoneal fluid may also be obtained from the cul-de-sac. These additional cultures are helpful as it is not uncommon for several kinds of organisms to be involved or for an organism cultured from the cervix to differ from that found in the upper genital tract. Several different types of antibiotics may then be necessary to treat the infection effectively.

An infection, once introduced into the upper genital tract, may travel along several routes (see Fig. 85–3). Tuberculosis, a rare cause of PID, travels through the blood and affects the fallopian (uterine) tubes and sometimes the ovaries, uterus, and pelvic peritoneum. The symptoms are those of PID combined with those of pulmonary tuberculosis (see Unit XVI). It is treated with antituberculosis drugs. The excreta are contaminated until the drugs have become effective.

Gonococcus and staphylococcus organisms spread along the uterine endometrium to the fallopian tubes, where they cause an acute *salpingitis* (inflammation of the fallopian (uterine) tubes) and thus the characteristic symptoms. The tubes become partially occluded and may drain pus, leukocytes, and other debris into the pelvic cavity, causing *pelvic peritonitis*, or the material may form a pocket around the ovary, causing a *tubo-ovarian abscess*. Streptococci spread in a similar fashion, except they tend to travel via the uterine or cervical lymphatics across the parametrium to the tubes or ovaries. Here they may cause *pelvic cellulitis* and sometimes *thrombophlebitis* of the major pelvic veins, with the inherent danger of embolic episodes.

The third route of spread of infection is from the pelvic cavity itself. Organisms such as *E. coli* may be extruded from a ruptured viscus, causing peritonitis.

Treatment. *Treatment* of the acute phase of PID may occur on an outpatient basis or may

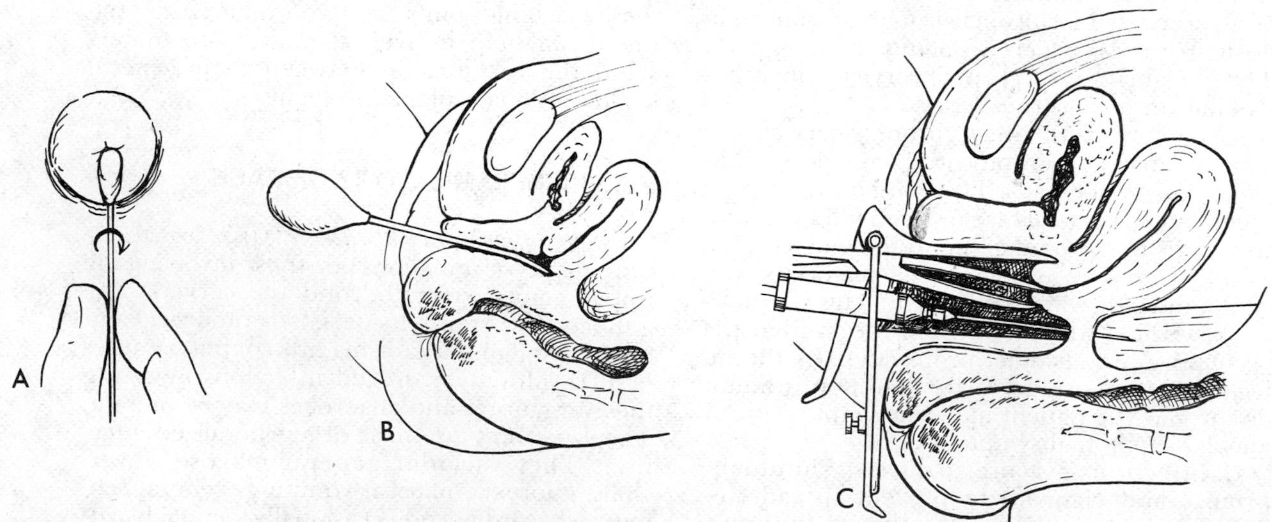

Some procedures used to diagnose PID. **A.** Swabs may be obtained from the cervix, urethra, and rectum. **B.** The vaginal pool is aspirated. **C.** Culdocentesis may be performed. Gram stains of cervical secretions show gram-negative intracellular diplococci. Cultures are placed on Thayer Martin medium. Negative stains and cultures do not rule out gonococcal disease.

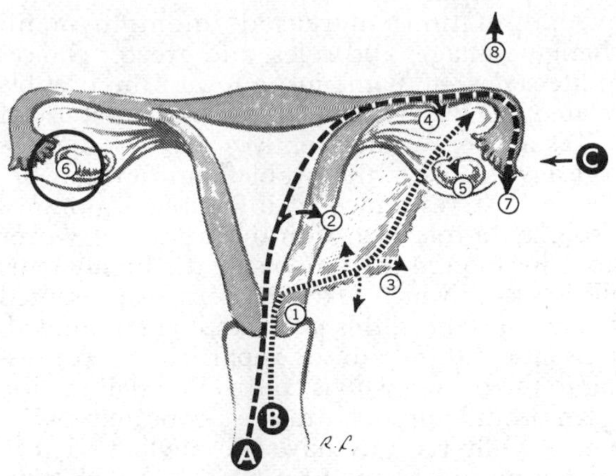

Figure 85–3. The routes of spread of PID: (*A*) staphylococcus, gonococcus; (*B*) streptococcus; (*C*) *E. coli.* (*1*) Endocervicitis. (*2*) Endometritis. (*3*) Parametritis. (*4*) Salpingitis. (*5*) Oophoritis. (*6*) Tubal ovarian abscess. (*7*) Pelvic abscess. (*8*) Systemic spread. (From Behrman, S. J., and J. R. Gosling: *Fundamentals of Gynecology.* 2nd ed. New York: Oxford University Press, 1966, p. 173.)

require hospitalization. The outpatient is given the appropriate antibiotics and is cautioned to avoid sexual relations, douches, and other activities that might exacerbate the infectious process. If the patient's condition deteriorates or her symptoms continue, she is asked to return and is then generally hospitalized. If the patient is improving with treatment, she is given a return appointment in about one week to be sure that the infection is gone. If a patient with PID requires hospitalization, she is usually quite ill.

Antibiotics appropriate to the offending organism are given in maximal doses. The woman is placed in semi-Fowler's position to promote downward drainage. Heat, applied periodically to the lower back or abdomen, or sitz baths may decrease the pain, as do analgesics and sedatives. Douches should be avoided to prevent spreading the infection. The amount, color, odor, and appearance of the vaginal discharge are recorded and frequent perineal cleansing should be done. Depending on the organism, the patient may be isolated.

Supportive therapy such as intravenous nutrition and treatment for pain may also be necessary in treating PID. During this period, it is important for nurses to watch for indications of complications and provide emotional support for the woman.

While septic shock and other catastrophic problems can occur, *the most common complication is the development of a pelvic abscess*. While some such abscesses are treated relatively easily, some may require surgical intervention or may rupture, causing peritonitis. The type of surgical intervention and its timing (acute or after a "cooling off" period) varies somewhat with the philosophy of the physician and the presenting problem. At times, an abscess can be drained without resorting to laparotomy. However, in treating some women it may be necessary to resort to laparotomy and removal of the infection as well as removal of the uterus, ovaries, and tubes. If surgery is done while the patient's condition is acute, the operative risk is increased. However, this risk is balanced against that inherent in continuing conservative medical therapy that has not succeeded. These patients are also at higher risk for developing chronic PID (discussed below). Frequently, patients are not able to bear children after the infection is gone.

Much of nursing care often needs to be directed toward providing specific patient teaching and emotional support. One of the most important factors that the nurse must consider in caring for a woman with PID is how the patient feels about the disease and about herself. Because PID is often caused by venereal disease, there may be guilt feelings and family-related problems centered around the patient's contracting the infection. Important nursing interventions may sometimes include the patient's significant others.

Nurses need to be careful that their personal attitudes toward sexually transmitted diseases do not become an additional burden to patients. Some patients experience a loss of the ability to have children, which may be an emotional burden needing discussion. Each patient can benefit from factual information about the infection, how to identify recurrences, and general hygiene measures that can help in preventing new infections. Moreover, patients need to know when they can resume intercourse and other activities. Pragmatic discussions of these areas sometimes also assist the woman to cope more effectively with emotional reactions that she may be experiencing.

Chronic PID. Chronic PID can occur if the acute phase of the illness does not respond to therapy or if therapy is inadequate. The symptoms include chronic pelvic discomfort, disturbances of menstruation or dysfunctional uterine bleeding, constipation, malaise, and periodic recurrence of the acute symptoms. Sterility, one of the more serious complications, is the result of destruction of part of the fallopian tubes and loss of their patency. The sterility is usually irreversible.

Treatment of PID is aimed at removing the offending organism and improving the general health status of the woman. If treatment is unsuccessful, removal of the pelvic organs may be necessary.

SEXUALLY TRANSMITTED DISEASES (STD, VENEREAL DISEASES)

It is estimated that up to 10 million people in the United States contract one of the sexually transmitted diseases each year. Moreover, there has been a steady rise in the number of cases of reported venereal diseases. The United States government allocates increasing funds (e.g., $45 million in fiscal 1979) toward controlling this national epidemic. Much of this money is spent in trying to educate the public. Moreover, local governments spend large amounts in community services to detect and treat these diseases.

> *The three venereal diseases most commonly seen are gonorrhea, syphilis, and genital herpes.*

Genital herpes has only recently increased in incidence. Many authorities estimate that it is secondary only to gonorrhea in frequency. Genital herpes is caused by a virus; currently we are without a specific cure. While gonorrhea is known to be curable with penicillin, the dosages required for cure have increased rapidly. Moreover, resistant strains have begun to be identified. Concerned authorities point to an increasing risk of losing more ground to the venereal disease epidemic.

The traditional venereal disease (gonorrhea, syphilis, chancroid, donavania, granulomatosis, and lymphogranuloma venereum) and, more recently, genital herpes are included with other infectious genital diseases such as trichomoniasis in a broader category called the *sexually transmitted diseases*—STD. These diseases share several characteristics: (1) They are sexually transmitted. (2) Both sexual partners need to be evaluated for treatment. (3) They frequently coexist in the same patient. The latter characteristic may be partly responsible for some treatment failures, e.g., syphilis and gonorrhea may coexist. Generally, the high doses of penicillin used to treat gonorrhea are also adequate to treat syphilis. However, if the patient is allergic to penicillin, the alternative therapy used for gonorrhea may be inadequate for syphilis. Current treatment guidelines for venereal diseases are available in the United States from the Center for Disease Control of the National Institutes of health.[167] This organization assumes responsibility for testing established treatment regimens as well as for studying the effectiveness of new antibiotics.

The increased incidence of venereal diseases is due to a number of problems, some of which are only incidently related. In the last decade, society has changed, with increased mobility, increased sexual freedom, increased crime rates, overpopulation, increased unemployment, changing images and roles, and greater choices in life styles—to name just a few of the possible related factors. In addition, the increased use of IUD's and oral contraceptives may also be biologically related to the problem as they may decrease host resistance to infection. Ignorance also plays a role and, with the controversy over sex education in the schools or the highly moralistic way in which sexual material is presented in some instances, this problem is compounded. This latter attitude to sex is particularly confusing to the person who is confronted daily by the "glamorous" approach to sex advocated by the media. Only recently have the media and concerned organizations begun to deal with education about sex and venereal diseases in a manner calculated to have greater appeal for the young, and hence provide education for this age group.

The nurse needs to be well informed about sex and venereal diseases, and to separate morality from appropriate educational processes in order to help combat these major public health problems. The following information is presented to provide some of the basic facts about sexually transmitted diseases. The nurse working with patients who have these diseases or those who are at high risk of contracting them may wish to consult other textbooks for additional information on this subject.

Gonorrhea

Gonorrhea (also called by lay persons "white," "the drips," "the strain," "clap," and "the dose") can be divided into two groups: local infections and disseminated infections. *Local infections* include those involving the mucosal surfaces of the urethra, rectum, cervix, pharynx, and conjunctiva. *Disseminated infections* are those that occur due to local extension of the infection into adjacent organs or those due to septicemia, which can result in dermatitis, arthritis, endocarditis, or meningitis.

Gonorrhea is caused by the gram-negative diplococcus *Neisseria gonorrhoeae*. The disease is easy to transmit; it has a variable incubation time (usually 3 to 8 days); there is no lasting immunity; and there is a large carrier population who are asymptomatic. Gonorrhea is seen commonly in women with trichomoniasis and also with syphilis. A variety of strains of gonorrhea are being studied. *Unfortunately, increasing resistance to standard therapy has been developing, requiring increasingly large doses of penicillin or even the use of other antibiotics.*

Gonorrheal infection is transmitted sexually in almost all cases. Exceptions are that a child may develop gonorrhea when in close contact with the discharge from an infected mother, and medical personnel who have lacerations

TABLE 85–1. POTENTIAL SITES OF GONOCOCCAL INFECTION

	Genitourinary	
Women	Skene's glands	Bartholin's glands
	Urethra	Cervix
	Vagina	Fallopian tubes
	Endometrium	
Men	Glands of Tyson	Urethra
	Prostate	Seminal vesicles
	Epididymis	
	Extragenital	
Women and Men	Meninges	Eyes
	Heart	Joints
	Liver	Peritoneal cavity
	Skin	Pharynx

Modified from Crespo, J. H., and M. W. Rytel: Venereal diseases. *American Family Physician,* 18:90, Aug. 1978.

may develop gonorrhea if they are not careful in disposing of infected discharges. However, these instances are rare, since the organism does not survive very long outside the body.

The initial infection in females may involve the vestibular glands, the urethra, the anus, and the endocervix. The adult vagina is resistant to the infection, although the prepubertal child's is not. Symptoms, when present, can include a red, swollen and sore vulva; a minor, purulent, yellow discharge; dysuria; frequency; pruritus; and a rectal discharge. The Bartholin glands (and other vestibular glands) may be involved, with symptoms such as those described earlier in this chapter. The infection can progress to pelvic inflammatory disease, and the first symptoms may be related to this problem. (Chapter 82 discusses symptoms of gonorrhea in men.)

There are no blood serology tests currently available to establish the *diagnosis* of gonorrhea (although research is being done to develop one). Therefore, the diagnosis is based on the history, physical findings, and identification of the organism on cultures or smears. Occasionally, the fluorescent tagged antibody method is used to establish the diagnosis. The cultures or smears should be obtained from the cervix, the urethra, the vestibular glands, the ducts, and the anus (Fig. 85–4). Additionally, some physicians now advocate obtaining throat cultures. All these tests can be done during the menstrual period. The woman should be instructed not to void, douche, or clean the vulva for 2 hours before the examination. The organism may disappear after a short time, and the cultures may thus be sterile even though the infection is still present.

Characteristics and treatment of infection at various sites include the following;

▶ The treatment of *simple genital gonorrhea* is the administration of large doses of penicillin given with probenecid. If penicillin cannot be used because a patient is allergic to it, tetracyline, spectinomycin, or ampicillin may be given. Treatment schedules are changing rapidly owing to the appearance of increasingly resistant strains of gonorrhea. Treatment failures or partial failures are appearing with greater frequency. Thus, it is important that the patient return for follow-up cultures 7 to 14 days after treatment is completed and again at 6 weeks.

▶ *Gonococcal pharyngitis* occurs in women and in homosexual men who practice fellatio. The relationship between cunnilingus and pharyngeal infection is less well documented. The infection is usually asymptomatic, and in 10 to 20 per cent of the patients this is the only site of infection. When symptoms are present, they resemble those seen with either a strep throat or viral throat infection. The diagnosis is established by a specialized type of throat culture. The treatment is the same as that given for genital gonorrhea. Alternative therapy with ampicillin or spectinomycin has a high failure rate. Because this type of gonorrhea is more difficult to treat, follow-up cultures are essential.

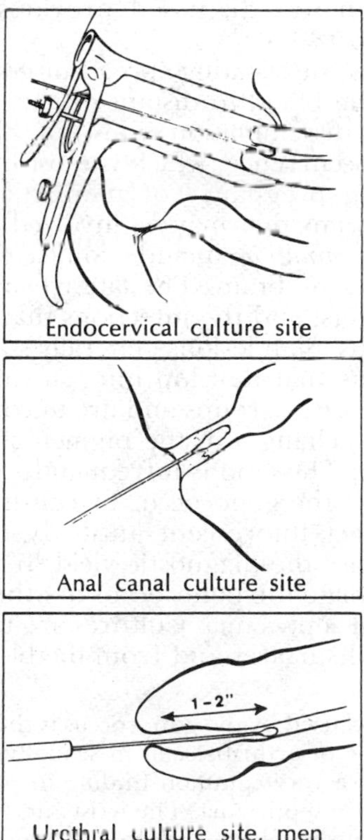

Figure 85–4. Specimen collection techniques for diagnosis of gonococcal infections. (From Crespo, J. H., and M. W. Rytel: Venereal diseases. *American Family Physician,* 18:90, Aug. 1978.)

- *Gonococcal proctitis* occurs in females with a cervical gonorrhea—presumably as an extension of that infection—and in those who practice anal intercourse. A small number of persons who have rectal gonorrhea are asymptomatic. When present, symptoms can include a rectal discharge, itching, and pain with defecation. The area may appear erythematous. The infection is diagnosed by culture; these cultures should be done routinely in evaluating patients with gonorrhea. The treatment and follow-up regimen is the same as that for simple genital gonorrhea.
- *Infection of the eyes* can occur in an adult through transfer of infectious exudate to the eyes from other infected areas. However, this type of gonorrhea is more common in the neonate, before birth, during birth, or after birth. Initially there is a serous conjunctival discharge, which becomes purulent. This is followed by edema and ultimately by corneal ulceration. The diagnosis is established by gram staining the exudate. Treatment is with local and systemic antibiotics.

As mentioned above, gonorrhea can also spread from its initial lower genital tract focus to the upper genital tract. This causes *gonococcal PID*, which was discussed previously in this chapter (p. 1891).

The most devastating spread of gonorrhea is through the blood to distant organs, i.e., hematogenous dissemination. This is a relatively infrequent occurrence, which is most likely to occur during pregnancy or menstruation. The various organs that may be involved in the *septicemic dissemination* include joints, skin, heart valves, and the brain. The latter two are infrequent targets, and the infections that result are very serious. Skin lesions generally start as macular lesions that develop into pustules. These tend to occur in groups and are uncomfortable. Permanent changes in the pigmentation of the skin result. The lesions infrequently allow identification of the gonococcus by culture or gram stain. Direct fluorescent antibody techniques may increase the diagnostic yield. It is also difficult to isolate the gonococcus in other types of gonococcal septicemia. Cultures are taken from all mucosal surfaces and from the blood.

- *Arthritis* caused by the gonococcus is the most common type of arthritis seen in sexually active people. It is a very common finding in patients with gonococcal septicemia. The wrist and knee are the usual joints involved, and the symptoms vary from mild arthralgias to severe arthritis. The fluid in the joint can be serous or purulent, but aspiration and culture of the fluid for the gonococcus is only diagnostic about half of the time. If the infection proceeds undetected, the body structures may atrophy and the cartilage erodes. The end result can be one of very disabling arthritis.
- *Gonococcal endocarditis* is a very serious infection that can result in the death of the patient from a septic embolus or permanent valve damage and progressive heart failure. Emboli can cause acute nephritis or cerebrovascular accidents. The diagnosis and treatment is similar to that of other types of endocarditis (see Chapter 38).
- *Meningitis* of gonococcal origin is manifested in the same way as other bacterial meningitis infections. It is most closely related to meningococcal meningitis. The diagnosis and treatment are similar to other forms of meningitis (see Chapter 26).

The treatment schedules for disseminated gonococcal infections involve the use of large doses of penicillin or alternate drugs over a more prolonged period of time. Hospitalization may be necessary.

The treatment of gonorrhea is subject to change, as resistant organisms become more prevalent. It is important for nurses to keep informed about current regimens. Moreover, many patients are not aware that the doses of penicillin used to treat gonorrhea are much greater than those used with most other infections. Hence, some people may believe that an antibiotic taken for some other problem (a respiratory infection, for example) will also "cure" gonorrhea if present. The nurse can help correct this misinformation and can assist in active efforts to make the general public more aware of facts about gonorrhea—its transmission, symptoms, and treatment. Public education is one essential component in fighting the current epidemic of venereal diseases. Persons receiving treatment must learn the importance of taking the complete course of recommended medications and of returning for follow-up evaluation. (See table on page 1898.)

Syphilis

Syphilis ("bad blood," "lues," "pox," "syph"), while less common than gonorrhea, has potentially severe late complications including blindness, insanity, paralysis, heart disease, and death. Caused by a spirochete, *Treponema pallidum*, syphilis is typically transmitted through sexual intercourse. Rarely, infection of an open wound is possible. Syphilis can occur alone or in conjunction with other venereal diseases, and has a variable incubation period of 10 to 90 days, the average being 20 to 30 days.

Stages of Syphilis. There are several stages of syphilis, which are frequently referred to as the primary, secondary, and tertiary stages. However, in other classifications the primary and secondary stages are together called *infectious syphilis*, and the tertiary stage is called *latent* *stage*, which is followed by another stage, *late clinical syphilis*. Late syphilis may also be called the *noninfectious stage*.

Primary Syphilis. Primary syphilis has two principal symptoms, the appearance of a chancre and lymphadenopathy. The *chancre* is usually located on the genitalia or in the mouth, but it can appear anywhere, as the spirochetes can penetrate intact skin. The presence of several chancres is rare, although possible. Chancres in women commonly are not noticed. Typically, the chancre is an oval shaped sore with a raised border, which feels hard under the skin. It does not readily bleed and is painless unless infected. Local lymph glands near the chancre swell painlessly, i.e., *lymphadenopathy* occurs.

Secondary Stage. If untreated, the chancre heals within 4 to 6 weeks. The patient is then often asymptomatic for a time. However, between 2 weeks and 6 months after the chancre disappears, the *secondary stage* begins. Manifestations of this stage include: a generalized rash, generalized lymphadenopathy, mucous patches and condylomata lata, various general symptoms, and loss of patches of hair. The rash and cutaneous lesions can resemble a wide variety of illnesses. The rash is typically described as maculopapular, nonpruritic, and uniquely present on the palms and soles of the feet (Fig. 85–6). Few diseases cause a rash in these particular locations. The hair loss generally occurs in the eyebrows and scalp. The mucous patches occur in the mouth and may be accompanied by a sore throat. Condylomata lata (not the same thing as venereal warts) may develop in warm, moist areas of the body—most commonly on the labia, anus, or at the corners of the mouth. While all of the skin lesions are infectious, the condylomata are the most infectious. The generalized symptoms can include nausea; anorexia; constipation; headaches; muscle, joint, and bone pain; and a chronically elevated temperature. All of the symptoms generally disappear within 2 to 6 weeks. This heralds the beginning of disease latency in about three fourths of the people afflicted. The other quarter experience relapses into the primary or secondary stages during the first 2 years of the latent stage.

Tertiary Stage. The latent phase, or tertitary stage, is asymptomatic. It occurs approximately 2 or more years after the appearance of the primary lesion and can last for up to 50 years. About two thirds of the patients remain in this stage without further problems. They may develop granulomatous destructive

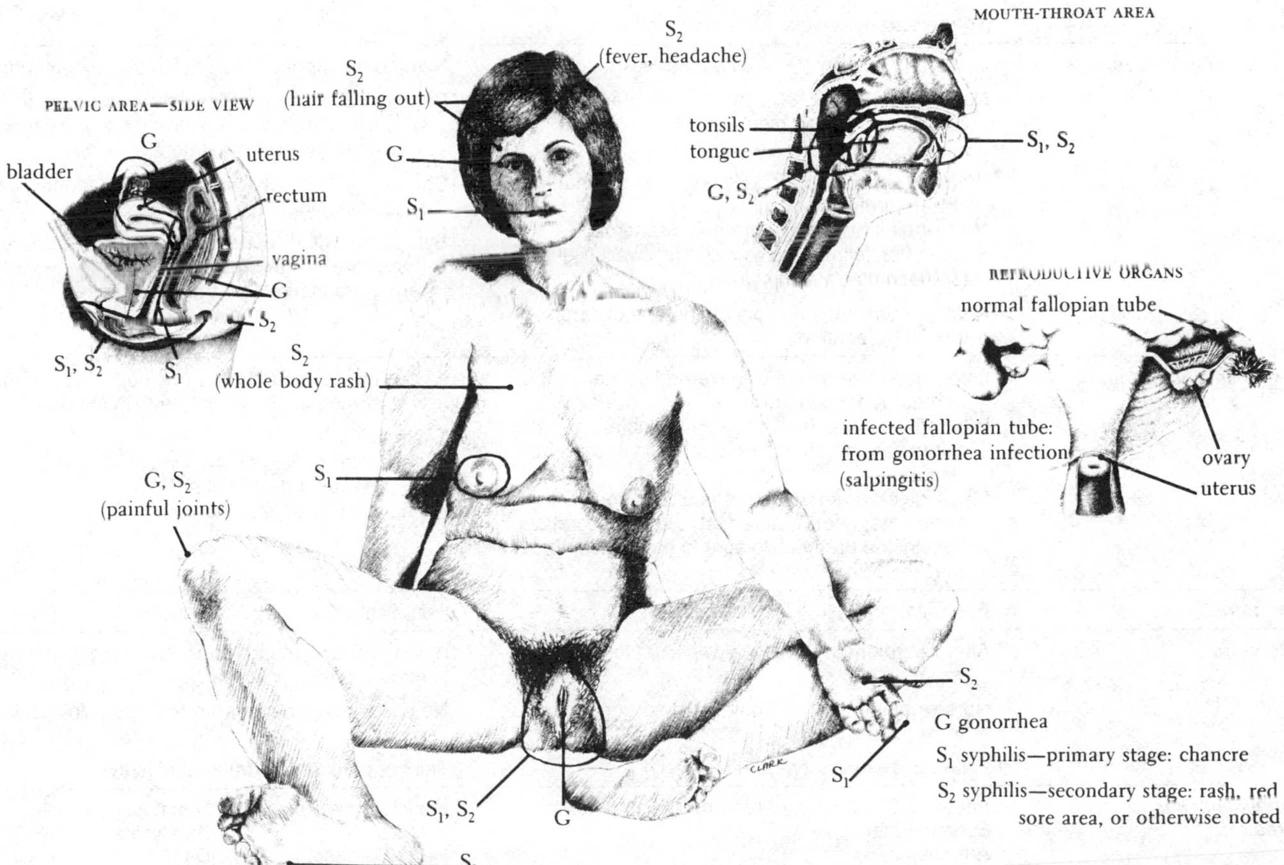

Figure 85–5. Where venereal disease symptoms show up. From Boston Women's Health Book Collective: *Our Bodies, Ourselves*, 2nd ed. New York: Simon and Schuster, 1976, p. 174.)

lesions called *gummas*, which are painful and are located in bone, skin, nervous, and cardiovascular tissues.

Late Clinical Syphilis. About one third of persons who have been in the latent phase develop late clinical syphilis, which is devastating. The complications developed at this time are irreversible. Manifestations may include: chronic inflammation of the bones and joints; cardiovascular problems, including valvular involvement and aneurysms; skin lesions; and CNS problems including insanity, slurred speech, ataxic gait, paralysis, judgment loss, and senility. While this stage is not infectious, if the disease is not treated, it may be terminal. (Refer to Chapter 27 for discussion of CNS manifestations.)

Diagnosis. The *diagnosis* of syphilis is based on a careful history, a search for the characteristic findings and a variety of laboratory studies.

VENEREAL DISEASE

	Gonorrhea	**Syphilis**
Other names:	Clap, drip, a dose, a case, strain, whites, morning dew, gleet.	Siff, pox, lues, bad blood, Old Joe.
How you catch it:	Sexual intercourse (vaginal, anal, oral-genital) with someone who has it; In eyes, from contact with discharge of infected person; Infant's eyes infected in birth canal of infected mother. *Not* spread by towels, toilet seats, objects.	Sexual intercourse (vaginal, anal, oral-genital) with someone who has it; If fluid from syphilitic sore or rash gets on your skin; Fetus infected in womb of infected mother.
How to tell you have it:	Symptoms appear 1–14 days after sexual contact. No symptoms for 80% of the infected women, 5–20% of infected men. If there are symptoms: Women—greenish or yellow-green vaginal discharge, irritation of vulva; Men—painful urination, urethral discharge; Both—after fellatio, sore throat or swollen glands (sometimes no symptoms). Anal gonorrhea: irritation of anus, discharge, or painful defecation.	Symptoms appear 9–90 days after sexual contact. Primary: Chancre (painless sore) appears at spot where syphilis bacteria entered body, disappears 1–5 weeks without treatment. Secondary; rash, flu-like symptoms, mouth sores, patchy balding. Symptoms will disappear after some months even if you are not treated; disease then attacks internal organs in 1/3 of untreated cases.
How to find out for sure:	If you have symptoms or have had sexual contact with someone who might have gonorrhea: Women—culture test (80–90% reliable); be sure culture taken from cervix, anus (and throat if necessary); Men—quick gram stain test is often enough. If no symptoms, need culture test: swab of secretions from inside urethra. Be sure to have anus, throat checked if indicated.	If you have symptoms or have had sexual contact with someone who might have syphilis: Tests are— examination of fluid of chancre; blood test (after 4–6 weeks); lumbar puncture (later stages).
Treatment:	Penicillin, or, if allergic, a substitute.	Penicillin, or, if allergic, a substitute.
Follow-up:	After treatment, have a weekly culture test until two are negative. No sexual intercourse from first suspicion until you know you're cured. Tell your sex partner(s) immediately!	Blood test one month after treatment, once every three months for a year. No sexual intercourse from first suspicion until you know you're cured. Tell your sex partner(s) immediately!
Complications if untreated:	Severe inflammation of reproductive organs. Eventual sterility. Arthritis. Blindness.	Muscle incoordination. Insanity. Heart Disease. Blindness. Deafness. Paralysis. Death.

From 2nd ed. Boston Women's Health Book Collective: *Our Bodies, Ourselves*. New York: Simon and Schuster, 1976, p. 179.

These tests are direct or indirect. Once lesions have appeared, they can be scraped, and organisms may be located with the darkfield microscope technique. *Darkfield examination*, a direct test, allows identification of the spirochetes of *T. pallidum* but must be done by an expert, as there are other types of spirochetes present in the oral and genital areas. This test is used to provide confirmation of the diagnosis of syphilis in the primary stage, when other tests are generally negative, and in the secondary stage.

The remaining tests, the so called *serologic tests for syphilis* (STS), all rely on the presence of antibodies to *T. pallidum*. Early in the primary stage, sufficient time for antibody formation has not passed, so these tests are often negative. There are a number of different tests, but two common ones are the VDRL (a nontreponemal test) and the FTA-ABS (a treponemal test).

The *VDRL* tests for nonspecific antibodies.

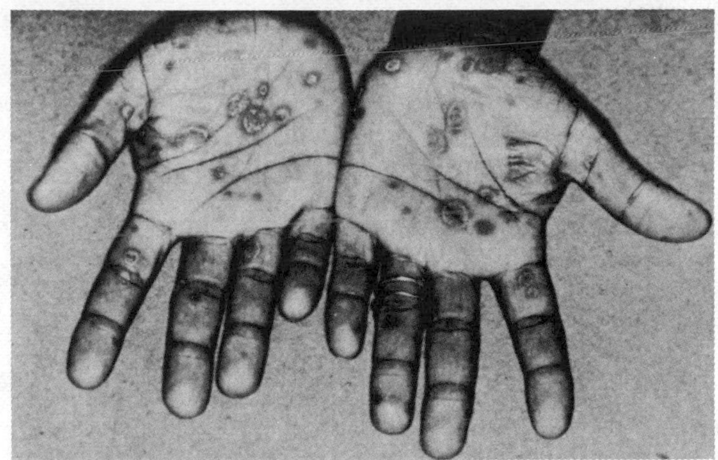

Figure 85–6. The palmar rash of secondary syphilis consists of symmetrical bilateral hyperpigmented, scaling macular lesions. (From: If it looks like Ca, give a thought to VD. *Emergency Medicine*, 9:209, June 1977.)

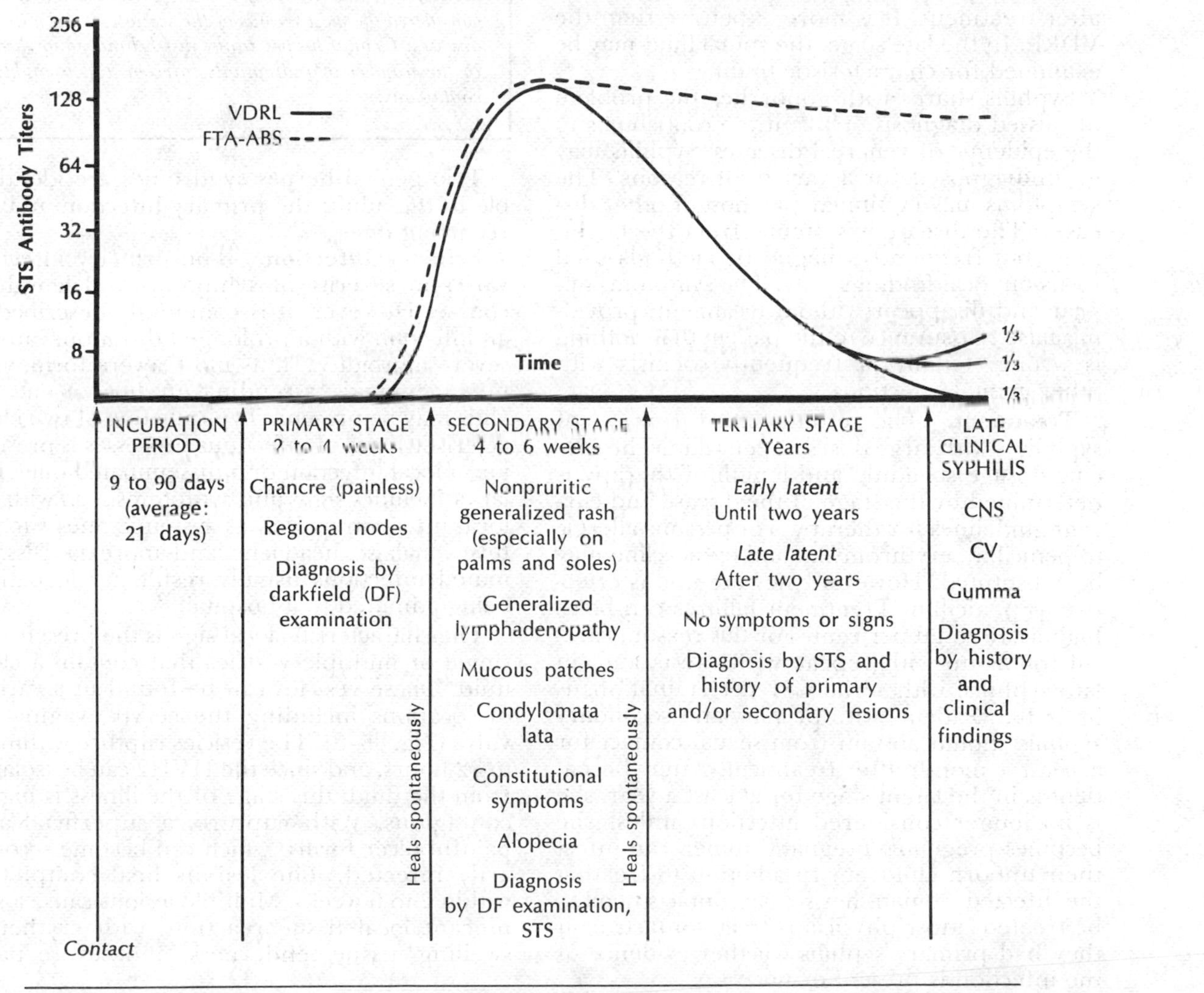

STS Antibody Titers: 256, 128, 64, 32, 16, 8

VDRL ——
FTA-ABS - - -

Time

1/3
1/3
1/3

INCUBATION PERIOD	PRIMARY STAGE 2 to 4 weeks	SECONDARY STAGE 4 to 6 weeks	TERTIARY STAGE Years	LATE CLINICAL SYPHILIS
9 to 90 days (average: 21 days)	Chancre (painless)	Nonpruritic generalized rash (especially on palms and soles)	*Early latent* Until two years	CNS
	Regional nodes	Generalized lymphadenopathy	*Late latent* After two years	CV
	Diagnosis by darkfield (DF) examination	Mucous patches	No symptoms or signs	Gumma
		Condylomata lata	Diagnosis by STS and history of primary and/or secondary lesions	Diagnosis by history and clinical findings
		Constitutional symptoms		
		Alopecia		
		Diagnosis by DF examination, STS		

Contact

Heals spontaneously

Heals spontaneously

Figure 85–7. Clinical course of untreated syphilis. (From Crespo, J. H., and M. W. Rytel: Venereal disease. *American Family Physician*, 18:90, Aug. 1978, p. 97.)

The qualitative test (antibodies are present or not) is the most commonly used screening test for syphilis. The test will be positive about 4 to 6 weeks after the onset of syphilis. False positive reactions are found in acute febrile illnesses, in heroin users, after smallpox vaccination, in collagen vascular disease and in autoimmune diseases. The VDRL can also be used to validate a cure in most instances (except late syphilis). As the antibody titre decreases, the quantitative (how much antibody is present) will decrease.

A more specific test, the *FTA-ABS* (fluorescent treponemal antibody absorption test), measures specific antibodies to *T. pallidum*. It can be used sooner than the VDRL or when there are no signs and symptoms and the VDRL is positive. It cannot be used to test for a cure, as it usually remains positive for about 2 years after treatment. It is more expensive than the VDRL. In the late stage, the spinal fluid may be examined for characteristic findings.

Syphilis shares with gonorrhea the problem of missed diagnosis. Thus, it too contributes to the epidemic of venereal diseases. Syphilis may go undiagnosed for a variety of reasons. The symptoms may be similar to a host of other diseases. The disease is systemic from the beginning, but frequently, diagnostic methods used focus on local findings only. The symptoms appear and disappear without treatment, providing false reassurance to the patient that nothing is wrong. Finally, it frequently coexists with other genital infections.

Treatment. The recommended *treatment* of syphilis is with large doses of penicillin. The specific dosage schedule and length of therapy is determined by the stage of the disease and current guidelines for therapy. For persons allergic to penicillin, erythromycin and tetracycline may be substituted. However, they are not as effective as penicillin. Treatment failures can be as high as 10 to 20 per cent. For this reason, careful follow-up with repeat VDRL tests and, in late syphilis, with serial CSF determinations is indicated. Patients with primary and secondary syphilis should abstain from sexual contact for at least 1 month after treatment. After the patient is in the latent stage for at least a year, she is no longer considered infectious unless she becomes pregnant. Pregnant women can infect their unborn children. In addition to treating the infected woman, her sexual contacts need to be treated. Most physicians treat contacts as if they had primary syphilis whether evidence of the infection is present or not.

As with the other diseases discussed in this chapter, the nurse's role in treating a patient with syphilis is principally one of teaching the patient about the disease and providing supportive therapy, including emotional support.

Genital Herpes Infections

Genital herpes, a disease recognized for centuries, has recently received renewed attention because of its epidemic incidence. Caused by a virus, *Herpesvirus hominis* (HVH) type II, the infection is closely related to other herpes infections,* e.g., the classic "cold sore." The latter is caused by *Herpesvirus hominis*, type I. Type I herpes is principally a nongenital infection occurring above the waist (often on oral structures), whereas type II occurs primarily below the waist, often in sexually transmitted genital infections. It is, however, possible for cross-over infections to occur.

> *A genital herpes infection causes severe morbidity, recurs, and has no cure. For the third reason, it is considered the most serious of the sexually transmitted diseases. Genital herpes ranks just behind gonorrhea in the number of individuals infected and is highly contagious.*

Two genital herpes syndromes are identifiable in the adult: the primary infection and the recurrent one.

Primary Infection. The primary infection varies in severity of symptoms and length of course. However, it is commonly described as an infection with a prolonged duration, causing severe morbidity. In its most severe form, viremia, meningitis, ascending myelitis, or encephalitis may be present. Typically one of two characteristic types of infectious processes is present, i.e., a local infection or a disseminated one. The latter includes signs and symptoms seen with the local infection as well as systemic ones such as fever, malaise, headache, and anorexia. Disseminated infections usually result in the patient being admitted to a hospital.

The characteristic local sign is the presence of single or multiple vesicles that contain a clear fluid. These vesicles can be found in a variety of locations including the cervix, vagina, or vulva (Fig. 85–8). The vesicles rupture within 24 to 72 hours, and since the HVH2 can be isolated from the fluid, this stage of the illness is highly contagious. With rupture, a superficial and painful ulcer forms, which can become secondarily infected. The lesions heal completely within 2 to 6 weeks. Multiple lesions cause a significant local tissue reaction, with erythema, swelling, tissue tenderness, and severe pain.

*Herpes simplex is discussed in Chapters 60 and 79: herpes zoster is discussed in Chapters 27 and 79.

The common reasons the patient seeks care, are that she is unable to void, experiencing dyspareunia or has a very painful genital area. Other local signs and symptoms can include: inguinal lymphadenopathy; other urinary tract symptoms such as dysuria; vaginal discharge; paresthesias and a burning sensation in the local tissues.

Indications of a genital herpes infection generally appear 3 to 7 days (up to 20 days) after sexual contact with an infected individual. Although widely variable in its effect on the individual patient, the primary syndrome often produces a significant and noticeable impact, lasting up to 6 weeks.

Recurrent Infection. Recurrent genital herpes infection is generally a much less devastating problem physically than the primary infection. Emotionally, however, many patients find recurrent genital herpes very difficult to cope with. Common problems are that this infection is not curable, and prediction of recurrences is not possible. Reappearance of the infection has a significant impact on the patient's sex life. Recurrence can also be a particular problem for the pregnant patient, as discussed later in this section.

The recurrent syndrome occurs in about half of infected persons. It is thought that the herpes virus lies dormant in the body, probably the central nervous system, until it is somehow activated. Recurrent infections are known to be associated with a variety of life events, including systemic illnesses, fever, the menses, and emotional crises. Although these associations are known, not enough data exist to demonstrate a causative relationship between them and recurrent infections.

Characteristically, recurrent genital herpes causes local but not systemic symptoms. A prodrome of burning and paresthesias may appear in those areas where the vesicular lesions eventually develop. The vesicles have a tendency to reappear where they were previously. However, not all sites of previous infection will always be involved in recurrent ones. In most women, the recurrent lesion or lesions develop on a site such as the cervix and are unnoticed. Otherwise, these patients are asymptomatic. The remaining patients will have local symptoms similar to those seen with the primary infection, although usually less severe. The vesicles rupture in 24 to 48 hours, and the syndrome generally lasts 7 to 10 days. (See p. 1840 for discussion of genital herpes in men.)

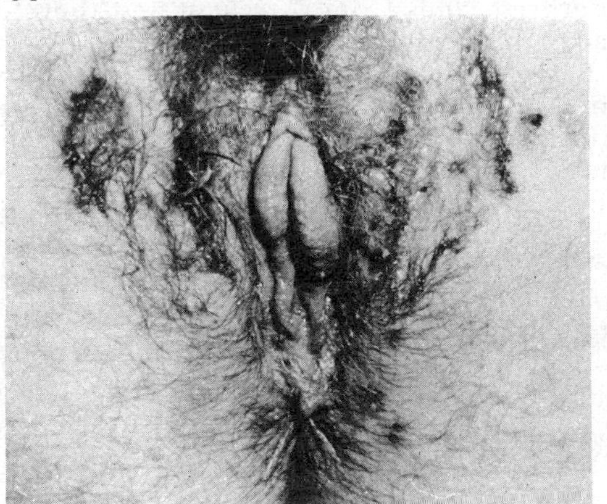

Figure 85–8. Herpes progenitalis. (From Webster, S. B.: Asymptomatic gonorrhea. *American Family Physician,* 16:121, Nov. 1977, p. 126.)

Diagnosis. The diagnosis of genital herpes is established from a history of the symptoms, the presence of vesicles, and from a variety of diagnostic tests. Most commonly, a Papanicolaou smear is done. The presence of multinucleated giant cells with or without inclusion bodies, although not direct evidence of a herpes infection, is characteristic. Direct evidence can be obtained by doing viral cultures. However, these tests are expensive and available only in major centers.

Treatment and Nursing Care. The treatment of genital herpes is symptomatic because no cure is known today.

Nursing care consists of providing symptomatic treatment, emotional support, and patient teaching. Symptomatic treatment may consist of using a variety of soothing lotions, heat lamps, and other general comfort measures. It is important that the infected area be kept clean and dry. Secondary infections may be preventable or minimized with careful cleaning. Some patients may require an indwelling bladder catheter to minimize pain and discomfort in the infected genital area.

> Remember: *When vesicles rupture, they release a highly contagious exudate. Careful handwashing technique by the patient and others is essential. Isolation may be necessary. Infected persons should not have sexual contact, in order to prevent spread of the infection.*

The emotional support required by the person with genital herpes varies, depending upon the patient's understanding of the infection and the effectiveness of the patient's coping mechanisms. The family or personal community of the patient can have a significant impact on the patient's emotional response to the illness. It is important for the nurse to assess this response and assist as necessary in providing education and helping these people be supportive of the patient.

The patients' teaching needs are basically those of understanding the illness, its sexual transmission and its treatment. Women with genital herpes also need to know that it is important for them to have regular gynecologic examinations, including a "Pap" smear test. There is a known association between genital herpes infections and an increased risk of cervical cancer. Lastly, *genital herpes can be a significant problem when associated with pregnancy*. The pregnant patient needs sensitive and experienced management throughout the pregnancy. It is possible for the fetus to be infected, and therefore amniocentesis may be done. If the virus is found, the patient may elect to have an abortion. If the pregnancy proceeds to term, frequently a delivery by Caesarean section is done. Not all infants delivered from a herpes-infected mother acquire the infection. However, it is a very serious infection if present and is potentially fatal.

In summary, genital herpes is one of the most serious of the sexually transmitted infections. As there is no known cure, it is becoming increasingly more common and has special seriousness for pregnant women. The nurse should watch the research literature for new developments in treating this illness.

Other Venereal Infections

We discuss here three other venereal diseases briefly. They are most commonly found in the tropics.

- *Granuloma inguinale* is a chronic infection which occurs more commonly in persons with poor hygienic habits. It is characterized by the development of papular lesions on the genitalia, which become ulcerated and cause tissue destruction. This infection is treated with antibiotics and may be difficult to differentiate from cancerous lesions. Discovery of Donovan's bodies in the lesions establishes the diagnosis.
- *Chancroid* is caused by *Hemophilus ducreyi* and is also associated with poor hygiene. A pustular ulcer develops, leading to ulceration of the vulva. This is often very painful but may heal spontaneously. The diagnosis is difficult to establish. Treatment is with antibiotics.
- *Lymphogranuloma venereum* is caused by a virus and may cause systemic symptoms. It is characterized by the development of a small pustule followed by involvement of the lymphatics along with vulvar edema. Eventually ulceration and extensive scarring may occur with marked deformity of the external genitalia. The diagnosis is based on the results of a variety of tests and treatment is with sulfonamides or antibiotics.

NURSING IMPLICATIONS

This section could be titled "health care," as nurses have made broad and valuable contributions to the attempts to eradicate these pandemic infections.

> *The focus of the attack on sexually transmitted diseases has been twofold: to educate the public about these diseases, and to identify and successfully treat infected persons.*

These goals have provided direction in the United States to a wide variety of community and national programs in which health care professionals have collaborated with lay people. In some instances, nurses have played a pivotal role by helping to identify the needs of the public as well as by helping to meet these needs. In doing so, nurses have stepped out of their more conventional roles and been more facile in working as team members.

It is mandatory for health care personnel working in the area of sexually transmitted diseases to examine their own attitudes toward sexuality and sexual behavior and to try to approach clients or potential clients in a nonjudgmental manner. While the individual's own moral values are important in guiding personal behavior, it has been found that these attitudes may interfere with the exchange of information between the client and the health care worker. The communication of professional bias and prejudice can be obvious or subtle. In any event it is not helpful to the client, who may feel judged and discounted. A prejudiced health professional easily misses or misinterprets clues from the client and therefore makes inaccurate assessments.

Besides actually treating clients, which nurses often do, nurses also obtain privileged/private information from patients and give them information about sexually transmitted diseases. Both activities may be difficult. Obtaining information may require that the health care personnel be extremely skilled at interviewing. Skilled epidemiologists spend many hours in this type of interviewing, and they can often provide valuable clues as to how to interact successfully with these patients.

The information* to be obtained (not necessarily by the nurse) typically includes:

- A comprehensive sexual history

*See also Chapter 14 for discussion of information gathering.

- A history of sexual contacts
- A history of previous infections, their treatment and test results
- A history of parental infections
- A history of recent use of antibiotics
- A history of allergy to antibiotics (including manifestations)
- A history of any signs or symptoms

It is important to remember when seeking information about sexual contacts that a patient's sexual partners may include people of the same sex as the patient.

After the organism or organisms have been identified, the patient with a sexually transmitted disease is usually treated with large doses of penicillin intramuscularly. Before administering the injections, the nurse should again *check for penicillin allergy*. The patient should be observed for a short time following the injection to be sure adverse reactions to the medication do not occur. Additionally, the nurse may suggest that the patient do mild exercises to decrease the pain at the site of the injection.

As previously stated, an important aspect of the treatment program is educating the patient and significant others. There are many myths about venereal diseases; often patients need solid factual information so they can avoid reinfection. The following topics should be included in teaching about sexually transmitted diseases:

- Modes of transmission
- Incubation periods
- Signs and symptoms of infection
- Asymptomatic problems
- Methods of treatment
- Consequences of lack of complete treatment
- Consequences of repeated infections

Examples of some questions patients may ask and suggested responses are:

Q: Will treatment protect me from getting this again?
A: No, immunity to reinfection is rare if it indeed exists. In other words, you could get infected again.

Q: Can I resume my sex life?
A: It is better to wait until the tests come back showing no organisms are present. If you wait, you will not be in danger of spreading the infection to your sexual partner.

Q: Do I have to come back?
A: We would like to see you again in ________ (give an appointment) to be sure that you are cured (especially with the resistant strains of gonorrhea).

Q: Since I didn't have any symptoms this time, how will I be able to tell if I have this again?
A: When you have your periodic "Pap" test ask your doctor to check you for venereal diseases. (Modify this answer for the male patient.)

These are only a few of the questions which patients may ask or be curious about but fail to ask. In all contacts with the patient, the nurse should continuously assess the patient's understanding of the infection and provide information as needed. To do this well, the informed nurse will seek additional knowledge by consulting more detailed sources of information.

Moreover, the nurse who plans to teach others about sexually transmitted diseases will need to seek knowledge about the kind of information that various types of people want. Community education lectures about these infections may be given by nurses. Requests may come from men's groups, women's groups, schools, the Boy Scouts, the Girl Scouts, and others. To meet the needs of each group requires versatility and understanding of the types of information needed, as well as an appreciation of the learner's maturity and life style.

In summary, the nurse who works with persons who have contracted a sexually transmitted disease will find a variety of patient needs. Providing comprehensive care involves far more than merely administering prescribed drugs. Because sexuality is such a private and personal matter, nurses need to examine their own attitudes toward sexuality and be nonjudgmental in approaching patients. Only in this way, can nurses provide a valuable service in educating and comforting patients during what may be a very distressing and guilt-ridden period of life.

CHAPTER 86

BENIGN GYNECOLOGIC CONDITIONS AND PROBLEMS

by Judith Atwood R.N., M.N., and Judy Johnson, R.N., M.A.

One important consideration in caring for the woman with a *benign* tumor of the genital tract is the *malignant potential* inherent in several of these tumors. Despite the fact that the malignant potential is low, women often are concerned about the possibility of having a malignancy. These are important concerns to take into account when planning nursing care. Malignant changes are often asymptomatic until late in the course of the disease, after metastasis has occurred. (See Unit IX for further discussion of cancer.)

In addition to benign tumors of the lower genital tract, several other conditions involving the organs in this area are discussed in this chapter, e.g., endometriosis and fistulas. These conditions bear a close relationship to sexuality and potential reproductive functions of affected women. Therapy may involve disruption of one or both of these entities; it is thus important for the nurse to consider these factors in planning individualized care.

The last part of this chapter discusses pelvic relaxation and displacement. Again, the areas of sexuality and reproductive function must be considered in planning care to meet individual patient's needs. Moreover, pelvic relaxation and/or displacement may be caused by malignancies, may be aggravated by malignancies, or may be the result of treatment to eradicate malignancies. Hence, these factors need to be incorporated as appropriate into the nursing process.

BENIGN TUMORS OF THE LOWER GENITAL TRACT

Benign tumors of the lower genital tract (below the cervix) are relatively uncommon and may result from chronic inflammation or from a variety of other causes. One classification used to differentiate types of benign tumors is cystic or solid tumors. *Cystic tumors* include granulomas from syphilis, granuloma inguinale, lymphogranuloma venereum, and glandular cysts (e.g., the Bartholin cyst). *Solid tumors* are not individually discussed because they occur infrequently. Suffice it to say that solid tumors are those that involve either endometrial or supporting tissues. Both types of tumors have a low malignant potential. Further details about particular types of tumors can be obtained from specialty textbooks.

Topics that nurses may discuss while caring for women with benign tumors of the lower genital tract include the following:

- Malignant potential of a tumor
- Symptoms produced by the tumor
- Nature of therapy planned
- Expected results of therapy

If symptomatic, many of these tumors are surgically excised. Nursing care is then similar to that given after any surgical procedure, with special attention to aseptic perineal care to maximize healing. (See Chapter 84 for nursing care related to specific gynecologic procedures.)

LEIOMYOMAS

Leiomyomas are the most common tumors of the female genital tract, occurring in more than 20 per cent of all women during the menstrual years. The incidence in black women of this age group approaches 50 per cent.

Frequently these benign tumors are asymptomatic. Symptoms that do appear are generally related to the size (very small to very large), location (see below), or number of tumors (they tend to be multiple). Additionally, abnormal bleeding, often hypermenorrhea, may be present. This is true because leiomyomas are thought to be hormone (estrogen) dependent, growing slowly during the reproductive years (except during pregnancy) and then atrophying after menopause.

Leiomyomas are known by a variety of names (some not technically correct) related to the tissues involved. Some of these are: fibroids, fibromas, fibroleiomyomas, myomas, fibromyomas, and "fireballs." These tumors are made up mainly of muscle and fibrous connective tissue.

Leiomyomas may be *classified according to location*, those occurring in the body of the uterus being most common. (See Fig. 86–1.) There are six types:

- *Intramural*—in the uterine wall, surrounded by myometrium. These tend to increase the size of the uterus and may cause bleeding and dysmenorrhea.
- *Submucous*—directly under the endometrium, involving the endometrial cavity. These may cause prolonged bleeding and cramps and may become *pedunculated* (grow on a stalk) and protrude through the cervix.
- *Subserosal*—on the outer surface (under the serosa) of the uterus. These tend to become *pedunculated*, "wander" (see below), and are likely to be multiple and large, with symptoms such as backache, constipation, and bladder problems.
- *Wandering or parasitic*—occurs when a leiomyoma which is *pedunculated* twists on its pedicle and "breaks off." It then attaches to other tissues, particularly the omentum, to obtain a blood supply.
- *Intraligamentary*—implants on the pelvic ligaments and may displace the uterus or involve the ureters.

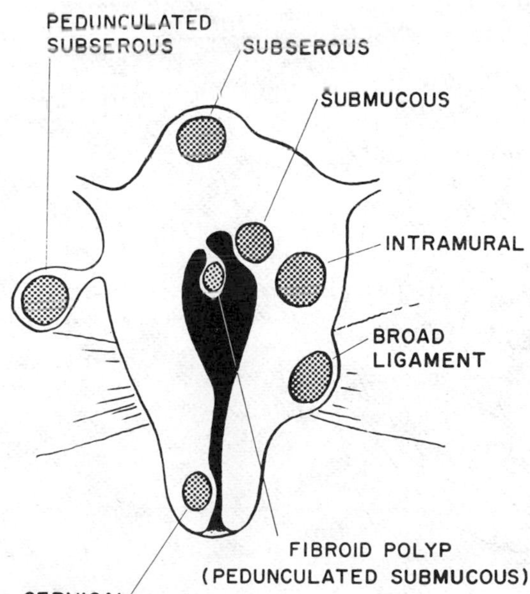

Figure 86–1. Diagram showing some locations of leiomyomas. (Modified from Ditts, P. V., J. W. Greene, and J. W. Roddick: *Core Studies in Obstetrics and Gynecology*. Baltimore: Williams & Wilkins Co., 1979.)

- *Cervical*—occurs infrequently. May obstruct the canal.

Secondary changes can occur with leiomyomas (all six categories). Types of changes can include:

- *Hyaline degeneration*—occurs when the tumor outgrows its blood supply.
- *Cystic degeneration*—tends to follow hyaline degeneration. The tumor becomes liquefied and ultimately cystic.
- *Calcification*—more common in large tumors.
- *Infection*—more common in submucous tumors.
- *Sarcomatous (malignant) degeneration*—rare. It should be suspected in rapidly enlarging tumors, in recurrent tumors, and when hemorrhage occurs in the presence of a known tumor.
- *Red (carneous) degeneration*—usually occurs during pregnancy. This type may be accompanied by acute pain over the area of the leiomyoma, fever, tachycardia, nausea, vomiting, and abdominal rigidity.
- *Fatty degeneration*—rare.
- *Acute torsion of the pedicle*—leads to acute disruption of the blood supply, with gangrenous changes and symptoms of an acute abdomen. (See *red carneous degeneration* above.)

Symptoms vary widely and occur in only half of patients with leiomyomas. When present, they are often related to the size, location, and number of leiomyomas. The onset of symptoms most commonly occurs in the patient's fifties. It is rare for symptoms to begin after menopause, as the leiomyomas tend to regress during this time. Should new symptoms develop during these years, other diagnoses such as cancer need to be ruled out.

The most common symptom is some type of abnormal uterine bleeding. This bleeding is excessive in amount or in duration. Frequently it is accompanied by anemia and is associated with feelings of tiredness, weakness, and lethargy. Urinary frequency is also common, occurring when the tumor location causes pressure on the bladder. Urinary retention may also occur. Constipation, hydroureter, and hydronephrosis occur less frequently. Abdominal pain and dyspareunia are also less common symptoms. Occasionally, the patient may have a vaginal discharge. Abdominal "pressure" is a complaint heard from patients with large tumors. These leiomyomas are large enough to cause the abdomen to be enlarged. They may also be palpable. Lastly, the patient may have problems with sterility and/or a history of one or more spontaneous abortions.

The presence of a characteristic history confirmed by abdominal and pelvic examination findings usually establishes the diagnosis. A number of other disorders, such as cancer or a problem pregnancy, need to be ruled out before a treatment plan is designed.

The *treatment* plan is formulated by considering the symptoms, the patient's age, the location and size of the tumor(s), the onset of complications, and the patient's desire to have additional children. If the patient is nearing menopause and the uterus is smaller than 12 weeks' gestation in size, the physician may elect to follow the patient closely (every 3 to 6 months) and simply allow the menopause to "solve the problem." Although malignant degeneration is rare, should such a woman show a rapid increase in the size of the leiomyomas more definitive therapy is necessary.

Younger, asymptomatic women may require no therapy. However, when definitive therapy is indicated, it typically includes *myomectomy* (removal of the tumor without removal of the uterus) if the tumor is small, or *hysterectomy* (removal of the uterus). Uterine leiomyomas are a common indication for hysterectomy. In rare instances irradiation may be used if a patient is unable to undergo surgery.

ENDOMETRIOSIS

The endometrium is the lining of the body of the uterine cavity. It is abnormal for this tissue to be located elsewhere; such a condition is called endometriosis. Usually confined to the pelvic cavity, the tissues can be found in a wide variety of other areas. Hence, sometimes bizarre symptoms are seen with this condition. Several theories as to the cause have been offered, but to date none has provided a satisfactory explanation. What is known is that the aberrant tissue is hormone dependent and subject to the same cyclic changes that occur in normal endometrial tissue. The highest incidence of this condition occurs in women between the ages of 25 and 45 who have never been pregnant.

Aberrant endometrial tissue may be found in: (a) ovaries (most common location), (b) fallopian (uterine) tubes, (c) ligaments, (d) cul-de-sac, (e) bladder or rectum, (f) rectovaginal septum, (g) appendix, and (h) bowel. Moreover, it may be found in the uterus itself, where it causes "*adenomyosis*" (see below). Rarely, the tissue may be

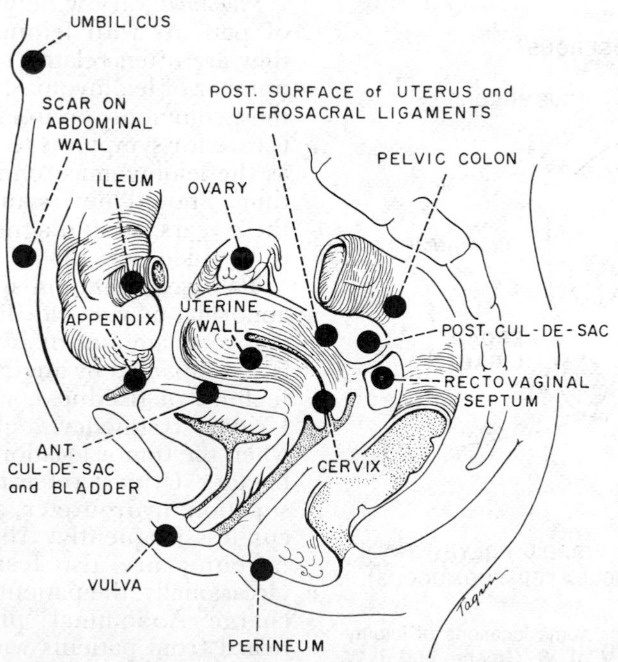

Figure 86–2. Sites of occurrence of endometriosis. (From T. H. Green, Jr.: *Gynecology: Essentials of Clinical Practice,* 3rd ed. Boston: Little, Brown and Company, 1977.)

found outside the pelvis—in surgical scars, the lungs, the extremities, or other areas.

Aberrant endometrial tissue responds to hormonal stimulation and "bleeds." Because the aberrant tissue is hormone dependent, endometriosis may be considered to be self-limited. With regression of ovarian function during the menopause, the tissue atrophies. It also regresses during pregnancy. Therefore, women who desire children are encouraged to become pregnant. Malignant changes are possible, though rare. Therefore, before treatment is undertaken, cancer should be ruled out.

The most characteristic symptom of endometriosis is pain. However, about one quarter of all patients are asymptomatic. The pain typically begins prior to the menstrual period and becomes progressively more severe. It lasts for the duration of menstruation and at times for several days thereafter. Usually pain is at its peak just prior to menstruation and during the first 1 or 2 days of the period. The pain is located in a variety of places, and it is this aspect that tends to make establishing the diagnosis difficult. Women with endometriosis may erroneously be thought to be neurotic!

Other symptoms are dyspareunia, menstrual irregularities, infertility without tubal obstruction, and severe pain if a cyst ruptures. Implants on the ureters may obstruct them; those involving the rectum may be associated with bleeding and obstruction. In any event, the symptoms do not necessarily coincide with the amount of disease present.

Definitive *therapy* for endometriosis is removal of the uterus, ovaries, tubes, and as many of the implants as possible. This therapy has the disadvantages of: (1) surgically inducing menopause and (2) causing permanent sterility. If the ovaries have not progressively been destroyed by endometrial implants, induced menopause often produces severe symptoms and morbidity in the patient (see Chapter 83). As this is such radical surgery, its use is generally limited to patients over 45 years of age. Less radical is the removal of the uterus, as many implants as possible, and some or none of the ovarian tissue (badly damaged tissue is removed). This procedure is most commonly used in women between 35 and 45 years who do not wish to retain childbearing ability. Conservative surgery is the usual treatment for women under 35 in whom medical management is not producing desirable results. This refers to the removal of as much of the aberrant endometrial tissue as possible. In all situations, the operation will be tailored to the particular needs of the patient.

The *nursing care* involves the standard care given pre- and postoperatively for a patient undergoing abdominal operation. (See Chapter 84 and Unit VIII.) In addition to specific pre- and postoperative care, the nurse needs to determine the expected outcome of the individual's operation. It is then possible to design a teaching plan to keep the patient apprised of these outcomes and specific problems which may develop postsurgically (Fig. 86–2).

Most patients have a long-term goal of pain relief. Some additionally desire pregnancy. Most statistics indicate that after conservative therapy pregnancy is achieved by less than half of the patients. Moreover, pain relief is rarely complete and other sequelae of the surgery may be unpleasant for the patient. The nurse can do much to help the patient to set and achieve realistic goals.

Nondefinitive *medical therapy* for endometriosis involves the use of a variety of hormonal drugs, including androgens, estrogens, or progestogens. The goal is to suppress ovulation either for a short time or indefinitely. In the former instance, symptom remission is induced by a state of "pseudo-pregnancy," which in turn may produce remission of the endometrial tissue. This has been thought to then enhance the possibility of pregnancy after withdrawal of the hormones. Unfortunately, this approach has not been very successful in infertile women. Indefinite use of hormones is reserved for those patients wishing to use these drugs for suppression of symptoms and for contraception. Pain relief occurs in 70 to 80 per cent of patients using this type of treatment. The side effects of the agents may, however, be most troublesome. (See sections on birth control and steroid hormones in Chapter 88.)

ADENOMYOSIS

Adenomyosis, or "internal endometriosis," is a condition caused by invasion of the myometrium by endometrial tissue. This disorder is more common in older women who have had children. It can be diffuse or be localized in the form of a tumor (*adenomyoma*). The uterus is enlarged and if the disease is extensive, the process may extend to involve adjacent organs.

Bleeding and even hemorrhage are characteristic *symptoms* of adenomyosis. Hypermenorrhea with dyspareunia is the most common combination of symptoms. Since the condition can occur in combination with endometriosis or with leiomyomas, the symptoms may be diffuse. Endometrial adenocarcinoma may develop in the uterus and present the same general symptoms. Therefore, the possibility of cancer is ruled out before a therapeutic course is chosen. Otherwise, the *treatment* is similar to that given for endometriosis. Nursing considerations are also comparable, except that patients with extensive disease may have significant bleeding, with resultant anemia. Therefore, part of the nurse's teaching responsibilities may be related to the care of persons with anemia. (See Unit XIV.)

POLYPS

Polyps (they may be called *fibroid polyps*) are pedunculated tumors that arise from the mucosa and extend into the opening of a body cavity. They are found primarily in the endometrium (uterus) and in the cervix. Cervical polyps may cause bleeding after intercourse and are subject to infection. Those in the uterus may cause hypermenorrhea, intermenstrual bleeding, and bleeding after menopause. They occasionally undergo malignant changes, particularly in postmenopausal women. Since cervical and endometrial polyps frequently co-exist, when cervical polyps are seen or felt, uterine polyps should be searched for.

OVARIAN TUMORS

Ovarian tumors may be roughly classified as non-neoplastic (physiologic) and neoplastic. Neoplastic tumors are either benign or malignant, and may have hormonal effects. Non-neoplastic tumors are solid or cystic. All of the neoplastic tumors and some of those that are non-neoplastic are subject to surgical removal. Surgery is indicated because of the potential interference with function of the pelvic organs caused by both types. Fortunately, the physiologic, and particularly the cystic, tumors are more common (Fig. 86–3).

There are a number of different types of ovarian tumors that are benign and rare. To obtain specific information about individual types of tumors, specialty literature should be consulted. The following information is presented to help you gain a general understanding of the implications of benign ovarian tumors.

Many ovarian tumors are asymptomatic until they become large enough to cause pressure *symptoms*, thus making early detection of malignancies difficult. Some smaller tumors may cause symptoms owing to their location. Symptoms related to location and/or size can include: painful defecation, constipation, dyspareunia, vague aching, heaviness, and sterility. Later symptoms include abdominal distention with dyspnea, peripheral edema, and anorexia. Pelvic pain may be present, particularly if the tumor is growing rapidly. If the tumor produces hormones, there may be menstrual irregularities and masculinizing or feminizing effects.

Complications of ovarian tumors include: hemorrhage into a cyst, with rupture and possibly infection; torsion of a cystic pedicle which may cause the former; and malignant changes. The first two complications cause symptoms similar to those discussed under uterine leiomyomas. Malignancy is suspected when there is a sudden rapid growth of a tumor, if the tumor is bilateral, or if it is large. The incidence of malignancy is higher in postmenopausal women.

Treatment is based on the type of tumor present. Cysts tend to regress in size and are therefore a type of tumor that allows the physician to watch the reproduction-age patient closely during one or two menstrual cycles. Tumors that are growing rapidly, those that disrupt the function of the pelvic organs or the ovary, those which are bilateral, and neoplastic tumors are removed surgically with or without the ovary. Therefore, surgery includes removal of the tumor; removal of the ovary or ovaries; or removal of the ovaries, tubes, and uterus. Nursing care is related to the type of surgery. If the patient is managed conservatively, the nurse should stress the importance of close follow-up. (Refer to Chapter 87 for a discussion of the types of surgery and related nursing care.)

BENIGN FALLOPIAN TUBE TUMORS

Tubal tumors are extremely rare and may be cystic or solid.

FISTULAS

Fistulas (abnormal tube-like passages within body tissue) are an extremely distressing and common problem in the genital and urinary tracts. They may occur: (a) when there is an abnormal opening between two adjacent organs, (b) as a result of the spread of a malignant lesion, (c) after irradiation for cancer, (d) after pelvic or radical surgery, or (e) after a prolonged and difficult labor and delivery. The last was formerly the most frequent cause, but improved labor and delivery techniques have changed this. Infrequently, fistulas may result from venereal and other inflammatory diseases. Some fistulas are congenital; others result from injury or diagnostic or therapeutic surgery.

Fistulas are *classified* by location. There are two general types: (1) vaginal fistulas and (2) urinary tract fistulas. *Urinary tract fistulas* are not the focus of this discussion, although much of the following information is relevant to this type

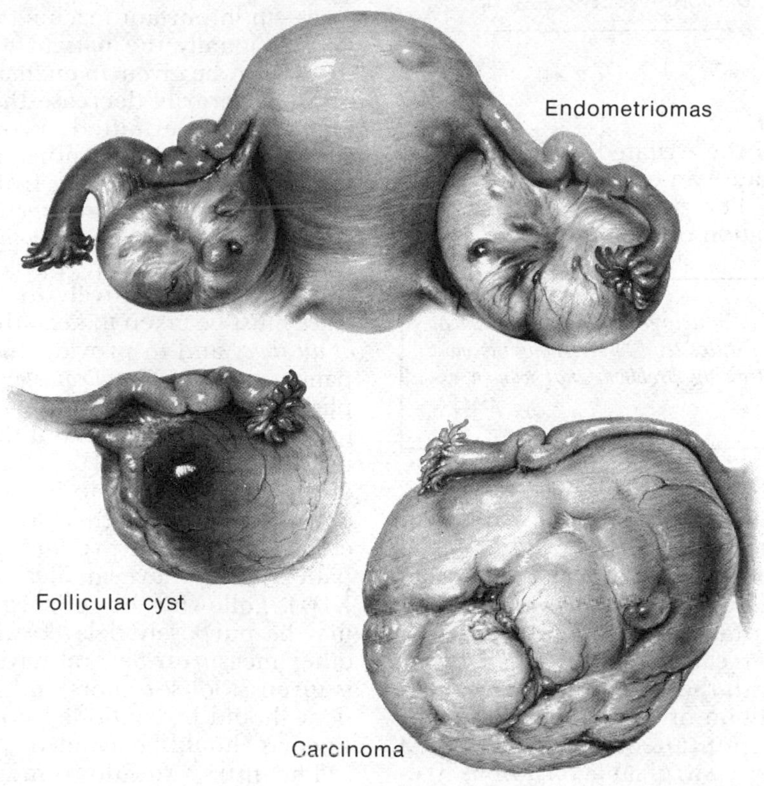

Figure 86–3. Ovarian tumors. (From Greiss, F. C., Jr.: Ovarian tumors. *American Family Physician,* 16:170, Oct. 1977, p. 171.) (Note: Cancer of the female genital tract is discussed in Chapter 87.)

of fistula. *Vaginal fistulas* include vesicovaginal (bladder), ureterovaginal (ureter), urethrovaginal (urethra), and rectovaginal (rectum) fistulas (Fig. 86–4).

All of the above vaginal fistulas cause some similar *symptoms*. Urine or flatus and feces leak into the vagina. Excoriation and irritation of the vaginal and vulvar tissues occur. Severe infec-

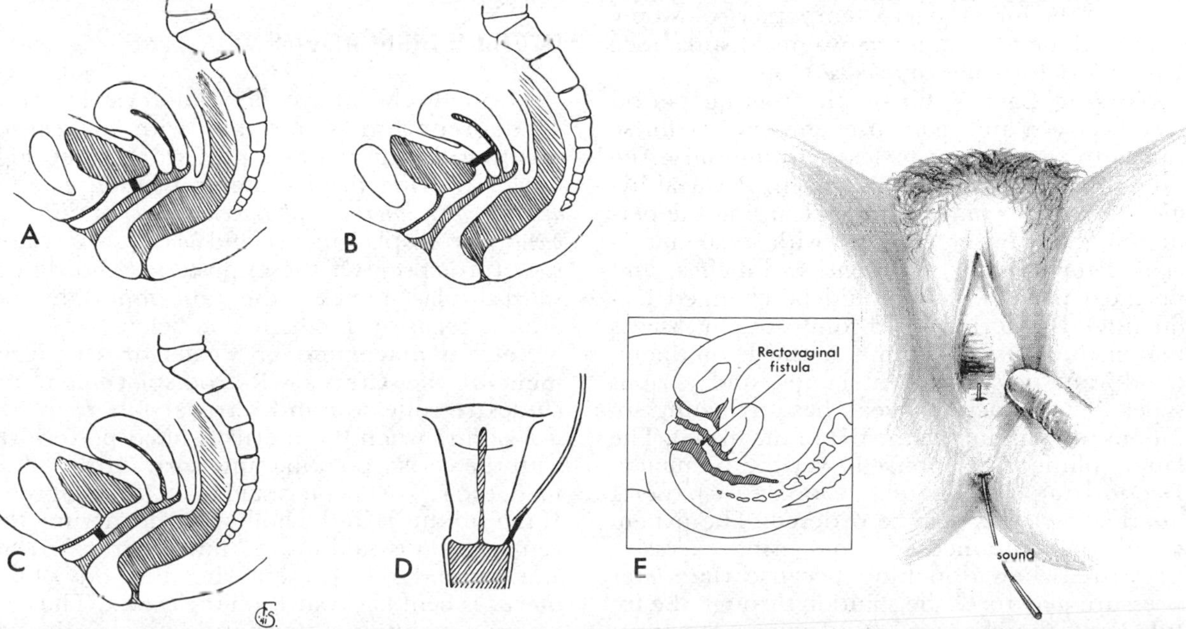

Figure 86–4. Diagram of chief varieties of vaginal fistula. (*A*) Vesicovaginal. (*B*) Vesicouterine. (*C*) Urethrovaginal. (*D*) Ureterovaginal. (*E*) Rectovaginal. (*A* to *D* from Novak, E. R., G. S. Jones, and H. W. Jones: *Gynecology.* Baltimore: Williams & Wilkins Co., 1971. *E* from Miller, N. F., and H. Avery: *Gynecology and Gynecologic Nursing,* 5th ed. Philadelphia: W.B. Saunders Co., 1965.)

tion may occur in the irritated area. Rectovaginal fistulas may cause an offensive, particularly unpleasant, odor. The patient experiences wetness and the sensation of feeling "dirty."

> *In addition to producing unpleasant physical symptoms, vaginal fistulas tend to be among the most psychologically distressing problems that women experience.*

Persons with these disorders frequently become social recluses, causing great disruption in their significant relationships and other social activities. Often they fail to consult a physician until the problem has become severe, and even then they are reluctant to discuss it.

Diagnosis and treatment may be difficult. *Treatment* varies with the location, extent, cause, and general condition of the patient. Small fistulas may heal spontaneously after 1 to 3 months. However, surgical excision is frequently required. Surgery is not always successful in curing the problem, and, for this reason, it is extremely important that the patient be in optimal condition before it is attempted. A waiting period of about 6 months is required while the inflammation and tissue edema subside. Treatment during this time is directed toward avoiding infection by performing thorough perineal hygiene and improving the overall health status of the individual. A temporary colostomy may be done to treat a rectovaginal fistula. (See Unit XVII for colostomy care.)

Nursing Care. During the waiting period *prior to surgery* and again after surgery, the nurse can help the patient to learn to minimize the symptoms and to care for herself. Perineal hygiene measures may include: cleansing the perineum about every 4 hours (with sterile materials after surgery), sitz baths, douches, and perineal pads (which should be changed frequently). Deodorizing and comforting measures may include using vitamin A and D ointment, deodorant powders, heat lamps, and various types of weak acid or weak base irrigating solutions (depending on the pH of the urine). The latter solutions are poured over the perineum. Deodorizing douches (e.g., Clorox, 1 tsp. per 1 quart water) may also be ordered. The patient should be cautioned to avoid using excessive pressure when douching because the water pressure may force the solution through the fistula tract, thereby causing infections. Some patients inadvisably restrict their fluid intake in an attempt to decrease drainage. This may actually increase the size of the fistula and cause infection—an important teaching point.

Occasionally the patient with a rectovaginal fistula may be given an enema to clean the bowel and temporarily decrease the drainage. When an enema is permitted, a soft rubber catheter should be used. The catheter should be gently inserted above and away from the fistula tract.

After surgery, care is directed toward two objectives: (1) *avoiding stress on the repaired area,* and (2) *preventing infection*. A Foley catheter may be in place postoperatively to drain the bladder. Care must be taken to keep the catheter *draining at all times* and to provide enough fluid for the patient so that *internal catheter irrigation* is accomplished. The catheter should not be routinely irrigated (externally), but if this is essential, minimal pressure should be used. Strict asepsis is essential in addition to maintaining dependent drainage. Some patients have a suprapubic catheter, and the same precautions are used. A few patients may have an ileal conduit (see Unit XIII). Following bowel surgery, the first stool may be purposely delayed with liquid diet and other measures. Several days later, the patient is given stool softeners and laxatives. The patient should be cautioned not to strain at stool. Enemas should be avoided.

The nurse should remember that expert nursing care, including the above measures, is extremely important, since surgical repair may not be successful even under optimal conditions. This is particularly true if the patient has extensive tissue damage from tumors or irradiation. Supportive nursing care is extremely important for persons experiencing this distressing disorder and for their significant others.

UTERINE DISPLACEMENT

Normally the uterus flexes anteriorly about 45 degrees and is movable, with the cervix pointing downward and posteriorly. (See Fig. 86–5.) Uterine displacements include *anterior displacement, lateral displacement, posterior displacement* (retrodisplacement), and *downward displacement* (prolapse). Of these, posterior and downward displacement are the most important and are the focus of the discussion below.

Retrodisplacement or Posterior Displacement of the Uterus. Retrodisplacement includes retroflexion and retroversion. *Retroversion* occurs when the uterus is tilted posteriorly with the cervix pointing anteriorly. If the tilt is mild, the retroversion is said to be "first degree." If the fundus is in the hollow of the sacrum, the retroversion is said to be "third degree." *Retroflexion* is said to be present when the body of the uterus is bent backwards on the cervix. The cervix may maintain a normal position in the vagina. (See Fig. 86–5.)

Retrodisplacement is caused by congenital or

acquired weakness of the pelvic support structures. These structures can be injured during surgery, during childbirth, by tumors, by inflammatory diseases, by endometriosis, and by other problems.

The majority of women with retrodisplacement are asymptomatic, and *symptoms*, when present, do not necessarily correlate with the amount of displacement. Backache (accentuated by standing a long time or occurring during the menses), secondary amenorrhea, infertility, a sense of pelvic pressure, and dyspareunia may be present. Pelvic congestion and adhesions may be the cause of some of these symptoms because the uterus is less mobile.

Treatment is directed toward the underlying cause if it can be determined. Some women, particularly those who have recently given birth, may be helped by *exercise therapy*. Assumption of the knee-chest position for a few minutes several times each day may correct mild retrodisplacement.

In other cases, the physician may elect to insert a *vaginal pessary* (Fig. 86–5*B*). After the uterus is manually placed in a normal position, the pessary is inserted. The pessary should maintain the uterine position by holding the cervix posteriorly, thus allowing the uterus to fall forward. Once it is correctly inserted the patient should not be aware of the pessary. Before leaving the physician's office, the patient should be checked to see that the pessary stays in place even during bodily movement and that she is able to void. A pessary irritates the vaginal mucosa; therefore, the patient should be instructed to douche regularly to remove excess vaginal debris. Four to 6 weeks following insertion of a pessary, the patient should return to the physician and report whether or not the presenting symptoms have been relieved. At that time, the physician checks to see that the pessary is not excessively irritating to the tissues, changing or removing it if indicated.

If left in place too long, a pessary may cause cervical erosion and adhere to the mucosa. The nurse should be sure that the patient understands the need for periodic check-ups.

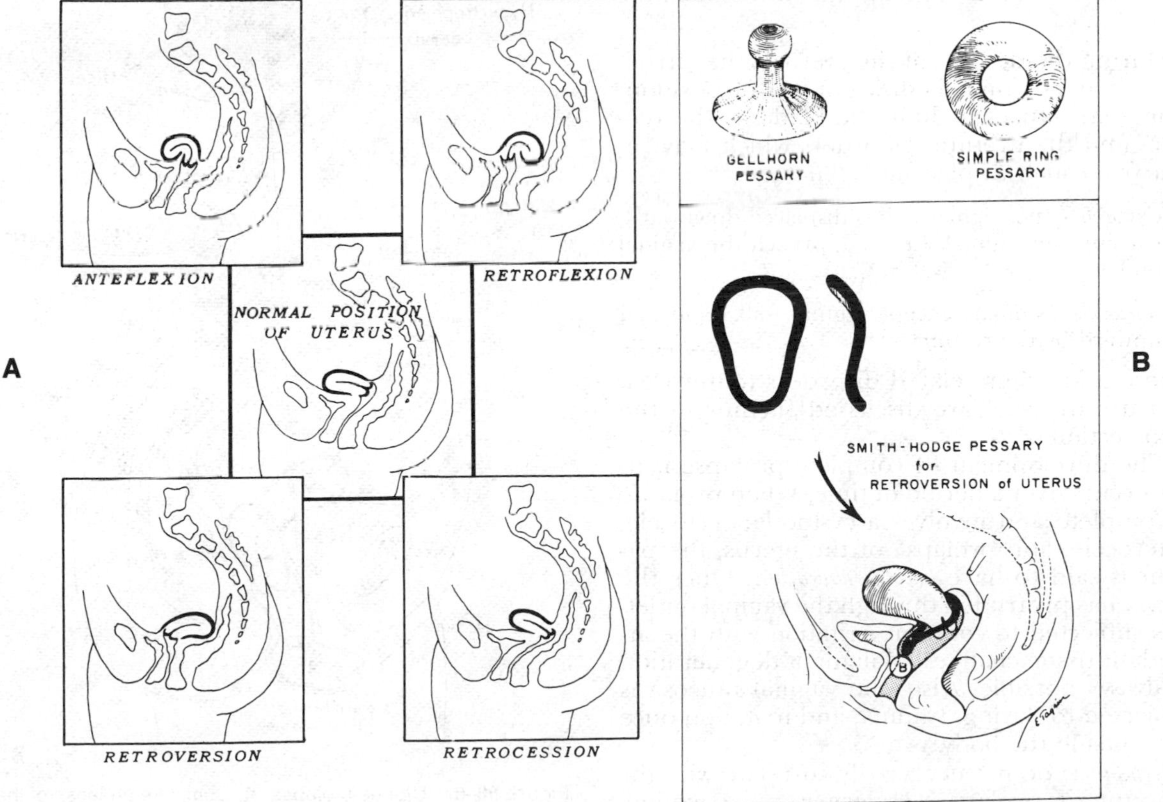

Figure 86–5. **A.** Degrees of uterine displacement. (From Miller, N. F., and H. Avery: *Gynecology and Gynecologic Nursing*, 5th ed. Philadelphia: W. B. Saunders Co., 1965.) **B.** Types of vaginal pessaries that are used in the conservative management of uterine prolapse. (From Green, T. H., Jr.: In Nardi, G. L., and G. D. Zuidema (Eds.): Surgery: *A Concise Guide to Clinical Practice*, 3rd ed. Boston: Little, Brown and Co., 1972.)

Occasionally, retroversion may be corrected by a surgical procedure called a *"uterine suspension."* More often, this procedure is not done alone but rather is performed in combination with another surgical procedure to correct another problem.

Prolapse or Downward Displacement of the Uterus. Uterine prolapse or downward displacement of the uterus into the vagina may be caused by weakening of the pelvic supports, including ligaments, fascia, and muscles. In addition, uterine prolapse may result from childbirth injuries, loss of elasticity due to aging, congenital weaknesses, or increased intra-abdominal pressure (e.g., from tumors or occupations requiring heavy lifting). When the pelvic floor relaxes, the uterus "sags" into the vaginal canal or through it to the outside of the body (Fig. 86–6).

Prolapse or descent of the uterus occurs in three stages:

1. First degree—uterus descends into the vaginal canal and the cervix reaches but does not go through the introitus.
2. Second degree—body of the uterus is still within the vagina, but the cervix protrudes through the introitus.
3. Third degree (also called "procidentia" or "complete prolapse")—the entire uterus and the cervix protrude through the introitus with inversion of the vaginal canal.

During the descent of the uterus, other structures may be "pulled" down or out of position. These structures include the bladder, the rectum, and the urethra. Disorders which may result from such displacements include:

- *Cystocele*—the vaginal wall is displaced downward, causing the vaginal wall to approach the vaginal outlet
- *Rectocele*—similar, except vaginal wall is pushed upward by the rectum

These and other related disorders (enterocele and urethrocele) are discussed further in the next section.

The development of complete prolapse usually occurs over a period of time. When prolapse is complete and involves a cystocele, rectocele, enterocele, and prolapse of the uterus, the patient is said to have *pelvic relaxation*. Once the cervix has protruded through the vaginal outlet, it is subjected to constant irritation with the attendant tissue changes. Malignant degeneration is always possible. Also, the vaginal mucosa is subjected to drying, trauma, and irritation once it is outside the body.

Symptoms do not necessarily correlate with the amount of prolapse. However, most women with a significant degree of prolapse are aware that "something is coming down in there." Additionally, patients may experience: dyspareunia; vague abdominal problems including a feeling of pressure, dragging and heaviness; backaches; and bladder and/or bowel problems if there is an associated cystocele or rectocele. Stress incontinence (discussed below) may be present.

Better than treatment is prevention, particularly through improved obstetric care (this has already decreased the incidence of prolapse). The nurse can assist in preventing uterine prolapse by (a) encouraging pregnant patients to seek qualified obstetric care, and (b) teaching patients after delivery to alternately tense and relax their gluteal muscles and the muscles of the pelvic floor (can she stop the urinary stream?). In some instances prolapse is treated with pessaries (see above). Various surgical procedures may be employed in selected women. One pro-

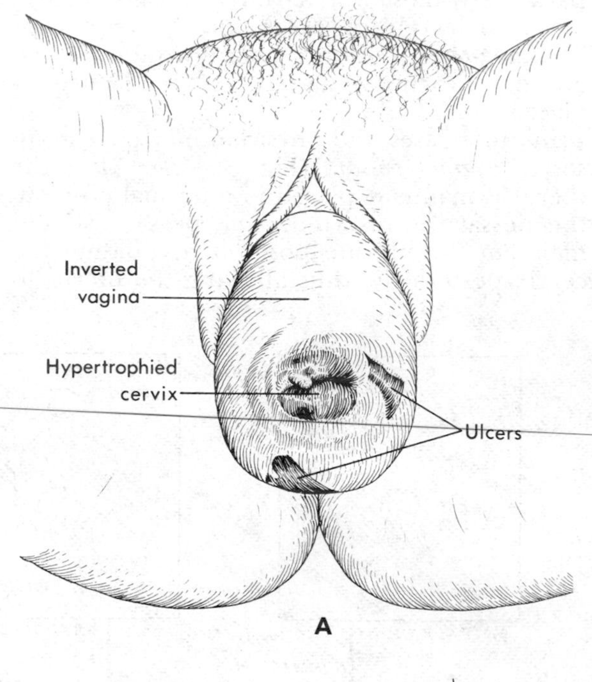

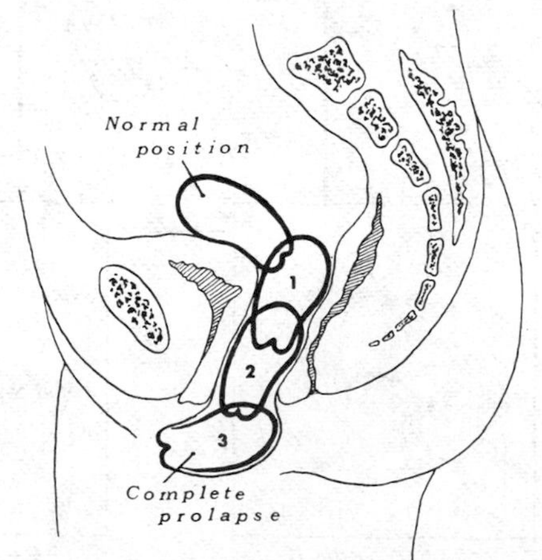

Figure 86–6. Uterine prolapse. **A.** Complete prolapse of the uterus, showing hypertrophy and ulceration of the cervix. **B.** Course followed by the uterus as it descends: 1 and 2, incomplete prolapse; 3, completed prolapse. (From Miller, N. F., and H. Avery: *Gynecology and Gynecologic Nursing,* 5th ed.)

cedure is vaginal hysterectomy with anterior and posterior colporrhaphy (repair of vagina and underlying fascia). Nursing care is related to the form of therapy.

Cystocele, Rectocele, Urethrocele and Enterocele. Caused by altered pelvic support as discussed above, these conditions occur together in some combination, separately, or in conjunction with prolapse of the uterus. As stated previously, *cystocele* develops when the bladder is displaced downward and causes the vaginal wall to approach the vaginal outlet. A *rectocele* is similar except the vaginal wall is pushed upward by the rectum. An *enterocele* involves the small bowel, and a *urethrocele* involves the urethra. (See Fig. 86–7.)

All of these disorders cause a sensation of pelvic pressure, backaches, or other vague *symptoms*. A cystocele (and urethrocele) may cause urinary symptoms including incontinence (often stress), frequency, urgency, urinary tract infections, and difficulty emptying the bladder. If the patient pushes the bladder back in place by pushing on the vaginal wall, she may notice that voiding is easier. A rectocele (and enterocele) causes bowel symptoms such as constipation and/or incontinence of feces and gas. Additionally, a rectocele may be associated with incomplete or complete tearing of the anal sphincter. Complications of these conditions include infection, cervical ulceration, hemorrhoids, and cystitis.

Perineal exercises may be prescribed as *treatment* for mild problems, and a pessary may be used with some patients (see above). A cystocele may be surgically treated with an *anterior colporrhaphy*. A rectocele is corrected with a *posterior colporrhaphy*. Other surgical procedures may be done to correct associated problems.

The postoperative care required by persons undergoing these surgical procedures is similar to that given after repair of uterine prolapse and fistula repair. The goals are the same: (a) *to prevent infection*, and (b) *to prevent pressure on the suture line*. Therefore, catheter care (or close observation of urine output), perineal care, and bowel care including avoiding straining at stool are very important. After discharge from the hospital, the patient may be instructed to douche and take mild laxatives as needed. Heavy lifting and prolonged periods of standing, walking, or sitting are contraindicated postoperatively. Additionally, the patient should avoid sexual intercourse until healing has occurred.

Stress Incontinence. Urinary continence is maintained by the junction of the bladder and the urethra, by support from the perineal floor, and by the muscle around the urethra. The angle between the urethra and the posterior bladder wall is acute and is obliterated by the process of voiding. With stress incontinence, this angle is obliterated by increasing the intravesical pressure. Such a pressure increase results from an increase in intra-abdominal pressure, e.g., during sneezing, coughing, heavy lifting. Stress incontinence is characterized by the loss of small amounts of urine during these activities.

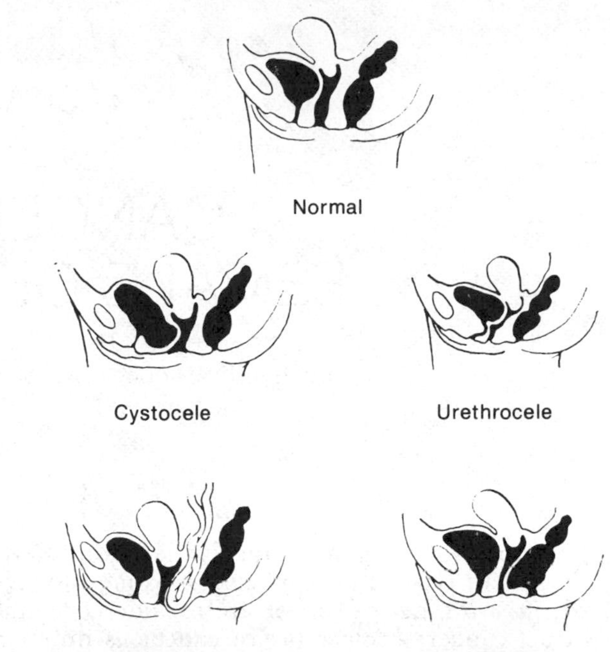

Figure 86–7. Sagittal view of normal pelvis compared to defects of cystocele, urethrocele, enterocele, and rectocele. (Modified from Dilts, P. V., J. W. Greene, and J. W. Roddick: *Core Studies in Obstetrics and Gynecology.* Baltimore: Williams and Wilkins Co., 1971.)

It is sometimes difficult to distinguish stress incontinence from other types of incontinence. Stress incontinence is due to many of the same problems that cause the previously discussed conditions and is usually made worse by the menopausal decrease in tissue elasticity. It can be caused by a cystocele, or can occur after a cystocele has been repaired.

Prevention is the most efficient care. Perineal exercises as previously discussed can help to cure mild cases. Patient education is thus important. Surgical procedures done to correct stress incontinence usually attempt to elevate the urethra and re-establish the normal angle between the urethra and the posterior bladder wall. Many of these procedures are the so-called *sling operations*. After surgery, the nurse should carefully observe the urinary output and take catheter precautions, if the patient has a catheter. If there is no catheter or it has been removed, the patient may find it beneficial to bend forward and put her feet on a support to loosen the abdominal muscles when trying to void.

CHAPTER 87

CANCER OF THE FEMALE GENITAL TRACT

by Judith Atwood, R.N., M.N., and Judy Johnson, R.N., M.A.

Cancer of the genital tract is the second most frequent type of cancer seen in women today. If in situ types of cancer are included, genital tract cancers replace breast cancer as number one in frequency. Genital tract malignancies have been studied more and for a longer time than other types of cancer in women. Basically they are malignancies that most commonly begin to appear in the middle years of life, with cervical cancer being the most common. Between the ages of 45 and 50 years, the incidence of cancer of the uterine body and of the ovary begins to equal that of cervical cancer. After the age of 55 years, the incidence of cervical cancer declines, and the other two types predominate.

> *A comprehensive cancer program consists of three parts: (1)* prevention *of cancer, (2)* early detection *of cancerous or pre-cancerous conditions, and (3)* treatment *of detected disorders. Annual, or possibly more frequent, gynecologic examinations are recommended. However, not all women follow this important health maintenance practice.*

Genital tract cancer is more commonly being treated today in major centers by gynecologists who have subspecialized in gynecologic oncology. These physicians are assisted by other cancer specialists including cancer nurse specialists, radiologists, and physicians specializing in chemotherapy. These specialists are usually actively involved in improving treatment.

One of today's major health care concerns is the encouragement of *preventive care*. It is not uncommon to hear some women say that they do *not* have gynecologic examinations because they are fearful of the findings, i.e., afraid that the examination will identify "something wrong." Clearly, an important nursing function is to provide women with support and teaching that will help them to obtain gynecologic examinations on a regular basis.

In this chapter we discuss the various types of malignancies, their symptoms, how they are diagnosed, and types of medical treatment employed. As you study the specific malignant conditions discussed in this chapter, you will find it helpful to refer to other parts of this book. Chapter 84 includes the nursing care related to the various gynecologic procedures used in diagnosing and treating malignant conditions. The unit on cancer is designed to increase your understanding of malignant properties of lesions and the type of treatment used with the appropriate nursing care considerations. Review Unit VIII as needed for general principles of nursing care for the patient experiencing surgery. Table 87–1 presents important terms related to treatment of female genital tract cancers. To avoid confusion in your studying and in clinical practice, learn to differentiate accurately among these terms.

CARCINOMA OF THE VULVA

Vulvar carcinoma is a form of malignancy found primarily in women over 50 years of age. It can arise from skin, urethra, glands, or subcutaneous tissues. Thus, there are a variety of types of tumors. Approximately 5 to 10 per cent of female genital cancers are primary vulvar tumors. Chronic vulvar dystrophies ("leukoplakia") have been implicated by some in the development of vulvar cancer. The *early symptoms* (pruritus, minimal soreness of the vulva, and tissue irritation with some bleeding) may be ignored by patients, as these symptoms differ little from those experienced with nonmalignant lesions of the vulva. As the disease progresses, the symptoms may include edema of the vulva and pelvic lymphadenopathy. Secondary infection may cause a foul-smelling discharge. Distant metastasis, infection, and gen-

TABLE 87–1. TERMINOLOGY RELATED TO CANCER OF THE FEMALE GENITAL TRACT

Sub-total hysterectomy	Removal of the uterus without removal of the cervix
Total hysterectomy	Removal of the uterus and the cervix
Panhysterectomy	Removal of the uterus, the cervix, the fallopian tubes, and the ovaries
Vaginectomy	Removal of the vagina
Simple vulvectomy	Resection of the vulva
Radical vulvectomy	Resection of the vulva, with superficial and deep lymph node dissection
Salpingo-oophorectomy	Removal of a uterine tube and ovary
Wertheim's operation	A panhysterectomy, a partial vaginectomy, and dissection of the lymph nodes in the pelvis
Lymphadenectomy	Excision of lymph nodes
Intracavity irradiation	Radiation source placed within a cavity of the body, e.g., the uterus
External irradiation	Radiation source is outside the body
Exenteration operation	Wertheim operation, total vaginectomy, removal of the bladder with diversion of the urinary system, and resection of the bowel with colostomy
Anterior exenteration	Exenteration operation, except bowel is not resected
Posterior exenteration	Exenteration operation, except bladder is not removed
Chemotherapy	Treatment of a disease with drugs; in this instance treatment of cancer with drugs specific to the type of lesion

eral disability are the usual causes of death when the disease is extensive.

The early malignant lesion may be of the in situ variety, or it may be invasive. If invasive, extensive local spread occurs, particularly into the lymphatic channels, both deep and superficial. If the lesion is of the in situ type, a *simple vulvectomy* (resection of the vulva) may be adequate treatment. However, more often a *radical vulvectomy* with superficial and deep lymph node dissection is indicated. Because the vulvar resection is of necessity extensive, some type of plastic repair procedure may be needed to close the excised area. The surgery may be done in either one or two stages. In either instance, both patient and nurse may find that the mutilation of this area is very unpleasant to look at. The nurse should be particularly careful not to respond in such a way that increases the patient's distress. Vulvectomy is a very difficult surgery to experience (see also p. 1883).

Irradiation is not generally used, since the tissues do not tolerate it well. Irradiation and chemotherapy are used less commonly than is surgery. The prognosis is poor with invasive lesions.

CARCINOMA OF THE VAGINA

Primary invasive carcinoma of the vagina is a rare lesion of older women. Most recently adenocarcinoma of the vagina and cervix has been seen in young women whose mothers ingested stilbestrol during their pregnancy. It seems to appear in these young women regardless of the *dosage* of stilbestrol taken by their mothers. Primary in situ vaginal malignancy is also rare, but when it occurs, it is usually part of an in situ vulvar lesion. Metastasis or secondary carcinoma may result from several causes, e.g., trophoblastic disease (discussed later in this chapter). Secondary carcinoma is also rare. Primary invasive carcinoma tends to involve the anterior, the posterior, or both of the vaginal walls, with resultant complications of bowel or bladder function such as fistula formation. The *signs and symptoms* of vaginal carcinoma include vaginal discharge and bleeding, presence of a mass in the vagina, and pain. The usual treatment consists of *radiation therapy*, both externally and intravaginally. Despite active therapy, the prognosis is generally poor, and the complications tend to be distressing.

CARCINOMA OF THE CERVIX

Early cervical carcinoma is usually termed *in situ* or *pre-invasive*. It is most prevalent in women between the ages of 30 and 40. *In situ and invasive carcinoma of the cervix are the most common genital tract malignancies in women*.

The majority of cervical carcinomas are of the squamous cell type (about 95 per cent). While adenocarcinoma does exist it is more difficult to diagnose. Squamous cell carcinoma usually begins at the squamocolumnar junction near the external os of the cervix, while adenocarcinoma involves the endocervical glands.

Potentially, 100 per cent of patients with in situ cervical cancer (that is, before it becomes invasive) can be cured. For this reason, one of the most important roles of nurses is encouraging women to have annual check-ups including a Papanicolaou smear. Although there is no general agreement among authorities as to the age when these check-ups should begin, it is safe to say that all women over 30 should be checked.

> *There is general agreement that invasive cervical carcinoma can be prevented by early diagnosis and treatment, while the cancer is still confined to the pre-invasive stage.*

There is also general agreement that 5 to 10 years may elapse between the pre-invasive and invasive stages, and that cervical cancer is rare before the age of 20.

Several factors have been identified that seem to correlate with the incidence of cervical carcinoma. The presence of several of the following conditions might indicate that a woman should be followed earlier than 30 years of age, as her risk is higher: early marriage; early, frequent intercourse (before age 20); multiple sexual partners; multiple pregnancies; postpartum lacerations; untreated chronic cervicitis; indications of hereditary predisposition; and a history of genital herpes. Although these factors do not actually cause cancer, there seems to be some increased risk of cervical carcinoma in women to whom some or all of these factors are relevant. In any event, the nurse should make every effort to see that each woman understands the importance of and reason for annual Pap tests. Remember, knowledge of the importance of such tests does not necessarily mean that a woman will follow through and actually obtain the test. Thus, the nurse must also consider individual women's motivations. Stressing the positive outcomes resulting from early diagnosis and treatment may help increase motivation.

Invasive carcinoma of the cervix is more prevalent between the ages of 40 and 50. Recently, there have been indications that cervical carcinoma is being diagnosed more commonly prior to the invasive stage (while in situ) or while invasion is confined to the cervix. This is encouraging because once invasion has gone beyond the cervix, the prognosis rapidly deteriorates.

Cancer of the genital organs is divided into several stages according to a variety of classification systems. The World Health Organization system is presented in Table 87–2. An estimate of 5-year survival rates is included.

Invasive Stages. From the early in situ stage, the malignancy may spread into the stroma of the cervix, over the epithelial surfaces of the cervix to the vagina and/or the uterus, into the bladder and/or rectum, into the parametrial tissue (tissue around the broad ligament), along the lymphatic pathways to the pelvic wall, and eventually into the pelvic blood vessels. Extension within the pelvis eventually leads to fixation of the pelvic organs; involvement of the blood vessels may precipitate hemorrhage; invasion of nerve tissue will lead to pain, and invasion of the rectum and/or bladder leads to the development of fistulas or obstruction of these organs.

Distant metastases are late events and may occur in a variety of organs including the liver, lungs, and bones. General debilitation (cachexia) and emotional deterioration are common, and death occurs from a variety of problems, usually within two to four years after the onset of invasive carcinoma. These events can

TABLE 87–2. WORLD HEALTH ORGANIZATION INTERNATIONAL CLASSIFICATION (CARCINOMA OF THE CERVIX)

Stage	Extent	Treatment	Prognosis For 5-year Survival (%)
Stage O (pre-invasive)	Carcinoma in situ (also called pre-invasive intraepithelial); focal in nature, confined to epithelial layer of cervix	Cervical conization; total hysterectomy with partial vaginectomy	95–100*
Stage I (invasive—Stages I to IV)	Confined to cervix, but has invaded into cervical tissue; small lesion may be present	Wertheim's hysterectomy; irradiation	75–85
Stage IIa	Has extended to vaginal mucosa but not to lower one third	Irradiation; Wertheim's hysterectomy	65–75
Stage IIb	Has extended to parametrial tissue (tissues around the broad ligament) but not to pelvic wall, or has extended to corpus of uterus	Irradiation	50–65
Stage III	Has reached pelvic wall or lower one third of vagina	Irradiation	20–30
Stage IV	Has invaded bladder and/or rectum or distant metastasis	Irradiation; surgery, e.g., exenteration	1-10

*Statistics are compiled from a variety of references. Those most generally agreed upon are used.

include death from the following conditions: pulmonary metastasis with pneumonia or other sequelae, peritonitis due to gastrointestinal obstruction and perforation, hemorrhage due to erosion of major blood vessels, or urinary tract obstruction (usually from blockage of the ureters) and subsequent uremia.

Symptoms. There are no symptoms early in the course of cervical carcinoma. When symptoms develop, a vaginal discharge and bleeding occur first. Metrorrhagia, postmenopausal bleeding, and polymenorrhea may be present. However, early bleeding may also be in the form of spotting or contact bleeding from trauma to the cervix secondary to sexual intercourse, douching, or other such causes. This early minimal bleeding increases in amount and duration as the disease progresses and usually means that the disease process involves the lymphatics.

Vaginal discharge is usually watery and becomes dark and foul smelling as the disease advances. With infection of the neoplastic area, the discharge becomes more profuse and malodorous. Moreover, the concurrent bleeding adds to the unpleasantness. Other symptoms that develop are related to the areas involved in the malignant process. Occurring late, these include pressure on the bowel and/or bladder, bladder irritation and rectal discharge, symptoms of ureteral obstruction, heavy aching abdominal pain, and fistula formation when the malignancy has eroded through the walls of adjacent organs. Pain is another late symptom and usually becomes a difficult problem with the onset of the general wasting (cachexia) that accompanies the terminal stage of cancer.

Diagnosis and Treatment. In the presence of a suspicious-appearing lesion (as viewed either by the naked eye or through a *colposcope*), or a positive Pap test, the physician will obtain a *cervical biopsy* to determine if the patient has carcinoma. This frequently allows the diagnosis to be established early, when the prognosis for eradicating the malignancy is best. (For further discussion of diagnostic procedures, see Chapter 84.) The nurse may assist with the biopsy procedure, which, if done in the office, is a minor one, causing relatively little discomfort to the patient. The procedure is relatively painless because the cervix has few nerve endings.

Most commonly the biopsy is performed through a *colposcope* (a magnifying instrument used for closer inspection of the tissues). Much less commonly a *Schiller test* may be done prior to the biopsy. This consists of cleaning debris off the cervix and then painting the tissue with an iodine preparation. Abnormal tissue which is glycogen-depleted will not stain. The biopsy is then performed by removing a bit of tissue from various areas, including all of those which are not stained.

Occasionally, the biopsy may be obtained by doing a *cold conization*. This may be done in cases where the colposcope examination is not believed to be adequate. Cold conization involves obtaining a cone-shaped section of the cervix with a scalpel. This procedure provides more tissue for analysis, thus increasing the chance that any area of invasive carcinoma will be identified, since invasive and in situ carcinoma may coexist in the same patient. It is particularly helpful if nonvisible areas, e.g., the endocervical glands, may be involved.

Conization may also be the only type of therapy needed if analysis of the tissue demonstrates that a wide area of normal tissue surrounds the excised malignancy. The result is that the patient may retain the capacity to reproduce, which in some instances is an important consideration. *Cautery* or *freezing of the cervical tissues* may also be done for those women who wish to retain the ability to become pregnant. However, it is *extremely* important that the patient recognize the necessity for close follow-up care, including serial Pap tests, since conization, cauterization, or freezing is not always adequate therapy. A total *hysterectomy* with removal of part of the vaginal cuff is a safer type of treatment for those women who do not wish any future pregnancies.

Irradiation is also used as primary therapy for early cervical carcinoma. It is usually curative treatment but induces menopause rapidly. Thus unpleasant symptoms may occur. Moreover, it makes the identification of invasive carcinoma difficult or impossible.

The nursing care following conization, cauterization or freezing is similar to that following any type of minor vaginal surgery but also includes that given after a vaginal or abdominal hysterectomy for other problems. It is important for the nurse to remember, however, that this is a patient with cancer, in addition to a gynecologic disorder. Therefore, this is a patient who is likely to be undergoing a stress response to the knowledge that she has a potentially lethal disease and that the treatment for the disease may alter her reproductive status.

The emotional responses to cancer and the nurse's function in helping patients to cope with them are discussed more fully in Unit IX. One of these responses, that of denial, may have serious implications for the patient who has had treatment designed to preserve reproductive capacity. Should she feel quite well after the treatment and fail to obtain adequate follow up care, she could remain uncured. Without frightening the patient, the importance of adequate follow-up care must be stressed.

Early invasive carcinoma is treated by removing

or destroying the involved areas and lymphatic drainage in addition to the adjacent uninvolved tissue. This is done with external and/or internal irradiation or surgery. At times, both types of therapy are used in the same patient. Stage I cervical cancer is frequently treated by panhysterectomy, partial vaginectomy, and dissection of the pelvic lymph nodes. If the disease has spread to the parametrial tissues and/or to the pelvic wall, surgery is less valuable, and irradiation is the usual treatment of choice. However, irradiation is not always effective in sterilizing the involved lymph nodes. Advanced cases are irradiated except in rare instances, when a partial or total exenteration may be done. The latter carries with it a high surgical mortality rate.

Treatment for the Terminally Ill Patient. Some patients will become terminally ill despite vigorous therapy. In this instance, the treatment goals change and are directed toward promoting physiologic and psychologic comfort, and relieving pain. The latter may be accomplished through the use of conventional drug therapy, including narcotics, sedatives, and, at times, sedation. When these agents do not produce the desired results, palliative irradiation (which also helps to achieve hemostasis when this is a problem) or selective nerve blocks may help. In some instances, various neurosurgical procedures, including cordotomy (destruction of spinal sensory pathways), give some relief. Other procedures may become necessary, e.g., a colostomy to relieve a bowel obstruction. The patient's course may be complicated by a variety of problems including fistulas, bowel and bladder obstruction, persistent pain, and cachexia. Death results within a relatively short time after the onset of the terminal phase of the illness.

CARCINOMA OF THE ENDOMETRIUM (UTERUS)

Endometrial carcinoma is the second most common genital malignancy, being second only to cervical carcinoma.

As with cervical carcinoma, if endometrial carcinoma is diagnosed early, the prognosis is relatively good. Unlike cervical malignancy, the cell type is usually adenocarcinoma (involving the glands), and is more common in older females, the average age of patients being 57 years. The adenocarcinoma is a relatively slow-growing tumor and metastasizes late. However, once it has spread to the cervix, significantly invaded the myometrium, increased the size of the uterus, or spread outside the uterus, the prognosis is seriously altered, being somewhat grim.

Although the relationship is indirect, women who are obese, hypertensive (or have cardiovascular problems), or diabetic or have not had children seem to have a higher incidence of endometrial carcinoma. Those women with a history of abnormal bleeding before menopause and/or menstrual abnormalities at the time of the menopause also have a higher incidence of this type of cancer. Exposure to radiation and the prolonged use of exogenous estrogen therapy also correlate with an increased incidence of carcinoma of the endometrium. It has been postulated that a prolonged period of abnormal endogenous estrogen stimulation not opposed by endogenous progesterone plays a role in the development of cancer.

This malignancy tends to be slow in spreading to other organs. Most commonly, the carcinoma invades the uterus itself, entering into either the cavity or the myometrium from where it can progress to involve other peritoneal structures including the lymphatics and blood vessels. From there, it can spread to the vagina, through the lymphatics, to other areas and occasionally to distant structures such as the brain and lungs. The carcinoma may extensively invade the uterus itself, causing it to become enlarged. Moreover, the extension of the cancerous process may occur along the endometrial surface to either the cervix or the tubes and ovaries. After invasion of the cervix, further spread resembles that seen with cervical carcinoma. Death may result from problems similar to those seen with cervical malignancy.

The Pap test is not reliable in ruling out endometrial carcinoma. Thus, this carcinoma is usually discovered only after the first symptom has appeared. This first and most important symptom is some type of abnormal uterine bleeding. Most frequently it is postmenopausal bleeding, since the average patient is in this stage of her reproductive life. As with cervical carcinoma, pain occurs relatively late, and other symptoms are related to invasion and/or metastasis to other organs.

The *diagnosis* of endometrial carcinoma is most frequently established by doing an examination under anesthesia and with dilatation and curettage. The latter yields tissues for analysis by the pathologist. A Pap test rarely helps in establishing the diagnosis. Women at high risk may undergo periodic sampling of the uterine contents by means of insertion of a device to irrigate, to aspirate, to brush, or to biopsy the uterine contents. *Hysterosalpingography* (an x-ray study using a contrast medium to show the uterus and tubes) and *hysteroscopy* (use of an instrument to visualize uterine contents) are occasionally used as diagnostic aids.

The *treatment* is similar to that employed with cervical carcinoma. Early endometrial carcinoma is treated by removing the uterus (with the cervix), the fallopian tubes, the ovaries, and a part of the vaginal cuff. This may be preceded or followed by irradiation either externally (e.g., with cobalt) or internally. Another form of treatment which may be used in some situations, particularly with recurrent disease, is progesterone therapy. A variety of synthetic progesterone agents may be used in large doses. Other combinations may be used. Chemotherapy is less effective in this disease than in other types of cancer therapy, e.g., that given with many types of nongenital cancer.

As recurrence of carcinoma of the uterus usually happens within 5 years, the 5-year survival rates are fairly good indicators of the overall cure rate. Age (younger patients do better), the absence of other significant medical diseases, the degree of tumor differentiation (more differentiated tumors generally have a better prognosis), the size of the uterus (generally the more abnormally enlarged the uterus the poorer the prognosis), and the absence of significant myometrial invasion all affect the prognosis positively.

CARCINOMA OF THE FALLOPIAN TUBES

The fallopian tubes are the least likely gynecologic site of *primary* carcinoma. If it occurs, the patient is generally 45 to 60 years old. *Secondary* tubal carcinoma is somewhat more common and generally is an extension from ovarian or uterine sites. Both primary and secondary tubal cancers—like ovarian carcinoma—remain asymptomatic until late in the course of the malignancy. Late symptoms seen most frequently are pain, abnormal bleeding and a watery discharge. Generally a "mass" can be felt in the pelvis. However, symptoms can be variable, causing confusion in establishing the diagnosis.

Unfortunately, due to the late appearance of symptoms, treatment is also often begun late. The cancer is relatively widespread, and the prognosis is poor. The primary treatment is with total abdominal hysterectomy and bilateral salpingo-oophorectomy. This is commonly followed by irradiation postoperatively. Chemotherapy is occasionally given to patients with widespread or recurrent disease. It is becoming more popular in some centers as the secondary treatment of choice.

CARCINOMA OF THE OVARY

> *Ovarian carcinoma is the leading cause of death in women who have genital cancer.*

It is the fourth leading cause of cancer death in American women. These poor survival rates are thought to be due to a variety of factors.

Cancer of the ovary is not a single disease but rather a collection of various types of tumors. Etiologic factors are unknown, but there is a high familial incidence. More important is the fact that the disease is *asymptomatic* until late in its course. When they first come to a physician with symptoms, more than two thirds of the patients have disease that has spread!

Ovarian carcinoma tends to grow and spread silently (without symptoms) until it causes pressure on adjacent organs or abdominal distention. When the pressure phenomena finally appear, the malignancy has usually spread to the tube, uterus, and ligaments, and the potential is great for rapid spread to the opposite ovary and its associated tissues. Moreover, the malignancy may have invaded bowel surfaces, including the omentum and other organs. The pelvic blood vessels may become involved, with resultant distant metastasis. The usual routes of spread include lymphatic, hematogenic, local extension, and peritoneal seeding.

As stated above, during the early stages there are *no symptoms* with ovarian carcinoma. The symptoms—abdominal distention, urinary frequency and urgency, constipation, ascites with dyspnea, bleeding from the uterus, and ultimately pain—do not occur until the malignancy is well established, and frequently not until it has spread. Usually, the patient eventually develops symptoms of terminal cancer, e.g., cachexia, anorexia, nausea, vomiting, and weight loss, unless the malignancy is diagnosed early—in its asymptomatic phase.

Early *diagnosis* is best accomplished by routine pelvic examination. The examiner may palpate a mass in the ovarian area and if it is suspicious will elect to do a *laparotomy* to establish the diagnosis. If the mass turns out to be a malignancy, the standard treatment is carried out: a panhysterectomy.

If early spread is suspected, this will either regress with removal of the primary tumor or be treated by postoperative *chemotherapy*. In some cases, even in the face of advanced disease, the physician may elect to remove as much of the malignancy as possible, not to cure the patient but rather to make her more comfortable. This procedure is usually followed by palliative *irradiation* and/or chemotherapy.

Compounding the problems faced by an already sick patient, *complications* such as hemorrhage and/or infection of the tumor mass are not uncommon. Though not a true complication, the rapid onset of a surgical menopause in younger patients produces various uncomfortable sequelae of the menopause. (The menopause is discussed in Chapter 83.)

GENITAL TRACT SARCOMAS

Constituting a very small percentage of the genital tract malignancies in women (about 2 to 5 per cent), sarcomas are most commonly found in the uterus and ovaries. *Uterine leiomyomas* are one type of tumor which may undergo *sarcomatous degeneration*, although this is rare in relation to the total incidence of leiomyomas in women.

Sarcomatous lesions tend to develop in younger women (20 to 30 years old) and grow very rapidly. They metastasize, particularly to the lungs, and may result in death from pulmonary causes. Treatment usually includes wide excision of the involved area and normal surrounding tissue, at times followed by irradiation. The prognosis is poor.

GESTATIONAL TROPHOBLASTIC DISEASE

Gestational trophoblastic disease, GTD, refers to a continuum of a single neoplastic disorder. The various disease forms are called *hydatidiform mole, invasive mole* (chorioadenoma destruens), and *choriocarcinoma* (chorionepithelioma). On the spectrum, these disorders range from nonmalignant trophoblastic disease (NMTD) to highly malignant trophoblastic disease (MTD). All share several properties:

1. They come from the trophoblast of human pregnancy (trophoblast is a type of embryonic tissue which aids in deriving nourishment for the developing embryo from the maternal uterus).
2. They represent invasion of the maternal host by fetal chorionic tissue.
3. The fetal chorionic tissue produces a protein hormone called human chorionic gonadotropin (HCG).
4. This hormone is produced in direct proportion to the amount of tumor present.
5. Potential cure is possible with chemotherapy.

Hydatidiform Mole. All of the entities are quite rare, the most common being the *hydatidiform mole*, which occurs in one out of every 2000 to 2500 pregnancies. Of these moles, about 80 to 85 per cent are benign; the remainder develop into one of the malignant conditions. Although hydatidiform moles can occur during any of the reproductive years, they are more common in either the early or late years. It is distressing but not uncommon to have a very young patient with a so-called *molar pregnancy*. The *signs and symptoms* of a mole include:

- Intermittent bleeding in the first trimester, which sometimes contains some of the characteristic grape-like tissue (such tissue should be sent to the pathologist for analysis)
- Excessively rapid growth of the uterus
- Absence of fetal heart tones, a fetal skeleton, and fetal movement
- Spontaneous abortion at about 14 to 18 weeks of gestation

There is a high correlation with bilateral ovarian cysts, hyperemesis gravidarum, and toxemia, particularly during the first or early in the second trimester.

DIAGNOSIS. The *diagnosis* of a hydatidiform mole is made from a specimen submitted to pathology, obtained either by spontaneous passage or by dilatation and curettage. A persistently elevated HCG (human chorionic gonadotropin) level in blood or urine is diagnostic and allows monitoring of the effects of treatment. When the diagnosis is uncertain, ultrasonography, angiography of the uterine vessels, pelvic x-rays (which show absence of a fetal outline), amniography and serial HCG determinations help to clarify the problem. Some of these measures must be used with caution lest there be a viable fetus present.

TREATMENT. Hydatidiform moles are treated by evacuating the uterus. This may be done by dilatation and curettage, suction curettage, or hysterectomy.

The *follow-up care* is of particular importance and must be meticulous. HCG titer levels are checked frequently and usually return to normal within a week of evacuation of the uterus. During the early care, the titers are followed weekly, then every other week, and finally monthly for a year to be sure that metastatic invasion has not occurred. In some centers, patients are also treated with a course of *chemotherapeutic agents* in an effort to insure that invasion has not occurred.

Invasive Mole. *Invasive mole* (*chorioadenoma destruens*) is a neoplasm of the chorion with grossly visible invasion of the myometrium and sometimes of the adjacent tissues. Metastases rarely occur, and the disease is often benign. This disorder was previously *treated* with hysterectomy; however, drugs (e.g., methotrexate and actinomycin D) are the treatment of choice today. For this reason, a precise diagnosis is difficult to obtain, since tissue studies cannot be done.

Choriocarcinoma. A malignant neoplasm

of the chorion, characterized by its tendency to metastasize early, rapidly, and widely, choriocarcinoma is an extremely malignant, necrotic tumor, with its usual primary site in the uterus. The primary site may also occur in the ovaries (or in the testes in men). These forms of the disease are associated with a grim prognosis and are not the focus of this discussion.

The clinical course of choriocarcinoma is capricious and, without intervention, is rapid. Without therapy, it is often fatal within 6 to 12 months, although a few patients may experience spontaneous disappearance of the disease without therapy. The presenting symptoms may include heavy vaginal or abdominal bleeding or may be related to metastasis; e.g., the patient may present with lung problems. Death typically occurs as a result of respiratory embarrassment, hemorrhage into the tumor, and so forth. The prognosis is directly related to the duration of the illness and to the HCG titer level on admission. If the duration has been short and the titers are low, then with careful management of the patient's drug regimen, prognosis may be excellent. Metastases occur to the following organs: (1) lungs, (2) vagina, (3) brain or central nervous system (these respond poorly to treatment), (4) liver (responds poorly), (5) kidney, and (6) spleen. Metastasis to the lungs is the most common occurrence and responds quite well to the drug program. The tumor is not radiosensitive.

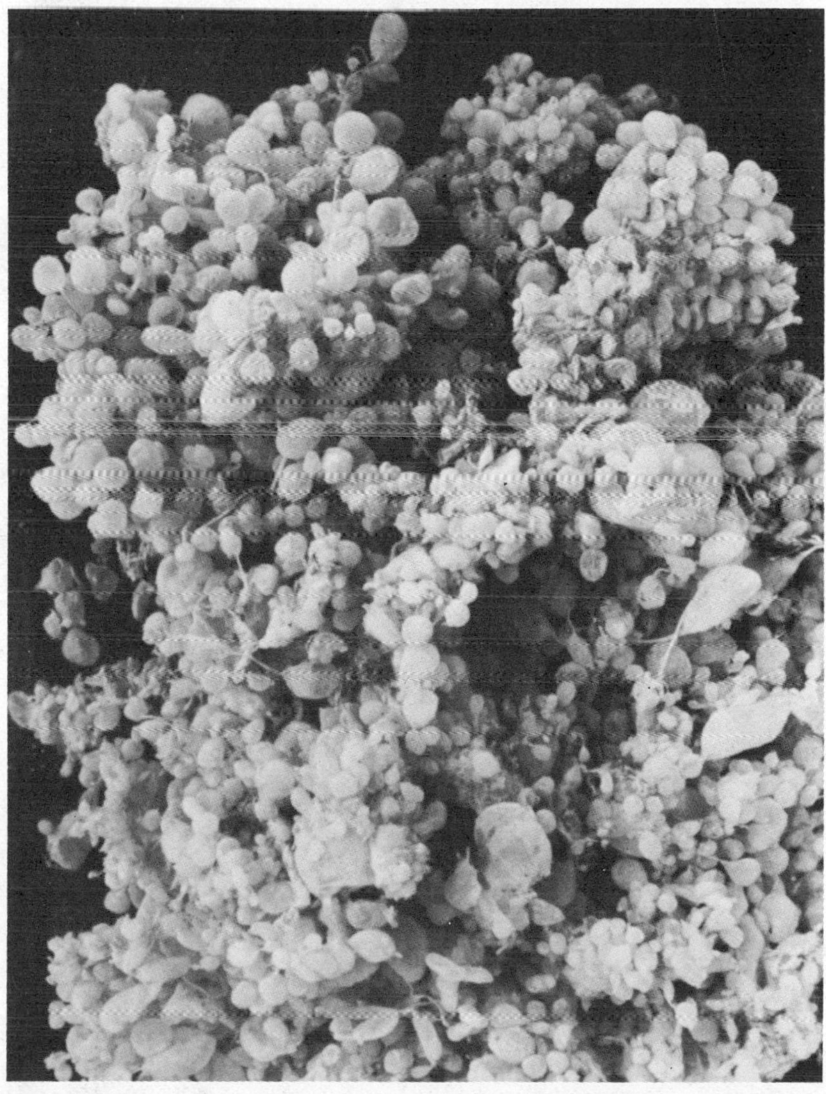

Figure 87–1. Grapelike vesicular pattern of hydatidiform mole. (Courtesy of Dr. Jan Smalbraak, Bloemendaal, The Netherlands.) (From Novak, E., G. S. Jones, and H. W. Jones: *Gynecology.* Baltimore: Williams and Wilkins Co., 1975.)

Methotrexate and *actinomycin D* are the drugs of choice in treating trophoblastic disease. For this very malignant tumor, they are given in very high doses, with 1 to 2 week rest periods between courses of therapy. The response of the patient is measured by various laboratory studies and by serial HCG determinations. When the HCG titer level has returned to normal for about two courses of therapy, the patient is discharged and followed closely as an outpatient.

Nursing care of patients with GTD is extremely challenging and requires extensive planning. In addition to the daily need for psychologic support through what is often a long therapeutic period, the patients are usually extremely ill because of the toxic effects of the drugs used. The nurse must be a keen observer and able to revise and improvise to meet the many needs of the patient. The drug side effects, which are discussed in Unit X, are potentially life threatening, thus making meticulous attention to all details of care important in order to avoid losing the patient to the therapy.

Summary

Consideration of each of the types of malignancy discussed in this chapter makes it apparent that the key elements in treating malignancies of the female genital tract are early discovery and prevention of the more serious forms of these diseases. The nurse—in contacts with patients in a variety of settings—is in an excellent position to help educate and motivate women to meet this goal.

CHAPTER 88

BIRTH CONTROL AND ISSUES AND DISORDERS RELATED TO REPRODUCTIVE FUNCTION

by Judith Atwood, R.N., M.N., and Judy Johnson, R.N., M.A.

The topic of controlling birth is not a new one, having been a matter of concern to individuals for many years. However, what is relatively new is the concern of the society as a whole about such social issues as population control, the rights of women, and ecology. Intimately linked to these three issues is the rapid increase in medical technology which has markedly increased the life span of individuals while decreasing the infant mortality rate in many countries.

Thus, as our world population has grown, concern over its growth has been expressed, first by scientists, ecologists, and demographers and then by large groups of society and the mass media. One proposed solution to the population problem is to voluntarily limit the number of children to two per each family unit. This solution has, of course, pointed up the need for adequate methods of voluntarily avoiding conception, and a great deal of effort has been expended to perfect such methods.

In this chapter we discuss topics that for many people are controversial and emotion-laden—including methods of contraception, induced abortions, and sterilization. We also discuss sexual assault (including sexual abuse, physical abuse, and in particular, rape). These areas have all become linked within the broad social context of women's rights—women's rights to control their own lives and their own bodies. These issues can tap intense feelings in almost everyone—especially individuals with a high level of personal involvement.

Abortion on demand has been particularly controversial, with extreme emotional commitment both from people who oppose abortion and people who believe it is an option women have the right to choose.

In the mid 1970's in the United States, a Supreme Court decision and state legislative actions rendered abortion on demand easier to obtain as a health care service. More recently, however, groups that oppose abortion have reopened the issue of abortion on demand, hoping to reverse the current position. Currently, a focus of controversy is the use of public funds for abortions. Whatever the controversy, the reality is that abortions *are* being performed and nurses *are needed* to care for patients during and after abortion. This can be particularly difficult for nurses who personally find pregnancy termination distasteful or immoral. Each individual nurse must clarify his or her own value system carefully or less than useful nursing care may be offered to clients.

A personal negative attitude toward abortion—coupled with a sincere professional commitment to respect the individuality of the patient and her right to make decisions for herself—may cause a nurse to feel intense conflict. This conflict can be partially resolved by having only those who choose to do so care for patients during and after abortions.

However, this solution is not totally satisfactory, as extenuating circumstances may prevail. For this reason, every nurse may come into contact with a woman undergoing an abortion, and must consider how to best cope with such an eventuality. Moreover, nurses and other health care personnel must work together to avoid allowing differing feelings to cause intrastaff conflict and thus diminish the quality of care given to the patients.

Nurses may also find themselves giving nursing care to rape victims. Again, nurses who have stereotyped beliefs or limited knowledge about women who have been sexually assaulted may give less effective and sensitive comprehensive nursing care than more informed professionals.

In this chapter we discuss also three topics which can be thought of as "involuntary birth control": *ectopic pregnancy, infertility*, and *spontaneous abortion.* These conditions prevent pregnancy or delivery of a child and may be, in some women, accompanied by psychologic trauma. Accurate psychosocial assessment by the nurse of a woman experiencing any of these conditions is essential to good nursing care.

ECTOPIC PREGNANCY

Implantation of a fertilized ovum outside the uterine cavity is called an *ectopic pregnancy*. Usually the implantation occurs in the ampulla of the fallopian (uterine) tube, although other tubal sites are possible. Implantation may rarely occur in the cervical os, the ovary, or the abdomen. A small number of abdominal implantations have been reported to be carried to term. Delivery is accomplished by laparotomy in such cases.

Approximately one of every 250 to 300 pregnancies is ectopic in nature and many of these patients have been pregnant before. In addition, patients who have experienced one ectopic pregnancy are more likely to have another. There also appears to be a higher incidence of ectopic pregnancy in women using IUD's. (IUD's, i.e., intrauterine devices, are discussed on p. 1932.)

The *causes* of ectopic pregnancy or faulty implantation are many. Blockage of the fallopian tubes, or abnormal tubal peristalsis, impedes or slows down the passage of the ovum through the tube, thus promoting tubal fertilization.

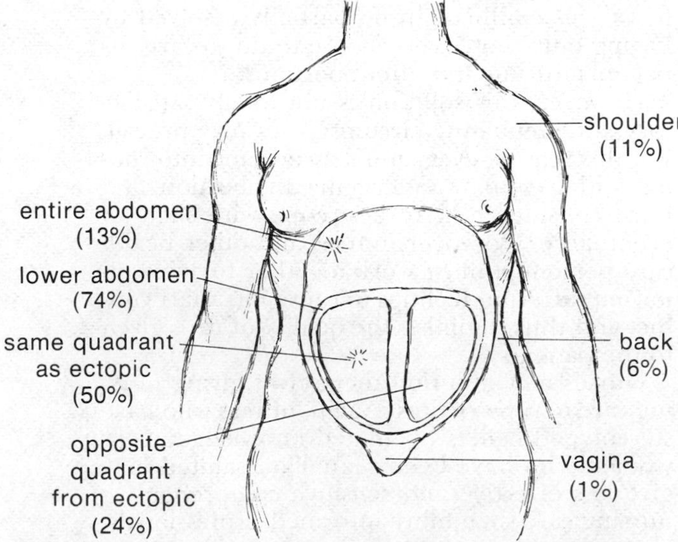

Figure 88–1. Location of pain in an ectopic pregnancy. (From Taber, B.: *Manual of Gynecologic and Obstetric Emergencies.* Philadelphia. W.B. Saunders Co., 1979, p. 314.)

Adhesions, other residuals of inflammatory problems, large leiomyomas, endometriosis, and other causes of tubal distortion or disease may also result in delayed passage of the ovum through the tubes. Once implantation has occurred in one of the tubes, one or more of the blood vessels eventually erode and bleeding results. Usually the fetus dies. The process of growth and erosion may continue through the tubal wall with bleeding into the abdominal cavity. Blood collects in the abdominal cavity and in the cul-de-sac, the latter site giving rise to a *pelvic hematocele*. In other situations, the fetus extrudes through the end of the tube or is retained in the tube.

Diagnosis. The *diagnosis* may be very difficult to establish, as the clinical picture resembles other conditions, and often the patient is not yet aware that she is pregnant. Somewhat more frequently, the typical presumptive signs of pregnancy are present. Scanty vaginal bleeding is a frequent early sign in most patients, even those with a recent history of amenorrhea. This can occur from a few days to 2 weeks before the onset of lower abdominal pain. Bleeding, abdominal pain, and pain during examination of the cervix are considered a useful diagnostic triad. Diagnosis of the condition may be made by palpation, arteriography, and ultrasound.

The signs and symptoms of an *acute tubal rupture* are usually rapid in onset and the patient is suddenly acutely ill. She may go into shock if the blood extruded rapidly into the abdominal cavity is sufficient in amount. Early symptoms (often before the onset of shock, if it occurs) may include intermittent pain localized on the involved side. The pain gradually increases in intensity. An episode of sharp, localized pain may follow, and then, as the tube ruptures, the pain becomes generalized and involves the lower abdomen. This latter type of pain is pre-

DIAGNOSIS OF ECTOPIC PREGNANCY

	Subjective Symptoms
Menses	Missed or decreased followed by spotting
Pain	Unilateral cramps before rupture
Syncope	Possible
Vaginal discharge	Brownish, bloody
	Objective Findings
Abdominal tenderness	Unilateral
Pelvic exam	Unilateral tenderness especially on cervical motion; possible unilateral mass
White blood count	Up to 15,000
Hematocrit	Decreased or dropping
Temperature	Normal
Blood pressure	Normal or decreased
Sedimentation rate	Normal

Extracted from Taber, B.: *Manual of Gynecologic and Obstetric Emergencies.* Philadelphia: W. B. Saunders Co., 1979.

sumably due to blood entering the peritoneal cavity and irritating the peritoneal membranes. The pain may be referred to the shoulder. The patient may double over, vomit, and go into hypovolemic shock rapidly, as manifested by the classic signs and symptoms. (Shock is discussed in Chapter 13.) This represents an emergency, and may present a particular problem if the diagnosis is still in doubt. Surgical intervention is usually undertaken as soon as the patient's condition is stabilized. It is sometimes preceded by culdocentesis in an attempt to find blood in the cul-de-sac and establish the diagnosis. The surgical intervention involves removal of the fetus and control of the hemorrhage. This frequently requires a salpingectomy.

In *less acute situations*, the patient continues to have intermittent pain. In addition to the abdominal pain, she may experience pain on defecation because of the blood in the cul-de-sac (an excellent diagnostic cue). Five to seven days after the onset of the pain, vaginal bleeding may occur. This is presumably due to the death of the fetus with subsequent loss of hormonal support of the uterine lining which is then shed. Earlier bleeding in the form of spotting may also have been present. Again, the treatment is surgical, although the need for urgency is diminished.

Nursing Care. Nursing care of a patient who loses an ectopic pregnancy depends on the condition of the patient and how she feels about the loss. If the diagnosis is in question, nursing observations are extremely important in helping to establish one. If the diagnosis has been determined, observations are more critical in the early identification of problems. Acute care may involve rapid preparation of a patient for surgery and helping to control shock. As these patients usually have a major abdominal operation, postoperative general care is similar to that given to other patients who have undergone abdominal surgery. (See Chapter 20.)

It is important to assess each patient's emotional response to the whole experience and to help her to cope with the process as well as she can. This involves understanding the physician's interpretation of the potential effects on the patient's ability to have future normal pregnancies, and the extent of the surgery done. The more serious *postoperative complications* include hemorrhage and peritonitis.

INFERTILITY

Infertility refers to the inability of a couple to conceive after 12 months of adequate exposure without the use of contraceptives. *Sterility* implies the absolute inability to procreate, e.g., the woman who has had a hysterectomy cannot have children.

Factors involving the male partner's ability to reproduce are almost as frequently the cause of infertility (about 40 per cent) as are those factors involving the female partner's ability to reproduce (about 50 per cent). A small percentage of couples are unable to reproduce owing to factors involving the couple as a unit (about 10 per cent).

Usually, a single cause for infertility cannot be identified, and the cause is presumed to be multiple factors. In any event, an *infertility diagnostic work-up* must involve both partners. Infertility is not uncommon. Between 20 and 50 per cent of couples can be helped.

Since a variety of minor and major health problems can contribute to infertility, the evaluation usually begins with an assessment of the general health status of the two individuals. The work-up may be difficult, time consuming, and expensive. Couples seeking such evaluation are wise to choose their physician carefully, seeking out a specialist, particularly one with expertise and special interest in the problem of infertility. In many instances the work-up will involve using the services of more than one specialist, e.g., a gynecologist, a urologist, an endocrinologist, and at times, a psychiatrist.

A comprehensive list of the various *causes* of infertility is beyond the scope of this discussion. However, the following list of possible causes of infertility in a *woman* demonstrates the complexity of the evaluation:

1. Loss of organ patency, e.g., tubal adhesions and occlusion
2. Glandular malfunction, e.g., pituitary, thyroid, adrenal
   a. Impairment of ovarian function
   b. Loss of secretory endometrium
3. Ovarian failure, e.g., polycystic ovarian disease
4. Organ infection, e.g., with changes in pH of cervical and vaginal secretions
5. Organ displacement, e.g., of the uterus
6. Obesity and debilitating diseases
7. Marital, sexual, psychologic maladjustment or lack of knowledge about reproductive functioning
8. Psychologic stress

The evaluation itself may "cure" the patient who presumably has a psychologic cause for infertility. It is thought that the decrease in tension is a major contributing factor. For this reason, as well as others, it is very important for the couple and the physician to have a satisfactory relationship. Other health team members should also relate well with the couple if they are to contribute effectively to the care.

Special Tests

As part of the extensive work-up, there are several *special tests* which may be performed to evaluate the cause of infertility in a woman. Some of these are discussed below.

Basal Body Temperature Record. This test is done in an effort to document ovulation and the development of a secretory endometrium. Other tests done before or in conjunction include *cervical and serial vaginal smears, analysis of the urine for pituitary gonadotropins*, and an *endometrial biopsy* on about day 21 or 22 of the cycle.

The basal body temperature is one of the less expensive tests used to determine when ovulation occurs. The woman takes a daily rectal temperature before arising, smoking, drinking, eating, or moving about, i.e., in a "basal state." This is charted on a graph (see Fig. 88–2); such records are kept for several months. At approximately midcycle, the basal temperature drops slightly, followed by a rise of 0.5 to 0.7 degree under the influence of progesterone. Ovulation is thought to occur just before, at the time, or just after the low temperature. The temperature charts may be somewhat confusing and the doctor should help the patient to interpret them. Those patients who wish to become pregnant should have intercourse during this time of ovulation, while those who wish to avoid pregnancy should practice abstinence (the "rhythm method" of birth control is discussed on p. 1931). Verification of ovulation can be accomplished by an endometrial biopsy on the first day of the menstrual period.

Rubin Test. This is one of several tests used to evaluate tubal patency. Carbon dioxide or compressed air is introduced into the uterus and through the tubes into the peritoneal cavity under pressure. The amount of pressure is measured with a mercury manometer, the pressure being measured when gas is heard, via a stethoscope, swishing through the abdomen. If the pressure is less than 180, then the tubes are open; if it is over 200, they are considered to be closed. If the finding is between these two values, the test results are less conclusive and some other type of test is usually indicated. Atropine may be given to minimize tubal spasm. After the test, an x-ray may be taken to see if there is gas under the diaphragm.

After the test is completed, the patient should rest for about 3 hours. She may experience cramping pain, dizziness, shoulder pain, vomiting, and nausea. These symptoms are minimized by having the woman lie on her abdomen with her pelvis higher than her head (either the knee-chest position or Trendelenburg position) so that the gas will rise in her pelvis. One additional value of the Rubin test is that it may treat a partial tubal obstruction by "blowing" it out.

Hysterosalpingography. This is an x-ray study of the uterus and tubes. An aqueous radiopaque substance is injected into the genital tract and x-rays are taken to see the outline of the various structures. Among other things, the patency of the tubes and the presence of uterine pathology can be determined. The patient is usually asked to take a laxative the night before the test, and sometimes an enema the day of the test. This is to prevent distention and gas shadows which make the x-ray films difficult to read. The patient may experience some discomfort after

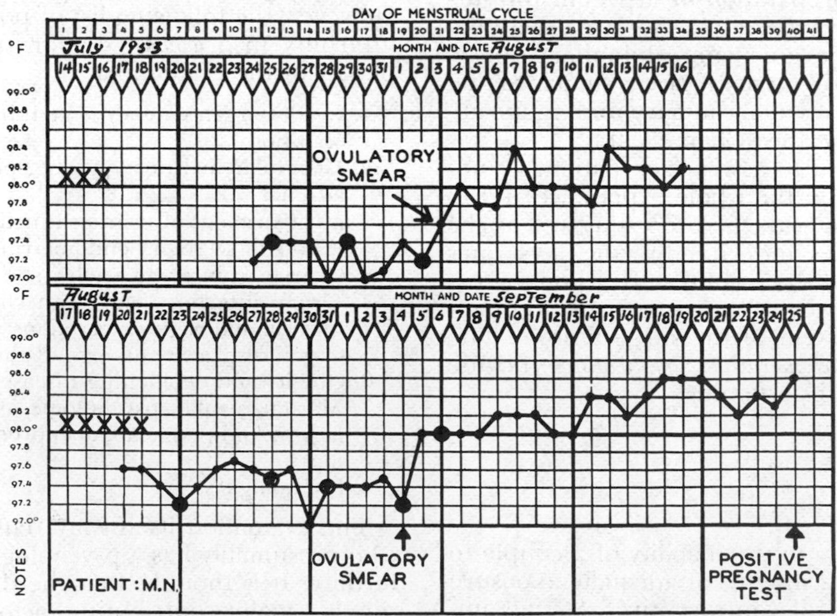

Figure 88–2. Basal body temperature chart. Upper curve represents type obtained with normal ovulatory cycle. Lower curve reveals first an ovulatory response, followed by leveling off due to pregnancy. (From Miller, N. F., and H. Avery: *Gynecology and Gynecologic Nursing*, 5th ed. 1965.)

this test and should be watched for the appearance of dye sensitivity. The symptoms of dye sensitivity are similar to those of an allergic reaction to other substances, and the discomfort is similar to that experienced after the Rubin test.

Sims-Huhner Test. Usually done at about the time of ovulation, cervical and vaginal pool secretions are aspirated and a smear is made. These secretions are obtained at a specified time after the woman has had intercourse. The time may vary from one to several hours, depending on the physician's instructions. The secretions are then checked for the presence of viable spermatozoa. Failure to find any sperm suggests faulty intercourse technique, while failure to find any viable sperm in the cervical or vaginal secretions, or both, implies that the environment is not conducive to them. Vaginal infections with a resultant change in pH are one cause of the latter problem. The patient should wear a perineal pad, and avoid douching or bathing before coming to the office for the test. Moreover, it is helpful if she remains on her back with her hips elevated for about one half hour after intercourse.

Treatment of Infertility

The *treatment* of infertility depends on the cause. Some of the more common treatments are presented below.

As already mentioned, *insufflation* of the tubes may open them. If this does not occur, plastic operations are sometimes done to restore patency. Laparoscopic or culdoscopic examination can be used for diagnosing infertile women with no detectable cause for infertility, especially if *tuboplasty* is being considered as a form of treatment. However, the overall results of tuboplasty (the surgical insertion of patent polyethylene tubes replacing nonpatent portions of fallopian tube), as measured in terms of subsequent successful pregnancies, show a low rate of success, ranging from 16 to 22 per cent. It is unfortunate that this surgery is frequently unsuccessful and, in fact, may result in tubal pregnancy.

At times, *improving the general health* of a patient may help. This is particularly true if the patient has either a debilitating disease or a chronic one. *Improving the patient's emotional outlook* also helps, as previously stated.

Still other patients may receive *hormonal therapy*. One drug, Clomid (clomiphene), may be given to stimulate the oocyte to mature. An artificial gonadotropin such as Pergonal may be given to stimulate the hypothalamic-pituitary-ovarian cycle. This latter drug may result in ovarian cyst development. Both drugs may cause multiple pregnancy.

Another method for treating infertility is *artificial insemination*, an inexpensive, simple, and often successful procedure. Legal, religious, and personal reasons often preclude couples from using this method of conception. Male sterility is most often, but not always, the reason for considering insemination. Donors should be screened for medical and genetic history, sperm count, and blood type. In addition, it is recommended that the donor and the child's legal father have the same blood type. The pregnancy rate using this procedure is between 60 and 70 per cent. Another method being used to treat infertility is the insemination of a woman with frozen sperm specimens that are aggregates of several specimens from a man with a deficient sperm count.

The newest and most revolutionary form of treating infertility occurred in Great Britain in the late 1970's, when conception occurred outside the human body in a laboratory environment. The fertilized ovum was next implanted in the natural mother's uterus, with subsequent birth of a healthy child after approximately normal gestation. Women with nonpatent fallopian tubes perhaps may opt for this unique intervention in the future, though ethical debate persists about moral implications.

It is important to remember that an infertility evaluation and treatment program may be very time consuming. Thus, *no matter what the outcome*, patients undergoing such a process should be allowed to talk, and they should receive ongoing and understanding support.

SEXUAL ASSAULT AND RAPE

Social thought concerning rape and sexual assault is gradually changing from the once popular Freudian view of a masochistic woman desiring and even precipitating rape to the view of a woman (or man in "homosexual rape") being victimized by an aggressor demonstrating the ultimate expression of scorn and attendant humiliation.

Possibly no crime has been viewed more negatively than rape. Recently, in many countries rape victims have become the focus of increased social attention. Today many medical centers offer specific medical and psychological services to rape victims. Woods defines *rape* as intrusion of the male genitalia into the female without permission, while *sexual assault* is defined as oral, genital or manual contact with the victim's genitalia.[177] Rape or sexual assault can occur between men (i.e., "homosexual rape"). However, females, either adult or children, are most often the victims. (For this reason the patient is referred to as female throughout this section. The discussion applies to male rape victims as well, however.)

Sexual assault and rape are emotionally humiliating experiences for the victim. The experience, the medical examination, and any participation in legal proceedings may contribute to long-lasting emotional trauma for the victim. Currently, there is emphasis on encouraging the victim to fight back, using both physical and emotional resistance if possible and using every available legal power to prosecute the offender.

Estimates are that one out of five rapes in the United States is reported. Approximately one half of the offenders are apprehended, three fourths of them prosecuted, and one half of these cases dismissed. About one third of the assailants use a weapon, a knife or gun, when committing the crime. The usual places of occurrence are either the victim's or rapist's home or car. Rape most often is committed against women in their twenties, followed by adolescent girls. Young children who are raped or assaulted are usually acquainted with the offender; this most commonly involves an adult male and a young girl.

Physical consequences of rape may include: genital and body trauma, pregnancy, and venereal disease. The *psychologic impact* of the trauma often affects the victim's sexual functioning and intimate relationships.

The comprehensive aim when nursing rape or sexual assault victims is efficient and sensitive care, from assessment through discharge planning. The nurse also assists in gathering medical-legal evidence should the victim wish to prosecute. Assessment of the patient should include examining the entire body, as bruises or lacerations may be found in many areas. Woods comments that genital bruising may not be apparent until twenty-four hours after the assault.[177]

Other data gathered include a physical examination, history of the assault, and a sexual history. It is important to remember that information from the patient may be necessary to prosecute the assailant. Therefore, it is necessary to know if the patient has bathed, douched, or was wearing a tampon during the rape. The date of the last menstrual period and of last sexual intercourse is also important.

Laboratory tests, including gonococcal smears, vaginal aspiration for sperm, and pregnancy tests, are done. A pelvic examination is com-

RAPE PROTOCOL

The history should be taken with no one present but the examiner and the patient. The physical examination should be done with a nurse in attendance. The social worker may be present.

I. Initial observation before examination
- Mental state:
- Physical state:
  - Clothing:
  - Dirt:
  - Debris:

II. History
- History of incident:
  - Where contacted:
  - Circumstances of the rape:
  - What happened afterward:
- Specific questions:
  - Any physical violence?
  - Any threats?
  - Any weapons seen or alluded to?
  - Has the patient cleaned up or bathed or douched since the episode?
  - Condom on assailant?
  - Douche used before the episode?
- Prior Ob-Gyn history:
  - History of serious illnesses, including venereal diseases:
  - Date of last menstrual period:
  - Pregnancy protection, if any:
  - Date of last prior sexual intercourse:

III. Physical examination (The patient's entire body should be scanned for injuries. Note the approximate age of the injuries.)
- Superficial examination:
  - Cuts:
  - Scrapes:
  - Bruises:
  - Debris:

III. Physical examination (cont'd)
- Pelvic examination:
  - Debris:
  - Lacerations:
  - Bleeding:
  - Introitus:
  - Vagina:
  - Cervix:
  - Uterus:
  - Adnexa:

IV. Laboratory cultures to be obtained (All slides should be labeled by the physician or by the nurse in the physician's presence.)
- ☐ Two dry slides, air dried
- ☐ One slide preserved in ethyl alcohol bottle
- ☐ One wet mount to be checked by the examining doctor
- ☐ Transgrow® culture medium
- ☐ Vaginal vault wash: 10 cc. sterile saline; placed in rubber-top blood container tube
- ☐ VDRL

  Laboratory tests placed in refrigerator by__________________

V. Other considerations (The patient should be prophylactically treated for venereal disease.)
- Drugs used and doses:
- Prophylaxis for pregnancy prevention; pregnancy test:
- Any torn or bloody clothing is considered evidence and should be saved until released by the police.
- ☐ Follow-up arranged
  With whom?_______________________

Figure 88–3. Rape Protocol. (From Hunt, G. R.: Rape: An organized approach to evaluation and treatment. *American Family Physician*, 15:154, Jan. 1977).

pleted, often a traumatic experience for the patient, by re-creating memories of the rape. It is essential that a supportive person be with the patient at all times, as physical assessment may re-create some of the trauma of the actual experience for the patient.

A sample "Rape Protocol" is shown in Figure 88–3.

Before discharge the nurse should give clear verbal and written instructions about medications to be used and their side effects as well as follow-up instructions. Prophylaxis against venereal disease may be given in the form of an appropriate antibiotic. A diethylstilbestrol regimen, known as the "morning after pill," may be prescribed to prevent pregnancy. The nurse also ascertains if someone will be with the victim after discharge to lessen fears of abandonment and listen to her should she wish to verbalize feelings.

Crisis intervention can assist the rape victim with feelings of anger, guilt, and fear so she need not view herself as basically helpless, permanently degraded and stigmatized. Counseling begins with helping the patient to verbalize angry feelings toward the assailant. People experiencing discomfort talking about their anger may become depressed and find it difficult to discuss their feelings of shame about the trauma. Should this occur, development of insight can be hindered and future intimate relationships may be jeopardized. Counseling assists the patient in integrating a new self-concept and planning for the future by anticipating potential problem areas such as future sexual relationships. Counseling often includes the family and other significant others, especially if a child or adolescent is the victim. Many communities have services (e.g., Rape Relief) which can be contacted for help and/or information.

CONTRACEPTION AND BIRTH CONTROL

Prior to reading the following discussions, review Figure 88–4, showing pathways of sperm and ovum in the female reproductive organs.

For every 100 women who are proved fertile and who do not use some means of contraception, about 80 women will become pregnant in one year. Family planning, therefore, is seen as a responsibility by some in our society. There is increasing need for the distribution of information about contraceptives and for the contraceptives themselves. Nurses are often expected to be well informed about the various techniques of contraception and how they are used. Thus, nurses need to keep up to date on the latest developments in this field and know about appropriate community resources in order to

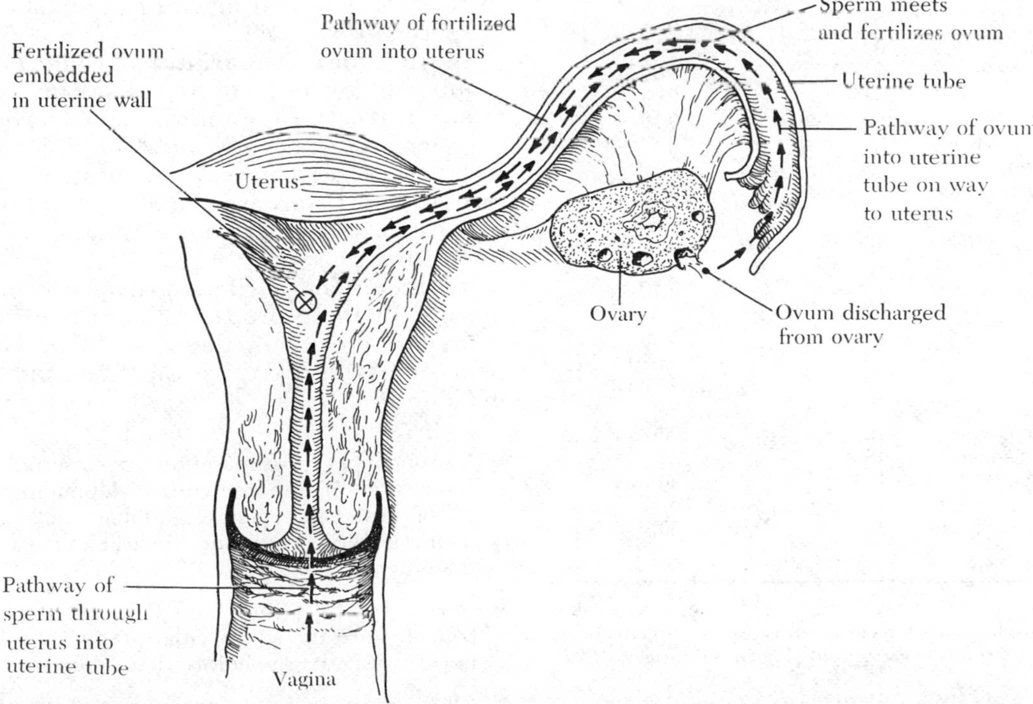

Figure 88–4. Pathways of sperm and ovum in the female reproductive organs. (Modified from Miller, B. F., and C. B. Keane: *Encyclopedia and Dictionary of Medicine, Nursing, and Allied Health,* 2nd ed. Philadelphia: W.B. Saunders Co., 1978.)

refer people who wish to obtain contraceptives. One such resource in most communities is Planned Parenthood (or some other family planning clinics). In addition, nurses need to be able to provide literature to those who request it.

The *choice of a contraceptive* is usually made either by the client or by the client and consulting physician or nurse practitioner.

> *The contraceptive chosen should be effective, in keeping with the patient's moral views, aesthetically acceptable, easy to use, reversible, and one that can be used consistently. More importantly, it should reflect the choice of the patient.*

With some methods of contraception, the patient should also choose an alternative method to be used in emergencies. For example, the patient who forgets to take several of her "pills" may use foam and have her male partner use a condom.

APPROXIMATE FAILURE RATE OF CONTRACEPTIVE METHODS (PREGNANCIES PER 100 WOMAN-YEARS)

	Theoretical Failure Rate	Actual Use Failure Rate
Abortion	0 +	0 +
Abstinence	0	?
Hysterectomy	0.0001	0.0001
Tubal ligation	0.04	0.04
Vasectomy	Less than 0.15	0.15
Oral contraceptives (combined)	Less than 1.0	2-5
I.M. long acting Progestin	Less than 1.0	5-10
Condom + spermicidal agent	1.0	5
Low-dose oral progestin	1-4	5-10
IUD	1-5	6
Condom	3	15-20
Diaphragm	3	20-25
Spermicidal foam	3	30
Coitus interruptus	15	20-25
Rhythm (calendar)	15	35
Lactation for 12 months	15	40
Chance (sexually active)	80	80

Note: Extensive references, often conflicting, are available on the complicated subject of contraceptive effectiveness, including 14 references in *Contraceptive Technology, 1973-1974*.

From *Our Bodies, Ourselves*. The Boston Women's Health Book Collective. New York: Simon and Schuster, 2nd ed. 1976, p. 185.

None of the methods of contraception presently available is totally effective, although all are more effective than nothing. Some of them have *side effects* that can be quite serious. However, it should be remembered that pregnancy may also be a risk for some women, frequently exceeding the risk from the form of contraception chosen for these individuals.

Douches. Douches under high pressure may actually force spermatozoa into the uterus. They are not an effective birth control method.

Coitus Interruptus. The *"withdrawal" method* is presumably the oldest form of birth control known to humans. As ejaculation becomes imminent, the man quickly withdraws his penis from the vagina in order that the spermatozoa be deposited outside the woman's body. Care must be taken to avoid depositing seminal fluid on the vulva where it could conceivably enter the vagina. Withdrawal requires that the male partner be highly motivated as well as aware of, and in control of, ejaculation. Many men feel that this method makes coitus less enjoyable, as there is a need for conscious control of the male impulse of deep penetration at the time of ejaculation. This need for self-control is contrary to the desire for self-abandonment at this time.

Coitus interruptus may be preferred by some persons, rather than practicing no birth control method. However, the pregnancy rate can be relatively high and it is possible to have "accidents." Moreover, the contribution of the Cowper's glands to the seminal fluid may contain sperm which may be deposited in the vagina prior to ejaculation. Also, the first few drops of the ejaculate contain much of the total deposit of spermatozoa.

Spermicidal Preparations. There are a number of different types of creams, jellies, foams, aerosols, suppositories, and tablets that are chemicals with a spermicidal action (i.e., destructive to spermatozoa). Of these, the jellies, creams, and foams are usually the most effective. All must be inserted into the vagina before intercourse.

It is important to tell the patient who plans to use one of these preparations to read the instructions and follow them carefully. The patient should also receive the following information:

- Various types of preparations are inserted at different times before intercourse, depending on the properties of the agent; e.g., tablets need time to melt and should be inserted earlier than some of the other preparations.
- Avoid douching for about 6 hours after intercourse, since the spermicidal preparation should not be washed away before that time.
- Check to see if another application of the product is necessary if coitus occurs more than once in a short interval. Vigorous intercourse can force

most of the agent out of the vagina, thus negating its action.

These spermicidal products are considered to be quite effective when used properly. Some are viewed as being better than others. They are frequently used in combination with another form of contraception, such as a condom or diaphragm. Alone or with one of these other methods, the spermicidal agents provide additional lubrication for coitus. Some people do not like the fact that their use may be "messy."

All of these preparations can be bought without a prescription. They are inexpensive and easy to use. There are virtually no side effects, with the possible exception of irritation, particularly in the male.

Condoms. Condoms (often called "rubbers," "French letters," "skins," "safes," or "prophylactics") are widely used and provide a mechanical barrier for the spermatozoa, as well as against organisms causing some venereal diseases. They are readily available, relatively inexpensive, and do not require a prescription. When properly used, they are highly effective.

Condoms are made from a variety of synthetic materials and have a ring around the open end. They must be put on the penis *after* the male has an erection, and, for this reason, many men consider them a nuisance. Additionally, some men feel that they lessen pleasurable sensation during coitus.

Because men lose penile erection after intercourse, the penis size decreases. Thus, at this time, a condom may not retain its fit and semen can leak into the vagina. Also, if the male fails to grasp the ring of the condom as he removes his penis from the vagina, the condom may come off in the vagina. The third way that semen can leak into the vagina is rupture or perforation of the condom. This latter event can frequently be avoided by using condoms that have a built-in dead space to collect the ejaculate. They are slightly more expensive.

Condoms are frequently used in combination with a spermicidal agent inserted in the woman's vagina at the appropriate time. This procedure provides lubrication as well as additional protection against pregnancy.

The Rhythm Method *(Calendar Method)*. This is the only form of birth control approved by all religions in some circumstances. It is based on *abstinence from coitus during ovulation*. Ovulation is most frequently said to occur about 14 days before the next menstrual period, and only once each month or cycle. An ovum is said to live about 24 hours unless it is fertilized, and spermatozoa supposedly live about 72 hours. (Review Chapter 83 as necessary.) Unfortunately, all of these postulates are not necessarily true. However, they are the basis for using a period of abstinence as a form of birth control.

The primary problem with using the rhythm method is pinpointing the event of ovulation. This is most commonly attempted by using the basal body temperature records (described on p. 1926.) Many physicians request that a woman keep these records for 6 months to 1 year. From these records they use a formula to calculate the "safe period" for intercourse. This usually means abstinence from intercourse for about 8 days each month during approximately midcycle. (See Fig. 88–5.)

As can be seen, to be effective, a couple using the rhythm method must be highly motivated. In addition, the woman's cycle must be relatively regular. Variations in the cycle can be caused by stress, illness, fever, medications, travel, and other such events. These variations may disrupt the effectiveness of this method of contraception. However, despite all of these potential pitfalls, the rhythm method is quite effective for some couples.

A variation of natural birth control methods is the *ovulation method* first described by Doctors John and Evelyn Billings in 1952. The method is based on the assumption that cervical mucus formation accompanies ovulation, necessary for the motility and viability of sperm. With this method, women are taught to evaluate their sensation of vaginal "wetness" or "dryness" each evening. Prior to ovulation, thick, yellow or cloudy mucus is typically secreted. The closer to ovulation, the clearer the mucus. This clear, watery mucus can be stretched into a fine thread and signals the peak of ovulation. Women are instructed to avoid sexual contact on "wet" days. "Safe" days are considered to be 10 days prior to menstruation and approximately 2 days postmenstruation. Persons using the ovulation method are advised to keep a record of mucus observations and a basal temperature graph for more accurate prediction of ovulation.

While safety, lack of cost, and reversibility are advantages of this method, it is not very reliable in preventing pregnancy.

Diaphragm. A *diaphragm*, another means of mechanical contraception, *fits over the cervical os*. (Fig. 88–6*B*.) It must be fitted to the woman by her physician and is made from a synthetic material or rubber with a flexible ring or coil around the outside. The woman inserts some spermicidal agent in the dome of the diaphragm, folds it over and inserts it sometime before sexual activity occurs. It is removed and cleaned afterward. Some women may then reinsert it the subsequent day, repeating the routine. *In any event, the diaphragm should not be removed for at least six hours after intercourse*. In addition to using the spermicidal agent in the dome, women may also use the same agent intravaginally before intercourse for extra protection.

A diaphragm is not difficult to insert. However, some women may find insertion awkward at first. For this reason, when a woman is fitted with a diaphragm, she should be carefully checked to see that she can insert it and remove it. She should also be taught to check the diaphragm to be sure the position when inserted is correct.

The size of a diaphragm should be checked several months after it is initially used, with every pregnancy, and periodically to be sure that it is still appropriate.

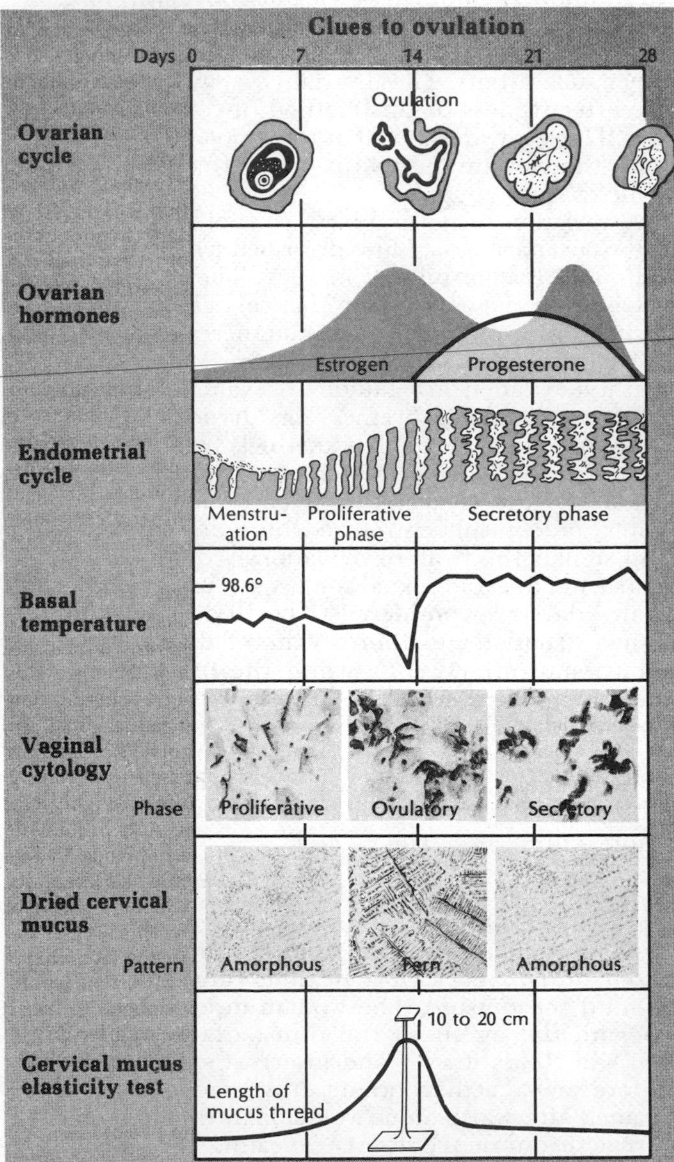

Figure 88–5. Clues to ovulation. (From Worley, R. J.: How to manage consistent failure to ovulate. *Consultant,* 17:101, Oct. 1977.)

If properly inserted, neither partner should be aware of the diaphragm. Well-fitting diaphragms are effective in preventing pregnancy in the majority of well-motivated, properly instructed women. A few with uterine descent or other pathology may not be able to use this type of contraceptive.

Intrauterine Devices (IUD). IUD's were used for camels as early as Biblical times. They were used to prevent pregnancy, especially while crossing the desert. They were first used in humans in the late 1800's but did not become popular until more recently.

An IUD is an object of varying shape made of inert plastic and/or some metal *which is placed in the uterus to prevent pregnancy.* The mechanism of action of the device is not really known. It has been postulated that IUD's: (a) interfere with implantation and cause rapid contraction of the tubes so that the ovum is transported through too rapidly to be fertilized, or (b) increase the number of inflammatory cells in the endometrium and intrauterine fluid. This precipitates either an out-of-phase endometrium not conducive to implantation or phagocytosis of the fertilized ovum.

IUD's are made in a variety of shapes and sizes, and from a variety of materials. Nurses should be familiar with the types used in their community. Such information may include: knowledge of the side effects, rate of complications, and other characteristics of the particular device. No effort has been made here to discuss the various brands available, as this is an area of rapid development. (See Fig. 88–6*A*.)

An IUD is inserted and removed by a physician. Insertion involves sounding the uterus for size and placement and then inserting the IUD through the cervix with a plunger or inserter. This may be done as a sterile outpatient procedure. Many IUD's have strings attached to them that are left in the vagina in order that the presence of the device can be checked. The patient is taught to check these strings frequently, and especially after a menstrual period. Insertion may cause discomfort, including cramping. Patients are encouraged to rest after the insertion and may be given an analgesic. Some women, frequently those who have never been pregnant, may not be able to retain an IUD or have it inserted. Expulsion can be expected to occur during the first year following insertion. Thus, another type of contraception must be used.

Should women using IUD's become pregnant, they are generally advised to have the IUD removed because of the risk of septic abortion with a retained IUD. However, other considerations may be taken into account in individual situations.

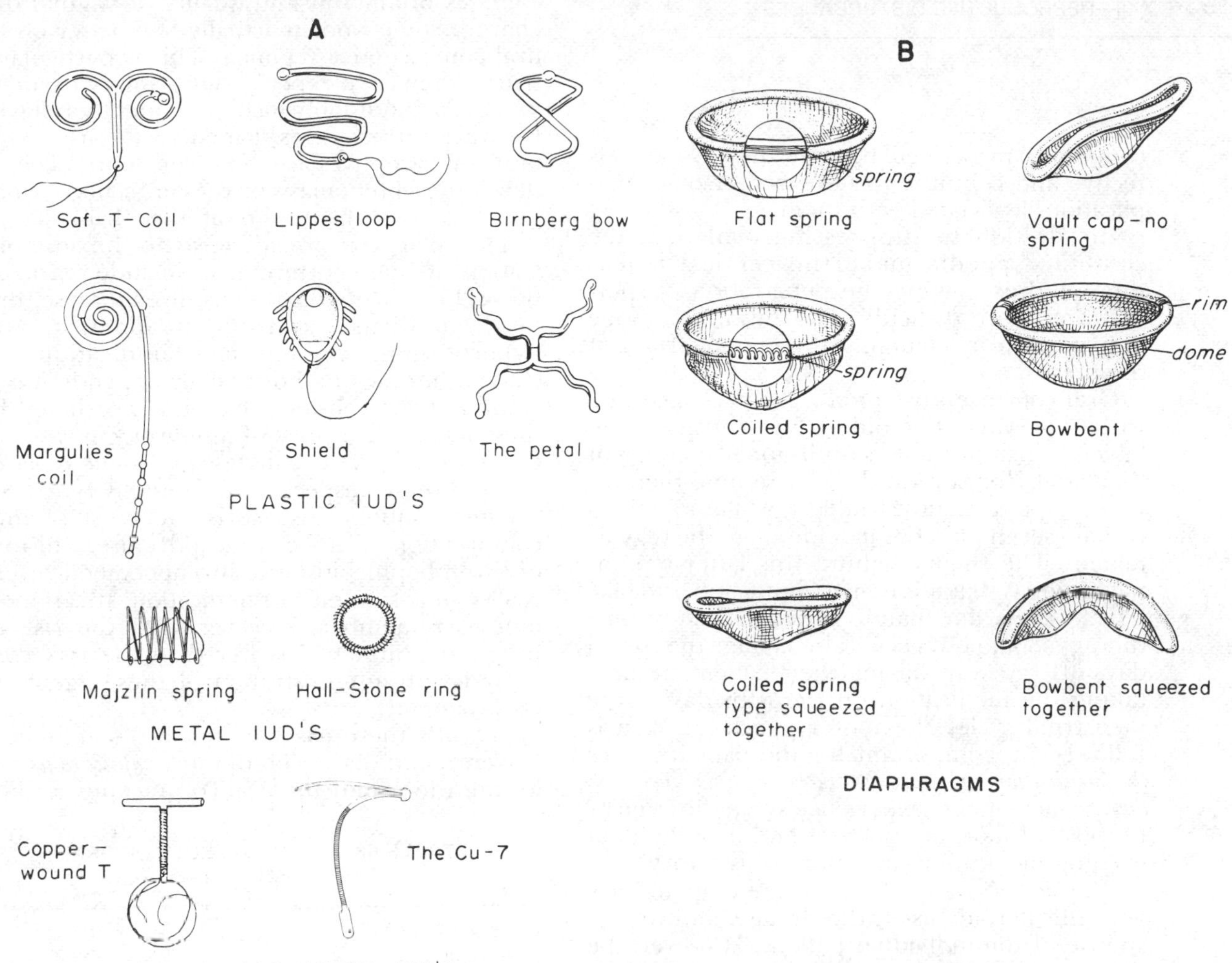

Figure 88–6. Birth control devices. **A.** Intrauterine devices. **B.** diaphragms. (From Hubbard, C. W.: *Family Planning Education*. St. Louis: C. V. Mosby Company, 1973.)

> *In any event it is important for the woman with an IUD to be closely supervised medically because of possible complications.*

Complications of these devices include expulsion of the device, cramping, spotting, heavy bleeding with menstrual periods, infection, an increase in vaginal discharge, and rarely, perforation of the uterus. There is also an increased incidence of ectopic pregnancy in women using IUD's for more than 1 year. IUD's are quite effective, although the pregnancy rate is somewhat higher than that for the contraceptive pill.

It is imperative that women using IUD's have normal uterine sensation so that pain (symptom of pelvic inflammatory disease or perforation) is perceived. For this reason, IUD's are not appropriate for some disabled women (see also p. 576).

While an IUD is in place, the patient should have her usual annual examination. At this time some physicians will remove the IUD and replace it. About 20 per cent of women fitted with an IUD find them unacceptable either because of cramping or because of other side effects. These women are usually better advised to use some other form of birth control.

Oral Contraceptive Agents. Oral contraceptive agents (the "pill") are *the most effective method of birth control available today, short of sterilization*. They are synthetic steroid preparations designed to suppress ovulation by inhibiting the production of pituitary gonadotropins. There are several types of these preparations. However, the combined agents are the most effective and therefore the most commonly used. (This discussion focuses on these agents.) The *combined agents* consist of synthetic estrogens and progesterone. The other two types of agents are the *sequentials*, which contain a progesterone preparation only in the last seven tablets, and the *"mini" pill*, which is a microprogestational low-dose agent. The latter two types are not commonly prescribed because they are less effective and continue to have bothersome complications associated with them.

In addition to suppressing ovulation, the combined agents make the cervical mucus thicker, thus making the penetration of spermatozoa more difficult. They also discourage implantation by changing the endometrium of the uterus.

Oral contraceptive agents are packaged in a variety of ways. The oldest type consists of 20 tablets which are taken until gone; the patient then waits for several days to resume therapy. Other types contain 21 tablets, while still others contain seven placebos in addition to the regular tablets. The theory behind this latter type of packaging is that it is easier to remember to take a tablet every day than to stop and then resume therapy. Some physicians also change the "seven days off" cycle by having their patients resume taking the medication on the fifth day of the menstrual cycle. No matter which regimen is followed, it is important for the patient to *take the medication at approximately the same time each day*. Some patients experience symptoms similar to those of morning sickness and may find that evening medications are more satisfactory.

The *side effects* of the combined agents vary with the steroids used, the dosage, and the response of the individual patient. However, the patient should know that menstrual periods may be shorter and the amount of flow diminished. The period usually occurs between 2 and 4 days after the last tablet. An occasional period may be missed; however, should this happen repeatedly, the patient should notify her physician. Some women will experience breakthrough bleeding (i.e., spotting bleeding between menstrual periods), particularly if taking the lower dosage preparations. The physician should be notified of this and usually will increase the dosage. It is also possible to forget to take one tablet; this usually causes no problem. The woman should take the tablet when she remembers the omission. Should she forget more than one, however, she should notify her physician and/or use an alternative method of contraception for the rest of the cycle. However, the chances of pregnancy with the combined type of therapy remain low.

Minor and annoying *side effects* are experienced by many women as they begin taking oral contraceptives. These effects are rarely serious in an otherwise healthy woman. They include: nausea, vomiting, enlargement and tenderness of the breasts, minor depression, vaginal spotting, weight gain, acne, changes in libido, and changes in amount and quality of vaginal discharge. Some women actually feel better on an oral contraceptive regimen. This is particularly true if they have experienced primary dysmenorrhea, a condition which is frequently relieved by oral contraceptives. Patients who are taking oral contraceptives are, however, more likely to develop trichomoniasis or yeast infections which may be very difficult to treat. (See Table 88–1.)

The relative *contraindications* to the administration of oral contraceptives include: varicosities, a history of convulsions, liver disease, diabetes mellitus, migraine headaches, and hypertension. Absolute contraindications include a history of a hormonally dependent carcinoma, hypertension which is exacerbated by these agents, a history of a neurologic vascular event, or gall bladder disease and some types of heart disease, especially congestive types. As thromboembolic disease is the most serious complication of oral contraceptive use, a history of thrombophlebitis or a thromboembolic event is also an absolute contraindication. It is important to remember, however, that the risk of pregnancy may be greater than the risk connected with administration of these agents in most patients.

Recently there has been much research, controversy, and discussion of *rare complications* following the use of the oral contraceptives. The

TABLE 88–1. SIDE EFFECTS OF ORAL CONTRACEPTIVES

Estrogen Excess:
- Nausea
- Edema and leg cramps
- Vertigo
- Leukorrhea
- Increase in leiomyoma size
- Chloasma
- Uterine cramps

Estrogen Deficiency:
- Irritability, nervousness
- Hot flushes
- Uterine prolapse
- Monilial vaginitis
- Early and midcycle bleeding
- Decreased amount of menstrual flow

Progestin Excess:
- Increased appetite and weight gain
- Tiredness and fatigue
- Depression, change in libido
- Oily scalp, acne
- Loss of hair
- Cholestatic jaundice
- Decreased length of menstrual flow

Progestin Deficiency:
- Late breakthrough bleeding and spotting
- Heavy menstrual flow and clotting
- Delayed onset of menses

From Balin, H.: Oral contraceptives. *American Family Practitioner*, Jan. 1976, p. 113.

last word has by no means been spoken, but the research has emphasized the need for an adequate health evaluation of the woman who wishes to use oral contraceptives. No authority has yet suggested that the oral agents are not useful. However, *approximately 15 per cent of women using oral contraceptives are considered at high risk for serious complications.*

> *Women over age 40 years, particularly if they are smokers, overweight, have diabetes, or have cardiovascular disease, are considered the high risk group most susceptible to complications from oral contraceptives.*

Other birth control options are usually explored with women in the above groups. British researchers found a significant morbidity and mortality rate among women over forty who smoked, with death due to myocardial infarction. Obviously, adequate screening procedures are essential.

Women using oral contraceptives should be taught about indications of possibly serious problems. (See Table 88–2.)

The nurse's knowledge of pill types, dosages, expected side effects, and possible complications is necessary for patient teaching and follow-up. Pills prescribed should be in the lowest effective dose range possible. It is important to remember that the estrogen and progesterone in various oral contraceptives do not have the same potency per milligram or microgram. Patients are often cautioned to discontinue pill use 4 weeks before major surgery in order to lower the incidence of clot formation. Oral contraceptives are generally discontinued approximately 3 months before attempting pregnancy, as use during the first trimester may harm the cardiovascular development of the fetus. In addition, mothers who breast feed may be advised to use other types of contraception because synthetic hormones appearing in the breast milk can interfere with the baby's liver function.

In 1972, Wood[177] reviewed significant British and American studies on the effects of oral contraceptives on the cardiovascular system. In 1973, the Duke cooperative study[31] presented data related to the cerebrovascular effects of oral contraceptives, specifically the incidence of stroke. These and other population studies completed as recently as 1977 have pointed out the rare but serious effects of these agents. Below, a synopsis of the findings is presented, using the framework of Wood.[177]

Wood noted the following cardiovascular physiologic effects of the oral contraceptives:

- Blood vessels—". . . the net effect . . . is that of producing stasis of flow in the veins of the lower extremities."[177]
- Clotting—" . . . the net effect is to increase the tendency of blood to clot."[177]
- Renin-angiotensin-aldosterone system—"the net effect is an increase in angiotensin and thus aldosterone with a potential exaggeration of hypertension."[177]

Clinically the following conclusions have been drawn from various studies and cited by Wood and the Duke study.[31,177]

Thromboembolism—the incidence of this problem was cited as being 12 times as high as that in a comparable population not taking these agents in the British studies. The incidence of thrombophlebitis was eight times as high. These problems are frequently manifested clinically by pulmonary emboli and deep vein thrombosis. Wood concluded that these data demonstrated that these agents were not suited to patients suffering from some forms of heart disease.[177]

Varicose veins—since the physiologic effect of these agents was venous dilatation of the legs, Wood concluded that those patients with varicosities who could use another type of birth control ought to do so.

Migraine headaches—those suffering from migraine are better treated with another type of birth control measure, according to Wood.[177]

Cerebrovascular disorders—the Duke population study revealed that the incidence of thrombotic stroke was nine times greater in those on oral contraceptive agents than in matched controls.[31] The evidence for a correlation between hemorrhagic stroke and oral contraceptives was less conclusive. The study did not report the incidence of other risk factors for stroke (e.g., diabetes mellitus) in either the study group or the control group. Vessey, in an editorial commenting on this study, stated: "Although the increase in risk of thrombotic stroke among women using oral contraceptives has been found to be large in this study, in relative terms, *it must be remembered that the absolute risk to the individual woman is extremely small*." He cited this risk at about five deaths per one million users per year.[92]

TABLE 88–2. POSSIBLE PROBLEMS WITH ORAL CONTRACEPTIVES

Five Signals	Possible Problem
Abdominal pain (severe)	Gallbladder disease, hepatic adenoma, blood clot
Chest pain (severe) or shortness of breath	Blood clot in lungs or myocardial infarction
Headaches (severe)	Stroke or hypertension
Eye problems: blurred vision, flashing lights, or blindness	Stroke or hypertension
Severe leg pain (calf or thigh)	Blood clot in legs

From Hatcher, R., et al.: *Contraceptive Technology 1978–1979*, 9th ed. New York: Irvington Publishers, Inc., 1978.

Hypertension—there is evidence that, in some women, hypertension may be exacerbated with these agents. The changes occur early and reverse soon after the oral contraceptives are discontinued.

Summarizing the collected data, Wood points out the need for individual evaluation: "As in all branches of medicine, the physician must balance these risks against other potentially more substantial risks."[177]

Two additional synthetic steroid contraceptive preparations available to women are diethylstilbestrol and medroxyprogesterone. *Diethylstilbestrol* (DES), a nonsteroid synthetic estrogen known as the "morning after pill," is most often prescribed for women who have been sexually assaulted. DES prevents implantation of the ovum, owing to high levels of estrogen. This treatment regimen is instituted within 72 hours of unprotected intercourse. Because of the high hormone dose used, nausea and vomiting may be severe. An antiemetic agent, particularly of the type used during pregnancy, may be prescribed. This type of contraceptive has limited use.

Long-acting progesterone injections of *medroxyprogesterone* are often used by women who have difficulty remembering to take oral contraceptives. The injections are given every 3 months to inhibit ovulation. Some women experience spotting and irregular periods. The injections are especially useful for some women with serious blood dyscrasias or for those who absolutely should not become pregnant.

Careful medical follow-up is important for users of synthetic steroid preparations, including annual pap smears and regular breast examination. When seeking medical help for any illness or condition, the patient is advised to tell health care providers that she uses oral contraceptives. Many physicians advise discontinuing birth control pills every 2 years for 1 month. The nurse may assist the patient at this time with information on use of a different method of birth control. Patient teaching may also include instruction regarding dietary supplements such as folic acid or vitamin B_6.

With more women using oral contraceptives for longer periods of time, nurses will be increasingly responsible for providing current, relevant information about types of synthetic steroids available, dosages, side effects, and contraindications. Given the complexities of birth control technology, the nurse's role includes helping patients to examine both the advantages and disadvantages of contraceptive use on an individual basis.

Contraception by means of synthetic steroid preparations, usually in oral form, is the most widely used method of birth control in the United States.

STERILIZATION

Sterilization is the termination of the reproductive capacity of a man or woman.

In the male, sterilization through *vasectomy* is an easier procedure than any of the methods currently employed in women. Sterility is achieved through bilateral excision of portions of the vas deferens. Vasectomy is quickly done in a doctor's office or clinic. Vasectomy does not affect a man's sexual hormones nor sexual functioning. Although various attempts have been made to reverse the procedure, results have been mixed, and vasectomy at this time should be considered a permanent procedure. Vasectomy is gaining increasing popularity.

In women, incidental sterilization can be accomplished through several of the procedures discussed in Chapter 84. The most common procedure to produce sterility without other untoward effects in women is *tubal ligation*. This procedure is done without disruption of either ovulation or the menstrual function. However, with these two functions continuing, failure of the tubal procedure can result in pregnancy. The patient and her partner should be aware of this, as the tubes may recanalize or in other ways allow for pregnancy.

Recently the laws governing sterilization have become more liberal in some countries and increasing numbers of patients are taking advantage of this. Despite the legal status in a given community, the woman and her partner should both understand the potential effects of any proposed procedure before they consent to its being done.

Tubal ligation can be done vaginally or through the abdomen. The latter approach is used more commonly. When done vaginally, it is usually in combination with a vaginal repair procedure. Abdominally, tubal ligation is performed through an incision in the lower abdomen or through a laparoscope. The fallopian tube is freed from surrounding tissues and a loop is brought up. The loop is then ligated and either the area around the ligation is crushed or the ligated segment is excised. In some instances metal clips have been used in an experimental effort to provide temporary sterility. The more common techniques for tubal ligation are the *Pomeroy and Irving techniques*.

In healthy women, tubal ligation is associated with few *complications*. However, when complications do occur, they may include pulmonary embolism, hemorrhage, infection, and tubal pregnancy.

Another controversial aspect of sterilization is the right of people not to be sterilized without their full knowledge and understanding. The social and ethical implications of forced sterilization are tremendous. As a nurse, you should be aware of the ongoing legal developments in the area of "informed consent," e.g., the reproductive rights of mentally retarded persons.

ABORTION

As noted in the beginning of this chapter, abortion arouses many and conflicting emotions in people. It is not uncommon to discover that many people hold stereotyped emotions which they feel a woman undergoing abortion "ought to" experience. Conflicting emotions may also be present. When nurse-patient interaction breaks down, it is often because nurses have failed to separate their own individual moral values and emotions from those of patients and from those they expect patients to experience. This may be the experience of the nurse who has contact with patients who have experienced an induced or a spontaneous abortion. It is very important for the nurse to keep in mind how easy it is to confuse and transfer emotions and to attempt to understand these processes carefully so that the care provided will be psychologically therapeutic for the patient.

Abortion may be defined as the spontaneous or induced expulsion of the products of conception before the fetus is legally viable. "Viability" as defined legally varies between 20 and 28 weeks of gestation and between 500 and 1000 gm. of weight. *Miscarriage* is the lay term for a spontaneous abortion. After the viable period has been reached and before term pregnancy is reached, there is a period when expulsion of the fetus is termed *premature labor*. The incidence of spontaneous abortion is somewhere between 10 and 15 per cent of all pregnancies. The incidence of induced abortion is quite high; however, these figures are very difficult to obtain. With spontaneous abortion, the incidence of either fetal or maternal abnormalities is also quite high.

A number of *classifications of types of abortion* are presented below. First, a review of the major *symptoms* is pertinent. These include the presence of pregnancy with its signs and symptoms, spotting and then vaginal bleeding, cramping pain which becomes intense during the actual separation of the fetal tissues, and low back pain which frequently accompanies dilatation of the cervix and heralds the onset of inevitable abortion.

Threatened Abortion. This condition may be present when the patient shows early labor-like signs, including a small amount of bleeding. The cervix is not dilated. The patient is put to bed immediately for about 24 hours, after which her activity is restricted. Sedation may be used. Cathartics and vaginal examinations are avoided. Hormones such as progesterone preparations may be given to maintain implantation, although their use is controversial. If abortion is successfully averted, the patient is asked to report any subsequent symptoms immediately.

Inevitable Abortion. Inevitable abortion is said to occur when the symptoms of threatened abortion have progressed to the point where expulsion is unavoidable. These symptoms usually include bleeding, cramping, and dilatation of the cervix.

Complete Abortion. When inevitable abortion results in the expulsion of all of the products of conception, complete abortion results. The uterus is emptied of both the fetus and the placental tissues in their entirety.

Incomplete Abortion. This type of abortion is said to occur when the patient continues to bleed after the fetus and other tissues have been expelled. It is usually due to retention of part of the placenta and is treated either with drugs, such as oxytocin, or by dilatation and evacuation (D and E) of the uterus under anesthesia.

Septic Abortion. A septic abortion usually results when tissue is retained and then becomes infected. It is associated with symptoms such as abdominal pain or tenderness, fever, a foul discharge, and laboratory evidence of infection. It is treated with antibiotics in large doses and D and E. Occasionally the serious complication of septic shock may occur with septic abortion. Fluid, electrolyte, and blood replacement often must be instituted and monitored carefully. Occasionally, renal cortical necrosis may occur and may result in renal failure. The use of large doses of steroids and possibly vasopressors may be necessary to preserve the patient's life. Further discussion of septic shock is found in other sections of this text (See Chapter 13.)

Missed Abortion. This disorder is present when a dead fetus weighing less than 500 gm. is retained in the uterus for more than 4 weeks. It can occur after the administration of progesterone preparations to maintain a threatened fetus. It is characterized by the disappearance of signs and symptoms of pregnancy. It is usually treated by evacuating the uterus. Nursing care involves monitoring indicators of blood loss. Bleeding may be severe owing to a decrease in clotting factors and subsequent uterine nonresponsiveness to oxytocin. Signs and symptoms are similar to those seen in any patient with severe blood loss.

Habitual Abortion. Three or more consecutive abortions without an intervening successful pregnancy constitute the criteria for habitual abortion. The abortion usually occurs early in the course of the pregnancy. The treatment of such a condition is based on discovery of the cause, which may be a complex process. One cause which has received attention is an incompetent cervical os. In this instance, a purse string suture may be placed in the cervix until labor

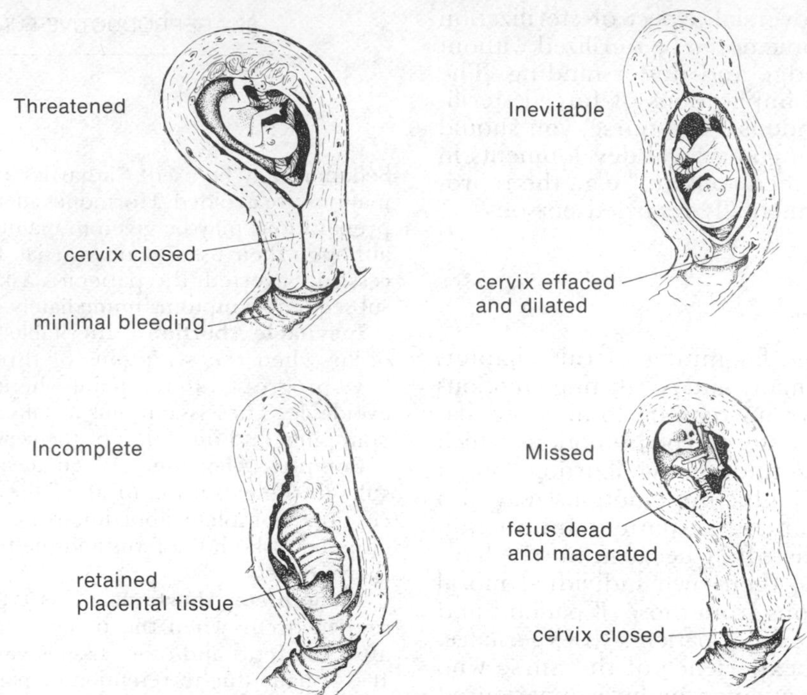

Figure 88–7. Types of abortion. (From Taber, B.: *Manual of Gynecologic and Obstetric Emergencies*. Philadelphia: W.B. Saunders Co., 1979.)

begins. At time of delivery, it is important that the patient let the medical team know that such a suture is in place. Another major cause of habitual abortion is thought to be a defect in either the endometrium or an anatomical defect in the fetus.

Habitual abortion is usually manifested by the painless onset of dilatation of the cervix, with rupture of the membranes and expulsion following quite rapidly. If bleeding and pain are present, they are late symptoms.

Therapeutic and Criminal Abortion. The distinction between these types of abortion is a legal one and is not very clear, owing to the changing laws. In a practical sense, criminal abortion is frequently associated with a clandestine and often unsafe abortion.

Techniques of Induced Abortion

Abortion may be *induced* in a variety of ways.

Suction Curettage (Dilatation and Evacuation). *Suction curettage* is a popular method of inducing early abortion before 12 weeks of gestation. The cervix is dilated and "cleaned out" with a suction curettage which is much safer than the older, more conventional type of curettage. The procedure takes only a few minutes and complications are quite rare. Suction curettage is usually conducted in an outpatient setting with local anesthetic such as a paracervical block, making the procedure less costly than if done in a hospital. Nursing care postabortion involves monitoring vital signs and blood loss until the patient is able to leave the health care setting, usually within 2 to 6 hours.

Dilatation and Curettage. Abortion performed from the twelfth to the sixteenth week of gestation usually necessitates a *D & C* with general anesthesia, a costlier procedure with a higher incidence of complications (blood loss and uterine injury). Moreover, a short hospitalization may be required.

Saline Abortion. *Saline abortion* is usually done between 14 and 20 weeks of gestation and involves the replacement of amniotic fluid with hypertonic saline. The amniotic fluid is withdrawn through a spinal needle which has been placed through the fetal membranes. The saline is injected through the same needle and results in the death of the fetus within about one hour of the injection. Labor usually begins within 24 hours and the products of conception are expelled. When carefully done on appropriately selected patients, the procedure results in few complications.

> *A rare but significant occurrence associated with saline abortion is cardiac failure. The saline solution may be accidentally injected into a major blood vessel, causing symptoms of hypernatremia.*

During the procedure the patient is asked to inform the staff immediately if she feels extremely hot, thirsty, or dizzy or has a headache. If this happens, it occurs during the injection or right after and should be treated with dextrose in water intravenously to reverse the hypernatremia. Hypernatremia may also result from leakage of the saline into the peritoneal cavity and is treated in the same fashion. If the saline is inadvertently injected into the bladder, sloughing of the epithelium may occur. This is treated with immediate bladder irrigation with normal saline. An occasional patient may develop *water intoxication* secondary to the administration of oxytocics to induce labor. This is treated with lactated Ringer's solution intravenously or with another electrolyte preparation. The other two complications of saline abortion are *amniotic fluid embolism* and *retained placental tissues*, the latter being treated with curettage.

Other Types of Abortion. A recent technique for inducing abortion after the first trimester is the administration of a hormone-like substance called *prostaglandin*.

Hysterectomy is done occasionally for late abortions.

Nursing Care

Nursing care of the patient experiencing a *second trimester abortion* includes gathering health history data, with specific information about previous pregnancies, RH factor, Pap smear, breast examination, and gonorrhea cultures. History of liver or kidney pathology, cardiac failure, hypertension, or sickle cell anemia usually precludes the use of saline for a second trimester abortion.

Twelve hours prior to abortion, a *Laminaria tent* may be inserted into the cervix. Laminaria, a form of seaweed, swells, absorbs fluid, and helps dilate the cervix. It should not be left in longer than 12 hours, as infection may develop.

Nursing care of the patient may also involve assisting the physician with instillation of the substance inducing the abortion, monitoring the patient's labor, assisting with the expulsion of fetal and placental contents, and monitoring the patient's recovery phase. The nurse may assist the patient with breathing techniques used for contractions similar to those experienced in full term labor. For management of labor, consult an obstetrics text book.

Usually the patient delivers the fetus in bed. Of course, this event is often a traumatic moment. Nursing care includes assisting the patient in resolving ambivalent feelings about whether or not to look at the expelled fetus, whether or not to ascertain the sex of the fetus, and whether or not to be given information about fetal normality or abnormality. The nurse can expect women experiencing a second trimester abortion to have more ambivalent feelings about the procedure than with earlier abortions. Usually the patient has felt the fetus move; often the fact the patient waited beyond the time when a D & C or D & E could have been performed is an indicator of mixed feelings about pregnancy termination. In addition, the discomfort of labor and fear of the procedure may cause considerable anxiety in a woman who may view herself negatively for deciding to abort her fetus. It is vitally important that nursing staff not give verbal or nonverbal messages indicating that they may view the patient negatively. Osofsky and Osofsky state that though severe postabortion depression is rare, occurrence is more usual during the second trimester than during the first.

Instructions postprocedure are necessary for preventing complications. Before discharge, patients may be advised not to douch, use tampons, have intercourse, or take tub baths for 2 weeks after the procedure. Birth control information may be shared at this time. In addition, the patient may also be advised to take her temperature daily for 5 days. If the temperature rises above 38°C. (100.4°F.), she is usually advised to contact her health care provider.

Postabortion counseling is part of the nursing care plan and includes assessing the patient's understanding of and feelings about the procedure. Follow-up counseling may greatly diminish possible feelings of guilt and fear and lead to a more rapid recovery.

> *Part of comprehensive nursing care of patients having an abortion of any kind includes helping the patient express her feelings and concerns. Postabortion nursing care includes sharing information about possible indications of complications, resumption of sexual activity, and birth control measures. The nurse also gives the patient the name of an emergency person to contact should symptoms of infection, pain, or significant blood loss occur.*

Summary

This chapter has, in a limited way, discussed the more controversial aspects of gynecology. The scope of the presentation does not permit extensive discussion of the controversies or of the solutions that have been presented. However, there are many excellent articles and books about these subjects. A good beginning source of references is provided in this unit's bibliography.

BIBLIOGRAPHY (Chapters 83 through 88)

1. A closer look at uterine bleeding. *Emergency Medicine*, 9:58, Aug. 1977.
2. A safer abortion. *Emergency Medicine*, 10:223, Jan. 1978.

3. A way out of the estrogen-ca bind. *Emergency Medicine*, 10:193, June 1978.
4. Abortion under attack. *Newsweek*, June 5, 1978, pp. 36–47.
5. Adams, H. G., et al.: Genital herpetic infection in Menard Women: Clinical course and effect of topical application of adenine arabinoside. *Journal of Infectious Diseases*, 133, 1976.
6. After abortion: Abscess. *Emergency Medicine*, 9:210, Apr. 1977.
7. Anapol, D., and N. N. Wagner: Patient provider preferences and the pelvic examination. *Nurse Practitioner*, 3:13, July–Aug. 1978.
8. Anderson, F. D., et al.: Recurrent herpes genitalis: Treatment with Mycobacterium Bovis (BCG). *Obstetrics and Gynecology*, 43:797, June 1974.
9. Avery, W., C. Gardner, and S. Palmer: Vulvectomy. *American Journal of Nursing*, 74:453, Mar. 1974.
10. Balin, H.: Evaluation of the infertile couple. *American Family Physician*, 13:96, June 1976.
11. Barber, H.: Ovarian carcinoma: *Etiology, Diagnosis and Treatment*. New York: Masson Publishing, Inc., 1978.
12. Bartosik, D.: Oral contraceptives—an update. *American Family Physician*, 19:149, May 1979.
13. Beaton, J. H.: How to treat—and cure—vaginitis. *Consultant*, 17:159, Sept. 1977.
14. Beard, R. J. (Ed.): *The Menopause*. Baltimore: University Park Press, 1976.
15. Beecham, C. T.: Endometriosis: When is surgical treatment indicated? *Postgraduate Medicine*, 63:221, Mar. 1978.
16. Behrman, S. J., and J. R. G. Gosling: *Fundamentals of Gynecology*, 2nd ed. New York: Oxford University Press, 1966.
17. Benton, B. D. A.: Stilbestrol and vaginal cancer. *American Journal of Nursing*, 74:900, May 1974.
18. Brown, J. R., and M. E. Brown: Psychiatric disorders associated with the menopause. *In*: Beard, R. (Ed.) *The Menopause*. Baltimore: University Park Press, 1976.
19. Brown, M. S.: Syphilis and gonorrhea: An update for nurses in ambulatory settings. *Nursing 76*, 76:71, Jan. 1976.
20. Brown, W. S., and S. J. Kraus: Gonococcal colony types. *Journal of the American Medical Association*, 228:862, May, 1974.
21. Brueschke, E., J. T. Archie, and G. D. Wilbanks: Hysteroscopy. *American Family Physician*, 15:126, Apr. 1977.
22. Burgess, A., and L. Holmstrom: Rape trauma syndrome. *American Journal of Psychiatry*, 131:981, Sept. 1974.
23. Burgess, A., and L. Holmstrom: *Rape: Victims of crisis*. Bowie, Maryland: R. J. Brady Co., 1974.
24. Burgess, A. W., and A. T. Laszlo: Courtroom use of hospital records in sexual assault cases. *American Journal of Nursing*, 77:64, Jan. 1977.
25. Chen, S. S.: Current concepts in gynecologic oncology. *Geriatrics*, 32:47, Apr. 1977.
26. Chow, A. W., et al: The bacteriology of acute pelvic inflammatory disease. *American Journal of Obstetrics and Gynecology*, 122:876, Aug. 1975.
27. Christian, C. D.: Maternal deaths associated with an intrauterine device. *American Journal of Obstetrics and Gynecology*, 119:441, 1974.
28. Cibilo, L. A.: *Gynecologic Laparoscopy*. Philadelphia: Lea & Febiger, 1975.
29. Clark, T.: Primary health care: Counseling victims of rape. *American Journal of Nursing*, 76:1964, Dec. 1976.
30. Cleary, R., and L. Green: Dysfunctional uterine bleeding. *American Family Physician*, 15:130, Mar. 1977.
31. Collaborative Group for the Study of Stroke in Young Women: Oral contraceptives and increased risk of cerebral ischemia and thrombosis. *New England Journal of Medicine*, 288:871, Apr. 1973.
32. Colón, V. F., and G. B. Schumann: Gynecologic cytology. *American Family Physician*, 18:135, Nov. 1978.
33. Cook, R. J., and B. M. Dickens: A decade of international change in abortion law: 1967–1977. *American Journal of Public Health*, 68:637, July 1978.
34. Cunningham, F. G., and L. C. Gilstrap, III: 10 questions physicians most often ask . . . about drug therapy in acute pelvic inflammatory disease. *Consultant*, 18:109, Oct. 1978.
35. Curran, J. W., et al.: Female gonorrhea: Its relationship to abnormal uterine bleeding, urinary tract symptoms and cervicitis. *Obstetrics and Gynecology*, 45:195, Feb. 1975.
36. Curettage with comfort. *Emergency Medicine*, 9:107, Oct. 1977.
37. Curry, S. L., et al.: Hydatidiform mole: Diagnosis, management and long term follow-up of 347 patients. *Obstetrics and Gynecology*, 45:1, Jan. 1975.
38. Curtin, L. L., and J. A. Petrick: Reproductive manipulation: Technical advances, options, and ethical ramifications. *Nursing Forum*, XVI:7, No. 1, 1975.
39. Cusumano, C., and G. R. Monif: A word of caution concerning photodynamic inactivation therapy for herpes virus hominis infections. *Obstetrics and Gynecology*, 45:335, Mar. 1975.
40. Dawood, Y. M., et al.: Human chorionic gonadotropin and its subunits in hydatidiform mole and choriocarcinoma. *Obstetrics and Gynecology*, 50:172, Aug. 1977.
41. DeAlvarez, R. R. (Ed.): *Textbook of Gynecology*. Philadelphia: Lea & Febiger, 1977.
42. DePalma, J. R.: The ubiquitous anaerobe: Cause for concern in OBG. *RN*, 38:61, Dec. 1975.
43. de Prosse, C. A., and W. C. Keettel: Office gynecology: The missed menstrual period. *Postgraduate Medicine*, 61:251, Jan. 1977.
44. Dickey, R. P.: Menstrual problems of the adolescent. *Postgraduate Medicine*, 60:183, Oct. 1976.
45. Dillon, P., and J. Seashoetz: Oral contraceptives and myocardial infarction. *Cardiovascular Nursing*, 15 (2):5, Mar.–Apr. 1979.
46. Dilts, P. V., Jr., J. W. Greene, and J. W. Roddick, Jr.: *Core Studies in Obstetrics and Gynecology*, 2nd ed. Baltimore: Williams and Wilkins Co., 1978.
47. Dolin, R., et al.: Genital herpes simplex virus type II infection: Variability in modes of spread. *Journal of American Venereal Disease Association*, 2:13, Dec. 1975.
48. Drusin, L. M.: The diagnosis and treatment of infectious and latent syphilis. *Medical Clinics of North America*, 56:1161, Sept. 1972.
49. Easterling, W. E.: Managing the menopause. *American Family Physician*. 7:136, Mar. 1976.
50. Enos, W. F., and J. C. Beyer: Management of the rape victim. *American Family Physician*, 18:97, Sept. 1978.
51. Eschenbach, D., et al.: Pathogenesis of acute pelvic inflammatory disease: Role of contraception and other risk factors. *American Journal of Obstetrics and Gynecology*, 128:838, Aug. 1977.
52. Estok, P. J.: Abortion attitude of nurses: A cognitive dissonance perspective. *Image*, 10:70, Oct. 1978.
53. Fallopian tubes run both ways. *Emergency Medicine*, 9:117, Dec. 1977.
54. Feeley, E., and H. Pyne: The menopause: Facts and misconceptions. *Nursing Forum*, XIV:74, *No. 1*, 1975.
55. Feeling the loss of a uterus. *Emergency Medicine*, 11:225, June 1979.
56. Fleshman, R. P. (Ed.): Symposium: The young adult

in today's world. *Nursing Clinics of North America*, 8:1, Mar. 1973.

57. Flint, M.: The menopause: Reward or punishment? *Psychosomatics*, XVI:161, Oct.–Nov.–Dec., 1975.
58. Freeman, W. S.: Not all PID is GC. *Emergency Medicine*, 10:47, Sept. 1978.
59. Friedrich, E. G., Jr.: Office gynecology: Vulvar pruritus—A symptom, not a disease. *Postgraduate Medicine*, 61:164, June 1977.
60. Friedrich, E. G., Jr.: Relief for herpes vulvitis. *Obstetrics and Gynecology*, 41:74, Jan. 1973.
61. Galloway, K.: The change of life. *American Journal of Nursing*, 75:1006, June 1975.
62. Gedan, S.: Abortion counseling with adolescents. *American Journal of Nursing*, 74:1856, Oct. 1974.
63. Gellman, D. D.: Cervical cancer screening programs. *Canadian Medical Association Journal*, 114:1003, June 1976.
64. Getting the bugs out of vaginitis. *Emergency Medicine*, 19:119, Nov. 1978.
65. Gilbert, S.: Artificial insemination. *American Journal of Nursing*, 76:259, Feb. 1976.
66. Gordon, G., and B. Greenberg: Exogenous estrogens and endometrial cancer. *Postgraduate Medicine*, 59:66, June 1976.
67. Graber, E. A., and H. R. K. Barber: The case for and against estrogen therapy. *American Journal of Nursing*, 75:1766, Oct. 1975.
68. Greenblatt, R. B.: Estrogens and endometrial cancer. *In* Beard, R. J. (Ed.): *The Menopause*. Baltimore: University Park Press, 1976, pp. 247–265.
69. Greenblatt, R. B.: Estrogens and endometrial cancer: Gross exaggeration or fact. *Geriatrics*, 32:60, Nov. 1977.
70. Greiss, F. C., Jr.: Ovarian tumors. *American Family Physician*, 16:170, Oct. 1977.
71. Guzick, D. S.: Efficacy of screening for cervical cancer: A review. *American Journal of Public Health*, 68:125, Feb. 1978.
72. Hamilton, A., and P. Kelley: An education program for hysterectomy patients. *Supervisor Nurse*, 10:19, Apr. 1979.
73. Hamilton, M. S., and N. B. Schlapper: Pelvic exenteration. *American Journal of Nursing*, 76:266, Feb. 1976.
74. Hammond, C. B., et al.: Treatment of metastatic trophoblastic disease: Good and poor prognosis. *American Journal of Obstetrics and Gynecology*, 115:451, Feb. 1973.
75. Hammond, D. O.: How to manage dysfunctional uterine bleeding in the woman over 40. *Consultant*, 18:91, Oct. 1978.
76. Hatcher, R. A., G. Steward, F. Stewart, F. Guest, P. Stratton, and A. Wright: *Contraceptive Technology 1978–1979*. New York: Irvington Publications, Inc., 1978.
77. Haufrect, E. J., and A. L. Kaplan: Answers to questions on pelvic inflammatory disease. *Hospital Medicine*, 12:6, Dec. 1976.
78. Haynes, D. M.: *Essentials of the gynecologic history and examination*. Philadelphia: Smith, Kline and French Laboratories, 1965.
79. Hertz, R.: *Choriocarcinoma and Related Gestational Trophoblastic Tumors in Women*. New York: Raven Press, 1978.
80. Hildebrand, B. (Ed.): *The Nursing Clinics of North America, 13:1*, June 1978, Symposium on the nursing management of the cancer patient receiving chemotherapy.
81. Hill, E. C.: Carcinoma of the cervix: Diagnostic guide. *Hospital Medicine*, 12:31, May 1976.
82. Holmes, K. K., and D. Martin: Sexually transmitted diseases: Advances in management. *Postgraduate Medicine*, 64:121, Sept. 1978.
83. Homesley, H. D.: Evaluation of the Abnormal Pap Smear. *American Family Physician*, 16:190, Sept. 1977.
84. Holmstrom, L. L., and W. Burgess: Assessing trauma in the rape victim. *American Journal of Nursing*, 75:1288, Aug. 1975.
85. Hoover, R., L. Gray, P. Cole, and B. MacMahon.: Menopausal estrogens and breast cancer. *New England Journal of Medicine*, 295:401, Aug. 1976.
86. Horosak, I.: Learn to fight rape—without hang-ups. *RN*, 39:52, July 1976.
87. Huffman, J. W.: Office gynecology: Examining the child. *Postgraduate Medicine*, 60:159, Aug. 1976.
88. Huffman, J. W.: Office gynecology: Some facts about the clitoris. *Postgraduate Medicine*, 60:245, Nov. 1976.
89. Hunt, G. R.: Rape: An organized approach to evaluation and treatment. *American Family Physician*, 15:154, Jan. 1977.
90. Huxley, L.: Today's pill and the individual woman. *American Journal of Maternal Child Nursing*, Nov.–Dec. 1977, pp. 359–363.
91. Ibrahim, M. A.: The case for cervical cancer screening. *American Journal Public Health*, 68:114, Feb. 1978.
92. Inman, W. H. W., M. P. Vessey, B. Westerholm, and A. Engelund: Thromboembolic disease and the steroidal content of oral contraceptives: A report to the Committee on Safety of Drugs. *British Medical Journal*, 2:203, Apr. 1970.
93. Jacobs, H. S.: Prolactin and amenorrhea. *New England Journal of Medicine*, 295:954, Oct. 1976.
94. Jick, H., and R. N. Watkins, et al.: Replacement estrogens and endometrial cancer. *New England Journal of Medicine*, 300:218, Feb. 1979.
95. Josey, W. E.: Vaginitis: Reducing the number of refractory cases. *Postgraduate Medicine*, 62:171, Sept. 1977.
96. Josey, W. E.: The sexually transmitted infections. *Obstetrics and Gynecology*, 43:465, March 1974.
97. Kalbarcyk, J. A.: Cancer of the vulva. *Nursing '75*, 5:28, Aug. 1975.
98. Karney, W. W., et al.: Spectinomycin versus tetracycline for the treatment of gonorrhea. *The New England Journal of Medicine*, 296:889, Apr. 1977.
99. Kaufman, R. H., et al.: Clinical features of herpes genitalis. *Cancer Research*, 33:1446, June 1973.
100. Kaufman, R., and H. Gardner: Relation of herpesvirus type 2 and carcinoma of the cervix. *Clinical Obstetrics and Gynecology*, 15:919, Dec. 1972.
101. Kennedy, D. (Ed.): Update on estrogens and uterine cancer. *F.D.A. Drug Bulletin*, February-March, 1979, 9:2–3, Department of Health, Education and Welfare, Rockville, Maryland.
102. Klingbeil, K. S., S. C. Anderson, and L. Vontver: Multidisciplinary care for sexual assault victims. *Nurse Practitioner*, 1:21, July–Aug. 1976.
103. Knapp, R. C., and R. S. Berkowitz: Gynecologic cancer: Guide to diagnostic approach. *Hospital Medicine*, 14:88, Mar. 1978.
104. Ledger, W. J., and M. A. Child: The hospital care of patients undergoing hysterectomy. *American Journal of Obstetrics and Gynecology*, 117:423, Oct. 1973.
105. Ledger, W. J., et al.: Guidelines for antibiotic prophylaxis in gynecology. *American Journal of Obstetrics and Gynecology*, 121:1038, Apr. 1975.
106. Ledger, W. J.: *Infection in the Female*. Philadelphia: Lea & Febiger, 1977.
107. Lee, L., and J. D. Schmale: Ampicillin therapy for Corynebacterium vaginale (Hemophilus vaginalis) vag-

initis. *American Journal of Obstetrics and Gynecology*, 115:786, Mar. 1973.
108. Louka, M. H., and G. C. Lewis, Jr.: Obstetric and gynecologic bleeding. *Hospital Medicine*, 12:44, Aug. 1976.
109. Manisoff, M.: Family planning democratized. *American Journal of Nursing*, 75:1660, Oct. 1975.
110. Manisoff, M. T.: Intrauterine devices. *American Journal of Nursing*, 73:1188, July 1973.
111. Martin, L. L.: *Health Care of Women*. Philadelphia: J. B. Lippincott Co., Mar. 1978.
112. Massey, L. K., and M. A. Davison: Effects of oral contraceptives on nutritional status. *American Family Physician*, 19:119, Jan. 1979.
113. Masters, W. H., and V. E. Johnson: *Human Sexual Response*. Boston: Little, Brown and Company, 1966.
114. May, W. J.: Current status of estrogen replacement therapy. *American Family Physician*, 16:108, Dec. 1977.
115. McDonough, P. G.: Ten steps in the management of primary adolescent amenorrhea. *Consultant*, 16:124, Aug. 1976.
116. McGowan, L.: *Gynecologic Oncology*. New York: Appleton-Century-Crofts, 1978.
117. McGuire, L. S., and A. K. Sorley: Understanding and preventing the menopausal crisis. *Nurse Practitioner*, 3:15, July–Aug. 1978.
118. Merkatz, R., D. Smith, and P. Seitz: Preoperative teaching for gynecologic patients. *American Journal of Nursing*, 74:1072, June 1972.
119. Metzger, D.: It is always the woman who is raped. *American Journal Psychiatry*, 133:405, Apr. 1976.
120. Milligan, C., D. Cummings, and V. Williamson: Screening for cervical cancer. *American Journal of Nursing*, 75:1343, Aug. 1975.
121. Mims, F. (Ed.): Symposium on human sexuality. *Nursing Clinics of North America*, 10:517–587, Sept. 1975.
122. Moran, S.: Vaginal Hysterectomy. *RN* 42:53, Apr. 1979.
123. Morrow, C. P., et al.: Clinical and laboratory correlates of molar pregnancy and trophoblastic disease. *American Journal of Obstetrics and Gynecology*, 128:424, June 1977.
124. Nahmias, A. J., and B. Roizman: Infection with herpes simplex viruses 1 and 2. *New England Journal of Medicine*, 289:667, 1973.
125. Neeson, J.: Special feature: Herpesvirus genitalis: A nursing perspective. *Nursing Clinics of North America*, 10:598, Sept. 1975.
126. New guidelines against gonorrhea. *Emergency Medicine*, 11:55, Apr. 1979.
127. News AFP: Management of vaginitis. *American Family Physician*, 20:143, July 1979.
128. *Newsweek*: About that baby. August, 1978, pp. 67–70.
129. Newton, M.: 9 questions physicians most often ask . . . about uterine bleeding. *Consultant*, 18:87, May 1978.
130. Niswander, K.: *Obstetrics*. Boston: Little, Brown and Company, 1976.
131. Notelovitz, M.: Gynecologic problems of menopausal women: Part 1. Changes in genital tissue. *Geriatrics*, 33:24, Aug. 1978.
132. Notelovitz, M.: Gynecologic problems of menopausal women: Part 2. Treating estrogen deficiency. *Geriatrics*, 33:35, Sept. 1978.
133. Notelovitz, M.: Gynecologic problems of menopausal women: Part 3. Changes in extragenital tissues and sexuality. *Geriatrics*, 33:51, Oct. 1978.
134. Novak, E., G. S. Jones, and H. W. Jones: *Gynecology*. Baltimore: Williams and Wilkins Co., 1975.
135. *Our Bodies, Ourselves*, 2nd ed. Boston Women's Health Collective. Simon & Schuster, New York, 1976.
136. Parsons, L., and S. C. Sommers: *Gynecology*, 2nd ed. Philadelphia: W. B. Saunders Co., 1978.
137. Pastorfide, G. B., et al.: Serum chorionic gonadotropin activity after molar pregnancy, therapeutic abortion, and term delivery. *American Journal of Obstetrics and Gynecology*, 118:293, Jan. 1974.
138. PID and the IUD. *Emergency Medicine*, 10:170, 1978.
139. Programmed instruction: Patient assessment: Examination of the female pelvis. Part I. *American Journal of Nursing*, 78:PI1, Oct. 1978.
140. Programmed instruction. Patient assessment: Examination of the female pelvis. Part II. *American Journal of Nursing*, 78:PI1, Nov. 1978.
141. Public welfare. The joys of hysterectomy. *Human Behavior*. 6:38, May 1977.
142. Quirk, B. and L. K. Huxall: VD, the equal opportunity disease. *Nursing Digest*, 6:69, Winter 1976.
143. Rogers, R. E.: Vaginal discharge: Guide to diagnosis and management. *Hospital Medicine*, 13:68, Nov. 1977.
144. Rudel, H. W.: Safety and effectiveness of a new low-dose oral contraceptive: A three-year study of 1,000 women. *The Journal of Reproductive Medicine*, 21:79, Aug. 1978.
145. Russo, N. G.: Protocol: Women's health assessment. *Nurse Practitioner*, 3:23, July–Aug. 1978.
146. Rx After Rape. *Emergency Medicine*, 9:218, Mar. 1977.
147. Sabin, H. B.: Misery of recurrent herpes: What to do? *New England Journal of Medicine*, 293:986, Nov. 1975.
148. Schaefer, J. L., R. A. Sullivan, and F. L. Goldstein: Counseling sexual abuse victims. *American Family Physician*, 18:85, Nov. 1978.
149. Schrader, E. S.: Counseling helps gyn patients handle surgery. *AORN*, 30:233, Aug. 1979.
150. Schwartz, A. D., U. Zor, H. Lindner, and S. Neor: Primary dysmenorrhea alleviation by an inhibitor of prostaglandin synthesis and action. *Obstetrics and Gynecology*, 4:709, Nov. 1974.
151. Seaman, B., and G. Seaman: *Women and the Crisis in Sex Hormones*. New York: Bantam Books, 1977.
152. Seiler, J. C.: Estrogens for the menopause. *Postgraduate Medicine*, 62:73, Sept. 1977.
153. Simone, C. M.: The transsexual patient. *RN*, 40:37, Mar. 1977.
154. Smith, D. R., P. D. Thompson, and W. Herrman: Association of exogenous estrogen and endometrial carcinoma. *New England Journal of Medicine*, 293:1164, Dec. 1975.
155. Sredl, D. R., and M. Rojkind: Offering the rape victim real help. *Nursing 79*, 9:29, July 1979.
156. Stanhope, C. R., and F. J. Hofmeister: Axioms on the detection, diagnosis and treatment of uterine cancer. *Hospital Medicine*, 14:91, Jan. 1978.
157. Stillman, M. J.: Nursing decisions: Helping your patient through elective hysterectomy. *RN*, 42:75, Feb. 1979.
158. Sullivan, R. A., J. L. Schaefer, and F. L. Goldstein: Child molestation. *American Family Physician*, 19:127, Mar. 1979.
159. Symonds, M.: The rape victim: Psychological patterns of response. *The American Journal of Psychoanalysis*, 36:27, Spring 1976.
160. The absence of ovulation. *Emergency Medicine*, 11:239, Feb. 1979.
161. The case for a second smear. *Emergency Medicine*, 10:42, Nov. 1978.
162. The compleat pelvic. *Emergency Medicine*, 11:233, Feb. 15, 1979.
163. The feminine condition. *Emergency Medicine*, 11:215, Feb. 1979.

164. Timby, B. K.: Ovulation method of birth control. *American Journal of Nursing*, 76:928, June 1978.
165. Tovell, H., and L. Dank: *Gynecologic Operations*. Hagerstown, Md.: Harper & Row. 1978.
166. Tyson, M. C.: Let's talk about menopause. *Nursing '78*, 8:34, Aug. 1978.
167. USPHS Center for Disease Control, Atlanta: Gonorrhea: Recommended treatment schedules, 1978. *American Family Physician*, 19:169, Mar. 1979.
168. Vessey, M. P. and R. Doll: Investigation of relation between use of oral contraceptives and thromboembolic disease: A further report. *British Medical Journal*, 2:651, June, 1969.
169. Vessey, M. P.: Oral contraceptives and stroke. *New England Journal of Medicine*, 288:906, Apr. 1973.
170. Walz, M. A., et al.: Effect of immunization on acute and latent infections of vaginouterine tissue with herpes simplex virus, types 1 and 2. *Journal of Infectious Disease*, 135:744, May 1977.
171. Weideger, P.: *Menstruation and Menopause*. New York: A Delta Book—Dell Publishing Company, 1975.
172. Welch, M. S.: Rape and the trauma of inadequate care. *Nursing Digest*, 5:50, Spring 1977.
173. Whisnant, L., and L. Zegans: White middle-class adolescent girls' attitudes toward menarche. *Nursing Digest*, 4:52, Winter 1976.
174. Williams, M. A.: Easier convalescence from hysterectomy. *American Journal of Nursing*, 76:438, Mar. 1976.
175. Wind, J.: Abortion, ethics, and biology. *Perspectives in Biology and Medicine*, 21:492, Summer 1978.
176. Wiser, W. L., et al.: Management of bladder drainage following vaginal plastic repairs. *Obstetrics and Gynecology*, 44:65, July 1974.
177. Wood, J. E.: The cardiovascular effects of oral contraceptives. *Modern Concepts of Cardiovascular Disease*, 16:37, Aug. 1972.
178. Woods, N. F.: *Human Sexuality in Health and Illness*. St. Louis: C. V. Mosby Company, 1975, pp. 95–107.
179. Worley, R. J.: How to manage consistent failure to ovulate. *Consultant*, 17:100, Oct. 1977.
180. Yankauer, A.: Abortions and public policy. *American Journal of Public Health*, 67:604, July 1977.
181. Yen, S. S. C.: Estrogen and the menopause. *American Family Physician*, 16:87, July 1977.
182. Zier, H., and W. Finkle: Increased risk of endometrial carcinoma among users of conjugated estrogens. *New England Journal of Medicine*, 293:1167, Dec. 1975.

UNIT XXIII

NURSING PEOPLE EXPERIENCING DISTURBANCES OF THE EYE AND EAR

INTRODUCTION AND STUDY GUIDE

EYE

Sight is one of the human senses most people rely on for accurate information about the environment. We live in a visual world. It is estimated that 90 per cent of our information reaches our brain by way of the eyes. Ocular disorders are common and can pose serious problems for people experiencing them. It is thus not surprising that patients with ocular disorders are frequently anxious.

Nurses have an important role in detecting ocular disorders and referring patients for medical assessment. Practices vary concerning treatment of disorders of the eye; we shall discuss some of those more commonly accepted. We have concentrated on those disorders that are particularly important (recognizing, of course, that any disorder is important for the person experiencing it).

Ophthalmology refers to the sum of knowledge concerning the eye and ocular diseases. Much confusion exists concerning terminology related to occupations in the field of eye care. Some important terms are clarified below:

- ► *Ophthalmologist* or *oculist* refers to an M.D. who has taken special training in care of the eye and management of ocular disorders, and who is qualified to give complete eye care, i.e., refraction and medical and surgical therapy.
- ► *Optometrist (or O.D.)* does *not* have a medical degree, but is qualified to measure the refractive error of the eyes *without* the use of eyedrops. The optometrist cannot diagnose or treat ocular or systemic disease.
- ► *Orthoptist* is a medical technician who assists an ophthalmologist in examining and caring for patients with disorders of ocular movement. An orthoptist may direct ocular exercises.
- ► *Optician* is a technician who grinds and fits lenses according to prescription.
- ► *Ocularist* is a technician who makes ophthalmoscopic prostheses, e.g., artificial eyes.

Study Guide

1. Review anatomy, physiology, pharmacology, and nursing fundamental procedures in greater detail as necessary, in addition to content included in Chapter 89.*
2. What are some common ocular symptoms and their significance?

---

*For nursing fundamentals, see particularly Sorensen and Luckmann, *Basic Nursing: A Psychophysiologic Approach.*

3. What are some basic preventive measures for protection of the eyes?
4. What are some common groups of ocular medications, and what are the major functions of each group? Be certain you know the differences between mydriatics and miotics; name some examples of each, some conditions they are used for, and some contraindications to their use.
5. Why should atropine never be put in an eye unless ordered by a physician? How should eyedrops and eye ointments be administered?
6. Define the following: diplopia, amblyopia, cycloplegic, scotoma, photophobia, hyphema, iridocyclisis, enucleation, proptosis, exenteration, nystagmus, emmetropia, presbyopia, exophthalmos, ptosis, hordeolum, chalazion, ectropion, dacryocystitis, iritis, panophthalmitis.
7. What is accommodation? What is binocular vision? Diagram and explain the rays of light converging in the normal eye, the myopic eye, and the hypermetropic eye. Illustrate and explain how lenses correct myopia and hyperopia.
8. Common specific disorders that should receive special emphasis as you study include strabismus, conjunctivitis, ophthalmia neonatorum, trachoma, keratitis, corneal ulcer, corneal opacity, retrolental fibroplasia, retinal detachment, glaucoma, cataract, errors of refraction, trauma, and enucleation. What are major symptoms of a cataract? of glaucoma? of detached retina? Where are cataracts formed? Why do patients need a corrective lens following cataract surgery?
9. Identify major nursing functions related to intraocular surgery.
10. Familiarize yourself with services for the blind in your community.

EAR

The ear is a complex, extraordinarily delicate sense organ which consists of two functional units: the *acoustic* apparatus, concerned with the exteroceptive sense called "hearing"; and the *vestibular* apparatus, concerned with the special proprioceptive sense involved with posture and equilibrium. The acoustic apparatus is innervated by the cochlear nerve; the vestibular apparatus is innervated by the vestibular nerve. Collectively these two nerves form the eighth cranial nerve (also called the vestibulocochlear, acoustic, auditory, or statoacoustic nerve). The ear translates sound of between some 16 to 20,000 cycles per second into nerve impulses. Although the ear can perceive sound waves of up to 16,000 cycles, 250 to 6000 cycles covers most of the speech range. Much is known about how the ear works, but the phenomenon of hearing (which involves auditory centers in the brain) has long been one of the mysteries of physiology.

A nurse's role in the prevention, detection, and treatment of hearing and vestibular disorders is highly diversified. Such disorders are common and may occur at any age. By teaching others how to properly care for their ears, the nurse works to prevent aural damage. Also, nurses are often in a position to encourage persons with aural disorders to seek appropriate medical assessment and help. Infections of the ear and related structures can have serious complications, and should thus receive early treatment before irreparable damage occurs. In many settings nurses participate in the case-finding of persons with hearing disorders and in the rehabilitation of these individuals. In the physician's office, clinic, and hospital nurses contribute to the medical and surgical treatment of aural disorders.

Chapter 90 focuses on some of the more common diagnostic procedures used to investigate disorders of the ear, the more common types of aural disorders, and the usual treatment of these problems. General ear care, protection of the ear, and common nursing procedures related to ear care are also discussed. Ear surgery and rehabilitation of the deaf individual are considered only briefly.

Otology refers to the sum of knowledge concerning the ear and ear diseases. An *otologist* is a physician who has specialized in studying and treating aural disorders. An *otolaryngologist* treats ear problems, but is also a specialist in problems of the throat and nose. *Audiology* refers specifically to the study of hearing. An *audiologist* is a person who specializes in the evaluation of individuals who have hearing problems and in the rehabilitation of these individuals. Generally the audiologist has an M.A. or Ph.D. degree and not an M.D. degree.

Study Guide

1. *Review* anatomy, physiology, pharmacology, and nursing fundamentals* procedures in greater detail as necessary, in addition to content included in Chapter 90. You may find it helpful to draw an anatomic picture of the ear (cross section, horizontally). Label the significant parts in addition to stating the major function of each part.
2. *Define* the following terms in your own words: otoscope, tuning fork, audiogram, furuncle, otitis media, mastoiditis, myringotomy, myringoplasty, tympanoplasty, otosclerosis, stapedectomy, fenestration, cold caloric test, presbycusis, conductive hearing loss, sensori-neural hearing loss, cerumen, vertigo, tinnitus, and nystagmus.
3. *Review* Meniere's syndrome and acute labyrinthitis. These disorders were discussed in Unit X.
4. *Familiarize* yourself with services for the deaf in your community. Familiarize yourself with various hearing aids by examining different types, if possible.

OBJECTIVES

After studying the material presented in this unit and applying it in clinical experience you can expect to be able to:

1. Describe the structure and function of the human ear and eye.
2. Appreciate the significance of the senses of sight, hearing, and balance for those who have them and for those who have such senses impaired in some way,
3. Understand and perform (or assist in performing) diagnostic assessment techniques relating to the eye and ear.
4. Discuss accurately the pathophysiology involved in common disorders of the eye and ear.
5. Prepare and implement a learning program emphasizing sound care of the eyes and ears and prevention of disorders of the eyes and ears.
6. Offer appropriate and sensitive physical, social, and emotional support to those undergoing surgery or other treatment of the eyes and ears.
7. Carry out nursing and delegated medical care skillfully for people experiencing disorders of the eyes and ears.
8. Offer sound and appropriate preventive and rehabilitative teaching for patients and significant others.

---

*For nursing fundamentals, see particularly Sorensen and Luckmann, *Basic Nursing: A Psychophysiologic Approach.*

CHAPTER 89*

DISORDERS OF THE EYE AND RELATED STRUCTURES

BASIC ANATOMY AND PHYSIOLOGY

The eye and its adnexa represent a complex anatomic structure. Included within the small space of these structures are examples of almost all the tissues found in the rest of the body. Additionally the eye contains avascular structures not duplicated elsewhere in the body, e.g., cornea, lens, and vitreous. Physiologically the eye is also complex.

Specific details of the anatomy and physiology of the eye and related structures are discussed as appropriate throughout this chapter. The following outline summarizes basic facts which will help orient you to the anatomy and physiology of the eye and related structures as a whole. Study this outline and the associated illustrations carefully.

I. *Description of the eyes* (see Fig. 89–1): The eyes are a pair of spherical organs located in bony cavities *(orbits)* in the front of the head. The eyes are the body's organs of vision. The orbits protectively surround each eye completely except for a relatively small area which is anteriorly exposed. The eyes are each about 1 inch in diameter, have a clear circular window *(cornea)* in front to allow entrance of light, and have *muscles* originating at the back of the orbit which are inserted around the outer circumference, thereby supporting the eye and enabling it to be rotated in various directions to view the environment. From the back of each eyeball, an *optic nerve* passes through the posterior portion of the orbit, carrying impulse messages to the brain from the eye's light-sensitive tissues in the *retina.*

II. *Protection of the eye:* The eye is protected by:
   A. The *bony skull orbit,* which dorsally surrounds the eyeball, and *pads of fat* lying under each eyeball over the base of the orbit.
   B. The *eyelids (palpebrae)* and *eyelashes* which close over the eye.
   C. The *lacrimal apparatus,* i.e., lacrimal gland and its ducts and passages, which produces tears to wash over the eye's surface, thus lubricating the eye and washing off foreign particles.
   D. A delicate mucous membrane *(conjunctiva)* which lines the eyelids and is also reflected over the eyeball's exposed surface.

III. *External structures of the eye:* orbital cavity; extrinsic ocular muscles; eyelids and eyelashes; conjunctiva; lacrimal apparatus.

IV. *Internal structures of the eye:*
   A. *Three separate coats or "tunics" of the eyeball:*
      1. *Outer fibrous protective layer* composed posteriorly of the *sclera* and anteriorly of the *cornea.* The sclera is white and opaque, i.e., "the white of the eye," and is composed of firm, tough connective tissue. The cornea, or "window of the eye," is a forward continuation of this outer fibrous protective layer and is transparent and colorless.
      2. *Middle vascular layer* consists of the *choroid* posteriorly, the *ciliary body* and *iris* anteriorly. The choroid is highly vascular and darkly pigmented, thus preventing internal reflection of light. The muscles of the ciliary body serve to change the shape of the lens, allowing changes in the focal distance of the eye. The iris is a diaphragm with a circular opening in the center, i.e., *pupil,* which regulates the amount of light admitted to the eye's interior. With strong light and near vision, the pupil contracts; with dim light and far vision, the pupil enlarges. The choroid, ciliary body, and iris are also collectively called the *uveal tract.*
      3. *Inner neural layer* called the *"retina"* includes some ten different layers of nerve cells, including those photosensitive receptive end-organs called rods and cones. The retina translates light waves into neural impulses.
         a. *Rods:* receptors concerned with twilight vision. Rods are sensitive to dim light.
         b. *Cones:* receptors concerned with daylight and color vision.
   B. *Refracting media:*
      1. *Cornea* (previously mentioned).
      2. *Aqueous humor,* a watery fluid filling the eyeball's *anterior chamber,* i.e., cavity in

*Heather Boyd-Monk, R.N., B.S.N., and Walter C. Petersen, M.D., critically reviewed and assisted with the revision of this chapter.

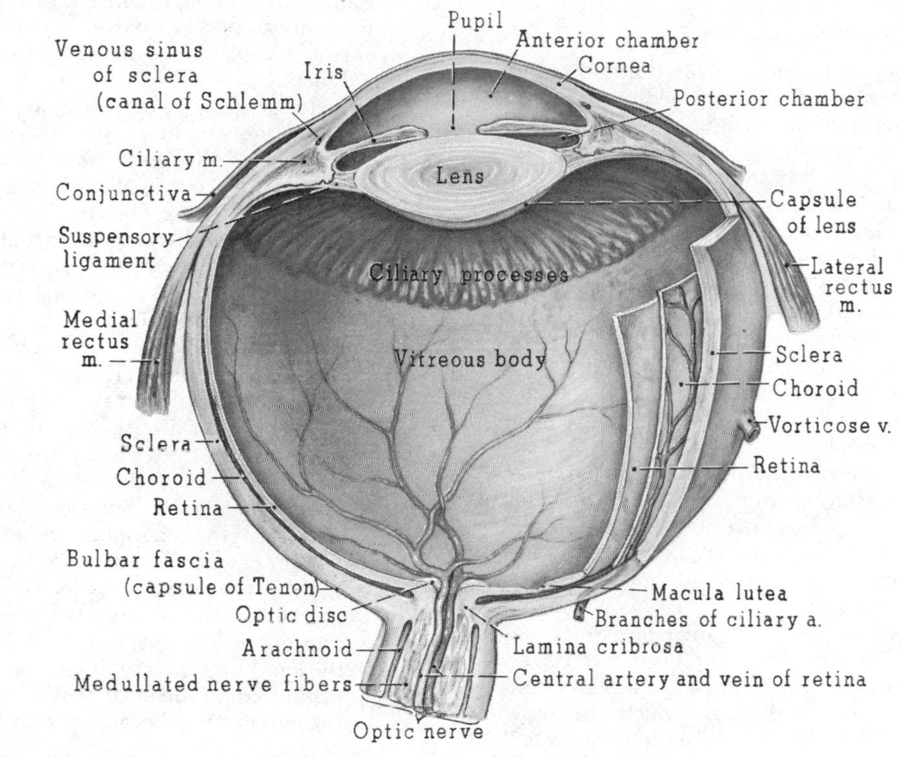

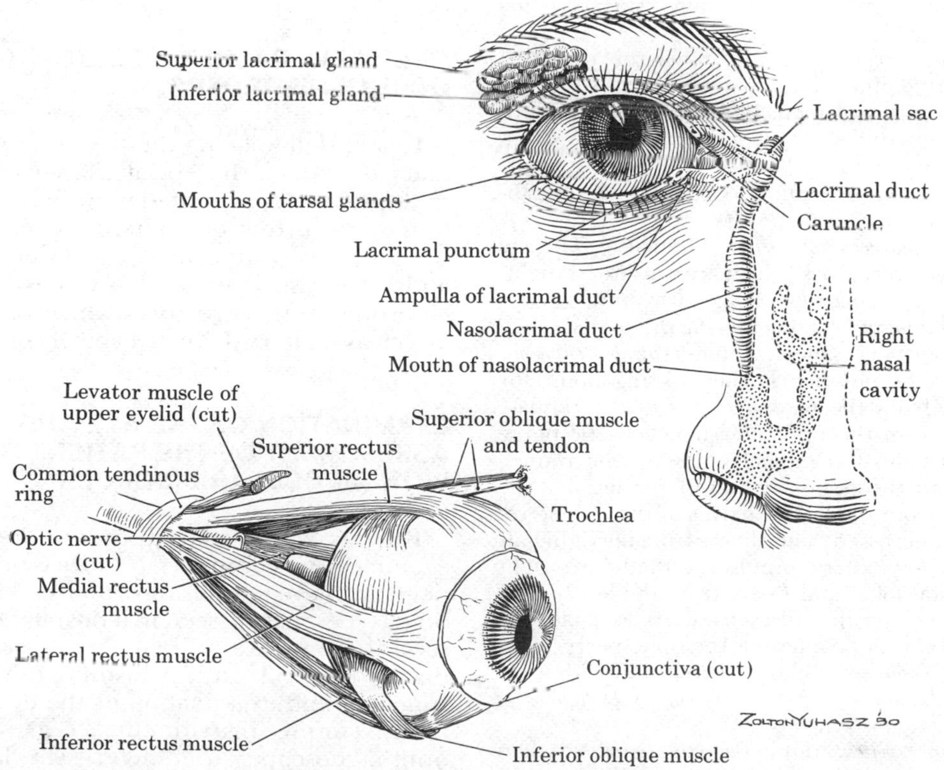

Figure 89–1. **A.** Mid-sagittal section through the eyeball, showing layers of retina and blood supply. **B.** The eye and related structures. (*A* from Jacob, S. W., C. A. Francone, and W. J. Lossow: *Structure and Function in Man*, 4th ed. *B* from *Dorland's Illustrated Medical Dictionary*, 25th ed.)

front of the lens. This fluid not only serves as a refracting medium but also helps maintain a slight forward curve in the cornea.

3. *Lens,* i.e., *"crystalline lens,"* a biconvex crystalline body enclosed in a transparent elastic capsule suspended by suspensory ligaments. The shape of the lens changes to focus the image.
4. *Vitreous humor,* a jellylike material filling the posterior cavity of the eye behind the lens. The vitreous humor not only serves as a refracting medium but also maintains the eyeball's spherical shape.

V. *Muscles of the eye:*
   A. *Intrinsic muscles:* the iris; the ciliary body.
   B. *Extrinsic muscles:* four straight (rectus) muscles, i.e., superior, inferior, lateral, and medial; two oblique muscles, i.e., superior and inferior.

VI. *Nerve supply to eye:*
   A. *Optic nerve* (second cranial nerve) carries visual impulses, received by the rods and cones, to the brain. The sclera has an opening posteriorly through which the optic nerve enters the eyeball. Within the eyeball the nerve spreads out over the posterior two thirds of the globe's inner surface, thus forming the retina.
   B. *Ophthalmic nerve* (a branch of the fifth "trigeminal" cranial nerve) carries sensory impulses of pain, touch, and temperature from the eye and its surrounding structures.
   C. *Motor nerve:* oculomotor, trochlear, and abducens.

VII. *Sensory pathway for vision* (summary): The *rod* and *cone* receptors, which are sensitive to light, initiate *nerve impulse messages* which travel over the *optic nerves.* Upon entering the cranial cavity the optic nerves meet, forming the *optic chiasma.* The optic chiasma is the crossing point for fibers from the medial halves of the retinae. That is, in the optic chiasma the optic nerve fibers from the medial halves of the retinae cross to the opposite side of the brain while those from the lateral halves of the retinae remain uncrossed. Thus fibers from the right half of each eye carry impulses to the brain's right occipital lobe, and fibers from the left half of each eye carry impulses to the left occipital lobe. From the optic chiasma the optic nerves continue, as *optic tracts,* to the cerebrum. Within the brain, visual *impulses are interpreted as sight.*

VIII. *Reflexes of the eye:*
   A. *Light reflex:* pupil becomes smaller when light is flashed in the eye (see Unit X).
   B. *Accommodation reflex:* pupil becomes smaller when gaze is shifted from distant to near objects.

IX. *Physiology of binocular vision* (summary): Binocular vision is the normal simultaneous use of both eyes, which results in depth perception and enables a larger visual field. In order for binocular vision to occur, images must be brought to focus on identical points on the two retinae. The coordinated processes necessary to achieve this goal include:
   A. *Convergence of visual axes,* i.e., the coordinated movement of the two eyes toward fixation of the same near point, e.g., together the two eyeballs turn slightly inward to focus on close objects. The eyeballs are parallel when looking at distant objects.
   B. *Regulation of pupil size,* i.e., regulating the amount of light entering the eyes by changes in pupil sizes.
   C. *Refraction of light rays* through the cornea, the aqueous humor, the lens, and the vitreous humor until the rays are focused on the retinae. The rays are bent or refracted as they pass through media of varying densities.
   D. *Accommodation,* i.e., the process by which the lens strength is changed for viewing objects near or distant. This is achieved by contractions of the ciliary muscle. For near vision the ciliary muscle contracts, lessening the tension on the suspensory ligaments, and the lens bulges, becoming more convex. For distant vision the ciliary muscle relaxes and the lens flattens, because the suspensory ligaments are taut.

OVERVIEW: BASIC TYPES OF OCULAR DISORDERS

In addition to being the site of numerous primary disorders, the eye also *secondarily* reflects multiple disorders located elsewhere in the body (discussed further on). There are many possible ways of classifying primary disorders of the eye and related structures. One way is to list them according to the structures which they basically affect, as we have done in Table 89–1.

EXAMINATION OF THE EYE AND ASSESSMENT OF THE PATIENT WITH AN OCULAR DISORDER*

Patients with ocular disorders are generally examined in the physician's office or clinic. Patients with eye injuries or ocular emergencies of other types may be seen in a hospital emergency service. Most cases of acute eye disease can be diagnosed by a careful history, tests of visual function, and examination of the eye with relatively simple instruments, e.g., flashlight, ophthalmoscope, tonometer, slit lamp. The physician examines the eye both externally and

*See also Chapter 15, pp. 322–327.

internally, in addition to testing the eye's ability to perform. Assessment of vision is made not only by the objective findings of the examination but also by the subjective comments a patient makes about his or her vision.

History

When taking an ophthalmic history, the examiner pays particular attention to the nature of the visual symptoms, the occurrence of previous trouble, and the possibility of an injury. The patient is questioned to obtain a possible history of the reason for a difference in visual acuity in what should be a normal eye. *Pain and loss of vision are always important ocular symptoms.*

In taking an ocular history it is also of importance to determine the presence of any systemic diseases and to take a family history. Some systemic disorders which may cause ocular disease are diabetes, thyroid disease, and connective tissue disease. A strong hereditary tendency characterizes certain tumors, various degenerative disorders, strabismus, and myopia.

External Examination

Eyelids, Eyelashes, Lacrimal Apparatus, Conjunctiva. As part of the external examination of the eye, the physician examines the *eyelids* to determine if (a) the lids close effectively to protect the eyes; (b) the lids indicate systemic disease (e.g., lid edema may be caused by heart failure, nephrosis, allergy, or thyroid deficiency); (c) the lids are affected by a local disorder (e.g., tumor); or (d) the lids are malpositioned (e.g., roll out or roll in). The lids are gently palpated to determine the presence of enlargements due to glandular infections and are inspected for crusting or scales.

The *eyelashes* are observed to see if they are properly placed or if the eyelashes abnormally turn in toward the eye, thereby irritating the cornea.

A portion of the *lacrimal gland* may be observed beneath the retracted upper lid when the patient looks down. The region of the "tear sac" is examined for swelling. By pressing on the lacrimal sac (inside of the lower inner orbital rim), the physician can check for obstruction of the nasolacrimal duct and can express any infected material which may be present.

The *conjunctiva* consists of the palpebral conjunctiva (which lines the posterior lid surface) and the bulbar conjunctiva (which covers the eyeball up to the limbus, i.e., the junction of the cornea and sclera). The palpebral conjunctiva is examined by everting the eyelid; the bulbar conjunctiva is examined by widely separating the lids and having the patient look up, down, and to-

TABLE 89–1. EXAMPLES OF DISORDERS OF EYE AND RELATED STRUCTURES

Areas Involved	Examples of Disorders
Eyelids	Blepharitis (inflammation of lid margin); chalazion (cystic dilation of meibomian gland); edema; hordeolum (sty); positional defects of lids (e.g., entropion, ectropion, ptosis); trichiasis (eyelashes turning in against cornea); tumors; virus infections
Lacrimal structures	Dacryocystitis (inflamed tear sac); hyposecretion of lacrimal fluid (dry eye); hypersecretion of lacrimal fluid (lacrimation); tumors
Bony orbit and eyeball	Orbital fractures; inflammatory diseases of orbit; lesions of orbital bones; tumors; displacement of eyeball (e.g., enophthalmos, exophthalmos, proptosis); hyperopia (error of refraction due to short anteroposterior diameter of eyeball); myopia (error of refraction due to long anteroposterior diameter of eyeball)
Extraocular muscles	Strabismus or "squint" (deviations of eye); diplopia (double vision); nystagmus (rhythmic involuntary oscillation of eyes); ophthalmoplegia (paralysis of eye muscles)
Conjunctiva, cornea, sclera	Conjunctivitis (inflammation of conjunctiva); subconjunctival hemorrhage; trachoma (blinding viral infection); keratitis (corneal inflammation); keratoconus (cone-shaped distortion of central cornea); corneal opacity; astigmatism (various irregularities in corneal curvature which cause optical distortion); scleritis (inflammation of sclera); ophthalmia neonatorum (acute purulent conjunctival infection in newborn); tumors
Uveal tract (iris, ciliary body, choroid)	Uveitis (inflammation of uvea); iritis (inflammation of iris); choroiditis (inflammation of choroid); cyclitis (inflammation of ciliary body); choroidocyclitis (inflammation of choroid and ciliary process); choroidoiritis (inflammation of choroid and iris); tumors
Retina	Retinitis (inflammation of retina); retinal hemorrhages; retinal detachment; retrolental fibroplasia (destructive overgrowth of retina in premature infants placed in high concentrations of oxygen); tumors
Lens	Opacity of lens (cataract); loss of elasticity of lens (presbyopia)
Ocular chambers and humors	Increased intraocular pressure (glaucoma)

ward either side. The conjunctival surfaces of the eyelids are inspected for any change in color, smoothness, or thickness and for the presence of secretions or foreign bodies.

Cornea. Superficial corneal irregularities are searched for by oblique moving illumination, with a small flashlight directed at the eyeball from the side. Corneal abrasions are difficult to see unless they are stained with a drop of sterile fluorescein solution. This stains abrasions a bright greenish color. Dropper bottles of fluorescein solution easily become contaminated with *Pseudomonas aeruginosa* and are thus unsafe. Therefore, individually packaged strips of filter paper are used which are saturated with fluorescein solution, dried, and sterilized. For use, the drug strip is wetted with a drop or two of sterile saline or sterile water, or the paper is touched to the patient's lower cul-de-sac so tears will dissolve the fluorescein and disperse it over the eyeball. The paper is momentarily placed in the lower fornix, and the patient is directed to shut the eyes and then quickly look up and down to distribute the stain. Excess stain may be washed out of the eye with sterile saline solution. Then, if a corneal abrasion is present, it is clearly marked by the stain.

The *corneal reflex* is a test of corneal sensitivity (an activity governed by the fifth cranial nerve). Nurses frequently perform this test on patients with neurologic disorders and altered states of consciousness (as discussed in Unit X). If the eyelids do not completely close to protect the cornea, or if the corneal reflex is absent (e.g., in an unconscious patient), the unprotected cornea may become dry and injured, resulting in loss of vision due to a corneal ulcer.

Eye care is not only of importance in unconscious patients; it also should be performed on all patients with *corneal anesthesia* or *facial palsy* and on all patients *following section of the fifth cranial nerve.* Conscious patients with the preceding conditions are taught to frequently and regularly inspect their eyes each day for signs of irritation or the presence of foreign bodies, e.g., eyelashes, cinders. Such persons must learn to live with their anesthetized, denervated corneas and protect their vision. Protective glasses or goggles may be advisable when out of doors or performing tasks hazardous to vision, e.g., sanding, working in areas with heavy dust in the air, chopping wood. These persons should be particularly careful when using aerosol products that spray does not get into their eyes. Additionally, these patients are instructed to:

1. Frequently blink the affected eye to help it cleanse itself.
2. Never rub the affected eye, because this could seriously damage the cornea, particularly if a foreign body is present.
3. Avoid irritating the cornea when pulling on clothing and from contact with cold compresses, washcloths, sheets.
4. Irrigate the eye and use protective drops or ointments as prescribed.
5. Always wash their hands before examining the eye or performing eye care.

Pupil. Pupils are normally equal in size, are perfectly round, and visibly constrict during accommodation and when exposed to light. Each of these characteristics of the normal pupil is evaluated during the ocular examination. It is important for nurses to be familiar with normal and abnormal pupillary findings and how they are obtained. In the hospital setting nurses often evaluate the pupils of neurologic patients (see Unit X).

Enlargement of the pupil is called mydriasis; *constriction of the pupil is called* miosis. Mydriatics *are drugs which enlarge the pupil;* miotics *are drugs which constrict the pupil.*

It is always important to know if either a mydriatic or miotic has been used on the patient's eye before the eye is examined. Irregularity of the *contour* of the pupil is always an abnormal finding. It may indicate such disorders as trauma, central nervous system syphilis, congenital defects, or iritis.

The *reaction to accommodation* is tested by holding one fingertip directly in front of the eye being tested, about 4 inches from the eye. The patient is then asked to look alternately at the fingertip and at the far wall directly beyond the finger, thus using both near and distant vision. *Direct pupil reaction to light* refers to constriction of a pupil when it is receiving increased illumination. Such a light reflex should not be checked by approaching a flashlight from straight ahead, but rather by bringing the light in from the side. *Consensual pupil reaction* refers to constriction of the pupil in the eye opposite the eye being illuminated. Such a pupillary reaction normally occurs, even though the opposite eye does not receive an increase in illumination.

Placement of the Eyeball in the Orbit. The physician may use a special instrument called an "*exophthalmometer*" to measure the height of the summit of the cornea of each eye, from the outer margin of each eye's orbital rim in the skull. The physician thus determines the placement of the eye in the orbit, e.g., whether the eye is pushed forward (exophthalmos, proptosis) or is sunken (enophthalmos). If an exophthalmometer is not available, the doctor may measure with a millimeter ruler.

Extraocular Muscles. The mobility of the eyeball is assessed to determine if the two eyes move together and whether the visual lines meet at the object of fixation. The physician tests the ability of both eyes to follow a test object smoothly and synchronously as it is moved to various positions of gaze (see Fig. 89–2). Deviations in mobility are investigated to ascertain whether there is loss of motion in any direction (paralysis or paresis) or a disorder of muscle balance, either latent *(heterophoria)* or obvious *(strabismus).*

Straightness of the two eyes is tested by observing the reflection of a light upon the cornea. A flashlight is held directly in front of the examiner's eyes, and the patient is asked to gaze directly at the light. Normally reflection of the light symmetrically occurs in the two pupils. If one eye deviates, the light reflex is asymmetric.

Some patients' eyes develop a rhythmic twitching motion, called *"end-positional nystagmus,"* when looking to the side. In this benign condition the quick portion of the movement is always in the direction of the gaze and is followed by a slow drift back. *Pathologic nystagmus* is that in which the quick component of the movement is always in the same direction, regardless of the direction of the patient's gaze. Nystagmus may be defined as "rhythmic involuntary oscillation of the eyes due to abnormal innervation or to lifelong reduced vision."[56] The movement of the eyeball may be horizontal, vertical, rotary, or mixed, i.e., of two varieties. The direction of the nystagmus is designated by the direction of the quick component of the movements. Nystagmus is closely related to the oculovestibular mechanisms and concerns the function of the vestibular nerve (discussed in the section pertaining to the ear and in Unit X). There are numerous kinds of nystagmus, of which end-positional nystagmus is but one.

Visual Fields. (See also p. 323). The integrity of the visual pathways may be roughly determined by testing the peripheral extent of the field of vision. Such an examination may be made by *confrontation testing.* Peripheral vision refers to side vision or vision other than central reading vision. Peripheral vision is highly important for safety and guidance. With confrontation testing the patient is directed to cover one eye and look steadily straight ahead at the examiner. The examiner then takes a small object, e.g., pen, and slowly moves it. Beginning by holding the object beyond the limits of the field of vision, the examiner gradually advances it toward the center of the patient's gaze to the point at which the patient first reports seeing the object approaching from the periphery. The visual field may be altered by central nervous disorders, e.g., brain tumors or syphilis, and by ocular disorders, e.g., glaucoma. Normally the visual field of each eye is such that the patient can see about 60 degrees nasalward, 50 degrees upward, 90 degrees temporally, and 70 degrees downward.

Intraocular Pressure. The intraocular pressure is routinely examined in all patients over age 40 and in all others known to have, or suspected to have, a pressure increase.

> *Measurement of intraocular pressure is important because elevated intraocular pressure (called "glaucoma") may cause blindness by slowly destroying nerve fibers. (Glaucoma is discussed later in this chapter.)*

An approximate measurement of intraocular pressures may be obtained by tonometry. Two common methods of measurement are *indentation* (Schiøtz) and *applanation* (most commonly Goldmann type). In indentation, Schiøtz tonometry, the eye is anesthetized with a topical anesthetic and, with the patient supine, the lids are gently separated without pressing upon the eyeball. The tonometer is placed gently on the center of the cornea and allowed to rest there by its own weight. The physician translates the needle deflection of the Schiøtz tonometer to a scale of millimeters of mercury (see Fig. 89–3).

Applanation tonometry (Goldmann) is performed with the patient sitting at the slit lamp. The cornea is anesthetized with a fluorescein-anesthetic solution, and the applanation tonometer is applied to the cornea. More precise measurements of intraocular pressure are obtained

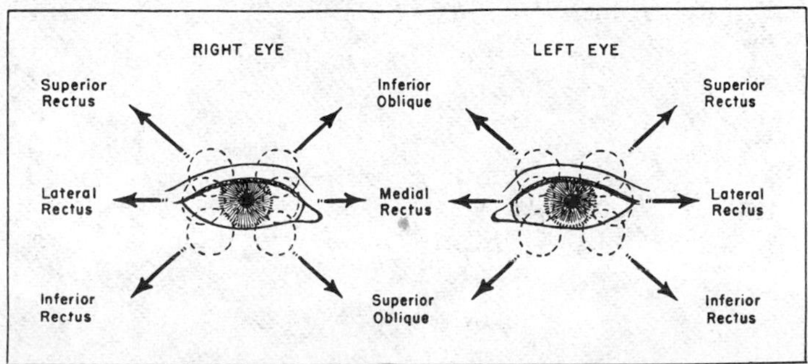

Figure 89–2. Diagram showing the muscles acting predominantly in the six cardinal directions of gaze. The six cardinal directions of gaze are: (1) right; (2) left; (3) up and right; (4) up and left; (5) down and right; and (6) down and left. (From Allen, J. W. (ed.): *Diseases of the Eye,* 24th ed. Baltimore: Williams & Wilkins Co., 1968.)

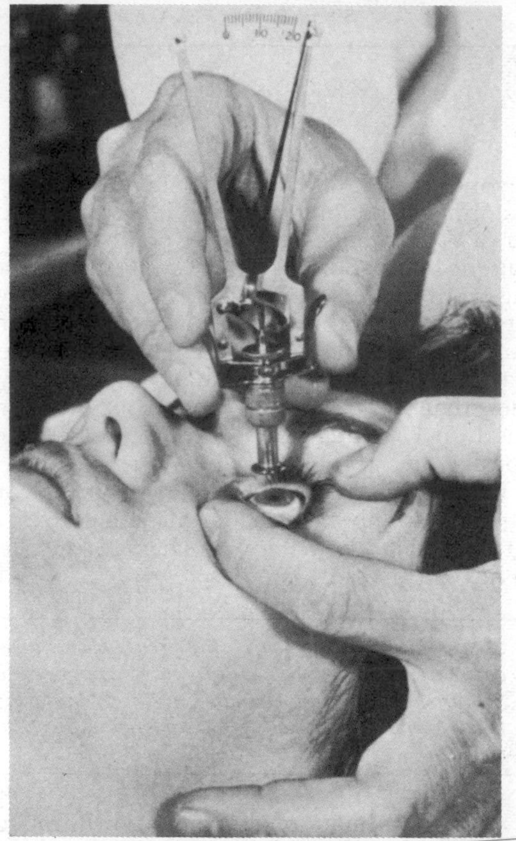

Figure 89–3. Technique for applying Schiøtz tonometer. (From Abrahamson, I. A., Jr.: Introcular pressure tonometry. *American Family Physician,* 17:75, June 1978.)

by applanation tonometry than by Schiøtz tonometry (see Fig. 89–4).

> *The average intraocular pressure is approximately 17 mm. Hg., with the normal range considered from 12 to 25 mm. Hg.*

CLEANING OF TONOMETERS. Although neither a Schiøtz nor a Goldmann tonometer can be boiled, the Schiøtz tonometer may be gas sterilized, using an ethylene oxide gas sterilizer. If this is unavailable, the tonometer should be dismantled; the footplate may be washed in soap and water. The tonometer should then be soaked in 70 per cent isopropyl alcohol, ether, or acetone for 20 minutes. When it is removed from the solution it should be dried (the center lumen can be dried with a pipe cleaner). The pieces should then be carefully reassembled. Care should be taken that the screw holding the plunger in place is fitted like a hat, with the crown uppermost; otherwise, when the extra weights are placed on the tonometer they could fall into the patient's eye because they are improperly fitted.

The tonometer tip used for the applanation procedure is easily removed and may be soaked in a bacteriocidal and viricidal solution. It should then be rinsed thoroughly in a solution of normal saline or sterile water.

Visual Acuity. Visual acuity is examined in one eye at a time while the patient is comfortably seated. Always start with the right eye, as this will prevent the possibility of error in recording. The

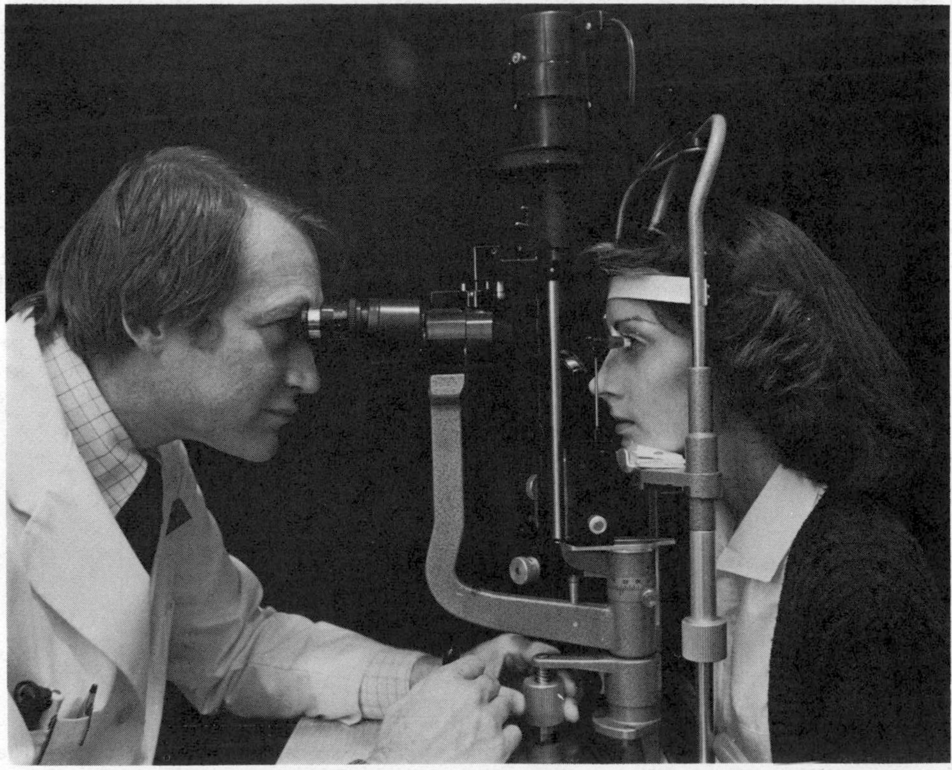

Figure 89–4. Applanation or Goldmann tonometry. (Photograph courtesy of Walter C. Petersen, M.D.)

eye not being tested is kept covered with an occluder or opaque card.

Distant visual acuity is measured with a standardized *visual acuity chart*, e.g., *Snellen's chart* (Fig. 89–5). Nurses may be asked to perform this test in ophthalmologists' offices, schools, industry, or other settings. The chart is imprinted with a series of block letters or numbers (the letter E at different angles is successfully used if the patient is illiterate or is a child) in gradually decreasing sizes; the sizes are identified according to distances at which they are ordinarily visible, e.g., the largest letters can be read at a distance of 200 feet by persons with unimpaired vision. The chart is placed 20 feet from the patient and the examiner points to the line of letters the patient is to read.

Visual acuity is recorded as a fraction. The fraction's numerator represents the distance to the chart; the denominator represents the distance at which a "normal eye" can read the line. For example, 20/30 means the patient is 20 feet away from the chart and can read the line that a normal eye should read at 30 feet. Thus, the larger the denominator, the poorer the patient's visual acuity.

Patients with vision so poor that they cannot see even the largest numbers on the Snellen chart are given additional tests to determine if they can see well enough to (a) count fingers (C.F.); (b) perceive hand movements (H.M.); or (c) perceive light (L.P.) N.L.P. indicates no light perception. An ophthalmologist does not consider a patient to be *"blind"* unless that patient cannot even perceive light. *However, legally "blindness" is defined as vision (corrected by eyeglasses) of 20/200 or less, or less than 20 degrees of visual field in the better eye.*

Near visual acuity is not routinely tested unless the patient is over 40 years of age or complains specifically of having difficulty reading. With increasing age *presbyopia* frequently occurs, i.e., the lens of the eye becomes less flexible. As a result the person loses accommodation for near vision and therefore experiences difficulty with close reading without backing away from the material.

> *People who cannot read newspaper print at a distance of one foot, with their own glasses on, should be advised to have an ophthalmologic examination and refraction.*

Refraction. "Refraction" refers to the state of focus of the eye. When a patient is examined for refraction, the physician clinically measures the error of focus in the eye and then prescribes lenses to correct the error and thereby bring light rays into correct focus on the retina. Refraction is tested by the Snellen chart (previously discussed) and trial corrective lenses. Refraction is a common eye examination performed in the ophthalmologist's office. Correction of errors of refraction is discussed on pages 1996–2002.

Ophthalmoscopic Examination. Examination of the fundus (posterior eye) is usually performed with an ophthalmoscope (Fig. 89–6). The ophthalmoscope has been of great value in clinical medicine.

With an ophthalmoscope the blood vessels of the interior eye, as well as other structures, can be visualized and magnified. *The fundus is the only area of the body in which blood vessels can be directly observed.* Thus ophthalmoscopic examination not only is useful in diagnosing diseases of the eye and aberrations in the refractive mechanism, but also is extremely valuable in diagnosing many systemic and intracranial disorders. For example, arteriosclerosis, nephritis, brain tumor, and other disorders cause characteristic changes in the retina which can be recognized by the trained observer. Examination of the details of the posterior eye with an ophthalmoscope is part of every complete physical examination as well as ocular examination.

Ophthalmic examination may be performed by a direct method (Fig. 89–6), an indirect method (Fig. 89–7), or by slit lamp biomicroscopy. In the *direct method,* the instrument is held close to the patient's eye, with a system of lenses to correct the refractive error of either the patient or the observer. This method gives a magnification of approximately 13 times, in an upright image.

The *indirect method* usually includes stereoscopic evaluation, the light source emanating from a head-mounted light and observation system. An objective lens is then held approximately 2 inches from the patient's eye and an inverted

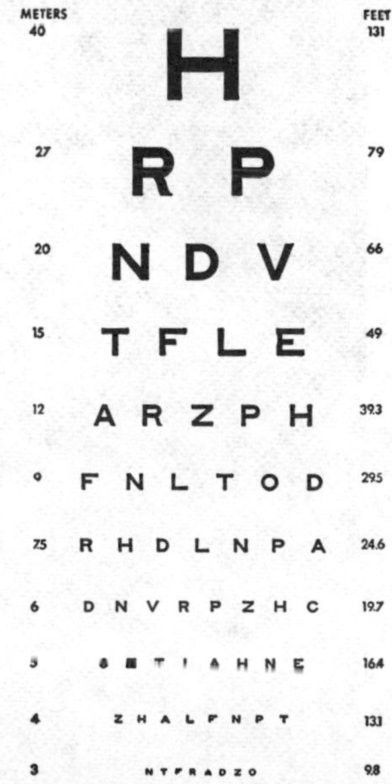

Figure 89–5. Snellen chart. (From Scheie, H. G., and Albert, D. M.: *Textbook of Ophthalmology,* 9th ed., Philadelphia: W. B. Saunders Co., 1977.)

reversed image is seen by the observer. The magnification of the image may be varied by utilizing differing objective lenses.

The third common method of fundus evaluation utilizes the *biomicroscope (slit lamp)* and contact lens placed on the patient's eye. (An alternative method is a lens mounted to the biomicroscope in the space in front of the patient's eye.) This method results in very high magnification and the ability to observe very fine detail of the posterior aspect of the eye.

With ophthalmoscopic experience the physician can often study the retina and optic nerve head without dilating the pupil. However, at times the physician may use a mydriatic to dilate the pupil so the retina (including the macula), blood vessels, and optic disk can be observed more clearly. After completing examination of the fundus, the physician can use the ophthalmoscope to visualize the vitreous body, lens, iris, aqueous humor, and cornea.

An ophthalmoscope should not be boiled, autoclaved, or soaked in solution but may be wiped off with a 70 per cent alcohol solution. The instrument itself does not touch the patient's eye, but rather is held about 1 inch away from the eye. The nurse should see that the battery handle ophthalmoscope has fresh batteries and an operable bulb. A variety of self-luminous electric ophthalmoscopes are in use. The room should be darkened during ophthalmoscopy.

Other Procedures. Some additional procedures which are not routinely used in examination of the eye but are used as indicated are discussed in this section.

The *biomicroscope*, i.e., *slit lamp microscope*, is an

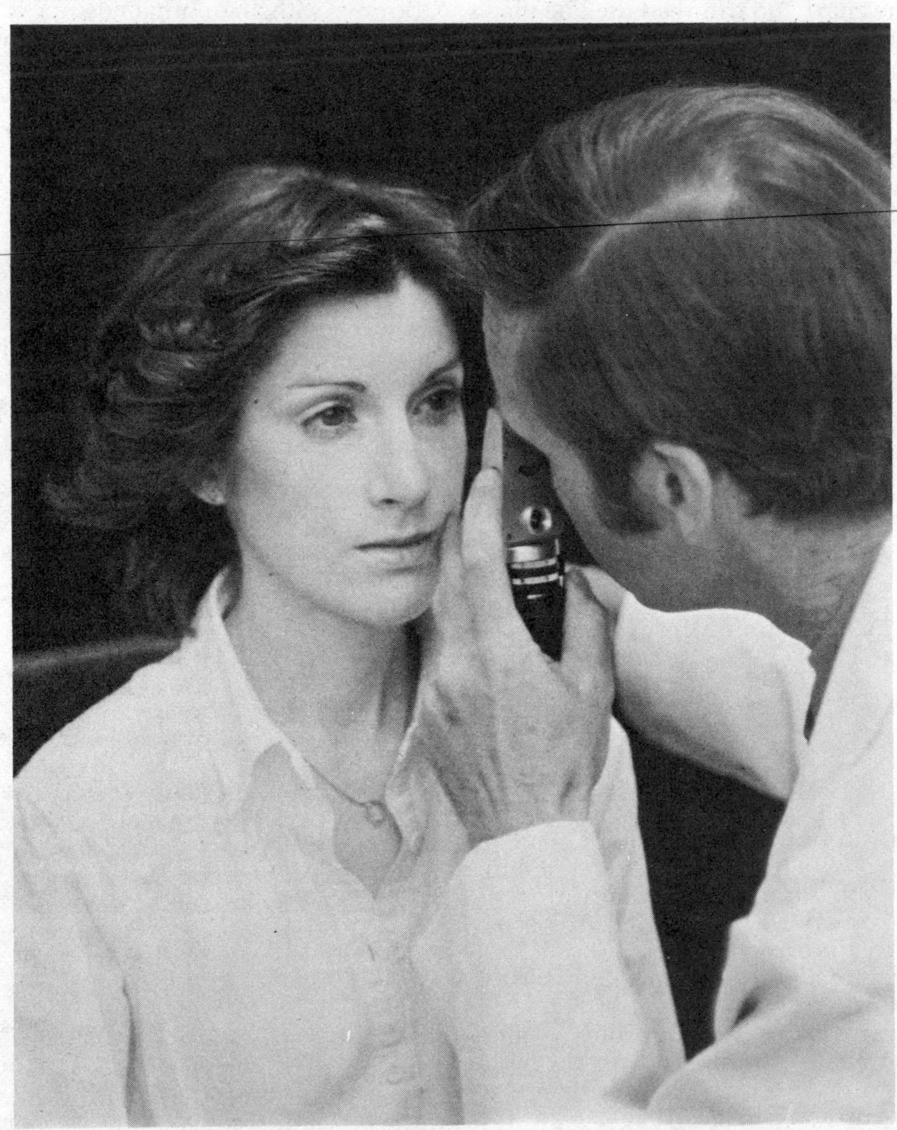

Figure 89–6. Direct ophthalmoscopy. (Photograph courtesy of Walter C. Petersen, M.D.)

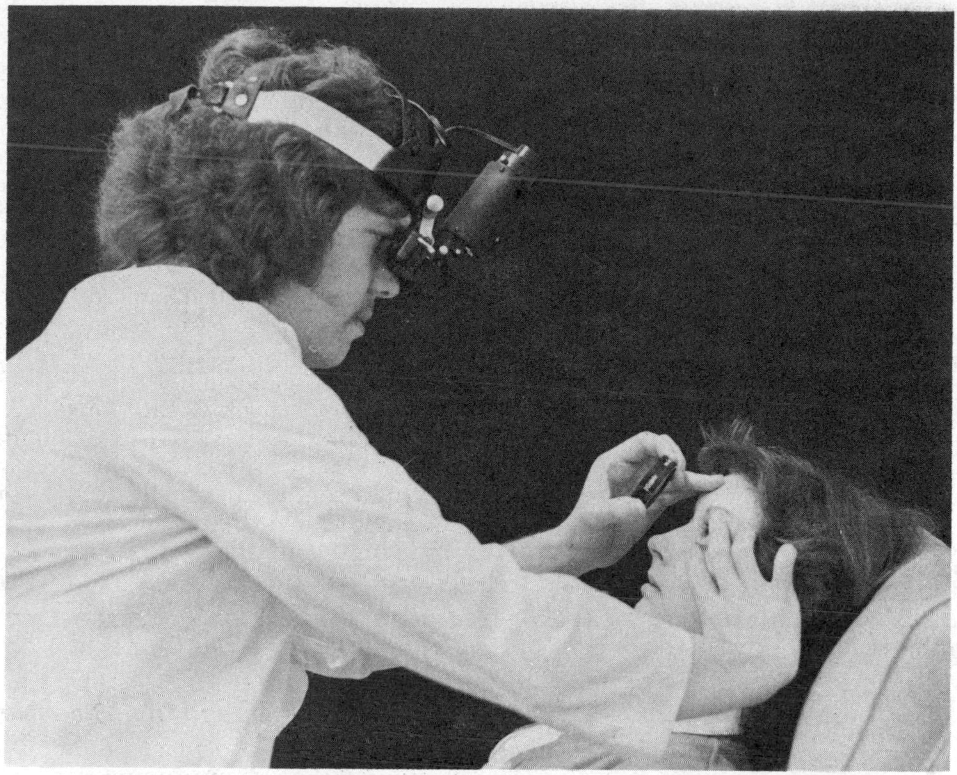

Figure 89–7. Indirect ophthalmoscopy. (Photograph courtesy of Walter C. Petersen, M.D.)

instrument used in examining the *anterior* portion of the eye under high magnification and in optical section (obtained by a finely focused slit of brilliant light which may be focused in various ways) (Fig. 89–8). By combining intense illumination and magnification, the slit lamp and biomicroscope make it possible to study microscopic changes in the eyeball's anterior portion. By adding a strong concave lens to the slit lamp, the *posterior* vitreous and retina can be examined with the biomicroscope. The biomicroscope is used in a darkened room. The slit lamp is highly useful in determining the location of a foreign body or the depth of a corneal ulcer and in diagnosing inflammatory conditions of the eye.

We discussed on page 1953 the method of confrontation which serves to roughly determine peripheral visual fields. More precise methods of evaluation of the visual field may be used when additional investigation appears indicated. These methods may include use of a perimeter or tangent screen. A *perimeter* is a curved metallic device into which the patient looks. Inside, a test object is systematically moved along the inner surface of the arc, and the patient's peripheral vision is then outlined upon a diagram of a normal visual field. A similar principle is utilized with the *tangent screen*. In this procedure the test object is systematically moved across a large black curtain supported by a framework, and the visual field is mapped.

Precise evaluation of the peripheral and central visual fields is particularly important in examining patients with neurologic disorders, glaucoma, or retinal detachment and in making postoperative evaluations. A *scotoma* is an area of depressed vision or loss of vision within the visual field. There are various types of scotomas. Everyone has a normal physiologic scotoma

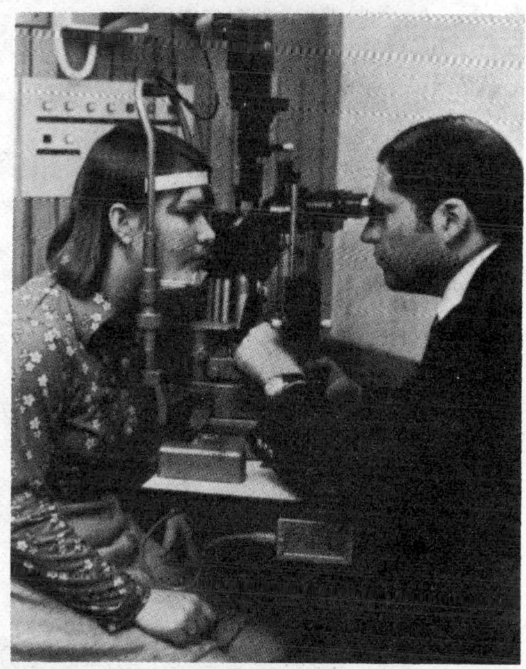

Figure 89–8. Slit lamp bimicroscopic examination. (From Scheie, H. G., and D. M. Albert: *Textbook of Ophthalmology*. 9th ed., 1977.)

which is often called the "blind spot." This is the area of the *optic disk*. In this area the optic nerve enters the eyeball and there are no photosensitive receptors. The axons converge, after several synapses within the retina, and leave the eyeball as the optic nerve. The area of a scotoma may be plotted out, just as the normal visual field is mapped out.

The *color sense*, i.e., the faculty of distinguishing different colors, is tested by a variety of methods. The *central* perception of color is evaluated with color plates or samples of colored wool. The *peripheral* perception of color is tested in ways similar to those discussed for testing the visual field (e.g., confrontation, perimeter, tangent screen), except that the test objects are colored rather than white. The visual field for colors is smaller than that for white, but it has the same general shape. The visual field varies for different colors. The points measured in this test are those at which the colors are recognized, rather than those at which the patient merely perceives the moving test object coming into the visual field.

Gonioscopy is a specialized type of examination to evaluate the angle of the anterior chamber (the angle created by the juncture of the iris and the peripheral cornea) (see Fig. 89–9). Two types of gonioscopy are performed: Koeppe and slit lamp. With Koeppe examinations, a large dome-shaped contact lens is placed on the cornea, with the patient in the supine position. A magnifying device and light source are used together to illuminate and observe the angle through the contact lens. The second method, utilizing the slit lamp, requires the patient to be seated at the slit lamp with a contact lens applied that has a special internal mirror surface. Via the angled mirror, the angles may be observed. Gonioscopy is especially important in evaluating patients with glaucoma.

An *electroretinogram* (ERG) is a record of the changes in the retina's electric potential following stimulation by light. The ERG is clinically useful in some patients with retinal disease. An ERG is obtained by placing a contact lens electrode on the anesthetized cornea. The potential recorded on the cornea is identical with the response which would be obtained if the electrodes were placed directly upon the surface of the retina.

Ocular Symptoms and Their Significance

Some common ocular symptoms and their possible meanings are summarized below:

▶ *Pain:* Two serious eye disorders which cause pain are iritis and acute glaucoma. If these are not present, the patient may have an acute lid infection, corneal abrasion, or foreign body. The patient with a corneal ulcer or foreign body will note that the eye

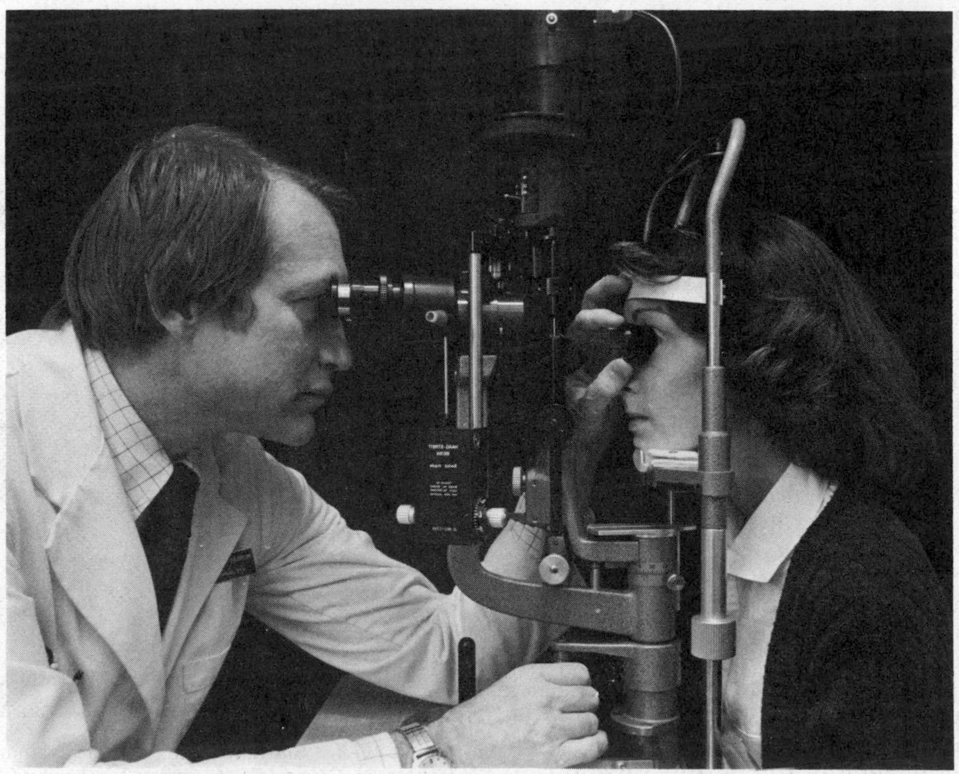

Figure 89–9. Gonioscopy. (Courtesy of Walter C. Petersen, M.D.)

is more comfortable closed; blinking increases discomfort. Deep-seated pain occurs with intraocular inflammation; frequently the pain is referred to the trigeminal nerve's cutaneous distribution. This pain is often worse at night. Sinusitis often causes pain referred to the eyes.

- *Foreign body sensation:* may indicate superficial corneal erosions, e.g., actinic keratitis (inflammation of the cornea resulting from the action of ultraviolet light) or erosions secondary to the wearing of contact lenses.
- *Subconjunctival hemorrhages* (gross extravasations of blood over the underlying sclera which are spontaneously absorbed within about two weeks): are asymptomatic, may occur at any age, generally follow coughing, sneezing, and other straining efforts. Subconjunctival hemorrhages may be a sign of hypertension; therefore, people who develop them should have their blood pressure checked. Subconjunctival hemorrhages follow most types of ocular surgery; these are of no significance and clear within several weeks.
- *Retinal hemorrhages:* are always of importance, generally indicating such underlying systemic diseases as diabetes, blood dyscrasias, renal disease, or hypertension.
- *Vitreous hemorrhages* (extravasations of blood into the vitreous humor): commonly due to diabetes or rupture of a peripheral retinal vessel by a surrounding area of choroiditis.
- *Scotoma* (blind spot or area of loss of vision within visual field): when occurring in front of one eye is due to damage to optic nerve or retina, e.g., hemorrhage or choroiditis. When occurring in same area of both eyes it is commonly a quadratic defect due to a lesion involving the optic pathways.
- *Exophthalmos* (abnormal displacement of the eye forward out of the orbit in such a manner that the eye appears to be "bulging" forward): may be caused by thyroid disease or orbital disease.
- *Blurred vision:* may indicate refractive error, corneal opacities, cataract, retinal detachment, optic neuritis, optic atrophy, vitreous clouding, or macular degeneration.
- *Sudden loss of vision:* could be due to central retinal artery occlusion or central retinal vein thrombosis, both of which are true ocular emergencies.
- *Photophobia* (abnormal intolerance of light): suggests keratitis, iritis, corneal ulcer, ocular albinism, or conjunctivitis, although usually photophobia is without significance. Blondes or lightly pigmented persons are often easily disturbed by glare or light.
- *Conjunctival discharge:* generally results from viral or bacterial conjunctivitis.
- *Nausea and vomiting:* may be presenting symptoms of acute glaucoma.
- *"Halos" or "rainbows" around lights:* may indicate acute glaucoma.
- *"Eyestrain" and headache:* are common complaints. "Eyestrain" usually refers to eye discomfort associated with prolonged periods of close work or reading. Head pain related to the eye is discussed in Unit X. Causes of eyestrain and ocular headache include inadequate illumination; significant refractive error; early presbyopia; phoria, i.e., latent tendency to ocular deviation (usually exophoria with poor convergence).
- *Diplopia* (double vision): results from muscle imbalance or paralysis of an extraocular muscle, e.g., hemorrhage or inflammation of a nerve. It may also result from trauma. This is a common complication of diabetes. These muscle pareses usually recover within six months.
- *"Spots" or "floaters":* "Spots before the eyes" or "floaters" in the visual field (accentuated in bright light) are vitreous opacities which generally have no clinical significance and come and go. They are more prevalent in highly myopic, i.e., "nearsighted," and older persons. Single spots or floaters are usually benign; however, the sudden appearance of multiple floaters may indicate posterior uveitis, impending retinal detachment, or intraocular hemorrhage from diabetes or retinal detachment). *Frequently retinal detachment is preceded by a shower of "sparks"* in one quadrant of the visual field (diagnostically opposite to the tear in the retina), *followed by a sensation of a curtain moving across the eye.*

GENERAL EYE CARE AND PROTECTION OF VISION

Nurse's Role

Nurses are in a key position to teach others about general eye care and the protection of vision. Also, a nurse may be the person called upon to administer first aid following ocular injuries or to offer advice concerning the need for referral of a patient to a physician. In schools and industrial settings nurses may perform cursory procedures of visual testing to identify persons requiring further professional evaluation. Often it is a nurse who instills medication into the eyes of newborn infants to protect their vision. These are all important responsibilities which may ultimately prevent ocular disorders or improve or preserve vision. Foremost in a nurse's thoughts should be the remembrance that *blindness is often preventable* with proper care. With the appropriate application of medical knowledge, many ocular disorders can be prevented or successfully treated.

Incidence of Impaired Vision

While the United States has the lowest incidence of blindness of all the major nations, there is much work still to be done if the goal of elimination of preventable blindness is to be attained. World Health Organization surveys indicate that the United States has 200 blind persons per 100,000 population (approximately 400,000 persons).

Protection of Vision

One means of preventing blindness and other less severe visual losses is through *teaching* the public proper general eye care, safety precautions, first-aid for eye injury, and the warning symptoms of eye disease.

Seven Eye Danger Signals. Seven eye danger signals which indicate the need for medical evaluation are:

1. *Persistent redness* of the eye.
2. *Continuing pain or discomfort* around the eye or in the eye, particularly following injury.
3. *Visual disturbances*, such as difficulty seeing near or at a distance; fogginess or rainbow-colored halos around lights; sudden development of floating spots before the eyes; loss of side vision; or persistent double vision.
4. *Crossing of the eyes* (particularly in children).
5. *Growths* on the eye or eyelids or *opacities* noticeable in the normally transparent portions of the eye.
6. *Continuing discharge, crusting, or tearing* of the eyes.
7. *Pupil irregularities* (unequal size in the two pupils or distorted shape).

Self-treatment of ocular disorders may be disastrous! Unfortunately, vision has been lost in many eyes through inappropriate self-treatment, e.g., instillation of contaminated or contraindicated drops or ointments. Encourage individuals with any of the above symptoms to seek professional care.

It is recommended that *the eyes be routinely examined* at the following times:

1. At birth (to detect infections, injuries, or malformations.
2. Between ages 2½ and 5 (to detect "lazy eyes," which need correction prior to school entrance).
3. At age 10 and in early adolescence.
4. Every five years during young adulthood.
5. Every 2 to 5 years after age 40 (because the highest incidence of blindness is in older age groups and also because after age 40 the lens becomes less resilient).
6. Upon the appearance of ocular symptoms. When a history of glaucoma occurs in a patient's family, the patient's intraocular pressure should be measured annually.

Because the eyes' health is related to an individual's general state of health, regular total physical examinations (which include examination of the eyes) are important in eye care and visual protection. Blindness may be caused by such general disorders as hypertension, diabetes, poisoning, and disorders of the nervous system, e.g., brain tumors. Such conditions may first be recognized if the physician notes changes occurring in the patient's eyes at the time of a routine annual physical examination.

The eyes are more likely to be healthy if the total body is in a good nutritional state and has regular periods of exercise and rest.

Vision is also protected in the following ways:

- *Enforcement of safety regulations and standards,* e.g., shatterproof automobile glass and lenses in eyeglasses; safety goggles in industry; safety standards concerning protective sports equipment, e.g., face masks for hockey goalies and baseball catchers.
- *Outlawing dangerous toys, BB guns, arrows, fireworks.*
- *Early identification and treatment of strabismus in children.* This can prevent the blindness of disuse (amblyopia) which occurs in the deviating eye of a child with strabismus.
- *Routine programs of eye examinations in schools.*
- *Early consultation and treatment when eye symptoms occur.*
- *Instillation of appropriate drops in the eyes of every newborn infant.* This procedure is routinely carried out (by law) to prevent ophthalmia neonatorum (see p. 1976), a bacterial infection of the eyes which has in the past blinded numerous unprotected infants.
- *Performance of blood tests during pregnancy to identify syphilis* so it can be treated and thus prevent blindness in the newborn.
- *Vaccination against smallpox, where indicated.* At one time smallpox was the leading cause of blindness because it produced blinding scars. The World Health Organization believes it has now isolated the last cases of this disease or perhaps eliminated it.
- *Performance of inoculation against rubella.* During the first trimester of pregnancy, rubella can be responsible for the interruption of the embryonic formation of the eyeball and the development of congenital cataracts in the infant at birth.
- *Regulation of oxygen concentrations administered to premature infants.* If the oxygen concentration given to premature infants is too high, blindness results from the development of retrolental fibroplasia (see p. 1984). It is estimated that in the United States 5000 premature infants were blinded before the cause of this disorder was identified.
- *Prevention of ocular infections by properly treating injuries of the eye and other ocular disorders.*

Daily General Eye Care

Some factors of importance in the *daily general care of the eyes* are summarized below:

- *Do not habitually rub the eyes.* Rubbing may introduce bacteria or cause irritation of the eyes. The hands are generally best kept away from the face and eyes unless they are washed and brought up to the face for some specific purpose. Habits of rubbing and picking at the face and eyes, and having the hands up around the eyes, hair, and mouth should be broken; such gestures are unsightly and unhealthy.

- *Supervise and instruct children regarding eye protection and eye care.* Children should be taught the dangers of (a) fireworks; (b) throwing rocks, dirt, and so forth; (c) poking, throwing, or running with sticks; (d) throwing or shooting paper wads, rubber bands, tin can lids, paper airplanes, slingshots, BB guns or other pellet guns, arrows, darts, and so forth; and (e) looking directly into the sun, eclipses, sun lamps, or other bright lights.
- *Reduce eyestrain.* While eyestrain (i.e., strain of the ciliary muscles when accommodation is difficult) does not permanently damage the eyes, it does cause discomfort and may slow down or impair performance of visual tasks. Eyestrain can be reduced by (a) having adequate lighting which is placed in such a manner that a shadow is not cast on the object being illuminated; and (b) periodically resting the eyes when engaging in prolonged periods of close work, reading, or televison watching. The eyes may be rested by pausing occasionally to look at distant views, e.g., out the window or across the room, and by resting the head and closing the eyes occasionally. While prolonged television watching does not appear to damage vision, it is not advisable to sit too close to the set.
- *Reduce glare and wear protective goggles as indicated.* Shatterproof or unbreakable sunglasses should be worn in bright light, e.g., sunny days when snow is on the ground or when the sun is shining on a body of water. Ultraviolet rays can cause serious eye damage. Excessive exposure to sun lamps can be highly dangerous, producing not only serious skin burns but also eye injury.
- *Keep glasses clean, protected from scratching and breakage, and properly aligned.* If the glasses seem to tilt and not sit straight across the bridge of the nose and not at an even distance from both eyes, they should be readjusted by a specialist.
- *Do not use eyewashes, eyedrops, or any medications in the eyes unless they are prescribed by a physician.* The normal, healthy eye is bathed by protective conjunctival secretions which should not be washed off. *Eyecups* can spread infection or cause injury and thus should not be used.
- *Never use a soiled washcloth to wash around the eyes.* When cleaning matter from the eye's canthi, do not use the same tissue for both eyes.
- *Eat a well-balanced diet* with adequate vitamins A, B, and C. *Maintain a general state of good health.*
- *Exercise caution when using aerosol spray products.* Be certain the nozzle is pointing away from the eyes before pressing the spray button. Shut the eyes when using hair sprays.
- *Exercise caution when using solvents, lye solutions, ammonia, caustic solutions,* and so forth, to avoid splashing or spilling them into the eyes.

OCULAR EMERGENCIES AND OCULAR FIRST AID

Ocular emergencies include acute (angle closure) glaucoma; foreign bodies; corneal abrasions; contusions; actinic keratitis; corneal ulcers; chemical conjunctivitis and keratitis (e.g. chemical burns); gonococcal conjunctivitis; sudden loss of vision; lacerations; and orbital cellulitis. These conditions require immediate referral to an ophthalmologist. (See Chapter 95.)

GENERAL GUIDELINES, COMMON NURSING PROCEDURES, AND MEDICATIONS RELATED TO EYE CARE

General Guidelines Related to Eye Care

- Always wash before and after performing procedures related to the eye. If attending to both eyes, treat the least infected eye first to minimize chances of accidentally infecting it from the other eye. Use a clean piece of cotton or tissue for each eye.

  Maintain aseptic technique to protect an unaffected eye from cross-contamination. Prevent cross-contamination between the two eyes not only by washing and treating the least infected eye first but also by having separate equipment for use on each eye, e.g., separate eye compress set-ups, if eye compresses are ordered for both eyes. When active infection is present, it is imperative to prevent cross-contamination from medication droppers, ointment tubes, and so forth.
- Be gentle when giving eye care of any kind. Do not exert pressure over the eyeball when performing ocular procedures. A pressure dressing may be specifically used following removal of the eyeball, i.e., enucleation, after retinal surgery, lid surgery, or a corneal erosion. However, a pressure dressing is never applied to a viable eyeball without a physician's order. Remember that the eye is a sensitive structure and that the patient has a natural tendency to protectively withdraw from ocular procedures. You can minimize this tendency if you tell patients what you are going to do and how they can help you. At times you need to steady the head by having the patient rest it against the back of a chair or lie down to prevent the person from pulling away as you treat the eye.
- Protect a patient's eyes as indicated. We have mentioned protection from cross-contamination and steadying patient's head during ocular procedures. Other protective measures include prevention of corneal irritation if the patient's eyelid does not completely close. Do not touch the eyeball, or even the eyelashes or lids, e.g., with the tip of an eyedropper, ointment tube, irrigating syringe, or your fingers. Never direct forceful streams of solutions or ointments into the eye. Use low pressure for such procedures and direct the stream towards the nasal side of the eyeball, have the patient tilt the head so that the stream runs over the surface of the eyeball, then ask the patient to look up and down, as the case may be.
- Open the eyelids by pressing against the bony orbit rather than directly against the eyeball.

- Keep all strong solutions, which should *not* be used on the eye, away from the bedside of a patient with an ocular disorder and away from the area where ocular medications are stored.
- Find out from partially sighted people how well they can see and then provide appropriate care related to each person's level of vision. Make certain all staff members are aware of those patients with visual losses so appropriate care can be given.
- Post a sign on the patient's bed which clearly states any contraindicated activities, e.g., restricted positions or movements, activity limitations, dietary restrictions.
- Familiarize yourself with agencies which provide services for the blind and with other aspects of the rehabilitation of blind persons. Then make appropriate referrals for blind patients.
- Provide appropriate safety measures for the blind or partially sighted (including patients with eye dressings). For example, supervise smoking if it is allowed and assist the ambulatory patient to prevent bumps and falls. When the patient is in bed, keep siderails up, the bed in low position, and the call bell within easy reach and always located in the same place. Do not rearrange the patient's belongings or the furniture in the room; keep things orderly so the person always knows where to find them. Maintain a safe environment around the patient's bed and chair, e.g., see that no electric cords run across the floor where the patient could fall over them. Keep footstools pushed under other furniture; keep casters locked on moveable furniture; keep the floor clean, picked up, and dry. Handrails are useful in bathrooms and along hallways.
- Place only sterile materials in the eye.
- Always have adequate light when performing ocular procedures; however, avoid directing light unnecessarily into the patient's eye. At times the patient's room is kept dimly lit, e.g., if the patient is photophobic.
- Familiarize yourself with standard abbreviations used with reference to the eye. Particularly be certain you know that "O.D." (R. or R.E.) refers to oculus dexter or right eye; "O.S." (L. or L.E.) means oculus sinister or left eye; and "O.U." means oculus uterque or both eyes.
- Cleanse eyelids by moving in a direction from the inner to the outer canthus.
- Instruct patients to never touch their eyes, eye dressings, or eye shields. If the dressing needs adjusting, instruct the patient to call a nurse to attend to it.
- Familiarize yourself with general guidelines concerning ocular medications and with specific eye medications.
- Familiarize yourself with ocular first aid and teach basic principles to others.
- Teach patients how to correctly use contact lenses and eyeglasses.
- Attempt to prevent disorientation in the patient who has both eyes covered or in the newly blinded patient. Such patients experience sensory deprivation which may cause them to become disoriented, hallucinate, and so forth. Frequent drop-in visits, a radio softly playing for an hour or so (not steadily all day), and physical contact with the patient (e.g., gently holding the person's hand while talking) are all measures which help minimize the ill effects of such sensory deprivation.
- Encourage persons with ocular disorders to seek professional evaluations and treatment.
- Familiarize yourself with basic ocular disorders, their symptoms and common treatments (medical and surgical).

Common Nursing Procedures Related to the Eye

Common nursing procedures related to eye care include eversion of the upper eyelid; ocular irrigations; cleansing of the eyelids; instillation of eye drops and ocular ointments; application of hot and cold compresses; application and care of eye dressings; and removal and care of an artificial eye.

Eversion of the Upper Eyelid. Eversion of the upper eyelid is necessary to inspect the palpebral conjunctiva and is accomplished as follows:

1. Instruct the patient to look down (this relaxes the levator muscle, making eversion possible).
2. Instruct the patient not to squeeze the lids shut but to gently close the eyelids.
3. Grasp the eyelashes of the upper lid between the thumb and forefinger, then with an applicator stick held horizontally against the outer eyelid push down and fold the eyelid on itself.
4. As soon as the lid is everted, appose the fingers and hold the lashes up against the eyebrow. It may be necessary to evert the eyelid to remove foreign objects from the palpebral conjunctival region (see Fig. 89–10).

Ocular Irrigation. Cleansing and irrigating solutions of various kinds may be ordered to flush the conjunctival sac and remove chemicals accidentally splashed in the eye or secretions, e.g., preoperatively or in various inflammatory conditions. Examples of such solutions are normal saline solution and lactated Ringer's solution. Cleansing and irrigating solutions should be bland and at room temperature when used. The solutions may be applied (a) by using the IV tubing in the case of flushing for chemical burns when copious irrigation is necessary; (b) by using commercial sterile ophthalmic solutions, e.g., Blinx, Dacriose, contained in a plastic irrigating bottle; (c) by using a soft rubber bulb syringe or (d) by being poured from an undine.

The patient may be either sitting up with the head tilted slightly to the side that is being irrigated, to prevent contamination of the other eye, or lying flat in bed. If the patient's head is tilted

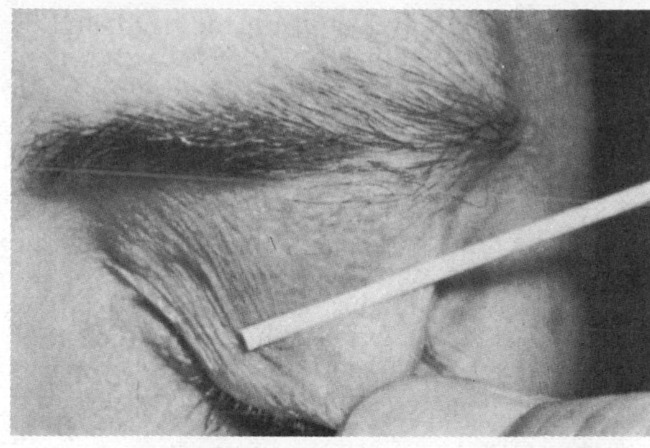

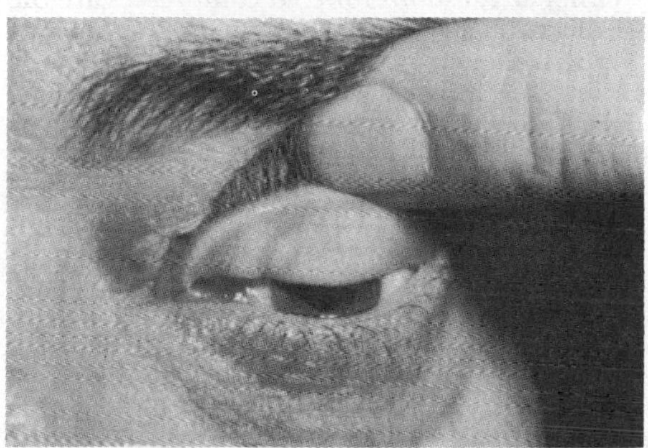

Figure 89–10. Technique for everting the eyelid. (From Carr, R. E.: Look them in the injured eye. *Emergency Medicine,* 9:53, Nov. 1977.)

toward the side of the eye to be irrigated, the solution will flow away from the eye's inner canthus and will not flow across the bridge of the nose into the other eye. A handful of cotton balls or a clean towel is held against the patient's cheek to prevent the flow of water from going down the patient's neck. A small curved basin can also be placed against the patient's cheek to catch the fluid; however, this is useful only when the patient is lying down.

The nurse then holds the patient's eyelids apart with one hand (because the patient will instinctively try to close the eye) and asks the patient to look upward with both eyes. The nurse directs the flow of solution toward the inner canthus onto the conjunctiva. Because of the head tilt, the stream of irrigating solution will flow over the eyeball, from the inner to the outer canthus. Do not direct the stream forcefully onto the eyeball itself and do not contaminate the irrigating apparatus by touching the eye's structures. The procedure is continued until obvious secretions are removed from the eye, and then the area around the eye is gently dried with cotton.

It is desirable for each patient to have individualized irrigating equipment and irrigating solution. With the use of isotonic solutions, the necessary electrolytes are not removed from the eye's secretions.

Cleaning the Eyelids.* It is important to clean a patient's eyelids before applying compresses, before removing or inserting an artificial eye, before instilling medication into the eye, or if lids are crusted or have discharge on them following removal of dressings.

Instillation of Eyedrops and Ocular Ointments.* Be certain you have the *correct patient,* the *correct medication,* and the *correct eye.*

Application of Hot and Cold Eye Compresses. Wet compresses to the eye are a socially clean procedure; the equipment in the hospital setting should be sterile. When compresses are to be sterile, or if the eye has copious discharge, a new compress is used each time one is changed. If both eyes are to have compresses applied, use separate equipment for each eye and wash between the treatment of each eye to avoid cross-contamination.

Hot moist compresses may be applied to the eye to cleanse the eye, to relieve pain, and to increase circulation. This may reduce tension and increase absorption in the treatment of superficial infections and inflammation of the eye or eyelid, as well as such deep-seated disorders as iritis.

To prepare the patient for the application of hot compresses, a sterile bowl and gauze are used in the hospital setting. The patient is seated where there is access to a warm water faucet; the patient's chest is draped with a towel. Warm water from the faucet is permitted to run into the bowl onto the gauze. The patient is directed to squeeze the excess moisture out, then hold the warm wetted gauze against the closed eyelid until it cools. The gauze is then discarded, and the patient repeats the procedure for 15 to 20 minutes. If the water cools, the patient may be directed to run more warm water into the bowl. Most eye patients are ambulatory; however, if this is not the case the bowl will have to be brought to the patient's bedside, and a nurse will be responsible for keeping the water at a warm temperature. The patient should be warned not to use water hot enough to burn the skin and to lift the compress off if it feels too hot. Warm compresses are usually prescribed four times a day.

If the patient is to apply hot compresses at home, water from the hot water faucet may be used, or a pan of water may be heated on the

*See Sorensen and Luckmann, *Basic Nursing: A Psychophysiologic Approach,* for detailed descriptions of these topics.

stove or hot plate until it is hot, but not hot enough to burn. A clean face cloth or other cloth should be placed in the water, wrung out, and held against the eye as directed above.

Should the patient have impaired innervation to the eyelids, great care should be taken not to burn the eyelids with the hot compress. The patient should test the compress against the back of the hand before placing it against the eye.

Cold compresses may be used to (a) reduce swelling; (b) relieve pain; (c) relieve itching; (d) prevent or control edema; and (e) help control bleeding. Some feel that it may retard bacterial growth and prevent the spread of infection. The cold produces capillary constriction. Cold compresses are used in such conditions as inflammatory and allergic conjunctivitis and following ocular injuries and ocular surgery. Cold compresses are contraindicated in deep-seated ocular inflammations because the cornea's nutrition is impaired when capillary constriction is produced.

To prepare a cold compress, something soft to rest against the eye and something that will hold ice chips or pellets are needed; a small amount of chipped ice can be placed in a small plastic bag and the bag knotted at the end. Explain the procedure to the patient, then have him or her lie down, close both eyes, and tilt the head slightly toward the side opposite to the area that is to receive the compress. Moisten a piece of 3 × 4 gauze in the center with a small amount of the sterile irrigating solution; place this over the affected eye, then gently rest the bag containing the ice on the moistened gauze. The corner of the bag can be taped to the patient's forehead. The cold will go through the moistened area of the gauze, and any condensation will be collected by the dry part of the gauze. The small amount of ice will take 15 to 20 minutes to melt, which is usually the length of time prescribed for a cold compress.

Other suggestions for cold compresses are the use of a rubber glove filled with a small amount of chipped ice and placed over the eye as mentioned above. Ice chips can also be placed in a clean washcloth and gently held against the eye (see Fig. 89–11).

When applying any compress to the eye, be careful not to exert pressure on the eye. Following compresses, the eye is gently dried.

Application and Care of Eye Dressings. Eye dressings may be applied for various reasons, e.g., to apply pressure to the eye (following enucleation); to protect the eye from light, infection, or injury; to cover a deformity of the eye; to eliminate double vision; to limit movement of the eye and prevent usage of the eye (following surgery or trauma); and to absorb secretions and blood. *Unless specifically ordered to do so, do not apply pressure to the eye when applying an eye dressing.* However, do apply the dressing firmly enough to

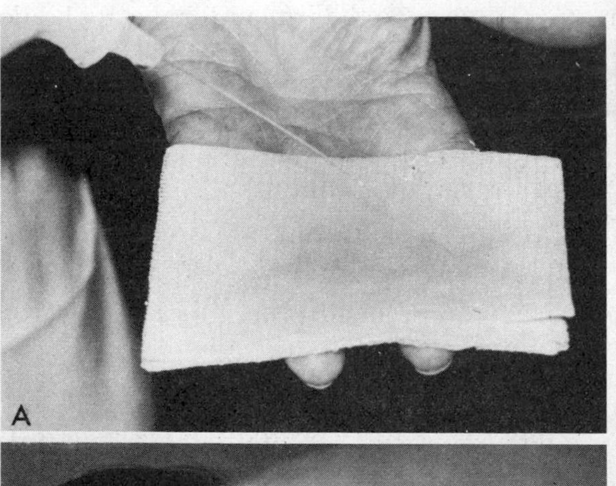

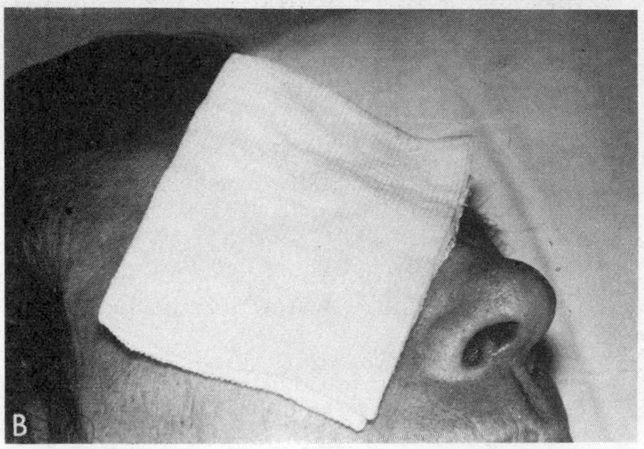

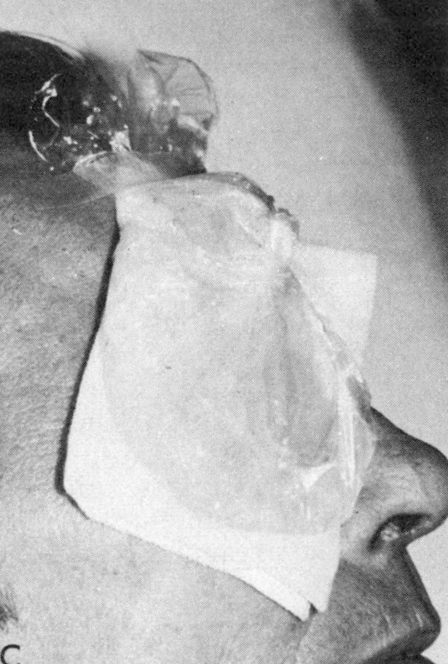

Figure 89–11. Cold compresses. **A.** Moisten center of sterile gauze. **B.** Place over patient's closed eye; have patient tilt head slightly toward the unaffected side. **C.** Tape small ice-filled plastic bag onto patient's forehead for 15–20 minutes. (Courtesy of Wills Eye Hospital, Philadelphia.)

hold the eyelid fairly securely against the cornea. If pressure is desired, two or three eye pads are applied. Occasionally additional pressure is obtained with a wrap-around head dressing.

> *An eye with a surface bacterial infection should not be covered with a dressing because covering promotes bacterial growth.*

Eye pads are composed of a layer of absorbent cotton between two layers of gauze. The pads are oval and are held in place with two narrow strips of Scotch tape or nonallergenic plastic adhesive tape. The eyelids must be closed if an eye pad or pads are to be applied to the eye. If the eye is not closed upon application of the dressing, the cornea will be abraded by the gauze of the eye pad.

At times, e.g., following surgery, it is desirable to protect the eyeball from pressure or rubbing. To accomplish this protection a metal or plastic eye shield is bent so it rests upon the bony prominences of the brow, cheek, and nose without touching the underlying dressing. The shield is taped in place as shown in Figure 89–12.

Protective covering and care of the eyes of unconscious patients is discussed in Unit X.

When removing an eye dressing loosen the tape first by pulling the tape gently off the forehead, then support the cheek with a finger and remove the tape and the dressing together with the other hand. Should the eye pad be contaminated it can be folded over with the contaminated part innermost. Do not slide it across the eye. Do not change eye dressings unless the physician has instructed you to do so.

Removal, Insertion, and Care of an Artificial Eye; Care of Eye Socket. Artificial eyes are hollow or shell-shaped structures made of plastic or glass and painted to match the patient's normal eye. Shell-shaped prostheses are more common but the type varies with the surgery performed. The artificial eye is generally fitted over a solid plastic sphere, i.e., "implant," which remains in the eye socket to prevent contracture of the socket tissues and to maintain the normal contour of the eyelids by filling the eye's socket. (See discussion of enucleation, p. 2004–2005.)

Artificial eyes are *removed* by pulling down the lower lid and pressing on the bony orbital rim with the fingers of one hand, while cupping the other hand under the eye to catch the prosthesis as it falls out of place (Fig. 89–13). After slipping the lower edge of the shell-like prosthesis out over the edge of the lower eyelid, ask the patient to squeeze the lids, and if the fingers are placed on the upper eyelid and gently pushed down the prosthesis will be squeezed into the waiting hand below. It is advisable to remove the eye over a soft surface, e.g., a folded towel or pillow, so if you fail to catch the prosthesis as it drops out of place, it does not break as it falls.

To *insert* the artificial eye, the following steps are performed: (a) the eye is wetted; (b) the prosthesis is held with the apex pointing toward the nasal side and gently slid under the patient's upper eyelid; (c) with the other hand the lower eyelid is pulled down; and (d) the patient is asked to blink. The artificial eye will slip into place. Before inserting an artificial eye, be certain you are holding the prosthesis in the correct position; otherwise, only the white of the eye will be showing, and the eye will have to be removed and replaced.

Occasionally a patient who wears an artificial eye has a small rubber suction device to place and remove the prosthesis. To *remove* the eye, the suction cup is moistened, squeezed, placed against the iris of the artificial eye, and twisted somewhat counterclockwise (after the lower lid is pulled down with the index finger). After the eye

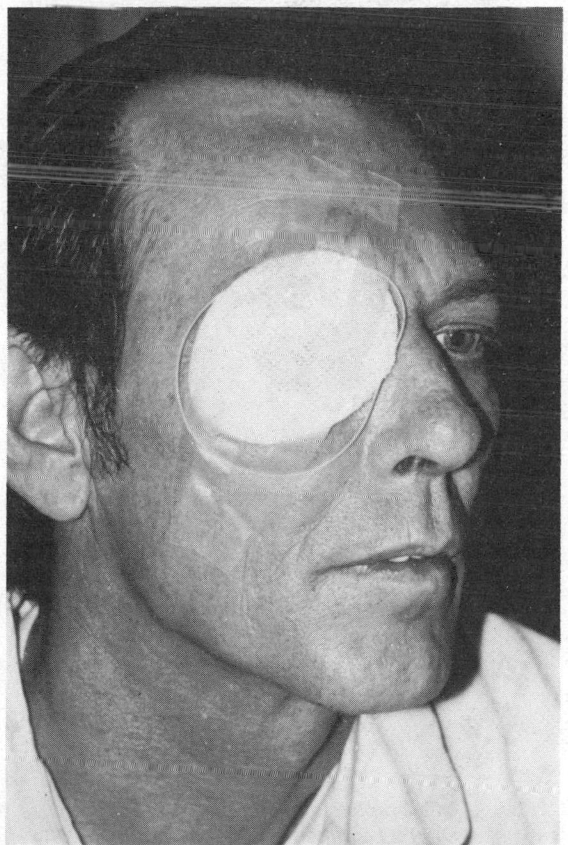

Figure 89–12. Eye patch and plastic shield. Tape is placed diagonally from forehead to cheek. (Courtesy of Wills Eye Hospital, Philadelphia.)

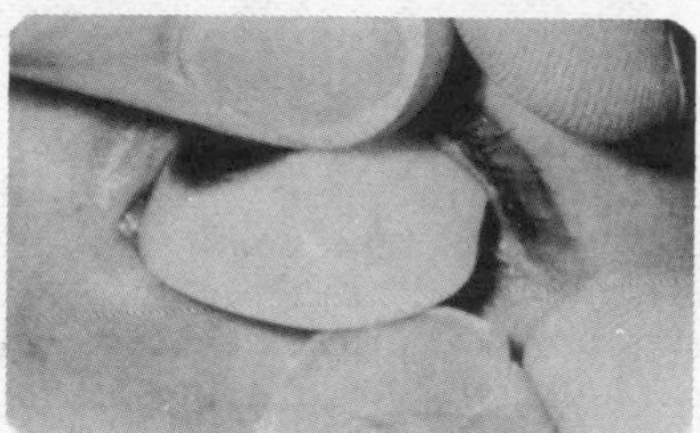

***Depressing** lower lid allows prosthesis to slide out and down.*

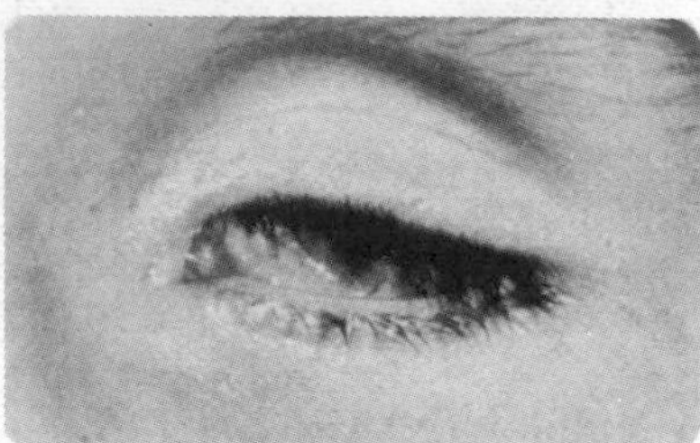

***Socket** after removal; wash off external matter and encrustations.*

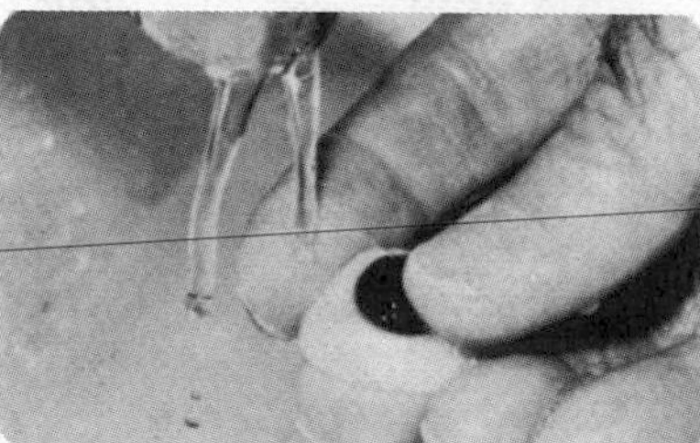

***Wash prosthesis** with soap and water; scrub with thumb and finger.*

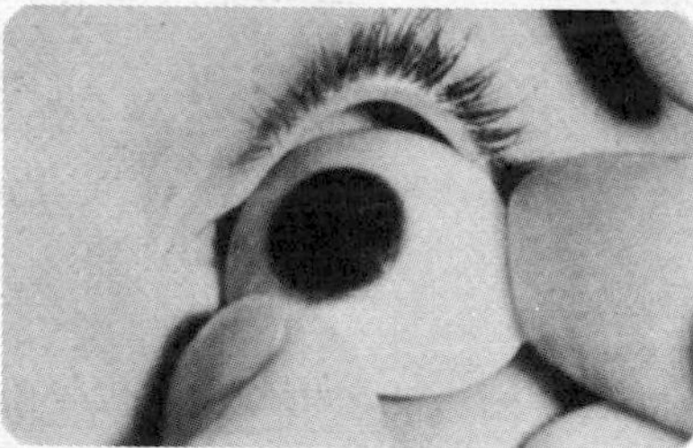

***Lift upper lid,** depress lower lid, and slip artificial eye in place.*

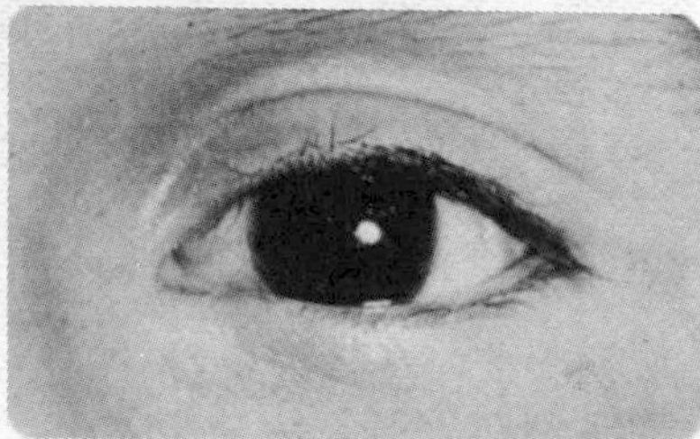

***Once prosthesis** is in place, eye should be wiped toward the nose.*

Figure 89–13. Care of an artificial eye. (From Zucnick, M.: Care of an artificial eye. *American Journal of Nursing,* 75:835, May 1975.)

is placed on a soft surface, the suction is broken by squeezing the suction cup slightly. The device is then removed from the prosthesis. To *replace* the eye by using a suction device, first moisten the tip of the suction cup, squeeze it, and place it over the iris. Then retract the upper lid and place the eye as discussed in the preceding paragraph. Remove the suction device from the properly positioned eye by applying a small amount of pressure on the eye with one finger while squeezing and removing the suction cup.

Because it is important to maintain a clean socket and prevent infection, it is essential that one's hands be washed before insertion and removal of the eye. Following removal of an artificial eye, the socket may be irrigated with a solution as ordered.

Artificial eyes are to be removed only for routine cleansing. After the prosthesis is removed, it is placed in a gauze pad and may be washed under running water. The prosthesis is then stored in a safe place on a clean piece of gauze or in a labeled envelope. Since it is kept dry, it will need to be moistened before reinsertion. When handling and cleaning the artificial eye, take care not to scratch or chip its surface or edges. Do not use alcohol or other corrosive chemicals to clean plastic artificial eyes.

To minimize the formation of secretions in the socket, the prosthesis may be lubricated with a commercially prepared ophthalmic solution. If the patient develops sinusitis or a head cold, the amount of socket secretions may increase. When secretions are increased, it is desirable to remove the eye more frequently and cleanse the eye and socket.

The patient with an artificial eye requires instruction as follows:

- How to remove, cleanse, inspect, and replace the prosthesis, and how to care for the socket. Weekly, the prosthesis's edges and surface should be inspected for rough places. If damaged, rough, or scratched, the eye should not be reinserted but should be taken to an ocularist for possible repair.

- Do not vigorously rub the eye when the prosthesis is in place. Rubbing may displace the prosthesis (perhaps causing it to fall out) or may injure the socket (by forcibly pushing the hard edge of the prosthesis against the socket rims).

- When the prosthesis is in place, if it is necessary to wipe the eyelid, do so in a direction *from the inner to the outer canthus, or just blot the canthi.* The prosthesis should fit tightly enough so that normal gentle irrigations will not displace it. If it is not being held in place adequately by the lids, the patient is probably a candidate for assessment by either an ocularist or a plastic surgeon.

In addition to instructing the patient about prosthesis care, the nurse of course practices these appropriate activities when caring for a patient with a prosthesis who is unable to care for the eye or socket alone.

Common Ocular Medications

Numerous medications are used in ophthalmology. Some of the more common groups of these medications and some examples of specific medications in each group are briefly summarized in the following outline.

I. *Local anesthetics:* act to anesthetize the eye and thus prevent pain during various ocular procedures. Both topical and injectable anesthetics are available for use in ophthalmology.
   A. *Topical anesthetics:* proparacaine hydrochloride (Ophthaine, Ophthetic), 0.5 per cent; benoxinate hydrochloride (Dorsacaine), 0.4 per cent; tetracaine hydrochloride (Pontocaine), 0.5 per cent; cocaine hydrochloride, 2 to 10 per cent.
   B. *Injectable local anesthetics:* lidocaine hydrochloride (Xylocaine), 1 and 2 per cent; procaine hydrochloride (Novocaine), 1 and 2 per cent.

II. *Parasympathomimetic drugs,* i.e., drugs which produce effects resembling those of stimulation of parasympathetic nerves. Used as miotics to control intraocular pressure in glaucoma by widening filtration angle and permitting outflow of aqueous humor. Also used to treat certain types of strabismus.
   A. *Group I: Cholinergic drugs* which act directly on myoneural junction; produce strong contractions of iris (i.e., miosis) and ciliary body musculature (accommodation). Sympathomimetic agents will reverse the action of these drugs.
      1. *Examples* of cholinergic drugs: pilocarpine hydrochloride, 0.5 to 6 per cent; carbachol (Doryl), 1.5 to 3 per cent; acetylcholine chloride (Miochol), 1 per cent.
   B. *Group II: Cholinesterase inhibitors* (i.e., anticholinesterase drugs). Action of these drugs is difficult to reverse.
      1. *Examples* of cholinesterase inhibitors: echothiopate iodide (Phospholine iodide), 0.03 to 0.125 per cent; physostigmine salicylate (eserine), 0.25 and 0.5 per cent; isoflurophate (di-isopropyl fluorophosphate, DFP, Floropryl), 0.25 per cent ophthalmic ointment and 0.1 per cent ophthalmic solution.

III. *Parasympatholytic drugs* (anticholinergic drugs), i.e., those which produce effects resembling those of interruption of parasympathetic nerve supply to a part. Used to facilitate ophthalmoscopic examination and refraction; also used in treatment of uveitis (to rest eye in inflammatory conditions). Parasympatholytic medications cause smooth muscle of ciliary body and iris to relax, thus producing mydriasis (i.e., extreme pupillary dilatation) and cycloplegia (i.e., paralysis of ciliary muscle, resulting in paralysis of accommodation). *Note:* In predisposed persons pupillary dilatation can precipitate acute glaucoma, which can result in blindness if untreated.
   A. *Mydriatics:* e.g., eucatropine hydrochloride (Euphthalmine), 2 to 5 per cent.
   B. *Cycloplegics,* e.g., atropine sulfate, 0.5, 1, and 2 per cent; scopolamine hydrobromide (hyoscine), 0.25 to 5 per cent; homatropine hydrobromide, 1 to 5 per cent; cyclopentolate hydrochloride (Cyclogyl), 1 and 2 per cent; tropicamide (Mydriacyl), 0.5 and 1 per cent.

IV. *Sympathomimetic drugs (adrenergic drugs),* i.e., drugs which produce effects similar to those of impulses carried by adrenergic postganglionic fibers of sympathetic nervous system, are used in ophthalmology primarily to produce mydriasis and vasoconstriction; do not cause cycloplegia. Vasoconstriction appears to decrease rate of formation of aqueous humor. Also these drugs may increase outflow of aqueous humor, thus reducing intraocular pressure. Although used in treating some forms of glaucoma, adrenergic drugs are contraindicated in treatment of narrow angle glaucomas (dilation of pupil causes closure of anterior chamber angle and may markedly increase intraocular pressure).
   Examples of sympathomimetic drugs: epinephrine hydrochloride (Adrenaline), 1:1000; epinephrine bitartrate or epinephrine borate 0.5 to 2 per cent; phenylephrine hydrochloride (Neo-Synephrine), 0.125 to 10 per cent; hydroxyamphetamine hydrochloride ophthalmic solution (Paredrine), 1 per cent.

V. *Dyes:* Various dyes are used to stain cornea to identify corneal disorders, e.g., abrasions, ulcerations.
   Examples of dyes used in ophthalmology: sterile fluorescein sodium ophthalmic solution (sterile papers or single-dose containers of 2 per cent solution); rose bengal, 1 per cent.

VI. *Irrigating solutions:* Irrigating solutions used on an injured eye must be sterile and for single-patient use. If corneal epithelial tissues and sclera are intact, sterile nonirritating solutions may be used on more than one patient from same bottle.

VII. *Antibiotics:* They may be used locally or systemically, depending upon disorder being treated.
   Examples of topical antibiotics: chloramphenicol (Chloromycetin), topically as 1 per cent ointment, or 0.25 to 0.5 per cent solu-

tion; combination of neomycin, polymyxin, and bacitracin (Neosporin).

Examples of systemic antibiotics: penicillin, tetracycline, gentamicin, Keflin.

VIII. *Sulfonamides:* Sulfonamides are perhaps the most commonly used medications in treating conjunctivitis.

Examples of sulfonamides: sulfisoxazole (Gantrisin), 4 per cent ointment and 4 per cent solution; sulfacetamide sodium (sodium sulamyd), 10 per cent ointment and 10, 15, and 30 per cent solution.

IX. *Adrenal corticosteroids:* Steroids are effective in treating nonpyrogenic inflammations, allergic reactions, and severe ocular injuries. They are useful in decreasing vascularization and scarring following chemical burns, trauma, and severe inflammation. They may increase ocular susceptibility to fungus infection; prolonged ocular steroid therapy may cause increased intraocular pressure and cataracts. Corticosteroids come in various forms for ocular use and are available in various strengths and in combination with various antibiotics.

Examples of corticosteroids available for ocular use: cortisone acetate; hydrocortisone; methyl-prednisolone; prednisone; prednisolone; dexamethasone; betamethasone; triamcinolone acetonide; Medrysone.

X. *Carbonic anhydrase inhibitors:* Carbonic anhydrase inhibitors may be administered in treatment of glaucoma (where intraocular pressure is abnormally high) to reduce formation of aqueous humor and thus reduce intraocular pressure. Diuresis is produced.

Examples of carbonic anhydrase inhibitors: acetazolamide (Diamox); dichlorphenamide (Daranide, Oratrol); ethoxyzolamide (Cardrase, Ethamide); methazolamine (Neptazane).

XI. *Other materials:*

Silicone fluids: Used to lubricate the eye socket when an artificial eye is worn. These fluids reduce irritation, increase comfort, prevent crusting on the lids, and give a lifelike effect to the prosthesis.

Methylcellulose, 0.5 to 2 per cent: This solution, sometimes called "artificial tears," provides moisture and lubrication to the eye when normal tear production is impaired or lid closure is incomplete.

Space does not permit detailed discussion of the various drugs used in ophthalmology. Familiarize yourself with details as necessary by referring to a textbook of pharmacology and watch for the development of side effects when caring for patients receiving these medications. Remember the importance of minimizing absorption of ocular medications through the lacrimal system during instillation of eye drops.

The following additional *guidelines* are important in the use of ophthalmic medications:

- *Never instill medication into the eye unless it is ordered by a physician.*
- *Do not use "old" medications,* i.e., those that have been on the shelf for a long while. Check the expiration date on the medication. Two weeks is a reasonable time to use a solution before discarding it. Date the bottle at the time it is procured from the pharmacy.
- *Before using ocular solutions,* e.g., "eye drops," *inspect them,* e.g., for cloudiness, discoloration, and precipitation. If precipitate is present or if the solution is cloudy or discolored, do not use it.
- *Follow package instructions concerning proper storage of eye medications.*
- *Use no stock solutions.* Medications should be either the patient's own medication or individual "one-time" packaging.
- *Ophthalmic solutions must be sterile.* They are prepared and handled with the same degree of caution against contamination that is given to fluids intended for IV administration. Use sterile medications supplied in sterile, disposable, single-use eyedropper units.
- *Use eyedroppers correctly.* Do not use the same eyedropper to instill two different medications. Do not allow medication in an eyedropper to flow back into the dropper's bulb, and do not return medication remaining in the eyedropper back into the bottle after instillation. Such practices cause contamination of the medication.
- *Check carefully which medication is to be inserted in which eye.* Different medications may be ordered for each of the two eyes.
- *Familiarize yourself with specific eye medications.* Certain medications are definitely contraindicated for certain eye disorders.
- *Never substitute a solution or medication of one strength for that of another strength without permission from the physician.* Also, never substitute one eye medication for another without permission.
- *Carefully read instructions and labels for all ocular medications* (and any other ocular treatment). If labels are smeared or otherwise unreadable, discard them or return them to pharmacy for relabeling.
- *Never use an unlabeled solution or ointment on the eye or around the eye.*

GENERAL FACTORS CONCERNING SURGERY ON THE EYE

Introduction

Eye surgery accounts for 10 per cent of the operations performed in the United States on persons over age 65. While some ocular surgeries (e.g., surgery on extraocular muscles) are performed under general anesthesia, most eye surgeries are performed under local anesthesia. In many hospitals the anesthesiologist is responsible for the sedation of the patient; therefore, small amounts of sedation tend to be ordered preoperatively and supplemented by the anesthesia department during surgery. Topical eye medications and local anesthesia, including facial nerve blocks or retrobulbar injections, are used. *Local anesthetics are preferred* to a general anesthetic for eye surgery when possible because restlessness may follow administration of general anesthesia; a restless patient may accidentally cause eye injury. During local anesthesia, depending on anesthesia policy, the patient may be permitted to keep dentures in place to maintain facial contour. But more often the dentures are removed; they can be replaced in the patient's mouth as soon as he or she has recovered enough to ask for them. During surgery the surgeon can enlist the help of the patient who has only had a local anesthetic. For example the patient can be asked to "look up," "look down," or follow other directions.

Strong solutions of germicides are not tolerated by the eye; otherwise the rules of asepsis and antisepsis which govern general surgery are also indicated for ophthalmic surgery. To prepare the operative area, the physician may preoperatively order prophylactic antibiotics (eyedrops or systemic), cleansing of the face, ocular irrigations, and cutting of the eyelashes. Many eye surgeons prefer to prepare the eye, e.g., irrigate it, cut lashes, and so forth, in surgery rather than having these procedures performed on the ward.

Psychologic care is highly important for patients who are hospitalized for eye surgery. Fear and depression are common reactions. Many patients are apprehensive about having their eyes operated on while they are "awake." The possible loss of vision is of real concern. Older patients easily become confused or disoriented.

The techniques of ocular surgery have greatly improved over recent decades. Three major advances have been in the therapy of retinal detachment, the treatment of corneal scarring, and cataract extraction. The details of specific ocular surgeries have been discussed throughout the unit. Here we briefly discuss some general preoperative and postoperative considerations pertaining to eye surgery.

Preoperative Care

Because the patient's vision may be absent or impaired following eye surgery (e.g., due to eye dressings and eye medications as well as the trauma of the operative procedure), it is particularly important to preoperatively orient the patient to the environment and to introduce the patient to other staff members as well as those patients in the same room. Familiarizing the patient with the surroundings preoperatively not only makes the patient generally more comfortable psychologically but also may specifically lessen postoperative disorientation. This appears particularly true of elderly persons.

Before surgery attempt to identify and discuss the patient's operative concerns. Patients often are fearful are of pain which may occur with operative procedures on the eye. Also, many patients are particularly tense about having any surgery performed on the eye because of emotional feelings about the eye and its importance. Tell patients if the eyes will be bandaged after surgery so they will be prepared for this. Discuss with them ways in which you will help during the time they have the eye (or eyes) bandaged. At an appropriate time before surgery, teach the patient about postoperative procedures and necessary restrictions. Be sure to tell the patient not to lean over the edge of the bed after surgery because this increases intraocular pressure. Inform the patient that medication will be available after surgery for pain and that a medication may be ordered to prevent nausea if necessary. Additionally, medications may be ordered to suppress coughing and to facilitate bowel movements (to prevent straining). Emphasize that patients should feel free to tell the nurse how they are feeling so medications and other appropriate care can be given to keep them comfortable. If a local anesthetic is to be used instruct the person to hold the head still during surgery and not to squeeze the eye shut. Tell the patient that the doctor will be talking during surgery and will be giving directions as to what the patient should do.

Specific preoperative orders vary, depending upon the physician, hospital policies, the procedure to be performed, and the type of anesthetic to be used. Check orders carefully for each patient. Preoperative orders may specify for male patients to shave closely before surgery. Shampooing of the hair should be done before hospital admission for eye surgery, for these activities are going to be restricted for a time postoperatively to protect the eye. In some cases the condition of the patient's eye does not allow these activities even preoperatively. It may be advisable to comb and braid the patient's hair if it is long. Cleansing enemas are usually not ordered before ocular surgery since local anesthetics are predominantly used. However, sometimes enemas are ordered preoperatively if straining is contraindicated after surgery.

Give eye medications *at the precise time* they are ordered preoperatively, so the eye will be in a state of readiness at the time of surgery. Medications may be ordered to dilate or constrict the pupil. Other preoperative medications may include: pentobarbital sodium (Nembutal), chloral hydrate, or meperidine hydrochloride (Demerol). Currently, oral diazepam (Valium) is very much in vogue, but this, like the administration of atropine sulfate, will depend upon the policies of the anesthesia department. As mentioned earlier, usually topical anesthetics are instilled in the operating room, and a local nerve block may also be administered.

The surgeon may wish to cut off the eyelashes in preparation for surgery on the eye. The blades of the scissors are lubricated with petrolatum jelly so the cut lashes will adhere to the blade surface rather than falling into the eye. Before surgery begins, the eyebrows and area of the skin around the eye are cleaned, and the eye is irrigated. Sometimes a mark is made on the forehead over the eye to be operated on so the correct eye is easily identified. At the time of surgery the operative team checks carefully to ensure that surgery is performed on the correct eye.

Preoperative charting should include comments concerning the patient's attitude toward the surgery to be performed, as well as charting regarding preparation of the patient for surgery.

Postoperative Care

As with preoperative orders, considerable variation exists concerning postoperative orders following ocular surgery. Usually few if any restrictions are placed on the activity of patients who have *not* had intraocular procedures. However, postoperative attempts are made to minimize the stress on the eye that has had intraocular surgery, because while the intact, healthy eye can tolerate numerous stresses upon it, the eye which is weakened or damaged by intraocular surgery is highly vulnerable. Following intraocular procedures, the eye is in a delicate condition for several weeks or months. Below are details relevant to postoperative care following *intraocular* surgical procedures.

Following intraocular surgery the major goals of care are to (a) prevent hemorrhage; (b) prevent stress on the suture line; (c) prevent increased intraocular pressure; (d) minimize jerky movements of the patient's head; (e) prevent infection; (f) minimize sensory deprivation; and (g) prevent complications of immobility and anesthesia.

When the patient is being transferred from the operating table onto a bed or stretcher, the patient's body is lifted in horizontal alignment, often using a lifter. However, if local anesthesia is used, the patient may be encouraged to slide onto the bed while a nurse supports the head. Patients are seldom totally immobilized after ocular surgery these days, but they may be positioned depending on the procedure that has been performed. A general guideline is that a patient may lie on the back or on the unoperated side after returning from the operating room. If a different position is to be used, this will be written as a postoperative order, e.g., "head of bed up 45 degrees" or "lie on stomach in a face-down position as much as possible." A small pillow may be given for comfort.

Once the patient is correctly positioned in bed, put up the siderails and give the patient the call bell. Always tell patients who you are and reorient them to the surroundings and to the time of day. Avoid bumping the bed while giving care, and keep the immediate area free of bright lights. Keep a record of intake and output and observe for urinary retention and abdominal distention. The current trend is to discontinue the intravenous infusion as soon as it is completed; encourage the patient to start taking fluids when recovered sufficiently from the anesthesia, and permit the person to go to the bathroom with help as soon as he or she is awake enough to be safe. It has been found that this early mobilization cuts down on urinary retention and abdominal distention, and the psychologic fear of using a bedpan. Following ocular surgery the patient is *not* urged to routinely cough, but rather is encouraged to frequently and regularly take deep breaths to expand the lungs and to keep the tracheobronchial tree clear of secretions. Coughing is contraindicated because it increases intraocular pressure. If the patient is on bed rest, to improve circulation while in bed and prevent fatigue, supervise and see that the patient regularly performs active range-of-motion arm and leg exercises without moving the head. Some physicians prescribe isometric exercises.

Check the physician's orders before giving care to a patient following intraocular surgery to determine restrictions on activities. Are the following allowed: (a) head elevation (how much); (b) turning (both sides or one side); (c) shaving; and (d) tooth brushing? (It may be more judicious to have the patient use only a mouth wash in the immediate postoperative period.) Secure the physician's permission before allowing the patient to read, smoke, brush teeth, shave. Usually the patient is discouraged from hair washing until after discharge and the first postoperative office visit.

Following intraocular surgery the patient must learn to prevent pressure upon the globe until the incision in the eye has healed and the eye can again tolerate the stresses of normal daily activities. The patient and significant others are instructed concerning positions which the patient may and may not assume, and activities which are permitted or are contraindicated.

Following surgery on the eye, use restraints only if the safety of the patient is in jeopardy. Straining against anything, including restraints, is to be avoided, as it may elevate the intraocular pressure. When used, explain to the patient why the restraint is being used ("to prevent you from hurting your eye") and tell the patient restraints will be used for only a short time. Carefully observe the restrained patient; do not assume the attitude that because the person is restrained he or she is "O.K." The disoriented or mentally retarded patient may continually touch the operated eye, and light wrist restraints may be needed, but often repeated touching of the eye is an indication that the patient is not comfortable or has pain. Generally speaking, most patients can be encouraged not to handle their eye patch. Frequent skin care and frequent position changes are important aspects of care for any restrained patient.

Lying on the unoperated side keeps the operated eye free from pressure and also prevents possible contamination of the dressing if the patient vomits. If the patient does vomit after intraocular surgery, do not raise the head, but rather hold the head toward the unoperated side. Most patients return from the operating room with an antiemetic order to cover the first signs of nausea and so prevent emesis and the straining that accompanies retching.

Frequently patients are allowed out of bed on the first postoperative day. The current trend is to ambulate patients earlier and earlier. Generally activities which would increase venous pressure in the head and thus would increase intraocular pressure are restricted for several weeks.

Activities which increase intraocular pressure, and are thus contraindicated, include excessive energy exertion, extreme emotion, sudden jerky movements, sneezing, coughing, running, jumping, straining at bowel movements, bending over, lifting or pushing heavy objects, rubbing the eyes, and tightly closing the eyes. Teach the patient to try to avoid coughing by deep breathing when he or she feels a need to cough and to keep the mouth open while coughing (this reduces pressure inside the head). Instruct the patient to immediately notify a nurse if he or she feels nauseated. An antiemetic is administered as soon as a patient feels nauseated. Do not wait until a patient vomits before giving the medication. Also, tell the patient not to forcefully squeeze the eyelids shut or to rub or press on the eye or eye dressing.

Because understanding is an important aspect of patient acceptance of restrictions, be certain to *tell the patient why activity is being temporarily limited.* When emphasizing to the patient the need for postoperative restrictions, tell the patient that eye tissue requires more time to heal than other body tissues.

Observe sterile technique for all procedures performed on the eye following intraocular surgery. The development of intraocular infection is a serious complication.

Conveniently arrange items on the patient's bedside stand so the person can easily reach them without straining. Then place the bedside stand on the unoperated side so the patient is not tempted to turn onto the operated side.

Keep the patient as comfortable as possible postoperatively by frequent slight position changes, by providing back and skin care, and by giving analgesics as indicated. Generally postoperative eye pain can be controlled with Demerol, Darvon, or aspirin. Avoid opiates for pain control if possible, since they may cause vomiting.

Because sneezing and coughing are especially hazardous for patients following intraocular surgery, in some hospitals these patients are not allowed to have pepper on their trays (since it may make them sneeze or may cause them to choke and cough). The use of talcum powders or other similar products, which could cause sneezing and coughing, may also be prohibited. Care should be taken not to expose patients to substances to which they are known to be or may be allergic, e.g., foods, drugs, plants. Nurses should be watchful for any indications of the development of an upper respiratory infection in a patient who has intraocular surgery. Indications of such a condition should be reported to the physician.

The dressings must never be removed from a patient's eye for inspection during the immediate postoperative period by anyone but the ophthalmologist, unless the physician has given specific orders for a nurse to do so. If an eye dressing comes loose, it should be gently replaced, including the protective shield. Remind the patient to keep both eyes closed when this is being done so as not to abrade the cornea of the patched eye. Normally a small amount of serous drainage occurs postoperatively. Additionally the eyelid may be edematous for a few days, and subconjunctival hemorrhages may be present.

Notify the physician at once of any indications of complications. Prompt treatment may prevent serious eye injury. The physician should be informed of coughing, marked restlessness, sharp eye pain or eye pain which is not relieved by analgesics, disorientation, symptoms of an upper respiratory infection (e.g., rhinitis) [remember that as the operative eye tears, the nostril on that side will also drip, so don't confuse this with a U.R.I.—the drip is unilateral], obvious hemorrhage, disturbance of the dressing, and the patient assuming contraindicated postures or activities. Feelings of sharp pain or pressure in the eye suggest hemorrhage; sharp pain may also indicate possible infection.

Marked restlessness most often occurs when a patient has both eyes bandaged and when the patient is an older person. Since both eyes turn together, the surgeon may bandage both eyes to provide rest for the operated eye. Sometimes the physician leaves an order for the unoperated eye to be uncovered if the patient becomes quite restless or during meals. Usually removal of this one dressing helps the patient to become calmer and to become reoriented if the person is disoriented. Minor mental symptoms which patients with bilateral eye patches may develop (as a result of sensory deprivation) include restlessness, mental clouding, perceptual disorientation, mood changes, and thinking disturbances. More serious mental symptoms include memory impairment, confusion, disorientation, and vivid hallucinations. These symptoms frequently increase in the evening when patients have bilateral eye patches. Patients experiencing these mental changes as a result of bilateral patching may also perform actions which they have been told are contraindicated, e.g., they may pull off their eye dressings and assume contraindicated postures. It is obviously desirable to minimize sensory deprivation following intraocular surgery, to prevent the above problems.

In an attempt to keep the patient oriented postoperatively and to combat sensory deprivation, the patient should be:

1. Placed in a room where there is an oriented and active patient
2. Observed closely for indications of disorientation (especially older persons)
3. Stimulated frequently verbally and physically (e.g., by frequently talking with the patient, and by touching the patient's hand or arm while talking)
4. Visited frequently by nurses and visitors, to decrease isolation

If a general anesthetic is given, it is important to begin to reorient the patient as soon as the person begins to recover from the anesthesia. Always tell the patient who has bilateral dressings (and thus cannot see) when you enter or leave the room and when you are about to touch the patient.

Following intraocular surgery, it is helpful if relaxing diversional activities are provided for the patient during recovery. Such activities must be in keeping with the patient's interests and abilities.

The patient with impaired vision must be protected from accidental injury postoperatively. Keep siderails up on all patients with bilateral eye dressings and on all disoriented patients. Also be sure the patient's protective eye shield is properly positioned and secured in place. Following surgery observe the patient carefully to be certain the eye patch is not accidentally removed and thus the eye possibly injured. Do not allow the patient to smoke unsupervised, because it is easy for a lighted ash to fall unnoticed by the patient with impaired vision. Keep the patient's call bell in place at all times. Keep everything in its proper and familiar place so the patient will be less likely to have an accident while reaching for something or otherwise moving about. Once the patient can be out of bed, assist with ambulation so the person does not bump, fall, or otherwise become injured. When assisting the patient with food or drink, be careful to prevent choking and aspiration.

Following intraocular surgery eating may be resumed as soon as the patient desires and once he or she is able to take and retain adequate fluids. Some physicians believe that abdominal distention and discomfort are reduced if the patient receives a diet which requires moderate chewing.

When feeding a person who cannot see, be certain you first describe the food on the tray to the patient. Patients who cannot see what they are being fed frequently say that all food tastes the same to them. Descriptions of the food being fed helps to improve perceptions of that food. Attempt to make the meal time a pleasant, unhurried experience for the person who must be fed. Try to understand how difficult it is for a person to eat without being able to see and having to be fed. You might practice helping a sightless person to eat by blindfolding and feeding a classmate. Then reverse roles and take your turn as the patient.

If a patient must remain on *prolonged bed rest* following eye surgery, it is important that isometric or other exercises be performed frequently. Other appropriate care can be administered to prevent the complications of prolonged inactivity. Frequent deep breathing sessions (not coughing) to clear the lungs and frequent position changes are also highly important (see also Unit VIII). Of course, it is necessary to maintain the patient's fluid-electrolyte and nutritional status. Constipation due to inactivity must be prevented since straining at stool may cause a hazardous rise in intraocular pressure. A laxative of choice may be ordered to minimize straining with bowel movements. Many eye surgeons allow bathroom privileges with help, believing the effort is less for the patient in the bathroom than with the bedpan.

Significant others can be very helpful following eye surgery. For example, they may be able to sit with the patient and watch to see that the person stays properly positioned and does not disturb the eye dressing. Also, they may visit with and read to the patient and thus help keep the person oriented. By being available to hand things to the patient, family members or friends may prevent the person from lifting the head, reaching, straining, and possibly injuring the eye. Visitors can also help by feeding the patient. However, today's patients are encouraged to resume active daily living tasks as soon as they can postoperatively.

Prior to discharge be sure the patient (and significant others) understands restrictions which are necessary to prevent elevation of intraocular pressure, and see that they are familiar with home care procedures, e.g., instillation of eye drops. Sponge baths may be necessary for a period of time at home, and it may be desirable for the patient to wear a metal or plastic eye shield at night or when lying down, to protect the eye. Dark glasses may be worn if the patient is photophobic; shading the room from sunlight also helps the patient to feel more comfortable. All patients receiving dilating drops may need dark glasses. Instruct the patient who will be wearing any type of glasses postoperatively to hold glasses by the tips of their bows when putting them on to avoid accidentally poking the eyes. Teach the patient how to properly care for eyeglasses or contact lenses or both. Instruct the patient to grasp both arms of a chair before sitting down, to prevent slipping and possibly falling. Emphasize to the patient that eyes must not be rubbed or wiped with a soiled handkerchief. Be certain the patient realizes the importance of keeping follow-up appointments with the physician and the necessity for contacting the doctor whenever untoward symptoms develop. If enucleation has been performed, the patient must be instructed regarding the use and care of an artificial eye.

COMMON SPECIFIC DISORDERS OF THE EYE AND RELATED STRUCTURES AND THEIR CLINICAL MANAGEMENT

Disorders of the Eyelids

Common disorders of the eyelids and their treatment are summarized below. The eyelids normally function to protect the eyes (from foreign bodies, external injury, undue exposure, excessive light) and to lubricate the eyeball by distributing secretions over the eyeball (thus washing away dust and keeping the cornea moist and transparent).

Blepharitis. Blepharitis is an inflammation of the lid margins, sometimes called "granulated eyelids." The patient experiences irritation, burning, and itching of the eyelids; the lid margins are "red-rimmed" in appearance and have scales or "granulations" clinging to them. In some cases the lid margins are ulcerated and the eyelashes tend to fall out. *Treatment* consists of (a) removal of scales from the lids daily with a damp cotton applicator; (b) cleanliness of the scalp, eyebrows, and lid margins; (c) application of an antibiotic or sulfonamide eye ointment once daily to the lid margins with a cotton applicator to prevent build-up of the scales on the lids.

Chalazion. A chalazion is a granulomatous enlargement of the meibomian gland resulting from occlusion of the gland's duct. Most frequently a chalazion points toward the lid's conjunctival side. The patient notices a painless, slow-growing, hard, nontender, round mass growing on the eyelid. The skin can be moved loosely over the growth; the conjunctiva in the region of the chalazion is elevated and red. Vision is distorted if the lesion is large enough to impress the cornea. *Treatment* consists of excision, or incision and curettage (performed in the physician's office or clinic) if the chalazion does not spontaneously absorb or recede following the application of hot compresses and topical steroid-antimicrobial therapy. After surgical removal, an eye pad may be worn from 8 to 24 hours, then warm compresses may be restarted, and an antibacterial ointment, e.g., neomycin sulfate, may be applied to the conjunctiva.

Hordeolum (Stye). A hordeolum is a pustular inflammation of an eyelash follicle or sebaceous gland on the lid margin. Hordeola (styes) are common painful disorders of the eyelid. The intensity of the pain is directly related to the amount of swelling. Staphylococci are typically the causative organisms. Common in all age groups, styes often propagate a "crop" of infections along the lid margins which may last for long periods of time when the skin's resistance to staphylococci is reduced. Patients with styes should be instructed not to "squeeze" at the lesion, since this spreads the infection. The disorder typically begins with local irritation, redness, and swelling and progresses to an acutely tender abscess formation which points "outwards" from the lid margin. Usually styes discharge after 3–4 days. *Treatment* consists of application of warm, moist compresses to hasten suppuration. Usually if compresses are used the stye opens and drains without surgery.

Virus Infections. *Herpes simplex* is an acute viral infection which produces superficial clear cutaneous vesicles that heal without scarring. When such vesicles occur on the eyelid, one must be cautious not to inoculate their contents onto the cornea. Such inoculation could produce a dendritic corneal ulcer. These corneal ulcers commonly occur. Corticosteroid treatment is *contraindicated* in the treatment of acute herpes simplex corneal infection, since it can cause spread of the infection (resulting in the formation of disabling corneal scar tissue).

Herpes zoster involving the eye typically has a unilateral trigeminal distribution (see Unit X). These skin lesions are deeper than those of the herpes simplex infection, Also, they are painful, tend to become secondarily infected, and often leave permanent scars. Ophthalmic herpes zoster is treated vigorously with mydriatic, antibiotic, and corticosteroid ointment. Skin lesions should be kept clean of infection and crusts by means of antibiotic ointment, mechanical cleansing, and hot soaks.

Disorders of the Extraocular Muscles

Introduction. *Binocular vision,* i.e., the normal simultaneous use of both eyes which results in depth perception, was discussed briefly on page 1950 (see also pp. 2000 and 2001). In order to maintain binocular vision, simultaneous binocular movements of both eyes are necessary. Such movements require the coordinated use of the extraocular muscles. The eyes need to be properly aligned in order for corresponding retinal areas to be stimulated by the same object. Thus, convergence is necessary for near vision so that both macular areas can fixate on a single object. Normally anatomically corresponding areas in each retina have a common visual direction in space; the principal corresponding points of the retinas are the right and left *foveae.* The fovea is the central portion of the retina with the highest visual acuity.

The two pictures received from the eyes may be used within the brain in three different ways: (1) normal fusion may occur; (2) diplopia may occur; or (3) suppression may occur. In normal vision *fusion* occurs. "Fusion" refers to the cerebral synthesis of the two ocular pictures into a single mental image. Fusion occurs when the two eyes are perfectly aligned so that both foveae are aimed exactly at the same point. When disparate rather than corresponding retinal points are stimulated, the retinal images cannot be fused into a single mental impression. In such a situation *diplopia* results. "Diplopia" refers to double vision. Usually diplopia is caused by faulty alignment of the two eyes. "Suppression" refers to the phenomenon of one mental image being ignored if the two eyes send two different mental images to the brain. If you are able to use a monocular microscope effectively with both eyes open you are practicing normal suppression. Although the brain is receiving both the image of the table or surface upon which the microscope sits (from one open eye) and the image seen through the microscope (i.e., the magnified field), the brain focuses only on the image of the magnified field and suppresses the other image. Suppression may irreversibly damage vision in the deviating eye at an early age, usually before the age of four years. The latter visual loss is termed *suppression amblyopia.*

Strabismus. "Strabismus" refers to a deviation of an eye which the patient cannot overcome. Thus, the two eyes are not straight when fixing on an object, i.e., the visual axes do not remain parallel. While one eye (the fixing eye) looks directly at the object of attention, the other eye (the deviating eye) does not. Synonyms for strabismus include "squint," "tropia," and "heterotropia." Usually the various forms of strabismus are spoken of as "tropias," and their direction is indicated by an appropriate prefix, e.g., *esotropia* (inward or convergent deviation), *extropia* (outward or divergent deviation), *hypertropia* (upward), and *hypotropia* (downward). The preceding terms are listed in order of frequency. In all these forms, fusion is lacking.

Strabismus is easily observed and is a common symptom of ocular as well as central nervous and general systemic disorders. Strabismus may be paralytic or nonparalytic in orgin. *Paralytic strabismus* usually is the result of nerve damage (e.g., cranial nerves III, IV, or VI); however, the lesion itself may be of the extraocular muscles. Paralytic strabismus occurs in such disorders as encephalitis, brain tumor, cerebral vascular accident, intracranial aneurysm, myasthenia gravis, orbital cellulitis, and thyrotoxic and exophthalmos. *Nonparalytic strabismus* is not the result of a paralyzed extraocular muscle, but rather results from a defect of position of the two eyes relative to each other. Usually the tendency to develop nonparalytic strabismus is inherited; however, this type of ocular deviation may additionally be caused by serious disease of the brain or eye, e.g., retinoblastoma.

As discussed previously (see p. 1953), the effectiveness of the extraocular muscles is tested by having the patient rotate the eyes into the six cardinal positions of gaze. A "cardinal position" of the eye refers to a position which the eye cannot reach without the action of a specific extraocular muscle. If the eye fails to attain one of the cardinal positions of gaze, it may mean that that specific muscle is paralyzed. Paralytic strabismus is thus identified by this procedure. Paralysis of the ocular muscles, as occurs in paralytic strabismus, is termed "*ophthalmoplegia.*"

Nonparalytic strabismus is a positional defect of the two eyes relative to each other. This defect has been compared to that of a car with its front wheels out of alignment; the abnormal relationship of the front wheels to each other is not corrected no matter which way the steering wheel is turned. Thus, in nonparalytic strabismus the amount of crossing of the eyes does not change as the eyes are rotated through the six cardinal positions of gaze. When evaluating nonparalytic strabismus precise measurements of the amount of ocular deviation are made with prisms. Nonparalytic strabismus may be monocular or alternating. With monocular strabismus, the deviating eye is always the same one, while with alternating strabismus either eye may be used for fixation.

An estimated 5 per cent of children are born with or develop strabismus. Routine preschool examinations of visual acuity can detect almost all cases of amblyopia due to strabismus. Suppression amblyopia commonly occurs; *an estimated 0.5 per cent of patients have lost good vision in one eye because of suppression amblyopia. It is important for strabismus to be treated early in a child's life.* Generally by age six the brain has developed such severe suppression, when strabismus is present, that the condition will not respond readily to therapy.

As indicated earlier, esotropia, i.e., inward or convergent strabismus, is the most common form of strabismus. About one third of these patients have what is called "accommodative" esotropia, and the remaining two thirds have "nonaccommodative" esotropia. Accommodative esotropia responds well to correction of hyperopia (farsightedness) with eyeglasses if treatment is instituted within 6 months of onset. Occasionally, long-acting miotics are useful. However, these drugs must be stopped two weeks before surgery because of systemic absorption and the potential danger of respiratory distress during anesthesia.

In general, the treatment of all forms of nonparalytic strabismus is complex and requires the supervision of an ophthalmologist. While different combinations of treatment are used for the various specific disorders, some other aspects of treatment of strabismus are listed below:

- *Assessment* of the condition to rule out cerebral or ocular disease. Such assessment includes *cycloplegic refraction* to detect and correct refractive disorders.
- *Orthoptic assessment and training.* The angle of strabismus is measured under various conditions; this is necessary to determine the method of surgical correction (if surgery is being considered) or to assess progress under nonsurgical management. Orthoptic training and eye exercises help restore fusion ability.
- *Occlusion* to restore good vision if suppression amblyopia has developed. Constant occlusion of the "good" eye often helps restore vision in the "bad" eye; however, after age six occlusion is useless.
- *Surgery* is necessary if the previous steps are insufficient. However, surgery does not help amblyopia. Surgery is performed to restore muscle balance.

The major types of surgery performed on extraocular muscles to correct strabismus are (a) *advancement, resection* (Fig. 89–14*A*), *and tucking* and (b) *tenotomy and recession* (Fig. 89–14*B*). These various procedures rotate the eye to a different position than it was in preoperatively. The direction of rotation depends upon the procedure performed and the muscle or muscles which are the surgical target. "Tenotomy" refers to the cutting of a tendon. "Recession" consists of tenotomy and the suturing of the severed muscle back onto the sclera at a selected point *in back* of its original attachment (Fig. 89–14*B*). The muscle is thus actually moved back farther on the eyeball. With "advancing" procedures the opposite effect is obtained. In general, advancement refers to any surgical procedure which increases the action of a selected extraocular muscle. Three varieties of advancing procedures are (1) advancement, in which a muscle is reattached on the eyeball *ahead* of its original point of attachment; (2) resection, in which a muscle is shortened by actually cutting out a piece of the muscle (see Fig. 89–14*A*); and (3) muscle tucking, in which the muscle is shortened by making a permanent fold in the muscle, i.e., by taking a "tuck" in the muscle.

Postoperatively following extraocular muscle surgery, the patient is typically cared for as follows:

- *Immediately:* (a) an antibiotic ointment is applied to the operated eye following closure of the conjunctiva; (b) no patch is used unless two or more muscles are cut on the same eye; then a patch may be applied on the operated eye only with adult patients; (c) the patient is reminded not to rub eyes; (d) the patient is ambulated as soon as possible; and (e) to prevent nausea and vomiting following general anesthetic, only carbonated beverages, Jell-O, and soda crackers are permitted for the first 24 hours.

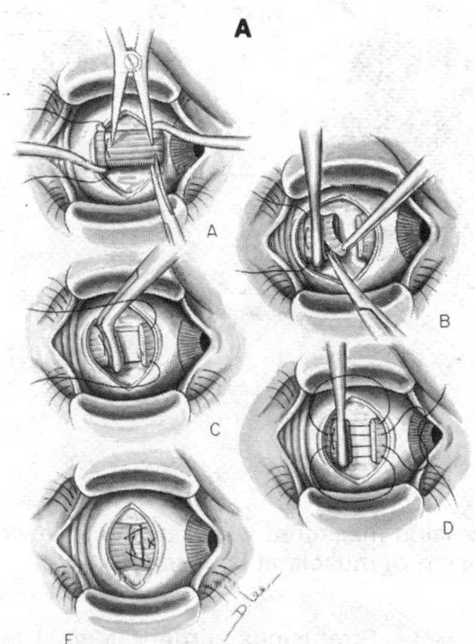

Figure 89–14A. Resection of rectus muscle. This procedure generally is the same for each muscle. Operation on the right medial rectus muscle is illustrated. (From Dyer, J. A.: *Atlas of Extraocular Muscle Surgery,* 1970.) *Continued on next page.*

B

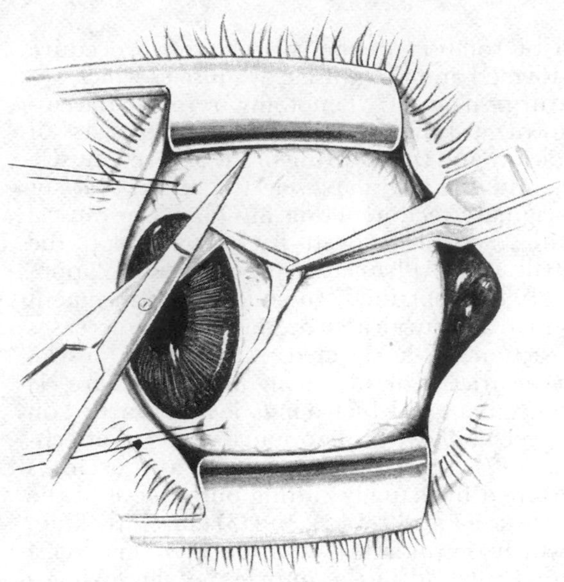

1
Conjunctival incision following peritomy near limbus. Globe abducted with 6-0 PERMA-HAND silk.

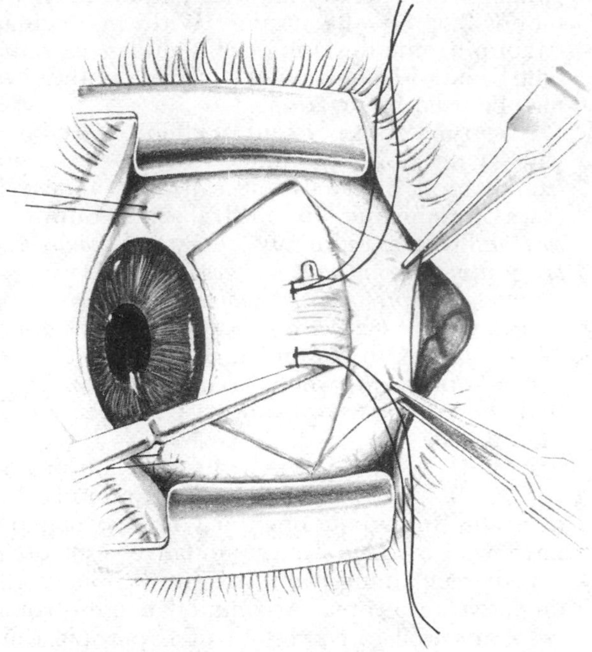

2
6-0 absorbable sutures locked at muscle borders following exposure of medial rectus muscle.

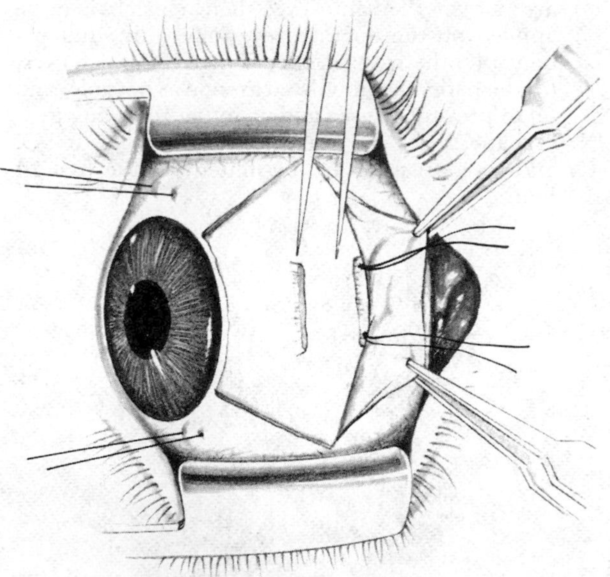

3
Recession measured with calipers following excision of muscle at its insertion.

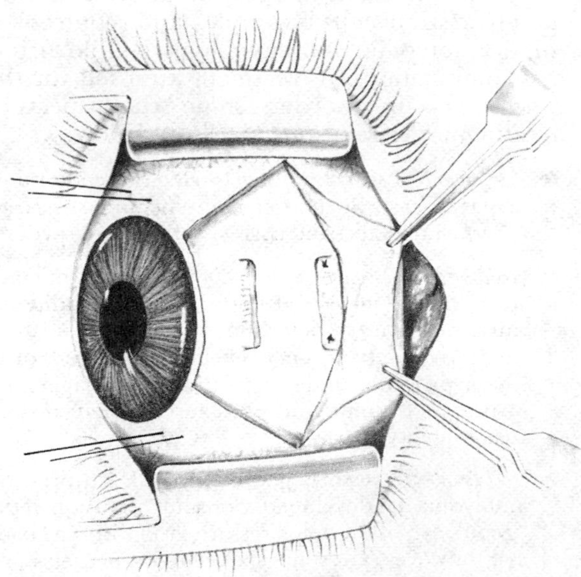

4
Needle bites in superficial sclera with knots carefully tied.

Figure 89–14B. Strabismus surgery. Medial rectus recession. (From Ethicon, Inc.: *Wound Closure in Eye Surgery*. Reproduced by permission of Ethicon, Inc.)

- *Muscle* surgery procedures are being done on a short-stay basis; parents are permitted to stay with the children before and after surgery. As soon as the child is fully reactive and has recovered sufficiently from anesthesia, has voided, and has taken and retained some fluids, he or she may be discharged. Eye patches are infrequently used. Cleaning the eye is discussed with the parents; some serous sanguineous fluid may drip down the child's cheek, and this should be wiped from the cheek only. If the patient is to have eye drops, the parents are shown how to instill them in the child's eye.
- *Adults* are discharged if they feel well enough (orders are given for follow-up visits to physician). Dark glasses are prescribed for adults for a few days if required. Patients are permitted to use eyes as tolerated. Antibiotic-steroid drops may be prescribed for adults (t.i.d. for 7–10 days).
- *Later:* (a) patient is reexamined periodically until all reaction subsides and eyes attain a stable position; (b) hot packs and steroid drops are prescribed for 3–4 days if suture reaction occurs after 10 days to 4 weeks; and (c) antibiotic-steroid drops are stopped when the eye is healing well.

Disorders of the Conjunctiva, Sclera, and Cornea

Conjunctivitis. Inflammation of the conjunctiva is called "conjunctivitis."

> *Conjunctivitis is the most common eye disease in the Western Hemisphere. It may be acute or chronic.*

Generally conjunctivitis is exogenous and the result of bacterial or viral infection. Conjunctivitis may also result from endogenous inflammation, allergy (commonly associated with hay fever), chemical irritations, and fungal or parasitic infections. Regardless of the cause, the symptoms typically include redness, swelling, lacrimation, and pain. Discharge varies in amount and nature, depending upon the causative organism.

Acute bacterial conjunctivitis is a benign, self-limited disease commonly called *"pink eye."* This condition is *highly contagious*, particularly among children. Thus, precautions must be taken to prevent spreading the infection to other persons and to the patient's unaffected eye. Teach and practice thorough handwashing. Instruct the patient not to touch or rub the eyes and make certain clean towels and washcloths are available and the person does not share these with others.

Remember: not all red eyes are cases of "pink eye" or conjunctivitis. Thus, the nurse should refer all persons with red eyes to a physician for assessment. A careful differential diagnosis is important to distinguish between acute conjunctivitis (generally a self-limited condition with no serious side effects) and such serious disorders as iritis, keratitis, or glaucoma (Table 89–2). One of the most common errors of diagnosis is that of conjunctivitis when the disorder is actually glaucoma or corneal ulcer.

Gonococcal conjunctivitis is not a self-limited, benign form of conjunctivitis. This condition constitutes a *medical emergency* which can cause serious complications, e.g., corneal ulceration, possibly resulting in blindness. Gonococcal conjunctivitis causes copious purulent secretions and is *highly contagious*. The gonococcus is one of the few pyogenic bacteria that are capable of attacking an intact corneal epithelium. This condition is easily transmitted to the eyes of nurses and others unless careful handwashing is practiced. The Credé method of instilling 1 per cent silver nitrate into the eyes of newborn infants was developed to destroy gonoccocci acquired during delivery. Such instillation must be carefully performed with the correct solution. Cases of permanent and severe eye injury are reported following the accidental substitution of ammoniacal silver nitrate solution (25–30 per cent) for the 1 per cent strength.[48]

The specific treatment of the various types of conjunctivitis depends upon the causative factor. However, generally the patient does best in a darkened room. The physician's orders may include orders for (a) specific antibacterial drugs locally and systemically; (b) eye irrigations; (c) hot moist compresses; and (d) eye drops or ointments. *Corticosteroids are contraindicated* in the presence of infectious conjunctivitis since they reduce ocular resistance to bacteria. Also, *eye-dressings are contraindicated* since covering an eye which has a surface bacterial infection promotes bacterial growth. When the cause of conjunctivitis is allergic in origin (e.g., associated with hay fever, allergic rhinitis, or asthma) rather than bacterial, topical steroids may be ordered and may effectively relieve symptoms.

Ophthalmia Neonatorum (Conjunctivitis Neonatorum). This disorder is any purulent conjunctivitis of the newborn which is acquired from an infected birth canal. While most cases originally were due to gonococcal infections (discussed above), staphylococci, streptococci, pneumococci, and other bacteria and viruses may also be the causative organisms.

> *Trachoma causes more blindness throughout the world than any other condition.*

Trachoma. Although relatively rare in the United States (except among American Indians and Mexicans), trachoma has a worldwide distribution which is estimated to affect some 15 per cent of the world's population. This disease is especially prevalent in the Orient, Middle East, Africa, and South America, because of unsanitary conditions. Trachoma is a chronic infectious disease of the conjunctiva and cornea caused by an organism which appears to be an intermediate between the virus and the rickettsia. Trachoma is *highly communicable* and if untreated may result in *blindness*. Known cases must be isolated and treated. Teaching regarding personal cleanliness is also important in eliminating this disorder since it is spread by direct contact. The World Health Organization is helping eliminate trachoma throughout the world; however, much work remains. Vaccines are being developed. Trachoma responds well to treatment with local and systemic sulfonamides or local antibiotics (tetracyclines) or both. Corticosteroids activate trachoma viruses. (It is noteworthy that almost all fungi also grow better when corticosteroids are given, since these drugs inhibit host defenses. Since the advent and widespread use of corticosteroids, severe fungous eye infections are more common.)

Scleritis. "Scleritis" refers to inflammation of the sclera. It may be superficial, i.e., *episcleritis*, or deep. Bulging and thinning of the sclera occur in the latter form. Scleritis causes the eye to be very red, and movement is usually painful. Generally iritis accompanies scleritis. Scleritis and iritis are treated similarly. (See discussion of iritis on pp. 1982–1983.)

Keratitis (Corneal Inflammation) and Corneal Ulcer. Inflammations of the cornea (i.e., keratitis) generally are characterized by the following symptoms: pain, photophobia, lacrimation, blepharospasm (i.e., the involuntary contraction of the orbicularis muscle), and interference with vision. Corneal inflammations may be divided into (a) superficial keratitis, (b) deep keratitis, and (c) corneal ulcer.

There are numerous different types of keratitis. Keratitis may be acute or chronic, superficial, or deep. *Dendritic keratitis* is a *superficial* corneal ulceration caused by the herpes simplex virus which can result in permanent corneal scarring unless properly treated. Idoxuridine (IDU) is almost the specific therapy for this condition. If this fails after eight days, adenine arabinoside (Vira-A) or trifluorothimidine can be used. Mechanical or chemical debridement may be indicated in resistant cases. Topical cortical steroids are contraindicated in the early stages of dendritic keratitis (unless covered with antiviral medications). *Disciform keratitis* is a deep, disk-shaped corneal inflammation, with accompanying iritis, which often follows dendritic keratitis. Treatment consists of atropine, 1 per cent, to dilate the pupil, and topical or systemic corticosteroids, or both, with antiviral medications to prevent recurrence of dendritic keratitis.

Corneal ulcers constitute a medical emergency, because of the potential danger of perforation of the cornea, corneal scarring, or intraocular infection. Such complications can cause permanent visual impairment. Corneal ulcers may result from many causes, e.g., following exposure or trauma, or as a result of allergy, vitamin deficiency (avitaminosis A), lowered resistance (e.g., diabetes mellitus), or infections, e.g., bacterial, viral, or fungal. The commonest bacterial

TABLE 89–2. DIFFERENTIAL DIAGNOSIS OF COMMON CAUSES OF INFLAMED EYE*

	Acute Conjunctivitis	Acute Iritis †	Acute Glaucoma ‡	Corneal Trauma or Infection
Incidence	Extremely common	Common	Uncommon	Common
Discharge	Moderate to copious	None	None	Watery or purulent
Vision	No effect on vision	Slightly blurred	Markedly blurred	Usually blurred
Pain	None	Moderate	Severe	Moderate to severe
Conjunctival injection	Diffuse; more toward fornices	Mainly circumcorneal	Diffuse	Diffuse
Cornea	Clear	Usually clear	Steamy	Clarity change related to cause
Pupil size	Normal	Small	Moderately dilated and fixed	Normal
Pupillary light response	Normal	Poor	None	Normal
Intraocular pressure	Normal	Normal	Elevated	Normal
Smear	Causative organisms	No organisms	No organisms	Organisms found only in corneal ulcers due to infection

*From Krupp, M. A., and Chatton, M. J.: Current Medical Diagnosis and Treatment. Los Altos, California, Lange Medical Publications, 1974.

† Acute anterior uveitis.

‡ Angle closure glaucoma.

cause of corneal ulcer is *Staphylococcus aureus* or *Pseudomonas aeruginosa.* Local therapy with antibiotics is usually effective. Early, vigorous treatment is imperative to try to preserve vision. Topical administration of antibiotics in the form of eyedrops, ointments, subconjunctival injections, or, sometimes, systemic antibiotics is used. It is mandatory to perform scrapings or smears, culture, and sensitivity tests before any therapy is instituted. *Herpes simplex virus is a more common cause of corneal ulceration than any bacterium.* Herpes simplex has been discussed on page 1973.

The outline of a corneal ulcer may be visualized by using sterile fluorescein to stain the cornea. The specific treatment of a corneal ulcer depends upon its specific cause. Some of the treatment measures that may be employed include (a) instillation of atropine sulfate or scopolamine to keep the pupil dilated (this puts the ciliary body and iris at rest, favors healing of the ulcer, and decreases pain); (b) antibiotics topically, by subconjunctival injection, or systemically, or a combination of these; and (c) corticosteroids once the infection is under control to decrease inflammation and prevent scarring.

Topical anesthetics should not be used more than absolutely necessary for pain relief and are not prescribed for home use owing to their deleterious effects on the cornea. Dressings are not used on infectious suppurative lesions because they favor bacterial multiplication and prevent the free flow of discharge from the eye. However, with superficial epithelial erosions and clean corneal abrasions, a dressing may be useful and may relieve pain.

Perforation of the cornea is a serious complication of corneal ulcer which may rapidly occur. Intraocular hemorrhage may follow sudden perforation and destroy vision. Perforation occurs spontaneously, or it may be caused by increased pressure (e.g., from blepharospasm, straining, or force exerted during examination). Following perforation the aqueous humor escapes (often prolapsing the iris and carrying it into the wound); the lens may become dislocated; the eye feels soft; the anterior chamber is obliterated; and the pupil constricts (even though previously it may have been dilated with atropine). After spontaneous perforation of an ulcer, atropine is instilled, a firm dressing is applied, and the patient is placed on *complete* rest and is instructed to avoid straining.

> *Corneal scarring or perforation of the cornea due to corneal ulceration is a major cause of blindness throughout the world.*[114]

Because most forms of corneal ulceration are amenable to therapy, it is important that a patient with symptoms of corneal ulceration rapidly be given medical treatment.

Corneal Opacity. A perfectly smooth and transparent cornea is a necessary component of good vision. Normally the cornea is invisible except for reflections from its surface. "Corneal opacity" refers to a lack of transparency of the cornea resulting from inflammation, ulceration, or injury. Corneal opacities reduce vision when they encroach upon the pupil; disfigurement is caused from dense opacities.

In some patients, who have only superficial corneal opacity, vision may be improved by the surgical removal of the opaque corneal layers; this procedure is called "*superficial keratectomy.*" If the opacity entirely occludes the pupillary area, but there are still other regions of the cornea which are clear, an optical *iridectomy* (i.e., excision of a part of the iris) may be performed to create an *artificial pupil.* The new opening (coloboma) is made opposite a clear part of the cornea. When the entire cornea is opaque and vision is greatly reduced, the surgical procedure of *corneal transplantation,* i.e., *keratoplasty,* may be performed in selected patients.

Corneal Transplantation (Keratoplasty). Keratoplasty may be performed not only to repair a corneal opacity but also to correct *keratoconus,* i.e., a condition in which there is a cone-shaped distortion of the central cornea (Fig. 89–15). Additionally many ophthalmic surgeons now advocate corneal transplants when perforation of a corneal ulcer is imminent.

There are various types of corneal transplant procedures (Figs. 89–16 and 89–17). For example, a *lamellar keratoplasty* is a corneal graft which involves replacement of only some of the cornea's five layers, while a *penetrating keratoplasty* is a procedure in which all five layers of the cornea are replaced with a graft. A penetrating corneal transplant extends into the anterior chamber.

A donor eye for corneal transplantation is obtained from a cadaver, or a patient whose eye has been removed surgically (provided that the cornea is normal). In working with cadavers, the donor's eye must be removed as soon after death as possible because the cornea begins to deteriorate after death. At the time of death (when a patient is known to have donated eyes), the cornea is preserved and protected by closing the eyelids over the cornea and placing on the lids pieces of gauze moistened with normal saline. Nothing is placed directly on the cornea itself.

Ideally a donated eye should be removed from the body within 2 to 4 hours following death; however, it may still be viable if removed up to 12 hours after death provided the body has been refrigerated. Also, ideally the cornea should be transplanted into the recipient's eye immediately after it is removed from the donor. However, this is not always possible. The fresh eye may be transplanted up to 48 hours after death if it is

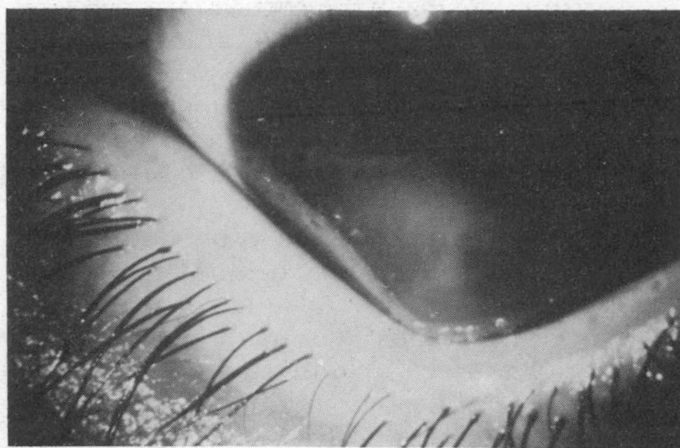

Figure 89–15. Keratoconus. Anterior protrusion of the cornea with central scar. Photograph of Munson's sign. As the patient looks down the cone indents the lower eyelid. (From Boyd-Monk, H.: Helping the corneal transplant patient to see again. Reprinted with permission from the February issue of *Nursing 78,* copyright © 1978. Intermed Communications, Inc., Horsham, PA 19044.)

kept in a sterile container (in an upright position on a piece of gauze soaked in normal saline) and placed in the cool part of a standard household refrigerator (a temperature of 4°C. is recommended for storage). Recently numerous successful *lamellar* transplants have been performed with corneas which have been stored for months in a frozen state or in glycerine. Until quite recently it was only possible to perform *penetrating* keratoplasties with fresh corneas (transplanted within 48 hours after removal from the donor);

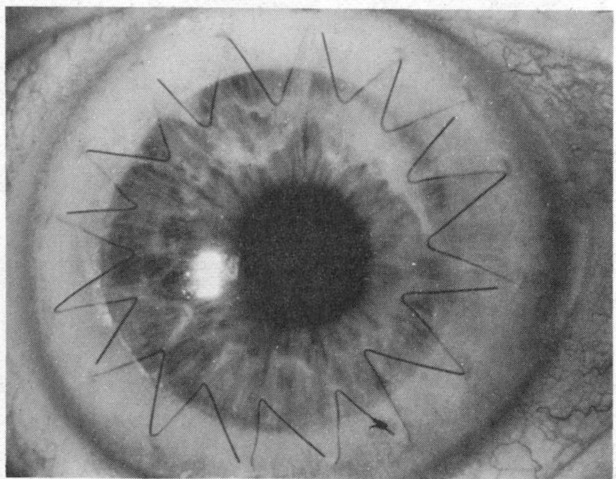

Figure 89–16. A corneal transplant with the donor button sutured in place using continuous suture. Trephine was used to remove the central portion (button) of donor's cornea as well as the button of recipient's eye. The suture can be removed in about 1 year. (From Boyd-Monk, H.: Helping the corneal patient to see again. Reprinted with permission from the February issue of *Nursing 78.* Copyright © 1978. Intermed Communications, Inc., Horsham, PA 19044.)

however, frozen grafts have now also been successfully transplanted with this procedure. In some cases in which corneal transplants are prone to failure—for example, the corneal diseases characterized by a dry, opaque cornea, such as ocular pemphigoid, Stevens-Johnson syndrome, and alkali burns—a *prosthokeratoplasty* has been used successfully. This is a small optical cylinder that is passed through the cornea and the upper lid. The prosthesis is fixed to the cornea with multiple sutures; the eyelid is sutured closed, and remains that way permanently.

Anyone wishing to do so can make arrangements (through a physician or by writing the national eye bank) to give legal permission for eyes to be donated for use by a qualified ophthalmologist. To contact the eye bank write: Eye Bank Association of America (EBAA), 3195 Maplewood Avenue, Winston-Salem, North Carolina, 27103. Telephone: (919) 765-0932. In the United States, further information can be obtained by contacting state agencies for the blind. Because eye banks cannot meet the demands of sightless persons wishing to have corneal transplants performed, there are currently lists of names of persons waiting to receive grafts.

Corneal transplantations are intraocular surgical procedures. Nursing care varies according to the type of transplant performed, but the general pre- and postoperative care of a patient is discussed on pages 1969 to 1973. A partial lamellar graft requires less conservative postoperative care than a total penetrating transplant, which widely and completely opens the eyeball. Combination graft and cataract extraction may be done. Preoperative preparation includes dilating the eye for this procedure.

Preoperative preparation of the patient varies, depending upon the anesthetizing procedure selected. Local or general anesthesia may be used, depending upon the patient. Typically a miotic, e.g., pilocarpine, is preoperatively instilled to constrict the pupil. Miotics, by elongating and flattening the iris and extending it over the lens, help reduce the possibility of damage to this area during the course of the operation. During surgery a round section of clear cornea is removed from the donor eye with a trephine (an instrument which has a structure and function similar to that of a cookie cutter). The same trephine is used on the donor cornea to remove the opaque area of the cornea from the recipient eye. The donor cornea is then carefully sutured into place.

Postoperatively, because the operated eye has been temporarily weakened and damaged, nursing care emphasizes preventing pressure increases upon or within the eye, which could put stress on the suture line. Other postoperative nursing care goals include making the patient as comfortable as possible, since these patients often have a great deal of pain on their postoperative night; promoting healing by allowing

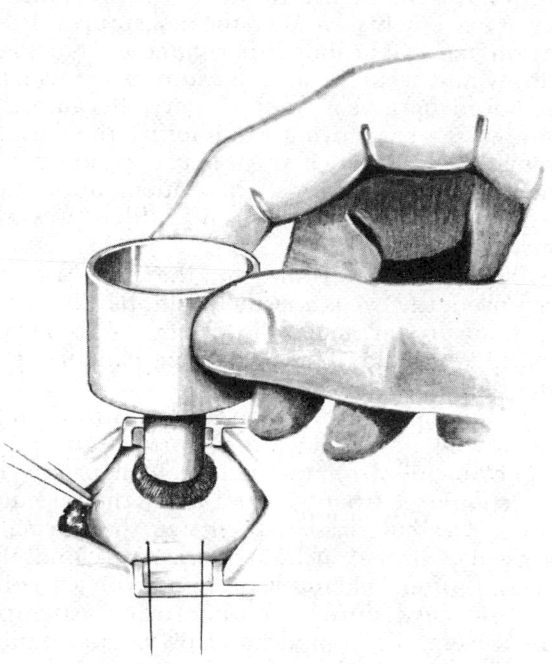

1
Corneal trephination under magnified visual control.

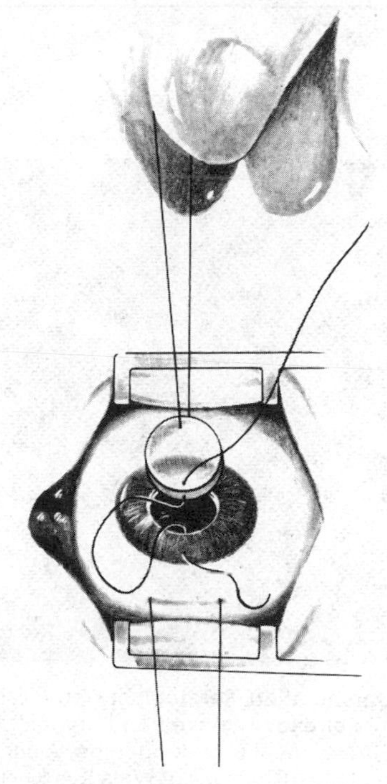

2
First stabilizing suture carefully placed to avoid rubbing donor endothelium.

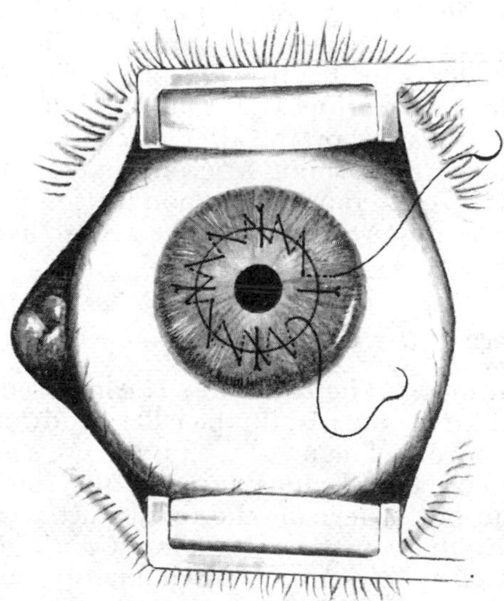

3
Wound closed with continuous 10-0 ETHILON suture. GS-10 or GS-14 needle facilitates deep placement of suture.

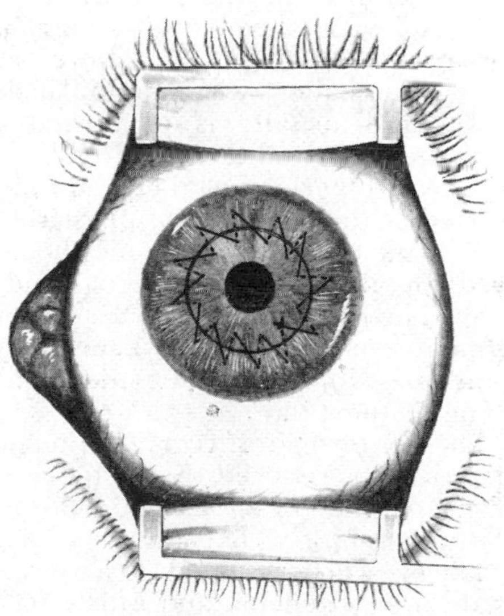

4
Continuous suture adjusted for watertight wound. Single knot placed in needle track. Stabilizing silk sutures removed.

Figure 89–17. Corneal surgery. Penetrating keratoplasty. (From Ethicon, Inc.: *Wound Closure in Eye Surgery.* Reproduced by permission of Ethicon, Inc.)

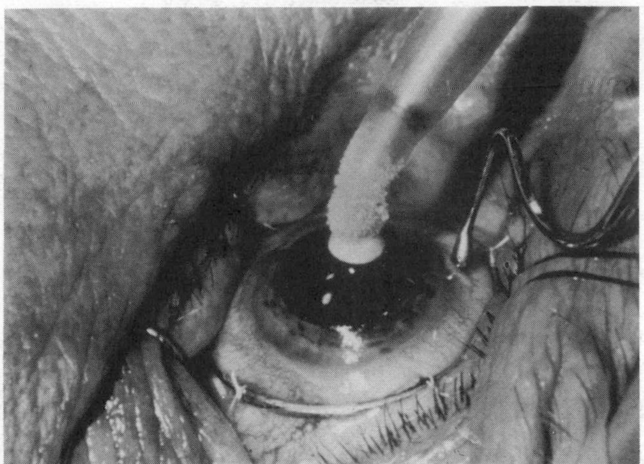

Figure 89–18. Combination keratoplasty and cataract. Photograph shows cornia already removed and cryoextraction of cataract lens through the corneal button opening. A donor cornea will then be sutured in place. (Courtesy of Wills Eye Hospital, Philadelphia.)

the eye to completely rest; and preventing infection.

Postoperative orders vary with the extent of the procedure and with the wishes of the physician. Following a penetrating keratoplasty, the patient may wear a unilateral eye patch for 24 hours. The patient will be ambulated within 24 hours and usually is permitted bathroom privileges after the first dressing. Dressing changes are performed daily, and the eye is inspected at this time by the physician, who may instill a dilating drop (atropine should never be used) or a combination steroid and antibiotic drop. The nurse will be requested to instill subsequent eye medications. Lamellar grafts are sometimes done, and the patients may be sent home the next day.

The use of microsurgery and modern suture materials has reduced the postoperative period of hospitalization necessary following keratoplasty to as little as five days.

The eye will be irritated for a week or two, and as the wound edema and inflammatory conditions gradually subside, vision will improve and photophobia will decrease. To protect the eye once the dressing is removed, the patient may be instructed to wear dark glasses (while convalescing and while photophobia is still present) and to wear a protective eye shield at night (to protect the healing eye from accidental injury). Care of the patient following intraocular surgery is discussed on p. 1970. Following corneal transplant, strong corrective lenses are not necessarily needed, unless a combination cataract and transplant procedure was done. Otherwise, the patient is corrected with regular spectacles or contact lenses.

Because the cornea is avascular, corneal healing is extremely slow. With the new sutures (10–0 nylon) corneal healing is permitted to take place slowly and securely, and the sutures are usually removed by a year after surgery. Because the cornea is weak during the interim, the danger remains of intraocular pressure pushing the healing graft forward. The patient must thus learn to protect the eye from sudden pressure increases.

When the time comes for the sutures to be removed, the eye is anesthetized topically with a drop of proparacaine; the sutures are removed by the ophthalmologist while the patient sits at the slit lamp.

Sometimes, unfortunately, after functioning for a while, a proportion of corneal grafts become opaque (from the immunologic process of rejection) (see Chapter 11). During the rejection process vascularization occurs in the normally avascular cornea. Such vascularization clouds the cornea, often making it necessary for a second grafting procedure to be undertaken. Attempts to prevent the complication of vascularization include steroid administration immediately.

Because corneal transplantation is an elective procedure, the patient must be in a state of general good health preoperatively, and the affected eye needs to be improved to its maximum. Corneal transplantation is usually not performed unless the physician believes there is a reasonable chance of success. However, in all cases there is the possibility that vision will only slightly improve (even though the procedure was technically excellent), or that the transplant will be rejected after several weeks or months. Follow-up visits are thus important after discharge. The feasibility of performing a second operation if the graft is rejected depends upon the condition of the patient's eye, as well as the availability of donor eyes.

Disorders of the Uveal Tract

Definitions. The *uveal tract* is composed of three parts: (1) the iris; (2) the ciliary body; and (3) the choroid. The uveal tract is the eye's middle vascular layer, contributing to the retina's blood supply. Externally the uveal tract is protected by the cornea and sclera. *"Uveitis"* is a general term referring to inflammatory disorders of the uveal tract. *"Anterior uveitis"* is the term generally used to refer to *iritis* and *iridocyclitis.* "Iritis" refers to inflammation of the iris; when the ciliary body is involved, the condition is called "iridocyclitis." *"Posterior uveitis"* is the term generally used to refer to *choroiditis* and *chorioretinitis,* i.e., inflammation of the choroid, and inflammation of the choroid and overlying retina.

Uveitis. Inflammation of the uveal tract may be caused by numerous factors, e.g., local or systemic disease, injury, or unidentified factors.

The inflammation may involve only one portion of the tract or may simultaneously involve all three parts. *The most frequent form of uveitis is acute anterior uveitis (iritis)*. Usually this is unilateral and is characterized by a history of pain, blurred vision, and photophobia. The pupil is typically small and the eye is red without purulent discharge. Uveitis may be either granulomatous or nongranulomatous.

Treatment of uveitis may involve such measures as:

- *Mydriatics*, e.g., atropine sulfate, 1 per cent, or 0.25 per cent scopolamine, to keep the pupil dilated. This prevents adhesion formation between the anterior capsule of the lens and the iris, relieves pain and photophobia, reduces congestion, and keeps the iris and ciliary body at rest.
- *Moist, hot compresses* several times each day to reduce pain and inflammation; applied for 10 minutes 3–4 times each day.
- *Local and systemic steroid therapy* is helpful in uveitis by reducing inflammation.
- *Bed rest* may be prescribed during acute episodes.
- *Dark glasses* are worn to relieve photophobia.
- *Analgesics* are administered for pain relief, e.g., aspirin, acetaminophen or propoxyphene, as indicated.
- *Treatment of associated systemic disease* is important in the therapy for granulomatous uveitis.

Treatment is generally more satisfactory for nongranulomatous uveitis than for the granulomatous form; however, recurrences are common. Serious complications can result from uveitis. Among these are glaucoma, cataract, and retinal detachment. Such complications can cause loss of vision. Obviously uveitis is a condition which must have the careful attention of an ophthalmologist. Granulomatous uveitis may be highly resistant to treatment.

Sympathetic Ophthalmia (Sympathetic Uveitis). This is a rare, severe, bilateral, granulomatous uveitis of unknown etiology which occurs anytime from 10 days to as long as several years *following a penetrating injury near the ciliary body* (or following a retained foreign body). The injured eye (exciting eye) becomes inflamed first, then the other eye (sympathizing eye) also becomes red and photophobic, and vision becomes blurred. The *preventative* removal (enucleation) of any severely injured eye (with perforation of the sclera and ciliary body, with loss of vitreous humor and retinal damage) is the treatment of choice. (Enucleation is discussed on p. 2004.) However, such preventative treatment is difficult for some patients to accept. Ideally the severely injured eye should be enucleated within 10 days following injury. Once sympathetic ophthalmia begins, systemic and local steroid therapy may be useful, plus local atropine. Corticosteroids are continued for at least a year. Once inflammation is advanced in the sympathizing eye, it is not advisable to remove the exciting eye, since that eye may eventually prove to be the better of the two impaired eyes. *If untreated this devastating disorder slowly and relentlessly progresses until the patient is bilaterally blind*. Blindness occurs in a period of months or years. Very rarely sympathetic ophthalmia follows uncomplicated intraocular surgery for glaucoma or cataract.

Disorders of the Retina

The retina, the most essential part of the eye, is equivalent in function to the film in a camera; all the other structures of the eye exist only to nourish and protect the retina and to focus light rays upon it.[114]

The *retina*, the most complex of the ocular tissues, is a direct outgrowth of the central nervous system (an expansion of the optic nerve) and is thus not capable of regeneration. The rods and cones are the receptor cells of the retina. The retina is a thin, delicate, transparent membrane, which is said to have the highest rate of respiration (oxygen consumption per unit weight) of any of the body's tissues. The retina is attached to the underlying choroid at the optic nerve border posteriorly and at the ora serrata anteriorly. Between these two points, the retina is in contact with the choroid but is not attached to it.

The *"fundus"* of the eye is the eye's internal surface, including the retina, the optic disk, and the choroidal or scleral details visible through the retina. A variety of systemic disease are reflected in the appearance of the fundus, e.g., diabetes, hypertension, arteriosclerosis, and blood dyscrasias. Thus, by carefully studying the retina with an ophthalmoscope the physician can learn much of importance not only about the condition of the patient's eye, but also about the patient's general physical condition. A discussion of the eye and other bodily disorders, e.g., systemic disorders, is presented on p. 2004. Here we focus on specific disorders which primarily affect the retina.

Retinal disorders are diagnosed by history, testing visual acuity, ophthalmoscopy, and testing visual fields. The retina is designed to receive visual images and transmit them to the brain via the optic nerve. Thus, most disorders of the retina cause blurred vision. Because the retina contains no pain fibers, there is no pain with retinal disease. Also, the eye does not become red or inflamed.

Retinitis. *"Retinitis"* refers to inflammatory disease of the retina. However, inflammatory disease is seldom limited to the retina, but rather is commonly associated with disease of the choroid, i.e., *"chorioretinitis,"* and *"neuroretinitis."* Prior to the antibiotic era, retinitis was caused by bacteria, fungi, and related organisms. Since the advent of antibiotics, most retinitises include toxoplasmosis, cytomegalovirus retinitis, and others. Retinitis may be bilateral and may last several weeks or even months.

There are no external symptoms of retinitis; the typical retinal changes are observable only with an ophthalmoscope. The patient may notice diminution in visual acuity, changes in the visual field, alterations in the shape of objects, a feeling of discomfort in the eyes, and photophobia.

Retinitis may completely subside without impairing useful vision, or it may cause considerable visual loss or even blindness as a result of scarring and atrophy. Treatment of retinitis centers on treatment of the constitutional condition causing the retinal disorder. Local treatment includes providing *total rest for the eyes*, protection from light (smoked glasses may be worn), and frequently the use of atropine.

Retrolental Fibroplasia (Retinopathy of Prematurity). This condition is a cause of blindness occurring usually in premature infants of low birth weight, before age 3 months. Bilateral retrolental fibroplasia results from exposure of the infant to a high concentration of oxygen while incubated in a nursery for premature infants, though it can occur even in the absence of supplementary oxygen. Fortunately now this type of vision loss is rare.

Retinal Detachment (Retinal Separation). Retinal detachment refers to actually splitting of the retina. The "retinal detachment" occurs between the rod and cone layer and the pigment epithelial layer of the retina. The pigment epithelium is closely applied to the choroid and does not separate with "retinal detachment." The separation or detachment is usually partial at first, but if untreated will eventually involve the entire retina, with subsequent total loss of vision.

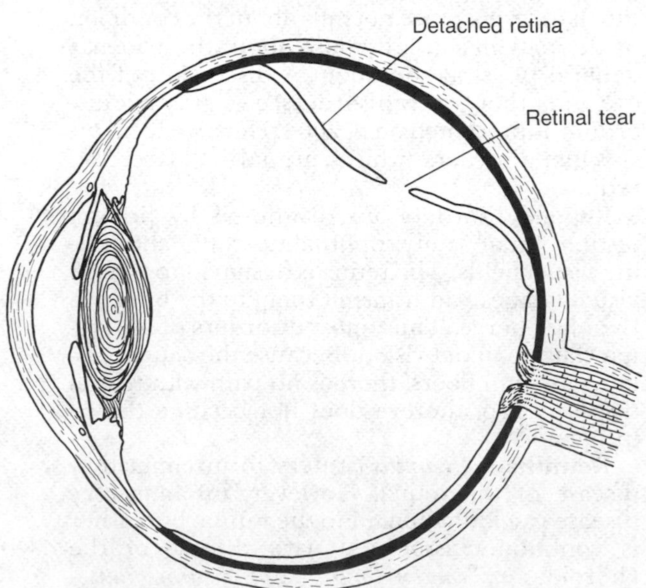

Figure 89–19. Detachment of retina caused by retinal tear.

The retina is not firmly attached in position except at the optic nerve head and at the ora serrata. Thus, if the retina is torn or if a hole develops in it, fluid from the vitreous cavity (mixed with a transudate from the choroidal vessels) can seep through the opening, run behind the retina, and elevate the retina away from the pigment epithelium and choroid (Fig. 89–19). The portion of the retina which is thus separated from its choroidal nutrition becomes blind. *Early treatment is important* before irreparable damage occurs, resulting in irreversible blindness. If the condition is treated early enough, surgical repair may be able to successfully restore vision by reapproximating the retina and choroid.

Retinal detachment may occur as a *primary event* (from a break in the continuity of the retina, i.e., a hole or tear) or may occur *secondary* to various intraocular disorders. Traction phenomena can cause retinal tears which pull the retina away from its normal position. Retinal detachment may occur following surgery on the eye, e.g., cataract removal. Also it may occur following contrecoup injuries or following loss of vitreous humor, e.g., from perforating injuries. The most common predisposing causes of retinal datachment are aphakia (absence of lens) and myopia. In the myopic eye (see p. 2000) the retina may be thinner; the retina does not stretch at the same rate as the sclera, and it tears because of vitreous bands.

Retinal detachment most commonly occurs after age 40 and usually occurs spontaneously. Spontaneous detachments are ultimately bilateral in 10 to 25 per cent of cases.[24] Unless treated, retinal detachment usually becomes total within 1–6 months. Retinal detachment may occur slowly or suddenly. The patient may notice the sudden appearance of flashes of light or floating spots before one eye, followed days or months later by the loss of a portion of the visual field, as if a curtain were descending over one of the eyes. The floating spots are caused from pigment or blood cells freed into the vitreous at the time the retina tears. The streaks and flashes of light are caused by vitreous traction on the retina. Vision is blurred in the affected eye and becomes progressively worse. No pain or redness occurs in the eye with retinal detachment. The area of visual loss depends upon the area of detachment, e.g., if the retina's upper portion is detached, visual field loss will be inferior. Ophthalmoscopic examination reveals a portion of the retina hanging like a gray cloud in the vitreous and one or more retinal tears (usually crescent-shaped and red or orange in color). The vitreous may appear cloudy. The physician may examine the eye by using a binocular indirect ophthalmoscope and a scleral depressor.

Surgery is necessary to reattach the retina. The surgical procedures by which retinal detachments are corrected are numerous and varied. However, these procedures all have in common the goals of closing the retinal breaks and of reapproximating the retina and choroid. Procedures performed to correct retinal detachment include the following:

- *Retinal surgery* involves the sealing of retinal breaks by the production of localized chorioretinal adhesions associated with transscleral drainage of subretinal fluid. The production of an exudative sterile choroiditis may be accomplished at and immediately surrounding the retinal break in various ways. Freezing, i.e., *cryotherapy*, does not significantly damage the sclera. It can be applied to a wet surface. The *photocoagulator* and *laser beam* incite a thermal inflammatory response in the pigment epithelium and choroid by focusing an external source of radiant energy through the eye's refracting media onto a relatively small area of retina.

  After an exudative choroiditis is produced, the retina must be brought back into apposition with the underlying choroid so that the inflammatory reaction will involve it and produce a firm adhesion, i.e., chorioretinal scar, which will hold the retina in place. Draining fluid from the subretinal space (by perforating the sclera and choroid) helps make it possible for the retina to return to its normal position. However, in addition to *subretinal fluid drainage*, other mechanical procedures may be performed.
- *Scleral buckling* is currently the most common procedure for repairing a retinal tear; it is designed to *mechanically* restore the contact of the retina with the pigment epithelium by depressing the area of sclera that lies over the retinal defect. By indenting the defect inward toward the vitreous, the retina and choroid are brought together. Either an *explant* or an *implant* may be used to depress the sclera. A Silastic explant may be sutured over the outside of the sclera with mattress sutures; local intrascleral implants of various materials, e.g., Silastic sponge (fascia lata and preserved sclera can be used, while polyviol, polyethylene, and gelatin have been used in the past but only rarely today) may be placed within the scleral layers (within a surgically created scleral pocket), and the external layers are then sutured back in place over the implant. A similar result used to be obtained with an infolded segment of sclera (*"scleral infolding technique"*), rather than an artificial implant, used to act as a tampon, but this is an infrequent technique.
- *Circling procedures* are those in which the entire globe has a Silastic strip and band tied around it so it tightly encircles the globe and indents it over the retinal defect. A circling strip of material is passed beneath the extraocular muscles and is fixed to the eye with anchoring sutures. The ends of the band are then tied together. The encircling element is often used to overlie and support a scleral implant.
- *Intravitreal injections* push the retina up against the choroid by increasing the pressure within the globe. Injections of balanced salt solution[25] or air may be made into the vitreous cavity if the eye is hypotonic following surgery. Experimental gases that increase their volume following injection into the eye are being used. They help continue the pressure exerted on the retina from the inside of the globe (but FDA approval has to be obtained for the use of SF6).

Over the past 25 to 30 years diagnosis and treatment of retinal detachment have improved considerably. Diagnosis by means of the binocular indirect ophthalmoscope and treatments by the various scleral buckling procedures have improved the statistics from an approximate 45 per cent success rate to reattachment in 90 per cent of cases. The duration of hospitalization and bed rest has been dramatically reduced from total immobility of 21 to 28 days 30 years ago to bed rest for one day in many cases and average hospitalization of less than one week.

Patients should always be told by the physician before surgery that there is a possibility that the surgery will not be successful. If the retina is still attached two months postoperatively, the patient can be reassured that the condition will probably remain corrected and that recurrence is unlikely.

Preoperatively, both eyes may be bandaged. During this period of tension and confinement before surgery, emotional care is important for the patient's general well-being. The patient is kept positioned preoperatively as ordered by the physician. Generally the patient is positioned in such a manner that the area of detachment is in a dependent position. *Carefully check orders concerning the position of a patient who has a detached retina* and inform the patient of positions which he or she can and cannot assume. Sedatives and tranquilizers may be prescribed during the preoperative period to help keep the patient comfortable and relaxed and to minimize strain on the eye. The patient is cautioned against straining and making sudden movements, e.g., sneezing, coughing, sitting up in bed, and so forth. Never allow the patient with a detached retina to lie with the face down or to stoop or bend over. Warn the patient not to rub or touch the eyes. If the patient has bilateral patches on the eyes, keep the siderails up and the call bell within easy reach. When approaching this patient, speak first so that the person knows you are there; visit frequently and anticipate the person's needs. Some physicians permit the bilaterally patched patient to have the patch off the unaffected eye while eating. This also helps to decrease the patient's anxiety level; otherwise the nurse must feed the patient cautiously. (Choking, coughing, or vomiting may cause further retinal detachment.) Stool softeners may be administered to prevent straining at stool. In the past, pinhole glasses were worn instead of bandages to decrease eye movements. Such glasses have only a small circular opening in the center of the lens through which the patient can see.

Prior to surgery for retinal detachment the pupil is dilated widely with mydriatics: 10 per cent phenylephrine (Neo-Synephrine) and cycloplegics (1 per cent Cyclogyl and ¼ per cent scopolamine eye drops); this facilitates visualization of the retina. Surgery is usually performed under general anesthesia.

Postoperatively, following scleral buckling procedures, antibiotic ointment is instilled and a pressure dressing is applied using eye pads and plastic tape.

During the immediate postoperative period, it is advisable to keep the patient's head and eyes at rest and instruct the person to avoid straining (which increases venous pressure in the head). Antiemetics are frequently ordered to prevent emesis if the patient is nauseated, e.g., prochlorperazine 10 mg. I.M., benzquinamide (Emetecon 50 mg. I.M.), or trimethobenzamide (Tigan 200 mg. I.M.). Medications to relieve pain are also ordered. Often a narcotic, such as Demerol, is ordered for the first 48 hours, because these patients do experience pain in the immediate postoperative period.

The current trend is for only the surgical eye to be patched when the patient returns from surgery. This patch will remain in place until the following day, when it will be removed by the surgeon. At this time dilating drops will be resumed, a combination antibiotic-steroid eye drop will be added to the regimen, and cold compresses will be started if the eyelids are swollen. The patient may lie supine or on the unoperated side unless specific instructions request a contrary position, in which case the patient may be positioned with the hole (retinal tear) dependent.

The patient is placed on bed rest with bathroom privileges and may be up to the bathroom when fully recovered from anesthesia. The patient will, of course, need assistance the first time out of bed. During the first postoperative day this is usually the only activity that is permitted, but by the second postoperative day the person may begin to resume all reasonable aspects of active daily living. Most patients are discharged to home care on the fourth or fifth postoperative day. To relieve discomfort mild analgesics may be prescribed. Cold compresses applied for 15–20 minutes help alleviate discomfort too. Shaving, hair care, bathing, dressing, and ambulation are permitted at home. The dressing on the operated eye may or may not be used once discharge and excessive swelling disappear. Television watching is permitted, but reading may or may not be allowed for 2–3 weeks. Light work is allowed after 3 weeks, and fully normal activity may be resumed within 6 weeks. The patient is told to be careful not to bump the head.

The postoperative routine described in the preceding paragraph is that recommended by one author in accordance with current trends in a large retina department. Postoperative orders given by other physicians may differ from this recommended routine; thus orders are checked carefully for each patient, especially the physician's orders concerning positioning allowed or forbidden activities. Some physicians recommend longer periods of postoperative bedrest; some may still (although it is not common) prescribe the use of pinhole glasses after dressings are removed; and some tell their patients to avoid heavy lifting and deep bending or stooping forward for the remainder of their lives. Wearing of dark glasses may be advisable during the time mydriatics are used.

Increased Intraocular Pressure (Glaucoma)

Introduction. Glaucoma is not one disease, but rather a complex of ocular disorders, all of which share the characteristic symptom of increased intraocular pressure. Over a period of time elevated intraocular pressure causes visual impairment, producing typical defects in the visual field due to atrophy of the retinal ganglion cells and atrophy of the optic nerve. If uncorrected, blindness may result.

Glaucoma is responsible for 12 per cent of blindness in the United States. This condition is often referred to as a "thief in the night" because in its most common form glaucoma steals away vision, without the person really being aware of it. Glaucoma is the second most frequent cause of blindness. It is estimated that two persons in every 100 over age 40 now have glaucoma, but *do not realize they have it!* Routine tonometer measurements are thus important, since this is the only way to identify glaucoma before the eye is permanently damaged from the increased pressure within it. It is recommended that a tonometer reading be performed with every routine *general* physical examination, as well as with every routine ocular examination in persons over age 40. Because of the hereditary tendency associated with the most common forms of glaucoma, persons with a family history of glaucoma should have their intraocular pressures measured routinely every year.

Pathophysiology. Normally, the *aqueous humor* fills the anterior and posterior chambers and permeates the vitreous humor. Aqueous humor is produced by the ciliary body and is crystal clear. In addition to serving as a refractive medium, the aqueous humor furnishes nutritional support to the avascular lens and cornea and contributes to the maintenance of intraocular pressure.

The *intraocular pressure* is determined by the

rate of aqueous humor production and the resistance to outflow of aqueous humor from the eye. Normally an almost constant balance is maintained between the rate of formation and the rate of absorption of aqueous humor. From the posterior chamber, the aqueous humor passes between the iris and lens and leaves the posterior chamber through the pupil (Fig. 89–20). Emerging from the pupil into the anterior chamber, a portion of aqueous humor then passes through the trabecular meshwork of the chamber angle into the canal of Schlemm and out through the collector channels or aqueous veins into the anterior ciliary veins. This is the major direction of outflow of aqueous humor. Additionally, however, a portion of the aqueous humor is absorbed through the iris vessels, and some diffuses into the vitreous humor to leave the eye by posterior drainage routes.

Glaucoma (increased intraocular pressure) results from obstruction of the trabecular network and the canal of Schlemm, thus interfering with the mechanism of outflow in the angle of the anterior chamber. While many causes and types of obstruction exist (as we shall see), the *most common* is genetic loss of trabecular permeability, resulting in chronic simple glaucoma.

TYPES OF GLAUCOMA

The various types of glaucoma can be broadly classified as follows:

A. Adult primary glaucoma
   1. Chronic open angle (wide angle, simple, chronic simple) glaucoma
   2. Angle closure (narrow angle, closed angle, acute congestive) glaucoma
      a. Acute
      b. Chronic
B. Secondary glaucoma
C. Congenital glaucoma
D. Absolute glaucoma

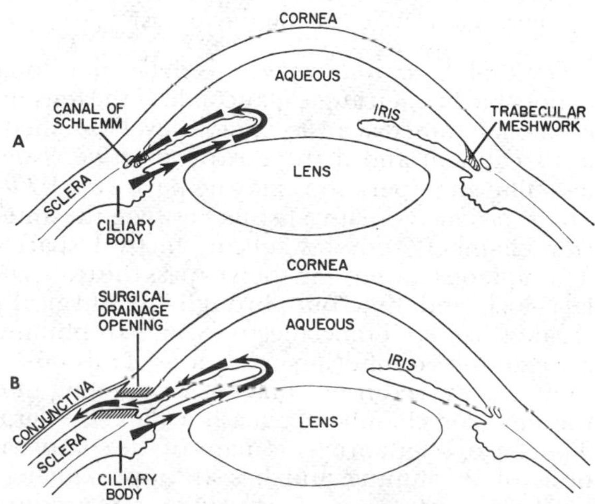

Figure 89–20. Normal flow of aqueous humor and creation of new channel with glaucoma surgery. (From Havener, W. H.: *Synopsis of Ophthalmology,* 3rd ed. St. Louis, C. V. Mosby Co., 1971.)

Absolute glaucoma may be the end result of any form of glaucoma and refers to any blind eye (with no light perception) in which intraocular pressure is elevated. To relieve the discomfort of the eye, a retrobulbar injection of absolute alcohol may be given, but ultimately the only cure for a blind, painful eye is enucleation. *Congenital glaucoma* occurs in an eye during its early period of growth and development and usually makes its appearance within the first 6 months of life. *Secondary glaucomas* may develop from numerous causes, e.g., uveitis, neovascular disorders, trauma, tumors, postoperatively, degenerative diseases of the eye. Our discussion focuses on adult primary glaucomas.

Hereditary factors appear to play an important role in *adult primary* glaucomas, particularly in *open angle glaucoma,* which is the most common of the primary glaucomas. Open angle glaucoma occurs in persons who appear to have normal "open" chamber angles but have a resistance to the flow of aqueous humor out of the chamber angle. This resistance may be in the meshwork, in Schlemm's canal, or in the aqueous veins. With *angle closure glaucoma,* which is much less common, there is a forward displacement of the last roll and root of the iris against the cornea. This narrows (or perhaps entirely closes) the chamber angle, thus obstructing the outflow of aqueous humor. Complete closure of the angle, and thus complete obstruction of the aqueous, may occur in a person who has a narrowed angle as a result of sudden dilation of the pupil (administration of mydriatics is thus hazardous in the presence of a narrowed angle); swelling of the lens; swelling of the iris (from inflammation); or slight forward movement of the lens and iris. Mydriatic and cycloplegic medications should not be used until the anterior chamber angle has been evaluated by gonioscopy. Such precautionary practice can prevent accidental precipitation of an acute attack of glaucoma.

Open Angle (Chronic Simple) Glaucoma. This most common form of glaucoma is usually bilateral and may progress to complete blindness without ever producing an acute attack. Although usually painless, open angle glaucoma occasionally causes a slight aching in the eyes. No symptoms appear in the early stages, and the disease progresses insidiously (usually in older persons).

There may be times when the patient notices foggy vision and diminished accommodation with open angle glaucoma. Occasionally, mild aching in the eyes or nondescript ocular discomfort, which the patient may interpret as a need for a change of glasses, is the presenting complaint. Over a period of years peripheral vision is gradually, often unnoticeably, lost. Because central vision typically remains effective for a longer period of time, the patient may be unaware that the ability to see peripherally is being lost. The chronic elevation of intraocular pressure eventually destroys the eye's ability to function.

Late symptoms occur only after severe and irreversible eye damage has taken place:

1. Visual field losses
2. Reduced visual acuity uncorrectable with glasses
3. Cupping and atrophy of the optic disk (as viewed with an ophthalmoscope)
4. Markedly elevated intraocular pressure which is detectable with a crude finger tension estimation. "Halos around lights" do not occur unless the intraocular tension is markedly elevated. Because these are late findings, it is obvious that case-finding of glaucoma is dependent upon careful specific measurements of intraocular pressure through the simple screening procedure of *tonometry.*

In addition to tonometry, other *diagnostic tests* which may be used to diagnose glaucoma include (a) *tonography* (an electric tonometer is allowed to rest on the patient's eye for 4 minutes while a record of the pressure is made); (b) various *provocative tests* to evaluate the effects of various conditions or agents upon intraocular pressure (such tests are explained in texts of ophthalmology and include procedures such as the water drinking test, the dark room test); (c) *visual field* evaluation; (d) *ophthalmoscopy* (to evaluate the optic nerve head); and (e) *gonioscopy* (to examine the angle of the anterior chamber).

If untreated, chronic open angle glaucoma which begins at age 40–45 will probably result in complete blindness by age 60–65. Useful vision can be preserved in most patients whose glaucoma is diagnosed early and controlled medically. It is important that the patient with glaucoma (of any type) realize that it is a condition which (like diabetes) requires *treatment for the rest of the person's life.* Periodic reevaluations of the patient's condition are important. Glaucoma is a condition which is controlled rather than cured; in this sense it is comparable to diabetes.

The treatment of choice for open angle glaucoma is medical rather than surgical. The objective of the management of all forms of glaucoma is to decrease the intraocular pressure to a level at which progression of the disease is halted. However, surgery is necessary for some patients. The majority of patients with chronic, open angle glaucoma are treated with the following medications (in individualized combinations and dosages):

► *Miotics* (e.g., pilocarpine, 1–4 per cent) cause constriction of the pupil (miosis) and contraction of the ciliary musculature; contraction of the ciliary musculature is thought to be responsible for lowering intraocular pressure by facilitating aqueous outflow. It should be noted that the change in the size of the pupil has no effect on aqueous outflow, except in patients with acute angle closure glaucoma. Thus by constricting the pupil intraocular pressure is controlled. Physostigmine (a *parasympathomimetic* drug) may occasionally be used in combination with pilocarpine. Miotics often cause a temporary dimness of vision for 1–2 hours following instillation. Stronger miotics, e.g., echothiophate, can cause retinal detachment or insidious cataract formation or both. Periodic reevaluation is thus important for patients receiving anticholinesterase medications; annually they should have their pupils carefully dilated and their lenses and fundi examined.

Until recently miotics could be administered only in eyedrop form. Such drops need to be instilled three or four times a day. Pilocarpine is now available in a *wafer or disk form* (Ocusert). A thin, flexible, rate-controlling disk made of ethylene vinyl acetate copolymer and surrounding pilocarpine can be simply placed beneath the eyelid. Pilocarpine is then available to the eye at a constant rate of 20 or 40 μg per day for a week.

► Timolol (timoptic) is a relatively new drug which is available as eyedrops. It has several advantages over pilocarpine: (a) less is needed to maintain normal intraocular pressure without fluctuations; (b) the undesirable effects of miotics are reduced (e.g., loss of accommodation, miosis, and cataractogenesis); and (c) the drug is administered less frequently (b.i.d.).

► *Carbonic anhydrase inhibitors,* e.g., acetazolamide (Diamox), ethoxyzolamide (Cardrase), decrease the rate of aqueous humor production. Epinephrine eyedrops (*sympathomimetic* drug) also decrease aqueous humor production, but this should not be used in narrow angle glaucoma because it also causes pupillary dilatation (mydriasis).

Generally, *surgical treatment* is delayed as long as possible in open angle glaucoma. If the tension is not maintained at an acceptable level with medical treatment and if there is progressive visual loss, filtering operations may be performed. *Filtering operations* create a fistula between the anterior chamber and the subconjunctival spaces. The aqueous humor can then bypass the trabecular block and flow out through the surgically created fistula. Trabeculectomy and trephining are examples of filtering operations. Trabeculectomy is a procedure of making an opening into the anterior chamber beneath a flap of sclera. The flap of sclera prevents many of the complications of trephining and has an approximately similar rate of success. *Trephining* is a procedure in which a small button of sclera is removed to permit aqueous outflow through the tunnel thus created. In both these procedures the aqueous humor flows out into the sub-Tenon's space.

There, within the subconjunctival space, the aqueous drainage is absorbed. Other filtering operations are sclerectomy and cyclodialysis. *Sclerectomy* permits aqueous humor to escape through a notch cut from the sclera. *Cyclodialysis* is an operation which separates the ciliary body from the sclera, thus forming a new exit for the aqueous. *Cyclodiathermy* and *cyclocryopexy* or *-therapy* are also procedures used in the surgical treatment of glaucoma.[8] The patient who has a cyclocryopexy treatment will have extreme pain after this procedure, and the nurse should be aware of the patient's need to be medicated for this. These procedures directly reduce the amount of aqueous formation by damaging the ciliary body (by diathermy or cryosurgery).

Any of the antiglaucoma operations discussed above may speed up cataract formation. Thus, if lens opacity is present, *lens extraction* may be the first procedure performed in the treatment of glaucoma. Lens extraction is discussed later in this chapter. Frequently lens extraction alone favorably affects the course of glaucoma; miotics may control the intraocular pressure following cataract surgery when they have been unable to do so prior to the surgery. Postoperative nursing care following these procedures is similar to that following other intraocular surgery. Very often after trabeculectomy the patient may be positioned with the head elevated to ensure that nothing will block the new filtering site; however, following cyclocryopexy the patient may be ambulatory immediately following surgery. Relatively few restrictions on activity are necessary. Check the doctor's orders carefully.

Angle Closure (Narrow or Closed Angle) Glaucoma. *Acute* angle closure glaucoma is a medical emergency. *The principal aim of the treatment of angle closure glaucoma (acute or chronic) is to open the closed chamber angle and thus permit outflow of aqueous humor.* While this goal may sometimes be achieved medically, *usually surgery is eventually required.*

Angle closure glaucoma may produce *prodromal symptoms* in which the patient experiences transitory attacks characterized by diminished visual acuity, colored halos around lights, and some head and eye pain. These *transitory attacks* may last only a few hours, recurring at intervals of weeks or years before the patient experiences full-blown typical prolonged attacks of acute glaucoma. Clinically, a typical angle closure attack occurs unilaterally either in a darkened environment, which causes dilatation of the pupil, or under conditions of emotional stress.

Three basic mechanisms involved in the pathogenesis of an *acute* angle closure glaucoma attack are (1) the anatomically narrowed angle; (2) a relative pupil block; and (3) pupillary dilatation (which increases the thickness of the root of the iris, thus further blocking the angle and thwarting outflow of the aqueous humor).

When angle closure glaucoma occurs acutely, definite symptoms present themselves (unlike the asymptomatic picture of open angle glaucoma). A sudden rise in intraocular pressure results from closure of the angle, and this pressure elevation causes striking symptoms. Edema and congestion occur in the iris and ciliary process. Usually the patient with an *acute attack of glaucoma* rapidly seeks treatment. The eye is typically red, the cornea is steamy, the anterior chamber is shallow, the aqueous is turbid, the intraocular pressure is greatly elevated, and the pupil is moderately dilated and does not react to light. The patient also typically experiences blurred vision, halos around lights, or a rapid loss of vision. Excruciating pain (of a throbbing nature) occurs in the eye and radiates over the sensory distribution of the fifth cranial nerve. Nausea and vomiting also frequently occur. Usually attacks are unilateral. Following treatment the symptoms usually subside; however, after each acute attack the patient's vision and visual field worsen. Only surgery (peripheral iridectomy, to be discussed) will prevent further attacks.

Unless it is relieved, the excessive intraocular pressure which occurs with acute angle closure glaucoma will cause permanent damage to the eye, resulting in *absolute glaucoma.* Complete and permanent blindness will result within 3–5 days after symptoms appear. Emergency medical treatment is first given to reduce intraocular pressure, and then surgery is performed.

Medically the first objective is to establish miosis, since constriction of the pupil will pull the iris out of the chamber angle and thus open the outflow path for the aqueous. (Remember that with angle closure glaucoma the problem centers in the closure of the angle and not in the trabecular meshwork and Schlemm's canal. These structures will function normally once the angle is reopened.) Prior to surgery the intraocular pressure is lowered by (a) the local use of *miotics* (pilocarpine 4 per cent may be instilled as often as every 5–10 minutes until the pupil is constricted during an acute attack); (b) *osmotic agents* administered systemically (mannitol or urea may be given IV; glycerol is given orally in iced lemon juice); and (c) *carbonic anhydrase inhibitors* given systemically to restrict the action of the enzyme necessary to produce aqueous humor (in two to four times the normal dose). Medical treatment also directs itself at controlling nausea and relieving the intense pain associated with this acute eye disorder. Meperidine (Demerol) may be necessary to control pain.

The above medical treatment regimen reduces intraocular pressure within 4–6 hours; *surgery* is best deferred for a day or so until the eye is less inflamed. Surgery is necessary because the high pressure causes death of nerve fibers. A *peripheral iridectomy* is the surgical procedure of choice once the acute episode has been relieved. In this procedure a small portion of the iris is excised, thus leaving a hole in the iris through which aqueous humor can bypass the pupil. Iridectomy allows the iris to fall back and thus deepens the anterior chamber. The iridectomy is performed in the upper segment of the iris for cosmetic as well as functional reasons. Since the upper eye lid normally covers the upper segment of the cornea, it covers the iridectomy, thus occluding it and preventing the discomfort which accompanies an accessory pupil. Additionally, there is less likelihood of infection, since the flow of tears is gravitational, thereby carrying bacteria into the tear fluid which collects in the lower cul-de-sac.

If extensive peripheral anterior synechiae appear to have developed in the eye (and they will as a result of repeated glaucomatous attacks), a filtering operation, such as a trabeculectomy, may be indicated.

Peripheral iridectomy is usually prophylactically performed on the fellow eye before the patient is discharged from the hospital (e.g., within a week after surgery on the originally operated eye). *Prophylactic peripheral iridectomy* is recommended because the glaucoma is a bilateral disorder, and thus an acute attack is likely to occur (or recur) in either eye. An acute attack occurs in the second eye in at least 50 per cent of cases, even though the patient may be conscientiously carrying out prophylactic miotic treatment. Peripheral iridectomy is thus desirable since well-controlled peripheral iridectomies have little operative risk and result in "true cure of angle-closure glaucoma if permanent anterior synechias have not formed."[114] Since permanent medical control of chronic angle closure glaucoma is generally impossible, it is desirable to have peripheral iridectomy performed as soon as possible. The earlier in the course of the disease that the surgery is performed, the better the prognosis. Once the disease has progressed to the point that a filtration operation is necessary, the long-term visual prognosis becomes more greatly guarded.

Postoperative care following peripheral iridectomy consists of mobilization of the pupil, often by alternate dilatation and constriction, to prevent development of posterior synechiae. The patient is usually ambulated immediately, and no dressings are worn. The postoperative care for filtering procedures typically is concerned with maintaining a "quiet" eye by use of local steroids and dilatation of the pupil. Some surgeons recommend massage of the eye to encourage continued flow of fluids through the surgical opening.

Patient Teaching. Patient teaching is an important role for the nurse in caring for patients who have glaucoma. We have emphasized that case-finding and *early* diagnosis and treatment are highly important in preventing blindness from glaucoma. Also, we have stressed the importance of regular tonometry measurements on all persons with a family history of glaucoma. These are general facts of importance concerning protection of vision which nurses should emphasize to all persons whenever possible.

Now let us review some important areas which the nurse should plan to cover during planned teaching sessions with glaucoma patients and significant others when appropriate.

- *Follow your doctor's specific orders concerning your case.* Today most doctors impose few limitations on their patients, but some doctors may advise you to (a) avoid excessive fluid intake; (b) attempt to remain reasonably calm and avoid highly upsetting situations which cause excessive worry, anger, excitement, or fear; and (c) avoid heavy lifting or excessive straining.
- *Take only those medications prescribed for you and faithfully use them as directed.* Do not substitute medications, do not use "old" medications, and do not miss even one instillation of eyedrops. Teach the patient important rules concerning ocular medications. Teach the patient how to properly instill medications into the eye (remember to teach about occluding the tear duct to prevent excessive systemic absorption of very strong preparations). Describe the important side effects of medications. Emphasize that the patient should contact the doctor at once if these symptoms develop. Instruct the person to use eye medications *only* in the eye for which they are specifically ordered (accidental use of a mydriatic, e.g., atropine, in glaucomatous eye may precipitate an attack of acute glaucoma resulting in blindness).
- *Maintain regular contact with your physician, even though you may have had surgery performed on your eye.* Surgery does not necessarily correct glaucomatous conditions. Artificial pathways may become obstructed or closed, or other new problems may develop in the eye which require medical evaluation and treatment. Emphasize to the patient that glaucoma is a condition which will require lifelong medical supervision. Tell the patient to contact the doctor at once if ocular symptoms develop.
- *Inform others of your condition and emphasize to them that you need medication regularly* (if it is ordered for you). It is advisable to carry a card with you or wear an identification tag at all times which states that you have glaucoma. Thus, in case of accident, your condition will be recognized by persons caring for you and you will be given the medications necessary to preserve your vision. When you are admitted to a hospital for any reason, always inform your nurse at

once that you have glaucoma, and tell him or her if you need medications regularly and the times of day when you are ordered to take your medication. It is usually advisable to continue this routine in the hospital unless the physician decides to change the pattern.

- *Keep an extra bottle of medication with you at all times* when away from home and keep an extra bottle at home.
- *Establish and maintain general health practices.* For example, protect your vision by having adequate light. Establish regular elimination habits which avoid constipation (straining at stool increases intraocular pressure). Exercise moderately to promote general circulation but avoid excessive exertion. Practice good habits of personal cleanliness.
- *Practice good safety habits.* Because mydriasis does not occur when miotics are being used, the patient will have difficulty seeing in dark places while using miotics. Instruct the patient to add extra lights at home, as they are needed. Teach the person to be particularly cautious when walking or driving in the dark. Instruct the patient to always use handrails when on stairs. Loss of accommodation makes added problems, e.g., the patient will have difficulty watching fast-moving objects.

As you plan your teaching sessions with a patient who has glaucoma (and with the patient's significant others), remember that during the few minutes you spend with such people you will be teaching them how to live with a disorder which will affect them for the remainder of their lives. Your teaching may prevent future blindness. Your teaching may make it easier for them to adjust. Do not impose unnecessary restrictions. If you do so the patients, and maybe their significant others, may become uncooperative and not perform those activities which are essential to management of glaucoma. Be certain to *individualize* your teaching plan. Base it on the doctor's suggestions for this particular patient. Encourage the patient to express concerns and to ask questions, and then plan accordingly to help him or her understand the condition.

Opacity of the Lens (Cataract)

A cataract is a clouding or opacity of the normally transparent crystalline lens. When the lens becomes opaque, it becomes milky or whitish in color; thus the *normally unobservable lens becomes noticeable,* and the normal black pupil may appear whitish.

Normal Lens. The lens is a biconvex, colorless, and almost completely transparent structure which is suspended behind the iris by the zonular fibers (which connect it to the ciliary body). The aqueous humor is anterior to the lens; the vitreous body lies posterior to it. Devoid of blood vessels (except in fetal life), the lens derives its nourishment from the intraocular fluids. The lens capsule is a semipermeable membrane (slightly more permeable than a capillary wall) which admits water and electrolytes. The lens consists of about 65 per cent water, a trace of minerals, and about 35 per cent protein (the highest protein count of any body tissue). The lens has no pain fibers. With aging, subepithelial lamellar fibers are continuously produced; gradually the lens undergoes a loss of water and an increase in density, and it becomes larger and less elastic throughout life. The adult lens consists of a peripheral portion (cortex) and a central portion (nucleus). With advancing years, the nucleus increases in size and the cortex diminishes in proportion. In old age the entire lens is hard and unyielding. Thus, with aging, the lens undergoes a gradual reduction in its accommodative power. Accommodation, you will recall, is the focusing of near objects upon the retina by the lens. The only function of the lens is to focus light rays upon the retina. To accomplish such focusing the lens shape is altered by the actions of the ciliary muscles as they relax or contract.

Cataract Formation. Some degree of cataract formation is expected in individuals over age 70. The precise cause of senile cataracts has not yet been identified; however, it appears to be a change in the metabolism of the lens and changes in the metabolism of the physical and chemical processes in its colloids. While senile cataract is the most common type, not all cataracts are associated with aging. In general there are two major groups of cataracts: (1) *developmental cataracts,* e.g., congenital and juvenile cataracts; and (2) *degenerative cataracts,* e.g., senile cataracts; toxic cataracts (resulting from ingestion of certain toxic substances or use of certain medications); radiation, lightning, electric, and heat ray cataracts; traumatic cataracts (most often due to a metallic intraocular foreign body striking the lens); complicated cataract (resulting from intraocular disease, e.g., severe recurrent uveitis); and cataract associated with systemic disease (e.g., diabetes). Senile cataracts pass through four stages: (1) incipient stage; (2) swelling stage; (3) mature stage (cataract can easily be separated from lens capsule); and (4) hypermature stage. *Formerly it was necessary to wait until the mature stage was reached (the cataract was referred to as being "ripe") before surgery could be performed. This waiting period is no longer necessary.* Today the favorable time for extraction of senile cataracts is when the vision of the better-seeing eye has failed so greatly that it causes interferences with the patient's comfort and normal daily activities. Cataract extraction can safely be performed on aged persons.

While cataracts are usually bilateral, they generally progress at different rates of speed in each eye. It is never advisable to perform bilateral surgery for cataract removal during one operation. If surgery is indicated, visual acuity improves in about 95 per cent of cases following lens extraction followed by corrective refraction to replace the removed lens. The remaining 5 per cent are not benefited by surgery because they either have preexisting retinal damage or develop postoperative complications, e.g., infection, retinal detachment, glaucoma, or hemorrhage.

The physician examines for disorders of the lens by testing visual acuity and by observing the lens with an ophthalmoscope, a hand flashlight, or a slit lamp or loupe. It is more helpful if the pupil can be dilated for examination. Cataracts vary markedly in their size, degree of density, and location. Cataracts are usually not noticeable externally until they reach the mature or hypermature stage and cause blindness. The retina becomes increasingly difficult to visualize as the cataract matures; ultimately the fundus reflection is absent, and the pupil is white when the cataract is mature. The patient with a cataract notices blurred vision which progressively worsens over months or years. The degree of visual loss corresponds to the opacity of the lens. No pain or redness of the eye is associated with cataract formation.

Cataract Surgery. Currently medical treatment is ineffective in stopping the changes which cause lens opacity. Thus, surgical treatment is the only available treatment. In cataract surgery the lens is removed from the eye, i.e., a lens extraction is performed. The two major methods of extracting the lens are (1) intracapsular extraction, and (2) extracapsular extraction. *Intracapsular extraction* has become the procedure of choice. In this procedure the lens is removed in toto, i.e., within its capsule.

The lens may be delivered from the eye by means of *cryoextraction* (Fig. 89–21). In this form of cryosurgery, a supercooled metal probe is applied to the lens to be removed. The probe

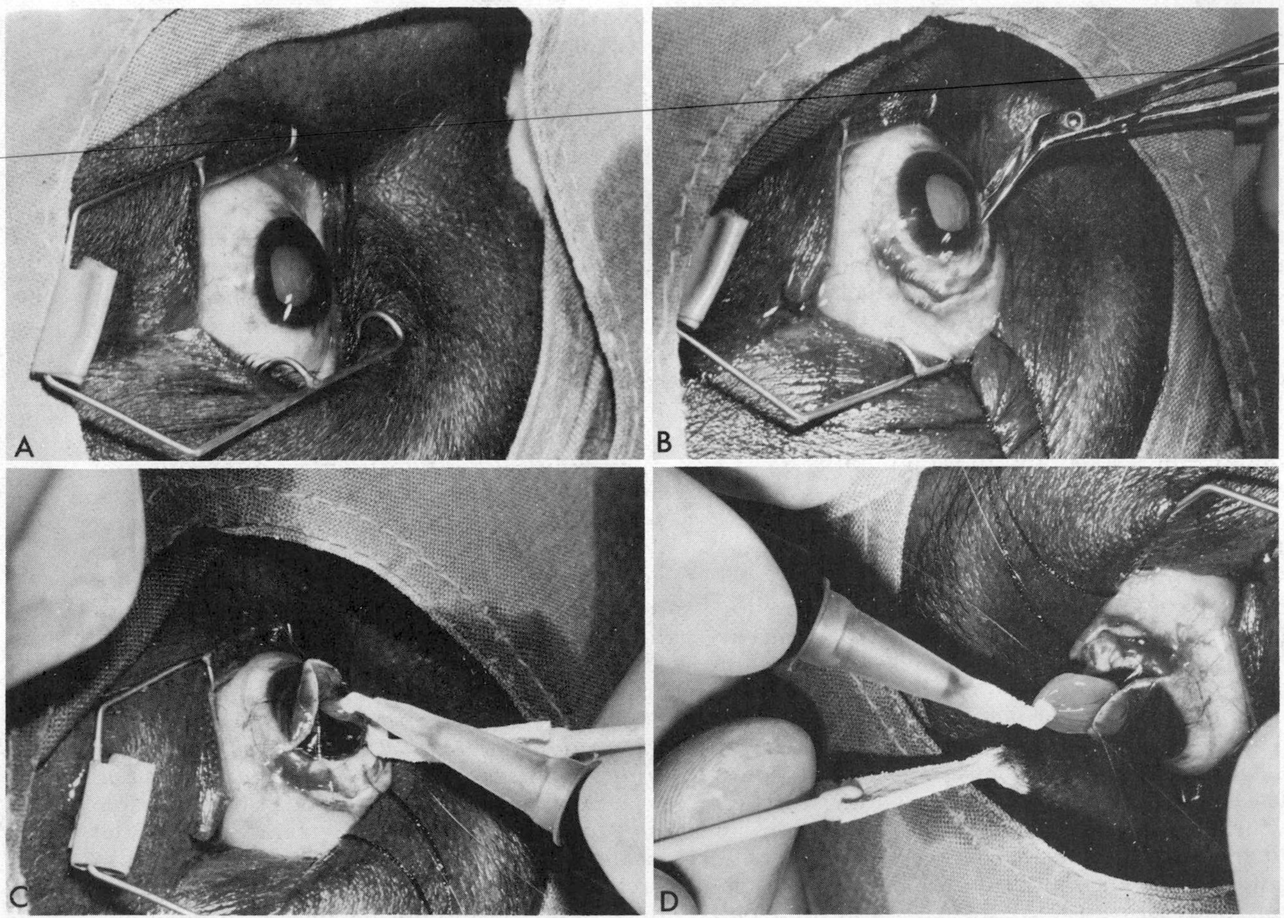

Figure 89–21. Cataract extraction by cryosurgery (cryoextraction). **A.** Eyelids retracted immediately preoperatively, showing mature cataract. **B.** Making a 120°–180° arc at the limbus preparing for insertion of cryoprobe. **C.** Applying the cryoprobe to the cataractous lens. **D.** Easy removal of the intact, cooled lens and capsule. (From Boyd-Monk, H.: Cataract surgery. Reprinted with permission from June issue of *Nursing 77,* copyright © 1977. Intermed Communications, Inc., Horsham, PA 19044.)

then becomes firmly adherent to that area on the lens because an ice ball forms at the point of contact on the lens capsule and adjacent crystalline substance, i.e., the cold metal adheres to the wet, moist lens capsule. The bond forms in a matter of seconds, and the lens is then delivered from the eye by a gentle upward and then sideward pull. With cyroextraction the lens capsule is less likely to tear than with routine delivery with a forceps. Cryosurgery makes removal of a cataract safer and makes possible safe removal of immature lenses before they seriously interfere with vision.

During surgery, extraction of the lens may be made considerably easier by injecting some chymotrypsin (a fibrinolytic and proteolytic enzyme) into the eye's posterior chamber under the iris. This procedure is called *enzymatic zonulolysis*. The material is left in place 2–3 minutes before the lens is extracted. Then, because the material has a specific lytic action on the zonules, the lens can be lifted out more easily. Acetazolamide (Diamox) is given postoperatively following zonulolysis because it prevents secondary glaucoma which chymotrypsin can cause.

Extracapsular extraction is performed in the treatment of some types of congenital and traumatic cataract. In this procedure the capsule's anterior portion is first ruptured and removed, and then the lens cortex and nucleus are expressed from the eye. The posterior capsule of the lens is left in the eye.

A type of extracapsular extraction is performed through a small (3.0 mm.) incision. The procedure is called phacoemulsification (see Fig. 89–22). Through the 3 mm. incision, a probe, which is hollow and able to vibrate at ultrasonic speed, is introduced into the nucleus of the lens after opening of the anterior capsule. The nucleus is "emulsified" by the ultrasonic energy and aspirated via the hollow tip of the instrument. Cortical material is then removed by aspiration. This procedure may be done at any age but is generally used in persons under 70. A secondary membrane develops in the eye which later requires severance (i.e., *discission*) in about one third of patients.

In some cases, a "lens implant" is performed at the time of surgery; and in others a "secondary" implant is performed at a later time. Because of the relative difficulty in use of the cataract glasses (peripheral vision is limited owing to the thickness of the lenses) the lens implant offers an alternative to contact lenses. Contact lenses are infrequently successful in the patient over 70 years of age. The implanting of lenses to replace cataract is becoming a more common procedure in the United States.

Cataract surgery is usually performed under local anesthesia, but sometimes general anesthesia may be used. Heavy sedation used to be prescribed preoperatively, but the current trend is to give the patient a premedication of diazepam (Valium p.o.). The anesthetist, then, is responsible for inducing the state of neuroleptanalgesia, in which the patient is awake but has a decreased response to pain and decreased motor activity. Sympathomimetic drugs (e.g., homatropine and Neo-Synephrine or Mydriacil and Neo-Synephrine) may be instilled in the eye preoperatively to accomplish mydriasis and vasoconstriction. To reduce the intraocular pressure two different agents may be used. Oral glycerol (Glyrol 120 ml may be poured over ice chips—a dash of concentrated lemon juice cuts the sweetness). This, however, is often preceded by an IM antiemetic, since some patients have difficulty retaining this syrupy mixture. A unit of Mannitol 20 per cent (urea is still ordered occasionally) may be given by IV infusion.

Postoperatively the patient's operated eye is patched and covered with a protective eye shield.

In some instances, nurses may be requested to change the dressing about 6 hours after surgery and at that time instill the eye medication; these will include atropine 1 per cent and also a combination steroid and antibiotic eyedrop (scopolamine ¼ per cent may be used instead of the atropine). Otherwise the dressing remains in place until the first postoperative day, when it is removed by the surgeon. At this time the surgeon will examine the eye at the slit lamp, and if the patient has poor vision in the other eye or is aphakic (without a lens) may order temporary, thick, convex cataract glasses to be worn im-

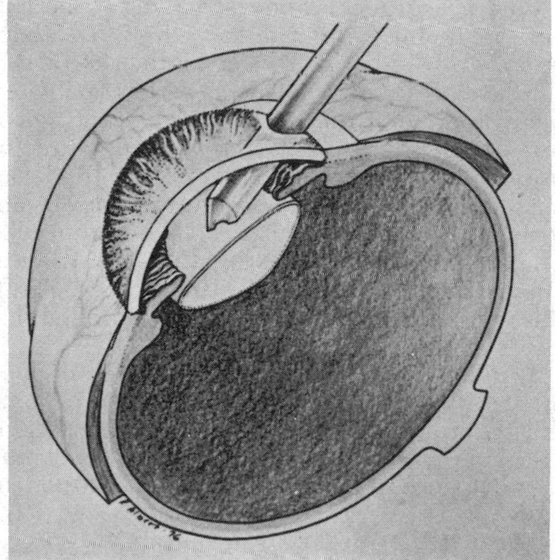

Figure 89–22. Phacoemulsification. Diagram showing cross section of an eyeball with a phacoemulsifier inserted at the limbus. Note that tip of the probe is directed toward the anterior capsule in order to perform an extracapsular catract extraction (E.C.C.E.). (Courtesy of Donaldson Manley, M.D., Wills Eye Hospital, Philadelphia.)

mediately. The patient should be instructed to protect the eye at all times either with the glasses during the day or with the shield. The shield should be worn at night for a period after the time of discharge, for the patient could damage the eye by accidentally rubbing it very hard while still asleep.

Postoperative restrictions following cataract surgery are very few these days. The patient is permitted up to the bathroom with assistance as soon as he or she has recovered from anesthesia. Tell the patient it is all right to lie on the back and on the unoperated side following surgery. Usually there is no contraindication to the patient having a pillow or to elevating the head if it is more comfortable. Many patients who have their surgery in the morning are sufficiently recovered to eat a regular diet by the evening. Nurses should be able to distinguish between pain and discomfort (which can be controlled by a mild analgesic such as aspirin or acetaminophen). One symptom a nurse may observe on the first postoperative day occurs in the patient who has a raised intraocular pressure. The patient asks for a pain pill, has breakfast, and then shortly after breakfast is nauseated and vomits. The pain does not subside. The doctor should be informed of this episode. It will be necessary to carefully check the intraocular pressure and prescribe an osmotic agent, such as Glyrol p.o. or mannitol IV, to decrease the intraocular tension.

Cataract surgery is done by making an incision into the limbus; conventionally this is a 180 degree cut through which the lens is then extracted. The use of a supracooled probe has facilitated the technique of removing the lens and its capsule. This procedure is referred to as an intracapsular cataract extraction (I.C.C.E.). The incision is then sutured. The sutures may be absorbable or silk. The latter need to be removed at a later date in the doctor's office after topical anesthesia has been instilled into the eye. With this type of procedure the patient's hospital stay varies from two to four days.

If phacoemulsification (P.E.) is used only one or two sutures are required. The total hospital stay required for this procedure may be as little as 48 hours. There is a possibility of performing cataract surgery in the future on an out-patient basis.

Because the surgery is an intraocular procedure, the patient should be cautioned to avoid placing strain on the eye and to avoid any heavy lifting and any straining during bowel movements. Encourage the patient to bend the knees if it is necessary to retrieve something from the floor. Resumption of sexual activity should be discussed with the doctor postoperatively, at the time that the eye and suture line are checked.

Because the eye cannot function well without a lens, the patient must be given a corrective lens to replace the opaque lens which was surgically removed.

The patient must be prepared to spend several weeks learning to adjust to the new glasses. This adjustment period will be a time of frustration during which the patient will need the understanding and support of significant others and health professionals. Great patience is necessary during the period of adjusting to cataract glasses. While the patient is still in the hospital, the nurse may be able to discuss the best use the patient can make of glasses once he or she has them. Helpful hints concerning adjustment to cataract lenses include the following pointers:

- *Initially use the new glasses only while sitting down, because there is considerable distortion which must be adjusted to.* A cataract lens in glasses magnifies everything by one third. If surgery has been performed on only one eye, binocular vision is no longer possible with spectacles, and the patient must use only one eye at a time to prevent diplopia. If both eyes are aphakic, i.e., without a lens, binocular vision is possible since both eyes can be used simultaneously.
- *Practice looking through the center portion of the cataract corrective glasses' lenses; turn the head rather than only the eyes when looking to the side.* Clear vision is possible only through the center of the lens; a ring of blind area occurs in the periphery of the visual field. Peripheral vision is poor owing to the optical distortions created by strong lenses, e.g., curvature and distortion of detail occur. *New safety practices must be learned,* e.g., remember to turn the head and not the eyes in both directions before stepping off a curb.
- *Practice manual coordination with assistance initially until new spatial relationships become familiar.* Practice walking, going up and down steps, and so forth with assistance until these abilities are safely relearned. Teach the patient to always use handrails when they are available. The patient may practice finely coordinated movements alone, e.g., practice picking up scattered buttons, practice pouring into and reaching for a cup or glass, practice writing; suggest that when pouring water from a pitcher that the person bring the glass and pitcher together before pouring so as to prevent spilling the liquid.
- *Have your glasses checked if they are dropped, are bumped, or do not seem to be fitting your head correctly.* In order to effectively focus an image within the eye, the lenses must sit at the correct distance and at the correct angle with relation to the eye.
- *Wear your glasses at all times once you are accustomed to them.* Help the patient to understand that now the light can get into the eye it can only be focused properly when wearing the glasses.
- *Do not be surprised to find that the color of objects seen with the operated eye is much brighter.*

Usually the patient learns to adjust to new eyeglasses by the time the permanent expensive glasses are ordered; permanent glasses may be ordered from 2–12 months postoperatively (typically 2 months). Permanent lenses are not prescribed until the cornea's curvature stops changing (it changes continuously during healing). Loss of the lens (aphakia) causes the eye to have a high degree of hyperopia and usually to have a considerable astigmatism. Additionally the aphakic eye has loss of accommodation, a deep anterior chamber, and usually a tremulous iris.

It is now possible to obtain *plastic cataract eyeglass lenses* rather than the heavy glass lenses. The advent of these plastic lenses makes quite a change in the aphakic patient's postoperative care. Currently, the cost of plastic lenses is about double that of the glass lenses. However, if patients can afford and use these plastic lenses, they are worth the investment. Advantages of the plastic eyeglass lenses are that they are two thirds lighter than glass and do not cause pressure lesions under the nose pads.

Some patients (mostly younger persons) wear a corrective *contact lens* rather than corrective eyeglasses. Because a contact lens is worn closer to the retina than a lens in the eyeglass frame, the magnification is reduced to only about 5 per cent. This of course varies depending on the patient's own refractive error. Binocular vision is possible if the patient with a unilateral lens extraction is capable of wearing a contact lens. Older persons are sometimes unable to learn to adjust to contact lenses and to properly insert, remove, and care for such lenses. Thus, unfortunately some older persons cannot use contact lenses even though their vision would be greatly facilitated if they could do so. A new extended wear contact lens is available for the aphacric eye. It is changed every 6 months in the ophthalmologist's office. Corneal contact lenses allow almost normal vision without the degree of distortion or magnification or the reduced peripheral vision attendant to the use of thick convex eyeglasses. Corneal contact lenses are especially helpful to those patients who have had cataract removal on only one eye, since the use of the contact lens makes binocular vision possible. (Contact lenses are discussed further on pp. 1997–2000.)

Recently it has become possible to insert a plastic (polymethyl methacrylate) lens *into* the eye at the time of surgery to replace the lens which was removed. Insertion of an *intraocular* lens removes the need for either a contact lens or eyeglasses postoperatively. Use of the intraocular lens enables the patient to see almost immediately and also permits binocular vision—if there is good vision in the other eye. With this intraocular lens the patient may see well at a distance but may have to wear reading glasses to read and write. The person may even be able to participate in sports that were not possible with the heavy glasses. (See Fig. 89–23.)

Before the patient is discharged home following cataract surgery he or she (and a significant other) must be taught how to instill eyedrops. Limitations of activity which the doctor advises are also explained to the patient. The sexually active patient may be requested to abstain for up to 6 weeks after cataract and intraocular lens implant surgery in order to prevent dislocation of the lens; the pupils are known to dilate during orgasm. Also, depending on the type of lens used, the patient may be required to instill Pilocarpine 2 per cent to prevent this pupillary dilatation. A pair of sunglasses or an eye shield may be advisable to protect the eye from injury until permanent glasses are worn.

Complications. Various serious *postoperative complications* can follow cataract surgery. Early postoperative complications, which may be apparent at the first dressing change (24 hours following surgery), include prolapse of the iris and a flat anterior chamber. *Iris prolapse* occurs at a site of rupture in the cataract incision; *wound rupture* may be due to the loosening of a suture, but it can also be due to pressure exerted on the eye by the patient. With modern suture materials this is rare. Bulging of the wound or a pear-shaped pupil are indicative of prolapse of the iris and should be reported if the nurse notices these at the time of dressing change. (Some physicians prefer to always change the dressing themselves so they can inspect the eye.) But the competent ophthalmologic nurse may be given the responsibility of changing this dressing and giving initial eyedrops. Wound rupture is a serious complication which may result in such problems as corneal opacity, infection, uveitis, or glaucoma. Prolapsed iris is thus immediately treated. The prolapsed portion of iris may be excised or reposited, and the area of the wound where the pro

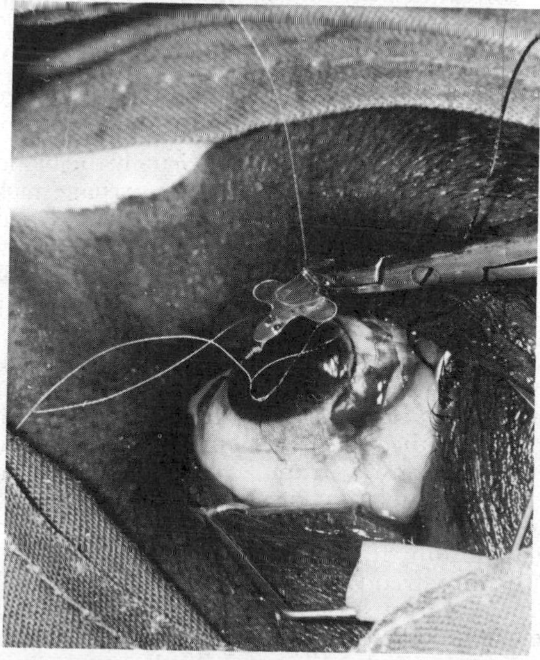

Figure 89–23. Copeland intraocular lens about to be inserted inside the eye, after cataract extraction.

lapse occurred is carefully sutured. A *flat anterior chamber* is carefully evaluated to determine if it is due to a leaking wound. If this is found to be the cause the eye is put at rest by dilating the pupil. A pressure patch may be applied for 24 hours. If the chamber is allowed to remain flat for a prolonged period of time, adhesions tend to form between the peripheral iris and the cornea (since the iris is in contact with the cornea owing to lack of fluid in the anterior chamber). Such adhesions obliterate the drainage angle and cause the subsequent development of *aphakic secondary angle closure glaucoma.*

Hemorrhage into the anterior chamber, i.e., *hyphema,* occasionally occurs spontaneously during the postoperative period; the nurse should be aware of the signs and symptoms, which include a sudden sharp pain in the eye. If a flashlight is beamed into the eye to inspect it, a nurse may see a half-moon of blood in a dependent position in the anterior chamber. If this occurs ask the patient to rest quietly in bed, elevate the head of the bed, offer the patient something for pain, and then notify the doctor. At this time the granulation tissue which is healing the wound is highly vascularized and the capillaries are fragile. Hemorrhage can injure the eye's delicate structures by causing pressure on them. This is an ocular emergency. The patient should also be aware that if he or she experiences sharp eye pain after discharge the doctor should be contacted quickly. Mild pain or aching of the eye is not uncommon postoperatively. Hyphema may be precipitated by strain on the eye (e.g., if the patient tightly squeezes the eye or otherwise exerts pressure on the eye), or it may occur for no apparent reason. Treatment consists of bedrest and keeping the pupil dilated. Usually the blood is rapidly reabsorbed. Severe hemorrhage may necessitate surgery to wash out the blood and debris. IV mannitol or IM Diamox may be ordered if the angle is blocked by blood and debris and the intraocular pressure thus secondarily rises.

Postoperative infection, i.e., *endophthalmitis,* usually appears about 3–4 days postoperatively if it is going to develop. Vigorous treatment is necessary to save the eye. Treatment may include local administration of atropine, subconjunctival injection of antibiotics, parenteral antibiotics, parenteral steroids, and perhaps Diamox or related carbonic anhydrase inhibitors.

Loss of vitreous is another possible complication of cataract surgery. Vitreous loss increases the likelihood of complications developing, such as glaucoma, uveitis, and retinal detachment. Vitreous strands may develop, and as these bands of scar tissue contract, they exert tension on the retina which will tear a retina undergoing degeneration.

Because of the *postoperative iritis* which usually occurs (mildly) following cataract surgery, there is a possibility that the eye may form *adhesions* between the iris and the vitreous face. The pupil is kept dilated unless the patient has had an intraocular lens inserted, in which case it is constricted. (Dilating drops accidentally instilled into an eye in which the lens is being held in place by the pupil initially may be the cause of a dislocated intraocular lens, with all its surgical ramifications.) Some sources recommend instillation of a cycloplegic drop daily for 1–2 months following cataract extraction. One prophylactic measure for the potential complication of *pupillary block glaucoma* following cataract surgery is to start the drops shortly after the patient has returned from the operating room. At the time of surgery, iridectomy is usually performed as a prophylactic measure to prevent secondary pupillary block glaucoma and to minimize chances of the iris prolapsing postoperatively. Iridectomy facilitates the flow of aqueous humor from the posterior chamber into the anterior chamber in a situation that could result from forward movement of the vitreous humor in the globe (blocking the pupil and causing pressure against the iris; this is referred to as an iris bombé).

Tumors of the Eye and Related Structures

The eye and its related structures may be the site of both benign and malignant tumors. Often such tumors can be visualized early in their development since they are readily apparent, displace the eyeball, or interfere with vision. Secondary (metastatic) tumors are the most common intraocular malignancies, but they are often not seen clinically because patients with advanced cancer do not have an eye examination. When they do occur, x-ray or other treatment may relieve the condition; however, it is hopeless to try to cure the metastatic cancer by enucleation.

The early diagnosis of tumors related to the eye is of importance and in some instances may mean the difference between cure or only palliation. Biopsies are taken of all suspicious accessible lid and conjunctival lesions. ^{32}P uptake studies may help detect intraocular tumors and facilitate differentiation between benign and malignant neoplasms. Retinoblastomas and malignant melanomas are the most common primary intraocular tumors. Cancer is discussed in detail in Unit IX.

Errors of Refraction

Errors of refraction are the most common type of ocular disorder.

General Considerations. "Refraction" refers clinically to an examination of the eye performed to determine the eye's refractive state. Refraction also refers to the bending of light as it passes through the eye's optical structures. The eye's refractive media include the cornea, the aqueous humor, the lens, and the vitreous body. The purpose of these structures is to bend light rays so they ultimately focus on the retina. The eye's refractive media are all normally transparent. When light obliquely strikes a transparent substance, while passing from one medium to another of different density, it is bent or deflected at the interface; this is the process of "refraction."

It is not possible to discuss in this text the precise mechanism of refraction. Such details are presented in specialized textbooks of ophthalmology. In general, the procedures of refraction may be classified as either being "cycloplegic" or "noncycloplegic."

Cycloplegic refraction determines the refractive state of the eye *at rest*. To obtain this state, various solutions may be instilled into the eye's conjunctival sac to produce cycloplegia, i.e., reduction of the accommodative power and weakening of the ciliary muscle. Coincidentally mydriasis occurs, i.e., pupillary dilation. This dilation makes ophthalmoscopic examination of the fundus easier. Patients should be told that their vision will be blurred temporarily after leaving the physician's office and that they should wear sunglasses in bright light until the eye returns to its normal state.

During cycloplegic refraction, while the eye is in a state of rest, the eye may be examined objectively and/or subjectively. *Objective evaluation* includes performance of *retinoscopy*. In this procedure a beam of light is directed into the pupil (from a retinoscope) and the movement of a reflected light "shadow" in the fundus is neutralized by placing appropriate lenses before the eye. The observed patterns of movement emerging from the patient's eye are easily recognized by the trained observer as being characteristic of the various refractive errors, e.g., myopia, hyperopia, or astigmatism. *Subjective evaluation* includes having a patient look through various lenses and then asking the person to identify the lens which gives best visual sharpness. The patient thus chooses the best of a series of corrective lenses. Cycloplegic refraction is most frequently used on children and young adults. With aging, weakening of the power of accommodation occurs.

Noncycloplegic refraction is accomplished, as the name indicates, without the use of cycloplegics. Both objective and subjective evaluation of refraction are then made as described above, and allowances are made for the action of accommodation. Accommodation is highly active in youth and then diminishes with age as the eye becomes presbyopic.

Eyeglasses; Contact Lenses. Once the physician has completed a refractive examination, he or she knows whether or not the patient requires corrective lenses and, if so, what strength and type of lens are necessary. The two major reasons for wearing corrective lenses are (a) to improve visual acuity and (b) to provide relief from the symptoms which refractive errors can cause. Refractive errors not only cause visual disorders but also cause many other associated symptoms, such as rubbing the eyes, blinking, frowning, closing one eye, photophobia, injection, tearing, head tilting, clumsiness, eyestrain, headache, dizziness, and occasionally nausea. Visual acuity is improved by selecting a lens which will correctly focus images on the retina. Corrective lenses may be either contact lenses or lenses worn in eyeglasses.

Prescription *eyeglasses* are available with case-hardened, shatterproof glass or plastic lenses. Plastic lenses are of lighter weight but scratch more easily and are more expensive. Persons who need to wear eyeglasses should use their glasses as prescribed and should keep the lenses clean and free from scratches. (The nurse should see that patients who need corrective glasses have them and that the glasses are clean.) When not in use, eyeglasses should be safely stored in a protective glasses case.

It is advisable for persons needing prescription glasses to have an extra pair of glasses (in case of breakage or loss) and to have prescription sunglasses or dark lenses to clip over their regular prescription lenses. Because of the variety of ocular refractive disorders which exist, it is important that eyeglasses be individually prescribed. The practice of buying "dime-store glasses" or of borrowing other persons' glasses should be discouraged.

Special bifocal or trifocal lenses may be prescribed to provide correction for vision at several different distances within one pair of lenses. *Bifocal lenses* are double lenses which are generally prescribed for persons with poor powers of accommodation, e.g., older persons; the lower portion of the lens provides correction for near vision while the upper portion enables focusing for distances. *Trifocal lenses* are triple lenses. Each lens is divided into three segments; the lower is for near vision, the middle is for intermediate distance, and the upper is for distant vision. It is helpful to instruct people when they are first learning to adjust to bifocal lenses to be sure to drop the head down (by tucking chin down and flexing the neck) when going down stairs or stepping off a curb. By merely lowering the eyes (as we are accustomed to doing), a person wearing bifocals will look through the bottom portion of the lens (which is designed for near vision) and will not be able to focus clearly on the stairs or curb.

Children, and all patients with severely limited vision or those who have had eye surgery, should learn how to safely put on their eyeglasses in a manner which reduces the likelihood of their eyes being poked by the bows of the glasses. This may be accomplished by picking up the glasses with both hands (one hand over the tip of each bow) and then guiding the bows past the eyes and along either side of the head to the ears.

A *contact lens* is essentially a small, thin, polished disk of plastic that is ground on the outer side to correct or improve vision while the inner side is designed to correspond to the surface shape of the eye. There are numerous sizes and shapes of contact lenses, but most are basically variations of two main types: (1) scleral lenses and (2) corneal lenses. *Scleral lenses,* sometimes called "haptic" lenses, cover most of the visible portion of the eye. This type of lens is about 1 inch in diameter and rests on the sclera. Scleral lenses have been used for several types of eye disorders since they cover and protect the eye's entire anterior segment. For example, scleral lenses may be used immediately after thorough irrigation of the eye when chemical burns have occurred to the eye; the scleral lens prevents the lids from adhering to the cornea and conjunctiva. Scleral lenses will keep fluid in contact with the eye when the eye is dry from lack of tears. Also, if the cornea is severely ulcerated and has thin areas, the scleral lens acts as a splint, protecting the thin zone until it has healed.

The *corneal contact lens* is the type of contact lens most frequently used. This lens is usually tinted grey, light blue, light green, or brown. A corneal lens covers only the major area of the cornea and is about ⅓ inch in diameter. The corneal contact lens is held in place on the cornea by the surface tension of the eye's natural fluid or tears. Surface tension is the phenomenon which makes it difficult to pull two flat plates of glass apart if they are wet. Thus contact lenses actually tend to float on a tear. The capillary attraction of tears and the upper lid loosely holds the lens in place. The flow of tears over all surfaces not only provides the necessary lubricating fluid but also is important in refraction. Centered over the cornea, the lens moves with the eye.

Contact lenses are safe to wear if they are professionally prescribed, ground, and adjusted to the patient, and provided the patient uses the lenses as directed. Periodic check-ups are always of importance for the person who wears contact lenses, and the person should see a physician if any problems occur between scheduled check-ups. Corneal lenses can now be worn comfortably for longer periods of time than formerly; however, they still should be worn only intermittently. *The lenses should not be worn when the eye shows symptoms of marked inflammation or infection, or if the vision is blurred.* If superficial scratches are present on the cornea and foreign bacteria are introduced with the lens, an infection may develop which requires immediate attention. Corneal contact lenses are available in two types: (1) methyl methacrylate and (2) so-called "soft lenses" of various chemical compositions. The so-called "hard" contact lens is usually smaller in size, lasts longer, and is easier to care for. The "soft lens" is more fragile, requires more frequent replacement, and needs more meticulous care.

In recent years corneal contact lenses have become quite popular. Most frequently these lenses are fitted for cosmetic reasons (because the patient feels more attractive than with eyeglasses) or because they are better than eyeglasses for a patient's activities (corneal lenses do not "fog" from rain, steam, or perspiration). Other *advantages* of contact lenses are as follows: (a) improved peripheral vision; (b) safe for many athletic events (low incidence of breakage); (c) unobstructed vision when sighting through cameras, microscopes, binoculars; (d) less distortion and more realistic size of objects viewed; (e) usually require changing less often than eyeglasses; (f) automatically cleaned as the eye is blinked; (g) enable the eyes to more efficiently work together in some instances; and (h) greatly improve the postoperative status of patients with cataracts by replacing heavy cataract eyeglass lenses. Generally patients have reduced corneal sensation following cataract surgery and can wear the corneal contact lens all day.

In addition to being useful in unilateral aphakia (where the greater discrepancy in image size which occurs while wearing eyeglass lenses interferes with binocular vision), corneal contact lenses are also useful in (a) some types of astigmatism; (b) the presence of turned-in eyelashes; (c) absence of the iris (aniridia); (d) congenital absence of pigment; (e) treating hyperopia (near-vision is increased and visual field is larger); and (f) treating keratoconus. Keratoconus is a degenerative thinning and anterior protrusion of the central cornea; in this condition a satisfactory correction of the refractive error is impossible with eyeglasses. High myopics also benefit from contact lenses, because of increase in image size and visual field.

Some *disadvantages* of contact lenses are (a) they are relatively more expensive than eyeglasses; (b) they can be lost more easily than eyeglasses; (c) they require more care than eyeglasses; (d) they are more difficult to insert into the eye than eyeglasses are to place on the head; (e) several office visits are necessary for prescription and adjustments of the lens; (f) usually sensitivity to light increases while wearing contact lenses; (g) not all visual disorders can be corrected with contact lenses; (h) not all persons can adjust physically or psychologically to contact lenses; and (i) semiannual evaluations are necessary.

Not all ophthalmologists believe in the general use of contact lenses. All potential candidates for contact lenses should have a thorough assessment of their visual problems by an ophthalmologist, whose recommendations should be followed. It is generally agreed that contact lenses should not be prescribed for persons who exhibit poor personal hygiene (e.g., dirty fingernails), or who are not responsible, cooperative, and intelligent. Increasingly eyes are being damaged as a result of carelessly wearing contact lenses, e.g., wearing the lens when the eye is inflamed or infected. Contact lenses are contraindicated in the presence of inflammatory and allergic conditions, presbyopia, severe exophthalmos, abnormal overflow of tears (epiphora), local neoplasm, and pterygium. They cannot be worn if there is insufficient circulation of tears under the lenses. Contacts are hazardous during accidental chemical injury of the eye, since some of the chemical may seep under the lens and severely burn the cornea before the lens can be removed. Also, care must be taken by wearers of contacts to prevent dust or dirt from collecting behind the lens where it can cause corneal damage. Contact lenses are prohibited for workers in some occupations where these hazards are particularly great.

Because contact lenses are actually foreign bodies in the eye, it takes a while for the eye to adjust to wearing corneal lenses. Definite metabolic changes occur in the cornea when contact lenses are initially introduced, e.g., edema, decreased corneal sensitivity. To facilitate adjustment of the eye to the lenses, the contact wearer is instructed to initially wear the lenses for only brief periods of time. Gradually the length of time is increased until the lenses are worn for the prescribed length of time. Hard lenses are worn maximally for 10–16 hours. They should never be worn during sleep. Contact with the cornea by hard lenses for excessive periods of time will cause corneal damage. Corneal abrasion is the most common complication from wearing contact lenses. However, the incidence of permanent eye damage from wearing contact lenses is low, considering the large number of persons wearing these lenses.

Patient teaching is an important part of preparing an individual for contact lenses. Once the patient's lenses have been properly fitted, it is the patient's responsibility to give the lenses and eyes the daily care which will ensure prevention of complications. The patient is taught the proper technique for applying and removing the lenses, in addition to the correct method of caring for the lenses. Unless cleaned, stored, and inserted in the recommended manner, the lenses may carry bacteria to the cornea. Before touching the lenses (for removal, insertion, or cleaning), the hands are washed. Lenses are cleaned prior to insertion with a recommended sterile, noncaustic solution. A wetting agent, e.g., methylcellulose, is applied to the lenses just before inserting them into the eye. Saliva should never be used as a wetting or cleaning agent; because the mouth contains pathogens, an infection can be introduced into the eye if there is a corneal abrasion present or if the person is passing through a period of low immunity. Stale, contaminated solutions used to clean, wet, or store the lenses must be discarded. After removal from the eye, hard lenses are wiped dry of lid secretions and may be stored in a dry, well-ventilated case or stored in a prescribed solution. Soft lenses are always stored in solution. Because individual lenses are ground for each eye, the lenses should be stored in a labeled container, i.e., "right," "left."

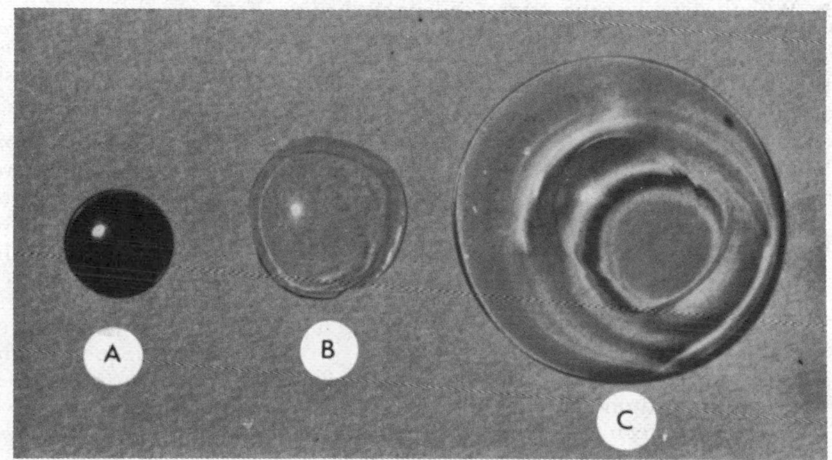

Figure 89–24. Three types of contact lenses are worn today. The most widely used is the hard contact lens *(A)* which is available either clear or tinted. Hard lenses come in three shades of blue, and in green, grey, pink, and brown. The soft contact lens *(B)* is the kind most recently developed, and is gaining in popularity. But, its use is limited to persons with low astigmatism. The scleral lens *(C)* is used least often because wearing time is limited to about four hours. Athletes use this lens during contact sports. (From Gould, H: How to remove contact lenses from comatose patients. *American Journal of Nursing,* 76:1483, Sept. 1976.)

Remember: Do not use force to remove a contact lens. If the lens can be seen but cannot be removed, gently slide if off the cornea, completely onto the sclera. It can safely remain on the sclera until the physician is available. Never try to remove a contact lens from an injured eye!

It is necessary for the nurse to *know how to remove contact lenses from a helpless patient,* e.g., an accident victim. Persons wearing contact lenses should carry a card or wear an identification tag stating they wear contact lenses. Unconscious persons or persons suffering serious injury should be checked for such a card or medallion, and should also have their eyes checked for contact lenses. To look for a contact gently separate the eyelids and shine a small light into the eye from the side to obliquely view the cornea. If present, contacts must be removed so the cornea will not be damaged from prolonged contact with the lens. Always remove contact lenses before sending a patient to surgery. In an emergency situation if you suspect that contact lenses are in the patient's eyes, but you have not had the time to remove them or you believe it is unsafe for you to try to remove them (e.g., if the eye is injured), apply a strip of adhesive tape labeled "CONTACT LENSES" to the patient's forehead and inform the physician. Do not attempt to remove a contact lens without expert help if the cornea of the patient's eye is not visible upon opening the eyelids.

A corneal contact lens can usually be removed from a helpless person in the following manner:

- With clean hands, gently position one thumb on the upper eyelid and one thumb on the lower eyelid. Have the tips of the thumbs near the lids' margins but rest the thumbs themselves over the eye's bony orbit.
- Gently separate the eyelids. Do not apply pressure directly on the eye, but rather pull the lids (up or down) toward the orbital rim.
- A visible lens should slide easily with a gentle movement of the eyelid. A lens may be found correctly positioned over the cornea, on the sclera only, or on both the sclera and cornea. If the lens is not over the cornea, slide it to this position with an appropriate movement of the eyelids. The lens must be positioned over the cornea if it is to be safely removed.
- With the lens over the cornea, widen the opening of the eyelids beyond the top and bottom edges of the lens and maintain this opening.
- Press both eyelids gently but firmly against the eye.
- Move the lower eyelid margin to a position barely touching the bottom edge of the lens.
- Next bring the upper eyelid margin down to the top edge of the lens, while keeping both eyelids firmly pressed on the eye.
- By pressing slightly harder on the lower eyelid, move it underneath the bottom edge of the lens. This movement should cause the lens to tip outward from the eye by pivoting the top edge and flipping out on the bottom edge.
- Once the lens has tipped slightly, begin moving the eyelids toward one another. The lens should then slide out between the eyelids where it can safely be retrieved.

The Nature of Refractive Error. Refractive errors tend to be inherited, but in no definitely predictable manner. Numerous variables influence refraction, e.g., corneal curvature, depth of the anterior chamber, shape of the lens, and length of the eye. Upon entering the eye, a ray of light passes through the cornea, the aqueous humor, the anterior and posterior surfaces of the lens, and the vitreous to focus upon the retina's fovea.

The ideal refractive condition of the eye is called *emmetropia.* In this "ideal" condition the unaccommodated eye (with the lens perfectly at rest) focuses parallel light rays from a distant source (of 6 meters or more) into a sharp image on the fovea. This condition of emmetropia ("sight in proper measure") refers to production of an image on the retina and has no relationship to vision produced. That is, despite emmetropia there may be cataract, retinal scarring, or nerve damage preventing normal vision. As emphasized, this is actually an ideal rather than a normal condition, since most adults have some degree of refractive disorder. *Ametropia* ("sight not in proper measure") refers to all variations from the emmetropic state which are not due to opacities or disease. Among the variations of ametropia are *aniseikonia* (difference in image size in the two eyes) and *anisometropia* (variation in the refractive errors of the two eyes). The most commonly encountered variations of ametropia are discussed below (Fig. 89–25).

- *Hyperopia (hypermetropia, "farsightedness"):* In this condition parallel rays of light are brought to a *focus behind the retina* when accommodative powers are relaxed. Typically vision is normal beyond 20 feet, but near-vision is poor. Hyperopia may result from shortness of the anteroposterior dimension of the eyeball or weakness of the refractive power of the cornea or lens. Hyperopia may be corrected with the use of a *convex lens,* which increases the angle of incidence of the light rays entering the cornea and lens, thus focusing the light rays on the surface of the retina.

- *Myopia ("nearsightedness"):* In this condition parallel rays of light are brought to a *focus in front of the retina,* i.e., before reaching the retinal surface. Typically near vision is normal, but distant vision is defective. Myopia is caused by an abnormally long anteroposterior dimension of the eyeball or by an increase in the strength of the refractive power of the media. Heredity is highly important in myopia. The most common symptom is inability to distinguish objects clearly at a distance. The patient frequently frowns or squints in an effort to sharpen visual acuity by making the lid aperture smaller; a smaller opening eliminates peripheral rays of light from entering the eye. Myopia may be corrected with *concave* (minus) lenses which diverge the light rays so they will focus correctly on the retina. Myopia usually increases in the teens and levels off at about age 25. In the 40's presbyopic symptoms develop, necessitating reading glasses or bifocals.

► *Presbyopia ("old sight"):* As discussed earlier, this is a disorder in which a *lessening of the effective powers of accommodation* occurs as a result of hardening of the lens due to the aging process. Loss of accommodation is manifested by blurring of near objects or visual fatigue when doing "close work." Presbyopia may be corrected with a lens which corrects any basic refractive error and which also has a proper *convex reading addition* for close work. This lens brings the near point within suitable range for focusing on the retina. Usually first reading lenses are necessary between ages 42–45. Presbyopia does not mean a worsening of hyperopia, but is merely a reduction of the powers of accommodation.

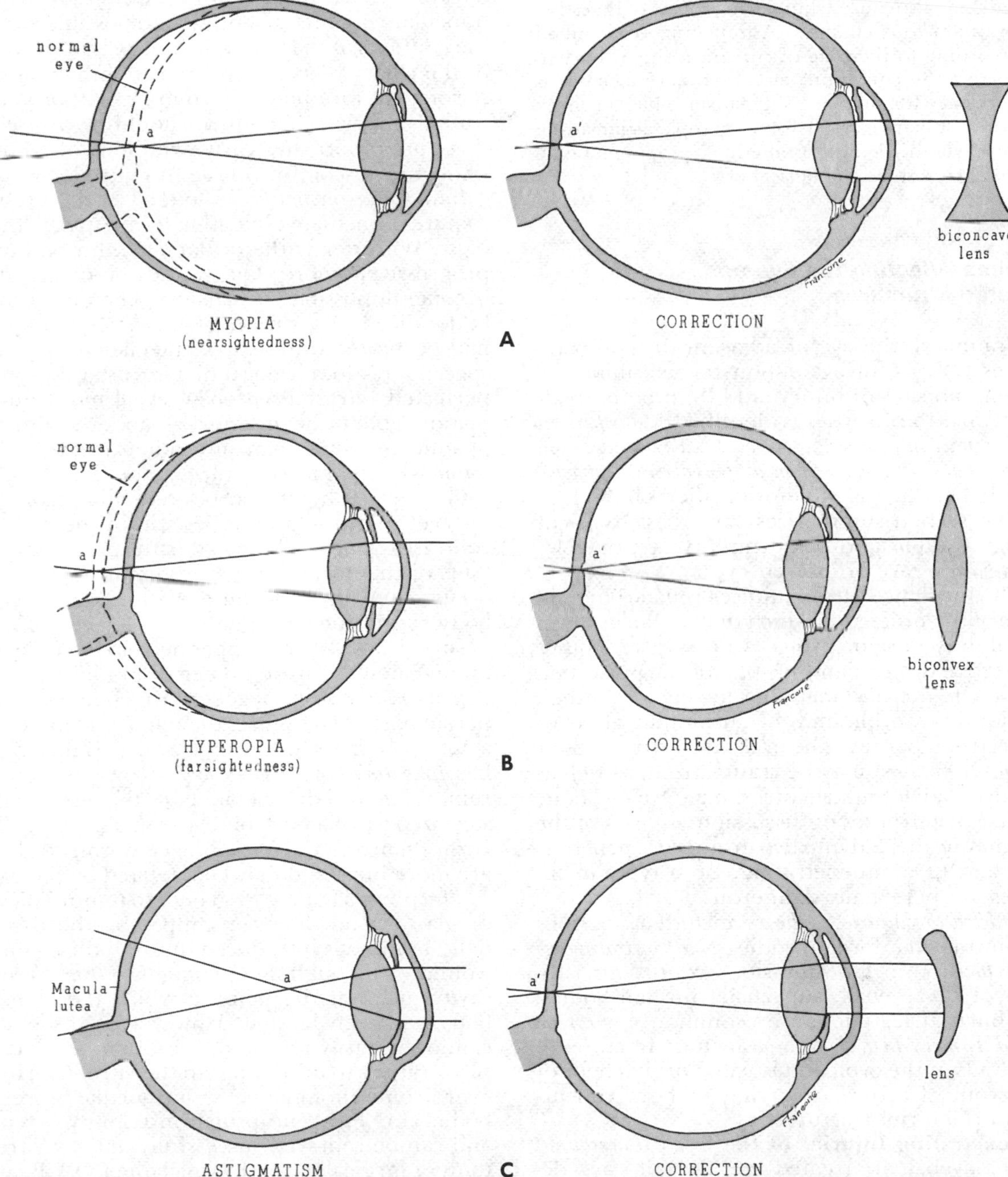

Figure 89–25. Common variations of ametropia and their correction. (From Jacob, S. W., C. A. Francone, and W. J. Lossow: *Structure and Function in Man.* 4th ed., 1978.)

► *Astigmatism ("distorted vision"):* Astigmatism refers to vision which is "not at a point." Astigmatism is distorted vision caused by a *variation in refractive power along different meridians of the eye.* The optical distortion is most often caused by irregular corneal curvature, which prevents the clear focus of light from any point; i.e., rays in the horizontal and perpendicular planes do not focus at the same point. The lens may also cause astigmatism, e.g., in old age, due to cataractous changes. Astigmatism is identified according to the type of *cylindric lens* necessary to correct the condition; e.g., a concave cylinder is necessary for myopic astigmatism, while a convex cylindric lens is used for hyperopic astigmatism. The cylindric lens is oriented in a proper meridian (axis) to restore a spherical effect.

Trauma Affecting the Eye and Related Structures

Trauma to the eye or adjacent structures requires (a) careful evaluation to determine the extent and sites of injury, and (b) prompt treatment once the disorder is identified. *Many persons with serious injury of the eye can have useful vision salvaged if they receive immediate, correct treatment.* Gentle handling is imperative. (See Ch. 95.)

This section summarizes some basic types of ocular trauma and some important principles concerning care of injured eyes.

The incidence of eye injuries remains high in spite of the protection which the eye can be given through the use of protective glasses and other protective devices, and in spite of the protection which the eye has anatomically, e.g., eyelashes, eyelids, bony orbit, and the cushioning effect of the retrobulbar fat. The eye's deep structures or its outer surface may be traumatized, as well as the eye's adjacent structures, e.g., eyelids, bony orbit. For purposes of discussion, injuries of the eye may be divided into two groups: (1) penetrating, and (2) nonpenetrating. Both types of injuries are potentially dangerous.

Penetrating injuries to the eye include lacerations and intraocular foreign bodies. *Nonpenetrating injuries to the eye* include abrasions, contusions, rupture of the eyeball, superficial foreign bodies, and burns. Lacerations are a common *injury of the eyelid. Injuries to the bony orbit* include fractures of the walls of the orbit and isolated orbital floor or "blowout" fracture occurring without concurrent orbital rim fracture.

Penetrating Injuries of the Eye. *Lacerations* of the eyeball are treated in different ways, depending upon whether or not prolapse of tissue has occurred. Generally a wound can be repaired surgically if the eyeball has been penetrated anteriorly, if there is no obvious evidence of prolapse of intraocular contents, and if the wound is clean and grossly free of contamination. The wound may also be surgically repaired if only a small portion of iris or only small amounts of uveal tissue have prolapsed. Following closure of such surgical repairs, a mydriatic is used, an antibiotic solution is instilled into the conjunctival sac, and a patch and shield cover the eye. The patient is then usually kept on bedrest with bathroom privileges for a day or two, and systemic antibiotics are employed prophylactically. Enucleation is indicated when the wound is extensive and has resulted in significant loss of intraocular contents. In addition to possible loss of the contents of the eye, if the injury is in the area of the ciliary body, sympathetic ophthalmia is a serious but rare potential complication of penetrating injuries. The nurse should be aware of this and report any early symptom of photophobia or discomfort in the uninjured eye.

Intraocular foreign bodies lodged in the eyeball require immediate evaluation by an ophthalmologist. With delay, the ocular medium becomes progressively more cloudy, and the object may become impossible to visualize. The object may be localized in a variety of ways. Metal objects may be located with a special metal detector, and special x-ray localizing studies are used. Recently perfected ultrasonic probes reveal more information about the interior of an eye with an opaque medium than any other method. *Ultrasonography* projects (upon the front of a cathode ray tube) the echoes returning from interfaces of varying densities within the eye. In contrast to the oscilloscopic pattern of the contents of the normal eye, a prominent echo peak occurs as a result of the presence of a foreign body within the eye.[30]

Particles of iron or copper need to be removed immediately to prevent later disorganization of ocular tissues from degenerative changes. Copper, in particular, ionizes the retina and indicates a poor prognosis for the injured eye. If the object has magnetic properties, e.g., iron or steel, its removal may be facilitated by the use of the sterilized tip of a portable electromagnet, e.g. the Bronson magnet. Some of the newer metal alloys are more inert and may be tolerated by the eye.

The physician may try at once to remove pieces of glass, wood, lead, or copper by the use of delicate forceps introduced through the original wound or through an opening into the vitreous cavity made at the point at which the foreign body has been located. However, if the object cannot be easily removed, it is often best left in place rather than stirring up the vitreous. However, some nonmagnetic intraocular foreign bodies (I.O.F.B.) encapsulate in a cloudy vitreous and can be removed successfully only by vitrectomy, a surgical means by which the I.O.F.B. and the vitreous body are removed. The hydrostatic pressure of the eye is maintained by the introduction of a basic salt solution; air or SF6 gas may be inserted, and as the gas expands it holds the retina in place. The nurse is responsible for positioning the patient postoperatively as prescribed by the physician. This patient may have to lie in a face-downward position or alternatively may sit up in a chair and rest the head on the arms of a bedside table; a pillow may be placed on the table for patient comfort. This position relieves the discomfort of lying in one position for an extended period of time, e.g., 3–4 days, until the gas or air absorbs. Some inert substances are well tolerated by the eye. It is usually more hazardous and more destructive to try to surgically remove such foreign bodies than it is to allow the continued presence of such inert material in the eye. Dirty wood splinters often promote endophthalmitis (intraocular infection), and toxins are contained in many varieties of thorns. Extensive systemic antibiotic therapy will be necessary to combat this.

If a foreign body causes a retinal hole in the far posterior portion, the hole may be sealed prophylactically by using a photocoagulator (providing the media are clear). Retinal detachment is one of the most serious complications involving an intraocular foreign body. Usually such detachments occur several months following the injury. Visual prognosis is usually poor with intraocular foreign bodies.

Important practices when caring for patients with penetrating eye injuries include the following:

1. Wash your hands thoroughly before approaching the eye.
2. Refer the patient to an eye specialist immediately for care.
3. Avoid applying pressure on the eye, and keep the patient from applying pressure to the eye.
4. Penetrating injuries may be covered with a plastic or metal eye shield to protect the eye until the patient reaches the physician.
5. Instruct the patient not to perform activities which will increase ocular pressure, e.g., not to bend the head down to get into a car and not to pull the car door closed (loss of intraocular contents could result).
6. Remember to use sterile medications and sterile technique whenever a penetrating injury has occurred.

Tetanus prophylaxis is given routinely to all patients with penetrating eye injuries. Because surgical repairs of penetrating injuries are usually performed under general anesthesia, advise the patient not to eat or drink until the physician gives permission to do so.

Nonpenetrating Injuries of the Eye. *Abrasions* of the lids, cornea, or conjunctiva may be treated with an antibiotic ointment prophylactically and an eye bandage applied with firm, gentle pressure. *Contusions* of the eyeball are carefully evaluated. Those contusions which are severe enough to cause intraocular hemorrhage, e.g., hyphema or vitreous hemorrhage, may eventually cause intractable glaucoma and damage to the eyeball. Patients with intraocular hemorrhage may be put on complete bed rest for 4–5 days. Both eyes may be patched or just the injured eye, and the patient may wear dark glasses as well in an attempt to minimize the chance of further bleeding. It may be necessary to administer acetazolamide (Diamox), mannitol, or other systemically administered agents to lower intraocular pressure. Also, a short-acting cycloplegic, e.g., 5 per cent homatropine and/or a steroid eyedrop, may be administered. *Rupture of the eyeball* can be surgically repaired in some cases; in others, enucleation of the eye is necessary, followed by implantation of a plastic sphere (to act as a space-filler and to assist in movement of the artificial eye). *Corneal and conjunctival foreign bodies* have been discussed previously. Foreign bodies on the cornea must be removed by a physician. A sterile local anesthetic is instilled into the eye, and the object is removed with special spuds, a scalpel blade, or a hypodermic needle. Untreated corneal infection is serious.

> *Foreign bodies and corneal abrasions are the most frequent causes of eye injury.*

Thermal burns of ocular structures are treated essentially the same as burns of the skin structures elsewhere, as far as lid involvement is concerned. (Burns are discussed generally in Unit XXI.) The lid surface is gently cleansed and greased thoroughly with an antibiotic ointment. If the lid is kept covered with ointment, dressings are not necessary. However, if lid closure is impaired (because of severity of the burn), the exposed cornea must be kept constantly covered with generous amounts of an ointment, or eyedrops such as methylcellulose natural tears, may be instilled every hour. Gentle, mechanical swabbing or warm, moist compresses are used to remove crusting and discharge. If corneal tissue sloughs off, permanent damage usually results. *Infrared exposure* seldom causes an ocular reaction. However, permanent visual impairment can result from viewing the sun or an eclipse of the sun without an adequate filter. Excessive exposure to *nuclear devices* or *radiation* (x-ray) may cause cataractous changes which may not appear until several months have passed following exposure. Even moderate exposure to *ultraviolet radiation* (e.g., ultraviolet keratitis, actinic keratitis) produces a highly painful keratitis. Such exposure may come from exposure to a welding arc ("welder's flash), excessive sunlight, sunlight on snow ("snow blindness"), or an artificial sunlamp.

> *Chemical burns of the eye are treated immediately by continuous irrigation of the eyes for 15 to 20 minutes. Do this immediately, without pausing to call for aid.*

Poisoning and the Eye. Lead, arsenic, carbon bisulfide, quinine, methyl alcohol, and tobacco are among the various toxins and chemical poisons which may affect the eye. *Ocular symptoms of poisoning* include:

- Miotic pupil (morphine addiction).
- Papilledema (vitamin A intoxication, lead poisoning).
- Reddened conjunctiva (alcoholic intoxication).
- Cataract formation (paradichlorobenzene poisoning, prolonged systemic corticosteroids, strong parasympathomimetic medications, excessive radiation exposure).
- "Yellow vision" (digitalis intoxication).

Posterior subcapsular lens opacities may develop if systemic corticosteroids are given for longer than 6 months in large or moderate doses. While these changes usually do not progress to cause an advanced cataract, they do cause some irreversible impairment of usual visual function.

Tobacco amblyopia may result from smoking of heavy tobacco in a pipe for many years. This condition results from disturbance of retinal ganglion cells and causes bilateral visual failure. Visual failure is typically first in color appreciation, especially the color red. Sometimes the condition is associated with excessive alcohol consumption (alcohol-tobacco amblyopia); it is more severe in patients who are also diabetic.

Injuries to the Eyelids. Eyelid lacerations should be treated by an ophthalmologist who can assess possible damage to the eye. It is important to repair lacerations of the canaliculus as a primary procedure, especially those involving the lower canaliculus. If this is not done, the resultant lacrimal obstruction is often very difficult to correct without more extensive surgery. Lacerations may be sutured after foreign materials are removed and bleeding is controlled.

Injuries to the Bony Orbit. Concussion injuries to the orbital contents may produce hemorrhage or subsequent tissue atrophy, with enophthalmos.

Hemorrhage into the orbit often accompanies trauma to the eye or surrounding tissues. The result is a *hematoma ("black eye")* of the lids and surrounding skin. Such bleeding generally stops spontaneously, but it is helpful to apply cold compresses initially to help reduce the bleeding and swelling. Hot compresses may help to speed absorption of the blood after the initial 24 hours. Medications may also be given to help absorb the hematoma. All patients with ecchymosis around the eye and orbital structures are examined for possible skull fractures. When *traumatic subconjunctival hemorrhage* occurs, the pupil is usually dilated so that a complete ophthalmoscopic examination can be performed.

The Eye and Other Bodily Disorders

Because the eye is intimately connected with the rest of the body, it provides large amounts of knowledge about the body as a whole. Since the eyes and their supporting structures are favorably exposed to easy inspection, the physician can learn a great deal about a patient's state of health by performing a thorough ocular examination.

Many objective signs of abnormality can be found by examining the eye. Examination of the eye's portal can reveal not only disorders of the eye itself but also manifestations of many other disorders affecting the rest of the body. Ocular involvement occurs as part of the morbid process or as a complication of numerous disorders, which affect the body as a whole or which affect a particular system, e.g., nervous system, cardiovascular system, or endocrine system. Ocular symptoms may be the first manifestations of some of these diseases; in other instances, the ocular symptoms (by their evolution and course of resolution) are significant prognostic indications of the general disease. Characteristic fundus pictures occur with some conditions, such as hypertension, diabetes, blood dyscrasias, and arteriosclerosis.

Nurses do not usually examine the eye's interior, e.g., with an ophthalmoscope, to look for ocular symptoms of disease. However, nurses should be aware that the following *external* ocular symptoms may indicate systemic or nervous system diseases: edema, conjunctival jaundice, xanthelasma (flattened, yellowish orange, slightly raised, lipoid plaques deposited in the lids' skin); bilateral subconjunctival hemorrhage; redness of the eyes; pupil disorders; paralysis of an extraocular muscle; and exophthalmos. Persons with these undiagnosed symptoms should be encouraged to seek a complete physical examination, which includes an ocular examination. Nurses can perform valuable health teaching by emphasizing that the general state of the body's health is reflected in the health of the eyes, and that because of this relationship general health practices (e.g., balanced nutrition, adequate rest and exercise, cleanliness) are important for eye health.

Removal of the Eyeball (Enucleation)

Some indications for enucleation, i.e., removal of the eyeball, are severe infections, malignant tumors, irritating foreign bodies which cannot be removed, management of severe pain in a blind eye, absolute glaucoma, cosmetic improvement of a blind and disfiguring eye, and extensive trauma to the eye. Prophylactically enucleation may be performed when sympathetic ophthalmia is likely to occur.

Enucleation may be performed under local or general anesthesia. During enucleation, the tendons of the rectus muscles are isolated and divided close to the globe. The muscles may be sutured to each other around a synthetic sphere. This builds up the eye to look similar to the other, providing a better cosmetic appearance.

Implants are balls made of such materials as plastic or Teflon. Following enucleation a "conformer" is placed in the socket until later when a prosthesis (artificial eye), designed to be identical to the opposite eye, is placed beneath the lids. Usually the artificial eye is not placed until edema subsides, i.e., several days or weeks. Insertion, removal, and care of artificial eyes and care of the socket have been discussed previously. The physician discusses with the patient whether the prosthesis should be removed or not.

Following enucleation a firm pressure dressing is applied for 24–48 hours. Usually the patient is allowed out of bed with no restrictions on activity on the first postoperative day. Possible complications following enucleation include hemorrhage and infection. Infection may be indicated by pain and headache on the side of the enucleation, or a temperature elevation. Occasionally infection results in abscess, thrombosis, or meningitis. Because the possibility of meningitis is increased if an actively suppurating eyeball is enucleated, panophthalmitis is a contraindication to enucleation. Usually panophthalmitis necessitates evisceration of the eyeball.

Evisceration is a surgical procedure in which the entire contents of the eyeball, and sometimes the cornea are removed but the sclera remains. Evisceration with the removal of the cornea is used in the presence of panophthalmitis. Some physicians prefer evisceration with retention of the cornea in a case requiring enucleation when there is no sign of neoplasm. Recovery is less rapid following this procedure than it is following enucleation. Reaction and pain are greater. However, good support is left for use of an artificial eye following evisceration.

Exenteration is a procedure which is more radical than either enucleation or evisceration. With exenteration the eyelids, eyeball, and orbital contents are removed. Because of disfigurement it is usually necessary for a black patch to be worn, or if glasses are worn, they may be fitted with a side goggle-type covering to prevent the curious stares of onlookers; a prosthesis is unsatisfactory in this area.

The patient who has had to have an eye surgically removed needs help in (a) understanding why it was necessary to remove the eye; (b) adjusting to a new body image; (c) learning how to care for, insert, and remove an artificial eye if one is used; (d) learning how to care for the eye socket; (e) adjusting to vision with only one eye; and (f) learning how to protect vision in the remaining eye. Nurses may provide help in all these areas. A normal period of depression usually follows removal of an eye. Typically satisfactory adjustment occurs to loss of the eye. The physician may recommend that the patient wear a safety glass over the remaining eye.

REHABILITATION OF THE BLIND INDIVIDUAL

Blindness may be present at birth or it may develop suddenly or slowly at any time during an individual's life. Because vision is highly important, its absence initially represents a great loss and presents a serious disability.

The majority of blind persons lose their vision after 20 years of age. Thus they must make major adjustments in their adult years to learn to live without vision. Rehabilitation of the newly blinded person frequently begins in the hospital; however, extensive rehabilitation continues after the patient is discharged home or after transfer to a special rehabilitative facility for the blind. The patient's physician and a nurse or social worker help the patient and significant others to contact appropriate agencies which will participate in the rehabilitative process.

It is important for the newly blinded person to be immediately introduced to the various national, state, and private agencies which will assist with rehabilitation before psychologic attitudes develop which could cause the patient unnecessary difficulties. Today rehabilitation is directed toward helping the blind to live as normal a life as possible. Blind persons are thus encouraged to live in their home community rather than in special settings where they associate primarily with other blind persons. Periods of stay at special schools for the blind may be helpful, but permanent residence in a facility for the blind is undesirable.

Lack of vision is all that blind persons have in common. Otherwise *they differ from one another as greatly as the members of any heterogeneous group differ.* If one emphasizes the loss, there is then the detrimental tendency to mentally lump all blind persons together as a group, and thus not to consider them as individuals. Also, emphasis on the loss of vision (rather than on the remaining capabilities of the blind) tends to foster dependence rather than independence for blind persons. Instead of assuming that the needs and problems of all blind persons are similar, the personalized problems of blind *individuals* need to be identified. Each blind person's uniqueness should be considered during the rehabilitative process, as well as during day-to-day contacts with blind persons.

Rehabilitative Facilities and Procedures

Government legislation provides many benefits for blind persons. The newly blinded person needs to be informed of these benefits and other services which are available. All United States local and state agencies and their special services may be found listed in the *Directory of Agencies Serving Blind Persons in the United States* (available from the American Foundation for the Blind, Inc., 15 W. 16th St., New York, N.Y. 10011). This voluntary agency also distributes a catalogue of *Aids and Appliances* for blind persons which is distributed free of charge. A braille edition of the catalogue is also available on request.

The National Society for the Prevention of Blindness, 79 Madison Ave., New York, N.Y. 10016, is a voluntary agency specializing in education, preventive services, and research. Pamphlets, films, and a quarterly publication *(The Sight Saving Review)* are available from this agency.

The newly blind individual may be advised to contact the State Welfare Department Division for the Blind. The federal government (through the Social and Rehabilitation Services Administration of the United States Department of Health, Education, and Welfare) allocates on a formula basis funds provided by Congress to be added to state funds for vocational rehabilitation programs within each state. These resources may be used by the blind to further their rehabilitation efforts and to obtain additional training.

Many blind persons benefit from contact with the closest library facility for the blind. These libraries provide numerous services, among which are books, magazines, and newspapers in braille, and "talking books," i.e., books, magazines, and so forth which have content read aloud and recorded for blind persons to listen to. Information concerning library resources for sightless persons can be obtained from the Library of Congress, Division for the Blind, Washington, D.C. Recordings of textbooks and educational materials, as well as the other recorded materials mentioned, are all available free of charge to blind persons. Talking book machines are loaned free of charge to the legally blind. Information may also be obtained from the national organizations for the blind mentioned previously, from public libraries, or from Recordings for the Blind, Inc., 215 East 58th St., New York, N.Y. 10022.

Blind children may be educated in special facilities, located in public or parochial schools, or in residential schools. Most states have a school for the blind. Students learn through the braille system and auditory instruction. Additionally the blind person can take a variety of correspondence courses with such schools as the Hadley Correspondence School for the Blind in Berwyn, Illinois. While older sightless persons may have difficulty learning braille (if they have some reduction in the ability to learn and in their tactile sense), many blind persons can be taught to read and write braille. Once this basic tool is learned, many avenues of study are open to the patient. Tape recorders are useful for the blind student to record lectures. Today it is not unusual for blind students to attend colleges and universities. There they may study with the help of braille notes, braille books, tape recorders, and readers. They are usually exceptional students because they concentrate their whole auditory attention on the subject matter being presented.

Blind persons can learn numerous occupations and may become completely self-sufficient if given adequate rehabilitative help. Total rehabilitation may require the assistance of an occupational therapist, physical therapist, social worker, and psychiatrist in addition to the patient's personal physician and nurses in various agencies.

Appropriate timing is highly important for successful rehabilitation. The accomplishment of new performances may markedly improve the patient's spirits. Failure, however, may intensify depression. For example, if braille is introduced too early and the patient fails to learn the technique, he or she may become seriously depressed.

The first steps made by a blind individual in regaining self-sufficiency involve learning how to feed, dress, and groom and to walk about in a small area. When blind people are learning to feed themselves they may find it helpful to practice once or twice with an empty spoon to gauge the distance from the plate to the mouth before trying to handle food on the spoon. Practice with an empty cup and empty glass is also useful at first. Establishing a routine placement for the various table pieces, e.g., plate, utensils, glass, cup and saucer, helps the blind person to have a familiar orientation at every meal. It is important to always set up the blind individual's tray or table in the same pattern. If changes are made, the patient should be informed. Beverages should be served in vessels which are not easily overturned. The glass or cup should not be excessively full. If the person mentally visualizes the plate as a clock or compass face, it is then possible to consistently place certain foods in the same location. For example, the patient may be told that meat will always be located at "six o'clock" or "south" (i.e., on the portion of the plate closest to the patient). Other foods may then also be placed consistently in other areas which the patient can visualize, e.g., potatoes at "three o'clock" or "East." Another useful way to orient blind people to the surroundings is for the nurse to take the patient's hand and permit his or her fingertips to touch the area the nurse is describing, e.g., the edge of the tray, and the spatial relationship between this and the edge of the plate or the glass containing liquid. This also prevents the embarrassment of accidents. Privacy should be provided until the patient learns to eat independently reasonably well.

During the rehabilitation process, blind people learn to groom themselves and learn in other ways not to call unnecessary attention to their lack of vision. For example, if a patient appears to be developing unnecessary postural attitudes or mannerisms, e.g., grimacing, gently tell the person of these tendencies and help him or her to correct them.

If blind people are going to be independent and have a reasonable amount of privacy, it is essential that they be able to get about by themselves and not rely on another person to guide them. Through a mobility training program blind people can be taught to increase the usefulness of remaining intact senses to help orient them to the surroundings. It is particularly helpful to increase the skillful use of hearing and object sense. Blind people may become quite sensitive to tones of voice; this helps them to communicate more effectively with others since they cannot see facial expression or other nonverbal cues.

Blind people may be trained to become more sensitive to *facial perception*. Facial perception is an echo interpretive factor which helps one to recognize the presence of such solid obstacles as high walls and fences. By becoming more sensitive to air currents in a room, sightless people may obtain some idea about the placement of doors, windows, and so forth. By developing the sense of touch in the hands, it is possible for blind people to more easily identify objects in the surroundings. Blind people benefit from learning to listen with greater acuity. Changes in the pitch of sound may help them navigate by tapping a cane as they walk. A variety of canes are available and are usually selected according to the height of the blind individual. Specialists teach proper use of the cane during the rehabilitative process.

Some blind persons are suited to having a guide dog. Various guide dog schools are located throughout the country. Dogs are furnished free of charge to the blind. The sightless person who has selected to receive a dog lives in residence at the school for several weeks. At the school the person and dog learn to work with and care for one another.

Younger persons are especially suited to guide dog training. Canes are particularly useful for older persons or persons who for other reasons cannot walk rapidly enough to use a guide dog. When possible the blind person should use both cane and guide dog travel. The cane is useful when the dog is not in harness or when the blind person is temporarily without a dog. The individual who is properly trained to use a cane can become as mobile and independent as a person trained to use a dog.

By learning to use white canes, guide dogs, braille writing, and other helpful devices and by participating in appropriate training and educational programs, blind people can attain remarkable self-sufficiency if they are well motivated.

Regular physical examinations are encouraged for blind people (and for guide dogs). Hearing problems should be treated early, since hearing defects pose serious problems for the blind. General nutritional status and physical condition require periodic evaluation and correction to maintain the optimal state of health necessary to help blind people compensate their visual loss.

Courtesies Toward the Blind Individual

In the previous section we have discussed some of the compensatory techniques that blind persons may learn in order to help themselves. Now let us consider some of the ways in which other persons can help the blind individual.

When blind persons are hospitalized they should have a call bell available at all times. Attempts should be made to keep newly blinded patients oriented. They may be placed in a ward with other patients. It is helpful if you explain noises which they may wonder about. Show patients around the room. Walk with them and have them touch various objects in the room, e.g., table, chair, window, door, sink, radio. Once patients are able to walk about the halls, walk with them, showing them where the nurses' station, elevator, visitors' lounge, telephone, rest rooms, and so forth are located. Try to help prevent patients from feeling neglected, e.g., by frequently dropping in to visit briefly, by performing procedures on time. When walking with blind patients have them take hold of your forearm and walk so that you are a half step in front of them. This way they feel the movement of your gait. Some blind patients who are totally independent prefer to walk next to the person showing them around, merely permitting elbows to touch, and become amazingly adept in following the tiniest deviation along a pathway.

Introductions are always important; this is particularly true with blind persons. Upon approaching blind individuals, speak to them so they know someone is nearby. When introduced to a blind person, speak to them, saying something about who you are, e.g., "I am a student of nursing. I will be taking care of you this morning." If the patient extends a hand, take it and shake hands. Speak clearly, yet quietly and calmly. When with blind persons do not try to avoid use of such words as "see" and do not avoid discussing the appearance of things. Do not apologize for the fact that you can see, e.g., "I feel guilty that I can see these lovely flowers and you cannot." When you are addressing a blind person in a group of people, use the person's name to make it clear whom you are talking to. Blind people, of course, cannot see eye contact. Always speak to blind persons when you approach them or enter or leave the room. Also tell them before you touch them. Prepare the blind person for what is going to happen next. This is particularly important when performing nursing procedures. Make smooth movements rather than sudden jerky ones. Attempt to appear relaxed and unhurried. Rushing blind people may be confusing to them.

As emphasized previously, do not change the location of objects in the room or environment of a sightless person without describing the change. Keeping things in familiar places adds to the patient's independence and thus to a sense of security. A blind patient's

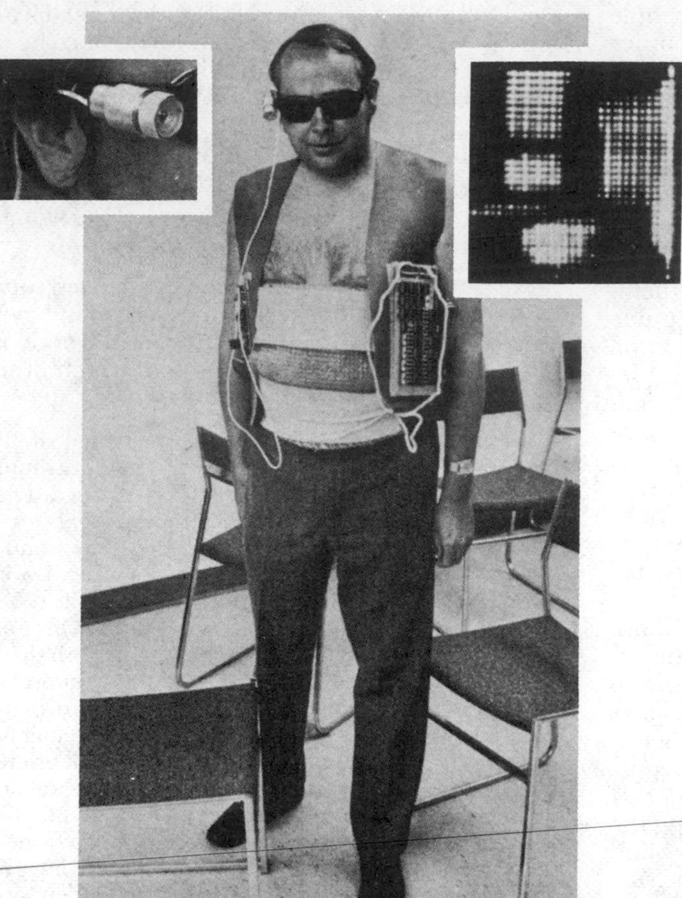

Figure 89–26. An example of advances being made in aids that can assist visually impaired people to become more independent. This device can help a person navigate more quickly than with a cane. The device consists of a minicamera (worn on the frame of eye glasses); about 1000 electrodes sewn into an elastic garment and worn on the abdomen, and a "commutator," which is worn over the elastic garment. The minicamera sends visual images to the "commutator," which converts the images to electrical impulses. The person feels vibrations on the skin when the impulses reach the electrodes. These vibrations conform to the image shape picked up by the camera. With practice, the person is able to identify objects in the environment by the pattern felt on abdominal skin. (From Clarke. M.: Medicine. Electronic eyes. *Newsweek,* May 24, 1976.)

environment should be kept well lit and pleasant. Patients should learn to put lights on when awake and moving about, even though they cannot benefit from them. This prevents others from being startled by meeting a person in the dark.

In the hospital it is advisable to take special precautions to ensure the safety of blind patients. For example, it is advisable to supervise smoking, keep at least one siderail up, assist patients when walking, and keep dangerous objects away from the bedside, e.g., chairs that can be knocked over if they are left in an unaccustomed place after visiting hours are over. Restrictions may be greater for the newly blind than for patients who have become accustomed to blindness. Never leave doors partially open, because blind persons may walk into them. Either completely open the door or completely shut it. Teach patients to take hold of both armrests of a chair before sitting down.

Nurses should discuss safety factors with significant others of the newly blinded patient. Advise them how they can rearrange the home to make it possible for the patient to more easily and more safely move about. The visiting nurse may be helpful in this aspect of planning or in making home visits for other purposes. Significant others must learn that an overprotective attitude toward the patient is harmful.

Do not rush up and offer help to a blind person unless it is clear that the person wants help. When you decide to offer help, don't sneak up on the blind person, but rather walk firmly up (approaching on the side opposite the cane or dog) and ask in a clear, friendly voice if help is needed. Do not take hold of the person before speaking. This is most important if the person has a guide dog. The guide dog is a disciplined worker, and when a dog is on duty it should not be disturbed. Do not try to touch or give directions to the guide dog while it is working. Do not touch or speak to the dog until you have asked the owner for permission to do so.

When walking with a sightless person, offer your arm rather than grasping the person's arm. The blind individual has a better sense of balance and direction of movement by holding your arm and if you walk slightly ahead. Tell the person when you are approaching stairs, a curb, an incline, and so forth. Then pause briefly before beginning to step up or down.

Visitors, friends, or family members may ask your advice about gifts for the blind patient. Suggest gifts which appeal to senses other than vision, e.g., a new record, scented flowers, cologne, or, if the patient is newly permanently blinded, objects which will help the person to regain independence.

BIBLIOGRAPHY (Chapter 89)

1. A cataract is not necessarily a calamity. *Health*, 9:10, Mar., 1972.
2. *A Glimpse of Vision*. (Pamphlet) Guide Dogs for the Blind, Inc., San Rafael, California, 94902.
3. Abrahamson, I. A., Jr.: Chalazion. *GP*, 38:83, July 1968.
4. Abrahamson, I. A., Jr.: Intraocular pressure tonometry. *American Family Physician*, 17:75, June 1978.

5. Abrahamson, I. A., Jr.: Management of ocular foreign bodies. *American Family Physician*, 14:81, Sept. 1976.
6. American Foundation for the Blind: *Directory of Agencies Serving Blind Persons in the United States*. 15th ed. New York, The William Byrd Press, Inc., 1967.
7. Andriola, M. J.: When visual disturbances are linked to neurologic disorders. *Geriatrics*, 31:109, Mar. 1976.
8. Appen, R. E., and C. F. Hutson: Traumatic injuries. Office treatment of eye injury. 1. Injury due to foreign materials. *Postgraduate Medicine*, 60:233, Oct. 1976.
9. Appen, R. E., and C. F. Hutson: Traumatic injuries. Office treatment of eye injury. 2. Injury from sharp instruments or blunt trauma. *Postgraduate Medicine*, 60:237, Nov. 1976.
10. Arentsen, J.: Changing indications for keratoplasty: *American Journal of Ophthalmology*, 81:313–318, 1976.
11. Barsam, P. C.: Specific prophylaxis of gonorrheal ophthalmia neonatorum: a review. *New England Journal of Medicine*, 274:731, Mar. 1966.
12. Baum, J. L.: Current concepts in ophthalmology, ocular infections. *New England Journal of Medicine*, 299:28–31, 1978.
13. Bellows, A. R., and W. Grant: Cyclocryotherapy. *American Journal of Ophthalmology*, 75:679–684, April 1973.
14. Bellows, J. G.: Understanding cataracts. *AORN Journal*, 7:64, May 1968.
15. Bergersen, B. S.: *Pharmacology in Nursing*. 12th ed. St. Louis, C. V. Mosby Co., 1973.
16. Bixler, D. P.: Bacterial decontamination and cleaning of contact lenses. *American Journal of Ophthalmology*, 62:324, Aug. 1966.
17. Bledsoe, C. W., and R. C. Williams: The vision needed to nurse the blind. *American Journal of Nursing*, 66:2432, Nov. 1966.
18. Bonnett, K.: Adjusting to blindness. *Nursing Mirror*, 126:21, Feb. 1968.
19. Boyd-Monk, H.: Cataract surgery. *Nursing 77*, 7:56, June 1977.
20. Boyd-Monk, H.: Helping the corneal transplant patient to see again. *Nursing 78*, 8:47, Feb. 1978.
21. Boyd-Monk, H.: Screening for glaucoma. *Nursing 79*, 9:42, Aug. 1979.
22. Boyd-Monk, H.: Taking a closer look at contact lenses. *Nursing 78*, 8:39, Oct. 1978.
23. Branson, H. K.: The blind mother. *American Journal of Nursing*, 75:414, Mar. 1975.
24. Brief consultation: Is surgery indicated for congenital nystagmus? *Consultant*, 18:153, Mar. 1978.
25. Cardona, H.: Restoring vision by prosthokeratoplasty. *Nursing Mirror*, 125:4, Nov. 1967.
26. Carr, R. E.: Look them in the injured eye. *Emergency Medicine*, 9:53, Nov. 1977.
27. Clark, M.: Medicine: electronic eyes. *Newsweek*, May 24, 1976, p. 83.
28. Cohen, K. L., and R. A. Hydniuk: Ocular emergencies. *American Family Physician*, 18:178, Oct. 1978.
29. Coleman, D. J., L. Katz, and F. L. Lizzi: Isometric, three-dimensional viewing of ultrasonagrams. *Archives of Ophthalmology*, 93:1362–1365, Dec. 1975.
30. Condl, E. D., et al.: Ophthalmic nursing. *Nursing Clinics of North America*, 5:449, Sept. 1970.
31. Coodley, E. L. (ed.): Therapeutic conference. Problem: acute loss of vision. *Emergency Medicine*, 10:60, Jan. 1978.
32. Cullin, I. C.: Techniques for teaching patients with sensory defects. *Nursing Clinics of North America*, 5:527, Sept. 1970.
33. Davis, M. D., P. A. Segal, and A. MacCormick: The natural course followed by the fellow eye with rhegmatogenous retinal detachment. *In* Pruett and Regan (eds.): *Retina Congress*, 56:643–660. New York, Appleton-Century-Crofts, 1972.
34. Delaney, W. V., Jr.: Intravitreal saline in retinal detachment. *American Journal of Ophthalmology*, 74:241, Aug. 1972.
35. Delaney, W. V., Jr.: Preventable blindness. *GP*, 38:121, Nov. 1968.
36. Delaney, W. V., Jr., and R. P. Oates: Retinal detachment in the second eye. *Archives of Ophthalmology*, 96:629–634. Apr. 1978.
37. Drance, S. M.: Visual field defects. *In* Duane, T. (ed.): *Clinical Ophthalmology*. Vol. III, Ch. 49. New York, Harper & Row, 1976.
38. Dyer, J. A.: *Atlas of Extraocular Muscle Surgery*. Philadelphia, W. B. Saunders Co., 1970.
39. Eddy, D. M.: Vitrectomy. *American Journal of Nursing*, 78:608, Apr. 1978.
40. Ehrlich, D. R., and R. H. Keates: What to do when the elderly patient complains of external eye problems. *Geriatrics*, 33:34, July 1978.
41. Emery, J. M., G. K. von Noordeen, and D. A. Schlernitzauer: Management of orbital floor fractures. *American Journal of Ophthalmology*, 74:299, Aug. 1972.
42. Epstein, D. L., and D. Paton: Keratitis from misuse of corneal anesthetics. *New England Journal of Medicine*, 279:396, Aug. 1968.
43. Fenwick, E., et al.: Traumatic blindness: a flexible approach for helping a blind adolescent. *Nursing 79*, 9:37, Jan. 1979.
44. Fernsebner, W.: Early diagnosis of acute angle-closure glaucoma. *American Journal of Nursing*, 75:1154, July 1975.
45. Fulton, M., et al.: Helping diabetics adapt to failing vision. *American Journal of Nursing*, 74:54, Jan. 1974.
46. Gass, J. D. M.: Differential diagnosis of intraocular tumors. St. Louis, C. V. Mosby Co., 1974.
47. Geary, R. P.: Journey into fog. *American Journal of Nursing*, 78:246, Feb. 1978.
48. Giffin, R. B., Jr.: Eye damage in newborns from use of strong silver nitrate solutions. *California Medicine*, 107:178, Aug. 1967.
49. Glaser, J. S.: How to recognize ischemic optic neuropathy—and what to do about it. *Geriatrics*, 33:68, Aug. 1978.
50. Gould, H.: How to remove contact lenses from comatose patients. *American Journal of Nursing*, 76:1483, Sept. 1976.
51. Grant, W. M.: *Toxicology of the Eye*. 2nd ed. Springfield, Ill., Charles C Thomas, 1974.
52. Guyton, A. C.: *Textbook of Medical Physiology*. 4th ed. Philadelphia, W. B. Saunders Co. 1971, Chs. 52 to 54.
53. Hamilton, M. J.: What the nurse should know about eye banks. *Nursing Clinics of North America*, 5:483, Sept. 1970.
54. Hassani, S. N.: Evaluating the eye through ultrasonography. *Geriatrics*, 32:94, Oct. 1977.
55. Havener, H.: *Ocular Pharmacology*. 3rd ed. St. Louis, C. V. Mosby Co., 1974.
56. Havener, W. H.: *Synopsis of Ophthalmology*. 3rd. ed. St. Louis, C. V. Mosby Co., 1971.
57. Havener, W. H., and S. L. Gloeckner: *Atlas of Diagnostic Techniques and Treatment of Intraocular Foreign Bodies*. St. Louis, C. V. Mosby Co., 1969.
58. Hickman, J. W., W. C. Edwards, and E. Torczynski: Nonthyropathic exophthalmos. *American Family Physician*, 16:99, Oct. 1977.
59. Hiles, D. A.: Strabismus. *American Journal of Nursing*, 74:1082, June 1974.
60. How to Remove Contact Lenses From an Unconscious Person. (Kit) American Optometric Association, 7000 Chippewa St., St. Louis, Mo. 63119.
61. Jackson, C. R. S.: *The Eye in General Practice*. 5th ed. London; E. & S. Livingstone, Ltd., 1969.
62. Jacob, S. W., C. A. Francone, W. J. Lossow: *Structure and Function in Man*, 4th ed. Philadelphia, W. B. Saunders Co., 1978.
63. Jaffee, N. S.: Current concepts in ophthalmology, cata-

ract surgery—modern attitude toward a technologic explosion. *New England Journal of Medicine*, 299:235–238, 1978.
64. Keeney, A. H.: Trauma of the globe, Adnexa, and orbital walls: prophylaxis and immediate therapy. *In* Harley, R. D. (ed.), *Pediatric Ophthalmology*. Philadelphia, W. B. Saunders Co., 1975.
65. Kent, S.: Continuous drug delivery methods reflect progress in therapy for chronic diseases. *Geriatrics*, 32:146, Sept. 1977.
66. Leopold, I. H., and M. A. Mosier: Four common ocular complications of diabetes—and how to treat them. *Geriatrics*, 33:33, Nov. 1978.
67. Levenson, L., and J. Levenson: Corneal transplantation. *American Journal of Nursing*, 77:1160, July 1977.
68. McDonald, L. L.: Are you ready for contact lenses? *Family Health*, 4:32, May 1972.
69. Magoon, R. C., and R. Sexon: Wet or dry contact lens storage. *Archives of Ophthalmology*, 77:197, Feb. 1967.
70. Marmor, M. F.: The eye and vision in the elderly. *Geriatrics*, 32:63, Aug. 1977.
71. Mechner, F.: Programmed instruction. Patient assessment: examination of the eye. Part 1. *American Journal of Nursing*, 74:1–24, Nov. 1974.
72. Mechner, F.: Programmed instruction. Patient assessment: examination of the eye. part 2. *American Journal of Nursing*, 75:1–24, Jan. 1975.
73. Medical News: System may let blind "see with their skins." *Journal of the American Medical Association*, 207:2204, Mar. 1969.
74. Morse, P. H.: Ocular symptoms and signs of diabetes. *Geriatrics*, 31:59, Oct. 1976.
75. Mummah, H.: Fingers to see. *American Journal of Nursing*, 76:1608, Oct. 1976.
76. Neu, C.: Coping with newly diagnosed blindness. *American Journal of Nursing*, 75:2161, Dec. 1975.
77. Newell, F. W.: *Ophthalmology: Principles and Concepts*. 2nd ed. St. Louis, C. V. Mosby Co., 1969.
78. Nordstrom, W.: Adjusting to cataract glasses. *American Journal of Nursing*, 66:1578, July 1966.
79. Ohno, M. I.: The eye-patched patient. *American Journal of Nursing*, 71:271, Feb. 1971.
80. Okamura, I. D.: Implants in retinal surgery. *In* Pruett and Regan (eds.): *Retina Congress*. 24:319–324. New York, Appleton-Century-Crofts, 1972.
81. Okun, E., G. P. Johnston, and I. Boniuk: *Management of Diabetic Retinopathy*. St. Louis, C. V. Mosby Co., 1971.
82. Ostler, H. B., et al.: Opportunistic ocular infections. *American Family Physician*, 17:134, April 1978.
83. Palumbo, P. J., and J. M. Munoz: Diabetic retinopathy. *American Family Physician*, 14:60, July 1976.
84. Patton, D., and J. A. Craig: Glaucomas: diagnosis and management. *Clinical Symposia*, 28:2, 1976.
85. Patz, A.: Current concepts in ophthalmology, retinal vascular disease. *New England Journal of Medicine*, 298:1451–1454, 1978.
86. Pilgrim, M., and B. Sigler: Phaco-emulsification of cataracts. *American Journal of Nursing*, 75:976, June 1975.
87. Rabb, M. F.: The present status of corneal transplantation. *Nursing Clinics of North America*, 5:477, Sept. 1970.
88. Rakusin, W.: Traumatic hyphema. *American Journal of Ophthalmology*, 74:284, Aug. 1972.
89. Rodreguez, M. N., and J. A. Shields: Iris metastases from a bronchial carcinoid tumor. *Archives of Ophthalmology*, 96:77–83, 1978.
90. Rosborough, J. F.: Ocular emergencies. *Hospital Medicine*, 7:46, Nov. 1971.
91. Sarnat, L. A.: Contact lenses: separating fact from fancy. *Postgraduate Medicine*, 64:125, July 1978.
92. Scheie, H. G., and D. M. Albert: *Adler's Textbook of Ophthalmology*. Philadelphia, W. B. Saunders Co., 1969.
93. Schepens, C.: Rationale of surgical procedures. *In* Pruett and Regan (eds): *Retina Congress*. 23:297–318. New York, Appleton-Century-Crofts, 1972.
94. Seaman, F. W.: Nursing care of glaucoma patients. *Nursing Clinics of North America*, 5:489, Sept. 1970.
95. Shafer, D. M.: Vitrectomy. *New England Journal of Medicine*, 295:836, Oct. 1976.
96. Shields, J. A. and R. S. Stephens: Metastatic cases to the uvea, in press.
97. Shiery, S.: Insight into the delicate art of eye care. *Nursing 75*, 5:50, June 1975.
98. Smith, J.: Focusing your care for the patient with an intraocular lens implant. *RN*, 41:46, Mar. 1978.
99. Smith, J. F., and D. Nachazel: Retinal detachment. *American Journal of Nursing*, 73:1530, Sept. 1973.
100. Sochocy, S.: Giant cell arteritis and blindness. *American Family Physician*, 16:120, 1977.
101. Soll, D. B., and T. M. Obrotka: Antiviral drugs for herpes simplex keratitis. *American Family Physician*, 16:116, Dec. 1977.
102. Soll, D. B., and K. T. Oh: Industrial ocular injuries. *American Family Physician*, 16:115, Nov. 1976.
103. Soothing a child's angry eye. *Emergency Medicine*, 11:173, Apr. 1979.
104. Sussman, W.: A guide to common eye problems. Part 1: Foreign bodies, corneal abrasions and ulcers. *Consultant*, 16:148, Oct. 1976.
105. Sussman, W.: A guide to common eye problems. Part 2. conjunctivitis, iritis, and episcleritis. *Consultant*, 16:93, Nov. 1976.
106. Sussman, W.: A guide to common eye problems. Part 3. Penetrating injuries, burns, lacerations, and other eye injuries. *Consultant*, 16:131, Dec. 1976.
107. Sussman, W.: A guide to common eye problems. Part 4. Acute glaucoma, pinguecula, phlyctenule, and pterygium. *Consultant*, 17:188, Jan. 1977.
108. Sutton, A. L.: *Bedside Nursing Techniques in Medicine and Surgery*. 2nd ed. Philadelphia, W. B. Saunders Co., 1969.
109. Tasman, W.: Coats' disease. *American Family Physician*, 15:107, Apr. 1977.
110. The emergent eye. *Emergency Medicine*, 10:25, Sept. 1978.
111. Tiefert, J. W.: Orbital auscultation. *American Family Physician*, 18:117, Dec. 1978.
112. Vaughan, D.: Common ocular disorders. *Hospital Medicine*, 7:22, Oct. 1971.
113. Vaughan, D.: Eye. *In* Krupp, M. A., and M. J. Chatton (eds.): *Current Diagnosis and Treatment*. Los Altos, California, Lange Medical Publications, 1972.
114. Vaughan, D., and T. Asbury: *General Ophthalmology*. 8th ed. Los Altos, California, Lange Medical Publications, 1977.
115. Veirs, E.: The lacrimal system. *In* Duane, T. (ed.): *Clinical Ophthalmology*. Vol. 4, Ch. 3. New York, Harper and Row, 1977.
116. Weinstein, G. W.: Electrophysiologic examination of the retina. *In* Duane, T. (ed.): *Clinical Ophthalmology*. Vol. 3. New York, Harper and Row, 1977.
117. Weinstock, F. J.: Emergency treatment of eye injuries. *American Journal of Nursing*, 71:1928, Oct. 1971.
118. Weinstock, F. J., Glaucoma: how to treat and when to refer. *Geriatrics*, 33:31, Oct. 1978.
119. Weinstock, F. J.: What your aging patient may want to know about cataracts. *Geriatrics*, 33:57, Dec. 1978.
120. Wertz, R.: Alternatives to standard cataract surgery. *Postgraduate Medicine*, 64:96, July 1978.
121. What's new in drugs. *RN*, 42:49, Jan. 1979.
122. Your cataract. *Geriatrics*, 33:67, Dec. 1978.
123. Zimmerman, L. E.: Changing concepts concerning the malignancy of ocular tumors. *Archives of Ophthalmology*, 78:166, Aug. 1967.
124. Zucnick, M.: Care of an artificial eye. *American Journal of Nursing*, 75:835, May 1975.

CHAPTER 90*

DISORDERS OF THE EAR AND RELATED STRUCTURES

OVERVIEW OF ANATOMY AND PHYSIOLOGY OF THE EAR AND RELATED STRUCTURES

If you require an extensive review of these topics, consult an anatomy and physiology text. You should reacquaint yourself with the ear's basic anatomy, the path for sound, and the mechanism governing equilibrium. The following outline summarizes outstanding areas for review.

I. *Description:* The ears are a pair of sensory organs, located on either side of the head, which participate in both hearing and position sense. "Hearing" is the sense by which sounds are appreciated. "Position sense" includes orientation of the head in space and movement of the body through space: its balance and equilibrium. Each ear is divided into three main sections: (1) external ear; (2) middle ear; and (3) internal ear (Fig. 90–1).

II. *External ear:* Includes outer projection of ear, a canal, and tympanic membrane. Functions to receive sound waves and direct them to tympanic membrane.
   A. *Pinna* or *auricle:* Projecting, visible part of ear composed of cartilage covered by skin.
   B. *External auditory canal:* A passage from the outer projection of the ear extending inward, forward, and downward in adult for approximately 1–1½ inches. First part of canal contains *ceruminous glands* which form *cerumen,* i.e., wax. Normally cerumen is protective.
   C. *Tympanic membrane* or *eardrum:* Located at end of auditory canal. Divides meatus and middle ear cavity. Normally eardrum vibrates with incoming sound waves.

III. *Middle ear:* Small, flattened space containing air and three small bones, i.e., ossicles.
   A. *Ossicles:* Three bones joined in such a manner that they amplify sound waves received by tympanic membrane, then transmit the sound waves to fluid in inner ear. First bone, *malleus* ("hammer"), has handlelike portion attached to tympanic membrane and headlike portion which connects with second bone, *incus* ("anvil"). Incus connects with third bone, *stapes ("stirrup").* Footplate of stapes fits into the *oval window* (also called *"vestibular window"*), which is a small opening in the wall between middle and inner ear. Oval window's membrane vibrates and conducts sound waves to fluid in inner ear. Normally ossicles have freely movable joints between them, thus forming a bony lever system.
   B. *Eustachian tube* or *auditory tube:* Brings air into middle ear, thus equalizing pressure on both sides of the eardrum (tympanic membrane). Middle ear's mucosal lining is continuous with that of nasopharynx via eustachian tube.
   C. *Mastoid air cells:* Air-filled spaces in a portion of skull's temporal bone. Middle ear communicates posteriorly with mastoid air cells.

IV. *Inner ear* or *labyrinth:* Included is a system of tubes and spaces within a hollowed-out temporal bone, collectively called the *bony labyrinth.* Within the bony labyrinth is the *endolymph*-containing *membranous labyrinth,* which is, in turn, surrounded by *perilymph.*
   A. *Vestibule:* Entrance space next to oval window; communicates with cochlea (toward front) and semicircular canals (toward back). In vestibule are vestibular receptors (called *utricle* and *saccule*) for position of head as it relates to pull of gravity.
   B. *Cochlea:* Bony tube shaped like snail shell. Cochlear portion contains *organ of Corti,* the receptor end-organ of hearing.
   C. *Semicircular canals:* Contain sensory organs related to equilibrium. These receptor end-organs are stimulated by changes in rate or direction of movement.
   D. *Acoustic (eighth cranial) nerve:* Two parts: (a) *cochlear nerve,* connecting cochlea to the brain, and (b) *vestibular nerve,* connecting semicircular canals, saccule, and utricle with the brain.

BASIC TYPES OF DISORDERS OF THE EAR

The ear is subject to many of the same types of disorders that occur in other parts of the body.

*Jonathan Chinn, M.D., critically reviewed and assisted with the revision of this chapter.

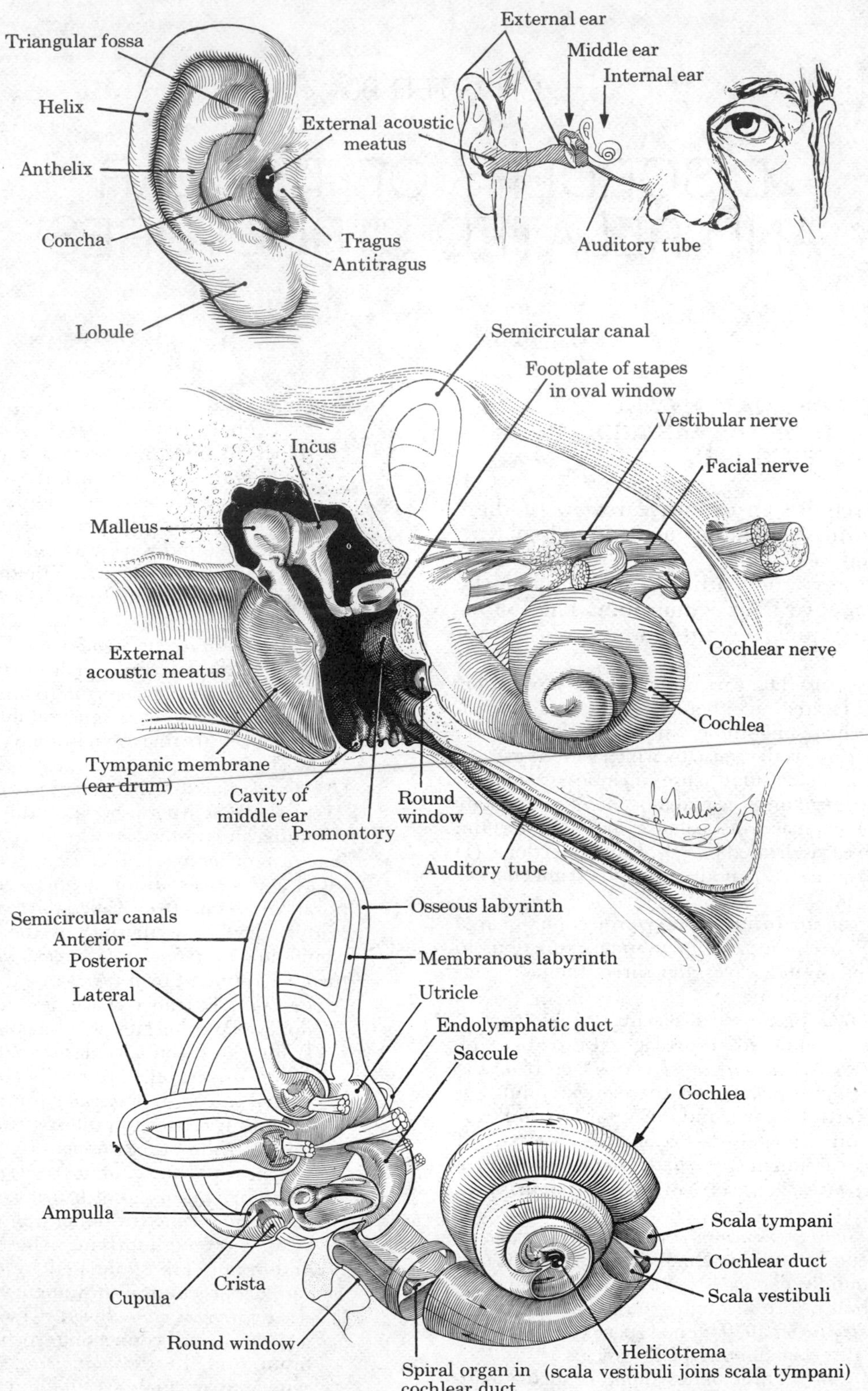

Figure 90–1. External and internal structures of the ear. (From *Dorland's Illustrated Medical Dictionary*, 25th ed. 1974.)

These include:

- *Obstructions:* of the external auditory canal or eustachian tube.
- *Trauma:* may affect all parts of the ear, or parts of the brain that connect or interpret auditory messages.
- *Inflammation and scarring:* of the tympanic membrane or ossicles.

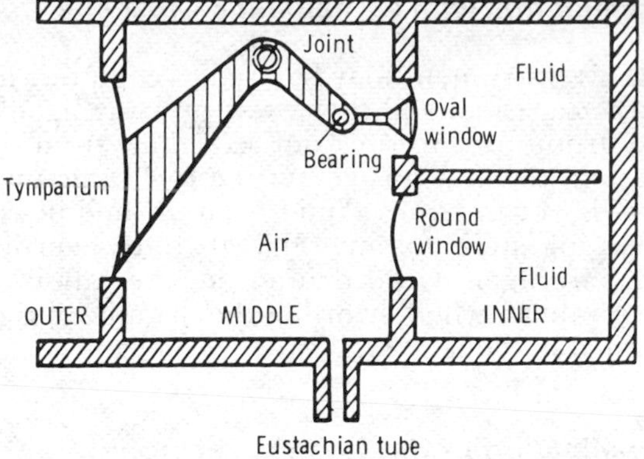

Figure 90–2. Diagrammatic representation of the transmission of vibrations from the outer to the inner ear. (From Lippold, O. C., and F. R. Winton: *Human Physiology,* 6th ed. Longman, 1972.)

- *Skin disorders:* of the external auditory canal.
- *Infection:* of the external ear, middle ear, the mastoid air cells, or the inner ear.

In addition, there are certain types of disorders peculiar to the ear:

- *Disturbances of balance:* Meniere's syndrome, acute labyrinthitis (see below); vertigo (e.g., Meniere's disease, acute vestibular neuronitis, benign positional nystagmus).
- *Disturbances of hearing:* conductive or transmission deafness; sensorineural or perceptive deafness; central deafness.
- *Tinnitus* (ringing in the ear); may be subjective or objective.

EXAMINATION OF THE EAR* AND ASSESSMENT OF THE PATIENT WITH A DISORDER OF THE EAR

Examination of the External Ear

The external ear can be visualized directly; the middle ear and inner ear cannot be evaluated in this manner. In examining the external ear canal, the condition of the ear's epithelium is assessed. Great care and gentleness are important in performing procedures in this area to prevent pain and bleeding. The first half of the ear canal is cartilaginous. About halfway to the eardrum, the cartilage stops and the supporting wall becomes osseous. Epithelium lining this bony portion of the canal is quite thin and *is highly sensitive.* One must be especially gentle in cleaning the inner half of the ear canal. This area is as sensitive as the drumhead's outer surface. (*Note:* it is not advisable for anyone but a physician to perform cleaning of the inner half of the canal or of the drumhead. Cleaning of the ear is discussed further below.)

To look most easily into the ear, tip the patient's head sidewise (toward the opposite shoulder when sitting up). This tipping is necessary because of the oblique direction of the ear canal.

Frequently the ear canal and drumhead are cleansed by a physician prior to examination of the ear. This cleansing is performed to remove accumulated cerumen, particulate matter, pus, and secretions which may otherwise impair visualization of the canal's epithelium and the drumhead. Cleansing may be accomplished with a cotton-tipped applicator, with a small angulated sucker tip, with a cerumen spoon, or by irrigation. (Irrigation is discussed on p. 2020.) When a cerumen spoon is used, it is inserted beyond the impacted wax and then is carefully withdrawn.

After cleansing of the ear, the auricle is inspected and palpated. Next the external auditory canal and tympanic membrane are visualized. The examination is started by *"straightening the ear canal,"* i.e., the auricle is pulled upward and backward and the tragus forward. Nurses should know how to straighten the canal, since they may need to do this before performing nursing procedures on the ear, such as instilling eardrops or performing ear irrigations. Straightening the canal makes it possible to see more easily into the canal. Also, straightening the canal enables solutions or medication to be introduced into the canal (see also p. 2020).

Various instruments may be used to inspect the ear canal and drumhead. Among these are the (a) aural speculum, (b) otoscope, and (c) operating microscope.

When an *aural speculum* is used to examine the eardrum (Fig. 90–3), light is reflected into the ear from a *head mirror.* Ear specula are plain, metal funnels which come in various sizes. One is selected which approximates the size of the patient's external auditory meatus. The speculum used is the largest which will fit the ear canal. The speculum is inserted to straighten and slightly dilate the cartilaginous ear canal.

The eardrum may be magnified for visualization by fitting a lens to the speculum or by using an operating microscope or an otoscope. Increasingly the operating microscope is being used by otologists to examine the ear diagnostically (it is also used during ear surgery). This instrument gives the examiner binocular vision, magnification (6× to 40×), and brilliant illumination.

The normal, healthy drumhead is very slightly conical (with concavity externally), quite shiny, and pearly gray in color. With respect to the ear

*Refer also to Chapter 15, pp. 328–332.

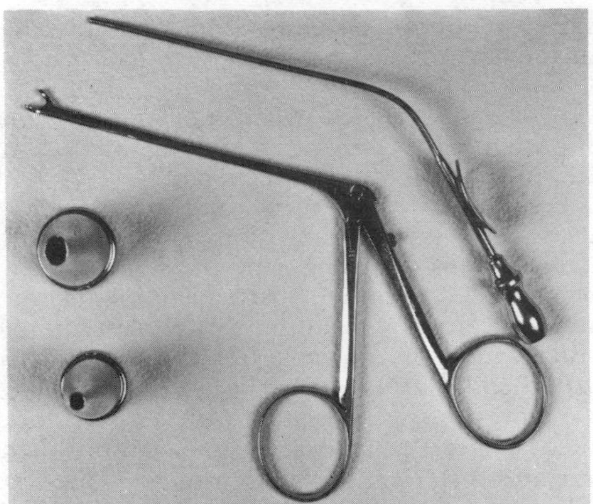

Figure 90–3. Two ear specula (always use the largest that will fit); an aural forceps and a small angulated sucker. (From Paparella, M. M., and D. A. Shumrick: *Otolaryngology.* Vol. I. Philadelphia, W. B. Saunders Co., 1973.)

canal, the position of the drumhead is oblique. In the presence of disease, the drumhead's color changes. Blue indicates hemotympanum, a hemorrhagic exudation into the drum cavity of the ear; yellow or amber, serum in the middle ear; red or pink, infection of the middle ear. The eardrum itself may be infected, sometimes with blood blebs (hemorrhagic bullous myringitis).

Upon examination of the drumhead, not only changes in color may be seen but also other abnormalities, such as (a) perforation or scars; (b) white plaques or flecks (usually indicative of old, healed disease); (c) bulging outward of the drumhead (indicative of pus in the middle ear); or (d) a retracted drumhead (resulting from reduced intratympanic pressure, e.g., from obstruction of the eustachian tube in association with too-rapid a descent in air travel).

Demonstration of Function of the Eustachian Tube

Several tests have been developed to evaluate eustachian tube function. They are important in assessing people with symptoms indicative of occlusion of the eustachian tube, e.g., fluid in the middle ear, pressure in the ear, deafness, or tinnitus (ringing, buzzing, clicking, or roaring noises). The simplest test is to have the patient perform a Valsalva maneuver (hold the nose and blow with the mouth closed) and observe the eardrum for motion. If the eustachian tube is patent the eardrum may be seen to move, and/or the patient will feel a pressure change in the ear.

Examination with a Pneumatic Otoscope

This instrument may be used to compress air in the ear canal and thus exert pressure against the drumhead; to suck out secretions from the mastoid antrum (in patients with chronic mastoiditis); or to remove fluid from the middle ear following myringotomy (Fig. 90–4). By exerting pressure against the drumhead, the physician can evaluate whether or not the drumhead is of normal flaccidity.

Examination of the Nose and Throat

Examination of the ear is accompanied with examination of the nose and throat because infection of these areas may be a contributing factor in ear disorders. Examination of the nose and throat is discussed in Unit XXIV.

A

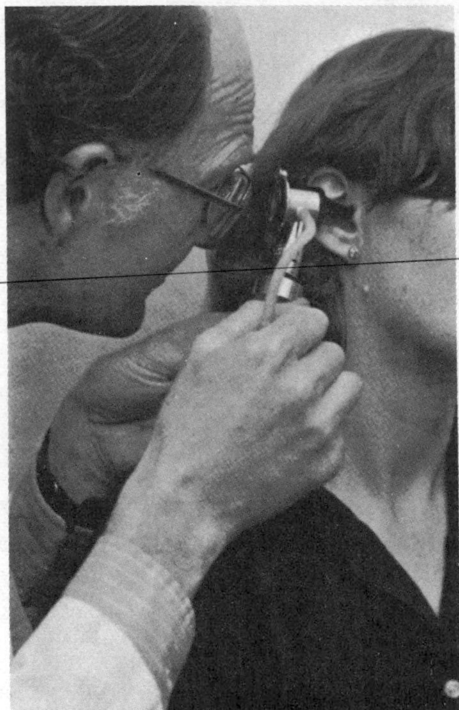

B

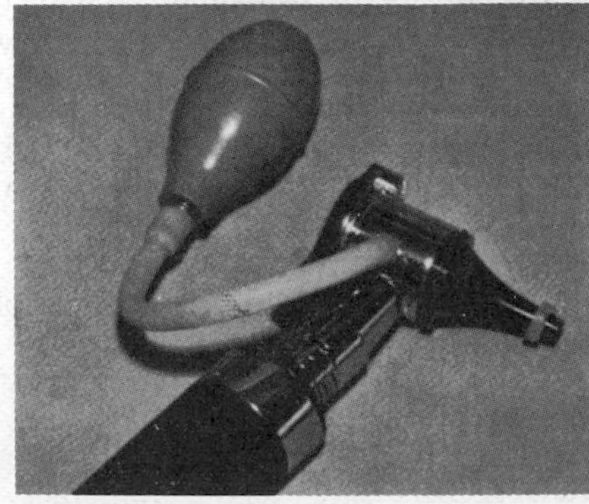

Figure 90–4. A. Assessment of a person's ear with a pneumatic otoscope. **B.** Pneumatic otoscope. An airtight seal is produced by fitting rubber tubing over the speculum. (From Donaldson, J. A.: How to recognize and manage middle ear fluid. *Consultant,* 16:99, Aug. 1976.)

X-Ray Examination of the Mastoid

Patients with acute infections of the middle ear who do not respond to treatment, or who have chronic middle ear suppuration may have x-rays taken to further assess their conditions. X-ray examination of the temporal bone may be necessary to confirm the diagnosis of acute or chronic mastoiditis. In such a case the characteristic findings are clouding of the mastoid air cells and decalcification of the bony walls between the air cells. Most patients with chronic suppurative otitis media have a small, contracted and acellular mastoid which can be demonstrated with roentgenograms of the mastoid. Also, cholesteatomas (see p. 2027) (a special type of chronic middle ear condition which is pathologically identical to epidermoid inclusion cysts) may enlarge, expand into the mastoid antrum, and eventually cause bony destruction with erosion into important adjacent structures. This erosion can be visualized by x-ray examination of the temporal bone.

An added dimension to the x-ray assessment of the ear is polytomography. By use of this specialized technique the fine structures of the middle and inner ear can be visualized.

Assessment of Hearing

Classification of Types of Hearing Loss. Types of hearing losses may be classified in various ways. One classification is the following:

- *Conductive deafness* (transmission deafness): resulting from disturbances of the sound transmission mechanism of the external or middle ears, which prevents sound waves from reaching the inner ear.
- *Sensorineural deafness* (perceptive or "nerve" deafness): results from disturbances of the inner ear neural structures or nerve pathways leading to the brainstem.
- *Central deafness:* results from damage to the brain's auditory pathways or auditory center, e.g., from a cerebrovascular accident. (See Unit X.)
- *Mixed type deafness:* results from disturbances in both the conductive and nerve mechanisms.
- *Functional deafness* (psychogenic or nonorganic deafness): hearing loss for which no organic lesion can be detected.

Currently *conductive deafness* is the only type of organically caused deafness that can be effectively treated. If the basic disorder cannot be corrected, hearing aids that amplify sound are highly beneficial in conductive deafness, because the inner ear and organs that perceive sound are not damaged (see below).

Perceptive deafness commonly results from exposure to excessive noise, such as industrial noise or gunfire. Recently this condition has appeared in teenagers as a result of electric amplification of modern music; this condition is termed *"rock and roll" deafness. Presbycusis* refers to hearing loss due to aging. Presbycusis is a progressive, bilateral type of perceptive deafness. Since sensorineural forms of deafness cannot generally be effectively treated, prevention of such hearing losses is highly important, when possible, as discussed on p. 2018. Hearing aids may be of considerable benefit.

Deafness may also be classified as *congenital* (present at time of birth) or *acquired* (occurring at the time of birth or thereafter). So-called "congenital deafness" may be caused by such factors as ototoxic drugs, familial predisposition, or prenatal causes, such as exposure of the mother during the first trimester of pregnancy to viral diseases (German measles). "Neonatal" causes of perceptive deafness include anoxia during delivery, Rh incompatibility, and birth trauma (e.g., use of forceps during delivery).

Hearing acuity may be determined in various ways. A *gross assessment* may be made by examining the patient's ability to hear a whispered or spoken voice or the ticking of a watch; a *precise assessment* may be made by employing special equipment, such as an audiometer. Additional methods of assessment include tuning fork tests and a bevy of specialized assessment techniques. See Chapter 15, pp. 329 and 330, for discussion of the measurement of hearing acuity by whispered or spoken voice test, watch tick test, and tuning fork tests.

Audiometry. Most quantitative measurements of hearing are made with an audiometer. Pure tones and/or speech are used in testing.

The pure tone audiometer produces pure tones which can be varied according to frequency and intensity. A chart is made of the patient's test results by plotting the intensity against the frequency (audiogram). Frequency of vibration of sound waves is measured in cycles per second; intensity is measured in decibels. The greater the number of cycles per second, the higher the pitch of a sound (Fig. 90–5).

The patient sits in a soundproof room for the audiometry tests, and listens to the sounds produced by the machine by listening through headpiece earphones. The patient is instructed to signal on first hearing each sound by pressing a button or raising a finger. Seven frequencies are tested (from 125 to 8000 cycles per second) by first presenting the tone loud enough for the patient to clearly hear it and then seeking the threshold for that frequency. The "threshold" is the lowest intensity at which the pure tone is heard. Each ear is tested, and both air and bone conduction measurements are made at the threshold levels. A bone oscillator, which produces mechanical vibrations of the skull, is placed against the head to test bone conduction. Hearing is normally most acute in the human ear at about 1000 cycles. Audiometers are equipped with a masking device which can be varied in intensity.

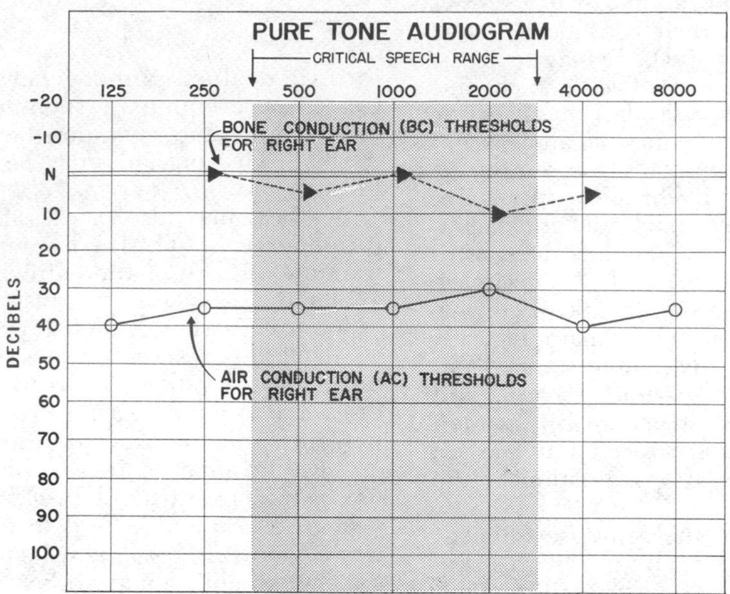

Figure 90–5. An audiogram presents a graphic outline of the individual's hearing as measured by tones of different pitches ranging from 125 through 8000 cycles per second (cps or Hz). Thresholds for these different tones as heard by air and bone conduction are plotted on this graph. The information is important for determining the type of hearing loss. Also, by testing through the critical speech range (approximately 300 to 3000 cps), one can predict how much difficulty there may be in hearing and understanding speech. (From Nilo, E. R.: Hearing impairment. *In* Saunders, W. H., *et al.: Nursing Care in Eye, Ear, Nose and Throat Disorders*, 2nd ed. St. Louis: C. V. Mosby Co., 1968.)

TABLE 90–1. DEGREE OF HEARING LOSS AND RELATIONSHIP TO COMMUNICATIVE SEQUELAE

Pure-tone Average of the Better Ear	Effect of Hearing Loss on Communicative Skills	Aural Rehabilitation Requirements
27 to 40 db† (slight)	May only have difficulty with hearing faint speech	May benefit from a hearing aid when loss approaches 40 db Needs preferential seating and lighting May need lip-reading instructions
41 to 55 db (mild)	Understands conversational speech when face to face May miss as much as 50 per cent if voices are faint May exhibit anomalies in language and speech	Individual hearing aid evaluation and training in its use Needs preferential seating Attention to language skills Lip-reading instruction Speech conservation and correction Child should be referred to special education
56 to 70 db (marked)	Will only understand loud conversation Is likely to have defective speech Child is likely to be deficient in language usage and comprehension Will have limited vocabulary	Individual hearing aid evaluation and auditory training Lip-reading instruction Speech conservation and correction Special help in language development Child should be referred to special education
71 or more db (severe)	Will hear only very loud voices May be able to identify some loud environment sounds May be able to discriminate vowels but not all consonants Relies on vision rather than hearing as primary avenue for communication Speech and language defective and likely to deteriorate	Individual hearing aid evaluation Auditory training Child should be referred to full-time special program for deaf children, with emphasis on all language skills, concept development, lip-reading, and speech Continuous appraisal of needs in regard to oral and manual communication

From Harrison, R. J.: Current concepts in the management of hearing loss. *American Family Physician, 19*:135, Jan. 1979.
†All decibel ranges according to American National Standards Institute, 1969 norm.

Specialized Tests. Additional tests to assess hearing include (a) assessment of such special auditory phenomena as *recruitment* (an abnormally rapid increase in loudness), *diplacusis* (the perception of a single auditory stimulus as two sounds), and *loss of aural discrimination* (ability to properly distinguish between speech sounds; a measurement of how meaningfully or accurately the patient hears, not how keenly the person hears). There are a number of other specialized tests of hearing function described in textbooks of otology.

Assessment of Equilibrium

When a patient is troubled by dizziness or vertigo, it is useful to find out if the labyrinths are functioning normally. This information can be obtained by *performing tests which artificially stimulate the semicircular canals. The Barany test and cold caloric tests are examples of tests used to assess labyrinthine reactions.* The findings of these tests are then compared with the known normal reaction.

Nystagmus may be produced by ocular abnormalities and disturbances of the central nervous system, as well as disturbances of the labyrinth. In labyrinthine nystagmus, the movement of the eye is rhythmic; i.e., a slow movement of the eye in one direction is followed by a rapid compensatory movement in the opposite direction. In optic nystagmus, both excursions of the eye are of equal amplitude, the amplitude is greater, and the motion is of a wandering or pendulous nature rather than in the form of rhythmic excursions. It is not always possible, however, to differentiate between labyrinthine nystagmus and optic nystagmus. *In fact, a battery of tests are needed to thoroughly assess disequilibrium.*

As mentioned, stimulation of the labyrinth also normally produces *past pointing* and *falling,* in addition to nystagmus. Both past pointing and falling always occur in the direction of flow of the endolymphatic fluid, as does the slow component of the nystagmus. Severe reactions to labyrinth stimulation include *dizziness* or *vertigo, nausea,* and *vomiting.* "Dizziness" refers to a disturbed sense of relationship to space in which the patient experiences a subjective sensation which is alarming and disturbing. Often patients have difficulty describing exactly how they feel. They may have a feeling of turning or whirling or may experience less clearly defined symptoms, such as weakness, giddiness, confusion, blankness, or unsteadiness. "True vertigo" is characterized by a sensation of true turning or whirling (sometimes defined as a "hallucination of motion"). For example, patients may have a sense of the outside world turning or they may have a sense that they themselves are turning.

When a person experiences nystagmus, past pointing, and falling it may be suspected that a problem with equilibrium exists. Detailed testing is needed for more specific diagnosis.

Nurses may care for patients experiencing dizziness or vertigo. Important *observations* include the following:

- ► Whether or not the patient experienced true whirling or turning sensations. The direction of the sense of turning and the influence of the position of the head on the sensations.
- ► Does the patient have paroxysmal attacks or is the sensation continuous? What time of day did the sensation occur? Is it related to a change in position? Is the patient's standing or walking affected? Is there an apparent relationship to occupation, menstrual periods, trauma, or medications?
- ► How severe is the sensation or attack? Did nausea or vomiting occur? Was there any associated hearing loss or tinnitus? If so, was it unilateral or bilateral? Was the episode followed by pallor, slow pulse, and sweating?
- ► Was nystagmus present? If so, in what direction?

Barany Test. This test of labyrinthine function was formerly widely used but is currently used only under special circumstances. The Barany test involves the use of a chair which is especially designed to (a) turn in a complete circle, and (b) hold the patient's head in different positions. To perform the test the chair is turned at a predetermined rate of speed, e.g., 10 turns in 20 seconds, and then is suddenly stopped. The endolymph continues to move (because of its momentum) even though the patient's body is stopped. The result is falling, past pointing, nystagmus, and vertigo. This test stimulates both labyrinths simultaneously and is thus not as valuable as the caloric tests in which each labyrinth is separately tested.

Caloric Tests. (See also Chapter 25.) The introduction of water or air (above or below body temperature) into the external auditory canal stimulates the semicircular canals. The most common caloric tests are those in which cold water or ice water is used. Cold caloric tests may be performed to induce either maximal or minimal stimulation.

Maximal stimulation is obtained by performing a cold caloric test *by douche.* A one-quart canister is filled with cold water, the patient's head is tipped 30 degrees forward, and the water (at 20° C.) is directed through a rubber tube into the ear canal. Water flowing out of the ear is caught in an emesis basin held under the patient's ear. Irrigation is terminated when nystagmus begins.

Minimal stimulation of the semicircular canals is obtained by directing ice water against the eardrum through an ear speculum. This procedure is called the *"Kobrak caloric test."* The patient wears 20-

diopter glasses over the eyes and sits with the head tipped forward at a 30 degree angle. A Luer-Lok syringe fitted with a 22-gauge needle is then used to direct 4–5 ml. of ice water against the eardrum for 15 seconds. Labyrinthine reactions typically begin after a short time. If they do not the test is repeated using 10 ml. of ice water. If a reaction still does not occur, the test is repeated using 15, 20, or 30 ml. of ice water. The *labyrinth is considered to be dead if no reaction occurs* with 30 ml.

Regardless of whether the maximal or minimal method of stimulation is used, the patient is allowed to rest for 10–15 minutes between the tests on the two ears. The expected reactions to both kinds of cold caloric test are (a) nystagmus in the direction opposite from the ear being stimulated; and (b) past pointing and falling toward the ear stimulated. Thus, the physician observes the direction of the nystagmus and tests the patient for past pointing following injection of cold water. The nurse should be prepared to steady or catch the patient as he or she falls toward the ear being stimulated. Before the test, in addition to assembling equipment for the test, the nurse protectively drapes the patient's shoulders with a water-repellent cover. Detailed explanations of what to expect during the test are not given to the patient, as they may foster false responses. However, the patient is briefly told that some cold water will be placed in the ear. Because maximal stimulation may precipitate vomiting, an emesis basin and tissues should be close at hand.

Warm caloric tests produce reactions which are opposite to those obtained by cold caloric tests, i.e., the induced nystagmus is in the opposite direction. Regardless of whether cold or warm tests are being performed, both ears are tested separately, and stimulation of opposite ears gives opposite directions to the labyrinthine reactions.

A more quantitative method of recording the labyrinth responses to caloric stimulation has recently gained widespread popularity. The technique is called *electronystagmography* and involves electronically recording eye movement (i.e., nystagmus) during ear irrigations.[44]

CARE AND PROTECTION OF THE EAR

Nurse's Role

Nurses have numerous opportunities to teach others how to care for and protect the valuable sensory apparatus located in the ear. Such teaching opportunities arise among the nurse's own family members, friends, and neighbors, as well as in the professional setting in which the nurse practices. In schools and industries nurses may participate in auditory screening programs directed at identifying persons with impaired hearing.

The nurse encourages persons with symptoms of auditory disorders to seek professional assessment and care. For example, during home visits the community health nurse may observe a person who is hard-of-hearing or a child with a draining ear. As a result of a nurse's intervention these individuals may receive treatment.

In homes, hospitals, clinics, and physicians' offices, nurses participate in the diagnosis and clinical care of persons with auditory disorders. When giving clinical care the nurse observes the general guidelines related to ear care to be discussed below.

Incidence of Impaired Hearing

It is estimated that there are between 13 and 14 million people in the United States with hearing loss sufficient to cause some difficulty with everyday activities.[50] Hearing problems most commonly occur among the elderly. However, only 35 per cent of persons over age 65 who have a hearing loss have had their condition checked by a doctor. The hard-of-hearing may not accept the fact that they have a hearing loss. Rehabilitation of the hard-of-hearing or deaf individual is discussed later in this chapter. It is important for deafness to be prevented, if possible, by adequate protection of the ear.

Protection of the Ear

Protection of the ear involves five major activities: (1) proper general hygiene of the ear (discussed below); (2) prompt, adequate treatment of infections which could involve the ear (e.g., upper respiratory infections) or which already do involve the ear (e.g., acute purulent otitis media); (3) prevention of trauma to the ear; (4) early detection of hard-of-hearing individuals; and (5) periodic ear examinations.

Middle ear infection occurs more often in children than in adults because the eustachian tube is more horizontal in the child. In the adult the tube tends to slant toward the pharynx, thus making it somewhat more difficult for infected material to pass from the pharynx into the middle ear. Because many hearing defects begin in childhood, a child should receive prompt medical care when respiratory infections develop or if the child shows symptoms of ear discomfort or ear infection. Adequate clinical care at this time may prevent a hearing disorder. Middle ear infections are discussed in greater detail later in this chapter.

Prevention of trauma to the ear encompasses such activities as: (a) preventing children from injuring their ears with sharp objects or foreign bodies; (b) teaching children and adults never to poke into their ears with any small or sharp object, (c) preventing occupational hearing loss in industry or other occupations; and (d) preventing excessive environmental noise levels in all settings.

In the industrial setting the nurse may participate in teaching about the proper use of protective ear devices, e.g., ear plugs. Occupational hearing loss may result from loud noise, intense heat, explosions, or accidents involving the head. Trauma may result in fracturing of the ear canal; destruction of the eardrum; disruption of the ear ossicles; paralysis of the facial nerve; or inner ear damage affecting hearing and balance. The most common and most important type of occupational hearing loss is that caused by loud noise. Unions and individual workers have in recent years filed suits totaling millions of dollars for compensation for hearing loss caused by noise in job settings. Currently many industries require pre-employment audiometric examinations and periodic retesting. In the United States, OSHA* has established by federal regulation acceptable levels of noise in work environments.

Persons working in areas of high noise levels may wear protective ear plugs made of rubber or malleable plastic. Ear plugs come in several sizes or may be custom-made (molded to the individual's ear canal dimensions by impression techniques). In settings with extremely high noise levels (e.g., jet engine factories), the workmen not only wear ear plugs but also ear muffs and a large shield over the entire head.

Sound *intensity,* i.e., the pressure exerted by sound, is measured in *decibels.* Ordinary speech is about 50 decibels, heavy traffic is about 70 decibels. Above 80 decibels sound becomes quite uncomfortable to the human ear. Prolonged exposure (for months or years) to industrial noise levels greater than 85 to 90 decibels causes cochlear damage. In jet engine factories the sound level may reach 140 decibels.

Noise is often quite irritating to sick persons. The nurse strives to keep the environment of the ill quiet to enhance their rest and mental comfort.

The early detection of hard-of-hearing individuals is facilitated by *audiometric screening programs* in schools, industries, and other settings. Some nurseries test the hearing of newborn infants. Meconium may be sucked into the middle ear with the first breath of life, causing ear problems. Developmental defects may also be present. Early detection of hearing problems is then followed up by early assessment and treatment.

Many communities have screening programs to test the hearing of preschool and school-aged children. Hearing defects seriously interfere with a child's ability to learn. Children who have difficulties learning to speak and who do not follow instructions properly may have hearing disorders which make it virtually impossible to learn. Periodic evaluation of hearing is also important in elderly persons because with aging degenerative changes frequently occur in the ear as well as in other body tissues. Persons of all ages should periodically have their ears examined. Examination of the ears is a routine part of a general complete examination. If a problem appears to be present, the patient is referred to a specialist for further assessment and treatment.

* Occupational Safety and Health Administration.

General Ear Care

Excessive cleaning of the ear is undesirable. The ear is generally "self-cleaning." Ear wax lubricates the ear's skin and entraps foreign material entering the canal. Because ear wax serves a protective function, attempts should not be made to clean all wax out of the canal. Excessive, repetitive cleaning of the ear canal results in loss of wax formation. In the absence of the protective wax, serious ear problems can develop. Too little cerumen may be more annoying than excessive cerumen. With an inadequate amount of cerumen the ear canal is dry and scaly, and itching may occur. While this disorder is not easily cured, the application of suitable ear ointments may improve the condition.

The following factors are important aspects of *routine, general ear care:*

- *It is generally recommended that the ear be cleansed only with a wet washcloth over the tip of a finger.* Nothing smaller than a finger should be inserted into the ear for routine care. Cotton tipped applicators should not be used. Items such as hairpins, matchsticks, or toothpicks should never be used to clean the ear since they may scratch the skin, thus creating a lesion which could become infected. *Nothing should be inserted into the ear canal beyond the extent of vision;* to do so could result in accidental puncture of the eardrum. When washing a patient's ears, observe for indications of irritation, infection, or other problems.
- *Protection of the ear from contamination from water when bathing, swimming, or diving is important if the patient has a history of ear infection.* This is particularly important if perforation of the drum has occurred. The ear should be plugged with lamb's wool or cotton which is saturated with petrolatum; additionally a swimming cap should be worn when swimming.
- *During acute upper respiratory infections ("colds") the nose should not be blown hard or douched.* Preferably the patient should blow the nose while keeping both nostrils open and mouth open. Excessive pressure forces contaminated material up the eustachian tube into the middle ear.

GUIDELINES AND COMMON NURSING PROCEDURES IN EAR CARE

General Guidelines

The following are important guidelines to remember when caring for a patient with a disorder of the ear.

▶ Always wash your hands before and after caring for the patient's ear, and wash between caring for the two ears to prevent cross-contamination. If one ear is infected, care for the noninfected ear first.
▶ Observe strict asepsis when the middle ear or inner ear has been opened surgically or has been accidentally opened by trauma. The introduction of infection may cause suppurative labyrinthitis or meningitis.
▶ Have good light so you can see exactly what you are doing. An adjustable light is best.
▶ Straighten the ear canal as necessary for good visualization and so medications instilled will go into the ear canal. (See p. 2013 for discussion of how to straighten the adult ear canal.) In infants and young children the ear canal is straightened by pulling the auricle downward.
▶ Place nothing in a patient's ear without an order.
▶ Solutions used for irrigations of the ear (see below) and eardrop solutions should be at body temperature before they are instilled into the ear. Hot or cold temperatures easily stimulate the inner ear, causing vertigo and occasionally nausea and vomiting.
▶ Avoid traumatizing the ear. Be sure glass-tipped medication droppers are not chipped on the tip.
▶ Be gentle. Some conditions make the ear extremely sensitive. Also, as discussed earlier, the inner ear canal is normally very tender.
▶ Never obstruct the ear canal during instillation of medications or during irrigations. Do not obstruct the ear canal with cotton or gauze unless ordered to do so. Obstruction may cause a dangerous pressure increase against the eardrum.
▶ Use every appropriate opportunity to teach people how to properly care for their own ears.
▶ When caring for a patient who has vertigo, instruct the person to slow down movements, and thereby reduce the possibility of precipitating an attack. Assist and protect the patient as necessary, as in getting up or walking, and keep siderails on bed. Keep your movements slow and unhurried.

Common Nursing Procedures Related to Ear Care

Routine cleansing of the ears, instillation of ear drops, softening and removal of wax deposits, irrigation of the ear, use of dry wipes, and insertion and removal of ear wicks are procedures which nurses commonly perform. Remember to wash before and after each procedure; to identify the patient and which ear is to be treated before beginning; to explain to the patient what you are going to do and how the person can help; and to chart after each procedure.

Instillation of Eardrops. Various eardrop solutions are instilled into the auditory canal to produce such local effects as anesthesia, destruction of microorganisms, destruction of an insect lodged in the ear canal, or to soften ear wax.* (*Note:* As an emergency measure in the home, if an insect is in the ear canal, try holding a flashlight to the ear to see if this will attract the insect to the light. If this is unsuccessful, a few drops of mineral oil or olive oil can be placed in the ear canal to smother and immobilize the insect. The movements and wingbeating of an insect in the ear canal are very distressing. A physician must then remove the insect.)

Softening and Removal of Wax Deposits. Impacted, dry accumulations of ear wax may be softened for easy removal by daily instilling a few drops of hydrogen peroxide or warmed glycerine. Carbamide (urea) peroxide in glyceryl (Debrox) is another softening agent which may be instilled. After this is done for 2–3 days, the ear is irrigated to wash out the softened wax. This procedure should not be undertaken without the approval of the physician. The physician may use a cerumen spoon to remove ear wax plugs. Removal of wax with this instrument requires skill and the use of an ear speculum for direct vision.

Ear Irrigations. The ear may be irrigated to (a) cleanse the external auditory canal; (b) remove impacted wax; (c) apply heat to the ear; (d) apply antiseptic solutions for their local action; or (e) remove foreign bodies. (*Note:* Because moisture causes vegetable matter to swell, this procedure is never used to remove such foreign objects as beans, corn, and so forth.) The nurse does not irrigate a patient's ear unless a physician orders the treatment. Irrigations are typically not used if a patient's eardrum is punctured, since the irrigation could cause additional middle ear infection. The physician orders the solution to be used, e.g., tap water, normal saline, antiseptic solution, solution of bicarbonate of soda. The solution should be warmed to body temperature prior to instillation or else vertigo will occur owing to vestibular stimulation. The irrigation may be performed with a rubber bulb syringe, a glass Asepto syringe, or a metal Pomeroy syringe (Fig. 90–6). Ear irrigations may also be performed with an irrigating can with tubing and an ear tip.† Some physicians use a Water-Pik at very low pressure.

To perform an ear irrigation: (1) Protectively drape the patient, position the person so the head is tilted slightly forward and toward the side of the affected ear (the procedure may be performed with the patient sitting up or lying down; sitting up is easiest), and position the light. (2) Have the patient hold a basin beneath the ear and against the face to catch the irrigating solution. (3) Cleanse external ear with gauze wipes and some of the solution. (4) Fill syringe and expel air from the rubber tubing. (5) Straighten ear canal. (6) Place tip of syringe

---

*The correct technique for instillation of eardrops is discussed in Sorensen and Luckmann, *Basic Nursing: A Psychophysiologic Approach.*

†A *Glass ear tip* has two extensions: one for the solution to enter the ear, the other for it to leave the canal. Inspect tip for breakage prior to use.

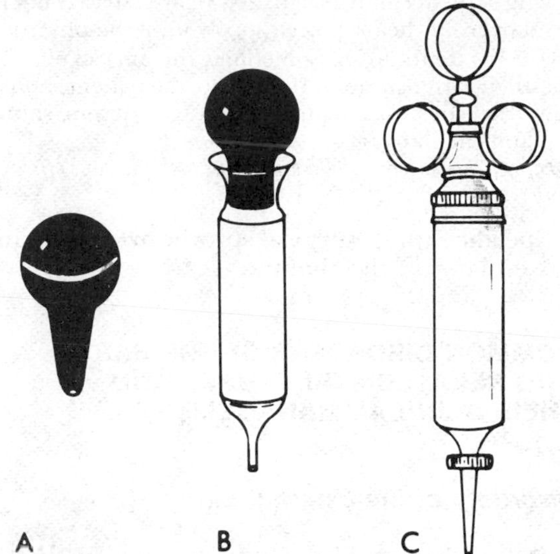

Figure 90–6. Three types of syringes used to irrigate the ear: **A,** rubber bulb syringe; **B,** glass Asepto syringe; and **C,** metal Pomeroy syringe. (Drawn by K. C. Sorensen.)

or tube just inside meatus and direct a slow, steady stream of solution against *roof* of auditory canal (directing the stream upward prevents forcing plugging materials further into the canal and prevents injury of tympanic membrane). (7) Do not use excessive force (if tubing is used do not elevate can higher than is necessary to remove the secretions). The least force results from use of a rubber bulb syringe; the Pomeroy syringe must be cautiously used because it can exert great pressure. (8) Do not occlude the auditory canal with the irrigating tip (the force of the stream will not damage the eardrum if space is left around the syringe to allow the fluid to escape). (9) Use approximately 500 ml. of irrigating liquid. (10) After the irrigation is completed, the ear canal should be carefully dried with a sterile cotton applicator (the physician may use a small length of cotton inserted with bayonet forceps). (11) Have the patient lie on the irrigated side for a few minutes after the treatment is complete so any remaining solution will drain out of the ear by gravity.

When charting following an ear irrigation, be certain to comment on the nature of the drainage, e.g., "Returning solution contained particles of brown wax."

Use of Dry Wipes. "Dry wipes" may be ordered to periodically clean the ear canal if a patient has ear discharge. The wipe is performed with a dry, sterile cotton-tipped applicator. Often applicators are especially prepared by hospital central services departments for use in the ear since commercial applicators are usually too stiff for such usage.

To perform the procedure: (1) position the patient laterally with the affected ear uppermost and position the light; (2) straighten the ear canal; (3) gently insert and rotate the applicator; (4) withdraw the applicator; and (5) note the appearance of discharge and discard the applicator. Generally it is necessary to use several applicators. Use a new, sterile applicator each time the canal is entered; never go repeatedly in and out with the same applicator.

Insertion and Removal of Ear Wicks. Wicks of small pieces of cotton or single pieces of gauze (picked up in the center, twisted, and sterilized) may be used as drains in the ear to encourage exudate drainage or following instillation of eardrops. The wick is gently inserted into the canal only as far as it is possible to see. The loose ends of the wick are left extending out of the canal. Wicks are changed frequently to prevent them from obstructing drainage flow or hardening or both. A number of commercially made wicks are now available. These, like most wicks, are most effective if *aqueous* instead of oil-base eardrops are used.

GENERAL CARE OF THE PATIENT HAVING AURAL SURGERY

The following guidelines are important in the nursing care of any patient having ear surgery.

▶ *Preoperatively assess the patient's understanding* of the surgery and the possible results of that surgery. Then provide appropriate answers to the patient's questions and see that the person receives necessary explanations. If a procedure is being performed to improve hearing, inform the patient that improvement may not be noticeable for several weeks, until swelling leaves the operative area and dressings, packings, and so forth are removed.

▶ *Preoperatively review with the paient common postoperative restrictions.* For example: (a) discuss restrictions concerning positioning and movements; (b) tell the patient not to blow the nose, but rather to wipe off the end of the nose as necessary; (c) inform the patient not to sneeze or strenuously cough since such activities (including blowing the nose) may disrupt the delicate structures of the ear before healing occurs (e.g., may loosen the eardrum or dislocate a prosthesis) or may force air and possibly infected material into the eustachian tube; and (d) instruct the patient not to touch the ear or the ear dressing.

▶ *Prepare the ear for surgery as ordered.* The physician often prefers to clean the ear personally to prevent scratching or otherwise irritating the ear's tissues. A scratch could become infected. Prior to surgery topical and systemic antibiotic chemotherapy is ordered if a patient's ear has frequent or continuous discharge.

▶ *During surgery and postoperatively practice aseptic technique to prevent infection.* Infection is especially hazardous because of the ear's close proximity to the brain. Observe for symptoms of infection: temperature elevation, drainage from the ear, headache.

▶ *Administer antibiotics as ordered.* Assist with ear cultures if the physician takes them.

▶ *Postoperatively position the patient as ordered,* e.g., on side with operated ear up (to prevent displacement of grafts) or with operated ear down (to enhance drainage). In some cases the head of the bed is ordered flat or elevated 30 degrees. Some orders state the patient may lie on whichever side causes less vertigo. Lying on the unoperated side sometimes minimizes nausea and vomiting. The patient may be on a strict bedrest for 24–48 hours.

▶ *Provide pain relief as ordered.*

▶ Reinforce external bandage if necessary, but *do not disturb the inner ear dressing.*

▶ *Never apply pressure* to the ear or ear dressing. To do so could dislodge a graft or prosthesis.

▶ *Protect and help the patient with nausea and vertigo.* Vertigo and nausea commonly follow surgery on the ear (owing to trauma and edema) and may be extemely uncomfortable as well as hazardous to the patient's safety. Discuss these symptoms with the patient. Explain that they result from a *temporary* disturbance to the ear's balancing functions. Inform the patient that discomfort can be minimized by (a) remaining positioned as ordered; (b) avoiding contraindicated activities or movements; (c) moving slowly; and (d) avoiding sudden turning. Keep siderails up while the patient is in bed and assist the person with moving about. Also, encourage the patient to use handrails in the halls and bathrooms to help keep steady. Be careful not to bump or jar the patient or bed when giving care. Do not rush the patient. The nauseated patient may obtain relief by taking slow, deep breaths through the open mouth. Give medications as ordered to minimize nausea and vertigo, e.g., Dramamine.

▶ *Provide nourishment as ordered.* A light or liquid diet may be ordered to prevent nausea or vomiting or to make it more comfortable for the patient to eat (if chewing is painful).

▶ *Observe for and report symptoms of postoperative complications.* Symptoms of infection have been discussed. Observe also for (a) fluctuations in hearing; (b) tinnitus; (c) vertigo (if vertigo is present, look for nystagmus also. Record the direction and dependency on position.); (d) gait disturbance; (e) bleeding (do not attempt to stop bleeding by applying pressure to the ear); or (f) indications of injury to the facial nerve, i.e., inability to frown, wrinkle the forehead, close the eyes, bare the teeth, or pucker the lips. During ear surgery the facial nerve may be injured temporarily (due to edema) or permanently. Paralysis resulting from edema may not appear for 12–24 hours postoperatively. The physician may loosen the ear dressing and order anti-inflammatory medications in an attempt to relieve the pressure of edema. Protective eye care is sometimes indicated if the facial nerve is injured.

▶ *Prior to discharge tell the patient how to protect and care for the ear.* For example, the patient may be advised not to get the ear wet from showering, shampooing, or swimming. Infection could result from water in the ear. Contact with persons who have upper respiratory infections should be avoided because of the danger of the patient acquiring the infection and possibly developing a middle ear infection. Some patients, e.g., following stapedectomy (see p. 2033), are advised not to bend over, lift heavy objects, or fly until the physician says it is safe to do so. Sometimes the auricle may be anesthetic after surgery. If this is so, the patient should be warned of possible injury from hair dryers, showers, and the like.

▶ *Inform the patient of follow-up visits to the doctor's office or clinic.*

Specific aural surgical procedures are discussed later in the chapter.

COMMON DISORDERS OF THE EAR AND RELATED STRUCTURES AND THEIR CLINICAL MANAGEMENT

Disorders of the External Ear

Deformities. The external ear may be deformed as a result of trauma ("cauliflower" ears associated with boxing), congenital malformation (atresia—absence or closure of the ear canal), or abnormal size or protrusion of the auricle. Often such disorders are amenable to corrective plastic surgery.

Foreign Bodies. As briefly mentioned earlier, foreign materials may become lodged in the ear canal. Poor technique in the removal of these objects can cause damage to the canal or tympanic membrane and possible middle ear infection, resulting in deafness. Thus, a physician should be consulted. Irrigation is contraindicated for substances which will swell when in contact with moisture and for pointed objects. Cautious removal by instrumentation is necessary in such cases. Removal of insects from the ear was discussed on p. 2020. Objects may be inserted into the ear by psychotic or mentally retarded individuals and by children.

Impacted Cerumen (Ear Wax). Some persons produce large quantities of cerumen. Impacted cerumen may cause conductive deafness. In addition to diminished hearing, other symptoms of impacted cerumen are itching or irritation of the ear canal; and feelings of plugging or discomfort in the ear. After examination of the ear the physician may advise that hard wax be softened and then removed by irrigation. If perforation of the eardrum is present, irrigation is contraindicated, and the physician must remove the wax with a curet. While accumulated earwax is usually hard, when mixed with water (as from swimming) it may soften and become a culture medium for bacteria, producing external otitis. The nurse should remember that accumulations of earwax are not necessarily indicative of poor personal hygiene. Patients who consider their condition as a sign of uncleanliness may be embarrassed to seek professional help.

External Otitis. "External otitis" is a general term used with reference to inflammatory disorders of the auricle and external auditory canal. These disorders may be caused by either infections or a dermatosis, or both. External otitis varies in severity from a diffuse mild eczematoid dermatitis to cellulitis or even furunculosis of the ear canal. In many cases there is no infection, and the reaction is a contact dermatitis (e.g., from earrings, earphones) or a variant of seborrheic dermatitis. Either bacteria or fungi may produce the infectious type. Usually infections of the ear canal are bacterial (staphylococcal and gram-negative rods); however, a few cases are caused by fungi *(Aspergillus, Mucor, Penicillium)*. Predisposing factors include (a) moisture in the ear canal in a warm, moist climate or as a result of swimming; (b) trauma resulting from attempts to clean or scratch the itching ear; and (c) seborrheic and allergic dermatitis. Clinical findings include scaling, crusting, erythema, edema, and pustule formation. Major symptoms are itching and pain in a dry, scaling ear canal. Additional symptoms may include a watery or purulent (sticky yellow) discharge, intermittent deafness, adenopathy, and fever. Severe pain may occur if the ear canal becomes completely occluded with debris and edematous skin.

Special mention of a lethal variety of otitis externa, called *malignant otitis externa,* should be made. It is a rampant infection of the outer ear in diabetes, which rapidly involves all contiguous structures and causes a mortality of 50 to 75 per cent unless recognized and treated quickly (see Fig. 90–7).

Treatment may include systemic analgesics for pain and systemic antibiotics if fever or lymphadenopathy is present. Local treatments may include (a) 70 per cent alcohol to control itching in a dry, scaling ear canal; (b) topical corticosteroids (to help control the underlying dermatitis and help decrease inflammatory edema); (c) topical antibiotic ointments and eardrops (e.g., neomycin, polymyxin, bacitracin) applied to the ear canal with a cotton wick for 24 hours, followed by eardrops twice daily to help control infection; (d) compresses of Burow's solution (aluminum acetate solution) or 0.5 per cent acetic acid may be used with acute weeping infected eczema; and (e) use of glycerite of peroxide with urea drop eardrops t.i.d. to help remove debris. Debris may also be removed by gently wiping the ear canal with a cotton applicator, with suction, or occasionally by irrigation. During all local procedures be careful not to traumatize the area. Frequent gentle debridement is important to remove debris and to allow medicaments to reach the diseased tissue. Because the ear is often extremely sensitive, cool or warm compresses may be ordered to minimize discomfort. Touching or moving the auricle may produce intense pain, and thus patients may be naturally resistant to treatments which necessitate movement of the ear.

External otitis occurs in both acute and chronic forms. External otitis may be refractory to treatment and frequently recurrences occur. Thorough drying of the ear after swimming, bathing, or shampooing helps prevent infections. Persons having chronic external otitis often are advised against swimming and are instructed to protect their ear canals from water when bathing or shampooing. Acute external otitis frequently follows swimming. With "swimmer's ear" the patient gets contaminated water in the ear; frequently the patient has wax in the ear which then absorbs the contaminated water, macerates the skin, and provides the basis for infection. In contrast to acute external otitis, with chronic otitis there is usually no pain when the auricle or tragus is manipulated. In chronic external otitis, itching rather than pain is the major discomfort, and the epithelium of the auricle, ear canal, and drum may become thickened, red, and quite insensitive. Frequently aural discharge is present.

Furunculosis. Furunculosis is a form of localized external otitis in the outer half of the ear canal. In this area glands and hair follicles may become infected and form furuncles (boils). Even a small furuncle causes *severe pain* until it either spontaneously breaks or is surgically drained. Furuncles on the canal floor and anterior wall cause pain upon mastication. Pain also occurs from movement of the auricle, and from pressure on the tragus. Onset may be acute. In addition to pain, the patient may notice a feeling

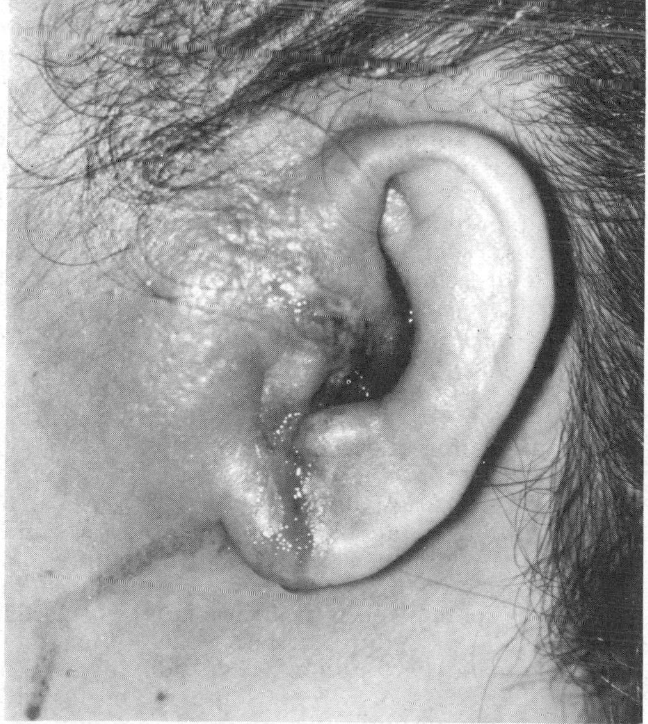

Figure 90–7. Malignant otitis externa. (Courtesy of Jonathan Chinn, M.D.)

of fullness in the ear, impaired hearing, adenopathy, and postauricular swelling. The area involved is red and may be severely swollen. At times the entire canal is obliterated.

Treatment generally includes insertion of a small gauze wick into the canal and wetting of this wick every few hours with 10 drops of half-strength Burow's solution. This helps relieve pain. A piece of cotton saturated with the solution may also be applied to the external meatus. This therapy is continued for 48 hours. Usually local heat applications also help provide relief and hasten recovery. Once fluctuation is well developed the apex is incised. Pain may be controlled with codeine. Systemic antibiotics are also given, especially in the presence of fever or cellulitis of adjacent tissues. Keeping the auditory canal dry, reasonably clean, and trauma-free are all important measures in the prevention of furuncles in this region.

Malignant Tumors. The external auditory meatus may be the site of both basal cell carcinomas and squamous cell carcinomas. Basal cell carcinomas invade the meatus and ear canal from the external ear. Squamous cell carcinomas may come from (a) the parotid gland; (b) skin of the auricle or epithelium of the external ear canal; (c) middle ear; or (d) mastoid. Symptoms include hearing loss, ear drainage, deep boring pain, and (late) peripheral facial paralysis. If the tumor is confined to the cartilaginous canal, the prognosis of carcinoma is reasonably good. Cure may result from wide local excision and skin grafting. The cure rate is greatly reduced if the osseous portion of the canal is invaded. Once the bone is involved, radical mastoidectomy and subsequent deep roentgenotherapy are usually employed in treatment of the cancer. In selected cases, total removal of the temporal bone may be attempted to cure the cancer. There seems to be a higher incidence of cancer of the ear in the presence of chronic ear infections. (Cancer is also discussed in Unit IX.)

Perforation of the Eardrum

The eardrum may be perforated as a result of infection (acute or chronic suppurative otitis media) or trauma (skull fracture, compression, burns, punctures). Usually accidental perforations spontaneously heal; sometimes corrective surgical procedures are necessary. While most traumatic perforations heal spontaneously in several days or weeks, some physicians give prophylactic antibiotics.

Some physicians advise patients with perforated eardrums not to dive, swim, or shower because of danger of water entering the middle ear and producing infection. In other cases the patient is advised to wear custom-molded ear plugs under a bathing cap to prevent water from entering the ear.

A perforated eardrum leaves a patient susceptible to chronic ear infections and their possible complications. Also, chronic perforations of the eardrum may cause conductive hearing loss. It is thus desirable for the eardrum to be repaired surgically, i.e., *myringoplasty*, if the tympanic membrane does not heal by itself. Various techniques of myringoplasty may be employed. One method is to cauterize the edges of the wound and insert a piece of blood-soaked Gelfoam. New tissues then grow over the Gelfoam patch, filling in the hole. In other procedures the eardrum's opening is enlarged surgically, and a graft of skin, vein, or fascia is sutured over the hole. Gelfoam or clotted blood may be used to support the graft and keep it positioned (see also p. 2031).

The presence of an active infection of the middle ear is an obvious contraindication to the surgical closure of perforations of the eardrum.

Disorders of the Middle Ear

"Otitis media" refers to inflammation of the middle ear. There are several types of otitis media.

Serous (Catarrhal) Otitis Media. This condition may be acute or chronic, may occur at any age, and is characterized by the accumulation of sterile fluid (serous or mucoid) in the middle ear. Serous otitis media may be caused by[11] (a) an obstruction of the eustachian tube which prevents normal ventilation of the middle ear and subsequent transudation of serous fluid; (b) incomplete resolution of the exudate of purulent otitis media; or (c) an allergic exudate of serous fluid into the middle ear. Serous otitis media is distinguished from acute purulent otitis media by *absence of* fever, pain, and toxic symptoms. Symptoms of serous otitis media include a full plugged feeling in the ear, hearing loss, and an unnatural reverberation of the patient's voice.

Acute serous otitis media may occur spontaneously without symptoms of other disease, or it may accompany or follow virus diseases or episodes of allergy. Additionally, it may occur following sudden changes in atmospheric pressures, as during flying. Air moves out from the middle ear, through the eustachian tube, upon ascending from a high atmospheric pressure to a low atmospheric pressure. With descent, however, if the air is unable to pass back through the tube into the middle ear, feelings of discomfort develop. This condition is particularly likely to occur if the individual travels by air while experiencing an upper respiratory infection. It is advisable when flying to suck on hard candy, chew gum, or yawn several times during the plane's descent. These activities help open the eustachian tube and thus facilitate the entrance of air into the middle ear. Upon examination the patient displays a conductive hearing loss, and the eardrum is retracted. Air-fluid bubbles or a fluid level may be visible through the eardrum.

The *treatment* of acute serous otitis media may include such measures as (a) inflation of the eustachian tube; (b) myringotomy, i.e., incision of the tympanic membrane (eardrum), and sucking out of fluid in the middle ear; or (c) removal of fluid from the middle ear by needle aspiration (needle paracentesis of the eardrum with aspiration of middle ear contents). Additionally, such nasal decongestants as 0.25 per cent phenylephrine nasal spray or phenylpropanolamine, orally, may be prescribed. If there are indications of contributing nasal allergy, antihistamines are given.

Chronic or recurrent serous otitis media can cause a serious threat to hearing. Chronic serous otitis media may be caused by (a) inadequate treatment of acute or subacute suppurative otitis media (inadequate chemotherapy with antibiotics has caused an increase in chronic serous otitis media); (b) allergy of the nose and nasopharynx; (c) overgrowth of lymphoid tissue in the nasopharynx; (d) chronic sinus infection; (e) hypometabolism; (f) lowered resistance to infection (evidenced by low gamma globulin in the blood plasma); or (g) carcinoma of the naso-

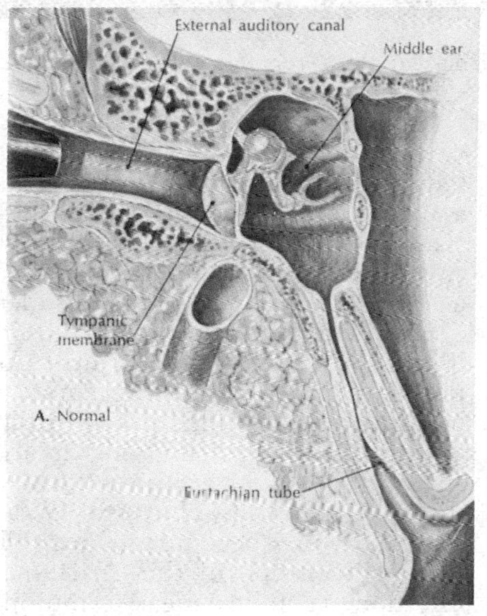

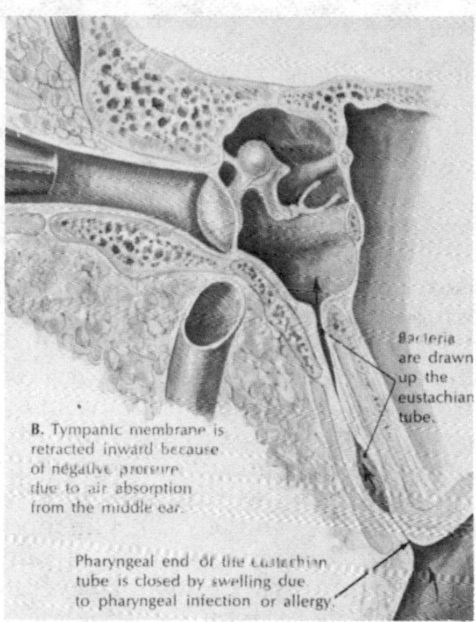

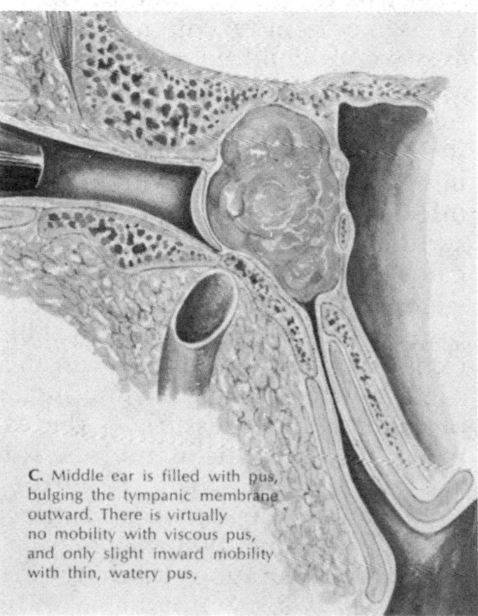

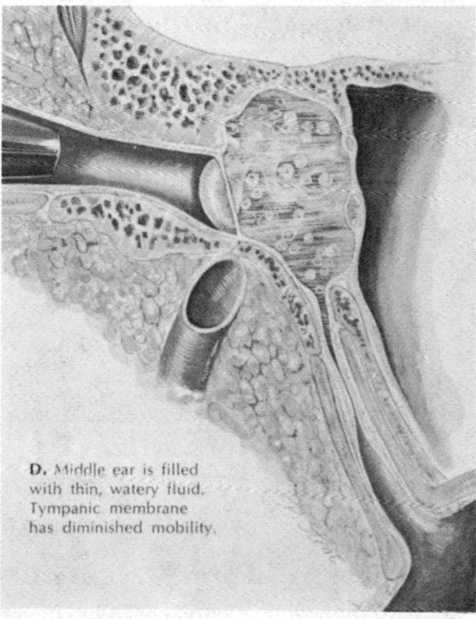

Figure 90–8. Pathogenesis of otitis media. (From Schwartz, R. H.: New concepts in otitis media. *American Family Physician*, 19:91, May 1979.)

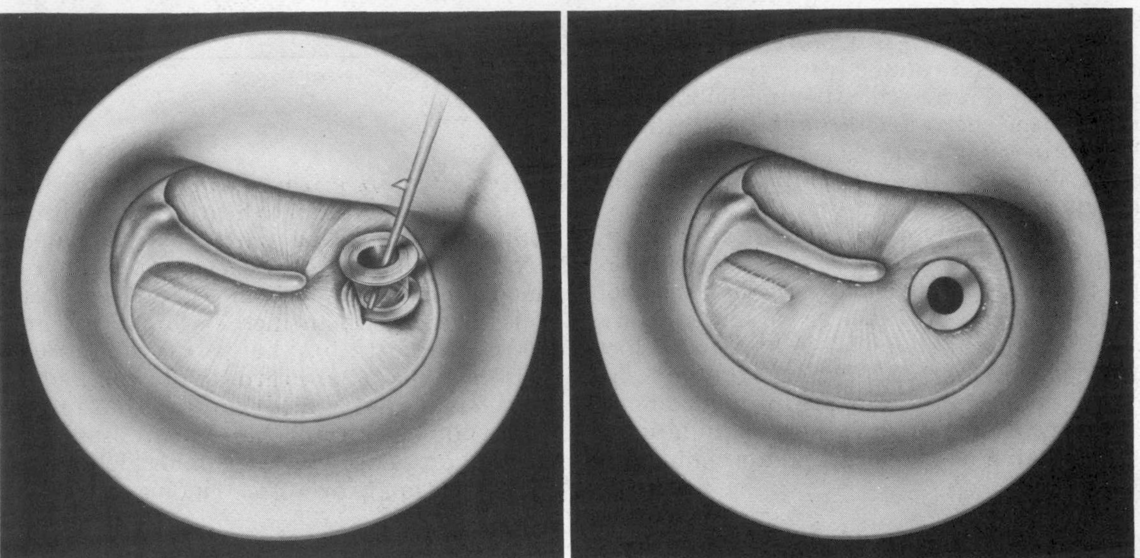

Figure 90–9. Insertion of Sheehy Button (left), and button in place (right). (From Paparella, M. M., and D. A. Shumrick: *Otolaryngology.* Vol. II. 1973.)

pharynx in the adult. Cancer of the nasopharynx must be ruled out in adult patients with persistent unilateral serous otitis media.

Chronic serous otitis media presents only minimal symptoms. There is no discharge from the ear. The most common symptom is hearing loss, which may fluctuate. *Treatment* is directed at control of possible systemic disease and removal of fluid from the ear. Numerous myringotomies may be necessary. Sometimes a myringotomy is performed, and a polyethylene tube or a Teflon button is inserted through the eardrum and into the middle ear (Figs. 90–9 and 90–10). The tube makes it possible for secretions to drain out or be suctioned out over a period of several weeks. The tube also allows aeration of the middle ear and seems to hasten recovery of the eustachian tube obstruction. The myringotomy heals around the tube or button after a few hours. Tubes may be left in place for several months or until they extrude spontaneously from the ear.[12] In persistent cases local or systemic corticosteroids may be administered. Underlying factors must be corrected by tonsillectomy, adenoidectomy, control of nasal allergy, and treatment of nasal or sinus infections. Because hearing loss can result from untreated recurrent serous otitis media, the patient requires early treatment and follow-up supervision.

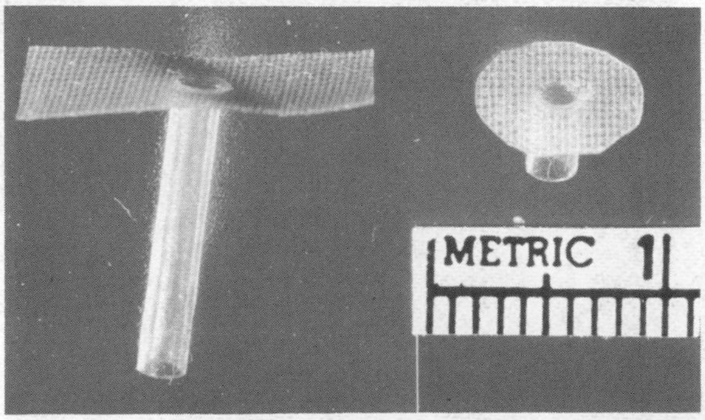

Figure 90–10. Silastic tube with siliconized Teflon mesh flange. The tube on the right has been trimmed for use. (From Crabtree, J. A.: *Otolaryngologic Clinics of North America,* 3:61–65, 1970.)

Suppurative (Purulent) Otitis Media. Normally the middle ear is sterile. An acute suppuration (pus formation) occurs when virulent bacteria enter the middle ear. Infections and inflammations of the middle ear are caused by spread of infection, via the eustachian tube, from the nose and nasopharynx. Occasionally the middle ear may become infected following traumatic perforation of the eardrum. Middle ear infection may follow measles, mumps, influenza, scarlet fever, pneumonia, or the common cold. Otitis media most commonly occurs in infants and young children because during the early stages of life the straight position of the eustachian tube favors the conduction of infection into the middle ear. Otitis media may also result from improper, forceful blowing of the nose (forcing infected material into the middle ear) and from swimming in contaminated water (if the water gains entrance to the middle ear).

Acute suppurative otitis media is characterized primarily by severe deep throbbing ear pain. Other symptoms include fever, deafness, chills, slight dizziness, nausea, vomiting, and a feeling of fullness and pressure in the ear. If unruptured, the tympanic membrane is fiery red and bulging. If the eardrum ruptures, discharge is found in the ear canal, and after the canal is cleaned a pulsing discharge may be seen coming from the perforation. Discharge from the ear is called "*otorrhea.*" ("Otorrhagia" refers to hemorrhage from the ear.) Usually the white count is increased. Culture of the drainage identifies the infecting organism (commonly *Steptococcus,*

Pneumococcus, or *Hemophilus influenzae*). Hearing tests show a conductive hearing loss. Possible *complications* which can result from extension of the disease into adjacent structures include mastoiditis, periostitis, meningitis, lateral sinus thrombosis, brain abscess, labyrinthitis, and facial nerve paralysis.

Treatment of acute suppurative otitis media includes both local and systemic measures. Systemic treatment includes bed rest and systemic antibiotics. Antibiotics are given in full dosage, and the patient is instructed to take the prescribed medication for as long as it is ordered, even though the symptoms of the infection may have disappeared. Inadequate treatment results if the full course of antibiotics is not taken. Penicillin is the drug of choice for the older child and adult. In children under three years there is a significant incidence of *Hemophilus influenzae* infection, and ampicillin is the drug of choice. There has been a recent emergence of an ampicillin-resistant *Hemophilus influenzae* however, and the trend is to use sulfonamide compounds in treatment. If sensitivity to penicillin is known to be present, the patient may be given sulfonamides, erythromycin, tetracyclines, or broad-spectrum antibiotics. Usually antibiotics are continued for at least 7 days to minimize the possibility of recurrence of an incompletely resolved infection after a latent period. Antibiotics are continued in full dosage until the ear is dry, the eardrum looks normal, and hearing is normal. Nasal decongestants (systemic and topical) help restore function of the eustachian tube. After rupture or myringotomy, sterile cotton is loosely placed in the outer ear to prevent the discharge from infecting the skin of the face and neck and the ear lobule. Usually medication for pain relief is not necessary once the eardrum has ruptured or has been lanced. However, if analgesics are required, codeine or acetylsalicylic acid may be ordered. Sometimes local cold applications relieve pain. Generally eardrops are of limited value. Local heat may be ordered to speed up resolution. Usually fluids are forced if the patient is febrile and is not vomiting or nauseated.

With modern chemotherapy, acute otitis media seldom reaches a highly painful stage. If it does, the condition usually resolves if it is adequately treated with antibiotics and myringotomy. Myringotomy is important when the infection does not promptly resolve or when bulging of the eardrum indicates that a discharge is present and is under pressure. Additional indications for myringotomy include continued pain or fever, increasing hearing loss, or vertigo. Complicating mastoiditis develops in cases which have received no treatment or in those inadequately treated. It is important to examine the ears and test hearing following otitis media to prevent persistent conductive hearing loss. Persistent conductive hearing loss (with or without fluid in the middle ear) may occur following incomplete resolution of the infection.

Chronic suppurative otitis media is usually preceded by neglected or recurrent acute otitis media and acute mastoiditis. *With chronic infection of the middle ear there is a permanent perforation of the eardrum.* Eventually a chronic change occurs in the mucosa of the ear, and the ossicles may be destroyed. Usually chronic suppurative otitis media results in a contracted, acellular, "sclerotic" mastoid. Chronic suppurative middle ear infection occurs most commonly in persons who had ear disease in early childhood.

Chronic suppurative otitis media is characterized by recurrent painless discharge from the ear. The discharge may be foul-smelling or nearly odorless, and frequently worsens with upper respiratory infections. Hearing loss is always present. Pain or vertigo may indicate impending complications, e.g., pus under pressure, irritation of dura, brain abscess, irritation, or erosion of labyrinth.

A *cholesteatoma* is a special chronic condition of the middle ear and mastoid. It consists of squamous epithelium that has become trapped in the tympanum or mastoid or both. The epithelium continues to desquamate, forming a cystic mass that is locally destructive. Cholesteatomas can become quite extensive, eroding bone and exposing the inner ear and dura overlying the temporal lobe.

Treatment of chronic suppurative otitis media may be medical or surgical or both. *Medical treatment* consists of such measures as (a) carefully cleaning the ear with cotton and carefully removing granulation tissue, polyps, and visible cholesteatomas to allow medications to more effectively reach the areas of infection; (b) blowing various powders into the middle ear (performed by the physician); (c) instilling eardrops containing topical antibiotics and corticosteroids to help eliminate fetid discharge, break up debris, and promote healing; (d) systemically administering an appropriate antibiotic if the organism is known or if an acute exacerbation occurs in a chronically infected ear; and (e) instilling dilute aluminum acetate solution into the ear as drops.

The *surgical treatment* of chronic suppurative otitis media may involve a *mastoidectomy* (simple, modified radical, or radical) if there is evidence of continued suppuration, mastoiditis, or other complications. If a cholesteatoma is present, it is surgically removed as is all diseased tissue. Frequently it is desirable to attempt to reconstruct the sound-conducting mechanism in an effort to restore the hearing loss. Examples of such reconstructive operations are *myringoplasty* (repair of defects such as perforation of the tympanic membrane), and *tympanoplasty* (rebuilding of the middle ear structures or replacement of these structures with prostheses).

The possible complications of chronic suppurative otitis media are similar to those mentioned earlier for the acute form of this middle ear disorder. In the absence of pain or symptoms of complications, the local medical therapy of chronic suppurative otitis media may continue for months or years. Generally systemic antibiotics are not helpful unless there is a superimposed acute process.

Serious infections of the middle ear are preventable with early medical treatment of ear disorders. *Earaches should always be professionally treated* as should other symptoms of disorders of the ear. Fortunately severe ear infections and their serious complications occur less commonly today than previously. This reduced incidence is attributable to improved treatment of acute infections (e.g., with antibiotics) and improved methods of follow-up evaluation. Because antibiotic therapy may mask symptoms, the patient should be periodically evaluated by the otologist. All new symptoms should be promptly investigated. The virulence of the infecting organism, the patient's state of resistance, and the presence or absence of the organisms' resistance to chemotherapy are all factors influencing a patient's response to therapy.

Death from ear infections commonly occurred prior to the development of antimicrobial medications. Patients who did survive an ear infection often were left with extensive damage to the ear. Currently infections of the ear can usually be effectively treated before the ear is severely damaged. However, serious sequelae may develop if ear infections do not receive early, thorough treatment. Inadequate treatment with antibiotics results in the development of drug-resistant microorganisms which then make resolution of the infection problematical. Following some procedures, e.g., tympanoplasties, infection caused from resistant organisms may be treated by instilling topical antibiotics into a small catheter placed in the wound.

Mastoiditis. "Mastoiditis" refers to inflammation of the mastoid antrum and mastoid cells, usually by direct extension from a middle ear infection. *Acute* mastoiditis, a complication of acute suppurative otitis media, seldom occurs since chemotherapeutic treatment became available for otitis media. When it does occur, however, bony necrosis of the mastoid process and breakdown of the bony intercellular structure occur in the second and third weeks of the acute suppurative otitis media infection. Drainage continues from the ear if a perforation has occurred, and there is mastoid tenderness and bone destruction on x-ray examination. Also, there are systemic manifestations of illness, such as fever and headache. If the earache is severe, analgesics and an ice bag may be ordered for pain relief. Possible *complications* include paralysis of facial muscles, meningitis, epidural or brain abscess, sigmoid sinus thrombosis, suppurative labyrinthitis, and subperiosteal abscess.

Before antibiotics, the *treatment* of acute mastoiditis almost always was surgical. Currently the disease may be cured with wide myringotomy and massive doses of antibiotics if only clouding of the mastoid air cells and early decalcification of bone are visible. However, a *simple mastoidectomy* must be surgically performed if bone destruction is apparent.

Chronic mastoiditis is a complication of chronic suppurative otitis media. Usually antibiotics are of limited usefulness in clearing chronic infection of the mastoid, but they may help treat complications. The presence of a cholesteatoma in the middle ear or mastoid, paralysis of the facial nerve, and/or evidence of labyrinthine irritation are indications for mastoid and/or middle ear surgery. Other therapy is local cleansing of the ear and instillation of antibiotic powders or solutions, as previously discussed for chronic purulent otitis media.

Otosclerosis. Otosclerosis is the formation of spongy bone in the capsule of the labyrinth of the ear. Dystrophy occurs in the bony labyrinth, and normal bone is replaced by highly vascular otosclerotic bone which tends to grow over the normal bony labyrinth. As the otosclerotic bone advances in growth, it causes progressive *fixation of the footplate of the stapes,* eventually locking it in the oval window. Normally as the footplate of the stapes rocks in the oval window, sound pressure is transmitted directly to the perilymph of the inner ear. With obstruction of the oval window (by an ankylosed stapedial footplate), hearing by air conduction is reduced, since sound pressure is no longer effectively transmitted to the hair cells.

Otosclerosis is the most common cause of conductive deafness.

While otosclerosis generally produces pure conductive hearing loss, it can cause a mixed hearing loss or a sensorineural hearing loss if the condition involves neural elements. The loss of hearing typically first occurs in the late teens or early twenties. Usually the patient notices difficulty hearing softly spoken tones. Tinnitus may occur. Otosclerosis appears to have a familial tendency and affects women more than men. In the United States, 10 per cent of the adult white population have otosclerotic foci, and 10 per cent of those develop conductive hearing loss.[2]

Audiometric testing is used to diagnose otosclerosis. A tuning fork test will confirm that bone conduction is greatly superior to air conduction.

Patients with otosclerotic deafness may be advised to try to improve their hearing by the use of a hearing aid or to undergo surgery on the ear. Surgical procedures may improve the patient's hearing in the presence of otosclerosis if cochlear function is normal. Surgical procedures used on the otosclerotic ear include fenestration, stapes mobilization, and stapedectomy (most common).

Disorders of the Inner Ear

Inner ear disorders are due to a number of problems. The following conditions may produce disturbances in the inner ear mechanism:[2] (a) suppurative labyrinthitis, arising primarily from acute or chronic otitis media; (b) cochlear otosclerosis; (c) trauma associated with brain concussion; (d) cardiovascular diseases, e.g., arteriosclerosis, vasomotor disturbances; (e) congenital malformations; (f) allergy (a possible cause of Meniere's disease): (g) endogenous or exogenous toxins, including ototoxic medications (e.g., kanamycin, neomycin, streptomycin, dihydrostreptomycin, nitrofurantoin, acetylsalicylic acid), and bacterial products from foci of infection; (h) blood dyscrasias; and (i) aging. Usually disorders of the inner ear are difficult to treat.

Typical symptoms of labyrinthine disease include deafness, tinnitus, vertigo, nausea, and vomiting. Other symptoms may include blurred vision, nystagmus, past pointing, and a tendency to fall in a certain direction. *Meniere's disease* is a common labyrinthine disorder; it is discussed in Chapter 27. *Acute labyrinthitis* also is discussed in Chapter 27.

Inner ear deafness is of the sensorineural type. Many cases of nerve deafness result from intense noise, especially with high frequency components.

AURAL SURGICAL PROCEDURES

Included in this section are discussions of (a) paracentesis of the middle ear (needle aspiration, myringotomy); (b) mastoidectomies (simple, radical, modified radical); (c) tympanoplasties (including myringoplasty); (d) stapedectomy; (e) stapes mobilization; and (f) fenestration. The indications for these various procedures have been discussed throughout the chapter. Comments concerning the general care of the patient having aural surgery also have been presented; these aspects of clinical care are not repeated in this section.

Unfortunately, surgical procedures performed for the purpose of restoring or improving hearing are not always successful. Rarely the patient's hearing is even worsened by the surgical intervention. The physician preoperatively discusses with each patient the surgical risk. Remember that in the presence of infection the primary objective of surgery is the control of infection; hearing preservation or improvement of hearing becomes secondary.

Paracentesis

Draining fluid from the middle ear is called "paracentesis." This may be accomplished by needle aspiration or by an incision of the tympanic membrane (myringotomy).

Needle Aspiration. Needle paracentesis of the middle ear is performed with a 2-ml. syringe and a short-bevel 10-gauge needle. After the tympanic membrane is punctured with the needle, the fluid is withdrawn into the syringe.

Myringotomy. Myringotomy is an incision made in the tympanic membrane to relieve pressure and pus in the middle ear. Although still performed, this procedure is less commonly necessary in acute infections now owing to antibiotic therapy. Usually a myringotomy heals rapidly with only slight scarring and does not affect hearing. Lay persons often incorrectly believe myringotomy causes hearing loss.

To perform a myringotomy the physician needs good light, a head mirror, an aural speculum, and a myringotomy knife with a *very sharp* blade. The physician may elect to incise the eardrum under general anesthesia, local anesthesia, or no anesthesia. Local anesthesia may be obtained by moistening a small piece of cotton with Bonain's solution and placing it against the eardrum for 5 minutes. Myringotomy is carefully performed to avoid injuring the middle ear's medial wall. The incision is best made posteriorly and inferiorly, where no ossicles can be injured and the eardrum can be easily seen. A suction tip may be used to remove fluid from the middle ear after the incision is made. Cultures of the fluid may be taken. Following myringotomy drainage may continue for several days. Usually antibiotics are continued for several days following termination of drainage.

After myringotomy has been performed, the following aspects of care are important:

- ▶ *Maintain free drainage.* The physician may order eardrops to enhance drainage. Do not stuff plugs of cotton into the ear canal.
- ▶ *Keep external ear dry and clean.* A small piece of sterile cotton may be loosely placed in the external ear to absorb some drainage. Replace this cotton when it becomes moist to minimize possible secondary in-

fection. Dry wipes may be ordered to remove excess drainage. Cleanse external ear frequently as ordered. To prevent excoriation of the skin from the drainage, apply petrolatum around the external ear.

- *Prevent contamination from the ear drainage.* Because the discharge may be infectious, wash after giving ear care.
- *Prevent infection of the wound.* Wash prior to caring for the ear and use only sterile cotton.
- *Observe for and report symptoms of complications,* e.g., headache, temperature elevation, disorientation, increasing ear pain (sometimes myringotomy must be performed again).

Mastoidectomies

Three types of mastoidectomy are simple, radical, and modified radical. These procedures are summarized below:

- *Simple (complete) mastoidectomy:* Performed through postaural (behind ear) or endaural (from ear canal) incision (Fig. 90–11). All of the infected mastoid cells are removed. A small drain may be inserted. The middle ear is not disturbed except that a myringotomy may be performed to drain the middle ear. Hearing is not affected. Usually complete healing occurs within 7 to 10 days. Postoperatively antibiotics are continued.
- *Radical mastoidectomy:* Performed through postaural or endaural incision. All mastoid air cells are removed, then the posterior wall of the external auditory canal is removed. Next the remnants of the eardrum, the ossicles (except the stapes), and all of the middle ear's mucosa are removed. The stapes is left in position to protect the entrance to the inner ear. The tensor tympani muscle is removed, and the middle ear orifice of the eustachian tube is cleaned of infected mucosa and plugged. Thus the middle ear and mastoid space are converted into one cavity. The cavity which results heals within 2–3 months by ingrowth of epithelium from the skin of the external canal. In some cases grafts of skin, fascia, or muscle are made to facilitate closure of the space. If a graft is used, the wound is packed to hold the graft in position and to ensure hemostasis and patency of the external meatus. Eventually the packing is removed postoperatively through the external ear. Following radical mastoidectomy some patients may be able to hear with a hearing aid; others permanently lose hearing in the operated ear.
- *Modified radical mastoidectomy:* Differs from radical mastoidectomy because eardrum and middle ear structures are preserved. Hearing is better than following a radical mastoidectomy. The eardrum is left attached posteriorly to the external auditory canal's skin. Thus the middle ear is sealed from the mastoid cavity.

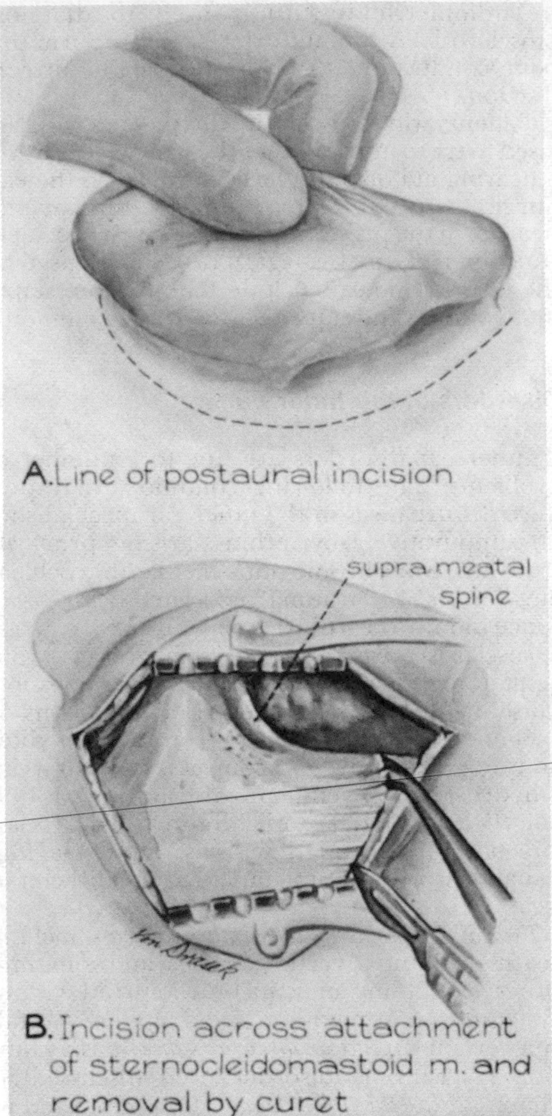

Figure 90–11. Incision and exposure for simple mastoidectomy. (From Shambaugh, G. E., Jr.: *Surgery of the Ear*, 2nd ed. 1967.)

Postoperatively following mastoidectomy a firm, bulky dressing is applied over the ear and a circling bandage is placed around the head to hold the ear dressing in place and thus provide hemostasis. Some serosanguineous drainage may seep through the dressing. If this happens, the dressing is reinforced with *sterile* dressings. Such reinforcement prevents contamination of the wound through the damp dressing.

> *Because mastoid surgery is performed close to the brain, meningitis is a serious possible complication. Sterile dressing technique is essential.*

The nurse should not change a mastoid dressing. Usually the physician does this daily or every other day. Report at once the appearance of bright blood on the dressing or any symptoms of possible complications, e.g., stiff neck, excessively tight dressing (from edema), facial paralysis, vomiting, dizziness, disorientation, headache. Postoperative complications include facial nerve injury, meningitis, brain abscess, lateral sinus thrombosis, chronic purulent otitis media, hemorrhage, and wound infection.

Sedatives and analgesics may be ordered for a while postoperatively following mastoidectomy. After radical mastoidectomy, if a graft was taken from the arm or leg, be certain to check the donor site for indications of infection (e.g., temperature elevation, yellow or foul-smelling drainage through dressing) and reinforce the dressing as necessary. Packing may be removed entirely after 3 to 4 days. Fluids are forced postoperatively as tolerated. Usually the patient is allowed out of bed 24 to 48 hours after surgery. Vertigo may occur for several days as a disturbance to the inner ear.

Tympanoplasties

"Tympanoplasty" is a term which collectively refers to a variety of reconstructive surgical procedures performed on deformed or diseased middle ear structures. Tympanoplasty may be useful in the presence of defects in the tympanic membrane, necrotic destruction of the ossicles, otosclerosis, stenosis, or the formation of deposits, fibrous or bony plaques, granulomas, or polyps.

Tympanoplastic procedures may include reconstruction of the eardrum utilizing grafts (also called "myringoplasty"); removal of scar tissue and/or granulation which interferes with ossicular function; replacement of diseased ossicles with prostheses (see discussion of stapedectomy); and formation of fenestra (see discussion of fenestration).

Myringoplasties and tympanoplasties involve precise work on minute, delicate structures. Thus, the surgeon requires effective illumination of the operative field and high magnification (obtained with an operating microscope). By reconstructing or preserving the middle ear's conductive mechanism, hearing may be improved or maintained.

Tympanoplasty may be performed with mastoidectomy or following mastoidectomy in an attempt to restore middle ear function. The ear must be free of infection before tympanoplasty is performed.

Reconstructive procedures on the ear are highly individualized for each patient. A postauricular or an endaural approach may be used. After the middle ear has been exposed and the extent of mechanical derangement has been visualized, the surgeon decides on the method of reconstruction to be used. Materials which may be utilized in the reconstructive process may include grafts (of fascia, skin, or vein), cartilage, bone, perichondrium, silicones, Teflon, and stainless steel wire. The necessary tissues may be obtained from the ear itself or from nearby sites or homografts may be used. For example, at times a piece of Silastic or Gelfoam may be placed in the middle ear to create an air channel from the eustachian tube to the round window. In other cases, fresh tissue (a vein, a piece of perichondrium, or fascia) may be used to repair or replace the tympanic membrane and seal off a pocket of air in front of the round window. A sliding skin graft may be fashioned from the ear canal's inner part.

Some tympanoplasties are carried out in two stages. The first operation is performed to remove diseased tissue and to leave the middle ear dry and healed. Next, after the middle ear has been dry for 2–3 months, the reconstructive surgery is performed to restore the conductive mechanism necessary for hearing.

Myringoplasty (Type I Tympanoplasty). A myringoplasty is performed by grafting epithelium from the ear canal, fascia from the temporal muscle, or portions of vein from the hand or forearm to reconstruct the tympanic membrane. Gelfoam soaked in saline may be used to maintain the graft's position against the eardrum, and a gauze strip is placed in the ear canal. Hospitalization is a maximum of 3–4 days. One week after surgery the strip is removed. About 12 days postoperatively the Gelfoam and debris may be gently removed from the ear canal with suction.

Postoperative medications typically include antibiotics, Neosporin or Chloromycetin-boric powder topically, and an antihistamine medication with an ephedrine derivative. Postoperative care is directed at keeping the graft in place, promoting healing, preventing infection or contamination, e.g., from water, and preventing pressure on the healing drum.

Myringoplasty not only seals off the middle ear cavity (with a graft over the tear or hole in the eardrum) but also improves hearing by restoring the function of the eardrum in sound conduction. Closing the tympanic membrane prevents contamination of the middle ear with water.

Stapedectomy, Stapes Mobilization, Fenestration. Currently stapedectomy is the surgical procedure of choice in the treatment of otosclerosis. On rare occasions, mobilization may be attempted prior to stapedectomy. Occasionally fenestration is still advisable.

Summarized below are the major characteristics of fenestration, stapes mobilization, and stapedectomy and some specific possible postoperative complications of each of these surgical procedures.

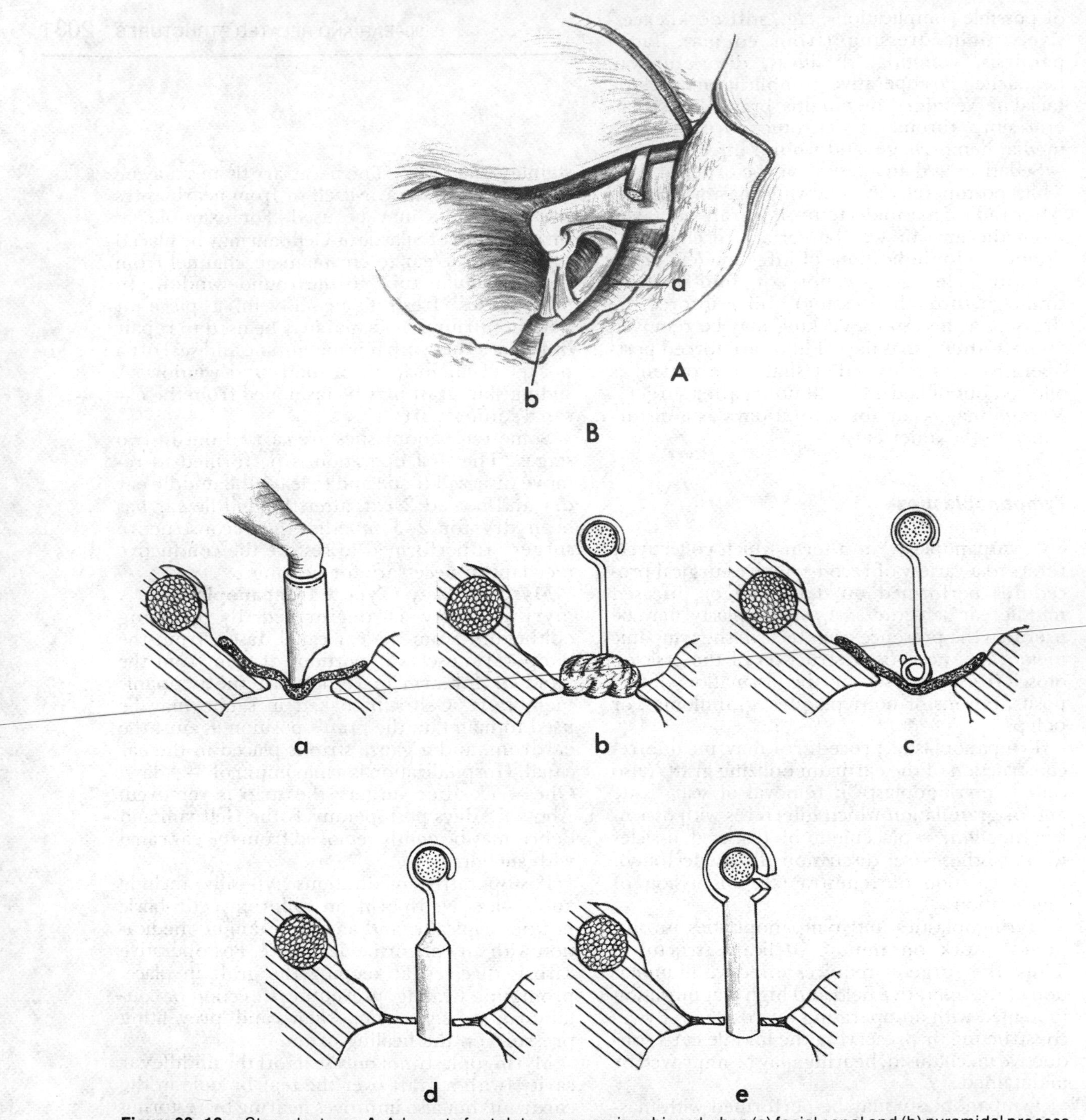

Figure 90–12. Stapedectomy. **A,** Adequate footplate exposure is achieved when (a) facial canal and (b) pyramidal process are seen. **B,** Stapedectomy prosthesis (a) vein-polyethylene strut (Shea); (b) wire fat (Schuknecht) (connective tissue preferred by author); (c) wire on compressed Gelfoam (House); (d) wire Teflon piston; (e) Teflon piston (Shea). (From Paparella, M. M., and Shumrick, D. A.: *Otolaryngology*. Vol. II. 1973.)

▶ *Fenestration:* Bypasses the fixed stapes and creates a new window which serves as a substitute for the immobile oval window. Thus a new pathway for sound is established. *Postoperative complications:* Some patients develop reduced hearing again 6–12 months postoperatively if sterile labyrinthitis develops or if fibrous or bony closure of the new window occurs.

▶ *Stapes mobilization:* Reestablishes the normal pathway of sound to the cochlea by freeing or remobilizing the fixed stapes. *Postoperative complications:* Approximately half the successful cases develop refixation of the stapes either by healing of the fractured footplate margin or by new otosclerotic growth.

▶ *Stapedectomy:* Reestablishes the normal sound pathway by using various prostheses to replace the stapes (Fig. 90–12). *Postoperative complications:* External otitis, otitis media, or labyrinthitis may develop. Displacement or rejection of the graft or prosthesis is possible. Also, incomplete closure of the oval window may allow perilymph to leak around the prosthesis and into the middle ear. This may cause tinnitus, fluctuating hearing, and/or vertigo. (These are reportable postoperative symptoms.)

FENESTRATION. Although fenestration is seldom performed currently, it is still occasionally employed in an attempt to relieve deafness caused by otosclerosis. The fenestration operation does not alter the disease process but merely creates a new window into the labyrinth. The new window serves the function of the obstructed oval window and bypasses the fixed stapes and immobile oval window. In the fenestration procedure a window is surgically created in the horizontal semicircular canal. This new arrangement restores hearing because it again permits sound pressure to displace hair cells. (The hair cells must be stimulated by physical distortion or displacement for hearing to take place.)

The patient who is the best candidate for fenestration is one who has lost effective hearing in both ears and who requires hearing improvement to comfortably participate in daily life. A thorough audiometric examination is performed prior to fenestration. Following fenestration 90 per cent of properly selected patients again have serviceable hearing. Postoperative edema temporarily obscures the final possible benefits of the surgery. The patient is told to be prepared to wait 4–6 weeks before the effects of surgery can be determined.

Fenestration is a major surgical procedure usually performed under general anesthesia. During surgery asepsis is essential because the labyrinth's perilymphatic space is opened and the perilymphatic fluid is exposed.

Following fenestration *severe vertigo* may be present for 2–4 days, and the patient may be kept on bedrest for 3–4 days. Nausea may also occur, as well as pain upon moving the jaws. Analgesics may help the patient eat more comfortably. Postoperatively position the patient as ordered (usually on the back or operated side). If positioned on the unoperated side, drainage from the operative area may enter the ear. As the patient's vertigo lessens and as the condition otherwise improves, the person's activities are gradually increased. The cavity usually heals completely after 6–10 weeks.

STAPES MOBILIZATION. Under magnification the stapes may be mobilized in various ways during surgery. These methods include (a) applying pressure and manipulating various portions of the stapes; (b) prying or chiseling the otosclerotic bone around the footplate of the stapes; and (c) fracturing a portion of the stapes and cutting across the footplate to mobilize the posterior part of the footplate. Stapes mobilization may produce immediate, indeed dramatic, hearing improvement at the time of surgery if good mobilization is obtained. Stapes mobilization requires a briefer hospitalization than fenestration and only minimal postoperative care. Also, it may result in better hearing than that obtained following fenestration. Local anesthesia is usually used.

STAPEDECTOMY. In performing stapedectomy, a local anesthetic and operating microscope (Fig. 90–13) are used to remove the otosclerotic lesion at the footplate of the stapes and to insert a tissue implant and prosthesis. Prostheses used to replace the stapes may be fashioned from a number of materials, including tissue and autoplastic materials alone or in combination. One

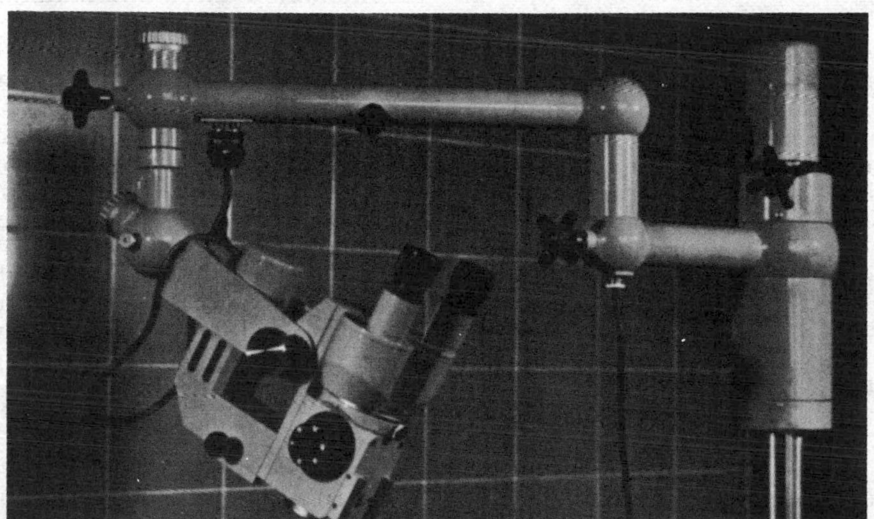

Figure 90–13. Operating microscope used during stapes mobilization, fenestration, and tympanoplasty procedures. Lens system allows magnification change from 6 to 10 times without change in distance between microscope and ear. (From DeWeese, D. D., and W. H. Saunders: *Textbook of Otolaryngology*, 5th ed. St. Louis: The C. V. Mosby Co., 1977.)

end of the prosthesis is attached to the incus, the other to the graft or plug in the oval window to transmit sound to the inner ear. After surgery the ear is packed.

The success of stapedectomy cannot be determined during the immediate postoperative period. Following stapedectomy the patient's hearing is affected for a while owing to postoperative edema and packing in the ear. Unless these reasons for diminished hearing are explained, the patient may be worried about why hearing is not as effective immediately following surgery as it initially was in the operating room. Usually the ear packing is removed on the fifth or sixth day after surgery. Once the packing is removed the patient may be instructed to gently place a piece of cotton loosely in the meatus (not into the ear canal) to protect the ear for a few days. Be certain to tell the patient to change the cotton once or twice each day.

Usually the patient is off work for about 2 weeks and is hospitalized 3–4 days. The physician discusses postoperative restrictions with the patient. To prevent the prosthesis from moving out of place, the patient may be advised not to fly while experiencing an upper respiratory infection and not to engage in deep-water diving. With these exceptions normal activities are usually permitted once the ear has healed, e.g., swimming and showering are allowed.

REHABILITATION OF THE HARD-OF-HEARING OR DEAF INDIVIDUAL

Hearing loss affects a significant number of people. Hearing impairments occur in varying degrees. Persons with slight or moderate hearing loss are often refered to as *"hard-of-hearing,"* while those with severe hearing loss are termed *"deaf."* Technically, "hard-of-hearing" persons are those whose hearing is defective but is serviceable with or without a hearing aid, while "deaf" persons have hearing which is nonfunctional for ordinary life.

Recognizing the Need for Help

The nurse can do much to identify persons with impaired hearing and to encourage them to seek professional diagnosis and treatment. Indications of impaired hearing include (a) excessive loudness or softness of speech; (b) abnormal awareness of sounds (dulled awareness or heightened awareness); (c) a strained facial expression or tilt of the head when listening; (d) the need for frequent clarification of conversation or inappropriate interpretation of the content of conversation; and (e) apparent inattentiveness or lack of response when spoken to.

Persons with hearing loss should not be falsely encouraged about the possible benefits of surgery or hearing aids. Professional assessment of hearing loss is always necessary so that correct advice may be obtained about a person's individual disorder.

Often the person with difficulty in hearing tries to conceal the problem. The person may refuse to acknowledge the need for professional help even when others mention that the need is obvious. Attempts at self-diagnosis and self-treatment may cause the hard-of-hearing person to try "quack cures" or fraudulent devices. The patient may buy a hearing aid without finding out the cause of the hearing loss or whether or not a hearing aid is necessary or will help. Perhaps the patient's reduction in hearing is merely caused by accumulated ear wax which is plugging the ear canal and can be easily removed; or perhaps the loss of hearing is the result of irreversible nerve damage. Only the physician can diagnose the condition. We have previously discussed the medical and surgical methods which may be employed in some cases to improve hearing. Here we focus on other aspects of rehabilitation.

Rehabilitative Facilities and Procedures

> *Rehabilitation of the hard-of-hearing or deaf individual is directed at obtaining maximum use of any remaining hearing ability and teaching the patient more effective use of the senses of vision, touch, and vibrations.*

Rehabilitation is affected by a patient's age and the severity of impairment. Rehabilitation is more difficult if the patient is older and has some visual reduction. Infants and children with hearing disorders require the rehabilitative efforts of specialists who help them to learn and to communicate. (Technically the process is one of *"habilitation"* rather than rehabilitation if the infant is born deaf or acquires deafness in early childhood and thus is unable to normally develop speech and language.) Rehabilitative or habilitative problems are compounded for the deaf-blind and deaf-retarded; however, if appropriate help is given, the talents of these individuals can also be developed.

Special educational facilities are available for the deaf. Instructors are professional persons especially trained to work with the deaf. These settings have equipment designed to enhance communication with the deaf, e.g., earphones, microphones.

Successful rehabilitation of the adult requires the patient's acceptance of the fact that he or she does not hear well and needs help. As with other forms of rehabilitation, those patients who are the most successful are those who work diligently as directed and who have a high degree of motivation.

A careful, complete assessment of the patient's abilities and disabilities is the first step in the rehabilitative process. Part of this assessment is the administration of thorough audiometric studies, including a hearing aid assessment. If useful, a suitable *hearing aid* is selected.

Deaf and hard-of-hearing people must learn various compensatory techniques to offset the effects of their disability. *Speech-reading* (also called "lip-reading") is one of these techniques. Speech-reading is the ability to understand speech through observation of lip and tongue movements, facial expression, gestures, and body movements. *Sign language* is another tool which makes possible fluent communication by means of hand signals. The technique of sign language (e.g., the various hand signals which represent different letters of the alphabet, words, and so forth) is taught by specialists. Not all deaf persons are capable of learning sign language. However, it is highly rewarding for those who can. Sometimes entire families learn sign language and communicate in this way in the presence of a deaf family member.

Patients with hearing disabilities may have speech problems which need correction through *speech therapy*. Speech problems develop when the deaf individual cannot hear his or her own voice or the voices of others (to mimic their sounds). Speech training may be directed at developing or conserving speech or both.

As mentioned, any hearing ability which remains is capitalized upon in the rehabilitative process. *Auditory training* is another aspect of rehabilitation which emphasizes speech discrimination and listening skills.

The employable person with impaired hearing may require *vocational training* as part of rehabilitation. Some deaf persons have the additional problems of poor balance (resulting from damage to the inner ear's vestibular portion) and unusual sensitivity to noise (even though hearing is inadequate for normal conversation). Consideration is given to the presence of these problems in selecting appropriate work for a deaf individual.

The deaf individual may additionally benefit by having a *specially trained dog* which, in effect, serves as "ears" for the person (in the way that seeing-eye dogs serve as "eyes" for a blind person). The dog is trained not to go forward or step off a curb if hearing an approaching sound (e.g., a car or siren). Also, in the home the dog gains the person's attention when someone knocks at the door or rings the doorbell or when the telephone rings.

Numerous *local and national agencies* are available which offer a variety of services for persons with impaired hearing.

Hearing Aids

The otologist determines whether a patient's hearing can be improved medically, surgically, or mechanically (with a hearing aid). Hearing aids can help some deaf or hard-of-hearing individuals to reestablish or maintain communication. *A hearing aid is any kind of mechanical or electrical device which improves hearing.* While hearing aids may improve a patient's hearing, they never restore hearing to a normal level; hearing aids amplify sound but do not improve the ear's ability to hear.

Patients with middle ear problems usually do well with a hearing aid. Patients with nerve damage, on the other hand, may be advised to rent a hearing aid for a month before purchasing one, to be certain that the hearing aid will actually be helpful. Amplification from a hearing aid may be uncomfortable in the presence of sensorineural hearing loss (i.e., nerve damage), because with this disorder there is typically an intolerance for loud sounds, hearing loss in the higher frequencies, and difficulty in understanding speech. Frequently older persons have sensorineural hearing losses. With some types of hearing loss an *ear trumpet* actually provides the best type of amplification.

Speech audiometry is useful in prescribing an appropriate hearing aid. If the hearing aid selected is suitable for the patient's needs and is properly fitted, used, and maintained, it may help and please the person greatly. In the past some deaf people were sold hearing aids that were inappropriate for their type of hearing loss and became discouraged with their hearing aids. A hearing aid is as much a prescription item as eyeglasses are, and federal law (in the United States) now requires a medical assessment prior to the fitting of a hearing aid.

The retail cost of hearing aids is a deterrent for some persons. The cost may exceed $600 if both ears require a hearing aid. Additionally there are maintenance costs.

Electric hearing aids have the following parts to properly amplify sound: (a) a microphone to convert sound waves into electric energy; (b) an amplifier; (c) a receiver to convert electric energy back into sound waves; and (d) a power source (batteries) to run the system.

While a variety of electric hearing aids are available, they are of two basic types: (1) *bone conduction receivers* (worn behind the ear against the skull); and (2) *air conduction receivers* (worn in

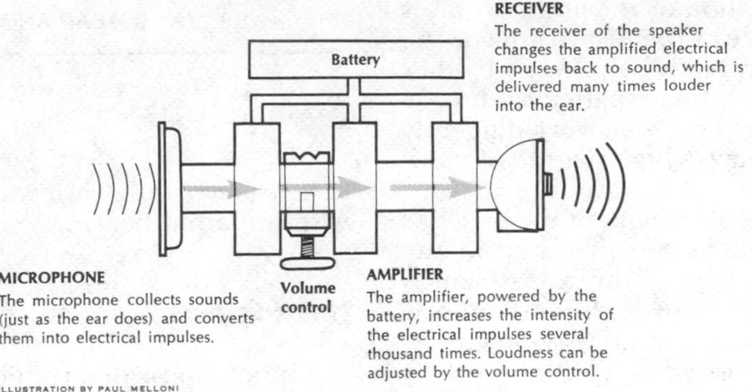

Figure 90–14. Basic components of a hearing aid. (From Gardner, G.: Hearing aids. *American Family Physician*, 15:94, June 1977.)

a mold made to fit into the auditory canal). The design of hearing aids was formerly conspicuous and bulky. Today, hearing aids are frequently inconspicuous and small. Reductions in the size and weight of these instruments are possible owing to the use of transistors in place of vacuum tubes. The size and design of a patient's hearing aid is determined by the nature of the specific disorder.[2]

Whatever type of hearing aid is prescribed, the patient needs instruction and psychologic preparation for its use. The patient is taught about the particular instrument: its use, maintenance, what to do if it doesn't work, and what it will and will not do. It may take several months for the patient to learn how to obtain maximum benefit from the aid.

Hearing aids have adjustable tone and volume controls. Several adjustments may be necessary before the aid is correctly set for the individual's needs. Initially the person wearing a hearing aid may find that amplified background noises are disturbing. The aid is not selective in amplifying sounds; it amplifies background noises as well as those sounds which the wearer wants to concentrate on. The problem of amplified background noise is alleviated somewhat by wearing hearing aids in both ears, i.e., *binaural aids.* Binaural hearing aids may be built into the stems of eyeglasses.

Some sources recommend that the patient initially wear a hearing aid for only short periods of time. By gradually lengthening the time the aid is worn, the patient can become accustomed to a "new world of sound."

Instruct the patient who wears a hearing aid to handle the instrument carefully. The ear mold should be washed daily in soap and water. A pipe cleaner or small applicator is used to clean the cannula. The mold is snapped into the receiver after it is thoroughly dry. It is advisable to carry an extra cord and battery.

If the hearing aid fails to work:
1. *The on-off switch is checked.*
2. *The ear mold is cleaned.*
3. *The battery position is checked.*
4. *The cord plug-in is checked.*
5. *The cord is inspected for breaks.*
6. *A new battery and new cord are tried.*

If these activities do not correct the mechanism, it must be taken to a local service agency.

It is not uncommon to meet people who are reluctant to wear a hearing aid because of cosmetic reasons. These persons require patient counseling about the benefit of the instrument and the fact that improved hearing will add to their social acceptance and pleasure. Wearing the hearing aid notifies others that difficulty in communicating is not necessarily due to an intellectual deficit. A hearing aid may serve the useful additional function of making others aware of the need to speak more clearly. A person's inability to hear may be a social detriment; this hearing impairment cannot be "covered up" by not wearing a hearing aid and "faking" an understanding. The patient needs to realize that a hearing aid actually makes others more comfortable in communicating with him or her than they are if the person does not improve hearing with the hearing aid. Of course, the patient will also be able to lead a more normal life by taking advantage of the improved hearing which a hearing aid will provide.

The person who has a hearing disorder may find that speech-reading (lip-reading) is useful, even while using a hearing aid.

When a hospitalized patient has a hearing aid, it becomes the nurse's responsibility to store the instrument safely when it is not in use. Encourage significant others to bring a patient's hearing aid to the hospital if the patient does not already have it.

Problems Associated with Hearing Loss

We could do much to ameliorate the tragedy of deafness if we changed some of our attitudes toward it. Blindness evokes our instant sympathy, and we go out of our way to help the blind person. But deafness often goes unrecognized. If a deaf person misunderstands what we say, we are apt to attribute it to a lack of intelligence instead of to faulty hearing. Very few people have the patience to help the deafened. To a deaf man the outside world appears unfriendly. He tries to hide his deafness, and this only brings on more problems.[57]

While blind people are often pitied, the deaf are frequently reacted to with ridicule and impatience. Perhaps one explanation for such reactions is the fact that generally deafness is not an obvious disability, while blindness is usually readily noticeable.

It is not surprising that the hard-of-hearing or deaf person frequently feels depressed, insecure, and removed from many of life's activities and pleasures. Additionally it is not unusual for such people to feel that others are whispering or talking about them when they observe people talking but cannot understand the conversation.

The individual with a hearing loss loses the multiple benefits of verbal communication and environmental sounds. Hearing loss in the infant and child removes valuable verbal learning clues. Deaf children cannot hear the speech of others and so cannot imitate speech patterns and learn to talk. At any age, hearing loss impairs the abilities to protect oneself and to communicate. Environmental sounds not only may be pleasant and help orient us to our surroundings but also may warn of impending danger, e.g., an approaching car.

Hearing helps maintain contact with reality and the environment. The inability to hear may cause disorientation and depression to a suicidal degree. In fact, *deafness may cause more serious emotional difficulties than blindness.* Persons with impaired hearing often tend to withdraw from social contacts. Sometimes this behavior is incorrectly interpreted as "aloofness." The patient may be increasingly excluded from conversation and social gatherings. The more this occurs, the more difficult it becomes for the person to once again resume these activities. Friends and family often need help in understanding the feelings, behavior, and needs of a person who has a hearing impairment. The nurse may explain considerations which are important in communicating with such a person. Everyone (including the patient) must *accept the patient's disability* and make necessary adjustments.

In the hospital setting it is important to identify a patient who has difficulty hearing. The nurse then makes a special effort to clearly communicate with the patient. Such patients require additional attention to be certain that they understand important directions and that they understand procedures being performed. If they do not know what is happening or what is expected, patients may appear to be uncooperative and resistant to care. Anxiety may reduce even further a patient's ability to hear.

Courtesies Toward the Individual with Hearing Loss

The following considerations are important in communicating with a person whose hearing is impaired:

- Do not rely on an intercommunication system, as from the nursing station in a hospital, to communicate with patients who are deaf. Rather, go to them in person. Then, before speaking gain the person's attention if he or she has not seen you enter the room. Try to avoid startling patients or giving the impression that you are "sneaking up" on them. If the patient is wearing a hearing aid, allow time to adjust it if necessary before you speak.
- Concentrate on communicating with the patient. Direct your complete attention to what you and the patient are saying and doing. Provide adequate light so the patient can see you clearly, and look directly at the patient when speaking. Speech-reading may help the person understand you. Do not cover your mouth and do not eat, smoke, or chew gum when talking (these movements interfere with speech-reading).
- Employ nonverbal cues to help convey your meaning, e.g., facial expressions, hand gestures, writing, pointing.
- It may be helpful to slightly raise your voice. Do not drop your voice at the end of sentences. Speak slowly and distinctly rather than shouting. Excessive loudness distorts the voice and may actually impair understanding. Patients who wear a hearing aid are quite sensitive to loud noises and speaking loudly may be uncomfortable as well as ineffective. If necessary, rather than shouting at patients try speaking through a rolled-up newspaper or magazine. In some instances a patient may be given a stethoscope to wear while the nurse speaks into the amplifying end of it.
- When telling something to a person whose hearing is impaired, first state the major topic of discussion and then go ahead with the details. For example: "Breakfast (pause). Do you want eggs or cereal?"
- Be calm and patient if the person cannot understand you. If the person does not appear to understand you, use different words to restate your message. Some words are more easily understood than others. If it is necessary to introduce new or unfamiliar words, pronounce them carefully or write them out. Remember that many medical and nursing words are unfamiliar to patients. If you remain uncertain about whether your message is understood, always write out your statement. Keep paper and pen or a magic slate placed close to the patient for this purpose.
- If patients speak too loudly help them learn to properly modulate the voice. Tactfully tell them when they are speaking too loudly and encourage them to try again.
- When deaf people have a speech disorder, attempt to understand the main message of what they are saying. After you have identified the main message,

PATIENT-FAMILY TEACHING GUIDE*

Suggestions for Patients with Hearing Loss	Suggestions for Spouse or Friends of Patients with Hearing Loss	How to Take Care of a Hearing Aid
1. Initiate conversations rather than waiting for others to speak to you first. 2. Position yourself so that your better ear is toward the speaker. 3. Install a telephone amplifier at home. The amplifier is attached to the receiver and has a volume control. 4. Ask your spouse or a friend to tell you when the topic of conversation changes. Knowing the topic of conversation reduces the guesswork. 5. Always position yourself so that good light is on the face of the speaker. 6. When dining in a restaurant, give the waiter your complete order and thus avoid having to answer the waiter's questions, which may be difficult to understand. 7. If you rely on lip-reading, avoid dining by candlelight. Better lighting is necessary for good communication.	1. Talk at a moderate rate. 2. Talk in a normal tone of voice. Shouting does not make your voice more distinct. 3. Use longer phrases that tend to be more easily understood. 4. Keep your voice at about the same volume, without dropping it at the end of each sentence. 5. Do not overarticulate. 6. Be certain that the hearing-impaired person follows changes in the topic of conversation.	1. The life of the battery will vary with users, depending on how many hours a day the instrument is used and the power requirements of the aid. Batteries generally last from two days to two weeks. 2. Turn off the instrument when not in use. 3. Open the battery compartment at night to avoid accidental draining of the battery. 4. Be sure the battery is inserted properly. This and a "dead" battery are the two most common problems of nonfunctioning aids. 5. Check to make sure earmold is not clogged with wax. 6. If the hearing aid "whistles" the earmold is probably not inserted properly into the ear canal or a new earmold needs to be made.

* From McCartney, J. H., and G. Nadler: How to help your patient cope with hearing loss. *Geriatrics, 34*:69, Mar. 1979.

it then becomes easier to recognize associated details. If you do not understand the patient's communication, do not act as if you have understood. Ask for clarification. It may be necessary for the person to write out the message.

► Encourage the patient's attempts to compensate for hearing loss. Give appropriate praise.

BIBLIOGRAPHY (Chapter 90)

1. Ballenger, J. J.: *Diseases of the Nose, Throat and Ear.* Philadelphia, Lea & Febiger, 1977.
2. Berkow, R. (ed.): *The Merck Manual.* 13th ed. Rahway, New Jersey, Merck, Sharp & Dohme Research Laboratories, 1977.
3. Bohne, B. A., P. H. Ward, and C. Fernández: Rock music and inner ear damage. *American Family Physician,* 15:117, May 1977.
4. Brown, M. S.: The Gordons needed all the help they could get. *Nursing 77,* 7:40, Oct. 1977.
5. Carney, A. E.: Management of sensorineural hearing loss. *Postgraduate Medicine,* 62:135, Oct. 1977.
6. Caulfield, C.: Hearing screening in children: a self study guide for nurse practitioners. *Nurse Practitioner,* 1:22, March–April 1976.
7. Cohen, N. L.: The ears, the nose, and the throat. *Emergency Medicine,* 9:63, Nov. 1977.
8. Conover, M., and Cober, J.: Understanding and caring for the hearing impaired. *Nursing Clinics of North America,* 5:497, Sept. 1970.
9. Cullin, I. C.: Techniques for teaching patients with sensory defects. *Nursing Clinics of North America,* 5:527, Sept. 1970.
10. Daroff, R. B.: Vertigo. *American Family Physician,* 16:143, Oct. 1977.
11. Deatsch, W. W.: Ear, nose, and throat. *In* Krupp, M. A., and Chatton, M. J. (eds.): *Current Diagnosis and Treatment.* Los Altos, California, Lange Medical Publications, 1972.
12. De Weese, D. D., and W. H. Saunders: *Textbook of Otolaryngology.* 3rd ed. Saint Louis, C. V. Mosby Co., 1977.
13. Dolowitz, D. A.: An appraisal of genetics in clinical otology. *Annals of Otology, Rhinology and Laryngology,* 80:264, Apr. 1971.
14. Donald, P. J.: Guide to the diagnosis and management of eustachian otitis. *Hospital Medicine,* 12:44, Mar. 1976.
15. Donaldson, J. A.: How to recognise and manage middle ear fluid. *Consultant,* 16:99, Aug. 1976.
16. Fairbanks, D. N. F.: How to remove middle ear fluid without surgery. *Consultant,* 18:112, Sept. 1978.
17. Farrell, D. E.: Hearing loss in the geriatric patient. *Nurse Practitioner,* 3:30, Nov.-Dec. 1978.
18. Fee, W.: Earlobe to cochlea. *Emergency Medicine,* 10:43, Feb. 1978.
19. Gardner, G.: Hearing aids. *American Family Physician,* 15:94, June 1977.
20. Hall, I. S., and B. H. Colman: *Diseases of the Nose, Throat and Ear.* 9th ed. London, E. & S. Livingstone, Ltd., 1976.
21. Harrison, R. J.: Current concepts in the management of hearing loss. *American Family Physician,* 19:135, Jan. 1979.
22. Herth, K.: Beyond the curtain of silence. *American Journal of Nursing,* 74:1060, June 1974.
23. Holm, C. S.: Deafness: common misunderstandings. *American Journal of Nursing,* 78:1910, Nov. 1978.
24. Holt, G. R., and J. R. Thomas: Vertigo. *American Family Physician,* 14:84, Oct. 1976.
25. Keane, J. R.: Vertigo as a vestibular symptom. *Hospital Medicine,* 14:76, Nov. 1978.
26. Keim, R. J.: How aging affects the ear. *Geriatrics,* 32:97, June 1977.
27. Keim, R. J.: Medical practice today. Common ear diseases. *Postgraduate Medicine,* 61:72, May 1977.
28. Konigsmark, B. W.: Hereditary congenital severe deafness syndromes. *Annals of Otology, Rhinology and Laryngology,* 80:269, Apr. 1971.
29. Konopa, V. O., et al.: Noise—the challenge of the future. *Journal of School Health,* 42:172, Mar. 1972.
30. Larsen, G.: Removing cerumen. *American Journal of Nursing,* 76:264, Feb. 1976.
31. Lowell, S. H.: The vertiginous patient: getting the world to stand still. *Geriatrics,* 34:39, Aug. 1979.
32. Ludman, H.: Modern surgery of deafness. *Nursing Mirror,* 134:36, May 1972.
33. McCartney, J. H., and G. Nadler: How to help your patient cope with hearing loss. *Geriatrics,* 34.69, Mar. 1979.
34. McCurdy, J. A.: Middle ear effusion: current concepts. *American Family Physician,* 17:107, Apr. 1978.
35. McMicken, D. B.: After the emergency. *Emergency Medicine,* 11:129, May 1979.
36. Mamaril, A. P.: Sudden deafness. *American Journal of Nursing,* 76:1992, Dec. 1976.
37. Mechner, F.: Programmed instruction. Patient assessment: examination of the ear. *American Journal of Nursing,* 75:PI1, Mar. 1975.
38. Meyerhoff, W. L.: Medical management of hearing loss. *Postgraduate Medicine,* 62:103, Oct. 1977.
39. Meyerhoff, W. L., and M. M. Paparella: Diagnosing the cause of hearing loss. *Geriatrics,* 33:95, Feb. 1978.
40. Meyers, A. D.: Practical ENT. Managing Cerumen Impaction. *Postgraduate Medicine,* 62:207, July 1977.
41. Myers, D., et al: *Otologic Diagnosis and the Treatment of Deafness* Clinical Symposia. CIBA Pharmaceutical Co., 1970.
42. Onion, D. K., and C. Taylor: The epidemiology of recurrent otitis media. *American Journal of Public Health,* 67:472, May 1977.
43. Paparella, M. M.: Hearing loss—a common medical responsibility. *Postgraduate Medicine,* 62:93, Oct. 1977.
44. Paparella, M. M., and D. A. Shumrick: *Otolaryngology.* Vols. 1–3. Philadelphia, W. B. Saunders Co., 1973.
45. Perron, D. M.: Deprived of sound. *American Journal of Nursing,* 74:1057, June 1974.
46. Potsic, W.: Middle ear effusions. *Hospital Medicine,* 14:20, Oct. 1977.
47. Pulec, J. L.: Surgically treatable sensorineural hearing loss. *Postgraduate Medicine,* 62:121, Oct. 1977.
48. Richardson, R. J.: Abnormal patency of the eustachian tube. *Postgraduate Medicine,* 63:187, Feb. 1978.
49. Roberts, J.: Mechanics of hearing. *Nurse Practitioner,* 3:34, Dec. 1978.
50. Rowland, H. S. (ed.): *The Nurse's Almanac.* Germantown, Maryland, Aspen Systems Corporation, 1978.
51. Ryan, R. E.: Common and uncommon causes of head and face pain. *Consultant,* 18:90, Nov. 1978.
52. Saunders, W. H., and M. M. Paparella: *Atlas of Ear Surgery.* St. Louis, C. V. Mosby Co., 1971.
53. Schuknecht, H. F.: Gelfoam as an implant in oval window following stapedectomy. *Annals of Otology, Rhinology and Laryngology,* 80:415, June 1971.
54. Schwartz, R. H.: New concepts in otitis media. *American Family Physician,* 19:91, May 1979.

55. Stewart, T. W., Jr.: Common otolaryngologic problems of flying. *American Family Physician,* 19:113, Feb. 1979.
56. Thornell, W. C.: Swimmer's ear. *Consultant,* 17:72, July 1977.
57. von Békésy, G.: The ear. *Scientific American,* Aug. 1957.
58. Wever, E. G.: The mechanics of hair-cell stimulation. *Annals of Otology, Rhinology and Laryngology,* 80:786, Dec. 1971.
59. What makes Johnny spin? *Emergency Medicine,* 10:257, Jan. 1978.
60. Wolfson, R. J., et al.: *Vertigo.* Clinical Symposia. CIBA Pharmaceutical Co., 1965.
61. Wright, J.: Deaf but not mute. *American Journal of Nursing,* 76:795, May 1976.

UNIT XXIV*

NURSING PEOPLE EXPERIENCING DISTURBANCES OF THE NOSE, SINUSES, PHARYNX, AND LARYNX

INTRODUCTION AND STUDY GUIDE

This unit is divided into three chapters. *Chapter 91* focuses on disorders of the nose and sinuses; *Chapter 92* considers disorders of the pharynx; and *Chapter 93* discusses disorders of the larynx. Anatomy, physiology, and diagnostic procedures are discussed as appropriate in these chapters.

Two highly important areas of clinical care are considered in detail in this unit. These are (1) care of people experiencing cancer of the larynx; and (2) care of people who require tracheal intubation, i.e., intubation of the airway with a tracheostomy or endotracheal tube. Many of the disorders discussed in this unit occur quite frequently. Often nurses are asked by friends to give advice about problems affecting these structures, or nurses may be required to give emergency care in the presence of nosebleeds, aspirated foreign bodies, nasal fracture, or acute laryngeal edema.

Examples of some disorders affecting the nose, sinuses, pharynx (throat), and larynx are summarized below:

- *Disorders of the nose and sinuses:* rhinitis (simple acute rhinitis, allergic rhinitis, nonallergic vasomotor rhinitis); nasal polyps; hypertrophied turbinates; foreign bodies; epistaxis (nosebleed); deviated nasal septum; nasal fracture; infected and hypertrophied adenoids; and acute and chronic sinusitis.
- *Disorders of the pharynx:* acute pharyngitis; acute follicular pharyngitis; diphtheria; chronic pharyngitis; quinsy (peritonsillar abscess); tonsillitis; and aspirated foreign bodies.
- *Disorders of the larynx:* laryngeal spasm; laryngeal edema; laryngeal paralysis; laryngeal injury; laryngitis; and cancer of the larynx.

Objectives

After studying the material presented in this unit and applying it during clinical experience you can expect to be able to:

1. Discuss clearly the structure and function of the human nose, sinuses, pharynx, and larynx.
2. Understand the pathophysiology involved in common disorders of the nose, sinuses, pharynx, and larynx.

---

*Jonathan Chinn, M.D., critically reviewed and assisted in the revision of this unit. The material was also reviewed by Mark Robinson, R.N.

3. Perform and assist in the performance of some diagnostic assessment techniques relating to the status of the nose, pharynx, and larynx.
4. Be familiar with the usual medical and surgical treatments available for disorders of the nose, sinuses, pharynx, and larynx.
5. Carry out nursing and delegated medical care skillfully for people experiencing tracheal intubation and other conditions of the nose, sinuses, pharynx, and larynx.
6. Recognize the psychosocial stress felt by patients and their significant others experiencing disorders of the nose, sinuses, pharynx, and larynx and be able to offer supportive care.
7. Offer sound and appropriate preventive and rehabilitative teaching for patients and significant others.

STUDY GUIDE

The following *study guides* may help you when working toward achievement of these objectives.

Disorders of the Nose and Sinuses

A. *Answer the following questions:* What are the major functions of the nose? What purposes do the turbinate bones, vibrissae, and mucous blanket serve? Why is Kiesselbach's plexus ("Little's area") of clinical importance? What are some possible complications of the common cold? What is the common name for allergic rhinitis? Is nonallergic vasomotor rhinitis an acute or a chronic disorder? How are nasal polyps treated? What symptom most typically indicates the presence of a foreign object in the nose? Why is prompt treatment important following nasal fracture? What information should be included in preoperative patient teaching prior to nasal surgery? Why is positioning of the patient important in the administration of nose drops? What is the "rebound effect" which can occur with nasal vasoconstricting medications? Is air conditioning helpful to persons with sinusitis? Why is early treatment of sinusitis important? How might surgery be helpful in treating chronic sinusitis?

B. *Define the following terms:* ozena, coryza, submucous resection, rhinoplasty, "mustache dressing," Proetz position, Parkinson position, multisinusitis, pansinusitis, Caldwell-Luc procedure.

C. *Perform the following activities:*
   1. Identify actions of importance in the clinical care of patients with nasal packs and in postoperative care following nasal surgery.
   2. Review instructions which should be given to a patient when teaching how to use a nasal atomizer or when preparing a patient for a nasal irrigation.
   3. State the basic mechanical causes of sinusitis and some possible complications of acute and chronic sinusitis.
   4. List the essentials of treatment of acute sinusitis and chronic sinusitis.

Disorders of the Pharynx

A. *Answer the following questions:* What microorganisms most commonly cause acute follicular pharyngitis? Tonsils are primarily composed of what type of tissue? What first aid should be given to a person who has aspirated a foreign object into the throat? Why is aspiration of organic foreign objects often more potentially serious than aspiration of nonorganic objects? What factors are of importance to ensure that a tracheostomy tube properly fits a patient? How is extubation accomplished in a patient with a tracheostomy? What aspects of patient teaching are emphasized to a patient with a permanent tracheostomy? How is mouth-to-neck resuscitation performed? How is endotracheal extubation accomplished? Why is it difficult or impossible for a patient with a tracheostomy to cough effectively? Is suctioning through a tracheal stoma a sterile procedure? Why is it important for cuffed tracheostomy and cuffed endotracheal tubes to periodically be deflated? Why should the upper airway be suctioned before the cuff is deflated?

B. *Define the following terms:* "Dick positive," tracheotomy, tracheostomy, tracheostoma, endotracheal tube.

C. *Perform the following activities:*
   1. Name the microorganism which causes diphtheria.
   2. Identify potential hazards associated with adenotonsillectomy and discuss important aspects of postoperative care following this procedure.
   3. Review the procedures for throat sprays and throat irrigations.
   4. List four purposes of tracheotomies.
   5. Familiarize yourself with the parts of tracheostomy tubes and summarize nursing care associated with each piece of equipment, e.g., procedures for cleaning the tracheostomy tube and changing neckties.
   6. Review indications for tracheotomy and list groups of patients who may benefit from tracheotomy.
   7. Familiarize yourself with the operative procedure for performing tracheotomy.
   8. Summarize complications which may develop following tracheotomy. Identify symptoms of these complications and review appropriate clinical care.
   9. State, in your own words, some advantages and disadvantages of tracheostomies and summarize essential aspects of clinical care for patients with tracheostomies.
   10. Identify some advantages, disadvantages, and complications of endotracheal intubation with an orotracheal or nasotracheal tube.
   11. Familiarize yourself with the procedure of suctioning through a tracheal stoma. Refer back to material on suctioning in Unit XVI as necessary for review, e.g., review potential hazards associated with tracheal suctioning and the prevention of these hazards.
   12. Summarize some advantages and disadvantages of cuffed tracheostomy and cuffed endotracheal tubes.

Disorders of the Larynx

A. *Answer the following questions:* What factors predispose to cancer of the larynx? What is a radical neck dissection? What postoperative complications may follow laryngectomy? What is esophageal speech?

B. *Define the following terms:* laryngoscopy, laryngoscope, laryngectomy, hemilaryngectomy.

C. *Perform the following activities:*
   1. State the functions of the larynx.
   2. List symptoms of laryngeal disease.
   3. Identify disorders which may produce acute laryngeal edema. Review appropriate emergency clinical care.
   4. Summarize factors of importance in preoperative and postoperative clinical care with laryngectomy. Consider carefully the emotional trauma associated with this surgery.

CHAPTER 91

DISORDERS OF THE NOSE AND SINUSES

ANATOMY

Air enters the nose through two nostrils (nares), separated in the middle by the *nasal septum*. This septum is composed of both cartilage and bone. Usually it is straight in adults but may deviate from the midline and thus appears dislocated into one nasal vestibule. The *nasal cavities* are located between the roof of the mouth and the frontal, ethmoid, and sphenoid bones. The walls of the nasal cavities are composed of bone covered with mucous membrane. On the lateral walls of each nasal cavity are three projections (superior, middle, and inferior) called *"turbinate bones"* (or "conchae," meaning "shell-shaped" structures). These structures greatly increase the mucous membrane surface area over which air travels as it passes through the nasal passages and into the *nasopharynx*. The turbinates also partially obstruct the air flow entering the body (Figure 91–1).

The *vestibule* of the nose is lined with skin which contains *nasal hairs* (*vibrissae*). The nose is lined with *respiratory mucosa* (except for the skin in the vestibule and olfactory epithelium far superiorly). *Mucus* secreted from this mucosa is carried back into the nasopharynx by *ciliary movements*. Nasal mucosa is normally redder in appearance than oral mucosa. This is because the lining of the nasal cavities is actually a *vascular membrane* which contains numerous blood vessels. The blood carries moisture and heat to the mucosa (the functions of these elements are discussed in the section on physiology). The blood supply to the nose comes from both the *external and the internal carotid systems*. The blood and nerve supply of the nasal septum is illustrated in Figures 91–2 and 91–3.

The *paranasal sinuses* are cavities, lined with mucous membrane, located in facial bones surrounding the nasal cavities. The sinuses drain into the nasal cavities through openings located in grooves between the turbinates. The sinuses are located in the frontal, sphenoid, ethmoid, and maxillary bones. The *maxillary sinuses* (or antra) are the largest and most accessible to treatment; they are located on either side of the nose in the maxillary bones. The *frontal sinuses*

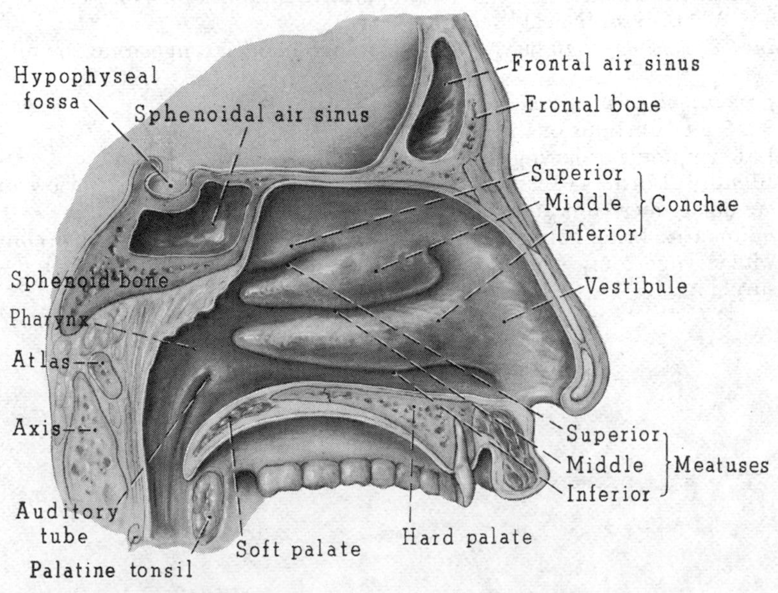

Figure 91–1. Nasal septum removed, showing lateral aspect of nasal cavity with conchae (turbinates). (From Jacob, S. W., C. A. Francone, and W. J. Lossow: *Structure and Function in Man*, 4th ed. 1978.)

are located in the lower forehead between and above the eyes. The *sphenoid sinuses* are placed at the rear of the nasal cavity, and the *ethmoid sinuses* lie between the eyes and nose. The sinuses function to lighten the weight of the skull and to give resonance and timbre to the voice.

Olfactory sense organs (i.e., those associated with the sense of smell) are located in the olfactory membrane covering the roof of the nose and the floor of the anterior cranial fossa. The *nasolacrimal duct* is a small duct that communicates indirectly with the lacrimal glands which produce tears, and the nose. Hence, when tears flow the nose "runs."

PHYSIOLOGY

Major functions of the nose are *olfaction* (the act or process of smelling) and *air conditioning* (temperature control, humidity control, and particle removal in preparation for the air's entrance to the trachea, bronchi, and lungs). Of these two functions the air conditioning functions of inspired air are the most important. These activities are truly remarkable. Inspired atmospheric air varies widely in its temperature, humidity, and particulate matter content. For example, (a) atmospheric temperature may be below zero (−17.7° C.) or above 100° F. (37.7° C.); (b) humidity of atmospheric air may vary from less than 1 per cent to more than 90 per cent; and (c) the air may be relatively clean and free of particulate matter or may be heavily laden with it (as in a dust storm).

The inspired air reaches the nasopharynx in about one fourth of a second; during this brief period of time, the nose "conditions" the air for its inspiration into deeper respiratory structures. By the time the inspired air reaches the nasopharynx, its temperature will be adjusted to between 96.8 (36° C.) and 98.6° F. (37°C.) and it will have a constant relative humidity of 75–80 per cent. Temperature control is accomplished by enlargement or contraction of "blood spaces" or "swell spaces" located in the turbinates' erectile tissues. When inspired air is cold and dry, large amounts of water are absorbed by it from the nasal mucosa. A blanket of serum and mucus covers the surface of the nasal mucosa. As much as 1000 ml. of moisture can be evaporated from the nose during 24 hours of normal breathing. The submucosal glands replenish the moisture as it is evaporated.

Particle control is achieved by the *mucous blanket* which runs continuously throughout the nose, sinuses, pharynx, trachea, bronchi, and bronchioles. Airborne particles cling to this viscid blanket on contact with it. The blanket-secretion contains lysozyme, an enzyme which causes most bacteria to disintegrate on contact. The beating action of cilia carries the blanket (with its ensnared particulate matter) back toward the pharynx, where it is swallowed. Any residual bacteria are then destroyed by gastric juice and hydrochloric acid.

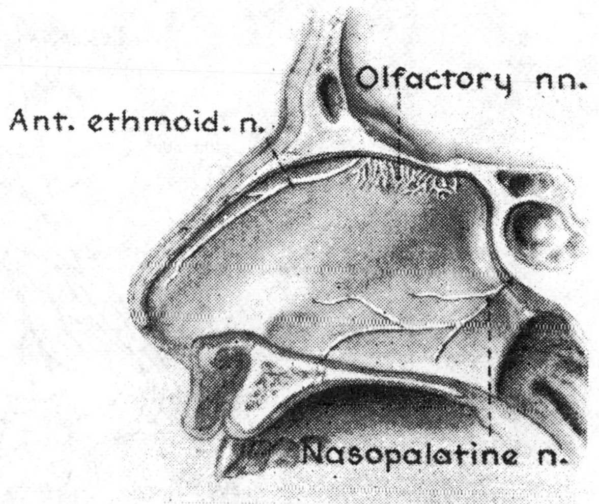

Figure 91–2. Nerve supply of the nasal septum. (From Adams, G. L., L. R. Boies, Jr., and M. M. Paparella: *Boies's Fundamentals of Otolaryngology*, 5th ed. Philadelphia: W. B. Saunders Co., 1978.)

DIAGNOSIS OF DISORDERS

Examination of the Nose, Nasopharynx, and Paranasal Sinuses

Nasal chambers are examined anteriorly with a nasal speculum (Figures 91–4 and 91–5) and posteriorly with a postnasal mirror. Bright, well-focused light is important. Shrinkage of the nasal mucosa is frequently a necessary part of a complete intranasal inspection. This is accomplished by topical application of vasoconstrictor, e.g., ephedrine, cocaine.

The *nasopharynx* is best examined with a postnasal mirror while the tongue is depressed with a tongue blade or gauze. The mirror is warmed prior to placing it in the mouth (to prevent fogging of the mirror). After it is cool the mirror is held next to one side of the uvula and light is focused on it. A small part of the nasopharynx can be observed with a nasal speculum. Specialists may use a nasopharyngoscope to examine the nasopharynx.

The *paranasal sinuses* are assessed by (a) inspection and palpation of the soft overlying tissues; (b) observation of the location of purulent secretions in the nose (it is possible to determine which sinus is infected according to where purulent discharge appears in the nose); and (c) transillumination of the maxillary and frontal sinuses. Transillumination of maxillary sinuses is performed by shining a bright light in the patient's mouth with the lips closed around a special bulb. The frontal sinuses are transilluminated by shining a shielded beam of light through the floor of the sinus, e.g., below the eyebrow. The light inside the closed mouth shines through the sinuses.

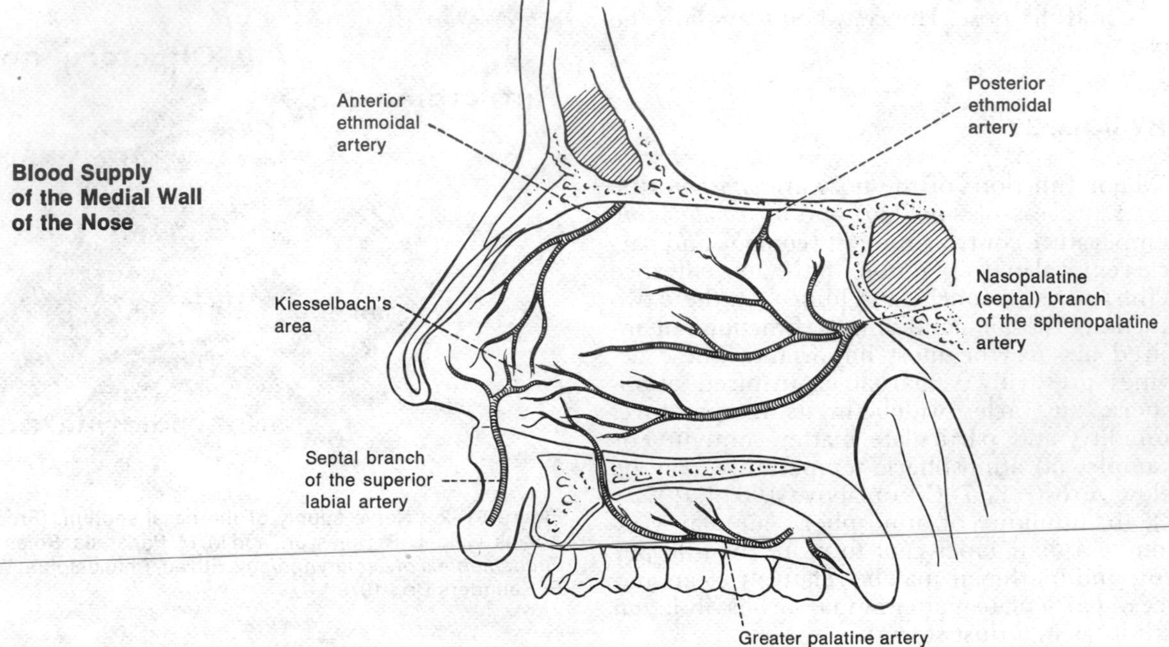

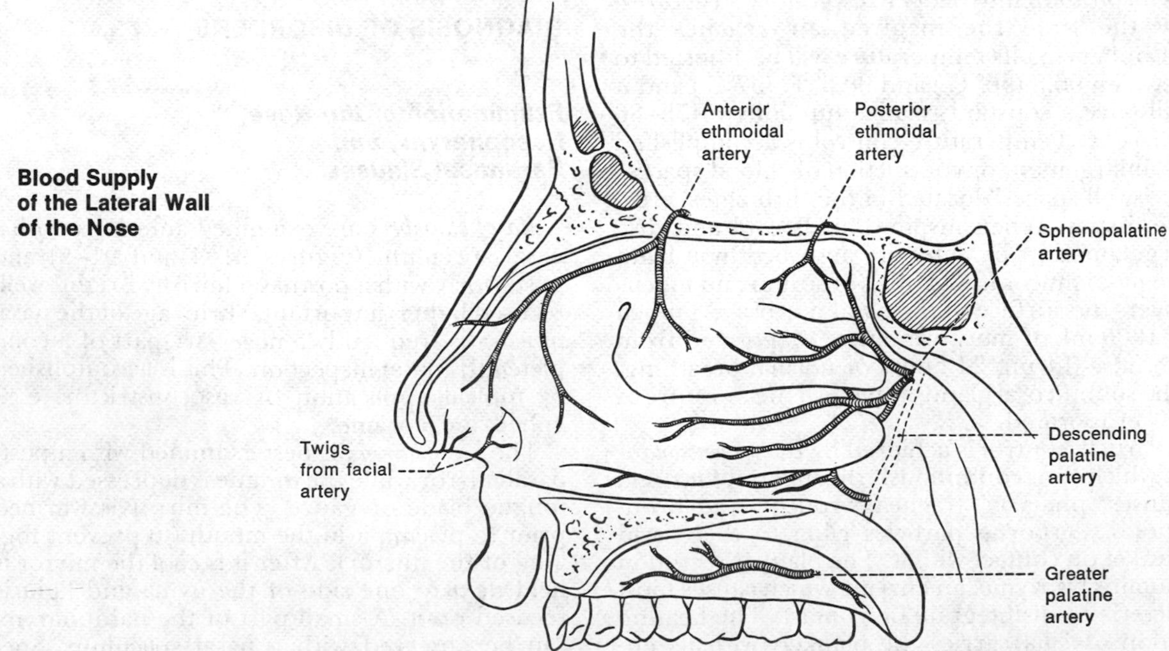

Figure 91–3. Blood supply of the nose. (From Lingeman, R. E.: Epistaxis. *American Family Physician.* 14:79, Dec. 1976.)

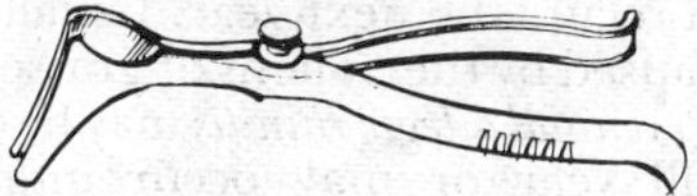

Figure 91–4. One kind of nasal speculum. (From Sutton, A. L.: *Bedside Nursing Techniques in Medicine and Surgery,* 2nd ed. Philadelphia: W. B. Saunders Co., 1969.)

These areas can be identified when the patient sits in a darkened room. If a sinus contains pus, the light is blacked in that region.

In order to more completely assess sinus conditions, *sinus x-rays* may be taken. The air which is normally present in the sinuses causes shadows to appear on the films; these shadows are then interpreted in the developed x-ray film.

Nose and Throat Cultures

Often it is diagnostically helpful for the physician to know which bacteria are present in a patient's nose and throat. This information is obtained by culturing material from the nose and throat. Many bacteria are normally present, including such organisms as streptococci, staphylococci, pneumococci, *Hemophilus influenzae,* and *Klebsiella pneumoniae.* The appearance of other organisms is definitely abnormal, e.g., those causing diphtheria or tuberculosis. In reading culture results, the physician considers other findings and decides if the appearance of certain organisms in the nose and throat is related to the patient's illness.

A sterile cotton swab is used for collecting material from the nose and throat for culture. After these areas have been swabbed, the swab is placed in a sterile culture tube. In some institutions the swab is suspended in a tube which contains 2 ml. of *broth* (to keep air in the tube moist and prevent evaporation and subsequent drying of the specimen); the broth is not a culture medium, and hence the swab should *not* touch the broth. (An exception, when the medium *should* touch the swab, is when a special culture tube containing Loeffler's medium is used, i.e., when diphtheria is suspected.) Sometimes culture tubes *without broth* are used if the specimen is taken immediately to the laboratory. In the laboratory the swab is streaked across a culture plate.

RHINITIS

"Rhinitis" refers to inflammation of the mucous membrane of the nose. Only the more common causes of this inflammation are considered here: simple acute rhinitis, allergic rhinitis, and nonallergic vasomotor rhinitis. Rhinitis may be an acute or chronic disorder. In acute cases the nasal mucous membrane becomes temporarily swollen, edematous, and congested. Chronic rhinitis causes the nasal mucous membrane to become thickened by connective tissue. Frequently nasal spurs and polyps develop. Some patients eventually develop an offensive-smelling nasal discharge, i.e., *ozena.*

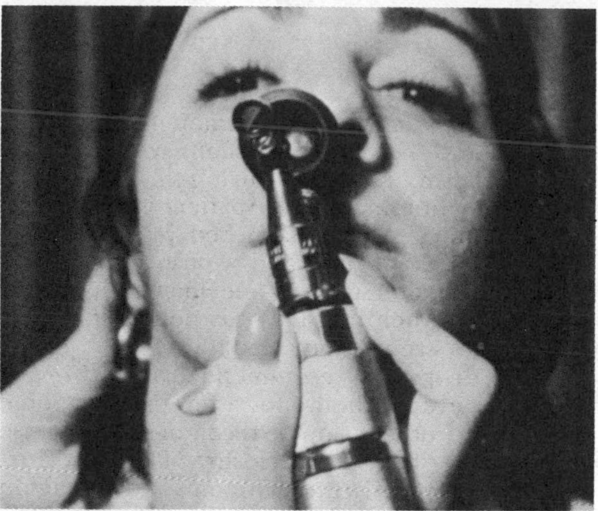

Figure 91–5. Use of nasal speculum. The patient's head is tilted backward to allow for easy viewing of the nasal passage. (From Sherman, J. L., Jr., and S. K. Fields: *Guide to Patient Evaluation,* 2nd ed. Flushing, New York: Medical Examination Publishing Co., 1976.)

Patients with rhinitis are instructed not to blow the nose too hard or unnecessarily. The nose should always be blown with the mouth open slightly and with both nostrils open. This prevents excessive pressure and the forcing of infected matter into the eustachian tubes.

The Common Cold. *Simple, acute rhinitis* is also called *"coryza"* or the *"common cold."* The common cold is the most frequent cause of acute rhinitis. Caused by a filterable virus, the common cold is spread by droplet contact from sneezing. The condition is contagious for the first 2–3 days. Although the patient should avoid contact with others during this time, few people will remain in isolation. It is advisable for the person with a cold to avoid crowds, cover the nose and mouth when coughing and sneezing, and use disposable tissues.

Great diversity exists among agents known to cause the common cold. Among them are the rhinoviruses (30 different serologic types are currently identifiable); adenovirus; ECHO virus; Coxsackie virus; influenza viruses; parainfluenza viruses; and mycoplasmal organisms.

A sore throat does *not* usually occur with a common cold. Symptoms which do occur include a feeling of burning and irritation in the nasopharynx; these symptoms are closely followed by sneezing, chilliness, copious nasal discharge, muscular aching, malaise, and mild fever. Headache may occur during the first 2 days, and as the condition progresses the nasal discharge becomes purulent and increasing nasal obstruction occurs.

If *uncomplicated*, the common cold is self-limited, and the patient is usually symptom-free after about 6 or 7 days. During this time treatment is symptomatic. The patient is advised to avoid chilling and to take bed rest, adequate fluids, a general diet, and aspirin if required. Warm salt water gargles and moist inhalations may also be helpful. There is no specific cure. Antibiotics are not indicated.

Nose drops are recommended for *infrequent* use (e.g., every 4 hours for a few days) by some physicians; others do not recommend their use because they believe that closure of the nose during the period of acute symptoms and contagion may be a protective device which prevents spread of the infection elsewhere in the body. Examples of nose drops which may be used if the physician so recommends are naphazoline hydrochloride (Privine), 0.1 per cent; ephedrine sulfate, 1 per cent; or phenylephrine hydrochloride (Neo-Synephrine hydrochloride), 0.25 to 1 per cent. When applied locally these medications constrict capillaries and reduce hyperemia, thus relieving nasal congestion. Continued use beyond 3 to 5 days may lead to "rebound" phenomenon of the nasal mucosa, actually making the symptoms *worse*.

While antihistamines may minimize such symptoms of the common cold as tearing of the eyes and sneezing, they also produce drowsiness and should therefore be taken cautiously if the patient is attempting to work, drive a car, and so forth.

Secondary invasion of virulent bacteria may *complicate* the common cold, causing symptoms to persist and become worse. Possible complications are pneumonia, bronchitis, sinusitis, and otitis media.

Persons who have frequent colds should consult a doctor for a thorough physical examination. Additionally any person with a cold should be advised to see a physician if a temperature elevation occurs or if symptoms last longer than a week.

Allergic Rhinitis. *Allegic rhinitis* (frequently called "*hay fever*") may be seasonal and acute, or perennial and chronic. Common symptoms are sneezing, nasal obstruction, tearing, recurrent thin nasal discharge, frontal headache, and itching of the eyes and nose. Allergic rhinitis typically causes the turbinates to be pale and edematous. The posterior ends of the inferior turbinates can become so enlarged that they intrude into the nasopharynx. Nasal mucosa appears smooth and glistening.

Seasonal allergic rhinitis occurs as an acute episode lasting for several weeks before it disappears and recurs the next year. Usually the condition is caused by the pollens of grasses, flowers, or trees. *Perennial allegic rhinitis* may be constantly present all year or may occur intermittently without any set pattern over a period of many years. Frequently perennial allergic rhinitis is associated with allergic sinusitis. Generally perennial allergic rhinitis is caused from sensitivity to contacts which are constantly present in our environment, e.g., domestic animal hair and dandruff, mohair, newspaper, wool, house dust, foods, tobacco. The symptoms of this form of allergic rhinitis are less severe than those of seasonal allergic rhinitis; however, its treatment is more problematic since it is usually difficult to specifically identify the allergen.

The specific *treatment* for allergic rhinitis is to identify the specific allergen and then eliminate it, or desensitize the patient to the allergen. If skin tests are refused or cannot be performed, then some less specific measures may be tried:

1. Eliminate or limit intake of chocolate, milk, and eggs.
2. Cover mattress and pillows with plastic.
3. Do not have domestic animals in the house.
4. Use nonallergenic cosmetics.
5. Cover overstuffed furniture.
6. Use antihistaminics as directed.
7. Install air conditioning in the house.
8. Avoid use of wool bedding. (Immunity, hypersensitivity, and allergy are discussed in Unit V, Chapter 11.)

Nonallergic Vasomotor Rhinitis. *Nonallergic vasomotor rhinitis* is a condition in which the patient has *chronic*, intermittent nasal obstruction or nasal stuffiness accompanied frequently by nasal discharge. These nasal symptoms may result from stress, nervousness, tension, or some endocrine disturbances. Symptoms may be aggravated by changes in environmental temperature, such as on stepping into the cold from a heated room. Treatment starts with sympathomimetics, such as pseudoephedrine, and progresses to surgery if symptoms are severe enough.

NASAL POLYPS

Nasal polyps gradually form from recurrent, localized swellings of the nasal or sinus mucosa. Once fully developed, they appear as smooth, pale tumors with pedunculated bases; the tumors themselves can be moved back and forth (Figure 91–6). Usually nasal polyps are multiple and insensitive to touch. They most frequently develop in patients who have allergic rhinitis. Symptoms of nasal obstruction occur when the polyps become large enough to obstruct the airway. Some benefit may be derived from steroid nasal sprays or injections of steroids into the polyps, but large persistent polyps must be removed surgically (polypectomy). Each polyp is avulsed with a wire snare. The procedure is performed under local

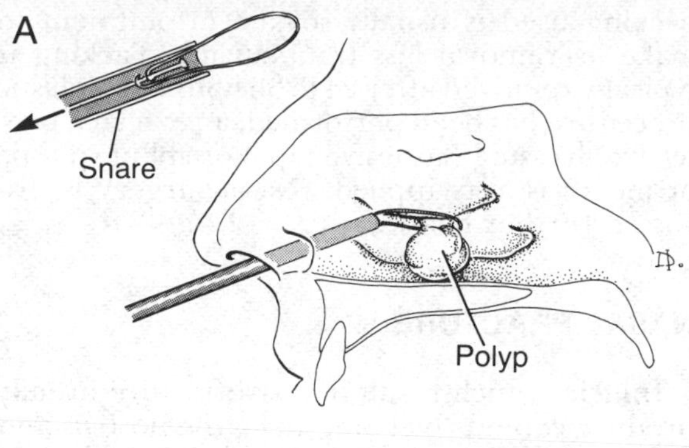

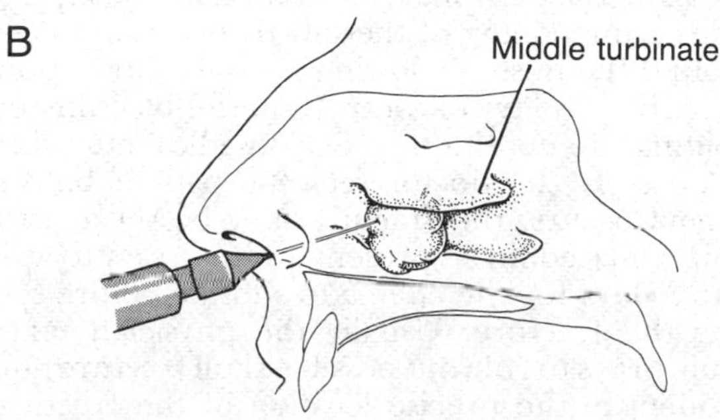

Figure 91–6. Removal of a nasal polyp. *A,* After anesthetizing the nose with tetracaine 2 per cent or cocaine 10 per cent, a nasal snare is slipped around the polyp and the polyp is transected. The polyp is then removed with a forceps. Usually more polyps will be seen after the initial ones have been removed. These should be excised in a similar fashion. *B,* The nasal polyp is visualized and a 25-gauge needle inserted into the polyp. A small amount of steroid solution (Depo-Medrol) is injected into the polyp. Usually 0.25–0.5 ml. is sufficient for this purpose. (From Hill, G. J., II: *Outpatient Surgery.* 1973.)

anesthesia. If the underlying allergy cannot be well controlled, polyps tend to recur. Polyps may develop in the sinuses as well as in the nose. The most common site in the nose is the middle meatus. Occasionally it is necessary to remove polyps from the paranasal sinuses by an external operation. Sinus surgery is discussed later in this chapter.

HYPERTROPHIED TURBINATES

Patients with chronic forms of rhinitis may develop enlarged turbinates in addition to nasal polyps. Astringent applications may be used to treat hypertrophied turbinates. These solutions act by shrinking the turbinates back against the side of the nose.

At times surgical correction of hypertrophied turbinates is indicated. An *anterior inferior turbinectomy* consists of removal of the anterior end of the inferior turbinate in order to restore respiration and proper drainage. It is performed preliminary to an antrum operation if the opening is to be made through the antral wall in the inferior meatus. ("Antrotomies" are discussed later in this chapter.) *Inferior turbinectomy* consists of the removal of the greater part of the lower border of the inferior turbinate. Hypertrophy of this structure causes pressure against the floor of the nose and interferes with drainage and respiration. *Anterior middle turbinectomy* consists of the removal of the anterior end of the middle turbinate body to restore proper drainage. Since there is some evidence that turbinectomy may lead to atrophic rhinitis (after many years), some surgeons are cautious and selective in recommending this form of surgery.

FOREIGN BODIES

Just as children often poke foreign objects into their ears, they likewise may poke them into their noses. Typically the presence of a foreign object in the nose causes unilateral purulent nasal discharge. Usually there is no pain, thus parents may be unaware of the accident. Objects most commonly poked into the nose are paper wads, rubber erasers, peas, beans, and pebbles. Sometimes a foreign body remains in the nose for years and eventually becomes encased in calcium. To remove a foreign body from the nose the physician may shrink the nose with a vasoconstrictor and then use a special grasping forceps or other instrument to dislodge it. In small children, general anesthesia may be required so the patient will hold still enough to remove the foreign body.

NOSEBLEED (EPISTAXIS)

Nosebleed may result from disease or trauma, or it may be spontaneous. Minor trauma, e.g., picking off crusts inside the nose, is the most common cause. More severe trauma, a deviated nasal septum, a perforated nasal septum, acute sinusitis, or local cancer may also cause nosebleed. Other more obscure causes include the presence of such diseases as arterial hypertension, sclerotic blood vessels, acute rheumatic fever, purpura, and leukemia.

Severe epistaxis is a highly stressful condition for a patient to experience and for persons in attendance to observe. The patient's appearance is usually very bloody; the person's emotional state is generally anxiety-ridden and fearful. In addition to blood flowing from the nares and being expectorated, occasionally blood appears in the auditory canal (as a result of passing up the eustachian tube and through a perforated eardrum) or in the corners of the patient's eyes (having passed through the lacrimal ducts). See Chapter 95 for further discussion of patient management during epistaxis (p. 2209). See also p. 2051 for discussion of nasal packs.

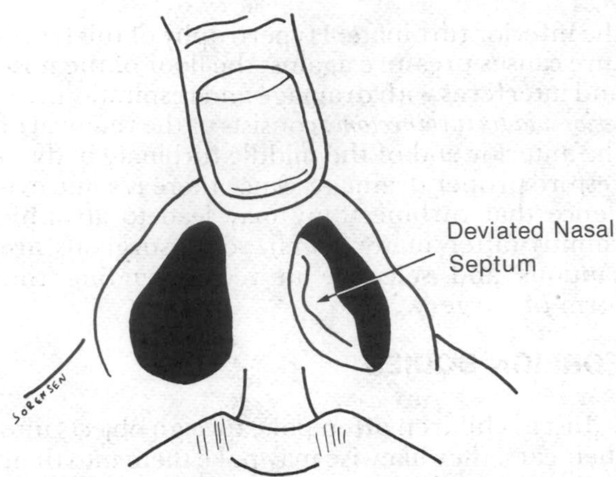

Figure 91–7. Deviated nasal septum, as viewed when tip of nose is pushed back. Dislocation of the columellar end of the septal cartilage has occurred, causing deflection of that portion of cartilage into left nostril. Note obstruction of nasal airway on that side.

DEVIATED NASAL SEPTUM

A deviated nasal septum inevitably causes some degree of nasal obstruction (Figure 91–7). Other conditions which may or may not be present are headache, sinusitis, or nosebleeds. Inspection of the nose shows the septum to be bent or inclined towards one side (or sometimes both sides if an S-shaped curve is present). In addition to deviating from the midline, the nasal septum may contain rounded humps or sharp projections (ridges or spurs). Further, the septum may be dislocated off the maxillary crest. If such deviations or irregularities interfere with respiration by obstructing the airway, they may require surgical correction by a procedure called *"submucous resection"* (SMR) or *"nasal septal reconstruction."* These procedures are carried out in numerous different ways technically, but the goal of all of them is to straighten out the septum and thus relieve airway obstruction or other problems possibly related to deviation of the septum. During this surgery great care is taken not to perforate the septum and not to weaken the structure of the nose so much that the bridge will be deformed.

Following local anesthesia an incision is made internally in the nose from the top to the bottom of the nasal septum on one side. After the mucous membrane is elevated, portions of bone and cartilage are removed, the mucous membrane is returned to its normal position, and plastic surgery is performed as necessary. Both sides of the nose are tightly packed postoperatively not only to prevent bleeding but also to serve as a splint and to hold the mucosa in place. The gauze packing used is usually soaked in ointment to make its removal less traumatizing. Packing is typically removed after 24 to 36 hours. If a plastic procedure has been performed, an external protective dressing (adhesive tape) or splint (plastic or metal) is also applied. (Nasal surgery is discussed further below.)

NASAL FRACTURE

Injuries which result in nasal fracture usually produce copious bleeding from the nostrils and back into the nasopharynx. Soon after the injury, disfiguring edema of the soft tissues also occurs around the nose. Following a nasal injury apply an ice bag and try to control anterior bleeding by holding the nose tightly. Seek medical attention at once. If the doctor sees the patient before edema occurs, the fracture may be set at that time. Once edema is present it is necessary to wait 2 to 3 days for the edema to subside before setting the fracture. Usually the physician takes skull x-rays to rule out possible skull fracture and to identify the precise location of the fracture and bone fragments. If the nose is not set, it heals in improper alignment and may cause later disorders, e.g., facial deformity, nasal obstruction (deviated nasal septum), chronic rhinitis, chronic sinusitis.

A nasal fracture is reduced under intravenous anesthesia, local anesthesia or general anesthesia. Once the displaced fragments of bone are pushed into proper alignment, they are held in place with intranasal packing and/or external dressings (adhesive tape) or nasal splints (Figure 91–8). If an external splint is worn, check the underlying skin periodically for indications of excess pressure. If observed, the physician needs to readjust the splint to prevent pressure necrosis. To minimize nasal swelling after reduction, have the patient sit with the head elevated in bed and apply ice compresses. Usually the physician removes the splint or dressing daily to again properly align the nose. Nasal fractures are usually stable enough to remove the splint in 7 to 10 days.

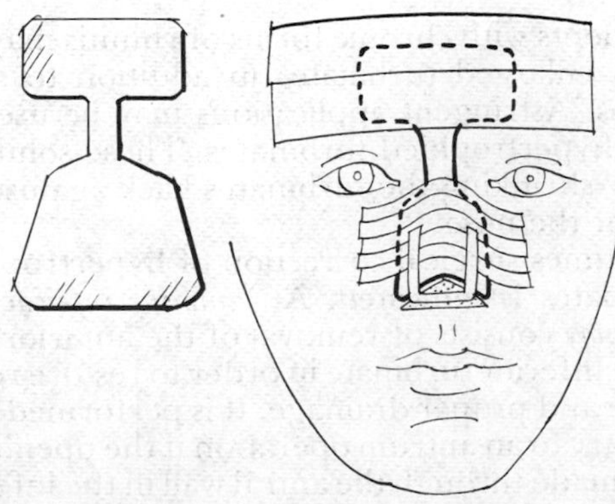

Figure 91–8. Nasal splint. (From Sutton, A. L.: *Bedside Nursing Techniques in Medicine and Surgery,* 2nd ed. 1969.)

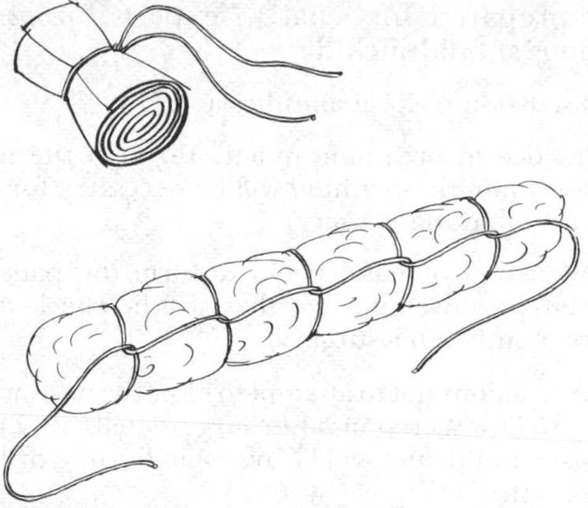

Figure 91–9. Postnasal packs. (From Sutton, A. L.: *Bedside Nursing Techniques in Medicine and Surgery*, 2nd ed. 1969.)

THERAPEUTIC PROCEDURES PERFORMED ON THE NOSE

Nasal Packs

Local nasal packs consist of a small piece of petrolatum gauze or a small cotton ball soaked in epinephrine. The pack is placed with a small hemostat or bayonet forceps. After 1 to 2 days the physician removes the pack. *Conventional postnasal packs* are made of gauze which has strong silk sutures sewn through it to give it the desired shape and to provide traction (Figure 91–9). The pack may be impregnated with petrolatum or an antibiotic ointment. Sometimes a tampon may be used for a nasal pack. When this is used the string is taped to the patient's face to prevent the pack from slipping back into the throat and obstructing the airway.

To place a postnasal pack the physician first passes a soft rubber catheter through one nostril (the bleeding nostril in epistaxis) into the pharynx, and then pulls it partially out of the mouth (Figure 91–10). Next the physician attaches two of the pack's strings onto the tip of the catheter coming out of the mouth and, pulling the catheter back out of the nose, also pulls these two strings out of the nose and pulls the postnasal pack into the mouth and then up into the nasopharynx and choana behind the soft palate. Care is taken not to roll the uvula upward beneath the pack. Once the pack is correctly positioned, the physician packs the anterior part of the nostril with a long strip of petrolatum gauze. The two strings are tied and brought out of the nostril from the pack, around the gauze or around a gauze bolster placed at the anterior nares. The third string (used later to pull the pack out) is left coming out of the mouth and is taped to the face, or it is cut about 4 inches long and is allowed to dangle in the pharynx.

Initially a patient may panic after nasal packing is placed because he or she feels unable to breathe. Quietly encourage the patient to breathe through the mouth. A patient with a nasal pack is told to gently expectorate any blood accumulating in the nasopharynx and not to swallow it. The position of a postnasal pack is periodically checked by the nurse with a flashlight directed into the patient's mouth.

> *Airway obstruction can occur if a postnasal pack accidentally slips back out of place.*

In this emergency situation the nurse may save the patient's life by quickly cutting the strings on the pack and pulling it out of the patient's mouth with a hemostat. Always keep scissors, a flashlight and a hemostat available *at the bedside* for emergency care when a patient has a postnasal pack in place. Also, see that the patient's signal bell is close by and is in proper working order so the patient can rapidly summon help if necessary. Of course, close observation of the patient is

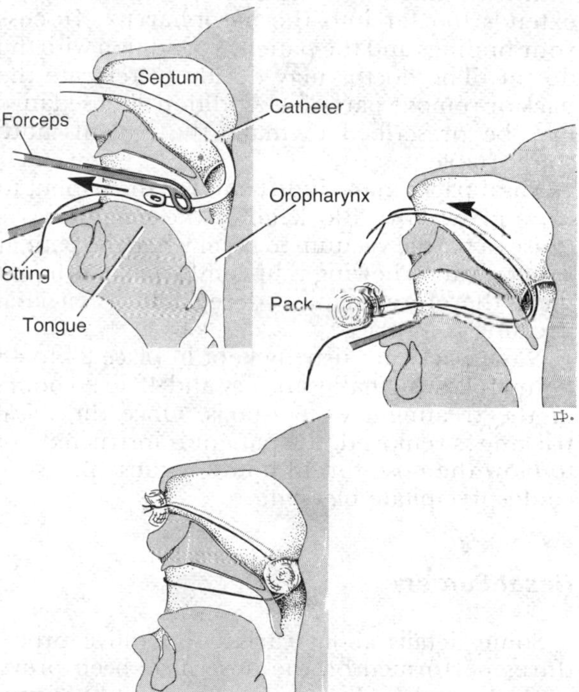

Figure 91–10. Posterior nasal pack. A pack is inserted after the nose has been anesthetized. A small rubber catheter (No. 10 French) is passed through the nose into the oropharynx where it is grasped and pulled through the mouth with a forceps *(A)*. A pack is fashioned from a roll of gauze with three 18-inch lengths of string tied about it. The pack is then tied to the catheter with one of the strings, and the catheter and string are pulled through the nasopharynx, nasal cavity, and external naris. This procedure is repeated on the opposite side. With steady traction on the nasal strings and pressure from the index finger, the pack is directed into the nasopharynx *(B)*. The third string is left hanging from the mouth and taped to the cheek to allow easy removal of the pack *(C)*. (From Hill, G. J., II: *Outpatient Surgery*, 1973.)

also important. Don't rely on the patient to call you; check periodically yourself.

Rectal temperatures are taken whenever a patient has a nasal pack. Since the person must rely on mouth breathing, the patient is unable to keep the mouth closed around an oral thermometer. Nasal packs usually cause a slight temperature elevation. However, fever generally subsides after packing is removed. Temperature elevations are always reported to the physician since they may also indicate infection. The pack may obstruct the eustachian tube and cause such ear disorders as otitis media or hemotympanum. The nurse thus reports any ear symptoms. The physician inspects the ear every day that a postnasal pack is in place.

If a patient with a postnasal pack appears to have excessive discomfort, check the position of the pack (by looking at the patient's nasopharynx with a flashlight). Sometimes part of the pack extends too far into the nasopharynx. Discuss your findings and the patient's condition with the doctor. The doctor may decide to relocate the pack or remove part of it. Additionally a sedative may be prescribed to make the patient more comfortable.

Nasal packs make it difficult for the patient to eat and swallow. Blockage of the nasal airways causes a partial vacuum to form when the patient swallows and chewing is uncomfortable. A liquid diet is therefore usually ordered as long as a nasal dressing is in place.

Nasal packs are usually kept in place 24 to 48 hours following nasal surgery and 48 to 96 hours in the treatment of epistaxis. Once the nasal packing is removed, the patient is instructed not to blow the nose for 48 hours because pressure could precipitate bleeding.

Nasal Surgery

Some details about various operative procedures performed on the nose have been previously discussed. Here we focus on aspects of general importance in the care of all patients undergoing nasal surgery.

Nasal surgery is typically performed with a local anesthesia, and the patient is premedicated with a sedative and narcotic. Remember to keep siderails up when a patient is sedated. Because nausea and vomiting can occur postoperatively, the patient usually is not allowed oral intake for 2 to 6 hours before surgery.

Preoperative Teaching. Preoperative teaching is an important aspect of nasal surgery. The patient will be less apprehensive and generally more comfortable during and after surgery if well prepared for what to expect. *Preoperative teaching* should include

- ▶ Discussion of local anesthesia
- ▶ Practice in breathing quietly through the mouth (since mouth breathing will be necessary for a few days following surgery)
- ▶ Discussion of nasal packs (inform the patient of their purpose and that they will be checked very frequently after surgery)
- ▶ Instructions not to attempt to blow the nose and not to swallow secretions after surgery (tell the person a basin and tissues will be available for him or her to spit into)
- ▶ Discussion of some postoperative reactions likely to occur, e.g., some postoperative bleeding, discoloration around the eyes, swelling of the operative area, and possible tarry stools
- ▶ If nasal plastic surgery is going to be performed, discussion of the fact that the final cosmetic result may not be apparent for several weeks. Effective preoperative teaching may help minimize postoperative bleeding since anxiety tends to increase bleeding.

Anesthesia. *Topical anesthesia* of the nose is created by inserting into the nostrils cotton pledgets with cocaine. Local anesthetic is then injected (1 per cent Xylocaine with 1:100,000 epinephrine) to complete anesthesia. Patients are often highly anxious about having nasal surgery performed "while they are awake." Emotional support is thus important. During local anesthesia the patient may not be aware of the presence of blood trickling down the throat, i.e., the person does not reflexly swallow. Thus it cannot be assumed that blood is not entering the stomach simply because the patient is conscious and is not swallowing. Of course, with *general anesthesia* the patient is unconscious and thus does not have a swallow reflex.

Postoperative Considerations. The nostrils (one or both) are usually packed following nasal surgery. After the packing is in place, a folded piece of gauze is taped across the nostrils to catch any drainage which may leak past the packing. This external dressing is called a "*mustache dressing.*" Packing stimulates mucus production, and the patient should be prepared for the additional postnasal drip.

Postoperatively following nasal surgery, (a) observe for hemorrhage; (b) change the mustache dressing as necessary; (c) periodically check the position of nasal packs; (d) observe for respiratory difficulty (e.g., due to airway obstruction from a displaced nasal pack); (e) administer fluids as ordered; (f) periodically assess vital signs, e.g., for indications of shock or infection; (g) encourage relaxation and administer sedation as ordered and as indicated; (h) provide for frequent oral hygiene and mouth care; (i) provide ice compresses over the nose as ordered (to minimize pain, edema, discoloration, and bleeding); (j) position the conscious patient with the head elevated in mid-Fowler's position (to reduce local edema, promote drainage, minimize discomfort, and facilitate respiration); (k) observe for pressure areas on the skin if an external nasal splint is present; (l) foster the patient's appetite (appetite is reduced due to inability to smell, difficulty swallowing, presence of postoperative blood and secretions, and the general discomfort of nasal packs); (m) reduce pain (e.g., by reducing the patient's anxiety, providing ice packs, promoting drainage, administering analgesics, and keeping the patient generally comfortable); and (n) administer a mild cathartic if ordered. Nasal surgery is usually not acutely painful.

Following nasal surgery *oral hygiene* is important to combat the offensive odor and taste in the mouth resulting from bleeding and postnasal discharges. Also, the mouth becomes dry owing to mouth breathing. Sometimes the throat is anesthetized with cocaine when nasal surgery is performed. Be certain such anesthesia is not still present (test the gag reflex) before giving oral hygiene or liquids postoperatively. If the gag reflex has not returned, serious aspiration of liquids may occur.

A cathartic may be ordered because the patient probably swallowed blood during the operative procedure and postoperatively. Because of the presence of this blood in the gastrointestinal tract, it is not unusual for stools to be tarry for a day or so following nasal surgery.

Postoperatively observe the patient closely for *indications of hemorrhage*, as mentioned. With a flashlight periodically look at the back of the patient's throat to see if blood is trickling down. Other indications of hemorrhage are (a) soaking with blood of the mustache dressing or nasal packing; (b) hemoptysis or hematemesis or both; (c) frequent swallowing; (d) belching (resulting from blood accumulating in the stomach); and (e) systemic symptoms of hemorrhage, e.g., rapid pulse. While some bleeding is expected following nasal surgery, unusual symptoms or excessive bleeding should not occur, and thus should be reported immediately. It is not unusual for 2–3 mustache dressings to be saturated after nasal surgery.

Following surgery remind the patient not to try to blow the nose. Explain that the feeling of fullness in the nose results from swelling and packing, and therefore attempts to blow the nose will not relieve the condition.

Usually a liquid diet is given on the operative day and a general diet is ordered thereafter. Sedation may help keep the patient comfortable until the nasal packs are removed.

Self-care is encouraged once the patient is able. For example, the patient may take care of oral hygiene and ice compresses if the necessary equipment is placed at the bedside and the person is given the necessary instructions. Remember to check, however, to be certain that the treatments ordered are actually carried out as scheduled. The patient may need your friendly reminder from time to time; your responsibility for the necessary treatments does not cease merely because the patient is assigned to self-care.

PLASTIC SURGERY ON THE NOSE (RHINOPLASTY)

Facial disfigurement resulting from gross nasal deformity may be a source of great unhappiness. Nasal deformity may be congenital in origin or acquired from disease or injury. "Rhinoplasty" refers to the surgical reconstruction of the nose using local tissues or distal tissue or both supplemented with alloplastic material as needed. The results not only may cosmetically improve the patient's appearance, but also may make the nose function better if nasal airway obstruction was present.

Rhinoplasty is usually performed under local anesthesia. Incisions are made which are inconspicuous after healing. Many variations exist in rhinoplastic techniques. In performing plastic surgery on the nose, the physician may add or remove tissue, and may lengthen or straighten the nose. Some individuals require grafting procedures. Silicone rubber (Silastic) is a synthetic substance used not only for rhinoplasty but also for surgical augmentation of the chin. More recently Proplast has been added to the materials available to the plastic surgeon. These products cause very little postoperative reaction, and the prosthesis can be cut into whatever shape is needed or wanted. Figure 91–11 shows an example of results following rhinoplasty.

Nose Drops

Oil base solutions are usually not used for nose drops, since they interfere with normal ciliary action and may cause pneumonitis if aspirated. Anesthetics and antiseptics may be used locally in the nose. However, *the medications most often instilled into the nose are vasoconstrictors,* e.g., phenylephrine, used mainly to reduce nasal congestion. If such nose drops are used over a long period of time or if they are used too frequently or in excessive amounts, they become ineffective and, in fact, may actually worsen a patient's nasal congestion. A *rebound effect* occurs in which the stuffiness worsens after each successive dose. This occurs in the following way. The state of engorgement of the turbinates is controlled by the autonomic nervous system. Because vasoconstrictors stimulate the sympathetic nerves, a compensatory relaxation of the turbinal vessels occurs after the effect of the nose drop medication has stopped. Relaxation of these vessels is

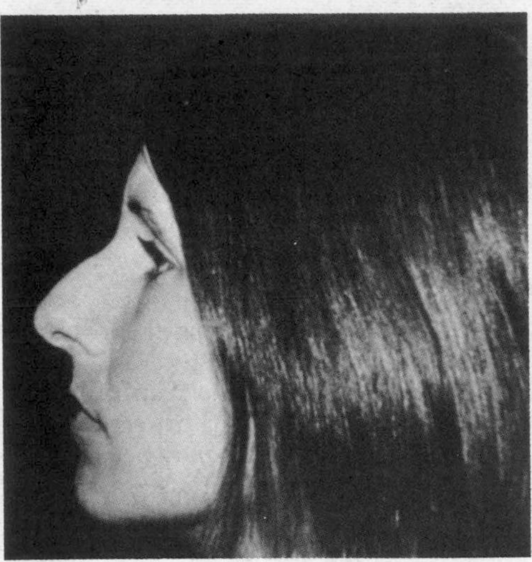

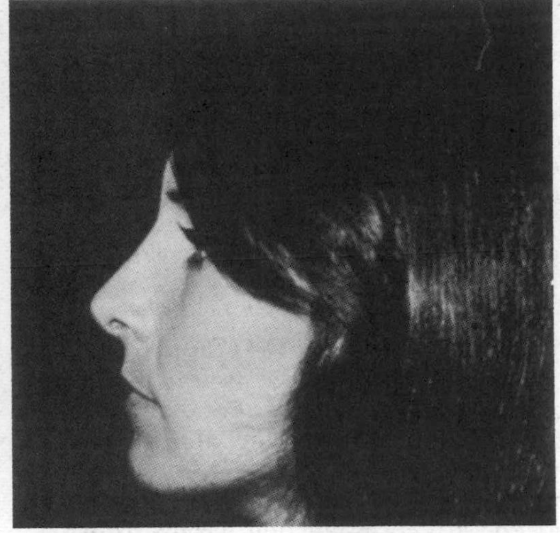

Figure 91–11. Lateral views. Note the reduction in excess nasal-tip projection as well as the more obvious hump reduction. *(Left)* Preoperative appearance. *(Right)* After rhinoplasty. (From Johnson, C. M.: When the patient wants facial cosmetic surgery. *American Family Physician,* 16:170, Sept. 1977.)

accompanied by nasal stuffiness. Thus, after a period of temporary relief from the nose drops, the nose becomes more stuffy than it was before. The only cure is for the patient to go without any type of vasoconstrictor for 2 to 3 weeks. During that interval the nose is stuffy, but eventually the normal reflexes should return, and the nose will again function properly.

Some nose drops contain drugs which may cause distressing symptoms, e.g., restlessness, heart palpitations, and tension. Patients need instructions so they will most effectively use nose drops and will not suffer rebound or side effects. Because vasoconstrictors can be systemically absorbed, they should be used by hypertensive patients only if prescribed by a physician.

Another word of caution! Various solutions are used in the examination and treatment of disorders of the nose and throat.

> *Take care to accurately identify a solution before using it or before handing it to a physician for use.*

For example, *distinguish between procaine and cocaine*. While procaine is an injectable local anesthetic, cocaine is highly toxic if injected and thus is used only by surface application. Additionally, be certain you are using a concentration of the correct strength of an ordered medication, e.g., Neo-Synephrine may be ordered in strengths of 0.125 to 1 per cent.

Procedure for Instilling Nose Drops

When possible, direct nose drops toward the area of disease by positioning the patient in such a manner that the drops will flow toward the affected area once they are introduced into the nares.

For example, (a) place the patient flat on the back with the head tilted slightly to the affected side if the drops should reach the eustachian tube's opening; (b) place the person with the head slightly over the edge of the bed and turned toward the affected side (Parkinson position) if the drops are to be directed toward the maxillary sinuses, the frontal sinuses, and nasal passages; and (c) place the person with the head hanging straight back over the edge of the bed (Proetz position) to treat the ethmoid and sphenoid sinuses (Figure 91–12). If the patient is unable to hang the head over the edge of the bed to assume the Parkinson or Proetz position, instruct the person to lie down with a *large* pillow under the shoulders so the head tips well back over the shoulders. Positioning the patient over the edge of the bed or over a pillow allows the solution to flow back into the nares. If the patient's head is merely tilted slightly back, the procedure is ineffective since the drops simply run down into the throat and are swallowed.

If a dropper is used, withdraw enough solution into it for instillation into both nostrils. Insert the tip of the dropper just inside the nares (about ⅓ inch) without touching the sides of the nostrils (to do so may cause sneezing). Instill no more than 3 drops of the prescribed solution into each nostril, unless the physician has specifically ordered a larger dose. Larger doses may be used in treating sinus disorders. Ask the patient to remain as positioned for at least 5 minutes after the drops are instilled. This prevents the escape of the solution from the anterior nares and gives the medication time to constrict the mucous membranes in the anterior portion of the nose. Then the solution can drain back into the posterior nose. Provide a basin for the patient to expectorate solution which runs into the oropharynx and mouth. Also have tissues available to wipe excess solution from the external nares and face.

Nasal Sprays or Inhalers

Medications are ordered to be administered by nasal spray, e.g., nebulizer or hand atomizer, when the physician wishes them to be diffused over the nose's inner surface. Generally the pa-

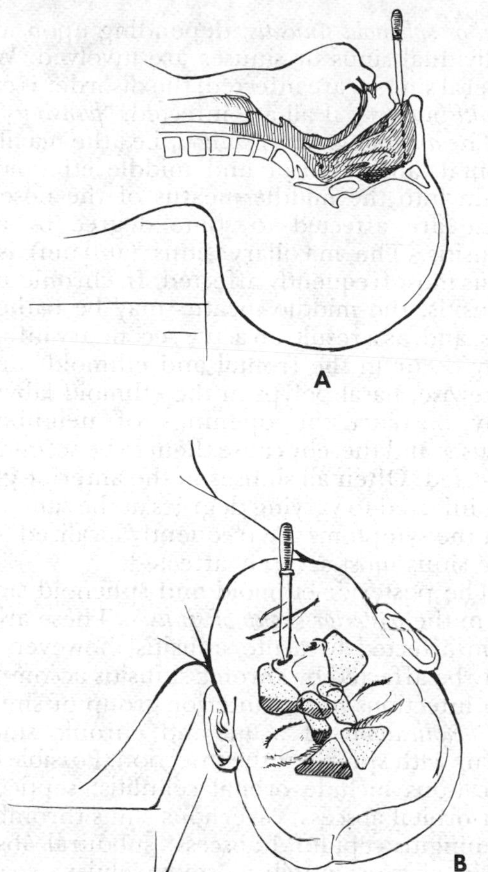

Figure 91–12. Two effective positions for administering nose drops. *A*, Proetz position, for treating ethmoid and sphenoid sinuses. *B*, Parkinson position, for treating frontal and maxillary sinuses and nasal passages. (From Sutton, A. L.: *Bedside Nursing Techniques in Medicine and Surgery*, 2nd ed. 1969.)

tient is instructed how to administer treatments. Nebulization is most effective if the patient sits upright and tilts the head slightly backward. After the nebulizer is inserted into one nostril, the other nostril is held closed (by pressing against the side of the nose with one finger) and the patient inhales (breathes through the nose with the mouth open). Similar procedures are used with a hand atomizer or inhaler. To insert medication with an atomizer, the end of the nose is pushed slightly up and the tip of the nozzle is inserted just inside of the nostril and directed backward. The bulb is squeezed as the patient inhales. This may be repeated three times for each nostril. Excessive force is avoided in spraying medication into the nose since it may force contaminated matter into the eustachian tubes or sinuses or both. Medications used for nose drops may also be applied with a spray.

Nasal Irrigations

Occasionally nasal irrigations are ordered to cleanse the nose, e.g., of crusts blocking sinus drainage. Solutions (normal saline, antiseptic solutions) are used at body temperature. Normal saline is most commonly used. Patients with chronic atrophic rhinitis may be ordered to perform nasal irrigation at least once each day. At times the physician orders nasal irrigation with an alkaline solution (e.g., sodium bicarbonate) prior to the local application of an estrogenic compound. Patients are taught to do their own nasal irrigations if this procedure is used to treat chronic nasal conditions. However, nasal irrigations are not commonly ordered because of the potential danger of forcing infected matter into the patient's eustachian tubes or sinuses or both. Aspiration is also a potential hazard.

INFECTED AND HYPERTROPHIED ADENOIDS

The adenoid (pharyngeal tonsil) is a collection of lymphoid tissue which grows from the roof and posterior wall of the nasopharynx. This tissue is present in all children and in only a few adults. Normally adenoids atrophy during puberty. In children acute infections of the adenoids usually accompany acute tonsillitis. If repeated adenoid infection occurs, the tissue becomes hypertrophied.

Hypertrophied adenoids obstruct the eustachian tubes and posterior nares and cause changes in the eustachian tubes and ears. Chronically infected and hypertrophied adenoids that obstruct the eustachian tubes may lead to ear complications such as conductive hearing loss (perhaps deafness), mastoid infections, earaches, draining ears, and middle ear infections (serous or purulent otitis media). (Disorders of the ear are discussed in Chapter 90.) Large adenoids are also associated with nasal obstruction, noisy respirations, snoring, mouth breathing, difficulty swallowing, voice impairment ("nasal" voice), fetid breath, poor rest at night, bronchitis, and frequent head colds.

Adenoid hypertrophy indicates the need for surgical removal of the adenoid tissue. If indications of chronic infection of the tonsils is also present, the tonsils and adenoids are removed together. (Tonsillectomy and adenoidectomy are discussed on pp. 1065–1067.)

SINUSITIS

As previously stated, the sinuses are cavities filled with air and lined with mucous membranes. "Sinusitis" refers specifically to inflammation of a sinus which produces an inflammatory change in the mucosa. Much of the head pain and mucoid nasal discharge commonly attributed to chronic sinusitis is actually caused by other disorders. Out of every 100 patients who consult an otolaryngologist because of "sinus trouble," fewer than 10 actually have sinusitis.

Mechanically the basic causes of sinusitis are (a) spread of infection from the nasal passages to the sinuses; and (b) blockage of normal routes of sinus drainage. Normally the sinuses drain through openings *(ostia)* into the meatuses (under the turbinates) (Figure 91–13). Obstructions cause a backup of secretions in the sinuses and produce pain in the region of the affected sinuses. Secretions trapped in the sinuses become foci for infections.

Blockage of sinus openings may result from disorders (e.g., a deviated nasal septum, nasal polyps resulting from allergy, edema of the turbinates) causing chronic nasal infections. Infection or allergy may cause swelling of the turbinates. Sinusitis often follows common colds and other respiratory infections, such as influenza. Infections easily spread from the nasal passages into the sinuses because the mucous membranes lining the nose are continuous with those lining the sinuses. If the openings remain patent, acute sinus infections usually subside quite rapidly. In the presence of obstruction, however, severe acute infection or prolonged secondary infection may occur.

Susceptible persons (e.g., those with an allergy, frequent colds, or a deviated nasal septum) may have recurrent episodes of sinusitis. Sinusitis may be *purulent* or *nonpurulent, acute* or *chronic.* Sinusitis is referred to as *ethmoid, frontal, maxillary, or sphenoid sinusitis,* depending upon which individual sinus or sinuses are involved. When several sinuses are infected, the disorder is called *"multisinusitis"*; if all are infected, *"pansinusitis."*

The *anterior group of sinuses,* i.e., the maxillary, frontal, and anterior and middle ethmoid, all drain into the middle meatus of the nose. All these are affected to some degree by acute sinusitis. The maxillary sinus (antrum) is the sinus most frequently affected. In chronic antral sinusitis, the middle meatus may be bathed in pus, and, as a result, an acute secondary infection may occur in the frontal and ethmoid sinuses. Likewise, nasal polyps in the ethmoid labyrinth may obstruct the openings of neighboring sinuses and thereby cause them to be secondarily infected. Often all sinuses in the anterior group are infected to varying degrees at the same time, but the symptoms are frequently localized to the one sinus most severely affected.

The posterior ethmoid and sphenoid sinuses form the *posterior group of sinuses.* These are seldom affected by acute sinusitis; however, they may be affected by chronic sinusitis accompanying infections in the anterior group of sinuses.

Complications of acute and chronic sinusitis occur with spread of the infection. Possible complications include orbital cellulitis; septicemia; periorbital abscess; cavernous sinus thrombosis; meningitis; epidural abscess; subdural abscess; brain abscess; osteitis; osteomyelitis; oroantral fistula (connecting the maxillary sinus with the oral cavity); choanal polyp; nasal obstruction; mucocele; pyocele; unilateral conductive deafness (due to edema of the eustachian tube).

All persons with sinusitis, whether acute or chronic, benefit from (a) not smoking (smoking causes further irritation to the sinus mucous membranes and inhibits the normal self-cleaning ciliary action of the mucosa); (b) avoidance of cold, damp conditions and chilling; and (c) a constant room temperature and room humidity

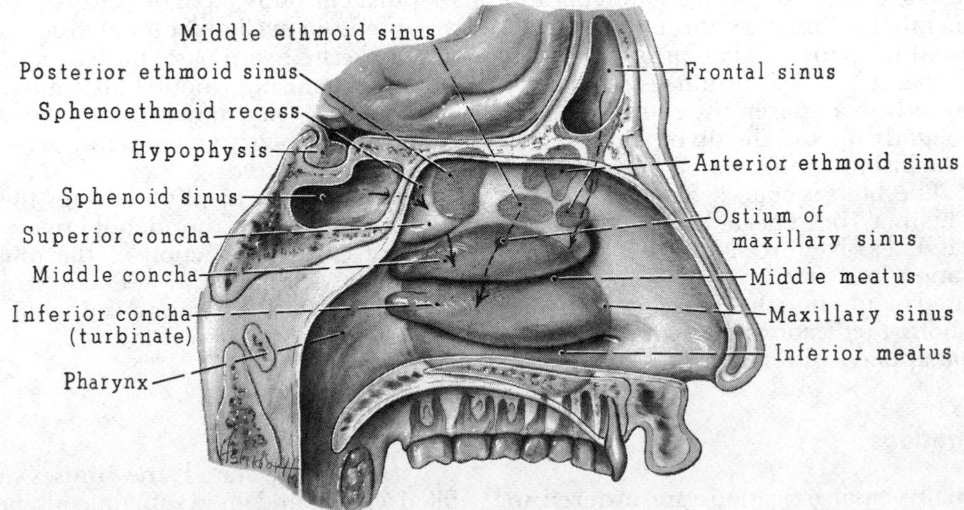

Figure 91–13. Sagittal section of the nasal cavity showing anatomy of the sinuses and direction of normal drainage. (From Jacob, S. W., C. A. Francone, and J. W. Lossow: *Structure and Function in Man,* 4th ed. 1978.)

of 40 to 50 per cent. Air conditioning tends to aggravate sinusitis. Some patients benefit from living in a warm, dry climate.

Acute Sinusitis

This inflammatory sinus condition is caused by infections (pneumonia, influenza, rhinitis) passing into the sinuses via the nasal passages. Frequently acute sinusitis accompanies or follows upper respiratory infections. Other causes of acute sinusitis are allergy, the presence of abscessed teeth, and tooth extraction. The *early treatment of acute sinusitis is important* to prevent chronic sinusitis or possible complications or both.

Symptoms of acute sinusitis include malaise; lack of appetite; nausea; nasal obstruction and congestion; purulent nasal discharge (if the duct remains open); cough and sore throat (from postnasal drainage); orbital edema or swelling over the sinuses involved; fever; feelings of pressure over the involved sinuses; and pain. Temperature elevations vary, according to the severity of the infection and whether the sinus remains open and draining or becomes occluded. Usually fever is low-grade. With complete sinus obstruction and a severe infection, the temperature may elevate to as high as 40° C. (104° F.).

Pain manifests itself in acute sinusitis as a severe, constant headache, as well as pain over the region of the infected sinuses. The location of pain is diagnostically important and thus is charted by the nurse. Pain increases with even slight pressure over the infected sinus, e.g., when the patient stoops over. Involvement of the *ethmoid* and *sphenoid* sinuses causes frontal headache with pain over the eyebrows, between the eyes, and occasionally at the vertex of the head. Infection of the *maxillary* sinuses causes pain in the cheek below the eyes and lateral to the nose and behind the eyes; occasionally the upper teeth also ache on the affected side. Sometimes swelling and redness occur over the involved sinuses, causing the patient's face to appear asymmetrical and "puffy." The nasal mucosa may appear swollen and red upon examination, and pus may or may not be found in the nasal cavity or nasopharynx. Transillumination may show the sinus to be opaque; x-rays may be taken.

In general, *treatment* of acute sinusitis is directed at (a) relieving pain; (b) promoting sinus drainage; (c) controlling infection; and (d) strengthening resistance. Essentials of treatment include the following:

- ► *Pain may be relieved* by the administration of such analgesics as acetylsalicylic acid (aspirin), codeine, meperidine (Demerol), or morphine sulfate. Pain relief may also be enhanced by the application of heat over the infected sinus, e.g., by heat lamp or hot, moist packs (see Unit XI).
- ► *Sinus drainage* is promoted by ensuring adequate fluid intake and by inhalation of moist steam; a room vaporizer may be used. Be certain windows are kept closed if a vaporizer is used. Drainage is also improved by the administration of medications which cause vasoconstriction and reduce hyperemia. These medications are administered by inhalation or as nose drops, and may be ordered to be given as often as every 1 to 4 hours until drainage occurs. Care is taken, however, to avoid excessive use of nose drops because of possible rebound effects. Shrinkage of the edematous turbinates allows drainage through the openings beneath the turbinates. Mucolytic agents (e.g., plain normal saline or Alevaire) may be administered by inhalation. Mucolytic agents destroy or dissolve mucus.
- ► *Infection control* is obtained by giving the patient specific medications to which the infecting organism is sensitive, e.g., broad-spectrum antibiotic, such as tetracycline or ampicillin. Chemotherapy is directed at speeding recovery and preventing complications.
- ► *Bed rest, intake of a nutritious diet,* and *mental rest* are advised to *heighten resistance.*

Very early in the course of sinusitis, an oral *antihistamine* may be prescribed for symptomatic relief. However, these medications are given cautiously since (by thickening nasal secretions) they may prevent adequate sinus drainage.

Sometimes it is necessary for the physician to *manually irrigate the frontal or maxillary sinuses* to promote drainage and removal of purulent matter. Normal saline may be inserted through the sinuses' normal openings with a trocar and cannula. If insertion is not possible through the normal opening, the physician may perform trephination of the frontal sinus or an antrum puncture to irrigate the maxillary sinus. *Trephination of the frontal sinus* is accomplished by drilling a small hole into the frontal sinus and inserting a small tube into this hole to allow drainage and to provide a path by which medications can be directly instilled into the sinus.

An *antrum puncture* is accomplished by pushing a trocar through the *maxillary sinus* wall. Irrigation is then performed with warm, normal saline. The patient catches drainage from the puncture in a basin held under the nose. Antral puncture is not a dangerous procedure and is believed by some specialists to be the most beneficial method of treatment for subacute and early chronic suppurative sinusitis. This procedure can be repeated numerous times without permanently damaging the nose or maxillary sinus. Antral puncture may be performed for diagnosis as well as treatment. If pus is withdrawn, the presence of active infection is established.

Two precautions are important: (a) the patient

should be taking antibiotics at the time of the puncture because of the possibility of causing an osteomyelitis; (b) air is *never* used to clear sinuses since it can be rapidly absorbed through inflamed mucosa and picked up by the venous system to cause a fatal air embolus.

Unlike the maxillary sinus, the *ethmoid and sphenoid sinuses* cannot be irrigated directly. Removal of retained purulent matter from these sinuses is accomplished by a procedure called the *"Proetz displacement method."* Details of this procedure are discussed in textbooks of otolaryngology. Let us briefly say that the procedure utilizes the principle of gravity displacement of one fluid by another. Thick, purulent secretions are partially suctioned into the nose and a thinner fluid (isotonic saline solution containing a vasoconstrictor) is introduced into the sinus faster than the thick material can reenter.

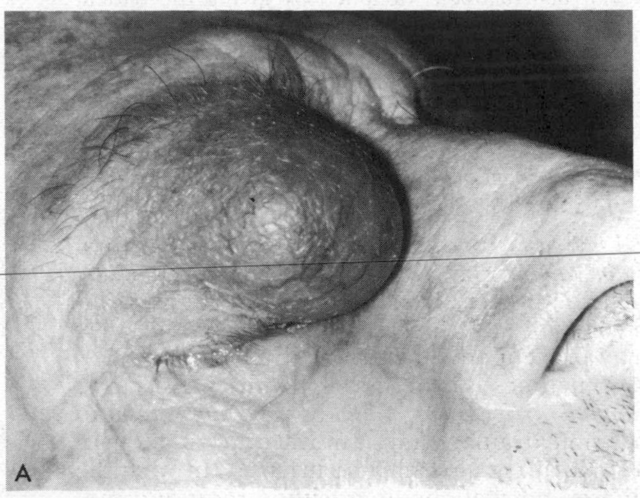

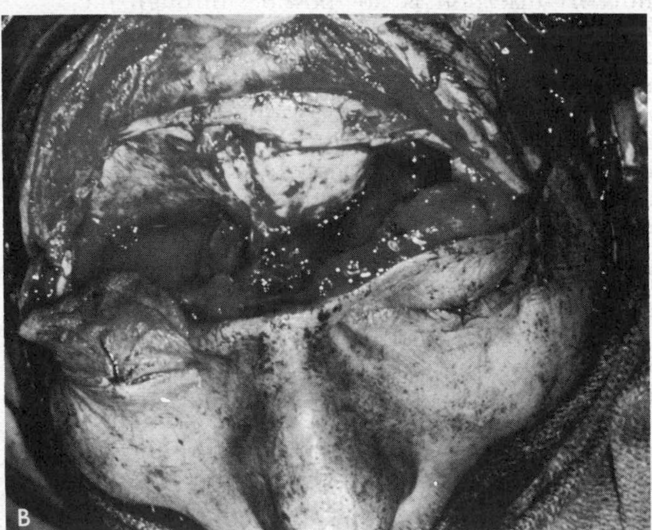

Figure 91–14. A. Mucopyocele of frontal sinus presenting as a facial abscess. **B.** At definitive surgery, dura overlying the brain is exposed. Once evacuated, the frontal lobe is exposed. (Courtesy of Jonathan Chinn, M.D.)

The frontal and sphenoid sinuses, because of their proximity to the brain, represent the greatest risk of significant complications (CNS) and need to be treated aggressively.

Chronic Sinusitis

Repeated or sustained sinus infections cause the mucous membrane lining a sinus to become thickened, and a chronic sinusitis develops which is difficult to treat effectively. In addition to the measures discussed above for the treatment of acute sinusitis, the treatment of chronic sinusitis is directed at correcting underlying disorders, e.g., removing polyps, eradicating dental infections, straightening a deviated nasal septum. If allergy is an underlying cause of chronic sinusitis, treatment is directed at that cause. The physician also investigates and treats general systemic conditions which adversely lower resistance to infection, e.g., anemia, malnutrition, hypometabolism, and lowered plasma gamma globulin. Nasal irrigations may be ordered as part of chronic sinusitis therapy, e.g., with sterile Ringer's solution. While a few patients may be cured by repeated irrigation or displacement and antihistaminics or antibiotics as indicated, most patients require surgical treatment.

Symptoms of chronic sinus infection include lethargy; difficulty sleeping; chronic cough (due to postnasal drip); chronic purulent nasal discharge; inability to smell (if nasal obstruction occurs); and a chronic sinus headache. Typically sinus headaches are dull head pains which are present upon awakening (due to the accumulation of secretions in the sinus during sleep). Movements during the day eventually help the sinus to drain so the headache typically is relieved after a while, only to reappear the following morning. Contrary to popular opinion, chronic infection of the paranasal sinuses is not a common cause of recurrent headache. Far more common causes of headache in the frontal region or between the eyes are allergic rhinitis and swelling of nasal tissue. Polyps commonly occur with allergic rhinitis. Also, with allergic rhinitis it is usual for the lining of the sinuses to undergo the same changes as those occurring in the nose.

Sinus Surgery

As mentioned, surgery may be part of the treatment for repeated episodes of sinusitis. Basically, this surgical treatment may be directed at (a) *correction of nasal deformities* which may be causing obstruction of sinus openings (correction of hypertrophied turbinates, submucous resection, or removal of nasal polyps); (b) *removal of diseased mucous membrane;* and/or (c) *enlargement of or creation of sinus openings to improve drainage.* The goal of every sinus operation is to eradicate the infection while leaving contiguous structures normal.

Generally sinus surgery is performed during the subacute stage of infection. Various surgical approaches are used under local or general anesthesia. The maxillary, sphenoid, and ethmoid sinuses can be approached through a nostril although the surgeon may wish added exposure of the sinuses through external approaches.

The maxillary sinus can be approached through the nostril or by an incision made through the gum tissues under the upper lip (above the level of the roots of the maxillary teeth). This oral incision is called a *Caldwell-Luc procedure* or *a radical antrum operation* (see Fig. 91–15). The antrum may be packed with gauze after surgery to control bleeding. This packing is removed (after 24 to 48 hours) through the nose and the nasoantral window which has been created. It is not unusual for numbness of the upper lip and teeth to occur for several months postoperatively following a Caldwell-Luc procedure.

Sinus surgeries frequently cause a black eye and swelling of the operative area for a week or so postoperatively. Antibiotics may be administered prophylactically during the postoperative period. During this time the nurse reports indications of postoperative infection or insufficient sinus drainage, e.g., temperature elevation, tenderness, or pain in the area of the sinus.

Immediately after sinus surgery, if a general anesthetic was given, the patient is turned well over onto the side to prevent aspiration of bloody drainage before consciousness returns. Following return to consciousness or following local anesthesia, the patient is positioned with the head elevated 45 degrees to encourage drainage and to minimize postoperative edema. Remind the patient to (a) breathe through the mouth (because of nasal packing); (b) not blow the nose (nasal packs are in place and also the pressure of blowing may traumatize the sinus); and (c) spit out drainage accumulating in the nasopharynx. Observe for indications of hemorrhage. If the patient swallows frequently, hemorrhage may be occurring and he may be swallowing the blood.

Postoperatively an ice bag or ice compresses may be ordered to relieve pain and constrict blood vessels (thus minimizing edema and bleeding). Cool or warm vapor inhalations may also be ordered. Mouth care is important during the postoperative period because nasal packing forces the patient to breathe through the mouth and because of the unpleasant taste of postoperative secretions. Oral hygiene also helps prevent infections. This is particularly true if an oral incision was made. Set up an oral hygiene tray at the patient's bedside and schedule the procedure as a treatment to be regularly performed. The tray should include not only refreshing aromatic solutions for rinsing the mouth but also petrolatum for application to the lips. Oral hygiene before meals improves the patient's appetite. Encourage fluid intake during the postoperative period. Following an oral incision the patient is usually given a liquid diet for 24 hours or so and then a soft diet for a few days to minimize oral trauma.

FACIAL TRAUMA AND RECONSTRUCTION*

In recent years, ear, nose, and throat surgeons have become extensively involved in the repair and reconstruction of faces damaged in accidents or assaults. Nursing considerations of facially traumatized people are briefly discussed here. As skills are refined and newer techniques are de-

*This section was written by Mark Robinson, R.N.

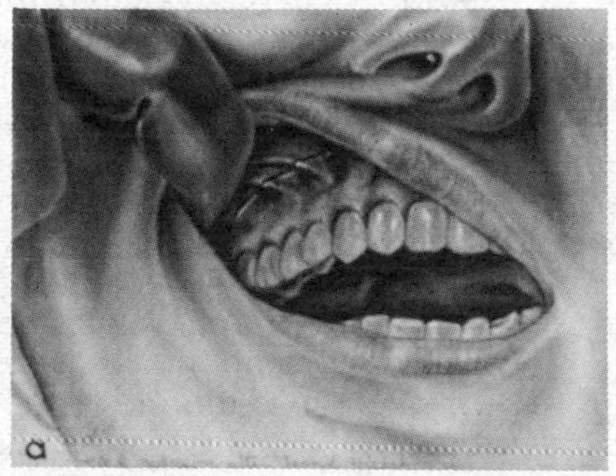

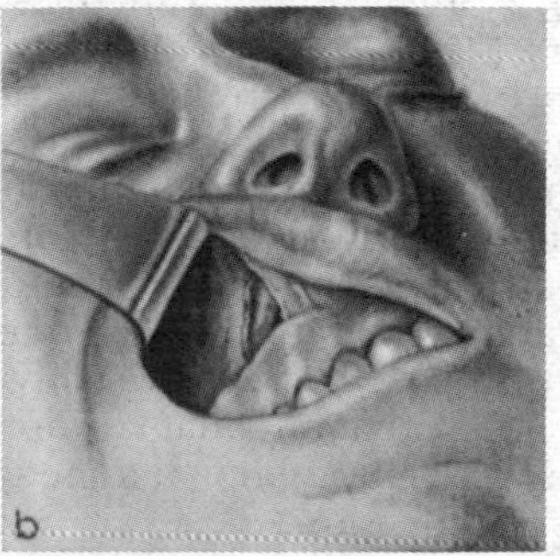

Figure 91–15. The purpose of the Caldwell-Luc ("radical antrum") operation is to clean out under direct vision the diseased tissue in the sinus. A horizontal incision *(a)* is made in the canine fossa, the soft tissue is elevated, the sinus is entered through its anterior wall, and enough of the wall is removed to provide adequate exposure. Then the diseased membrane in the sinus is removed and a large window made under the inferior turbinate *(b).* The incision in the canine fossa is then sutured. (From Adams, G. L., L. R. Boies, Jr., and M. M. Paparella: *Boies's Fundamentals of Otolaryngology,* 5th ed. Philadelphia, W. B. Saunders Co., 1978.)

veloped, normal or near-normal appearance can be restored. Very often, however, the process is long and drawn out, requiring more than one surgical procedure. Patients may go home between operations and must face the world with ego-traumatizing disfigurements.

The role of nurses in these cases is twofold: (a) physical care while patients are undergoing often painful surgery and convalescence and (b) psychologic care of patients (and their significant others) with serious body image problems.

Physical Care

Nursing care for patients with facial trauma consists of all the usual considerations of generalized patient care along with some specific factors that depend on the nature of the injuries.

Airway Maintenance. Patients with facial trauma may have compromised airways from a variety of sources, i.e., direct injury to the larynx, laryngospasm, swelling and edema, subcutaneous emphysema, aspiration, wired jaws. When possible, consent for tracheostomy should be obtained. A tracheotomy tray should be kept at the bedside. All patients with wired jaws should have suction and wirecutters at bedside.

Neurologic Problems. (See also Unit X.) Severe head trauma often accompanies facial trauma and is always a consideration in patient care. Neuro checks should be done regularly, including checks of pupillary action, grip strength, and ability to smile, wrinkle forehead, open and close eyes, and move extremities. Changes in sensorium or increasing lethargy should be reported to the physician immediately. Any cerebrospinal fluid rhinorrhea or otorrhea should be reported. (CSF may be easily recognized by collecting a small quantity of the discharge on a tissue or piece of gauze. CSF shows a characteristic pattern, with a central red or pink spot surrounded by a halo much lighter in color.) Presence of CSF indicates direct communication with the brain or meninges, and special care must be taken to prevent bacteria from ascending these pathways. Patients are cautioned to keep their hands away from nose and ears. Usually no dressings are applied, so that adequate drainage is maintained and secretions are not dammed up to provide a focus of infection.

Skin Grafts. (See also Chapter 80.) Skin grafting is becoming more and more common in facial reconstruction. There are several types: split-thickness, full-thickness, flap, rotation, pedicle, and mesh. Pigskin is often used as a temporary dressing on abraded tissue. There are two principal objectives in nursing patients with skin grafts: maintenance of circulation and prevention of infection. Failure of either can result in loss of the graft.

Maintenance of circulation often requires improvisation to keep pressure off the source of blood flow. Positioning, sandbags, loose dressings, and sometimes restraints may be necessary. Always look for the donor site, which may be far removed from the graft site, and requires care similar to that of the graft itself. Strict sterile technique must be observed when caring for graft and donor sites. Any purulence, odor, or color change should be reported. Dressing changes are usually done by the doctor, but if nurses are required to do this, strict adherence to the doctor's orders and asepsis can spell the difference between success and failure of the graft.

Nutrition. Maintaining adequate nutrition usually poses problems in patients with facial injuries, ranging from difficulty in chewing or swallowing through wired jaws to nasogastric tube feeding. Pureed, mechanically soft diets are usually adequate for those with problems chewing or swallowing. These diets should be made as tasty as possible, since their usually bland nature discourages good appetite.

The patient with wired jaws may require special consideration. While some may be able to drink from a cup, many need to use straws or syringes. A very useful device consists of a 50- or 60-ml catheter-tip syringe with eight or 10 inches of red Robinson catheter cut off at a slight bevel, which may be inserted inside the cheek alongside the mandible. Many patients find this the easiest way to take fluids.

Tube Feeding. (See also Unit X.) Nasogastric tube feeding is common with patients who have had facial injuries. Care should be taken to see that the tube causes a minimum of pressure on the nares. Tapes should be changed frequently and benzoin applied to minimize skin problems. The tube should be aspirated and checked for proper positioning with each feeding. When possible, the oropharynx should be checked with tongue blade and flashlight to see that the tube has not been regurgitated into the mouth. Patients must always be fed in an upright position to prevent aspiration. Diarrhea is a common problem with tube-fed patients. Dilution of milk or meat-base liquids with 50 percent water, frequent small feedings, and antidiarrhetic drugs help prevent this problem. As soon as possible, patients should be encouraged to feed themselves, as they are usually better able to judge comfortable amounts and participating in their own care raises morale.

Safety. Patients with facial trauma require extra safety precautions. Very often, eyes are swollen shut or damaged. Apply the same precautions as you would for blind patients. Confusion and disorientation are frequently present. Siderails should be up and frequent observations made. Postoperative patients may have to be prevented from lying on the operative site, and face guards should be maintained in place.

*Psychologic Care**

Patients with facial trauma have extraordinary body image problems. The emphasis on youth and beauty in our culture may give rise to profound emotional disturbances in patients with potentially disfiguring injuries. Suicidal tendencies are often present and at times may have been the cause of the injuries. Suicide precautions are always in order. Trauma victims pick up expressions of distaste and horror, so nurses must be matter-of-fact, accepting, and supportive. Family and friends should be cautioned that their loved ones may appear terribly mutilated and should be taught to be calm and helped to maintain an optimistic outlook. In the early stages, until the patient becomes accustomed to a drastically changed appearance, do not use a mirror with the person. Realistic reassurance that satisfactory reconstruction is possible goes a long way in maintaining patient morale. Before-and-after pictures of similar patients can assist the patient over periods of depression. Most important of all, patients and significant others must be allowed to express their feelings and concerns. If patients must go home between reconstructive procedures, they may face often traumatic encounters with the public. If family and friends have been encouraged in acceptance of the person's appearance and nursing has been supportive and friendly, these encounters may be considerably softened. Above all, the patients must be assured (by words and deeds) that they are esteemed for themselves and not for their appearance. (A comprehensive text on maxillofacial trauma is that by R. H. Mathog: Symposium of maxillofacial trauma. *Otolaryngologic Clinics of North America,* 9, pp. 313–538, 1976.)

*See also discussion of psychosocial factors affecting the burned person, p. 1804, Chapter 80.

CHAPTER 92

DISORDERS OF THE PHARYNX

"Pharynx" is the Greek word for "throat." The pharynx is the space behind the oral cavity which extends downward from the base of the skull to the larynx. The pharynx is subdivided into three sections: (1) *nasopharynx* (epipharynx), the area above the margin of the soft palate; (2) *oropharynx,* the area visible when the tongue is depressed with a tongue blade; and (3) *hypopharynx* (laryngopharynx), inferior to the base of the tongue.

ACUTE PHARYNGITIS

This disorder is the most common throat inflammation. Viral or bacterial in origin, acute pharyngitis may precede the common cold or other communicable disease. Typical symptoms include mild fever, mild sore throat, hacking cough, and some difficulty swallowing. If uncomplicated, the symptoms remain mild and the throat returns to normal after 4 to 6 days.

Treatment for acute pharyngitis commonly includes rest, a liquid or soft diet, aspirin, and warm saline gargles or throat irrigations (see below). An ice collar may be worn and lozenges may be sucked which contain mild anesthetics. Moist inhalations may relieve the dry throat. Additionally the patient is encouraged to drink at least 2500 ml. of liquid per day. Oral hygiene and mouth care are refreshing for the patient and help prevent drying and cracking of the lips and oral pyoderma. If the patient has a distressing cough, an antitussive may be ordered.

ACUTE FOLLICULAR PHARYNGITIS

The throat is commonly afflicted with *streptococcal or staphylococcal infections.* Symptoms usually occur suddenly and may include temperature elevation (103° F. [39.4° C.,] or more), chills, flushed face, headache, muscle and joint pain, general malaise, inflammation of the throat, and severe sore throat. The throat's mucous membrane appears acutely inflamed and is "studded" with white or yellow "follicles." Follicular exudate does not cover the tonsillar pillars or the soft palate. Possible serious complications may develop, e.g., cervical adenitis, sinusitis, otitis media, mastoiditis, acute rheumatic fever, and acute glomerulonephritis. In addition to being a severely distressing condition, acute follicular pharyngitis may be quite debilitating and highly dangerous. Some of the most serious infections are those caused by the Group A streptococci. The typical rash of scarlet fever may develop in persons infected with this organism who are "Dick-positive," i.e., are not immune to the organism's exotoxin. A blood leukocyte count exceeding 12,000 is also not unusual.

Mention should be made of *acute infectious mononucleosis.* This presents as acute pharyngitis in older children, adolescents, and young adults. It is important because the liver and spleen become involved, and potentially disastrous spontaneous or traumatic rupture of these organs is possible. The patient should be advised to be extremely careful not to have any abdominal injury and should abstain from hepatotoxins (i.e., alcohol).

Treatment for acute follicular pharyngitis includes those measures discussed above for acute pharyngitis. In addition, antibiotics are prescribed as indicated by the findings of throat, nasal, and blood cultures. *Early antibiotic therapy* is especially important in treating hemolytic streptococcal infections, to prevent possible serious complications. While penicillin (IM) is the drug of choice, penicillin-sensitive patients may be treated with other antibiotics, e.g., tetracycline, erythromycin, or cephalosporin. Antibiotics are continued for 24 to 48 hours after visible throat inflammation subsides, to prevent recurrence (usually a total of 7 to 10 days). Because the throat pain may be severe, codeine sulfate may be necessary as an analgesic. A barbiturate may be prescribed as a soporific at night, e.g., Nembutal.

Some patients require hospitalization for fluid therapy if their throats become too swollen and painful to permit them to swallow. Intravenous feedings are given until the acute inflammation subsides, e.g., 24 to 72 hours. In the hospital medical asepsis is carefully practiced to prevent spread of infection. Morning and evening temperatures are taken until the patient is completely recovered. Generally patients are not allowed to resume full activity until they have been out of bed for as many days as they were on bed rest. Because complications may develop 2 to 3 weeks after the pharyngitis has apparently disappeared, the patient is advised to see the doctor promptly if indications of possible complications develop.

CHRONIC PHARYNGITIS

Chronic pharyngitis usually occurs in persons who (a) are habitual users of tobacco and alcohol; (b) have a chronic cough; (c) are employed in or live in dusty environments; or (d) use their voices excessively. Chronic pharyngitis may cause relatively few symptoms (cough, dry throat, thick mucus in the throat which is expelled with difficulty, and an irritated, full feeling in the throat), or recurrent, more severe, acute episodes may occur, with sore throat, mild mucosal swelling, hyperemia, and thick, tenacious mucus in the hypopharynx.

Chronic pharyngitis is treated by (a) restricting irritants, e.g., tobacco, alcohol, spicy foods; (b) treatment of underlying disorders, e.g., infections of the nose, sinuses, or tonsils or other pulmonary infections; (c) voice rest; (d) local removal of tenacious secretions with suction or saline irrigation and application of 2 per cent silver nitrate; (e) nasal sprays or instillations to relieve nasal congestion; and (f) administration of an antihistaminic to treat allergy. Some patients benefit from aspirin or acetophenetidin for malaise.

DIPHTHERIA

Diphtheria, a severe disease of the throat that most often affects children, is caused by the bacillus *Corynebacterium diphtheriae.*

There has been a recent resurgence of cases of diphtheria that has been attributed to a decline in emphasis on childhood immunization. Further, recent outbreaks have been identified in indigent populations (Bowery or "skid row" inhabitants). Commonly the skin is the site of infection.

Because diphtheria is highly contagious, isolation technique is employed during treatment. (See discussion of prevention of spread of airborne organisms in Unit XVI.) Diphtheria may be transmitted directly via infected droplets of moisture (ejected from an infected person's throat, nose, or mouth) or via objects used by the patient, such as eating utensils, towels, handkerchiefs. Additionally, diphtheria may be spread by "carriers," i.e., healthy persons who carry the organisms even though they are not ill. An infected person may have bacilli in the throat 2 to 4 weeks following recovery from the acute effects of the infection.

Immunization programs have caused the incidence of diphtheria to decrease rapidly in the past 40 to 50 years, although, as mentioned above, there is some recent change in this trend. *Preventative measures should not be relaxed.* Artificial immunization is achieved by the administration of weakened toxins, given by injection in combination with pertussis ("whooping cough") and tetanus immunizing agents. These combined injections are commonly called "DPT" immunizations, i.e., diphtheria-pertussis-tetanus immunizations. See Table 11–2 (p. 139) for an immunization schedule.

The incubation period for diphtheria is typically 2 to 5 days, but may be longer. Diphtheria produces a white or gray membrane in the throat which advances rapidly and may cover all three sections of the pharynx and extend down into the trachea. A bleeding base becomes visible if one attempts to remove the membrane. The throat is swollen, and breathing and swallowing may be impaired. (Emergency tracheostomy may be required to prevent asphyxiation).

Pseudomembranous inflammation develops on mucosal surfaces as an acute inflammatory response to a powerful necrotizing toxin, that is, the diphtheria exotoxin. The surface epithelial cells undergo necrosis and desquamation, and a fibrino-suppurative exudate pours forth. Robbins observes: "As the fibrin coagulates and traps the necrotic cellular debris, it produces a dirty gray-white, rubbery membrane which layers the inflamed, eroded surfaces."[88]

The patient infected with diphtheria is severely ill and has a rapid, thready pulse. However, the body temperature seldom goes higher than 101° F. (38.3° C). Early symptoms include sore throat, headache, nausea, and temperature elevation. Diagnosis is confirmed by culture of a specimen swabbed from a portion of bleeding base after a piece of membrane is lifted up (see Chapter 91). A special culture medium, such as Loeffler's, is required to grow the bacillus. In addition to possible tracheostomy, treatment focuses on bed rest, large doses of penicillin, and intravenous and intramuscular injections of specific diphtheria antitoxin. Oxygen may be given to relieve cyanosis and dyspnea. Early treatment is important to prevent serious complications such as paralysis or cardiac complications. Permanent neurologic or cardiac damage may result from toxin produced by the diphtheria bacillus as this toxin spreads throughout the body. Prognosis is affected by the administration of antitoxin and the severity of the infection. The risk of mortality progressively increases as the infection spreads from the nose down into the lungs. With pulmonary involvement the mortality is in excess of 85%. It is desirable for the antitoxin to be administered *early* in the course of the illness. A prolonged period of recovery is often advisable.

PERITONSILLAR ABSCESS (QUINSY)

Acute streptococcal or staphylococcal tonsillitis (see below) may cause a peritonsillar abscess to form as a result of infection of tissue between the tonsil and the fascia covering the superior constrictor muscle (Figure 92–1). Typically the patient has tonsillitis for several days, appears to be improving, and then develops increasing pain on one side of the throat (and ear) and has difficulty swallowing. Usually the patient's voice is described as a "hot potato voice" since the speech is muffled. Often the person sits with the mouth partially open so he or she can drool rather than having to try to swallow. Thick secretions are "hawked" up with difficulty. A peritonsillar abscess causes extensive swelling of the soft palate. The uvula may be pushed to one side; half of the pharyngeal opening may be occluded by this swelling. The tonsil is pushed forward, downward, and toward the midline of the throat; this displacement is the result of pus forming in the fascial space.

A peritonsillar abscess may rupture spontaneously (causing pus to drain through the anterior pillar), or it may need to be surgically incised to provide good drainage (Fig. 92–1). Other therapeutic measures are topical anesthetic throat sprays or local anesthetic injections, narcotics, application of an ice collar, antibiotics, hot saline throat irrigation, or saline or alkaline mouthwashes or gargles (105–110° F [40.5° C–43.3° C]). The patient may be able to swallow more easily when drinking if someone stands behind him or her and pulls upward on the sides of the throat while the person swallows.

If antibiotics, e.g., penicillin, are given early and in a high dose, abscess formation (and possible surgical incision and drainage) may be avoided. However, if incision is necessary, the patient is positioned sitting up to make it easier to expectorate pus and blood.

Usually it takes at least 1 month for the infection of a peritonsillar abscess to subside. Then a tonsillectomy is frequently advised to prevent recurrence.

A

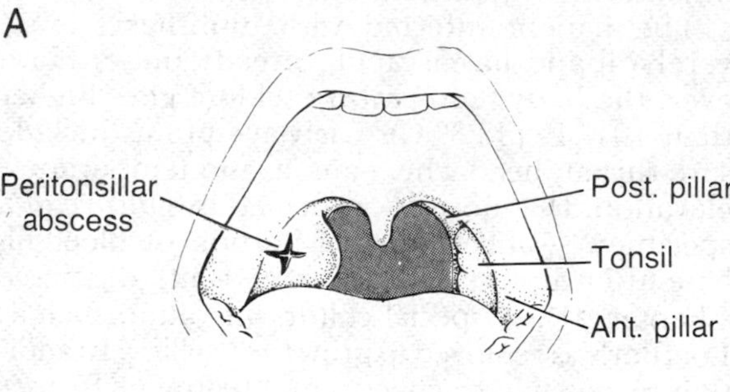

B

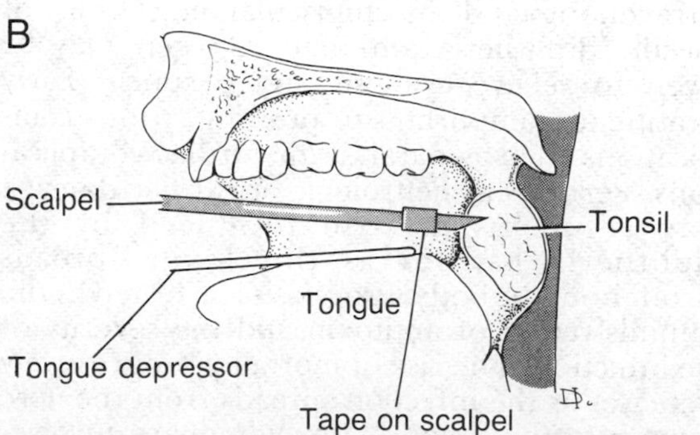

Figure 92–1. Peritonsillar abscess. The incision is made near the anterior pillar through the area of greatest fluctuance. Local anesthesia is usually quite adequate for this operation. (From Hill, G. J., II (Ed.): *Outpatient Surgery*, 2nd ed. Philadelphia: W. B. Saunders Co., 1980.)

TONSILLITIS

"Tonsillitis" means inflammation of a tonsil. The tonsils are masses of lymphatic tissue located on either side of the oropharynx. Normally the palatine (or faucial) tonsils do not project much beyond the limits of the tonsillar pillars, and they are approximately the same color as the rest of the oral mucosa. A pillar retractor may be used to withdraw the anterior pillar during examination. Each tonsil is a small, almond-shaped mass composed primarily of lymphoid tissue which is covered by mucous membrane. Within the tonsil are many crypts and lymph follicles which supply phagocytes to the mouth and pharynx.

Several decades ago undue emphasis was placed on sequelae which could possibly result from infected tonsils and adenoids. As a result, during the 1930's the removal of the tonsils and adenoids was the most common surgical procedure performed and represented almost 35 per cent of all operations. Currently fewer of these operations are performed, as it is realized that (a) the throat's lymphoid structures are important in immunity; (b) the incidence of upper respiratory disease is not lowered significantly by removal of tonsils and adenoids; and (c) a disservice may actually be done to the patient if tonsils and adenoids are indiscriminately removed in hopes of some future benefit.

Acute Tonsillitis. Acute tonsillitis begins as a sore throat accompanied by fever, anorexia, chills, muscular pain, and headache. Swollen, tender anterior cervical lymph glands are also usually present. The malaise and discomfort of uncomplicated tonsillitis increase for 24 to 72 hours before slowly subsiding over a period of 7 to 10 days. The tonsils appear enlarged and brightly inflamed. Pus or exudate is present on the tonsils or in the crypts. The tonsils are studded with yellow follicles if the infection is streptococcal. Throat cultures identify the infecting organism. Acute tonsillitis frequently elevates the white blood cell count and causes cervical lymph nodes to be swollen and tender.

The usual treatment for acute tonsillitis is bed rest, hot saline gargles or throat irrigations, and maintenance of adequate fluid intake. Severe cases may be given antibiotics. Once started, the antibiotics are continued for 24 to 48 hours after subsidence of symptoms for a total of 7 to 10 days. Pain may be relieved by an ice collar, aspirin, or codeine sulfate if necessary. (There is some thought that acetaminophen [Tylenol] should be given instead of aspirin, because of the platelet dysfunction reported with aspirin administration.) Repeated acute attacks of tonsillitis are not indicative of the need to remove the tonsils surgically unless indications of persistent infection remain. Bed rest is recommended for 48 hours after the temperature returns to normal, to help prevent complications. Complications which may develop from streptococcal tonsillitis include pneumonia, nephritis, osteomyelitis, and rheumatic fever. Complications which can result from local extension of the infection are chronic tonsillitis, acute otitis media, acute rhinitis, acute sinusitis, and peritonsillar abscess or other deep neck abscesses.

Acute tonsillitis is usually a bacterial infection and is most often due to streptococci. This contagious airborne or food-borne infection occurs most often in children but can occur at any age. If uncomplicated, acute tonsillitis typically resolves spontaneously after 5 to 7 days. Treatment is encouraged, since it not only makes the patient more comfortable and hastens recovery but also may prevent serious complications.

Chronic Tonsillitis. Chronic tonsillitis is not as common as formerly believed. Recurrent sore throat is the most frequent symptom. Between episodes of acute tonsillitis the throat remains uncomfortable. The tonsils often appear enlarged and, if infected, a sharp line may be seen between the color of the buccal mucosa and the tonsillar pillar. The most reliable indication of chronic tonsillitis is the ability to express purulent material from the tonsil crypts with a wooden tongue blade. Once chronic tonsillitis is proved, surgical removal of the tonsils is the recommended treatment. Surgery is contraindicated during periods of acute tonsillar infection, although tonsillectomy may be performed during acute peritonsillar abscess.

Adenotonsillectomy ("T & A")

Surgical removal of the tonsils ("tonsillectomy") and of the adenoids ("adenoidectomy") is collectively called "adenotonsillectomy" and is abbreviated "T & A." While the tonsils or adenoids may be removed in separate procedures, most often they are removed during one surgical operation. *Contraindications* for T & A are (a) the presence of any acute infection (surgery is canceled if there is any indication that the patient may be developing an upper respiratory infection); (b) active tuberculosis; and (c) the presence of such disorders as hemophilia, aplastic anemia, purpura, or leukemia. *Potential hazards* associated with tonsillectomy and adenoidectomy include (a) failure to secure *obscure bleeding points;* (b) *airway obstruction* resulting from blood and secretions collecting in the airway during surgery (note: this can cause hypoxia, cardiac arrest, excessive bleeding); and (c) *aspiration.*

Because hemorrhage is a potential threat following T & A, the patient's hemostasis is carefully assessed preoperatively.

In addition to checking bleeding and clotting times, urinalysis and blood count are performed. Preoperatively atropine is always given to reduce mucous secretions if a general anesthesia is to be administered.

During surgery the patient is placed in the dorsal position if general anesthesia is to be given. If local anesthesia is used, the patient is in a sitting position. Adults are usually given a local anesthetic, and the patient is typically premedicated with a barbiturate, a narcotic, and atropine. General anesthesia is used for some adult T & A's. The most common operative method of removing the tonsils is by dissection and snare (Figure 92–2); however, some surgeons prefer the guillotine method. The main mass of adenoid tissue is removed with an adenotome or an adenoid curette. Remaining adenoid remnants are removed with a biting punch forceps.

During (and following) tonsillectomy, blood frequently passes into the stomach.

Postoperative Care. If local anesthesia was used, the patient is positioned with the head elevated 45 degrees for postoperative care. Following general anesthesia, to prevent aspiration position the patient with the face partially down and with a pillow under one shoulder, or have the patient lie prone with the head turned to one side. In these positions secretions are easily expelled from the mouth. The airway is left in place until the patient is able to handle his or her own secretions, i.e., is conscious enough to swallow. Have gauze wipes available to wipe the patient's nose and mouth and have a towel placed under the head. Keep the patient positioned well over onto the side with a towel and emesis basin under the mouth to catch secretions until the person is fully conscious. Then position the person with the head elevated 45 degrees.

During the first postoperative hour take the patient's pulse and blood pressure every 15 min-

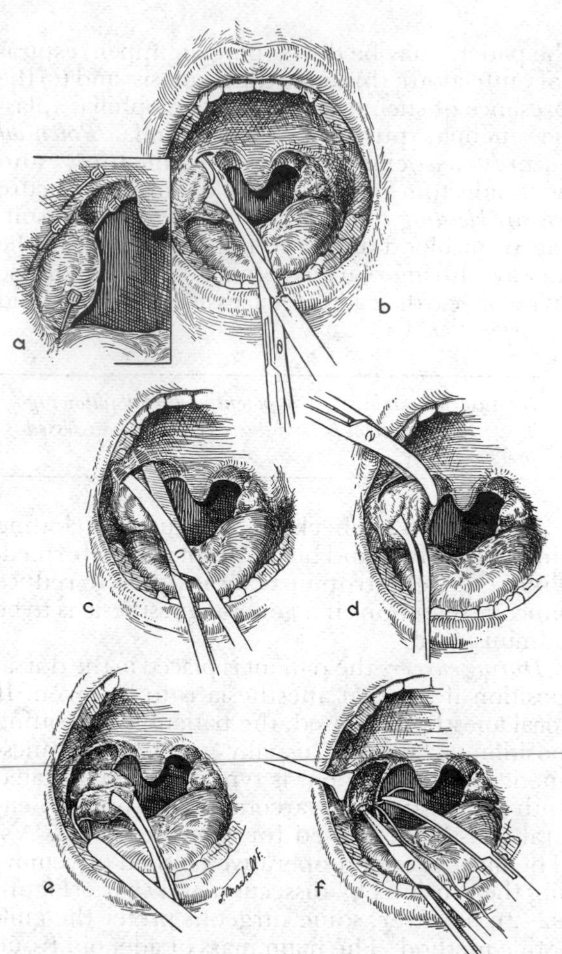

Figure 92–2. A method of dissection tonsillectomy. **A.** Points of infiltration for local anesthesia. **B.** Start of incision with tonsil knife at attachment of anterior pillar to the tonsil superiorly. **C.** Separation by scissor dissection of the superior pole of the tonsil. **D.** Continuation of dissection of tonsil from its attachment to pillars and bed of tonsillar fossa. **E.** Separation of the tonsil by snare at the lower pole, including the plica triangularis. **F.** Hemostasis. (From Adams, G. L., L. R. Boies, and M. M. Paparella: *Fundamentals of Otolaryngology*, 5th ed. Philadelphia: W. B. Saunders, Co., 1964.)

utes; then every half hour for several hours. Take the temperature rectally (as with any patient who has oral surgery). A slight temperature elevation is not unusual for a day or so postoperatively.

Instruct the patient not to try to clear the throat or cough, since these actions could precipitate bleeding. Also advise the patient to rest the throat by not talking excessively. Give analgesic medication as ordered and apply an ice collar around the throat. An ice collar may provide some comfort for the patient and is believed by some to minimize postoperative bleeding.

The nurse observes the patient for possible postoperative hemorrhage because emergency treatment may be indicated. It is not unusual for a patient to vomit a *small* amount of blood following adenotonsillectomy or to have a *small* amount of dark bloody drainage. However, hemorrhage may be indicated by the vomiting of *large* amounts of swallowed blood (brown in color), by the expectoration of bright red colored blood, or by large amounts of bloody drainage. A gradually increasing pulse rate, restlessness, a falling blood pressure, and pallor are other possible indications of hemorrhage. Notify the surgeon of these symptoms. Remember to save emesis specimens for the surgeon to inspect. Since external evidence of bleeding is not always present, inspect the throat periodically with a flashlight to look for blood trickling down the back of the throat; it is particularly important to do this if the patient is sleeping or is not fully conscious. Sometimes the surgeon can stop postoperative bleeding by simple procedures such as pressure or local applications of vasoconstrictors. If this fails, the patient is returned to surgery and reanesthetized, and vessels are sutured or cauterized as necessary.

Once full consciousness has returned and if there is no bleeding, the patient is allowed ice chips or liquids. Orange juice, grapefruit juice, and tomato juice are avoided because they cause burning sensations in the throat. Lukewarm water is less irritating than ice water to drink. Encourage the patient to take large swallows of fluid (rather than small swallows) because this causes less discomfort and also enables a greater fluid intake. The patient is *not* given a straw, since sucking can start bleeding, and also the careless or stuporous patient could injure the throat with a straw. Gradually the patient's diet progresses to include soft foods, e.g., custards, ice cream, mild-flavored cream soups, bland cereals, poached eggs. Hot liquids, spicy foods, and rough foods should be avoided for a week. If sutures were placed during tonsillectomy, a liquid or soft diet may be necessary until suture absorption has occurred, because swallowing is more painful with sutures in the throat.

Alkaline mouthwashes are offered to the patient. Not only are they refreshing, but also they help clear away viscous mucus.

Usually following T & A the patient is kept on bed rest for 24 hours and is discharged on the first postoperative day. However, some patients are discharged the evening of surgery. All patients are kept hospitalized for at least a few hours because of the potential danger of postoperative bleeding. If serious bleeding occurs, it usually happens a few hours following surgery. Thus this dangerous period is over before the patient is discharged.

Discharge, Instructions, and Self-Care. In preparation for discharge, the patient is told the doctor's orders and is given instructions for home care. (Sometimes written instructions are given to the patient and/or significant others.)

Instructions for control of pain are variable. Typically pain is not severe beyond the second postoperative day. *Prolonged* pain should be investigated, since it may indicate secondary complications. The discomfort experienced during swallowing can interfere with obtaining adequate food and fluid intake. It is thus important to provide adequate analgesia and appetizing, nonirritating food and liquids (e.g., jello, custard, cream of wheat, creamed potatoes). Orange and grapefruit juices and raw fruits and vegetables should be avoided for the first postoperative week. In addition to instructions concerning pain relief and diet, the patient is given recommendations for rest and follow-up appointments. Frequently following T & A the patient is advised to stay indoors for several days and to avoid strenuous exercise and sunbathing. Activities containdicated because of the risk of starting bleeding include sneezing, coughing, clearing the throat, and vigorous nose blowing. (The patient should avoid contact with other people who have respiratory infections.)

Not all bleeding problems following T & A occur *immediately* after surgery; *sometimes bleeding problems are delayed and do not occur until the fifth to tenth postoperative day.* Delayed bleeding results from the premature separation of the white "scab" that forms postoperatively over the areas from which the tonsils and adenoids were removed. Between 5 and 10 days following surgery, the membrane which has formed over the operative area begins to slough off. As this occurs, the throat is usually quite sore, and there is danger of possible hemorrhage. If the patient eats rough foods or if infection is present, the scab may come off; the surface vessels and small capillaries then begin to bleed.

Before discharge the patient is told that a very small percentage of patients have some bleeding after 5 to 6 days and that if this happens the best thing to do is to (a) remain calm, since the bleeding is usually only minor; (b) gently gargle the throat with ice water; (c) lie quietly down and gently spit the blood out; and (d) call the physician if the bleeding does not stop promptly. Although rarely dangerous, if a soft clot has formed, its removal by a physician is required. It takes about 3 weeks for the mucous membrane to heal completely.

Ear pain 2 to 3 days after a tonsillectomy is a common accompaniment of the surgery and does not necessarily indicate an ear infection. The patient (and/or significant others) should be warned to expect the discomfort and should report it to the doctor if it persists or is accompanied by an elevated temperature.

Blood swallowed during surgery may cause the patient's stool to be tarry for a day or so following adenotonsillectomy. This is expected, and the patient should be told about this. Occasionally a mild laxative is necessary. Increasing fluid intake helps relieve constipation and also the unpleasant mouth odor which follows oral surgery. Additionally, the fluid intake helps compensate for the slight temperature elevation which may occur for a few days.

ASPIRATED FOREIGN BODIES

Foreign bodies may be aspirated into the pharynx, larynx, or trachea. These objects may result in dyspnea or asphyxia (due to airway obstruction), and they may also cause serious tracheobronchial irritation if aspirated deeper into the tacheobronchial tree. Heimlich's maneuver is used to dislodge the foreign body (see p. 2151, Chapter 95). If the object is not coughed up after attempts at dislodgement, emergency laryngoscopy or tracheotomy is indicated.

In addition to severe dyspnea and other symptoms of respiratory distress, the presence of a foreign body may be indicated by such symptoms as hemoptysis, mucus expectoration, or a croupy or whistling cough. In the presence of acute respiratory distress, the examiner attempts to remove a foreign body lodged in the pharynx with a finger. Emergency tracheotomy is indicated if the obstruction is lower in the airway (see below). When time permits, an x-ray is taken to confirm the presence of a foreign object and to localize the object. While nonorganic objects may sometimes be tolerated in the tracheobronchial tree for years without causing marked symptoms, organic matter, e.g., peanuts, may rapidly swell or cause serious infection, e.g., pneumonia. Foreign bodies may be removed in some cases by the use of special instruments inserted through a bronchoscope or laryngoscope.

THROAT SPRAYS AND IRRIGATIONS

Anesthetics and antiseptics may be applied to the throat by *spraying*. Medications commonly prescribed for use as throat sprays may come prepackaged in plastic, squeezable bottles attached to a spray tip. To spray the larynx properly, the patient is given the following instructions: (a) be certain the spray tip used turns down at the tip so the medication will be directed down into the throat rather than merely at the back of the throat; (b) open the mouth and gently place the spray tip at the back of the throat, behind the tongue; and (c) spray the medication down into the throat as you deeply inhale once or twice. Greater force is necessary when using a throat spray than when instilling a nasal spray.

The resolution of acute or chronic throat inflammations is often speeded up by periodic "bathing" of the throat with warm or hot normal saline. Other solutions which may be used are

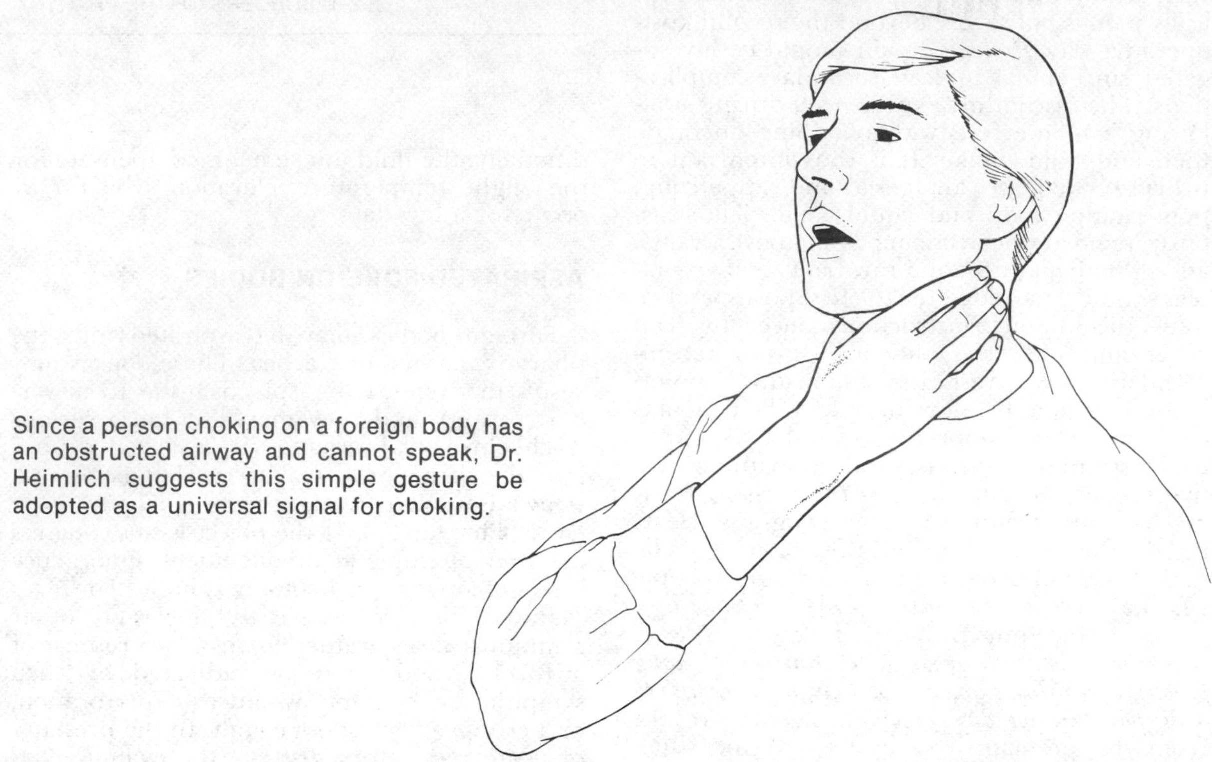
Since a person choking on a foreign body has an obstructed airway and cannot speak, Dr. Heimlich suggests this simple gesture be adopted as a universal signal for choking.

Figure 92–3. A universal signal for choking. (From Bartlett, P. C.: Aliens in the ENT. *Emergency Medicine,* 11:279, Feb. 1979, p. 282.)

mild antiseptics or sodium bicarbonate. The latter is especially effective when secretions are tenacious. "Bathing" of the throat may be accomplished by *throat irrigations* or *gargling.* Throat irrigations are usually more effective than gargling, since gargling does not reach all the parts of the throat. Also, gargling is more uncomfortable, since it produces tension and stretching of the inflamed, painful throat tissues. However, either process not only provides comfort to the patient but also cleanses the throat (loosens and removes secretions) and increases surface blood supply by causing vasodilation. The degree of heat applied is important. Solutions are used as hot as a patient can tolerate them, but never hotter than 120° F. (48.8° C.).

Throat irrigations may be ordered 2 to 3 times daily or as often as every 1 or 2 hours while the patient is awake, depending upon the condition of the patient's throat. Throat irrigation is accomplished by attaching a rubber tube (with a clamp) and a plastic or glass irrigating tip onto an irrigating can or hot-water bottle. Before use, inspect the tip to be certain it is not chipped or cracked. The container is filled with the prescribed irrigating solution at the desired temperature. The container is then hung above the patient's head. Recommendations for the height at which the can should be hung vary from 2 to 3 feet[21] above the patient's head to only slightly above the level of the patient's mouth. The patient leans over a washbasin or collecting basin so fluid will run back out of the mouth. The person then opens the mouth and inserts the nozzle without touching the base of the tongue or uvula, since this could cause gagging. Then, while holding the breath to prevent aspiration, the patient directs the solution so that all parts of the throat are irrigated. Periodically it is, of course, necessary to clamp the tubing to breathe and rest. Approximately 1500 to 2000 ml. of irrigating fluid are used.

TRACHEOTOMY; TRACHEOSTOMY CARE

The trachea may be intubated in two basic ways: (1) by passing a tube through the nose or mouth into the trachea, i.e., *endotracheal intubation;* or (2) by making a surgical incision into the trachea via the throat, i.e., *tracheotomy,* and then inserting a tube through that incision into the trachea. Clinical care of the patient with tracheal intubation is considered in detail because this is an important aspect of modern nursing practice.

Definition of Terms

A *tracheotomy* is an incision into the trachea through the second, third, or fourth tracheal ring. This surgical procedure is performed for such purposes as exploration, removal of a foreign body, removal of a local lesion (e.g., tumor), to obtain a biopsy specimen, or most

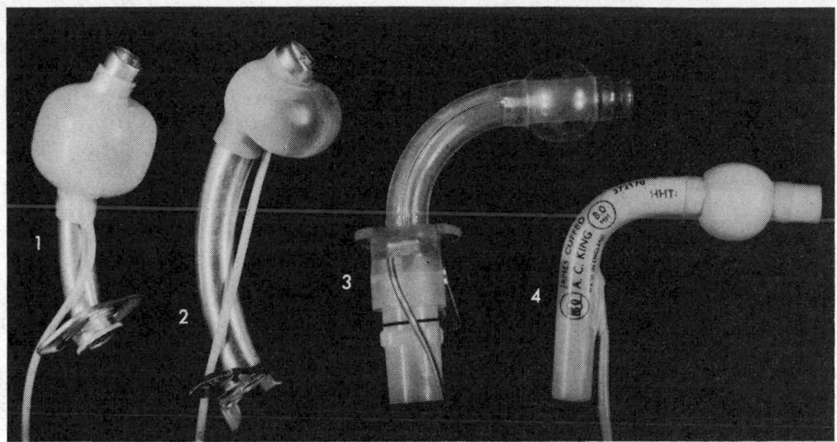

Figure 92–4. Tracheostomy tubes (from left to right): (1) The Hollinger tracheostomy tube with separately attached "Sof-Cuf" cuff. Note the relatively shallow curve of the tube and the evenly inflated (low-pressure) cuff; (2) The Jackson tracheostomy tube with separately attached cuff. Note the relatively sharp angle of the tube and the eccentrically inflated (high-pressure) cuff; (3) The Portex plastic tracheostomy tube with attached cuff which inflates evenly at relatively high pressure; and (4) The James tracheostomy tube with attached cuff which inflates evenly; this tube is occasionally used in short-necked patients. (From Sanderson, R. G. (Ed.): *The Cardiac Patient.* Philadelphia: W. B. Saunders Co., 1972.)

commonly to gain access to the airway for purposes of assisting oxygenation.

The opening which results from a tracheotomy is called a *"tracheostomy."* A tracheostomy may be a permanent or temporary opening. An indwelling tube (e.g., tracheostomy tube or laryngectomy tube) may be inserted through this opening to facilitate the removal of tracheobronchial secretions or to make the passage of air easier or both. Tracheostomies (a) facilitate prolonged artificial ventilation; (b) bypass serious upper respiratory obstructions (e.g., due to edema); (c) prevent aspiration of blood, secretions, or food into the lungs (e.g., when normal swallowing is impossible because of a reduced state of consciousness or muscular paralysis or in the presence of hemorrhage); and (d) provide easier access to the lower airways than is possible through the nose or mouth.

Tracheostomy Tubes

As Figures 92–4 and 92–5 demonstrate, a variety of tracheostomy tubes are available. Space does not permit detailed discussion of the techniques for using each of these tubes; consult specialized texts and equipment information for these details as necessary. Tracheostomy tubes may be made of various substances, e.g., disposable plastic, stainless steel, or sterling silver.

Tracheostomy tubes may consist of several separate pieces or only one piece. *Metal tubes* typically have three parts which are kept together as one set and are not interchangeable with other tube sets. These three parts are (1) an outer tube (also called "outer cannula"); (2) an inner tube ("inner cannula"); and (3) an olive-tipped "obturator." When tracheostomy tubes have three pieces, the *outer tube* remains held in place by a *ribbon* or *tie* which is passed through loops on either side of the tube's opening. (Tracheostomy neck ties or tapes are further discussed later in this section.)

The *obturator* is slipped into the outer tube before the tube is inserted into the trachea. The obturator's position in the outer tube is such that it extends beyond the tube's end and thus serves as a blunt, smooth guide while the tube is slipped

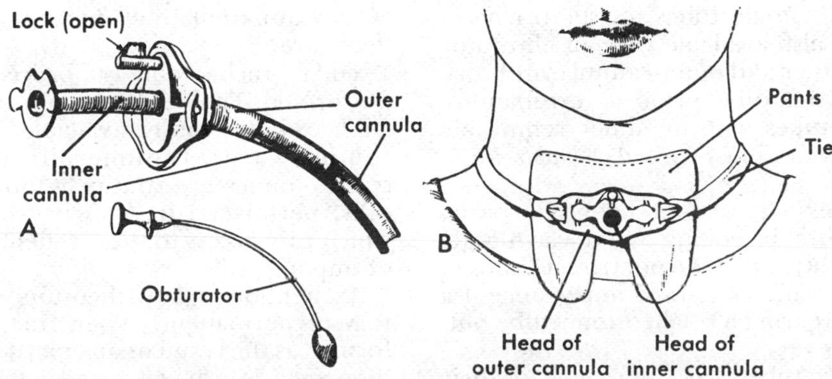

Figure 92–5. **A.** Parts of metal tracheostomy tube. **B.** Tracheostomy ties and gauze pants in place. (From Work, W., and M. F. W. Smith: *Postgraduate Medicine*, 34:479, Nov. 1963.)

into the trachea. Following insertion, the obturator is immediately removed, since it occludes the tube's lumen and thus prevents the exchange of air between the lungs and the atmosphere. *The obturator is kept at the patient's bedside in a place where it is easily seen in case the tube is expelled* and another sterile tube set is not available. In such a situation, the obturator is slipped into the expelled tube, and the tube may be immediately reinserted (see below). Because the obturator for a metal tracheostomy tube is part of a matched set, care is taken not to lose it or to separate it from the other pieces of the set. If one piece is lost, the entire set becomes useless.

The *inner tube* fits inside the outer tube and is removed periodically for cleaning. Upon initial insertion of the outer tube, the inner tube is placed as soon as the obturator is removed. After it is slipped inside the outer tube, the inner tube is held in place by a small flip *lock* (located on the top part of the outer tube's face plate). *The inner tube is left out of place only during the period in which it is being cleaned.* If left out longer, secretions begin to form into crusts and other debris collects inside the outer tube's lumen.

Silver tracheostomy tubes are carefully handled because silver is a soft metal which dents easily. Dents may cause trauma to the patient, cause a poor tracheal fit, or make it impossible for the various pieces of the matched set to fit together.

Tracheostomy tubes made of *synthetic materials* (e.g., nylon, plastic, polyethylene) are increasingly replacing the more traditional silver tubes. Some synthetic tubes consist of a *single tube* which has one or two balloons affixed to the outer surface of the end of the tube which lies in the trachea. Some metal tracheostomy tubes also have balloons. Metal and plastic tracheostomy tubes (and endotracheal tubes) which have balloons of this sort are referred to as "cuffed" tubes (see below).

In addition to single tubes, plastic tracheostomy tubes are also available with an obturator ("pilot tube"), inner and outer cannula, and cork (used to plug the tube prior to extubation). Tracheostomy tubes with an inner removable cannula are sometimes called *"double-wall" tracheostomy tubes.*

Synthetic tubes (a) have interchangeable parts; (b) can be sterilized by boiling or autoclaving; (c) are of light weight; and (d) do not frost if exposed to cold air. The latter fact is of importance if a patient will be wearing a tracheostomy tube out-of-doors.

Tracheostomy tubes vary not only in their composition and number of separate parts but also in their *shapes* and *sizes.* The size and type to be used is carefully determined before the tracheotomy procedure is started. A tracheostomy tube's *diameter* should be sufficiently smaller than the trachea that it lies comfortably within the trachea's lumen. It should be possible for air to pass between the trachea's wall and the outer wall of the tube. Jackson tracheostomy tubes are available in 14 different sizes (from No. 00 through No. 12). Silver tubes No. 6 and No. 7 are most commonly used for adults; No. 00 is used for premature infants.

In addition to the tracheostomy tube's diameter, *its length* and *curve* are also of importance. Tracheostomy tubes may be long (e.g., the Hollinger tube) or short (end tracheostomy) and may be angulated from 50 to 90 degrees. The most frequently used tracheostomy tubes are the shorter tubes with a 60-degree angle. Within the trachea the tube's length should be such that it prevents dislodging into the paratracheal areas as the patient turns the head or coughs; the tube's lower end should remain above the carina. The tracheostomy's curve should be such that, when in position, the inner opening of the tube points directly in line with the trachea and does not press against either the trachea's anterior or posterior walls. If the tube tilts against the posterior wall (or if the incision is made too low), injury and obstruction may result; if it tilts against the anterior wall, erosion of the innominate artery may occur. Frequently the position of the tube is checked by x-ray after insertion to prevent such complications.

Other criteria met to ensure a properly fitting tracheostomy tube are being certain that (a) the patient can breathe easily through the tube; (b) the tube's lumen is such that it can easily be suctioned with a catheter; and (c) the tube's faceplate does not cause pressure on the skin of the neck, yet is flush with the skin.

Indications for Tracheotomy

Medical history cannot definitely document when someone first had the courage and foresight to attempt to improve respiration by cutting through the neck into the trachea. However, the life-saving value of this procedure is readily apparent to all persons involved in patient care.

Today tracheotomy is a procedure commonly performed. Tracheotomy trays are kept at hospital bedsides, readily available, as part of the routine care of numerous patients. Also, tracheotomies are routinely, often prophylactically, performed in a variety of conditions in which easy access to the tracheobronchial tree is of importance.

As mentioned, a tracheostomy may be temporary or permanent. When tracheotomy is performed as the result of an emergency procedure, the stoma is usually closed later when normal respiration has been restored. Under certain circumstances, however, usually as the result of trauma or surgery, the stoma must remain open permanently to permit respiration to take place (see section on permanent tracheostomy below).

Because tracheotomy was once feared and indicated a serious prognosis, it is important that patients who are going to have tracheotomies performed (and their significant others) be told that the procedure will be of benefit and that it does not necessarily indicate worsening of physical condition. If the patient is unconscious and cannot be given such an explanation before the procedure, explanation of the tracheostomy should be given as the person regains consciousness.

> *Apnea, respiratory obstruction, circulatory arrest, and exsanguinating hemorrhage are all medical emergencies which may require tracheotomy as part of their treatments.*

Patients with any of the above conditions are *immediately* observed for indications of the possible need for tracheotomy. The patient's neck, thorax, and upper abdomen are uncovered and observed for retraction of the soft spots surrounding the thoracic cage. Such retraction serves as an index of the degree to which intrapleural pressure must be reduced in order to move air through an obstructed lumen. Simultaneously the patient's pulse is taken and is assessed both qualitatively and quantitatively. The patient's facial expression is rapidly scanned for evidence of fatigue, anxiety, and apprehension. If it is determined that tracheotomy is not indicated, appropriate therapy is instituted, and the nurse is frequently left to continue assessment of the patient's ability to maintain ventilation satisfactorily. The nurse's vigilance must be constant during this period, because the condition may worsen so rapidly that the patient is unable to summon help.

Major indications of respiratory insufficiency include apprehension, restlessness, agitation, confusion, inability to sleep, increasing exhaustion, motor dysfunction, and a rising pulse or respiratory rate. Diaphoresis, headache, and flapping tremor may also occur. Even more serious symptoms of respiratory obstruction are chest wall retractions, stridor, and increasing tachycardia accompanied by a decreasing rate of respirations. Another late, ominous symptom is cyanosis due to impaired oxygenation of the blood. The physician is promptly notified if any of these symptoms begin to appear.

The nurse's complete assessments and reports are highly important. Nurses need to be skilled observers and summon the physician at the appropriate time. The trachea is intubated when doubt exists about the necessity for the procedure, rather than waiting until it is obvious that the procedure is unquestionably necessary.

In all situations in which tracheotomy may be indicated, attempts are made to perform the procedure before conditions become desperate. For example, the physician does not wait until cyanosis develops before performing a tracheotomy. In the presence of arterial unsaturation, the patient may die before tracheotomy can be performed. Proctor and Safar warn that ". . . cyanosis is a notoriously unreliable sign. Its apparent absence should never be counted as reliable evidence of adequate ventilation."[85] Likewise, in patients with upper airway obstruction, the decision to perform the tracheotomy is not postponed until the patient displays a lower arterial pO_2 or elevated pCO_2. It may be too late once such ventilatory failure has started. *Performance of an early tracheotomy is often the key to successful respiratory therapy.* When a tracheotomy is performed on this basis, the patient is ensured of greater comfort and safety.

Types of patients who may benefit from tracheotomy include the following:

▶ *Patients requiring prophylactic tracheotomy.* As discussed, instead of waiting for patients to develop acute respiratory difficulties before performing tracheotomy, it is desirable to carry out this procedure prophylactically in various situations. For example, prophylactic tracheotomy is indicated preoperatively when a patient's ventilatory capacity is severely reduced and postoperatively following some intrathoracic surgeries (e.g., cardiopulmonary procedures) and some neurosurgical procedures (e.g., those which could result in unconsciousness, impaired swallowing, or impaired respiration). Additionally, prophylactic tracheotomy is indicated in some patients with severe respiratory disease, critical illnesses (of various kinds), and radical neck surgery, and in patients receiving irradiation therapy for laryngeal tumors encroaching on the airway. Most permanent stomas would of course be performed on a prophylactic, nonemergency basis.

▶ *Apneic patients.* Artificial respiration is indicated (see Unit XII). If cardiac arrest is also present, tracheotomy is deferred until circulation is restored. In the interim, endotracheal intubation is employed. Tracheotomy is hazardous during external cardiac compression.

▶ *Unconscious patients with inadequate ventilation.* Attempts are rapidly made to determine the cause of the inadequate ventilation, e.g., obstruction of the airway, respiratory depression.

▶ *Patients in respiratory failure* who apparently will require respiratory assistance for periods longer than 1 to 2 days.

▶ *Patients with head, neck, or chest injuries.* Following throat trauma, airway obstruction may result from hemorrhage, unconsciousness, edema, muscular paralysis, or submucosal hematoma. Fracture of the larynx or trachea produces subcutaneous emphysema and may cause sudden airway obstruction. Following crushing chest injuries (resulting in "flail chest," i.e., an unstable chest wall), tracheotomy enables easier aspiration of blood and secretions and makes it possible to "splint" the chest from inside by using intermittent positive pressure ventilation. Other benefits are reduction of paradoxical movement and prevention of exhaustion from the effort of breathing in the presence of pain and an impaired respiratory system. (Chest injuries are discussed in Unit XVI.)

▶ *Patients with fulminating infections of the mouth, pharynx, or throat,* e.g., diphtheria, Ludwig's angina.

▶ *Conscious patients with upper airway obstruction.* In these patients tracheotomy is performed if there is evidence of severe obstruction or of the patient tiring in attempts to overcome the obstruction to breathe. Emergency tracheotomy may be necessary if a foreign body is present in the hypopharynx or larynx.

▶ *Patients with accumulations of secretions in the lower tracheobronchial tree which could cause hypoxia or atelectasis or both.* Tracheotomy is commonly indicated when a patient cannot comfortably clear tracheobronchial secretions from the lower airways.

▶ *Patients with severe burns, especially around the head and face.* Laryngeal edema and pulmonary edema may develop, seriously jeopardizing patency of the airway. Tracheotomy helps overcome upper airway obstruction; it also helps assist ventilation and control secretions.

▶ *Patients who have had thyroidectomy or radical neck resection* may hemorrhage into the soft tissues of the neck. Pressure is then exerted on the trachea by the blood in the soft tissues. Tracheotomy may be indicated to prevent or relieve upper airway obstruction.

▶ *Patients with neurologic disorders* which impair respiratory muscles or the act of swallowing, e.g., head injuries, drug overdose, bulbar paralysis, cerebrovascular accidents. Also, patients with prolonged episodes of convulsive seizures.

▶ *Patients with severe pulmonary edema* who have poor gas transport across the alveolar capillary membrane.

▶ *Patients with severe emphysema* for whom it is desirable to reduce dead space because of impaired tidal volume.

▶ *Weak, feeble patients* for whom it is desirable to reduce the work of breathing. Tracheostomy reduces the work of breathing by reducing the volume of the anatomical dead space air by as much as 50 per cent.

▶ *Postoperative patients with laryngeal edema due to prolonged intubation.* This emergency frequently occurs during recovery from anesthesia or following endotracheal extubation, and may cause airway obstruction. Before tracheotomy is resorted to, attempts may be made to correct the situation by using epinephrine, antihistamines, steroids, and high-humidity oxygen.

Performing Tracheotomy

A tracheotomy may be performed either as an emergency or as an elective surgical procedure. In emergency situations the incision may be made at the scene of an accident (if necessary with such crude instruments as a penknife) or at the patient's bedside (with an emergency tracheotomy set). The procedure for performing tracheotomy is discussed in detail, since nurses often assist with this procedure on wards and in emergency rooms as well as in surgery. In the hospital if an emergency tracheotomy is anticipated, a *basic emergency tracheotomy tray* is kept available at the patient's bedside. Usually these trays are preassembled and kept sterilized for immediate use. Items on the tray vary from hospital to hospital; basic items include the following: scalpel, dissecting scissors, hemostat, suture material, suction tip, syringes, needles, curved blunt bistoury (long, narrow surgical knife), two retractors, tracheal dilator, gauze sponges, sterile gloves, and tracheostomy tubes. Necessary antiseptic solutions and local anesthetics are also required.

Tracheotomies are less frequently employed as emergency measures now than formerly, owing to increasing use of emergency endotracheal intubation. Tracheotomy results are far superior when the procedure is performed electively in an operating room. In this setting, asepsis is more complete, and a general anesthetic may be administered if advisable. The procedure described in this section is that of a planned, orderly, elective tracheotomy.

Generally an orotracheal tube is passed before tracheotomy is performed. Passage of such a tube is desirable for the following reasons: (a) normal pulmonary ventilation may be rapidly restored; (b) time is obtained to perform tracheotomy more safely as an orderly surgical procedure; (c) after an adequate airway is established, a general anesthetic may be given (if indicated) to perform the tracheotomy; and (d) it is usually possible to eliminate the most common complications of tracheotomy, i.e., pneumothorax and mediastinal emphysema. In some cases orotracheal intubation may be impossible prior to tracheotomy. Some authorities feel that orotracheal intubation is contraindicated prior to tracheotomy because stimulation of the vagus nerves may result in the "vasovagal reflex," causing cardiac arrest.

In preparation for tracheotomy, all necessary equipment is selected and made ready for use. A tracheostomy tube of the appropriate size and type is selected. If a cuffed tube is to be used, the cuff is checked for patency and uniformity of expansion when inflated. Adaptors are available for artificial ventilation, should it become necessary. During the procedure respiration is assisted as indicated (by mask or tracheal tube).

The patient is positioned on the back with neck extended so the trachea becomes prominent. To accomplish this, a pillow or blanket roll is placed under the patient's shoulders. Following appropriate skin preparation and draping, a local or general anesthetic is administered and a skin incision is made. Either a horizontal or a vertical incision may be used. Generally, for a temporary tracheostomy a horizontal incision will ultimately yield the less conspicuous scar.

Dissection is carried out until the thyroid isthmus is identified. The isthmus is surgically divided over the trachea and is sutured back from the midline. Next the first tracheal ring is identified, and the trachea is incised through the second and third rings. A small window may be cut in the trachea. If an endotracheal tube is in place during the procedure, it is partially withdrawn before the trachea is entered to prevent accidental cutting of the tube. (The endotracheal tube is not completely removed until the tracheostomy tube is properly functioning.) Before the tracheostomy tube is inserted into the tracheotomy, the trachea is thoroughly aspirated to remove secretions and blood. Once properly positioned, the tube is secured in place with a tie around the neck.

Some surgeons place two loose black silk sutures through the lateral tracheal edges and tape these sutures to the chest skin before completing the procedure; others suture a small flap of the tracheal edge to the neck skin. These actions may be taken so the trachea can easily be identified again if the tracheostomy tube becomes dislodged during the first few postoperative days (before an adequate tract has formed). Without such a flap or sutures, it may be difficult to find the trachea to replace the tube, because the trachea may become submerged as the various incised layers close over it. After a few days the path into the trachea becomes more clearly established and the tracheostomy tube can be more easily replaced. The sutures make it possible to pull the trachea up to the skin incision and thus ensure an airway until the tracheostomy tube can be properly reinserted.

If the tracheotomy is to be permanent, the margins of the entire tracheal opening are sutured to the skin so a permanent stoma will form. This facilitates replacing tubes. Eventually, once healing occurs, a tube may not be necessary to keep the stoma open.

Upon completion of tracheotomy, the incision is sealed with a plastic spray, or a sterile, dry dressing is placed over the incision around the tracheostomy tube to absorb secretions and protect the incision.

Recently a new emergency tracheostomy procedure has been developed which is performed *percutaneously* by inserting a small catheter into the trachea. The trachea is first punctured with a small needle, and then a special device is used to insert the catheter into the hole used to localize the trachea. The procedure can be rapidly performed. For details refer to Jacobs[47] and Toy and Weinstein.[116]

Complications of Tracheotomy

Possible complications to be aware of while giving post-tracheotomy care include subcutaneous emphysema, pneumothorax, or mediastinal emphysema (see Unit XVI); obstruction of the tracheostomy tube; respiratory insufficiency; displacement of the tube from its position in the trachea's lumen; hemorrhage; pulmonary infection; atelectasis; and tracheoesophageal fistula. These complications may develop slowly or suddenly. Their *early detection* requires a nurse's vigilance. The nurse should be familiar with possible complications, systematically observe for their possible development, and institute appropriate early action if complications develop.

Respiratory insufficiency may develop in the tracheotomized patient for various reasons, one of which is tracheobronchial obstruction occurring at a level lower than that of the tracheostomy tube. Evidence of such respiratory insufficiency includes unequal respiratory movements on the two sides of the chest; marked respiratory effort; and retraction of all the soft spots surrounding the thoracic cage, e.g., supraclavicular, intercostal, and substernal retraction.

The airway may be obstructed (completely or partially) by such factors as external pressure, foreign bodies, swelling (edema) of the mucous membrane lining the tracheobronchial tree, or excessive secretions occluding respiratory lumina. A tracheostomy tube may be obstructed by accumulations of encrustations or by thick, dry secretions or by both.

If suctioning does not relieve obstruction of the tube, immediately call for the physician. In some cases the patient's life may be saved by removing the obstructed tube and holding the patient's trachea open with a tracheal dilator and hook.

Ask the attending physician ahead of time whether you have permission to remove the entire tracheostomy tube if the patient becomes obstructed and suctioning the tube does not relieve the obstruction. Make it clear that you will not do this if a physician is immediately available.

Accidental expulsion of a single cannula tracheostomy tube or the outer cannula of a double-walled tube occasionally occurs. When this happens, stay at the bedside and hold the tracheal incision open with a dilator (or hemostat) until help arrives and another tube is properly reinserted. A Trousseau tracheal dilator (or hemostat) and a tracheal hook are kept at the bedside of a tracheostomized patient at all times in case of this emergency (Figure 92–6). The nurse remembers during this emergency to reassure the patient and to act calmly.

Never try to forcefully push a "blown-out" tracheostomy tube back into place. Frantic attempts to do so may have tragic results due to compression of the trachea and misplacement of the tube. The tube may accidentally be pushed through the incision into soft tissues of the neck or mediastinum rather than into the trachea. Asphyxia may result because the trachea is compressed and any air being forced into the tracheostomy tube (e.g., by

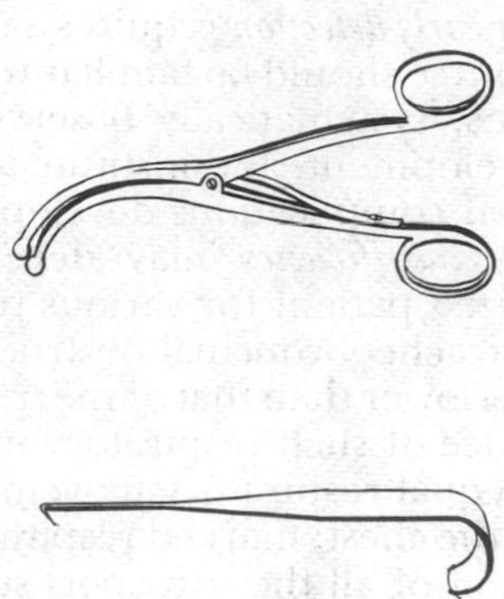

Figure 92–6. Tracheal dilator and hook. (From Sutton, A. L.: *Bedside Nursing Techniques in Medicine and Surgery*, 2nd ed. Philadelphia: W. B. Saunders Co., 1969.)

controlled ventilation) is forced into the soft tissue space. Attempts at reinsertion of a tracheostomy tube should be made only by persons qualified to do so and then only with adequate light, adequate retraction, and a tracheal hook and Trousseau dilator.

Accidental expulsion of the tube is rare, but it can happen as a result of neck ties not being properly secured or as a result of violent coughing. Caution is necessary when changing ties on a tracheostomy tube while the tube is in place to prevent accidental expulsion of the tube if the patient should suddenly cough or turn the head. As the wound heals, the possibility decreases of being unable to reinsert the tube easily if it is dislodged. Expulsion of the tube in infants carries a very high mortality because it is extremely difficult to replace a tracheostomy in such a tiny airway. The risk from expulsion is also increased in patients with short, fat necks, again because tube replacement becomes very difficult.

Inflammation and *infection* are other possible complications of tracheostomy. *Wound infection* can easily occur because of contact with tracheobronchial secretions. The wound is inspected frequently for indications of infection, and good preventative technique is used whenever tracheostomy care is given. The incision is kept as clean and dry as possible. *Tracheal perichondritis* may occur because some degree of local infection is usually present. "Tracheal perichondritis" refers to inflammation of the white, fibrous membrane (i.e., perichondrium) which covers the surface of tracheal cartilage. This inflammation may also involve the walls of such major blood vessels as the innominate and carotid arteries. Vessel erosion may result in exsanguinating hemorrhage.

Intubation (endotracheal or tracheostomy) causes reduction in a patient's ability to build up the intrapulmonary pressure necessary for an effective, expulsive cough. This *inability to cough up secretions* predisposes to *pulmonary infection* and *atelectasis.* A chest x-ray may be taken daily for several days following tracheostomy. For other measures for the detection of pulmonary complications, see Unit XVI.

Following tracheotomy *hemorrhage* may become manifest by bleeding around the tube at the incision site, by frank blood or bright blood-tinged tracheobronchial secretions, or by both. Other indications of hemorrhage are a rapid pulse rate and increasing restlessness. (Remember the latter two symptoms are also indicative of possible hypoxia.) While it is not unusual for tracheostomy secretions to have some blood mixed with them immediately following tracheotomy, it is abnormal for frank blood to appear or for secretions tinged with bright blood to persist longer than 6 to 8 hours postoperatively. Notify the physician if these abnormal findings occur. Massive hemorrhage from the innominate artery can result from erosion of the trachea's anterior wall by a malpositioned tracheostomy cannula (Figure 92–7).

Sometimes a tracheotomized patient develops a *tracheoesophageal fistula* caused by erosion

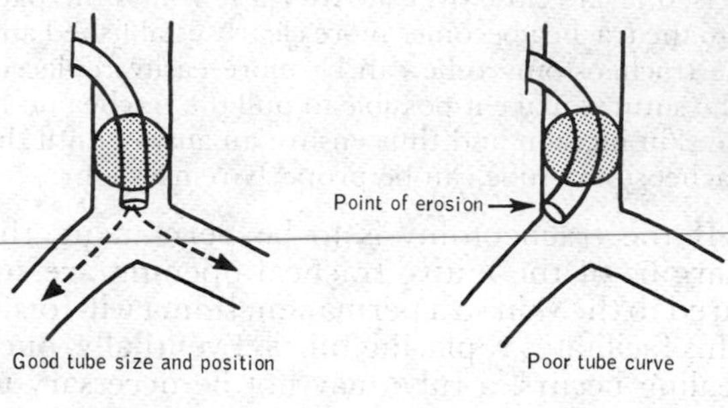

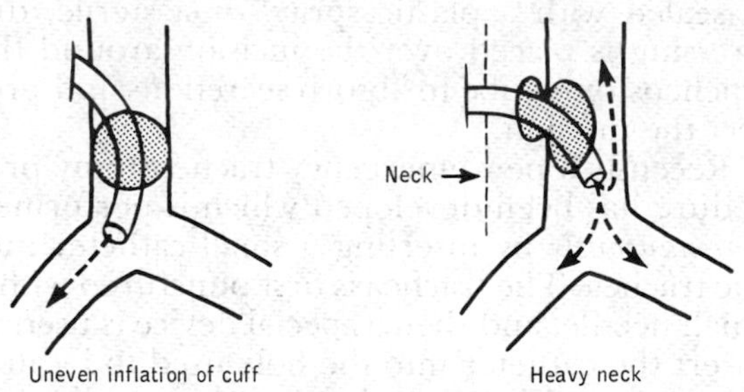

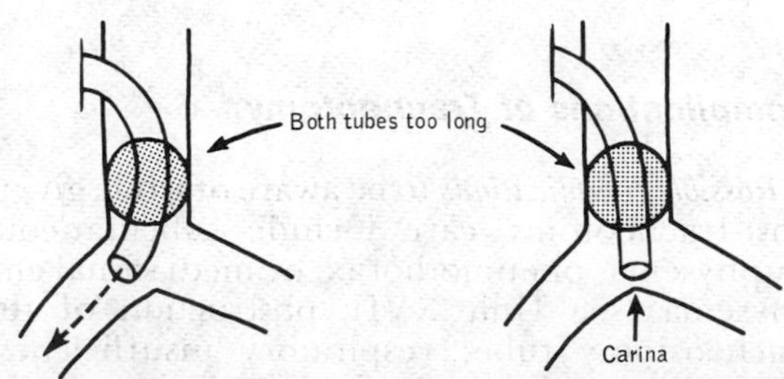

Figure 92–7. Tracheostomy tube positions and factors affecting them. (From Murphy, E. R.: Intensive nursing care in a respiratory unit. *Nursing Clinics of North America* 3:433, 1968.)

through the trachea's posterior wall. Important symptoms of the possible presence of a fistula of this nature include coughing or choking when eating or drinking, and aspiration of or leakage of food or liquids from the tracheostomy. Report these symptoms immediately.

The complications of tracheoesophageal fistula and hemorrhage may result from (a) improper angulation of the tube; (b) improper cannula length; (c) improper fixation of the tube; and (d) an incorrect tracheostomy site (see Fig. 92–7).

In addition to the possible development of the previously discussed complications, tracheostomy has certain inherent *disadvantages.* These include (a) loss of the cough reflex; (b) reduction or loss of the ability to speak normally; and (c) loss of the upper air passages' normal functions of warming, filtering, and humidifying inspired air. Loss of the latter three functions means that (a) microorganisms and foreign particles, e.g., dust, lint, may be directly inspired into the lungs; and (b) mucosa in the lower tract becomes irritated and dry, and tracheobronchial secretions become dry, tenacious, and difficult to raise (owing to normal lack of warming and humidification of inspired air).

Obviously, nursing care must be directed at minimizing the effects of loss of the normal functions described above. Part of the nursing care of the tracheostomized patient therefore includes:

- ▶ Recognition that the cough reflex cannot be relied upon to protect the tracheobronchial tree or to move secretions within that system
- ▶ Provision for communication and instruction of the patient in communicating
- ▶ Protection of the artificial tracheal opening to prevent introduction of microorganisms or foreign particles
- ▶ Ensuring humidification of inspired air.

These and other aspects of clinical care are discussed more completely in the following section.

Clinical Care of the Tracheostomized Patient

Important factors in the clinical care of any tracheostomized patient include those listed below. Some of these aspects of clinical care are discussed in detail in following sections.

▶ *Maintain an open airway.* Suction and clean the tube as indicated. Prevent aspiration, e.g., of water, solutions, and so forth, through the tracheostomy. Keep materials which may occlude the tracheostomy tube away from the opening (e.g., clothing, bed sheets).

▶ *Observe the patient carefully for indications of respiratory difficulty,* e.g., alterations in respiratory rate, noisy respirations, restlessness, pallor, cyanosis, intercostal and substernal retraction, labored respirations.

▶ *Practice asepsis.* Fatal infection may be introduced directly into the tracheobronchial tree unless asepsis is maintained by *all* persons caring for the patient's tracheostomy.

▶ *Observe for complications of tracheostomy and take appropriate action should they develop.*

▶ *Ensure maximal humidification of inspired air and appropriately warm inspired air.*

▶ *Provide adequate hydration to help liquefy pulmonary secretions.* At least 3000 ml. of fluid intake is typically desirable daily. Intravenous fluids are ordered if adequate oral intake is not possible.

▶ *Maintain fluid-electrolyte balance.* Keep an accurate intake-output record and periodically evaluate the record.

▶ *Be gentle.* The tracheal mucosa can easily be traumatized, e.g., during suctioning. Also, because of its sensitivity, procedures involving the trachea may be quite uncomfortable for the patient, e.g., movement of the tube is extremely uncomfortable.

▶ *Keep appropriate equipment at the bedside.*

▶ *Prevent pressure trauma to the tracheobronchial tree.* If a cuffed tube is being used, see that the cuff is deflated as ordered to relieve pressure periodically on the trachea's wall.

▶ *Periodically inspect the tracheostomy for indications of trauma or infection.*

▶ *Ensure use of a fresh tracheostomy tube as needed.* Clean the inner cannula of mucus and encrustations as indicated. Assist with outer tube changes as scheduled or change the tube yourself *if* you are qualified to do so and you have the physician's permission.

▶ *Change dressing and tracheostomy ties as necessary.*

▶ *Provide appropriate skin care.* Keep skin clean and dry.

▶ *Provide frequent mouth care,* to minimize possible infection and to relieve halitosis. Set up an oral hygiene tray at the bedside and schedule mouth care as a treatment to be performed at definite times. Drinking large amounts of water is also important for oral hygiene.

▶ *Provide adequate nourishment.*

▶ *Administer medications as ordered.* Tracheostomy usually does not cause acute pain. Medications which depress the respiratory center, e.g., narcotics and sedatives, are usually avoided or given very cautiously if indicated. Mild tranquilizers or mild sedatives may initially be ordered if the patient is quite apprehensive.

▶ *Provide appropriate education for the patient and significant others,* preoperatively and predischarge. If the patient is to be discharged with a tracheostomy tube in place, it is vital that both the patient and significant others know how to care for it.

▶ *Alleviate the patient's apprehension.* This may be accomplished in such ways as being readily available; closely observing the patient; providing care in a calm yet efficient manner; talking about what you are doing and how the patient can help; keeping the patient's signal bell within reach; helping the patient communicate.

It is very important that you try to *anticipate* the needs of the tracheostomized patient, who is frequently under great stress and is attempting to adjust to a highly dependent situation. The patient should not be additionally subjected to the frustration of having to try to communicate obvious needs.

Bedside Tracheostomy Equipment. Equipment kept available in the room of a patient with a tracheostomy includes suction equipment; oral hygiene tray; respirator; self-inflating bag (Ambu bag); humidification equipment; extra sterile tracheotomy tray (complete with a sterile tracheostomy tube of proper size to replace the tube being used if necessary); sterile obturator of tube currently in use; sterile forceps, tracheal hook, and Trousseau tracheal dilator; sterile gauze squares appropriate for use on tracheostomy; sterile scissors; tracheostomy ties; appropriate solutions (clearly labeled) for cleansing the tube and for cleansing around the incision; roller gauze; small tube brush and pipe cleaners for cleansing the inner cannula; syringe and hemostat for inflating tube of cuffed tubes.

Suctioning Through a Tracheal Stoma. Always remember that during suctioning the patient is apneic since you are also suctioning the air out of the patient's lungs. As a test hold your own breath while suctioning the patient; when you run out of oxygen, so has the patient! Generally, suctioning of a tracheostomy tube is performed only when secretions are audible, not just "routinely." It is, of course, desirable if the patient can cough and move bronchopulmonary secretions up into the trachea so the secretions either may be expelled from the tube by the force of the cough or can be removed by only superficial suctioning. Postural drainage with clapping (see Unit XVI) is useful to help move secretions into the trachea so they can easily be removed by suction. These techniques of respiratory physical therapy can be used on patients being artificially ventilated, as well as on those with spontaneous respirations. Some positions of postural drainage are contraindicated in intubated patients, e.g., extreme head-low positions are contraindicated with tracheostomy.

An effective cough may be difficult or impossible with a tracheal stoma, because endotracheal pressure cannot be elevated by forcing expiration against a closed glottis. The nurse's encouragement to cough is often needed by the patient, since coughing requires energy which may be difficult for the patient to expend. Tracheostomized patients who are debilitated or have copious secretions often require suctioning, since they often are unable to clear their tracheobronchial trees of secretions without assistance. During the first 24 to 48 postoperative hours following tracheostomy, it may be necessary to suction a patient as often as every 15 to 30 minutes. Frequently, strong, cooperative tracheostomized patients can cough up their own secretions if they take a deep breath and momentarily occlude the tracheostomy tube opening. This maneuver substitutes for the "glottal stop" normally used to increase intrathoracic pressure and thus move secretions up in the tracheobronchial tree. Some tracheostomized patients can be taught to suction their own mouths to remove oropharyngeal secretions. Self-care permits patients to be more independent and also enables them to keep themselves more comfortable than they might be when others attempt to anticipate their need for suctioning.

Various items are recommended to be kept at the bedside for purposes of suctioning. It is desirable to *set up a suction tray* and to change the items on this tray every 8 hours to prevent possible usage of contaminated equipment. Some *sterile* items which may be kept on the suction tray are suction catheters, towels, forceps, gloves, gauze squares, disposable cups, and appropriate solutions. Paper bags or a covered (foot pedal) waste can should be conveniently placed for disposal of used disposable equipment. The suction tube is kept attached to the wall suction outlet or suction machine in readiness for immediate use, and a Y-connector is attached to the suction catheter so the catheter can be inserted without applying suction during insertion.

It is advisable to use disposable sterile catheters and gloves for tracheal suctioning to minimize possible contamination of equipment.

The above are discarded after each suctioning. The ideal suction catheter is a disposable one with a thumb valve. If it is not possible to use disposable catheters, a catheter may be kept submerged in a basin of solution (e.g., 70 per cent alcohol, which is rinsed off the catheter with sterile normal saline or sterile water before use); this catheter is discarded when the tracheal care tray is changed. Some sources recommend changing the tray and its contents (for a fresh supply of sterile equipment and solutions) every 4 hours when a catheter is kept stored in solution and is repeatedly used. Let us emphasize that the repeated use of a single catheter stored in a "sterile" solution is a procedure to be used *only* if it is *absolutely* impossible to use disposable catheters. Catheter storage solutions left at the bedside and believed to be "sterile" may actually introduce infection. Adaptors and introducers may be kept in an antiseptic noncorrosive solution, e.g., NP solution (neomycin, 1 mg./ml., plus polymyxin B, 0.1 mg./ml.).

Suction catheters for tracheostomies should (a) be smooth; (b) have a cone-shaped, noncollapsible proximal end for the adaptor; (c) have an opening at the tip and possibly a smaller opening 1 to 2 cm. above the tip on the side; and (d) have a slight curve at the tip. Unless the catheter is slightly curved, it has a tendency to pass into the right main bronchus. It is best for catheters of several sizes to be kept on the suctioning tray. The catheter size should be much smaller than the diameter of the tracheostomy tube, so that it passes easily into the lumen of the tube without completely obstructing it. For adults, a No. 14 or No. 16 (Fr.) whistle tip catheter is frequently used.

If the patient has tenacious sputum, which is difficult to remove, the physician may order a few milliliters of sterile normal saline or sterile water to be inserted into the tube prior to suctioning. Sterile normal saline instilled into the trachea helps loosen secretions and stimulate coughing. This procedure should be used, however, only when indicated, since anything entering the tracheal tree is a potential source of infection. The normal saline may be obtained from a 30-ml. bottle or a 150-ml. IV bottle, depending upon how much may be required over an 8-hour period. Be certain to discard the bottle of solution at the end of each shift and use careful sterile technique when withdrawing solution from the bottle. Make every attempt to keep the solution sterile. Always remove the needle from the syringe before instilling the solution into the tube in the trachea. A needle not only is sharp but also may come loose and fall into the trachea.

It is important that the right and left mainstem bronchi each be suctioned separately. Position the patient with the head turned to the appropriate side to reach the desired bronchus; i.e., turn the head to the right to suction the left mainstem bronchus, vice versa for the right bronchus.

The suction procedure is essentially as follows:

▶ *Auscultate the chest* before and after suctioning to evaluate effectiveness.

▶ *Wash hands* and use sterile gloves or use a "no-touch" technique (i.e., with sterile forceps). Usually the catheter can be handled more easily with a gloved hand than with sterile forceps when suctioning.

▶ Place a sterile towel across the patient's chest, just below the tracheostomy tube.

▶ Clean the skin around the tube and the adaptors with a recommended antiseptic, noncorrosive solution, e.g., NP solution.

▶ Select catheter, attach it to the Y-connector (if one is necessary), lubricate the catheter with sterile normal saline in a disposable cup, and gently insert it into the tracheostomy tube. After it is inserted 6 to 8 inches, the obstruction created by the tracheal bifurcation (carina) may be felt. If deep suctioning is indicated, insert the tube as far as it can easily be inserted into one mainstem bronchus. Do not apply suction during insertion, i.e., keep the Y-vent open. Pull the catheter back slightly (1 to 2 cm.) to avoid completely blocking the bronchial lumen. Slowly withdraw the catheter while rotating or twirling it and intermittently apply suction by putting the thumb off and on the vent opening. Suctioning should generally not be continued for longer than 5 seconds at one time to prevent hypoxia and other complications. If necessary, suction again after oxygenating the patient. *Note:* successive reinsertions with the same catheter during one suctioning period are possible only if you have not contaminated the catheter. If in doubt, take another sterile catheter. *The tracheostomized patient is highly susceptible to infection; do not risk this complication.*

▶ After suctioning, discard the cup of saline rinsing solution as well as catheter and gloves. Do not leave a "sterile" bowl of normal saline at the bedside for repeated use to rinse or lubricate catheters. While rinsing the catheter to clear the tubing of secretions, note the amount and character of secretions aspirated.

▶ *Wash hands upon completion of procedure.*

If the suction catheter seems to be pulling or attaching to the tracheal wall when you are applying suction, immediately release the suction (i.e., open the vent) so you do not traumatize the tracheal wall. Begin to remove the catheter when it stimulates forceful coughing. If the catheter is not removed, the effects of the coughing are negated (since the tube obstructs the trachea or bronchus). Also, the patient must exert extra effort to create enough pressure to cough around the catheter. By suctioning as you remove the catheter, you will suction out some of the secretions being moved upward in the respiratory tree by the cough. Once the suction catheter is removed, be prepared to wipe away secretions which are coughed out of the tracheostomy tube opening. Plain gauze squares may be used to gently wipe away the expelled secretions. Be careful that threads in the gauze do not catch and pull on the tube's protruding pieces. *Never use facial tissues to wipe secretions away from the tube's orifice* because they contain lint which may be aspirated. Some cellulose tissues (e.g., Chix) may be used if they contain no lint. Mucus which is only partially expelled from the tube should be quickly wiped away before it can be drawn back into the trachea with the patient's next inspiration. Remember when the patient is coughing to keep your face away from the tube's opening as much as possible because of possible contagion.

Secretions may be ejected from the tracheal opening not only by coughing stimulated by suctioning but also during forceful expirations. Additionally, some patients are able to cough up secretions through the tracheostomy tube by themselves, i.e., they do not require tracheal stimulation. If a patient has copious secretions, place a face-towel bib under the tracheostomy tube to protect the patient's gown and bed linens. Teach the patient to hold either side of the tracheostomy tube during vigorous coughing to prevent possible accidental displacement or expulsion of the tube. If a patient cannot stabilize the tube, a nurse should do this.

In addition to tracheal suction, nasopharyngeal suction is important in patients with tracheal stomas. *After* suctioning the trachea, you may use the catheter to suction the mouth and nose before discarding the catheter and other disposable equipment. If disposable catheters are not available, be certain to store the catheter used for nasopharyngeal suction in a clearly labeled container separate from that used for suction of the tracheal stoma.

Secretions should be cultured 2 to 3 times each week to evaluate the effectiveness of the sterile suctioning technique. The presence of *Pseudomonas* in the specimen does not by itself mean the patient is infected. Observations should also be made for clinical indications of infection, e.g., elevated white blood count, elevated temperature.

Tracheal suctioning is associated with numerous potential hazards, some of which may be fatal. These hazards and their prevention (e.g., keeping the patient oxygenated prior to, during, and following the procedure if necessary) are discussed in Unit XVI. Factors of general importance in tracheal suctioning also are presented in that unit. For an excellent illustrated summary of suctioning tracheostomized patients, review Tyler and Synnestvedt.[121]

Cleansing the Inner Cannula. The tracheostomy tube is inspected frequently to determine the need for suctioning and cleaning. The inner cannula of a double-walled tracheostomy tube is removed and *cleaned as often as necessary* to keep it clear of secretions which cannot be removed by suctioning and encrustations of dried mucus. Sometimes crusts may be coughed out of the tube or may be removed with forceps. However, if this does not work, the tube is removed and cleaned. Immediately following the tracheotomy procedure, the inner tube may need cleaning approximately every half hour. While "routine" tracheostomy care (i.e., cleaning the inner cannula, changing dressings and ties as necessary) usually is *scheduled* every 2 to 4 hours, it is given more often as indicated. Some patients need the tube cleaned hourly; others may need this done only every 6 to 8 hours.

Various procedures are reported for cleansing the inner cannula of a tracheostomy tube. Among these are (a) washing the inner cannula with a small test-tube brush and a cold solution of half-strength hydrogen peroxide, sterile normal saline, or sterile 2 per cent sodium bicarbonate solution, then next washing with detergent; (b) simply using cold running water and gauze strips or pipe cleaners (pulled through the tube) to clean the inside of the tube; and (c) cleaning the inner cannula with soap and hot water. (Some sources recommend not using hot water to clean the tube because heat coagulates mucus.) After cleaning, hold the tube up and look through its lumen to be certain it is clear. Next, sterilize the cannula by submerging it in boiling water for 3 to 5 minutes and then transfer it to sterile gauze with a sterile hemostat, so it can cool before being reinserted. If boiling is not possible (it damages some synthetic tubes), submerge the cannula in 70 per cent alcohol, then place it on a sterile gauze to dry; replace the cannula when the alcohol has evaporated. Wear sterile gloves when replacing the cannula.

Silver tubes must be cleaned carefully, since they are easily bent or dented. Prior to sterilization, tarnish can be removed from silver tubes by using silver polish.

Before reinserting the inner cannula, suction and clean the outer cannula (without removing it). After reinserting the inner cannula be certain to lock it securely onto the outer cannula.

Do not leave the inner cannula out for longer than 5 to 10 minutes when removing it for cleaning. If left out longer, secretions and crusts begin to form in the outer cannula, making it difficult to reinsert the inner cannula.

Some tracheostomy tubes have two inner cannulas or identical interchangeable inner cannulas, so while one is removed for cleaning another can be inserted.

Some of the newer synthetic tracheostomy tubes, e.g., those made from Silastic and other synthetic substances, do not need an inner cannula, since encrustations do not tend to form on them as easily as on metal tubes. Occasionally, however, crusts do form in them, e.g., owing to insufficient humidification, and then the entire tube must be changed.

Connectors; Adaptors. Numerous types of adaptors are available for use with tracheostomy tubes. Some are part of the inner cannula; others are separate pieces which may or may not have accordion tubing. If the tracheostomy tube is to be connected to a mechanical respirator, a flexible swivel connector (e.g., Mörch swivel) is used to hook up the "trach" tube with the respirator's ventilatory tube. A connector of this sort minimizes the possibility of displacing the tube when turning or moving the patient. For example, use of a threaded swivel connector makes it possible to turn the patient into the semiprone position without dislodging the tube. By removing the threaded swivel cap, the nurse can suction the trachea without disconnecting the patient's oxygen supply. A connector is cleaned or replaced with a sterile one at the time routine tracheostomy care is given. If the patient is on a respirator, a sterile substitute inner cannula or adaptor is inserted into the outer cannula to continue ventilation while the tube or the removed connector or both are being cleaned.

Tracheostomy Tube Changes. Generally it takes 4 to 5 days for a tracheostomy tract to be well established. During this interval, the outer (main) cannula should be changed only by a physician with the help of an assistant. Difficulty changing the tube is most likely to occur within 48 hours after tracheotomy. Problems also frequently occur in imperfectly performed tracheostomies and in apneic respirator patients. Ideally the outer tube should be changed every 24 to 48 hours.

Prior to tube removal, oxygen is administered. The nurse assembles the following *equipment for the tube change:* tracheal intubation equipment; bag-mask unit; sterile gloves; tracheal hook; retractor; Trousseau dilator; water-soluble lubricating jelly; tube ties; one replacement tube the same size as that currently in place; and another replacement tube one size smaller than that currently being used. Cuffs on replacement tubes are checked prior to their insertion. A spotlight is also essential equipment to have at the bedside.

If the channel from the skin to the tracheal opening is not clearly established as yet, the physician may insert a gloved finger into the incision and then slip a tracheal hook alongside the finger until he or she catches the trachea. Traction is then exerted on the edge of the tracheal incision, and the new tube is inserted. Sometimes the physician elects to intubate the patient from above the tracheostomy before the tracheostomy tube is changed. Then in case of difficulty, the patient's respirations can be maintained.

The nurse may be given permission to change outer tubes after approximately 10 postoperative days, or once the tract is established.

Skin Care: Dressing Changes. Keep the area around the tracheostomy clean and dry. Moisture encourages skin maceration and infection. Change dressings and ties as necessary to keep them clean and dry. *Skin* around the tracheostomy may be antiseptically cleansed with prescribed solutions, e.g., sterile normal saline, mild antiseptics, hydrogen peroxide, or a recommended soap solution. Be careful not to allow the solution to enter the stoma and be aspirated during the cleansing procedure. Generally it is not practically possible to mechanically cleanse the stoma itself. However, the area is kept generally clean. Crusting may occur on the skin around the stoma. After these crusts are lubricated with a prescribed ointment, they are gently removed with tweezers. Care is taken that the crusts are not aspirated. A small amount of antibiotic ointment may be prescribed for application when the tracheostomy tube is changed.

Report indications of irritation of the skin or stoma. Although it rarely happens, some patients develop allergic skin reactions to the composition of various types of tracheostomy tubes. This condition is usually relieved once a different kind of tube is used.

The *tracheostomy dressing* is most easily placed between the incision and the back of the tube's faceplate before the tapes are tied. When replacing the dressing be careful not to dislocate or unnecessarily move the tube. Normally wound drainage is minimal, but the dressing may require changing owing to dampness or soilage from secretions.

Gauze squares may be used for tracheostomy dressings; these fit easily around the tube if they are cut halfway through, i.e., from the center of one edge into the center of the square (Fig. 92–8). The edges of these squares are bound to prevent loose strings being aspirated. Usually prepackaged, sterile tracheostomy dressings are available. In addition to not having loose strings, tracheostomy dressings must be made of gauze squares which do *not* have a layer of absorbent cotton; loose pieces of cotton could accidentally enter the tracheostomy tube. In some settings, cut 4 × 4's are not used for tracheostomy dressings because of the danger of loose threads. Instead the 4 × 4 is opened and folded into a long strip, and the strip is then folded over in the center and placed around the tracheostomy tube in the shape of an inverted "V."

If the tracheostomy tube is left open, e.g., is not connected to a respirator, the tube's opening may be protectively covered with a layer of gauze to reduce the risk of aspiration of foreign particles. Gauze used for this purpose should not have any absorbent or loose threads. If dampened, this gauze layer helps humidify inspired air. The gauze should not be so wet, however, that drops could enter the tracheostomy. (Humidification is discussed in Unit XVI.) For cosmetic reasons, some patients like to keep a piece of gauze over their tracheostomies to conceal the tube or opening somewhat.

Tracheostomy Neck Ties or Tapes. Ties or tapes holding the tracheostomy tube in place are checked frequently to be certain they are clean and dry and neither too loose nor too tight. *Always keep scissors* at the bedside to cut the ties if

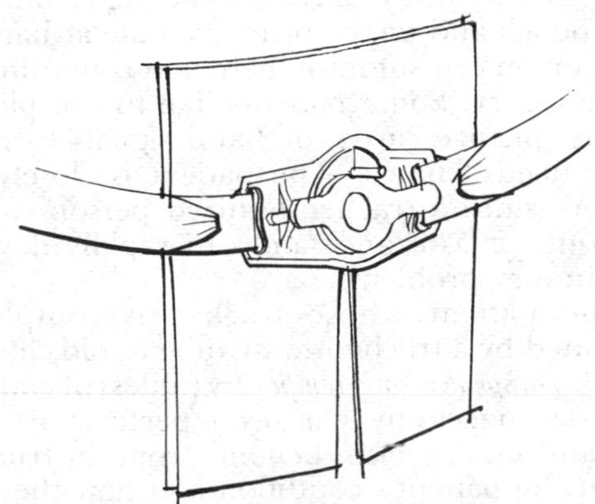

Figure 92–8. Gauze square cut to serve as tracheostomy dressing. (From Sutton, A. L.: *Bedside Nursing Techniques in Medicine and Surgery,* 2nd ed. Philadelphia: W. B. Saunders Co., 1969.)

they become too tight or if the tube must be removed. If the tube is partially coughed out, the tape is cut at once.

Tracheostomy tie tapes may be made of 16-inch long pieces of ¾-inch twill tape. One tie is fastened to each loop of the outer cannula. This is accomplished by making a horizontal cut through a portion of the tape about 1 inch from one end of the tape. Then this end of the tie is pulled through the tube's loop. Next, open the cut you have made in the tape, take the other end of the tape and pull it through the loop until the tie secures itself. This method of fastening the tie onto the faceplate's loops avoids the use of knots which could cause uncomfortable pressure on the patient's neck. The two ties are brought together and tied. The tie should be snug but not so uncomfortably tight that it obstructs veins. The tie is knotted on the side of the neck, not on the back of the neck where it would be uncomfortable and could not easily be observed. A secure knot is used (not a bow) to prevent the tube from accidentally being dislodged during coughing.

Two nurses are needed to safely adjust or change the ties on a tracheostomy tube while the tube is in place. One nurse gloves and holds the tube in place by placing the fingers of one hand on either side of the tube's faceplate, and places the other hand firmly behind the patient's neck. The other nurse then fixes the ties. The ties should be replaced as often as necessary.

If the patient is wearing a hospital gown, there is danger that the tracheal ties could accidentally be untied instead of the gown's ties. To prevent this possibility the gown is placed on the patient so it ties in front. The top tie is left open and the gown is secured by the second tie.

Communication. The tracheostomized patient should always have a signal light, tap bell, and pencil and paper or magic slate at hand so the person can summon help and communicate as necessary. Some patients like to use picture charts, picture cards, or hand signals to make their needs known. The patient is closely observed, since a tracheostomized person cannot call out for assistance and can rapidly develop respiratory problems.

The patient whose trachea is completely occluded by a tracheostomy tube is told that the *inability to speak is only temporary* (unless of course a total laryngectomy has been performed). Significant others also benefit from instruction about the patient's condition and how they can make communication with the patient less tiring for both their loved one and themselves by not asking the patient questions which require detailed answers.

Before helping the patient to talk, ask the physician's permission. In some conditions voice rest is important, e.g., if the larynx is edematous, in the presence of other laryngeal disorders, or following laryngeal surgery. Some patients are allowed to use a cork to obstruct the tracheostomy opening for purposes of speaking. Other patients (without laryngectomy) can speak by taking a breath and then covering the tube with a finger while speaking. Only a word or two may be spoken before it is necessary to remove the finger to continue breathing. Speaking may be tiring; thus the nurse makes every attempt to understand the patient's communication and to anticipate needs.

Oral Intake. An intake-output record is maintained for tracheostomized patients. Typically intravenous fluids are given for 24 hours following tracheotomy to ensure adequate hydration and nutrition; some patients may be allowed fluids orally a few hours after tracheotomy. Sometimes diet is ordered as tolerated, beginning the first postoperative day. It may be desirable for a few days to avoid serving foods which are hard to swallow.

When the tracheostomized patient first begins oral intake, coughing may occur and the person may fear aspiration. However, the patient rapidly learns how to eat and drink safely with the tube in place. Nonetheless, the nurse remains prepared to suction as necessary because the patient may cough or aspirate while eating and drinking.

Care of the Newly Tracheostomized Patient

Clinical care of the patient who has a tracheostomy requires scrupulous, uncompromising attention to detail 24 hours a day by all persons caring for the patient. Careless technique or the omission of necessary activities can seriously jeopardize the patient's chances of recovery. The newly tracheostomized patient is totally dependent upon others and thus requires constant supervision and alert care. The importance of excellent nursing care for the patient with a tracheostomy cannot be overemphasized.

Because newly tracheostomized patients require constant attendance, they are frequently cared for in an intensive care unit. The nurse carefully monitors the patient's general condition (pulse and respiratory rates, rhythms, and characters; blood pressure; skin and mucous membrane color), observing for indications of shock, respiratory insufficiency, hemorrhage, and other possible complications. While carrying out these activities, the nurse also works constantly to maintain the patency of the tracheostomy tube, to provide adequate humidification, and to protect the tracheotomy wound. The wound itself is periodically inspected. Aseptic technique is practiced when giving tracheostomy care.

Vital signs are checked at least every half hour for the first 24 to 48 postoperative hours. Additionally, during the postoperative period the patient's tidal and minute volumes are periodically assessed. After the patient's pulse and blood pressure have stabilized and if conscious, the patient is positioned with the head elevated approximately 45 degrees to enhance comfortable breathing.

Frequent suctioning and cleaning of the inner cannula of double-walled tubes are usually necessary for the first 12 to 24 hours postoperatively owing to tracheobronchial hypersecretion. The trauma caused to the trachea by the surgical procedure of tracheotomy causes the trachea to react by producing increased secretions. While the newly tracheostomized patient may require suctioning every few minutes, eventually, as the amount of mucus subsides, suctioning may be needed only every few hours.

In order to assess the patient's condition completely, the nurse listens to the chest with a stethoscope for sounds of pulmonary congestion and periodically uncovers the patient's chest to look for such symptoms of respiratory distress as (a) uneven movements of the two sides of the chest; (b) exaggerated respiratory movements; and (c) retraction of tissues in the supraclavicular spaces and the suprasternal notch, intercostal soft tissues, and epigastric tissues. Cuffed tubes are cared for as ordered (see below).

Reportable situations during the postoperative period following tracheotomy include (a) tube displacement; (b) indications of shock, hemorrhage, respiratory insufficiency, hypoxia, and other possible complications (see earlier discussion); (c) respiratory obstruction (report immediately such symptoms as respiratory distress not relieved by suctioning, increasing respirations accompanied by rales, crowing, or wheezing); and (d) excessive restlessness or apprehension or both (these conditions influence cardiopulmonary actions in addition to serving as possible clues to other complications). Restlessness and apprehension are carefully assessed as possible indications of hemorrhage or hypoxia.

The patient's mucous membranes and fingertips are closely observed for cyanosis. If *oxygen administration* is necessary, it may be given via a tent or via a clear plastic tracheal mask (or collar or funnel) into the tracheostomy tube. Because humidification of inspired air is essential, the oxygen device is connected to a humidity apparatus. A catheter is never used to administer oxygen into a tracheostomy, since it sends a jet of oxygen directly into the trachea and dries the mucosa and secretions. Obviously oxygen administered via nasal catheter does not help a patient who has a tracheostomy, since the upper airway does not effectively connect with the lower airway.

Complete charting is among the nurse's important contributions to the care of the newly tracheostomized patient. Remember to include comments about the character of secretions and the appearance of the incision and the skin around it.

The newly tracheostomized patient is often upset by frequent, brassy-sounding episodes of coughing which are productive of *mucus*. The patient is taught to wipe mucus away from the tracheostomy after coughing it up and to hold a piece of gauze (not tissue) protectively in front of the opening (rather than in front of the mouth) when coughing. The copious amounts of mucus initially present are due to the tracheobronchial tree's attempts to compensate for bypassage of the respiratory mucosa in the nose (which normally warms and humidifies inspired air). Increased tracheobronchial secretions and the noises they cause often make patients fearful that the tube is obstructing and that they may drown in their own secretions. Gradually the tracheobronchial mucosa adapts to the upper respiratory tract bypassage, and the cough becomes less frequent and less productive.

Rhinorrhea also occurs with a tracheostomy. Rhinorrhea, the frequent tendency to cough, and the copious production of mucus all cause newly tracheostomized patients to think that they may have a cold. Gentle suctioning is necessary to remove nasal secretions. Eventually rhinorrhea ceases as the body adjusts to its altered physiology.

Tracheostomy breathing differs from normal nasal-oral breathing in that the sensation of breathing is absent. Also there is loss of the Valsalva maneuver, making effective coughing impossible. These changes from normal physiologic experiences may also initially frighten the patient.

Often newly tracheostomized patients need *frequent reassurance* that the *tube is open* and that they *can breathe* through it. Patients may be afraid to go to sleep for fear of suffocation. The nurse's verbal reassurance and constant attention are helpful in relieving this fear until patients gain confidence in those caring for them and until they become less anxious about the tube.

Extubation (Decannulation)

The process of removing the tracheostomy tube is called "extubation" or "decannulation." Patients with temporary tracheostomies are helped to return *gradually* to normal breathing before the tube is removed; the patient must learn again to breathe through the upper respiratory tract. Extubation is a time of fear and anxiety for many patients. They have learned that they can safely breathe through their tracheostomies, and now they are concerned that independent respiratory function may no longer be possible.

When the physician believes that the patient is able to begin to breathe without respiratory assistance, orders are given to begin to reduce the lumen of the tracheostomy tube for a day or so and then to partially obstruct the tracheostomy tube's outer opening for varying lengths of time. Eventually the patient is able to tolerate complete occlusion of the tracheostomy opening.

Occlusion of the tracheostomy tube (either partially or completely) is accomplished in various ways. For example, a special tube with a small opening may be inserted into the main tracheostomy tube; tape may be placed over the tube's opening; or corks of gradually increasing size may be inserted into the tube's opening until it is eventually completely occluded. Corks used are either plastic or pure rubber (natural cork could crumble and bits could be aspirated). The corks are secured to the tracheostomy tube with braided threads. *Remember, corking or other occlusion of the tracheostomy opening must be preceded by deflation of cuffed tubes and insertion of a fenestrated or smaller diameter tube.* If you fail to remember this and occlude the opening of the tracheostomy tube, you totally obstruct the patient's airway! During the "trial" periods of occlusion of the tracheostomy tube, the patient is closely observed and his or her tolerance of the procedure charted. Immediately remove the obstruction upon any evidence of respiratory difficulties. Once the patient has been able to comfortably tolerate complete plugging of the tube for 24 hours, the tracheostomy tube is removed.

Close nursing supervision continues following extubation, and pO_2 and pCO_2 levels are typically assessed for several days. After tube removal, the incision is allowed to close by secondary intention (i.e., spontaneously from below). Wound edges may be loosely approximated with tape to help create a more favorable scar. Closure which is too tight promotes deep infection. Following tube removal, an air leak occurs for a while at the area of the incision. This reduces the effectiveness of the patient's cough (because it makes it difficult to create high intrathoracic pressures) and can pose problems in maintaining a patent airway. (These problems do not occur following removal of an endotracheal tube, since an incision was not made.) Teach the patient to hold a dressing firmly over the stoma's incision line when coughing until the incision is healed. Pressure of this sort can help the patient increase intrathoracic pressure and hence cough more effectively. Some physicians cover the incision with petrolatum gauze to seal the area and prevent air leak. It takes several days for the tracheostomy wound to heal sufficiently to stop air from leaking through it.

Generally it is advisable for any patient who has had a tracheostomy to continue under medical supervision for at least a year following extubation. Tracheal scarring and tracheal stricture are problems which can develop and are watched for during this period.

A *Kistner button* is sometimes used as an intermediate step between use of a standard tracheostomy tube and complete extubation. This device is a short, straight tracheostomy tube which fits into the tracheostomy stoma but does not project down into the tracheal lumen. The Kistner button has a removable cap which has a one-way flap inside. Inhalation is possible through the cap's opening, but exhalation is not possible, since the force of the air being exhaled pushes the flap over the cap's opening. When the cap is on the tube, the patient can talk. The cap is removed for suctioning of the stoma. A Kistner button cannot be used with a ventilator but may be used in place of a standard tracheostomy tube in patients with retained secretions who do not require ventilatory assistance. In these patients the button is substituted for the standard tube once a well-established tracheostomy tract has formed. Less airway resistance is created with a Kistner button than with a plugged standard tracheostomy tube. Breathing is therefore easier. Artificial humidification of inspired air is necessary with a Kistner button (as with any type of tracheostomy tube), since the natural airway is bypassed.

Permanent Tracheostomy

Some patients are not decannulated but instead have a permanent tracheostomy. Most patients with permanent tracheostomies have had a laryngectomy. (See discussion of laryngectomy, Chapter 93.) A small percentage are victims of injury, burns, or infection.

Patient education regarding tracheostomy care is started early during the course of hospitalization if a patient is going to be discharged with a permanent tracheostomy. Instructions for self-care include care of the tracheostomy tube, skin care of the stoma, suctioning, and care of suction catheters. It is desirable to teach a significant other as well as the patient. Supervise the patient's self-care until the person is skilled enough to act without supervision. Teaching self-care early is the best means of assuring rapid care for the patient if airway obstruction should occur. The patient and a significant other need to be confident of their ability to give tracheostomy care before the patient is discharged.

Provide a mirror for patients when they are learning to care for their own tracheostomy. Instruct ambulatory patients with a tracheostomy to carry scissors (to cut the neck tie) and a hemostat (to hold the tracheostomy open until help arrives) and teach them what to do if the tube becomes dislodged.

Some persons with permanent tracheostomies do not need to wear any type of appliance in their tracheostomy stomas; others wear a tracheostomy or laryngectomy tube; still others wear small plastic tracheostomy "buttons" which are hollow in the center and have a flange on each side to anchor the button just at the neck's skin surface (Figure 92–9).

It is psychologically desirable for persons with permanent tracheostomies to cover the tracheostomy tube or stoma. Murphy and Ogura comment:[72] "Display of either the bib or . . . of the open stoma itself represents a public proclamation of 'difference' or disability not in keeping with the achievement of the most normal functioning possible." Shirts or blouses buttoned at the neck or scarves are means of effectively covering (and protecting) the tracheostomy opening and yet enabling easy accessibility to the stoma when necessary. Covering the opening helps warm and filter inspired air. High-necked, properly fitted collars and neck scarves also help conceal the disfigurement resulting from unilateral or bilateral radical neck dissection when these procedures have been performed.

Teach patients with permanent tracheostomies that they must prevent accidental aspiration through the tracheostomy stoma, e.g., when washing hair, bathing, and so forth. Swimming is prohibited. When bathing in a tub, a towel should be placed around the neck to prevent water from entering the stoma. Likewise a mirror is always used when washing the face to prevent the accidental entrance of soap and water into the stoma. Tub baths should be taken with the drain open to prevent accidental drowning if the patient falls asleep. When showering, the patient is told to direct the stream of water at chest height and to wear a special protective shower-shield to cover the stoma. If a shield is not available, the person can hold a washcloth between the teeth with one end protectively hanging over the stoma. Special care is necessary when using after-shave lotions on the neck or any powder or spray (aerosol) product directed at the upper half of the body, e.g., aerosol shaving lathers, hair sprays, deodorants, to prevent accidentally directing them toward the stoma. When receiving haircuts, the patient needs to inform the operator to take care not to allow falling hair to enter the stoma, e.g., when shaking off the cape or brushing off the patient's shoulders. When aspiration does occur, it precipitates violent coughing which is not only uncomfortable but also frightening. Airway damage may occur, and, of course, at times aspiration may be fatal. (*Note:* these precautions are important for any patient with a tracheostomy, permanent or temporary.)

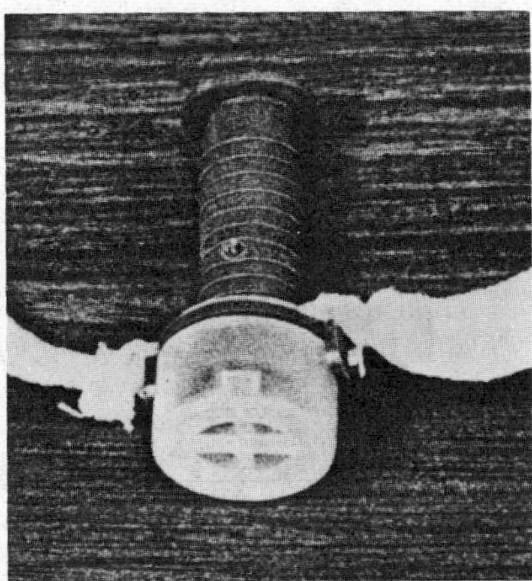

Figure 92–9. Kistner tracheal button occludes the stoma without obstructing the airway. (From Adams, N. R.: The nurse's role in systematic weaning from a ventilator. *Nursing 79,* 9:35, Aug. 1979.)

If suctioning is necessary, the patient is informed that many local chapters of the American Cancer Society have suction machines available for home use; machines can also be rented from hospital equipment rental firms. A list of necessary supplies for home care is given to the people the patient lives with along with information about where the equipment can be purchased.

Instructions for home care also include emphasizing that the patient should not have contact with persons who have respiratory infections. Additionally, a significant other person should be taught how to give emergency mouth-to-neck resuscitation to the patient if the patient experiences respiratory depression or respiratory arrest.

Mouth-to-Neck Resuscitation

Emergency mouth-to-neck, i.e., "mouth-to-tracheostomy," resuscitation may be necessary if the tracheostomized patient experiences respiratory depression or respiratory arrest. Patients with tracheostomies are important exceptions to the standard emergency mouth-to-mouth artificial method. Cardiopulmonary resuscitation is discussed in detail in Unit XII.

> *Immediately upon finding any unconscious person, check the neck to determine if the person is a "neck-breather," i.e., has a tracheostomy.*

The nurse must be prepared to administer and to teach emergency resuscitation for neck-breathers and partial neck-breathers. This technique is discussed and illustrated in "First Aid for (Neck-Breathers) Laryngectomees," published by the American Cancer Society.[29]

It is possible to give emergency neck resuscitation mechanically with a rubber or plastic inflatable bag (e.g., Ambu bag) fitted with a baby-sized mask. However, mouth-to-neck breathing is more efficient and safer. Pressure of the mask on the neck's major blood vessels may interfere with circulation to the brain (cerebral circulation); also, it is difficult to maintain a tight seal over the tracheostomy with a mask.

ENDOTRACHEAL INTUBATION

An endotracheal tube is inserted by the physician into a patient's trachea through the nose or mouth. An *orotracheal tube* is passed through the mouth into the trachea; a *nasotracheal tube* is passed into the trachea via the nose.

Endotracheal intubation is used for reasons similar to those for tracheostomy, that is, to deliver oxygen (or anesthetics, since this is the primary mode of administering general anesthesia), to remove secretions, or to facilitate ventilation.

Advantages and Disadvantages

Advantages of endotracheal intubation over tracheostomy are that (a) the intubation can be done rapidly, and (b) surgical trauma is avoided. Orotracheal or nasotracheal tubes may be used instead of a tracheostomy in patients whose conditions are expected to be *self-limited* within a day or so. Also, endotracheal intubation is preferred rather than tracheotomy in managing *emergency* situations. For example, patients with exsanguinating pulmonary hemorrhage may have their lives saved if it is possible to carry out orotracheal intubation and suctioning rapidly. In most emergency situations orotracheal intubation is preferable to nasotracheal intubation or tracheostomy. *Orotracheal intubation is more advantageous than nasotracheal intubation* for the following reasons: (a) its results are more predictable; (b) it is less time-consuming to perform; (c) no nasal bacteria are introduced into the trachea; and (d) it is potentially less traumatic. (Nasotracheal intubation may precipitate epistaxis.)

Endotracheal tubes have several *disadvantages*. While it is possible to suction through an endotracheal tube, it is not as effective as suctioning through a tracheostomy. Usually frequent suctioning (with a sterile catheter) is necessary when an endotracheal tube is in place. An endotracheal tube cannot be passed in some conditions, e.g., severe burns, laryngeal edema. *Endotracheal tubes can be more damaging to the airway than tracheostomy tubes. Therefore, endotracheal tubes are generally not left in place for longer than 24 to 48 hours.* After this time, a tracheostomy is necessary if the patient cannot maintain adequate respiratory function. Nasotracheal or orotracheal tubes can cause extensive and permanent damage to the larynx and airway after 24 hours or more. Thus, when *long-term* airway care is necessary, tracheotomy becomes the procedure of choice because it is safer, it facilitates nursing care, and it is more comfortable for the conscious patient.

Complications

Complications which may be associated with usage of endotracheal tubes include (a) *vocal cord damage* (the tube keeps the cords open); (b) *laryngeal erosion* and eventual *stricture* (resulting from friction); (c) *pressure ulceration of the lip* (if an orotracheal tube is used); (d) *laryngeal edema* (following tube removal); and (e) *pulmonary infection* (resulting from inability to cough effectively or introduction of pathogens via the tube or both). Respiratory infection may easily occur when endotracheal intubation removes the normal protective barrier against bacteria which the glottis usually provides for the airway. Additionally, bacterial exposure may be increased if contaminated ventilator equipment is used. Gram-negative organisms tend to grow easily in this equipment; therefore, all equipment must be changed daily, including the vaporizer, tubes, and valves. Infection of the respiratory tract may also be minimized by using isolation precautions to prevent cross-infection and by employing an aseptic suctioning technique.

Other complications of endotracheal intubation include (a) *tracheal injuries;* (b) *hypoxia;* and (c) *cardiac arrhythmias.* Tracheal injuries, e.g., tracheoesophageal fistula and tracheal stenosis, result from local tissue trauma. This trauma may result from such factors as (a) use of an excessively large tube; (b) prolonged inflation or overinflation of a cuff; (c) excessive movement of the endotracheal tube (e.g., due to improper fixation of the tube); (d) traumatic suctioning; and (e) "dragging" on the indwelling tube (e.g., due to lack of support of the cannula and its connecting tubes). Hypoxemic complications, e.g., cardiac arrhythmias, may result from prolonged endotracheal suctioning or dislodgment, plugging, or malposition of the endotracheal tube. Complications of endotracheal intubation can be fatal.

Malfunctioning of an endotracheal tube can result from such problems as displacement or obstruction of the tube. *Malfunctioning of an endotracheal tube is a medical emergency, since asphyxiation can rapidly occur. Tube displacement* can occur into either the esophagus or a mainstem bronchus (usually the right). Any tube placed in the trachea has a tendency to enter the right mainstem bronchus, because this bronchus separates from the trachea at a smaller angle than in the left mainstem bronchus. If an endotracheal tube enters the right mainstem bronchus, only the right lung is intubated; consequently, the left lung is not ventilated. The inflated cuff of a cuffed tube placed too low in the trachea can completely block off a bronchus. Displacement of an endotracheal tube into the right mainstem bronchus results in hypoxia and may lead to asphyxiation.

Displacement of the tube into the esophagus causes inflation of the stomach if a respirator is used. If the patient is capable of spontaneous respirations, he or she can continue to breathe if the tube is in the esophagus. However, if the patient must rely on a respirator, esophageal tube displacement results in asphyxiation. Gastric distention alone impairs respiration, and acute gastric distention can precipitate cardiopulmonary arrest.

Obstruction of an endotracheal tube may be detected not only by observable respiratory distress but also by auscultation of both lungs. Failure to hear breath sounds in either or both lungs can indicate obstruction. Endotracheal tube obstruction can result from such factors as (a) displacement of the inflated cuff over the tube's orifice; (b) tube kinkage; or (c) tube compression due to the patient's biting the tube (prevent this by using "bite-block" or an oropharyngeal airway). Secretions are also a common cause of tube obstruction.

Types of Endotracheal Tubes

A wide variety of endotracheal tubes are available for orotracheal or nasotracheal intubation (Figure 92–10). All endotracheal tubes are available with inflatable cuffs near their tips. Because considerable variety exists in cuff design, the physician selects one which (a) requires minimal cuff inflation pressure; (b) inflates evenly and uniformly over a broad area; and (c) is composed of material which is nonirritating to tissue and not subject to leakage. Before insertion into the trachea, the balloon or cuff of an endotracheal tube is tested for uniform inflation and for possible leakage. (Cuffed tubes are further discussed below.)

Orotracheal tubes are somewhat larger than nasotracheal tubes and thus enable more effective suctioning. Of course, care is taken not to use a tube which is excessively large and will injure the larynx and mucosa. *While mucosal damage can result from an overinflated cuff, it most commonly results from use of too large a tube or trauma during intubation.* Generally it is most desirable to select a tube whose outside diameter is three fourths that of the inside diameter of the trachea. Oral endotracheal tubes are commonly more uncomfortable than nasal endotracheal tubes.

Endotracheal tubes do not have inner cannulae which can be removed for cleaning (as do many tracheostomy tubes).

Bedside Endotracheal Intubation

Nurses often participate in bedside endotracheal intubation. Equipment necessary to insert a cuffed endotracheal tube includes (a) endotracheal tube; (b) syringe to inflate the cuff; (c) laryngoscope (to visualize the larynx, depress the tongue, and lift the jaw); (d) adequate bedside lighting; (e) a flexible copper stylet (may be employed to give the tube greater rigidity during

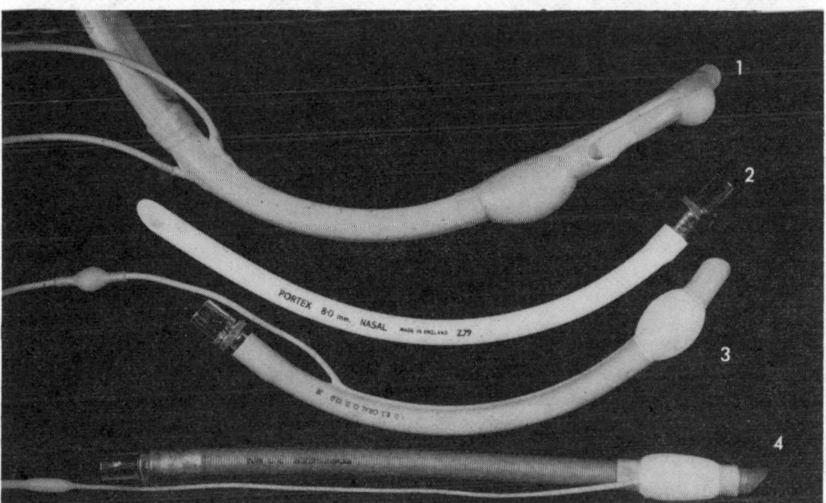

Figure 92–10. Endotracheal tubes (from top to bottom): (1) The Robert-Shaw double-lumen tube to isolate the flow to each lung. Note the individual inflatable cuffs for the trachea and the left bronchus; (2) The Portex nasotracheal tube, without attached cuff; (3) An orotracheal tube with attached inflatable cuff (very commonly used); and (4) The LA (Latex-Armored) tube. Note the spiral winding to prevent kinking. (From Sanderson, R. G. (Ed.): *The Cardiac Patient.* Philadelphia: W. B. Saunders Co., 1972.)

insertion); and (f) syringes, needles, and medications. Sometimes a muscle relaxant medication is administered intravenously to facilitate intubation. Be certain to precheck the light in the laryngoscope to be certain it is properly functioning. Steps in endotracheal intubation are shown in Figure 92–11.

Because endotracheal intubation is difficult for the conscious patient to tolerate, carefully explain purposes of the procedure prior to intubation. Attempts to enlist the patient's cooperation make it easier for the patient to tolerate an uncomfortable but essential procedure.

If possible, prior to intubation topical anesthesia is applied between periods of assisted ventilation. If the patient is unconscious or if the airway must immediately be established, the orotracheal intubation is performed without the topical anesthesia. A nasopharyngeal airway should be lubricated with anesthetic jelly prior to insertion. The airway may then be left in place for up to a week. Orotracheal intubation is best performed by direct laryngoscopy with the patient supine. To obtain maximum laryngeal exposure in the supine patient, the patient's occiput is elevated and the head is tilted slightly backward at the atlanto-occipital joint so the person appears to be in a "sniffing position."

The physician can most effectively intubate a patient by standing or sitting on a stool directly behind the patient's head. If time permits, it is desirable for a patient in a standard hospital bed

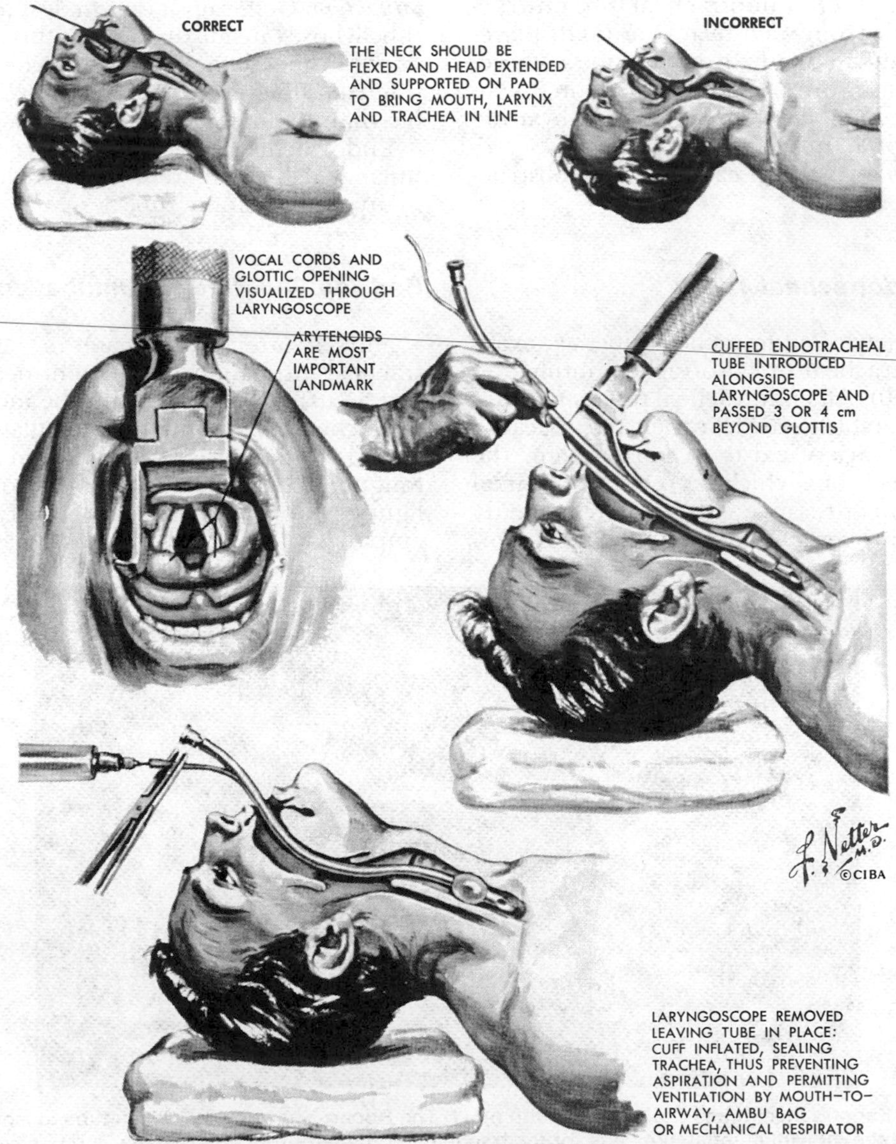

Figure 92–11. Endotracheal intubations. (© Copyright 1970 CIBA Pharmaceutical Company. Division of CIBA-GEIGY Corporation. Reproduced, with permission, from the CLINICAL SYMPOSIA illustrated by Frank H. Netter, M.D. All rights reserved.)

to be positioned with the head at the foot of the bed, so the head can more easily be reached.

During the intubation, an assistant can additionally facilitate exposure by retracting the right corner of the patient's mouth and pressing the patient's larynx backward or by further raising the occiput. The attending physician holds the laryngoscope in the left hand and inserts it into the right corner of the patient's mouth. Once the scope is positioned so the larynx can be visualized, the doctor passes the tube (with the right hand) while looking through the blade. A stylet is used to guide the tube's tip in difficult intubations; however, it is not "routinely" used because it can injure glottic structures.

Immediately after the tube is passed, its correct location is assured by observing the patient's breathing through it or by artificially inflating the patient's lungs. Auscultation of the chest may also be performed to rule out bronchial obstruction, and x-rays are taken to ensure the tube's correct location. Finally the cuff is inflated (a cuffed tube is preferred in adults). The tube is firmly fixed to a bite-block or pharyngeal tube and then to the patient's face. The patient is given continued ventilatory assistance as indicated.

Frequently endotracheal tubes are used with a respirator, and the cuff is therefore inflated. To prevent pressure damage to the tracheal walls, a very slight air leak may be allowed, and the cuff is routinely deflated periodically (see discussion of cuffed tubes below). Ventilation therapy becomes inaccurate and ineffective if *uncontrolled air leaks* occur around endotracheal tubes, and alveolar ventilation may be inadequate. Air leaks make volume respirators particularly difficult to use with accuracy; thus these respirators are almost always used with cuffed tubes.

Following endotracheal intubation, care is taken to *provide adequate humidification* and to *prevent contamination of inhaled air.*

With proper endotracheal intubation, *both* sides of the thorax rise evenly during inspiration. Frequent observation of the intubated patient's chest is thus important in addition to using a stethoscope to listen for airflow in *both* lungs. To *prevent displacement,* the endotracheal tube must be anchored adequately exteriorly and care taken while giving care (e.g., turning the patient) not to exert traction on the tube. The position of the tube may be checked periodically with x-ray and is always checked immediately if displacement is suspected.

Secure oral endotracheal tubes to the patient's face in the following manner: (a) carefully apply tincture of benzoin to the patient's cheeks where the tape will be placed; cover the patient's eyes during this application; (b) wrap adhesive tape around the tube and extend the tape over the face on both sides; (c) tape the tube and slip-joint tightly to the bite-block; and (d) if the patient is especially active, place the tape loosely around the patient's neck and place sandbags on either side of the patient's head to help immobilize the head. The patient's chest should be padded for protection, and the respiratory apparatus stabilized on the chest to prevent "dragging" or misplacement of the endotracheal tube.

Mild sedation may be necessary for the conscious patient who has endotracheal intubation because of discomfort, gagging, difficulty in swallowing, and so forth. Some conscious patients are unable to tolerate an endotracheal tube, even with sedation.

Give frequent mouth care to the patient who has an endotracheal tube in place, and suction as necessary. The tube may cause excessive oropharyngeal secretions which must be periodically removed by suctioning. *A catheter used for oropharyngeal suctioning is never used for tracheal suctioning,* since it could introduce pathogens into the tracheobronchial tree. (Suctioning is discussed in Unit XVI.) When suctioning an endotracheal tube, make certain the suction catheter is long enough to reach beyond the length of the tube and touch the bronchial mucosa. This mucosal stimulation elicits coughing and thus helps the patient clear the tracheobronchial tree of secretions. Rubber suction catheters sometimes slide more easily in plastic endotracheal tubes than do plastic suction catheters. Periodically the endotracheal tube is repositioned (if it is an orotracheal tube) to prevent pressure necrosis on the lip. An emergency tracheostomy tray and an extra sterile endotracheal tube of correct size are always kept at the bedside of an intubated patient for emergency use. Inspect the nasal mucosa periodically for erosion when a nasal endotracheal tube is being used.

Patients with endotracheal tubes are not allowed anything orally; intravenous or nasogastric feedings are given.

"Crash Intubation." "Crash intubation" procedures are often necessary in emergency rooms. In these settings patients often present numerous problems which are clinically challenging to the resuscitating team. For example, the patient may be comatose, convulsing, cyanotic, vomiting, obstructed, and have head injury or trismus. Initially attempts may be made to suction quickly the patient's nose and mouth. If the patient does not have head injuries, this suctioning is best done with the patient supine and the head turned to one side. Then the patient is positioned with the head elevated about 45 degrees (to counteract passive regurgitation and cerebral congestion) and with the legs elevated (to avoid postural hypotension). In this V-position, attempts may be made to start an intravenous infusion and to oxygenate the patient by use of bag and mask. If ventilation with bag and mask is inadequate, the immediate goal of care becomes intubation (of a well-oxygenated patient when possible).

In a patient with trismus (spasm of masticatory muscles producing difficulty opening the jaws, i.e., "lockjaw") and asphyxia, orotracheal intubation may be possible only after rapid muscle paralysis with succinylcholine. The larynx is rapidly exposed (with suction ready), the trachea is intubated, and the cuff is inflated. If the patient's airway is open and if time permits, it is desirable to hyperoxygenate, e.g., by the inhalation of 100 per cent oxygen (high flow) with bag and mask for at least 2 minutes. If the patient is conscious prior to paralysis, he or she is rapidly anesthetized lightly, e.g., with thiopental, halothane, or cyclopropane. If it has not been possible to carry out preliminary oxygenation under spontaneous breathing, positive pressure ventilation is instituted after paralysis is achieved. Paralyzing agents must be used with caution. A patient may have marginal oxygenation with great effort. If such a patient is paralyzed and then unable to be intubated, a disaster occurs.

Endotracheal Extubation

Accidental removal of an endotracheal tube can occur (a) if the tube is not properly secured in place; (b) from a confused patient pulling at the tube; or (c) from traction exerted on the tube when giving patient care. Because the endotracheal tube is probably the only means by which the patient is getting oxygen, further accidental extubation is hazardous because of possible aspiration, tracheal trauma, laryngeal edema, laryngeal spasm, or respiratory arrest.

Prior to *planned endotracheal extubation,* some physicians order steroids intravenously in an attempt to prevent laryngeal edema. The physician performs the extubation after determining that the patient's respiratory status is satisfactory. In reaching this decision, the physician assesses blood gas values, vital capacity, and other measurements of respiratory function. Before an endotracheal tube is removed, the nurse checks the emergency respiratory equipment at the bedside. It may be necessary to reintubate the patient or to use resuscitatory equipment, e.g., Ambu bag. Sometimes tracheotomy is required. If laryngospasm occurs, muscle relaxants may be administered.

When possible, the patient is placed in semi-Fowler's position for extubation. It is desirable to maintain this position or place the patient in high-Fowler's position after the tube is removed to improve alveolar ventilation and to encourage chest expansion.

The pharynx is suctioned before the cuff is deflated on the endotracheal tube. Thus secretions which have accumulated above the cuff will not be aspirated when the cuff is deflated.

Following endotracheal intubation, the patient is generally given mist treatment (by mask or tent) and is *closely observed* for indications of *respiratory distress or laryngeal edema,* e.g., upper airway obstruction, laryngeal stridor. The nurse remains prepared to assist with reintubation or tracheotomy if necessary.

CUFFED TUBES

Previous sections have focused on tracheostomy and endotracheal tubes in general. Here our emphasis is on *cuffed* tracheostomy and endotracheal tubes. Inflation of the cuff with air (once the tube is properly positioned in the trachea) firmly fixes the tube in the trachea and forms a seal which prevents leakage of air around the tube or possible aspiration of food or secretions into the lungs (Figure 92–12). Most tubes are cuffed today. Some tubes have cuffs that are applied around the tube separately, but most have a cuff built into the tube, i.e., the tube and cuff are all-in-one.

Cuffed tubes are used for various reasons. As mentioned above, cuffed tubes help prevent aspiration of pharyngeal and regurgitated gastric contents by forming a seal between the tube and tracheal wall. Also, inflated cuffs are necessary for controlled positive pressure mechanical ventilation, since these cuffs prevent air leak around the tube. Thus, when controlled positive pressure ventilation cannot be given effectively by mask, endotracheal intubation or tracheostomy is performed with a cuffed tube, and the mechanical ventilator is attached to the tube. (Ventilators are discussed in Unit XVI.)

While cuffed tubes are advantageous in some situations, they also can cause serious *complications* unless properly used. (Many of these complications have been discussed in detail earlier in this chapter.) Pressure of the inflated cuff impairs blood supply to tracheal tissue; also, the presence of the cuff irritates the tracheal wall. After cuff inflation, tissue changes may begin as soon as 48 hours. Complications which can result from *overinflation or prolonged inflation* of cuffs include tracheal necrosis, erosion, or ulceration; tracheo-innominate fistula; tracheoesophageal fistula; tracheomalacia; tracheal stenosis (from scarring and irritation); tracheitis above the site of the cuff (due to pooling of secretions there); and herniation of the tracheal wall over the distal portion of the tube (producing tube obstruction). *Misplacement* of a cuffed tube (such that the end of the tube is on the carina or in a mainstem bronchus) will produce airway obstruction, i.e., air will not flow in and out of the bronchus and lung opposite the side intubated. Following insertion of a cuffed tube, the chest is periodically auscultated (as previously mentioned) on both sides to make certain that airflow is occurring in both lungs.

Soft *low-pressure cuffs* are now available which help minimize trauma. Also, some cuffs are now designed as an *elongated cuff* rather than the traditional more rounded cuff. Advocates of the elongated cuffs maintain that this type of cuff distributes pressure over a greater surface area and thus minimizes pressure in any one place on the tracheal wall. Prestretching cuffs and periodically deflating them are techniques used to help minimize cuff trauma. These procedures are discussed in following paragraphs.

Cuffed tubes may be prestretched *and* periodically deflated *in an attempt to prevent tracheal complications associated with excessive cuff pressure.*

Prestretching an inflatable cuff makes the cuff more pliable. The cuff, therefore, conforms more readily to the rings of the trachea and does not excessively distort or compress the tracheal wall. A cuffed tracheostomy tube can be prestretched by (a) placing the tube in 95° C. sterile water; (b) gently inflating the cuff with 20 to 30 ml. of air; and (c) removing the tube from the water after 10 minutes and allowing it to cool.

A cuff should be inflated prior to insertion and examined to be certain it is uniformly rounded, i.e., does not have abnormal bulges or indentations. Discard the tube if its cuff is lopsided when inflated. A lopsided cuff is unsafe, since a bulged area may herniate over the distal end of the tube when in place in the trachea and obstruct the airway.

Deflation of the Cuff

The cuff of a cuffed tube is deflated periodically to allow blood to circulate through the affected area and thus prevent damage to the trachea caused by prolonged cuff pressure. Deflation routines vary with the doctor's orders and the patient's condition. Ideally the cuff should be deflated for 1 minute every 20 to 30 minutes. However, in practice this is sometimes not possible because of the patient's condition. During periods of deflation the patient is constantly attended to prevent aspiration. Deflating the cuff for 5 minutes every hour is not adequate.

If a patient with a cuffed tracheal tube develops sudden respiratory distress, the cuff should be immediately deflated until the problem has been identified. Also, the cuff should be deflated during suctioning (as described in the following paragraph). *If an acute airway emergency develops in an intubated patient,* Tyler and Synnestvedt recommend the following actions:[121] *first,* disconnect the mechanical ventilator and manually ventilate

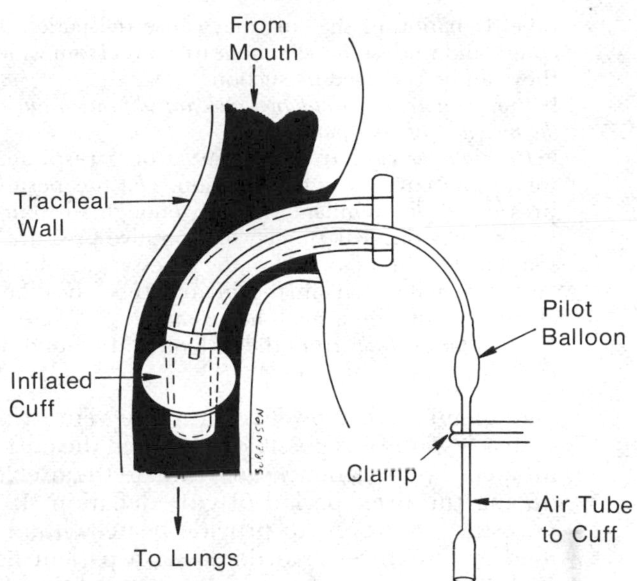

Figure 92–12. Cuffed tracheostomy tube with cuff inflated.

the patient (the problem may be in the ventilating machine); *second,* pass a catheter rapidly to clear any plugs from the lumen of the tube or from the tube's distal end (a plug at the end of a tube may permit inhalation but may obstruct the tube during exhalation—thus causing increasing trapping of air and distention of lung tissue); *third,* almost simultaneously deflate the cuff completely (a dislodged or herniated cuff may be obstructing the airway); and *finally,* remove the tube while summoning help *if* the preceding steps fail to relieve the emergency immediately. While waiting for help, continue ventilating with a self-inflating bag and mask. To prevent the escape of air through a tracheostomy stoma during ventilation, tightly cover the stoma.

Some important steps to remember when *deflating* cuffed tubes are:

▶ *Before deflating the cuff, suction the upper airway,* i.e., the nasal and oral pharynx, to remove secretions which have accumulated above the inflated cuff. Unless removed, these secretions may be aspirated when the cuff is deflated. *The tracheal tube is also suctioned before the cuff is deflated and again as the cuff is deflated* (to suction out any secretions which have accumulated on top of the inflated cuff).

▶ *Next, deflate the cuff.* Using a syringe, release the air slowly from the small tube leading to the pilot balloon and cuff. *While doing this maintain positive pressure* from an Ambu bag or ventilator. The positive pressure prevents pulmonary aspiration by forcing accumulated secretions in the upper trachea and larynx into the mouth (where they can be removed by suctioning).

▶ *After deflating the cuff, suction the lower airway* to remove secretions accumulated around the cuff and tube. Deflation of the cuff may cause the patient to cough and raise some secretions to a level from which they can be removed by suction.

▶ *Provide adequate ventilation and humidification during the time the cuff is deflated.*

▶ *Reinflate the cuff.* If the patient is on a respirator, inflate the cuff during inspiration, i.e., the positive pressure cycle. Reinflate with only enough air to prevent an obvious leak of air when positive pressure is reapplied to the airway. After the necessary amount of air has been inserted into the inflating tube, the tube is clamped shut with a small hemostat.

▶ *Check for air leaks* from the balloon and around the cuff.

Remember that positive pressure ventilation with a respirator is possible only when the cuff is inflated. Some patients can ventilate themselves during the brief period of cuff deflation. It is necessary, however, to provide heated, humidified gas mixtures as ordered. If a patient has such high airway resistance that manual ventilation is impossible, he or she must be kept on a respirator and have the cuff frequently deflated for only a few seconds at a time, e.g., 30 to 60 seconds if the patient's condition permits. The apneic patient should not be kept off the respirator for longer than 15 seconds or cardiac arrhythmias or cardiac arrest may develop.

If a patient is severely hypoxic and is on prolonged, controlled, ventilatory assistance, it is most desirable to deflate the cuff when the patient needs to be off the respirator for some other aspect of care, e.g., for endotracheal suctioning. The patient is hyperoxygenated prior to suctioning, i.e., the percentage of oxygen he or she receives from the respirator is increased for a few minutes. During this period of hyperoxygenation, the patient is given naso- or oropharyngeal suctioning. The cuff is then deflated, and simultaneously the trachea is suctioned. Two nurses work together to rapidly carry out hyperoxygenation, cuff deflation, endotracheal suctioning, and cuff reinflation. Another method is to leave the patient on the respirator while carrying out naso- or oropharyngeal and tracheal suctioning. Next, deflate the cuff and let oxygen from the respirator push any secretions pooled above the cuff up into the pharynx, where they can easily be removed by suctioning.

Before adding more air to an inflated cuffed tube, be certain to suck out the air that is in the cuff. This is necessary to prevent excessively filling the cuff by adding air to the air which is left in the cuff. Air will not empty out of a stretched cuff by itself; it must be withdrawn.

An *automatic intermittent cuff inflator* has been developed which can be used with either a pressure or volume-controlled respirator. The volume to which the cuff is to be inflated is set on the machine. The machine is then connected to (a) an oxygen power source; (b) the cuff inflation tube; and (c) the respirator's exhalation valve. Then the cuff is automatically deflated with each expiration and is inflated to the preset volume with each inspiration. If a patient is likely to aspirate or vomit, have a nasal gastric tube in place as a precaution against aspiration while the cuff is deflated.

The risk of tissue damage is especially great when a patient has both a tracheal tube and a nasogastric tube. The nurse closely observes for symptoms of tracheoesophageal fistula. If the nasogastric tube is to be used for tube feedings, prior to the feedings the patient is placed in semi-Fowler's position, and the cuff is inflated to prevent possible aspiration of regurgitated food. The patient is kept in the semi-Fowler's position during the feeding and for about 20 minutes after the feeding (to permit the contents of the feeding to pass through the stomach).*

Cuffed Tracheostomy Tubes

In adults cuffed tracheostomy tubes are useful in the following situations: (a) in patients who are likely to aspirate (e.g., those who lack the swallowing reflex, those in coma and/or with bulbar paralysis, and those with upper airway bleeding or abdominal distention); (b) in patients requiring assisted or controlled positive pressure ventilation (these two points have been discussed in the previous section); and (c) routinely for the first few hours after tracheostomy to prevent blood from leaking into the lungs.

In some patients a cuffed tracheostomy tube is in place prophylactically, and the cuff is not inflated unless necessary. Therefore, always check the physician's orders concerning inflation of a cuff. If the cuff is to be inflated, this is accomplished by introducing air into the cuff via a syringe connected to a fine tube which leads into the cuff. Near the proximal end of this small inflating tube is a "pilot balloon" (see Figs. 92–4 and 92–12). The introduction of air into the air-tube inflates both the cuff and the pilot balloon. If a leak occurs anywhere in the "tube-balloon-cuff" system, the pilot balloon becomes noticeably deflated. Thus the nurse frequently observes the pilot balloon to determine patency of the cuff seal. If the cuff is not inflating adequately and is to be inflated, the physician is notified and the tube is replaced. (*Note:* a nurse does not replace a tracheostomy tube unless she or he is trained to do so and has the physician's order.) It is also possible to detect a leak around a

*Tube feedings are discussed in Chapters 26 and 59. For a detailed description of procedures, see Sorensen and Luckmann, *Basic Nursing: A Psychophysiologic Approach.*

cuff by (a) briefly blocking off the tracheostomy tube and listening carefully for the sound of escaping air; (b) placing your hand in front of the patient's mouth or nose and having the patient blow against your hand (a leak is present if you can feel air moving); or (c) listening for a harsh oral sound during the inspiratory phase when the patient is on ventilatory assistance.

Check with the physician whether or not a patient's tracheostomy tube cuff is to be inflated or deflated while the patient eats or drinks. Some doctors prefer a deflated cuff at these times because they believe inflation of the cuff makes swallowing more difficult (owing to the pressure exerted on the esophagus by the inflated cuff). Other doctors prefer cuff inflation to prevent possible aspiration of oral intake.

With careful technique it is possible to use cuffed tracheostomy tubes for several months without causing tracheal trauma. Proctor and Safar[85] recommend observing the following precautions:*

► In managing patients who are in danger of aspirating, use a *"no-leak"* or *"full-seal" technique* which allows no air to leak around the tube or escape through the nose or mouth.

► In treating conscious respirator patients, employ a *"minimal-leak" technique* in which the cuff is slowly inflated until all audible leakage is abolished and then is deflated slowly.

► Never inflate the cuff without simultaneously applying positive pressure through the tube to prevent overinflation of the cuff.

► Practice asepsis and use optimal humidification. Increasing the moisture content of inspired air prevents drying of the tracheal mucosa and facilitates removal of secretions. Disposable rubber gloves and disposable suction catheters are used with aseptic technique during suctioning to protect the patient from foreign microorganisms. *Remember:* A tracheostomy is a possible portal of entry for infectious microorganisms which may cause pulmonary infection.

The minimal-leak inflation technique does not make it possible to obtain an accurate measurement of tidal volume; before this measurement is taken, the cuff must be fully inflated.

The *constant-leak* technique is one in which the cuff is deflated until a leak is detected during the inspiratory cycle. A clamp is then applied to prevent further deflation of the cuff. The constant-leak technique is used on patients being ventilated with volume ventilators. Also it may be possible with pressure ventilators which have terminal flow settings. This technique is useful when a tube has a cuff which is stiff (and is thus producing high intracuff pressures), but the tube cannot be immediately replaced. With constant-leak technique, it is important to check the patient's exhaled tidal volume frequently. A respirometer attached to the ventilator's exhalation manifold is used to obtain this measurement. Increases in the ventilator's volume or pressure may be necessary to compensate for air being leaked past the cuff. The constant-leak technique is helpful when indicated because it (a) minimizes lateral tracheal wall pressure; (b) enables some patients to talk with the leaked air; and (c) carries secretions out of the trachea on leaking air and thus prevents pooling of secretions above the cuff.

The physician's orders serve as a guide for the pattern of periodically deflating and reinflating the cuff of a tracheostomy tube. These orders should specify the frequency with which the cuff is to be deflated, the interval of time it should remain deflated, and the amount of air to be reinserted to inflate the cuff. The nurse records the time of inflation of the tube, the interval of deflation, and the amount of air reintroduced. Generally insertion of 2 to 10 ml. of air inflates the cuff and produces a seal without creating a hazardous amount of pressure. The amount of air necessary to inflate a cuffed tube properly varies with the stiffness of the cuff, the tracheostomy tube size, and the size of the patient's trachea. Smaller tracheostomy tubes require more air than do larger tracheostomy tubes. Usually a leak-free closed system is obtained by inflating the cuff with from 2 to 5 ml. of air.

The nurse assesses serially the amounts of air recorded as necessary to inflate the cuff. A pattern of *decrease* in the amounts necessary may indicate that the trachea's lumen is being decreased owing to swelling and edema. A pattern of *increase* may indicate air leaking around the tube or tracheal damage. Increasing amounts of air necessary in the cuff may also indicate overdistention of the trachea. This situation produces tracheal necrosis and eventually tracheal stenosis. *Significant changes in the amounts of air required to inflate the cuff should be reported.*

Sometimes orders are given for a patient's tracheostomy opening to be obstructed during periods of deflation. This may be ordered when it is desirable for the patient to begin to breathe again through the upper airway, e.g., in preparation for extubation.

According to some sources, cuffed tracheostomy tubes which do not have inner cannulas may be used for days without changing. Others state that tracheostomy tubes should be changed every other day. Some physicians prefer use of cuffs inflated only by inspiratory positive pressure from the respirator or double cuffs. Double cuffs alternate the site of inflation. By inflating and deflating each balloon at predetermined intervals, the sites of tracheal irritation and pressure are alternated.

*This procedure is recommended for use with the silver tube with the Mörch modification (swivel adaptor) and a narrow, double-walled, seamless, slip-on cuff.

CHAPTER 93

DISORDERS OF THE LARYNX

ANATOMY OF THE LARYNX

The larynx forms the upper extremity of the trachea. The entire *nerve supply* to the larynx is from the *vagus nerve*. Most of the *blood supply* to the larynx comes from the *superior and inferior laryngeal arteries*. The larynx is composed of several cartilages which are connected below with the trachea and above with the hypopharynx through a wide opening (Figure 93–1). The cartilages are held together with muscles and ligaments. The larynx lies in front of the 4th, 5th, and 6th cervical vertebrae in an adult and somewhat higher in children. In front of the larynx the *thyroid cartilage* protrudes, forming what is commonly called the "Adam's apple." The *cricoid cartilage* lies just below the thyroid cartilage. The *hyoid bone* lies just above the thyroid cartilage,

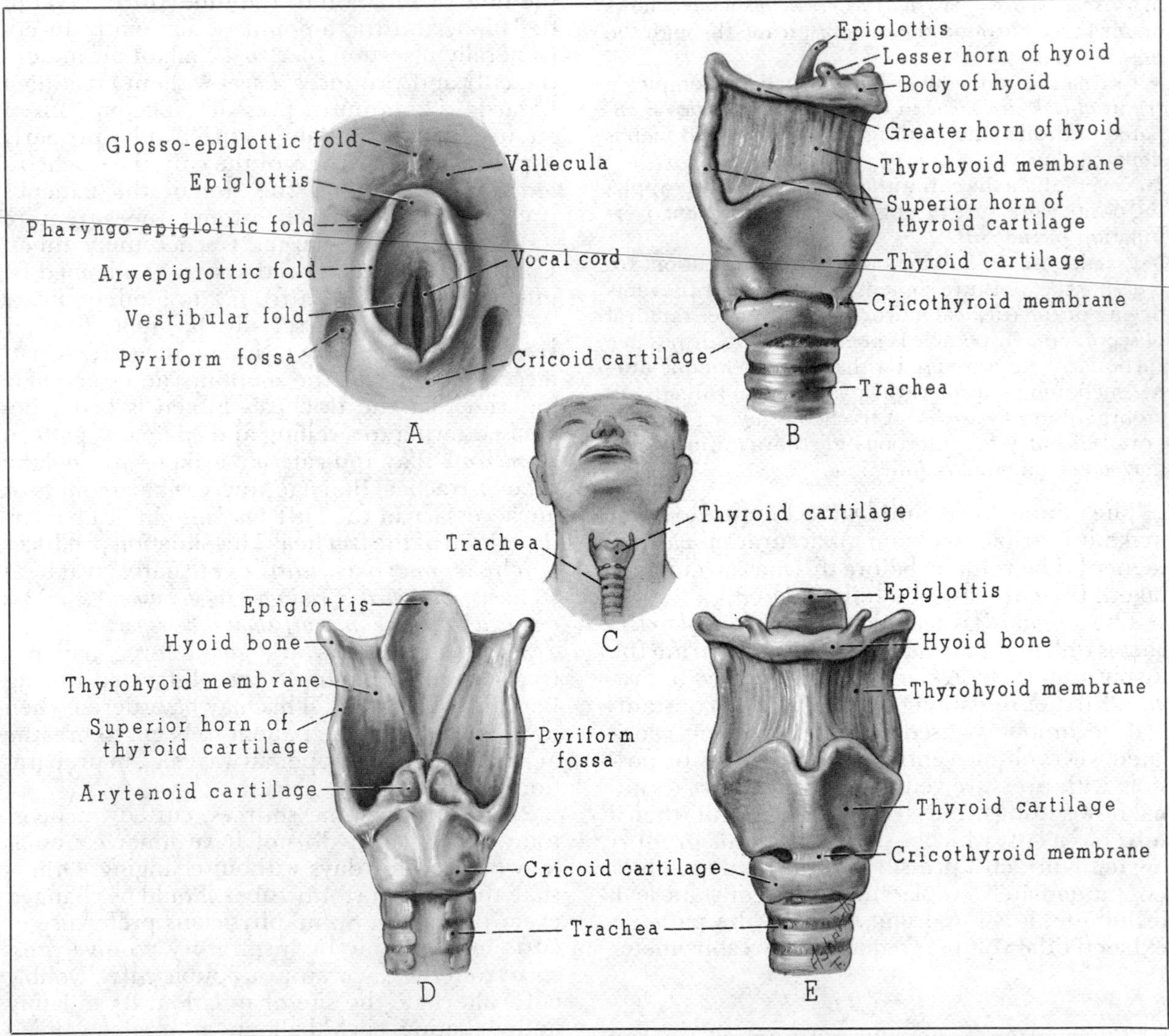

Figure 93–1. The larynx. (From Jacob. S. W., C. A. Francone, and W. J. Lossow: *Structure and Function in Man,* 4th ed. Philadelphia: W. B. Saunders Co., 1978.)

forming an attachment for the larynx and for the tongue and other muscles. The hyoid bone can be excised surgically if necessary without causing any great deformity or physiologic problems.

The cricoid cartilage articulates not only with the thyroid but also with *arytenoid cartilages.* The latter swing in and out, opening and closing the *glottis,* i.e., the space between the vocal cords. The *epiglottis* is a cartilaginous structure attached to the base of the tongue and the thyroid and arytenoid cartilages.

FUNCTIONS OF THE LARYNX

The chief function of the larynx is *not* that of producing speech sounds, i.e., *phonation,* but rather it is to act efficiently as an *airway* between the trachea and pharynx. While the trachea is merely a tube (the walls of which have ciliary action), the larynx is an organ with important *sphincteric actions* which help to (a) *prevent aspiration;* and (b) *increase intrathoracic pressure.* Aspiration is prevented during swallowing because the larynx closes tightly to keep food out of the trachea. Likewise the glottis closes if a foreign body drops in the throat. The *cough reflex* (called "watchdog of the lungs") is triggered whenever a foreign body touches the highly sensitive laryngeal mucosa. By increasing intrathoracic pressure, the larynx assists during straining efforts, e.g., coughing, lifting. The increased pressure gives added advantage to the use of the muscles of the shoulders and thorax. The vocal cords are adducted for coughing as well as for speech.

> Remember: *Following local anesthesia of the larynx, e.g., for laryngoscopy or bronchoscopy, the patient is not allowed to take anything orally for 2 to 3 hours because the person may aspirate through the anesthetized larynx.*

Commonly called the "voice box," the larynx creates sounds as a result of vocal cord vibrations. The sounds are then formed into speech patterns by the pharynx, palate, tongue, teeth, and lips. Thus, words are not actually formed in the larynx. During phonation numerous changes occur within and around the larynx. For example, (a) the larynx moves up and down, changing the length of the air columns above and below the larynx; (b) the edges of the vocal cords are relaxed and firmed; and (c) the length of the cords varies. The air column and vibrations are changed by these as well as other actions. As the vibrating column of air comes up from the larynx, the palate, tongue, and lips mold words.

EXAMINATION OF THE LARYNX

As part of a complete examination of the larynx, the neck is palpated externally, and the larynx is visualized internally, e.g., by direct or indirect laryngoscopy.

Direct Laryngoscopy. This is performed with a laryngoscope, i.e., a hollow, rigid metal tube lighted at its distal end. The patient is given a preoperative sedative, and food and fluids are withheld for a specified number of hours before the procedure to prevent regurgitation and possible aspiration. The patient's eyeglasses and dentures are removed, and the patient is transported to the operating room. Laryngoscopy may be performed with local or general anesthesia. While the patient lies motionless on the back, the laryngoscope is passed through the mouth and down to the larynx. The illuminated structures of the larynx are then directly observed. Minor surgical procedures may be performed through the laryngoscope, e.g., biopsy.

Following laryngoscopy the patient is allowed nothing to eat until the gag reflex returns. (The procedure by which the nurse tests the gag reflex is discussed in Unit X.) After the gag reflex returns, allow the patient to drink water first, since it is least damaging if accidentally aspirated. Following laryngoscopy the patient is drowsy or asleep because of the preoperative sedation. The nurse therefore provides safeguards as necessary, e.g., siderails, and provides a restful environment. The patient is observed for any of the following reportable symptoms during the postoperative period:

1. Apprehension (possibly due to bleeding or laryngeal edema).
2. Coughing or spitting blood or blood-tinged mucus.
3. Pain in the throat or chest.
4. Swelling in the throat and neck.

Nursing care following laryngoscopy is similar to that given following bronchoscopy. (See Chapter 52.)

Indirect Laryngoscopy. With this procedure the larynx is viewed in a laryngeal mirror; light is directed onto the mirror as it is held in the pharynx (Figure 93–2). To prevent unnecessary "gagging" during inspection of the larynx, the patient is approached calmly and gently. The patient sits *very* erect for the examination, with the chin drawn forward and both feet on the floor with knees drawn together. The tongue is protruded as far as possible and firmly grasped with a piece of gauze. A mirror (No. 5 for adults) is warmed over an alcohol lamp to prevent fogging, tested on the back of the examiner's hand for heat, and inserted with its back side against the tip of the uvula. The patient is told to breathe quietly through the mouth, or "pant like a dog" to prevent gagging. If indicated, biopsy can be performed via indirect laryngoscopy.

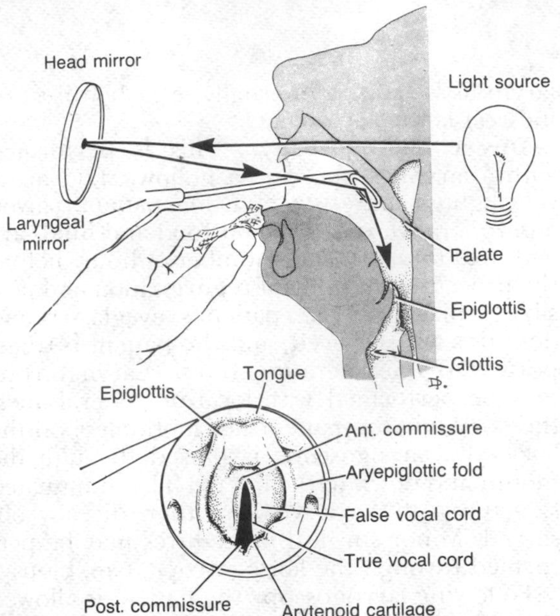

Figure 93–2. Indirect laryngoscopy. (From Hill, G. J., II: *Outpatient Surgery*, 2nd ed., Philadelphia: W. B. Saunders Co., 1980.)

The vocal cords are examined during quiet respiration and during phonation. Phonation causes adduction of the cords, and they can be seen to vibrate as sound is produced. Normally there is perfect approximation of the cords (Figure 93–3). In the aged, however, there is a small space which cannot be closed; thus older people may have quavering voices. With cord paralysis, the paralyzed cord (or cords) do not move.

SYMPTOMS OF LARYNGEAL DISORDERS

The larynx is easily examined. Thus, if a patient reports symptoms soon after they occur, an early diagnosis of laryngeal disorders is generally possible. Among the symptoms of laryngeal disease are:

▶ *Hoarseness:* the most important and most common symptom. Usually caused from improper approximation of the vocal cords, inflammation of the larynx, or laryngeal paralysis. *The larynx should be carefully inspected whenever a patient is hoarse longer than 2 weeks.*

▶ *Cough:* a common symptom of laryngeal disorders.

▶ *Dyspnea:* an ominous symptom indicative of severe airway obstruction. Slowly developing laryngeal obstruction is tolerated far better than an equally severe sudden obstruction. Unlike the patient with asthma, the patient with laryngeal dyspnea can expire air easily. However, inspiration is difficult. *Tracheotomy or passage of an endotracheal tube may be necessary to restore the airway in the presence of dyspnea or stridor or both.*

▶ *Stridor* (harsh respiration): an ominous symptom. Stridor associated with laryngeal disorder is usually inspiratory.

> *Encourage patients with dyspnea and stridor to try to relax and breathe quietly. Use of narcotics and sedatives is dangerous.*

▶ *Dysphagia:* fairly uncommon symptom of laryngeal disorders. However, it may occur secondary to laryngeal inflammation or tumor obstruction. Tube feedings may be indicated.

▶ *Pain:* occurs occasionally as an early symptom of acute pharyngeal inflammatory disorders and as a late symptom of neoplasms. At times narcotics are indicated. Generally chronic laryngeal inflammtory disorders are not painful.

Laryngeal disorders are potentially serious because they may cause airway obstruction or constriction. *Symptoms of laryngeal obstruction* include dyspnea, stridor, cyanosis, and increased, ineffective inspiratory effort which produces retraction of soft tissues around the thoracic cage. *Sudden laryngeal obstruction* may result from trauma,

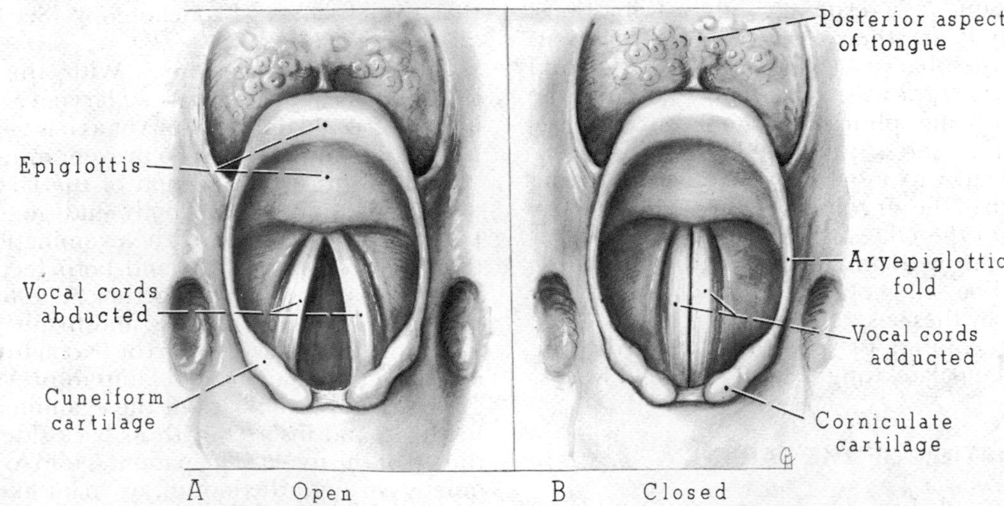

Figure 93–3. Superior view of vocal cords. (From Jacob, S. W., C. A. Francone, and W. J. Lossow: *Structure and Function in Man*, 4th ed. Philadelphia: W. B. Saunders Co., 1978.)

an allergic response in a hypersensitive individual, serious inflammatory diseases (scarlet fever, diphtheria), laryngeal edema, laryngeal spasm, or aspiration of a foreign body. In these conditions emergency treatment (e.g., endotracheal intubation or tracheotomy) may be necessary to save the patient's life.

LARYNGEAL SPASM

Occasionally following use of some general anesthetics, a spasm of laryngeal muscle tissue may occur, seriously jeopardizing the airway. Patients with low blood calcium levels also occasionally develop muscle tetany, which causes not only laryngeal spasm but also other skeletal muscle hyperirritability and spasm. In an attempt to relieve laryngeal muscle spasm, calcium chloride or calcium gluconate is given intravenously.

LARYNGEAL EDEMA

Because the larynx is a rigid structure, the airway size is reduced if edema occurs within the larynx (or glottis). *Acute* laryngeal edema requires immediate restoration of the airway. An endotracheal tube or tracheotomy may be necessary. Laryngeal edema is a potential medical emergency in the following disorders: anaphylaxis (i.e., angioneurotic edema); urticaria; acute laryngitis; direct injury to the larynx during surgery or intubation; and serious inflammatory conditions of the throat, such as erysipelas and scarlet fever. If laryngeal edema is caused by an allergic reaction, treatment may include (a) local application of ice to the neck; (b) administration of an adrenal corticosteroid; or (c) epinephrine (Adrenaline), 1:1000 subcutaneously (see also Unit V, Chapter 11).

Chronic laryngeal edema is usually less of a medical emergency because the patient has adjusted somewhat to the breathing disorder. Tracheotomy may be necessary, however. Chronic laryngeal edema may result from irradiation treatment of the larynx, tumors of the neck, and infections obstructing the laryngeal lymphatics. In the presence of laryngeal edema, the larynx may be sprayed with vasoconstrictors and steroids prior to tracheal intubation. This procedure, in addition to the use of systemic steroids, may alleviate the need for tracheotomy.[85]

LARYNGEAL PARALYSIS

Generally laryngeal paralyses result from peripheral disorders, but they occasionally can also result from central nervous system disorders. Complete laryngeal paralysis rarely occurs. Among the peripheral causes of laryngeal paralysis are aortic aneurysm, mitral stenosis, carcinoma of the thyroid gland, neck injuries, tuberculosis, tumors (e.g., of bronchi, lungs, mediastinum), metallic poisons (lead), and infectious diseases (diphtheria). Trauma during thyroidectomy is one of the most common causes of laryngeal paralysis. These disorders cause paralysis by affecting the recurrent laryngeal nerve in a variety of ways (it may be stretched, eroded, crushed, or cut).

Either one or both vocal cords may be paralyzed. If only one cord is affected, the airway is adequate and the patient's only symptom may be hoarseness (sometimes not even this is present). With bilateral paralysis, the voice is weak (though adequate), and a poor airway causes incapacitating dyspnea and stridor upon exertion. If the paralyzed cords are bilaterally adducted, an emergency tracheotomy may be necessary. Numerous types of surgical procedures exist to open the glottis. One transoral procedure is called an *arytenoidectomy,* in which one or both arytenoid cartilages are removed and the vocal cord(s) held in an open position.

LARYNGEAL INJURY

The larynx is seldom injured even though it appears to be relatively unprotected. Occasionally, however, fracture of the thyroid cartilage occurs, causing the mucosa and other soft tissues inside the larynx to be torn or causing hematoma formation. A tracheotomy may be necessary as a result of such airway damage. Before tracheotomy the patient may appear cyanotic, have a tender, swollen, and ecchymotic neck, and have stridor. Subcutaneous emphysema may contribute to the swelling.

By themselves, tracheobronchial cartilages cannot effectively maintain the normal caliber of airways within the thorax. Such normal caliber is mainly dependent upon elastic fibers in the lungs which are kept stretched by the chest wall's elastic ability to expand. While these forces act within the thorax to maintain adequate tracheobronchial lumina, at the upper end of the airway an adequate tracheal lumen is maintained only by attachment of the trachea to the cricoid cartilage. This cartilage forms the only complete circle in the lower airway. Dangerous *tracheal stenosis* thus typically follows injury of the cricoid.[85]

Laryngeal (and tracheal) trauma may result from a patient's neck striking the steering wheel during an automobile accident. Severe trauma which completely cuts off the airway rapidly causes death unless tracheotomy is performed immediately. If the patient survives after tracheotomy, the larynx and tracheal airway must be surgically restored. In addition to fracture of the larynx, other laryngeal injuries include those resulting from inhalation of hot gases or the aspiration of caustic liquids.

LARYNGITIS

Acute laryngitis is a common laryngeal disorder which may occur (a) as an isolated infection involving only the vocal cords; (b) as part of a general upper respiratory infection; or (c) as a result of vocal abuse. No infection is present in the last-named condition. Hoarseness is the main symptom of acute laryngitis and may progress to aphonia, i.e., complete voice loss. Other possible symptoms are cough, pain, and rough or tickling feelings in the throat. Patients with severe, acute laryngitis may develop stridor or dyspnea as a result of massive laryngeal edema. Hospitalization, even tracheotomy, may be necessary. Patients with laryngitis are advised not to smoke. Those with persistent cough, stridor, or fever are treated with steam or aerosol therapy, voice rest, and antibiotics if infection is present. Pain may be relieved with throat lozenges containing a topical anesthetic.

Chronic laryngitis refers to long-term inflammatory changes in laryngeal mucosa. Among the many causes of chronic laryngitis and factors contributing to this condition are constant use or misuse of the voice, repeated episodes of acute laryngitis, smoking, syphilis of the larynx, alcohol consumption, laryngeal tuberculosis (associated with far-advanced pulmonary tuberculosis), and allergic and hypometabolic states. Persons with chronic laryngitis should always have a laryngoscopic examination performed to rule out possible cancer of the larynx.

The main symptom of chronic laryngitis is hoarseness. Other symptoms are frequent cough; voice fatigue; and a tired, aching throat. Pain is usually only minimal or absent. When possible, treatment focuses on removing the cause. Treatment of chronic laryngitis is far more difficult than treatment of acute laryngitis. Often the cause is difficult to identify. Additionally, with chronic laryngitis tissue changes may be irreversible, and the causes of the disorder may be difficult to remove. Effective treatment measures include inhalation of unmedicated steam, stopping smoking, and *total* temporary voice rest (in which the patient does not speak at all). However, often patients who smoke will not stop, and total voice rest is difficult to maintain. Explain the term "voice rest" to the patient. Tell the person it is important not to talk or even whisper for a while. Give the patient a writing pad and pencil or magic slate for communication and a tap bell for attracting attention.

Relying on writing and hand signals for communication is difficult for many patients. Nurses can help patients who must maintain complete voice rest if they (a) post a sign clearly on the bed stating the patient is to rest his or her voice and not speak; (b) keep other means of communication close at hand for the patient; (c) instruct the patient's significant others about the need for voice rest and ways in which they can help the patient not to speak; and (d) anticipate the patient's needs.

CANCER OF THE LARYNX

"For thousands of years, man died as a result of cancer of the larynx and because of other laryngeal disorders and injuries. Today, the well-informed layman has some knowledge of the importance of the larynx in terms of its functions as a valve to protect the lungs and as a means of communication, but he is not always well enough informed to save his life or at best his voice from the ravages of cancer. We use the term *he* on purpose, for approximately ten men to one woman will have cancer of the larynx."[110]

Benign as well as malignant tumors of the larynx occur. As with carcinoma anywhere in the body, *early recognition is the key to the successful treatment of cancer of the larynx.* The longer the cancer remains undetected and untreated, the more radical surgical treatment needs to be and the greater the possibility of treatment failure. Radical surgery on the larynx (total laryngectomy) results in loss of important functions, e.g., loss of the ability to talk and breathe normally. (The effects of total laryngectomy are discussed more completely later in this chapter.) Important improvements have been made in the surgical treatment of cancer of the larynx, however. Today, if cancer of the larynx is recognized early, the patient has an excellent chance for being cured by surgery and for retaining a good residual voice.

Cancer of the larynx is the most common upper respiratory malignancy; cancer of the tonsil is the second most common. Most laryngeal malignancies are squamous cell carcinomas. In 1977 (in the United States) an estimated 9000 new cases of cancer of the larynx were predicted to occur and 3350 deaths were estimated from this cancer.[89] (8000 cases were predicted to occur in men and only 1000 in women.)

Approximately 30,000 persons with laryngectomies (sometimes called "laryngectomees") live in the United States. Predisposing factors in cancer of the larynx are irritants, e.g., alcohol, cigarette smoke, and other noxious fumes. Three of four patients with cancer of the larynx are smokers. Relationships appear to exist between cancer of the larynx and a familial predisposition to cancer. The condition also appears to occur more often in persons who have chronic laryngitis or frequently abuse their voices.

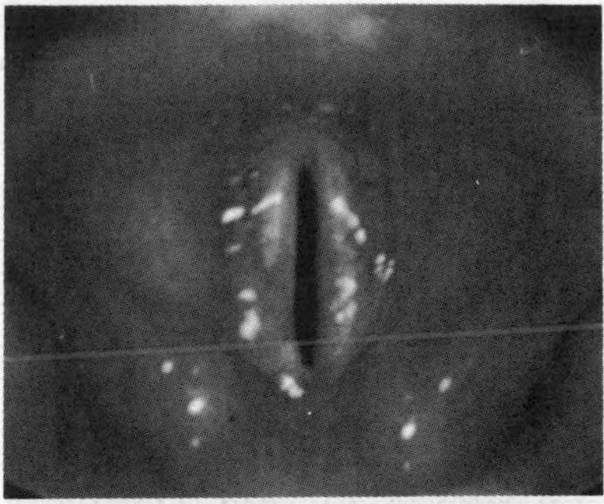

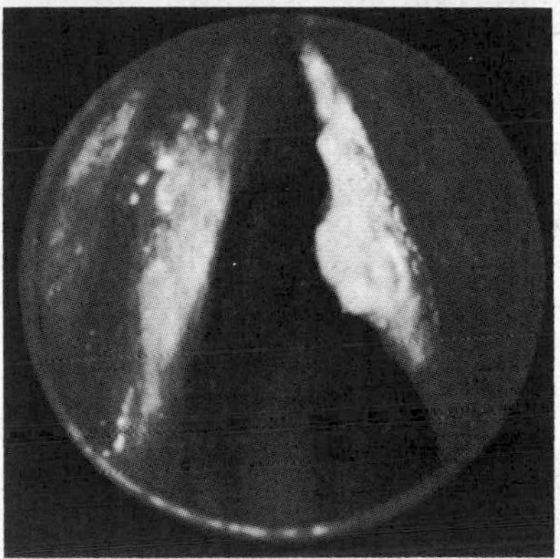

Figure 93–4. **A.** View in the laryngeal mirror of a normal larynx during phonation of "eee." Vocal cord edge vibrations are detected even in this 1/100 second exposure time. **B.** Cancer of the larynx, which began as painless, slowly progressive hoarseness without other symptoms. (From Holinger, P. H.: Why worry about hoarseness? *Consultant,* 16:21, Aug. 1976.)

Cancer of the larynx most often occurs in white males, at about age 60.

Cancer may develop within the larynx on the true vocal cord (intrinsic cancer) or in some other part of the larynx (extrinsic cancer).

Intrinsic cancer produces hoarseness very early; thus early diagnosis can be made if the patient promptly consults a physician and has the larynx examined.

> *With early treatment the prognosis for intrinsic cancer of the larynx is very good, and the treatment is not seriously disabling.*

Hoarseness occurs with tumors of the true cords because accurate approximation of the cords during phonation is not possible owing to the space-occupying tumor.

In contrast to intrinsic cancer of the larynx, *tumors of the extrinsic larynx do not produce early symptoms.* One of the first symptoms of extrinsic cancer of the larynx is pain and burning of the throat when drinking hot liquids, orange juice, and so forth. A lump in the neck is another symptom due to metastasis. Late symptoms include dysphagia (difficulty swallowing), dyspnea, hoarseness, muffled voice, weight loss, general debility, and foul breath. Other symptoms of cancer of the larynx are cough and expectoration of blood.

If the cancer involves only the vocal cords, it grows slowly and metastasizes slowly (because of the area's paucity of lymph vessels). However, if the cancer involves other portions of the larynx, it typically grows and metastasizes rapidly. *Symptoms indicative of metastasis* include dysphagia and the sensation of a "lump" in the throat, dyspnea, cough, enlarged cervical lymph nodes, and pain radiating to the ear.

Cancer of the larynx is most easily *diagnosed* by mirror (indirect) laryngoscopy. Direct laryngoscopy may also be performed. A biopsy may be obtained by either method. Biopsy is performed with either local or general anesthesia. Staining the larynx with 2 per cent toluidine blue dye helps pinpoint the most likely area for a positive biopsy in early carcinoma. Carcinoma in situ takes up the dye which is applied to the larynx through a direct laryngoscope with fiberoptic illumination.

Other diagnostic procedures which may be employed include special roentgenographic techniques to help define the tumor's borders; e.g., after the larynx is cocainized, a radiopaque dye, such as Lipiodol, is instilled and an x-ray is taken. X-ray examination by tomography and routine barium esophagograms may also be helpful. Once a physician has determined the precise area of involvement, he or she recommends the form of treatment that seems likely to be most effective for the particular patient, i.e., surgery or irradiation.

In *early intrinsic* cancer of the larynx, the cure rate is about the same whether the patient is treated surgically by partial laryngectomy or receives irradiation therapy. Surgery is usually the more effective treatment in more advanced cancer, e.g., with extrinsic involvement, neck involvement by metastases, and so forth. Preoperative irradiation may slightly increase cure rates in surgery for laryngeal cancer.[11]

Some cancers of the head and neck are too advanced for surgical therapy. Persons with these cancers may be treated palliatively by procedures such as intra-arterial infusion with methotrexate or vinblastine, followed by deep x-ray therapy. Soft lesions respond more readily to such treatment than do lesions involving bone.[39]

Surgical Treatment of Cancer of the Larynx

Basically there are three types of operations for carcinoma of the larynx. These are briefly summarized below. Many variations of these basic procedures are performed.

▶ *Partial laryngectomy:* useful in early, intrinsic lesions, e.g., a lesion on the true cord on one side may be excised along with a wide margin of normal tissue. Following surgery the patient is still able to talk and has a normal airway. Sometimes a *hemilaryngectomy* is performed, i.e., half of the thyroid cartilage is excised along with the soft tissue on the inside of the larynx. Some of the simpler partial laryngectomy procedures are *laryngofissure* or *thyrotomy,* in which the thyroid cartilage is split in the midline (to gain access to the interior of the larynx), and then the tumor-bearing portion is removed and the larynx closed.

▶ *Conservation laryngectomy:* useful in selected extrinsic tumors. Enough of the larynx remains to function, but the diseased part is removed and a *radical neck dissection* may be performed on the involved side. Broadly speaking, a "radical neck dissection" means the surgical dissection and removal of lymph nodes and tissues adjacent to the larynx.

▶ *Total laryngectomy:* the best known operation related to cancer of the larynx. (See Fig. 93–5.) Necessary with far-advanced lesions; contraindicated in patients with distant metastases and in persons with unresectable local lesions. Along with the entire larynx, the hyoid bone, pre-epiglottic space, strap muscles, and one or more tracheal rings are removed. A total laryngectomy deprives the patient of two important factors necessary for speech: (1) a motor mechanism to blow a blast of air; and (2) a vibratory mechanism to vibrate the air wave into a sound wave. After the necessary excision of tissue is made, the trachea's pharyngeal opening is closed, and the distal portion of the trachea is formed into a *permanent tracheostomy.* The latter opening becomes the patient's permanent airway. A *radical neck dissection* may also be performed. The effects of total

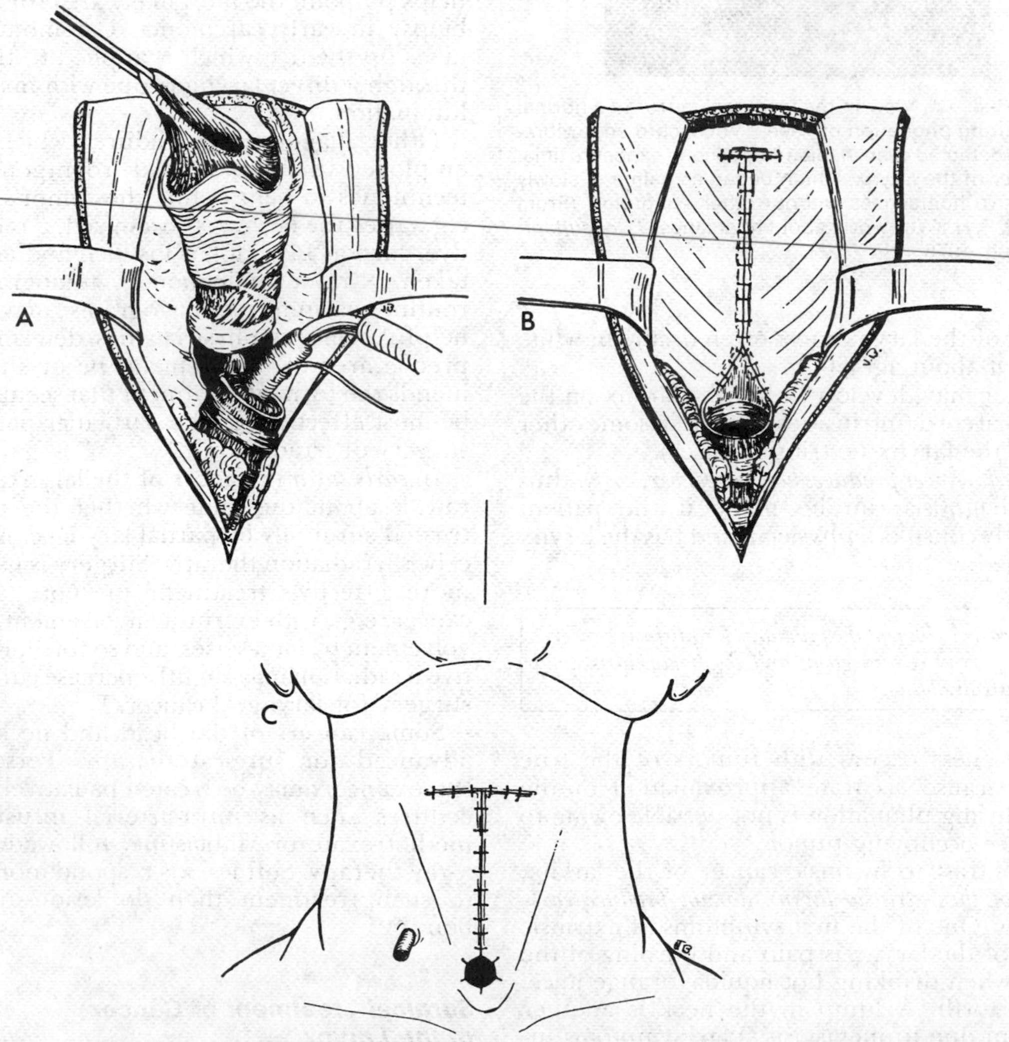

Figure 93–5. Total laryngectomy. **A.** Usually one or two tracheal rings and hyoid bone are included with specimen. **B.** Mucous membrane and muscles of pharynx are closed in layers. **C.** Tracheostomy—trachea is sutured to skin. (From DeWeese, D. D., and W. H. Saunders: *Textbook of Otolaryngology.* 5th ed. St. Louis: The C. V. Mosby Co., 1977.)

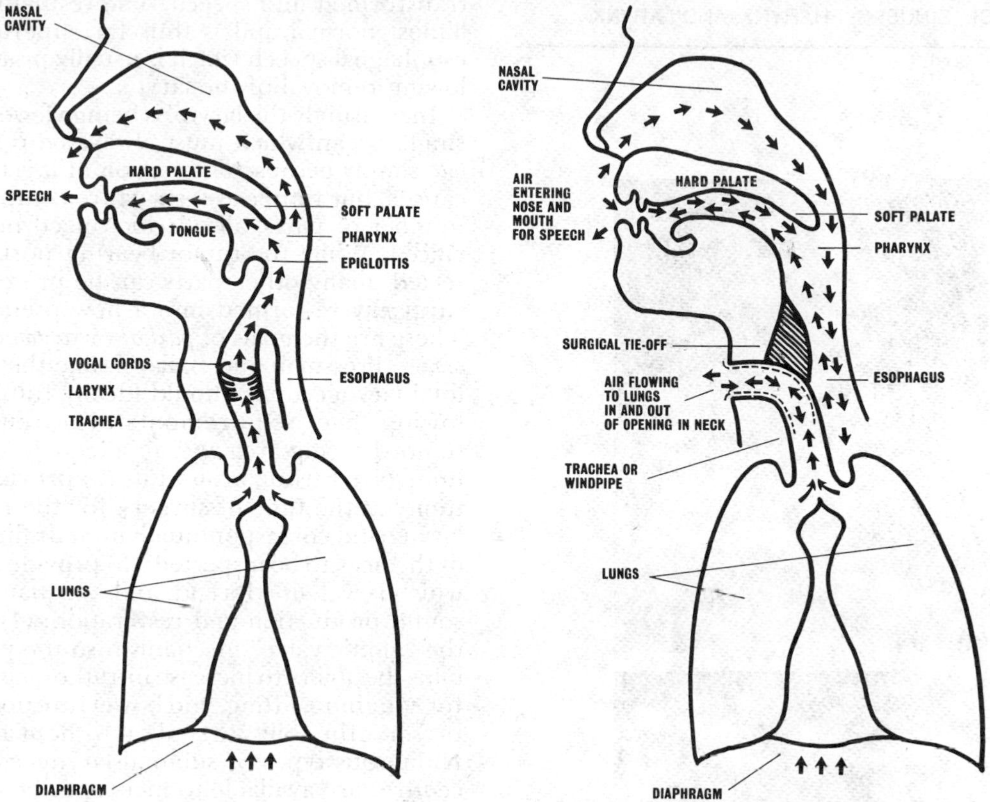

Figure 93–6. **A.** Physiology of respiration and speech in a person with normal anatomic laryngeal structures. **B.** The effect of laryngectomy on the physiology of respiration and speech. (Courtesy of American Cancer Society, Inc.)

laryngectomy on the physiology of respiration and speech are pictured in Figure 93–6.

Let us briefly explain more completely what a *radical neck dissection* is and why this surgical procedure is performed. When cancer is believed to have spread to the lymph nodes of the neck, all removable structures of the involved side of the neck (or both sides) are surgically excised. A radical neck dissection may be performed on the same side as the cancer, even though lymph nodes are not palpable and metastases cannot definitely be proved. This is done because as many as 35 per cent of patients with cancer of the larynx have had cervical lymph node metastases. When a total laryngectomy is performed with a radical neck dissection, in addition to removing the larynx and attached ribbon muscles, other structures may be removed, e.g., the sternocleidomastoid and omohyoid muscles; the muscles of the floor of the mouth together with the stylohyoid and digastric muscles; the submaxillary gland; sometimes the ipsilateral (same side) half of the thyroid gland; the parathyroid glands of the affected side; the fat pad of the posterior triangle of the neck; the internal jugular vein and some of its branches; the external carotid artery and some of its branches; and the deep cervical chain of lymph nodes together with their lymphatic channels. (See Fig. 93–7.)

Following radical neck dissection, patients may experience paralysis of the trapezius muscle, shoulder pain, and sensory loss in a large area of the shoulder and into the chest and back. The loss of muscle function is due to loss of the spinal accessory nerve (CN XI) and results in considerable loss of strength in the ipsilateral shoulder. When postoperative sensory loss occurs, it is important for the patient to be taught appropriate safety measures to prevent accidental trauma to the "numb" area, e.g., cutting while shaving. Occasionally the phrenic nerve is injured during radical neck surgery, producing paralysis of the hemidiaphragm. Often people with laryngectomies with accompanying radical neck dissections have more difficulty learning esophageal speech than those people with laryngectomies who did not require radical neck dissection.[53]

During laryngeal surgery it is essential for an adequate airway to be maintained. If endotracheal intubation is not possible, a tracheotomy is performed preoperatively so the anesthetist can intubate the patient through the stoma.

Following standard widefield laryngectomy the continuity between the oral cavity and upper esophagus is re-established. Tube feeding is maintained until suture lines have healed. In extended laryngectomy with cervical esophagectomy, reconstruction may require multiple staged procedures necessitating prolonged tube feeding.

Surgical research is constantly attempting to

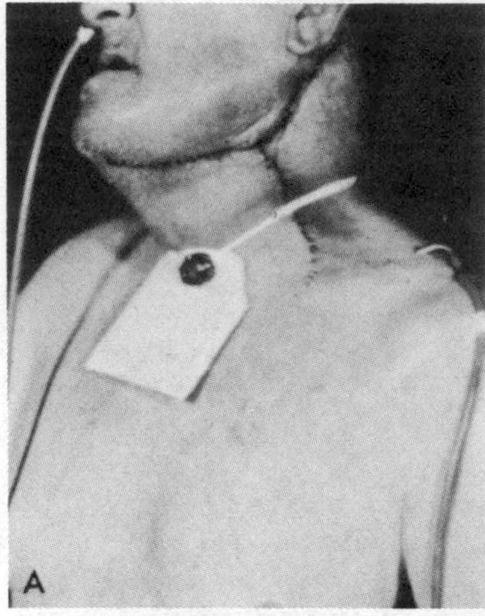

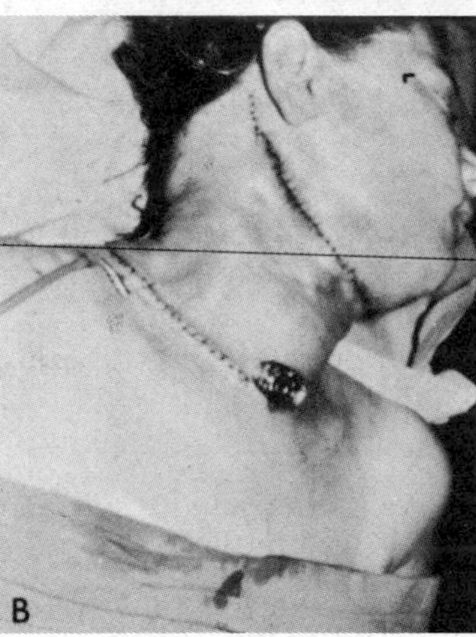

Figure 93–7. **A.** Postoperative appearance following radical neck dissection. Note suction catheter, feeding tube, tracheostomy. **B.** Postoperative appearance following radical neck dissection for metastasis from a primary tongue cancer. Note suction catheter and tracheostomy. (From McConnell, E. A.: How to truly help the patient with a radical neck dissection. *Nursing 76,* 6:58, Nov. 1976.)

perfect operations for cancer of the larynx which permit more nearly normal speech than is possible following total laryngectomy. One new type of *total laryngectomy with laryngoplasty* has been developed which enables vocal rehabilitation of the laryngectomized patient. The procedure is a delicate three-stage operation called the *Asai operation* (named for the surgeon who developed the surgery).[108] Basically in this procedure a dermal tube is constructed from the upper end of the trachea into the hypopharynx. By closing the lower tracheal fistula (i.e., the permanent tracheostomy opening) with a finger, the patient can expire air up the dermal tube and into the pharyngeal cavity. The sound produced there is transformed into speech. The resultant voice is almost normal and is thus far superior to the esophageal speech which is usually practiced following removal of the larynx.

Increasingly the larynx is being viewed not as a single organ which must always be removed *in toto* simply because one section of it is the site of cancer, but rather as a structure composed of a number of parts, all of which need not be sacrificed. While the tumor-bearing portion is resected, many other parts can be preserved and surgically re-formed into a new pseudolarynx. These are the goals of *partial* or *subtotal laryngectomies*. Pressman and Bailey[84] state that any subtotal laryngectomy should ideally fulfill the following five requirements: (1) remove the tumor-bearing area and an adequate margin of uninvolved tissue around it; (2) provide opportunity at the time of surgery for the remaining larynx and corresponding lymph drainage areas of the neck to be inspected; (3) provide an airway which is well lined, rigid, and adequate for both sound production and respiration; (4) preserve the "glottic valve" mechanism so the patient retains the ability to increase intrathoracic pressure for coughing, lifting, and bowel function; and (5) preserve the ability to swallow without aspiration. Numerous types of subtotal laryngectomy procedures are available to meet specific purposes.

Previously it was thought that subtotal laryngectomy procedures should always be limited to small unilateral carcinomas. More recently, however, some surgeons have been able to resect large tumors involving both sides of the larynx and leave sufficient parts of the larynx which can be reconstructed, resulting in adequate voices and adequate respiratory exchange. Significant surgical advances are being made, and many patients previously considered as requiring total laryngectomy have been spared the disability of loss of the normal airway by less radical but more sophisticated techniques. These accomplishments are being made without lessening the cure rate.

Some *postoperative complications* which may follow partial or total laryngectomies are (a) *fistula formation,* between the reconstructed hypopharynx and the skin; (b) *infection*, particularly in the postradiation and/or debilitated patient; (c) *carotid artery rupture* (occurs most often in patients who have had radical neck surgery or preoperative radiation therapy); and (d) *stenosis of the tracheostomy* (occurs weeks or months after surgery). The use of wound suction under the skin flaps postoperatively tends to prevent fistula formation. If they occur, fistulas are usually left to close by themselves, but a few are closed surgically. In the event of carotid artery hemorrhage, attempt to stop the bleeding by compressing the neck wound, suction as necessary, and get help *at once* so the patient can immediately be taken to surgery for carotid ligation. An immediate transfusion is given, and attempts are made to maintain blood pressure. This is vitally important so the remaining carotid artery has a maximal chance of perfusing the brain. Stoma stenosis may result from a fistula, fibrosis, or infection. Stenosis of the tracheostomy may be treated surgically (the opening is enlarged) or by fitting the patient with successively larger tracheostomy tubes (eventually a large one is left in place for many months or perhaps permanently).

Other possible complications are *atelectasis* and *pneumonia.* These complications can be warded off by careful nursing care during the immediate postoperative period and the first few postoperative days, e.g., suctioning, humidification, positioning, tracheostomy care.

Surgery on the larynx may be performed under general or local anesthesia.

PREOPERATIVE PREPARATION FOR TOTAL LARYNGECTOMY*

Total laryngectomy is a radical surgical procedure—one which is naturally difficult for a patient to accept. Psychologic care of the patient with cancer of the larynx is therefore an important aspect of total care. Pause to think for a moment about the many anxieties and fears which the patient may have when thinking about the forthcoming surgery, e.g., possible suffocation, choking, death, mutilation, recurrence of cancer, inability to speak or work, rejection by friends and loved ones. The patient, the people in the household, and friends all need the skilled emotional support and teaching that a nurse can offer during the preoperative period and throughout the patient's hospitalization. An excellent nurse is particularly careful to provide opportunities for the patient to discuss concerns during the preoperative period. Such a nurse realizes that it is especially important that this be accomplished *before* surgery, since it will be several weeks following surgery until the patient can learn to communicate verbally once again.

During the preoperative period the physician discusses with the patient what the postoperative results are expected to be, and the nurse discusses with the patient what will happen during the immediate postoperative period, e.g., suctioning, care of the laryngectomy tube, feeding methods, vital sign measurements. When appropriate, significant others should be included in the preoperative teaching sessions. Both physician and nurse attempt before surgery to give the patient a realistic description of the sensations and apprehensions which the patient will experience upon awakening from anesthesia. Reassurance is also given at this time concerning the patient's safety. *Plentiful reassurance is one of the most necessary components of total care for the patient hospitalized for laryngectomy.*

It is important that the nurse and physician first discuss *together* what the results are expected to be following a patient's surgery. This is especially important when the larynx is going to be operated upon, since there are numerous surgical procedures producing various results. Obviously physician and nurse should both be describing the same expected results or the patient will be confused and frightened. For example, you would certainly not want to tell a patient that he or she will not be able to speak after surgery if this is not true.

If a *total* laryngectomy is to be performed, the physician tells the patient that the surgery will cause loss of (a) normal speech (since the larynx is completely removed); (b) normal respiratory patterns through the nose and mouth; and (c) the ability to inspire and expire air through the nose and mouth. Be sure to tell patients about to have a laryngectomy how they will be able to breathe through a permanent tracheostomy and how they will learn to care for the tracheostomy alone when they are able. Patients are also informed that there are other methods of speech which they will be helped to learn, i.e., esophageal speech or the use of a mechanical or electrical device. (Speech therapy is discussed more completely later in this chapter.) If the surgeon expects to perform radical neck dissection, this surgery is discussed with the patient.

Often it is difficult for a lay person to understand the new physiologic relationships which will result after a total laryngectomy. The patient may be unable to comprehend all of what the physician explains and may ask the nurse for further clarification. It is therefore desirable for the nurse to be present when the physician talks preoperatively with the patient. As with any patient-education program, it is never assumed that patients *understand* what they have been told merely because they "were told." Follow-up discussions are planned to explore further questions or concerns which patients and their significant others may have about information given them by the physician or nurse.

Voice loss is referred to as a "temporary" voice loss when discussing it with patients and their significant others since the patient will learn new methods of speaking after surgery. Care is also taken not to discuss esophageal speech in terms which may be upsetting to some patients. For example the thought of "belching up air to speak with" may be disgusting to some persons.

Some physicians like to arrange for a person who has had a laryngectomy and who has been successfully rehabilitated to visit preoperatively patients who are about to have a laryngectomy performed. Other physicians do not follow this

* For a general discussion of preoperative care, refer to Unit VIII.

practice. Some patients gain courage from meeting a person who can speak with an esophageal voice and who has successfully survived the procedure they are about to have performed on them. On the other hand, other patients are frightened by such a visit and may even cancel surgery after seeing what a tracheostomy stoma is like and after hearing an esophageal voice. It is best, then, to discuss such a visit with the patient and the patient's physician before making arrangements. The physician may ask the nurse to arrange for a visitor to come from one of the clubs established for persons who have had laryngectomies, e.g., a "New Voice Club" or a "Lost Chord Club." Lost Chord Club members distribute literature pertinent to laryngectomies; descriptions of their services and activities may be obtained by writing to the International Association of Laryngectomees in care of the American Cancer Society, Inc.

Preoperatively some patients benefit by a visit from a speech therapist. The therapist may teach patients how to take air into the esophagus so they can practice this before surgery, while they still have a voice to ask questions of the therapist. Not all patients are able to begin speech rehabilitation before surgery. Some are too anxious to learn effectively at this time.

If postoperative tube feedings will be used, an explanation of this procedure is given to patients before surgery. Included is explanation of the fact that normal eating will be possible after removal of the tube. If tube feedings are used, they tend to be used for a much shorter interval of time now than formerly, perhaps only for a couple of days.

Be certain to establish with patients preoperatively a means by which they can communicate with staff members after surgery. Inform them that a call bell will always be available to them in addition to writing materials. If the patient cannot write, discuss nonverbal communication, e.g., hand signals. Tell the patient that a nurse will be present immediately following surgery and that the patient will not be left alone until quite able to care for himself or herself again.

Preoperatively antibiotics may be ordered to minimize the possibility of infection. Oral hygiene is also important at this time. (General preoperative care is discussed in Unit VIII.)

POSTOPERATIVE CARE FOLLOWING TOTAL LARYNGECTOMY*

Psychologic Care

"However vivid one's imagination, it is difficult to prepare for the impact of finding oneself entirely voiceless. Upon awakening, the postoperative laryngectomy patient is suddenly confronted with the utter impossibility of making himself heard—of being unable to cry for help. It can be a profoundly frightening feeling. . . . Immediately upon awakening from surgical anesthesia, the patient discovers just how isolated he is without the ability to speak. His new way of breathing "through a hole in the neck" may also be alarming since the sensation of breathing is lacking."[72]

A total laryngectomy causes numerous "losses" of normal physiologic abilities. Sometimes socioeconomic losses also occur. All these losses result in profound disturbances in body image. Men may associate loss of the larynx, i.e., "Adam's apple," with loss of masculinity. It is not unusual for loss of the larynx thus to be viewed by many as a form of castration. Loss of the voice means not only loss of a primary means of communicating thoughts but also loss of a highly individual characteristic. Human beings are recognized as individuals by others to a large extent by the personal qualities of their voices. Often we can identify whom we are listening to if we can hear the other person speak only one or two words. Also, vocal abilities help to express emotions, e.g., a curt tone of voice indicates impatience, while laughter is indicative of merriment. It is not unusual for a voice to be described as "sexy." Thus, loss of the voice may change an individual's sexual self-image and methods of sexual expression. A laryngectomy also causes loss of the normal means of breathing. Some patients are unable to continue with their presurgery means of employment following laryngectomy. In addition to losing the sense of smell, the person can often no longer blow his or her nose, blow air from the mouth, sip soup, suck on a straw, gargle, whistle, or lift heavy objects. (The larynx makes it possible to lift and hold heavy objects by acting as a fixator factor for the thorax.)

The personal impact of the losses associated with the radical surgery of a total laryngectomy vary from individual to individual. However, postoperatively the patient normally experiences grief over loss of self and depression of varying degrees. The period of depression is commonly most intense about the third or fourth postoperative day. Severe, prolonged depression is not a "normal" reaction. Persons caring for the patient are alert to indications of severe depression, and these symptoms are reported when observed. Remember that the severely depressed person may be suicidal. Professional skills are necessary in caring for the severely depressed patient, and psychiatric help may be helpful.

Women usually react with greater despondency than do men when threatened with removal of the larynx. Appearance may be so shocking postoperatively that some patients faint. Some women are embarrassed at the low pitch of esophageal speech.

Postoperatively, even though patients may know that the surgery was necessary, they may bitterly resent the bodily changes that have been surgically produced. It is not uncommon following total laryngectomy for a patient's moods to

* For a general discussion of postoperative care, see Unit VIII.

fluctuate from expressions of anger, bitterness, and fear to apathy, bewilderment, and depression. Significant others also experience a gamut of emotions as they witness the effects of surgery on their loved one. The excellent nurse draws on all resources available to provide skilled, effective emotional care during this period of psychologic suffering and intense feelings. *This is vital care.*

Because surgery on the larynx reduces or entirely removes a patient's ability to communicate orally (until new methods are learned or healing has taken place), *the patient requires constant attendance during the early postoperative period.* Life-threatening respiratory obstruction can rapidly develop. In addition to attentive nursing care (including frequent observations), the patient is given a tap bell and signal light to summon help and a magic slate or pad and pencil to write requests upon. *Remember not to start IVs in the arm the patient needs to use for writing.*

It is frustrating, tiresome, and time-consuming to patients to have to write out everything they wish to communicate. Naturally at times patients appear obviously upset, perhaps angry, because they cannot speak. If the nurse can anticipate many of a patient's needs, the person's frustrations due to the inability to speak can be greatly reduced. Try to make it easier for the patients by carefully reading their written statements. To protect the privacy of the patient's communications with you, be certain to destroy written notes in the person's presence before leaving the room. A magic slate reduces clutter and also helps to ensure privacy, since patients can erase statements whenever they wish.

Unknowingly, staff members and visitors may add to a postlaryngectomy patient's communication problems in various ways. For example, (a) they may raise the tone of their voices as if the patient were hard-of-hearing; (b) they may be tempted to complete sentences verbally which the patient has started to write out (it is best to let the patients complete their own thought); and (c) they may talk nervously and excessively because of their own discomfort with the patient's silence.[81]

Some patients cannot read and write, and thus, following total laryngectomy, they are unable to communicate by writing. These patients are even more completely prisoners of silence than are literate patients until they learn esophageal speech or another method of artificial speech. Nonverbal communication, e.g., hand and facial gestures, is their only means of communication, and therefore they need to be closely observed by nurses for indications of their needs.

If an intercom system exists between patient rooms and the nursing station, be certain to post a note on the control board to inform staff members that patients cannot use the intercom following total laryngectomy because they cannot speak.

Postoperatively all clinical care and procedures, e.g., suctioning, changing the laryngectomy tube, and so forth, are carefully explained to patients before care is started. This is helpful since such patients cannot speak to ask questions, and they may justifiably panic if they do not know what is going to be done.

Clinical Care. Immediately following surgery the patient is positioned on the side until consciousness is regained. Then, if the blood pressure is stable, the person's head is elevated 30 to 45 degrees to promote drainage, facilitate respirations, prevent uncomfortable strain on the suture lines, and minimize edema. When moving the patient about in bed or helping the person to sit up, be certain to support the back of the neck with both hands. This gives the person a feeling of security and prevents painful tension on the sutures. Also, particularly if a radical neck dissection has also been performed, the neck musculature has been severed and so some loss of control and support of the head has gone. (When patients begin to help themselves, teach them to support their own heads in this manner.) Initially patients are usually highly restless and anxious upon regaining consciousness. Positioning the patient with the head slightly flexed prevents tension on the suture line and possible wound dehiscence.

On return from surgery a tube may or may not be in the tracheostomy and the patient may or may not have a neck dressing. If a tube is in place in the tracheostomy, it is a *laryngeal or laryngectomy tube* or a *cuffed tracheostomy tube.* A laryngectomy tube is shorter and slightly larger in diameter than a tracheostomy tube; however, the tube care is the same for either tube (see Chapter 92).

Suctioning is discussed in detail in Unit XVI and in Chapter 92. Here we mention only a few points of importance in suctioning laryngectomized patients:

1. Suction nasally as well as through the tracheostomy, since the patient can no longer blow the nose (air can no longer be forced up through the nose to "blow" it).
2. Use a size 14 catheter for suctioning through a laryngectomy tube if one is in place.
3. Do not use the same catheter to suction the nose and trachea.
4. Suction the mouth gently.
5. Do not attempt deep suction through the nose or mouth without permission; you could accidentally penetrate the suture line.

Artificial humidification must be provided for the patient with a permanent tracheostomy (see Unit XVI).

In giving postoperative care following laryngectomy, the nurse gives tracheostomy care as indicated and also observes for *indications of postoperative complications,* e.g., respiratory distress (cyanosis, dyspnea), hemorrhage, hemoptysis, excessive coughing, symptoms of shock. Vital signs are checked every 15 minutes until stable. Observe for hemorrhage from the wound and from the tracheostomy tube. (General postoperative care is discussed in Unit VIII.)

Other nursing activities commonly performed during the early postoperative period following laryngectomy are (a) evaluation and recording of fluid intake and output; (b) regulation of *intravenous feedings* or administration of *tube feedings;* (c) administration of medications, such as analgesics, vitamins, and antibiotics (postoperative wound contamination and infection may easily occur); and (d) administration of *frequent oral hygiene.* Oral hygiene is given frequently to prevent infection and to keep the patient more comfortable. Apply Vaseline to the patient's lips if they are dry. If diarrhea occurs, the patient is carefully evaluated to prevent fluid and electrolyte imbalances (see Unit V, Chapter 12).

Following surgery, *drainage catheters* are usually inserted under the wound's skin flaps; they are then connected to *Gomco suction* or to a *Hemovac,* i.e., a small plastic device which creates its own suction. These drainage catheters are used to remove fluid from the potential dead space left after removal of the larynx and related structures. When wound suction is used, it is usually kept on constantly unless otherwise ordered; do not discontinue suction to measure contents without permission. Care is taken to maintain free drainage within the suction system. Drainage systems are potential sources of infection, since bacteria can ascend the tubes and get directly into the wounds. Drainage systems must therefore be handled so their contents remain sterile. Wound drainage catheters are usually removed on about the third postoperative day. Dressings may not be present if wound drainage catheters are being used. If the catheters are not used, *pressure dressings* may be present to minimize serous fluid accumulation or hematoma formation under the skin flaps. Following radical neck dissection, drains may be left in the wound and pressure dressings applied. Check the dressings frequently for drainage and be certain they are not excessively interfering with the patient's respirations.

Narcotics are used with caution in patients with head and neck surgery, since they depress respirations and inhibit coughing.

Fortunately laryngectomy typically does not produce severe postoperative *pain.* Minimal postoperative pain occurs following laryngectomy because sensory nerve endings are cut by the skin flap incisions. Analgesics, such as buffered aspirin or dextropropoxyphene (Darvon), are usually adequate to relieve discomfort. These medications can be dissolved in water and given via the feeding tube or per rectum if the patient cannot take them orally. Occasionally, small doses of opiates may be ordered. When they are given, watch carefully for indications of respiratory depression and immediately report such findings if they occur. Hypoventilation and hypotension should be avoided.

Pain does occur during the immediate postoperative period following laryngectomy when the patient attempts to swallow. Gentle oral suctioning and allowing the patient to expectorate saliva rather than swallowing it are measures which give relief during this period of painful swallowing. While incisional pain is minimal, the patient may have a headache or other discomfort, e.g., sore throat due to the presence of a nasogastric tube.

A *nasogastric tube* may or may not be present postoperatively for *tube feedings.* Maintain patency of the tube. Some patients are given intravenous nourishment until the third postoperative day; then they may be allowed oral nourishment. Other patients are given oral fluids as early as the first postoperative day. Still other patients have a nasogastric feeding tube for several days following total laryngectomy. Gastric suction may be ordered if tube feedings cause nausea.

Possible advantages of tube feedings are (a) reduction of possible incision contamination, (b) prevention of fistula formation by relieving the tension which swallowing places on the pharyngeal suture line, and (c) enhancement of the healing process by avoiding the muscular activity necessary for swallowing. As discussed earlier, in some patients the anterior wall of the esophagus is reconstructed at the time laryngectomy is performed (this portion of esophagus connects with the posterior wall of the larynx). In such a situation, postoperative tube feedings minimize the esophageal irritation which swallowed food causes.

If a nasogastric tube is used for very long, patients may be instructed how to pass a tube and feed themselves. This is done with the physician's approval postoperatively. Nasogastric tube feedings should never be performed when the patient is reclining or the formula will be regurgitated. During feedings the patient should be awake and sitting erect with the feet over the side of the bed. If the tube is not in place when the patient returns from surgery, the doctor passes the tube the first time (usually on the first postoperative day). A nurse should never attempt to reinsert a nasogastric tube following laryngeal surgery without the physician's permission, because of the potential danger of rupturing the internal suture line. Once a patient can safely swallow, the physician may allow the person to take sips of water. The nasogastric tube is removed once the patient is able to take oral nourishment satisfactorily.

Following laryngectomy the patient's first attempts to take liquids orally are carefully supervised. Initial attempts to swallow may cause a choking feeling and severe coughing. Water is given until the patient can confidently swallow, then other fluids may be introduced. The nurse remains calm as the patient learns to swallow and is prepared to suction as necessary, since coughing may raise secretions. Food inhalation is not possible orally following total laryngectomy because the food passage (esophagus) and breathing passage (trachea) are separate, i.e., the tracheal opening is sutured to the skin of the neck. If aspiration does occur or feedings return through the tracheostomy, then an internal fistula exists. This must be reported to the physician. Before oral feedings are started, the patient may be given some fluid to swallow which contains methylene blue dye if a fistula is suspected. Confirmation of a fistula usually means that tube feedings will be continued until the fistula is healed.

When the surgeon thinks it is advisable, the patient may begin to practice belching after oral feedings, e.g., an hour after eating. This is preliminary training for the explosive movement of air out of the esophagus which is necessary for esophageal speech.

Self-Care and Patient Teaching. *Self-care is started early in the postoperative course* following laryngectomy. As mentioned, if a nasogastric tube is in place, patients may be given instructions about how to give their own feedings as soon as they are able. On the first postoperative day patients are usually taught to suction the tracheostomy tube (be sure to provide a mirror). Normally patients are also helped to get up for a while on this day, since early ambulation assists rapid recovery. Within 4 to 5 days after surgery, patients are usually ambulatory as desired, able to feed and bathe themselves, and are not only suctioning the laryngectomy tube but also removing and cleaning the inner cannula if one is present. Much of the nurse's time with a patient during these first few postoperative days is spent in teaching the patient self-care and in supervising a patient's early attempts at performing nursing procedures.

Because a considerable amount of the patient's care centers on teaching, it is necessary to *have a detailed care plan to be certain all aspects of patient education are covered.* Typically it is not possible for the same nurse to conduct all the necessary teaching sessions with one patient. A care plan makes it possible for several nurses to participate in the teaching process without duplicating their efforts and without overlooking some areas which should be covered.

As patients begin to gain self-confidence following a laryngectomy, they can be left alone for gradually longer periods of time. *However, the call signal must always be answered immediately*, and nurses continue to make frequent "drop-in" visits so patients feel secure in the knowledge that they are being watched out for by concerned people. Praise is freely given to patients as they progress in the difficult readjustments necessary. Remembering that a patient's self-esteem and self-image are dealt a severe blow by surgery as radical as that of a laryngectomy, the excellent nurse utilizes every opportunity to show respect for the patient. If a speech therapist is visiting the patient, the nurse coordinates the plan of care with the goals of speech therapy.

Sometimes a patient's course of progress is slowed down by the development of an esophageal fistula during the postoperative period. This complication most often develops in those persons who have been treated with radiotherapy (see Unit IX).

Prior to *discharge* patients and persons who will be with them at home need detailed teaching about tracheostomy care and other aspects of care following surgery on the larynx. Humidification must be set up in the home before discharge. Air conditioning may provide air which is excessively cool or dry and thus is undesirable. Patients are instructed how to remove and replace the entire laryngectomy tube if one is still being worn. Generally suctioning is not necessary once patients are ready for discharge. However, an occasional patient may need to have a suction machine available at home. (The local chapter of the American Cancer Society may help the patient obtain a suction machine.)

To insert a laryngectomy tube the patient breathes in, holds the breath, inserts the tube, and then resumes normal breathing. Tell the patient not to hyperextend the neck when inserting the tube, since this is not helpful but will instead cause the stoma to become smaller. The laryngectomy tube is cleaned in a manner similar to cleaning a tracheostomy tube (see Chapter 92). The tube is cleaned at least once daily.

While an occasional patient needs to wear a laryngectomy tube permanently, most patients wear one only for the first 3 to 8 postoperative weeks until the stoma has permanently formed. A few patients are advised to wear the tube part of the time, e.g., at night if the stoma tends to collapse or does not provide adequate air exchange during sleeping.

Patients are taught precautions which must be taken to prevent accidental cutting of the neck and to prevent aspiration through the tracheostomy stoma. Caution is necessary when shaving because it takes about 6 months for the sensory nerve endings which were cut at the time of surgery to regenerate. Accidental cutting can easily occur during this interval. Precautions necessary with a permanent tracheostomy were discussed in Chapter 92.

Before returning home, patients must be given appropriate *dietary instructions*. Usually the diet progresses from liquid to soft to general. Muscular tonus is important for esophageal speech. Often the entire muscular mechanism, necessary for esophageal speech, is weak and flaccid because of the soft and liquid foods which the patient's diet has been limited to before, during, and sometimes even after hospitalization. Some speech therapists will not begin to teach a person esophageal speech until he or she is on a full and normal diet. While observing necessary dietary restrictions (as ordered by the physician), it is important as soon as possible for the patient to chew and swallow a normal diet so the throat and abdominal musculature will regain tonus. Desirable foods from this standpoint include raw vegetables, rough dry cereals, raisins, peanuts, and not-too-tender meats cut in moderately small pieces.

Rehabilitation. Every attempt is made to minimize feelings of difference and to help the person reestablish a normal life pattern. Significant others are counseled not to treat the patient as an invalid and never to apologize to others for the patient's condition. Expressions of embarrassment accentuate differences, place the patient in the role of an invalid, and tend to foster reclusive and depressive tendencies.

It is desirable for the patient to return to employment as soon as possible, even before esophageal speech is fully mastered. Steady employment is one of the strongest motivations for regaining speech and as such is important in speech rehabilitation as well as total rehabilitation. Following total laryngectomy a patient is often able to return to work within 4 to 8 weeks after hospitalization.

Occasionally it is necessary for a patient to make an occupational change following laryngectomy, e.g., if previous employment is highly voice-dependent or is in a dusty environment. However, often patients are able to continue with their presurgery type of employment. Some patients manage quite well, even in sales positions which require a lot of talking.

Rehabilitation is the rule rather than the exception following laryngectomy. However, in spite of the generally good prospects for rehabilitation, some patients fail to regain a good occupational or social adjustment, or the adjustment is delayed many months.

Before hospital discharge the person is informed of rehabilitative agencies which are available to help. The *International Association of Laryngectomees* (IAL) is an autonomous agency, supported by the American Cancer Society, which has about 175 member clubs in the U.S. and various parts of the world. The IAL focuses on both social and educational aspects of cancer of the larynx. Bimonthly the *IAL News* is printed and distributed free of charge to more than 18,000 persons in 55 countries. While local *Lost Chord Clubs* and *New Voice Clubs* are now often affiliated with the IAL, they also continue to maintain their local autonomy and service to "laryngectomees." The IAL publishes a "Directory of Sources of Supply for Items of Benefit to Laryngectomees." This directory lists such items as tracheostomy equipment, humidifiers, artificial larynxes, amplifiers for weak voices, films, exhibits, publications, and emergency instructions.

Other rehabilitation resources in the community which the patient should be made aware of are (a) a local or regional branch of the *American Cancer Society;* (b) a local, regional, or state university or college with a speech and hearing center; (c) the *American Speech and Hearing Association;* and (d) the state office of vocational rehabilitation (helpful when a change of occupation is necessary). The American Speech and Hearing Association publishes a booklet listing persons especially qualified to teach esophageal speech. This association is active in speech research, therapy, and education.

Before discharge the person is given an identification card which states that he or she has no vocal cords and also gives information for *artificial respiration* if needed. Because the person breathes through a tracheostomy rather than through the nose and mouth, mouth-to-mouth resuscitation is ineffective. Effective first aid measures include mouth-to-neck resuscitation (see Chapter 92) and the administration of oxygen through the tracheostomy. The patient's head should not be turned to the side, since this may obstruct the tracheostomy. On the back of the identification card the person's name and the name of the person he or she wishes notified in case of emergency should be written. Official identification cards for persons who have had laryngectomies are obtainable from the International Association of Laryngectomees.

Many postlaryngectomy patients benefit from associating with other persons who have had this operation. Membership in clubs like the Lost Chord Club helps give these persons social confidence and helps with their voice development. Other individuals who have had laryngectomies do not enjoy belonging to clubs of this nature, but rather they prefer dealing privately with the new situation. *Thus, the most desirable rehabilitation program is the one which meets the needs of a given patient and gives recognition to his or her individual pattern of best adapting to changes.*

Although patients are usually advised not to smoke following laryngectomy, some continue to do so. Following total laryngectomy the smoke is no longer directly inhaled into the throat or lungs. Nonetheless the smoke-laden air is inhaled, to some extent, through the tracheostomy. There are even some people who place the cigarette over the tracheostomy and "smoke" directly into their lungs! Such a practice should be discouraged.

POSTOPERATIVE CARE FOLLOWING PARTIAL LARYNGECTOMY

In the previous section we discussed at length clinical care given following *total* laryngectomy. Here let us briefly consider significant aspects of clinical care following *partial* laryngectomy.

During surgery a tracheostomy tube is placed. Postoperatively this tube is removed after tissue edema subsides. Following partial laryngectomy the patient is typically given nourishment by vein or nasogastric tube for the first 2 postoperative days. Oral fluids are usually then permitted.

A partial laryngectomy, e.g., laryngofissure, leaves the patient with a husky but useful voice. Postoperatively the patient is instructed not to attempt speaking until the doctor advises it. Voice rest is usually continued for the first 2 to 3 postoperative days. The patient may then be allowed to begin to whisper. Gradually, after further healing occurs. the patient is allowed to begin to use the voice again.

The adequacy of the airway is even more critical than with total laryngectomy and must be observed carefully. Further, people who have had partial laryngectomy have a high incidence of aspiration and require some adjustment to swallowing.

Speech Rehabilitation Following Laryngectomy

Following conservative or total laryngectomy, speech therapy is indicated to either (a) teach the patient how to correct speech problems resulting from surgery (if some ability to speak is retained); or (b) teach the person esophageal, i.e., alaryngeal, speech or other methods of artificial speech (if without the ability to speak).

As mentioned previously, preoperatively the physician, speech therapist, and nurse all reassure the patient that after the larynx is removed either esophageal speech or some type of artificial larynx as a new sound source will be possible. Nonetheless, the patient must accept the fact that the normal voice is lost forever. This loss causes noticeable reactions in others (as they listen to the patient's new voice) and changes in the patient's own self-image. The patient must adjust to the reactions of others and to the necessary change in his or her own self-image. Initially patients may seem "somewhat like a stranger" to themselves and to persons who were familiar with their normal voice.

The physician gives orders for speech rehabilitation to begin. Speech therapy may begin while the patient is hospitalized and usually continues after the patient is discharged. Esophageal speech can best be learned by attending a speech clinic or working individually with a speech therapist. Some highly motivated patients are able to learn esophageal speech within 2 to 3 weeks of instruction. Because motivation is highly important in speech therapy, the patient benefits from enthusiastic encouragement from significant others as well as the speech therapist, physician, and nurse. Discouragement comes easily because of the repeated efforts necessary before esophageal speech can be effectively used. In addition to instruction, the patient needs opportunity to practice privately as well as in the presence of others. Patients should be told that their new voice will continue to improve over many months of practice.

Most people who have had laryngectomies are capable of learning esophageal speech if given good instruction. In spite of being highly motivated, a few people cannot learn esophageal speech. Advanced age prevents some patients from learning esophageal speech, e.g., hearing problems may be present which prevent effective learning. An aged person may also lack the motivation and strength necessary for esophageal speech. Occasionally esophageal speech is impossible because of other physical problems, e.g., esophageal stenosis, emphysema, asthma. Individuals who cannot learn esophageal speech may benefit from the use of an artificial larynx. Some people learn to use both esophageal speech and an artificial larynx. Then they are able to use whichever method best meets their needs in various situations.

Esophageal Speech. "Esophageal speech" is a method of speaking in which the patient learns to take air in through the mouth, hold it in the upper esophagus, and then form words while expelling the air back out of the mouth in a controlled flow. In other terms, esophageal speech is somewhat similar to a controlled belch. With practice, up to 6 to 10 words may be spoken after each intake of air. Vibration at the top of the gullet replaces that from the lungs. (The "gullet" is the passage to the stomach, including both the pharynx and the esophagus.)

When possible, it is most desirable for a patient to begin to learn esophageal speech *before* surgery. This enables the person to ask questions more readily during the learning process, and it helps to minimize the psychologic impact of losing the natural voice, i.e., the person knows that successful communication is possible with esophageal speech postoperatively.

The basic act in learning esophageal speech is the "charging" and "releasing" of air from the upper portion of the esophagus. The esophagus has an elastic wall and thus can stretch with the intake of air. Most patients find it more difficult to take air into the esophagus, i.e., to "charge" the esophagus, than it is to release the air. There are three well-established methods of charging air.[109]

1. The suction, "breathing," or inhalation method.
2. Air injection by tongue and related structures.
3. The glossopharyngeal press or plosive-injection method.

Details of these methods are beyond the scope of this text. However, the goal of all of them is to take air rapidly into the esophagus so it can then be released and its force can be used to create the sounds of speech.

With practice the air-charge necessary for esophageal speech can be taken in in about one half to one fourth of a second. This is actually less time than that of a normal speaker inhaling for an intraphasal breath pause. Expert esophageal speakers speak relatively easily and are no more conscious of the "breathing" function than normal speakers, i.e., they are not consciously aware of the process of taking an air-charge.

Air is held only briefly in the top half or third of the esophagus. The air intake should be immediately followed by the speech sound. Relaxation is necessary in order to get air into the top of the esophagus and to release it.

Diaphragmatic action and the exhalation of lung air facilitate expulsion of air from the esophagus. Pushing the head back when releasing air often helps improve loudness and quality. Voicing usually takes place in the cricopharyngeal area. A segment of the gullet and the top of the gullet vibrate. Esophageal voice sounds are somewhat hoarse and are more low-pitched than laryngeal voice sounds. However, the qualities of speech provided by the use of the nasopharynx are still present.

Practice enables the esophageal speaker to develop a speech which flows quite smoothly and is easily understood. Also, the person learns to speak an increasing number of words with each swallow of air. Small amplifiers are available for the esophageal speaker to use when addressing conferences.

Temporary digestive problems may occur when a patient first begins to learn esophageal speech. These problems are related to nervous tension, tension placed on abdominal muscles, and air swallowing. Some persons are excessively troubled with flatulence as a result of air swallowing when using esophageal speech. Once efficient esophageal speech is learned, these disorders usually no longer occur.

The person who speaks with an esophageal voice needs to avoid excessive fatigue; it is more difficult to speak this way when tired. Also, the person's spouse should have his or her hearing evaluated. If the spouse is even a marginal candidate for a hearing aid, he or she should wear one. A hearing aid may make it easier for the spouse to understand the esophageal speech. While the effective esophageal speaker has sufficient loudness for the normal listener, shouting is not possible.

Artificial Larynx. If a patient has not been able to learn esophageal speech after 2 to 3 months of instruction and practice, or if the person initially is obviously not a potential candidate for artificial speech, the speech therapist may recommend use of an artificial larynx. Also, many speech therapists advise use of an artificial larynx to get the patient communicating soon after surgery and thus to make the learning of esophageal speech easier. A wide variety of mechanical and electrical instruments are available to replace the phonation functions of the removed larynx. Basically three types of artificial larynxes are available: (1) the reed-type artificial larynx; (2) an electronic throat vibrator aid; and (3) an electronic aid which vibrates directly in the mouth.

The *reed-type artificial larynx* is perhaps best

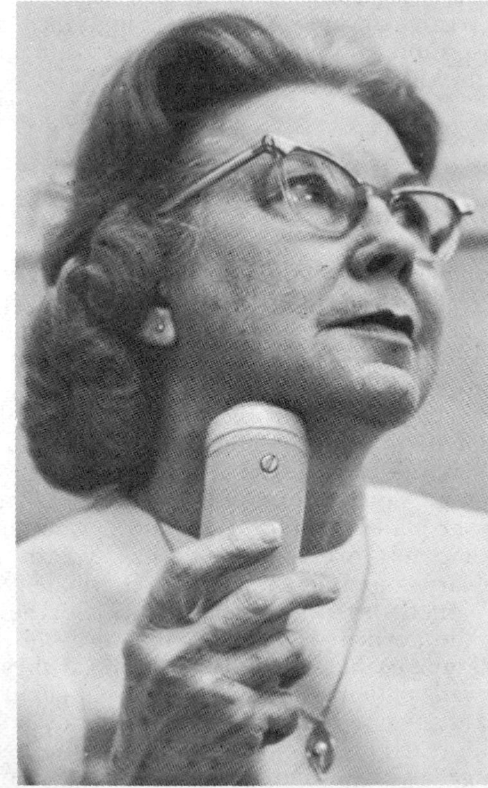

Figure 93–8. Western Electric artificial larynx. (From Flowers, A. M.: *Nursing Clinics of North America,* 3:529, 1968.)

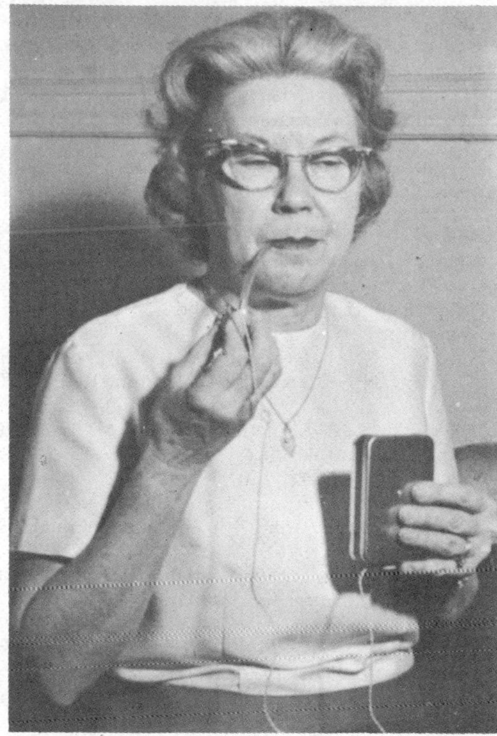

Figure 93–9. Cooper-Rand electronic speech aid. (From Flowers, A. M.: *Nursing Clinics of North America,* 3:529, 1968.)

represented by the instruments developed by Western Electric. One of these instruments is powered by breath from the tracheal stoma; the air passes through a loop of tubing from the neck to the mouth. In the mouth the air is pushed out through a reed at the end of the tubing. Some believe the skilled user of this instrument can develop speech superior to that of esophageal speech. Others believe this instrument is superseded by newer instruments, e.g., the Western Electric Electronic Larynx *throat vibrator.* The latter instrument is an inexpensive, light-weight, transistorized device which is economic in its utilization of batteries. It is available in a model for the male voice and a model for the female voice. While the Western Electric Electronic Larynx is somewhat lacking in loudness, it has manual, continuous control of pitch modulation which provides some simulation of the complex changes in pitch which characterize the normal voice (Figure 93–8). Often a throat vibrator instrument cannot be used in the immediate postoperative period because the neck wounds are too sensitive at that time.

Two other throat vibrator electrolarynxes are (1) the Aurex larynx (highly favored by many persons with laryngectomies); and (2) the Kett, Mark III larynx. Although somewhat heavy, the Kett, Mark III aid is rechargeable and is particularly useful when a loud voice is desirable.

Throat-vibrating artificial larynxes all are somewhat less favorable than superior esophageal speech, because even the newest and best of them are somewhat noisy. These devices all basically operate by a pulsating disk which sets the throat tissues vibrating.

Another type of aid is one that *vibrates directly in the mouth,* e.g., the Cooper-Rand Electronic Speech Aid (Fig. 93–9). This pipes sound into the mouth through a small plastic tube held in the corner of the mouth.

The design of artificial larynxes continues to improve. While some of the first models produced speech which sounded highly mechanized, monotonous, and artificial, modern artificial larynxes are capable of producing speech which more naturally fluctuates in volume and pitch.

Let us emphasize that the acquisition of an artificial larynx does not guarantee that clear and intelligible speech will automatically be possible. The patient needs to be properly instructed in the use of the particular instrument. Speech therapy is therefore desirable.

Space does not permit a detailed discussion of speech rehabilitation after laryngectomy. Nurses, patients, and other interested persons can obtain additional information about esophageal (alaryngeal) speech and artificial larynxes by contacting local chapters of the American Cancer Society, the International Association of Laryngectomees, or the American Speech and Hearing Association.

BIBLIOGRAPHY (Unit XXIV)

1. A *non*indication for tonsillectomy. *Emergency Medicine,* 10:211, Oct. 1978.
2. Adams, N. R.: The nurse's role in systematic weaning from a ventilator. *Nursing 79,* 9:35, Aug. 1979.
3. . . . And beat him when he wheezes—But not for too long. *Emergency Medicine,* 9:98, May 1977.
4. Anderson, H. A., B. J. Rice, and R. W. Cantrell: Effects of injected deposteroid on posttonsillectomy morbidity. *Archives of Otolaryngology,* 101:86, Feb. 1975.
5. Arlen, H.: Microlaryngoscopy. *AORN Journal,* 16:37, Aug. 1972.
6. Audible woes. *Emergency Medicine,* 10:153, Oct. 1978.
7. Barness, L. A., and F. I. Marlowe: Is tonsillectomy indicated? *Consultant,* 18:62, Feb. 1978.
8. Bartlett, P. C.: Aliens in the ENT. *Emergency Medicine,* 11:279, Feb. 1979.
9. Bartlett, P. C., et al.: Q and A on ENT. *Emergency Medicine,* 10:85, Feb. 1978.
10. Barton, N. W., S. H. Miller, and W. P. Graham: Managing lacerations of the parotid gland, duct and facial nerve. *American Family Physician,* 13:130, Apr. 1976.
11. Beattie, E. J., and Economou, S. G.: The current status of radical laryngectomy. *Nursing Clinics of North America,* 3:515, Sept. 1968.

12. Beeson, P. B., and McDermott, W. (Eds.): *Textbook of Medicine.* 13th ed. Philadelphia, W. B. Saunders Co. 1971, pp. 865–946.
13. Beland, I. L.: *Clinical Nursing: Pathophysiological and Psychosocial Approaches,* 2nd ed. New York: The Macmillan Co., 1970.
14. Block, P. L.: Dental health in hospitalized patients. *American Journal of Nursing,* 76:1162, July 1976.
15. Boyle, M. T., Sr., and A. Kaufman: Strep screening to prevent rheumatic fever. *American Journal of Nursing,* 75:1487, Sept. 1975.
16. *1973 Cancer Facts and Figures.* New York, American Cancer Society, 1973.
17. Chobin, N., J. Kangos, and J. Miller: From project to ongoing program. *American Journal of Nursing,* 75:1489, Sept. 1975.
18. Conner, G. H., et al.: Tracheostomy. *American Journal of Nursing,* 72:68, Jan. 1972.
19. Deatsch, W. W.: Ear, nose and throat. *In* Krupp, M. A., and M. J. Chatton (Eds.): *Current Diagnosis and Treatment.* Los Altos, Cal.: Lange Medical Publications, 1972.
20. Detour, adenoids. *Emergency Medicine,* 9:143, July 1977.
21. DeWeese, D. D., and W. H. Saunders: *Textbook of Otolaryngology,* 3rd ed. St. Louis: C. V. Mosby Co., 1968.
22. Dobie, R. A.: Rehabilitation of swallowing disorders. *American Family Physician,* 17:84, May 1978.
23. Don't be quick to cut a throat. *Emergency Medicine,* 10:85, Dec. 1978.
24. Dyer, E. D., M. A. Monson, and M. J. Cope: Dental health in adults. *American Journal of Nursing,* 76:1156, July 1976.
25. Elusive aspirations. *Emergency Medicine,* 9:49, Aug. 1977.
26. Epiglottitis grows up. *Emergency Medicine,* 9:174, Aug. 1977.
27. Epiglottitis, another view. *Emergency Medicine,* 9:67, Jan. 1977.
28. Ewing, D. M.: Electronic larynx for aphonic patients. *American Journal of Nursing,* 75:2153, Dec. 1975.
29. *First Aid for (Neck-Breathers) Laryngectomees.* New York, American Cancer Society, 1971.
30. Getting the teeth into trauma. *Emergency Medicine,* 10:143, June 1978.
31. Goldman, S. M., and J. O. Salik: Acute epiglottitis in adults. *American Family Physician,* 18:99, July 1978.
32. Grant, H., and R. Murray: *Emergency Care.* Washington, D.C.: Robert J. Brady Co., 1971.
33. Greenberg, L. W., and R. Schisgall: Acute epiglottitis in a community hospital. *American Family Physician,* 19:123, Feb. 1979.
34. Guyton, A. C.: *Physiology of the Human Body,* 5th ed. Philadelphia: W. B. Saunders Co., 1979.
35. Harrison, T. R., et al. (Eds.): *Principles of Internal Medicine,* 6th ed. New York: McGraw-Hill Book Co., 1970.
36. Harrold, C., J. Terry, and W. Stingle: Common surgical problems of the head and neck. *Postgraduate Medicine,* 62:162, Nov. 1977.
37. Hayes, T. P., J. P. Atkins, and A. Raventos: Carcinoma of the larynx: Diagnosis and treatment by surgery or irradiation. *Annals of Otology, Rhinology and Laryngology,* 80:627, Oct. 1971.
38. Heimlich, H. J.: The Heimlich maneuver: Where it stands today. *Emergency Medicine,* 10:89, July 1978.
39. Helman, P., et al.: Intra-arterial cytotoxic therapy and x-ray therapy for cancer of the head and neck. *American Journal of Surgery,* 112:606, Oct. 1966.
40. *Helping Words for the Laryngectomee.* International Association of Laryngectomees, 1964. (Distributed by The American Cancer Society, Inc.)
41. Henderson, B. E., et al.: Risk factors associated with nasopharyngeal carcinoma. *The New England Journal of Medicine,* 295:1101, Nov. 1976.
42. Herzon, F. S.: Bacteremia and local infections with nasal packing. *Archives of Otolaryngology,* 94:317, Oct. 1971.
43. Holinger, P. H.: Why worry about hoarseness? *Consultant,* 16:21, Aug. 1976.
44. Holvey, D. N., et al. (Eds.): *The Merck Manual,* 12th ed. Rahway, N.J.: Merck Sharp & Dohme Research Laboratories, 1972.
45. Jabaley, M. E., R. L. Clement, and W. M. Bryant: Recognizing oral lesions. *American Family Physician,* 13:60, May 1976.
46. Jacob, S. W., C. A. Francone, and W. J. Lossow: *Structure and Function in Man,* 4th ed. Philadelphia: W. B. Saunders Co., 1978.
47. Jacobs, H. B.: Emergency percutaneous transtracheal catheter and ventilator. *Journal of Trauma,* 12:50, Jan. 1972.
48. Jacobson, S.: Errors in emergency practice. Nasal trauma. *Emergency Medicine,* 11:239, May 1979.
49. Jacquette, G.: To reduce hazards of tracheal suctioning. *American Journal of Nursing,* 71:2362, Dec. 1971.
50. Jaffe, B. F.: *Diseases and Surgery of the Nose.* Clinical Symposia. Volume 26. Summit, N.J.: CIBA Pharmaceutical Co., 1974.
51. Kearns, B.: Tracheostomy suctioning technique. *Canadian Nurse,* 66:44, Feb. 1970.
52. Kennedy, T. J., et al.: The team approach to treatment of the cleft lip and palate. *American Family Physician,* 18:74, July 1978.
53. King, P. S., et al.: Effect of radical neck dissection on total rehabilitation of the laryngectomee. *American Journal of Physical Medicine,* 52:1, Feb. 1973.
54. Kolz, C.: Microlaryngoscopy: The nurse's role. *AORN Journal,* 16:42, Aug. 1972.
55. Kormorn, R. M.: Laryngectomy and surgical vocal rehabilitation. *AORN Journal,* 17:73, June 1973.
56. Langer, A.: Oral signs of aging and their clinical significance. *Geriatrics,* 31:63, Dec. 1976.
57. Lawless, C. A.: Helping patients with endotracheal and tracheostomy tubes communicate. *American Journal of Nursing,* 75:2151, Dec. 1975.
58. Lewy, R .M.: Preventing mumps and its complications. *American Family Physician,* 16:119, Oct. 1977.
59. Linet, O. I., and C. Metzler: Practical ENT. Incidence of palpable cervical nodes in adults. *Postgraduate Medicine,* 62:210, Oct. 1977.
60. Lingeman, R. E.: Epistaxis. *American Family Physician,* 14:79, Dec. 1976.
61. Loeb, W. J.: Experiences with a modified cuffed tracheostomy tube. *Annuals of Otology, Rhinology and Laryngology,* 80:549, Aug. 1971.
62. Lucente, F. E.: Aspirin and the otolaryngologist. *Archives of Otolaryngology,* 94:443, Nov. 1971.
63. Lyons, H. A.: Guide to acute upper airway infections. *Hospital Medicine,* 12:94, June 1976.
64. Marcott, M.: There's more to post-op extubation than just pulling out a tube. *RN,* 40:43, Sept. 1977.
65. McCarthy, P. L.: How to recognize and treat leukoplakia. *Consultant,* 18:68, Oct. 1978.
66. McConnell, E. A.: How to truly help the patient with a radical neck dissection. *Nursing 76,* 6:58, Nov. 1976.
67. McGurdy, J. A., Jr.: The tonsillectomy-adenoidectomy dilemma. *American Family Physician,* 16:137, Sept. 1977.

68. McGovern, F. H., et al.: The hazards of endotracheal intubation. *Annuals of Otology, Rhinology and Laryngology,* 80:556, Aug. 1971.
69. Mechner, F., L. J. Saffioti, and L. Holman: Programmed instruction. Patient assessment: Examination of the head and neck. *American Journal of Nursing,* 75:P.I.1, May 1975.
70. Millen, D. L.: Aspiration—Foiling a silent killer. *RN,* 41:34, Aug. 1978.
71. Miller, B. F., and C. B. Keane: *Encyclopedia and Dictionary of Medicine and Nursing,* 2nd ed. Philadelphia: W. B. Saunders Co., 1978.
72. Murphy, G. E., and J. Ogura: Rehabilitation following laryngectomy. *Geriatrics,* 22:119, Dec. 1967.
73. Nicholson, E. M.: Personal notes of a laryngectomee. *American Journal of Nursing,* 75:2157, Dec. 1975.
74. Olson, N. R., and W. K. Miles: Treatment of acute blunt laryngeal injuries. *Annals of Otology, Rhinology and Laryngology,* 80:704, Oct. 1971.
75. On tracheal trauma. *Emergency Medicine,* 11:117, Jan. 1979.
76. Pagana, K. D.: Teaching your tracheostomy patients to cope at home. *RN,* 41:63, Dec. 1978.
77. Parvulescu, N. F.: Care of the surgically speechless patient. *Nursing Clinics of North America,* 5:517, Sept. 1970.
78. Passey, V., and W. C. McMaster: Foreign bodies in the throat, nose and ear, *Hospital Medicine,* 13:8, July 1977.
79. Peres, C. A., et al.: Irradiation of early carcinoma of the larynx. *Archives of Otolaryngology,* 93:465, May 1971.
80. Pilgrim, M. C., and D. Sands: Reconstructive nasal surgery. *American Journal of Nursing,* 73:451, Mar. 1973.
81. Pitorak, E.: Laryngectomy. *American Journal of Nursing,* 68:780, Apr. 1968.
82. Podgore, J. K., and C. G. Ray: Axioms on croup in children and adults. *Hospital Medicine,* 12:50, Dec. 1976.
83. Potter, B. E., C. T. Yarington Jr., and J. W. Walike: Management of intraoral injuries. *American Family Physician,* 18:96, Nov. 1978.
84. Pressman, J. J., and Bailey, B. J.: The surgery of cancer of the larynx with especial reference to subtotal laryngectomy. *In* Snidecor, J. C. (Ed.): *Speech Rehabilitation of the Laryngectomized,* 2nd ed. Springfield, Ill.: Charles C Thomas, Publisher, 1969.
85. Proctor, D. F., and P. Safar: Management of airway obstruction. *In* Safar, P. (Ed.): *Respiratory Therapy.* Philadelphia: F. A. Davis Co., 1965.
86. Reed, G. F.: Sinusitis: Treat or tolerate? *Consultant,* 17:30, Sept. 1977.
87. Reid, J. M., and J. A. Donaldson: The indications for tonsillectomy and adenoidectomy. *Otolaryngologic Clinics of North America,* 3:339, June 1970.
88. Robbins, S. L., and R. S. Cotran: *Pathologic Basis of Disease,* 2nd ed. Philadelphia: W. B. Saunders Co., 1979.
89. Rowland, H. S. (Ed.): *The Nurse's Almanac.* Germantown: Aspen Systems Corporation, 1978.
90. Roy, A., C. De la Rosa, and Y. A. Vecchio: Bleeding following tonsillectomy. *Archives of Otolarygology,* 102:9, Jan. 1976.
91. Ryan, R. E.: How to recognize headaches arising from the nose and sinuses. *Consultant,* 17:31, Dec. 1977.
92. Sabiston, D. C. (Ed.): *Davis-Christopher Textbook of Surgery: The Biological Basis of Modern Surgical Practice,* 11th ed. Philadelphia; W. B. Saunders Co., 1977.
93. Schindler, R. A.: The bloody nose. *Emergency Medicine,* 10:34, Feb. 1978.
94. Score 26 or more for strep. *Emergency Medicine,* 9:214, Nov. 1977.
95. Secor, J.: *Patient Care in Respiratory Problems.* Philadelphia: W. B. Saunders Co., 1969.
96. Sessions, R. B.: Cosmetic rhinoplasty today. *AORN Journal,* 15:35, Feb. 1972.
97. Shan, N.: Epistaxis. *Nursing Mirror,* 134:28, Mar. 10, 1972.
98. Shan, N.: Foreign bodies in ENT. *Nursing Mirror,* 134:39, Mar. 17, 1972.
99. Shan, N.: Respiratory obstruction tracheosotomy. *Nursing Mirror,* 134:35, Mar. 31, 1972.
100. Shank, J. C.: Streptococcal infection and the chronic carrier state. *American Family Physician.* 15:87, Jan. 1977.
101. Shires, T.: Initial care of the injured patient. *The Journal of Trauma,* 10:940, Nov. 1970.
102. Sinusitis: When the eyes have it. *Emergency Medicine,* 9:108, Dec. 1977.
103. Sladen, A.: Maintenance of a patent airway. *Hospital Medicine,* 13:56, Aug. 1977.
104. Slattery, J.: Dental health in children. *American Journal of Nursing,* 76:1159, July 1976.
105. Smith, C.: Infections of the mouth and pharynx. *Nursing Times,* 68:566, May 11, 1972.
106. Smith, M. L.: Parotidectomy. *American Journal of Nursing,* 76:422, Mar. 1976.
107. Smith, R. L., et al.: Metastatic malignancies of the parotid gland. *American Family Physician,* 16:139, Nov. 1977.
108. Snidecor, J. C.: Speech therapy for those with total laryngectomy. *In* Snidecor, J. C. (Ed.): *Speech Rehabilitation of the Laryngectomized,* 2nd ed. Springfield, Ill.: Charles C Thomas, Publisher, 1969.
109. Snidecor, J. C.: The charging and expulsion of esophageal air. *In* Snidecor, J. C. (Ed.): *Speech Rehabilitation of the Laryngectomized,* 2nd ed. Springfield, Ill.: Charles C Thomas, Publisher, 1969.
110. Snidecor, J. C.: The nature of the problem. *In* Snidecor, J. C. (Ed.): *Speech Rehabilitation of the Laryngectomized,* 2nd ed. Springfield, Ill.: Charles C Thomas, Publisher, 1969.
111. Stivers, F. E., and C. T. Yarington, Jr.: Indications for tonsillectomy and adenoidectomy. *American Family Physician,* 3:72, Mar. 1971.
112. Taub, S.: A different way of seeing the larynx and nasopharynx. *AORN Journal,* 16:50, Dec. 1972.
113. Teirney, E. A.: Accepting disfigurement when death is the alternative. *American Journal of Nursing,* 75:2149, Dec. 1975.
114. The bloody nose. *Emergency Medicine,* 4:74, Apr. 1972.
115. Thomas, A. N.: Respiratory care. *In* Sanderson, R. G. (Ed.): *The Cardiac Patient.* Philadelphia: W. B. Saunders Co., 1972.
116. Toy, F. J., and J. D. Weinstein: Percutaneous tracheostomy device. *Surgery,* 65:384, Feb. 1969.
117. Tracheostomy is trauma. *Emergency Medicine,* 4:169, May 1972.
118. Trodahl, J. N., et al.: White lesions of the mouth. *Hospital Medicine,* 7:6, Nov. 1971.
119. Trowbridge, J. E.: Caring for patients with facial or intraoral reconstruction. *American Journal of Nursing,* 73:1930, Nov. 1973.
120. Trowbridge, J. E., and W. Carl: Oral care of the patient having head and neck irradiation. *American Journal of Nursing,* 75:2146, Dec. 1975.
121. Tyler, M. L., and N. Synnestvedt: Artificial airways. *Nursing '73,* 3:21, Feb. 1973.
122. Up-to-date survey of tracheal tubes. *Nursing 76,* 6:66, Nov. 1976.

123. Ventura, M. R.: Care after nasal surgery. *Nursing 74,* 4:87, Sept. 1974.
124. Wang, R. M.: Streptococcal sore throat. *American Journal of Nursing,* 77:1796, Nov. 1977.
125. When infection strikes the salivaries. *Emergency Medicine,* 10:80, Sept. 1978.
126. White, H. A.: Tracheostomy: Care with a cuffed tube. *American Journal of Nursing,* 72:75, Jan. 1972.

UNIT XXV

NURSING PEOPLE EXPERIENCING DEPENDENCY ON ALCOHOL AND OTHER DRUGS

by Kathleen Smith-DiJulio, R.N., M.A.

INTRODUCTION AND STUDY GUIDE

Persons who abuse alcohol and other drugs have always needed nursing care and medical treatment. In the past, however, attention has been focused on immediate physical problems, e.g., gastritis, cirrhosis, or nerve damage. While nurses and physicians may have known that the root of these problems was the excessive intake of alcohol or other drugs, the subject was not openly discussed with the person. There have been at least three reasons for this: (1) ignorance as to how to discuss these problems, (2) lack of knowledge about the effects of drugs, and (3) a prevailing belief that dependence on drugs results from moral weakness and therefore that little can be done about it. When abuse problems are not recognized and treated, many patients continue drug abuse. Consequently, they return repeatedly with similar problems to health care facilities. Nurses generally become frustrated in such situations and prefer, when possible, to avoid these persons who make them feel helpless and ineffective. Patient care, as a result, is often inadequate.

Fortunately, today, this sequence of events is being interrupted. The social view of alcohol and other drug abuse is beginning to change. Health professionals are beginning to see drug-dependent people in a new light.

> *Alcoholism, as a prototype of drug dependency, is now recognized as a disease. Persons experiencing this problem are no longer labeled as morally weak. Alcoholism and other drug addictions are coming to be viewed as treatable, which implies a hope for change.*

To be sure, treatment and care are still difficult, as nurses know. However, now there are options. The nurse with knowledge of alcoholism and other drug abuse can more effectively assess patients' needs and can plan and implement patient care to meet these needs.

The long-term treatment of drug-dependent people is beyond the scope of this chapter. In most communities today there are specialized agencies that provide this kind of treatment. These include self-help groups, inpatient residential treatment programs, outpatient services, and "halfway houses." By becoming knowledgeable about the resources in your own locality, you can provide patients and their significant others with information about available treatment services most appropriate to their needs.

Stopping the intake of drugs in many cases requires a person to make significant attitude and life style changes. The prognosis for either decreasing or totally stopping drug abuse is related to many factors, including the duration of drug dependence and the addicted person's physical and psychosocial well-being. All forms of drug dependence are chronic disorders and are thus prone to relapse. The rate of relapse is highest during the first 6 months after treatment, drops at 6 months, and decreases even further at 1 year. About 90 percent of people doing well at 1 year are still doing well at 2 years.[41]

In general, *early diagnosis of a person's problem is the key to successful treatment.* It is important to identify drug-dependent persons while their social resources (e.g., family, friends, job) are still intact. Thus, one of the purposes of this chapter is to help you *recognize the indications of drug dependence.*

A second purpose of this chapter is to *encourage you to examine your own attitudes about drugs and drug dependence.* Consider the following questions before reading the chapter. They are designed to help you think honestly about alcohol and other drugs and to become aware of your own value system.

- ▶ Do I use alcohol or other drugs? If so, when, where, how much, how often, and for what reasons?
- ▶ What did I learn about alcohol and other drugs when I was growing up?
- ▶ What do the words "alcoholism" and "heroin addiction" mean to me?
- ▶ What do I experience when I see an intoxicated man? An intoxicated woman?
- ▶ What do I believe about *why* people drink or take other drugs?
- ▶ How do I decide upon my drug consumption patterns? Do I emulate my parents? My peers?
- ▶ What words do I use to describe drug-dependent people?

This last question is of particular importance in recognizing your own attitudes. We have often in this text discussed the importance of not labeling people.* Perhaps in no other area of nursing practice are examples of labeling so extreme. The terms "junkie," "drunk," "wino," "addict," and many others are commonly used in society. While such terms should be understood by nurses, they should not be used in nursing practice. It is important to remember that *people* use drugs, *people* abuse drugs, and *people* need nursing care.

A crucial issue in the treatment of drug-dependent persons is confidentiality.

People who abuse drugs may hesitate to seek treatment if they believe that information about them will not be kept confidential. In the United States there are, in fact, quite specific federal regulations concerning confidentiality and drug treatment. These were developed in response to a need for protection of the identities of persons seeking treatment. Since some people who abuse drugs, especially those addicted to illicit drugs, are wanted for criminal offenses, treatment personnel are not to divulge any information about a client (not even to state whether or not an individual is in treatment) to a law enforcement officer. Of course, discussing patients in casual conversation with persons not involved in their treatment is *never* acceptable nursing practice.

---

*See especially Chapter 14, Psychosocial Assessment, and p. 578, on language and the disabled person.

Objectives

After studying the material in this chapter, you should be able to do the following:

- ▶ Define drug use, abuse, and addiction and describe how these entities are related.
- ▶ Discuss theories about the causes of drug dependence, with emphasis on psychosocial, cultural, and biologic factors.
- ▶ Describe the effects of the following psychoactive drugs: alcohol and other sedative-hypnotic drugs, heroin, stimulants, cocaine, cannibas derivatives, hallucinogens, and organic solvents.
- ▶ Recognize clinical problems resulting from drug dependence and describe the actions a nurse can take in planning and implementing care for these patients.

Study Guide

1. As you read this chapter, familiarize yourself with the following terms:

drug use
drug abuse
drug addiction
drug dependence
tolerance
withdrawal
physical dependence
psychologic dependence
zero-order kinetics
first-order kinetics
blood levels
polyneuropathy
Wernicke-Korsakoff syndrome
"tracks"
"skin-popping"
polydrug abuse
fetal alcohol syndrome

2. As you study, try to answer the following questions:

a. How do drug use, abuse, and addiction differ? How are they related?

b. What are some of the psychosocial, cultural, and biologic factors that contribute to drug dependence?

c. How does the combination of the *person consuming the drug, the characteristics of the drug* itself, and the *environment* in which it is consumed influence the development of patterns of abuse or addiction?

d. What is the most abused drug in the Western world?

e. What are the three primary routes of drug administration?

f. What are some nursing implications of the development of tolerance and physical dependence?

g. What is "withdrawal"? How can you prevent a severe withdrawal episode in a person you are caring for? What nursing actions are helpful for a person suffering from a withdrawal reaction?

h. What are some initial physiologic reactions to each group of drugs discussed?

i. What are some of the clinical problems associated with alcohol abuse?

j. How might a nurse plan patient care for a person suffering from alcoholic malnutrition and associated disease entities?

k. What are some etiologic factors involved in the majority of clinical problems associated with heroin addiction? What are some controversial issues in regard to the clinical course and the treatment of heroin addiction?

l. What are some special problems of a drug-dependent person who is undergoing surgery?

m. What is the current state of knowledge about the effects of alcohol ingestion by a pregnant woman on the unborn child?

CHAPTER 94

NURSING PEOPLE EXPERIENCING DEPENDENCY ON ALCOHOL AND OTHER DRUGS

Any psychoactive drug is potentially harmful to the individual. The effects depend on the agent; the user; the environment in which the drug is used; and the intensity, frequency, and duration of use. Once heavy drug use is started, a cyclical pattern develops. Drug use to relieve discomfort ultimately causes more discomfort, thus necessitating more drugs. This pattern is not broken until alternative methods for relieving discomfort are found.

Nursing drug addicted persons is often a very difficult, challenging, experience. It is difficult to shift such a person's preoccupation with drugs to more constructive matters. Recidivism is high. However, it can be highly rewarding to see persons succeed in becoming drug free.

DEFINITIONS

Throughout this chapter, the term "drug" refers to *all mood-affecting substances* (including alcohol) *that are a potential or real threat to the health of an individual.* Table 94–1 provides an overview of abused substances other than alcohol. It is essential to clarify between drug use, drug abuse, and drug addiction.

- *Drug use*: the moderate intermittent taking of drugs for social or recreational purposes. Persons usually take drugs for their mood-altering effects, e.g., to relax with significant others. Drugs are used in a social context. Their use is most commonly designed to facilitate social interaction.
- *Drug abuse*: encompasses such features as (a) frequent intoxication; (b) consumption for the purpose of blotting out reality, or finding short-term solutions to a problem; and (c) disruption of normal social behavior patterns, e.g., problems with spouse or relatives, friends or neighbors, employers, and police.[38]
- *Drug addiction*: chronic, progressive, and potentially fatal use of drugs. Drug consumption becomes a dominant necessity for the individual.[8] In any drug-taking episode, an addicted person cannot predict the duration of the episode or the quantity of drug to be consumed. The drug-taking pattern is usually continuous but may be intermittent. Drug addiction may be characterized by tolerance and/or pathologic organ changes. An exacerbation of the disruption of normal social patterns that occurs with abuse is noted. Addiction is also termed *physical dependence.*

The *characteristics of developing dependence* on drugs are summarized here.[15] These apply to all dependence-producing drugs.

- An overpowering desire or need (compulsion) to continue taking the drug and to obtain it by any means
- A tendency to increase the dose
- A psychologic dependence on the drug's effects
- Detrimental effect on the individual and/or society

> *All dependence-producing drugs are capable of creating a state of mind in certain individuals which is termed psychic dependence . . . a psychic drive which requires periodic or chronic admininstration of the drug. . . .*[67]

Drug use, abuse and addiction lie on a continuum. Thus, drug use may begin as a normal part of being a member of a drug-oriented society. In some individuals, use proceeds to drug abuse and finally addiction. The process from use to addiction is a gradual, progressive one and may be interrupted at any point along the continuum.

Overview

There is evidence of drug use to alter consciousness throughout history. Reasons for drug use are individualized and include psychosocial, cultural, and biologic factors.

Psychosocial Factors. Throughout the ages the use of drugs has been a way of coping with the anxiety produced by life's stresses. Advice such as that in Proverbs 31:6, "Give . . . wine unto them that be of heavy hearts" has been passed down through the generations.

Anxiety is an uncomfortable feeling, and drugs allay anxiety, at least temporarily. This message is communicated to children through parents and the media, perhaps most strongly through television. Parents who require alcohol to "unwind" convey the desirability of alcohol use for tension relief. Advertisements encourage us to relieve discomfort through medications to dissipate tension or give energy. The mood alteration that occurs with initial drug consumption is immediately reinforcing. Repeated, immediate reinforcement of a desirable state can lead to addiction.[2] Other *coping styles* (e.g., relaxation techniques, meditation, problem solving) provide more delayed reinforcement and thus are less likely to be repeated. (Stress is discussed in Unit III.)

Among young people, perhaps the most influential determinant of drug-taking is the *peer group.* For an adolescent attempting to disengage from parents, this group is very important. Participation in certain groups may be contingent upon drug use. Individuals may gravitate to those groups that support their particular drug preferences, thereby reinforcing drug dependency.

Adults may begin taking drugs for *self-medication,* e.g., to relieve depression or lose weight. People may use drugs to reduce anxiety and tension, alleviate fatigue, influence mood, change activity level, or facilitate social interaction.[30] Many persons seek a physician's help with some of these problems. Doctors can and do *prescribe* a variety of drugs for treatment, with the result that for many persons, abuse of and addiction to, tranquilizers, sleeping pills, and amphetamines becomes a problem. Prescribing these drugs is a quick way to treat vague complaints, and many physicians succumb to the practice.

> *It is essential that health professionals offer alternatives to drugs, in order to reduce the frequency of iatrogenic health problems resulting from abuse of and addiction to these agents.*

Social roles also greatly influence the pattern of drug taking. Truck drivers, for example, often choose amphetamines to help them make long trips in the shortest possible time. Doctors and nurses have ready access to a variety of drugs, including narcotics, and may abuse them.

Steffenhagen[34] maintains that social theories on drug misuse fail to explain why some individuals become addicted and others do not. While social group is important in determining an individual's experimentation with drugs, he believes that *low self-esteem* is the key factor in determining misuse of drugs.

There are a myriad of potential psychosocial reasons for drug use. It is virtually impossible to effectively generalize about psychosocial etiologic factors. Each person must be understood as an individual.

Cultural Factors. In caring for persons experiencing drug dependency — as in so many areas of nursing practice — it is important to be aware of one's own cultural attitudes and how they differ from the cultural background of persons needing care. In the United States, society includes many subcultures (e.g., ethnic, racial, or religious groups) with particular attitudes toward or problems with drug use. If you are working as a nurse in a setting in which you have contact with persons of a different cultural background — for whom alcohol or other drug usage represents different values than your own — it is essential that you learn (e.g., through reading or continued education) about the cultural norms around you.

While it is difficult to generalize about any particular group's drug abuse problems, research does support some conclusions. For example, among *black Americans,* frustration, prejudice, and the desire to escape reality may lead to drug abuse. Discrimination leads to inadequate education and to social and economic injustices — stresses many blacks would rather avoid. Alcohol is the most used and abused drug among black Americans. *In general,* alcohol abuse in black communities is more widespread and devastating than is alcohol abuse in nonblack communities.[19] (On the other hand, *religious influence* in black communities is an important factor mitigating against drug use, abuse, and addiction. Certain strong religious groups ban all alcohol use.) Another factor in black American drug abuse is the fact that many blacks live in urban ghettos where organized crime thrives and illicit drugs are available. This combination of drug influences results in a greater likelihood of black alcoholic persons begin addicted also to other drugs, as compared to white alcoholics. In general, the implications of research on drug use in black communities

TABLE 94–1. CONTROLLED SUBSTANCES: USES AND EFFECTS

	Drugs	Often Prescribed Brand Names	Medical Uses	Dependence Potential	
				Physical	Psychological
Narcotics	Opium	Dover's Powder, Paregoric	Analgesic, antidiarrheal	High	High
	Morphine	Morphine	Analgesic	High	High
	Codeine	Codeine	Analgesic, antitussive	Moderate	Moderate
	Heroin	None	None	High	High
	Merperidine (Pethidine)	Demerol, Pethadol	Analgesic	High	High
	Methadone	Dolophine, Methadone, Methadose	Analgesic, heroin substitute	High	High
	Other narcotics	Dilaudid, Leritine, Numorphan, Percodan	Analgesic, antidiarrheal, antitussive	High	High
Depressants	Chloral Hydrate	Noctec, Somnos	Hypnotic	Moderate	Moderate
	Barbiturates	Amytal, Butisol, Nembutal, Phenobarbital, Seconal, Tuinal	Anesthetic, anticonvulsant, sedation, sleep	High	High
	Glutethimide	Doriden	Sedation, sleep	High	High
	Methaqualone	Optimil, Parest, Quaalude, Somnafac, Sopor	Sedation, sleep	High	High
	Meprobamate	Equanil, Meprospan, Miltown Kesso-Bamate, SK-Bamate	Anti-anxiety, muscle relaxant, sedation	Moderate	Moderate
	Other depressants	Dormate, Noludar, Placidyl, Valmid	Anti-anxiety, sedation, sleep	Possible	Possible
Stimulants	Cocaine*	Cocaine	Local anesthetic	Possible	High
	Amphetamines	Benzedrine, Biphetamine, Desoxyn, Dexedrine	Hyperkinesis, narcolepsy, weight control	Possible	High
	Phenmetrazine	Preludin	Weight control	Possible	High
	Methylphenidate	Ritalin	Hyperkinesis	Possible	High
	Other stimulants	Bacarate, Cylert, Didrex, Ionamine, Plegine, Pondimin, Pre-Sate, Sanorex, Voranil	Weight control	Possible	Possible
Hallucinogens	LSD	None	None	None	Degree unknown
	Mescaline	None	None	None	Degree unknown
	Psilocybin-Psilocyn	None	None	None	Degree unknown
	MDA	None	None	None	Degree unknown
	PCP†	Sernylan	Veterinary anesthetic	None	Degree unknown
	Other hallucinogens	None	None	None	Degree unknown
Cannabis	Marihuana, Hashish, Hashish oil	None	None	Degree unknown	Moderate

*Designated a narcotic under the U.S. Controlled Substances Act.
†Designated a depressant under the U.S. Controlled Substances Act.

From Langer, J.H.: Drugs of abuse. *Drug Enforcement* (Special Issue) 2:70, Spring 1975.

seem to be that not until prejudice, discrimination, and poverty are dealt with can the issues of drug abuse among black Americans be effectively addressed.[19]

Among *North American Indian groups,* alcoholism is one of the most significant and urgent health problems today.[1] Probably no other condition so adversely affects the quality of life in their communities. When alcohol was introduced to North American Indian groups in the 16th and 17th centuries, socially disruptive patterns of drinking quickly developed that persist today. These include periodic and explosive drinking, group binge drinking, and the ab-

TABLE 94–1. CONTROLLED SUBSTANCES: USES AND EFFECTS

Tolerance	Duration of Effects *(in hours)*	Usual Methods of Administration	Possible Effects	Effects of Overdose	Withdrawal Syndrome
Yes	3 to 6	Oral, smoked	Euphoria, drowsiness, respiratory depression, constricted pupils, nausea	Slow and shallow breathing, clammy skin, convulsions, coma, possible death	Watery eyes, runny nose, yawning, loss of appetite, irritability, tremors, panic, chills and sweating, cramps, nausea
Yes	3 to 6	Injected, smoked			
Yes	3 to 6	Oral, injected			
Yes	3 to 6	Injected, sniffed			
Yes	3 to 6	Oral, injected			
Yes	12 to 24	Oral, injected			
Yes	3 to 6	Oral, injected			
Probable	5 to 8	Oral	Slurred, speech, disorientation, drunken behavior without odor of alcohol	Shallow respiration, cold and clammy skin, dilated pupils, weak and rapid pulse, coma, possible death	Anxiety, insomnia, tremors, delirium, convulsions, possible death
Yes	1 to 16	Oral, injected			
Yes	4 to 8	Oral			
Yes	4 to 8	Oral			
Yes	4 to 8	Oral			
Yes	4 to 8	Oral			
Yes	2	Injected, sniffed	Increased alertness, excitation, euphoria, dilated pupils, increased pulse rate and blood pressure, insomnia, loss of appetite	Agitation, increase in body temperature, hallucinations, convulsions, possible death	Apathy, long periods of sleep, irritability, depression, disorientation
Yes	2 to 4	Oral, injected			
Yes	2 to 4	Oral			
Yes	2 to 4	Oral			
Yes	2 to 4	Oral			
Yes	Variable	Oral	Illusions and hallucinations (with exception of MDA); poor perception of time and distance	Longer, more intense "trip" episodes, psychosis, possible death	Withdrawal syndrome not reported
Yes	Variable	Oral, injected			
Yes	Variable	Oral			
Yes	Variable	Oral, injected, sniffed			
Yes	Variable	Oral, injected, smoked			
Yes	Variable	Oral, injected sniffed			
Yes	2 to 4	Oral, smoked	Euphoria, relaxed inhibitions, increased appetite, disoriented behavior	Fatigue, paranoia, possible psychosis	Insomnia, hyperactivity, and decreased appetite reported in a limited number of individuals

sence of a social sanction for appropriate drinking behavior.[24] Investigators have attempted to determine if there are physiologic differences in response to alcohol among various Indian groups. However, there is no valid evidence today that North American Indians do differ in their response to alcohol.[15]

Drug dependency is not currently a major problem among *Asian groups* in the United States.

In general, white American populations have low rates of opiate addiction.[41] Recently marijuana has made inroads across age and social class barriers. *Marijuana is the second most frequently used drug among white Americans. Alcohol still ranks number one.* It is difficult to generalize about drug use among white Americans because so many subcultures exist. These subgroups have different ways of introducing drug use to their members (usually *only* alcohol use is sanctioned) and different social standards for drug consumption and misuse. For example, Italian groups, who commonly use wine with meals and who scorn intoxication, have relatively low rates of alcoholism.[38]

Biologic Factors. Individual variations in reaction to drugs are readily observable. It is not known whether some innate physiologic difference causes susceptibility to the development of patterns of abuse or addiction.

Studies of *genetic links* have produced some interesting findings. For instance, studies of adopted children indicate that children of alcoholic parents are more likely to have alcohol problems than children of nonalcoholics, even when separated from their parents early in life.[17] Also, identical twins have been found to be more concordant for heavy drinking than fraternal twins. While biologic variations in responses to alcohol appear to be genetic in origin, there is no direct evidence that innate factors contribute to the development of alcohol abuse and alcoholism. Little is known about the possible genetic role in other addictive processes.

Development of Drug Use

No one factor can singly account for the development of patterns of drug abuse or addiction. What seems crucial to this development is a combination of (1) *characteristics of the person (host)* consuming the drug, (2) *properties of the drug (agent)* itself and (3) the *environment* in which the drug consumption takes place (Fig. 94–1). Prevention and treatment efforts are likely to be ineffective unless these three *influences are taken into account.*

The Host. Characteristics of the person consuming a drug include the psychosocial and biologic

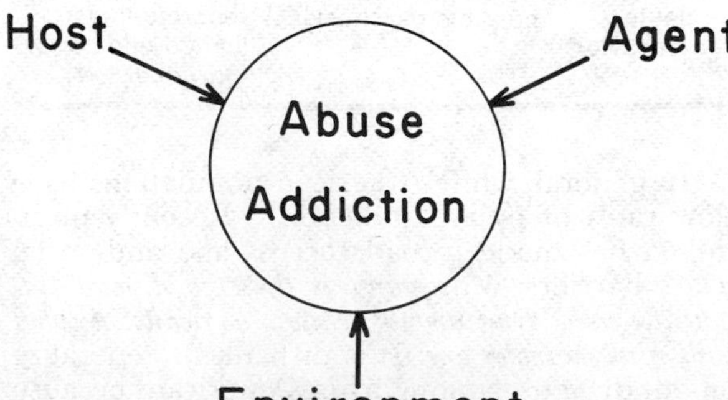

Figure 94–1. Dynamic factors influencing the development of abuse and addiction.

factors discussed. The interplay between a chemical substance and the reaction of an individual to the substance leads to psychic dependence. Certain personality features have been identified that seem to be characteristic of addicts. Some of these features are ". . . emotional immaturity, a strong wish to turn one's back on reality, a low frustration tolerance, an unwillingness or inability to endure and to cope with tension, or to stick for long to a given course of activity (low staying power). . . ."[15] Susceptibility may be determined not only by personality but also by genetic influences, or perhaps by a combination of both.

The Agent. In addition to characteristics of the "host," the *pharmacologic properties* of a given drug can play a decisive role in the addiction process. For example, the opiates rapidly lead to both physiologic and psychologic dependence for most users. In contrast, alcoholic beverages are used by many persons, but only a small proportion of users become dependent, and this dependence usually develops slowly. *Method of administration* also contributes to the likelihood of dependence. Injectable drugs (especially intravenous) produce dependence more readily than those which can be taken only orally.

The Environment. The particular *environment* in which an individual consumes a drug plays a role in the development of dependence. Environmental influence can most readily be illustrated by persons who relapse into drug-taking after a period of abstinence. These persons usually attribute the resumption not to physiologic or psychologic dependence but to returning to their former environment — centered around drug abuse. The influence of the environment thus has implications for post-treatment planning. Assisting the former addict to find other living accommodations and friends who do not take drugs may be essential for recovery.

Environmental influences also include the *social and cultural factors* discussed. In addition, differences between men and women in the consumption of various drugs may be a result of *sex roles* dictated by society. *Economic factors* are important as well. What drug a person uses, how much drug is used, and how often it is used may be determined by cost and available money.

> *The distinctions between drug abuse and addiction are not clear-cut. Different forms of abuse and addiction occur in different individuals. Probably in all cases of dependence, complex interacting forces are at work. Awareness of this interplay can help you to avoid stereotyping drug-dependent persons.*

Assessment will be more accurate when you look for individual differences and needs. In addition, implementation of a plan of care will be more effective when treatment is tailored to a patient's uniqueness.

TOOLS IN ASSESSING DRUG ABUSE

Space does not permit detailed discussion of the assessment and diagnosis of drug abuse.

Michigan Alcoholism Screening Test

Questions	Answers with weighted scoring	
1. Do you feel you are a normal drinker? If patient denies any use of alcohol, check here ————.)	Yes ____	No 2
2. Have you ever awakened the morning after some drinking the night before and found that you could not remember a part of the evening before?	Yes 2	No ____
3. Does your spouse (or a parent) ever worry or complain about your drinking?	Yes 1	No ____
4. Can you stop drinking without a struggle after one or two drinks?	Yes ____	No 2
5. Do you ever feel bad about your drinking?	Yes 1	No ____
6. Do friends or relatives think you are a normal drinker?	Yes ____	No 2
7. Do you ever try to limit your drinking to certain times of the day or to certain places?	Yes 0	No ____
8. Are you always able to stop drinking when you want to?	Yes ____	No 2
9. Have you ever attended a meeting of Alcoholics Anonymous (AA)?	Yes 5	No ____
10. Have you gotten into fights when drinking?	Yes 1	No ____
11. Has drinking ever created problems with you and your spouse?	Yes 2	No ____
12. Has your spouse (or other family member) ever gone to anyone for help about your drinking?	Yes 2	No ____
13. Have you ever lost friends or dates because of drinking?	Yes 2	No ____
14. Have you ever gotten into trouble at work because of drinking?	Yes 2	No ____
15. Have you ever lost a job because of drinking?	Yes 2	No ____
16. Have you ever neglected your obligations, your family or your work for two or more days in a row because you were drinking?	Yes 2	No ____
17. Do you ever drink before noon?	Yes 1	No ____
18. Have you ever been told you have liver trouble? Cirrhosis?	Yes 2	No ____
19. Have you ever had delirium tremens (DTs) or severe shaking, heard voices or seen things that weren't there after heavy drinking?	Yes 2	No ____
*20. Have you ever gone to anyone for help about your drinking?	Yes 5	No ____
*21. Have you ever been in a hospital because of drinking?	Yes 5	No ____
*22. Have you ever been a patient in a psychiatric hospital or on a psychiatric ward of a general hospital where drinking was part of the problem?	Yes 2	No ____
*23. Have you ever been seen at a psychiatric or mental health clinic or gone to a doctor, social worker or clergyman for help with an emotional problem in which drinking had played a part?	Yes 2	No ____
24. Have you ever been arrested, even for a few hours, because of drunk behavior?	Yes 2	No ____
25. Have you ever been arrested for drunk driving or driving after drinking?	Yes 2	No ____

*—*Do not include this hospital episode or any outpatient consultation that led to this hospital episode.*

The questions are weighted in scoring from one to five points, with the exception of Question 7, which is worth 0 points, regardless of how it is answered. Among patients scoring five points or more, the alcoholic patients scored a significantly higher number of "alcoholic responses" than the nonalcoholic patients.

From Glass, G.S.: Recognizing and Managing the Outpatient Alcoholic. *American Family Physician.* 15:176, Mar. 1977, p. 179.

The use of screening questions to determine the presence of drug problems needs to become a part of all routine intake information wherever patients are seen. A number of useful screening tools for assessing alcohol abuse are available. This is less true for other drugs of abuse.

Instruments available to aid in the identification of alcohol abuse include: (1) *"What Are the Signs of Alcoholism?"*, a checklist published by the National Council on Alcoholism, which is designed to help individuals determine whether they have a problem with alcohol.[42] (2) The short *Michigan Alcoholism Screening Test,* questions useful in identifying alcohol problems. This is considered to be a valid and reliable tool for diagnosing alcohol abuse and alcoholism.[33]

Of course, as when using any assessment tool, a thorough understanding of scoring and interpretation processes is imperative. A listing of drug use assessment tools is available in *The Drug Abuse Instrument Handbook,* published by the National Institute on Drug Abuse.

Any history must include a thorough exploration of social, emotional, and physical aspects of the life of the person abusing drugs. It must provide information about past and present drug consumption habits, including the amount and type of drug consumed, frequency of use, situations in which the drug is used, self-perception of drug taking behavior, and the effects of the drug on performance.

In addition to initial screening and history-taking, *physical assessment* is used in diagnosing drug abuse. It serves to broaden the base of clues that lead to identification of physiologic problems coexisting with, or consequent to, drug abuse. Such potential problems are discussed in some detail later in this chapter. (See Chapters 14 and 15 for discussion of psychosocial and physical assessment.)

Drug abuse and addiction are usually not effectively diagnosed. Some reasons for failure to recognize these problems are: (a) low professional awareness of the problems; (b) shielding of the affected person by significant others, and (c) problems of differential diagnosis.

PREVALENCE

Alcohol is the most used drug in the Western world. It has been estimated that one in ten users develops a problem with abuse and addiction.

> *Alcohol abuse and addiction are the number one drug problems today.*

In recent years, there has been an increase in alcohol abuse among teenagers. However, alcoholism still tends to occur most frequently among those 35 to 55 years of age. The ratio of women to men alcoholics is 1:3. This probably reflects traditional social constraints on heavy drinking among women. As women's roles and images change, this ratio is decreasing and may well reach 1:1 in years to come.

In studies of people *who seek medical aid* and are diagnosed as drug abusers, women frequently outnumber men.[41] This may be because of the high incidence of abuse and addiction to *prescription drugs* among women. Perhaps women prefer to get their emotional relief from prescription drugs, which are socially acceptable, rather than from heavy drinking or from illegal drug use.[15]

A particular drug abuse pattern practiced by a small number of young people is the *inhalation of substances containing organic solvents,* such as airplane glue or gasoline.

Besides legally available substances, there is a wide variety of illegal, mood-altering drugs potentially available for use, abuse and addiction. These include heroin, amphetamines, cocaine, marijuana, and hallucinogens. In general, *the use of illegal drugs* is not as widespread as the use of legal drugs.[30] A few trends can be noted. Men become dependent on illegal drugs more often than women, and most persons dependent on illegal drugs are young adults or middle-aged.[40]

EFFECTS OF PSYCHOACTIVE DRUGS

The onset of a drug's effect depends on *characteristics of the drug* itself in addition to the *route of administration* and the *adequacy of the circulatory system.*

The magnitude of drug effects depends upon the concentration of the drug at the neuron. Generally, the greater the amount of a drug that is consumed, the greater will be the observed behavioral response. Expectations and beliefs about the effect that the drug will produce are also important.

The drug is delivered to the neuron via the blood stream. There are three primary ways the drug *enters the blood stream:* (1) oral ingestion, (2) injection, and (3) inhalation. If a drug is taken *orally,* it must diffuse or be actively transported into capillaries from cells that line the stomach and small intestine. On the other hand, a drug immediately enters the blood stream if *injected* into a vein. With an intramuscular or subcutaneous injection, the drug enters the blood stream by diffusion from the intracellular space where it was deposited.[30] *Inhalation* efficiently delivers some drugs, since the capillary walls are very accessible in the lungs. The drug then quickly enters the blood stream.

Drug effects can be additive. Different drugs can act on the same system.[30] Even though each is ingested in low doses, the combination of drug effects may be the same as a high dose of a single drug. An example of a drug combination that has additive effects is alcohol and the barbiturates. Taken together, their combined depressant effects can be lethal. Drug interactions of this type are discussed later in the chapter.

Blood assays can indicate whether a certain drug is present in the system at a particular time. But they are of no value in assessing the long-term drug history.

Tolerance, Dependence, and Withdrawal

Tolerance is the process whereby the central nervous system adapts to the continued presence of the abused drug. It permits high drug concentrations in the blood. As a result, the person has to take increasing quantities of the drug in order to get the desired effect. This phenomenon results in physical dependence and pathologic changes in the tissues of organs.

> *Evidence of tolerance and physical dependence is necessary for the diagnosis of pharmacologic addiction.*

Dependence, as defined previously, may be psychologic as well as physiologic. Addicted persons have an overwhelming psychologic desire to continue consuming their drug of choice. Susceptible individuals can become psychologically dependent on any and all drugs.

Tolerance and dependence are important to understand. They help explain the phenomenon of *withdrawal.* Withdrawal is a consistent pattern of physical responses that appears when regular drug use is discontinued. When a person who is *physically dependent* on drugs abruptly stops drug consumption (or even decreases the daily amount), withdrawal signs and symptoms can occur. Not all drugs produce physical dependence. We discuss this for specific drugs later in this chapter.

In general, drug withdrawal reactions tend to produce the opposite effect of the ingested drug. A depressant drug, for example, causes hyperactivity in a withdrawing abuser.

> *The intensity and progression of withdrawal symptoms is proportional to the quantity and duration of drug consumption.*

Nurses encounter persons withdrawing from drugs in various settings. For example, such a person may be admitted to a hospital for surgery or as a result of illness or traumatic injury. The staff, if unaware of the heavy drug intake, are "caught by surprise" when symptoms of withdrawal begin. It is essential that assessment of drug intake be an integral part of initial nursing histories for all patients.

It is important to obtain accurate *historical information* from patients or significant others about the quantity of drug consumed, how long the person has been taking drugs, and when the last drug was ingested. It is also useful to discuss past withdrawal episodes in order to be alert to possible adverse reactions. With knowledge of a patient's drug history, nurses can be alert to indications of impending withdrawal. If drug abuse or addiction is not detected and treated, a patient may progress to a severe state of withdrawal that may be difficult to treat.

> *In order to prevent a severe withdrawal episode, the usual* treatment for physically dependent persons *is to gradually decrease the amount of the drug they are dependent on. Another drug, with which the addictive drug is cross-tolerant, may be given in initially intoxicating doses and the dosage gradually decreased.*

An appropriate nursing action is to encourage *long-term treatment* for the drug-dependent person. This might consist of residential treatment, half-way house placement, long-term counseling, or any combination of these.

Having discussed general drug effects and nursing management, let us consider some individual psychoactive drugs: (1) alcohol and other sedative-hypnotics, (2) stimulants, (3) opiates, (4) cannabis derivatives, (5) hallucinogens, and (6) solvents.

Alcohol and Other Sedative-Hypnotic Drugs

Alcohol (ethyl alcohol, ethanol, C_2H_5OH) belongs to the pharmacologic class of drugs known as sedative-hypnotics. These drugs relieve anxiety at one level (sedative) and produce sleep at another, higher, level (hypnotic).[43] *Most drugs of abuse are sedative-hypnotics* which are commonly prescribed. Besides alcohol, this group includes tranquilizers, barbiturates, and other central nervous system depressants. (Neuroleptics are excluded from this category.) Table 94–1 lists common brand names of depressants. Among the slang terms used for these drugs are:

Barbiturates	barbs, block busters, blues, downers, pink ladies, rainbows, reds, red devils, yellows, sleeping pills
Methaqualone	quads, soapers
Glutethimide	C.D., Cibas

ALCOHOL

Alcohol is a simple molecule. It is taken orally, requires no digestion, and is absorbed readily from the stomach and the initial part of the small intestine. The *rate of absorption* primarily depends on the concentration in the stomach, and duodenum, but can be altered. For example, soda water speeds up the absorption of alcohol by increasing the rate at which alcohol enters the bloodstream. Food, on the other hand, especially protein, takes longer to digest and slows down the absorption of alcohol. Thus alcohol consumed with or shortly after a meal or snacks is absorbed more slowly. Once absorbed into the blood, alcohol passes almost immediately through the *liver.*

A fixed amount of alcohol can be metabolized at any given time. This is known as *zero-order kinetics.* The metabolism rate will not increase no matter how much alcohol is consumed. The "average" person metabolizes about 6 Gm. of pure ethanol per hour. This is equivalent to 30 ml. of "hard" liquor or whiskey (vodka, gin, etc.), which contains 40 to 50 per cent alcohol; 150 ml. of table wine (12 per cent alcohol); or 400 ml. of beer (5 per cent alcohol). (See Figure 94–2.)

When a person drinks at a rate faster than alcohol can be metabolized, alcohol accumulates in the blood in ever higher concentrations. This results in evidence of intoxication.

Blood Levels and Behavior. The relationship between blood alcohol levels and behavior in a "naive" drinker are shown in Table 94–2. Except when death occurs, these effects are temporary. They subside as alcohol consumption is stopped and as the liver has time to metabolize the alcohol present in the blood. These relationships between blood alcohol levels and behavior are not valid, however, in the person who has developed tolerance to alcohol.

Tolerance. Chronic consumption of large amounts of alcohol over long periods of time results in *tolerance*, by altering the state of sensitivity of the central nervous system. Alcohol-dependent people who have developed tolerance can drink large quantities without obvious impairment. They can accurately perform complex behavioral tasks at blood alcohol levels several times as great as those that would lead to behavioral impairment in moderate and heavy drinkers. By combining knowledge about symptoms expected at certain blood alcohol levels in the naive drinker with an individual's blood alcohol level and symptoms, a nurse can estimate the person's level of tolerance. For example, a patient exhibiting symptoms of stupor with a blood alcohol level of 0.60 per cent shows high tolerance to alcohol.

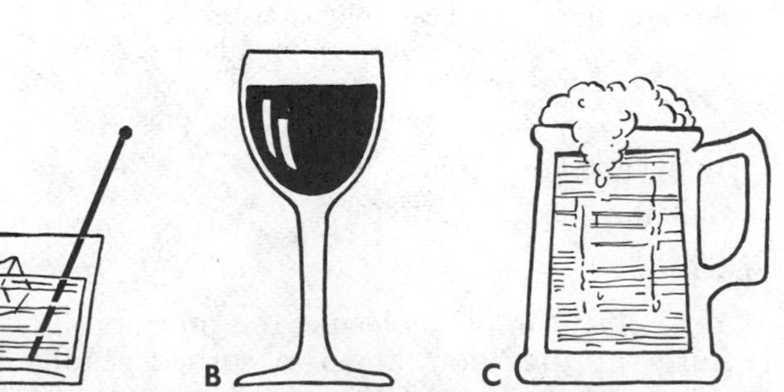

Figure 94–2. In a 150 lb. (68.2 kg.) male, alcohol is metabolized at the rate of approximately one drink per hour. The "typical" drink–25 ml. of pure alcohol–is provided by the following: **A.** A "shot" of spirits (30 ml. of 40–50% alcohol). **B.** A glass of table wine (150 ml. of 12% alcohol). **C.** A pint of beer (400 ml. of 5% alcohol).

TABLE 94–2. THE RELATIONSHIP BETWEEN BLOOD ALCOHOL LEVELS AND BEHAVIOR IN A NAIVE DRINKER

Blood Levels (%)	Behavior
0.05	Perceptible changes in mood and behavior. Judgment and restraint are loosened. The individual feels carefree.
0.10	Voluntary motor action becomes clumsy. Legal evidence of intoxication in most states.
0.20	The function of the entire motor area of the brain is measurably depressed, causing staggering. The individual may be easily angered, and may shout or weep.
0.30	Confusion; stupor.
0 40	Coma.
0.50	Death due to respiratory blocking effects on the medulla.

Withdrawal. Alcohol is a sedative-hypnotic. The removal of alcohol from the body, or withdrawal,* results in psychomotor agitation. The earliest and most common features of withdrawal are anxiety, anorexia, insomnia, and tremor. The patient appears hyperalert and manifests jerky movements, irritability, and a tendency to be easily startled. The subjective distress is often described as internal shaking. This set of problems develops within a few hours of cessation of drinking and peaks about 24 hours afterwards.[12] The pulse and blood pressure are typically elevated and are useful indicators of progress through withdrawal. Diaphoresis is manifest in some persons. A brief, mild disorientation, particularly to time, may also occur. *Alcoholic hallucinosis* may develop. It is benign and does not induce fear in the patient. Orientation remains intact.

During the first 48 hours of withdrawal, self-limiting grand mal convulsive seizures may develop. *Delirium tremens* (DT's) may occur about 72 hours after cessation of drinking. They are

**Detoxification* is the process whereby a longer acting sedative-hypnotic drug is substituted for alcohol and the dose tapered gradually downward so that withdrawal occurs in a slow, predictable fashion.

characterized by severe psychomotor agitation, confusion, disorientation, frightening hallucinations, metabolic dysfunction, and increased autonomic activity, i.e., fever, tachycardia, profuse diaphoresis.

Figure 94–3 graphically depicts the usual time course of alcohol withdrawal symptoms. Individual reactions can differ extensively from this model. Also, symptoms of "minor" and "major" withdrawal often overlap.

The time when withdrawal symptoms can be expected to appear after cessation of alcohol intake can be predicted. For example, after 6 to 8 hours tremulousness develops. Then, after 10 to 30 hours convulsions and hallucinations may occur. As mentioned, delirium tremens may appear about 72 hours after drinking has stopped. Variations do occur. However, these estimates provide a guide to the nurse in anticipating the severity of symptoms.

Nursing Actions. An estimated 30 per cent of hospitalized patients are alcohol abusers.[23] It is thus important for a nurse to elicit an alcohol consumption history from patients and to observe them for indications of alcohol problems or withdrawal.

> *The more critical withdrawal reactions – seizures and delirium tremens – can be avoided with anticipatory observations and intervention.*

The pulse and blood pressure, which provide the most accurate clues to the degree of psychomotor agitation, are frequently assessed. If the *pulse* reaches 110 or more and the *blood pressure* 150/90 or greater in the absence of concurrent illnesses such as fever, hypovolemia or chronic hypertension, further assessment should be carried out. The presence or absence of *tremors* or *diaphoresis* should be noted. If no history of alcohol intake has been obtained, it should be acquired now. Evaluate the reason the patient is seeking health care. Many illnesses are highly suggestive of excessive alcohol intake. (See section on clinical problems, pp. 2133–2140.) In addition, traumatic injuries occur more frequently in people who abuse drugs. (See Ch. 95.)

When you suspect an impending *withdrawal reaction,* the physician must be notified. Orders may then be given for a drug that is cross-tolerant with alcohol. The *benzodiazepine class of sedatives* (e.g., Librium, Valium) is most frequently used because of the large margin of safety between the effective and lethal dose.[32] The goal is to prevent the withdrawal reaction from becoming severe. Large, frequent doses of sedatives may be required to keep agitation minimal. Remember that alcoholic persons have acquired tolerance to depressant drugs and thus may need greater, more frequent doses than nonalcoholic people.

Dosages are adequate when withdrawal symptoms are suppressed. The pulse and blood pressure should decrease; frequent and accurate monitoring is essential. As vital signs stabilize, the drug dosage is slowly and steadily decreased until the drugs can be totally discontinued. This usually takes 3 to 5 days.

A *quiet, calm, environment* is also useful in minimizing reactions such as alcoholic hallucinosis and seizures. Excessive stimuli may precipitate either of these two conditions in an agitated, hyperexcitable person. Lewis stresses that even the profound hallucinations of delirium tremens can be totally avoided with knowledgeable nursing care.[25] Minimizing intrusions, moving slowly and deliberately instead of hurriedly and brusquely, and calmly informing the

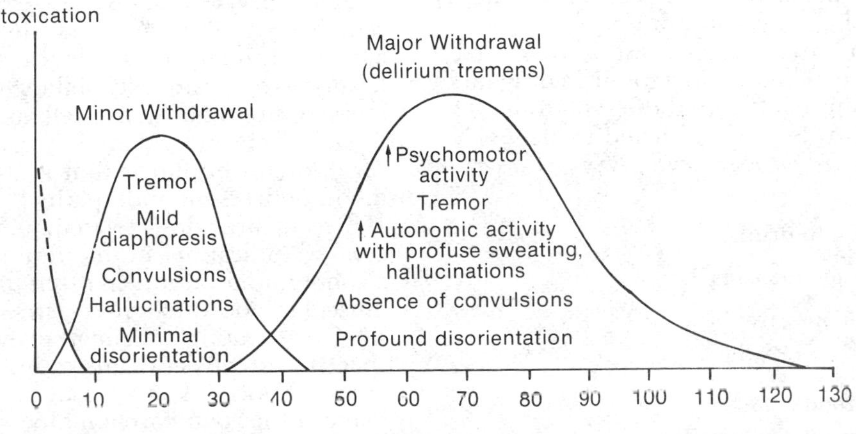

Figure 94–3. Clinical findings during the minor (early) alcohol withdrawal syndrome and the major withdrawal syndrome (delirium tremens). (From Wolfe, S.M., and M. Victor: The physiological basis of the alcohol withdrawal syndrome. *In* Mello, N., and J.H. Mendelson (Eds.): *Recent Advances in Studies of Alcoholism.* Rockville, Md.: National Institute on Alcohol Abuse and Alcoholism, 1971, p. 189.)

patient of what you are doing are some of the measures employed to create a therapeutic environment. In addition, keeping lighting even and bright enough to minimize the chance of creating shadows but not so bright as to cause glare is also helpful. A significant other may be asked to sit quietly in the patient's room and to be available for answering questions, reorienting the person if necessary, and calling a nurse if a problem should arise.*

In summary, nurses can do much to minimize the agitation of alcohol withdrawal. By maintaining a calm, supportive environment and medicating appropriately, alcohol withdrawal need not be life-threatening.

Clinical Course of Alcoholism. Characteristically, drinking in the early stages is intermittent, becoming more frequent and gradually more prolonged.

Early significant landmarks of ensuing alcoholism are:

- Constant drinking for relief of tension and anxiety
- Psychologic dependence
- Onset of memory blackouts
- Surreptitious drinking
- Urgent need to drink
- Increasing physical dependence on alcohol, manifested by increasing tolerance

With the persistence of continued heavy drinking, withdrawal symptoms such as tremors and agitation become manifest if the person stops drinking. Then the person drinks again in order to obtain relief from these symptoms. The person has now become addicted to alcohol.

Progress toward the chronic stages in characterized by:

- Inability to stop drinking
- Loss of outside interests
- Work and money troubles
- Difficulties with significant others
- Neglect of food
- Feelings of guilt, remorse, depression
- Intense loneliness

A stage of continuous drinking develops. The person remains in a more or less constant state of inebriation, or goes through a vicious cycle of drinking bouts that end in acute withdrawal and lead to another bout. *Progression to chronicity characteristically takes from 12 to 20 years.*

Tolerance decreases during the chronic stage and numerous pathologic conditions are demonstrable. Although poorly understood, the mechanism for decreased tolerance is believed to be related to diffuse brain damage.[96]

OTHER SEDATIVE-HYPNOTIC DRUGS

The most frequent route of administration for sedative-hypnotic drugs is oral, but they can be injected either intramuscularly or intravenously. The drugs are manufactured in both tablet and injectable form. Street *"mainliners"* (the term used for persons who inject drugs intravenously) often dissolve tablets in warm water for injection purposes.

Sedative-hypnotics are readily absorbed. The *time of onset* of action varies from 15 minutes to 1 hour. The *duration of action* ranges from 2 hours to more than 10 hours, depending on the preparation and route of administration.

Deactivation occurs in the liver and is mediated by the microsomal enzymes. Sedative-hypnotic drugs are handled by the body in a *first order kinetic way* (as are all other drugs except alcohol). This means that a fixed percentage of the drug remaining in the body is handled per unit of time. First order kinetic drugs have measurable half lives; the amount handled per unit of time proportional to the amount in the body.[43] Thus, the more that is ingested, the more that is deactivated. This process seems to be characteristic of the microsomal enzyme system.

Behavioral Changes. Effects of the other sedative-hypnotics are very similar to those of alcohol. Initially these drugs cause a general lowering of brain excitability, resulting in decreased inhibitions, as well as mild sedation. Relief of tension and anxiety produces a temporary state of euphoria, but it also may produce mood depression and apathy.

Effects are dose-related. As the dose increases, indications of intoxication are similar to alcohol intoxication. An often unrealized loss of muscular coordination occurs. Mental confusion, a "floating" feeling, drowsiness, slurred speech and physical unsteadiness (ataxia) may be experienced. Large doses can disrupt performance of certain psychomotor, intellectual, and perceptual functions, e.g., driving motor vehicles and operating machinery. People do, of course, differ in their response to these drugs. In some, increased aggression rather than the

*See Sorensen and Luckmann, *Basic Nursing: A Psychophysiologic Approach,* for discussion of a safe, therapeutic environment; promoting rest and sleep; and disorganized behavior and thought processes accompanying illness.

usual calming effect has been observed. Characteristics of individual drugs within this category also vary. Variations are reported in achieved blood levels, metabolism, and the rate at which the drug is stored in body tissues.[30]

Because additive central nervous system effects occur, the clinical evidence of intoxication may be much greater than the evidence of intake, from history or blood levels, would suggest. *Whenever a patient appears more intoxicated than the history given would indicate, drug intake should be further clarified.* Sedative drugs, singly or in combination, may induce stupor, coma, and possible death.

Tolerance and Physical Dependence. In addition to CNS tolerance, it is likely that an increased rate of deactivation caused by the stimulation of the liver's microsomal enzymes is also involved in the development of tolerance and physical dependence. Besides increasing drug intake capacity, tolerance to sedative-hypnotics narrows the range between an intoxicating and lethal dose. Thus, the tolerance to a lethal dose does not increase as rapidly as does the tolerance to an intoxicating dose. A person who is unaware of the dangers of increasing dependence may seek prescriptions from several physicians concurrently, thus increasing the daily dose up to 10 or 20 times the recommended amount.

Withdrawal. People who abruptly stop taking or sharply curtail the amount of a sedative-hypnotic that they have become physically dependent on will experience severe withdrawal symptoms. The severity and course of the withdrawal syndrome is influenced by the particular drug used, the pattern and duration of use, and individual susceptibility. In its *mildest form*, withdrawal is characterized by anxiety, agitation, and apprehension. It is accompanied by loss of appetite, nausea, vomiting, tachycardia, diaphoresis, insomnia, fainting, tremulousness, and muscle spasms. If the individual is dependent on a large amount of the drug, *severe withdrawal* may occur, with delirium, psychotic behavior, convulsions, or even death. As an example, the spectrum of barbiturate withdrawal signs and symptoms is presented in Figure 94–4.

In view of the possible severity of the withdrawal syndrome, hospitalization is recommended for *treatment*. A long-acting barbiturate is usually substituted for the sedative-hypnotic of abuse, in gradually decreasing doses. The process is usually completed in 10 to 14 days. Withdrawal from sedative-hypnotics takes longer than withdrawal from alcohol because they are eliminated from the body more slowly.

The goal of withdrawal management is to provide safe treatment of the physical dependence. *The onset, intensity, and progression of withdrawal symptoms can be predicted* by obtaining the patient's drug history and ascertaining blood levels.

Nursing Actions. Withdrawal signs or symptoms and toxic symptoms must be carefully monitored. The drug dosage is initially kept high to keep signs of withdrawal minimal. If toxic symptoms develop, the drug dosage will need to be decreased. The specific management is virtually the same as that described for alcohol.

Clinical Course. Progression to severe forms of drug abuse with sedative-hypnotics is typically a gradual process. Ingestion begins intermittently and, in some persons, becomes gradually more frequent and prolonged. Early significant *landmarks of abuse* are:

▶ Increase in drug tolerance, physical dependence

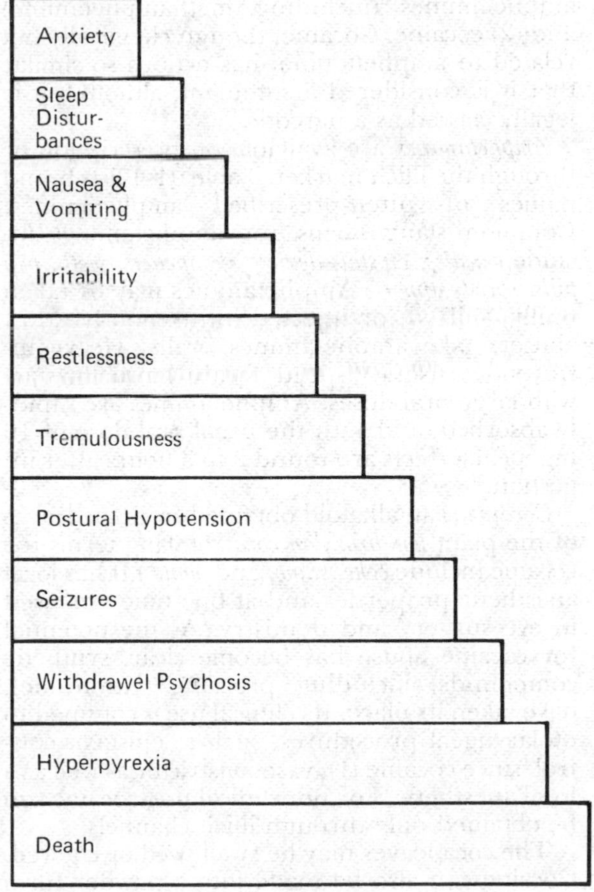

Figure 94–4. The spectrum of barbiturate withdrawal signs and symptoms. (From Bourne, P. G. (Ed.): *A Treatment Manual for Acute Drug Abuse Emergencies.* Rockville, Md.: National Clearinghouse for Drug Abuse Information Publication, No. 16, 1974.)

- ▶ Constant drug use to relieve anxiety and tension
- ▶ Psychologic dependence

Physical dependence becomes manifest with persistent drug consumption. As little as 600 mg. of short-acting barbiturate taken daily for 30 days has been shown to be sufficient to produce withdrawal seizures in some persons.[44] Marked physical dependence is an indicator of addiction. For example, any person who chronically takes short-acting barbiturates in excess of 1500 mg. per day can be assumed to have a marked physical dependency.[5]

Stimulants

Stimulants are classified into two types: (1) the amphetamines (including methamphetamine) and (2) cocaine. Cocaine, though chemically not related to amphetamine, has actions so similar that it is considered a stimulant, although it is legally classed as a narcotic.

Amphetamines are available on prescription or through the illicit market. Table 94–1 lists brand names of often-prescribed amphetamines. Common slang terms for amphetamines include *bennies, crystal, dexies, eye openers, meth, pep pills, speed, uppers*. Amphetamines may be taken orally, sniffed, or injected intravenously. Most abusers take amphetamines orally. Heavy intravenous users ("speed freaks") usually start with large oral doses. Amphetamines are rapidly absorbed, and with the usual oral dose of 10 mg. peak effects are found 2 to 3 hours after ingestion.[30]

Cocaine is an alkaloid obtained from the leaves of the plant *Erythroxylon coca*.[15] (Slang terms for cocaine include *coke, snow,* and *white*.) It has local anesthetic properties and at one time was used in eye surgery and dentistry. As the potential for cocaine abuse has become clear, synthetic compounds, including procaine (Novacaine), have taken its place. Its clinical use is confined to otolaryngeal procedures, such as epistaxis control, since cocaine is a vasoconstrictor as well as a local anesthetic. For nonclinical use, cocaine can be obtained only through illicit channels.

The coca leaves may be swallowed or chewed. Cocaine can also be made into a powder form and is either mainlined or snorted (inhaled, sniffed). It readily passes into the blood stream from any of these administration routes.

The major difference between the amphetamines and cocaine is the duration of action. The effects of cocaine are very transient, as it is rapidly destroyed in the body.[15] It must be injected every 15 minutes or snorted every hour to maintain the state of exhilaration.[30] Thus, very large amounts may be taken throughout the day. Amphetamine needs to be injected every 2 to 4 hours, as it is excreted from the body fairly slowly.[15] The duration of action would be longer if the drug were taken orally.

Behavioral Changes. Stimulants increase the activity of the reticular activating system as well as other areas in the central nervous system. Behavioral output and responsiveness to sensory input is increased. Stimulants are considered to be agents that improve mental and physical performance when a person is fatigued or bored. They also suppress appetite. In the past, amphetamines were prescribed for these purposes. As the potential for abuse has become known, limits have been placed on manufacture of the substances. Many physicians believe that the only legitimate use of amphetamines is in the treatment of narcolepsy or hyperactive children.

When stimulants are injected intravenously, a "flash" or sudden feeling of intense pleasure is experienced. It probably represents the delivery of a very high blood concentration of the drug to the brain.[30]

Amphetamine abusers are usually remarkably alert, with an extended wakefulness. They may appear euphoric, exhilarated, hyperactive, overly enthusiastic and extremely talkative. This overactivity may be followed by an unpleasant period of depression, lethargy, and fatigue known as "crashing." Since the depression can be counteracted by taking more stimulants, the abuse pattern becomes increasingly difficult to break. Heavy abusers may take stimulants every few hours, a process sometimes continued to the point of delirium, psychosis, or physical exhaustion. Abusers demonstrate tremulousness and a marked tendency to agitation, apprehension, and irritability. They may become hostile and aggressive.

Sustained stimulant use may lead to a paranoid psychosis manifested by delusions and hallucinations, usually visual or auditory. Withdrawal from stimulants leads to a marked improvement of symptoms.

High doses of stimulants may cause "cocaine bugs." These are tactile hallucinations, the feeling that insects are crawling under one's skin. The sensation may be so distressing that the person may try anything to "get them out." The basis for this experience is probably a drug-induced stimulation of nerve endings in the skin; however, the mechanism is not yet clear.[9]

Amphetamine effects on body systems can be extensive. Acute physiologic reactions may complicate debilitation from chronic use.

Initial Physiologic Reactions. Excessively dry mouth, diaphoresis, dilated pupils, brisk reflexes, and tremors are usually present on examination of a stimulant abuser. Tachycardia and hypertension may initially be present but may be absent in a chronic tolerant user. Respiratory rates are increased. Malnutrition with weight loss is common. Teeth may be worn and the lips and tongue ulcerated.[5] Needle marks and tracks may be present.

Because of its vasoconstrictor properties, individuals who have been snorting cocaine may have a perforated nasal septum. High levels of cocaine delivered intravenously may stop the heart because of a direct action of cocaine on the heart muscle.[30]

Tolerance. Tolerance to the effects of stimulants occurs rapidly, increasing the probability of stimulants is considerable. Whether or not pressant effect occurs first, generally within 4 weeks. This is followed by tolerance to the cardiovascular effects, tachycardia, and hypertension. Lastly, tolerance to the central nervous system effects of arousal and euphoria develops.

Dependence. The risk of development of psychologic dependence with the sustained use of stimulants is considerable. Whether or not physical dependence is produced by these drugs is still open to question. Profound apathy and depression, lethargy and fatigue, prolonged sleep (e.g, up to 20 hours a day), and overeating characterize the immediate withdrawal syndrome. This may last for several days.

Abrupt cessation of regular high doses of stimulants is not life-threatening, and convulsions never occur.[30] *Treatment* is nonspecific and is based on a careful history of drug use as well as observable symptoms.

Nursing Actions. Environmental safety measures (including frequent observations) are important for hyperactive, euphoric patients. Realistic limits must be set on behavior. A person on stimulants is agitated and may easily be provoked into aggressive, violent behavior. A calm approach is necessary.

As the stimulant effects subside, lethargy, fatigue, hunger, and depression may become manifest. Extra calories and a lot of sleep may be needed for a few days. Depression usually clears with time, a good diet, and rest. In severe cases, however, tricyclic antidepressants may be prescribed.

Amphetamine abusers may seek health care following a real or suspected *overdose*. Dizziness, tremor, agitation, hostility, panic, headache, flushed skin, chest pain with palpitations, diaphoresis, vomiting, and abdominal cramps are among the symptoms of a sublethal overdose. Without medical intervention, hyperpyrexia, convulsions, and cardiovascular collapse may precede the onset of death. Death is due in part to the consequences of a marked increase in body temperature. Therefore, physical exertion and a high environmental temperature may increase the hazards of stimulant use.

Opiates

Morphine is extracted from *opium*, which comes from the oriental poppy, *Papavar somniferum*. *Heroin* is only a minor chemical change from morphine. The effects of morphine and heroin are identical except that heroin acts faster. *Codeine*, also derived from opium, is abused largely by addicts who cannot get heroin. Codeine's euphoric and analgesic effects are very slight. Its major appeal is that it may be more readily available, particularly in combination with cough medicine.

Heroin is the most commonly abused opiate. Thus it is the focus of this discussion. Much of what is said about heroin also applies to morphine. (Since morphine is available only by prescription, it is primarily abused by health professionals, especially physicians and those closely related to physicians.)

Slang terms for heroin include *big H, H, horse, junk, and smack*. Heroin comes in powder form. To administer, it is mixed with water and heated, usually in a spoon. The solution is then drawn into a syringe or eye dropper through cotton, to filter out the major impurities. The person injects the solution intravenously. The effects are felt within seconds. The drug can also be injected subcutaneously ("skin popping").

Behavioral Changes. Heroin acts on the CNS, providing a sense of calm, relaxation, and euphoria because of the relief of physical or psychic suffering. Soon the user goes "on the nod," an alternately waking and drowsy state during which the world is forgotten The dose required for the pleasant effects, "the high," may induce nausea and vomiting because of effects on lower brain centers. As the dose is increased, respiratory depression becomes progressively more marked and may be fatal. With very large doses the following occur: the person cannot be roused, the pupils are contracted to pinpoints, the skin is cold, moist, and bluish, the body is limp, the jaw relaxed. Risk of death is high on the street, where contents of a "hit" cannot be accurately gauged.

Tolerance. Tolerance develops quickly. Possibly an alteration in general neuronal metabolism is directly responsible for both tolerance and physical dependence.[30]

Withdrawal. Symptoms are most frequently described as like those of gastric flu. The sequence of symptoms and the time of their appearance after the last dose of narcotics are shown in Table 94–3.

The first withdrawal signs are usually experienced shortly before the time of the next scheduled dose. Uneasiness, "craving," complaints, pleas, and demands by the addict are prominent. These increase in intensity, peak between 36 and 72 hours after the last dose, and then gradually subside. Symptoms such as lacrimation, rhinorrhea, yawning, and perspiration appear about 8 to 12 hours after the last dose. Thereafter, the person may fall into a restless sleep. As withdrawal progresses, restlessness, irritability, loss of appetite, insomnia, piloerections, tremors and finally violent yawning and severe sneezing occur. The patient is weak and depressed, with nausea and vomiting. Stomach cramps and diarrhea are common. Heart rate and blood pressure are elevated. Chills alternating with flushing and diaphoresis are also characteristic symptoms. Pain is experienced in the bones and muscles of the back and extremities. Muscle spasm and kicking movements occur. These may be the source of the expression "kicking the habit." The individual may become suicidal. Without treatment, most symptoms disappear in 7 to 10 days. Withdrawal from heroin is rarely a life-threatening process, as it can be with alcohol and other sedative-hypnotics.

Treatment is usually symptomatic, similar to treatment for gastric flu. The process of recovery may take months. Major persisting symptoms are sleeplessness, depression, and inability to concentrate.[15] Withdrawal symptoms are more severe the more rapidly the drug is withdrawn. Thus, if possible, the drug should be withdrawn gradually, over a period of 1 to 3 weeks. Oral methadone is often given as a substitute for heroin during this period. (Methadone is discussed below, in *Clinical Course*.)

Nursing Actions. Nurses most frequently encounter persons addicted to heroin during withdrawal. These patients may be very uncomfortable and need a lot of supportive nursing care. A thorough knowledge of indications of heroin withdrawal is important for assessment. Addicted persons may be quite manipulative when attempting to obtain medication to relieve suffering. *The nurse bases therapeutic decisions on knowledge of the physiologic events taking place as well as on assessment of each individual patient.*

Assessing pupil size is helpful in gauging adequacy of drug doses during withdrawal. Constricted pupils indicate adequate blood levels; dilated pupils indicate withdrawal is occurring. Thus, if an addicted person expresses withdrawal discomfort and asks for medication, the drug dosage can be judged as adequate if the pupils are constricted.

Support and sympathetic listening by the nurse are more important than medication during withdrawal. The discomfort of withdrawal can be better tolerated if a patient trusts the nurse. Anxiety may be reduced by therapeutic communication.

It takes a minimum of about one week for medically supervised detoxification of a heroin addict.[4] Adequate nutrition is important. Food may have been neglected while "fixing." In addition, constipation may be a problem since heroin (1) impairs digestion by decreasing the secretion of essential digestive juices, (2) decreases peristaltic activity, and (3) enhances water absorption from intestinal material.[30]

Clinical Course. As with all addictions, heroin addiction is progressive. The clinical course for heroin addiction may vary between countries. Note, for example, the differences between the clinical course of heroin addiction in Britain and the United States. In America, heroin can be obtained only illicitly at extreme prices. Thus, an addicted person's entire day is typically spent attempting to procure the desperately needed drug. It becomes impossible to hold down a job or engage in any constructive activity. Basic needs, e.g., nutrition and hygiene, are neglected. Thus, the person becomes under-

TABLE 94–3. SEQUENCE OF APPEARANCE OF SOME OF THE HEROIN ABSTINENCE SYNDROME SYMPTOMS

Signs	Approximate hours after last dose		
	Heroin	*Morphine*	*Methadone*
Craving for drugs, anxiety	4	6	12
Yawning, perspiration, running nose, teary eyes	8	14	34 to 48
Increase in above signs plus pupil dilation, goose bumps (piloerection), tremors (muscle twitches), hot and cold flashes, aching bones and muscles, loss of appetite	12	16	48 to 72
Increased intensity of above, plus insomnia; raised blood pressure; increased temperature, pulse rate, respiratory rate and depth; restlessness; nausea	18 to 24	24 to 36	
Increased intensity of above, plus curled-up position, vomiting, diarrhea, weight loss, spontaneous ejaculation or orgasm, hemoconcentration, increased blood sugar	26 to 36	36 to 48	

From Ray, O.: *Drugs, Society and Human Behavior.* St. Louis: C. V. Mosby Co., 1972, p. 203.

nourished and prone to infections. These vocational and medical problems do not stem from the drug or its regular use, but from the subculture that surrounds illegal drug use. Physicians and biomedical people may become addicted yet continue their normal activities for years because they have access to their drugs.[30]

In Britain, persons addicted to heroin can be registered and receive their drug legally by prescription. They know each day that their drug will be supplied, and the cost is negligible. Thus it is possible to spend their time working and spend their money on food and other basic needs.

This same rationale supports the use of methadone in treatment of heroin addiction. Methadone is an addicting substance designed to substitute for, not eliminate, heroin dependencies. A heroin-addicted person may be *maintained* on methadone, receiving consistent daily doses. There is much controversy about the use of methadone. Some advantages attributed to this form of treatment are: (a) the addicted person has a regular, pure supply and does not have to commit crimes to obtain drugs; (b) there is less chance of overdose because the supply is regulated; and (c) the addicted person has a greater chance of social integration, since time and energy are not exclusively devoted to drug procurement.

Opponents of methadone believe that such treatment simply commits people to drug dependence for the rest of their lives.

Cannabis Derivatives

Marijuana and *hashish* are cannabis derivatives. The psychoactive agent is concentrated in the resin of the *Cannabis sativa* plant. Hashish, or hash, is resin from the flowering tops and is highly potent. Marijuana is much less potent. It consists chiefly of leafy material and fine stems. Hashish and marijuana are taken either orally or by inhalation of smoke from cigarettes ("joints") or from a pipe. The time of onset of effect is more rapid with inhalation.

Terms used to describe marijuana include *pot, tea, weed, grass, Acapulco gold, reefer,* and many others, which vary with social group and geographic location.

Behavioral Changes and Initial Physiologic Reactions. The expected or usual *effects of marijuana* include the following:

- Euphoria, elation, relaxation, well-being, dreaminess, self-confidence, laughing, silliness (in short, a "high" feeling)
- Feelings of detachment, clarity, cleverness, wittiness, disinhibition, depersonalization
- Impaired logical thinking because of irrelevant thoughts, disturbed associations, altered reality testing, decreased concentration and attention span, altered sense of identity
- Speech changes—rapid, impaired, flighty speech, characterized by difficulty with sequential thoughts and poor short-term memory
- Impaired ability to drive a car or perform other complex tasks, as a result of alterations in thinking and memory
- Altered concepts of time, e.g., feeling that more time has passed than actually has
- Suggestibility; rapidly changing emotions
- Increased appetite and thirst
- At a later stage, quietness, reflectiveness, sleepiness
- Dizziness
- Lightness, numbness and weakness of limbs; sensation of floating; paresthesias; changes in body sensations and body image
- Restlessness, ataxia, tremor
- Dry mouth, tachycardia, injected conjunctiva
- With larger doses, sharpened or distorted perceptions of sound, color, and other sensations; slow and confused thinking

In very large doses, the effects may be similar to hallucinogens, e.g., confusion, excitement and hallucination. These effects may cause anxiety, panic, or paranoia or may even precipitate a psychotic episode.

The effects of cannabis derivatives usually last a few hours. Evidence shows that with repeated use less of the drug is needed to produce the same effects. It has been shown that the agent persists in the body as an active metabolite as long as 8 days after use.[30] Therefore, less of the drug would be needed to produce the same effects during this time. *Physical dependence*, exhibited by withdrawal symptoms, does not occur.

Like most toxic substances, this agent is metabolized in the liver. Cannabis derivatives, however, are relatively safe drugs and death associated with their use have not been reported.

Nursing Actions. Professionally, a nurse is likely to encounter an intoxicated cannabis user in the context of an adverse reaction to the drug experience. (There are no completely safe drugs.) Care related to the presenting symptoms is appropriate. Most effects will disappear in 5 to 8 hours as the drug wears off. A frank psychosis may occur, however, and require treatment. Probably the most effective way to help persons experiencing adverse reactions to marijuana is to spend time talking with them in supportive, positive, and concerned ways. Reassurance that the reaction is temporary, that the person is not alone, and that nothing terrible is likely to happen is often remarkably helpful. In order to prevent another adverse reaction, avoidance of drugs should be recommended.

Clinical Course. The addiction pattern itself is one of psychologic dependence, since marijuana does not seem to be addictive in a pharmacologic sense. It has not yet been shown to produce a withdrawal syndrome, and the evidence for tolerance is lacking. Thus the personality of the user rather than characteristics of the drug seems to be the major factor in development of abuse and addiction to cannabis. With the exception of a few individuals, marijuana use does not seem to lead to use of "harder" drugs like heroin.

Cannabis derivatives seem to have become the drugs of choice for a number of persons. They have become an integral part of many social circles and will probably persist as social drugs for some time.

Hallucinogens

The hallucinogenic drugs are substances, both natural and synthetic, that distort perception of objective reality. They produce sensory illusions, making it difficult for a person to distinguish between fact and fantasy. If taken in large doses, they cause hallucinations. Senses of direction, distance, and time become disoriented. Restlessness and sleeplessness are common until the drug wears off. *The greatest hazard of the hallucinogens is that their effects are unpredictable each time they are taken.*

Hallucinogens include the following substances:

- *Mescaline* (*mesc, buttons, cactus*) is obtained by grinding buttons of the peyote cactus. Ingestion is a part of religious ceremonies of certain Indian tribes.
- *Psilocybin* (*magic mushroom*) is derived from types of mushrooms, grown primarily in Mexico. It also has been a traditional part of certain Indian tribes' rites.
- *Phencyclidine* (PCP, *angel dust, hog*) is a synthetic drug that can be smoked, injected or taken orally. It is currently legally marketed as a general anesthetic in veterinary medicine.
- *Lysergic acid diethylamide* (*LSD,* acid) is an extremely potent synthetic compound. Absorption is rapid. It has a half life of 3 hours, so blood levels decrease fairly rapidly also.

The use of hallucinogens appears to have been a fad or social phenomenon in some subcultures. With the exception of PCP few people persist in the abuse of these drugs, hence they are not discussed in detail here.

The peak of LSD use occurred in the late 1960's, and usage today is on the wane for a variety of reasons. One is the possible risk of genetic and chromosomal damage, which has been debated in recent years. Another is the frequency of reports of bad trips associated with use of this drug. Milder hallucinogens, such as mescaline and peyote, have become more popular.

As in other types of drug abuse, the personality of the user seems to be especially important in establishing dependence. Hallucinogens have, for example, been used historically in religious ceremonies and rituals by American Indian tribes. No risk of drug dependence occurred in this context. The secularization of these agents and their use by emotionally unstable and socially maladjusted people resulted in a rise in abuse of these substances.

Solvents

Substances used for inducing an inhalation "high" include gasoline, model airplane glue, paint and paint thinner, lighter fluid, cleaning fluids and nail polish remover. These fat-soluble organic solvents pass the blood-brain barrier quickly.

Behavioral Changes. Short-term effects, which usually wear off in about an hour, include exhilaration, disorientation, confusion, slurred speech, dizziness, distortions of perception, visual and auditory hallucinations, and poor muscular control. With larger doses, drowsiness and unconsciousness can occur.[15] Physical exertion by someone affected by large doses of solvents may produce death from heart failure. An inhalation psychosis may develop. Hallucinations and paranoid delusions are the most characteristically reported clinical features.[5]

Tolerance and Dependence. Tolerance to these agents does not seem to develop. Psychologic dependence, which includes craving and habituation, can occur. Physical dependence has not been definitely established. A withdrawal syndrome consisting of restlessness, anxiety, and irritability has been noted.

Nursing Actions. The acute form of an inhalation psychosis is seldom seen by nurses since it is of relatively brief duration. If a patient does present for treatment, it would be important to provide a supportive, protective environment. Stimuli should be kept at a minimum and frequent observation made.

Most often, however, the nurse will come into

contact with the solvent abuser because of some physiologic damage. For example, a person may be burned on the hands and face because the flammable substance accidentally ignited. Appropriate nursing intervention may include exploring with patients the reason for their solvent abuse and referral for counseling if indicated.

Clinical Course. The pattern of solvent abuse is usually experimental and of limited duration. The abuser either stops abuse of psychoactive substances altogether or chooses different drugs. When chronicity does develop, it can be considerable.[5]

PHYSICAL AND PSYCHOSOCIAL PROBLEMS ASSOCIATED WITH ALCOHOL ABUSE

Multiple, serious pathophysiologic disturbances result from chronic alcohol abuse. Serious disturbances occur in the nervous, gastrointestinal, cardiovascular, respiratory, and musculoskeletal system (Table 94–4 and Figure 94–5). The development of tolerance is in part responsible for these effects. As discussed previously, tolerance is characterized by a reduced sensitivity of cells to the effects of a drug. This permits large quantities of the drug to be consumed and to circulate in the blood stream. Cell damage is a consequence of prolonged exposure to high drug concentrations.

*Neurologic System**

Alcohol's most profound effects are on the nervous system.

> *Nutritional deficiencies are the major etiologic factor in neurologic disorders associated with chronic alcoholism.*

The daily activities of a "steady drinker" are focused on obtaining alcohol, not food. Even a "binge drinker" suffers serious nutritional deficits, because, during the time of drinking, eating is not high priority. While alcohol provides a ready source of calories (and thus energy), it has absolutely no nutritional value. Thus, people who obtain most of their daily caloric requirements from alcohol lack vitamins and other essential nutrients. Persons who continue to consume a normal amount of food while drinking heavily will become overweight.

Poor dietary habits contribute to nutritional deficits, which may lead to *anemias, beriberi heart disease, cheilosis* (fissuring and scaling of the lips and corners of the mouth), and other secondary pathologic changes.

*See also Unit X.

Nutritional deficits alter the normal metabolic activity of the nervous system. The absorption, intestinal transport, tissue storage, utilization, and conversion of vitamins to metabolically active forms may be curtailed.[22] In addition to causing abnormal vitamin metabolism, chronic alcholism may profoundly affect mineral, carbohydrate, protein, and lipid metabolism.[12] If an alcoholic person becomes ill or otherwise severely stressed, metabolic demands increase and thus nutritional deficits are exacerbated. *Alcoholic polyneuropathy and the Wernicke-Korsakoff syndrome are the most commonly seen clinical sequelae to alcohol abuse and inadequate nutritional intake.*

Alcoholic Polyneuropathy. Polyneuropathies are most frequently seen in the fourth

TABLE 94–4. ALCOHOL-RELATED DISORDERS AND THEIR CAUSES

Disorder	Cause
Hypoglycemia	Inhibition of gluconeogenesis, depletion of glycogen stores, low-carbohydrate diet
Hyperlipidemia	Increased lipoprotein production, increased lipoprotein clearance, mobilization of non-hepatic fat stores
Hyperuricemia	Decreased renal clearance of uric acid
Esophagitis	Direct toxic effect, vomiting
Gastritis	Increased secretin and histamine production, direct toxic effect
Duodenal ulceration	Increased secretin and histamine production
Steatorrhea and malabsorption	Pancreatic insufficiency, thiamine deficiency, hyperperistalsis
Fatty liver	Triglyceride accumulation in hepatocytes
Alcoholic hepatitis	Inflammation and necrosis in hepatocytes
Cirrhosis	Scarification of liver parenchyma
Pancreatitis	Increased secretin production, malnutrition
Various anemias	Direct toxic effect, malabsorption, malnutrition, decreased transferrin synthesis
Beriberi heart disease	Thiamine deficiency
Cardiomyopathy	Direct toxic effect, malnutrition
Skeletal myopathies	Direct toxic effect

From Cohen, S.: The pharmacology of alcohol. *Postgraduate Medicine,* 64:97, Dec. 1978.

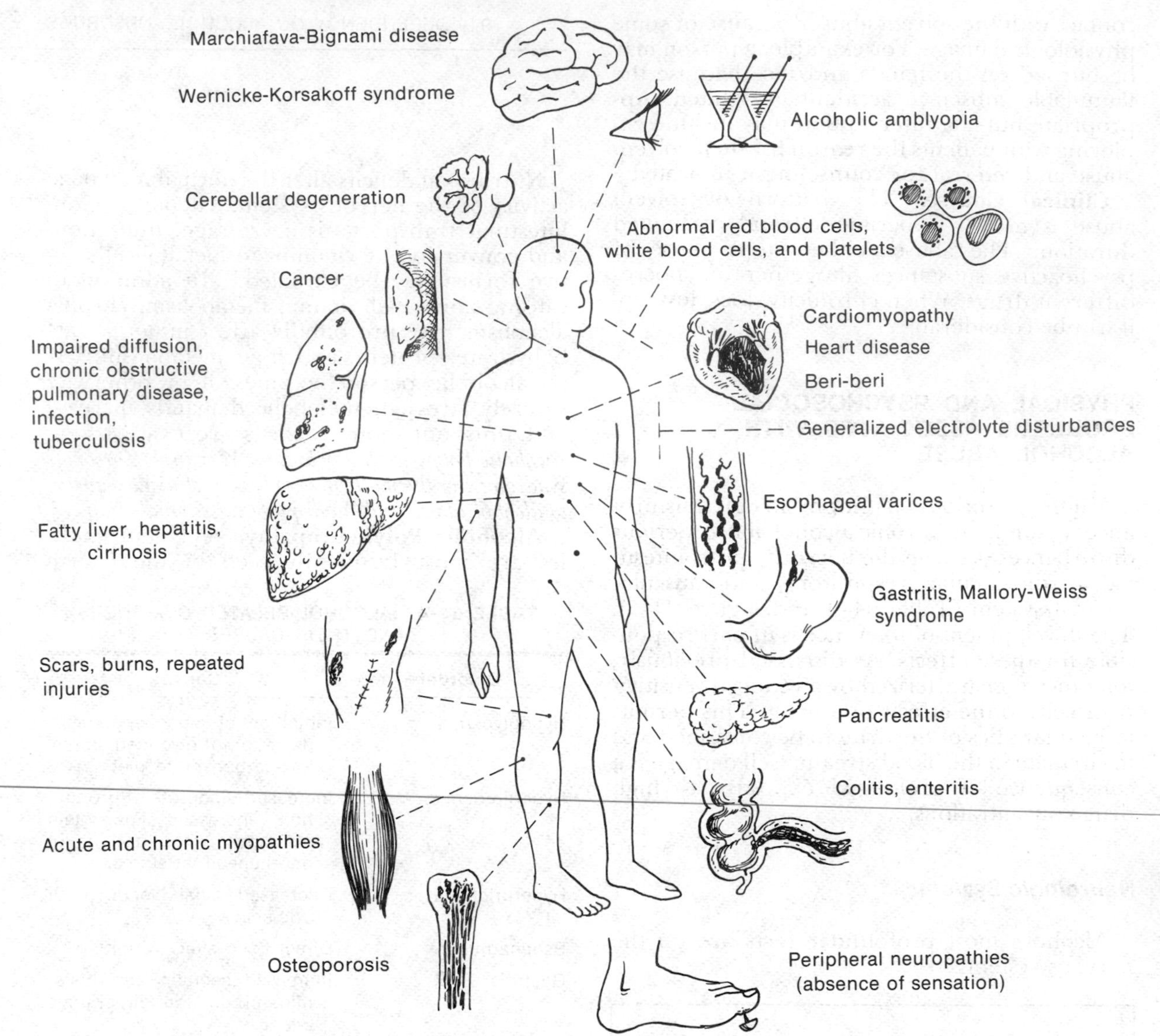

Figure 94–5. Clinical problems resulting from alcohol abuse.

through seventh decades of life, largely because the onset is slow, progressive, and insidious. The pathological process is a degenerative one, always involving multiple nerves.[16, 22]

Some persons with polyneuropathies may be asymptomatic. Findings evident on neurologic examination consist of varying degrees of motor, reflex, and sensory loss, which typically occur in the feet before the hands, and move from distal to proximal. The sensory symptoms appear first and are usually described as tingling, pricking, burning, or numb sensations. Occasionally, there are dull or sharp pains. Calf muscles may be tender to touch. The person's senses of pain, temperature, and vibration are usually diminished. Because of diminished sensation and weak muscles, the patient may present with a wide stance gait.

Recovery is a slow process and depends on a nutritious diet with supplemental vitamins as well as stopping or decreasing the intake of alcohol. Thiamine replacement is particularly important, because thiamine is essential for the conversion of glucose to metabolically active forms and nerve cell function depends upon glucose.

Safety measures are very important for persons with diminished sensation. Teach the person to be especially careful in smoking, cooking, and moving about in order to prevent burns and bruises. Teach foot care and other appropriate hygenic measures. In severe cases, prevent skin breakdown, contractures, muscle wasting and atrophy.

Wernicke-Korsakoff Syndrome. The Wernicke-Korsakoff syndrome is usually superimposed on peripheral neuropathies. It is the more progressive phase of the same nutritional deficiency. This syndrome was formerly viewed as two separate entities: (1) Wernicke's encephalopathy and (2) Korsakoff's psychosis. It is now recognized as one entity, since the two aspects have the same etiologic basis and usually occur together.

The symptoms of the *Wernicke* component consist of ocular disturbances, horizontal nystagmus on lateral gaze and ophthalmoplegia, as well as an ataxic gait. There may be palsy of the sixth cranial nerve, which is usually bilateral, though not symmetrical, and results in diplopia. The ataxia is of stance and gait and may be obscured by polyneuropathies. In the condition's severest form, the affected person is literally unable to stand unaided, walking steps are short and uncertain, and the gait wide-based and reeling.[23] The patient may show disinterest and lassitude.

Korsakoff's psychosis is the mental component of the same process causing Wernicke's disease. A disturbance in memory function, predominantly for recent events, is the most common manifestation. In severe cases remote memory may also be impaired. *Confusion* is manifested in part by an inability to think with usual speed and efficiency. *Confabulation* (filling in gaps in memory by reciting imaginary experiences) may occur in an attempt to respond to questions regarding recent events.

The speed and extent of recovery from Wernicke-Korsakoff's syndrome vary but are generally slow and incomplete. (This is a characteristic of nerve cell recovery.)

Indications of nutritional depletion, as in polyneuropathies and the Wernicke-Korsakoff's syndrome, may be masked by withdrawal symptoms during the acute phase. Careful nursing assessment is required to determine etiology.

Specific guidelines for the *management of alcoholic malnutrition* and associated disease entities are the following:

- Treatment should be started as soon as possible, to prevent irreversible damage.
- Initially, high doses of thiamine and perhaps other vitamins should be given.
- Abstinence, or at least diminished drinking, will help reverse the problem.
- A good diet fortified with vitamins is essential. Diet planning must be individualized and realistic. Follow-up is helpful so that ongoing adjustments can be made.
- To promote safety, major environmental adjustments may be necessary for persons whose recovery is incomplete. Unfortunately, many persons with Wernicke-Korsakoff's syndrome do not recover completely and may require supervisory care for the rest of their lives.

Other Neurologic Disturbances. Other neurologic conditions that have been associated with chronic, heavy alcohol intake include *alcoholic amblyopia, Marchiafava-Bignami disease,* and *alcoholic cerebellar degeneration.* They are relatively rare, of uncertain etiology, and are not discussed here.

Esophagus, Stomach, Intestines*

Alcohol affects nearly every organ in the gastrointestinal system. To appreciate this fact, consider the path of alcohol as it is consumed, i.e., from the esophagus through the GI tract and then to the other abdominal organs.

Esophageal pathology is secondary to other clinical problems associated with alcohol. *Esophageal varices,* for example, are a symptom of portal hypertension secondary to cirrhosis of the liver. (See Chapter 66.) Esophageal varices that rupture and bleed can be a *life-threatening emergency.* The *Mallory-Weiss syndrome,* a tearing of the gastroesophageal mucosa with severe upper GI bleeding, may occur in persons who vomit forcefully. *This is a medical and surgical emergency.* The bleeding must be controlled to prevent shock, coma, and death.

Alcohol has a direct corrosive effect on the *stomach,* part of which is concentration-dependent. Alcohol destroys the mucosal barrier that protects the stomach from autodigestion. The only other substance presently known that has the same effect is aspirin. Thus,

> *Do not suggest aspirin as an analgesic to a person who consumes alcohol excessively.*

There is some question whether alcohol also increases acid production, which would tend to exacerbate the process of autodigestion.[12] The presence of either of these two conditions or both may result in an *acute gastritis,* which may be *hemorrhagic.* The symptoms are the same as gastritis from any cause, as are the potential complications of perforation or obstruction. *Gastric and duodenal ulcers* may also occur. Again, signs, symptoms, and possible complications are the same as with ulcers of any etiology.

> *Alcohol requires very little digestion. Some of it is absorbed directly from the stomach into the blood stream.*

*Refer also to Unit XVII.

The largest portion, however, is absorbed from the small intestine, principally the duodenum. Alcohol has an irritant effect, increasing motility and producing an outpouring of fluid. This frequently causes *enteritis* or *colitis. Malabsorption* of essential nutrients from food may result.

Hemorrhoids are the only disorder in the large intestine related to alcohol abuse. These are secondary to the impaired blood flow resulting from portal hypertension.

Liver*

After alcohol is absorbed from the stomach and small intestine, it is carried via the blood stream to the liver for detoxification.

> *A specific, progressive syndrome of alcoholic liver disease, which is the direct result of the toxic effects of alcohol, has been identified and described. The syndrome begins with fatty liver, and may progress to alcoholic hepatitis and, finally, cirrhosis.*

- The first manifestation of liver damage is *fatty liver.* Fat is deposited in the liver during the course of alcohol metabolism. The liver in an alcoholic may become enormously enlarged by the accumulation of fat. This extreme accumulation may be associated with functional deficit. Abstinence from alcohol early in the course of liver changes results in complete reversal of pathologic processes, with a return of normal liver function.
- If drinking continues, some persons develop *alcoholic hepatitis,* a toxic, necrotic, inflammatory condition of the liver. The inflammation is caused by the death of liver cells, which incites polymorphonucleocyte response. The person severely ill with alcoholic hepatitis has typically been drinking heavily for weeks or months and is anorexic, jaundiced, and febrile. Hepatomegaly and hepatic pain are usually present. Treatment during the acute stage is symptomatic. Long-term recovery depends upon abstinence. Even then reversibility is variable, depending upon the severity and chronicity of the hepatitis.[12]
- The final stage of alcoholic liver disease is *cirrhosis,* a progressive form of fibrosis of the liver. Signs in cirrhosis are divided according to the mechanism of liver impairment and are presented in Table 94–5.

*Refer to Unit XVIII for complete discussion of liver disorders.

TABLE 94–5. SIGNS OF CIRRHOSIS

Signs of Cirrhosis
Related to Inadequate Functioning Liver Mass
Jaundice
Fluid retention—edema and ascites
Spider angiomas
Palmar erythema
Breast atrophy (women)
Gynecomastia (men)
Loss of body hair
Testicular atrophy
Amenorrhea, anovulatory
Clubbing
Related to Portal Hypertension
Ascites (without edema)
Abdominal collateral veins or varices
Splenomagaly
Confusion, tremor
Cyanosis
Related to Liver Process
Hepatomegaly
Hardness of liver
Fever
Wide pulse pressure

Extracted from Whitfield, C. L., and K. Williams (Eds.): *The Patient with Alcoholism and Other Drug Problems.* Whitfield and Williams, 1976, p. 124.

Alcohol is a common cause of cirrhosis. For example, about 85 per cent of all cases of liver cirrhosis in the United States are due to alcohol. It is imperative, then, that persons with cirrhosis be asked about alcohol use and given information about physiologic effects and treatment options, so they can have some choice as to outcomes. The only treatment at this point is to remove the underlying cause, alcohol, and to maximize the possibilities for tissue regeneration.

Complications of cirrhosis are difficult to treat and should be prevented whenever possible. They include portal hypertension, ascites, esophageal varices, and hepatic encephalopathy.

Pancreas

Alcoholism is a factor in 50 per cent or more of cases of pancreatitis. *Acute alcoholic pancreatitis* is most often seen in men 25 to 65 years of age who have been drinking heavily for 5 to 10 years or more.[22] There often is no characteristic clinical picture. Usually the outstanding symptom is *severe, constant epigastric pain,* which frequently radiates to the back. Nausea and vomiting are common. The patient usually looks ill, and there may be signs of abdominal tenderness and distention. The hallmark of this syndrome is the relationship of onset of symptoms to alcohol ingestion. The symptoms usually begin 1 to 2 days after a drinking bout.

Again, it is essential to remove the underlying cause — the consumption of alcohol — in order to expect any improvement in this condition. Treatment of pancreatitis is discussed in detail in Chapter 70.

Effective treatment of all alcohol-related disorders of the GI tract depends upon the patient. The patient must stop drinking alcohol and must start eating a nutritious diet. Without these changes, no treatment can be effective.

Cardiovascular System*

Alcohol exerts many direct as well as indirect effects on the cardiovascular system. The heart's mechanical performance is decreased with alcohol consumption. The heart rate and cardiac output increase with very small amounts of alcohol. However, heart rate slows and cardiac output decreases with increasing doses, as a result of stimulation of the vagus nerve. Slowing of the heart rate produces an accumulation of lactic acid in the peripheral vascular system. This causes dilation of these vessels and an ensuing tachycardia. Blood pressure is variable. Very large amounts of alcohol interfere with nerve conduction in the heart and can result in decreased myocardial contractility and eventually cardiac failure.[22]

If a person has evidence of myocardial disease and there is no evidence of other heart disease, then the patient's alcohol intake must be assessed. Most likely, the myocardial disease is due to heavy alcohol intake. Physical examination may reveal little cardiac disturbance. One clue to *alcohol-related myocardial disease* is an inappropriate tachycardia, especially if associated with extrasystoles.[22] Symptoms that infrequently present include: shortness of breath, palpitations, decreased exercise tolerance, increased heart size, atrial fibrillation, excessive nocturnal diaphoresis, a narrow pulse pressure, intermittent paroxysmal nocturnal dyspnea, and edema.[40] Symptoms of *congestive heart failure (CHF),* edema, dyspnea and/or orthopnea, become the predominant clinical findings as cardiac damage increases. Nursing care is the same as for CHF of any cause. (See Chapter 34.) Supportive care is essential. The patient needs rest in addition to the prescribed medical regimen. Prognosis is usually good when the diagnosis is made early. Complete, permanent recovery may be possible in the early stages; however, it depends upon abstinence from alcohol. Depending on the severity of cardiac damage, some degree of impairment may persist.

Triglycerides accumulate in the myocardial cell secondary to increased triglyceride extraction by the myocardium. In addition, since cell permeability is changed, a variety of electrolytes and enzymes leak with elevated blood alcohol levels (200 mg./100 ml.).[12] The resulting syndrome has been called *alcoholic cardiomyopathy* and seems to occur as a direct result of the toxic effects of alcohol on heart muscle. Cardiac conduction abnormalities and rhythm disturbances are common clinical findings.[13] The mode of action for these changes is still unclear. Alcoholic cardiomyopathy is a long-term development, usually appearing after many years of alcohol consumption.

Many factors associated wtih heavy alcohol intake lead to *indirect cardiac effects.* The alcohol withdrawal reaction, for example, puts a heavy workload on the heart. For example, *sinus tachycardia* and *hypertension* typically occur.

A prolonged, severe detoxification may lead to an extreme state of fatigue and possibly to sudden death through such mechanisms as cardiogenic shock, cardiac standstill, ventricular fibrillation, and flutter or abrupt left-sided heart failure.[22]

Careful observation and attentive management of patients during detoxification can usually prevent such catastrophes from occurring, or at least can lead to rapid institution of restorative measures if complications do occur. *Detoxification is an extremely stressful process, which places great demand on the heart.* Minimizing stress can do much to insure adequate cardiac functioning. The implications of excessive stress in an alcoholic person with compromised cardiac function have been largely overlooked.

In order to allow heavy drinkers to make an informed choice about whether or not they choose to continue an excessive alcohol intake, they need to be instructed about the harmful effects alcohol has on the heart (and other body systems) and how their activity levels may be limited.

Beriberi heart disease, caused by thiamine deficiency, occurs in many alcoholic persons. Peripheral neuropathies are present in addition to the increased cardiac output and decreased circulation time secondary to marked reduction in peripheral vascular resistance. This latter is characteristic of the disease. These clinical findings are the opposite of the decreased cardiac

*Refer to Unit XII for further discussion of cardiovascular disorders.

output and increased circulation time seen in alcoholic cardiomyopathy.[12] Treatment consists of vigorous thiamine replacement, a nutritious diet, and abstinence from alcohol.

Peripheral blood vessels dilate with alcohol intake. This increases the heat loss from the body and makes the drinker feel warm. However, alcohol should not be given to individuals suffering from extreme cold or shock. Under these conditions, blood is needed in the central parts of the body and heat loss must be diminished.[30]

Other Physiologic Effects of Alcohol

Respiratory System*. There is a high incidence of *chronic, obstructive pulmonary disease* among alcoholic persons. The mechanism appears to be due to a combination of (1) direct toxic effects of alcohol on pulmonary tissue and (2) impaired clearance of bacteria from the lungs, resulting from alcohol ingestion. The lungs become more susceptible to chronic bronchial infections and more vulnerable to the effects of cigarette smoke or other toxic agents. Once a certain degree of pulmonary injury takes place, function may not be restored to normal even in spite of abstinence from alcohol.[11]

Another common lung abnormality in chronic alcoholism is *impaired diffusion.* In most cases, abstinence from alcohol restores diffusion to normal. There is also a high association of *tuberculosis* with alcoholism. It is important to regularly screen all suspected or known alcoholics for possible tuberculosis.

Fluid and Electrolyte Balance†. The popular belief that alcohol is a *diuretic* is true only while the blood alcohol level rises and as it stabilizes. As blood alcohol levels fall, an antidiuretic effect occurs, resulting in fluid retention.[3] Thus, *alcoholics are more likely to be overhydrated than dehydrated (except, of course, when experiencing vomiting or diarrhea).*

The frequent nursing practice of forcing fluids during the withdrawal phase is contraindicated, except perhaps in cases of chronic malnutrition. Adding fluid to an overhydrated person whose cardiac muscle may not be working well could result in severe, potentially fatal, congestive heart failure.

* Disorders of the respiratory system are discussed in detail in Unit XVI.

†See also Chapter 12 for discussion.

Impaired electrolyte balance also has secondary cardiac effects. Serum potassium levels are often decreased with heavy alcohol intake. The implications of this *hypokalemia* are potentially severe. This is especially true for those alcoholic persons receiving digitalis preparations to treat CHF secondary to alcoholic cardiomyopathy. The sensitivity of the myocardium to these preparations will be increased.

Hypomagnesemia is frequently encountered in alcoholics, since alcohol selectively increases the urinary excretion of magnesium. This has cardiac implications as well as significance for the course of withdrawal. It has been suggested that hypomagnesemia is the implicating factor in the etiology of *withdrawal seizures.*[46] The policy in many alcoholic treatment programs is to give magnesium whenever blood tests reveal low or borderline serum magnesium levels.

Routine blood tests should be performed on all alcoholic persons seen by health professionals in order to allow for quick correction of possible electrolyte disturbances.

Hematologic System*. Adverse effects of alcohol on hematopoiesis result in abnormalities of red blood cells, white blood cells, and platelets. Virtually no aspect of blood cell development, survival, or function escapes the physiologic and biochemical toxicities of alcohol.[12] Abnormalities may result in *anemias,* and *difficulties in counteracting infections* and may *interfere in the clotting mechanism.*[12] The patient shows symptoms of severe infections and frequently has hematomas. Complete blood counts provide evidence as to the existence of anemias and abnormal white blood cell counts.

Close observation is particularly necessary when an alcoholic person is receiving anticoagulant therapy. Frequent monitoring of prothrombin time is indicated. In addition, protection from infections is crucial.

Probably one of the most important effects of alcohol on the hematologic system is the *inhibition of folate metabolism.* Alcohol interferes with the delivery of folate to marrow precursors. Depending on the duration and level of alcohol consumption, ineffective cell production, thrombocytopenia, megaloblastic hematopoiesis, leukopenia, and anemia may result.[12] With abstinence from alcohol and proper nutrition, these abnormalities are reversible. Short-term folate supplementation may be required.

Musculoskeletal System†. Alcohol ingestion may have a deleterious effect on skeletal muscle, resulting in acute or chronic alcoholic myopathy or subclinical alcoholic myopathy.[55]

*Unit XIV discusses disturbances of the blood and blood-forming organs.

†See also Unit XX.

The pathologic process is the same as in alcohol cardiomyopathy.

- *Acute alcoholic myopathy* is a syndrome of muscle pain, tenderness, and edema occurring after acute excesses of alcohol ingestion. Proximal muscles of the extremities, the pelvic and shoulder girdle, and the muscles of the thoracic cage are most commonly affected. The symptoms usually subside in 1 to 3 weeks but may recur with repeated alcohol ingestion. Treatment consists of abstinence from alcohol and a well-balanced diet with supplemental vitamins.
- *Chronic alcoholic myopathy* is a syndrome of muscle weakness and wasting involving the muscle groups described above. There is no history of pain or tenderness and onset is slow and insidious. Treatment is the same as for acute alcoholic myopathy.
- *Subclinical alcoholic myopathy* is an acute myopathy in which symptoms are absent or are obscured by either the effects of intoxication or withdrawal. Treatment is the same as that of acute alcoholic myopathy.

Alcoholism contributes to *skeletal complications* in at least two ways. A syndrome of *nontraumatic osteonecrosis of the hip* is being recognized in alcohol consumers. It may be caused by fat emboli blocking end arteries.[26]

Another common complication of alcohol abuse is an increased incidence of *fractures and other injuries secondary to trauma and falls.* Impaired coordination due to high blood alcohol levels is a contributing factor.

Skin*. Skin lesions are common in alcoholic persons. Many, such as *generalized pruritus, gray skin pigmentation,* and *rosacea,* are linked to liver disease.[163] Others may be associated with nutritional deficiencies, e.g., *glossitis* secondary to folate deficiency. Some conditions that may be present in the general population flare up with drinking bouts. These include *psoriasis* and *seborrheic dermatitis.* A person who is drinking heavily usually neglects basic hygenic measures. Skin infections and lesions may result. Treatment consists of the establishment of good hygiene, a nutritious diet, and abstinence from alcohol. Referral to a dermatologist may be necessary for more severe cases.

Cancer. An association between alcohol abuse and cancer of the *oropharynx, larynx,* and *esophagus* (where there is direct contact of tissues with alcohol) and the *liver* (where there is serious organ damage) has been clinically observed for many years. In addition, heavy drinking may be implicated in the genesis of cancer of the *pancreas* and *prostate.*[43] Cancer in these sites should be a clue to a possible alcohol problem. Smoking and malnutrition, which usually accompany heavy drinking, may increase the risk of cancer in certain organs, especially the *lung.*

*Diseases of the skin are discussed further in Chapter 79.

The reasons for the association of cancer with alcohol abuse are unclear, but among the possibilities are (1) the prolonged effects of alcohol on body tissues and (2) the presence of carcinogenic substances in some alcoholic beverages.[38] (For additional discussions of cancer refer to Unit IX and to other chapters describing disorders in specific body areas.)

Psychosocial Deterioration

Repeated, heavy alcohol abuse eventually leads to upheavals in relationships with significant others. The alcoholic person's behavior alienates others and may lead to social isolation.

Alcoholism has been called a "family illness" because the entire family suffers the consequences of even one member's severe alcohol consumption. The family with alcoholism falls short of achieving its primary functions of socializing children and providing security for adults, because of major difficulties in communication, sexual interaction, and role fulfillment.[12]

Communication with a person who is frequently intoxicated is exasperating. Intoxicated people often are not held responsible for their words or actions. As a result, they set the rules in their social interactions. In response, others eventually cease trying to communicate. The use of defense mechanisms such as projection and rationalization also contributes to destructive interactions. The alcoholic person increasingly tries to escape through alcohol while his or her significant others either retreat into activities that exclude the alcoholic or become apathetic.

An "alcoholic marriage" is rarely free of *sexual problems.*[35] For example, a nonalcoholic woman may begin to see her alcoholic partner as undesirable and may avoid intimacy. This rejection then causes the alcoholic person to feel a failure. This feeling is compounded by alcohol's direct effects on sexual functioning. The porter in *Macbeth* described it well: "Drink . . . provokes the desire but takes away the performance."

Since an alcoholic family member is not able to function within the family as expected, the spouse and children alter their behavior (*role performances*) in an effort to keep the family functioning. They often take on the neglected duties of the alcoholic person. This places an additional burden on them, especially on the children, who frequently assume adult responsibilities at a young age. In addition, the children often suffer from parental emotional neglect since both parents are too preoccupied with the alcoholism to spend much time with the children.

> *Recovery from alcoholism requires help for the alcoholic person and significant others. The impact that alcoholism has had on them individually and as a unit must be acknowledged. Only then will the social deterioration begin to be repaired.*

An alcoholic person's economic status is complicated by heavy drinking. The purchase of alcoholic beverages may be a severe financial drain. Income may be threatened because deteriorating job performance may result in job loss. Increased rates of illness, injury, and traffic accidents among alcoholic persons further deplete their monetary resources. Economic referrals may be appropriate.

Alcohol abuse is costly to society. Illness, traffic accidents, and reduced productivity secondary to alcohol abuse cost the United States, for example, about 15 billion dollars in 1971.[38] The costs of an alcoholic person's involvement in the criminal justice and social welfare systems is high. Alcohol-related programs and research run the economic costs even higher.

Summary

Complications of both a physiologic and psychosocial nature result from prolonged consumption of alcohol. It is important for nurses to have a high level of awareness of the risks of alcoholism and the associated clinical problems which may occur. Initial nursing care may focus on symptom relief in order to assist the patient through an acute crisis. Fairly early in treatment, however, the person should be taught about the role alcohol plays in his or her impairment. Long-term management requires the cessation of alcohol abuse patterns. As mentioned earlier, specific techniques of long-term management are beyond the scope of this text.

CLINICAL PROBLEMS ASSOCIATED WITH HEROIN ADDICTION

Virtually none of the clinical problems resulting from heroin addiction are the direct consequence of the drug itself (Figure 94–6). Rather they are the indirect results of such things as multiple unsterile injections, sharing needles, and adulterants.[4] Since heroin is an analgesic, the addict may not be aware of discomfort due to illness. Often this results in severe problems developing before treatment is sought.

Physiologic Problems. Disorders associated with heroin addiction include: tetanus, duodenal ulcers, hepatitis, bacterial endocarditis, atrial and ventricular arrhythmias, pneumonias, respiratory depression (can be fatal), pulmonary edema, septic pulmonary embolism secondary to septic thrombophlebitis, bronchiectasis, acute nephritis, nephrotic syndrome, acute tubular necrosis, renal failure, urinary tract infections, gonorrhea, pelvic inflammatory disease, septicemia, osteomyelitis, septic arthritis, cellulitis and abscesses.

Addicts may have thin, scarred, collapsed veins, owing to the repeated trauma of intravenous injection with unsterile equipment. It may be difficult for a nurse to take blood from or administer intravenous fluids to these patients. Any accessible vein may be utilized. The entire body should be searched in an attempt to find one. The patient may know where his or her most accessible veins are.

Psychosocial Deterioration. A heroin addict's significant others suffer as a result of the addicted person's preoccupation with drugs. Significant others may suffer from anxiety, worry, and guilt — wondering what they might have done to cause the drug problem or what they might possibly do to solve it. If their efforts are always futile or are continuously rejected by the addicted person, they may come to feel isolated and alienated from someone they care about very much. Intimate relationships suffer, since addicted people rapidly lose sexual desire and interest.[20a] They receive more pleasure from their drugs. Gradually, the behavior of addicted persons drives away their significant others.

As more and more of an addicted person's time becomes occupied with attempts to procure drugs, the time available to work for legitimate income becomes negligible. This occurs at the same time that the need for money to procure drugs is becoming more acute. The addict then begs or turns to illegal activities (e.g., "cons," steals, forges checks, becomes a pimp or prostitute) in order to get the money to obtain drugs.

Nursing Actions. Nurses most frequently encounter heroin addicts in acute care settings. A nurse's immediate concern is focused on the presenting symptoms. Once the acute physiologic crisis has passed, the nurse can focus on the patient's primary problem, the heroin addiction.

Persons addicted to heroin are usually more willing to give a history of drug use than are alcoholic persons. Heroin addicts want health care providers to know they use drugs so that they can receive medication and not suffer the discomfort of the withdrawal symptoms. As stated previously, people experiencing drug addiction can be extremely manipulative, and working with them is often frustrating. An effective nurse must be highly skilled in assessing addicted persons and must be familiar with the language of the drug user's subculture.

When an addicted person stops taking heroin, the physiologic effects usually abate. Such people require supportive care over time. Prolonged patterns of social isolation result in poor communication skills and make establishment of helpful interpersonal relationships difficult. It is important that a nursing approach to an addicted person be fair, firm, and consistent. After caring for the physiologic needs, and with the establishment of a trusting relationship, the nurse can begin to explore psychosocial concerns. Referral to an appropriate drug treatment program is often the most desirable intervention.

CLINICAL PROBLEMS RESULTING FROM ABUSE OF OTHER SUBSTANCES

Many of the physiologic complications resulting from abuse of other substances are similar to those already described, e.g., nutritional deficiencies, reduced resistance to disease, and problems secondary to injection of foreign substances. Discussion of these problems is not repeated here. Some additional complications that may appear include the following:

- Prolonged use of *amphetamines* often leads to a broad range of illness. The chronic "speed freak" suffers dehydration and weight loss and has a higher than normal rate of liver and cardiovascular diseases, hypertensive disorders, and psychiatric problems.[6] Cerebrovascular complications (stroke and coma) as well as intracerebral and subarachnoid hemorrhage have been reported in young intravenous amphetamine abusers.[15] Hypertensive crises and vascular damage appear to be responsible for these complications.
- *Stimulants* and *hallucinogens* lead to psychiatric crises more often than to medical-surgical crises.[159]
- Retinovascular damage has been found to occur in intravenous *methylphenidate hydrochloride (Ritalin)*

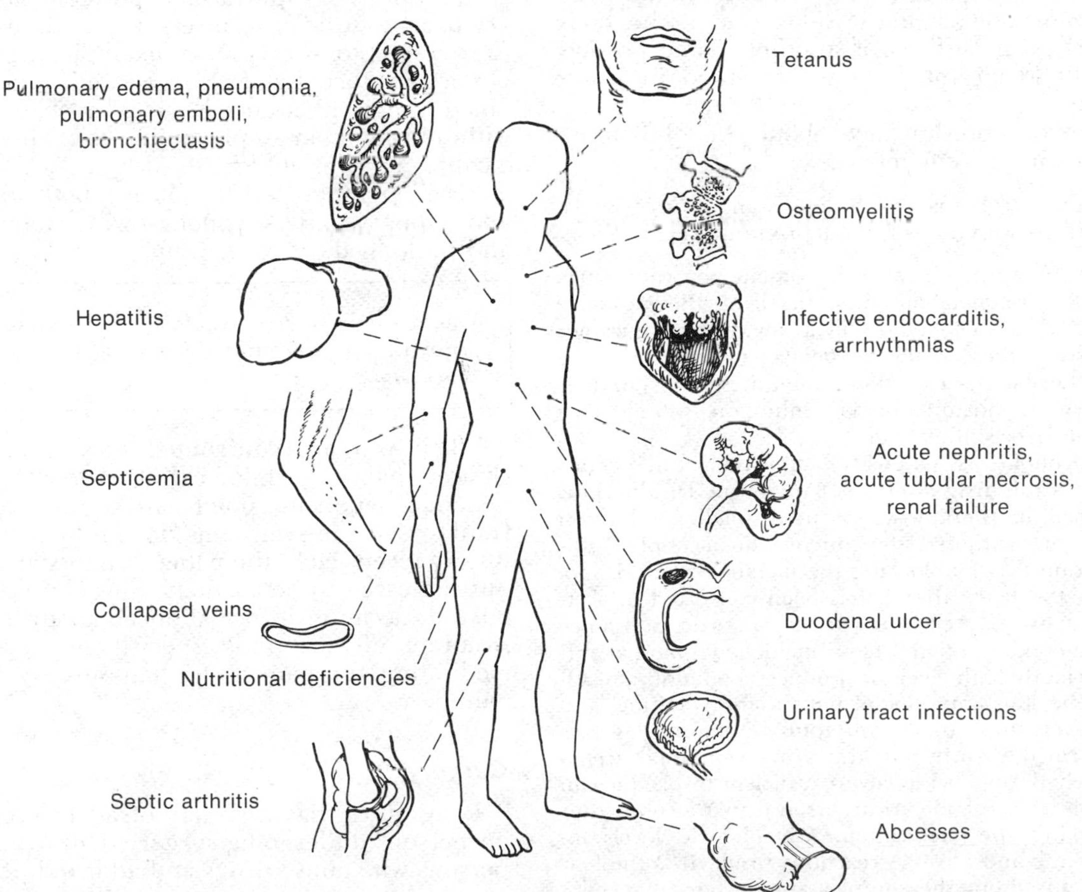

Figure 94–6. Clinical problems resulting from heroin addiction.

abusers. Abscesses, often in parts of the body other than the injection site, are common.

- Heavy use of *marijuana* has been associated with a variety of lung problems, including acute and chronic bronchitis and pneumonias.
- Extensive exposure to *solvents* may lead to liver and kidney damage.[16]

Nursing Actions. The nurse's initial contact with persons abusing these substances is often in an acute care setting, and care is focused on acute physiologic or psychiatric problems. The care is similar to that previously described for persons addicted to alcohol and heroin. Referral to specialized agencies for long-term follow-up and treatment is usually appropriate.

SPECIAL PROBLEMS

Consideration is given here to drug interactions and polydrug abuse, the surgical patient who is a drug abuser, and the fetal alcohol syndrome.

Drug Interactions and Polydrug Abuse

A *drug interaction* occurs whenever the presence of one chemical substance in the body changes the effects of another. Some possible alcohol-drug interactions are listed in Table 94–6.

Some important facts about alcohol-drug interactions to remember are:

- Since alcohol is a CNS depressant, it has additive effects with other CNS depressant drugs.
- When alcohol is taken in combination with drugs that are metabolized in the liver, the inductive effect of alcohol on liver microsomal enzymes causes these drugs to be less effective. On the other hand, drugs that inhibit these liver enzymes (e.g., monoamine oxidase inhibitors) will enhance the effects of alcohol.[18]
- Alcohol has extensive unpleasant interactions with the drug *disulfiram* (Antabuse). Disulfiram is used in therapy aimed at dissuading a person from continued dependence on alcohol. Disulfiram acts by blocking the metabolism of alcohol in the body after it has been converted to acetaldehyde. Acetaldehyde is a toxic substance (chemically related to formaldehyde), and at sufficiently high levels, it produces a pounding headache, flushing, violent nausea and vomiting, and other unpleasant symptoms. Disulfiram is prescribed in sufficient doses to keep blood acetaldehyde just below levels sufficient to produce an adverse reaction. If a person drinks alcohol after taking the medication, acetaldehyde levels increase and adverse reactions result. It is the fear of sustaining these unpleasant reactions that keeps a person who is on disulfiram from consuming alcohol. Nurses need to understand the effects of disulfiram so that they can accurately assess patients' symptoms and can teach patients about the consequences of drinking alcohol while taking disulfiram.

It is surprising how unaware people are of the many dangerous, even lethal, interactions of alcohol with other drugs. When a person is taking a therapeutic drug, the safest rule is to take the least possible amount of other drugs. Since drug abusers are not likely to follow this rule, nurses must obtain thorough drug histories and be alert to clinical evidence of possible drug interactions. If you learn that a patient has a substance abuse problem, give this information to the physician who is prescribing additional drugs.

A nurse must be aware that some people abuse more than one drug. Often, the drugs have opposite effects. Polydrug abuse is not confined to abusers of illicit substances. For example, a person who appears to be functioning normally may (a) take prescription "uppers" to get going in the morning, (b) consume alcoholic beverages at lunch for a temporary sedative effect, and (c) consume prescription or over-the-counter drugs to get to sleep at night. The consumption of multiple substances makes clinical diagnoses difficult and also may result in complicated and dangerous drug effects.

Indications of withdrawal in polydrug abusers are usually difficult to assess, as multiple withdrawal symptoms occur. For example, the autonomic hyperactivity of alcohol withdrawal combined with the need to "crash" upon withdrawing from amphetamine abuse presents a confusing clinical picture. Also, the withdrawal reaction for a person abusing both alcohol and other sedative-hypnotics will be delayed and prolonged.

> *When obtaining a drug use history, do not assume a person uses only one drug. Ask what other drugs the patient uses.*

When you are confronted by a confusing clinical picture while caring for a drug-dependent person, point out to the patient frankly that the symptoms do not fit the drug history given. Help the patient understand that nursing care can be adequate only if it is based on full, accurate information about drug use. Accurate information is especially important in medicating for pain and when surgery is required.

*Surgery**

Drug abuse has a variety of adverse effects on persons undergoing surgery. Unfortunately persons who abuse drugs and addicted persons

*Nursing care of persons experiencing surgery is discussed in detail in Unit VIII.

are at a high risk for both emergency and non-emergency conditions that necessitate surgery. *Traumatic injuries,* which often require surgery, are frequent. For example, about 50 per cent of all fatal automobile accidents are related to alcohol, as are about one third of all head injuries seen in hospital emergency rooms.[43]

Caring for persons who abuse drugs and are undergoing surgery is challenging. Frequent observations are required to differentiate between disorders caused by drugs and those caused by neurosurgical lesions. In addition to the problems caused by their injuries or illness, addicted persons needing surgery may have the following problems:

- ▶ Poor general health
- ▶ Impaired liver function (secondary to chronic alcoholism, malnutrition, or hepatitis from the use of unsterile needles)

TABLE 94-6. DRUG INTERACTIONS WITH ALCOHOL

Drug	Effect	Probable Mechanism
Antabuse	Abdominal cramps, flushing, vomiting, psychotic episodes, confusion	Inhibits intermediary metabolism of alcohol
Anticoagulants, Oral	Diminished anticoagulant effect with chronic alcohol abuse	Enhanced microsomal enzyme activity
	Enhanced anticoagulant effect with acute intoxication	Reduced metabolism
Anticonvulsants		
diphenylhydantoin (Dilantin; and others)	Diminished anticonvulsant effect with chronic alcohol abuse	Enhanced microsomal enzyme activity
	Enhanced anticonvulsant effect with acute intoxication	Reduced metabolism
Antimicrobials		
chloramphenicol (Chloromycetin; and others)	Minor Antabuse-like symptoms	Inhibits intermediary metabolism of alcohol
isoniazid (many brands)	Diminished effect with chronic alcohol abuse	Enhanced microsomal enzyme activity
metronidazole (Flagyl)	Minor Antabuse-like symptoms	Inhibits intermediary metabolism of alcohol
quinacrine (Atabrine)	Minor Antabuse-like symptoms	Inhibits intermediary metabolism of alcohol
Hypoglycemics		
chlorpropamide (Diabinese)	Minor Antabuse-like symptoms	Inhibits intermediary metabolism of alcohol
phenformin (DBI; Meltrol)	Lactic acidosis	Synergy
tolbutamide (Orinase)	Diminished hypoglycemic effect with chronic alcohol abuse	Enhanced microsomal enzyme activity
	Enhanced hypoglycemic effect with ingestion of alcohol, particularly in fasting patients	Suppression of gluconeogenesis
	Minor Antabuse-like symptoms	Inhibits intermediary metabolism of alcohol
MAO Inhibitors	Hypertensive crisis	Inhibit metabolism of tyramine in Chianti wine and some other alcoholic beverages
Salicylates	Gastrointestinal bleeding	Additive
Sedatives and Tranquilizers		
barbiturates	Diminished sedative effect with chronic alcohol abuse	Enhanced microsomal enzyme activity
	Enhanced central nervous system depression with acute intoxication	Additive; reduced metabolism
chloral hydrate (Noctec; and others)	Prolonged hypnotic effect	Mutual potentiation
diazepam (Valium)	Enhanced central nervous system depression	Additive
meprobamate (Miltown; and others)	Diminished sedative effect with chronic alcohol abuse	Enhanced microsomal enzyme activity
	Enhanced central nervous system depression with acute intoxication	Additive; reduced metabolism

Reprinted with permission from *The Medical Letter,* 56 Harrison Street, New Rochelle, N.Y. 10801, 16:92, October 25, 1974.

- Inaccessible veins (which may be life-threatening)
- Effects of recent drug ingestion
- Withdrawal symptoms
- Agitation; inability to cooperate

The presence of any combination of these factors makes the entire surgical course difficult. When emergency surgery is required, there is little time to obtain a thorough history of drug use, and health professionals must be especially alert to signs of drug-associated problems.

Since persons addicted to central nervous system depressants are cross-tolerant to pharmacologically related *anesthetic agents,* larger amounts of anesthetics are needed to achieve adequate sedation. On the other hand, if the patient has liver dysfunction, anesthetic agents are not metabolized efficiently. The resulting accumulation of drugs in the blood stream may alter and prolong sedation. Careful monitoring of patients during and after surgery contributes much to their safety.

In itself, drug abuse does not indicate or contraindicate any specific anesthetic technique or agent.[4] Side effects of some anesthetic agents, however, preclude their use with the abuse of certain drugs. For example, inhalation agents such as cyclopropane and halothane often decrease hepatic blood flow, a danger in an alcoholic patient whose circulating blood flow is already reduced by peripheral vasodilation.[43]

During surgery, persons addicted to drugs are prone to cardiac and respiratory depression, depleted catecholamines, and hemorrhage. Careful *postoperative monitoring* is necessary, because these patients have a high risk or complications. Respiratory complications are likely; therefore, frequent turning, coughing, and deep breathing are a must. Intermittent positive pressure breathing may be required. Cardiac problems such as congestive heart failure and atrial fibrillation are more common in alcoholic patients. In addition, patients with cirrhosis may have concomitant urinary retention, so it may be necessary to run intravenous fluids at a slower than normal rate. Also, the postoperative risks of bleeding and of infection are increased in drug-dependent persons.

A problem particular to drug-dependent people is *postoperative withdrawal from the drug of abuse.* The onset of the withdrawal from CNS depressant drugs (e.g., alcohol) may be delayed for up to 5 days postoperatively because of the cross-tolerance with anesthetics and pain medications. Cross-tolerance also affects the amount of pain medication required. Dosages may need to be increased. It is important to evaluate requests for pain medication, give increased doses if indicated, and to gradually, but steadily, withdraw the drugs, according to the plan of care for the individual person.

Fetal Alcohol Syndrome

Some newborns of alcoholic women have been shown to have a number of abnormalities. These include pre- and postnatal growth deficiency, developmental delay, microcephaly, short palpebral fissures, maxillary hypoplasia, cardiac anomalies, deficient motor development, altered palmar creases, and hip dislocations.[20b] Furthermore, an infant's growth and development seem to be permanently impaired, with small height and low weight persisting into childhood. Impaired mental development is also noted, the severity of which is related to the severity of the physical characteristics.[34a]

> *That alcohol is a fetotoxin is clear. What is not known is the amount of alcohol required to produce abnormalities.* Until more is known, the best course of action is to encourage women to abstain from alcohol during pregnancy.

BIBLIOGRAPHY (Unit XXV)

1. Alcohol and the Indians. *Medical Times,* 103(6):124, June 1975.
2. Arieti, S.: *American Handbook of Psychiatry.* Volume 1. New York, Basic Books, Inc., 1969.
3. Beard, J.D., and D.H. Knott: Fluid and electrolyte balance during acute withdrawal in chronic alcoholic patients. *Journal of the American Medical Association,* 204:133, 1968.
4. Bourne, P.G. (Ed.): *Acute Drug Abuse Emergencies: A Treatment Manual.* New York: Academic Press, 1976.
5. Bourne, P.G. (Ed.): *A Treatment Manual for Acute Drug Abuse Emergencies.* Rockville, Maryland: National Clearinghouse for Drug Abuse Information Publication No. 16, 1974.
6. *Do You Know the Facts About Drugs?* Miami, Fla.: Health Communications, Inc., 1977.
7. Done, A.K.: The toxic emergency. An abused drug by any other name. *Emergency Medicine,* 10:116, July 1978.
8. Edwards, G.: The meaning and treatment of alcohol dependence. *British Journal of Psychiatry,* Special Publication No. 9:239–51, 1975.
9. Ellinwood, E.H., Jr.: Amphetamine psychosis: A multidimensional process. *Seminars in Psychiatry,* 6:208, May 1969.
10. Ellinwood, E.H., Jr., and S. Cohen: Amphetamine abuse. *Science,* 171:420–1, Jan. 1971.
11. Emirgil, C., and B. Sobol: Pulmonary function in former alcoholics. *Chest,* 72(1):45, July 1977.
12. Estes, N.J., and M.E. Heinemann (Eds.): *Alcoholism: Development, Consequences and Interventions,* St. Louis: C.V. Mosby Co., 1977.

13. Ettinger, P.O., M. Lyons, H.A. Oldewurtel, T.A. Regan: Cardiac conduction abnormalities produced by chronic alcoholism. *American Heart Journal,* 91(1):66, Jan. 1976.
14. Gilbert, J.A.L., and O. Schaeffer: Metabolism of ethanol in different racial groups. *Canadian Medical Association Journal,* 116:476, May 1977.
15. Glatt, M.M.: *A Guide to Addiction and Its Treatment.* New York: John Wiley and Sons, Inc., 1974.
16. Glatt, M.M.: Alcoholism. *Nursing Times,* 71:936, June 12, 1975.
17. Goodwin, D.W.: *Is Alcoholism Hereditary?* New York: Oxford University Press, 1976.
18. Griffin, J.P., and P.F. D'Arcy: *A Manual of Adverse Drug Interactions.* Bristol: John Wright and Sons, Ltd., 1975.
19. Harper, F.D. (Ed.): *Alcohol Abuse and Black America.* Alexandria, Virginia: Douglass Publishers, Inc., 1976.
20. Hollan, E.L.: Alcohol withdrawal: The unexpected post-op syndrome. *RN*. 39:40, Feb. 1976.
20a. Jessup, M.A.: Heroin and Methadone: Their impact on human sexuality. *The American Journal of Maternal-Child Nursing,* 4:367, Nov.–Dec. 1979.
20b. Jones, K.L., and D.W. Smith: Recognition of the fetal alcohol syndrome in early infancy. *Lancet,* 2:999, 1973.
21. Kissin, B., and Begleiter, H. (Eds.): *The Biology of Alcoholism.* Volume 3. Clinical Pathology. New York: Plenum Press, 1974.
22. Kissin, B., and Begleiter, H. (Eds.): *The Biology of Alcoholism.* Volume 2. Physiology and Behavior. New York: Plenum Press, 1972.
23. Knott, D.H., R.D. Fink, and J.D. Beard: Unmasking alcohol abuse. *American Family Physician,* 10(4):28–33, Oct. 1974.
24. Leland, J.: *Firewater Myths.* New Brunswick, New Jersey, Publication Division, Rutgers Center of Alcohol Studies, 1976.
25. Lewis, L.W.: The hidden alcoholic: A nursing dilemma. *Nursing 75*, 5(7):20, Sept. 1975.
26. Lieber, C.S.: *Metabolic Aspects of Alcoholism.* Baltimore: University Park Press, 1977.
27. Luke, B.: Maternal alcoholism and fetal alcohol. *American Journal of Nursing,* 77:1924, Dec. 1977.
28. Luke, B.: The nutritional implications of alcohol abuse. *RN,* 39:32, Apr. 1976.
29. *Marijuana and Health.* Sixth Annual Report to the Congress by the Department of Health, Education and Welfare, 1976.
30 Ray, O.S.: *Drugs, Society and Human Behavior.* St. Louis: C.V. Mosby Company, 1972.
31. Schnoll, S.H.: Guidelines for the care of the drug abusing patient. *Hospital Medicine,* 12:85, Oct. 1976.
32. Seixas, F.A.: Alcohol and its drug interactions. *Annals of Internal Medicine,* 83:86, 1975.
33. Selzer, M.L., et al.: A self-administered short Michigan Alcoholism Screening Test. *Journal of Studies on Alcohol,* 36:117, Jan. 1975.
34. Steffenhagen, R.A.: Toward a self-esteem theory of drug dependence: A position paper. *Journal of Alcohol and Drug Education,* 22(2):1, Feb. 1977.
34a. Streissguth, A.P.: Psychological handicaps in children with the fetal alcohol syndrome. *Work in Progress on Alcoholism,* Annals of the New York Academy of Sciences, 273:140, May 1976.
35. Thiel, D.H., and R. Lester: Sex and alcohol: A second peek. *The New England Journal of Medicine,* 295:835, Oct. 1976.
36. Ufer, L.: How to recognize and care for the alcoholic patient. *Nursing 77,* 7:37, Oct. 1977.
37. United States Department of Health, Education and Welfare. First Special Report to the U.S. Congress on Alcohol and Health from the Secretary of Health, Education and Welfare. DHEW publication (HSM) 73-9031. Washington, D.C., 1971.
38. United States Department of Health, Education and Welfare, Second Special Report to the U.S. Congress on Alcohol and Health from the Secretary of Health, Education and Welfare, DHEW publication (ADM) 74-124. Washington, D.C., 1971.
39. Vourakis, C., and G. Bennett: Angel dust: Not heaven sent. *American Journal of Nursing,* 79:649, Apr. 1979.
40. Welch, C.C.: Alcoholic heart disease. *Postgraduate Medicine,* 61(5):138–44, May 1977.
41. Westermeyer, J.: *Primer on Chemical Dependency.* Baltimore: Williams and Wilkins Company, 1976.
42. *What Are The Signs of Alcoholism?* National Council on Alcoholism, 733 Third Avenue, New York, N.Y. 10017.
43. Whitfield, C.L., and K. Williams (Eds.): *The Patient with Alcoholism and Other Drug Problems.* Illinois: Whitfield and Williams, 1976.
44. Wilder, A.: Diagnosis and treatment of drug dependence of the barbiturate type. *American Journal of Psychiatry,* 125:758, 1968.
45. Wiley, L.: Managing a hospitalized drug addict. *Nursing 77,* 7:47, June 1977.
46. Wolfe, S.M., and M. Victor: The relationship of hypomagnesemia and alkalosis to alcohol withdrawal symptoms. *Annals of the New York Academy of Sciences,* 162:973, Aug. 1969.
47. Zinberg, N.E.: Marijuana. *Psychology Today,* 10:45, Dec. 1976.

UNIT XXVI

NURSING PEOPLE EXPERIENCING MEDICAL-SURGICAL EMERGENCIES

by Margaret M. McMahon, R.N., B.S.N., CCRN, EMT

INTRODUCTION AND OBJECTIVES

Emergency situations which threaten the health and well-being of individuals occur daily. Nurses are expected to respond appropriately and function effectively in a variety of emergencies, regardless of the setting in which they occur.

This chapter provides general principles governing the emergency care of adult disorders. Emphasis is placed on assessing and managing problems that are life-threatening or frequently encountered in emergency care settings. Since many of the conditions discussed here are also addressed in other sections of this text, a simplified, step-by-step approach is used. Psychiatric, pediatric, and obstetric disorders are not covered. An attempt has been made to prioritize suggested assessment and possible management, since *the ability to establish priorities of care is an essential skill of all emergency care providers.* Because the content of this chapter is limited, the reader is encouraged to consult other sections of this text as well as specialized sources for more information.

Objectives

This unit is included with the expectation that by studying it carefully and applying it in supervised clinical practice you will develop the skills to be able to:

- ▶ Make and report quickly and accurately appropriate observations of people in emergency circumstances.
- ▶ Prioritize emergency patient management logically and safely.
- ▶ Act quickly, safely, and appropriately in emergency situations.
- ▶ Make sound nursing interventions to alleviate the physical and psychosocial stress impinging on people in emergency circumstances.
- ▶ Commit yourself to an ongoing professional responsibility to remain current and competent in a knowledge of emergency management.

It is also expected that you will recognize the need to be thoroughly familiar with emergency and disaster management systems operating in your own community and health center. You should also be aware of any emergency situations unique to your own locality (e.g., drowning in communities near bodies of water; natural emergencies such as snake or spider bites specific to a geographic location) and be particularly skillful in their management.

The immediate management of patients with life-threatening problems involves many actions which often must be initiated simultaneously. Thus, nurses involved in emergency care may function in extended and expanded roles. By functioning under established protocol and standing orders, they may initiate diagnostic and/or therapeutic measures which, in other circumstances, may be physician responsibilities. In some settings, particularly in rural communities, nurses may be the only qualified care providers immediately available. Management approaches discussed in this unit include both medical and nursing care. Even when nurses are working side by side with physicians, knowledge of the normal medical management of specific problems enhances delivery of efficient, effective emergency care for the patient and significant others.

The nature of emergency nursing demands that nurses be very knowledgeable about emergency medications and their dosages. For this reason, the dosages of commonly used emergency medications are included whenever appropriate. *Although every effort has been made to insure that the dosages are accurate and current, changes in medical therapy, specific patient considerations, and physician preference may dictate dosages different from those listed in the text. Therefore, it is imperative that all drug dosages be verified with current literature and specific orders prior to medication administration.*

Unit Contents

CHAPTER 95

MEDICAL-SURGICAL EMERGENCY NURSING

In all emergencies the nurse must keep perfectly calm; she should think what has happened and what should be done, and then do it quietly. If she gets excited and loses her presence of mind, the life of the patient may be lost.

EMILY A. M. STONEY, 1906[131]

WHAT IS AN EMERGENCY?

Basically, an emergency exists when a patient (or the patient's significant others) believes that his or her physical or emotional well-being is in jeopardy.

Failure to appreciate a patient's perspective of his or her problem often results in frustration and less than ideal care. In patients with clearly non-emergency problems, it may be a nursing responsibility to help the patient find other sources of health care, once the presenting problem has been assessed and dealt with. *It is important that no patient be refused care.* People under stress, even from a *minor* illness or injury, are often unable to focus their attention on any area other than that which is making them uncomfortable. Once the immediate problem has been attended to, the patient is often more receptive to considering health care in a broader context.

WHAT IS EMERGENCY NURSING?

Emergency nursing has been defined as "the nursing care of individuals of all ages with perceived physical and/or emotional alterations which are undiagnosed and may require prompt intervention. Emergency nursing care is unscheduled and most commonly occurs in a specific setting, i.e., an emergency department, a mobile unit, or a suicide prevention center. Thus, the nursing care is episodic, primary, and acute in nature."[7]

The scope of emergency nursing is broad, requiring knowledge and skill in areas ranging from the detection and management of life-threatening arrhythmias to finding food and shelter for homeless transients.

Since less than 20 per cent of the persons seeking emergency care have life-threatening problems, a major role of the nurse is client teaching. Disease detection and health promotion must be embraced as vital roles of the nurse in emergency care. Finally, since a patient's first impressions of the health care system are often molded by experiences in an emergency department, nurses must be skilled at public relations, stress management, and creative problem solving.

PSYCHOLOGIC NEEDS

As shown, the word "emergency" implies a sense of danger, a crisis, an experience with the unknown. This feeling may be shared by patients, significant others, and emergency care personnel.

Emergency patients *are* unique. They differ from in-hospital patients in that they often have not accepted the "patient role." *Emergency patients* are usually anxious, fearful and confused because of the suddenness of their problems. Occasionally they are angry. They may experience a loss of control, a loss of individuality, and possibly a loss of dignity. In order to provide effective, compassionate care, nurses need to be aware of patient's feelings, needs, and concerns.

The needs of a patient's *significant others* must also be given special attention. In instances when these people are summoned to the emergency care setting, their lives may be suddenly and dramatically disrupted. They may be completely unaware of circumstances surrounding the emergency. They want desperately to see and talk with their loved one. Advising a patient's significant others of the patient's presence in the emergency service by phone requires tact and sensitivity. When appropriate, you may preface the conversation by saying that the patient asked you to call. Exercise caution as you discuss the urgency of the situation. It is not uncommon for persons to be injured or killed as they rush to hospitals to be with loved ones. You may suggest that neighbors or friends help with driving to the hospital. State clearly information such as the name of the hospital, its location, phone number, and directions. Directions may need to be repeated several times.

Notification of significant others and/or their presence in the emergency department is communicated to the team members and is often also recorded on the patient's clinical record. If a patient's condition is serious and the religion is unknown, this information is obtained as tactfully as possible from a family member.

As soon as possible, permit at least one significant other to see the patient. This is especially important when the patient is seriously ill or injured.

Provide visitors with support and information about the patient's condition and appearance, particularly when there is disfigurement and/or loss of ability to communicate. Also prepare visitors for the presence of tubes, equipment, and other devices.

Significant others may be better able to respond to, and cope with, an emergency if provided with a private waiting area. *A support person from the hospital staff should remain with the family, providing continuous support and information. Additionally, it is important that the nurse actually caring for the patient periodically visit to facilitate understanding of the patient's progress.* When the prognosis is grave, frequent updating of information about the patient's condition provides an opportunity for "anticipatory grieving."*

Feelings experienced by *staff* during an emergency usually result from the unpredictability of emergency problems, and concerns about possibly being unable to handle problems effectively. Insecurity may be related to lack of knowledge about management of a particular problem, or inability to perform a technical skill. Although a little apprehension is helpful in emergency situations (because it increases epinephrine flow and thus the ability to respond quickly), repeated anxiety and nervousness are destructive and interfere in effective care. The best way to cope with these feelings is to be fully prepared to deal with potential problems, both clinically and technically. Gaining knowledge and acquiring competence in the performance of specific skills comes with obtaining thoughtful experience. Once uncertainties are eliminated, the urgency of an emergency diminishes. Finally, it may be helpful for emergency personnel to remember that the emergency is the patient's, not the staff's.[31]

*See Sorensen and Luckmann, *Basic Nursing: A Psychophysiologic Approach* for an extended discussion of the grief process.

ESTABLISHING PRIORITIES OF CARE*

The goal of emergency care is prompt, effective resuscitation and stabilization of the critically ill or injured. How do you know which patient is the most critically ill or injured? While a massively injured person is not hard to recognize, the urgency and priority for care of other patients is often not as obvious. The system of identifying patients at greatest risk and initiating treatment is called *triage.* Table 95–1 lists the indications for assigning patients priority for treatment.

These guidelines shown may vary according to the nature of the problems commonly encountered in a particular emergency care setting. Since a complete assessment is impossible when seeing a patient initially, it is wise to err on the side of assigning a *higher* triage priority than a lower one.

The process of triage is not static, but fluid. Patients should be reassessed at frequent intervals, and the priority of care altered as needed.

Initial Assessment. When first confronted with a seriously ill or injured person, gain as much information as possible in a short time. This information can be gained by carrying out a rapid, two minute, physical assessment. The goals are (a) to identify if immediate life-sustaining measures are needed and (b) to identify what injuries or problems are present.

The *steps in an initial patient survey* are:

- ▶ *Assess the airway.* (See also Unit XVI and Chapter 93.) Place your face over the patient's face, with your head turned sideways to visualize the chest and assess chest wall excursion. The patient's air exchange should be felt against your cheek. If patient is not ventilating, position head and neck as for CPR (see Chapter 35), and reassess ventilations. If still no air exchange, initiate airway man-

*See references 114, 116, 122, 129, and 148.

TABLE 95–1. INDICATIONS FOR PRIORITY IN CARE

- ▶ Altered levels of consciousness
- ▶ Respiratory distress
- ▶ Chest pain, especially in the patient over 35 years
- ▶ Elderly or very young patient
- ▶ Severe pain
- ▶ Alterations in body temperature (less than 35°C or more than 40°C)
- ▶ Injuries that will most likely be worsened by movement
- ▶ Shock
- ▶ Bleeding that cannot be controlled by direct pressure
- ▶ Behavior that is disturbing to others, e.g., dangerous, very noisy, hysterical
- ▶ Chemical burns
- ▶ Significant alterations in vital signs
- ▶ Symptomatology which is vague, but which causes concern

agement techniques. If airway obstruction due to a bolus of food *("a cafe coronary")* is suspected, carry out either a chest thrust or an abdominal thrust. An *abdominal thrust,* also known as the *Heimlich maneuver,* is illustrated in Figure 95–1. An alternative action, believed by some to be safer, is the *chest thrust.* To accomplish chest thrust: (a) stand behind victim and encircle victim's chest with your arms under his or her axilla; (b) make a fist with your right hand and place your left hand on top of your right hand, (c) position your fist above the patient's xiphoid and (d) give four quick inward thrusts. This should cause the food bolus to be expelled. If the action is ineffective, deliver four back blows between shoulder blades and repeat chest or abdominal thrust.

If all attempts fail, a *cricothyroidotomy (coniotomy)* may be necessary. This fairly simple procedure requires more courage than skill. The location of the cricothyroid membrane and the technique are illustrated in Figure 95–2. If you are reluctant to use a scalpel to penetrate the membrane, one or more large bore teflon IV catheters may be used.[48] *If an incision is made, the opening must be kept patent.* A tracheotomy tube, plastic tubing or, in a field situation, the cartridge end of a ball point pen (with cartridge removed) may be used. This provides a "tube-like" device with a hole in both ends. Whatever device is used must be stabilized until a tracheotomy can be done.

Other aids to airway maintenance include *intubation of the trachea or the esophagus.* Although this skill is appropriate and necessary for emergency nurses to possess, complete discussion of endotracheal intubation is beyond the scope of this

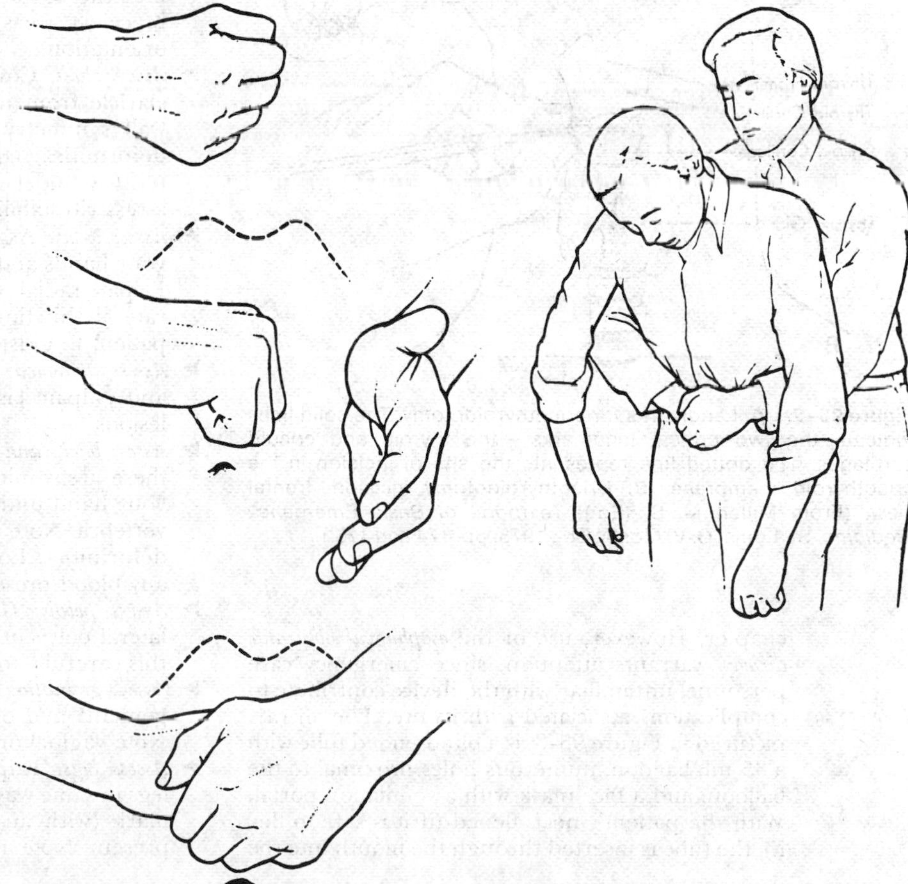

Figure 95–1. Use of the Heimlich maneuver (abdominal thrust) to relieve airway obstruction. The maneuver uses air in the lungs to force an obstruction out of the airway. To move the air you have to apply sudden pressure below the rib cage, which forces the diaphragm up and compresses the lungs. The basic technique (left) begins with a fist. Note the knob formed by the thumb and index finger – that's what helps push the diaphragm upward. Place your fist thumbside against the abdomen, slightly above the navel and below the rib cage. Then grasp your fist with your free hand and press into the abdomen with a quick upward thrust. Do this while standing or kneeling behind a standing or sitting victim with your arms wrapped around his waist (right). Repeat this procedure several times if necessary. (From: To save a choking victim. *Emergency Medicine,* 11:287, Feb. 1979.)

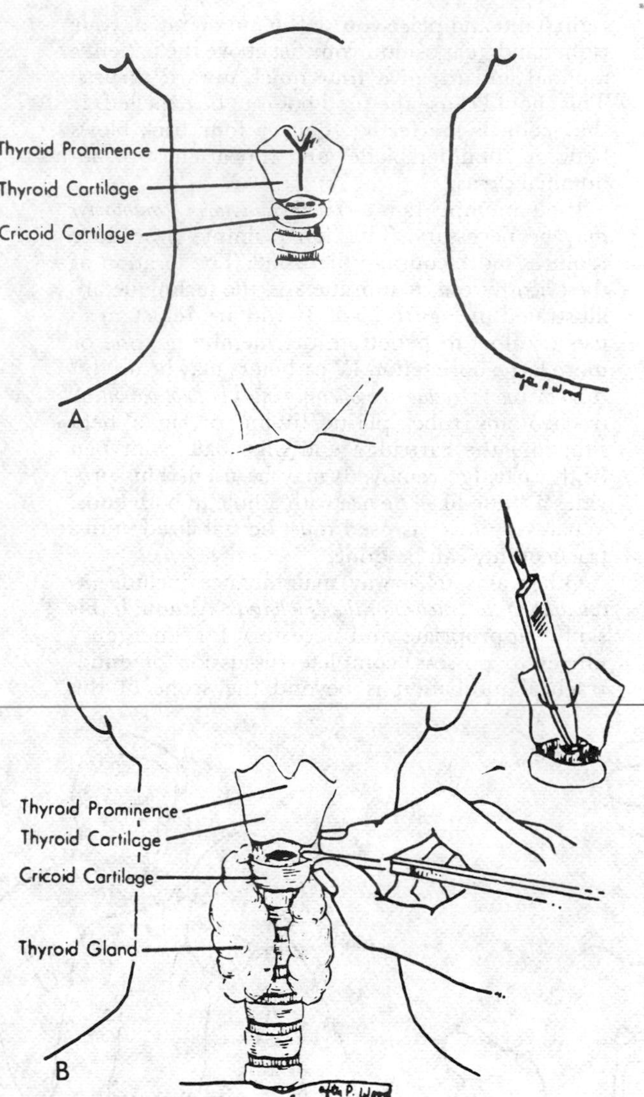

Figure 95–2. **A.** Landmarks for cricothyroidotomy. The solid lines indicate the two critical landmarks – the thyroid and cricoid cartilages. The dotted line represents the site of incision in the cricothyroid membrane. **B.** Cricothyroidotomy incision, frontal view. (From Miller, M. S. (Ed.): *Textbook of Basic Emergency Medicine.* St. Louis: C. V. Mosby Co., 1975, pp. 174 and 175.)

chapter. However, use of the *esophageal obturator airway* warrants attention, since emergency care personnel unfamiliar with the device contribute to complications associated with its use. The airway, pictured in Figure 95–3, is a blind-ended tube with a 35 ml. balloon, numerous holes proximal to the balloon, and a face mask with a ventilation portal. With the patient's neck flexed (if it is safe to flex it), the tube is inserted through the mouth into the esophagus and the balloon inflated. The patient is ventilated and breath sounds are auscultated. When the airway is properly positioned, air exits the holes and enters the trachea. Since the distal esophagus is occluded, the problem of emesis and subsequent aspiration is minimized. A newer model allows for nasogastric (NG) tube insertion and suction as needed.

Some *hazards* of an esophageal obturator include: tracheal intubation, esophageal laceration, and aspiration of gastric contents upon tube removal.[76] *It is recommended that a cuffed endotracheal tube be inserted before an esophageal obturator airway is removed.* An esophageal obturator airway is an effective adjunct to airway management when used by properly trained personnel.

- ▶ *Once the airway has been established, note the rate, rhythm, and volume of respirations.* Do not stop to count the rate at this time. Initiate ventilatory support as needed.
- ▶ *Stop major bleeding,* using direct pressure, pressure dressing or, rarely, a tourniquet.
- ▶ *Assess head and neck:* Palpate cervical spine without moving head, palpate skull, observe for drainage from ears and nose, observe for ecchymosis of mastoid process, palpate facial bones, check pupils, look in mouth and check teeth alignment, have patient smile and observe for ptosis or weakness. If cervical spine (C-spine) injury is suspected, apply cervical collar and initiate traction. (See Unit X.)
- ▶ At the same time, *gather data* concerning illness or injury, patient data (name, allergies, MD's name, medical problems, etc.), look for medical alert bracelets, areas of pain, level of consciousness and orientation.
- ▶ *Assess chest:* Cover sucking chest wounds, palpate clavicle from sternum to shoulder, observe chest wall symmetry and presence of ecchymoses or deformities, compress anterior chest wall posteriorly and lateral chest wall toward midline to assess rib stability, listen to breath sounds.
- ▶ *Assess arms:* Assess each arm by encircling it with your hands and palpating from shoulder to hand. Palpate radial pulses but do not stop to count pulse rate at this time. Test motor function by asking patient to grasp your fingers.
- ▶ *Assess abdomen:* Observe first, auscultate second, and palpate last. Observe for distention, masses, lesions.
- ▶ *Assess back, and thoracic and lumbar spines:* Palpate these areas initially while patient is supine. Slide your hand under patient's back and palpate each vertebra. Note presence of pain, muscle spasm or deformities. Look at your hands to see if there is any blood present.
- ▶ *Assess pelvis: Gently* compress pubic bones and lateral pelvis in order to detect pelvic fracture. Do this carefully to avoid causing further injury.
- ▶ *Assess genitalia:* Note obvious injuries to external genitalia and observe urethral meatus for blood. Note vaginal or urethral discharge.
- ▶ *Assess legs:* Palpate femoral pulses and examine legs in same way as arms. Palpate pedal pulses and mark (with an "X" with a pen) if an injury is present. Note any edema.

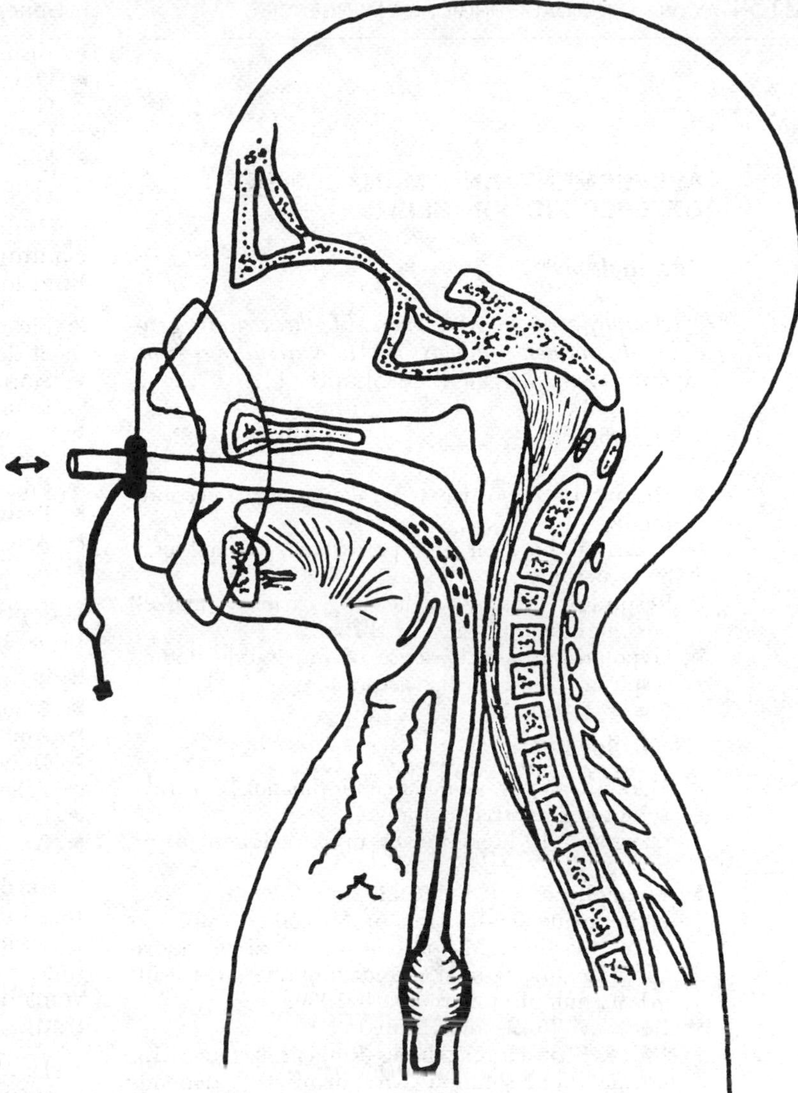

Figure 95–3. The esophageal obturator airway in place. (From Johnson, K. R., et al.: Esophageal obturator airway: Use and complications. *Journal of the American College of Emergency Physicians,* 5:36, Jan. 1976, p. 37.)

- *Assess back and buttocks:* If spinal, pelvic, or femoral fracture is *not* suspected, turn patient onto one side and inspect and palpate back and buttocks. In patients with gunshot wounds with no wound of exit, separate and inspect the buttock fold; exit wound may thus be located. Pelvic fracture or retroperitoneal hematoma may cause ecchymoses of back or flank. Infections or trauma to the kidney may cause tenderness at the costovertebral angle *(CVA tenderness).*

Following the initial physical assessment, assess *complete vital signs.* Note respiratory rate and temperature. Take postural vital signs whenever volume depletion is suspected, if this maneuver is safe. Patients with chest pain or chest trauma have blood pressure measurements taken on both arms, because of possible aortic aneurysm.

Although they vary from patient to patient, some of the more *common treatment assessment priorities* are listed in Table 95–2.

TABLE 95–2. COMMON TREATMENT/ASSESSMENT PRIORITIES IN EMERGENCIES

- Oxygen
- IV fluids; draw appropriate lab studies from IV catheter before attaching IV tubing
- Cardiac monitor
- Diagnostic studies: X-ray, ECG, etc.
- Nasogastric tube, e.g., #18 Fr. Salem Sump tube
- Foley catheter
- Repeated assessment, e.g., VS q̄ 5 minutes for unstable patient
- Measure girth of abdomen and extremities as needed
- Splint fractures, apply ice packs, and elevate extremities
- Clean, repair and dress wounds
- Medications: pain relief, tetanus booster, etc.
- Comfort measures, patient/significant others reassurance

ASSESSMENT AND MANAGEMENT OF SPECIFIC PROBLEMS

Anaphylaxis[98]

(Anaphylactic shock) a severe, life-threatening, generalized antigen-antibody reaction resulting from exposure to an allergen. (See Chapter 11.)

Recognition

- History of exposure (e.g., bee sting, injection, food).
- Urticaria, perioral and periorbital edema, total body swelling.
- Respiratory distress, wheezing, stridor, hoarseness, tightness in chest or throat.
- Hypotension, shock, sense of impending doom, respiratory and cardiac arest.

Management

- Maintain airway — may need intubation, cricothyroidotomy, or tracheotomy.
- Oxygen 6–10 liters/min by mask (if tolerated) or prongs.
- Epinephrine — 0.3–0.5 ml. of *1:1000* sq or IM; epinephrine 0.5–1.0 ml. of *1:10,000* IV for extreme reactions. May also apply tourniquet above sting or injection site and infiltrate area with 0.1–0.3 ml. of epinephrine 1:1000.
- Benadryl 25–50 mg. IM or IV.
- IV (#18 or larger), hang Ringer's lactate (RL), normal saline solution (NSS) or 5% D/W depending on condition.
- Steroids such as dexamethasone or Solu Medrol, given IV.
- Aminophylline 250–500 mg. given IV push *very slowly,* or IV drip over 20 minutes. Patient should be on a cardiac monitor.
- Gastric lavage if secondary to ingestion.
- Cardiac monitor.
- Constant nursing observation with vital signs (VS) q 5 minutes.
- IPPB with Isuprel or racemic epinephrine may be used.
- Reassurance. Note: Patients often hear what personnel say even though they appear unconscious.
- Arrange for ICU bed.
- *Patient/family teaching:* Wearing of medical alert band; how to use a bee sting kit (with return demonstrations); avoidance of allergen; use of meat tenderizer for stings (reduces reaction).

Shock

Includes hypovolemic, septic, cardiogenic, and neurogenic shock. (See Chapter 13.)

General Management

- Insure adequate airway.
- Oxygen 6–10 liters/min. unless patient has COPD.
- Cardiac monitor and/or 12 lead ECG.
- Start at least one IV, preferably a 14 or 16 gauge.

Hypovolemic. Characterized by cool, clammy skin, hypotension, history of blood or fluid loss, diaphoresis, flat neck veins, etc.

- Elevate legs (*Note:* Recent studies dispute the value of this maneuver).
- Start a second IV; hang Ringer's lactate or normal saline; albumin or whole blood later.
- Draw blood: CBC, Lytes, BUN, sugar, coagulation screen, type and crossmatch if blood loss.
- Pressor agents (rarely used).
- Prepare for or insert a CVP line.
- Arterial blood gases.
- Anti-shock trousers (see p. 283)

Septic. History of instrumentation, infections, fever, warm skin, flushed, diaphoretic.

- Steroids.
- Blood cultures q 20 minutes × 3.
- Antibiotics given after blood cultures drawn.
- Draw blood as above.
- Foley catheter; urine for UA, C&S.
- Locate source of infection.
- Anti-shock trousers.

Cardiogenic. May be due to myocardial infarction, ventricular rupture, pericardial tamponade, ruptured chordae tendineae, arrhythmias, etc. Characterized by distended neck veins; patient may have chest pain or history of trauma.

- IV 5% D/W with a microdripper — no more than a 500 ml. bag.
- Antiarrhythmics and digitalis.
- Diuretics (Lasix).
- CVP line, Swan-Ganz catheter.
- Anti-shock trousers as a reversible fluid challenge.
- Pressor agents: dopamine, Levophed, etc.
- Admit to CCU.

Neurogenic. Results from loss of vasomotor tone and vasodilation following spinal cord injury or spinal anesthesia: may also be psychogenic/vasovagal.

- Elevate legs.
- IV may be started.
- Usually self-limiting.

The Unconscious Patient[24, 97, 117]

The causes of unconsciousness are many, and treatment is specific for each cause. Management discussion in this section covers only general guidelines. One way of categorizing coma for evaluation is: (1) metabolic, (2) structural, (3) intoxication, and (4) functional. (See Ch. 26.)

Metabolic: (a) hypoglycemia; (b) hyperglycemia; and (c) uremia.

Structural: (a) Hemorrhages, including subdural, epidural, subarachnoid, intracerebral, and brain stem; (b) infectious processes, including meningitis, encephalitis, and brain abscesses; (c) seizures; and (d) vascular insufficiency secondary to cardiac arrhythmias, CVA, TIA and carotid artery occlusion.

Intoxication: (a) alcohol; (b) drugs; and (c) poisons, e.g., carbon monoxide, organophosphate insecticides.

Functional: Psychogenic.

Recognition

- Variable according to the cause. However, color of skin, respiratory pattern, pupillary reaction, motor function, odors, nuchal rigidity, and posturing may aid in identifying the cause.

Management

- Suspected narcotic overdose, e.g., presence of pinpoint pupils, needle marks, etc. Narcan 0.4 mg. IV may be given and repeated × 3.
- Suspected hypoglycemia, 50 ml. 50% dextrose given *after* drawing blood sugar.
- With head trauma history, suspected C-spine (cervical spine) injury.
- Insure airway.
- Position patient on side or in swimmer's position to allow secretions to drain after C-spine or other possible injury is ruled out.
- Oxygen may be appropriate by mask.
- Eye care.
- Frequent VS and continuous nursing assessment.
- Draw appropriate lab work; consider toxicology if drugs or alcohol suspected.
- Foley catheter; monitor urine output; UA to lab.
- Safety — side rails up, locked.

Acute Respiratory Insufficiency*

Asthma (Acute Attack). Characterized by bronchial spasm, mucosal edema, and increased secretions. (See also Unit XVI.)

Recognition

- Respiratory distress, tachypnea, wheezing (especially expiratory wheezing), air hunger, use of accessory muscles for breathing.
- Anxiety, apprehension.
- Usually history of asthma.
- Evidence of sympathetic effect: elevated blood pressure, tachycardia, cool and moist skin.
- Fever may be present.

*See references 28, 43a, 121, 132, 134.

Caution: *The inability to ausculate wheezing initially in an asthmatic patient with acute respiratory distress is sometimes an ominous sign. It may indicate that the small airways are* so constricted *that not enough air is being exchanged to create a wheezing sound. This patient may be critically ill, requiring more aggressive medical management.*

Management

- Find out if patient recently used a medi-haler containing Isuprel or epinephrine.
- Oxygen via prongs.
- Epinephrine 1:1000 in dose of 0.3–0.5 ml. given sc unless patient has: pulse greater than 140, diastolic BP greater than 100, history of hypertension or cardiac problems, or unless epinephrine has not been effective in the past. Epinephrine may be given every 20 minutes for a maximum of three doses. Listen to breath sounds to see if breathing has improved (i.e., wheezes gone) before giving subsequent injections.
- Aminophylline is used if epinephrine is not indicated (see above). The initial dose is usually 250–500 mg. IV, given either IV push *slowly* or IV drip in 50–100 ml. 5% D/W. If wheezing continues, the patient may be given 0.6 to 0.9 mg./kg./hour of aminophylline added to 1000 ml. 5% D/W.

Caution: *Aminophylline, when administered in large doses to a patient with hypoxemia, may precipitate cardiac arrhythmias. The use of a cardiac monitor may be desirable in selected patients.*

- Reassurance; hydration with oral fluids.
- IPPB with normal saline, bronchodilators, etc.
- Sputum specimen; arterial blood gases; spirometry; chest x-ray.
- Corticosteroids if patient not responding to standard treatments or if patient routinely takes steroids daily. If steroids are required, hospital admission usually indicated.
- Sodium bicarbonate IV for profound respiratory acidosis.
- VS every 15 to 30 minutes in initial treatment period, retake temperature at least once.

Status Asthmaticus.[121, 137] Asthma attack that is refractory to the usual treatments. (See Unit XVI.) Management includes above items as well as endotracheal intubation and mechanical ventilation when exhaustion and significant respiratory acidosis present. Admit to ICU.

> Caution: *Rule out other causes of respiratory failure, including foreign body, pulmonary edema, pulmonary embolus, pneumothorax, and anaphylaxis with atypical or unresponsive asthma attack.*

Emphysema. Development of acute respiratory failure in a person with emphysema is often the result of a pulmonary infection. (See Unit XVI.)

Recognition

- ▶ Increasing dyspnea, easily fatigued.
- ▶ Barrel chest with increased AP diameter.
- ▶ Use of accessory muscles to breathe.
- ▶ Prolonged expiratory phase through pursed lips.
- ▶ Characteristic sitting position, leaning forward with arms propped on knees or table.
- ▶ Altered levels of consciousness, e.g., confusion or agitation.
- ▶ Face may be flushed ("pink puffer") or cyanotic ("blue bloater").
- ▶ Elevated blood pressure, tachycardia, cardiac arrhythmias.
- ▶ Arterial blood gases indicate hypoxemia, hypercarbia, and respiratory acidosis.

Management

- ▶ Arterial blood gases, sputum specimen, spirometry.
- ▶ Low flow oxygen via a Venturi mask.

> Caution: *Unlike other persons (whose stimulus to breathe is rising CO_2 levels), the respiratory drive in a person with COPD is activated by O_2 levels. Thus, if supplemental oxygen is administered in large amounts and without frequent observation, the patient with COPD may cease to breathe.*

- ▶ Bronchodilators, e.g., aminophylline, Isuprel, Bronchosol.

> Caution: *It is preferable that aminophylline and Isuprel be administered alternately rather than concurrently, in order to minimize side effects such as tachycardias and arrhythmias.*

- ▶ Hydration, IV fluids.
- ▶ Chest physiotherapy and/or postural drainage.
- ▶ Be prepared to intubate and ventilate.
- ▶ Antibiotics may be used.

*Near Drowning**

The condition of persons initially surviving submersion in water. Major problems are: hypoxia, hypercarbia and acidosis resulting in cardiopulmonary arrest. Bronchospasm, from water in the lungs, causes most drowning deaths. A few victims have "dry drowning" due to laryngospasm. Pulmonary edema is common in victims of either salt water or fresh water submersion. In *salt water* aspiration, water aspirated into the lungs is hyperosmolar and fluid is pulled from the vascular tree into the alveoli to achieve equilibrium. In *fresh water* near drowning, there is a washout of pulmonary surfactant and the alveoli collapse. This results in a negative interalveolar hydrostatic pressure and subsequent fluid accumulation.

Fluid and electrolyte abnormalities may be present, depending upon the volume and kind of water aspirated. Victims of fresh water aspiration may be hypervolemic, have hemodilution, and have red cell lysis, since the water is absorbed into the circulation within a few minutes.

Other problems associated with near drowning include pneumonia and lung abscesses (due to aspiration of foreign matter) and hyaline membrane disease. Hypothermia may be present if submersion occurred in a cold climate; however, the decreased metabolic demand and oxygen consumption associated with hypothermia may protect the patient to some degree. Bradycardia may also play a role in decreasing metabolic need.

Recognition

- ▶ History of submersion
- ▶ Cardiopulmonary arrest.
- ▶ Cyanosis.
- ▶ Pulmonary edema.
- ▶ Fluid and electrolyte abnormalities.
- ▶ Hypothermia

Management

> Caution: *In cardiac arrest, CPR should always be initiated, regardless of the estimated length of a person's submersion.*

- ▶ Vigorous, prolonged CPR — possibly for several hours.
- ▶ Do not waste time trying to remove water from lungs; ventilate with 100% oxygen and 5–10 cm. of PEEP.
- ▶ Arterial blood gases, CBC, electrolytes, STAT portable chest film.
- ▶ IV line with NSS; however, fluid of choice may vary.

*See references 18, 33, 67, 120, 134a.

- CVP line.
- Diuretics and other appropriate therapies if pulmonary edema present (management of pulmonary edema discussed later).
- Foley catheter, frequent urine measurement.
- Nasogastric tube to remove swallowed water.
- Evaluate for other injuries — suspect C-spine injury if patient unconscious.
- Try to treat causes of near drowning, e.g., myocardial infarction, drug overdose.
- Perform appropriate toxicological studies for suspected drug and/or alcohol ingestion.
- Core rewarming.
- Steroids may be used (controversial).
- Antibiotics may be used.
- Admit and observe for 24–48 hours; repeat chest film after 24 hours; psychologic support.

> Caution: *Near drowning victims may have subclinical pulmonary edema. Even minimal exertion may precipitate an acute episode. Complete bed rest is advised initially.*

Pneumonia

Infectious pulmonary process caused by various organisms or by aspiration. (See also Chapter 55.)

Bacterial Pneumonia

Recognition

- History of minor recent URI.
- Chest pain, usually in lateral lung fields, increasing with respiration.
- Shaking chills; possibly fever.
- Sputum may appear green, yellow, rust colored or blood tinged.
- Dyspnea and/or tachypnea.
- Skin flushed, patient may look toxic but usually alert and oriented.
- Chest exam: decreased tactile fremitus, dullness, decreased breath sounds, presence of rales or rhonchi.

Management

- Position for comfort, usually high Fowler's.
- Humidified oxygen; hydration (possibly IV).
- Sputum specimen for gram stain and C&S, blood for CBC.
- ABG's if severe respiratory distress.
- Appropriate antibiotics.
- Chest PT, postural drainage or IPPB.
- Patient/family teaching about taking antibiotics.

Aspiration Pneumonia

Recognition

- Hypoxia, cyanosis, tachypnea, pulmonary edema.
- Commonly seen in patients with decreased or absent gag reflex, e.g., overdose, neurologic disorder, following general anesthesia, etc.

Management

- Quickly turn patient onto one side.
- Suction airway; administer 100% oxygen by mask.
- Endotracheal intubation and mechanical ventilation; PEEP.
- Sputum culture.
- Broad-spectrum antibiotics.
- Steroids, e.g., hydrocortisone 1 gm. IV and/or 1 gm. through endotracheal tube.
- Bronchodilators.
- Arterial blood gases.

Pulmonary Embolism (PE)[69, 150]

Usually due to a thrombus mobilized from elsewhere in the body. However, it may also result from amnionic fluid or fat emboli. (See also Chapter 49.) Symptoms are variable.

Recognition

- Hyperventilation, wheezing, hemoptysis, tachycardia, extreme apprehension; feeling of chest tightness or pleuritic chest pain.
- Pleural effusion, pleural friction rub.
- Predisposing histories include: prolonged immobilization, trauma, post partum, thrombophlebitis, oral contraceptives, previous pulmonary embolism, arrhythmias.
- Hypoxemia, cyanosis, hypotension if massive.
- ECG changes compatible with PE.

Management

- Oxygen by mask or prongs; arterial blood gases.
- 12 lead ECG, cardiac monitor, treat arrhythmias.
- Routine blood work, including coagulation screen.
- Chest x-ray, lung scan, pulmonary arteriography.
- Pain relief — Demerol rather than morphine.[30]
- Anticoagulation — done as inpatient procedure.

Air Embolism[121, 143]

This life-threatening problem may result from pulmonary barotrauma in divers, in patients with large CVP or hyperalimentation lines, and during mechanical ventilation. Indications of air embolism vary and may be unimpressive; however, prompt treatment is needed.

Recognition

- Compatible history.
- Chest pain; cyanosis; cough.

- CNS signs: disorientation, vertigo, tingling of limbs, sudden loss of consciousness, convulsions, same-sided spastic or flaccid paralysis of arm and leg, visual disturbances.

Management

- Quickly turn patient onto left side, lowering head of the bed into Trendelenberg position to minimize chance of air bubbles entering cerebral circulation.
- 100% oxygen.
- Rapidly transport patient to recompression chamber.[106] (Chapter 13, briefly discusses hyperbaric oxygen therapy.)
- Additional therapy may include: IV line, chest tube(s), sodium bicarbonate.
- For air transport, a plane capable of pressurizing is ideal; however, transport should not be delayed for this reason.

Pneumothorax[16, 105]

An accumulation of air in the pleural space, resulting in partial or complete collapse of the lung on that side. (See also Unit XVI.) A tension pneumothorax is a life-threatening problem requiring immediate intervention. (See p. 1342.)

Recognition

- Sudden, sharp chest pain; dyspnea or tachypnea.
- Tachycardia
- Decreased or absent breath sounds on affected side; hyperresonance or tympany to percussion.
- Tension pneumothorax may cause severe respiratory distress, shock, tracheal deviation, distended neck veins, cyanosis.

Management

- Oxygen, high Fowler's position, chest film.
- Immediate needle aspiration for suspected tension pneumothorax. A large needle, 3-way stop cock and a syringe can be used. A simple device made from a spinal needle and finger cot is also highly effective. This device, pictured in Figure 95–4, should be readily available in every emergency department (ED) and CCU. The needle is inserted between the second and third interspace, midclavicular line on the side of the pneumothorax. Significant improvement should be noted immediately after evacuation of the air.
- Small chest tube (16–20 F.) inserted in second or third intercostal space, midclavicular line and attached to chest drainage. (See p. 1367 for a discussion of chest drainage.)

Caution: *A chest tube should be clamped only with a physician's order. If air is allowed to accumulate in the pleural space, a tension pneumothorax may develop.*

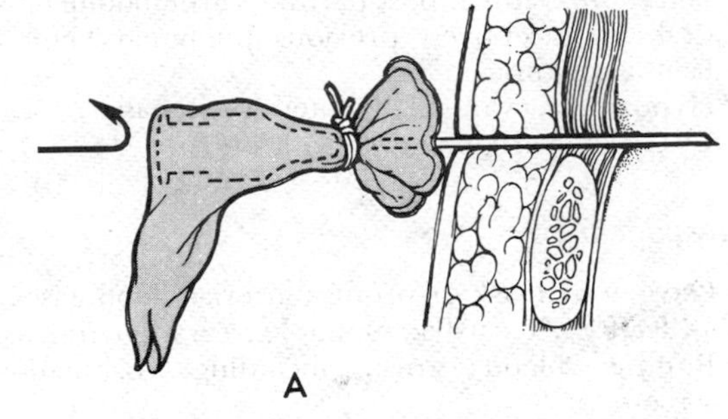

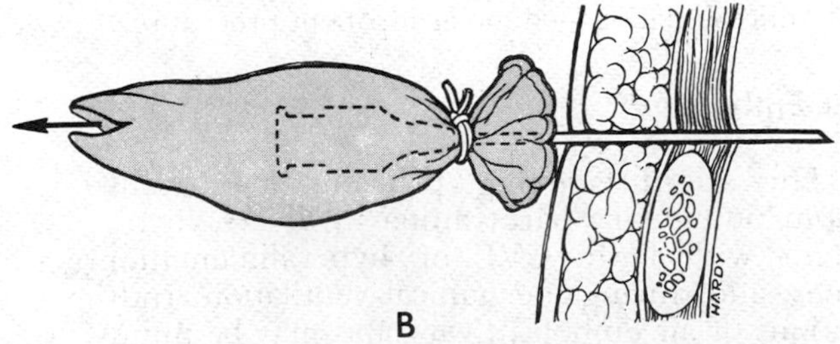

Figure 95–4. Flutter valve device used in the relief of a tension pneumothorax. The device consists of a finger cot, the end of which has been cut, tied onto the hub of a large needle. **A.** On inspiration, the finger cot collapses, preventing air from entering the pleural cavity. **B.** On expiration, air trapped in the pleural space is expelled through the end of the finger cot. (From Cosgriff, J. H., Jr., and D. L. Anderson: *The Practice of Emergency Nursing.* Philadelphia: J. B. Lippincott Company, 1975, p. 278.)

Pulmonary Edema*

An accumulation of fluid in the alveoli. Treatment is directed toward decreasing the transudation of fluid into the alveoli and resolving the underlying cause. Pulmonary edema is a medical emergency. (See also Chapters 34 and 57.)

Recognition

- Severe dyspnea, tachypnea, cyanosis, cough, rales, wheezes.
- Frothy, occasionally blood tinged, sputum. Distended neck veins and other signs of heart failure; hyper- or hypotension, tachycardia, possible arrhythmias.
  Altered level of consciousness (e.g., confusion, agitation).
  Peripheral edema.
- Compatible history, e.g., MI, CHF, hypertension, narcotic overdose, previous cardiac surgery such as valve replacement, arrhythmias, near drown-

*See references 48, 62, 74, 93, 121, 134, and 137.

ing. Chest film compatible with pulmonary edema, e.g., fluffy white infiltrates.

Management

- High Fowler's position or allow patient to dangle legs.
- High flow oxygen by mask if tolerated.
- IPPB with or without alcohol; arterial blood gases.
- IV with 250–500 ml. of 5% D/W with a microdripper, *to keep vein open only.*
- STAT portable chest film.
- Diuretics, e.g., furosemide (Lasix) is most often used. Dose depends on whether patient is taking the drug at home. If the patient is taking Lasix at home, twice the daily dose is administered IV. If the patient is not on Lasix, the loading dose is 40–80 mg. IV. This drug should be given *slowly.* The onset of action, when it is administered IV, is usually within 3 to 5 minutes.
- Morphine sulfate 4–8 mg. IV *slowly;* use cautiously because it is a respiratory depressant.
- Foley catheter; accurate I & O.
- Cardiac monitor; 12 lead ECG.
- Rotating tourniquets, manually or via machine.[50]
- Phlebotomy (uncommon).
- Digitalis preparations.
- Aminophylline 250–500 mg. IV over 15 to 20 minutes.
- Treat cause, e.g., give Narcan if narcotic or propoxyphene (Darvon) overdose; diazoxide (Hyperstat) if hypertensive crisis.
- Continued reassurance and psychologic support.
- Be prepared for endotracheal intubation and ventilation.
- Hemodialysis may be needed with renal failure.
- Admit to ICU or CCU.

CARDIAC EMERGENCIES

Cardiac dysfunctions vary widely, from "cardiac arrest" to mild "palpitations." (See Unit XII and reference 62.) Emphasis here is on the differential diagnosis and management of a person with chest pain, with a brief review of the most life-threatening cardiac arrhythmias.

*Differential Diagnosis of Chest Pain**[66, 69]

The patient with chest pain represents a true diagnostic and management challenge since there are many causes of chest pain, some life-threatening and others relatively benign. Effective triage depends upon recognizing problems which may cause chest pain. Causes of chest pain can be divided into four categories: cardiovascular, musculoskeletal, pleuritic or pulmonary, and gastrointestinal. A fifth category, psychogenic, is used occasionally. Some conditions commonly associated with chest pain are listed in Table 95–3.

*See also Chapter 33.

In *assessing chest pain,* specific questions which should be asked include:

- When did the pain start? How long did it last? Have you had this kind of pain before? What was the problem diagnosed as the last time you had the pain? Is this pain worse, less or the same as before? Have you had a chest injury?
- Where is the pain located? Point with one finger to where it bothers you the most. Does the pain go (radiate) anywhere, e.g., back, shoulders, arm, jaw, etc?
- Describe the pain on a scale of 1 to 10, with 1 being minimal pain, and 10 being the worst possible pain you can imagine. What number would you give this pain?
- What were you doing when the pain started, or what had you been doing right before it started?
- Did you notice anything else beside the pain, e.g., nausea, vomiting, sweating, dizziness, etc.?
- Does anything cause the pain or make the pain worse? Does anything make it better? What have you tried to relieve the pain?
- Do you take any medications now, and have you taken any in the past? Do you have any problems with your heart?

Objective Information

- Presence of adrenergic influence, e.g., elevated BP, tachycardia, diaphoresis, dilated pupils, anxiety.
- Presence of cholinergic influence, e.g., bradycardia, nausea, vomiting.
- Complete vital signs with BP taken on both arms.
- Reassurance is vital.
- Chest examination.
- Apply defibrillator paddles with a "through-the-

TABLE 95–3. CONDITIONS COMMONLY CAUSING CHEST PAIN

Cardiovascular
Myocardial infarction
Angina pectoris
Pericarditis
Dissecting aneurysm of the thoracic aorta
Musculoskeletal
Rib fractures
Costochondritis, including Tietze's syndrome
Muscle strain
Pleuritic or Pulmonary
Pulmonary embolism
Pneumothorax
Pneumonia
Pleurisy
Gastrointestinal
Esophagitis
Peptic ulcer
Hiatal hernia
Cholecystitis
Pancreatitis

paddles-look" to the chest *after explaining* to the patient that this will give you an idea of the heart rate and rhythm. Many patients have either experienced or observed defibrillation and may become unduly alarmed.

- If the patient is stable and does not have a dangerous arrhythmia, assessment and management can be carried out as discussed below.

CARDIOVASCULAR

Myocardial Infarction (MI). (See also p. 852.)

Recognition

Sudden onset of substernal, midline or left anterior chest pain, possibly radiating to neck, back, shoulder, jaw, abdomen, or down one or both arms. Dyspnea may be present. Pain lasts minutes to hours and is described as squeezing, vicelike, crushing, stabbing, someone sitting on my chest, etc. Pain is associated with nausea, vomiting, dizziness, anxiety, sense of impending doom and is usually only relieved with narcotics. Vital signs: BP may be normal, elevated or lowered; pulse may be normal, rapid or slow.

> Caution: *The person with an acute MI may have none of the above symptoms and may merely "just not feel right." Thus, maintain a high index of suspicion in caring for patients with vague complaints.*

Management

- Oxygen via prongs; cardiac monitor; 12 lead ECG; treat arrhythmias; chest film.
- IV of 500 ml. 5% D/W with a microdripper TKO.
- Draw blood (when inserting the IV) for CBC, electrolytes, BUN, sugar, cardiac enzymes, coagulation screen, etc.
- Pain relief — morphine 5–15 mg. given *IV only.* This insures absorption in a vasoconstricted patient and decreases the possibility of falsely elevated enzyme levels due to muscle damage from IM injections.
- Provide frequent reassurance; tell about all procedures before beginning them.
- Admit to CCU with continuous nursing assessment and cardiac monitoring *en route* (bring along lidocaine, atropine, and a resuscitation bag/mask). Advise CCU staff of patient's condition before leaving ED and give full report to nursing staff once patient is settled in CCU. Include ECG and other remarkable tracings with record or send for official readings.

> Caution: *Never discard an ECG done in the ED on a patient with chest pain, even if the patient is discharged and the ECG is believed to be normal.*

Angina Pectoris. (See also p. 849.)

Recognition

Sudden or gradual onset of substernal or left anterior chest pain. Pain may not be sharply localized, and may radiate. Pain description may be the same as for an MI, or may be described as a "tightness." Character and pattern of pain are similar to previous episodes. Typically pain is precipitated by exertion, relieved by rest and usually lasts only a few minutes (usually no more than 30 minutes, often less than five minutes). Adrenergic or cholinergic symptoms may be present.

Management

- R/O MI, e.g., by history, by ECG.
- Reassurance.
- Nitroglycerin sublingually. (*Note:* A burning sensation of the sublingual mucosa and headache are normal effects of nitroglycerin.)
- Patient/family teaching: (a) what angina is, (b) how to take nitgroglycerin and when to get a new supply, (c) when and how to seek professional help.

Pericarditis. (See also p. 890.)

Recognition

- Sudden onset of continuous dull or sharp left anterior or substernal chest pain which may radiate to the back. Pain increases with talking, respiraton, movement, or lying flat and is relieved somewhat by sitting up and leaning forward.
- Vital signs: may have fever; lowered, normal or elevated blood pressure, tachycardia, and dyspnea.
- Chills, sweating, malaise and history of mild viral illness, e.g., URI. Pericardial friction rub may be present. Heart sounds may be muffled.

Management[126]

- Position of comfort, usually with head of bed elevated and patient leaning forward on an over-the-bed table.
- Oxygen by prongs; sedation.
- 12 lead ECG (classic findings: sinus tachycardia and 1–3 mm. ST segment elevation in all leads except AVR and AVL).
- Routine blood work including ESR (erythrocyte sedimentation rate) and CBC.
- Pain relief: Nitroglycerin is ineffective with pain of pericarditis but may be used for differential diagnosis; narcotics for pain relief.
- Pericardiocentesis if volume of fluid interferes with normal cardiac function, or to determine etiology of the effusion.

Dissecting Aneurysm of the Thoracic Aorta. This life-threatening problem is associated with severe chest pain. The person often appears similar to a person with MI. Recognition and management of dissecting aortic aneurysm is discussed later (p. 2201.)

*Cardiac Arrhythmias**

ATRIAL ARRHYTHMIAS

Sinus Tachycardia

Recognition

- Atrial and ventricular rate of 100–150; normal QRS complex with normal intervals, usually associated with another problem, e.g., fever.

Management

- Treat underlying cause; carotid sinus massage may differentiate sinus tachycardia from more significant arrhythmias.

Paroxysmal Atrial Tachycardia (PAT)

Recognition

- Usually begins and ends abruptly.
- Atrial and ventricular rate usually 150–250.
- P waves may be abnormally shaped. P waves may be superimposed on T waves.
- Heart rate usually regular; hypotension with prolonged PAT.

Management

- Depends on cause and effect on cardiac output.
- Sedation; digitalization.
- Stimulate mammalian diving reflex by placing face in cold water.
- Valsalva maneuvers; carotid sinus massage; cardioversion.
- Edrophonium chloride (Tensilon) 5 mg. given IV over 30–60 seconds with patient on a cardiac monitor, or
- Propranolol hydrochloride (Inderal) 1–3 mg. given IV at the rate of 1 mg./min. with patient on cardiac monitor; stop drug when patient converts to NSR.
- Metaraminol (Aramine) or levarterenol bitartrate (Levophed) may be used to suddenly raise the blood pressure, causing vagal stimulation in the aortic arch and carotid sinus, thus slowing heart rate.
- Phenylephrine hydrochloride (Neo-Synephrine) given IV.

Atrial Flutter

Recognition

- Atrial rate 250 to 350; characteristic "sawtooth" flutter waves.
- Some degree of AV block is present, so ventricular rate is variable (usually below 160) but is slower than atrial rate and is usually regular; e.g., in a 2:1 conduction there may be an atrial rate of 300 with a ventricular rate of 150.

Management

- Digitalization or cardioversion.

Atrial Fibrillation

Recognition

- P waves are irregular, usually not discernible and the isoelectric line appears wavy.
- Atrial rate ranges from 380–600 (usually cannot be counted).
- Ventricular rate usually irregular and PVC's may be present.
- May precipitate embolic conditions.

Management

- Digitalization with rapid acting digitalis preparation; quinidine may be used with digitalis preparation.
- Cardioversion after anticoagulation (inpatient).

VENTRICULAR ARRHYTHMIAS

Premature Ventricular Contractions (PVC's or VPC's)

Recognition

- May be benign but have the potential to precipitate ventricular tachycardia or ventricular fibrillation. May be due to hypoxia.
- Premature, wide (greater than 0.12 second), bizarre complex with the T wave often pointing in a direction opposite the QRS.
- P wave usually absent.
- Often followed by a compensatory pause.
- May arise from a single focus (unifocal) or from several foci (multifocal).
- May occur in a rhythmic pattern, e.g., bigeminy, trigeminy, etc.
- May precipitate ventricular tachycardia or ventricular fibrillation if the R of the PVC falls on the preceding T wave — called "R on T phenomena."

Management

- PVC's are treated under the following circumstances: (1) more than 6/minute; (2) runs or bursts of 3 or more, called a burst of V tachycardia; (3) R on T phenomena; (4) multifocal (*Note:* If the ventricular rate with PVC's is below 60, atropine may be given to increase the rate before PVC's are treated. Increasing rate abolishes PVC's in some cases.

*See also Chapter 35.

- ▶ Insure adequate oxygenation.
- ▶ Lidocaine 1% 50-100 mg. IV push and lidocaine drip of 2 Gr. added to 500 ml. 5% D/W; run at a rate of 1–4 mg./minute (15–60 microdrops/minute).
- ▶ Procainamide hydrochloride.
- ▶ Dilantin to treat digitalis-induced PVC's.

> Caution: *Lidocaine used to treat PVC's should be "cardiac" lidocaine rather than the lidocaine used for local anesthesia. The latter contains a variety of preservatives which may be undesirable when used in the large amounts required for treatment of PVC's.*

Ventricular Tachycardia. A life-threatening tachyarrhythmia which interferes with cardiac output and may progress to ventricular fibrillation.

Recognition

- ▶ Wide, bizarre, QRS complexes.
- ▶ Rate usually 120–250.
- ▶ Rhythm usually regular.
- ▶ Atria beat independently of ventricles and P wave often not discernible.
- ▶ Patients may be unconscious.

Management

- ▶ Precordial thump if episode monitored and witnessed; call for help.
- ▶ Lidocaine bolus and drip; bretylium (Bretylol) in selected cases.
- ▶ Defibrillate if lidocaine not effective and patient unconscious.
- ▶ Other measures for cardiac arrest (see later).

Ventricular Fibrillation. A form of cardiac arrest in which ventricles are not contracting effectively and there is little or no cardiac output.

Recognition

- ▶ Rate 150–300; fine or coarse waves in no organized pattern.
- ▶ Patient unconscious, with absent pulse and respiration.

Management

- ▶ Precordial thump if arrest is witnessed and monitored; defibrillate at 400 watt seconds; CPR.
- ▶ Endotracheal intubation when feasible.
- ▶ Start 2 IV's and hang 5% D/W.
- ▶ Sodium bicarbonate 1–2 amps (44.64 mEq/amp) STAT. Repeat as needed according to arterial blood gas values, usually every 10 minutes. (*Note:* The amount of sodium bicarbonate required in managing cardiac arrest is controversial; caution must be exercised to prevent over-alkalinizing and causing a metabolic alkalosis.)
- ▶ Epinephrine 5–10 ml. of a 1:10,000 solution given either IV or IC (intracardiac) if fine ventricular fibrillation is present and does not convert with defibrillation.
- ▶ Lidocaine 50–100 mg. IV or Dilantin 100 mg. IV slowly if patient is digitalis toxic.
- ▶ Bretylium (Bretylol) may be used if other therapies fail.
- ▶ Continue CPR.
- ▶ Start either a dopamine, Levophed or Aramine drip.
- ▶ Defibrillate as needed; make sure patient is well oxygenated.
- ▶ Lidocaine drip continued after ventricular fibrillation reversed.
- ▶ Arterial blood gases as needed.
- ▶ Foley catheter.
- ▶ Admit to CCU when stable; physician and nurse should accompany patient.

ASYSTOLE (CARDIAC STANDSTILL)

Recognition

- ▶ Patient unconscious, apneic.
- ▶ No electrical activity of the ECG.

Management

- ▶ Call for help.
- ▶ Precordial thump if arrest is monitored and witnessed.
- ▶ Defibrillate if rhythm is unknown.
- ▶ Start CPR; start IV's.
- ▶ Sodium bicarbonate 1–2 amps STAT and as needed.
- ▶ Epinephrine 5–10 ml. of 1:10,000 solution IV or IC.
- ▶ Calcium chloride 5–10 ml. of a 10% solution; calcium gluconate (10%) can be used in "approximately 2 to 3 times the dose of calcium chloride.[62]
- ▶ Endotracheal intubation when feasible.
- ▶ Arterial blood gases.
- ▶ Isuprel 0.2 mg. given IV push or IC and/or 1 mg./250 ml. 5% D/W to increase the heart rate.
- ▶ Start a Levophed, dopamine or Aramine drip.
- ▶ Atropine may also be used to increase rate.
- ▶ Transvenous or transthoracic pacemaker may be inserted.
- ▶ Continue CPR and other treatments as needed.
- ▶ Admit to CCU when stable.

HEART BLOCK (AV BLOCK)

Interference with normal conduction of atrial stimulus to ventricle. Heart block may be incomplete or complete and may be temporary or permanent. (See also Chapter 35.)

First Degree Block

Recognition

- ▶ Prolonged PR interval; heart rate usually within normal limits.

Management

- Observe; treat bradycardias or arrhythmias as needed.

Second Degree Block – Mobitz Type I (Wenckebach)

Recognition

- Progressive prolongation of the PR interval until there is finally a dropped beat (i.e., a P wave and no QRS); patient may experience irregular heart beats; variable rhythm.

Management

- Observe; temporarily discontinue cardiac depressant drugs.

Second Degree Block – Mobitz Type II

Recognition

- AV junction fails to respond to every stimulus from SA node.
- PR interval constant when P waves are followed by a QRS complex. QRS width may be normal or widened. Ventricular rate usually regular, often slow.
- "Patient may be aware of slow, forceful heart beats."[62]
- Usually associated with heart disease.
- May progress to complete AV block.

Management

- Discontinue digitalis if patient receiving this drug.
- Atropine to increase heart rate.
- Isuprel to increase heart rate.
- Pacemaker may be inserted.
- CPR if cardiac output inadequate to perfuse patient.
- Admit to CCU or unit with monitoring capability.

Third Degree or Complete Heart Block

Recognition

- All stimuli are blocked at AV junction.
- QRS complexes may appear wide.
- Slow ventricular rate.
- Regular P waves and regular QRS complexes but atrial rate is faster than ventricular rate.
- PR interval variable; a normal PR interval is coincidental.
- Syncope (Adams-Stokes syndrome) may occur.

Management

- Dependent upon symptomatology.
- Atropine 0.5–1 mg. IV.
- Isuprel drip 1 mg./500 ml. 5% D/W.
- Temporary pacemaker.
- CPR as needed while preparations made for pacemaker insertion.
- Steroids theoretically helpful in reducing inflammation around AV junction.
- PVC's should not be treated with cardiac depressant drugs until pacemaker has been inserted.

ABDOMINAL EMERGENCIES

Abdominal pain is common and the causes are numerous. Serious emergencies requiring immediate assessment and management must be identified. The term *acute abdomen* is used to describe a patient with a sudden onset of abdominal pain.

> *Although most patients with an acute abdomen requiring surgical intervention can wait for more complete evaluations, those with intra-abdominal catastrophes such as a ruptured aortic aneurysm or laceration of the aorta must be identified and managed within minutes.*

Because of the urgency associated with some problems causing abdominal pain, a nurse must be adept at performing an abdominal assessment and obtaining rapid, reliable information.

Specific information which should be elicited includes:

- What is the nature of the pain? (See Chapter 29.) Where is the pain located; pinpoint the pain with one finger. How long has the pain lasted? Has the patient ever experienced pain like this before? Is there a history of injury?
- Is there a history of nausea, vomiting or loss of appetite? Did nausea accompany the vomiting? What is the character of the emesis?
- When did the patient last have a bowel movement? What was the character of the stool? When did the patient last have something to eat? What was eaten?
- Has the patient taken any medications or other remedies in an attempt to relieve the pain? Is the patient currently taking any medications, including over-the-counter drugs?

Physical assessment of a patient with abdominal pain includes at least the following:

INSPECTION

- What position is the patient assuming? A patient lying quietly with flexed knees often has an inflammatory process (e.g., peritonitis) while the person constantly moving about trying to find a comfortable position may have colic-type pain (e.g., ureteral calculi).
- Is the patient distended? Distention can be de-

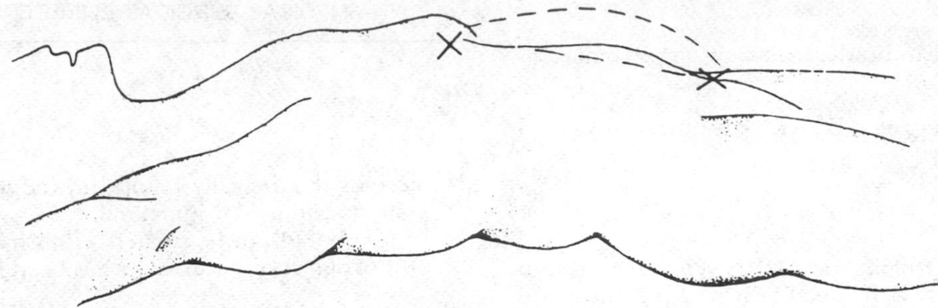

Figure 95–5. Assessing abdominal distention in a supine patient. Distention is present if the umbilicus is above an imaginary line drawn from the xiphoid process to the symphysis pubis. (From Sproul, C. W., and P. J. Mullanney: *Emergency Care: Assessment and Intervention.* St. Louis: C. V. Mosby Co., 1974, p. 335.)

tected using the technique illustrated in Figure 95–5. With the patient lying supine, draw an imaginary line from the xiphoid process to the symphysis pubis. If the umbilicus is above that line, the patient is distended.[126] If distention is present, measure abdominal girth at frequent intervals, especially in the trauma patient.

- ▶ Are there any masses, protrusion of the umbilicus, or discoloration around the flank or umbilicus?
- ▶ Is there evidence of trauma, penetrating or blunt?

AUSCULTATION

- ▶ Identify whether bowel sounds are normal, hypoactive, hyperactive, high pitched (tinkling) or absent.

PALPATION

- ▶ Have the patient pinpoint the area most painful. Avoid palpating that area until last. Does the pain increase with direct palpation? Is there rebound or referred pain?

Numerous problems may cause an acute abdomen: (1) inflammation, with or without perforation; (2) obstruction of a hollow viscus; (3) gastrointestinal hemorrhage; and (4) abdominal trauma, blunt or penetrating. Some common disorders characterized by abdominal pain in specific quadrants are summarized in Table 95–4.

Inflammatory Problems

Perforated Peptic Ulcer. (See also Chapter 62.)

Recognition

- ▶ Sudden onset of sharp, severe, upper, possibly left quadrant abdominal pain.
- ▶ Possible history of ulcer disease or frequent antacid use or long term and/or frequent use of aspirin or aspirin-containing substances.
- ▶ Abdominal rigidity; absent bowel sounds; hypotension.

Management

- ▶ IV (Ringer's lactate or saline)
- ▶ Draw blood: for CBC, electrolytes, BUN, sugar, type and cross match (T&C).
- ▶ Flat and upright abdomen films; possible lateral decubitus film.
- ▶ NG tube (preferably 18 F. Salem sump tube) aspirate gastric contents, test for blood, connect to suction.
- ▶ Frequently assess vital signs.
- ▶ Prepare for surgery.

Cholecystitis. Gall bladder inflammation, often associated with gallstones (cholelithiasis). (See also Chapter 69.)

Recognition

- ▶ More common in women.
- ▶ History of discomfort (fullness) or pain after eating, especially after eating greasy or fatty foods.
- ▶ Pain often in right upper quadrant, may be referred to the shoulder and increased by respiration.
- ▶ Patient may appear pale, diaphoretic and in severe pain; may present like MI.
- ▶ Mass may be palpated.
- ▶ Stones may be seen on X-ray film or ultrasound.

Management

- ▶ IV with at least an 18 gauge catheter; hang RL or saline solution.
- ▶ Lab studies: CBC, electrolytes, BUN, sugar, amylase, bilirubin, SGOT, UA.
- ▶ X-ray: flat and upright views of abdomen; possible chest film.
- ▶ NG tube (Salem sump).
- ▶ Pain relief *only after surgeon evaluates patient;* narcotics, e.g., Demerol, usually indicated.
- ▶ Patient/family teaching if discharged: dietary counseling, observation of worsening symptoms, e.g., increased pain, fever, etc.

Acute Cholangitis. Inflammation of the bile ducts outside the gall bladder. (See also Chapter 69.)

Recognition

- ▶ High fever; icterus (jaundice); severe RUQ abdominal pain.

TABLE 95–4. DIFFERENTIAL DIAGNOSIS OF ACUTE ABDOMINAL PAIN BY LOCATION

Right upper quadrant
- Acute cholecystitis
- Perforated duodenal ulcer (forme fruste)
- Acute pancreatitis (bilateral pain)
- Acute hepatitis
- Acute congestive hepatomegaly
- Pneumonia with pleural reaction
- Acute pyelonephritis
- Angina pectoris

Left upper quadrant
- Ruptured spleen
- Perforated gastric or marginal ulcer
- Acute pancreatitis (bilateral pain)
- Ruptured aortic aneurysm
- Perforated colon (tumor, foreign body)
- Pneumonia with pleural reaction
- Acute pyelonephritis
- Acute myocardial infarction

Central (periumbilical)
- Intestinal obstruction
- Appendicitis
- Acute pancreatitis
- Mesenteric thrombosis
- Strangulated groin hernia
- Dissecting or rupturing aortic aneurysm
- Diverticulitis (small intestine or colon)
- Uremia

Right lower quadrant
- Appendicitis
- Acute salpingitis, tubo-ovarian abscess
- Ruptured ectopic pregnancy
- Twisted ovarian cyst
- Mesenteric adenitis
- Incarcerated, strangulated groin hernia
- Meckel's diverticulitis
- Cecal diverticulitis
- Regional ileitis
- Perforated cecum (tumor, foreign body)
- Psoas abscess
- Ureteral calculus

Left lower quadrant
- Sigmoid diverticulitis
- Acute salpingitis, tubo-ovarian abscess
- Ruptured ectopic pregnancy
- Twisted ovarian cyst
- Incarcerated, strangulated groin hernia
- Perforated descending colon (tumor, foreign body)
- Regional ileitis
- Psoas abscess
- Ureteral calculus

From Condon, R. E., and L. M. Nyhus: *Manual of Surgical Therapeutics,* 3rd ed. Boston: Little, Brown and Company, 1975.

- ▶ Hypotension or shock.
- ▶ History of gall bladder disease, pale (acholic) or pasty stools, and dark urine.
- ▶ Diagnosis confirmed by lab data: elevated bilirubin and alkaline phosphatase; SGOT and LDH may be normal or elevated.

Management

- ▶ Restore circulating volume — large bore IV with RL or saline.
- ▶ NG tube (Salem sump).
- ▶ Pain relief *after* surgical evaluation (e.g., Demerol).
- ▶ Lab studies: above plus CBC, obtain urine for UA.
- ▶ Antibiotics.
- ▶ Cardiac monitoring if hypotensive.
- ▶ Prepare for possible surgery.

Pancreatitis. Inflammation of the pancreas. (See also Chapter 70.)

Recognition

- ▶ Severe, continuous, boring pain located in epigastrium (and often both upper quadrants); pain often radiates to back; pain often occurs after a meal, dietary indiscretion, or alcohol use. Patient acutely ill — may be in shock due to plasma volume depletion. Fever, nausea, vomiting, severe retching, abdominal spasm or rigidity, decreased or absent bowel sounds and possible rebound tenderness may be present.
- ▶ X-rays: abdominal film may demonstrate paralytic ileus, calcific densities in pancreas, or dilation of the loop of jejunum near the pancreas. Chest film may show pleural effusion.

Management

- ▶ Cardiovascular support; vigorous fluid resuscitation; large bore IV with Ringer's lactate.
- ▶ Lab studies: CBC, serum amylase (elevated amylase is expected), bilirubin, SGOT, electrolytes, BUN, sugar, calcium (hypocalcemia is commonly seen) and phosphorus; obtain urine for amylase and UA; type and cross match for whole blood.
- ▶ NG tube (Salem sump) connected to suction.
- ▶ Pain relief — Demerol is preferred narcotic; morphine may increase pain.
- ▶ Further management varies, e.g., surgical, medical.

Appendicitis. Most common cause of acute abdomen and results from obstruction and subsequent inflammation of the appendix. (See also Chapter 63.)

Recognition

- ▶ Nausea, vomiting, low-grade fever.
- ▶ Abdominal discomfort which may be peri-umbilical or located in RLQ at McBurney's point; pain gradually sharpens and signs of peritoneal irritation occur.
- ▶ Elevated white count; urine may have elevated specific gravity and acetone.

Management

- ▶ CBC, UA.
- ▶ IV (Ringer's lactate, normal saline or solutions containing dextrose).

- Salem sump tube connected to suction.[94, 95]
- Prepare for surgery.
- *Patient/family teaching* if discharged: temperature taking, observation of worsening symptoms, when to return to ED.

Regional Enteritis or Ileitis. Acute or chronic inflammation of the small bowel. (See also Chapter 63.)

Recognition

- RLQ abdominal pain; symptoms similar to appendicitis; may have symptoms of chronic disease, e.g., diarrhea, bloody stools, abdominal cramps, weight loss, etc.

Management

- Same as for appendicitis unless diagnosis can be made. GI series when symptoms subside.

Acute Diverticulitis. Inflammation of diverticulum (abnormal outpouching of bowel). (See also Chapter 63.)

Recognition

- Left lower abdominal pain or cramping; elevated WBC. History of chronic bowel problems including constipation.

Management

- IV fluid to restore circulating volume.
- Salem sump tube.
- Lab studies: CBC, abdominal X-ray (usually not diagnostic).
- Prepare for surgery (perforation or abscess).

Obstruction of a Hollow Viscus[89, 128]

Small Bowel Obstruction. (See also Chapter 63.)

Recognition

- Vomiting; fever, hypotension; abdominal distention; hyperactive, high pitched bowel sounds.
- Crampy abdominal pain; severe pain may indicate vascular impairment.
- Possible history of previous abdominal surgery may be present.

Management

- IV with large bore catheter – vigorous fluid resuscitation may be needed.
- CVP line if volume status unstable.
- NG tube or long intestinal tube (Miller–Abbott).
- Draw blood for: CBC, electrolytes, BUN, sugar, T&C.
- X-rays of abdomen.
- Monitor urine output.
- Prepare for possible surgery.

Large Bowel Obstruction. (See also Chapter 63.)

Recognition

- History may be compatible with diverticulitis or malignancy.
- Volume depletion; distention; high-pitched bowel sounds.
- Fecal emesis — late sign.
- Enlarged colon on X-ray.

Management

- Fluid replacement; lab studies as for small bowel obstruction.
- X-rays: flat and upright abdomen.
- NG or intestinal tube.[94]
- Surgical decompression.

Incarcerated or Strangulated Hernia. An incarcerated hernia cannot be manually reduced; a strangulated hernia is irreducible and has a compromised blood supply.

Recognition

- Localized pain, fever, elevated WBC, decreased or absent bowel sounds.

Management

- IV fluids; NPO; Salem sump tube, prepare patient for surgery.

Gastrointestinal Bleeding[58, 91, 109]

The causes of GI bleeding are many. Only a few are discussed here. Immediate management goals are to: (1) provide cardiovascular stabilization; (2) identify bleeding source; and (3) attempt to stop bleeding. Additionally, psychological support to the patient and significant others is of great importance because massive bleeding is incredibly frightening and because many procedures, which may be uncomfortable, are carried out rapidly in the initial phase of care.

Gastritis. Inflammation of gastric mucosa.

Recognition

- Burning epigastric pain. Emesis or gastric aspirant may be coffee ground colored or grossly bloody. History not suggestive of ulcer disease.

Management

- R/O more significant problem, e.g., peptic ulcer.

- ▶ Antacids; refrain from causative agent; take medications with meals or milk; dietary counseling.

Peptic Ulcer. May be gastric or duodenal; symptoms vary according to location.

Recognition

- ▶ Hematemesis; guaiac positive stool. History of ulcer symptoms or prolonged use of aspirin or aspirin-containing compounds; frequent use of antacids.
- ▶ Possible postural hypotension or profound shock.

> Caution: *Patients with peptic ulcers often have no pain when bleeding occurs. There is an axiom that "penetrating ulcers don't bleed and bleeding ulcers don't penetrate." Penetrating ulcers are usually painful.*

Management

- ▶ Start 1 or 2 large bore (14–16g) IV's; hang Ringer's lactate.
- ▶ Draw blood: CBC, T&C, electrolytes, BUN, sugar, coagulation screen.
- ▶ Treat for shock; administer whole blood as needed.
- ▶ Large bore (30–36 Fr.) Ewald tube to evacuate clots and lavage stomach with iced saline until fluid returns clear.
- ▶ Endoscopy possibly; occasionally gastric angiography used to pinpoint bleeding source; catheter(s) may be left in place to administer vasopressin (Pitressin) to stop bleeding.
- ▶ Further management may be medical or surgical.
- ▶ Admit patient to ICU if unstable.

Esophageal Varices. Varicosities in the distal esophagus and upper stomach. Blood loss in esophageal varices is sudden, massive, and often fatal. (See also Chapters 61 and 67.)

Recognition

- ▶ History of alcohol abuse or hepatitis; symptoms of portal hypertension and/or cirrhosis. Blood often wells up in throat; hematemesis; melena or bright red rectal bleeding. Shock.

Management

- ▶ Treat shock: start two large bore IV's, hang RL; blood and/or other plasma expanders.
- ▶ Draw blood: CBC, T&C, electrolytes, BUN, sugar, liver function studies, coagulation screen.
- ▶ Sengstaken-Blakemore (Blakemore) tube inserted by MD (Figure 95–6).
- ▶ Gastric lavage with iced saline.
- ▶ Vitamin K (Aquamephyton) may be administered.
- ▶ Admit to ICU.

Other Abdominal Emergencies. In summary, there are many abdominal emergencies which are manifested by abdominal pain or gastrointestinal bleeding. In addition to the conditions discussed previously, a person with either *penetrating or blunt trauma* to the abdomen may also present with these symptoms, therefore, a careful history must be obtained. Likewise, persons with a *non-traumatic intra-abdominal vascular emergency* may have pain of varying intensity.

Awareness of psychological needs of patients and their significant others is an important part of nursing care. Basins of blood or bloody lavage fluid should be disposed of promptly or at least kept out of the patient's vision. Although often difficult, nurses should attempt to provide a comfortable and aesthetic environment. The

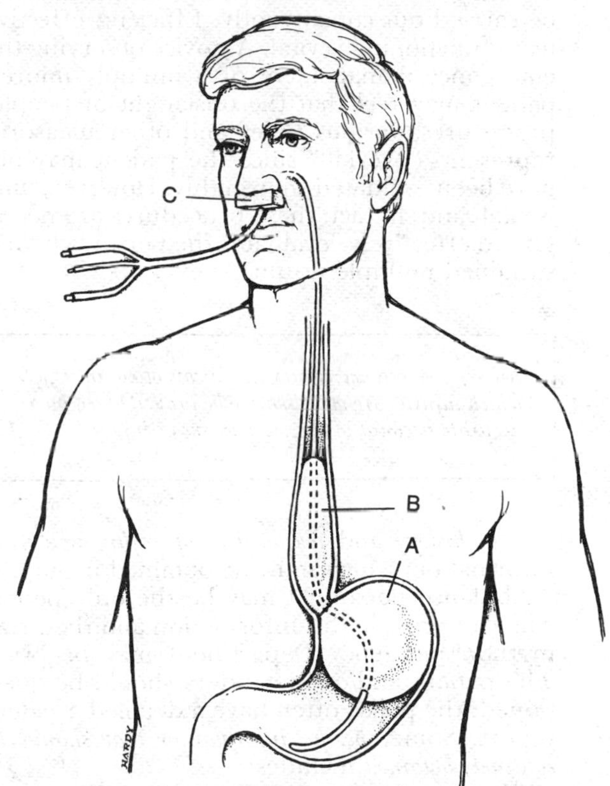

Figure 95–6. Sengstaken-Blakemore tube in place. The gastric balloon (*A*) and the esophageal balloon (*B*) are inflated. Traction is maintained by a foam sponge placed about the tube at the external nares and held by tape (*C*). The foam sponge also prevents ulceration of the nasal skin and cartilage. The three open tube ends are then connected: The one marked gastric balloon is closed with a screw clamp. The esophageal balloon is connected to a mercury or aneroid sphygmomanometer, and pressure is maintained at 40 mm. Hg. The third tube is connected to an intermittent nasogastric suction machine. (Note: It is helpful to have the patient wear a football helmet and to secure the tube to the mouth guard, thus sustaining traction.) (From Cosgriff, J. H., Jr., and D. L. Anderson: *The Practice of Emergency Nursing.* Philadelphia: J. B. Lippincott Co., 1975, p. 327.)

room may need to be warmer than usual since patients often become chilled during iced saline lavage and transfusions of cool blood. (Warm blood is preferable.) Mouth care is important for patients with hematemesis. As with all seriously ill or injured patients, record carefully and complete flow sheets.

CARE OF THE PERSON WITH MULTIPLE TRAUMA*

Patients with multiple trauma are highly challenging. Instant recall by the nurse of all possible injuries which may be associated with a specific mechanism of injury is essential. Various diagnostic and therapeutic measures must be carried out concurrently. Efficient, effective team functioning is vital. A novice observing the emergency management of a multiply injured patient may feel that the onslaught of people, procedures, various tubes and other measures represents "overkill" since the patient may not have been evaluated thoroughly. However, time is vital, and, in fact, these procedures are necessary to effectively "evaluate" the person who has sustained multiple trauma.

> *An experienced emergency nurse can often anticipate which injuries are most likely to be present based on an accurate account of the mechanism of injury.*

The *history* and *mechanism of injury* are vital information, which must be obtained promptly. Ambulance personnel may be the only people who can provide this information and their stay in the Emergency Department may be brief. The patient and/or bystanders should be questioned; the police often have a detailed accident report. Some *specific information that should be routinely obtained* includes:

- *Mechanism of injury* — what happened?
- *Auto accident*: occupant or driver; what was the car's speed; where did the car travel after impact; what was the car's position when it stopped, e.g., overturned or upright; how long ago did the accident occur and was extrication (removal from the car) prolonged? Were seat belts in use?[71] If the patient was a pedestrian, was he/she thrown and if so, how far? Did the victim hit anything while being thrown?
- *Gunshot wounds*: kind of gun/bullet; distance from gun; protective clothing or other covering worn by victim; what was the bullet's direction; where is bullet, i.e., did it exit the patient?
- *Stab wounds*: distance of victim from assailant; assailant's sex (females may stab typically downward and males stab upward); assailant's height; kind of knife (or weapon); length of weapon; where is the weapon; what clothing was the patient wearing?
- *Falls/jumps from high places*: how far did victim fall; how did victim land and on what surface; was anything hit while falling; why did the fall occur, e.g., chest pain, electrical injury, loss of consciousness, etc.?

*See references 16, 19, 37, 47, 56, 60, 68, 71, 84, 103, 104, 112, 140, 142.

Recognition and Management

- Insure adequate airway and good air exchange.
- Stop hemorrhage with direct pressure, pressure dressing, or tourniquet. (*Note*: Tourniquet used only as last resort.)
- Assess and immobilize C-spine as needed.
- Completely undress the patient. Do rapid initial assessment (see p. 2150); remember to assess back and buttocks.

> *"If it is forgotten that a patient has a back as well as a front, important wounds may be missed."*[140]

- Oxygen by prongs or mask.
- Take vital signs and start a flow sheet (Fig. 95–8).
- Start 1–2 large bore IV's; hang Ringer's lactate; run fluid rapidly if hypotensive.

> Caution: *If patient has massive chest injuries and possible disruption of the superior vena cava,* one *IV may be placed in a lower extremity. In most other circumstances, IV's should* not *be inserted in the legs or feet because of potential thrombophlebitis and subsequent pulmonary embolism.*

- Insert CVP line; measure CVP every 5–15 minutes.
- Draw appropriate blood studies: CBC, electrolytes, BUN, sugar, amylase, T & C, coagulation screen, possible drug and/or alcohol levels, creatinine if renal trauma suspected.
- Blood replacement; autotransfusion if situation is extreme and banked blood is not readily available.[60, 68]
- Anti-shock trousers if appropriate.
- Cardiac monitor[112, 142]; arterial blood gases.
- Foley catheter; UA, monitor output every 15–30 minutes. Salem sump tube (18F); test aspirant for blood; connect to suction. Keep patient npo. 12 lead electrocardiogram.
- Tetanus booster if wounds present.
- Measure girth of abdomen and extremities if injuries present. Mark extremity pulses if injuries present.

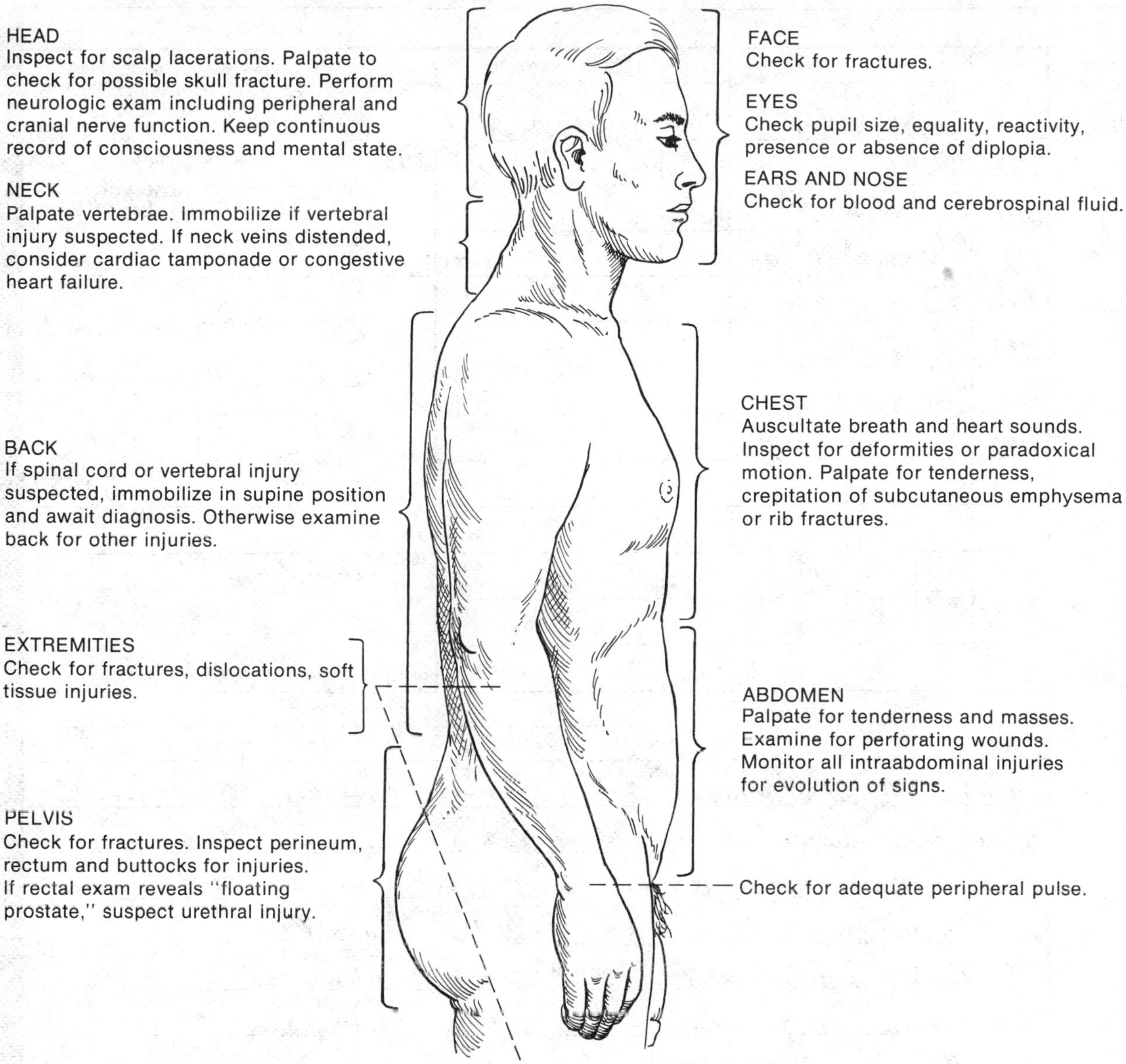

HEAD
Inspect for scalp lacerations. Palpate to check for possible skull fracture. Perform neurologic exam including peripheral and cranial nerve function. Keep continuous record of consciousness and mental state.

NECK
Palpate vertebrae. Immobilize if vertebral injury suspected. If neck veins distended, consider cardiac tamponade or congestive heart failure.

FACE
Check for fractures.

EYES
Check pupil size, equality, reactivity, presence or absence of diplopia.

EARS AND NOSE
Check for blood and cerebrospinal fluid.

BACK
If spinal cord or vertebral injury suspected, immobilize in supine position and await diagnosis. Otherwise examine back for other injuries.

CHEST
Auscultate breath and heart sounds. Inspect for deformities or paradoxical motion. Palpate for tenderness, crepitation of subcutaneous emphysema or rib fractures.

EXTREMITIES
Check for fractures, dislocations, soft tissue injuries.

ABDOMEN
Palpate for tenderness and masses. Examine for perforating wounds. Monitor all intraabdominal injuries for evolution of signs.

PELVIS
Check for fractures. Inspect perineum, rectum and buttocks for injuries. If rectal exam reveals "floating prostate," suspect urethral injury.

Check for adequate peripheral pulse.

Figure 95–7. Checklist for rapid evaluation of the injured person after immediate treatment priorities have been covered. Following initial examination the state of consciousness and vital signs are frequently monitored while x-ray and laboratory findings are being obtained.

- ▶ X-rays: chest, abdominal films and other films. Coordinate X-ray studies so patient makes only one trip to X-ray department.
- ▶ Other diagnostic procedures according to injuries, e.g., chest tube insertion, stabilization of flail chest, endotracheal intubation, peritoneal lavage, etc.
- ▶ Constant nursing assessment and repeated vital signs at a minimum of every 15 minutes until stable; record on flow sheet.
- ▶ Give emotional support to the patient and significant others; allow significant others to visit patient as soon as feasible; keep them informed, especially when prognosis is grave.
- ▶ Splint fractures; apply ice and elevate area(s). Clean and dress wounds; wounds are repaired only after patient stable or in OR.
- ▶ Priorities of *multisystem injury requiring surgical intervention* are (1) chest, (2) abdomen, (3) head and neck, (4) genito-urinary, (5) fractures and (6) soft tissue.
- ▶ Avoid moving patient suddenly; rapid position changes may precipitate cardiovascular collapse. Remain with patient until in the OR or admitted to a nursing unit; give full report to nurses assuming care.
- ▶ Pain medication is commonly *not* used in a patient with multiple trauma and an unstable cardiovascular system. If narcotics are given, they are administered IV in small doses; coordination with the anesthesia department is important if immediate surgery is anticipated.
- ▶ Insure that patient's clothes and valuables are safeguarded, using the proper chain of custody (discussed later), especially if criminal or suspicious acts were associated with the trauma.[40, 42, 61]
- ▶ Provide patient opportunity for spiritual support,

1/12/78

TIME	BP	P	R	CVP	OUTPUT TYPE VOLUME	TIME	MEDICATIONS
2110	70/palp	140	28			2140	Keflex 2 Gm IV [illegible] given
2115	80/50	130	28				
2118	90/56	128	24				
2130	90/60	120	24	6	urine 500 cc		
2135	90/60	120	24	8			
2137	100/60	116	24	8			
2140	100/60	116	24	8			
2145	100/60	116	24	8	urine 20 cc		

LAB WORK

TIME		BLOOD GAS
2115	CBC Hct 30 Wbc 14.8	#1 - 2130 pH 7.38, pO_2 96 pCO_2 26 Bicarb 25 O_2 Sat 99%
	ESR	
	M-12	
	LYTES	
	BUN	TYPE & CROSS:
	GLUE	10 MIN ✓ NO. UNITS 6
	AMYLASE	2 HR ___ No. UNITS ___
	ENZYMES	
	TOX. SCREEN	UA 4+ blood; Sg
	ETOH PRO. TIME	A neg, pH 6 GRAVINDEX

ALLERGIES Penicillin

DIP-TET. 0.5 CC given 2140 [illegible]

OBSERVATIONS
T 36.8 (R) 28 B, male c̄ .38 GSW abd,
no exit wound, awake but con-
fused, ? ETOH on breath; feet ↑
2111 - O_2 via prongs @ 10 l/min
2130 (L) subclav inserted; foley
cath #16 inserted → 4+ blood
2142 - #18 Salem sump → guaiac neg.
Family here; priest here - sacraments
given. 2145 → urine clearing
2147 TO OR in critical condition
Clothes to police / M. A. Taylor, RN/CEN

IV RECORD

TIME	NO.	SITE	VOL-TYPE	TIME	VOLUME RECEIVED
2112	1	#14 g. (L) arm	1000 RL	2130	1000 cc
2114	2	#14 g (R) arm	1000 RL	2135	1000 cc
2130	3	(L) arm	1000 RL	2145	1000 cc
2130	4	subclav. (L) CVP	1000 RL		
2135	5	(R) arm	#81-0003 W. blood O neg		
2145	6	(L) arm	#81-0072 W. blood O neg		

8-8-06-42-93

SMITH, JAMES N.

UNIVERSITY OF WASHINGTON HOSPITALS
HARBORVIEW MEDICAL CENTER
UNIVERSITY HOSPITAL
SEATTLE, WASHINGTON

EMERGENCY ROOM FLOW SHEET

1-74-325

UH FORM M—10, REV. 2/74

EMERGENCY ROOM FLOW SHEET

Figure 95–8. Emergency care flow sheet completed for patients with critical medical or surgical problems.

especially if immediate surgery or death is anticipated.

NEUROLOGIC AND NEUROSURGICAL EMERGENCIES*

Head Trauma

A cautious emergency nurse gives all patients with head trauma thorough neurologic assessment even though a patient seems "fine" when first seen. To understand the importance of careful nursing assessment of a patient with head trauma, recall central nervous system (CNS) structures and develop a working knowledge of common injuries associated with craniocerebral trauma. (Refer back to Unit X as necessary.) Head injuries may involve the skull, meninges, blood vessels, or the brain substance itself. Changes indicative of increased intracranial pressure may be subtle and easily missed unless frequent reassessment is done. Even slight head trauma, without obvious external signs, may result in significant brain contusion.

Neurologic assessment of the person with *head trauma* includes:

- ▶ Level of consciousness.
- ▶ Orientation.
- ▶ Response to commands or painful stimuli.
- ▶ Motor and sensory function in all extremities.
- ▶ Pupil size and reaction.
- ▶ Reflexes.
- ▶ Complete vital signs.
- ▶ Doll's head eyes maneuver (may be carried out).

As you recall, although the brain is surrounded by bone, it floats in cerebrospinal fluid (CSF) and can thus move or turn if there is significant force against the skull. This movement of the brain, plus the damage to tissues directly beneath the blow, are responsible for the symptoms associated with head injury.

With a moderate or severe blow the brain may move about considerably, twisting the stationary (fixed) brain stem structures. Damage to the brain stem is manifest by loss of consciousness. Loss of consciousness of short duration is said to be due to a *concussion*. More severe brain stem damage, causing hemorrhage and tissue destruction, results in more prolonged unconsciousness and is called a *contusion*. Injury may also cause a contusion of the brain itself (i.e., a cerebral contusion); however, unconsciousness usually does not occur from this alone. Such damage may cause a *subdural hematoma* or an *epidural hematoma*.

Because of motion of the brain, a person with a blow to the head may have both a direct injury at the site of initial impact and also an injury on the brain's opposite side. The direct injury is called a *coup injury* and the other *contrecoup*. Remember this, because patients may have varying and confusing neurologic findings in the presence of two such, possibly different, injuries.

Deterioration in neurologic status, especially with localization of symptoms, may indicate development of an *intracranial hemorrhage*.

The most common hemorrhages associated with head trauma are discussed next. (See p. 662 for illustration and detailed discussion.) Table 95–5 summarizes the classification and treatment of various head injuries.

Epidural Hematoma. A rapidly developing accumulation of blood between the skull and the dura mater. The bleeding is commonly associated with skull fracture. Since the bleeding is arterial, the hematoma expands quickly and exerts significant pressure on surrounding brain tissue. *Rapid management is vital.*

Recognition

- ▶ Typical history of brief unconsciouness *immediately* after injury, then often awake and alert soon thereafter.
- ▶ Headache; rapidly deteriorating neurologic signs (confusion, coma, death); signs of increased intracranial pressure; loss of motor function in extremities on side *opposite* injury; pupil on *same side* as injury may react sluggishly initially and later become fixed and dilated.

Management

- ▶ Maintain airway.
- ▶ Skull films, echoencephalogram, cerebral arteriogram, CAT scan.
- ▶ Burr holes (see p. 664).
- ▶ Steroids, e.g., dexamethasone (Decadron) 10 mg. IV push.
- ▶ IV (large bore); hang isotonic solution and attach microdripper to IV. *Run IV very slowly.*
- ▶ Mannitol or furosemide (Lasix).
- ▶ Foley catheter.
- ▶ NG tube.
- ▶ Intubation and hyperventilation (CO_2 is cerebral vasodilator).

Subdural Hematoma. Slower developing acute or chronic collection of blood between the dura mater and the arachnoid mater. Often caused by a venous injury.

Recognition

- ▶ Same as epidural hematoma, but slower onset. Possibly only slight behavioral changes with chronic disorder.

*See references 10, 24, 78, 102, 108, 110, 133, 139, 149.

Management

- Same as for an epidural hematoma; however, burr holes are typically a less emergent procedure.

Subarachnoid Hemorrhage. Bleeding into the subarachnoid space. Rarely results from trauma; usually due to rupture of congenital aneurysm.

Recognition

- Sudden onset of occipital or retro-ocular headache.
- Nausea and vomiting; nuchal rigidity; photophobia.
- Back pain later — due to blood in spinal subarachnoid space; blood in CSF.
- Altered levels of consciousness.

Management

- Maintain adequate airway.
- Prevent rebleeding if possible by providing calm, quiet environment and absolute bed rest with all care provided by staff. Restrict visitors. Darkened room may be comfortable; no smoking in room.
- Elevate head of bed 15 to 20 degrees.
- Cardiac monitor.
- Oral temperatures — nothing administered rectally.
- Avoid very hot or very cold food or fluids.
- Foley catheter if patient unconscious.
- Hypothermia and antihypertensive therapy.
- Diagnostic studies, e.g., arteriogram, CAT scan, etc. (after patient is stable).
- Surgical repair of aneurysm (usually done on nonemergency basis).
- Cautious use of pain medications and/or sedatives.

Tentorial Herniation. Forcing of brain tissue through the tentorial notch, because of pressure exerted by an expanding mass lesion or swelling of one or both cerebral hemispheres.

TABLE 95–5. CLASSIFICATION OF VARIOUS TYPES OF ACUTE HEAD INJURIES AND TREATMENT

Anatomic Location	Type of Injury	Usual CNS Signs or Symptoms	Treatment
Skull	Linear fracture	Those of underlying brain injury	Observation if uncomplicated
	Depressed fracture	Same as linear fracture	Surgical decompression with brain débridement or hemorrhage evacuation as indicated
	Frontal basilar fracture	Cerebrospinal fluid rhinorrhea, periorbital ecchymoses, pneumocephalus	Elevation of head, antibiotics, surgical closure if rhinorrhea persists for more than 1 week or if recurrent episodes of meningitis occur
	Petrobasilar fracture	May be associated with CN VII and CN VIII dysfunction, otorhinorrhea, Battle's sign	Observation, possibly antibiotics
Meninges and their spaces	Epidural hemorrhage	"Lucid interval," progressive deterioration, ipsilateral dilated pupil, skull fractures crossing meningeal artery groove	Urgent decompression
	Dural laceration	Those of underlying brain injury, venous oozing (if compound injury) from lacerated dural sinus	Elevation of head and packing of wound, surgical débridement and closure
	Subdural hemorrhage	Those of underlying brain injury, progressive deterioration, may be acute or chronic	Evacuation of hemorrhage
	Subarachnoid hemorrhage	May be mild or severe depending on brain injury and presence or absence of associated arterial spasm	Observation if uncomplicated by collection of blood or other surgical CNS lesion
Brain	Concussion	Mild headache, nausea, vomiting, dizziness; no focal signs or unconsciousness	Observation
	Contusion	History of unconsciousness, transient focal signs, prolonged elevated intracranial pressure, possibly signs of severe focal damage with cerebral edema	Observation if mild or transient; steroids, hyperventilation, intracranial pressure monitoring, internal decompression if severe
	Laceration	As with contusion	Exploration and débridement if suspected; often an incidental finding during decompression
	Intracerebral hemorrhage	Usually associated with deepened consciousness and focal signs of damage	Evacuation of clot; if in frontal, occipital, or temporal lobe, subtotal lobectomy

From Zsoche, D. (Ed.): *Mosby's Comprehensive Review of Critical Care.* St. Louis: C. V. Mosby Company, 1976.

Results in compression of blood vessels and other tissues, including the brain stem, and further complicates increasing intracranial pressure.

> *Tentorial herniation is a life-threatening problem, which must be handled promptly and aggressively.*

Recognition

- ▶ Decreased level of consciousness; headache, nuchal rigidity; dilation of one or both pupils.
- ▶ Signs of brain stem involvement: Cheyne-Stokes respirations, elevated blood pressure, bradycardia and/or arrhythmia.
- ▶ Changes occur rapidly; symptoms vary depending upon kind of herniation.

Management

- ▶ Maintain effective airway; may intubate and hyperventilate.
- ▶ Start IV.
- ▶ Steroids, e.g., dexamethasone (Decadron) 10 mg. IV; mannitol.
- ▶ Surgery — burr holes; other supportive measures.

Skull Fractures. The major concern is not with the skull fracture itself, but rather with associated damage, e.g., infection, tissue damage, hematoma formation. Skull fractures can be classified as: (a) *Simple linear skull fractures* which do not require treatment. Asymptomatic patients may be sent home with head trauma precautions and instructions. (b) *Depressed skull fractures,* which are usually managed surgically to elevate or remove bone fragments. (c) *Basilar skull fractures,* which occur at the skull's base and may be associated with C-spine injury or cord injury.

Although difficult to *diagnose* radiographically at times, classic signs of basilar skull fracture are: ecchymosis of the mastoid process (Battle's sign), periorbital ecchymosis without direct trauma (raccoon eyes), blood behind the tympanic membrane, and CSF rhinorrhea or otorrhea. (*Note*: Determine if such drainage is CSF by testing it for sugar with a Clinistix. A blue color usually indicates that CSF is present.)

Management

- ▶ Elevate head of bed 30 degrees unless C-spine injury is suspected.
- ▶ Caution patient not to blow, pack or pick nose.
- ▶ Be cautious when inserting an NG tube. If the fracture communicates with nose or posterior pharynx, it is possible to insert tube through fracture site and into brain tissue.[27, 149]
- ▶ Careful, frequent observation.

Key Points in the Management of Patients with Head Trauma. (See Fig. 95–9 and p. 656.)

- ▶ Hypoxia and CO_2 accumulation complicates cerebral edema.
- ▶ Maintain adequate airway; hyperventilate if necessary. Draw arterial blood gases if unconscious.
- ▶ Suspect C-spine injury in head injured patients especially if unconscious.
- ▶ Shock usually not due to head injury, but rather due to blood loss elsewhere, e.g., chest, abdomen.
- ▶ Never place head injured patients in head low position. Keep head of bed elevated 30 degrees to minimize cerebral edema. Position patient to allow for drainage of secretions.
- ▶ Frequent neurologic assessment; record carefully.
- ▶ *Eye care*; (1) locate and remove contact lenses,[63] (2) prevent corneal abrasion by using artificial tears and tape lids closed if necessary, (3) if dilating drops are used, record this information on a piece of adhesive tape and place on patient's forehead.
- ▶ Safety — siderails up, locked.
- ▶ Be prepared for seizures; note posturing.
- ▶ Talk to unconscious patient as though patient were awake.
- ▶ Keep significant others informed; provide necessary support; provide for religious needs as desired.
- ▶ Organs which may later be used for transplants (in event of death) must be perfused.
- ▶ *Patient/family teaching* if patient discharged home: (1) Wake patient every 2 hours (for the next 8 hours) and check level of consciousness and orientation; (2) Give only liquids initially for the first 8 hours, then progress to regular diet; (3) Aspirin or acetaminophen for headache. If stronger medication required, contact physician (*Note:* emphasize this because patients may have narcotics from previous illnesses. They must understand that narcotics are contraindicated in head injury); (4) Notify physician or return to ED if any of the following occur: one or both pupils becomes dilated and nonreactive; level of consciousness decreases; inability to use an arm or leg; seizure(s) or continued vomiting. *These instructions should be written, since anxious people often have difficulty remembering what they are told verbally.* Have the patient/significant other sign the chart, indicating that they have received a copy of the instructions, that the instructions have been explained to them and that they understand the instructions. Include an appropriate phone number on the take-home instruction sheet.

Other Neurologic Emergencies

Status Epilepticus. Continuing seizure lasting more than 5 minutes or repeated seizures with no recovery interval (see p. 645).

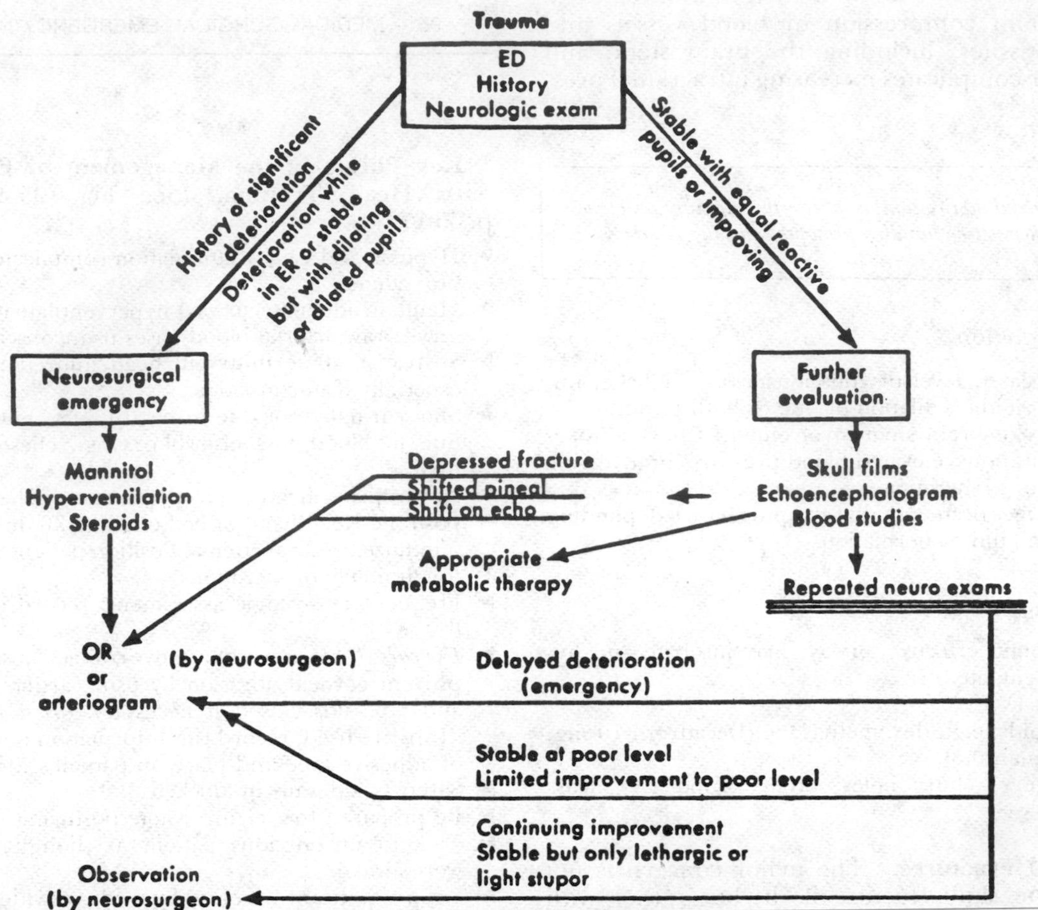

Figure 95–9. Acute management of a head injury in the emergency department. (From Sproul, C., and P. Mullanney, (Eds.): *Emergency Care: Assessment and Intervention.* St. Louis: C. V. Mosby Co., 1974, p. 237.)

Management

- ▶ Protect patient but *do not attempt to restrain.*
- ▶ Maintain airway; suction as needed.
- ▶ Start IV promptly.
- ▶ Give IV medications slowly.
- ▶ Medications commonly used: Valium 5–10 mg. IV *slowly* (*Note:* Have resuscitation bag close by) or phenobarbital 60–240 mg. IV slowly or Sodium Amytal 150–250 mg. IV. Dilantin 100–150 mg. may be given IV or IM, usually after one of the above medications has been given. 50 per cent dextrose if hypoglycemia is suspected as the cause.
- ▶ Administer high flow oxygen by mask.
- ▶ Identify and treat cause.
- ▶ General anesthesia sometimes required.

Meningitis. Inflammation of the meninges caused by a variety of organisms; often bacterial in etiology. (See p. 594.)

Recognition

- ▶ Fever, headache, photophobia; nausea; vomiting; stiff neck (nuchal rigidity), Kernig's and Brudzinski's signs.
- ▶ Petechial rash (check ankles) in meningococcal meningitis.
- ▶ Changes in level of consciousness; possible shock.

Management

- ▶ Maintain airway.
- ▶ Start IV (fluid depends on vital signs).
- ▶ Treat shock.
- ▶ Draw appropriate lab studies: CBC, cultures, electrolytes, BUN, sugar, etc.
- ▶ Lumbar puncture (send specimen for C & S, cell count, protein, sugar).
- ▶ Antibiotics.
- ▶ Isolation if meningococcal or etiology unknown.
- ▶ Other nursing care appropriate for a comatose patient.
- ▶ Arrange for intensive nursing care.

Myasthenic Crisis. Characterized by muscle weakness, often affecting specific muscle groups. Respiratory insufficiency associated with myasthenia gravis is termed a *myasthenic crisis* (see p. 633).

Recognition

- ▶ Muscle weakness becoming progressively worse as the day goes on; somewhat improved after rest.

- Blank look on face. Head tilted back in order to see (because of eyelid ptosis).
- Regurgitation of fluids from nose; inability to swallow.
- Nasal tone to voice.
- Respiratory arrest.

Management

- Respiratory support; ventilate if needed.
- Edrophonium chloride (Tensilon) 2–10 mg. IV; then neostigmine (Prostigmin) 1–2 mg. IM.
- Symptoms rapidly reverse with Tensilon. However, reversal lasts only a few minutes.
- Reevaluation of medications if patient is taking anticholinesterases.
- *Note: Cholinergic crisis* may develop from excessive anticholinesterase medication. Symptoms of this are often difficult to distinguish from myasthenic crisis. This is why Tensilon is usually used first to make the diagnosis. The treatment for cholinergic crisis is atropine sulfate 1 mg. IV as needed to control symptoms.

Neck and Spinal Injuries.[81] The roles of nurses in emergency care are: (a) to prevent further injury by careful handling of the patient and (b) to provide life support measures. Nurses are also actively involved in consumer teaching programs designed to prevent injuries to the spine and spinal cord.

The *mechanisms of injury* commonly associated with spinal injuries involving the cervical area include hyperflexion, hyperextension, flexion compression and acceleration whiplash (see Figure 95–10). In addition to obvious cord injury from complete or partial transection, edema, hemorrhage and impairment of vertebral artery circulation may result in permanent spinal cord damage.

Recognition

- *Suspect C-spine* (cervical spine) *injury in all unconscious trauma patients*; bruised forehead or chin suggests hyperextension injury.

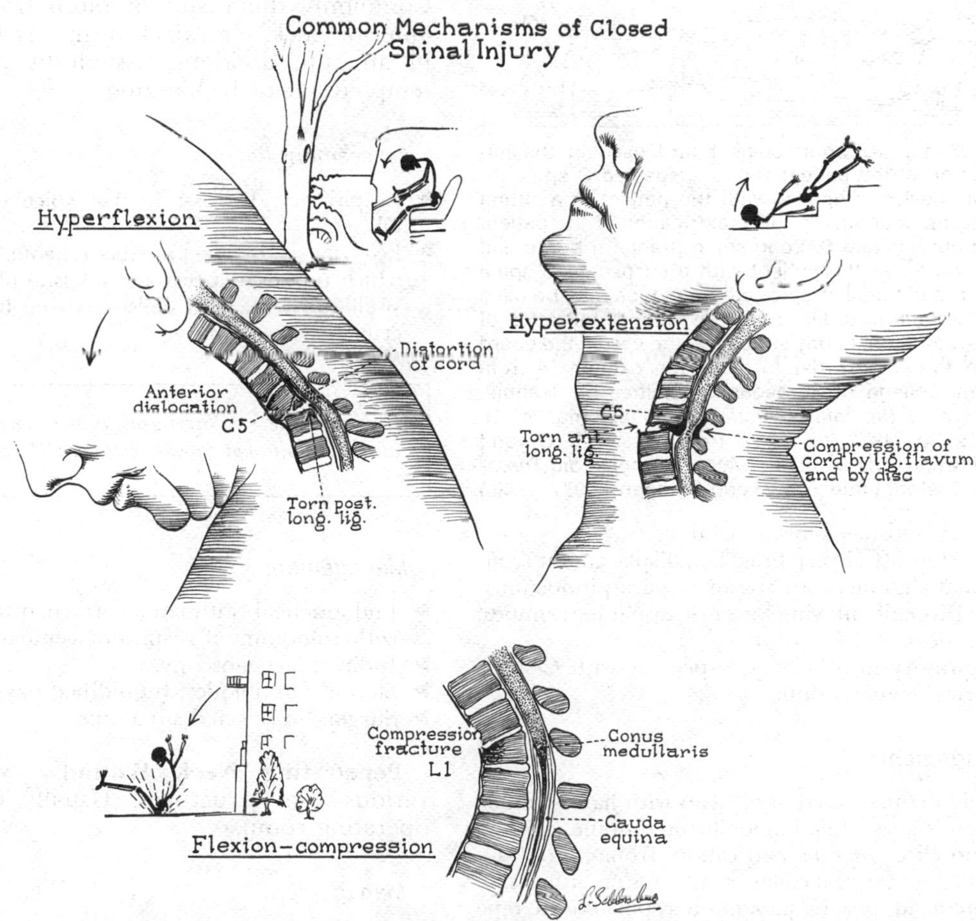

Figure 95–10. Schematic illustrations of closed spinal injury mechanisms. The cervical hyperflexion and hyperextension diagrams represent a composite of possible factors, any number of which may occur in a particular case. (From Ballinger, W. F., II, R. B. Rutherford, and G. D. Zuidema, (Eds.): *The Management of Trauma.* Philadelphia: W. B. Saunders Co. 1973, p. 194.)

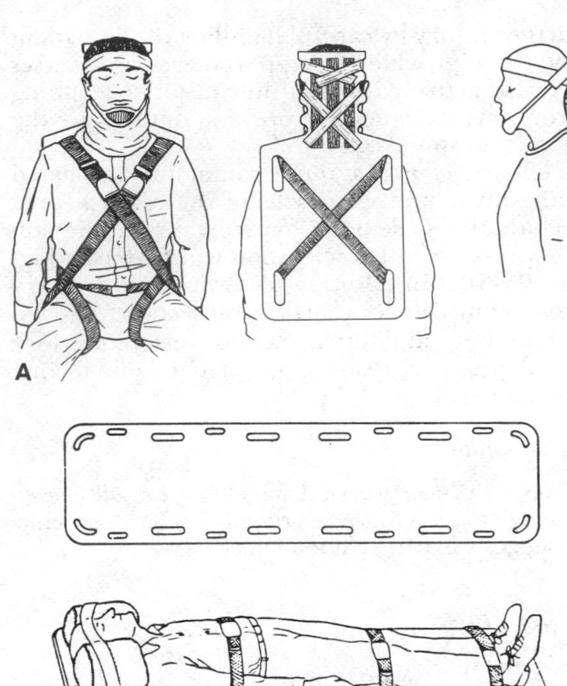

Figure 95–11. **A.** Short spine board used in the immobilization of the patient with a suspected C-spine injury. This device is applied with the patient in a sitting position and is applied prior to extrication of the patient from an automobile. **B.** Long spine (fracture) board and immobilization of the patient with a suspected C-spine injury. An additional strap or adhesive tape may be used across the chin in order to provide more stabilization of the neck. Additional body straps may be used if the board must be turned in order to move the patient. (*A* from American College of Surgeons Committee on Trauma. *Early Care of the Injured Patient.* Philadelphia: W. B. Saunders Co., 1972, p. 192. *B* from Iversen, L. D., and D. K. Clawson: *The Manual of Acute Orthopaedic Therapeutics.* Boston: Little, Brown and Company, 1977, p. 46.)

- History and mechanism of injury.
- Pain, step-off of vertebrae, i.e., displacement from normal alignment, or spasm of paraspinous muscles. Difficulty moving lower or upper extremities, numbness.
- Respiratory insufficiency, especially with C-spine injuries. Hypotension.

Management

- Apply manual traction to head with hands under patient's jaws while immobilizing C-spine
- Immobilize *prior to* extrication from auto (Fig. 95–11) by: cervical collar; sand bags on either side of the head; placing patient on a spine board, tape sand bags and head to fracture (spine) board; use a chin halter device if appropriate. *Caution the patient not to turn or move his/her head.*
- Ultimately patient will be placed in skeletal traction using devices such as Crutchfield, Gardner-Wells or Vinke tongs at 10–25 pounds of traction.
- Maintain airway — jaw thrust technique may be needed, i.e., apply forward traction at angle of mandibles to push jaw forward. Blind endotracheal intubation or esophageal obturator airway placement may be necessary.
- Start IV with Ringer's lactate or normal saline; a solution with 5 per cent dextrose may be desired.
- Treat hypotension.
- Oxygen by prongs or mask.
- *Slow, careful, cautious movement.*
- Cross-table lateral film of the neck *before any other films are done*; (carried out without moving patient's neck). It may be necessary to apply traction on the arms in order to visualize entire C-spine.
- Foley catheter.
- Patient may initially be placed on a Stryker frame or circOlectric bed.
- Continuous psychologic support for patient and significant others.
- Assess and treat for other injuries.
- Admit to a spinal cord center.

Laryngeal Fracture or Laceration.[16, 140] Commonly the result of blunt trauma to the anterior neck, e.g., neck hitting steering wheel in an auto accident, assault by choking, attempted suicide by hanging.

Assessment

- Respiratory distress; hoarse voice or unable to talk.
- Ecchymosis of neck; subcutaneous emphysema which rapidly dissects along tissue planes causing swelling of ace and chest — tissue has a crackly, crunchy sensation.

> Caution: *Severe laryngeal injury may be associated with minimal initial symptoms.*[140]

Management

- Endotracheal intubation, tracheostomy, or cricothyroidotomy if respiratory embarrassment.
- Indirect laryngoscopy.
- Steroids; antibiotics; humidified oxygen.
- Surgery in selected situations.

Penetrating Neck Wounds. May involve various vital structures. Usually explored in operating room.

Management

- Insure airway; treat shock; stop bleeding with direct pressure (do not clamp bleeding vessels), and prepare for prompt surgery.

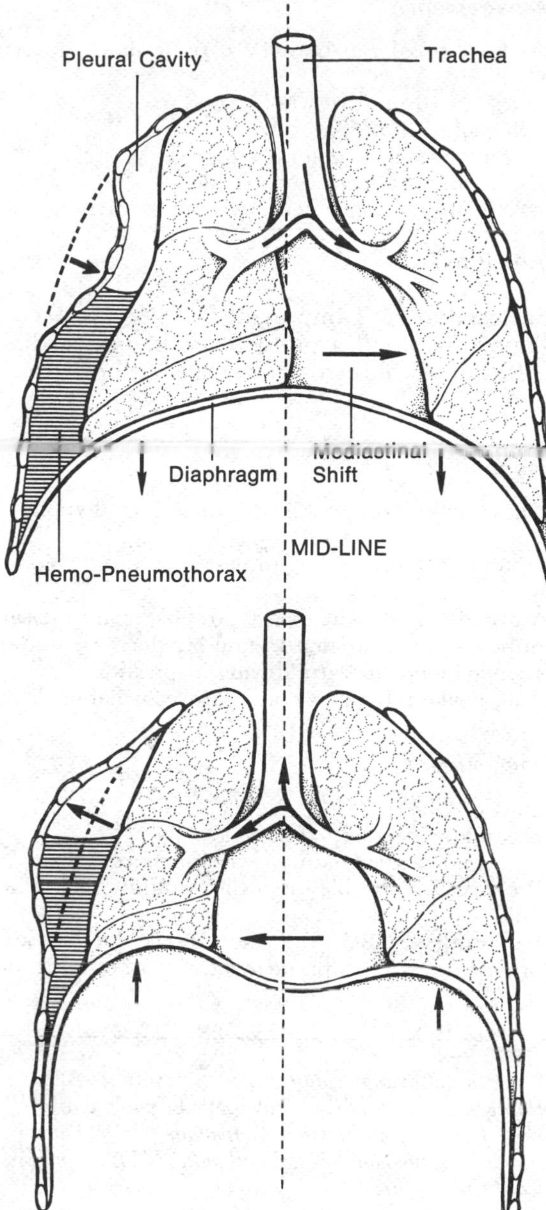

Figure 95–12. Respiration in a flail chest. Diagram on top shows flail area of right chest wall, which moves in with inspiration. Air moves into the left (normal) lung from the right bronchial tree as well as via normal tracheal inflow. Ventilation of the right lung is compromised. The mediastinum shifts to the uninjured side, further compromising exchange on the normal side. On expiration (bottom), air is driven out through the trachea and into the right (injured) side. This movement of air from one lung to the other is known as "pendulum movement." which leads to further deoxygenation. Hemopneumothorax further compromises oxygen exchange. (From Cosgriff, J. H., Jr., and D. L. Anderson: *The Practice of Emergency Nursing.* Philadelphia: J. B. Lippincott Co., 1975, p. 281.)

CHEST INJURIES — PENETRATING AND BLUNT

Flail Chest. Results from fracture of several ribs in more than one place or fractures of the ribs at the junction of sternum (flail sternum). Rigidity of the chest wall is lost. Changes in intrapleural pressure result, causing respiratory insufficiency due to inadequate oxygenation of lung tissue involved in the flail segment. (See p. 1345.)

Recognition

- Paradoxical respirations: the flail segment sinks in with inspiration and bulges during exhalation (Fig. 95–12).
- Respiratory distress; deformity of the chest wall, and chest pain.

Management

- Oxygen.
- Immobilize flail segment by: turning patient on affected side; applying sandbags to chest wall, bridging flail segment; traction to flail segment by placing towel clips on several of ribs involved in the flail (Fig. 95–13).
- Endotracheal intubation and mechanical ventilation (preferred treatment).

Hemothorax. Accumulation of blood in the pleural space. Result of blunt or penetrating trauma to major vessels or heart. (See p. 1341.)

Recognition

- Respiratory distress; decreased breath sounds; history of trauma; hypotension or shock; fluid level on chest film.

Management

- Oxygen.
- IV (Ringer's lactate or normal saline).

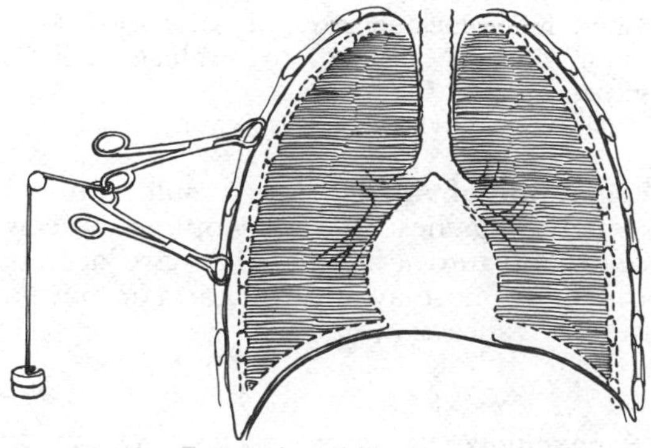

Figure 95–13. External stabilization of a flail chest, using towel clips and traction. This method may be used if mechanical ventilatory support is not available. (From Ballinger, W. F., II, R. B. Rutherford and G. D. Zuidema (Eds.): *The Management of Trauma.* Philadelphia: W. B. Saunders Co., 1973, p. 348.)

- Chest tube inserted – large (30 to 36° F.) low (6th intercostal space), and lateral (anterior, mid or posterior axillary line); connect to suction.
- Autotransfusion (with own blood) may be lifesaving if massive hemothorax.
- Lab studies: CBC, T & C, arterial blood gases (optional).
- Observe volume and consistency of chest drainage, report promptly if volume increases or changes color.
- Chest film.
- Prepare for surgery if indicated (not responding to chest suction or losing large amounts of blood).
- Insure proper suction; milk chest tubes as needed. Tape all connections to chest tube and drainage system.
- CVP line may be inserted.

Pneumothorax. Accumulation of air in pleural space, often from penetrating (sucking) chest wounds. Pressure of the air causes collapse of the lung on the same side as the injury initially but can become a tension pneumothorax if untreated. (See Chapter 56, also p. 2158.)

Recognition

- Respiratory distress; chest pain; hyperresonance or tympany to percussion; whistling sound in sucking chest wound; x-ray evidence of partial or complete lung collapse.

Management

- Cover sucking wounds with air tight dressing (Vaseline gauze or cellophane wrap, gauze, sponges, wide adhesive tape) and label "sucking chest wound" on the dressing.
- Chest film.
- Chest tube to underwater seal and suction.
- Chest film repeated after tube in place. Repeat chest film as needed to evaluate lung re-expansion.
- Tetanus prophylaxis if open wound.

Laceration of Aorta. May result from blunt or penetrating chest trauma. Commonly seen in deceleration auto accidents. May have laceration of only innermost layer of the aorta or may have complete transection.

Recognition[22, 113]

- History of trauma; hypotension, shock or cardiac arrest; chest pain; respiratory distress; widening of mediastinum on chest film.

Management

- At least two large bore IV's; treat shock, insert CVP line.
- T & C 5–10 units of whole blood.
- CBC; chest film.
- Urgent surgery if deteriorating.
- Dye studies of aorta when stable.
- Avoid sudden movement, twisting or turning patient.
- Admit to ICU.

Pericardial Tamponade.[39, 55, 84, 112] Accumulation of blood around heart in pericardial sac. Result of blunt or penetrating chest trauma.

Recognition

- Chest pain; progressively worsening hypotension.
- Distended neck veins (unless profound blood loss).
- Muffled or distant heart sounds; paradoxical pulse — greater than a 15 mm Hg decrease in the systolic blood pressure during inspiration.[16]
- Tall, peaked T waves noted in precordial leads

Management

- Start one or two IV's; insert CVP line.
- Oxygen as needed; chest x-ray.
- ECG and cardiac monitor; pericardiocentesis.
- Prepare for possible open thoracotomy in ED or OR.
- Lab studies: CBC, T & C, arterial blood gases, other studies appropriate to location of other trauma.

> Caution: *Cardiac contusion with resulting ECG changes and arrhythmias may occur in patients with chest trauma even without tamponade.*[101, 112] *Thus, initiate cardiac monitoring in all patients with significant chest trauma.*

Traumatic Asphyxia.[78a] Results from sudden, massive compression of chest with blood forced into face, neck and upper chest. Commonly accompanied by massive chest injuries.

Recognition

- History of crushing injury; shock.
- Severe respiratory distress; cyanotic head, neck and upper chest.
- Protrusion and ecchymosis of the eyes; swollen, cyanotic tongue and lips.

Management

- Establish and maintain airway (intubation and ventilation often necessary); high flow oxygen.
- IV fluids (because of possible disruption of major

vessels, it may be necessary to place one IV in a lower extremity).

- ▶ Stabilize chest wall (bilateral flail chest common).
- ▶ Arterial blood gases, CBC, other routine studies.
- ▶ Foley catheter; frequent check of urine output.

> Caution: *In any patient with a crush injury, there may be massive muscle damage and accumulation of myoglobin in the kidney causing renal failure. Thus, monitoring of urine output is essential. There may also be massive release of potassium from damaged muscles, thus monitoring of urine output, cardiac status and serum potential is essential.*

ABDOMINAL INJURIES

May be blunt or penetrating trauma and associated with significant organ injury. With low velocity blunt trauma (e.g., a fist) there is usually single organ injury. High velocity blunt abdominal trauma often produces multiple organ involvement. Likewise, small caliber bullets generally produce single organ injury while larger bullets create a shock wave and a path of destruction involving many organs. In general, solid organs (e.g., liver and spleen) are more vulnerable to injury than hollow organs with blunt abdominal trauma.

Recognition

- ▶ History or evidence of injury. Abdominal pain; abdominal distention. Muscle guarding; decreased or absent bowel sounds; obliteration of psoas muscle shadow on X-ray; nausea and/or vomiting; hypotension or shock.

Management

- ▶ Start two large bore IV's — hang Ringer's lactate.
- ▶ Draw blood: CBC, T & C, amylase, SGOT.
- ▶ Foley catheter; urine for UA.
- ▶ 18 g Salem sump tube; test aspirate for blood and connect to suction.
- ▶ CVP line inserted if not responding to IV fluids.
- ▶ Peritoneal lavage or 4 quadrant tap to determine presence of blood in abdominal cavity.[19]
- ▶ Dye studies (sinogram or stabogram) of wound tract in penetrating abdominal wound.
- ▶ Culdocentesis may be done in female patients.[56]
- ▶ X-rays: flat, upright and lateral decubitus views of abdomen.
- ▶ Frequent measurement of vital signs and abdominal girth. (*Note*: Include postural vital signs if safe).
- ▶ IVP in patients with hematuria.
- ▶ Prepare for urgent surgery in selected patients.

Retroperitoneal Hematoma. Blood accumulated in retroperitoneal space, often caused by pelvic fracture.

Recognition

- ▶ Hypotension; falling hematocrit.
- ▶ Abdominal and/or back pain; ecchymosis of the flank.
- ▶ Hypoactive bowel sounds; increasing abdominal girth; obliteration of psoas muscle shadow on X-ray.

Management

- ▶ Fluid and blood replacement.
- ▶ Draw blood: CBC, T & C, other studies.
- ▶ Immobilize pelvis if fracture suspected.
- ▶ Foley catheter.
- ▶ Frequent vital signs and measurement of abdominal girth.
- ▶ Surgery may be required.

HEAT AND COLD INJURIES

Burns*. Burns are also discussed in Chapter 80.

Recognition

- ▶ Area may be reddened, white, charred black. Pain is usually present unless the burn is full thickness. "Hair test" — a hair can be easily pulled out with full thickness burns, but not in partial thickness burns.

Management

- ▶ Learn why burn occurred; consider possible multiple trauma, electrical injury, etc.
- ▶ Stop burning process; remove clothing and jewelry.
- ▶ Irrigate chemical burns copiously with water or appropriate agent. Specific antidotes or neutralizing agents may be used and are listed in Table 95–6.
- ▶ Maintain airway; administer humidified oxygen (especially if: (a) soot around nose or mouth; (b) facial burns, or (c) history of smoke inhalation).[46]
- ▶ Relieve pain. Apply moist packs or immerse the part in tepid (not cold) water or normal saline. (*Note:* This may be appropriate only for minor, not major, burns). Morphine or Demerol given in small doses IV for major, or IM for minor burns.
- ▶ Establish IV line (14 or 16 g) upper extremities are preferred sites; start two IV lines with greater than 40 per cent BSA (body surface area) burn. Ringer's lactate used initially.
- ▶ Estimate degree of burn and per cent BSA.

*See references 45, 46, 52, 75, 77, 78, 88, 96, 135, 138.

TABLE 95–6. COMMONLY USED NEUTRALIZING AGENTS FOR CHEMICAL BURNS

Type of Burn	Neutralizing Agent
Alkali burns Potassium hydroxide Sodium hydroxide Ammonium hydroxide	Acetic acid 0.5% to 5% (1 teaspoon vinegar per pint of water) or ammonium chloride 5%
Tear gas or mace	Sodium bicarbonate solution
Phosphorus	Copper sulfate soaks*
Acid burns Hydrochloric acid Sulfuric acid Nitric acid Trichloroacetic acid	Sodium bicarbonate solution (1 teaspoon baking soda per pint of water) or sodium bicarbonate paste
Hydrofluoric acid	Sodium bicarbonate solution or paste and local injections of calcium gluconate
Phenol	Ethyl alcohol followed by sodium bicarbonate solution or paste

*Actually, the copper sulfate soak does not neutralize the phosphorus but it is used to give color to the phosphorus, which must be manually removed, thoroughly and painstakingly.

From Jacoby, F. G.: *Nursing Care of the Patient With Burns.* St. Louis: C. V. Mosby Company, 1976.

- Foley catheter; UA to lab; monitor output every 15–30 minutes.
- Salem sump (16–18 F.).
- Lab studies: CBC, electrolytes, BUN, sugar, creatinine, arterial blood gases.
- Tetanus prophylaxis.
- Wound care. Clean area gently with a 1:1 solution of NSS or Tis-U-Sol and povidone-iodine (Betadine) solution, debride loose tissue, and irrigate well. Topical agent, e.g., silver sulfadiazine (Silvadene), may be applied after wound cleaning. (*Note*: Amount of wound cleaning and use of topical agents depends on where patient will be treated. If to be transferred promptly to burn unit or burn center, extensive wound care is unnecessary and a topical agent should not be applied). Wound care should be carried out under aseptic technique; personnel wear gowns, masks and hats.
- Cover patient with *sterile* sheets and blankets to minimize contamination and heat loss.
- Psychologically support patient and significant others.
- Transfer patient to *burn center* or *burn unit* if: 2nd or 3rd degree burn greater than 20 per cent BSA; patient under age 2 or over 60 years; burns over joints; burns involve face, neck, or perineum; electrical burns; or patient at risk due to preexisting disease. Patients requiring transfer should be accompanied by a nurse and/or a physician and possibly a respiratory therapist.
- Frequently assess pulses in burned extremities and chest wall excursion; escharotomy may be necessary.
- Have available extra supplies of narcotics, IV fluids, and oxygen as well as escharotomy and airway maintenance equipment during transfer.
- A transfer summary sheet and copies of patient records should accompany patient; receiving facility should accept the patient prior to transport, i.e., be certain to telephone ahead.

Heat Cramps. Muscle spasms of arms, legs, and occasionally of abdomen due to excessive sodium depletion during perspiration. Treated by removing patient from the hot environment and administering oral fluids containing salt, e.g., one teaspoon of salt per quart of water.

Heat Exhaustion

Recognition

- Headache, dizziness, faintness; loss of appetite and nausea; skin may be cool and clammy. Normal vital signs.

Management

- Remove patient from source of heat and place in cool environment.
- Administer oral or IV fluids.

Heat Stroke

Recognition

- Extremely elevated temperature; warm, dry skin; depressed level of consciousness; possible coma, hypotension or shock.

Management

- Cool patient rapidly (immerse in or sponge with cool water); hypothermia blanket.
- Start IV; provide other cardiovascular support.
- Cardiac monitor; frequent vital signs.
- Foley catheter unless recovery is prompt.

Hypothermia. Lowered core body temperature, usually below 34.4° C. (94° F.) May occur in divers, persons exposed to cold weather and near drowning victims.[15, 125]

Recognition

- Some patients appear deathlike yet have feeble pulse; pupils may be fixed and dilated.
- Symptomatology depends on patient's core temperature:
  34.4° C. (94° F) — amnesia or sluggishness.
  32.2° C (90° F) — cardiac arrhythmias, especially ventricular premature contractions.
  30° C. (86° F) — loss of muscle coordination, possible unconsciousness.
  25° C. (77° F.) — cardiac arrest.

Management

- Initiate CPR when indicated; endotracheal intubation.

- Insert esophageal thermometer or rectal thermometer probe.
- Start one peripheral line and a CVP; add other IV lines as needed.
- Draw blood for: CBC, electrolytes, BUN, sugar, creatinine, coagulation screen, amylase, arterial blood gas analysis.
- *Core rewarming* using heated oxygen, gastric, urinary bladder and peritoneal lavage with heated fluids.

> Caution: *Heat externally applied to a profoundly hypothermic patient causes vasodilation and further cardiovascular collapse. Peripheral warming is usually delayed until the patient's core temperature has been raised.*

- Hyperthermia blanket may be used *very cautiously after* core rewarming.
- Standard cardiac arrest treatment; 12 lead ECG — a "J" wave or Osborn wave may occur. (*Note:* An Osborn wave is a "positive deflection of the terminal 0.04 seconds of the QRS complex."[125])
- Insert Foley catheter; monitor urine output every 30 minutes.

> Caution: *There is often a great deal of water on the floor during immediate resuscitation of a person with profound hypothermia. Use a battery powered defibrillator, rather than one connected to a higher voltage wall outlet, in order to protect the staff from electrical hazard.*

Frostbite. Damage to tissues and blood vessels as a result of prolonged cold exposure. Fingers, toes, nose and ears commonly affected.

Recognition

- Numbness, paresthesia and pallor of part initially. Severe pain, swelling, erythema and blistering (similar to second degree burn) once in a warm environment. Necrosis and gangrene in severe cases.

Management

- Handle tissues gently.
- Rewarm part in tepid water bath (about 105° F.).
- Debridement of blisters is controversial.
- Bulky dressings permit drainage and provide protection; bed cradle may be needed.
- Arteriography to determine extent of injury or to try to open up vasoconstricted vessels.
- Vasodilators and/or nerve block.
- *Patient/family teaching:* dressing changes; body part will be hypersensitive to cold in future, so additional clothing will be needed.

MUSCULOSKELETAL TRAUMA

Promptly assess musculoskeletal trauma before swelling makes evaluation difficult. Be gentle and careful. A history of the mechanism of injury as well as the patient's description of sounds or sensations experienced is particularly important. Additionally, obtain history of previous injury or pre-existing disease. (See also Unit XX.)

A *fracture* is a break in bone continuity. It may be open or closed, transverse, oblique, spiral, comminuted, or impacted. A *dislocation* is a complete disruption of two articulating surfaces. A *subluxation* involves only partial disruption of two articulating surfaces. A *sprain* is a ligamentous injury (graded one through four according to the amount of damage to the tissue fibers). A *strain* involves damage to muscle body or a tendon attachment. Sprains are more severe injuries than strains and are often associated with joint instability. (See Chapter 77.)

Characteristics of a fracture are: (a) point tenderness, (b) swelling, (c) crepitus, (d) deformity, (e) false motion, and (f) restricted use of the extremity.

> *Although fractures are important in themselves, it must be remembered that a force capable of causing a fracture also causes soft tissue damage. Accompanying neurovascular damage may have more significance than the actual fracture.*

Detailed evaluation of the patient's neurovascular and motor function is vital. Whenever an injury is within a confined space (e.g., forearm, lower leg) edema fluid may accumulate in fascial compartments. The resulting neurovascular impairment may be permanent. *Compartmental syndrome* is characterized by pain that is excessive for the injury sustained, severe pain with passive movement of the injured part, tissue swelling and tenseness, erythema, and often diminished neurovascular function. *If compartmental syndrome is suspected, do not elevate the part. Elevation would further impede blood supply to the area.* Notify the physician promptly; surgical decompression may be necessary.

General guidelines for care with a fracture are:

- Always check and mark pulses.
- Splint extremities, including the joint above and below the suspected fracture site.
- Do not straighten out joints which are injured.
- Do not relocate dislocated joints unless vascular compromise is evident.

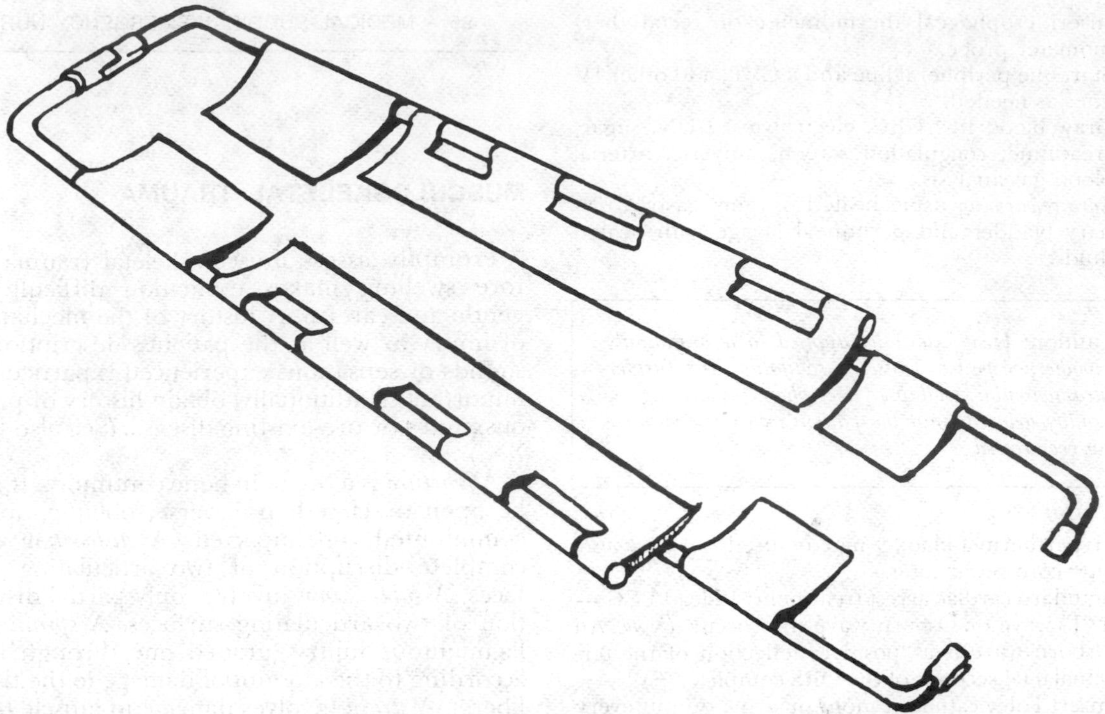

Figure 95–14. Scoop or clamshell stretcher used in immobilizing and transporting patients with musculoskeletal trauma. The device is divided into halves lengthwise, with locking devices at each end. One side of the stretcher is positioned under the patient and then the other side positioned. The halves are joined together at the ends of the stretcher and are locked in place. Securing straps are then applied. (From American Academy of Orthopaedic Surgeons: *Emergency Care and Transportation of the Sick and Injured,* 2nd ed. Menasha, Wis.: George Banta Company, Inc., 1977, p. 391.)

- Apply ice bags around the site, not just on top of it; incorporate ice bags into the splint if necessary. Remove rings or other constrictive jewelry.
- Frequently reassess neurovascular status and motor function.

Only fractures associated with significant blood loss (Table 95–7), respiratory or vascular embarrassment, or disability are discussed.

Dislocation of the clavicle at the sternoclavicular joint. Posterior dislocation of the clavicle may result from blunt trauma. Pressure exerted by the dislocation may cause respiratory or vascular impairment. In an emergency situation, dislocation can be reduced by applying traction using a towel clip placed around the clavicle's proximal portion.

TABLE 95–7. ESTIMATES OF LOCALIZED BLOOD LOSS ASSOCIATED WITH ADULT FRACTURES

	Liters
Humerus	1.0–2.0
Elbow	0.5–1.5
Forearm	0.5–1.0
Pelvis	1.5–4.5
Hip	1.5–2.5
Femur	1.0–2.0
Knee	1.0–1.5
Tibia	0.5–1.5
Ankle	0.5–1.5

From Iversen, L. D., and D. K. Clawson: *Manual of Acute Orthopaedic Therapeutics.* Boston: Little, Brown and Company, 1977.

Fracture of the Middle Third of the Clavicle. May cause laceration of major vessels, requiring prompt surgical repair. Observe for hematoma formation, check pulses distal to the injury, and avoid inserting an IV catheter in arm on side of injury.

Humerus. Damage to the radial nerve (resulting in wrist drop) and artery is a major concern, especially in fractures involving the middle portion of the humerus. This injury is common in the elderly, often resulting from falls on an outstretched hand. Frequently assess pulses and neurologic function. The injured area is initially immobilized by sling and swathe. (See Chapter 77.)

Hand Injuries. Because of the superficial nature of many structures in the hand, damage to tendons, nerves and bones is common. Detailed assessment is important. Since hand lacerations are a common type of surface trauma, the steps in evaluating hand injuries are discussed in the surface trauma section. (See p. 2183.)

Pelvis. As shown in Table 95–7, the potential blood loss associated with pelvic fractures may be profound. Goals of care are: (1) cardiovascular stabilization, (2) minimizing blood loss by immobilization, and (3) preventing organ injury. Pelvic fractures commonly occur with deceleration accidents.

Recognition

- ▶ Mobility and grating of pelvic bones with compression; pain upon pelvic movement; back pain.
- ▶ Hypotension or shock.
- ▶ Ecchymosis of flank; hematuria with GU trauma.

Management

- ▶ Immobilize patient on fracture board; have pelvic sling on stretcher if time permits.
- ▶ Start IV, draw blood (CBC and T&C), hang Ringer's lactate.
- ▶ Foley catheter (urethra or urinary bladder injuries are common). Listen to bowel sounds – fractures of iliac crest may be associated with adynamic ileus.
- ▶ Apply covered ice pack to fracture site.
- ▶ Pain relief.
- ▶ Anti-shock suit to decrease blood loss and immobilize pelvic fracture.

Femur. Midshaft fractures are commonly caused by high velocity blunt trauma, e.g., auto accidents. (See Chapter 77.)

Recognition

- ▶ Significant pain at fracture site; spasm of thigh muscles; spasm or damage to femoral artery; hypotension or shock may be present.

Management

- ▶ Apply traction around ankle until a traction splint is applied.
- ▶ Immobilize and provide traction with half ring Thomas splint or Hare traction splint (Fig 95-15) and an ankle hitch. Maintain traction until a pin can be surgically placed through the distal femur.
- ▶ Palpate dorsalis pedis pulse before and after applying traction splint; reassess frequently.
- ▶ Apply ice pack; elevate leg.
- ▶ Measure thigh girth to estimate blood loss; frequently remeasure.
- ▶ Start IV if hypotensive or distal pulse is absent.
- ▶ Lab studies: CBC, T&C, arterial blood gases. (*Note:* ABG values sometimes used to monitor for fat embolism.)
- ▶ Observe for respiratory insufficiency or changes in consciousness level (associated with fat emboli).

Knee. Knee dislocation often results from blunt trauma and is a *very serious injury.* Often there is associated blood vessel, nerve, or ligament disruption.

Recognition

- ▶ Distal portion of femur not aligned with tibia/fibula; distal pulses diminished or absent.
- ▶ Significant pain.
- ▶ Knee joint often flexed and patient unable to straighten it out.

Management

- ▶ Notify physician promptly. Do not try to straighten out knee; splint in flexion (if that is joint's position) with knee supported on pillows.
- ▶ Apply ice pack.
- ▶ Start IV so medications needed in relieving pain during relocation of knee can be administered; give pain medications.
- ▶ Frequently reassess distal pulses and sensation; a Doppler device (see Chapter 18) may help assess vascular integrity.
- ▶ Keep patient NPO until further treatment decided.

Calcaneus. Often calcaneus (heel) fractures are relatively minor injuries. However, they often result from falls from high places with the victim landing on the feet. The shock wave generated may cause compression fracture of thoracic or lumbar spine. Hence, careful assessment of these areas is indicated. A person with an isolated calcaneal fracture is usually discharged home with instructions to wear a hard soled shoe for several weeks.

SURFACE TRAUMA

Damage to skin and soft tissues is often encountered in emergency settings. Responsibility for providing total care is often a nursing activity. Types of surface trauma included here are: contusions, abrasions, avulsions, lacerations, puncture wounds, insect bites and stings, animal, human and snake bites, and wound infections. Goals of care are to: (1) promote optimal wound healing, (2) minimize scarring, and (3) assist the patient to return to normal function (see also Chapter 80.)

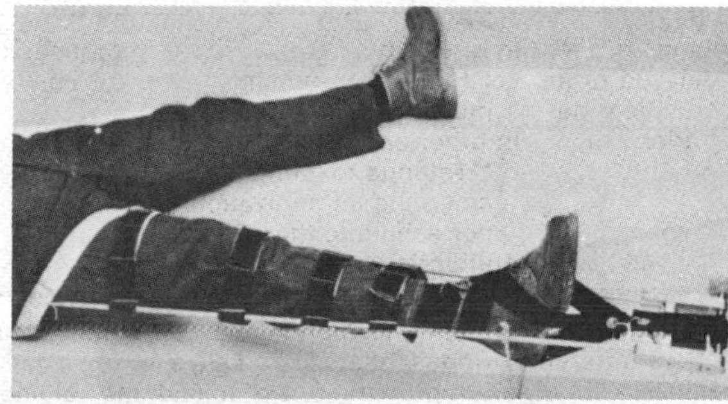

Figure 95–15. Thomas splint and ankle hitch traction device used in the immobilization of a suspected fracture of the femur. (Courtesy Rockford Safety Equipment Company, Rockford, Ill.)

Nursing management of persons with surface trauma:

- Attention to total patient - ABC's (airway, breathing, circulation).
- Provide psychologic support.
- Stop bleeding by direct pressure or pressure dressing.
- Identify mechanism of injury; length of time since injury occurred; allergies; immunization status. (See Table 95–8.)
- Assess range of motion and sensation in part distal to wound; assess patient's occupation and how injury may affect activities of daily living.
- Assess wound: location; size and depth; degree of contamination; other structures involved; amount of tissue loss and viability of wound edges and of amputated tissue.

*Key points in cleaning and dressing wounds:**

- Provide adequate anesthesia after assessing motor and sensory function.
- Avoid putting soaps, disinfectants, or other strong chemicals in wounds:[53] *"Chemical antiseptics and antimetabolites effective in killing bacteria also kill cells which either contribute to the local defense mechanism or participate in other ways in the healing process."*[111]
- Clean area *around* wound with a suitable agent, e.g., povidone-iodine (Betadine scrub solution), but keep the wound itself covered to prevent solution from entering wound.
- Irrigate wound with physiological solution (e.g., Tis-U-Sol or normal saline) using 30–50 ml. syringe and blunt tipped 14–18 gauge needle.[130, 146] Lift up wound edges with gloved finger and irrigate copiously. A good rule is to use a minimum of 50 ml. of irrigation solution per inch of wound per hour since the injury. For example, a 2″ laceration that is also 1″ deep requires a minimum of 150 ml. of irrigation, providing the wound is less than one hour old. Add another 50 ml. for each hour since the wound occurred.
- After wound repair, dress wound in layers: Owen's silk or fine mesh gauze, coarse mesh sponges, Kling or Kerlix, elastic net or bias stockinet and adhesive tape. (*Note:* Adhesive tape placed over draining wounds inhibits drainage and provides an environment optimal for bacterial growth. Place adhesive tape *around* wounds, not over them). The work done by Noe and Kalish [105c] is an excellent resource on wound care and dressings.
- Immobilize the joint; place the fingers in the position of function unless there is a burn involving the fingers (Fig. 95–16).
- Tetanus prophylaxis; give patient immunization record.
- Patient/family teaching: (1) Wound healing, in-

*See also Sorensen and Luckman, *Basic Nursing: A Psychophysiologic Approach,* Chapter 42.

TABLE 95–8. PROPHYLACTIC TREATMENT OF TETANUS*

Type of Wound	Patient Not Immunized or Partially Immunized	Patient Completely Immunized Time Since Last Booster Dose		
		1 to 5 years*	*5 to 10 years*	*10 years +*
Clean minor	Begin or complete immunization per schedule; tetanus toxoid, 0.5 cc.	None	Tetanus toxoid 0.5 cc.	Tetanus toxoid 0.5 cc.
Clean major or tetanus prone	In one arm: **Human tetanus immune globulin 250 mg. In other arm: **Tetanus toxoid 0.5 cc., complete immunization per schedule	Tetanus toxoid 0.5 cc.	Tetanus toxoid 0.5 cc.	In one arm: **Tetanus toxoid 0.5 cc. In other arm: **Human tetanus immune globulin 250 mg.
Tetanus prone, delayed or incomplete debridement	In one arm: **Human tetanus immune globulin 500 mg. In other arm: **Tetanus toxoid 0.5 cc., complete immunization per schedule thereafter. Antibiotic therapy	Tetanus toxoid 0.5 cc.	Tetanus toxoid 0.5 cc. Antibiotic Therapy	In one arm: **Tetanus toxoid 0.5 cc. In other arm: **Human tetanus immune globulin 500 mg. Antibiotic Therapy

*No prophylactic immunization is required if patient has had a booster within the previous year.
**Use different syringes, needles and sites.
NOTE: With different preparations of toxoid, the volume of a single booster dose should be modified as stated on the package lable.
From American College of Surgeons Committee on Trauma: *Early Care of the Injured Patient.* Philadelphia: W. B. Saunders Co., 1976.

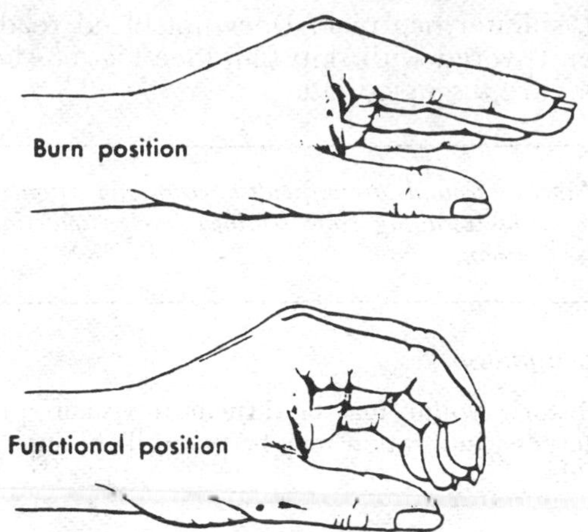

Figure 95–16. Positioning the hand in dressings. (From Sproul, C. W., and P. J. Mullanney (Eds.): *Emergency Care: Assessment and Intervention.* St. Louis: The C. V. Mosby Co., 1974, p. 164.)

struct that a wound often looks worse after suture removal than it did when first injured. Wounds mature, flatten out, and fade. The process may take 6 months. Decisions concerning plastic surgery for scar revision are usually withheld until at least that time. (2) Tissue swelling continues 8–12 hours after the injury. Thus, keep on a pressure dressing, elevate the injured area and apply cool packs to prevent cross hatching of tissues from sutures. (3) Keep dressings on, clean and dry. Return for dressing change if above not followed. Wound check (check for healing, infection and suture intactness) and dressing change may or may not be indicated. If required, tell where and when this is to be done. (4) Supplies and technique for dressing change if to be done at home. (5) Importance of suture removal, when and where this is to be done. (6) How to take medications (e.g., antibiotics, analgesics, etc.). (7) Return if signs of infection occur, e.g., swelling, pain, redness, drainage, fever. (8) How to carry out activities of daily living with dressing in place, e.g., use rubber gloves, place plastic bag over injured extremity while showering or bathing, etc. (9) Expected reaction to tetanus or diphtheria tetanus booster, e.g., redness, swelling, discomfort around the site is normal. Slight fever may occur. Aspirin or acetaminophen can be used for comfort. The patient should *wait in the ED at least 20 minutes after receiving the immunization;* allergic reactions should be obvious during that time.

Contusion. Blunt trauma to the skin without penetrating tissues, i.e., a bruise. (Fig. 95–17*A*.)

Recognition

- Ecchymosis; pain, swelling, may compromise distal circulation if severe).

Management

- Clean area; apply ice pack; assess neurovascular status; may need to measure extremity girth.
- Elevate unless compartment syndrome is developing; administer mild analgesia.
- *Contused nailbed (subungual hematoma):* Often very painful. May require evacuation by making a hole in the nail with the end of a heated paper clip or by using a special device (Fig. 95–18). Gentle pressure on the nail will then evacuate hematoma. Apply dressing to absorb drainage and prevent infection. Tetanus booster may be given.
- *Patient/family teaching:* ice, elevation, circulation checks.

Abrasion. Wound associated with loss of epidermis and occasionally part of dermis. (See Fig. 95–17*B*.) Result of friction or shearing force. Failure to properly clean may result in a permanent tatto that can not be removed by plastic repair.[2]

Recognition

- Denuded area with weeping of serous fluid; extremely painful; often grossly contaminated with imbedded dirt.

Management

- Provide anesthesia by applying lidocaine jelly directly into wound (or with a gauze pad) or by infiltrating area with 1% lidocaine.
- Scrub area with soft brush and normal saline. Use forceps to remove imbedded foreign material; excise wound if needed. Irrigate wound copiously with NS.
- Apply thin layer of Neosporin or Vaseline to prevent crusting; leave open if area small. If area large or friction would result, dress with fine mesh

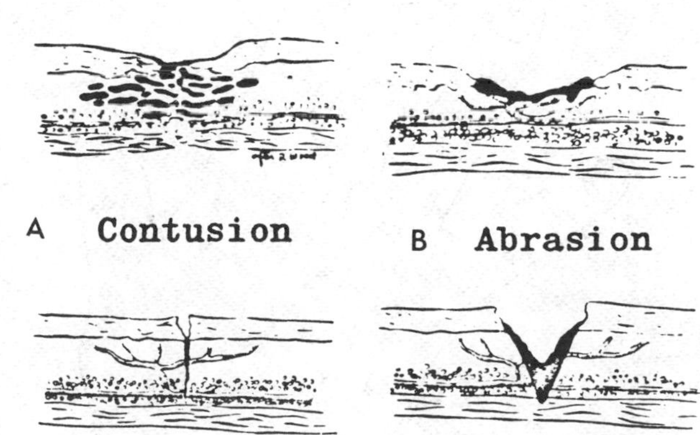

Figure 95–17. Types of surface trauma. (Modified from Miller, R. H. (Ed.): *Textbook of Basic Emergency Medicine.* St. Louis, C. V. Mosby Co., 1975, p. 155.)

gauze, then coarse mesh gauze and covered with an outer wrap; *avoid applying adhesive tape over wound.*

- Tetanus prophylaxis.
- Patient/family teaching: (1) Observe for signs of infection (pseudomonas infections are common). (2) If open, wash off and then reapply Neosporin or Vaseline petroleum 4 times a day.[146] (3) If closed, change dressing daily or PRN serous drainage. (4) Explain that there may be temporary decrease in pigment after healing.

Puncture Wound. Narrow, penetrating wound resulting from small objects, e.g., tooth, nail, splinter, ice pick. Does not bleed readily; often covered with skin flap (See Fig. 95–17C). (Bites are discussed later.)

Puncture wounds are difficult to clean and irrigate. Infections resulting from retained foreign material are common.

Recognition

- History; wound may be difficult to visualize; tenderness; induration may be noted if the injury is old.

Management

- R/O fracture or foreign body. Be especially cautious of foot puncture wounds in persons wearing

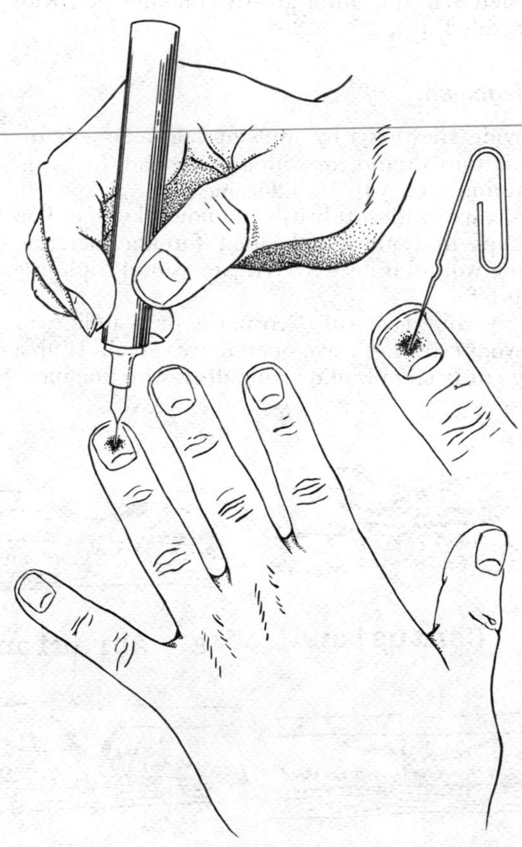

Figure 95–18. Evacuation of a subungual hematoma through a hole placed in the nail by a heated paper clip, a drill or a battery operated cautery. (From Grabb, W. C., H. E. Kleinert, and C. L. Puckett: *Techniques in Surgery: Facial and Hand Injuries.* Ethicon, Inc., 1976, p. 27.)

tennis shoes; rubber plugs (from shoe sole) may be deeply imbedded. Severe osteomyelitis may occur following puncture wounds of the foot.[85]

- Debride and open up the wound; cleanse wound meticulously and irrigate copiously.
- Remove *wood splinters before* cleansing area. Liquids cause wood to become very soft, making removal difficult.
- *Fish Hook removal: Push* barbed end through skin (do not try to pull out) or make an incision over barbed end. Cut off hook shaft below barb. Pull remainder of hook out.
- *Splinters under the nail* may require removal of V-shaped portion of nail to remove splinter.
- *Sewing needles* imbedded in tissue are very difficult to remove without fluoroscopy.
- Tetanus prophylaxis.
- Patient/family teaching: Observe for signs of infection; warm soaks 4 times a day for several days.

Avulsion or avulsed laceration. A wound with tissue loss. Wound edges cannot be easily approximated, e.g., loss of finger tip.

Recognition

- Freely bleeding wound with many exposed small vessels; loss of tissue; generally painful; may be associated with crush injury.

Management

- Direct pressure to stop bleeding.
- Appropriate anesthesia; topical agents often effective. Nerve block or local infiltration may be needed.
- Clean wound gently; irrigate well. Management may include: (1) hemostasis with topical thrombin or Gelfoam, (2) granulation healing by secondary intention), (3) skin grafting, and (4) reimplantation of avulsed part (see below).
- Dressings: fine mesh gauze or Owen's silk, coarse mesh fluffs, pressure dressing with tubular gauze if finger or toe, protect fingertips with aluminum splint.
- Tetanus prophylaxis.
- *Care of avulsed/amputated body part: At home:* roll up tissue so subcutaneous tissue is on inside and is protected from drying; place tissue in airtight container; place container on ice. *In ED:* place body part in container containing sterile normal saline or Tis-U-Sol and keep it cool or refrigerate.

> Caution: *An amputated part should* not *be placed in water or other non-isotonic solutions. This may cause further damage to injured cells.*

- *Patient/family teaching:* (1) Dressings often left in place longer than with other wounds (10–14 days) when wounds healing by granulation. (2) First dressing change is often by physician; soak off these dressing if adherent to wound. *Pulling the dressing may cause loss of granulation tissue.* (3) Dressings must be kept clean and dry; patients must return for dressing changes and *not* do them at home (*Note:* If dressing *must* be changed prematurely, fine mesh gauze or Owens silk usually left in place.) (4) Observe for signs of infection. Discuss regional or systemic signs of infection since patient will not have access to the wound to observe it for local indications of infection.

Laceration. An incised wound usually made by a sharp object such as a knife, glass, etc. (See Fig. 95–17*D*.)

Recognition

- Obvious wound, often freely bleeding; possible fractures. History with careful attention to the mechanism of injury.
- Degree of contamination (e.g., foot laceration from garden rake is highly tetanus-prone wound and will probably not be sutured closed). Presence of foreign bodies.
- Time of injury. Wounds more than 12 hours old often not sutured because of high incidence of infection associated with primary closure.
- Circulation and sensory-motor function in part distal to wound.
- Position of part when laceration occurred. (*Note:* If flexed when lacerated, transected tendons may be retracted and not visible in wound.)

Management

- Stop bleeding by direct pressure or pressure dressing; tourniquets rarely needed.
- Shave area around wound if necessary; *do not shave eyebrows.*
- Clean area around wound; irrigate well.
- Anesthesia may be needed to clean wound properly. Lidocaine 1% *without* epinephrine is used on fingers, toes, nose, ears, penis and for elderly people with thin skin; it may also be used in persons with cardiovascular disease. Lidocaine *with* epinephrine is used on other areas to minimize bleeding and/or prolong anesthesia.

> *Persons administering lidocaine should be aware of the maximum dosage for the weight/size of the patient and be familiar with the side and toxic effects. Allergic reactions to lidocaine rarely occur.*

- Tetanus prophylaxis.
- *Wound closure – noninvasive technique:* accomplished with adhesive strips often reinforced with nylon thread. Strips used instead of sutures to approximate wound edges in small or superficial wounds not subject to a great deal of tension and easily

approximated. Adhesive strips also used with sutures, to reinforce wound edges after suture removal (especially in plastic repairs), and to close skin when subcutaneous sutures have been inserted. There is less trauma to the tissues and decreased incidence of infection when strips are used in properly selected patients. Major disadvantages of closure with adhesive strips are: (1) potential for wound edge inversion, (2) strips come off easily if skin not prepared properly and (3) strips easily removed by unreliable patients, e.g., young child. Substances which enhance adhesiveness (e.g., benzoin) may be used; however, allergic reactions may occur. Inquire about allergy history.

To apply adhesive strips:

(1) dry area with sponge, (2) apply tincture of benzoin around wound (but not on wound), (3) start on one side of wound and place one edge of strip on skin across wound edges and then place other end of strip on skin, applying tension so wound edges close. Avoid inverting wound edges; forceps may help keep wound edges up. Apply enough strips so that wound edges do not gap. Apply additional strips approximately ¼ inch from and parallel to wound to redistribute tension (See Figure 95–19). Additional strips may be placed at ends of the strips (again parallel to wound) to minimize curling or lifting of strip ends.

- For wound closure by suturing (invasive technique) see Chapter 80, p. 1776.
- Splint the joint if a laceration is over a joint; movement of joint will create undue tension on the suture line and may cause the sutures to pull out.
- *Patient/family teaching:* The best repair of a wound will be useless if the patient/significant others fail to receive and understand instructions concerning proper wound care, dressing changes, etc. Include the following information in teaching: (1) how to keep dressing clean and dry, (2) how and when to change dressings, (3) supplies needed for dressing changes and where to get them, (4) indications of infection, (5) what to do if dressing becomes too tight, (6) arrangements for wound checks, (7) arrangements for suture removal.

Bee Stings. May result in localized and/or generalized reactions. Management of generalized anaphylactic reactions has been discussed previously (see p. 2154 and Chapters 11 and 13). Only *local wound care* is included here.

Recognition

- History; stinger(s) may be seen; local erythema, edema and pain.

Management

- Remove stinger by gently scraping with scalpel blade or needle. *Do not use tweezers, as more venom may be deposited into tissues by squeezing stinger. (Note:* stinger should be removed because walls of the sac continue to contract and release venom long after separation of stinger from the insect.)
- Clean area. Put liquid meat tenderizer on a 2 × 2 and place directly on site. If only powdered meat tenderizer is available, make paste by mixing ¼ teaspoon of powder with one teaspoon of water; apply paste directly to site. (*Note:* Use of meat tenderizer is most effective if begun *immediately* after sting.) Apply ice pack over meat tenderizer. Remove ice pack after twenty minutes. Clean area and dress as needed.
- Stings around the eye may cause perforation of globe; carry out standard eye/assessment (see p. 1950) including visual acuity. Ophthalmologic consultation may be indicated.
- Serum sickness following bee stings may occur.
- *Patient family teaching:* (1) Prevention of stings, (2) meat tenderizer and ice as a home remedy, (3) local symptoms may last for several days; warm soaks applied 4 times a day may provide comfort, (4) mild analgesia with aspirin or acetaminophen as needed, (5) antihistamines, e.g., Benadryl, are of little value in reducing swelling but may help relieve itching, (6) signs of infection including lymphadenitis and lymphangitis, and (7) where to receive follow up care if needed.

Spider Bites, Scorpion Bites, Fish-Related Injuries. Discussion of spider bites,[72, 136] scorpion bites,[39] and fish-related injuries (e.g., stingray barb injuries, shark bites) is beyond the scope of this chapter. Some of these injuries

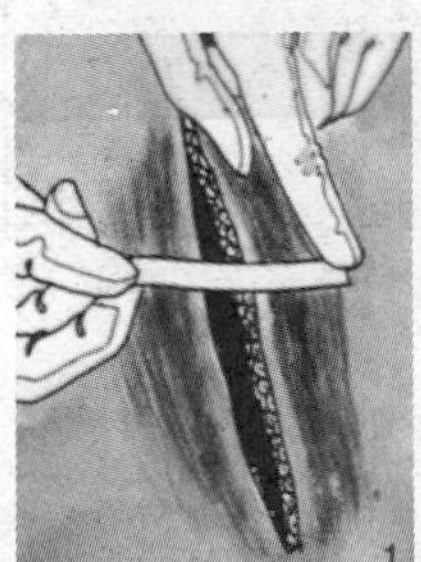

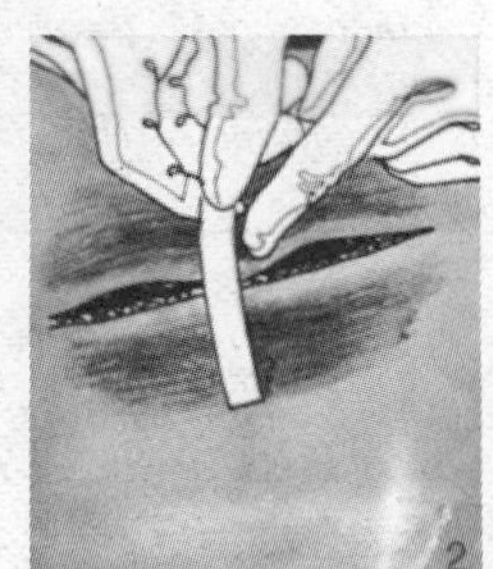

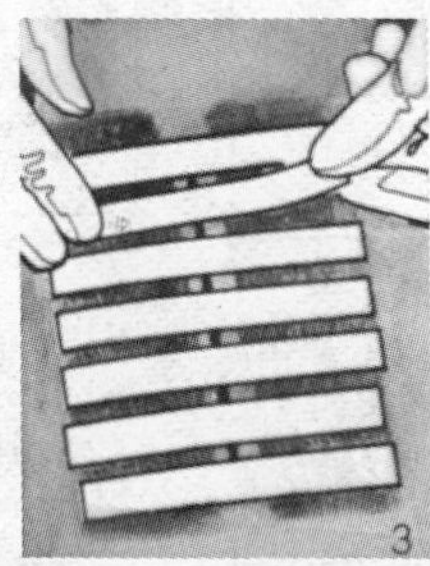

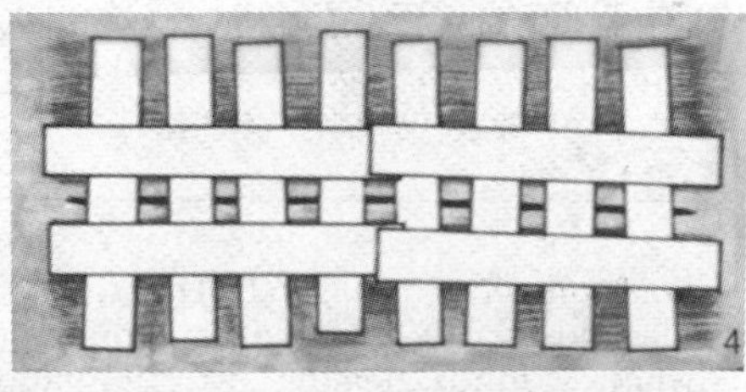

Figure 95–19. Steps in applying skin closure strips. (Courtesy the 3M Company, Surgical Products Division, St. Paul, Minn.)

may be *very* serious, possibly fatal because of CNS involvement. Familiarize yourself with the kinds of potential "injuring agents" in your geographical location and learn how to manage such injuries should they occur. For example, in the United States emergency management is needed for bites from *Latrodectus mactans* ("black widow") and *Loxosceles reclusa* ("brown recluse") spiders.

Snake Bites.[31, 99, 118, 136, 141] Familiarize yourself with poisonous snakes in your region and with the emergency management of bites from these snakes. Poisonous snakes may be found in most states in the United States.

PIT VIPER BITES. Pit vipers (Crotalidae family) are responsible for most snake bites seen in the United States. These include rattlesnakes, copperheads and water moccasins. Coral snakes account for only 2 per cent of snake bites in the United States.

Recognition

- *Description of pit viper:* Pit vipers have a pit or depression between the eye and nostril; pupils are elliptical or slit-like; head usually triangular. Fangs are long and tubular, can be retracted against roof of mouth. There are usually two fangs, longer than the rest of the teeth.
- Not all persons attacked by a pit viper are bitten. Not all persons bitten are envenimated. Snake bites in spring may be more severe, because venom is more concentrated then.
- Classically, bite of pit viper is different from that of a nonpoisonous snake (Fig. 95–20).
- Envenination is graded 0 through 4, with 0 being no envenination and 4 being severe involvement.
- Local reactions: intense burning pain immediately after the bite; swelling and copious bleeding; two puncture wounds above and two bites below. (*Note*: This is not always seen.) Blisters and blebs develop within 1 hour and become large and hemorrhagic; significant swelling.

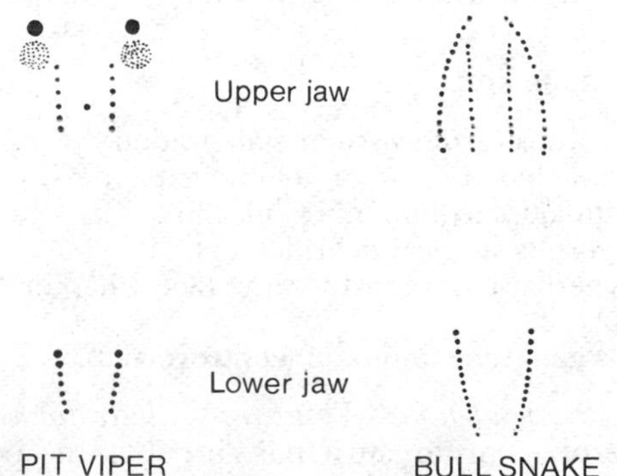

Figure 95–20. Characteristic bite patterns for poisonous and non-poisonous snakes. The pattern on the left is made by a pit viper, with the black dots representing the puncture wounds made by the fangs. The strippled area below the fangs is where the venom is deposited. The pattern on the right is that of a non-poisonous bull snake. (From American College of Surgeons Committee on Trauma: *Early Care of the Injured Patient.* Philadelphia: W. B. Saunders Company, 1972, p. 77.)

- Generalized reactions: muscle twitching and fasciculation, especially around the mouth; metallic taste in mouth; nausea and vomiting, GI bleeding; diaphoresis, tachycardia, hypotension; syncope and coma; shallow respirations progressing to respiratory arrest.

Management

- Act calmly and reassure patient; put patient at rest, placing the involved part at heart level if possible. Apply a constricting band above site; *this is to minimize lymphatic and venous return only.*
- Wash skin, incise and suction wounds. (*Note:* Incision done only within 20 minutes after bite; beyond that time, probably ineffective. Incisions should be no larger than ¼ inch long and ⅛ inch deep (preferably along the long axis of the body part). The usefulness of incision is controversial.
- *Do not* apply ice or cool packs.
- Start one or two large bore IV's and hang Ringer's lactate.
- Lab studies: CBC, T&C, coagulation screen, electrolytes, BUN, sugar, ESR, UA. (*Note:* If whole blood is needed, fresh blood, rather than stored blood, should be used.)
- Steroids possibly used for anaphylactic reactions, but contraindicated in routine treatment of snake bite, as may enhance absorption of venom or block action of antivenin.
- Excision of the enveninated tissue may be done.
- Antivenin: Antivenin (Crotalidae) Polyvalent (Wyeth) most commonly used. Made from horse serum, so patients must be skin (or eye) tested before administration. Dosage ranges from 3 to 40 vials, depending upon degree of envenination and age of patient. Antivenin added to IV fluid and given IV drip in less than 1 hour.

Caution: *Children may require larger doses of antivenin than adults.*

- Measure girth of the extremity proximal to bite every 15–30 minutes. This is guide for additional antivenin.
- Tetanus prophylaxis.
- Cardiovascular stabilization; cardiac monitor and intensive nursing care.
- Pain relief: aspirin or codeine for mild cases; Demerol indicated in more severe situations. Observe for respiratory depression from narcotics.
- Limit initial wound care to cleansing and dressing with large, absorbent, bulky dressings.

Human Bites.[65] Include *self-induced* (e.g., laceration of tongue during grand mal seizure), *dental abrasions* (usually superficial hand abrasion at the MCP joint — often incurred during a fist fight if knuckle hits opponent's tooth), and *penetrating bites* causing puncture wounds and tissue loss. Assess neurovascular and musculoskeletal function carefully. Fractures and tendon lacerations, especially of the hand, not uncommon.

> *Human bites can cause severe necrotizing infections and require vigorous management.*

Recognition

- History; puncture wounds, lacerations, superficial abrasions, large tissue loss; increased pain over site may indicate fracture.

Management

- Reassure victim and significant others.
- Careful neurovascular and musculoskeletal assessment; possibly x-rays.
- Careful wound cleansing; vigorous irrigation; open and debride puncture wounds. Wounds usually not sutured unless large or located on face; loosely placed sutures or adhesive closure strips may be used.
- Broad-spectrum antibiotics; tetanus prophylaxis.
- Repeated wound checks are important; more radical debridement may be necessary.
- Persons with human bites may be admitted to hospital for at least 24 hours.
- Warm soaks four times daily.
- Patient/family teaching: Stress importance of follow-up and when and where it will be done, (2) how to take antibiotics, (3) how to dress wound, (4) signs of infection.

Animal Bites.[32] Generally less dangerous than human bites. However, problem of infection (e.g., *Pasteurella multocida*) is significant. Assess possibility that the biting animal is rabid. Incidence of rabies in domesticated animals is very low in United States.

Recognition

- History: (1) type of animal, (2) who owns animal, (3) description of incident, i.e., provoked or unprovoked, and (4) location of animal, its immunization history, and its state of health.
- Type of wound, e.g., puncture wound, skin loss, etc. Neurovascular and musculoskeletal assessment.

Management

- Psychologic support for patient and significant others; in their anger they may destroy the animal.
- X-rays if indicated, especially hand and head bites.
- Careful wound cleansing, debridement, and copious irrigation.
- Dressings: (1) bulky, fluffy and absorbent, (2) place fingers in burn position (refer to Figure 95–16); place other areas in position of function.
- Tetanus prophylaxis; Antibiotics.
- Duck Embryo Vaccine (DEV) used only if high index of suspicion or rabid animal. Commonly DEV causes both localized and generalized reactions. Rabies hyperimmune serum now available.
- Hospital or family contact Public Health officials or animal control.
- Patient/family teaching: (1) signs of infection, (2) daily wound check, (3) dressing changes. Animal management: (1) do *not* destroy animal; confine and observe for 10–14 days, (2) if animal *must* be destroyed, avoid damaging its head, (3) try to locate owner of domestic animal.

Significant Infections or Disorders Associated with Surface Trauma

Clostridium perfringens – Gas Gangrene.[80] This anaerobic organism produces endotoxin affecting cells around wound site. Normal incubation period is 1 day to 6 weeks. May be massive tissue destruction; generalized sepsis. (*Note:* Gas gangrene may occur after hypodermic injections, especially epinephrine given SC, and after minor trauma to an old scar containing clostridial spores.)

Recognition

- Local reactions: severe, sudden pain in injured part. Distal portion of limb becomes cold and edematous. Drainage of thin, watery, brown or brown-grey liquid. Tissue palpation crepitant, produces crunchy, bubbly sensation which may be heard with a stethoscope before it is palpable.
- Systemic reactions: temperature usually below 38.3° C. (101° F.), pulse often greater than 120; anorexia; vomiting; profuse watery or bloody diarrhea; delirium; coma; death.

Management

- Vigorous cardiovascular stabilization.
- Whole blood or other volume expanders.
- Antibiotics (commonly penicillin).
- Vigorous surgical debridement.
- Hyperbaric oxygen therapy. (See Chapter 13, p. 282.)
- Gas gangrene antitoxin (controversial).

Clostridium tetani – Tetanus: *Clostridium tetani* (anaerobic organism) has incubation period ranging from 2 days to several months, perhaps longer. Organism releases *two toxins: tetanospasmin* and *tetanolysin.* Tetanospasmin acts on spinal cord's anterior horn cells, which inhibit motor activity. Result is exaggerated motor activity, spasticity of skeletal muscles, and seizures. Once toxin combines with certain receptors it cannot be released. Tetanolysin causes lysis of erythrocytes and leukocytes, thus contributing to development of tetanus by causing local tissue necrosis and interfering with phagocytosis. It also affects cardiac muscle.

Many patients who develop tetanus have wounds considered so trivial they either did not seek medical attention or the health care provider was not impressed enough to carry out good wound care or to immunize the patient.

Nurses also have a role in promoting immunization programs for school age children and the public at large.

Recognition

- Headache, restlessness. Muscle pain and spasm, especially of jaw and mastication (trismus) giving face a classic distorted grin called *risus sardonicus.*
- Difficulty swallowing, stiff neck, opisthotonos. Generalized muscle rigidity and spasm. Generalized seizures precipitated by almost any stimuli, e.g., noise, injections.
- Patient awake, alert but restless and in pain from spasms.
- Respiratory insufficiency may ensue. Temperature normal or slightly elevated.

Management

- Maintain airway (possible tracheostomy).
- Minimize stimuli by gentle care, and quiet, dark environment.
- Muscle relaxants.
- IV fluids for nutrition.
- Tetanus immune globulin (TIG) may be given in doses of 3000–6000 units (*Note*: Dose used in treating tetanus is much larger than the 250 units used in tetanus *prophylaxis.*); *Tetanus anti-toxin (TAT)* rarely, if ever, used in tetanus management in the United States.
- Foley catheter (urinary retention common).
- Active immunization against tetanus is initiated.
- Local wound care; antibiotics.
- Long-term intensive nursing care.

Wound Botulism. Although extremely rare, botulism may occur following a wound or soft tissue trauma with skin penetration. Since *Clostridium botulinum* is a spore-forming anaerobe it is believed the organism may be present from an old injury and be activated with reinjury. Symptoms are similar to those with botulism following ingestion of contaminated food, e.g., weakness, blurred vision, difficulty speaking and swallowing, dilated pupils, respiratory arrest. Treatment focuses on: airway maintenance and support; use of *botulism antitoxin,* and intensive nursing care. Recovery often slow, requiring prolonged hospitalization.

EMERGENCIES INVOLVING THE GENITOURINARY TRACT[15, 51]

Renal Trauma*. Blunt and penetrating kidney trauma accounts for approximately half of all GU tract injuries, and may be classified as minor, major or severe.[16] Contusion of a kidney without disruption of a capsule or laceration of the collecting system is a *minor injury.* A *major injury* involves laceration of the capsule and renal parenchyma with continuation of the laceration into the collection system, resulting in hematuria. A severe *(critical) renal injury* has avulsion or transection of portions of the kidney from the pedicle.

Recognition

- History of trauma; also obtain history of previous GU tract injury or disease.
- Flank pain, tenderness, ecchymosis. Shock. Hematuria, which usually resolves quickly with minor injuries but continues or worsens when with major or critical injury. (*Note*: Hematuria may be absent in presence of renal artery thrombosis or severe avulsion injuries.)
- Obliteration of psoas (muscle) shadow on abdominal x-ray may occur. Fractures of lower ribs or lumbar vertebral transverse processes indicates possible renal injury.

Management

- Cardiovascular stabilization (start IV, hang Ringer's lactate or normal saline).
- Routine blood studies; creatinine and T&C may be appropriate.
- Foley catheter, obtain urine for UA, monitor output every 15–30 minutes (*Note*: Use 18 or 20 F. catheter.) Maintain catheter patency; irrigate as needed.
- Observe and measure borders of flank mass if present.
- Diagnostic studies; IVP (*Note*: Normal blood pressure necessary to adequately visualize kidney; IVP usually unsuccessful if systolic blood pressure below 60 mm. Hg.), excretory urogram, retrograde pyelogram, renal arteriogram.
- Surgery if cannot stabilize vital signs or if enlarging flank mass; surgery typical with critical injury.

Bladder Trauma:* Injuries to urinary bladder, ranging from contusion to rupture. Result usually from auto accidents. Commonly occur with pelvic fractures. An empty urinary bladder

*See also Unit XIII.

is relatively well protected. Bladder rupture often caused by direct blow to a full bladder.[16]

Recognition

- Hematuria. Signs of peritoneal irritation with intraperitoneal perforation.
- Back or flank pain and/or ecchymosis if extravasation (escape of blood or other substance) is extraperitoneal.
- Suprapubic pain; pain upon attempts to void. Inability to void.
- Pelvic fractures, diminished or absent femoral pulses and/or loss of sciatic nerve function — all commonly associated with bladder trauma.

Management

- Cardiovascular stabilization.
- Immobilize on fracture board if pelvic fracture suspected.
- Foley catheter may or may not be inserted; some believe catheter causes additional trauma if urethra injured.
- Surgery indicated with intraperitoneal bladder rupture; with extraperitoneal bladder rupture patient may be admitted for observation.

Urethral Injuries. Result most commonly from pelvic fractures due to auto accidents; are associated with bladder injuries. Males have a higher incidence of urethral injuries than females.

Recognition

- Suprapubic hematoma; hematuria or continuous blood flow from urethral meatus.
- Inability to void if urethra transected.
- Swelling of perineum, scrotum or penis due to extravasation of urine.

Management

- Cardiovascular stabilization.
- Diagnostic studies: excretory urogram; retrograde cystourethrogram.
- Foley catheter (controversial).

> Caution: *If urethral transection is suspected, an experienced physician, preferably a urologist, should insert the urethral catheter. The trauma of catheterization may convert a partial urethral transection into a complete one.*

- Other supportive care.
- Treatment may involve primary surgical anastomosis of transected urethral ends or initial insertion of a suprapubic tube for urinary diversion, with urethroplasty several months later.

Ureteral Calculi (Stones)

Recognition

- Severe, intense, stabbing flank pain, often radiating around to abdomen and into groin. Patient may be too uncomfortable to remain still; may pace in an effort to manage pain.
- Nausea, vomiting (usually due to pain).
- Tachycardia, diaphoresis, blood pressure elevation.
- Hematuria (gross or microscopic).
- Possible history of previous calculi.

Management

- R/O other disorders associated with abdominal pain.
- Pain relief with large dosages of narcotics. (*Note:* Since these patients often walk around because of intense pain, take precautions to prevent patient injury; ask significant other to stay with patient.)
- Obtain clean catch urine for UA: possible C & S.
- *Strain all urine* for stones; send stones for analysis.
- Lab studies: CBC, urea, calcium, phosphorus, uric acid, acid phosphatase, serum protein, chloride and CO_2.
- X-ray studies: abdominal film — KUB (kidneys, ureter and bladder), IVP.
- Cystoscopy depending upon stone location.
- *Patient/family teaching*: (1) How to strain urine, e.g., using gauze sponges stretched over a container, a tea strainer or a commercially available urine strainer; (2) need to increase fluid intake; cranberry juice may be ordered; (3) how to take medications, e.g., narcotics and antibiotics; (4) need for follow up, when and where provided; (5) what to look for, e.g., fever, increased pain.

Testicular Torsion*. Twisting of testis and epididymis on a pedicle, resulting in venous thrombosis and occlusion. Most often occurs in young boys, may also occur in young adult males. Torsion usually spontaneous, can also result from trauma.

Recognition

- Severe testicular or groin pain unrelieved with rest. Swelling, cyanosis, or hyperemia of scrotum or testicle. Lower abdominal pain.
- Nausea, vomiting; lower abdominal pain; faintness.

Management

- Manual manipulation to relieve torsion and emergency surgical repair if manipulation unsuccessful.

---

*See also Chapter 82.

- Psychological support to patient and significant others; may be little time for detailed explanations because of urgent need for surgery. Patient or partner may not completely understand what the surgery will involve, i.e., that the procedure is not disfiguring and normal sexual function is usually preserved.
- Standard emergency surgery procedure.

Pyelonephritis. Infection involving renal parenchyma. Appropriate recognition and management important to prevent permanent tissue damage and renal failure.

Recognition

- Lower back pain, CVA tenderness, high fever.
- White blood cells, casts, bacteria and possibly red cells in urine.
- Nausea, vomiting, diarrhea or constipation; symptoms of cystitis.

Management

- Obtain clean catch, midstream urine specimen for UA, C&S, colony count, gram stain.
- Ampicillin commonly prescribed.
- Pregnant patients (in third trimester) or debilitated patients may be admitted.
- *Patient/family teaching*: (a) Importance of taking antibiotic for *full course*, usually ten days; (b) need to increase fluid intake; (c) how to take medications; (d) importance of follow-up care and repeat urine examinations.

Cystitis.[9] Inflammation of urinary bladder caused by a variety of organisms. (*E. coli* most common.)

Recognition

- Suprapubic pain and tenderness. Dysuria, frequency, urgency.
- Possible hematuria (gross or microscopic).

Management

- Obtain clean catch urine as above (*Note*: If patient is menstruating, may have her insert tampon into vagina to prevent menstrual blood from mixing with urine.) Send specimen for UA, C&S, colony count; possible gram stain.
- Antibiotics (sulfa preparations, ampicillin).
- Urinary analgesics.
- *Patient/family teaching*: As listed above and: (a) inform urine may be unusual color if analgesics used; (b) prevention includes voiding immediately after sexual intercourse, and careful perineal care.

Abortion

Termination of gestation before fetus is viable, usually 20 weeks. An abortion may be spontaneous or induced; therapeutic or criminal. (See also Chapter 88.)

Threatened Abortion. The pregnancy may or may not be sustained.

Recognition

- Positive pregnancy test; varying degrees of vaginal bleeding; crampy lower abdominal pain; closed cervical os.

Management

- Obtain blood or urine specimen for pregnancy test if pregnancy unconfirmed.
- Cardiovascular stabilization usually not required.
- Sedation; bed rest.
- *Patient/family teaching*: Pad counts; nothing in vagina (e.g., no tampons, intercourse, tub baths, or douching); need for follow-up care.

Inevitable Abortion. The pregnancy will terminate but has not yet done so.

Recognition

- Varying amounts of vaginal bleeding; crampy lower abdominal pain; nausea, vomiting (usually secondary to pain); cervical os is open, but tissue has not been passed.

Management

- Start IV: draw blood: CBC, Type, Rh.
- Pitocin may be added to IV; start infusion slowly.
- Rhogam given for Rh incompatibility as needed.
- Curettage.
- Pad count.
- Frequent vital signs.

Incomplete Abortion. Part, but not all, of the products of conception have been expelled. Often fetus has been delivered but placental fragments remain.

Recognition

- Often massive vaginal bleeding. History of passing tissue.
- Hypotension or profound shock. Crampy lower abdominal pain.
- Cervical os is open.

Management

- Start 1–2 large bore IV's; draw blood: CBC, T&C.
- Pitocin 20–40 units often added to IV bag; start infusion *slowly* to avoid sudden, severe contractions.
- Frequent vital signs with postural (if safe).
- Pad count.

- ▶ Psychologic support: discuss patient's feelings about what is happening; some patients may be relieved while others are saddened. Feelings of guilt are common; it may be of some comfort to know that spontaneous abortions often occur when the fetus is imperfect.
- ▶ Save all tissue passed for physician inspection, then send for pathology analysis.
- ▶ If patient habitually aborts, the products of conception may be sent for genetic studies. In this case place specimen in normal saline rather than formaldehyde; special arrangements must be made for genetic studies.
- ▶ Arrange for administration of Rhogam if necessary.
- ▶ Curettage may be done on either an outpatient or inpatient basis.
- ▶ *Patient/family teaching*: (1) pad count — bleeding usually is similar to menstrual bleeding and should taper off within a few days; (2) take temperature every 6 hours for 2 days; return for care if elevated temp; (3) how to take pain medications; (4) no tampons, intercourse, douching or tub baths until bleeding has stopped; (5) patient usually advised to wait at least 6 months before attempting to become pregnant; (6) where to get Rhogam if needed; (7) call or return if: increased bleeding, pain, fever greater than 38.3°C. (101°F.), foul-smelling discharge; (8) where to get follow-up care.

Septic Abortion. Abortion associated with infection (sepsis). May be associated with spontaneous abortions or therapeutic abortions. Sepsis following abortion is most commonly seen following "criminal" abortions, i.e., abortions done outside of legitimate medical settings. Septic abortion is common in areas which do not allow legal abortions; maternal death is not an uncommon outcome.

Devices used to induce a criminal abortion include such items as household cleaning products, coat hangers, knitting needles, and catheters.

Symptoms vary greatly, according to (a) method used and (b) time lag between onset of symptoms and obtaining medical care.

Recognition

- ▶ Elevated temp; abdominal pain, possible peritonitis; foul smelling vaginal discharge.
- ▶ Cardiovascular collapse, other symptoms of septic shock.
- ▶ Free air in abdomen if uterus perforated.
- ▶ Renal failure, especially if nephrotoxic chemicals used.
- ▶ Clotting disorders and disseminated intravascular coagulation (DIC). Elevated WBC, anemia.

Management

- ▶ Cardiovascular stabilization; one or more large bore IV's; vigorous fluid resuscitation with crystalloid and/or colloid.
- ▶ Draw blood: CBC, T&C, coagulation studies, creatinine, electrolytes, BUN, sugar, cultures.
- ▶ Pressor agents may be necessary, e.g., dopamine, Levophed.
- ▶ Cultures of vaginal discharge.
- ▶ Foley catheter; urine for UA, C&S; monitor output carefully.
- ▶ Broad-spectrum antibiotics.
- ▶ NG tube inserted if bowel sounds decreased.
- ▶ Suction evacuation of uterine contents (uterine walls often too friable to use a standard metal curette).
- ▶ Psychologic support and understanding.
- ▶ Arrange for intensive nursing care; usually these patients cannot go in an open ICU (because of sepsis).

Ectopic Pregnancy

Pregnancy located outside uterus. May be anywhere in abdominal cavity; however, most are implanted in fallopian (uterine) tube. (See also Chapter 88.)

Recognition

- ▶ Dull or sharp lower abdominal pain (usually unilateral until rupture and intra-abdominal bleeding occur). Shoulder pain — Kehr's sign.
- ▶ Postural hypotension or severe shock if ruptured.
- ▶ Pregnancy test may or may not be positive.
- ▶ Vaginal bleeding may be present.

Management

- ▶ One or two large bore IV's; Ringer's lactate initially.
- ▶ Blood for CBC, T&C; urine for pregnancy test.
- ▶ Diagnosis made by evacuating nonclotting blood from cul de sac (culdocentesis). Nursing preparation of patient for culdocentesis is important; brief, sudden, severe pain is experienced. By patient not moving during the procedure, the period of pain can be significantly shortened. A self-administered, short-acting anesthetic agent, e.g., Trilene or Penthrane, may help.
- ▶ Diagnostic laparoscopy (alternative to culdocentesis).
- ▶ NPO until diagnosis made.
- ▶ Emergency pre-operative care.
- ▶ Frequent vital signs.

Nursing Assessment and Management of Patient with Vaginal Bleeding[12]

Vaginal bleeding may result from various problems in addition to those mentioned above. The amount of bleeding varies. The following *guidelines* may be appropriate, regardless of the etiology.

- ▶ Promptly place patient in a room with exam table with stirrups. Help patient undress; provide perineal pad and items for perineal care.
- ▶ Determine amount of bleeding, e.g., how many pads, tampons, towels, etc., used in last hour.
- ▶ Assess vital signs, including postural vital signs.
- ▶ Initiate IV fluid therapy (if hypotensive or significant postural changes).
- ▶ Obtain history concerning: (1) duration of bleeding; (2) presence of pain; (3) last menstrual period; (4) is patient pregnant; any previous pregnancies? (5) sexual history; (6) birth control measures used; (7) is this really vaginal bleeding (rectal or urethral bleeding may be mistaken for vaginal bleeding); (8) previous history of vaginal bleeding; (9) allergies and medical history.
- ▶ Obtain appropriate laboratory studies, e.g., CBC, pregnancy test.
- ▶ Initiate flow sheet (record vital signs and pad count).
- ▶ Reassess vital signs frequently if bleeding significant.
- ▶ Observe and save all tissue passed.
- ▶ Report promptly presence of excess bleeding, tissue passed, hypotension.
- ▶ Provide comfort measures/psychologic support.

Sexual Assault*

Sexual assault and rape are common crimes, which often are not reported. (See Chapter 88 for definitions of assault and rape. Remember that males, especially young boys, may be victims of sexual assault.) Victims often experience both acute and long-term physical and psychologic trauma in addition to lengthy legal proceedings, public humiliation, and destruction of social relationships.

> *The emergency department role in caring for victims of sexual assault is to provide sensitive, thorough physical care coupled with empathetic psychologic support and careful gathering of vital information, which is usually legally evaluated.*

Recognition

- ▶ Patient, significant others or authorities may report the assault.
- ▶ Some patients have massive trauma with loss of consciousness; the possibility of sexual assault may not be obvious; consider possibility of sexual assault in unconscious trauma patient when history is unknown or suspicious.
- ▶ Common signs include: ecchymotic areas, especially of face or neck; trauma to larynx and/or fracture (with or without dislocation) of mandible; multiple contusions and lacerations.
- ▶ Clothing may be stained, torn or disheveled.
- ▶ Affect variable; do not assume that lack of concern or relative calm means the assault did not occur or victim is "handling it well." Feelings of guilt, humiliation (especially after meeting with police), and fear may stop many patients from expressing themselves.

Management

- ▶ Attention to ABC's.
- ▶ Psychologic support.
- ▶ High care priority — place patient in private (GYN) exam room; have someone stay with her. Expedite registration process. Insure patient privacy; do not give information over phone, to media, etc.
- ▶ Explain to patient not to wash, gargle, douche, etc., until necessary specimens obtained.
- ▶ Encourage patient (or parents) to report assault to authorities if unreported.
- ▶ Contact sexual assault counselor(s) if available if not already done; obtain patient's permission for this.
- ▶ Clothes may be used as court evidence; handle them carefully (*Note*: Clothes often are taken by police, so make arrangements for clean clothes to be brought.) Place clothes in paper, not plastic bag.
- ▶ Detailed history and physical exam after explaining need for detail. Take history immediately and only once. Patients report that giving a history is almost as traumatic as the assault. Record history in detail, using the patient's own words; many agencies have a special form for such history and physical examination. Record extent, location and treatment of all injuries. Pictures may be included. A gynecological exam should be carried out *only once*, preferably by a licensed physician who will be available for court trial, i.e., not intern or resident. Protect patient privacy during exam.
- ▶ Lab data: Cultures for gonorrhea; hanging drop analysis and smears for presence of sperm and their motility; acid phosphatase of vaginal secretions; foreign pubic hairs analyzed by police laboratory; serology or FTA.
- ▶ Provide patient with opportunity to bathe *after* examination.
- ▶ "Morning after pill," Diethylstilbesterol (DES), may be given if possibility of pregnancy. (*Note*: Use of DES is controversial.) Many hospitals thus ask patient to sign a statement that she will have an abortion if pregnancy occurs while receiving DES. DES is taken in doses of 25 mg. BID for 5 days and should be started within 72 hours. DES often causes nausea; antiemetic may be prescribed. It is important that patient complete full 5 day course.
- ▶ VD prophylaxis. Penicillin 4.8 million units administered IM 30 minutes after 1 Gr. of probenecid (Benemid) given orally.

---

*See references 12, 29, 30, 35, 90, 127.

- Suggest someone stay with patient for several days.
- *Patient/family teaching*: (1) importance of completing DES treatment; (2) follow up care in 4–6 weeks for test results, pregnancy test, and psychological support; (3) name and number of person to contact if patient unwilling or unable to utilize counseling resources; (4) discussion of some emotional responses to this type of trauma. (5) menses should start within 7 days after completing DES; if this does not occur D & C is arranged.
- Hospital records often placed in "security file" because of possibility they will be used in court. Release of records and information should be only by medical records department and only to credentialed authorities.

*Infectious Disorders of Reproductive System**

Pelvic Inflammatory Disease (PID).[34, 38, 90] Bacterial infection of pelvic organs, commonly uterus, ovaries and fallopian (uterine) tubes. Although gonococcal PID is common, various other organisms may be responsible.

Recognition

- Bilateral, lower abdominal pain often associated with rebound tenderness; lower back pain may be present. Adenexal tenderness on pelvic exam.
- Foul smelling, thick, purulent vaginal discharge.
- Patients often walk slowly, doubled over, with little movement of pelvic girdle ("PID shuffle").
- Elevated WBC; fever. Presence of IUD.

Management

- Evaluate and treat peritonitis.
- Gram stains and cultures of cervical and vaginal secretions; rectal and/or pharyngeal cultures may also be done. (*Note*: Evaluated for GC [Gonococcus] as well as other organisms. The GC requires a special culture medium; these specimens should be taken promptly to lab.)
- Draw blood for: CBC, VDRL, and possibly FTA (fluorescent treponemal antibody absorption) and TPHA (*Treponema pallidum* hemagglutination); draw blood cultures if disseminated GC.
- Procaine penicillin 4.8–6.0 million units given IM 30 minutes after probenecid is given orally in a dose of 1 Gr; Ampicillin in doses of 3.5 Gr. PO STAT, followed by 500 mg. QID for 10 days may be used instead of procaine penicillin.
- Venereal disease report form initiated; form is completed and submitted to Public Health authorities if cultures are positive for *Neisseria gonorrheae.*
- *Patient/family teaching*: (1) importance of taking meds for full course of therapy; (2) bed rest; (3) how to take pain meds and prevent future infections; (4) necessity of informing contacts about need for treatment if cultures are positive for GC; (5) refrain from intercourse until therapy completed, or at least 7 days; (6) arrange follow-up care.

*See also Chapters 82 and 85.

Herpes Simplex Type II[38] (Herpes Progenitalis). A viral infectious disease transmitted sexually. Incidence becoming epidemic in United States. Symptom exacerbation is self-limiting. Organism remains dormant and recurs during stressful periods, e.g., trauma, menstruation. Treatment is symptomatic; no effective cure. Genital herpes in a pregnant woman at term is of particular concern. Infant delivered vaginally may develop herpes meningoencephalitis. Staff may develop herpetic infections of fingers, hands, face, or other areas which may have come in contact with organism.

Recognition

- Extremely painful vesicular lesions of genital area. Vesicles may not be present; Small ulcerated areas surrounded by edema.
- Enlarged inguinal nodes.
- Dysuria due to urine passing over lesions. Volume depletion due to self-imposed fluid restriction because of dysuria.
- Temperature elevation.

Management

- Primarily supportive; no readily accepted "cure."
- Warm or cold sitz baths or sitting on moistened towel.
- Pain medication, e.g., codeine with aspirin; possible hospitalization for pain relief.
- Foley catheter may be used until lesions less painful.
- Antibiotics for secondary infections.
- Rehydration with oral or IV fluids.
- Toilet isolation important to prevent spread and/or reinfection; disinfect toilet with suitable agent.
- Pap smear, viral cultures and other special studies.
- Application of Congo Red to lesions followed by UV light exposure (controversial).
- *Patient/family teaching*: (1) hydration; (2) treatments; (3) isolation; (4) follow-up appointments for repeat treatments; (5) prevention.

METABOLIC EMERGENCIES*

Hypoglycemia[14]. Significant lowering of the blood sugar may result from various causes.

*See also Unit XIX and references 13, 14, 64, and 147.

Drug induced hypoglycemia, i.e., insulin administration associated with inadequate caloric intake, is the most common hypoglycemia requiring ED management.

Recognition

- Symptoms vary with blood sugar level. *CNS symptoms* include: irritability, confusion, tremors, blurring of vision, coma, seizures.
- Skin is cool and clammy; diaphoresis.
- Hypotension, tachycardia.
- May be difficult to differentiate from hyperglycemia; however, patient initially treated as if hypoglycemic.

Management

- Insure patient airway.
- Liquids containing additional sugar if patient awake. If unconscious, start IV with at least 18g catheter, draw blood from site for blood sugar. Advise lab of urgent need for blood sugar results.
- 50 ml. 50% dextrose IV given after blood sugar drawn. IV of 5–10% dextrose/water.
- Most patients are awake during or after the first dose of 50% dextrose; some require second dose.
- If IV cannot be started, place glucose paste under tongue.
- Glucagon or epinephrine IM may also raise blood sugar (reserved for use when IV cannot be started).

> Caution: *Lab sticks which measure blood glucose may be used as indicator of blood glucose level. However, they may be inaccurate, especially if old or exposed to the environment. When in doubt about accuracy of lab sticks, rely on your clinical assessment of a patient.*

- Cardiac monitor and/or 12 lead ECG.
- Repeat blood sugar in 1–2 hours.
- Determine and treat cause.

Diabetic Ketoacidosis.[3, 13, 14] Results from incomplete metabolism of glucose due to lack of circulating insulin. Characterized by hyperglycemia, osmotic diuresis, hypovolemia, ketonemia secondary to lipolysis, and electrolyte abnormalities.

Recognition

- Polyuria progressing to oliguria, polydipsia, polyphagia.
- Dehydration, dry mucous membranes, depressed and soft eyeballs.
- Warm, dry skin; elevated temperature.
- Vomiting, malaise, weakness, chest and/or abdominal pain.
- Hypotension, tachycardia.
- CNS symptoms: headache, drowsiness, stupor, coma.
- Lab data; elevated blood sugar (usually above 450 mgm/100 ml); serum and urine ketones; normal or low sodium; potassium low, normal or elevated; BUN normal or elevated; lowered serum bicarbonate; increased serum osmolality; arterial blood gases indicate metabolic acidosis with a respiratory alkalosis (compensation attempt); the WBC and hematocrit may be elevated.

Management

- Maintain patent airway.
- Start IV, draw blood for above studies; then give 50/ml 50% dextrose if diagnosis unclear.
- Vigorous fluid resuscitation with normal saline or 0.45% NaCl.
- Cardiac monitor with 12 lead ECG. (*Note*: Acute myocardial infarction common precipitating cause of DKA.)
- Regular insulin may be given IM, IV bolus, IV drip or SC:[3, 13, 14]

  IV bolus: 150–200 units of regular insulin may be given every hour until blood sugar is 250 mg. or one half of original value. At this time, 5% D/NSS is added to IV to prevent hypoglycemia.

  IV drip: 0.05–1 unit/kg. of regular insulin via continuous IV drip, with infusion pump on line, until blood sugar is as listed above.[13]

  IM: 20 units of regular insulin given IM STAT, followed by 10–15 units every hour until blood sugar lowered to level discussed above.

> Caution: *When IM insulin is administered, needle must be long enough to insure that the medication is delivered IM. Needle on prepackaged insulin syringes is not usually long enough for IM use.*

- Potassium, 40 mEq/liter/hour, is started as soon as patient has satisfactory urine output. (*Note*: Although a patient may have a normal or elevated serum K initially, remember this value does not reflect intracellular K; treatment of DKA causes significant shifts of K back into cells and hypokalemia may develop rapidly if K replacement is not included in therapy.)
- Bicarbonate, given as sodium bicarbonate, may be used if pH less than 7.0; usually added to first two liters of IV fluid.
- Intensive nursing care with frequent vital signs and repeated nursing assessment. *Complications of therapy* include hypoglycemia, hypokalemia and cerebral edema. Treatment of cerebral edema is dexamethasone (Decadron) 10 mg. administered IV.
- Foley catheter if patient obtunded; measure output at least hourly and test urine for sugar, ketones and specific gravity.
- Laboratory studies often repeated hourly until patient stable.

- CVP line may be inserted if patient is elderly and large amounts of fluid are required for resuscitation.
- Identify and treat (if possible) precipitating cause, e.g., myocardial infarction, pulmonary or urinary tract infections, etc.

Hyperglycemic, Hyperosmolar Non-Ketotic (HHNK) State.[13, 147] HHNK is characterized by severe hyperglycemia (blood sugars as high as 3000 mg./100 ml.), dehydration, increased serum osmolality, and no ketonemia. Most commonly seen in adult onset diabetics, often those taking oral hypoglycemia agents. High mortality rate.

Recognition

- Signs of dehydration: dry mucous membranes; soft, depressed eyeballs. Polyuria progressing to oliguria. Hypotension or shock, tachycardia.
- Elevated temperature; altered levels of consciousness.
- Lab findings: elevated blood sugar and serum osmolality; electrolytes usually normal but sodium may be lowered; normal or minimally elevated plasma ketones; arterial pH normal; phosphate may be lowered.

Management

- Differentiate from DKA.
- Lab studies as above drawn and repeated every hour until patient stable.
- Vigorous fluid replacement usually with 0.45% Na Cl; several liters given in first several hours.
- CVP line.
- Regular insulin, doses similar to those for DKA.
- K replacement started after adequacy of renal function established, usually after second or third liter of fluid. Large doses may be necessary but should not exceed 40 mEq/hour.
- Cardiac monitor; 12 lead ECG.
- Other studies as appropriate, e.g., chest x-ray, cardiac enzymes, blood cultures.
- Frequent monitoring of vital signs, urine output, etc.

Acute Adrenal Insufficiency.[13, 36, 145] *Adrenal crisis*. A life-threatening situation resulting from inadequate amounts of aldosterone and cortisol.

Recognition

- Hypovolemia, hypotension, frank shock; epigastric pain, nausea; hyperthermia; petechiae or ecchymosis.
- Fatigue, weakness progressing to coma, death.
- Lab data: serum sodium/potassium ratio less than 30; hyperkalemia; normal or lowered sodium; elevated eosinophil count; normal or decreased plasma cortisol.

Management

- Insure adequate airway and ventilation.
- Start 1–2 large bore IV's and hang 5% D/NSS; fluids given rapidly, e.g., one liter/1 to 2 hours.
- Lab studies: CBC with attention to eosinophil count, electrolytes, BUN, sugar, coagulation screen, fibrinogen level and fibrin split products, plasma cortisol level, blood and urine cultures, other studies as appropriate.
- Steroids, e.g., hydrocortisone succinate (Solu-Cortef) 100–200 mg. IV STAT and 50–100 mg. every 2–4 hours.[13]
- Pressor agents, e.g., dopamine, Neo-Synephrine.
- Cardiac monitor; 12 lead ECG.
- CVP line.
- Foley catheter; measure output at least every hour.
- Frequent nursing assessment and monitoring of vital signs.
- Arrange for an ICU bed.

Hyperthyroid Storm.[13,36,64,115] A rare, life-threatening emergency seen with hyperthyroidism.

Recognition

- Hypermetabolic state with fever, tachyarrhythmias. Possible pulmonary edema.
- Warm, diaphoretic, thin, smooth skin. Nausea, vomiting, diarrhea.
- Blood pressure may elevate significantly at first, but may drop precipitously.
- Large, tender thyroid gland.
- Ophthalmoplegia or exophthalmos.
- CNS irritability, agitation, convulsions, coma, psychotic behavior.
- Lab findings: elevated T_3 and T_4, elevated BUN.

Management

- Decrease synthesis of thyroid hormones by administration of propylthiouracil (PTU) or methimazole (Tapizole).
- Sodium iodide 1–2 Gr. slowly IV drip; Lugol's (iodine) solution orally 30 gtt/day.
- Propranolol (Inderal) to slow heart rate.
- Frequent vital signs monitoring.
- Lab studies: CBC, electrolytes, BUN, sugar, plasma ketones, T_3 and T_4, chest x-ray, blood cultures; other studies as necessary to identify precipitating cause.
- Congestive heart failure treated with diuretics and digitalis preparations.
- Oral and IV hydration.
- Treat hyperthermia – ASA, cooling blanket, etc.
- Steroids may be ordered.
- Arrange for ICU bed.

Myxedema Coma.[13, 36, 64] A life-threatening state often diagnosed in patients with long-standing, often unrecognized, hypothyroidism, or in patients receiving radioactive iodine to treat hyperthyroidism. May also occur in patients following thyroidectomy.

Recognition

- Hypothermia — may be profound. Hypoventilation; hypotension.
- CNS depression, lethargy, coma.
- Low pitched, deep, coarse voice.
- Dry skin; pallor; thin, coarse hair. Abdominal distention.
- Paranoid or delusional behavior.
- Pleural, pericardial and/or joint effusions.
- Thyroidectomy scar may be present.
- Lab data: respiratory acidosis; hyponatremia; hypoglycemia; ECG shows bradycardia with low voltage and flattened or inverted T waves; elevated SGOT, CPK, LDH.

Management

- Directed at replacing thyroid hormone and at identifying and treating etiology and complications.
- Airway maintenance; possibly mechanical ventilation and oxygen.
- Start an IV, draw appropriate blood studies (see later), hang glucose-containing fluid.
- Restrict fluids to treat hyponatremia.
- Cardiac monitor; 12 lead ECG.
- Thyroid replacement with L-thyroxine.
- Treatment of hypotension with pressor agents is most effective if thyroid replacement has been initiated first; phenylephrine (Neo-Synephrine) is commonly administered by IV bolus or IV drip.
- Rewarm patient *slowly*.
- Hydrocortisone sodium succinate (Solu-Cortef) given IV drip in doses of 200–300 mg./day to control secondary adrenal insufficiency.[13]
- Lab studies: CBC, electrolytes, BUN, sugar, T_3 and T_4, thyroid binding globulin (TBG), arterial blood gases, SGOT, CPK, LDH, plasma cortisol levels, urine and blood cultures.
- Frequent vital signs, measurement of urine output and CNS function.
- Arrange for ICU with respirator capability.

HYPERTENSIVE CRISIS[36, 62]

A life-threatening situation characterized by extreme elevations of both the systolic and diastolic blood pressures. Some *common hypertensive emergencies* requiring prompt management include:

1. Hypertensive encephalopathy.
2. Pre-eclampsia and eclampsia.
3. Dissecting aortic aneurysms.
4. Pulmonary edema secondary to severe hypertension.
5. Hypertensive emergencies associated with increased intracranial pressure and hemorrhage.
6. Hypertensive emergencies associated with sudden release of catecholamines.
7. Hypertensive crisis associated with renal disease, e.g., pyelonephritis.
8. Transient ischemic attacks (TIA's) associated with hypertension.
9. Hypertensive patients with severe bleeding.[36]
10. Hypertensive patients with myocardial infarction.[36]

Recognition

Symptoms vary greatly; patient may not appear very ill. Symptoms include: headache, initially occipital then quickly generalized; blurred vision; nausea or vomiting; confusion, lethargy, memory defects, coma, convulsions; papilledema and hemorrhagic exudates of eyegrounds.

Management

Treatment goal is to lower blood pressure as quickly and safely as possible. Medication depends upon etiology and urgency of the situation.

- Bed rest in position of comfort, with head of bed elevated.
- Explain procedures to minimize patient's stress.
- Start IV of 5% D/W with a microdrip.
- Treat immediate problems, e.g., pulmonary edema.
- Administer medications as ordered, with continuous monitoring of vital signs. Medications used for management of hypertensive crisis are summarized in Table 95–9. Antihypertensive medications administered by IV infusion should be "piggy backed" to the main IV line. They should not be the sole IV line in case there is a need to quickly discontinue medication.
- A microdripper should be used on all IV lines; infusion pumps are usually not used in an ED (because patient is not there long enough); may be added when patient is in ICU.
- Diagnostic studies to determine etiology carried out after patient is stable.

VASCULAR EMERGENCIES*

May include acute or chronic processes involving either the arteries or the veins, and may be occlusive (embolic) or exsanguinating. (See also Chapters 48 and 49.)

Traumatic Vascular Emergencies. May be caused by either blunt or penetrating trauma, e.g., "aortic rupture occurs in 15–20% of patients killed in vehicular accidents."[22] Hemor-

*See references 22, 44, 57, and 113.

TABLE 95–9. MEDICATIONS USED IN THE MANAGEMENT OF HYPERTENSIVE EMERGENCIES

Agent	Dose and Route of Administration	Special Considerations
Diazoxide (Hyperstat)	300 mg. or 5 mg./kg. IV *PUSH quickly.* Dose may be repeated after 30 minutes.	*Must be given as quickly as possible.* When given slowly IV, it binds with serum albumin and is rendered ineffective. Causes Na^+ and H_2O retention: diuretics may be given before hand. Can cause hyperglycemia. May precipitate angina or myocardial infarction. Maximal fall in BP should occur within 5 minutes after administration. Sudden and severe hypotension may occur, especially in an MI patient. Continuous BP monitoring for first 5 to 10 minutes after administration.
Sodium Nitroprusside (Nipride)	50 mg. vial added to 500 or 1000 ml. 5% D/W. Average IV drip dose is 3 *micrograms*/kg./minute with a range of 0.5 to 8.0 micrograms/kg./minute.*	Use a microdripper and an infusion pump. Solution is light sensitive: container and IV tubing are covered with aluminum foil. Solution stable only for 4 hours after mixing; must be discarded after 4 hours. BP must be monitored constantly. May cause chest or abdominal pain, GI disturbances, psychosis.
Trimethaphan Camsylate (Arfonad)	500 mg. vial added to 500 ml. 5% D/W. Start with 4 mg./min. for one minute then stop the drip and check the BP. Titrate the drip to the desired BP.	*Action is very rapid,* e.g., within a few seconds; continuous BP monitoring is essential. Pressor agents and resuscitation equipment should be available at bedside. Causes dilated pupils. (NOTE: When pupils dilated and non-reactive, an increase in the dose will not lower the BP any further.) Must be piggy-backed to main IV, should not be the only IV. Extreme caution is exercised when this drug is used becaused of its potency and rapid onset of action.
Phentolamine mesylate (Regitine)	5 mg. IV push slowly.	Used both for diagnosis of pheochromocytoma, and for acute hypertensive emergencies associated with this tumor. Also used for hypertensive crisis associated with MAO inhibitors, as well as for decreasing vasoconstriction in patients in shock. May be infiltrated around IV site in the event of extravasation of a Levophed drip in order to prevent sloughing of tissue. May cause angina, hypotension, shock, or acute MI. May activate a peptic ulcer. Hypotension may be treated with Levophed.

*Note that the dosage is *micrograms,* not milligrams.

rhage or occlusion are initial concerns. However, prevention of complications (e.g., such as arteriovenous fistulas and false aneurysms) is also important.

Recognition

- ▶ Blood loss usually obvious but may be concealed in closed injuries, e.g., fractures. (*Note*: if artery completely severed and the ends have contracted, bleeding may have stopped.)
- ▶ History of mechanism of injury.
- ▶ Hypotension or profound shock.
- ▶ Pallor, mottled cyanosis, coolness, pulselessness of extremity distal to the injury. These findings difficult to evaluate with profound shock or with pre-existing peripheral vascular disease.
- ▶ Numbness, tingling, nerve pain.
- ▶ Widening of mediastinum on chest x-ray with thoracic aortic disruption.
- ▶ Increase in abdominal girth, back pain, ecchymosis of flank, with damage to abdominal aorta.

Management

- ▶ Insure adequate airway.
- ▶ Assess wound for bleeding, foreign bodies, etc.
- ▶ Stop bleeding by: applying direct pressure for at least several minutes; using a pressure dressing, or applying pressure at pressure points. Tourniquet may be used as last resort. Blind clamping of a vessel is generally contraindicated.
- ▶ Insert 1 or 2 large bore IV catheters; hang Ringer's lactate; avoid inserting IV on same side as injury.
- ▶ Lab studies: CBC, T&C, clotting studies, arterial blood gases if hypotensive.
- ▶ Type-specific, uncrossmatched blood or O positive blood may be needed with massive blood loss.
- ▶ Vital signs every 5–10 minutes until stable; assess and mark (with an X) pulses; re-evaluate frequently.
- ▶ Ultrasound to evaluate vessel integrity.
- ▶ Assess motor and sensory function.
- ▶ Measure abdominal girth if abdominal aortic laceration suspected.

- Tetanus prophylaxis if a wound is present.
- Antibiotics usually started if penetrating wound.
- Arteriography may be indicated if time permits.
- Surgery may be done urgently or within 12 hours.
- Fasciotomy may be carried out if signs of compartmental syndrome develop.

Degenerative Vascular Disorders

The most common disorders of this type requiring emergency management are (a) arterial and venous occlusion, and (b) leaking or dissecting aortic aneurysms.

Arterial Occlusion. Often caused by an embolus — usually at the bifurcations of major vessels, e.g., femoral, popliteal, carotid arteries. (See Figure 48–6, p. 1105.) Patients over age 50 years with arteriosclerotic peripheral vascular disease and cardiac dysrhythmias, especially atrial fibrillation, are at greater risk. Measures to restore distal blood flow must be carried out promptly.

Recognition

- Sudden onset of pain, pallor, pulselessness, paresthesia, and coolness of affected extremity. Numbness, difficulty moving involved extremity.
- CVA-like symptoms in carotid artery occlusion.
- Doppler exam shows diminished or absent blood flow.
- Collapsed veins, decreased capillary refill in affected limb. Tenderness at site of occlusion.

Management

- Prompt surgical repair to prevent gangrene.
- Frequent assessment of extremity's color and temperature.
- Lab studies: ECG, CBC, clotting studies, T&C, etc.
- Cardiac monitor; treat cardiac arrhythmias.
- Arteriography to identify occlusion site and to evaluate collateral circulation.
- Prepare patient for surgery.
- Keep extremity straight; if femoral occlusion is suspected, keep patient flat with no bending at hips.

Ruptured or Dissecting Aortic Aneurysm. An aneurysm is an outpouching of a vessel wall, usually resulting from arteriosclerotic changes or trauma involving the tunica media (the muscular layer of an artery). The abdominal aorta is commonly affected, most often in males over age 60. Aneurysms may be saccular or fusiform and may leak, rupture, or dissect. (See Figure 48–1, p. 1100.) A *saccular aneurysm* balloons out to one side, whereas a *fusiform aneurysm* encircles the vessel. In a *dissection*, blood separates the vessel layers and a larger portion of the vessel may be affected.

> *Few emergencies require as rapid and efficient recognition and management as a dissecting or ruptured aneurysm; effective team functioning and communication is vital.*

Recognition (Abdominal Aortic Aneurysm)

- Extremely severe abdominal pain and back pain if aneurysm is leaking. Back pain often due to irritation, as blood accumulates in retroperitoneal space. *Extreme pain* is experienced, indicating a catastrophic event. Narcotics may be of no value in pain relief but may be administered liberally.
- Enlarging abdominal girth; palpable pulsatile abdominal mass.
- Leg numbness, tingling, loss of motor function.
- Mottled cyanosis below level of aneurysm.
- Hematuria; reduced urine output.
- Profound hypotension is typical; however, occasionally initial hypertension.
- Normal or diminished distal pulses. (*Note*: If the aneurysm dissects upward into the thoracic aorta, blood pressure on one arm may differ significantly; chest pain is also usually present.)
- Extreme apprehension, anxiety, and restlessness.

Management

- Speed is vital.
- Start oxygen (usually only nasal prongs tolerated).
- Start 2–4 large bore IV's and hang Ringer's lactate; avoid fluid overloading.
- CVP line and arterial line.
- Lab studies: CBC, *T&C for 10–20 units of whole blood,* electrolytes, BUN, sugar, creatinine, coagulation screen, UA, ABG's; ECG; portable chest and abdominal films.
- Vital signs at least every 5 minutes.
- Foley catheter (monitor output every 15–30 minutes).
- Cardiac monitor.
- Antihypertensive agents used with a dissection to minimize extension of the dissection.
- *Psychologic support.* Even though critically ill, these patients are often awake, alert and agitated; provide reassurance, explanations, and opportunity to see significant others and clergy if desired.
- Inform operating room and lab of urgency of this problem.
- If diagnosis unclear and patient somewhat stable, aortogram may be done; a nurse must provide care during this procedure.
- Transport to operating room quickly, with resuscitative personnel in attendance and emergency laporotomy tray on stretcher.
- Occasionally (and hopefully rarely!) if a patient arrests, and is thus unconscious, there may be no

time to reach the OR, and the abdomen or chest may be opened in the ED in hopes of saving a patient by cross clamping the aorta. Insure that necessary instruments are readily available. (*Note*: All nursing units that might have patients with abdominal aneurysms should have a large, sterile, pre-assembled, scalpel blade and handle immediately available.)

POISONING AND OVERDOSE*

Accidental or intentional poisonings requiring emergency care frequently occur.

Also, phone inquiries are often directed to ED staff. It is thus important that nurses responsible for emergency care be knowledgeable about the management and complications of poisonings and overdoses. Various resources are available, e.g., Poison Control Centers, Poison Index, and toxicology texts. An emergency nurse should have a working knowledge of those agents commonly used or abused, especially those street drugs currently popular.

*See references 11, 28, 77, 80, 83, 87, 92, 95, 124, 139, 140, 142a.

TABLE 95–10. ANTIDOTES COMMONLY USED IN MANAGING POISONED OR OVERDOSED PERSONS

Antidote	Substance
Atropine	Cholinesterase inhibitors, e.g., organophosphate insecticides, nerve gases
Deferoxamine	Iron
Dextrose 50%	Insulin
Dimercaprol (BAL)	Mercury, arsenic, lead
Ethanol	Methanol
EDTA (Ethylenediamine tetra acetic acid)	Lead
Levallorphan (Lorfan)	Narcotics and narcotics derivatives
Nalorphine (Nalline)	Narcotics, e.g., opiates
Naloxone (Narcan)	Narcotics and narcotic derivatives
Nitrates and nitrites	Cyanide
Oxygen	Carbon monoxide
2 PAM (Protopam)	Cholinesterase inhibitors
Physostigmine (Antilirium)	Atropine, scopolamine, tricyclic anti-depressants
Sodium thiosulfate	Cyanide
Vitamin K	Anticoagulants, e.g., warfarin, coumadin

NOTE: Acetylcysteine (Mucomyst), administered orally, has recently been found to be effective in minimizing liver damage following acetaminophen ingestion; however, its use is currently experimental.

TABLE 95–11. SIGNS AND SYMPTOMS ASSOCIATED WITH VARIOUS TOXINS

Physical Signs or Symptoms	Toxins To Be Considered
Vomiting, nausea, diarrhea	Heavy metals (lead, arsenic); alcohols (ethanol, methanol, ethylene glycol); salicylates; digitalis; morphine and its analogs
Coma	Barbiturates; chloral hydrate; paraldehyde; bromide; ethchlorvynol; carbon monoxide; salicylates; atropine; scopolamine; ethanol
Delirium, agitation	Atropine; scopolamine; alcohol; amphetamine; barbiturates; physostigmine
Convulsions	Phenothiazines; strychnine; propoxyphene; amphetamines; alcohols (ethanol, methanol, ethylene glycol); salicylates; carbon monoxide; cholinesterase inhibitors; hydrocarbons
Dilated pupils	Amphetamines; glutethimide; alcohols; belladonna group; meperidine; cocaine; ephedrine; sympathomimetics; parasympatholytics; cyanide; botulin toxin
Constricted pupils	Morphine; propoxyphene; barbiturates; chloral hydrate
Partial or total blindness	Methanol
Pink skin	Carbon monoxide; cyanide; atropine (skin flushed and dry); phenothiazine
Kussmaul respiration	Salicylates; methanol; ethanol; ethylene glycol
Dry mouth	Belladonna group; botulin toxin; antihistamines; morphine; phenothiazines; tricyclic antidepressants
Hematemesis	Mercuric chloride; salicylates; phosporus; fluoride
Diaphoresis	Alcohol; insulin; fluoride; salicylates physostigmine
Extrapyramidal tremor	Phenothiazines

From Cohen, A. S., R. B. Freidin, and M. A. Samuels: *Medical Emergencies: Diagnostic and Management Procedures from Boston City Hospital.* Boston: Little, Brown and Company, 1977.

A discussion of the signs, symptoms, management and complications of the many agents involved in overdoses or poisonings is beyond the scope of this text; however, general guidelines for the management of overdosed/poisoned persons are summarized. Information about commonly used antidotes is listed in Table 95–10. Signs and symptoms associated with various toxins are included in Table 95–11.

Guidelines for the Care of an Overdosed/Poisoned Patient

The acronym "SIRES" is an aid to remembering the essential care in cases of poisoning:

Stabilize the patient's condition.
Identify the toxic substance.
Reverse its effect.
Eliminate the substance from the patient's body.
Support the patient (physically and psychologically).

- Stabilize patient: ABC's, respiratory support, O_2.
- Rapid physical exam, start IV's, obtain appropriate lab studies including toxicology, cardiac monitor, Foley catheter, ECG, CVP, etc.
- Obtain accurate history: was the substance inhaled, injected, ingested, sniffed, or confined to skin surfaces? How long ago, how much, what kind of environment was patient found in? Associated incidents, e.g., fire, trauma, near drowning, etc. History of prescribed medications, allergies, medical problems, state of physical and mental health.

> Caution: *Despite careful fact finding and detailed questioning, a history of the nature, amount, and time since ingestion of a toxic substance may be grossly inaccurate. Patients may exaggerate or minimize the conditions of an overdose in order to achieve their own goals. The history is considered in planning care; however, reliance on physical findings is also important.*

- Select appropriate means of *reversing* or *eliminating* toxic substance: shower or wash off externally applied substances, e.g., organophosphate insecticides, radioactive substances. Injected substances such as heroin are treated with antidotes, e.g., Narcan. Ingested substances are treated with emesis, lavage, adsorptives, purgatives or cathartics. Induced emesis is used to treat alert patients with a good gag reflex who recently ingested the substance. *Although induced emesis is more effective than gastric lavage, it is contraindicated in patients with depressed levels of consciousness and in persons who have ingested corrosives. It is controversial in the management of hydrocarbon (petroleum based) substances.* Emesis may be produced by: (1) syrup of Ipecac or (2) apomorphine.
- *Syrup of Ipecac* is a safe, effective emetic when used in properly selected patients. The dose is 15–30 ml. (depending upon patient's age) administered orally, preceded or/and followed by several hundred milliliters of water or other solution, e.g., juice. Walk the patient if safe to do so; this may enhance the emetic's action. Emesis usually occurs within 15–20 minutes; however, a second dose can be given 20 minutes after the first dose. More than two doses of syrup of Ipecac should not be given. It is important that enough oral fluids (several glasses) be given to prevent retching and possible esophageal tears. Save emesis for possible toxicological analysis; note presence or absence of pill particles.

> Cautions in the Use of Ipecac:
>
> 1. *Use only syrup of Ipecac, not Ipecac Fluid Extract.*
> 2. *Always check patient's gag reflex before giving Ipecac. Do not assume the physician has done this.*
> 3. *Ipecac may be ineffective in inducing emesis following phenothiazine ingestions, since phenothiazines have antiemetic properties.*
> 4. *Ipecac, in large doses, may be cardiotoxic; lavage should be done if emesis does not occur.*
> 5. *Frequently reassess the patient; someone who was awake when the Ipecac was administered may be obtunded when emesis occurs and aspiration may result.*
> 6. *Ipecac is most effective when adequate amounts of oral fluids are administered.*

- *Apomorphine* is a rapid-acting emetic administered SC or IM in doses of 0.1 mg/kg.[107, 142b] Emesis usually begins within 10 minutes after administration. Only one dose is recommended. As with Ipecac, oral fluids should be provided. Apomorphine is a sedative and a respiratory depressant. It is contraindicated in persons with CNS and/or respiratory depression. The depressant effects of apomorphine may be reversed with naloxone (Narcan) as soon as adequate emesis is achieved.

Gastric Lavage. Gastric lavage involves insertion of a large bore (30–36 Fr. in adults) Ewald tube through the nose or mouth and then washing out the stomach contents using normal saline, half saline (0.45% NaCl), or tap water. (*Note:* Difference of opinion exists concerning appropriate fluid.) Gastric lavage is believed to be less effective than emesis in removing ingested substances from the stomach. Thus, gastric lavage is reserved for use in patients with CNS depression, diminished or absent gag reflex, or patients unable to cooperate with emetic therapy. *Gastric lavage is contraindicated in patients who have ingested corrosives, because of the danger of esophageal perforation by the tube.* The volume of each "run" of fluid instilled into the stomach varies from patient to patient; recommendations range from 250 ml. to 500 ml. Volumes in excess of 500 ml. should be avoided because large volumes may foster passage of the ingested substance into the duodenum. Lavage is carried out until the fluid return is clear and, although larger amounts are sometimes used, the normal volume rarely exceeds 10 liters.

An effective, time-saving, and accurate system for gastric lavage is illustrated in Figure 95–21. The system includes bags of NS irrigation fluid, tubing, a Y connector, clamps, and a collecting system. When such a system is utilized, gastric lavage can safely and effectively be carried out by one person with a minimum of difficulty.

Gastric lavage is not without hazard. Death due to inadvertent pulmonary placement of the tube and subsequent instillation of lavage fluid has been reported, and bradyrhythmias and aspiration of gastric fluid are not uncommon complications of this procedure.

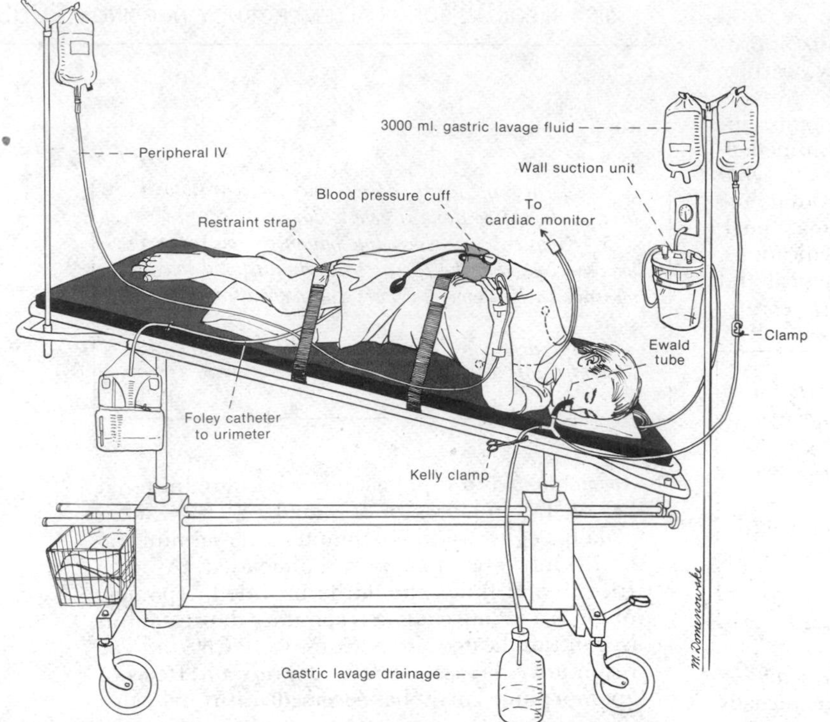

Figure 95–21. Position of the patient and location of equipment during gastric lavage in poisoning/overdose management. The patient is shown uncovered for illustration purposes.

Precautions that should be considered during tube placement and gastric lavage include:

- ▶ Explain the procedure and try to elicit patient cooperation.
- ▶ Place an endotracheal tube, with cuff inflated, prior to insertion of the Ewald tube in patients with CNS depression or diminished gag reflex.
- ▶ Lubricate Ewald tube end liberally with water-soluble jelly when inserting tube nasally. An anesthetic agent, e.g., lidocaine jelly, may make insertion more comfortable for a responsive patient.
- ▶ Insert Ewald tube *slowly* and *gently*; forceful insertion may cause significant tissue trauma and epistaxis.
- ▶ Emesis often occurs when the Ewald tube reaches the posterior pharynx. Be prepared to immediately suction the airway using a firm suction tip, such as a Yankauer or tonsil tip suction device.
- ▶ Vagal stimulation and subsequent cardiac arrhythmias may occur during tube passage in the posterior pharynx. Continuous cardiac monitoring is indicated and atropine may be administered prophylactically.
- ▶ Once the tube has passed the posterior pharynx, it is customary to position patient on the left side in a three-quarter prone position, with the stretcher in Trendelenburg. It is believed this position minimizes passage of gastric contents into the duodenum and also prevents aspiration of stomach contents into the lung in the event of emesis.
- ▶ Secure Ewald tube with adhesive tape; insert bite block if tube placed orally.
- ▶ *If* patient restraint is *necessary* during the procedure, secure all four extremity restraints on the same side of the stretcher; *avoid restraining a patient in a "spread eagle" position as quick turning onto one side may be very difficult in the event of emesis.*
- ▶ Aspirate stomach contents to insure proper tube placement; save all gastric aspirate for possible toxicological analysis.
- ▶ Clamp outflow tubing and allow a maximum of 500 ml. of fluid to enter stomach. Carefully observe patient's response to fluid inflow. Stop inflow if retching, vomiting, tachycardia, or other signs of intolerance occur.
- ▶ When recommended amount of fluid has been instilled into stomach, clamp inflow tubing and unclamp outflow tubing, allowing gastric drainage to flow to drainage container.
- ▶ Note whether outflow volume equals inflow volume and reposition tube if outflow volume is significantly less than inflow volume.
- ▶ Continue to lavage until return fluid is clear; save lavage fluid for possible analysis.
- ▶ Record total fluid volume instilled and note any discrepancies in total volume returned. Advise physician of any differences in inflow and outflow volumes.
- ▶ When large volumes of lavage fluid are necessary, serum electrolytes and/or arterial blood gases may be obtained during, or at completion of, gastric lavage.
- ▶ Frequently re-evaluate patient, including vital signs, urine output, cardiac rhythm, level of consciousness, etc., at least every 15 minutes.
- ▶ When tube is placed orally, many patients have increased oral secretions, and frequent suctioning may be necessary; apply gentle suction on Ewald tube as it is withdrawn.

Gastric lavage is employed when emetic therapy cannot be used. It is not a deterrent to future overdose attempts and should not be used as a punitive measure.

- *Gut lavage*[21] is a fairly new therapy sometimes used in managing selected poisonings. Presently it is not routinely used for persons who have ingested toxic substances. Gut lavage is carried out by instilling a warmed electrolyte solution into the stomach via a tube and is regulated by a peristaltic pump delivering approximately 75 ml./min. The goal of gut lavage is to rid the bowel of toxic substances.
- *Adsorptives*. Activated charcoal powder, usually mixed with water, is administered in dosages of 15–30 Gr. to adsorb any remaining particles of toxic substance. This may be administered orally or inserted through the Ewald tube. Since it is black and does not easily mix in water, activated charcoal may be mixed with cherry syrup or similar substances to make it more appealing, especially for children. Although it would seem ideal to mix the charcoal with ice cream, this binds approximately 25% of the charcoal.
- When cathartics are indicated as part of treatment, charcoal may be mixed with the cathartic. *Ipecac and charcoal should not be administered together*, since ipecac is inactivated by the charcoal. Additionally, insure that emesis has ceased before administering the activated charcoal.
- *Cathartics* may be administered in order to hasten excretion of a toxic substance and thus minimize further absorption from the bowel. Commonly used cathartics are magnesium sulfate, sodium sulfate and magnesium citrate. Oil-based cathartics (castor oil) are contraindicated because of the danger of aspiration pneumonitis.
- *Antidotes/Antagonists*. Only a few agents are used as antidotes in managing toxic substance ingestion. Some are used for diagnosis as well as treatment. The most dramatic is Narcan for opiate overdoses. Remember that although an antidote may produce significant results *initially*, the half life of the ingested substance may be longer than that of the antidote. Thus, a patient who responds well to Narcan initially may become obtunded as the Narcan wears off. *Patients receiving antidotes/antagonists must hence be observed for several hours before being discharged*. The more commonly used antidotes are listed in Table 95–10.
- *Other measures*. Depending upon the: (a) patient's condition, (b) nature of ingested substance, and (c) length of time since ingestion, a variety of other treatment measures may be employed, including: diuresis, fluid loading, cooling or warming measures, anticonvulsive therapy, antiarrhythmic therapy, hemodialysis, hemoperfusion, or exchange transfusions.

Nursing care involves frequent assessment of many parameters, carrying out therapies, and providing supportive care.

Some professionals have difficulty dealing with people who intentionally overdose, and they are ill at ease with these patients. The patient and significant others need empathy and understanding. Vindictive or hostile attitudes toward the patient are destructive and maximize the patient's feelings of guilt and low self-esteem. If the patient is awake, one way of fostering communication is to say, "You must have been feeling badly to do this." The patient may then feel able to talk about problems and be more receptive to psychiatric help. Remember that suicidal attempts may be repeated while the patient is receiving care for the overdose; suicide precautions should be exercised.

Psychiatric evaluation is indicated for all persons who intentionally overdose or whose intentions were unclear. The evaluation should occur before discharge. Also, plans for follow-up care should be well established. Available support systems should be investigated and utilized. Someone should stay with the patient for the next several days. Provide a phone number for the crisis team or clinic.

Patient/Family Teaching. Capitalize on the opportunity to prevent future accidental poisonings, especially in small children. The following aspects of teaching might be appropriate:

- Syrup of Ipecac should be readily available in all households where children live or visit. Although usually available without a prescription, consider providing the family with a bottle of Ipecac and insure that directions for use are well understood.
- Give phone number of nearest Poison Control Center or other appropriate care facility.
- Discuss location of household cleaners and poisonous substances with parents. Such agents are often stored under kitchen or bathroom sinks — readily accessible to a young child. Encourage parents to move dangerous substances to high shelves and/or install sturdy, "childproof" locks on doors of these cabinets. It is helpful if "Mr. Yuk" or other warning stickers are available in the ED and are given to parents with the recommendation that these stickers be placed on all containers containing dangerous substances. These stickers may be available at such places as Poison Control Centers, some drug stores, and government health agencies.
- *Childproof caps*. The incidence of ASA "aspirin" ingestion among young children has significantly decreased in communities using childproof caps for medicine bottles. However, many adults find the caps cumbersome and leave them off bottles. Encourage proper use of safety caps and the locking of medicines in high cupboards.
- Avoid placing or storing toxic substances in containers normally used for food items.
- Advise family that many house, garden and wild plants are poisonous and should be removed from children's environments. Familiarize yourself with poisonous plants in your area.

OCULAR EMERGENCIES*

These common emergencies (involving the eye and surrounding structures) range from mild corneal abrasions to avulsion of the eye. Ocular emergencies have a high priority. *General guidelines* used in assessing ocular trauma include: (1) history, including mechanism of injury, presence of foreign body, possibility of chemical burns; (2) amount of pain; (3) visual acuity with and without corrective lenses (if possible); (4) need to adequately anesthetize the eye to perform adequate evaluation and treatment; (5) need to evert upper eyelid to assess for foreign bodies; and (6) awareness that there may be associated injuries to other structures. (See also Chapter 89.)

Chemical Burns of the Eye. Prompt attention is needed to minimize eye damage caused by chemicals. Often, assessment and management are concurrent. *Speed is vital, especially in alkali burns, which continue to penetrate and destroy tissue.*

Recognition

- Acids immediately coagulate protein; an area of demarcation may be noted.
- Alkali substances continue to damage tissue after initial contact; opacification of corneal tissue sometimes occurs, e.g., with strong alkali burns.
- Conjunctiva often reddened; severe pain.
- Copious tearing unless deeper structures involved.
- Patient history important.

Management

- Tell patient your plans; immediately irrigate eye *copiously* with normal saline, water, or other mild solution. The eye's pH may be frequently tested and used to guide irrigation; irrigation may be continued until pH is in range of 6–7.
- Often necessary to use a short acting local anesthetic in order to adequately irrigate the eye.
- Evert upper lid in order to observe for and remove chemical particles; this is especially important in alkali burns.
- Alkali burns may need continuous irrigation for many hours; special irrigation lens devices are available. A pulsation lavage at the lowest possible setting, e.g., Water Pik, is sometimes used for eye irrigation.
- Antibiotic drops, ointments, or irrigants may be used.
- Pain with eye injuries often due to blepharospasm; a mydriatic (e.g., Homatropine, Cyclogel) may relieve pain.
- Patch both eyes if necessary to immobilize one eye. (Eye patch application discussed on p. 2208.)
- Patient safety is important (e.g., stretcher siderails up and secured; call light within patient's reach).
- Significant burns, e.g., alkali burns, are usually referred to ophthalmologist; hospital admission not uncommon.
- *Patient/family teaching*: (1) remind that eye patch reduces peripheral vision, thus patient should not operate an automobile or other machinery; (2) how to instill drops or ointments; (3) proper eye patching technique and where to obtain necessary supplies; (4) importance of follow-up care, usually within 24 hours.

Flash Burns. Flash burns or welder's burns result from exposure to ultraviolet light and commonly occur in persons using sun lamps or welding torches without eye protection.

Recognition

- Extreme pain and photosensitivity to even low, diffuse light; copious tearing. Multiple, small, puncture lesions of cornea noted with fluorescein staining.

Management

- Darken room for comfort.
- Anesthetic drops to obtain an adequate visual acuity and a satisfactory examination.
- Mydriatic agent (e.g., Homatropine or Clyclogel) to relieve blepharospasm; cool, moist packs are also helpful.
- Oral sedatives and/or narcotic analgesics.
- Bilateral patching.
- *Patient/family teaching*: same as for chemical burns; however, many welders have their own supply of anesthetic drops.

> *It is essential that the patient understand that while anesthetic agents relieve pain, they also prevent healing of the cornea. Thus, they may facilitate further eye injury, and should be used only on recommendation of a physician. Topical anesthetic agents are rarely prescribed for home use.*

Foreign Bodies. Include surface, imbedded, and impaled objects. Usually only surface foreign bodies are managed by a nurse. Obviously imbedded or impaled objects are managed initially by immobilizing the eye and head, immobilization of the impaled object, and protection of any exposed ocular tissue with moist saline dressings and an airtight covering.

Recognition

- Sensation of "something in the eye." Often history is compatible with a foreign body. Pain and tearing may be present.

*See references 41, 50, 63, 123.

- Insure removal of contact lenses.
- Apply local anesthetic drops.
- Inspect eye using magnifying glass. Double evert eyelid to look for foreign body.
- Stain eye with fluorescein dye by moistening the end of a fluorescein strip with a drop of irrigating fluid and touching lower conjunctival sac with the strip; dye will flood into eye.
- Darken room and examine cornea using a blue light or a Wood's lamp. This turns the orange fluorescein green, and the dye concentrates in the area of any irritated corneal tissue.

> Caution: *(1) Never apply fluorescein to an eye with a soft contact lens in place. Fluorescein may permanently stain and discolor lens. (2) Make sure fluoroscein is rinsed out after examination; failure to do so may result in a chemical conjunctivitis.*

- Remove small *foreign bodies* with a moistened cotton tip applicator; stop if unable to remove them after a few tries.
- Small foreign bodies that cannot be removed with an applicator may be *very gently and carefully* removed with the point of a small hypodermic needle, e.g., 25 or 27 gauge, or with an "eye spud," a fine-pointed instrument designed specifically for this purpose.
- After removal of the foreign body, corneal abrasion is treated if present. Treatment includes antibacterial eye drops or ointment and patching of the eye; a mydriatic is indicated if there is significant pain. Follow-up in 24 hours, if pain still present.
- Assessment of visual acuity should be completed and recorded before patient leaves the ED.
- *Impaled foreign bodies* are left intact until removed by an ophthalmologist. Stabilize the object by applying dressings (moistened with normal saline) around the base of the object and securing the object to the patient's head. Avoid exerting pressure on the globe and immobilize the patient's head.
- Do not attempt to stop bleeding from the eye or eyelids by applying direct pressure – this can cause further injury.
- *Contact lenses* may become dislodged, making removal by the patient very difficult. (See also Chapter 89.) The lenses are often found under the upper eyelid. If the lens is a *hard lens* and cannot be slid back over the cornea, a suction device can be used.[63] A *soft contact lens* is removed by sliding the lens off the cornea laterally and, since it is flexible, pinching the lens and removing it from the eye. The suction device is not used on soft lenses, because it may damage them. Unlike hard lenses, soft lenses do not have markings indicating whether they are for the left or right eye, so it is important that they be placed in well marked containers. The container should contain sterile saline solution *without preservative* since soft lenses become brittle and crack when allowed to dry.

Avulsion of the Eye. Avulsion of the eye from its socket may result from either blunt or penetrating trauma. Even with rapid and expert care, the probability of preserving vision in the affected eye is slim.

Recognition

- Extrusion of eye from orbit; gross deformity; pain. Loss of visual acuity may or may not be present.

Management

- Protect eye from drying by gently applying sterile dressing moistened with warm saline.
- Apply an eye protector (e.g., cone, shield, or paper cup) and secure it gently to patient's head using Kling or Kerlix.
- Patch unaffected eye and immobilize head.
- Provide reassurance but do not give false hopes about saving the eye.
- Promptly refer to ophthalmologist.
- Prepare patient for surgery; keep NPO.

Retinal Detachment. (See also p. 1984.)

Recognition

- History of flashes of light, floating black spots, curtain-like defects causing diminished peripheral vision.
- Central visual acuity may be normal. Detachment may be noted upon ophthalmoscopic examination.

Management

- Place patient at bed rest; immobilize head; patch both eyes.
- Prompt evaluation by ophthalmologist.

Hyphema. Accumulation of blood in the anterior chamber of the eye, often resulting from blunt trauma. Glaucoma and permanent loss of vision are concerns.

Recognition

- History of blunt or penetrating eye trauma.
- Blood/fluid level in eye's anterior chamber is usually fairly obvious upon direct and lateral visualization of the eye (Fig. 95–22). In severe cases, entire chamber may be filled with blood.
- Degree of vision loss depends on size of the hyphema.
- Somnolence, unrelated to head injury.[16]
- Elevated intraocular pressure.

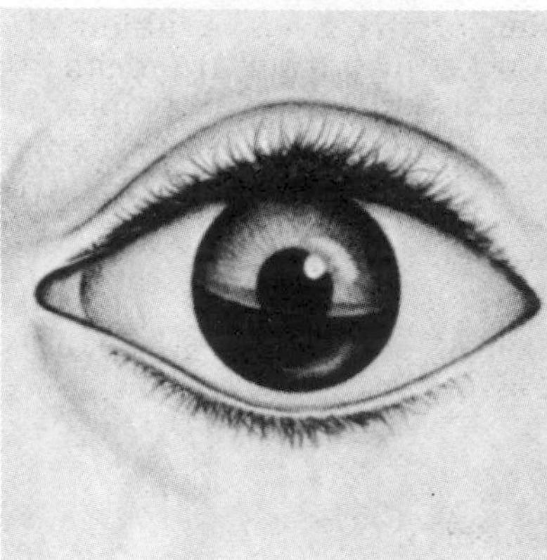

Figure 95–22. A hyphema is an accumulation of blood in the anterior chamber of the eye, often as a result of trauma to the orbit caused by a blunt object. The blood usually collects at the bottom of the eye and a fluid level is easily noted. (From DuPont, J.: What to do for common eye emergencies. *Nursing 76*, 6(5):17, May, 1976.)

Management

- Initially no dilating or constricting drops should be used; they may promote bleeding.
- Patch both eyes.
- Sedation sometimes used to minimize movement and prevent further bleeding.
- Bed rest; head of bed elevated 30 degrees.
- Restriction of activities for 4 or 5 days to foster absorption of the hyphema and prevent further bleeding; hospitalization may be appropriate.
- Medications such as Diamox may be administered to reduce intraocular pressure.
- Frequent re-evaluation by ophthalmologist is extremely important.

Blow Out Fracture of the Orbit. Results from blunt trauma to the eye, with a force that causes fracture of the floor of the orbit, the weakest part of the bony structure of the eye. The inferior rectus and the inferior oblique muscles are easily trapped in the fracture and restriction of eye movement may result.

Recognition

- Usually associated with significant eye trauma; contusion, ecchymosis may be present.
- Deformity of lower orbital rim; i.e., affected eye may appear to be lower than normal eye. Patient is usually unable to look upward; diplopia may be present.

Management

- X-ray to confirm diagnosis. Special views may be needed to visualize the fracture; inform x-ray technician of possible diagnosis.
- Surgical repair and support of orbital floor by ophthalmologist.

Applying Eye Patches. Eye patches are applied to limit eye movement, to promote healing, and to protect the eye. Carefully applied patches aid in patient recovery, whereas poorly applied patches may cause further damage.

Insure that all makeup (e.g., mascara, eye shadow) has been removed and the area cleaned. Place patient in supine position with table or stretcher at a good working height. Have all equipment readily available on a Mayo table or other stand. Instill any prescribed medication and dry area around eye. Have patient close both eyes normally.

Apply patch in the following steps:

- Fold one eye patch in half lengthwise and place folded patch in hollow of affected socket. Have patient hold patch in place while you obtain the second patch.
- Place second patch over first patch, on the diagonal, again conforming patch to eye socket.
- Apply strips of paper tape over patch, starting at forehead, and placed diagonally across patch down toward side of face in front of ear.
- Repeat above step until 6 to 8 strips have been placed over the patch; some *gentle* pressure may be appropriate unless there is a possibility of a fluid leak or a foreign body in eye.
- A skin tackifier, e.g., tincture of benzoin, may be used on the face to promote sticking of adhesive tape used to keep the patch in place, but should be used with caution because of possible allergic reactions. Also take care *not* to get such substances in the eye. Apply the skin tackifier *after* the patch is placed over the eye and *before* applying tape.
- If patch is secure, patient will be unable to open the eye or raise the eyelid.
- Extra adhesive (paper) tape can be removed once the patch is secure.
- Some practitioners believe that more even pressure is obtained if placement of strips is alternated, e.g., first strip is started on forehead and second started in front of ear.

If a patient is to instill medications into the eye, show a significant other proper techniques both for medication administration and for repatching of eye. New eye patches should be used each time. Ensure that the necessary supplies are available.

ENT AND FACIAL EMERGENCIES*

Priorities of Care

- *Open and maintain adequate airway*. Special maneuvers may be necessary to maintain airway in persons with maxillofacial trauma. (1) Fracture of mandible may require application of a towel clip to the tongue and use of gentle, forward traction in order to open airway. (2) Airway obstruction

*See also Chapter 91.

Figure 95–23. Fractures of the maxilla. Mobility of the maxilla when pushing or pulling on the anterior alveolar process indicates a fracture of the maxilla. In a LeForte III fracture, the whole of each infraorbital rim moves with the maxilla. In a LeForte II fracture, only the medial section of each infraorbital rim moves with the maxilla. In a LeForte I fracture, the whole orbital complex remains stable. (From American College of Surgeons Committee on Trauma: *Early Care of the Injured Patient.* Philadelphia: W. B. Saunders Co., 1972, p. 113.)

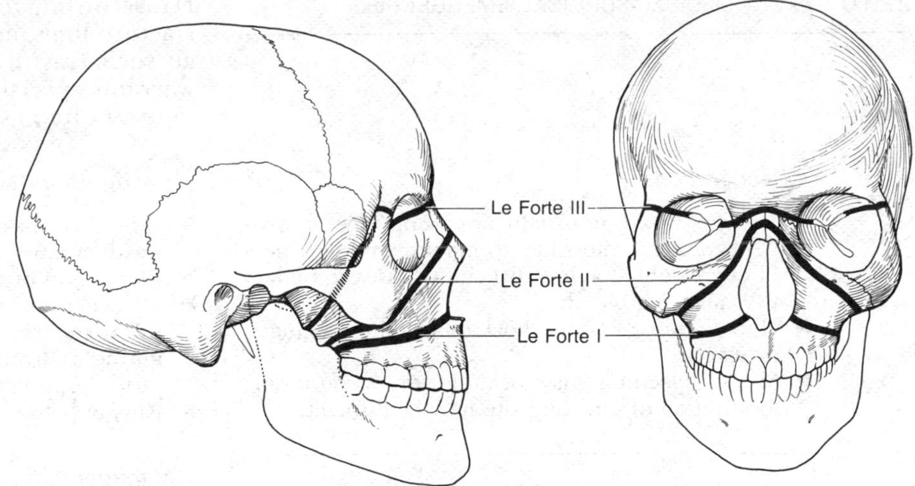

may occur with maxillary fractures due to posterior displacement of bone and soft tissue. This is especially true in a *LeFort III fracture* (Fig. 95–23), known as a "mid-face mash," with fracture of the maxilla, nasal bones, and zygoma and "complete separation of the facial bones from their cranial attachments."[84] Airway obstruction may be relieved by applying gentle forward traction against the soft palate. (3) In severe maxillofacial trauma with much tissue destruction, it may be necessary to perform a *cricothyroidotomy (coniotomy)* or a *tracheotomy.* (Refer to Fig. 95–2, p. 2152.)

> Caution: *Patients with maxillofacial trauma may also have cervical spine injury. Thus, usual airway positioning maneuvers may be dangerous in these patients.*

- ▶ Be alert for head, spinal, and other injuries.
- ▶ *Control bleeding*, using one of the following methods: (1) elevate head of bed, (2) apply firm gentle pressure, (3) pinch nostrils together if safe to do so, (4) insert nasal packing, or (5) insert balloon tamponade device (Fig. 95–24).
- ▶ Physical assessment includes:
  1. Examine oral cavity; check occlusion of teeth.
  2. Gently palpate facial bones.
  3. Evaluate integrity of cranial nerves 3 through 7.*
  4. Examine ear; note presence of blood behind TM.
  5. Look for ecchymosis of mastoid process (Battle's sign), which may be associated with basilar skull fracture; lacerations of ear canal.
  6. Test nasal drainage for CSF.
  7. Assess visual acuity.
- ▶ X-rays of facial bones often require special views.

Epistaxis. Bleeding from the nose; onset may be spontaneous or secondary to trauma.

*See Chapter 25 (p. 496) for assessment of cranial nerves.

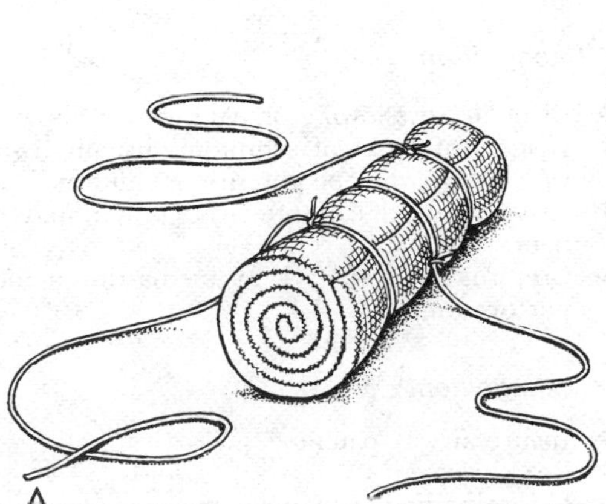

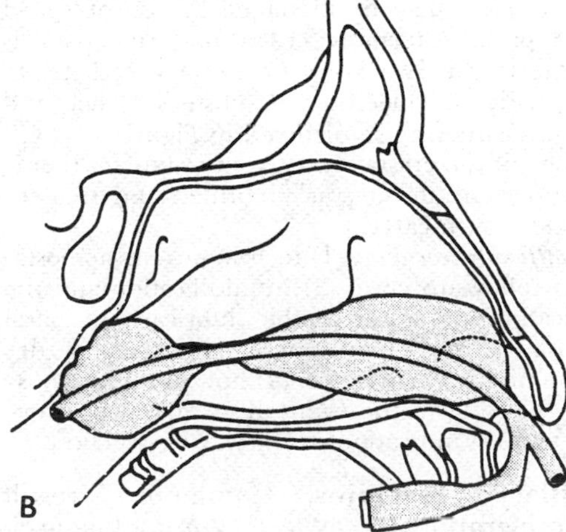

Figure 95–24. Devices used in the management of posterior epistaxis. **A.** A posterior pack made of rolled gauze. **B.** A ballooned anterior and posterior epistaxis catheter. (*A*, Cosgriff, J. H., Jr. and D. L. Anderson: *The Practice of Emergency Nursing.* Philadelphia: J. B. Lippincott Co., 1975, p. 429.) (*B*, courtesy Perry Co., a division of Affiliated Hospital Products, Inc., Massillon, Ohio.)

Recognition

- ▶ History. Bleeding usually apparent; however, patients often swallow blood, making an assessment of degree of blood loss difficult. Nausea secondary to swallowing blood.
- ▶ Hypotension or frank shock if bleeding prolonged or severe.
- ▶ Site of bleeding may be anterior or posterior; localization of bleeding site may be difficult.

> Caution: *Epistaxis may be the presenting symptom in a patient with a hypertensive crisis.*

Management

- ▶ Position patient in a sitting position unless hypotensive.
- ▶ Pinch nostrils together to apply pressure.
- ▶ Obtain postural vital signs.
- ▶ Protect patient's clothing.
- ▶ Hematocrit or hemoglobin ordered if bleeding significant; whole blood replacement sometimes necessary.
- ▶ Locally applied vasoconstrictors, e.g., cocaine or epinephrine, often used to control bleeding; silver nitrate cautery used occasionally.

> Caution: *Epinephrine applied locally for hemostasis should be used with caution; monitor vital signs carefully.*

- ▶ Nasal packing with nonadherent gauze, e.g., Vaseline gauze, often used for anterior bleeding; posterior bleeding may be managed by use of rolled gauze pack. Alternative to a posterior pack is short-term use of a Foley or epistaxis catheter to tamponade the bleeding. A posterior pack and epistaxis catheter are pictured in Figure 95–24.
- ▶ Etiology of the epistaxis, e.g., anticoagulant therapy, hypertension, etc., is identified and treated.
- ▶ Provide mouth care.
- ▶ *Patient/family teaching:* (1) techniques for hemostasis, (2) follow-up care, (3) humidification and the application of water-soluble lubricant to nasal mucosa if the environment is extremely dry may minimize recurrence, (4) how to remove posterior packing in the event of an airway obstruction, and (5) indications of airway obstruction.

Maxillary Fractures. Commonly result from deceleration forces, e.g., automobile accidents and plane crashes, where significant force is directed at the mid-face. These fractures may be classified as LeFort (or Le Forte) I, II, and III, according to the number and location of the fracture lines, as shown in Figure 95–22. While all such fractures are important, a LeFort III warrants special mention because of the serious injuries often associated with it.

Recognition (LeFort III)

- ▶ "Mid-face mash" — structures may be forced inward, creating a "dish-face" deformity.
- ▶ Elongation of face.
- ▶ Malocclusion of teeth. Significant edema and/or soft tissue trauma. Fractured segment may be very movable. Commonly associated with other injuries, especially CNS trauma.
- ▶ Airway patency may be compromised.

Management (LeFort III)

- ▶ Relieve airway obstruction due to posterior dislocation of fracture segment by applying gentle forward traction against soft palate.
- ▶ Start an IV and hang Ringer's lactate or 5% D/RL.
- ▶ Manage hemorrhage with catheters and/or packing.
- ▶ Ice packs to minimize swelling.
- ▶ Neurologic assessment.
- ▶ Attention to other injuries, e.g., head or orbital trauma. Usually repaired surgically by experienced team of physicians, often composed of ophthalmologist, otolaryngologist, and oral surgeon; surgeon specializing in plastic repair may also be included.

> Caution: *Fractures of this type rarely occur in isolation; other, more serious, injuries may be present and have priority once airway patency and hemorrhage management have been established.*

Foreign Body in the Esophagus. Commonly caused by bolus of meat or other substance containing bone. Esophageal perforation is a major concern.

Recognition

- ▶ Difficulty swallowing or pain with swallowing.
- ▶ History of onset of symptoms usually associated with eating, may be obscure in children.
- ▶ Area involved can often be pinpointed by patient.
- ▶ Crepitus around neck or mediastinum indicates perforation.

Management[4, 59]

- ▶ Insure airway patency.
- ▶ Reassurance.
- ▶ If foreign body is boneless piece of meat, and the obstruction just occurred, patient may be asked to swallow liquid meat tenderizer. This often softens meat enough so it can be swallowed.

Caution: *Since liquid meat tenderizer may act on traumatized esophageal tissue, it is* not *used if the foreign body has been present for some time or if perforation of esophagus is suspected, or may occur.*

- IV glucagon, which relaxes esophageal sphincters, has been proposed.[59]
- Neck or chest film.
- Barium swallow to localize foreign body if it is not readily visible, and to demonstrate tissue damage.
- Esophagoscopy.
- Surgical exploration and treatment if perforation demonstrated.

Caustic Substances Ingestion. Accidental or intentional ingestion of substances that cause significant tissue destruction, often involving mouth, posterior pharynx, esophagus and stomach. While both acids and alkaline substances may be caustic, alkali substances cause more damage, with deep tissue penetration and necrosis. Even with early, aggressive therapy, significant morbidity often results.

Recognition

- Accurate history; obtain container in which caustic substance was stored; ascertain pH of the caustic substance if possible.
- Examine patient's face, nose, mouth and posterior pharynx.

Caution: *The extent of esophageal and gastric injury cannot be determined by the amount of tissue damage to the lips and oral cavity.*[92]

Management

- Insure airway patency.
- Neutralizing agents such as milk or antacids may be administered; other "antidotes" may liberate heat of neutralization, resulting in further tissue damage.

Caution: *Information listed on the container of a caustic substance may be unreliable concerning treatment; contact a Poison Control Center for current management guidelines.*

- Soapy water, often listed as a neutralizing agent, is now believed to be contraindicated because it stimulates emesis, thus re-exposing the esophagus and posterior pharynx to the caustic substance; plain water may be used.
- Cardiovascular stabilization.
- A nasogastric tube (if indicated) should be inserted only by a physician, preferably an otolaryngologist; perforation of friable esophageal tissue is a hazard.
- Keep patient NPO except for antacids.
- Endoscopy is used to determine extent of damage.
- Steroids and antibiotics may be administered.
- Admission and observation for 24 hours may be recommended, even though the burns may appear minor.
- Psychiatric evaluation if ingestion was intentional.
- *Patient/family teaching* about prevention if ingestion was accidental.

DEATH AND DYING

Unlike deaths encountered elsewhere in the hospital, death in an emergency department is often sudden, dramatic, completely unanticipated, and particularly painful. The victims are often young previously healthy adults stricken in the prime of life. An emergency department death, called *D.I.E. (death in emergency)*, may be a student's first experience with death. There is often little time to interact with the patient, to provide grief and loss counseling. Because of the suddenness of the situation, patients and significant others probably will not have time for anticipatory grieving. Both patients and families often have denial; however, behaviors range from rage and physical violence to quiet acceptance.

Because the patient and significant others have not had time to prepare, talk, share ideas, resolve conflicts, and reaffirm love for one another, there may be remorse and anger about "not enough time" and "unfinished business." It is vitally important, then, that patients and significant others be given opportunities to be together and say the things they need to say. If, for example, endotracheal intubation is anticipated, and the patient is able to talk, allow the patient to talk with those who mean so much, if only for a moment, prior to intubation if possible.

Recently researchers have proposed a phenomenon of separation of the body and the spirit at the time of death, so called *"out of body experiences."* Persons who have been resuscitated from cardiac arrest may give accurate, vivid accounts of the resuscitation procedure, along with repeating verbatim words spoken by staff members during this time. The meaning and validity of such accounts is unclear; however, possible nursing implications are far-reaching. We must be concerned with our verbal communication, and with the value of touch, during these stressful times.

Many persons, regardless of whether they were deeply religious before, find comfort in religion at the time of death. Every opportunity should be provided for religious support if desired by the patient or significant others. Persons who are members of the Roman Catholic Church, or whose religion is unknown, may be given the Sacraments of the Sick. For some significant others, knowledge that the sacraments were received (either before or after death) is a source of comfort.

As mentioned earlier, it is important that significant others be aware of the seriousness of a patient's illness or injury so they can prepare themselves in some way for dealing with an inevitable death. Likewise, these individuals should be afforded privacy, comfort, and staff support, as well as assistance in anticipatory grieving and in making necessary preparations. *Viewing the body, particularly in instances of sudden death or trauma, is encouraged. This removes any doubt that the deceased actually was their loved one, and it facilitates the grieving process.* Since preservation of legal evidence (discussed later) is often important in sudden death, the significant others are advised beforehand of the various tubes and devices that are present on the patient. Also, the patient may not be cleaned prior to examination by the medical examiner.

Although it is often difficult for the staff, the significant others should be asked about the patient's wishes concerning organ donation. It is a source of comfort for some persons to know that others will be able to see or to have a kidney transplant and live a fuller life because of organ transplants. (*Note*: The patient's wallet or purse is checked for an organ donor card.) Since many emergency department deaths fall under the jurisdiction of the Medical Examiner or the Coroner, information concerning funeral arrangements is coordinated through that office.

It may be therapeutic for both the staff and significant others if a follow-up phone call or visit is planned. After several days the family may have questions or concerns relating to the emergency department activities, and they should be encouraged to call or visit if needed.

The use of tranquilizers for significant others is generally unwise. Such agents may actually delay the grieving process and resolution of death. The nurse may be more effective by assisting the significant others to explore and utilize their own support systems.

The emergency department staff likewise needs support. Personnel must be given the opportunity to express and share their angers, concerns, and frustrations. If at all possible, those involved in the resuscitation efforts should be offered this opportunity immediately after the event; feelings that are unexpressed for days are often destructive. There is a need for reinforcement that each member functioned well in the emergency and that everything possible was done for the patient. The expertise of a psychiatric clinical nurse specialist may also be used to assist staff in dealing with their feelings and concerns.

MEDICAL/LEGAL IMPLICATIONS OF EMERGENCY CARE*

> *In addition to providing physical care and psychologic support, the emergency department staff has a responsibility to protect the legal rights of individuals.*

The most common way this occurs is through preservation of evidence, particularly in instances of death, assault, and intoxication. While laws governing evidence vary from one jurisdiction to another, there are some common aspects. The following discussion centers around: (1) cases of Medical Examiner/Coroner jurisdiction; (2) handling of bullets; (3) collection of specimens for legal purposes; and (4) reportable conditions.

Medical Examiner/Coroner Jurisdiction. A medical examiner, a physician with special training in forensic pathology, is concerned with determining the manner and cause of death. Deaths associated with the following are *reported* to the medical examiner's office: (1) suspected suicides or homicides; (2) deaths in which the deceased had not been attended by a physician within 24 hours prior to death; (3) suspicious deaths; (4) deaths due to accidents; (5) deaths following surgery; (6) deaths associated with firearms or other weapons; (7) deaths occurring as a result of crime; (8) stillborns; (9) deaths resulting from drugs; (10) deaths possibly associated with hazards to public safety, e.g., infectious diseases that may cause epidemics.

When notified of a death, the medical examiner may accept or decline jurisdiction for determining the manner and cause of death. If jurisdiction is accepted, the medical examiner may conduct an autopsy or other investigation, or may grant the hospital caring for the patient permission to perform an autopsy. Permission of the family for post mortem examination in these cases is not required.

When the medical examiner plans to conduct the autopsy, it is important that *all evidence* be

*See references 40, 42, 61, 69.

preserved. This means that all tubes, instruments, devices, etc., are left in place, especially IV catheters. The patient is not washed, nails are not cleaned, and any body fluids on the patient at the time of death are left on the patient. Clothing is left on the patient. Clothing that has been removed is carefully folded and place in a *paper*, not a plastic, bag. (Plastic allows for decomposition of the clothing and obscures evidence.) When removing clothing, do not cut through the bullet holes or stab wound tears, or other tears. Do not wash the clothes. All valuables and clothing must be inventoried with the medical examiner's staff; only they may release these items to significant others. A receipt for valuables and clothing is given to the ED staff and should be included with the patient's medical record. The name and badge number of the medical examiner's staff or the police officers who take clothing and effects is written on the patient's medical record. A copy of the emergency department record is given to the medical examiner's staff. The record must be detailed, with special attention given to injuries, marks, etc., noted on arrival of the patient as well as a description and location of tubes, surgical incisions, venipunctures, and other therapeutic interventions.

Bullets. Bullets removed from a patient's body or recovered from clothing are handled with great care. When a bullet is removed from a person's body, the physician usually makes a mark on the bottom of the bullet. This identifying mark may be referred to later during an investigation or trial. The bullet is then placed in a bag. The bag is sealed so that removal of a seal will be obvious, labeled, and given to proper authorities. If a bullet must be kept in the emergency department for any reason, it is kept in a locked, secure place. All persons having access to the bullet must sign for it, thus maintaining a *chain of custody*. This information is also included on the patient's clinical record.

Specimens. Specimens obtained for legal purposes, as opposed to those obtained for medical purposes, are most often *blood alcohol levels,* and items obtained during the examination of a patient with alleged *sexual assault*, e.g., alleged rape. When a blood alcohol determination is desired by either the patient or legal authorities, the patient's written permission must be obtained before the specimen is drawn. A patient may not be forced into having a blood alcohol drawn. In many instances, police officers have a kit with the necessary equipment for drawing the specimen.

It is important that you do not use isopropyl alcohol or any antiseptic solution containing alcohol as a skin preparation prior to drawing a blood alcohol specimen. This may falsely elevate the blood alcohol and render the test invalid.

Once the specimen is drawn, it is handed to a police officer, who signs that the specimen has been received. The tube is sealed with an identifying mark placed on the seal. The chain of custody is similar to that listed above. Documentation of the procedure on the patient's clinical record, along with the nurse's signature and the name and badge number of the officer, is important. (Sexual assault is discussed on p. 2195.)

Reportable Conditions. Conditions that must be reported to medical or legal authorities vary from one locality to another. The following are most often reported: (1) gunshot or shotgun wounds; (2) stab wounds; (3) assault; (4) automobile accidents; (5) attempted homicide/suicide; (6) venereal disease; (7) contagious diseases (to the Center for Disease Control); (8) food-borne illnesses, e.g., salmonella, botulism; (9) suspected child abuse/neglect. Consult your agency's policy and procedure manuals to determine reportable instances and the method of reporting.

CONCLUSION

Providing emergency care is exciting, challenging, and gratifying. Because of the many problems requiring emergency care, nurses must assume responsibility and accountability for continually updating knowledge and skill. By possessing a knowledge of the principles of emergency care, nurses can function effectively, regardless of the environment in which the care is delivered. A nurse must also be constantly aware of the psychologic stresses experienced by the patient/significant others during emergency situations. Expert technical skill does not replace the need for the "caring" component of emergency care.

BIBLIOGRAPHY

1. *Accidental Death and Disability: The Neglected Disease of Modern Society.* National Academy of Sciences, Division of Medical Sciences, Washington, D.C., 1966.
2. Agris, J.: Traumatic tattooing. *Journal of Trauma,* 16:798, Oct. 1976.
3. Alberti, K. G.: Low dose insulin in the treatment of diabetic ketoacidosis. *Archives of Internal Medicine,* 137:1637, Oct. 1977.
4. Allen, T.: Suspected esophageal foreign body – choosing appropriate management. *JACEP,* 8:101, Mar. 1979.
5. American Academy of Orthopaedic Surgeons: *Emergency Care and Transportation of the Sick and Injured,* 2d ed. Menasha, Wis.: George Banta Company, 1977.
6. American College of Surgeons Committee on Trau-

ma: *Early Care of the Injured Patient.* Philadelphia: W. B. Saunders Co., 1976.

7. American Nurses' Association – Emergency Department Nurses Association: *Standards of Emergency Nursing Practice.* Kansas City, Missouri. American Nurses' Association, 1975.
8. Anderson, D. M., and J. H. Anderson: Epistaxis. *Journal of Emergency Nursing*, 2:9, July–Aug. 1976.
9. Anderson, E. R.: Women and cystitis. *Nursing 77*, 7:50, Apr. 1977.
10. Ansbaugh, P.: Emergency management of intoxicated patients with head injuries. *Journal of Emergency Nursing*, 3:9, May-June 1977.
11. Aronow, R., and A. K. Done: Phencyclidine overdose: an emerging concept of management. *JACEP*, 7:56, Feb. 1978.
12. Avila, S. M., et al.: Emergency management of vaginal bleeding. *Journal of Emergency Nursing*, 1:16, Nov.–Dec. 1975.
13. Bacchus, H.: *Metabolic and Endocrine Emergencies – Recognition and Management.* Baltimore: University Park Press, 1977.
14. Baker, F. G., II, et al.: Diabetic emergencies: hypoglycemia and ketoacidosis. *JACEP*, 5:119, Feb. 1976.
15. Bangs, C. C., M. P. Hamlet, and W. J. Mills: Help for the victim of hypothermia. *Patient Care,* 11:46, Dec. 1977.
16. Ballinger, W. F., II, R. B. Rutherford, and G. D. Zuidema (Eds.): *The Management of Trauma.* Philadelphia: W. B. Saunders Co., 1973.
17. Bates, B.: *A Guide to Physical Examination.* Philadelphia: J. B. Lippincott Co., 1978.
18. Bennett, R. M.: Drowning and near-drowning: Etiology and pathophysiology. *American Journal of Nursing*, 76:6, June 1976.
19. Berg, B., and D. Danzl: Peritoneal lavage and scintigraphic evaluation of blunt trauma. *JACEP*, 6:397, Sept. 1977.
20. Berry, J. (Ed.): *Emergency Nursing.* New York: McGraw-Hill Book Company, 1978.
21. Boba, A.: Management of drug overdosage. Rapid whole gut evacuation. *Illinois Medical Journal*, 155:156, Mar. 1979.
22. Bodily, K., et al.: The salvageability of patients with post-traumatic rupture of the descending aorta in a primary trauma center. *Journal of Trauma*, 17:754, Oct. 1977.
23. Boedeker, E., and J. Dauber (Eds.): *Manual of Medical Therapeutics.* Boston: Little, Brown and Company, 1974.
24. Bolin, K. L.: Assessing the status of neurological patients. *American Journal of Nursing*, 77:1478, Sept. 1977.
25. Botsford, T. W., and R. E. Wilson: *The Acute Abdomen: An Approach to Diagnosis and Management.* Philadelphia: W. B. Saunders Co., 1977.
26. Botulism hits the dirt. Emergency Medicine, 6:194, Jan. 1974.
27. Bouzarth, W. F.: Intracranial nasogastric tube insertion. *Journal of Trauma,* 18:818, Dec. 1978.
28. Budassi, S. A.: An emergency nurse's guide to drawing arterial blood gases. *Journal of Emergency Nursing*, 3:24, Jan.–Feb. 1977.
29. Burgess, A. W., and L. L. Holmstrom: Sexual assault: Signs and symptoms. *Journal of Emergency Nursing*, 1:10, Mar.–Apr. 1975.
30. Burgess, A. W., and A. T. Laslo: Courtroom use of hospital records in sexual assault cases. *American Journal of Nursing*, 77:64, Jan. 1977.
31. Bush, S.: Snakebite. *Emergency*, 11:72, May 1979.
32. Callaham, M. L.: Treatment of common dog bites: Infection risk factors. *JACEP*, 7:83, Mar. 1978.
33. Caudle, J. T.: Emergency nursing of the near-drowning victim. *American Journal of Nursing*, 76:6, June 1976.
34. Center for Disease Control, U.S. Public Health Service: Newest Treatment Schedules for Gonorrhea. *Medical Times*, 107:15d, Mar. 1979.
35. Clark, T. P.: Counseling victims of rape. *American Journal of Nursing,* 76:1964, Dec. 1976.
36. Cohen, A. S., et al.: *Medical Emergencies: Diagnostic and Management Procedures from Boston City Hospital.* Boston: Little, Brown and Company, 1977.
37. Condon, R. E., and L. M. Nyhus (Eds.): *Manual of Surgical Therapeutics.* Boston: Little, Brown and Company, 1975.
38. Cooke, C. W.: *Handbook of Gynecologic Emergencies. A Guide For Emergencies In Gynecology.* Flushing, New York: Medical Examination Publishing Company, Inc., 1975.
39. Cosgriff, J. H., Jr., and D. L. Anderson: *The Practice of Emergency Nursing.* Philadelphia: J. B. Lippincott Co., 1975.
40. Creighton, H.: Your legal risks in emergency care. *Nursing 78,* 8:52, Feb. 1978.
41. D'Acuti, D. L.: Eyes, ears, nose and throat emergencies: Triage and treatment. *Journal of Emergency Nursing,* 1:34, May-June 1975.
42. Davis, R. W., and J. E. Hooker: If the patient is a criminal. *American Journal of Nursing*, 7:1250, July 1979.
43. De Muth, W. E., et al.: Buckshot wounds. *Journal of Trauma,* 18:53, Jan. 1978.

43a. Delaney, M. T.: Examining the chest, Part I: the lungs. *Nursing 75*, 5:12, August, 1975.

44. De Santis, R.: How to spot a dissecting aneurysm. *Emergency Medicine*, 6:241, May 1974.
45. Dimick, A. R.: Emergency management of the acutely burned patient. *JACEP*, 3:23, Jan.–Feb. 1974.
46. Donovan, L.: Polyvinyl chloride. Fighting the secret killer in fires. *RN*, 41:58, Feb. 1978.
47. Drury, L. R.: Evacuation and early care of the trauma patient. *Heart and Lung*, 7:249, Mar.–Apr. 1978.
48. Dunlap, L. B.: A modified, simple device for the emergency administration of percutaneous transtracheal ventilation. *JACEP*, 7:42, Feb. 1978.
49. Dunphy, J. E. (Ed.): *Wound Healing. A MEDCOM Update for the 70's.* Pearl River, New York: Davis & Geck, American Cyanamid Company, 1971.
50. Dupont, J.: What to do for common eye emergencies. *Nursing 76,* 6:17, May 1976.
51. Dushoff, I. M.: A stitch in time. *Emergency Medicine*, 5:21, January, 1973.
52. Edlich, R. F., et al.: Emergency department treatment, triage and transfer protocols for the burn patient. *JACEP*, 7:152, Apr. 1978.

52a. Epidural hematoma. *Nursing 75*, 5:35, Mar. 1975.

53. Faddis, D., et al.: Tissue toxicity of antiseptic solutions: A study of rat articular and periarticular tissues. *Journal of Trauma*, 17:895, Dec. 1977.
54. Finnerty, F. A., Jr.: Aggressive drug therapy in accelerated hypertension. *American Journal of Nursing,* 74:2176, Dec. 1974.
55. Frey, C.: *Initial Management of the Trauma Patient.* Philadelphia: Lea and Febiger, 1976.
56. Generelly, P., et al.: Delayed splenic rupture: Diagnosed by culdocentesis. *JACEP*, 6:369, Aug. 1977.
57. Gill, S. S., et al.: Arterial injuries of the extremities. *Journal of Trauma*, 16:766, Oct. 1976.
58. The G. I. bleeder — seldom as safe as he seems. *Nursing '75*, 5:48, Sept. 1975.

59. Glauser, J., et al.: Intravenous glucagon in the management of esophageal food obstruction. *JACEP*, 8:228, June 1979.
60. Glover, J. L., et al.: Autotransfusion of blood contaminated by intestinal contents. *JACEP*, 7:142, Apr. 1978.
61. Godley, D. R., and T. K. Smith: Some medicolegal aspects of gunshot wounds. *Journal of Trauma*, 17:866, Nov. 1977.
62. Goldberger, E., and M. W. Wheat, Jr.: *Treatment of Cardiac Emergencies*, 2d ed. St. Louis: The C.V. Mosby Company, 1977.
63. Gould, H.: How to remove contact lenses from comatose patients. *American Journal of Nursing*, 76:1483, Sept. 1976.
64. Hallal, J.: Thyroid disorders. *American Journal of Nursing*, 77:418, Mar. 1977.
65. Heinrich, J. J., et al.: Human bites. *Journal of Emergency Nursing*, 2:23, Jan.–Feb. 1976.
66. Hersch, A. T.: Postmyocardial infarction syndrome. *American Journal of Nursing*, 79:1240, July 1979.
67. Hoff, B. H.: Multisystem failure: A review with special reference to drowning. *Critical Care Medicine*, 7:310, July 1979.
68. Hollingsworth, P.: Autotransfusion in the emergency department. *Journal of Emergency Nursing*, 3:9, July–Aug. 1977.
69. Houser, D.: What to do first when a patient complains of chest pain. *Nursing 76*, 6:54, Nov. 1976.
70. Howe, J. R.: *Patient Care in Neurosurgery*. Boston: Little, Brown and Company, 1977.
71. Huelke, D. F., et al.: The hazard of the unrestrained occupant. *Journal of Trauma*, 16:383, May 1976.
72. Hutchinson, R.: What to do when treating stings and bites. *Nursing 77*, 7:69, June 1977.
73. Iversen, L. D., and D. K. Clawson: *Manual of Acute Orthopaedic Therapeutics*. Boston: Little, Brown and Company, 1977.
74. Isacson, L. M., and K. Schultz: Treating pulmonary edema. *Nursing 78*, Feb. 1978.
75. Jacoby, F. G.: *Nursing Care of the Patient With Burns*. St. Louis: C.V. Mosby Company, 1976.
76. Johnson, F. R., Jr., et al.: Esophageal obturator airway: Use and complications. *JACEP*, 5:36, Jan. 1976.
77. Jones, C. A., and I. Feller: Burns: What to do during the first crucial hours. *Nursing 77*, 7:22, Mar. 1977.
78. Jones, C. A., and I. Feller: Burns: Avoiding and coping with complications. *Nursing 77*, 7:72, Nov. 1977.
78a. Jones, M. J., and E. C. James: The management of traumatic asphyxia: Case report and literature review. *Journal of Trauma*, 16:235, Mar. 1976.
79. Kaplan, B. C., et al.: The military anti-shock trouser in civilian pre-hospital care. *Journal of Trauma*, 13:843, Oct. 1973.
80. Kerner, M., et al.: Gas gangrene complicating limb trauma. *Journal of Trauma*, 16:106, Feb. 1976.
81. Kline, N. S., et al.: *Psychotropic Drugs*. Oradell, NJ: Medical Economics Company, 1974.
82. Krenzelok, E. P., and J. E. Vlinton: Esophageal and gastric erosion without evidence of oral burns following detergent ingestion. *JACEP*, 8:194, May 1979.
83. Krieger, D.: The therapeutic touch. *American Journal of Nursing*, 75:784, May 1975.
84. Lance, E., and H. Sweetwood: Chest trauma: When minutes count. *Nursing 78*, 8:28, Jan. 1978.
85. Land, A. G., and H. A. Peterson: Osteomyelitis following puncture wounds of the foot in children. *Journal of Trauma*, 16:993, Dec. 1976.
86. Larrabee, J.: The person with spinal cord injury. Physical care during early recovery. *American Journal of Nursing*, 77:1320, Aug. 1977.
87. Lazoritz, S., B. S. Saunders, and W. M. Bason: Management of acute epiglottitis. *Critical Care Medicine*, 7:285, June 1979.
88. Lenoski, E. F., and K. A. Hunter: Specific patterns of inflicted burn injuries. *Journal of Trauma*, 17:842, Nov. 1977.
89. Literte, J. W.: Nursing care of the patient with intestinal obstruction. *American Journal of Nursing*, 77:1003, June 1977.
90. London, R. S., et al.: P.I.D. treatment: A growing problem for urban E.D.'s. *RN*, 38:OR-6, Aug. 1975.
91. Long, G. D.: G. I. bleeding: What to do and when. *Nursing 78*, 8:44, Mar. 1978.
92. Manzi, C. C.: Edema: How to tell if it's a danger signal. *Nursing 77*, 7:66, Apr. 1977.
93. Manzi, C. C.: Cardiac emergency! How to use drugs and CPR to save lives. *Nursing 78*, 8:30, Mar. 1978.
94. McConnell, E.: All about gastrointestinal intubation. *Nursing 75*, 5:30, Sept. 1975.
95. McConnell, E. A.: Insuring safer stomach suctioning with the Salem sump tube. *Nursing 77*, 7:54, Sept. 1977.
96. McKinley, J. C., et al.: Call for help: An algorithm for burn assessment, triage and acute care. *JACEP*, 5:13, Jan. 1976.
97. McVan, B. (Ed.): Odors: What the nose knows. *Nursing 77*, 7:46, Apr. 1977.
98. Mefford, E. D.: Allergic reactions: Plan ahead! *Journal of Emergency Nursing*, 1:36, Sept.–Oct. 1975.
99. Menton, S. A., Jr., et al.: Snakebite? Get the facts, then hurry. *Patient Care*, 10:48, June 1976.
100. Millam, D. A.: How to insert an IV. *American Journal of Nursing*, 79:1268, July 1979.
101. Miller, M. S., and F. C. Scott: Cardiac contusion and right bundle branch block. *JACEP*, 6:504, Nov. 1977.
102. Mitchell, P. H., and N. Mauss: Intracranial pressure: fact and fancy. *Nursing 76*, 6:53, June 1976.
103. Molyneux-Luick, M., and J. W. Knecht: The emergency that supercedes all other duties: Hypovolemic shock. *Nursing 77*, 7:32, Nov. 1977.
104. Molyneux-Luick, M.: The ABC's of multiple trauma. *Nursing 77*, 7:30, Oct. 1977.
105. Morgan, C. V., and T. W. Orcutt: The care and feeding of chest tubes. *American Journal of Nursing*, 72:305, Feb. 1972.
105a. Noe, J. M., and S. Kalish: *Wound Care*. Greenwich, Conn.: Chesebrough-Pond's Inc., 1975.
106. Norkool, D. M.: Current concepts of hyperbaric oxygenation and its application in critical care. *Heart and Lung*, 8:728, July–Aug. 1979.
107. O'Dell, A. J.: Emergency care in establishing an effective airway. *Nursing Clinics of North America*, 8:413, Sept. 1973.
108. O'Riordan, W. D., and D. V. Hubbel: Compound depressed skull fracture. *JACEP*, 5:123, Feb. 1976.
109. Palmer, E. D.: Upper gastrointestinal hemorrhage. *JAMA*, 231:853, Feb. 1975.
110. Parsons, L. C.: Respiratory changes in head injury. *American Journal of Nursing*, 71:2187, Nov. 1971.
111. Peacock, E. E., Jr., and W. Van Winkle, Jr.: *Wound Repair*, 2d ed. Philadelphia: W. B. Saunders Co., 1976.
112. Pearce, W., and E. Blair: Significance of the electrocardiogram in heart contusion due to blunt trauma. *Journal of Trauma*, 16:136, Feb. 1976.

113. Pickard, L. R., et al.: Transection of the descending aorta secondary to blunt trauma. *Journal of Trauma,* 17:749, Oct. 1977.
114. Pool, M.: Triage nursing as problem solving. *Journal of Emergency Nursing,* 2:25, Nov.–Dec. 1976.
115. Rexilius, B. G.: *Chest Drainage and Suction.* Philadelphia: F. A. Davis Co. 1977.
116. Riley-Kesler, A.: Pitfalls to avoid when interviewing outpatients. *Nursing 77*, 7:70, Sept. 1970.
117. Rudy, E.: Early omens of cerebral disaster. *Nursing 77*, 7:58, Feb. 1977.
118. Sabback, M. S., et al.: A study of the treatment of pit viper envenomization in 45 patients. *Journal of Trauma,* 17:569, Aug. 1977.
119. Schroeder, S. A.: The increasing use of emergency services: Why has it occurred? Is it a problem? *Western Journal of Medicine*, 130:67, Jan. 1979.
120. Schuman, S. H., et al.: Risk of drowning: An iceberg phenomenon. *JACEP*, 6:139, Apr. 1977.
121. Shibel, E. M., and K. M. Moser: *Respiratory Emergencies.* St. Louis: C. V. Mosby Co., 1977.
122. Shields, J. E.: Making triage work: The experience of an urban emergency department. *Journal of Emergency Nursing,* 2:37, July–Aug. 1976.
123. Shiery, S.: Insight into the delicate art of eye care. *Nursing 75*, 5:50, June 1975.
124. Sinte, R. J.: Accietal hypothermia. *JACEP*, 6:413, Sept. 1977.
125. Speich, P.: Brought back to life: A case study in hypothermia. *Journal of Emergency Nursing,* 3:9, Mar.–Apr. 1977.
126. Sproul, C. W., and P. J. Mullanney (Eds.): *Emergency Care: Assessment and Intervention.* St. Louis: C. V. Mosby Co., 1974.
127. Sredl, D. R., et al.: Offering the rape victim real help. *Nursing 79,* 9:38, July 1979.
128. Stahlgren, L. H., and N. W. Morris: Intestinal obstruction. *American Journal of Nursing,* 77:999, July 1977.
129. Stephany, T.: What I learned from a question I didn't think to ask. *RN*, 38:53, Nov. 1975.
130. Stevenson, T. R., et al.: Cleansing the traumatic wound by high pressure syringe irrigation. *JACEP*, 5:17, Jan. 1976.
131. Stoney, E. A. M.: *Practical Points in Nursing for Nurses in Private Practice.* Philadelphia: W. B. Saunders Co., 1906.
132. Sweetwood, H.: Acute respiratory insufficiency: How to recognize it . . . how to treat it. *Nursing 77*, 7:24, Dec. 1977.
133. Swift, N.: Head Injury. *Nursing 74*, 4:27, Sept. 1974.
134. Tinker, J. H.: Understanding chest x-rays. *American Journal of Nursing,* 76:54, Jan. 1976.
134a. Tintinalli, J. E.: Near-drowning. *JACEP*, 4:346, July–Aug. 1975.
135. Tintinalli, J. E.: Hydrofluoric acid burns. *JACEP,* 7:24, Jan. 1978.
136. *Treatment Guide: Common Biting and Stinging Insects and Other Arthropods Causing Allergic or Toxic Reactions.* West Point, Penn.: Merck, Sharp, and Dohme. Division of Merck and Company, Inc., 1977.
137. Wade, J. F.: *Respiratory Nursing Care: Physiology and Technique.* St. Louis: C.V. Mosby Co., 1973.
138. Wagner, M. M.: Emergency care of the burned patient. *American Journal of Nursing,* 77:1788, Nov. 1977.
139. Wahl, S.: Only a concussion. *Nursing 76*, 6:44, Aug. 1976.
140. Walt, A. J., and R. F. Wilson: *Management of Trauma: Pitfalls and Practice.* Philadelphia: Lea and Febiger, 1975.
141. Watt, C. H., Jr.: Snakebite: Don't cool it. *Emergency Medical Services,* 8:10, May–June 1979.
142. Weisz, G. M., et al.: Electrocardiographic changes in traumatized patients. *JACEP*, 5:329, May 1976.
142a. What an unconscious patient can tell you. *Emergency Medicine*, 6:96, July 1974.
142b. When you talk about poison. *Emergency Medicine,* 10:35, May 1978.
143. Whitecraft, D. D., et al.: Air embolism and decompression sickness in scuba divers. *JACEP*, 5:355, May 1976.
144. White, K. M.: Evaluating the trauma of gunshot wounds. *American Journal of Nursing,* 77:1589, Oct. 1977.
145. Wintrobe, M. M., et al.: *Harrison's Principles of Internal Medicine.* New York: McGraw-Hill Book Co., 1970.
146. Wischman, J., and M. M. McMahon: *The Patient With Surface Trauma* (Unpublished).
147. Witt, K.: HHNK. *Nursing 76*, 6:66, Feb. 1976.
148. Wolcott, B. W., LTC: What is an emergency? Depends on whom you ask. *JACEP*, 8:241, June 1979.
149. Wyler, A. R., and A. F. Reynolds: An intracranial complication of nasogastric intubation: A case report. *Journal of Neurosurgery,* 47:297, Aug. 1977.
150. Wyper, M.: Pulmonary embolism: Fighting the silent killer. *Nursing 75*, 5:31, Oct. 1975.

INDEX

Page number in *italics* indicate illustrations; page numbers followed by t indicate tables.